VOLUME 1

FOURTH EDITION

SILVERBERG'S

Principles and Practice of

SURGICAL

PATHOLOGY and

CYTOPATHOLOGY

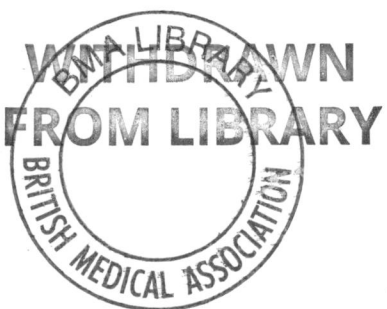

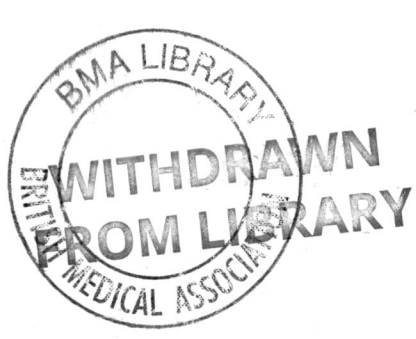

Silverberg's Principles and Practice of Surgical Pathology and Cytopathology

ELSEVIER CD-ROM LICENSE AGREEMENT

SILVERBERG'S
Principles and Practice of
SURGICAL PATHOLOGY and CYTOPATHOLOGY

VOLUME 1

FOURTH EDITION

Editor in Chief

Steven G. Silverberg MD

Clinical Professor of Pathology, Department of Pathology, University of Maryland
School of Medicine, Baltimore, Maryland

Associate Editors

Ronald A. DeLellis MD

Professor and Associate Chair, Department of Pathology and Laboratory Medicine,
Brown Medical School; Pathologist-in-Chief,
Rhode Island Hospital and The Miriam Hospital, Providence, Rhode Island

William J. Frable MD

Professor of Pathology, Virginia Commonwealth University, Richmond, Virginia

Virginia A. LiVolsi MD

Professor of Pathology and Laboratory Medicine and Otolaryngology, Head and Neck
Surgery, Department of Pathology and Laboratory Medicine,
University of Pennsylvania Medical Center, Philadelphia, Pennsylvania

Mark R. Wick MD

Professor of Pathology, Division of Surgical Pathology and Cytopathology, University
of Virginia Health System, Charlottesville, Virginia

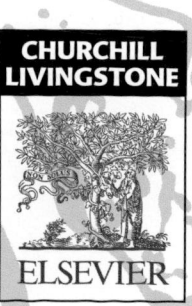

CHURCHILL LIVINGSTONE

ELSEVIER

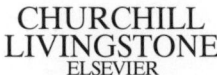

CHURCHILL
LIVINGSTONE
ELSEVIER

An imprint of Elsevier Inc.

© 2006, Elsevier Inc. All rights reserved.
Chapter 34 © William M Murphy

First edition 1983
Second edition 1990
Third edition 1997
Fourth edition 2006

ISBN 0443066221

British Library Cataloguing in Publication Data
A catalogue record for this book is available from the British Library

Library of Congress Cataloging in Publication Data
A catalog record for this book is available from the Library of Congress

Notice
Medical knowledge is constantly changing. Standard safety precautions must be followed, but as new research and clinical experience broaden our knowledge, changes in treatment and drug therapy may become necessary or appropriate. Readers are advised to check the most current product information provided by the manufacturer of each drug to be administered to verify the recommended dose, the method and duration of administration, and contraindications. It is the responsibility of the practitioner, relying on experience and knowledge of the patient, to determine dosages and the best treatment for each individual patient. Neither the Publisher nor the editors nor contributors assume any liability for any injury and/or damage to persons or property arising from this publication.

The Publisher

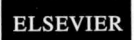
Commissioning Editor: *Michael J Houston*
Project Development Manager: *Agnes Byrne*
Project Manager: *Susan Stuart*
Senior Designer: *Sarah Russell*
Illustration Manager: *Mick Ruddy*
Illustrator: *Richard Prime*
Marketing Manager(s) (USA/UK): *Ethel Cathers/Leontine Treur*

Printed in China
Last digit is the print number : 9 8 7 6 5 4 3 2 1

Contents

Preface   ix
List of Contributors   xi

VOLUME 1

SECTION 1: General principles

1. General philosophy and principles of surgical pathology and cytopathology, including quality and malpractice issues   3
Steven G. Silverberg, Mark R. Wick

2. General and special techniques in surgical pathology and cytopathology   15
Ronald A. DeLellis, Murray Resnick, William J. Frable

SECTION 2: Conditions involving multiple organs

3. Infectious disease pathology   57
Margie A. Scott, Washington C. Winn, Jr, William J. Frable

4. Pathology of immunologically mediated diseases and transplantation   113
Edward C. Klatt, M. Elizabeth H. Hammond

5. Iatrogenic lesions   135
Robert E. Fechner, Guy E. Nichols, I-Tien Yeh

6. Differential diagnosis of metastatic tumors   167
Tarik M. Elsheikh, Jan F. Silverman

SECTION 3: Skin, soft tissue, and breast

7. Surgical pathology of non-neoplastic skin disease   193
Bruce R. Smoller

8. Cutaneous tumors and tumor-like conditions   241
Mark R. Wick, David J. Glembocki, Mark W. Teague, James W. Patterson

9. Soft tissue tumors   307
Elizabeth Montgomery

10. The breast   419
James L. Connolly, Timothy W. Jacobs

SECTION 4: Hematopoietic system

11. Lymph nodes and spleen   507
Karen L. Chang, Daniel A. Arber, Karl K. Gaal, Lawrence M. Weiss

12. Bone marrow   609
Nora C.J. Sun, Jun Wang, Eric F. Glassy

SECTION 5: Skeletal system

13. Non-neoplastic diseases of bones and joints   677
Peter G. Bullough

14. Neoplastic and tumor-like lesions of bone   701
G. Petur Nielsen, Lester J. Layfield, Andrew E. Rosenberg

SECTION 6: Upper respiratory system

15. Sinonasal and nasopharyngeal surgical pathology   787
Margaret Brandwein-Gensler

16. Larynx and trachea   833
William J. Frable

SECTION 7: Pulmonary and cardiovascular systems and serosal membranes

17. Diffuse lung diseases   859
Kevin O. Leslie, Nestor L. Müller, Thomas V. Colby

18. Localized diseases of the bronchi and lung   935
Arthur S. Patchefsky, Hormoz Ehya, Hong Wu

19. Pleura, pericardium, and peritoneum   1005
Victor L. Roggli, Philip Cagle

20. The cardiovascular system   1041
Allen Burke, Renu Virmani

21. The thymus and mediastinum   1091
Mark R. Wick, Celeste N. Powers

SECTION 8:   Oral cavity and salivary glands

22. The oral cavity   1137
Robert O. Greer, Jr, Sherif Said

23. Major and minor salivary glands   1203
Paul L. Auclair, Gary L. Ellis, Michael W. Stanley

VOLUME 2

SECTION 9:   Gastrointestinal system

24. The esophagus   1281
Mary P. Bronner, Kim R. Geisinger

25. The stomach   1321
A. Scott Mills, Melissa J. Contos, Rajat Goel

26. Non-neoplastic diseases of the small and large intestines   1373
John Hart

27. Neoplastic diseases of the small and large intestines   1419
Robert D. Odze, Amy E. Noffsinger

SECTION 10:   Hepatobiliary system and pancreas

28. Medical diseases of the liver   1467
Zachary D. Goodman, Kamal G. Ishak

29. Surgical diseases of the liver   1527
Linda D. Ferrell, Kim R. Geisinger

30. The pancreas and extrahepatic biliary system   1549
Ralph H. Hruban, Pedram Argani, Syed Z. Ali

SECTION 11:   Genitourinary system

31. Medical diseases of the kidney   1597
Guillermo A. Herrera, Xin Gu

32. Surgical diseases of the kidney   1661
David J. Grignon, Gregg A. Staerkel

33. The urinary bladder, urethra, renal pelves, and ureters   1707
William M. Murphy

34. The testis, paratesticular structures, and male external genitalia   1731
Satish K. Tickoo, Mahul B. Amin, Harvey M. Cramer, Lara R. Harik, Thomas M. Ulbright

35. The prostate gland   1791
Peter A. Humphrey

SECTION 12:   Female reproductive system

36. The uterine cervix   1831
Olga B. Ioffe, Michael R. Henry

37. The vulva and vagina   1885
Edward J. Wilkinson, Ashraf M. Hassanein

38. The uterine corpus   1933
Steven G. Silverberg, Sana O. Tabbara

39. The ovary and fallopian tube   1987
Charles Zaloudek, Brenda W. Ng

40. The placenta, products of conception, and gestational trophoblastic disease   2063
Rebecca N. Baergen, Kurt Benirschke

SECTION 13:   Endocrine system

41. The pituitary gland   2093
Sylvia L. Asa

42. The thyroid gland   2119
Zubair W. Baloch, Virginia A. LiVolsi

43. The parathyroid glands   2149
Gerardo Guiter, Ronald A. DeLellis

44. The adrenal gland   2169
Jacqueline A. Wieneke, Ernest E. Lack

SECTION 14:   Peripheral and central nervous system

45. Muscle and peripheral nerve pathology   2213
Richard A. Prayson

46. The ear   2267
Leon Barnes

47. The eye and ocular adnexa   2289
Ralph C. Eagle, Jr

48. The central nervous system   2329
Kymberly A. Gyure, Brock Kaya, John M. Hardman

Index

Preface

This edition of *Silverberg's Principles and Practice of Surgical Pathology and Cytopathology* follows the pathway established by the three previous editions, especially the Third Edition of 1997, which for the first time added full coverage of cytopathology to what had formerly been a classical surgical pathology text. In the new millennium, molecular pathways have become an important part of the study of the mechanisms of origin and development of most disease processes and are being incorporated into the practical diagnostic, prognostic, and therapeutic workup of many of them. Our current knowledge of these pathways, and particularly their adaptation where appropriate into current diagnostic practice, receives more emphasis in this Fourth Edition than ever before.

The format, established in the First Edition of 1983, of having an introductory section (the "Principles") followed by organ-based chapters (the "Practice"), is continued, but my talented Associate Editors and authors have enabled the former to be combined into two rather than ten chapters, allowing a more integrated approach. As in all previous editions, the chapter authors are world-recognized experts in their fields, and the progress in surgical pathology and cytopathology in the past 22 years is indicated by the fact that 45 of the authors are newly added since the Third Edition, and only nine are veterans of the First Edition. The year of publication of this edition happens to coincide with the year in which a record number of American medical graduates are choosing to enter training in pathology programs, and so it is appropriate to dedicate this edition at least in part to these pathologists of the future, both in the United States and in other countries around the world.

In addition to Drs. DeLellis and Frable, who joined me in the Third Edition, the current edition welcomes Drs. Mark Wick and Virginia LiVolsi as new Associate Editors. It is my hope that these talented pathologists, and others like them, will carry this work through subsequent editions with which I will no longer be associated. They certainly have made my life easier – and the final product a great deal better – with regard to this edition.

As in the past, friends, colleagues, and relatives have continued to inspire us. My own mentors, as mentioned in previous editions, have included the late Drs. Abou Pollack, Harry Greene, Averill Liebow, Fred Stewart, and Frank Foote. Sadly, Dr. Saul Kay, a wonderful pathologist, leader, and friend, passed away and joined them last year. Drs. Claude Gompel and Leopold G. Koss are, fortunately, still active and contributing to our field. My colleagues and friends at the University of Maryland are a continuing source of personal support. Susan Boeshore has served tirelessly and ably as Editorial Assistant. The editorial and production staff members at Elsevier – notably but not exclusively Natasha Andjelkovic, Agnes Byrne, Susan Stuart, and Michael Houston – have combined to make me feel as if this were the only book in their domain. Finally, my wife Kiyoe has provided her usual cheerful help and encouragement, as she has been doing for the past 39 years.

Steven G. Silverberg

It has been both a great pleasure and inspiration to be associated with Dr. Silverberg and the many fine authors who have brought this book through four editions, adding to the advancement of the art and science of surgical pathology and cytopathology.

Ronald A. DeLellis
William J. Frable
Virginia A. LiVolsi
Mark R. Wick

List of Contributors

Syed Z. Ali, MD
Associate Professor of Pathology and Radiology
Department of Pathology
The Johns Hopkins Medical Institutions
The Sol Goldman Pancreatic Cancer Research Center
Baltimore, Maryland

Mahul B. Amin, MD
Director of Surgical Pathology,
Professor of Pathology, Urology, Hematology, and Oncology
Associate Director, Cancer Pathogenomics
Winship Cancer Institute
Emory University School of Medicine
Emory University Hospital
Atlanta, Georgia

Daniel A. Arber, MD
Professor of Pathology
Department of Pathology
Stanford University Medical Center
Stanford, California

Pedram Argani, MD
Associate Professor of Pathology and Oncology
The Johns Hopkins Medical Institutions
The Sol Goldman Pancreatic Cancer Research Center
Baltimore, Maryland

Sylvia L. Asa, MD, PhD
Professor
Laboratory Medicine and Pathobiology
University of Toronto,
Pathologist-in-Chief
University Health Network and
Toronto Medical Laboratories
Toronto, Ontario

Paul L. Auclair, DMD, MS
Attending Pathologist
Department of Pathology and Laboratory Medicine
Maine Medical Center and Mercy Hospital
Portland, Maine

Rebecca N. Baergen, MD
Professor of Clinical Pathology and Laboratory Medicine
New York-Presbyterian Hospital
Weill Cornell Medical Center
New York, New York

Zubair W. Baloch, MD, PhD
Associate Professor of Pathology and Laboratory Medicine
Department of Pathology and Laboratory Medicine
University of Pennsylvania Medical Center
Philadelphia, Pennsylvania

Leon Barnes, MD
Professor of Pathology and Otolaryngology
Department of Pathology
University of Pittsburgh Medical Center
Presbyterian Hospital
Pittsburgh, Pennsylvania

Kurt Benirschke, MD
Professor Emeritus of Pathology and Reproductive Medicine
Department of Pathology
University of California, San Diego
San Diego, California

Margaret Brandwein-Gensler, MD
Professor of Pathology and Otolaryngology
Montefiore Medical Center
Albert Einstein College of Medicine
New York, New York

Mary P. Bronner, MD
Director, Gastrointestinal and
Hepatic Pathology Fellowship Program
Co-Section Head, Molecular Morphologic Pathology
The Cleveland Clinic Foundation
Cleveland, Ohio

Peter G. Bullough, MB ChB
Professor of Pathology
Weill Medical College of Cornell University
Director of Laboratory Medicine
Hospital for Special Surgery
New York, New York

Allen Burke, MD
Associate Professor of Pathology
University of Maryland School of Medicine
Baltimore, Maryland

Philip Cagle, MD
Professor of Pathology
Weill Medical College of Cornell University,
Director of Pulmonary Pathology
Department of Pathology
The Methodist Hospital
Houston, Texas

Karen L. Chang, MD
Director of Clinical Pathology
City of Hope National Medical Center
Duarte, California

Thomas V. Colby, MD
Professor of Pathology
Department of Laboratory Medicine and Pathology
Mayo Clinic Scottsdale
Scottsdale, Arizona

James L. Connolly, MD
Professor of Pathology
Harvard Medical School
Director of Anatomic Pathology
Beth Israel Deaconess Medical Center
Boston, Massachusetts

Melissa J. Contos, MD
Associate Professor
Department Pathology
Section of Gastrointestinal and Hepatobiliary Pathology
Virginia Commonwealth University Medical Center
Richmond, Virginia

Harvey M. Cramer, MD
Associate Professor of Pathology
Department of Pathology
Indiana University School Of Medicine
Wishard Hospital
Indianapolis, Indiana

Ronald A. DeLellis, MD
Professor and Associate Chair, Department of Pathology and
Laboratory Medicine, Brown Medical School;
Pathologist-in-Chief, Rhode Island Hospital and
The Miriam Hospital, Providence, Rhode Island

Ralph C. Eagle, Jr., MD
Professor of Ophthalmology and Pathology
Jefferson Medical College
The Noel T. and Sara L. Simmonds Professor
of Ophthalmic Pathology
Director, Department of Pathology
Wills Eye Hospital
Philadelphia, Pennsylvania

Hormoz Ehya, MD
Senior Member and Director of Cytopathology
Fox Chase Cancer Center
Adjunct Clinical Professor
Jefferson Medical College
Philadelphia, Pennsylvania

Gary L. Ellis, MD, DDS
Director, Oral and Maxillofacial Pathology
Centers of Excellence
ARUP Laboratories
Salt Lake City, Utah

Tarik M. Elsheikh, MD
Director of Cytology
Ball Memorial Hospital
Pathologists Associated
Muncie, Indiana

Robert E. Fechner, MD
Professor Emeritus
Department of Pathology
University of Virginia School of Medicine
Charlottesville, Virginia

Linda D. Ferrell, MD
Professor, Vice Chair, Department of Pathology
Director of Surgical Pathology
Department of Anatomic Pathology
University of California, San Francisco
San Francisco, California

William J. Frable, MD.
Professor of Pathology
Virginia Commonwealth University
Richmond
Virginia

Karl K. Gaal, M.D.
Pathologist
Department of Pathology
City of Hope National Medical Center
Duarte, California

Kim R. Geisinger, M.D.
Director of Surgical Pathology and Cytology
Professor of Pathology
Wake Forest University School of Medicine
Winston-Salem, North Carolina

Eric F. Glassy, MD
Medical Director, Department of Pathology
Little Company of Mary Hospital
Torrance, California

David J. Glembocki, MD
Staff Pathologist and Dermatopathologist
Scottsdale Pathology Associates
Scottsdale, Arizona

Rajat Goel, MD
Staff Pathologist
Pathology Associates of Central Pennsylvania
Harrisburg, Pennsylvania

Zachary D. Goodman, MD PhD
Chief, Division of Hepatic Pathology
Armed Forces Institute of Pathology
Washington, D.C.

Robert O. Greer, Jr., DDS, ScD
Professor
Department of Pathology
University of Colorado School of Medicine
Professor and Chairman
Division of Oral and Maxillofacial Pathology
University of Colorado School of Dentistry
Denver, Colorado

David J. Grignon, MD
Professor and Chairman
Department of Pathology
Detroit Medical Center
Barbara Ann Karmanos Cancer Institute
Wayne State University
Detroit, Michigan

Xin Gu, MD
Assistant Professor of Pathology
Department of Pathology
Louisiana State University Health Sciences Center
Shreveport, Louisiana

Gerardo Guiter, MD
Assistant Professor of Pathology
Department of Pathology and Laboratory Medicine
Brown Medical School
Providence, Rhode Island

Kymberly A. Gyure, MD
Assistant Professor of Pathology
Director, Division of Neuropathology
University of Maryland School of Medicine
Baltimore, Maryland

M. Elizabeth H. Hammond, MD
Medical Director, Office of Research
Intermountain Health Care
Professor of Pathology and
Adjunct Professor of Internal Medicine
University of Utah School of Medicine
Department of Pathology
LDS Hospital
Salt Lake City, Utah

John M. Hardman, MD
Professor of Pathology
John A. Burns School of Medicine
University of Hawaii
Honolulu, Hawaii

Lara R. Harik, MD
Fellow, Surgical Oncologic Pathology
Department of Pathology
Memorial Sloan-Kettering Cancer Center
New York, New York

John Hart, MD
Professor
Sections of Surgical Pathology and Gastroenterology
Department of Pathology
The University of Chicago
Pathologist
The University of Chicago Hospitals
Chicago, Illinois

Ashraf M. Hassanein, MD, PhD
Associate Professor of Pathology and Dermatology
Department of Pathology, Immunology and Laboratory Medicine
University of Florida College of Medicine
Gainesville, Florida

Michael R. Henry, MD
Associate Professor of Pathology
Director of Cytopathology
Department of Pathology
University of Maryland Medical Center
Baltimore, Maryland

Guillermo A. Herrera, MD
Professor of Pathology, Medicine,
Cellular Biology and Anatomy
Chairman, Department of Pathology
Louisiana State University Health Sciences Center
Shreveport, Louisiana

Ralph H. Hruban, MD
Professor of Pathology and Oncology
The Johns Hopkins Medical Institutions
The Sol Goldman Pancreatic Cancer
Research Center
Baltimore, Maryland

Peter A. Humphrey, MD, PhD
Professor of Pathology and Immunology
Department of Pathology and Immunology
Washington University School of Medicine
St. Louis, Missouri

Olga B. Ioffe, MD
Assistant Professor of Pathology
Department of Pathology
University of Maryland School of Medicine
Baltimore, Maryland

Kamal G. Ishak, MD, PhD
Chairperson
Department of Hepatic and Gastrointestinal Pathology
Armed Forces Institute of Pathology
Washington, D.C.

Timothy W. Jacobs, MD
Deputy Chief of Pathology
Department of Pathology
Virginia Mason Medical Center
Seattle, Washington

Brock Kaya, MD
Associate Professor of Pathology
Department of Pathology
John A. Burns School of Medicine
University of Hawaii
Honolulu, Hawaii

Edward C. Klatt, MD
Professor and Academic Administrator
Department of Biomedical Sciences
Florida State University
College of Medicine
Tallahassee, Florida

Ernest E. Lack, MD
Director of Anatomic Pathology
Department of Surgical Pathology
Washington Hospital Center
Washington, D.C.

Lester J. Layfield, MD
Professor of Pathology
Director of Surgical Pathology
Vice President, Anatomic Pathology Division
ARUP Laboratories,
Department of Pathology
University of Utah School of Medicine
Salt Lake City, Utah

Kevin O. Leslie, MD
Consultant and Professor of Pathology
Department of Laboratory Medicine and Pathology
Mayo Clinic Scottsdale
Scottsdale, Arizona

Virginia A. LiVolsi, MD
Professor of Pathology and Laboratory Medicine and
Otolaryngology, Head and Neck Surgery, Department of Pathology
and Laboratory Medicine, University of Pennsylvania Medical
Center, Philadelphia, Pennsylvania

A. Scott Mills, MD
Professor of Pathology
Department of Pathology
Section of Gastrointestinal and Hepatobiliary Pathology
Virginia Commonwealth University Medical Center
Richmond, Virginia

Elizabeth Montgomery, MD
Associate Professor of Pathology and Oncology
Department of Pathology
Johns Hopkins Medical Institutions
Baltimore, Maryland

Nestor L. Müller, MD
Professor and Head
Department of Radiology
University of British Columbia
Vancouver, British Columbia

William M. Murphy, MD
Consultant in Urologic Pathology
Emeritus Professor of Pathology
University of Florida College of Medicine
Gainesville, Florida

Brenda W. Ng, MD
Attending Pathologist
Department of Pathology
El Camino Hospital
Mountain View, California

Guy E. Nichols, MD, PhD
Chairman and Medical Director
Bon Secours Richmond Regional Laboratory System
Richmond, Virginia

G. Petur Nielsen, MD
Associate Pathologist
James Homer Wright Laboratories
Department of Pathology
Massachusetts General Hospital,
Associate Professor
Harvard Medical School
Boston, Massachusetts

Amy E. Noffsinger, MD
Associate Professor of Pathology
Department of Pathology
University of Chicago
Chicago, Illinois

Robert D. Odze, MD, FRCPC
Associate Professor of Pathology
Chief, Gastrointestinal Pathology Service
Brigham and Women's Hospital
Boston, Massachusetts

Arthur S. Patchefsky, MD
Chairman, Department of Pathology
Fox Chase Cancer Center
Philadelphia, Pennsylvania

James W. Patterson, MD
Professor of Pathology and Dermatology
Department of Pathology
Division of Surgical Pathology and Cytopathology
University of Virginia Health System
Charlottesville, Virginia

Celeste N. Powers, MD, PhD
Professor and Chair, Division of Surgical Pathology and
Cytopathology
Director of Anatomic Pathology Services
Medical College of Virgina/Virginia Commonwealth University
Health System
Richmond, Virginia

Richard A. Prayson, MD
Professor of Pathology
Cleveland Clinic Lerner College of Medicine
of Case Western Reserve University
Section Head of Neuropathology
Department of Anatomic Pathology
Cleveland Clinic Foundation
Cleveland, Ohio

Murray Resnick, MD, PhD.
Professor of Pathology
Brown University Medical School
Director of Surgical and Gastrointestinal Pathology
Rhode Island Hospital
Providence, Rhode Island

Victor L. Roggli, MD
Professor of Pathology
Department of Pathology
Durham VA and Duke University Medical Centers
Durham, North Carolina

Andrew E. Rosenberg, MD
Associate Pathologist
James Homer Wright Laboratories
Department of Pathology
Massachusetts General Hospital
Associate Professor of Pathology
Department of Pathology
Harvard Medical School
Boston, Massachusetts

Sherif Said, MD
Assistant Professor and Director of Head and Neck Pathology
Department of Pathology
University of Colorado Health Science Center
Denver, Colorado

Margie A. Scott
Vice Chair of Pathology and Associate Professor
Department of Pathology
University of Arkansas for Medical Sciences
Central Arkansas Veterans Healthcare System
Little Rock, Arkansas

Steven G. Silverberg, M.D.
Clinical Professor of Pathology
Department of Pathology
University of Maryland School of Medicine
Baltimore, Maryland

Jan F. Silverman, MD
Professor and Chairman
Department of Pathology and Laboratory Medicine
Allegheny General Hospital
Pittsburgh, Pennsylvania

Bruce R. Smoller, MD
Professor and Chair
Department of Pathology
College of Medicine
University of Arkansas for Medical Sciences
Little Rock, Arkansas

Gregg A. Staerkel, MD
Professor, Division of Cytopathology
Department of Pathology
University of Texas MD Anderson Cancer Center
Houston, Texas

Michael W. Stanley, MD
Pathologist
Hospital Pathology Associates
Professor of Pathology and Laboratory Medicine
University of Minnesota
Minneapolis, Minnesota

Nora C. J. Sun, MD MSc
Professor Emeritus
Department of Pathology and Laboratory Medicine
David Geffen School of Medicine
University of California, Los Angeles
Harbor-UCLA Medical Center
Torrance, California

Sana O. Tabbara, MD
Chief, Surgical Pathology
George Washington University Medical Center
Washington, D.C.

Mark W. Teague, MD
Staff Pathologist
Pathology Associates
Huntsville, Alabama

Satish K. Tickoo, MD
Associate Attending Pathologist
and Associate Member
Memorial Sloan-Kettering Cancer Center
Department of Pathology
New York, New York

Thomas M. Ulbright, MD
Director of Anatomic Pathology
Clarian Health Partners
Lawrence M. Roth Professor of Pathology
Indiana University School of Medicine
Indianapolis, Indiana

Renu Virmani, MD
Medical Director
CVPath
International Registry of Pathology
Gaithersburg, Maryland

Jun Wang, MD
Associate Professor of Pathology
Chief, Hematopathology Section
Department of Pathology and Human Anatomy
Loma Linda University School of Medicine
Loma Linda, California

Lawrence M. Weiss, MD
Chairman
Department of Pathology
City of Hope National Medical Center
Duarte, California

Mark R. Wick, MD
Professor of Pathology
Division of Surgical Pathology and Cytopathology
University of Virginia Health System
Charlottesville, Virginia

Jacqueline A. Wieneke, MD
Pathologist
Department of Endocrine and Otorhinolaryngologic-
Head and Neck Pathology
Armed Forces Institute of Pathology
Washington, D.C.

Edward J. Wilkinson, MD
Professor and Vice Chairman
Director and Chief
Division of Anatomic Pathology
University of Florida
Department of Pathology, Immunology and Laboratory Medicine
Gainesville, Florida

Washington C. Winn, Jr., MD
Professor of Pathology
Department of Pathology and Laboratory Medicine
University of Vermont College of Medicine
Burlington, Vermont

Hong Wu, MD, PhD
Staff Pathologist, Dermatopathology
Associate Member
Department of Pathology
Fox Chase Cancer Center
Philadelphia, Pennsylvania

I-Tien Yeh, MD
Associate Professor
Department of Pathology
University of Texas Health Science Center at San Antonio
San Antonio, Texas

Charles Zaloudek, MD
Professor of Pathology
Department of Pathology
University of California, San Francisco
San Francisco, California

General principles

General philosophy and principles of surgical pathology and cytopathology, including quality and malpractice issues

Steven G. Silverberg   Mark R. Wick

What is surgical pathology? Probably the best definition is that surgical pathology is the discipline that deals with the anatomic pathology of tissues removed from living patients. Many surgical pathologists expand this definition to include smears, aspirates, and body fluids as well, so cytopathology is usually considered within the domain of surgical pathology. Indeed, it has been my (SGS) philosophy for many years that it is difficult to be an excellent surgical pathologist without also practicing cytopathology, and virtually impossible to be an excellent cytopathologist – especially in the era of fine needle aspiration of almost every organ – without also obtaining and retaining expertise in general surgical pathology.

By the above definition, surgical pathology differs from autopsy pathology in (1) the nature of the specimens seen most frequently, and (2) the usual immediacy of the decisions to be made and their relation to the subsequent management of an individual patient. The latter distinction is perhaps more immediately apparent. The diagnosis made by the surgical pathologist or cytopathologist often precedes the treatment of the patient and, in fact, in such instances usually influences or even determines what such treatment will be. On the other hand, the role of the autopsy pathologist, or morbid anatomist, invariably begins after treatment has ended and includes an assessment of the appropriateness and adequacy of the therapeutic regimens employed.

The first difference listed above between surgical and autopsy pathology is also an important one to remember, however. As an example, diagnostic material from the heart forms a fairly small (but currently increasing) portion of the workload of the surgical pathologist, whereas it is a major (if not the major) consideration in the practice of autopsy pathology. By contrast, the skin and the female genital tract are usually not studied extensively at autopsy, yet together they comprise more than one-half the specimens seen in most practices of surgical pathology. Thus, it is apparent that the reading and continuing education that must be undertaken to keep up to date in the two fields is quite different, almost justifying their characterization as entirely separate disciplines. By contrast, the basic skills essential to the practice of surgical pathology are the same as those learned in the performance of autopsies, and there are few practicing surgical pathologists who do not continue their involvement with autopsy pathology as well.

PRACTICE OF SURGICAL PATHOLOGY

Whether working in an academic medical center or a small community hospital, the surgical pathologist always functions as a teacher and often as a researcher. The main role of the surgical pathologist, however, is still essentially the practice of medicine,[1] which is sometimes easy to forget, particularly for the pathologist who does not regularly see living patients. The results of such

distance may be disastrous for both the pathologist and the patient. The role of the surgical pathologist should be that of a consultant to the clinician for the ultimate benefit of the patient, and this role must be remembered even when the pathologist is in the laboratory, far from direct contact with either the clinician or the patient.

Furthermore, despite the traditional name of the field (surgical pathology), the practitioner soon learns that service to, and contact with, general and specialty surgeons comprises only a small part of the total practice. Because the workload of the modern surgical pathologist also includes specimens from dermatologists, gynecologists, gastroenterologists, pediatricians, nephrologists, and physicians in many other specialties, the pathologist must have some familiarity with each of these fields and the clinical problems encountered therein. Thus, the formative and continuing education must consist of training not only in morphologic interpretation but also in the clinical practice of medicine.

This need for clinical competence is even more apparent for cytopathologists who perform their own fine needle aspiration biopsies (FNABs). We have found that sometimes interventional cytopathologists can localize and aspirate small masses after repeated failures by even very experienced clinicians. Exact knowledge by the cytopathologist of the clinical context of the aspirated mass can be extremely useful in making the correct diagnosis, as well as in knowing whether a paucicellular aspirate is representative of the lesion and diagnosable as benign or is truly insufficient for diagnosis. Cytopathologists who perform FNABs are also well aware of the clinical effort involved in obtaining pertinent historic data, in reassuring the patient, and in dealing with the fortunately rare complications of the procedure.

CONSULTATIVE ROLE OF THE SURGICAL PATHOLOGIST

By recalling the relationship between the surgical pathologist and the clinician and patient, the general principles of the approach to a specimen are greatly simplified. Surgical pathologists should deal with each specimen as if they were the clinician – or, better yet, the patient – awaiting the surgical pathology report. Questions such as whether to photograph a gross specimen, how many sections to submit of a particular lesion, how carefully to search for lymph nodes in a radical procedure, whether to order recuts or special stains, whether to write or dictate a microscopic description, and so forth, all become answerable in terms of the single basic question, 'Were I either the clinician or the patient in this case, what information would I need about this specimen, and how can that information best be supplied?'

In addition to this common-sense approach, numerous published guidelines now exist for the reporting (and processing) of common surgical pathology specimens. In the United States, the best known of these have been promulgated by the Association of Directors of Anatomic and Surgical Pathology (ADASP) and the College of American Pathologists (CAP). The American College of Surgeons (ACS) Commission on Cancer, which accredits cancer centers in the US, has recently recommended adopting these or similar reporting formats,[2] although synoptic reporting,[3] which is now utilized in many institutions and is preferred by ADASP,[2] will not be required. Where appropriate, these guidelines or modifications of them for specific organs are included in the corresponding chapters of this book.

Since the approach to any specimen received in the surgical pathology laboratory obviously depends on the specific clinical problem to be resolved by the interpretation of that specimen, it is essential that each specimen be accompanied by an adequate description of what it represents, as well as an appropriate clinical history. The surgical pathologist should design the request form so the clinician filling out the form is sure to appreciate the need for supplying this information. Recent progress toward some degree of standardization of the surgical pathology report may aid in making the information more universally available.[3] If adequate clinical information is not received with a particular specimen, the surgical pathologist is completely justified in not processing that specimen until the appropriate information is obtained. The telephone should also be an important part of the surgical pathologist's equipment. Submitting physicians should be called promptly if any question exists about a specimen submitted.

Similarly, the responsibility of the surgical pathologist does not end when a diagnosis has been made and recorded on the surgical pathology report. If the diagnosis differs significantly from what was clinically suspected, or if it requires any immediate response by the clinician, the clinician should be contacted promptly rather than waiting for the report to reach him or her by the usual route of distribution. If the diagnosis made is an uncommon one, the significance of which is not likely to be understood by the clinician, the surgical pathologist should be sure that the meaning of the term is explained and a pertinent reference provided, either verbally or in the body of the surgical pathology report (preferably by both means).

The importance of communication between the clinician and the pathologist is often underestimated by both parties. This is particularly true of surgical pathologists, who perhaps become too familiar with the 'What do you think of this slide without any history?' type of quiz they often receive during residency. It is essential to remember, however, that the practice of surgical pathology is not an intellectual game, but rather a serious facet of the practice of medicine, often with life or death implications. Thus, when dealing with any living patient, all the available clinical information should be presented to the surgical pathologist responsible for the case. This is obviously of less importance in some cases than in others, but it is easier to invoke it as a general rule to which occasional exceptions will be made than to face a constant struggle in obtaining clinical information when it is urgently needed.

These comments pertaining to communication between the clinician and the surgical pathologist are indicative of the role of the surgical pathologist as a clinical consultant. The clinician would certainly not think of calling in a gynecologist as a consultant to evaluate a possible pelvic mass without providing both adequate clinical data and the reason for the consultation; similarly, the clinician should not obtain a consultation from the surgical pathologist without the same courtesy. To continue the same analogy, just as the clinician would not demand that the gynecologic consultant perform a specific diagnostic or therapeutic procedure, the surgical pathologist should not be required to perform a particular stain, a frozen section,

or any other procedure on the tissues submitted. The other side of the coin is that it then becomes the role of the surgical pathologist to decide what special stains or other studies to perform based on an interpretation of all the clinical and pathologic data available in a given case, and it is the surgical pathologist's responsibility to be sure that all this information has indeed been supplied, as well as to use special studies in a judicious and cost-effective manner.[4]

In cytopathology as well, the issue of communication is extremely important and (as mentioned above in association with the performance of FNAB) may involve the patient directly as well as through the medium of the clinician. The problem of communicating the result of a suspicious Papanicolaou (Pap) smear to the submitting clinician and ultimately to the patient, and of ensuring timely and appropriate follow-up, is one that becomes even more obvious when it results in malpractice litigation.[5] If the cytopathologist does not also personally see the tissue specimen accompanying or following a Pap smear, a bronchial wash, an FNAB, or some other cytologic specimen, communication with the surgical pathologist who receives that tissue specimen also becomes crucial in the process of quality assurance. This process is obviously a two-way street, and the surgical pathologist equally needs to compare the tissue diagnosis with cytopathologic material from the same patient.

INTERPATHOLOGIST CONSULTATION IN SURGICAL PATHOLOGY

The question of consultations in surgical pathology is frequently puzzling for the novice. It is always difficult to find the proper middle ground between the hesitancy to ever ask for a consultation and the temptation to seek consultation on virtually every case that is not entirely routine. We who practice surgical pathology are fortunate that it is far easier to transport slides to an expert consultant than to transport the patient; therefore, there is never really an excuse for not obtaining a consultation in situations in which it is indicated, and thus we are safer in erring on the side of overutilization rather than underutilization of this service.

Internal consultation should always be used in questionable cases.[6] Thus, if three members of a group at a particular institution practice surgical pathology, all three should review such a case, and the final report should express the consensus diagnosis. If such a consensus is unobtainable, or if doubt remains, outside consultation is then sought.[7,8] A good general rule to follow is that one outside consultant should be used for each case. Nothing is more disturbing to the practicing pathologist than to send slides from a case to three different eminent consultants and get three different answers. The consultant should be chosen for expertise in a particular field of surgical pathology or because the referring pathologist has had previous favorable experience with that consultant – not because the consultant is located at a famous institution, although the person chosen may lack the credentials of an expert consultant in the particular case to be referred.

Having chosen the consultant, it is essential to provide that individual with the same courtesies that we expect our clinicians to provide to us.[9] Thus, the name, age, and sex of the patient, the hospital and/or surgical pathology number, and the pertinent clinical history should be submitted, as well as a copy of the surgical pathology report in which the gross pathologic features of the case are described. The slides submitted should be adequate in both quantity and quality, since the function of a consultant is not to overcome someone else's inadequate histotechnique. Specially stained slides, if pertinent, should also be submitted, or at least unstained slides or paraffin blocks on which consultants may perform the stains they deem necessary. The need for performing – and often repeating – immunostains in consultation cases involving cancer has recently been demonstrated.[10] Referring pathologists should always include their own diagnoses, or the differential if a final diagnosis has not been reached. If questions about the clinical management of the case exist, these should be asked directly in the referring letter. Unless there is some compelling reason for wanting these slides returned (such as the lesion being seen on only one slide or the block being unavailable), the consultant should be permitted to retain the submitted slides. When the report of the consultant is received by the referring pathologist, it should always be made available to the clinician, even (or especially) if it is at variance with the referring pathologist's original diagnosis.

The surgical pathologist should always be willing to send a case for consultation if so requested by the clinician, but certainly the surgical pathologist is free to state that a consultation is not really necessary if such is the case. If the clinician requests a specific consultant, and the pathologist believes that that individual is inappropriate for the case in question, the clinician should be so informed. If the clinician still insists on that consultant, the pathologist should probably acquiesce but is certainly entitled to send the case to another consultant as well. This is one of the few acceptable reasons for violating the 'one consultant per case' rule mentioned earlier.

If slides or clinical data submitted in consultation are in any way inadequate, consultant pathologists should feel free to make the same demands of the referring pathologist that they would make of their clinicians or of their laboratory, and they should not make a diagnosis on the basis of inadequate clinical or pathologic data. They may need to request the paraffin blocks or fixed tissues for processing in their own laboratory; the fear of insulting the referring pathologist by asking for this material should not outweigh the responsibility to the patient of rendering a diagnosis only on optimal preparations.

Consultations on cytopathologic material sent to pathologists outside one's own institution are more problematic, since no paraffin block exists (except in the case of material processed as a cell block) from which to cut additional slides, and the referring pathologist may therefore hesitate to risk loss or breakage of the only glass slide showing a worrisome finding. Photomicrographs may be useful in this situation, and even more immediacy is provided by the rapidly developing field of telepathology, by which high-quality photographic images can be transferred virtually instantaneously to the consultant.[11–13] This technology is clearly available – but perhaps less necessary – for tissue consultations as well, and may be of particular value in obtaining rapid help with interpretation of a difficult frozen section.[14]

INTRAOPERATIVE CONSULTATION IN SURGICAL PATHOLOGY

The question of false-positive diagnoses is particularly relevant with respect to intraoperative consultations, exemplified by frozen section examinations. Older reports of frozen section results in breast lesions, for example, have generally indicated that the frequency of false-positive diagnoses (something being called cancer that in reality is benign) should be zero, that false-negative diagnoses comprise about 1% of cases, and that diagnosis must be deferred to permanent sections in 1–2% of the cases.[15–17] Several points should be emphasized with reference to these figures. First, authors who publish results of frozen section examination (or, for that matter, of

anything) are invariably those who have a great deal of experience with the technique; the surgical pathologist who performs 100 frozen section examinations a year is likely to have considerably poorer results than one who performs 1000 a year. Second, the frequency of false-positive diagnoses is inversely related to that of deferred diagnoses, so the attempt to 'force' a diagnosis in a difficult situation is likely to lead to the feared result of a false-positive interpretation. Thus, there should be no shame in equivocating in such a situation, and sometimes (e.g. for intralobular and intraductal mammary lesions, questionable lymphomas), discretion is usually the better part of valor. Third, most false-negative interpretations are probably due to sampling error and are thus unavoidable. Despite our competence in gross pathology, when one or two sections are taken from a 10-cm specimen, we will invariably encounter situations in which the definitive diagnosis is not made until many more sections are examined the following day.

Finally, recent changes have occurred in both the indications for frozen section examination and the specimens most frequently encountered.[18,19] In almost one-half of our own cases, the examination is performed not primarily for a diagnosis, but rather to comment on the adequacy of the specimen for subsequent diagnosis, to select tissue for special studies (e.g. lymphoid cell markers, flow cytometry), or to demonstrate gross pathology and thus ensure better communication. Thus, the proportion of cases with a deferred diagnosis has increased considerably since the early reports. Similarly, the proportion of breast cases in which a diagnosis is requested (always the most common intraoperative consultation type in past series) has decreased remarkably after publication of recommendations that frozen sections not be performed in these instances.[20,21]

In actuality, 'frozen section' examination is a poor term, since many intraoperative consultations (the preferred term) do not result in performance of frozen section examinations. It is the responsibility of the surgical pathologist, as the consultant in this situation, to decide exactly what needs to be done; if the gross appearance of the specimen is characteristic, or if the diagnosis can be made by the imprint or smear technique alone, the performance of a frozen section examination may be unnecessary. Similarly, freezing of tissues may not only be unnecessary but may actually be contraindicated in certain situations. For example, if the specimen submitted is so small that frozen section examination would be likely to exhaust the tissue completely, and if the frozen section diagnosis is likely to be either difficult to make or unnecessary for the immediate management of the patient, then certainly this procedure should not be performed.

Special mention should be made of the surgical practice of requesting frozen section examination to determine the adequacy of margins in a resection for cancer. This is done most frequently in the head and neck area: such tissues are often difficult to freeze and section because of the high fat content. In addition, it is apparent that in a large resection specimen, only a limited number of frozen section examinations can be performed perpendicular to the tumor and its resection margins while the patient is still waiting under anesthesia. Thus, a report of a positive margin is of great value, but a negative report does not by any means guarantee that tumor will not be found when permanent sections of the adjacent tissues are examined.

Margins on tumor resections, incidentally, are one of those situations in which cytologic preparations do not add significantly to the information obtained by performing a classic frozen section examination. Unless massive amounts of tumor are present at a resection margin (usually enough to be visible grossly), the results of the imprint or smear will probably still be negative for tumor cells. By contrast, we have found these preparations of considerable assistance as a complement to frozen section examination in many situations; in some cases, they even supplant the frozen section examination itself.[18,19,22–25] For example, false-negative results on a lymph node containing a small volume of metastatic cancer are more likely to be obtained from a frozen section examination than from a smear preparation of that lymph node. The main reason is that multiple cut surfaces of the node can be processed on one slide using the cytologic technique, as opposed to the multiple frozen sections that would be necessary to examine the node as thoroughly without the use of smears. Also, since freezing artifact is not a factor in the smear preparation, a few cancer cells are more easily distinguished from the surrounding population of lymphocytes and histiocytes than they are in the artifactually distorted frozen section. Imprints or smears also are often of more value than the classic frozen section in the case of a tumor that is largely necrotic, in which a few malignant cells can be lost in the sea of necrosis on the frozen section but are usually easily visible on the cytologic preparation.

There are relatively few other situations in which the imprint is of more value than the frozen section examination, but many situations exist in which it is of equal (or at least complementary) value. When only a small tissue sample is provided and the possibility exists that a frozen section examination would exhaust the specimen and leave none available for permanent sections, a positive imprint can preclude the necessity of performing the frozen section examination and can thus preserve the tissue in its entirety. Since imprints and smears are also quicker to perform, time (an essential consideration) is saved in the operating room. Toward this end, we have used them extensively in the intraoperative evaluation of cases of hyperparathyroidism and have found that they are at least as accurate as the frozen section examination in distinguishing parathyroid tissue from thyroid, lymph node, thymus, or adipose tissue.[26] Indeed, we can also distinguish normal or atrophic from hyperfunctioning parathyroid glands in almost all cases.[27] In other non-neoplastic situations as well, the cytologic technique has been helpful; for example, we have been able to identify ganglion cells in smears from sympathetic ganglia that were submitted for intraoperative evaluation. A more complete summary of the technique and our experience with it is available elsewhere.[19]

Before leaving the topic of intraoperative cytology entirely, it is worth mentioning that this technique can prepare the surgical pathologist for the interpretation of fine needle aspiration specimens. An excellent way for surgical pathologists to prepare for reading specimens of this sort is to perform touch preparations or smears on all tumors received fresh in the operating room, and for that matter even to perform needle aspirations of these tissues themselves before beginning to accept in vivo specimens from their clinicians. As in the case of frozen section examinations, discretion is often the better part of valor, and the results of an aspiration should never be reported as positive without absolute certainty that tumor is indeed present. As in other cytologic techniques, the emphasis should be on reporting in terms of the anticipated histopathologic diagnosis, rather than using a 'negative-suspicious-positive' or numeric grading system.

THE SURGICAL PATHOLOGY REPORT

The subject of special stains and their uses and abuses is obviously important in surgical pathology. The question of which (if any) special stains to use in a particular case is best resolved by a consideration of the clinical significance of the report in that case. Since special stains are performed most frequently in the search for and interpretation of either infectious or neoplastic disease, their use in these two situations is covered in more detail in Chapters 3 and 6, respectively. General principles of histochemistry and immunohistochemistry are discussed in Chapter 2. Similarly, questions of how many sections to submit from a particular gross specimen, how these sections should be taken and labeled, whether multiple or serial sections are required, and similar considerations are best decided with reference to an individual case. Thus, such questions are dealt with in the individual chapters of this text relating to specific organs and organ systems. In general terms, however, perhaps the most important single consideration is that of consistency in the practice of surgical pathology within a given laboratory. Thus, if one surgical pathologist in the laboratory does not use the letter 'I' as a designation for tissue sections because of its possible confusion with the Roman numeral 'I' none of the pathologists submitting tissue in that laboratory should use that designation. If one pathologist uses a particular designation for resection margins, then all colleagues should use the same designation. Only in this manner can submitting clinicians be guaranteed that the terms of a surgical pathology report they receive on a Monday will mean the same as the terms of the report they receive on Tuesday. Similarly, when all the surgical pathologists in that laboratory have gone elsewhere, their successor or successors will be able to review old slides and old reports and be aware of exactly what they signify.

This brings us to the topic of the correct way to prepare a surgical pathology report; the best statement that can be made is that there is no single best way. The most important aspect to remember is that the report should be prepared with the best interests of the clinician and the patient in mind. Thus, the most important features are clarity, brevity, and careful attention to those details that may influence the management of the patient. In general terms, those portions of the clinical history that are relevant to the specimen should always be included in the final report, as should the exact source of the specimen and the condition in which it is received (e.g. in formalin, fresh, unfixed and poorly preserved, intact, or previously opened). All necessary measurements should be performed before the specimen is dissected, and these measurements (including weight) should be recorded. The description of the gross pathology encountered should proceed from the general to the specific; for example, the presence of a tumor must be noted before its characteristics are described in detail. In general terms, the portion of a specimen (or multiple specimens) described first should be that in which the clinician is most interested, although there may be exceptions to this rule (e.g. when peripheral specimens are received first for frozen section examination and thus are described first in the gross description). If anything has been done to the specimen before its gross examination and sectioning, this should be mentioned in the surgical pathology report. Thus, if a frozen section examination has been performed, the final report should mention this fact, should contain the exact (i.e. word-for-word) frozen section report rendered to the clinician, and should indicate who performed the frozen section examination and rendered the report (in many instances, the pathologist who performed the frozen section examination may not be the same one who cuts, examines, and eventually signs out the case). Similarly, if portions of tissue have been removed for electron microscopic examination, virologic or other cultures, or any study other than histologic examination, this should also be noted in the final report. This is particularly true when a portion of a specimen has been submitted (with the consent of the patient) for one or more research studies. The ethical[28] and tissue quality[29] issues involved in research using human tissues continue to be discussed, and the surgical pathologist should be aware of these issues and of his/her own role in obtaining tissue for research while maintaining specimen quantity and quality to provide 'routine' diagnostic and prognostic information. The continuing importance of standard morphology in the molecular era has been discussed eloquently by Rosai.[30]

If the gross specimen is a complex one, a photograph may add immeasurably to the dictated or written gross description. Photographs should be taken before the specimen is extensively dissected and may be repeated if necessary during and after the process of dissection as well. Important gross details should be adequately labeled in the photograph; a Polaroid, digital, or other instant photographic technique may be extremely valuable for this purpose. Finally, the gross dictation should always include the eventual disposition of the specimen, since this is the only way that future reviewers of the case will have of knowing what each slide represents. This rule should be followed whether the specimen is a single, small piece of tissue that is submitted in toto, or a radical resection for cancer, in which 100 or more sections may be submitted, with the relationship of the label for each section to its exact source duly recorded in a 'slide key' accompanying the gross description.

In addition to the possible benefit mentioned earlier for future reviewers, the advantage of a careful recording of the disposition of the gross specimen may be more immediate. Thus, in the unfortunate event that a specimen is lost or confused with another specimen, the gross dictation and slide key may resolve the possible serious confusion resulting in this situation. Similarly, if the gross description indicates that four pieces of tissue were submitted from a particular biopsy, and only three appear on the slide produced by the histotechnologist, the pathologist knows instantly that the block should be inspected and deeper levels ordered.

The same rules of reason that pertain to gross descriptions and dictations apply equally to both the microscopic description and the final diagnosis. In both sections of the report, the clinically most significant lesions should precede the incidental findings, even if the portion of the specimen containing the latter was processed grossly before the former. As a general rule, what is visible with the scanning lens of the microscope should be described before what is visible with the high-power objective. For example, the pushing versus infiltrating character of the margin of a tumor should always be described before its degree of nuclear pleomorphism or mitotic activity. The microscopic description should be just that, rather than a diagnosis or prognostic commentary. Thus, a phrase such as 'a tumor that appears to be of low-grade malignancy' should never appear in the microscopic description but should be reserved for a comment appended to the final diagnosis. Information included in the microscopic description should be as specific as possible; thus 'vascular invasion' should be replaced by an exact characterization of the type of vessel (e.g. artery, vein, capillary, lymphatic) invaded, and 'chronic inflammation' should yield to an enumeration of the specific cells (lymphocytes, histiocytes, plasma cells) comprising the infiltrate.

Similarly, the final diagnosis should be as specific as possible, should list diagnoses in their order of clinical importance, and should be inclusive of all the specimens received (not forgetting, for example, the unremarkable appendix received with the hysterectomy specimen for cervical cancer). Terminology will vary with the individual laboratory, but again some attempt should be made at standardization. For example, tumors may be subdivided as well, moderately, or poorly differentiated or as grade I, II, or III, but not as both on different days or by different pathologists. The diagnosis should also be clinically relevant, so for some malignant tumors (for example, serous carcinoma of the endometrium), no grade is given, while for others an entity-specific grading system (such as the Gleason system for prostatic adenocarcinoma) is more appropriate. If terminology used is likely to be confusing to the clinician, it should be clearly defined in an appended comment, perhaps with a suitable bibliographic reference. Better yet, clinicians should also be contacted in person or by telephone to be sure they fully understand the information the pathologist is seeking to convey.[31]

Although the essentials of a microscopic description have been detailed above, it should be noted that there has been a great deal of debate in recent years over the necessity for any microscopic description at all in a surgical pathology report. At the University of Maryland, my colleagues and I (SGS) have adopted the middle ground between those who demand a microscopic description on every specimen and those who consider it totally unnecessary. Normal appendices, cervical biopsy specimens showing only chronic cervicitis, unremarkable hernia sacs, and the like are described grossly and given a diagnosis, with the microscopic features omitted; the time thus saved is put to good use in ensuring that the microscopic descriptions for diagnostic biopsy specimens, tumor resections, and other 'nonroutine' specimens are complete to the point of containing all the pertinent observations.

As mentioned previously, a current trend exists toward standardization of the surgical pathology report, not just within each institution but between different institutions as well.[3] One such useful technique is use of computerized checklists to ensure that the clinically relevant information (e.g. tumor size, histologic type, grade, status of resection margins, involvement of lymphatic and blood vessels, and so forth) is always included in the same format in every report.

Standardization of cytopathology reports is also rapidly becoming the rule rather than the exception. The Bethesda System for reporting Pap smears has already become the standard in the United States. In this system (discussed in greater detail in Chapter 36), not only are diagnostic impressions recorded in a checklist fashion, but statements concerning the adequacy of the specimen are standardized as well. Similar systems have been proposed for the reporting of breast and thyroid FNAB results, as well as other types of cases.[32,33]

NEW ADJUNCTS TO THE PRACTICE OF SURGICAL PATHOLOGY AND CYTOPATHOLOGY

The history of the field of surgical pathology contains innumerable techniques that were initially developed as basic research tools and subsequently became adapted to the diagnostic armamentarium. Many of the techniques we now consider as routine (e.g. cryostat procedures for frozen section preparation, electron microscopy, immunohistochemistry, and fine needle aspiration cytology) were at one time a novelty – to our antecedents, or even to us. In previous editions of this book, this section briefly discussed a few of the new adjuncts already in place in some surgical pathology laboratories and some that were anticipated to become commonplace while that volume was still in use. The main subjects discussed were flow cytometry, various molecular biologic techniques, morphometry, computerization, and telepathology. With the exception of morphometry, which, because it is still both expensive for start-up equipment and time and labor intensive, has remained largely a research tool, the other fields have become so much a part of the routine practice of surgical pathology and cytopathology that they are now covered in detail elsewhere in the current edition. The reader is referred to Chapter 2 for more complete discussions.

TRAINING IN SURGICAL PATHOLOGY AND CYTOPATHOLOGY

It is difficult to be specific about training without first defining the ultimate goal of the individual to be trained. For example, the resident who desires to become an academic surgical pathologist/cytopathologist should spend a minimum of 3 years of training in anatomic pathology, with at least 2 of those years devoted to surgical pathology and cytology. Ideally, at least 1 more year is advisable, as is training in more than one institution (both because of the variety of specimens seen in different institutions and because of the exposure to several different philosophies). A prolonged period of exposure to specialized techniques (such as electron microscopy, immunohistochemistry, FNAB) and/or fields of study (dermatopathology, hematopathology, gynecologic pathology) is also advisable. The neophyte academic surgical pathologist is also well advised to undertake and complete some research project or projects during training and to experience the difficulties and triumphs resulting from the presentation and publication of the results thereof.

On the other hand, the training program in surgical pathology for the resident who spends a total of 2 years (or less) each in anatomic and clinical pathology before taking the board examinations and entering clinical practice must, by virtue of the length of time on surgical and cytopathology rotations, be considerably different. At institutions in which training is received in several different hospital laboratories, many residents follow the latter path. Although the nature of the workload differs both quantitatively and qualitatively from one laboratory to the next within such training programs, the directors of these laboratories should believe that the principles to be learned by the trainee are similar in each laboratory. Fundamentals that residents are expected to master during their training include:

1. Cognizance of their own role in the clinical situation in relation to both the clinician and the patient. Residents are responsible for the surgical specimen from the time it is obtained from the patient until the final report is received by the clinician. They should ensure that the specimen is received in time and in proper condition for processing, that the slides are prepared to their satisfaction, and that the diagnosis is received and understood as early as possible by the clinician.
2. Ability to perform in a reasonable time a technically adequate frozen section examination and to deliver an appropriate interpretation. In this situation, residents should be able to communicate with the surgeon to obtain and deliver pertinent information. Residents should also be aware of the limitations of frozen section technique, should know when a diagnosis must be deferred, and should be able to apply special techniques such as smears and imprints, which complement or supplant the frozen section examination.
3. Ability to identify, describe, and submit appropriate sections from specimens commonly encountered in surgical pathology practice. Trainees should establish which cases need to be processed first in a day's workload. They should be able to dictate the gross descriptions of the great majority of cases in final form at the cutting table; to identify the specimens received, how they are processed, and what each section submitted represents, in clear enough fashion that this information is immediately evident to anyone subsequently reading the report; and to recognize the importance of maintaining the specimen for subsequent diagnostic work-up and for teaching.
4. Cooperation with investigators studying human tissues, to the extent that patient care is not compromised.
5. Ability to determine whether slides received are adequate in number and quality and to take appropriate remedial steps if they are not. Residents should be aware of uses and abuses of special stains, recuts, and similar techniques; should be able to assign priorities for the earlier and more extensive investigation of more important cases; and should be able to write a clinically relevant, concise but complete, organized, and intelligible microscopic description on every case for which such a description is required.
6. Ability to diagnose correctly the great majority of commonly encountered lesions, awareness of the existence of other lesions, and knowledge of when and how to seek consultation. Trainees should develop a systematic approach to slide examination, to ensure that lesions, even if they are not always correctly interpreted, will at least not be overlooked. They should also be able to relate the histologic findings to the clinical and gross features of the case.
7. Cognizance of specialized techniques in such fields as histochemistry, electron microscopy, immunopathology, molecular biology, and specimen radiography and their applications to diagnostic surgical pathology. It is important to have knowledge of when it is appropriate to submit tissues for these and other studies, and in what form the tissue must be submitted for the studies to be successful.
8. Understanding the clinical manifestations and natural history of lesions encountered. This demands independent reading, beginning with standard textbooks (especially, we hope, this one) and progressing to familiarity with and critical reading of current clinical and pathologic literature.
9. Familiarity with the technical aspects of histopathology as related to surgical pathology. This includes techniques of sectioning, embedding, and staining, comparative values of different fixatives, operation and servicing of microtomes and cryostats, and similar problems.

Although this list of goals might easily be modified in different institutions that train residents in surgical pathology, we believe that goals should be established by each institution for its own training program. Both trainees and those who are responsible for their training should be aware of these goals and should monitor the program carefully to be sure they are being met. Similarly, the wording should be changed somewhat to apply to training in cytopathology, but very similar goals will still apply. For example, the reference to frozen sections will be altered to rapid interpretation of FNAB specimens, and the emphasis on gross pathology will change to clinical localization of masses for FNAB. Nevertheless, training overall should emphasize the similarities rather than the differences between the two disciplines, and opportunities to compare cytologic and tissue pathologic manifestations of the same lesions should always be provided.

New program requirements developed by the Accreditation Council for Graduate Medical Education (ACGME) in the United States have demanded defined education programs for trainees in all medical specialties, based on six areas of competency: patient care, medical knowledge, practice-based learning and improvement, interpersonal and communication skills, professionalism, and systems-based practice. All training programs are required to develop both curricula and evaluation systems to evaluate each resident's competence in each of these areas, emphasizing increased expectations with increased time in the program for the resident. An attempt to adapt the traditional Anatomic Pathology training objectives to this system has recently been developed and published by the Association of Directors of Anatomic and Surgical Pathology (ADASP).[34] Similar 'professional performance indicators' for practicing pathologists in the United Kingdom have been published by the Royal College of Pathologists.[35] Together, these two documents provide valuable information on the currently accepted standards of practice in these two countries.

A word should also be said about training in surgical pathology for nonpathologists. Although it is our strong conviction that surgical pathology should be practiced by pathologists, we also believe that, just as the pathologist with advanced clinical experience is often a better pathologist, the general surgeon, gynecologist, dermatologist, or other clinical specialist who has been exposed to a rotation in surgical pathology during training is often the better for this experience as well. These rotations by clinical trainees through the surgical pathology service will often be limited to one or a few months, and the goals of the training in this situation should be as follows: (1) to instill an appreciation of the role of the surgical pathologist as a consultant in the appropriate clinical field; (2) to develop a recognition of the importance of adequate communication (including the provision by the clinician of appropriate clinical histories and specimen descriptions) in the performance of this consultative role of the surgical pathologist; (3) to develop a respect for the specimen as the primary vehicle for this communication, together with an appropriate appreciation of proper techniques of fixation and submission of specimens; (4) to develop a realization of what surgical pathologists cannot do, so as to expect fewer miracles from them in subsequent clinical practice; (5) to develop some concept of basic principles of gross pathology, so that inflammatory, neoplastic, traumatic, and other processes can be distinguished in the operating room or the clinic; and (6) to develop the same sort of familiarity with microscopic interpretation, and with the clinical and pathologic significance of the main entities encountered in the individual field of clinical practice, so that a surgical pathology report may be interpreted and slides reviewed with the surgical pathologist with more confidence in the future.

QUALITY ISSUES IN ANATOMIC PATHOLOGY

In the relatively recent past, issues of quality in the hospital laboratory were tied entirely to the professional self-respect and discretion of the staff pathologists. The natural tendency of physicians is to be at the forefront of development in their chosen fields, and to compete with their peers for accomplishment and the concomitant esteem of their fellows. Indeed, this is still a powerful force that is often underestimated or disregarded by administrative or regulatory personnel in the healthcare industry. In the 1980s, when the latter individuals began to control the overall functioning of medical centers at a level theretofore exercised only by persons with formal medical educations, pathologists were suddenly faced with the need to familiarize themselves with 'corporate' concepts that were often new to them – 'quality control,' 'quality assurance,' 'continuous quality improvement,' 'cost-effectiveness,' and 'outcomes analysis.'[36–47] Indeed, in the current business that is Medicine, formal adherence to those principles is expected on all fronts. However, because pathology deals more than other specialties with the generation of quantifiable data, it lends itself more readily than other areas to the application of standards. Particularly when considered in the context of *anatomic* pathology, quality issues concern the generation of diagnostic reports that are timely, complete, accurate, and understandable, and that are based on optimal tissue preparation and processing. All of these components of 'quality' can be addressed

at least semiquantitatively, and, in the present climate of medical 'accountability,' it is expected that they will be measured and recorded on a regular basis.

'Quality control' (QC) is an ongoing evaluation process that is designed to assess the activities of personnel and the functioning of equipment and materials.[39] Its purpose is to provide evidence that the laboratory is functioning in a consistent manner, or, if not, that prescribed corrective actions are being applied in a predictable fashion. On the other hand, 'quality assurance' (QA) has a more subjective association, because it is aimed at showing that the delivery of patient care-related services occurs in a manner that assesses 'excellence' in medical practice.[37] QA principles encompass 'preanalytical' factors such as specimen procurement, transportation, and accessioning; 'analytical' variables such as the technical handling of tissue preparations, the interpretation thereof, and the use of standardized reporting formats; and 'postanalytical' factors such as medical transcription, prompt and thorough review of reports by pathologists, and timely delivery of final reports to clinical physicians and hospital departments.[47] 'Continuous quality improvement' (CQI) has interfaces with both QC and QA, in that it represents the structuring of an organized plan for effecting increasing quality in all aspects of both areas.[36,44] CQI deals principally with the evaluation and enhancement of 'systems' in the laboratory and the hospital, in other words, the sequences of activity that culminate in the production of a final product, the diagnostic report. Accordingly, when problems are identified, CQI-related interventions are applied which are intended to ensure that the defects are systematically prevented or eradicated.

The matrix of data-recording activities that attends the monitoring of QA, QC, and CQI functions is complex. Fortunately, with the advent of computer-based anatomic pathology practices, it is now relatively easy to record such information as the interval between the accessioning of a specimen and delivery of the diagnostic report to which it is attached; the turnaround time for disposition of cases by individual pathologists; the number of reports that are returned over a given period of time for correction by transcriptionists; the number of intramural or extramural consultations obtained by the pathology staff; and many others. The details of necessary procedures in this realm of laboratory medicine can be found in other treatises that are devoted entirely to quality issues,[48–58] and will not be recounted here for the sake of brevity. However, that is not to imply that such actions are unimportant; indeed, failure to attend to them would result in serious problems regarding laboratory accreditation.

Other facets of QC, QA, and CQI in anatomic pathology are either common to all scientific endeavors, or, conversely, unique to that discipline. For example, in the first of those categories, it is necessary to develop and update detailed procedure manuals for use in each subdivision of the hospital laboratory; these must be reviewed and initialed by responsible pathologists at regular intervals. Likewise, instrument maintenance must be scheduled and documented consistently. In the second category, one can consider such topics as cytologic-histologic correlations,[59] review of specimens from outside hospitals that accompany referral cases,[60] and the degree of concordance between frozen section diagnoses and final interpretations.[61] All of these should be accompanied by consistent matrices for monitoring, and documented appropriately.

The assessment of the subjective quality of histologic or cytologic preparations is an area that still has been left largely to the judgments of individual pathologists. That is curious, inasmuch as poor-quality slides are certainly an important source of diagnostic mistakes, or, at least, an impediment to proper interpretation. There is currently no systematic program for interinstitutional evaluations along such lines, in which, for example, sections would be prepared from specimens distributed by a central organization and sent back to it for critical analysis and grading. Absent that, it is important for all pathologists to initiate intralaboratory plans to address such details. A representative group of histologic sections (stained with hematoxylin and eosin as well as other common histochemical dyes), immunohistologic preparations, and cytologic specimens should be reviewed together qualitatively, by pathologists and technologists, on a regular schedule. The outcome of such assessments can then be recorded, along with written plans to remedy any deficiencies that are identified. An even more ambitious approach would be to trade specimens with a 'reference' laboratory and compare the results.

One of the most difficult topics in quality management in anatomic pathology concerns the measurement of interobserver agreement between pathologists, or between pathologists and cytotechnologists.[62] Several approaches have evolved to accomplish this task, including mandatory review by a second pathologist of any new diagnosis of malignancy; record-keeping of the interpretative concordance between pathologists who are presenting cases at interdepartmental conferences and the person originating the diagnosis; predefined cross-sectional reviews of a percentage of diagnoses by a second observer in the same practice group; and referral of a prescribed proportion of cases to an extramural consultant over any given time period. Each of these has its own advantages and disadvantages, which principally center on the issues of timeliness and expense. At present, there is no perfect or universally applicable approach to this subject, but it can be said that *some* form of interobserver validation must take place in all laboratories.

Along the same lines, some professional organizations have developed subscription programs for the evaluation of diagnostic competency. In these (e.g. the Performance Improvement Program for pathologists offered by the College of American Pathologists; CheckPath and CheckSample, provided by the American Society for Clinical Pathology; an Immunohistochemistry Quality Assurance program of the College of American Pathologists; and various societal or governmentally sponsored programs for diagnostic cytopathology), 'test' cases are distributed to participating institutions or individuals, who then answer prescribed questions. Their performances are graded by the originating agency, which may also provide a certification of ongoing proficiency. The shortcomings of these programs have been summarized by Cramer et al.[63] One is the definition of which diagnoses are 'correct' and which are 'incorrect' and the selection of proper experts to make such determinations. A second is the even more problematic assessment of which 'misdiagnoses' would have a measurable and significant effect on patient care and case outcome. Despite these problems, it is recommended that all pathology laboratories should indeed participate in extramural programs for the review of professional proficiency.

Another controversial area concerns the structure of diagnostic reporting formats.[64] Many laboratories have now embraced the use of predefined 'synoptic' reports in surgical pathology, especially for malignancies.[65–67] These offer the user prescribed choices that cover virtually all interpretative possibilities pertaining to any given organ site and a particular set of diagnoses. Those applying to the case at hand can then be selected by the pathologist from checklists and compiled by transcriptionists into a final report. The same concept has been extended to non-neoplastic diseases as well. For example, at one of the authors' institutions, a synoptic reporting format is available for colonic biopsies in suspected cases of Hirschsprung's disease, to make certain that information desired by attending pediatricians is always provided. Moreover, 'templates' have also been developed for dictation of gross findings or descriptions of histologic observations, wherein one 'fills in the blanks' to provide information that is unique to a particular case. The rewards of this approach are those of greater consistency and completeness of reporting, and it should also be understood that *ad libitum* comments can still be appended to synoptic reports or templates as desired. Realistically, the only drawback of such formats is a limitation of the 'personal freedom' of the pathologist, and that factor is actually antithetical to many principles of QC.

Given the litigious climate of medical practice in the United States, there has been considerable concern over which, if any, of the QC, QA, and CQI activities mentioned in this section would be 'discoverable' (provided to the court mandatorily via a *subpoena*) if a malpractice action were initiated against a particular pathologist or laboratory. At present, there is no uniform answer to that question, because the law pertaining to it varies from state to state. Nonetheless, some principles can be enumerated to minimize risk in this context. First, all QC/QA/CQI documents should be anonymized with regard to patient and case identities, as much as possible. Second, the identities of pathologists and technologists may also be encoded by a dispassionate observer in the hospital administration, who then is responsible for keeping records on the performance of those individuals. This provision maintains privacy but still supports the function of a meaningful self-assessment program. The latter goal is really all that should concern the courts, at least arguably. Third, it is critical that laboratory directors in anatomic pathology obtain the advice of their local hospital counsels and risk-management personnel to guide them through this process.

LAWSUITS IN ANATOMIC PATHOLOGY

The topic just mentioned provides the nexus for a broader discussion of malpractice actions in anatomic pathology. Unfortunately, unless some sort of tort reform occurs in this country in the future, most, if not all, pathologists now in practice can anticipate that they will likely be named in at least one malpractice claim during their working careers. Often, the only 'fault' that applies is that the pathologist's name appears somewhere in the medical record as a 'treating' physician (anyone involved in the care of the patient). This is true because some plaintiffs' attorneys will indiscriminately name any and all such persons in the legal 'bill of complaint' that is issued against the caregivers.

In that regard, one should remember that two important requirements exist to justify a claim of malpractice against any physician. The practitioner must be shown to be culpable of 'negligence' – defined by 'expert' testimony as medical practice that breaches the regional or national standard of care (behavior expected of a 'prudent, careful, and informed physician') for his or her specialty – and also to have caused a definable 'injury' (an adverse consequence that is objectively documented and judged to be directly tied to putative medical negligence). Many claims made against physicians are grossly lacking in one or both of those proofs, but there is currently no penalty that can be levied against injudicious attorneys or plaintiffs for bringing such deficient allegations to the court.

There are several other factors that help to explain the proliferation of malpractice lawsuits in the last 20 years. First, the popular press has become enamored of the idea that doctors and hospitals are hotbeds for mistakes, despite published scientific data to the contrary.[68] Second, the pervasive attitude of 'entitlement' in our society fosters the notion that adverse life events must inevitably be tied to blame and monetary compensation. Third, relatively few states have legislated reasonable 'caps' on financial judgments against physicians and hospitals in malpractice actions, and where these do exist, their numerical values vary (e.g. in Virginia, the cap is $1.8 million per event per practitioner, whereas it is $0.75 million in Texas). That fact has a direct bearing on the system of remuneration for plaintiffs' attorneys, who are still allowed to work on a contingency basis. In many locales, lawyers collect up to 33% of any monetary judgment levied by the court in a malpractice case. Last, some states even allow plaintiffs to file separate civil lawsuits against a physician's *personal* assets in malpractice actions, apart from any judgment that may be made against his or her insurance carrier.

Just how many clinically significant diagnostic 'errors' are made in anatomic pathology? The published rates for such mistakes have been between 0.25% and 6% of cases,[69] but it is difficult to know how the terms 'error' or 'clinically significant' were defined in some of those studies. There is still a paucity of definitive diagnostic criteria for many pathologic conditions, and at least a proportion of published 'errors' have been based on adequate interpretative proficiency but misleading clinical data that were provided to the pathologist. Those factors are difficult to quantify or integrate in considerations of true diagnostic mistake-making. Sadly, that point is considered irrelevant in the public's perception and that of the plaintiffs' bar, both of whom expect a 0% standard of error by physicians.

In absolute numbers, claims against pathologists comprise a relatively small fraction of all medical malpractice suits. For example, in a 3-year period, Troxel reported that 218 pathology-related actions were handled by one sizable insurer.[70,71] Although this total is substantially smaller than the number associated with general surgeons, obstetricians, anesthesiologists, and other specialists, it is growing. That fact may have multifactorial underpinnings, including greater visibility of pathologists produced by public education activities of various societies and misrepresentation of the power of certain laboratory tests (especially cervical Papanicolaou [Pap] smears) to laypersons. For example, in a novel entitled *A Case of Need*, author Michael Crichton – himself a physician – quite erroneously stated that 'the Papp [sic] smear is the most accurate diagnostic test in all of medicine.'[72]

If confronted with a bill of complaint, physicians should immediately consult their hospital risk management department (RMD) to obtain formal assistance and procure legal services. Under no circumstance is it ever advisable to respond by speaking with the plaintiff or his or her attorney. Conversations with RMD personnel are typically protected by the same level of confidentiality as that attending attorney–client privilege. Indeed, if one even suspects that a lawsuit *may* be initiated over a particular case, it is wise to contact the RMD early to make them aware of the details. The adage 'forewarned is forearmed' applies to such situations. Once legal representation has been secured in a malpractice action, the attorney's roles are to gather as much information as possible, serve as the ultimate liaison between the contestants (and the court), and advise the physician-client of the best course of legal action based on existing statutes and case law. After this process is completed, the pathologist usually makes the final decision on whether a case should be litigated at a trial or settled instead. However, the prudent approach is certainly to follow legal advice regarding that issue.

Along the way, there are some important guidelines to remember. First, one should never answer questions from the opposing legal counsel without having one's own attorney present. Second, discussion of the case with other persons named in the bill of complaint is a bad idea, and it would be even more damaging to try to influence their views. Third, attempts to deflect one's own potential liability by impugning the actions of other physicians are unprofessional and virtually always unsuccessful. Fourth, it is obvious that it is never permissible to alter, discard, or conceal pertinent medical records or diagnostic materials (e.g. glass slides or paraffin blocks) relating to the case in question. Finally, beware of 'legalese' that can be employed by attorneys to an adverse end. For example, the words 'expert,' 'authority,' and 'authoritative' have special meanings in the law, implying infallibility.[73] Therefore, if one stipulates that Dr. X is indeed an expert, anything written or said by that person potentially has the patina of absolute truth, in the eyes of the court.

The specific areas of anatomic pathology that are most often substrates for malpractice suits include the alleged misinterpretation of Pap smears, failure to diagnose cutaneous melanoma, errors in the interpretation of breast biopsies, mistakes in the diagnosis of hematopathologic specimens, problems attending the performance and interpretation of fine needle aspiration biopsies, frozen section errors, and misinterpretation of prostate needle biopsies.[70,71] One response to this list would be to require surgical pathology subspecialists to review all cases in the cited topic areas. However, that would, in fact, offer no absolute guarantee against commitment of errors, and it also would be patently unfeasible for most practice groups. Instead, particular QA practices can be aimed at the topics in question, to maximize interobserver review and focus continuing-education activities on those particular areas. The use of extramural consultations is also a consideration in regard to the types of specimens listed above.

There are also some 'hidden' sources of legal liability in the laboratory. An important example concerns specimen accessioning, prosection, and processing.[52,74] If grossly similar specimens (e.g. prostatic needle biopsies) are transposed during these steps, disaster may follow. Similarly, contamination of one specimen by tissue from another may have serious consequences. This potentially may occur in the gross room, the cytology preparation area, the histology autoprocessing machines, or the paraffin embedding station. A case example follows.

A 53-year-old woman complained of persistent dyspepsia and underwent esophagogastroduodenoscopy. The gastroenterologist saw only 'mild gastritis' visually, but he obtained several random biopsies of the gastric mucosa. These unexpectedly demonstrated the presence of an enteric-type adenocarcinoma in one of three tissue fragments (Figs 1.1–1.4); the other pieces of gastric mucosa were histologically normal. A total gastrectomy was performed. There was no evidence of malignancy in the resection specimen, despite the fact that the entire mucosal surface was submitted for histologic examination. Because a transposition of tissue was then suspected in regard to the original biopsy, immunostains for blood group isoantigens were obtained on that specimen.[75] They continued the suspicion that contamination had occurred; the fragments of non-neoplastic gastric mucosa were labeled for blood group isoantigen A, whereas the fragment showing carcinoma stained for isoantigen B. Review of the surgical pathology log revealed that a colonic adenocarcinoma with an identical appearance had been prosected in the gross laboratory on the same day the gastric biopsies were received, and the patient with that carcinoma had blood type B.

Another area of uncertainty concerning legal liability is the use of adjunctive diagnostic technology in anatomic pathology. The version of the Clinical Laboratory Improvement Act (CLIA) that was issued in 1988 has the potential to certify selected laboratories to perform 'complex testing' such as immunohistochemistry, in situ hybridization, the polymerase chain reaction assay, and other 'molecular' analyses.[76] However, there are no codified guidelines

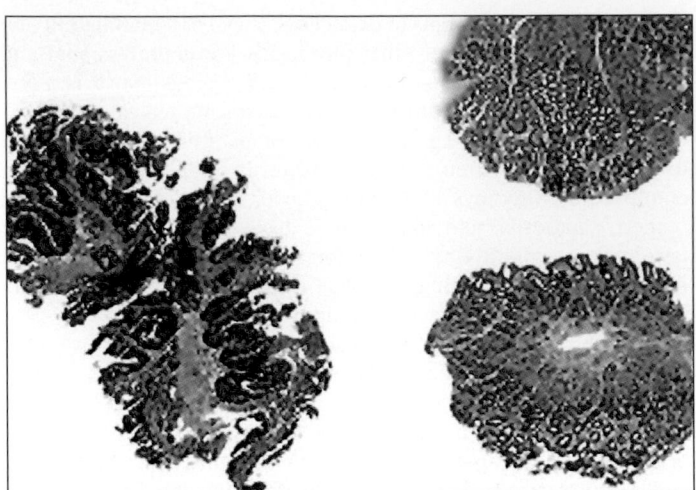

Fig. 1.1 Gastric biopsy specimen from a middle-aged woman with dyspepsia and no macroscopic abnormalities on endoscopy. It shows two fragments of histologically normal mucosa and one containing enteric-type adenocarcinoma.

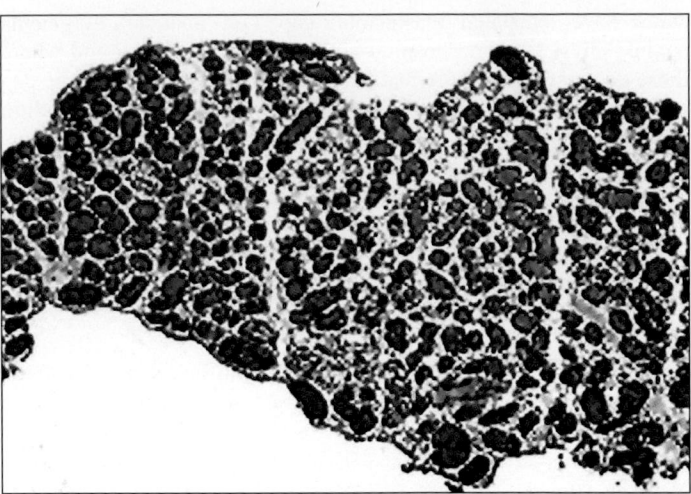

Fig. 1.3 Immunostaining for blood group isoantigen A on the original biopsy (Fig. 1.1) showed strong epithelial and endothelial labeling for that marker in the non-neoplastic tissue (shown here), but not in the carcinomatous fragment.

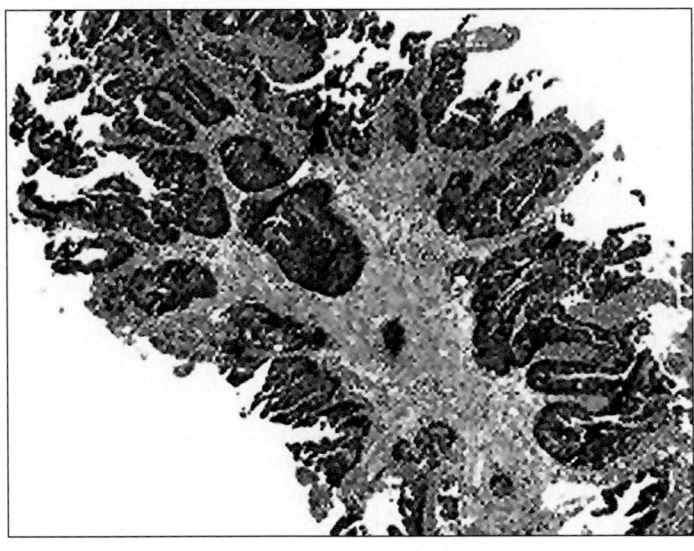

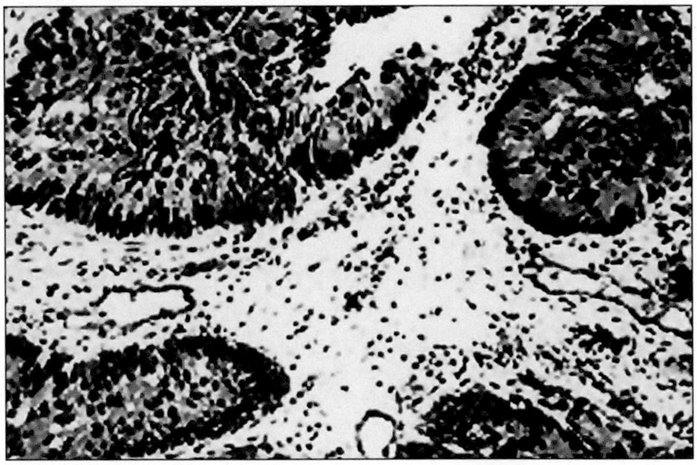

Fig. 1.2 The enteric-type adenocarcinoma shown in Fig. 1.1 is seen at higher magnification. On the basis of its presence in the specimen, a gastrectomy was performed, histologic examination of which revealed no evidence of malignancy.

Fig. 1.4 Immunostaining for blood group isoantigen B showed epithelial and endothelial labeling in the fragment of tissue containing carcinoma in the original biopsy (Fig. 1.1), confirming the suspicion that it represented a 'floater'.

that enumerate universally accepted technical details for those procedures or which provide methods for QC/QA/CQI pertaining to them. Therefore, the issue of whether or not adjunctive studies constitute 'standard of practice' in relation to particular pathologic diagnoses is murky. In 1998, the US Food and Drug Administration issued a determination on which immunohistochemical reagents were recognized under its authority,[77] resolving a difficult situation wherein those reagents had been used for years beforehand with no formal governance. However, other adjuvant testing methods still have not been addressed in the same way. That circumstance sets the stage for legal problems which relate to whether a technology could or should have been applied to pathologic evaluations at a particular point in time. The following case is illustrative.

A 41-year-old man presented in 1993 with rapidly worsening abdominal pain, and imaging studies showed a cecal mass with a thickened bowel segment flanking the ileocecal junction. He underwent laparotomy and resection of the distal ileum and proximal colon. A 6-cm mass was found in the cecum, histologic sections of which were interpreted as showing anaplastic carcinoma. Regional lymph nodes and the liver were uninvolved by the tumor, and no adjuvant chemotherapy was administered. Eight months later, the patient returned with diffuse lymphadenopathy and hepatosplenomegaly. Lymph node biopsies done at that time revealed large cell non-Hodgkin's lymphoma. Review of the intestinal specimen and retrospective immunostaining for CD45 showed that it too had contained lymphoma instead of carcinoma (Figs 1.5–1.7). The pathologist was sued because of a 'failure to employ available diagnostic methods in a timely manner,' and for

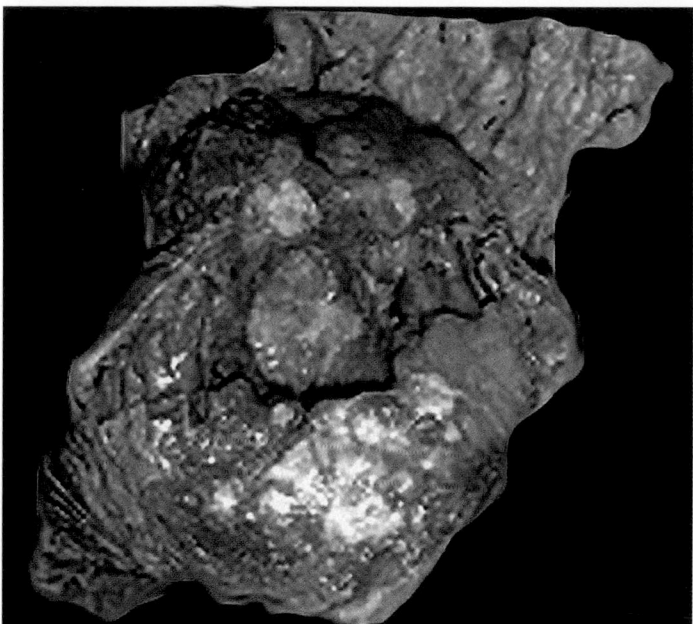

Fig. 1.5 This cecal mass was detected radiographically in a 41-year-old man with abdominal pain.

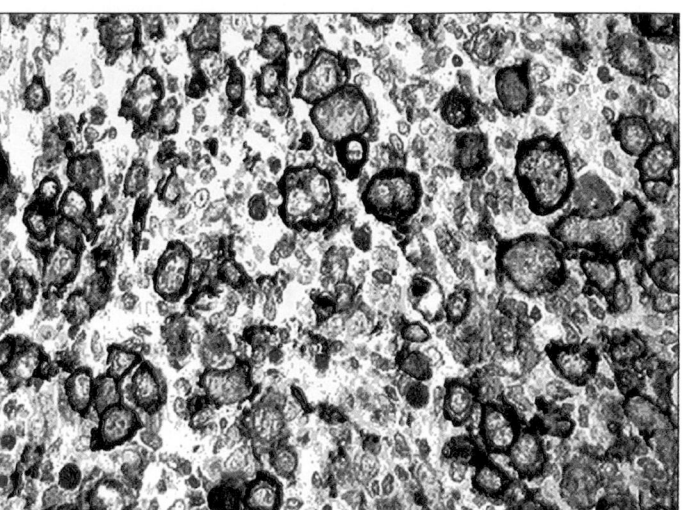

Fig. 1.7 After the patient returned with lymphadenopathy and organomegaly, the original biopsy (Fig. 1.5) was immunostained for CD45, yielding the strong reactivity shown here. The amended diagnosis was that of large cell non-Hodgkin's lymphoma. However, because the case had been seen before immunostains were accredited for clinical application, there was no mandate, according to existing standards of care, that immunohistochemical procedures should have been performed.

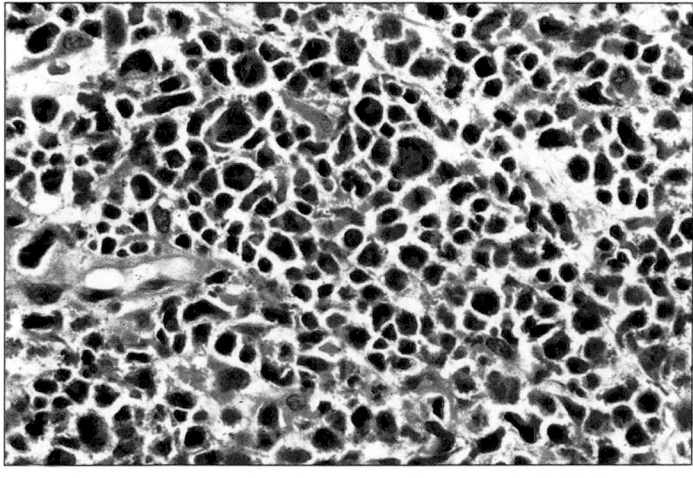

Fig. 1.6 Histologically, the mass shown in Fig. 1.5 was comprised by large undifferentiated polygonal cells, admixed with inflammatory elements. It was interpreted as an undifferentiated carcinoma.

putative damage caused by that omission in regard to the delay of optimal therapy.

The plaintiff's attorney in the latter action claimed that immunostains for CD45 were available in 1993 and should have been used by the pathologist, according to the existing 'standard of practice.' However, it was successfully argued in rebuttal that immunohistochemistry was not formally accredited as a diagnostic procedure at that time; indeed, all antibody reagents marketed through 1998 were accompanied by a manufacturer's disclaimer stating that they were 'for investigational use only.'

The use of systematic intramural and extramural QC and QA programs is a feasible response to the nebulous state of affairs regarding technological procedures in anatomic pathology. Even if a particular technique is not 'accredited,' it can be shown by those means to perform consistently and to correlate with the results of a validating diagnostic method. Standardized statements to that effect can be placed in diagnostic reports to reflect the presence of an institutional program for technological control.

REFERENCES

1. Jenkins D, Philips Z, Grisaffi K, et al. The boundaries of cellular pathology: how pathologists see their clinical role. J Pathol 2002; 196: 356–363.

2. Connolly JL, Fletcher CDM. What is needed to satisfy the American College of Surgeons Commission on Cancer requirements for the pathologic reporting of cancer specimens? Am J Clin Pathol 2003; 119: 629.

3. Association of Directors of Anatomic and Surgical Pathology. Standardization of the surgical pathology report. Am J Surg Pathol 1992; 16: 84–86.

4. Murphy WM. Ethical issues in anatomic pathology. Are we going the way of the financial sector? Am J Surg Pathol 2003; 27: 392–395.

5. Greening SE, Somrak TM. Medicolegal issues in cytology: legal principles and liability outlook. In: Cytopathology annual 1994. Chicago: ASCP Press; 1994: 65–81.

6. Renshaw AA, Pinnar NE, Jiroutek MR, et al. Quantifying the value of in-house consultation in surgical pathology. Am J Clin Pathol 2002; 117: 751–754.

7. Tomaszewski JE, Bear HD, Connally JA, et al. Consensus conference on second opinions in diagnostic anatomic pathology. Am J Clin Pathol 2000; 114: 329–335.

8. Azam M, Nakhleh RE. Surgical pathology extradepartmental consultation practices. A College of American Pathologists Q-Probes study of 2746 consultations from 180 laboratories. Arch Pathol Lab Med 2002; 126: 405–412.

9. Association of Directors of Anatomic and Surgical Pathology. Consultations in surgical pathology. Am J Surg Pathol 1993; 17: 743–745.

10. Wetherington RW, Cooper HS, Al-Saleem T, et al. Clinical significance of performing immunohistochemistry on cases with a previous diagnosis of cancer coming to a national comprehensive cancer center for treatment or second opinion. Am J Surg Pathol 2002; 26: 1222–1230.

11. Weinstein RS, Descour MR, Liang C, et al. Telepathology overview: From concept to implementation. Hum Pathol 2001; 32: 1283–1299.

12. Cross SS, Dennis T, Start RD. Telepathology: current status and future prospects in diagnostic histopathology. Histopathology 2002; 41: 91–109.

13. Williams BH, Hong IS, Mullick FG, et al. Image quality issues in a static image-based telepathology consultation. Hum Pathol 2003; 34: 1228–1234.

14. Kaplan KJ, Burgess JR, Sandberg GD, et al. Use of robotic telepathology for frozen-section diagnosis: A retrospective trial of a telepathology system for intraoperative consultation. Mod Pathol 2002; 15: 1197–1204.

15. Ackerman LV, Ramirez GA. The indications for and limitations of frozen section diagnosis. Br J Surg 1959; 46: 336–350.

16. Holaday WJ, Assor D. Ten thousand consecutive frozen sections. Am J Clin Pathol 1974; 61: 769–777.

17. Nakazawa H, Rosen P, Lane N, et al. The frozen section experience in 3000 cases. Am J Clin Pathol 1968; 49: 41–51.

18. Oneson RH, Minke JA, Silverberg SG. Intraoperative pathologic consultation: an audit of 1,000 recent consecutive cases. Am J Surg Pathol 1989; 13: 237–243.

19. Nochomovitz L, Sidawy M, Silverberg SG, et al. Intraoperative consultation. a guide to smears, imprints, and frozen sections. Chicago: ASCP Press; 1989.

20. Oberman HA. A modest proposal. Am J Surg Pathol 1992; 16: 69–70.

21. Association of Directors of Anatomic and Surgical Pathology. Current controversy: frozen section examination of nonpalpable or small palpable breast lesions. Pathol Case Rev 1996; 1: 2–5.

22. Sidawy MK, Silverberg SG. Intraoperative cytology: back to the future? Am J Clin Pathol 1991; 96: 1–3.

23. Mair S, Lash RH, Suskin D, et al. Intraoperative surgical specimen evaluation: frozen section analysis, cytologic examination, or both? A comparative study of 206 cases. Am J Clin Pathol 1991; 96: 8–14.

24. Blumenfeld W, Hashmi N, Sagerman P. Comparison of aspiration, touch and scrape preparations simultaneously obtained from surgically excised specimens. Effect of different methods of smear preparation on interpretive cytologic feature. Acta Cytol 1998; 42: 1414–1418.

25. Shidham V, Gupta D, Galindo LM, et al. Intraoperative scrape cytology: comparison with frozen sections, using receiver operating characteristic (ROC) curve. Diagn Cytopathol 2000; 23: 134–139.

26. Geelhoed GW, Silverberg SG. Intraoperative imprints for the identification of parathyroid tissue. Surgery 1984; 96: 1124–1130.

27. Sasano H, Geelhoed GW, Silverberg SG. Intraoperative cytologic evaluation of lipid in the diagnosis of parathyroid adenoma. Am J Surg Pathol 1988; 12: 282–286.

28. Furness PN. Research using human tissue – a crisis of supply? J Pathol 2001; 195: 277–284.

29. Jewell SD, Srinivasan M, McCart LM, et al. Analysis of the molecular quality of human tissues. An experience from the Cooperative Human Tissue Network. Am J Clin Pathol 2002; 118: 733–741.

30. Rosai J. The continuing role of morphology in the molecular age. Mod Pathol 2001; 14: 258–260.

31. Powsner SM, Costa J, Homer RJ. Clinicians are from Mars and pathologists are from Venus: clinician interpretation of pathology reports. Arch Pathol Lab Med 2000; 124: 1040–1046.

32. Sneige N, Staerkel GA, Caraway NP, et al. A plea for uniform terminology and reporting of breast fine needle aspirates. Acta Cytol 1994; 38: 971–972.

33. The Papanicolaou Society of Cytopathology Task Force on Standards of Practice. Guidelines of the Papanicolaou Society of Cytopathology for the examination of fine needle aspiration specimens from thyroid nodules. Mod Pathol 1996; 9: 710–715.

34. Association of Directors of Anatomic and Surgical Pathology. Curriculum content and evaluation of resident competency in anatomic pathology. Am J Clin Pathol 2003; 120: 652–660.

35. Professional Standards Unit, Royal College of Pathologists. Professional performance indicators for pathology specialties. Bull Royal Coll Pathol 2002; July,119: 21–22.

36. Zarbo RJ. Improving quality in pathology and laboratory medicine. Am J Clin Pathol 1994; 102: 563–564.

37. Howanitz PJ. Quality assurance measurements in departments of pathology and laboratory medicine. Arch Pathol Lab Med 1990; 114: 1131–1135.

38. Rickert RR. Quality assurance goals in surgical pathology. Arch Pathol Lab Med 1990; 114: 1157–1162.

39. Bachner P. Quality assurance: an accreditation perspective. Lab Med 1989; 20: 159–162.

40. Langley FA. Quality control in histopathology and diagnostic cytology. Histopathology 1978; 2: 3–18.

41. Murthy MSN, Derman H. Quality assurance in surgical pathology: personal and peer assessment. Am J Clin Pathol 1981; 75: 462–466.

42. Travers H. Quality assurance in anatomic pathology. Lab Med 1989; 20: 85–92.

43. Association of Directors of Anatomic and Surgical Pathology. Recommendations on quality control and quality assurance in anatomic pathology. Am J Surg Pathol 1991; 15: 1007–1009.

44. Berwick DM. Continuous improvement as an ideal in health care. N Engl J Med 1989; 320: 53–56.

45. Zarbo RT. Monitoring anatomic pathology practice through quality assurance measures. Clin Lab Med 1999; 19: 713–742.

46. Raab SS. Cost-effectiveness analysis in pathology. Clin Lab Med 1999; 19: 757–771.

47. Stanley MW. Cost benefit and outcomes analysis for fine needle aspiration: why do we know so little? Clin Lab Med 1999; 19: 773–796.

48. Cowan DF. Quality assurance in anatomic pathology: an information system approach. Arch Pathol Lab Med 1990; 114: 129–134.

49. Ramsay AD. Locally organized medical audit in histopathology. J Clin Pathol 1991; 44: 353–357.

50. McBroom HM, Ramsay AD. The clinicopathologic meeting: a means of auditing diagnostic performance. Am J Surg Pathol 1993; 17: 75–80.

51. Travers H, ed. Quality improvement manual in anatomic pathology. Northfield, IL: College of American Pathologists; 1993.

52. Nakhleh RE, Zarbo RJ, Surgical pathology specimen identification and accessioning. Arch Pathol Lab Med 1996; 120: 227–233.

53. College of American Pathologists Commission on Laboratory Accreditation, Inspection checklist I, laboratory general. Northfield, IL: College of American Pathologists; 1994.

54. College of American Pathologists Commission on Laboratory Accreditation. Inspection checklist VIII, anatomic pathology & cytopathology. Northfield, IL: College of American Pathologists; 1994.

55. Zarbo RJ, Gephardt GN, Howanitz PI. Intralaboratory timeliness of surgical pathology reports: results of two College of American Pathologists Q-Probes studies of biopsies and complex specimens. Arch Pathol Lab Med 1996; 120: 234–244.

56. Duckworth JK. Laboratory licensure and accreditation. In: Howanitz PJ, Howanitz JH, eds. Laboratory quality assurance. New York, NY: McGraw-Hill; 1987: 334–353.

57. Joint Commission on Accreditation of Health Care Organizations. Accreditation manual for hospitals. Chicago, IL: Joint Commission on Accreditation of Health Care Organizations; 1992.

58. Joint Commission on Accreditation of Health Care Organizations. Monitoring and evaluation in pathology & medical laboratory services. Chicago, IL: Joint Commission on Accreditation of Health Care Organizations; 1989.

59. Clary KM, Silverman JF, Liu Y, et al. Cytohistologic discrepancies: a means to improve pathology practice and patient outcomes. Am J Clin Pathol 2002; 117: 567–573.

60. Abt AB, Abt LG, Olt GJ. The effect of interinstitution anatomic pathology consultation on patient care. Arch Pathol Lab Med 1995; 119: 514–517.

61. Zarbo RJ, Schmidt WA, Bachner P, et al. Indications and immediate patient outcomes of pathology intraoperative consultations: a College of American Pathologists/Centers for Disease Control and Prevention outcomes working group study. Arch Pathol Lab Med 1996; 120: 19–25.

62. Glaessgen A, Hamberg H, Pihi CO, et al. Interobserver reproducibility of percent Gleason grade 4/5 in total prostatectomy specimens. J Urol 2002; 168: 2006–2010.

63. Cramer SF, Roth LM, Ulbright TM. The mystique of the mistake: with proposed standards for validating proficiency tests in anatomic pathology. Am J Clin Pathol 1991; 96: 774–777.

64. Association of Directors of Anatomic and Surgical Pathology. Standardization of the surgical pathology report. Am J Surg Pathol 1992; 16: 84–86.

65. Rosai J. Standardized reporting of surgical pathology diagnosis for the major tumor types: a proposal. Am J Clin Pathol 1993; 100: 240–255.

66. Robboy SJ, Bentley RC, Krigman H, et al. Synoptic reports in gynecologic pathology. Int J Gynecol Pathol 1994; 13: 161–174.

67. Markel SF, Hirsch SD. Synoptic surgical pathology reporting. Hum Pathol 1991; 22: 807–810.

68. Blendon RJ, DesRoches CM, Brodie M, et al. Views of practicing physicians and the public on medical errors. N Engl J Med 2002; 347: 1933–1940.

69. Lee TH. A broader concept of medical errors. N Engl J Med 2002; 347: 1965–1967.

70. Troxel DB. Diagnostic errors in surgical pathology uncovered by a review of malpractice claims. Part I: General considerations. Int J Surg Pathol 2000; 8: 161–163.

71. Troxel DB. Diagnostic pitfalls in surgical pathology – discovered by a review of malpractice claims. Int J Surg Pathol 2001; 9: 133–136.

72. Crichton M. A Case of need, New York, NY: Signet Publishers; 1968.

73. Internet Reference. URL = http://dictionary.law.com

74. Gephardt ON, Zarbo RJ. Q-Probe-94-03; extraneous tissue in surgical pathology slides: data analysis and critique. Northfield, IL: College of American Pathologists; 1995.

75. Ritter JH, Sutton TD, Wick MR. Use of immunostains to ABH blood group antigens to resolve problems in identity of tissue specimens. Arch Pathol Lab Med 1994; 118: 293–297.

76. Ferreira-Gonzalez A, Garrett CT. Pitfalls in establishing a molecular diagnostic laboratory. Hum Pathol 1996; 27: 437–440.

77. Taylor CR. Report from the Biological Stain Commission: FDA issues final rule for classification/ reclassification of immunohistochemistry (IHC) reagents and kits. Biotech Histochem 1998; 73: 175–177.

General and special techniques in surgical pathology and cytopathology

2

Ronald A. DeLellis   Murray Resnick   William J. Frable

INTRODUCTION

The disciplines of surgical pathology and cytopathology have witnessed a remarkable growth and development over the past several decades. Many of the advances in these fields have resulted directly from conceptual and technical discoveries in the basic sciences of immunology, molecular and cellular biology, and biochemistry. The resultant techniques have not only revolutionized the daily practice of pathology but also have served as cornerstones for the development of novel clinical and pathological concepts. Although some of these techniques can be performed on routinely processed surgical pathology and cytology specimens, others require special processing (Table 2.1). It is imperative, therefore, to develop a plan of action upon receipt of a specimen in order to maximize the amount of information that can be obtained with the submitted cytological sample or biopsy. In this regard, frozen sections or imprints of tumors or rapid cytological examination of aspirates are of particular value prior to the triage of samples for morphological analysis and special studies (see Table 2.1). It is also essential to develop a close working relationship with the responsible clinician in order to determine the specific information to be derived from the patient samples.

The purpose of this chapter is to highlight these techniques in addition to providing overviews of tissue fixation, standard staining methodologies, and cytological techniques, including fine needle aspiration biopsy.

TISSUE FIXATION

Adequate fixation is a prerequisite to all cell and tissue staining methods. The purposes of fixation are to inhibit autolysis and bacterial overgrowth, to prevent solubility of cellular components, to preserve their localization at the sites in which they occur in living cells, and to provide optimal conditions that will permit their visualization with specific indicator reagents.[1] Additionally, fixation is required to facilitate sectioning and slide preparation. Components of various fixatives differ with respect to their effects on cells and tissues. While some components cause cell shrinkage, others may result in cell swelling. Over the years, mixtures of components of fixatives have been devised to circumvent many of these effects.

Optimal fixation can be achieved only when tissues are adequately prepared. Tissues must be placed in fixatives as soon as they are obtained and must be sufficiently thin to permit thorough penetration of the fixative solution. Generally, tissues must be less than 2 mm thick and should be placed in at least 20 times their own volumes of fixative solution.

Fixatives are usually classified as cross-linking or precipitating types.[2–5] The most commonly used fixative in surgical pathology

Table 2.1 Special techniques in surgical pathology and cytopathology

Techniques	Cell/tissue preparative methods
General histochemistry	Formalin-fixed paraffin-embedded sections (other fixatives or frozen sections as indicated); air-dried or alcohol-fixed smears; cell blocks
Enzyme histochemistry	Snap frozen tissues; air-dried or alcohol-fixed smears; formalin-fixed paraffin-embedded sections for some enzymes (e.g. chloroacetate esterase)
Immunofluorescence	Snap frozen tissues; air-dried smears
Immunohistochemistry	Formalin-fixed paraffin-embedded sections for most applications (other fixatives or frozen sections as indicated); air-dried or alcohol-fixed smears; cell blocks
Flow cytometry (cell surface and selected cytoplasmic markers)	Fresh tissue/cells
Flow cytometry (ploidy analysis, S-phase)	Fresh tissue/cells; formalin-fixed paraffin-embedded samples
Cytogenetics	Fresh tissue/cells
Molecular technologies	
Southern blot	Snap frozen tissues/cells; aspirates
PCR, RT-PCR	Snap frozen tissues/cells; formalin-fixed paraffin-embedded sections; smears
ISH, FISH, CGH	Snap frozen tissues/cells; formalin-fixed paraffin-embedded sections; smears and imprints
DNA microarrays	Snap frozen tissues/cells; formalin-fixed paraffin-embedded samples

PCR, polymerase chain reaction; RT-PCR, reverse transcriptase polymerase chain reaction; ISH, in situ hybridization; FISH, fluorescence in situ hybridization; CGH, comparative genomic hybridization.

laboratories is formaldehyde, a prototypic cross-linking fixative. Formaldehyde is a gas that is available as a solution containing 37–40% by weight of the gas dissolved in water, and is generally used as a 10% neutral buffered solution (Formalin) which is equivalent to 4% formaldehyde. Formalin solutions can also be prepared from the solid polymer (paraformaldehyde).[3] The use of buffered formalin solutions is critical because of the formation of formic acid with prolonged storage of unbuffered aqueous solutions. The pigment that results from the action of Formalin on hemoglobin is known as Formalin pigment (acid hematein) and is particularly prominent in bloody tissue. This pigment is birefringent and can be distinguished from many other pigment

Table 2.2 Cell and tissue staining methods

Component	Stain	Result
Nucleic acids		
DNA	Feulgen reaction (fuchsin-sulfuric acid)[12,13]	DNA – red purple; RNA – uncolored
	Acridine orange[12]	DNA – green; RNA – orange
Nucleolar organizing regions(AgNORs)	Aqueous silver nitrate[14]	DNA loops – black
RNA	Methyl green pyronin Y[12]	RNA – red; DNA – green
Fibrous proteins, amyloid, fibrin		
Collagen, muscle	Van Gieson (acid fuchsin, picric acid)[15]	Collagen – red; muscle and red blood cells – yellow
	Mallory's trichrome (acid fuchsin, orange G, aniline blue, phosphomolybdic acid) (Fig. 2.1)	Collagen and reticulin – blue; muscle and fibrin – red
	Masson's trichrome (Ponceau acid fuchsin, phosphomolybdic acid, aniline blue, or light green)	Collagen and reticulin – blue (aniline blue) or green (light green); muscle, fibrin, red blood cells – red
	Gomori's trichrome (chromotrope 2R, fast green or aniline blue, phosphotungstic acid)	Collagen – green (fast green) or blue (aniline blue); muscle red blood cells, fibrin – red
Reticulin	Gordon-Sweet (silver diamine, potassium permanganate)[15] (Fig. 2.2)	Reticulin – black
Basement membranes	Hexamine silver (Jones), (alkaline hexamine silver salt, periodic acid)[15] (Fig. 2.3)	Basement membranes – black
Elastic tissue	Verhoeff (iodine, ferric chloride, hematoxylin)[15] (Fig. 2.4)	Elastic fibers – black
	Weigert (resorcin fuchsin)	Elastic fibers – blue to black
	Aldehyde fuchsin	Elastic fibers – purple
	Orcein	Elastic fibers – dark brown
Amyloid	Congo red[16] (Fig. 2.5)	Amyloid fibers – orange to red (apple green in polarized light)
	Thioflavin T[17]	Amyloid – yellow/green fluorescence
Fibrin	Mallory's phosphotungstic acid hematoxylin[15]	Fibrin – blue
Carbohydrates		
Glycoproteins, glycolipids, mucins, glycogen	Periodic acid–Schiff (PAS) (periodic acid–Schiff's reagent)[18] (Fig. 2.6)	Glycoproteins, glycolipids, glycogen, neutral mucins, acid mucins (containing sialic acid) – magenta (glycogen can be distinguished from other PAS positive substances on the basis of its susceptibility to diastase digestion)
Sialylated and sulfated mucins	Alcian blue (Fig. 2.6)	All acidic glycoproteins and glycosaminoglycans (pH 2.5) – blue At pH 1.0, both weakly and strongly sulfated acid mucosubstances – blue Treatment of the sections with testicular hyaluronidase prior to staining will remove hyaluronic acid, hyaluronosulphate and chondroitin sulfates A and C At pH 0.2, strongly sulfated mucosubstances – blue
Sulfated mucins	High iron diamine (diamine salts, ferric chloride) for sulfated mucins[19]	Sulfate ester groups – black to brown
Acid and neutral mucins	Mucicarmine (Fig. 2.7)	Acid mucins – red; neutral mucins are negative or weakly positive; strongly sulfated mucosubstances are variably positive
Lipids		
Unsaturated hydrophobic lipids, triglycerides, cholesterol	Oil Red O[20] (Fig. 2.8)	Lipids – orange-red; phospholipids – pink
Unsaturated lipids, cholesterol esters, triglycerides, phospholipids	Sudan black B	Lipids – black
Myelin	Luxol fast blue (Fig. 2.9)	Myelin – blue
Phosphates	Von Kossa (Fig. 2.10)	Phosphates – black
Calcium	Alizarin red	Calcium deposits – orange-red
Argentaffin and argyrophil cells	Masson-Hamperl	Argentaffin cells – black
	Grimelius (Fig. 2.11)	Argyrophil cells – black

Table 2.2 Cell and tissue staining methods (*cont'd*)

Component	Stain	Result
Urates	Polarized light	Birefringent (alcohol is fixative of choice)
	De Galantha stain	Urates – black
Bacteria	Gram (crystal violet, iodine, safranin)[22–24]	Gram positive – blue; Gram negative – pink
	Fite acid fast	*Nocardia*, atypical mycobacteria – red
	Ziehl-Neelsen acid fast[22]	*Mycobacteria* – red
	Warthin-Starry[22]	*H. pylori*, spirochetes, organisms of cat scratch disease – black
	Steiner[22]	*H. pylori*, spirochetes – black
	Dieterle[22]	*Legionella* – black
	Auramine O-rhodamine B[22]	*Mycobacteria* – red to yellow fluorescence
Fungus	Grocott methenamine-silver[22]	Organisms – black
	Periodic acid–Schiff	Organisms – magenta
	Mucicarmine	*Cryptococcus* – red (capsules)
Virus	Orcein[25]	Hepatitis B infected cells – red-brown

types on the basis of this property (Table 2.3). Formalin pigment can be removed by placing sections in alcoholic picric acid or alcoholic ammonium hydroxide prior to staining with hematoxylin and eosin or other stains.

The reactions of formaldehyde with proteins are numerous and complex since this fixative can react with a number of functional end-groups (amino, imino and amido, peptide, guanyl, hydroxyl, carboxyl, sulfhydryl, aromatic rings) to form methylene bridges.[1] The extent of the resultant cross-linking is dependent on many factors, the most important of which is duration of fixation. Although formalin penetrates tissues rapidly, complete fixation requires relatively prolonged time periods. Tissues fixed in formalin for short time periods become completely fixed only as a result of their subsequent exposure to alcohol during the dehydration process. Glutaraldehyde and acrolein are also classified as cross-linking fixatives.

Both ethanol and methanol are precipitating fixatives which have the capacity to denature proteins.[1,2–5] Both of these reagents rupture hydrogen bonds, which are responsible for maintaining the tertiary structure of proteins. Ethanol may be combined with formalin to produce alcoholic formalin, which penetrates tissue more rapidly than formalin alone. Carnoy's fluid, which is composed of an admixture of ethanol, chloroform, and acetic acid, is also a precipitating fixative. Carnoy's fluid causes lysis of red cells and is associated with considerable tissue shrinkage. Picric acid, a major component of Bouin's solution (picric acid, formalin, glacial acetic acid) is also classified as a precipitating fixative and forms picrates with the basic groups of proteins.

Mercuric chloride is also a commonly used fixative, particularly in the form of formol sublimate (B5). It combines with the hydroxyl and carboxyl groups of proteins and with the phosphoric acid of nucleoproteins. In addition, mercury has a selective affinity for thiol groups. Since formol sublimate penetrates tissues very slowly, samples must be sectioned very thinly prior to fixation. Overfixation will result in excessive tissue hardness.[5] Zenker's fixative includes a combination of potassium dichromate, mercuric chloride, and glacial acetic acid. Chromium-containing fixatives have both cross-linking and precipitating effects. Because of their oxidizing effects, chromate fixatives convert adrenaline and noradrenaline into adrenochrome and noradrenochrome pigments (chromaffin reaction). Osmium tetroxide, which was formerly used as a lipid stain, is now employed primarily as a fixative for electron microscopy. The mechanism of fixation is not well understood, although some cross-linking appears to be involved. This fixative penetrates tissues slowly, and its use is limited to very small blocks.

In addition to standard liquid fixatives, vapor fixation following freeze drying has also been used to preserve certain diffusible components such as catecholamines and small peptides.[6] Microwave fixation has been advocated for very rapid fixation, and this subject is covered in detail in several reviews.[7,8] Morales and coworkers have developed a microwave-based method which circumvents the use of formalin and xylene.[9] This procedure (continuous throughout processing method, CTPM) utilizes common histology reagents such as isopropanol, acetone, polyethylene glycol, mineral oil, paraffin, and small amounts of glacial acetic acid and dimethyl sulfoxide. The CTPM procedure permits preparation of paraffin blocks in approximately 1 hour and allows continuous flow of specimens at 15-minute intervals. Histological, histochemical, and immunohistochemical results are comparable to standard preparative methods; moreover, the preservation of RNA has been reported to be superior to that obtained with standard fixation and embedding protocols.[9]

STAINING METHODS

Despite their continuous use for more than a century in pathology laboratories throughout the world, the specific mechanisms underlying most of the commonly used staining methods are poorly understood (Table 2.2) (Figs 2.1–2.12). Staining occurs as a result of a complex series of interactions of cell and tissue components with single dyes or complex mixtures of dyes.[10–25] Differing affinities between the dyes and tissue binding sites result in selective staining of certain cell constituents. Reaction conditions may be adjusted to emphasize these selective affinities, thereby providing maximal contrast between intensely stained and less stained (or negative) components. For example, varying the pH and electrolyte concentrations of certain cationic dyes will permit the distinction of classes of acidic mucosubstances. Patterns of staining can be further modified by tissue fixation, selective blocking or extraction methods

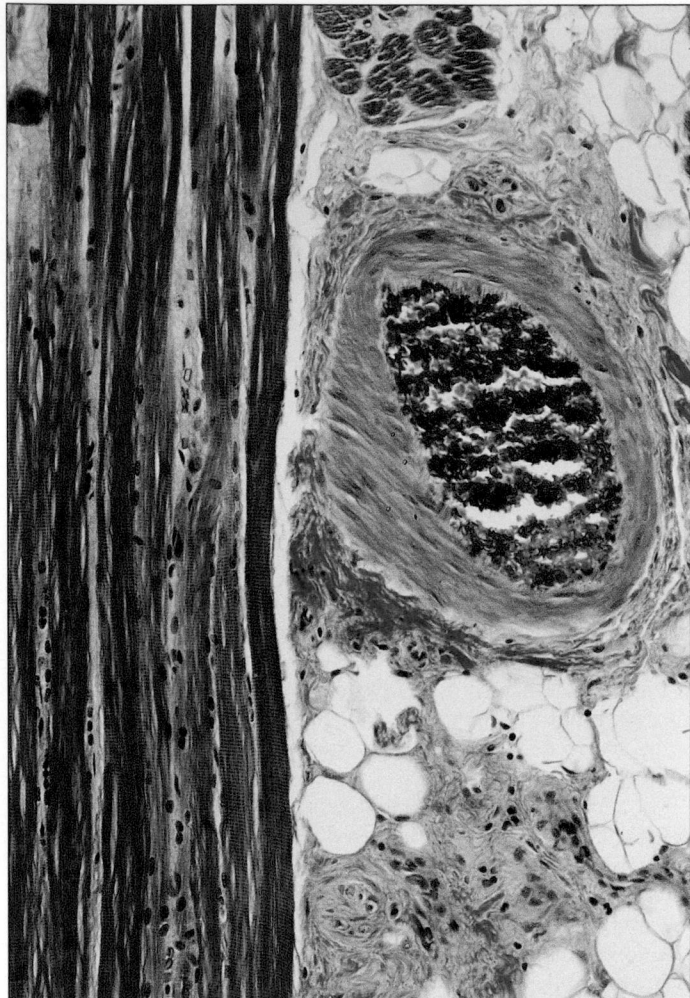

Fig. 2.1 Gomori's trichrome stain. Collagen is stained blue, and skeletal muscle fibers are stained red.

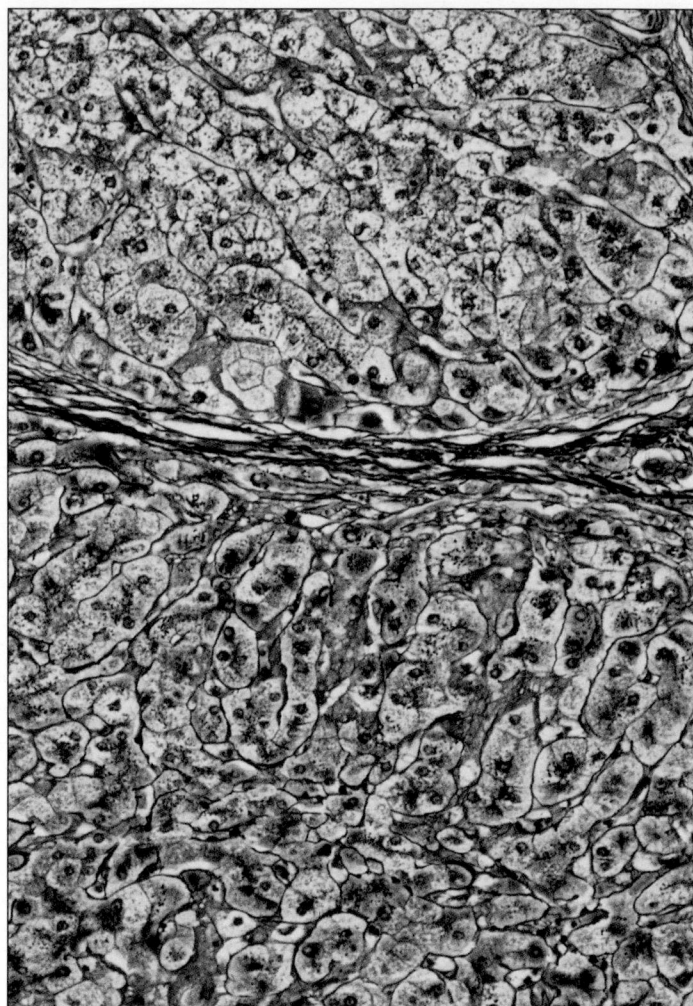

Fig. 2.2 Gomori's reticulin stain. Reticulin fibers surrounding cords of liver cells are stained black.

(e.g. diastase digestion to remove glycogen), and post-staining differentiation procedures.[10,11]

Dyes can bind to cell and tissue components by a variety of mechanisms including electrostatic forces, hydrogen bonding, van der Waal's forces, covalent binding, and hydrophobic interactions, as exemplified by the preferential solubility of oil red O in lipid droplets.[10,11] Staining may occur through the action of an intermediary binding agent, which is referred to as a mordant. The latter term most commonly refers to metal ions that bind covalently to dye molecules to form dye-metal complexes. For example, aluminum potassium sulfate serves as a mordant for hematoxylin in Mayer's hematoxylin procedure. In fact, the oxidation product of hematoxylin, which is known as hematein, has a very low affinity for nuclei without the addition of the metal mordant. Alternatively, certain cellular and tissue components may have a direct affinity for metal salts. The Gordon-Sweet reticulin stain, for example, takes advantage of this phenomenon. Staining of a specific cellular component may also result from the formation of a colored compound in situ, as in the case of enzyme histochemistry.

Basic (cationic) dyes carry a net positive charge which permits them to react with a variety of tissue-bound anionic sites, including phosphate groups of nucleic acids, sulfate groups of glyco-

saminoglycans, and carboxyl groups of proteins. The reaction of basic dyes with anionic sites is a pH-dependent phenomenon. At high pH, phosphate, carboxyl, and sulfate groups will stain positively. At acidic pH, only sulfate groups will be reactive. Thus, staining at controlled pH can provide important data on the chemical composition of the cell.

When some basic dyes react with tissue components, a color shift in the dye is produced. This phenomenon, which is termed metachromasia, reflects the presence of polyanions that are sufficiently close to form dimeric and polymeric aggregates of dye molecules. Absorption properties of aggregated dye molecules differ from those of the nonaggregated dye, resulting in the characteristic color shift.

In contrast to basic (cationic) dyes, acidic (anionic) dyes carry a net negative charge which permits them to react with tissue-bound cationic moieties. In addition to electrostatic forces, additional factors that are important in the reactions of anionic dyes include size and aggregation of the dye molecules and the permeability or texture of the tissue components.[11] Acidophilic components include cytoplasmic filaments of various types, intracellular membranous components (e.g. mitochondria), and extracellular fibrous proteins.

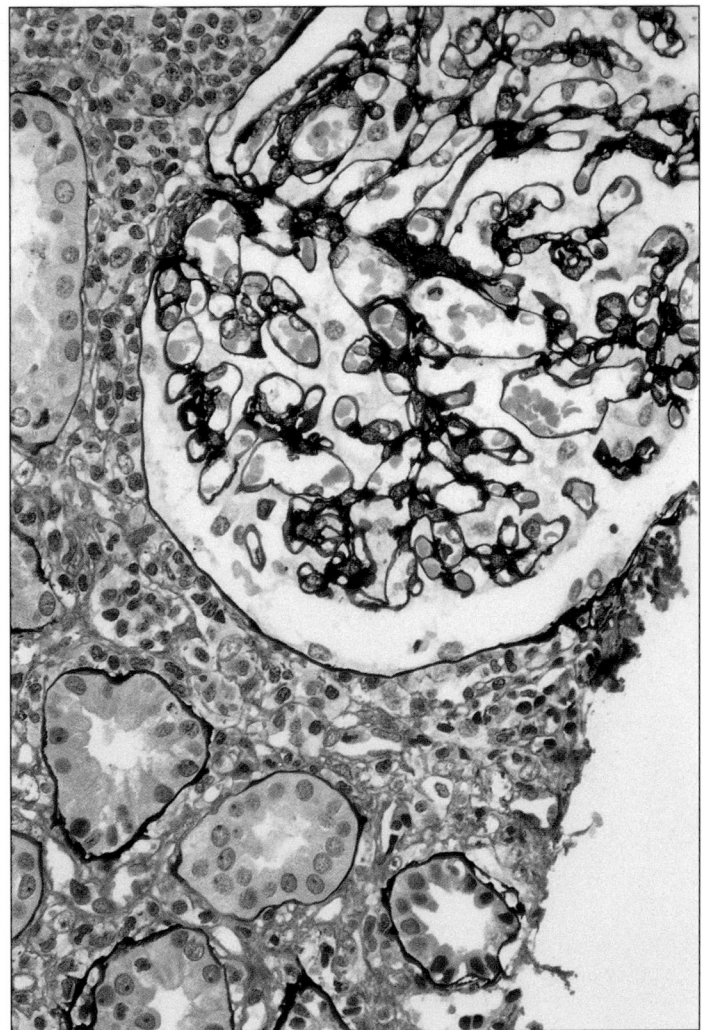

Fig. 2.3 The Jones modified hexamine silver technique. The renal glomerular capillary basement membranes and the tubular basement membranes are stained black.

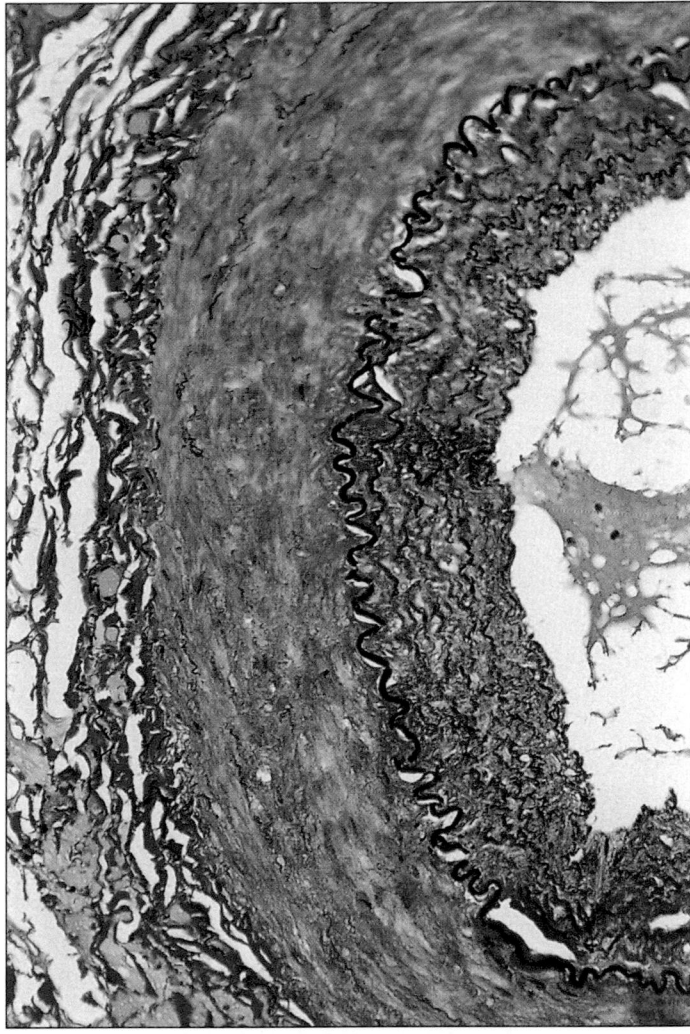

Fig. 2.4 Verhoeff's elastic fiber stain. The elastic fibers in the arterial wall are stained black.

A variety of pigments may also occur in normal and pathological conditions.[26] The properties and histochemical characteristics of the various pigment types are summarized in Table 2.3.

Histochemistry has provided a successful approach for demonstration of a wide variety of oxidative and hydrolytic enzymes.[27] A positive reaction results from the formation of a colored product in situ. Numerous methods, including metal precipitation reactions, simultaneous coupling procedures, and postincubation staining methods, have been developed. With few exceptions, procedures for the demonstration of enzymes must be performed on fresh frozen tissue samples. Chloroacetate esterase is one clinically useful enzyme that can be demonstrated in formalin-fixed paraffin-embedded samples in cells of granulocytic lineage and mast cells.[28]

Currently, enzyme histochemistry is used primarily for evaluation of muscle biopsies and for classification of leukemias.[29] The myofibrillar ATPase reaction, for example, is the most reliable method for the distinction of muscle fiber types (Fig. 2.12).[30] At alkaline pH, for example, type 1 muscle fibers stain lightly for ATPase while type 2 fibers stain darkly. At acid pH, type 1 fibers stain darkly, type 2A fibers stain lightly, and type 2B fibers stain with intermediate intensity. Oxidative enzymes such as NADH are present in high concentrations in type 1 fibers but are present in low to intermediate concentrations in type 2 fibers. Phosphorylase, on the other hand, is present in high concentrations in type 2 fibers but in low concentrations in type 1 fibers.

CYTOLOGICAL SAMPLES AND FINE-NEEDLE ASPIRATION BIOPSY

Fixation is critical for maintaining cytologic detail in smears prepared from different body sites. Since chromatin is well preserved with alcohol fixatives, wet fixation with 95% ethanol is generally recommended for most cytologic preparations.[10] In wet fixation, a freshly prepared slide is submerged immediately into fixative for 15–30 min prior to staining. Other fixatives that have been used include methanol and isopropanol. Ten percent formalin has also been used, but considerable loss of chromatin detail is usually apparent. In some instances, air-dried preparations are used for subsequent Romanowsky-type staining procedures.

Table 2.3 Pigments

Types	Properties
Formalin	Yellow to black microcrystalline deposits; birefringent; iron negative (properties are identical to malarial pigment).
Pseudomelanin (melanosis coli pigment)	Yellow to brown; nonbirefringent; yellow to orange autofluorescence. Acid fast and iron negative.
Lipofuscins	Golden-brown; nonbirefringent; iron negative; autofluorescent; PAS positive; variably acid fast; Sudan black B positive.
Melanin	Brown to black; nonbirefringent; nonautofluorescent. Can be bleached with hydrogen peroxide, chlorine water, chromic acid or potassium permanganate. Negative for iron and PAS negative. Fontana-Masson, argentaffin, and Schmorl's ferric ferricyanide stains are positive.
Hemosiderin	Yellow-brown; nonbirefringent; nonautofluorescent. Perls' Prussian blue stain is positive (ferric iron reacts with potassium ferrocyanide to produce ferric ferrocyanide). Acid fast and PAS negative.
Hematoidin/bilirubin	Hematoidin pigment is birefringent. Both hematoidin and bilirubin are iron negative and are nonautofluorescent. Nitric acid oxidizes the pigment to red, purple and blue green products (Gmelin reaction). Bilirubin can be oxidized by iodine to form the green biliverdin pigment (Stein reaction).
Porphyrin	Yellow to brown black if present in sufficient quantities. Autofluorescent: orange-red (quickly fades).
Copper	Forms a green-black pigment with rubeanic acid (Uzman reaction). Can also be demonstrated with a modified orcein stain or with rhodamine.

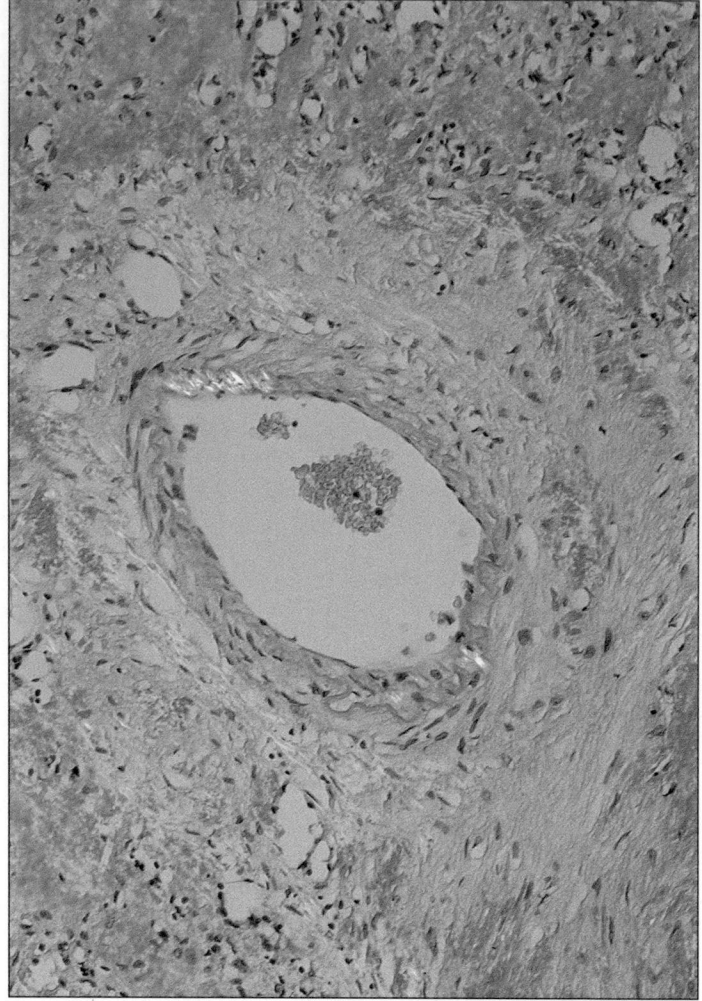

Fig. 2.5 Congo red stain photographed in partially polarized light. The amyloid deposits exhibit green birefringence.

Coating fixatives containing ethanol or its substitute and polyethylene glycol are also used frequently, particularly for cervicovaginal smears.[31] Coating fixatives are commercially available as spray fixatives, or they may be prepared directly in the laboratory. Polyethylene glycol is a wax-like substance that coats and protects the cells on the slide. Before staining, however, this coat must be dissolved by placing the slide in ethanol.

Transport of sputum, urine, cerebrospinal fluid, cyst fluid, effusions, and brushing and washing specimens to the laboratory should be immediate to prevent autolytic changes and bacterial overgrowth. If a delay in transporting or processing occurs, specimens should be refrigerated; alternatively, 50–70% ethanol may be added to the specimen in a 1:1 ratio.[31] It is important to note that when fixatives are added to fluid specimens, cells may have a decreased adherence to glass slides.

Body fluids are usually centrifuged prior to subsequent preparative procedures.[31] After centrifugation, direct smears may be made from the cell pellet. One method is to use a pipette to aspirate and expel several drops of the cell button onto a slide; smears are then prepared by placing a second glass slide on top and gently pulling them apart.[32] This procedure effectively disperses the cells. If the specimen is clear or scanty, or both, and does not produce a pellet, cytocentrifugation or filter monolayer preparations may be the methods of choice.

Filter preparations are designed to produce a thin uniform dispersion of cells on a slide with minimal cell overlapping. Either a cellulose membrane filter or a polycarbonate filter may be used; both have slightly different characteristics. The ThinPrep process is a monolayer technology and first requires transfer of cells into a preservative solution (Cytolyte or PreserveCyte). The cells are then automatically collected on a polycarbonate filter and transferred to a glass slide.[33–35]

Technical problems may exist with sputum, urine, and bloody specimens. Sputum produced by a deep cough is extremely viscous and difficult to concentrate by centrifugation. Commercially available mucolytic agents or 8% hydrochloric acid may be added to dissolve the mucus and facilitate the centrifugation. Others, however, prefer to make direct smears without mucolytic agents based on the belief that tumor cells are concentrated in the mucus. Blood and white-tinged areas are usually sampled selectively. A second problematic specimen is voided urine, which is a hostile environment with low pH, high osmolality, and the potential for bacterial contamination and

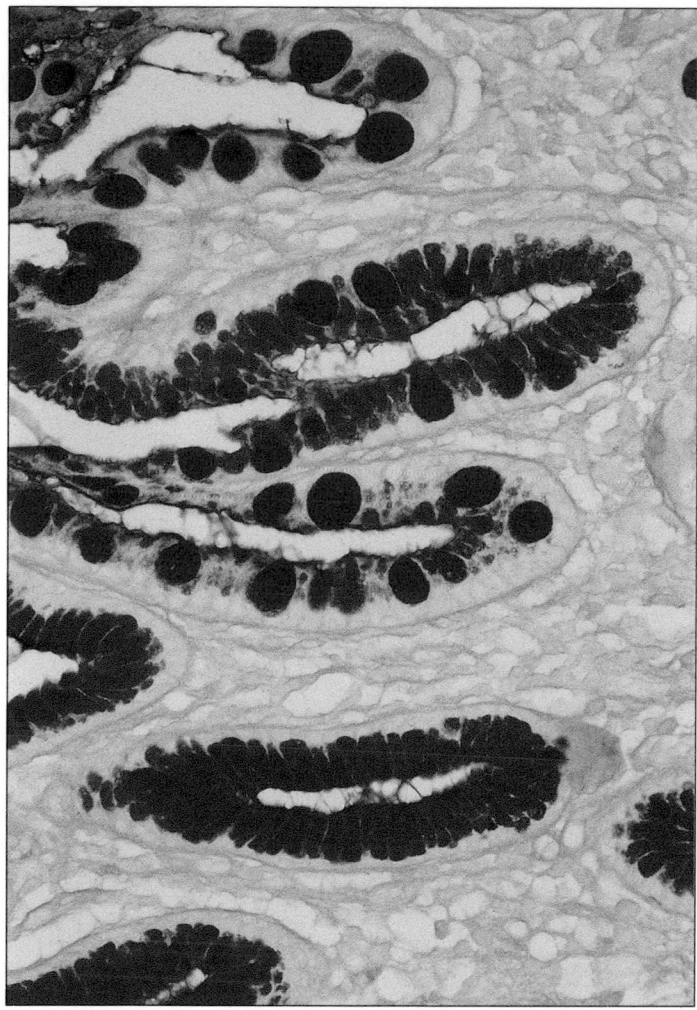

Fig. 2.6 Alcian blue/periodic acid–Schiff stain (pH 2.5) of stomach with complete intestinal metaplasia. The mucous cells are magenta (periodic acid–Schiff positive), and the goblet cells are purple, indicating a mixture of acidic and neutral mucins.

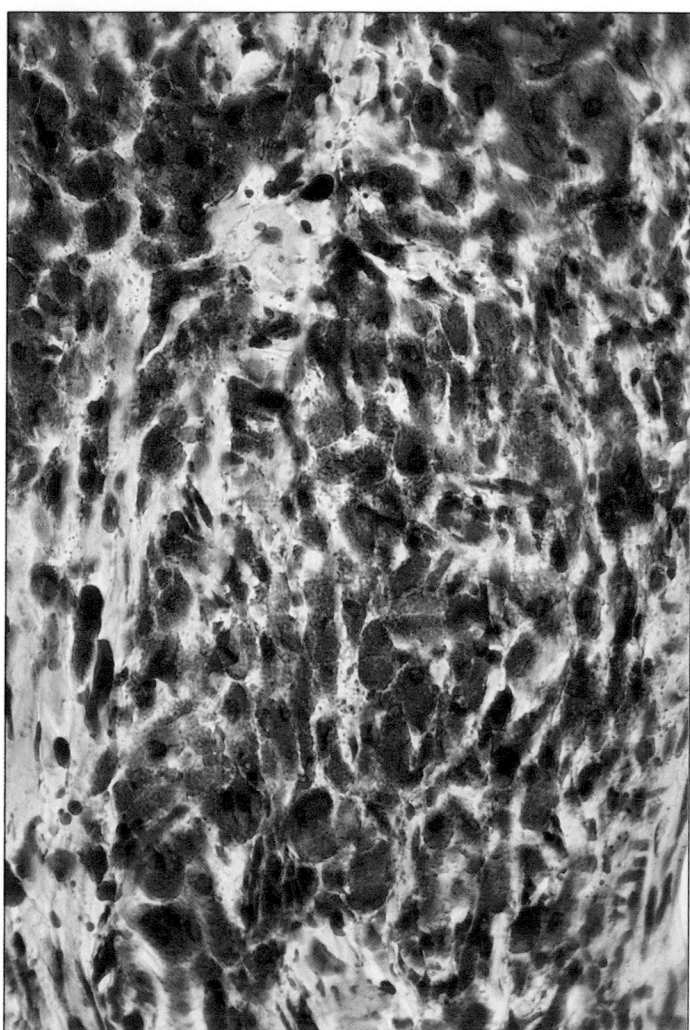

Fig. 2.8 Oil red O stain of skin biopsy from a patient with hyperlipoproteinemia. Lipid deposits are stained red.

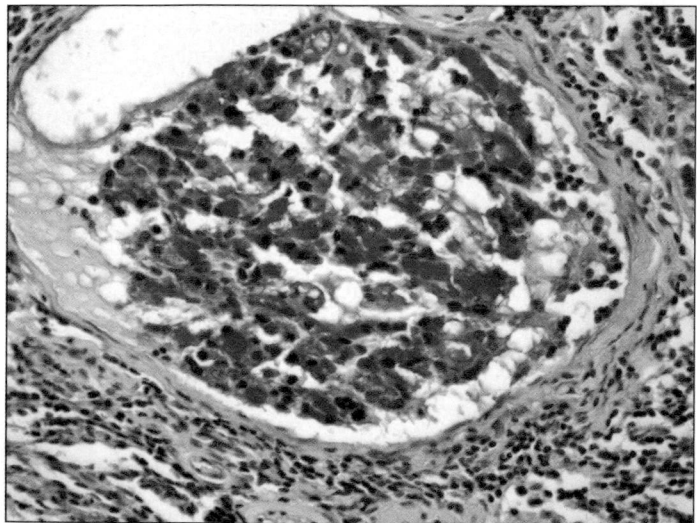

Fig. 2.7 Mucicarmine stain of gastric adenocarcinoma. Mucin deposits are stained red.

overgrowth. Because the first voided morning specimen usually has the most degenerative changes, the second urine specimen of the day preceded by hydration and vitamin C ingestion is recommended.[36–38]

Bloody specimens cause diagnostic problems when red cells overlap and obscure cells of interest. To eliminate or diminish this problem, a variety of lysing agents may be used.[31] One technique involves placing the glass slide into 50–70% ethanol or into modified Carnoy's fixative followed by 95% ethanol. Alternatively, after fixation in 95% ethanol, the slide may be placed into a urea solution or acid alcohol followed by 95% ethanol.

Cell blocks are often diagnostically useful and may provide architectural information not readily apparent from cell smears. They also offer the possibility of providing material for histochemical, immunohistochemical, or in situ hybridization studies. The cell block is prepared by centrifuging the specimen, pouring off the supernatant, fixing the cell pellet, and submitting it for paraffin embedding and sectioning. Ten percent buffered formalin is used most commonly, although other fixatives may also be employed for specific indications.[31] Cell blocks may also be prepared from material fixed in Cytolyte or PreserveCyte.

Imprint preparations, made by touching a slide to the cut surface of a tissue, provide important cytologic detail that may not be readily

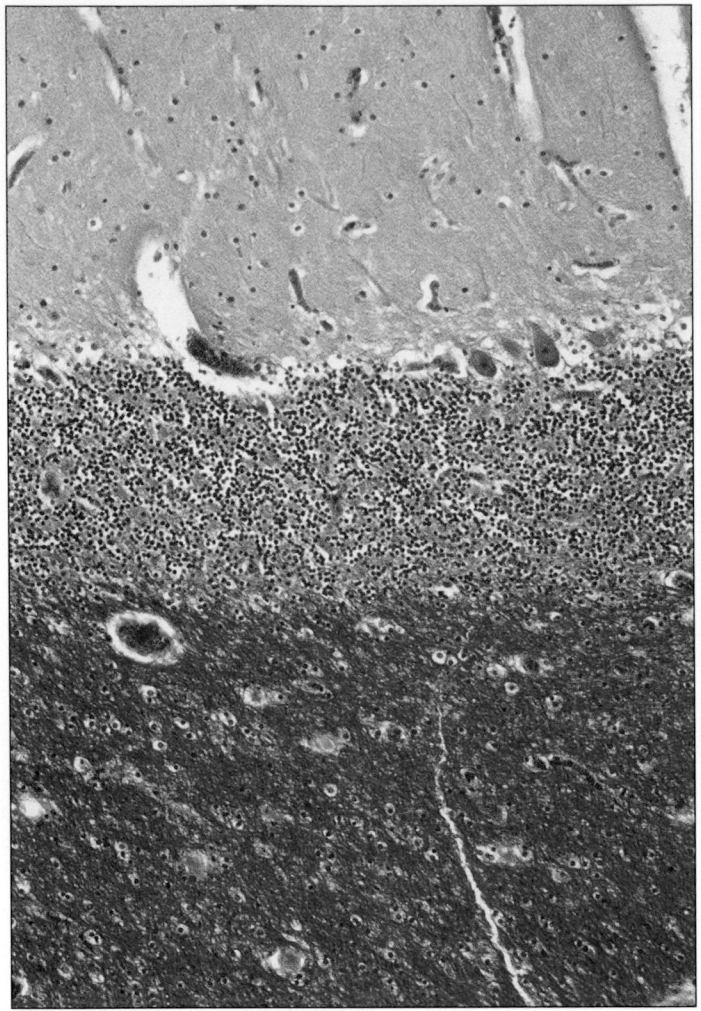

Fig. 2.9 Luxol fast blue stain of brain. The myelin deposits are stained blue.

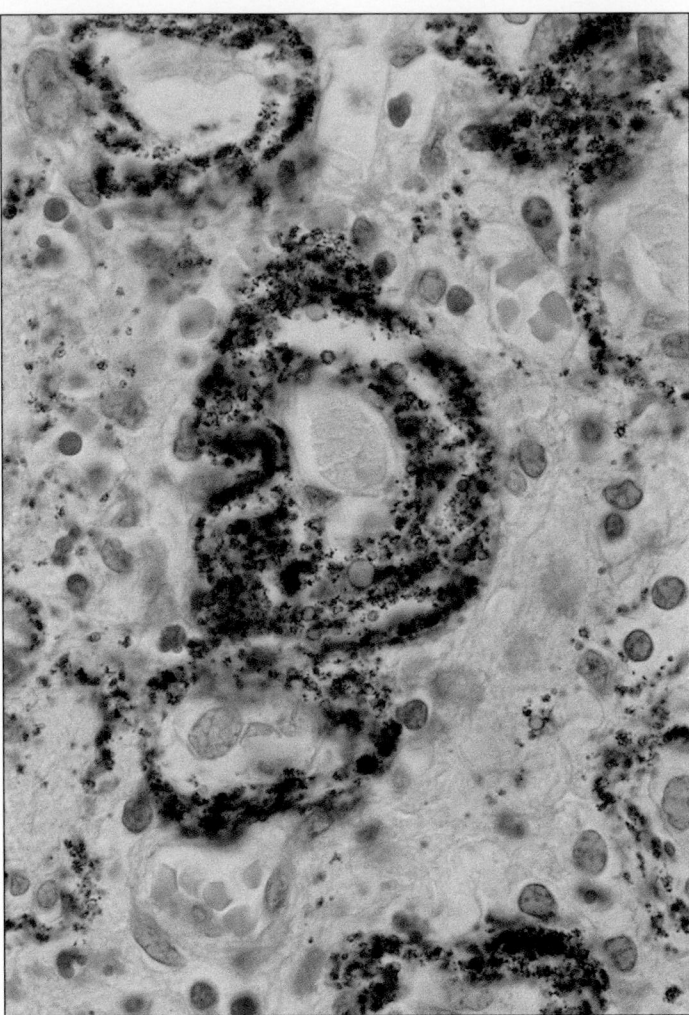

Fig. 2.10 Von Kossa's stain of kidney with nephrocalcinosis. Phosphate and carbonate deposits are stained black.

apparent on frozen section or even permanent sections. In addition, a rapid diagnosis may be rendered by a touch preparation without having to prepare a frozen section.

FINE-NEEDLE ASPIRATION BIOPSY

Aspiration biopsy, aspiration cytology, or fine-needle aspiration biopsy (FNAB) has come of age in the past 25 years and has contributed substantially to the timely and cost-effective diagnosis of neoplastic and non-neoplastic disease.[39] Common clinical targets for FNAB are masses in the breast, thyroid, and enlarged lymph nodes while the widespread use of sophisticated radiologic imaging techniques has been successful in the detection of clinically silent lesions that can also be sampled.[40,41] High-resolution mammography and stereotactic needle placement allow sampling of nonpalpable breast lesions and transrectal ultrasound guided thin-core needle biopsies have become standard for detecting prostate cancer discovered by abnormalities in prostatic specific antigen (PSA) levels.[42,43]

Martin and Ellis were the first to report a systematic study of tumors sampled by means of small gauge needle and aspiration.[44]

Although the method became quite popular at Memorial Sloan-Kettering Cancer Center in the 1950s, the procedure did not gain general acceptance by other major medical centers in the United States. A group of Swedish clinicians with special expertise in hematology and oncology reinvented aspiration biopsy cytology in post-World War II Europe.[45–48] Clinicians and pathologists from the United States studied in Sweden in the early 1970s, and with their support and enthusiasm, FNAB again came to be recognized as an efficient and cost-effective method for diagnosing tumors.[49,50] Close cooperation between clinicians, surgeons, and cytologist is essential for the success of this technique. Stewart's comment from 70 years ago still holds true today: 'Aspiration biopsy is as good as the combined intelligence of the clinician and pathologist makes it.'[51]

A pathology department may decide to develop an aspiration biopsy service. Abele and Miller detail the evolution of a free-standing clinic from a hospital-based FNAB service.[52] Proving the utility of FNAB to clinicians is accomplished by providing on-demand service that includes hospitalized patients, outpatients, and patients in attending physicians' offices. It is essential to obtain documented informed consent for FNAB. Potential complications are bleeding and infection, although both are quite rare. Consent

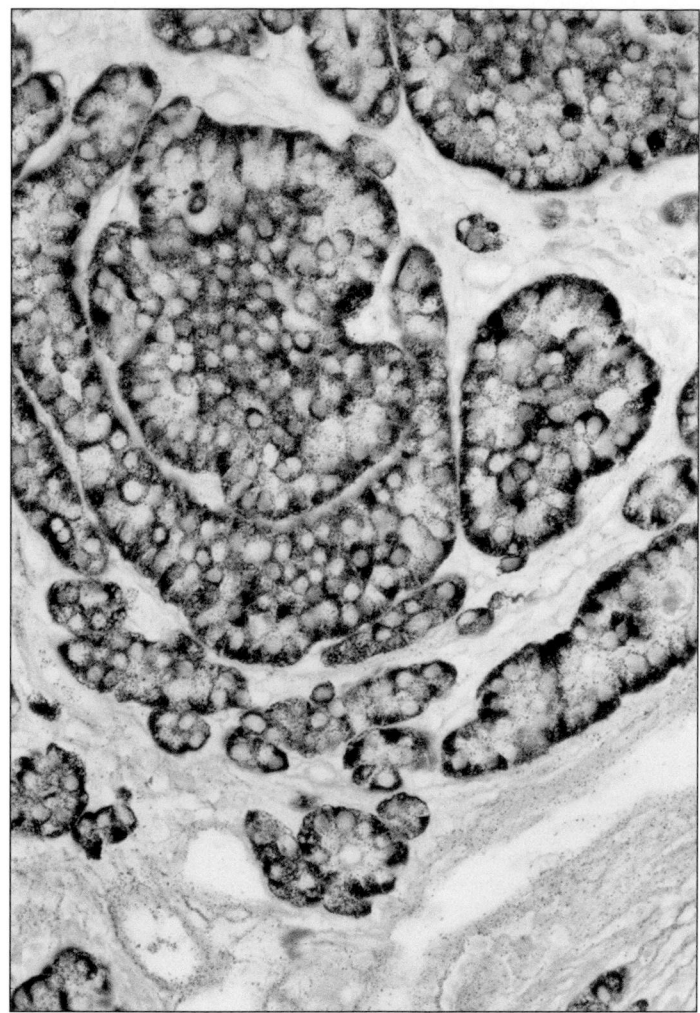

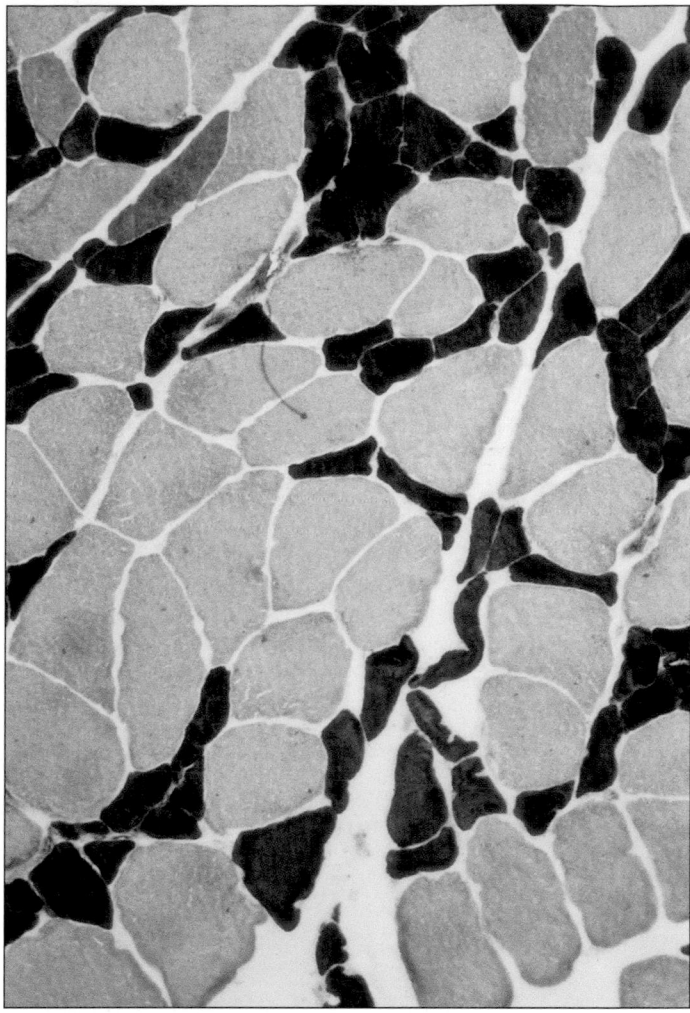

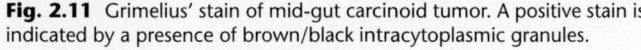

Fig. 2.11 Grimelius' stain of mid-gut carcinoid tumor. A positive stain is indicated by a presence of brown/black intracytoplasmic granules.

Fig. 2.12 ATPase reaction in muscle biopsy with evidence of type 2 fiber atrophy. The type 2 fibers are stained black.

should be witnessed, and, for children, written consent should be obtained from parents and/or guardians.

When clinicians or surgeons are performing FNABs, success will be obtained only as a result of a close working relationship between the clinician and pathologist. This is essential if the pathologist does not have the opportunity to examine the patient directly. A detailed description of the location of the lesion, its consistency upon aspiration, the clinical history, and the differential diagnosis should be either clearly recorded or personally communicated to the pathologist.[53] The pathologist's responsibility is to render a meaningful report to the clinician, and the final interpretation must make sense within the context of the clinical presentation. The quality of the aspirate should be reported and no attempt should be made to provide a definitive interpretation from an inadequate aspirate or even from a good aspirate when important clinical information is missing. Caution is advised when the initial cytologic interpretation does not fit the clinical situation. No major therapeutic decisions should be made on the basis of the cytologic findings alone[40,54] The necessary equipment for the performance of an FNAB is listed in Table 2.4.

FNAB may be repeated enough times to procure suitable amounts of aspirated material both for diagnostic purposes and for special studies.[55–66] It is important to take time to explain the procedure to the patient as this should allay the fear of needles or any medical procedure. Under no circumstances should an uncooperative patient undergo aspiration biopsy. Some degree of restraint or light sedation may be necessary in children, with appropriate parental permission.

The medical history should be reviewed and the relationship of the clinical problem to the lesion to be biopsied should be determined.[41] The location of the lesion in relationship to the surrounding structures should be assessed and an optimal approach to the performance of the biopsy should be planned. A deeply located mass is best approached directly and perpendicularly to the skin surface while superficial lesions are best approached by penetrating the skin at a nearly horizontal plane while feeling for the lesion when advancing the needle tip. The patient should be placed in a comfortable position for the FNAB with the mass readily palpable and easily stabilized. This is particularly important in head and neck lesions where the prominence of a mass is dependent on the position of the patient.

The basic aspiration technique is summarized in Table 2.5. Radiologists performing FNAB prefer to place a guide needle, usually 18 gauge, to the surface of the target, check its position by imaging, then insert the actual aspiration biopsy needle through the guide needle,

Table 2.4 Equipment needed for FNAB

1. Cameco syringe pistol (Precision Dynamics, San Fernando, CA), or some type of aspiration gun handle.
2. 10 or 20-ml disposable plastic syringes with straight or Leur-Lock Tips (Becton Dickenson, Rutherford, NJ), depending on the gun handle size.
3. 22, 23, 25, 27-gauge 0.6–1.0 mm. External diameter disposable needles, 3.8, 8.8, 15 and 20 cm long, with or without stylus.
4. Alcohol sponges; Betadene sponges for deeper aspirations, transabdominal, transthoracic, bone or deep soft tissue.
5. Sterile gauze pads.
6. Microscopic glass slides with frosted ends.
7. Small vial of balanced salt solution or RPMI tissue culture transport media, or both; RPMI media may be used for sample to be sent for flow cytometry or other special studies.
8. Suitable alcohol spray fixative for immediate fixation of wet smears.
9. Vial of local anesthetic, 1–2% lidocaine (optional); topical spray anesthesia for aspirate in children or Intraoral aspirations.
10. Small vial of buffered glutaraldehyde for fixing aspirate for electron microscopy, if required.

A small plastic tray will conveniently hold all the equipment. Some pathologists and clinicians prefer to inject a local anesthetic at the site of the aspiration in all patients. Equipment used by dentists is available from dental supply houses: 30-gauge disposable needles, 2.0-ml disposable cylinders of 2% lidocaine hydrochloride, with or without epinephrine, and a reusable metallic injection handle, dispenses anesthesia along the planned needle tract without tissue distortion that might affect palpation of the target for aspiration. This method generally avoids anesthesia burn. With permission from Abele et al.[52]

Table 2.5 Performing the aspiration

1. Grasp the lesion with one hand, usually between two fingers, or push it into a position where it seems fixed and stable.
2. Prepare the skin with an alcohol sponge as for a venipuncture.
3. Lay the syringe pistol with attached needle against the skin at the determined puncture site and angle.
4. With a quick motion insert the needle through the skin and advance the needle into the mass.
5. Puncture of the target may be tested by differences in resistance, by feeling that a capsule was penetrated, or by moving the syringe pistol very slightly laterally and detecting a corresponding movement of the mass beneath the palpating fingers.
6. Apply suction to the aspirating syringe, usually about one-third the length of the syringe barrel.
7. Move the needle back and forth within the tumor with short, quick strokes and in slightly different directions.
8. Note at all times the junction of the needle and the hub of the syringe for the appearance of any specimen.
9. At the first appearance of any sample at the junction of the syringe and needle, release the trigger of the syringe pistol and let the vacuum in the syringe equate to normal.
10. With the air pressure in the syringe equalized, withdraw the needle from the mass.*
11. Apply gentle pressure to the puncture site with a sterile gauze pad; the patient or an assistant may apply pressure to the puncture site while the aspirator prepares smears.

*Never withdraw the needle from the mass with any vacuum in the syringe pistol, as the small aspiration sample will be drawn into the syringe where it begins to dry and is quite difficult to recover. If a cyst is encountered, it should be evacuated as completely as possible. After aspiration of any cyst, it is essential that the patient be re-examined for any residual mass. If one is detected, a repeat FNAB of that residual lesion should be performed.

checking its position in the target by imaging.[41] The position of the needle is monitored continuously for aspirates performed using ultrasound guidance, currently a growing method of FNA through an endoscope.[67,68]

The amount of suction should be modified in accordance with the type of target. In the thyroid, for example, little or no suction is often sufficient to obtain a biopsy, since the thyroid is quite vascular. The exceptions are some neoplasms and chronic forms of thyroiditis with significant fibrosis.[69,70] Reactive lymph nodes and some cases of chronic sialoadenitis also produce excessive blood in the aspirate if too much suction is applied. The 'needle only' method may prove quite useful for aspiration of the thyroid, lymph nodes, and when the target lesion is quite small.[69,70]

Aspiration is most effective when one describes with the needle a small cone, with the apex at the point where the needle penetrates the skin. If the target is large, multiple separate aspirates describing overlapping cones are indicated. It is critical to keep the aspirate within the needle and not to aspirate excessive blood or fluid, which dilutes the cellular composition of the specimen. Excellent instructional videos and texts are now available emphasizing these points and others.[71,72] Practicing on surgical specimens, including normal tissue, develops these skills and provides a reference collection of smears for comparison with actual patient material. The technique of smear preparation is summarized in Table 2.6.[40]

Some aspirates are diluted by excessive blood or fluid. For example, most specimens from non-neoplastic goiter of the thyroid are largely composed of blood and/or colloid, with relatively few follicular cells. Inexperienced interventional radiologists often provide samples that are essentially all blood. It is quite difficult to make good smears from this type of specimen. The liquid nature of the aspirates results in smears that occupy most of the slide surface with any cells that might be present being dispersed to the edges of the smear. The blood may start to clot quickly, pulling any diagnostic cells together into the clot and further compromising good smear preparation. The procedures for working with bloody or diluted aspirates are summarized in Table 2.7.[41]

When deep aspirations or intraoperative aspiration biopsies consist mostly of blood and all the blood is pulled into the syringe, it is best to process this part of the sample as a cell block. Only the portion of the specimen left within the needle should be used to prepare smears. Even a few milliliters of blood drawn up into the syringe can result in the rapid formation of a clot that will greatly interfere with good smear preparation. The clotting of blood traps cells and small tissue fragments, evenly spread smears cannot be prepared, and heavy and uneven staining of any cells present occurs (Fig. 2.13).[53]

Samples for cell blocks may be handled by one of several techniques: simple centrifugation, addition of 10% neutral buffered formalin to the cell button, addition of thromboplastin or bacterial agar to the cell button, or the use of a commercially available cytoblock system. Material collected in Cytolyte may also be used for cell-block preparation. With any cell-block method or very small biopsy fragments, it is important to work closely with the histotechnologist so

Table 2.6 Smear preparation

1. Immediately after completing the aspiration biopsy, detach the needle from the syringe; then pull back on the syringe pistol trigger, filling the syringe with air.
2. Reattach the needle and place the tip of the needle in the center of a plain glass slide, touching the needlepoint to the surface, bevel side down.
3. Advance the plunger of the syringe to express a small drop of sample, approximately 2–3 mm in diameter, onto the slide.
4. Quickly continue this procedure over a series of slides (usually 4–6).
5. Invert a second plain glass slide over the drop; as the drop spreads, pull the two slides apart horizontally in a single gentle motion.
6. An alternative smear method, when the drop spreads between the two slides, is to pull the two slides apart vertically (compression smears or pop smears).
7. Repeat the above procedure quickly for all slides; fix some as prepared immediately in 95% ethyl alcohol or other suitable fixative depending on preference for staining.
8. Allow unfixed smears to air-dry for Romanowsky-type stains (most popular currently is Diff-Quik)

It is quite important to place the bevel of the needle against the slide as the sample is expressed so that no air gap exists between the end of the needle and the slide surface. Splattering of the biopsy over the surface of the slide is prevented, as is excessive air-drying of the sample prior to making the smear and fixation. By practicing smear-making methods it is possible to place nearly all the aspirated material, normally 4 or 5 drops, within a 3.8-cm (1½-in) needle over a small series of slides and then begin smear preparation. With the rapid Papanicolaou staining method of Yang and Alvarez[73] all smears may be allowed to air-dry. The most important point is to have the smear occupy only a small area of the slide. With good smear technique, a tissue-like pattern is created and the area of the smear that must be reviewed by the cytopathologists is reduced.

Table 2.7 Smear preparation for bloody or diluted samples

1. Place the drop of bloody fluid on the slide as described previously; because of the liquid nature of the aspirate the drop will probably measure 5–10 mm in diameter.
2. Hold the slide with the drop of aspirate sample in the left hand and horizontal.
3. Take a second slide in the right hand and bring the edge of that slide at about a 45° angle up to the drop noting that it will spread along the edge of the slide in the right hand. Push the slide in the right hand, keeping it in contact with the slide in the left hand, toward the end of the slide in the left hand farthest from the drop of biopsy's original position. This maneuver is analogous to making a blood smear.
4. Reaching the halfway point as described in step 3, lift the spreader slide (slide in the right hand) straight up off the slide in the left hand.
5. Immediately tilt the smear slide (slide in the left hand), away from the leading edge of the smear; note that the blood runs back and away from that leading edge.
6. Next, start smear preparation with the clean lateral edge of the slide in the right hand (spreader slide) from the leading edge of the smear on the slide in the left hand, pulling toward the farther end of the smear slide (slide in the left hand).
7. Make a second smear using a third clear slide from the edge of the spreader slide (slide in the right hand) as described in step 6.
8. Tissue particles that may be present at the edges of these two slides (smear and spreader slide) should be found in the two smears prepared as described in steps 6 and 7.

The method of smear preparation outlined above is difficult to perform, and takes practice and dexterity. If the aspirate is largely fluid, then it is appropriate to handle it as one would handle any fluid specimen submitted to the cytology laboratory. Even with a cyst aspiration there are a few drops of fluid retained in the aspirating needle. Smears can be prepared from them in the standard fashion and can provide some preliminary idea of what the cyst might represent.

that paraffin blocks are trimmed and sectioned carefully to preserve ribbons of thin sections. Some of the cell-block slides should be stained initially while reserving others for special stains if needed. Cell-block sections provide more consistent results for immunohistochemistry with the exception of lymphoproliferative disease, where cytospins provide good preparations for immunohistochemistry if enough cells are obtained from the aspirate (Fig. 2.14).[74]

The tip design of the Franseen needle, used principally for transthoracic and transabdominal FNAB, seems to result in the procurement of microcores. As imaging has improved, interventional radiologists and clinicians performing endoscopic ultrasound-guided biopsies have gone to larger needles, more frequently obtaining small tissue cores in preference to aspirates. Inserting the stylus into the needle dislodges the small cores. The radiologist should not discard the stylus when they are performing the aspirate. These cores should not be smeared since that will result in distortion of cells and poor diagnostic yield.[53] To provide a provisional interpretation, one or two smears should be prepared by rolling the core over the slide surface in a small area. The core should then be placed in suitable fixative and processed as a small biopsy. A knowledgeable histo-technologist is required to handle core biopsies in order to achieve good sections. It is anticipated that thin-core biopsies will replace the more conventional larger-core biopsies and may also supplant aspiration biopsy, although the two procedures are complementary.

FNAB may obtain fluid that is clear and yellow in color, usually from breast cysts. This fluid does not need to be examined cytologically and can be discarded. Cyst fluid that is cloudy should be sent for cytologic examination. Following evacuation of a cyst, re-examination for any residual mass is very important and a repeat FNAB of that residual mass should be performed. When aspirating masses in and around the thyroid, a cyst with water-clear fluid may be encountered. This is diagnostic of a parathyroid cyst.[75] A portion of that fluid may be submitted for determination of parathyroid hormone levels, which are usually quite high.

A rare and challenging lesion is cystic papillary carcinoma of the thyroid. Clinical clues to this condition are fresh blood aspirated from a thyroid cyst, a residual mass after aspiration of a thyroid cyst, or a cyst that immediately refills following aspiration[76] For the vast majority of thyroid cysts that refill, from non-neoplastic goiter, the re-accumulation of fluid takes place very slowly. Use of thyroid suppression therapy may keep that process in check. A reasonable policy is to aspirate a thyroid cyst two or three times. If it continues to refill while the patient is on suppression therapy, it should be excised. Occasionally, such a case will prove to be cystic degeneration in a follicular neoplasm.

Fixation and stains for FNABs

Air-dried smears are stained by the Romanowsky method or one of a number of variations.[40] The Diff-Quik stain is currently very popular. This stain is composed of methyl alcohol, a fixative, eosin Y and azure A. Smears fixed initially in alcohol (95% ethyl, methyl, or isopropyl) are stained with the Papanicolaou (Pap) stain or one of its

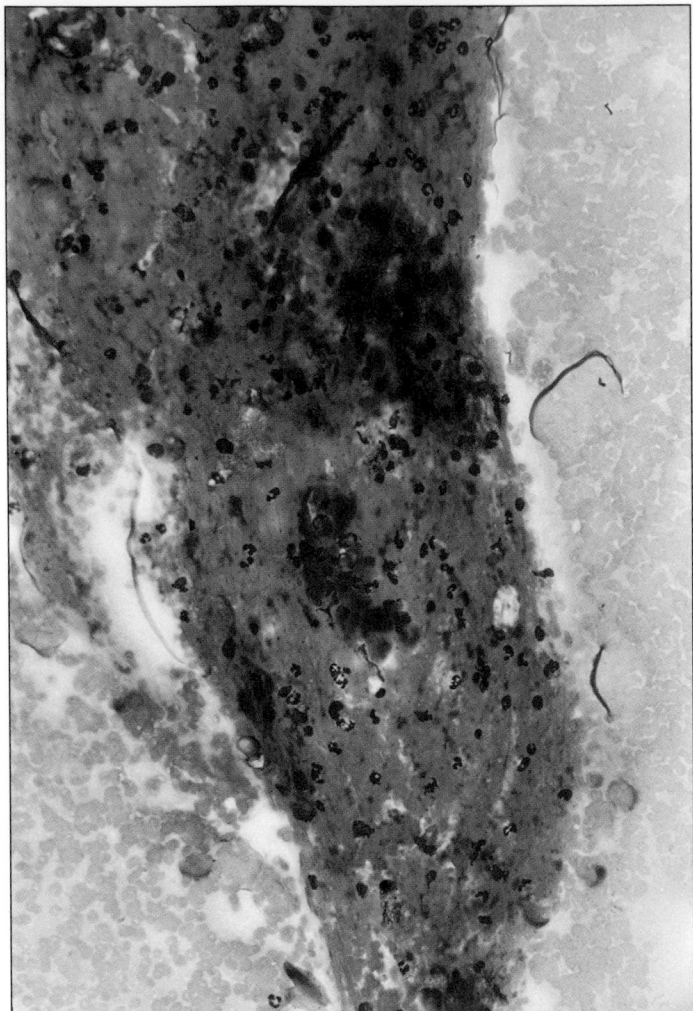

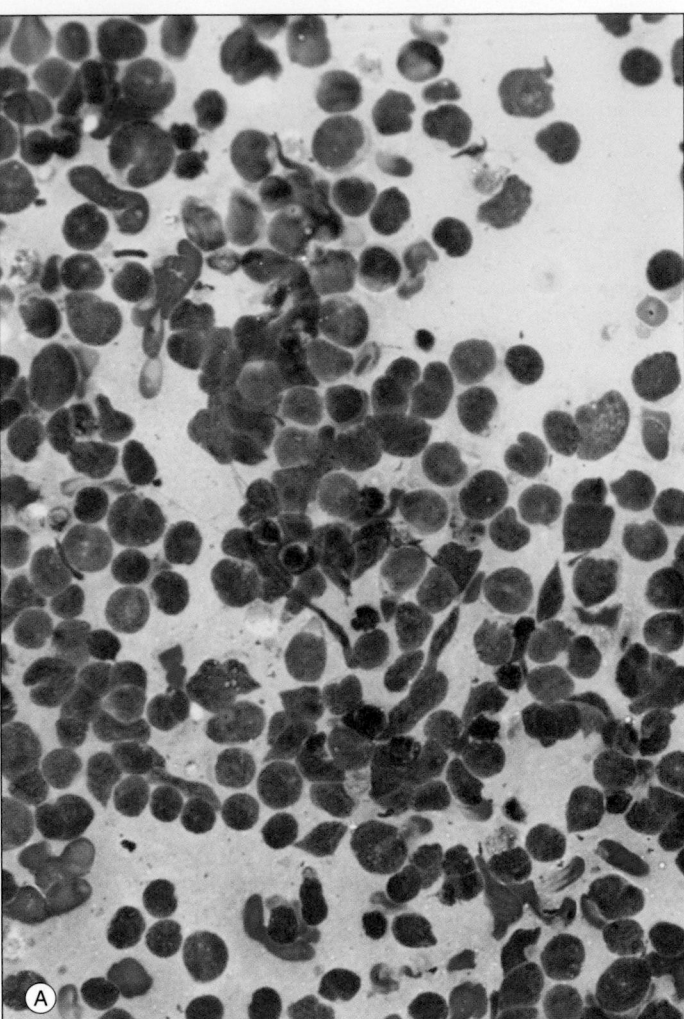

Fig. 2.13 Effects of prior clotting of blood on preparation of smears from an aspiration biopsy. Blood that has partially clotted traps cells, disrupting the pattern of the smear and obscuring details of individual and groups of cells (Diff-Quik).

modifications. The Papanicolaou stain consists of an admixture of cationic and anionic dyes.[31] Nuclei are first stained with hematoxylin. Slides are then rinsed in water and are dehydrated with ethanol for cytoplasmic staining with orange G (OG) and EA solutions. Orange G contains a monochromatic dye and stains keratin orange. EA is a label that was given by Papanicolaou to a mixture of eosin, light green, and Bismark brown. The role of Bismark brown is poorly understood and it is rarely included in current staining protocols. Eosin stains the cytoplasm of mature squamous cells and nucleoli pink and light green stains the more immature squamous cells and columnar cells green to blue. It should be stressed that the pink and green colors are not reliable by themselves in predicting the superficial versus the more immature nature of the squamous cells. Poorly understood factors such as fixation and pH may affect the colors; therefore, superficial cells should be recognized as those cells with a low nuclear cytoplasmic ratio and a pyknotic nucleus with cut-off corners of the cytoplasm regardless of the cytoplasmic coloration. Cell loss during fixation and staining is markedly reduced with the rapid Pap staining method developed by Yang and Alvarez.[73] The rehydration step also lyses red blood cells,

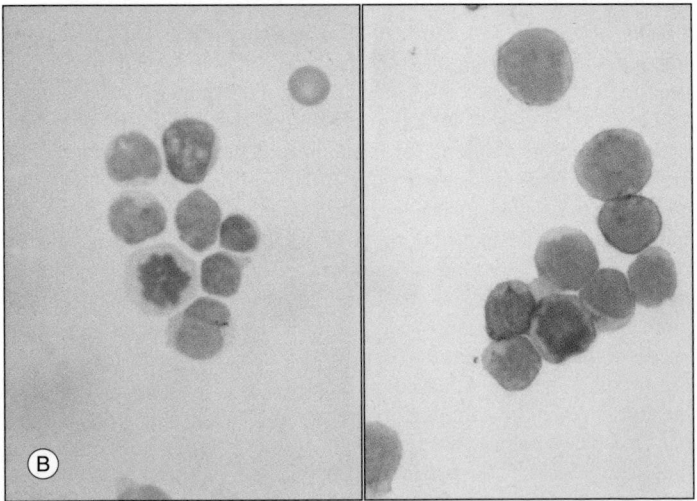

Fig. 2.14 (A) FNA smear and **(B)** cytospin of FNA of an enlarged supraclavicular mass in a 9-year-old patient. Interpretation of the smears indicated acute lymphoblastic lymphoma (A, Diff-Quik). Pan B-cell marker was negative (left) while CD1a, a T-cell marker, was strongly positive (B, peroxidase-antiperoxidase) (right). With the use of cytospins for immunohistochemistry, the smear background is quite clean.

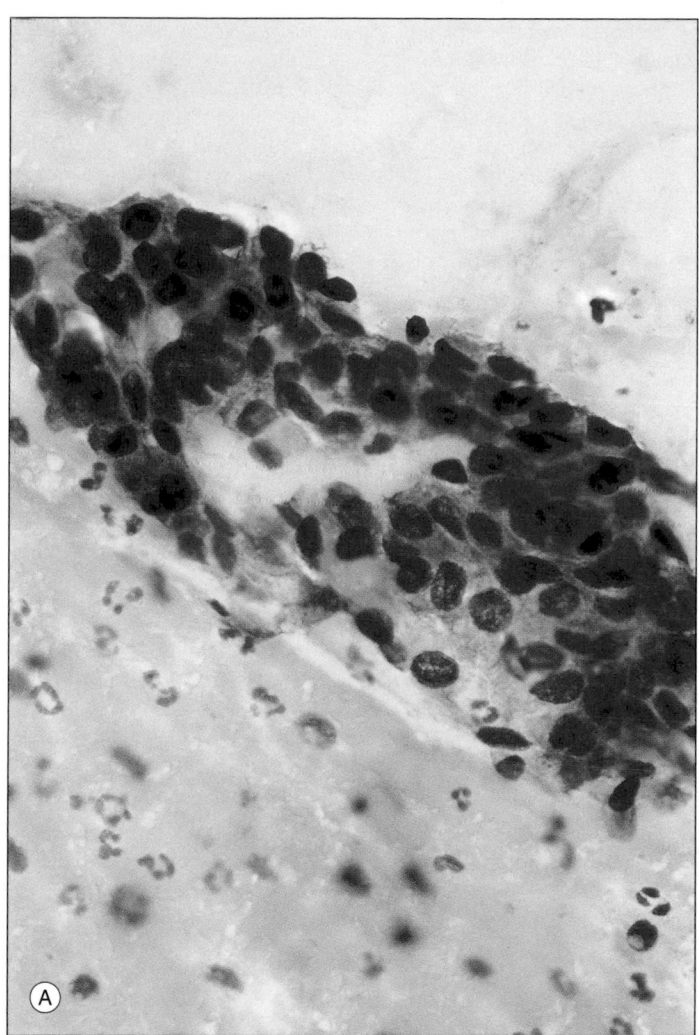 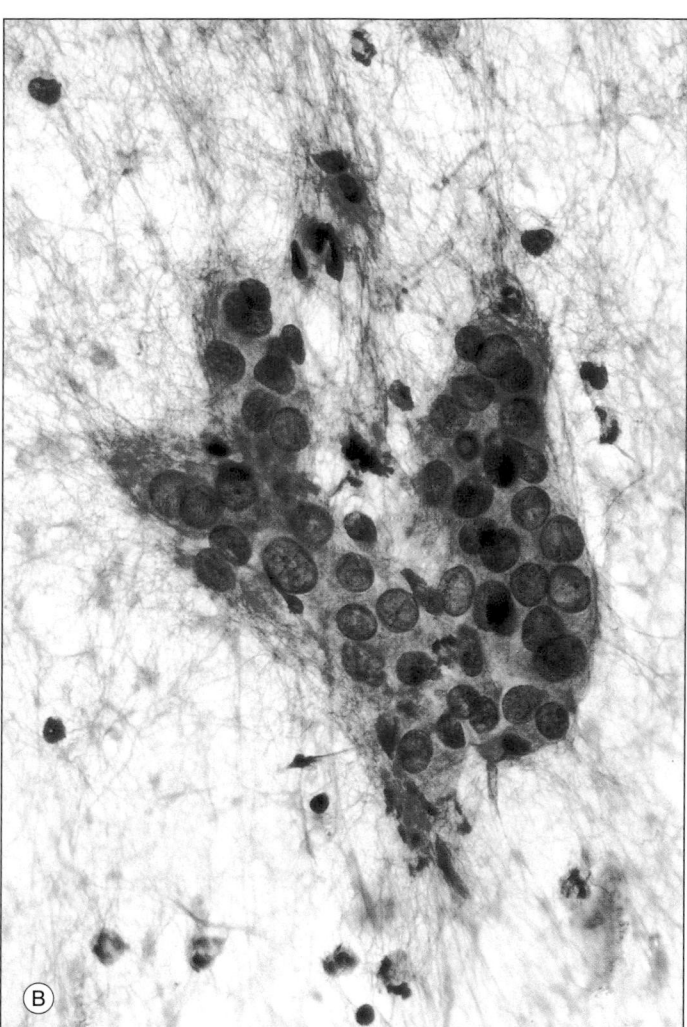

Fig. 2.15 Comparison of Diff-Quik and rapid Papanicolaou stains in FNAB of thyroid mass (papillary carcinoma of the thyroid). **(A)** Diff-Quik-stained smear reveals clusters of cells with elongated nuclei. The pattern suggests papillary carcinoma, but the nuclear features (grooves or intranuclear inclusions) are not convincing (Difff-Quik, ×600). **(B)** Rapid Papanicolaou stain shows the same pattern of cell clusters, but the nuclear features, (grooves and inclusions) are much more evident (Rapid Papanicolaou, ×600).

eliminating their effects on staining and clearing the background of the smears.

It has been helpful in some cases to have the rapid Pap-stained smears to compare with air-dried Diff-Quik-stained smears. For example, nuclear grooves and intranuclear inclusions may be easier to observe in some cases of papillary carcinoma of the thyroid (Fig. 2.15). An added advantage is that clinicians performing their own aspiration biopsies do not have to consider the details of fixation of smears; rather, the laboratory can decide which smears should be stained by the rapid Pap method and which can be optimally prepared for the use of other stains. If smears are fixed with a spray fixative it is important to allow them to dry for at least 1 hour prior to staining.

If a rapid hematoxylin and eosin stain is used, smears should be fixed by immersion for a few seconds in equal parts of 50% ethyl alcohol and 10% neutral buffered formalin. When staining with a quick hematoxylin and eosin method, hot (tap) water should be used in the rinsing steps. This will improve the overall quality of the staining and sharpen cell detail.

Personal preference and experience dictates which stain or stains will be used on aspiration biopsy smears. Cytopathologists with an orientation toward surgical pathology may prefer a rapid hematoxylin and eosin stain.[77] Those with a major experience in cytopathology most often prefer the Pap stain.[55] Individuals influenced by training in hematology prefer the Romanowsky, May-Grunwald-Geimsa, straight Giemsa, or Wright's stain, or in the United States, Diff-Quik.[40,45–47,78] All of these stains result in a contrasting metachromasia between cellular elements and stroma. Moreover, they are quite rapid, allowing immediate evaluation of the quality of the aspirate, an immediate diagnosis or differential diagnosis, and the opportunity to obtain additional samples for ancillary studies during the same procedure. Table 2.8 compares properties of air-dried versus wet-fixed smears and the contrast in staining features emphasized by Romanowsky versus the conventional Pap stain.[78]

Important components included in a complete FNAB report are demographics of the patient, history, and the precise procedure performed. These data are provided by the aspirator.[53] The microscopic features and interpretation are the responsibility of the cytopathologist. The final interpretation should include the site as well as the morphology as observed; for example, 'benign mixed tumor of right parotid salivary gland.' The cytologic interpretations are formatted

Table 2.8 Comparison of air-dried and wet-fixed smears

	Air-dried smear, Romanowsky stain	Wet-fixed smear, Papanicolaou stain
Dependence on smear technique	Strong	Moderate
Dry smear	Good fixation	Drying artifacts common
Wet smear	Artifacts common	Good fixation
Tissue fragments	Cells poorly seen, heavy ground substance staining	Individual cells clearly seen
Cell and nuclear area	Exaggerated, differences enhanced	Comparable to tissue section
Cytoplasmic detail	Well demonstrated	Poorly demonstrated
Nuclear detail	Different pattern from Papanicolaou stain	Excellently demonstrated
Nucleoli	Not always discernible	Well demonstrated
Stromal components	Well demonstrated and often differentially stained	Poorly demonstrated
Partially necrotic tissue	Poor definition of cell detail	Good definition of single intact cells

(From Orell et al.[54] with permission)

in the same way as standard surgical pathology interpretations. If a definite diagnosis cannot be made, this needs to be stated in the report. Examples would be 'atypical cells of undetermined type and significance, from aspirate of left cervical lymph node' or 'nondiagnostic aspirate of right breast mass.' A cytologic description of what is felt to be present should be part of these reports but does not constitute a diagnosis.

Recommendations for appropriate additional studies are an important part of the report and may include a request for repeat aspiration, core needle biopsy, open biopsy, or another management plan.[53] These various recommendations are dependent on the degree of certainty of the cytopathologists in reporting of the aspiration biopsy coupled with a synthesis of the clinical information and results of physical examination of the lesion, including how it felt during the FNAB. An intraoperative frozen section should be specifically suggested if, after aspiration biopsy, the cytopathologist cannot make a definitive malignant diagnosis and major surgery is planned. With respect to the current medical malpractice climate in the United States, it may be advisable to confirm any malignant aspiration biopsy diagnosis by frozen section where a major surgical procedure is to be performed.

Most 'lumps and bumps' in patients who present for FNAB are superficially located and are not in direct relationship to anatomic structures hazardous for biopsy. Complications from properly performed FNAB of superficial masses are few and of little consequence.[50] They include some minor discomfort in the region of the aspiration, usually of no more than a few hours' duration, some minimal ecchymosis of the aspiration site, and (rarely) small hematomas.[53] Complications are directly related to needle size, with figures of less than 0.03% when needles of finer gauge than 20 have been used.[79] Tumor cells seeding the needle tract have been reported only rarely with fine needles. Most reported cases of that complication are poorly documented. Our laboratory (WJF) has observed no cases of needle tract seeding in over 20 000 superficial and deep aspirations performed since 1972.

Reports have documented tissue damage or the displacement of tumor cells causing confusion in the interpretation of subsequent surgical biopsies or inability to make a diagnosis on the surgical specimen. Careful examination of these cases indicates the use of a larger needle than 22 gauge or thin needles with a tip design that ensures damage to tissue. Other reports suggest that an ill-trained or inexperienced clinician performing FNAB accounts for most or all of the cases in a given series.[80,81]

While taking a superficial FNAB, particularly in the area of the head and neck, some patients may experience lightheadedness or actual syncope.[44] Most of these patients have a past history of vasovagal responses to needle puncture. This information can be uncovered prior to biopsy, allowing appropriate precautions to be taken. A very rare complication with breast aspiration, and occasionally with sampling of a supraclavicular or high axillary lymph node, is pneumothorax.[82] When performing FNAB of the mammary gland in patients with small breasts, or a mass deeply placed at the margin of the breast, the aspiration needle should be directed away from the chest wall to avoid this complication.

In addition to complications of the procedure, FNAB is vulnerable to medical legal risk in two areas. These are a false-positive diagnosis of malignancy or false-negative diagnosis when a malignant tumor is present.[40] A false-negative diagnosis may arise in several ways: failure to recognize or find malignant cells that are present; poorly prepared or inadequate samples; not actually sampling the tumor; and intrinsic features of some tumors (e.g. marked sclerosis), which makes them unsuitable for aspiration biopsy. The first problem, failure to recognize malignant cells, is entirely the responsibility of the cytopathologist. The remaining problems are those of the aspirator and focus on the importance of attention to details in every part of the aspiration biopsy method.[53]

FNAB of the breast more than other sites presents the potential problem of the false-negative result.[41,50] Patients may be aspirated by clinicians for vague 'thickenings' of the breast. These changes in the breast do not constitute a defined mass and are rarely suspicious for malignancy.[53] The entire breast is found to be 'lumpy.' Following a benign aspiration biopsy report, and a benign appearance of the mammogram, the risk of a breast cancer being overlooked is very small. Most of these patients can be followed safely at regular intervals by physical examination of the breast for any appearance of a definite mass. Serial mammography may be performed as well, as an added safeguard. If a documented plan of follow-up is established and is understood by the patient, the rare small carcinoma that may be missed for a time should not cause any change in prognosis once the diagnosis is established. Emphasis should be placed on a defined plan for follow-up of this group of patients with negative FNAB to avoid a potential adverse effect of an unrealistically long-term sense of security from a false-negative result. Ultimately, the clinician must decide for each patient the likelihood that an FNAB is representative of the lesion, the degree of confidence in the FNAB interpretation, and whether to accept a diagnosis of negative for malignancy as the final step in the patient's evaluation.[53]

Invariably, false-positive interpretations are the result of over-reading atypical cells. If an FNAB diagnosis of malignancy does not fit the clinical picture, the clinician must ask for a review of the slides, specifically with that information in mind. Even with good sampling, masses that consistently yield few cells, regardless of the suspicion of malignancy, are nearly always benign. One notable exception is from aspiration biopsy of the breast, where both fibroadenomas and benign phyllodes tumors often exhibit large numbers of atypical cells.[83] Tumor cells from fibroadenoma and benign phyllodes tumors may even appear to infiltrate fat that is found on the smears, thus simulating a pattern of invasive breast carcinoma. Myoepithelial cells are usually present in these cases, frequently in large numbers. When they are present in an FNAB of the breast, this always indicates either a benign mass or at least one in which the pathologist should not report anything more than a suspicion of a malignant breast tumor. Myoepithelial cells may be few in number and easily overlooked by the cytopathologist in some cases (see Figs 2.10, 2.11). When the typical patterns of breast cancer are not easily recognized on FNAB, it is important to be cautious with the final interpretation

The most common pitfall for the clinician is failure to procure a good specimen.[53] It is not appropriate to judge this from the total volume of the aspirate but rather from the number of cells found and their pattern of distribution on the slide. A large volume of sample is not better when most of it is only blood or cyst fluid. The target for the FNAB must be clearly identified. A clinical differential diagnosis should be transmitted to the pathologist. The important questions are as follows: what is the indication for this aspiration biopsy, and what do I wish to learn from it to influence my management of this patient?

The pathologist's most common difficulty is trying to read too much into a limited FNAB, particularly with insufficient clinical information. The seven golden rules of aspiration biopsy are: (1) be aware of the limitations of FNAB for the body site being sampled; (2) obtain cellular samples that are adequate and well prepared; (3) be aware of the diagnostic pitfalls for each body site sampled; (4) correlate cytologic impressions with the patient's history and physical findings; (5) live within your limitations; (6) compare the cytology of FNAB with tissue samples whenever they are available; (7) maintain good lines of communication among clinicians, cytopathologists, and patients.[84]

ELECTRON MICROSCOPY

The implementation of electron microscopy laboratories in many departments of pathology in the late 1960s revolutionized the diagnosis and classification of renal diseases and other immunologically mediated disorders. Additionally, this modality was used extensively for the classification of tumors and tumor-like conditions both in adult and pediatric patients. The enhanced resolution of the electron microscope permitted cells to be characterized on the basis of particular organelles, cell products, and other structures which could not be visualized by standard light microscopic techniques.

Although the use of electron microscopy has decreased progressively with the development of immunohistochemistry, there remain a considerable number of diagnostic applications of this technique.[85–87] Current applications include selected aspects of tumor classification (Table 2.9) (Fig. 2.16), characterization of renal glomerular and interstitial diseases, classification of ciliary abnormalities (e.g. Kartagener's syndrome), and characterization of metabolic (storage) diseases.[85] In addition, electron microscopy is of value for the analysis of nerve and muscle biopsies, the characterization of endomyocardial biopsies, and for the rapid identification of viruses.

Glutaraldehyde is the fixative of choice for electron microscopy with postfixation in osmium tetroxide.[88] Generally, fresh tissue blocks measuring not more than 1 mm^3 are fixed in buffered glutaraldehyde for 1–4 hours. Following fixation, tissues are transferred to buffer prior to dehydration and further processing. Tissues are subsequently embedded in resin followed by the preparation of semithin sections which are stained with toluidine blue. These sections are used to select the most appropriate blocks for ultrastructural studies.

Table 2.9 Selected applications of electron microscopy in tumor diagnosis

Tumor type	Ultrastructural features
Squamous cell carcinoma	Tonofilaments, desmosomes
Adenocarcinoma (lung)	Short microvilli with glycocalyx, intracellular lamellar bodies/myelin bodies; intratubular nuclear inclusions
Adenocarcinoma (colon)	Short microvilli with glycocalyx, rootlets and tight junctions
Mesothelioma (epithelioid)	Elongated microvilli without glycocalyx
Small cell (neuroendocrine) carcinoma	Dense core (small <100 µm) secretory granules
Acinic cell carcinoma	Large (600–900 µm) secretory granules
Endocrine tumors (e.g. pancreas)	Intermediate sized (100–400 µm) secretory granules
Adrenal cortical tumors	Abundant smooth endoplasmic reticulum, mitochondria with tubulovesicular cristae
Melanoma	Premelanosomes, melanosomes
Neuroblastoma	Cell processes, dense-core secretory granules
Leiomyosarcoma and other smooth muscle tumors	Thin (6–8 µm) filaments with focal densities and attachment plaques
Angiosarcoma and other vascular tumors	Weibel-Palade bodies
Clear cell sarcoma of soft parts	Premelanosomes
Alveolar soft part sarcoma	Crystalloids
Schwann cell tumors	Cell processes with extensive basal lamina
Synovial sarcoma	Cell junctions, villus-like filopodia, microvilli, basal lamina
Langerhans cell histiocytosis	Birbeck granules

Ultrathin sections are then stained with uranyl acetate followed by lead citrate prior to examination.

Although tissues fixed in formalin may be used for electron microscopy, there is often considerable disruption of intracellular architecture. There are several methods for using material previously embedded in paraffin for ultrastructural studies, but preservation of structural detail is usually quite poor.[88] Nonetheless, the latter approach may be of value for the identification of certain organelles such as premelanosomes and neuroendocrine secretory granules.

Electron microscopy has also proven to be effective for studies of material obtained by fine needle aspiration biopsy (Fig. 2.17).[89–91] Generally, preparative techniques designed to remove red blood cells and concentrate the remaining cellular material are particularly effective in increasing the cellular yield.[92] In general, these studies have underscored the fact that electron microscopy can provide clinically relevant information in aspirated samples.

Microprobe analysis is performed with an electron microscope equipped with an energy dispersive X-ray spectrometer and is commonly referred to as electron probe X-ray microanalysis.[93] Elements with an atomic number equal to or greater than beryllium can be detected and quantitated. The most commonly studied clinical problems that can be evaluated by this methodology include the

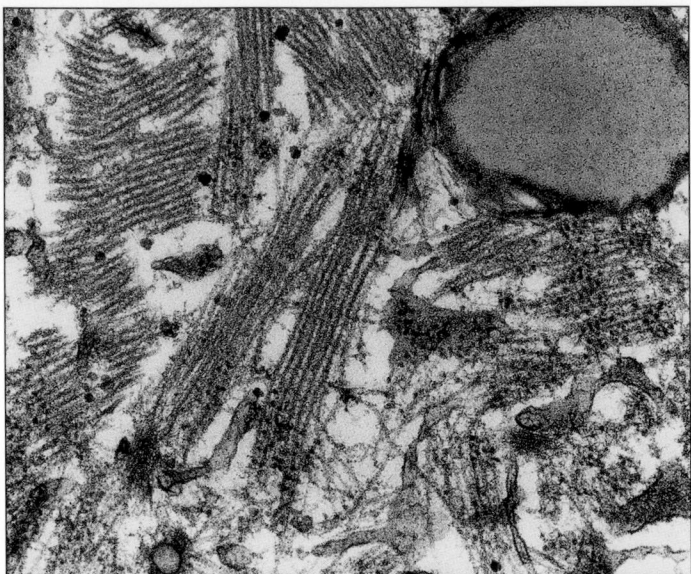

Fig. 2.16 Rhabdomyosarcoma in a 46-year-old man. Perineal mass attached to bulbar urethra showed poorly differentiated sarcoma on light microscopy. Electron microscopy revealed the minimal criteria for diagnosis of a rhabdomyosarcoma, myosin-ribosome complexes (×44 330). With permission from Gurley et al.[85]

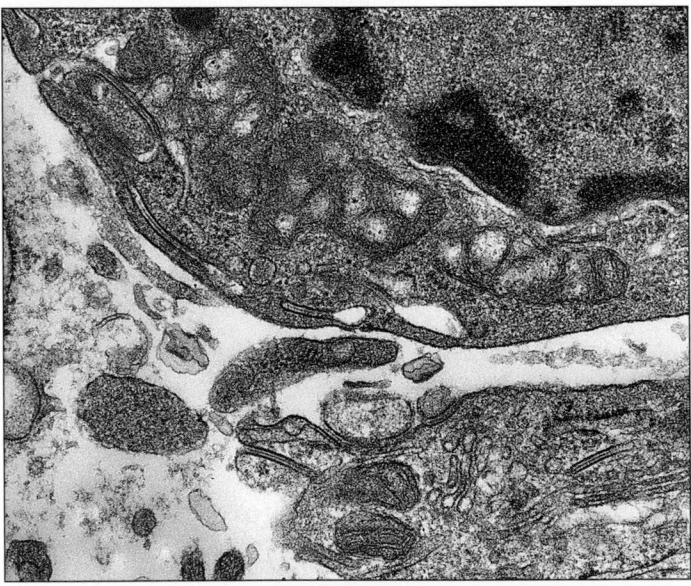

Fig. 2.17 Langerhans cell histiocytosis in a 11-year-old boy. Fine needle aspirate of T5 vertebral body mass. Electron microscopy revealed classic Birbeck's granules (×35 000). With permission from Gurley et al.[85]

pneumoconioses (e.g. asbestosis), 'hard metal' pulmonary fibrosis, and other mineral-induced pneumoconioses. Specific identification of the material has the potential to permit recognition of sources of exposure and the development of strategies to eliminate potential exposures. Laser microprobe mass analysis (LAMMA) and secondary ion mass spectrometry (SIMS) have considerably greater sensitivity than electron probe X-ray microanalysis. Moreover, these

techniques have capabilities for isotopic separation and the ability to detect and localize molecules and molecular fragments.[93]

Both immunocytochemistry and in situ hybridization procedures may be performed at the ultrastructural level.[94,95] However, there are relatively few current diagnostic applications of these methodologies.

IMMUNOHISTOCHEMISTRY

The development and implementation of immunohistochemical methods have revolutionized the practice of surgical pathology and cytopathology over the past four decades. This phenomenon has occurred because of the development of an extensive array of polyclonal antisera and monoclonal antibodies (Table 2.10), together with increasingly more sensitive immunological staining sequences and detection methods. Moreover, standardized antigen retrieval methods have permitted the detection of many antigens, even in suboptimally fixed tissue samples. In the realm of tumor pathology, immunohistochemistry has proven to be a remarkably powerful tool for the classification of undifferentiated and poorly differentiated malignant tumors, the classification of small round blue cell tumors, the determination of sites of origin of unknown primaries, and the subclassification of lymphomas and leukemias. In addition to its diagnostic applications, immunohistochemistry is being used increasingly for the prognostic assessment of tumors of various types. Detailed reviews of the applications of these methods will be discussed in the subsequent chapters of this text.

Immunohistochemistry is best described as that branch of immunology (or histochemistry) that deals with the identification of cellular components through the use of antibodies. Although immunofluorescence techniques were first utilized in the 1940s, they did not gain widespread acceptance until the following decade when they became critically important tools in experimental immunology.[96] These methods have since been used extensively in the classification of renal diseases and other immunologically mediated disease processes. Principal drawbacks to the more widespread adoption of these methods included a relatively low sensitivity, the need for fresh frozen tissues, lack of sufficient morphological detail, impermanence of the preparations, and the need for a fluorescence microscope.

Techniques utilizing antibodies conjugated to enzymes (horseradish peroxidase alkaline phosphatase, glucose oxidase) were introduced in the mid-60s as an alternative to immunofluorescence methods.[97] Sites of antibody binding were visualized by incubation with substrate (H_2O_2) and a chromogen (diaminobenzidine) when horseradish peroxidase was used as the enzyme conjugate to produce a colored and insoluble reaction product. Although this approach did not provide greater sensitivity than corresponding immunofluorescence methods, its major advantage was that results could be studied directly with a light microscope.

The field of immunohistochemistry was revolutionized in the 1970s by the development of the immunoglobulin enzyme bridge[98] and peroxidase antiperoxidase methods[99] which could be performed on formalin-fixed paraffin-embedded sections. The peroxidase antiperoxidase method involves the sequential application of primary antiserum (or monoclonal antibody), a bridge or secondary antigen with specificity directed to the globulin faction of the primary antiserum, and a soluble peroxidase antiperoxidase complex prepared in the same species as the primary antiserum. The peroxidase antiperoxidase method possesses considerably higher sensitivity than the conjugate methods due to the virtual absence of background staining with a resultant high signal to noise ratio. Since

Table 2.10 Classes of markers for immunohistochemisty*

Adhesion Proteins
Cadherins, ICAM-1, NCAM (CD56), fibronectin, integrins, catenins

Calcium Binding Proteins
S-100, calmodulin, calretinin, calbindin

Connective Tissue Proteins
Collagens, laminin, fibronectin

Cytoskeleton Associated Actin Binding Proteins
Caldesmon, calretinin, villin, calponin

Cytotoxic Drug Metabolism
Multidrug resistance associated proteins, P-glycoprotein, heat shock proteins

Endothelial Proteins
CD31, CD34 (QBEND), Factor VIII-related antigen

Enzymes
Prostatic acid phosphatase, myeloperoxidase,deoxynucleotidyl terminal transferase (TdT), placental alkaline phosphatase, cathepsins, alpha-methylacyl-CoA racemase, prostate specific antigen (kallikrein family of serine proteases), tyrosinase, mismatch repair enzymes, telomerase, matrix metallo-proteinases.

Fusion Proteins
ALK-1 (for NPM-ALK protein), PAX8-PPAR-gamma

Growth Factors (GF) and GF Receptors(R)
Her2 neu (c-erbB2), epidermal growth factor (EGF) and EGFR, platelet derived growth factor (PDGF), vascular endothelial growth factor (VEGF)

Hormones
Peptides, glycoproteins, steroids, amines

Hormone Receptors
Estrogen receptor, progesterone receptor, androgen receptor, somatostatin receptor

Immunoglobulins
Heavy and light chains, J-chain

Intermediate Filaments
Cytokeratins, vimentin, neurofilaments, glial fibrillary acidic protein, peripherin, lamins, desmin

Melanocytic Proteins
HMB-45, MiTF (microphthalmia transcription factor), MART-1 (melan A)

Mucin and Glycoprotein Antigens
B72.3, CEA, CA19-9, MUC 1, MUC 2, CA125, BCA-225, thyroglobulin

Muscle and Contractile Proteins
Myoglobin, actin, myosin, dystrophin

Neuroendocrine Secretory Granule Matrix Proteins
Chromogranins/secretogranins

Oncogene Proteins
Abl, bcl-2, bax, c-myc, c-kit (CD117), bcl-6

Proliferation Markers/Cell Cycle Regulators/Apoptosis Markers
Cyclins, PCNA, MIB-1(Ki-67), p27 (kip 1), bcl-x, caspases, topoisomerases

Protease Inhibitors
Alpha-1-antitrypsin, alpha-1-antichymotrypsin

Synaptic Vesicle and Synaptic Plasma Membrane-Associated Proteins
Synaptophysin, synaptic vesicle protein 2, vesicle associated membrane protein
Synaptosomal associated protein of 25kD (SNAP-25)

Transcription Factors
Thyroid transcription factor-1(TTF-1), CDX2, Bcl-6, pituitary transcription factor-1, (pit-1),myoD1, myogenin, WT-1, FLI-1

Table 2.10 Classes of markers for immunohistochemisty* (cont'd)

Transmembrane Glycoproteins
CD3, CD4, CD5, CD8, CD20, CD30, CD45 (LCA), CD99 (MIC2)

Tumor Suppressor Gene Proteins
Retinoblastoma (Rb), deleted in colon cancer (DCC), adenomatous polyposis coli (APC) protein, maspin, p63, p53, PTEN, p16

Other Markers
Alpha fetoprotein (AFP), epithelial membrane antigen (EMA), gross cystic disease fluid protein (GCDFP), hepatocyte specific marker, renal cell carcinoma antigen (RCC), surfactant apoprotein, uroplakins

Viral and bacterial antigens
Herpes simplex, CMV, HPV, Hepatitis B, adenovirus, *H. Pylori*

*Selected examples of markers are listed under each heading.

this method could be applied to routinely processed material, it was adopted rapidly by pathology laboratories throughout the world.

The peroxidase antiperoxidase method has been largely replaced by avidin- or streptavidin-based methods. Avidin is a 68-kD glycoprotein which has four binding sites for the low molecular weight vitamin, biotin.[100] The interaction of biotin with avidin has an association constant that is several million times greater than that of antigen–antibody interactions. In the labeled avidin biotin (LAB) or labeled streptavidin biotin (LSAB) methods, the reaction sequence includes primary antibody, a biotinylated secondary or bridge antibody, and peroxidase labeled avidin or streptavidin.[100] The avidin biotin peroxidase complex method involves sequential incubations with a primary antibody, a biotinylated secondary or bridge antibody, and preformed complexes of avidin or streptavidin and biotin horseradish peroxidase (ABC technique).[101] The intensity of the staining is due to the formation of a lattice-like structure containing multiple peroxidase antibodies. Similar to avidin, streptavidin also possesses a high affinity for biotin, and because of the absence of carbohydrates, non-specific binding due to electrostatic interactions is considerably less than with avidin-based methods because of streptavidin's lower isoelectric point.[102] These features result in very high signal to noise ratios. In most diagnostic immunohistochemistry laboratories streptavidin procedures have replaced avidin-based methods.

A variety of methods employing natural or synthetic polymer carriers to increase the number of enzymes or ligands that are coupled to linker antibodies have been developed.[103–106] Polymeric carriers that have been used include dextran, polypeptides, dendrimers, and DNA branches. In the direct enhanced polymer, one step staining (EPOS) system, primary antibodies and horseradish peroxidase are coupled to a divinyl sulfone-activated dextran polymer. An indirect polymer method has also been developed by Dako laboratories (En Vision™ +). With this procedure, tissues are first incubated with the primary antibody and are then incubated with a polymeric conjugate consisting of a large number of peroxidase and secondary antibody molecules bound to an activated dextran backbone. The polymeric conjugates hold up to 100 enzyme molecules and up to 20 antibody molecules per backbone.[104] The indirect system provides considerably greater flexibility than the direct method since the primary antibody can be varied. The use of this polymer-based approach circumvents false-positive staining due to endogenous biotin.[107] Comparative studies indicate that the polymer-based En Vision method possesses a sensitivity which exceeds that of the ABC or labeled streptavidin methods.[104] This method has been adapted for use with frozen sections and is potentially capable of detecting a broad range of antigens in less than 13 minutes.[106]

Some studies have suggested that the sensitivity of these methods for the detection of certain antigens may be decreased because of the spatial hindrance afforded by the high molecular weight of the dextran carrier. In order to circumvent this problem, Shi et al. have utilized a more compact enzyme linker antibody conjugate with a high number of enzyme molecules attached to each linker antibody with minimal increase in molecular size (Power Vision System).[105] The Power Vision reagent is derived from small multifunctional, polymerizable linkers that are used to activate a mixture of enzymes and linker antibodies with polymerization occurring under controlled conditions.[105] The result of this polymerization process is an enzyme linker antibody with a more compact molecular shape than other types of polymers, thereby allowing the attachment of multiple conjugates in close proximity to one another. This procedure also circumvents problems with endogenous biotin.

Protein A-based methods are not generally used in diagnostic immunohistochemistry laboratories;[108] however, these methods are of particular value for ultrastructural immunohistochemistry when combined with colloidal gold.[109] The catalyzed reporter deposition (CARD) method, which is also known as the tyramide amplification technique (TAT), depends on the ability of horseradish peroxidase to catalyze the dimerization of biotinylated tyramine (tyramide), thereby permitting the deposition of a large number of avidin-biotin-peroxidase complexes or peroxidase-labeled streptavidin molecules.[110–112] Although this method possesses very high sensitivity, it has not been generally adopted in routine diagnostic immuno-histochemistry laboratories

Diaminobenzidine is the most commonly employed chromogen in immunoperoxidase-based systems.[102] Its many advantages include a distinct brown color, its insolubility in organic solvents, its high substantivity (lack of diffusion from sites of deposition) and its stability in sections stored for prolonged time periods. However, because of its potential carcinogenicity, a variety of other chromogens have been developed, including aminoethylcarbazole and 4-chloro-1-naphthol, which produce red and blue reaction products, respectively. Both of these chromogens are soluble in aqueous solutions, tend to fade with prolonged storage, and are also potential carcinogens. Although peroxidase-based systems are used in most diagnostic laboratories, other enzymes (e.g. alkaline phosphatase, glucose oxidase) have also been used in immunohistochemical formats.[113,114]

Ten percent formalin is the most commonly employed fixative in diagnostic immunohistochemistry laboratories; however, other fixatives have also been used successfully, including alcohols, picric acid-containing solutions, and mercury-based fixatives such as formol sublimate (B5) and Zenker's fixative.[102,115] Some of these fixatives provide optimal results for certain classes of antigens. For example, alcohol-based fixatives are particularly useful for the demonstration of intermediate filament proteins while picric acid containing fixatives and B5 provide optimal results for peptide hormones and lymphoid markers (including immunoglobulins), respectively. Most currently available antibodies and staining techniques, however, have been optimized for formalin-fixed tissues.

Tissues that have been decalcified with nitric or formic acids or with EDTA have been used successfully for the demonstration of many antigens.[116] However, if a negative result is obtained, a decalcified sample of tissue known to contain the antigen should be stained concurrently. This step is necessary to rule out the possibility that the decalcification step may have destroyed the antigen. While routine processing and embedding has proven to be effective for the demonstration of most antigens, these procedures may lead to the destruction of certain epitopes. In these instances, fresh frozen tissue should be used to determine if the epitope(s) are susceptible to processing and embedding steps. Certain epitopes may deteriorate in previously sectioned stored tissue samples. If a negative result is obtained with this type of material, freshly sectioned tissue should be tested for reactivity with the particular antibody.

While many earlier immunohistochemical studies were performed with polyclonal antisera, more recent studies have used monoclonal antibodies almost exclusively.[102,115] Polyclonal antisera contain many different antibodies of varying specificities and affinities. Repeated immunizations with the same antigen generally results in the production of antisera containing high-affinity antibodies. Advantages of polyclonal antisera include the presence of a complex mixture of high- and low-affinity antibodies to different epitopes with a resultant increased probability of antigen–antibody interactions. As a result, more antibodies will be deposited per antigen molecule. In order to provide reagents that are effective in immunohistochemical formats, antisera must be absorbed with unwanted antigens and should be affinity purified. Pre-immune sera are invaluable controls to detect the presence of pre-existing antibodies.

Monoclonal antibodies are restricted in their specificity to a single epitope and can be produced in limitless supply.[102,115] Since monoclonal antibodies recognize a relatively short amino acid sequence, there is a real potential for unexpected cross-reactivities. A higher level of sensitivity is needed when antigens are present in low concentrations; however, mixtures of monoclonal antibodies (cocktails) can be used to circumvent this problem. Selective masking of epitopes resulting from fixation and processing may also lead to significant loss of binding monoclonal antibodies.

ANTIGEN (EPITOPE) RETRIEVAL METHODS

It is well recognized that suboptimal preservation of epitopes is a major factor leading to staining inconsistencies in immuno-histochemical formats.[102] The deleterious effects of formalin fixation can be reversed to some extent by prolonged washing of tissues in water or buffer. Proteolytic enzyme digestion prior to staining has been particularly effective for the unmasking of some formalin-sensitive epitopes; however, other epitopes may be particularly susceptible to the effects of various proteases and may be completely destroyed even after relatively brief treatments.[117] The mechanism of protease-induced retrieval most likely results form the breakage of formaldehyde-induced cross-links in the antigen with exposure of cryptic epitopes or hydrolysis of adjacent micro-molecular complexes that may have masked the epitope(s) of interest. Optimization of the length of proteolysis is more crucial to the success of this approach than the particular enzyme used.[117] In general, tissue fixed for prolonged time periods require the most extended periods of enzyme digestion.

Microwave-induced antigen retrieval is currently the method of choice for the detection of most antigens of interest to pathologists.[118] Moist heat can lead to disruption of formalin-induced bonds between proteins and calcium ions, thereby exposing 'hidden' or cryptic epitopes.[119] The most commonly used approach utilizes microwave heating in 10-mM/L citrate buffer at pH 6.0. Alternatively, other moist heating methods using pressure cookers and rice steamers have been found to be equally successful or even superior to microwave methods.[120,121] A 'test battery' approach has been suggested by Shi et al. to determine optimal retrieval conditions.[120]

Heat-induced antigen retrieval methods have several potentially serious pitfalls. For example, since most monoclonal antibodies

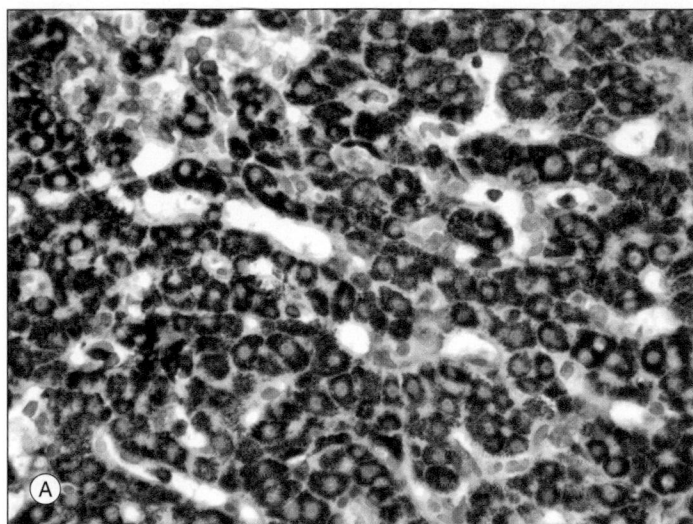
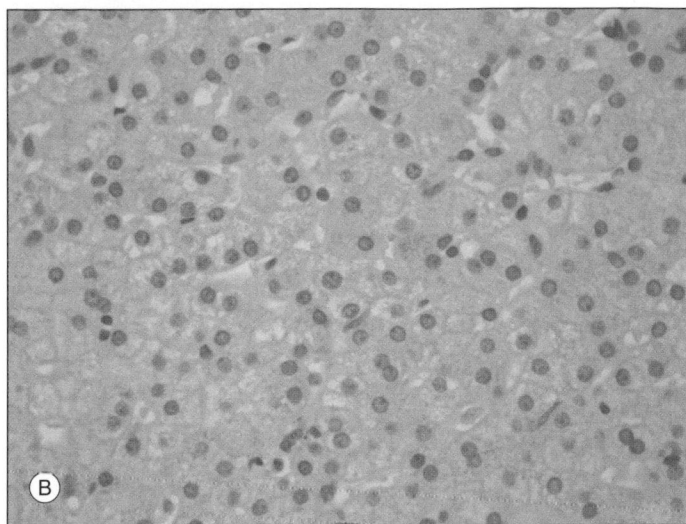

Fig. 2.18 (A) Formalin fixed and paraffin embedded liver biopsy stained for CD3 with the streptavidin biotin peroxidase method following microwave antigen retrieval without biotin blocking. There is intense granular cytoplasmic reactivity with the hepatocytes indicative of endogenous biotin. **(B)** Same specimen with prior blocking of endogenous biotin. The hepatocytes are completely negative.

react with epitopes containing 3–8 amino acids, these methods could expose unwanted epitopes of identical sequence in unrelated antigens. Heat-induced antigen retrieval may also result in enhanced reactivity of endogenous biotin, which is particularly problematic in mitochondrion-rich cells (Fig. 2.18).[122]

Background staining

A large number of factors may contribute to unwanted background staining in immunohistochemical preparations and these factors may lead to considerable interpretative difficulties.[102,115,123] Hydrophobic interactions (van der Waals forces), for example, may lead to non-specific staining of collagen and other connective tissue elements, fat cells, and squamous epithelium. One of the most commonly used approaches to reduce hydrophobic interactions is the use of a blocking protein, either as a separate step, or by its incorporation into the antibody diluent. In most laboratories, 1% bovine serum albumin is used as the blocking protein. Ionic interactions can also lead to substantial non-specific background staining. This problem can generally be circumvented by the use of diluent buffers of relatively high ionic strengths. Endogenous peroxidase activity may also lead to unacceptable levels of background staining, but this problem can be largely avoided by pretreatment of sections with hydrogen peroxide or a mixture of hydrogen peroxide and methanol.

The presence of unwanted naturally occurring antibodies in polyclonal antisera is another potential source of background staining. Generally, this problem can be circumvented by employing high dilutions of the primary antiserum or brief incubation times. The presence of unwanted antibodies induced by immunization with impure antigens can generally be avoided by the use of high dilutions of the antiserum or by the use of affinity-purified antibodies. Cross-reactivity of polyclonal antisera and monoclonal antibodies result from the sharing of epitopes by unrelated proteins. These problems can generally be avoided for monoclonal antibodies by selecting clones that do not possess the unwanted patterns of cross-reactivity. With polyclonal antisera, absorption with the 'unwanted' antigen will generally eliminate this problem.

Endogenous biotin is a source of non-specific staining when avidin or streptavidin are exposed.[102,115,122,123] Considerable endogenous biotin activity may be enhanced following microwave retrieval and it is particularly important to use the appropriate blocking step with these types of preparations (Fig. 2.18). Non-specific binding due to Fc receptors may be problematic in frozen sections and smears. In general, this type of interaction can be circumvented by the use of $F(ab')_2$ fragments in place of the intact IgG molecules and by careful screening of monoclonal antibodies. Complement-mediated binding may also occur, particularly in frozen sections, but this phenomenon may be avoided by the use of decomplemented sera. Diffusion of antigens from their sites of synthesis or storage into adjacent cells and tissues may lead to considerable non-specific staining. Generally, this occurrence may be circumvented by the use of rapidly fixed tissues.

INTERPRETATION OF RESULTS AND CONTROLS

Interpretation of immunohistochemical results is based on meticulous staining techniques, the use of appropriate controls, and knowledge of the cellular distribution of various antigens. For example, some antigens (e.g. Her 2 neu) have a predominant plasma membrane distribution (Fig. 2.19) while others such as p53, TTF-1 (Fig. 2.20), CDX2 (Fig. 2.21), and MIB-1 have an exclusive nuclear distribution. Cytokeratins, on the other hand, may be present diffusely throughout the cytoplasm (Fig. 2.22) or may be localized to particular cytoplasmic regions such as the paranuclear regions of certain small cell carcinomas (Fig. 2.23). Some cytoplasmic antigens such as melan-A (A103) have a granular cytoplasmic distribution (Fig. 2.24). Other antigens, such as S-100 protein and calretinin, are present both within the nucleus and cytoplasm (Fig. 2.25). As noted by Nadji and Morales, the most important quality of a true positive reaction is heterogeneity in distribution among a group of cells or throughout a neoplasm.[115] When using diaminobenzidine, the reaction should be present as distinct brown staining. Diffuse pale brown or yellow staining most likely represents a non-specific reaction. False-positive staining may occur under a number of circumstances. For example, crushed cells or

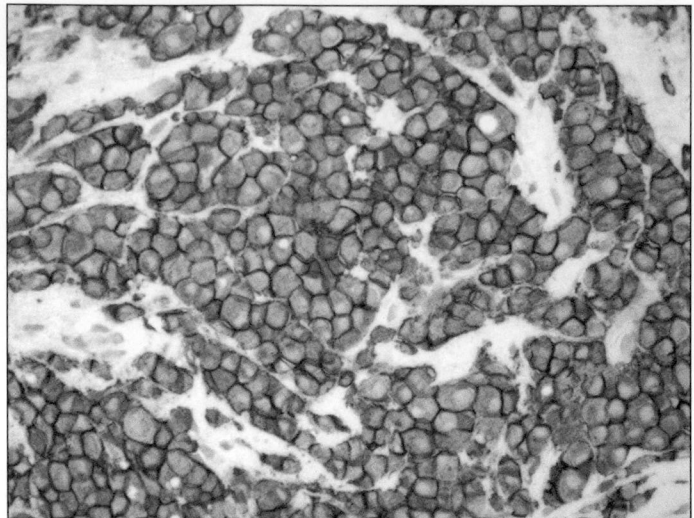

Fig. 2.19 Invasive ductal breast carcinoma stained for Her2 neu. There is strong positive staining of the plasma membranes of the cells.

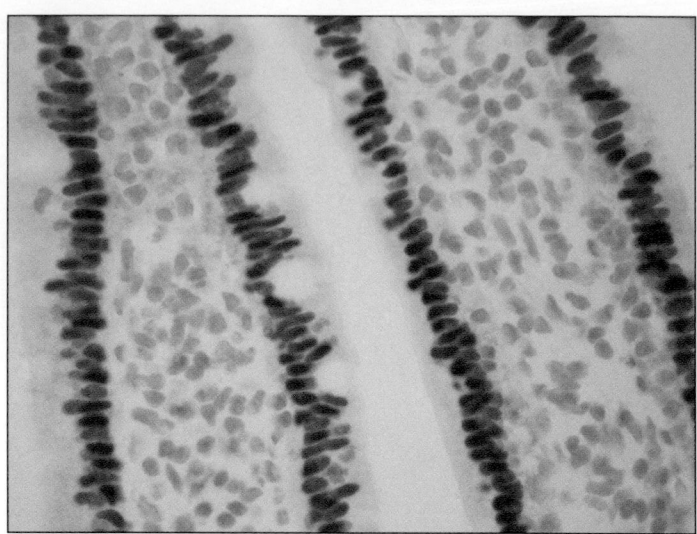

Fig. 2.21 Normal small intestinal mucosa stained for CDX2. Staining is confined to the nuclei of the epithelial cells.

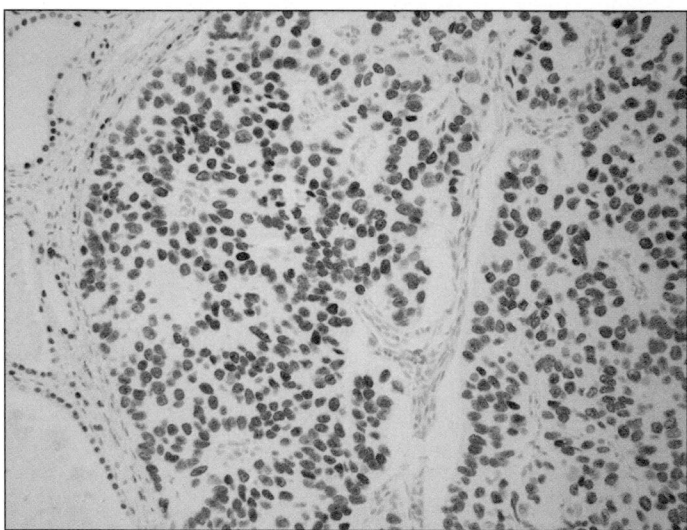

Fig. 2.20 Poorly differentiated thyroid carcinoma stained for TTF-1. The nuclei of the tumor cells are strongly stained. In addition, there is nuclear staining of the adjacent normal follicular cells.

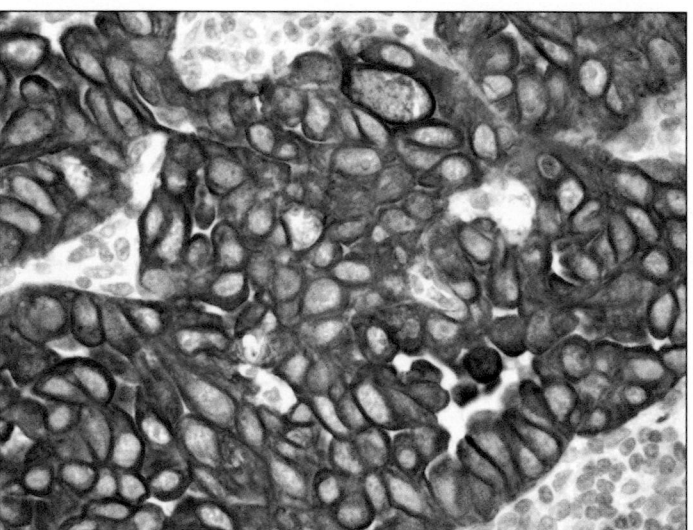

Fig. 2.22 Poorly differentiated adenocarcinoma of the lung stained for cytokeratin 7. Staining is present diffusely throughout the cytoplasm.

necrotic cells may exhibit considerable non-specific staining, especially when polyclonal antisera are used. Edges of sections may also show false-positive reactions and this phenomenon may be particularly problematic in small-core biopsies. False-negative staining may result from a prozone-like phenomenon. This occurs when the tissue contains high concentrations of the antigen such that the antigen–antibody reaction does not occur unless the antibody is diluted. This type of problem occurs more commonly when polyclonal antisera are used.

Both positive and negative controls should be used in conjunction with the patient test samples.[102,115] The positive control should of course contain the antigen of interest and should be fixed and processed in the same manner as the test samples. In addition, the positive controls should be subjected to the same antigen retrieval procedure as the test samples. A positive control slide should produce staining that is distinct in the areas know to contain the antigen while the adjacent areas should be negative. For example, insulin immunoreactivity should be present in a subset of pancreatic islet cells and should be absent from other islet cell types, acinar cells, and stromal elements. Control slides provided by the manufacturer are best used to validate reagent performance and generally should not be used in place of controls prepared in the laboratory that is performing the testing. Negative controls are performed by eliminating the primary antibody from the staining sequence. This can be accomplished by substituting the primary antibody with the antibody diluent and carrier protein or with the same concentration of nonimmune immunoglobulin derived from the same species as the primary antibody. Alternatively, a class-matched irrelevant antibody can be used as a negative control. Although absorption controls were used commonly in the past,

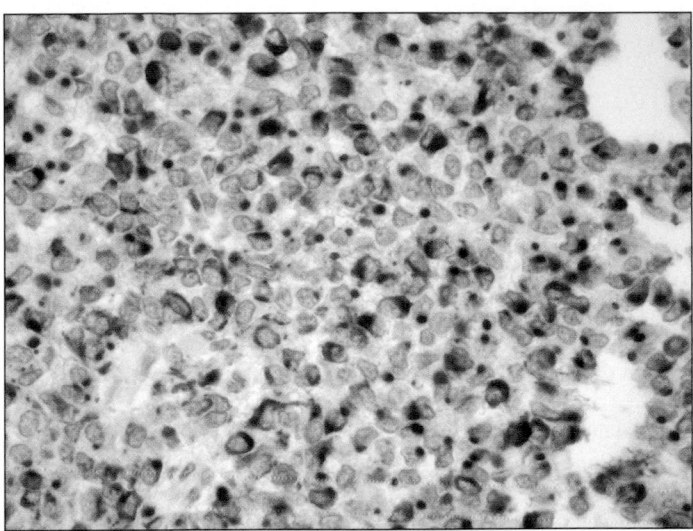

Fig. 2.23 Small cell bronchogenic carcinoma stained with a cytokeratin 'cocktail.' Immunoreactivity has a dot-like distribution, corresponding to paranuclear areas.

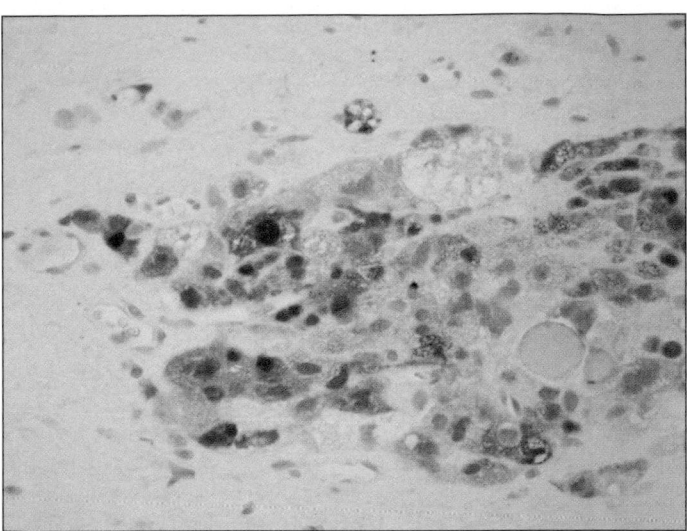

Fig. 2.25 Adrenal cortical adenoma stained for calretinin. Staining is present both within the cytoplasm and nuclei.

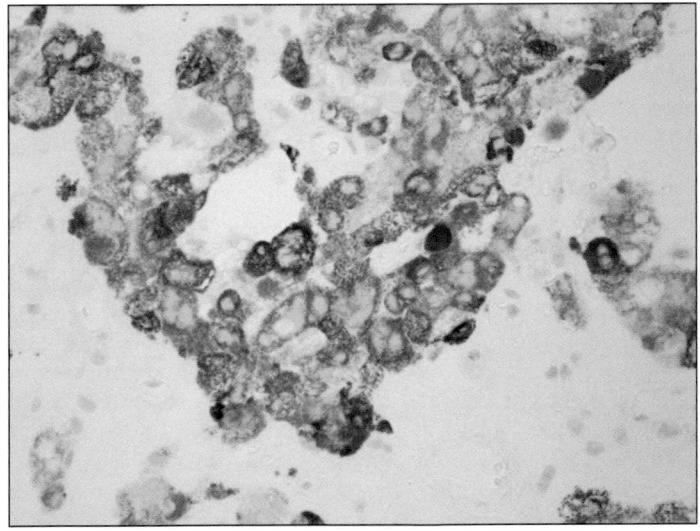

Fig. 2.24 Adrenal cortical adenoma stained for Melan-A (A103). Immunoreactivity has a granular cytoplasmic distribution.

particularly for polyclonal antisera, they do not provide the requisite specificity for tissue-bound antigens that have been altered by fixation.[102]

CYTOLOGICAL SAMPLES

Immunohistochemistry can be performed on most cytological samples, including exfoliated cells, effusions and FNABs. For FNABs, cytospins can be made from the needle rinse and may be either air-dried or fixed in 95% ethyl alcohol. Direct smears or cytospins, either air-dried or fixed for immunohistochemistry, may be preserved in a deep freezer for up to 4 weeks. Slides prepared by the Thin Prep procedure are also useful for immunohistochemical studies. As noted previously, cell blocks are of particular value for studies of cytological samples. Either fixed or snap-frozen aspirate samples are also suitable for certain molecular diagnostic methods.

Immunohistochemical staining may be performed directly on smears, on microcore biopsies or cell-block samples and on cytospin preparations of aspirates (see Fig. 2.14). Immunohistochemistry applied to direct smears may result in significant background staining.[124] If the cells in question are stained intensely, this represents a positive reaction to the applied antibody. The detection of a terminally differentiated protein, such as gastrin or prostate-specific antigen, is quite reliable on direct smears because of this high intensity of staining. Any background positive staining can be ignored. To obtain a clean background, and in cases of lymphoproliferative disease, cytospin preparations provide good differentiation between positive and negative staining for various types of lymphoid cells and may be used to determine clonality and identify the predominant cell type.[125] Flow cytometry may be used in the same manner to segregate various populations of lymphoid cells.[126] Fluorescent in situ hybridization (FISH) can be used on FNAs to detect numeric chromosome abnormalities. The method described by Cajulis and Frias-Hidvegi[66] has good sensitivity and specificity and has particular value when only a few tumor cells are present in a given specimen.

REGULATORY ISSUES

Most antibodies used in pathology laboratories are classified by the FDA as analyte specific reagents (ASRs) and class I medical devices which exempt them from premarket notification.[127,128] This ruling is based on the fact that most immunostains do not provide 'stand-alone' results. The results are incorporated into a surgical pathology or cytopathology report as one component of the entire diagnostic evaluation. Class III medical devices include those immunostains (e.g. estrogen and progesterone receptors) which do not have routine morphological correlates but which have substantial and widely accepted scientific validation. Class III devices include reagents that are not part of the surgical or cytopathological diagnostic process and may result in an independent report (e.g. Her Cep™ test). These tests require premarket notification and FDA approval. Reports should include a statement to the effect that responsibility for assuring quality of the immunostains rests with the individual laboratory and not the manufacturer of the reagents.

According to the National Committee for Laboratory Standards, the results of immunohistochemistry should be incorporated into the final pathology report. When this is not possible, the immuno-histochemical findings should be reported as an addendum. The report should include a description of the specimen, the type of fixative, and the antibody (clone number and generic description).

AUTOMATION AND TISSUE MICROARRAYS

Automated immunohistochemistry instrumentation has improved dramatically over the past 10 years.[102] The greatest advantage of this technology is improved intra- and interlaboratory reproducibility. This fact is of particular importance in view of the increasing number of assays that have been developed for prognostic assessment of patients with malignancies of various types. In addition, automation has permitted the completion of significantly larger workloads in considerably shorter times as compared with the manual methods. As noted by Taylor et al., additional advantages include the use of microliter amounts of reagents, 'walk-away' functionality, increased biosafety by reducing exposure to and facilitating disposal of hazardous chemicals, and computer-driven accountability and reporting of each procedural step.[102]

Automated image analysis by digital microscopy is a useful approach for quantitative immunohistochemistry[129–131] and is further discussed in the section on Image Cytometry.

Tissue microarrays provide an invaluable approach for analyzing many different tissues on a single slide by immunohistochemistry or other analytical approaches.[131] In this technique, small tissue cylinders are removed from multiple tissue blocks and are then assembled into an array-like format. The small diameters of the cores maximizes the number of samples that can be analyzed with a minimum of damage to the original block. Comparative studies have revealed an excellent concordance between the intact blocks and the cores, provided that 2–3 representative cores are obtained from the donor blocks. Several different types of tissue microarrays have been developed. 'Prevalence' microarrays are designed to evaluate the prevalence of a particular marker in tumors of either the same or different types. 'Progression' microarrays focus on different stages of one particular tumor type (e.g. in situ, invasive, and metastatic carcinoma). 'Prognosis' microarrays contain tumor samples from patients with known clinical follow-ups and are particularly valuable to relate patterns of gene expression with prognosis. Microarrays can also be constructed to represent a series of positive and negative controls that can be used in conjunction with clinical samples for diagnostic immunohistochemical studies.

FLOW AND IMAGE CYTOMETRY

Flow cytometry (FCM) and image cytometry are commonly used methods to analyze surface antigen expression and DNA content in histologic and cytologic specimens.[132] This section briefly reviews technical aspects of specimen preparation, staining, cytometric analysis, data handling and interpretation, and quality control.

FLOW CYTOMETRY

Flow cytometry rapidly measures the intensity of fluorescence emitted by dyes that have been excited, most commonly by an argon-

ion laser, to emit light at a higher wavelength. This technique has great value in the immunophenotyping of hematopoietic proliferations present in peripheral blood, bone marrow, lymph nodes, effusions, and aspiration specimens (see Chapters 11 and 12). The discussion in this section is limited to the consideration of methods in the analysis of ploidy and proliferative fraction of solid tumors.

FCM allows the detection of gross changes in ploidy of interphase cells. It is able to resolve DNA content abnormalities when an excess or deficiency of at least two of the largest chromosomes exists. Because the finding of DNA aneuploidy is suggestive but not specific for the presence of malignant cells, DNA analysis has been investigated primarily for its potential prognostic impact. The value of ploidy and S-phase fraction (SPF) as prognostic factors for patients with solid tumors is currently limited, reflecting the discordant results recorded in hundreds of articles in the literature. Sources for the disparate data are numerous and include variations in patient selection, specimen type and number, use of fresh versus archival material, methods of tumor disaggregation and staining, criteria for histogram interpretation, data analysis, and therapy. Many of these variables relate to the lack of standardization in FCM methodology and lack of correlative data. For example, when examining the value of ploidy and proliferative fraction for invasive mammary carcinomas, FCM results must be analyzed in comparison with tumor size, axillary lymph node status, histologic grade, and histologic type in multivariate statistical analysis.[132,133]

In providing guidelines for the implementation of clinical DNA cytometry, a Consensus Conference was held in 1992 to evaluate the state of knowledge of the clinical utility of DNA analysis and to formulate recommendations regarding its methodology.[134–140] A panel of flow cytometrists formulated a framework for the development of standards for DNA analysis. The participants also reviewed the literature to determine whether FCM had clinical value for patients with neoplasms of the breast,[136] bladder,[138] colon or rectum,[139] prostate,[137] or hematopoietic system.[140] Unfortunately, the Consensus Conference had few or no representatives from surgical pathology, surgical or medical oncology, or other disciplines whose members routinely participate in the diagnosis or management of patients with cancer. Ultimately, the evaluation of DNA analysis by FCM as an important clinical tool requires prospective studies of large numbers of patients who are uniformly diagnosed, staged, and treated, and who are evaluated after long-term follow-up intervals.

Basic principles and instrumentation

A flow cytometer measures the fluorescence from particles (labeled whole cells or nuclei) as they pass single-file in a fluid sheath through a light beam.[132] The light source is most often an argon-ion laser. Thousands of particles may be analyzed in a few seconds or minutes. A series of optical filters and mirrors separates and reflects the wavelengths of light. The light falls on detectors that produce analog signals. These signals are digitized and displayed at specific channels in the histogram. The numbers generated correlate with the amount of fluorescence emitted or light scattered by individual particles. In a single parameter histogram, the amount of fluorescence (channel numbers) is plotted on the x axis, and the number of particle counts per channel is plotted on the y axis. The critical requirement for accurate measurement of a single cell suspension is laminar flow. Forward-angle light scatter of a sample particle is proportional to its size. Ninety-degree light scatter is indicative of cell granularity.

Argon-ion lasers produce a strong light at a wavelength of 488 nm. Fluorescent dyes absorb the laser light and emit light at a longer wavelength. With more than one fluorochrome, the emission spectra

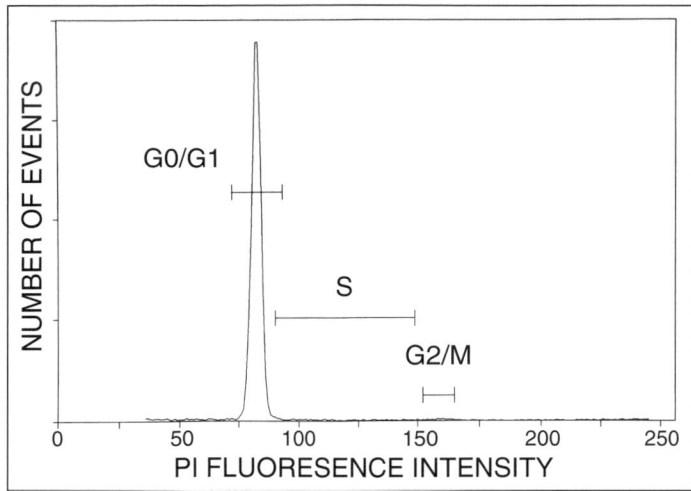

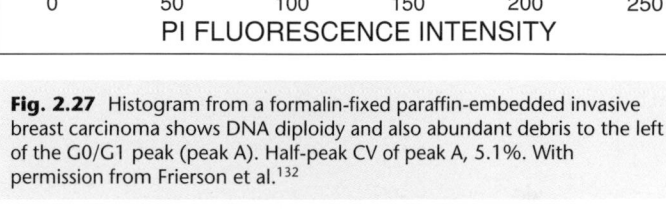

Fig. 2.26 Flow cytometric analysis allows the determination of ploidy (DNA diploidy in this histogram) and the number of cells in G0/G1 S, and G2/M phases of the cell cycle (propidium iodide stain). Half-peak CV of G0/G1 peak, 2.5%. With permission from Frierson et al.[132]

Fig. 2.27 Histogram from a formalin-fixed paraffin-embedded invasive breast carcinoma shows DNA diploidy and also abundant debris to the left of the G0/G1 peak (peak A). Half-peak CV of peak A, 5.1%. With permission from Frierson et al.[132]

of each must have no or very minimal overlap. Two-color analysis has become a standard procedure for surface marker analysis of lymphocytes. Labeled particles of interest in a histogram may be sorted into gates (windows). Data gathered for light scatter and fluorescence intensity are stored in a computer for subsequent analysis. Sorting of cells by the instrument after they pass through the laser beam has become more efficient over the last several years with improvements in reagents, electronics, and computer power.

Specimen disaggregation and preanalytic preparation

Tissue (biopsy and excision specimens) and cytologic samples are suitable for FCM analysis (Fig. 2.26). Results from fresh samples are superior to those for samples that have been fixed and embedded in paraffin. Fresh samples can be analyzed immediately or they can be stored frozen as small tissue blocks or as disaggregated cells in a cryoprotective agent. They may also be fixed in ethanol for subsequent analysis.[141–144] False DNA aneuploidy has been observed in normal tissues that have undergone autolysis.[145] Therefore, prompt submission of fresh samples for analysis is important. Fresh tissue specimens can be transported to the laboratory in a suitable medium such as RPMI-1640 culture medium, 5% fetal calf serum, and 1% penicillin-streptomycin.[146]

A variety of mechanical and enzymatic methods of dissociation have been used to disaggregate tissue samples. Mechanical procurement of single cells from solid tissues is usually preferred over enzymatic methods. This may be accomplished by mincing, scraping, or ex vivo fine needle aspiration.[147–152] Heterogeneity of ploidy and S-phase fraction (SPF) occur within solid tumors. The extent differs according to the particular study, tumor type, and specimen type.[153] As an extreme example, many studies have found that approximately 60–65% of invasive breast carcinomas are DNA aneuploid and that 5–20% are DNA multiploid.[154-157] In regard to heterogeneity of SPF, a 45% disagreement rate was found when each of four samples of mammary carcinoma was analyzed.[158] Although some degree of intratumoral heterogeneity certainly exists in breast, colon and rectum, lung, bladder, and prostate carcinomas, among others, the clinical importance of this finding is largely unknown.[135] The ploidy

status of a primary tumor, however, is essentially a reflection of that for its metastasis.[147]

Although the use of fresh samples usually leads to superior FCM results, hundreds of retrospective studies have utilized archival formalin-fixed, paraffin-embedded tissue specimens. A good correlation is often seen between the ploidy results for fresh and fixed specimens, although fixed specimens typically have much more debris, leading to poorer resolution of peaks (and hence a lower frequency of detection of DNA aneuploidy) and higher values for SPF (Fig. 2.27).[142,153,159–161] The quality of histograms for paraffin-embedded samples is affected by tissue damage prior to fixation, amount of debris, and section thickness.[142] For paraffin-embedded tissues, formalin has been shown to be the most suitable fixative for FCM analysis.[162] The best results for formalin-fixed tissues occur with fixation times between 8 and 24 hours, as deterioration in histogram quality occurs with more prolonged fixation.[163] For simultaneous staining of DNA, intracellular proteins, and cell surface antigens, paraformaldehyde has been found to be a suitable fixative.[164]

The initial procedure for FCM analysis of formalin-fixed, paraffin-embedded specimens was published by Hedley and colleagues in 1983.[159] With this method, 30-μm thick sections are dewaxed in xylene, rehydrated in decreasing concentrations of ethanol, washed in distilled water, and incubated with 0.5% pepsin, pH 1.5, at 37°C for 30 minutes. Paraffin blocks that contain well-preserved cells with little necrosis should be selected for analysis. Normal cells must also be present in the blocks to serve as an internal DNA diploid standard. Numerous modifications of Hedley's original technique have been described (Table 2.11).[152,160,162,165–174] In one of the most important modifications, paraffin sections 50 μm thick or greater were found to yield better histograms, as decreased section thickness resulted in an increase in debris and a decrease in relative height of the DNA aneuploid peak.[165] No standardized and generally accepted methodology for FCM analysis of formalin-fixed, paraffin-embedded specimens currently exists.

Isolation of nuclei or whole cells and staining

In addition to mechanical methods, enzymatic (collagenase, pepsin, pronase, trypsin), detergent (Triton X-100, NP-40), and chemical

Table 2.11 Modifications of Hedley's method[a] for flow cytometric analysis of formalin-fixed, paraffin-embedded specimens

Authors	Procedure
Schutte et al. 1985[160]	Substituted trypsin for pepsin
Stephenson et al. 1986[165]	Recommended >50 μm sections
Sickle-Santanello et al. 1988[166]	Dewaxed and rehydrated sections in cassettes in specially designed container
Amberson et al. 1988[167]	Sections in cassettes dewaxed and rehydrated in automatic tissue processor
Babiak and Poppema 1991[168] Heiden et al. 1991[169] Hedley 1989[162]	Substituted Histoclear (National Diagnostics, Somerville, NJ) for xylene
Heiden et al. 1991[169]	Used subtilisin Carlsberg (pronase, Sigma protease XXIV) and then stained without washing and centrifugation
Wang et al. 1993[170]	For keratinized squamous cell carcinomas, pretreatment with 85% formic acid/0.3%H$_2$O$_2$ followed by subtilisin Carlsberg
Carlsberg Crissman et al. 1988[152]	Increased pepsin incubation time
Pollack et al. 1993[171] Ciancio et al. 1993[172] Zalupski et al. 1993[173]	Substituted trypsin or pronase for pepsin for sarcomas
Albro et al. 1993[174]	Substituted proteinase K and heat for pepsin for liver tissue

[a]For Hedley's method, see Hedley et al.[159]

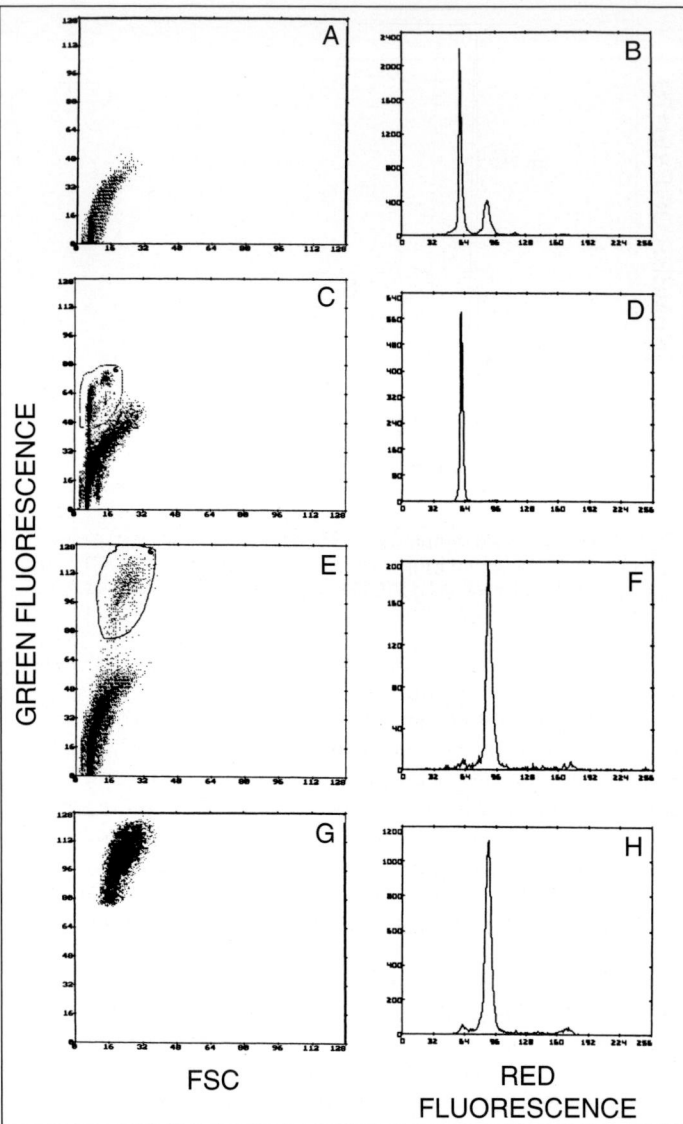

Fig. 2.28 This DNA aneuploid breast carcinoma was stained with the one-shot, two-color method. Left column, forward angle light scatter versus log green fluorescence dot-plots show binding of FITC-bound monoclonal antibody. Right column, the DNA content of the specific tumor subpopulations. **(A)** Non-specific FITC fluorescence is seen using staining with nonimmune mouse IgG-FITC propidium iodide (PI). **(B)** The corresponding ungated histogram shows two distinct G0/G1 peaks. **(C)** The CD45+ cells are indicated in the CD45-FITC/PI-stained aliquot. **(D)** The histogram of the CD45+ cells defines the DNA diploid population as the lower of the two peaks in the ungated histogram. **(E)** The cytokeratin (CK)-positive cells are indicated in the CK-FITC/PI-stained sample. **(F)** The cytokeratin-positive cells show the DNA aneuploid cells as a single peak. **(G)** 'Live' gating of the CK-FITC/PI-stained sample allows the acquisition of only those cells that are CK positive. **(H)** The corresponding histogram is composed of 220 000 CK-positive events. (From Zarbo et al.[189] with permission.)

(EDTA, EGTA) treatments have been used for the dissociation of cells from fresh or frozen tissue specimens.[135] Depending on the particular method employed, differences may be found in cell recovery, viability, and histogram quality.[175] Loss of DNA aneuploid cells in squamous cell carcinomas has been reported for mechanically dissociated cells, whereas reduction in DNA aneuploid cells has been observed in enzymatic preparations of colonic adenocarcinomas.[176] Collagenase has been found to be useful for the enzymatic release of cells from soft tissue neoplasms, but it is unsatisfactory for prostate tissue specimens.[177–180]

Multiparameter (especially multicolor) FCM analysis assists in improving the detection and analysis of neoplastic cells in heterogeneous populations. Reagents that preserve membranes and cytoplasm for multicolor analysis include buffered formaldehyde acetone,[181] paraformaldehyde and ethanol,[182] lysolecithin,[183] and saponin.[184] With two-color DNA analysis, whole cells are released from tissue mechanically, fixed in 50% ethanol, stained with propidium iodide, and labeled with either FITC-cytokeratin or FITC-leukocyte common antigen (CD45) antibodies (Fig. 2.28).[185–189] For analyzing epithelial cells in specimens that also contain inflammatory and stromal cells, this dual labeling with a DNA-binding dye and an FITC-conjugated antibody to cytokeratin assists in detecting small DNA aneuploid peaks and also renders a more accurate assessment of SPF.[185–190] Dual labeling is particularly helpful for SPF determination in DNA diploid neoplasms, because both neoplastic and non-neoplastic cells fall in the same G0/G1, S, and G2/M peaks in the histogram. The DNA content of lymphoid cells is easily assessed when the DNA dye is used along with an FITC-conjugated antibody to CD45. Although only a few laboratories have routinely used two-color analysis for fresh specimens, the use of whole-cell preparations instead of bare nuclei from fresh tissue samples has been recommended by participants in the 1992 Consensus Conference.[135] Future multiparametric measurements of solid tumors will also likely include

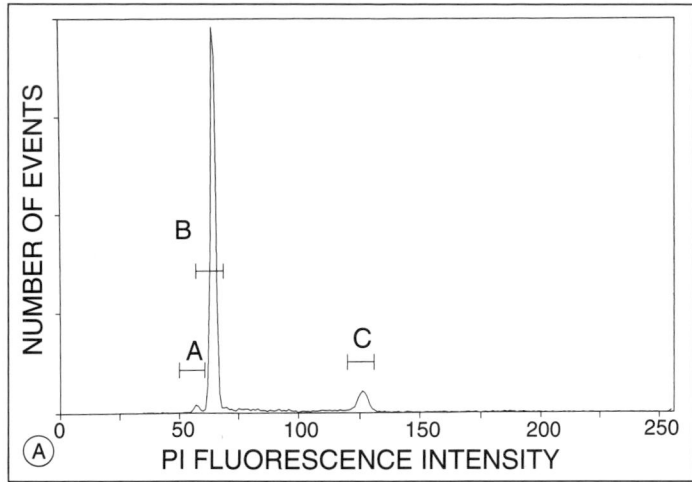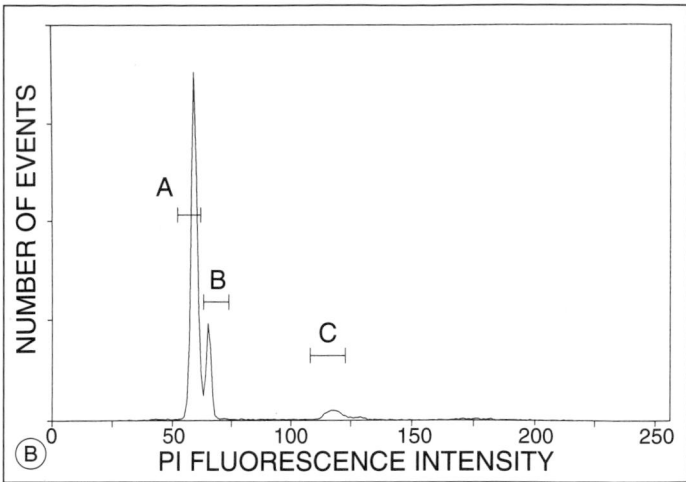

Fig. 2.29 **(A)** In this sample containing cells from an adrenal neuroblastoma only 1.8% of the cells were in G0/G1, peak A. **(B)** With the addition of normal human peripheral blood lymphocytes, peak A is determined to represent the G0/G1 peak of DNA diploid cells, whereas peak B represents neoplastic G0/G1 cells with a DNA index of 1.13. Half-peak CV of peak A, 2.0% and peak B, 1.7%. With permission from Frierson et al.[132]

assessments of proliferation-associated antigens, oncoproteins, and surface antigen determinants.

Several fluorochromes that bind to DNA have been found useful in FCM analysis,[135,191] including propidium iodide, ethidium bromide, acridine orange, DAPI, and Hoechst 33342 and 33358. DAPI and the Hoechst dyes are DNA base pair affinity-specific stains, whereas the others intercalate into double-stranded nucleic acids. Since propidium iodide, ethidium bromide, and acridine orange bind to double-stranded RNA, cells must be pretreated with RNAse. Stoichiometric binding to DNA may be affected by several variables including acid concentration and enzymatic treatments. Propidium iodide has been, by far, the most popular dye in clinical FCM. Acridine orange has been used for the assessment of RNA content.[192]

For the assessment of ploidy and calculation of the DNA index, the DNA diploid standard is quite important. The most appropriate DNA diploid standard consists of internal non-neoplastic cells present in the clinical specimen that also contains the neoplastic cells. At times, it is useful to add biologic standards (chiefly normal human peripheral blood lymphocytes) to fresh specimens as a control to identify the DNA diploid peak (Fig. 2.29). It is critical that such control cells be prepared in the same manner as the sample cells and that they be added prior to staining, since variations in dye binding occur when stained control cells are added to stained sample cells.[193,194] For formalin-fixed, paraffin-embedded specimens, no control cells of any kind should be mixed with the sample.

Cell quantity and analysis

The measurement of DNA content is affected by numerous conditions that include laser power, fluorochrome binding, salt concentration of the cell suspension, instrument sensitivity, and amplification of signal. Poorly controlled processing or instrument/analytic variables may lead to differences in channel location for peaks.[195] Beads of varying fluorescence intensity are typically used to provide instrument linearity.[135] Just before FCM analysis, cells must be monodispersed, which can be accomplished by vortexing the suspension, syringing through small (27-gauge) needles, or sonication.[196] It is recommended that at least 10 000 events be collected during analysis, but DNA aneuploid peaks may be clearly visible during analysis of fewer cells.[135] Samples should contain at least 20% tumor cells, but DNA

aneuploidy can be observed in specimens that contain less than this.[135] Obviously, a high percentage of tumor cells leads to a more accurate SPF determination.

Ploidy assessment and histogram interpretation

As a percentage of total autosomal DNA, the DNA content of chromosomes ranges from 4.3% (chromosome 1) to 0.8% (chromosome 21). The DNA content of female cells is 1.5% higher than that of male cells. The minimal difference in DNA content required for the appearance of a bimodal peak is twice the coefficient of variation.[179] Hence, for the detection of a DNA content difference of 4%, each of the two resolved peaks would need to have a coefficient of variation of approximately 2%. In clinical samples, most cells are present in the G0/G1 peak, while fewer cells are in S-phase or in the postsynthetic (G2) or mitotic phase (M).

Visual inspection of the histogram is an important indication of its quality. In addition, inspection of the fluorescence/light scatter dot-plot may provide assistance in its evaluation.[180] Some histograms are inadequate for assessment because there is too much debris or a high coefficient of variation of the G0/G1 peak. DNA aneuploidy (abnormal DNA stemline) should be reported only when two separate G0/G1 peaks are present (with the corresponding additional S-phase and G2/M peak). The DNA index is calculated by dividing the mean relative DNA content (channel number) of diploid G0/G1 cells into the mean relative DNA content (channel number) of DNA aneuploid G0/G1 cells.[193] Hence, the DNA index for a DNA diploid peak is 1.0, whereas that for an abnormal stemline is less or more than 1.0. By convention, the first G0/G1 peak for paraffin-embedded samples is considered DNA diploid; with this guideline, DNA hypodiploidy cannot be determined for formalin-fixed, paraffin-embedded specimens (DNA hypodiploidy, however, occurs in only approximately 2% of neoplasms). In addition to the coefficient of variation, the proportion of cells in each peak is important for peak separation.[197] In general, 2–5% of all cells must be present in a particular channel location before a small peak becomes manifest. Peridiploid DNA aneuploid peaks may be difficult to resolve, particularly when abundant debris is seen in formalin-fixed, paraffin-embedded specimens.[161] Problematic G0/G1 peaks are broad or asymmetric. Such peaks may harbor unresolvable peridiploid DNA aneuploid peaks. A skewing to

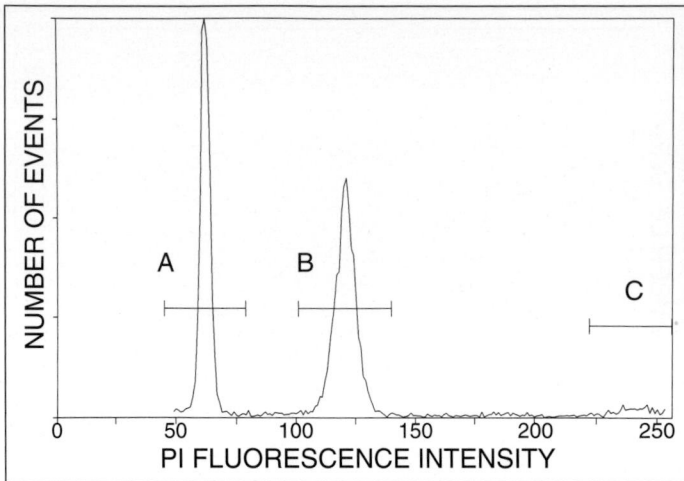

Fig. 2.30 Invasive breast carcinoma histogram. Peak B contains DNA tetraploid cells (DNA index, 1.95), whereas peak C represents the corresponding G2/M peak. Half-peak CV of peak A, 2.8% and peak B, 3.0%. With permission from Frierson et al.[132]

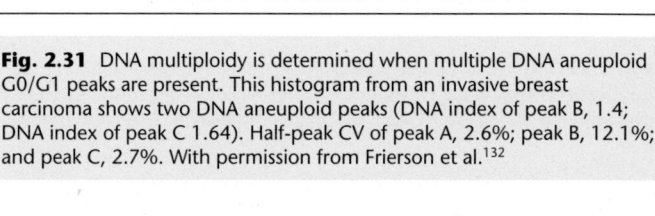

Fig. 2.31 DNA multiploidy is determined when multiple DNA aneuploid G0/G1 peaks are present. This histogram from an invasive breast carcinoma shows two DNA aneuploid peaks (DNA index of peak B, 1.4; DNA index of peak C 1.64). Half-peak CV of peak A, 2.6%; peak B, 12.1%; and peak C, 2.7%. With permission from Frierson et al.[132]

the right of the DNA diploid peak simulating an abnormal stemline, however, occurs in bladder barbotage specimens that contain numerous polymorphonuclear leukocytes. For autolyzed specimens, a shoulder to the right of the DNA diploid G0/G1 peak, a false DNA aneuploid peak with a small coefficient of variation (CV), or a broad peak with a high CV may be seen. False peaks are rarely seen in poorly fixed surgical material that has been embedded in paraffin.[198]

The definition of DNA tetraploidy has not been uniform.[198] As presently defined, DNA tetraploid cells have a DNA index ranging from 1.9 to 2.1 (Fig. 2.30). A DNA tetraploid population is present when a larger number of cells appears in the DNA diploid G2/M peak than the G2/M cells of the normal tissue counterpart.[135] Previous authors have defined DNA tetraploidy using arbitrary cutoff values for the number of cells in G2/M such as at least 15–20% of all events, or they have used a statistical approach of more than 2 or 3 standard deviations above the G2/M mean for the cells of the normal tissue counterpart.[135] If a DNA tetraploid peak is truly present, then a G2/M peak at 8N should be apparent, and corresponding cells should appear in the SPF. Some software programs assist in eliminating cell aggregates from analysis. Two-color FCM analysis may be especially useful when histograms show increased numbers of cells in G2/M.[185–188]

The definition of DNA multiploidy has also varied, which is part of the reason for the differences in multiploidy frequency reported for particular neoplasms. DNA multiploidy has usually been defined as the presence of multiple DNA aneuploid G0/G1 peaks (Fig. 2.31). DNA multiploidy is probably best defined as the presence of two or more DNA aneuploid G0/G1 peaks in the same histogram.[154–156] Neoplasms exhibit heterogeneity of DNA content not only when they are multiploid but also when DNA aneuploidy is observed in one sample of a particular neoplasm and only DNA diploid detected in another area of the same tumor.

It is clear that histograms may be difficult to classify and that classification is to some extent subjective.[199] Lack of agreement in histogram interpretation was shown by Joensuu and Kallioniemi,[200] who circulated histograms from paraffin-embedded samples among six investigators. In this study designed to contain many different and sometimes difficult types of histograms, in only 44% of histograms was ploidy agreed on by all; in 85% concordance was reached by five of the six participants.

Coefficient of variation

The coefficient of variation (CV) of the G0/G1 peak is the single most important parameter of histogram quality.[180] It is influenced by differences in sample preparation and staining and instrument performance. It is quite important for studies to report the mean and range of CV values for controls and tumor samples and the method of CV calculation in order that the quality of results can be ascertained.[193] For fresh tissue samples, the goal for the CV for the DNA diploid G0/G1 peak should be less than 5%, whereas for formalin-fixed, paraffin-embedded samples the goal for diploid CVs should be no higher than 8%. Neoplasms with CVs less than 8% are recommended for useful SPF determination.[135] Higher CVs may render SPF determination inaccurate.

S-phase fraction

The number of cells in S (synthetic)-phase has been recommended for the reporting of the proliferative component, although the number of cells in S+ G2/M is also reflective of the proliferative fraction.[135] In DNA aneuploid tumors, the SPF for the DNA aneuploid peak should be reported. When it is impossible to completely resolve the proliferating DNA aneuploid cells from the DNA diploid population, either the weighted average value for SPF of both peaks can be reported or it can be assumed that all cells in S-phase are neoplastic cells. It is the consensus opinion that the former approach is preferable to the latter.[135]

The major source of error in SPF determination is debris which results from necrosis, mechanical disaggregation, or enzymatic dissociation. This is nearly always a more severe problem for paraffin-embedded material than for fresh specimens.[201] The correlation of SPF with the thymidine-labeling index is better for DNA aneuploid than for DNA diploid neoplasms, since non-neoplastic diploid cells contaminate the DNA diploid peak.[202]

Types of histograms that result in difficult or impossible SPF determination include those with skewed DNA diploid or peridiploid

Table 2.12 Sources of variation in S-phase fraction determination by flow cytometry

Fresh vs. paraffin-embedded samples

Debris

Particle aggregates

Debris subtraction methods

Number of neoplastic cells

Analytic techniques

Software algorithms for modeling

Single parameter vs. two-color analysis

Intratumoral heterogeneity

Coefficient of variation of G0/G1 peak

Table 2.13 Algorithms used for calculation of S-phase fraction by flow cytometry

Mathematical model	Algorithm
Model of Baisch et al.[208]	Simple rectangle without functions for debris subtraction
Polynomial (Dean-Jett model[206,207]	Series of rectangles without background subtraction
Histogram-dependent exponential function (Multicycle*, Modfit†)[250]	Nonlinear least-squares fitting with background subtraction
Classic exponential function (Lampariello model)[251]	Maximum likelihood as parameter estimation with back ground subtraction

* Pheonix Flow Systems, San Diego CA.
† Verity Software House, Topsham, ME.

peaks, multiple DNA aneuploid peaks, overlapping peaks, small peaks, and high CVs. Table 2.12 lists the numerous sources of variation in SPF analysis. Higher values for SPF are typically seen for paraffin-embedded specimens compared with fresh samples. Specimens in which tumor cells comprise less than 15–20% of the total population are unsatisfactory for SPF, while histograms that contain greater than 20% aggregates and debris are also unsatisfactory.[135] Background aggregates and debris are an important software calculation in the accurate assessment of SPF. It is the ratio of the estimated number of aggregates and debris to the total number of particle events over the region from the lowest G0/G1 mean to the highest G2/M mean.[135] A paucity of neoplastic DNA diploid cells leads to a particularly inaccurate assessment of SPF. Two-color multiparametric analysis is helpful for the calculation of SPF for DNA diploid neoplasms, since keratin-positive epithelial cells may be analyzed separately. Using this two-color approach, however, neoplastic epithelial cells cannot be distinguished from those epithelial cells that are non-neoplastic.

Algorithms for debris compensation have evolved from single models to more complex nuclear cutting models. A good correlation in SPF for frozen and paraffin-embedded tissues is seen when debris is subtracted with multi-cut or single-cut algorithms.[203] Debris compensation models allow more accurate SPF estimates than uncompensated histograms.[204] It is probable that debris compensation should be performed for histograms from all types of specimens including those having only 5% debris or less.[205] The calculation of SPF depends greatly on the particular methodology employed (Table 2.13).[206] Sophisticated mathematical modeling software programs such as Multicycle (Phoenix Flow Systems, San Diego, CA)[207] and Modfit (Verity Software House, Topsham, ME)[208] are currently recommended for SPF analysis (Fig. 2.32).[135] They include nuclear cutting and exponential debris compensation algorithms. An algorithm has recently been reported for fully automated SPF determination.[209] Although this type of automated analysis does not replace human supervision, it does serve as a guideline for less experienced users, facilitates interlaboratory comparisons, and assists in extensive recalculations of large datasets.

Studies comparing SPF with prognosis have generally divided SPF values into two or three groups. The establishment of cutoff values is to some degree artificial, since SPF is a continuous variable. For each particular type of neoplasm, individual laboratories must set their own range of SPF values, establishing the cutoff points for low, intermediate, and high SPF. Values set by one laboratory should not be adopted by another, since interlaboratory differences in type of

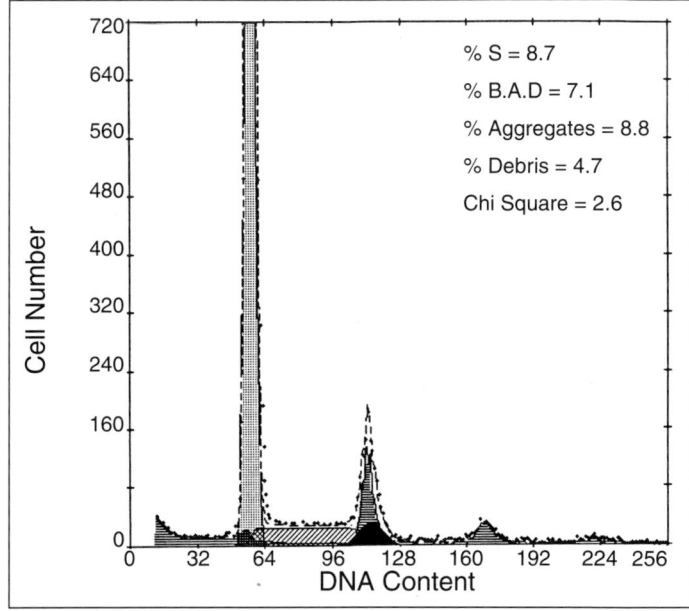

Fig. 2.32 Using Multicycle (Phoenix Flow Systems, San Diego, CA), an accurate assessment of S-phase and the amount of background aggregates and debris can be made. (Courtesy of Richard J. Zarbo, M.D., D.M.D., Detroit, MI).

specimen, data analysis, and methodology usually exist. Studies using the most sophisticated modeling techniques along with multiparametric analysis are needed to fully evaluate the prognostic importance of SPF.[210] Fluorescent antibodies to Ki-67, proliferating cell nuclear antigen, or the various cyclins can be used to determine the percentage of nonquiescent cells, but these antibodies have been used sparingly in FCM analysis.

Quality control

Lack of standardization of FCM procedures for DNA analysis has largely been responsible for nonuniformity of results among laboratories. Variations in methodology and measurement of ploidy and SPF by FCM are numerous and include type of specimen analyzed, specimen disaggregation and staining, instrument calibration, data analysis and interpretation, and quality control. Wheeless and colleagues[211] identified three sources of variation affecting FCM in general and its transportability: (1) interlaboratory variation that is constant across time (generally reflecting stable differences in instrument set-up and laboratory techniques); (2) differences that are not constant across time (inconsistencies in preparation of samples, staining, and analysis); and (3) measurement variability (affecting sensitivity of technique). These important sources of variation were discovered in studies from the Bladder Cancer Flow Cytometry Network established by the National Cancer Institute, in which replicate samples were analyzed in five different laboratories.[211–214] Several other groups of investigators have also examined issues of reproducibility for FCM analysis.[215,216] In a study of 43 Italian laboratories each of which used their own staining and measurement protocols, good intralaboratory reproducibility was found for ploidy, but statistically significant differences were noted among laboratories for DNA index and CV.[216]

In 1988, the College of American Pathologists introduced a proficiency testing program for DNA content analysis for clinical laboratories.[217] In a report published in 1994, results of ploidy analysis obtained from a mean of 241 participating laboratories on 19 unknowns from 1990 to 1992 showed a mean correct response rate of 86% (range, 58–97%) for modal number of DNA aneuploid peaks.[218] Incorrect responses were most commonly associated with near DNA diploid and DNA tetraploid unknowns, while some laboratories demonstrated consistent deviations from the mean of DNA index determination, which probably indicates problems in instrument linearity. SPF results for five specimens revealed wide interlaboratory variation, although the means were close to reference values. The largest range for SPF was 0–97%. These results clearly reveal the extent of differences for obtaining reproducible results for SPF among clinical laboratories. Reproducibility for SPF can be improved if laboratories use the same mathematical model for calculation.[206] The optimal and most reproducible mathematical approach for calculating SPF needs to be defined and agreed on.

The value of DNA analysis of ploidy and SPF as prognostic determinants will be clarified when the most highly developed FCM methods are employed in large prospective studies of fresh specimens from uniformly treated patients.[219] In addition, the impact of FCM analysis can only be assessed when each of the most important time-tested prognostic parameters has been incorporated into the multivariate statistical model. It is anticipated that in addition to ploidy and SPF determination, FCM will be used to study the clinical importance of a myriad of oncogene products. Multiparameter analysis by FCM will permit the study of surface membrane components, cytoplasmic proteins, receptors, and nuclear factors that may ultimately be shown to impart useful clinical information.[220]

LASER SCANNING CYTOMETRY

DNA analysis of ethanol-fixed, propidium iodide-stained imprints or smears can be performed by a microscope slide-based automatic laser scanning cytometer (CompuCyte Corporation, Cambridge, MA). In a comparison with FCM and image cytometry, the laser scanning cytometer showed concordance for ploidy in over 90% of 53 cancers.[221] Good correlation in SPF was also seen between the laser scanning cytometer and the flow cytometer. Similar to the flow cytometer, the laser scanning instrument is automated and leads to rapid and reliable SPF determination. Similar to image cytometry, it has a minimal tissue requirement and the potential for visual selection of cells to be measured. In addition to DNA content analysis, the

applications include the quantitation of cell receptors and oncoproteins, immunophenotyping of hematolymphoid cells, and determining chromosome copy number by fluorescence in situ hybridization.

IMAGE CYTOMETRY

Image cytometry, also termed *image analysis*, has similarities to and differences from flow cytometry.[222] Image cytometry has relative strengths and weaknesses compared with flow cytometry, depending on the particular application or the specimen type being analyzed. Image cytometry broadly refers to the quantitative measurement of morphologic features in histologic tissue sections or cytologic preparations. Measurements may be made on individual cells or noncellular tissue components, or on the relationships between cells. A variety of parameters can be measured using different physical techniques (e.g. laser-induced fluorescence, stoichiometric binding of dyes, enzymatic reduction of chromogens). The most common application of image cytometry is the quantitation of DNA content. Comments cited earlier in this chapter relating to the determination of ploidy by flow cytometry also apply to image cytometry. The most critical issues relate to the lack of standardization in both specimen processing and interpretation of data.[223]

Basic principles and instrumentation

Computers and video technology are central to all applications of image cytometry.[224] The technique depends on the initial capture of an image in digital format, which can then be subjected to mathematical analysis.[225] Image capture is usually performed with a video camera mounted on a light or fluorescent microscope. The analog signal from the camera is converted to digital form through an analog-to-digital conversion process. The resulting digital data can reside in the computer memory or on other memory media. In this format it can be displayed on a computer monitor, or manipulated or analyzed by computer software.

A concept central to image cytometry is the notion of a *pixel* or picture element. This is represented by a discrete digital value in the computer memory. The number of pixels that comprise an image is determined by the quality of the video camera and the rate that the video signal from the camera is sampled by the analog-to-digital converter. Depending on the camera and the software configuration, images may be captured in black and white or in color. Numeric values, either 0–255 (gray scale) or red, green, and blue wavelengths, so-called RBG color, can be assigned to the light intensity that a camera simultaneously captures. Color-sensitive cameras are useful for the analysis of DNA ploidy as well as quantitative immuno-histochemistry, which relies on colored chromogens.

Preanalytic preparation

Specimens suitable for image cytometry include thin tissue sections or cytologic preparations (cell smears or cytocentrifuge or monolayer preparations). Most of the sample preparative techniques previously cited for cell suspensions for flow cytometric analysis work equally well for image cytometry. The primary goal of cytopreparation is the depositing of cells onto a glass slide with a minimum of cell overlap. This greatly facilitates the measurement of morphologic features of individual cells.

For the measurement of DNA content, image cytometry can be performed on nuclei stained with fluorochromes or other dyes. With the exception of laser scanning microscopy, a hybrid between image and flow cytometry, fluorochromes are rarely used. The major reagent used for DNA quantitation is the Feulgen stain, which binds to DNA in a stoichiometric fashion. Quantitative immunohistochemistry, the other major clinical application of image cytometry, may utilize the entire gamut of monoclonal antibodies that mark antigens expressed within, or on the surface of cells, or to other tissue components (see section on Immunohistochemistry).

Image analysis

The digital image can be subjected to a variety of measurements by various software tools. Fundamentally, image analysis is achieved by the assessment of the mathematical values of individual pixels that comprise the image. These measurements might include the pixel intensity, the relationship of the pixels to each other, or the number of pixels. Through such measurements it is possible to describe morphometric features of cells, such as nuclear shape, size, texture, or the relationship between cells (so-called contextual karyometry). It is also possible to sum the optical density of specific regions of the cell, such as the nucleus, that has been stained by a specific chromogen. DNA content is determined in this fashion. The Feulgen staining intensities of cells under examination are compared with normal human diploid cells (that are known to have a mass of 7.14 picograms of DNA per nucleus). Through the use of a standard curve, cells with unknown DNA content can be identified. When image cytometry is performed on histologic tissue sections of neoplasms, normal cell nuclei are often included in the same tissue section. These normal nuclei have been subjected to the same fixation, sectioning, and staining as the neoplasm being measured and can serve as internal controls.

Ploidy assessment

The measurement of the optical density of the population of cells allows the preparation of a DNA histogram plotting the DNA mass in picograms on the horizontal axis relative to the number of cells on the vertical axis. In a normal human sample, most cells will have a mass of 7.14 pg/cell nucleus, reflecting the G0/G1 peak. A smaller number of cells will be G2 or mitotic phase, so-called G2/M peak. The intervening distance between the G0/G1 peak and the G2/M peak corresponds to the SPF. This is analogous to flow cytometry; however, the number of cells in S-phase are usually too few to measure by image cytometry, unless monoclonal antibodies are used that specifically mark cells in the DNA synthetic phase. Debris, inflammatory cells, or specimen autolysis can affect the shape of and the ability to interpret the histogram.

Despite technical differences between flow and image cytometry, a high concordance exists between ploidy measurements obtained by the two techniques.[226–231] Depending on the source of the sample and methodology used in analysis, concordance exceeds 90%.[232,233] Thus, the choice of technique for clinical applications is often a matter of personal preference. Conceptually, flow cytometry is the preferred analytic tool for fluid samples, such as blood and body fluids. Flow cytometric methods allow the measurement of large numbers of cells, thus achieving high statistical reliability in a relatively short time. However, cells that are infrequent in the population may be un-detectable.[234] Image cytometry typically involves the measurement of a few hundred cells. While this is slower, and potentially more labor intensive, it allows the morphologic visualization of cells so that individual cells with specific attributes can be selected for measurement.[226,235] DNA ploidy may be prognostically significant or useful in planning therapy.[235–237]

Quantitative immunohistochemistry

The number of cells that are usually analyzed by image cytometry is too few for accurate assessment of cell proliferation. S-phase determination is one example in which immunohistochemical stains can be combined with the quantitative power of image cytometry.[238] Several monoclonal antibodies specifically bind to nuclear antigens expressed on cells in the proliferating phase of the cell cycle.[239] These include MIB-1, Ki-67, antibodies to DNA polymerase alpha, and proliferating cell nuclear antigen.[240,241] Individual cells, or tissue sections stained by the immunohistochemical technique, can be examined by image cytometry to determine the proportion of cells in a sample that mark with the antibody. These antibodies provide an alternative to the counting of mitoses, which is classically performed in surgical pathology. Tissue sections that have been treated with these monoclonal antibodies may be examined to determine the relative proportion of cells that are in the proliferative phase of the cell cycle. Thus, a proliferating cell fraction is determined that is comparable to the SPF of the DNA histogram obtained by flow cytometry. Depending on the software program, the percentage of positive nuclei may be determined, or a percentage of the total nuclear area present in the tissue section. These determinations may require the simultaneous assessment of DNA content in the tissue section.

A more common application of quantitative immunohistochemistry is the measurement of estrogen or progesterone receptor expression in carcinomas of the breast or other organs.[242–244] Depending on antibodies used in the analysis, immunohistochemical staining can either be performed on fresh frozen, imprint, or formalin-fixed materials. By using standard curves, the mass of receptor protein in nuclei can be determined (usually expressed as femtomoles). A good correlation exists between the immunohistochemical determination of receptors and standard biochemical methods of analysis. The immunohistochemical method has distinct advantages, notably that it requires far less tissue than the biochemical method, and it is possible to visualize the tumor cells. This latter point can be particularly useful in a sample having a relatively small proportion of tumor, in which erroneous results may be obtained from normal breast tissue that either does or does not express receptors.

Quantitative immunohistochemistry has been used to measure the protein product of oncogenes such as p53 and HER-2/*neu*. The expression of such oncoproteins from various tumors as well as their prognostic significance is currently under evaluation.[245] Comparison of digital microscopy assisted scores and manual scores of Her2 neu immunostaining of breast cancer cells, for example, revealed better concordance with gene copy number as analyzed by FISH for the digital approach.[129] As noted by Bloom and Harrington, the use of digital automated microscopy permits the observer to achieve color recognition to 255 levels of intensity as compared to 4 (0–3+) for the human eye when using manual microscopy for Her2 neu quantitation.[129] This approach has also proven to be useful for the detection of rare cells (e.g. single tumor cells) in lymph node biopsies and cytospin preparations of bone marrow and peripheral blood.[131]

The potential of measuring resistance of tumors to chemotherapy by quantitating P-glycoprotein has been demonstrated.[246]

MORPHOMETRY

Classic morphometric measurement is not widely used in the daily practice of pathology with the exception of measurement of muscle or nerve fiber size and shape which is used as a diagnostic adjunct by some neuropathologists.[247] Likewise, some investigators have advocated the determination of nuclear contour in some T-cell lymphomas.[240]

CYTOLOGY AUTOMATION

Efforts to automate the examination of the cervical vaginal Papanicolaou smear have fueled many of the advances in image cytometry.[248,249] Since the introduction of the Papanicolaou smear in the 1950s, research efforts have been focused on application of image cytometry for screening and also for diagnostic interpretation of cytologic materials. After many years of frustration, recent improvements in computer technology, software design, and slide preparation techniques have made automated cytology feasible. Several commercial instruments measure various cell parameters to classify cells as normal or abnormal. Approaches include the classic measurement of nuclear size, shape, and texture, as well as the use of nonalgorithmic neural networks. Studies show that they give favorable results in the identification and classification of abnormal cells.

CYTOGENETICS

Nonrandom chromosomal abnormalities are common in many malignant tumors with more than 600 recurrent balanced aberrations having been identified to date.[252] They have been identified in many hematopoietic tumors[253] and are being recognized with increasing frequency in nonhematopoietic tumors of various types, particularly soft tissue sarcomas.[254] Moreover, many carcinomas at the time of diagnosis have a wide array of chromosomal abnormalities acquired during tumor progression. As a result, the distinction between early and pathogenetically essential changes and secondary changes accumulated during progression is considerably more difficult than in hematopoietic and soft tissue neoplasms. Moreover, karyotypic analysis of carcinomas have been hampered because of problems with chromosomal quality.

Chromosomal aberrations detectable by standard cytogenetic methods include deletions, amplifications (as manifested by homogeneously stained regions and double minutes), inversions, and translocations. The identification of genes at breakpoints or deletions has been of particular value for the identification of oncogenes and tumor suppressor genes. In addition, identification of these changes has been of value for the diagnosis of tumors of specific types. Some of the common translocations recognized in hematopoietic, soft tissue and bone tumors are listed in Table 2.14. In a significant proportion of these cases, the translocation is the sole abnormality, reflecting its probable causal role in the development of these tumors.

Material for cytogenetics must be obtained fresh and in sterile conditions.[255] The material can be stored in standard culture media, such as RPMI, or in phosphate buffered saline for up to 36 hours prior to culture, but the best results are obtained when the material is cultured as soon as possible following excision.

MOLECULAR BIOLOGY

Over the past 20 years molecular biological techniques have become an integral part of the practice of surgical pathology.[256] This process has accelerated in recent years with the development of high-throughput molecular technologies and global initiatives such as the human genome project. It is crucial for the modern surgical pathologist to be well versed in molecular biology terminology, and have a basic understanding of the techniques involved including their strengths and limitations. It is also critical for the contemporary

Table 2.14 Common chromosomal translocations in selected hematopoietic and soft tissue/bone tumors

Tumor	Translocations	Involved genes
Chronic myeloid leukemia	t(9;22) (q34;9-11)	ABL/BCR
Burkitt lymphoma	t(8;14) (q24;q23)	C-MYC/IgH
Mantle cell lymphoma	t(11;14) (q13;q32)	CYCLIN D1/IgH
Follicular lymphoma	t(14;18) (q32;q21)	IgH/BCL-2
Alveolar rhabdomyosarcoma	t(2;13) (q35;q14)	PAX3/FKHR
	t(1;13) (p36;q14)	PAX7/FKHR
Ewing tumor/PNET	t(21;22) (q24;q12)	EWS/FLI1
	t(21;22) (q22;q12)	EWS/ERG
	t(7;22) (p22;q12)	EWS/ETV1
	t(17;22) (q12;q12)	EWS/E1AF
	t(2;22) (q33;q12)	FEV/EWS
Clear cell sarcoma	t(12;22) (p12;q12)	ATF1/EWS
Congenital fibrosarcoma and mesoblastic nephroma	t(12;15) (p13;q25)	ETV6/NTRK3
Extraskeletal myxoid chondrosarcoma	t(9;22) (q22;q12)	EWS/CHN (TEC)
	t(9;17) (q22;q11)	RBP56/CHN(TEC)
	t(9;15) (q22;q21)	TEC/TCF12
Myxoid liposarcoma	t(12;16) (q13;p11)	TLS (FUS)/CHOP
	t(12;22) (q13;q12)	EWS/CHOP
Desmoplastic round cell tumor	t(11;22) (p13;q12)	WTI/EWS
Synovial sarcoma	t(X;18) (p11;q11)	SYT-SSX1
		SYT-SSX2

surgical pathologist to be able to integrate molecular biological results with both the morphologic and clinical findings in generating a more precise diagnosis as well as predicting prognosis whenever possible.

Currently, molecular techniques have proven to be invaluable primarily in two areas of surgical pathology, oncology and infectious disease. The main focus of this chapter will be on techniques used in molecular oncology with references to infectious disease when applicable. Each technique will be followed by a list of commonly used applications, which by no means is meant to be all-inclusive.

Molecular techniques used in diagnostic tumor biology are based on the fact that cancer is a genetically determined disease which occurs as a result of DNA mutations in oncogenes (overexpression) and tumor suppressor genes (loss of function).[257,258] These mutations are either germline, somatic, or a combination of the two in origin. Types of DNA alterations commonly involved in oncogenesis include gene amplifications, translocations, deletions, and point mutations. Different neoplasms possess a wide array of mutational complexities varying from simple translocations seen in hematologic and soft tissue neoplasms to the complex array of mutations seen in many common solid tumors.

Molecular pathology allows for the establishment of a more definitive diagnosis and classification of neoplasms based on specific mutational profiles. Due to their extreme sensitivity molecular techniques are also commonly used for the detection of minimal residual disease and for the early detection of malignancies. Molecular pathology is also useful in the assessment of molecular prognostic factors. The same molecular techniques used for identification of mutational profiles are also utilized to assess clonality and to determine susceptibility to cancer by tracing closely linked genes or chromosomal regions to as yet uncharacterized genes by linkage analysis.

NUCLEIC ACID ANALYSIS

Extraction of nucleic acids

Fresh or snap frozen tissue is preferred for the extraction of both RNA and DNA; however, in recent years the methodologies for extraction of nucleic acids from formalin-fixed paraffin-embedded tissues have been greatly improved.[259] DNA, as opposed to RNA, is extremely physiochemically stable. DNAses, the catalytic enzymes responsible for DNA degradation, are present ubiquitously in tissues but can be easily neutralized by heat or chemical agents. RNAses are also present ubiquitously in tissues and throughout the laboratory environment, including the hands of the extractor. RNAses are much more stable than DNAses and thus great care must be taken in creating an RNAse-free environment when extracting and amplifying RNA. Nucleic acids are typically fragmented during tissue processing; therefore, for archival tissue the DNA and RNA target fragments should be kept small, 500 bp or less for DNA and 200 bp or less for RNA. RNA obtained from archival tissue can be amplified by reverse transcriptase polymerase chain reaction (RT-PCR) (as discussed subsequently), whereas DNA may be amplified by the polymerase chain reaction (PCR).

Nucleic acid hybridization

The majority of molecular techniques are dependent on nucleic acid hybridization, which enables the identification of a specific nucleic acid sequence within a complex mixture of sequences. Hybridization is based on the formation of a double-stranded complex between the target DNA or RNA and its complementary probe. Hybridization may be performed in a solution (e.g. PCR), on solid supports such as nitrocellulose or nylon membranes (e.g. Southern blots) or at the cellular or subcellular level (in situ hybridization).[260]

Probes

Nucleic acid probes are segments of DNA or RNA of variable length that may be labeled either radioisotopically or with a variety of nonisotopic reporter molecules and revealed with a colorimetric reaction.[260] In routine molecular diagnostics, nonisotopic probes are rapidly replacing radiolabeled probes because they are safe and easy to manipulate, have a long shelf life, and do not require radioisotopic containment facilities. The types of probes that are commonly used include: (1) short (up to 50 bp) single-stranded synthetic oligo-nucleotides used primarily in PCR reactions, and in allele-specific filter hybridization to detect point mutations and in in situ hybridization; (2) complementary RNA probes of intermediate size (commonly ranging 200–800 bp in length) used for in situ hybridization and in Northern blots; (3) long (one to several thousand bases in length) double-stranded DNA probes utilized in solid support hybridization assays and in fluorescent in situ hybridization (FISH).

MOLECULAR TECHNIQUES

Southern blotting

Southern blotting, first described by Edwin Southern (hence the name) in 1975, is based on the transfer of nucleic acids from separation gels to a transfer membrane.[261] In this method the DNA is first digested by restriction enzymes which introduce highly specific

Table 2.15 Limitations of Southern blotting

Requirement for fresh tissue
Requirement for a relatively larger quantity of DNA (5–10 micrograms)
Technically demanding and relatively slow (may take up to 1 week)
Commonly based on radioactive probes
Abnormality must be present in 2–5% of cells in a heterogeneous sample in order to be detectable
Abnormalities can be identified only in defined genes or sequences with available probes
Translocations may be detected only if the breakpoints in one of the chromosomes are clustered within a 15-2-kb region

breaks in the DNA by recognizing sequences of four to eight bases. The digested sequences of DNA generated, ranging in size from 100 to 30 000 bp, are separated by conventional agarose gel electrophoresis. Following denaturation, the single-stranded pieces are transferred (blotted) to a solid support (such as nitrocellulose filter or nylon membrane) thus immobilizing the DNA. The specific DNA sequence of interest is then detected by hybridization with a complementary single-stranded labeled probe. The detection process is then carried out by autoradiography or colorimetry, depending on the probe, and the band or series of bands is localized to a specific-size fragment. The limitations of Southern blotting compared to other more advanced molecular techniques are summarized in Table 2.15.

Southern blotting is commonly applied to the detection of gene amplifications such as N-myc in neuroblastoma,[262] and in determining DNA rearrangements such as heavy chain for B-cell and the T-cell receptor for T-cell lymphomas.[263] It is also used for the detection of specific chromosomal translocations such as those found in sarcomas and for the detection of gene deletions and point mutations.[264,265]

Restriction fragment length polymorphisms

Although Southern blotting is not useful as a screening tool for DNA mutations it has been commonly used for the identification of base pair mutations which result in altered size fragments following treatment with specific restriction enzymes commonly known as restriction fragment length polymorphisms (RFLP).[266] RFLP analysis is used in the establishment of a link between a specific chromosomal region to a disease. It has been commonly used in familial studies of inherited diseases and in identifying regions of the genome containing somatic mutations.

Polymerase chain reaction

Polymerase chain reaction (PCR) is a very sensitive method for the detection of specific nucleic acid sequences based on the exponential in vitro amplification of a segment of DNA.[267] PCR is one of the techniques which has most revolutionized molecular biology since its discovery in 1986 by Mulis.[268] The technique is based on the function of a DNA polymerase enzyme to create a new complementary DNA strand from a native template strand. The method requires a pair of oligonucleotide primers, usually about 20 nucleotides in length, that complement both ends of each strand of a target sequence. The target DNA must first be denatured by heating and the reaction mixture cooled to allow the complementary sequences of the primers to anneal to target. Heat resistant Taq-DNA polymerase synthesizes new strands of DNA based on the nucleotide template between the primers. This cycle is then repeated, usually 20 to 50 times, resulting in exponential amplification of the target sequence. Thus, within a few hours one can increase the target DNA to 10^{8-9} copies. PCR may be performed virtually on all types of pathological specimens including formalin-fixed paraffinized tissue, cytological fluids, and laser microdissected sections.[269]

The major advantages of PCR and its variants are:

1. Very few target cells are required, allowing for diagnostic use on limited biopsy or cytological samples;
2. May be performed on formalin-fixed paraffin-embedded tissues;
3. Extremely sensitive and may detect chromosomal aberrations in one out of a million cells.

One of the major disadvantages of PCR methodology is its extreme sensitivity. Special care must be taken to avoid the introduction of exogenous sequences. For this reason, within a molecular lab it is important to geographically separate the area where the experiments are set up from the area where the analytical phase is performed.

The number of PCR applications in diagnostic contemporary surgical pathology is enormous and a comprehensive listing is beyond the scope of this chapter; however, some of its major uses include: (1) the identification of chromosomal translocations for diagnostic purposes and for the detection of minimal residual disease after treatment; (2) the detection of gene amplifications such as c-erbB-2, N-myc;[270] (3) the identification of point mutations in oncogenes and tumor suppressor genes such as ras and p53;[271] (4) determination of lymphoma clonality via immunoglobulin and T-cell receptor gene rearrangements.[272] PCR techniques are also commonly employed in the detection of viruses,[273] mycobacteria,[274] and other microorganisms.

PCR variants

Many variants of PCR have been developed to suit specific needs. Some of these variants and their uses in molecular pathology are briefly described below.

Multiplex PCR

In this technique two or more different sets of primers are added to the same reaction mixture.[275] This allows for the screening of multiple sequences from one sample. Accordingly, the reaction products must be of different sizes in order to permit their identification by gel electrophoresis. Multiplex PCR is used commonly in screening clinical specimens for translocations. It is also used to screen clinical samples for various bacterial and fungal infections.

Reverse-transcriptase RT-PCR

Reverse-transcriptase PCR is based on the unique ability of reverse transcriptase enzyme to make a DNA copy (cDNA) from a target mRNA molecule.[276,277] The cDNA transcript is then amplified using standard PCR. RT-PCR is especially useful for identification of translocations where the breakpoints are scattered over large regions of DNA. In these situations, although the DNA translocation products may vary, the chimeric RNA transcribed from the translocated chimeric gene remains constant from case to case. RT-PCR is extremely sensitive, being able to detect one tumor cell within ten million normal cells.[278] It requires significantly less starting material than other techniques such as Northern blotting or cDNA array analysis. RT-PCR can be semi-quantitative by comparing to a known standard[279,280] or purely quantitative when the copies of the amplified target sequence are measured.

Applications of RT-PCR include quantification of RNA viruses (such as HCV and HIV) in clinical specimens,[281] detection of circulating cells in peripheral blood using tumor-specific protein expression such as tyrosinase for melanomas and prostate specific antigen (PSA) for adenocarcinoma of the prostate, and the detection of chimeric DNA products.[278]

Real-time PCR and RT-PCR

Real-time PCR is a modification of the PCR technique used for more accurate quantification of transcripts by measuring the product following each round of amplification.[282,283] Fluorescent dyes are used to allow monitoring of the product within each well. Real-time PCR is used for quantification of viral loads such as HIV, HCV, and CMV to monitor therapy.[284]

Nested PCR

Nested PCR is more sensitive and specific than simple PCR and is used frequently when the quality of the starting sample is suboptimal. In nested PCR, two rounds of amplification are performed; in the first a large reaction product is generated that is used as a template for the second round. Because of its high level of sensitivity, nested PCR is prone to contamination and false-positive results.

In situ PCR

In situ PCR is a potentially powerful technique whereby oligonucleotide primer pairs are used on tissue sections to amplify target sequences in situ. Thus, the signal may be localized within a specific cellular subtype. Unfortunately, this technique has not proven to be reproducible among laboratories and very few have perfected it.[285]

In situ hybridization

In situ hybridization (ISH) refers to the hybridization of specific DNA or RNA probes to complementary nucleic acid sequences in target cells. This technique is ideal for visualization and localization of specific nucleic acid sequences in tissue sections or cell preparations such as bone marrow aspirations and cytological specimens.[286] The greatest advantage of ISH over other molecular techniques is the ability to correlate cellular morphology with the detection of the nucleic acid sequence. For example, ISH allows for the localization of her2neu amplification in neoplastic as opposed to benign mammary epithelial cells in breast biopsies containing heterogeneous populations.

Under the appropriate conditions, the molecular probe will hybridize (through the establishment of hydrogen bonds) to the target DNA in the nucleus or RNA in the cytoplasm and be visualized by either radioactive or nonradioactive labels incorporated into the probe. Nonradioactive probes are based on the presence of a reporter molecule introduced chemically or enzymatically, which is detectable by affinity cytochemistry.[287,288] Common reporters include tagging with peroxidase, digoxigenin, and biotin. Nonradioactive probes are highly stable, safe, and approach the level of sensitivity of isotopically labeled probes. Common molecular probes for ISH include cloned RNA and DNA probes and synthetic oligonucleotide probes. The type and length of probe (RNA or DNA, single- or double-stranded) and the reaction conditions must be individualized for each application. DNA probes, being less sensitive than RNA probes, are more effective when the target is abundant, such as viral DNA, or when a high labeling efficiency is required to visualize single targets such as FISH. RNA probes are preferentially used when the target is present in low copy numbers such as mRNA detection. As cross-hybridization and non-specific probe binding may result in false-positive results, hybridization conditions, and appropriate controls have to be individualized for each application. In studies employing in situ mRNA the sense probe is frequently used as the negative control.

Since formaldehyde is a protein cross-linker, a permeabilization step, usually enzymatic, is included when performing ISH on formalin-fixed tissues. RNA is not as stable as DNA in tissues, so delayed fixation may lead to target loss by endogenous ribonucleases. Although more easily performed on frozen sections, mRNA ISH may be applied to formalin-fixed tissue. In certain situations, such as post-translational modifications, protein secretion or transport, mRNA ISH may prove to be more sensitive than immunohistochemistry for the identification of protein synthesis

ISH for DNA is used to detect viral infection including HPV, CMV, HIV, EBV, and HHV-8,[289–295] fungal infections,[296] and oncogene amplification in tumors such as c-erB2 and N-myc.[297,298]

mRNA ISH is used to detect light chain restriction in lymphomas,[299] the determination of specific tumor subtype via protein, such as albumin in hepatocellular carcinoma,[300] or peptide hormone synthesis[301] and gene expression in tumor biology or prognostics.[286]

Fluorescent in situ hybridization

Fluorescent in situ hybridization (FISH) is a high-resolution technique which permits the detection of numerous chromosomal alterations in tissue sections or cytological preparations. This approach is especially suitable for the detection of chromosomal aberrations in solid tumors and may be performed on metaphase spreads and nuclei in interphase (interphase cytogenetics). The technique allows the identification of translocations, deletions, loss of heterozygosity, gene amplification, changes in chromosome number, rearrangements, and assignment of genetic loci to newly cloned genes.[302] A major advantage of FISH over classic cytogenetic techniques is the ability to analyze intact, nondividing tumor cells. FISH is also cheaper and faster than cytogenetics and may be performed on paraffin-embedded tissue.

FISH analysis is based on hybridization with a fluorescently labeled nucleic acid probe. Different probes are suitable for the detection of specific chromosomal abnormalities; tandem repeat (centromeric or satellite) probes are used for assessing chromosome copy number, regional- or locus-specific probes for the detection of translocations, deletions, and amplifications; and whole chromosome probes are useful for identifying structural rearrangements (Fig. 2.33).[302–304] Multiple probes can be assessed simultaneously using various fluorochromes.[305]

Chromogenic in situ hybridization

Chromogenic in situ hybridization (CISH) is a relatively new development which is based on enzymatic detection similar to immunohistochemistry.[306] The major advantage of CISH over FISH is that the analysis is performed by bright-field microscopy allowing for easier correlation of tumor morphology with the cytogenetic changes and does not require a fluorescent microscope.

COMPARATIVE GENOMIC HYBRIDIZATION

Comparative genomic hybridization (CGH) is a rapid and powerful screening technique which permits the detection of chromosomal aberrations without the need to culture tumor cells.[307] In this technique metaphase spreads are prepared from a normal donor. Target tumor DNA and normal DNA are isolated and labeled with different contrasting colored fluorochromes. The labeled DNAs are mixed together at equal ratios and hybridized with the normal metaphase preparation and scored with a fluorescent microscope. Regions of chromosomal loss (deletions) will appear the color of the normal DNA and regions of chromosomal gain (duplications) the color of the target tumor DNA. A major limitation of this methodology is that it is not able to detect alterations smaller than 20 megabases.

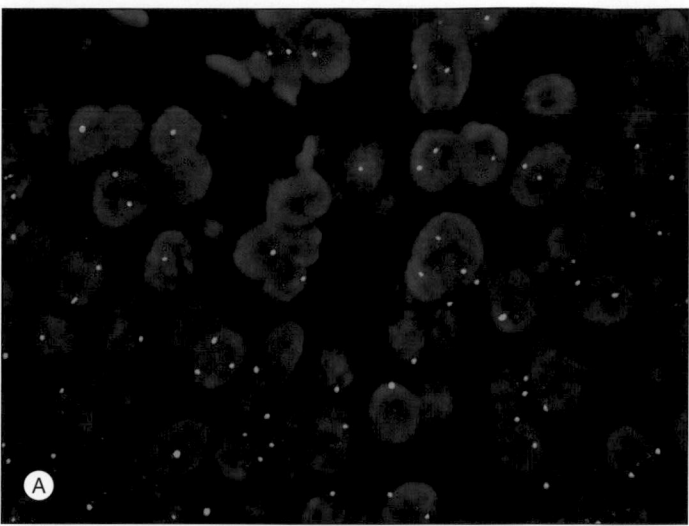

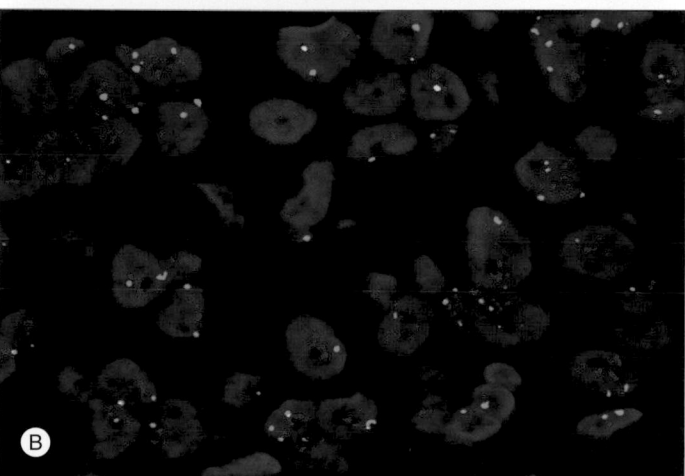

Fig. 2.33 FISH. Formalin fixed paraffin embedded sections of invasive breast carcinoma. The green signal represents a centromeric probe for chromosome 17 while the red signal is the gene specific probe for Her2/neu. **(A)** is from a case with no evidence of amplification. **(B)** shows her2/neu amplification. (Courtesy of Dr. Umadevi Tantravahi, Director of the Division of Genetics, Women and Infants Hospital, Providence, RI.)

GENE EXPRESSION MICROARRAYS

An emerging area of research in the field of tumor markers and prognostication is transcriptional profiling via microarray expression analysis (Fig. 2.34).[308–312] In this method, gene expression rather then DNA copy number is measured. These microarray chips carry thousands of oligonucleotides representing up to 60 000 human genes and expressed sequence tags (ESTs). Alternatively, cDNA fragments may be mounted on glass slides. To these microarray chips or glass slides a mixture of fluorescently labeled RNA prepared from extracted total RNA is hybridized. Commonly, the RNA from two tissues (frequently tumor and adjacent normal tissue) is analyzed simultaneously by labeling each RNA extract with different fluorochromes. The ratio of signal intensities for each spot is measured, providing relative levels of gene expression in each pair of tissues. The vast quantity of data generated are analyzed using specialized 'data mining' software.[313]

There are numerous applications of microarray expression in the fields of pathology and oncology, including the differentiation of

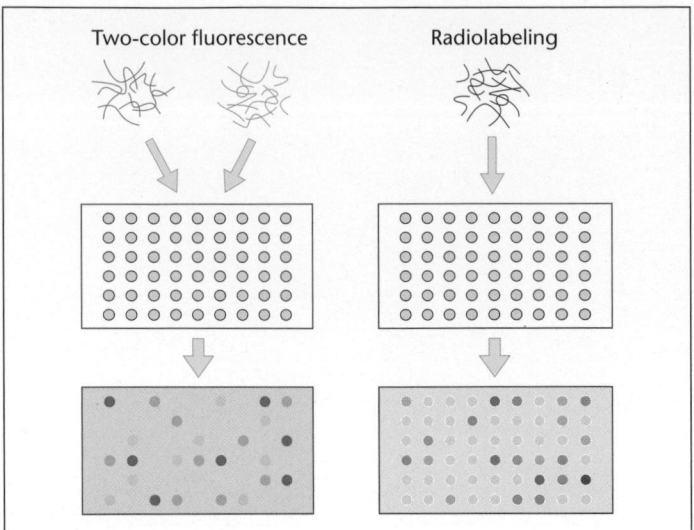

Fig. 2.34 Principles of gene expression measurements using arrays. RNA samples are labeled in a reverse transcription reaction using fluorescent nucleotides (left) or radioactive nucleotides (right), and hybridized to arrays representing multiple different genes. For fluorescent labeling, two or more samples labeled with differently colored fluorescent markers (e.g. red and green) are cohybridized to an array. Level of RNA for each gene in the sample is measured in intensity of fluorescence or radioactivity binding to the specific spot. With fluorescence labeling, relative levels of expressed genes in two samples can be directly compared with a single array. (Reproduced with the permission of the United States Academy of Pathology and Modern Pathology.[311])

primary from secondary tumors, identification of diagnostic and prognostic markers, comparing different stages of cancer progression, monitoring resistance to chemotherapy, and others. For example, gene expression profiling of diffuse large B-cell lymphomas identified a specific gene expression profile that predicted survival better than existing histopathological and clinical criteria.[314]

DNA MICROARRAYS

DNA arrays are a novel technique applicable to oncology used to identify chromosomal aberrations such as gene polymorphisms and mutations of individual nucleotides.[315] In this method the sample DNA is hybridized to an array of oligonucleotides with different combinations of base pair substitutions and nucleic acid polymorphisms. The strongest signal will be generated where the target DNA hybridizes to the most complementary sequence. This method is used for screening mutations in specific genes such as p53[316] and in the detection of antimicrobial resistance alleles.[317]

MICROSATELLITE ANALYSIS AND INSTABILITY

Scattered throughout the human genome are a huge number of short, 2–6 nucleotide reiterations ranging from tens to several hundreds.[318] The function of these microsatellite repeats is unclear. These sites are relatively stable in healthy individuals. However, they are heterozygous for any given locus as the pattern of microsatellite repeats from the maternal alleles differs from that seen in the paternal alleles. This heterozygosity is used frequently in genetic mapping.

Many neoplasms possess increases and decreases in the lengths of these repeated elements relative to the patient's normal DNA. This phenomenon is termed microsatellite instability (MSI).[319] MSI has been shown to result from mutations in DNA repair genes whose function is to correct errors made by DNA polymerase during replication. Somatic microsatellite instability has been detected in numerous cancer types.[320,321] For example, MSI can be detected in approximately 90% of tumors from individuals with hereditary nonpolyposis colorectal cancer (HNPCC) as well as up to 30% of sporadic colon cancers.[322]

Analysis of MSI is useful in the identification of hereditary cancer syndromes, as a screening technique to detect cancer and monitor recurrence.[323]

EPIGENETIC (METHYLATION) ANALYSIS

Over the past two decades increasing evidence has shown that epigenetic regulation plays a critical role in carcinogenesis.[324] The three primary types of epigenetic information include cytosine DNA methylation, genetic imprinting. and histone modification. Cytosine DNA methylation is the covalent transfer of a methyl group to the 5′ position of the cytosine ring in CpG residues by a family of cytosine methyltransferases. Throughout the genome the distribution of CpG is nonrandom and infrequent except for CpG islands at the promoter and the 5′ ends of gene. DNA methylation plays an important regulatory role in development, X-chromosome inactivation, genetic imprinting, and suppressing of parasitic DNA sequences. Hypo- or hypermethylation of the promoters of specific oncogenes or tumor suppressor genes may lead to malignant transformation.

Various methods have been devised to determine DNA methylation patterns, including Southern hybridization and PCR-based methods utilizing methylation-sensitive enzymes.[325] Determining the methylation status of specific genes has been used as a marker for cancer detection and screening.[326]

ANALYSIS OF CLONALITY AND LOSS OF HETEROZYGOSITY

It is sometimes difficult, based on morphologic criteria alone, to determine whether a cellular population is neoplastic or reactive in origin. In these situations, information may be gained by determining clonality, as all neoplastic processes are clonal. Differentiating lymphomas from reactive lymphoid processes is frequently performed through clonality assessment of either Ig or the T-cell receptor gene rearrangement for B- and T-cell lymphomas, respectively.[263]

Determination of loss of heterozygosity (LOH) in a sample may be applied to the determination of clonality in neoplasms. LOH is based on the principle that certain DNA sequences are expressed heterozygously in human cells. In order to define a state of LOH, a marked decrease of more than 50% has to be present in one allele of the tumor sample as compared to the normal tissue sample of the same patient. Common methods of determining LOH include detection of chromosome X inactivation, PCR-based RFLP, and microsatellite analysis.[327]

ACKNOWLEDGMENT

The authors thank Ms Joanne Harker for her invaluable assistance in the preparation of this chapter.

REFERENCES

1. Pearse AGE. The chemistry and practice of fixation. In: Histochemistry. Theoretical and applied, 4th edn. Vol. 1. Edinburgh: Churchill Livingstone; 1980: 97–158.

2. Hopwood D. Fixation and fixatives. In: Bancroft JD, Stevens A, eds. Theory and practice of histological techniques. Edinburgh: Churchill Livingstone; 1990: 21–42.

3. Kiernan JA. Histological and histochemical methods. Theory and practice. Oxford: Pergamon; 1981.

4. Baker JR. Introduction to fixation. In: Cytological Technique: The principles underlying routine methods, 5th edn. London: Science Paperbacks and Methuen; 1966: 14–30.

5. Banks PM. Technical aspects of specimen preparation and introduction to special studies. In: Jaffe ES, ed. Surgical pathology of the lymph nodes and related organs. Philadelphia: WB Saunders; 1995: 1–21.

6. Pearse AGE. Freeze drying of biological tissues. In: Histochemistry. Theoretical and applied, 4th edn. Vol. 1. Edinburgh: Churchill Livingstone; 1980.

7. Leong ASY, Daymon ME, Milios J. Microwave irradiation as a form of fixation for light and electron microscopy. J Pathol 1985; 146: 313–332.

8. Hopwood D. Cell and tissue fixation, 1972–1982. Histochim J 1985; 17: 389–442.

9. Morales AR, Essenfield H, Essenfield E, et al. Continuous-specimen-flow, high-throughput, 1-hour tissue processing. A system for rapid diagnostic tissue preparation. Arch Pathol lab Med 2002; 126: 583–590.

10. Bancroft JD, Cook HD. Manual of histochemical techniques and their diagnostic applications. Edinburgh: Churchill Livingstone; 1994.

11. Horobin RW. An overview of the theory of staining. In: Bancroft JD, Stevens A, eds. Theory and practice of histological techniques. Edinburgh: Churchill Livingstone; 1990: 93–105.

12. Stevens A, Bancroft JD. Proteins and nucleic acids. In: Bancroft JD, Stevens A, eds. Theory and practice of histological techniques. Edinburgh: Churchill Livingstone; 1990: 143–153.

13. Pearse AGE. Nucleic acids and nucleoproteins. Histochemistry. Theoretical and applied. 3rd edn. Vol. 1. Boston: Little, Brown; 1968: 248–293.

14. Ploton D, Menager M, Jeannesson P, et al. Improvement in the staining and in the visualization of the argyrophilic proteins of the nucleolar organizing regions at the optical level. Histochem J 1986; 18: 5–14.

15. Bradbury P, Gordon KC. Connective tissues and stains. In: Bancroft JD, Stevens A, eds. Theory and practice of histological techniques. Churchill Livingstone; Edinburgh: 1990: 119–142.

16. Puchtler H, Sweat F, Levine M. On the biding of Congo red by amyloid. J Histochem Cytochem 1962; 10: 355.

17. Vassar PS, Culling FA. Fluorescent stains with special reference to amyloid and connective tissue. Arch Pathol 1959; 68: 487–498.

18. Cooke HC. Carbohydrates. In: Bancroft JD, Stevens A, eds. Theory and practice of histological techniques. Edinburgh: Churchill Livingstone; 1990: 1177–213.

19. Sorvari TE. Histochemical observations on the role of ferric chloride in the high iron diamine technique for localizing sulphated mucosubstances. Histochem J 1972; 4: 193–204.

20. Bayliss-High OB. Lipids. In: Bancroft JD, Stevens A, eds. Theory and practice of histological techniques. Edinburgh: Churchill Livingstone; 1990: 215–244.

21. Grimelius LA. A silver nitrate stain for A_2 cells of human pancreatic islets. Acta Soc Med Upsal 1968; 73: 243–270.

22. Stevens A. Microorganisms. In: Bancroft, JD, Stevens A, eds. Theory and practice of histological techniques. Edinburgh: Churchill Livingstone; 1990: 289–308.

23. Noda Y, Toei K. A new bacterial staining method involving Gram stain with theoretical considerations of the staining mechanism. Microbios 1992; 70: 49–55.

24. Glynn JH. The application of the Gram stain to paraffin sections. Arch Pathol 1935; 20: 896–899.

25. Shikata T, Uzawa T, Yoshiwara N, et al. Staining methods for Australian antigen in paraffin sections – detection of cytoplasmic inclusion bodies. Jpn J Exp Med 1974; 44: 25–36.

26. Stevens A. Pigments and minerals. In: Bancroft JD, Stevens A, eds. Theory and practice of histological techniques. Edinburgh: Churchill Livingstone; 1990: 245–267.

27. Bancroft JD, Cook HC. Enzyme histochemistry. Manual of histological techniques and their diagnostic application. Edinburgh: Churchill Livingstone; 1994: 289–322.

28. Leder LD. Uber die selektive fermentcytochemicsche Darstellung von neutrophilen myeloischen Zellen Gewebsmastzellen in Parafinschnit. Kurze wissenschaftliche Mitteilungen. Klin Wochenschr 1964; 42: 553.

29. Stevens A. Enzyme histochemistry. Diagnostic applications. In: Bancroft JD, Stevens A, eds. Theory and practice of histological techniques. Edinburgh: Churchill Livingstone; 1990: 401–412.

30. Dubowitz V. Muscle biopsy: a practical approach. London: Baillière Tindall; 1985.

31. Keebler CM, Somark TM. Cytopreparative techniques. In: The manual of cytotechnology. 7th edn. Chicago: ASCP; 1993: 412–447.

32. Woronzoff-Dashkoff KP. The Ehrlick-Chenzinsky-Plehn-Malachowski-Romanowsky-Nocht-Jenner-May-Grünwald-Leishman-Reuter-Wright-Giemsa-Lillie-Roe, Wilcox stain. The mystery unfolds. Clin Lab Med 1993; 13: 759–771.

33. Wilbur DC, Cibas ES, Meritt S, et al. ThinPrep processor. Clinical trials demonstrate an increased detection rate of abnormal cervical cytologic specimens. Am J Clin Pathol 1994; 101: 209–214.

34. Hutchinson ML, Agarwal P, Denault T. A new look at cervical cytology: ThinPrep multicenter trial results. Acta Cytol 1992; 36: 499–504.

35. Hutchinson ML, Isenstein LM, Goodman AK, et al. Homogeneous sampling accounts for the increased diagnostic accuracy using the ThinPrep processor. Am J Clin Pathol 1994: 101: 215–219.

36. Ro JY, Staerkel GA, Ayala AG. Cytologic and histologic features of superficial bladder cancer. Urol Clin North Am 1992; 19: 435–453.

37. Hossein M, Yazdi MB. Genitourinary cytology. Clin Lab Med 1991; 11: 369–377.

38. Koss LG. Diagnostic cytology and its histopathologic bases. 4th edn. Philadelphia: Lippincott-Raven; 1992.

39. Frable WJ. Needle aspiration biopsy: past, present, and future. Hum Pathol 1989; 20: 504–517.

40. Stanley MW, Lowhagen T. Fine needle aspiration of palpable masses. Boston: Butterworth-Heinemann; 1993: 3–5.

41. Koss LG, Woyke S, Olxzewski W. Aspiration biopsy. Cytologic interpretation and histologic bases. 2nd edn. New York: Igaku Shoin; 1992: 12–53;193–196.

42. Helbich TH, Matzek W, Fuchsjager MH. Stereotactic and ultrasound-guided breast biopsy. Eur Radiol 2004; 14: 383–393.

43. Zhou M, Epstein JI.. The reporting of prostate cancer on needle biopsy: prognostic and therapeutic implications and the utility of diagnostic markers: Pathology 2003; 35: 472–479.

44. Martin HE, Ellis EB. Biopsy by needle puncture and aspiration. Ann Surg 1930; 92: 169–181.

45. Lopes Cardozo P. Clinical cytology. Leiden: Stafleu; 1954.

46. Zajicek J. Aspiration biopsy cytology. part 1. cytology of supradiaphragmatic organs. Vol. 4. Monographs in clinical cytology. New York: S. Karger; 1974: 1–15, 20–26.

47. Soderstrom N. Fine needle aspiration biopsy. Stockholm: Almqvist & Wiksell; 1966: 13–18.

48. Dahlgren SE, Nordenstrom B. Transthoracic needle biopsy. Stockholm: Almqvist & Wiksell; 1966.

49. Frable WJ. The history of fine needle aspiration biopsy: The American experience. In: Schmidt W, ed. Cytopathology annual 1994. Chicago: ASCP Press; 1994: 91–100.

50. Frable WJ. Thin-needle aspiration biopsy. Vol. 14. In: Bennington JL, ed. Major problems in pathology. Philadelphia: WB Saunders; 1983: 184, 184, 231, 232.

51. Stewart FW. The diagnosis of tumors by aspiration biopsy. Am J Pathol 1933; 9: 801–812.

52. Abele JS, Miller TR. Implementation of an outpatient needle aspiration biopsy service and clinic: a personal perspective. In: Schmidt W, ed. Cytopathology annual 1993. Chicago: ASCP Press; 1993: 43–71.

53. Frable WJ. Fine needle aspiration biopsy. In: Banks P, Kraybill WB, eds. Pathology for the surgeon. Philadelphia: WB Saunders; 1996: 33–45.

54. Orell SR. The two faces of fine-needle biopsy: its role in the teaching hospital and in the community. Diagn Cytopathol 1992; 8: 557–558.

55. Dabbs DJ. Immunocytology. In: Dabbs DJ, ed. Diagnostic immunohistochemistry. Philadelphia: Churchill Livingston; 2002: 625–639.

56. Akhtar M, Iqbal MA, Mourad W, et al. Fine-needle aspiration biopsy diagnosis of small round cell tumors of childhood: A comprehensive approach. Diagn Cytopathol 1999; 81–91.

57. Johnson DE, Powers CN, Rupp GN, et al. Immunocytochemical staining of fine-needle aspiration biopsies of the liver as a diagnostic tool for hepatocellular carcinoma. Mod Pathol 1991; 5: 117–123.

58. Young NA, Al-Saleem T. Diagnosis of lymphoma by fine-needle aspiration cytology using the revised European-American classification of lymphoid neoplasms. Cancer 1999; 87: 325–345.

59. Katz RI, Hirsch-Ginsberg C, Childs C, et al. The role of gene rearrangements for antigen receptors in the diagnosis of lymphoma obtained by fine needle aspiration: a study of 63 cases with concomitant immunophenotyping. Am J Clin Pathol 1991; 96: 479–490.

60. Saboorian MH, Ashfaq R. The use of fine needle aspiration biopsy in the evaluation of lymphadenopathy. Semin Diagn Pathol 2001; 18: 110–123.

61. Dabbs DJ, Silverman JF. Selective use of electron microscopy in fine needle aspiration cytology. Acta Cytol 1988; 32: 880–884.

62. Boon ME, Schut JJ, Suurmeijer AJH, et al. Confocal microscopy of false-negative breast aspirates. Diagn Cytopathol 1995; 12: 42–50.

63. Masood S, Bui MM. Prognostic and predictive value of HER2/neu oncogene in breast cancer. Microsc Res Tech 2002; 59: 102–108.

64. Kube MJ, McDonald DA, Quin JW, et al. Use of archival and fresh cytologic material for the polymerase chain reaction. Analyt Quant Cytol Histol 1994; 16: 174–182.

65. Udayakumar AM, Sundareshan TS, Goud TM, et al. Cytogenetic characterization of Ewing tumors using fine needle aspiration samples. a 10-year experience and review of the literature. Cancer Genet Cytogenet 2001; 127: 42–48.

66. Cajulis RS, Frias-Hidvegi D. Detection of numerical chromosomal abnormalities in malignant cells in fine needle aspirates by fluorescent in situ hybridization of interphase cell nuclei with chromosome-specific probes. Acta Cytol 1993; 37: 391–396.

67. Jhala NC, Jhala D, Eltoum I, et al. Endoscopic ultrasound-guided fine-needle aspiration biopsy: A

powerful tool to obtain samples from small lesions. Cancer Cytopathol 2004; 102: 239–246.

68. Schwartz MR. Endoscopic ultrasound-guided fine-needle aspiration: Time, diagnostic challenges, and clinical impact. Cancer Cytopathol 2004; 102: 203–206.

69. Zajdela A, Zillhardt P, Voillemot N. Cytological diagnosis by fine needle sampling without aspiration. Cancer 1987; 59: 1201–1205.

70. Kinney TB, Lee MJ, Filomena CA, et al. Fine-needle biopsy: prospective comparison of aspiration versus non-aspiration techniques in the abdomen. Radiology 1993; 186: 549–552.

71. Ljung B. Thin needle aspiration biopsy: an instructional video. San Francisco, CA: Department of Cytopathology, University of California, San Francisco; 1992.

72. Grohs HK. Fine needle aspiration and smear making techniques: an instructional video. Manchester, MA: International Institute for Applied CytoScience; 1992.

73. Yang GCH, Alvarez II. Ultra-fast Papanicolaou stain: an alternative preparation for fine-needle aspiration cytology. Acta Cytol 1995; 39: 55–60.

74. Shield PW, Perkins G Wright RG: Immunocytochemical staining of cytologic specimens. How helpful is it? Am J Clin Pathol 1996; 105: 157–162.

75. Silverman JF, Khazanic PG, Norris HT, et al. Parathyroid hormone (PTH) assay of parathyroid cysts examined by fine needle aspiration biopsy. Am J Clin Pathol 1986; 86: 776–780.

76. Davidson HG, Campora RG. Thyroid. In: Bibbo M, ed. Comprehensive cytopathology. Philadelphia: WB Saunders; 1991: 660–662.

77. Hadju SI. The value and limitations of aspiration cytology in the diagnosis of primary tumors. Acta Cytol 1989; 33: 741–790.

78. Orell SR, Sterrett GF, Walters Max N-I, et al. Manual and atlas of fine needle aspiration cytology. 2nd edn. New York: Churchill Livingstone; 1992: 8–32.

79. Powers CN. Fine needle aspiration biopsy: Perspectives on complications. The reality behind the myths. In: Schmidt W, ed. Cytopathology annual 1996. Chicago: ASCP Press; 1996: 71–98.

80. Lee KC, Chan JKC, Ho LC. Histologic changes in the breast after fine-needle aspiration. Am J Surg Pathol 1994; 18: 1039–1047.

81. LiVolsi VA, Merino MJ. Worrisome histologic alterations following fine needle aspiration of thyroid. WHAFFT. Pathol Ann 1994; 29(pt2): 99–120.

82. Powers CN, Frable WJ. Fine needle aspiration biopsy of the head and neck. Boston: Butterworth-Heinemann; 1996.

83. Dusenbery D, Frable WJ. Fine needle aspiration cytology of phyllodes tumor. Potential diagnostic pitfalls. Acta Cytol 1992; 36: 215–221.

84. Frable WJ. Fine needle aspiration biopsy (Chapter 10). In: Silverberg SG, DeLellis RA, Frable WJ, eds. Principles and practice of surgical pathology and cytopathology, 3rd edn. New York: Churchill Livingstone; 1997: 137–154.

85. Gurley AM, Cluroe AD, Roberts EC. Electron microscopy (Chapter 9). In: Silverberg SG, DeLellis RA, Frable WJ, eds. Principles and practice of surgical pathology and cytopathology, 3rd edn. New York: Churchill Livingstone; 1997: 127–135.

86. Dardick I, Herrera GA. Diagnostic electron microscopy of neoplasms. Hum Pathol 1998; 29: 1335–1338.

87. Llombart-Bosch A. Introduction (electron microscopy of tumors). Seminars Diagn Pathol 2003; 20: 21–24.

88. Hyatt MA. Principles and techniques of electron micrsocopy. 3rd edn. New York: MacMillan Press; 1989.

89. Willis EJ, Carr S, Philips J. Electron microscopy in the diagnosis of precutaneous fine needle aspiration specimens. Ultrastruct Pathol 1987; 11: 361–387.

90. Dardick I, Yazdi HM, Brosko C. et al. A quantitative comparison of light and electron microscopic diagnoses in specimens obtained by fine needle aspiration biopsy. Ultrastruct Pathol 1991; 15: 105–129.

91. Dabbs DJ, Silverman JF. Selective use of electron microscopy in fine needle aspiration cytology. Acta Cytol 1998; 32: 880–884.

92. Akhtar M, Bakry M, Nash EJ. An improved technique for processing aspiration biopsy for electron microscopy. Am J. Clin Pathol 1986; 85: 57–60.

93. Howell DN, Payne CM, Miller SE, et al. Special techniques in diagnostic electron microscopy. Hum Pathol 1998; 29: 1339–1346.

94. Herrea GA. Ultrastructural immunolabeling: A general overview of techniques and application. Ultrastruct Pathol 1992; 16: 37–45.

95. Trembleau A, Bloom FE. Enhanced sensitivity for light and electron microscopic in situ hybridization with multiple simultaneous non-radioactive oligodeoxynucleotide protein. J Histochem Cytochem 1995; 43: 829–841.

96. Coons AH, Creech HJ, Jones RN. Immunological properties of an antibody containing a fluorescent group. Proc Soc Exp Bull Med 1941; 47: 200–202.

97. Nakane PK, Pierce GBJ. Exzyme labeled antibodies for the light and electron microscopic localization of tissue antigens. J Cell Biol 1967; 33: 307–318.

98. Mason TE, Phifer RF, Spicer SS, et al. An immunoglobulin-enzyme bridge method for localizing tissue antigens. J Histochem Cytochem 1969; 17: 563–569.

99. Sternberger LA, Hardy PH, Cuculis JJ, et al. The unlabeled antibody enzyme method of immunohistochemistry: preparation and properties of soluble antigen-antibody complex (horseradish peroxidase-anti-horseradish peroxidase) and its use in identification of spirochetoses. J Histochem Cytochem 1970; 18: 315–333.

100. Guesdon JL, Ternynck T, Avrameas S. The use of avidin biotin interaction in immunoenzymatic techniques. J Histochem Cytochem 1979; 27: 1131–1139.

101. Hsu S-M, Raine L, Fanger H. Use of avidin biotin peroxidase complex (ABC) in immunoperoxidase techniques: A comparison between ABC and unlabeled antibody (PAP) procedures. J Histochem Cytochem 1981; 29: 577.

102. Taylor CR, Shi S-R, Barr NJ, et al. Techniques of immunohistochemistry: principles, pitfalls and standardization (Chapter 1). In: DJ Dabbs, ed. Diagnostic immunohistochemistry. New York: Churchill Livingstone; 2002: 3–44.

103. Vanderloos CM, Naruko T, Becker AE. The use of enhanced polymer one step staining reagents for immunoenzyme double labeling. Histochem J 1996; 28: 709–714.

104. Sabattini E, Bisgaard K, Ascani S, et al. The EnVision++ System: A new immunohistochemical method for diagnostics and research. Critical comparison with the APAAP, Chem Mate, CSA, LABC and SABC techniques. J Clin Pathol 1998; 51: 506–511.

105. Shi S-R, Guo J, Cote RJ, et al. Sensitivity and detection efficiency of a novel two step detection system (Power Vision) for immunohistochemistry. Appl Immunohistochem Mol Morphol 1999; 7: 201.

106. Kammerer U, Kapp M., Gassel AM, et al. A new rapid immunohistochemical staining technique using the EnVision antibody complex. J Histochem Cytochem 2001; 49: 623–630.

107. Vyberg M, Nielsen S. Dextran polymer conjugate two step visualization system for immunohistochemistry. Appl Immunohistochem 1998; 6: 3.

108. Hsu SM, Raine L. Protein A, avidin and biotin in immunohistochemistry. J Histochem Cytochem 1981; 29: 1349–1353.

109. DeLellis RA, May L, Tashjian AJ Jr, et al. C-cell granule heterogenicity in man. An ultrastructural immunocytochemical study. Lab Inves 1978; 38: 263–269.

110. Bobrow MN, Shaughnessy KJ, Litt GJ. Catalyzed reporter desposition: a novel method of signal amplification. II. Application to membrane immunoassay. J Immunol Methods 1991; 137: 103–112.

111. Toda V, Kono K, Abiru H, et al. Application of tyramide signal amplification system to immunohistochemistry: A potent method to localize antigens that are not detectable by ordinary method. Pathol Int 1999; 49: 479–483.

112. Von Wasielewski R, Mengel M, Gignac S, et al. Tyramine amplification technique in routine immunohistochemistry. J Histochem Cytochem 1997; 45: 1455–1459.

113. Cordell JL, Falini B, Erber WN, et al. Immunoenzymatic labeling of monoclonal antibodies using immune complexes of alkaline phosphatase and monoclonal anti-alkaline phosphatase (APAAP complexes). J Histochem Cytochem 1984; 32: 219–229.

114. Gown AM, Garcia R, Ferguson M, et al. Avidin-biotin immunoglucose oxidase: use in single and double labeling procedures. J Histochem Cytochem 1986; 34: 403–409.

115. Nadji M, Morales A. Immunohistochemical techniques (Chapter 5). In: Silverberg SG, DeLellis RA, Frable WJ, eds. Principles and practice of surgical pathology and cytopathology. 3rd edn. New York: Churchill Livingstone; 1997: 63–75.

116. Mukai K, Yoshimura S, Anzai M. Effects of decalcification on immunoperoxidase staining. Am J Surg Pathol 1986; 10: 413–419.

117. Battifora H, Kopinski M. The influence of protein digestion and duration of fixation on the immunostaining of keratins. A comparison of formalin and ethanol fixatives. J Histochem Cytochem 1986; 34: 1095–1100.

118. Shi S-R, Key M, Kalra KL, et al. Antigen retrieval in formalin fixed paraffin embedded tissue: an enhancement method for immunohistochemical staining based on microwave heating of tissue sections. J Histochem Cytochem 1991; 39: 741–748.

119. Morgan JM, Navabi H, Jasani B. Role of calcium chelation in high temperature antigen retrieval at different pH values. J Pathol 1997; 182: 233–237.

120. Shi S-R, Cote RJ, Taylor CR. Antigen retrieval immunohistochemistry: past, present, future. J Histochem Cytochem 1997; 45: 327–344.

121. Miller RT, Swanson PE, Wick MR. Fixation and epitope retrieval in diagnostic immunohistochemistry: A concise review with practical considerations. Appl Immunohistochem Mol Morph 2000; 8: 228–235.

122. Bussolati G, Gugliotta P, Volante M, et al. Retrieved endogenous biotin: a novel marker and a potential pitfall in diagnostic immunohistochemistry. Histopathology 1997; 31: 400–407.

123. Boenisch T. Handbook immunohistochemical staining methods. 3rd edn. Dako Corporation: 2001.

124. Abendroth CS, Dabbs DJ. Immunocytochemical staining of unstained versus previously stained cytologic preparations. Acta Cytol 1995; 39: 379–386.

125. Skoog L, Tani E, Svedmyr E, et al. Growth fraction in non-Hodgkin's lymphomas and reactive lymphadenitis determined by Ki-67 monoclonal antibody in fine needle aspirates. Diagn Cytopathol 1995; 12: 234–239.

126. Young, NA, Al-Saleem T. Cancer: Diagnosis of lymphoma by fine-needle aspiration cytology using the revised European-American classification of lymphoid neoplasms. 1999; 87: 325–345.

127. Taylor CR. FDA issues final rule for classification and reclassification of immunohistochemistry reagents and kits. Am J Clin Pathol 1999; 111: 445–448.

128. Swanson PE. Labels, disclaimers and rules (oh, my!). Analyte specific reagent and practice of immunohistochemistry. Am J Clin Pathol 1999; 111: 445–448.

129. Bloom K, Harrington D. Enhanced accuracy and reliability of her-2/neu immunohistochemical scoring using digital microscopy. Am J Clin Pathol 2004; 121: 620–630.

130. Pierga J-Y, Bonneton C, Vincent-Salomon A, et al. Clinical significance of immunocytochemical detection of tumor cells using digital microscopy in peripheral blood and bone marrow of breast cancer patients. Clin Cancer Res 2004; 10: 1392–1400.

131. Simon R, Mirlacher M, Sauter G. Tissue microarrays. Bio Techniques 2004; 36: 98–105.

132. Frierson HJ Jr, Linder J. Flow and image cytometry (Chapter 7). In: Silverberg SG, DeLellis RA, Frable WJ, eds. Principles and practice of surgical pathology and cytopathology. 3rd edn. New York: Churchill Livingstone; 1997: 95–111.

133. Frierson HF Jr. Ploidy analysis and S-phase fraction determination by flow cytometry of invasive adenocarcinoma of the breast. Am J Surg Pathol 1991; 15: 358–367.

134. Hedley DW, Shankey TV, Wheeless LL. DNA cytometry consensus conference. Cytometry 1993; 14: 471.

135. Shankey TV, Rabinovitch PS, Bagwell B, et al. Guidelines for implementation of clinical DNA cytometry. Cytometry 1993; 14: 472–477.

136. Hedley DW, Clark GM, Cornelisse CJ, et al. Consensus review of the clinical utility of DNA cytometry in carcinoma of the breast. Cytometry 1993; 14: 482–485.

137. Shankey TV, Kallioniemi O-P, Koslowski JM, et al. Consensus review of the clinical utility of DNA content cytometry in prostate cancer. Cytometry 1993; 14: 457–500.

138. Wheeless LL, Badalament RA, deVere White RW, et al. Consensus review of the clinical utility of DNA cytometry in bladder cancer. Cytometry 1993; 14: 478–481.

139. Bauer KD, Bagwell CB, Giaretti W, et al. Consensus review of the clinical utility of DNA flow cytometry in colorectal cancer. Cytometry 1993; 14: 486–491.

140. Duque RE, Andreeff M, Braylan RC, et al. Consensus review of the clinical utility of DNA flow cytometry in neoplastic hematopathology. Cytometry 1993; 14: 492–496.

141. Vindelov LL, Christensen IJ, Keiding N, et al. Long-term storage of samples for flow cytometric DNA analysis. Cytometry 1983; 3: 317–322.

142. Alanen KA, Klemi PJ, Joensuu H, et al. Comparison of fresh, ethanol-preserved, and paraffin-embedded samples in DNA flow cytometry. Cytometry 1989; 10: 81–85.

143. Alanen KA, Klemi PJ, Taimela S, et al. A simple preservative for flow cytometric DNA analysis. Cytometry 1989; 10: 86–89.

144. Frierson HF Jr. Ploidy and proliferative fraction analysis of cytologic specimens. In: Keren DF, Hanson CA, Hurtubise P, eds.: Flow cytometry and clinical diagnosis. Chicago: ASCP Press; 1994: 596–613.

145. Alanen KA, Joensuu H, Klemi PJ. Autolysis is a potential source of false aneuploid peaks in flow cytometric DNA histograms. Cytometry 1989; 10: 417–425.

146. Torres FX, Mackowiak PG, Brown RD, et al. Comparison of two methods of mechanical disaggregation of scirrhous breast adenocarcinomas for DNA flow cytometric analysis of whole cells. Am J Clin Pathol 1995; 103: 8–13.

147. Frankfurt OS, Slocum HK, Rustum YM, et al. Flow cytometric analysis of DNA aneuploidy in primary and metastatic human solid tumors. Cytometry 1984; 5: 71–80.

148. Eliasen CA, Opitz LM, Vamvakas EC, et al. Flow cytometric analysis of DNA ploidy and S-phase fraction in breast cancer using cells obtained by ex vivo fine-needle aspiration: an optimal method for sample collection. Mod Pathol 1991; 4: 196–200.

149. Bach BA, Knape WA, Edinger MG, et al. Improved sensitivity and resolution in the flow cytometric DNA analysis of human solid tumor specimens. Use of in vitro fine-needle aspiration, and uniform staining reagents. Am J Clin Pathol 1991; 96: 615–627.

150. Cornacchiari A, Grigolato PG, Facchetti F, et al. Usefulness of the scraping method for DNA flow cytometry in breast tumors. Cytometry 1995; 19: 263–266.

151. Lee TK, Wiley AL Jr, Esinhart JD, et al. Variations associated with disaggregation methods in DNA flow cytometry. Anal Quant Cytol Histol 1993; 15: 195–200.

152. Crissman JD, Zarbo RJ, Niebylski CD, et al. Flow cytometric DNA analysis of colon adenocarcinomas. A comparative study of preparatory techniques. Mod Pathol 1988; 1: 198–204.

153. Kallioniemi O-P. Comparison of fresh and paraffin-embedded tissue as starting material for DNA flow cytometry and evaluation of intratumor heterogeneity. Cytometry 1988; 9: 164–169.

154. Beerman H, Smit VTHBM, Kluin PM, et al. Flow cytometric analysis of DNA stemline heterogeneity in primary and metastatic breast cancer. Cytometry 1991; 12: 147–154.

155. Kute T. Response to Beerman et al.: flow cytometric analysis of DNA stemline heterogeneity in primary and metastatic breast cancer (letter). Cytometry 1991; 12: 155.

156. Beerman H, Cornelisse CT. Response to Dr. Kute's letter to the editor (letter). Cytometry 1991; 12: 156.

157. Wersto RP, Liblit RL, Deitch D, et al. Variability in DNA measurements in multiple tumor samples of human colonic carcinoma. Cancer 1991; 67: 106–115.

158. Ferno M, Baldetorp B, Ewers S-B, et al. One or multiple samplings for flow cytometric DNA analyses in breast cancer – prognostic implications? Cytometry 1992; 13: 241–249.

159. Hedley DW, Friedlander ML, Taylor IW, et al. Method for analysis of cellular DNA content of paraffin-embedded pathological material using flow cytometry. J Histochem Cytochem 1983; 31: 1333–1335.

160. Schutte B, Reynders MMJ, Bosman FT, et al. Flow cytometric determination of DNA ploidy level in nuclei isolated from paraffin-embedded tissue. Cytometry 1985; 6: 26–30.

161. Frierson HF Jr. Flow cytometric analysis of ploidy in solid neoplasms: comparison of fresh tissues with formalin-fixed paraffin-embedded specimens. Hum Pathol 1988; 19: 290–294.

162. Hedley DW. Flow cytometry using paraffin-embedded tissue: five years on. Cytometry 1989; 229–241.

163. Esteban JM, Sheibani K, Owens M, et al. Effects of various fixatives and fixation conditions on DNA ploidy analysis. A need for strict internal DNA standards. Am J Clin Pathol 1991; 460–466.

164. Schmid I, Uittenbogaart CH, Giorgi JV. A gentle fixation and permeabilization method for combined cell surface and intracellular staining with improved precision in DNA quantification. Cytometry 1991; 12: 279–285.

165. Stephenson RA, Gay H, Fair WR, et al. Effect of section thickness on quality of flow cytometric DNA content determinations in paraffin-embedded tissues. Cytometry 1986; 7: 41–44.

166. Sickle-Santanello BJ, Farrar MB, DeCenzo JF, et al. Technical and statistical improvements for flow cytometric DNA analysis of paraffin-embedded tissue. Cytometry 1988; 9: 594–599.

167. Amberson JB, Wersto RP, Agarwal V, et al. Preparation of paraffin-embedded tissue for flow and image cytometric analysis: an improved and more efficient procedure (abstract). Cytometry 1988; Suppl. 2: 34.

168. Babiak J, Poppema S. Automated procedure for dewaxing and rehydration of paraffin-embedded tissue sections for DNA flow cytometric analysis of breast tumors. Am J Clin Pathol 1991; 96: 64–69.

169. Heiden T, Wang N, Tribukait B. An improved Hedley method for preparation of paraffin-embedded tissues for flow cytometric analysis of ploidy and S-phase. Cytometry 1991; 12: 614–621.

170. Wang N, Pan Y, Heiden T, et al. Improved method for release of cell nuclei from paraffin-embedded cell material of squamous cell carcinomas. Cytometry 1993; 14: 931–935.

171. Pollack A, Ciancio G, Terry NHA, et al. Recognition and reduction of artifacts from autolysis in paraffin-embedded tissue using DNA/nuclear protein flow cytometry. Cytometry 1993; 14: 565–568.

172. Ciancio G, Pollack A, Block NL. Flow cytometric analysis of DNA and nuclear protein in paraffin-embedded tissue. Cytometry 1993; 14: 205–209.

173. Zalupski MM, Maciorowski Z, Ryan JR. DNA content parameters of paraffin-embedded soft tissue sarcomas: optimization of retrieval technique and comparison to fresh tissue. Cytometry 1993; 14: 327–333.

174. Albro S, Bauer KD, Hitchcock CL, et al. Improved DNA content histograms from formalin-fixed, paraffin-embedded liver tissue by proteinase K digestion. Cytometry 1993; 14: 673–678.

175. Chassevent A, Daver A, Bertrand G, et al. Comparative flow DNA analysis of different cell suspensions in breast carcinoma. Cytometry 1984; 5: 263–267.

176. Ensley JF, Maciorowski, Z, Hassan M, et al. Variations in DNA aneuploid cell content during tumor dissociation in human colon and head and neck cancers analyzed by flow cytometry. Cytometry 1993; 14: 550–558.

177. Zalupski MM, Ryan JR, Ensley JF, et al. Development and optimization of tissue preparative methodology for DNA content analysis of soft tissue neoplasms. Cytometry 1993; 14: 922–930.

178. Konig JJ, van Dongen JW, Schroder FH. Preferential loss of abnormal prostate carcinoma cells by collagenase treatment. Cytometry 1993; 14: 805–810.

179. Vindelov LL, Christensen IJ, Jensen G, et al. Limits of detection of nuclear DNA abnormalities by flow cytometric DNA analysis. Results obtained by a set of methods for sample-storage, staining and internal standardization. Cytology 1983; 3: 332–339.

180. Vindelov LL, Christensen IJ. A review of techniques and results obtained in one laboratory by an integrated system of methods designed for routine clinical flow cytometric DNA analysis. Cytometry 1990; 11: 753–770.

181. Slaper-Cortenbach ICM, Admiraal LG, Kerr JM, et al. Flow cytometric detection of terminal deoxynucleotidyl transferase and other intracellular antigens in combination with membrane antigens in acute lymphatic leukemias. Blood 1988; 72: 1639–1644.

182. Lakhanpal S, Gonchoroff NJ, Kazmann JA, et al. A flow cytofluorometric double staining technique for simultaneous determination of human mononuclear cell surface phenotype and cell cycle phase. J Immunol Methods 1987; 96: 35–40.

183. Schroff RW, Bucana CD, Klein RA, et al. Detection of intracytoplasmic antigens by flow cytometry. J Immunol Methods 1984; 70: 167–177.

184. Jacob MC, Favre M, Bensa J-C. Membrane cell permeabilization with saponin and multiparametric analysis by flow cytometry. Cytometry 1991; 12: 550–558.

185. Zarbo RJ, Visscher DW, Crissman JD. Two-color multiparametric method for flow cytometric DNA analysis of carcinomas using staining for cytokeratin and leukocyte-common antigen. Anal Quant Cytol Histol 1989; 11: 391–402.

186. Zarbo RJ. Quality control issues and technical considerations in flow cytometric DNA and cell cycle analysis of solid tumors. In: Keren DF, Hanson CA, Hurtubise P, eds. Flow cytometry and clinical diagnosis. Chicago: ASCP Press; 1994: 425–469.

187. Brown RD, Zarbo RJ, Linden MD, et al. Two-color multiparametric method for flow cytometric DNA analysis. Standardization of spectral compensation. Am J Clin Pathol 1994; 101: 630–637.

188. Van der Linden JC, Herman CJ, Boenders JGC, et al. Flow cytometric DNA content of fresh tumor specimens using keratin-antibody as second stain for two-parameter analysis. Cytometry 1992; 13: 163–168.

189. Zarbo RJ, Brown RD, Linden MD, et al. Rapid (one-shot) staining method for two-color multiparametric

DNA flow cytometric analysis of carcinomas using staining for cytokeratin and leukocyte common antigen. Am J Clin Pathol 1994; 101: 638–642.

190. Ramaekers FCS, Beck HLM, Fritz WFJ, et al. Application of antibodies to intermediate filament proteins as tissue-specific probes in the flow cytometric analysis of complex tumors. Anal Quant Cytol Histol 1986; 8: 271–280.

191. Myc A, Traganos F, Lara J, et al. DNA stainability in aneuploid breast tumors: comparison of four DNA fluorochromes differing in binding properties. Cytometry 1992; 13: 389–394.

192. Darzynkiewicz Z, Traganos F, Sharpless T, et al. Conformation of RNA in-situ as studied by acridine orange staining and automated cytofluorometry. Exp Cell Res 1975; 95: 143–153.

193. Heidemann W, Schumann J, Andreeff M, et al. Convention on nomenclature for DNA cytometry. Cytometry 1984; 5: 445–446.

194. Iverson OE, Laerum OD. Trout and salmon erythrocytes and human leukocytes as internal standards for ploidy control in flow cytometry. Cytometry 1987; 8: 190–196.

195. Price J, Herman CJ. Reproducibility of FCM DNA content from replicate paraffin block samples. Cytometry 1990; 11: 845–847.

196. Gonchoroff NJ, Ryan JJ, Kimlinger TK, et al. Effect of sonication on paraffin-embedded tissue preparation for DNA flow cytometry. Cytometry 1990; 11: 642–646.

197. Benson NA, Braylan RC. Evaluation of sensitivity in DNA aneuploidy detection using a mathematical model. Cytometry 1994; 15: 53–58.

198. Joensuu H, Alanen KA, Klemi PJ, et al. Evidence for false aneuploid peaks in flow cytometric analysis of paraffin-embedded tissue. Cytometry 1990; 11: 431–437.

199. Joensuu H, Alanen K, Falkmer UG, et al. Effect of DNA ploidy classification on prognosis in breast cancer. Int J Cancer 1992; 52: 701–706.

200. Joensuu H, Kallioniemi O-P. Different opinions on classification of DNA histograms produced from paraffin-embedded tissue. Cytometry 1989; 10: 711–717.

201. Haag D, Feichter G, Goerttler K, et al. Influence of systematic errors on the evaluation of the S phase portions from DNA distributions of solid tumors as shown for 328 breast carcinomas. Cytometry 1987; 8: 377–385.

202. Meyer JS, Coplin MD. Thymidine labeling index, flow cytometric S-phase measurement, and DNA index in human tumors. Am J Clin Pathol 1988; 89: 586–595.

203. Weaver DL, Bagwell CB, Hitchcox SA, et al. Improved flow cytometric determination of proliferative activity (S-phase fraction) from paraffin-embedded tissue. Am J Clin Pathol 1990; 94: 576–584.

204. Kallioniemi O-P, Visakorpi T, Holli K, et al. Improved prognostic impact of S-phase values from paraffin-embedded breast and prostate carcinomas after correcting for nuclear slicing. Cytometry 1991; 12: 413–421.

205. Wersto RP, Stetler-Stevenson M. Debris compensation of DNA histograms and its effect on S-phase analysis. Cytometry 1995; 20: 43–52.

206. Silvestrini R. Quality control for evaluation of the S-phase fraction by flow cytometry: a multicentric study. The SICCAB Group for Quality Control of Cell Kinetic Determinations. Cytometry 1994; 18: 11–16.

207. Rabinovitch PS. Practical considerations for DNA content and cell cycle analysis. In: Bauer KD, Duque RE, Shankey TV, eds. Clinical flow cytometry: principles and applications. Baltimore: Williams & Wilkins; 1993: 117–142.

208. Bagwell CB. Theoretical aspects of flow cytometry data analysis. In: Bauer KD, Duque RE, Shankey TV, eds. Clinical flow cytometry: principles and applications. Baltimore: Williams & Wilkins; 1993: 41–61.

209. Kallioniemi O-P, Visakorpi T, Holli K, et al. Automated peak detection and cell cycle analysis of flow cytometric DNA histograms. Cytometry 1994; 16: 250–255.

210. Zarbo RJ, Nakhleh RE, Brown R, et al. Prognostic significance of flow cytometry (FCM) synthetic phase fraction (SPF) in 168 cytokeratin (CK) stained colorectal carcinomas (abstract). Mod Pathol 1995; 8: 71A.

211. Wheeless LL, Coon JS, Cox C, et al. Measurement variability in DNA flow cytometry of replicate samples. Cytometry 1989; 10: 731–738.

212. Coon JS, Deitch AD, de Vere White RW, et al. Interinstitutional variability in DNA flow cytometric analysis of tumors. The National Cancer Institute's Flow Cytometry Network experience. Cancer 1988; 61: 126–130.

213. Coon JS, Deitch AD, de Vere White RW, et al. Check samples for laboratory self-assessment in DNA flow cytometry. The National Cancer Institute's Flow Cytometry Network experience. Cancer 1989; 63: 1592–1599.

214. Wheeless LL, Coon JS, Cox C, et al. Precision of DNA flow cytometry in interinstitutional analyses. Cytometry 1991; 12: 405–412.

215. Kallioniemi O-P, Joensuu H, Klemi P, et al. Inter-laboratory comparison of DNA flow cytometric results from paraffin-embedded breast carcinomas. Breast Cancer Res Treat 1990; 17: 59–61.

216. Danesi DT, Spano M, Altavista P. Quality control study of the Italian Group of Cytometry on flow cytometry cellular DNA content measurements. Cytometry 1993; 14: 576–583.

217. Homburger HA, McCarthy R, Deodhar S. Assessment of interlaboratory variability in analytical cytology. Results of College of American Pathologists flow cytometry study. Arch Pathol Lab Med 1989; 113: 667–672.

218. Coon JS, Paxton H, Lucy L, et al. Interlaboratory variation in DNA flow cytometry. Results of the College of American Pathologists' survey. Arch Pathol Lab Med 1994; 118: 681–685.

219. Frierson HF Jr. The need for improvement in flow cytometric analysis of ploidy and S-phase fraction 9 (editorial). Am J Clin Pathol 1995; 95: 439–441.

220. Brotherick I, Lennard TWJ, Cook S, et al. Use of the biotinylated antibody DAKO-ER ID5 to measure oestrogen receptor and cytokeratin positive cells obtained from primary breast cancer cells. Cytometry 1995; 20: 74–80.

221. Martin-Reay DG, Kamentsky LA, Weinberg DS, et al. Evaluation of a new slide-based laser scanning cytometer for DNA analysis of tumors. Comparison with flow cytometry and image analysis. Am J Clin Pathol 1994; 102: 432–438.

222. Weinberg DW. Relative applicability of image analysis and flow cytometry in clinical medicine. In: Bauer KD, Duque RE, Sharkey TV, eds. Flow cytometry: principles and applications. Baltimore: Williams & Wilkins; 1993: 359–371.

223. Gill J. Image analysis in pathology: what are the issues? Hum Pathol 1989; 20: 203–204.

224. Inoue S. Video microscopy. New York: Plenum; 1986.

225. Wells WA, Rainer RO, Memoli VA. Basic principles of image processing. Am J Clin Pathol 1992; 98: 493–501.

226. Bauer TW, Tubbs RR, Edinger MG, et al. A prospective comparison of DNA quantitation by image and flow cytometry. Am J Clin Pathol 1990; 93: 322–326.

227. Chabanas A, Rambeaud JJ, Seigneurin D, et al. Flow and image cytometry for DNA analysis in bladder washings: improved concordance by using internal reference for flow. Cytometry 1993; 14: 943–950.

228. Claud RD, Weinstein RS, Howeedy A, et al. Comparison of image analysis of imprints with flow cytometry for DNA analysis of solid tumors. Mod Pathol 1989; 2: 463–467.

229. Colombel MC, Pous MF, Abbou CC et al. Computer assisted image analysis of bladder tumour nuclei for

230. Wilbur DC, Zakowski MF, Kosciol CM, et al. DNA ploidy in breast lesions: a comparative study using two commercial image analysis systems and flow cytometry. Anal Quant Cytol Histol 1990; 12: 28–34.

231. Wojcik EM, Katz RL, Johnston DA, et al. Comparative analysis of DNA ploidy and proliferative index in fine needle aspirates of non-Hodgkin's lymphomas by image analysis and flow cytometry. Anal Quant Cytol Histol 1993; 15: 151–157.

232. Danque PO, Chen HB, Patil J, et al. Image analysis versus flow cytometry for DNA ploidy quantitation of solid tumors: a comparison of six methods of sample preparation. Mod Pathol 1993; 6: 270–275.

233. Dawson AE, Norton JA, Weinberg DS. Comparative assessment of proliferation and DNA content in breast carcinoma by image analysis and flow cytometry. Am J Pathol 1990; 136: 1115–1124.

234. Taylor SR, Zachariah S, Chakraborty S, et al. Ploidy studies by image analysis on fine needle aspirates of the breast. Acta Cytol 1993; 37: 923–928.

235. Pindur A, Chakraborty S, Wheeler TM. DNA ploidy measurements in prostate cancer: differences between image analysis and flow cytometry and clinical implications. Prostate 1994; 25: 189–198.

236. Bauer KD, Merkel DE, Winter JN, et al. Prognostic implications of ploidy and proliferative activity in diffuse large cell lymphomas. Cancer Res 1986; 46: 3173–3178.

237. Michie BA, Black C, Reid RP, et al. Image analysis derived ploidy and proliferation indices in soft tissue sarcomas: comparison with clinical outcome. J Clin Pathol 1994; 47: 443–447.

238. Weinberg DS. Proliferation indices in solid tumors. Adv Pathol Lab Med 1992; 5: 163.

239. Bravo R. Synthesis of the nuclear protein cyclin (PCNA) and its relationship with DNA replication. Exp Cell Res 1986; 163: 287–293.

240. Schwartz BR, Pinkus G, Bacus S, et al. Cell proliferation in non-Hodgkin's lymphomas: digital image analysis of Ki-67 staining. Am J Pathol 1989; 134: 327–336.

241. Pesce CM. Defining and interpreting diseases through morphometry. Lab Invest 1987; 56: 568–575.

242. Allred DC, Bustamante M, Daniel CO, et al. Immunocytochemical analysis of estrogen receptors in human breast carcinomas: evaluation of 130 cases and a review of the literature regarding concordance with the biochemical assay and clinical relevance. Arch Surg 1990; 125: 107–113.

243. Auger M, Katz RL, Johnston DA, et al. Quantitation of immunocytochemical estrogen and progesterone receptor content in the fine needle aspirates of breast carcinoma using the SAMBA 4000 image analysis system. Anal Quant Cytol Histol 1993; 15: 274–280.

244. Bacus S, Flowers JL, Press MF, et al. The evaluation of estrogen receptor in primary breast carcinoma by computer-assisted image analysis. Am J Clin Pathol 1988; 90: 233–239.

245. Bacus SS, Chin D, Stern RK, et al. HER-2/neu oncogene expression, DNA ploidy and proliferation index in breast cancers. Anal Quant Cytol Histol 1992; 14: 433–445.

246. Grogan T, Dalton W, Rybski J, et al. Optimization of immunocytochemical P-glycoprotein assessment in multidrug-resistant plasma cell myeloma using three antibodies. Lab Invest 1991; 63: 815–824.

247. Castleman KR, Chui LA, Martin TP, et al. Quantitative muscle biopsy analysis. Monogr Clin Cytol 1984; 9: 101.

248. Wied GL, Bartels PH, Bahr GF, et al. Taxonomic intracellular system (TICAS) for cell identification. Acta Cytol 1968; 12: 180–204.

249. Wied GL, Bartels PH, Bibbo M, et al. Image analysis in quantitative cytopathology and histopathology. Hum Pathol 1989; 20: 549–571.

250. Baisch H, Goehde W, Linden W. Analysis of PCP-date to determine the fraction of cells in the various phases of the cycle. Radiat Environ Biophys 1975; 12: 31–37.

251. Dean P, Jett J. Mathematical analysis of DNA distributions derived from flow microfluorometry. J Cell Biol 1974; 60: 523–527.

252. Mitelman F. Recurrent chromosome aberrations in cancer. Mutation Rea 200; 462: 247–253.

253. Chen Z, Sandberg AA. Molecular cytogenetic aspects of hematological malignancies. Clinical implications. Am J Med Genetics 2002; 115: 130–141.

254. Sandberg AA. Cytogenetics and molecular genetics of bone and soft tissue tumors. Am J Med Genetics (Semin Med Genet) 2002; 115: 189–193.

255. Gosden JR. Chromosome analysis protocols (methods in molecular biology). Totawa, NJ: Humana Press; 1994.

256. Loda M., DeLellis RA. Molecular diagnostic techniques (Chapter 6). In: Silverberg SG, DeLellis RA, Frable WJ, eds. Principles and practice of surgical pathology and cytopathology. 3rd edn. New York: Churchill Livingstone; 1997: 77–94.

257. Hanahan D, Weinberg R. The hallmarks of cancer. Cell 2000; 100: 57–70.

258. Knudson AG. Antioncogenes and human cancer. Proc Natl Acad Sci USA 1993; 90: 10914–10921.

259. Dubeau L, Chandler LA, Gralow JR, et al. Southern blot analysis of DNA extracted from formalin-fixed pathology specimens. Cancer Res 1986; 46: 2964–2969.

260. Wright CF, Reid AH. Hybridization and blotting techniques. In: O'Leary, ed. Advanced methods in pathology. principles, practice and protocols. Philadelphia: Saunders; 2003: 3–91.

261. Southern E. Detection of specific sequences among DNA fragments separated by gel electrophoresis. J Mol Biol 1975; 98: 503–517.

262. Seeger RC, Brodeur GM, Sather H, et al. Association of multiple copies of the N-myc oncogene with rapid progression of neuroblastomas. N Engl J Med 1985; 313: 1111–1116.

263. Cossman J, Zehnbauer B, Garrett CT, et al. Gene rearrangements in the diagnosis of lymphoma/leukemia. Guidelines for use based on a multiinstitutional study. Am J Clin Path 1991; 95: 347–354.

264. Ladanyi M, Bridge JA. Contribution of molecular genetic data to the classification of sarcomas. Human Pathol 2000; 31: 532–538.

265. El-Naggar A. Methods in molecular surgical pathology. Sem Diag Pathol 2000; 219: 56–72.

266. Blomek B, Shields PG. Laboratory methods for the determination of genetic polymorphisms in humans. IARC Sci Publ 1999; 148: 133–147.

267. Erlich HA, Gelfand D, Sninsky JJ. Recent advances in the polymerase chain reaction. Science 1991; 252: 1643–1651.

268. Holland PM, Abramson RD, Watson R, et al. Detection of specific polymerase chain reaction product by utilizing the 5' exonuclease activity of thermus aquaticus DNA polymerase. Proc Natl Acad Sci USA 1991; 88: 7276–7280.

269. Liu H, Huang X, Zhang Y, et al. Archival fixed histologic and cytological specimens including stained and unstained materials are amenable to RT-PCR. Diagn Mol Pathol. 2002; 11: 222–227.

270. Sestini R, Orlando C, Zentilin L, et al. Gene amplification for c-erbB-2, c-myc, epidermal growth factor receptor, int-2 and N-myc measured by quantitative PCR with a multiple competitor template. Clin Chem 1995; 41: 826–832.

271. Cerutti P, Hussain P, Pourzand C, et al. Mutagenesis of the H-ras protooncogene and the p53 tumor suppressor gene. Cancer Res 1994; 54(7 Suppl): 1934s–1938s.

272. Griesser H. Applied molecular genetics in the diagnosis of malignant non-Hodgkin's lymphoma. Diagn Mol Pathol 1993; 2: 177–191.

273. Hodinka RL. The clinical utility of viral quantitation using molecular methods. Clin Diagn Virol 1998; 10: 25–47.

274. Osaki M, Adachi H, Gomyo Y, et al. Detection of mycobacterial DNA in formalin-fixed, paraffin embedded tissue specimens by duplex polymerase chain reaction: application to histopathologic diagnosis. Mod Pathol 1997; 10: 78–83.

275. Edwards MC, Gibbs RA. Multiplex PCR: advantages, development and applications. PCR Methods Appl 1994; 3: S65–S75.

276. Wang A, Doyle M, Mark DF. Quantitation of mRNA by the polymerase chain reaction. Proc Natl Acad Sci USA 1989; 86: 9717–9721.

277. Salomon RN. Introduction to reverse transcriptase polymerase chain reaction. Diag Mol Pathol 1995; 4: 2–3.

278. Ghossein RA, Rosai, J. Polymerase chain reaction in the detection of micrometastases and circulating tumor cells. Cancer 1996; 78: 10–16.

279. Loda M. Polymerase chain reaction-based methods for the detection of point mutations in oncogenes and tumor suppressor genes. Hum Pathol 1994; 25: 564–571.

280. Crotty PL, Staggs RA, Porter PT. Quantitative analysis in molecular diagnostics. Hum Pathol 1994; 25: 572–579.

281. Sandin RL, Greene JN. Diagnostic molecular pathology and infectious disease. Cancer Control 1995; 2: 255–257.

282. Loda M, Giangaspero F, Badiali M, et al. P53 gene expression in medulloblastoma by quantitative polymerase chain reaction. Diang Mol Pathol 1992; 1: 36–41.

283. Gibson UE, Heid CA, Williams PM. A novel method for real-time quantitative RT-PCR. Genome Res 1996; 6: 995–1001.

284. Abravaya K, Huff J, Marshall R, et al. Molecular beacons as diagnostic tools: technology and applications. Clin Chem Lab Med 2003; 41: 468–474.

285. Nuovo GJ. Co-labeling using in-situ PCR: A review. J Histochem Cytochem 2001; 49: 1329–1339.

286. DeLellis RS. In situ hybridization techniques for the analysis of gene expression. Applications in tumor pathology. Human Pathol 1994; 25: 580–585.

287. Yap EPH, Martinez-Montero JC, McGee JO'D. mRNA detection in clinical samples by non-isotopic in situ hybridization. In: Herrington CS, McGee JO'D, eds. Diagnostic molecular pathology. a practical approach. Oxford: IRL Press; 1992.

288. Holm R, Karlsen F, Nesland JM. In situ hybridization with non-isotopic probes using different detection systems. Mod Pathol 1992; 5: 315–319.

289. McDougall JK, Myerson D, Beckmann AM. Detection of viral DNA and RNA by in-situ hybridization. J Histochem Cytochem 1986; 34: 33–38.

290. Niedobitek G, Finn T, Herbst H, et al. Detection of viral DNA by in situ hybridization using bromodeoxyuridine labeled probes. Am J Pathol 1988; 131: 1–4.

291. Park JS, Kurman RJ, Kessis TD, et al. Comparison of peroxidase-labeled DNA probes with radioactive RNA probes for detection of human papilloma-viruses by in situ hybridization in paraffin sections. Mod Pathol 1991; 4: 81–85.

292. Hilborne LH, Nieberg RK, Cheng L, et al. Direct in-situ hybridization for rapid detection of cytomegalovirus in bronchial lavage. Am J Clin Path 1987; 87: 766–769.

293. Shapsak P, Sun NC, Resnick L, et al. The detection of HIV by in situ hybridization. Mod Pathol 1990; 3: 146–153.

294. Bashir R, Hochberg F, Singer RH. Detection of Epstein-Barr virus by in situ hybridization. Progress towards development of a non-isotopic diagnostic test. Am J Pathol 1989; 135: 1035–1044.

295. Li JJ, Huang YQ, Cockerell CJ, et al. Localization of human herpes-like virus 8 in vascular endothelial cells and perivascular spindle-shaped cells of Kaposi's sarcoma lesions by in situ hybridization. Am J Pathol 1996; 148: 1741–1748.

296. Hayden RT, Isotalo PA, Parrett T, et al. In situ hybridization for the differentiation of Aspergillus, Fusarium and Pseudallescheria species in tissue sections. Diagn Mol Pathol 2003; 12: 21–26.

297. Slamon DJ, Godolphin W, Jones LA, et al. Studies of the Her-2/neu proto-oncogene in human breast and ovarian cancer. Science 1989; 244: 707–742.

298. Walker RA, Senior PV, Jones JL, et al. An immunohistochemical and in situ hybridization study of c-myc and c-erbB2 expression in primary human breast carcinomas. J Pathol 1989; 158: 97–105.

299. Weiss LM, Movahed LA, Chen YY, et al. Detection of immunoglobin light chain mRNA in lymphoid tissues using a practical in situ hybridization method. Am J Pathol 1990; 137: 979–988.

300. Krishna M, Lloyd RV, Batts KP. Detection of albumin messenger RNA in hepatic and extrahepatic neoplasms. A marker of hepatocellular differentiation. Am J Surg Pathol 1997; 21: 147–152,.

301. Lloyd R. Introduction to molecular endocrine pathology. Endocr Pathol 1993; 4: 64–72.

302. Wolman SR. Fluorescence in situ hybridization. A new tool for the pathologist. Hum Pathol 1994; 25: 586–590.

303. Lee W, Han K, Harris CP, et al. Use of FISH to detect chromosomal translocations and deletions. Analysis of chromosome rearrangements in synovial sarcoma cells from paraffin embedded specimens. Am J Pathol 1993; 143: 15–19.

304. Shapiro DN, Valentine MB, Rowe ST, et al. Detection of N-myc gene amplification by fluorescence in situ hybridization. Diagnostic utility for neuroblastoma. Am J Pathol 1993; 142: 1339–1346.

305. Strefford JC, Lillington DM, Young BD, et al. The use of multicolor fluorescence technologies in the characterization of prostate carcinoma cell lines: A comparison of multiplex fluorescence in situ hybridization and spectral karyotyping data. Cancer Genet Cytogenet 2001; 124: 112–121.

306. Tanner M, Gancberg D, Di Leo A, et al. Chromogenic in situ hybridization: a practical alternative for fluorescence in situ hybridization to detect HER-2/neu oncogene amplification in archival breast cancer samples. Am J Pathol 2000; 157: 1467–1472.

307. Kallioniemi A, Kallioniemi OP, Sudar D, et al. Comparative genomic hybridization for molecular cytogenetic analysis of solid tumors. Science 1992; 258: 818–821.

308. Golub TR, Slonim DK, Tamayo P, et al. Molecular classification of cancer: class discovery and class prediction by gene expression monitoring. Science 1999; 286: 531–537.

309. Emmet-Buck MR, Strausberg RL, Kritzman DB, et al. Molecular profiling of clinical tissue specimens. Feasibility and applications. J Mol Diagn 2000; 2: 60–66.

310. Rosenwald A, Wright G, Chan WC, et al. The use of molecular profiling to predict survival after chemotherapy for diffuse large B-cell lymphoma. New Engl J Med 2002; 346: 1937–1947.

311. Gabrielson E, Berg K, Anbazhagan R. Functional genomics, gene arrays and the future of pathology. Mod Pathol 2001; 14: 1294–1299.

312. Giordano TJ, Shedden KA, Swartz DR, et al. Organ-specific molecular classification of primary lung, colon and ovarian adenocarcinomas using gene expression profiles. Am J Pathol 2001; 159: 1231–1238.

313. Bassett DE Jr, Eisen MB, Boguski MS. Gene expression informatics – it's all in your mind. Nature Genet 1999; 21(1 Suppl): 51–55.

314. Alizadeh AA, Eisen MB, Davis RE, et al. Distinct types of diffuse large B-cell lymphoma identified by gene expression profiling. Nature 2000; 403: 503–511.

315. Bertucci F, Viens P, Tagett R, et al. DNA arrays in clinical oncology: promises and challenges. Lab Invest 2003; 83: 305–316.

316. Ahrendt SA, Halachmi S, Chow JT, et al. Rapid p53 sequence analysis in primary lung cancer using an oligonucleotide probe array. Proc Natl Acad Sci USA 1999; 96: 7382–7387.

317. Kozal MJ, Shah N, Shen N, et al. Extensive polymorphisms observed in HIV-1 clade B protease gene using high-density oligonucleotide arrays. Nat Med 1996; 2: 753–759.

318. Jeffreys AJ, Wilson V, Thein SL. Hypervariable 'minisatellite' regions in human DNA. Nature 1985; 31: 467–472.

319. De la Chapelle A. Microsatellite instability. New Engl J Med 2003; 349: 209–210.

320. Wooster R, Cleton-Jansen AM, Collins N, et al. Instability of short tandem repeats (microsatellites) in human cancers. Nature Genet 1994; 6: 152–156.

321. Loeb LA. Cancer cells exhibit a mutator phenotype. Adv Cancer Res. 1998; 72: 25–56.

322. Liu B, Nicolaides NC, Markowitz S, et al. Mismatch repair gene defects in sporadic colorectal cancers with microsatellite instability. Nature Genet 1995; 9: 48–55.

323. Naidoo R, Chetty R. The application of microsatellites in molecular pathology. Pathol Oncol Res 1998; 4: 310–315.

324. Jones PA, Baylin SB. The fundamental role of epigenetic events in cancer. Nat Rev Genet 2002; 3: 415–428.

325. Liu ZJ, Maekawa M. Polymerase chain reaction-based methods of DNA methylation analysis. Anal Biochem 2003; 317: 259–265.

326. Jones PA. Epigenetics in carcinogenesis and cancer prevention. Ann NY Acad Sci 2003; 983: 213–219.

327. Diaz-Cano SJ, Blanes A, Wolfe HJ. PCR techniques for clonality assays. Diagn Mol Pathol 2001; 10: 24–33.

Conditions involving multiple organs

Infectious disease pathology

Margie A. Scott   Washington C. Winn, Jr.   William J. Frable

3

The importance of infectious disease pathology for the practicing anatomic pathologist has grown enormously over the past 25 years. This is primarily due to the ever-expanding number of moderate to severely immunocompromised patients within the general population that we serve. Modern life-sustaining technologies, expanding chemotherapeutic protocols, immunosuppressive drugs and transplantation medicine has forced us to consider many infectious agents, previously thought to be innocent bystanders, as potential life threatening pathogens.[1] The discovery of the human immunodeficiency virus (HIV) as the causative agent of the acquired immunodeficiency syndrome (AIDS) in 1983 by Montagnier and Gallo represents a critical milestone in re-establishing the importance of infectious disease pathology. The anatomic pathologist now faces yet another type of medical emergency – the need for rapid, reliable, criteria-based diagnosis of unculturable agents such as HIV, hantavirus, *Pneumocystis jirovecii (carinii), Microsporidium* and *Cyclospora*. In fact, the 'at risk' population of immunosuppressed patients continues to grow each year as medical protocols designed for treatment of autoimmune disorders and maintenance of both bone marrow and solid organ transplantation continue to evolve.[2] With the advent of new imaging technology such as spiral CT scans, smaller and smaller nodules are being targeted for needle aspiration or surgical resection with frozen section to rule out malignancy. Sometimes these lesions turn out to be granulomas or abscesses excised without rapid assessment, thus missing the opportunity for fungal and mycobacterial cultures. In the cytology laboratory, as clinicians embrace the rapid and reliable technique of fine-needle aspiration, we find ourselves called upon to aspirate lymph nodes and superficial nodules which may represent a bacterial abscess, mycobacterial granuloma, or the ever-elusive cat-scratch disease. The charge for the anatomic pathologist in today's era of infectious disease pathology is three-fold; we are expected to:

1. optimize opportunities to intervene and guide in collection of appropriate cultures based upon rapid evaluation techniques within the surgical pathology and cytology laboratories;
2. maximize availability of limited tissue samples for multiple diagnostic modalities, including molecular techniques, by using a systematic approach to the laboratory work-up; and
3. formulate final anatomic diagnoses that correlate clinical history with histologic findings, special stains, immunohistochemistry, follow-up cultures, and molecular studies.

THE PATHOLOGY-BASED INFECTIOUS DISEASE TEAM: MICROBIOLOGIST, CYTOPATHOLOGIST, AND SURGICAL PATHOLOGIST

The goals and approaches used by the microbiologist, cytopathologist, and surgical pathologist are more similar than many realize. In this modern age of computer technology and information access, we should maximize the opportunity to share our expertise in order to provide the most complete final diagnostic summary possible. No longer are we required to walk down the hall or to another building in order to determine what the microbiology direct smears or cultures have revealed. A simple computer click, and the information is instantly available for review. The 'old-fashioned' telephone call is still quite appreciated by many because it allows communication of details and pending follow-up testing. The unique goals and the common roles of each of these three counterparts of the diagnostic pathology infectious disease team are illustrated below.

The microbiologist is an expert in the subcellular realm of the pathogen, meticulously tracking and exploring intracellular or extracellular single-cell pathogens and highlighting phenotypic characteristics that allow clinicians to eradicate an organism and thus thwart a human disease. The microbiologist deals routinely with body fluids, aspirate samples, and tissue samples. The first goal is usually a direct search for organisms using Gram stain methods, which allows for rapid evaluation of both the tissue inflammatory background and whether Gram-positive or Gram-negative organisms are present. The distribution of these organisms and the inflammatory background help guide the microbiologist in determining whether additional stains, medias, or culture conditions should be added to the work-up. Without conscience effort, the microbiologist has traversed the boundary that crosses into the realm of surgical pathology and cytopathology. Primary microbiology evaluation tools include the Gram stain, acid-fast stain, KOH prep, and calcofluor white stain. The second goal of the microbiologist is to ensure a homogeneous sampling of the submitted tissues and fluids in order to allow uniform inoculation onto all medias, broths, and types of culture environments needed for the case. In a sense this is similar to the goals of the cytopathologist and surgical pathologist as we try to ensure all appropriate representative materials are sampled and submitted for processing and microscopic evaluation. The third goal of the microbiologist is to use colony morphology, phenotypic biochemical expression, and antimicrobial sensitivities for a definitive organism identification and characterization to guide antimicrobial therapy.

The cytopathologist is the expert at the cellular reaction level. Cytopathology adds to the depth of infectious disease assessment by evaluating in great detail the cellular response patterns, noting inflammatory components, cytopathic effects, and the presence or absence of organisms. An ever-present first goal of the cytopathologist is to ensure that samples are evaluated for the possibility of malignancy. Samples submitted for cytopathology are usually easily collected with minimal risk to the patient. Basic tools of the cytopathologist include rapid staining methods such as the Wright stains, hematoxylin and eosin stains, and toluidine blue stains. The second goal of the cytopathologist is to ensure that the specimens submitted are adequately sampled and processed in a timely fashion. Fine-needle aspiration samples or generously cellular body fluids are easily assessed using a combination of smears, cytospin preparations, and cell blocks. All of these can be used for a host of routine and special staining techniques. In the event that an infectious etiology is suspected, additional air-dried smears or cytospin preparations can be set aside for organism stains. The final goal is for cytopathologists to apply their unique expertise for a complete descriptive diagnosis reflecting the cellular changes and, when possible, the infectious etiologic agent. When a definitive agent is not identified, the cellular changes, such as ciliocytophthoria (characteristic ciliated respiratory epithelial cell breakage pattern associated with respiratory viral infections) with parainfluenza infection or proteinaceous alveolar casts of *Pneumocystis jirovecii (carinii)* infection, can narrow the etiologic categories for a more focused work-up. Like the microbiologist, the cytopathologist focuses on the organism in question, but takes s step further with an analysis of the cellular background in which the organism resides.

The surgical pathologist is the expert of the tissue reaction pattern and host response level, patching together the overall histologic picture and in the ideal circumstances visualizing the offending pathogen. The surgical pathologist plays a pivotal role in the recognition of infectious agents, particularly those that are rare, unexpected, and unculturable. It is usually in emergent situations or when the patient care team has exhausted all other methods for clarifying the diagnosis, that the invasive step of a tissue biopsy is undertaken. When infection is suspected, both cytology sampling and cultures usually accompany tissue biopsies. Sometimes, however, the clinical picture is heavily biased towards malignancy and tissue biopsies are obtained and immediately fixed, negating the possibility of cultures for that particular sample. Under these circumstances when the window of opportunity has passed, and cultures are not obtained, it is still possible for the surgical pathologist to make a definitive diagnosis. It is dependent upon demonstration of the causative agent, recognition of the incited host immune response, and a systematic approach of tissue examination, using both routine and special stains. The expertise of the surgical pathologist is key in solving many of the uncommon, but clinically critical mysteries. In the spectrum of infectious diseases, the microbiologist, cytopathologist, and surgical pathologist are all seeking the same final answer. Their evaluation paths overlap and strengthen each other in many aspects and their final goal is to make a definitive diagnosis of the infectious disease and causative pathogen at hand.

The diagnosis of infectious diseases is truly a multidisciplinary cooperative endeavor involving the surgical pathologist, cytologist, microbiologist, and the clinician, especially the infectious disease consultant. A clinician faced with classic chickenpox in an immunocompetent patient does not require laboratory support for the diagnosis. The microbiologist who isolates *Mycobacterium tuberculosis* knows that the etiology of a disease has been established and understands the public health concerns leading to the subsequent infection control measures. Similarly, the surgical pathologist who views the diagnostic spherules of *Coccidioides immitis* can define the etiologic agent as well as describe the host response and anticipated extent of disease. Far more often, however, the activities of the principal players are complementary and synergistic.

This chapter is designed to consider infectious disease pathology from three distinct but equally important interconnecting viewpoints. Part one considers diagnostic techniques and approaches to organism identification and some unique aspects inherent to specific infectious disease agent groups or families. Part two considers the host defense mechanisms and expected host tissue reactions in response to each of these groups. Part three examines unique infectious disease pathology considerations within most major organ systems. All of these viewpoints are mutually dependent and intricately linked to the daily practice of infectious disease pathology for both the cytopathologist and surgical pathologist. The final part will consider unique opportunities for optimizing diagnostic certainty through the practical use of molecular techniques.

PART I: DIAGNOSTIC TECHNIQUES AND UNIQUE ASPECTS OF INFECTIOUS AGENTS

The microbial world is composed of a vast spectrum of organisms. Only a small number of these organisms interfere with normal human daily activities and function. Bacteria are an integral part of our existence and our normal human host defense mechanisms could not operate effectively without them. Within days of birth, our gastrointestinal system becomes colonized with mixed aerobic and anaerobic bacterial forms that aid in our ability to produce sufficient quantities of vitamin K, which facilitate the production of coagulation factors. The normal bacterial flora of the oropharynx, nasopharynx, skin, and mucocutaneous surfaces help ward off potential pathogens that we may accidentally encounter during our daily activities. Even mucocutaneous fungal forms, such as *Candida*, in sparing quantities, can be beneficial to maintaining normal healthy surface conditions. Many infectious agents that perplex the anatomic pathologist, actually represent 'accidental encounters' of a human instead of the intended animal host. Examples of these include the vector transmitted encephalitis viruses such as eastern equine encephalitis virus (EEE), western equine encephalitis virus (WEE), and Venezuelan equine encephalitis virus (VEE).

DIAGNOSTIC TECHNIQUES

Approaches to the establishment of an etiology for an infectious process are summarized in Table 3.1. The clinical impression leads to the formulation of an initial hypothesis that is communicated to others on the team in hopes of expediting confirmation of the leading diagnosis. Once the specimens have been collected, the microbiologist, cytopathologist, and surgical pathologist focus on the tasks within their areas of expertise.

Gross examination
Careful inspection and gross examination of the specimen submitted includes: documenting that the specimen is properly labeled and attributed to the patient in question; examining the specimen to search for areas of heterogeneity so that all lesional areas within the submitted specimen are thoroughly sampled; and submitting the most appropriate tissues for expeditious initiation of cultures, cytology and/or surgical pathology.

Rapid direct examination
Touch imprints, direct smears, tissue scrape, or squash preps can all be used for preparation of either fixed or air-dried slides. Air-dried slides can be set aside and reserved for potential use for Gram stains, acridine orange stains, and Wright stains. Fixed slides can be used for rapid assessment with hematoxylin and eosin stains or toluidine blue stains. When making direct touch preparations from specimens such as solid organ wedge biopsies, it is often helpful to first gently blot the surface with an absorbent material, to remove excessive blood and tissue fluid that may obscure the cellular surface underneath that one needs to examine. It is essential that an adequate number of

Table 3.1 Approaches to the etiologic diagnosis of infectious diseases

Diagnostic method	Technique	Specimen required	Advantages	Disadvantages	Comments
Clinical diagnosis	Clinical history, travel history, occupational, history, other data	None	Provides clues to exposure or risk factors	Rarely provides etiologic diagnosis	
Morphologic diagnosis	Histologic sections: H&E	Fresh or fixed tissue	Essential information on host response and other disease processes	Usually not etiologically specific	
Morphologic diagnosis	Histologic sections or smears; histochemistry	Fresh or fixed tissue or smears	Defines morphology of some agents and relation of agent to host response	Often provides only a presumptive diagnosis	Non-specificity an advantage if the likely agent is not known
Immunologic diagnosis	Histologic sections or smears: immuno-fluorescence or immunoenzyme assay	Fresh or fixed tissue or smears	Definitive identification of some agents	Must know target antigens; limited library of commercial reagents	Some antigens altered by fixation, especially with fluorescence, requiring pretreatment
Molecular diagnosis	Histologic sections or smears; in situ hybridization	Fresh or fixed tissue or smears	Definitive identification of some agents	Limited availability of commercial reagents	Must know precise target; costly
Molecular diagnosis	Amplification techniques (e.g. PCR, LCR)	Fresh tissue or paraffin blocks	Definitive identification	Limited availability	Must know precise target; costly; some still in research stages

H&E, hematoxylin and eosin; PCR, polymerase chain reaction; LCR, Ligase chain reaction.

touch preparations be made before the specimen is placed into formalin. There is no turning back once the specimen is plunged into fixatives. It is often easier to examine a thin smear or touch preparation for infectious agents than to search through the planes of a 3–5-μm thick section with a histochemical stain.

Histochemical stains

A variety of histochemical stains can be used for evaluation of infectious agents.[3] None is specific, but in combination with the morphology of the organism, the host response, and the clinical history, a presumptive etiologic diagnosis may often be rendered with a high level of certainty. The Gram stain remains the most useful rapid diagnostic technique in the microbiology laboratory. Similarly, the hematoxylin and eosin (H&E) stain remains the mainstay of the histology laboratory and surgical pathologist. For the cytologist the Wright stain and Papanicolaou stains are the mainstay. The most common histochemical stains used for detection of infectious agents in smears and tissues are summarized in Table 3.2. An excellent reference book for the histology laboratory is the text by Prophet et al.[4] A great deal of care and expertise goes into the preparation of high-quality special stains and each histology laboratory is challenged by the diversity of stains ordered in any one given day by a busy pathology department. Whenever possible, it is best to use a limited number of special stains and order them often in order to hone the skills of the histology team and provide a consistent reliable product for review and interpretations by the pathologist.

Bacteria

The premier method for histochemical detection of bacteria in smears and tissues remains the Gram stain, described over 100 years ago by a Danish microbiologist, Hans Christian Gram. The advantage of this simple method is that it differentiates bacteria into two groups: Gram-positives (those that retain crystal violet after treatment with iodine and decolorization with alcohol); and Gram-negatives (those that release crystal violet upon decolorization with alcohol). Saffranin, a red counterstain, is then applied to color the cellular material and the Gram-negative bacteria. Addition of 0.05% acid fuchsin to the counterstain enhances the staining of pale, fastidious Gram-negative bacteria. Several modifications of the Gram stain exist and each has its own particular strengths. The Brown-Hopps[5] is acclaimed by many as the best stain to use when searching for the elusive fastidious Gram-negative rods of organisms such as *Yersinia* and *Bartonella*. The Gram-positive organisms are easily identified in comparison to the small Gram negatives. Other Gram stains that may be employed include the Brown Brenn, MacCallum-Goodpasture, and the Twart methods. A good test of the sensitivity of the Gram stain method is to use tissue infected with *Brucella* or *Legionella* as a control. The easiest control may be colonic tissues to display *Enterobacteriacea*; however, visualization of these organisms does not ensure that one will be able to detect the fastidious small Gram-negative rods. Also, it is good to remember that tissue section Gram stains will display more stain variability with the Gram-positives compared to culture smears. As the Gram-positive organisms die within the tissue, they lose the ability to retain crystal violet in their cell walls, thus leaching out the crystal violet to become 'pinkish' Gram-positives. This is simply a phenomenon caused by the degeneration of the cell wall and should not be reason to suspect mixed infection or poor histology techniques. Tissue section Gram stains are thin slices through three-dimensional specimens, thus cross-sections, longitudinal sections, and oblique sections of organisms will artifactually enhance the degree of organism morphologic variability.

The second important group of bacterial stains comprises the silver impregnation stains, originally designed for *Treponema pallidum* that do not stain by the Gram method. The Warthin-Starry, Levaditi, Dieterle, and Steiner methods provide essentially similar results. Any one of these stains may help in identifying the fastidious

Table 3.2 Histochemical stains for demonstrating infectious organisms

Stain	Cytologic (C) or histologic (H)	Intended organisms	Other possible organisms	Artifacts	Comments
Gram stain	C	Bacteria	Some yeasts and molds; rarely *Pneumocystis*	Stain debris (Gram-positives) fibrin (Gram-negatives)	First choice for demonstration of bacteria
Gimenez stain	C, H (frozens)	Bacteria, rickettsiae			Uncommonly used
Brown and Brenn	H	Bacteria	Some yeasts and molds	Mast cell granules; cell debris (Gram-positive); fibrin, cell membranes (Gram-negative)	Best for Gram-positives
Brown-Hopps	H	Bacteria	Some yeasts and molds	See Brown and Brenn	Best for Gram-negatives
MacCallum-Goodpasture	H	Bacteria	Some yeasts and molds	See Brown and Brenn	Uncommonly used
Silver impregnation stains (Warthin-Starry, Dieterle, Levaditi, Steiner)	C, H	*Treponema Leptospira Borrelia*	Bacteria (e.g. *Bartonella*; *Helicobacter*)	Carbon; cell debris	Very sensitive but nonspecific
Ziehl-Neelsen, Kinyoun	C, H	Mycobacteria	Schistosomal eggs; some partially acid-fast organisms	Lipfuscin; debris; carbol fuchsin crystals	Cytology and histology complement each other
Modified Ziehl-Neelsen or Kinyoun (Putt, Fite, Fite-Farraco)	C, H	Nocardia	Mycobacteria (rapid growers and *M. leprae*); schistosomal eggs, *Legionella micdadei*, *Rhodococcus equi*	See Ziehl-Neelsen	Putt stain false positivity for *Actinomyces*
Periodic acid-Schiff	C, H	Fungi	Bacteria (e.g. *Tropheryma whippeliae*)	*Pneumocystic* exudates; glycogen; Russell bodies	
Gomori methenamine silver	C, H	Fungi	Bacteria, including *Nocardia, Actinomyces* spp.	Fibrin, elastin, collagen, erythrocytes, capillaries	Preferred for fungi
Gridley stain	H	Fungi	See periodic acid-Schiff	See periodic acid-Schiff	Counterstain contrast good
Hematoxylin and eosin	C, H	Some parasites, molds, yeast; viral inclusions			Routine stain histology
Papanicolaou stain	C	Some parasites, yeasts, viral inclusions	Bacteria; molds		Routine stain cytology
Giemsa stain	C, H	Some parasites, dimorphic fungi	Bacteria	Phagocytized debris	

Gram-negative bacilli such as *Bartonella henselae*, *Fransicella tularensis*, *Yersinia enterocolitica*, *Yersinia pseudotuberculosis*, or *Helicobacter pylori*.[6–8] It must be remembered that the silver impregnation stains are non-specific and are best applied in combination with other stains such as the Gram stain and acid-fast stains. This non-specific, yet very sensitive stain can actually be advantageous when searching for an unknown agent. Morphologic details will be limited and it cannot be determined if the organism identified is Gram positive, Gram negative, or even acid-fast.

Other stains that may be used in identification of bacterial forms include the carbol fuchsin-based Gimenez stain for rickettsiae, the methylene blue stain for chlamydia, the Giemsa, Gomori methenamine silver (GMS), and H&E.

Mycobacteria

The principle of the acid-fast stain is that the wall of the mycobacteria, which has a high content of lipid rich mycolic acids, retains carbol fuchsin dyes that are not subsequently removed by acid or acid-alcohol solutions. The traditional stains are the Ziehl-Neelsen and the Kinyoun stains. Acid-fast organisms are red, slightly curved, beaded bacilli with variable pleomorphism depending upon which

species is being observed. An alternative approach for staining mycobacteria is using a fluorochrome dye, such as auramine, rhodamine, or a combination of the two. Acid-fast organisms appear yellow (auramine), red (rhodamine), or orange (auramine-rhodamine) when viewed with a fluorescence microscope. The fluorochrome dyes are best detected with an epifluorescence microscope and a halogen light source; mercury vapor lamps are not required. Microbiology laboratories use the fluorochrome method as the initial screen because it has a tenfold increased sensitivity. Positive fluorochrome slides are directly restained with a carbol fuchsin method to assess morphology of the acid-fast forms and to count organisms per high-power field for reporting purposes. Both the fluorochrome and the carbol fuchsin slides retain staining characteristic well during storage.

Some mycobacteria, particularly the rapid growers *Mycobacterium fortuitum* and *M. chelonae*, do not stain reliably with the traditional acid-fast stains.[9] For these organisms it is better to use a modified acid-fast method such as the Fite stain that incorporates peanut oil into the xylene solutions for a more gentle decolorization step. This method also works quite well for other bacterial forms that are weakly acid fast such as *Nocardia*, *Rhodococcus equi*, and select corynebacteria. A word of caution to note is that the Putt stain has been reported to color the filaments of *Actinomyces israelii* red, thus potentially classifying this organism incorrectly as an acid-fast filamentous bacterium such as *Nocardia*.[10,11]

Mycobacteria may be visualized occasionally with other stains, particularly if they are in a rapid growth phase. When visualized in this state they will appear weakly Gram positive, PAS positive, and GMS positive. Most of the time these organisms will be displayed as a 'negative image' resisting color uptake as the surrounding background takes on the tincture of the counterstain used.

Fungi

Two major groups of stains are in use for detection of fungi: stains for the chitin in the cell walls of fungi and anialine dyes that emphasize the cellular detail of the organisms. The two most commonly used procedures for staining cell walls are the GMS and PAS stains. Both of these stains may be used with smears or histologic sections. The fungal cells appear black with the silver stain and bright pink with the PAS technique. The material in the cell walls is not glycogen, and the PAS reaction is thus resistant to diastase digestion. A modification of the PAS method by Gridley makes most fungi stand out clearly against a yellow background. The calcofluor white stain method uses calcofluor to bind fungal cell wall chitin and fluoresces blue-white when exposed to ultraviolet light.[12,13]

Stains that reveal cellular detail used for staining fungi include the Giemsa stain, Wright stain, Papanicolaou, and the H&E. The Romanowsky blue stains, such as the Wright-Giemsa, are particularly helpful when distinguishing the subtle differences between *Leishmania* and *Histoplasma capsulatum*. Most yeast forms stain well with Gram stain, revealing an intense dark blue Gram-positive appearance. It should be noted that heavily encapsulated *Cryptococcus neoformans* can either fail to stain at all, forming ghost-like empty spaces, or may preferentially take up the iodine and stain as blotchy brown yeast forms. Both of these staining characteristics make the organism very difficult to visualize, particularly if one is not aware of this unique possibility. Occasionally even the experienced eye will miss *Cryptococcus* on a Gram stain because of this resistance to staining.

Other histochemical stains are important for highly selected situations. Mucicarmine or Alcian blue stains for the mucopolysaccharide capsules of heavily encapsulated fungi, especially *Cryptococcus neoformans*, are useful. The melanin pigment in the walls of dematiaceous molds and in *C. neoformans* can be demonstrated with the Fontana-Masson stain.[14]

Pneumocystis jirovecii (carinii) cyst walls may also be detected with the toluidine O stain, the Gram-Weigert stain, the calcofluor white stain, and the favorite for most pathologists the GMS stain.[15–18]

To detect the intracystic bodies of *Pneumocystis jirovecii (carinii)* it is necessary to use a Romanowsky stain, such as the Giemsa or Diff-Quik stains.

Viruses and parasites

The most important stains for recognition of viral inclusions and parasites in the surgical pathology and cytopathology laboratories are the routine H&E and the Papanicolaou stains. In addition, the Giemsa stain and trichrome stains are useful for observing the fine details of some protozoa in both smears and histologic sections. In most instances a well-trained eye looking at a properly processed thin tissue section with routine H&E can provide ample diagnostic information for appropriate clinical follow-up and treatment.

Quality control

Selection of appropriate material for quality control of histochemical stains is critical for assurance that staining characteristics are appropriate and reliably sensitive. Although historically many histology laboratories have developed and banked their own control blocks, this requires considerable time, thought, and attention to detail.[19–21] Many laboratories now rely on commercially prepared control slides. Commercial controls provide tissues that have been carefully characterized for distribution of organisms and ease of detection using many different methods; these can be a tremendous time saver for the busy histology laboratory. The ideal controls have the following characteristics.

1. The source of the controls matches the source of the test material (e.g. using both bronchoalveolar lavage and histologic sections containing *P. jirovecii (carinii)*;
2. The control organism either matches the organism sought in the test material, or has similar staining qualities;
3. When staining variability is anticipated, controls may combine organisms (one that stains easily and one that is resistant to staining). This allows confirmation that the stain is not over colorizing and that it is sensitive enough to detect the more resistant organisms. (e.g. *L. pneumophila* in addition to *Escherichia coli* for the Gram stain);
4. The positive control slide should contain enough organisms to be found without an extended time-consuming search, but should not have masses of organisms;
5. Use of a negative control only if it provides additional information.

The normal tissue of histologic sections can serve as a negative control in most situations, including tissue Gram stains and GMS, PAS, and mucicarmine stains. It is important to recognize that having a separate negative control does not substitute for experience in evaluating and recognizing artifacts and staining irregularities, because no single block of tissue will contain all possible distracters. Negative control slides to screen for potential contamination is recommended for silver impregnation stains and acid-fast stains. It is acceptable to store unstained paraffin sections for positive controls, but the negative control slides should be sectioned from the block each time controls are used in order to screen for possible water bath and line container contamination. Suggested quality control material for various types of stains are listed in Table 3.3.

Immunologic detection

Direct immunologic detection of infectious agents in smears and tissue provides increased specificity and sensitivity as well as an additional level of certainty for the definitive identification of infectious disease agents. This must be done in combination with the clinical history and knowledge of the appropriate inflammatory reaction in the tissues under investigation. Techniques used for this purpose include direct or indirect immunofluorescence assays and enzyme linked immunochemistries. The marker for these immunochemistry methods may be horseradish peroxidase, alkaline phosphatase, or biotin-avidin compounds. Commercial reagents are available for immunologic detection of many viruses, such as HIV, herpes simplex virus, cytomegalovirus, hepatitis C, and adenovirus; for bacteria, such as *Legionella* spp. and *T. pallidum*; and for parasites, such as *Toxoplasma gondii*.[22–25]

Although immunologic techniques allow more definitive identification of infectious agents that cannot be differentiated by morphologic means, we must always be aware of potential cross-reactivity which is an inherent risk with any antigen antibody-based reaction. Users must always scrutinize the specificity of commercial agents on an ongoing basis, particularly when the identified agent does not fit the clinical scenario or the pattern of reactivity is unusual.

Table 3.3 Quality control for histochemical stains

Type of organism	Type of stain	Positive control	Negative control
Bacteria	Gram	1. Staphylococcal or pneumococcal infection	Optional
		2. Enteric Gram-negative bacillus infection	
		3. *Legionella* pneumonia	
	Silver impregnation	1. Cat-scratch disease	
		2. *Legionella* pneumonia	Uninfected tissue
Spirochetes	Silver impregnation	*Treponema pallidum*	Uninfected tissue
Fungi	Gomori methenamine silver		
	Periodic acid-Schiff		
	Gridley	*Aspergillus* or zygomycetes infection	Optional
	Mucicarmine	*Cryptococcus neoformans*	Mucin-negative *Blastomyces*
	Fontana-Masson	*Cryptococcus neoformans*	*Aspergillus* spp.
Pneumocystis	Gomori methenamine silver; Gram-Weigert	*Pneumocystis jirovecii (carinii)* infection	Uninfected lavage or tissue
Various	Giemsa	*Toxoplasma* or *Leishmania* infection	Optional

It is well known that the reagents for herpes simplex type I and type II show considerable cross-reactivity. Reagents for CMV can also occasionally cross-react with other members of the herpes family viruses such as HHV 6, giving a nucleolar pattern of reactivity.

In certain situations, the specificity of the reactions may be compromised not only by immunologic cross-reactions, but also by environmental contamination. This is particularly true of the fluorescent methods. Direct fluorescent antibody (DFA) stains for *Legionella* or any other bacterial rod, can be interpreted incorrectly as positive if one of the autofluorescent organisms is in the sample being tested. The three bacterial rods most notable for autofluorescence are *Pseudomonas aeruginosa*, *Pseudomonas fluorescens*, and *Pseudomonas putida*. Non-specific antibody cross-reactivity can be seen with the fluorescent methods as well and can have tremendous epidemiological impact.[26] One of the authors had a patient referred to hospital for a 'positive' *Bordetella pertussis* DFA; the patient happened to be a healthcare provider in a very busy hospital setting. After epidemiologists called back over 100 employees and patients, none of whom had the symptoms of whooping cough or positive follow-up cultures, it was determined that the positive test was caused by misinterpretation of a cross-reactive *Staphylococcus aureus*! The well-seasoned microbiologist would have been able to avoid this infectious disease misadventure, but unfortunately the test was performed in a small laboratory without the advantage of a microbiologist's eye. The best way to avoid these pitfalls is to ensure that the organism morphology, the inflammatory reaction incited, and the clinical history all support the diagnosis rendered.

Several fungal forms also have the unique characteristic of autofluorescence, including the dimorphic systemic fungi and *Aspergillus*.[27] The intensity of the autofluorescence is quite variable, but some is intense enough to be detected after routine processing and H&E staining. The autofluorescence of *Aspergillus* is the reason a direct fluorescent confirmation test has never been developed for rapid identification of this opportunistic pathogen. Most of the systemic dimorphic fungi are also autoflorescent to various degrees. Interestingly, some have used the predictable autofluorescence as a tool to further confirm they are dealing with a dimorphic fungal form. Likewise, autofluorescence in an organism with dichotomous acute angle branching would further support the diagnosis of *Aspergillus*.[28] Papanicolaou staining has been documented to enhance the fluorescence of *Aspergillus* hyphae form. Autofluorescent fungi may interfere in any test method dependent upon fluorescent scope visualization. Confirmatory methods for fungal organisms in tissue sections or cell blocks requires use of a colorimetric signal. Limited colorimetric in situ hybridization (CISH) methods have been developed to use for confirmation of autofluorescent fungi.[29]

The forgotten culture

Optimal patient care occurs when the clinician can combine information from the microbiology, cytology and surgical pathology laboratories. Alas, sometimes the surgeons obtaining the biopsy or the healthcare providers ordering cytology specimens simply forget or overlook the need for cultures. It is prudent for the pathologist to ensure that cultures have been initiated when dealing with a case that appears to be infectious in nature. The pathologist examining fresh endocardial leaflets or open lung biopsies at the grossing bench may quickly surmise through touch prep or frozen section the possibility of an infectious etiology and should check to ensure cultures have been obtained. Although the surgical pathology and cytology laboratories are not an ideal location to try to sequester a culture, it can be attempted, particularly for fungal and mycobacterial cultures. It is also sometimes helpful to freeze a small portion of a potential infectious disease specimen, just in case additional studies for a rare, previously unsuspected agent are desired in the future. Many infectious disease agents tolerate freezing and thawing fairly well.

PART II: HOST DEFENSE MECHANISMS AND TISSUE RESPONSES

Although there are thousands of potentially infectious agents we may encounter, there are a very limited number of immune responses to those agents. A particular type of pathogen usually elicits a predictable response based on the mediators and potentiators provided by the organism and the composition of the cytokine response to the invading pathogen. The local tissue injury occurring with the initial contact may also cause further injury and potentiation of the inflammatory response. The lipopolysaccharide component of the Gram-negative bacilli external membrane stimulates an intense release of IL-1, tumor necrosis factor, IL-6, and IL-8 leading to a predominately neutrophilic response. On the other hand, invasion of an obligate intracellular pathogen, such as a virus or a rickettsial

Table 3.4 Tissue responses to infectious agents

Tissue reaction pattern*	Injury mechanisms	Potential etiologic agents	Methods for confirmation
Exudative inflammatory reaction	NF-κBpathway; IL-1; TNF; IL-6;IL-8; IFN-γ	Pyogenic bacteria; rapid growing organisms; *Legionella*	Culture; H&E; tissue Gram; silver impregnation stain; PAS
Necrotizing inflammatory reaction	Toxins; leukocidins and NF-κB pathway	*Clostridium*; *Legionella*; *Pseudomonas*; pyogenic bacteria; *E. histolytica*	Culture; H&E; tissue Gram; trichrome; PAS
Granulomatous inflammatory reaction	TH-1;IL-1, IL-2; TNF; IL-6; IL-8; IL-10.	Mycobacteria; fungi; rare gram negatives; helminth larvae/eggs	Culture; H&E; GMS; AFB; Gram; PAS; trichrome; molecular
Mononuclear, predominately foamy macrophage reaction	IL-1; IL-2; IL-6; IL-8; MCP; MIP; IL-12, IL-15	Fungal, intracellular and intravascular agents; *Rhodococcus*; *Pneumocystis jirovecii (carinii)*	Culture; H&E; gram; Giemsa; AFB, GMS; molecular; serology
Interstitial, predominately lymphocytic reaction	IL-1; IL-2; IL-6; IL-8; MCP; MIP; IL-12, IL-15	Fungal, intracellular organisms bacteria; protozoa	Culture; H&E; Gram; Giemsa; AFB, GMS; PAS; molecular; serology
Cytopathic/direct injury reaction	Apoptosis; receptor entry; NK, CT cells	Viral agents; parasitic infections; toxin producing agents	Culture; H&E; immunohistology; molecular
Paucity or 'absent' reaction (consider immune status of host)	Low virulence and cellular mimicry	Latent viruses; toxin producing agents; low virulence bacteria; mycobacteria; parasites	Culture; H&E: Gram; Giemsa; AFB, GMS; PAS; molecular; serology

*Note: In cases demonstrating overlap features, first consideration should be given to the overriding pattern.
H&E, hematoxylin & eosin; PAS, Periodic acid-Schiff; GMS, Gomori methenamine silver; AFB, acid-fast bacilli stain.

organism stimulates the release of IL-1, IL-2, and interferon leading to a mononuclear cell mediated response. Because there are predictable responses with specific categories of infectious agents, we can make certain generalizations that provide a framework that narrows and focuses our search when dealing with an unknown infectious disease pathogen. It comes as no surprise that there are exceptions when using this approach. Nonetheless, we can begin an immune response-guided systematic approach to identification of the unknown pathogen. Seven major types of histologic responses can be delineated as follows:

- Exudative acute inflammatory reaction
- Necrotizing inflammatory reaction
- Granulomatous inflammatory reaction
- Mononuclear, predominately foamy macrophage reaction
- Lymphoplasmacytic reaction
- Cytopathic/direct injury reaction
- Paucicellular or 'absent' reaction

Attention to tissue responses is critical when considering what type of infectious agent to target and often provides the initial clues in the search for causality. Tissue reactions allow pathologists to categorize injury patterns and then group potential infectious agents. The search is then narrowed by application of a vast array of identification methods. Table 3.4 provides an overview of the types of inflammatory responses, some of the cytokines responsible for those responses, types of infectious agents to consider, and recommended diagnostic tools to narrow in on the offending organism.

It should also be noted that some infections are not associated with a recognizable cellular reaction in the affected tissue. The most common explanation for serious infections without an inflammatory response is that the pathogenic mechanism of the infection is production of a toxin that exerts its effects biochemically. Two examples are cholera, which is a disease of intestinal fluid secretion, and botulism, which is a disorder of neuromuscular transmission. A second completely diverse explanation is that the immune system of the infected host is either severely suppressed or they are anergic. Both of these settings could result in the paucicellular or 'absent' response pattern.

THE ACUTE INFLAMMATORY RESPONSE

The acute inflammatory response, represented at the cellular level by the polymorphonuclear neutrophil (PMN), is the basis of the body's reaction to almost any injury. It is an intricate component of the wound repair process. The PMN has two main types of granules, primary (azurophilic) and secondary (specific) granules. The primary granules are designed for intracellular pathogen killing with release into the cell membrane protected phagolysosome space. These granules contain numerous proteases for bacterial digestion, mannosidase for fungal wall digestion, and an acidic background to enhance killing. The secondary granules of the PMN are designed to potentiate the inflammatory response with granules containing chemotactic substances such as the C5a fragment of complement being released into the extracellular space along with soluble mediators such as lactoferrin and vitamin B12 binding proteins to inhibit bacterial growth. All of these factors contribute to a crescendo-like immune response resulting in a dense influx of neutrophils. If this continues over time, abscesses or empyemas may form. If the invading pathogen produces a leukocidin exotoxin (e.g. *Staphylococcus aureus* or *Pseudomonas*) to inhibit and kill neutrophils, the likelihood of abscess development is even greater.

The major clinical and pathologic presentations of acute bacterial infection are acute inflammation, cellulitis, abscess formation, empyema formation, and localized gas accumulation. Acute inflammation is the hallmark of pyogenic bacterial infection. The most common infectious agents are the major Gram-positive agents: staphylococci; streptococci, including *Streptococcus pneumoniae* and *Enterococcus* spp.; the Gram-negative bacilli, including *Haemophilus* spp., the enteric bacilli, and nonfermenting bacilli, such as pseudo-

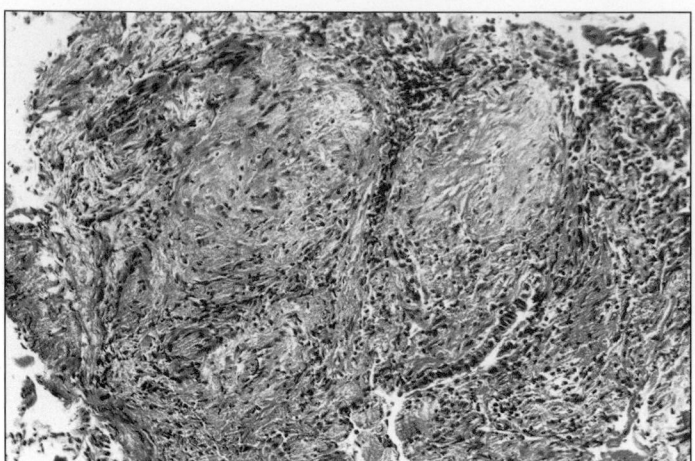

Fig. 3.1 *Mycobacterium tuberculosis*. Noncaseating granulomas with multinucleated giant cells in the submucosa of a bronchus. Transbronchial biopsy (H&E, ×100, *Mycobacterim tuberculosis* isolated in cultures).

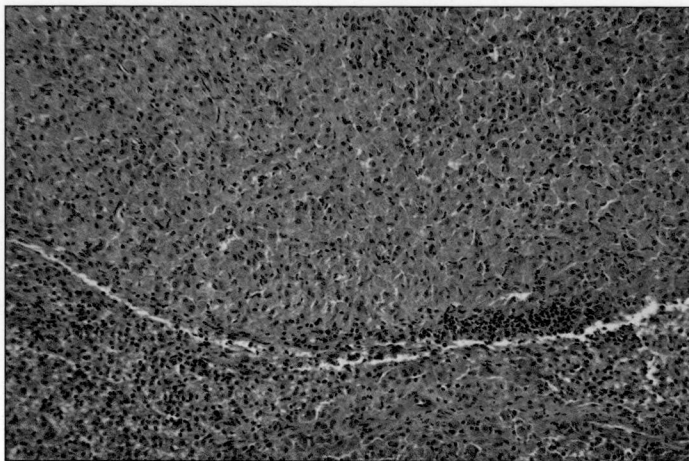

Fig. 3.2 Disseminated infection in the spleen of a patient infected with human immunodeficiency virus. Masses of macrophages with abundant cytoplasm replace the splenic tissue and resemble the lesion of Whipple's disease (H&E, ×200, *Mycobacterium avium* complex isolated in culture). (Courtesy of David Walker, MD)

monads and *Acinetobacter* spp.; and a variety of anaerobic bacteria. *Clostridium* spp. are often participants in mixed bacterial infections that may associated with a varying degree of gas formation.

There are a limited number of nonbacterial pathogens that mimic the acute inflammatory tissue response. These are often associated with tissue necrosis, and it is unclear how much of the response is due to the organism and how much is secondary to direct tissue injury. Examples include invasive *Candida* spp., the parasites *T. gondii* and *Leishmania* spp., and members of the herpes family of DNA viruses such as herpes simplex virus and adenovirus.

THE GRANULOMATOUS AND MACROPHAGE RICH RESPONSES

When the initial review of an H&E stain or a Papanicolaou stain shows a macrophage-rich tissue or granulomatous response, the initial step must be to rule out a mycobacterial and fungal infectious process. Granulomas are organized collections of macrophages that may take the form of epithelioid histiocytes and Langhans giant cells, which typically have nuclei marginated at the cell membrane. Granulomas may be poorly formed, well formed and intact, or may display several forms of central necrosis. The necrosis may be caseous with cellular debris and ghost cells; intensely eosinophilic-resembling fibrinoid necrosis as seen in collagen vascular diseases; or microabscess-like with a stellate appearance as seen in tularemia and cat-scratch disease. Although certain pathogens are associated with particular types of necrosis, there is too much overlap to rely upon this feature. For instance, tuberculosis commonly elicits a caseating granulomatous response, but some infections may be characterized by noncaseating granulomas that are indistinguishable from those seen in sarcoidosis (Fig. 3.1).

Mycobacterium avium complex infections in the moderate to severely immunosuppressed host are characterized by a dense macrophage-rich response. Large collections of macrophages distort and replace normal tissue (Fig. 3.2), and the cells are often stuffed with mycobacteria (Fig. 3.3).[30–32] Because *M. avium* complex bacteria are stained with the PAS procedure, these nongranulomatous lesions may resemble Whipple's disease, particularly in the gastrointestinal

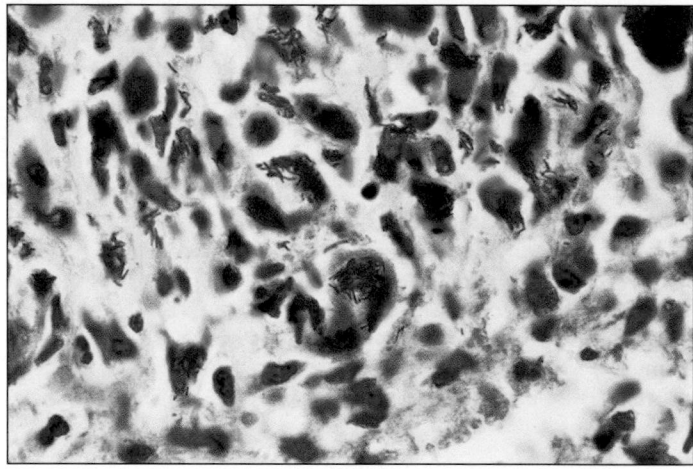

Fig. 3.3 Acid-fast stain of the tissue show in Fig. 3.2. The cells are packed with mycobacteria (AFB, ×1,000).

tract and in lymphoid tissue.[32] An even greater challenge for the surgical pathologist is presented by the spindle cell pseudotumor that is caused by *M. avium* complex in HIV-infected patients (Fig. 3.4).[33] These lesions may be found in skin, lymphoid tissue, soft tissues, or bone. The cells resemble a fibroblastic neoplastic proliferation but are clearly histiocytes by immunohistochemical staining. They often contain large numbers of mycobacteria (Fig. 3.5). This spindle cell pseudotumor appearance of the macrophage-rich reaction has also been associated with chronic *Rhodococcus equi* infections, particularly within soft tissues.[34]

If the conventional acid-fast stain fails to demonstrate bacilli in lesions with morphology suggestive of mycobacterial or nocardial disease, a modified stain should be used. The Fite method is preferred in tissue sections. Partial or variable acid fastness indicates that a portion of the bacterial population will be stained or, in the case of *Nocardia* spp., that portions of individual organisms will stain positively.

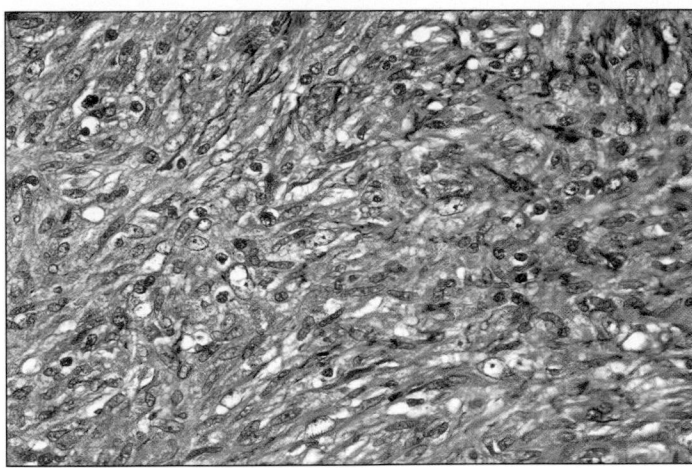

Fig. 3.4 Spindle-cell lesion of soft tissue in a patient infected with human immunodeficiency virus. Despite the elongated appearance of the cells, suggesting an origin from fibroblasts, immunohistochemical stains confirm that they are macrophages (H&E, ×500). (Courtesy of Ann-Marie Nelson, MD)

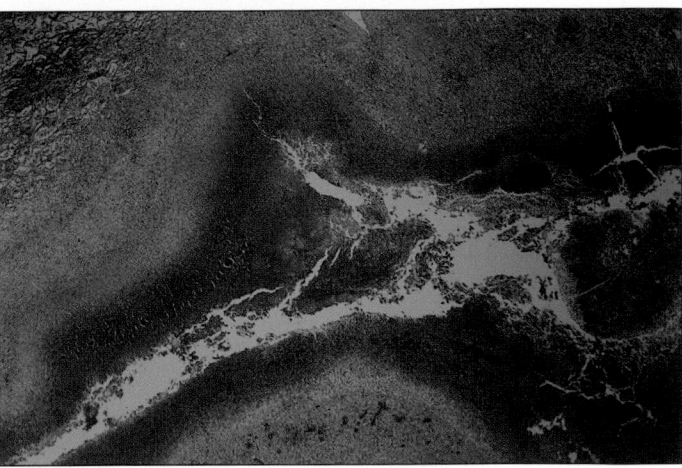

Fig. 3.6 *Rhodococcus equi* pneumonia. A large necrotizing granuloma with microabscess is present. Other areas show an unorganized infiltrate of plump hypereosinophilic macrophages (H&E, ×45, *Rhodococcus equi* isolated in culture).

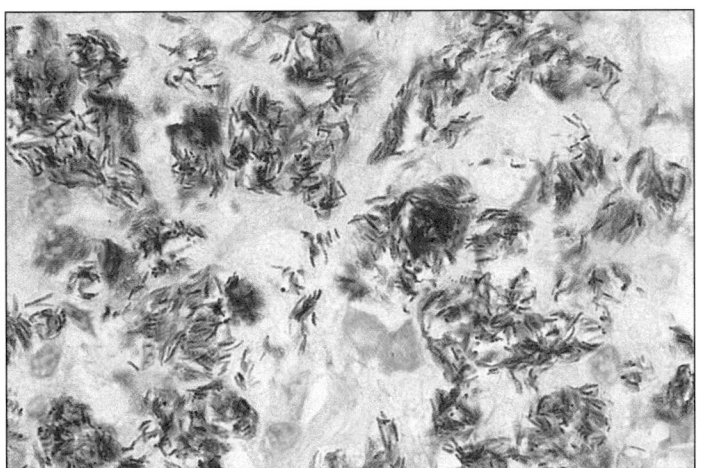

Fig. 3.5 Acid-fast stain from the tissue shown in Fig. 3.4. The cells are packed with acid-fast bacilli characteristic of *Mycobacterium avium-intracellulare* complex (Ziehl-Neelsen, ×1000). (Courtesy of Ann-Marie Nelson, MD)

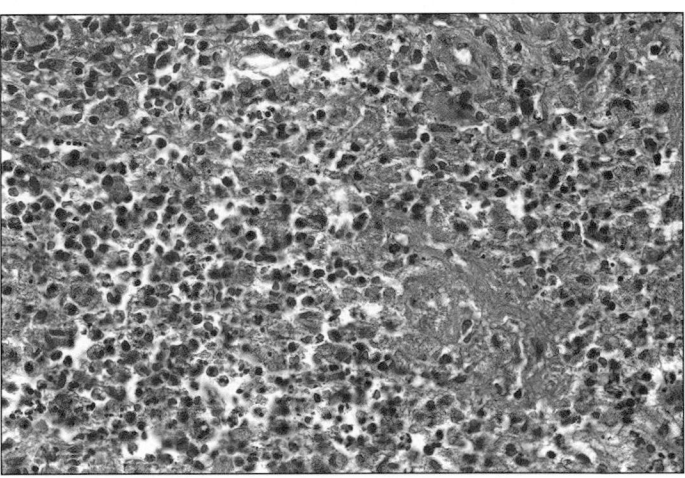

Fig. 3.7 Rapid-grower mycobacterial infection of soft tissue. Necrotizing inflammation consisting of macrophages and a minor component of polymorphonuclear neutrophils (H&E, ×400, *Mycobacterium abscessus* isolated in culture).

Several less commonly encountered bacterial species, such as *Rhodococcus equi* and *Legionella micdadei*, elicit a prominent macrophage response accompanied by PMNs. *Rhodococcus* organisms produce foamy macrophage-rich infiltrates that may include focal granulomas and may persist and evolve into a focus of malacoplakia. (Fig. 3.6).[34–37] *L. micdadei* and *Rhodococcus* are both variably acid fast, and tend to loose this property after isolation and subculturing.[38]

Poorly formed granulomas combined with mixed PMNs and lymphocytes may be associated with *M. fortuitum*, *M. chelonae*, and *M. abscessus* (Fig. 3.7), and are also typical of nocardial and actinomycete infections.[39,40] The lesions of leprosy may be granulomatous (Fig. 3.8) in patients with active cell-mediated immune responses or may consist of aggregates of poorly organized macrophages when cellular immunity is less aggressive. The numbers of mycobacteria also reflect the efficacy of the host response. In tuberculoid (granulomatous) leprosy, organisms are sparse may be very difficult to find, whereas the macrophages (Lepra cells) of lepromatous leprosy may be stuffed with acid-fast bacteria.

Fungi and yeasts

Fungi may take two distinctive morphologic forms: plump budding yeasts and plant-like filamentous molds. Some species are considered dimorphic because they produce both forms, concurrently or separately depending on the temperature of the environment in which they are growing. Two helpful references for the identification of clinically important fungi are the textbooks by Larone and by deHoog et al.[41,42] The vast majority of fungi exist as filamentous, septate molds. If these septate hyphae are essentially colorless, as in the majority of cases, they are referred to as hyaline molds. A small group of fungi contain melanin pigment in their septae; these are

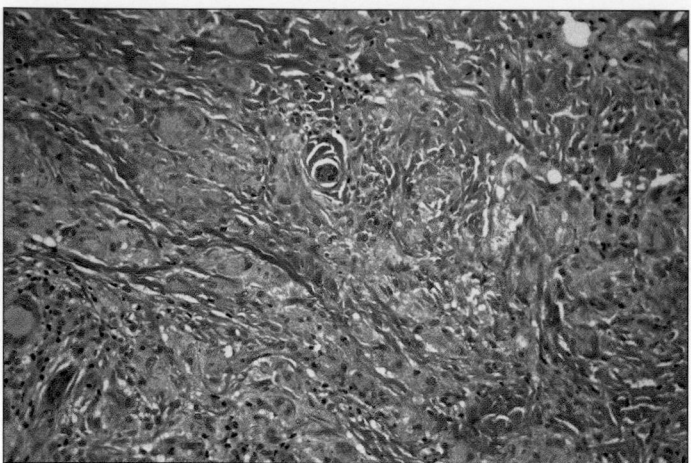

Fig. 3.8 Cutaneous leprosy. The dermis is infiltrated with epithelioid macrophages organized into confluent granulomas. Small numbers of acid-fast bacilli are present (H&E, ×200).

known as dematiaceous molds. Table 3.5 is a helpful comparison of the morphologic characteristics of filamentous molds as seen in cytologic smears and tissue sections. Yeasts or blastoconidia are single-celled organisms that reproduce by a process called budding. An excellent reference for morphologic identification of fungi in tissue is the atlas assembled by Chandler and Watts.[43]

The systemic dimorphic fungi include *Histoplasma capsulatum*, *Blastomyces dermatitidis*, *Coccidioides immitis*, *Sporothrix schenckii*, *Penicillium marneffii*, and some dematiaceous fungi. When grown at 37°C in the laboratory or in the body of an infected host, the form is a budding yeast *(Histoplasma, Blastomyces, or Sporothrix)*, a yeast-like form *(P. marneffii* and some dematiaceous fungi), or a spherule (sporangium) with endospores *(C. immitis)*.

The best overall stain for yeast in tissue is the routine H&E procedure. Even if a special stain is needed to detect fungi, the H&E stain provides diagnostically important cytologic clues as to the identification. Several additional clues can be used to facilitate the identification of yeast in tissue (Table 3.6). The size of the yeast provides an important clue for identification. Approximate sizes may be inferred by comparison with adjacent cells. Some yeasts are extremely uniform in size and shape, while others such as *Cryptococcus neoformans* shows extensive variability in size. Another important clue is the character of the bud. With most yeasts the mother cell in the process of division develops a small appendage bud that increases in size until it is mature and ready for separation. The connecting point between the mother cell and the daughter cell is characteristically very narrow. In *Blastomyces dermatitidis* this is not the case; the interface between the mother and daughter cell with *Blastomyces dermtitidis* is characteristically very broad. This extremely broad connecting point is present as the daughter bud forms and is maintained until the point of separation. Often, the very early buds of *Blastomyces dermtitidis* with a broad-based connection are the most striking examples of this phenomenon. This, along with other features, can be used to help characterize the invasive fungal forms when seen in tissue sections or cytologic preparations. Clinical history, the organ(s) infected, and the tissue response to the yeast may be useful clues. Finally, in some instances histochemical stains may be useful for differentiation of certain yeasts.

THE LYMPHOCYTE RICH RESPONSE

When a predominately lymphocytic response is encountered as the primary tissue reaction, the focus should initially be narrowed to first consider the obligate intracellular pathogens. The vast majority of

Table 3.5 Morphologic characteristics of filamentous molds in smears and tissue

Mold	Size (μm)	Cellular detail	Staining	Histologic response	Vascular invasion	Yeast forms	Comments
Zygomycetes	5–20	Broad, ribbon-like Hyphae; rare sepatations; right-angle branching	H&E±; BH±; GMS±; PAS±; FM−	PMNs; abscesses hemorrhage, necrosis	Yes	No	Cross-sections may resemble yeast; *Rhizopus* most common
Aspergillus	3–6	Thin hyphae; septate; acute angle branching	H&E±; BH±; GMS+, PAS+, FM−	PMNsl abscesses; macrophages; granulomas; hemorrhage, necrosis	Yes	No	Cross-sections may resemble yeast; calcium oxalate crystals with *A. niger*
Hyaline molds	2–8	Thin hyphae; septate; acute angle branching	H&E±; BH±; GMS+, PAS+, FM−	PMNs, abscesses; macrophages; hemorrhage, necrosis	Yes	No	Cross-sections may resemble yeast; most common are *Pseudallescheria; Fusarium*
Candida	2–6	Hyphae and pseudohypha, blastoconidia	H&E±; BH±; GMS+, PAS+, FM−	PMNs, abscesses, macrophages, granulomas	Rare	Yes	Cannot differentiate species
Dematiaceous	2–6	Thin hyphae	H&E±; BH±; GMS+,PAS+, FM+	PMNs, abscesses, necrosis, granulomas, macrophages	No	Yeast-like sclerotic bodies with *Chromomycosis*	Tissue response varies

H&E, hematoxylin and eosin; BH, Brown-Hopps; GMS, Gomori methenamine silver; PAS, periodic acid-Schiff; FM, Fontana-Masson; PMNs, polymorphonuclear leukocytes.

Table 3.6 Identification of yeasts in smears and tissue

Yeast	Size (μm)	Cellular detail	Staining	Histologic response	Location	Tissue hyphae	Comments
Histoplasma capsulatum	3–5	Thin wall; budding ±; single nucleus; large distorted forms in old granulomas	H&E+, GMS+, PAS+, mucin–, FM–	Macrophage, granulomas, necrosis ±	Intracellular, extracellular in necrosis	No	Must differentiate from *Candida*, *Torulopsis*, small blasto forms
Histoplasma duboisii	8–15	Same as above	Same as above	Same as above	Macrophage, giant cell	No	Found in Africa
Blastomyces dermatitidis	8–15	Thick wall; broad buds; multiple nuclei	H&E+, GMS+, PAS+, mucin±, FM–	Macrophage, granulomas, microabscess	Macrophages, giant cells, extracellular in necrosis	No	Differentiate from *Coccidioides* and *Cryptococcus*
Coccidioides immitis	5–30	Thin wall; endospores; no budding	H&E+, GMS+, PAS+, mucin–, FM–	Macrophage, granuloma	Macrophages, giant cells	Rare	Differentiate from blasto
Sporothrix schenckii	2–6	Thin wall; cigar shaped buds	H&E+, GMS+, PAS+, mucin–	Macrophage, granuloma	Macrophages, giant cells	No	Splendore-Hoeppli
Candida spp. (*Torulopsis*)	2–6	Thin wall; budding pseudohyphae (except *C. glabrata*)	H&E+, GMS+, PAS+, mucin–, FM–	PMNs, ± abscesses, stellate granuloma	Extracellular, (except for *C. glabrata*)	Yes	Differentiate from histo
Cryptococcus neoformans	2–20	Thin wall; budding; variable sizes	H&E+, GMS+, PAS+, mucin+, FM+	Macrophage, paucicellular, granulomas	Macrophages, giant cells	Rare	Differentiate from blasto
Malassezia furfur	2–5	Thin wall buds; division by septation	H&E+, GMS+, PAS+, mucin–, FM–			No	Rare; primarily in infants with lipid infusions
Penicillium marneffi	2–5	Thin wall; division by septation					
Chromomycosis	5–12	Division by septation					

H&E, hematoxylin and eosin; GMS, Gomori methenamine silver; PAS, periodic acid-Schiff; FM, Fontana-Masson; PMNs, polymorphonuclear leukocytes.

obligate intracellular pathogens causing human disease are viruses. It should be remembered, however, that organisms from other groups such as the bacteria and parasitic categories may also exist as obligate intracellular pathogens. A good systematic approach would be to first consider viral etiologies with careful examination of other 'clues' such as viral inclusions or characteristic cytopathic effects; then to continue on to consider pathogens such as rickettsial form, ehrlichia and intracellular protozoans such as *Toxoplasma*.

Although viral infections are known to cause the largest number of human illness each year, they are often mild or even subclinical and as such are rarely encountered by the anatomic pathologist. Viral infections do not often result in invasive diagnostic procedures because the diagnosis can be made by culturing accessible secretions, testing serum for antibodies, or simply by characteristic clinical findings.

The list of viruses that infect hospitalized or immunocompromised patients is relatively short. Some of the most lethal viruses that produce all too abundant pathologic material, such as the arenaviruses (e.g. Lassa virus) and filoviruses (e.g. Ebola virus) occur in remote parts of the world, and are unlikely to be encountered in the United States.

A single viral agent, the human immunodeficiency virus (HIV), is responsible for an explosion of interest and concern about many of the infectious agents discussed in this chapter. HIV does cause disease other than destruction of the immune system, but it is the secondary infectious agents, rather than HIV itself that results in the submission of a surgical specimen. Viruses exert their effects at the cellular level, and the cellular reaction is a response to damage done to individual cells. Although some important exceptions are seen, the primary lesion is individual cell death and the tissue response is mononuclear, predominately lymphocytic in nature.

The anatomic pathologist is able to contribute diagnostic information primarily in those infections in which masses of viral particles are sufficiently large to be seen with the light microscope in the form of viral inclusions. Viruses contain either RNA or DNA, not both. As a general rule the inclusions of DNA-containing viruses are found in the nucleus, whereas RNA-containing viruses are assembled in the cytoplasm (Table 3.7). Several treatises on the cellular morphology of viral infections are available.[44,45]

An excellent reference for the practicing surgical pathologist that describes the tissue section morphology of all types of pathogens is the textbook by Connor et al. entitled *Pathology of Infectious Diseases*.[46]

PART III: AN ORGAN-BASED APPROACH TO INFECTIOUS DISEASES

SKIN, MUCOCUTANEOUS SURFACES, AND SOFT TISSUE

The skin, mucocutaneous surfaces, and soft tissue represent the largest organ system of the human body. Fortunately, these surfaces

Table 3.7 Viral inclusions

Virus	Nucleic acid	Location	Staining	Comments
Herpes simplex virus	DNA	Intranuclear	Eosinophilic	Multinucleated giant cells; cannot be differentiated from varicella-zoster virus
Varicella-zoster virus	DNA	Intranuclear	Eosinophilic	Multinucleated giant cells; cannot be differentiated from herpes simplex virus
Cytomegalovirus	DNA	Intranuclear and cytoplasmic	Amphophilic to basophilic	Cytomegaly, cytoplasmic inclusions variably present
Epstein-Barr virus	DNA	Intranuclear	Eosinophilic	Only rarely present
Smallpox virus	DNA	Intracytoplasmic	Eosinophilic	Guarneri bodies
Parvovirus B19	DNA	Intranuclear	Basophilic	Erythroid precursors
JC virus	DNA	Intranuclear	Basophilic	Present in oligodendroglia
Measles virus	RNA	Intranuclear and cytoplasmic	Eosinophilic	Inclusions present in epithelioid giant cells; not present in Warthin-Finkeldey giant cells
Respiratory syncytial virus	RNA	Intracytoplasmic	Eosinophilic	Syncytial giant cells
Parainfluenza virus	RNA	Intracytoplasmic	Eosinophilic	Irregularly present in type 2 and 3 strains; syncytial giant cells
Rabies virus	RNA	Intracytoplasmic	Eosinophilic	Negri bodies; irregular staining

are designed to resist abrasion, puncture, and hostile environmental conditions. When these anatomic defense layers are breached we see infections of the skin and underlying soft tissues, primarily in the form of a cellulitis, fasciitis, myositis, or abscess formation. A second important aspect to consider is that some diseases manifesting as a skin or soft tissue nodule may reflect a systemic infection with dissemination through the vasculature, or a systemic disease such as systemic mastocytosis, hematopoietic neoplasia, or any number of autoimmune and collagen vascular disorders. Skin lesions should first be categorized by the combination of the clinical findings, distribution of the lesions, nature of the lesions grossly (macule, papule, maculopapular, vesicular), and by the inflammatory cell response noted microscopically. Careful examination of the state of the overlying epidermis and any junctional changes such as spongiosis or thickened basement membranes will also provide important etiologic clues. The underlying dermis and soft tissue should always be inspected for the possibility of foreign materials, such as splinters, tick mouth parts, or fragments of glass; this can easily be accomplished by performing a rapid screen under polarized light. Several serious and complex disease states, such as lymphomatoid papulosis, cutaneous Hodgkin's disease, and the cutaneous leukemias and lymphomas may present for evaluation to the anatomic pathologist. This chapter will only deal with the most commonly encountered infectious etiologies.

Cellulitis

Cellulitis is a superficially spreading infection of skin and immediate underlying soft tissues that is usually associated with bacterial infection and generally incites a pure acute inflammatory polymorphonuclear neutrophilic response (Fig. 3.9). The classic pathogens that cause cellulitis are *Staphylococcus aureus* and *Streptococcus pyogenes* (group A beta-hemolytic streptococcus). The lesion is an aggressive acute inflammatory response that dissects through fascial planes.

Classic group A beta-hemolytic streptococcal cellulitis causes an impetigo clinical presentation with little or no necrosis. Since the 1980s there have been selected strains of group A beta-hemolytic streptococci with markedly upregulated necrosis-inducing enzymes such as hyaluronidase that cause a presentation hailed by the media

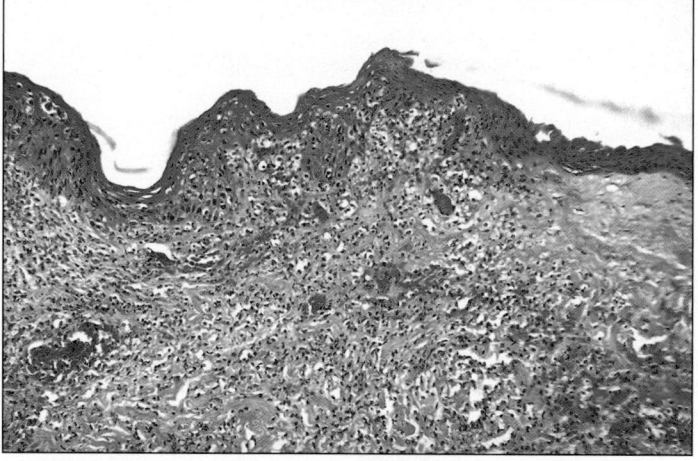

Fig. 3.9 Streptococcal dermatitis and cellulitis. An acute inflammatory response with polymorphonuclear neutrophils and edema disrupting the basal layer of the epidermis, the dermis and the subcutaneous tissue (H&E, ×50, *Streptococcus pyogenes* isolated in pure culture from the tissue).

as 'flesh eating bacteria.' These may be life threatening and are often cause for emergent surgical debridement. Occasionally the surgical pathologist will be called upon to render the edge of the debridement 'clear' of offending pathogens and necrosis – a line that should be crossed with great trepidation.

Mixtures of anaerobic bacteria or mixtures of aerobic and anaerobic bacteria, which may result in synergistic gangrene, also produce necrotizing cellulitis/fasciitis with or without myositis, particularly in persons who have other risk factors such as diabetes mellitus or severe peripheral vascular disease.

Some bacterial species not usually associated with cellulitis, such as members of the *Enterobacteriaceae*, may produce this lesion.

Cellulitis and fasciitis may take on special characteristics and ominous implications when they occur in certain anatomic locations.

The two most dramatic are Ludwig's angina and Fournier's gangrene (perineal phlegmon). In both conditions polymicrobial infection that includes anaerobic bacteria dissects rapidly through tissue planes and may cause uncontrollable, life-threatening infection. Ludwig's angina is caused by a mixture of oral bacteria and begins in the floor of the mouth or retropharyngeal space. The infection may end fatally, with compromise of the airway. Fournier's gangrene is a variant of synergistic infection that is caused by a mixture of perineal bacteria of fecal origin. Spread of the disease through the pelvis into the peritoneum may occur so rapidly that even aggressive antimicrobial therapy and surgical debridement cannot salvage those affected.

Gas-forming Infections

Gas-forming infections are most commonly caused by clostridial species, of which the most common are *Clostridium perfringens* and *C. septicum*.[47-49] Clostridial cellulitis and particularly myonecrosis are often characterized by minimal cellular inflammation, being associated with tissue necrosis, a proteinaceous exudate, and bubbles of gas in the tissues. *C. septicum* causes necrotizing infection in the gastrointestinal tract (Fig. 3.10). Distant foci of myonecrosis caused by this pathogen should prompt a search for neoplastic disease in the gastrointestinal tract, which provides a portal of entry for the bacilli. Rarely, hemolytic exotoxins produced by *C. perfringens* produce a syndrome of fatal, massive intravascular hemolysis, particularly after gallbladder surgery. Histologically, numerous bacterial rods are easily seen with routine H&E stains, there is extensive necrosis with empty pockets caused by gas release from bacterial metabolism, and there is a paucity of neutrophils when compared to the extent of damage caused. This is due to the production of an intense leukocidin by this group of organisms. Frozen section evaluation that show foci of necrosis and gas formation, even without the presence of neutrophils, should still be considered involved. This can be a very difficult call for the pathologist. Of course, absolute 'clearance' cannot be made until cultures are finalized, long after the surgical procedure has been completed.

Abscess and empyema formation and necrotizing infection

Necrotizing infection and formation of abscesses or empyema are features of pyogenic bacterial pathogens except for *Haemophilus* spp. and *S. pneumoniae*. The classic abscess-forming pathogen is *S. aureus*, but a variety of Gram-negative facultatively anaerobic and strictly anaerobic bacilli must also be considered. *Pseudomonas* is an important Gram-negative nonfermenter that produces multiple exotoxins resulting in abscess formation. The cytology of abscesses is usually directed toward the bacterial pathogen with a Gram smear rather than toward the host cell, but fine-needle aspiration (FNA) is performed occasionally on pyogenic lesions when the nature of the process has not been clear to the clinician (Fig. 3.11).

Actinomycosis

Actinomycosis is caused by one of several species of *Actinomyces*, most commonly *Actinomyces israelii*. These bacteria are normal inhabitants of the upper respiratory tract, gastrointestinal tract, and female genital tract. The associated infections occur in organs or soft tissue adjacent to these structures: cervicofacial, thoracic, abdominal, and pelvic actinomycosis.[50,51] The infection was first described in cattle as lumpy jaw, caused by *A. bovis*. Similar human disease may be caused by *A. israelii*. *Rothia dentocariosa*, and other species of *Actinomyces* may also produce the infection.

The hallmarks of the infection are extensive chronic inflammation and fibrosis that produces firm, tumor-like nodules. Intermixed in the

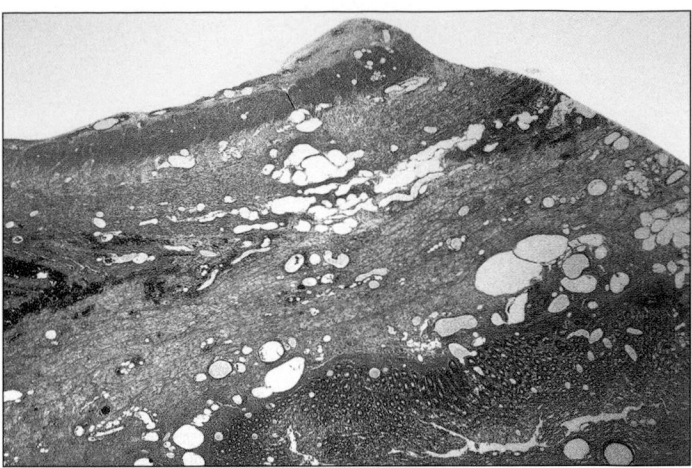

Fig. 3.10 *Clostridium* necrotizing infection of the colon. Scant inflammation and edema disrupt the wall of the colon and coat the serosal surface. The most prominent feature is the accumulation of gas within the soft tissue. It is noted by the appearance of clear spaces in levels of the mucosal wall that fat does not exist (H&E, ×50, *Clostridium septicum* isolated in culture). (Courtesy of Stephen Allen, MD)

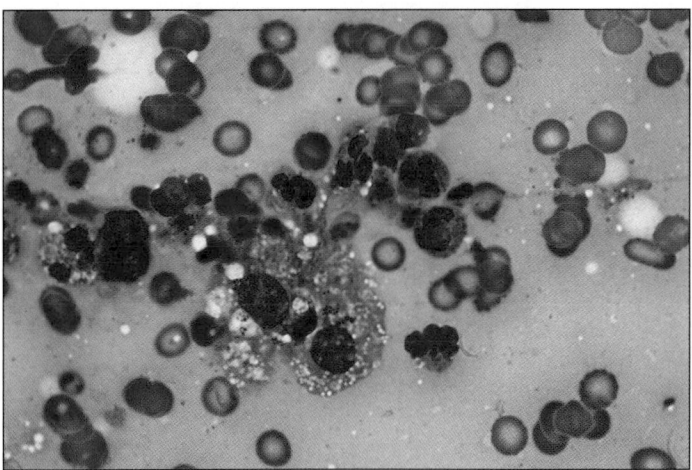

Fig. 3.11 Staphylococcal abscess, lymph node aspirate. Erythrocytes and polymorphonuclear neutrophils are seen in an edematous background. Some of the neutrophils contain ingested cocci and show the vacuolated degenerative changes due to bacterial byproducts (Giemsa, ×1000, *Staphylococcus aureus* isolated from the lymph node).

chronic inflammatory masses are islands of neutrophilic inflammation that result in draining sinuses. The characteristic actinomycotic sulfur granules, named for their macroscopic appearance, are found in the middle of the neutrophilic pools (Fig. 3.12). Sulfur granules consist of a mass of filamentous, branching Gram-positive bacteria enmeshed in an eosinophilic matrix of uncertain composition. At the edge of the granules are eosinophilic club-shaped structures, an example of the Splendore-Hoeppli phenomenon. Polymorphonuclear neutrophils often cling to the edge of the granules, which may measure several millimeters in size and be visible to the naked eye. The sulfur granules are well demonstrated by H&E stains, but the bacteria cannot be seen without special stains. Tissue Gram stain, particularly the Brown and Brenn stain, or the methenamine silver technique reveal tangled

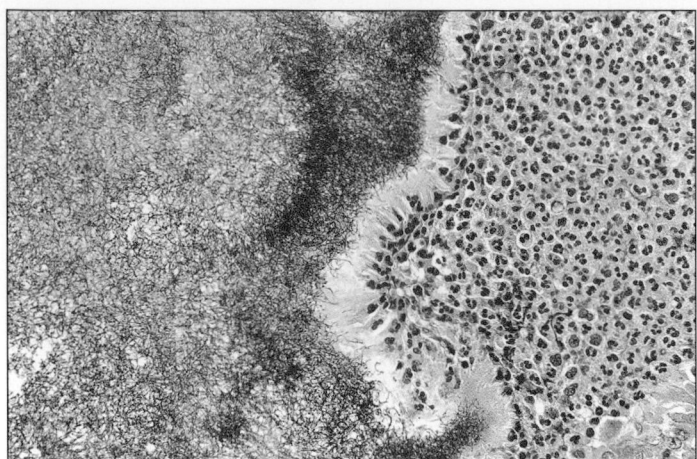

Fig. 3.12 Sulfur granule of *Actinomycosis* with well-demonstrated sulfur granule composed of thin, delicate branching bacilli visible on H&E. The bulk of the granule is composed of amorphous material. (H&E, ×450.)

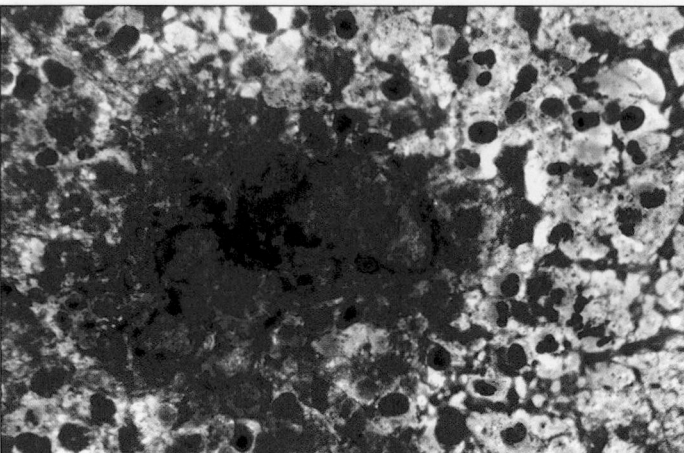

Fig. 3.13 *Actinomycosis*. Fine needle aspiration of an enlarged and partially fixed neck mass thought clinically to be carcinoma. Large ball-like cluster of organisms with filaments and clubs on the surface seen in a background of marked acute inflammation (Diff-Quik, ×400).

bacterial filaments coursing throughout the granule (Fig. 3.12). The actinomycetes are not colored by the PAS or Gridley techniques. Sulfur granules are distinct from colonies of various bacteria, without the proteinaceous matrix or peripheral clubs, which may be seen in a variety of infections or as colonizing flora in the crypts of the tonsils. Pelvic actinomycosis has been associated with the use of intrauterine contraceptive devices and suggests a more chronic, recalcitrant course than similar infections lacking actinomycetes.[52,53]

Botryomycosis

Botryomycosis is an uncommon disease process that resembles actinomycosis clinically and pathologically but is caused by bacteria other than *Actinomyces*.[54–56] The most common bacterial pathogen is *S. aureus*, but several Gram-negative bacteria and other Gram-positive bacteria may be the etiologic agents. Grains of bacterial colonies may be present, or the structures may appear identical to actinomycotic sulfur granules. Diagnosis is made by culture or by demonstration of cocci or bacilli in the granules instead of filamentous Gram-positive bacilli.

Cytologic Diagnosis: Actinomycosis may also be recognized on aspiration biopsies and has been seen frequently in the past in cervical/vaginal smears in patients who have intrauterine contraceptive devices (IUDs).[57] The appearance of the organisms is similar in both situations: a relatively amorphous mass of material with some filamentous club-like structures on the surface surrounded by polymorphonuclear leukocytes (Fig. 3.13) within a background of heavy acute inflammation. The organisms may be few in number, requiring a thorough search of the smears whenever a very heavy inflammatory exudate is present. Clinically, enlarged nodes or masses in the neck may be very indurated and suggest an advanced head and neck carcinoma. In patients with IUDs a large pelvic mass with induration of the vagina may stimulate an advanced ovarian or uterine carcinoma. Since IUDs have largely been abandoned, these cases are now quite rare, as is the identification of this organism in cervico-vaginal smears.

Syphilis

Syphilis is an age-old disease caused by *T. pallidum* subsp. *pallidum*. The lesions of primary and secondary syphilis are characterized by

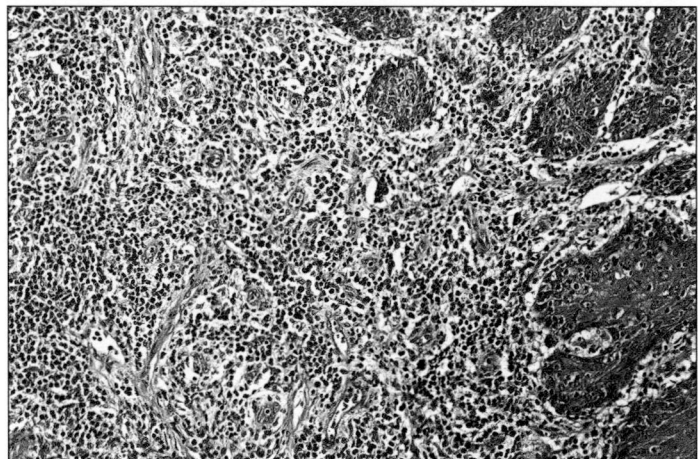

Fig. 3.14 Secondary syphilis. Pseudoepitheliomatous hyperplasia, proliferation and arborization of capillaries are seen, as well as a dense mononuclear infiltrate that includes numerous plasma cells (H&E, ×500).

prominent endothelial cells in proliferating small blood vessels and by a mononuclear inflammatory infiltrate that is rich in plasma cells (Fig. 3.14). In the placenta there is also often relative villous immaturity.[58] The lesions of primary and secondary syphilis are less commonly granulomatous.[59,60] Fully formed granulomas, known as gummas, are a feature of late syphilis and fortunately are rarely, if ever, encountered by the anatomic pathologist in the United States. In an age that has witnessed an unfortunate resurgence in syphilis, it is important to think of this possibility in unusual granulomatous lesions or inflamed foci that have a high proportion of plasma cells or vascular proliferation. The spirochetes can be demonstrated by silver impregnation techniques, such as the Warthin-Starry or related techniques (Fig. 3.15) or by staining with fluoresceinated antibodies.[61]

Candida Species: *Candida* spp. are the most common causes of fungal infection in hospitalized patients and those who are immuno-suppressed.[62] *Candida albicans* is by far the most common pathogen,

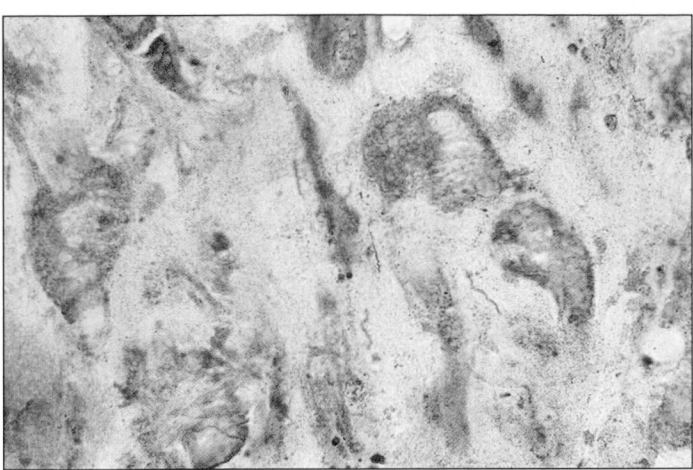

Fig. 3.15 Congenital syphilis. Tightly coiled spirochetes establish the diagnosis. Fluoresceinated antibodies are also available for an immunologically specific diagnosis (Warthin-Starry, ×1,000).

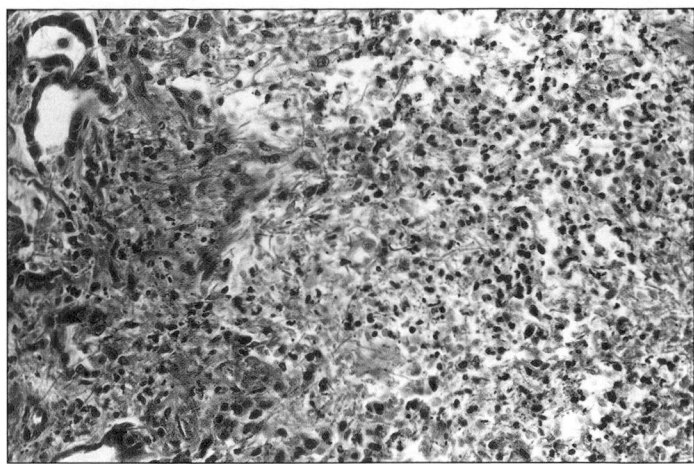

Fig. 3.17 Candida mucosal infection. A necrotizing mucosal infection includes a neutrophilic and mononuclear inflammatory response. Pseudohyphae, which can be seen coursing through the tissue, are too large to be bacterial forms (H&E, ×45).

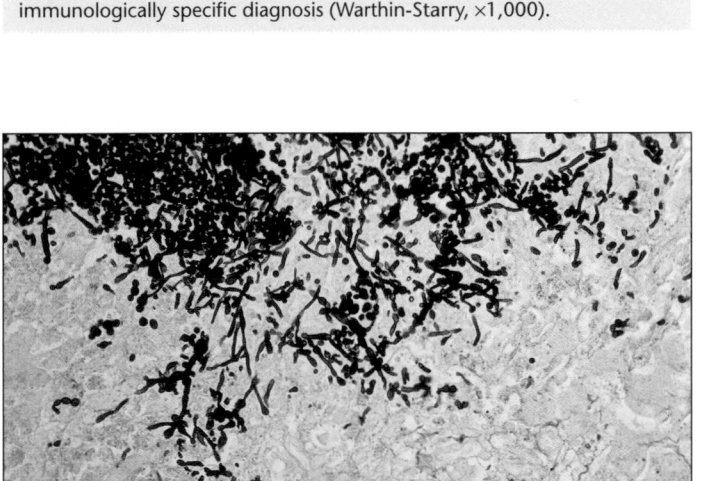

Fig. 3.16 Candida liver abscess. A combination of budding yeast and pseudohyphae makes the most likely etiologic diagnosis candidiasis (GMS, ×45, *Candida albicans* isolated in culture).

but in some locations *C. tropicalis* has been equally or more frequent as a nosocomial pathogen.[63] Other species that may be encountered with some frequency are *C. guilliermondii*, *C. parapsilosis*, and *C. krusei*,[64,65] which is especially important because of its intrinsic resistance to the imidazole class of antifungal agents. *T. (Candida) glabrata* is a small yeast that produces urinary tract infections, fungemia, and endocarditis.

Candida spp. are small elliptical yeasts that measure 3–6 µm in size. They commonly produce pseudohyphae both in vivo and in vitro, which differentiates them from most of the other commonly encountered yeasts. The yeast cells stain well with H&E, Gram stain, methenamine silver, and PAS techniques. The pseudohyphae consist of budding yeast cells that have not separated, producing elongated structures that have nonparallel walls at the cellular junctions (Fig. 3.16). True hyphae, which are also produced by *C. albicans*, have parallel cell walls.

Candida spp. produce a variety of clinical infections, most commonly of the skin, nails, vagina, and mucocutaneous areas. More serious infections include oral candidiasis (thrush); disease of the gastrointestinal tract (Fig. 3.17), especially the lower esophagus; endocarditis; and disseminated infection that may involve any organ.[66,67] Infection of the central nervous system and primary infection of the lungs are uncommon.[68,69] The portals of entry are usually the skin or the gastrointestinal tract. The histologic response is usually pyogenic (Fig. 3.17), but granulomatous lesions or mixed acute and chronic inflammation may result. The development of the triazole agents, beginning with fluconazole, that can be administered effectively both orally and parenterally, has significantly decreased the mortality and morbidity of persistent, recurrent, and disseminated candidal infections.[70]

The differential diagnosis on initial analysis usually includes bacterial pathogens (which may also be present). Once the presence of yeasts and pseudohyphae is recognized, the diagnosis is usually obvious (see Fig. 3.16). If yeasts alone are present, they must be differentiated from dimorphic yeasts, which usually have different clinical and pathologic presentations. The pseudohyphae must be differentiated from hyaline molds, such as *Aspergillus* spp.

Sporothrix schenckii: *S. schenckii* is a small, round to oval yeast that measures 2–6 µm in size. The yeasts are rarely seen in histologic sections, both because they are sparse and because they stain poorly with H&E. Likewise, the characteristic elongated, 'cigar-shaped' cells are not commonly encountered. A characteristic, but not diagnostic feature of sporotrichosis is the asteroid body, an eosinophilic structure measuring up to 100 µm. The asteroid body is produced by accretion of proteinaceous material around a yeast cell, the Splendore-Hoeppli phenomenon.[71] Unfortunately, the asteroid bodies, which were frequently reported in early cases from South African miners, are not commonly seen in the United States. *S. schenckii* stains well with the methenamine silver and PAS techniques. A potential pitfall is the presence of cigar-shaped structures in sarcoid-like granulomas in lymph nodes, known as Hamazaki-Wesenberg bodies.[72,73] These nonbiologic structures can be differentiated from yeast cells by their inherent yellow-brown pigmentation.

The distribution of *Sporothrix* is worldwide. Epidemics in the United States have been associated particularly with agricultural products, particularly sphagnum moss.[74,75] The classic description of the patient as an alcoholic rose gardener is not often accurate, but a modern analogy was contributed by a group of beer-guzzling fraternity brothers who acquired their infection when they were passing straw-packed bricks along a chain line as they constructed a masonry wall.[76] The portal of entry is usually the skin, resulting in a local lesion that may be followed by lymphangitis and proximal lesions in skin or lymph nodes, or both. Disseminated infection occurs uncommonly, primarily to the lymph nodes, skeletal system, and solid organs, often accompanied by a history of possible primary pulmonary exposure.[77] In developed countries the therapy has shifted away from potassium iodide to itraconazole as the antimycotic agent of choice. The occasional entry of *S. schenckii* into the respiratory tract results in a primary granulomatous pneumonia that must be differentiated from other fungal and mycobacterial processes.[78] Histologically, the process is granulomatous, with both caseating and noncaseating lesions. A component of acute inflammation and microabscesses may be present. The differential diagnosis of sporotrichosis clinically and pathologically includes swimming pool granuloma caused by *Mycobacterium marinum*, tularemia caused by *Francisella tularensis* (which may also result in lymphangitis and proximal lesions), blastomycosis, and neoplastic disease. Because the causative microbes are rarely demonstrated in tissue, the etiology must often be resolved by culture or an exhausting search of submitted tissues.

Chromoblastomycosis: Chromoblastomycosis is a chronic infection of skin and subcutaneous tissue that is caused by several genera of dematiaceous (pigmented) fungi, particularly *Fonsecaea pedrosoi* as well as *Cladophialophora* and *Ramichloridium*.[79] The infection is most prevalent in tropical and subtropical regions. In the United States it is uncommon but is most often documented in the southern states and is associated with steam baths. As the name implies, the clinical and histologic appearance of the lesions resembles blastomycosis most closely. The chronic lesions are caused by direct inoculation of the fungi, so they are most often seen on exposed parts of the lower extremities. The histologic response is granulomatous, with the inclusion of microabscesses and a profound pseudoepitheliomatous hyperplasia that accounts for the verrucous, tumor-like skin masses. The hallmark of the infection is the presence of dark-brown, thick-walled muriform cells that measure 5–12 µm (Fig. 3.18). These structures, which are diagnostic of the infection, are referred to as sclerotic bodies. Special stains are not necessary because of the intrinsic pigmentation. As is true in blastomycosis, the yeast-like cells are found in the microabscesses surrounded by polymorphonuclear neutrophils. The sclerotic bodies divide by septation, which may be visualized in the brown cells. Infections with these pigmented fungi are typically very refractory to therapy, and as such, no single treatment of choice has been identified. Therapy often requires systemic antimycotic agents such as itraconazole or terbinafine used at high doses for periods extending up to 12 months. If combined with local thermotherapy (locally applied heat or cryosurgery), results may be enhanced in particularly resistant cases.[80]

Prototheca species: *Prototheca* spp. are achlorophyllous algae that occasionally cause infection of the skin and subcutaneous tissue and often infect bursae, especially that of the olecrenon.[81–83] They are considered with the fungi because of their morphologic and cultural similarities. The diagnostic form is a sporangium that contains up to 20 endospores (Fig. 3.19). The sporangia of the two most common species, *P. wickerhamii* and *P. zopfii*, measure 2–12 µm and 10–25 µm in diameter, respectively.[84] Crowding of the endospores, each of which has a single nucleus and its own cell wall, causes molding of the endospores that may resemble septation. The

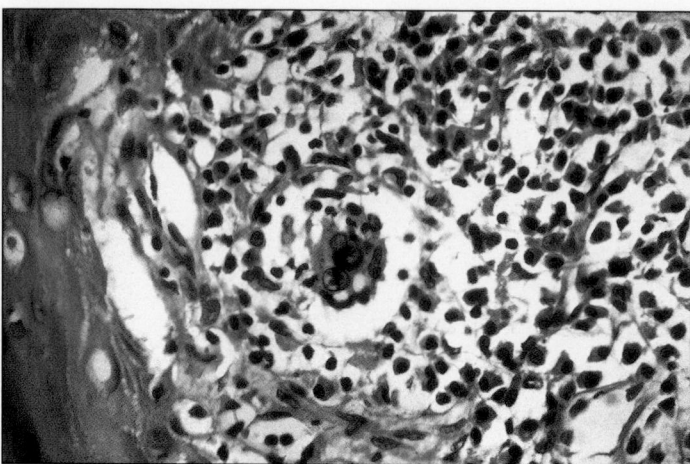

Fig. 3.18 Chromoblastomycosis. Yellow-brown yeast-like cells are present in a mononuclear infiltrate within the upper dermis. The yeast-like cells, some of which have septae, are referred to as sclerotic bodies. They are produced by several species of dematiaceous fungi (H&E, ×450).

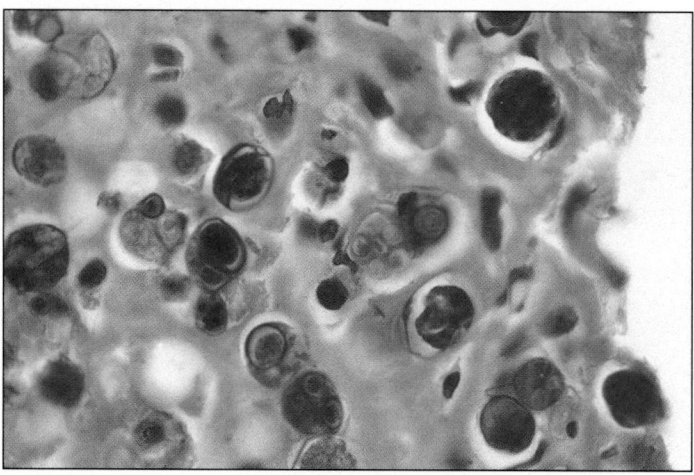

Fig. 3.19 Protothecosis. The inflammatory lesion contains numerous sporangia with internal spores. The cells of these achlorophyllous algae can be misinterpreted as multinucleated cells with inclusions (H&E, ×1000, *Prototheca wickerhamii* isolated from culture).

sporangia of *P. wickerhamii* may assume the form of a morula – a central endospore surrounded by peripheral endospores. The sporangia and endospores are stained well with H&E, although in some cases only the walls of the individual endospores are colored. The structures are also demonstrated well with the methenamine silver and PAS techniques.

The histologic response in cutaneous lesions is a scant mononuclear infiltrate with focal necrosis and many interspersed sporangia. Inflammation of the bursa may include granulomas with or without necrosis (Fig. 3.20). The differential diagnosis is not difficult if the observer is familiar with this organism. Other organisms that form sporangia, such as *C. immitis*, are considerably larger. In H&E-stained sections the sporangia may be mistaken for strange multinucleated host cells. Rare reports of disseminated protothecosis have been documented, but these have been restricted to the immuno-

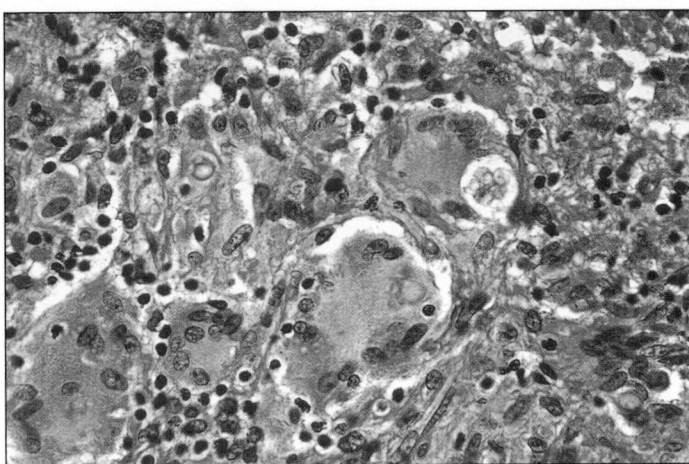

Fig. 3.20 Protothecosis. After resection of the lesion shown in Fig. 3.19, recurrent disease was characterized by few organisms and a granulomatous inflammatory response. The algae are present in the cytoplasm of multinucleated giant cells (H&E, ×500).

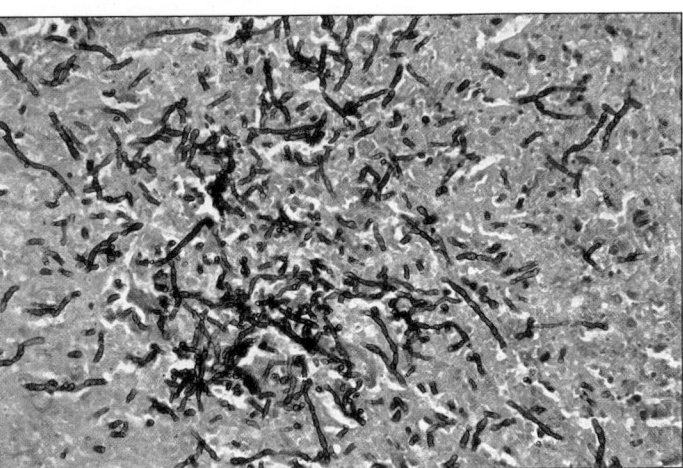

Fig. 3.22 Phaeohyphomycosis of the brain. Septate, branching hyphae in a necrotic lesion. The hyphae are colored by demonstration of melanin in their walls (Fontana-Masson method, ×400, *Cladosporium bantianum* isolated from cultures).

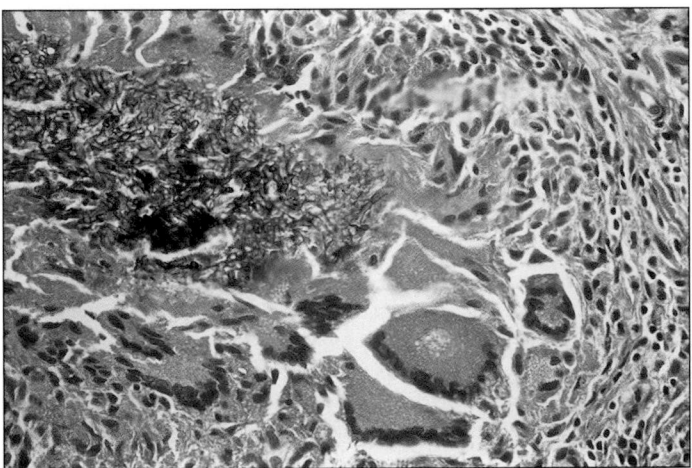

Fig. 3.21 Phaeohyphomycosis. An inoculation lesion of the subcutaneous tissue includes a granuloma with multinucleated giant cells. A mass of brown pigmented hyphae is contained in the granulomas. The fungus is identified by the pigment as dematiaceous, but the specific identification cannot be made from the morphology. (H&E, ×400.)

compromised host, particularly those with neutrophil functional defects.[85]

Phaeohyphomycosis: *Phaeohyphomycosis* is a term used to describe cutaneous or systemic infections caused by dematiaceous (naturally pigmented) molds.[86] The most common lesions are localized subcutaneous infections that result from direct entry of the fungus through the skin (Fig. 3.21). Many of these molds are commonly found in nature, associated with vegetation. Occasionally, the vehicle for entry – usually a splinter or thorn – may be seen in the lesion. Granulomatous inflammation in the subcutaneous tissue is the hallmark of the infection, and the epidermis is usually uninvolved. As a result the clinical presentation is ordinarily a firm or fluctuant nodule. The fluctuance results from the formation of cystic spaces in the granulomas, producing a phaeomycotic cyst. The infecting fungus cannot be identified specifically without culture. *Exophiala*

spp. and *Phialophora* spp. are the most common causes of phaeomycotic cyst, and diffuse granulomatous inflammation is commonly caused by *Bipolaris* spp., *Wangiella* spp., and *Alternaria* spp. The therapy is simple excision of the lesion.

Systemic infection, which is very uncommon, usually affects the central nervous system and is most often caused by *Cladosporium (Xylohypha) bantianum*.[87] A review of 101 cases of central nervous system phaeophyphomycosis over a 34-year period, revealed that more than 50% of the patients had no known immunocompromised state and that mortality rates are high, regardless of immune status. The portal of entry is probably the lung, but pulmonary infection is not evident. A destructive infection with tissue necrosis is the result, and the inflammatory response may include either granulomas or purulent inflammation. The remarkable trophism for the brain is unexplained. Septate hyphae, some with bizarre swollen forms, and occasionally yeast-like cells are found in the necrotic material or abscesses (Fig. 3.22). Aggressive treatment of disseminated disease usually includes amphotericin B, one or more azoles such as flucytosine and itraconazole, and surgical debridement. Phaeohyphomycosis occurring in the transplant population can be refractory to therapy, particularly if infection is acquired during the high-dose immunosuppression phase. In one well-documented case, the fungal infection was irradicated by the combination of amphotericin B, flucytosine, and itraconazole.[88] In vitro testing of the fungal isolate confirmed a synergistic effect of the combined antimycotic agents.

The diagnosis of phaeohyphomycosis is established by demonstration of yellow-brown, septate hyphae in the lesions. Special stains are not usually necessary because of the naturally occurring pigment, but methenamine silver and PAS techniques stain the fungi well. In fact, an unstained section is sometimes useful for demonstration of the hyphae unobscured by histochemical staining. The dematiaceous fungi contain melanin. If the pigmentation of the hyphae is slight and the identification is in doubt, the Fontana-Masson stain may be used to document the nature of the organisms (Fig. 3.22).

Mycetoma

Mycetoma is a chronic, tumorous infection of the skin and subcutaneous tissue, usually of the lower extremities.[89] The pathogens

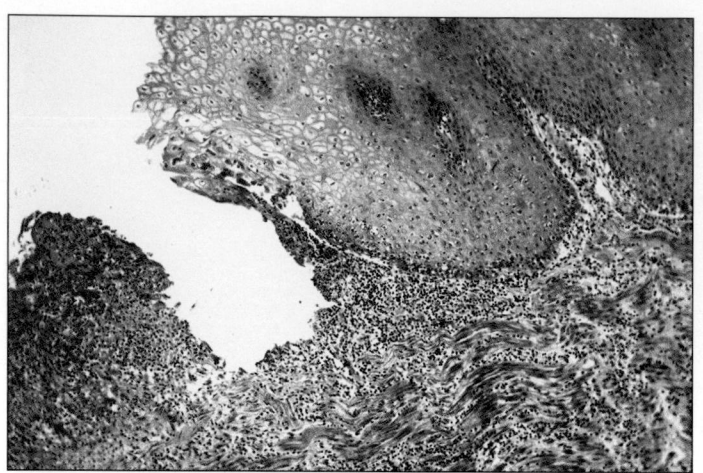

Fig. 3.23 Herpes simplex esophagitis. There is intense mixed inflammation beneath the ulcerated epithelium. Several epithelial cells at the edge of the ulcer contain intranuclear inclusions (H&E, ×50).

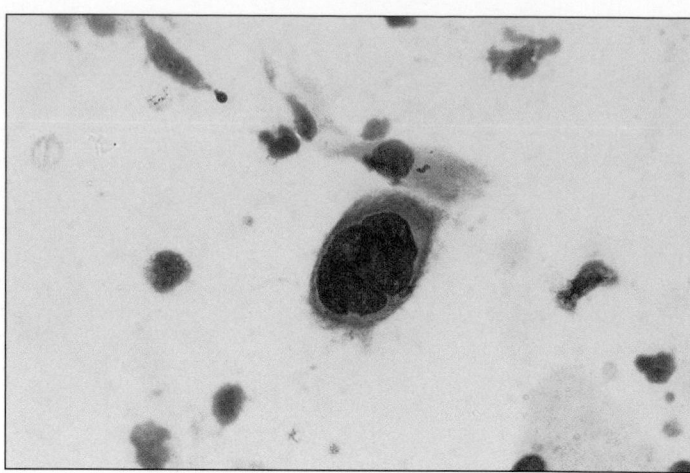

Fig. 3.24 Tsanck preparation. A multinucleated giant cell is demonstrated in this scraping from the base of a vesicular lesion. Intranuclear inclusions are not readily seen, but the molding of the nuclei is clearly demonstrated. It is not possible to distinguish between herpes simplex and varicella-zoster viruses with this technique (Diff-Quik, ×1000).

are introduced directly into the host through the skin by trauma.[90] Histologically, a mixture of acute and chronic inflammation with grains of varying morphology is seen, depending on the etiologic agent. Mycetoma may be caused by aerobic actinomycetes, particularly *Actinomadura* spp. (causing the designation Madura foot), *Nocardia* spp. (including *N. asteroides), Nocardiopsis* spp., and *Streptomyces somaliensis*.[91,92] Eumycotic mycetomas are caused by a variety of hyphomycetes (white grain mycetoma) and dematiaceous fungi (black grain mycetoma). The differentiation is made by demonstration of bacteria or fungi in the grains with appropriate special stains.

Herpes simplex virus

Herpes simplex virus is ubiquitous and extremely versatile in its ability to cause human disease. Type 1 strains, which predominantly infect the upper half of the body, are found in people of all ages, beginning in early childhood. Sexually transmitted type 2 strains make their appearance in adolescence and almost exclusively infect the genitourinary systems and skin of the lower body. Pathologists are most likely to encounter herpes simplex virus in cytologic preparations of genital lesions (type 2) or skin (either type). The primary lesions on the skin or mucosa are maculopapules followed quickly by vesicles, caused by infection of squamous epithelium and subsequent disruption of the keratinocytes. Keratinolysis produces intraepidermal bullae, and multinucleated giant cells are present in the adjoining intact epithelium. Mucosal lesions ulcerate so quickly that the vesicles are less commonly seen (Fig. 3.23). Cytologic preparations are obtained by scraping the base of an ulcer or unroofed vesicle. Smears may be air dried and stained with a Romanowsky or H&E stain (Fig. 3.24), a procedure known as a Tsanck preparation. Alternatively, the smear may be fixed and stained by the Papanicolaou technique. The inclusions of herpes simplex virus are homogeneous and often fill the nucleus, pushing the normal nucleoprotein to the periphery of the nuclear envelope. In formalin-fixed H&E-stained sections, artifactual shrinkage of the inclusion produces a halo between the eosinophilic inclusion and the more basophilic peripheralized chromatin. It is easy to miss inclusions that do not have a halo. In cytologic preparations inclusions are often difficult to

discern, but molding of the nuclei in multinucleated cells assists in differentiating the virally infected cell from its normal neighbors.

The sensitivity of cytologic diagnosis is very high in skin lesions, but unfortunately not so high in infections of the female genital tract. The specificity of cytologic diagnosis by experienced investigators is also high, but atypical, reactive cells have been misinterpreted as herpes-infected cells in cytologic preparations. Herpes simplex and varicella-zoster viruses produce inclusions that cannot be differentiated by morphologic criteria. Use of dual antibodies with different fluorescent labels has been successfully evaluated as a means of diagnosing vesicular skin lesions.[93] Anomalous immunostaining with antisera to herpes simplex virus has been described in optically clear nuclei in gestational endometrium, leading to an erroneous diagnosis of intrauterine herpes infection.

Type 1 herpes simplex virus is the most common cause of sporadic viral encephalitis, and type 2 virus also causes serious life-threatening systemic infection in neonates whose mothers have active genital infections at the time of vaginal delivery and in patients whose host defenses are compromised. Diagnosis of herpes simplex infection in brain biopsies was once a prerequisite for therapy, but the advent of effective, nontoxic drugs has reduced the necessity of obtaining brain tissue. In a large study of diagnostic methods for herpes encephalitis, histologic examination was only 56% sensitive and 86% specific.[94] Both sensitivity and specificity were improved by use of immunofluorescence.

Disseminated infection may cause destructive disease in many organs, particularly the liver (Fig. 3.25), if the patient is immunocompromised. Necrotizing infection in the liver, adrenal glands, or other organs is typically seen in severely immunosuppressed patients, such as recipients of organ transplants and in neonates who have disseminated gestational infection (Fig. 3.25). Herpetic esophagitis is characterized by ulcerating lesions that may be coinfected with *Candida* spp. In other situations compromise of physical defenses may increase the risk of herpes simplex virus infection. Cutaneous disease is associated with damage to the normal epidermis by physical abrasions in wrestling matches ('herpes gladiatorum') or by thermal burns. Similarly, destructive corneal infection results from direct inoculation of herpes simplex virus into the eye. Intubated

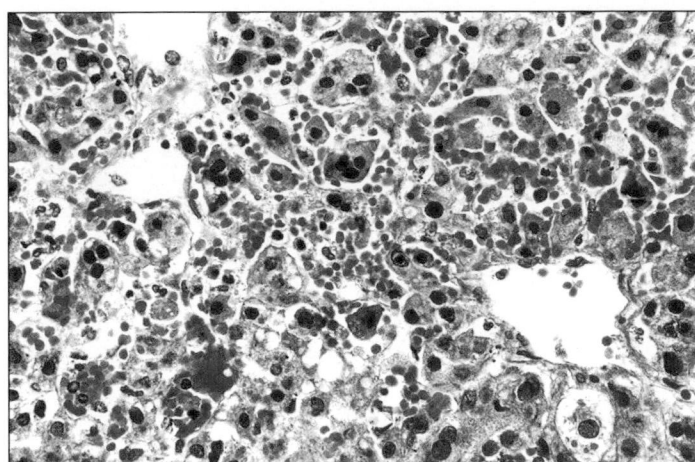

Fig. 3.25 Herpes hepatitis in disseminated neonatal infection. Extensive necrosis and hemorrhage are seen in the hepatic cords. Most of the intact cells shown here at the edge of the necrotic lesions contain eosinophilic intranuclear inclusions. The inclusions vary from homogeneous masses that fill the nucleus to condensed aggregates of viral nucleoprotein that are separated from the surrounding nuclear membrane. Multinucleated giant cells with inclusions are present. It is not possible to distinguish between herpes simplex viruses (type I and II) or varicella-zoster viruses by histologic findings (H&E, ×500, herpes virus Type II isolated by culture).

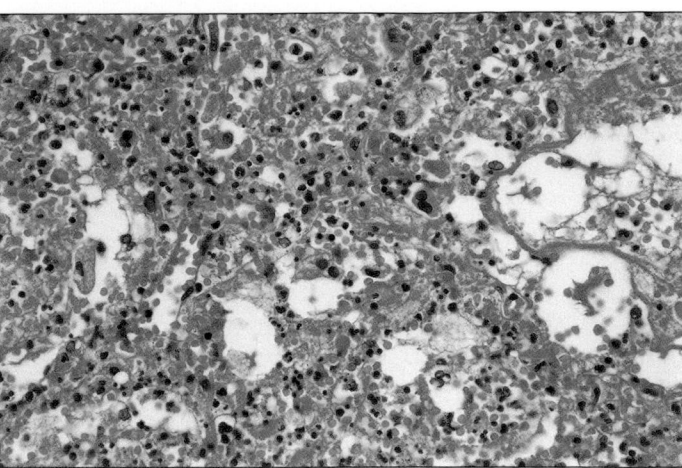

Fig. 3.26 Herpes simplex virus pneumonia. Extensive necrosis and acute inflammation are seen. The inflammatory response initially suggests a bacterial etiology, but the correct diagnosis is rendered when the eosinophilic intranuclear inclusions are identified. These can be confirmed by immunoperoxidase studies or by culture (H&E, ×200 herpes virus Type I isolated by culture).

patients at risk of repetitive aspiration have a higher than normal incidence of herpetic infection in the lower respiratory tract. The virus is usually type 1 and probably enters the lungs from where it may be shed asymptomatically. The distribution of inflammation in the lungs is patchy. By contrast, viremic type 2 infection in neonates or type 1 infection in immunosuppressed adults usually results in multifocal, punctate pulmonary lesions.

The unitary lesion in herpetic infections is the accumulation of damaged cells, which may result in extensive necrosis as the cells rupture. The inflammatory response includes mononuclear cells, and a pattern of diffuse alveolar damage is often found. In addition, however, an intense polymorphonuclear neutrophilic response is elicited by the extensive necrosis (Fig. 3.26).[95] The exuberance of the acute inflammatory response may mislead the observer into assuming that the etiology is bacterial. Careful observation of the section will reveal the presence of inclusions in epithelium.[96] Multinucleated giant cells are often present but are not as dramatic as in some other viral infections.

Cytologic Diagnosis of Female Genital Tract Herpes Infections: Infection of the female genital tract by the herpes virus is quite symptomatic on the external genitalia but clinically silent when involving the cervix. Characteristic ground-glass changes or cells with definite inclusion bodies (or both) may be seen in cervico-vaginal smears stained by the Papanicolaou method (Fig. 3.27). Detection of herpes virus inclusions in the cervical smear can be important in the pregnant patient near term, as a vaginal delivery may result in increased risk of infection of the newborn, with devastating results.[97]

Varicella-zoster virus

Varicella-zoster virus causes chickenpox on initial contact and shingles when the virus in spinal ganglia is reactivated. The diagnosis is usually obvious clinically, and difficult cases can be resolved without recourse to biopsy. In immunosuppressed patients and in

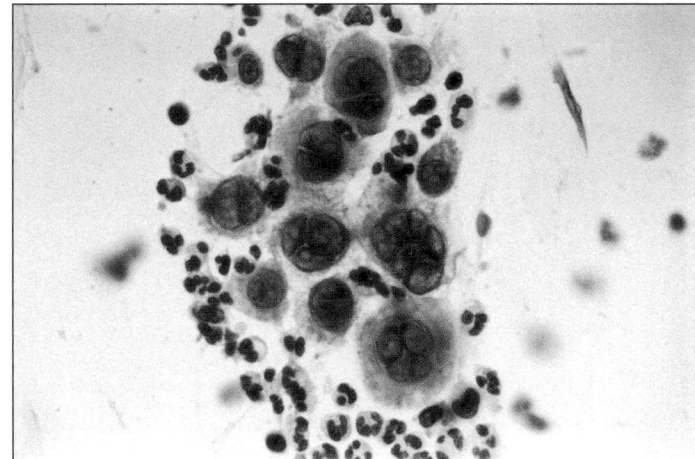

Fig. 3.27 Herpes virus in cervical vaginal smear. Multinucleated giant cells with ground-glass nuclear inclusions (Papanicolaou, ×600).

pregnant women varicella-zoster virus can produce severe pneumonia and disseminated infection.[98] The lesions and the viral inclusions closely resemble those of herpes simplex (Fig. 3.28), so the etiology must be determined by culture or by detection of specific viral antigens or nucleic acids.

Papoviruses

Papoviruses consist of papillomaviruses, which cause human warts, papillomas, and epithelial neoplasia; polyomaviruses, which cause disease in immunosuppressed patients; and vacuolating agents, which do not cause human disease.[99] The most important poly-omaviruses, SV40 and JC virus, cause progressive multifocal leukoencephalopathy, a disease that is more likely to be seen by the autopsy pathologist than the surgical pathologist. Multiple foci of demyelination without inflammation are produced in the subcortical

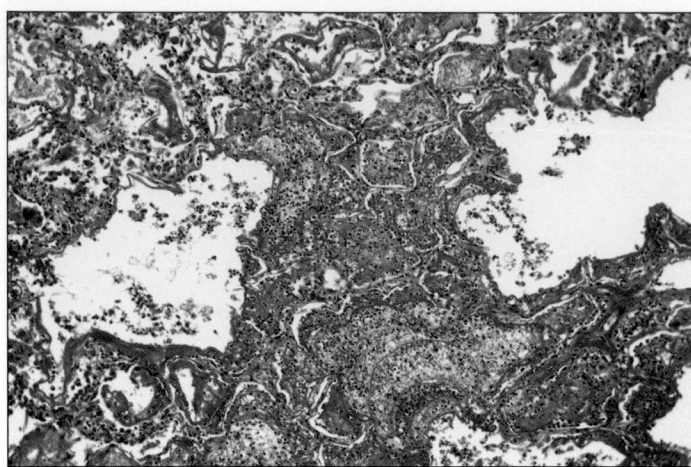

Fig. 3.28 Varicella-zoster pneumonia. Interstitial mononuclear infiltrates and an intense alveolar inflammatory exudates are seen. Note neutrophils, intra-alveolar fibrin, and hyaline membrane formation (H&E, ×50).

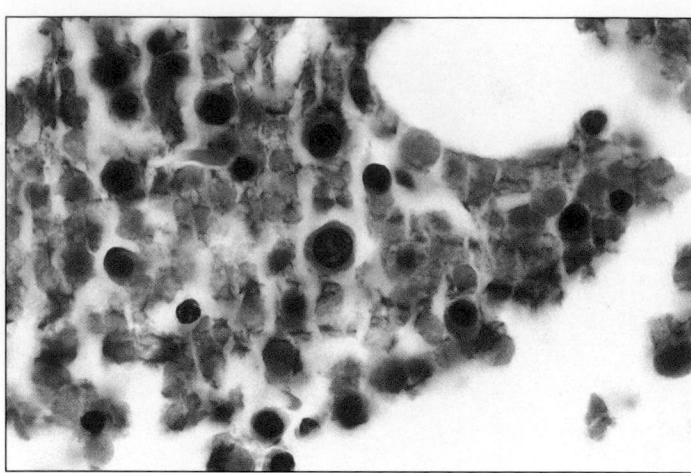

Fig. 3.30 Parvovirus B19 infection in a young black female with a hemoglobinopathy. Autopsy bone marrow demonstrated extensive necrosis and there was widespread fat embolization in the brain, lungs, and kidneys. Some enlarged remaining erythroids show intranuclear inclusions (H&E, ×600).

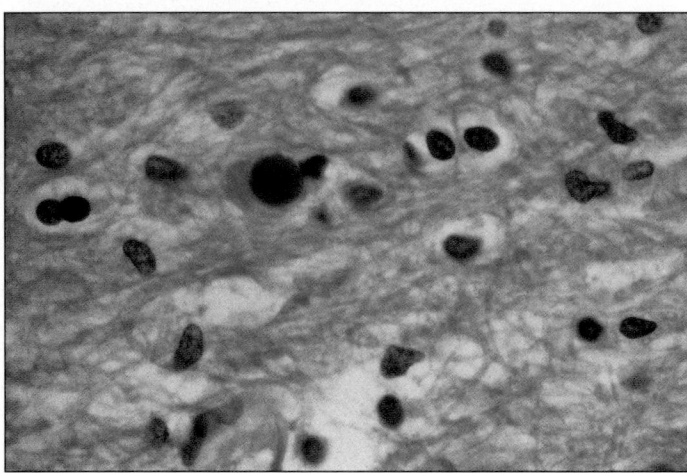

Fig. 3.29 Progressive multifocal leukoencephalopathy. An infected oligodendroglial cell contains a basophilic inclusion that fills the nucleus. The loose neuropil reflects accompanying demyelination. The polyomavirus (usually JC virus) are very difficult to culture, but the diagnosis can be confirmed by documenting the virions ultrastructurally (H&E, ×1000).

white matter.[100] Oligodendroglia are the target cells, in which accumulation of virions produce a basophilic intranuclear inclusion (Fig. 3.29).

Human parvovirus 19

Human parvovirus 19 produces erythema infectiosum (fifth disease) in children, nonimmune hydrops in pregnant women, and acute arthritis in adults. Parvovirus infections are most likely to be seen by surgical pathologists in bone marrow biopsies from patients with hemoglobinopathies and chronic hemolytic anemia.[101] Parvovirus B19 may cause aplastic crisis in these patients accompanied by extensive marrow necrosis, and basophilic intranuclear inclusions can be demonstrated in erythroid precursors (Fig. 3.30).

Molluscum contagiosum

Molluscum contagiosum is the only poxvirus that is likely to be encountered in the surgical pathology laboratory.[102] A distinctive raised, umbilicated skin lesion(s) provides little diagnostic challenge and is not usually biopsied unless the nodules are atypical. The elevated mass consists of enlarged, proliferated keratinocytes that contain large masses of eosinophilic cytoplasmic inclusions. Although treatment is controversial and usually directed towards limiting local spread or autoinnoculation, care must be taken when exposure to immunocompromised patients is a possibility.

Leishmania Species: Leishmania spp. are protozoan parasites that are distributed widely throughout the Old and New Worlds. Travel to Mexico, Central and South America, and the Persian Gulf is responsible for most cases seen in the United States.[103] Leishmaniasis, including visceral disease, was one of the infectious diseases most commonly noted in veterans of the recent Gulf War.[104] Leishmaniasis occurs as relatively benign, but unsightly cutaneous disease; potentially disfiguring mucocutaneous infection; and disseminated, potentially fatal infection, known as kala-azar. The type of infection is roughly associated with the country of origin, but molecular techniques are now available for definitive characterization of the risks if the protozoan can be isolated in culture. Disseminated infection may occur more frequently in severely immunosuppressed patients.[105,106]

Leishmania spp. are intracellular parasites that are associated prominently with macrophages as amastigotes. There is no flagellated form in tissue. The histologic response in cutaneous and mucocutaneous disease consists of accumulations of macrophages; noncaseating granulomas with giant cells may also be present. It is not uncommon to find an intermixed acute inflammatory response with microabscesses. Pseudoepitheliomatous hyperplasia of the overlying dermis may be present. The differential diagnosis of the skin lesions includes other mixed inflammatory infections, such as blastomycosis or chromoblastomycosis. Once the amastigotes are recognized they must be differentiated from other parasites and from *H. capsulatum* (Fig. 3.31). Demonstration of the kinetoplast in the amastigotes narrows the differential diagnosis to *T. cruzi* (Fig. 3.32).[107]

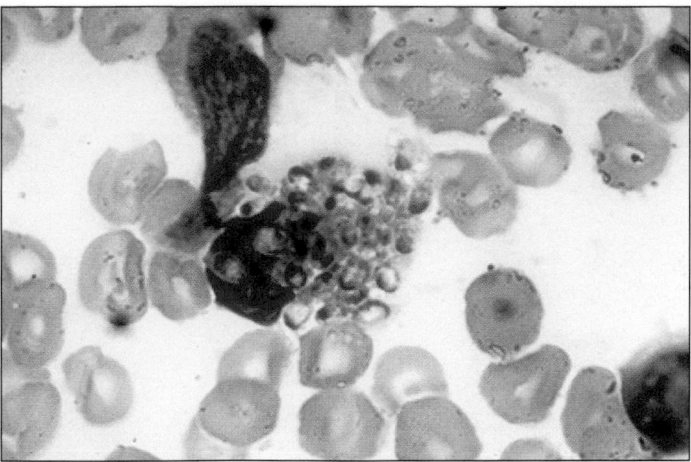

Fig. 3.31 This Wright-stain smear of a patient with disseminated histoplasmosis shows the morphology that is most difficult to differentiate from leishmaniasis. Each organism has only one nuclear body that is pushed to the edge of the cell wall (Wright, ×1000).

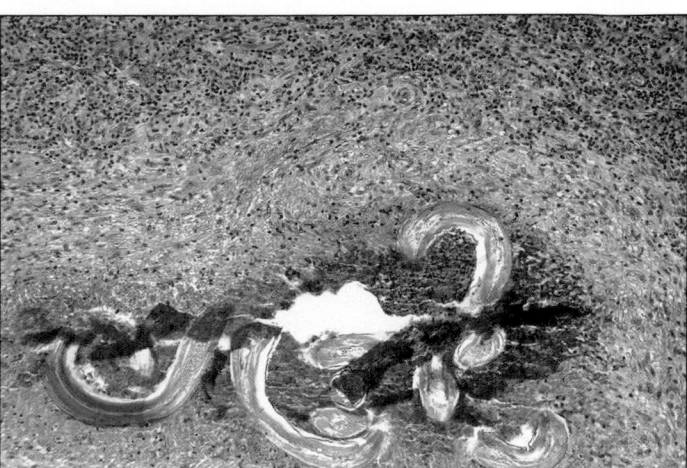

Fig. 3.33 Visceral larvae migrans. A degenerating nematode larva is trapped in a lymph node. The worm is surrounded by a granuloma, and frequent eosinophils are present in the adjacent tissue (H&E, ×160). (Courtesy of Sandy Dorman, MD)

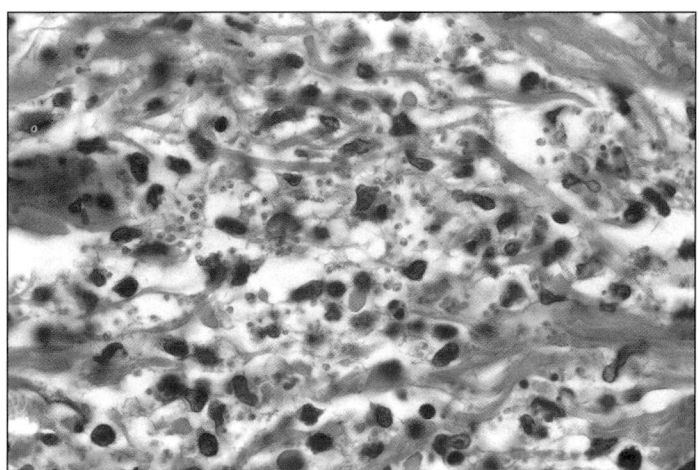

Fig. 3.32 Cutaneous leishmaniasis. Numerous amastigote forms of *Leishmania* are contained in macrophages. Other areas of the biopsy contained a neutrophilic inflammatory response. Despite the numerous organisms, the etiology was not recognized at the time of the initial interpretation (H&E, ×500).

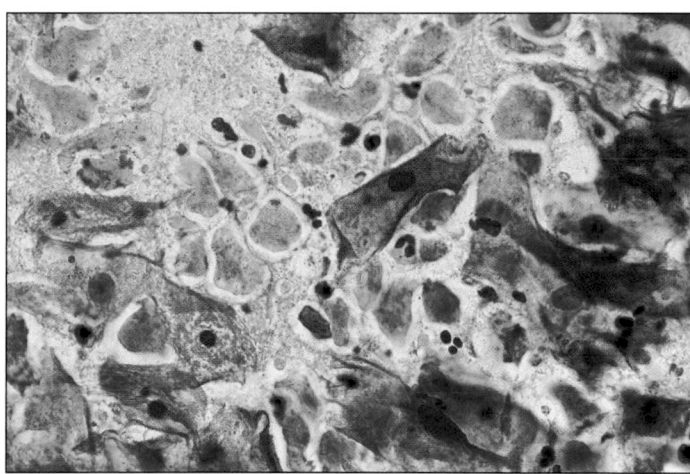

Fig. 3.34 *Trichomonas vaginalis* in a cervical vaginal smear. Many gray-green vaguely outlined organisms are seen between scattered superficial squamous cells (Papanicolaou, ×600).

Visceral Larva Migrans: The migrating larvae of nonhuman nematodes, most commonly *Toxocara canis* and *T. cati*, cause visceral larva migrans.[108] In human roundworm infections such as *Ascaris lumbricoides*, a human host ingests eggs that develop into larvae in the gastrointestinal tract; the larvae migrate through the wall of the gastrointestinal tract, to the liver, through the lungs, and back into the gastrointestinal tract, where they develop into mature worms. The tissue phase of the life cycle is transient, and, although symptoms may be provoked, only rarely is tissue damage seen. In contrast, the larvae of nonhuman ascarid worms wander through the tissues of the body until they come to rest in an organ, where they die and produce an inflammatory response. The tissue response consists of chronic, granulomatous inflammation with many eosinophils. The dying larvae are present in the center of the lesion, but serial sections may be necessary to demonstrate them (Fig. 3.33). Excision of the lesion is curative.

Cytologic Diagnosis of Common Female Genital Tract Infections: Pathogens commonly encountered in the routine pap smear review process include *Trichomonas* infection (Fig. 3.34) and bacterial vaginitis (Fig. 3.35), neither of which is a problem for the practicing cytopathologist.

THE NASOPHARYNX AND UPPER RESPIRATORY SYSTEM

The upper respiratory tract is composed of the nose, paranasal sinuses, nasopharynx, larynx, and middle ear with associated mastoid air spaces. These anatomic sites are exposed to innumerable airborne and fomite-borne infectious organisms as well as numerous

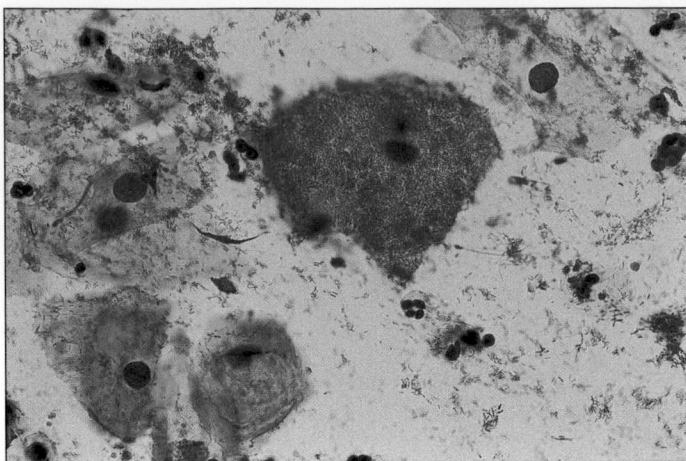

Fig. 3.35 Bacterial vaginitis, cervical vaginal smear. Squamous cell covered with small coccobacillary organisms with many additional organisms in the background. These cells are referred to as 'clue' cells, indicating a bacterial overgrowth of mixed-type vaginal flora (Papanicolaou, ×600).

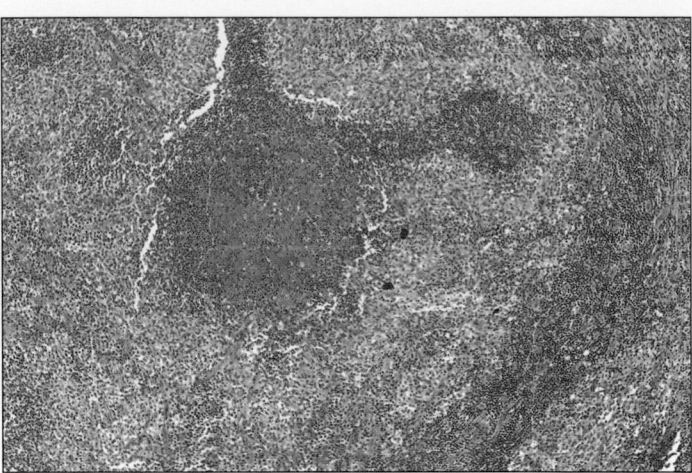

Fig. 3.36 Section from a child with oculoglandular cat-scratch disease with no history of a scratch. Note typical necrotizing granuloma with stellate central microabscess formation (H&E, ×250).

allergens, toxins, and carcinogens. The oropharynx and nasopharynx host a myriad of microorganisms, most of which are harmless under normal conditions in the healthy host. In fact, the mere presence of colonizing mixed bacterial flora serves a protective purpose as surface and nutrient competitors to 'would-be' pathogens.

Common bacterial infections such as group A beta-hemolytic *Streptococcus*, *Streptococcus pneumoniae*, and *Hemophilus influenza* cause readily diagnosable conditions within the upper respiratory tract and the need for biopsies is usually avoided. Likewise, most viral infections of the head and neck do not require biopsy for appropriate therapy. However, select viral, bacterial, mycobacterial, fungal, and protozoal pathogens may present diagnostic dilemmas pushing clinicians to obtain biopsies to determine if the process is reactive, neoplastic, or infectious. A few pathogen look-alikes that may be encountered in the upper respiratory system include cholesterol granulomas, teflon granulomas, myopherulosis, localized laryngeal amyloidosis, and pyogenic granulomas.

Actinomycosis

Actinomycosis is a chronic suppurative infection of the soft tissue caused by the delicate branching Gram-positive bacteria within the Actinomycetales group. Although once thought to be a fungal agent, we now know these are anaerobic bacterial pathogens that normally reside within the tonsils and gingival surfaces of the oropharynx. Dental and periodontal disease and intra-oral traumatic injury often initiates the infectious disease we have come to know as 'lumpy jaw.' Lesions may arise anywhere in the upper nasopharyngeal area including presentation as a solitary laryngeal nodule with or without ulceration.[109] Classic clusters of organisms seen grossly as 'sulfur granules' incite a suppurative tissue reaction, soft tissue necrosis, and tunneling, the end result of which may be a cutaneous draining fistula. If left untreated, this infection may extend directly into adjacent sinuses, bone, and to distant sites. The organisms must be distinguished from eumycotic mycetomas, as well as *Nocardia* that are partially acid fast.

Oculoglandular cat-scratch disease

Oculoglandular cat-scratch disease (CSD) of Parinaud is caused by *Bartonella henselae*, a fastidious Gram-negative bacillus which is

difficult to culture using routine methods.[110] The tissue response is a necrotizing granulomatous reaction with microabscess formation identical to that we have come to recognize with the more common CSD peripheral lymph node presentation occurring predominantly on the extremities of children (Fig. 3.36). Oculoglandular CSD usually occurs without a history of a cat scratch or skin papule.[111] The most likely route of entry in these cases is via the conjunctival membrane with subsequent spread to the preauricular lymph node.

Klebsiella rhinoscleromatis

Rhinoscleroma is a rare chronic granulomatous destructive infection of the orofacial soft tissues caused by the Gram-negative bacteria *Klebsiella rhinoscleromatis*.[112,113] This organism is NOT a normal inhabitant of the nasal flora. As the infection progresses, an intense fibrotic reaction develops, hence the term 'scleromatous' nodules. These nodules eventually may result in destruction of the soft palate, nose, and uvula. Rhinoscleroma progresses through three stages histologically: the rhinitis stage, the granulomatous stage, and the fibrotic stage. The rhinitis stage is non-specific and diagnosis in this stage is unlikely. The failure of resolution often brings these patients back for a second biopsy during the granulomatous or fibrotic stage. In both of these, the mucosal surface epithelium is hyperplastic with an intense submucosal inflammatory infiltrate rich in plasma cells and large foamy histiocytes called 'Mikulicz cells.' The bacteria may be identified within the cytoplasm of these histiocytes and can best been seen using precipitation silver methods such as the Steiner or Warthin-Starry stains. If bacteria are plentiful, they may be seen with the H&E stain. After histologic review and suggestion of rhinoscleroma within the differential diagnosis, repeat biopsy for culture identification is recommended. Squamous cell carcinoma has been reported as a complication of this rare infectious disease.

Noma

Noma, also known as cancrum oris, gangrenous stomatitis, and necrotizing ulcerogingivostomatitis, is a rare chronic destructive bacterial infection predominantly of children usually caused by *Pseudomonas aeruginosa*.[114] Beginning as an aphthous mucocutaneous

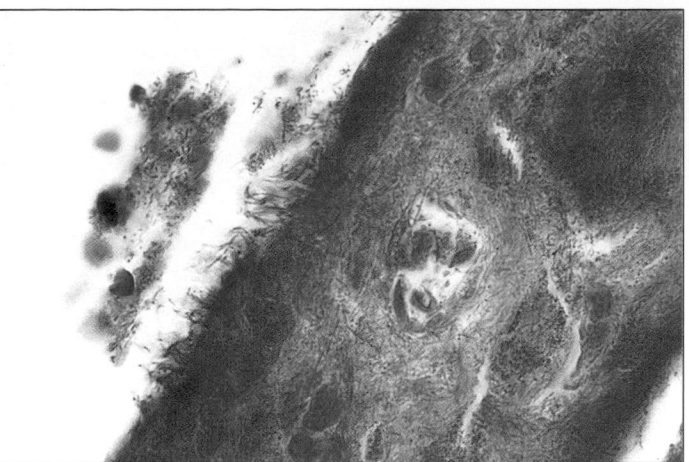

Fig. 3.37 Destructive oral mucositis in neutropenic child undergoing chemotherapy shows extensive surface overgrowth of *Pseudomonas*. Note edge of mucosa with 'hair on end' appearance of the bacilli (H&E, ×100).

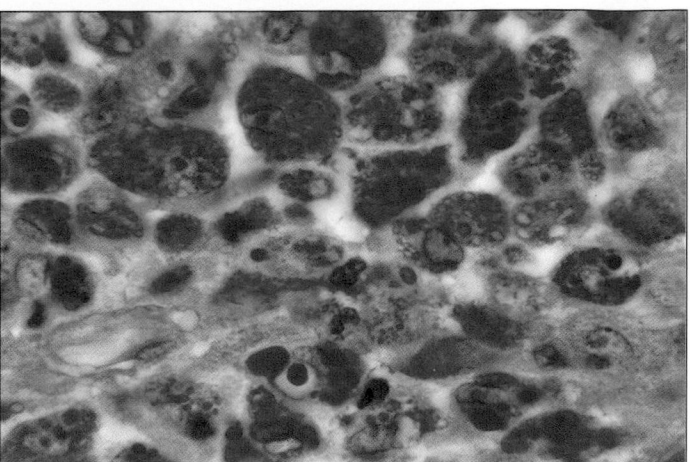

Fig. 3.39 *Rhodococcus equi*. Longstanding infection in a renal transplant patient who developed multiple soft tissue masses and a nasopharyngeal mass, in addition to his pulmonary lesions. Note intense periodic acid–Schiff (PAS)-positive histiocytes and the intracellular PAS-positive Michaelis-Gutmann (MG) bodies (PAS, ×600).

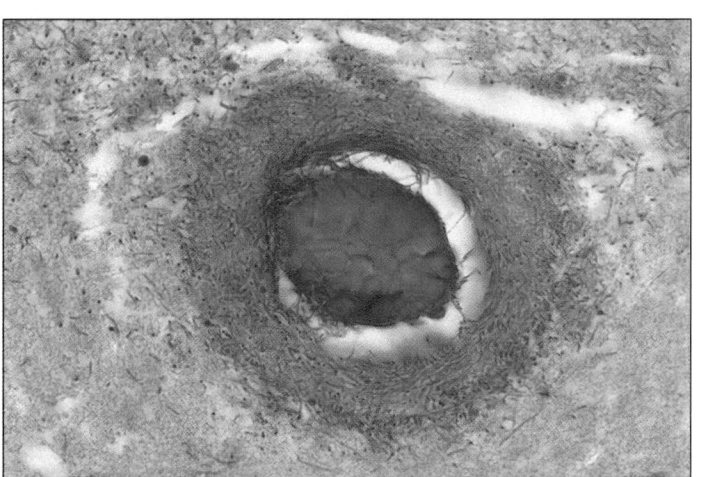

Fig. 3.38 In addition to the aggressive soft tissue invasion noted in Fig. 3.37, *Pseudomonas* can actively invade the underlying blood vessel walls in a pattern sometimes called '*Pseudomonas* vasculitis' (H&E, ×450).

pulmonary infection is usually the presentation, rare nasopharyngeal presentations that mimic carcinoma have been reported.[34] This bacteria enters via the respiratory route and establishes a chronic histiocyte-rich immune response that progresses to malacoplakia and mass formation. The histiocytes contain organisms in both intact and partially degenerated forms. Organisms stain well with PAS, tissue Gram stains, and fungal silver stains such as the GMS. The Michaelis-Gutmann (MG) bodies have rounded concentric layers and measure up to 10–12 μm in diameter (Fig. 3.39). The MG bodies stain with PAS, GMS, Geimsa, von Kossa, and Prussian blue. Culture recognition is difficult as this organism has the morphology of a 'diphtheroid' and may be discounted as normal flora in routine bacterial cultures.[115] They are often recovered retrospectively when they grow on mycobacterial media where the experienced microbiologist easily recognizes their salmon-pink color and colony morphology. The acid-fast nature of these bacteria is best demonstrated in fresh culture isolates and is difficult to reproduce with tissue AFB stains.

Mycobacterial infections

Mycobacterium tuberculosis as well as 'mycobacterium other than tuberculosis' (MOTT) infections may be encountered in the head and neck. Often, by the time this occurs, disease has manifested itself elsewhere and treatment has been initiated. Nonetheless, the alert surgical pathologist should always include mycobacterial infections in the evaluation of any granulomatous disease process encountered in the head and neck. Subtle presentations with initial diagnoses have been reported from biopsies of oral mucosal lesions as well as laryngeal lesions.

Systemic mycoses

Any of the systemic mycoses may present with head and neck lesions. As with tuberculosis, the work-up of all granulomatous or mixed inflammatory lesions should include the possibility of the systemic fungi blastomycosis, paracoccidiodomycosis, histoplasmosis, cryptococcosis, and coccidioidomycosis.[116–120] Of particular interest is the presentation of laryngeal blastomycosis that can masquerade as laryngeal squamous cell carcinoma, resulting in unnecessary

ulcer, this infection progresses to erode large areas of soft tissue and even underlying bone (Fig. 3.37). Cultures of the necrotic tissue usually grow a mixture of bacterial forms. This infection is rare in North American, but is still common in Africa, Asia, and South America. Within the United States this infection is usually associated with the immunosuppressed. Recognition of the unique histologic picture of numerous adherent bacterial rods oriented perpendicular to the soft tissue or bone surface, vascular invasion, and an obvious absence of neutrophils leads to proper diagnosis of this infectious disease (Fig. 3.38). Antibiotics combined with surgical debridement and correction of nutritional or immunodeficiency state is required for resolution of this infection. Disfiguring scar formation is common.

Rhodococcus equi

Rhodococcus equi is an aerobic, Gram-positive partially acid-fast coccobacillary zoonotic infection of man. Although chronic cavitary

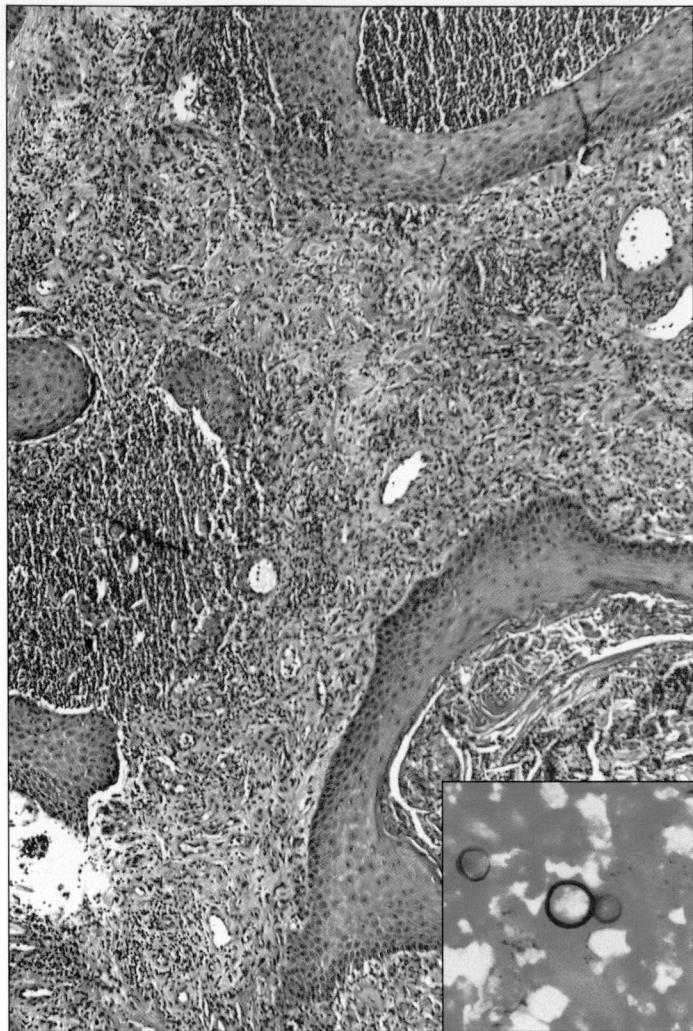

Fig. 3.40 Exuberant pseudoepitheliomatous hyperplasia can be mistaken for well-differentiated squamous cell carcinoma (H&E, ×100). Inset shows GMS silver stain with broad-based budding yeast characteristic of blastomycosis (GMS, ×600).

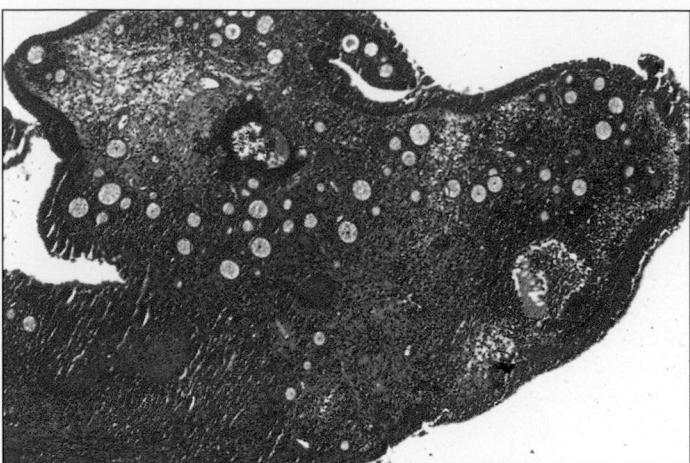

Fig. 3.41 *Rhinosporidium*. One of the largest fungal forms can easily be seen in this nasopharygeal polyp (H&E, ×20).

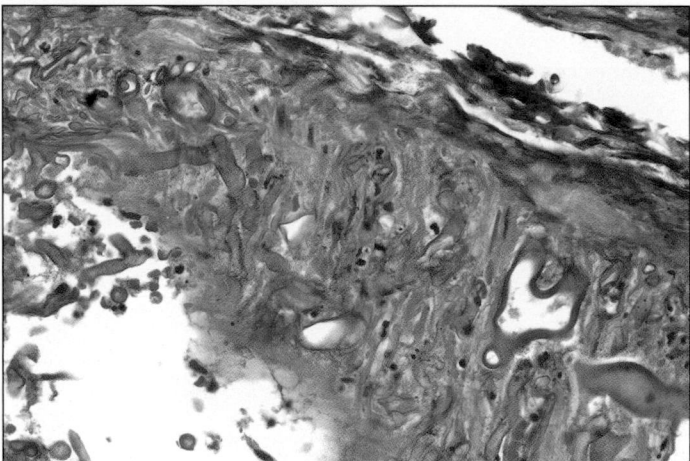

Fig. 3.42 The irregular thick and thin hyphae of the mucorales group organisms aggressively invade blood vessels as seen in this photo, as well as adjacent nerves (H&E, ×100).

surgical intervention. The granulomatous nature of laryngeal blastomycosis is not always as apparent as the other systemic fungi. The histologic response may be driven towards exuberant pseudoepitheliomatous hyperplasia with secondary irritation resulting in nuclear atypia. Careful H&E examination along with silver stains should be used to exclude this possibility (Fig. 3.40). The strict hospital policy of requiring outside pathology slides to be reviewed prior to definitive surgical excision of tumors has, in the experience of one author, saved a patient from a completely unnecessary total laryngectomy.

Rhinosporidiosis

Rhinosporidium seeberi is one of the largest fungal forms encountered in human infection. Essentially unculturable, diagnosis is dependent upon histologic evaluation. Rhinosporidiosis presents as a friable nasopharyngeal mass or polyp with occasional involvement of the larynx.[121] The organisms vary from small spores to mature, thick, double-walled sporangia that contain thousands of spores (Fig. 3.41). The organisms induce a mixed inflammatory response of

neutrophils, lymphocytes, and plasma cells. Although common in India and Sri Lanka, only rare cases have been reported from lifelong US residents.

Zygomycetes

Zygomycetes are hyaline fungi with broad, sparsely septate hyphae that branch haphazardly, often at right angles (Fig. 3.42). They measure 5–20 μm in width. The most common human pathogen is *Rhizopus* spp. Other members of the *Mucorales* group include *Mucor* spp., *Rhizomucor* spp., *Absidia* spp., and *Cunninghamella* spp. Rhinocerebral zygomycosis (often incorrectly referred to by clinicians as mucormycosis) is a life-threatening infection of the nose and paranasal sinuses that may extend into the orbit or cerebrum. Risk factors are diabetic ketoacidosis and malignancies, particularly of the hematopoietic system.

A characteristic feature of zygomycosis is invasion of the hyphae into the walls of blood vessels, producing thrombosis and infarction. Vascular invasion is the mechanism of dissemination (Fig. 3.43). The infections are, therefore, usually necrotizing and hemorrhagic.

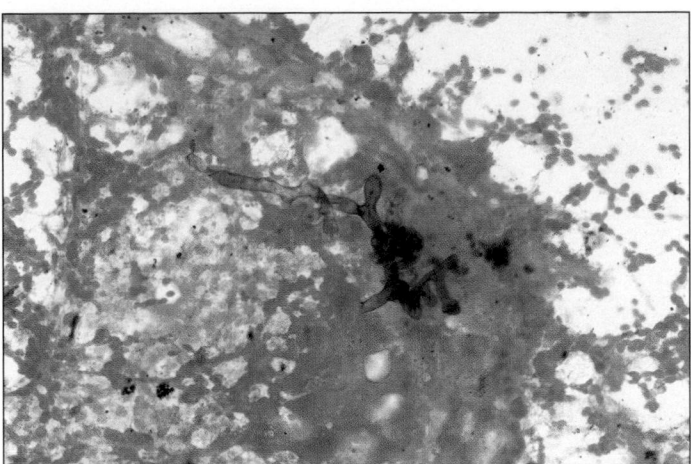

Fig. 3.43 Zygomycetes in a fine needle aspiration of a liver abscess. Large, somewhat crumpled ribbon-like hyphae branch at right angles and do not have septae. Notice that folding of the hyphae produce transverse densities that may resemble septae. This group of fungi often stains as well or better with H&E than with special stains (GMS, ×400).

The thin walls of the hyphae result in distortion and collapse of the structures. Sparse septae may be seen, and collapsed folded hyphae may mistakenly be taken for septae. The zygomycetes must be differentiated from hyphomycetes, such as *Aspergillus* spp., in which the width of the hyphae is at the lower end of the range. Swollen hyphae or hyphae cut in cross-section can be mistaken for yeast. The zygomycetes usually stain well with H&E, PAS, and GMS.

Infection of the upper respiratory system by members of the Mucorales order represent one of the rare surgical pathology emergencies, often requiring frozen section for immediate diagnosis followed by debridement and aggressive antifungal therapy. These pauciseptate fungi with irregular thick-and-thin hyphal contours will be seen aggressively invading blood vessels and nerves. There will be acute thrombosis and extensive tissue necrosis along with an intense acute inflammatory response. Occasionally the response may be granulomatous, or 'paucicellular.' When examining frozen sections it is sometimes helpful to lower the light condenser, which helps highlight the refractile edges of these hyphal forms. Complications include orbital enucleation, meningoencephalitis, and cerebral infarction.

Other hyphomycetes that produce serious infection are numerous. The most commonly identified agents are *Scedosporium (Pseudoallescheria) boydii* and *Fusarium* spp.[122–124] These fungi produce invasive infection; mycetomas, especially of the paranasal sinuses; ulcerative keratitis; and rarely dermatomycosis. Virtually any fungus can be pathogenic in a host with the requisite risk factors, emphasizing the importance of culturing all specimens when an infectious etiology is a possibility.

Opportunistic fungal sinus infections

Noninvasive fungal-ball formation within the sinuses may be due to a host of opportunistic organisms including *Aspergillus, Bipolaris, Fusarium, and Cunninghamella*. Tissue reaction may be minimal to completely absent. Careful examination to confirm the noninvasive nature of the process is essential. Precise identification may not be possible unless fruiting bodies are present. Simple surgical curettage is often curative.

THE RESPIRATORY SYSTEM

Respiratory tract infections continue to be a leading cause of morbidity and mortality worldwide. For the pathologist dealing with transbronchial biopsies, bronchoalveolar lavage, bronchial wash samples, and open lung biopsies, the goal is always to establish the etiologic agent as rapidly as possible. The search may be narrowed by consideration of the tissue response and application of a vast array of identification techniques.

The clinical history is of paramount importance when evaluating lung tissue from a patient with respiratory predominant symptoms. It goes without saying that the easy, straightforward cases of respiratory infections with common agents such as *Streptococcus pneumoniae, Klebsiella pneumoniae, Pseudomonas*, and *Staphylococcus aureus* are diagnosed by blood or respiratory cultures and never make it to the bronchoscopy and/or operating suite. The pathologists are left to deal with culture resistant or unculturable organisms. Known risk factors, zoonotic exposures, tick/insect exposures, work exposures, age, and immune status are some of the critical clinical elements required to expedite the final diagnosis.

The complexity increases when we consider infections of the immunocompromised host. *Pneumocystis jirovecii (carinii)* in classic form with abundant protein-rich alveolar casts and abundant organisms is not usually a diagnostic challenge. However, given the unusual presentations of hyaline membrane-rich type, granulomatous and interstitial paucireactive, the pathologist can be caught off guard unless pertinent history is provided. The patient with suppressed immune status may produce no granulomas or poorly formed granulomas in the setting of overwhelming *Mycobacterium tuberculosis* and systemic fungal infections. One must also consider a much broader differential in the immunocompromised host, giving consideration for agents such as *Rhodococcus equi* in the setting of a patient presenting with cavitary lung lesions, but negative mycobacterial cultures. In the transplant patient population, consideration must be given to viral-induced lymphoproliferations due to Epstein-Barr virus infection.

Legionella species

Legionella spp., particularly *L. pneumophila*, causes an acute lobular pneumonia known as Legionnaire's disease that is more common and more severe in patients who have compromised immunologic or pulmonary defense mechanisms. A second clinical syndrome, Pontiac fever, is self-limited and will not be seen by surgical pathologists. The airspaces in Legionnaire's disease are packed with fibrin and acute inflammatory cells, but paradoxically a productive cough develops in only approximately 50% of patients. Leukocytoclasis of the airspace exudate is characteristic, but not diagnostic (Fig. 3.44). The bacteria, which are both extracellular and intracellular within macrophages, can be demonstrated with the Warthin-Starry or other silver impregnation staining method (Fig. 3.45). Direct immunofluorescence can be performed on cytologic smears or open biopsy touch preparations. Fixation of the tissue in formalin is not detrimental to the relevant antigens. Abscesses are demonstrable in as many as 20% of autopsied lungs, but are not usually evident ante-mortem.[38]

Nocardia asteroides

Nocardia asteroides is an aerobic actinomycete that produces mycetoma and acute infection of the lung, particularly in immunocompromised patients.[39,40] Dissemination from the lung, especially to the brain, may result. The inflammatory response is usually purulent, and abscesses may result (Fig. 3.46), but nocardial pneumonia may also be chronic, in which case fibrosis and granulomas may be found (Fig. 3.47). *N. asteroides* is readily demonstrable as branching,

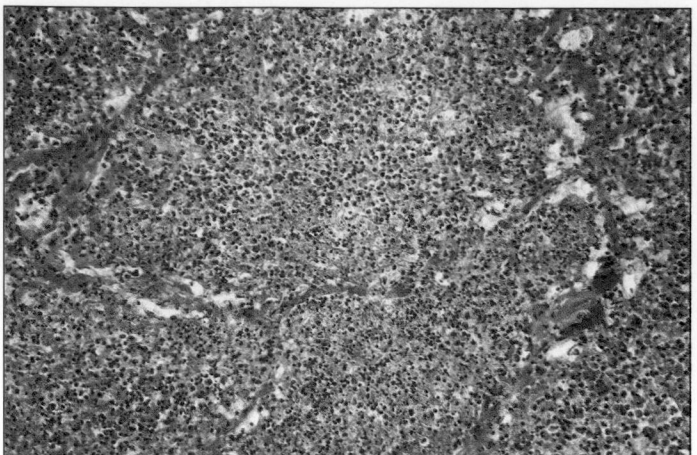

Fig. 3.44 *Legionella pneumophila* pneumonia. The exudates in the alveoli consist of edema, fibrin, and polymorphonuclear neutrophils, many of which have undergone leukocytoclasis, producing a dusty appearance (H&E, ×100, *Legionella pneumophila* isolated from cultures).

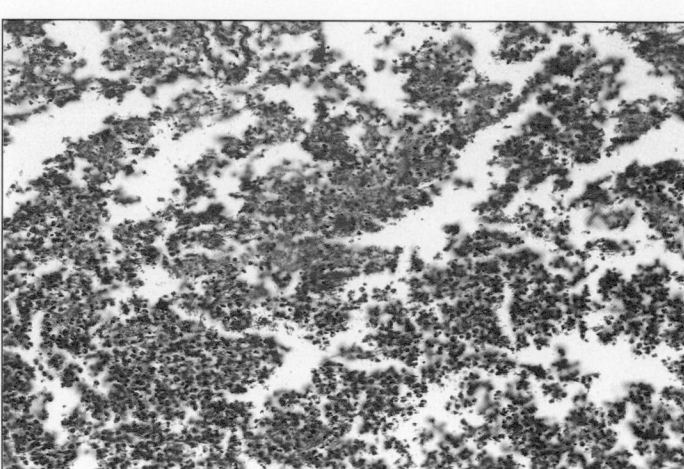

Fig. 3.46 *Nocardia* pneumonia in an immunosuppressed patient. Necrotizing inflammation with formation of abscesses has destroyed pulmonary parenchyma. The exudates consists of masses of polymorphonuclear neutrophils (H&E, ×45, *Nocardia asteroides* isolated in cultures).

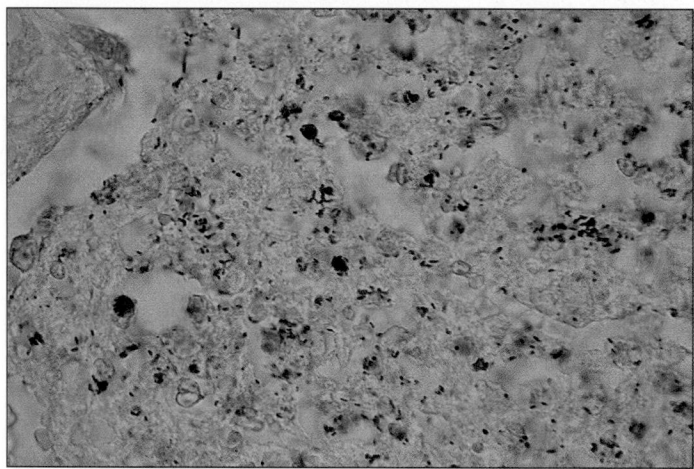

Fig. 3.45 *Legionella pneumophila* pneumonia. Numerous bacteria are demonstrated by silver impregnation stain, which distorts and enlarges the outlines of the bacilli. Clusters of organisms reflect their position within the cytoplasm of macrophages. The Gram reaction cannot be determined with this stain (Dieterle, ×1000, *Legionella pneumophila* isolated from cultures).

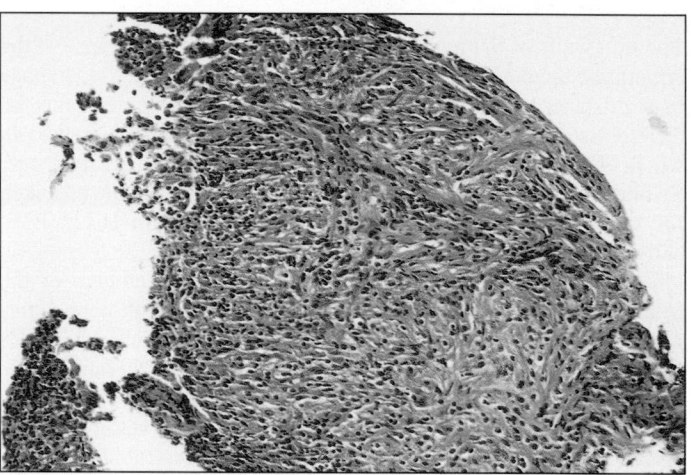

Fig. 3.47 *Nocardia* pneumonia. A well organized, noncaseating granuloma is present in the interstitium. Transbronchial biopsy (H&E, ×200, *Nocardia asteroides* isolated in cultures).

filamentous Gram-positive bacilli (Fig. 3.48), which also stain well with the methenamine silver technique. The documentation of filaments and branching is important, because other Gram-positive bacilli may be filamentous or may display rudimentary branching, or both. Differentiation of *Nocardia* from *Actinomyces* can be made by evaluation of the clinical presentation, the absence of sulfur granules in systemic infection, and the demonstration of partial acid fastness in the bacilli. Modified acid-fast stains such as the Fite stain are best used to demonstrate this feature.

Coxiella burnetii

Coxiella burnetii is a rickettsia-like bacterium that causes pneumonia (Q fever) and endocarditis. It is associated with dairy products and body fluids of a variety of animals.[125,126] Laboratory workers have developed Q fever after exposure to infected sheep.[127] Hepatitis with noncaseating granulomas may be encountered by the surgical pathologist in liver biopsies.[128,129] So-called fibrin ring granulomas consist of macrophages and lymphocytes around a central hole. They are distinctive findings in Q fever but may be seen in several other infections.[130,131]

Mycobacterium tuberculosis

Pulmonary tuberculosis caused by *Mycobacterium tuberculosis* (Mtb) continues to be a leading cause of worldwide morbidity and mortality. Any pulmonary biopsy or cytology specimen demonstrating granulomas is immediately suspect of being tuberculosis until proven otherwise. The work-up includes exclusion of Mtb as well as the systemic dimorphic fungi. The histologic hallmark is the centrally necrotic granuloma, or 'tubercle' (Fig. 3.49). Acid-fast stains reveal the classic long, slightly curved, beaded rods characteristic of

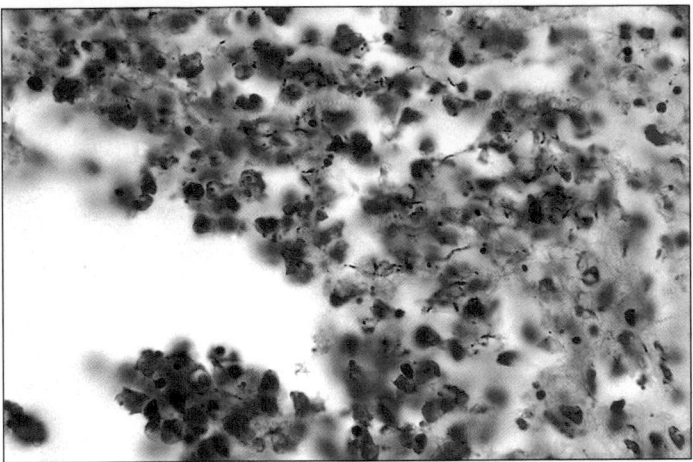

Fig. 3.48 *Nocardia* pneumonia. Thin, branching, irregularly staining Gram-positive bacilli course through necrotic pulmonary tissue (Brown-Hopps Gram, ×1000).

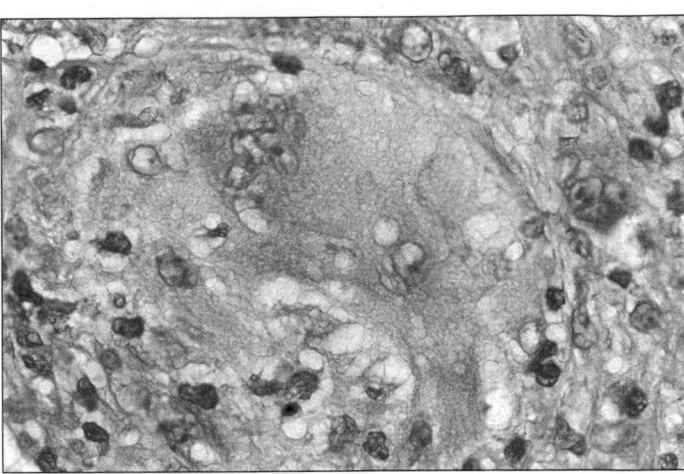

Fig. 3.50 Identifying acid-fast bacilli can be time consuming; note the single acid-fast form in this giant cell in a patient in active tuberculosis (Ziehl-Neelsen, ×1000).

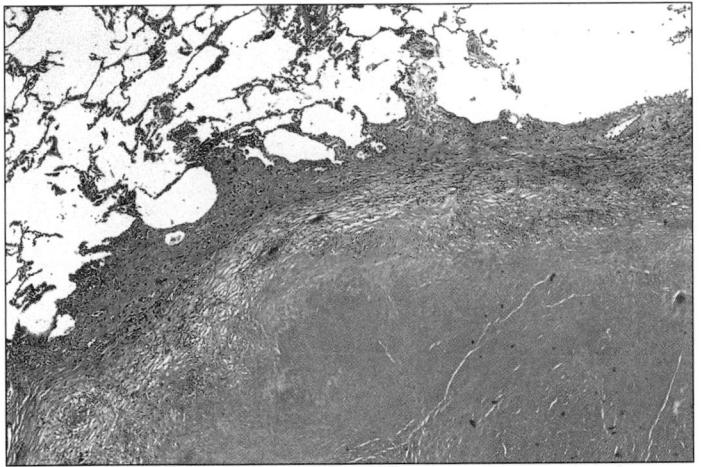

Fig. 3.49 The characteristic lesion of tuberculosis is the 'tubercle' seen in this photo; a single granuloma with a necrotic center and thin rim of lymphocytes, histiocytes, and occasional giant cells (H&E, ×20).

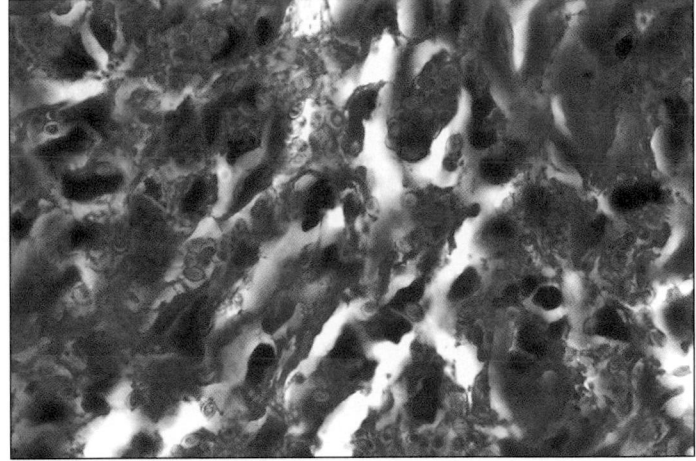

Fig. 3.51 Mucosal histoplasmosis. The infiltrate consists of macrophages that are packed with small oval yeasts. The clear space around the nuclear material is not a true capsule. A single nuclear mass can be seen in some yeast cells (H&E, ×1000, *Histoplasma capsulatum* isolated in culture).

Mycobacterium tuberculosis (Fig. 3.50). These small tubercles expand to the size of millet seeds that may then coalesce, forming large zones of cheesy central necrosis noted grossly as caseous necrosis. Long-standing tubercles may undergo regression and fibrosis, or calcification. Active or indolent lesions within the lungs caused by Mtb, generally cause no major problem for the anatomic pathologist. In addition to acid-fast stains, immunoperoxidase methods and molecular methods are now available for confirmation of Mtb infection in suspected tissues. Culture identification along with sensitivity studies remains the gold standard for this diagnosis. Molecular genotyping continues to expand our knowledge of the pathogenesis and epidemiology of tuberculosis.[132]

Histoplasma capsulatum

Although *Histoplasma capsulatum* is a small yeast measuring 3–5 μm, yeast forms in old caseous lesion may be moderate to very

large and quite distorted. *H. capsulatum* has a close association with macrophages and is usually found intracellularly in active infections. Macrophages in which the cytoplasm is packed with small oval structures suggested to early investigators that the organism was a protozoan parasite similar to *Leishmania*, hence the name *Histoplasma* (tissue plasmodium). The clear spaces that may be seen around the yeast are artifacts of fixation that yielded the species name (Fig. 3.51). *H. capsulatum* is typically oval, has a single nucleus in H&E-stained sections, and buds via a narrow base. Both viable and nonviable yeast cells stain well with methenamine silver (Fig. 3.52) and the PAS technique after diastase digestion.

Histoplasmosis occurs in a variety of forms, depending on the immune status of the host.[133] The most common clinical manifestation is asymptomatic or minimally symptomatic infection. In the hyper-endemic areas of the US – roughly the Ohio and Mississippi River valleys and the central Appalachian Mountains – as many as 90% of

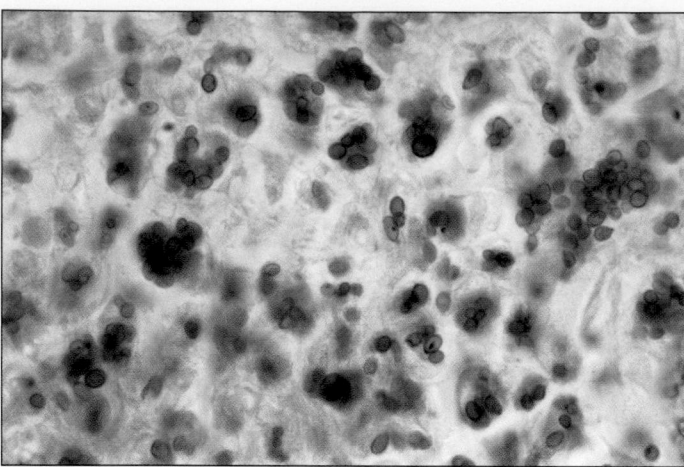

Fig. 3.52 The small uniform budding yeasts of *H. capsulatum* are well demonstrated by silver precipitate staining. Although the background cellular elements are not well stained, the intracellular location of the yeasts are betrayed by the clustering (GMS, ×1000).

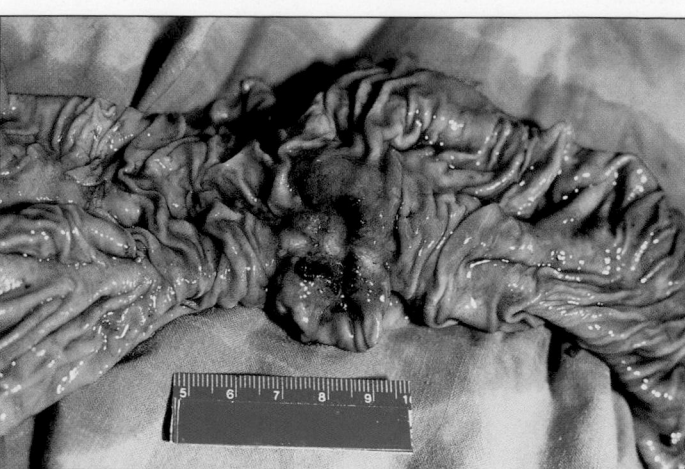

Fig. 3.54 Colonic mass in disseminated histoplasmosis in patient infected with the human immunodeficiency virus. The inflammatory mass resembles an annular, constricting carcinoma (*H. capsulatum* isolated in cultures) (Courtesy of David Walker, MD).

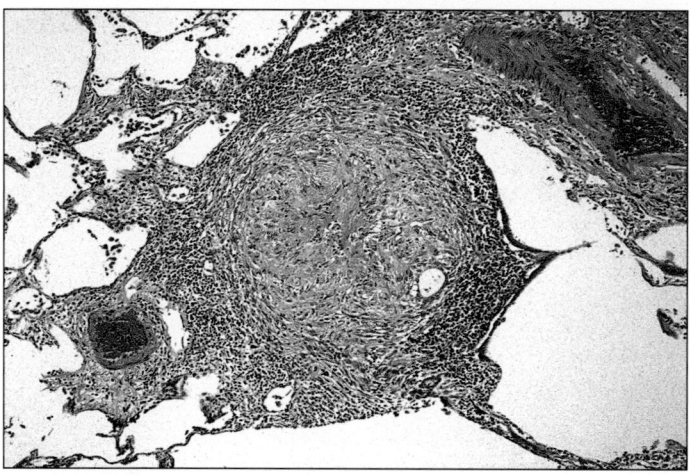

Fig. 3.53 Miliary histoplasmosis of the lung. A well-formed interstitial granuloma with slight central necrosis is surrounded by an abundant mantle of lymphocytes (H&E, ×25, *Histoplasma capsulatum* DNA sequences confirmed by polymerase chain reaction) (Courtesy of James Smith, MD).

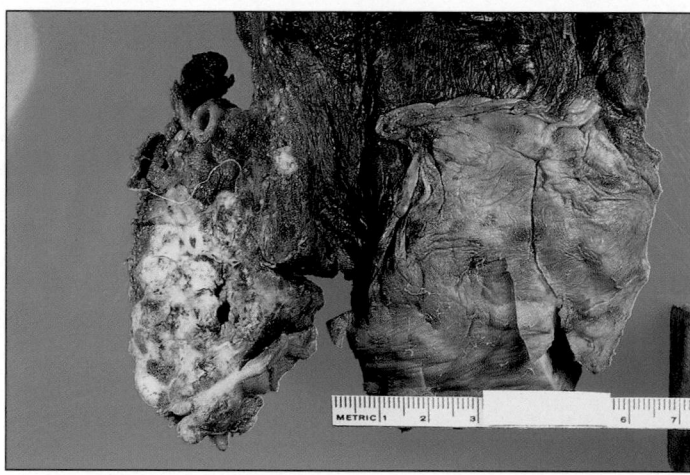

Fig. 3.55 Chronic pulmonary histoplasmosis. A lobectomy specimen, obtained because of the suspicion of carcinoma, demonstrates dense parenchymal, granulomatous inflammation with fibrosis, a cavitary lesion, and overlying dense pleural fibrosis. Postoperatively, a sputum specimen obtained 6 weeks previously yielded *Histoplasma capsulatum*.

the population may show immunologic evidence of prior infection. Immunocompetent patients may experience an acute self-limited pneumonia, in which granulomas may not be prominent initially. The tissue response may be noncaseating granulomas, caseating granulomas with an organization that varies from quite loose to very tight (Fig. 3.53), or unorganized collections of macrophages. A continuum exists from the macrophage collections to the loosely organized granulomas. The histologic response appears to correspond to the extent to which cellular immunity is operative.

Dissemination of yeast throughout the reticuloendothelial system often follows the pulmonary infection. The end result of the primary encounter is usually a healed granuloma in the lung, lymph nodes, liver, or spleen. Concentric rings of calcification in a solitary lung nodule, which may be demonstrable in chest radiographs, are highly suggestive of histoplasmosis. Disseminated infection occurs most often in immunosuppressed patients.[134–136] Lesions are most common in organs of the reticuloendothelial system and the gastrointestinal tract. Unimpeded growth of yeast in HIV-infected patients may produce gastrointestinal lesions that resemble neoplasms macroscopically (Fig. 3.54). Skin infections are not uncommon.[137]

Chronic pulmonary disease occurs primarily in patients with chronic obstructive lung disease, resembling cavitary tuberculosis (Fig. 3.55).[138] Lesions may consist entirely of infected macrophages when infection disseminates in immunosuppressed individuals. Infected circulating mononuclear cells may be demonstrated, particularly in HIV-infected individuals. Whenever tuberculosis enters the differential diagnosis, histoplasmosis should be close behind. Fibrosing mediastinitis is often attribute to *H. capsulatum*, but it is

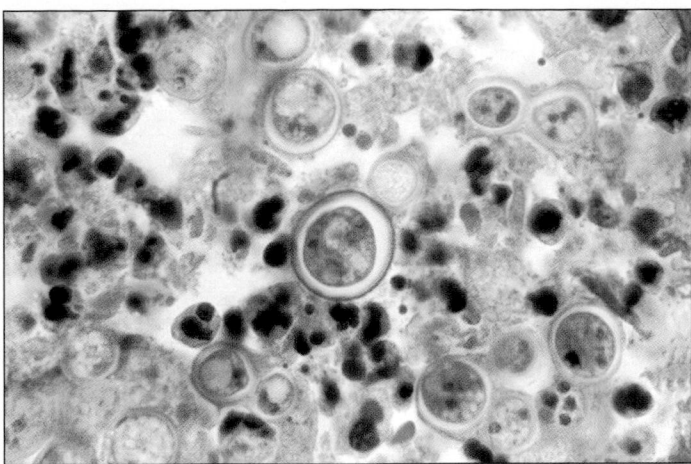

Fig. 3.56 Localized blastomycosis was an incidental finding in an autopsy. Yeast cells of *Blastomyces dermatitidis* demonstrate multiple nuclei, thick cell walls, broad-based budding, and an artifactual separation of the cytoplasm from the cell wall (H&E, ×1000).

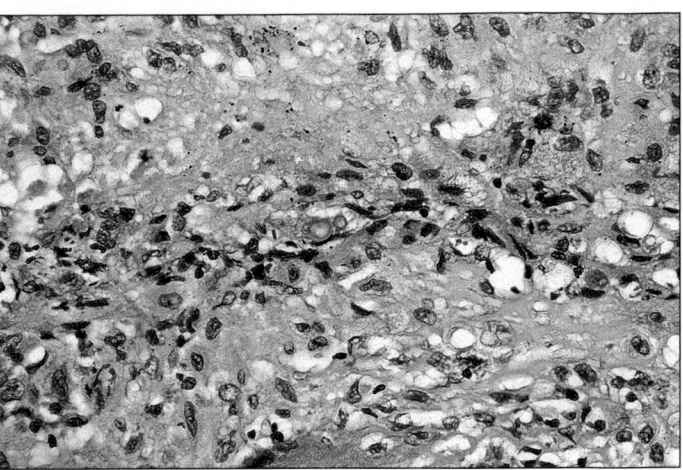

Fig. 3.57 Yeast cells of *Blastomyces dermatitidis* in a granulomatous lesion are colored by the mucicarmine stain. The correct diagnosis must be made by careful morphologic study of the yeast or by fungal culture, or by both (Mucicarmine, ×250).

extremely difficult to identify the organisms in sections.[139,140] The differential diagnosis of *Histoplasma* in tissues and smears includes protozoan parasites, a rare small form of *B. dermatitidis*, *P. jirovecii (carinii)*, and other small yeasts. The protozoa may be differentiated because they do not stain with methenamine silver. The small forms of *B. dermatitidis* retain their broad-based budding and have multiple nuclei if examined closely. *Candida* spp. usually produce a neutrophilic inflammatory response with or without granulomas, are often accompanied by hyphae or pseudohyphae, and are most commonly extracellular. *Torulopsis (Candida) glabrata* overlaps *Histoplasma* in size but is a rare cause of tissue infection. Particularly in older or florid lesions, in which the yeast cells of *H. capsulatum* demonstrate greater variation in size and morphology, confusion with the cysts of *P. jirovecii (carinii)* may result. We have seen a case that was variously diagnosed as histoplasmosis or granulomatous pneumocystosis by experienced pathologists. Molecular amplification studies eventually established the etiology of the infection as *H. capsulatum*.

Blastomyces dermatitidis

Blastomyces dermatitidis is a medium-sized yeast that measures 8–15 μm. It is roughly spherical or subspherical in shape and has a distinctive thick cellular wall that may almost appear refractile in H&E-stained sections, and a single broad-based bud. *B. dermatitidis* has multiple nuclei and is usually demonstrated well with H&E stains (Fig. 3.56). The yeasts are also stained well with methenamine silver and the PAS technique. Some strains are weakly or moderately mucicarmine positive, a point to remember when depending on this technique for documentation of *C. neoformans* (Fig. 3.57).

The endemic zone for blastomycosis covers much of the eastern United States and overlaps that of histoplasmosis. This infection is much less common than histoplasmosis and almost always occurs as single, sporadic cases, whereas histoplasmosis more commonly causes epidemic disease. Infection is almost always contracted through the respiratory system, resulting in asymptomatic infection, self-limited pneumonia, or localized infection which may be mistaken for neoplastic disease.[141,142] Disseminated infection usually results in cutaneous and skeletal disease. Chronic, ulcerating, hyperkeratotic skin lesions may suggest the possibility of squamous cell carcinoma

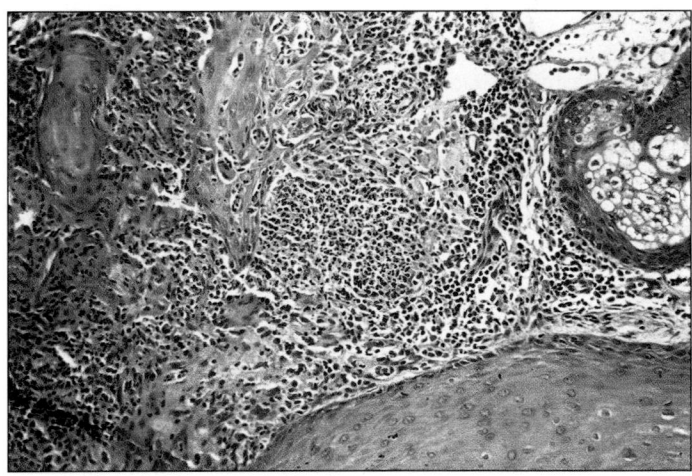

Fig. 3.58 Cutaneous blastomycosis is characterized by prominent pseudoepitheliomatous hyperplasia, granulomatous inflammation, and microabscess formation with abundant polymorphonuclear neutrophils (H&E, ×45).

(Fig. 3.58). Aggressive, systemic infection has been observed in immunosuppressed patients.[143] The histologic response in blastomycosis is granulomatous, often with a characteristic mixture of acute inflammation including microabscesses. In the skin, a pronounced overlying pseudoepitheliomatous hyperplasia is frequently seen (Fig. 3.58). Yeast cells are usually found in macrophages or multinucleated giant cells and in the microabscesses (see Figs 3.56 and 3.58). *B. dermatitidis* must be differentiated from *C. neoformans*, from developing spherules of *C. immitis*, and in parts of Africa from *Histoplasma duboisii*. The yeast cells of *Cryptococcus* are more uniformly round and more variable in size, have a thin wall, and bud with a narrow base. The capsule of *C. neoformans* is always stained by the mucicarmine and Fontana-Masson methods, whereas *Blastomyces* organisms are usually negative with the former and always negative with the latter (although we have seen a case in which a false-positive

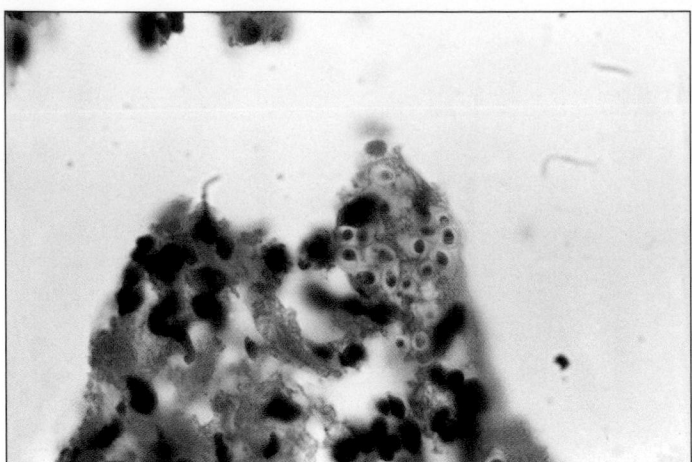

Fig. 3.59 *Blastomyces dermatitidis.* Small form in a macrophage, resembling the yeast cells of *Histoplasma capsulatum.* The correct identification can be made by notation of the multiple nuclei and broad-based budding, and by culture (H&E, ×1000).

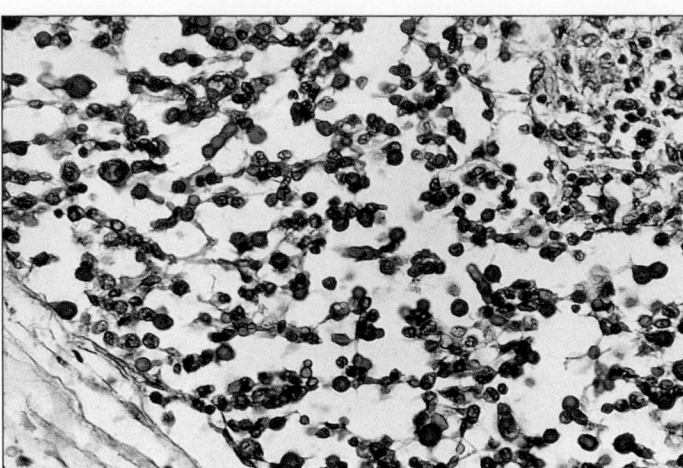

Fig. 3.60 The mucopolysaccharide capsules of *Cryptococcus neoformans* in a mediastinal lymph node are well demonstrated. There is minimal inflammation. The yeast cells are round to oval in shape and vary in size. The capsule closest to the cell wall is stained. A few short pseudohyphae can be seen (Mucicarmine, ×400).

Fontana-Masson stain led to an incorrect diagnosis). *Coccidioides* can be eliminated if budding yeast cells are demonstrated; in their absence the differentiation can be accomplished by evaluation of the thick cell wall and the search for more completely developed spherules. Extremely rarely hyphal forms of *B. dermatitidis* have been reported in lung tissue and sputum obtained from immunosuppressed patients.[144] The unusual small form of *B. dermatitidis* (Fig. 3.59) must be differentiated from *H. capsulatum*.[145,146]

Cryptococcus neoformans

Cryptococcus neoformans is a variably sized yeast that ranges 2–20 μm in diameter, with a preponderance of cells measuring 4–8 μm. The sexual form of the fungus, *Filobasidiella neoformans*, which is not found in human tissue or demonstrated in clinical laboratories, is a basidiomycete – the closest thing we have to an infectious mushroom. Other species of *Cryptococcus* are only rarely, if ever, human pathogens.

C. neoformans has a thin wall and a narrow-based bud. The great variability in size and the uniformity in shape of the spherical cells are useful clues to the diagnosis. The yeasts are moderately well stained by the H&E stain and are well displayed with the methenamine silver and PAS techniques. Staining of the often abundant polysaccharide capsule with the mucicarmine stain (Fig. 3.60) and demonstration of a melanin pigment with the Fontana-Masson stain are useful histochemical clues to the correct etiology. Most strains of *C. neoformans* are heavily encapsulated in tissue, although they may lose much of the polysaccharide after isolation in the clinical laboratory. The large capsule, which does not stain with H&E, often produces a clear zone around the yeast cell, the in vivo equivalent of the India ink preparation in the clinical laboratory. The mucicarmine stain usually colors the area of the capsule directly around the cell wall, leaving the mass of capsule comparatively unstained (Fig. 3.60). Some strains of *C. neoformans* are poorly encapsulated, both in vivo and in vitro. In these cells the mucicarmine stain produces a thin rim of staining at the cell wall. Very rarely, pseudohyphae of *C. neoformans* may be demonstrated in tissue (Fig. 3.60).[147]

Cryptococcosis is a worldwide cosmopolitan infection, which is primarily acquired through the respiratory tract. The pulmonary–

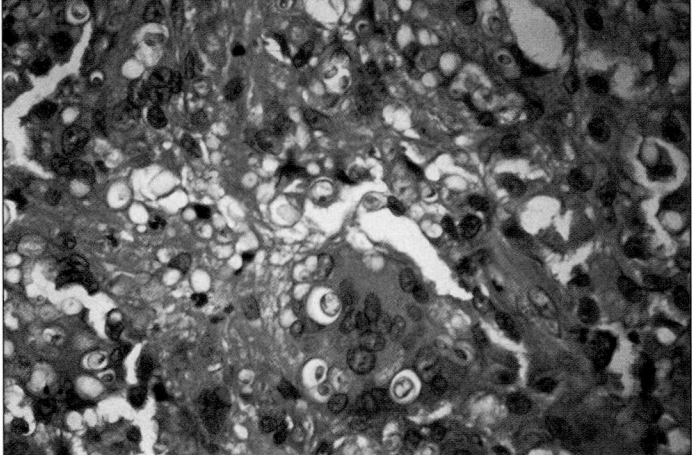

Fig. 3.61 Cryptococcal osteomyelitis. A poorly encapsulated strain of *Cryptococcus neoformans* has elicited a granulomatous reaction. Variably sized, round yeast cells are present in macrophages and multinucleated giant cells (H&E, ×400, *Cryptococcus neoformans* isolated in culture).

lymph node complex is demonstrated only rarely.[148,149] Active pulmonary infection may result, but the clinical manifestations are dominated by disseminated infection, especially to the central nervous system.[150] Much less commonly, primary inoculation into the skin may produce localized cutaneous infection, which resembles the chronic, crusted lesions of blastomycosis or may present as cellulitis.[151] Cryptococcal infections are frequently seen in HIV-infected patients.[152] The histologic response appears to depend on the degree of encapsulation of the yeast cells. Most often, the fully encapsulated cells produce a relatively noninflammatory process in which the encapsulated yeasts produce a gelatinous mass. It is easy to miss the fungal nature of the infection if poorly staining yeast are missed in an H&E-stained section (Fig. 3.61). Minimally encapsulated strains elicit a granulomatous inflammatory response with multinucleated giant

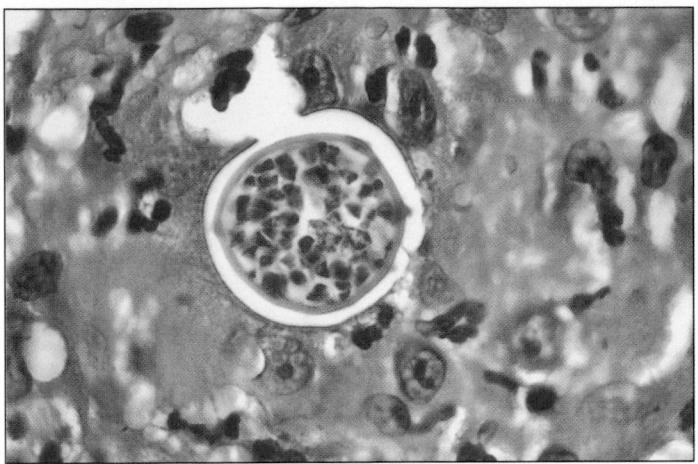

Fig. 3.62 *Coccidioides immitis* mature spherule in a multinucleated giant cell. The thick wall of the spherule encloses many endospores. Among the commonly seen systemic fungal infections, the spherule is distinctive and diagnostic (H&E, ×1000). (Courtesy of Louis Rosati, MD)

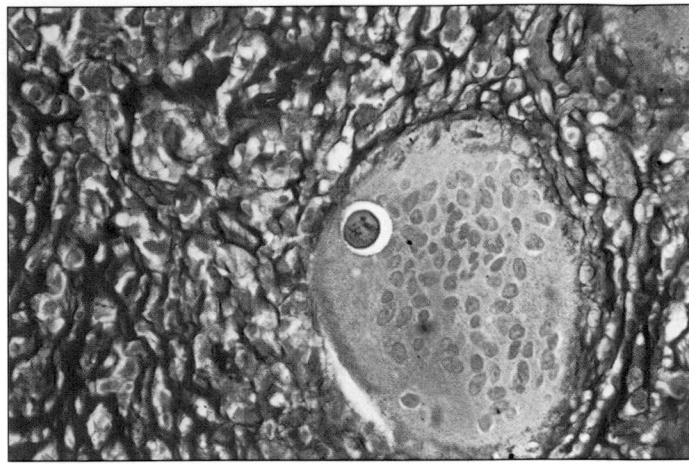

Fig. 3.63 Coccidioidomycosis. A developing spherule of *Coccidioides immitis* is located within a multinucleated giant cell. The primary differential at this stage of development is with *Cryptococcus neoformans* and *Blastomyces dermatitidis* (Periodic acid-Schiff, ×250).

cells (Fig. 3.61).[153] The yeasts are located intracellularly in macrophages and giant cells.

The primary differential diagnosis of cryptococcosis is with blastomycosis and coccidioidomycosis.[154] The inflammatory response, the relatively uniform shape, and the greatly variable size of the yeast cells should suggest the correct diagnosis. Histochemical stains are useful, particularly the mucicarmine and Fontana-Masson stains.[155] Combination of these two stains has been described.[156] The possibility that *B. dermatitidis* may stain with the mucicarmine stain must be remembered.

Coccidioides immitis

Coccidioides immitis is a dimorphic fungus that reproduces in vivo and at 37°C by endosporulation rather than by budding. A mature spherule contains many endospores (Fig. 3.62), which are released when the spherule ruptures. Each of the endospores enlarges and develops into a new spherule. The smallest endospores measure 5 μm, whereas the mature spherules range from 30 to 100 μm in size, occasionally reaching 200 μm. Spherules and their endospores are stained well by H&E. Spherules that are developing from released endospores may also be visible but are more reliably seen after staining by the methenamine silver or PAS techniques (Fig. 3.63). The endospores also stain with the special stains, but the wall of the spherule is not stained by the PAS technique and is only variably stained with methenamine silver. In pulmonary cavitary disease, oxygenation of the cavity may lead to the development of the filamentous phase of the fungus. The arthroconidia of the mold phase are the infective form. Thus, certain surgical specimens are at least theoretically infectious, whereas the yeast phase of dimorphic fungi is infectious only if inoculated directly into tissue.

The distribution of *C. immitis* is limited to the southwestern United States, but the disease is increasingly seen throughout the country because of increasing travel.[157] The arthroconidia are so infectious that a brief sojourn in an endemic area may result in infection. Recent increases in the frequency of infection in California may be related to more favorable conditions for dissemination of the arthroconidia during periods of drought.[158] Infection, which is acquired through the respiratory tract, is usually asymptomatic or minimally symptomatic. Acute or chronic pneumonia may result, and progressive, disseminated disease may occur, particularly in immunocompromised patients.[159,160] The organs most commonly involved are the skin, bones, and central nervous system.[161] The inflammatory process in coccidioidomycosis is granulomatous, but acute inflammation and microabscesses may also be seen. Granulomas may be either caseating or noncaseating.

As the endospores of *C. immitis* develop, they overlap *Histoplasma*, *Cryptococcus*, and *Blastomyces* in size. The lesions most closely resemble those of blastomycosis, and, as has been mentioned, the developing spherules may resemble the yeast cells of *Blastomyces*. Developing spherules may be found in macrophages, in multinucleated giant cells, or extracellularly. Endosporulation documents *Coccidioides*, whereas demonstration of budding yeast eliminates the possibility of this fungus. The differential diagnosis may be very difficult when few nondiagnostic forms are present. Immunofluorescence has been used successfully to confirm identity. Cultures are definitive, but it is wise to inform the microbiology laboratory if *Coccidioides* is suspected, as this organism carries an increased risk of transmission to laboratory workers.

Pneumocystis jirovecii (carinii)

Pneumocystis jirovecii (carinii) is a fungus that contains a cyst stage in which eight intracystic bodies develop. After maturity these intracystic bodies are released into the surrounding tissues. The mature intracystic bodies (trophozoites) measure 2–4 μm in size and can be stained by Romanowsky stains, such as the Giemsa or Diff-Quik stain. They are difficult to visualize in small numbers because of their small size and faint staining quality. The cysts measure 5–8 μm and are roughly spherical but frequently appear partially collapsed, producing the so-called helmet-shaped form (Fig. 3.64). A thickening of the cyst wall often produces a darker comma-shaped area of staining with the methenamine silver technique. With electron microscopy studies it has been demonstrated that this focal thickening represents the portal through which the mature intracystic bodies are released.

The cysts stain poorly or not at all with H&E or Giemsa stains, but occasionally the cysts may be outlined as ghosts, and internal

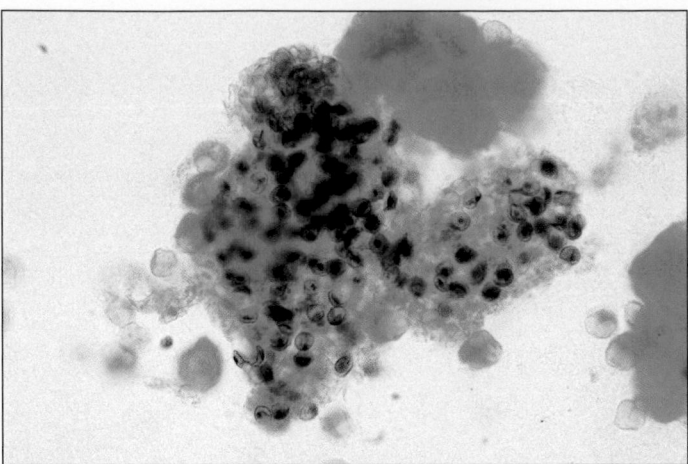

Fig. 3.64 *Pneumocystis* pneumonia. Clusters of cysts are present in the foamy alveolar exudates. Collapsed cysts produce the 'helmet' shape. The focal thickening of the cyst wall is seen as intracystic comma or parenthesis marks (GMS, ×450).

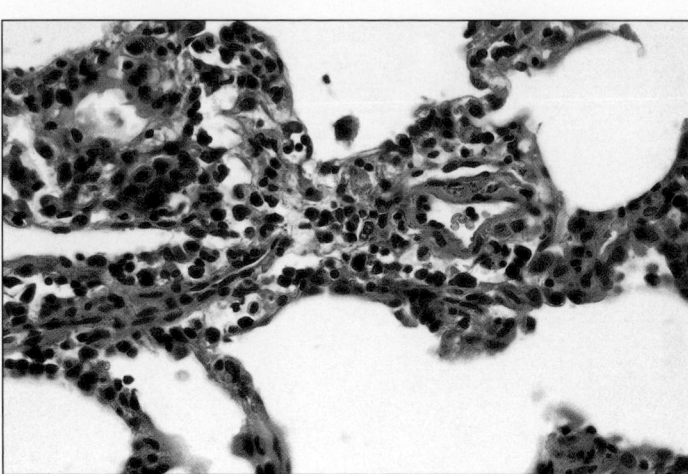

Fig. 3.66 *Pneumocystis* plasma cell pneumonia. The original presentation of this infection. An interstitial mononuclear infiltrate including many plasma cells is not accompanied by a significant inflammatory response within the alveoli (H&E, ×250).

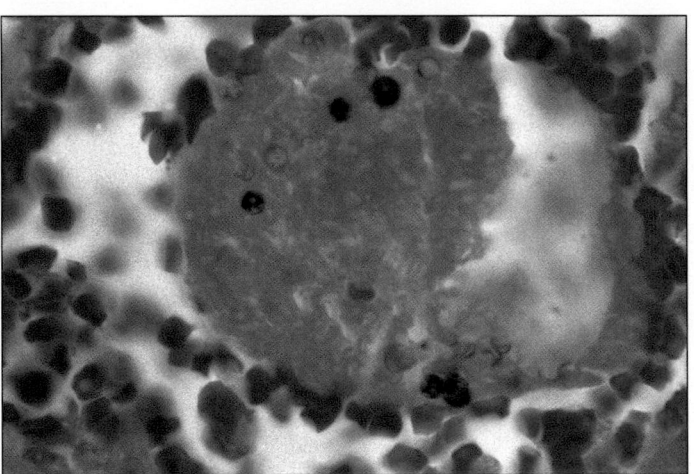

Fig. 3.65 *Pneumocystis* pneumonia. Cysts are demonstrated in the foamy background of the proteinaceous alveolar exudates (Gram-Weigert, ×1000).

intracystic bodies appears as tiny 'stippled' foci.[162] The PAS technique does not color the cysts but does stain the 'foamy exudate' in which the cysts are often enmeshed and that is thought to be elaborated by the organism. The cysts are well stained by the methenamine silver procedure, but the optimal staining times are slightly longer than what is typically used for other fungi. The cysts also stain using Gram-Weigert (Fig. 3.65), calcofluor white, and toluidine blue. *Pneumocystis* cysts fluoresce when smears are stained by the Papanicolaou technique and examined in a fluorescence microscope.[163] Fluoresceinated monoclonal antibodies to *P. jirovecii (carinii)* are commercially available and have been used to help with difficult cases, particularly when organisms are few in number.[164–166] Pneumocystosis is distributed worldwide and usually occurs as sporadic infection, but small outbreaks have been described.[167] The portal of entry is the respiratory tract, and the predominant organ affected is the lung. Subclinical infection is not commonly recognized but is probably a

frequent occurrence as judged by the prevalence of antibody[168] and occasional demonstration of the organisms in lung tissue of patients without symptoms referable to the lower respiratory tract. Symptomatic infection occurs almost invariably in immunosuppressed individuals. The infection was first described in malnourished infants in Europe, but steroid therapy and neoplastic disease, particularly of the hematopoietic system, were the most important risk factors before the appearance of HIV infection.[169] Pneumocystosis was the infection that initially defined AIDS, and most infections now occur in HIV-infected individuals.[170,171] Coinfecting organisms, particularly cytomegalovirus, may be present.[172] The institution of prophylactic therapy with trimethoprim-sulfamethoxazole has significantly reduced the incidence of this infection.[173] Disseminated infection was rare in the pre-AIDS era, but infection of virtually every organ system has been reported in HIV-infected patients.[174]

The histologic response to *P. jirovecii (carinii)* is quite varied. An interstitial pneumonia rich in plasma cells was described in malnourished children (Fig. 3.66) but is not often seen in its pure form. The most typical reaction is a modest mononuclear infiltrate in the interstitium accompanied by a prominent intra-alveolar accumulation of foamy material that is colored by the PAS technique (see Fig. 3.65). This exudate may calcify.[175] The other common inflammatory response is diffuse alveolar damage (Fig. 3.67) with mononuclear interstitial inflammation, proliferation of pneumocytes, and accumulation of fibrin with hyaline membranes in the airspaces.[176] Less common histologic responses include granulomatous inflammation,[177] vascular invasion, vasculitis, and cavitary lesions, especially in patients infected with HIV.[178] Most cases of disseminated infection are characterized by pools of 'foamy exudate' that disrupt the normal architecture of the organ and in which large numbers of cysts are present. The efficacy of bronchoalveolar lavage and cytologic examination has resulted in fewer biopsy samples being submitted for evaluation.[179]

If the classic foamy exudate is present, there is little difficulty in establishing the correct diagnosis. Diffuse alveolar damage calls into play a large differential of infectious and noninfectious etiologies. The cysts must be differentiated from small yeasts, such as *Candida* spp. or *H. capsulatum*. Erythrocytes that have been overstained with

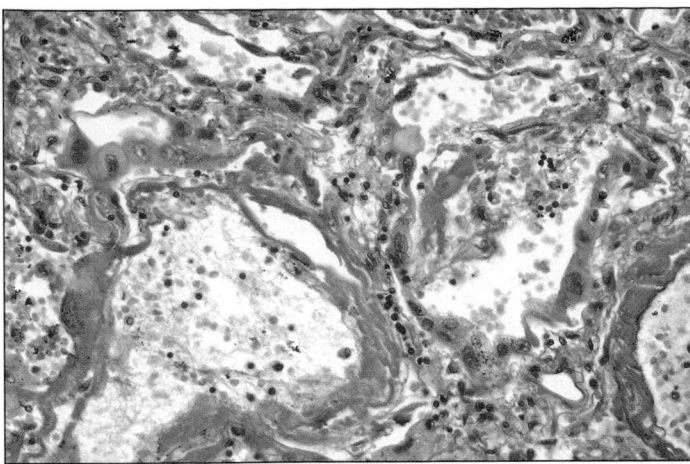

Fig. 3.67 Pneumocystis pneumonia. The histologic response is characterized by diffuse alveolar damage, including mononuclear interstitial inflammation and exudation of fibrin into the airspaces with hyaline membranes (H&E, ×200).

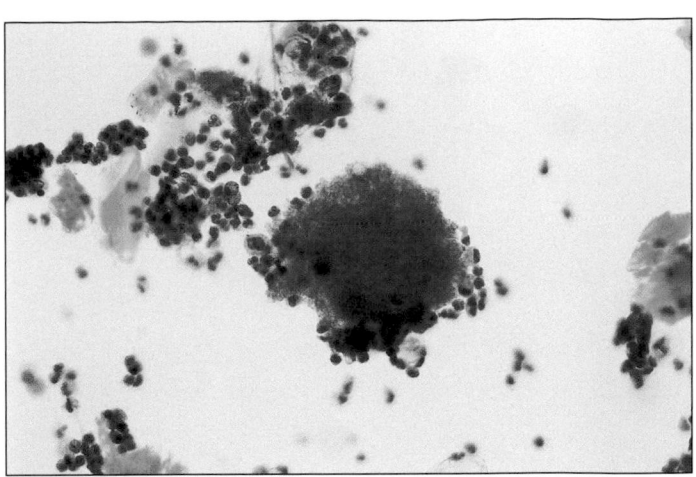

Fig. 3.69 *Pneumocystis* in bronchial washing. Clusters of organisms enmeshed in fibrin and surrounded by a few inflammatory cells. There is a vague outline of small cysts, but trophozoites are not seen with the Papanicolaou stain (Papanicolaou, ×1000).

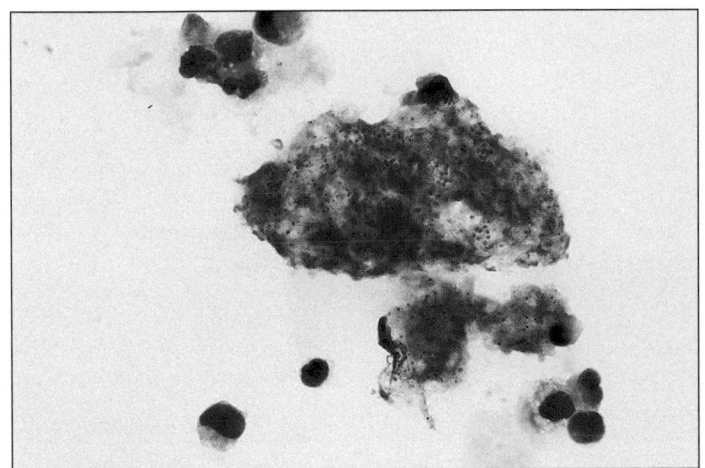

Fig. 3.68 *Pneumocystis* pneumonia. The smear from a bronchoalveolar lavage contains clusters of trophozoites and cysts in a clump of foamy alveolar exudates. The intracystic trophozoites are visible (Giemsa, ×1000).

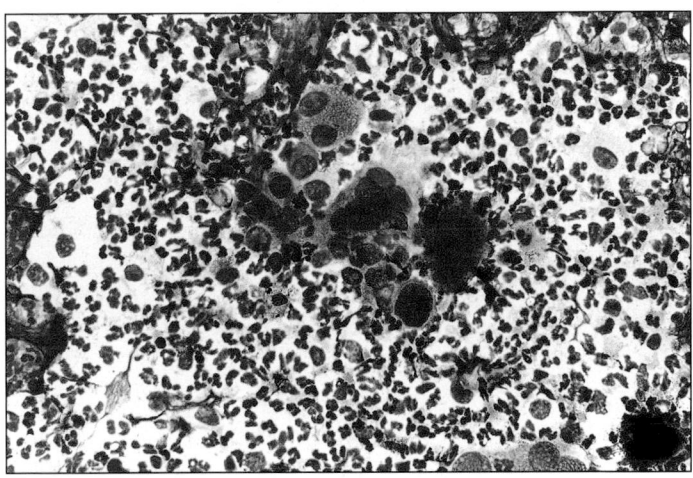

Fig. 3.70 *Pneumocystis* pneumonia and herpesvirus pneumonia in a bronchial wash. Small fibrin masses of *Pneumocystis* organisms are seen mixed with enlarged ground-glass nuclei of herpesvirus in bronchial cells. Note the acute inflammatory background. The patient suffered from the acquired immunodeficiency syndrome (Diff-Quik, ×250).

the methenamine silver method also provide a challenge for the unwary observer.

Cytologic Diagnosis: The most common infection of the respiratory tract seen both in patients with AIDS and in other immunocompromised patients is *P. jirovecii (carinii)*.[180] This organism is tightly bound within the alveolar framework of the lung, produces little or no inflammatory reaction, and can be difficult to detect in respiratory tract specimens unless direct sampling is used (i.e. bronchial lavage, brushings, washings, and FNA biopsies). In air-dried smears stained by Romanowsky methods (Wright's stain, May-Grünwald, Giemsa, and the most popular of these stains, Diff-Quik), the morphology is a metachromatic tangled mass of fibrin-like material containing the dark small trophozoites. (Fig. 3.68). At high magnification there is a suggestion of separate cyst walls

surrounding the trophozoites, the whole mass of material reproducing a cast of the alveolus. In the Papanicolaou stain (Fig. 3.69) the individual trophozoites do not stain, but the cyst walls of multiple cysts embedded in the fibrin matrix are more apparent. The inflammatory reaction to *Pneumocystis* organisms is usually minimal unless, as often happens, another pathogen is present. Figure 3.70 demonstrates both *Pneumocystis* and herpes inclusions in material obtained by bronchial washing from an area of infiltrate detected radiographically in the lung. This patient suffered from AIDS, in which multiple infections are not uncommon.

Penicillium marneffii

Penicilllium marneffii is an opportunistic fungal infection that is endemic in Asia.[181–183] Immunocompetent patients have been infected,

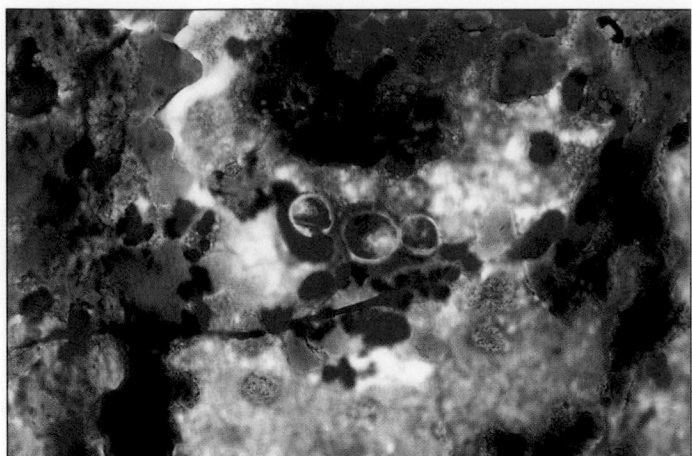

Fig. 3.71 Blastomycosis of the lung. Fine needle aspirate of a lung mass clinically suspected to be carcinoma demonstrates organisms with broad-based budding in a background of acute inflammation (Diff-Quik, ×1000).

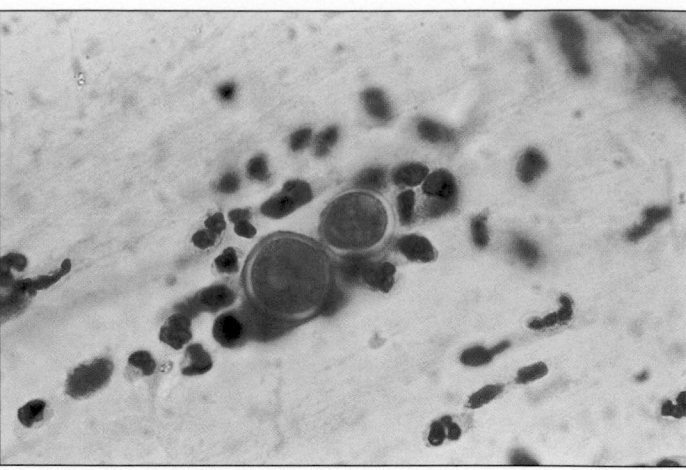

Fig. 3.72 Blastomycosis of the lung. Bronchial washing in a patient suspected of having carcinoma demonstrates yeasts with broad-based buds in an acute inflammatory background (Papanicolaou, ×1000).

but most patients have been immunocompromised. In the United States most patients have been HIV-infected individuals who have traveled to Asia. The portal of entry is thought to be the lung, resulting in a chronic pneumonia and on occasion dissemination to peripheral organs, particularly the liver. Accumulations of macrophages, which may undergo necrosis, form the basic histopathologic response. Numerous intracellular yeast-like cells that measure 2–5 μm in size resemble *H. capsulatum* most closely. If budding yeast cells are identified, the possibility of *Penicillium* infection can be eliminated. The yeast-like cells of *P. marneffii* divide by septation. Occasionally, elongated, sausage-shaped cells with septa can be demonstrated, establishing the diagnosis in conjunction with the clinical presentation and histologic response.

Cytologic diagnosis of dimorphic fungal infections

Primary mycotic infections may occur in the respiratory tract and initially be mistaken clinically and radiographically for a lung neoplasm. The budding organisms of blastomycosis found in the FNA biopsy of a lung mass are seen in Figures 3.71 and 3.72, stained with Diff-Quik and Papanicolaou reagents, respectively. The organisms of blastomycosis have an internal structure that resembles a nucleus, at least in its staining characteristics, and is called a nuclear body. This is in contrast to the cytomorphology of *Crypto-coccus* (Fig. 3.73), which has a narrow-based, teardrop-shaped budding and an opaque or homogeneous center bounded by a thick capsule. *Cryptococcus* organisms may show a flattened surface and a crystalline-like center, which is actually an artifact of coverslipping Papanicolaou-stained slides. Most of these yeast-like organisms are rigid, and the irregularly flattened side of *Cryptococcus* may trap a very small air bubble, which when viewed in the microscope will refract light, giving the appearance of a small crystal in the center of the organism (Fig. 3.74). An interesting case of the use of FNA biopsy is illustrated in Figures 3.75 to 3.77. This patient was suffering from Addison's disease and was found to have bilateral adrenal masses (Fig. 3.75). Aspiration demonstrated organisms of *Cryptococcus* (Fig. 3.76) stained with mucicarmine to demonstrate the capsule and with GMS (Fig. 3.77) to illustrate the size range and narrow-based budding of these organisms.

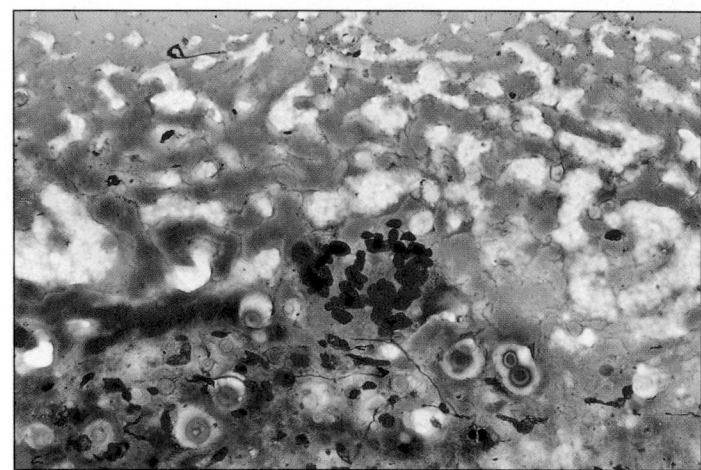

Fig. 3.73 *Cryptococcus neoformans* infection of lung. Patient with acquired immunodeficiency syndrome and pulmonary infiltrates. Many round yeast are present and show thick capsules and narrow-based budding (Diff-Quik stain, ×600).

An example of coccidiomycosis is seen in a sputum sample in a patient who had AIDS but who was also from the dusty desert area of the southwestern United States, where the organism is commonly found. The irregularity of the spherules of this organism may appear as debris contaminating the sample (Fig. 3.78). Figure 3.79 shows a single small early spherule with a thin but distinct capsule. Such a structure may be ignored as plant material or some other contaminant in the sample. When these organisms are seen in a background of granuloma formation, more distinctly in an FNA biopsy, the diagnosis is much easier.

H. capsulatum is rarely identified in sputum, bronchial washing, or brushing specimens as the organism is either not present or is present in very small numbers when only a single or several granulomas are present. In children, who may acquire a very disseminated form in the lung, the organisms may be found within multiple

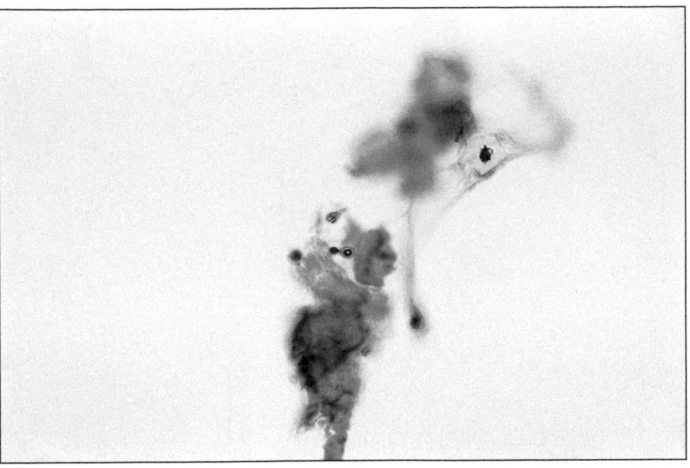

Fig. 3.74 *Cryptococcus neoformans* infection of the meninges. Morphology of *Cryptococcus* organisms demonstrating crystalline-like center, which is an artifact due to the flattened shape of some of the organisms (Papanicolaou stain, ×200).

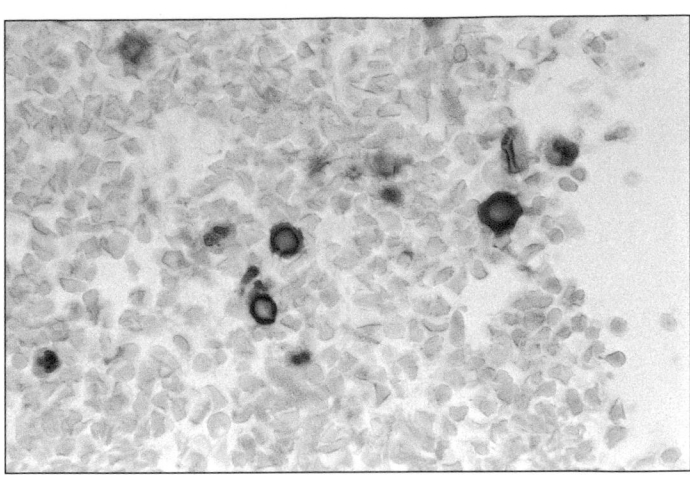

Fig. 3.76 *Cryptococcus neoformans* infection of the adrenal glands. Organisms show mucicarmine positive capsule (Mucicarmine, ×1000).

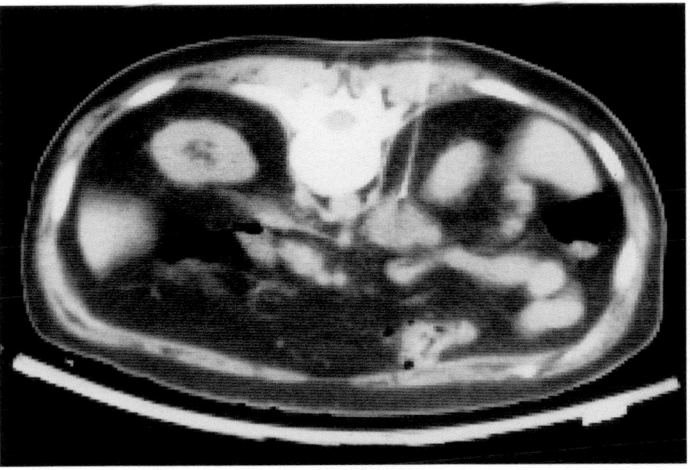

Fig. 3.75 *Cryptococcus neoformans* infection of the adrenal glands in a patient with Addison's disease. Fine-needle aspiration was performed to determine the cause of Addison's disease in a patient with bilateral adrenal gland enlargement. Metastatic carcinoma was suspected clinically. Computerized tomography scan shows aspiration needle in place.

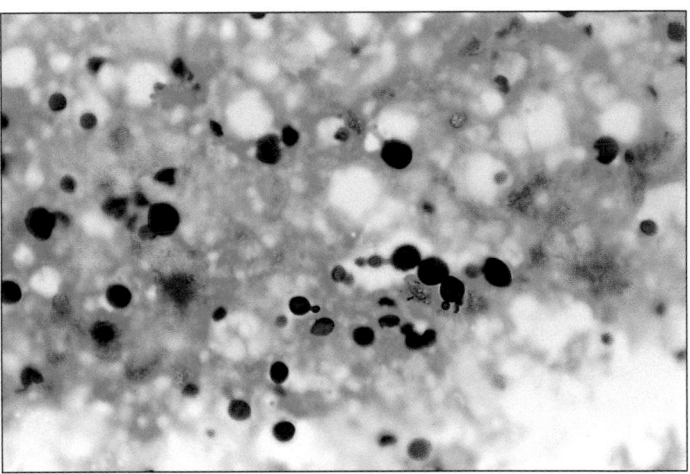

Fig. 3.77 *Cryptococcus neoformans* infection of the adrenal gland. Multiple round narrow-based budding yeasts seen on silver precipitate stain (GMS, ×1000).

histiocytes.[184] An example of the aspiration of a solitary lung mass demonstrates these small organisms in a large multinucleated giant cell as small symmetrical clear round spaces with very small central darker dot-like structures (Fig. 3.80). Special stains, such as the methenamine silver or PAS with light green techniques, are usually required to identify or confirm the presence of this small organism. The cell block from this lung aspirate (Fig. 3.81) demonstrates a small granuloma with a multinucleated giant cell. On close examination, very small round clear areas are seen in the cytoplasm of some cells making up the granuloma. A barely detectable small slightly darker dot is present in some of these clear areas. These two features together characterize the yeast cells of *H. capsulatum*.

Aspergillus species

Aspergillus spp. are hyaline, septate hyphae that branch dichotomously. The most common human pathogens are *A. fumigatus, A.*

flavus, and *A. niger*. The hyphae measure 3–6 μm in width. They stain moderately well with H&E and are well demonstrated by methenamine silver and PAS techniques.

Aspergillosis comes in three forms: allergic bronchopulmonary disease, mycetoma, and invasive disease. Allergic bronchopulmonary aspergillosis has several manifestations.[185,186] Chronic eosinophilic pneumonia is characterized by macrophages and eosinophils in the interstitium and airspaces, sometimes Charcot-Leyden crystals, and aggregation of the eosinophils into microabscesses. In the distal airways, impaction of mucus and endobronchial inflammation may be present. If hyphae are not demonstrated, the lesion cannot be differentiated from other causes of eosinophilic pneumonia. Mucoid impaction is characterized by inspissated plugs of mucus with eosinophils and Charcot-Leyden crystals in the lumens of large bronchi. Fungal hyphae may be difficult to demonstrate. A similar pathologic process has been described in the paranasal sinuses.[187]

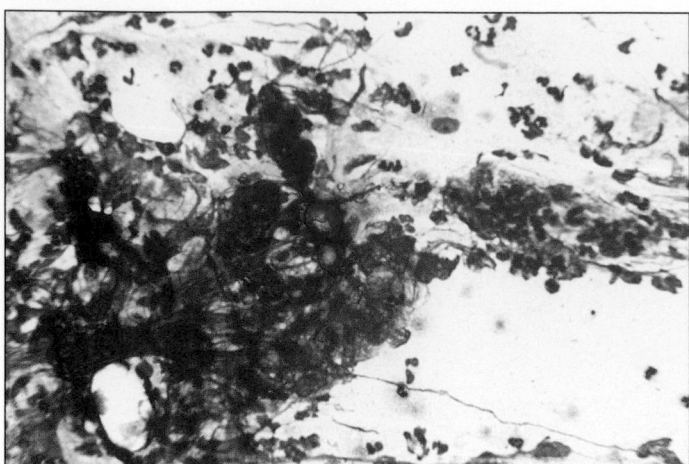

Fig. 3.78 *Coccidioides immitis* in sputum. Two round blue-staining spherules are seen in a background of marked acute inflammation (Diff-Quik stain, ×400).

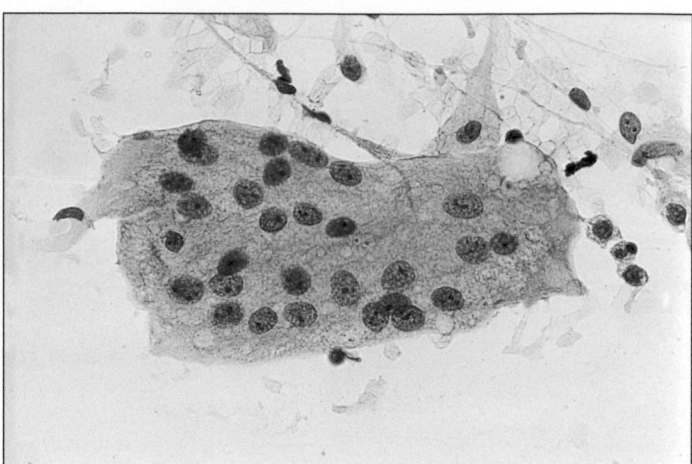

Fig. 3.80 Histoplasmosis of lung. Fine needle aspiration of a lung nodule demonstrated the pattern of granulomatous inflammation. Large multinucleated giant cell in this figure has small round clear areas (some with a faint central dot) that represents the organisms (Papanicolaou, ×600).

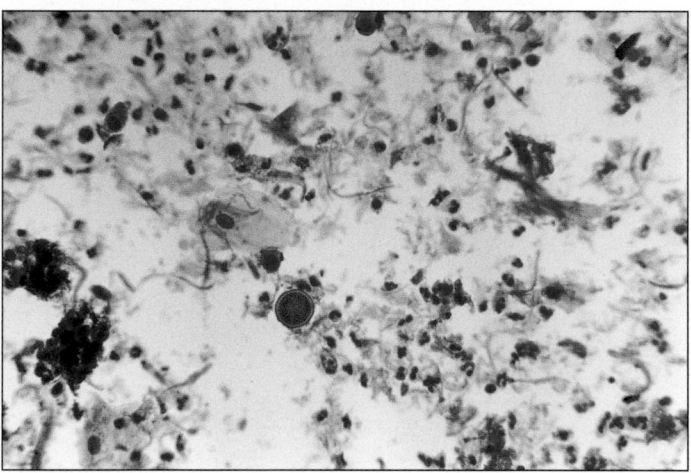

Fig. 3.79 *Coccidioides immitis* in sputum. Same case as Fig. 3.78, with larger orange-staining spherule in a background of acute inflammation (Papanicolaou, ×400).

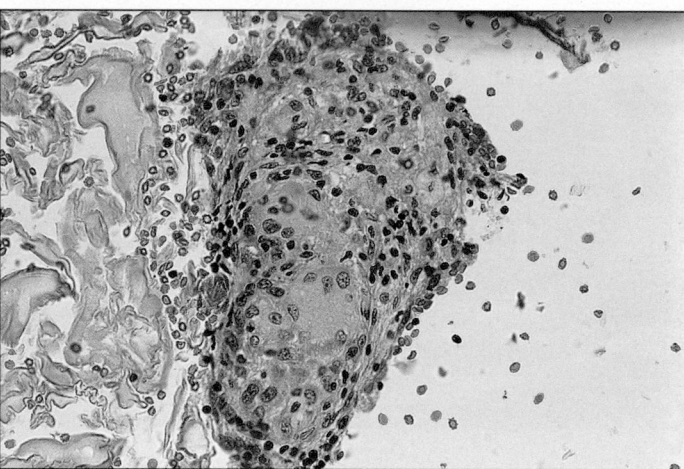

Fig. 3.81 Histoplasmosis of lung. Cell block from case seen in Fig. 3.80. Small granulomas are present with multinucleated giant cells. Organisms of histoplasmosis were easily demonstrated with special stains (H&E, ×400).

Allergic bronchocentric granulomatosis is a chronic granulomatous process that partially or completely destroys the walls of bronchi and bronchioles. The inflammation commonly involves adjacent arterioles and arteries but is clearly centered on the bronchial tree. Hyphal fragments are present in the bronchial lumens but do not invade the parenchyma. In the nonasthmatic patient, other causes of granulomatous inflammation, such as mycobacteria, *H. capsulatum*, and *B. dermatitidis*, should be considered.[188]

Mycetomas (aspergillomas) occupy pre-existing cavities in the lung, usually produced by tuberculosis, or the cavities of the paranasal sinuses (Fig. 3.82). Masses of hyphae, many of which are distorted, stain poorly and are presumably dead; they occupy the cavity but do not invade tissue. Cavities are also produced in the course of invasive aspergillosis, but they have a much more sinister implication in this setting (Fig. 3.83). A form of minimally invasive disease that is

somewhere between pure mycetoma and invasive aspergillosis does occur. The major complication is erosion of the infiltrating hyphae, surrounding chronic inflammation, or superimposed acute inflammation into adjacent blood vessels. The mycetoma cavities are usually exposed to the air, which allows the development of fruiting heads, asexual reproductive structures that are ordinarily seen only in the microbiology laboratory. The presence of conidiophores with swollen vesicles, phialides, and chains of conidia confirms the genus and may even allow identification of the infecting species (Fig. 3.84). Calcium oxalate crystals may be seen in the tissue adjacent to mycetomas caused by *A. niger*. They are well demonstrated with polarized light and provide strong presumptive evidence as to the etiology (Fig. 3.85).

Invasive aspergillosis, the most serious clinical form, occurs primarily in patients who are immunocompromised, especially those

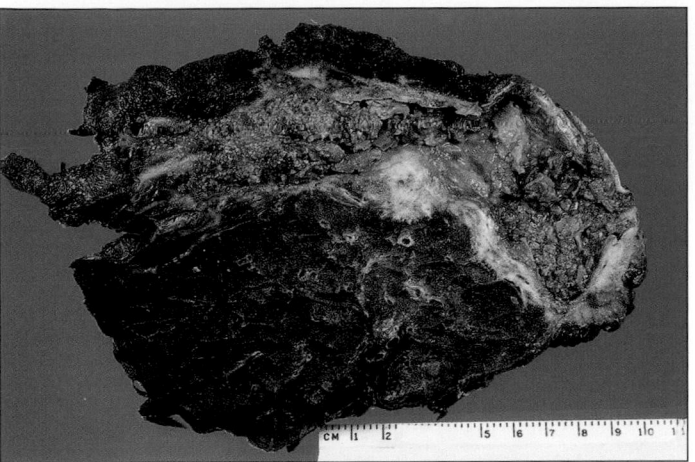

Fig. 3.82 *Aspergillus niger* mycetoma of lung. A large, thick-walled cavity contains brown grumous material due to masses of hyphae.

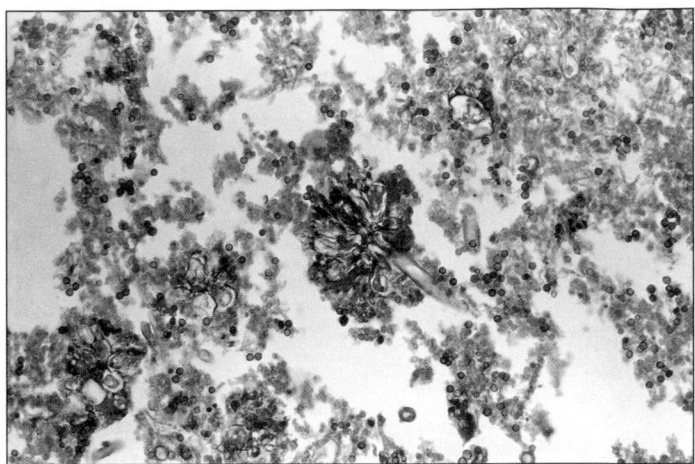

Fig. 3.84 *Aspergillus niger* fruiting bodies in a mycetoma. A condiophore supports elongated phialides. Small dark spores and pieces of other phlalides are present in the surrounding tissue. Although the spores and fruiting heads are colored, the hyphae are not pigmented. These asexual structures occur when the mold grows within an air-filled space, such as a pulmonary cavity (H&E, ×400).

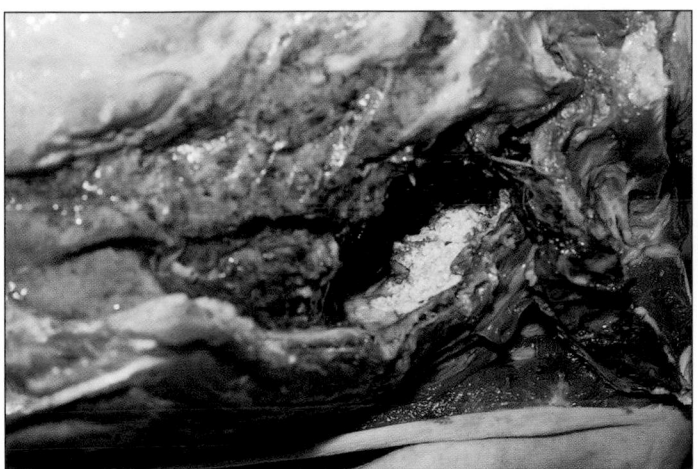

Fig. 3.83 *Aspergillus fumigatus* invasive disease with cavitation. The necrotizing infection has produced cavities in which masses of white mold are growing. The clinical implication of the 'mycetomas' is that of the underlying invasive infection.

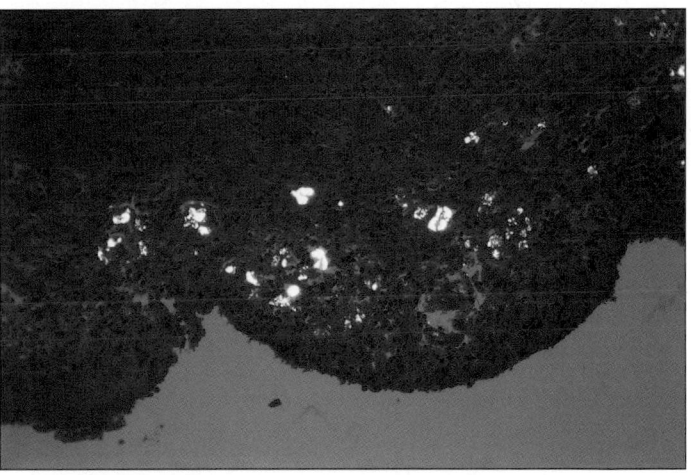

Fig. 3.85 Calcium oxalate crystals in an *Aspergillus niger* mycetoma of the lung. The presence of these crystals provides a presumptive diagnosis of the infecting fungal species (H&E with polarized light, ×40).

who are neutropenic. The portal of entry is usually the lung, but it may be through compromised skin or gastrointestinal epithelium. *Aspergillus* spp. are angioinvasive and produce destructive, necrotizing lesions analogous to those produced by the zygomycetes. Cavitary lesions in the lung may be produced by infarction and then overgrowth by the invading fungi (see Fig. 3.83).

The histopathology of invasive aspergillosis is dominated by hemorrhage and necrosis, and acute inflammation is common if the patient has adequate circulating neutrophils. Less commonly, the inflammatory response in smoldering infection is granulomatous. The diagnosis of hyphomycete infection can be made by recognition of thin, septate, dichotomously branching hyphae (Fig. 3.86). The differential diagnosis includes thin hyphae of zygomycetes and pseudohyphae of *Candida* spp. The presence of numerous septae, which may be best seen with special stains, differentiates these hyphae from those of the zygomycetes. Differentiation of *Candida* pseudohyphae from irregular mold hyphae is usually not difficult,

and the presence of budding yeast cells establishes the diagnosis. *Aspergillus* spp. cannot be differentiated in tissue from other hyphomycetes that are less common, but sufficiently common to warrant circumspection in the report (Fig. 3.87). A firm diagnosis of aspergillosis is not possible. A report of 'hyphomycete (or mold) such as *Aspergillus* spp.' is more accurate.

Influenza virus

Influenza virus is an RNA-containing myxovirus that causes sporadic and epidemic respiratory disease. Influenza viruses types A and B are the primary causes of epidemic respiratory infection, and influenza A virus is the only agent that produces pandemic disease. The most common manifestation is a syndrome of fever, nonproductive cough, and intense myalgias known as 'the flu.' Secondary bacterial pneumonia is a feared complication that is caused most

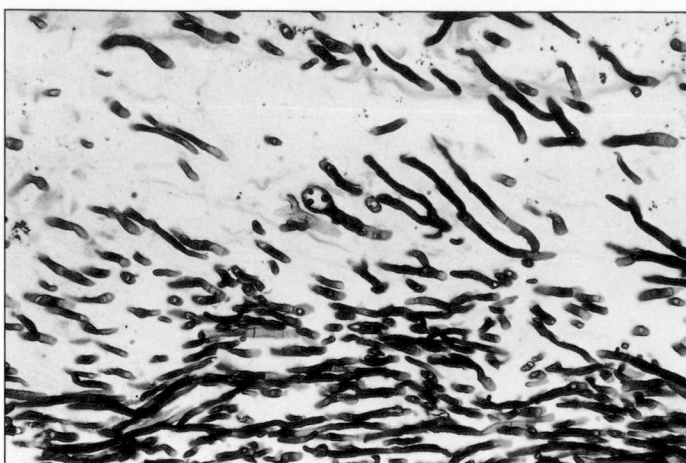

Fig. 3.86 *Aspergillus* morphology. The thin, regular hyphae are septate and branch at acute angles (dichotomously). A single swollen hyphal segment is present. On the basis of this morphology *Aspergillus* cannot be differentiated from other hyphomycetes (GMS, ×400).

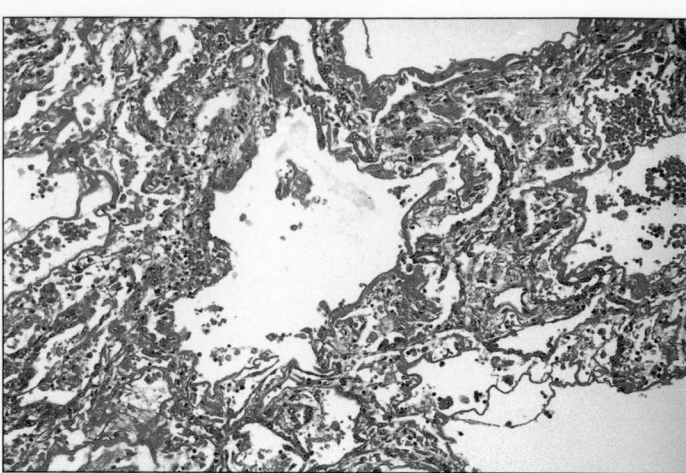

Fig. 3.88 Influenza virus pneumonia. The histologic reaction is manifested by acute alveolar damage with mononuclear interstitial infiltrate and exudation of fibrin and hyaline membranes in the alveoli. The diagnosis can be suspected from the clinical history, but must be confirmed by either culture or serologic confirmation (H&E, ×50).

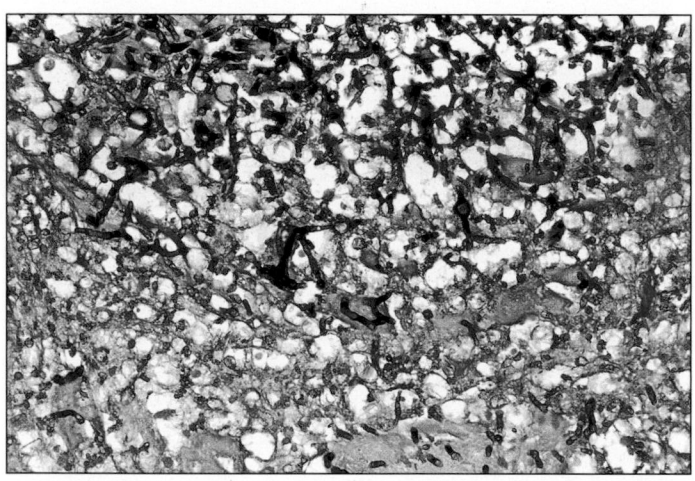

Fig. 3.87 *Pseudoallescheria boydii (Scedosporium apiospermum)* myocarditis. The thin septate hyphae with dichotomous branching cannot be differentiated from *Aspergillus* (GMS, ×400) (Courtesy of David Walker, MD).

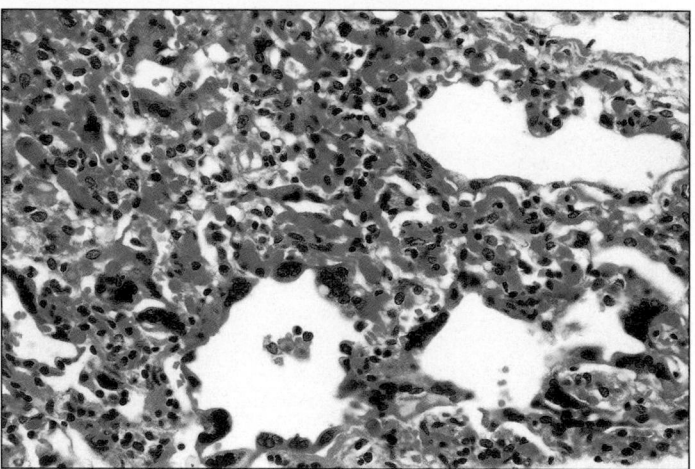

Fig. 3.89 Giant cell pneumonia caused by parainfluenza virus 3 infection. There is a mononuclear interstitial infiltrate. The virus has produced numerous multinucleated syncytial giant cells. Inclusions are not appreciated (H&E, ×200, parainfluenza virus type 3 isolated from cultures).

commonly by *S. aureus*, *Streptococcus pneumoniae*, and *H. influenzae*. In epidemics, primary influenza virus pneumonia is a cause of fatal infection. The hallmark of influenza infection of the lower respiratory tract is diffuse alveolar damage, a host response that is shared by most other viral respiratory pathogens. Mononuclear interstitial inflammation is accompanied by proliferation of pneumocytes and accumulation of fibrin with hyaline membranes in the airspaces (Fig. 3.88). Inclusions are not found, and the diagnosis must be made by demonstration of viral antigen or by culture. Rarely, influenza virus may cause myositis (sometimes with myoglobinuria) and myocarditis.[189]

Parainfluenza viruses

Parainfluenza viruses are of four serotypes. They usually cause upper respiratory tract infection or croup (laryngotracheobronchitis) but may produce bronchiolitis and pneumonia, which are especially common in infections caused by serotype 3 strains. Diffuse alveolar damage may be accompanied by multinucleated syncytial giant cells in type 2 and type 3 infection (Fig. 3.89). Inclusions are not usually seen. The histologic appearance of lung tissue infected with parainfluenza viruses that produce giant cells and inclusions is identical to the host reaction to respiratory syncytial virus.

Respiratory syncytial virus

Respiratory syncytial virus is the most common cause of bronchiolitis and pneumonia in infants and young children but may also produce serious infection and epidemic disease in adults.[190,191] Peribronchiolar inflammation and diffuse alveolar damage are accompanied by syncytial giant cells, which may contain eosinophilic intranuclear inclusions (Fig. 3.90).

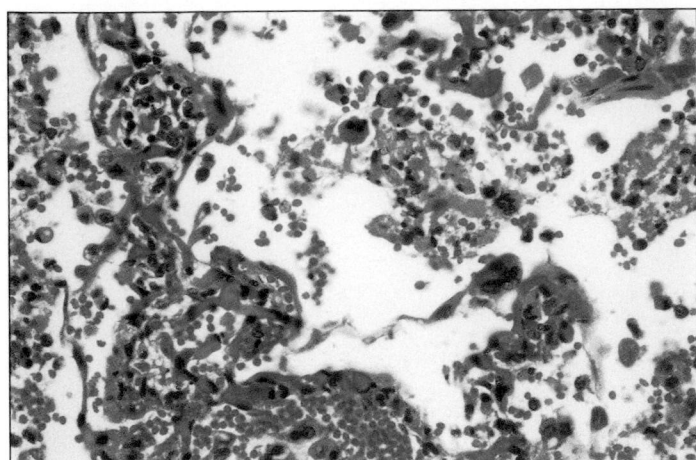

Fig. 3.90 Giant cell pneumonia caused by respiratory syncytial virus (RSV) infection. The histologic response resembles that seen in parainfluenza virus infection. Multinucleated giant cells may contain eosinophilic intracytoplasmic inclusions; however, this is difficult to appreciate in this photomicrograph (H&E, ×200, RSV isolated from cultures).

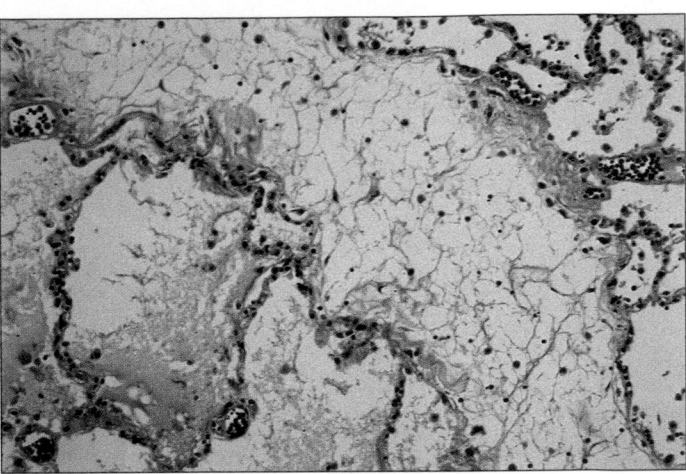

Fig. 3.92 Hantavirus pulmonary syndrome. The histologic reaction is relatively noninflammatory, consisting of edema in the interstitium and airspaces as a result of viral infection of the vascular endothelium. Large immunoblastic cells are often present (H&E, ×200, Sin Nombre virus demonstrated in tissue). (Courtesy of Sherif Zaki, MD)

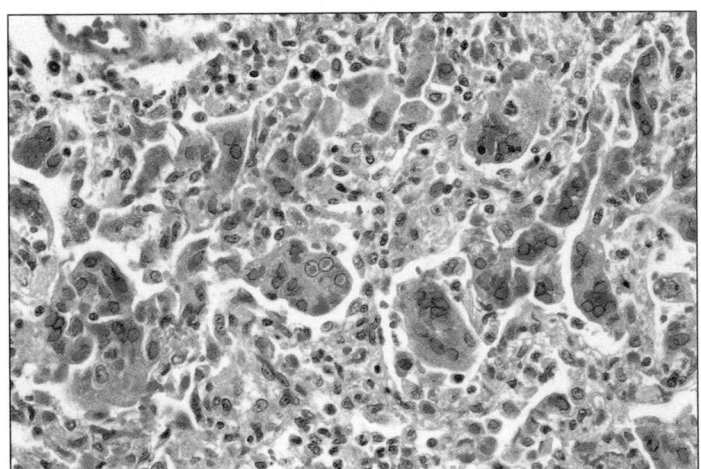

Fig. 3.91 Giant cell pneumonia caused by measles virus infection. There is a mononuclear infiltrate in the interstitium and the airspaces. Numerous multinucleated syncytial giant cells contain eosinophilic intranuclear and intracytoplasmic inclusions (H&E, ×400).

Measles virus

Measles virus enters the body through the upper respiratory tract, after which it disseminates through the body. The maculopapular skin rash is the most familiar manifestation of infection. The most serious complications are pneumonia and encephalitis.[192] In the lung, diffuse alveolar damage is accompanied by syncytial giant cells (the original giant cell pneumonia). The giant cells contain intranuclear inclusions and occasionally cytoplasmic inclusions (Fig. 3.91). Warthin-Finkeldey giant cells in lymphoid tissue may have a different pathogenesis and do not contain inclusions.

Hantaviruses

Hantaviruses classically produced hemorrhagic fever, such as Korean hemorrhagic fever, and a milder infection called nephropathia endemica. The spectrum of disease expanded considerably in the 1990s when acute respiratory disease in the Four Corners area of the American southwest was attributed to a new hantavirus, now known as Sin Nombre virus. Other related viruses have been discovered in the eastern United States, but very few infections have so far been attributed to these agents. The infection presents as acute respiratory failure, and the pulmonary pathology includes prominent pulmonary edema and enlarged immunoblastic lymphoid cells (Fig. 3.92).[193,194] The capillary leakage is produced by viral infection of the endothelium.

Severe acute respiratory syndrome virus

Severe acute respiratory syndrome (SARS) was initially described in November of 2002 during an outbreak in southern China, which subsequently spread to Hong Kong and then to many countries including Canada.[195,196] The etiology is linked to a unique coronavirus that has been named the SARS-associated coronavirus, spread by respiratory droplet transmission. The pathology is that of an acute lung injury pattern with edema, interstitial mononuclear inflammation, fibrinous exudates, and organizing pneumonia. Some cases progressed to a diffuse alveolar damage pattern and no viral inclusions were identified. Viral particles were confirmed using electron microscopy.[197]

Viral mimics

The most important infection in the mimic group is pertussis, which will rarely be seen by the surgical pathologist. *Bordetella pertussis* elicits a lymphocytic response in the epithelium of the respiratory tract from the larynx to the lower airways. Rare fatal cases are characterized by lymphocytic infiltrates in the peribronchial and peribronchiolar mucosa.

Dirofilaria species

Dirofilaria spp. are common parasites of a variety of animal species and are transmitted to new hosts by the bite of a mosquito. When the filaria enters a human host, localized nodules are produced, most commonly in the skin (typically *Dirofilaria tenuis* from raccoons) or

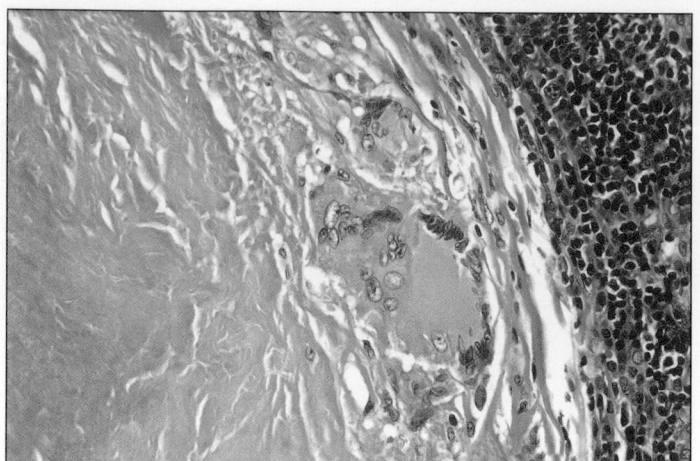

Fig. 3.93 The coin lesions of dirofilariasis are often thought to represent pulmonary tumors clinically. The edges of these lesions are often accompanied by a subtle granulomatous reaction (H&E, ×250).

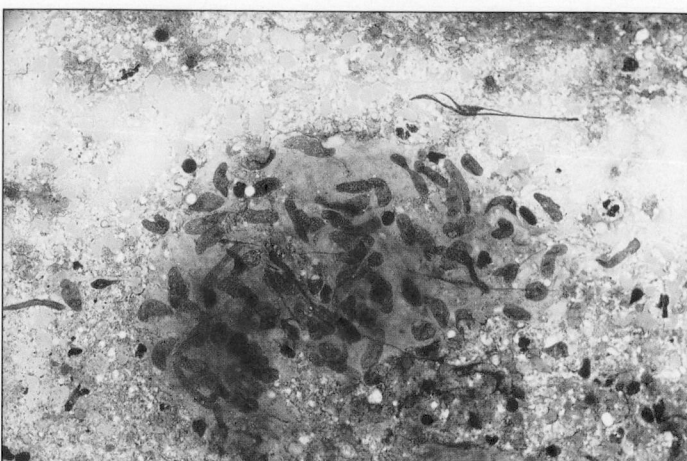

Fig. 3.94 Tuberculosis of the lung. Fine needle aspiration of a lung mass demonstrates epithelioid granuloma in a granular necrotic background. The same type of granuloma, most often in a clear smear background, can be seen in sarcoidosis (Diff-Quik, ×400).

in the lungs (typically *Dirofilaria immitis* from dogs). The histologic response is granulomatous, with a component of acute inflammation in the early lesions. In pulmonary coin lesions, which are often resected because of the possibility of neoplastic disease,[198,199] the association of the process with a pulmonary artery may be detectable (Fig. 3.93). The species of *Dirofilaria* can be differentiated (at least by experts) in histologic sections.[200]

LYMPH NODE INFECTIONS

Cytologic diagnosis of mycobacterial infections

Tuberculosis, still a predominant infection in Third World countries, is making a resurgence in the United States with the identification of drug-resistant strains. This infection may be encountered and diagnosed or at least suspected from the interpretation of cytologic samples principally obtained by FNA biopsy.[201] Several examples have been seen in FNA of enlarged cervical lymph nodes, particularly in children. Sometimes, there may be a picture of necrosis and relatively acute inflammation but without well-formed granulomas. The background of relatively homogeneous necrosis in the absence of any atypical cells suggesting a neoplasm is the morphologic clue that leads to performance of special stains to identify the organisms. Careful search of additional smears is often necessary to find them. The same picture may appear in an aspiration biopsy of the lung, but more intact granulomas may also be found within the necrotic background (Fig. 3.94).

With infection by atypical mycobacteria in patients with the acquired immunodeficiency syndrome (AIDS), the cytologic and histologic picture is quite different. Many histiocytes are seen that in air-dried smears stained with Romanowsky methods appear like Gaucher cells. They have been termed pseudo-Gaucher cells and were described in bone marrow smears and originally in an aspirate of an inguinal lymph node from a patient who had been injected with bacille Calmette-Guérin to treat superficial carcinoma of the bladder. Few to many clear, thin, slightly curved areas appear in these smears both in the background and within the histiocytic cells, so-called negative images (Fig. 3.95).[202] These areas that do not stain with water-based stains represent the atypical mycobacteria that are easily stained

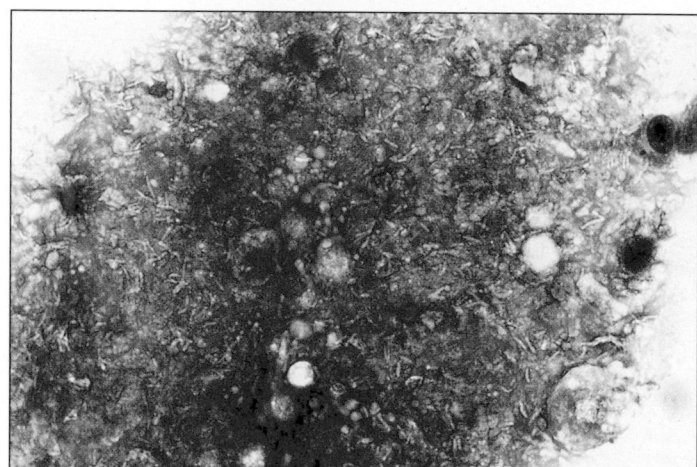

Fig. 3.95 Atypical mycobacterial infection in a mediastinal lymph node. Fine needle aspiration of the enlarged nodes show homogeneous metachromatic material with only a few inflammatory cells. Note the curved short clear spaces seen throughout the smear, 'negative images' that represent the large number of organisms. Patient suffered from the acquired immunodeficiency syndrome (Diff-Quik, ×400).

with acid-fast stains and that usually occur in profusion in such smears (Fig. 3.96).

Cat-scratch fever

Cat-scratch fever is caused by *Bartonella (Rochalimaea) henselae*. A primary lesion at the site of the scratch, usually of a kitten, is often not visible, and the disease is dominated by regional lymphadenitis.[203,204] The basic lesion is a necrotizing granuloma that has an irregular zone of stellate necrosis. The interior of the granuloma is composed of degenerating mononuclear and polymorphonuclear inflammatory cells. Palisading epithelioid histiocytes and multinucleated giant cells followed by a zone of lymphocytes with surrounding fibrosis complete the picture (Fig. 3.97). The intense inflammatory reaction often extends through the capsule of the lymph nodes and

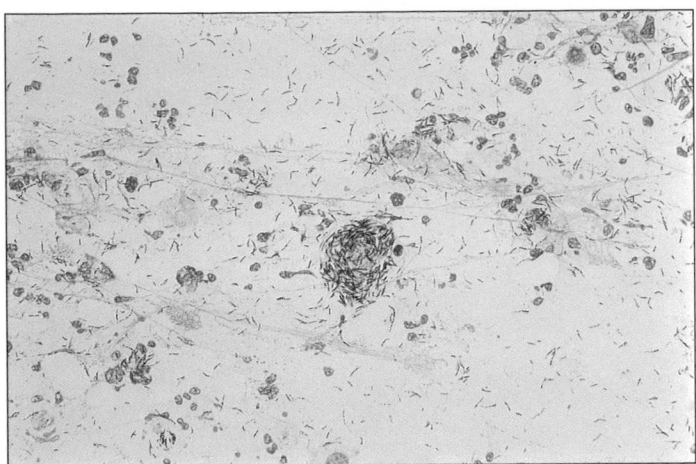

Fig. 3.96 Atypical mycobacterial infection of cervical lymph node as seen in fine-needle aspirate smear (AFB, ×600).

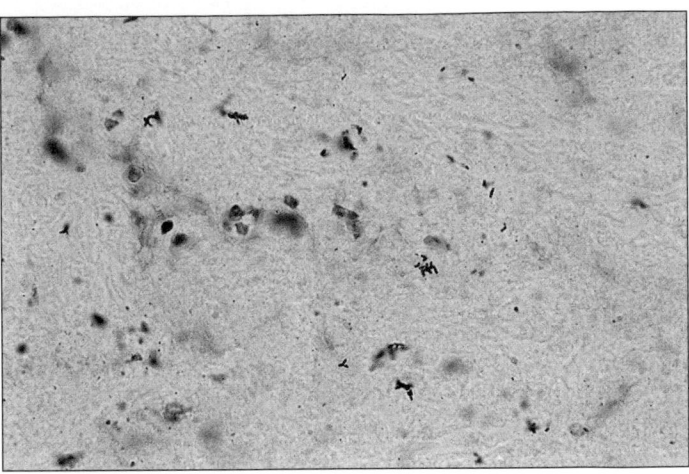

Fig. 3.98 Short, plump pleomorphic bacilli of *Bartonella henselae*. The morphology is obscured by the silver deposition (Warthin-Starry, ×1000).

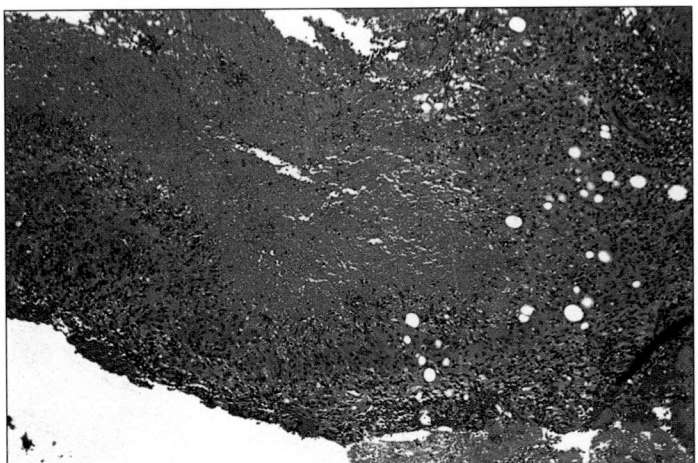

Fig. 3.97 Cat-scratch disease caused by *Bartonella henselae*. A large geographic necrotizing granuloma is present in the lymph node that drained the site of the initial cutaneous cat-scratch site. The patient had elevated antibodies and polymerase chain reaction was positive for *Bartonella henselae*-specific DNA sequences (H&E, ×20).

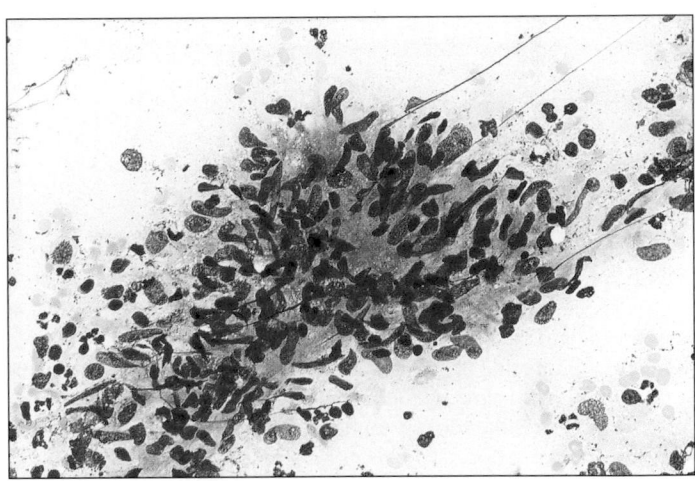

Fig. 3.99 Cat-scratch disease. Fine-needle aspirate of an enlarged cervical lymph node with a reactive pattern of mixed lymphoid cells. Clinical correlation is required, as the aspiration findings are non-specific. Polymerase chain reaction confirmation for *Bartonella henselae* DNA can be performed on cell-block material (Diff-Quick, ×400).

into the adjacent soft tissue. The differential diagnosis of necrotizing granulomas with stellate necrosis includes tularemia *(F. tularensis)*, *Yersinia* infection, and lymphogranuloma venereum *(Chlamydia trachomatis)*. The causative organism is usually not visualized in these infections, so the diagnosis may be suggested by the clinical presentation and the organ system involved, but the definitive diagnosis must be made by culture or molecular techniques. Granulomas with caseous necrosis may also be present, expanding the differential diagnosis to include mycobacterial and fungal infection. Severe, prolonged disease and systemic infection have been reported.[205,206]

Bartonella organisms are not demonstrated by tissue Gram stains but may be visualized by the Warthin-Starry or related silver impregnation techniques.[207] Short, pleomorphic bacilli, the morphology of which is distorted by the silver salts, are present in early lesions, particularly in vascular areas (Fig. 3.98). In our experience

the bacilli are more often photographed than seen. The etiologic agents can be recovered in culture, but the necessary procedures are difficult, tedious, and not often accomplished in microbiology laboratories.[208]

Cytologic Diagnosis of Lymph Node Cat-scratch Infections: Enlarged lymph nodes are a frequent target for aspiration biopsy. Historically, aspiration of lymph nodes was used to diagnosis sleeping sickness in the early 1900s.[209] Today a variety of infections may be encountered in such samples, and certain aspiration patterns, while not specific, may suggest an infectious etiology in the appropriate clinical setting. The most frequently encountered of these is cat-scratch disease. Smear patterns are of three types: an early phase with a hyperplastic reactive pattern and few granulomas (Fig. 3.99); a middle phase with many granulomas of stellate shape and suppuration (Fig. 3.100); and a late phase that is largely a

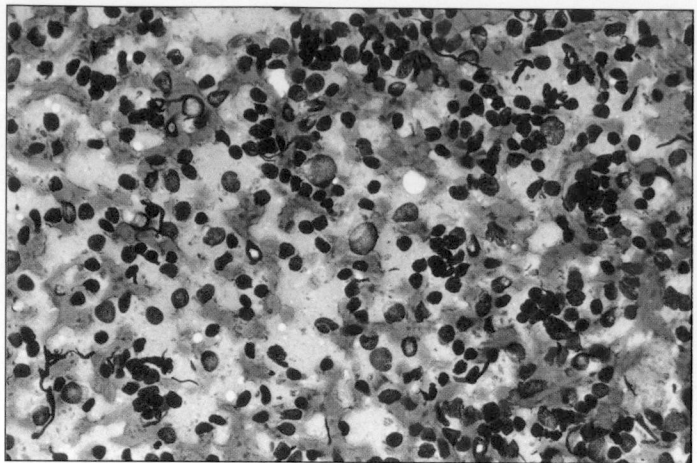

Fig. 3.100 Cat-scratch disease. Fine needle aspiration of an enlarge lymph node showing evidence of stellate granulomas and abundant acute inflammatory exudates. Clinical correlation along with serologic studies and molecular or immunohistochemical confirmation is required for a definitive diagnosis (Diff-Quik, ×600).

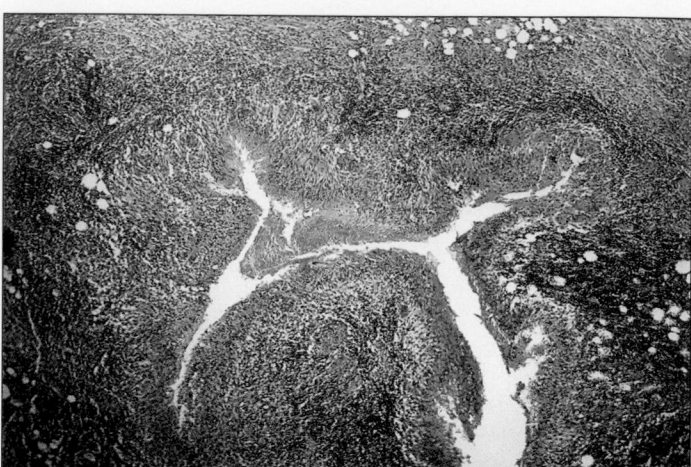

Fig. 3.101 Oculoglandular tularemia. A large geographic granuloma with prominent palisading of epithelioid histiocytes and central necrosis occupies a cervical lymph node. The patient had inoculated her eye when she squashed an engorged tick, after which she developed conjunctivitis followed by lymphadenopathy. Tularemia titers were positive and she responded to antibiotic therapy (H&E, ×15).

necrotic smear pattern obscuring many granulomas.[210] It has not been possible to identify the organisms with special stains on smears, and identification of the organisms with special stains on section is quite problematic.

Tularemia

Tularemia, a zoonotic infection that is caused by *Francisella tularensis*, is widely distributed through the United States, and most heavily endemic in Arkansas.[211–216] Infection is acquired from direct contact with infected animals, particularly rabbits (rabbit fever), but ticks may also transmit the infection. Several clinical forms of the infection may result. Most common is ulceroglandular tularemia, which resembles sporotrichosis clinically. An inflammatory lesion at the site of injury is followed by lymphangitic spread and involvement of regional lymph nodes. The basic inflammatory lesion is a necrotizing granuloma that resembles the lesion of cat-scratch disease and must be differentiated from the same differential diagnoses (Fig. 3.101). Less common forms of infection include oculoglandular tularemia, a typhoidal form without an obvious portal of entry, and primary tularemia pneumonia.

Yersinia species

Yersinia spp. produce varied clinical disease depending on the species. *Yersinia pestis*, which is the most venerable and most virulent pathogen, causes human plague, which in many respects resembles tularemia.[217,218] Fleas from infected rodents transmit the infection to the human host. Historically, rats have been the primary host, but indigenous infection in the southwestern United States is associated with contact with infected prairie dogs. The most common type is ulceroglandular, which is dominated by enlarged, fluctuant lymph nodes draining the primary inoculation site. Primary lesions and lymphangitic spread are not prominent. Histologically, the lymph nodes, which are more likely to be aspirated than surgically resected, are replaced by necrotizing granulomas and acute inflammation. The bacteria can be demonstrated in the lesions with methylene blue or Gram stain, and they are easily cultured. Primary plague pneumonia,

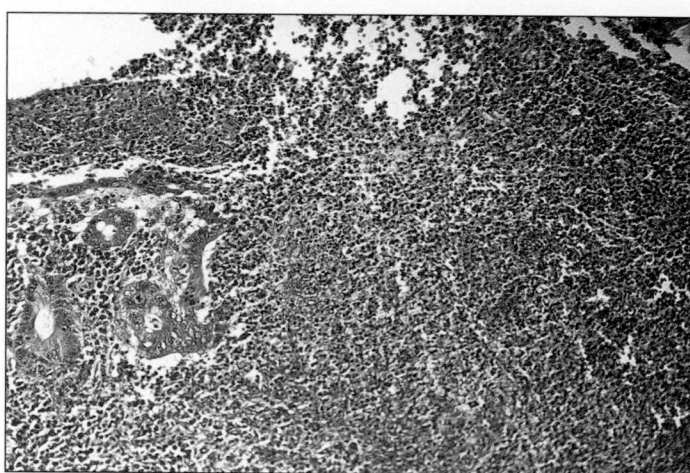

Fig. 3.102 *Yersinia* appendicitis. An ulcerated lesion is populated by mononuclear cells and polymorphonuclear neutrophils. The surface lesion communicated with a large submucosal stellate granuloma (H&E, ×30, *Yersinia enterocolitica* isolated from culture).

which can result in human-to-human spread, has a high mortality and is the most feared form of the disease.

Y. enterocolitica and *Y. pseudotuberculosis* produce acute disease in the gastrointestinal tract and the draining mesenteric lymph nodes.[219–223] Necrotizing granulomas may cause ulceration in the mucosa of the ileum or appendix (Fig. 3.102). Alternatively, a syndrome of granulomatous mesenteric lymphadenitis may occur without primary lesions in the gastrointestinal tract (Fig. 3.103). Clinically, mesenteric lymphadenitis resembles acute appendicitis, but the surgeon finds fluctuant, matted mesenteric nodes and a normal appendix. *Y. enterocolitica* is more often associated with primary gastroenteritis and ulcerating intestinal lesions, whereas *Y. pseudotuberculosis* is associated more closely with mesenteric lymphadenitis. Multinucleated giant cells may be seen with either

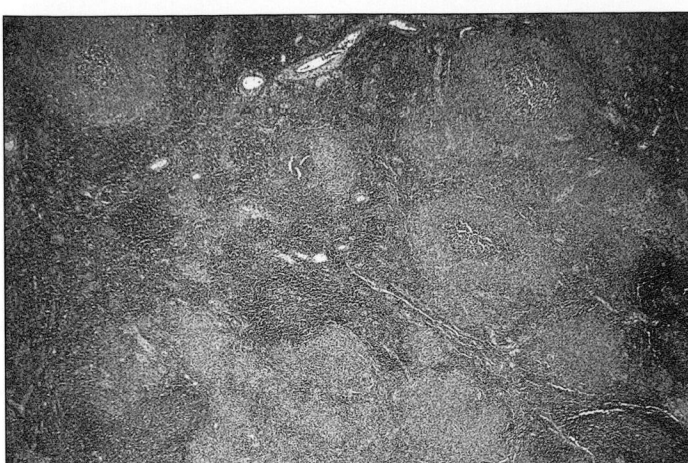

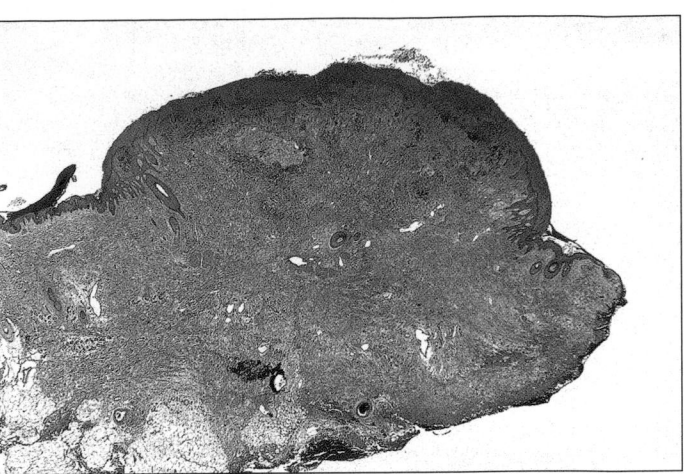

Fig. 3.103 *Yersinia* mesenteric lymphadenitis. Multiple stellate granulomas with central necrosis replace a mesenteric lymph node. The inflammation extends into the surrounding perinodal fat. The preoperative diagnosis was acute suppurative appendicitis, but the appendix was macroscopically and microscopically normal (H&E, ×5, *Yersinia pseudotuberculosis* isolated from cultures).

Fig. 3.105 Bacillary angiomatosis. A nodular cutaneous lesion consists of inflammatory cells and proliferating small blood vessels. The lesions resemble a pyogenic granuloma (H&E, ×5) (Courtsey of Ann-Marie Nelson, MD).

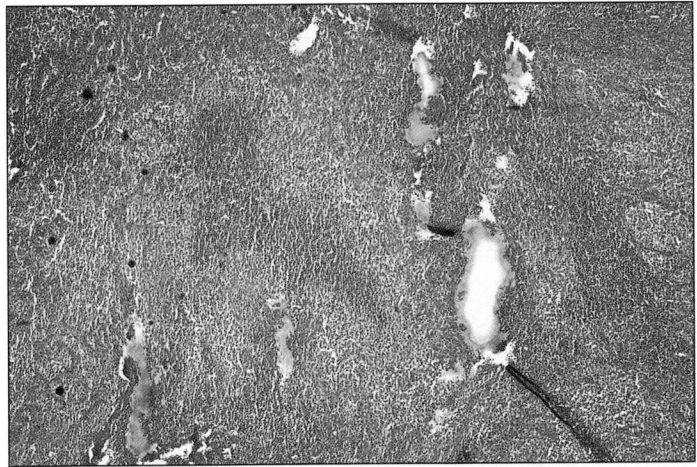

Fig. 3.104 Lymphogranuloma venereum. A large portion of an inguinal lymph node is replaced by suppurative granulomas filled with necrotic debris and polymorphonuclear leukocytes. Such lymph nodes often appear fluctuant on physical examination (H&E, ×5).

species. Both species can cause septicemia in immunosuppressed patients and in individuals with iron overload syndromes.

Lymphogranuloma venereum

Lymphogranuloma venereum, which is caused by the L1 to L3 serotypes of *Chlamydia trachomatis*, is a sexually transmitted infection that results in enlarged inguinal lymph nodes.[224] The lymph nodes are fluctuant because of extensive necrotizing granulomas with stellate necrosis (Fig. 3.104). Extension of the chronic inflammation into the perirectal tissues can result in fibrosis and strictures. Lymphogranuloma venereum serotypes can also cause granulomatous proctitis, most often described in homosexual men.[225] Other serotypes produce genital infection in men and women.

THE CARDIOVASCULAR AND SKELETAL SYSTEMS

The vascular system is involved primarily or secondarily in many infectious diseases. Bacterial intravascular infections occur as secondary infections of damaged endothelium – bacterial endocarditis and mycotic aneurysm. The neutrophilic inflammatory response is differentiated from thrombus by the intensity of the neutrophilic response and the demonstration of bacteria in the lesions. The endothelium is the primary target for *Rickettsia rickettsii*, the causative agent of Rocky Mountain spotted fever. Vasculitis may also be seen in meningococcemia, which may be associated with disseminated intravascular coagulation. *Pseudomonas aeruginosa* occasionally produces a 'vasculitis' in which bacterial colonies obliterate the walls of blood vessels and may contribute to the necrotizing character of the infections.

Bartonella (Rochalimaea) quintana is the historic agent of trench fever.[226] This bacterium was first demonstrated by molecular techniques to be the etiologic agent of two non-neoplastic diseases of vascular proliferation that occur in HIV-infected individuals.[227] Bacillary angiomatosis consists of capillary proliferation, leukocytoclastic debris, and amorphous material that represents colonies of bacteria.[228] The lesion resembles pyogenic granuloma histologically (Fig. 3.105). The bacteria can be demonstrated with the Warthin-Starry stain or related silver impregnation procedures (Fig. 3.106). The lesions of bacillary angiomatosis have also been demonstrated in lymph nodes.[228] Similar lesions in the viscera, especially the liver, are known as peliosis (Fig. 3.107).

Vascular invasion is an important component of fungal infections caused by the zygomycetes and certain hyphomycetes, such as *Aspergillus* spp., as discussed previously. Certain viruses also have an attraction for the vasculature, in this case endothelial cells. The most important of these viruses for surgical pathologists is the new group of respiratory hantaviruses. Other hemorrhagic fever viruses that are not indigenous to the United States also affect the endothelium. Cytomegalovirus and varicella-zoster virus are common viral agents that infect the endothelium, and the histopathology may be influenced by this tropism.

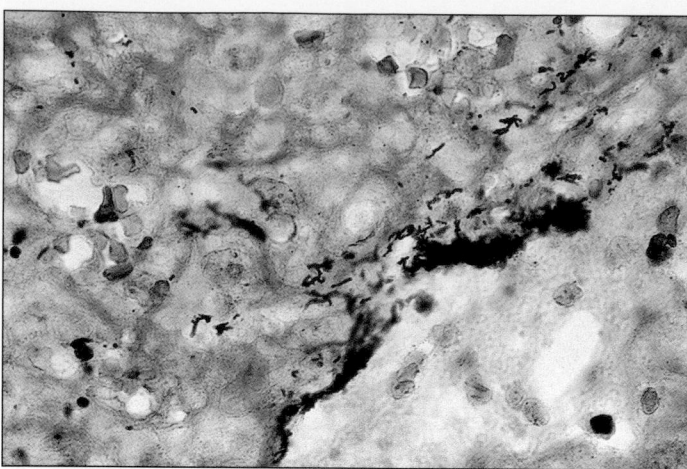

Fig. 3.106 Bacillary angiomatosis. Multiple bacilli are demonstrated in the vascular lesion. The morphology of these tiny Gram-negative bacilli are distorted by the silver impregnation staining techniques. (Warthin-Starry stain, ×1000) (Courtsey of Ann-Marie Nelson, MD).

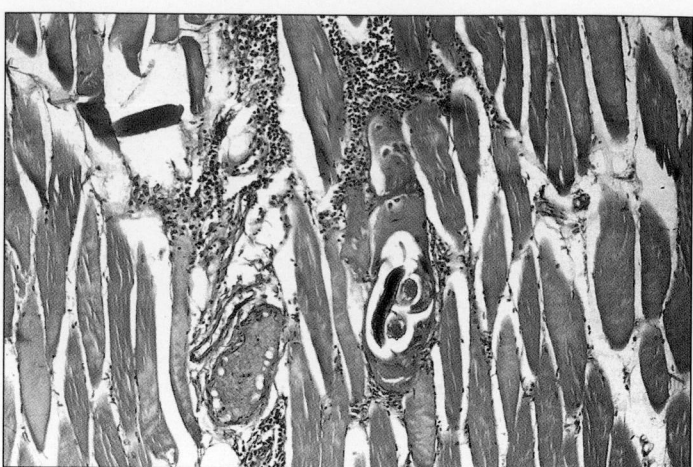

Fig. 3.108 *Trichinella spiralis* myositis. A nematode larva has encysted in a skeletal muscle fiber. The diagnosis can be made from the characteristic location of the worm. Intense focal inflammation reflects the acute nature of the lesion with reaction to encysting or dying larvae. Eventually the larvae will calcify (H&E, ×200).

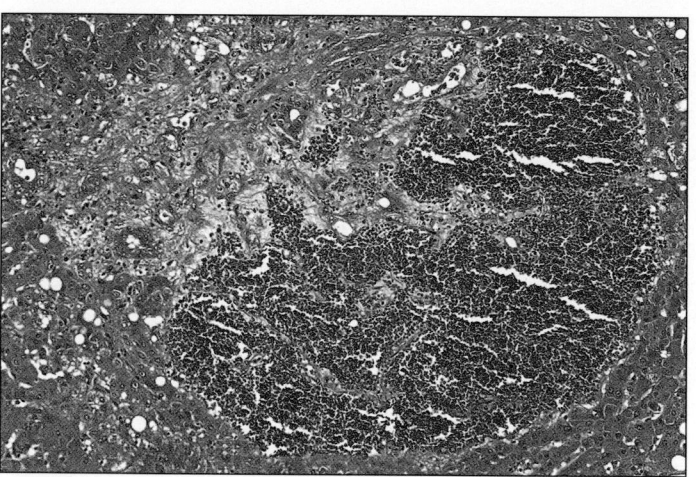

Fig. 3.107 Peliosis hepatis. A noninflammatory vascular lesion in the liver of a patient infected with the human immunodeficiency virus is caused by *Bartonella henselae* (H&E, ×30) (Courtsey of Ann-Marie Nelson, MD).

Trypanosoma cruzi

Trypanosoma cruzi is a protozoan parasite of the New World that produces both acute and chronic infection, known as Chagas' disease. It is unusual in the United States but may be seen particularly in the states that border Mexico. The parasite has both flagellated (trypomastigotes) and nonflagellated (amastigotes) forms. In tissue the amastigote is usually encountered. The most serious consequences of acute infection are myocarditis and encephalitis, which may be more frequent in immunosuppressed patients.[229] Amastigotes, which are round to oval and measure 1.5–4 µm, accumulate in myofibers or in glial cells, evoking an intense acute inflammatory response. In chronic Chagas' disease, the amastigotes multiply in the autonomic ganglia of the gastrointestinal tract, resulting in megaesophagus and megacolon.

The amastigotes of *T. cruzi* are differentiated from *T. gondii* and the yeast cells of *H. capsulatum* by the presence of a cellular kinetoplast in

addition to a nucleus, although this structure may be difficult to visualize in histologic sections. Staining of the yeast cells of *H. capsulatum* with the methenamine silver technique provides an additional clue to that pathogen. The amastigotes of *Leishmania* spp. are similar to those of *Toxoplasma*, but the former predominantly infect cells of the skin, mucous membranes, liver, and spleen, whereas the latter predominantly affect the brain, myocardium, and smooth muscle.

Trichinella spiralis

Trichinella spiralis naturally infects swine, rats, and a variety of wild animals, such as bears and cougars. The larvae of *T. spiralis* infect only striated muscle, where they mature and are encapsulated by the host. They may remain viable for many years, but eventually die and calcify. The symptoms of the infection include muscle aches and tenderness, myocardial dysfunction, and periorbital edema from involvement of ocular muscle.[230] An acute inflammatory response may be demonstrated in muscle early in the disease (Fig. 3.108). Later the larvae calcify, and the infection becomes quiescent. The infection is transmitted only when one carnivorous animal eats the flesh of the other, releasing the larvae, which then burrow into the intestinal epithelium of the new host. Trichinosis elicited such paranoia in nineteenth-century Europe that it is said there were more meat inspectors than soldiers in Bismarck's Germany. The infection has been virtually eliminated in the United States by stopping the practice of feeding offal to swine. Most infections are now associated with consumption of inadequately cooked game. The larvae can be identified specifically by their morphologic characteristics, but the typical clinical presentation and cellular location are virtually diagnostic.

THE GASTROINTESTINAL SYSTEM AND LIVER

Many infections of the gastrointestinal tract manifest as acute self-limited gastroenteritis and may be of bacterial (salmonella and shigella) or viral (rotavirus, Norwalk virus) origins. Seldom do these result in biopsy and when they do, non-specific acute inflammation is all that will be apparent (Fig. 3.109).

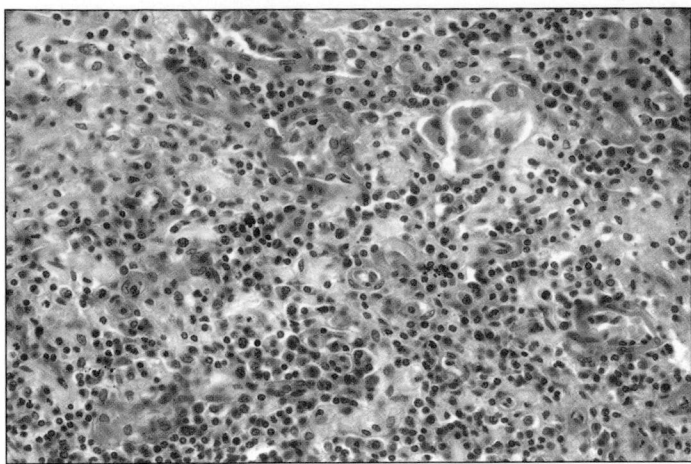

Fig. 3.109 This biopsy was inadvertently obtained prior to the completion of cultures which revealed *Salmonella typhi*. Note non-specific acute inflammation (H&E, ×20).

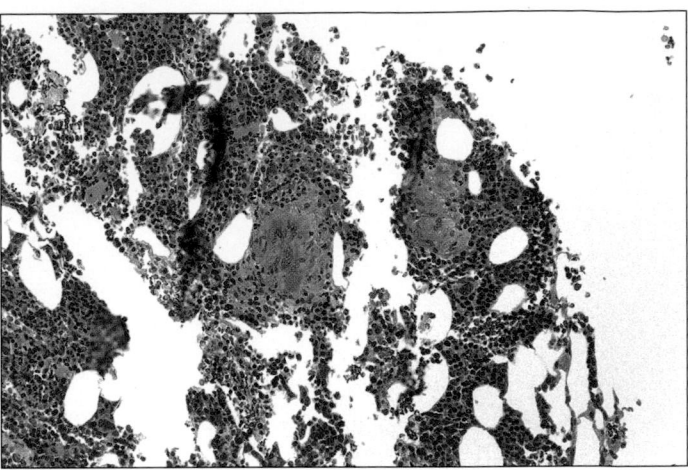

Fig. 3.111 Brucellosis. Several small noncaseating granulomas are present in the bone marrow of a patient with an unexplained febrile disease. He was not aware of exposure to *Brucella* in over 30 years (H&E, ×40, *Brucella suis* isolated from blood cultures).

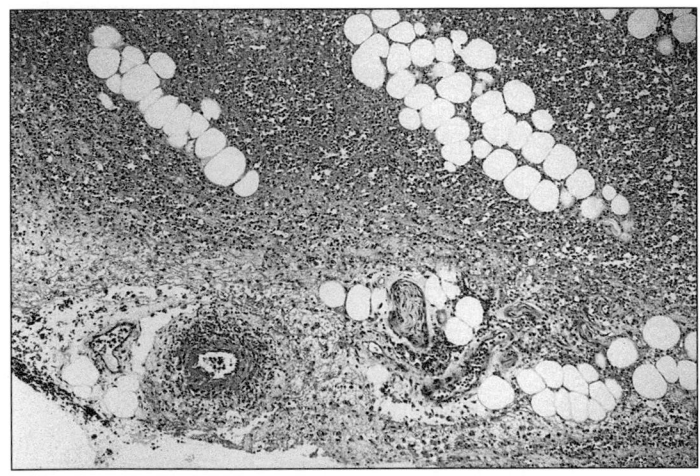

Fig. 3.110 *Vibrio* necrotizing inflammation in soft tissue. An intense acute inflammatory response destroys the subcutaneous tissue. Involvement of a small artery can be seen (H&E, ×45, *Vibrio vulnificus* isolated from culture) (Courtesy of David Walker, MD).

Vibrio species

Vibrio cholerae causes a toxin-mediated, noninflammatory infection that is limited to the intestinal epithelium. Other *Vibrio* spp., particularly *V. vulnificus*, cause necrotizing infection of the skin and soft tissues (Fig. 3.110) after introduction of the bacteria into the skin or gastrointestinal tract by salt water or shellfish that have been harvested from contaminated water.[231,232] The infections have occurred most commonly in Gulf Coast states but have also been described in patients who have been exposed to water in the interior of the United States.[233] *Aeromonas* spp. cause similar infections after exposure to fresh water.[234] Disseminated infection, which may be fatal, occurs in some cases.

Brucella species

Brucella spp. produce disseminated infection after exposure to infected milk products, or animal parts, of goats *(Brucella melitensis)*,

cattle *(B. abortus)*, or swine *(B. suis)*.[235,236] The reticuloendothelial system is a particular target of these bacteria, which usually produce multiple, small, noncaseating granulomas (Fig. 3.111).[237–239] Larger granulomas with necrosis may occasionally result. Calcified, healed granulomas in the spleen have been described in patients who have been infected with *B. suis*.

Epstein-Barr virus

Epstein-Barr virus is important as a cause of both infectious mononucleosis and certain neoplasms. Mononucleosis is usually diagnosed serologically, and the participation of the virus in neoplasms must be evaluated with molecular techniques. Occasionally, a liver biopsy will be obtained if hepatitis occurs in a patient who does not have other classic findings of mononucleosis. A non-specific mononuclear infiltrate is present in the parenchyma, and extensive hepatocellular necrosis is not seen (Fig. 3.112). Rarely, inclusions that resemble those of herpes simplex have been reported.

Cytomegalovirus

Cytomegalovirus is the virus most often seen by surgical pathologists because of its ubiquity and its prominence in infections of immunocompromised patients. Infection of virtually any organ may occur. Interstitial pneumonitis, myocarditis, and hepatitis have classically presented the most common clinical problems.[240–243] The pneumonia is usually diffuse, but focal and even miliary lesions have been described.[244]

The dilemma with cytomegalovirus is less to document the presence of infection in an individual patient than to establish that this virus, which persists for many years in tissues, has caused the clinical disease. Multiple cells that have been infected with this virus may be demonstrated in tissues that display no inflammatory reaction. For decades many pathologists believed that cytomegalovirus did not cause gastrointestinal disease, but that infected macrophages or endothelial cells populated ulcerating lesions previously caused by other agents. Experience with HIV-infected patients has convinced all observers that cytomegalovirus does cause ulcerative disease in the gastrointestinal tract from the esophagus through the colon.

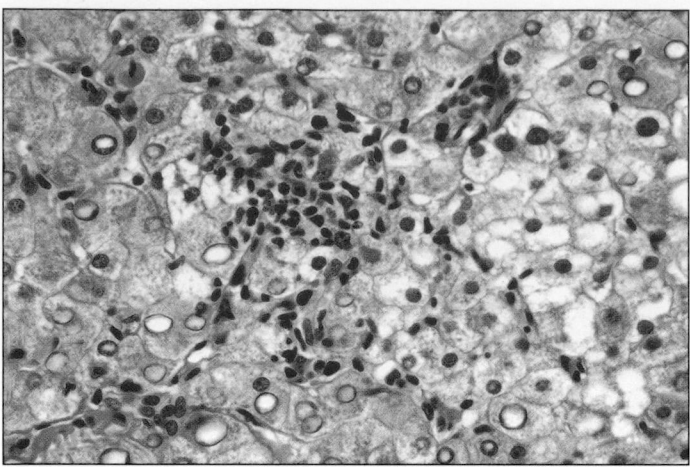

Fig. 3.112 Epstein-Barr virus hepatitis. A focus of hepatocellular necrosis and mononuclear infiltrates is seen. Mild hepatitis is common in infectious mononucleosis, but clinical illness that leads to biopsy is unusual (H&E, ×400).

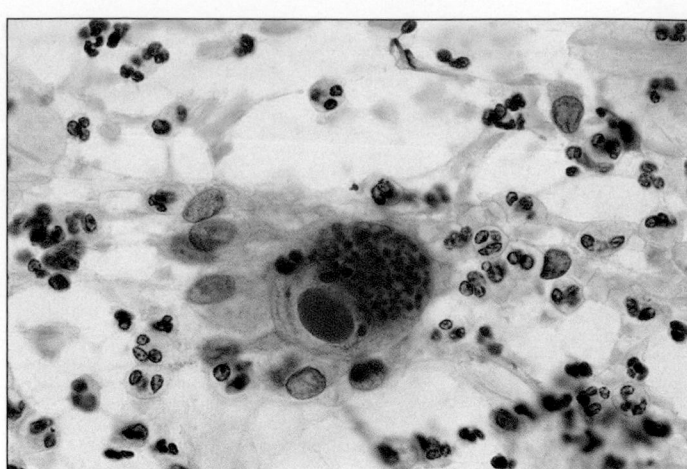

Fig. 3.114 Cytomegalovirus inclusion in a cervical vaginal smear. There is a single, probably endocervical cell with a large intranuclear inclusion and many smaller intracytoplasmic inclusions (Papanicolaou, ×1000).

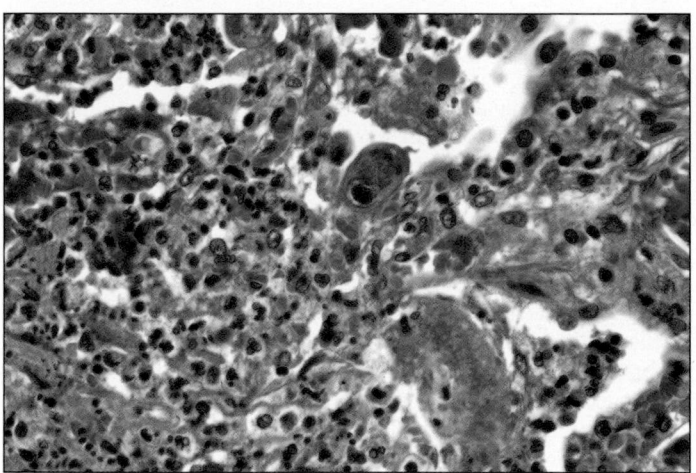

Fig. 3.113 Cytomegalovirus pneumonia. Mononuclear interstitial inflammation, focal tissue necrosis, and nuclear fragmentation are seen in the airspaces. A large cytomegalic cell with an amphophilic intranuclear inclusion surrounded by a halo and irregular, granular, basophilic cytoplasmic inclusions is present. Several clumps of eosinophilic exudates indicate an accompanying infection with *Pneumocystis* (H&E, ×500).

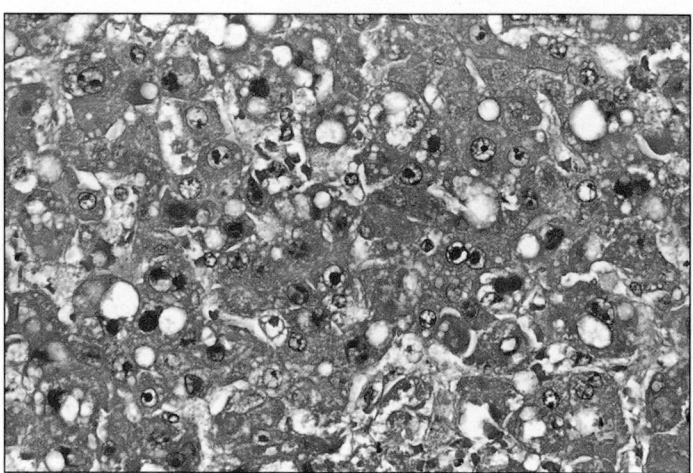

Fig. 3.115 Adenovirus hepatitis. Extensive hepatocellular necrosis and many cells with intranuclear viral inclusions are seen. Some inclusions have an artifactual halo between the inclusion and the nuclear membrane. Other inclusions are more basophilic, filling the nucleus with a 'smudge cells' appearance (H&E, ×250).

The histologic response to cytomegalovirus is principally mononuclear. The infected cell is globally enlarged, with a large, amphophilic to basophilic intranuclear inclusion (Fig. 3.113). Granular basophilic inclusions are present in the cytoplasm of many infected cells (Fig. 3.114). Multinucleated giant cells are not produced by cytomegalovirus.

Adenovirus

Adenovirus causes disease of virtually every organ system. Specific serotypes are associated with some adenovirus infections, most of which cause morbidity but not mortality. Disseminated infection and severe hepatitis have been documented in recipients of organ transplants. Cells infected with adenovirus contain intranuclear inclusions that initially resemble the eosinophilic inclusions of herpes

viruses. As the inclusion matures it becomes more basophilic and increasingly fills the nucleus (Fig. 3.115). Eventually the inclusion may obscure the outline of the nuclear membrane, producing a 'smudge cell.' The early adenovirus inclusions must be differentiated from herpes simplex and varicella-zoster viruses. The late inclusions can resemble those of cytomegalovirus and must also be differentiated from degenerated cells.

Protozoa

Entamoeba histolytica: *Entamoeba histolytica* is a protozoan parasite that is transmitted by the fecal–oral route.[245,246] The pathologic tissue form is the trophozoite, which measures 10–60 μm in size. Trophozoites in tissue are usually 20 μm or greater in diameter. The most common disease is acute infection of the gastrointestinal tract, known

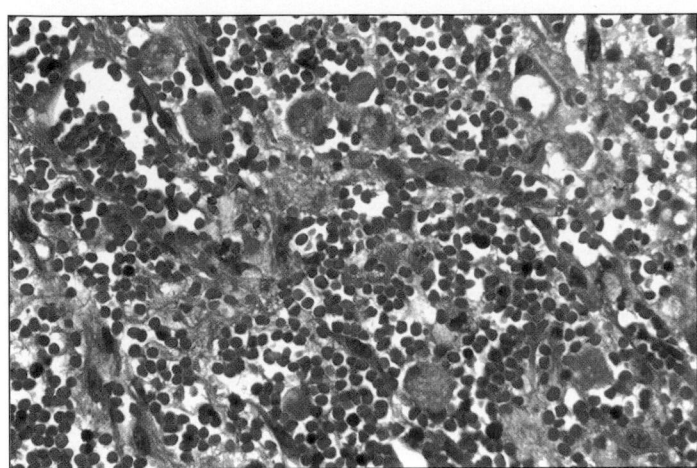

Fig. 3.116 *Entamoeba histolytica* liver abscess. Multiple amebae with fine cytoplasm are present in a hemorrhagic, necrotic exudate. The nuclei are small with a small karyosome (nucleolus) and fine nuclear chromatin. (H&E, ×1000).

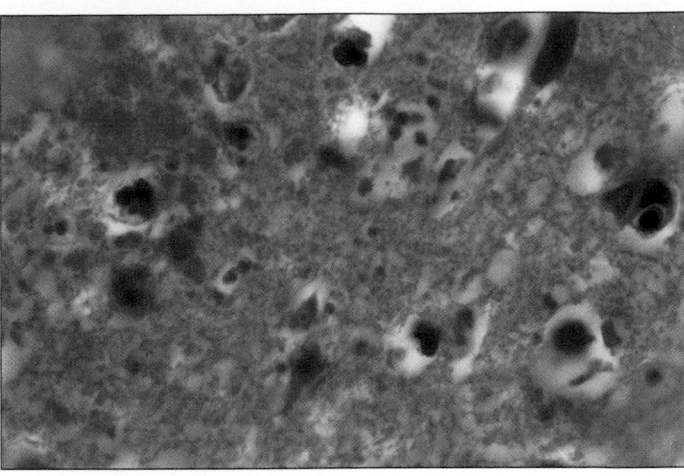

Fig. 3.117 Cerebral toxoplasmosis. Multiple oval *Toxoplasma gondii* tachyzoites are present in a necrotic lesion. The nuclei and cytoplasm are demonstrated, but the kinetoplast cannot be appreciated in this preparation (H&E, ×1000).

as amebic dysentery. Systemic infection usually results in infection of the liver, but other organs may be involved. Active gastrointestinal disease is often not present in patients with hepatic amebic abscesses. The frequent occurrence of amebae in asymptomatic homosexual men has concentrated attention toward the varying pathogenicity of intestinal amebae.[247] A small form of *Entamoeba*, *Entamoeba hartmanni*, resembles *E. histolytica* but measures less than 10 μm in size and is not pathogenic. A proposal has been put forward to place avirulent strains that resemble *E. histolytica* morphologically in a separate species.[248]

The tissue response to *E. histolytica* is necrotizing and hemorrhagic, but without appreciable acute inflammation (Fig. 3.116). The designation of the destructive liver lesions as amebic abscess is, therefore, something of a misnomer. Trophozoites are usually demonstrated in the necrotic lesions without difficulty if the possibility is considered. The amebae are irregular in shape, reflecting their motility by formation of pseudopods. Trophozoites are often positioned in clear lacunae that are produced by pulling away of the adjacent inflammatory exudate, calling attention to the protozoa (Fig. 3.116). The amebic nucleus measures 3–4 μm in size with a punctate central karyosome (nucleolus), whereas the cytoplasm has a vacuolated appearance and may contain ingested erythrocytes. If trophozoites are not clearly visualized in H&E-stained sections, the PAS technique may be applied to make the amebae stand out against the necrotic background. Amebae must be differentiated from macrophages, which are also stained by the PAS technique, by close examination of the cellular morphology, and by analysis of the nuclear detail in the H&E-stained sections.

Toxoplasma gondii: *T. gondii* is a coccidian parasite that undergoes sexual replication in the gastrointestinal tract of cats. After the oocysts develop in the environment, humans may ingest the resulting sporozoites, which disseminate throughout the body. Rapidly multiplying parasitic forms are referred to as tachyzoites. *T. gondii* is an intracellular pathogen, but a very nondiscriminating one, as virtually any nucleated cell in the body may be infected. The dividing tachyzoites fill the infected cell, eventually producing a pseudocyst. Within this pseudocyst the more slowly developing forms are referred to as bradyzoites. Individual tachyzoites are crescent shaped and

measure approximately 2 by 6 μm (Fig. 3.117). Tissue cysts are round to subspherical and measure from 5 to 100 μm in size and are packed with hundreds of bradyzoites. All the forms stain with H&E or Giemsa, but careful search may be required to detect them. Bradyzoites stain well with the PAS technique, but tachyzoites stain less well. The cyst wall stains weakly by the PAS technique but is intensely colored with the methenamine silver technique. The tachyzoites and bradyzoites, by contrast, do not stain with silver impregnation techniques. As previously noted, use of immunofluorescence or immunoenzyme techniques facilitates detection of parasites in necrotic lesions.

Acute infection is most often manifested by a syndrome that resembles Epstein-Barr virus disease. The characteristic pathology in the affected lymph nodes includes follicular hyperplasia with tingible bodies and small, noncaseating, epithelioid granulomas in follicular centers and in interfollicular areas. Peripheral sinuses are crowded with macrophages, and plasma cells are common. *Toxoplasma* cysts are found in lymph nodes only with great rarity.[249] Parasites were not detected in a group of serologically documented cases even when molecular techniques were employed.[250] A more serious result of acute infection is chorioretinitis, which is usually diagnosed by serology and clinical presentation. In pregnant women transplacental migration of the protozoa to the fetus may produce severe or fatal intrauterine infection.

In immunosuppressed patients, severe disease may be produced by accelerated multiplication in many organs, most importantly the brain and the lung.[251] The cyst forms do not elicit a pathologic reaction, but their rupture to release tachyzoites produces an acutely necrotizing and hemorrhagic inflammatory process. The inflammatory response and the degree to which cerebral lesions are encapsulated are determined, however, by the immunologic status of the host.[252] In the lung an interstitial pneumonitis and diffuse alveolar damage may precede the necrotizing phase.[253]

The pseudocysts of *Toxoplasma* must be differentiated from other coccidian and microsporidian parasites, which produce larger cysts, predominantly in the heart and skeletal muscle. Macrophages infected with *H. capsulatum* must not be mistaken for *Toxoplasma*. If doubt exists, demonstration of the yeast cells with methenamine silver will resolve the issue.

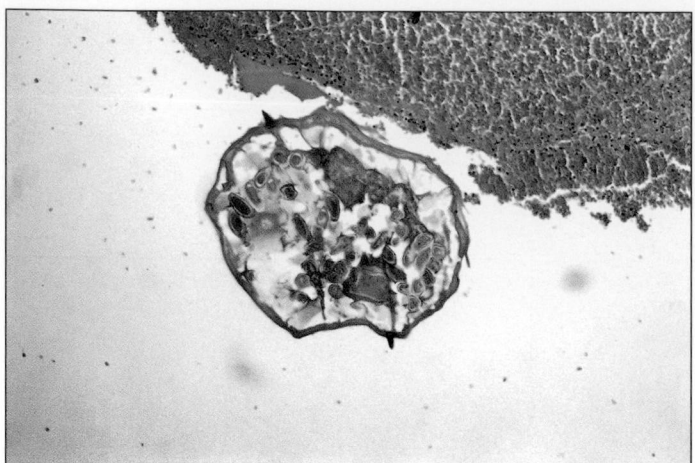

Fig. 3.118 *Enterobius vermicularis* in the lumen of an appendix is an incidental finding. Symptoms occur when the gravid female migrates to the perianal area to lay her eggs. The worm is identified as a nematode by the characteristic 'tube within a tube' morphology combined with the prominent lateral alae. In this case, a specific identification can be made because the characteristic pinworm eggs can also be seen within the section (H&E, ×250).

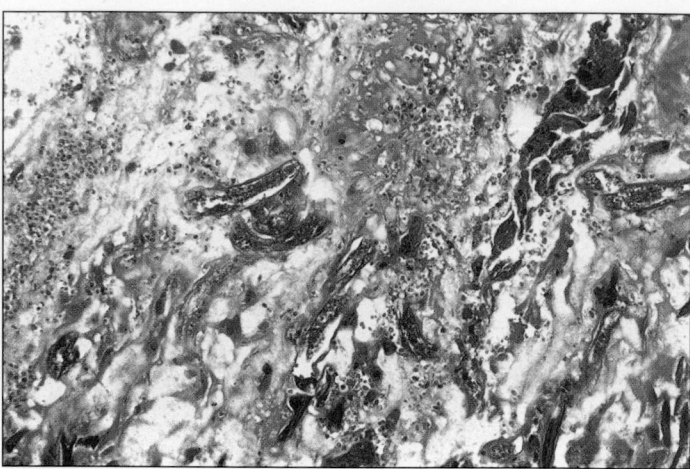

Fig. 3.119 *Strongyloides stercoralis* hyperinfection in the small intestines. Many sections of larvae are present in the necrotic mucosa, intermixed with large numbers of yeasts. The worms can be identified as nematodes, but not characterized more specifically from this morphology alone. Careful study of multiple sections or visualization of intact worms in the feces can establish the diagnosis (H&E, ×100).

Nematodes

A variety of roundworms infect humans, but few reside sufficiently long in tissue to be seen in surgical specimens. Some features permit characterization of the roundworms in histologic sections, but identification of the infecting parasite requires considerable experience. The nematodes are worm-like, nonsegmented, bilaterally symmetric, and pseudocoelomate. The cuticle consists of three distinct layers, which may be exaggerated in degenerating worms. A thin superficial epicuticle may also be present. The cuticle of most nematodes contains transverse striae or annulations, which may impart the appearance of segmentation. Longitudinal ridges, called alae, ranging from one to three in number, are termed cervical, longitudinal, or caudal depending on their location. The presence, number, and morphology of the alae are useful clues to the nature of the worm. Nematodes also contain a hypodermis, muscles, digestive system, reproductive system, and nervous system.

Enterobius vermicularis: The pinworm causes its clinical symptoms as ova hatch and migrate into the perianal area. The mature worms live in the cecal area and may migrate into the appendix, where they are occasionally seen incidentally in the lumen of appendectomy specimens. The cuticle with its transverse striations and lateral alae suggests that the specimen is a nematode (Fig. 3.118). If the section happens to include an ovary with eggs, a definitive identification is easy.

Strongyloides stecoralis: *Strongyloides stercoralis* differs from hookworm in that it can produce autoinfection of humans, because the eggs do not require a stage of development in the environment before infective larvae hatch. Chronic *Strongyloides* infection may occur in immunocompetent individuals, but severe disease is found primarily in immunosuppressed individuals, who may have been infected many years earlier.[254] As the infective rhabditiform larvae migrate from the gastrointestinal tract through the lungs, they may produce large accumulations of larvae in the gastrointestinal tract. Systemic symptoms result, and ulceration of the gastrointestinal tract may occur (Fig. 3.119).

Cestodes

Cestodes include the fish tapeworm, *Diphyllobothrium latum*; the pork tapeworm, *Taenia solium*; the beef tapeworm, *Taenia saginata*; and the dog tapeworm, *Echinococcus granulosus*. The adult tapeworm consists of a 'head' (scolex) that contains a groove (*Diphyllobothrium*), suckers (*T. saginata*), or suckers and hooklets (*T. solium* and *E. granulosus*). A short undifferentiated 'neck' connects the scolex to a long series of segments, also called proglottids. Each proglottid contains male and female genital systems. The genital systems become increasingly mature as the proglottids progress caudally. Microscopically, the proglottids of cestodes contain an acellular, homogeneous tegument beneath which is a layer of nuclei and thin bands of longitudinal and circular muscle. Most of the segment is composed of a loose network of fluid and cells. Distinctive round to oval calcareous bodies that contain calcium carbonate identify the worm as a cestode.

When a human intermediate host ingests an embryonated egg of *T. solium* or *E. granulosus*, the larval form penetrates the intestinal wall and migrates to a variety of organs, depending on the species. Larvae of the pork tapeworm develop into a cysticercus, which consists of the larva in a fluid-filled space that is referred to as a bladder. The most common site for development of cysticerci is the skin and subcutaneous tissue, where the larvae become encapsulated, die, and eventually calcify. Next in frequency is the retina and the central nervous system, where the cysticerci are not encapsulated and cause significant morbidity and mortality, sometimes years after the primary infection. *T. solium* infection is common in Mexico, so cases of cysticercosis are most likely to be seen in states along the southern border of the US.[255] Fully developed cysticerci are round or oval and measure 5–15 mm in length by 4–12 mm in diameter. The 'bladder worms,' therefore, form a space-occupying lesion that may cause symptoms by pressure on adjacent brain. If the larva dies, an intense inflammatory response may be produced, causing an acute exacerbation of symptoms. The larva can be seen in the clear fluid of the cysticercus and can be identified, at least to being a cestode, by general morphology including calcareous bodies. If a larva is not found, documentation of the nature of the lesion is difficult.

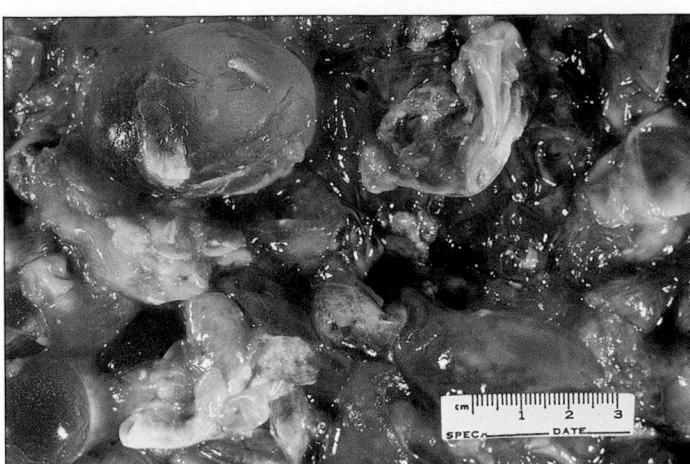

Fig. 3.120 Echinococcal cyst of the liver. Eight liters of cysts and daughter cysts were present in a cyst that had slowly enlarged over a period of 10 to 20 years. Hydatid sand can be seen as granular material in the clear cyst fluid.

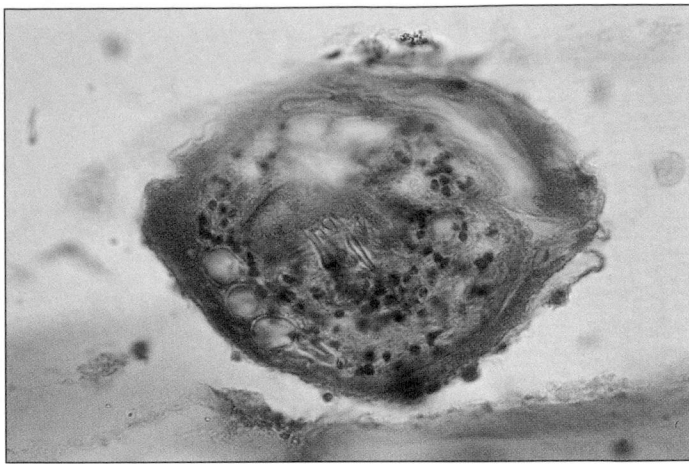

Fig. 3.121 A protoscolex of *Echinococcus granulosus*, including the refractile hooklets, is demonstrated (H&E, 2 ×50).

When humans ingest an egg of the dog tapeworm, *E. granulosus*, the larval form migrates to an organ, usually the liver or lung, where it develops into a hydatid cyst. A germinal layer of the hydatid cyst gives rise to brood capsules that eventually result in new cysts, called daughter cysts, producing an enlarging mass of increasingly complicated cysts. The final result resembles a giant balloon that is filled with myriads of tiny balloons (Fig. 3.120). Within each daughter cyst are numerous protoscoleces, which have an invaginated head complete with hooklets. Degenerated brood capsules, scoleces, and hooklets floating in the cyst fluid are referred to as hydatid sand. Large hydatid cysts may measure 20 cm or more in size and may take years to develop.

In histologic sections, the germinal epithelium of the cyst wall and the protoscoleces can be demonstrated, complete with hooklets and calcareous corpuscles typical of cestodes (Fig. 3.121). As long as the cyst is intact, the symptoms relate primarily to the effects of a large space-occupying lesion. When a cyst ruptures, an anaphylactic reaction may occur, and, if the patient survives, new cysts may form from the scoleces released from the ruptured cysts.

The most common natural cycle of *E. granulosus* includes development of hydatid cysts in herbivores, such as sheep, and mature worms in the intestinal tract of carnivores, such as dogs. Humans function as incidental, 'dead end' intermediate hosts. Many human infections in the United States are seen in patients who were infected years previously in sheep-raising areas of the Old World. Basque sheepherders brought the infection to the western United States, however, and indigenous foci remain well established.

Trematodes

Schistosomes: The most important flukes in the United States are the schistosomes, which have a complex life cycle. Human species are endemic throughout the world, but none exists in the continental United States. The final developmental stage of schistosomes, the fork-tailed cercariae, swims freely in water and penetrates the skin of human hosts. Avian schistosomes, which are found in the continental United States, proceed no further than the skin, where they produce a disease known as swimmer's itch. The clinical disease and pathology produced by schistosomes depends on the species and the

stage of disease.[256,257] *Schistosoma mansoni* migrates through the body, eventually lodging in the hemorrhoidal venous plexus. Eggs migrate into the intestinal tract and are excreted.

Gastrointestinal symptoms including diarrhea, and even dysentery may result. The most serious manifestations of infection result from migration of eggs to the liver and spleen. *S. mansoni* occurs in Africa, the Arabian peninsula, Brazil, and the Caribbean, including Puerto Rico. *S. japonicum*, the oriental blood fluke, migrates to the superior mesenteric or portal veins. Eggs are deposited in the gastrointestinal tract, especially the small bowel, and the liver. *S. haematobium*, which is endemic in Africa, southern Europe, the Middle East, and parts of India, localizes in the vesicle and pelvic venous plexuses. Eggs migrate through the wall of the bladder and are excreted in the urine.

Mature worms are only rarely identified in histologic specimens. The chronic infection is dominated by the tissue reaction to the eggs. A cellular infiltrate of neutrophils and eosinophils is followed by a granulomatous reaction including multinucleated giant cells. Fibrosis eventually results. Eggs in the intestine, liver, and spleen are most likely to be *S. mansoni* or *S. japonicum*. Typically, *S. japonicum* produces the largest egg burden, and the eggs are most likely to calcify. Many of the eggs are difficult to identify, because of distortion, collapse, or calcification. The classic lateral spines of *S. mansoni* or the terminal spines of *S. haematobium* may be demonstrated in some eggs, however. The end result of extensive fibrotic response to deposited eggs in the intrahepatic biliary system is referred to as pipestem cirrhosis. Eggs in the bladder represent infection with *S. haematobium*. Visualization of the eggs in tissue with acid-fast stains has been described.

THE CENTRAL NERVOUS SYSTEM

Free-living Amebae: Free-living amebae include *Acanthamoeba* spp., which cause destructive infections of the skin, cornea, and central nervous system, and *Naegleri fowleri*, which causes an acute destructive meningoencephalitis.[258,259] Recently, a new genus, *Balamuthia*, has been defined; this organism is believed to be responsible for some infections previously attributed to *Acanthamoeba*.[260,261] Both genera occur in warm fresh and brackish water

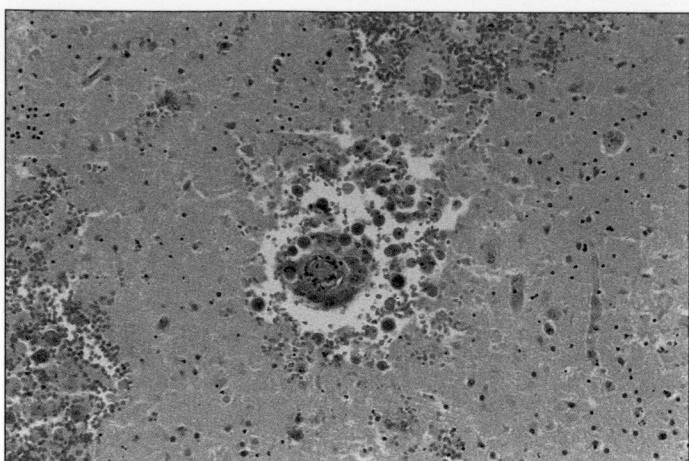

Fig. 3.122 *Acanthamoeba* encephaltitis. Multiple amebae are present in a Virchow-Robin space. At higher magnification the amebic nuclei contain a large karyosome and coarse chromatin. There is necrosis and hemorrhage in the surrounding brain (H&E, ×500).

Table 3.8 Comparison of microbiologic and molecular criteria for causality

	Causality criteria for infectious diseases	
Step	Koch (1882)	Falkow (1988)
1	ID organism in lesion	ID unique phenotype or trait associated with virulent strains
2	Culture organism from lesion	Isolate gene responsible for phenotype or trait
3	Inoculate organism into experimental model to re-create lesion	Inactivate gene and inoculate organism into experimental model to show 'lack' of virulence
4	Re-isolate organism from lesion	Restore 'wild-type' gene and demonstrate recurrence of virulence

and in soil, from which sources they enter the human host directly. The path to the central nervous system is believed to be through the nasal cavity for *Naegleria*, whereas *Acanthamoeba* reaches the brain through the bloodstream after entry into the respiratory tract.

Morphologically, the two genera overlap sufficiently that definitive diagnosis of trophozoites is impossible without culture or immunochemical stains. *Acanthamoeba* spp., but not *Naegleria* spp., however, produces cysts in tissue. The trophozoites of *Acanthamoeba* measure 15–35 µm in size. Actively motile trophozoites of *Naegleria* measure 15–30 µm by 6–9 µm, whereas rounded trophozoites measure 9–15 µm in diameter. The amebae contain a single nucleus with a prominent central karyosome (Fig. 3.122). The cysts of *Acanthamoeba* measure 15–20 µm in diameter, but they may measure up to 30 µm. Cysts have a thick double wall, which varies in morphology by species. Nuclear morphology is difficult to discern, but cytoplasmic globules can often be seen in histologic sections. The trophozoites must be differentiated from macrophages on the basis of nuclear morphology. If the nucleus is not present in the plane of section, differentiation is not possible.

The histologic response to *Acanthamoeba* is granulomatous with multinucleated giant cells. *Naegleria* encephalitis is an acute infection, and the meninges are infiltrated with polymorphonuclear neutrophils and macrophages intermixed with amebae, which may be difficult to distinguish without careful study.

PART IV: PRACTICAL APPLICATION OF MOLECULAR TECHNIQUES

Evolving technology has driven clinical laboratorians to a new level of service in the realm of infectious disease pathology. Culture and sensitivity techniques continue to be refined and molecular applications provide a rapid method for determining organism load, virulence factor traits, and invaluable genomic information. Although culture still remains the gold standard, molecular diagnostics allows us to confirm the presence of the 'unculturable' agents and to tremendously improve the turn-around time for those organisms requiring prolonged incubation times and tedious confirmation steps.

In addition, when the histologic features suggest an unsuspected infectious process, molecular techniques can confirm special stain findings in the absence of available cultures.

As Koch in 1882 established criteria for infectious disease causality using cultures, Falkow in 1988 proposed molecular criteria for establishing causality. Although the guidelines for Falkow's system are not applicable in all settings, they give us a solid reference point in determining if an organism is indeed the etiologic agent, or just an innocent bystander. Table 3.8 compares the system as outlined in 1882 by Koch and the modern molecular version proposed by Falkow in 1988.[262]

When considering any new test methodology or technology it is always helpful to step back and consider the basics of laboratory medicine. What are the strengths and limitations of a new technology? All tests, even molecular amplification methods, have limitations. Other considerations include cost, expertise, and added value. The National Committee for Clinical Laboratory Standards (NCCLS) has developed a set of recommendations to consider specifically when evaluating new molecular technology.[263] Although the healthcare industry looks to the FDA as the final sanctioning body for new testing methodologies, the FDA simply has not been able to keep up with the vastly expanding numbers of new molecular tests and methodologies. We must scrutinize each of these new applications carefully prior to adopting them for our patient populations. We must compare and contrast sensitivity, specificity, precision, accuracy, method-specific limitations, and cost for every new test we consider utilizing. This puts a tremendous burden on the pathologist who is expected to be the expert for all laboratory testing methodologies.

OVERVIEW OF MOLECULAR METHODS

Molecular microbiology methods can be divided into four main categories:

1. Direct detection methods;
2. Amplification methods;
3. Enzyme digestion and electrophoretic separation methods; and
4. Sequencing methods.

Direct Detection Methods: Direct detection methods are very rapid and useful when the target is present in the tissue or sample in ample quantity. Most commonly used are the direct nucleic acid probes and in situ hybridization. Nucleic acid probes are short sequences of single-stranded nucleic acid that represents a 'complementary match' and can thus bind directly to the target (hybridize). Probes can be constructed for either DNA or RNA detection. In situ hybridization allows utilization of direct probe (DNA or RNA) technology to glass slides. Histologic tissue sections are treated and then exposed to the designed probe that is tagged for microscopic detection. If a 'match' is present, the signal is read in a similar fashion as reading paraffin immunoperoxidase slides. This allows not only confirmation of the presence of an infectious disease pathogen, but allows the pathologist to describe the distribution of the organisms histologically. In situ hybridization techniques are most often used when evaluating tissues for the presence of viral pathogens, such as human papillomavirus (HPV) in cervical biopsies.

Amplification Methods: Amplification represents the most commonly utilized molecular testing method. Amplification techniques are much more sensitive than direct probe methods. Several variations of amplification exist and the following lists those one may encounter:

Polymerase chain reaction (PCR);
Nested PCR;
Multiplex PCR;
In situ PCR;
Ligase chain reaction (LCR); and
Branched chain DNA (bDNA).

APPLICATION OF MOLECULAR METHODS

The question of when to order a molecular test is driven largely by clinical impact. If a molecular method is the only way available to confirm a diagnosis, then it is most reasonable to use this technology. Inappropriate utilization must be minimized if we are to keep healthcare costs down. This, unfortunately, becomes the responsibility of the pathologists in charge of the laboratory budget.

Sometimes a molecular method results in markedly improved turn-around times (TATs) and thus timelier treatment of the patient. Not only does the patient get appropriate therapy faster, but exposure and potential spread of the infection is minimized. Molecular techniques have become a standard component in many TB and fungus laboratories.

Cost-effectiveness sometimes extends beyond the walls of the laboratory. Rapid confirmation of MTB in sputum samples may eliminate the need for a bronchoscopic examination in a critically ill patient. Confirmation of *Bartonella henselae* DNA in the fine needle aspirate of a lymph node often allows definitive treatment without excisional biopsy. All aspects of the patient care impact should be considered when evaluating the cost efficiency of a molecular technique. Tables 3.9 and 3.10 lists infectious disease pathogens, methods available for molecular testing, and the intended application of these methods. This list is not intended to be all-inclusive, as the list continuously expands.

Table 3.9 Bacterial pathogens that may be confirmed using molecular methods

Bacterial pathogen	Detection method	Application
Aureobacterium sp.	PCR	ID culture isolate
Bartonella henselae	PCR, SB	Direct detection in body fluids and biopsies
Bartonella quintana	PCR, SB	Direct detection in body fluids and biopsies
Bordetella pertussis	PCR, Probe	Direct specimen (NP) detection
Bordetella parapertussis	PCR Direct	specimen (NP) detection
Borrelia burgdorferi	Nested PCR	Direct detection in urine samples
Brucella sp.	PCR	Laboratory confirmation
Burkholderia pseudomallei	PCR	Direct specimen detection
Campylobacter sp.	PCR-RFPL	Speciation of culture isolate
Chlamydia trachomatis	PCR	Direct detection in urine samples
Corynebacterium diphtheriae	PCR	Culture confirmation of toxogenic strains
Ehrlichia chaffeensis	PCR	Direct detection in blood and biopsy samples
Escherichia coli O157:H7	Multiplex PCR	Culture confirmation of isolates
Haemophilus ducreyi	Multiplex PCR	Direct detection in specimens
Helicobacter pylori	PCR	Direct detection in gastric biopsy
Mycobacterium avium	PCR	Culture ID of M. avium vs M. intracellulare
Mycobacterium avium-intracellulare complex	Probe	ID culture isolate
Mycobacterium gordonae	Probe	ID culture isolate
Mycobacterium kansasii	Probe	ID culture isolate
Mycobacterium tuberculosis complex	Probe, PCR	ID culture isolate; direct detection in body fluids & biopsy
Neisseria gonorrhoeae	LCR	Direct detection in specimens
Treponema pallidum	Multiplex PRC	Direct detection in specimens
Tropheryma whipplei	PCR	Direct detection in biopsies
Yersinia enterocolitica	PCR	Direct detection in specimens and biopsies
Yersinia pseudotuberculosis	PCR	Direct detection in specimens and biopsies

PCR, polymerase chain reaction; SB, Southern blot; RFLP, restriction fragment length polymorphism: LCR, ligase chain reaction.

Table 3.10 Fungal, viral, and protozoan pathogens that may be confirmed using molecular methods

Pathogen	Detection method	Application
Fungal		
Aspergillus sp.	PCR	Direct detection in bronchial specimens
Blastomyces dermatiditis	Probe	Culture confirmation
Candida sp.	Probe, PCR	Direct detection and culture ID
Coccidiodes immitis	Probe	Culture confirmation
Cryptococcus neoformans	Probe	Culture confirmation
Histoplasma capsulatum	Probe	Culture confirmation
Pneumocystis jiroveci (carinii)	PCR	Direct detection in bronchial specimens
Viral		
Adenovirus	PCR	Culture confirmation and typing
Cytomegalovirus	PCR	Direct detection in body fluids
Enteroviruses	PCR	Direct detection in body fluids
EBV	PCR, LCR, in situ	Direct detection
Hantavirus	PCR	Direct detection in respiratory samples
Hepatitis B	PCR	Direct detection in blood; viral load analysis
Hepatitis C	PCR, bDNA	Direct detection in blood; viral load analysis and genotyping
Herpes simplex virus 1 & 2	Multiplex PCR	Direct detection in specimens
Human immunodeficiency virus (HIV)	PCR, bDNA, NASBA, LPA sequencing	Direct detection in blood and body fluids; viral load analysis; genotyping for resistance mutations
Human papillomavirus	In situ PCR	Detection and typing in biopsies
Human parvovirus B19	PCR	Detection in blood and biopsies
Measles	PCR, in situ PCR	Direct detection in urine and biopsies
Respiratory syncytial virus	PCR	Direct detection in samples and biopsies
Rubella	PCR	Direct detection in samples
Severe acute respiratory syndrome virus (SARS)	PCR, multiple	Direct detection in samples
Protzoan		
Enterocytozoon bieneusi	PCR	Direct detection in samples and biopsies
Encephalitozoon hellem	PCR	Direct detection in samples and biopsies
Plasmodium sp.	PCR	Direct detection in blood
Toxoplasma gondii	PCR	Direct detection in samples and biopsies
Trichomonas vaginalis	PCR, probe	Direct detection in samples
Trypanosoma cruzi	PCR	Direct detection in biopsies

PCR, polymerase chain reaction; LCR, ligase chain reaction; bDNA, branched chain DNA; LPA, line probe assay; NASBA, nucleic acid sequence based amplification,

All methods and diagnostic tools used by the pathologist in both the clinical and anatomic realm have their limitations in sensitivity and specificity. Even when an amplification molecular method is 'negative' it cannot completely rule out the presence of an organism. Organisms don't always follow the rules, and although targeting the 'most likely pathogen' based on immune response and tissue reaction pattern makes perfect sense, it doesn't always disclose the precise etiologic agent. When the history of a patient is known and discussed by the pathologist and internist in advance, the best outcome will occur. This will allow for advanced planning to include the most appropriate cultures, including bacterial, fungal, mycobacterial, and comprehensive viral cultures; touch preparations for rapid stains, as clinically needed; and ordering of appropriate special stains at the time of tissue processing to improve final turn-around time. The need for additional studies such as flow cytometry can quickly be assessed via touch preparation, scrape preparation, or frozen section. And finally, consideration may be given to set tissue aside frozen for direct fluorescent stains and/or molecular studies should they be needed after review of the routine and special stains from the case.

REFERENCES

1. Procop GW, Wilson M. Infectious disease pathology. Clin Infect Dis. 2001; 32(11): 1589–1601.
2. Singh N. Fungal infections in the recipients of solid organ transplantation. Infect Dis Clin North Am 2003; 17(1): 113–34, viii.
3. Woods GL, Walker DH. Detection of infection or infectious agents by use of cytologic and histologic stains. Clin Microbiol Rev 1996; 9: 382.
4. Prophet EB, Mills B, Arrington JB, et al, eds. Laboratory methods in histotechnology. Washington: American Registry of Pathology; 1992.
5. Brown RC, Hopps HC. Staining of bacteria in tissue sections: a reliable Gram stain method. Am J Clin Pathol 1973; 60: 234.
6. Wear DJ, Margileth AM, Hadfield TL, et al. Cat scratch disease: a bacterial infection. Science 1983; 221: 1403.
7. Chandler FW, Hicklin MD, Blackmon JA. Demonstration of the agent of Legionnaires' disease in tissue. N Engl J Med 1977; 297: 1218.
8. Marshall BJ. Unidentified curved bacilli on gastric epithelium in active chronic gastritis. Lancet 1983; 2: 1273.
9. Woods GL, Meyers WM. Mycobacterial diseases. In: Damjanov I, Linder J, eds. Anderson's pathology, 10th edn.. St. Louis: CV Mosby; 1996: 843–865.

10. Robboy SJ, Vickery AL Jr. Tinctorial and morphologic properties distinguishing actinomycosis and nocardiosis. N Engl J Med 1970; 282: 593.

11. Lowe RN, Azimi PH, McQuitty J. Acid-fast *Actinomyces* in a child with pulmonary actinomycosis. J Clin Microbiol 1980; 12: 124.

12. Monheit JE, Brown G, Kott MM, et al. Calcofluor white detection of fungi in cytopathology. Am J Clin Pathol 1986; 85: 222.

13. Monheit JE, Cowan DF, Moore DG. Rapid detection of fungi in tissues using calcofluor white and fluorescence microscopy. Arch Pathol Lab Med 1984; 108: 616.

14. Wood C, Russel-Bell B. Characterization of pigmented fungi by melanin staining. Am J Dermatopathol 1983; 5: 77.

15. Baselski VS, Robison MK, Pifer LW, et al. Rapid detection of *Pneumocystis carinii* in bronchoalveolar lavage samples by using Cellufluor staining. J Clin Microbiol 1990; 28: 393.

16. Gosey LL, Howard RM, Witebsky FG, et al. Advantages of a modified toluidine blue O stain and bronchoalveolar lavage for the diagnosis of *Pneumocystis carinii* pneumonia. J Clin Microbiol 1985; 22: 803.

17. Rosen PP, Martini N, Armstrong D. *Pneumocystis carinii* pneumonia. Diagnosis by lung biopsy. Am J Med 1975; 58: 794.

18. Kim YK, Parulekar S, Yu PK, et al. Evaluation of calcofluor white stain for detection of *Pneumocystis carinii*. Diagn Microbiol Infect Dis 1990; 13: 307.

19. Elston HR. Synthetic controls for microbiological stains in histopathology. Lab Med 1986; 17: 750.

20. Tseng CH, Tseng C. Laboratory method for producing tissue controls for fungal stains. Lab Med 1991; 22: 637.

21. Jung WK. In vitro positive controls for histochemical stains of bacteria and fungi. Am J Clin Pathol 1985; 84: 342.

22. Sickel JZ, di Sant'Agnese PA. Anomalous immunostaining of 'optically clear' nuclei in gestational endometrium. A potential pitfall in the diagnosis of pregnancy-related herpesvirus infection. Arch Pathol Lab Med 1994; 118: 831.

23. Nuovo GJ, Silverstein SJ. Comparison of formalin, buffered formalin, and Bouin's fixation on the detection of human papillomavirus deoxyribonucleic acid from genital lesions. Lab Invest 1988; 59: 720.

24. Sun T, Greenspan J, Tenenbaum M, et al. Diagnosis of cerebral toxoplasmosis using fluorescein-labeled antitoxoplasma monoclonal antibodies. Am J Surg Pathol 1986; 10: 312.

25. Conley FK, Jenkins KA, Remington JS. *Toxoplasma gondii* infection of the central nervous system. Use of the peroxidase-antiperoxidase method to demonstrate toxoplasma in formalin fixed, paraffin embedded tissue sections. Hum Pathol 1981; 12: 690.

26. Neinstein LS, Rabinovitz S. Detection of *Chlamydia trachomatis*. A study of the direct immunofluorescence technique and a review diagnostic limitations. J Adolesc Health Care 1989; 10(1): 10–15.

27. Mann JL. Autofluorescence of fungi: an aid to detection in tissue sections. Am J Clin Pathol 1983; 79(5): 587–590.

28. Hettlich C, Kupper TH, Wehle K, et al. Aspergillus in the Papanicolaou stain: morphology, fluorescence and diagnostic feasibility. Cytopathology 1998; 9(6): 381–388.

29. Schroder S, Hain M, Sterflinger K; Colorimetric in situ hybridization (CISH) with digoxigenin-labeled oligonucleotide probes in autofluorescent hyphomycetes. Int Micrbiol 2000; 3(3): 183–186.

30. Horsburgh CR Jr. *Mycobacterium avium* complex infection in the acquired immunodeficiency syndrome. N Engl J Med 1991; 324: 1332.

31. Klatt EC, Jensen DF, Meyer PR. Pathology of *Mycobacterium avium-intracellulare* infection in acquired immunodeficiency syndrome. Hum Pathol 1987; 18: 709.

32. Gillin JS, Urmacher C, West R, et al. Disseminated *Mycobacterium avium-intracellulare* infection in acquired immunodeficiency syndrome mimicking Whipple's disease. Gastroenterology 1983; 85: 1187.

33. Umlas J, Federman M, Crawford C, et al; Spindle cell pseudotumor due to *Mycobacterium avium-intracellulare* in patients with acquired immunodeficiency syndrome (AIDS). Positive staining of mycobacteria for cytoskeleton filaments. Am J Surg Pathol 1991; 15: 1181.

34. Scott MA, Graham B, Verrall R, et al. *Rhodococcus equi*. An increasingly recognized opportunistic pathogen: report of 12 cases and review of 65 cases in the literature. Am J Clin Pathol 1995; 103(5): 649–655.

35. Emmons W, Reichwein B, Winslow DL. *Rhodococcus equi* infection in the patient with AIDS: literature review and report of an unusual case. Rev Infect Dis 1991; 13: 91.

36. van Etta LL, Filice GA, Ferguson RM, et al. *Corynebacterium equi*: a review of 12 cases of human infection. Rev Infect Dis 1983; 5: 1012.

37. Lasky JA, Pulkingham N, Powers MA, et al. *Rhodococcus equi* causing human pulmonary infection: review of 29 cases. South Med J 1991; 84: 1217.

38. Winn WC Jr, Myerowitz RL; The pathology of the *Legionella* pneumonias. A review of 74 cases and the literature. Hum Pathol 1981; 12: 401.

39. Simpson GL, Stinson EB, Egger MJ, et al. Nocardial infections in the immunocompromised host: a detailed study in a defined population. Rev Infect Dis 1981; 3: 492.

40. Javaly K, Horowitz HW, Wormser GP; Nocardiosis in patients with human immunodeficiency virus infection. Report of 2 cases and review of the literature. Medicine 1992; 71: 128.

41. Larone DH. Medically important fungi – A guide to identification. 3rd edn. Washington, DC: ASM Press; 1995.

42. de Hoog GS, Guarro J, Gene J, et al. Atlas of clinical fungi, 2nd edn. The Netherlands: Centraalbureau voor Schimmerlculture; 2000.

43. Chandler FW, Watts JC. Pathologic diagnosis of fungal infections. Chicago: ASCP Press; 1987.

44. Strano AJ. Light microscopy of selected viral diseases (morphology of viral inclusion bodies). Pathol Ann 1976; 11: 53.

45. Cheville NF. Cytopathology in viral diseases. Basel: S Karger; 1975.

46. Connor DH, Chandler FW, Schwartz DA, et al. Pathology of infectious diseases. Stamford, CT: Appleton & Lange; 1997.

47. Stevens DL, Musher DM, Watson DA, et al. Spontaneous, nontraumatic gangrene due to *Clostridium septicum*. Rev Infect Dis 1990; 12: 286.

48. Kaiser CW, Milgrom ML, Lynch JA. Distant nontraumatic clostridial myonecrosis and malignancy. Cancer 1986; 57: 885.

49. Narula A, Khatib R. Characteristic manifestations of clostridium induced staphylococcus gangrenous myositis. Scand J Infect Dis 1985; 17: 291.

50. Brown JR; Human actinomycosis: a study of 181 subjects. Hum Pathol 1973; 4: 319.

51. Sudhakar SS, Ross JJ. Short-term treatment of actinomycosis: two cases and a review. Clin Infect Dis. 2004; 38(3): 444–447.

52. Schmidt WA. IUDs, inflammation, and infection: assessment after two decades of IUD use. Hum Pathol 1982; 13: 878.

53. Bhagavan BS, Gupta PK. Genital actinomycosis and intrauterine contraceptive devices. Cytopathologic diagnosis and clinical significance. Hum Pathol 1978; 9: 567.

54. Wilson DJ. Botryomycosis. Am J Pathol 1959; 35: 153.

55. Greenblatt M, Heredia R, Rubenstein L, et al. Bacterial pseudomycosis ('botryomycosis'). Am J Clin Pathol 1964; 41: 188.

56. de Vries HJ, van Noesel CJ, Hoekzema R, et al. Botryomycosis in an HIV-positive subject. J Eur Acad Dermatol Venereol 2003; 17(1): 87–90.

57. Burkman RT, Schlesselman S, McCaffrey L, et al. The relationship of genital tract *Actinomyces* and the development of pelvic inflammatory disease. Am J Obstet Gynecol 1982; 143: 585.

58. Qureshi F, Jacques SM, Reyes MP. Placental histopathology in syphilis. Hum Pathol 1993; 24: 779.

59. Murray FE, O'Loughlin S, Dervan P, et al. Granulomatous hepatitis in secondary syphilis. Ir J Med Sci 1990; 159: 53.

60. Wu SJ, Nguyen EQ, Nielsen TA, et al. Nodular tertiary syphilis mimicking granuloma annulare. J Am Acad Dermatol 2000; 42(2 Pt 2): 378–380.

61. Ito F, Hunter EF, George RW, et al. Specific immunofluorescence staining of *Treponema pallidum* in smears and tissues. J Clin Microbiol 1991; 29: 444.

62. Saral R. *Candida* and *Aspergillus* infections in immunocompromised patients: an overview. Rev Infect Dis 1991; 13: 487.

63. Wingard JR, Merz WG, Saral R. *Candida tropicalis*: a major pathogen in immunocompromised patients. Ann Intern Med 1979; 91: 539.

64. Weems JJ Jr. *Candida parapsilosis*: epidemiology, pathogenicity, clinical manifestations, and antimicrobial susceptibility. Clin Infect Dis 1992; 14: 756.

65. Goldman M, Pottage JC Jr, Weaver DC. *Candida krusei fungemia*. Report of 4 cases and review of the literature. Medicine (Baltimore) 1993; 72: 143.

66. Johnson TL, Barnett JL, Appelman HD, et al. Candida hepatitis. Histopathologic diagnosis. Am J Surg Pathol 1988; 12: 716.

67. Ostrosky-Zeichner L, Rex JH, Bennett J, et al. Deeply invasive candidiasis. Infect Dis Clin North Am 2002; 16(4): 821–835.

68. Haron E, Vartivarian S, Anaissie E, et al. Primary *Candida* pneumonia. Experience at a large cancer center and review of the literature. Medicine (Baltimore) 1993; 72: 137.

69. Parker JC Jr, McCloskey JJ, Lee RS. Human cerebral candidosis – a postmortem evaluation of 19 patients. Hum Pathol 1981; 12: 23.

70. Cha R., Sobel JD. Fluconazole for the treatment of candidiasis: 15 years experience. Expert Rev Anti Infect Ther 2004; 2(3): 357–366.

71. Lurie HI; Histopathology of sporotrichosis. Notes on the nature of the asteroid body. Arch Pathol 1963; 75: 421.

72. Ro JY, Luna MA, Mackay B, et al. Yellow-brown (Hamazaki-Wesenberg) bodies mimicking fungal yeasts. Arch Pathol Lab Med 1987; 111(6): 555–559.

73. Takemura T, Eishi Y, Matsui Y. An autopsy case of sarcoidosis followed up for 27 years, with special reference to pulmonary fibrosis. Acta Pathol Jpn 1988; 38(7): 909–920.

74. Grotte M, Younger B; Sporotrichosis associated with sphagnum moss exposure. Arch Pathol Lab Med 1981; 105: 50.

75. Coles FB, Schuchat A, Hibbs JR, et al. A multistate outbreak of sporotrichosis associated with sphagnum moss. Am J Epidemiol 1992; 136: 475.

76. Sanders E. Cutaneous sporotrichosis. Beer, bricks, and bumps. Arch Intern Med 1971; 127: 482.

77. Morris-Jones R. Sporotrichosis. Clin Exp Dermatol 2002; 27(6): 427–431.

78. England DM, Hochholzer L. Primary pulmonary sporotrichosis. Report of eight cases with clinicopathologic review. Am J Surg Pathol 1985; 9: 193.

79. De Hoog GS, Queiroz-Telles F, Haase G, et al. Black fungi: clinical and pathogenic approaches. Med Mycol 2000; 38 Suppl 1: 243–250.

80. Bonifaz A, Paredes-Solis V, Saul A. Treating chromoblastomycosis with systemic antifungals. Expert Opin Pharmacother 2004; 5(2): 247–254.

81. Kantrow SM, Boyd AS. Protothecosis. Dermatol Clin 2003; 21(2): 249–255.

82. Nosanchuk JS, Greenberg RD. Protothecosis of the olecranon bursa caused by achloric algae. Am J Clin Pathol 1973; 59: 567.

83. Chandler FW, Kaplan W, Callaway CS. Differentiation between *Prototheca* and morphologically similar green algae in tissue. Arch Pathol Lab Med 1978; 102: 353.

84. Holcomb HS 3d, Behrens F, Winn WC Jr, et al. *Prototheca wickerhamii* – an alga infecting the hand. J Hand Surg [Am] 1981; 6: 595.

85. Wirth FA, Passalacqua JA, Kao G. Disseminated cutaneous protothecosis in an immunocompromised host: a case report and literature review. Cutis 1999; 63(3): 185–188.

86. Brandt ME, Warnock DW. Epidemiology, clinical manifestations, and therapy of infections caused by dematiaceous fungi. J Chemother Suppl 2003; 2: 36–47.

87. Revankar SG, Sutton DA, Rinaldi MG. Primary central nervous system phaeohyphomycosis: a review of 101 cases. Clin Infect Dis 2004; 38(2): 206–216.

88. Clancy CJ, Wingard JR, Hong Nguyen M. Subcutaneous phaeohyphomycosis in transplant recipients: review of the literature and demonstration of in vitro synergy between antifungal agents. Med Mycol 2000; 38(2): 169–175.

89. McGinnis MR. Mycetoma. Dermatol Clin 1996; 14(1): 97–104.

90. Fahal AH. Mycetoma: a thorn in the flesh. Trans R Soc Trop Med Hyg 2004; 98(1): 3–11.

91. Venugopal PV, Venugopal TV. Actinomadura madurae mycetomas. Australas J Dermatol 1990; 31(1): 33–36.

92. Boiron P, Locci R, Goodfellow M, et al. Nocardia, nocardiosis and mycetoma. Med Mycol 1998; 36 Suppl 1: 26–37.

93. Brumback BG, Farthing PG, Castellino SN. Simultaneous detection of and differentiation between herpes simplex and varicella-zoster viruses with two fluorescent probes in the same test system. J Clin Microbiol 1993; 31: 3260.

94. Nahmias AJ, Whitley RJ, Visintine AN, et al. Herpes simplex virus encephalitis: laboratory evaluations and their diagnostic significance. J Infect Dis 1982; 145: 829.

95. Pollara G, Katz DR, Chain BM. The host response to herpes simplex virus infection. Curr Opin Infect Dis 2004; 17(3): 199–203.

96. Drew WL, Buhles W, Ehrlich KS. Herpesvirus infections (CMV, HSV, VZV). Infect Dis Clin North Am 1986; 2: 495–505.

97. DeMay RM. The art & science of cytopathology. Chicago: ASCP Press; 1995.

98. Gurevich I. Varicella-zoster and herpes simplex virus infections. Heart Lung 1992; 21(1): 85–91.

99. Kazory A, Ducloux D. Renal transplantation and polyomavirus infection: recent clinical facts and controversies. Transpl Infect Dis 2003; 5(2): 65–71.

100. Aksamit AJ Jr. Progressive multifocal leukoencephalopathy: a review of the pathology and pathogenesis. Microsc Res Tech 1995; 32(4): 302–311.

101. Bultmann BD, Klingel K, Sotlar K, et al. Parvovirus B19: a pathogen responsible for more than hematologic disorders Virchows Arch 442(1): 8–17. Epub 2002 Nov 14, 2003.

102. Bikowski JB Jr. Molluscum contagiosum: the need for physician intervention and new treatment options. Cutis 2004; 73(3): 202–206.

103. Melby PC, Kreutzer RD, McMahon-Pratt D, et al. Cutaneous leishmaniasis: review of 59 cases seen at the National Institutes of Health. Clin Infect Dis 1992; 15: 924.

104. Magill AJ, Grögl M, Gasser RA Jr, et al. Visceral infection caused by *Leishmania tropica* in veterans of Operation Desert Storm. N Engl J Med 1993; 328: 1383.

105. Fernandez-Guerrero ML, Aguado JM, Buzon L, et al. Visceral leishmaniasis in immunocompromised hosts. Am J Med 1987; 83: 1098.

106. Berenguer J, Moreno S, Cercenado E, et al. Visceral leishmaniasis in patients infected with human immunodeficiency virus (HIV). Ann Intern Med 1989; 111: 129.

107. Olivier M, Badaro R, Medrano FJ, et al. The pathogenesis of Leishmania/HIV co-infection: cellular and immunological mechanisms. Ann Trop Med Parasitol 2003; 97 Suppl 1: 79–98.

108. Kayes SG. Human toxocariasis and the visceral larva migrans syndrome: correlative immunopathology. Chem Immunol 1997; 66: 99–124.

109. Bennhoff DF. Actinomycosis: diagnostic and therapeutic considerations and a review of 32 cases. Laryngoscope 1984; 94: 1198–1217.

110. Cunningham ET, Koehler JE. Ocular bartonellosis. Am J Ophthalmol 2000; 130(3): 340–349.

111. Carithers HA. Cat scratch disease. A overview based on a study of 1200 patients. Am J Dis Child 1985; 139: 1124–1133.

112. Attia OM. Rhinoscleroma and malignancy: two cases of rhinoscleroma associated with carcinoma. J Laryngol Otol 1958; 72: 412–415.

113. Lenis A, Ruff T, Diaz JA, et al. Rhinoscleroma. South Med J 1988; 81(12): 1580–1582.

114. Juster-Reicher A, Moligner BM, Levi G, et al. Neonatal noma. Am J Perinatol 1993; 10: 409–411.

115. Linder R. *Rhodococcus equi* and *Arcanobacterium haemolyticum*: two 'coryneform' bacteria increasingly recognized as agents of human infection. Emerg Infect Dis 1997; 3(2): 145–153.

116. Hanson JM, Spector G, El-Mofty SK. Laryngeal blastomycosis: a commonly missed diagnosis. Report of two cases and review of the literature. Ann Otol Rhinol Laryngol 2000; 109(3): 281–286.

117. Sant'Anna GD, Mauri M, Arrarte JL, et al. Laryngeal manifestations of paracoccidioidomycosis (South American blastomycosis). Arch Otolaryngol Head Neck Surg 1999; 125(12): 1375–1378.

118. Wolf J, Blumberg HM, Leonard MK. Laryngeal histoplasmosis. Am J Med Sci 2004; 327(3): 160–162.

119. Boyle JO, Coulthard SW, Mandel RM. Laryngeal involvement in disseminated coccidioidomycosis. Arch Otolaryngol Head Neck Surg 1991; 117(4): 433–438.

120. Nadrous HF, Ryu JH, Lewis JE, et al. Cryptococcal laryngitis: case report and review of the literature. Ann Otol Rhinol Laryngol 2004; 113(2): 121–123.

122. Wheeler MS, McGinnis MR, Schell WA, et al. Fusarium infection in burned patients. Am J Clin Pathol 1981; 75: 304.

123. Louie T, el Baba F, Shulman M, et al. Endogenous endophthalmitis due to Fusarium: case report and review. Clin Infect Dis 1984; 18: 585.

124. Gamis AS, Gudnason T, Giebink GS, et al. Disseminated infection with Fusarium in recipients of bone marrow transplants. Rev Infect Dis 1991; 13: 1077.

125. Reimer LG. Q fever. Clin Microbiol Rev 1993; 6: 193.

126. Spelman DW. Q fever. A study of 111 consecutive cases. Med J Aust 1982; 1: 547.

127. Hall CJ, Richmond SJ, Caul EO, et al. Laboratory outbreak of Q fever acquired from sheep. Lancet 1982; 1: 1004.

128. Srigley JR, Vellend H, Palmer N, et al. Q-fever. The liver and bone marrow pathology. Am J Surg Pathol 1985; 9: 752.

129. Pellegrin M, Delsol G, Auvergnant JC, et al. Granulomatous hepatitis in Q fever. Hum Pathol 1980; 11: 51.

130. Lobdell DH. 'Ring' granulomas in cytomegalovirus hepatitis. Arch Pathol Lab Med 1987; 111: 881.

131. Ruel M, Sevestre H, Henry-Biabaud E, et al. Fibrin ring granulomas in hepatitis A. Dig Dis Sci 1992; 37: 1915.

132. Barnes PF, Cave MD. Molecular epidemiology of tuberculosis. N Engl J Med 2003; 349(12): 1149–1156.

133. Goodwin RA, Des Prez RM; Pathogenesis and clinical spectrum of histoplasmosis. South Med J 1973; 66: 13.

134. Johnson PC, Khardori N, Najjar AF, et al. Progressive disseminated histoplasmosis in patients with acquired immunodeficiency syndrome. Am J Med 1988; 85: 152.

135. Reddy P, Gorelick DF, Brasher CA, et al. Progressive disseminated histoplasmosis as seen in adults. Am J Med 1970; 48: 629.

136. Wheat LJ, Connolly-Stringfield PA, Baker RL, et al. Disseminated histoplasmosis in the acquired immune deficiency syndrome: clinical findings, diagnosis and treatment, and review of the literature. Medicine (Baltimore) 1990; 69: 361.

137. Studdard J, Sneed WF, Taylor MR Jr, et al. Cutaneous histoplasmosis. Am Rev Respir Dis 1976; 113: 689.

138. Goodwin RA, Owens FT, Snell JD, et al. Chronic pulmonary histoplasmosis. Medicine (Baltimore) 1995; 55: 413.

139. Loyd JE, Tillman BF, Atkinson JB, et al. Mediastinal fibrosis complicating histoplasmosis. Medicine (Baltimore) 1988; 67: 295.

140. Goodwin RA, Nickell JA, Des Prez RM. Mediastinal fibrosis complicating healed primary histoplasmosis and tuberculosis. Medicine (Baltimore) 1972; 51: 227.

141. Sarosi GA, Hammerman KJ, Tosh FE, et al. Clinical features of acute pulmonary blastomycosis. N Engl J Med 1974; 290: 540.

142. Witorsch P, Utz JP. North American blastomycosis: a study of 40 patients. Medicine (Baltimore) 1968; 47: 169.

143. Pappas PG, Threlkeld MG, Bedsole GD, et al. Blastomycosis in immunocompromised patients. Medicine (Baltimore) 1993; 72: 311.

144. Atkinson JB, McCurley TL. Pulmonary blastomycosis: filamentous forms in an immunocompromised patient with fulminating respiratory failure. Hum Pathol 1983; 14: 186.

145. Case Records of the Massachusetts General Hospital. Case 49-1988: *Histoplasma capsulatum* or *Blastomyces dermatitidis*? N Engl J Med 1989; 320: 1699.

146. Lemos LB, Baliga M, Guo M. Blastomycosis: The great pretender can also be an opportunist. Initial clinical diagnosis and underlying diseases in 123 patients. Ann Diagn Pathol 2002; 6(3): 194–203.

147. Freed ER, Duma RJ, Shadomy HJ, et al. Meningoencephalitis due to hyphae-forming *Cryptococcus neoformans*. Am J Clin Pathol 1971; 55: 30.

148. Salyer WR, Salyer DC, Baker RD. Primary complex of *Cryptococcus* and pulmonary lymph nodes. J Infect Dis 1974; 130: 74.

149. Baker RD. The primary pulmonary lymph node complex of cryptococcosis. Am J Clin Pathol 1976; 65: 83.

150. McDonnell JM, Hutchins GM. Pulmonary cryptococcosis. Hum Pathol 1985; 16: 121.

151. Anderson DJ, Schmidt C, Goodman J, et al. Cryptococcal disease presenting as cellulitis. Clin Infect Dis 1992; 14: 666.

152. Chuck SL, Sande MA. Infections with *Cryptococcus neoformans* in the acquired immunodeficiency syndrome. N Engl J Med 1989; 321: 794.

153. Farmer SG, Komorowski RA. Histologic response to capsule-deficient *Cryptococcus neoformans*. Arch Pathol 1973; 96: 383.

154. Perfect JR, Casadevall A. Cryptococcosis. Infect Dis Clin North Am 2002; 16(4): 837–874; v–vi.

155. Ro JY, Lee SS, Ayala AG. Advantage of Fontana-Masson stain in capsule-deficient cryptococcal infection. Arch Pathol Lab Med 1987; 111: 53.

156. Lazcano O, Speights VO Jr, Bilbao J, et al. Combined Fontana-Masson-Mucin staining of *Cryptococcus neoformans*. Arch Pathol Lab Med 1991; 115: 1145.

157. Stevens DA. Coccidioidomycosis. N Engl J Med 1995; 332: 1077.

158. Pappagianis D. Marked increase in cases of coccidioidomycosis in California: 1991, 1992, and 1993. Clin Infect Dis 1994; Suppl. 1,19: S14.

159. Galgani JN, Ampel NM. Coccidioidomycosis in human immunodeficiency virus-infected patients. J Infect Dis 1990; 162: 1165.

160. Fish DG, Ampel NM, Galgiani JN, et al. Coccidioidomycosis during human immunodeficiency virus infection. A review of 77 patients. Medicine (Baltimore) 1990; 69: 384.

161. Vincent T, Galgiani JN, Huppert M, et al. The natural history of coccidioidal meningitis: VA-Armed Forces cooperative studies, 1955–1958. Clin Infect Dis 1993; 16: 247.

162. Macher AM, Shelhamer J, MacLowry J, et al. Pneumocystis carinii identified by Gram stain of lung imprints. Ann Intern Med 1983; 99: 484.

163. Ghali VS, Garcia RL, Skolom J. Fluorescence of Pneumocystis carinii in Papanicolaou smears. Hum Pathol 1984; 15: 907.

164. Wolfson JS, Waldron MA, Sierra LS. Blinded comparison of a direct immunofluorescent monoclonal antibody staining method and a Giemsa staining method for identification of Pneumocystis carinii in induced sputum and bronchoalveolar lavage specimens of patients infected with human immunodeficiency virus. J Clin Microbiol 1990; 28: 2136.

165. Midgley J, Parsons PA, Shanson DC, et al. Monoclonal immunofluorescence compared with silver stain for investigating Pneumocystis carinii pneumonia. J Clin Pathol 1991; 44: 75.

166. Kovacs JA, Gill V, Swan JC, et al. Prospective evaluation of a monoclonal antibody in diagnosis of Pneumocystis carinii pneumonia. Lancet 1986; 2: 1.

167. Singer C, Armstrong D, Rosen PP, et al. Pneumocystis carinii pneumonia: a cluster of eleven cases. Ann Intern Med 1975; 82: 772.

168. Pifer LL, Hughes WT, Stagno S, et al. Pneumocystis carinii infection: evidence for high prevalence in normal and immunosuppressed children. Pediatrics 1978; 61: 35.

169. Walzer PD, Perl DP, Krogstad DJ, et al. Pneumocystis carinii pneumonia in the United States. Epidemiologic, diagnostic, and clinical features. Ann Intern Med 1974; 80: 83.

170. Gottlieb MS, Schroff R, Schanker HM, et al. Pneumocystis carinii pneumonia and mucosal candidiasis in previously healthy homosexual men. Evidence for a new acquired cellular immunodeficiency. N Engl J Med 1981; 305: 1425.

171. Masur H, Michelis MA, Greene JB, et al. An outbreak of community-acquired Pneumocystis carinii pneumonia. Initial manifestation of cellular immune dysfunction. N Engl J Med 1981; 305: 1431.

172. Wang NS, Huang SN, Thurlbeck WM. Combined Pneumocystis carinii and cytomegalovirus infection. Arch Pathol 1970; 90: 529.

173. Schneider MME, Hoepelman AIM, Schattenkerk JKME, et al. A controlled trial of aerosolized pentamidine or trimethoprim-sulfamethoxazole as primary prophylaxis against Pneumocystis carinii pneumonia in patients with human immunodeficiency virus infection. N Engl J Med 1992; 327: 1836.

174. Telzak EE, Cote RJ, Gold JW, et al. Extrapulmonary Pneumocystis carinii infections. Rev Infect Dis 1990; 12: 380.

175. Lee MM, Schinella RA. Pulmonary calcification caused by Pneumocystis carinii pneumonia. A clinicopathological study of 13 cases in acquired immune deficiency syndrome patients. Am J Surg Pathol 1991; 15: 376.

176. Askin FB, Katzenstein AL. Pneumocystis infection masquerading as diffuse alveolar damage: a potential source of diagnostic error. Chest 1981; 79: 420.

177. Cupples JB, Blackie SP, Road JD. Granulomatous Pneumocystis carinii pneumonia mimicking tuberculosis. Arch Pathol Lab Med 1989; 113: 1281.

178. Travis WD, Pittaluga S, Lipschik GY, et al. Atypical pathologic manifestations of Pneumocystis carinii pneumonia in the acquired immune deficiency syndrome. Review of 123 lung biopsies from 76 patients with emphasis on cysts, vascular invasion, vasculitis, and granulomas. Am J Surg Pathol 1990, 14: 615.

179. Golden JA, Hollander H, Stulbarg MS, et al. Bronchoalveolar lavage as the exclusive diagnostic modality for Pneumocystis carinii pneumonia. A prospective study among patients with acquired immunodeficiency syndrome. Chest 1986; 90: 18.

180. Johnson WW, Elson CE. Respiratory tract. In: Bibbo M, ed. Comprehensive cytopathology. Philadelphia: WB Saunders; 1991: 340–352.

181. Jones PD, See J. Penicillium marneffei infection in patients infected with human immunodeficiency virus: late presentation in an area of nonendemicity. Clin Infect Dis 1992; 15: 744.

182. Deng ZL, Connor DH. Progressive disseminated penicilliosis caused by Penicillium marneffei. Report of eight cases and differentiation of the causative organism from Histoplasma capsulatum. Am J Clin Pathol 1985; 84: 323.

183. Cooper CR Jr, Haycocks NG. Penicillium marneffei: an insurgent species among the penicillia. J Eukaryot Microbiol 2000; 47(1): 24–28.

184. Butler JC, Heller R, Wright PF. Histoplasmosis during childhood. South Med J 1994; 87: 476.

185. Bosken CH, Myers JL, Greenberger PA, et al. Pathologic features of allergic bronchopulmonary aspergillosis. Am J Surg Pathol 1988; 12: 216.

186. Katzenstein AL, Liebow AA, Friedman PJ. Bronchocentric granulomatosis, mucoid impaction, and hypersensitivity reactions to fungi. Am Rev Respir Dis 1975; 111: 497.

187. Katzenstein AL, Sale SR, Greenberger PA. Pathologic findings in allergic aspergillus sinusitis. A newly recognized form of sinusitis. Am J Surg Pathol 1983; 7: 439.

188. Myers JL, Katzenstein AL. Granulomatous infection mimicking bronchocentric granulomatosis. Am J Surg Pathol 1986; 10: 317.

189. Engblom E, Ekfors TO, Meurman OH, et al. Fatal influenza A myocarditis with isolation of virus from the myocardium. Acta Med Scand 1983; 213: 75.

190. Englund JA, Sullivan CJ, Jordan MC, et al. Respiratory syncytial virus infection in immunocompromised adults. Ann Intern Med 1988; 109: 203.

191. Takimoto CH, Cram DL, Root RK. Respiratory syncytial virus infections on an adult medical ward. Arch Intern Med 1991; 151: 706.

192. Duke T, Mgone CS. Measles: not just another viral exanthem. Lancet 2003; 361(9359): 763–773.

193. Nolte KB, Feddersen RM, Foucar K, et al. Hantavirus pulmonary syndrome in the United States: a pathological description of a disease caused by a new agent. Hum Pathol 1995; 26: 110.

194. Zaki SR, Khan AS, Goodman RA, et al. Retrospective diagnosis of hantavirus pulmonary syndrome, 1978–1993: implications for emerging infectious diseases. Arch Pathol Lab Med 1996; 120: 134.

195. Sampathkumar P, Temesgen Z, Smith TF, et al. SARS: epidemiology, clinical presentation, management, and infection control measures. Mayo Clin Proc 2003; 78(7): 882–890.

196. Yu IT, Sung JJ. The epidemiology of the outbreak of severe acute respiratory syndrome (SARS) in Hong-Kong – what we do know and what we don't. Epidemiol Infect 2004; 132(5): 781–786.

197. Cheung OY, Chan JW, Ng CK, et al. The spectrum of pathological changes in severe acute respiratory syndrome (SARS). Histopathol 2004; 45(2): 119–124.

198. Mizrachi HH, Lieberman PH, Tolui SS, et al. Pulmonary dirofilariasis: mimicry of well-differentiated squamous carcinoma. Hum Pathol 1989; 20: 818.

199. Ro JY, Tsakalakis PJ, White VA, et al. Pulmonary dirofilariasis: the great imitator of primary or metastatic lung tumor. A clinicopathologic analysis of seven cases and a review of the literature. Hum Pathol 1989; 20: 69.

200. Gutierrez Y. Diagnostic features of zoonotic filariae in tissue sections. Hum Pathol 1984; 15: 514.

201. Metre MS, Jayaram G. Acid-fast bacilli in aspiration smears from tuberculous lymph nodes: an analysis of 255 cases. Acta Cytol 1987; 31: 17.

202. Maygarden SJ, Flanders EL. Mycobacteria can be seen as 'negative images' in cytology smears from patients with acquired immunodeficiency syndrome. Mod Pathol 1989; 2: 239.

203. Margileth AM, Hayden GF. Cat scratch disease. N Engl J Med 1993; 329: 53.

204. Schwartzman WA. Infections due to Rochalimaea: the expanding clinical spectrum. Clin Infect Dis 1992; 15: 893.

205. Margileth AM, Wear DJ, English CK. Systemic cat scratch disease: report of 23 patients with prolonged or recurrent severe bacterial infection. J Infect Dis 1987; 155: 390.

206. Miller Catchpole R, Variakojis D, Vardiman JW, et al. Cat scratch disease. Identification of bacteria in seven cases of lymphadenitis. Am J Surg Pathol 1986; 10: 276.

207. Lamps LW, Gray GF, Scott MA. Hepatic cat scratch disease – The histologic spectrum of changes in confirmed Bartonella henselae infection. Am J Surg Pathol 1996; 20: 1253–1259.

208. Scott MA, McCurley TL, Vnencak-Jones CL, et al. CAT SCRATCH DISEASE – detection of Bartonella henselae DNA in archival biopsies from patients with clinically, serologically and histologically defined disease. Am J Pathol 1996; 149(6): 2161–2167.

209. Cohen MB, Miller TR, Bottles K; Classics in cytology; note on fine needle aspiration of the lymphatic glands in sleeping sickness. Acta Cytol 1986; 30: 451.

210. Stastny JF, Wakely PE Jr, Frable WJ. Cytologic features of necrotizing granulomatous inflammation consistent with cat-scratch disease. Diagn Cytopathol 1996; 15: 108.

211. Pullen RL, Stuart BM. Tularemia analysis of 225 cases. JAMA 1945; 129: 495.

212. Stuart BM, Pullen RL. Tularemic pneumonia. Review of American literature and report of 15 additional cases. Am J Med Sci 1945; 210: 223.

213. Mille RP, Bates JH. Pleuropulmonary tularemia. A review of 29 patients. Am Rev Respir Dis 1969; 99: 31.

214. Brooks GF, Buchanan TM. Tularemia in the United States – epidemiologic aspects in the 1960s and follow-up of the outbreak of tularemia in Vermont. J Infect Dis 1970; 121: 357.

215. Evans ME, Gregory DW, Schaffner W, et al. Tularemia: a 30-year experience with 88 cases. Medicine (Baltimore) 1985; 64: 251.

216. Lamps LW, Havens JM, Sjostedt A, et al. Histologic and molecular diagnosis of tularemia: a potential bioterrorism agent endemic to North America. Mod Pathol 2004; 17(5): 489–495.

217. Reed W, Palmer D, Williams RC Jr, et al. Plague in the southwestern United States – a review of recent experience. Medicine (Baltimore) 1970; 19: 465.

218. Reilly CG, Kates ED. The clinical spectrum of plague in Vietnam. Arch Intern Med 1970; 126: 990.

219. Sternby NH. Morphologic findings in appendix in human Yersinia enterocolitica infection. Contrib Microbiol Immunol 1973; 2: 141.

220. Gleason TH, Patterson SD. The pathology of Yersinia enterocolitica ileocolitis. Am J Surg Pathol 1982; 6: 347.

221. Finlayson NB, Fagundes B. Pasteurella pseudotuberculosis infection: three cases in the United States. Am J Clin Pathol 1971; 55: 24.

222. Hubbert WT, Peteny CW, Glasgow LA. Yersinia pseudotuberculosis infection in the United States: septicemia, appendicitis, and mesenteric lymphadenitis. Am J Trop Med Hyg 1971; 20: 679.

223. Lamps LW, Madhusudhan KT, Greenson JK, et al. The role of Yersinia enterocolitica and Yersinia pseudotuberculosis in granulomatous appendicitis: a

histologic and molecular study. Am J Surg Pathol 2001; 25(4): 508–515.

224. Scieux C, Barnes R, Bianchi A, et al. Lymphogranuloma venereum: 27 cases in Paris. J Infect Dis 1989; 160: 662.

225. Klotz SA, Drutz DJ, Tam MR, et al. Hemorrhagic proctitis due to lymphogranuloma venereum serogroup L2 – diagnosis by fluorescent monoclonal antibody. N Engl J Med 1983; 308: 1563.

226. Maurin M, Raoult D. *Bartonella (Rochalimaea) quintana* infections. Clin Microbiol Rev 1996; 9: 273.

227. Relman DA, Loutit JS, Schmidt TM, et al. The agent of bacillary angiomatosis. An approach to the identification of uncultured pathogens. N Engl J Med 1990; 323: 1573.

228. LeBoit PE, Berger TG, Egbert BM, et al. Bacillary angiomatosis. The histopathology and differential diagnosis of a pseudoneoplastic infection in patients with human immunodeficiency virus disease. Am J Surg Pathol 1989; 13: 909.

229. Oddo D, Casanova M, Acuna G, et al. Acute Chagas' disease (*Trypanosomiasis americana*) in acquired immunodeficiency syndrome: report of two cases. Hum Pathol 1992; 23: 41.

230. Pinals RS. Fever, eosinophilia, and periorbital edema. Hosp Pract (Off Ed) 1980; 23: 55–74.

231. Beckman EN, Leonard GL, Castillo LE, et al. Histopathology of marine vibrio wound infections. Am J Clin Pathol 1981; 76: 765.

232. Woo ML, Patrick WG, Simon MT, et al. Necrotising fasciitis caused by *Vibrio vulnificus*. J Clin Pathol 1984; 37: 1301.

233. Tacket CO, Barrett TJ, Mann JM, et al. Wound infections caused by *Vibrio vulnificus*, a marine vibrio, in inland areas of the United States. J Clin Microbiol 1984; 19: 197.

234. Joseph SW, Daily OP, Hunt WS, et al. Aeromonas primary wound infection of a diver in polluted waters. J Clin Microbiol 1979; 10: 46.

235. Pfischner WCE, Tshak KG, Neptune EM. Brucellosis in Egypt. A review of experience with 228 patients. Am J Med 1957; 22: 915.

236. Buchanan TM, Faber LC, Feldman RA. Brucellosis in the United States 1960–1972. An abattoir-associated disease. Part 1. Clinical features and therapy. Medicine (Baltimore) 1974; 53: 403.

237. Hunt AC, Bothwell PW. Histological findings in human brucellosis. J Clin Pathol 1967; 20: 267.

238. Simpson WM. Undulant fever (brucellosis) – a clinicopathologic study of ninety cases occurring in and about Dayton, Ohio. Ann Intern Med 1930; 4: 238.

239. Spink WW, Hoffbauer FW, Walker WW, et al. Histopathology of the liver in human brucellosis. J Lab Clin Med 1949; 34: 40.

240. Fend F, Prior C, Margreiter R, et al. Cytomegalovirus pneumonitis in heart-lung transplant recipients: histopathology and clinicopathologic considerations. Hum Pathol 1990; 21: 918.

241. Craighead JE. Cytomegalovirus pulmonary disease. Pathobiol Ann 1975; 5: 197.

242. Myers JD, Spencer HCJ, Watts JC, et al. Cytomegalovirus pneumonia after human marrow transplantation. Ann Intern Med 1975; 82: 181.

243. Heurlin N, Brattstrom C, Tyden G, et al. Cytomegalovirus the predominant cause of pneumonia in renal transplant patients. A two-year study of pneumonia in renal transplant recipients with evaluation of fiberoptic bronchoscopy. Scand J Infect Dis 1989; 21: 245.

244. Beschorner WE, Hutchins GM, Burns WH, et al. Cytomegalovirus pneumonia in bone marrow transplant recipients: miliary and diffuse patterns. Am Rev Respir Dis 1980; 122: 107.

245. Adams EB, MacLeod IN. Invasive amebiasis-amebic dysentery and its complications. Medicine (Baltimore) 1977; 56: 315–324.

246. Adams EB, MacLeod IN. Invasive amebiasis-amebic liver abscess and its complications. Medicine (Baltimore) 1977; 56: 325–334.

247. Sorvillo FJ, Strassburg MA, Seidel J, et al. Amebic infections in asymptomatic homosexual men, lack of evidence of invasive disease. Am J Publ Health 1986; 76: 1137.

248. Diamond LS, Clark CG. A redescription of *Entamoeba histolytica* (Schaudinn, 1903; emended Walker, 1911) separating it from *Entamoeba dispar* (Brumpt, 1925). J Euk Microbiol 1993; 40: 340.

249. Cohen C, Trapuckd S. Toxoplasma cyst with toxoplasmic lymphadenitis. Hum Pathol 1984; 15: 396.

250. Weiss LM, Chen YY, Berry GJ, et al. Infrequent detection of *Toxoplasma gondii* genome in toxoplasmic lymphadenitis: a polymerase chain reaction study. Hum Pathol 1992; 23: 154.

251. Oksenhendler E, Cadranel J, Sarfati C, et al. *Toxoplasma gondii* pneumonia in patients with the acquired immunodeficiency syndrome. Am J Med 1990; 88: 5–18N.

252. Falangola MF, Reichler BS, Petito CK. Histopathology of cerebral toxoplasmosis in human immunodeficiency virus infection: a comparison between patients with early-onset and late-onset acquired immunodeficiency syndrome. Hum Pathol 1994; 25: 1091.

253. Nash G, Kerschmann RL, Herndier B, et al. The pathological manifestations of pulmonary toxoplasmosis in the acquired immunodeficiency syndrome. Hum Pathol 1994; 25: 652.

254. Kaye D. The spectrum of *Strongyloidiasis*. Hosp Pract (Off Ed) 1988; 23: 111–126.

255. Shandera WX, White AC Jr, Chen JC. Neurocysticercosis in Houston, Texas: a report of 112 cases. Medicine (Baltimore) 1994; 73: 37.

256. King CH. Acute and chronic schistosomiasis. Hosp Pract (Off Ed) 1991; 26: 117–130.

257. Smith JH, Christie JD. The pathobiology of *Schistosoma haematobium* infection in humans. Hum Pathol 1986; 17: 333.

258. Ma P, Visvesvara GS, Martinez AJ, et al. *Naegleria* and *Acanthamoeba* infections: a review. Rev Infect Dis 1990; 12: 490.

259. Tan B, Weldon-Linne CM, Rhone DP, et al. Acanthamoeba infection presenting as skin lesions in patients with the acquired immunodeficiency syndrome. Arch Pathol Lab Med 1993; 117: 1043.

260. Visvesvara GS, Martinez AJ, Schuster FL, et al. Leptomyxid ameba: a new agent of amebic meningoencephalitis in humans and animals. J Clin Microbiol 1990; 28: 2750.

261. Deol I, Robledo L, Meza A, et al. Encephalitis due to a free-living amoeba (*Balamuthia mandrillaris*): case report with literature review. Surg Neurol. 2000; 53(6): 611–616.

262. Falkow S. Molecular Koch's postulates applied to microbial pathogenicity. Rev Infect Dis 1988; 10: S274.

263. Enns RK and the NCCLS Subcommittee on Molecular Microbiology. Molecular diagnostic methods for infectious diseases: proposed guideline. NCCLS medical microbiology – proposed standard, 3-P, vol. 14, No. 4, 1994.

Pathology of immunologically mediated diseases and transplantation

4

Edward C. Klatt   M. Elizabeth H. Hammond

AUTOIMMUNE DISEASES

Loss of self-tolerance and inappropriate activation of the immune system can lead to a variety of autoimmune conditions. The MHC expression by many cells plays an important role in this process, along with T lymphocytes. Many pathologic lesions seen with autoimmune diseases are a consequence of immune hypersensitivity reactions, particularly immune complex mediated disease. Immune complexes can be identified by immunofluorescence with staining for IgG, C1q, C3d and C4d. The serum antinuclear antibody (ANA) test is positive in many cases. Differential features of the major autoimmune conditions are detailed in Table 4.1.[1–5]

Endocrine autoimmune diseases may include type 1 diabetes mellitus, thought to result from alteration of beta cells in islets of Langerhans by viral or chemical factors followed by abnormal MHC expression and autoimmune destruction mediated via T lymphocytes and cytokine release. Microscopically, there is a lymphocytic insulitis with edema culminating in loss of islets.[6] Addison's disease is most commonly an autoimmune process, and initially there are lymphocytic infiltrates with adrenal cortical destruction, followed by fibrosis and atrophy.[7] Lymphocytic hypophysitis is a rare disorder seen most often postpartum women that can account for pituitary failure.[8]

PRIMARY IMMUNODEFICIENCY DISEASES

These congenital conditions have a variety of molecular mechanisms, many of which are now known to be associated with specific genetic defects. The differential features of the most important of these diseases are given below.[9–11]

X-LINKED (BRUTON'S) AGAMMAGLOBULINEMIA

A mutation in the Bruton tyrosine kinase (Btk) gene results in failure of pre-B cells to differentiate into B cells. With time, about 20% of affected persons will develop an autoimmune disease such as rheumatoid arthritis, systemic lupus erythematosus, or dermatomyositis. There are normal numbers of circulating T cells with low to absent B cells, <100 mg/dL of IgG and absent IgA and IgM. Grossly atrophic lymph nodes and tonsils have rare follicles lacking germinal centers and plasma cells, but normal thymus and T cell numbers are present. Recurrent bacterial infections with *Hemophilus influenzae*, *Streptococcus pneumoniae*, and *Staphylococcus aureus* are frequent, beginning in infancy when passively acquired maternal antibody diminishes. *Giardia lamblia* diarrhea, vaccine-associated poliomyelitis, echovirus meningoencephalitis, and arthritis of large joints from *Ureaplasma urealyticum* infection also occur.[12]

DIGEORGE ANOMALY

A 22q11 chromosome deletion leads to abnormal morphogenesis of structures formed from 3rd and 4th pharyngeal pouches. The complete variant has a lack of thymic cortex and medulla, with only scattered Hassall's corpuscles and a few small lymphocytes. Lymph nodes have follicles but decreased numbers of T cells in paracortical and mantle zones, and periarteriolar cuffs of lymphocytes in spleen are virtually absent. The partial variant shows decreased numbers of T cells in thymus and other lymphoid regions, with absent or decreased circulating T cells but normal levels of immunoglobulin, though serum IgE may be increased and IgA decreased. There are great vessel and cardiac anomalies, parathyroid hypoplasia or agenesis (with hypocalcemia) and facial anomalies.[11,12]

SEVERE COMBINED IMMUNODEFICIENCY (SCID)

Half of cases result from an X-linked mutation in the IL2RG gene encoding for the common gamma chain of interleukin-2, which forms a receptor for many cytokines needed for T-cell development. Normal or increased numbers of B lymphoyctes may be present. Half of cases result from autosomal recessive mutation in the adenine deaminase (ADA) gene, leading to accumulation of purine metabolites toxic to T cells. In both forms of SCID, though T cells are primarily involved with greater decrease in cell mediated immunity than in humoral immunity, there is secondary impairment of B-cell function so that affected persons have diminished IgG levels and no IgA or IgM, leading to increased susceptibility to virtually all infectious organisms. Affected infants have markedly decreased circulating lymphocytes (<1000/microliter), though NK cells may be normal or increased.

The thymus in SCID does not develop beyond initial embryogenesis, does not descend to the anterior mediastinum, and has virtual absence of lymphocytes and Hassall's corpuscles. Lymphoid tissues throughout the body are hypoplastic. Infants develop *Candida* skin rashes and thrush, persistent diarrhea, severe respiratory tract infections with *Pneumocystis carinii* and *Pseudomonas* soon after birth, and failure to thrive after 3 months of age. Severe viral infections can occur. Maternal T lymphocytes crossing the placenta may produce fetal graft-versus-host disease.[11–13]

SELECTIVE (ISOLATED) IGA DEFICIENCY

About 1 in 500 persons of European descent has either a virtual lack of circulating IgA (<50 mg/dL) as well as secretory IgA, or has partial IgA deficiency (>50 mg/dl but >2 standard deviations below normal). There are normal numbers of T and B cells but

Table 4.1 Autoimmune diseases

Disease	Autoantibodies (specific)	Distinguishing features
Systemic lupus erythematosus (SLE)	dsDNA, Smith	Skin rash with leukocytoclastic vasculitis and basal hydropic degeneration, arthralgia without joint inflammation or deformity, myalgia without myopathy, cytopenias, hemolytic anemia, serositis with pleural/pericardial/peritoneal effusions, Libman-Sacks endocarditis, splenic periarteriolar fibrosis ('onion skinning'), lupus nephritis can lead to renal failure, antiphospholipid antibody with vascular thromboses or hemorrhage, vasculitis involving any organ (e.g., lupus cerebritis)
Drug-induced SLE	histone	Features similar to SLE, but without severe vasculitis or extensive organ involvement
Discoid lupus erythematosus (DLE)	ANA positive in only 30%	Skin rash with vasculitis only in sun-exposed areas, without major internal organ involvement; some cases progress to SLE
Rheumatoid arthritis (RA)	Rheumatoid factor (RF)	Arthritis mainly of small joints of hands and feet with pannus formation with mononuclear infiltrates including many plasma cells in synovium with joint destruction and deformity; rheumatoid nodules (localized fibrinoid necrosis) at pressure points in subcutaneous and visceral organ locations. A very high titer RF, an autoantibody (mostly IgM) formed against the Fc portion of autologous IgG, can be seen with vasculitis similar to polyarteritis nodosa but involving mainly small peripheral arteries. Associated with HLA-DR4.
Scleroderma, diffuse	DNA topoisomerase I (Scl-70)	Minimal inflammation; mainly fibrosis. Sclerodactyly with extensive dermal fibrosis, esophageal dysmotility and stricture, gastrointestinal submucosal fibrosis with malabsorbtion, renal vasculopathy with hyperplastic arteriolosclerosis with concentric intimal endothelial proliferation in small arcuate and interlobular arteries can lead to severe hypertension and arteriolar fibrinoid necrosis with cortical microinfarcts, pulmonary alveolitis may proceed to interstitial fibrosis with restrictive lung disease.
CREST syndrome	Centromere	More limited features than diffuse scleroderma, without major renal or pulmonary disease (C=calcinosis; R=Raynaud phenomenon; E=esophageal dysmotility; S=sclerodactyly; T=telangiectasias)
Polymyositis	Jo-1	Myalgia with myopathic changes (inflammation with degeneration and regeneration) in skeletal muscles, along with skin findings similar to SLE
Dermatomyositis	Jo-1	Skin rash with dermatitis in addition to myalgia with myopathy
Sjögren syndrome	SS-A, SS-B	Xerostomia and xerophthalmia with chronic inflammation of salivary and lacrimal glands; a predilection for coexistence of other autoimmune diseases and for development of lymphoid malignancies
Mixed connective tissue disease (MCTD)	U1-RNP	Overlap syndrome with milder features of SLE, scleroderma, rheumatoid arthritis, and polymyositis but generally without serious organ involvement leading to renal or pulmonary failure

absent IgA-secreting plasma cells and deficiencies in IgG subclasses 2 and/or 4, while IgG subclasses 1 and 3 are increased. The cause is either failure in final differentiation of IgA-secreting B cells into plasma cells or decreased survival of plasma cells. Some patients may develop common variable immunodeficiency, suggesting a similar defect in B-cell maturation and function.

Increased susceptibility to respiratory, urinary, and gastrointestinal infections (bacterial and *Giardia lamblia* with mild diarrhea) is present in some cases, typically when other antibody deficiencies are present, and half of IgA deficient persons have systemic anaphylaxis with blood transfusion from circulating IgA antibodies. Atopy with asthma can be present. More severely affected persons may have a sprue-like illness with malabsorbtion. Concomitant autoimmune diseases, particularly systemic lupus erythematosus and rheumatoid arthritis, can occur. The gross and microscopic architecture of lymphoid organs appears normal.[14–16]

COMMON VARIABLE IMMUNODEFICIENCY (CVID)

This heterogeneous group of disorders has an incidence of 1 per 100 000 and can involve both humoral and cell mediated immunity, including failure of B-cell maturation to plasma cells, excessive T-cell suppression, or defective T-helper cell function. A selective abnormality of T-cell activation, demonstrated by decreased synthesis of interleukins has been identified in some cases. Other cases have T- and B-cell autoantibodies, or have a decreased CD4/CD8 ratio. In two-thirds of cases, normal numbers of circulating B lymphocytes are present. There is a decrease in immunoglobulins, generally in all classes, more often IgG and IgA, but sometimes only of IgG. Normal numbers of T cells are present. It may be linked to selective IgA deficiency in families.

Half of CVID cases are diagnosed before age 21, but in some cases complications do not develop until adulthood. At least two of the three main serum immunoglobulin isotypes are decreased. Persons with CVID are prone to recurrent bacterial infections, particularly sinusitis, bronchitis, pneumonia, bronchiectasis, and otitis. *Bordatella pertussis* infections occur in childhood. Viral infections are uncommon, though recurrent herpes simplex with eventual herpes zoster is an exception. Giardiasis is common. There is an increased incidence of autoimmune diseases, particularly hemolytic anemia, thrombocytopenia, pernicious anemia, celiac disease, and Crohn disease. The risk for gastric adenocarcinoma and small intestinal lymphoma is increased. Some patients develop multiorgan noncaseating granulomas similar to sarcoidosis.[14,17–19]

Grossly, thymic and lymphoid tissues develop normally, but lymphadenopathy, gastrointestinal lymphoid hyperplasia, and splenomegaly are often present. Microscopically, germinal centers of lymphoid follicles can appear hyperplastic with increased B lymphocytes. Nodal and extranodal lymphoid proliferations range from reactive to atypical lymphoid hyperplasia. There is an increased tendency for non-specific noncaseating sarcoid-like granulomas to be present in liver, spleen, lymph nodes, and bone marrow. Hodgkin's disease, non-Hodgkin's lymphomas, gastric carcinoma, and inflammatory bowel diseases are more frequent. Some affected persons develop amyloidosis.[20]

WISKOTT-ALDRICH SYNDROME

Wiskott-Aldrich syndrome (WAS) results from an X-linked mutation in the gene coding for WAS protein that may function in maintaining lymphoid cell and platelet cytoskeleton and in apoptosis. There are normal to low numbers of circulating T cells and normal B cells, but usually normal levels of serum IgG, along with a decrease in IgM, but often an increase in both IgA and IgE. Grossly, thymus and lymph nodes appear normal. Microscopically, there can be T-lymphocyte depletion in paracortical areas of lymphoid tissues. There are normal numbers of megakaryocytes in bone marrow. More severe forms of WAS have thrombocytopenia, eczema, diarrhea, recurrent infections, hemolytic anemia, vasculitis, arthritis, and increased risk for malignancies, including Epstein-Barr virus driven lymphomas.[14]

The initial onset of WAS in early childhood is accompanied by recurrent bacterial infections, particularly to encapsulated bacteria such as *Streptococcus pneumoniae*, with development of pneumonia, meningitis, and septicemia. Later, failure of T-lymphocyte function may predispose to recurrent herpetic infections and to *Pneumocystis carinii* pneumonia. Thrombocytopenia may result in a bleeding diathesis. A milder form of the disease with platelet abnormalities is known as X-linked thrombocytopenia (XLT).[11,12,21]

ATAXIA-TELANGIECTASIA

Mutations in DNA repair genes lead to several related syndromes: ATM gene in ataxia-telangiectasia (A-T); gene on chromosome 8 in Nijmegen syndrome; BLM gene in Bloom syndrome. There is thymic atrophy with lymphocyte depletion and absence of Hassall's

corpuscles. Lymph nodes demonstrate T-cell depletion in paracortical areas and mantle zones, and eventually become atrophic. Recurrent pulmonary infections lead to bronchiectasis and pulmonary fibrosis. The neoplasms that occur with A-T are often lymphomas (usually B cell) and leukemias, but there is also an increased risk for solid tumors.

The symptoms usually begin between 9 months and 2 years of age. There is a triad of progressive cerebellar ataxia, mucocutaneous telangiectasias, and recurrent respiratory tract infections with a variety of bacterial and fungal organisms. Immunoglobulin deficiencies, particularly IgA and/or IgE, may be present, though serum IgM is usually elevated. The related Nijmegen breakage and Bloom syndromes are also characterized by risk for malignancy and radiation sensitivity.[22,23]

HYPER IGM SYNDROME

Genetic mutations in the CD40 ligand (CD154) induce failure in B cells that produce immunoglobulin. There is hypogammaglobulinemia with low IgG, IgA, and IgE levels but increased IgM. In infancy and childhood there is an increased risk for severe infections (often respiratory) with bacterial and viral agents and opportunistic agents such as *Pneumocystis carinii*. There is neutropenia, recurrent diarrhea, oral or perirectal ulcerations.[11]

X-LINKED LYMPHOPROLIFERATIVE (XLP) DISEASE

A mutation in the gene at Xq25 encoding for an adapter protein in T cells and NK cells that interferes with binding of signaling lymphocyte activation molecule leads to failure to control proliferation of cytotoxic T cells with Epstein-Barr virus (EBV) infection in XLP disease (Duncan syndrome). As a consequence, EBV infection in early childhood leads to fatal infectious mononucleosis from hepatic necrosis. The few survivors develop hypogammaglobulinemia, aplastic anemia, and non-Hodgkin lymphomas.[12,14]

CHRONIC GRANULOMATOUS DISEASE

Chronic granulomatous disease (CGD) results from mutations in genes coding for proteins in the NADPH oxidative killing pathway for microorganisms ingested by granulocytes. Two-thirds of cases are X-linked and the rest autosomal recessive. The incidence is 1 in 200 000. There are normal numbers of circulating leukocytes, but a defect in flow cytometry respiratory burst assay. Beginning in childhood affected persons have lymphadenopathy with granulomatous inflammation from recurrent infections with *Aspergillus*, *Staphylococcus*, *Serratia*, *Nocardia*, and *Pseudomonas*.[10] Half of persons with CGD develop Crohn disease. Relatives of affected persons have an increased risk for discoid lupus.[14]

CHÉDIAK-HIGASHI SYNDROME

There is a mutation in a gene on chromosome 1q42 that encodes for a protein involved in intracellular trafficking of proteins. The abnormal fusion of lysosomes forms giant granules in peripheral blood leukocytes that fail to function. Soft tissue abscesses with *Staphylococcus aureus* are frequent. Other affected cells include platelets (bleeding), melanocytes (albinism), Schwann cells (neuropathy), and NK and cytotoxic T cells (aggressive lympho-proliferative disorder).[10]

LEUKOCYTE ADHESION DEFICIENCY

There are autosomal recessive mutations in CD18, the common beta chain of cellular integrins which aid in binding of leukocytes to endothelium prior to diapedesis into inflamed tissues. Affected persons have leukocytosis, but absence of suppurative inflammation in areas of tissue necrosis and ulceration caused by *Staphylococcus aureus* and gram-negative enteric bacteria.[10] Persistent leuko-cytoclastic vasculitis may occur.[14]

AMYLOIDOSIS

Regardless of underlying disease, amyloid appears with H&E stains as a homogeneous eosinophilic material between the cells of tissues distinguished from other pink amorphous 'hyaline' deposits by its staining with alkaline Congo red. In routine histologic sections from formalin-fixed and paraffin-embedded tissues, the Congo red dye will line the amyloid fibrils so that they not only appear reddish-orange by light microscopy, but also will have an 'apple-green' birefringence under polarized light. By electron microscopy, amyloid appears as a beta-pleated sheet composed of fibrils ranging from 7.5 to 10 nanometers in width that are nonbranching and of indefinite length and associated with a P component (similar to serum C reactive protein) which is donut shaped and pentagonal. Staining with thioflavin T will demonstrate amyloid by fluorescence microscopy in the blue–violet range.[24]

Sites for diagnosis of amyloidosis with a high (>75%) yield include: heart, liver, skin, kidney, small intestine, sural nerve, rectum, and tongue. Immunohistochemical staining can be done to subclassify the amyloid proteins present.[25] Subclassification is based upon the nature of the proteinaceous material forming the amyloid fibrils and the disease states that coexist with it. Amyloidosis can also be classified as systemic or localized. Amyloid deposited extracellularly interferes with organ function as it occupies space and displaces normal cellular constituents. Amyloid is often deposited in vascular walls. The classification and features of major amyloidoses are shown in Table 4.2.[26–29] The characteristic microscopic features of amyloid are shown in Figures 4.1 to 4.3.

ACQUIRED IMMUNODEFICIENCY SYNDROME (AIDS)

The human immunodeficiency virus (HIV) is a retrovirus of the lentivirus family that causes AIDS. HIV infection leads to relentless destruction of the immune system that puts all HIV-infected persons at risk for illness and death from opportunistic infectious and neoplastic complications. The great majority of AIDS cases are caused by HIV-1.[30] HIV primarily infects cells with CD4 cell-surface receptor molecules, including cells of the mononuclear phagocyte system, principally CD4 lymphocytes, blood monocytes, tissue macrophages, dendritic cells, and microglial cells. HIV has the additional ability to mutate easily because its reverse transcriptase enzyme introduces a mutation approximately once per 2000 incorporated nucleotides. The rapid turnover of HIV and CD4 lymphocytes promotes origin of new strains of HIV that can resist immune attack, are more cytotoxic, can generate syncytia more

Table 4.2 Amyloidosis

Type of amyloidosis	Underlying or related disease	Composition	Distribution
Immunologic	Plasma cell dyscrasia (multiple myeloma, Waldenstrom's macroglobulinemia) Primary systemic amyloidosis	Immunoglobulin light chains	Anywhere, but liver, spleen, kidney, peripheral nerve, and adrenal are most common
Reactive systemic	Chronic infections, autoimmune diseases, malignancies	Serum amyloid associated (SAA) or amyloid A (AA) protein	Anywhere
Heredofamilial	Familial Mediterranean fever	Serum amyloid associated (SAA) protein	Anywhere
Familial	A variety of autosomal dominant conditions	Serum prealbumin transthyretin (ATTR) protein	Heart, kidney, eye
Hemodialysis-associated	Chronic hemodialysis	Serum beta-2-microglobulin	Mainly in joints
Localized (nodular)	Chronic inflammation with plasma cells	Immunoglobulin light chains	Single site, most commonly in lungs, larynx, skin, urinary bladder, or tongue
	Medullary thyroid carcinoma	Polypeptide hormones secreted by the neoplasm	Thyroid, or other endocrine neoplasm
	Type II diabetes mellitus	Amylin protein	Islets of Langerhans
Cardiac	Infiltrative cardiomyopathy	Serum prealbumin transthyretin (ATTR) protein	Heart – interstitial and vascular
'Senile' cardiac	Seen with aging	Atrial natriuretic peptide	Atrial appendages
Cerebral	Alzheimer's disease	Beta-amyloid (A4) protein	Cortical neuritic plaques, cortical cerebral arteries
	Idiopathic, in elderly persons	Serum prealbumin transthyretin (ATTR) protein	Cortical cerebral arteries
	Spongiform encephalopathies	Prion protein	Cortical cerebral arteries

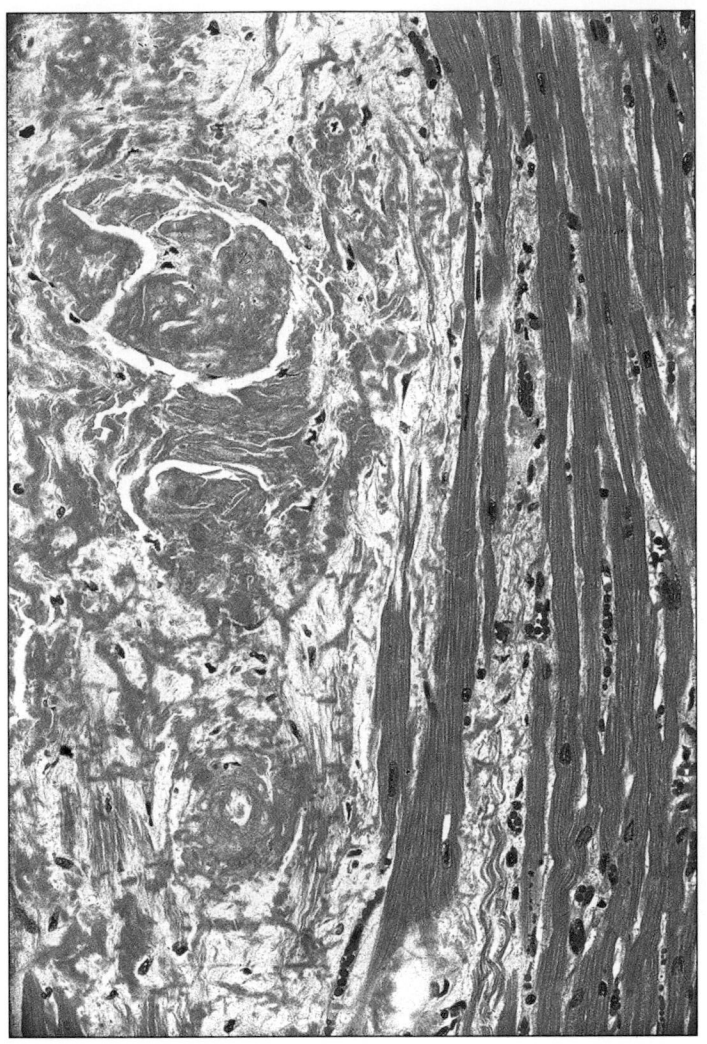

Fig. 4.1 Amyloid. Amorphous pink deposits of amyloid are seen in the heart.

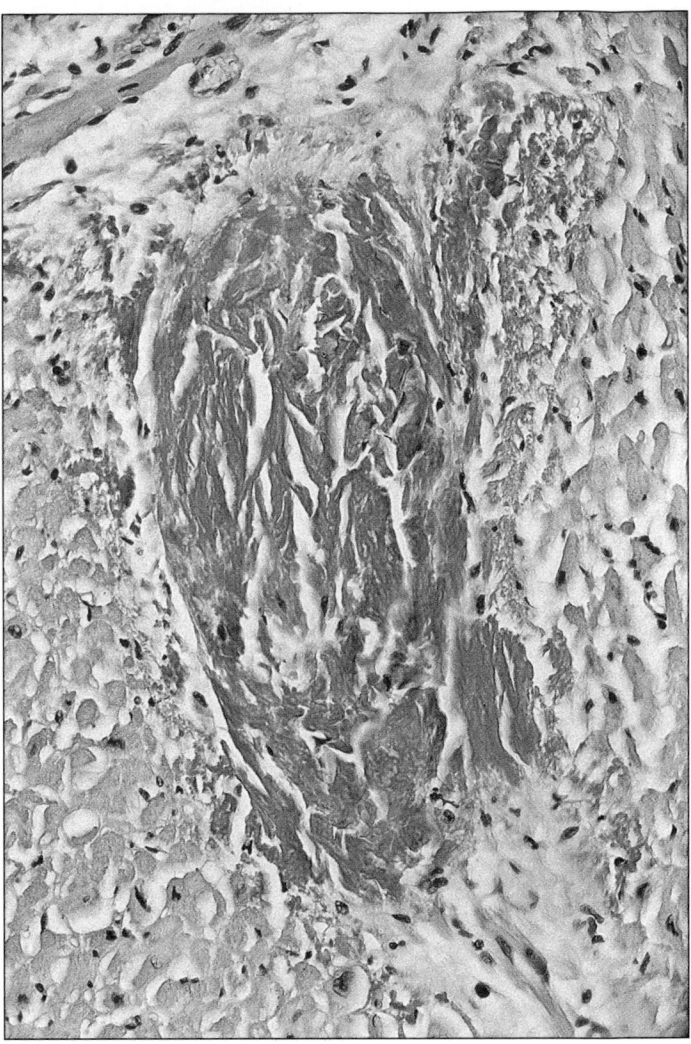

Fig. 4.2 Amyloid. An orange-red appearance with Congo red stain is seen in cardiac muscle.

readily, can resist drug therapy, or result in variability of pathologic lesions as different cell types are targeted or different cytopathic effects are elicited during the course of infection. The biologic properties of HIV can vary even within an individual HIV-infected person.[31,32]

Replication of HIV may first occur within inflammatory cells or peripheral blood mononuclear cells near the site of infection, but quickly shifts to lymphoid tissues including lymph nodes, spleen, liver, and bone marrow. Besides nodes, the gut-associated lymphoid tissue is a substantial reservoir for HIV. Macrophages and Langerhans cells in epithelia such as the genital tract are important both as reservoirs and vectors for spread of HIV because they can be HIV infected but are not destroyed. Within lymph nodes, HIV virions are trapped in the processes of infected follicular dendritic cells where they may infect migrating CD4 lymphocytes. Presence of HIV in genital secretions and in blood, and to a lesser extent breast milk, is significant for spread of HIV, but transmission via saliva, urine, tears, and sweat does not routinely occur because of the low concentration of HIV in these fluids.[33]

Acute HIV infection may produce a mild disease for 1 to 2 months that resembles infectious mononucleosis. Fever, lymphadenopathy,

pharyngitis, diffuse erythematous rash, arthralgia/myalgia, diarrhea, and headache are the commonest symptoms. Biopsied lymph nodes reveal reactive changes.[34,35] Generally, within 2 weeks to 3 months an immune response is accompanied by a simultaneous decline in HIV viremia and presence of positive serologic HIV tests. The CD4 lymphocytes rebound in number, but not to pre-infection levels.[36]

A clinically latent period of HIV infection lasts on average from eight to ten years during which time enough of the immune system remains intact to prevent most infections, but viral replication actively continues in lymphoid tissues.[37] A decrease in the total CD4 count below 500/microliter presages the development of clinical AIDS, and a drop below 200/microliter not only defines AIDS, but also indicates a high probability for the development of AIDS-related opportunistic infections and/or neoplasms, or death.[38] Plasma HIV-1 RNA increases as plasma viremia becomes more marked. For perinatally acquired HIV infection, latency before clinical AIDS may be shorter than in adults.[39]

HIV-related lymphadenopathy (HIVL) can be seen with primary HIV infection or at any time during progression through AIDS. Loss of normal nodal architecture as the immune system fails is marked by development of generalized lymphadenopathy with nodes that vary

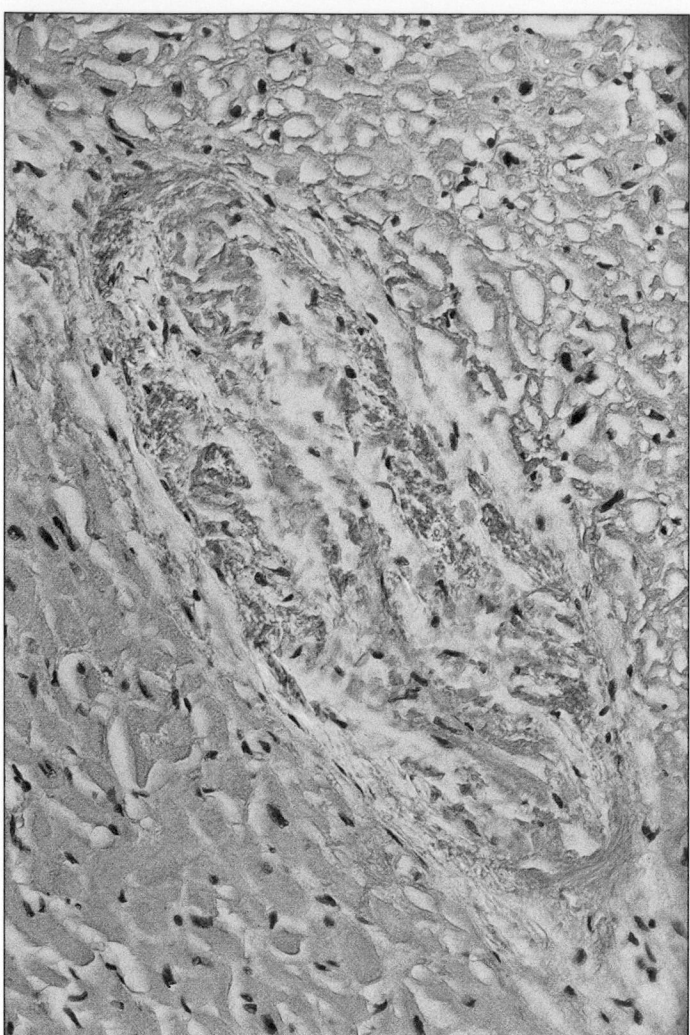

Fig. 4.3 Amyloid. When stained with Congo red and viewed under polarized light, the amyloid deposits in cardiac muscle demonstrate an apple-green birefringence.

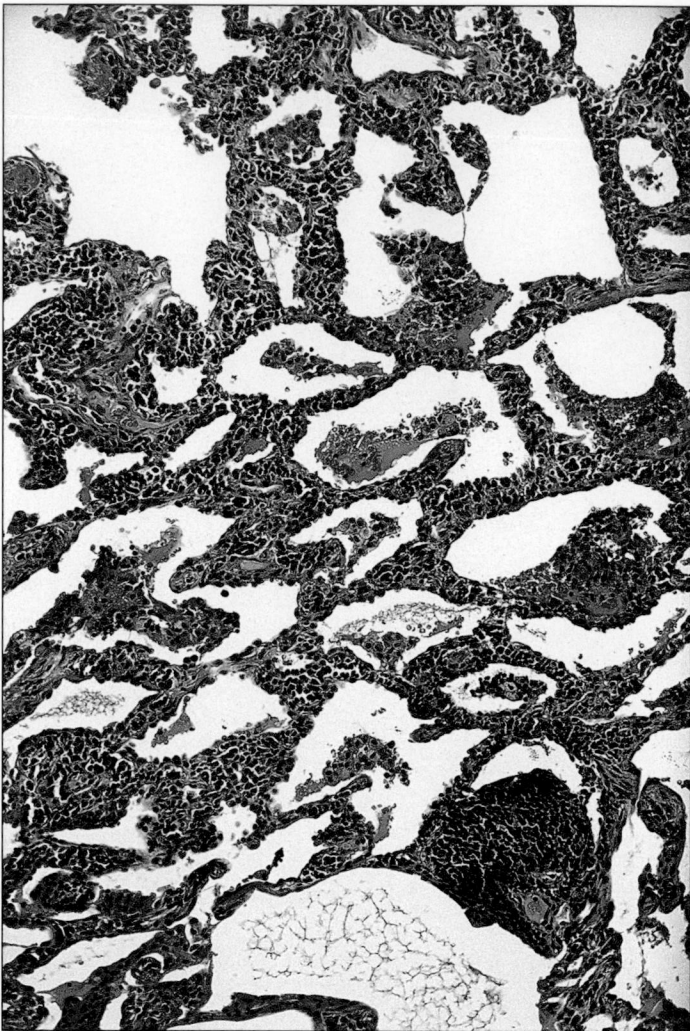

Fig. 4.4 Lymphoid interstitial pneumonitis (LIP). There is a diffuse interstitial infiltrate of lymphocytes, plasma cells, and histiocytes along with a small lymphoid aggregate.

in size over time but usually do not exceed 3 cm. This condition, called persistent generalized lymphadenopathy (PGL), appears in at least 25% of persons with AIDS.[40] HIVL can be grouped into four major patterns that follow in sequence and parallel the decline in CD4 lymphocytes.[41]

At least 10% of HIV-1 infected persons are 'long survivors' who show little or no marked progressive decline in immune function. In addition, their nodal architecture is maintained without either the hyperplasia or lymphocyte depletion common with progression to AIDS. Though peripheral blood mononuclear cells contain detectable HIV-1 and viral replication continues, their viral burden is low. Variations in cellular chemokine receptors may explain variability in progression of HIV.[42]

Lymphoid interstitial pneumonitis (LIP) is a diagnostic criterion for AIDS in childhood but is not frequently seen in adults. Peripheral blood may show plasmacytosis and eosinophilia. Diagnosis is made by open lung biopsy because bronchoscopic biopsies are frequently nondiagnostic.[43] The earliest microscopic finding is aggregates of lymphocytes and plasma cells in a bronchovascular distribution with minimal interstitial inflammation. In more advanced lesions, all lung

fields demonstrate a diffuse interstitial infiltrate of lymphocytes, plasma cells, and histiocytes (Fig. 4.4). Additional features can include lymphoid aggregates with germinal centers, intraluminal fibrosis, and increased alveolar macrophages. Advanced cases may demonstrate confluent pulmonary nodules several centimeters in size. Rarely, poorly formed granulomas may be present, but progressive pulmonary interstitial fibrosis is rare. Immunohistochemical staining will demonstrate a polyclonal cellular proliferation.[44]

Accompanying LIP may be a pattern of pulmonary lymphoid hyperplasia (PLH) characterized by lymphoid follicles with or without germinal centers that often surround bronchioles. The most florid form of lymphoid hyperplasia involving the lung in HIV-infected children is known as polyclonal B cell lymphoproliferative disorder (PBLD) in which there are nodular infiltrates of polyclonal B lymphocytes and CD8 cells. Other organs may be involved by PBLD.[45]

HIV infection of microglia and macrophages residing in the brain, particularly in patients with dementia, leads to a variety of changes seen on brain biopsy. Microscopic examination often reveals HIV encephalitis consisting of multiple foci with small macrophages, microglia, and multinucleated giant cells often seen

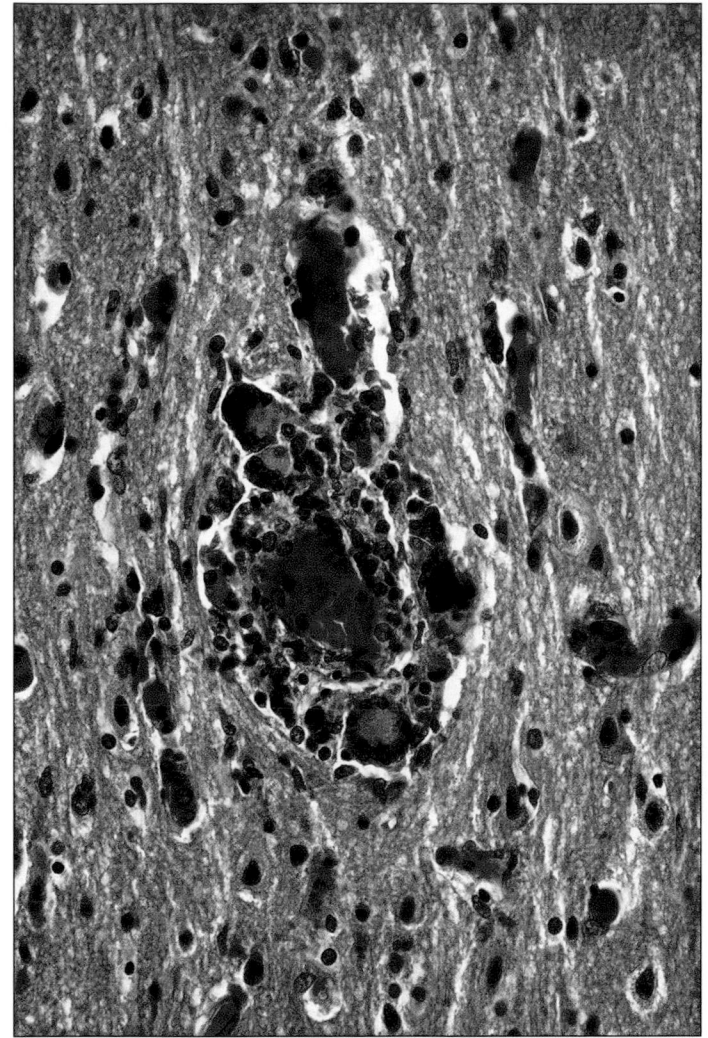

Fig. 4.5 HIV encephalitis. The cerebral cortex has perivascular inflammatory infiltrates containing prominent multinucleated cells.

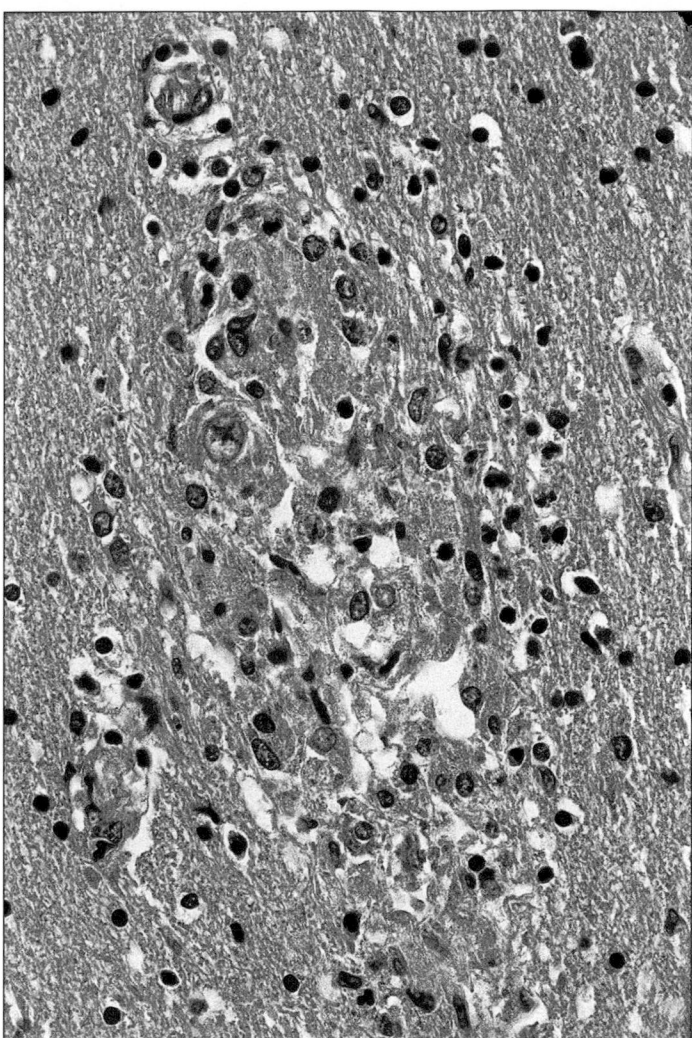

Fig. 4.6 HIV encephalitis. A microglial nodule contains plump reactive astrocytes and inflammatory cells, including macrophages.

near small blood vessels (Fig. 4.5). They appear less commonly scattered in the gray matter or leptomeninges. The multinucleated giant cells, often numerous, are the hallmark of HIV infection involving the CNS, and HIV can be demonstrated in their cytoplasm by immunocytochemistry.[46–48]

HIV leukoencephalopathy, which overlaps with HIV encephalitis, produces diffuse bilateral damage to cerebral and cerebellar white matter. Grossly, the lesions are similar to multiple sclerosis plaques. Microscopically, the predominantly perivascular lesions demonstrate myelin debris in macrophages, reactive astrocytosis, hemosiderin in macrophages, multinucleated giant cells, and little or no inflammation. Vacuolar myelin swellings can appear, as well as axonal damage. Oligodendroglial cells appear normal. Without the presence of multinucleated giant cells, the diagnosis depends upon the finding of HIV antigen in macrophages.[49]

Microglial nodules are frequent with HIV infection in both gray and white matter and are collections of plump reactive astrocytes and inflammatory cells, including macrophages (Fig. 4.6). They are often located near small capillaries that may have plump endothelial cells with nearby hemosiderin-laden macrophages. Sometimes the

macrophages can give rise to multinucleated cells. Small foci of necrosis may be seen in or near these nodules. Microglial nodules are not specific for HIV infection. Etiologic agents including fungi, cytomegalovirus inclusions, and *Toxoplasma gondii* organisms can sometimes be identified. Some microglial nodules contain HIV by immunohistochemical staining.[47,49]

Progressive multifocal leukoencephalopathy (PML) from human papovavirus infection (designated JC virus) targets myelin-producing oligodendrocytes. Cerebrospinal fluid analysis is typically normal, though some patients have mild protein elevations along with mononuclear cell pleocytosis and oligoclonal bands. PML affects primarily white matter along the gray–white junction with adjacent cortical gray matter, leading to focal areas of granularity a few millimeters in size that may coalesce. Microscopically, the lesions centered around capillaries demonstrate demyelination with perivascular monocytes, T cells, astrocytosis with bizarre or enlarged astrocytes (with occasional mitotic figures), and lipid-laden macrophages. At the periphery are large 'ballooned' oligodendrocytes that have enlarged 'ground-glass' nuclei containing JC viral antigen (Fig. 4.7) that can be identified with immunohistochemical

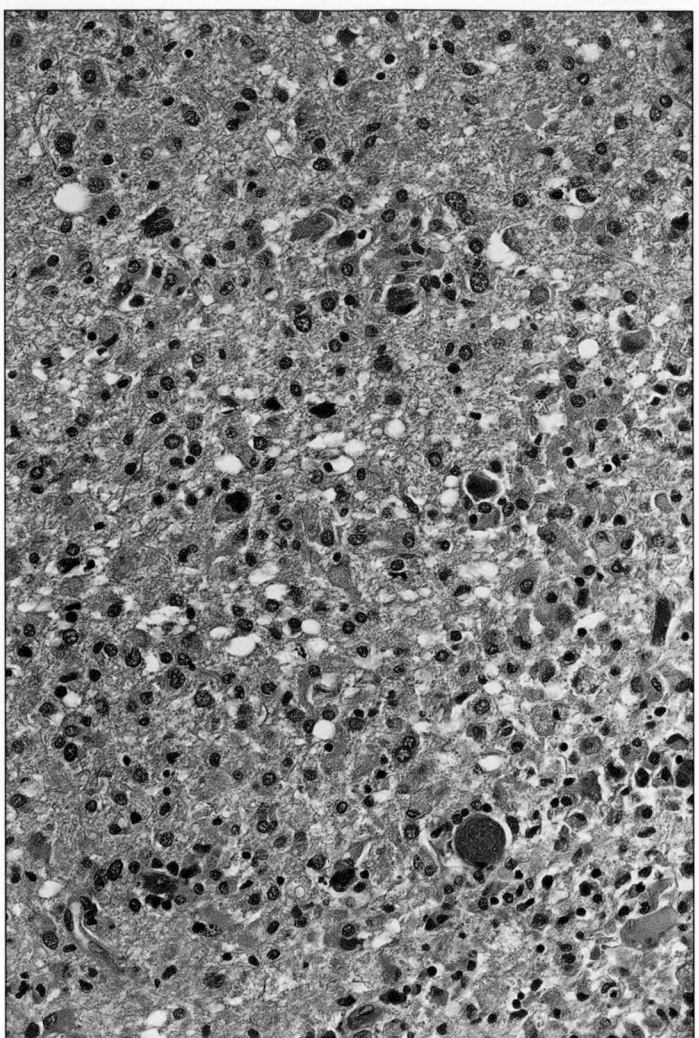

Fig. 4.7 Progressive multifocal leukoencephalopathy (PML). There is astrocytosis with bizarre astrocytes, macrophages, and several large oligodendrocytes that have ground-glass nuclei

staining. Multinucleated giant cells containing HIV may also be present.[50,51]

A variety of neoplasms are associated with HIV infection and AIDS. These are detailed in Table 4.3.[52–61]

MECHANISMS OF HUMAN ALLOGRAFT REJECTION

Although our understanding of mammalian immune regulation has been much more clearly defined in the last few years, the precise importance of various mechanisms underlying human allograft rejection is still open to considerable speculation. In humans, the ABO and HLA antigen systems play the most important roles in transplantation. The ABO system is the most important in solid organ transplantation, while the HLA system is the major determinant of bone marrow transplant success.[62] The following discussion summarizes the current state of our knowledge concerning allograft rejection with the above caveats in mind.

When an allograft is introduced, specific T-lymphocyte responses against the foreign histocompatibility (HLA) antigens of the donor are initiated. T cells recognize foreign HLA class II antigens and are activated to proliferate, differentiate, and secrete a panel of soluble growth differentiation factors called cytokines. These cytokines induce further expression of HLA class II antigens on grafted tissue, stimulate B lymphocytes to produce antibodies against determinants on the transplant, and facilitate the development of specific effector functions, including cytotoxicity and cytokine-mediated effector functions (similar to delayed hypersensitivity responses) mediated by CD4+ lymphocytes and macrophages. Damage to the allograft occurs by direct parenchymal injury or indirectly by vascular damage in the allograft leading to ischemic changes.[63–65]

HLA MOLECULES AND ANTIGEN RECOGNITION

Allograft rejection is based upon the major histocompatibility complex (MHC),[66] called the HLA (human leukocyte antigen) complex, which contains multiple genes in about 4000 kb on the short arm of chromosome 6 encoding class I molecules (HLA-A, -B, and -C and class I-like molecules HLA-F, -G, -H, and -J), and class II molecules (HLA-DP, -DQ, and -DR), which determine antigen recognition by T lymphocytes.[67] Class I molecules are constitutively expressed by most cells and tissues, most strongly by the vascular endothelium and lymphoid cells.[68] Class II molecules are constitutively expressed only by a small number of cell types, including B lymphocytes, monocytes, follicular dendritic cells, and capillary endothelial cells. However, class II antigen expression can be induced on a variety of cells by cytokines such as interferon-gamma (IFN-gamma) and tumor necrosis factor-alpha (TNF-alpha).[64,65,68,69]

Cells whose class II molecules are upregulated under such circumstances include activated T lymphocytes, endothelial cells, renal tubular epithelial cells, liver bile duct epithelial cells, and pancreatic beta cells. Direct T-cell recognition of alloantigen requires the expression of MHC molecules of the allograft and host along with the foreign peptide of the allograft.[69] Thus, the surfaces presented by foreign HLA peptide complexes to host T-cell receptors will be different in both the HLA molecules and the bound peptide. This property, coupled with the diversity of bound peptides, probably accounts for the high number of T lymphocytes that are stimulated by foreign HLA antigens.[70] The great polymorphism of MHC molecules expressed by a person expands the range of peptides that can be bound and broadens T-cell responsiveness. Class I and class II loci are highly polymorphic; most humans express six different molecules of each class. Thus, it is likely that unrelated humans will have different HLA types, and transplant rejection is an indirect consequence of the advantage to the species of having more HLA types so that the likelihood of encountering a pathogen against which all members of a population have a poor response generally decreases.[69,71] Foreign MHC antigens may also be recognized by host T lymphocytes as processed peptides, a mechanism called indirect presentation, which is especially important during chronic rejection. Soluble proteins, endocytosed by antigen presenting cells, then activates CD4 T lymphocytes. Minor MHC are thought to be exclusively recognized by this mechanism.[69,70]

IMMUNE ACTIVATION

Antigen-presenting cells (APCs) in the allograft, including dendritic reticulum cells, macrophages, and endothelial cells, are critical to the

Table 4.3 Neoplasms with AIDS

Neoplasm	Biology	Distribution	Features
Kaposi's sarcoma (KS)	Associated with human herpesvirus 8 infection. Spindle cells of KS have features of both endothelium and smooth muscle, with immunohistochemical staining for CD34, CD31, and/or Factor 8-related antigen. All KS lesions demonstrate positivity for vimentin.	Skin in virtually all cases; visceral organ involvement in up to 75% of cases	Proliferation of fusiform to epithelioid cells with eosinophilic cytoplasm and prominent round, oval, or fusiform nuclei. Helpful findings include individually necrotic cells, a mononuclear cell infiltrate, epithelioid cells, dilated irregular vascular spaces, and perivascular distribution. Red blood cells in the slit-like spaces, hemosiderin granules either free or within macrophages, and hyaline globules.
Non-Hodgkin's lymphoma, high-grade B-cell (small noncleaved) Burkitt-like lymphomas (in the REAL classification)	$1/3$ of AIDS lymphomas, called intermediate grade and classified as small noncleaved-cell (SNCLL) lymphomas (Burkitt or Burkitt-like) in working formulation classification. Demonstrate c-myc activation in all cases, p53 mutation in some cases, and Epstein-Barr virus (EBV) infection in a minority of cases.	Extranodal sites are common, including brain, GI tract, liver, and lungs. May also involve lymph nodes and bone marrow.	Cells have round nuclei, one or more prominent nucleoli, and scant cytoplasm and comprise diffuse sheets that form a discreet mass or irregularly infiltrate normal tissues without significant necrosis. Within sheets are uniformly distributed macrophages, and occasional mitoses. Plasmablastic features include eccentric nuclei and well-defined Golgi zone.
Non-Hodgkin's lymphoma, diffuse large B-cell lymphoma (in the REAL classification)	$2/3$ of AIDS lymphomas, which can be either large cell immunoblastic lymphomas or large noncleaved-cell lymphomas in working formulation classification. Arise from an expansion of EBV-infected B lymphocytes.	Nodal and extranodal sites can be involved, but brain involvement is not frequent.	Immunoblastic types have moderate to large amounts of cytoplasm with or without plasmacytic features of eccentric nuclei and basophilic cytoplasm, large round to oval nuclei, and prominent single nucleoli. Large cell types have less cytoplasm and nuclei with one or more peripheral nucleoli and finely dispersed chromatin. Necrosis is often prominent and mitoses frequent.
Primary body cavity-based lymphomas	Associated with human herpesvirus 8 infection, as well as c-myc and EBV infection	Appear as malignant pleural, pericardial, or peritoneal effusions	Are high-grade large cell lymphomas but often mark as null cells
Mucosa-associated lymphoid tissue (MALT) lesions	Appear to follow an indolent course in children. Unlike MALT lesions in other immunocompromised adults that regress when immune suppression is reduced, those in adults with AIDS have an aggressive course with a poor prognosis.	Extranodal sites such as the gastrointestinal tract, bronchi, and salivary glands	MALT lesions have been described in association with both adult and pediatric AIDS.
Cutaneous non-Hodgkin's lymphomas	Two types are seen with AIDS: CD30+ T-cell lymphomas and high-grade B-cell lymphomas.	Skin	Cutaneous T-cell lymphomas are like those in non-HIV-infected persons and often present as localized nodules that may spontaneously regress. Diffuse large B-cell cutaneous lymphomas may remain localized for months without extracutaneous spread, but do not regress.
Squamous dysplasias and carcinomas	Related to human papillomavirus (HPV) infection	In women, cervical squamous dysplasias and carcinomas. In men having sex with men, anal squamous dysplasias and carcinomas.	Squamous cell carcinomas are more likely to be multifocal and extensive with HIV infection.
Lung cancer	May not be a strong link with immunosuppression	Most are adenocarcinomas, but often stage III or IV	Not a diagnostic criterion for AIDS, but seen more frequently. Tend to occur at a younger median age than in the general population.
Hodgkin's disease	Shows an association with EBV infection	Compared to non-AIDS cases, are more likely to be stage III and IV, have a mixed cellularity or lymphocyte depletion histologic subtype, have numerous Reed-Sternberg cells, and have non-contiguous spread.	Not a diagnostic criterion for AIDS, but seen more frequently. Have an aggressive course. Tend to present earlier in the course of HIV infection than non-Hodgkin's lymphomas.
Smooth muscle tumors	Associated with EBV infection of smooth muscle cells	Both leiomyomas and leiomyosarcomas can occur	Most often seen in children, but can occur in adults

process of T-cell activation.[72,73] A full T-cell response (proliferation and differentiation) will only occur if T cells, in addition to the primary signal through their antigen specific receptor (TCR), also receive a secondary (accessory) signal provided by APCs. In humans, endothelial cells are potent APCs, providing MHC antigen recognition and accessory signaling. Since APCs derived from the allograft express MHC class II antigens, these cells can also directly activate CD4 TCR and the combination of the primary and accessory signal to CD4 lymphocytes leads to the production of interleukin-2 (IL-2), and to proliferation of CD4- and CD8-expressing cells.[64,69] Within seconds to minutes of their addition to T cells, alloantigens induce a variety of biochemical events that induce T cells to express higher affinity forms of IL-2 receptor, produce cytokines, proliferate, and differentiate. The initial events include activation of the calcium dependent calcineurin pathway, mitogen and stress-activated protein (MAP/SAP) kinase pathways, and the protein kinase C pathway. A single antigen-activated T cell can expand into a population of several hundred or thousand genetically identical cells bearing the same TCR, a phenomenon termed clonal expansion. The early consequences of T-cell activation also include expression of cytokines that act on a variety of cells, starting with IL-2.[73] A little later, IL-3 is produced and stimulates the proliferation of stem cells, which can in turn differentiate into granulocytes and macrophages. IFN-gamma and TNF-alpha are also produced, inducing APC activation, inflammation, and chemokine secretion. B-cell growth and the differentiation factors IL-4, IL-5, and IL-6 induce clonal expansion of B cells that have been stimulated by specific antigen, leading to the production of specific antibodies and activation of complement with acceleration of inflammation. After this burst of cytokine production, T cells divide under the influence of IL-2 and IL-4 and begin to assume different effector functions such as cytotoxicity.[74] Finally, a group of very late activation molecules is produced 7 to 14 days after stimulation. The CD4 subset of peripheral blood lymphocytes reacts preferentially with MHC class II molecules, whereas CD8 cells react preferentially with MHC class I molecules. These receptor–ligand pairs increase the avidity of interaction between the T cells and targets.[69,70, 73–77]

MECHANISMS OF EFFECTOR FUNCTION IN ALLOGRAFT REJECTION

SPECIFIC AND NONSPECIFIC CYTOTOXICITY

CD8+ cells can differentiate into cytotoxic cells that are specific for single cell surface antigens (cytotoxic T lymphocytes, or CTL). However, this process is triggered by recognition of MHC class I specificities in concert with the T cell receptor.[63–65,69,74,78–80] Such mature CTLs then specifically bind to their target tissue and deliver a lethal hit. Three potential mechanisms of this cytotoxicity are under investigation: pore formation in target cells produced by pore-forming proteins (perforin, granzyme A and B, fas ligand, and granulysin); release of cytokines such as TNF-alpha that enhance MHC class I expression on target cells, enhancing sensitivity; or release of proteolytic enzymes such as serine esterases that may damage the cell membrane directly or initiate apoptotic cell death.[64,65,69,78] Nonspecific cytotoxic cells such as macrophages and natural killer (NK) cells may bind to target parenchymal cells in the allograft via Fc receptors of specific IgG bound to such cells. Macrophages cause cytocidal activity via secretion of proteases. They also accelerate inflammation and repair. This mechanism,

known as antibody-dependent cell-mediated cytotoxicity, may be activated with or without participation of complement.[79,80]

CYTOKINE-MEDIATED EFFECTOR FUNCTION (DELAYED-TYPE HYPERSENSITIVITY)

CD4+ sensitized cells that have recognized the antigen on antigen-presenting cells or vascular endothelium in association with MHC class II molecules secrete cytokines (IL-1, IL-2), which recruit other CD4+ cells and recruit and activate macrophages and endothelial cells.[81,82] Graft destruction is then instigated by microvascular injury, ischemia, and macrophage cytotoxicity. Such mononuclear phagocytes are an essential component of graft inflammatory responses. They produce a variety of cytokines that amplify the immune response, including IFN-gamma, TNF-alpha, IL-1, IL-6 and degradative enzymes, reactive oxygen intermediaries and other free radicals such as nitrous oxide. IFN-gamma transforms blood-borne monocytes into mature tissue macrophages. IL-1 mobilizes polymorphonuclear leukocytes (particularly eosinophils) and acts as a potent fibroblast-activating factor.[83,84]

IFN-gamma and IL-1 produced by activated endothelial cells, which in addition produce platelet activating factor (PAF), amplify the inflammatory consequences of cytokine-mediated reactions.[81–83] IL-1, IL-2, IL-4, IL-5, IL-6, IFN-gamma, and TNF have all been found in rejection allografts as opposed to nonrejection allografts. The expression of these factors in infection as opposed to rejection has not been described.[84–86] IL-2 and IL-2 receptor also appear in the blood and urine during acute rejection. Studies have evaluated the diagnostic utility using serum enzyme-linked immunosorbent assays and found no significant value because levels are similarly elevated in the presence of infection of the allograft.[87]

ANTIBODY-MEDIATED EFFECTOR FUNCTION

Specific sensitization of CD4+ cells and generation of IL-2, IL-4, and IL-5 promote B-cell differentiation and generation of antigraft antibodies, which can promote graft destruction via antibody-dependent cell-mediated cytotoxicity or complement-mediated cytotoxicity, or both mechanisms.[88] Activation of mononuclear phagocytes leads to activation of the arachidonic acid pathway, leading to thrombocyte aggregation and accumulation. Finally, such activation also leads to activation of the extrinsic coagulation pathway via tissue factor. These effects ultimately lead to vascular endothelial injury, fibroblast proliferation, and occlusive vasculopathy with tissue ischemia. The contribution of these factors to chronic rejection is therefore very important.[79,80,89,90]

PATHOLOGIC MANIFESTATIONS OF ACUTE ALLOGRAFT REJECTION

ACUTE CELLULAR REJECTION OF ALLOGRAFTS

The most common manifestation of allograft rejection is the infiltration of the allograft by large numbers of activated lymphocytes (accompanied by macrophages) infiltrating parenchymal structures of the allograft, such as the kidney tubules, the cardiac myocytes, the bronchioles, or the bile ducts.[91–94] The lymphoid infiltrate may be

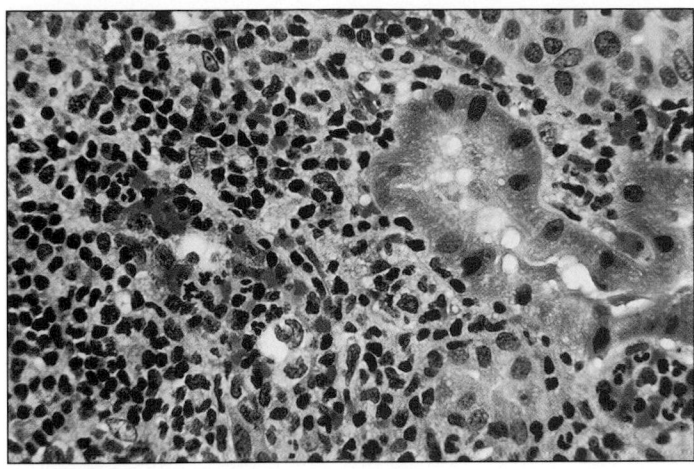

Fig. 4.8 Renal biopsy with acute cellular rejection and lymphoid cells invading the renal tubules.

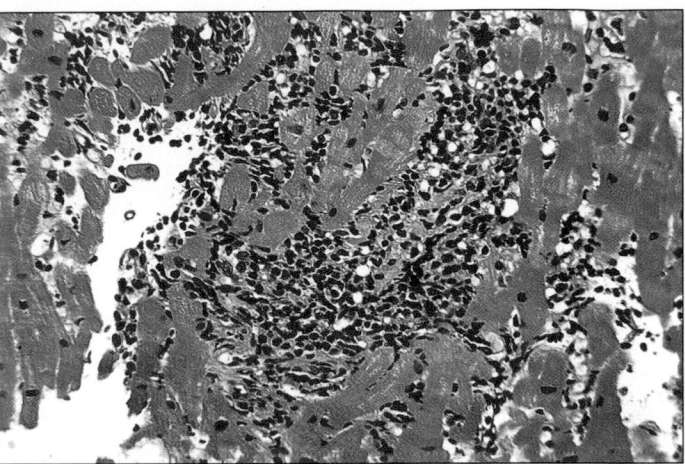

Fig. 4.9 Cardiac biopsy illustrating moderate cellular rejection (ISHLT grade 3A) with architectural distortion of myocytes by infiltrates with prominent lymphoid cells and inconspicuous macrophages. The distorted arrangement of myocytes indicates myocyte damage.

accompanied by small numbers of other inflammatory cells such as neutrophils or eosinophils. The process of acute cellular rejection in bone marrow is not often appreciated pathologically and is manifested by lack of adequate numbers of leukocytes in the circulation and of precursor cells in the marrow.[95] The pathologic features of allograft rejection are illustrated in Figures 4.8 to 4.10.

Since the infiltrating cells arrive in the allograft via the blood, adherence and penetration of the capillaries, arterioles, and venules by lymphoid cells is often considered a part of the rejection process.[96–98] The notable exception to recognition of this involvement of the microvasculature in the rejection process is the pathologic classification of acute rejection in the heart.[99] In other solid organ allografts, endothelialitis (endothilitis) is a well-recognized part of acute rejection, making the diagnosis of significant allograft rejection more certain. In the kidney the involvement of arteries or arterioles is found in 50% of acute cellular rejection, is designated

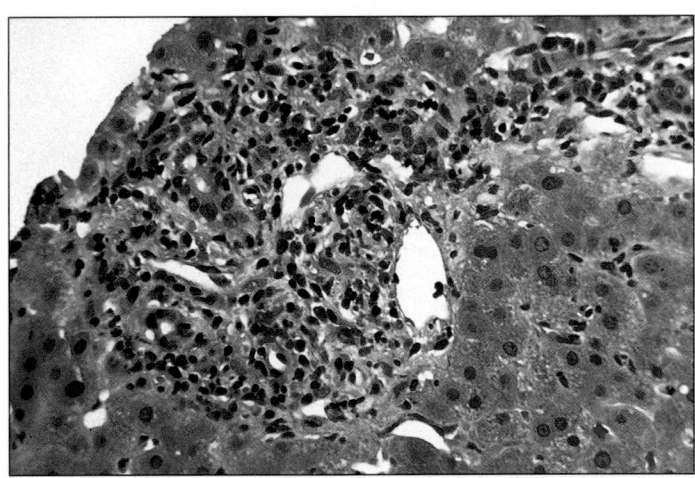

Fig. 4.10 Liver biopsy illustrating moderate cellular rejection based upon endothelialitis (only one adherent is seen) and a mixed infiltrate of lymphoid cells and eosinophils, seen in >50% of portal triads. Parenchyma at the lower right is unaffected.

Table 4.4 Acute cellular rejection features

Organ	Primary target	Endothelial target	Differential diagnosis
Kidney	Tubular epithelial cells	Microvasculature, arterioles (50% of acute rejection involves arterioles)	Infection, ischemia, cyclosporine toxicity, acute tubular damage, interstitial nephritis
Heart	Myocytes	None specified as part of process; arteriolitis rarely seen on biopsy	Ischemia, biopsy site artifact, Quilty lesion, infection
Liver	Bile duct epithelium	Venulitis of portal and central veins; endothelialitis secures diagnosis of rejection	Hepatitis, drug toxicity, bile duct obstruction, sepsis, ischemia, hyperalimentation toxicity
Lung	Bronchioles, alveolar lining cells	Arteriolitis/venulitis necessary for diagnosis of moderate rejection	Infection, BALT, biopsy site, ischemia
Pancreas	Acini and ductal epithelium	Venulitis; arteriolitis is diagnostic for moderate vascular rejection	Infection, ischemia
Bone marrow (GVHD)	Keratinocytes, intestinal lining cells, bile duct epithelium, salivary glands	None known	Chemotherapy, radiation effects

GVHD, graft-versus-host disease; BALT, bronchus-associated lymphoid tissue

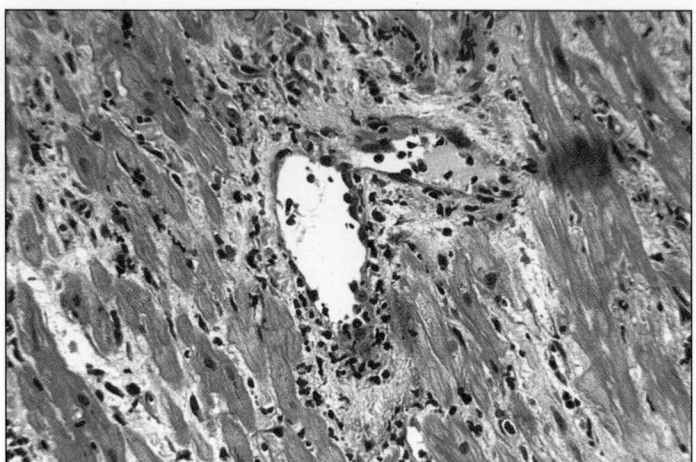

Fig. 4.11 Cardiac biopsy showing moderate vascular rejection with lymphoid cells infiltrating a venule (venulitis), along with interstitial edema, but no appreciable cellular rejection.

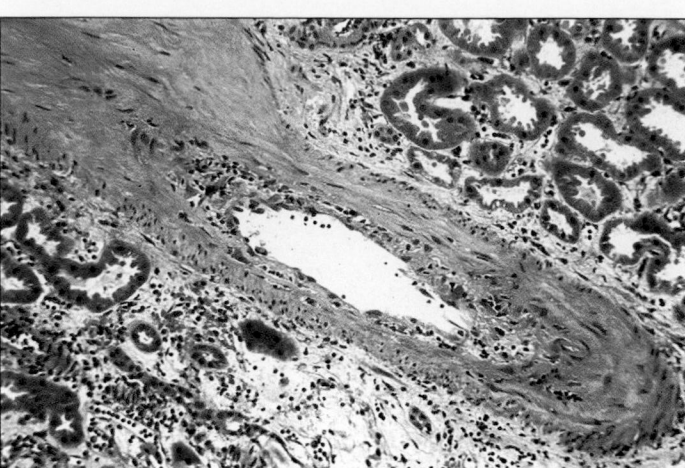

Fig. 4.13 Renal biopsy with obvious vasculitis involving an interlobular artery.

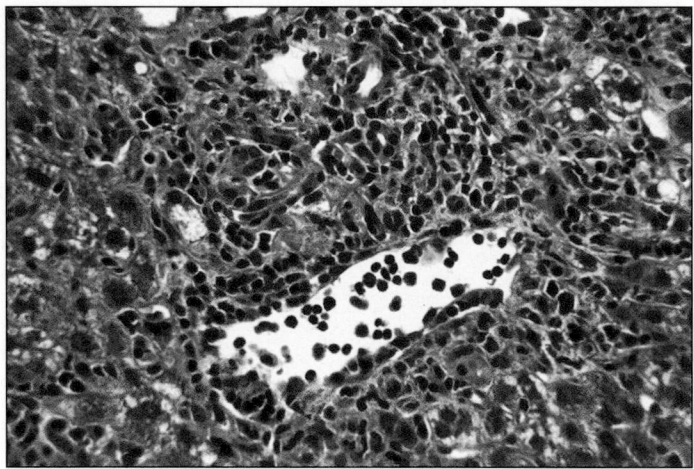

Fig. 4.12 Liver biopsy showing lymphoid cells infiltrating beneath endothelium. Endothelialitis is commonly identified involving veins and arterioles.

as a pathognomonic feature, and is considered a poor prognostic feature.[96] In the liver, the endothelialitis involving venules is necessary to exclude other causes of inflammation of portal regions.[100] Table 4.4 illustrates the differences in the rejection findings in various solid organ allografts. Figures 4.11 to 4.13 illustrate the pathologic features in heart, kidney, and liver allografts.

The major differential diagnosis of allograft rejection is infiltration by lymphocytes for other reasons, such as renal tubular epithelial infection.[101] In the heart, lymphocytes are very uncommon, and are only found, associated with scarring, at the sites of previous biopsy or associated with ischemic damage related to transplantation.[102] In the lung, bronchiolar and interstitial inflammation is also associated with pulmonary infections such as pneumonia.[103] In liver allografts, a portal infiltrate of lymphocytes is nonspecific.[104]

For each type of allograft, the rules for grading rejection are somewhat different, but all depend on an evaluation of the extent and severity of the lymphocytic infiltration process determined by the amount of associated parenchymal damage. Grading schemes

for the various allografts are given in Tables 4.5 to 4.10, and the reader is referred to the references for further information.[97–106]

ACUTE ANTIBODY-MEDIATED REJECTION OF ALLOGRAFTS

Hyperacute rejection

In virtually all allografts, deposition of preformed alloantibody directed against the graft on the microvascular endothelium of the newly ingrafted organ can occur. Such rejection responses are usually rapid and occur in situations in which the recipient has circulating alloantibodies at the time of transplantation, typically against HLA antigens of the donor.[107,108] Donors and recipients are HLA typed prior to allografting, and cross-matches are performed to detect reactivity of recipients' serum antibodies directed against donor peripheral blood cells as antigens. These procedures are common for kidney transplants, but cardiac and lung transplant recipients are often transplanted before cross-match results are available because of the short length of time that hearts and lungs can be perfused prior to transplantation. Patients with circulating levels of panel-reactive antibodies greater than 20% are very likely to have positive cross-matches to many donors and are therefore prospectively cross-matched to prevent hyperacute rejection.[109] This makes the availability of organs much more limited for these patients. Liver transplant recipients rarely experience hyperacute rejection even in the presence of a positive cross-match, although hyperacute rejection has been reported. The cause of this resistance to hyperacute rejection is unknown, but it may relate to the availability of Kupffer cells to process large amounts of antigen-antibody complexes.[100,110]

The non-specific pathology of hyperacute rejection depends on the time after transplant at which a biopsy is performed and how it is examined. Often, the organ is not biopsied and is received by the surgical pathologist as an explanted organ or is examined only at post-mortem examination. Gross descriptions of the events by the surgeon may provide important clues to the correct diagnosis. Often, the organ immediately appears well perfused and pink, after which it suddenly blanches and ceases to function. Attempts during surgery to improve graft perfusion are usually unsuccessful. In the case of

Table 4.5 Grading schema for acute rejection of kidney allografts

Grade	Banff designation	Description
Normal	g0, i0, t0, v0	No infiltrates or minimal ones; no tubulitis
Suspicious for rejection	g0, i1, t1, v0	Focal tubulitis and interstitial inflammation with < 4 cells/ infiltrated tubule
Mild rejection IA	g0-1, i2, t2, v0	Infiltrate of lymphocytes occupying >25% of cortex with moderate tubulitis (>4 cells/tubule)
Mild rejection IB	g0-1, i2, t3, v0	Infiltrate of lymphocytes occupying >25% of cortex and severe tubulitis (10 cells/tubule)
Moderate rejection IIA	g1-2, i1-3, t1-3, v1	Mild to moderate arteritis of at least one artery; infiltrate of lymphocytes occupying variable extent of cortex; variable tubulitis
Moderate rejection IIB	g1-2, i1-3, t1-3, v2	Severe intimal arteritis with at least 25% luminal narrowing in one artery; variable infiltrate and tubulitis
Severe rejection III Probably a manifestation of accelerated antibody mediated rejection	g1-3, i1-3, t1-3, v3	Transmural arteritis and/or fibrinoid necrosis of arterial wall; variable interstitial infiltrate and tubulitis
Antibody mediated rejection Hyperacute (immediate–hours) Accelerated rejection (delayed–days/weeks)	g1-3, i0-1, t0-1, v0-3	Findings related to time post transplant; interstitial edema, hemorrhage, arterial thrombosis, glomerular thrombosis; immunofluorescence will show Ig, C(esp C4d) and Fibrin in vessels, including microvascular capillaries and arteries

g = glomerulopathy score; i = interstitial infiltrate score; t = tubulitis score; v = vasculitis score; Ig = immunglobulin; C = complement components
Adequacy of biopsy for interpretation: 2 cores with 10 glomeruli and 2 arteries; minimally adequate: 1 core with 7 glomeruli and 1 artery.

Table 4.6 Grading schema for acute rejection of heart allografts

Grade	ISHLT designation	Description
No rejection	0	No rejection
Focal mild	1A	One focus of interstitial lymphocytes in one fragment
Diffuse mild	1B	Diffuse infiltrate of lymphocytes in one or more pieces
Focal moderate	2	One focus of space-occupying lymphoid infiltrate with architecturally distorting myocyte damage
Multifocal moderate	3A	Multiple foci of space-occupying infiltrates of lymphocytes causing architectural distortion of myocytes with myocyte damage
Borderline severe	3B	Diffuse space-occupying infiltrates of lymphocytes in >75% of area
Severe	4	Polymorphic infiltrate of lymphocytes and neutrophils associated with edema, hemorrhage, and vasculitis
Antibody mediated rejection (microvascular rejection)	Not recognized by ISHLT system; 0	Interstitial edema, endothelial activation with/without capillaritis, arteritis. Immunofluorescence demonstrates Ig and C within capillaries; fibrin accumulation in longstanding or severe cases.

ISHLT, International Society for Heart and Lung Transplantation. Ig = immunglobulin; C = complement components
Adequacy of biopsy for interpretation: 4–6 pieces for myocardium, each containing at least 50% evaluable myocardium; 2 pieces considered minimal for evaluation with disclaimer that if negative, rejection cannot be ruled out; 1 piece considered inadequate for interpretation.

Table 4.7 Grading schema for acute cellular rejection of liver allografts

Grade	Description
No rejection	No significant mixed infiltrates in portal triads
Indeterminate	Mixed infiltrate of lymphocytes and eosinophils in portal triads which fails to meet criteria for rejection
Mild rejection	Mixed infiltrate of lymphocytes and eosinophils in <50% of portal triads; bile duct damage, with/without endothelialitis of venules and central veins. RAI <4
Moderate rejection	Mixed infiltrate involving >50% of triads with/without endothelialitis of venules. RAI 4-6
Severe rejection	As above for moderate, with spillover into periportal areas and moderate to severe perivenular inflammation that extends into the hepatic parenchyma and is associated with perivenular hepatic necrosis. RAI > 6
Antibody mediated rejection	Criteria not defined; ischemic hepatic necrosis and arterial thrombosis are seen in hyperacute rejection

RAI, Rejection Activity Index, similar to scoring for chronic hepatitis, utilizing component scores for portal inflammation, bile duct inflammation and damage, and venous endothelial damage.
Adequacy of biopsy for interpretation: core biopsy with at least 5 triads.

Table 4.8 Grading schema for acute cellular rejection of lung allografts

Grade	ISHLT designation	Description
Minimal rejection	A1	Perivenular lymphoid infiltrates
Mild rejection	A2	Perivascular infiltrates of lymphocytes and eosinophils with endothelialitis and bronchiolitis
Moderate rejection	A3	Perivascular and alveolar infiltrates including neutrophils, endothelialitis, endothelial hyperplasia
Severe	A4	Confluent diffuse infiltrates with vasculitis and alveolar damage, necrosis, and hemorrhage
Lymphoid bronchitis	B1[a]	Lymphocytic infiltration of bronchi
Lymphoid bronchiolitis	B2[a]	Lymphocytic infiltration of terminal and respiratory bronchioles

ISHLT = International Society for Heart and Lung Transplantation
[a] B lesions are not part of acute rejection; these lesions may be precursors to chronic rejection.

Table 4.9 Grading schema for acute cellular rejection of pancreatic allografts

Grade	Designation	Description
Normal	Grade 0	Normal pancreatic histology
Borderline	Grade 1	Changes consisting of rare lymphocytic septal infiltrates while the acinar parenchyma is free of inflammation
Mild	Grade 2	Mixed inflammatory septal infiltrates with focal involvement of acinar parenchyma (ductal inflammation and/or venulitis are often seen)
Moderate	Grade 3	Septal inflammation with multifocal involvement of acinar parenchyma associated with single-cell injury, such as vacuolization, necrosis, or apoptosis
Moderate, vascular	Grade 4	Moderate rejection with arterial endotheliitis or vasculitis
Severe	Grade 5	Extensive inflammatory infiltrates with confluent acinar necrosis

Table 4.10 Features of chronic allograft rejection

Organ	Incidence at 5 years	Organ-specific features	Common features
Kidney	Up to 40%	Renal tubular atrophy, glomerulopathy	Arteriopathy, interstitial fibrosis
Heart	25–60%	Ischemic cardiomyopathy; acute myocardial infarction	Arteriopathy, interstitial fibrosis
Liver	3–17%	Portal ductopenia	Arteriopathy, interstitial fibrosis
Lung	28% (single) 45% (double)	Bronchiolitis obliterans	Arteriopathy, interstitial fibrosis
Pancreas	30–70%	Acinar loss	Arteriopathy, interstitial fibrosis

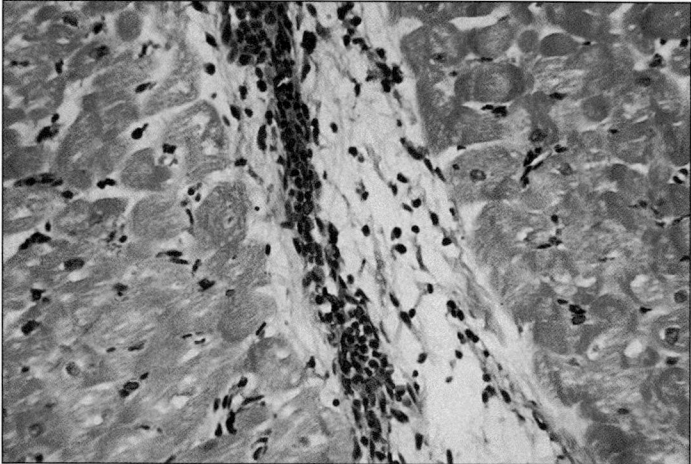

Fig. 4.14 Cardiac biopsy demonstrating significant interstitial edema associated with hyperacute rejection. There is marked endothelial activation and adhesion of leukocytes and platelets to the endothelium.

kidney allografts the organ is removed, but in liver, lung, or cardiac allografts, circulatory support for the allograft is often undertaken because the consequence of removal is a need for immediate retransplantation.

Microscopically, humorally mediated hyperacute rejection shows a paucity of findings, with interstitial edema and hemorrhage, and perhaps margination of neutrophils in capillaries and venules, being seen. If the process is prolonged, the allograft will show evidence of ischemia with parenchymal necrosis. Occasionally, thrombosis is seen. If frozen tissue is available, the allograft may be examined immunocytochemically to detect antibody and associated complement attached to capillaries, venules, and arterioles.[110,111] Fibrin may or may not be present in the vessels and interstitium, depending on the duration of the post-transplant period. The mechanism of such responses is well characterized in animal models. Antibody is deposited on the vascular endothelium, which is rich in the HLA antigen(s) to which the antibody is directed. This deposited antibody fixes complement components that attract neutrophils and promote tissue damage and destruction of the vessel walls. Such antibody and complement deposition also leads to elaboration of cytokines by the vascular endothelium, which aggravates the damage by increased inflammatory responses. The result of this reaction is the destruction of the microcirculation of the allograft, leading to ischemic damage and allograft loss.[88,96,100,103,111,112] An example of the vascular manifestation of hyperacute cardiac rejection is shown in Figure 4.14.

Accelerated antibody-mediated rejection

Antibody-mediated (humoral) reactions in allografts are uncommon. Though recipients may lack high levels of circulating antibodies at

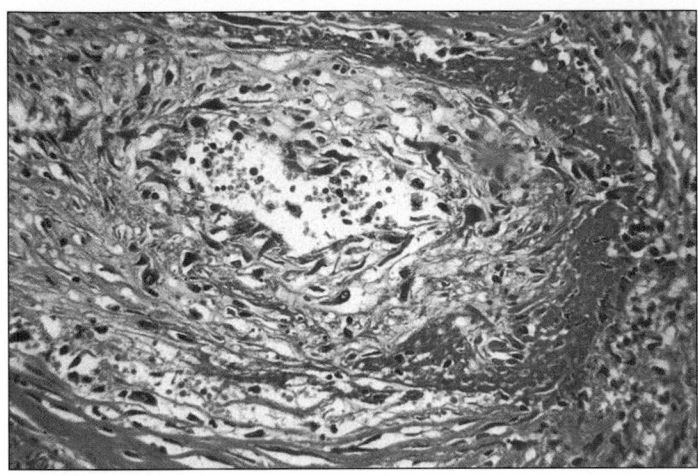

Fig. 4.15 Kidney biopsy shows arterial fibrinoid necrosis associated with severe accelerated rejection.

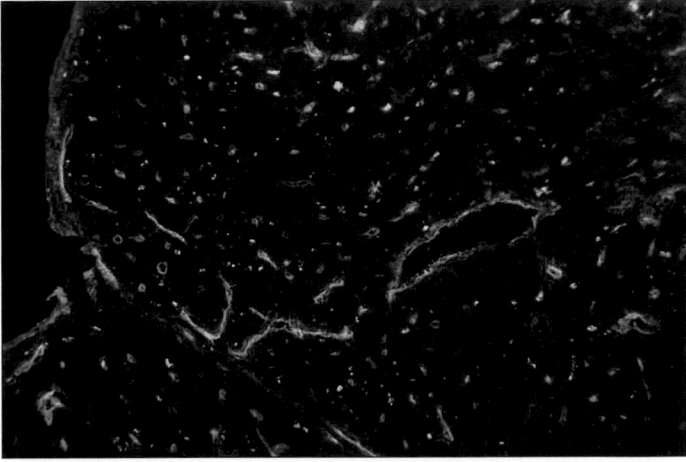

Fig. 4.16 Cardiac biopsy demonstrating vascular (humoral) rejection with vascular deposition of C4d by immunofluorescence. There was also positive staining with antibody to HLA-DR, IgG, and C3.

the time of transplantation, they develop them later in response to the massive antigen shedding from the microvascular endothelium that takes place shortly after transplantation as a result of perfusion and storage-related ischemia. Complement activation is a prominent feature of ischemic injury and serves to accelerate the inflammatory response whether or not antigen antibody complexes are formed.[88] Alternatively, these antibodies may accumulate slowly and may damage the allograft in a more subtle fashion. Common immunosuppressive regimens do not effectively modulate alloantibody responses or complement activation. Microscopically, such rejection reactions resemble vasculitis or capillaritis, because they are manifested by adherence to and penetration of vascular walls by neutrophils, eosinophils, macrophages, and lymphocytes and are associated with endothelial injury and fibrinoid necrosis of vascular walls.[99,110,113] Immunocytochemically, in frozen sections of the allograft, the humoral nature of the process is demonstrated by the finding of immunoglobulin and complement components especially C4d within the microvasculature.[112,113] In kidney transplants, immunoglobulin deposits within the peritubular capillaries are difficult to discriminate and the diagnosis rests on the finding of C4d within these vessels or the finding of fibrinoid necrosis of arteries and arterioles; in cardiac vessels, deposits are found in the microvasculature. Figures 4.15 and 4.16 illustrate the pathologic features of accelerated rejection in renal and cardiac allografts.

CHRONIC ALLOGRAFT VASCULOPATHY (CHRONIC REJECTION)

The long-term survival of solid organ allografts is compromised by the development of chronic vasculopathy, a form of chronic rejection in which large arteries are slowly narrowed by concentric intraluminal fibrosis.[114–116] This process develops slowly over time and eventually results in allograft loss due to vascular compromise. In cardiac transplantation, up to 10% of patients develop allograft vasculopathy each year after transplantation. Ultimately, chronic rejection causes allograft loss in most long-surviving transplant recipients. In each allograft the consequences of allograft vasculopathy are those of chronic ischemic damage, although the pathologic manifestations are organ specific.[117–119]

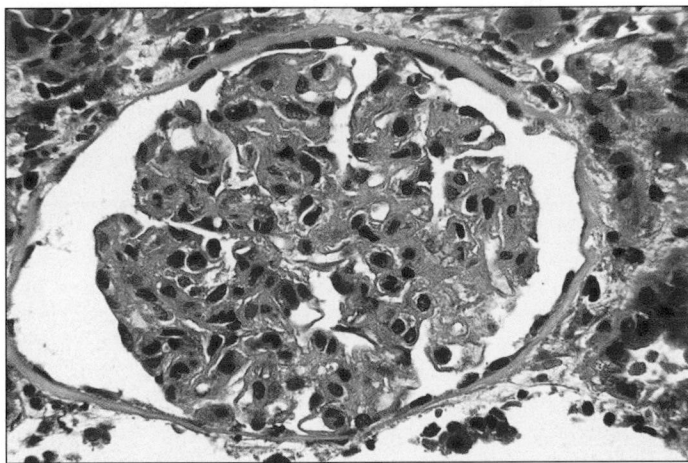

Fig. 4.17 Kidney biopsy with glomerulopathy of chronic allograft rejection. The biopsy also showed interstitial fibrosis and tubular atrophy as well as arterial fibrous proliferation.

KIDNEY ALLOGRAFTS

In kidney allografts chronic vascular nephropathy or chronic rejection is characterized by proliferative vasculopathy which involves the arteries and arterioles of the kidney. Arteries have concentric subintimal fibrosis without reduplication of the elastic lamina and infiltration by macrophages and lymphocytes, a pattern reminiscent of malignant hypertensive vascular changes. The kidney parenchyma shows ischemic damage with patchy interstitial fibrosis, tubular damage and atrophy, and periglomerular fibrosis, in descending order of frequency. Glomeruli commonly show collapse of tufts and may display a prominent glomerulopathy with marked reduplication of capillary membranes and slight increase in mesangial matrix, which is non-specific. The extent of reduplication of capillary basement membranes is usually greater in allograft vasculopathy than in recurrent glomerulonephritis.[115,116] (Fig. 4.17) The principal differential diagnosis is cyclosporine nephrotoxicity, which may

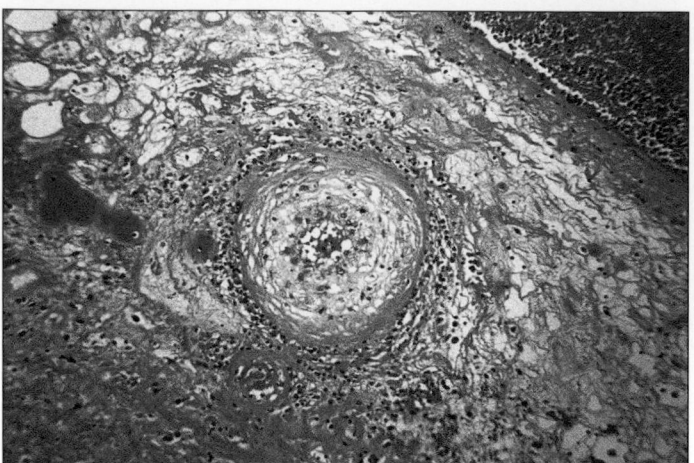

Fig. 4.18 A coronary artery at autopsy has prominent concentric subintimal fibrosis 10 months after transplant. The patient died from acute myocardial infarction.

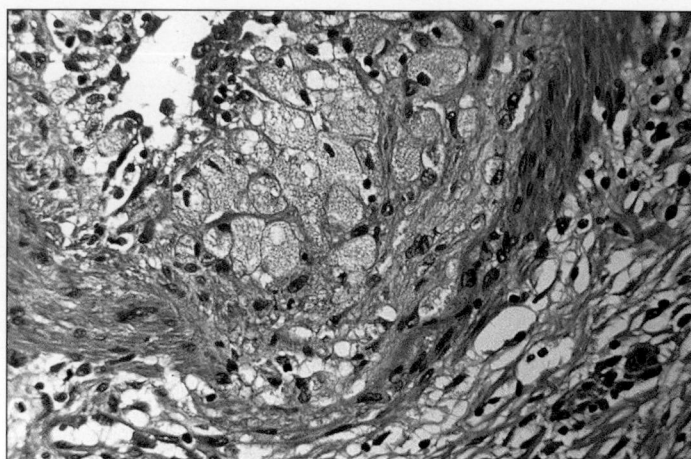

Fig. 4.19 A section of liver from autopsy with chronic rejection shows subintimal fibrosis and fat-laden macrophages within the wall of a central artery.

produce a similar vasculopathic lesion that can occur earlier after transplantation and is associated with significantly more acute tubular damage. Tacrolimus, another macrolide immunosuppressive agent, can also produce vasculopathy.[120–122]

HEART ALLOGRAFTS

The chronic rejection process in cardiac allografts produces progressive, uniform concentric narrowing of coronary vessels. Patients eventually develop heart failure and allograft loss or die of acute painless myocardial infarction or arrhythmia. The grafts show concentric subintimal fibrosis (Fig. 4.18) associated with infiltration of the arterial wall by lymphocytes and macrophages. Accumulation of lipid-laden macrophages is not a feature. On endomyocardial biopsy, the features of ischemic damage are irregular hypertrophy, interstitial scarring, and myocyte vacuolization. These features are not specific but are highly suggestive.[99,111]

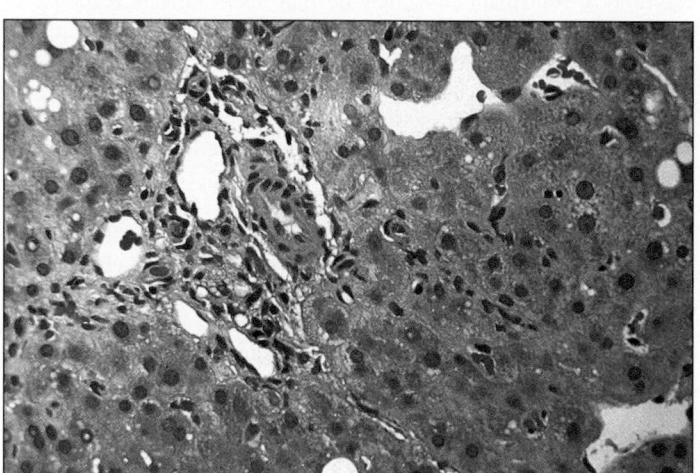

Fig. 4.20 Vanishing bile duct syndrome accompanied the vascular findings shown in Figure 4.19. A shrunken portal tract lacks a bile ductule.

LIVER ALLOGRAFTS

Chronic rejection or vasculopathy is evidenced by clinical findings of progressive liver failure. The vasculopathic lesions are known as obliterative endarteritis, are seen only in the larger arteries of the liver, and are not found in needle biopsies. Histologically, lipid-laden macrophages or fibrosis accumulate in the subendothelial area of the vessel, with subsequent narrowing and occlusion. Grossly, the vessel may be yellow because of the accumulated lipid (Fig. 4.19). The obliterative endarteritis leads to central hepatic parenchymal ischemic changes with ballooning degeneration and eventual confluent dropout of hepatic cells. Multinucleated giant hepatic cells indicate regenerative activity. Lipochrome is prominent. Central fibrosis and collapse may be seen; only rarely does micronodular cirrhosis occur. A rare type of chronic hepatic ischemic damage, thought to follow episodes of acute cellular rejection, is vanishing bile duct syndrome, which is characterized by complete absence of bile ducts in the portal triads. The portal triads appear fibrous, and no significant inflammatory infiltrate is present (Fig. 4.20). Vanishing

bile duct syndrome is occasionally reversible if not accompanied by vascular insufficiency.[123–125]

LUNG ALLOGRAFTS

In lung allografts, chronic rejection is chiefly manifested by chronic interstitial fibrosis and obliterative bronchiolitis as a consequence of ischemic damage produced by large vessel vasculopathy.[126–131] This process appears to develop through a sequence of epithelial injury leading to submucosal scarring and finally total obliteration of both membranous and respiratory bronchioles. This fibrotic scarring process may be eccentric or concentric, with a residual lumen in the early stages.[130] Ultimately, the airway lumen is totally obliterated by fibrous tissue. The smooth muscle layers of the bronchioles may be destroyed by extension of the fibrous tissue into the peribronchiolar interstitium, associated with mononuclear cell infiltration of all layers of the bronchiolar wall in the active phase. Epithelial damage with lymphocytic infiltration may be present, in addition to the fibrosis.[131]

Alternatively, the epithelium may be ulcerated, with subepithelial granulation tissue growing into the lumen in a polyploid fashion prior to scarring. During the active phase of obliterative bronchiolitis, perivascular infiltrates are noted in the adjacent parenchyma. In lung biopsies, bronchiolar scarring may only be evident on elastic stains demonstrating proximity of the fibrosed structure to the pulmonary arterioles and delineating the extent of luminal narrowing by submucosal fibrosis.[103,130] Extensive patchy peribronchiolar fibrosis associated with destruction of the smooth muscle may result in extrinsic compression of the lumen in a constrictive form of obliterative bronchiolitis. Features of chronic rejection are a frequent occurrence in nontransplant patients with immunologic lung disease, including collagen vascular diseases, and in bone marrow transplant recipients who have experienced graft-versus-host disease (GVHD).[126–131]

PANCREAS ALLOGRAFTS

There is severe acinar inflammation, acinar fibrosis, and vascular luminal narrowing with chronic rejection. This correlates significantly with a poor outcome. Acute and chronic vascular thrombosis in large and small vessels may commonly be seen any time following transplantation, but the appearance of chronic organized thrombosis is strongly associated with chronic rejection.[106]

GRAFT-VERSUS-HOST DISEASE

Graft-versus-host disease (GVHD) in bone marrow transplant (BMT) recipients is a syndrome of dermatitis, panenteritis, hepatitis, scleroderma, and immunodeficiency that results from allogeneic donor lymphoid cells which attack recipient epidermis, bowel epithelium, and liver cells. The precise immunologic mechanisms are poorly understood, but the severity of GVHD is clearly linked to the degree of HLA mismatch between donor and recipient. Direct damage to recipient lymphocytes in sites such as the thymus results in immunodeficiency.[132,133] Apoptosis of skin, gut, and bile duct epithelium results from direct cytotoxicity or indirectly through cytokine-mediated damage. Recent studies suggest that IL-1 and TNF play an important role in this process.[134,135]

Acute GVHD is a triad of dermatitis, enteritis, and hepatitis occurring within the first several weeks after BMT. Pathologically, the lesions are composed of individual or groups of apoptotic parenchymal cells accompanied by minimal to moderate lymphocytic infiltrates. In the skin, bulla formation occurs in moderately severe cases and progresses to total epidermal loss. Without serial biopsies, the lesions are difficult to distinguish from erythema multiforme, early herpetic skin infections, direct acute toxicity of chemotherapy or radiation, or lichen planus. In the gut, the lesions consist of apoptotic crypt cells with associated lymphoid infiltration. Eventually, crypt abscesses develop associated with lamina propria edema. Complete epithelial necrosis can occur, with fatal bleeding. In the liver, apoptosis in bile duct epithelial cells leads to cholestatic hepatitis, with eventual hepatocellular and cholangiolar cholestasis and hepatocytolysis. Endothelialitis can be seen but is not common, leading to diagnostic difficulties in distinguishing hepatic GVHD from chronic active hepatitis, cytomegalovirus hepatitis, and veno-occlusive disease occurring as a result of chemotherapy or radiation toxicity. Oral mucositis caused by chemotherapy or radiotherapy, or both, clouds interpretation of mucositis for up to about 30 days after transplant.[136–141]

Chronic GVHD occurring 80 to 100 days after transplant involves autoimmunity superimposed on immunodeficiency. The skin, the most frequently involved organ, has lesions resembling lichen planus and hypertrophic lupus erythematosus. Active GVHD is diagnosed based on findings of epithelial cell necrosis (basal layer vacuolar degeneration or rare eosinophilic bodies even without inflammatory cells) around appendages or in the epidermis. Fibrous remodeling of the dermis occurs within weeks to months, leading to widening of the papillary dermis and ultimately scleroderma-like changes. A patient with a lichen planus pattern has a significantly increased death hazard ratio, so evaluation of these biopsies is very important. Biopsies should be taken from areas of rash or from the forearm and be full thickness so that intradermal changes can be evaluated.[141,142]

The sicca syndrome (dry gland) involving mouth, eyes, nose, vagina, and urethra affects 80% of patients with chronic GVHD. Oral chronic GVHD is more difficult to diagnose histologically because of non-specific findings that range from pronounced lichenoid reaction to mucosal atrophy. A negative biopsy, which must include both lip mucosa and salivary gland, does not exclude GVHD. By contrast, a positive lip biopsy in conjunction with other evidence of chronic GVHD prompts specific immunosuppressive therapy. Kerato-conjunctivitis, a common manifestation of sicca syndrome, is best diagnosed clinically using slit lamp examination and decreased tear production (Schirmer's test). Other manifestations of chronic GVHD include difficulty in swallowing, reminiscent of scleroderma, due to mucosal ulcerations with submucosal fibrosis and destruction of submucosal glands. Patients can also develop renal vasculopathy and bronchiolitis obliterans, indistinguishable from chronic allograft rejection.[141–146]

OTHER ALLOGRAFT INJURIES

PERFUSION INJURY

Allografts must be kept in a perfusing solution for variable lengths of time, depending upon allograft type, prior to transplantation for purposes of transport and logistics. Kidney allografts can be kept successfully for 12 to 24 hours, livers can be kept for 36 hours, and heart and lung allografts must be transplanted within 4 hours. Organs with prolonged exposure to cold perfusing solutions show a variety of pathologic features related to the relatively ischemic state and the length of time of perfusion. In most cases, the histologic features resolve within 1 to 3 weeks after transplantation. Rarely, the graft is incapable of recovering from this ischemic insult, and primary graft failure results.

Renal allograft perfusion injury is manifested by acute tubular damage with tubular dilation and tubular epithelial cell sloughing, giving the luminal border a ragged appearance. This process must be distinguished from cyclosporine nephrotoxicity, which can produce similar tubular damage (Fig. 4.21). A glomerulitis may also occur, manifested by infiltration of glomeruli by neutrophils.[96]

Heart allograft perfusion injury may show focal areas of myocytolysis or contraction band necrosis (or both) as a manifestation of early ischemic damage (Fig. 4.22). Hearts undergoing prolonged perfusion can also require heightened amounts of catecholamines early after transplantation. Catecholamine effects on the heart are seen in the form of punctate ischemic myocytes surrounded by neutrophils.[97]

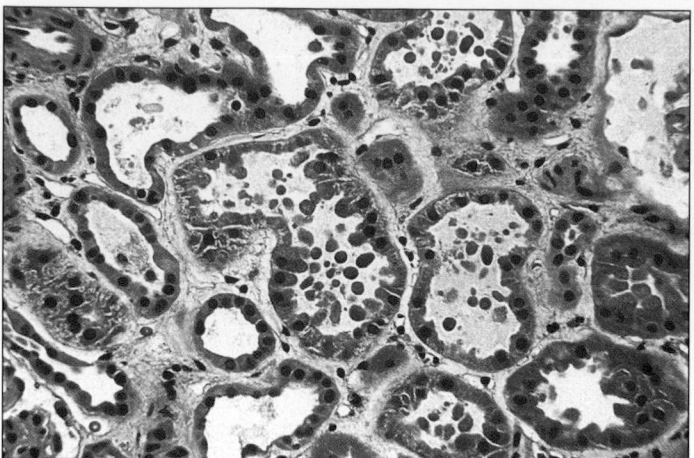

Fig. 4.21 Renal biopsy demonstrating acute tubular damage associated with acute cyclosporine nephrotoxicity. The tubular epithelial cells are desquamating. Since this biopsy was performed several months following transplantation, such acute tubular damage is unlikely from perfusion-related acute tubular necrosis.

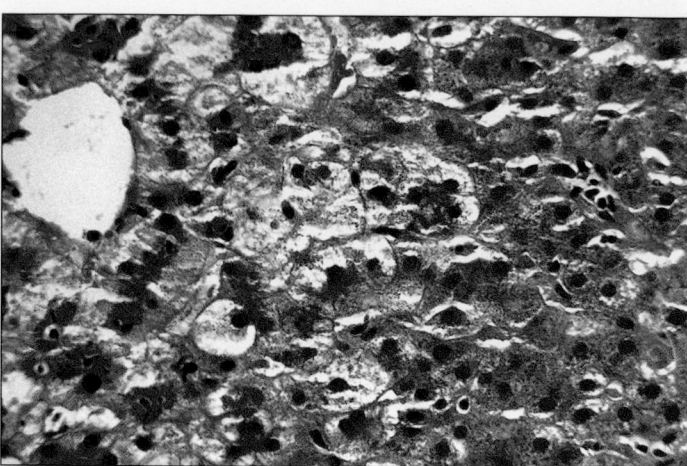

Fig. 4.23 Centrolobular balloon degeneration of liver cells is seen in this liver shortly after transplant, a manifestation of perfusion injury.

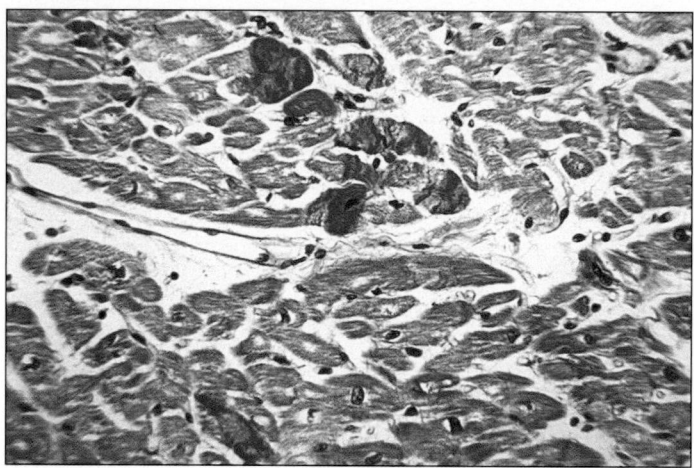

Fig. 4.22 Cardiac biopsy shows contraction band necrosis associated with perfusion injury. This change was noted one week following transplantation and resolved spontaneously without sequelae. If such changes are seen after the initial month after transplant, they suggest humoral rejection or allograft vasculopathy causing ischemia.

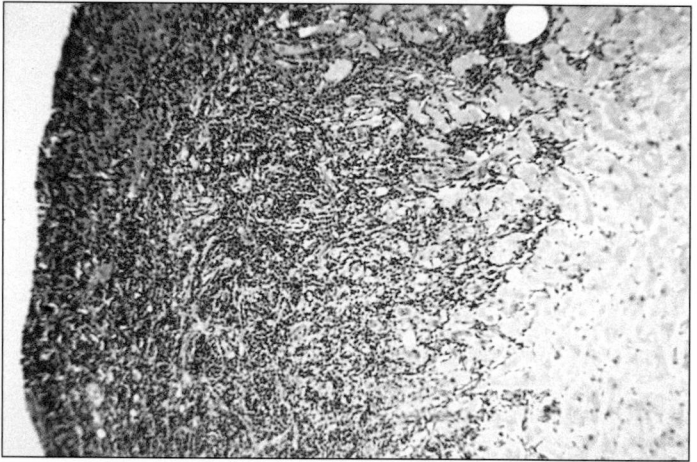

Fig. 4.24 Cardiac biopsy with endocardial lymphocytic infiltrate (Quilty).

Liver allografts often have widespread perfusion effects manifested by balloon cell degeneration of hepatocytes, especially in central areas (Fig. 4.23). Infiltration of neutrophils may also be seen in liver lobules, a condition known as surgical hepatitis.[100]

Lung allografts show diffuse alveolar damage as a manifestation of perfusion injury. Neutrophils may be associated with the damage, and desquamation of the alveolar lining cells associated with interstitial edema and hemorrhage occurs if the process is severe.[103]

INFLAMMATION AND REPAIR

Although the inciting events in allograft rejection are almost certainly immunologic, these responses are amplified in various ways by inflammatory stimuli. All the cells, plasma proteins and vascular constituents of the inflammatory process are present in the allograft.[147–149] Many of the vascular and cellular responses of inflammation are mediated by chemical factors derived from the action of the inflammatory stimulus.[147–150] Figure 4.24 illustrates the Quilty phenomenon, an endocardial inflammatory process seen in cardiac allografts. The change occurs in biopsies with and without acute rejection.

Early after transplantation, a potent inflammatory stimulus is always present – ischemia, induced by the necessary removal from the donor and delay prior to reimplantation. Such ischemia is of variable extent depending on circumstances; however, some parenchymal cell necrosis always exists, which triggers elaboration of inflammatory mediators.[150] In all solid organ allografts in the early post-transplant period, hallmarks of acute inflammation include vasodilation and vascular permeability, slowing of the circulation, and leukocyte margination, adhesion, and emigration. These changes are protean in the first few biopsies and are not manifestations of allograft rejection, but rather are manifestations of the perfusion injury that all allografts sustain.

ROLE OF IMMUNOSUPPRESSIVE DRUG TOXICITY

CYCLOSPORINE TOXICITY

In all solid allograft patients, nephrotoxicity can occur with cyclosporine use, manifested by acute tubular damage with isometric vacuolization of tubules and dystrophic calcification. Cyclosporine is also toxic to endothelial cells and can produce a thrombotic process involving arteries and glomeruli, similar to hemolytic uremic syndrome, in rare patients. Past use of higher doses of cyclosporine produced a vasculopathy with prominent medial hyalinosis of arteries and arterioles. Currently, this is a rare phenomenon. With chronic cyclosporine use, a chronic form of nephropathy with persistent tubular damage and interstitial fibrosis is difficult to distinguish from chronic allograft rejection in kidney transplant recipients, and it may coexist with chronic vasculopathy or may exacerbate it. In cardiac transplant recipients, no specific cardiac toxicity is seen, although the Quilty phenomenon is more frequent in patients treated with cyclosporine and was originally attributed to a drug effect.[96]

TACROLIMUS TOXICITY

Tacrolimus, another macrolide immunosuppressive drug, can also result in nephrotoxicity, although the extent of the problem and the frequency are less than with cyclosporine. Patients with kidney allografts develop an acute and chronic form of toxicity similar to that of cyclosporine. Isometric vacuolization of tubules is more prominent with this agent. No specific effects of tacrolimus on heart, lung, or liver allografts have been described.[96,122]

REFERENCES

1. Boumpas DT, Austin HA 3rd, Fessler BJ, et al. Systemic lupus erythematosus: emerging concepts. Part I. Ann Intern Med 1995; 122: 940–950.

2. Perez MI, Kohn SR. Systemic sclerosis. J Am Acad Dermatol 1993; 28: 525–547.

3. Smith JB, Haynes MK. Rheumatoid arthritis – a molecular understanding. Ann Intern Med 2002; 136: 908–922.

4. VonMuhlen CA, Tan EM. Autoantibodies in the diagnosis of systemic rheumatic diseases. Semin Arthritis Rheum 1995; 24: 323–358.

5. Kalovidouris AE. Immune aspects of myositis. Curr Opin Rheumatol 1992; 4: 809–814.

6. Durinovic-Bello I. Autoimmune diabetes: the role of T cells, MHC molecules and autoantigens. Autoimmunity 1998; 27: 159–177.

7. Kong MF, Jeffcoate W. Eighty-six cases of Addison's disease. Clin Endocrinol 1994; 41: 757–761.

8. Koshiyama H, Sato H, Yorita S, et al. Lymphocytic hypophysitis presenting with diabetes insipidus: case report and literature review. Endocr J 1994; 41: 93–97.

9. Puck JM. Primary immunodeficiency diseases. JAMA 1997; 278: 1835–1841.

10. Segal BH, Holland SM. Primary phagocytic disorders of childhood. Pediatr Clin North Am 2000; 47: 1311–1338.

11. Buckley RH. Advances in immunology: primary immunodeficiency diseases due to defects in lymphocytes. New Engl J Med 2000; 343: 1313–1324.

12. Rosen FS, Cooper MD, Wedgwood RJ. The primary immunodeficiencies. New Engl J Med 1995; 333: 431–440.

13. Stephan JL, Vlekova V, LeDeist F, et al. Severe combined immunodeficiency: a retrospective single-center study of clinical presentation and outcome in 117 patients. J Pediatr 1993; 123: 564–572.

14. Arkwright PD, Abinun M, Cant AJ. Autoimmunity in human primary immunodeficiency diseases. Blood 2002; 99: 2694–2702.

15. Koskinen S, Tolo H, Hirvonen M, Koistinen J. Long-term persistence of selective IgA deficiency in healthy adults. J Clin Immunol 1994; 14: 116–119.

16. Sandler SG, Mallory D, Malamut D, Eckrich R. IgA anaphylactic transfusion reactions. Transfus Med Rev 1995; 9: 1–8.

17. Eisenstein EM, Sneller MC. Common variable immunodeficiency: diagnosis and management. Ann Allergy 1994; 73: 285–292.

18. Herbst EW, Armbruster M, Rump JA, et al. Intestinal B cell defects in common variable immunodeficiency. Clin Exp Immunol 1994; 95: 215–221.

19. Cunningham-Rundles C. Clinical and immunologic studies of common variable immunodeficiency. Curr Opin Pediatr 1994; 6: 676–681.

20. Sander CA, Medeiros LJ, Weiss LM, et al. Lymphoproliferative lesions in patients with common variable immunodeficiency syndrome. Am J Surg Pathol 1992; 16: 1170–1182.

21. Rengan R, Ochs HD. Molecular biology of the Wiskott-Aldrich syndrome. Rev Immunogenet 2000; 2: 243–255.

22. Savitsky K, Bar-Shira A, Gilad S, et al. A single ataxia telangiectasia gene with a product similar to PI-3 kinase. Science 1995; 268: 1749–1753.

23. Gatti RA. Ataxia-telangiectasia. Dermatol Clin 1995; 13: 6.

24. Stone MJ. Amyloidosis: a final common pathway for protein deposition in tissues. Blood 1990; 75: 531–545.

25. Strege RJ, Saeger W. Diagnosis and immunohistochemical classification of systemic amyloidoses. Virchs Arch 1998; 433: 19–27.

26. Rocken C, Shakespeare A. Pathology, diagnosis, and pathogenesis of AA amyloidosis. Virchs Arch 2002; 440: 111–122.

27. Ohashi K. Pathogenesis of beta2-microglobulin amyloidosis. Pathol Int 2001; 51: 1–10.

28. Yamada M. Cerebral amyloid angiopathy: an overview. Neuropathology 2000; 20: 8–22.

29. Tan SY, Pepys MB. Amyloidosis. Histopathology 1994; 25: 403–414.

30. Levy JA. Pathogenesis of HIV infection. Microbiol Rev 1993; 57: 183–289.

31. Hogan CM, Hammer SM. Host determinants in HIV infection and disease. Part 1: cellular and humoral immune responses. Ann Intern Med 2001; 134: 761–776.

32. Hogan CM, Hammer SM. Host determinants in HIV infection and disease. Part 2: genetic factors and implications for antiretroviral therapies. Ann Intern Med 2001; 134: 978–996.

33. Centers for Disease Control. First 500,000 AIDS cases – United States, 1994. MMWR 1995; 44: 849–853.

34. Sinicco A, Palestro G, Caramello P, et al. Acute HIV-1 infection: clinical and biological study of 12 patients. J Acquir Immune Defic Syndr 1990; 3: 260–265.

35. Henrard DR, Daar E, Farzadegan H, et al. Virologic and immunologic characterization of symptomatic and asymptomatic primary HIV-1 infection. J Acquir Immune Defic Syndr Hum Retrovirol 1995; 9: 305–310.

36. Coutlee F, Olivier C, Cassol S, et al. Absence of prolonged immunosilent infection with human immunodeficiency virus in individuals with high-risk behaviors. Am J Med 1994; 96: 42–48.

37. Fauci AS, Pantaleo G, Stanley S, Weissman D. Immunopathogenic mechanisms of HIV infection. Ann Intern Med 1996; 124: 654–663.

38. Centers for Disease Control. Guidelines for national human immunodeficiency virus case surveillance, including monitoring for human immunodeficiency virus infection and acquired immunodeficiency syndrome. MMWR 1999; 48(RR13): 1–31.

39. Tovo PA, deMartino M, Gabiano C, et al. Prognostic factors and survival in children with perinatal HIV-1 infection. Lancet 1992; 339: 1249–1253.

40. Baroni CD, Uccini S. The lymphadenopathy of HIV infection. Am J Clin Pathol 1993; 99: 397–401.

41. Ost A, Baroni CD, Biberfeld P, et al. Lymphadenopathy in HIV infection: histological classification and staging. Acta Pathol Microbiol Immunol Scand Suppl 1989; 8: 7–15.

42. Pantaleo G, Menzo S, Vaccarezza M, et al. Studies in subjects with long-term nonprogressive human immunodeficiency virus infection. N Engl J Med 1995; 332: 209–216.

43. Moran CA, Suster S, Pavlova Z, et al. The spectrum of pathological changes in the lung in children with the acquired immunodeficiency syndrome. Hum Pathol 1994; 25: 877–882.

44. Travis WD, Fox CH, Devaney KO, et al. Lymphoid pneumonitis in 50 adult patients infected with the human immunodeficiency virus: lymphocytic interstitial pneumonitis versus nonspecific interstitial pneumonitis. Hum Pathol 1992; 23: 529–541.

45. Joshi VV, Kauffman S, Oleske JM, et al. Polyclonal polymorphic B-cell lymphoproliferative disorder with prominent pulmonary involvement in children with acquired immunodeficiency syndrome. Cancer 1987; 59: 1455–1462.

46. Gray F, Lescs MC. HIV-related demyelinating disease. Eur J Med 1993; 2: 89–96.

47. DeGirolami U, Smith TW, Hénin D, Hauw JJ. Neuropathology of the acquired immunodeficiency syndrome. Arch Pathol Lab Med 1990; 114: 643–655.

48. Achim CL, Wang R, Miners DK, Wiley CA. Brain viral burden in HIV infection. J Neuropathol Exp Neurol 1994; 53: 284–294.

49. Bell JE. The neuropathology of adult HIV infection. Rev Neurol (Paris) 1998; 154: 816–29.

50. von Einsiedel RW, Fife TD, Aksamit AJ, et al. Progressive multifocal leukoencephalopathy in AIDS:

a clinicopathologic study and review of the literature. J Neurol 1993; 240: 391–406.

51. Hair LS, Nuovo G, Powers JM, et al. Progressive multifocal leukoencephalopathy in patients with human immunodeficiency virus. Hum Pathol 1992; 23: 663–667.

52. Knowles DM. Molecular pathology of acquired immunodeficiency syndrome-related non-Hodgkin's lymphoma. Semin Diagn Pathol 1997; 14: 67–82.

53. Gaidano G, Pastore C, Lanza C, et al. Molecular pathology of AIDS-related lymphomas: biologic aspects and clinicopathologic heterogeneity. Ann Hematol 1994; 69: 281–290.

54. Raphael M, Gentilhomme O, Tulliez M, et al. Histopathologic features of high-grade non-Hodgkin's lymphomas in acquired immunodeficiency syndrome. Arch Pathol Lab Med 1991; 115: 15–20.

55. Joshi VV, Gagnon GA, Chadwick EG, et al. The spectrum of mucosa-associated lymphoid tissue lesions in pediatric patients infected with HIV: a clinicopathologic study of six cases. Am J Clin Pathol 1997; 107: 592–600.

56. Wotherspoon AC, Diss TC, Pan L, et al. Low grade gastric B-cell lymphoma of mucosa associated lymphoid tissue in immunocompromised patients. Histopathology 1996; 28: 129–134.

57. Beylot-Barry M, Vergier B, Masquelier B, et al. The spectrum of cutaneous lymphomas in HIV infection. Am J Surg Pathol 1999; 23: 1208–1216.

58. Moore PS, Chang Y. Detection of herpesvirus-like DNA sequences in Kaposi's sarcoma in patients with and those without HIV infection. N Engl J Med 1995; 332: 1181–1185.

59. Antman K, Chang Y. Kaposi's sarcoma. N Engl J Med 2000; 342: 1027–1038.

60. Niedt GW, Myskowski PL, Urmacher C, et al. Histology of early lesions of AIDS-associated Kaposi's sarcoma. Mod Pathol 1990; 3: 64–70.

61. Kao GF, Johnson FB, Sulica VI. The nature of hyaline (eosinophilic) globules and vascular slits of Kaposi's sarcoma. Am J Dermatopathol 1990; 12: 256–267.

62. Rydberg L. ABO-incompatibility in solid organ transplantation. Transfusion Medicine 2001; 11: 325–342.

63. Krensky AM, Weiss A, Crabtree G, et al. T-lymphocyte-antigen interactions in transplant rejection. N Engl J Med 1990; 322: 510–517.

64. Arakelov A, Lakkis FG. The alloimmune response and effector mechanisms of allograft rejection. Semin Nephrol 2000; 20: 95–102.

65. Cuturi MC, Blancho G, Josien R, Soulillou JP. The biology of allograft rejection. Curr Opin Neph Hyper 1994; 3: 578–584.

66. Sachs DH, Hansen TH. The major histocompatibility complex. In: Paul WE, ed. Fundamental immunology. Philadelphia: Lippincott-Raven; 1989: 445–488.

67. Rogers NJ, Lechler RI:. Allorecognition. Am J Transplant 2001; 1: 97–102.

68. Watschinger B, Gallon L, Carpenter CB, Sayegh MH. Mechanisms of allo-recognition. Recognition by in vivo-primed T cells of specific major histocompatibility complex polymorphisms presented as peptides by responder antigen-presenting cells. Transplantation 1994; 57: 572–576.

69. Dengler TJ, Pober JS. Cellular and molecular biology of cardiac transplant rejection. J Nucl Cardiol 2000; 7: 669–685.

70. Le Moine A, Goldman M, Abramowicz D. Multiple pathways to allograft rejection. Transplantation 2002; 73: 1373–1381.

71. Gregersen PK. HLA class II polymorphism: implications for genetic susceptibility to autoimmune disease. Lab Invest 1989; 61: 5–19.

72. Wagner CR, Vetto RM, Burger DR. Subcultured human endothelial cells can function independently as fully competent antigen-presenting cells. Hum Immunol 1985; 13: 33–47.

73. Steiniger B, Stehling O, Scriba A, Grau V. Monocytes in the rat: phenotype and function during acute allograft rejection. Immunol Rev 2001; 184: 38–44.

74. Wever PC, Boonstra JG, Laterveer JC, et al. Mechanism of lymphocyte mediated cytotoxicity in acute renal allograft rejection. Transplantation 1998; 66: 259–264.

75. Parnes JR. Molecular biology and function of CD4 and CD8. Adv Immunol 1989; 44: 265–311.

76. Colvin BL, Thomson AW. Chemokines, their receptors, and transplant outcome. Transplantation 2002; 74: 149–155.

77. Vierling JM. Immunology of acute and chronic hepatic allograft rejection. Liver Transpl Surg 1999; 5(4 Suppl 1): S1–S20.

78. Royer HD, Reinherz EL. T lymphocytes: ontogeny, function, and relevance to clinical disorders. N Engl J Med 1987; 317: 1136–1142.

79. Miltenburg AM, Meijer-Paape ME, Weening JJ, et al. Induction of antibody-dependent cellular cytotoxicity against endothelial cells by renal transplantation. Transplantation 1989; 48: 681–688.

80. Hayry P. Generation and breakdown of a vicious cycle in context of acute allograft rejection. Transplant Proc 1986; 18: 52–62.

81. Cotran RS. New roles for the endothelium in inflammation and immunity. Am J Pathol 1987; 129: 407–410.

82. Pober JS. Immunobiology of human vascular endothelium. Immunol Res 1999; 19: 225–232.

83. Dvorak HF, Galli SJ, Dvorak AM. Cellular and vascular manifestations of cell-mediated immunity. Hum Pathol 1986; 17: 122–137.

84. Leon MP, Bassendine MF, Gibbs P, et al. Hepatic allograft rejection: regulation of the immunogenicity of human intrahepatic biliary epithelial cells. Liver Transpl Surg 1996; 2: 37–45.

85. Hoffmann MW, Wonigeit K, Steinhoff G, et al. Production of cytokines (TNF-alpha, IL-1-beta) and endothelial cell activation in human liver allograft rejection. Transplantation 1993; 55: 329–335.

86. Ruan XM, Qiao JH, Trento A, et al. Cytokine expression and endothelial cell and lymphocyte activation in human cardiac allograft rejection: an immunohistochemical study of endomyocardial biopsy samples. J Heart Lung Transplant 1992; 11: 1110–1115.

87. Colvin RB, Preffer FI, Fuller TC, et al. A critical analysis of serum and urine interleukin-2 receptor assays in renal allograft recipients. Transplantation 1989; 48: 800–805.

88. Baldwin WM 3rd, Qian Z, Ota H, et al. Complement as a mediator of vascular inflammation and activation in allografts. J Heart Lung Transplant 2000; 19: 723–730.

89. Mannik M. Mechanisms of tissue deposition of immune complexes. J Rheumatol 1987; 14 (Suppl 13): 35–42.

90. Libby P, Pober JS. Chronic rejection. Immunity 2001; 14: 387–397.

91. Hall BM. Cellular infiltrates in allografts. Transplant Proc 1987; 19: 50–56.

92. Billingham ME. Diagnosis of cardiac rejection by endomyocardial biopsy. Heart Transplant 1982; 1: 25–30.

93. Higgenbottam T, Stewart S, Penketh A, Wallwork J. Transbronchial lung biopsy for the diagnosis of rejection in heart-lung transplant patients. Transplantation 1988; 46: 532–539.

94. Snover DC, Freese DK, Sharp HL, et al. Liver allograft rejection: an analysis of the use of biopsy in determining outcome of rejection. Am J Surg Pathol 1987; 11: 1–10.

95. Sale GE, Buckner CD. Pathology of bone marrow in transplant recipients. Hematol Oncol Clin North Am 1988; 2: 735–756.

96. Colvin RB. Kidney transplantation. In: Colvin RB, Bhan AT, McCluskey RT, eds. Diagnostic immunopathology. Philadelphia: Lippincott-Raven; 1995: 329–366.

97. Hammond EH. Cardiac transplantation. In: Colvin RB, Bhan AT, McCluskey RT, eds. Diagnostic Immunopathology. Philadelphia: Lippincott-Raven; 1995: 367.

98. Batts KP. Acute and chronic hepatic allograft rejection: pathology and classification. Liver Transpl Surg 1999; 5(4 Suppl 1): S21–29.

99. Hammond MEH, Renlund DG. Cardiac allograft vascular (microvascular) rejection. Curr Opin Organ Transplant 2002; 7(3): 233–239.

100. Demetrius AJ, Batts KP, Dhillon AP et al. Banff schema for grading liver allograft rejection: an international consensus document. Hepatology 1997; 25: 658–663.

101. Racusen LC, Solez K, Colvin RB, et al. The Banff 97 working classification of renal allograft pathology. Kidney Int 1999; 55: 713–723.

102. Billingham ME, Cary NR, Hammond EH, et al. A working formulation for the standardization of nomenclature in the diagnosis of heart and lung rejection: Heart Rejection Study Group. The International Society for Heart Transplantation. J Heart Transplant 1990; 9: 587–592.

103. Yousem SA, Berry GJ, Cagle PT. Revision of the 1990 working formulation for the classification of pulmonary allograft rejection: Lung Rejection Study Group. J Heart Lung Transplant 1996; 15: 1–15.

104. Demetris A, Adams D, Bellamy C. Update of the International Banff Schema for Liver Allograft Rejection: working recommendations for the histopathologic staging and reporting of chronic rejection. An International Panel. Hepatology 2000; 31: 792–799.

105. Bates WD, Davies DR, Welsh K, et al. An evaluation of the Banff classification of early renal allograft biopsies and correlation with outcome. Nephrol Dial Transplant 1999; 14: 2364–2369.

106. Dean DE, Kamath S, Peddi VR, et al. A blinded retrospective analysis of renal allograft pathology using the Banff schema: implications for clinical management. Transplantation 1999; 68: 642–645.

107. Myburgh JA, Cohen I, Gecelter L, et al. Hyperacute rejection in human-kidney allografts – Shwartzman or arthus reaction? N Engl J Med 1969; 281: 131–135.

108. Matas AJ, Scheinman JI, Rattazzi LC, et al. Immunopathological studies of the ruptured human renal allograft. Surgery1976; 98: 922–926.

109. Carpenter CB, Milford EL. HLA matching in cadaveric renal transplantation. Immunol Allergy Clin North Am 1989; 9: 45–60.

110. Demetris AJ, Jaffe R, Tzakis A, et al. Antibody-mediated rejection of human orthotopic liver allografts/a study of liver transplantation across ABO blood group barriers. Am J Pathol 1988; 132: 489–502.

111. Hammond EH, Hansen J, Spencer LS, et al. Vascular rejection in cardiac transplantation: histologic, immunopathologic and ultrastructural features. Cardiovasc Pathol 1993; 2: 21–34.

112. Collins AB, Schneeberger EE, Pascual MA, et al. Complement activation in acute humoral renal allograft rejection: diagnostic significance of C4d deposits in peritubular capillaries. J Am Soc Nephrol 1999; 10: 2208–2214.

113. Mauiyyedi S, Crespo M, Collins AB, et al. Acute humoral rejection in kidney transplantation: II. Morphology, immunopathology, and pathologic classification. J Am Soc Nephrol 2002; 13: 779–787.

114. Taylor DO, Yowell RL, Kfoury AG, et al. Allograft coronary artery disease: clinical correlations with circulating anti-HLA antibodies and the immunohistopathologic pattern of vascular rejection. J Heart Lung Transplant 2000; 19: 518–521.

115. Paul LC. Chronic allograft nephropathy: an update. Kidney Int 1999; 56:783–793.

116. Häyry P, Mennander A, Räisänen-Sokolowski A, et al. Pathophysiology of vascular wall changes in chronic allograft rejection. Transplant Rev 1993;7: 1–12.

117. Denton MD, Davis SF, Baum MA, et al. The role of the graft endothelium in transplant rejection: evidence that endothelial activation may serve as a clinical marker for the development of chronic rejection. Pediatr Transplant 2000; 4: 252–260.

118. Reed EF, Hong B, Ho E, et al. Monitoring of soluble HLA alloantigens and anti-HLA antibodies identifies heart allograft recipients at risk of transplant-associated coronary artery disease. Transplantation 1996; 61: 566–572.

119. Rose, ML. Role of antibodies in rejection. Curr Opin Organ Transplant 1999; 4: 227–233.

120. Clinton SK, Libby P. Cytokines and growth factors in atherogenesis. Arch Pathol Lab Med 1992; 116: 1292–1300.

121. Gordon D, Reidy MA, Benditt EP, Schwartz SM. Cell proliferation in human coronary arteries. Proc Natl Acad Sci USA 1990; 87: 4600–4604.

122. Morales JM, Andres A, Rengel M, Rodicio JL. Influence of cyclosporin, tacrolimus and rapamycin on renal function and arterial hypertension after renal transplantation. Nephrol Dial Transplant. 2001; 16(Suppl 1): 121–124.

123. Demetris AJ, Seaberg EC, Batts KP, et al. Chronic liver allograft rejection: a National Institute of Diabetes and Digestive and Kidney Diseases interinstitutional study analyzing the reliability of current criteria and proposal of an expanded definition. National Institute of Diabetes and Digestive and Kidney Diseases Liver Transplantation Database. Am J Surg Pathol 1998; 22: 28–39.

124. Ludwig J, Wiesner RH, Batts KP, et al. The acute vanishing bile duct syndrome (acute irreversible rejection) after orthotopic liver transplantation. Hepatology 1987; 7: 476–483.

125. Demetris AJ, Murase N, Lee RG, et al. Chronic rejection. A general overview of histopathology and pathophysiology with emphasis on liver, heart and intestinal allografts. Ann Transplant 1997; 2: 27–44.

126. Kramer MR, Stoehr C, Whang JL, et al. The diagnosis of obliterative bronchiolitis following heart-lung transplantation: low yield of transbronchial biopsy. J Heart Lung Transplant 1993; 12: 675–681.

127. Yousem SA, Burke C, Billingham ME. Pathologic pulmonary alterations in long-term human heart-lung transplantation. Hum Pathol 1985;16: 911–923.

128. Scott JP, Higgenbottam TW, Clelland CA. Natural history of chronic rejection in heart-lung transplant recipients. J Heart Transplant 1990; 9: 510–515.

129. Sibley RK, Berry GJ, Tazelaar HD, et al. The role of transbronchial biopsies in the management of lung transplant recipients. J Heart Lung Transplant 1993; 12: 308–324.

130. Stewart S. Pathology of lung transplantation. Semin Diagn Pathol 1992; 9: 210–219.

131. Milne DS, Gascoigne A, Wilkes J, et al. The immunohistopathology of obliterative bronchiolitis following lung transplantation. Transplantation 1992; 54: 748–750.

132. van den Brink MR, Burakoff SJ. Cytolytic pathways in haematopoietic stem-cell transplantation. Nat Rev Immunol 2002; 2: 273–281.

133. Muller-Hermelink HK, Sale GE, Borisch B, Storb R. Pathology of the thymus after allogeneic bone marrow transplantation in man. A histologic immunohistochemical study of 36 patients. Am J Pathol 1986; 129: 242–256.

134. Burakoff SJ, Degg HJ, Ferrara J, Atkinson K, eds. Graft-vs-host disease: immunology, pathophysiology, and treatment. New York: Marcel Dekker; 1990.

135. van Bekkum DW, de Vries MJ, van der Waay D. Lesions characteristic of secondary disease in germ free heterologous radiation chimeras. J Natl Cancer Inst 1967; 38: 223–231.

136. Sale GE, Lerner KG, Barker EA, et al. The skin biopsy in the diagnosis of acute graft-versus-host disease in man. Am J Pathol 1977; 89: 621–635.

137. Epstein RJ, McDonald GB, Sale GE, et al. The diagnostic accuracy of the rectal biopsy in acute graft-versus-host disease: a prospective study of thirteen patients. Gastroenterology 1980; 78: 764–771.

138. Parkman R, Champagne J, DeClerck Y, et al. Cellular interactions in graft-versus-host disease. Transplant Proc 1987; 19: 53–54.

139. McDonald GB, Shulman HM, Sullivan KM, Spencer GD. Intestinal and hepatic complications of human bone marrow transplantation. Part I. Gastroenterology 1986; 90: 460–477.

140. Shulman HM, Sharma P, Amos D, et al. A coded histologic study of hepatic graft-versus-host disease after human bone marrow transplantation. Hepatology 1988;8: 463–470.

141. Snover DC, Weisdorf SA, Ramsay NK, et al. Hepatic graft-versus-host disease: a study of the predictive value of liver biopsy in diagnosis. Hepatology 1984; 4: 123–130.

142. Nakhleh R, Miller W, Snover D. Significance of mucosal vs salivary gland changes in lip biopsies in the diagnosis of chronic graft-vs-host disease. Arch Pathol Lab Med 1989; 113: 932–934.

143. Jack MK, Jack GM, Sale GE, et al. Ocular manifestations of graft-v-host disease. Arch Ophthalmol 1983; 101: 1080–1084.

144. Janin-Mercer A, Saurat JH, Bourges M, et al. The lichen planus like and sclerotic phases of graft-versus-host disease in man: an ultrastructural study of six cases. Acta Derm Venereol 1981; 61: 187–193.

145. Wingard JR, Piantadosi S, Vogelsang G, et al. Predictors of death from chronic graft-versus-host disease after bone marrow transplantation. Blood 1989; 74: 1428–1435.

146. Parkman R. Chronic graft-versus-host disease. Curr Opin Hematol 1998; 5: 22–25.

147. Ryan G, Majno G. Acute inflammation. A review. Am J Pathol 1977; 86: 185–194.

148. Harlan JM. Consequences of leukocyte-vessel wall interactions in inflammatory and immune reactions. Semin Thromb Hemost 1987; 13: 434–444.

149. Gallin JI, ed. Inflammation: basic principles and clinical correlates. Philadelphia: Lippincott-Raven; 1992.

150. Cochrane CG, Gimbrone MA, eds. Biological oxidants: generation and injurious consequences. San Diego: Academic Press; 1992.

Iatrogenic lesions

5

Robert E. Fechner   Guy E. Nichols   I-Tien Yeh

The clinical application of hundreds of new therapeutic and diagnostic agents in the past few decades has added iatrogenic problems as a new dimension to the practice of medicine. Iatrogenic changes occur in diverse situations ranging from hyperplastic endometrium in women taking estrogen to life-threatening radiation-induced malignant tumors. The pathologist may be involved in the diagnosis of adverse drug reactions. In most cases of suspected adverse drug reaction, the diagnosis is made on clinical grounds but sometimes a biopsy is done in an effort to distinguish a drug-induced reaction from some other cause. A detailed discussion of the morphologic effects of drug therapy is beyond the scope of this chapter. We will largely limit the discussion to drug effects that cause or mimic neoplasia.

REACTION TO DIAGNOSTIC PROCEDURES

TRAUMA OF BIOPSY

Distortion of tissue due to the physical trauma at the moment of biopsy can alter the architectural pattern or the cytologic detail, or both. When a small piece of benign glandular mucosa is twisted or compressed, the evenly spaced distribution of normal glands is lost, and the irregular pattern may be worrisome. The problem is compounded if cytologic atypia is present, as in atrophic gastritis. Perhaps the most common mechanical distortion of glandular epithelium is seen in endometrial curettings, where telescoping of the epithelium may be mistaken for adenomatous hyperplasia. The loss of stroma between glands also gives a false impression of hyperplastic crowding (Fig. 5.1).

Mechanical compression and disruption of nuclei are especially common in small biopsy specimens along the edge of the tissue where cup forceps have severed the fragment from the parent organ. Lymphocytes and neutrophils are susceptible to this alteration, as well as epithelium. The cells of oat cell carcinoma of the lung are particularly prone to this type of damage. Nonetheless, even when much of the biopsy specimen is distorted, it is usually possible to identify a few intact cells and to make a cytologic diagnosis.

Tissue removed by surgical resection after a recent biopsy can have many alterations in the normal parenchyma and stroma at the biopsy site. The site is usually readily identified by the necrosis and hemorrhage along the edges of the incised tissue or needle track. In addition, changes may be present several millimeters away as a result of disruption of the blood supply beyond the area of direct trauma. Completely necrotic parenchyma is easily recognized but epithelium that is still viable can have enlarged nuclei and, when these cells are set in a degenerating collapsing stroma, the normal architecture may be severely altered. Reactive fibroblasts and

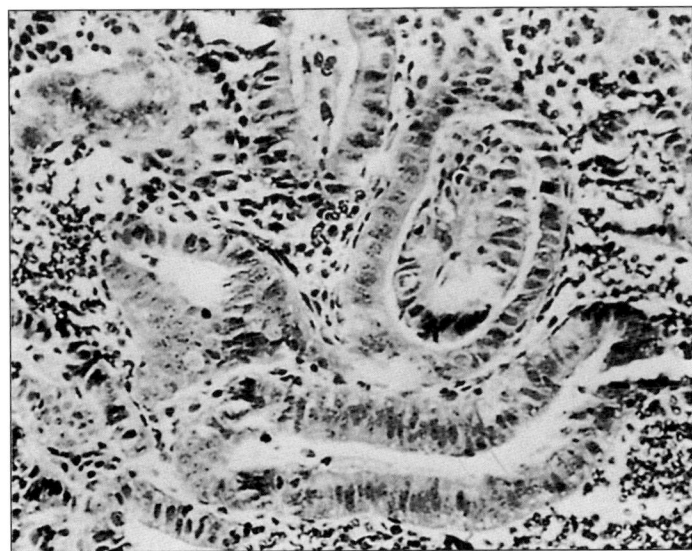

Fig. 5.1 Mechanical distortion of normal proliferative endometrium due to curettage. Note telescoping of epithelium within glandular lumens and loss of stroma between glands. No cytologic atypia is seen, nor is this the pattern of true architectural abnormality of hyperplasia.

endothelial cells further complicate the picture. The latter form small solid buds or cords of cells lacking a lumen or having an irregularly shaped lumen. The individual cells often have large vesicular nuclei with huge nucleoli and frequent mitoses. By cytologic criteria, the reactive cells raise the possibility of malignancy. Small aggregates of atypical cells in foci of hemorrhage or necrosis must not be diagnosed as epithelial unless unequivocal evidence exists of specialized functions such as keratin formation or mucin secretion. Even when they are recognized as epithelial, cells in these foci must be interpreted with extreme caution, since regenerative and degenerative changes of normal epithelium are often prominent.

Necrosis of fat after an incisional or needle biopsy may be confusing, especially in the breast. The nuclei of degenerating fat cells or reactive histiocytes range from hyperchromatic to vesicular but usually are small and lack the large nucleoli seen in reactive fibroblasts and endothelial cells. Occasionally, they are arranged in small nests or in a circular configuration that mimics adenocarcinoma. Cytologic smears of fat necrosis obtained by breast fine-needle aspiration (FNA) demonstrate numerous finely vacuolated macrophages in a hypocellular background of lymphocytes, multinucleated giant cells, and acellular debris.[1,2] Scarcity of branched epithelial groups distinguishes fat necrosis from intraductal papilloma

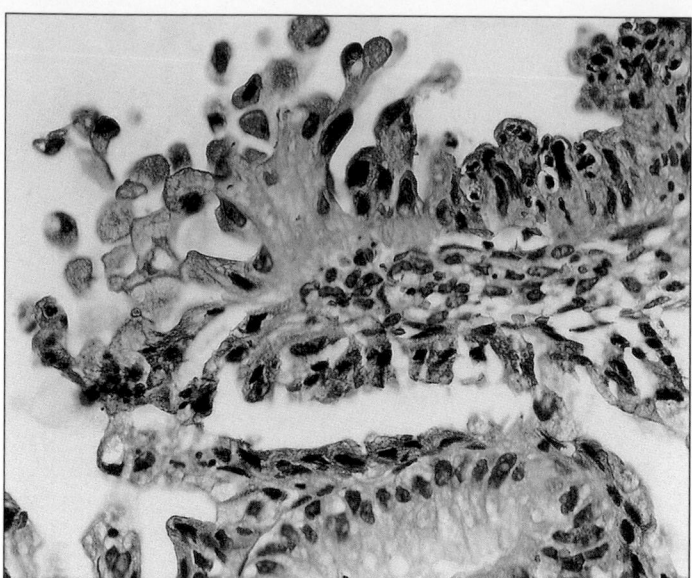

Fig. 5.2 Endocervical epithelium 12 days after endometrial curettage. Surface is lined by elongated cells with pleomorphic dense nuclei intermixed with neutrophils. Normal endocervical gland is at bottom.

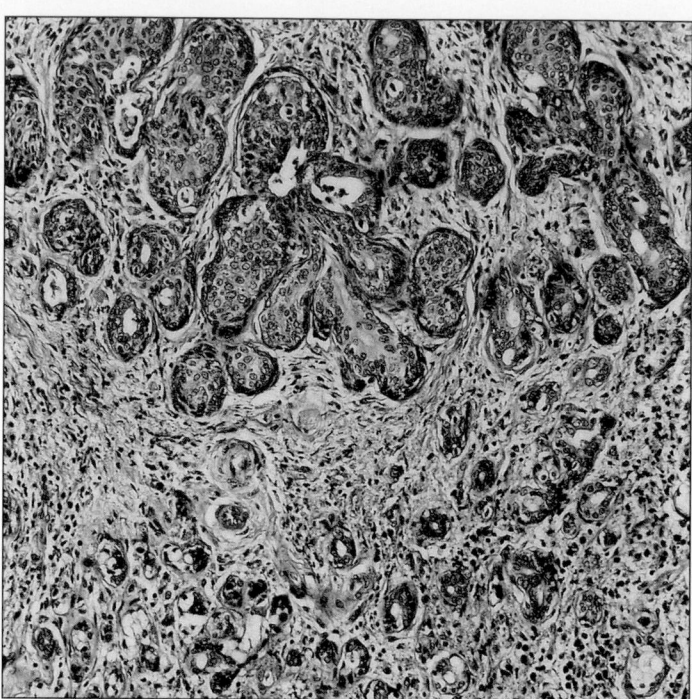

Fig. 5.3 Tissue from resection of palate showing squamous metaplasia in minor salivary gland tissue 8 days after incisional biopsy specimen detected squamous carcinoma. Degeneration of acini with loss of lobular pattern is seen in lower half of field, while squamous epithelium fills acini and ducts in upper half of field. The epithelium is cytologically bland.

of the breast, which also exhibits numerous foam cells in FNA specimens.[1]

Necrosis of parenchymal elements after a biopsy is often accompanied by vigorous repair. Re-epithelialization of the endometrium or endocervix after curettage is characterized by cells of variable size having nuclei that are dense and angulated and lack polarity (Fig. 5.2). These changes are most marked on the surface but may be seen in the underlying glands as well. The surface location of most of the atypical cells is the most helpful feature distinguishing them from adenocarcinoma. If the glands are involved, their even distribution with intervening stroma helps separate them from neoplastic glands, which are crowded, lack a regular pattern of distribution, and have little or no normal stroma between the glands.

Cytologic smears obtained after recent cervical biopsy or conization demonstrate reactive changes similar to those seen in histologic sections, but a lack of tissue architecture makes distinction from malignancy more problematic in smears. Reactive changes, generally referred to as reparative or regenerative in nature, are seen for up to 6 weeks after biopsy and consist of large sheets of glandular or metaplastic squamous cells with variably enlarged nuclei and enlarged, often multiple nucleoli.[3] In contrast to invasive cancers, reparative cells demonstrate fine, evenly distributed chromatin, only rare atypical single cells, and a lack of nuclear hyperchromasia. Because distinction of reparative change from malignant tumors can be difficult, cytologic follow-up should not be performed until at least 6 weeks after biopsy or conization.

In some cases, endocervical cytologic specimens can yield suspicious glandular cells for years after conization. In these cases, atypical groups and single glandular cells demonstrate hyperchromatic, irregular nuclear membranes and increased nuclear/cytoplasmic ratios that can be confused with adenocarcinoma in situ. These atypical glandular cells are distinguished from cells of adenocarcinoma in situ by a lack of nuclear enlargement and lack of nuclear crowding as well as pathologist awareness of conization history.[4] Their long-term persistence in endocervical

smears appears to result from postconization shortening of the endocervical canal or shifting of the squamocolumnar transformation zone that leads to sampling of low endometrial and high endocervical epithelium.[5] In addition, tubal and endometrioid metaplasia may occur, mimicking endocervical glandular dysplasia.[6]

Surgical specimens of mucosa from the oral cavity obtained after a biopsy may contain reactive changes in the minor salivary glands. The trauma of the original biopsy produces degeneration of the salivary gland lobules, which then undergo squamous metaplasia (Fig. 5.3). The squamous cells distend acini and ducts, forming complex branching arrangements that simulate either squamous or mucoepidermoid carcinoma. The cytologic blandness of the squamous cells, coupled with the surrounding remnants of degenerated acini, permit recognition of these changes as reactive rather than malignant. The appearance is identical to that described in the spontaneously occurring entity of necrotizing sialometaplasia of the palate.[7] Squamous metaplasia of acini has also been described in the major salivary glands after biopsy[8] and in the larynx.[9]

Hambrick[10] described the fate of colonoscopic polypectomy sites. Initially, there is acute inflammation in the submucosa and over a period of 2 weeks granulation tissue covers the defect as the inflammation subsides. By the end of 3 weeks, the site is completely resurfaced by normal colonic mucosa. Atypical epithelial changes are not mentioned. The radiologist may deliberately mark the site of a polypectomy site by an endoscopic clip or India ink tattoo.[11] The India ink may be seen in both intra- and extracellular locations within the lesion, as well as in surrounding normal tissues. Occasional cases with marked inflammatory reaction to tattoos have been reported.[12]

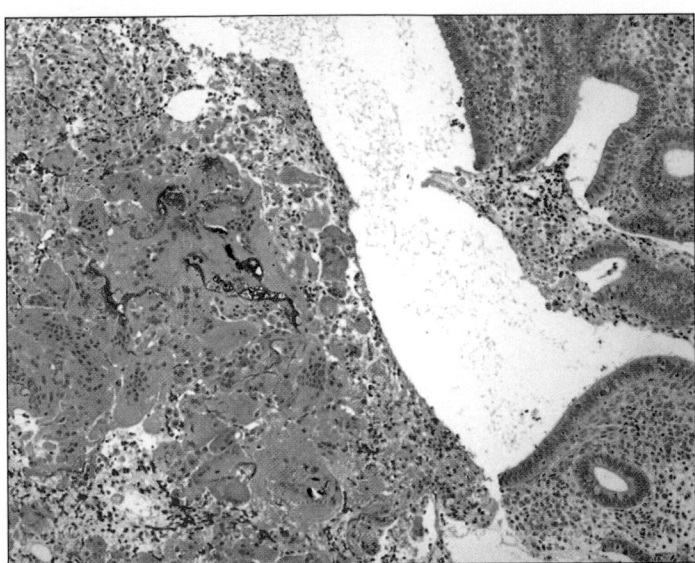

Fig. 5.4 Endometrial biopsy: posthysteroscopic ablation showing thermal residue and foreign body giant cell reaction.

THERMAL ARTIFACT

Thermal artifacts are found in a variety of cauterized specimens obtained by electrocautery or laser.[13] The changes are most severe at the edges but can reach the central portion of thin tissue fragments. It is sometimes possible to reach unaffected tissue by deeper sectioning beyond the peripheral thermal changes. The line of demarcation between the damaged area and normal tissue is quite abrupt. In one illustration of a high-power field of perineural invasion by prostatic carcinoma, half of the circumference of the nerve was uninterpretable due to thermal damage, whereas the other half had completely intact cells with good nuclear detail that allowed a firm diagnosis of carcinoma.[14] Tissue removed by laser will have a thin rim of thermal change identical to thermal changes from electrocautery.

Thermal artifact is often present extensively in transurethral resections. A signet ring configuration of lymphocytes and stromal cells in these resections, probably induced thermally, may be mistaken for carcinoma.[15]

Small colon polyps are routinely removed by electrothermal cautery, and the smaller the polyp the greater the percentage of cases with cytologic artifacts that preclude definitive diagnosis.[16]

Granulomas with a central necrobiotic zone surrounded by palisading histiocytes occur in various tissues including prostate, ovary, fallopian tube, cervix, and endometrium in patients who have had previous surgical procedures.[17–21] Electrocautery has been used in many of the operations, and various metals derived from the cutting loops[22] or laser housing[23] have been identified in some of the granulomas. This is sometimes referred to as *diathermy pigment*.[24] In the endometrium, hysteroscopic ablation may result in 'hard thermal residue' and foreign-body reaction[25] (Fig. 5.4). The differential diagnosis of this granulomatous response includes infectious etiologies, so special stains to rule out mycobacteria and fungi may be necessary.

The loop electrosurgical excision procedure (LEEP), also known as large loop excision of transformation zone (LLETZ) is being used more frequently to excise cervical squamous intraepithelial lesions, sometimes following cytologic diagnosis without confirming tissue biopsy. Thermal artifact from LEEP is identical to laser-induced thermal damage, consisting of a variably thick zone of densely eosinophilic coagulation–desiccation (approximately 0.1–0.5 mm) underlying a thin, superficial zone of carbonization (approximately 0.02 mm).[26,27] In the hands of experienced operators, LEEP thermal artifact does not limit accurate histologic evaluation of resection margins. In our experience, the usual LEEP artifact actually facilitates margin evaluation in fragmented specimens that can not be oriented and inked following excision. Occasionally, LEEP causes excessive tissue fragmentation and thermal damage that limits histologic evaluation of margins, presumably as a result of loop size or operator inexperience.[28]

IMPLANTATION OF NORMAL EPITHELIUM

Symptomatic intradural extramedullary squamous-cell-lined cysts measuring up to 2 cm in size have occurred at the site of lumbar punctures carried out 1–23 years previously. It appears that the pathogenesis is the use of needles with improperly fitting stylets that carry skin into the spinal canal.[29] Squamous epithelium has also been implanted in the meniscus of a joint.[30]

Mechanical transport of benign breast epithelial cells to axillary lymph nodes has been described after breast biopsy.[31] With sentinel node dissection being increasingly utilized for breast carcinoma, identification of metastatic carcinoma in these nodes should be confirmed as tumor by abnormal cytologic/molecular characteristics. Keratin positivity is not sufficient, as benign breast tissue will also be positive.

Though not strictly iatrogenic, other normal cells including hyperplastic mesothelial cells have been identified within lymph nodes, most probably dislodged from reactive serosal surfaces.[32,33] These nests have been confirmed to be mesothelial in origin by immunohistochemical and electron microscopic analyses. Mesothelial cells will be strongly keratin-positive; therefore, if keratin is the only immunostain done, these cells may be misinterpreted as metastatic carcinoma.

IMPLANTATION OF ABNORMAL EPITHELIUM

Clumps of adenomatous cells from tubular adenomas can be found in the submucosa 2–21 days after removal by forceps biopsy or polypectomy. If resection is carried out in this time span, it is possible to mistake this for adenocarcinoma. The cells eventually disappear but mucous pools are persistent.[34]

A surgical breast biopsy has often been subjected to one or more needling procedures such as FNA, core needle biopsy, needle localization, or infiltration with local anesthetic.[35–37] Irregular nests of epithelium dislodged into the stroma from ductal carcinoma in situ can mimic invasive carcinoma[36] (Fig. 5.5). Fragments of epithelium from ductal carcinoma in situ have also been seen in the subcapsular sinus of lymph nodes and in lymphovascular spaces within the breast.[37] Reports of sentinel lymph node metastases in 12–13%[38,39] of ductal carcinoma in situ cases may include some cases of epithelial displacement. Whether or not this has any potential for disseminated metastasis has not been determined. 'Pseudoinvasion' of vascular spaces has been attributed to needle injection of local anesthetic in the cervix.[40]

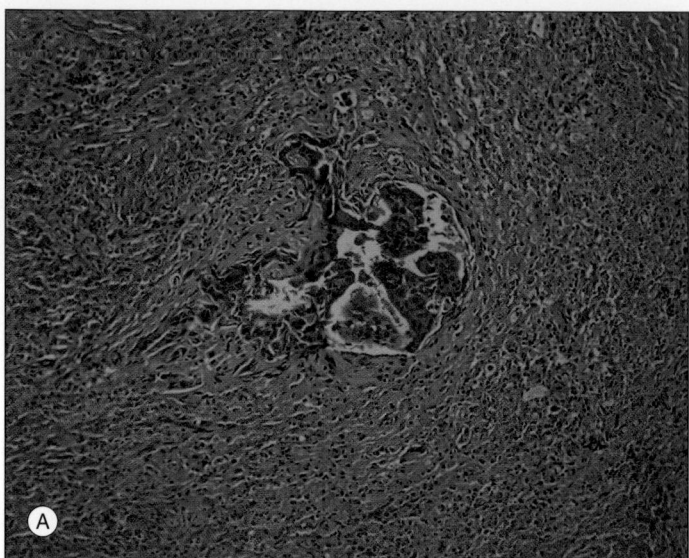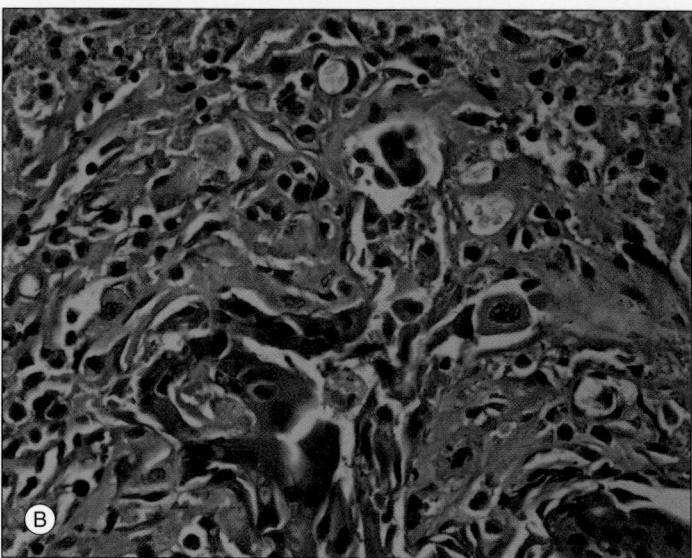

Fig. 5.5 Poststereotactic needle core biopsy specimen. The mastectomy showed extensive ductal carcinoma in situ (DCIS) throughout the entire breast. **(A)** The prior biopsy site shows a fibrohistiocytic reaction, with irregular clusters of displaced DCIS cells in the stroma, mimicking invasion. **(B)** Higher power of same area shows abnormal cell clusters in spaces, giving an impression of lymphovascular invasion.

FINE NEEDLE ASPIRATION CHANGES IN SUBSEQUENTLY EXCISED TISSUE

Previous lymph node FNA can produce hemorrhage, focal fibroblastic organization, and occasional nodal infarction but rarely limits subsequent histologic evaluation[41,42] FNA of kidney, thyroid, and salivary gland solid tumors rarely leads to extensive tumor necrosis.[43,44] After FNA, nearly 10% of breast biopsies have changes attributable to the procedure. These include infarction of fibroadenomas and papillomas as well as displaced epithelium.[45] Six days after an FNA, a 3-cm mesenteric mass with reactive fibroblasts was attributed to the FNA. It mimicked sarcoma at the time of frozen section.[46] Worrisome histologic alterations following FNA of the thyroid are seen in resected thyroid glands that have been previously aspirated. Acute changes such as inflammation, hemorrhage, and infarction are easily recognized. Chronic changes are potentially misleading and include pseudoinvasive tracking of epithelium through the capsule, atypical metaplasia, and nuclear clearing.[47]

NEEDLE-TRACK SEEDING

Ever since the introduction of needle aspiration, critics have claimed that it carries significant risk for dissemination of malignant tumors by needle-track seeding. Experiments in animals, early clinical experience with large-bore needles, and sporadic case reports continue to fuel these concerns.[48] However, an extensive survey of recent intraabdominal FNA experience using fine-bore needles, usually 22 gauge but up to 19 gauge, indicates that needle-track seeding of malignant cells is a rare complication. It occurs in less than 0.01% of total cases, although in a higher percentage of pancreatic cancers.[48] Risk of seeding appears to be related to the number of needle passes.[48,49] Peritoneal seeding is an even rarer complication of intra-abdominal FNA.[50] Some authors continue to warn against needle aspiration of ovarian cysts, based not on statistically significant data but on sporadic case reports of intraabdominal spread.[51] These concerns are also based largely on separate, controversial reports of malignant peritoneal implantation following surgical ovarian cyst rupture. The overall complication rate for ovarian cyst FNA of 1–2% is mostly due to pain, bleeding, and infection[52] and only rarely to tumor seeding. Cutaneous seeding may rarely occur following FNA of the thyroid.[48]

RADIOGRAPHIC MEDIA

Barium sulfate is seen on the enteric mucosa as chalky white strands. Microscopically it consists of fine, fairly uniform, golden granules. They are not doubly refractile. Barium elicits little inflammatory reaction when it reaches an extraluminal location through a perforated diverticulum or fistula. It lies free or is found in histiocytes. Rarely, foreign-body giant cells are seen but without well formed granulomas. When barium is found in areas of severe inflammatory and fibrous reaction, the response is due to concomitant fecal contamination rather than to barium per se. In one case, reaction was sufficient to cause ureteral obstruction.[53] Occasionally, barium is forced into the rectal mucosa at the time of barium enema and produces a polypoid mass.[54] In another report, barium entered the peritoneal cavity through a perforated duodenal ulcer and was still visible on radiographs 4 years later.[55]

Historically, the media used in hysterosalpingograms were oil-based iodine-containing compounds. The dye may be retained and has been reported to be visualized 25 years after a salpingogram.[56] In another patient, foreign body granulomas of the peritoneum were found that were attributed to extravasated medium.[57] The condition referred to as xanthomatous or lipoid salpingitis is characterized by a submucosal accumulation of foam cells; occasionally a history of salpingography will be obtained. Granulomatous meningitis has been described as a result of iodized oil used in myelography.[58] Currently, water-soluble radiologic contrast media are used, so that these conditions are rarely seen today.

REACTION TO PHYSICAL AND CHEMICAL AGENTS

STARCH, COTTON LINT, CELLULOSE, GELFOAM, AND TALC

Rubber surgical gloves were introduced by Halsted to protect the hands of his scrub nurse from irritating disinfectants used in the operating room and later were found to protect the patient from infection as well.[59] Talcum powder was used to facilitate the donning of the gloves. By the 1940s, it was clear that the powder caused intestinal adhesions, fecal fistulas, and delayed wound healing and occasionally led to death. Since the 1950s, cornstarch mixed with 2% magnesium oxide (Biosorb) has become the most widely used agent, but rice starch is also available and both can produce a granulomatous reaction.[60] Most symptomatic cases are due to peritonitis. Starch may be introduced into the abdomen by vaginal examination[61] and paracentesis[62] as well as at laparotomy. Granulomatous reactions have also occurred in the pleura, middle ear, oral cavity, and brain.[63]

Symptoms of starch peritonitis usually begin in the second or third week after an otherwise uneventful recovery from surgery. Low-grade fever and signs of peritonitis are often present; these gradually resolve after several days. If an exploratory laparotomy is done, the peritoneum is found to be focally or diffusely studded with granulomas ranging from 1 mm to more than 1 cm in size. Omental necrosis or matting of the fat into discrete masses may be found.

The histologic response to the starch ranges from scattered histiocytes, lymphocytes, and neutrophils to well formed granulomas containing foreign-body giant cells. The larger granulomas may have central necrosis.[62] The starch particles are seen on hematoxylin and eosin (H&E) sections as faintly eosinophilic particles averaging 3–10 mm in size. They stain deeply with periodic acid–Schiff (PAS) reagent and under polarized light have a Maltese-cross birefringence (Fig. 5.6). Peritoneal or pleural fluid contains the granules and the diagnosis can be made by examination with polarized light.[64] FNA of talc and starch granulomas demonstrate characteristic birefringent silicate crystals ranging in size from 2–100 μm[65] and Maltese-cross-shaped birefringent crystals,[66] respectively, within epithelioid histiocytes and multinucleated giant cells. Birefringent starch granules have also been detected extracellularly and intracellularly in cerebrospinal fluid filter preparations.[67] The well-documented problems with glove powders, along with the development of powder-free gloves, has led some authors to advocate discontinuing the use of powdered gloves during surgery.[68]

Lint from cotton gauze sponges also produces a granulomatous or fibrous reaction.[69] Initially, the fragments of lint are up to 50 mm in width and are several times longer. They are ragged, irregularly shaped particles that are refractile, pale pink or violaceous in H&E sections and are shown to better advantage with polarized light. Over time, they disintegrate and exist as tiny particles that require polarized light to be seen. At this stage, the distinction from starch granules is based on the formation of Maltese crosses in the latter, whereas the cotton lint lacks this property (Fig. 5.6).

Fibrous adhesions from patients who have had previous surgery almost invariably contain foreign material, whether it be glove powder or cotton lint.[69] Absorbable hemostatics and the vehicles of antimicrobial agents are other potential irritants that may enhance adhesion formation.[70]

Cellulose fibers are the major component of disposable surgical gowns and drapes. The fibers have produced symptomatic granulomatous peritonitis as well as other complications.[71] They are

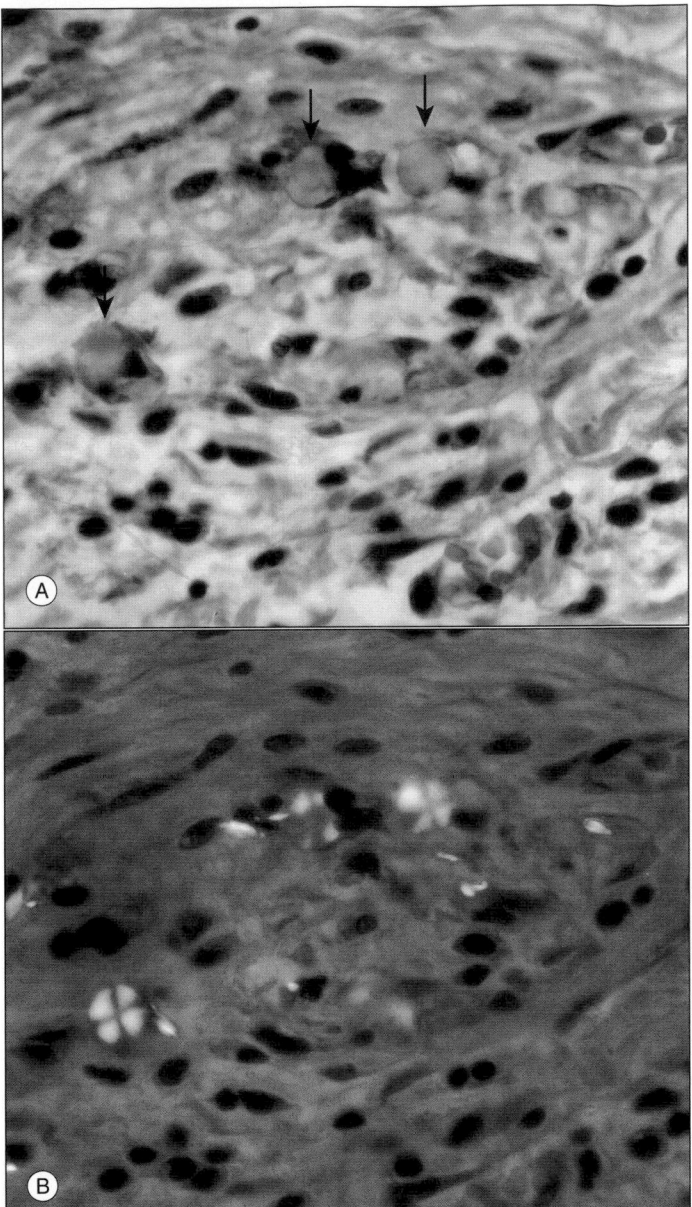

Fig. 5.6 Spherical particles of Biosorb (arrows) in subserosal fibrous tissue. **(A)** Specimen was obtained at time of closure of colostomy 5 weeks after previous surgery. Identical field under polarized light shows Maltese-cross configuration of Biosorb. **(B)** The small irregular shreds of doubly refractile material probably represent cotton lint from gauze sponges or packs.

5–15 μm in width and up to several hundred microns in length, with twists at many levels that result in obliquely transverse folds. On cross-section, they are doughnut-shaped, with a central empty space surrounded by the fiber wall. The material is faintly pink in H&E sections, PAS-positive, doubly refractile, and is found inside multinucleated giant cells or embedded in fibrous tissue.

EMBOLIZING AGENTS

Surgical pathologists encounter arterial embolization materials in resected vascular tumors that are preoperatively embolized to

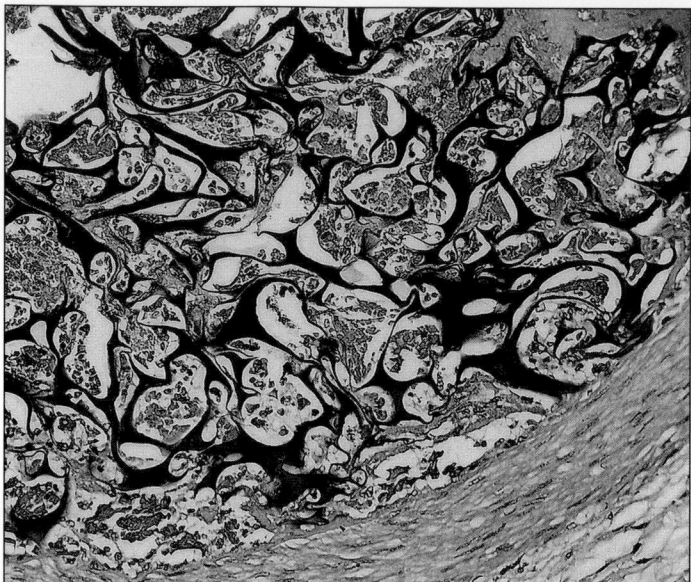

Fig. 5.7 Gelfoam has an irregular spiculated appearance. The material is in an artery injected before resection of a hemangioma in this region.

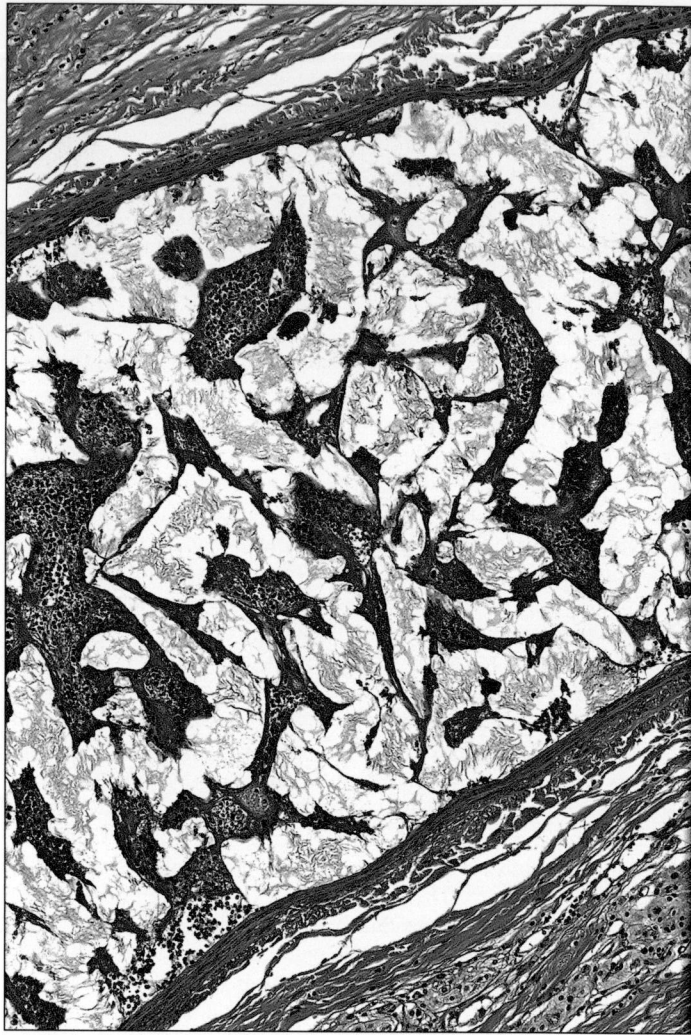

Fig. 5.8 Section from an intracranial meningioma following preoperative embolization and resection. Irregular, intravascular polyvinyl alcohol particles admixed with normal blood elements appear weakly basophilic by H&E staining.

optimize hemostasis or to shrink tumor size. Therapeutic arterial embolization of intractable epistaxis or hemoptysis is less likely to be detected in histologic sections.[72] A number of chemical embolization materials are used, sometimes in combination.[73,74] These include Gelfoam® (Pharmacia & Upjohn Co., Kalamazoo, MI), an absorbable gelatin that appears microscopically as basophilic, acellular, spiculated masses (Fig. 5.7). It may produce a severe foreign body reaction in the brain.[75] Avitene® (Davol, Inc., Cranston, RI) is a resorbable, microfibrillar collagen that forms intensely eosinophilic emboli that become rapidly endothelialized and recanalized and incite a minimal tissue reaction.[74] Surgifoam® (Ethicon, Inc., Somerville, NJ) is an absorbable gelatin sponge that is derived from porcine dermal gelatin. Microscopically, it appears as a meshwork of amorphous eosinophilic material. The tissue response to Surgifoam® is similar to that of Gelfoam®, consisting of a transient granulomatous response, but is slightly less.

Nonresorbable polyvinyl alcohol particles form irregular, intravascular emboli that are admixed with blood elements (Fig. 5.8). Polyvinyl alcohol particles are poorly stained by H&E but appear densely black on elastic stain.[76] They may induce an acute vasculitis and foreign-body reaction[77] but are essentially chemically inert, producing long-term vascular occlusion with recanalization and calcification.[78] The liquid embolization material bucrylate (isobutyl 2-cyanoacrylate) is partially dissolved during xylene tissue processing and is translucent by H&E staining. It is best demonstrated in tissue sections by ether-based oil-red O staining. Of the commonly used embolization materials, bucrylate appears to induce the most severe tissue reaction in the form of vasculitis, vessel necrosis, foreign body reaction, and occasional extravascular extrusion.[79]

Lipiodol-mediated delivery of cytotoxic drugs can be demonstrated in resected hepatocellular carcinoma by Sudan stain but not by H&E.[80] Microbead technology (Embogold®, Biosphere Medical, Inc., Rockland, MA) has recently been used to embolize smooth muscle tumors of the uterus. The material is spherical, made of an acrylic co-polymer cross-linked with gelatin. Microscopic sections show eosinophilic, spherical, acellular material in vessels, with foreign body reaction[81,82] (Fig. 5.9).

MYOSPHERULOSIS

In 1977, Kyriakos[83] reported that tissue removed from paranasal sinuses or the middle ear had small sacs containing spherules about the size of erythrocytes (Fig. 5.10). The name myospherulosis was chosen because of the identification of the findings with previously described cases from Africa, which occurred in muscle. All Kyriakos's patients had had previous operations that included packing with gauze impregnated with antibiotic ointment. Rosai[84] and Travis et al.[85] proved that the spherules are erythrocytes that become enveloped in a sac, so called 'endobodies.' Wheeler et al.[86] demonstrated that erythrocytes undergo the same change in vitro when incubated with human fat. This finding accounts for myospherulosis in soft tissues at injection sites.[87] Myospherulosis has also been demonstrated in the brain[88] and after portal vein

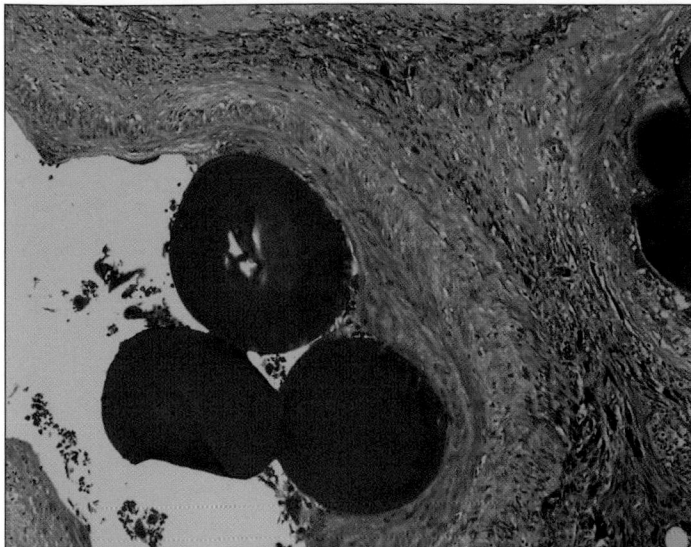

Fig. 5.9 Embogold® embolus in uterine vessel. Embolization was performed to shrink leiomyosarcoma prior to hysterectomy. The microbeads appear as round, eosinophilic, homogeneous material. Note the foreign-body reaction.

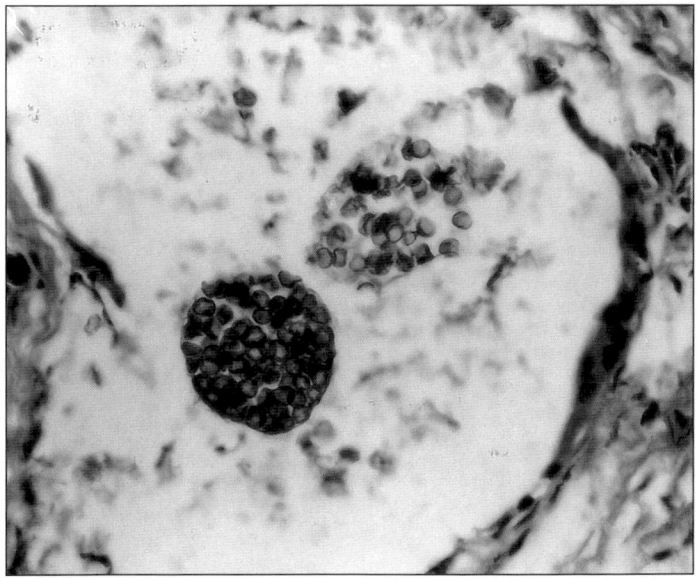

Fig. 5.10 Myospherulosis consists of an aggregate of altered red blood cells surrounded by a membrane. A fibrous and histiocytic inflammatory change is seen at the periphery. Patient had previous surgery for sinusitis that included packing with petroleum-impregnated gauze. (Courtesy of Dr Thomas M. Wheeler, Methodist Hospital, Houston, TX.)

embolization.[89] The 'endobodies' can be mistaken for fungi; however, PAS and Grocott stains are negative. An accurate, complete clinical history is extremely helpful.

In cytologic smears, the appearance of myospherulosis is essentially identical to its histologic image, isolated or sac-like aggregates of 4–7-μm spherules that presumably represent erythrocytes altered by previous lipid exposure. In addition to petroleum-based intramuscular injections, FNA detection of myospherulosis

has been associated with previous breast biopsy, fat necrosis, and invasive breast cancer.[90] Therefore, cytologic detection of myospherulosis indicates erythrocyte exposure to either endogenous or exogenous lipids and is a potential, albeit unusual, harbinger of underlying carcinoma.

STEROID INJECTION

A granulomatous reaction resembling rheumatoid nodules develops in the nasal mucosa after injection with steroids. The central amorphous area is apparently the injected substance itself.[91] A similar reaction occurs in keloids injected with steroids.[92] Rupture of tendons sometimes follows steroid injection but histologic findings are not specific.[93] Connective tissue steroid injection sites demonstrate similar deposits of amorphous, acellular material, but often no surrounding inflammatory reaction is present.[94]

OLEOGRANULOMA

Oleogranulomas (lipid granulomas, oleomas, paraffinomas) are reactive masses that occur as a reaction to a variety of oils that have been injected, topically applied, or used as a lubricant during dilatation of the cervix. Self-injection of sesame oil has been described in body builders, leading to soft tissue masses composed of multiple cystic spaces (lipid) surrounded by macrophages, giant cells, and fibrosis.[95] The histiocytic response may not produce a clinically detectable mass until years later, at which time rapid enlargement is possible.[96] Lesions have also been reported in the rectum, parametrium, and pleural space.[97,98]

LUBRICATING JELLIES AND CONTRACEPTIVE CREAMS

Lubricating jellies should not be used prior to obtaining cervicovaginal smears, since these can obscure cytologic detail and limit interpretation.[99] In addition, plant cellular materials found in some commercial lubricants may resemble neoplastic cells in cervicovaginal smears.[100]

TISSUE FILLERS

Tissue fillers include various substances that are either injected or surgically implanted, commonly for cosmesis in facial sites or the breast. In addition, there are many medical indications for tissue fillers, such as vocal cord paralysis or sphincter dysfunctions. Even cosmesis may be medically indicated, such as cleft lip/palate or postmastectomy for carcinoma. These substances include resorbable fillers, such as collagen (Zyderm®, INAMED, Santa Barbara, CA) and hyaluronic acid (Restylane®, Q-Med AB, Uppsala, Sweden); biodegradable substances, such as polylactic acid microspheres (New-Fill®, Biotech Industry SA, Luxembourg); and permanent fillers such as silicone, polymethylmethacrylate microspheres (Artecoll®, Rofil Medical International, Netherlands), acrylic hydrogel in hyaluronic acid (Dermalive®, Dermatech SA, Paris, France), and polytetrafluoroethylene (Teflon®, DuPont, Wilmington, DE). The histopathologic findings after injection/implantation range from almost no visible reaction to florid granulomatous inflammation.[101,102]

Silicone

Silicone is probably the most controversial of the tissue fillers. Silicones for medical use include: oil for coating needles and syringes, gel as implant material, elastomers in implanted prosthetic devices and intravenous fluid tubing. Soft tissue augmentation may use the liquid form of silicone, dimethylpolysiloxane.

Silicone injections of the breast are no longer used but many women still carry this substance and have symptoms that sometimes lead to biopsy. Silicone by itself causes little cellular reaction and may leak into adjacent tissues. Fibrosing agents were typically added to confine the silicone to localized areas. These agents cause a fibrohistiocytic reaction. Many of the histiocytes have an irregular configuration and the silicone produces a fine to coarse cytoplasmic vacuolization. Such cells may be mistaken for malignant lipoblasts.

More than 2 million silicone breast prostheses have been implanted in the United States alone since their introduction in the 1960s.[103] When the US Food and Drug Administration (FDA) began regulating medical devices in 1976, breast implants were 'grandfathered in,' with further investigations planned. Reports of increased autoimmune disease in patients with silicone breast implants surfaced, although no clear evidence of a linkage was proven.[104,105] The lack of safety data led the FDA to remove silicone implants from the market in 1992, except as investigational devices. Saline-filled implants remained on the market, although also lacking in safety information. The required safety information was subsequently submitted and the FDA approved saline breast implants in May 2000.[106]

Dense fibrous capsule formation or prosthetic rupture often leads to removal. Many of the fibrous capsules are lined with a cellular membrane histologically, immunohistochemically, and ultrastructurally identical to synovium.[107,108] This synovial metaplasia has been described in sutured skin, after repeated subcutaneous injections of air, and at the bone–cement interface of loosened hip prostheses.[109] The capsules and soft tissue beyond the capsule contain a variety of foreign material including droplets of silicone (Fig. 5.11), fragments of the prosthetic bag envelope, polyurethane, and talc.[110]

Silicone can appear in giant cells in the axillary nodes. Cytologic smears of silicone lymphadenopathy demonstrate refractile silicone fragments, both intracellular and extracellular, as well as asteroid bodies. FNA offers a relatively noninvasive method for excluding malignant lymphadenopathy in these patients.[111] Cases of carcinoma have been reported in patients with prostheses but no evidence thus far shows an increased incidence of cancer unless the patient had been irradiated.[112] Although needle aspiration in patients with silicone breast implants carries some risk of puncture, radiographically guided and unguided FNA attempts can still be performed to rule out malignant tumors. Cytologic smears in these cases occasionally detect silicone granulomas that exhibit loose aggregates of epithelioid histiocytes with variably sized, clear cytoplasmic vacuoles and little epithelium.[113]

Symptomatic splenomegaly due to macrophages filled with silicone has been reported in a patient undergoing hemodialysis. The silicone was presumably from the roller pumps.[114] It may also be found in the liver and kidney.

Silicone lymphadenopathy is seen in nodes draining joints that have silicone prostheses[115] (Fig. 5.12). The adenopathy can occur in the absence of synovitis or malfunction of the prosthesis.[116–18] However, cytologic demonstration of silicone elastomer microshards in fluids that accumulate adjacent to silicone joint prostheses may be an indication for removal of prostheses.[119]

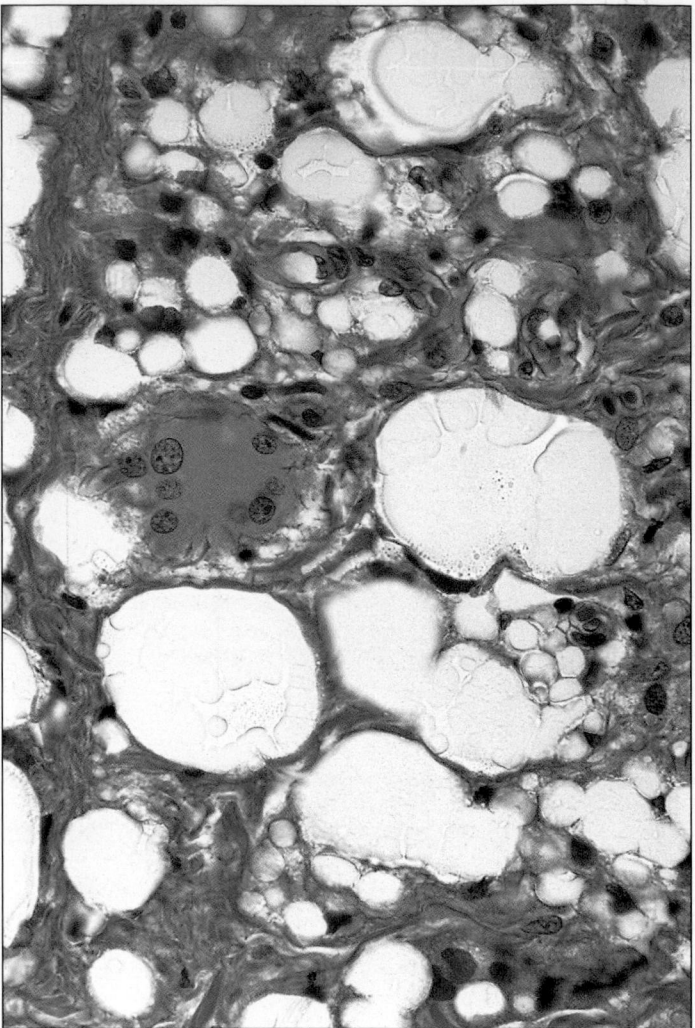

Fig. 5.11 Silicone in capsule of patient with silicone breast prosthesis removed because of contracture of fibrous capsule. Silicone gel is seen as variously sized droplets.

Teflon® paste and Proplast®

A paste containing the polymer polytetrafluoroethylene (PTFE, Teflon®) is used to correct vocal cord paralysis and for treatment of urinary incontinence.[120] Microscopically, it consists of shiny yellow particles in a myriad of shapes and sizes ranging from 6–100 mm (Fig. 5.13). The injected bolus becomes surrounded by a fibrous rim with some penetration between the particles. Mononuclear and multinucleated histiocytes also display a histiocytic response. In several patients treated for vocal cord paralysis, the material has entered the neck, resulting in a mass. Teflon® can be recognized on FNA.[121] The overlying epithelium of the vocal cord has not shown atypical changes nor have any other recognizable adverse reactions occurred despite the presence of small particles within the lymphatics or blood vessels.

Granulomatous foreign body reactions to Teflon® can be demonstrated by FNA. In one case, periurethral injection resulted in a macroscopic Teflon® cyst that yielded no giant cell or inflammatory infiltrate by FNA, only irregular, birefringent Teflon® particles.[122]

Proplast® (Vitek, Inc., Houston, TX) is a polymer of Teflon® and carbon or aluminum used mainly in cosmetic surgery for filling soft

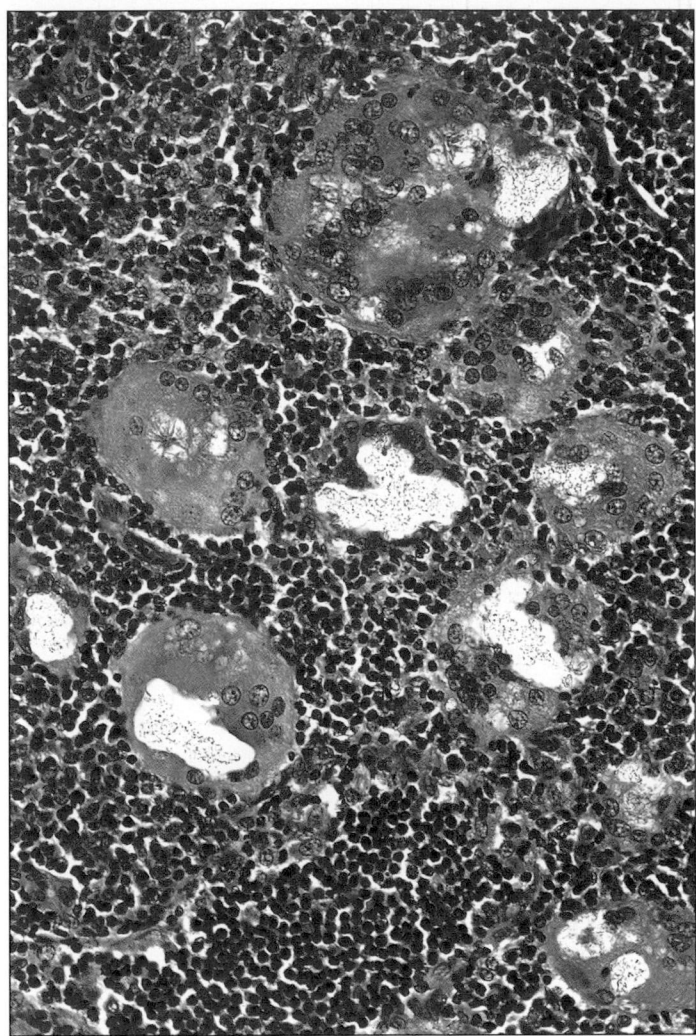

Fig. 5.12 Inguinal lymph node from patient with silicone prosthesis of hip joint. The translucent strands and globules of silicone are found within giant cells.

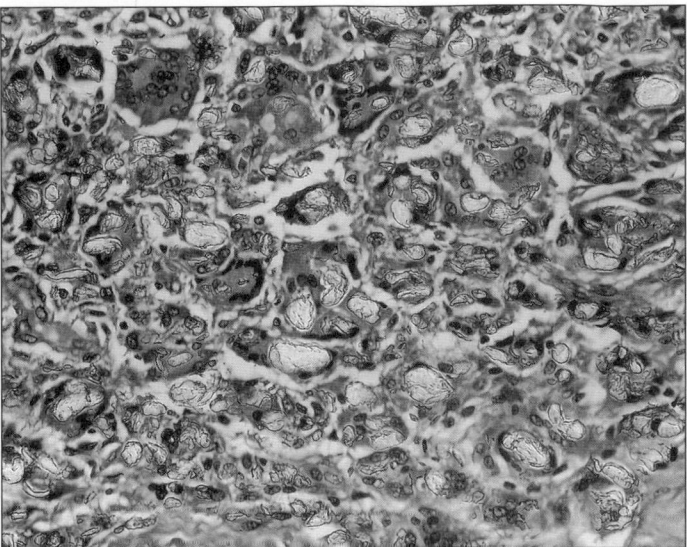

Fig. 5.13 Teflon paste within vocal cord. Irregular particles provoke a fibrous and histiocytic reaction.

tissue defects. Its porosity permits ingrowth of capillaries and connective tissue, which helps anchor the material in place. Occasionally the material may shift so the desired cosmetic effect is lost; the implant is then removed. The soft tissue around the prosthesis contains foreign body giant cells, some of which have small punctate particles of the carbon component.[123] Proplast® was also used in temporomandibular joint implants. With prolonged use, fragments of material may shear and cause a foreign body reaction.[124] Osseous destruction has also been reported, possibly due to release of hydrolytic enzymes by macrophages.[125] Similar to the silicone story, some patients alleged that autoimmune diseases were caused by this implant, without clear evidence. The material was taken off the market in 1991.[126]

INTRAUTERINE DEVICES

Intrauterine devices (IUDs) produce epithelial erosion and acute inflammation at the point of contact with the endometrium. Squamous metaplasia and foreign body granulomas are encountered

rarely.[127] Secretory development is delayed by 3 days or more in about 30% of women wearing these devices.[128]

Serious complications include perforation of the uterus and extrauterine infection, consisting usually of tubo-ovarian abscess. Inexplicably, the abscesses are nearly always unilateral, unlike 'ordinary' pelvic inflammatory disease, which is almost always bilateral.[129] Rarely, there is tubal migration of the IUD, which may lead to hydrosalpinx.[130] Disproportionate numbers of abscesses are secondary to *Actinomyces*, with its characteristic inflammatory response of a purulent exudate mixed with foamy histiocytes.

A constellation of cytologic abnormalities can be seen in the cervicovaginal smears of women using IUDs. In the early weeks after IUD insertion, smears show a prominent macrophage response followed by nonspecific reparative and degenerative changes similar to those that follow biopsy procedures.[131] Subsequent cellular changes that are specific for IUDs are easily confused with adenocarcinoma. These include shedding of glandular cells and occasional metaplastic squamous cells with prominent cytoplasmic vacuolization and variable degrees of nuclear enlargement, hyperchromasia, nucleolar prominence, nuclear membrane irregularity, and neutrophilic infiltration.[132,133] Less commonly, bizarre cells with high nuclear:cytoplasmic ratios and cytoplasmic protrusions can also be confused with malignancy. Pathologist awareness of IUD history helps to avoid a false diagnosis of malignant tumor.

In cytologic preparations, IUD-associated actinomycoses typically appear as irregular dense masses with radiating, filamentous bacterial organisms recognizable only at the periphery. Less commonly they appear as loose colonies of branched filaments. Similar but distinct filamentous aggregates surrounded by a dense rim of inflammatory cells are often inappropriately termed 'sulfur granules.' These can represent actinomycoses but are not specific, since they are also seen in other infections.[133] Fragments of IUD material, polarizable sulfa crystals from topical ointments, contraceptive creams, hematoidin crystals, and uncharacterized radiate crystals associated with pregnancy can also be confused with actinomycoses.[133,134] IUD usage is occasionally associated with calcifications and psammoma bodies in cervicovaginal smears, findings that otherwise would suggest the possibility of ovarian or endometrial adenocarcinoma.[135]

CRYOTHERAPY

Cryotherapy was first introduced in the 1960s and became standard therapy for many skin lesions and for the uterine cervix and vagina. The degree of damage to tissue by intense cold depends on the temperature and duration of application. In the uterine cervix, the epithelium becomes contracted and degenerates almost instantly. The sharp line of demarcation is only a few cells wide. Blood vessels regenerate a new endothelial lining after about 2 weeks. After a few months the only marker of previous cryosurgery is the hyalinized but patent blood vessels.[136]

In the immediate days following cervical and vaginal cryotherapy, smears contain a background of necrotic cellular debris and acute inflammation that should not be confused with malignant tumor diathesis. Early after cryotherapy, cytoplasmic vacuolization is seen that remains for weeks and occasionally for months.[137] Reparative changes identical to those seen in postbiopsy smears are seen following cryotherapy as well as electrocautery, laser ablation, and radiotherapy. In contrast to radiotherapy, cryotherapy changes lack significant nuclear and cytoplasmic enlargement and nuclear irregularity. In contrast to laser therapy and electrocautery, cryotherapy does not produce prominent epithelial cell elongation.[138] The duration of cytologic abnormalities that follow cryotherapy, electrocautery, and laser ablation varies with the mode of therapy, individual technique, and anatomic extent of treatment but generally lasts for 6 weeks or longer.[139] Cervical cryotherapy, electrocautery, and laser ablation can shift the squamocolumnar transformation zone superiorly into the endocervical canal, similar to conization, necessitating endocervical brush instead of cotton swab sampling of endocervical epithelium.[140]

In recent years, the development of thin cryoprobes aided by radiological procedures has allowed the freezing of deep tissue lesions with accuracy. This technique in being studied in a number of sites, especially in the prostate.[141]

Postcryotherapy histological changes in the prostate resemble those seen in the cervix. Early necrosis and inflammation is followed by granulation tissue, fibrosis, and focal re-epithelialization.[142] To minimize postcryotherapy complications, transrectal sonography is used to monitor hyperechoic periprostatic freeze damage as a signal for termination of therapy. Hyperechoic damage is not a good indicator of tumor destruction, since prostatectomy specimens removed 3–10 months following ultrasound-proven 'complete' freezing often contain viable carcinoma.[143]

ORTHOPEDIC HARDWARE

A variety of materials are used in prosthetic devices. The materials used and the tissue reactions are discussed in detail in Chapter 13. The carcinogenic effect of the various materials has been of concern, since the substances used in prostheses produce sarcomas in rodents. The relevance of these studies to humans remains to be determined. Thus far sarcoma has developed only rarely at the site of a prosthesis. The most frequent tumor to be diagnosed is malignant fibrous histiocytoma, with osteosarcoma, leiomyosarcoma, fibrosarcoma, chondrosarcoma, epithelioid sarcoma, synovial sarcoma,

angiosarcoma, and undifferentiated sarcoma also described.[144,145] Even if no cause-and-effect relationship exists in some of these cases, they attest to the rarity of neoplasms associated with the 300 000–400 000 total joint replacements inserted each year worldwide.[146]

Metallic components from hip prostheses can evoke a florid histiocytic response in the pelvic lymph nodes.[147] This alteration has been found in patients having pelvic lymphadenectomy for urinary bladder or prostatic cancer.[148] It has been confused with carcinoma.[149]

SUTURE MATERIALS

The thoughtful pathologist always removes suture material before submitting a block of tissue for embedding. Nevertheless, small fragments of suture may be buried in the middle of the block or may be in a stage of disintegration and not grossly detectable. A surgeon occasionally asks whether suture is present in an excised focus of inflammation; if so the surgeon may wish to know the type of material.

Sutures can be divided into two groups, absorbable and nonabsorbable. Absorbable sutures include catgut (derived from sheep or beef intestines), collagen, polyglycolic acid, polyglactin 910, polydioxone, and polyglyconate. The nonabsorbable sutures are polyamide (nylon), cotton, polyester, polypropylene, polybutester, and steel. Silk is generally placed in this category, although it disintegrates and eventually disappears after a period of many months to years.[150]

All sutures provoke a tissue response. Absorbable sutures generally incite a greater inflammatory response. Within a week, catgut is destroyed by the proteolytic enzymes of neutrophils and, therefore, requires inflammation to be absorbed. Chromic treatment to catgut delays proteolytic digestion for an additional week. The absorbable synthetic polymers are hydrolyzed by water and do not require enzymatic degradation but nonetheless they evoke a histiocytic and fibrous reaction.[151] The response to silk and cotton includes neutrophils, lymphocytes, or macrophages and eventually ends with a fibrous reaction accompanied only by macrophages. All the other materials excite a histiocytic response with minimal fibrosis.[152] Rarely, silk suture evokes a necrobiotic granuloma closely resembling rheumatoid nodules.[153]

On occasion, the inflammatory reaction to suture after resection of a portion of the gastrointestinal tract produces a mass sufficiently large to be seen as a filling defect on barium examination. A few patients have undergone re-exploration because the defect was believed to be a recurrence of neoplasm at the suture line or a new primary in another organ into which suture had migrated.[154,155]

Sutures may also be categorized by whether they are monofilamentous or multifilamentous (in general, monofilamentous sutures have a lower risk of infection, whereas multifilamentous sutures are easier to handle and tie). Silk, polyester and cotton are always multifilamentous. Nylon and steel are produced in either mono- or multifilamentous forms. Polypropylene is manufactured only as a monofilament. Catgut, whether plain or chromic, is a monofilamentous, homogeneous, faintly eosinophilic or amphophilic substance (Fig. 5.14). The multiple filaments of silk are of similar size but are round, square, or triangular when seen in cross-section (Fig. 5.15). Each of the filaments in the multifilament synthetic sutures is round and of identical size (Fig. 5.16). Randomly scattered tiny black specks are seen both in polyester and nylon. Polyglactin and polypropylene tend to have a glossy, transparent appearance.[152]

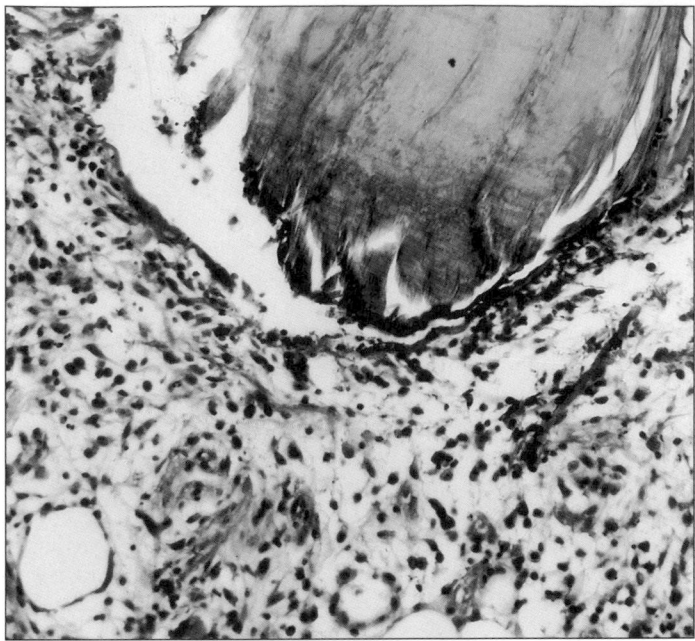

Fig. 5.14 Catgut suture is fairly homogeneous material with inflammatory response, including many neutrophils.

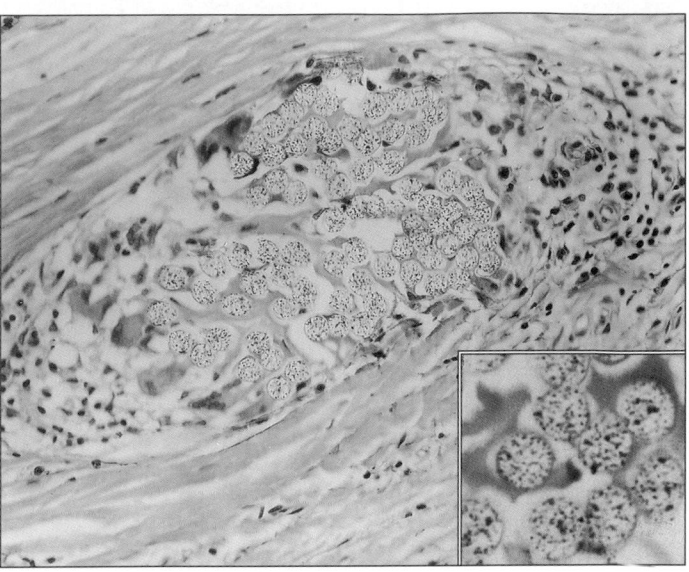

Fig. 5.16 Cross section of Dacron®, which had been in place for 2 years, showing foreign body giant cells between the individual filaments.

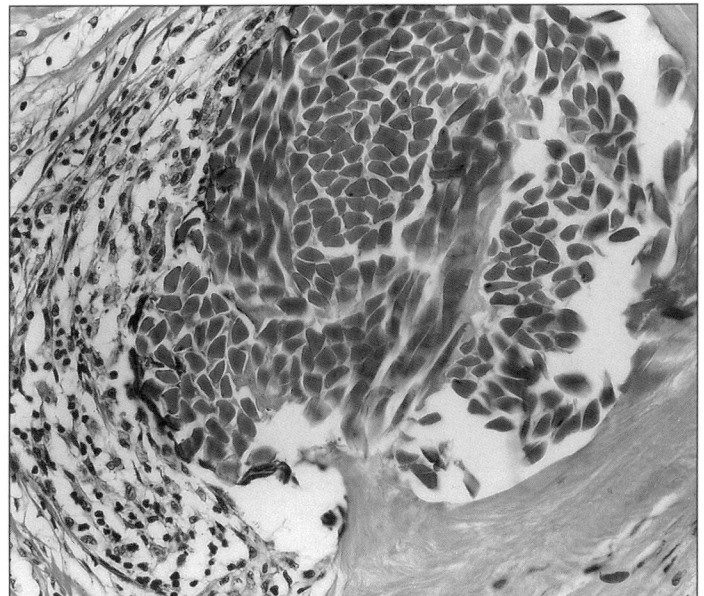

Fig. 5.15 Silk suture is always multifilamentous with irregularly shaped, dark filaments.

Some sutures are covered on the surface with Teflon® to decrease the abrasive effect, and minute fragments may be flaked off into the adjacent tissue.

On microscopic examination some sutures are always specifically identifiable (e.g. catgut), whereas others can only be placed in a general category (e.g. multifilamentous synthetic agents).

In sites of previous surgery for neoplasia, reactive suture granulomas can be clinically worrisome for recurrent disease.

Pathologic evaluation by needle aspiration typically demonstrates multinucleated giant cells with intracytoplasmic fragments of suture material, obviating the need for additional surgery. However, FNA smears of suture granulomas occasionally lack these diagnostic features and instead show a predominance of reactive spindle cells with mild nuclear pleomorphism. Depending on the histology of the original tumor, these findings can paradoxically augment suspicion for a malignant tumor and can necessitate rebiopsy.[156]

MONSEL'S SOLUTION

Monsel's solution (20% ferric subsulfate) is commonly used by dermatologists as a styptic or hemostatic after superficial skin biopsies. The compound may be in spindle cells with large vesicular nuclei[157] and may seep as deeply as skeletal muscle.[158] If the diagnosis on the biopsy specimen is melanoma and the area is subsequently excised, the interpretation of the depth of invasion is hampered by the distorted cells and pigment.[159] After excision of other skin lesions, the Monsel's artifact may mimic melanoma, and be a problem diagnostically, unless the pathologist is aware of the clinical history. Monsel's has also been used in the uterine cervix as a hemostatic agent in biopsies, causing problems in the interpretation of subsequent cone biopsies because of necrosis of the surface epithelium.[160]

VASCULAR PROSTHESES

Rare cases of sarcomas arising in the region of a vascular prosthesis graft have been reported, including angiosarcoma, malignant fibrous histiocytoma, and fibrosarcoma. Most of the tumors have high grade, with poor prognosis, with latency periods ranging from months to over 10 years.[161,162]

UNTOWARD RESULTS OF SURGICAL PROCEDURES

IMPLANTATION OF NORMAL TISSUE

Endometriosis is the classical example of implantation of normal tissue. Endometriosis occurring in a C-section scar has been mistaken for carcinoma, particularly if there is decidual reaction or myxoid change. The fallopian tube is sometimes caught in the incision at the time of vaginal hysterectomy and can produce a vaginal mass on subsequent examination. The biopsy specimen shows tubal architecture with its normal complement of cells; degenerative and regenerative cytologic alterations can be seen in the form of cells with enlarged or dense nuclei. Stratification of the cells can be prominent. Omentum has been implanted in the endometrium following operative perforation of the uterus.[163]

Normal colonic mucosa deep in the wall of the bowel was found when a colostomy was closed after 8 years. Presumably it was implanted at the original procedure.[164] Six of 19 patients with localized colitis cystica profunda of the rectum had a history of previous rectal surgery.[165] It is possible that the procedure implanted mucosa or altered the muscularis mucosae to permit downward extension of glands.

Thyroid tissue has been described in the lateral neck after prior surgery. The adjacent suture material suggests mechanical implantation.[166] Parathyromatosis, a syndrome consisting of parathyroid tissue scattered throughout the neck, is a complication of parathyroid surgery for parathyroid hyperplasia, presumably due to the implantation of parathyroid tissue in the neck during surgery.[167] Parathyromatosis has also been described after FNA of the parathyroid gland.[168]

ALTERATIONS DUE TO CARDIAC PROCEDURES

Fragments of tissue from suctioning of the pericardial cavity during surgery produces artifacts due to a mixture of adipose tissue, pericardial mesothelium, and foreign material.[169] Cardiac catheterization may also account for some of these mixtures of cells, and they may cause confusion with malignant neoplasm or endomyocardial biopsies.[170]

VENTRICULOPERITONEAL SHUNTS

Ventriculoperitoneal shunts are occasionally occluded by overgrowths of reactive inflammatory tissue, peritoneal mesothelium, or central nervous system (CNS) tissues including choroid plexus, glia, and meninges. Occluding tissues may be submitted for histologic examination to exclude recurrent neoplasia. Associated intraventricular inflammatory and foreign body reactions can be seen in cerebrospinal fluid.[171] Tissue from primary CNS tumors or, less commonly, benign choroid plexus may embolize through the shunt into the peritoneal cavity, where they appear cytologically positive or suggestive of malignant tumor, respectively.[172] Benign glial nodules as well as neoplasms have spread to the peritoneal cavity.[173,174]

ALTERATIONS AT THE SITE OF ANASTOMOSES

Numerous alterations, including adenocarcinomas, have been reported in the colon in the immediate area of ureterosigmoidostomies. Some are adenomatous polyps with prominent submucosal cysts resembling colitis cystica profunda. The carcinomas are weighted by undifferentiated and mucin-producing tumors. The neoplasms are closely related to the length of time that the patients have had the ureterosigmoidostomy (an average of about 20 years).[175] This argues strongly in favor of a causal relationship: the urinary stream produces premalignant changes, perhaps because of the high concentration of secondary amines with activation of *N*-nitroso compounds, and ultimately may produce a malignant neoplasm.[176,177] Carcinoma can occur even after early external diversion.[178]

Gastric polyps around gastroenterostomy stomas have included small discrete masses as well as completely circumferential proliferations, which on occasion have prolapsed into the lumen. Microscopically, dilated glands protrude through the muscularis and have been designated gastritis cystica polyposa.[179]

Even in the absence of a gross polyp, sections from the gastric mucosa at the anastomotic site may display abnormalities, including dilated glands and a decrease in chief and parietal cells. If an erosion or ulcer is present, the adjacent epithelium can have regenerating, immature cells with a high nuclear:cytoplasmic ratio that line irregular glands of variable sizes.[180,181] An increased incidence of gastric cancer exists in patients with gastroenterostomies,[182] and the tumors may arise in the polyps.[183] Some 37 years after a Billroth II resection, a squamous carcinoma developed in the gastric stump.[184]

POSTOPERATIVE ABDOMINAL CYSTS

Peritoneal cysts may develop several months to years after surgery, particularly in patients who have had a postoperative course with signs of peritonitis or wound infection.[185] Most patients are women with a previous history of pelvic or abdominal surgery, endometriosis, or pelvic inflammatory disease.[186] The cysts may be free-floating, embedded in the retroperitoneum, or attached to any of the abdominal viscera. They are unilocular or multilocular and contain clear, yellow, or green-brown fluid. The cysts are lined by low cuboidal or flattened mesothelium-like cells, squamous epithelium, or no cells at all. The wall is fibrous with variable vascularity and inflammation. The pathogenesis is not clear but possibly relates to walled-off areas of inflammation. The rapid growth that sometimes occurs may be due to osmotic forces secondary to hemorrhage.

In histologic sections, the cystic configuration, previous operative history, prominent chronic inflammation, stromal reaction, and mild to moderate degree of nuclear atypia indicate a reactive process.[186] Malignant mesotheliomas are rarely prominently cystic.[187] FNA of peritoneal inclusion cysts can yield reactive, hypertrophic mesothelial cells with nuclear enlargement and prominent nucleoli that suggest malignant tumor, especially after previous surgery for carcinoma. Wide variation in mesothelial cell size, cytoplasmic vacuolation, and multinucleation may be seen, identical to reactive mesothelial changes in other serous fluids. Fine chromatin, regular nuclear membranes, prominent but regular nucleoli, ruffled plasma membrane contours, and characteristic intercellular spaces or 'windows' generally allow distinction from recurrent malignant tumor. In difficult cases, panels of immunohistochemical stains performed on cytologic fluids, including the mesothelium-specific antibody ME1, or standard paraffin-based panels on cell block preparations are useful.[188,189]

The formation of lymphocysts is a complication of pelvic or renal surgery. The cyst contains a clear slightly yellow fluid and is devoid of lining cells. Symptoms are related to a mass compressing the ureter, bladder, colon, or vessels, resulting in edema of the lower extremities. The origin from lymphatic channels is documented by numerous reports in which lymphangiography medium has filled the mass.[190] Meticulous attention to ligation of lymphatic trunks at the time of the original surgery minimizes cyst formation.[191]

Mesenteric cysts, usually lined by luteal cells, can follow surgery of the ovary. Presumably minute portions of ovary are dislodged and implant on the peritoneum, where they survive and enlarge.[192]

REACTIONS RESEMBLING NEOPLASMS

Proppe et al.[193] described a highly cellular spindle cell proliferation with numerous mitotic figures that occurred in the vagina after a variety of surgical procedures. The largest mass was 4 cm in diameter. A similar proliferation has occurred in the prostatic urethra and urinary bladder following transurethral resections and in the endocervix.[194] The lesions appear 2 weeks to 3 months after surgery. Clinical history is essential since postoperative spindle cell nodules (PSCN) of the bladder and prostate can be histologically identical to spontaneous spindle-cell proliferations ('inflammatory pseudotumors'), which are sometimes associated with underlying carcinomas.[195] Focal immunohistochemical staining for cytokeratins in some PSCN may confound this differential. PSCN and spontaneous spindle-cell proliferations also share histologic features with two primary genitourinary tract cancers: spindle cell carcinoma and leiomyosarcoma. Accurate diagnosis frequently requires immunohistochemistry in addition to clinical history.[196] FNA smears of reparative mesenchymal proliferations, including PSCN and inflammatory pseudotumors, occasionally demonstrate sufficient spindle-cell hypercellularity and pleomorphism to be confused with cancer. A prominent inflammatory background in these cases should alert the pathologist not to make a definitive cytologic diagnosis of sarcoma.[197]

A highly cellular fibrohistiocytic proliferation with nuclear atypia resembling liposarcoma has occurred in sites in which sclerosing agents were used for the repair of hernia. Silica has been identified in these foci. Although this material is no longer used, the interval between injection and lesion has ranged up to 40 years; therefore, this lesion may still be seen.[198] A similar reaction has been described in the lip after use of liquid silicone for lip augmentation. The patient initially denied a history of intervention and only admitted to the injection procedure when confronted with the possibility of disfiguring facial surgery for 'liposarcoma.'[199]

Broad aggregates of histiocytes with eosinophilic granular cytoplasm may accumulate at the site of surgical trauma and resemble granular cell tumor. The granular cytoplasm is lipofuscin, which is usually acid-fast.[200]

Unilocular or multilocular cysts that raise the possibility of malignant neoplasm have been found in women who have undergone previous surgery.[201] Entrapped, markedly atypical mesothelial cells with mitotic activity mimic adenocarcinoma (Fig. 5.17).

MALIGNANT NEOPLASMS

A few malignant tumors have arisen at the site of previous surgery. One of the 200 malignant fibrous histiocytomas reported by Weiss and Enzinger[202] arose 8 years later at the excision site for a lipoma. Two additional cases, one at an amputation site and the other in a hernioplasty scar, have been reported.[203] Whether these are coincidental is arguable. Lymphangiosarcoma of the upper extremity (Stewart–Treves syndrome) is a rare complication of lymphedema following mastectomy with axillary dissection.[204]

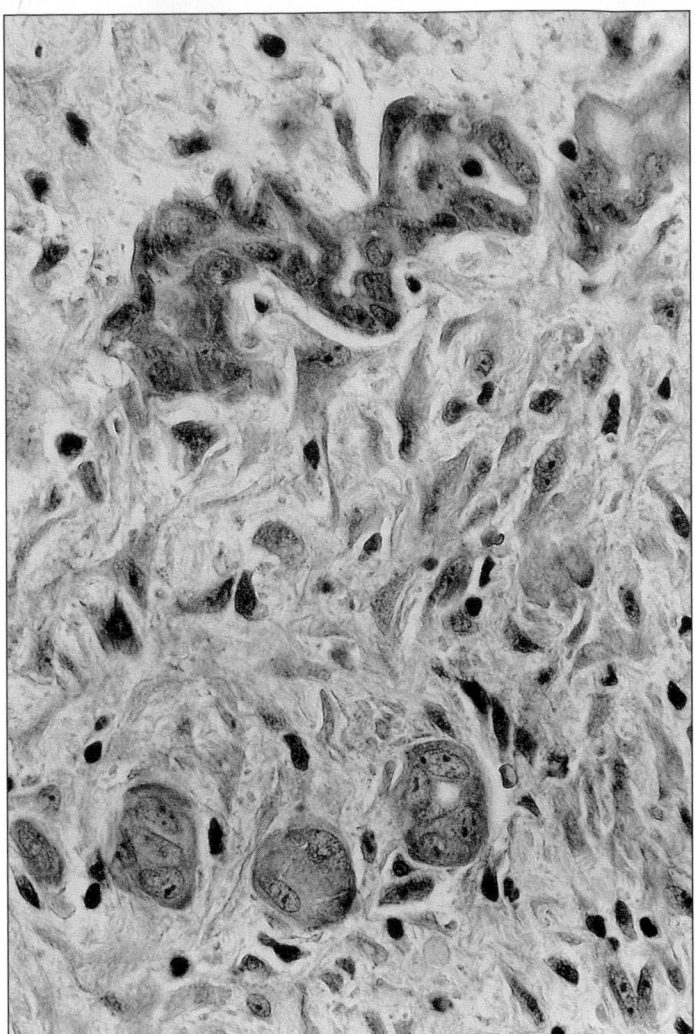

Fig. 5.17 Entrapped mesothelial cells mimic adenocarcinoma. This is from the wall of a postoperative peritoneal inclusion cyst. (Courtesy of Dr Philip B. Clement, Vancouver General Hospital, Vancouver, BC.)

REACTIONS TO CYTOTOXIC DRUGS AND IMMUNOSUPPRESSION

Chemotherapy for cancer and some nonmalignant conditions involves potent agents that may have morphologic as well as physiologic effects on a variety of normal tissues. The toxicity of the various agents is diverse. Much of the morbidity consists of gastrointestinal symptoms, bone marrow suppression, cutaneous alterations, and hepatic or renal impairment. The surgical pathologist is uncommonly involved in these problems, with some notable exceptions. For example, perforation of the small intestine in patients with widespread lymphoma was a rare event prior to chemotherapy but now occurs due to drug-induced massive necrosis of tumor within the bowel wall.[205] Some tumors also display behavioral changes such as unusual sites of metastases[206–208] or a more widespread distribution.[209–211] Whether this reflects immune suppression that facilitates spread of the tumor or is due to an increased duration of survival is uncertain. Cavitation of pulmonary metastases may occur that is due to chemotherapy and can be confused with inflammatory

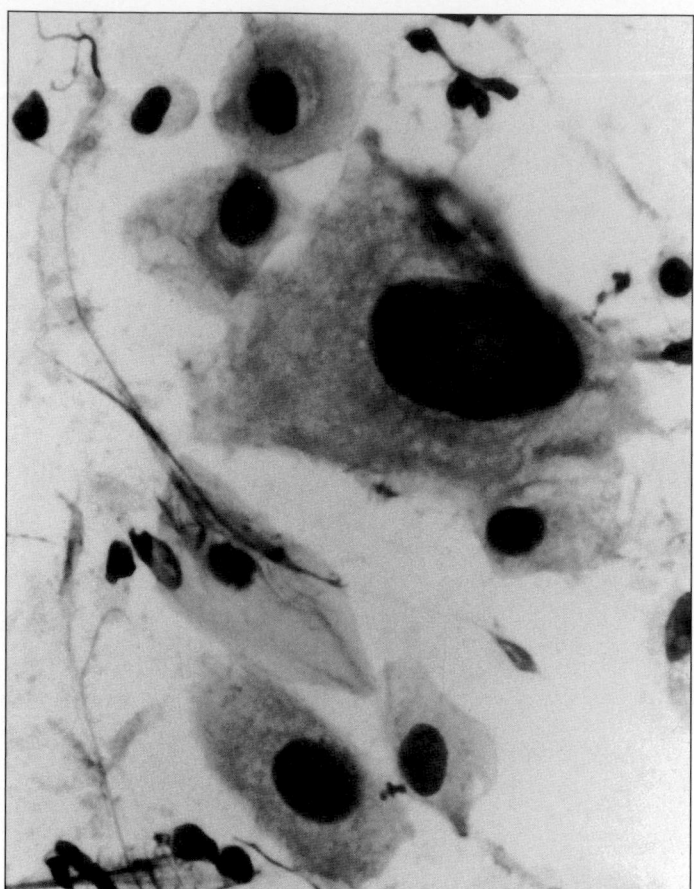

Fig. 5.18 Cells in sputum of a patient receiving busulfan for leukemia. He had pneumonia but no pulmonary neoplasm. The wide variation in size of qualitatively similar cells is the characteristic spectrum for this cytopathy.

lesions.[212] Hepar lobatum results from a chemotherapeutic effect on breast cancer metastatic to the liver.[213]

CHANGES IN NORMAL EPITHELIUM

Alkylating agents can induce epithelial abnormalities that mimic malignancy in many organs, notably lung, lower urinary tract, and cervix.[214–217] Multidrug chemotherapeutic regimens that include alkylating agents have produced marked epithelial atypia in diagnostic specimens from the breast[218,219] and esophagus.[220] Histologic effects of chemotherapy are usually seen in resected specimens following preoperative therapy.

Biopsies, FNAs, or cytologic smears of sputum, bronchoalveolar, urine, or cervicovaginal origin may contain identical abnormal cells, raising the possibility of metastases or a second primary neoplasm. Since alkylating agents can cause secondary solid tumors, this distinction is especially problematic. Cytologic changes due to alkylating agents mimic radiation-induced changes as well as cancers and include cytomegaly, increased nuclear size, increased nuclear:cytoplasmic ratio, bizarre shapes, cytoplasmic vacuolization, and occasionally hyperchromasia (Fig. 5.18). Morphometric image analysis of urine cytologies cannot clearly distinguish these toxic changes from malignancy.[221] A continuous spectrum of atypia from minimally enlarged, non-neoplastic cells to bizarre giant cells

and the detection of cilia on atypical pulmonary cells indicate drug-induced change.[221] However, in cases with extreme atypia, clinical history may be the most important discriminator.

Urine cytology is particularly affected by the alkylating agent cyclophosphamide,[222] which is concentrated in urine, and by intravesical cytotoxic therapy, although effects of the latter are less likely to resemble malignancy.[223] Nonalkylating agents such as bleomycin can cause changes similar to alkylating agents in the lung.[224]

Chemotherapy for mammary carcinoma may produce multi-lobated cells within otherwise normal ducts of the breast. These do not resemble the cells of carcinoma in situ and undoubtedly reflect chemotherapy effect.[225] Atrophy of lobules may be focally prominent. A teardrop appearance has been seen in some breasts treated with chemotherapy and may reflect hormonal (tamoxifen) therapy. Rarely, no residual carcinoma is detectable. The tumor site has been replaced by a nodular fibrous reaction accompanied by histiocytes.[224]

Extensive cytoplasmic vacuolization is found in glands of normal or hyperplastic prostate.[225] Involutional changes and basal cell hyperplasia may also be seen.

The effects of topical podophyllin therapy on condyloma acuminatum are frequently claimed to mimic high-grade squamous intraepithelial neoplasia. Acute post-therapy changes of edema, increased mitotic activity, and single cell keratinocyte degeneration and necrosis are followed by hyperkeratosis and mixed inflammation, all of which resolve within 2–6 weeks. Persistence of orderly maturation and lack of diagnostic nuclear atypia allow distinction from high-grade dysplasia.[226] By contrast, topical cytotoxic therapy with 5-fluorouracil can produce nonspecific chemical mucositis and nonhealing ulcers.[227]

Intravesical bacillus Calmette–Guérin (BCG) immunotherapy for transitional cell carcinoma or high-grade urothelial dysplasia induces a prominent granulomatous response in both the bladder and prostate. In addition to caseating and noncaseating granulomas, squamous metaplasia and a mixed inflammatory infiltrate are seen. Urine cytology demonstrates degenerating epithelial cell debris in a background of abundant mixed inflammation, but granulomatous features are not prominent. Prostatic FNA specimens taken after BCG therapy contain similar features but also demonstrate histiocytes and multinucleated giant cells, similar to prostatic FNA smears following transurethral resections.[217]

Toxic pulmonary effects of the antiarrhythmic drug amiodarone are morphologically striking, although they do not resemble malignancy. A prominent alveolar infiltrate of foamy macrophages and occasional vacuolated parenchymal cells demonstrates characteristic cytoplasmic lamellar inclusions by ultrastructural examination.[228] These toxic changes can be monitored by bronchoalveolar lavage[229] and are rarely seen in pleural fluids.[230]

CHANGES IN NEOPLASTIC EPITHELIUM

It is now common to give preoperative chemotherapy with or without radiotherapy prior to a surgical resection. The appearance of the treated cancer in the surgical specimen may have major implications for the type of additional therapy, as exemplified in the treatment of osteosarcoma. In this instance, the continuation of the preoperative chemotherapy regimen depends on the amount of viable tumor present in the resected tissue. Similarly, therapeutic judgments may be based on the appearance of neoplasm in patients who have received preoperative chemotherapy for carcinoma of the breast. In one study, the appearance of the tumor and the ability to grade it histologically were identical to the prechemotherapy biopsy in many instances.[231]

Kennedy et al[219] illustrated an extraordinary vacuolization of neoplastic cells such that they resembled foamy histiocytes. Epithelial markers were identified by immunohistochemistry, indicating that these were persistent epithelial cells.

Chemotherapy-induced changes in malignant tumors do not necessarily indicate a lethal effect. Morphologic and kinetic monitoring of pulmonary small cell carcinomas during multidrug chemotherapy demonstrates drug-induced vacuolization and nuclear enlargement that do not inevitably lead to cell death.[232]

HISTOLOGIC MATURATION AFTER CHEMOTHERAPY

Cytotoxic drug therapy may accentuate maturation of various elements in residual neoplasms. Testicular mixed germ cell tumors can have only benign-appearing elements in metastases after chemotherapy.[233] Many ovarian immature teratomas and a few adenocarcinomas have shown maturation after drug therapy.[234] A plausible explanation is based on the premise that neoplasms have heterogeneous subpopulations that react differently to the same therapeutic agent, with the less well differentiated component being more susceptible. This phenomenon has been reported frequently since the advent of chemotherapy, but it should be kept in mind that an identical maturation of metastatic germ cell tumors was reported prior to the chemotherapy era.[235]

Resected germ cell tumors that contain predominantly benign mature elements must be examined carefully, because they may also have small foci of malignancy. The malignancy can be present even when previously elevated serum markers have returned to normal.[233] Cytologic atypia, as opposed to obviously invasive cancer, does not seem to be an adverse prognostic factor in males.[236]

Residual rhabdomyosarcoma of childhood sometimes has a high proportion of rhabdomyoblasts and strap cells after chemotherapy. It occurs only when similar cells are focally present in the original tumor.[237,238] Other types of soft tissue sarcoma also have a lower histologic grade after chemotherapy (with or without concomitant radiotherapy).[239] This finding again suggests that high-grade populations of cells are more susceptible to therapy than low-grade clones.

Differentiation of neuroblastoma to ganglioneuroblastoma with a predominance of mature atypical ganglion cells and fewer immature malignant cells has been found after cytotoxic chemotherapy for neuroblastoma. Differentiation did not, however, correlate with prognosis.[240]

Hepatoblastomas may have small areas of osteoid in the original tumor, which may occupy large areas after chemotherapy. Such a predominance of 'benign tissue' does not seem to be a favorable prognostic sign, although this point is arguable.[241]

An autopsy study of patients with choriocarcinoma disclosed that a few patients had residua consisting only of atypical cytotrophoblasts.[242] Similar trophoblasts can be seen in surgically resected choriocarcinomas after chemotherapy. These cells resemble intermediate trophoblasts and may reflect an insensitivity of this stage of trophoblastic differentiation to chemotherapy.

Patients with Wilms tumor may receive preoperative chemotherapy. Up to 90% of the tumor mass may become necrotic, mainly in the replicating, undifferentiated elements.[243] Mature heterotopic elements such as cartilage, fat, and skeletal muscle persisted after therapy. A few tumors consisted almost entirely of skeletal muscle.[244] Favorable outcomes were associated with extensive tumor necrosis (>90%), low mitotic activity, and high degrees of differentiation of residual tumor.[244]

PERSISTENT NON-NEOPLASTIC TUMOR MASS

A tumor mass can persist after chemotherapy, radiotherapy, or a combination of the two. It can be interpreted as a therapeutic failure and result in additional, unnecessary therapy. After an adequate course of therapy, persistent tumor masses that are resected often consist only of inflamed fibrous tissue with necrotic areas lacking any neoplasm. It has been reported in lymph nodes from patients with Hodgkin's disease,[245] large-cell lymphoma,[246] and testicular embryonal carcinoma.[247,248] This phenomenon has also occurred in the spleen.[246]

THYMIC HYPERPLASIA

The thymus may become hyperplastic after chemotherapy and/or autologous stem cell transplantation and may mimic a mediastinal neoplasm.[249] A lesser degree of hyperplasia is not uncommon, occurring in 11% of 102 breast cancer patients in one study.[250] The cause is unknown but may be related to rebound hyperplasia after cytotoxic therapy.

NON-NEOPLASTIC LYMPHADENOPATHY

Enlarged lymph nodes following therapy for malignant neoplasm always raise the possibility of metastatic disease. In one instance, a man developed rapidly enlarging axillary nodes 1 month after completion of chemotherapy for lymphoma. The node consisted only of a narrow rim of lymphoid tissue surrounding normal mature fat.[251] Fatty replacement is commonly seen in nodes removed during axillary dissections for carcinoma of the breast, but rapid growth is not a feature of such nodes.[252]

Geis et al.[253] reported five renal transplant recipients in whom gigantic systemic lymphadenopathy developed shortly after transplantation. It rapidly resolved with no evidence of residual disease from 6–15 months later. These patients had received antithymocyte globulin and presumably had a transient reaction to this agent. The biopsies were indistinguishable from diffuse large cell lymphoma. In another report, a similar reaction developed in the soft tissue at the site of antilymphocytic globulin injection.[254] These may represent variant forms of post-transplantation lymphoproliferative disorders.

DRUG-ASSOCIATED NEOPLASMS

Secondary malignant tumors are attributed to a number of cytotoxic drugs, most notably the alkylating agents.[255] Alkylating agent therapy is associated with aggressive acute nonlymphocytic leukemias, which typically evolve through a myelodysplastic phase, occur 5–10 years following primary therapy, and are linked to toxins and genetic polymorphisms.[256] Among cases with chromosomal abnormalities, most are associated with deletions in chromosomes 5 and 7.[257] Acute leukemia has also been reported after alkylating agents were used in the treatment of rheumatoid arthritis or multiple sclerosis.[258] In contrast to alkylating agents, topoisomerase inhibitors lead to secondary acute nonlymphocytic leukemias that do not evolve through a myelodysplastic phase, occur 2–3 years following primary therapy, and demonstrate abnormalities of chromosomes 11q23.[259]

Second primary cancers have followed successful chemotherapy for Hodgkin's disease, non-Hodgkin's lymphoma, multiple myeloma, pulmonary small cell undifferentiated carcinoma, ovarian and breast carcinoma, and polycythemia vera. Within 20 years of therapy for Hodgkin's disease, second neoplasms include a predominance of solid tumors, mostly gastrointestinal and pulmonary carcinomas, in addition to earlier occurring acute leukemias and non-Hodgkin's lymphoma.[260] Adjuvant radiotherapy appears to play a role in the development of secondary solid tumors. By contrast, non-Hodgkin's lymphoma therapy carries a negligibly increased relative risk of development of solid tumors but is clearly associated with secondary acute leukemia.[261] Leukemia developed 30–90 months after the onset of therapy in 0.3% of nearly 6000 women treated for ovarian cancer.[262]

Carcinoma of the urinary bladder has occurred 1–10 years after chemotherapy. Most patients were being treated with cyclophosphamide for lymphoma. Dysplastic lesions, some interpreted as carcinoma in situ, were present in addition to invasive carcinoma. Some of the carcinomas were of unusual types, such as mucus-secreting carcinoma,[263] spindle cell carcinoma,[264] and a disproportionate number of squamous cancers.[265] A leiomyosarcoma of the bladder occurred in a 17-year-old boy treated at age 4 with cyclophosphamide.[266] A fibrosarcoma-like tumor has also been seen.[267]

Presumably, drug-induced secondary malignant tumors arise by direct, mutagenic effects of cytotoxic therapy, as evidenced by characteristic chromosomal abnormalities, or by immunosuppressive mechanisms that result in decreased tumor surveillance.

Immunosuppressed patients at increased risk of neoplasms include recipients of bone marrow and solid organ transplants who are on prolonged immunosuppressive therapy. One uncommon hazard is to receive a donor organ containing carcinoma and then develop metastases from the transplanted neoplasm.[268] More importantly, the risk of developing a primary neoplasm is estimated to be 80 times greater than in the general population.[269] Neoplasms have been reported in more than 2000 renal transplant recipients, occurring at a much younger age than in persons with similar tumors in the general population.[270] Malignant lymphoma, Kaposi's sarcoma, and squamous carcinoma of the cervix, lip, tongue, and anogenital region have been the main offenders. The squamous carcinomas, including the cutaneous tumors, are capable of widespread metastases. One sarcoma, malignant fibrous histiocytoma of bone, has been reported in a renal transplant patient.[271]

POST-TRANSPLANTATION LYMPHOPROLIFERATIVE DISORDERS

These represent a heterogeneous spectrum of Epstein–Barr virus (EBV)-related lymphoid proliferations. Incidence varies with the intensity of cyclosporine or monoclonal anti-T lymphocyte therapy and with the organ being transplanted. The vast majority of post-transplantation lymphoproliferative disorders (PTLDs) are B-cell proliferations arising in lymph nodes or extranodal sites, frequently the gastrointestinal tract or lung. Classification and prognostication are notoriously difficult because of wide variations in histomorphology, immunoglobulin light chain expression, and immunoglobulin gene rearrangements.[272,273] PTLDs are best classified by a molecular modification of Frizzera's morphologic scheme.[274,275] *Plasmacytic hyperplasias* are paracortical expansions of cytologically normal plasmacytoid lymphocytes and plasma cells with preservation of normal nodal architecture. They are polyclonal and regress following reduction of immunosuppression. *Polymorphic PTLDs* (formerly subdivided into polymorphic hyperplasia and polymorphic lymphoma) are polymorphous lymphocyte proliferations that efface normal nodal architecture and contain numerous immunoblasts. Further subclassification based on cytologic atypia or necrosis is not necessary. They are monoclonal, demonstrate clonal patterns of EBV infection and often regress following reduction of immunosuppression. Like the hyperplasias, they do not exhibit molecular oncogene abnormalities. *Lymphomas/myelomas* are monomorphous, cytologically malignant proliferations that are histologically identical to their non-transplantation-associated counterparts. They are monoclonal, demonstrate clonal patterns of EBV infection and less frequently regress following immunosuppression reduction. In contrast to polymorphic PTLDs, they demonstrate oncogene or tumor suppressor gene abnormalities, or both. T-cell lymphomas represent a minor fraction of PTLDs and exhibit more frequent cutaneous involvement, decreased response to immunosuppression reduction, and a lesser association with EBV.[276] Pediatric PTLDs are uncommon. They are more often associated with primary EBV infection and involvement of Waldeyer's ring.[277]

HORMONAL EFFECTS

Early in utero exposure to diethylstilbestrol (DES) results in vaginal adenosis, predominantly of the endocervical type, in most exposed women. Vaginal smears contain increased numbers of metaplastic squamous cells and endocervical-type columnar cells.[278] Approximately 0.1% of DES-exposed women develop vaginal or cervical clear cell adenocarcinoma.[279] Vaginal cytology has been used to follow patients for neoplasia but its reliability depends on sampling technique.[278] DES-exposed males occasionally develop benign epididymal cysts but they exhibit no cytologic abnormalities in urine or prostatic fluid.

Tamoxifen, an 'anti-estrogen' used for chemoprevention and treatment of breast cancer, has been shown to have estrogenic effects in the uterus, including polyp formation, adenomyosis, leiomyomas, endometrial metaplasia and hyperplasia, as well as endometrial carcinoma. The increased risk of endometrial cancer in tamoxifen-treated patients is approximately double that of an untreated population.[280]

Pure estrogen therapy, given as postmenopausal hormone replacement, is primarily of historical significance. When given alone, estrogens are clearly associated with endometrial hyperplasias and carcinomas, particularly at the doses given prior to the 1970s.[281] Subsequently, the dose of estrogens in postmenopausal hormone replacement therapy has been markedly reduced and patients even show a slight decrease in breast cancer.[282] Presently, estrogens are frequently combined with a progestational compound, which largely protects against the proliferative activity of estrogens in the uterus. A slightly increased risk of breast cancer was shown by the Women's Health Initiative (WHI),[283] when hormone replacement therapy was given for more than 5 years. Progesterone induces breast proliferative activity and may be the cause of the increased breast cancer incidence. Less widely publicized, there was a concomitant decrease in colon cancer incidence of about 33% in the patients who received hormone replacement therapy in the WHI trial. Microscopically, there is a wide range of histologic patterns, depending upon the dose, duration, and individual hormone receptor activity. Inactive endometrium, mixed proliferative and secretory patterns, endometrial metaplasia, and endometrial polyp formation as well as hyperplasia may be seen. When progesterone is given by itself, typically as a contraceptive or as

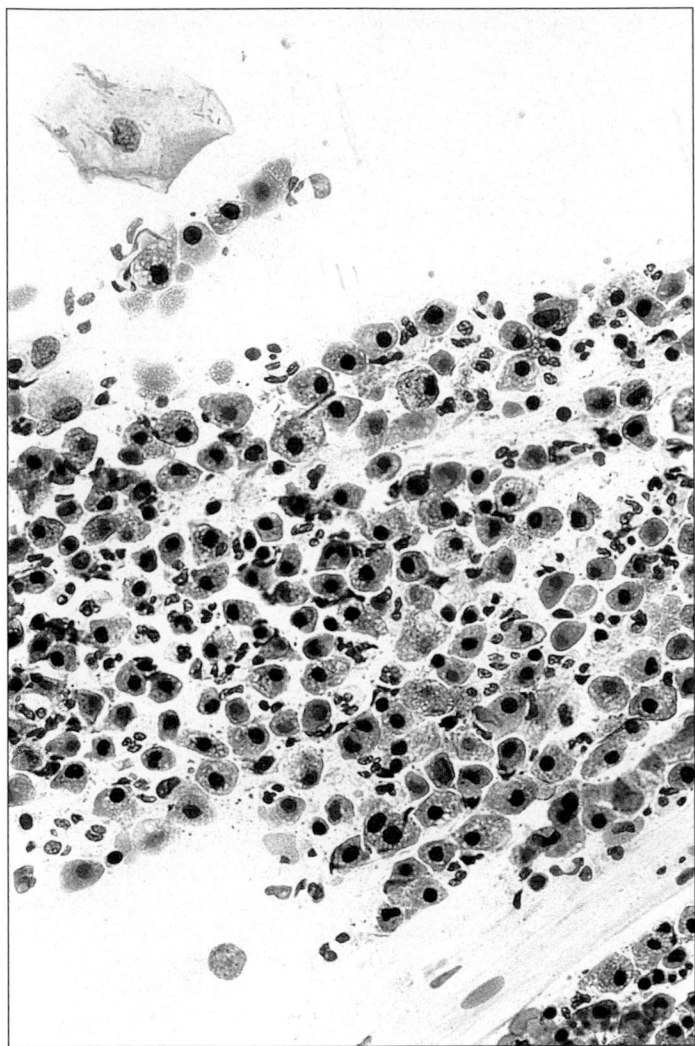

Fig. 5.19 'Pill effect.' Sheets of pseudoparakeratotic, small, metaplastic-appearing squamous cells with dense, pyknotic nuclei and fine cytoplasmic vacuolization in a cervicovaginal smear from a woman using oral contraceptives. Note superficial squamous cell (upper left); Papanicolaou stain.

therapy for hyperplasia, the endometrium shows a marked decidual reaction of the stroma, glandular secretions and mitotic arrest.[284]

Like estrogen replacement therapy, early forms of oral contraceptives contained relatively high doses of estrogens. With sequential forms that included progestins in the second half of the cycle, there were reported cases of endometrial hyperplasia and rarely carcinoma. Current combinations contain much lower doses of estrogens and progesterones. Endometrial effects include an inactive glandular appearance with decidualized stroma and thin-walled vessels. There is no significant increase in hyperplasia or carcinoma with the low-dose oral contraceptives. Pseudoparakeratosis is an unusual, infrequently described cytologic drug effect seen in the cervicovaginal smears of a minority of women using oral contraceptives.[285] It consists of focal groups of very small, discohesive, metaplastic-appearing cells with pyknotic nuclei and dense orangeophilic or cyanophilic cytoplasm with fine vacuolization (Fig. 5.19). Small cell size and vacuolization help to distinguish pseudoparakeratosis from high-grade dysplasia or parakeratosis.

Synthetic gonadotropin-releasing hormone agonists are used to shrink leiomyomas. Resected tumors often have hyaline degeneration and marked cytoplasmic contraction with crowded nuclei, imparting a hypercellular appearance. This is not accompanied by nuclear atypia or mitotic activity. The endometrium becomes atrophic.[284,286]

Multiple forms of preoperative endocrine therapy for prostatic adenocarcinoma produce neoplastic gland shrinkage, cytoplasmic vacuolization, nuclear degeneration, and inflammation that can limit postprostatectomy tumor grading. In some instances, tumor cells have voluminous vacuolated cytoplasm mimicking histiocytes, as described above in mammary carcinoma. Benign prostate glands exhibit atrophy, squamous and transitional cell metaplasia, vacuolization, and basal hyperplasia. Preoperative endocrine therapy does not completely ablate tumor but does appear to decrease involvement of surgical resection margins and extent of prostatic intraepithelial hyperplasia.[287–289]

Squamous metaplasia of normal prostatic glands occurs during estrogen therapy. In addition, several cases of adenocarcinoma with a malignant squamous element (adenosquamous carcinoma) have been diagnosed after 2–9 years of estrogen therapy for pure adenocarcinoma in the original biopsy.[290,291]

RADIATION RECALL BY DRUGS

The radiation recall phenomenon is defined by an inflammatory reaction within an irradiated area during subsequent drug treatment. The changes produced by the drug are clinically and pathologically indistinguishable from radiation damage occurring in the absence of drug therapy. Reported drugs causing this phenomenon include chemotherapeutic agents, as well as antituberculosis drugs and tamoxifen. Radiation recall has been described most often as erythema or necrosis in the skin but has also been described in virtually any radiated site, such as the gastrointestinal tract, central nervous system, lung, and lymphatic and musculoskeletal systems.[292]

IONIZING RADIATION

The pathologist receives irradiated tissue in four main clinical situations: (1) planned surgical resections in patients treated with preoperative radiation; (2) biopsy specimens from patients treated by radiation with the intent to cure but who have possible postirradiation persistent tumor; (3) non-neoplastic tissue resected because of late radiation damage; and (4) resection or biopsy specimens of postirradiation neoplasms.

High-energy radiation capable of producing ionization within living cells is generated either in the form of X-rays from a vacuum tube external to the body or in the form of beta and gamma rays emitted from the nuclei of radioactive atoms that are placed into the organ containing the neoplasm. The physiologic and morphologic changes are identical regardless of the source.

Radiation in therapeutic doses injures every living tissue to some degree. The beneficial result in cancer therapy is based on the difference in the sensitivity and regenerative capacity of normal versus malignant cells. Indeed, it is the deleterious effect of radiation on non-neoplastic tissue that limits the radiation dose.

The clinical effect of radiation on normal tissue can be divided into early and late phases. The temporal cutoff is arbitrary, but early is variably defined as any alteration occurring from 8 weeks to 6 months after initiation of therapy, and late is any time thereafter. Late changes may follow continuously on early changes, or a

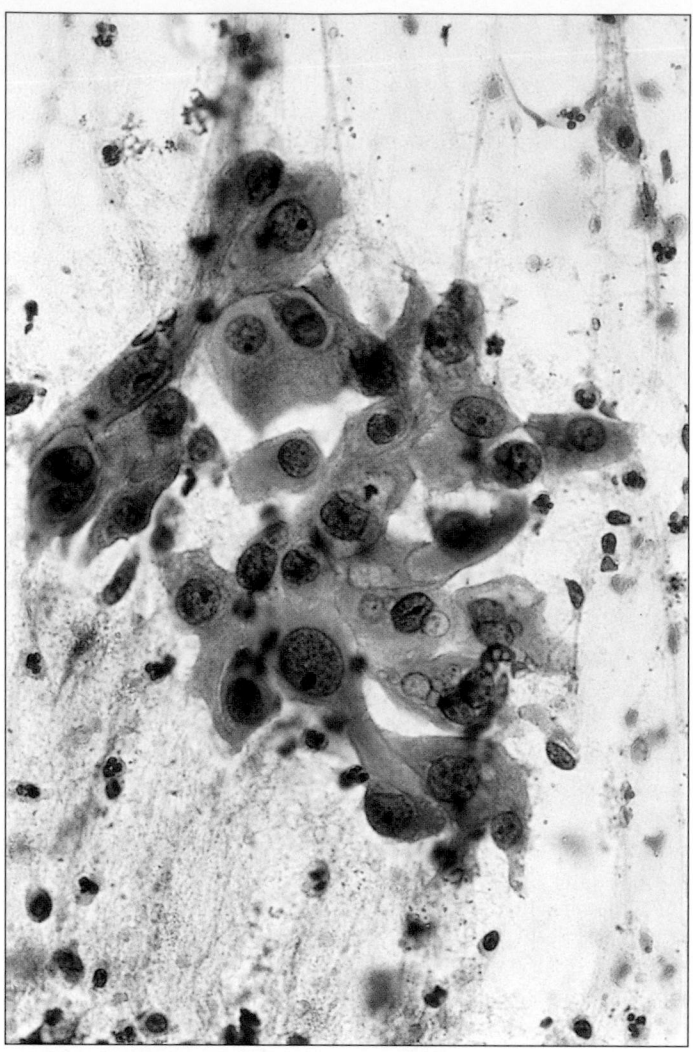

Fig. 5.20 Acute cellular changes of ionizing radiation in a cervicovaginal smear include nuclear and cytoplasmic enlargement and vacuolization, multinucleation, prominent nucleoli, amphophilic cytoplasmic staining, and irregular cell shapes. (Papanicolaou stain.)

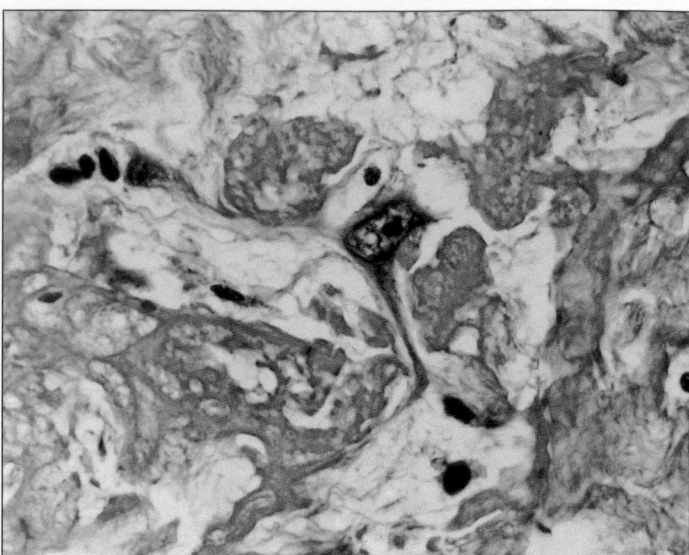

Fig. 5.21 Greatly enlarged fibroblasts with long cytoplasmic processes are typical, but not pathognomonic, of radiation damage. The stroma shows the splotchy, amorphous, hyalinized stroma characteristic of radiation effect.

symptom-free interval of weeks to many years may elapse before late changes declare themselves clinically.

The histologic alterations during the early phase include epithelial damage and connective tissue changes. Exquisitely sensitive cells such as those in the crypts of the small intestine show nuclear swelling and clumping of chromatin within minutes after receiving 50–100 cGy. Acute cellular changes include nuclear and cytoplasmic enlargement, cytoplasmic vacuolization, amphophilic cytoplasmic staining, nuclear membrane irregularity, multinucleation, prominent nucleoli, and occasional bizarre or 'tadpole' shapes[293] (Fig. 5.20). Although both nuclear and cytoplasmic enlargement is seen, the nuclear:cytoplasmic ratio may be slightly increased. Nuclear degeneration, including pyknosis and karyorrhexis, is seen but chromatin usually remains diffuse, fine, and normochromic. Occasional cells exhibit hyperchromasia. Acute radiation changes have been best described for cervical squamous epithelium but similar changes are seen in endocervical cells.[294] These changes correlate ultrastructurally with swelling of mitochondria, dilatation of the endoplasmic reticulum, the formation of vesicles, an accumula-

tion of lipid, and an increase in lysosome-like bodies. In addition, disintegration of the Golgi apparatus, mitochondria, cytoplasmic filaments, and centrioles may occur. Late epithelial radiation effects, which can last for many years, include persistent nuclear and cytoplasmic enlargement but not vacuolization. In cervical smears, elongated parabasal-like cells resembling atrophy and enlarged endocervical cells may demonstrate nuclear hyperchromasia. Reparative changes also occur in about one third of patients. The constellation of radiation changes resembles cancer, as evidenced by higher false-positive rates for malignant cytologic diagnoses in the postirradiation setting. Malignant cells are generally distinguished from benign radiation change by increased nuclear:cytoplasmic ratios and coarse, hyperchromatic chromatin.

Stromal changes are probably triggered by damage to the endothelium of capillaries.[295] The endothelial cytoplasm becomes swollen and vacuolated, and nuclear enlargement is present. These damaged cells result in an alteration of the histohematic barrier manifest by edema and a fibrinous exudate. A patchy fibrous reaction ensues, and the combination of collagen and persisting fibrin produces eosinophilic hyalinized areas. Ultrastructurally, the hyalinized areas are a mixture of collagen bundles and cytoplasmic fragments that are cemented together by an amorphous, finely granular protein substance. Large fibroblasts are often conspicuous, with proportionately enlarged nuclei that are either vesicular or hyperchromatic. Sometimes fibroblasts stand out as a result of basophilia secondary to abundant rough endoplasmic reticulum. Occasionally, angulated tapering cytoplasmic projections are seen, which have been called swallowtail fibroblasts or radiation fibroblasts (Fig. 5.21). Fibroblasts with this appearance are not found exclusively in irradiated tissue, however. Areas of intense inflammation due to any cause may display bizarre fibroblasts, especially when infection is present; radiation damage is not pathognomonic for this appearance.[296]

Endothelial damage is also seen in arterioles and muscular arteries but apparently does not acutely affect their function because

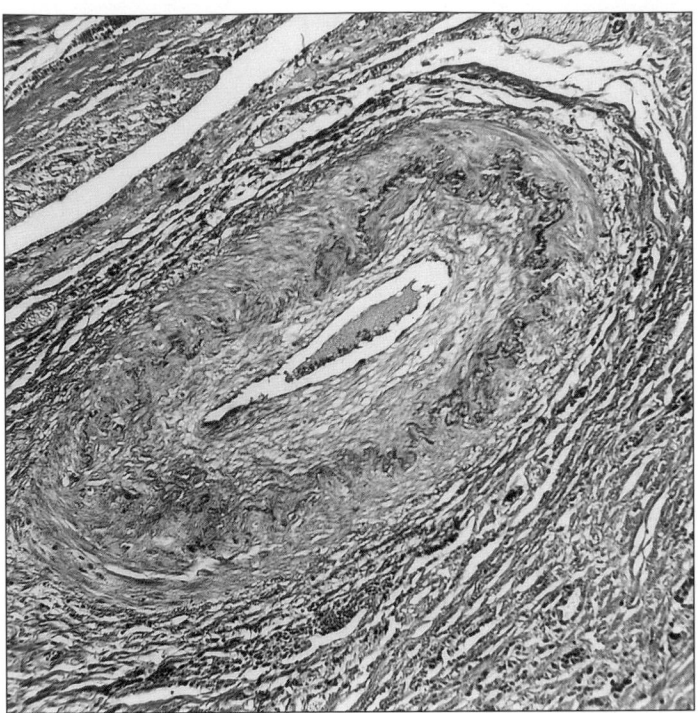

Fig. 5.22 Artery from soft tissue of neck 1 year after patient received 6000 cGy. The interna elastica is discontinuous, intimal fibrous thickening is seen, and the adventitia is fibrotic.

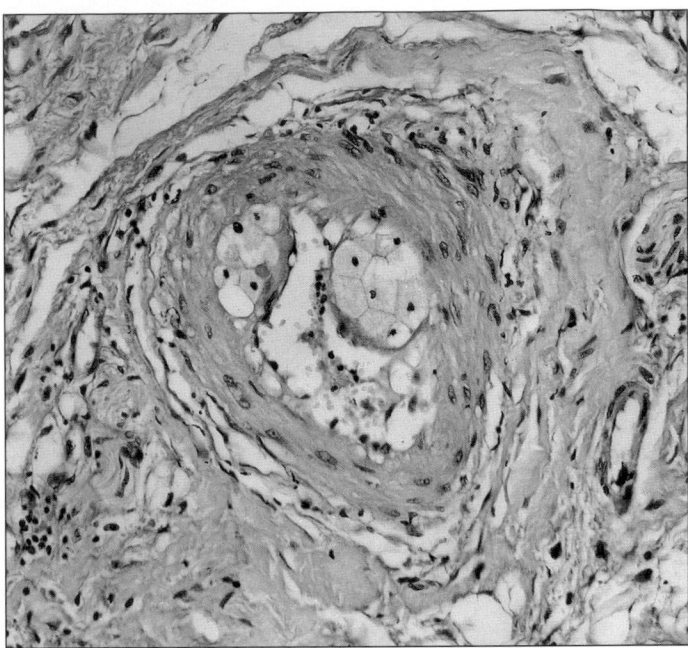

Fig. 5.24 Intimal foam cells are covered with endothelium. The change can be found at the completion of radiotherapy (as in this case) or can be seen many years later.

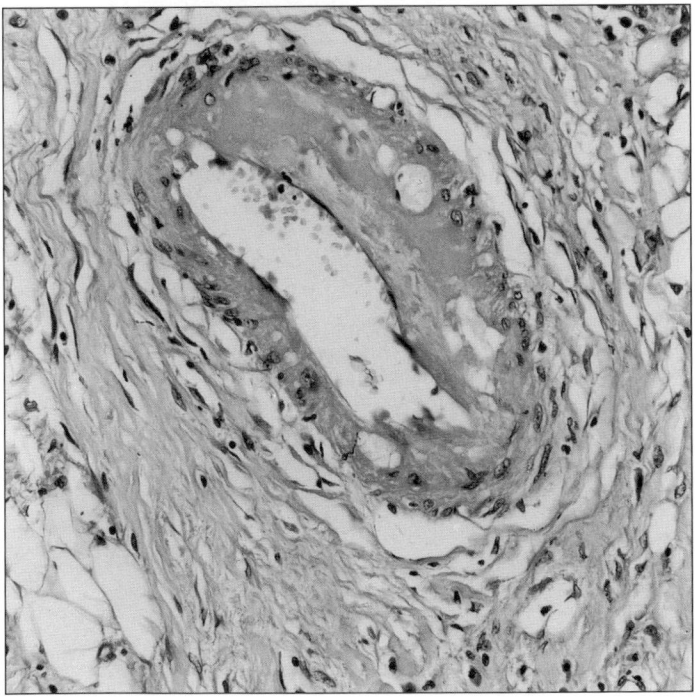

Fig. 5.23 Small artery with vacuolated and hyalinized media. This can be either an early or late radiation change.

of the large lumen. Within several weeks, however, intimal and medial fibrosis or hyalinization may drastically alter the configuration of the muscular arteries, and rarely an intimal accumulation of foam cells occurs, which compromises the lumen (Figs 5.22–5.24).

The changes along the course of a vessel may be spotty, so in any one tissue section relatively few sites of vascular damage are seen even though extensive connective tissue changes are evident. Arteries are affected far more often than veins, except for the unique sensitivity of hepatic veins.

Traditionally, late radiation damage has been attributed to progressive arterial sclerosis accompanied by stromal fibrosis. Many epithelial changes such as ulceration of the rectum or skin are considered secondary to vascular insufficiency rather than a persisting direct effect on the epithelial cells per se. The compromised vasculature presumably makes an irradiated tissue permanently susceptible to devastating damage if it becomes infected or is traumatized.[297]

EFFECT ON NEOPLASMS

The effect of radiation on the gross and microscopic appearance of a tumor is unpredictable. Attempts to predict tumor radiation response based on tumor differentiation (e.g. keratinizing vs nonkeratinizing squamous cancers) or cytologic changes in adjacent benign epithelium[298–300] have been unsuccessful.[301] For example, if two laryngeal squamous cancers with the same histologic pattern and clinical stage of disease are given preoperative radiotherapy, one tumor may be completely absent in the resected specimen whereas the other persists and is identical to the original biopsy. More often, the tumor is altered, with the most frequent change being necrosis. Many tumor cells undergo nuclear and cytoplasmic enlargement and vacuolization identical to that seen in normal epithelium. Sometimes the cells assume a gigantic size, with grotesquely shaped, densely hyperchromatic nuclei. The tumor pattern or degree of differentiation may be altered. Squamous carcinoma frequently has more keratin in the postirradiated tumor, which may or may not be associated with intact tumor cells.[302] This phenomenon probably reflects the sensitivity of poorly differentiated (immature) cells to radiation, whereas postmitotic cells are capable of maturing and carrying out specialized functions before dying. Increased pleomorphism and cytomegaly occur in the cells of undifferentiated nasopharyngeal carcinoma following radiotherapy. These are transient and usually disappear after 8 weeks.[303]

Generally, residual adenocarcinoma is histologically unchanged. This has been especially well documented for endometrial and prostatic carcinoma.[304,305] Occasionally, however, the malignant cells have grotesque cytologic features with gigantic nuclei and a degree of pleomorphism far greater than the original tumor (Fig. 5.25).

Squamous metaplasia has been described in adenocarcinomas of the breast and endometrium and in small cell undifferentiated carcinoma of the lung after irradiation.[306] However, squamous metaplasia can be seen in nonirradiated tumors of these types, and one must raise the question of sampling deficiencies in the small amounts of tissue available before irradiation. In an extensive study of irradiated uteri, Silverberg and DeGiorgi[304] found that squamous elements were first seen after irradiation in five cases but in three others the squamous elements were noted in sections of the initial biopsy specimen and not in sections of the uterus after hysterectomy. They concluded that this was more likely to be a result of sampling variation than a direct effect of irradiation.

Transitional cell carcinomas of the urinary bladder tend to have more nuclear pleomorphism after irradiation, whereas carcinoma in situ is not altered. Squamous differentiation in the carcinoma has been described but it raises the same questions as these described above.[307]

Residual carcinoma in a specimen resected as part of a combined radiotherapeutic and surgical approach is not unexpected because of the short interval between completion of radiotherapy and surgery. The prognostic significance of residual tumor in resected specimens is frequently raised, but few data answer this question. Residual carcinoma of the endometrium does not seem to affect the prognosis adversely if the tumor is in a favorable stage, namely, confined to the endometrium.[291] For laryngeal carcinoma, patients without residual tumor have a better survival but this again probably correlates with a more favorable initial clinical stage.[308]

A far more perplexing problem arises when intact tumor cells are found in tissue biopsies or cytologic smears from a patient irradiated for cure and for whom surgery was not planned. What is the reproductive capacity of these cells? Intact tumor cells with normal staining characteristics must be sufficiently metabolically active to maintain their appearance. Nonetheless, this intactness does not ensure their ability to complete the next cell division or the one after that. Suit and Gallager[309] showed that irradiated tumor samples histologically identical to the original tumor failed to grow when transplanted into other animals, whereas nonirradiated samples of the tumor grew when transplanted. Viability as measured by histologically intact cells is not to be equated with further growth potential. This has been demonstrated in uteri removed after irradiation[304] and in serial biopsies of patients with prostatic carcinoma who have been radiated.[305] Thus, the pathologist should limit the interpretation of tumor cells to the observation that 'morphologically intact tumor cells are present,' because an accurate prediction of future growth cannot be made. The significance of malignant cells in postirradiation cervicovaginal smears may depend on the post-therapy interval and degree of radiation change. In early postirradiation smears, malignant cells may be difficult to distinguish from acute, benign radiation change. This may explain conflicting reports regarding the clinical significance of malignant cells in the early

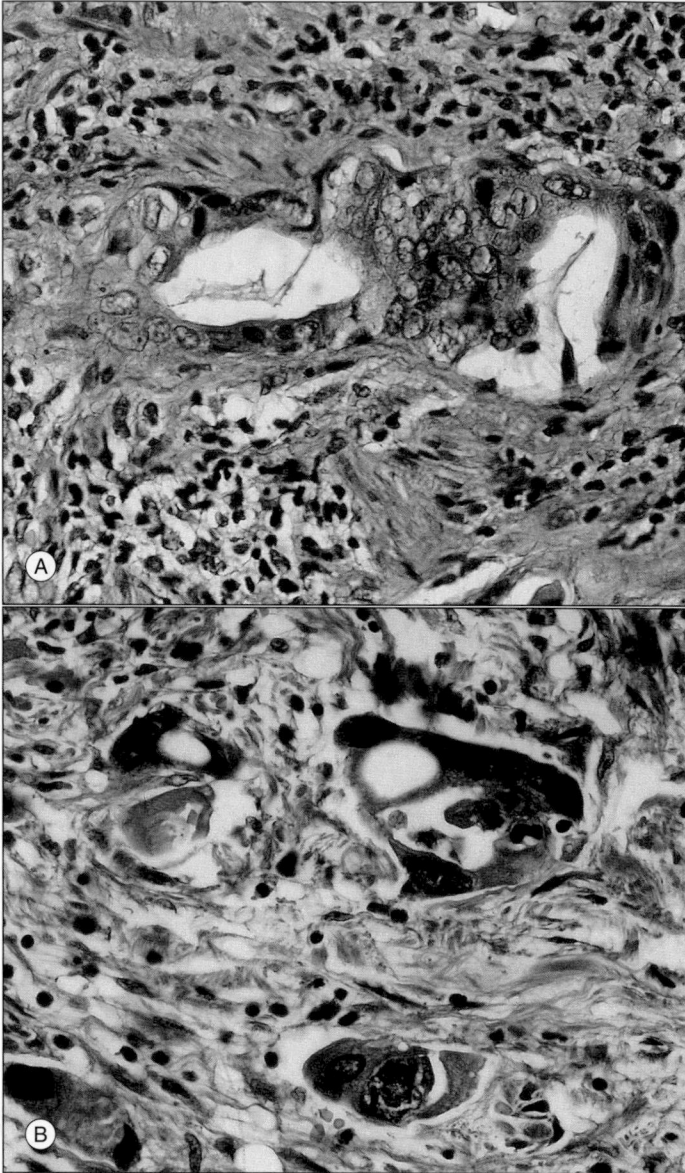

Fig. 5.25 (A) Well-differentiated adenocarcinoma of prostate before irradiation. **(B)** Immediately after the conclusion of 5500 cGy, the tumor in the resected specimen showed bizarre nuclei and minimal formation of lumens. The postirradiation section came from the immediate area of the original biopsy, and none of the residual tumor resembled the preradiation pattern. We have seen this change in needle biopsies more than 1 year after radiation in patients with normal prostatic serum antibody.

weeks after therapy. Malignant cells with marked acute radiation changes presumably have little or no potential for replication,[310] although some authors claim that any persistence is ominous.[311] Malignant cells exhibiting little to no radiation effect or those present for more than 1–4 months after therapy are an indication for aggressive clinical evaluation for residual disease.[293,310] Cervicovaginal cytology is only 50% sensitive in detecting cancer in those patients destined for recurrence, presumably because of limited sampling due to fibrosis.[293]

Postirradiation high-grade dysplasia of the cervix is difficult to detect clinically and occurs with higher frequency than dysplasia in nonirradiated patients. Whether reported cases of postirradiation dysplasia include patients with unrecognized invasive disease is uncertain but those who present within 3 years of completing therapy have a very high rate of recurrent invasive disease and poor survival.[293]

The problem of persistent tumor after irradiation for cure comes up most often in squamous cancers of the head and neck and cervix. Some carcinomas of the larynx undergo regression accompanied by mucosal healing but edema continues to be present at the site of the tumor. The difficulty in finding carcinoma in biopsy specimens from the edematous area is frustrating. Goldman et al.[312] found that tumor in postirradiation resected specimens often consisted only of scattered microscopic foci less than 0.5 mm in diameter. Furthermore, when the mucosa is intact, the tumor will not be reached unless a deep biopsy is performed. Even in the absence of tumor in a biopsy, progressive edema 3–6 months after radiotherapy may be an indication for surgical resection. Tumor will be found in almost all these resection specimens.[313,314]

Paradoxically, cutaneous metastases may be sharply confined to the field of previous irradiation. This may be due to increased vasculature secondary to the radiation.[315] The effects on normal tissues that are commonly irradiated will now be considered.

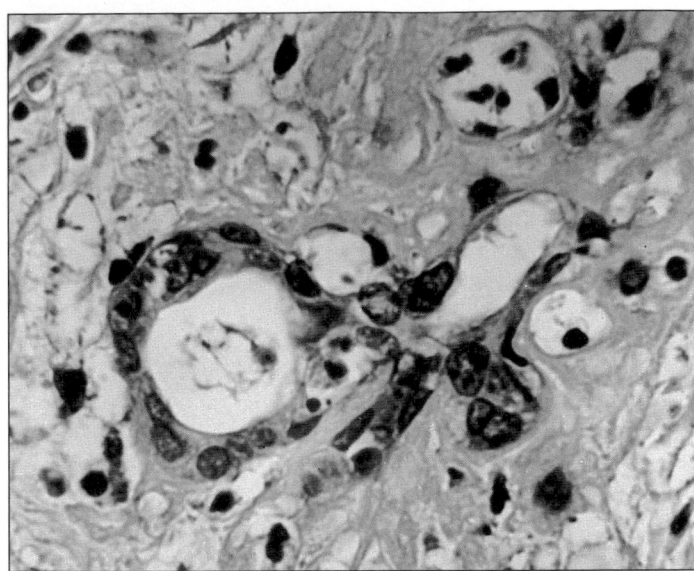

Fig. 5.26 Salivary gland at completion of 5800 cGy of therapy for carcinoma of the oral cavity. Most acini are destroyed and the remaining cells have pleomorphic nuclei.

SKIN AND MUCOUS MEMBRANES

The early phase of radiation dermatitis is occasionally seen when skin is excised en bloc after preoperative radiotherapy. The epidermis and dermis are edematous and the capillaries are dilated and lined by swollen endothelial cells. The cells of the pilosebaceous apparatus and sweat glands may be enlarged or focally necrotic.

In the late phase, the epidermis is atrophic in some areas and acanthotic in others. Hyperkeratosis is common. Atypical nuclei and individual cell keratinization are similar to those seen in solar keratosis. The dermal collagen bundles are swollen and often hyalinized, with variable staining. Fibrocytes associated with 'new' collagen are irregularly distributed. The capillaries are usually ectatic and appear to be held rigidly open by the dense stroma about them. The pilosebaceous apparatus is usually absent altogether, but sweat glands may persist. Inflammation is negligible unless the skin is ulcerated.[316] Mucous membranes show the same changes as the skin except for damage to the minor salivary glands in place of the skin appendages.

SALIVARY GLANDS

The acute effect of radiation on salivary glands is manifest clinically by mucositis; microscopically distention of the ducts and acini, with secretions, is seen. By the end of a course of radiotherapy, however, the lobular architecture is destroyed because of a loss of acini and a chronic inflammatory infiltrate. Ducts and acini may contain cells with enlarged nuclei (two to three times normal size), which may be either vesicular or hyperchromatic (Fig. 5.26). Fibrous tissue is increased, particularly within the lobules, but the broad bands of fibrosis seen in cases of obstruction are not attained.[317] It was also found that intralobular fat persisted in irradiated glands whereas it was absent in glands with obstructive disease. The epithelium of both ducts and acini may be partly replaced by squamous epithelium; occasionally, it irregularly distends the ducts and acini to a point where they may be confused with squamous carcinoma.[318] This may be particularly problematic if an enlarged, hard sub-

mandibular gland is removed because it is thought to be a lymph node with metastases.

INTESTINE

Either the small or large intestine may require surgical intervention for late radiation damage, which may appear within a few months after completion of therapy or may not be seen until more than 10 years later. Radiation enterocolitis manifests symptoms of obstruction due to a narrowed segment that ranges from 0.5–5 cm in length but is usually 1.5–2 cm long. Lesser degrees of edema and fibrosis extend away for 3–4 cm. The mucosa is usually ulcerated, but partial re-epithelialization may occur. Vascular damage is spotty but is invariably present within both the bowel wall and the adjacent mesentery. The circular muscular layer is particularly susceptible to destruction and fibrous replacement, whereas the outer longitudinal layer is almost always spared (Fig. 5.27). Since radiation damage is a progressive, continuing process, edema and inflammation are also present. In the small intestine, there can be villous atrophy, ulceration, atypical hyperplastic glands, cystic glandular inclusions, wall fibrosis and vascular sclerosis.[319]

Colonic glands may be located in the muscularis as a late change. The epithelium of the glands is normal or atrophic, and its appearance is identical to that seen in colitis cystica profunda.[320]

Modest doses (2000–2500 cGy) of preoperative radiation produce marked atypia in non-neoplastic colonic mucosa. The changes are not permanent, since biopsy specimens from colostomy sites after 2 months do not show the change even though the line of resection had atypia at the time of the operation.[321] Doses as low as 1000 cGy produce severe but transient alterations.

LIVER

Radiation damage to the liver is unique because the major site of vascular injury is to veins, i.e. the small radicles of the hepatic

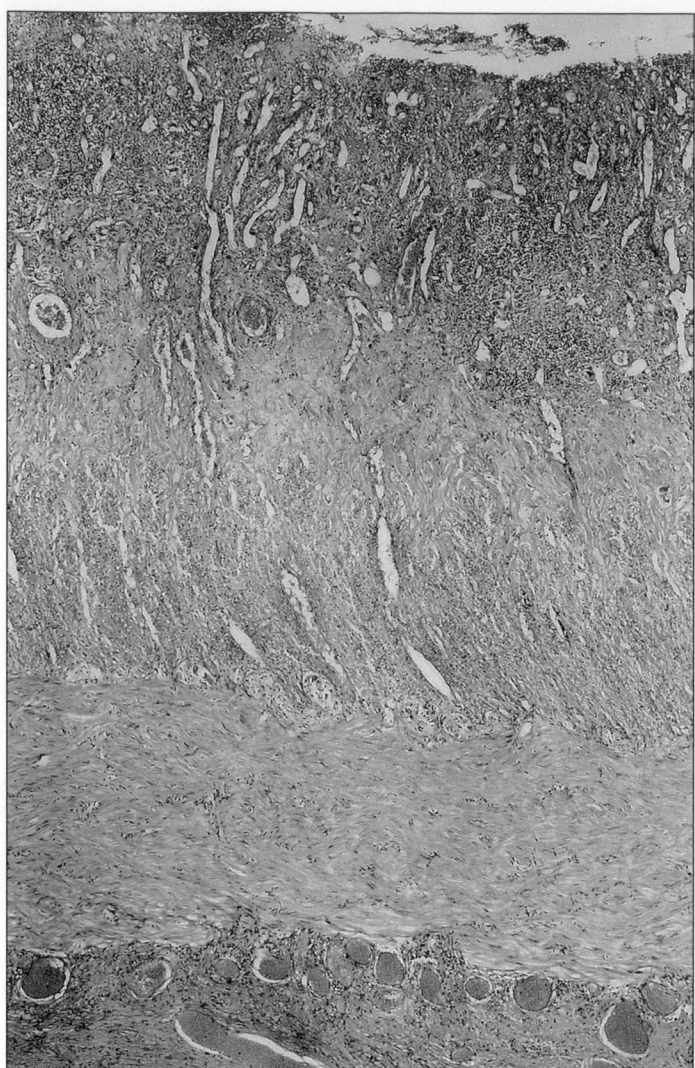

Fig. 5.27 Segment of obstructed small intestine removed 4 years after radiotherapy for carcinoma of cervix. The stenotic segment has ulcerated mucosa, greatly thickened and fibrotic submucosa, focal necrosis and fibrosis of the circular muscular layer, a normal longitudinal muscle layer, and serosal fibrosis with ectatic vessels.

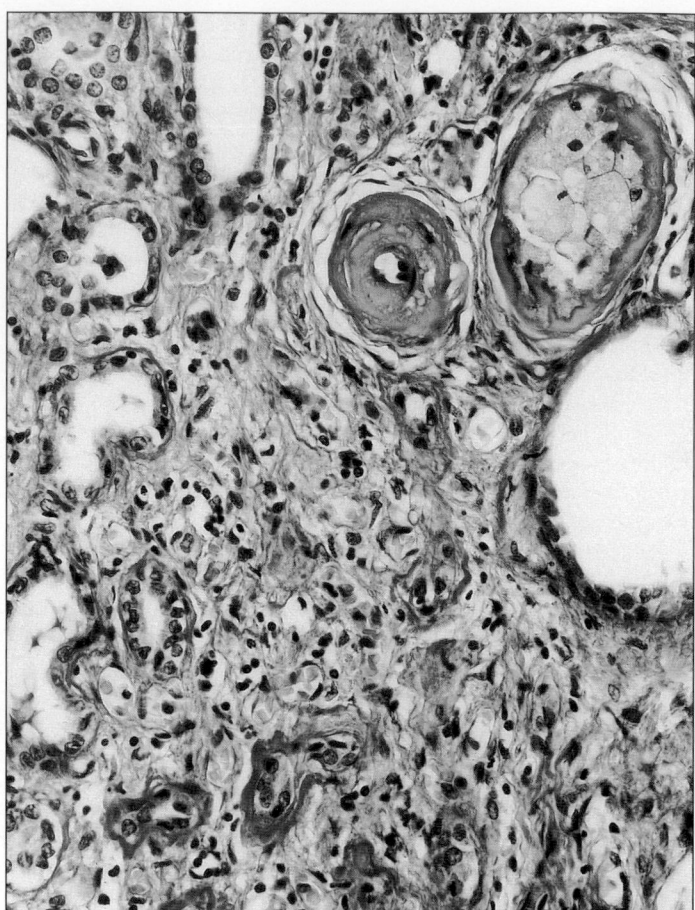

Fig. 5.28 Sclerosing nephrosis secondary to radiation consists of atrophic tubules separated by fibrous tissue. A markedly hyalinized arteriole is present, as well as an artery with intimal foam cells. The patient had been irradiated 10 years previously for testicular carcinoma.

venous system. Sclerosis of the portal vein is rare, and arterial lesions have not been reported.[322] The central veins and small sublobular hepatic veins undergo an intimal thickening that is unrelated to overt thrombosis.

KIDNEY

Radiation damage to the glomeruli, tubules, and vessels of the kidney is not accompanied by much inflammation; therefore the term 'radiation nephropathy' is preferable to the more widely used term 'radiation nephritis'. Luxton and Kunkler[323] followed 54 patients for up to 12 years and grouped them into five major clinical groups: (1) acute radiation nephropathy; (2) chronic radiation nephropathy; (3) asymptomatic proteinuria; (4) benign hypertension; and (5) malignant hypertension. From a morphologic viewpoint, Mostofi[324] divided radiation changes into four categories that serve to emphasize the different changes seen in the clinical groups. These categories are:

(1) mild sclerosing nephrosis; (2) severe sclerosing nephrosis with mild to severe nephrosclerosis; (3) mild to severe sclerosing nephrosis with hypertensive necrotizing vasculitis; and (4) nephroglomerulosis. Sclerosing nephrosis consists of small or collapsed tubules intermixed with interstitial fibrosis (Fig. 5.28). Nephroglomerulosis is predominantly a glomerular affliction; in contrast to most cases in the other groups, it begins within 3–12 months after irradiation. The dominant change is in the glomeruli, almost all of which have decreased lobulation and thickening of the capillary walls simulating membranous glomerulonephritis. By electron microscopy, disruption of hypertrophic endothelial and epithelial cells from the basement membrane is seen.[325] In a few instances, the affected zone has been sharply demarcated and the remainder of the kidney was normal, presumably because only a portion of the kidney was lying in the field of radiation. This possibility must be kept in mind because of the potential for sampling error at the time of needle biopsy.

URINARY BLADDER

Transitional epithelium is readily damaged by radiation, and almost all patients will exfoliate abnormal cells whether the therapy is directed to a primary cancer of the bladder or an adjacent pelvic organ. The cells and nuclei are enlarged and the cytoplasm is often vacuolated.[326] Nuclei are wrinkled, mildly hyperchromatic, enlarged more or less in proportion to the cytoplasm, and tend to be multiple. Radiation-induced changes, like postsurgical and cytotoxic drug effects, limit the accuracy of urine cytology.[327] This is especially true following low-grade transitional cell carcinoma. In a small number of cases, definitive distinction of cancer from benign radiation effect may be impossible, requiring further cytologic or histologic evaluation.[328] Radiation-induced alterations generally disappear within a few months after completion of therapy.[329] Abnormal cells noted beyond that time can be evaluated using standard criteria, especially if intervening urine cytologies are free of atypical cells. Recurrent high-grade transitional cell carcinomas demonstrate high nuclear:cytoplasmic ratios, marked hyperchromasia, and coarse chromatin. The presence of malignant-appearing cells in transitional epithelium from a patient who has been irradiated for primary bladder carcinoma probably reflects radioresistant invasive carcinoma or carcinoma in situ. The latter is a likely source for the later development of invasive carcinoma.[329,330]

The rich vasculature of the bladder and its abundant submucosal connective tissue renders this organ susceptible to late complications of radiation. Approximately 1–3% of long-term survivors will develop chronic devastating damage to the bladder in the form of deep ulceration, fibrotic contraction, or fistula formation in the absence of tumor. Patients undergoing cyclophosphamide therapy experience more frequent and severe toxicity when it is combined with pelvic irradiation.[331]

PROSTATE

Radiation-induced atypia in benign prostatic epithelium and stroma is similar to that described for other organs. In carcinoma, decreased numbers of irregularly distributed neoplastic glands limit accurate Gleason scoring, and tumor cell nuclear:cytoplasmic ratios may be decreased to the point of appearing anucleate. The significance of residual cancer in irradiated prostate gland biopsies is controversial but appears to indicate increased recurrence and spread of disease as well as decreased survival.[332]

Biopsies of men whose prostatic carcinoma has been radiated often show squamous metaplasia with marked cytologic atypia in the non-neoplastic glands, larger prostatic ducts, and prostatic urethra. In other glands, necrotic epithelium exposes corpora amylacea to the stroma, eliciting a giant cell reaction. The seminal vesicles become atrophic and fibrotic.[333]

UTERUS

Intracavitary radiation for endometrial carcinoma produces changes in the cervix, endometrium, and myometrium. The squamous lining of the exocervix is often obliterated, and only a fibrinous exudate lies on the surface. The endocervical epithelium may be pleomorphic, with either hyperchromatic or vacuolated nuclei that frequently lie in the middle or luminal end of the cell. Mucin is diminished. The distinction from adenocarcinoma involving the endocervix is readily made because, despite their cytologic changes, the glands are normally spaced.

Nuclear and cytoplasmic alterations are especially common in the endometrium treated with intracavitary radium. Markedly abnormal cells are found not only in the endometrium but in foci of adenomyosis. The latter might be diagnosed incorrectly as invasive adenocarcinoma. Misinterpretation can be avoided by knowing that residual endometrial

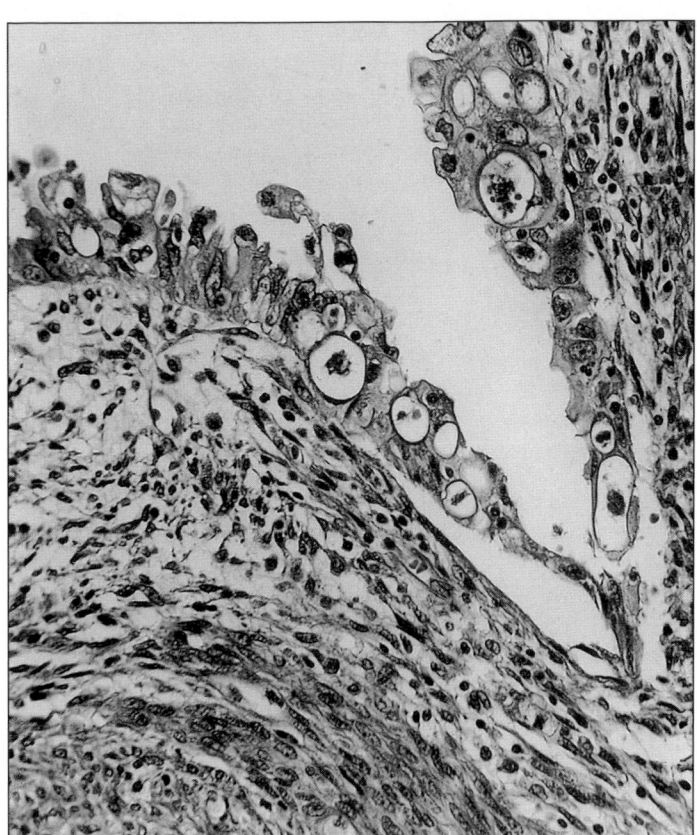

Fig. 5.29 Focus of adenomyosis after intracavitary radium therapy for endometrial carcinoma. The epithelium is stratified, and a few cells are attached only by a strand of cytoplasm. Many cells are vacuolated, and nuclear pleomorphism is present. The endometrial stroma beneath the epithelium is edematous and inflamed but the stromal cells are not atypical. Normal myometrium is at the bottom of the field.

adenocarcinoma characteristically shows little change when compared with preoperative biopsy material, whereas the non-neoplastic endometrium is severely altered.[304] The epithelium forms an irregular layer one to four cells thick with some cells protruding above the surface and attached to the epithelial lining only by a thin strand of cytoplasm (Fig. 5.29). Most cells are greatly enlarged and have a polygonal, round, or extremely attenuated shape rather than the normal cuboidal or low columnar configuration. The cytoplasm ranges from a powdery ground-glass appearance through a finely or coarsely eosinophilic granularity. Vacuolization is present in some cells as either tiny droplets or large vacuoles. Nuclei are occasionally normal, but most are enlarged and may be round, angulated, or have an irregular contour due to numerous folds and convolutions. Small nucleoli are frequent. The endometrial stromal cells do not undergo these cytologic changes although inflammation and edema are invariably present. Thus, the presence of bizarre endometrial cells adjacent to endometrial stromal cells is virtual proof that the epithelial cells are non-neoplastic. In rare cases, myometrial cells are enlarged and vacuolated after intracavitary radiation.[334]

THYROID

Numerous changes are found in the thyroid, including colloid nodules with foci of hyperplasia identical to those seen in nonirradiated thyroid. Small foci of hyperplasia are also scattered throughout the parenchyma, with the columnar cells forming small tufts. Occasionally, a nodule is composed of small fingers of thyroid tissue forming tiny lumens. Large, dense nuclei may be found either in hyperplastic nodules or within individual follicles. Oxyphilic cells are frequent and are often associated with a lymphocytic infiltrate.[335]

Many nodules have been classified as adenomas, since they have a trabecular pattern. When nuclear abnormalities are superimposed, the possibility of carcinoma is raised. In the absence of invasion, such nodules are probably best considered atypical adenomas.[336]

BREAST

Patients treated for breast cancer with primary radiotherapy may subsequently develop clinical or mammographic abnormalities that are biopsied. In some instances, fat necrosis has mimicked a primary tumor on physical examination. It may be located near the biopsy site and may result in fixation of the skin.[337] The most characteristic radiation effect is the presence of atypical epithelial cells in the terminal duct/lobular unit, accompanied by atrophy and lobular fibrosis. Occasionally, epithelial atypia is seen in larger ducts.[338] FNA smears from irradiated breasts typically demonstrate nuclear atypia, epithelial hypocellularity, and fat necrosis. Radiation-induced benign nuclear enlargement and prominent nucleoli may be difficult to distinguish from carcinoma but smears from recurrent cancer typically demonstrate abundant, discohesive malignant cells.[339]

LUNG

Radiation to the lungs is commonly given for lung carcinoma, and the lungs may be in the fields of radiation for other tumors such as lymphoma and breast malignancies. The pulmonary damage consists of pneumonitis and pulmonary fibrosis. The initial damage is to pneumocytes and endothelial cells, causing surfactant and exudates to be released into alveolar spaces and interstitium. An inflammatory response ensues. The late phase consists of interstitial fibrosis and obliteration of the alveolar spaces (pulmonary fibrosis).[340] Tumor cells show nuclear vacuolization, enlargement, loss of distinct chromatin, and rupture of the chromatin rim.[341] Similar cytologic atypia may be seen in benign lung, with nuclear and cytoplasmic vacuolization. The atypia may lead to a false positive diagnosis of malignancy. Metaplastic squamous cells, leukocytes and macrophages may be increased.[342]

RADIATION-ASSOCIATED TUMORS

Tumors associated with radiation have occurred in patients receiving high-dose therapy for cancer, low-dose therapy for benign conditions, multiple diagnostic exposures, and internal radiation due to deposition of isotopes used in diagnostic procedures (thorium dioxide) and therapeutic procedures (^{131}I).[343]

A threshold may not exist below which radiation has no effect, a concept summarized in the following manner by Rubin and Casarett:[344] (1) a finite probability exists that the smallest amount of radiation can cause a significant change in a cell such as gene mutation; (2) a finite probability exists that such a cell alteration may be an event in a complex multievent mechanism of carcino-

genesis; (3) the probability that such a single event will complete the carcinogenic mechanism in an individual of a population depends on the size of the exposed population and on the number of individuals in it that are so predisposed; and (4) it is therefore reasonable to assume that no threshold dose exists in a population in which there is not at least one patient who requires merely this one cell change to complete a carcinogenic event.

The following principles must be kept in mind when assigning radiation as the probable cause of a neoplasm. The new tumor must have been in the field of radiation. The organ in which it arises must have been previously documented as being normal. A symptom-free period should pass after radiation, which is conventionally considered to be at least 5 years. In point of fact, however, strong arguments can be made for radiation-induced tumors arising within 2–3 years after irradiation.

Most tumors attributed to radiation are malignant, although a few benign osseous and neurogenic neoplasms appear to have been radiation-induced.[344–346] Generally speaking, the gross and microscopic appearances of radiation-induced tumors are not distinctive, and their behavior parallels the course of disease that would be expected for the same histologic type of tumor arising in a nonirradiated organ. The few exceptions to these statements will be noted in the subsequent sections. Radiation damage to normal structures may or may not be found in the region of the tumor, and the presence of radiation damage in the surrounding non-neoplastic tissue is not a requisite for the diagnosis of a radiation-induced tumor.

SKIN

Ionizing radiation of the skin is most closely linked to basal cell carcinoma.[347] Postirradiation basal or squamous cell carcinomas of the skin are most common on the face and usually manifest 20 or more years after irradiation for benign conditions.[348] The latency period varies from 3–64 years, however.[349] The role of radiation is securely established by the occurrence of cancers in unusual locations such as the antecubital fossa or forearm after irradiation of these areas for dermatitis.[350] Multiple lesions are the rule, both synchronously and metachronously. Their number far exceeds the multiple lesions that are also characteristic of cutaneous cancers in nonirradiated patients. The squamous carcinomas are more aggressive than those arising in actinic keratosis. Nonetheless, skin damaged by radiation need not inevitably develop cancer even when the injury is severe enough to produce necrosis.[349]

Atypical fibroxanthomas have arisen in skin that had been irradiated.[351] Most appeared more than 15 years after irradiation, but a few were seen in less than 5 years. Angiosarcoma of the skin of the breast has occurred after lumpectomy and radiation.[352]

HEAD AND NECK

Radiation induced tumors of the head and neck include a variety of sarcomas, most commonly malignant fibrous histiocytoma.[353] Neoplasms may occur in pharynx, thyroid, or esophagus.[354] Clinical prognosis is poor.

Sinonasal small cell neoplasm after retinoblastoma has been reported in a few cases. In one case, immunohistochemical evidence suggested a primitive neuroectodermal tumor.[355] Another case was completely devoid of differentiation.[356]

Low-dose radiation to the head in childhood increases the incidence of mixed tumors of the salivary gland. In one study, two of

971 persons who received radiation had mixed tumors, whereas the expected number was 0.04 cases.[357] Other tumors include Warthin tumor, mucoepidermoid tumor, or unclassified carcinoma.[358–360] A few patients receiving high-dose radiotherapy for carcinoma have later developed malignant tumors of the parotid gland.[361]

In 1950, Duffy and Fitzgerald[362] suggested an association between thyroid carcinoma in childhood and a prior history of irradiation to the thymus in infancy. The practice of using radiation to treat benign conditions such as acne or tonsillitis had largely ceased by 1960, but thyroid cancer continues to occur in these patients. As many as 7% of the persons who received radiation to the head or neck have been found to have thyroid carcinoma.[363] In one report, 40% of the adults operated on for thyroid cancer between 1968 and 1972 had a history of irradiation.[364]

Virtually all the cancers have been classified as papillary, follicular, or mixed.[365] In one patient, medullary carcinoma was found in a gland also containing papillary cancer.[366] There is one report of a case of anaplastic carcinoma in a 32-year-old man who was irradiated at age 7.[367]

The thyroid gland removed from a patient with a history of irradiation almost always contains multiple nodules. As often as not, the clinically palpable nodule is either an adenoma or colloid nodule, and the carcinoma is present elsewhere. The cancers may be small, and in one series nearly one-half of the tumors were not found at the time of frozen section examination. Extensive sampling was required to disclose foci of carcinoma, which were 2–3 mm in size.[367] Frozen section interpretation is also complicated when non-neoplastic follicles with nuclear atypia are trapped within inflammatory fibrous areas. Multifocal bilateral cancers are common.[368]

Nearly a dozen cases of thyroid cancer have been reported in patients receiving relatively high doses of ^{131}I for Graves disease.[369] Nuclear pleomorphism, oncocytic change, and multiple small adenomas are also seen.[370]

Patients treated with radiation for medulloblastoma receive an estimated 200–3000 cGy to the thyroid, and several carcinomas have been reported.[371] Doses in excess of this are probably not associated with a markedly increased risk of cancer, perhaps because more of the injured thyroid cells are rendered incapable of division.[372] Nonetheless, several cases of papillary cancer have occurred after high-dose radiation for Hodgkin's disease.[373,374]

The possibility that low-dose irradiation may produce adenomas or hyperplasia in parathyroid glands has been raised. Several investigators have obtained a history of low dose irradiation in 14–30% of patients with hyperparathyroidism.[375] The irradiated glands do not have special histologic features, except for a possible increase in the proportion of oncocytes.[376] The latter has not been the subject of an adequately controlled study. The association of thyroid carcinoma and hyperparathyroidism (excluding medullary carcinoma and patients with syndromes of multiple endocrine adenomas) may in part be explained by irradiation. Nonetheless, in one series of 40 patients with coexistent parathyroid adenoma and thyroid carcinoma, only one had a history of prior irradiation.[376]

INTESTINE

Colorectal carcinomas have been reported in patients who had previous irradiation, usually of the uterine cervix. Castro et al.[377] analyzed 24 patients with colorectal carcinoma who were long-term survivors (5–28 years) of uterine cancer treated with radiotherapy. They found that in 13 cases the segment of bowel bearing the tumor had vascular and stromal changes consistent with radiation injury. Moreover, 13 patients had colloid carcinoma, which otherwise constitutes only about 10% of colon cancers. In another study, 17/32 patients with postradiation large bowel cancer showed mucinous differentition.[378] Qizilbash[379] described a treacherous combination wherein a papillary adenocarcinoma surrounded the margin of an ulcerated radiation-induced stricture. Colloid carcinoma has occurred in a child in the field of irradiation for Wilms tumor.[380]

Angiosarcoma of the small intestine developed in a woman 8 years after postoperative irradiation for ovarian carcinoma.[381] We have seen one case of small intestinal angiosarcoma 12 years after radiation for squamous cancer of the cervix.

UTERUS

Several hundred cases of endometrial cancer have been reported after irradiation of the uterus for endometrial bleeding from benign disease. It is uncertain how many of these are radiation-induced, since many of the cases received radiation for abnormal endometrial bleeding and may have been predisposed to adenocarcinoma. Furthermore, many of the postirradiation lesions were diagnosed as adenocarcinoma in situ, and the almost universal lack of illustrations leaves the exact nature of the lesions in question. It is possible that some of the cases may have been postirradiation cytopathy of normal endometrium.

The frequency of bona fide endometrial cancer in patients receiving radiation for squamous cancer of the cervix was studied by Fehr and Prem,[382] who found 12 examples in 2294 patients, which was more than double the expected number. The proportion of mixed müllerian tumors was striking. Looking at it from another direction, Norris and Taylor[383] found that 15% of 477 patients with uterine sarcomas had a history of irradiation. The tumors included carcinosarcomas, endometrial stromal sarcomas, and unclassified sarcomas. Leiomyosarcoma did not seem to be related. The behavior of postirradiation carcinosarcomas has been reported as more aggressive than spontaneous tumors in one study[384] but not in another study.[385] Postirradiation endometrial adenocarcinoma has a dismal outlook.[386]

BONE

Approximately 200 sarcomas have been reported at the site of a benign bone lesion that was irradiated. About three-quarters of these patients received what would now be considered unacceptably high doses. Moreover, most of the irradiated lesions (such as giant cell tumors) would currently be treated with newer surgical techniques. Postirradiation tumors have included osteosarcomas, fibrosarcomas, chondrosarcomas, and malignant fibrous histiocytomas.[387] The latent period has varied from slightly less than 3 years to 30 years with an average of 6 years for tumors occurring in weight-bearing bones and 14 years in non-weight-bearing bones.[388]

A new complication appears to be emerging from the successful treatment of Ewing sarcoma by local irradiation to the primary coupled with systemic chemotherapy. Four of 10 patients who had lived 5 or more years after the initial diagnosis of Ewing's sarcoma developed an osteosarcoma at the site of the original tumor.[389]

Postirradiation sarcoma in previously normal bone is a rare event. A review of about 6000 patients treated for malignant disease disclosed two osteosarcomas arising in bone that had been normal at the time of treatment 5 and 11 years previously.[390] This is 0.03% of all patients treated or 0.1% of the 5-year survivors. In another study, Tountas et al.[391] found 10 postradiation sarcomas, representing 0.035% of 5-year survivors. In children, genetic factors seem to play a role.[392]

Benign osseous tumors in the field of high-dose radiotherapy have all been osteochondromas. They occur when the radiation is given in childhood.[393]

SOFT TISSUE

Most sarcomas in irradiated soft tissues are on the chest or shoulder 4–16 years after radiation for breast carcinoma.[394] Most have metastasized. The lesions have had the conventional histologic patterns of angiosarcoma, lymphangiosarcoma, malignant fibrous histiocytoma, fibrosarcoma, chondrosarcoma, or a mixture of the latter two.[395–397] One fibrosarcoma had large, bizarre cells resembling so-called radiation fibroblasts interspersed among more typical foci of fibrosarcoma, a pattern that is occasionally seen even in the absence of prior radiation.[398] Postradiation sarcomas of the head and neck are rare. Malignant peripheral nerve sheath tumors have occurred in radiated soft tissues and have pursued a highly aggressive course. About one-half have been in patients with von Recklinghausen's disease.[399]

BREAST

Cancer of the breast has been reported in women in their 20s who received radiation to the chest during the first two decades of life, either for metastatic tumor[400] or for benign conditions[401] Adult women receiving radiation for mastitis or other benign breast disease have shown a twofold increase in frequency of breast cancer,[402] as have women undergoing repeated, prolonged fluoroscopic examination of the chest during therapy for tuberculosis.[403] Cancer of the breast appears to be slightly increased in patients treated with radiation for Hodgkin's disease.[404] Cancers in irradiated women tend to have less desmoplasia than cancers in controls.[405] Carcinoma of the male breast has been reported at age 46 after irradiation at puberty for gynecomastia[406] and at age 35 after low-dose irradiation in infancy.[407] The possible tumorigenic effect of repeated mammograms remains to be determined.[408]

CENTRAL NERVOUS SYSTEM

The most frequent radiation-induced tumor in the CNS is the so-called pituitary sarcoma, which is actually a fibrosarcoma with abundant collagen formation in some foci. Remnants of the irradiated adenoma are often scattered within the sarcoma. The latent period between irradiation and symptoms referable to the sarcoma ranges from 2.5–21 years, with an average of 7 years. The tumors do not metastasize, and death occurs from local growth.[409]

Donahue et al.[410] described two patients with neurofibromas of the spinal cord 11 and 13 years after radiation to the mediastinum in childhood.

Meningiomas have been found in a few patients receiving either high-dose or low-dose irradiation. Watts[411] reported meningiomas 15 and 25 years after therapeutic irradiation for glioma. Three meningiomas occurred in a group of more than 5000 patients receiving radiation to the scalp in childhood for tinea capitis, whereas none was present in the control group.[412] Radiation has been incriminated as a cause of malignant gliomas.[413] A spinal cord glioma arose in a region irradiated for Hodgkin's disease.[414]

MESOTHELIUM

Over 30 pleural or peritoneal mesotheliomas have been reported an average of 21 years after medium to high dose radiation, often for breast carcinoma or Hodgkin's disease.[415,416] An especially convincing argument for radiation as a causative agent can be made in mesothelioma developing after radiation in childhood.[417]

THORIUM DIOXIDE

Thorotrast is the trade name for a radioactive suspension of thorium dioxide used between 1930 and 1950 as a contrast medium. More than 50 000 persons received the agent,[418] including at least 4300 Americans.[419] More than 90% of the Thorotrast remains in the reticuloendothelial system for life, as brown, shiny granules. In the liver, it is found in Kupffer cells or in histiocytes. At the site of arterial injection, a progressive fibrous reaction around extravasated dye can continue for years, and sarcomas have been reported.[420,421] More than 200 neoplasms have been reported overall[422] and occasional cases continue to be reported.[423] More than one-half of the tumors are hepatic (approximately one-third angiosarcomas, one-third cholangiocarcinomas, and one-third hepatocellular carcinomas).[424] Rarely, all three types occur simultaneously.[425] The occurrence of tumors as long as 36 years after exposure indicates a lifelong risk.[426] Several osteosarcomas have been reported.[423,427] The actual sequence of carcinogenesis is poorly understood, but may involve p53 mutations.[428]

THERMAL THERAPY

Numerous studies on the use of hyperthermia have shown that it enhances radiotherapy or chemotherapy, or both.[429] Hyperthermia alone damages small vessels and presumably contributes to cytotoxic effects.[430] Alterations in experimental and human tumors are not specific. The quantity of necrosis or the frequency of absent tumor in the resected specimen may be increased when compared with resected specimens from patients treated with either radiation or chemotherapy alone.[431–433] Radiofrequency ablation and laser interstitial therapy involve the use of radio waves or laser light beams to produce heat.[434] The effect is in essence thermal ablation, necrosis and vascular damage of tissue.

REFERENCES

1. Maygarden SJ, Novotny DB, Johnson DE, et al. Subclassification of benign breast disease by fine needle aspiration cytology. Comparison of cytologic and histologic findings in 265 palpable breast masses. Acta Cytol 1994; 38: 115.

2. Feldman PS, Covell JL. Fine needle aspiration cytology and its clinical applications: breast and lung. Chicago: American Society of Clinical Pathologists Press; 1985: 47.

3. Vooijs GP. Benign proliferative reactions, intraepithelial neoplasia and invasive cancer of the uterine cervix. In: Bibbo M, ed. Comprehensive cytopathology, 2nd edn. Philadelphia: WB Saunders; 1997: 161–230.

4. Lee KR. Atypical glandular cells in cervical smears from women who have undergone cone biopsy. A potential diagnostic pitfall. Acta Cytol 1993; 37: 705.

5. Heaton RB, Harris TF, Larson DM, et al. Glandular cell derived from direct sampling of the lower uterine segment in patients status post-cervical cone biopsy. A diagnostic dilemma. Am J Clin Pathol 1996; 106: 511.

6. Yeh I, Bronner M, LiVolsi VA. Endometrial metaplasia of the uterine endocervix. Arch Pathol Lab Med 1993; 117: 734.

7. Fechner RE. Necrotizing sialometaplasia. A source of confusion with carcinoma of the palate. Am J Clin Pathol 1977; 67: 315.

8. Batsakis JG, Sneige N, El-Naggar AK. Fine-needle aspiration of salivary glands: its utility and tissue effects. Ann Otol Rhinol Laryngol 1992; 101: 185.

9. Walker GK, Fechner RE, Johns ME, et al. Necrotizing sialometaplasia of larynx secondary to atheromatous embolization. Am J Clin Pathol 1982; 77: 221.

10. Hambrick E. The fate of colonoscopic polypectomy sites. Dis Colon Rectum 1976; 19: 400.

11. Ellis KK, Fennerty MB. Marking and identifying colon lesions. Tattoos, clips and radiology in imaging the colon. Gastrointest Endosc Clin North Am 1997; 7: 401.

12. Lane KL, Vallera R. Washington K, et al. Endoscopic tattoo agents in the colon. Tissue responses and clinical implications. Am J Surg Pathol 1996; 20: 1266.

13. Yeh I. Atlas of microscopic artifacts and foreign materials. Baltimore: Williams & Wilkins; 1997.

14. Tannenbaum M. Differential diagnosis in uropathology. II. Urologic artifact and/or pathologist's dilemma. Urology 1974; 4: 485.

15. Alguacil-Garcia A. Artifactual changes mimicking signet ring cell carcinoma in transurethral prostatectomy specimens. Am J Surg Pathol 1986; 10: 795.

16. Goldstein NS, Watts JC, Neill JS, et al. The effect of electrothermal cautery-assisted resection of diminutive colonic polyps on histopathological diagnosis. Am J Clin Pathol 2001; 115: 356.

17. Evans SC, Goldman RL, Klein HZ, et al. Necrobiotic granulomas of the uterine cervix. Probable post-operative reaction. Am J Surg Pathol 1984; 8: 841.

18. Herbold DR, Frable WJ, Kraus FT. Isolated noninfectious granulomas of the ovary. Int J Gynecol Pathol 1984; 2: 380.

19. Balogh K. Palisading granuloma in the kidney after open biopsy (letter). Am J Surg Pathol 1986; 10: 441.

20. Spagnolo DV, Waring PM. Bladder granulomata after bladder surgery. Am J Clin Pathol 1986; 86: 430.

21. Epstein JI, Hutchins GM. Granulomatous prostatitis: distinction among allergic, nonspecific, and posttransurethral resection lesions. Hum Pathol 1984; 15: 818.

22. Henry L, Wagner B, Faulkner MK, et al. Metal deposition in post-surgical granulomas of the urinary tract. Histopathology 1993; 22: 457.

23. Thurrell W, Reid P, Kennedy A, Smith JHF. Necrotising granulomas of the peritoneum. Histopathology 1991; 18: 190.

24. Agel NM. Necrobiotic granulomas of the urogenital system. J Clin Pathol 1995; 48: 185.

25. Colgan TJ, Shah R, Leyland N. Post-hysteroscopic ablation reaction: a histopathologic study of the effects of electrosurgical ablation. Int J Gynecol Pathol 1999; 18: 325.

26. Baggish MS, Barash F, Noel Y, et al. Comparison of thermal injury zones in loop electrical and laser cervical excisional conization. Am J Obstet Gynecol 1992; 166: 545.

27. Chen R-J, Lee EF, Shih J-C. Does the loop electrosurgical excision procedure adversely affect the histopathological interpretation of cervical conization specimens? Acta Obstet Gynecol Scand 1994; 73: 726.

28. Montz FJ, Holschneider CH, Thompson LDR. Large-loop excision of the transformation zone: effect on the pathologic interpretation of resection margins. Obstet Gynecol 1993; 81: 976.

29. Batnitzky S, Keucher TR, Mealey J Jr, et al. Iatrogenic intraspinal epidermoid tumors. JAMA 1977; 237: 148.

30. Strauchen JA, Strefling AM. Epidermal inclusion cyst of the meniscus. J Bone Joint Surg 1982; 64A:290.

31. Carter BA, Jensen RA, Simpson JF, et al. Benign transport of breast epithelium into axillary lymph nodes after biopsy. Am J Clin Pathol 2000; 113: 259.

32. Brooks JS, LiVolsi VA, Pietra GG. Mesothelial cell inclusions in mediastinal lymph nodes mimicking metastatic carcinoma. Am J Clin Pathol 1990; 93: 741.

33. Isotalo PA, Veinot JP, Jabi M. Hyperplastic mesothelial cells in mediastinal lymph node sinuses with extranodal lymphatic involvement. Arch Pathol Lab Med 2000; 124: 609.

34. Dirschmid K, Kiesler J, Mathis G, et al. Epithelial misplacement after biopsy of colorectal adenomas. Am J Surg Pathol 1993; 17: 1262.

35. Youngson BJ, Cranor M, Rosen PP. Epithelial displacement in surgical breast specimens following needling procedures. Am J Surg Pathol 1994; 18: 896.

36. Tavassoli FA, Pestaner JP. Pseudoinvasion in intraductal carcinoma. Mod Pathol 1995; 8: 380–383.

37. Youngson BJ, Liberman L, Rosen PP. Displacement of carcinomatous epithelium in surgical breast specimens following stereotaxic core biopsy. Am J Clin Pathol 1995; 103: 598.

38. Cox CE, Nguyen K, Gray RJ, et al. Importance of lymphatic mapping in ductal carcinoma in situ (DCIS): why map DCIS? Am Surg 2001; 67: 513.

39. Klauber-DeMore N, Tan LK, Liberman L, et al. Sentinel lymph node biopsy: is it indicated in patients with high-risk ductal carcinoma-in-situ and ductal carcinoma-in-situ with microinvasion? Ann Surg Oncol 2000; 7: 636.

40. McLaughlin CM, Devine P, Muto M, Genest DR. Pseudo-invasion of vascular spaces: report of an artifact caused by cervical lidocaine injection prior to loop diathermy. Hum Pathol 1994; 25: 208.

41. Tsang WYW, Chan JKC. Spectrum of morphologic changes in lymph nodes attributable to fine needle aspiration. Hum Pathol 1992; 23: 562.

42. Behm FG, O'Dowd GJ, Frable WJ. Fine-needle aspiration effects on benign lymph node histology. Am J Clin Pathol 1984; 82: 195.

43. Kern SB. Necrosis of a Warthin's tumor following fine needle aspiration. Acta Cytol 1988; 32: 207.

44. Keyhani-Rofagha S, Kooner DS, Keyhani M, O'Toole RV. Necrosis of a Hürthle cell tumor of the thyroid following fine needle aspiration. Case report and literature review. Acta Cytol 1990; 43: 805.

45. Lee KC, Chan JKC, Ho LC. Histologic changes in the breast after fine-needle aspiration. Am J Surg Pathol 1994; 18: 1039.

46. Tabbara SO, Frierson HF Jr, Fechner RE. Diagnostic problems in tissues previously sampled by fine needle aspiration. Am J Clin Pathol 1991; 96: 76.

47. Livolsi VA, Merino MJ. Worrisome histologic alterations following fine-needle aspiration of the thyroid (WHAFFT). Pathol Annu 1994; 29: 99.

48. Karwowski JK, Nowels KW, McDougall IR, et al. Needle track seeding of papillary thyroid carcinoma from fine needle aspiration biopsy. A case report. Acta Cytol 2002; 46: 591.

49. Shenoy PD, Lakhkar BN, Ghosh MK, et al. Cutaneous seeding of renal carcinoma by Chiba needle aspiration biopsy. Case report. Acta Radiol 1991; 32: 50.

50. Pasieka JL, Thompson NW. Fine-needle aspiration biopsy causing peritoneal seeding of a carcinoid tumor. Arch Surg 1992; 127: 1248.

51. Trimbos JB, Hacker NF. The case against aspirating ovarian cysts. Cancer 1993; 72: 828.

52. Andersen WA, Nichols GE, Avery SR, Taylor PT. Cytologic diagnosis of ovarian tumors: factors influencing accuracy in previously undiagnosed cases. Am J Obstet Gynecol 1995; 173: 457.

53. Elliot JS, Rosenberg ML. Ureteral occlusion by barium granulomata. J Urol 1954; 71: 692.

54. Lewis JW Jr, Kerstein MD, Koss N. Barium granuloma of the rectum: an uncommon complication of barium enema. Ann Surg 1975; 181: 418.

55. Hayden RS. Perforation of duodenal ulcer during fluoroscopy. Disposition of barium sulfate in the abdominal cavity. Radiology 1951; 57: 214.

56. Fox RM, Malter IJ. Prolonged oviduct retention of iodized contrast medium. Obstet Gynecol 1972; 40: 221.

57. Kantor HI, Kamholz JH, Smith AL. Foreign-body granulomas following the use of Salpix. Report of a case simulating intraabdominal tuberculosis. Obstet Gynecol 1956; 7: 171.

58. Ruberu NN, Saito Y, Honma N, et al. Granulomatous meningitis as a late complication of iodized oil myelography. Neuropathology 2004; 24: 144.

59. Coder DM, Olander GA. Granulomatous peritonitis caused by starch glove powder. Arch Surg 1972; 105: 83.

60. Taft DA, Lasersohn JT, Hill JD. Glove starch granulomatous peritonitis. Am J Surg 1970; 120: 231.

61. Paine CG, Smith P. Starch granulomata. J Clin Pathol 1957; 10: 51.

62. Davies JD, Neely J. The histopathology of peritoneal starch granulomas. J Pathol 1972; 107: 265.

63. Aarons J, Fitzgerald N. The persisting hazards of surgical glove powder. Surg Gynecol Obstet 1974; 138: 385.

64. Sobel HJ, Schiffman RJ, Schwarz R, et al. Granulomas and peritonitis due to starch glove powder. Arch Pathol Lab Med 1971; 91: 558.

65. Housini I, Dabbs DJ, Coyne L. Fine needle aspiration cytology of talc granulomatosis in a peripheral lymph node in a case of suspected intravenous drug abuse. Acta Cytol 1990; 34: 342.

66. Tao LC, Morgan RC, Donat EE. Cytologic diagnosis of intravenous talc granulomatosis by fine needle aspiration biopsy. A case report. Acta Cytol 1984; 28: 737.

67. Reinhartz T, Lijovetzky G, Levij IS. Intracellular starch granules in cytologic material. Acta Cytol 1978; 22: 36.

68. Malinger G, Ginath S, Zeidel L, et al. Starch peritonitis outbreak after introduction of a new brand of starch powdered latex gloves. Acta Obstet Gynecol Scand 2000; 79: 610.

69. Sturdy JH, Baird RM, Gerein AN. Surgical sponges. A cause of granuloma and adhesion formation. Ann Surg 1967; 165: 128.

70. Saxen L, Myllarniemi H. Foreign material and postoperative adhesions. N Engl J Med 1968; 279: 200.

71. Dragan MJ. Wood fibers from disposable surgical gowns and drapes. JAMA 1979; 241: 2297.

72. Tomashefski J Jr, Cohen AM, Doershuk CF. Longterm histopathologic follow-up of bronchial arteries after therapeutic embolization with polyvinyl alcohol (Ivalon) in patients with cystic fibrosis. Hum Pathol 1988; 19: 555.

73. Novak D. Embolization materials. In: Diondelinger RF, Rossi P, Kurdziel JC, Wallace S, eds. Interventional radiology. New York: Thieme; 1990: 295–312

74. Schweitzer JS, Chang BS, Madsen P, et al. The pathology of arteriovenous malformations of the brain treated by embolotherapy. II. Results of embolization with multiple agents. Neuroradiology 1993; 35: 468.

75. Knowlson GTG. Gel-foam granuloma in the brain. J Neurol Neurosurg Psychiatry 1974; 37: 971.

76. Kepes JJ, Yarde WL. Visualization of injected embolic material (polyvinyl alcohol) in paraffin sections with Verhoeff-van Gieson elastica stain. Am J Surg Pathol 1995; 19: 709.

77. Germano IM, Davis RL, Wilson CB, et al. Histopathological follow-up study of 66 cerebral arteriovenous malformations after therapeutic embolization with polyvinyl alcohol. J Neurosurg 1992; 76: 607.

78. Davidson GS, Terbrugge KG. Histologic long-term follow-up after embolization with polyvinyl alcohol particles. Am J Neuroradiol 1995; 6(suppl. 4):843.

79. Lundie MJ, Ellyatt D, Kaufmann MB, et al. Staining procedure to aid in assessment of bucrylate histotoxicity in tissue sections. Arch Pathol Lab Med 1985; 109: 779.

80. Jinno K, Moriwaki S, Tanada M, et al. Clinicopathological study on combination therapy consisting of arterial embolization for hepatocellular carcinoma. Cancer Chemother Pharmacol 1992; 31: S7.

81. Spies JB, Benenati JF, Worthington-Kirsch RL, et al. Initial experience with use of tris-acryl gelatin microspheres for uterine artery embolization for leiomyomata. J Vasc Interv Radiol 2001; 12: 1059.

82. Uecker J, Postoak DW, Yeh I. A surgical alternative: microsphere embolization in uterine smooth muscle tumors. Pathol Case Rev 2003; 8: 115.

83. Kyriakos M. Myospherulosis of the paranasal sinuses, nose and middle ear. A possible iatrogenic disease. Am J Clin Pathol 1977; 67: 118.

84. Rosai J. The nature of myospherulosis of the upper respiratory tract. Am J Clin Pathol 1978; 69: 475.

85. Travis WD, Li C-Y, Weiland LH. Immunostaining for hemoglobin in two cases of myospherulosis. Arch Pathol Lab Med 1986; 110: 763.

86. Wheeler TM, Sessions RB, McGavran MH. 'Myospherulosis': a preventable iatrogenic nasal and paranasal entity. Arch Otolaryngol 1980; 106: 272.

87. White JT. Myospherulosis. South Med J 1979; 72: 485.

88. Mills SE, Lininger JR. Intracranial myospherulosis. Hum Pathol 1982; 13: 596.

89. Lui PCW, Luk ISC, Lee CKL et al. Hepatic myospherulosis complicating portal vein embolisation. J Clin Pathol 2004; 57: 155.

90. Shabb N, Sneige N, Dekmezian RH. Myospherulosis. Fine needle aspiration cytologic findings in 19 cases. Acta Cytol 1991; 35: 225.

91. Wolff M. Granulomas in nasal mucous membranes following local steroid injections. Am J Clin Pathol 1974; 62: 775.

92. Santa Cruz DJ, Ulbright TM. Mucin-like changes in keloids. Am J Clin Pathol 1981; 75: 18.

93. Ford LT, DeBender J. Tendon rupture after local steroid injection. South Med J 1979; 72: 827.

94. Balough K. The histologic appearance of corticosteroid injection sites. Arch Pathol Lab Med 1986; 110: 1168.

95. Georgieva J, Assaf C, Steinhoff M, et al. Bodybuilder oleoma. Br J Dermatol 2003; 149: 1289.

96. Hutton L. Oleothorax: expanding pleural lesion. AJR 1984; 142: 1107.

97. Hoare AM, Alexander-Williams J. Oleogranuloma of the rectum produced by Lasonil ointment. Br Med J 1977; 2: 997.

98. Ghosh A. Lipogranuloma of the uterine parametrium. Br J Obstet Gynecol 1976; 83: 409.

99. Keebler CM. Cytopreparatory techniques. In: Bibbo M, ed. Comprehensive cytopathology, 2nd edn. Philadelphia: WB Saunders; 1997: 889–917.

100. Avrin E, Marquet E, Schwartz R, et al. Plant cells resembling tumor cells in routine cytology. Am J Clin Pathol 1972; 57: 303.

101. Lombard T, Samson J, Plantier F, et al. Orofacial granulomas after injection of cosmetic fillers. Histopathologic and clinical study of 11 cases. J Oral Pathol Med 2004; 33: 115.

102. Lemperle G, Morhenn V, Charrier U. Human histology and persistence of various injectable filler substances for soft tissue augmentation. Aesth Plast Surg 2003; 27: 354.

103. Emery JA, Spanier SS, Kasnic G Jr, Hardt NS. The synovial structure of breast-implant-associated bursae. Mod Pathol 1994; 7: 728.

104. Gabriel SE, O'Fallon WM, Kurland LT, et al. Risk of connective-tissue diseases and other disorders after breast implantation. N Engl J Med 1994; 330: 1697.

105. Sanchez-Guerrero J, Colditz GA, Karlson EW, et al. Silicone breast implants and the risk of connective-tissue diseases and symptoms. N Engl J Med 1995; 332: 1666.

106. US Food and Drug Administration, Center for Devices and Radiological Health. Breast Implants, An Information Update 2000. Available on line at: www.fda.gov/cdrh/breastimplants/bioavail.html.

107. Hameed MR, Erlandson R, Rosen PP. Capsular synovial-like hyperplasia around mammary implants similar to detritic synovitis. A morphologic and immunohistochemical study of 15 cases. Am J Surg Pathol 1995; 19: 433.

108. Raso DS, Crymes LW, Metcalf JS. Histological assessment of fifty breast capsules from smooth and textured augmentation and reconstruction mammoplasty prostheses with emphasis on the role of synovial metaplasia. Mod Pathol 1994; 7: 310.

109. Edwards JCW, Sedgwick AD, Willoughby DA. The formation of a structure with the features of synovial lining by subcutaneous injection of air: an *in vivo* tissue culture system. J Pathol 1981; 134: 147.

110. Kasper CS. Histologic features of breast capsules reflect surface configuration and composition of silicone bag implants. Am J Clin Pathol 1994; 102: 655.

111. Tabatowski K, Elson CE, Johnston WW. Silicone lymphadenopathy in a patient with a mammary prosthesis. Fine needle aspiration cytology, histology and analytical electron microscopy. Acta Cytol 1990; 34: 10.

112. Frantz P, Herbst CA Jr. Augmentation mammoplasty, irradiation, and breast cancer. A case report. Cancer 1975; 36: 1147.

113. Dodd LG, Sneige N, Reece GP, et al. Fine-needle aspiration cytology of silicone granulomas in the augmented breast. Diagn Cytopathol 1993; 9: 498.

114. Bommer J, Ritz E, Waldherr R. Silicone-induced splenomegaly. Treatment of pancytopenia by splenectomy in a patient on hemodialysis. N Engl J Med 1981; 305: 1077.

115. Tabatowski K, Sammarco GJ. Fine needle aspiration cytology of silicone lymphadenopathy in a patient with an artificial joint. A case report. Acta Cytol 1992; 36: 529.

116. Christie AJ, Weinberger KA, Dietrich M. Silicone lymphadenopathy and synovitis. Complications of silicone elastomer finger joint prostheses. JAMA 1977; 237: 1463.

117. Christie AJ, Weinberger KA, Dietrich M. Recurrence of silicone lymphadenopathy. JAMA 1981; 245: 1314.

118. Travis WD, Balogh K, Abraham JL. Silicone granulomas: report of three cases and review of the literature. Hum Pathol 1985; 16: 19.

119. Friedlander GN, Potter GK, Tucker RS, et al. Silicone elastomer microshards in fluid from a painful metatarsophalangeal implant site. A case report. Acta Cytol 1995; 39: 586.

120. McKinney CD, Gaffey MJ, Gillenwater JY. Bladder outlet obstruction after multiple periurethral polytetrafluoroethylene injections. J Urol 1995; 153: 149.

121. Wenig BM, Heffner DK, Oertel YC, Johnson FB. Teflonomas of the larynx and neck. Hum Pathol 1990; 21: 617.

122. Hanau CA, Chancellor MB, Alexander A, et al. Fine-needle aspiration of a periurethral Teflon-filled cyst following radical prostatectomy. Diagn Cytopathol 1992; 8: 614.

123. Freeman BS. Proplast, a porous implant for contour restoration. Br J Plast Surg 1976; 29: 158.

124. Chuong R, Piper MA, Boland TJ. Recurrent giant cell reaction to residual Proplast in the temporomandibular joint. Oral Surg Oral Med Oral Pathol 1993; 76: 16.

125. Estabrooks LN, Fairbanks CE, Collett RJ, et al. A retrospective evaluation of 301 TMJ Proplast-Teflon implants. Oral Surg Oral Med Oral Pathol 1990; 70: 381.

126. US Food and Drug Administration. Vitek Jaw Implant. 91, 1991. Available on line at: www.fda.gov/bbs/topics/NEWS/NEW00249.html.

127. Ober WB. Effects of oral and intrauterine administration of contraceptives on the uterus. Hum Pathol 1977; 8: 513.

128. Czernobilsky B, Rotenstreich L, Mass N, et al. Effect of intrauterine device on histology of endometrium. Obstet Gynecol 1975; 45: 64.

129. McCormick JF, Scorgie RDF. Unilateral tubo-ovarian actinomycosis in the presence of an intrauterine device. Am J Clin Pathol 1977; 68: 622.

130. Sindou M, Pisal N, Setchell M, et al. Tubal migration: a rare complication of an intrauterine contraceptive device leading to formation of a hydrosalpinx. Am J Obstet Gynecol 2003; 188: 1109.

131. Sagiroglu N, Sagiroglu E. The cytology of intrauterine contraceptive devices. Acta Cytol 1970; 14: 58.

132. Fornari ML. Cellular changes in the glandular epithelium of patients using IUD's – a source of cytologic error. Acta Cytol 1974; 18: 341.

133. Gupta PK. Intrauterine contraceptive devices. Vaginal cytology, pathologic changes, and clinical implications. Acta Cytol 1982; 26: 571.

134. Zaharopoulos P, Wong JY, Edmonston G, et al. Crystalline bodies in cervicovaginal smears. Acta Cytol 1985; 29: 1035.

135. Barter JF, Orr JW, Holloway RW, et al. Psammoma bodies in a cervicovaginal smear associated with an intrauterine device – a case report. J Reprod Med 1987; 32: 147.

136. Ostergard DR, Townsend DE, Hirose FM. Treatment of chronic cervicitis by cryotherapy. Am J Obstet Gynecol 1968; 102: 426.

137. Gondos B, Smith LR, Townsend DE. Cytologic changes in cervical epithelium following cryosurgery. Acta Cytol 1970; 14: 386.

138. Holmquist ND, Bellina JH, Danos ML. Vaginal and cervical cytologic changes following laser treatment. Acta Cytol 1976; 20: 290.

139. Koss LG. Diagnostic cytology and its histologic basis. Philadelphia: Lippincott-Raven; 1992: 665.

140. Hoffman MS, Gordy LW, Cavanagh D. Use of the Cytobrush for cervical sampling after cryotherapy. Acta Cytol, 1991; 35: 7.

141. Onik G. Image-guided prostate cryosurgery: state of the art. Cancer Control 2001; 8: 522.

142. Grampsas SA, Miller GJ, Crawford ED. Salvage radical prostatectomy after failed transperineal cryotherapy: histologic findings from prostate whole-mount specimens correlated with intraoperative transrectal ultrasound images. Urology 1995; 45: 936.

143. Petersen DS, Milleman LA, Rose EF, et al. Biopsy and clinical course after cryosurgery for prostatic cancer. J Urol 1978; 120: 308.

144. Lucas DR, Miller PR, Mott MP, et al. Arthroplasty-associated malignant fibrous histiocytoma: two case reports. Histopathology 2001; 39: 620.

145. Fechner RE. Bone and joints. In: Riddell RH, ed. Pathology of drug-induced and toxic diseases. New York: Churchill Livingstone; 1982: 79.

146. Goldring SR, Schiller AL, Roelke M, et al. The synovial-like membrane at the bone-cement interface in loose total hip replacements and its proposed role in bone lysis. J Bone Joint Surg 1983; 65A:575.

147. O'Connell JX, Rosenberg AE. Histiocytic lymphadenitis associated with a large joint prosthesis. Am J Clin Pathol 1993; 99: 314.

148. Albores-Saavedra J, Vuitch F, Delgado R, et al. Sinus histiocytosis of pelvic lymph nodes after hip replacement. A histiocytic proliferation induced by cobalt-chromium and titanium. Am J Surg Pathol 1994; 18: 83.

149. Bjornsson BL, Truong LD, Cartwright J Jr, et al. Pelvic lymph node histiocytosis mimicking metastatic prostatic adenocarcinoma: association with hip prostheses. J Urol 1995; 154: 470.

150. Peacock EE Jr, Van Winkle W Jr. Wound repair, 2nd edn. Philadelphia: WB Saunders; 1976.

151. Postelthwait RW. Tissue reaction to surgical sutures. In: Dunphy JE, Van Winkle W Jr, eds. Repair and regeneration. The scientific basis for surgical practice. New York: McGraw-Hill; 1968: 263.

152. Salthouse TN, Matlaga BS, Wykoff MH. Comparative tissue response to six suture materials in rabbit cornea, sclera, and ocular muscle. Am J Ophthalmol 1977; 84: 224.

153. Alguacil-Garcia A. Necrobiotic palisading suture granulomas simulating rheumatoid nodule. Am J Surg Pathol 1993; 17: 920.

154. Shauffer IA, Sequeira J. Suture granuloma simulating recurrent carcinoma. AJR 1977; 128: 856.

155. Belleza NA, Lowman RM. Suture granuloma of the stomach following total colectomy. Radiology 1978; 127: 84.

156. Maygarden SJ, Novotny DB, Johnson DE, et al. Fine-needle aspiration cytology of suture granulomas of the breast: a potential pitfall in the cytologic diagnosis of recurrent breast cancer. Diagn Cytopathol 1994; 10: 175.

157. Amazon K, Robinson MJ, Rywlin AM. Ferrugination caused by Monsel's solution. Clinical observations and experimentations. Am J Dermatopathol 1980; 2: 197.

158. Olmstead PM, Lund HZ, Leonard DD. Monsel's solution. A histologic nuisance. J Am Acad Dermatol 1980; 3: 492.

159. Elenitsas R, Schuchter LM. The role of the pathologist in the diagnosis of melanoma. Curr Opin Oncol 1998; 10: 162.

160. Spitzer M, Chernys AE. Monsel's solution-induced artifact in the uterine cervix. Am J Obstet Gynecol 1996; 175: 1204.

161. Ben-Izhak O, Vlodavsky E, Ofer A, et al. Epithelioid angiosarcoma associated with a Dacron vascular graft. Am J Surg Pathol 1999; 23: 1418.

162. Weiss WM, Riles TS, Gouge TH, et al. Angiosarcoma at the site of a Dacron vascular prosthesis: a case report and literature review. J Vasc Surg 1991; 14: 87.

163. Armin A-R, Moradi A, Winters G. Posttraumatic intrauterine omental implantation mimicking lipomatous lesion 16 years later. Int J Gynecol Pathol 1987; 6: 89.

164. Rosen Y, Vaillant JG, Yerkmakov V. Submucosal mucous cysts at a colostomy site: relationship to colitis cystica profunda and report of a case. Dis Colon Rectum 1976; 19: 453.

165. Wayte DM, Helwig EB. Colitis cystica profunda. Am J Clin Pathol 1967; 48: 159.

166. Rosai J. Ackerman's surgical pathology. 7th edn. St Louis: CV Mosby; 1989.

167. Lee PC, Mateo RB, Clarke MR, et al. Parathyromatosis: a cause for recurrent hyperparathyroidism. Endocr Pract 2001; 7: 189.

168. Kendrick ML, Charboneau JW, Curlee KJ, et al. Risk of parathyromatosis after fine-needle aspiration. Am Surg 2001; 67: 290.

169. Courtice RW, Stinson WA, Walley VM. Tissue fragments recovered at cardiac surgery masquerading as tumoral proliferations. Evidence suggesting iatrogenic or artefactual origin and common occurrence. Am J Surg Pathol 1994; 18: 167.

170. Veinot JP, Tazelaar HD, Edwards WD, Colby TV. Mesothelial/monocytic incidental cardiac excrescences (cardiac MICE). Mod Pathol 1994; 7: 9.

171. Bigner SH, Elmore PD, Dee AL, et al. Unusual presentations of inflammatory conditions in cerebrospinal fluid. Acta Cytol 1985; 29: 291.

172. Bigner SH, Elmore PD, Dee AL, et al. The cytopathology of reactions to ventricular shunts. Acta Cytol 1985; 29: 391.

173. Hoffman HJ, Duffner PK. Extraneural metastases of central nervous system tumors. Cancer 1985; 56: 1778.

174. Lovell MA, Ross GW, Cooper PH. Gliomatosis peritonei associated with a ventriculoperitoneal shunt. Am J Clin Pathol 1989; 91: 485.

175. Huang A, McPherson GAD. Colonic carcinoma after ureterosigmoidostomy. Postgrad Med J 2000; 76: 579.

176. Harford FJ, Fazio VW, Epstein LM, et al. Rectosigmoid carcinoma occurring after ureterosigmoidostomy. Dis Colon Rectum 1984; 27: 321.

177. Iannoni C, Marcheggiano A, Pallone F, et al. Abnormal patterns of colorectal mucin secretion after urinary diversion of different types: histochemical and lectin binding studies. Hum Pathol 1986; 17: 834.

178. Schipper H, Deckter A. Carcinoma of the colon arising at uretero-implant sites despite early external diversion. Pathogenetic and clinical implications. Cancer 1981; 47: 2062.

179. Littler ER, Gleibermann E. Gastritis cystica polyposa. (Gastric mucosal prolapse at gastroenterostomy site, with cystic and infiltrative epithelial hyperplasia.) Cancer 1972; 29: 205.

180. Koga S, Watanabe H, Enjoji M. Stomal polypoid hypertrophic gastritis. A polypoid gastric lesion at gastroenterostomy site. Cancer 1979; 43: 647.

181. Stemmermann GN, Nayashi T. Hyperplastic polyps of the gastric mucosa adjacent to gastroenterostomy stomas. Am J Clin Pathol 1979; 71: 341.

182. Morgenstern L, Yamakawa T, Seltzer D. Carcinoma of the gastric stump. Am J Surg 1973; 125: 29.

183. Bogomoletz WV, Potet F, Barge J, et al. Pathological features and mucin histochemistry of primary gastric stump carcinoma associated with gastritis cystica polyposa. A study of six cases. Am J Surg Pathol 1985; 9: 401.

184. Ruck P, Wehrmann M, Campbell M, et al. Squamous cell carcinoma of the gastric stump. A case report and review of the literature. Am J Surg Pathol 1989; 13: 317.

185. Monafo W, Goldfarb W. Postoperative peritoneal cyst. Surgery 1963; 53: 470.

186. Ross MJ, Welch WR, Scully RE. Multilocular peritoneal inclusion cysts (so-called cystic mesotheliomas). Cancer 1989; 64: 1336.

187. Weiss SW, Tavassoli FA. Multicystic mesothelioma. An analysis of pathologic findings and biologic behavior in 37 cases. Am J Surg Pathol 1988; 12: 737.

188. O'Hara CJ, Corson JM, Pinkus GS, et al. A monoclonal antibody that distinguishes epithelial-type malignant mesothelioma from pulmonary adenocarcinoma and extrapulmonary malignancies. Am J Pathol 1990; 136: 421.

189. Nance KV, Silverman JF. Immunocytochemical panel for the identification of malignant cells in serous effusions. Am J Clin Pathol 1991; 95: 867.

190. Steinberg AO, Madayag MA, Bosniak MA, et al. Demonstration of 2 unusually large pelvic lymphocysts by lymphangiography. J Urol 1973; 109: 477.

191. Basinger GT, Gittes RF. Lymphocyst: ultrasound diagnosis and urologic management. J Urol 1975; 114: 740.

192. Payan HM, Gilbert EF. Mesenteric cyst-ovarian implant syndrome. Arch Pathol Lab Med 1987; 111: 282.

193. Proppe KH, Scully RE, Rosai J. Postoperative spindle cell nodules of genitourinary tract resembling sarcomas. A report of eight cases. Am J Surg 1984; Pathol 8: 101.

194. Kay S, Schneider V. Reactive spindle cell nodule of the endocervix simulating uterine sarcoma. Int J Gynecol Pathol 1985; 4: 255.

195. Lundgren L, Aldenborg F, Angervall L, et al. Pseudomalignant spindle cell proliferations of the urinary bladder. Hum Pathol 1994; 25: 181.

196. Wick MR, Brown BA, Young RH, et al. Spindle-cell proliferations of the urinary tract. An immunohistochemical study. Am J Surg Pathol 1988; 12: 379.

197. Powers CN, Berardo MD, Frable WJ. Fine-needle aspiration biopsy: pitfalls in the diagnosis of spindle-cell lesions. Diagn Cytopathol 1994; 10: 232.

198. Weiss SW, Enzinger FM, Johnson FB. Silica reaction simulating fibrous histiocytoma. Cancer 1978; 42: 2738.

199. Maly A, Regev E, Meir K, et al. Tissue reaction to liquid silicone simulating low-grade liposarcoma following lip augmentation. J Oral Pathol Med 2004; 33: 314.

200. Sobel HJ, Avrin E, Marquet E, et al. Reactive granular cells in sites of trauma. A cytochemical and ultrastructural study. Am J Clin Pathol 1974; 61: 223.

201. McFadden DE, Clement PB. Peritoneal inclusion cysts with mural mesothelial proliferation. A clinicopathologic analysis of six cases. Am J Surg Pathol 1986; 10: 844.

202. Weiss SW, Enzinger FM. Malignant fibrous histiocytoma: an analysis of 200 cases. Cancer 1978; 41: 2250.

203. Inoshita T, Youngberg GA. Malignant fibrous histiocytoma arising in previous surgical sites. Report of two cases. Cancer 1984; 53: 176.

204. Cozen W, Bernstein L, Wang F, et al. The risk of angiosarcoma following primary breast cancer. Br J Cancer 1999; 81: 532.

205. Sherlock P, Oropeza R. Jejunal perforations in lymphoma after chemotherapy. Arch Intern Med 1962; 110: 102.

206. Hartmann WH, Sherlock P. Gastroduodenal metastases from carcinoma of the breast. An adrenal steroid-induced phenomenon. Cancer 1961; 14: 426.

207. Mayer RJ, Berkowitz RS, Griffiths CT. Central nervous system involvement by ovarian carcinoma. A complication of prolonged survival with metastatic disease. Cancer 1978; 41: 776.

208. Gercovich FG, Luna MA, Gottlieb JA. Increased incidence of cerebral metastases in sarcoma patients with prolonged survival from chemotherapy. Report of cases of leiomyosarcoma and chondrosarcoma. Cancer 1975; 36: 1843.

209. Telles NC, Rabson AS, Pomeroy TC. Ewing's sarcoma: an autopsy study. Cancer 1978; 41: 2321.

210. Lockwood WB, Broghamer WL Jr. The changing prevalence of secondary cardiac neoplasms as related to cancer therapy. Cancer 1980; 45: 2659.

211. Espana P, Chang P, Wiernik PH. Increased incidence of brain metastases in sarcoma patients. Cancer 1980; 45: 337.

212. Thalinger AR, Rosenthal SN, Borg S, et al. Cavitation of pulmonary metastases as a response to chemotherapy. Cancer 1980; 46: 1329.

213. Qizilbash A, Kontozoglou T, Sianos J, et al. Hepar lobatum associated with chemotherapy and metastatic breast cancer. Arch Pathol Lab Med 1987; 111: 58.

214. Koss LG, Melamed MR, Mayer K. The effect of busulfan on human epithelia. Am J Clin Pathol 1965; 44: 385.

215. Nelson BM, Andrews GA. Breast cancer and cytologic dysplasia in many organs after busulfan (Myleran). Am J Clin Pathol 1964; 42: 37.

216. Koss LG. Diagnostic cytology and its histologic basis. Philadelphia: Lippincott-Raven; 1992: 675–681, 753–757, 920–926.

217. Walloch JL, Hong HY, Bibb LM. Effects of therapy on cytologic specimens. In: Bibbo M, ed. Comprehensive cytopathology, 2nd edn. Philadelphia: WB Saunders; 1997: 865–885.

218. Pinedo F, Vargas J, de Agustin P, et al. Epithelial atypia in gynecomastia induced by chemotherapeutic drugs. A possible pitfall in fine needle aspiration biopsy. Acta Cytol 1991; 35: 229.

219. Kennedy S, Merino MJ, Swain SM, et al. The effects of hormonal and chemotherapy on tumoral and nonneoplastic breast tissue. Hum Pathol 1990; 21: 192.

220. O'Morchoe PJ, Lee DC, Kozak CA. Esophageal cytology in patients receiving cytotoxic drug therapy. Acta Cytol 1983; 27: 630.

221. Stella F, Battistelli S, Marcheggiani F, et al. Urothelial toxicity following conditioning therapy in bone marrow transplantation and bladder cancer: morphologic and morphometric comparison by exfoliative urinary cytology. Diagn Cytopathol 1992; 8: 216.

222. Naryshkin S, Bedrossian C. Selected mimics of malignancy in sputum and bronchoscopic cytology specimens. Diagn Cytopathol 1995; 13: 443.

223. Forni AM, Koss LG, Geller W. Cytologic study of the effect of cyclophosphamide on the epithelium of the urinary bladder in man. Cancer 1964; 17: 1348.

224. Sharkey FE, Addington SL, Fowler LJ, et al. Efforts of preoperative chemotherapy on the morphology of resectable breast carcinoma. Mod Pathol 1996; 9: 893.

225. Armas OA, Aprikian AG, Melamed J, et al. Clinical and pathobiological effects of neoadjuvant total androgen ablation therapy on clinically localized prostatic adenocarcinoma. Am J Surg Pathol 1994; 18: 979.

226. Wade TR, Ackerman AB. The effects of resin of podophyllin on condyloma acuminatum. Am J Dermatopathol 1984; 6: 109.

227. Krebs HB, Helmkamp BF. Chronic ulcerations following topical therapy with 5-fluorouracil for vaginal human papillomavirus-associated lesions. Obstet Gynecol 1991; 78: 205.

228. Colgan T, Simon GT, Kay JM, et al. Amiodarone pulmonary toxicity. Ultrastruct Pathol 1984; 6: 199.

229. Martin WJ, Osborn MJ, Douglass WW. Amiodarone pulmonary toxicity: assessment by bronchial lavage. Chest 1985; 88: 630.

230. Stein B, Zaatari GS, Pine JR. Amiodarone pulmonary toxicity. Acta Cytol 1987; 31: 357.

231. Frierson HF, Fechner RE. Histologic grade of locally advanced infiltrating ductal carcinoma after treatment with induction chemotherapy. Am J Clin Pathol 1994; 102: 154.

232. Kuo SH, Luh KT. Monitoring tumor cell kinetics in patients receiving chemotherapy for small cell lung cancer. Acta Cytol 1993; 37: 353.

233. Tiffany P, Morse MJ, Bosl G, et al. Sequential excision of residual thoracic and retroperitoneal masses after chemotherapy for stage III germ cell tumors. Cancer 1986; 57: 978.

234. Hong SJ, Lurain JR, Tsukada Y, et al. Cystadenocarcinoma of the ovary in a four-year old: benign transformation during therapy. Cancer 1980; 45: 2227.

235. Willis GW, Hajdu SI. Histologically benign teratoid metastasis of testicular embryonal carcinoma: report of five cases. Am J Clin Pathol 1973; 59: 338.

236. Davey DB, Ulbright TM, Loehrer PJ, et al. The significance of atypia within teratomatous metastases after chemotherapy for malignant germ cell tumors. Cancer 1987; 59: 533.

237. Molenaar WM, Oosterhuis JW, Kamps WA. Cytological 'differentiation' in childhood rhabdomyosarcomas following polychemotherapy. Hum Pathol 1984; 15: 973.

238. Molenaar WM, Oosterhuis JW, Oosterhuis AM, et al. Mesenchymal and muscle-specific intermediate filaments (vimentin and desmin) in relation to differentiation in childhood rhabdomyosarcomas. Hum Pathol 1985; 16: 838.

239. Wilson RE, Antman KH, Brodsky G, et al. Tumor-cell heterogeneity in soft tissue sarcomas as defined by chemoradiotherapy. Cancer 1984; 53: 1420.

240. Ogita S, Tokiwa K, Arizono N, Takahishi T. Neuroblastoma: incomplete differentiation on the way to maturation or morphological alteration resembling maturity? Oncology 1988; 45: 148.

241. Saxena R, Leake JL, Shafford EA, et al. Chemotherapy effects on hepatoblastoma. A histological study. Am J Surg Pathol 1993; 17: 1266.

242. Mazur MT, Lurain JR, Brewer JI. Fatal gestational choriocarcinoma. Clinicopathologic study of patients treated at a trophoblastic disease center. Cancer 1982; 50: 1833.

243. Brisigotti M, Cazzutto C, Fabbretti G, et al. Wilms' tumour after treatment. Pediatr Pathol 1992; 12: 397.

244. Zuppan CW, Beckwith JB, Weeks DA, et al. The effect of preoperative therapy on the histologic features of Wilms' tumour. Analysis of cases from the Third National Wilms' Tumour Study. Cancer 1991; 68: 385.

245. Durkin W, Durant J. Benign mass lesions after therapy for Hodgkin's disease. Arch Intern Med 1979; 139: 333.

246. Stewart FM, Williamson BR, Innes DJ, et al. Residual tumor masses following treatment for advanced histiocytic lymphoma. Diagnostic and therapeutic implications. Cancer 1985; 55: 620.

247. Einhorn LH, Donohue J. Cis-diamminedichloroplatinum, vinblastine and bleomycin combination chemotherapy in disseminated testicular cancer. Ann Intern Med 1977; 87: 293.

248. Lamm DL, Wepsic HT, Feldman P, et al. Importance of alpha-fetoprotein in patients with seminoma. Urology 1977; 10: 233.

249. Mirsha SK, Melinkeri SR, Dabadghao S. Benign thymic hyperplasia after chemotherapy for acute myeloid leukemia. Eur J Haematol 2001; 67: 252.

250. Hara M, McAdams HP, Vredenburg JJ, et al. Thymic hyperplasia after high-dose chemotherapy and autologous stem cell transplantation: incidence and significance in patients with breast cancer. AJR 1999; 173: 1341.

251. Smith T. Fatty replacement of lymph nodes mimicking lymphoma relapse. Cancer 1986; 58: 2686.

252. Werbin N. Fatty changes and metastases in axillary lymph nodes. J Surg Oncol 1984; 25: 145.

253. Geis WP, Iwatsuki S, Molnar Z, et al. Pseudolymphoma in renal allograft recipients. Arch Surg 1978; 113: 461.

254. Deodhar SD, Kuklinca AG, Vidt DG, et al. Development of reticulum-cell sarcoma at the site of antilymphocyte globulin injection in a patient with renal transplant. N Engl J Med 1969; 280: 1104.

255. Boffetta P, Kaldor JM. Secondary malignancies following cancer chemotherapy. Acta Oncol 1994; 33: 591.

256. De Witte T, Oosterveld M, Span B, et al. Stem cell transplantation for leukemias following myelodysplastic syndromes or secondary to cytotoxic therapy. Rev Clin Exp Hematol 2002; 6: 72.

257. Olney HJ, Mitelman F, Johansson B, et al. Unique balanced chromosome abnormalities in treatment-related myelodysplastic syndromes and acute myeloid leukemia: report from an international workshop. Genes Chromosomes Cancer 2002; 33: 413.

258. Tchernia G, Mielot F, Subtil E, et al. Acute myeloblastic leukemia after immunodepressive therapy for primary nonmalignant disease. Blood Cells 1967; 2: 67.

259. Anderson MK, Christiansen DH, Jensen BA, et al. Therapy-related acute lymphoblastic leukaemia with MLL rearrangements following DNA topoisomerase II inhibitors, and increasing problem: report on two new cases and review of the literature since 1992. Br J Haematol 2001; 114: 539.

260. Varady E, Deak B, Molnar ZS, et al. Second malignancies after treatment for Hodgkin's disease. Leuk Lymphoma 2001; 42: 1275.

261. Ellis M, Lishner M. Second malignancies following treatment in non-Hodgkin's lymphoma. Leuk Lymphoma 1993; 9: 337.

262. Reimer RR, Hoover R, Fraumeni JR Jr, et al. Acute leukemia after alkylating-agent therapy of ovarian cancer. N Engl J Med 1977; 297: 177.

263. Dale GA, Smith RB. Transitional cell carcinoma of the bladder associated with cyclophosphamide. J Urol 1974; 112: 603.

264. Casko SB, Keuhnelian JG, Gutowski III, et al. Spindle cell cancer of bladder during cyclophosphamide therapy for Wegener's granulomatosis. Am J Surg Pathol 1980; 4: 191.

265. Wall RL, Clausen KP. Carcinoma of the urinary bladder in patients receiving cyclophosphamide. N Engl J Med 1975; 293: 271.

266. Seo IS, Clark SA, McGovern FD, et al. Leiomyosarcoma of the urinary bladder thirteen years after cyclophosphamide therapy for Hodgkin's disease. Cancer 1985; 55: 1597.

267. Carney CN, Stevens PS, Fried FA, et al. Fibroblastic tumor of the urinary bladder after cyclophosphamide therapy. Arch Pathol Lab Med 1982; 106: 247.

268. Peters MS, Stuard DI. Metastatic malignant melanoma transplanted via a renal homograft. A case report. Cancer 1978; 41: 2426.

269. Penn I, Starzl TE. Malignant tumors arising de novo in immunosuppressed organ transplant recipients. Transplantation 1972; 14: 407.

270. Penn I. Cancers of the anogenital region in renal transplant recipients. Analysis of 65 cases. Cancer 1986; 58: 611.

271. Barenfange J, Mazur JM, Mody N, et al. Malignant fibrous histiocytoma of bone in a renal-transplant patient. J Bone Joint Surg 1980; 62A:297.

272. Craig F, Gulley M, Banks P. Posttransplantation lymphoproliferative disorders. Am J Clin Pathol 1993; 99: 265.

273. Swerdlow S. Post-transplant lymphoproliferative disorders: a morphologic, phenotypic and genotypic spectrum of disease. Histopathology 1992; 20: 373.

274. Knowles D, Cesarman E, Chadburn A, et al. Correlative morphologic and molecular genetic analysis demonstrates three distinct categories of posttransplantation lymphoproliferative disorders. Blood 1995; 85: 552.

275. Harris NL, Jaffe ES, Diebold J, et al. The World Health Organization classification of neoplastic diseases of the haematopoietic and lymphoid tissues: Report of the Clinical Advisory Committee Meeting, Airlie House, Virginia, November 1997. Histopathology 2000; 36: 69.

276. Van Gorp J. Posttransplant T-cell lymphoma: a review. Adv Anat Pathol 1995; 2: 132.

277. Lones M, Mishalani S, Shintaku I, et al. Changes in tonsils and adenoids in children with posttransplant lymphoproliferative disorder: report of three cases with early involvement of Waldeyer's ring. Hum Pathol 1995; 26: 525.

278. Bibbo M, Ali I, Al-Nageeb M, et al. Cytologic findings in female and male offspring of DES treated mothers. Acta Cytol 1975; 19: 568.

279. Zaino RJ, Robboy SJ, Kurman RJ. Diseases of the vagina. In: Kurman RJ, ed. Blaustein's pathology of the female genital tract. New York: Springer-Verlag; 2002: 131–206.

280. Shapiro CL, Recht A. Side effects of adjuvant treatment of breast cancer. N Engl J Med 2001; 344: 1997.

281. Creasman WT. Estrogen and cancer. Gynecol Oncol 2002; 86: 1.

282. The Women's Health Initiative Steering Committee. Effects of conjugated equine estrogen in postmenopausal women with hysterectomy. The Women's Health Initiative randomized controlled trial. JAMA 2004; 291: 1701.

283. Writing Group for the Women's Health Initiative Investigators. Risks and benefits of estrogen plus progestin in healthy postmenopausal woman. Principal results from the Women's Health Initiative randomized controlled trial. JAMA 2002; 288: 321.

284. Deligdisch L. Hormonal pathology of the endometrium. Mod Pathol 2000; 13: 285.

285. Patten SF Jr. Diagnostic cytopathology of the uterine cervix. In: Weid GL, ed. Monographs in clinical cytology. 2nd edn, vol 3. New York: S Karger; 1978: 66–68.

286. Crow J, Gardner RL, McSweeney G, Shaw RW. Morphological changes in uterine leiomyomas treated by GnRH agonist goserelin. Int J Gynecol Pathol 1995; 14: 235.

287. Grignon DJ, Sakr WA. Histologic effects of radiation therapy and total androgen blockade on prostate cancer. Cancer 1995; 75: 1837.

288. Civantos F, Marcial M, Banks E, et al. Pathology of androgen deprivation therapy in prostate carcinoma. Cancer 1995; 75: 1634.

289. Van de Voorde W, Elgamal A, Poppel H, et al. Morphologic and immunohistochemical changes in prostate cancer after preoperative hormonal therapy. Cancer 1994; 74: 3164.

290. Devaney DM, Dorman A, Leader M. Adenosquamous carcinoma of the prostate: a case report. Hum Pathol 1992; 22: 1046.

291. Wernert N, Goebbels R, Bonkhoff H, et al. Squamous cell carcinoma of the prostate. Histopathology 1990; 17: 339.

292. Jeter MD, Janne PA, Brooks S, et al. Gemcitabine-induced radiation recall. Int J Radiat Oncol Biol Phys 2002; 53: 394.

293. Shield PW, Daunter B, Wright RG. Post-irradiation cytology of cervical cancer patients. Cytopathology 1992; 3: 167.

294. Frierson HF, Covell JL, Andersen WA. Radiation changes in endocervical cells in brush specimens. Diagn Cytopathol 1990; 6: 243.

295. Fajardo LF, Berthrong M. Vascular lesions following radiation. Pathol Annu 1988; 23: 297.

296. Fajardo LF, Berthrong M. Radiation injury in surgical pathology. Part I. Am J Surg Pathol 1978; 2: 159.

297. White DC. The histopathologic basis for functional decrements in late radiation injury in diverse organs. Cancer 1976; 37: 1126.

298. Graham RM, Graham JB. Cytologic prognosis in cancer of the uterine cervix. Cancer 1955; 8: 59.

299. Graham RM, Graham JB. Sensitization response in patients with cancer of the uterine cervix. Cancer 1960; 13: 5.

300. Zerne SRM, Morris JM. Prognostic significance of cytologic response in radiation of gynecologic cancer. Obstet Gynecol 1962; 19: 145.

301. Koss LG. Diagnostic cytology and its histologic basis. Philadelphia: Lippincott-Raven; 1992: 673.

302. Skolnik EM, Soboroff BJ, Tardy ME Jr, et al. Preoperative radiation of larynx. Analysis of serial sections. Ann Otol Rhinol Laryngol 1970; 79: 1049.

303. Nicholls JM, Sham J, Chan C-W, Choy D. Radiation therapy for nasopharyngeal carcinoma: histologic appearances and patterns of tumor regression. Hum Pathol 1992; 23: 742.

304. Silverberg SG, DiGiorgi LS. Histopathologic analysis of preoperative radiation therapy in endometrial carcinoma. Am J Obstet Gynecol 1974; 119: 698.

305. Cox JD, Stoffel TJ. The significance of needle biopsy after irradiation for stage C adenocarcinoma of the prostate. Cancer 1977; 40: 156.

306. Gray SR, Hahn IS, Cornog JL Jr. Short-term effect of radiation on human neoplasms. Arch Pathol Lab Med, 1974; 97: 7.

307. Neumann MP, Limas C. Transitional cell carcinomas of the urinary bladder. Effects of preoperative irradiation on morphology. Cancer 1986; 58: 2758.

308. Weymuller ER Jr. Prognostic importance of the tumor-free laryngectomy specimen. Arch Otol 1978; 104: 505.

309. Suit HD, Gallager HS. Intact tumor cells in irradiated tissue. Arch Pathol 1964; 78: 648.

310. Koss LG. Diagnostic cytology and its histologic basis. Philadelphia: Lippincott-Raven; 1992;666–673.

311. Campos J. Persistent tumor cells in the vaginal smears and prognosis of cancer. Acta Cytol 1970; 14: 519.

312. Goldman JL, Cheren RV, Zak FG, et al. Histopathology of larynges and radical neck specimens in a combined radiation and surgery program for advanced carcinoma of the larynx and laryngopharynx. Ann Otol Rhinol Laryngol 1966; 75: 313.

313. Flood LM, Brightwell AP. Clinical assessment of the irradiated larynx. Salvage laryngectomy in the absence of histological confirmation of residual or recurrent carcinoma. J Laryngol Otol 1984; 98: 493.

314. Calcaterra TC, Stern F, Ward PH. Dilemma of delayed radiation injury of the larynx. Ann Otol Rhinol Laryngol 1972; 81: 501.

315. Diehl LF, Hurwitz MA, Johnson SA, et al. Skin metastases confined to a field of previous irradiation. Report of two cases and review of the literature. Cancer 1984; 53: 1864.

316. Tessmer CF. Radiation effects in skin. In: Berdjis CC, ed. Pathology of irradiation. Baltimore: Williams & Wilkins; 1971: 146.

317. Harwood TR, Staley CJ, Yokoo H. Histopathology of irradiated and obstructed submandibular salivary glands. Arch Pathol Lab Med 1973; 96: 189.

318. Kashima HK, Kirkham WR, Andrews JR. Postirradiation sialadenitis. A study of the clinical features, histopathologic changes and serum enzyme variations following irradiation of human salivary glands. AJR 1965; 94: 271.

319. Somosy Z, Horváth G, Telbisz A, et al. Morphological aspects of ionizing radiation response of small intestine. Micron 2002; 33: 167.

320. Gardiner GW, McAuliffe N, Murray D. Colitis cystica profunda occurring in a radiation-induced colonic stricture. Hum Pathol 1984; 15: 295.

321. Weisbrot IM, Liber AF, Gordon BS. The effects of therapeutic radiation on colonic mucosa. Cancer 1975; 36: 931.

322. Lewin K, Millis RR. Human radiation hepatitis. A morphologic study with emphasis on the late changes. Arch Pathol Lab Med 1973; 96: 21.

323. Luxton RW, Kunkler PB. Radiation nephritis. Acta Radiol Ther Phys Biol 1964; 2: 169.

324. Mostofi FK. Radiation effects on the kidney. In: Mostofi FK, Smith DE, eds. The kidney. Baltimore: Williams & Wilkins; 1966: 338.

325. Kapur S, Chandra R, Antonovych T. Acute radiation nephritis. Light and electron microscopic observations. Arch Pathol Lab Med 1977; 101: 469.

326. Loveless KJ. The effects of radiation upon the cytology of benign and malignant bladder epithelia. Acta Cytol (Baltimore) 1973; 17: 355.

327. Wiener HG, Vooijs GP, van't Hof-Grootenboer B. Accuracy of urinary cytology in the diagnosis of primary and recurrent bladder cancer. Acta Cytol 1993; 37: 163.

328. Cowen PN. False cytodiagnosis of bladder malignancy due to previous radiotherapy. Br J Urol 1975; 47: 405.

329. Eposti PL, Edsmyr F, Moberger G, et al. Cytologic diagnosis in bladder carcinoma treated by supervoltage irradiation. Scand J Urol Nephrol 1969; 3: 201.

330. Tweeddale DN. Urinary cytology. Boston: Little, Brown; 1977.

331. Jayalakshmamma B, Pinkel D. Urinary-bladder toxicity following pelvic irradiation and simultaneous cyclophosphamide therapy. Cancer 1976; 38: 701.

332. Grignon DJ, Sakr WA. Histologic effects of radiation therapy and total androgen blockade on prostate cancer. Cancer 1995; 75: 1837.

333. Bostwick DG, Egbert BM, Fajardo LF. Radiation injury of the normal and neoplastic prostate. Am J Surg Pathol 1982; 6: 541.

334. Mazur MT, Kraus FT. Histogenesis of morphologic variations in tumors of the uterine wall. Am J Surg Pathol 1980; 4: 59.

335. Spitalnik PF, Straus FH. Patterns of human thyroid parenchymal reaction following low-dose childhood irradiation. Cancer 1978; 41: 1098.

336. Komorowski RA, Hanson GA. Morphologic changes in the thyroid following low-dose childhood radiation. Arch Pathol Lab Med 1977; 101: 36.

337. Clarke D, Curtis JL, Martinez A, et al. Fat necrosis of the breast simulating recurrent carcinoma after primary radiotherapy in the management of early stage breast carcinoma. Cancer 1983; 52: 442.

338. Schnitt SJ, Connolly JL, Harris JE, et al. Radiation-induced changes in the breast. Hum Pathol 1984; 15: 545.

339. Filomena CA, Jordan AG, Ehya H. Needle aspiration cytology of the irradiated breast. Diagn Cytopathol 1992; 8: 327.

340. Abratt RP, Morgan GW. Lung toxicity following chest irradiation in patients with lung cancer. Lung Cancer 2002; 35: 103.

341. Albright CD, Hafiz MA. Cytomorphologic changes in split-course radiation-treated bronchogenic carcinomas. Diagn Cytopathol 1988; 4: 9.

342. Longatto Filho A, Shirata NK, Maeda MY, et al. Cytology of pulmonary samples after cancer radiation therapy. Pathologica 1991; 83: 317.

343. Hutchison GB. Late neoplastic changes following medical irradiation. Cancer 1976; 37: 1102.

344. Rubin P, Casarett GW. Clinical radiation pathology. Philadelphia: WB Saunders; 1968.

345. Katzman H, Waugh T, Berdon W. Skeletal changes following irradiation of childhood tumors. J Bone Joint Surg 1969; 51A:825.

346. Schore-Freedman E, Abrahams C, Recant W, et al. Neurilemomas and salivary gland tumors of the head and neck following childhood irradiation. Cancer 1983; 51: 2159.

347. Shore RE. Radiation-induced skin cancer in humans. Med Pediatr Oncol 2001; 36: 549.

348. Van Vloten WA, Hermans J, van Daal WAJ. Radiation-induced skin cancer and radiodermatitis of the head and neck. Cancer 1987; 59: 411.

349. Martin H, Strong E, Spiro RH. Radiation-induced skin cancer of the head and neck. Cancer 1970; 25: 61.

350. Lazar P, Cullen SI. Basal cell epithelioma and chronic radiodermatitis. Arch Dermatol 1963; 88: 172.

351. Hudson AW, Winkelmann RK. Atypical fibroxanthoma of the skin: a reappraisal of 19 cases in which the original diagnosis was spindle-cell squamous carcinoma. Cancer 1972; 29: 413.

352. Moskaluk CA, Merino MJ, Danforth DN, Medeiros LJ. Low-grade angiosarcoma of the skin of the breast: a complication of lumpectomy and radiation therapy for breast carcinoma. Hum Pathol 1992; 23: 710.

353. Patel SG, See AC, Williamson PA, et al. Radiation induced sarcoma of the head and neck. Head Neck 1999; 21: 346.

354. Miyahara H, Sato T, Yoshino K. Radiation-induced cancers of the head and neck region. Acta Otolaryngol Suppl 1998; 533: 60.

355. Saw D, Chan JKC, Jagirdar J, et al. Sinonasal small cell neoplasm developing after radiation therapy for retinoblastoma: an immunohistologic, ultrastructural, and cytogenetic study. Hum Pathol 1992; 23: 896.

356. Frierson HF Jr, Ross GW, Stewart FM, et al. Unusual sinonasal small-cell neoplasms following radiotherapy for bilateral retinoblastomas. Am J Surg Pathol 1989; 13: 947.

357. Harzen RW, Pifer JW, Toyooka ET, et al. Neoplasms following irradiation of the head. Cancer Res 1966; 26: 305.

358. Walker MJ, Chaudhuri PK, Wood DC, et al. Radiation-induced parotid cancer. Arch Surg 1981; 116: 329.

359. Smith DG, Levitt SH. Radiation carcinogenesis: an unusual familial occurrence of neoplasia following irradiation in childhood for benign disease. Cancer 1974; 34: 2069.

360. Little JW, Rickles NH. Malignant papillary cystadenoma lymphomatosum. Report of a case, with a review of the literature. Cancer 1965; 18: 851.

361. Mark RJ, Poen J, Tran LM, et al. Postirradiation sarcomas. A single-institution study and review of the literature. Cancer 1994; 73: 2653.

362. Duffy BJ Jr, Fitzgerald PJ. Thyroid cancer in children: a report of 28 cases. J Clin Endocrinol 1950; 10: 1296.

363. Refetoff S, Harrison J, Karanfilski BT, et al. Continuing occurrence of thyroid carcinoma after irradiation to the neck in infancy and childhood. N Engl J Med 1975; 292: 171.

364. DeGroot L, Paloyan E. Thyroid carcinoma and radiation. A Chicago endemic. JAMA 1973; 225: 487.

365. Greenspan FS. Radiation exposure and thyroid cancer. JAMA 1977; 225: 4879.

366. Cerletty JM, Guansing AR, Engbring NH, et al. Radiation-related thyroid carcinoma. Arch Surg 1978; 113: 1072.

367. Komorowski RA, Hanson GA, Garancis JC. Anaplastic thyroid carcinoma following low-dose irradiation. Am J Clin Pathol 1978; 70: 303.

368. Schneider AB, Pinsky S, Bekerman C, et al. Characteristics of 108 thyroid cancers detected by screening in a population with a history of head and neck irradiation. Cancer 1980; 46: 1218.

369. McDougall IR, Kennedy JS, Thomson JA. Thyroid carcinoma following iodine-131 therapy. Report of a case and review of literature. J Clin Endocrinol 1971; 33: 287.

370. Sheline GE, Lindsay S, McCormack KR, et al. Thyroid nodules occurring late after treatment of thyrotoxicosis with radioiodine. J Clin Endocrinol 1962; 22: 8.

371. Roggli VL, Estrada R, Fechner RE. Thyroid neoplasia following irradiation for medulloblastoma. Report of two cases. Cancer 1979; 43: 2232.

372. Maxon HR, Thomas SR, Saenger EL, et al. Ionizing irradiation and the induction of clinically significant disease in the human thyroid gland. Am J Med 1977; 63: 967.

373. McDougall IR, Coleman CN, Burke JS, et al. Thyroid carcinoma after high-dose external radiotherapy for Hodgkin's disease: report of three cases. Cancer 1980; 45: 2056.

374. McHenry C, Jarosz H, Calandra D, et al. Thyroid neoplasia following radiation therapy for Hodgkin's lymphoma. Arch Surg 1987; 122: 684.

375. Russ JE, Scanlon EF, Sener SF. Parathyroid adenomas following irradiation. Cancer 1979; 43: 1078.

376. LiVolsi VA, LoGerfo P, Feind CR. Coexistent parathyroid adenomas and thyroid carcinoma. Can radiation be blamed? Arch Surg 1978; 113: 285.

377. Castro EB, Rosen PP, Quan SHQ. Carcinoma of large intestine in patients irradiated for carcinoma of cervix and uterus. Cancer 1973; 31: 45.

378. Shirouzu K, Isomoto H, Morodomi T, et al. Clinicopathologic characteristics of large bowel cancer developing after radiotherapy for uterine cervical cancer. Dis Colon Rectum 1994; 37: 1245.

379. Qizilbash AH. Radiation-induced carcinoma of the rectum. A late complication of pelvic irradiation. Arch Pathol Lab Med 1974; 98: 118.

380. Sabio H, Teja K, Elkon D, et al. Adenocarcinoma of the colon following treatment of Wilms' tumor. J Pediatr 1979; 95: 424.

381. Chen KTK, Hoffman KD, Hendricks EJ. Angiosarcoma following therapeutic irradiation. Cancer 1979; 44: 2044.

382. Fehr PE, Prem KA. Malignancy of the uterine corpus following irradiation-therapy for squamous cell carcinoma of the cervix. Am J Obstet Gynecol 1974; 119: 685.

383. Norris HJ, Taylor HB. Postirradiation sarcomas of the uterus. Obstet Gynecol 1965; 26: 689.

384. Meredith RF, Eisert DR, Kaka Z, et al. An excess of uterine sarcomas after pelvic irradiation. Cancer 1986; 58: 2003.

385. Varella-Duran J, Nochomovitz LE, Prem KA, et al. Postirradiation mixed müllerian tumors of the uterus. A comparative clinicopathologic study. Cancer 1980; 45: 1625.

386. Kwon TH, Prempree T, Tang C-K, et al. Adenocarcinoma of the uterine corpus following irradiation for cervical cancer. Gynecol Oncol 1981; 11: 102.

387. Huvos AG, Woodard HQ, Heilweil M. Postradiation malignant fibrous histiocytoma of bone. A clinicopathologic study of 20 patients. Am J Surg Pathol 1986; 10: 9.

388. Weatherby RP, Dahlin DC, Ivins JC. Postradiation sarcoma of bone. Review of 78 Mayo Clinic cases. Mayo Clin Proc 1981; 56: 294.

389. Chan RC, Sutow WW, Lindberg RD, et al. Management and results of localized Ewing's sarcoma. Cancer 1979; 43: 1001.

390. Phillips TL, Sheline GE. Bone sarcomas following radiation therapy. Radiology 1963; 81: 992.

391. Tountas AA, Fornasier VL, Harwood AR, et al. Postirradiation sarcoma of bone. A perspective. Cancer 1979; 43: 182.

392. Meadows AT, Strong LC, Li FP, et al. Bone sarcoma as a second malignant neoplasm in children: influence of radiation and genetic predisposition. Cancer 1980; 46: 2603.

393. Rutherford H, Dodd GD. Complications of radiation therapy: growing bone. Semin Roentgenol, 1974; 9: 1.

394. Oberman HA, Oneal RM. Fibrosarcoma of the chest wall following resection and irradiation of carcinoma of the breast. Am J Clin Pathol 1970; 53: 407.

395. Yap J, Chuba PJ, Thomas R, et al. Sarcoma as a second malignancy after treatment for breast cancer. Int J Radiat Oncol Biol Phys 2002; 52: 1231–237.

396. Bobin JY, Rivoire M, Delay E, et al. Radiation induced sarcomas following treatment for breast cancer: presentation of a series of 14 cases treated with an aggressive surgical approach. J Surg Oncol 1994; 57: 171.

397. Brady MS, Garfein CF, Petrek JA, Brennan MF. Post-treatment sarcoma in breast cancer patients. Ann Surg Oncol 1994; 1: 66.

398. Senyszyn JJ, Johnston AD, Jacox HW, et al. Radiation induced sarcoma after treatment of breast cancer. Cancer 1970; 26: 394.

399. Sordillo PP, Helson L, Hadju SI, et al. Malignant schwannoma – clinical characteristics, survival, and response to therapy. Cancer 1981;47: 2503.

400. Ivins JC, Taylor WF, Wold LE. Elective whole-lung irradiation in osteosarcoma treatment: appearance of bilateral breast cancer in two long-term survivors. Skeletal Radiol 1987; 16: 133.

401. Iknayan HF. Carcinoma associated with irradiation of the immature breast. Radiology 1975; 114: 431.

402. Baral E, Larsson LE, Mattsson B. Breast cancer following irradiation of the breast. Cancer 1977; 40: 2905.

403. Mackenzie I. Breast cancer following multiple fluoroscopies. Br J Cancer 1965; 19: 1.

404. Yahalom Y, Petrek JA, Biddinger PW, et al. Breast cancer in patients irradiated for Hodgkin's disease: a clinical and pathological analysis of 45 events in 37 patients. J Clin Oncol 1992; 10: 1674.

405. Dvoretsky PM, Woodard E, Bonfiglio TA, et al. The pathology of breast cancer in women irradiated for acute postpartum mastitis. Cancer 1980; 46: 2257.

406. Lowell DM, Martineau RG, Luria SB. Carcinoma of the male breast following radiation. Report of case occurring 35 years after radiation therapy of unilateral prepubertal gynecomastia. Cancer 1968; 22: 581.

407. Curtin CT, McHeffy B, Kolarsick AJ. Thyroid and breast cancer following radiation. Cancer 1977; 40: 2911.

408. Bailer JC III. Screening for early breast cancer: pros and cons. Cancer 1977; 39: 2783.

409. Powell HC, Marshall LF, Ignelzi AR. Post-irradiation pituitary sarcoma. Acta Neuropathol (Berl) 1977; 39: 165.

410. Donahue WE, Jaffe FA, Newcastle NB. Radiation-induced neurofibromata. Cancer 1967; 20: 589.

411. Watts C: Meningioma following irradiation. Cancer 1976; 38: 1939.

412. Modan B, Baidatz D, Mart H, et al. Radiation-induced head and neck tumours. Lancet 1974; 1: 277.

413. Marus G, Levin CV, Rutherford GS. Malignant glioma following radiotherapy for unrelated primary tumors. Cancer 1986; 58: 886.

414. Clifton MD, Amromin GD, Perry MC, et al. Spinal cord glioma following irradiation for Hodgkin's disease. Cancer 1980; 45: 2051.

415. Shannon VR, Nesbitt JC, Libshitz HI. Malignant pleural mesothelioma after radiation therapy for breast cancer. Cancer 1995; 76: 437.

416. Cavazza A, Travis LB, Travis WD, et al. Post-irradiation malignant mesothelioma. Cancer 1996; 77: 1379.

417. Pappo AS, Santana VM, Fuirman WL, et al. Post-irradiation malignant mesothelioma. Cancer 1997; 79: 192.

418. Grampa G. Radiation injury with particular reference to Thorotrast. Pathol Annu 1971; 6: 147.

419. Telles NC. Follow-up of thorium dioxide patients in the United States. Ann NY Acad Sci 1967; 145: 674.

420. Kamiho A, Okabe K, Hirose T. Thorium dioxide granuloma of the neck with resultant fatal hemorrhage. Arch Otol 1979; 105: 45.

421. Hasson J, Hartman KS, Milikow E, et al. Thorotrast-induced extraskeletal osteosarcoma of the cervical region. Report of a case. Cancer 1975; 36: 1827.

422. Levy DW, Rindsberg S, Friedman AC, et al. Thorotrast-induced hepatosplenic neoplasia: CT identification. AJR 1986; 146: 997.

423. Srinivasan R, Dean HA. Thorotrast and the liver – revisited. J Toxicol Clin Toxicol 1997; 35: 199.

424. Smoron GL, Battifora HA. Thorotrast-induced hepatoma. Cancer 1972; 30: 1252.

425. Kojiro M, Kawano Y, Kawasaki H, et al. Thorotrast-induced hepatic angiosarcoma, and combined hepatocellular and cholangiocarcinoma in a single patient. Cancer 1982; 49: 2161.

426. Underwood JCE, Huck P. Thorotrast associated hepatic angiosarcoma with 36 years latency. Cancer 1978; 42: 2610.

427. Sindelar WF, Costa J, Ketcham AS. Osteosarcoma associated with Thorotrast administration. Report of two cases and literature review. Cancer 1978; 42: 2604.

428. Iwamoto KS, Fujii S, Kurata A, et al. p53 mutations in tumor and non-tumor tissues of thorotrast recipients: a model for cellular selection during radiation carcinogenesis in the liver. Carcinogenesis 1999; 20: 1283.

429. Stewart JR, Gibbs FA Jr. Hyperthermia in the therapy of cancer. Perspectives on its promise and its problems. Cancer 1984; 54: 2823.

430. Badylak SF, Babbs CF, Skojal TM, et al. Hyperthermia-induced vascular injury in normal and neoplastic tissue. Cancer 1985; 56: 991.

431. Sugimachi K, Kai H, Matsufuji H, et al. Histopathological evaluation of hyperthermo-chemo-radiotherapy for carcinoma of the esophagus. J Surg Oncol 1986; 32: 82.

432. Sugaar S, LeVeen HH. A histopathologic study on the effects of radiofrequency thermotherapy on malignant tumors of the lung. Cancer 1979; 43: 767.

433. Skibba JL, Quebbeman EJ. Tumoricidal effects and patient survival after hyperthermic liver perfusion. Arch Surg 1986; 121: 1266.

434. Dick EA, Taylor-Robinson SD, Thomas HC, et al. Ablative therapy for liver tumours. Gut 2002; 50: 733.

Differential diagnosis of metastatic tumors

Tarik M. Elsheikh   Jan F. Silverman

6

There is an increasing emphasis on the diagnosis of metastases utilizing smaller fragments of tissue, particularly needle core biopsy and fine needle aspiration (FNA). FNA and effusion cytology examination have been shown to be highly accurate in the diagnosis of metastatic disease and may represent the initial procedures of choice in the work-up of metastases. In addition to establishing a diagnosis of metastatic malignancy, pathologists are increasingly asked to determine a possible primary site. This task can be especially challenging if there is no previous history of malignancy, prior pathology is not available for review, or there is an unpredictable pattern of metastasis. Accurate pathologic diagnosis of metastasis can significantly modify the management of patients and possibly prevent unnecessary radical surgery. In this chapter we will present a clinicopathologic approach for the pathologist to work up metastatic disease, which includes morphology, ancillary studies, and clinical patterns of metastasis. Recognition of subtle cytologic/histologic morphologic features of neoplasms and subclassifying them into diagnostic categories, that is, clear cell, granular cell, spindle cell, small cell, and large pleomorphic, will emphasize differential diagnostic considerations and may give valuable clues to possible primary sites. The use of ancillary studies such as molecular biology, electron microscopy, and particularly immunohistochemistry can be especially helpful in determining cell lineage and site of origin. Although pathologists may be familiar with the more usual patterns of metastasis to sites such as lung, liver, and lymph nodes, cancer may occasionally metastasize to unusual or uncommon sites such as breast, spleen, pancreas, and thyroid. This unpredictable pattern of metastasis may pose diagnostic problems for clinicians and pathologists and potentially result in erroneous diagnosis of a primary malignancy arising in these sites. Familiarity with the variable clinical patterns of metastasis and primary malignancies most commonly associated with those metastatic sites is crucial in narrowing down the possible origins of these neoplasms. We will also discuss the clinical significance and cost-effectiveness of the pathology work-up of metastases of unknown origin, and how oncologists may use this information to guide their management. Initially, however, we will review the biologic mechanisms believed responsible for the development of metastasis and the factors that may result in unusual metastatic patterns.

MECHANISMS OF METASTASIS

Metastasis is defined as the transfer of disease from one organ or part to another not directly connected to it.[1] The ability to metastasize is a characteristic of all malignant tumors. However, not all cells within a malignant tumor have metastatic capabilities. Only certain neoplastic clones develop a metastatic phenotype by acquiring irreversible structural and quantitative changes in genes and gene expression.[2] While alterations in c-oncogenes, tumor suppresser genes, and DNA repair enzymes are the key molecules involved in carcinogenesis, increased expression of proteases, motility factors, and altered expression of adhesion molecules are involved in metastasis. Metastasis develops through three major steps: (1) local invasion of extracellular matrix by malignant cells, (2) vascular dissemination, and (3) arrest and proliferation at a distant site.[3]

Malignant cells invade extracellular matrix (ECM) through loss of cell-to-cell adhesion, attachment to matrix components, and enzymatic destruction of basement membranes in host tissue. Adhesion molecules, such as E-cadherin, result in multicellular tumor cell aggregation (homotypic cell aggregation) and confinement of tumor cells to the primary site. Loss of E-cadherin expression is associated with detachment of tumor cells from each other and invasion into the surrounding stroma.[4] Attachment of tumor cells to matrix components is accomplished via a receptor–ligand interaction. One group of such cell surface receptors is the integrins, which specifically bind cells to laminin, collagen, or fibronectin of ECM.[5,6] Tumor progression has been associated with a gradual decrease of integrin expression, suggesting that the loss of integrins, coupled with the loss of E-cadherin, may facilitate detachment of cells from the primary neoplasm.[7] Degradative enzymes such as type IV collagenase and heparinase may be produced directly by the tumor cells or by surrounding host stroma.[8] The movement, then, of malignant cells within the degraded matrix and across degraded vessel walls is mediated by tumor cell-derived cytokines and motility factors.[9] The degraded components of ECM also act as chemotaxins for the neoplastic cells.[10,11]

Vascular dissemination is facilitated by angiogenesis, which is mediated by angiogenic growth factors that may be produced by the tumor cells or inflammatory cells infiltrating the tumor.[7] Many recent studies have concluded that increased angiogenesis is a significant and independent prognostic indicator in early-stage breast cancer and is associated with increased probability of metastatic disease.[12–15] After penetrating the vessel wall, detached tumor cells are free to circulate. However, only a small fraction of the circulating tumor cells (less than 0.01%) survive the harsh mechanical and immunologic insults encountered in the circulation. Cell survival is enhanced by homotypic aggregation (tumor cell to tumor cell) and heterotypic aggregation with fibrin and platelets, which protect malignant cells located within the center of the aggregate from destruction.[16]

Arrest and proliferation of tumor cell emboli at distant sites involves adhesion to the vascular endothelium and penetration of the basement membrane. This process is facilitated by adhesion molecules and proteolytic enzymes. Paracrine growth factors and inhibitors are produced by target organs in different types and amounts.[9] Site-specific metastasis may be explained by increased numbers of tumor cell receptors or increased affinities of tumor cell receptors for growth factors specifically produced by the target organ.[17] Paracrine growth inhibitors have been identified in certain organs, for example the kidney, and inhibit the growth of many metastatic tumors. The loss of paracrine growth inhibition may therefore account for metastatic progression and distribution of organ-specific metastasis.[18] Finally, genetic regulation of the metastatic process is the subject of many investigations. The *ras* oncogene is implicated in metastasis, in which ras-transformed cells show increased expression and activity of degradative enzymes and decreased expression of their inhibitors.[19] Further discussion of oncogene association (including tumor suppressor genes) with the metastatic phenotype of tumor cells is beyond the scope of this chapter.

CLINICAL PATTERNS OF METASTASIS

Although a previous history of malignancy and characteristic cytohistologic and immunohistochemical features are helpful in characterizing certain tumors, many metastatic malignancies lack a specific morphologic or immunohistochemical profile. Familiarity with the variable patterns of metastasis in conjunction with cytologic/histologic features and ancillary studies, when needed, will facilitate arriving at a more specific diagnosis. The clinical patterns of metastasis usually parallel the blood or lymphatic drainage of the primary neoplasm. Metastasis is, therefore, related to the anatomic localization of the primary tumor. The site where circulating tumor cells arrest may be related to mechanical tumor stasis, such as homotypic tumor cell aggregate arresting in a capillary bed as a result of its larger size. Neoplasms with a regional lymphatic metastatic pattern include squamous cell carcinoma of the head and neck, cervical carcinoma, and melanoma. Neoplasms also metastasize via characteristic anatomic venous pathways. The lung, for example, is the initial venous metastatic site for carcinomas of head and neck, bone, uterus, and kidney.[20] On the other hand, carcinomas of the pancreas, stomach, and colon often go to the liver as their initial venous site of metastasis. Prostate carcinoma metastasizes to the proximal axial skeleton via paravertebral veins. Subsequent widespread dissemination from that initial metastatic site (i.e. lung, liver, bone) is then believed to occur via the arterial system to the brain, endocrine organs, distal small bones, and spleen.[20] Some tumors have preferential distribution of metastasis not explainable by the natural pathways of drainage. This may be explained in part by the preferential interaction of tumor cell adhesion molecules with other adhesion molecules whose ligands are expressed on endothelial cells of the target organs.[21,22] Some target organs may also produce chemotactic agents that attract neoplastic cells to these sites. The fact that some of these tumors preferentially metastasize to specific organs, bypassing other organs along their route, seems to imply that distribution is at least partially due to selective homing to a specific organ.

METASTASIS OF UNKNOWN PRIMARY ORIGIN

Metastasis of unknown primary origin (MUO) constitutes 5% to 10% of all noncutaneous malignancies[23] and up to 15% of new referrals to hospital-based oncology centers.[24] Identification of the primary site is often the basis for predicting the expected behavior and prognosis and determining appropriate therapy; therefore, the absence of a primary origin can pose a major clinical challenge. The inability to identify a primary site also generates anxiety for the patient, who may feel that the physician's evaluation has been inadequate or that the prognosis would be improved if a primary could be established.[25] The finding of a primary site in MUO, however, can be challenging and made especially difficult by an atypical pattern of dissemination. For example, lung carcinoma metastasizes to bone in 30% to 50% of cases, but involves bone in only 5% of MUO cases. Prostate carcinoma metastasizes to the lung and liver in 15% of cases when the primary site is known, but in more than 50% of cases when presenting as MUO.[26] Bone metastases are uncommon in typical cases of pancreatic cancer but are frequent in pancreatic cancers presenting as MUO.[27] The types of neoplasms and/or primary sites in patients with MUO are also somewhat different from the frequency of various malignancies in the general cancer population. Germ cell, adrenal, hepatobiliary, pancreatic, and renal cancers are relatively overrepresented among MUO patients, whereas malignancies of the breast, endometrium, cervix, lung, and prostate are relatively underrepresented, because these latter tumors are more readily diagnosed by simple means such as physical examination and chest radiography.[27]

Adenocarcinoma and undifferentiated carcinomas account for up to 75% of MUO cases, followed by small cell carcinoma, squamous cell carcinoma, and melanoma. Metastatic adenocarcinoma, however, is the most difficult to accurately determine its origin since the cytologic/histologic features are often not specific for a certain primary site. When the primary site of MUO is ultimately found, carcinomas of the pancreas and the lung predominate, followed by colorectal, liver, and stomach.[28] Squamous cell carcinoma in the MUO syndrome most often originates in the head and neck or lung. Prognosis in MUO is generally poor, with an overall median survival of 3–4 months in older series,[29] and 9–12 months in more recent studies.[30–33] Subsets of patients with favorable prognosis include lymphoma, germ cell tumors, and thyroid cancer. A fair response to combination therapy can be expected in breast, ovarian, and prostate carcinoma. Metastatic gastrointestinal and urogenital carcinomas remain difficult to treat.[34] Many investigators have not included in their analysis the rare occasions when melanoma or soft tissue sarcoma present as MUO.[35]

COST ANALYSIS FOR PATHOLOGIC EVALUATION OF MUO

MUO is generally defined as a biopsy-confirmed malignancy in which the primary site remains unidentified after a rigorous, but limited initial clinical and radiographic evaluation.[36] There remains, however, considerable controversy surrounding the extent of evaluation required to accept the diagnosis of MUO and its cost-effectiveness. Basic clinical evaluation usually consists of history and physical examination (including breast palpation and pelvic exam in women, and testicular and prostate examination in men), laboratory studies including liver and renal function tests, chest X-ray, computed tomography (CT) of the abdomen and pelvis, mammography in women, and measurement of serum prostatic specific antigen (PSA) in men.[25] Depending on the clinical situation, additional studies might include CT of the chest, breast ultrasonography, positron emission tomography (PET) scan, magnetic resonance imaging (MRI) of the breast, intravenous pyelogram (IVP), and gastrointestinal endoscopy. Extensive radiological examinations and serum tumor markers, however, have turned out to be unsatisfactory means to establish the primary site in many of these cases.[34] Schapira and Jarrett[24] reported that among 56 patients with MUO, 410 clinical tests including endoscopic and radiological imaging studies were performed in order to identify the location of the primary site, with an average cost of approximately US$18 000 per patient (excluding physician charges). Primary cancer site was found in 4 of 56 (7.1%) patients, with only 4 (1.0%) tests correctly identifying the location of primary site. Other studies have documented a success rate of approximately 20% in locating the primary neoplasm, but only 1.0% of patients had malignancies deemed as potentially curable, such as lymphoma, germ cell tumor, or a hormonally sensitive carcinoma.[37-47] These investigators concluded that there was little justification to support extensive diagnostic evaluation of patients with MUO, once potentially curable malignancy has been excluded.[24]

There is little doubt that the search for the primary site utilizing pathologic evaluation, including performance of an extended panel of immunohistochemical stains, is more cost effective than other clinical diagnostic modalities. Wick et al.[48] as well as other investigators[49,50] reported that the success rate of immunohistochemistry (IHC) in determining primary site was between 65% and 75%, with an average cost of less than US$2000 per patient (Table 6.1). Using the aforementioned data, Raab[51] calculated that the cost-effectiveness ratio of IHC, expressed as the cost to determine the primary origin of MUO, would be approximately US$2900, which is considerably less than using clinical testing alone (Table 6.1). Using theoretical cost-effectiveness analysis, it was also concluded that selective use of IHC to refine diagnoses in MUO might increase life expectancy.[51] True cost-effectiveness studies of pathologic evaluation of patients presenting with MUO, however, have not been performed. Further studies are necessary to measure for costs and other outcomes across all alternatives such as cost per life-year saved and cost per major surgery avoided.

COMMON SITES OF METASTASIS

The most common sites of metastasis are lymph nodes, lung, large bones, and liver.[52] Other common sites discussed in this review include adrenal glands and salivary glands (Table 6.2).

LYMPH NODES

Lymph nodes are by far the most common site harboring metastatic disease. Utilization of FNA in the investigation of superficial lymphadenopathy is well documented in the literature.[53-55] Diagnostic accuracy for metastatic carcinoma is reported in the range of 82% to 99%.[55] Knowledge of exact location of the involved lymph node is of prime importance, as it can often shed light on the location of the primary site. For example, metastases involving the cervical spinal region are associated in the majority of cases with malignancies arising in the nasopharynx, followed by hypopharynx and base of tongue.[56] Submandibular metastases are usually derived from the anterior part of oral cavity and lips. Cervical lymph nodes are

Table 6.1 Cost effectiveness of IHC compared to clinical testing[24,48,51]

	Cost per patient	Success rate*	Cost-effectiveness ratio**
Clinical tests alone	US$18 000	20%	US$250 000
IHC panel	US$2000	70%	US$2900

IHC, Immunohistochemistry; MUO, Metastasis of unknown origin.
* Percentage of MUO patients in which a primary site can be determined
** Cost to detect a primary origin of MUO, i.e. for every US$250 000 or US$2900 spent, a primary site would be determined by only clinical tests or only IHC, respectively.

Table 6.2 Common and usual primary sites of metastases

Metastatic site	Probable primary site or malignancy
Lymph nodes	
Cervical	Head and neck, lung, melanoma, breast
Right supraclavicular	Lung, breast, lymphoma
Left supraclavicular	Lung, breast, cervix, prostate, lymphoma
Axillary	Breast, lung, arm, regional trunk, GIT
Inguinal	Melanoma, leg, cervix, vulva, trunk, anorectal, ovary, bladder, prostate
Lung	Breast, GIT (colon, pancreas, stomach), kidney, sarcoma, melanoma, prostate
Large bones	Prostate, breast, lung, kidney, thyroid
Liver	GIT (pancreas, colon, stomach), breast, lung, lymphoma, genitourinary, sarcoma, melanoma
Adrenal gland	Lung, breast, kidney, GIT (stomach, colon, pancreas), liver, melanoma, lymphoma
Brain	Lung, breast, melanoma, GIT
Skin and subcutaneous tissue	Lung, breast, melanoma, head and neck, GIT
Salivary glands	Head and neck, melanoma, lymphoma, lung, kidney

GIT: Gastrointestinal tract. Modified from Elsheikh TM, et al. Fine needle aspiration cytology of metastatic malignancies involving unusual sites. Am J Clin Pathol 1997; 108(Suppl 1): S12–S21.

commonly involved by squamous cell carcinoma metastatic from the head and neck region. Adenocarcinoma from supraclavicular (thyroid and salivary glands) and infraclavicular (lung, gastrointestinal tract, breast, ovary, prostate) primaries may also metastasize to cervical nodes.[52] Primary sites and types of malignancies that involve the left supraclavicular lymph nodes (LSC) are different from those that involve the right supraclavicular lymph nodes (RSC). We previously examined FNA of 96 supraclavicular nodes that were positive for malignancy.[57-60] Sixteen out of 19 pelvic tumors and all six abdominal malignancies metastasized to the LSC. However, thorax, breast, and head and neck malignancies showed no difference in their metastatic patterns to the LSC and RSC. The most common primary origins of metastases to RSC were thorax/breast, followed by lymphoma and pelvis/testis. The most common primary sites of metastases to LSC were thorax/breast followed by pelvis/testis and abdomen.[57-60] Large cell lymphoma may at times be difficult to distinguish cytologically from a small cell carcinoma or a poorly differentiated adenocarcinoma presenting in a predominantly discohesive pattern. Anaplastic large cell lymphoma (Ki-1 lymphoma) may also be confused cytologically with metastatic anaplastic carcinoma.[61] Obviously, malignant melanoma should always be considered in the differential diagnosis. IHC applied to surgical or FNA biopsies can be particularly helpful in this differential diagnosis. Common patterns of metastases to other lymph node regions are presented in Table 6.2.

LARGE BONES

Radiologic findings in metastatic diseases are seldom specific enough to allow for a definitive diagnosis. The differential diagnoses of bone lesions include reactive or inflammatory changes, sarcoma, myeloma, lymphoma, and metastatic carcinoma.[62,63] Bones of the axial and proximal appendicular skeleton with active hematopoietic marrow such as vertebral column, large bones, iliac bones, ribs and skull are more commonly involved by metastasis.[64] Metastatic carcinoma is by far the most common type of malignancy affecting the skeleton.[65] In most patients with osseous metastasis there is a known primary and multiple bone lesions are present; therefore, they are often not biopsied.[66] However, a bone biopsy is usually performed to establish a diagnosis when there is a solitary metastasis or no primary tumor is found. FNA is an excellent method for detecting metastasis and should be used as the initial diagnostic procedure in the evaluation of skeletal lesions of unknown origin, since it has a high diagnostic accuracy in diagnosing bone metastasis.[64] In a study of 110 patients who presented with malignancies involving large bones, the site and type of malignancy was correctly suggested in two-thirds of patients with metastatic carcinoma.[67] In this study, the primary site was suggested in the majority of metastatic tumors from kidney, prostate, and breast, while suggested in only half of the metastatic lung carcinomas. Most frequently encountered primary neoplasms that spread to the bone were prostate, breast, kidney, lung, and thyroid.[68] When the origin of the primary tumor is known, metastases are more often from breast or prostate. When the primary tumor is not known, however, lung and kidney are more likely sources of metastases.[68] Jorda et al. found lung followed by urinary tract, breast, head and neck, and gastrointestinal tract to be the most frequent sites of origin in 95 metastatic bone lesions.[64] In one-third of these cases, FNA cytology provided the initial diagnosis of malignancy. Symptomatic pathologic fractures of femur are usually due to carcinoma of the breast and occasionally due to lung carcinoma.[69] Skeletal metastases are usually osteolytic or osteoblastic, with the majority being osteolytic. Cancers of kidney, thyroid, lung, and gastrointestinal tract almost always cause osteolytic lesions. Metastatic prostate carcinoma, carcinoid tumors, and medulloblastoma almost always result in osteoblastic metastases, while metastatic breast cancer can be either osteolytic or osteoblastic.[70,71] Occasionally, osseous metastasis may have a spindle cell appearance, thereby mimicking a sarcoma. Therefore, metastatic spindle/sarcomatoid carcinoma, especially from kidney, and malignant melanoma should be excluded.[65] Some metastases may be associated with extensive osteoid formation or reactive osteoclastic proliferation simulating osteosarcoma or giant cell tumor. Careful attention should therefore be paid to the microscopic features to avoid making an erroneous diagnosis of a primary bone neoplasm.[65]

LUNG

Most common primary sites of lung metastases are breast and gastrointestinal tract, but almost any malignancy can metastasize to the lung.[52] Metastasis may present as multiple nodules, diffuse infiltrate, or a solitary nodule. Lung metastasis presents most commonly as multiple sharply circumscribed nodules having a miliary or cannonball appearance. In general, miliary nodules are common in metastatic malignant melanoma, renal cell carcinoma, thyroid medullary carcinoma, and ovarian carcinoma. Cannonball metastases are usually associated with sarcoma, renal cell carcinoma, melanoma, and colorectal carcinoma.[72] When metastasis presents as a diffuse infiltrate or a solitary coin lesion, distinction from a primary lung malignancy such as bronchioloalveolar carcinoma or adenocarcinoma, not otherwise specified, is problematic. Diffuse involvement of lung by metastasis typically occurs via extensive invasion of pulmonary lymphatics (lymphangitic metastasis), and accounts for

approximately 6–8% of all pulmonary metastases.[73] Lymphangitic metastases are most commonly associated with cancers of lung, breast, gastrointestinal tract, and pancreas. Lymphangitic metastases can often be diagnosed by transbronchial biopsy.[74] Approximately 3–9% of all solitary pulmonary nodules represent metastases, most often from malignant melanoma, breast, colon, renal cell carcinoma, sarcoma, and nonseminomatous germ cell tumors.[72,75] Some lung metastases show distinctive growth patterns such as lepidic growth, interstitial spread, and cavitation.[76] Up to 15% of metastatic colon adenocarcinoma may grow along the alveolar septa in a lepidic pattern simulating bronchioalveolar carcinoma.[77] The presence of dirty necrosis, however, combined with characteristic IHC staining pattern will help recognize a colon primay.[76] Predominant involvement of the pulmonary interstitium may be seen in metastatic sarcoma, lymphoma, carcinoma, carcinoid tumor, and malignant melanoma.[76] Cavitation may be seen in approximately 4% of metastatic malignancies arising in sites such as head and neck, cervix, colon, breast, bladder, and sarcoma.[78] When available, comparison with the previous cytology or surgical pathology material from the primary tumor is always indicated. Immunohistochemical studies are extremely helpful in suspected metastasis from certain organs such as breast, prostate, and thyroid. FNA of right lower lobe lung masses may inadvertently sample benign liver tissue, potentially leading to a false-positive diagnosis of well-differentiated carcinoma with clear and granular cell features such as renal cell carcinoma. Careful attention to the cytologic features, however, especially on fixed smears, and inquiry about exact site of lung FNA can prevent such a pitfall. Overall sensitivity and specificity of lung FNA are 89% and 96%, respectively.[52]

LIVER

Metastatic disease accounts for the great majority of malignant neoplasms in the liver. The liver is one of the most common recipients of metastatic malignancy.[52] Up to 40% of patients who die from cancer have liver metastasis, and 10% die from hepatic failure.[79] A diagnosis of metastases is best established by radiographically guided needle core biopsy or FNA. Specificity of liver FNA approaches 100%, while sensitivity is reported in the range of 85%.[52] The most common source of metastasis to the liver is the gastrointestinal tract, particularly colorectal and pancreas, followed by breast.[80] Hertz et al. reported their experience with 602 radiologically guided liver FNAs.[81] In their series, metastatic adenocarcinoma was the most commonly made diagnosis, accounting for approximately 40% of the cases, followed by hepatocellular carcinoma (24%), neuroendocrine carcinoma (7%), squamous cell carcinoma and lymphoma (4%).[81] Metastatic melanoma and leiomyosarcoma may also involve the liver, the latter more commonly arising in the uterus or GI tract (often GI stromal tumor).[52] Approximately three-fourths of metastatic neuroendocrine carcinomas arise in the lung, with the remaining cases arising from pancreas, unknown site, or representing a primary liver malignancy. Most metastatic squamous cell carcinomas originate in the head and neck, esophagus, and lung.[81] Distinguishing by biopsy between metastatic adenocarcinoma and cholangiocarcinoma is not possible in most instances. Adenocarcinoma with a small tubular or tubulopapillary architecture is most likely to arise from stomach, pancreas, or biliary tract, which are indistinguishable from each other by light microscopy or IHC. Metastatic colon adenocarcinoma will usually present with large well-formed glands and hyperchromatic cigar-shaped nuclei. The presence of dirty necrosis in the background is a helpful clue for a colon origin. Although colon and breast cancers frequently metastasize to the liver, they rarely present as occult primaries in the presence of clinically evident liver metastases.[82] IHC associated with elevated serum alpha-fetoprotein is helpful in distinguishing poorly differentiated hepatocellular carcinoma from metastatic poorly differentiated carcinoma. Metastatic melanoma may also be confused cytologically with hepatocellular carcinoma, in which case the predominantly discohesive cell pattern and IHC staining for S-100 and HMB-45 are characteristic for melanoma.[52] Metastatic renal cell carcinoma may also be confused with hepatocellular carcinoma; however, careful attention to architectural and IHC features as well as investigation for the presence of a kidney mass would facilitate arriving at the correct diagnosis.

ADRENAL GLANDS

The adrenal glands are the fifth most common site to harbor metastasis, surpassed in frequency only by metastases to lymph nodes, lung, liver, and large bones.[83] Since computed tomography (CT) and magnetic resonance imaging (MRI) are routinely used for staging of malignant neoplasms, detection of incidental adrenal cortical nodules has increased. These so-called 'incidentalomas' are found reportedly in 0.6–1.3% and 5–15% of patients without and with a known history of cancer, respectively.[84–87] In an autopsy study involving 1000 cases with evidence of malignancy, the adrenal glands were secondarily involved in 27% of the cases; breast, lung, kidney, stomach, pancreas, ovary, and colon accounted for most primary sites, in decreasing order of frequency.[83] In another autopsy study of 91 patients with lung cancer, adrenal metastases were found in 35% of the cases, with adenocarcinoma and squamous cell carcinoma representing the most frequent types.[88] We recently examined FNA of 162 adrenal masses where benign adrenocortical nodule (BACN) accounted for 33% and metastases for 31% of the cases.[89] Lung was by far the most common primary site, accounting for approximately 50% of malignancies. Other FNA series found lung to represent approximately 70% of metastases to adrenal glands.[90,91] In some instances small round cell malignancy, metastatic adenocarcinoma, renal cell carcinoma, and adrenocortical carcinoma may mimic BACN cytologically.[92–94] IHC may be helpful in these problematic cases, employing carcinoembryonic antigen (CEA) and epithelial membrane antigen (EMA). BACN is usually negative for both markers, metastatic adenocarcinoma positive for both markers, while renal cell carcinoma is negative for CEA and shows variable staining with EMA. Our series, however, only included high-grade adrenocortical carcinoma; therefore, distinguishing a well-differentiated adrenocortical carcinoma from BACN remains problematic. It is most important to verify that the tip of the sampling needle is within the adrenal nodule, since normal adrenal tissue is also indistinguishable from BACN. A cautionary note is not to confuse benign liver tissue for adrenal tissue, since liver parenchyma can occasionally mimic adrenal cortical tissue on FNA biopsies.[83]

SALIVARY GLANDS

Metastases to the salivary gland are not unusual, most commonly involving intraparotid or periparotid lymph nodes. Metastatic malignancies account for approximately 10% to 16% of all salivary gland malignancy.[95,96] Squamous cell carcinoma and melanoma from the head and neck make up the majority of metastases.[97–99] Primary sites below the clavicle are extremely rare, but come predominantly from lung, kidney, and breast.[100] Rarely, metastasis may be the initial manifestation of disease, mimicking primary salivary gland neoplasm, as most patients present with a known history of malignancy.[101,102] Certain metastatic tumors may be difficult to distinguish cytologically from primary salivary gland neoplasms. Metastatic squamous cell carcinoma, for example, may resemble primary high-grade mucoepidermoid carcinoma if glandular differentiation is not appreciated. Mucin positivity favors mucoepidermoid carcinoma, while abundant keratinization favors metastatic squamous carcinoma.[99] Primary squamous cell carcinoma of the salivary gland is extremely rare. Metastatic cystic squamous cell carcinoma that lacks significant atypia may be difficult, if not impossible, to differentiate on FNA from branchial cleft cyst or squamous metaplasia in Warthen's tumor. Primary clear cell carcinoma and small cell carcinoma may arise primarily in the salivary glands; however, metastatic renal and lung carcinomas must be excluded. As with other organ systems, metastatic poorly differentiated adenocarcinoma and undifferentiated carcinoma are difficult to separate from primary malignancies. Complete knowledge of clinical history, review of previous pathologic material and ancillary studies, when appropriate, are needed for accurate diagnosis of metastatic malignancies to the salivary glands.

UNUSUAL SITES OF METASTESIS

Since unusual sites of metastasis are not commonly encountered, they may pose diagnostic difficulties and lead at times to confusion with primary neoplasms arising in these sites. Unusual metastatic sites discussed in this chapter include breast, thyroid, pancreas, kidney, small bones, eye, spleen, and tumor-to-tumor metastasis. The most common primary malignancies metastasizing to these areas are shown in Table 6.3.

BREAST

Metastases to the breast from extramammary malignancies are quite rare, accounting for approximately 0.4–2.0% of all breast malignancies

Table 6.3 Unusual sites for metastases and their most likely primary sites

Metastatic site	Most common primary site or malignancy
Breast	
female	Contralateral breast, melanoma, lymphoma, lung, ovary, sarcoma, GIT, genitourinary
male	Prostate, lymphoma, lung, bladder
Thyroid	Kidney, lung, breast, melanoma
Pancreas	Lung, lymphoma, breast, kidney, liver, GIT, melanoma
Kidney	Lung, breast, GIT, lymphoma, melanoma
Small bones	Lung, kidney, breast, GIT, melanoma
Eye	Melanoma, breast, lung, lymphoma, GIT, kidney, prostate
Spleen	Lung, breast, melanoma

GIT, Gastrointestinal tract
Modified from Elsheikh TM, et al. Fine needle aspiration cytology of metastatic malignancies involving unusual sites. Am J Clin Pathol 1997; 108(Suppl 1): S12–S21.

in clinical studies.[103–105] Metastatic tumors in the breast are mostly seen in women with disseminated malignancies, and present more commonly as a solitary mass, thus mimicking a primary breast neoplasm. Metastasis may also present as multiple nodules or, rarely, may diffusely infiltrate the breast, simulating inflammatory carcinoma.[106,107] A large surgical pathology series of 51 patients found the most common extramammary primary tumors, in decreasing order of frequency, to be melanoma, lymphoma, lung carcinoma, ovarian carcinoma, and soft tissue sarcoma.[103] Another study of 60 secondary nonmammary neoplasms involving the breast found small cell carcinoma of lung, signet-ring adenocarcinoma of stomach, renal cell carcinoma, and cutaneous malignant melanoma to be the most frequent types; rare unusual sites of origin included thyroid, endometrium and pancreas.[108] Metastatic carcinoma should always be considered when the microscopic features are unusual for a primary breast carcinoma. Such may be the case with hematopoietic malignancies, pigmented malignant melanoma, and small cell carcinoma, among others. Distinguishing a primary from metastatic malignancy, however, may be difficult when the metastatic tumor does not show distinctive cytologic features such as metastatic poorly differentiated carcinoma or papillary carcinoma. Metastatic ovarian carcinomas are usually of the serous type; therefore, they can be mistaken for a primary papillary carcinoma.[109] Metastatic gastrointestinal tract mucinous carcinoma is histologically indistinguishable from primary breast mucinous carcinoma; however, adenocarcinoma of gastrointestinal tract, especially colon and rectum, rarely metastasizes to breast and often has a different IHC profile.[110] Surprisingly, metastatic carcinoid tumors of small bowel are frequently seen in breast metastases, and may be mistaken for lobular carcinoma or mammary carcinoma with neuroendocrine differentiation if a history of extramammary primary is not available.[111] Metastatic spindle cell malignancies such as malignant melanoma, sarcomatoid renal cell carcinoma, and sarcoma should be distinguished from primary metaplastic carcinoma. Some hematopoietic neoplasms, such as plasmacytoma and malignant lymphoma involving the breast, may resemble primary lobular carcinoma, in which case ancillary studies are needed for a definitive diagnosis. The presence of elastosis and in-situ carcinoma components in tissue samples support the primary nature of the malignancy, although its absence is not helpful in establishing the diagnosis.[112] Metastatic tumors often surround and displace normal-appearing breast parenchyma.[111] Other histologic features that have been reported to favor metastasis are sharp transition at the border of the lesion and presence in the subcutaneous rather than parenchymal breast tissue.[113] Knowledge of the clinical history of the extramammary malignancy and correlation of the previous cytologic/histologic material with current microscopic findings is crucial to arriving at an accurate diagnosis. Although it is unusual for metastatic malignancy to present as the initial finding of an unsuspected extramammary primary, this may occur in approximately one-fourth to one-half of the patients, particularly with metastatic pulmonary small cell carcinoma.[104] In contrast to metastasis in the female breast, metastatic neoplasms in the male breast represent approximately 55% of male breast malignancy.[114] Since gynecomastia accounts for approximately 70% of male breast lesions and may demonstrate epithelial hyperplasia and atypia, it represents the major differential diagnosis in FNA samples. Prostate carcinoma is reported as the most common primary site of breast metastasis in men.[115] Pursuing a complete work-up and excluding a metastatic lesion are indicated when a malignancy other than ductal carcinoma is suspected on biopsy of breasts in men.[114]

THYROID

The thyroid gland is a rare site for involvement by metastatic malignancy, with a reported prevalence of 1.3% to 25%.[116] Metastasis to the thyroid can present as multiple small nodules or as a solitary tumor mass, mimicking a primary neoplasm.[117] In some cases metastasis to the thyroid can become manifest long after the detection of primary cancer; this scenario may be encountered especially with renal cell carcinoma.[116] Breast and lung cancers are the most common primary tumors seen in autopsy studies, while the kidney is the most common site reported in surgical series.[118] The thyroid may also be involved by direct extension from carcinoma of the upper aerodigestive tract. Metastasis can be suspected when the microscopic features appear alien to the more common types of primary thyroid neoplasms such as papillary, follicular and medullary carcinoma. Michelow and Leiman reported 21 cases of metastases to the thyroid gland, in which only five patients had a known history of malignancy.[119] Metastatic clear cell carcinoma of the kidney is particularly difficult to differentiate from primary thyroid carcinoma with clear cell features.[120] IHC studies, including demonstration of thyroglobulin and thyroid transcription factor-1 (TTF-1) staining may aid in the differential diagnosis. Granular renal cell carcinoma may mimic Hürthle cell neoplasms; and plasmacytoma associated with amyloid may be misinterpreted as medullary carcinoma, especially on FNA specimens.[121] Recognition of metastatic malignancy may prevent inappropriate thyroidectomy and appropriately direct the search for the unsuspected or unknown primary malignancy.

PANCREAS

Neoplasms metastatic to the pancreas are uncommon and may be radiographically and clinically indistinguishable from primary pancreatic carcinoma. We described 19 cases of hematopoietic and other metastatic neoplasms involving the pancreas that clinically mimicked primary pancreatic carcinoma.[122] These cases represented 11% of all malignant pancreatic FNA diagnoses in this series. The most common primary sites reported in the literature are lung, breast, kidney, lymphoma, liver, and melanoma.[123–125] Primary cancers of adjacent organs such as stomach, intestine or biliary tract, may also directly extend to the pancreas.[126] Because the majority of primary pancreatic malignancies are ductal adenocarcinoma, recognition of unusual cytomorphologic features for a primary pancreatic carcinoma is a helpful clue toward suspecting metastatic disease. Small cell carcinoma in the pancreas is usually metastatic, most likely of pulmonary origin, as primary small cell carcinoma of the pancreas is quite rare.[127] While squamous differentiation may occur in primary pancreatic carcinoma as part of adenosquamous carcinoma, the presence of a pure squamous cell carcinoma in a pancreatic FNA is more suggestive of metastatic disease, possibly of pulmonary, esophageal, or cervical origin. Metastatic adenocarcinoma can be quite difficult to distinguish from primary adenocarcinoma of the pancreas.[123] Clearly, a history of adenocarcinoma at another site is essential in making an accurate diagnosis in these cases.

KIDNEY

Renal masses secondary to metastases are uncommon, accounting for approximately 8% to 13% of renal tumors.[128] The role of FNA biopsy in the diagnosis of renal masses remains controversial. Major indications for FNA include nonresectable tumor, radiographically indeterminate lesions, high surgical risk patients, metastatic tumors and drainage of benign cysts and abscesses.[129,130] Most metastases originate from lung, breast, stomach, pancreas, contralateral kidney, and melanoma in adults.[131] Metastatic malignancies are usually easily distinguished from renal cell carcinoma cytologically. It may be difficult, however, to distinguish occasional primary renal neoplasms such as collecting duct carcinoma from metastatic carcinoma.[130] Gattuso et al. recently described their experience with FNA of 28 metastatic tumors to the kidney.[130] Ninety percent of the patients in their series had a prior history of malignancy, most commonly of lung, liver, and lymphoma. Ten percent of their patients had no prior history of malignancy and showed metastatic adenocarcinoma of unknown origin.[130]

SMALL BONES

Although large bones are commonly involved by metastasis, involvement of small bones is exceptionally rare, accounting for less than 0.3% of all bone metastasis.[132,133] Clinically, small bone metastases may mimic a variety of infectious and inflammatory skeletal diseases, thereby leading to delayed diagnosis and treatment. Lung, kidney, and breast carcinomas are the most common neoplasms to metastasize to small bones of the hand and feet.[134] Although FNA cytology has been rarely used, it can play a significant role in the diagnosis of small bone metastasis. Metastases may present as part of a widely disseminated disease or as the first manifestation of an occult carcinoma, the latter being seen more commonly with lung metastasis. In two reports, 2 out of 5 patients had metastatic renal cell carcinoma to the calcaneus and metastatic pulmonary adenocarcinoma to small finger bones, as the initial presentations of occult malignancies.[132,134] The remaining three cases consisted of two squamous cell carcinomas from esophagus and floor of the mouth and a metastatic gastroesophageal adenocarcinoma. In general, subdiaphragmatic malignancies tend to metastasize to the bones of the feet, while malignancies arising above the diaphragm metastasize to the hand.[133] Small bone metastasis is usually associated with an extremely poor prognosis.

ORBIT

Another rare site for metastasis is the eye. FNA biopsy is not often used in the evaluation of intraocular neoplasms, but its diagnostic value has been demonstrated in selected reports.[135–138] Orbital metastatic tumors are different in children and adults. In children, they are most often of embryonal or undifferentiated type.[139] In adults, the most common metastatic epithelial malignancy is breast in women and lung in men.[140] Malignant melanoma is the most common nonepithelial tumor to metastasize to the orbit.[141] In a large series of transocular FNA biopsies, uveal metastasis was second only to uveal melanoma as the most common diagnosis encountered in transocular FNA.[142] We recently reported a high accuracy rate in the FNA diagnosis of orbital hematolymphoid lesions, especially when combined with appropriate ancillary studies.[138] FNA is recommended in those cases in which the diagnosis of malignancy is uncertain by clinical and radiographic studies, especially when differentiating between a primary and a metastatic neoplasm.[142]

SPLEEN

While splenic FNA is utilized rarely in the United States, core biopsy is contraindicated due to the potential of hemorrhagic complications. FNA of the spleen has been used predominantly for the diagnosis of lymphoma or non-neoplastic systemic diseases, such as sarcoidosis, amyloidosis, myeloid metaplasia, and infectious disease.[143–145] A limited number of reports described FNA cytology of metastatic disease to the spleen.[146–148] This may be due to the relative infrequency of splenic metastases and concerns about potential hemorrhagic complications following the FNA procedure.[149,150] Soderstrom, however, reported no hemorrhagic complications in his experience with more than 1000 splenic aspirates, using 22-gauge or smaller needle.[144] Metastatic neoplasms involving the spleen are uncommon and occur late in the course of disseminated disease. Metastatic carcinoma was found in 1.6% to 30% of patients in autopsy studies.[149,150] Lung, breast, and melanoma accounted for most of the primary sites. The spleen may also be involved by direct extension from pancreatic and retroperitoneal neoplasms. We previously described our experience with FNA biopsy of splenic neoplasms.[148] In a series of 11 patients with known epithelial or hematologic malignancies, FNA confirmed the presence of lymphoma in three out of seven patients. Metastatic malignancy (testicular embryonal carcinoma, bronchogenic large cell carcinoma, and ovarian papillary carcinoma) was confirmed in three of four patients with a history of malignancy.[148] Therefore, we believe that FNA biopsy can be a useful and safe procedure in the evaluation of diffuse and focal lesions and in the work-up of neoplastic and infectious splenic diseases.

TUMOR-TO-TUMOR METASTASIS

Tumor-to-tumor metastasis is extremely rare. Both benign and malignant tumors can act as hosts to metastatic malignancies. Adenomas of the thyroid and adrenal glands and meningioma are the most common recipient benign tumors.[151] Renal cell carcinoma has been reported to be the most common malignant recipient neoplasm, followed by sarcoma and lymphoma. The most common donor neoplasms are lung, prostate, and thyroid, in descending order of frequency.[52] Although tumor-to-tumor metastases are rare, the possibility should be entertained when two distinctly different cytomorphologic features are seen in patients with known or suspected second malignancy.[152] Immunohistochemical studies were reported to help establish the FNA diagnosis in metastatic breast, prostate, and neuroendocrine carcinomas to follicular adenomas and papillary carcinoma of the thyroid.[153,154] Tumor-to-tumor metastasis occurs through hematogenous dissemination, but the mechanism of metastasis is unclear at this time. It is suspected that hypervascularity of the recipient tumor and selective homing play major roles in this phenomenon.[155]

MORPHOLOGIC PATTERNS AND SPECIAL HISTOLOGIC FEATURES

In the work-up of a malignancy in a patient without a prior history of cancer, the differential diagnosis can include distinction of a primary cancer from metastatic disease. The most common type of malignancy in both settings is adenocarcinoma. The diagnostic approach for evaluation of metastatic as well as primary malignancies should begin with an attempt to determine cell lineage and/or assessment of the morphologic pattern/cell type, including specific histologic features that are encountered (Fig. 6.1). The major cell lineages are adenocarcinoma, squamous cell/urothelial carcinoma, lymphoma, sarcoma, and melanoma. We, as well as others, approach

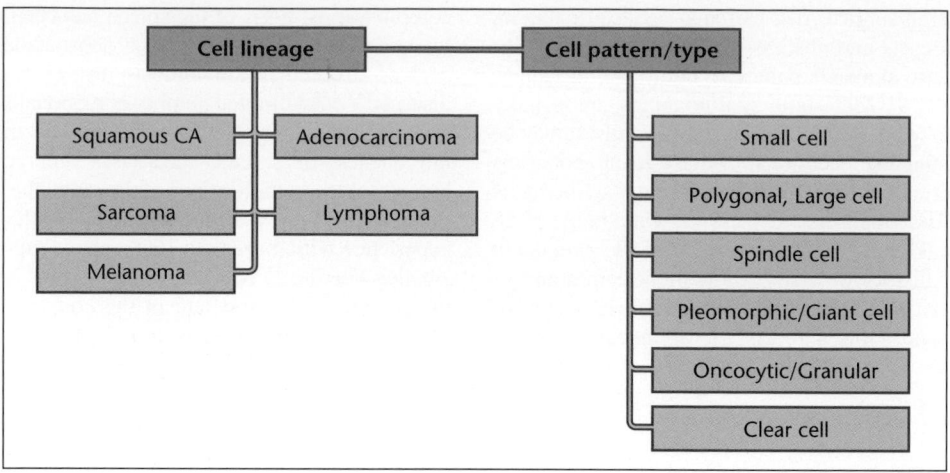

Fig. 6.1 Cytomorphologic patterns of metastases of unknown primary origin.

the assessment of morphologic patterns by categorizing the configuration of the cells based on their cytoplasmic qualities or size into the following groups: (1) small, round 'blue' cells, (2) large/polygonal cells, (3) spindle cells, (4) giant cell/pleomorphic cells, (5) eosinophilic or granular cells and (6) clear cells.[52,156,157]

Although the rubric 'small, round blue cell tumor' has been traditionally used to describe a variety of malignancies that occur in the pediatric age group, it can also be extended to neoplasms in the adult population.[158] All of these malignancies are characterized by a population of relatively small, round cells that are fairly nondescript, although certain types of malignancies may have specific diagnostic features that can suggest a more definitive classification. Types of malignancies that fall in the small, round cell tumor category include:

1. neuroendocrine tumors such as carcinoid and islet cell tumors (well-differentiated neuroendocrine carcinoma), as well as small cell carcinoma (poorly differentiated neuroendocrine carcinoma) (Fig. 6.2);
2. some poorly differentiated non-small cell carcinomas consisting of relatively small cells such as the occasional squamous cell carcinoma and less often, adenocarcinoma;
3. lymphomas and other hematopoietic malignancies;
4. small, round (blue) cell tumors of childhood;
5. some sarcomas such as the small cell variant of synovial sarcoma; and
6. the small cell variant of melanoma.

Occasionally, other malignancies considered within the small, round cell tumor category include lobular carcinoma of the breast, plasmacytomas, and granulosa cell tumor of the ovary.

When considering the diagnosis of one of the small, round cell tumors (SRCT) of childhood, the following entities are included: peripheral neuroectodermal tumor (PNET), Ewing's sarcoma, rhabdomyosarcoma, Wilms' tumor and neuroblastoma. PNET, Ewing's sarcoma and neuroblastoma generally consist of relatively uniform, small, round to oval cells with very high nuclear-to-cytoplasmic ratios. Usually, the nuclei of SRCTs are hyperchromatic, but lack prominent nucleoli. Rosette formation can be occasionally appreciated in PNET and neuroblastoma. In both Ewing's sarcoma and PNET, fine peripheral cytoplasmic vacuolization due to intra-

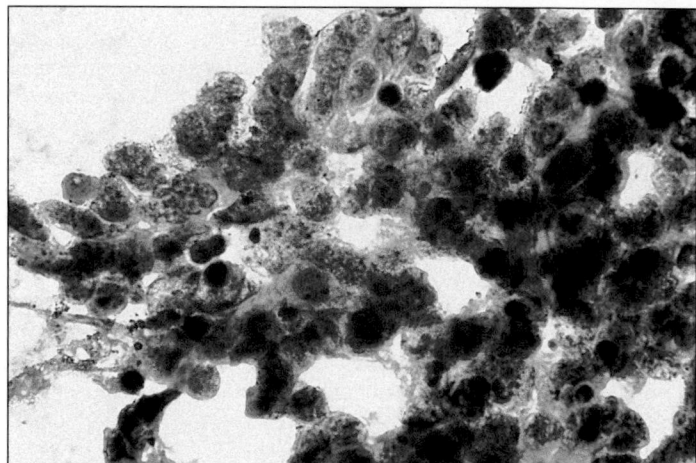

Fig. 6.2 Fine needle aspiration biopsy of pancreatic mass reveals a small cell malignancy. The cytologic findings suggest a metastasis from a small cell carcinoma, most likely of pulmonary origin. The neoplastic cells have very high nuclear-to-cytoplasmic ratios, nuclear angularity, salt-and-pepper type chromatin and lack prominent nucleoli. CT scan of the lung revealed a small lung mass (Papanicolaou stain ×400).

cytoplasmic glycogen can be present. The vacuoles are accentuated in air-dried, Romanowsky-stained preparations. Occasionally, cytoplasmic projections or neurites can be seen in the cytoplasmic material. Ancillary studies, including immunohistochemistry for a variety of neuroectodermal markers, as well as molecular studies for fusion transcripts and chromosomal translocations, can be helpful.[158] Non-Hodgkin's lymphoma often will be patternless in the tissue and have a strikingly dissociative pattern in the cytology smears. The nuclei tend to be irregular and nucleoli can be appreciated. So-called lymphoglandular bodies can be appreciated in both the alcohol-fixed, Papanicolaou preparation and air-dried, Romanowsky-stained smears. Again, immunocytochemistry for lymphoid markers can be of considerable help, as well as can flow cytometric and cytogenetic studies. The cells of rhabdomyosarcoma can show a range of morphologic features with a greater degree of nuclear atypicality

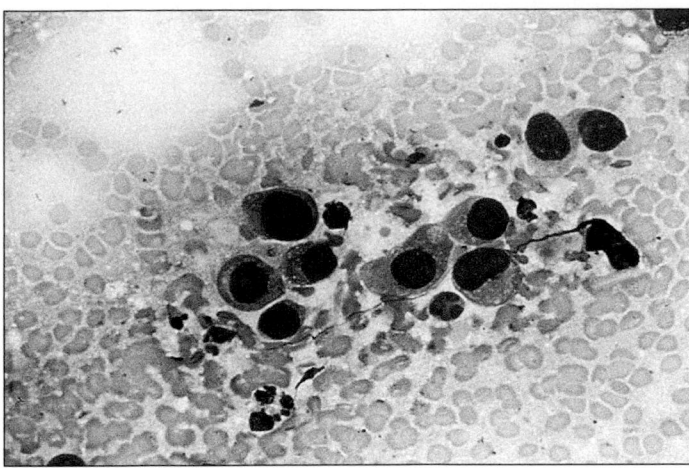

Fig. 6.3 FNA of splenic mass showing large polygonal cells arranged in a discohesive pattern. The malignant cells stained positive for cytokeratin and negative for CD45 and S-100, consistent with metastatic poorly differentiated carcinoma. A gastric primary was subsequently found (Diff-Quik ×400).

sections as well as the cytology smears. The sections can also show 'Azzopardi' effect characterized by DNA encrustation of intratumoral blood vessels. Lobular carcinoma of the breast consists of small malignant cells with high nuclear-to-cytoplasmic ratios. The cells are often arranged in a single-file pattern.

Tumors that have *large, round to polygonal cells* include a variety of carcinomas, lymphomas and melanoma (Fig. 6.3). It is in this setting especially that immunohistochemistry can be of value as well as attention to the H&E morphologic features.[52,156]

Neoplasms consisting of cells with *eosinophilic, granular cytoplasm* include:

1. a variety of adenomas as well as carcinomas that can involve the kidney, liver, salivary gland, cervix (glassy cell);
2. oncocytic and Hürthle cell neoplasms involving the kidney, thyroid, etc. (Fig. 6.4);
3. tumors of apocrine derivation involving the breast, sweat glands, and skin;
4. neuroendocrine tumors such as carcinoid and paraganglioma;
5. soft tissue tumors such as granular cell tumor and alveolar soft part sarcoma, etc.; and
6. melanoma and hilar/Leydig cell tumor.[52,156]

The cytoplasmic granularities can be due to increased numbers of mitochondria, smooth endoplasmic reticulum, lysosome-like bodies, secretory granules, and neuroendocrine-type granules. In the evaluation of these tumors, immunohistochemistry as well as electron microscopy can also help to sort out these various neoplasms.

In the *clear cell* tumor categories, a variety of carcinomas need to be considered, but conventional renal cell carcinoma should lead the list, followed by neoplasms of the ovary, liver, adrenal, salivary gland, lung, GYN, and thyroid (Fig. 6.5).[52,156] Other types of clear cell tumors include:

1. oncocytic neoplasms with clear cell change;
2. acinic/acinar cell tumors;
3. neuroendocrine tumors such as paraganglioma;
4. soft tissue tumors such as clear cell sarcoma; and
5. some germ cell tumors.

present than in the other small, round cell tumors of childhood.[158] This is one of the small, round cell tumors of childhood that can demonstrate larger cells having nuclei with prominent nucleoli.

The neuroendocrine neoplasms, carcinoid and islet cell tumors can show a variety of patterns in the tissue sections and a loosely cohesive and individually scattered pattern of small, uniform cells with a slight to moderate amount of granular cytoplasm and eccentrically placed nuclei with the characteristic salt-and-pepper type of chromatin in the cytology smears. In contrast, small cell carcinomas consist of small atypical cells having very high nuclear-to-cytoplasmic ratios with nuclear irregularity and molding. Due to nuclear fragility, DNA streaking can be appreciated in the tissue

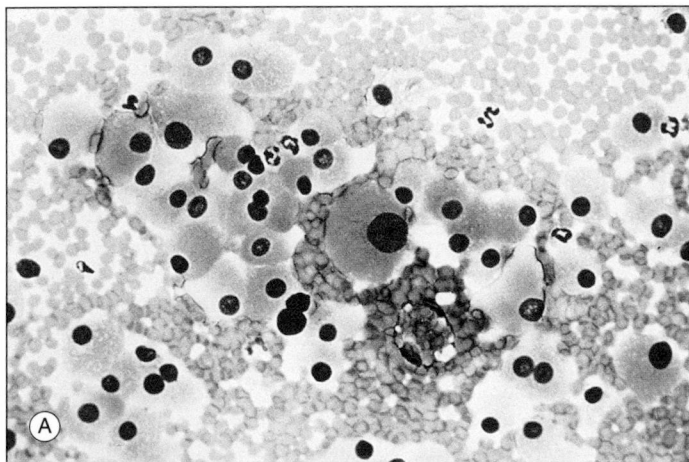

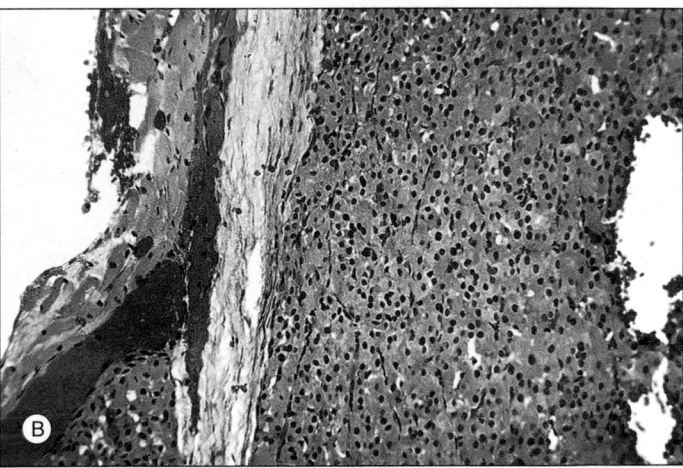

Fig. 6.4 A, FNA of a single lung mass demonstrated cells arranged in a loosely cohesive to dissociative pattern. The cells had round nuclei with small to prominent nucleoli and abundant eosinophilic, granular cytoplasm and showed considerable anisonucleosis. Diagnostic possibilities included a primary pulmonary neoplasm with oncocytic cells or a metastatic oncocytic or Hürthle cell malignancy (Diff-Quik ×200);
B, Physical examination revealed a thyroid mass which was resected. The thyroid neoplasm is consistent with a Hürthle cell carcinoma. Besides the characteristic Hürthle cells, vascular invasion was identified (H&E ×100).

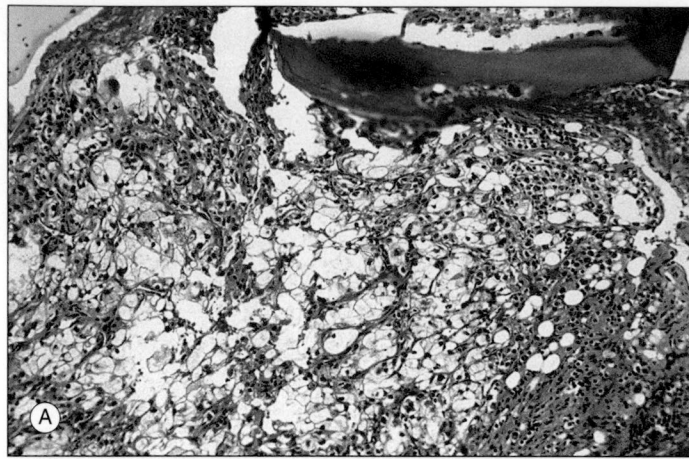

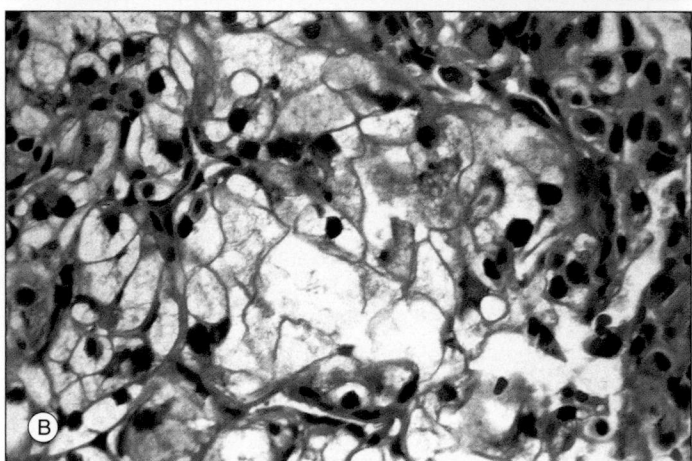

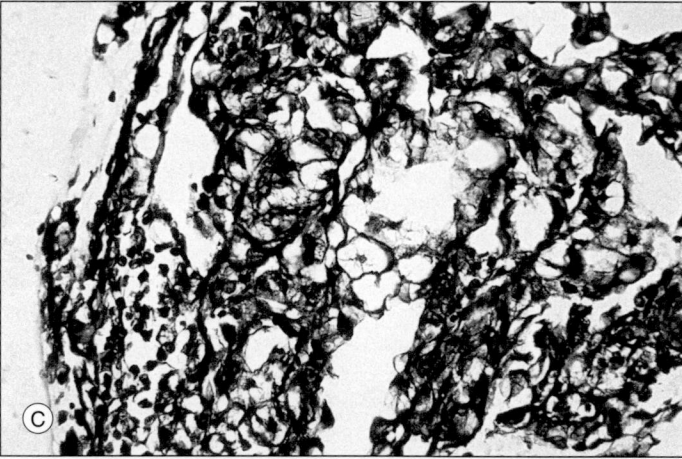

Fig. 6.5 A, This elderly patient presented with a destructive lesion of the acetabulum. The core biopsy revealed a clear cell neoplasm having a branching, chicken wire, vascular pattern that suggested a metastasis from a conventional clear cell carcinoma of the kidney (H&E ×100); **B**, High power of the malignancy revealed sheets of neoplastic clear cells having small, round nuclei. Abundant cytoplasm was noted as well as the delicate branching vasculature (H&E ×100); **C**, A panel of immunoperoxidase stains was performed which revealed positive staining of the clear cells for epithelial membrane antigen and vimentin. CD10, a marker that has shown to be positive in conventional clear cell carcinoma of the kidney, was strongly positive (CD10 immunoperoxidase stain ×200).

Very rarely, lymphomas and melanoma (balloon cell) can have clear cells. The clear cell appearance of some of these tumors may be due to: (1) intracytoplasmic glycogen or fat, (2) cells with a paucity of organelles, and (3) fixation artifacts or degeneration. Morphologic clues can often help to determine the primary site of a clear cell neoplasm. Cerilli and Wick approached the evaluation of malignant clear cell tumors by categorizing them into those with a nested architecture, sclerosing stroma or those lacking a consistent architectural pattern.[156] Conventional renal cell carcinoma often shows hemorrhage in the stroma or within the tubules, and the clear cells demonstrate fat and/or glycogen with special stains. Renal cell carcinomas also have a prominent vascular background. When glandular groups consisting of clear cells are present and the clear cells demonstrate a hobnail configuration, then a Müllerian origin should be suggested.[156] Clear cell variants of hepatocellular carcinoma as well as thyroid carcinoma will often show more conventional foci to suggest the correct diagnosis. Paragangliomas are arranged in small nests referred to as a zellballen pattern associated with a complex vasculature.

Sclerosing clear cell malignancies are usually of salivary gland origin.[156] Hyalinizing clear cell carcinoma of the minor salivary gland typically consists of solid sheets and cords of large malignant clear cells surrounded by hyalinized bands of collagen.[156] Acinar cell carcinomas often have cells with clear cytoplasm, but also can show foci with cells having a more amphophilic to basophilic granular cytoplasm. Tumors that may lack a distinctive architectural pattern but consist of clear cells include mucoepidermoid carcinoma, occasional adenocarcinomas and squamous cell carcinomas, malignant melanoma of balloon or signet-ring variant, and germ cell tumors. Immunohistochemistry can be very helpful in the work-up.

In the malignant *spindle cell* category the following entities should be considered:

1. sarcomas including fibrosarcoma and leiomyosarcoma;
2. sarcomatoid carcinomas such as spindle squamous cell carcinomas and renal cell carcinoma, etc.;
3. pseudosarcomas such as nodular fasciitis, fibromatosis and mesenchymal repair;
4. neuroendocrine tumors such as the occasional paraganglioma; and
5. melanoma.[52,156]

The evaluation of a spindle cell neoplasm is greatly influenced by the site of the involvement.[157] A malignant spindle cell lesion of soft tissue would most likely be a sarcoma, in contrast to a spindle cell lesion of the larynx in which a sarcomatoid (spindle) squamous cell carcinoma would be favored.[157] In cytologic preparations, lack of cohesion of the cells would favor a sarcoma or melanoma, in contrast to a spindle cell carcinoma (Fig. 6.6). Intracytoplasmic melanin and prominent nucleoli or intranuclear inclusions would favor a melanoma. It is in the work-up of spindle cell lesions of unknown primary that immunohistochemical markers can be invaluable. A typical IHC panel should include S-100 and HMB-45, etc., for melanoma, cytokeratin for carcinoma and specific soft tissue markers for a variety of sarcomas that can be encountered. Lastly, it is exceedingly unusual to have a spindle cell sarcoma account for a metastatic malignancy of unknown primary. More likely, the malignancy represents a spindle cell carcinoma or melanoma.[156]

In the evaluation of malignancies consisting of *pleomorphic and/or giant cells*, the following should be considered:

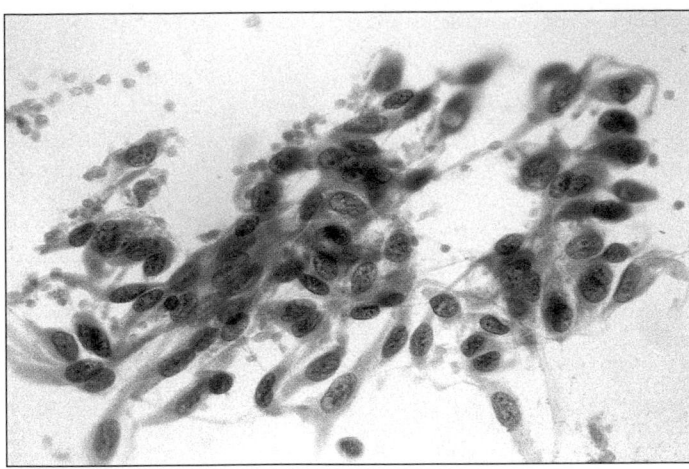

Fig. 6.6 FNA of one of many liver masses revealed loosely arranged and individually scattered atypical spindle cells having moderate amount of cytoplasm and nuclei possessing small but prominent nucleoli. Diagnostic considerations included metastatic melanoma, spindle carcinoma, and sarcoma. The cells showed strong staining with S-100 and HMB-45, consistent with metastatic melanoma (Papanicolaou stain ×400).

1. carcinomas such as giant cell carcinomas of lung, pancreas, liver, thyroid, etc. (Fig. 6.7);
2. high grade sarcomas such as malignant fibrous histiocytomas, etc.;
3. germ cell tumors such as choriocarcinoma;
4. neuroendocrine tumors such as pheochromocytomas;
5. a variety of lymphoreticular malignancies such as anaplastic large cell lymphoma and Hodgkin's disease; and
6. melanoma.[52,156]

An immunohistochemical panel for melanocytic, epithelial, soft tissue and lymphoid markers can be of value as well as can attention to the fine morphologic features of the cells.

In addition to the morphologic cell pattern, *specific histologic and cytologic features* can be present that can suggest the correct diagnosis. These features include the presence of either extracellular or intracytoplasmic mucin, intracytoplasmic hyaline globules, psammoma bodies and intranuclear cytoplasmic inclusions. For evaluation of mucinous neoplasms, the following entities should be considered: (1) colloid/mucinous neoplasms such as carcinomas of GI tract, breast, ovary, pancreas, (2) pseudomyxoma peritonei, usually of appendiceal origin, and (3) myxoid sarcomas. Mucin positivity virtually excludes lymphoma and leukemia, most sarcomas except for chordoma and, for all practical purposes, melanoma.[52] Intracytoplasmic hyaline globules can be seen in a variety of carcinomas, sarcomas, lymphomas, germ cell tumors and melanoma. When present in carcinomas, diagnostic considerations include hepatocellular carcinoma, renal cell carcinoma, germ cell malignancies, and ovarian carcinoma. When intracytoplasmic globules are eosinophilic and prominent, and the cells have nuclei with prominent nucleoli, then a 'rhabdoid' phenotype is present. Malignancies with a rhabdoid phenotype are usually poorly differentiated and aggressive in behavior.[156] Malignant melanoma may be one of the more common malignancies to show rhabdoid features.[36,53,159] The arrangement of the cells into groups that demonstrate papillary, microacinar, or single-file patterns can be helpful. Papillary neoplasms generally arise from the ovary, GI tract, pancreas, lung (especially bronchioloalveolar cell carcinoma), thyroid, and renal cell carcinoma. Tumors demonstrating microacinar complexes include those of prostate, thyroid, and carcinoid and islet cell tumors (Fig. 6.8). The microacinar pattern of carcinoid/islet cell tumors are referred to as rosettes. Malignancies that tend to show a single cell pattern especially include carcinomas of the breast and stomach, followed by pancreas, prostate, small cell carcinoma, mesothelioma, carcinoids, and melanomas. Those tumors that demonstrate prominent intranuclear cytoplasmic inclusions include papillary carcinoma of the thyroid, occasional bronchioloalveolar cell carcinomas of the lung, hepatocellular carcinoma, and melanomas, but many other types of neoplasms may demonstrate this nuclear morphologic feature (Table 6.4).

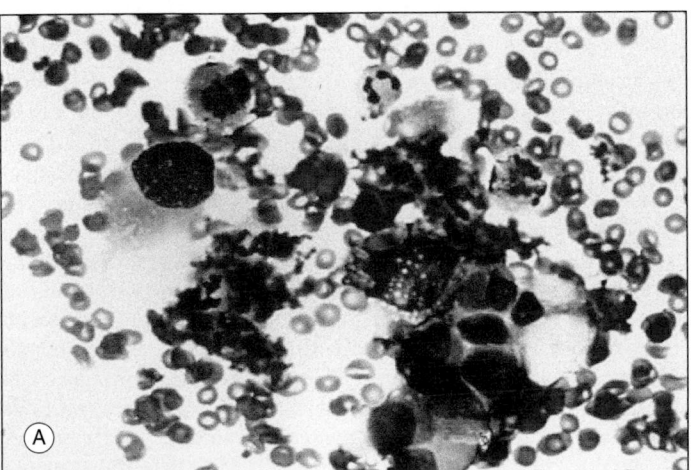

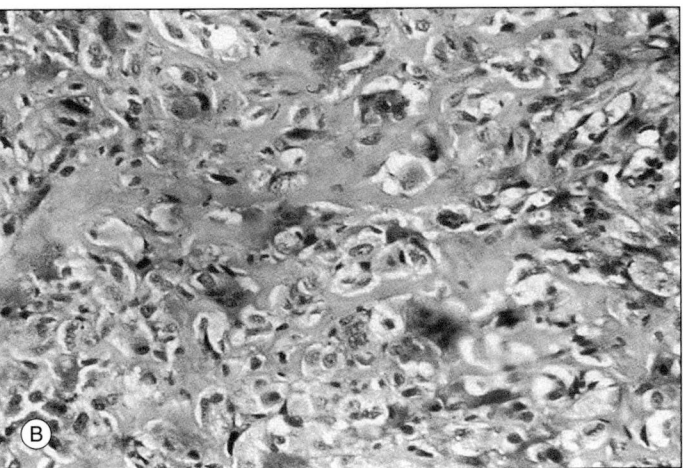

Fig. 6.7 **A**, FNA of pelvic mass from a 73-year-old man showing large, pleomorphic and giant malignant cells arranged as loosely cohesive clusters and singly scattered cells. (Diff-Quik stain ×400); **B**, The urinary bladder showed sarcomatoid carcinoma with cytologic features identical to those observed in the pelvic FNA (H&E ×200).

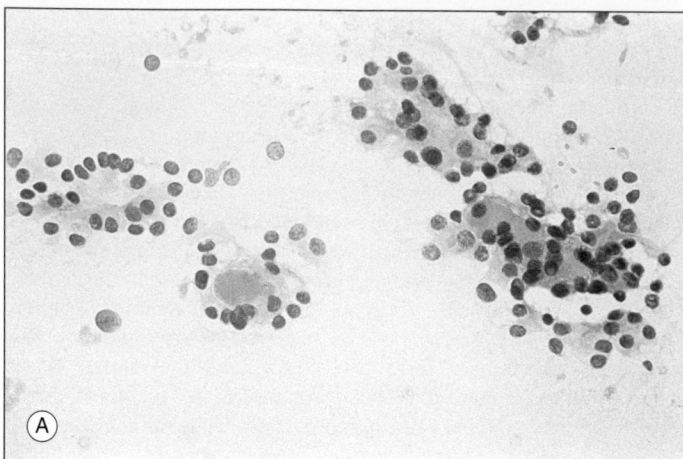

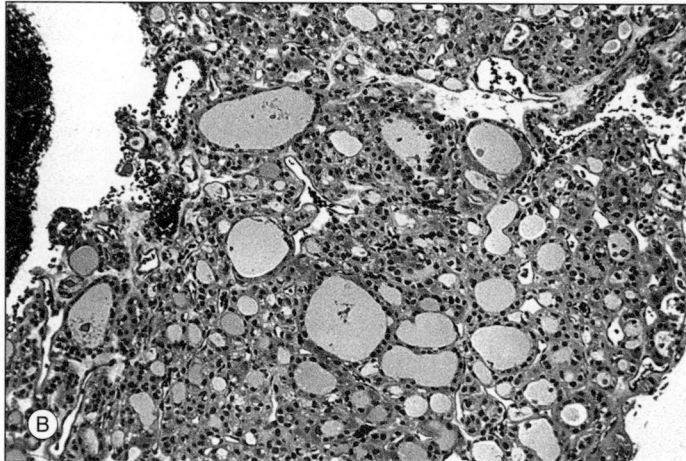

Fig. 6.8 A, FNA of humerus in which neoplastic cells are arranged in microacinar complexes. Within the lumen of these complexes, there is colloid-type material (Papanicolaou stain ×200); **B**, Core biopsy of the humerus revealed metastatic carcinoma consistent with a thyroid primary. Clinical examination revealed a thyroid mass which was confirmed as a follicular carcinoma following resection (H&E ×100).

Table 6.4 Morphologic patterns and associated primary sites

Morphologic pattern	Possible primary sites
Small cell	SBRCT, neuroendocrine tumors, PD/basaloid squamous carcinoma, PD adenocarcinoma, lobular carcinoma, lymphoma, sarcoma, melanoma
Oncocytic/Granular	Kidney, liver, salivary gland, thyroid, breast, neuroendocrine tumors, melanoma
Clear cell	Kidney, ovary, liver, adrenal, salivary gland, lung, GYN, thyroid, sarcoma, germ cell tumor, chordoma
Pleomorphic/Giant cell	PD carcinoma (lung, pancreas, thyroid, liver), sarcoma, choriocarcinoma, phaeochromocytoma, Hodgkin's lymphoma, anaplastic large cell lymphoma
Spindle cell	Sarcoma, sarcomatoid carcinoma (kidney, thyroid, lung, pancreas), neuroendocrine tumors, melanoma, lymphoma
Polygonal, large cell	PD carcinoma, melanoma, lymphoma, plasmacytoma, sarcoma
Papillary	Thyroid, ovary, endometrium, peritoneum, kidney, breast, lung
Mucinous	Breast, GIT, pancreas, ovary, lung, chordoma
Microacinar/Microfollicular	Thyroid, prostate, neuroendocrine tumors, granulose cell tumor, SBRCT

GIT, gastrointestinal tract; GYN, gynecologic; SBRCT, small blue round cell tumors; PD, poorly differentiated

IMMUNOHISTOCHEMISTRY

Ancillary studies are frequently utilized in the contemporary practice of surgical pathology and cytopathology to determine the primary site of a malignancy of unknown primary. Currently, immuno-histochemistry is the main ancillary study performed, with electron microscopy and molecular diagnostics less often or infrequently used. The performance of an immunohistochemical panel has been shown to be one of the most cost-effective procedures, when compared with other clinical and radiologic studies.[57] Immunohistochemical studies are frequently performed to determine either the primary site or cell lineage of the malignancy.

DeYoung and Wick, as well as others, have cautioned that there is no single immunohistochemical antibody that can provide a definitive diagnosis in most cases.[160] They also advise that in order for immunohistochemistry to be applied effectively, the following should occur: (1) processing of specimens should be under stringent conditions, (2) optimal dilutions of all antibodies used, (3) pathologists should standardize fixation, processing and staining in their laboratory, and (4) the interpretation of a panel of antibodies should be based on the pathologists' experience in their laboratory, as well as based on statistical analysis in the literature. However, most importantly, the antibodies chosen should be based on the morphologic and/or clinicopathologic features of the malignancies, in order for the evaluation to be meaningful. The pathologist should also be flexible in determining the appropriate IHC panel, since sometimes it appears that newer antibodies are becoming available almost on a daily basis. DeYoung and Wick strongly advocate an algorithmic interpretative approach that is based on entry points that have high predictive value followed by a decision tree based on binary branching of immunohistochemical markers with lesser predictive values to maximize results. The algorithm that DeYoung and Wick use has been shown to have an approximately two-thirds accuracy for the determination of the primary site of origin in the work-up of metastatic carcinoma of unknown primary. Others have used different algorithms with similar results.[161,162] Conceptually, these IHC algorithms attempt first to determine the major cell lines of differentiation, i.e., carcinoma, lymphoma, melanoma, sarcoma, or germ cell. The diagnosis can then be refined by using differential cytokeratins that are unique to certain tumor types.[163] The determination of vimentin coexpression positivity, plus analysis of specific epithelial or germ cell antigens, cell specific products, and/or hormone receptor analysis can also be included in the IHC panels.[163] The following is a brief discussion of the variety of immunohistochemical reagents that can be utilized in the algorithmic approach for the determination of the primary site of a metastatic cancer of unknown origin.

CYTOKERATINS

Determination of cytokeratin expression is often the starting point in the evaluation of the malignancy (Table 6.5). Cytokeratins that are often used are the simple cytokeratins 8 and 18, cytokeratin 19, AE1/3 cocktail, cytokeratin 7, cytokeratin 20, high molecular weight cytokeratin (antibody 34 βE12/keratin 903) and cytokeratin 5/6. DeYoung and Wick advocate the use of the cytokeratin cocktail consisting of a mixture of AE1/AE3, MAK-6 and CAM5.2 as an initial screening reagent. Cytokeratin 8 (CAM5.2) is a simple cytokeratin present in all simple nonstratified epithelium, ductal, and pseudostratified epithelial tissue.[163] Nearly all mesotheliomas and carcinomas are positive for CAM5.2 (except squamous cell carcinoma). Cytokeratin 7 is most often expressed in breast, lung, ovarian, pancreatic, and biliary tree carcinomas as well as transitional cell carcinoma, but is absent (or stains only a few cells) in colorectal and prostatic carcinomas.[163] Hepatocellular carcinoma, duodenal ampullary carcinomas, and adrenocortical neoplasms are usually negative for CK7. Cytokeratin 20 is expressed most often in colorectal, pancreatic, gallbladder, and urothelial carcinoma and Merkel cell carcinoma.[160,163] Breast carcinoma is generally negative for cytokeratin 20, although occasionally papillary and mucinous types can demonstrate positivity.[163] Although the literature reports

Table 6.5 Differential cytokeratin patterns

CK7+/20+
Transitional cell carcinoma (TCC) (TCC can be CK7+/20–)
Pancreatic carcinoma
Ovarian mucinous carcinoma
Occasional cholangiocarcinoma and gastric carcinoma

CK7–/CK20+
Colorectal carcinoma
Merkel cell carcinoma

CK7–/CK20–
Hepatocellular carcinoma
Prostate carcinoma
Renal cell carcinoma
Squamous cell carcinoma
Neuroendocrine carcinoma of lung
Adrenal cortical carcinoma
Germ cell malignancies
Thymomas

CK7+/CK20–
Ovary (nonmucinous)
Endometrial carcinoma
Breast carcinoma (papillary and mucinous types can be CK20+)
Lung carcinoma (mucinous type can be CK20+)
Mesothelioma (can also be CK20+)
Salivary gland tumors

CK5/6
Squamous cell carcinoma
Urothelial carcinoma
Mesothelioma

Modified from Dabbs DJ, Silverman JF. Pathology case reviews. 2001; July/August 6: 146–153.

that mesothelioma and prostate cancer are negative for cytokeratin 20, we have found cytokeratin 20 positivity in both of these malignancies.

Epithelial malignancies that are generally negative for cytokeratin 7 and 20 include hepatocellular carcinoma, renal cell carcinoma, squamous cell carcinoma, neuroendocrine carcinomas of the lung, adrenocortical carcinoma, most germ cell tumors, and thymomas.[162] Malignancies that can be positive for cytokeratin 5/6 include squamous cell carcinoma, urothelial carcinoma, and mesothelioma.

EPITHELIAL MEMBRANE ANTIGEN

Epithelial membrane antigen (EMA), a member of the milk fat globule glycoprotein family, is found on the surface of most epithelial cells.[160] Positive staining can be membranous with or without diffuse cytoplasmic staining. Most adenocarcinomas are positive for EMA, although hepatocellular carcinoma, adrenal cortical carcinoma, and most malignant germ cell neoplasms are negative, except for the occasional choriocarcinoma and teratoma.[162] Some neoplastic hematopoietic cells can also express EMA, such as cells from plasma cell dysplasia, erythroblasts, L & H cells of Hodgkin's disease, occasional B- and T-cell lymphomas and more than half of the anaplastic large cell lymphomas.[162] EMA staining is especially helpful as a supplement to cytokeratin evaluation to support an epithelial lineage.[164]

CARCINOEMBRYONIC ANTIGEN

Carcinoembryonic antigen (CEA) is often positive in adenocarcinomas of pulmonary, breast, and GI origin, but generally negative in cells from prostate, kidney, adrenal, endometrium, and serous ovarian carcinomas, as well as mesothelioma.[165] We prefer to use monoclonal CEA, since polyclonal CEA can at times be difficult to interpret due to considerable staining of cross-reacting antigens.[160] However, when evaluating the possibility of hepatocellular carcinoma, polyclonal CEA is utilized to demonstrate canalicular-pattern staining of the neoplastic liver cells.

VIMENTIN

Some carcinomas can coexpress vimentin, which can be a helpful finding in the work-up of a metastasis of unknown primary. Carcinomas that often coexpress vimentin include renal cell carcinoma, endometrial carcinoma, carcinomas of salivary gland or sweat gland origin, mesothelioma, thyroid carcinoma and sarcomatoid, or spindle cell carcinoma.[160,162] The neoplasm must express significant staining (> 25% of cells) to be of value. Vimentin coexpression is rarely seen in breast, nonserous ovarian, prostate, colon, and pulmonary non-small cell carcinoma.

GLYCOPROTEIN MEMBRANE ANTIGENS

There are a number of glycoprotein membrane-based antigens that are often used to distinguish adenocarcinomas from mesotheliomas. These include MOC-31, a 41 Kd glycoprotein and tumor-associated glycoprotein and TAG-72 (B72.3) that are positive in many adenocarcinomas, but generally negative in mesotheliomas, adrenal

Table 6.6 Cell line and site specific/associated antibodies

Antibody	Site
Cytokeratins, EMA	Adenocarcinoma, squamous cell carcinoma
	Urothelial carcinoma
PLAP, CD30, OCT-4, α-fetoprotein	Germ cell
HMB-45, Melan-A, S-100	Melanoma
Vimentin, desmin, S-100, CD34, myogenin	Sarcoma
MyoD1, HHF-35, etc.	
LCA, B and T cell markers	Lymphoma
Neuroendocrine markers	Small cell carcinoma, carcinoid/islet cell, paraganglioma, pheochromocytoma
Prostatic specific antigen (PSA) and prostatic acid phosphatase (PAP)	Prostate
Gross cystic disease fluid protein	Breast, salivary gland, skin adnexal
Thyroglobulin	Thyroid carcinoma
Thyroid transcription factor-1 (TTF-1)	Thyroid (nonmedullary) and lung
Uroplakin	Urothelial carcinoma
Hep Par-1	Liver, hepatoid carcinoma
Inhibin	Adrenal, ovarian stromal tumor, trophoblastic
CDX-2, Villin	Colorectal and occasional other GI tract/pancreas primaries
WT-1	Serious ovarian carcinoma, mesothelioma

PLAP, placental lactogen alkaline phosphatase; LCA, leukocyte common antigen.
From Pathology case reviews. Dabbs DJ, Silverman JF. 2001; July/August 6: 146–153.

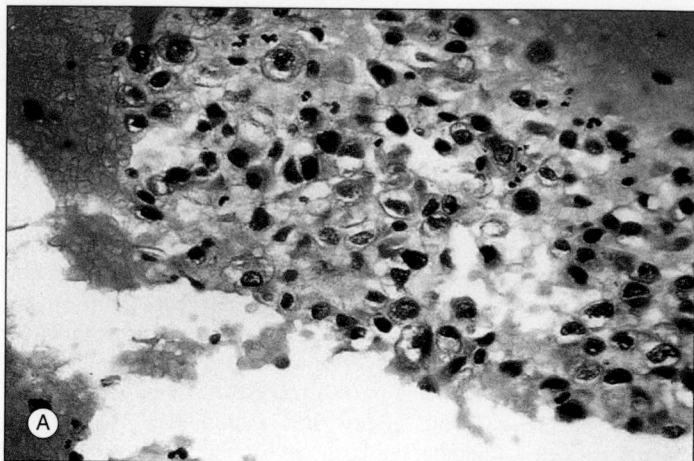

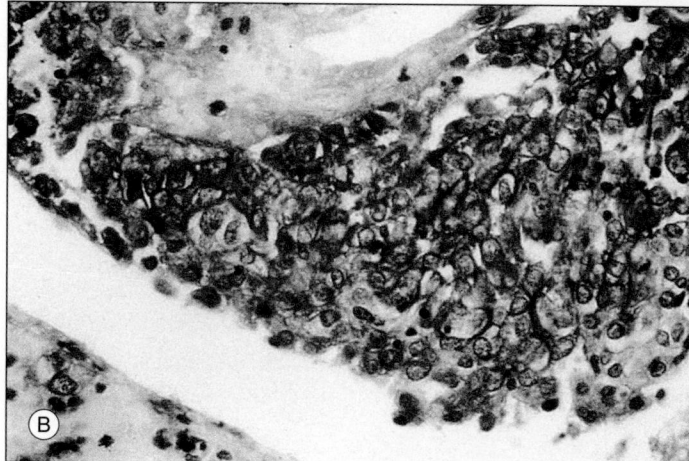

Fig. 6.9 **A**, FNA of mediastinal mass in a 27-year-old man showing cohesive clusters of large cells with abundant cytoplasm and clear cell features. The neoplastic cells showed round to oval nuclei with prominent nucleoli (Cell block H&E ×400); **B**, The malignant cells stained negative for AE 1/3, CD 45, S-100 and EMA. PLAP was strongly positive, consistent with the diagnosis of extragonadal germ cell tumor (PLAP immunoperoxidase stain ×400).

cortical carcinomas, hepatocellular carcinomas, renal cell carcinomas, nasopharyngeal carcinomas, thyroid carcinomas, and germ cell malignancies.[160,166–168] Other types of glycoprotein membrane antigens that are occasionally useful include CA-125, which is detected primarily in Müllerian tract neoplasms, and occasional neoplasms of the pancreas and biliary tract, but generally is negative in adenocarcinomas from other sites.[169–173] CA-19-9, a glycoprotein related to the Le^a blood group antigen, is positive in adenocarcinomas of GI tract, pancreas, biliary tract, urinary bladder, ovaries, and endometrium, but negative in most tumors from other sites.[174,175] Recently, IHC of genes coding for the protein expression of mucins (MUC1, MUC2, and MUC5AC) has also been studied for determining the primary site.[176]

CELL LINE AND SITE-SPECIFIC/ASSOCIATED ANTIBODIES

There is a variety of cell line and site-specific-associated antibodies that can be extremely useful in the work-up of a metastatic malignancy of unknown primary (Table 6.6). These antibodies can often be used in an IHC panel to identify the primary site. In the work-up of a germ cell neoplasm (Fig. 6.9), placental-like alkaline phosphatase (PLAP) is frequently positive,[160,163] and when used in conjunction with cytokeratins, epithelial membrane antigen, alpha-fetoprotein and human chorionic gonadotropin, can often establish the correct diagnosis.[163] Seminoma and embryonal carcinoma are generally negative for epithelial membrane antigen, while seminomas generally do not express cytokeratin.[177,178] Exceptions include the occasional extragenital seminomas, such as those occurring in the mediastinum, which can occasionally express simple cytokeratins such as CAM5.2, and EMA which can be positive in choriocarcinoma.[163] Alpha-fetoprotein is usually seen in yolk sac tumors, but can also be focally present in some embryonal carcinomas.[163,179–181] CD30 is expressed in embryonal carcinoma[182] and OCT4 in seminoma and embryonal carcinoma.[183]

Prostatic specific antigen (PSA), as well as prostatic acid phosphatase (PAP) with few exceptions, is very specific for a carcinoma of prostatic origin,[52,163] especially if monoclonal antibodies are utilized. However, PSA staining has occasionally been demonstrated in some salivary gland tumors, breast carcinomas, and periurethral and urinary bladder glandular lesions.[163,184–192] PAP has also been demonstrated in some hindgut carcinoid tumors.[193] There are also rare reports of PSA staining in metastatic melanoma.[194] Dual expression of PSA and PAP, however, will detect more than 95% of metastatic prostate carcinoma. Alpha-methylacyl-CoA racemase (P504S) positivity has also been demonstrated in prostatic carcinoma.[195]

Thyroglobulin is expressed in almost all thyroid carcinomas, with the exception of medullary carcinoma of the thyroid.[196,197] More recently, thyroid transcription factor-1 (TTF-1) has also been utilized to demonstrate carcinomas of thyroid origin, as well as a variety of lung malignancies (Fig. 6.10).[198,199] The IHC separation of these two malignancies can readily be performed, since carcinoembryonic antigen is often positive in non-small cell carcinomas of the lung, but negative in thyroid carcinomas with the exception of medullary carcinoma.

Gross cystic disease fluid protein-15 (GCDFP-15) is found in neoplasms expressing apocrine differentiation. Therefore, it is a good immunohistochemical marker for neoplasms of breast, salivary gland, and cutaneous apocrine origins.[160,163] Perhaps its greatest utility is its inclusion in a panel to identify metastatic malignancies of breast origin, since GCDFP-15 is expressed in approximately 60% of breast carcinomas.[200,201]

The panel should also include antibodies to estrogen receptor (ER) and progesterone receptor (PR) proteins. Expression of estrogen and progesterone receptor proteins are not restricted to carcinomas of the breast and Müllerian tract origin, as there are rare examples of positive tumors arising in other sites such as thyroid, carcinoid tumor, and skin sweat gland.[160,202,203] Some neoplasms are almost always negative for these receptors, which can be helpful in the differential diagnosis. Neoplasms that are usually negative for combined ER and PR proteins include gastrointestinal tract, lung, hepatocellular carcinoma, pancreas, thymoma, and transitional cell carcinoma.

In the work-up of neuroendocrine neoplasms, the IHC panel often includes neuron specific enolase (NSE), chromogranin and Leu-7 (CD57).[163] Based on our experience, we also include MAP-2.[204] A panel of neuroendocrine antibodies is recommended, since there are considerable differences in the sensitivities and specificities of these antibodies. Neuron specific enolase is quite non-specific, staining a variety of non-neuroendocrine tumors. However, the lack of NSE positivity should suggest that a neuroendocrine neoplasm is not present. Chromogranin is an excellent antibody for confirming an islet/carcinoid tumor, but is generally negative, in our experience, for small cell carcinomas due to the paucity of neuroendocrine granules present in many of these malignancies.[204] In our experience, synaptophysin and MAP-2 showed the greatest sensitivity for carcinoid tumors, small cell carcinomas, and large cell neuroendocrine carcinomas.[204] TTF-1 is also frequently positive in the poorly differentiated neuroendocrine carcinomas (small cell carcinoma and large cell neuroendocrine carcinomas) of the lung.

In the work-up for melanoma, a panel that consists of HMB-45 and S-100 can be invaluable. Although HMB-45 is quite specific for tumors of melanocytic origin (with a few exceptions), S-100 is less specific since it is expressed in a variety of different cell types besides melanocytes, such as histiocytes, cartilaginous cells, adipocytes, eccrine sweat glands, salivary glands, and myoepithelial cells, etc. The most frequent nonmelanocytic malignancies to express S-100 are carcinomas of the breast, genitourinary tract, salivary gland and sweat gland.[160,205–207] Other melanocytic markers that can be used include melan-A, tryosinase, microphthalmia transcription factor, and in our hands, MAP-2.[163,208,209]

A variety of other cell line and site-specific antibodies are also available including uroplakin for urothelial carcinomas, villin for GI tract carcinomas, and WT1 for serous ovarian carcinoma,[210] Hep

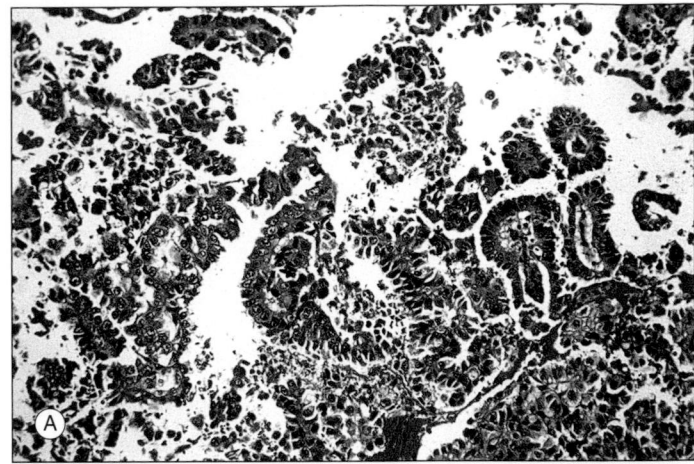

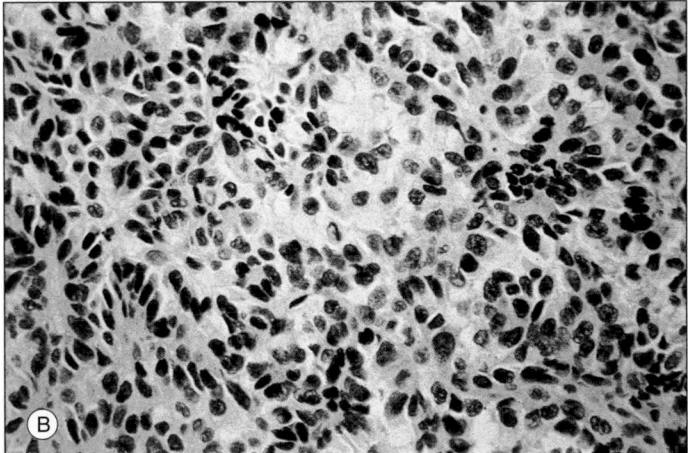

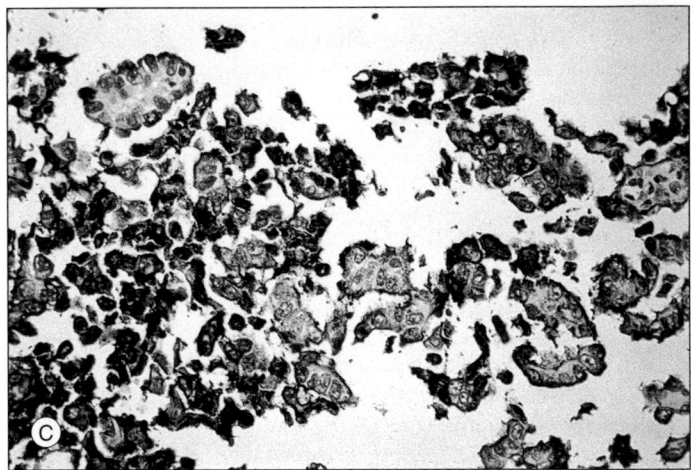

Fig. 6.10 **A**, A pleural-based mass consisting of uniform atypical cells arranged in a papillary pattern. The initial morphologic impression based on the H&E was that of a mesothelioma (H&E ×100); **B**, However, the neoplastic cells showed diffuse nuclear staining for TTF-1 consistent with either a lung or thyroid primary. A lung primary was suspected following examination of the CT scan which revealed a single small lung mass (TTF-1 immunoperoxidase stain ×200); **C**, The CEA positivity was also supportive of a lung rather than a thyroid primary (immunoperoxidase stain ×200).

Table 6.7 IHC work-up of undifferentiated/poorly differentiated malignancy

	AE-1/3	CD-45	S-100	PLAP	*Additional markers*
Carcinoma	+	–	±	–*	Differential keratins, EMA, etc.
Melanoma	–	–	+	–	HMB-45, Melan-A, etc.
Lymphoma	–	–	+**	–	CD20, CD3, CD30
Germ cell tumor	–***	–	–	+	EMA, etc. *

* Approximately 10% of non-germ cell carcinomas are PLAP +, and EMA +.
Nonseminoma germ cell tumors are keratin + and EMA –
** CD45 is very specific, but misses approximately 10% of large cell lymphoma including anaplastic large cell lymphoma. May include CD30 if suspect lymphoma with negative initial panel.
*** Seminoma and embryonal carcinoma are EMA –. Seminoma is CK –.

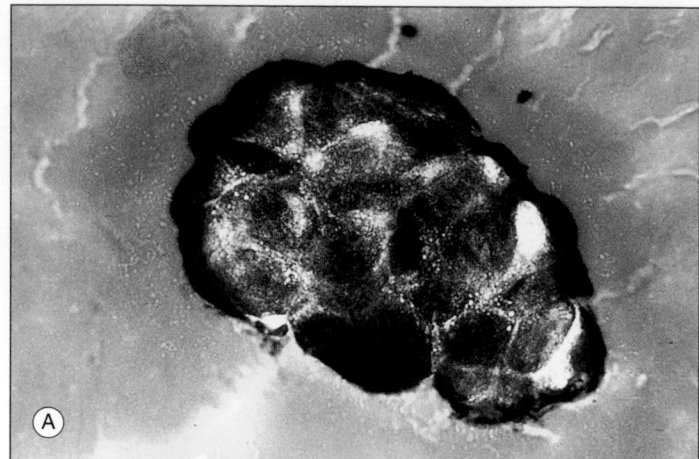

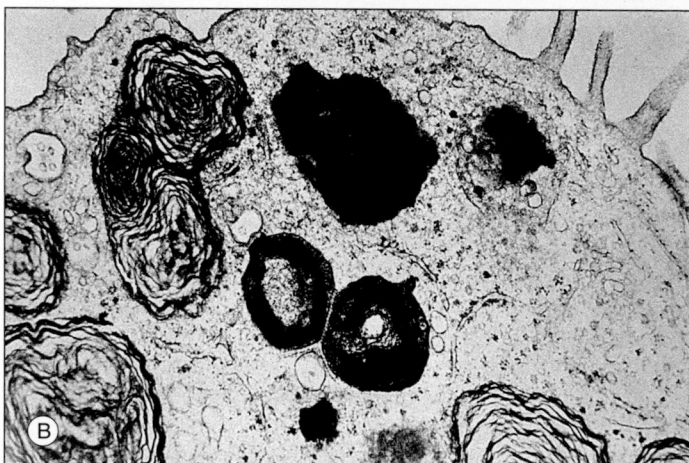

Fig. 6.11 A, Pericardial effusion specimen in which a cluster of neoplastic cells is present consistent with an adenocarcinoma (Diff-Quik ×400); **B,** Ultrastructural examination of the neoplastic cells in the pericardial fluid revealed surfactant-type granules consistent with pulmonary bronchioloalveolar cell carcinoma (electron microscopic examination).

Par-1 for hepatocellular carcinoma, inhibin for adrenal/ovarian stromal tumors and trophoblastic neoplasms, and a variety of hematopoietic markers for lymphoma.[162] Melan-A has also been utilized as a marker for adrenocortical neoplasms and some sex cord stromal tumors.[163,209] CD5 expression has been demonstrated in thymic carcinomas, and CD10 and RCC marker (GP200) can be useful for the diagnosis of renal cell carcinoma. CDX-2, a specific intestinal transcription factor which is especially expressed in colonic adenocarcinomas (but can occasionally be seen in other GI tract primaries) has also been demonstrated in GI tract neuroendocrine tumors.[211–214] It can be expected that additional new antibodies will be proposed in the future as useful in the work-up of metastatic malignancies of unknown primary origin.

In conclusion, when faced with a metastatic malignancy of unknown primary, ancillary immunohistochemical studies can be invaluable. It is recommended that a panel of antibodies be utilized if sufficient material is available. This is usually the case with tissue sections including needle biopsy, but only limited material may be available in a cytologic specimen. It is therefore recommended that an attempt be made to obtain either material for a cell block or to request the radiologist to procure a tissue core biopsy of the lesion, following the preliminary interpretation of the FNA biopsy, if a possible malignancy of unknown primary or a diagnostically challenging cytology case is encountered. Applications of an immunohistochemical pattern should be based on the morphologic findings, as well as the clinical scenario, in order to optimize the data. Similar to the axiom of 'junk in, junk out,' the ordering of immunohistochemical stains should be a thoughtful process in order to gain the relevant information to obtain the most definitive diagnosis. DeYoung and Wick as well as others have recommended that an algorithmic approach be employed with key entry points to initiate these studies. Often an 'entry point' for appropriate work-up includes obtaining some form of keratin study, which DeYoung and Wick refer to as first-tier study, especially for the work-up of a well to moderately differentiated adenocarcinoma, followed by second-tier and possibly third-tier immunoreactants to refine the diagnosis. If the morphologic feature is suggestive for a specific site or cell lineage, then the IHC work-up can be appropriately targeted and often shortened. For the initial work-up of an undifferentiated/poorly differentiated malignancy, an initial IHC panel often consists of cytokeratins, LCA, PLAP and/or S-100 (Table 6.7), which then may be followed by more specific markers. The reader is referred to the source material for a more complete discussion of these protocols.[160,163] Finally, the

role of electron microscopy is only briefly discussed, since currently this is not often used in most community hospital settings as well as tertiary/quaternary care institutions (with few exceptions) in the work-up of these cases. Occasionally, however, electron microscopy can help establish the diagnosis, if specific ultrastructural features of the neoplasm are present (Fig. 6.11). The reader is referred to other sources for a more complete discussion of the application of EM examination in this setting.[157] Lastly, it can be expected that molecular diagnostic/cytogenetic studies will be employed in the future as an aid for diagnosis, since specific molecular/cytogenetic abnormalities are associated with specific types of malignancies.[215–219] However, currently, there is a very limited role for these studies in the work-up of metastatic malignancies of unknown primary.

EFFUSION CYTOLOGY

Most patients with a malignant effusion have a known history of a prior malignancy, although a positive effusion cytology specimen may occasionally be the initial indication of cancer.[220] Monte et al. reported that positive cytologic studies were the first indication of malignancy in 7% of patients with malignant ascites and 14% of patients with malignant pleural effusions.[221] In this study, no patient with a malignant pericardial effusion had a positive specimen as the initial presentation of cancer, although we have seen this occurrence in our own clinical material. Malignant ascites, as expected, was predominantly seen in women, including those initially presenting with malignancies, while men more often presented with malignant pleural effusions.[221] In men, lung cancer was the most common primary site for the positive pleural effusion, including those initially presenting with malignancy. The ovary, in contrast, was the most common primary site for the initial presentation of malignancy in women with a positive peritoneal fluid specimen. In the experience of Monte et al., an unknown primary site was quite uncommon in patients having a positive pericardial effusion specimen.[221]

Adenocarcinoma is the most common histologic type of malignancy to be present in a positive serous effusion specimen.[52,222–227] Less commonly, squamous cell carcinoma, small cell carcinoma, a variety of hematopoietic malignancies, melanoma, sarcomas, and germ cell tumors can be seen in effusion specimens.[52,222,223] In the pediatric age group, small round cell type malignancies account for the vast majority of positive effusion specimens.[52,222,223]

Similar to the work-up of surgical pathology and FNA biopsy cases, the initial diagnostic approach to evaluating a malignant effusion specimen is to consider the site (i.e., pleural, pericardial, or peritoneal), sex, and age of the patient. Johnston has previously reported that men with malignant pleural effusions had primary sites or tumor types in the following descending order: lungs, lymphoma/leukemia, gastrointestinal (GI) tract, genitourinary tract ,and a variety of miscellaneous less common tumor types.[227] In Johnston's series, nearly 11% of the patients had an unknown primary site.[227] In women with a malignant pleural effusion and a known primary site, the most common locations or tumor types in descending order were: breast, female genital tract, lung, lymphoma/leukemia, GI tract, and a number of less common tumor types.[227] Approximately 9% of women with a positive effusion specimen had an unknown primary.[227] The most common primary sites in descending order in men with a positive peritoneal effusion were: GI tract, pancreas, prostate, and a variety of hematopoietic malignancies.[52] In women, the most common primary sites were: ovary, breast, uterus, GI tract, and hematologic malignancies. The most common malignancies accounting for a positive pericardial effusion in adults were: lung, breast, lymphoma/leukemia, and mesothelioma.[52] In the pediatric age group, the most common primary tumor types accounting for a positive pleural effusion were: hematopoietic malignancies, Wilms' tumor, neuroblastoma, and a variety of other small round cell tumors of childhood. In pericardial effusion specimens, hematopoietic malignancies, neuroblastoma, rhabdomyosarcoma, Wilms' tumor, and other small round cell tumors of childhood were most commonly present.

Murphy and Ng reported that the diagnostic sensitivity of effusion cytologic examination was 50–70% when the diagnosis was entirely based on morphology.[228] However, when the effusion site and the sex of the patient were known, the accuracy increased to 90%, which again validated the importance of clinical information and its correlation with the morphologic findings in making the most accurate diagnosis.

Similar to the metastatic carcinomas of unknown primary appreciated in surgical pathology and FNA specimens, metastatic carcinomas in effusions are often adenocarcinomas.[52,220] The low-power pattern of the cells in the effusion can occasionally be helpful in suggesting the primary site. Malignant cells can be arranged in large cell balls (cannonballs), clumps, papillary or gland-like acinar groupings. The number of cells within these groups is often much greater than what is found in clusters of reactive mesothelial cells, and it is not unusual to have clusters of more than 50 cells. The cell groups of metastatic carcinoma also tend to have a smooth peripheral community border, in contrast to the scalloped or knobby peripheral borders of clusters of benign and malignant mesothelial cells.

When papillary groups are appreciated, diagnostic considerations include ovarian epithelial neoplasms, papillary thyroid carcinoma, mesothelioma, transitional cell carcinoma, and mesothelial hyperplasia.[52,220,224] Three-dimensional clusters and/or large cannonball-type of groupings suggest breast cancer, pulmonary cancer, malignant mesothelioma, ovarian epithelial neoplasms, and mesothelial hyperplasias as diagnostic possibilities. Gland or acinar formation should suggest a diagnosis of colorectal adenocarcinoma, cholangiocarcinoma, ovarian epithelial neoplasms, lung adeno-carcinoma, endometriosis, and mesothelial hyperplasia. A linear arrangement of malignant cells with nuclear molding is quite characteristic of lobular carcinoma of the breast and small cell carcinoma. When malignant cells are associated with extracellular mucinous material causing pseudomyxoma peritonei, then an appendiceal and, less often, ovarian or another GI primary site should be considered.

Small cell types of malignancies having individually scattered cells in effusions should prompt the diagnostic consideration of small cell carcinoma, non-Hodgkin's lymphoma, carcinoid or islet cell tumor, lobular or ductal carcinoma of the breast, gastric adenocarcinoma, and a variety of pediatric small round cell tumors (Fig. 6.12).[220] When the tumor cells have eccentrically placed nuclei and granular cytoplasms, an islet cell/carcinoid tumor is possible. Signet-ring cells are seen especially with gastric and lobular carcinoma and tumor cells with very high nuclear-to-cytoplasmic ratios and salt-and-pepper type chromatin without nucleoli are typical of small cell carcinoma.

Individually scattered large cells in the effusion specimen should raise the possibility of malignant melanoma, hepatocellular carcinoma, squamous cell carcinoma, poorly differentiated adenocarcinomas, renal cell carcinoma, and adrenocortical carcinoma.[52,220] However, reactive mesothelial cells, as well as the occasional malignant mesothelioma, can have a predominantly single-cell pattern.[229] When multinucleated cells are noted in effusion specimens, the diagnostic possibilities include reactive mesothelial cells, giant cell carcinoma from various sites, hepatocellular carcinoma, malignant melanoma, sarcomas, and renal cell carcinoma. Rarely, carcinomas may even have associated osteoclast-like giant cells present. Extramedullary hematopoiesis with megakaryocytes, Hodgkin's disease, and some large cell lymphomas can also contain multinucleated atypical cells. It is in these settings that attention to the specific cytologic features and use of ancillary studies such as flow cytometry and immunohistochemistry can help in more accurately classifying the specific type of hematopoietic process.

When the atypical cells have intracytoplasmic vacuoles, diagnostic considerations include degenerating mesothelial cells and histiocytes, therapy-induced changes, signet-ring carcinoma of either breast or GI tract origin, and cytoplasmic microvacuolization in renal cell carcinoma.[220] Occasionally, the major differential is separating mucin producing adenocarcinoma from a mesothelioma having cells with vacuoles. Vacuoles in adenocarcinomas tend to be large with considerable variation in size and eccentrically located, often indenting the nucleus. These vacuoles often are positive for neutral mucin. Mesothelioma can have small uniform perinuclear

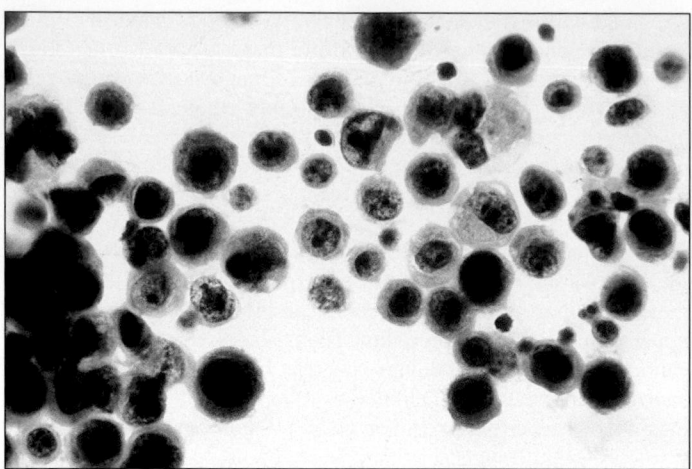

Fig. 6.12 Single-cell pattern was present in this pleural effusion specimen. The neoplastic cells were small to medium sized. Clinical examination revealed a breast mass which was confirmed as a poorly differentiated ductal carcinoma (Papanicolaou stain ×100).

lipid-rich vacuoles that tend to be small and indistinct, along with more peripherally located glycogen containing vacuoles. Occasionally, large vacuoles can be seen in mesothelioma, but they are positive for hyaluronic acid.[52] All types of vacuoles are best appreciated in air-dried Diff-Quik-stained material. Occasionally, cytoplasmic vacuoles can be seen in unusual neoplasms such as the balloon cell or signet-ring variants of melanoma.[230] Vacuoles can also be seen in degenerative mesothelial cells, as well as degenerating tumor cells of various types.[52,220]

Psammoma bodies are noted in a variety of benign and malignant effusions. These spherical basophilic microcalcifications are most often associated with papillary serous carcinomas, papillary carcinomas of the thyroid, mesotheliomas, and bronchioloalveolar cell carcinoma. They can also be present in benign entities such as endosalpingiosis.[231,232]

Pericellular lacunae have been suggested as a useful malignant cytologic feature.[233–236] However, most investigators believe that these lacunae are not a reliable indicator of malignancy.[234] Intercellular windows have been classically described as a feature of mesothelioma. Others, however, have found intercellular windows in metastatic carcinoma.[237]

When lymphoma is present in an effusion cytology specimen, it is most often seen late in the course of the disease when the patient has a widely disseminated malignancy. Rarely, however, a positive effusion specimen may be the initial presentation of a disseminated lymphoma or represent the primary site of involvement of primary body cavity or serous lymphoma.[239–240] These primary lymphomas are most often seen in patients with acquired immune deficiency syndrome (AIDS) who often have pre-existing Kaposi's sarcoma. Typically, they are large cell lymphomas of B-cell immunophenotype and are associated with human herpesvirus 8.[240] Lymphoid lesions are best evaluated in air-dried Diff-Quik preparations.

Ancillary studies can often be helpful in determining the site of origin of malignant cells present in an effusion cytology specimen.[241–256] The application of numerous antibodies has been reported in the literature, but we and others have found the most useful immunohistochemical panel for the confirmation of metastatic adenocarcinoma to consist of monoclonal CEA, *Ber*-EP4,

MOC-31, B72.3, *Leu*-M1 and TTF-1.[220,253,254,257] Recently, fairly specific positive markers for 'mesothelial' differentiation have become available, such as calretinin, HBME-1, thrombomodulin and CK5/6.[252–256] Epithelial membrane antigen (EMA) is an extremely sensitive marker for both adenocarcinomas and mesotheliomas, but is not specific since the vast majority of adenocarcinomas and mesotheliomas are positive.[256,258,259] However, in our experience, we usually do not see diffuse strong positive staining for EMA in reactive effusions.[258] In this study, EMA was positive in 100% of malignant cases and only 3.8% (3 of 78) of reactive cases.[258] Therefore, EMA could be a useful antibody in separating reactive, atypical mesothelial cells from metastatic carcinoma and mesothelioma. Leong et al. have previously reported that the staining pattern of EMA can be helpful in separating metastatic adenocarcinoma from mesothelioma.[259] In their experience, metastatic adenocarcinoma showed strong diffuse cytoplasmic staining, in contrast to the thick cell membrane pattern of mesothelioma.[259] Differential cytokeratins (CK) might also shed some light on the malignant cell of origin in the effusion specimen. We have found that mesotheliomas often express both CK7 and 20, while only a few types of adenocarcinoma present in the pleural fluid specimens are CK20 positive.

Although more recently there has been increased reliance on immunohistochemistry to help refine the diagnosis, special stains for neutral mucin such as mucicarmine can be beneficial.[220] Mucicarmine positivity is mainly seen in adenocarcinoma and only rarely present in mesothelioma. In contrast, the cells of mesothelioma can be positive for acidic mucin with the Alcian blue (pH 2.5) stain, that can be digested with hyaluronidase. Electron microscopy is also an excellent technique to separate adenocarcinomas from mesothelioma.[260] Ultrastructural features include true gland formation in adenocarcinoma, which is not seen in mesothelioma. Adenocarcinomas also demonstrate sparse intermediate filaments in contrast to the abundant filaments seen in mesothelioma. Adenocarcinomas have a limited amount to no glycogen, while mesotheliomas will demonstrate abundant intracytoplasmic glycogen. Most importantly, short microvilli having stubby roots are noted in adenocarcinoma, versus the characteristic long slender branching microvilli of mesothelioma.[52,220] The pathologic features contrasting adenocarcinoma with mesothelioma are detailed in Table 6.8.

WHAT THE ONCOLOGIST NEEDS TO KNOW

The treatment of patients with metastatic malignancy of unknown primary is contingent on the pathologic findings. Appropriate, specific therapy can be tailored when the malignancy is a lymphoma, sarcoma, melanoma, or a germ cell tumor.[36] Occasionally, local treatment with surgery and/or irradiation is beneficial when a single focus of metastatic disease is encountered; however, more commonly, systemic therapy is needed for disseminated disease of a metastatic adenocarcinoma or poorly differentiated/undifferentiated carcinoma of unknown primary.[36] Unfortunately, however, most of these patients have a suboptimal or minimal response to treatment. Recent series report the median survival of patients with metastatic carcinoma of unknown primary to be approximately one year, apparently more related to the performance status of the patient.[261,262] Poor survival is associated with male sex, increasing number of organs harboring metastatic disease, liver involvement, and the histologic diagnosis of adenocarcinoma.[263] In contrast, those patients having 'treatable' cancer had a median survival of twenty-three months.[264] Therefore, recognition of these favorable subgroups is critical. These favorable clinical subgroups include women with peritoneal carcinomatosis or

Table 6.8 Pathologic features of adenocarcinoma and mesothelioma

	Adenocarcinoma	Mesothelioma
Cell groupings	Community smooth borders	Irregular, knobby, scalloped borders
	Collagen cores rare	Collagen cores common
	Windows unusual	Windows common
	Usually dual population	Single population
Nucleus	Usually eccentric	Usually central or paracentral
	Often pleomorphic, occasionally bizarre	Often less pleomorphic not bizarre
	Less hyperchromatic	More hyperchromatic
	Micro- to macronucleoli	Macronucleoli
Cytoplasm	Delicate, homogeneous	Dense center with delicate, lacy edges
	Uniform staining	Two-tone staining
		Cytoplasmic blebs
Vacuoles	Large	Degenerative
	Random, irregular size	Perinuclear, small, uniform
Neutral mucin	Can be present	Rarely present
Acidic mucin	Often present	Positive, digested with hyaluronidase
PAS stain	May be positive (diffuse or focal)	Positive (peripheral) staining
	Often diastase resistant	Digested with diastase
IHC	EMA, CEA, Ber-EP4, MOC-31, LeuM1, B72.3 positive	EMA, calretinin, CK5/6 positive
EM	Short, stubby, unipolar microvilli, etc.	Long, slender microvilli around entire cell

Modified from Pathology case reviews. Dabbs DJ, Silverman JF. 2001; July/August 6: 146–153.

women who present with peritoneal carcinomatosis or positive axillary lymph nodes. In addition, HER2/neu should also be done on the axillary lymph node tissue. Other more favorable subgroups include patients with poorly differentiated carcinoma, including men with elevated beta-hCG or alpha-fetoprotein (AFP), poorly differentiated neuroendocrine tumors and patients with isolated cervical or inguinal lymph node involvement by squamous cell carcinoma.[36] Men with skeletal metastasis with or without increased PSA are treated with metastatic prostatic carcinoma protocols.[36] Patients with poorly differentiated adenocarcinoma and neuroendocrine carcinoma are often treated with cisplatin-based regimens, and men with poorly differentiated carcinoma with elevated beta-hCG or AFP are treated as having an extragonadal germ cell tumor. Those patients with metastatic squamous cell carcinoma can be treated with node dissection and/or radiation therapy. The clinicopathologic characteristics of these more favorable subgroups are outlined in Table 6.9.

Effective therapy does not currently exist for more than 60% of patients who present with a well-differentiated or moderately differentiated adenocarcinoma of unknown primary. However, some oncologists have tailored their chemotherapy strategy based on the histologic differentiation of the adenocarcinoma, especially with patients having well- or moderately differentiated adenocarcinoma.[265] Others have utilized an organ-specific management approach, and rely on accurate determination of the primary site, with preliminary data showing promising results.[160] Although metastatic melanoma is an aggressive malignancy, occasional patients may have a fairly reasonable survival, especially if a primary is not discovered after thorough evaluation and there is only one site of involvement, such as a single regional lymph node that can be treated by regional lymphadenectomy. This protocol has resulted in five year survivals in the range of 30–45%.[266]

Obviously, the medical oncologist's treatment strategy is based on the pathologic findings. Therefore, close collaboration between clinician and pathologist is critical in the management of these patients.

axillary nodal metastasis and men with skeletal metastasis with or without increased serum prostate specific antigen (PSA).[36] Women with peritoneal carcinomatosis are usually treated with ovarian carcinoma protocols, and women with positive axillary lymph nodes are treated as stage II breast cancer. Therefore, immunohistochemical studies for estrogen and progesterone receptors are of value for

CONCLUSION

Surgical and FNA biopsies as well as effusion cytology play major roles in the confirmation and diagnosis of known and unsuspected metastasis. Biopsy of a metastatic site is recommended early to establish the diagnosis and help direct further work-up. Besides

Table 6.9 Favorable clinical subsets in metastases of unknown primary

Cytologic diagnosis	Metastatic site	Sex	Suspected 1st site	Therapy	Median response rate/survival
*Adenocarcinoma	Peritoneal	F	Ovarian or peritoneal	Treat as stage III ovary	11–23 months
*Adenocarcinoma	Axillary nodes	F	Breast (55–75%)	Treat as stage II breast	Similar to breast
*Adenocarcinoma	Skeletal + elevated PSA	M	Prostate	Hormonal	18 months
PD NEC	Multiple	M/F	**Not lung	Chemotherapy	80%
Squamous carcinoma	Cervical or inguinal LN	M/F	Head & neck (20–50%) or anorectal/genital	Node dissection + irradiation	25–50% 5-year
PD carcinoma	Mediastinal/retroperitoneal	M	EG germ cell tumor	Chemotherapy	60%

LN, lymph node; PD, poorly differentiated; NEC, neuroendocrine carcinoma; EG, extragonadal
*Adenocarcinoma: well to moderately differentiated
**Multiple sites are usually involved. Lung primary is not considered favorable.

Table 6.10 General principles to be considered in analysis of suspected metastasis

1 Unusual cytology or histology for site
2 Clinical history of previous malignancy
3 Review of previous cytology/surgical pathology material
4 Ancillary studies in selected cases
5 Tissue confirmation in unresolved cases before definitive treatment

*Modified from Elsheikh TM, et al. Fine needle aspiration cytology of metastatic malignancies involving unusual sites. Am J Clin Pathol 1997; 108 (Suppl 1): S12–S21.

establishing a diagnosis of metastatic malignancy, pathologists are being asked more frequently to determine possible primary sites. Most metastatic malignancies, however, are adenocarcinomas and

may not show specific cytologic features that help establish the site of origin. For this reason, pathologists should also be familiar with the more usual patterns and presentations of common metastases to such organs as lung, liver, large bones, and lymph nodes. Also, metastases to unusual sites such as breast, pancreas, kidney, thyroid, and small bones may pose diagnostic problems on clinical and cytological examination, and may result in misdiagnosis. Familiarity with cytologic and histologic features of the common malignancies originating in a primary site are necessary. The recognition, then, of an uncharacteristic cytohistologic morphologic pattern for that site is the best clue to establishing a diagnosis of metastatic cancer. Previous clinical history of malignancy and review of surgical/cytologic material for comparison are essential in making a definitive diagnosis. Ancillary studies, especially IHC, can also be extremely valuable in selected cases (Table 6.10). A correct diagnosis of metastatic malignancy can substantially alter the therapeutic management of patients and possibly prevent unnecessary radical surgery.

REFERENCES

1. Dorland's Medical Dict. 27th edn. Philadelphia: WB Saunders; 1988.
2. Nicolson GL. Cancer progression and growth: relationship of paracrine and autocrine growth mechanisms to organ preference of metastasis. Exp Cell Res 1993; 204: 171–180.
3. Cotran RS, Kumar V, Robins SL. Robin's pathologic basis of diseases. 5th edn. Philadelphia: WB Saunders; 1994.
4. Schipper JH, Frixen UH, Behrens J, et al. E-cadherin expression in squamous cell carcinomas of the head and neck: inverse correlation with tumor dedifferentiation and lymph node metastasis. Cancer Res 1991; 51: 6328–6337.
5. Ruoslahti E. Integrins. J Clin Invest 1991; 87: 1.
6. Koretz K, Schlag P, Boumsell L, Moller P. Expression of VLA-alpha 2, VLA-alpha 6, and VLA-beta 1 chains in normal mucosa and adenomas of the colon, and in colon carcinomas and their liver metastases. Am J Pathol 1991; 138–741.
7. Fidler IJ. Cancer biology: invasion and metastasis. In: Abeloff MD, ed. Clinical oncology. 2nd edn. Philadelphia: Churchill Livingstone; 2000.
8. Liotta LA, Stetler-Stevenson WG. Tumor invasion and metastasis: an imbalance of positive and negative regulation. Cancer Res suppl 1991; 51: 5054s–5059s.
9. Elsheikh TM, Herzberg AJ, Silverman JF. Fine needle aspiration cytology of metastatic malignancies involving unusual sites. Am J Clin Path 1997; 108(suppl.1): S12–S21.
10. Jouanneau J, Tucker GC, Boyer B, et al. Epithelial cell plasticity in neoplasia. Cancer Cells 1991; 3: 525–529.
11. Stoker M, Gherardi E. Regulation of cell movement: the mitogenic cytokines. Biochem Biophys Acta 1991; 1072: 81–102.
12. Weidner N, Semple JP, Welch WR, Folkman J. Tumor angiogenesis and metastasis: correlation in invasive breast carcinoma. N Engl J Med 1991; 324: 1–8.
13. Weidner N, Folkman J, Pozza F, et al. Tumor angiogenesis: a new significant and independent prognostic indicator in early stage breast carcinoma. J Natl Cancer Inst 1992; 84: 1875.
14. Gasparini G, Harris AL. Clinical importance of the determination of tumor angiogenesis in breast carcinoma: much more than a new prognostic tool. J Clin Oncol 1995; 13: 765.
15. Toi M, Kashitani J, Tominaga T. Tumor angiogenesis is an independent prognostic indicator in primary breast carcinoma. Int J Cancer 1993; 55: 371.
16. Suzuki N. Centrifugal elutriation and characterization of tumor cells from venous blood of tumor-bearing

mice: possible relevance to metastasis. Cancer Res 1984; 44: 3505–3509.
17. Nicolson GL, Inoue T, VanPelt C, Cavanaugh PG. Differential expression of a Mr 90,000 cell surface transferrin-related glycoprotein on murine B16 metastatic melanoma sublimes selected for enhanced brain or ovary colonization. Cancer Res 1990; 50: 515–520.
18. Tucker RF, Shipley GD, Moses HL, Holley RW. Growth inhibitor from BSC-1 cells closely related to type beta transforming growth factor. Science 1984; 226: 705–707.
19. Chambers AF, Tuch AB. Ras-responsive genes and tumor metastasis. Critical reviews in oncogenesis. 1993; 4: 95–114.
20. Gilbert HA, Kagan AR, Rao A, et al. Considerations in the evaluation of cancer metastases to visceral organs. In: Grundman E, ed. Metastatic tumor growth. Stuttgart New York: Gustav Fisher Verlag; 1980: 223.
21. Matsushita Y, Cleary KR, Ota DM, et al. Sialyldemeric Lewis-X antigen expressed on mucin-like glycoproteins in colorectal cancer metastases. Lab Invest 1990; 63; 780–791.
22. Roos E, Roossien FF. Involvement of leukocyte function-associated antigen-1 (LFA-1) in the invasion of hepatocyte cultures by lymphoma and T-cell hybridoma cells. J Cell Biol 1987; 105: 553–559.
23. Haskell CM, Cochran AJ, Barsky SH, Steckel RJ. Metastasis of unknown origin. Curr Probl Cancer 1988; Jan-Feb 12(1): 5–58.
24. Schapira DV, Jarrett AR. The need to consider survival, outcome, and expense when evaluating and treating patients with unknown primary carcinoma. Arch Intern Med 1995; 155: 2050–2054.
25. Abbruzzese JL, Lenzi R, Raber M. Carcinoma of unknown primary. In: Abeloff MD, ed. Clinical oncology. 2nd edn. Philadelphia: Churchill Livingstone; 2000.
26. Nissenblatt MJ. The CUP syndrome (carcinoma unknown primary). Cancer Treat Rev 1981; 8: 211.
27. Ihde DC. Approach to the patient with metastatic cancer, primary site unknown. In: Goldman L, Bennett JC, eds. Cecil textbook of medicine. 21st edn. Philadelphia: W B Saunders; 2001.
28. Casciato DA, Tabbarah HJ, Rice DH. Metastases of unknown origins. In: Haskell CM, ed. Cancer treatment. 2nd edn. Philadelphia: WB Sanders; 1985: 225–243.
29. Newman KH, Nystrom JS: Metastatic cancer of unknown origin: non-squamous cell type. Semin Oncol 1982; 9: 427.

30. Greco FA, Vaughn WK, Hainsworth JD: Advanced poorly differentiated carcinoma of unknown primary site: recognition of a treatable syndrome. Ann Intern Med 1986; 104: 547.
31. Sporn JR, Greenberg BR: Empiric chemotherapy in patients with carcinoma of unknown primary site. Am J Med 1990; 88: 49.
32. Kambhu SA, Kelsen D, Fiore J, et al. Metastatic adenocarcinomas of unknown primary site. Am J Clin Oncol 1990; 13: 55.
33. Pasterz R, Savaraj N, Burgess M. Prognostic factors in metastatic carcinoma of unknown primary. J Clin Oncol 1986; 4: 1652.
34. Schlag PM, Hunerbein M. Cancer of unknown primary site. Ann Chir Gynaecol 1994; 83(1): 8–12.
35. Abbruzzese JL, Abbruzzese MC, Lenzi R, et al. Analysis of a diagnostic strategy for patients with suspected tumors of unknown origin. J Clin Oncol 1995; 13: 2094.
36. Lembersky BC. Metastatic malignancies of unknown primary: the medical oncologist's point of view. Path Case Rev 2001; 6: 178–184.
37. Nystrom JS, Weiner JM, Wolf AN, et al. Identifying the primary site in metastatic cancer of unknown origin. JAMA 1979; 241: 381–383.
38. Shildt RA, Kennedy PS, Clen TT, et al. Management of patients with metastatic adenocarcinoma of unknown origin: a Southwest Oncology Goup Study. Cancer Treat Rep 1983; 7: 77–79.
39. Stewart JF, Tattersall MN, Woods AL, Fox AM. Unknown primary adenocarcinoma: incidence of overinvestigation and natural history. BMJ 1979; 1: 1530–1533.
40. Hamilton CS, Langlands AO. ACUPS (adenocarcinoma of unknown primary site): a clinical and cost benefit analysis. Int J Radiol Biophys 1987; 13: 1497–1503.
41. Hainsworth JD, Greco FA. Treatment of patients with cancer of an unknown primary site. N Engl J Med 1993; 329: 257–263.
42. LeChevalier T, Cvi1kovic E, Kaille P, et at. Early metastatic cancer of unknown primary origin at presentation: a clinical study of 302 consecutive autopsied patients. Arch Intern Med 1988; 148: 2035–2039.
43. Smith PE, Krementz ET, Chapman W. Metastatic cancer without a detectable primary site. Am J Surg 1967; 113: 633–637.
44. Moertel CG, Aeitemeier AJ, Schutt AJ, Hahn AG. Treatment of the patient with adenocarcinoma of unknown origin. Cancer 1972; 30: 1469–1472.

45. Steckel AJ, Kagan AA. Metastatic tumors of unknown origin. Cancer 1991; 67: 1242–1244.

46. Karsell PA, Sheedy PF, O'Connell MJ. Computed tomography in search of cancer of unknown origin. JAMA 1982; 248: 340–343.

47. McMillan JM, Levine E, Stephens AH. Computed tomography in the evaluation of metastatic adenocarcinoma from an unknown primary site. Radiology 1982; 143: 143–146.

48. Wick MR, Ritter JH, Swanson PE. The impact of diagnostic immunohistochemistry on patient outcomes. Clin Lab Med 1999; 19: 797–814.

49. Brown RW, Campagna LB, Dunn JK, et al. Immunohistochemical identification of tumor markers in metastatic adenocarcinoma: A diagnostic adjunct in the determination of primary site. Am J Clin Pathol 1997; 107: 12–9.

50. Gamble AR, Bell A, Pearson D, et al. Use of tumor marker immunohistochemistry to identify primary site of metastatic tumor. Br Med J 1993; 306: 295–298.

51. Raab S. Cost analysis for pathologic evaluation of metastatic carcinoma of unknown origin. Path Case Rev 2001; 6: 173–177.

52. DeMay RM. The art and science of cytopathology. Chicago, IL: American Society of Clinical Pathologists Press; 1996.

53. Lioe TF, Elliott H, Allen DC, Spence RAJ. The role of fine needle aspiration cytology (FNAC) in the investigation of superficial lymphadenopathy; uses and limitations of the technique. Cytopathol 1999; 10: 291–297.

54. Prasad RRA, Narasimhan R, Sankaran V, Veliath AJ. Fine needle aspiration cytology in the diagnosis of superficial lymphadenopathy: an analysis of 2,418 cases. Diagn Cytopath 1996; 15: 382–386.

55. Nasuti JF, Yu G, Boudousquie A, Gupta P. Diagnostic value of lymph node fine needle aspiration cytology: an institutional experience of 387 cases observed over a 5-year period. Cytopathol 2000; 11: 18–31.

56. Molinari R, Cantu G, Chiesa F, et al. A statistical approach to detection of the primary cancer based on the site of neck lymph node metastases. Tumori 1977; 63: 267–282.

57. Cervin JR, Silverman JF, Loggie BW, Geisinger KR. Virchow's node revisited: analysis with clinicopathologic correlation of 152 fine-needle aspiration biopsies of supraclavicular lymph nodes. Arch Pathol Lab Med 1995; August 119: 727–730.

58. Nasuti JF, Mehrotra R, Gupta PK. Diagnostic value of fine-needle aspiration in supraclavicular lymphadenopathy: a study of 106 patients and review of literature. Diagn Cytopathol 2001; 25: 351–355.

59. Carson HJ, Candel AG, Gattuso P, et al. Fine-needle aspiration of supraclavicular lymph nodes. Diagn Cytopathol 1996; 14: 216–220.

60. McHenry CR, Cooney MM, Slusarczyk SJ, et al. Supraclavicular lymphadenopathy: the spectrum of pathology and evaluation by fine-needle aspiration biopsy. Am Surg 1999; 65: 742–746.

61. McCluggage WG, Anderson N, Herron B, Caughley L. Fine needle aspiration cytology, histology and immunohistochemistry of anaplastic large cell ki-1-positive lymphoma: a report of three cases. Acta Cytologica 1996; 40: 779–785.

62. Kreicbergs A, Bauer HCF, Brosjö O, et al. Cytological diagnosis of bone tumors. J Bone Surg [Br] 1996; 78-B: 258–263.

63. Bommer KK, Ramzy I, Mody D. Fine-needle aspiration biopsy in the diagnosis and management of bone lesions: a study of 450 cases. Cancer 1997; 81: 148–156.

64. Jorda M, Luis R, Hanly A, Ganjei-Azar P. Fine-needle aspiration cytology of bone: accuracy and pitfalls of cytodiagnosis. Cancer (Cancer Cytopathol) 2000; 90: 47–54.

65. Unni KK. Dahlin's bone tumors. General aspects and data on 11,087 cases. Philadelphia, PA: Lippincott-Raven; 1996.

66. Fechner RE, Mills SE. Tumors of the bone and joints. Atlas of tumor pathology, third series, fascicle 8. Washington DC: Armed Forces Institute of Pathology; 1993.

67. Wedin R, Bauer HCF, Skoog S, et al. Cytological diagnosis of skeletal lesions. J Bone Joint Surg 2000; 82-b: 673–678.

68. Brage ME, Simon MA. Evaluation, prognosis, and medical treatment considerations of metastatic bone tumors. Orthopedics 1992; May 15(5): 589–596.

69. Poigenfurst J, Marcove RC, Miller TR. Surgical treatment of fractures through metastases in the proximal femur. J Bone Joint Surg [Br] 1968; 50: 743–756.

70. Powell JM. Metastatic carcinoid of bone. Report of two cases and review of the literature. Clin Orthop 1988; 230: 266–272.

71. Vieco Pr, Azouz EM, Roeffel JC. Metastases to bone in medulloblastoma. A report of five cases. Skeletal Radiol 1989; 18: 445–449.

72. Filderman AE, Coppage L, Shaw C, Matthay RA. Pulmonary and pleural manifestations of extrathoracic malignancies. Clin Chest Med 1989; 10: 747–887.

73. Yang SP, Lin CC. Lymphangitic carcinomatosis of the lungs. The clinical significance of its roentgenologic classification. Chest 1972; 62: 170–187.

74. Wall CP, Gaensler EA, Carrington CB, Hayes JA. Comparison of transbronchial and open biopsies in chronic infiltrative lung diseases. Am Rev Respir Dis 1981; 123: 280–285.

75. Toomes H, Delphendahl A, Manke HG, Vogt-Moykopf I. The coin lesion of the lung. A review of 955 resected coin lesions. Cancer 1983; 51: 534–537.

76. Colby TV, Koss MN, Travis WD. Tumors of the lower respiratory tract. Atlas of tumor pathology, third series, fascicle 13. Washington DC: Armed Forces Institute of Pathology; 1995.

77. Rosenblatt MB, Lisa JR, Collier F. Primary and metastatic bronchioloalveolar carcinoma. Chest 1967; 52: 147–152.

78. Dodd GD, Boyle JJ. Excavating pulmonary metastases. Amer J Roentgenol 1961; 85: 277–293.

79. Pickren JW, Tsukada Y, Lane WW. Liver metastasis: analysis of autopsy data. In: Weiss L, Gilbert HA, eds. Liver metastasis. Boston: GK Rail; 1982: 2–18.

80. Craig JR, Peters, RL, Edmondson HA. Tumors of the liver and intrahepatic bile ducts. Atlas of tumor pathology. 2nd series, fascicle 26, Washington, DC: Armed Forces Institute of Pathology; 1989: 256–267.

81. Hertz G, Reddy VB, Freen L, et al. Fine-needle aspiration biopsy of the liver: a multicenter study of 602 radiologically guided FNA. Diagn Cytopathol 2000; 23: 326–328.

82. Ishak KG, Goodman ZD, Stocker JT. Tumors of the liver and intrahepatic bile ducts. Atlas of tumor pathology, third series, fascicle 31. Washington DC: Armed Forces Institute of Pathology; 2001.

83. Lack EE. Tumors of the adrenal gland and extra-adrenal paraganglia. Atlas of tumor pathology, third series, fascicle 19. Washington DC: Armed Forces Institute of Pathology; 1997.

84. Tao LC. Transabdominal fine-needle aspiration biopsy. New York: Igaku-Shoin; 1990: 218–248.

85. Suen KC. Atlas and text of aspiration biopsy cytology. Baltimore: Williams & Wilkins; 1990: 225–236.

86. Damjanov I, Linder J. Anderson's pathology, vol. 2, 10th edn. St. Louis: CV Mosby; 1995: 2020–2021.

87. Solcia E, Capella C, Günter K. Tumors of the pancreas. Atlas of tumor pathology, third series, fascicle 20. Washington, DC: Armed Forces Institute of Pathology; 1997.

88. Allard P, Yankaskas BC, Fletcher RH, et al. Sensitivity and specificity of computed tomography in the detection of adrenal metastatic lesions among 91 autopsied lung cancer patients. Cancer 1990; 66: 457–62.

89. Wu HH, Cramer HM, Kho J, Elsheikh TM. Fine needle aspiration cytology of benign adrenal cortical nodules. A comparison of cytologic findings with those of primary and metastatic adrenal malignancies. Acta Cytol 1998; 42: 1352–1358.

90. Katz RL, Shirkhoda A. Diagnostic approach to incidental adrenal nodules in the cancer patient. Cancer 1985; 55: 1995–2000.

91. Lee JE, Evans DB, Hickey RC, et al. Unknown primary cancer presenting as an adrenal mass: frequency and implications for diagnostic evaluation of adrenal incidentalomas. Surgery 1998; 124: 1115–1122.

92. Min KW, Song J, Boesenberg M, Acebey J. Adrenal cortical nodule mimicking small round cell malignancy on fine needle aspiration. Acta Cytol 1988; 32: 543–546.

93. Mitchell ML, Ryan FP, Shermer RW. Pulmonary adenocarcinoma metastatic to the adrenal gland mimicking normal adrenal cortical epithelium on fine needle aspiration. Acta Cytol 1985; 29: 994–998.

94. Sasano H, Shizawa S, Nagura H. Adrenocortical cytopathology. Am J Clin Pathol 1995; 104: 161–166.

95. Ellis GL, Auclair PL. Tumors of the salivary glands. Atlas of tumor pathology, third series, fascicle 17. Washington, DC: Armed Forces Institute of Pathology; 1996.

96. Gnepp DR. Metastatic disease to the major salivary glands. In: Ellis GL, Auclair PL, Gnepp DR, eds. Surgical pathology of the salivary glands. Philadelphia, PA: Saunders; 1991: 560–569.

97. Seifert G, Hennings K, Caselitz J. Metastatic tumors to the parotid and submandibular glands: analysis and differential diagnosis of 108 cases. Pathol Res Pract 1986; 181: 684–692.

98. Batasakis JG, Bautina E. Metastases to major salivary glands. Ann Otol Rhinol Laryngol 1990; 99: 501–503.

99. Elsheikh TM. Salivary gland aspiration cytopathology. In: Atkinson BF, Silverman JF, eds. Atlas of difficult diagnoses in cytopathology. Philadelphia, PA: WB Saunders; 1998: 451–480.

100. Zhang C, Cohen J, Cangiarella JF, et al. Fine needle aspiration of secondary neoplasms involving the salivary glands. Am J Clin Pathol 2000; 113: 21–28.

101. Bedrosian SA, Goldman RL, Dekelboum AM. Renal carcinoma presenting as a primary submandibular gland tumor. Oral Med Orl Pathol 1984; 58: 699–701.

102. Cantera JM, Hernandez AV. Bilateral parotid gland metastasis as the initial presentation of a small cell lung carcinoma. J Oral Maxillovac Surg 1989; 47: 1199–1201.

103. Hajdu SI, Urban JA. Cancers metastatic to the breast. Cancer 1972; 29: 1691–1696.

104. Silverman JF, Feldman PS, Covell JL, Frable WJ. Fine needle aspiration cytology of neoplasms metastatic to breast. Acta Cytol 1987; 31: 281–300.

105. Sneige N, Zachariah S, Fanning TV, et al. Fine needle aspiration cytology of metastatic neoplasms in the breast. Am J Clin Pathol 1989; 92: 27.

106. Page DL, Anderson TJ. Diagnostic histopathology of the breast. New York: Churchill Livingstone; 1987.

107. Palgon NM, Novetsky AD, Fogler RJ, Lichter SM. Lung carcinoma presenting as a breast tumor. NY State J Med 1983; 11–12: 1188–1189.

108. Georgiannos SN, Chin J, Goode AW, et al. Secondary neoplasms of the breast: a survey of the 20th century. Cancer 2001; 92: 2259–2266.

109. Elit LM, Cunnane MF. Breast metastasis from ovarian carcinoma: report of two cases and literature review. J Surg Pathol 1995; 1: 69–74.

110. Alexander HR, Turnbull AD, Rosen PP. Isolated breast metastasis from gastrointestinal tract carcinoma. J Surg Oncol 1989; 42: 264–266.

111. Rosen PP. Rosen's breast pathology. Philadelphia, PA: Lippincott-Raven; 1997.

112. Azzopardi JG. Problems in breast pathology. Major problems in pathology. Vol. 11. Philadelphia: WB Saunders; 1979.

113. Silverberg SG, Masood S. The breast. In: Silverberg SG, ed. Principles and practice of surgical pathology

and cytopathology. 3rd ed. New York: Churchill Livingstone; 1997: 660.

114. Sneige N, Holder PD, Katz RL, et al. Fine-needle aspiration cytology of the male breast in a cancer center. Diagn Cytopathol 1993; 9: 691–697.

115. Lo MC, Chomet B, Rubenstone AL. Metastatic prostatic adenocarcinoma of male breast. Urology 1978; 11: 641–646.

116. Baloch ZW, LiVolsi VA. Pathology of the thyroid gland. In: LiVolsi A, ed. Endocrine pathology. Philadelphia, PA: Churchill Livingston; 2002.

117. LiVolsi VA. Surgical pathology of the thyroid; major problems in pathology. Philadelphia: WB Saunders; 1990: 22.

118. Lernard TWJ, Wadehra V, Farndon JR. Fine needle aspiration biopsy in diagnosis of metastasis to thyroid gland. J R Soc Med 1984; 77: 196–197.

119. Michelow PM, Leiman G. Metastases to the thyroid gland: diagnosis by aspiration cytology. Diagn Cytopathol 1995; 13(3): 209–213.

120. Halbauer M, Kardum-Skelin I, Vranesic D, Crepinko I. Aspiration cytology of renal-cell carcinoma metastatic to the thyroid. Acta Cytologica 1991; 35(4): 443–446.

121. Bourtsos EP, Bedrossian CWM, De Frias DVS, Nayar R. Thyroid plasmacytoma mimicking medullary carcinoma: A potential pitfall in aspiration cytology. Diagn Cytopathol 2000; 23: 354–358.

122. Benning TL, Silverman JF, Berns LA, Geisinger KR. Fine needle aspiration of metastatic and hematologic malignancies clinically mimicking pancreatic carcinoma. Acta Cytol 1992; 36: 471–476.

123. Carson HJ, Green LK, Castelli MJ, et al. Utilization of fine-needle aspiration biopsy in the diagnosis of metastatic tumors to the pancreas. Diagn Cytopathol 1995; 12: 8–13.

124. Frias-Hidvegi D. Guides to clinical aspiration biopsy: liver and pancreas. New York: Igaku-Shoin; 1988: 205–321.

125. Kloppel G, Heitz PU. Pancreatic pathology. New York: Churchill Livingstone; 1984: 107–108.

126. Solcia E, Capella C, Kloppel G. Tumors of the pancreas. In: Atlas of tumor pathology, third series, fascicle 20. Washington DC: Armed Forces Institute of Pathology; 1997.

127. Banner BF, Myrent KL, Memoli VA, Gould VE. Neuroendocrine carcinoma of pancreas diagnosed by aspiration cytology. Acta Cytol 1985; 29: 442–448.

128. Abrams HL, Spira R, Goldstein N. Metastases in carcinoma: analysis of 1000 autopsied cases. Cancer 1950; 3(1): 74–85.

129. Kline TS. Handbook of fine needle aspiration biopsy cytology. 2nd edn. New York: Churchill Livingstone;1988: 495–465.

130. Gattuso P, Ramzy I, Truong LD, et al. Utilization of fine needle aspiration in the diagnosis of metastatic tumors to the kidney. Diagn Cytopathol 1992; 21: 35–38.

131. Bennington JL, Beckwith JB. Tumors of the kidney, renal pelvis, and ureter. In: Atlas of tumor pathology, second series, fascicle 12. Washington DC: Armed Forces Institute of Pathology; 1975: 162.

132. Knapp, Abdul-Karim FW. Fine needle aspiration cytology of acrometastasis: a report of two cases. Acta Cytol 1994; 38: 589–591.

133. Lisbon E, Bloom RA, Husband JE, Stoker DJ. Metastatic tumors of bones of the hand and foot: a comparative review and report of 43 additional cases. Skeletal Radiol 1987; 16: 387–392.

134. Healy JH, Turnbull ADM, Miedema B, Lane JM. Acrometastases: a study of twenty-nine patients with osseous involvement of the hands and feet. J Bone Joint Surg 1986; 68-A: 743–746.

135. Ausburger JJ, Shields JA. Fine needle aspiration biopsy of solid intraocular tumors: indications, instrumentation and techniques. Opthalmic Surg 1984; 15: 34–40.

136. Ausburger JJ, Shields JA, Folberg R. Fine needle aspiration biopsy in the diagnosis of intraocular cancer. Cytologic-histologic correlations. Ophthalmology 1979; 86: 19662–19678.

137. Palma O, Canali N, Scaroni P, Torri AM. Fine needle aspiration biopsy: its use in the management of orbital and intraocular tumors. Tumori 1989; 75: 589–593.

138. Nassar DL, Raab SS, Silverman JF, et al. Fine needle aspiration for the diagnosis of orbital hematolymphoid lesions. Diagn Cytopathol 2000; 23: 314–317.

139. Mclean IW, Burnier MN, Zimmerman LE, Jakobiec FA. Tumors of the eye and ocular adnexa. Atlas of tumor pathology, third series, fascicle 12. Washington DC: Armed Forces Institute of Pathology; 1993.

140. Font RL, Ferry AP. Carcinoma metastatic to the eye and orbit: III. A clinicopathologic study of 28 cases metastatic to the orbit. Cancer 1976; 38: 1326–1335.

141. Orcutt JC, Char DH. Melanoma metastatic to the orbit. Ophthalmology 1988; 95: 1033–1037.

142. Shields JA, Shields CL, Ehya H, et al. Fine needle aspiration biopsy of suspected intraocular tumors. Ophthalmology 1993; 100: 1677–1684.

143. Linsk JA, Franzen S. Diseases of the lymph node and spleen. In: Linsk JA, Franzen S, eds. Clinical aspiration cytology. 2nd edn. Philadelphia: JB Lippincott; 1989: 354–358.

144. Soderstrom N. Anatomy and histology of the spleen. In: Zajcek I, ed. Aspiration biopsy cytology. monographs in clinical cytology. 7th vol, 2nd pt. Cytology of infradiaphragmatic organs. Basal: S Karger; 1979: 224–247.

145. Taavitsainen M, Koivuniemi A, Helminen J, et al. Aspiration biopsy of the spleen in patients with sarcoidosis. Acta Radiol 1987; 28: 723–725.

146. Cristallini EG, Peciarolo A, Bolis GB, Valenti L. Fine needle aspiration biopsy diagnosis of a splenic metastasis from a papillary serous ovarian adenocarcinoma. Acta Cytol 1991; 35: 560–562.

147. Nosanchuk JS, Tyler WS, Terepka RH. Fine needle aspiration of spleen: diagnosis of a solitary ovarian metastasis. Diagn Cytopathol 1988; 4: 159–161.

148. Silverman JF, Geisinger KR, Raab SS, Stanley MW. Fine needle aspiration biopsy of the spleen in the evaluation of neoplastic disorders. Acta Cytol 1993; 2: 158–162.

149. Kline TS. Handbook of fine needle aspiration biopsy cytology. 2nd edn. New York: Churchill Livingstone; 1988: 495–465.

150. Wolf BC, Neiman RS, eds. Disorders of the spleen. Major problems in pathology. Philadelphia: WB Saunders; 1989: 199–204.

151. Richardson JF, Katayama I. Neoplasm to neoplasm metastasis: an acidophilic adenoma harboring metastatic carcinoma: a case report. Arch Pathol Lab Med 1971; 91: 135–139.

152. Khuraana KK, Powers CN. Basaloid squamous carcinoma metastatic to renal cell carcinoma: fine needle aspiration cytology of tumor-to-tumor metastasis. Diagn Cytopathol 1997; 17: 379–382.

153. Baloch ZW, LiVolsi VA. Tumor-to-tumor metastasis to follicular variant of papillary carcinoma of thyroid. Arch Pathol Lab Med 1999; 123: 703–706.

154. Ro JY, Guerrieri C, El-Naggar AK, et al. Carcinomas metastatic to follicular adenomas of the thyroid gland. Report of two cases. Arch Pathol Lab Med 1994; 118: 551–556.

155. Green LK, Ro JY, Mackay B, et al. Renal cell carcinoma metastatic to the thyroid. Cancer 1989; 63: 1810–1815.

156. Cerilli LA, Wick MR. Metastatic malignancies of unknown origin: a histologic and cytologic approach to diagnosis. Pathology Case Reviews 2001; July/August (6)4: 137–145.

157. Sidawy MK, Bosman FT, Orenstein JM, Silverberg SG. Differential diagnosis of metastatic tumors. In: Silverberg SG, DeLellis RA, Frable WJ, eds. Principles and practice of surgical pathology and cytopathology. 3rd edn. New York: Churchill Livingstone; 1997: 303–326.

158. Geisinger K, Silverman J, Wakely, Jr. P. Pediatric cytopathology. ASCP theory and practice of cytopathology 4. Chicago: American Society of Clinical Pathologists; 1994: 265–353.

159. Slagel DD, Raab SS, Silverman JF. Frequency, cytologic features, pitfalls and ancillary studies in fine needle aspiration biopsy of metastatic melanoma with 'rhabdoid' features. Acta Cytol 1997; 41: 1426–1430.

160. DeYoung BR, Wick MR. Immunohistologic evaluation of metastatic carcinomas of unknown origin: an algorithmic approach. Semin Diagn Pathol 2000; 17(3): 184–193.

161. Brown RW, Campagna LB, Dunn JK, et al. Immunohistochemical identification of tumor markers in metastatic adenocarcinoma: a diagnostic adjunct in the determination of primary site. Am J Clin Pathol 1997; 107: 12–19.

162. Dabbs DJ, Silverman JF. Immunohistochemical workup of metastatic carcinoma of unknown primary. Pathology Case Reviews 2001; July/August: 146–153.

163. Dabbs DJ. Carcinomatous differentiation and metastatic carcinoma of unknown primary. In: Dabbs DJ, ed. Diagnostic immunohistochemistry. Philadelphia: Churchill Livingstone; 2002: 163–196.

164. Pilieri S, Bocchia M, Baroni CD, et al. Anaplastic large cell lymphoma (CD30+/Ki1+): results of a prospective clinicopathologic study of 69 cases. Br J Haematol 1994; 86: 513–523.

165. Wick MR, Siegal GP. Monoclonal antibodies to carcinoembryonic antigen in diagnostic immunohistochemistry. In: Wick MR, Siegal GP, eds. Monoclonal antibodies in diagnostic immunohistochemistry. New York: Marcel Dekker; 1988.

166. Ruitenbeek CT, Gouw ASH, Poppema S. Immunocytology of body cavity fluids: MOC-31, a monoclonal antibody discriminating between mesothelial and epithelial cells. Arch Pathol Lab Med 1994; 118: 265–269.

167. Thor A, Ohuchi N, Szpak CA, et al. Distribution of oncofetal antigen tumor-associated glycoprotein-72, defined by monoclonal antibody B72.3. Cancer Res 1986; 46: 3118–3124.

168. Loy TS, Nashelsky MB. Reactivity of B72.3 with adenocarcinomas: an immunohistochemical study of 476 cases. Cancer 1993; 72: 2495–2498.

169. Bast RC, Feeney M, Lazarus H, et al. Reactivity of a monoclonal antibody with human ovarian carcinoma. J Clin Invest 1981; 68: 1331–1337.

170. Kabawat SE, Bast RC, Welch WR, et al. Immunopathologic characterization of a monoclonal antibody that recognizes common surface antigens of human ovarian tumors of serous, endometrioid and clear cell types. Am J Clin Pathol 1983; 79: 98–104.

171. Koelma IA, Nap M, Rodenburg CJ, et al. The value of tumor marker CA125 in surgical pathology. Histopathology 1987; 11: 287–294.

172. Loy TS, Quesenberry JT, Sharp SC. Distribution of CA125 in adenocarcinomas: an immunohistochemical study of 481 cases. Am J Clin Pathol 1992; 98: 175–179.

173. Haglund C. Tumor marker antigen CA125 in pancreatic cancer: a comparison with CA19-9 and CEA. Br J Cancer 1986; 54: 897–901.

174. Itzkowitz SH, Yuan M, Fukushi Y, et al. Immunohistochemical comparison of Le^a, monosialosyl Le^a (CA19-9) and disialosyl Le^a antigens in human colorectal and pancreatic tissues. Cancer Res 1988; 48: 3834–3842.

175. Gatalica Z, Miettinen M. Distribution of carcinoma antigens CA19-9 and CA15-3: an immunohistochemical study of 400 tumors. Appl Immunohistochem 1994; 2: 205–211.

176. Lau SK, Weiss LM, Chu PG. Differential expression of MUC1, MUC2, and MUC5AC in carcinomas of various sites: an immunohistochemical study. Am J Clin Pathol 2004; 122: 61–69.

177. Wick MR, Swanson PE, Manivel JC. Placental-like alkaline phosphatase reactivity in human tumors: an immunohistochemical study of 520 cases. Hum Pathol 1987; 18: 946–954.

178. Niehans GA, Manivel JC, Copland GT, et al. Immunohistochemistry of germ cell and trophoblastic neoplasms. Cancer 1988; 62: 1113–1123.

179. Fogel M, Lifschitz-Nercer B, Moll R. Heterogeneity of intermediate filament expression in human testicular seminomas. Differentiation 1990; 45: 242–249.

180. Cummings OW, Ulbright TM, Eble JM, et al. Spermatocytic seminoma: an immunohistochemical study. Hum Pathol 1994; 25: 54–59.

181. Mostofi FK, Sesterhenn RA, David CJJ. Immunopathology of germ cell tumors of the testis. Semin Diagn Pathol 1987; 4: 320–341.

182. Pallesen G, Hamilton-Dutoit SJ. Ki-1 (CD30) antigen is regularly expressed by tumor cells of embryonal carcinoma. A J Pathol 1988; 133: 446–450.

183. Jones TD, Ulbright TM, Eble JN, et al. OCT4 staining in testicular tumors: a sensitive and specific marker for seminoma and embryonal carcinoma. Am J Surg 2004; Pathol 28: 935–940.

184. Komoshida S, Tsutsumi Y. Extraprostatic localization of prostatic acid phosphatase and prostate specific antigen: distribution in cloacogenic glandular epithelium and sex dependent expression. Hum Pathol 1990; 21: 1108–1115.

185. Kote RJ, Taylor CR. Prostate, bladder and kidney. Philadelphia: WB Saunders, 1994.

186. Frazier HA, Humphrey PA, Burchette JL, et al. Immunoreactive prostate specific antigen in male periurethral glands. J Urol 1992; 147: 246–250.

187. Elgamaol A, van de Voorde W, van Poppel W, et al. Immunohistochemical localization of prostate-specific markers within the accessory periurethral glands of Calper, Lattre and Morgagni. Urology 1994; 434: 84–90.

188. Nowels K, Kent E, Ranshl K. Prostate specific antigen and acid phosphatase-reactive cells in cystitis cystica and glandularis. Arch Pathol Lab Med 1988; 112: 734–738.

189. Golz R, Shubert GE. Prostate specific antigen: immunoreactivity in urachal remnants. J Urol 1989; 141: 1480–1484.

190. Van Krieken JH. Prostate marker immunoreactivity in salivary gland neoplasms: a rare pitfall in immunohistochemistry. Am J Surg Pathol 1993; 17: 410–414.

191. Alanen KA, Kuopio T, Koskinen PT, et al. Immunohistochemical labeling for prostate specific antigen in nonprostatic tissues. Pathol Res Pract 1996; 192: 233–237.

192. Bostwick DG. Prostate specific antigen: current role in diagnostic pathology of prostate cancer. Am J Clin Pathol 1994; 102(Suppl): S31–S37.

193. Lowe FC, Trauzzi SJ. Prostatic acid phosphatase in 1993: its limited clinical utility. Urol Clin North Am 1993; 20: 589–596.

194. Bodey B, Birdie B, Kaiser H. Immunocytochemical detection of prostate specific antigen expression in human primary and metastatic melanomas. Anticancer Res 1997; 17: 2343–2346.

195. Tacha DE, Miller RT. Use of p63/P504S monoclonal antibody cocktail in immunohistochemical staining of prostate tissue. AIMM 2004; 12: 75–78.

196. Jiang C, Tan Y, Li E. Histopathological and immunohistochemical studies on medullary thyroid carcinoma. Chung Hua Ping Li Hsueh Tsa Chih 1996; 25: 332–335.

197. Kovacs CS, Mase RM, Kovacs K, et al. Thyroid medullary carcinoma with thyroglobulin immunoreactivity in sporadic multiple endocrine neoplasia type 2-B. Cancer 1994; 74: 928–932.

198. DiLoreto C, Pglisi F, DiLauro V, et al. Immunocytochemical expression of tissue specific transcription factor-1 in lung carcinoma. J Clin Pathol 1997; 50: 30–32.

199. Anwar F, Schmidt RA. Thyroid transcription factor-1 (TTF-1) distinguishes mesothelioma from pulmonary adenocarcinoma. Lab Invest 1997; 79: 181A.

200. Wick MR, Lillemoe TJ, Copland GT, et al. Gross cystic disease fluid protein-15 as a marker for breast carcinoma. Hum Pathol 1989; 20: 281–287.

201. Mazoujian G, Haagensen DE Jr. The immunopathology of gross cystic disease fluid proteins. Ann N Y Acad Sci 1990; 586: 188–197.

202. Perry A, Parisi JE, Kurtin PJ. Metastatic adenocarcinoma to the brain: an immunohistochemical approach. Hum Pathol 1997; 28: 938–943.

203. Kaufmann O, Deidesheimer T, Muehlenberg M, et al. Immunohistochemical differentiation of metastatic breast carcinomas from metastatic adenocarcinomas of other common primary sites. Histopathology 1996; 29: 233–240.

204. Liu Y, Sturgis CD, Grzybicki DM, et al. Microtubule-associated protein-2: A new sensitive and specific marker for pulmonary carcinoid tumor and small cell carcinoma. Mod Pathol 2001; 14(9): 880–885.

205. Drier J, Swanson PE, Cherwitz DL, et al. S100 protein immunoreactivity in poorly-differentiated carcinomas: immunohistochemical comparison with malignant melanoma. Arch Pathol Lab Med 1987; 111: 447–452.

206. Wick MR, Ockner DM, Mills SE, et al. Homologous carcinomas of the breasts, salivary glands and skin. Am J Clin Pathol 1998; 109: 75–84.

207. Matsushima S, Mori M, Adachi Y, et al. S100 protein-positive breast carcinomas: an immunohistochemical study. J Surg Oncol 1994; 55: 108–113.

208. Dawson RR, Saad RS, Silverman A, Liu YL, Silverman JF. A comparitive immunohistochemical study of microtubule associated protein (MAP-2) in spindle cell neoplasms of the skin. Mod Pathol 17 (1): 377, 2004.

209. Busam KJ, Jungbluth AA. Melan-A, a new melanocytic differentiation marker. Adv Anat Pathol 1996; 6: 12–18.

210. Shimizu M, Toki T, Takagi Y, et al. Immunohistochemical detection of the Wilms' tumor gene (WT1) in epithelial ovarian tumors. Int J Gynecol Pathol 2000; 19: 158–163.

211. Saad RS, Cho P, Silverman JF, Liu Y. Usefulness of Cdx2 in separating mucinous bronchioloalveolar adenocarcinoma of the lung from metastatic mucinous colorectal adenocarcinoma. Am J Clin Pathol 2004; 122: 421–427.

212. Saad RS, Essig D, Liu Y, et al. Diagnostic utility of CDX-2 expression in separating metastatic gastrointestinal adenocarcinoma from other metastatic adenocarcinoma in FNAC using cell blocks. Cancer 2004; 102(3): 168–73.

213. Hansel DE, Maitra A, Lin J, et al. Expression of Cdx1 and 2 distinguishes periampullary lesions by site of origin, tumor stage, metastatic potential, and patient outcome. Mod Pathol 2004; 17: 300.

214. Barbareschi M, Roldo C, Zamboni G, Capelli P, et al. CDX-2 homeobox gene product expression in neuroendocrine tumors: Its role as a marker of intestinal neuroendocrine tumors. Am J Surg Pathol 2004; 28: 1169–1183.

215. Huang J, Behrens C, Wistuba I, et al. Molecular analysis of synchronous and metachronous tumors of the lung: Impact on management and prognosis. Annal of Diagn Pathol 2001; 5: 321–329.

216. Leong PP, Rezai B, Koch WM, et al. Distinguishing second primary tumors from lung metastases in patients with head and neck squamous cell carcinoma. J Natl Cancer Inst 1998; 90: 972–977.

217. Van der Sijp JRM, Van Meerbeeck JPAM, Maat APWM, Zondervan PE, et al. Determination of the molecular relationship between multiple tumors within one patient is of clinical importance. J Clin Oncol 2002; 20: 1105–1114.

218. Su AI, Welsh JB, Sapinoso LM, et al. Molecular classification of human carcinomas by use of gene expression signatures Canc Res 2001; 61: 7388–7393.

219. Dennis JL, Vass JK, Wit EC, et al. Identification from public data of molecular markers of adenocarcinoma characteristic of the site of origin. Cancer Res 2002; 62: 5999–6005.

220. Silverman JF. Effusion cytology of metastatic malignancy of unknown primary. Pathol Case Reviews 2001; 6(4): 154–160.

221. Monte SA, Ehya H, Lang WR. Positive effusion cytology as the initial presentation of malignancy. Acta Cytol 1987; 31: 448–452.

222. Koss LG. Diagnostic cytology and its histopathologic bases. 4th edn. Philadelphia, PA: 1992: JB Lippincott; 1137–1174.

223. Bibbo M. Comprehensive cytopathology. 2nd edn. Philadelphia, PA: WB Saunders; 1997: 589–621.

224. Galindo LM. Effusion cytology. In: Atkinson BF, Silverman JF, eds. Atlas of difficult diagnosis in cytopathology. Philadelphia, PA: WB Saunders; 1998: 168–178.

225. Ehya H. Effusion cytology. Clin Lab Med 1991; 11: 443–467.

226. Bedrossian CWM. Diagnostic problems in serous effusions. Diagn Cytopathol 1998; 19: 131–137.

227. Johnston WW. The malignant pleural effusion. A review of cytopathologic diagnoses of 584 specimens from 472 consecutive patients. Cancer 1985; 56: 905–909.

228. Murphy WM, Ng AB. Determination of primary site by examination of cancer cells in body fluid. Am J Clin Pathol 1972; 58: 479–488.

229. Kho-Duffin J, Tao L-C, Cramer H, et al. Cytologic diagnosis of malignant mesothelioma, with particular emphasis on the epithelial noncohesive cell type. Diagn Cytopathol 1999; 20: 57–62.

230. Niemann TH, Thomas PA. Melanoma with signet-ring cells in a peritoneal effusion. Diagn Cytopathol 1995; 12: 241–244.

231. Fanning J, Markuly SN, Hindman TL, et al. False positive malignant peritoneal cytology and psammoma bodies in benign gynecologic disease. J Reprod Med 1996; 41: 504–508.

232. Sneige N, Fanning CV. Peritoneal washing cytology in women: Diagnostic pitfalls and clues for correct diagnosis. Diagn Cytopathol 1992; 8: 632–642.

233. Price BA, Ehya H, Lee JH. Significance of pericellular lacunae in cell blocks of effusions. Acta Cytol 1992; 36: 333–337.

234. Thomson T, Hayes MMM. Pericellular lacunae in the diagnosis of metastatic carcinoma in effusions: Is this a useful sign? Diagn Cytopathol 1996; 15: 193–196.

235. Finkel HI. An intriguing finding in malignant effusions. Diagn Cytopathol 1989; 5: 233–234.

236. McNeely TBD. Pericellular lacunae in effusions. Diagn Cytopathol 1993; 9: 503–507.

237. Yu GH, Sack MJ, Baloch ZW, et al. Occurrence of intercellular spaces (windows) in metastatic adenocarcinoma in serous fluids: A cytomorphologic, histochemical and ultrastructural study. Diagn Cytopathol 1999; 20: 115–119.

238. Jones D, Weinberg DS, Pinkus GS, et al. Cytologic diagnosis of primary serous lymphoma. Am J Clin Pathol 1996; 106: 359–364.

239. Ansari MQ, Dawson B, Nador R, et al. Primary body cavity-based AIDS-related lymphomas. Am J Clin Pathol 1996; 105: 221–229.

240. Ascoli V, Sirianni MC, Mezzaroma I, et al. Human herpesvirus-8 in lymphomatous and nonlymphomatous body cavity effusions developing in Kaposi's sarcoma and multicentric Castleman's disease. Ann Diagn Pathol 1999; 3: 357–363.

241. Frisman DM, McCarthy WF, Schleiff P, et al. Immunocytochemistry in the differential diagnosis of effusions: Use of logistic regression to select a panel of antibodies to distinguish adenocarcinomas from mesothelial proliferations. Mod Pathol 1993; 6: 179–184.

242. Lee JS, Nam JH, Lee MC, et al. Immunohistochemical panel for distinguishing between carcinoma and reactive mesothelial cells in serous effusions. Acta Cytol 1996; 40: 631–636.

243. Delahaye M, van der Ham F, van der Kwast TH. Complementary value of five carcinoma markers for the diagnosis of malignant mesothelioma, adenocarcinoma metastasis and reactive mesothelium in serous effusions. Diagn Cytopathol 1997; 17: 115–120.

244. Bedrossian CWM. Special stains, the old and the new: The impact of immunocytochemistry in effusion cytology. Diagn Cytopathol 1998; 18: 141–149.

245. Davidson B, Risberg B, Kristensen G, et al. Detection of cancer cells in effusions from patients diagnosed with gynaecological malignancies. Evaluation of five epithelial markers. Virchows Arch 1999; 435: 43–49.

246. Esteban JM, Yokota S, Husain S, et al. Immunocytochemical profile of benign and carcinomatous effusions. A practical approach to difficult diagnosis. Am J Clin Pathol 1990; 94: 698–705.

247. Bedrossian CWM, Bonsib S, Moran C. Differential diagnosis between mesothelioma and adenocarcinoma: A multimodal approach based on ultrastructure and immunocytochemistry. Semin Diagn Pathol 1992; 9: 124–140.

248. Nance KV, Silverman JF. The utility of ancillary techniques in effusion cytology. Diagn Cytopathol 1992; 8: 185–189.

249. Barberis MCP, Faleri M, Veronese S, et al. Calretinin: A selective marker of normal and neoplastic mesothelial cells in serous effusions. Acta Cytol 1997; 41: 1757–1761.

250. Riera JR, Astengo-Osuna C, Longmate JA, et al. The immunohistochemical diagnostic panel for epithelial mesothelioma. Am J Surg Pathol 1997; 21: 1409–1419.

251. Shield PW, Callan JJ, Devine PL. Markers for metastatic adenocarcinoma in serous effusion specimens. Diagn Cytopathol 1994; 11: 237–245.

252. Cury PM, Butcher DN, Fisher C, et al. Value of the mesothelium-associated antibodies thrombomodulin, cytokeratin 5/6, calretinin and CD44H in distinguishing epithelioid pleural mesothelioma from adenocarcinoma metastatic to the pleura. Mod Pathol 2000; 13: 107–112.

253. Jang KY, Kang MJ, Lee DG, Chung MJ. Utility of thyroid transcription factor-1 and cytokeratin 7 and 20 immunostaining in the identification of origin in malignant effusions. Analyt Quant Cytol Histol 2001; 23: 400–404.

254. Afify AM, Al-Khafaji BM. Diagnostic utility of thyroid transcription factor-1 expression in adenocarcinomas presenting in serous fluids. Acta Cytol 2002; 46: 675–678.

255. Ordonez NG. Value of thyroid transcription factor-1, E-cadherin, BG8, WT1 and CD44S immunostaining in distinguishing epithelial pleural mesothelioma from pulmonary and nonpulmonary adenocarcinoma. Am J Surg Pathol 2000; 24: 598–606.

256. Ordonez NG. Immunohistochemical diagnosis of epithelioid mesotheliomas: a critical review of old markers, new markers. Human Pathol 2002; 33: 953–967.

257. Silverman JF, Nance K, Phillips B, et al. The use of immunoperoxidase panels for the cytologic diagnosis of malignancy in serous effusions. Diagn Cytopathol 1987; 3: 134–140.

258. Singh HK, Silverman JF, Berns L, et al. The significance of epithelial membrane antigen in the workup of problematic serous effusions. Acta Cytol 1995; 13:3–7.

259. Leong AS-Y, Parkinson R, Milios J. Thick cell membranes revealed by immunocytochemical staining: A clue to the diagnosis of mesothelioma. Diagn Cytopathol 1990; 6: 9–13.

260. Sakuma N, Kamei T, Ishihara T. Ultrastructure of pleural mesothelioma and pulmonary adenocarcinoma in malignant effusions as compared with reactive mesothelial cells. Acta Cytol 1999; 43: 777–785.

261. Raber MN, Faintuch J, Abbruzzese JL, et al. Continuous infusion 5- fluorouracil, etoposide and cisplatin in patients with metastatic carcinoma of unknown primary origin. Ann Oncol 1991; 2: 519–520.

262. Hainsworth JD, Erland JB, Kalman LA, et al. Carcinoma of unknown primary site: Treatment with 1-hour paclitaxel, carboplatin, and extended-schedule etoposide. J Clin Oncol 1997; 5: 2385–2393.

263. Lenzi R, Hess KR, Abbruzzese MC, et al. Poorly differentiated carcinoma and poorly differentiated adenocarcinoma of unknown origin: Favorable subsets of patients with unknown-primary carcinoma? J Clin Oncol 1997; 15: 2056–2066.

264. Kirsten F, Chi HE, Leary JA, et al. Metastatic adeno- or undifferentiated carcinoma from an unknown primary site: Natural history and guidelines for identification of treatable subsets. Quart J Med 1987; 62: 143–161.

265. Saghatchian M, Fizazi K, Borel C, et al. Carcinoma of an unknown primary site: A chemotherapy strategy based on histological differentiation – results of a prospective study. Ann Oncol 2001; 12: 535–540.

266. Gupta T, Bowden L, Berg JW. Malignant melanoma of unknown primary origin. Surg Gynecol Obstet 1963; 117: 341–345.

Skin, soft tissue, and breast

Surgical pathology of non-neoplastic skin disease

Bruce R. Smoller

7

SPECIMEN PREPARATION

SHAVE BIOPSIES

The vast majority of skin specimens is received in formalin and represents one of three types of specimens. Presumed keratinocytic neoplasms are usually removed for diagnostic confirmation by means of a 'shave' or 'saucerization' biopsy. The resultant specimens are often no more than a millimeter in thickness and often curl up during fixation. The optimal method for processing these biopsy specimens is to attempt to flatten them and to divide them perpendicularly into several smaller pieces that can be oriented properly and embedded. Inking the specimens to assess for adequacy of margins is difficult, if not impossible, in these types of specimens, and is generally not indicated.

PUNCH BIOPSIES

The most common type of biopsy performed by clinicians seeking microscopic evaluation of inflammatory dermatoses is the punch biopsy. A core of tissue ranging from 2 mm to 6 mm in diameter is removed from the skin. Punch biopsies greater than 4 mm in diameter should be bisected (some authors recommend a slightly 'off-center' cut in order not to completely bisect a small, focal lesion) prior to final processing. Those of lesser diameter need not be bisected. Inking for margins is generally not necessary for these types of specimens.

ALOPECIA BIOPSIES

Punch biopsies taken from the scalp for the evaluation of alopecia may be processed in a different method. Transverse sectioning allows the pathologist to examine far more follicular units and enables enhanced diagnostic possibilities. In order to examine the tissue in this manner, the punch biopsy should be bisected parallel to its surface, approximately 1 mm from the skin surface and embedded en face by the histologic technician.

ELLIPTICAL EXCISIONS

The final type of skin biopsy specimen generally received in the gross pathology laboratory is an elliptical excision or biopsy. These larger specimens are often used for the removal of neoplasms or for the evaluation of subtle dermal or subcutaneous processes such as panniculitis or connective tissue nevi. If oriented by the clinicians, it is important to maintain proper orientation with the use of

multiple colors of ink prior to further specimen cutting. A bread-loaf technique is recommended for processing skin ellipses. The tips of the ellipse are so labeled and placed separately in cassettes, followed by sequential transverse 3 mm sections through the remainder of the tissue. Each successive section can be placed in a separate cassette, enabling relatively precise orientation, should this be essential. The older, 'cruciate' method of sampling elliptical specimens is no longer preferred, due to less complete sampling of surgical margins.

SPECIMENS FOR DIRECT IMMUNOFLUORESCENCE

Direct immunofluorescence examination is often helpful in establishing a diagnosis in inflammatory dermatoses. It is important to examine the correct sites in order to maximize the results. For blistering processes, it is important to examine perilesional skin. Examination of the blister itself results in false-negative readings, presumed to be due to degradation of immunoreactants by granulocytic enzymes. It is essential that the specimen be snap frozen or held in appropriate transport media (Michel's or Zeus's) prior to processing, as exposure to formalin immediately extinguishes any immunoreactivity. When evaluating for the presence of immunoglobulins in lupus erythematosus, it is important to examine biopsies from well-developed lesional skin. For lesions of presumed vasculitis, it is essential to examine lesions less than 24–38 hours old in order to prevent false-negative readings.

CLINICAL HISTORIES AND DESCRIPTIONS

As can be ascertained from the above paragraphs, appropriate clinical histories and physical findings are essential to the proper interpretation of biopsies of inflammatory dermatoses. Many dermatoses demonstrate similar, subtle histologic changes that can be helpful in making the correct diagnosis given the proper clinical settings. However, in the absence of such information, misleading or incorrect diagnoses may result. It is thus essential that clinical history be obtained pertaining to any inflammatory dermatosis, ideally before processing the specimen in the gross room.

NORMAL HISTOLOGY

EPIDERMIS

The epidermis, or outermost layer of the skin, consists of the stratum corneum, stratum granulosum (granular layer), stratum spinosum or Malpighian layer, and stratum basalis (basal layer). Keratinocytes account for the vast majority of cells that comprise the epidermis. Other types of cells residing in the epidermis include melanocytes, Langerhans cells and Merkel cells.

The stratum corneum normally has a basket-weave pattern and is orthokeratotic (absence of nuclei). On the palms and soles, the stratum corneum remains orthokeratotic, but has a compact appearance. A zone of clearing known as the lamina lucida is normally present under the orthokeratotic keratin in acral skin. Parakeratosis is never a normal finding in the skin, but is an expected finding on mucosal surfaces. The presence of parakeratosis overlying the skin surface is often a clue to either dysmaturation (such as is seen overlying actinic keratoses or squamous cell carcinomas) or keratinocyte hyperproliferation (such as is the case in psoriasis and various spongiotic dermatoses).

The granular layer normally occupies about 25% of the epidermal thickness. It is at this level that keratinocytes undergo terminal differentiation, develop keratohyalin granules, and begin to express the proteins necessary for the extrusion of their nuclei and evolution to stratum corneum. Changes in thickness of the granular layer can be helpful in making a diagnosis. Hypergranulosis is commonly seen in diseases such as lichen planus and lichen simplex chronicus, while hypogranulosis is characteristic of psoriasis and ichthyosis vulgaris.

The stratum spinosum is the zone of keratinocyte maturation. Basal layer keratinocytes are vertically oriented and have relatively high nuclear:cytoplasmic ratios. By the time the keratinocytes move upward through the spinous layer to the granular layer, they have become more horizontally oriented and have much smaller nuclear to cytoplasmic ratios. It is within this zone of the epidermis that Langerhans cells are found. These antigen-presenting cells appear as small dark nuclei with halos (not unlike melanocytes located within the basal layer). Only rarely are their dendritic processes apparent on routinely stained tissue sections. They constitute 3–5% of all epidermal cells and are present in greatly increased numbers in spongiotic processes.

The basal layer consists of small, cuboidal basal cells, melanocytes, and Merkel cells (that cannot be seen on routine sections). Mitotically active basal cells are present in this germinative layer of the epidermis (and may be seen rarely in keratinocytes in the one to two layers above the basal layer). In general, it takes approximately 28–30 days for a basal keratinocyte to move through the epidermis and desquamate from the stratum corneum.

Approximately every tenth cell along the basal layer is a melanocyte. These cells have smaller nuclei than do the keratinocytes and often have apparent halos on routine sections. The dendritic processes of epidermal melanocytes are only apparent in densely pigmented cells. Each melanocyte provides pigment to approximately 36 keratinocytes through these dendritic processes. In sun-exposed and normally hyperpigmented areas, the density of melanocytes may be slightly increased (every sixth or seventh cell), and in hypopigmented areas may be slightly less dense. Melanocyte density is unrelated to skin color, being approximately equal in all races. Skin color is a function of melanin production and distribution efficacy.

CUTANEOUS APPENDAGES

There are four types of cutaneous appendages derived from pluripotential keratinocytic stem cells. Hair follicles, apocrine glands, and sebaceous glands are embryologically related and form the 'pilosebaceous unit.' Eccrine glands are embryologically distinct.

Hair follicles are present on all skin surfaces except for palms and soles. They are not found on mucous membranes. In less 'hairy' body sites, many of the hairs are vellus, with the follicular epithelium giving rise to small, minimally pigmented hairs. In hirsute areas, the follicular epithelium gives rise to larger, pigmented terminal hairs. In the deep reticular dermis or subcutaneous fat, the hair bulb surrounds the hair papilla. The matrix is in immediate proximity to the papilla, allowing germination. The follicular epithelium is further differentiated into the inner and outer root sheaths. Each of these structures is readily identified in anagen phase hairs, but not in catagen or telogen phase hairs. In normal conditions, approximately 85% of hairs are actively growing (anagen phase). Approximately 12–13% of hairs are in the resting or telogen phase, and the remainder are actively involuting (catagen phase). Alterations in this ratio are seen in conditions giving rise to alopecia. Use of transverse sections in evaluating alopecia biopsies allows the observer to assess this ratio.

Sebaceous glands empty into the hair follicle at the level of the follicular infundibulum. These structures are most common on the face, but are found on all skin surfaces except the palms and soles. Ectopic sebaceous glands present on mucosal surfaces are known as *Fordyce spots*. The germinative layer of the sebaceous glands is at the periphery of the lobules, with the more mature sebocytes located centrally. Mature sebocytes have scalloped nuclei and cytoplasmic microvesicles. They are, at least in part, hormonally regulated and thus are most prominent in teenagers and young adults. They are small and inconspicuous in prepubertal children.

Apocrine glands are present within the axillae and groin but not normally within other body sites. Their function remains enigmatic. These large glands lined by cells with abundant eosinophilic cytoplasm originate in the deep reticular dermis. Apocrine ducts course upward through the dermis and empty into the hair follicle immediately beneath the epidermis. The presence of ectopic apocrine glands located on the scalp may be a helpful clue in making a diagnosis of *nevus sebaceus of Jadassohn*.

The eccrine glands are most common on acral surfaces. They are on most cutaneous surfaces and play a central role in thermoregulation. The eccrine glands are located in the deep reticular dermis and are surrounded by a thin rim of mature adipose tissue. The diameter of the eccrine glands is smaller than that of apocrine glands and the cytoplasm of the cells is less eosinophilic. The eccrine ducts empty directly into the epidermal surface through the acrosyringia.

DERMIS

Collagen is the main component of the dermis. The papillary dermis, defined as the portion of the dermis situated superficial to the superficial vascular plexus, has a high component of type III collagen admixed with type I collagen. The reticular dermis, comprising the vast majority of the dermal thickness and located deep to the superficial vascular plexus, is composed primarily of type I collagen. Elastic tissue fibers are present throughout the dermis. Increased amounts of elastic tissue fibers are present in the papillary dermis with prolonged sun-exposure.

The cutaneous vasculature is organized into superficial and deep vascular plexuses, with feeder vessels emanating from each. At the base of the reticular dermis, the deep vascular plexus courses parallel with the skin surface. Feeder vessels course vertically through the dermis bringing blood to and from the superficial vascular plexus that is also oriented parallel to the skin surface. Small vessels extend from the superficial plexus into the dermal papillae and provide nutrients to the epidermis. No blood vessels are present in the epidermis. The lymphatic system parallels this pattern.

Nerves are present throughout the skin. In addition to the Merkel cells that reside within the epidermis, there are autonomic nerves coursing with the vessels in so-called neurovascular bundles. Nerve fibers are also present surrounding cutaneous appendages and freely within the dermal collagen bundles. Specialized nerve endings have more restricted distributions. Pacinian corpuscles are found in the deep dermis of acral surfaces, while Meissner's corpuscles exist only in the dermal papillae of fingertips.

Inflammatory cells are present in small numbers throughout the dermis. They are situated primarily around blood vessels. Small numbers of lymphocytes, histiocytes, and mast cells are present in normal skin. In addition, several populations of immunocompetent spindle-shaped cells reside in the skin. Some of these cells label with S-100 protein and are related to intraepidermal Langerhans cells. Others label with factor XIIIa and are involved in antigen presentation. Another population of spindle-shaped cells expresses CD34 and invests cutaneous appendages. The function of these cells remains largely unknown. A final population of dermal spindle-shaped cells is fibroblasts. These cells are involved in collagen production.

SUBCUTIS

The subcutaneous fat is divided into lobules of adipocytes and fibrous septa. The large vessels and nerves course within the septa. Various panniculitides preferentially affect either the lobules or septa.

DEFINITIONS OF DERMATOPATHOLOGY TERMS

Acantholysis. A 'balling up' of keratinocytes due to the destruction of desmosomes. This finding is characteristic of pemphigus.

Acanthosis. Increased epidermal thickness due to increase in the thickness of the stratum Malpighii.

Apoptosis. Programmed cell death. Apoptotic cells demonstrate pyknotic nuclei and eosinophilic cytoplasm.

Bulla. Blister greater than 1 cm in diameter occurring within the epidermis or beneath it. Bullae can arise secondary to acantholysis, spongiosis, or trauma.

Colloid bodies. Dying keratinocytes usually found in the basal layer, also known as Civatte bodies or cytoid bodies. These are commonly found in lichen planus.

Dyskeratosis. Premature keratinization. Apoptotic cells are dyskeratotic.

Exocytosis. Presence of intraepidermal inflammatory cells accompanied by spongiosis. This is a prominent feature of many spongiotic, lichenoid, and interface dermatoses.

Hydropic degeneration. Destruction of keratinocytes secondary to intracytoplasmic vesicles. As these spaces enlarge and progressively fuse, the affected cells die. This finding is common in herpes virus infections.

Hyperkeratosis. Increased thickness of the stratum corneum with either orthokeratosis (normal keratinization pattern) or parakeratosis (with preservation of keratinocyte nuclei).

Interface change. Vacuolar degeneration of the basal layer of the epidermis accompanied by infiltrating lymphocytes. A reaction pattern seen in many collagen vascular diseases and erythema multiforme.

Leukocytoclasia. Degradation of leukocytes into small basophilic debris. This is a common finding in vasculitis.

Lichenoid. A tissue reaction pattern characterized by a band-like inflammatory infiltrate that obscures the dermal–epidermal junction and leads to destruction of basal keratinocytes, characteristic of lichen planus.

Microabscess. A small collection of inflammatory cells such as neutrophils (Munro's), lymphocytes (Pautrier's), or Langerhans cells. Microabscesses can be found in the stratum corneum, stratum Malpighii, or papillary dermis.

Orthokeratosis. The normal 'basket-weave' pattern of the stratum corneum. No nuclei are present.

Parakeratosis. See hyperkeratosis. Except on mucous membranes, parakeratosis is always associated with pathology, most commonly a hyperproliferative process or one of dysmaturation.

Pustule. A collection of neutrophils within a bulla or vesicle. May be found in the stratum corneum or stratum Malpighii (spongiform pustule of Kogoj).

Scale crust. Parakeratosis admixed with serum, neutrophils, and nuclear debris.

Spongiosis. Intercellular, intraepidermal edema. This is a characteristic histologic finding in all eczematous processes.

Ulcer. Full-thickness loss of the epidermis.

Vacuolar degeneration. Destruction of the basal layer keratinocytes characterized by the presence of intracytoplasmic vacuoles. This is usually seen in the presence of exocytosis and is characteristic of lupus erythematosus and other connective tissue diseases.

Vesicle. A small bulla, less than 1 cm in diameter.

DEFINITIONS OF CLINICAL DERMATOLOGY TERMS

Atrophy. Thinning of the skin. This can be due to epidermal thinning (such as in lupus erythematosus or old lichen sclerosis), dermal thinning (as is seen in focal dermal elastolysis), or atrophy of the subcutaneous fat (as in subcutaneous fat necrosis of the newborn).

Bullae. Blisters measuring greater than 1 cm in diameter. These may be filled with serum or inflammatory cells and may be tense or flaccid.

Crust. A scab.

Eczema. A non-specific term encompassing all spongiotic dermatoses. Clinically characterized by erythematous, weepy, oozing, erythematous patches and plaques.

Lichenification. Thickening of the skin with accentuated skin markings. Usually occurs secondary to chronic minor trauma.

Macule. A flat change in skin color.

Nodule. A raised lesion that is greater than 1 cm in diameter. A large papule.

Papule. A raised lesion that is less than 1 cm in diameter.

Patch. A large macule.

Plaque. A large, flat-topped papule.

Pustule. A vesicle filled with neutrophils.

Scale. Flakes of exfoliated epidermis.

Vesicle. A blister that is less than 1 cm in diameter. A small bulla.

INFLAMMATORY SKIN DISEASES

PREDOMINANTLY EPIDERMAL PROCESSES

Spongiotic dermatoses

Spongiotic dermatitides are the histologic correlate of the clinically eczematous dermatoses (Table 7.1). They are characterized clinically by erythematous, slightly scaly and oozing patches and plaques. Histologically, each of these processes demonstrates spongiosis and exocytosis, often in the presence of parakeratosis. Spongiotic

Table 7.1 Spongiotic dermatitis – histologic differential diagnosis

Allergic contact dermatitis
Atopic dermatitis
Autosensitization (id) reaction
Dermatophytosis
Dyshidrotic dermatitis
Incontinentia pigmenti (stage 1)
Nummular dermatitis
Pityriasis rosea
Pruritic urticarial papules and plaques of pregnancy
Stasis dermatitis
Urticarial bullous pemphigoid

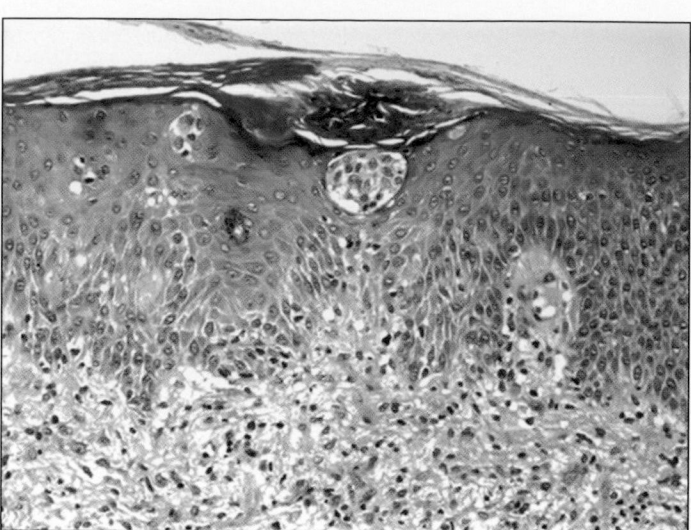

Fig. 7.1 Allergic contact dermatitis demonstrates an acute spongiotic dermatitis with flask-shaped abscesses of Langerhans cells and occasional eosinophils.

dermatoses can be categorized into acute, subacute, and chronic phases, each with slightly different histologic changes. Acute lesions are characterized by abundant spongiosis, often resulting in intra-epidermal vesicles, exocytosis, and a mild superficial perivascular lymphocytic inflammatory infiltrate. In the subacute phase, parakeratosis becomes more prominent and the amount of spongiosis is slightly diminished. The epidermis becomes slightly acanthotic. In the chronic stages, spongiosis is relatively minimal and is over-shadowed by acanthosis, parakeratosis, and occasionally papillo-matosis. Papillary dermal fibrosis is often seen and a lymphocytic infiltrate persists within the dermis.

Allergic contact dermatitis

Clinical features. Erythematous, oozing, scaly patches, often with an angulated appearance arise at the points of contact with an offending agent. The palms and soles are usually uninvolved, perhaps due to the protective effects of the thick keratin layer. The prototypical allergic contact dermatitis is 'poison ivy.'[1]

Histologic features. Allergic contact dermatitis is a typical spongiotic dermatitis. There is marked spongiosis accompanied by exocytosis in early lesions. A serum and neutrophilic crust may be present within the stratum corneum. Intraepidermal vesicles are common. Eosinophils may be present within the epidermis and in the underlying dermis. A superficial perivascular lymphocytic infiltrate is seen. In some cases, flask-shaped Langerhans cell microabscesses can be found in the upper portions of the epidermis (Fig. 7.1). These histologic changes may be present within 6–8 hours of exposure to an offending agent.[2]

Differential diagnosis. Clinical history is required to distinguish allergic contact dermatitis from a photoallergic type of drug eruption. Other spongiotic processes usually have fewer eosinophils, but there is great overlap and clinical history is essential in order to make a definitive diagnosis.

Irritant contact dermatitis

Clinical features. In contrast to allergic contact dermatitis, this reaction pattern requires no presensitization. Contact with offending agents such as soaps and detergents may result in the appearance of oozing, erythematous patches.

Histologic features. The histologic features of irritant contact dermatitis are similar to those of allergic contact dermatitis, but differ in the relatively lesser amounts of spongiosis, the absence of significant numbers of eosinophils, and the presence of occasional

dying keratinocytes. If necrosis is abundant, an overlying scale crust with neutrophils may be present.[3]

Differential diagnosis. Clinical correlation is required to distinguish irritant contact dermatitis from a phototoxic drug eruption. In some cases, it may be difficult to distinguish histologically a phototoxic drug eruption from erythema multiforme. Differences in clinical presentation help in these cases.

Nummular dermatitis (eczema)

Clinical features. Nummular dermatitis is characterized by the appearance of symmetrical, annular, coin-sized, oozing, erythematous patches, often on extremities. The dorsal surfaces of the hands are a frequent location for nummular dermatitis. The lesions are often extremely pruritic.[4,5]

Histologic features. Nummular dermatitis demonstrates the classic features of spongiotic dermatitis. While occasionally present, eosinophils are less abundant than in acute allergic contact dermatitis (Fig. 7.2).[5]

Differential diagnosis. The differential diagnosis of nummular eczema includes all of the other spongiotic processes, and clinical correlation is essential to make a definitive diagnosis.

Atopic dermatitis

Clinical features. Atopic dermatitis is most common in children and presents with pruritic, erythematous patches and follicular papules that often display secondary lichenification due to constant scratching. They are most common on flexural surfaces of extremities.[6]

Histologic features. Atopic dermatitis demonstrates the typical features of spongiotic dermatitis. The inflammatory infiltrate is relatively mild and microvesiculation uncommon. Occasional eosinophils and mast cells are seen. There are often superimposed changes of lichen simplex chronicus (see below).

Differential diagnosis. The differential diagnosis of atopic dermatitis includes all of the other spongiotic processes, and clinical correlation is essential to make a definitive diagnosis. The clinical presentation is markedly different than most of the other histologically similar entities.

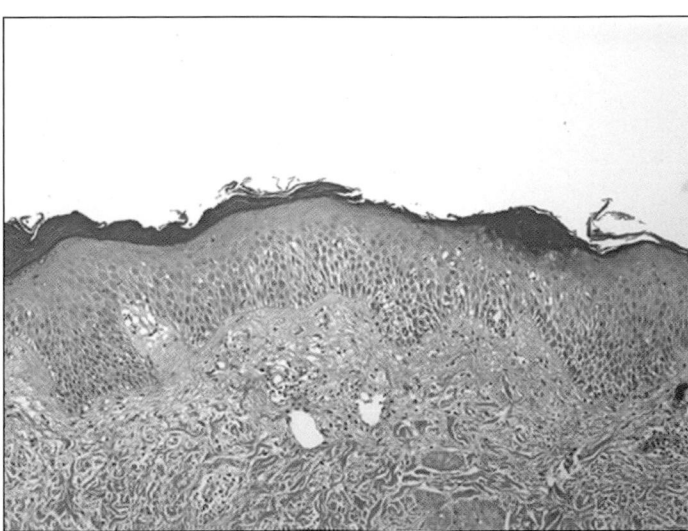

Fig. 7.2 Nummular dermatitis is characterized by spongiosis in the epidermis.

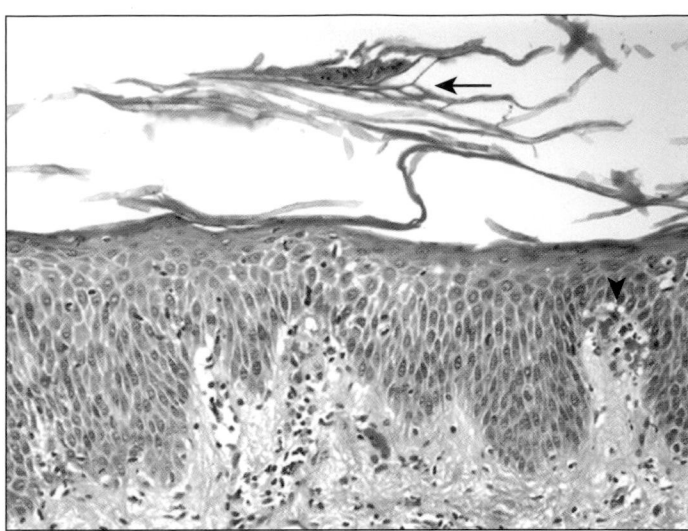

Fig. 7.4 Pityriasis rosea is characterized by a spongiotic dermatitis with tufts of parakeratosis (arrow) and intraepidermal hemorrhage (arrowhead).

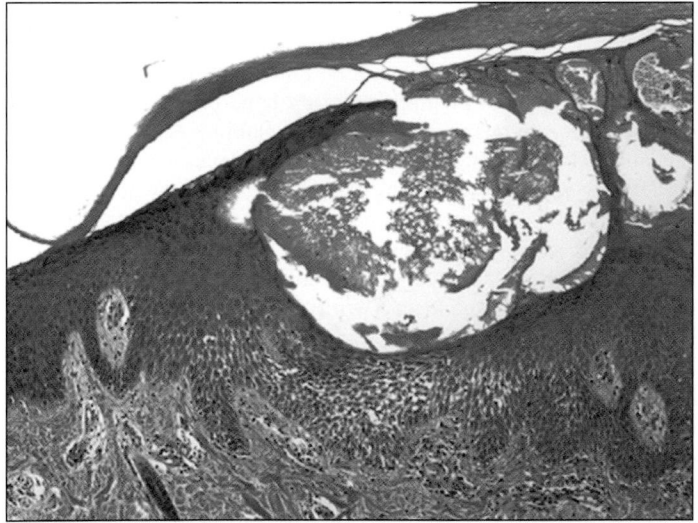

Fig. 7.3 Dyshidrosis represents a spongiotic dermatitis involving acral surfaces.

Dyshidrotic dermatitis (dyshidrotic eczema)

Clinical features. Dyshidrosis presents as multiple small, deep-seated vesicles with erythema and slight scale on acral surfaces. The margins of the fingers and toes are frequently involved. It is often quite pruritic. Dyshidrosis may be exacerbated by emotional stress.

Histologic features. The histologic changes of dyshidrotic dermatitis are those of spongiotic dermatitis occurring on acral skin. Micro-vesiculation is common. Eosinophils and plasma cells are only rarely encountered (Fig. 7.3).

Differential diagnosis. The differential diagnosis of dyshidrotic dermatitis includes all of the other spongiotic processes, and clinical correlation is essential to make a definitive diagnosis. The presence of an eczematous eruption largely limited to acral surfaces limits the differential diagnosis. Allergic contact dermatitis usually has a more

eosinophilic inflammatory infiltrate. A PAS stain with diastase pretreatment may be helpful in excluding a dermatophyte infection.

Pityriasis rosea

Clinical features. Pityriasis rosea (PR) is an idiopathic papulosquamous eruption that involves the trunk and extremities and is most common in young adults. An initial 'herald' patch occurring on the flank is often reported by afflicted patients. Shortly thereafter, there is a rapid appearance of symmetrically distributed, oval-shaped erythematous patches with a fine rim of scale at their periphery. The lesions form a 'Christmas tree-like' pattern over the back and chest. They may be asymptomatic or mildly pruritic and resolve without sequelae in 4–6 weeks. While a viral etiology has been postulated, the cause of PR remains unknown.

Histologic features. Focal mounds of parakeratosis (corresponding to the fine scale seen clinically) overlying small foci of spongiosis characterize pityriasis rosea. Exocytosis of lymphocytes is present in the areas of spongiosis. There is a slight perivascular lymphocytic infiltrate. Extravasation of erythrocytes into the epidermis and the superficial vascular plexus is characteristic and helps confirm the diagnosis (Fig. 7.4). Eosinophils and plasma cells are not common. The presence of plasma cells should raise the possibility of secondary syphilis (which clinically may resemble pityriasis rosea).

Stasis dermatitis

Clinical features. Stasis dermatitis occurs on the lower extremities of patients with peripheral vascular disease. Hyperpigmentation and a 'bound down' feel to the skin often progress to ulceration.

Histologic features. The epidermal changes of stasis dermatitis resemble those of the other spongiotic processes. The histologic differences include a proliferation of thick-walled and dilated blood vessels at all levels of the dermis. In addition, there is usually extravasation of erythrocytes and deposition of hemosiderin surrounding the vascular plexuses. Dermal fibrosis and loss of cutaneous appendages may also be observed. Florid cases may resemble Kaposi's sarcoma (pseudo-Kaposi's sarcoma, acral angiodermatitis). Slight changes in the walls of dermal blood vessels are seen on biopsies from the lower legs of most adults.

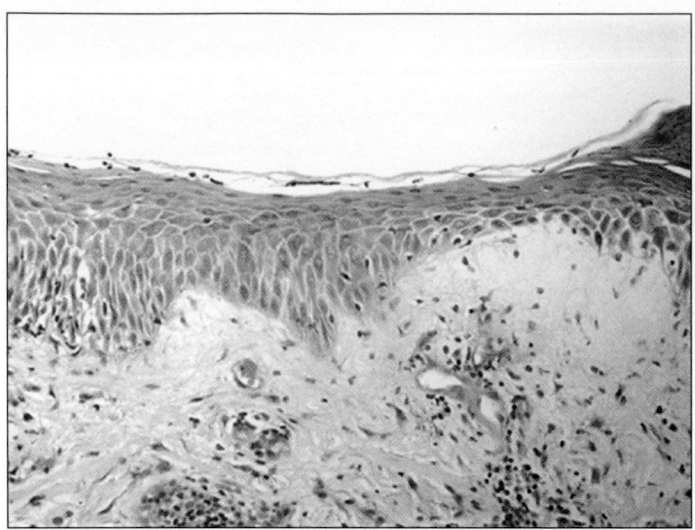

Fig. 7.5 A PAS stain with diastase pretreatment demonstrates hyphal and yeast forms within the epidermis, adjacent to clusters of neutrophils in this case of dermatophytosis.

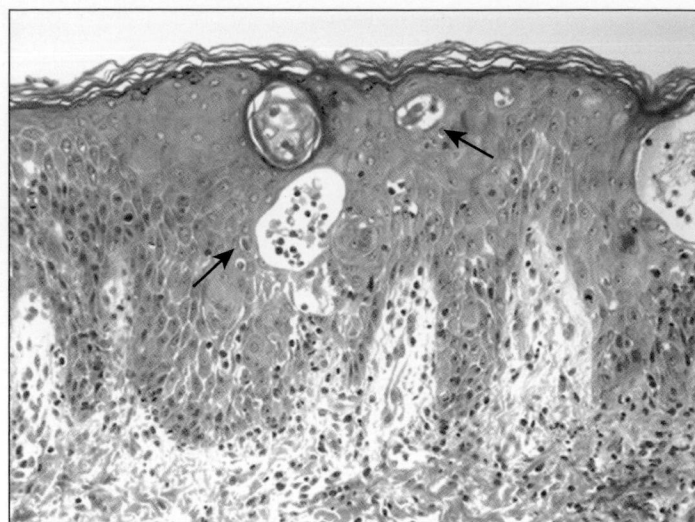

Fig. 7.6 The earliest stage of incontinentia pigmenti demonstrates eosinophilic spongiosis and dying keratinocytes (arrows).

Dermatophytosis

Clinical features. Patients with dermatophyte infections present with erythematous, scaling patches that can be widespread and pruritic. Other patients may demonstrate a vesicular eruption or less commonly, erythematous papules. Depending upon the body site(s) involved, the infections are named tinea capitis (scalp), tinea corporis (trunk), tinea manuum (palm), tinea cruris (groin), or tinea pedis (sole). 'Ringworm' is actually a dermatophyte infection.

Histologic features. The histologic changes are those of a relatively mild spongiotic dermatitis. Within the parakeratotic stratum corneum, slender hyphal forms can be found. These are best visualized with PAS (periodic acid–Schiff) stains with diastase pretreatment or with Gomori methenamine silver stains. Organisms are often found in areas adjacent to neutrophils (Fig. 7.5). For therapeutic reasons, it is important to distinguish dermatophytes from *Candida* infections and *Pityrosporum* species. Potassium hydroxide treated scrapings of the stratum corneum and/or tissue cultures are the best way to make a precise classification of the organisms.

Incontinentia pigmenti

Clinical features. Incontinentia pigmenti (IP) is a rare X-linked dominant genodermatosis that undergoes three stages of development. Newborn girls present with erythematous, linear eczematous patches, vesicles, and plaques that are distributed in a somewhat linear pattern on the trunk and extremities. (Boys are usually severely affected and abort in utero). Over a short period of time (2–6 weeks), the erythema and vesiculation are replaced by verrucous, hyperkeratotic papules that develop along this same pattern. In the final stage of the disease (12–26 weeks), whorls of hyperpigmentation develop along Blaschko's lines.[7] Up to 85% of affected children suffer concomitant neurological disorders, though not all of them are serious.[8,9]

Histologic features. In its earliest, spongiotic form, IP is characterized by a spongiotic dermatitis with abundant intraepidermal and dermal eosinophils.[10] The presence of intraepidermal eosinophils along with scattered necrotic keratinocytes in a newborn is very specific for the diagnosis of IP (Fig. 7.6). The histologic changes in the later stages of the disease are not as specific. In the middle stages of IP, verrucous epidermal hyperplasia is present. In the final stage, rare dying keratinocytes may still be found, but the most prominent changes are those of postinflammatory hyperpigmentation. Within the papillary dermis, aggregates of melanin-laden macrophages surround vessels of the superficial vascular plexus.

Differential diagnosis. In its earliest stages, it may be difficult to distinguish IP from acute contact dermatitis. The presence of widespread dying keratinocytes in IP is helpful in making this distinction. The middle stage, verrucous epidermal hyperplasia, is diagnostic only in conjunction with the clinical history. The final stage of IP, postinflammatory changes, is not specific and could be seen in a wide range of resolving interface dermatoses.

Pruritic urticarial papules and plaques of pregnancy

Clinical features. Pruritic urticarial papules and plaques of pregnancy (PUPPP) is an eruption of the third trimester of pregnancy. It occurs most commonly in first pregnancies and rarely recurs with subsequent ones. Patients present with intensely pruritic papules and plaques, often periumbilical and within striae. This eruption is not associated with any internal manifestations.

Histologic features. PUPPP represents a mild spongiotic dermatitis that is characterized by intraepidermal and dermal eosinophils. In extensive cases, microvesiculation may lead to small spongiotic blisters.

Differential diagnosis. The major differential diagnosis is herpes (pemphigoides) gestationis (see below). Herpes gestationis is an autoimmune disorder that demonstrates a subepidermal blister, also with abundant dermal eosinophils. Direct immunofluorescence examination and clinical history is often helpful in making this distinction. It can also be difficult to distinguish allergic contact dermatitis from PUPPP based purely on biopsy findings, but clinical history helps in these cases.

Adjuncts to diagnosis. Direct immunofluorescence examination is helpful in making the distinction between PUPPP and herpes gestationis. PUPPP is always negative while herpes gestationis demonstrates linear staining with C3 along the dermal–epidermal junction in most cases (see below).

Table 7.2 Psoriasiform dermatitis – histologic differential diagnosis

Acanthosis nigricans

Acrodermatitis enteropathica

Lichen simplex chronicus

Necrolytic migratory erythema

Pellagra

Pityriasis rubra pilaris

Prurigo nodularis

Psoriasis vulgaris

Reiter's syndrome

Seborrheic dermatitis

Syphilis (secondary)

Psoriasiform dermatoses

The psoriasiform dermatoses manifest themselves as scaly, erythematous patches and plaques (Table 7.2). These clinical features are reflected by the microscopic presence of alterations primarily within the stratum corneum and epidermis, including parakeratosis and regular acanthosis.

Psoriasis vulgaris

Clinical features. Psoriasis vulgaris is the most common psoriasiform dermatosis and one of the most common cutaneous eruptions.[11,12] Found primarily, but not exclusively in adults, patients present with erythematous patches with thick overlying silvery scales, most commonly on the extensor surfaces of the elbows and knees. The scalp and sacrum are also commonly involved. Koebnerization (spread of the eruption into slightly traumatized areas of the skin) is common in psoriasis. Rarely, patients develop exfoliative erythroderma. Psoriasis is associated with rapidly increased rates of keratinocyte proliferation and markedly shortened time for transit through the epidermis.[12] Both Reiter's syndrome and psoriasis are exacerbated by infection with HIV.

Histologic features. Diffuse, often thick, parakeratosis overlies an epidermis that is acanthotic. There is regular elongation of bulbous-appearing rete ridges. The granular layer is diminished or absent. Neutrophilic abscesses may be seen in the stratum corneum in about 75% of cases (Munro's microabscesses), or in the upper portions of the epidermis (spongiform pustule of Kogoj). There is usually only minimal spongiosis. Within the papillary dermis, there are ectatic blood vessels, frequently pressed up against the thinned suprapapillary plates. A slight, perivascular lymphocytic infiltrate is present surrounding the superficial vascular plexus (Fig. 7.7). Eosinophils and plasma cells are not abundant.

Variants. *Guttate psoriasis* presents acutely with smaller erythematous, scaly patches, often following a bacterial infection, most commonly β-hemolytic streptococcal infection.[13] The histologic features are similar, but not as well developed as those seen in classic psoriasis described above. The parakeratosis may be more focal than that seen in plaque-type disease. Patients with *pustular psoriasis* also have acutely explosive disease in which abundant pustules occur upon the psoriatic plaques. These pustules may be limited to palms and soles (pustular psoriasis of Barber) or widely disseminated (von Zumbusch).[14] In pustular psoriasis, classic changes of psoriasis are often not found. Intraepidermal neutrophilic abscesses (with possible dermal vascular ectasia) may be the only histologic changes.

Differential diagnosis. The differential diagnosis of psoriasis includes mainly the other entities with psoriasiform epidermal hyperplasia. Diffuse, thick parakeratosis and loss of the granular layer, with neutrophilic abscesses within the stratum corneum and superficial epidermis favor the diagnosis of psoriasis. In addition, suprapapillary thinning and vascular ectasia are not commonly seen in the other psoriasiform processes. Pustular psoriasis may be difficult, if not impossible to distinguish from other subcorneal pustular disorders (such as subcorneal pustular dermatosis of Sneddon-Wilkinson). Guttate psoriasis may be difficult to distinguish from pityriasis rosea

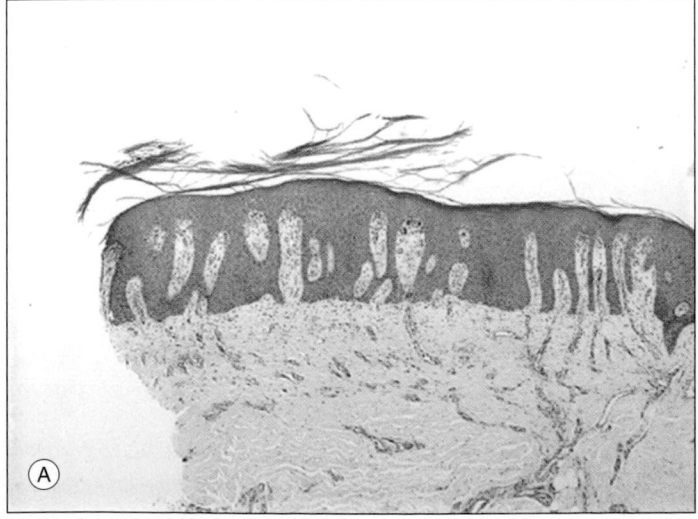
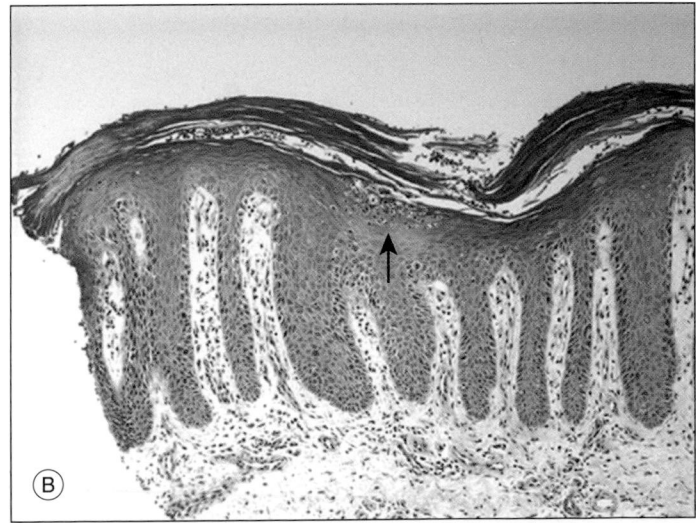

Fig. 7.7 **A**, Psoriasis is characterized by regular elongation of the rete ridges (pattern resembling a comb) with a slight perivascular lymphocytic inflammatory infiltrate; **B**, Munro's microabscesses and spongiform pustules of Kogoj (arrow) are clusters of neutrophils commonly seen within the epidermis and overlying parakeratotic stratum corneum in psoriasis.

and digitate dermatosis (small plaque parapsoriasis), but often the clinical history is helpful in making this distinction.

Seborrheic dermatitis

Clinical features. Seborrheic dermatitis is a very common inflammatory dermatosis, affecting 1%–3% of the population. It is most pronounced on the scalp and face, but can extend onto the chest and back. The disease affects newborns, adolescents, and adults. It presents as erythematous, greasy, and scaly patches and is characterized by extensive flaking ('dandruff').[15]

Histologic features. Seborrheic dermatitis is characterized by psoriasiform epidermal hyperplasia. Parakeratosis is present and is most prominent in the outflow tracts of follicles. A slight neutrophilic infiltrate is often seen in these outflow tracts. Spongiosis is present, unlike in most cases of psoriasis. Within the dermis, a lymphocytic infiltrate is seen within and around the follicular infundibulum. Eosinophils are not abundant (Fig. 7.8).[16]

Differential diagnosis. The major differential diagnostic entities are psoriasis, lupus erythematosus, and acne rosacea. Psoriasis does not demonstrate the proclivity for follicles and is generally less spongiotic. Lupus erythematosus has an interface dermatitis not seen in seborrheic dermatitis, peri-eccrine inflammation, and dermal mucin not seen in seborrheic dermatitis. Acne rosacea is the most difficult to distinguish from seborrheic dermatitis. Sebaceous hyperplasia, telangiectasia, and granulomatous inflammation all favor a diagnosis of acne rosacea, but in most cases, clinical correlation is necessary to make this distinction.

Pityriasis rubra pilaris

Clinical features. Pityriasis rubra pilaris (PRP) is a 'papulosquamous eruption' with five different clinical variants. Most cases occur in adults with erythematous folliculocentric patches and papules progressing in a cephalocaudal direction. There are characteristic islands of uninvolved skin that help in making a clinical diagnosis. Patients with PRP also display a characteristic yellowish keratoderma on their palms and soles.[17] Childhood forms of the disease are also well described.

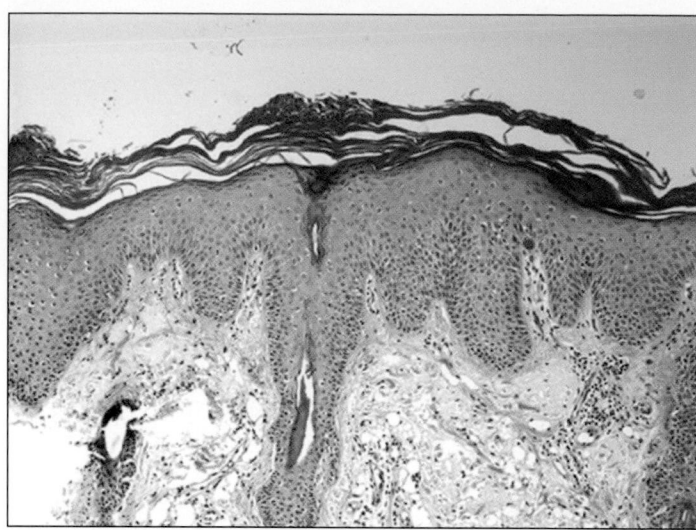

Fig. 7.8 Seborrheic dermatitis demonstrates psoriasiform epidermal hyperplasia, follicular spongiosis and neutrophils in the stratum corneum overlying the follicular ostium.

Histologic features. Parakeratosis is present focally around the follicular ostia (shoulders). The stratum corneum is otherwise orthokeratotic. The epidermis demonstrates only slight psoriasiform hyperplasia with no loss of the granular layer or suprapapillary thinning. Rare, small foci of acantholysis may be present. There is prominent follicular plugging in many cases. A minimal lymphocytic infiltrate is present surrounding the superficial vascular plexus (Fig. 7.9).[18]

Differential diagnosis. In general, the histologic changes, while resembling those seen in psoriasis, are much less impressive. Parakeratosis is focal and usually confined to the follicular ostia. A granular layer is present and there is minimal suprapapillary thinning. A definitive histologic diagnosis is possible in about half of the cases of PRP.

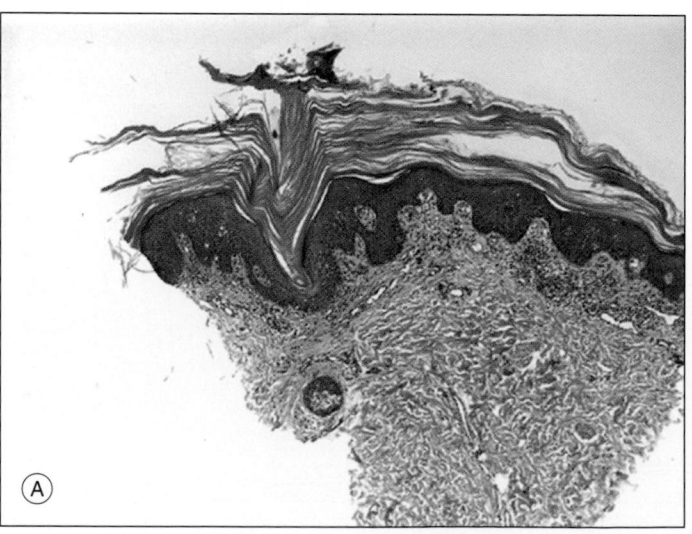

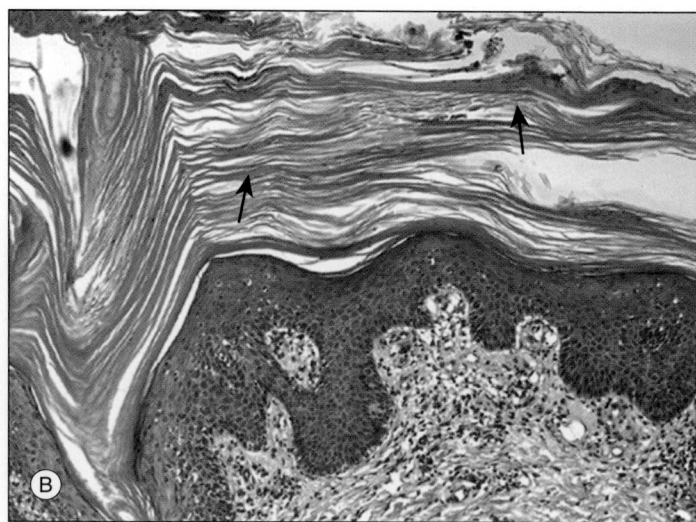

Fig. 7.9 A, Follicular plugging and psoriasiform hyperplasia characterize pityriasis rubra pilaris; **B,** Parakeratosis is present at the outflow tracts of hair follicles in pityriasis rubra pilaris (arrows).

Lichen simplex chronicus (prurigo nodularis, neurodermatitis)

Clinical features. In most cases, lichen simplex chronicus (LSC) is a secondary phenomenon, reflecting chronic irritation from rubbing or scratching. Patients develop a lichenified, or thickened, well-defined erythematous plaque with increased skin surface markings in an area of repeated mild local trauma. Prurigo nodularis represents the more nodular variant ('picker's nodule,' 'worry wart').[19]

Histologic features. The histologic changes in LSC resemble a combination of changes seen in psoriasis and those seen in lichen planus. The stratum corneum demonstrates hyperkeratotic orthokeratosis with variable parakeratosis and wedge-shaped hypergranulosis similar to changes seen in lichen planus. The epidermis demonstrates psoriasiform hyperplasia with bulbous-shaped rete ridges, similar to the pattern seen in psoriasis. Spongiosis is seen in acute lesions but is often absent from older ones. Increased papillary dermal fibrosis is present. A variable inflammatory infiltrate is present within the dermis depending upon the underlying pathologic condition, giving rise to the itch/scratch cycle (Fig. 7.10).[20] LSC is often the end result of chronic spongiotic dermatitis.

Differential diagnosis. The presence of thick orthokeratotic keratin, a pronounced granular layer, and papillary dermal fibrosis and expansion separate LSC from psoriasis histologically.

Secondary syphilis

Clinical features. Syphilis is known as the 'great imitator' on account of its protean clinical manifestations. Most cases of cutaneous involvement by secondary syphilis present as erythematous, slightly scaling annular patches on the trunk and extremities. Involvement of the palms and soles is characteristic and helps to distinguish secondary syphilis from pityriasis rosea and other papulosquamous disorders.[21] Secondary syphilis also gives rise to an alopecia that has been described as having a 'moth-eaten' appearance.

Histologic features. The histologic features of secondary syphilis vary widely. Most cases demonstrate psoriasiform epidermal hyper-

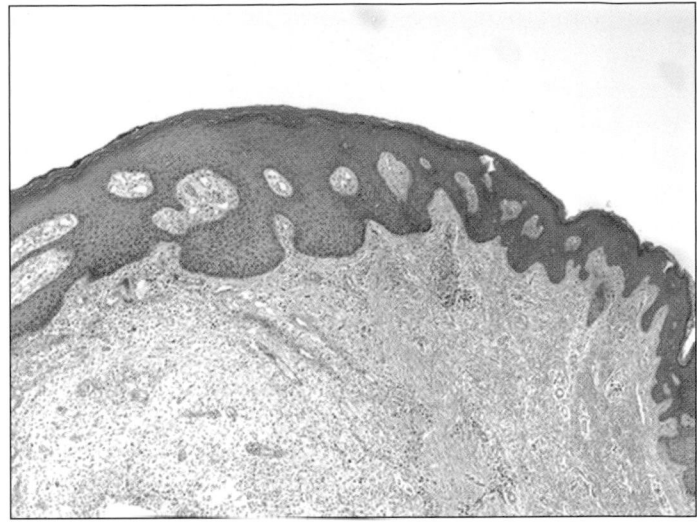

Fig. 7.10 Psoriasiform hyperplasia, hypergranulosis and hyperkeratosis characterize lichen simplex chronicus.

plasia with overlying parakeratosis. Basal keratinocyte vacuolization is seen in many cases. A band-like or even lichenoid inflammatory infiltrate, consisting of primarily lymphocytes and scattered plasma cells is present with focal exocytosis. The inflammatory infiltrate may also involve deeper portions of the dermis. Endothelial cell hypertrophy is frequently seen, but is not specific for syphilis and is rarely a helpful diagnostic feature.[22,23] Rare organisms may be detected, usually within the epidermis or around vessels of the superficial vascular plexus with silver stains (Fig. 7.11).[24] Syphilitic alopecia is a nonscarring process characterized by the presence of a lymphocytic and plasmacellular inflammatory infiltrate surrounding the vessels and the mid-portion of hair follicles.

Differential diagnosis. In some cases, histologic changes are distinguished from pityriasis rosea only by the presence of plasma

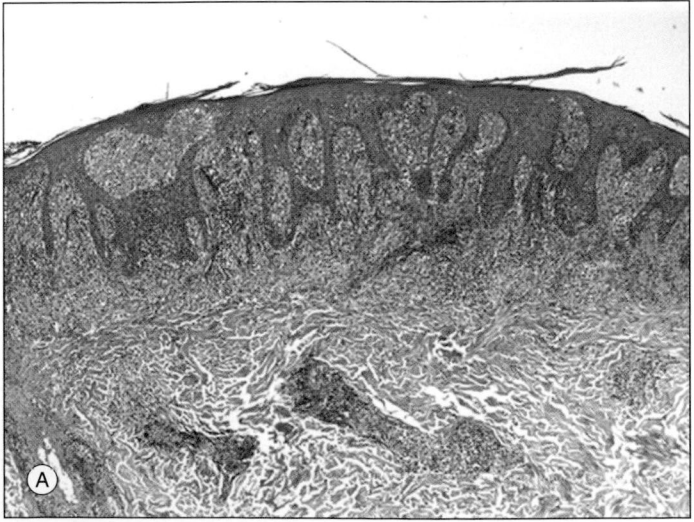
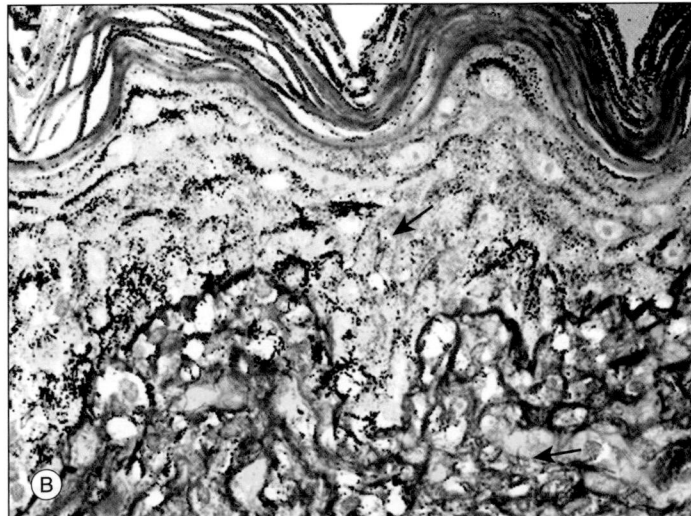

Fig. 7.11 A, Secondary syphilis demonstrates psoriasiform epidermal hyperplasia and a superficial and deep perivascular and lichenoid inflammatory infiltrate; **B,** A Steiner (silver) stain demonstrates multiple spirochetes in the epidermis and papillary dermis, in this case of secondary syphilis. Arrows demonstrate spirochetes.

Table 7.3 Lichenoid dermatoses – histologic differential diagnosis

Graft-versus-host disease (chronic)
Lichen nitidus
Lichen planus
Lichen striatus
Lupus erythematosus
Pityriasis lichenoides et varioliformis acuta
Syphilis (secondary)

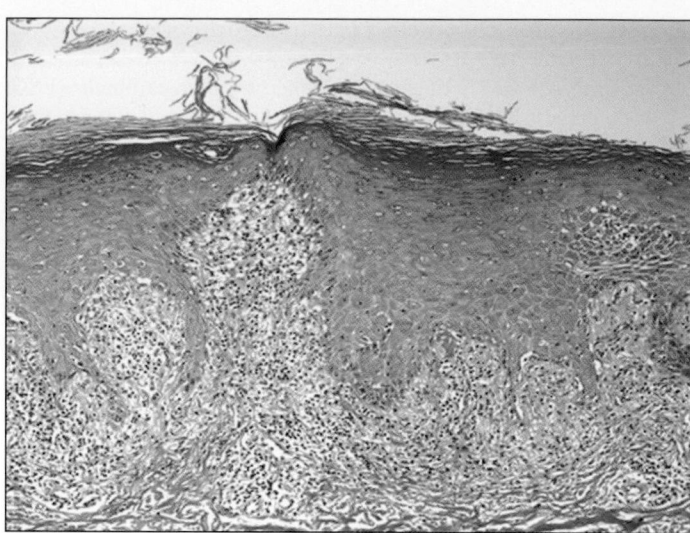

Fig. 7.12 Lichen planus demonstrates hyperkeratosis, hypergranulosis, acanthosis, saw-toothed rete ridges, a band-like dermal infiltrate of lymphocytes and many dying keratinocytes.

cells. In cases where this distinction cannot be made, serologic studies may be helpful.

EPIDERMAL AND DERMAL PROCESSES

Lichenoid dermatoses

The term 'lichenoid' refers to a band-like infiltrate of lymphocytes within the papillary dermis that abuts, obscures, and partially destroys the overlying epidermis (Table 7.3). The cytotoxic lymphocytes destroy basal keratinocytes through a process of vacuolar degeneration. Frequently, the dying basal cells release their pigment into the papillary dermis and the melanin is engulfed by macrophages, giving rise to the changes seen in postinflammatory hyperpigmentation. The lichenoid dermatoses are differentiated from the 'interface dermatoses' based upon an inflammatory infiltrate that is more dense and confluent than that seen in the latter disorders (though obviously there is some overlap).

Lichen planus

Clinical features. Lichen planus is the prototypical lichenoid dermatosis. It is characterized by the presence of flat-topped, pruritic, violaceous polygonal papules. Papules may demonstrate white lines (Wickham's striae) on their surfaces. Lichen planus is most common on the flexural surfaces of the wrists, but can be seen on any skin surface. It can also present in the oral cavity as a reticulated, lacy network of white streaks. Nails may also be involved. Koebnerization is common in lichen planus. The eruption spontaneously resolves within a year in most patients.[25] Lichen planus is either closely related to, or identical to, *lichen planopilaris* in which an identical histologic process involves the scalp hair, resulting in a scarring alopecia.[26] Other variants of lichen planus include an annular variant, which is more common in African-American patients, a hypertrophic variant, which occurs on the pretibial skin, and an atrophic variant, which is more closely associated with a Middle-Eastern population.

Histologic features. Lichen planus is characterized by hyperkeratotic orthokeratosis. Parakeratosis is not ordinarily seen in lichen planus and its presence may be a clue that another lichenoid process is present (i.e. lichenoid drug eruption, lichenoid keratosis). There is wedge-shaped hypergranulosis and the epidermis is acanthotic. Rete ridges have altered configurations and may take on a 'saw-toothed' appearance. There is squamatization of the basal layer and basal vacuolization may be present. Dying keratinocytes, known as Civatte bodies or cytoid bodies are present, usually most prominently near the basal layer. When extensive and confluent, destruction of the basal keratinocytes can give rise to a subepidermal blister cavity known as a 'Max Joseph space.' Within the dermis, there is a brisk, band-like

infiltrate of lymphocytes along the dermal–epidermal junction. The basement membrane zone is focally obscured and there is a brisk exocytosis. Macrophages may be present and may contain pigment lost from the overlying necrotic keratinocytes (Fig. 7.12). Eosinophils and plasma cells are uncommon and suggest the possibility of other lichenoid processes.[27]

Lichen planopilaris is characterized by identical changes surrounding the infundibular levels of affected hair follicles. There is relatively less inflammatory destruction of the intervening epidermis.[28] Some authors regard lichen planopilaris as identical to *pseudopelade of Brocq*, while others consider these to be separate, clinically distinct entities.

Differential diagnosis. A lichenoid drug eruption histologically may differ from lichen planus by the presence of parakeratosis and plasma cells. However, in some cases both of these features are absent, making the distinction impossible without the help of a clinical history. Many drugs have been implicated in causing a lichenoid drug eruption, but gold, thiazide diuretics, chloroquine and quinidine are the most commonly associated.[29] A lichenoid keratosis may also be histologically identical, but the clinical history of a single lesion resembling a basal cell carcinoma or a seborrheic keratosis clearly separates this from lichen planus. In some cases, it is difficult to distinguish lichen planus from lupus erythematosus. The presence of a deep and peri-appendageal infiltrate and dermal mucin favor the latter diagnosis.

Lichen nitidus

Clinical features. Lichen nitidus presents as crops of asymptomatic, tiny skin-colored to hypopigmented papules measuring less than 1 mm in diameter. It is most frequent in children and young adults. Common sites of involvement include the extremities and the genitals.[30]

Histologic features. Lichen nitidus gives rise to a 'ball and claw' type histologic configuration. Each of the clinical papules corresponds to a small focus of active disease in which small areas of parakeratosis overlie focally acanthotic epidermis. In these areas, adjacent rete ridges are abnormally elongated and envelop an

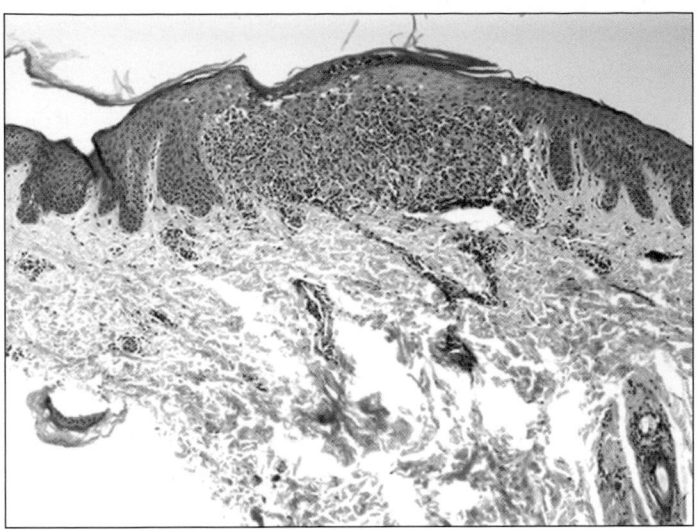

Fig. 7.13 Lichen nitidus demonstrates the 'ball and claw' pattern with focal epidermal hyperplasia enwrapping an aggregate of histiocytes and lymphocytes in the papillary dermis.

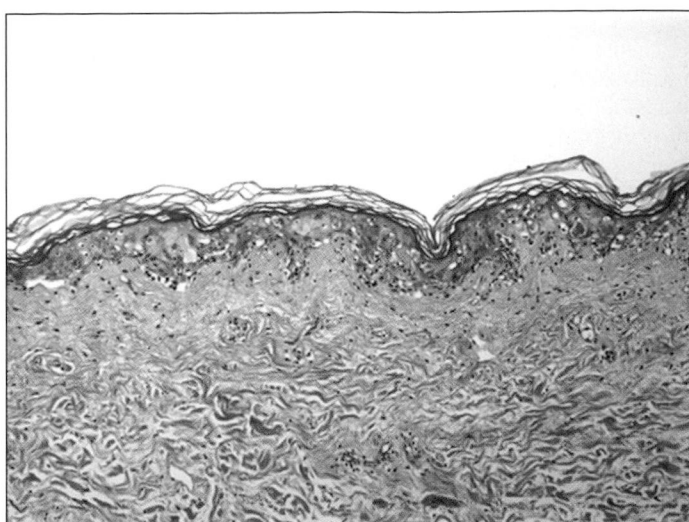

Fig. 7.14 Dying keratinocytes and a modest lymphocytic infiltrate with exocytosis are seen in erythema multiforme.

aggregate of lymphocytes and histiocytes that abuts and partially obscures the dermal–epidermal junction. Exocytosis is present. Scattered dying keratinocytes are often present. Occasional multinucleated giant cells may be seen (Fig. 7.13).[31]

Interface dermatoses

Interface dermatitis is a category that includes a wide range of inflammatory processes, including collagen vascular diseases, erythema multiforme, graft-versus-host disease, and pityriasis lichenoides et varioliformis acuta, amongst many others (Table 7.4). Each of these diseases demonstrates an acute phase during which erythematous lesions are present, and a chronic phase that is characterized by postinflammatory pigmentary alterations. All are characterized by a superficial perivascular lymphocytic infiltrate, exocytosis, and dying keratinocytes.

Erythema multiforme

Clinical features. Erythema multiforme is the prototypical interface dermatitis. Erythematous papules and macules develop central areas of necrosis and bullae. These 'targetoid' or 'iris' lesions are most common on the extremities and are slightly more common in young adults than in older patients. Erythematous plaques, vesicles and bullae are also seen in some cases, but are less specific than are the targetoid lesions.[32,33] Most cases are idiopathic, but many are related to infections with herpes virus or *Mycoplasma pneumoniae*, or ingested drugs.[34–36]

The more serious variant of erythema multiforme that involves at least two mucous membranes is known as Stevens-Johnson syndrome (SJS). SJS is most commonly related to therapeutic drugs and can be life threatening.[32]

Toxic epidermal necrolysis (TEN) is a bullous drug eruption. Large, flaccid bullae give rise to sheets of epidermis that rapidly desquamate following exposure to certain drugs in this idiopathic, life-threatening condition. While still controversial, most authors consider TEN to be a severe variant of erythema multiforme.[32,37]

Fixed drug eruption is a condition in which lesions recur at identical body sites with repeated exposures to inciting agents.

Table 7.4 Interface dermatoses – histologic differential diagnosis

Dermatomyositis

Erythema dyschromicum perstans

Erythema multiforme

Fixed drug eruption

Graft-versus-host disease (acute)

Lupus erythematosus

Pityriasis lichenoides chronica

Primary lesions may be erythematous patches or bullae and are most common on the face and the genitalia. The lesions become progressively hyperpigmented with each recurrence. Tetracyclines, barbiturates and phenolphthalein are commonly implicated agents.

Histologic features. Orthokeratotic keratin is present overlying an epidermis that is remarkable for the presence of scattered dying keratinocytes. There is papillary dermal edema along with exocytosis of lymphocytes in the areas of the dying cells.[38] There is a superficial perivascular lymphocytic infiltrate (Fig. 7.14). Eosinophils may present in drug-related cases. The absence of parakeratosis helps distinguish erythema multiforme from other interface dermatoses. The histologic features of SJS differ from classic erythema multiforme only by involving mucosal surfaces.

TEN demonstrates full-thickness epidermal necrosis and resultant subepidermal blister formation. The inflammatory infiltrate is often strikingly sparse. TEN must be differentiated from the clinically similar staphylococcal scalded skin syndrome. In the latter condition, the desquamated skin occurs high in the epidermis (within the granular layer), while in TEN there is full-thickness epidermal desquamation. This distinction can be made easily on frozen section of the strips of desquamated epidermis.

Fixed drug eruptions are histologically identical to erythema multiforme except that in recurrent lesions melanin-laden macrophages may be observed in the papillary dermis.

Differential diagnosis. It is often not possible to distinguish erythema multiforme from graft-versus-host disease; however, involvement of the acrosyringia (intraepidermal portions of eccrine ducts) may be more common in drug-related erythema multiforme than in graft-versus-host disease.[35] PLEVA (below) usually has a more intense inflammatory infiltrate than does erythema multiforme. In addition, the presence of diffuse parakeratosis, and epidermal and extensive dermal hemorrhage favor the diagnosis of PLEVA over that of erythema multiforme.

Adjuncts to diagnosis. Direct immunofluorescence demonstrates immunoglobulins and complement within vessels in the papillary dermis, but these findings are not specific for erythema multiforme.

Graft-versus-host disease

Clinical features. Graft-versus-host disease (GVHD) occurs in patients receiving allogeneic bone marrow transplants.[39] Less intense, but similar eruptions have been described in patients receiving autologous transplants and solid organ transplants.[40] Patients develop erythematous macules, most prominent on the trunk and extremities, usually more than two weeks following transplantation. Acute lesions most commonly develop within three months of transplantation, but can occur at more extended periods. With time, the eruption heals, often with postinflammatory changes. The chronic forms of the disease present as lichenoid papules and/or areas of dense sclerosis resembling scleroderma with overlying pigmentary alterations.[41,42]

Histologic features. The histologic features of acute graft-versus-host disease are quite similar to those seen in erythema multiforme. Scattered dying keratinocytes are present within the epidermis. There may be some keratinocyte dysmaturation secondary to recent chemotherapeutic intervention. There is a relatively slight superficial, perivascular lymphocytic infiltrate with slight exocytosis (Fig. 7.15). Plasma cells and eosinophils are not abundant.

Chronic GVHD has two histologic appearances. In some cases, changes that are essentially identical to lichen planus arise. There is hyperkeratosis, hypergranulosis and acanthosis, a lichenoid inflammatory infiltrate, and abundant dying keratinocytes. In other cases, a picture similar to scleroderma arises, characterized by markedly thickened and sclerotic dermal collagen.

Differential diagnosis. It is not possible to distinguish acute graft-versus-host disease from chemotherapy-induced changes prior to 21 days post-transplantation, and extreme caution should be exercised in making this diagnosis prior to that time. It is also usually difficult, if not impossible, to distinguish acute graft-versus-host disease from erythema multiforme.

Pityriasis lichenoides et varioliformis acuta

Clinical features. Pityriasis lichenoides et varioliformis acuta (PLEVA), also known as Mucha-Habermann disease, is a disease of adolescents and young adults. Patients present with erythematous papules and nodules that are scaly, hemorrhagic and may become ulcerated and necrotic. The individual lesions are most common on the trunk and extremities and last for several days to weeks. The individual lesions heal with scarring resembling smallpox (hence the name, varioliformis). The process is relatively asymptomatic to mildly pruritic. The entire eruption may last for months to years.

Histologic features. PLEVA is characterized by a confluent parakeratotic scale overlying an epidermis that may be acanthotic or slightly atrophic. Dying keratinocytes are abundant and may be surrounded by neutrophils. Extravasation of erythrocytes is present, possibly due to lymphocytic infiltration of dermal vascular walls. There is a brisk perivascular lymphocytic inflammatory infiltrate

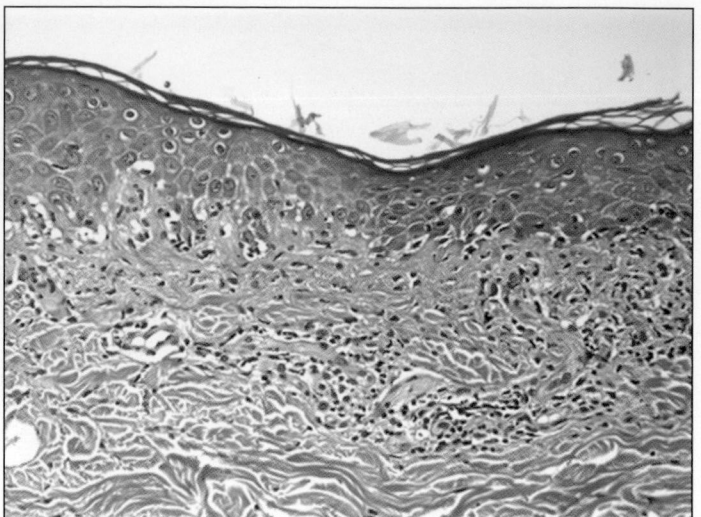

Fig. 7.15 A slight lymphocytic exocytosis and focal dying keratinocytes characterize graft-versus-host disease.

with abundant exocytosis. The inflammatory infiltrate may extend into the mid-reticular dermis. The infiltrate is more intense in the superficial dermis, giving it a wedge-like appearance (Fig. 7.16). Eosinophils and plasma cells are not commonly seen in PLEVA.

Differential diagnosis. The presence of parakeratosis, more extensive inflammation, and intra-epidermal and dermal extravasated erythrocytes help distinguish PLEVA from other interface dermatoses.

Pityriasis lichenoides chronica

Clinical features. Pityriasis lichenoides chronica (PLC) can be thought of as the milder variant of PLEVA. Individual lesions have a less pronounced, 'wafer-like' scale, rarely ulcerate, and tend to last for weeks. The disease process, which is relatively asymptomatic, may last for months to years.

Histologic features. PLC is characterized by bands of parakeratosis overlying epidermis that may be slightly acanthotic or atrophic. There is a relatively modest exocytosis and a superficial perivascular lymphocytic infiltrate. Dying keratinocytes are only rarely present, if at all. There is slight erythrocyte extravasation in most cases.

Differential diagnosis. The histologic differential diagnosis of PLC includes digitate dermatosis (small plaque parapsoraisis), guttate psoriasis, and pityriasis rosea. The presence of dying keratinocytes favors the diagnosis of PLC over these other entities. Tufts of parakeratosis and intra-epidermal hemorrhage favor the diagnosis of pityriasis rosea.

Lupus erythematosus

Clinical features. The cutaneous manifestations of lupus erythematosus are protean. Sharply demarcated, erythematous patches with overlying scale, telangiectasias and follicular dilatation and plugging in sun-exposed areas characterize discoid lesions. Discoid lesions may be present in discoid lupus erythematosus (DLE), in which the disease is limited to skin involvement, or in systemic lupus erythematosus (SLE). The scalp and ears are frequently involved. Cutaneous atrophy and hyperpigmentation are frequently seen in late lesions. Scarring is a common feature of DLE, but is not seen in patients with SLE. Some lesions may be verrucous.[43] DLE may be associated with a scarring alopecia. Patients

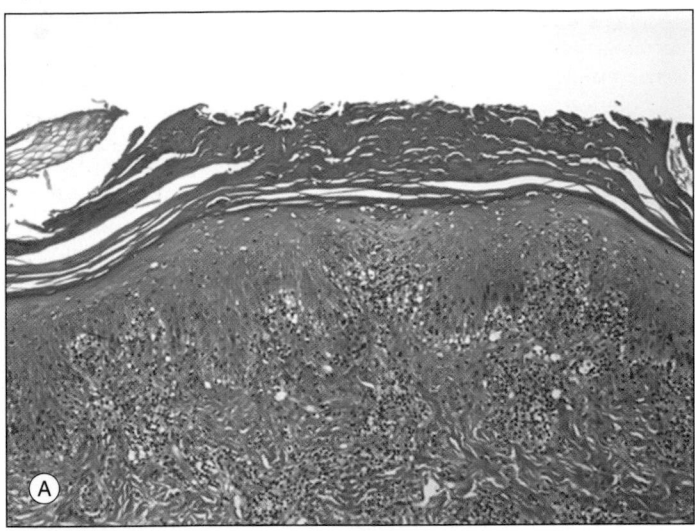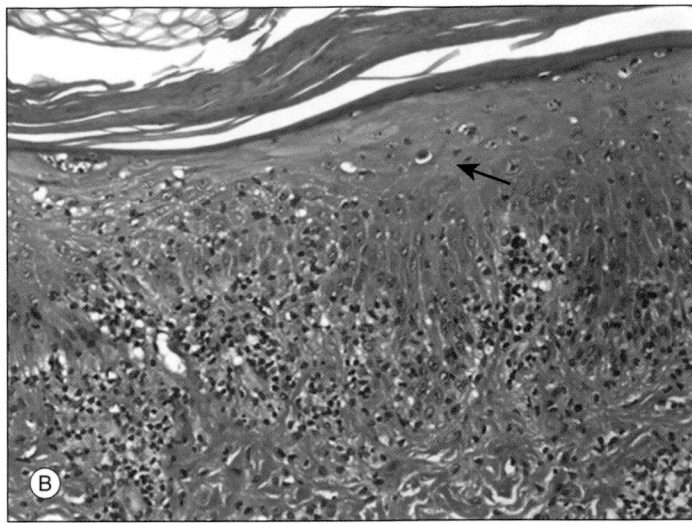

Fig. 7.16 A, Pityriasis lichenoides et varioliformis acuta demonstrates parakeratosis, exocytosis, and a superficial and deep perivascular lymphocytic infiltrate with hemorrhage; **B,** Dying keratinocytes are present in cases of pityriasis lichenoides et varioliformis acuta (arrow).

with SLE frequently display a pattern of malar erythema. Subacute cutaneous lupus erythematosus (SCLE) presents as psoriasiform or annular plaques on sun-exposed areas and is markedly photosensitive. SCLE does not heal with scarring.[44] Lupus panniculitis or lupus profundus show minimal skin changes, but present as deep dermal/subcutaneous nodules (see panniculitis, later in this chapter).[43]

Histologic features. The histologic features are as diverse as are the clinical variants. In general, lupus erythematosus is characterized by hyperkeratosis overlying an atrophic epidermis. Follicular plugging with orthokeratotic keratin is seen. (Patients with SLE may demonstrate less follicular plugging than do those with DLE). There is extensive vacuolization of the basal keratinocytes and exocytosis of lymphocytes. Scattered dying keratinocytes are present. Later lesions may demonstrate thickening of the basement membrane zone (accentuated with a periodic acid–Schiff stain). Melanin-laden

macrophages are usually present and may provide evidence of prior disease in late, burned out cases. There is a superficial and deep perivascular and peri-appendageal inflammatory infiltrate composed of lymphocytes and occasional plasma cells (Fig. 7.17A). Eosinophils are quite unusual in cases of lupus erythematosus. Increased mucin is found in the superficial reticular dermis in most cases, but is less pronounced than is seen in most cases of dermatomyositis.[45]

It is not possible to histologically subclassify cases of lupus erythematosus with any degree of precision.[46] In general, cases of subacute cutaneous lupus erythematosus demonstrate the most intense inflammatory infiltrate and have the greatest numbers of dying keratinocytes.[47] Cases of systemic lupus erythematosus frequently demonstrate the mildest changes.

Adjuncts to diagnosis. Direct immunofluorescence may be helpful in subtyping the various forms of lupus erythematosus. In

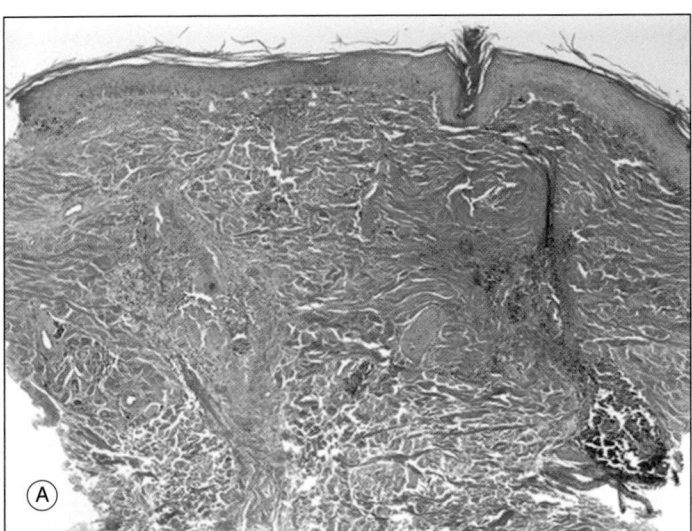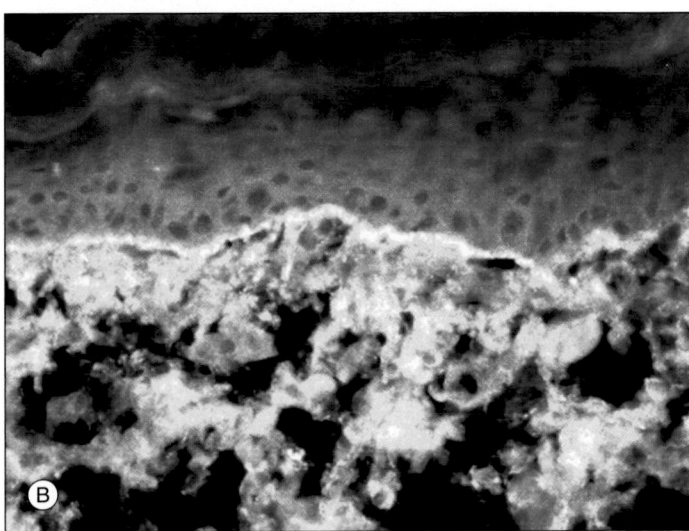

Fig. 7.17 A, Follicular plugging, hyperkeratosis, an interface dermatitis, and a superficial and deep perivascular and peri-appendageal inflammatory infiltrate characterize lesions of discoid lupus erythematosus; **B,** IgG is deposited in a granular pattern along the basement membrane zone in discoid lupus erythematosus.

DLE, nearly all lesional skin will demonstrate granular deposits of IgG, IgM, and C3 along the basement membrane zone (Fig. 7.17B). Nonlesional skin lacks immunoglobulin deposits. In SLE, lesional skin demonstrates similar immunoglobulin deposits. However, sun-exposed, nonlesional skin will demonstrate immunoglobulins in the majority of cases, and nonlesional, non-sun-exposed skin from these patients will also contain deposits in about half of cases. Patients with subacute cutaneous lupus erythematosus (SCLE) display a more varied pattern of immunoglobulin deposition. Lesional skin from about 60% of patients with SCLE demonstrates immunoglobulins. Nonlesional skin from sun-exposed areas from these patients demonstrates staining in about 40% of cases, and nonlesional, non-sun-exposed skin is invariably negative.

Dermatomyositis

Clinical features. Dermatomyositis may occur in patients of any age, but is most common in the elderly. Patients present with proximal muscle weakness in conjunction with a cutaneous eruption described as heliotrope erythema (periocular erythema and scaling), photo-distributed scaling, erythematous patches, and erythematous papules overlying the interphalangeal joints, known as Gottron's papules.[48] (Rarely, there may not be any muscle weakness or evidence of muscle disease.[49]) Later lesions appear poikilodermatous (epidermal atrophy, telangiectasia, and pigmentary mottling). There is a frequent association between dermatomyositis in adults and coexistent internal malignancy. This association is not found in the juvenile form of the disease. Some patients with juvenile dermatomyositis develop widespread calcification known as calcinosis universalis.

Histologic features. The histologic features of dermatomyositis resemble those of a very mild lupus erythematosus. An atrophic epidermis overlies an interface dermatitis with exocytosis, extensive vacuolization of basal keratinocytes, and a mild superficial perivascular lymphocytic infiltrate. Abundant dermal mucin is usually readily observed on routine sections, but may be accentuated with an Alcian blue or colloidal iron stain. Unlike lupus erythematosus, the inflammatory infiltrate rarely involves the deep dermis and there is no peri-appendageal involvement (Fig. 7.18).[50]

Differential diagnosis. The main differential diagnosis of dermatomyositis is lupus erythematosus. The presence of a deep and peri-appendageal inflammatory infiltrate favors the latter diagnosis. The clinical appearance of the cutaneous eruptions may also help with the diagnosis.

Adjuncts to diagnosis. Direct immunofluorescence does not demonstrate immune complexes along the basement membrane zone in patients with lupus erythematosus.[51] Deposition of the C5-9 membrane attack complex along the dermal–epidermal junction has been described as characteristic of dermatomyositis. Serologies are a useful adjunct to this differential diagnosis.

DERMATOSES INVOLVING PRIMARILY THE DERMIS

Superficial (and deep) perivascular dermatoses
(Table 7.5)

Polymorphous light eruption

Clinical features. Polymorphous light eruption (PMLE) is a condition in which patients present with a hypersensitivity to sunlight. The disease occurs in the early spring when afflicted

Table 7.5 Superficial (and deep) perivascular dermatoses – histologic differential diagnosis

Dermal hypersensitivity reaction
Erythema annulare centrifugum
Erythema gyratum repens
Erythema migrans
Pigmented purpuric eruption
Polymorphous light eruption
Urticaria
Viral exanthem

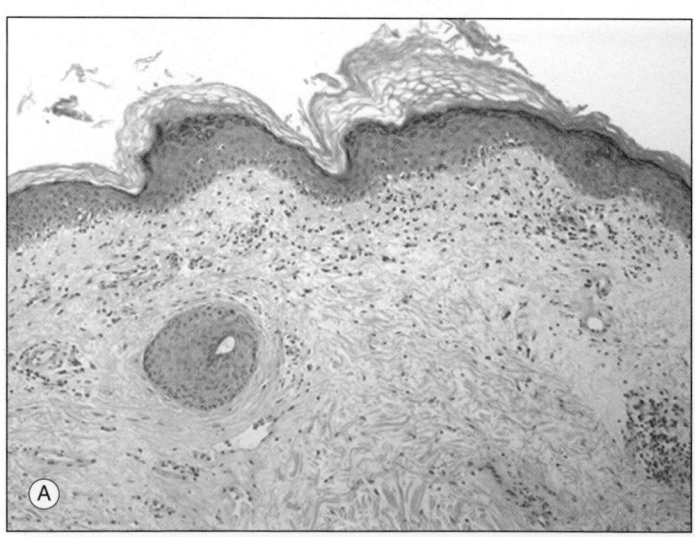
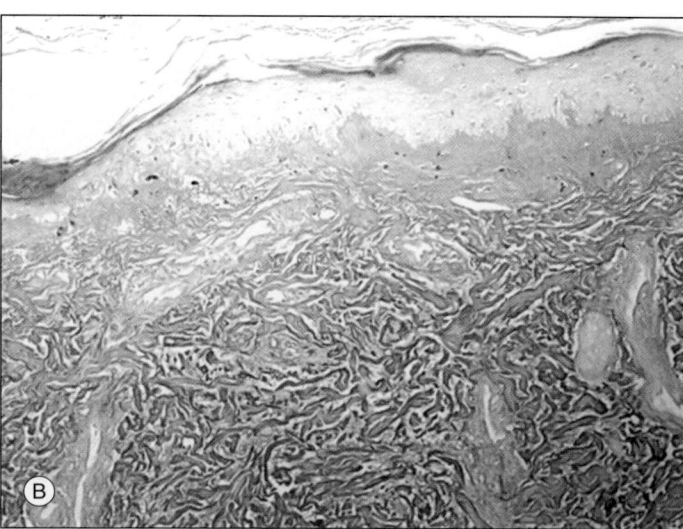

Fig. 7.18 A, A scant interface dermatitis and superficial dermal pallor characterize dermatomyositis, suggesting mucin accumulation; **B**, Colloidal Fe stains demonstrate increased dermal mucin in this case of dermatomyositis.

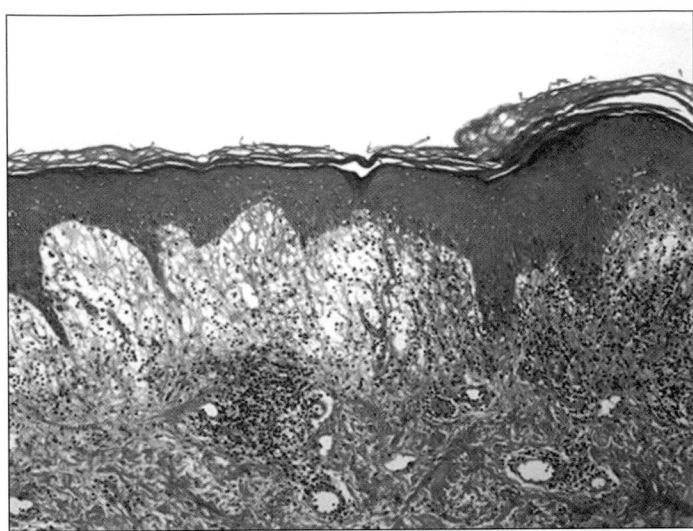

Fig. 7.19 Marked papillary dermal edema and a dermal lymphocytic infiltrate characterize polymorphous light eruptions.

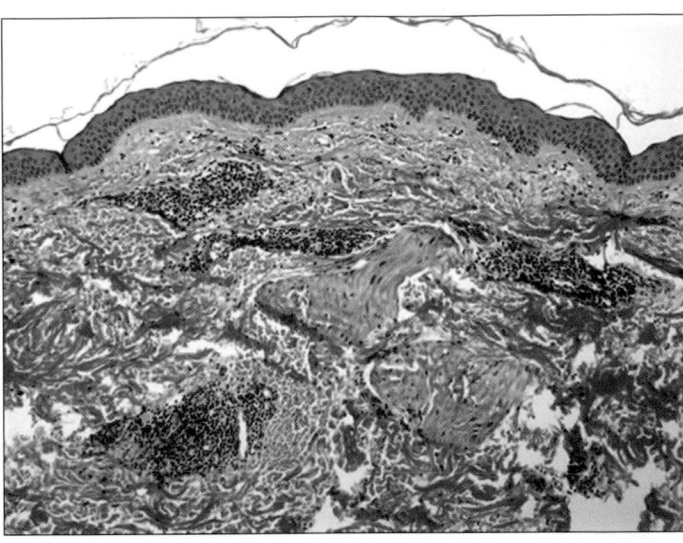

Fig. 7.20 A tightly cuffed perivascular lymphocytic infiltrate is characteristic of erythema annulare centrifugum.

patients are exposed to sunlight following a period of relatively less exposure. The individual lesions vary widely (hence the term polymorphous) and can be macules, papules, vesicles, or bullae. They occur in a photo-distribution. The eruption tends to fade within weeks to months and is usually not present during the summer and autumn months, only to recur the following spring. While the condition varies widely from patient to patient, each patient's presentation and clinical course remains remarkably consistent with each passing year.[52]

Histologic features. PMLE is characterized by a superficial and deep perivascular lymphocytic infiltrate. In the vesicular and bullous variants of the disease, there is marked papillary dermal edema, giving rise to the clinical presentations (Fig. 7.19). In other types of lesions, the papillary dermal edema is much less pronounced.[53]

Differential diagnosis. There is no interface dermatitis present and cutaneous appendages are not ordinarily involved, in contrast to lupus erythematosus, which is in the clinical differential diagnosis. In addition, there is no increase in reticular dermal mucin.

Digitate dermatosis (small plaque parapsoriasis)

Clinical features. The entire concept of parapsoriasis is a controversial one within the field of dermatology. While many observers feel that large plaque parapsoriasis and parapsoriasis variegata are variants or *formes fruste* of mycosis fungoides, most dermatologists are not as convinced that digitate dermatosis is as closely related.[54,55] Others, however, believe that it, too, is an early cutaneous T-cell lymphoma.[56] Patients present with yellowish red, asymptomatic thumb-print sized patches on their flanks. There is minimal overlying scale. The eruption persists for years without change and responds poorly to therapy.

Histologic features. The histologic features of digitate dermatosis are not specific. Focal parakeratosis is present overlying an epidermis that demonstrates small foci of spongiosis. Exocytosis is present only in the areas of spongiosis. There is a slight perivascular lymphocytic infiltrate around vessels of the superficial vascular plexus. Eosinophils and plasma cell are not abundant.[54]

Differential diagnosis. The histologic differential diagnosis of digitate dermatosis includes guttate psoriasis, pityriasis rosea, and pityriasis lichenoides chronica. The ectatic vessels and neutrophils within the stratum corneum that characterize psoriasis are not seen in digitate dermatosis. The intraepidermal hemorrhage often present in pityriasis rosea is not seen in digitate dermatosis, nor are the scattered dying keratinocytes characteristic of pityriasis lichenoides chronica. However, in most cases, the clinical history and presentation is essential in order to make these distinctions.

Gyrate erythemas (erythema annulare centrifugum, erythema gyratum repens, erythema migrans)

Clinical features. The most common gyrate erythema is erythema annulare centrifugum (EAC). EAC appears as one or several large annular erythematous patches on the trunk with delicate peripheral scaling.[57] In some cases, the peripheral scale may be absent. In many cases, EAC occurs in conjunction with a dermatophyte infection.[58] Erythema gyratum repens is an uncommon dermatosis that is frequently associated with internal malignancies.[59] Erythema gyratum repens appears as an eruption that resembles 'grains of wood.'[60] Erythema migrans is the clinical manifestation of Lyme disease. It appears as one or several annular, erythematous patches with slight peripheral scale surrounding the site of a tick bite.

Histologic features. If the periphery of a lesion of EAC is biopsied, a delicate tuft of parakeratosis can be found overlying a focally spongiotic epidermis with slight exocytosis of lymphocytes. In the more central portions of a lesion, epidermal changes are absent. A tightly cuffed, perivascular infiltrate of lymphocytes is present surrounding vessels of the superficial (and sometimes deep) vascular plexus (Fig. 7.20). Scattered eosinophils are present in some cases. The lack of interstitial and epidermal inflammation, in conjunction with the clinical presentation, are the defining features.

The histologic findings of erythema migrans are very similar to those of EAC.[61] Occasional plasma cells may be found in the infiltrate. Silver stains such as a Warthin-Starry or a Dieterle are helpful in identifying spirochetes within dermal blood vessel walls (as are antispirochetal antibodies). *Borrelia burgdorferi*, carried by the *Ioxedes dammini* tick, is the agent responsible for erythema migrans. There are no epidermal changes in this process.

The histologic features of erythema gyratum repens are not specific, but resemble those of the other gyrate erythemas. In some cases, the epidermis may be acanthotic and infiltrated by lymphocytes.

Pigmented purpuric eruptions

Clinical features. There are several clinical and histologic variants of pigmented purpuric eruptions (PPE). While there are subtle distinctions between these entities in terms of their clinical characteristics and the accompanying histologic changes, they have much in common and there seems little reason for the subdivisions. Nonblanching, purpuric papules and patches are present usually on the lower extremities. These erythematous patches have punctate areas of hemorrhage that resemble 'cayenne pepper' spots. Other types of PPE demonstrate surface changes such as spongiosis, annular configurations, or lichenoid changes. There is also a localized variant, known as lichen aureus. PPE are most common in the elderly and have been associated with therapeutic medications in some cases.[62] The eruptions tend to resolve slowly and without sequelae.

Histologic features. The histologic features common to all PPE are a superficial perivascular lymphocytic inflammatory infiltrate accompanied by extravasation of erythrocytes and the presence of hemosiderin-laden macrophages. Neutrophils and other features of vasculitis are not present in PPE (Fig. 7.21A). There may be associated epidermal changes in some types of PPE, but these are not found in all subtypes. A Perl's iron stain or Prussian blue stain may be helpful in confirming the nature of the pigment within the macrophages (Fig. 7.21B).[63]

Differential diagnosis. Clinically, most PPE are thought to be leukocytoclastic vasculitis (LCV). LCV is differentiated from PPE based upon the findings of true vascular destruction and a neutrophilic inflammatory infiltrate. The presence of hemosiderin is essential to differentiate PPE from acutely hemorrhagic processes. Lichen aureus, one type of PPE that is characterized by the above changes as well as a dense lichenoid inflammatory infiltrate, can be difficult to distinguish histologically from lichen planus, but has a very different clinical presentation.

Urticaria

Clinical features. Urticaria, or 'hives' can occur as an acute process or chronically. Acute episodes are more common in children, while the chronic form is seen more frequently in adults. Individual lesions appear rapidly as evanescent plaques of erythema with no overlying scale. By definition, individual plaques resolve without sequelae within 24 hours. Lesions with similar clinical appearances that persist for longer than 24 hours are classified as *urticarial vasculitis.*[64,65]

Histologic features. Urticaria has minimal histologic changes. The epidermis is uninvolved. There is a mild superficial perivascular inflammatory infiltrate that is characterized by a mixed infiltrate of lymphocytes, neutrophils, and eosinophils. Slight perivascular edema may be seen in some cases (Fig. 7.22). In cases of so-called urticarial vasculitis, extravasation of erythrocytes, more pronounced dermal edema, and a perivascular neutrophilic infiltrate are present, though definitive features of vasculitis are not seen.[66]

Dermal hypersensitivity reaction

Clinical features. There are no clinically distinctive features that correlate with this 'wastebasket' diagnosis. Most patients whose biopsies display these histologic changes have hypersensitivity reactions to arthropods or to drugs. The eruptions often consist of erythematous macules and papules, usually with no overlying scale. They may be widespread or localized. It is likely that this terminology correlates with the old term 'dermal erythema multiforme.'

Histologic features. A superficial and deep perivascular and diffuse inflammatory infiltrate characterize dermal hypersensitivity reaction. Lymphocytes are admixed with histiocytes, eosinophils, and occasional plasma cells. The infiltrate may extend into the subcutaneous fat. Except in areas of arthropod bite puncta, the epidermis is not involved. This diagnosis is best made only after consideration of more specific eruptions.

Viral exanthem

Clinical features. A viral exanthem generally presents as a morbilliform eruption. Erythematous macules and papules appear

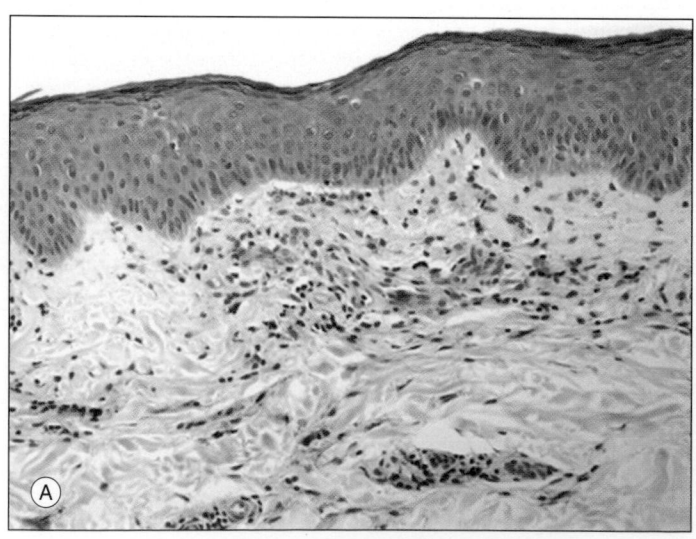 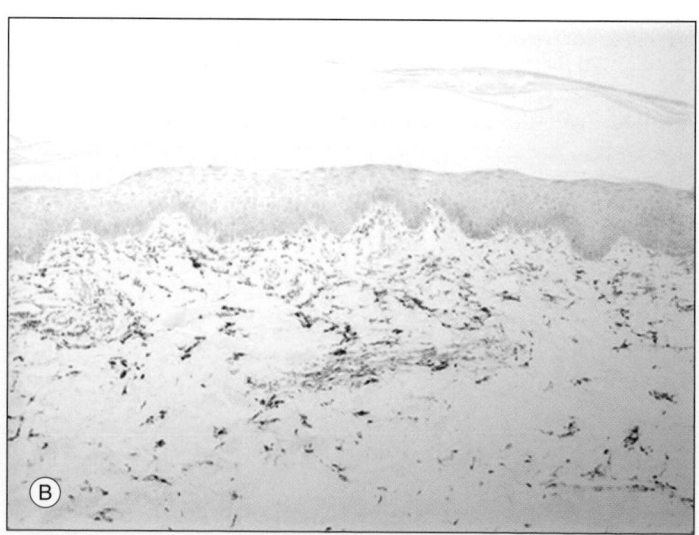

Fig. 7.21 A, Pigmented purpuric eruptions demonstrate perivascular lymphocytic inflammatory infiltrates, extravasated erythrocytes and hemosiderin-laden macrophages as are seen in this photomicrograph; **B,** Perl's stain for iron demonstrates extensive hemosiderin deposition in pigmented purpuric eruptions.

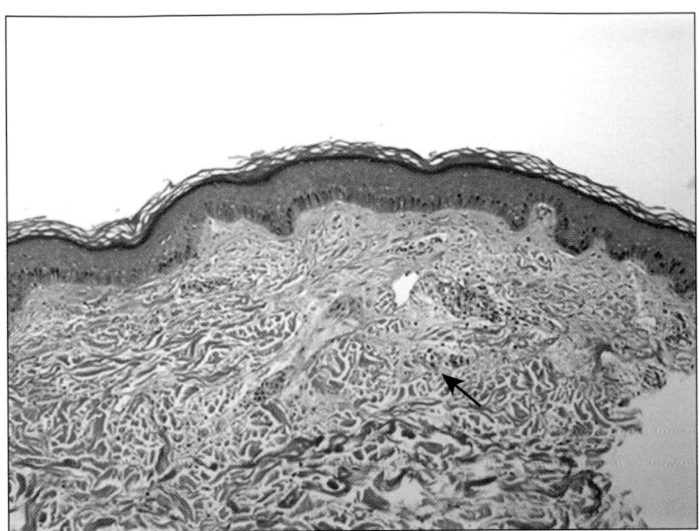

Fig. 7.22 A scant, mixed dermal inflammatory infiltrate including eosinophils (arrow) and slight papillary dermal edema characterize urticaria.

Table 7.6 Neutrophilic dermatoses – histologic differential diagnosis

Acute febrile neutrophilic dermatitis (Sweet's disease)
Cellulitis
Cryoglobulinemia (mixed type only)
Erythema elevatum diutinum
Erythema marginatum
Granuloma faciale
Leukocytoclastic vasculitis
Pyoderma gangrenosum
Rheumatoid papule
Urticarial vasculitis

on the trunk and extremities, usually sparing the face. Only minimal scaling is present until the lesions are resolving. A viral exanthem tends to resolve spontaneously without scarring within a few weeks.

Histologic features. The histologic features of a viral exanthem are non-specific. Minimal spongiosis is present in some cases. There is a slight lymphocytic inflammatory infiltrate surrounding the vessels of the superficial vascular plexus. Eosinophils and plasma cells are not abundant and should raise the possibility of other etiologies for the eruption.

Differential diagnosis. The differential diagnosis includes a drug eruption that most commonly has eosinophils or plasma cells in the inflammatory infiltrate. Other superficial perivascular lymphocytic infiltrates can usually be distinguished based upon the clinical histories and presentations.

VASCULITIDES AND VASCULOPATHIES

Vasculitis is defined as inflammation of the vessels. Histologically, the presence of inflammation within the vessel walls, giving rise to endothelial cell destruction, fibrin thrombi, and extravasation of erythrocytes are necessary to make the diagnosis. Vasculitis can be primarily neutrophilic, such as is seen in leukocytoclastic vasculitis and polyarteritis nodosa. It can also be granulomatous, as exemplified by allergic granulomatosis (Churg-Strauss) and Wegener's granulomatosis. The concept of lymphocytic vasculitis is more controversial. Some authors consider pityriasis lichenoides et varioliformis and pigmented purpuric eruptions to be examples of vasculitis (see discussions of these entities above). In most cases, biopsies from patients with Rocky Mountain spotted fever demonstrate a lymphocytic vasculitis.

Vessel caliber should also be considered when making a diagnosis of vasculitis. Leukocytoclastic vasculitis generally involves small capillaries and postcapillary venules. In contrast, polyarteritis nodosa shows similar changes of vasculitis involving the medium-sized muscular arteries in the deeper dermis and subcutis.

NEUTROPHILIC VASCULITIDES (Table 7.6)

Leukocytoclastic vasculitis

Clinical features. Leukocytoclastic vasculitis presents as palpable purpura. Hemorrhagic and purpuric patches, plaques, and nodules occur most commonly on the lower extremities. They fail to blanche with pressure, confirming the extravascular location of the erythrocytes. Ulceration is common in late lesions. Most cases of leukocytoclastic vasculitis are idiopathic.[67–69] The disease process is also seen in association with drug eruptions, collagen vascular diseases, and neoplasia. Henoch-Schönlein purpura is a specific type of IgA-mediated leukocytoclastic vasculitis that is much more common in children. It is associated with gastrointestinal and renal symptoms.[70]

Histologic features. Leukocytoclastic vasculitis is an inflammatory process that results in the destruction of small dermal blood vessels, most commonly the postcapillary venules. Histologic features include an inflammatory infiltrate with neutrophils present within and around blood vessel walls. Evidence of endothelial cell destruction is manifested by fibrin deposition within vessel walls and by extravasation of erythrocytes into the surrounding dermis. Karyorrhectic debris is usually present (Fig. 7.23). Deeper dermal blood vessels may be affected. Eosinophils are frequently seen, especially in drug-induced vasculitides.[69] Epidermal necrosis may become pronounced secondary to ischemia in lesions that have extensive vascular thrombosis. The neutrophilic infiltrate is replaced by lymphocytes and histiocytes within several days, leaving only extravasated erythrocytes, karyorrhectic debris, and fibrinous deposits in vessel walls as diagnostic clues.

Septic vasculitis is a subset of leukocytoclastic vasculitis. In general, cases with sepsis tend to be characterized by increased amounts of vascular occlusion and less inflammation than other causes of leukocytoclastic vasculitis. Neutrophilic abscesses may be present within the epidermis in some cases of septic vasculitis.

Urticarial vasculitis is a somewhat controversial entity that shares some features with leukocytoclastic vasculitis. Patients present with urticarial lesions that persist for greater than 24 hours (in contrast to urticaria). Purpura is only minimally present. The histologic changes demonstrate neutrophilic karyorrhectic debris, minimal extravasation of erythrocytes and mild dermal edema. While the changes are suggestive of a vasculitis, no definitive evidence for this diagnosis can usually be found.[65,71]

Differential diagnosis. It is important to distinguish true vasculitis from other entities in which neutrophils are present within the

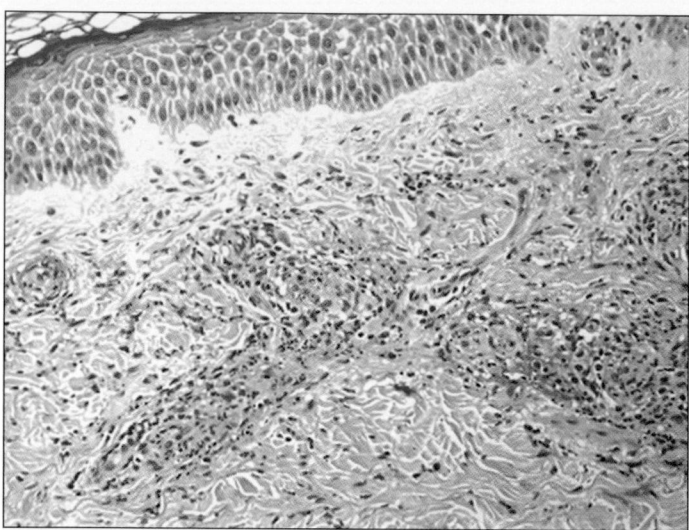

Fig. 7.23 A dense infiltrate of neutrophils is present within walls of the vessels in the superficial vascular plexus in leukocytoclastic vasculitis, resulting in destruction of vessel walls, fibrin deposition, and extravasation of erythrocytes.

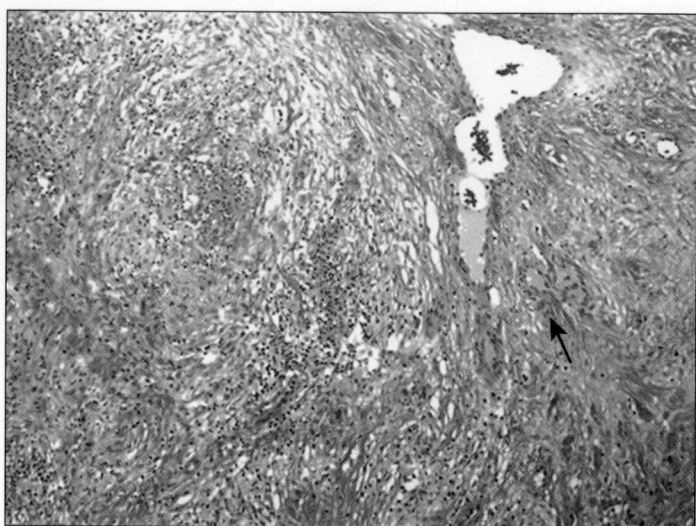

Fig. 7.24 Changes of leukocytoclastic vasculitis are juxtaposed with a histiocytic infiltrate (arrow) and fibrosis in erythema elevatum diutinum.

dermis, but are not attacking and destroying blood vessels (i.e. Sweet's syndrome). It is also important to note that a diagnosis of leukocytoclastic vasculitis should not be made in the setting of superficial ulceration, as neutrophils, karyorrhexis, and vascular destruction are expected in this setting.

Adjuncts to diagnosis. In some cases, direct immunofluorescence examination may be helpful in confirming a diagnosis of leukocytoclastic vasculitis. This process is mediated by circulating immune complexes, and deposition of IgG (or less commonly IgM) and C3 in vessel walls can be seen in lesions less than 24–48 hours old. IgA is present in vessel walls in cases of Henoch-Schönlein purpura.

Erythema elevatum diutinum

Clinical features. This unusual process presents with long-standing scaly, erythematous to brown patches that progress to plaques. Over time, the plaques evolve into firm yellowish nodules. Ultimately, lesions last for years. The extensor surfaces of the extremities are most commonly affected, as are the buttocks.[72] Erythema elevatum diutinum (EED) is often associated with monoclonal gammopathies, especially IgA.

Histologic features. EED is histologically indistinguishable from leukocytoclastic vasculitis in its earliest stages. Vessels within the superficial and mid-dermis are infiltrated by neutrophils, giving rise to endothelial cell destruction, fibrin deposition, and extravasation of erythrocytes. As the lesions evolve, an infiltrate of lipid-laden histiocytes appears in the intervening dermis, eventually accompanied by dense fibrosis (Fig. 7.24). It is the lipid ingested from dying inflammatory cells that gives rise to the late-developing yellow color of the lesions, and the fibrosis that contributes to the nodularity.[72]

Granuloma faciale

Clinical features. Granuloma faciale is a condition of adulthood that presents with one or several erythematous to violaceous plaques or nodules, almost always on the head and neck. The overlying skin surface is unremarkable. It is more common in males.[73]

Histologic features. The histologic features of granuloma faciale include an unremarkable epidermis and a prominent Grenz

zone (zone of sparing) in the papillary dermis and in the extensions of the papillary dermis around the cutaneous appendages (Fig. 7.25A). There is an intense inflammatory infiltrate that is concentrated around the dermal blood vessels. Neutrophils are present within and around vessel walls, and in some cases fibrin deposition and endothelial cell destruction is seen. Abundant eosinophils and lymphocytes are present in the interstitial collagen, and scattered plasma cells may be present (Fig. 7.25B).[73]

Differential diagnosis. The major differential diagnosis includes leukocytoclastic vasculitis. The prominent Grenz zone helps distinguish granuloma faciale from other leukocytoclastic vasculitides, as does the clinical history. Angiolymphoid hyperplasia with eosinophilia also enters the differential diagnosis, but the presence of abundant neutrophils and karyorrhectic debris is unusual in this entity.

Adjuncts to diagnosis. Direct immunofluorescence may demonstrate immune complex deposition within the vessel walls, identical to that seen in leukocytoclastic vasculitis.

Cryoglobulinemia

Clinical features. Patients present with small infarctions distally placed on acral skin.[74] These may or may not be painful and are exacerbated with cold temperatures.

Histologic features. The histologic features of most cases of cryoglobulinemia are those of an obstructive vasculopathy. The epidermis is unremarkable except in late lesions in which infarction may lead to necrosis. Within the dermis, there is plugging of many of the small vessels by PAS-positive eosinophilic material. In rare cases, the intravascular plugs may appear crystalline or angulated. Cases of mixed cryoglobulinemia frequently display an inflammatory response, but other types of cryoglobulinemia are not associated with inflammation, except as a secondary response in late lesions.[74]

Differential diagnosis. The differential diagnosis includes all entities that present with obstructive vasculopathies including lupus anticoagulant, protein C, or protein S deficiency, disseminated intravascular coagulation, septic emboli, and Waldenstrom's macro-

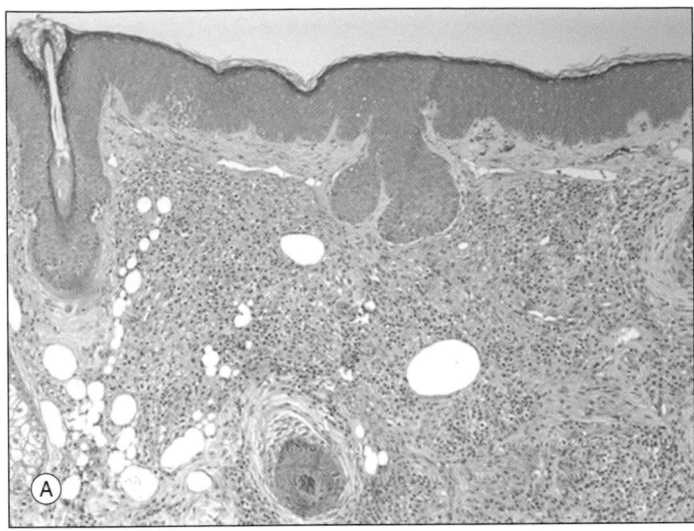
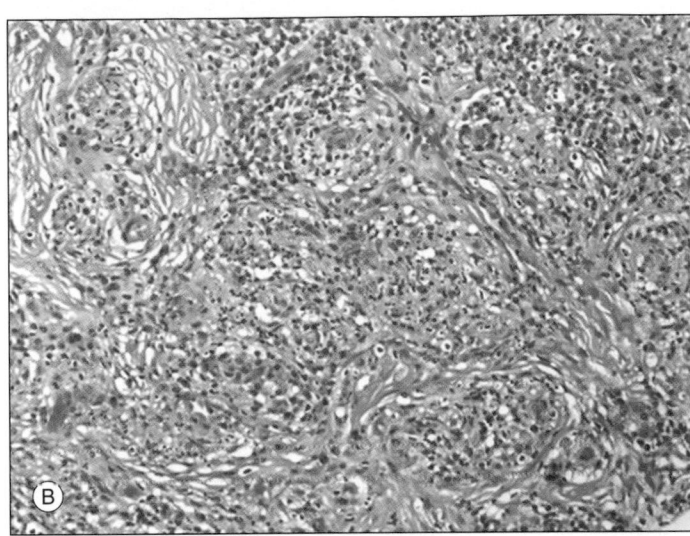

Fig. 7.25 A, A prominent *Grenz* zone is seen in granuloma faciale; **B**, Changes of leukocytoclastic vasculitis and abundant eosinophils are present in granuloma faciale.

globulinemia. These entities may be impossible to distinguish histologically, but clinical examination and other laboratory tests usually provide a more specific diagnosis.

Polyarteritis nodosa

Clinical features. Patients with polyarteritis nodosa (PAN) present with tender, erythematous nodules, most commonly on the lower extremities. The nodules may be linearly distributed, following deep vessels. Ulceration is common. A livedoid pattern may be present on the skin in some cases.[75] Classic polyarteritis nodosa is associated with systemic antigenemia, including most commonly hepatitis B or C.[76,77] A more limited, cutaneous form of the disease, *benign, cutaneous polyarteritis nodosa*, has also been described, and is also associated with systemic processes, though changes of vasculitis are largely limited to cutaneous involvement.[78,79] Rarely, the newly described form of the disease, microscopic polyarteritis nodosa, has been described in the skin.

Histologic features. PAN is a neutrophilic vasculitis. In the classic form of the disease, the changes of vasculitis are found both within the medium-sized arteries in the subcutis and the smaller postcapillary venules in the superficial dermis. If only a superficial biopsy is available, the changes are indistinguishable from leukocytoclastic vasculitis. Vascular destruction and thrombosis are prominent features, especially in the deeper, larger vessels (Fig. 7.26). Microscopic polyarteritis nodosa involves arterioles throughout the dermis, but is very uncommon.

Differential diagnosis. The differential diagnosis of PAN includes leukocytoclastic vasculitis. Involvement of larger vessels in the deep dermis and subcutis favors PAN, as does a clinical presentation of nodular lesions. It can be difficult to distinguish PAN from superficial migratory thrombophlebitis in some cases. In the latter entity, large veins within the subcutis demonstrate thrombosis and a marked neutrophilic infiltrate. An elastic tissue stain may be helpful in identifying an internal elastic lamina in making this distinction, but if the affected vessel is too extensively damaged, this may no longer be visible. Clinical correlation is essential in these cases.

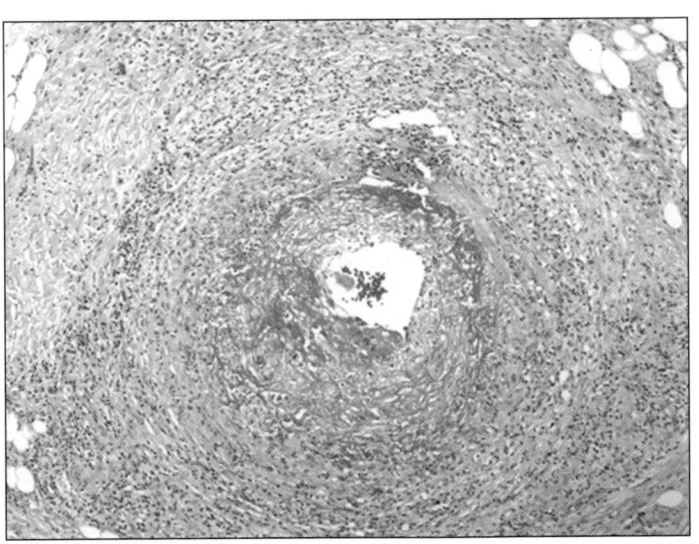

Fig. 7.26 A medium-sized artery in the deep dermis is overrun with neutrophils and is largely destroyed in this case of polyarteritis nodosa.

GRANULOMATOUS VASCULITIDES

Allergic granulomatosis (Churg-Strauss)

Clinical features. Allergic granulomatosis (AG) is a systemic disease that involves the lungs, kidneys, and skin in the majority of affected patients.[80] The cutaneous lesions are not specific.

Histologic features. Vasculitis with abundant eosinophils characterizes AG.[81,82] The vasculitis may also have a granulomatous quality. Small and medium-sized vessels are affected. Extravascular granulomas, usually with abundant degranulating eosinophils, are also commonly encountered in patients with AG.[82]

Differential diagnosis. If granuloma formation is scant, it can be difficult to distinguish AG from drug-induced leukocytoclastic vasculitis, in which eosinophils may be abundant. If eosinophils are not all that plentiful, the distinction from Wegener's granulomatosis can be difficult, and requires clinical correlation.

Wegener's granulomatosis

Clinical features. Wegemmer's granulomatosis (WG) is a systemic disease that involves the respiratory tract and kidneys in most affected patients.[83] Cutaneous involvement, as evidenced by necrotic ulcerations and purpuric macules, is seen in a minority of patients.[84,85] Lower extremities are preferentially affected.

Histologic features. The histologic findings of WG include leukocytoclastic vasculitis of the small vessels. On occasion, one encounters granulomatous vasculitis, in which aggregates of histiocytes comprise a part of the destructive inflammatory process. Granulomas are present within vessel walls. Extravascular granulomas with palisades of histiocytes surrounding areas of caseating necrosis and collagenous degeneration also may be present. Lesional biopsies may contain one or several of these changes.[85]

Differential diagnosis. Depending upon the histologic changes, the differential diagnosis includes leukocytoclastic vasculitis and infectious, granulomatous processes. In most cases, it is necessary to review stains for organisms in order to exclude an infectious process.

NEUTROPHILIC DERMATOSES

Sweet's syndrome

Clinical features. Patients with Sweet's syndrome present with erythematous and edematous papules and plaques.[86] In some cases, the edema results in 'pseudovesicles.' Sweet's syndrome is most common in middle-aged adults, is more common in women, and has been associated with acute myelogenous leukemia, inflammatory bowel disease, and rheumatoid arthritis. Most cases are idiopathic.[87–89]

Histologic features. The epidermis is unremarkable to mildly spongiotic. There is often pronounced papillary dermal edema, occasionally resulting in a subepidermal blister. A dense, diffuse infiltrate of neutrophils is present in the papillary dermis, extending into the superficial reticular dermis. Karyorrhectic debris may be present. There is no evidence of vascular destruction or infiltration of the vessel walls by the neutrophilic infiltrate (Fig. 7.27). Variable numbers of lymphocytes and eosinophils are present within the infiltrate, depending upon the age of the lesion biopsied.

Differential diagnosis. The differential diagnosis includes primarily leukocytoclastic vasculitis. It may also be helpful to get special stains to look for organisms, as an infectious process might also induce a diffuse dermal neutrophilic infiltrate.

Pyoderma gangrenosum

Clinical features. Pyoderma gangrenosum (PG) is a condition that presents with deep, sharply angulated ulcers with overhanging margins.[90] The legs are the most common sites, but PG can present in any location. Many patients have concomitant inflammatory bowel disease or rheumatoid arthritis. There is a weaker association with leukemia.[91] Some authors believe PG and Sweet's syndrome to be variants of the same process.[92] PG is characterized by a clinical condition known as *pathergy*. Any minor trauma to a lesion of PG results in expansion of the lesion; thus, debriding the ulcer cavity results in its expansion, rather than facilitating the healing process.

Histologic features. For the most part, the histologic findings in PG are non-specific. In a fortuitous section, it might be possible to

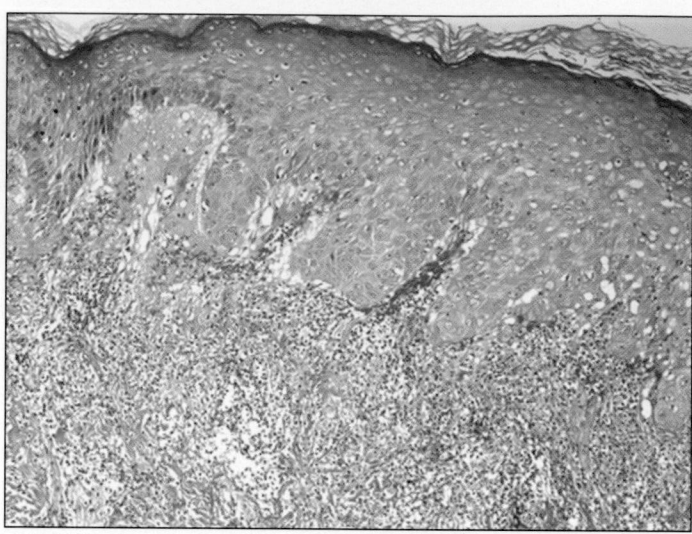

Fig. 7.27 Sweet's syndrome demonstrates marked papillary dermal edema and a brisk diffuse neutrophilic inflammatory infiltrate.

demonstrate an ulceration with adjacent intact epidermis overlying a dense inflammatory infiltrate apparently undermining the surface. The midst of the infiltrate is characterized by a dense mixed infiltrate including abundant neutrophils and lymphocytes. Occasional giant cells are often found. Some investigators believe that at the periphery of the lesion a lymphocytic vasculitis can be seen.

Differential diagnosis. The differential diagnosis includes non-specific ulceration, vasculitis, and infectious processes. In most cases, it is necessary to rule out infectious etiologies with special stains for organisms. As histologic changes indistinguishable from leukocytoclastic vasculitis may be seen immediately beneath ulcerated epidermis, it is important not to overdiagnose vasculitis in such a setting.

GRANULOMATOUS DERMATOSES

There are several types of granulomatous processes that affect the skin (Table 7.7). There are the granulomas that surround altered dermal connective tissue, whose clinical manifestations are primarily, if not exclusively, cutaneous. Systemic granulomatous processes, including infectious diseases and sarcoidosis, also affect the skin. Foreign body giant cell reactions also produce a granulomatous dermatitis.

Granuloma annulare

Clinical features. Granuloma annulare (GA) is a very common dermatosis that preferentially affects children and younger adults. One to two millimeter skin-colored papules appear in an annular configuration with a central area of clearing. There is minimal overlying scale. The dorsum of the hands is a commonly involved site, but annular plaques can occur at any location.[93,94] A disseminated form of the disease appears as individual papules that do not have the same annular distribution. The disseminated form of the disease is associated with pregnancy and diabetes mellitus.[95] A subcutaneous form of the disease is found in children. These lesions are deep-seated nodules. GA resolves without treatment in months to years.

Table 7.7 Granulomatous dermatoses – histologic differential diagnosis

Annular elastolytic granuloma

Foreign body granulomatous reaction

Granuloma annulare

Infectious processes
  Deep fungal infections
  Mycobacterial infections

Necrobiosis lipoidica

Necrobiotic xanthogranuloma (with paraproteinemia)

Rheumatoid nodule

Sarcoidosis

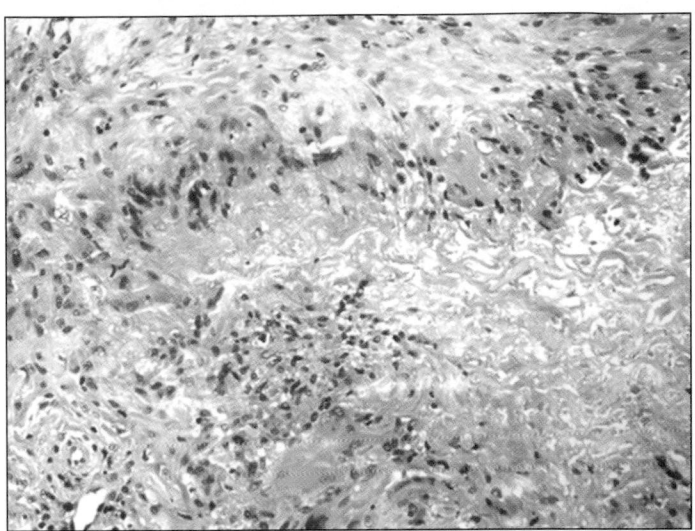

Fig. 7.29 Histiocytes and multinucleated giant cells in actinic granuloma (annular elastolytic granuloma) surround degenerating elastic tissue.

Annular elastolytic granuloma (AEG) (actinic granuloma, Miescher's granulomatosis) is a closely related, if not identical entity, that occurs on sun-damaged skin, especially the face. Annular, erythematous patches with yellowish color develop and spontaneously resolve.[96]

Histologic features. The histologic features of GA include small foci of granulomatous inflammation. Histiocytes palisade around collagen that is undergoing mucinous degeneration within the superficial portion of the reticular dermis. In well-developed lesions, increased dermal mucin is readily apparent on routinely stained sections. The histiocytes are arranged in sharply demarcated palisades. There is an associated perivascular inflammatory infiltrate that is predominantly lymphocytic. Multiple separate foci of collagenous degeneration can usually be seen on a single punch biopsy specimen (Fig. 7.28A).[97] Early lesions of GA display less-pronounced collagenous degeneration (Fig. 7.28B). In these cases, the histiocytes percolate individually between collagen bundles, but do not form true granulomas. Poorly formed granulomas or an increased number of interstitial histiocytes also characterize the disseminated form of the disease.[98] Subcutaneous GA demonstrates foci of collagenous

degeneration deeper within the reticular dermis. These foci are much larger than in classic GA.

Annular elastolytic granuloma has many histologic features in common with GA. However, in contrast to GA, instead of mucin accumulation associated with degenerating collagen, foci of elastolysis are present within the centers of the palisading histiocytes (Fig. 7.29). Further, intracytoplasmic elastic tissue fibers are often found within multinucleated giant cells.[96]

Differential diagnosis. The differential diagnosis of GA includes necrobiosis lipoidica and infectious granulomatous processes. Usually, the presence of mucin, absence of a brisk polymorphous inflammatory infiltrate, and clinical history preclude the need for special stains for organisms. Subcutaneous GA is difficult to distinguish from rheumatoid nodule. However, rheumatoid nodules occur exclusively in patients with known rheumatoid arthritis, so

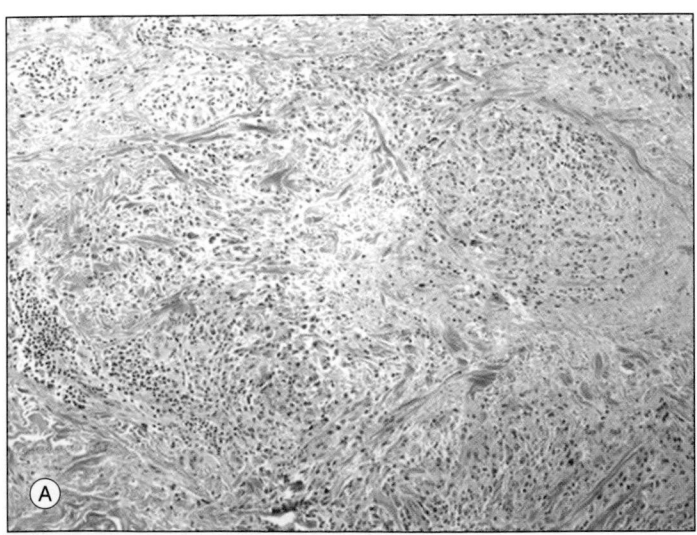
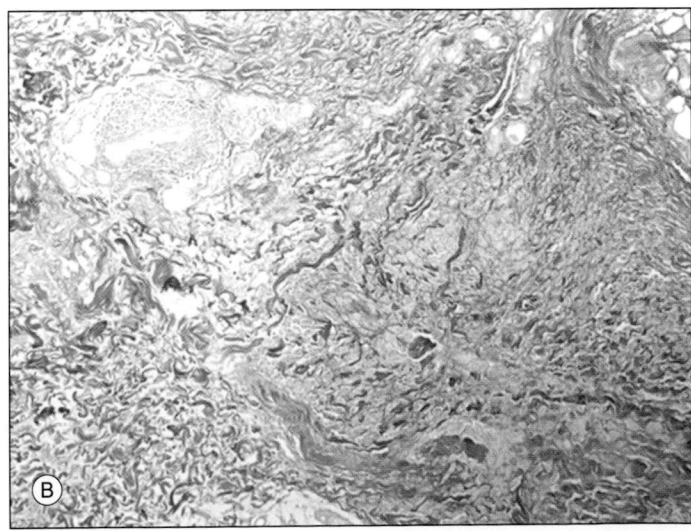

Fig. 7.28 A, Granuloma annulare is characterized by histiocytic infiltrates within the superficial portion of the reticular dermis; **B,** Colloidal iron demonstrates mucinous degeneration of the collagen bundles in granuloma annulare.

clinical history readily makes this distinction. Necrobiosis lipoidica is distinguished based upon the larger foci of degenerating collagen surrounded by larger areas of granulomatous inflammation, lack of mucin, and vascular changes seen in necrobiosis and not in GA. In addition, the foci of collagenous degeneration are located lower in the reticular dermis.

Necrobiosis lipoidica

Clinical features. Necrobiosis lipoidica (NL) is a disorder that occurs almost exclusively in patients with glucose metabolism abnormalities. About 75% of patients with NL have frank diabetes mellitus, yet NL occurs in only about 1% of those with diabetes. It is most common in women and about 67% of lesions occur on the lower extremities. Involvement of the face and other body sites has been reported less commonly. Patients develop erythematous annular patches that develop into atrophic yellow plaques. Overlying ulceration can be found in long-standing lesions.[99,100]

Histologic features. The epidermis is initially unremarkable, but becomes atrophic in long-standing lesions. The main pathology is within the reticular dermis. A large palisade of histiocytes surrounds zones of necrobiotic collagen. This affected collagen is pale-staining and hypocellular. The histiocytic infiltrate includes some multi-nucleated cells and many of the cells may have intracytoplasmic lipid. A lymphocytic and plasmacellular infiltrate is present in most cases and lymphoid nodules may be seen (Fig. 7.30). There is thickening of the dermal blood vessel walls, with narrowing of the vascular lumina.[101] In rare cases, well-formed sarcoidal granulomas may be present.

Differential diagnosis. Granuloma annulare also has a granulomatous dermal infiltrate, but the areas of altered collagen are much smaller, more superficially located, and contain mucin that is not seen in NL. Rheumatoid nodules are somewhat deeper in the dermis and subcutis and the altered collagen has a characteristic 'brick-red' appearance due to the fibrin deposition on the collagen. In rare cases, the granulomas in NL can be quite sarcoidal in appearance and distinction from sarcoidosis is possible only with clinical history and extensive systemic work-up.

Rheumatoid nodule

Clinical features. Rheumatoid nodules present as subcutaneous (or deep dermal) nodules that have no overlying epidermal changes. They are most prominent on protuberances overlying joints and may be related to repeated minor trauma. Rheumatoid nodules occur almost exclusively in patients with long-standing active rheumatoid arthritis.[102]

Histologic features. The histologic features of a rheumatoid nodule include a large area of altered collagen within the deep reticular dermis, frequently extending into the subcutis. A palisade of histiocytes surrounds the collagen. The central area often has a 'brick-red' tinctoral change due to fibrin present on the collagen bundles (Fig. 7.31).[102,103]

Differential diagnosis. The differential diagnosis includes necrobiosis lipoidica and subcutaneous granuloma annulare. Necrobiosis lipoidica demonstrates vascular wall thickening, pale-staining collagen, and a brisk inflammatory infiltrate and is usually centered in the reticular dermis. Subcutaneous granuloma annulare may be histologically identical to rheumatoid nodule, but occurs mainly in children who do not have rheumatoid arthritis.

Sarcoidosis

Clinical features. Cutaneous sarcoidosis can mimic many other entities in its myriad clinical appearances. Some patients present with skin-colored papules and nodules on the nose, in a distribution known as *lupus pernio*. In other patients, small papules are found along the margins of the eyelids. Some cases of sarcoidosis appear as flat-topped, lichenoid plaques.[104–106] Erythema nodosum is associated with some cases of acute-onset pulmonary sarcoidosis in a syndrome known as *Loeffler's syndrome* that usually resolves quickly.[107] In some patients with sarcoidosis, an acquired ichthyosis complicates the cutaneous features.[108]

Histologic features. Sarcoidosis within the skin resembles sarcoidosis in other affected organs. Well-formed, sharply demarcated granulomas are accompanied by little inflammation in most cases. The granulomas may be located within the papillary dermis, pushing up the epidermis and giving rise to the clinically apparent small papules.

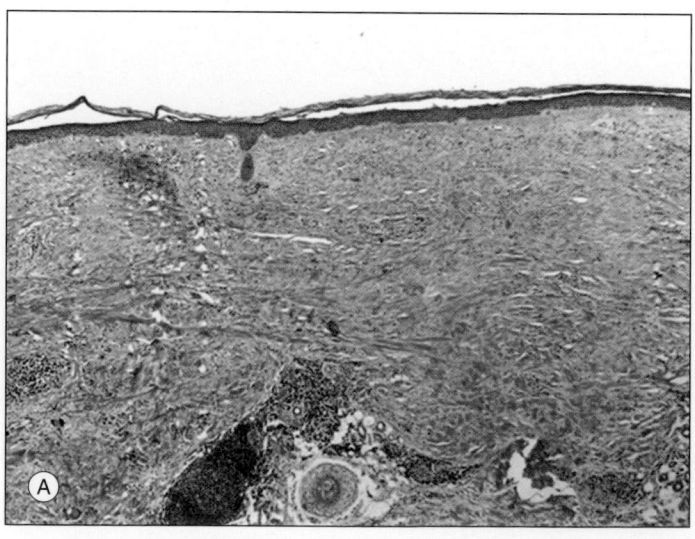
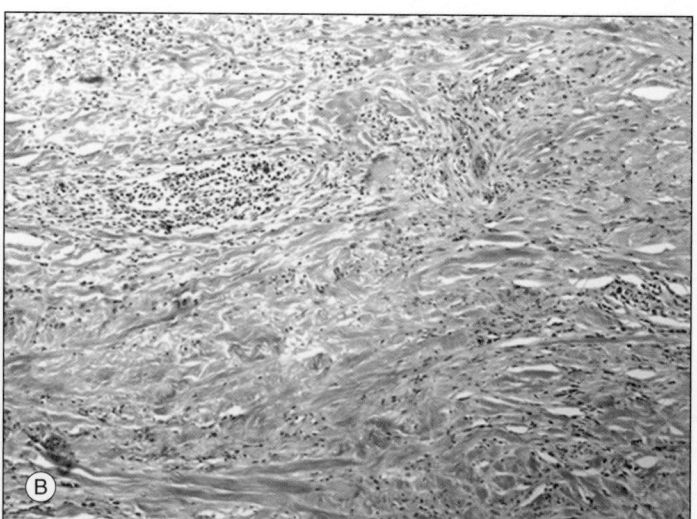

Fig. 7.30 A, Atrophic epidermis, pale-staining collagen bundles, and an infiltrate of histiocytes characterize NL. Lymphoid aggregates are present in many cases; **B,** Multinucleated giant cells are diffusely present throughout the dermis in NL.

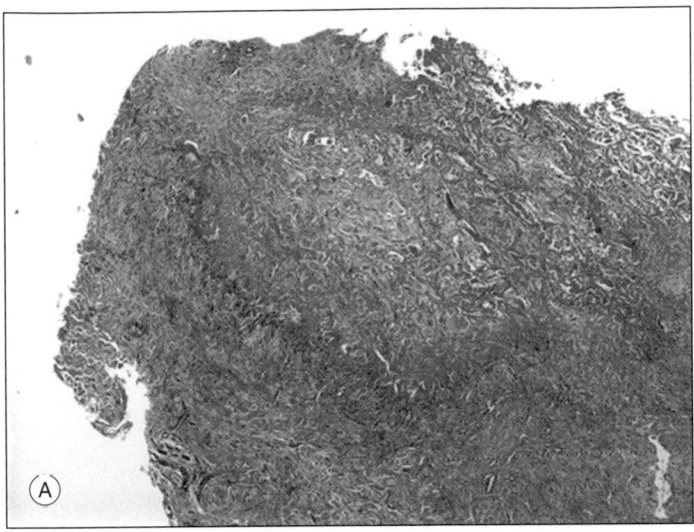
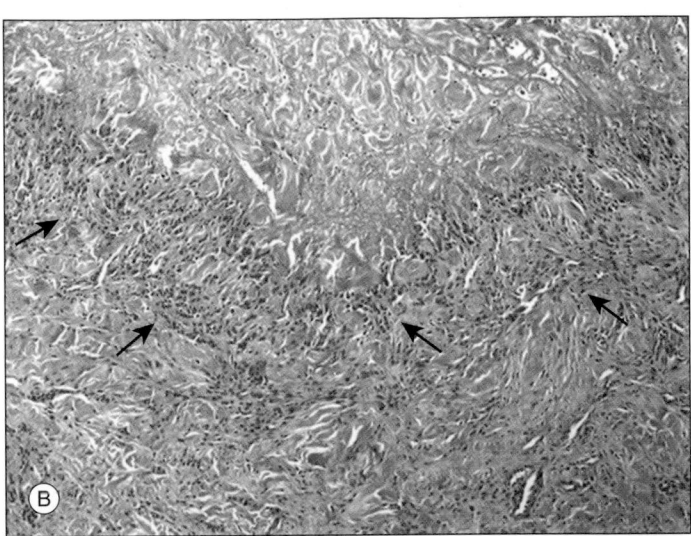

Fig. 7.31 **A**, A palisade of histiocytes in rheumatoid nodules surrounds deep-seated nodules of bright red collagen; **B**, A palisade of histiocytes (arrows) surrounds the altered collagen in rheumatoid nodules.

They may also be present throughout the reticular dermis and extending into the subcutis. The granulomas are not particularly associated with cutaneous appendages. Central caseation is unusual and is not seen in most cases of sarcoidosis (Fig. 7.32).

Differential diagnosis. Sarcoidosis is a diagnosis of exclusion. It is essential that infectious etiologies be excluded with special stains, cultures, and clinical correlation. It is often useful to polarize the tissue sections to exclude foreign body type granulomas. Acne rosacea is often in the differential diagnosis, but perifollicular localization of the granulomas and a more intense surrounding inflammatory response help to distinguish this from sarcoidosis in most cases.

Infectious processes

Clinical features. Clinical manifestations of each specific infectious disease are addressed elsewhere in this volume. Multiple deep fungi, including histoplasmosis, blastomycosis, coccidioidomycosis, cryptococcosis, sporotrichosis, and others can infect the skin. Some fungal infectious are associated with verrucous, hyperkeratotic plaques, while others appear more as erythematous patches, papules, and/or plaques.

Mycobacterium tuberculosis also can involve the skin in many ways, including direct inoculation (*tuberculosis verrucosa cutis*) that presents as a verrucous plaque,[109] miliary spread,[110] direct extension (*scrofuloderma*), and as *lupus vulgaris*, an erythematous, verrucous plaque on the face.[111] Atypical mycobacteria also infect the skin and may present as generalized eruptions or ulcerations at the sites of primary inoculation.[112] Erythema induratum (elsewhere in this chapter) most likely is related to tuberculosis infection.[113] *Papulonecrotic tuberculid* and *lichen scrofulosorum* represent cutaneous hypersensitivity reactions to tuberculosis infection in other body sites.[114]

Mycobacterium leprae also involves the skin, presenting as one or many erythematous to hypopigmented, annular patches with underlying anesthesia in some cases. Associated sensory neuropathies may be apparent on clinical examination. Tuberculoid and lepromatous forms of the disease both present with cutaneous lesions early in the course of the disease.[115,116]

Histologic features. Many deep fungal infectious of the skin demonstrate pseudoepitheliomatous hyperplasia. This is especially prominent in coccidioidomycosis, blastomycosis, and sporotrichosis infections. Similar epidermal hyperplasia is seen in tuberculosis verrucosa cutis and lupus vulgaris. Within the dermis, deep fungal and mycobacterial infections demonstrate granulomatous inflammation. Caseating necrosis is present within the centers of the granulomas and multinucleated giant cells are abundant. A dense, mixed inflammatory cell infiltrate is present in most cases.[117]

The reaction pattern is different in cutaneous leprosy and varies markedly with the subtype of leprosy. Tuberculoid leprosy is characterized by well-formed, sarcoidal granulomas that rarely display caseation. A moderately intense lymphocytic and plasma cellular inflammatory infiltrate is present. There is some tendency for nerve swelling, and the granulomas appear oblong as they parallel dermal nerves. Lepromatous leprosy demonstrates sheets of histiocytes with abundant granular cytoplasm that do not aggregate into granulomas. A prominent Grenz zone is characteristic. There is minimal surrounding inflammation.[118]

Adjuncts to diagnosis. Special stains such as PASD, Gomori methenamine silver, acid-fast, and fite stains are usually essential to make an accurate diagnosis.

Foreign body giant cell reactions

Clinical features. Erythematous nodules have variably present epidermal changes. Depending upon the foreign material, superficial discoloration may be apparent.

Histologic features. The histologic features of a foreign body giant cell reaction include variable epidermal changes, ranging from ulceration to pseudoepitheliomatous hyperplasia. Within the dermis, a diffuse, often dense inflammatory infiltrate is present. Abundant histiocytes, including multinucleated giant cells are present. Foreign material may be present within the cytoplasm of the giant cells or extracellularly (Fig. 7.33). In some cases, polarization is helpful in identifying foreign material.

Differential diagnosis. Infectious processes present the most difficult diagnostic challenge. Negative special stains and cultures

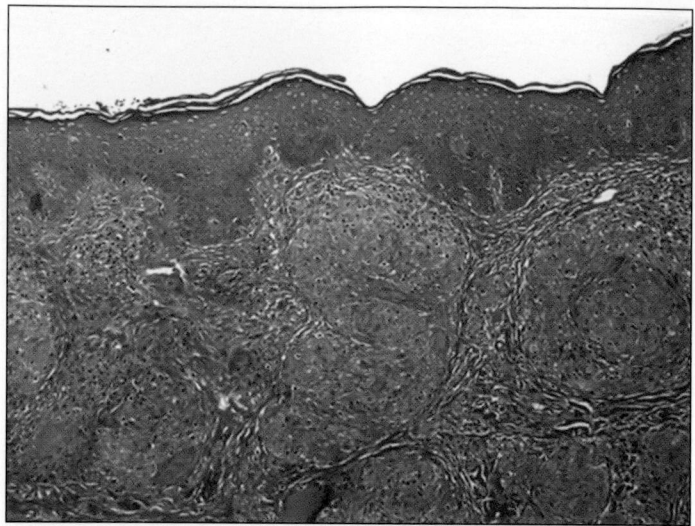

Fig. 7.32 Sarcoidosis is characterized by well-formed, 'naked' granulomas, often pushed high in the papillary dermis.

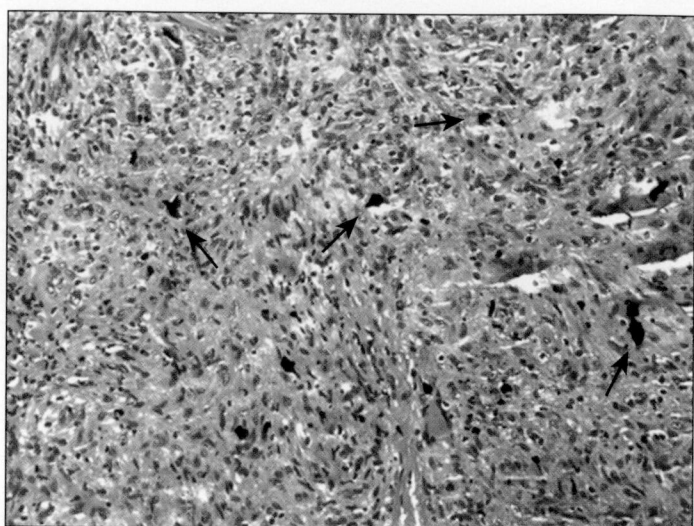

Fig. 7.33 Graphite particles (arrows) are seen within histiocytes in this traumatic tattoo surrounded by a foreign body giant cell reaction.

Table 7.8 Subcorneal blisters – histologic differential diagnosis

Candidiasis
Erythema toxicum neonatorum
Impetigo
Infantile acral pustulosis
Miliaria crystallina
Pemphigus erythematosus
Pemphigus foliaceus
Pustular psoriasis
Scabies
Staphylococcal scalded skin syndrome
Subcorneal pustular dermatosis
Toxic neonatal pustular melanosis

are helpful in excluding these types of processes, and identification of foreign material helps confirm the impression of a foreign body type of granulomatous reaction.

BULLOUS AND PUSTULAR DISORDERS

SUBCORNEAL BLISTERS (Table 7.8)

Subcorneal pustular dermatosis (of Sneddon and Wilkinson)

Clinical features. Subcorneal pustular dermatosis is characterized by an annular or serpiginous configuration of pustules appearing on an erythematous plaque. The most common location is the lower trunk. Intertriginous areas are also commonly involved. It is most common in middle-aged women.[119]

Histologic features. A subcorneal pustule filled with neutrophils overlies an otherwise unremarkable epidermis. The stratum corneum is unremarkable. Specifically, there is not an abundance of parakeratosis. Neutrophils may be present in small numbers within the papillary dermis, but this is not a constant finding (Fig. 7.34).[119]

Differential diagnosis. It is difficult, if not impossible, to distinguish subcorneal pustular dermatosis from pustular psoriasis based purely on histologic findings. However, the clinical presentation is different. Candidiasis and impetigo can be differentiated using special stains for organisms.

Adjuncts to diagnosis. IgA has been reported within the epidermis in some cases of subcorneal pustular dermatosis.[120] This test may be helpful, but is rarely employed. These cases probably represent the more recently described IgA pemphigus, and are not the same entity as the cases lacking IgA expression.

Scabies

Clinical features. The burrows formed by the female scabies mite can be seen in characteristic locations including the finger webs, the periumbilical area, and on nipples. The lesions are intensely pruritic. A florid form of the disease, Norwegian scabies, occurs in institutionalized and immunocompromised patients.[121]

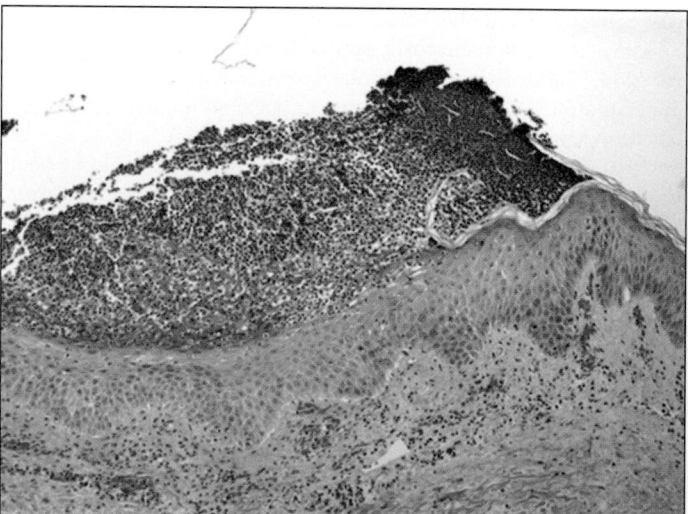

Fig. 7.34 Sneddon-Wilkinson subcorneal pustular dermatosis demonstrates a subcorneal pustule with no other changes to suggest psoriasis, and a minimal dermal inflammatory infiltrate.

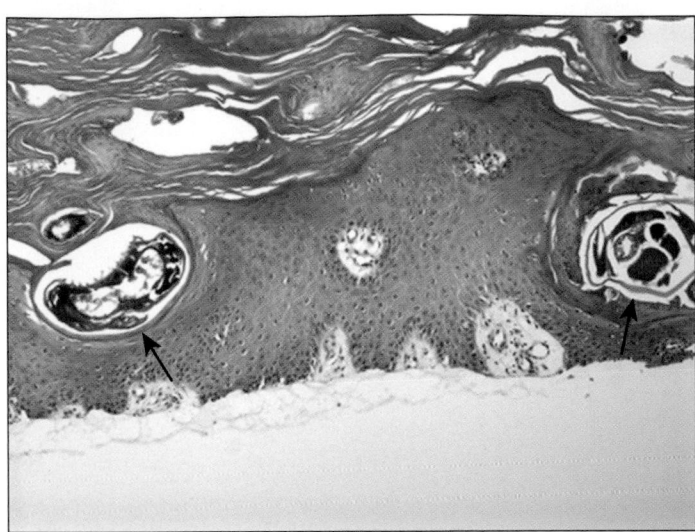

Fig. 7.35 Scabies mites are present within burrows (arrows) in the superficial epidermis in this case of Norwegian scabies.

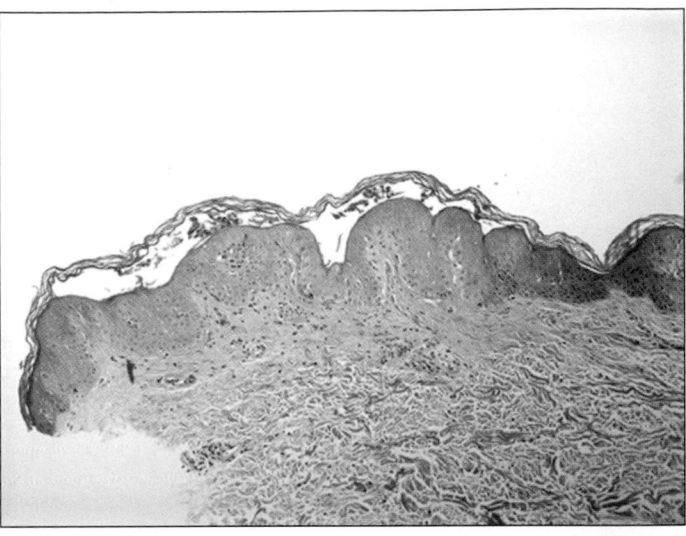

Fig. 7.36 A subcorneal blister in which many neutrophils are present characterizes impetigo. Acantholysis may be present, focally, at the edge of the blister.

Histologic features. Arthropod parts can occasionally be found within a cavity created in the stratum corneum. In other cases, focal serum and neutrophilic crust are seen in an otherwise unremarkable stratum corneum. The subjacent epidermis has marked spongiosis and exocytosis of lymphocytes and frequently eosinophils (Fig. 7.35). Langerhans cell microabscesses may be present in the area of the mite. The dermal inflammatory infiltrate is usually intense and is composed of lymphocytes, histiocytes, and abundant eosinophils. Inflammation extends into the subcutaneous fat. Large lymphoid nodules may persist long after the infestation is adequately treated.

Differential diagnosis. In long-standing lesions, activated lymphocytes become enlarged and can resemble those seen in a cutaneous lymphoma. This is especially the case in a so-called persistent nodular scabetic reaction in which the infestation has been successfully treated, organisms are no longer present, yet the hypersensitivity reaction persists.

Impetigo

Clinical features. In most cases, impetigo represents an infection with *Staphylococcus aureus*. Less commonly, streptococci are implicated in this process. Superficial pustules present most commonly on the hands and face. 'Honey-colored' serum and neutrophilic crusts are characteristic of this entity. It is more common in children and young adults.[122] When caused by group A streptococci, there may be associated glomerulonephritis.[123,124]

Histologic features. A superficial vesicle is present in the granular layer with adjacent parakeratosis. Neutrophils are usually seen within the vesicle, and there is surrounding spongiosis. Focal acantholysis is present at the edges of the blister cavity in some cases (Fig. 7.36). Neutrophils and lymphocytes are present in the epidermis and dermis.

Differential diagnosis. The differential diagnosis includes the other subcorneal pustular disorders. Clinical presentation, along with the detection of Gram-positive cocci within the tissue sections, help in confirming the diagnosis.

Candidiasis

Clinical features. Patients with candidiasis present with erythematous patches with superimposed pustular lesions. Characteristic satellite pustules are fairly typical of the clinical presentation, most often obviating the need for biopsy.[125] Candidiasis is common in intertriginous areas.

Histologic features. The histologic findings of candidiasis include a subcorneal pustule. The surrounding epidermis may be spongiotic or unremarkable. The underlying dermis generally displays a non-specific inflammatory host response. Special stains for fungi such as a PAS or GMS are helpful in establishing the diagnosis.

Differential diagnosis. The differential diagnosis of candidiasis includes all of the other subcorneal pustular dermatoses. The only other entity with PAS-positive organisms giving rise to subcorneal blisters is the rare bullous dermatophyte infection. In these cases, the PAS stain demonstrates mixed hyphal and yeast forms of the fungi.

Pemphigus foliaceus/pemphigus erythematosus

Clinical features. Pemphigus foliaceus and pemphigus erythematosus are indistinguishable clinically and histologically. Direct immunofluorescence examination is the only way to accurately distinguish between these two entities. Patients with both conditions present with superficial desquamation and scaling. There is slight erythema. No overt bullae or vesicles are seen in most patients. They are diseases of middle-aged to elderly patients and are most likely to involve the trunk and extremities. The face and scalp are frequently involved. Unlike pemphigus vulgaris, the oral cavity is rarely involved.[126] Both entities have been associated with drug ingestion.

Histologic features. The histologic features of pemphigus foliaceus and pemphigus erythematosus are identical. An acantholytic blister is present within the granular layer. In many cases, the roof of the blister is no longer present on the tissue sections and the major finding is that of an epidermis that is lacking a stratum corneum and part of the granular layer. With more intact specimens, acantholytic cells can be seen within the blister cavity or at its edges (Fig. 7.37). There is a minimal inflammatory infiltrate that may contain eosinophils.[127] Little dermal inflammation is seen.

Adjunct diagnostic tests. Direct immunofluorescence examination reveals intercellular deposits of IgG and C3 in both pemphigus foliaceus and pemphigus erythematosus. In addition, granular

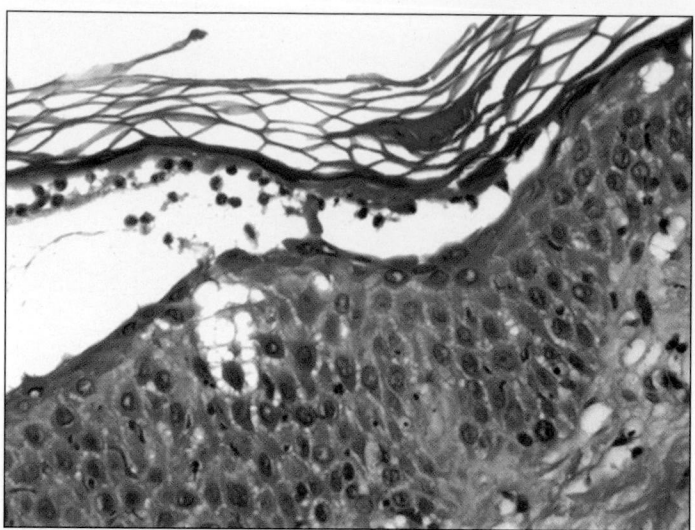

Fig. 7.37 Pemphigus foliaceus demonstrates an acantholytic blister at the level of the granular layer.

Fig. 7.38 Staphylococcal scalded skin syndrome is characterized by a blister at the level of the granular layer. The roof of the blister may remain adherent or desquamate, making the diagnosis difficult.

deposits of these immunoreactants are present along the dermal–epidermal junction in pemphigus erythematosus, but are not seen in pemphigus foliaceus.

Staphylococcal scalded skin syndrome

Clinical features. Staphylococcal scalded skin syndrome (SSSS) is a disease that occurs primarily in small children or in adults with renal insufficiency. Exfoliatin, a toxin produced by coagulase-positive *Staphylococcus aureus*, causes a superficial desquamative process with underlying erythema.[128,129] There is little inflammation associated with this process as no organisms are actually present within the lesion. SSSS is sometimes difficult to distinguish clinically from toxic epidermal necrolysis. As both are potentially medical emergencies, pathologists may be called upon to render a frozen section diagnosis (as discussed below).

Histologic features. SSSS is characterized by a very superficial separation beneath the stratum corneum or within the granular layer. There is little associated inflammatory reaction (Fig. 7.38). The changes are quite subtle and could be easily overlooked.[128,130]

Differential diagnosis. Distinguishing this process from toxic epidermal necrolysis is possible by simply preparing a frozen section of recently desquamated sheets of epidermis. In SSSS, only the stratum corneum and perhaps scant granular layer cells will be present, while in toxic epidermal necrolysis, the full thickness of the epidermis will be present.

INTRAEPIDERMAL BLISTERS

Each of the processes in this section is characterized by intra-epidermal blister formation (Table 7.9). In all of the cases, the blister cavities arise from acantholysis. The pathogenesis of the acantholysis differs, however, giving rise to a number of distinct pathologic processes.

Pemphigus vulgaris

Clinical features. Pemphigus vulgaris (PV) is primarily a disease of middle-aged to elderly patients who present with flaccid bullae

Table 7.9 Intraepidermal acantholytic blisters – histologic differential diagnosis

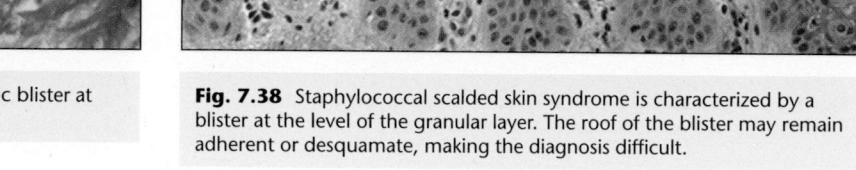

| Darier's disease (keratosis follicularis) |
| Grover's disease (transient acantholytic dermatosis) |
| Hailey-Hailey disease (benign familial pemphigus) |
| Herpesvirus infection |
| Paraneoplastic pemphigus |
| Pemphigus vegetans |
| Pemphigus vulgaris |

that progress to erosions. A positive Nikolski sign (ability to expand the size of the blister with gentle pressure) is present in most cases, in contrast to most other blistering disorders. Bullae expand rapidly and there is a high mortality rate if PV is left untreated. The oral cavity is frequently involved and is the initial site of involvement in at least a third of patients. Pemphigus vulgaris is associated with increased incidences of thymoma and myasthenia gravis.[131]

Histologic features. Histologic sections of PV demonstrate skin with a suprabasilar, acantholytic blister. The roof of the blister usually remains largely intact. The basal keratinocytes on the floor of the blister cavity remain firmly attached to the underlying basement membrane zone, but separate from each other (acantholysis), giving rise to a 'tombstone pattern' (Fig. 7.39). A mild inflammatory infiltrate is present and usually includes eosinophils. In early lesions, eosinophils may be seen within the epidermis in conjunction with spongiosis.

Differential diagnosis. The clinical presentation, positive direct immunofluorescence, and typical 'tombstoning' pattern of the basal layer keratinocytes help to distinguish PV from the other blistering disorders with a suprabasilar separation, including Darier's disease, Hailey-Hailey disease, and Grover's disease.

Adjuncts to diagnosis. PV is an autoimmune blistering disease in which autoantibodies directed against desmosomal protein

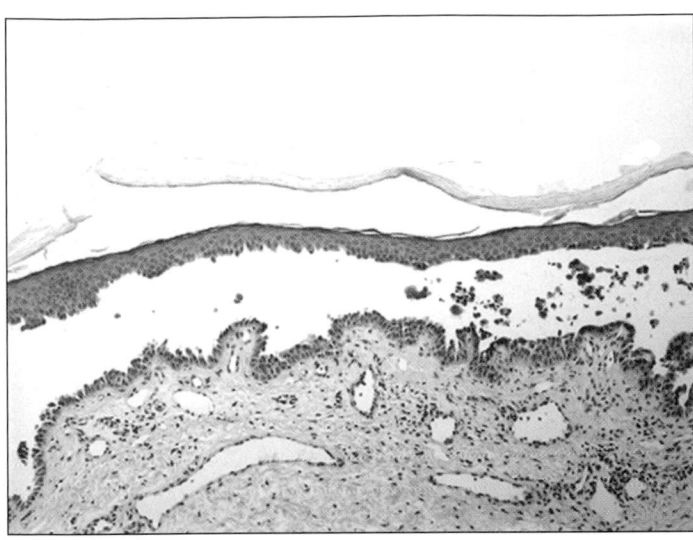

Fig. 7.39 Pemphigus vulgaris demonstrates a suprabasilar acantholytic blister with 'tombstone'-like basal keratinocytes.

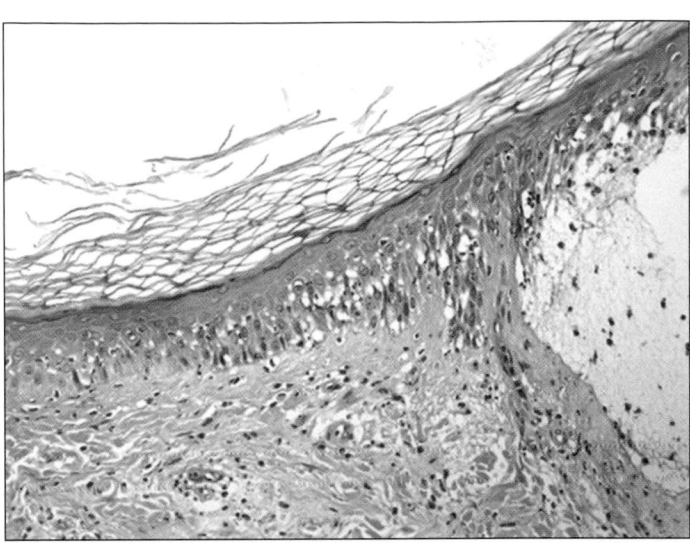

Fig. 7.40 There is often a brisk exocytosis in addition to the acantholysis in paraneoplastic pemphigus.

desmoglein-3 help to destroy desmosomes. Direct immunofluorescence examination reveals depositions of IgG (and C3) outlining epidermal keratinocytes and forming a 'chicken wire' staining pattern. A positive direct immunofluorescence examination is seen in greater than 90% of patients with PV. Indirect immunofluorescence examination demonstrates a similar staining pattern, revealing the presence of circulating IgG autoantibodies in afflicted patients. The titer of autoantibodies can be determined by this method and used to monitor disease progression.[132]

Paraneoplastic pemphigus

Clinical features. Patients present with erosions, occasionally preceded by clinically apparent flaccid bullae. Mucosal surfaces are usually affected and may result in severe clinical symptoms. In other patients, erythema multiforme-like targetoid erythematous patches are present, and in some, lichenoid papules have been described. Deeper mucosal surfaces including esophagus and bronchi may be involved and contribute to the extensive morbidity associated with this process.[133] Paraneoplastic pemphigus is associated with many types of malignancy, most commonly non-Hodgkin's lymphomas.[134–136] The disease remits with clinical remission of the underlying neoplastic process.[137]

Histologic features. A suprabasilar blistering process similar to that seen in pemphigus vulgaris is present in many, but not all cases. These changes may be focal and easily overlooked. In addition to the acantholytic cells, individual dyskeratotic cells may be present along the basal layer, with surrounding intraepidermal lymphocytes. This pattern is quite similar to the histologic changes seen in erythema multiforme (Fig. 7.40). In some cases, a lichenoid inflammatory response is present within the dermis and it may be difficult to distinguish paraneoplastic pemphigus from lichen planus.[138]

Differential diagnosis. The differential diagnosis includes pemphigus vulgaris. However, individual dyskeratotic cells, a lichenoid inflammatory response, and the clinical history serve to differentiate paraneoplastic pemphigus from pemphigus vulgaris. Erythema multiforme shares some histologic features, but acantholysis is not seen in this entity and the clinical appearance of

the eruption is different. Lichen planus also has a significantly different clinical history and is not characterized by acantholysis.

Adjuncts to diagnosis. Direct immunofluorescence may be helpful in making a diagnosis of paraneoplastic pemphigus; however, it is often very difficult to detect the autoantibodies. On indirect immunofluorescence examination, rat bladder has proven to be much more sensitive than monkey esophagus. The staining pattern is an intercellular staining pattern similar to that seen in pemphigus vulgaris. In addition, linear staining along the dermal–epidermal junction with IgG, similar to that seen in bullous pemphigoid, is present in most cases.[139]

Keratosis follicularis (Darier's disease)

Clinical features. Keratosis follicularis is an autosomal dominant genodermatosis that presents most commonly during adolescence as hyperkeratotic papules that become confluent. Skin on the neck, chest, and back is most commonly affected in a seborrheic-like distribution. The disease may be diffuse and widespread and in its most florid state is associated with an unpleasant odor (described as being similar to 'sweaty feet'). Despite the histologic features (described below), there are no clinically discernible blisters seen on patients with keratosis follicularis.[140]

Histologic features. Keratosis follicularis is characterized by prominent hyperkeratosis. A suprabasilar separation is present within the epidermis and abundant corps ronds and grains are found. Grains resemble 'fat' parakeratotic cells. These reflect the disordered keratinization that characterizes this disorder (Fig. 7.41). The epidermis demonstrates elongation of the rete ridges and the reciprocal papillary dermal tips resemble villous projections lined by single layers of basal keratinocytes.[141]

Differential diagnosis. Acantholysis is less prominent than is seen in PV, and corps ronds and grains more abundant. The hyperkeratosis and relatively little spongiosis also help to differentiate keratosis follicularis from PV and Hailey-Hailey disease. While transient acantholytic dermatosis can have a similar histologic appearance, the clinical presentation and the minute size of the affected areas of epidermal involvement distinguish it from keratosis follicularis. A

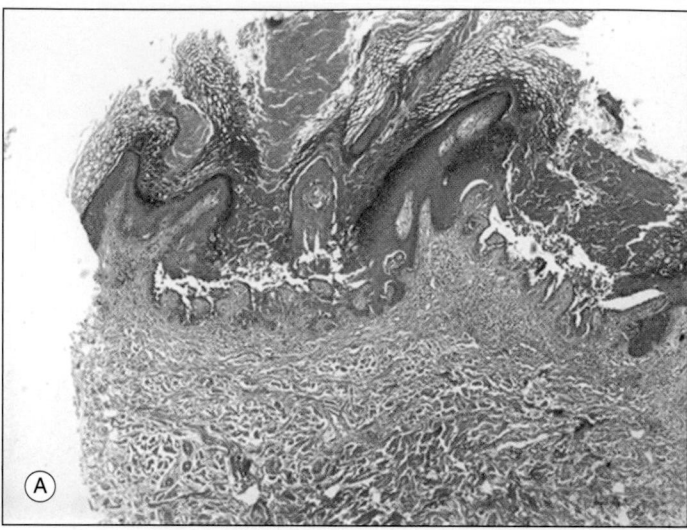

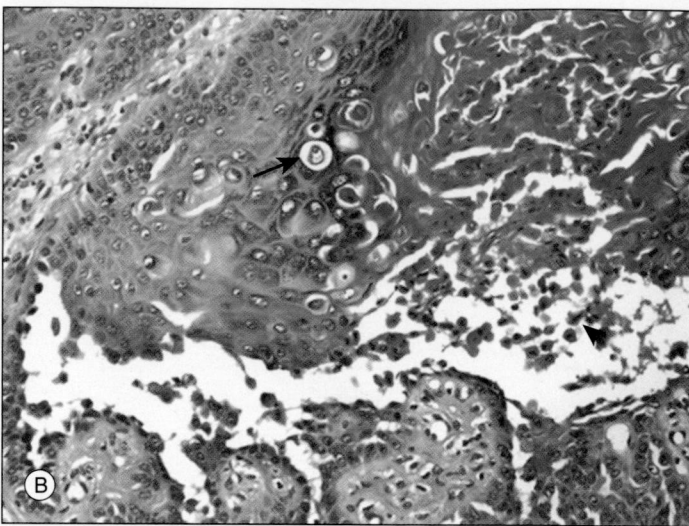

Fig. 7.41 A, Darier's disease (keratosis follicularis) demonstrates a suprabasilar blister and marked hyperkeratosis and papillomatosis; **B,** Abundant corps ronds (arrow) and grains (arrowhead) are present in most cases of Darier's disease (keratosis follicularis).

warty dyskeratoma has acantholytic changes similar to those seen in keratosis follicularis, but has a cup-shaped architecture and a markedly different clinical presentation. It is also important to evaluate the basal keratinocytes for atypia, as acantholysis is a common feature of actinic keratoses and squamous cell carcinomas, and these processes could be confused with Darier's disease or the other suprabasilar acantholytic blistering disorders.

Hailey-Hailey disease (benign familial pemphigus)

Clinical features. It is important to note that this disease is an autosomal dominant genodermatosis and not an autoimmune disease. Patients present early in life with erythematous, eczematous, and macerated patches in flexural and intertriginous areas. Intact bullae are rarely found. The disease tends to be exacerbated by heat and is worst in the summer months.[142]

Histologic features. An irregular, but primarily suprabasilar separation characterizes Hailey-Hailey disease. There is parakeratosis overlying the epidermis. The roof of the blister displays marked spongiosis and acantholysis, resulting in a 'dilapidated brick wall' appearance (Fig. 7.42). Corps ronds and grains may be seen, but are not common. A mild to moderate inflammatory infiltrate is present in the dermis, with focal exocytosis.[143]

Differential diagnosis. The epidermis on the roof of the blister cavity has a tendency to disintegrate in Hailey-Hailey disease in contrast to the other suprabasilar blistering processes. Unlike in keratosis follicularis, hyperkeratosis is not a feature of Hailey-Hailey disease. Direct immunofluorescence examination is negative in this process.

Transient acantholytic dermatotis (Grover's disease)

Clinical features. Transient acantholytic dermatotis (TAD) is a disease of middle-aged to elderly patients and is much more common in men. It presents as tiny, pruritic erythematous papules on the chest and back. It is often associated with conditions of increased body temperature. Lesions in TAD often persist for months to years, despite its name.[144]

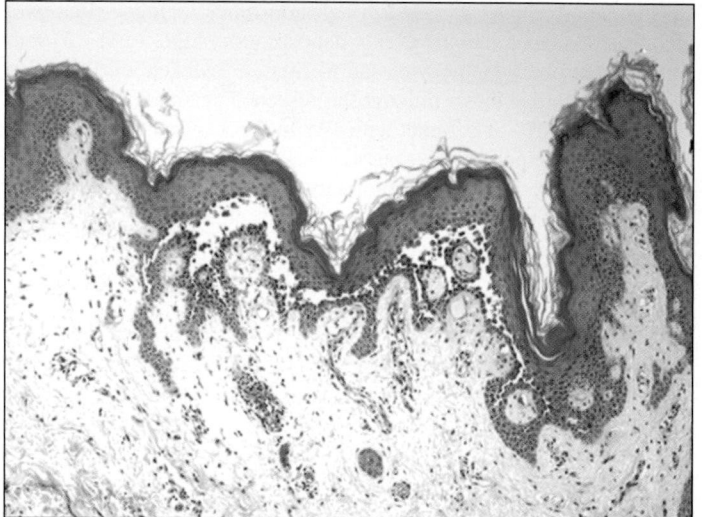

Fig. 7.42 A 'dilapidated brick wall' characterizes the roof of the blister in Hailey-Hailey disease (benign familial pemphigus).

Histologic features. Biopsies from patients with TAD can display several different histologic patterns. In some cases, features of spongiotic dermatitis are noted and there is no intraepidermal separation. In these cases, it is not possible to render a specific diagnosis. More typical cases demonstrate small foci of intraepidermal blister formation. These blisters may resemble those seen in pemphigus vulgaris, keratosis follicularis or Hailey-Hailey disease (Fig. 7.43). Blister spaces are quite small and it may require deeper sections through the block to identify them. There is a focal inflammatory infiltrate present in the papillary dermis in most cases. Scattered eosinophils are found in most cases.[145]

Differential diagnosis. The differential diagnosis of TAD includes the other suprabasilar blistering processes. Accurate diagnosis is made

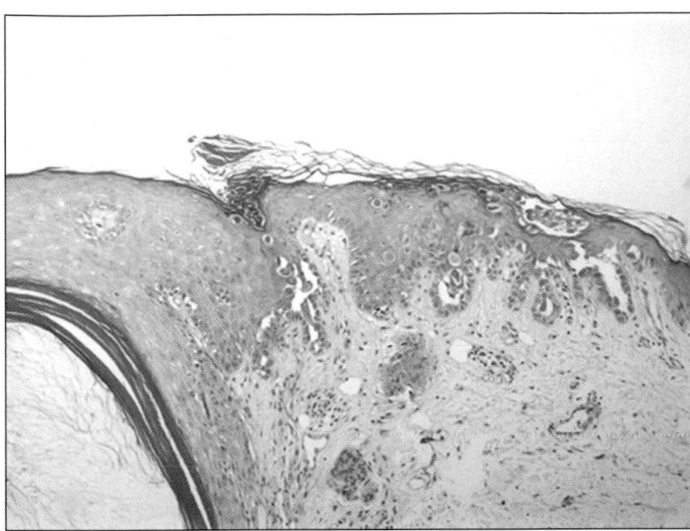

Fig. 7.43 Corps ronds and grains are present, along with a suprabasilar blister in this case of transient acantholytic dermatosis (Grover's disease).

based upon a classic clinical history for TAD (which is quite different from the other disorders in the histologic differential diagnosis) and by the minute sizes of the blisters. Direct immunofluorescence examination is invariably negative in TAD.

Herpetic dermatitis

Clinical features. Painful grouped vesicles with clear fluid based upon erythematous surrounding skin appear in a dermatomal distribution. Varicella-zoster, chickenpox, is most common in children. In this entity, the characteristic herpetic lesions appear most commonly on the face and trunk, with extremities involved to a lesser degree. Lesions of all stages of development can be seen simultaneously. Disease recurrence in the form of herpes zoster is seen in patients with altered immune status. The recurrences tend to

appear along a dermatomal distribution, as the viruses are harbored in nerve ganglia.[146–148] Herpes simplex types I and II infections present with similar appearing lesions. While type I lesions are most common on the face and type II infections more likely to be genital in distribution, there is extensive overlap. The lesions are often painful, especially with primary infections.

Histologic features. While the clinical manifestations of herpes simplex I, herpes simplex type II, and varicella-zoster virus infections differ, the histologic features are essentially identical. There is dissolution of the epidermis with reticular degeneration. It is difficult to precisely localize the level of the blister, as the epidermis appears to be falling apart at all levels within the affected areas. Ballooning degeneration of keratinocytes is prominent and herpetic inclusions are readily identified in most cases. 'Steel-gray' nuclei represent virally infected cells with margination of nuclear chromatin at the periphery (Fig. 7.44). Multinucleation and molding are other characteristics of affected keratinocytes. Follicular epithelium is involved in some cases.[149] There is a dense, polymorphous inflammatory infiltrate within the dermis. It is most pronounced in primary infections, but remains intense in all acute lesions. Vasculitis is present underlying many cases of herpesvirus infection. A granulomatous dermal inflammatory infiltrate has been described.[150]

Differential diagnosis. Herpes family viral infections can be reliably distinguished from other suprabasilar blistering processes based upon detection of the intranuclear inclusions, multinucleation of keratinocytes, and irregular site of the blister formation. In addition, there is often a much more intense inflammatory infiltrate within the dermis than is seen with the other intraepidermal blistering disorders.

SUBEPIDERMAL BLISTERING DISORDERS

Once it is established that a blister is occurring in a subepidermal location, it is important next to characterize the nature of the inflammatory response. Diseases with predominant eosinophils include bullous pemphigoid, bullous drug eruptions, and bullous

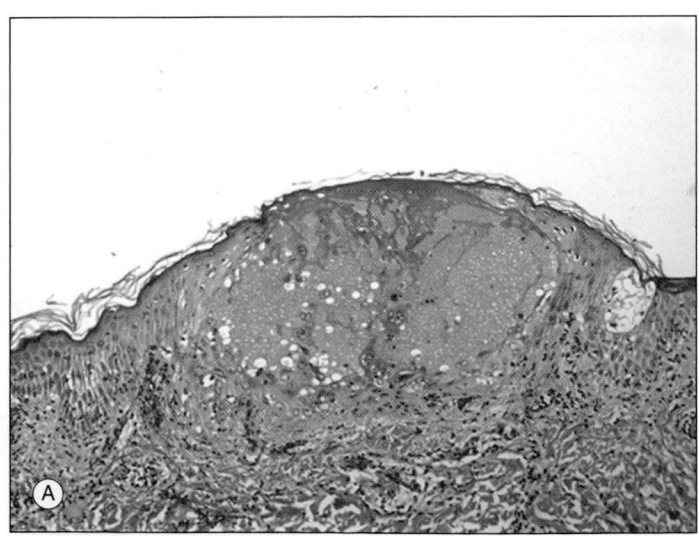
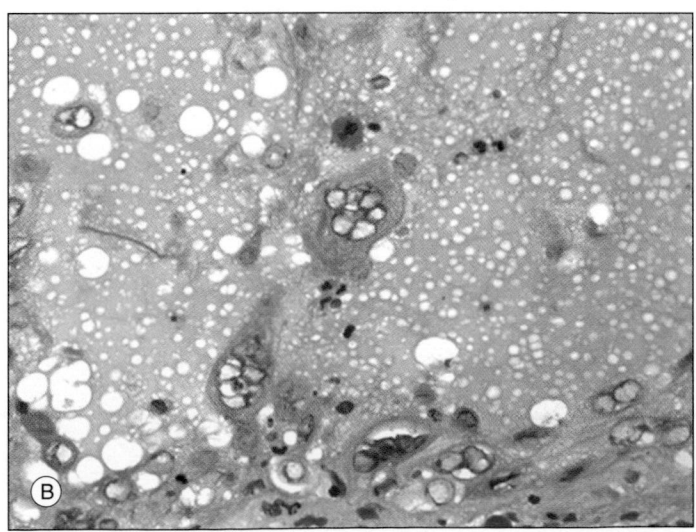

Fig. 7.44 A, An acantholytic blister, occurring at multiple levels of the epidermis is seen in herpes simplex infection; **B**, Multinucleated cells, 'steel-gray' nuclei, and nuclear molding characterize herpes simplex infection of the skin.

Table 7.10 Subepidermal blisters – histologic differential diagnosis

Inflammatory

Eosinophil predominant

   Bullous arthropod bite reaction

   Bullous pemphigoid

   Herpes (pemphigoides) gestationis

Neutrophilic predominant

   Cicatricial pemphigoid

   Dermatitis herpetiformis

   Epidermolysis bullosa acquisita

   Linear IgA bullous dermatosis (bullous dermatosis of childhood)

   Lupus erythematosus (bullous)

Lymphocytic

   Erythema multiforme

   Lichen planus

   Lichen sclerosis

Non-inflammatory

   Bullous dermatosis of hemodialysis

   Epidermolysis bullosa

   Porphyria cutanea tarda

   Scar

arthropod bites (Table 7.10). Those with abundant neutrophils include dermatitis herpetiformis, cicatricial pemphigoid, bullous lupus erythematosus, and some cases of epidermolysis bullosa acquisita. Non-inflammatory subepidermal blistering processes include inherited forms of epidermolysis bullosa and porphyria cutanea tarda. (Some cases of bullous pemphigoid may be paucicellular.) Most subepidermal blisters with lymphocytes as the predominant cell type are classified under interface dermatoses and are also characterized by dying keratinocytes, resulting in subepidermal blister formation.

These include lichen planus, erythema multiforme, and graft-versus-host disease.

Bullous pemphigoid

Clinical features. Bullous pemphigoid (BP) is primarily a disease of the elderly. Patients present with tense bullae occurring on erythematous bases. There may be associated pruritus. A Nikolski sign is absent in most cases (see pemphigus vulgaris). In some patients, tense bullae do not form, and the disease appears as urticarial plaques. About a third of patients with BP have involvement of the oral cavity.[151]

Histologic features. A subepidermal blister characterizes BP. There is no necrosis of overlying keratinocytes, except in secondarily ischemic older lesions. There is a dense, superficial inflammatory infiltrate with an abundance of eosinophils. The inflammatory cells are confined to the blister cavity and the papillary dermis (Fig. 7.45A). There is an urticarial form of BP in which no definitive bullae are detected clinically. In these cases, eosinophils are aligned along the dermal–epidermal junction, with some exocytosis of eosinophils into the overlying epidermis, but no subepidermal split is detected.

Differential diagnosis. The histologic differential diagnosis includes a bullous drug eruption and bullous arthropod bite reactions. The best way to distinguish these entities is with direct immunofluorescence examination. On purely histologic grounds, the presence of a deep inflammatory infiltrate suggests one of the two other processes over that of BP.[152]

Adjuncts to diagnosis. Direct immunofluorescence examination is very helpful in confirming a diagnosis of BP. Greater than 90% of biopsies demonstrate strong linear staining with IgG and C3 along the dermal–epidermal junction (Fig. 7.45B). Using the salt-split skin technique, these deposits can be further localized to the roof of the blister (within the lamina lucida). False-negative results are seen in biopsies taken from within the blisters themselves (possibly due to breakdown of immunoglobulins by the granulocytes) and on biopsies taken from lower extremities (for unknown reasons). Indirect immunofluorescence examination is also helpful, demonstrating a

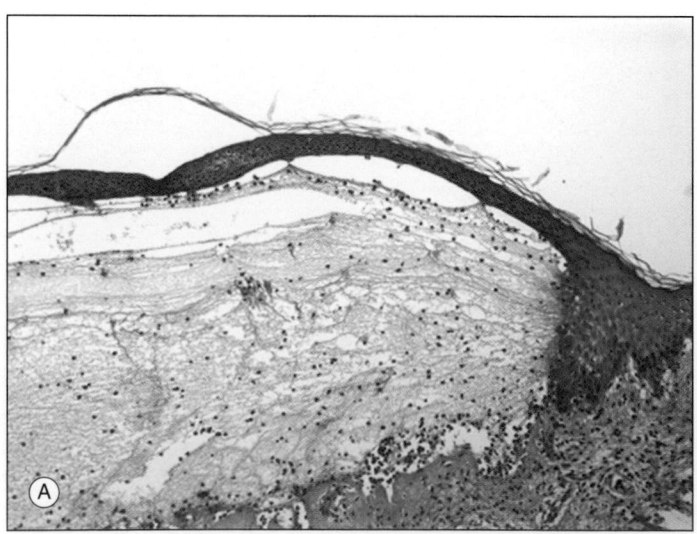
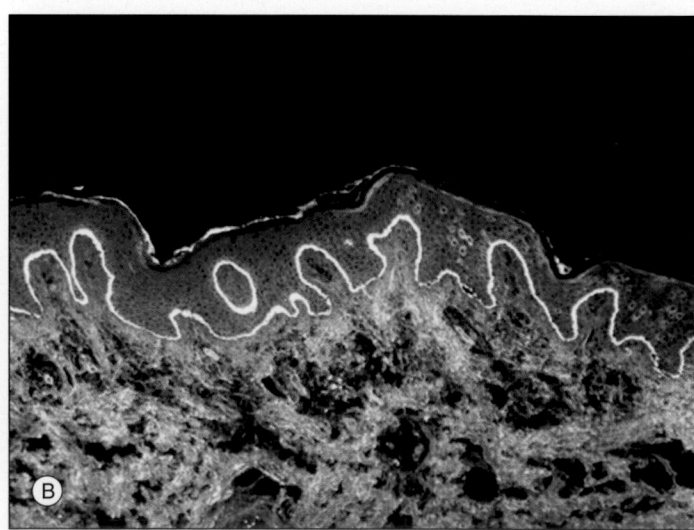

Fig. 7.45 A, A subepidermal blister with abundant eosinophils is seen in bullous pemphigoid; **B,** Strong linear staining with anti-IgG is present along the basement membrane in bullous pemphigoid.

similar staining pattern in the great majority of patients. However, unlike the case with pemphigus vulgaris, it is not always possible to monitor disease activity using antibody titers with indirect immunofluorescence.[152,153]

Herpes gestationis (pemphigoides gestationis)

Clinical features. Herpes gestationis (HG) is an autoimmune blistering disorder that is associated with pregnancy. It does not usually occur in first pregnancies, but when present, reappears with increased severity with each subsequent pregnancy. In the middle trimester, or later, patients develop tense blisters on erythematous bases. The autoantibodies may cross the placenta and cause a similar cutaneous eruption in newborn infants. However, the disorder is not associated with any long-term consequences for the infant or with increase in fetal mortality.[154]

Histologic features. The histologic features of HG are indistinguishable from bullous pemphigoid.[155]

Differential diagnosis. The major histologic differential diagnoses include bullous pemphigoid, which is most readily distinguished based upon clinical history, and linear IgA bullous dermatosis, which has more of a neutrophilic infiltrate as opposed to eosinophil predominant. The clinical differential diagnosis includes pruritic urticarial papules and plaques of pregnancy, which does not give rise to subepidermal blisters, but rather is a spongiotic disorder (see above).

Adjuncts to diagnosis. Direct immunofluorescence examination is often helpful in establishing the diagnosis of HG. A linear band of staining with complement is present along the dermal–epidermal junction. In many (but not all) cases, IgG is present in a similar pattern. In some cases, the antibodies used in the assay do not detect the subtype of IgG implicated in the pathogenesis of this auto-immune process and IgG may go undetected.[156]

Dermatitis herpetiformis

Clinical features. Patients with dermatitis herpetiformis present with symmetrically distributed, intensely pruritic papules, most commonly on the knees, elbows, and sacrum. It is a chronic and progressive disease of young to middle-aged adults. It is rare to find intact vesicles, as most of them are rapidly excoriated due to the intense pruritus. Dermatitis herpetiformis is associated with gluten-sensitive enteropathy. All patients have small intestinal involvement, though it is subclinical in many.[157,158]

Histologic features. Small subepidermal blisters characterize dermatitis herpetiformis. Neutrophilic microabscesses are present within the papillary dermal tips. It is important to find these in areas away from ulceration where neutrophils may be involved in the secondary pathology (Fig. 7.46). The deeper portions of the dermis demonstrate a perivascular lymphocytic inflammatory infiltrate. Occasional eosinophils may be present.[157,159]

Differential diagnosis. The differential diagnosis of dermatitis herpetiformis includes linear IgA bullous dermatosis, bullous lupus erythematosus, cicatricial pemphigoid, and epidermolysis bullosa acquisita. Linear IgA bullous dermatosis has a different clinical presentation, larger subepidermal bullae than are seen in dermatitis herpetiformis, and linear deposition of IgA along the dermal–epidermal junction. Bullous lupus erythematosus is characterized by other histologic features of lupus erythematosus not seen in dermatitis herpetiformis, in addition to the markedly different clinical presentation and direct immunofluorescence patterns. Cicatricial pemphigoid has larger subepidermal bullae and usually

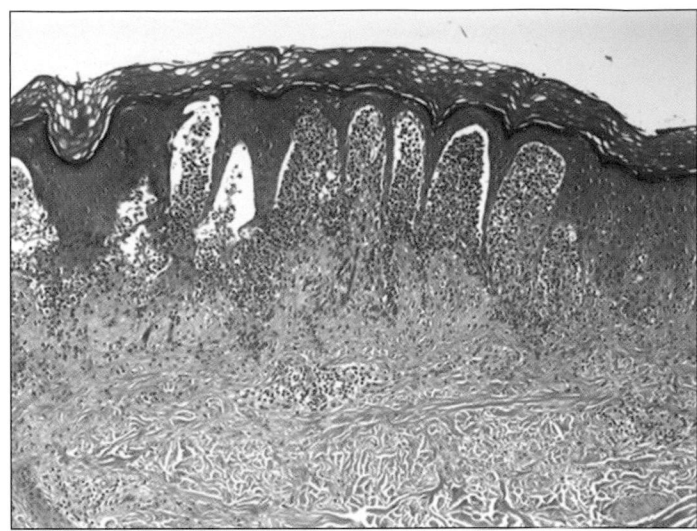

Fig. 7.46 Neutrophilic abscesses within the papillary dermal tips and small blisters characterize dermatitis herpetiformis.

involves mucosal surfaces, in contrast to dermatitis herpetiformis. Linear deposition of immunoglobulins is seen in this entity, in contrast to dermatitis herpetiformis. Epidermolysis bullosa acquisita affects different anatomic locations and is also characterized by linear deposition of immunoglobulins along the dermal–epidermal junction.

Adjuncts to diagnosis. Direct immunofluorescence examination is very helpful in confirming the diagnosis of dermatitis herpetiformis. Virtually all biopsies will demonstrate intense deposition of IgA in the papillary dermal tips, often with C3. This is most pronounced in perilesional skin, as the neutrophilic infiltrates within the lesions may degrade the immunoglobulins.

Linear IgA bullous dermatosis (bullous dermatosis of childhood)

Clinical features. Linear IgA bullous dermatosis and bullous dermatosis of childhood have similar histologic and clinical presentations, but occur in different settings. Linear IgA bullous dermatosis is a disease of adulthood that presents with many bullae occurring in an annular distribution on an erythematous patch. The pattern has been described as a 'cluster of jewels' appearance. This eruption is associated with many types of therapeutic drugs.[160–162] Oral and other mucous membranes are commonly involved. Bullous dermatosis of childhood gives rise to similar-appearing bullae in a similar distribution, but occurs in children.

Histologic features. Linear IgA bullous dermatosis (in both forms) demonstrates a subepidermal, inflammatory blister. Within the underlying dermis, there is a dense neutrophilic inflammatory infiltrate aligned along the dermal–epidermal junction without a tendency to aggregate in the papillary dermal tips (Fig. 7.47). Occasional eosinophils may be present. The deeper portions of the dermis are usually unremarkable.

Differential diagnosis. The differential diagnosis includes dermatitis herpetiformis, cicatricial pemphigoid, epidermolysis bullosa acquisita, and bullous lupus erythematosus. In dermatitis herpetiformis, the neutrophils are often clustered within the papillary dermal tips and the blisters are much smaller. The other entities in

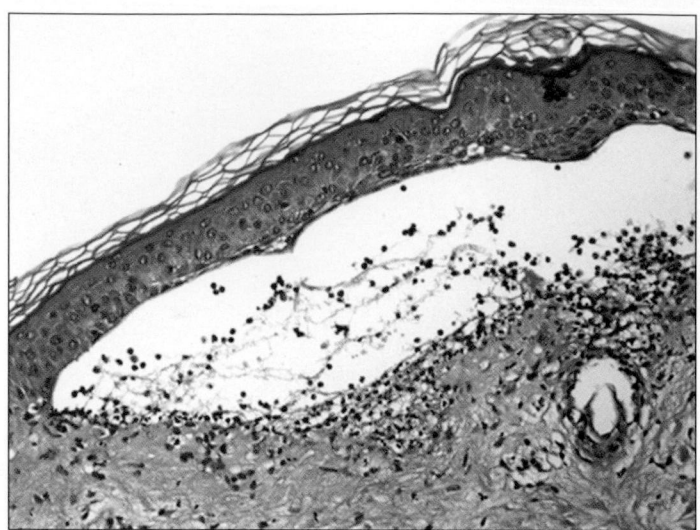

Fig. 7.47 Linear IgA demonstrates a subepidermal blister with abundant neutrophils in the blister cavity. The blisters are usually larger than those seen in dermatitis herpetiformis.

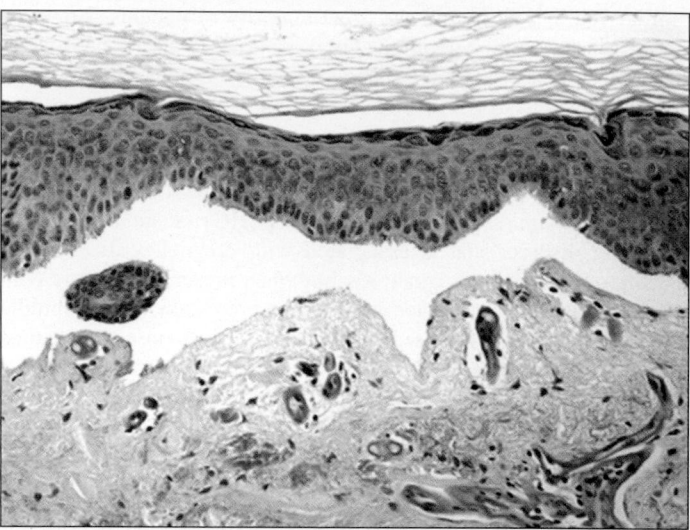

Fig. 7.48 A PAS stain with diastase pretreatment demonstrates a noninflammatory subepidermal blister with festooning and thickening of vessel walls in this case of porphyria cutanea tarda.

the differential diagnosis can be histologically indistinguishable from linear IgA bullous dermatosis, but the clinical histories and the direct immunofluorescence examination usually makes this separation straightforward.

Adjuncts to diagnosis. There is strong linear staining along the dermal–epidermal junction with IgA. C3 is present in most cases, and rarely IgM may be seen in a similar pattern. This pattern of immunoglobulin deposition is highly specific for this disease.

Cicatricial pemphigoid

Clinical features. Cicatricial pemphigoid (CP) is a bullous disorder that resolves with clinical scarring. Mucosal surfaces are frequently involved. This may result in blindness without rapid intervention. The very rare Brunsting-Perry variant of CP is most prevalent on the scalp and does not involve mucosal surfaces. A scarring alopecia may develop.[163]

Histologic features. Biopsies from patients with CP demonstrate skin with a subepidermal blistering process. An intact epidermis is present overlying a blister cavity that is filled with neutrophils and occasional eosinophils. The inflammatory infiltrate within the dermis remains relatively superficial. Scarring may be seen in well-developed lesions.[164]

Differential diagnosis. The differential diagnosis of CP includes other subepidermal blisters with neutrophilic inflammatory infiltrates. Linear IgA bullous dermatosis is best distinguished with direct immunofluorescence studies. Bullous pemphigoid has more abundant eosinophils and less prominent neutrophils in most cases, in addition to a different clinical presentation. Similarly, lupus erythematosus can usually be distinguished based upon the clinical presentation and the immunofluorescence findings. Clinical history and presentation best distinguish epidermolysis bullosa acquisita.

Adjuncts to diagnosis. Direct immunofluorescence examination reveals linear deposition of IgG and C3 (and less commonly IgM or IgA) along the dermal–epidermal junction. Performing the technique on salt-split skin reveals immunoglobulins on both the floor and roof of the blister space (in contrast to bullous pemphigoid

that demonstrates deposition on the roof). While most biopsies demonstrate immunodeposits on direct immunofluorescence, indirect immunofluorescence results are more variable in patients with CP.[165]

Porphyria cutanea tarda

Clinical features. Patients with porphyria cutanea tarda (PCT) demonstrate blisters on the dorsal aspects of their hands and fingers. The blisters tend to heal with scarring, and milia are prominent in many patients. Increased hirsutism, especially on the lateral sides of the face, is commonly seen. Many patients with PCT demonstrate extreme photosensitivity. PCT is associated with many systemic disorders, including hepatic insufficiency, hepatitis C, and alcoholism.[166]

Histologic features. A noninflammatory, subepidermal blister characterizes PCT. Within the dermis, there is extensive solar elastosis. Thickening of superficially located postcapillary venules that remain abnormally patent causes festooning of the papillary dermal tips. This thickening is demonstrated best with a PAS stain. A minimal inflammatory response is present in early lesions.[166]

Differential diagnosis. The differential diagnosis includes epidermolysis bullosa, in which festooning and solar elastosis are not present, nor is thickening of papillary dermal blood vessel walls (Fig. 7.48). In rare cases, bullous pemphigoid may be paucicellular, but the clinical presentation is usually helpful in making this distinction.

Adjuncts to diagnosis. Direct immunofluorescence examination reveals a linear band of IgG, IgM, and C3 along the dermal-epidermal junction and surrounding blood vessels in some cases. It is believed that this is not true immunoglobulin deposition, but represents non-specific trapping. The linear quality of the perivascular deposits helps distinguish this from the pattern seen in leukocytoclastic vasculitis.[152]

Epidermolysis bullosa

Clinical features. Epidermolysis bullosa (EB) is a rare family of related inherited mechanicobullous disorders. There are many

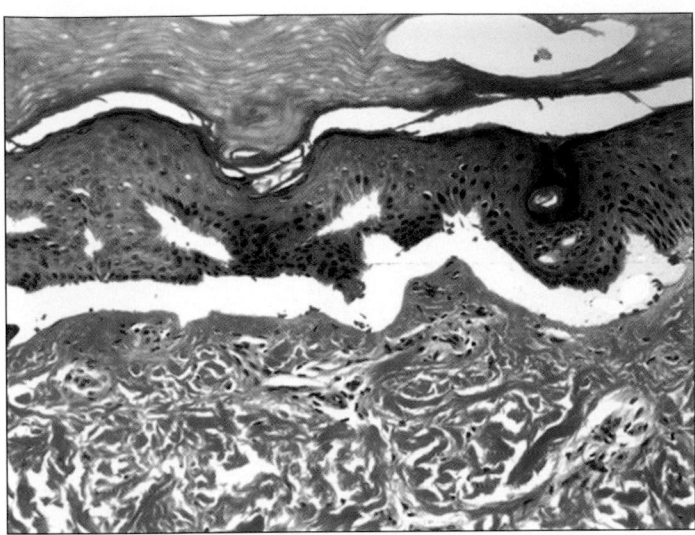

Fig. 7.49 A noninflammatory subepidermal blister without subjacent scar formation characterizes junctional epidermolysis bullosa.

clinical variants that are conveniently separated into three large categories.[167] *EB simplex* represents the group that demonstrates epidermal splitting through the basal keratinocyte (for the most part) due to abnormal keratins 5 and 14. These forms of the disease tend to be inherited in an autosomal dominant fashion, and are generally relatively mild. Small blisters develop, generally on acral surfaces and heal without clinical scarring. EB simplex tends to slowly become less symptomatic with age. There are many subtypes of EB simplex that are associated with other cutaneous and extracutaneous manifestations.[168]

Junctional EB is the form of EB that gives rise to blisters that occur within the lamina lucida portion of the basement membrane zone (Fig. 7.49).[169] Due to defects in the structural proteins that maintain the integrity of the zone, slight mechanical trauma gives rise to blisters. The *Herlitz* variant of this disease is associated with complete absence of some of these proteins and is associated with rapid progression to death. Less extensive variants exist that are associated with multiple cutaneous and extracutaneous manifestations. Junction EB is generally inherited in an autosomal recessive manner.

Dystrophic EB occurs in autosomal recessive and dominant inherited forms. Anchoring fibrils (type VII collagen) are either decreased (dominant) or absent (recessive), giving rise to blisters that occur beneath the basement membrane, high within the papillary dermis. These blisters heal with extensive scarring and result in flexion contractures and other severe physical deformities. Patients with the disease for decades are also predisposed to developing squamous cell carcinomas of the skin that have a high rate of metastasis. The recessive form of the disease is associated within significant shortening of life expectancy. Multiple variants have been described that are associated with a wide range of cutaneous and extracutaneous manifestations.

Epidermolysis bullosa acquisita (EBA) is a relatively recently described autoimmune blistering disease that presents with mechanically induced blisters at sites of minor trauma. Blisters are most common on extremities. The disease, whose onset is usually in adulthood, is very difficult to treat.[170]

Histologic features. The various subtypes of EB share many histologic features. On routine sections, they all appear as noninflammatory, subepidermal blisters (though in some cases of EB simplex, small fragments of basal keratinocyte can be detected at the base of the blister cavity). In the dystrophic forms of the disease, dermal scarring can be quite pronounced.

EBA is characterized by either a noninflammatory subepidermal blister or, in many cases, a densely inflammatory, neutrophilic subepidermal blister, greatly resembling bullous lupus erythematosus or linear IgA bullous dermatosis.[170]

Differential diagnosis. The differential diagnosis includes porphyria cutanea tarda that can be easily distinguished based upon clinical history, festooning, increased solar elastosis, and thickening of papillary dermal blood vessel walls.

Adjuncts to diagnosis. Direct immunofluorescence examination is negative in all inherited forms of EB, as these entities are not autoimmune mediated. EBA, in contrast, demonstrates a linear band of IgG and C3 along the dermal–epidermal junction, as it is caused by the deposition of autoantibodies directed against type VII collagen. On salt-split skin examination, the staining localizes to the floor of the blister, unlike in bullous pemphigoid.

Electron microscopic examination has, for many years, been the gold standard in establishing the precise level of the blister formation in the various subtypes of EB. In recent years, however, this technology has been largely supplanted by immunofluorescence examination using antibodies directed against specific basement membrane zone proteins. With these newer tests (which are not widely available yet), the precise biochemical defect can be ascertained, yielding extensive information about the disease process and its clinical prognosis.

INFLAMMATORY DISEASES OF THE HAIR FOLLICLES AND CARTILAGE

BACTERIAL AND FUNGAL FOLLICULITIS

Clinical features. Folliculitis appears as folliculocentric, erythematous papules. The disease is common on the trunk and extremities. Pustules are present in acute, suppurative stages of the disease. Pruritus is only variably present. Folliculitis is arbitrarily classified into a superficial type known as *impetigo of Bockhart* and a deeper type that is known as a furuncle. Multiple fused furuncles give rise to deep, inflamed sinuses known as carbuncles.[122] *Majocchi's granuloma* is a term for folliculitis caused by dermatophytes (most commonly *Trichophyton rubra*). A fungal folliculitis involving the scalp is known as a kerion. This can be the source of a scarring alopecia if not treated quickly and completely.

Histologic features. Folliculitis is characterized by an inflammatory infiltrate within and around hair follicles. In acute, suppurative cases, neutrophilic abscesses may be present within the follicular epithelium or in the outflow tract within the stratum corneum. In more extensive cases, follicular epithelial destruction results in granulomatous inflammation and scar formation. In subacute to chronic cases, plasma cells may be present within the inflammatory infiltrate. Fungal folliculitis is a diagnosis made based upon the recognition of fungi within the follicular epithelium (Fig. 7.50). Fungi can be within the hair shafts (endothrix) or outside (ectothrix). *Pityrosporum* is frequently present as a 'normal' inhabitant of the stratum corneum, and may not be pathogenetic. *Demodex* mites apparently give rise to some cases of folliculitis; however, these organisms are seen in biopsies from many patients with no evidence of folliculitis, so their role in causing disease remains unknown.

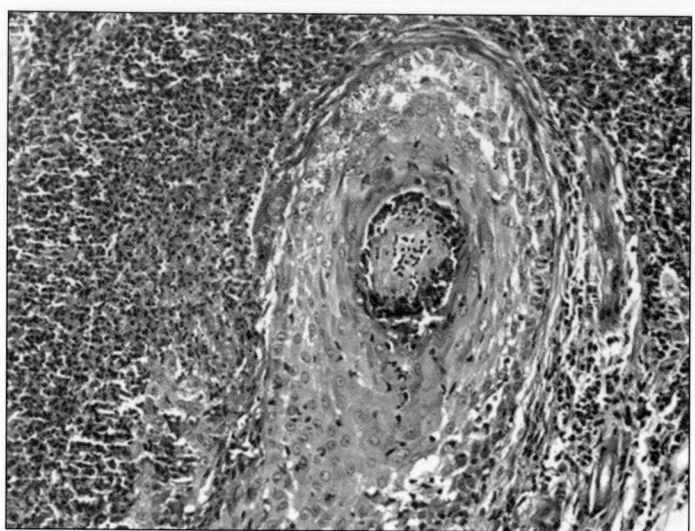

Fig. 7.50 PAS stain with diastase pretreatment demonstrates many yeast and hyphal forms within the infundibulum of the hair follicle in Majocchi's granuloma.

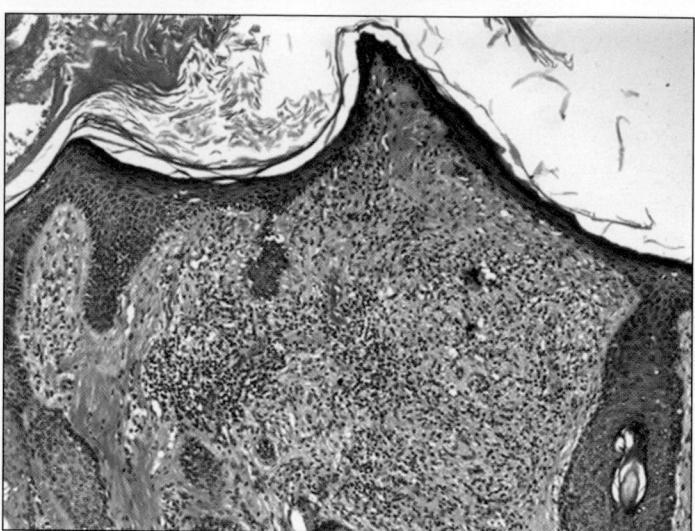

Fig. 7.51 A granulomatous folliculitis and perifolliculitis characterize acne rosacea.

Folliculitis decalvans is a neutrophilic folliculitis that rapidly progresses to a scarring alopecia. Multiple pustules are present on a diffusely erythematous and edematous base. Special stains fail to reveal organisms. Rapid clinical intervention is essential in order to prevent scarring alopecia.

Acne keloidalis nuchae is a folliculitis found primarily in young Afro-American adults. It presents as inflamed, erythematous nodules, most commonly on the back of the neck. These folliculocentric lesions heal with dense scar and keloid formation. The primary pathologic event is thought to be due to follicular epithelial rupture secondary to inwardly growing hairs. Unless there is superimposed infection, special stains and cultures are usually negative.

Differential diagnosis. Eosinophilic folliculitis should be distinguished from the usual case of folliculitis that may demonstrate scattered eosinophils within a predominantly lymphocytic inflammatory infiltrate.

ACNE (GRANULOMATOUS) ROSACEA

Clinical features. Acne rosacea (AR) is a disease of middle-aged people. It presents as papules and nodules on the face. Telangiectasias are prominent. One variant of the disease, known as rhinophyma, causes a bulbous nose secondary to hyperplasia of the sebaceous glands. While the eyelids are often spared, in the variant known as *lupus miliaris disseminatum faciei*, eyelid involvement may be prominent.[171]

Histologic features. Histologic findings of AR include a lymphocytic infiltrate surrounding and invading the follicular epithelium at the level of the infundibulum. In florid cases, the epithelium may be disrupted, giving rise to a granulomatous inflammatory infiltrate (Fig. 7.51). The granulomas are surrounded by a brisk infiltrate of lymphocytes. Ectasia of superficial blood vessels is present in some cases. Sebaceous hyperplasia may be present. In lupus miliaris disseminatum faciei, caseating granulomas are present adjacent to disrupted follicles.[171] Special stains fail to reveal organisms.

Differential diagnosis. The differential diagnosis includes lupus erythematosus and seborrheic dermatitis. An interface dermatitis, characteristic of the former, is not seen in acne rosacea. A psoriasiform, spongiotic process characteristic of seborrheic dermatitis is also not a feature, though it can sometimes be difficult to distinguish these entities without clinical history. In more granulomatous cases, sarcoidosis enters the differential diagnosis. The granulomas in sarcoidosis have relatively less inflammation and are not as intimately associated with hair follicles as is seen in acne rosacea. Lupus vulgaris (one form of cutaneous tuberculosis) can resemble lupus miliaris disseminatum faciei and special stains may be required to make this distinction.

FOLLICULAR MUCINOSIS

Clinical features. Follicular mucinosis (FM) presents as an erythematous, boggy plaque on the head or neck with grouped, patulous follicular openings. Hairs may be diminished or absent within the affected areas. The disease affects children and adults and is associated with mycosis fungoides in about half of the adult patients with it. It has also been associated with other types of lymphoma and non-neoplastic inflammatory conditions.[172] Idiopathic cases of FM resolve within months to two years.

Histologic features. Histologic features of FM include a dense infiltrate of lymphocytes within and around the follicular infundibular epithelium. Within the epithelium, there is abundant mucin deposition, most pronounced in the region of the insertion of the sebaceous glands. Colloidal iron and Alcian blue stains accentuate this finding (Fig. 7.52). Eosinophils may be abundant in some cases. Cases of FM associated with mycosis fungoides have lymphocytes with the characteristic neoplastic morphology in the lymphoid infiltrate; however, it is sometimes difficult to distinguish cases of follicular mucinosis with concomitant mycosis fungoides from idiopathic cases.

Differential diagnosis. The differential diagnosis includes folliculitis with abundant spongiosis. Other types of folliculitis fail to demonstrate intraepithelial mucin such as that seen in FM. Other

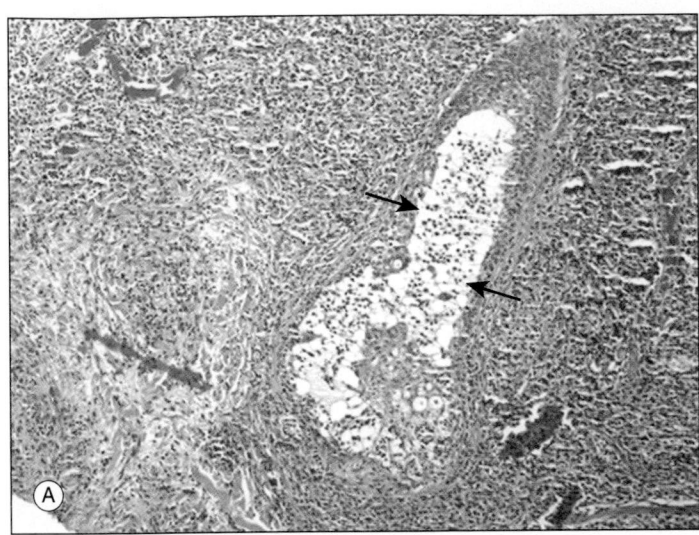
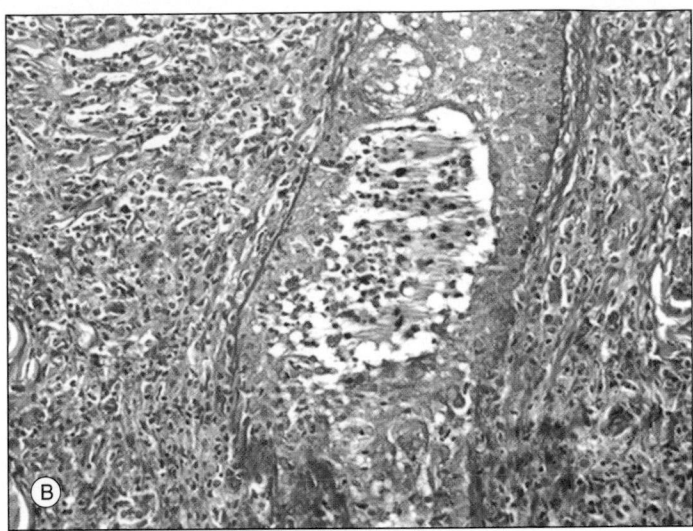

Fig. 7.52 A, Follicular mucinosis demonstrates abundant mucin within the follicular infundibulum (arrows), usually accompanied by a brisk lymphocytic infiltrate; **B**, Colloidal iron stain demonstrates abundant mucin within the follicular epithelium.

disorders with increased dermal mucin demonstrate the abnormal accumulations within the interstitium and not within the follicular epithelium.

EOSINOPHILIC FOLLICULITIS

Clinical features. Eosinophilic folliculitis is a generalized folliculocentric papular eruption. It occurs almost exclusively in patients suffering from AIDS and is intensely pruritic.[173] (There is a rare disease known as Ofuji's syndrome with similar histologic features that occurs exclusively in Japanese babies.[174]) The eruption is notoriously difficult to treat and a wide range of infestations and infections, including *Demodex* mites, *Pityrosporum* and bacteria has been implicated in its pathogenesis.

Histologic features. The histologic findings of eosinophilic folliculitis are essentially those of any type of folliculitis, except that the inflammatory infiltrate is comprised almost entirely of eosinophils. The infundibulum is the site of the most intense inflammation in most cases (Fig. 7.53). In some, but not all, cases, *Demodex* mites, or *Pityrosporum* organisms are present within the hair shaft cavity.[175]

Differential diagnosis. The differential diagnosis includes other types of infectious and noninfectious folliculitis that may include eosinophils as part of the inflammatory infiltrates. The clinical history of AIDS is helpful in arriving at the correct diagnosis.

CHONDRODERMATITIS NODULARIS HELICIS

Clinical features. Chondrodermatitis nodularis helicis (CNH) is a process associated with middle-aged to elderly patients. It occurs on the helix (usually) of the ear as a painful ulceration that does not heal. The clinical differential diagnosis includes basal cell carcinoma, actinic keratosis, and squamous cell carcinoma. The epidermal necrosis is caused by ischemic necrosis of the epidermis and underlying cartilage, caused by compression of dermal blood vessels by pressure during sleep.

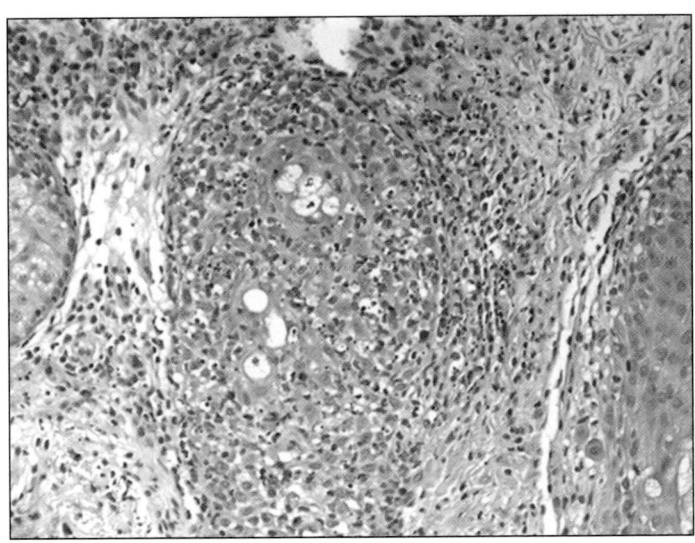

Fig. 7.53 Abundant eosinophils are present within the follicular epithelium in eosinophilic folliculitis.

Histologic features. Histologic findings of CNH include epidermal hyperplasia without atypia, hyperkeratosis, and focal central parakeratosis. Ulceration is usually present. There is fibrin along the dermal–epidermal junction. Within the dermis, many small vessels are present within dense collagenous stroma, giving a granulation tissue-like appearance. In deep biopsies, there is necrosis of the cartilage with a surrounding inflammatory infiltrate (Fig. 7.54). However, observation of cartilaginous destruction is not required to make the diagnosis.

Differential diagnosis. Relapsing polychondritis, a very uncommon autoimmune disease, may have similar histologic findings. In this entity, the epidermal changes associated with CNH are not present. There is a neutrophilic infiltrate within the cartilage and perichondrium that is not seen in CNH. Relapsing polychondritis is

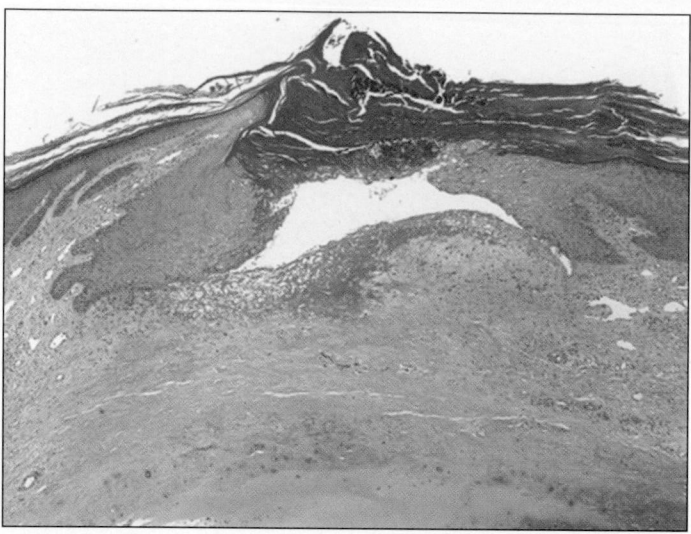

Fig. 7.54 Chondrodermatitis nodularis helicis demonstrates epidermal disruption with surrounding acanthosis, dermal fibrin deposition, and granulation tissue and, in deep biopsies, degeneration of the cartilage.

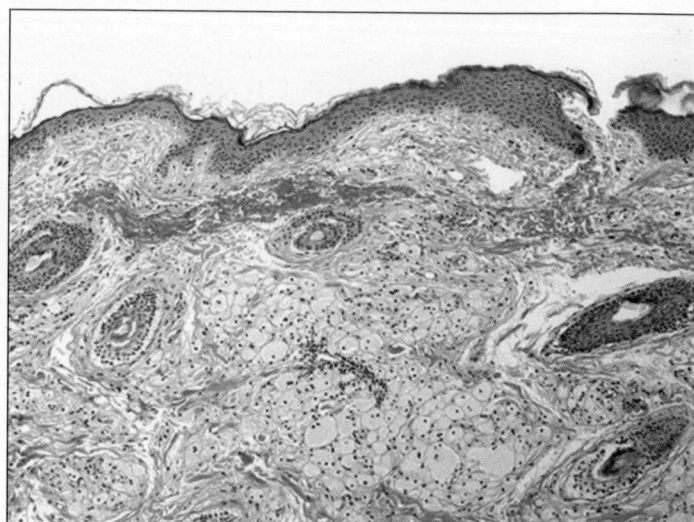

Fig. 7.55 Sheets of lipid-laden macrophages are present in the dermis in xanthelasma.

also associated with circulating antibodies directed against type II collagen.

DERMAL DEPOSITION DISORDERS

LIPIDOSES

Xanthelasma/xanthoma

Clinical features. Xanthomas have a range of different clinical features, depending upon the type. Xanthelasmata occur as yellow papules on the eyelids and are associated with hypercholesterolemia in about 33% of cases. Eruptive xanthomas appear as the sudden onset of multiple erythematous to slightly yellow papules. They are almost always associated with hypertriglyceridemia.[176,177] Tuberous xanthomas are yellow papules or nodules and are associated with hyperlipidemias in most cases.[178] Tendinous xanthomas have similar associations and appear as yellowish nodules within tendinous sheaths. Planar xanthomas are associated with biliary cirrhosis. Normolipemic planar xanthomas have also been described in patients with multiple myeloma.[179]

Histologic features. All xanthomatous processes are characterized by a dermal aggregation of lipid-laden macrophages. The degree of lipid correlates with the age of the lesion. Early lesions are more inflammatory and have lesser amounts of intracellular lipid. This pattern especially characterizes eruptive xanthomas. Well-developed xanthomas demonstrate sheets of lipid-laden cells, many of which may be multinucleated. Tendinous xanthomas are identified based upon their anatomic location in skin overlying fibrous tendons (that may be identified histologically in some biopsy specimens). Tuberous xanthomas are relatively large nodular lesions. Xanthelasmata are located on eyelids and biopsy specimens demonstrate lipid-laden histiocytes coursing in eyelid skin (Fig. 7.55).[180–182]

Differential diagnosis. Lepromatous leprosy could be confused with some types of xanthoma. Special stains and history, along with the prominence of nerves and plasma cells in leprosy, help to make this distinction. Juvenile xanthogranulomas may have extensive

Table 7.11   Cutaneous mucinoses

	Increased fibroblasts	**Normocellular dermis**
Superficial mucin	Lichen myxedematosus/ scleromyxedema	Pretibial myxedema
Deep mucin		Scleredema

lipidization, but present as single lesions, often in children, unassociated with hyperlipidemias.

MUCINOSES (Table 7.11)

Lichen myxedematosis/ scleromyxedema

Clinical features. Scleromyxedema and lichen myxedematosis (LM) have similar clinical appearances and may represent a spectrum of a single disease process. Affected patients present with crops of 2–4 mm, waxy, yellowish flat-topped papules. The face, hands, and dorsal extremities are commonly involved. In florid cases, the papules may coalesce into plaques, giving rise to a leonine facies. This is especially true of the scleromyxedema, the more extensive variant of this process. This disease affects middle-aged to elderly adults and is progressive. Scleromyxedema may also affect viscera and can be fatal.[183,184] It is occasionally associated with multiple myeloma or other gammopathies and an abnormal IgG light chain is almost always present.[185]

Histologic features. The epidermis is often atrophic, with diminution of rete ridges. The papillary and superficial reticular dermis contain increased amounts of mucin as detected on colloidal iron or Alcian blue stains. There is also an infiltrate of stellate-appearing fibroblasts. Minimal inflammation may be seen (Fig. 7.56). Some authors consider papular mucinosis to be a synonymous term.[186]

Differential diagnosis. The differential diagnosis includes other mucinoses. Pretibial myxedema also has increased mucin within the

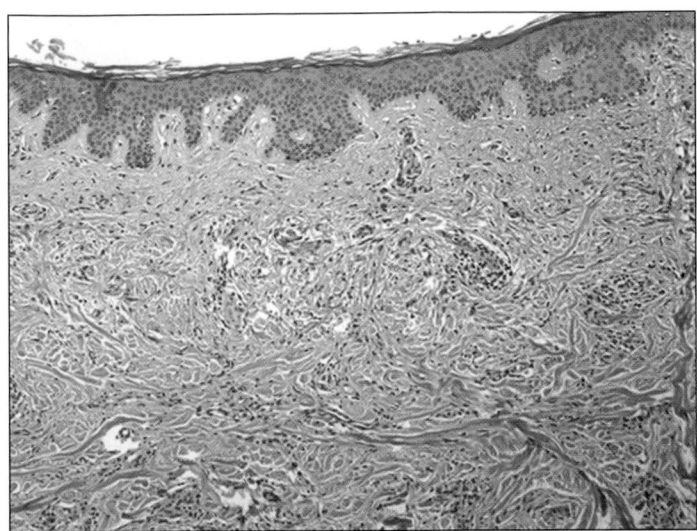

Fig. 7.56 Scleromyxedema is characterized by a proliferation of stellate-appearing fibroblasts coursing in a mucinous stroma in the superficial dermis.

superficial portion of the dermis, but is not associated with increased numbers of fibroblasts. Scleredema contains mucin primarily in the deep reticular dermis with no increase in fibroblasts. Dermatomyositis and lupus erythematosus both have prominent interface dermatoses in addition to superficially located dermal mucin.

Scleredema

Clinical features. There are two forms of scleredema. Both types present with diffuse thickening of the dermis on the face, shoulders, and upper back. The skin feels woody and tight. In children, scleredema most commonly occurs consequent to acute strep-tococcal infection and tends to resolve with time. In adults, the process tends to occur in patients with type II diabetes mellitus and is progressive.[187–189]

Histologic features. The striking histologic change is the marked thickening of the reticular dermis. The epidermis and papillary dermis are unremarkable. Collagen bundles are widely spaced throughout the deep reticular dermis. Often, the mucin is not detectable on routine stains, and may be difficult to see even with colloidal iron or Alcian blue stains (Fig. 7.57). There is no increase in numbers of fibroblasts.[190,191]

Differential diagnosis. The main histologic differential diagnosis is scleroderma. The dermal collagen bundles appear tightly packed with less interstitial space in scleroderma, whereas there is increased space between collagen bundles in scleredema. Scleroderma is also associated with a lymphoplasmacellular infiltrate not seen in scleredema, and does not have the increased mucin pathognomonic for scleredema. The other mucin deposition disorders demonstrate increased mucin in the upper dermis, unlike scleredema.

Pretibial myxedema

Clinical features. Patients suffering from thyroid disease may demonstrate waxy, yellowish, and somewhat edematous-appearing nodules and plaques on the lower extremities. The process is most common in patients with elevated LATS antibodies and Graves disease.[192,193]

Histologic features. The epidermis is hyperkeratotic and acanthotic. There is a *Grenz* zone within the papillary dermis. Increased amounts of dermal mucin are present within the superficial half of the reticular dermis (Fig. 7.58). Colloidal iron or Alcian blue stains enhance this finding. There is only a mild increase in numbers of dermal fibroblasts.[194,195]

Differential diagnosis. The differential diagnosis includes scleromyxedema/lichen myxedematosus. Clinical history is the easiest way to distinguish these entities. Pretibial myxedema has less of an infiltrate of fibroblasts. Generalized myxedema demonstrates only minimal increases in dermal mucin that are often difficult to detect, even with special stains.

Amyloidoses

Clinical features. Amyloidosis affects the skin in various ways. The most characteristic clinical manifestation is 'pinch purpura,'

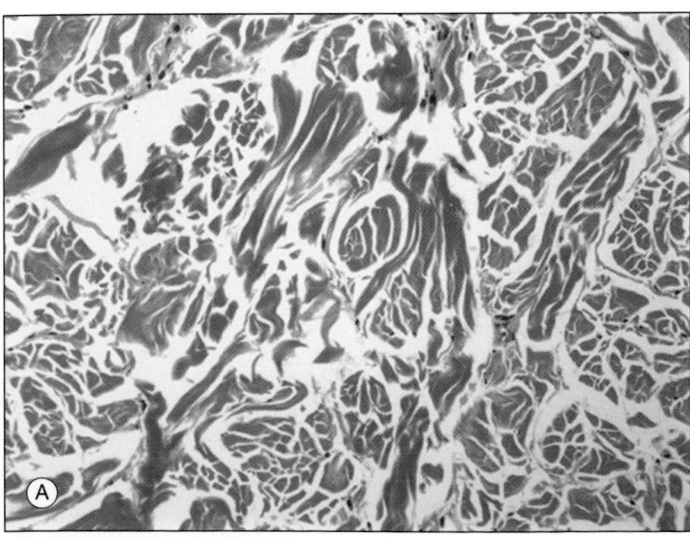

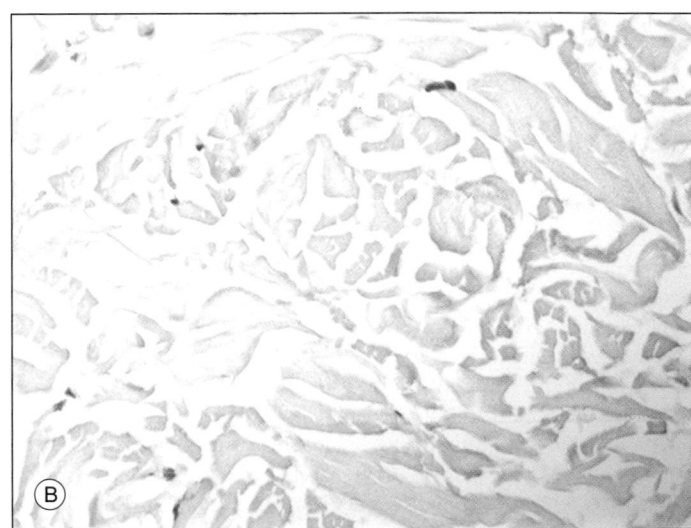

Fig. 7.57 A, Scleredema demonstrates increased amounts of clear space between adjacent deep reticular collagen bundles; **B**, Colloidal iron stain demonstrates abundant mucin within the reticular dermis in scleredema.

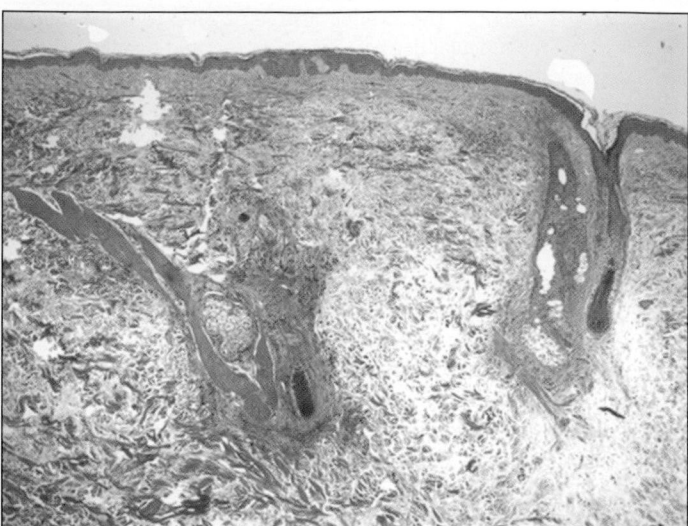

Fig. 7.58 Pretibial myxedema displays increased mucin in the superficial dermis with only a slight increase in numbers of fibroblasts.

purpuric patches, often around and on the eyelids. Waxy, yellow papules and nodules are also seen in some cases, as is thickening and apparent enlargement of the tongue. Primary amyloidosis, in which the amyloid is derived from degrading immunoglobulin light chains, involves the skin in patients with systemic or localized plasma cell dyscrasias.[196–198] Amyloidosis secondary to long-standing chronic inflammatory diseases does not manifest in the skin.

Lichen amyloidosis and macular amyloidosis are cutaneous processes in which the 'amyloid'-like material derives from degrading tonofilaments from degenerating keratinocytes. These closely related processes present as hyperpigmented, waxy patches or verrucous plaques (lichen amyloidosis) on body sites accessible to chronic rubbing or scratching. They are intensely pruritic and are most common in people from Southeast Asia.

Histologic features. The histologic features of amyloidosis vary with the types of lesion biopsied. Nodular amyloidosis appears as sheets of amorphous, amphophilic to eosinophilic material within the dermis that has a 'parched pavement' appearance. Crack-like clear spaces are present within the acellular masses of material (Fig. 7.59).[199,200]

In other cases, primary amyloidosis presents with similar-appearing eosinophilic material that is concentrated around dermal blood vessels and eccrine structures. In these cases, extravasation of erythrocytes is frequently seen.

In the primary cutaneous amyloidoses, small eosinophilic globules are present within the papillary dermis. These are derived from degrading keratinocytes. The epidermis may be acanthotic and hyperkeratotic (lichen amyloidosis) or relatively unremarkable (macular amyloidosis) (Fig. 7.60). Postinflammatory pigmentary incontinence is present in many cases, but there is minimal inflammation.

Differential diagnosis. The major differential diagnosis with nodular amyloidosis is colloid milium. The clinical history is helpful in making this distinction. In some cases, the dermal deposits in colloid milium have gray-blue color resembling elastic tissue, rather than the pinker color of the amyloid.

Adjuncts to diagnosis. While not usually necessary, antikeratin antibodies can be helpful in establishing a diagnosis of lichen

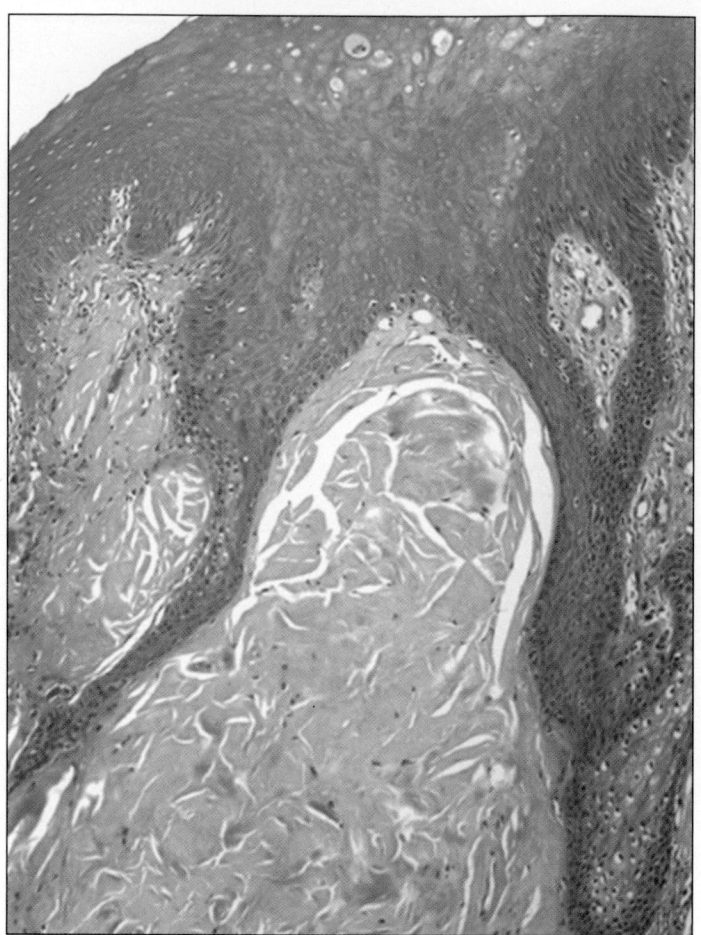

Fig. 7.59 Nodular amyloidosis is characterized by a 'cracked pavement' appearance in the dermis.

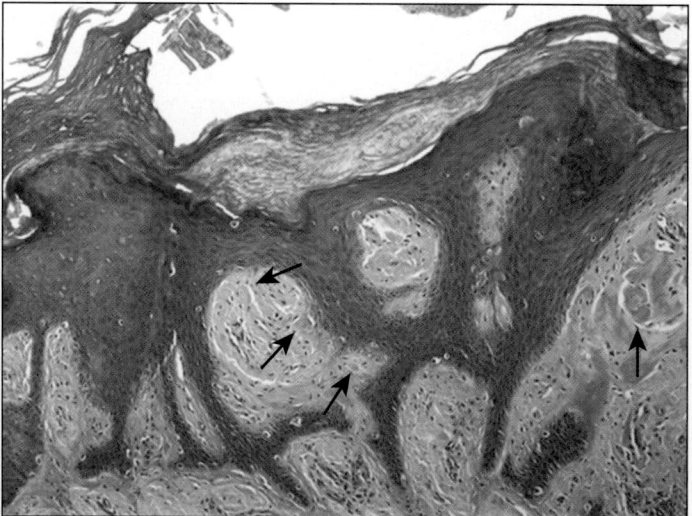

Fig. 7.60 Dying eosinophilic globules are present in the papillary dermis in lichen amyloidosis (arrows).

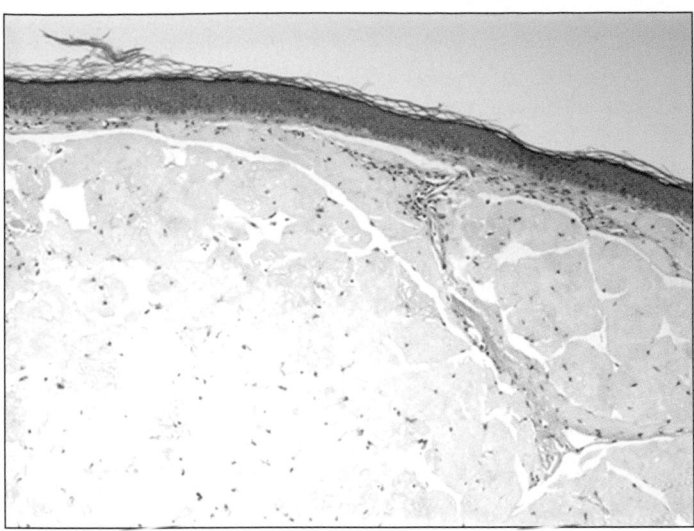

Fig. 7.61 Colloid milium displays a 'cracked pavement' appearance in the dermis, but the dermal material is usually more amphophilic than that seen in amyloidosis.

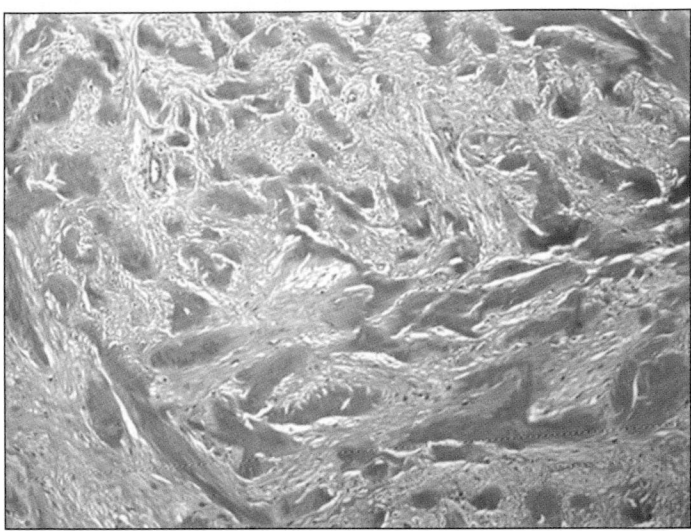

Fig. 7.62 A keloid is characterized by haphazardly arranged, enlarged and very eosinophilic collagen bundles.

amyloidosis or macular amyloidosis. Congo red and crystal violet stains may be helpful in identifying primary amyloid deposits (though occasionally, similar staining may be seen in colloid milium).

COLLAGEN DEPOSITION PROCESSES

Colloid milium

Clinical features. The adult form of colloid milium appears as 1–2 mm yellowish papules on sun-exposed areas of the hands, head, and neck. Degenerating elastotic material is believed to give rise to this process. A rare juvenile form of the disease is thought to be caused by abnormal breakdown of keratinocytes.

Histologic features. Sheets of amorphous, amphophilic material that is paucicellular largely replace the dermal collagen. It has a fissured appearance, similar to that seen in amyloidosis (Fig. 7.61).

Differential diagnosis. Colloid milium resembles nodular amyloidosis on routine histologic sections, but clinical history can usually distinguish these disorders. The abnormal dermal deposits may show weak congophilia.

Scar/hypertrophic scar/keloid

Clinical features. Scars are linear bands of fibrosis that occur at the sites of injury to the skin. They are flat to slightly raised and may be hypo- or hyperpigmented. Over time, they tend to become less prominent. Hypertrophic scars are raised scars. There is a more fibrotic response than that seen in ordinary scars. However, hypertrophic scars never extend beyond the boundaries of the original zone of injury and resolve spontaneously within two years. Keloids are aberrant scars in which large nodules appear at the sites of cutaneous injury. Keloids grow beyond the original site of injury and do not resolve spontaneously. They tend to recur with removal. Keloids are most common in young, Afro-American patients.

Histologic features. Ordinary scars are characterized by flattening of the rete rides and loss of cutaneous appendages within the area of scar. Linear, horizontally oriented collagen bundles extend parallel to the surface of the skin, admixed with increased numbers of fibroblasts within the dermis. As the lesions age, the number of fibroblasts diminishes. Vertically oriented, linear vessels are present throughout the region of the scar.

Hypertrophic scars appear as dome-shaped lesions. The epidermis is flattened by a nodular proliferation of collagen, which retains its linear orientation. Typical vertically oriented 'scar' vessels are present. Scant 'keloidal' collagen bundles, which are markedly thickened and eosinophilic, may be seen, but should not be prominent.

Significant amounts of altered collagen characterize keloids. Underlying a flattened epidermis, large nodules of haphazardly oriented collagen bundles are present. Many of the bundles are much thicker than ordinary collagen bundles and stain more intensely with eosin (Fig. 7.62). The number of fibroblasts decreases with the age of the lesion.

Differential diagnosis. Hypertrophic scars may resemble leiomyomas. A trichrome stain is helpful in distinguishing the slightly nodular, linear bundles of collagen from those of the smooth muscle proliferation. In connective tissue nevi, the collagen is haphazardly oriented, but no 'keloidal' collagen bundles are seen. In morphea/scleroderma, the collagen bundles are thickened, but maintain essentially normal orientation within the dermis (Table 7.12).

Scleroderma/morphea

Clinical features. Scleroderma is a systemic illness that is characterized by thickening of collagen within the skin and in internal viscera. Patients develop tight skin, with markedly decreased mobility, resulting in flexion contractures, sclerodactyly, and other cutaneous signs and symptoms.[201,202] Similar changes occur to vital organs, resulting in increased mortality. Renal-induced hypertension and esophageal dysmotility are common manifestations of the systemic illness. A more common variant of the process, morphea, demonstrates similar thickening of collagen bundles, but these changes are limited to the skin. Patients with morphea present with annular, sclerotic plaques that usually demonstrate tinctoral changes on the surface. Early lesions tend to be violaceous, especially at their periphery, and the lesions tend to become hyperpigmented over time. There are multiple subtypes of morphea that have various clinical presentations including *coup de sabre*, Perry-Romberg hemifacial

Table 7.12 Thickened dermal collagen – histologic differential diagnosis

Connective tissue nevus (collagenoma)
Keloid
Normal back/chest skin
Scleroderma/morphea
Scar

atrophy, and linear morphea, but all share similar histologic features. Unlike the systemic form of the disease, morphea is not associated with increased mortality, though it can be quite disfiguring.

CREST syndrome is a variant of morphea. The acronym describes the clinical features which include: *c*alcinosis, *R*aynaud's phenomenon (hypersensitivity to cold temperatures resulting in color changes and pain in fingertips), *e*sophageal dysmotility, *s*clerodactyly, and *t*elangiectasias. This form of the disease has a relatively good prognosis.

Histologic features. It is not possible to distinguish morphea from scleroderma histologically and the changes will be described together. The epidermis is usually unremarkable, but may demonstrate slight flattening of the rete ridges. The reticular dermis is characterized initially by increased edema and a mixed inflammatory infiltrate around vessels and appendages. Plasma cells are usually present along with lymphocytes and rare eosinophils. As the lesions progress, there is thickening of collagen bundles, diminution of interstitial edema, and a diminished inflammatory infiltrate. In late lesions, there is little space between collagen bundles and the dermis is markedly thickened. Cutaneous appendages are largely replaced, leaving arrector pili muscles without concomitant pilosebaceous units. Eccrine ducts become entrapped. Lymphoplasmacellular aggregates located around the eccrine glands and at the interface of the reticular dermis and the subcutaneous fat are characteristic of morphea/scleroderma (Fig. 7.63). Germinal centers may be seen in these aggregates. The fibrosis often extends into fibrous septa in the subcutaneous tissue.

Differential diagnosis. The differential diagnosis of scleroderma/morphea includes a connective tissue nevus, normal back skin, a scar, and scleredema. Scleredema is characterized by increased dermal mucin not seen in scleroderma or morphea. In a connective tissue nevus, thickened collagen bundles course through the dermis in a haphazard arrangement, often directly perpendicular to the skin surface. A scar has more linearly arrayed collagen and prominent, straight, vertically oriented vessels. In normal back skin, cutaneous appendages are present and normally distributed, as is the wispy connective tissue surrounding eccrine structures.

Lichen sclerosus (et atrophicus)

Clinical features. Lichen sclerosus (LS), which is now the preferred name for this entity, is seen most commonly in the perianal and genital regions. While it is most common in postmenopausal women, it can be seen in people of both sexes at any age. (More specific terms, *kraurosis vulvae* and *balanitis xerotica obliterans*, are not often used.) It also can be seen on any body location. The clinical appearance is that of a 'porcelain-white' hyperkeratotic patch overlying atrophic skin. Pruritus is a common symptom.[203]

Histologic features. The histologic features of LS vary greatly with the age of the lesion. Early lesions are characterized by a dense, band-like infiltrate of lymphocytes along the dermal–epidermal junction. There is extensive basal vacuolization, with scattered dying keratinocytes. As lesions progress, the epidermis becomes progressively atrophic. The lymphocytic infiltrate diminishes in intensity and is separated from the epidermis by pink, homogeneous material within the papillary dermis. Later lesions are identified by severe epidermal atrophy, marked homogenization of the papillary dermis, and a slight perivascular lymphocytic infiltrate deeper in the dermis (Fig. 7.64). As LS is clinically quite pruritic, changes of lichen simplex chronicus are often superimposed upon those of LS, obscuring the epidermal atrophy with psoriasiform hyperplasia, a prominent granular layer, and hyperkeratosis.[204]

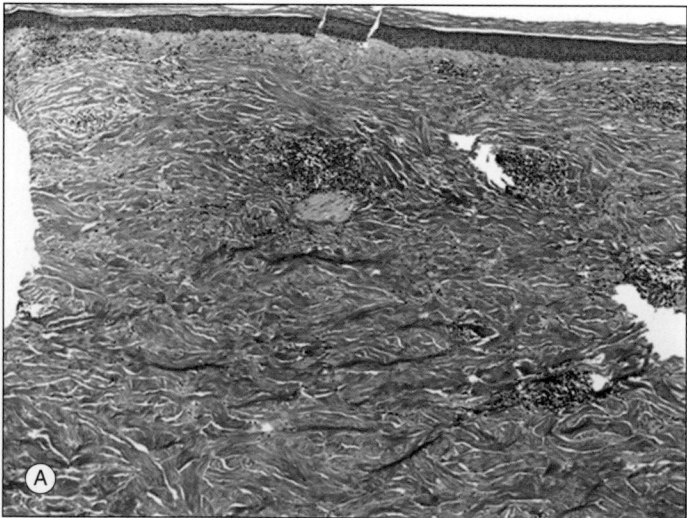
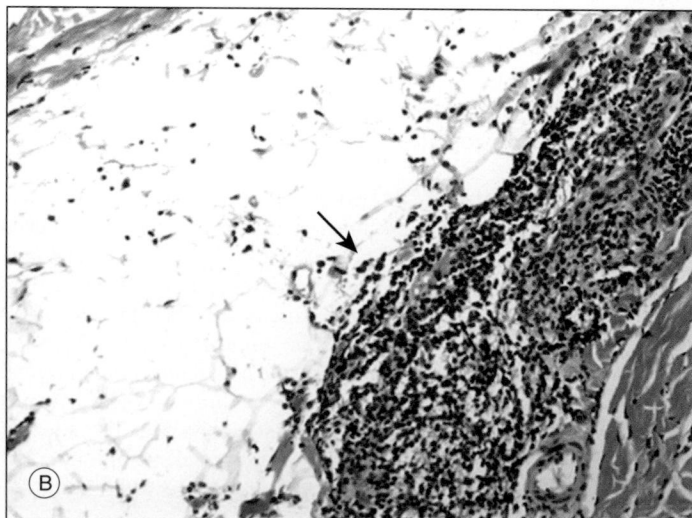

Fig. 7.63 A, Dense dermal sclerosis and a peri-appendageal and perivascular infiltrate are seen in morphea/scleroderma. There is also a loss of cutaneous appendages; **B,** At the junction between the reticular dermis and subcutaneous fat, there is a dense inflammatory infiltrate with plasma cells (arrow) in many cases of morphea/scleroderma.

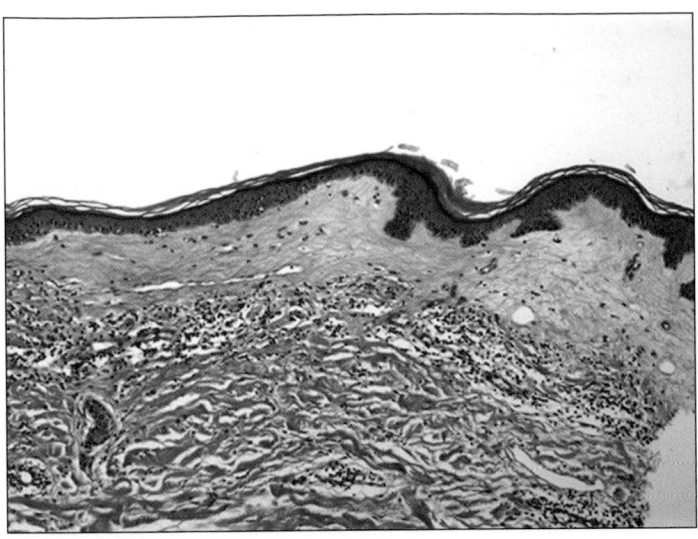

Fig. 7.64 Epidermal atrophy, expansion of the papillary dermis with homogeneous eosinophilic material, and a lymphocytic infiltrate characterize lichen sclerosis.

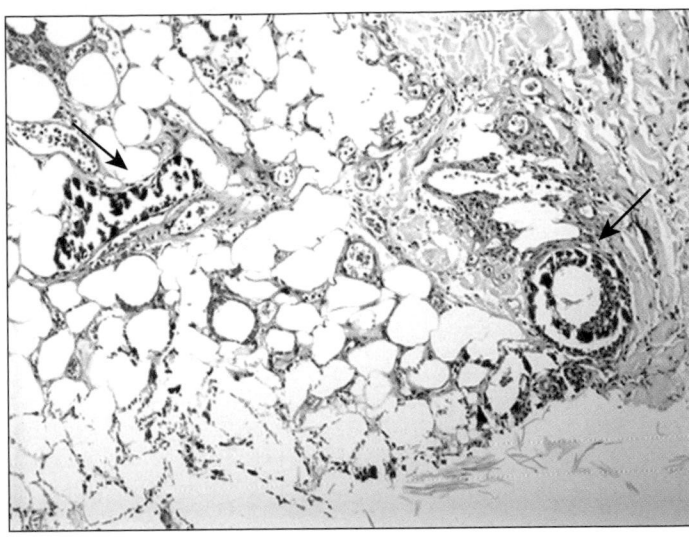

Fig. 7.65 Calcification (arrows) is present within vessels walls in calciphylaxis.

Differential diagnosis. In its earliest stages, LS is virtually indistinguishable from lichen planus on histologic sections. Clinical correlation is essential to make this distinction. Later lesions may resemble radiation dermatitis, though LS lacks the endothelial cell swelling and increased solar elastosis characteristic of the radiation-induced changes. LS may occur in conjunction with morphea. The changes of LS always involve the papillary dermis, primarily, and may extend only slightly into the reticular dermis. In contrast, morphea is a disease primarily of the reticular dermis.

CALCINOSES

Calcinosis cutis

Clinical features. Calcinosis cutis usually presents a non-specific, firm dermal nodule. It is most commonly associated with an antecedent inflammatory process such as acne vulgaris, with subsequent development of dystrophic calcification. Widespread calcification is an unusual sequel of juvenile dermatomyositis. Dystrophic calcification can also be present in appendage tumors such as pilomatricoma. Idiopathic tumoral calcinosis occurs in the scrotum as a dystrophic process. Metastatic calcification is quite rare, but can be seen in conditions with increased serum calcium levels including secondary hyperparathyroidism, milk alkalai syndrome, and hypervitaminosis D.

Histologic features. Calcinosis cutis appears as a well-circumscribed blue nodule within the dermis. There may or may not be a surrounding granulomatous inflammatory infiltrate. While usually unnecessary, the nature of the very hard material (as detected when cutting the sections) can be ascertained with an Alizarin red stain, or inferred from a von Kossa stain (which detects phosphates).

Differential diagnosis. Osteoma cutis is more eosinophilic than is calcinosis cutis, and gouty tophus demonstrates crystalline spaces.

Calciphylaxis

Clinical features. Calciphylaxis is a serious medical condition found in patients with end-stage renal disease and elevated calcium phosphate products in their blood. It presents as large areas of ulceration, most commonly on the extremities. This condition is quite serious and often fatal, and requires emergency intervention.[205,206]

Histologic features. Histologic sections of calciphylaxis demonstrate unremarkable epidermis, except in later lesions, in which case epidermal ischemia, necrosis, and ultimately ulceration are seen. Within the dermis and the subcutis, there is focal to extensive calcification of vessel walls (Fig. 7.65). Inflammation surrounds affected vessels in some cases.[207,208] While extravascular calcification may be present, it is not sufficient to make the diagnosis.

Differential diagnosis. The differential diagnosis includes stasis dermatitis with calcified vessel walls. This can be differentiated based upon clinical history, as well as upon the observation of markedly thickened and ectatic vessel walls throughout the dermis. Calcinosis cutis demonstrates calcium deposits in the dermal collagen, not in vessels as is seen in calciphylaxis.

Gout

Clinical features. Patients with chronically elevated serum uric acid levels are predisposed towards developing gouty tophi.[209] Tophi present as painful dermal nodules, often overlying joints on the toes or fingers. The great toe is the most common location. Tophi may also be found on ear lobes.[210] Gout is a disease of middle-aged to elderly people and is more common in men.

Histologic features. Uric acid crystals are dissolved with routine processing and can only be preserved with alcohol fixation and avoidance of other solvents throughout routine processing. However, it is not necessary to see the crystals in order to make a tissue diagnosis of a gouty tophus. The epidermis is unremarkable and within the dermis, areas of wispy material with alternating angulated, crystalline clear spaces are present (the sites of dissolved uric acid crystals). A dense granulomatous inflammatory response including many multinucleated giant cells surrounds these areas (Fig. 7.66).[210]

Differential diagnosis. The histologic differential diagnosis includes a rheumatoid nodule. Rheumatoid nodules are usually located deeper in the dermis than are tophi and demonstrate

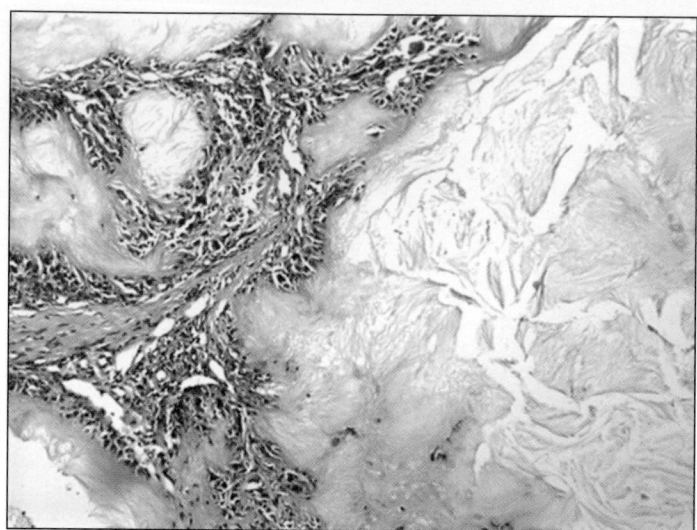

Fig. 7.66 Granulomatous inflammation surrounds wispy material in a gouty tophus.

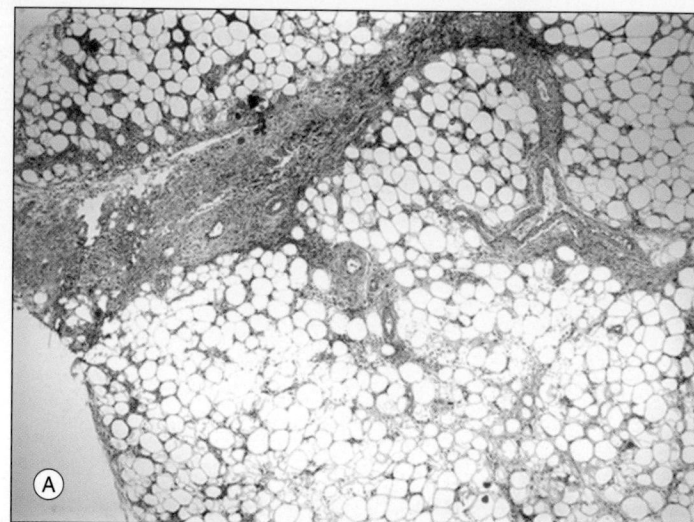

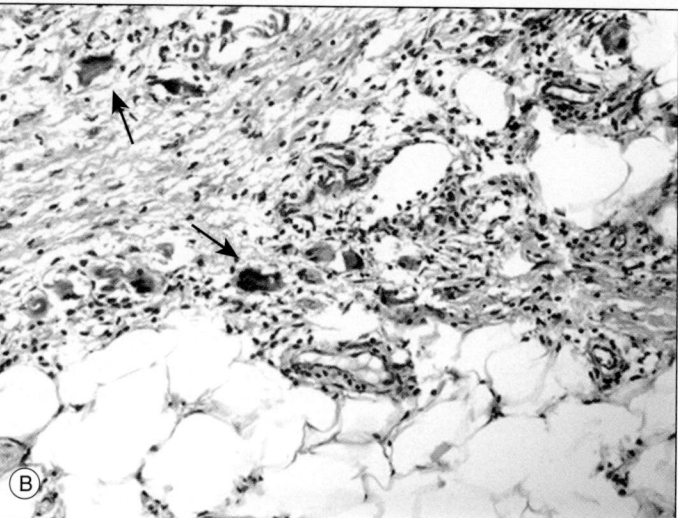

Fig. 7.67 A, Erythema nodosum is characterized by a septal panniculitis that spills slightly into the lobules of adipose tissue; **B**, Eosinophils and giant cells are seen within the inflammatory infiltrate in erythema nodosum (arrows).

fibrin-coated collagen in the centers of the granulomatous inflammation.

PANNICULITIS

The evaluation of a panniculitis is difficult as there is extensive histologic overlap in the various panniculitides. For the purpose of simplification and organization, it is useful to separate these entities into 'predominantly septal' or 'predominantly lobular' processes, and then to examine for the presence of vasculitis within these conditions. While this helps to more readily classify etiologies for panniculitis, it is imperative to recognize that the disease processes do not always fit exactly into one of these categories.

SEPTAL PANNICULITIS

Erythema nodosum

Clinical features. Erythema nodosum (EN) is a panniculitis that is most common in young women. It presents as one or several erythematous, tender 1–10 cm nodules, usually on the shins and thighs. Patients usually also have constitutional symptoms including fevers and arthralgias. Cutaneous lesions last for several weeks and resolve without sequelae in the more common acute variant. Associated overlying ulceration is most unusual.[211,212] A chronic form of the disease is also seen in which lesions continue to appear for months to years, but this is much less common.[213] EN is associated with oral contraceptives, multiple other medications, and a wide range of infectious processes including B-hemolytic streptococci. It is also associated with sarcoidosis. Most cases remain idiopathic.

Histologic features. EN is the prototypical septal panniculitis. The epidermis and dermis are usually completely unremarkable, though a slight perivascular lymphocytic infiltrate may be present around vessels in the dermal plexuses. Early lesions demonstrate septal edema and a mixed inflammatory infiltrate. Eosinophils are usually

present, and neutrophils may be seen (Fig. 7.67). As the lesions progress, the septa become fibrotic, with less edema. The inflammatory infiltrate becomes less intense, with a predominance of lymphocytes. Multinucleated giant cells are frequently seen.[211] They may aggregate into small granulomatous collections known as Miescher's granulomas.[214] In early, florid lesions, areas that are suggestive of leukocytoclastic vasculitis may be seen. Fibrin may be seen in blood vessel walls. The inflammatory infiltrate involves only the very peripheral parts of the lobules, and fat necrosis is not an expected finding in EN. In rare cases, the infiltrate may spill more extensively into the lobules.

Differential diagnosis. The differential diagnosis of EN includes other processes that involve the fibrous septa between the lobules of adipose tissue such as scleroderma and necrobiosis lipoidica. However, these entities more commonly display their main pathologic changes in the dermis and only secondarily extend into the subcutaneous tissues. The other panniculitides are primarily

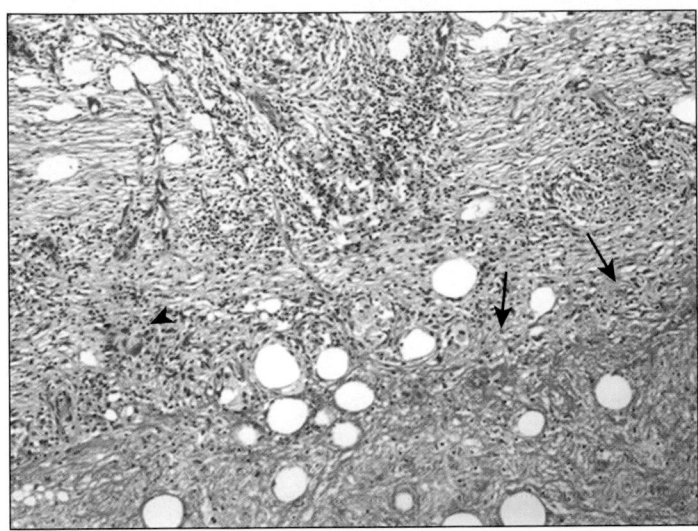

Fig. 7.68 Erythema induratum demonstrates a lobular panniculitis that may have central areas of caseation (arrows) and surrounding giant cells (arrowhead).

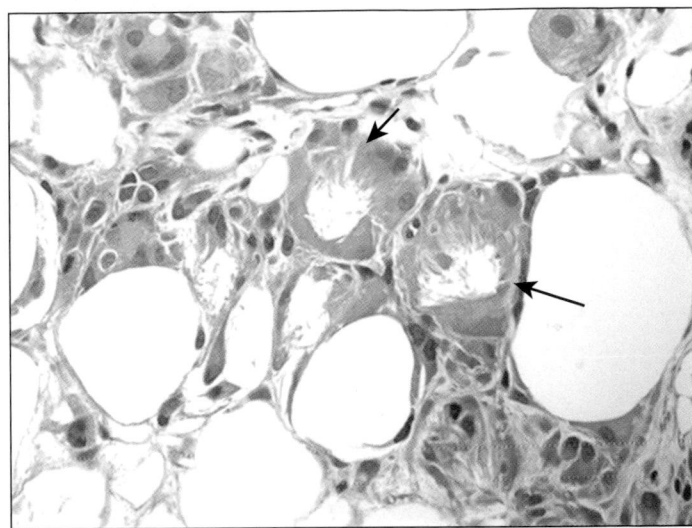

Fig. 7.69 Intracytoplasmic crystals are present within histiocytes adjacent to fat necrosis in subcutaneous fat necrosis of the newborn. The arrows demonstrate foci of calcification.

lobular and only secondarily involve the fibrous septa. Fat necrosis, if present, is a good way to make this distinction.

LOBULAR PANNICULITIS

Erythema induratum/nodular vasculitis

Clinical features. The distinction between erythema induratum (EI) and nodular vasculitis is not clear. Most dermatologists now regard EI as being a type of hypersensitivity reaction to *Mycobacterium tuberculosis* infection, with nodular vasculitis being an entity with an identical clinical and histologic presentation, but without the associated infection. Patients present with erythematous, tender nodules, most commonly on the calves. The lesions tend to have superficial ulceration and last for months. These entities occur most frequently in middle-aged women and are most prevalent in the colder months.[113]

Histologic features. The epidermis may be ulcerated, but is not otherwise involved in these processes. Within the dermis, there is often extensive inflammation, presumably extending up from the massively inflamed subcutaneous fat. The lobules of subcutaneous adipose tissue are overrun with a massive polymorphous inflammatory infiltrate. Abundant neutrophils and eosinophils, as well as lymphocytes, surround granulomas. Caseation may be present, giving the granulomas a tuberculoid appearance (Fig. 7.68). Fat necrosis is often pronounced. Vessels within the fibrous septa may be markedly inflamed. The apparent vasculitis may appear granulomatous.[113,215]

Differential diagnosis. Infectious processes such as tuberculosis and deep fungus infection are the main differential diagnostic entities. Special stains are required to exclude these conditions. The vasculitis also raises concerns about polyarteritis nodosa, in which there would be much less involvement of the adipose tissue, and Wegener's granulomatosis, which can be difficult to distinguish on purely histologic grounds. Vasculitis is not a prominent histologic feature of the other lobular panniculitides, nor are tuberculoid granulomas commonly seen in these other entities.

Adjuncts to diagnosis. Polymerase chain reaction technology has demonstrated mycobacterial DNA in some cases of EI, though AFB stains repeatedly fail to demonstrate organisms in most cases.

Pancreatic panniculitis

Clinical features. Pancreatic panniculitis is seen in patients with acute pancreatitis. Patients present with tender, erythematous plaques on the lower extremities with overlying ulceration and often an oily discharge. They also suffer from abdominal pain and arthralgias, and have elevated serum lipase levels. Patients are usually quite ill.[216,217]

Histologic features. The histologic features of pancreatic panniculitis include a diffuse florid infiltrate within the lobules of the subcutaneous fat. Neutrophils are the predominant cell type within the infiltrate. There is extensive fat necrosis. Ghost cells, i.e. cells with thickened cell walls and no nuclei, are a frequent histologic feature of pancreatic fat necrosis. Lesions later than a few days old also demonstrate extensive calcification and a brisk infiltrate of lipid-laden macrophages.[216,217]

Differential diagnosis. The main differential diagnosis is α-1 antitrypsin deficiency panniculitis that is most easily distinguished on clinical history.

Subcutaneous fat necrosis of the newborn

Clinical features. Subcutaneous fat necrosis of the newborn most commonly appears as a dimpling on the back, thighs, buttocks, arms, or cheeks. When discovered early, a tender, erythematous nodule may be detected. As the lesion involves, inflammatory changes abate, leaving only a depression caused by the resorbed necrotic adipocytes.

Histologic features. The epidermis and dermis are essentially unremarkable. Within the subcutaneous fat, there is a brisk infiltrate of lymphocytes and histiocytes within the lobules. Necrosis of adipocytes is diffuse. Abundant intracytoplasmic crystals are arranged radially within histiocytes (Fig. 7.69). In later lesions, calcification may be present. There is no vasculitis.

Differential diagnosis. The main differential diagnosis is sclerema neonatorum. Sclerema neonatorum is clinically diffuse and usually

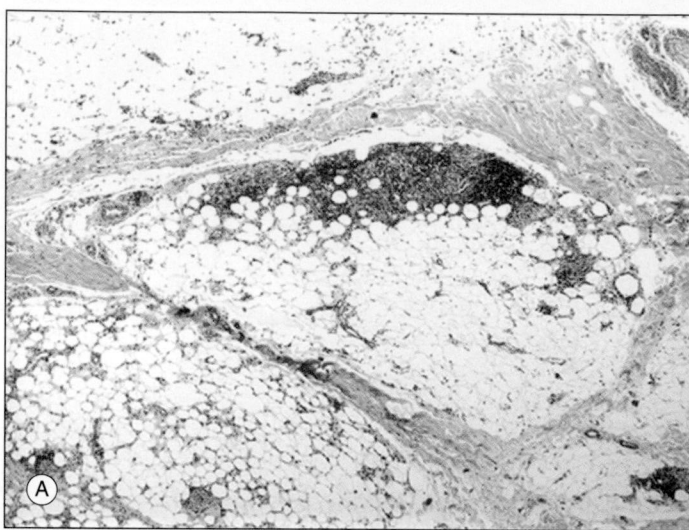
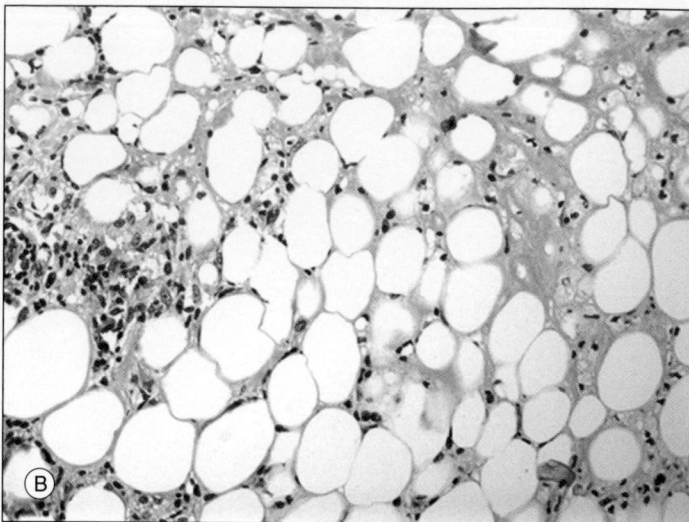

Fig. 7.70 A, A dense lymphocytic and plasmacellular infiltrate is present at the edge of the lobules in lupus panniculitis; **B,** Hyalinization of the fat is characteristic of lupus panniculitis.

fatal. Crystals are not seen within subcutaneous histiocytes and there is minimal inflammation and calcification.

Lupus panniculitis

Clinical features. Lupus panniculitis occurs most commonly in patients who have discoid lupus erythematosus. It is unusual in patients with the systemic form of the disease. Tender erythematous nodules may or may not demonstrate overlying surface scale. Proximal arms, face, and buttocks are frequent sites of involvement. Lupus panniculitis usually resolves with overlying atrophy, leaving a depression on the skin surface.[218–220]

Histologic features. In most cases, typical changes of lupus are not seen in the epidermis or dermis. In some cases, a mild interface dermatitis may be present. Within the dermis, there is a dense lymphocytic and plasmacellular infiltrate. Lymphoid follicles are present in a significant number of cases. The inflammatory infiltrate is most pronounced at the periphery of the lobules. Within the adipose tissue, a characteristic hyalinization is present in most cases. This change is relatively specific for lupus panniculitis (Fig. 7.70). In most cases, a slight lymphocytic infiltrate is present around, or even within, vascular walls in the deep dermis and subcutaneous septa. In more florid cases, leukocytoclastic vasculitis may be present.[221–223]

Differential diagnosis. The differential diagnosis includes other lobular panniculitides. Subcutaneous panniculitis-like T-cell lymphoma presents the greatest differential diagnostic challenge. In this entity, there is more extensive lymphocyte atypia, mitotic activity, and individual cell necrosis than that seen in lupus panniculitis. In some cases, it is necessary to resort to T-cell gene rearrangement studies to make the final distinction.

Adjuncts to diagnosis. Direct immunofluorescence examination is variably positive in lupus panniculitis. In cases with changes of lupus in the overlying skin, granular deposits of immunoglobulins and complement may be present along the dermal–epidermal junction. In cases without such changes, the immunofluorescence examination is usually negative.

Factitial panniculitis

Clinical features. As would be expected in a disease process caused by exogenous forces, there are no definitive clinical features of a factitial panniculitis. In most cases, sharply angulated ulcerations are present overlying tender dermal and subcutaneous nodules in readily accessible body sites.

Histologic features. The histologic features of factitial panniculitis are not specific and other causes of panniculitis must be excluded before making such a diagnosis. A dense inflammatory infiltrate including neutrophils and granulomas is seen. Factitial processes are less likely to respect anatomic demarcations, and thus irregular involvement of the lobules and fibrous septa is common. There is no evidence of vascular involvement in factitial panniculitis. Polarization occasionally reveals foreign material that has been introduced by the patient. The overlying epidermis is variably involved.

Differential diagnosis. The diagnosis of factitial panniculitis is one of exclusion and should only be made when other causes of panniculitis have been eliminated.

REFERENCES

1. Krasteva M. Contact dermatitis. Int J Dermatol 1993; 32: 547–560.

2. Taylor RM. Histopathology of contact dermatitis. Clin Dermatol 1986; 4: 18–22.

3. Nater JP, Hoedemaeker PJ. Histological differences between irritant and allergic patch test reactions in man. Contact Dermatitis 1976; 2: 247–253.

4. Hellgren L, Mobacken H. Nummular eczema – clinical and statistical data. Acta Derm Venereol 1969; 49: 189–196.

5. Sirot G. Nummular eczema. Semin Dermatol 1983; 2: 68–74.

6. Hanifin JM, Rajka, G. Diagnostic features of atopic dermatitis. Acta Derm Venereol (Suppl) 1980; 92: 44–47.

7. Zillikens D, Mehringer A, Lechner W, Burg G. Hypo- and hyperpigmented areas in incontinentia pigmenti. Light and electron microscopic studies. Am J Dermatopathol 1991; 13: 57–62.

8. O' Brien JE, Feingold M. Incontinentia pigmenti. A longitudinal study. Am J Dis Child 1985; 139: 711–712.

9. Aydingoz U, Midia M. Central nervous system involvement in incontinentia pigmenti: cranial MRI of two siblings. Neuroradiology 1998; 40: 364–366.

10. Takematsu H, Terui T, Torinuki W, Tagami H. Incontinentia pigmenti: eosinophil chemotactic activity of the crusted scales in the vesiculobullous stage. Br J Dermatol 1986; 115: 61–66.

11. Fry L. Psoriasis. Br J Dermatol,1988; 119: 445–461.

12. Stern RS, Wu J. Psoriasis. In: Arndt KA, LeBoit PE, Robinson JK, Wintroub BU, eds. Cutaneous medicine and surgery. Philadelphia: WB Saunders; 1996: 295–321.

13. Telfer NR, Chalmers RJG, Whale K, Colman G. The role of streptococcal infection in the intiation of guttate psoriasis. Arch Dermatol 1992; 128: 39–42.

14. Zelickson BD, Muller SA. Generalized pustular psoriasis. A review of 63 cases. Arch Dermatol 1991; 127: 1339–1345.

15. Webster G. Seborrheic dermatitis. Int J Dermatol 1991; 30: 843–844.

16. Barr RJ, Young EM Jr. Psoriasiform and related papulosquamous disorders. J Cutan Pathol 1985; 12: 412–425.

17. Griffiths WAD. Pityriasis rubra pilaris. Clin Exp Dermatol 1980; 5: 105–112.

18. Soeprono FF. Histologic criteria for the diagnosis of pityriasis rubra pilaris. Am J Dermatopathol 1986; 8: 277–283.

19. Shaffer B, Beerman H. Lichen simplex chronicus and its variants. Arch Deramtol 1951; 64: 340–351.

20. Ackerman AB. Subtle clues to diagnosis by conventional microscopy. Marked compact hyperkeratosis as a sign of persistent rubbing. Am J Dermatopathol 1980; 2: 149–152.

21. Crissey JT, Denenholz DA. Clinical picture of infectious syphilis. Clin Dermatol 1984; 2: 39–61.

22. Engelkens HJ, ten Kate FJ, Vuzevski VD, et al. Primary and secondary syphilis: a histopathological study. Int J STD AIDS 1991; 2: 280–284.

23. Carbia SG, Lagodin C, Abbruzzese M, et al. Lichenoid secondary syphilis. Int J Dermatol 1999; 38: 53–55.

24. Engelkens HJ, ten Kate FJ, Judanarso J, et al. The localisation of treponemes and characterisation of the inflammatory infiltrate in skin biopsies from patients with primary or secondary syphilis, or early infectious yaws. Genitourin Med 1993; 69: 102–107.

25. Boyd AS, Nelder KH. Lichen planus. J Am Acad Dermatol 1991; 25: 593–619.

26. Waldorf DS. Lichen planopilaris. Arch Dermatol 1966; 93: 684–691.

27. Ragaz A, Ackerman AB. Evolution, maturation, and regression of lesions of lichen planus. New observations and correlations of clinical and histologic findings. Am J Dermatopathol 1981; 3: 5–25.

28. Mehregan DA, Van Hale HM, Muller SA. Lichen planopilaris: clinical and pathologic study of forty-five patients. J Am Acad Dermatol 1992; 27: 935–942.

29. Van den Haute V, Antoine JL, Lachapelle JM. Histopathological discriminant criteria between lichenoid drug eruption and idiopathic lichen planus: retrospective study on selected samples. Dermatologica 1989; 179: 10–13.

30. Lapins NA, Willoughby C, Helwig EB. Lichen nitidus. A study of forty-three cases. Cutis 1978; 21: 634–637.

31. Bardach H. Perforating lichen nitidus. J Cutan Pathol 1981; 8: 111–116.

32. Fabbri P, Panconesi E. Erythema multiforme ('minus' and 'maius') and drug intake. Clinics in Dermatol 1993; 11: 479–489.

33. Tonneson M, Soter NA. Erythema multiforme. J Am Acad Dermatol 1979; 1: 357–364.

34. Shiohara T, Chiba M, Tanaka Y, Nagashima M. Drug-induced, photosensitive, erythema multiforme-like eruption: Possible role for cell adhesion molecules in a flare induced by Rhus dermatitis. J Am Acad Dermatol 1990; 22: 647–650.

35. Zohdi-Mofid M, Horn TD. Acrosyringeal concentration of necrotic keratinocytes in erythema multiforme: a clue to drug etiology. Clinicopathologic review of 29 cases. J Cutan Pathol 1997; 24: 235–240.

36. Huff JC, Weston WL, Tonnesen MG. Erythema multiforme: A critical review of characteristics, diagnostic criteria, and causes. J Am Acad Dermatol 1983; 8: 763–775.

37. Bastuji-Garin S, Rzany B, Stern RS, et al. Clinical classification of cases of toxic epidermal necrolysis, Stevens-Johnson syndrome and erythema multiforme. Arch Dermatol 1993; 129: 92–96.

38. Inachi S, Mizutani H, Shimizu M. Epidermal apoptotic cell death in erythema multiforme and Stevens-Johnson syndrome. Arch Dermatol 1997; 133: 845–849.

39. Ferrara JLM, Deeg HJ. Graft-versus-host disease. N Eng J Med 1991; 324: 667–674.

40. Hood AF, Vogelsang GB, Black LP, et al. Acute graft-versus-host disease: development following autologous and syngeneic bone marrow transplantation. Arch Dermatol 1987; 123: 745–750.

41. Chosidow O, Bagot,M, Vernant J-P, et al. Sclerodermatous chronic graft-versus-host disease. Analysis of seven cases. J Am Acad Dermatol 1992; 26: 49–55.

42. Freemer CS, Farmer ER, Corio RL, et al. Lichenoid chronic graft-vs-host disease occurring in a dermatomal distribution. Arch Dermatol 1994; 130: 70–72.

43. Tuffanelli DL. Lupus erythematosus. J Am Acad Dermatol 1981; 4: 127–142.

44. Harper JL. Subacute lupus erythematosus (SCLE): a distinct subset of LE. Clin Exp Dermatol 1982; 7: 209–212.

45. Clark WH, Reed RJ, Mihm MC. Lupus erythematosus. Histopathology of cutaneous lesions. Hum Pathol 1973; 4:157–163.

46. Jerdan MS, Hood AF, Moore GW, Callen JP. Histopathologic comparison of the subsets of lupus erythematosus. Arch Dermatol 1990; 126: 52–55.

47. Bangert JL, Freeman RG, Sontheimer RD, Gilliam JN. Subacute cutaneous lupus erythematosus and discoid lupus erythematosus. Comparative histopathologic findings. Arch Dermatol 1984; 120: 332–337.

48. Kovacs SO, Kovacs SC. Dermatomyositis. J Am Acad Dermatol 1998; 39: 899–920.

49. Euwer RL, Sontheimer RD. Amyopathic dermatomyositis (dermatomyositis sine myositis). J Am Acad Dermatol 1991; 24: 959–966.

50. Bowyer SL, Clark RA, Ragsdale CG, et al. Juvenile dermatomyositis: histologic findings and pathogenetic hypothesis for the associated skin changes. J Rheumatol 1986; 13: 753–759.

51. Magro CM, Crowson AN. The immunofluorescent profile of dermatomyositis: a comparative study with lupus erythematosus. J Cutan Pathol 1997; 24: 543–552.

52. Epstein JH. Polymorphous light eruption. J Am Acad Dermatol 1980; 3: 329–343.

53. Epstein JH. Polymorphous light eruption. Dermatol Clin 1986; 4: 243–251.

54. Lambert WC, Everett MA. The nosology of parapsoriasis. J Am Acad Dermatol 1981; 5: 373–395.

55. Haeffner AC, Smoller BR, Zepter K, Wood GS. Differentiation and clonality of lesional lymphocytes in small plaque parapsoriasis. Arch Dermatol 1995; 131: 321–324.

56. King-Ismael D, Ackerman AB. Guttate parapsoriasis/digitate dermatosis (small plaque parapsoriasis) is mycosis fungoides. Am J Dermatopathol 1992; 14:518–530.

57. Bressler GS, Jones RE Jr. Erythema annulare centrifugum. J Am Acad Dermatol 1981; 4: 597–602.

58. Mahood JM. Erythema annulare centrifugum: a review of 24 cases with special reference to its association with underlying disease. Clin Exp Dermatol 1983; 8: 383–387.

59. Boyd AS, Neldner KH, Menter A. Erythema gyratum repens: a paraneoplastic eruption. J Am Acad Dermatol 1992; 26: 757–762.

60. Caux F, Lebbe C, Thomine E, et al. Erythema gyratum repens. A case studied with immunofluorescence, immunoelectron microscopy and immunohistochemistry. Br J Dermatol 1994; 131: 102–107.

61. Jurca T, Ruzic-Sabljic E, Lotric-Furlan S, et al. Comparison of peripheral and central biopsy sites for the isolation of Borrelia burgdorferi sensu lato from erythema migrans skin lesions. Clin Infect Dis 1998; 27: 636–638.

62. Newton RC, Raimer SS. Pigmented purpuric eruptions. Dermatol Clin 1985; 3: 165–169.

63. Ratnam KV, Su WPD, Peters MS. Purpura simplex (inflammatory purpura without vasculitis): a clinicopathologic study of 174 cases. J Am Acad Dermatol 1991; 25: 642–647.

64. Black AK, Greaves MW, Champion RH, Pye RJ. The urticarias 1990. Br J Dermatol 1991; 124: 100–108.

65. Aboobaker J, Greaves MW. Urticarial vasculitis. Clin Exp Dermatol 1986; 11: 436–444.

66. Synkowski DR, Levine MI, Rabin BS, Unis EJ. Urticaria. An immunofluorescence and histopathology study. Arch Dermatol 1979; 115: 1192–1194.

67. Churg J, Churg A. Idiopathic and secondary vasculitis: a review. Mod Pathol 1989; 2: 144–160.

68. Fauci AS, Haynes BF, Katz P. The spectrum of vasculitis: clinical, pathologic, immunologic , and therapeutic considerations. Ann Intern Med 1978; 89: 660–676.

69. Lotti T, Ghersetich I, Comacchi C, Jorizzo JL. Cutaneous small-vessel vasculitis. J Am Acad Dermatol 1998; 39: 667–687.

70. Al-Sheyyab M, El-Shanti H, Ajlouni S, et al. The clinical spectrum of Henoch-Schönlein purpura in infants and young children. Eur J Pediatr 1995; 154: 969–972.

71. Strickland DK, Ware RE. Urticarial vasculitis: an autoimmune disorder following therapy for Hodgkin's disease. Med Pediatr Oncol 1995; 25: 208–212.

72. Yiannias JA, El-Azhary RA, Gibson LE. Erythema elevatum diutinum: a clinical and histopathologic study of 13 patients. J Am Acad Dermatol 1992; 26: 38–44.

73. Pedace FJ, Perry HO. Granuloma faciale. A clinical and histopathologic review. Arch Dermatol 1966; 94: 387–395.

74. Gorevic PD, Levo Y, Kassab H, et al. Mixed cryoglobulinemia: an immune complex disease often associated with hepatitis B. Trans Assoc Am Physicians 1977; 90: 167–172.

75. Thomas RHM, Black MM. The wide clinical spectrum of polyarteritis nodosa with cutaneous involvement. Clin Exp Dermatol 1983; 8: 47–59.

76. Cacaoub P, Lunel-Fablani F, Du LT. Polyarteritis nodosa and hepatitis C virus infection (letter). Ann Intern Med 1992; 116: 605–606.

77. Trepco CG, Zuckerman AJ, Bird RC, Prince AM. The role of circulating hepatitis B antigen/antibody immune complexes in the pathogenesis of vascular and hepatic manifestations in polyarteritis nodosa. J Clin Pathol 1974; 27: 863–868.

78. Minkowitz G, Smoller BR, McNutt NS. Benign cutaneous polyarteritis nodosa: relationship to systemic polyarteritis nodosa and hepatitis B infection. Arch Dermatol 1991; 127: 1520–1523.

79. Volk DM, Owen LG. Cutaneous polyarteritis nodosa in a patient with ulcerative colitis. J Pediatr Gastroenterol Nutr 1986; 5: 970–972.

80. Schwartz RA, Churg J. Churg-Strauss syndrome. Br J Dermatol 1992; 127: 199–204.

81. Lanham JG, Elkon KB, Pusey CD, Hughes GR. Systemic vasculitis with asthma and eosinophilia: a clinical approach to the Churg-Strauss syndrome. Medicine 1984; 63: 65–81.

82. Lie JT. The classification of vasculitis and a reappraisal of allergic granulomatosis and angiitis

(Churg-Strauss syndrome). Mt Sinai J Med 1986; 53: 429–439.

83. Fauci AS, Haynes BF, Katz P, Wolff SM. Wegener's granulomatosis: prospective clinical and therapeutic experience with 85 patients for 21 years. Ann Intern Med 1983; 98: 76–85.

84. Barksdale SK, Hallahan CW, Kerr GS, et al. Cutaneous pathology in Wegener's granulomatosis. A clinicopathologic study of 75 biopsies in 46 patients. Am J Surg Pathol 1995; 19: 161–172.

85. Daoud MS, Gibson LE, DeRemee RA, et al. Cutaneous Wegener's granulomatosis: Clinic, histopathologic, and immunopathologic features of thirty patients. J Am Acad Dermatol 1994; 31: 605–612.

86. Gunawardena DA, Gunawardena KA, Ratnayaka MRS, Vasanthanathan NS. The clinical spectrum of Sweet's syndrome (acute febrile neutrophilic dermatosis): report of eighteen cases. Br J Dermatol 1975; 92: 363–373.

87. Callen JP. Acute febrile neutrophilic dermatosis (Sweet's syndrome) and the related conditions of 'Bowel Bypass' syndrome and bullous pyoderma gangrenosum. Dermatol Clin 1985; 3: 153–163.

88. Cohen PR, Kurzock R. Sweet's syndrome and cancer. Clinics in Dermatol 1993; 11: 149–157.

89. Cohen PR, Talpaz M, Kurzock R. Malignancy-associated Sweet's syndrome: review of the world literature. J Clin Oncol 1988; 6: 1887–1897.

90. Powell FC, Su WPD, Perry HO. Pyoderma gangrenosum: classification and management. J Am Acad Dermatol 1996; 34: 395–409.

91. Powell FC, Schroeter AL, Su WPD, et al. Pyoderma gangrenosum: a review of 86 patients. Q J Med,1985; 55: 173–86.

92. Benton EC, Rutherford D, Hunter JA. Sweet's syndrome and pyoderma gangrenosum associated with ulcerative colitis. Acta Derm Venereol (Stockh) 1985; 65: 77–80.

93. Wells RS, Smith MA. The natural history of granuloma annulare. Br J Dermatol 1963; 75: 199–205.

94. Muhlbauer JE. Granuloma annulare. J Am Acad Dermatol 1980; 3: 217–230.

95. Dabski K, Winkelmann RK. Generalized granuloma annulare: Clinical and laboratory findings in 100 patients. J Am Acad Dermatol 1989; 20: 39–47.

96. O'Brien JP. Actinic granuloma. An annular connective tissue disorder affecting sun- and heat-damaged skin. Arch Dermatol 1975; 111: 460–466.

97. Umbert P, Winkelmann RK. Histologic, ultrastructural, and histochemical studies of granuloma annulare. Arch Dermatol 1977; 113: 1681–1686.

98. Dabski K, Winkelmann RK. Generalized granuloma annulare: Histopathology and immunopathology. J Am Acad Dermatol 1989; 20: 28–39.

99. Lowitt MH, Dover JS. Necrobiosis lipoidica. J Am Acad Dermatol 1991; 25: 735–748.

100. Binazzi M, Simonette V. Granuloma annulare, necrobiosis lipoidica, and diabetic disease. Int J Dermatol 1988; 27: 576–579.

101. Muller SA, Winkelmann RK. Necrobiosis lipoidica diabeticorum: Histopathologic study of 98 cases. Arch Dermatol 1966; 94: 1–10.

102. Yammamoto T, Ohkubo H, Nishioka K. Skin manifestations associated with rheumatoid arthritis. J Dermatol 1995; 22: 324–329.

103. Bennett GA, Zeller JW, Bauer W. Subcutaneous nodules of rheumatoid arthritis and rheumatic fever. Arch Pathol 1940; 30: 70–89.

104. Callen JP. Sarcoidosis. In: Dermatologic signs of internal disorders. Chicago: Year Book Medical Publishers; 1980:311–332.

105. Cronin E. Skin changes in sarcoidosis. Postgrad Med 1959; 46:507–509.

106. Sharma OP. Cutaneous sarcoidosis: Clinical features and management. Chest 1972; 61: 320–325.

107. Cancrini C, Angelini F, Colavita M, et al. Erythema nodosum: a presenting sign of early onset sarcoidosis. Clin Exp Rheumatol 1998; 16: 337–339.

108. Banse-Kupin L, Pelachyk JM. Ichthyosiform sarcoidosis. Report of two cases and review of the literature. J Am Acad Dermatol 1987; 17: 616–620.

109. Goette DK, Jacobson KW, Dory RD. Primary inoculation tuberculosis of the skin. Prospector's paronychia. Arch Dermatol 1978; 114: 567–569.

110. Daikos GL, Uttamchandani RB, Tuda C, et al. Disseminated miliary tuberculosis of the skin in patients with AIDS: report of four cases. Clin Infect Dis 1998; 27: 205–208.

111. Brown FS, Anderson RH, Burnett JW. Cutaneous tuberculosis. J Am Acad Dermatol 1982; 6: 101–106.

112. Tappeiner G, Wolf,K. Tuberculosis and other mycobacterial infections. In: Fitzpatrick TB, Eisen AZ, Wolff K, et al. Auseten, eds. Dermatology in general medicine. New York: McGraw-Hill; 1993: 2370–2391.

113. Schneider JW, Jordaan HF, Geiger DH, et al. A clinicopathological study of 20 cases and detection of mycobacterium tuberculosis DNA in skin lesions by polymerase chain reaction. Am J Dermatopathol 1995; 17: 350–356.

114. Victor T, Jordaan HF, Van Niekerk DJT, et al. Papulonecrotic tuberculid: identification of *M. tuberculosis* DNA by polymerase chain reaction. Am J Dermatopathol 1992; 14: 491–495.

115. Sehgel VN. Leprosy. Dermatologic Clinics 1994; 12: 629–644.

116. Sehgal VN. Clinical leprosy. 3rd edn. New Delhi: Jaypee Brothers; 1993.

117. del Carmen Farina M, Gezundez I, Pique E, et al. Cutaneous tuberculosis: a clinical, histopathologic, and bacteriologic study. J Am Acad Dermatol 1995; 33: 433–440.

118. Van Voorhis WC, Kaplan G, Nunes Sarno E, et al. The cutaneous infiltrates of leprosy. Cellular characteristics and the predominant T-cell phenotypes. N Engl J Med 1982; 307: 1593–1597.

119. Sneddon IB, Wilkinson DS. Subcorneal pustular dermatosis. Br J Dermatol 1979; 100: 61–68.

120. Takata M, Inaoki M, Shodo M, et al. Subcorneal pustular dermatosis associated with IgA myeloma and intraepidermal IgA deposits. Dermatology 1994; 189(suppl)1: 111–114.

121. Chouvet B, Ortonne JP, Perrot H, Thivolet J. Norweigian scabies: etiological grounds. Ann Dermatol Venereol 1979; 106: 569–574.

122. Darmstadt GL, Lane AT. Impetigo: an overview. Pediatr Dermatol 1994; 11: 293–303.

123. Adachi J, Endo K, Fukuzumi T, et al. Increasing incidence of streptococcal impetigo in atopic dermatitis. J Dermatol Sci 1998; 17: 45–53.

124. el Tayeb SH, Nasr EM, Sattallah AS. Streptococcal impetigo and acute glomerulonephritis in children in Cairo. Br J Dermatol 1978; 98: 53–62.

125. DeCastro P, Jorizzo JL. Cutaneous aspects of candidosis. Semin Dermatol 1985; 4: 165–172.

126. Koulu L, Stanley JR. Clinical, histologic, and immunopathologic comparison of pemphigus vulgaris and pemphigus foliaceus. Semin Dermatol 1988; 7: 82–90.

127. Kouskoukis CE, Ackerman AB. What histologic finding distinguishes superficial pemphigus and bullous impetigo? Am J Dermatopathol 1984; 6: 179–181.

128. Gemmell CG. Staphylococcal scalded skin syndrome. J Med Microbiol 1995; 43: 318–327.

129. Cribier B, Piemont Y, Grosshans E. Staphylococcal scalded skin syndrome in adults. A clinical review illustrated with a new case. J Am Acad Dermatol 1994; 30: 319–324.

130. Akiyama H, Yamasaki O, Kanzaki H, et al. Streptococci isolated from various skin lesions: the interaction with *Staphylococcus aureus* strains. J Dermatol Sci 1999; 19: 17–22.

131. Ahmed AR. Clinical features of pemphigus. Clin Dermatol 1983; 1: 13–21.

132. Moy R, Jorden RE. Immunopathology in pemphigus. Clin Dermatol 1983; 1: 72–81.

133. Osmanski JP 2nd, Fraire AE, Schaefer OP. Necrotizing tracheobronchitis with progressive airflow obstruction associated with paraneoplastic pemphigus. Chest 1997; 12: 1704–1707.

134. Chamberland M. Paraneoplastic pemphigus and adenocarcinoma of the colon. Union Med Can 1993; 122: 201–203.

135. Matz H, Milner Y, Frusic-Zlotkin M, Brenner S. Paraneoplastic pemphigus associated with pancreatic carcinoma. Acta Derm Venereol 1997; 77: 289–291.

136. Schlesinger T, McCarron K, Camisa C, Anhalt GJ. Paraneoplastic pemphigus occurring in a patient with B-cell non-Hodgkin's lymphoma. Cutis 1998; 61: 94–96.

137. Anhalt GJ. Paraneoplastic pemphigus. Adv Dermatol 1997; 12: 77–96.

138. Horn TD, Anhalt GJ. Histologic features of paraneoplastic pemphigus. Arch Dermatol 1992; 128: 1091–1095.

139. Helou J, Albritton J, Anhalt GJ. Accuracy of indirect immunofluorescence testing in the diagnosis of paraneoplastic pemphigus. J Am Acad Dermatol 1995; 32: 441–447.

140. Burge SM, Wilkdenson JD. Darier-White disease: a review of the clinical features in 163 patients. J Am Acad Dermatol 1992; 27: 40–50.

141. Rand R, Buaden HP. Commentary: Darier-White disease. Arch Dermatol 1983; 119: 81–83.

142. Palmer DD, Perry HO. Benign familial pemphigus. Arch Dermatol 1962; 86: 493–502.

143. Steffen CG. Benign familial pemphigus. Am J Dermatopathol 1987; 9: 58–73.

144. Grover RW. Transient acantholytic dermatosis. Arch Dermatol 1970; 101: 426–434.

145. Chalet M, Grover RW, Ackerman AB. Transient acantholytic dermatosis. Arch Dermatol 1977; 113: 431–435.

146. Juel-Jensen BE, MacCallum FO. Herpes simplex, varicella and zoster: Clinical manifestations and treatment. Philadelphia: J B Lippincott Co; 1972.

147. Hope-Simpson RE. The nature of herpes zoster: A long-term study and a new hypothesis. Proc R Soc Med 1965; 58: 9–20.

148. Goh CL, Khoo L. A retrospective study of the clinical presentation and outcome of herpes zoster in a tertiary dermatology outpatient referral clinic. Int J Dermatol 1997; 36: 667–672.

149. Muraki R, Iwasaki T, Sata T, et al. Hair follicle involvement in herpes zoster: pathway of viral spread from ganglia to skin. Virchows Arch 1996; 428: 275–280.

150. Rodriguez-Pereira C, Suarez-Penaranda JM, del Rio E, Forteza-Vila J. Cutaneous granulomatous vasculitis after herpes zoster infection showing polyarteritis nodosa-like features. Clin Exp Dermatol 1997; 22: 274–276.

151. Thivolet J, Barthelemy H. Bullous pemphigoid. Semin Dermatol 1988; 7: 91–103.

152. Ahmed AR. Diagnosis of bullous disease and studies in the pathogenesis of blister formation using immunopathological techniques. J Cutan Pathol 1984; 11: 237–248.

153. Weigand DA, Clements MK. Direct immunofluorescence in bullous pemphigoid: effects of extent and location of lesions. J Am Acad Dermatol 1989; 20: 437–440.

154. Holmes RC, Black MM. The specific dermatoses of pregnancy. J Am Acad Dermatol 1983; 8: 405–412.

155. Kertz KC, Katz SI, Maize J, Ackerman AB. Herpes gestationis. A clinicopathologic study. Arch Dermatol 1976; 112: 1543–1548.

156. Harrington CI, Bleehen SS. Herpes gestationis: immunopathological and ultrastructural studies. Br J Dermatol 1979; 100: 389–399.

157. Hall RP. Dermatitis herpetiformis. J Investig Dermatol 1992; 99: 873–881.

158. Reunala T, Salmi J, Karvonen J. Dermatitis herpetiformis and celiac disease associated with

Addison's disease. Arch Dermatol 1987; 123: 930–932.

159. Buckley DB, English J, Molloy W, et al. Dermatitis herpetiformis: A review of 119 cases. Clin Exp Dermatol 1983; 8: 477–487.

160. Whitworth JM, Thomas I, Peltz SA, et al. Vancomycin-induced linear IgA bullous dermatosis (LABD). J Am Acad Dermatol 1996; 34: 890–891.

161. Tonev S, Vasileva S, Kadurina M. Depot sulfonamid associated with linear IgA bullous dermatosis with erythema multiforme-like clinical features. J Eur Acad Deramtol Venereol 1998; 11: 165–168.

162. Camilleri M, Pace JL. Linear IgA bullous dermatosis induced by piroxicam. J Eur Acad Deramtol Venereol 1998; 10: 70–72.

163. Ahmed AR, Hombal SM. Cicatricial pemphigoid. Int J Dermatol 1986; 25: 90–96.

164. Person JR, Rogers RSI. Bullous and cicatricial pemphigoid. Clinical, histopathologic, and immunopathologic correlations. Mayo Clin Proc 1977; 52: 54 66.

165. Griffith MR, Fukuyama K, Tuffanelli DL, Silverman SJ. Immunofluorescent studies in mucous membrane pemphigoid. Arch Dermatol 1974; 109: 195–199.

166. Epstein JH, Tuffanelli DL, Epstein WL. Cutaneous changes in the porphyrias. A microscopic study. Arch Dermatol 1973; 107: 689–698.

167. Fine J-D, Bauer EA, Briggman RA, et al. Revised clinical and laboratory criteria for subtypes of inherited epidermolysis bullosa. J Am Acad Dermatol 1991; 24: 119–135.

168. Kitajima Y, Jokura Y, Yaoita H. Epidermolysis bullosa simplex, Dowling-Meara type. A report of two cases with different types of tonofilament clumping. Br J Dermatol 1993; 128: 79–85.

169. Valari MD, Phillips RJ, Lake BD, Harper JI. Junctional epidermolysis bullosa and pyloric atresia: a distinct entity. Clinical and pathological studies in five patients. Br J Dermatol 1995; 133: 732–736.

170. Woodley DT, Briggaman RA, Gammon WT. Review and update of epidermolysis bullosa acquisita. Semin Dermatol 1988; 7: 111–122.

171. Helm KF, Menz J, Gibson LE, Dicken CH. A clinical and histopathologic study of granulomatous rosacea. J Am Acad Dermatol 1991; 25: 1038–1043.

172. Sumner WT, Grichnik JM, Shea CR, et al. Follicular mucinosis as a presenting sign of acute myeloblastic leukemia. J Am Acad Dermatol 1998; 38: 803–805.

173. Soeprono FF, Schinella RA. Eosinophilic pustular folliculitis in patients with acquired immunodeficiency syndrome: report of three cases. J Am Acad Dermatol 1986; 14: 1020–1022.

174. Teraki Y, Konohana I, Shiohara T, et al. Eosinophilic pustular folliculitis (Ofuji's disease). Immunohistochemical analysis. Arch Dermatol 1993; 129: 1015–1019.

175. McCalmont TH, Altemus D, Maurer T, Berger TG. Eosinophilic folliculitis. The histologic spectrum. Am J Dermatopathol 1995; 17: 439–446.

176. Cooper PH. Eruptive xanthoma: a microscopic simulant of granuloma annulare. J Cutan Pathol 1986; 13: 207–215.

177. Crowe MJ, Gross DJ. Eruptive xanthoma. Cutis 1992; 50: 31–32.

178. Bulkley BH, Buja LM, Ferrans VJ, et al. Tuberous xanthoma in homozygous type II hyperlipoproteinemia. A histologic, histochemical, and electron microscopic study. Arch Pathol 1975; 99: 293–300.

179. Modiano P, Gillet-Terver MN, Reichert S, et al. Normolipemic plane xanthoma, monoclonal gammopathy, anti-lipoprotein activity, hypocomplementemia. Ann Dermatol Venereol 1995; 122: 507–508.

180. Zelger B, Cerio R, Orchard G, et al. Histologic and immunohistochemical study comparing xanthoma disseminatum and histiocytosis X. Arch Dermatol 1992; 128: 1207–1212.

181. Love JR, Dubin HV. Xanthomas and lipoproteins. Cutis 1978; 21: 801–805.

182. Braun-Falco O, Eckert F. Macroscopic and microscopic structure of xanthomatous eruptions. Current Problems in Dermatology 1991; 20: 54–62.

183. Gabriel SE, Perry HO, Oleson GB, Bowles CA. Scleromyxedema: a scleroderma-like disorder with systemic manifestations. Medicine (Baltimore) 1988; 67: 58–65.

184. Wright RC, Franco RS, Denton D, Blaney DJ. Scleromyxedema. Arch Dermatol 1976; 112: 63–66.

185. Kitamura W, Matsuoka Y, Miyagawa S, Sakamoto K. Immunochemical analysis of the monoclonal paraprotein in scleromyxedema. J Invest Dermatol 1978; 70: 305–308.

186. Dineen AM, Dicken CH. Scleromyxedema. J Am Acad Dermatol 1995; 33: 37–43.

187. Venencie PY, Powell FC, Su WPD, Perry HO. Scleredema: a review of thirty-three cases. J Am Acad Dermatol 1984; 11: 128–134.

188. Cohn BA, Wheeler CE, Briggman RA. Scleredema adultorum of Buschke and diabetes mellitus. Arch Dermatol 1970; 101: 27–35.

189. Cole GW, Headley J, Skowsky R. Scleredema diabeticorum: a common and distinct cutaneous manifestation of diabetes mellitus. Diabetes Care 1983; 6: 189–192.

190. Fleischmajer R, Lara JV. Scleredema. A histochemical and biochemical study. Arch Dermatol 1965; 92: 643–652.

191. Holubar K, Mach KW. Scleredema (Buschke). Histological and histochemical investigations. Acta Derm Venereol 1967; 47: 102–110.

192. Fatourechi V, Pahouhi, M, Fransway AF. Dermopathy of Graves disease (pretibial myxedema). Review of 150 cases. Medicine (Baltimore) 1994; 73: 1–7.

193. Kriss JP. Pathogenesis and treatment of pretibial myxedema. Endrocrinol Metab Clin North Am 1987; 16: 409–415.

194. Kind R, Hornstein OP. Clinical picture of pretibial myxedema and new aspects of diagnosis and pathogenesis. Hautarzt 1976; 27: 375–381.

195. Matsouka LY, Wortsman J, Uitto J, et al. Altered skin elastic fibers in hypothyroid myxedema and pretibial myxedema. Arch Intern Med 1985; 145: 117–121.

196. Brownstein MH, Helwig EB. Systemic amyloidosis complicating dermatoses. Arch Dermatol 1970; 102: 1–7.

197. Breathnach SM. Amyloid and amyloidosis. J Am Acad Dermatol 1988; 18: 1–16.

198. Barth WF, Willerson JT, Waldmann TA, Decker JL. Primary amyloidosis. Clinical, immunochemical and immunoglobulin metabolism studies in fifteen patients. Am J Med 1969; 47: 259–273.

199. Kyle RA, Bayrd ED. Amyloidosis: review of 236 cases. Medicine 1975; 54:271–299.

200. Kyle RA, Greipp PR. Amyloidosis (AL): clinical and laboratory features in 229 cases. Mayo Clin Proc 1983; 58: 665–683.

201. Livingston JZ, Scott TE, Wigley FM, et al. Systemic sclerosis (scleroderma): clinical, genetic, and serological subsets. J Rheumatol 1987; 14: 512–518.

202. Tuffanelli DL, Winkelmann RK. Systemic scleroderma: a clinical study of 727 cases. Arch Dermatol 1961; 84: 359–367.

203. Wallace HJ. Lichen sclerosus et atrophicus. Trans St John's Hosp Dermatol Soc 1971; 57: 9–30.

204. Barker LP, Gross P. Lichen sclerosus et atrophicus of the female genitalia. Arch Dermatol 1962; 85: 362–373.

205. Harris T, Schapiro B. Calciphylaxis. Med Surg Dermatol 1996; 3: 387–389.

206. Richens G, Piepkorn MW, Krueger GG. Calcifying panniculitis associated with renal failure: a case of Selye's calciphylaxis in man. J Am Acad Dermatol 1982; 6: 537–539.

207. Fischer AH, Morris DJ. Pathogenesis of calciphylaxis: Study of three cases with literature review. Hum Pathol 1995; 26: 1055–1064.

208. Ivker RA, Woosley J, Briggaman RA. Calciphylaxis in three patients with end-stage renal disease. Arch Dermatol 1995; 131: 63–68.

209. Tikly M, Bellingan A, Lincoln D, Russell A. Risk factors for gout: a hospital-based study in urban black South Africans. Rev Rheum Engl Ed 1998; 65: 225–231.

210. Seegmiller JE. Skin manifestations of gout. In: Fitzpatrick TB, Eisen AZ, Wolff K, et al., eds. Dermatology in general medicine. New York: McGraw-Hill; 1993: 1894–1900.

211. Bohn S, Buchner S, Itin P. Erythema nodosum: 112 cases. Epidemiology, clinical aspects and histopathology. Schweiz Med Wochenschr 1997; 127: 1168–1176.

212. Cribier B, Caille A, Heid E, Grosshans E. Erythema nodosum and associated diseases. A study of 129 cases. Int J Dermatol 1998; 37: 667–672.

213. Vilanova X, Pinol Aguade J. Subacute nodular migratory panniculitis. Br J Dermatol 1959; 71: 45–50.

214. Sanchez Yus E, Sanz Vico D, de Diego V. Miescher's radial granuloma. A characteristic marker of erythema nodosum. Am J Dermatopathol 1989; 11: 434–442.

215. Schneider JW, Jordan HF. The histopathologic spectrum of erythema induratum of Bazin. Am J Dermatopathol 1997; 19: 323–333.

216. Berman B, Conteas C, Smith B, et al. Fatal pancreatitis presenting with subcutaneous fat necrosis. J Am Acad Dermatol 1987; 17: 359–364.

217. Cannon JR, Pitha JV, Everett MA. Subcutaneous fat necrosis in pancreatitis. J Cutan Pathol 1979; 6: 501–506.

218. Martens PB, Moder KG, Ahmed I. Lupus panniculitis: clinical perspectives from a case series. J Rheumatol 1999; 26: 68–72.

219. Connolly K. Lupus erythematosus. In: Arndt KA, LeBoit PE, Robinson JK, Wintroub BU, eds. Cutaneous medicine and surgery. Philadelphia: WB Saunders; 1996: 260–278.

220. Watanabe T, Tsuchida T. Lupus erythematosus profundus: a cutaneous marker for a distinct clinical entity. Br J Dermatol 1996; 134: 123–125.

221. Peters MS, Su WPD. Eosinophils in lupus panniculitis and morphea profunda. J Cutan Pathol 1991; 18: 189–192.

222. Riccieri V, Sili Scavalli A, Spadaro A, et al. Lupus erythematosus panniculitis: an immunohistochemical study. Clin Rheumatol 1994; 13: 641–644.

223. Sanchez NP, Peters MS, Winkelmann RK. The histopathology of lupus erythematosus panniculitis. J Am Acad Dermatol 1981; 5: 673–680.

Cutaneous tumors and tumor-like conditions

Mark R. Wick   David J. Glembocki   Mark W. Teague   James W. Patterson

8

Cutaneous neoplasms comprise an extremely diverse and sizable collection of pathologic entities. Accordingly, consideration of such tumors in chapter format is a rather daunting task. The following discussion addresses those neoplastic skin lesions that are reasonably considered a part of general surgical pathology. By force of spatial constraint, more esoteric proliferations have been omitted; however, many excellent texts on dermatopathology that are now in print can be consulted for those problems. Similarly, clinical and epidemiological details of skin tumors covered here have largely been left to the contents of other monographs.

EPITHELIAL LESIONS

BENIGN PROLIFERATIONS OF SURFACE EPITHELIUM

Epidermal nevi are developmental abnormalities of the epidermis in which there is an excess of keratinocytes that may or may not show abnormal maturation. Typically, they are present at birth and have the clinical appearance of closely set verrucous papules, often in a linear arrangement.[1] Although the histopathology of these lesions is variable, the most common pattern is that of regular papillomatosis with acanthosis and overlying 'spiky' orthokeratosis (Fig. 8.1).[2] If the age of the patient is not known these lesions are often misdiagnosed as seborrheic keratoses. An uncommon version of the epidermal nevus is known by the acronym ILVEN or inflammatory linear verrucous epidermal nevus.[3,4] Clinically, these lesions are unilateral and have the appearance of a linear streak of psoriasis. Microscopically, there is psoriasiform epidermal hyperplasia with alternating areas of orthokeratosis and parakeratosis. Mild spongiosis and exocytosis and mild superficial perivascular lymphocytic infiltrate may be present.[5,6]

Verruca vulgaris (common wart) is a human papillomavirus (HPV) induced lesion that occurs in children and adults. In most cases it is associated with HPV type 2 but types 1, 4, and 7 may also be involved.[7] Clinically, the lesions are hard rough-surfaced papules that occur on the hands but may be spread to any body site by autoinoculation.[8] Microscopically, there is a variable amount of epidermal papillomatosis. Marked hyperkeratosis and columns of parakeratosis overlie the papillomatous projections. There is also elongation of rete ridges that often bow inward towards the center of the lesion. Cells in the granular layer contain large clumps of keratohyaline rather than the fine granules observed in normal epidermis. Another characteristic feature is the presence of large vacuolated cells (koilocytes) in the upper epidermis (Fig. 8.2).[9] This finding is often lost in older lesions.

Verruca plana (plane wart) occurs on the face or hand as a sessile flesh-colored papule. It lacks the papillomatous configuration of

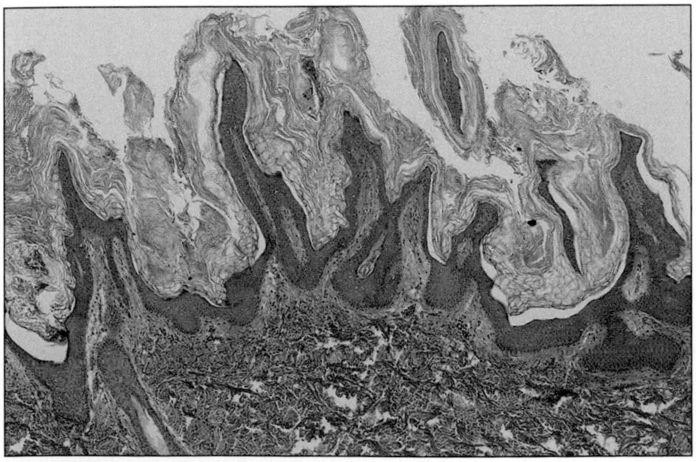

Fig. 8.1 Epidermal nevus. There is papillomatosis, acanthosis and overlying 'spiky' orthokeratosis.

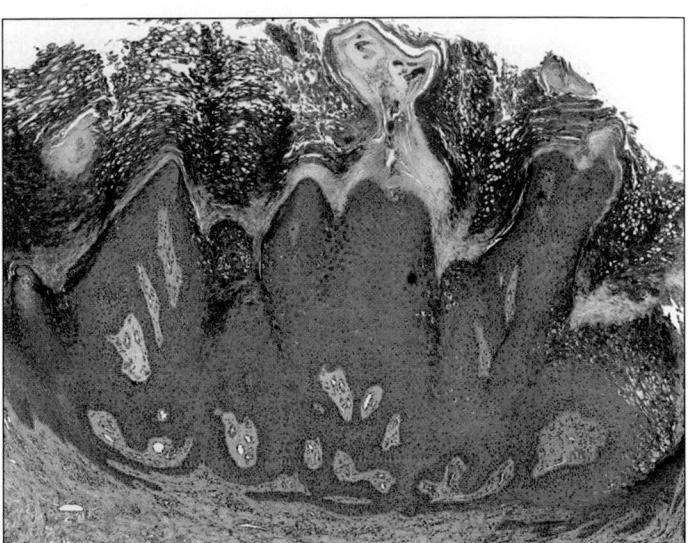

Fig. 8.2 Verruca vulgaris. Note the clumped keratohyaline granules, keratinocyte vacuolization and characteristic 'in-curving' of the rete ridges.

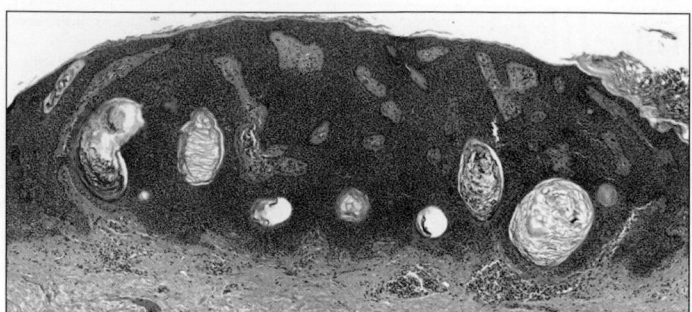

Fig. 8.3 Seborrheic keratosis.

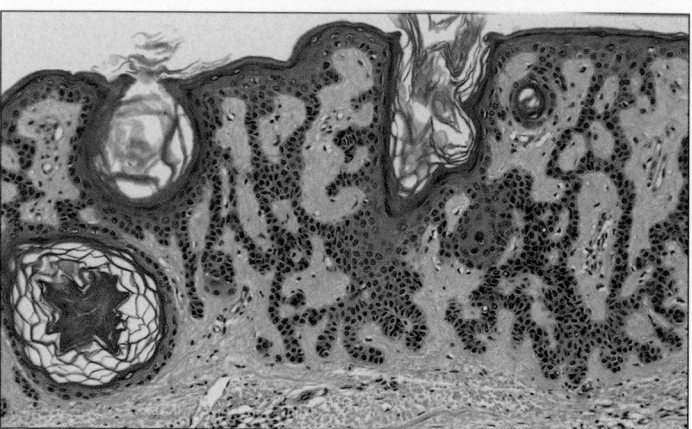

Fig. 8.4 Seborrheic keratosis, reticulated type. Interconnecting cords of basaloid cells are characteristic of this variant. Some of the basal cells also contain pigment.

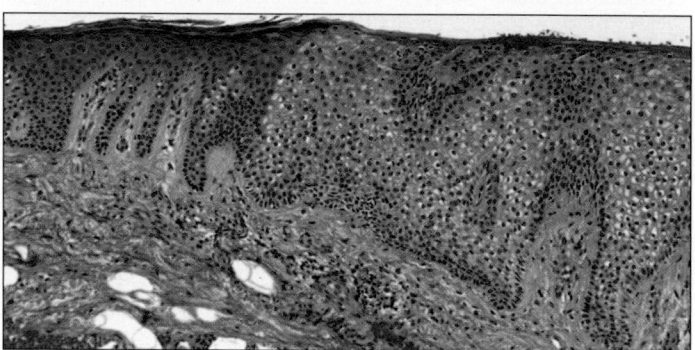

Fig. 8.5 Clear cell acanthoma. Normal epidermis abruptly becomes acanthotic with clear to pale cytoplasm seen in the keratinocytes.

verruca vulgaris. Instead, there is hyperkeratosis, acanthosis, and marked vacuolization of the granular layer keratinocytes.[9]

Verruca plantaris (plantar wart) occurs on the pressure points of the foot. Microscopically, there is endophytic growth of squamous epithelium with abundant keratohyaline granules and dense hyperkeratosis.[9]

In the genital regions of the body verrucous lesions are called *condyloma accuminatum* and are associated with HPV types 6 and 11. However, many other types have been reported, including those with oncogenic potential such as HPV-16.[10] See Chapters 34 and 37 for a complete discussion of this topic.

Epidermodysplasia verruciformis is an unusual form of generalized verrucae that presents in infancy or childhood. There are two recognized forms of the disease. In both forms patients have widespread plane warts that occasionally form plaques.[11] HPV types 3 and 10 are most frequently associated with the benign form of epidermodysplasia verruciformis, which does not progress to malignancy. The more aggressive form of epidermodysplasia verruciformis (EDV) may have an autosomal recessive or X-linked inheritance pattern.[12,13] Abnormalities in T-cell function have been implicated as one of the causes of this disease,[14,15] and it is associated with HPV types 5 and 8.[16,17] Transformation to squamous cell carcinoma occurs in roughly 25% of cases. Microscopically, the lesions of EDV demonstrate morphologic differences from the usual plane wart. There is usually less hyperkeratosis and acanthosis with marked enlargement of groups of keratinocytes in the epidermis; these have distinctive pale blue-gray cytoplasm. Perinuclear halos are also present.[18] However, the diagnosis cannot be reliably made by histology alone and requires clinicopathologic correlation. Lesions similar to those of EDV may occur in the setting of noninherited immunodeficiency such as HIV-1 infection.[19]

Seborrheic keratosis is an extremely common tumor that first presents at mid-life as a sharply demarcated brown to black lesion with a 'greasy' keratotic scale.[20] This tumor is characterized by small basaloid cells, which form an interconnecting trabecular image that follows the rete ridge pattern of the skin. Areas of squamoid differentiation are often present. Small keratin-filled cysts (horn cysts) are also a characteristic feature (Fig. 8.3). There are several recognized variants of seborrheic keratosis, including hyperkeratotic, acanthotic, reticulated (Fig. 8.4), clonal, and irritated-inflamed variants. Although the histologic pattern of each lesion is implicit in its name, inflamed seborrheic keratosis deserves special comment. That subtype is characterized by a heavy lichenoid inflammatory infiltrate that is often accompanied by striking squamous metaplasia, sometimes-alarming nuclear atypia, and mitotic activity. However, because such lesions retain the basic configuration of a seborrheic keratosis they should not be confused with carcinomas.[21,22] Rarely, several seborrheic keratoses will suddenly erupt in a patient with an internal malignancy. This combination of findings is known as the 'sign of Leser-Trelat.'[23]

Clear cell acanthoma is an uncommon benign tumor that presents as a red-brown papule on the lower legs of middle-aged and elderly individuals. Histologically, this lesion is characterized by psoriasiform epidermal hyperplasia and keratinocytes with clear or pale cytoplasm (Fig. 8.5). A hallmark feature of this tumor is the abrupt transition between the clear-pale cells and surrounding normal keratinocytes.[24]

Warty dyskeratomas are rare benign lesions that have a predilection for the head and neck in middle-aged or elderly individuals. Clinically, these lesions take the form of solitary nodules with a pore-like center that contains keratinous debris. Histologically, one sees a well-circumscribed cup-shaped invagination of acanthotic epidermis with a central plug of keratin (Fig. 8.6). Usually there is associated clefting of suprabasal epidermal cells and acantholysis as well.[25] The acantholytic cells may contain a ring of densely hypereosinophilic cytoplasm separated from a pyknotic nucleus by a thin clear halo. These elements are known as *corps ronds*. Many of the histologic findings in this entity are similar to those seen in Darier's disease, an autosomal dominant genodermatosis.[26]

Lichen planus-like keratosis (LPLK; benign lichenoid keratosis) is another solitary benign proliferation that microscopically resembles a

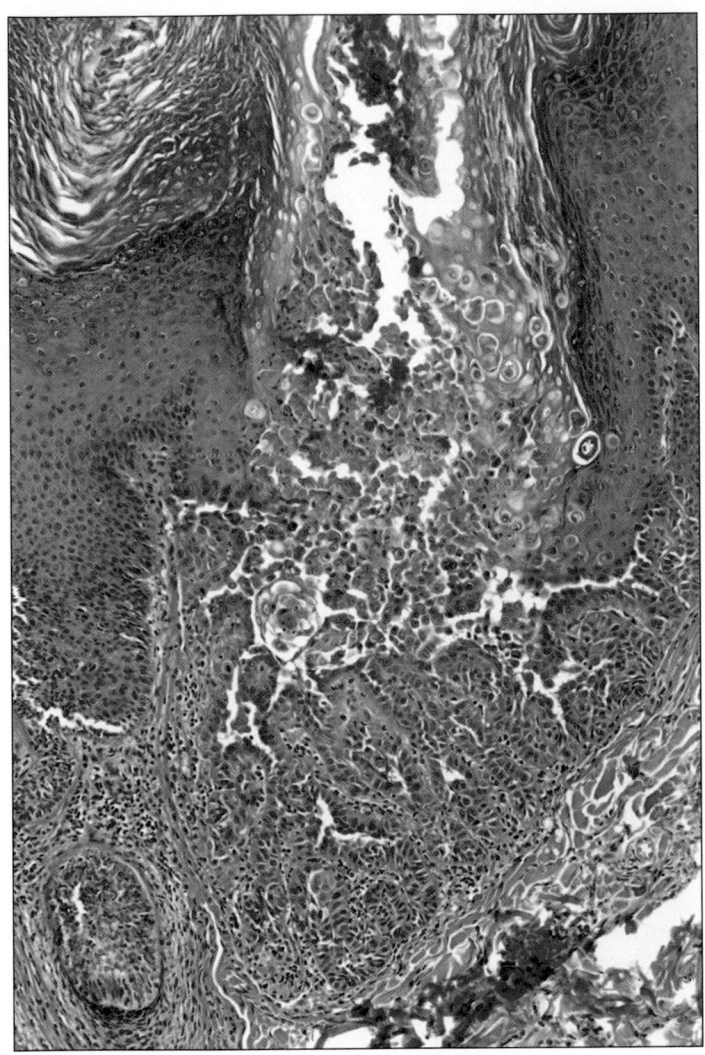

Fig. 8.6 Warty dyskeratoma. A cup-shaped invagination of epidermis contains a central keratin plug. Note the acantholytic keratinocytes (corps ronds) that contain a ring of densely hypereosinophilic cytoplasm separated from a pyknotic nucleus by a thin clear halo.

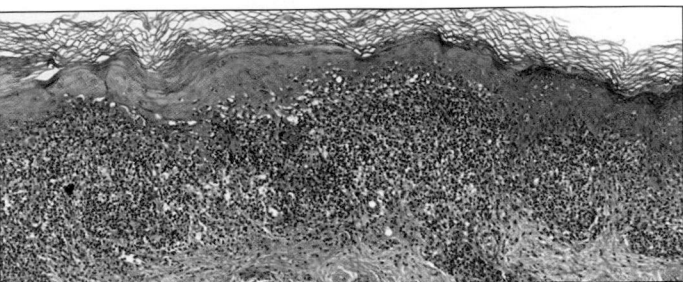

Fig. 8.7 Lichen planus-like keratosis. Lichenoid lymphocytic inflammation obscures the dermal—epidermal junction. There is also vacuolar change in the basal layer keratinocytes and numerous densely eosinophlic Civatte bodies.

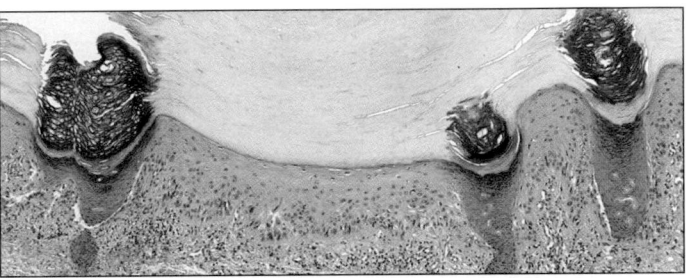

Fig. 8.8 Actinic keratosis. There is basal keratinocytic nuclear atypia with loss of an orderly epidermal maturation pattern. Note the alternating pattern of parakeratosis (over actinic epidermis) and orthokeratosis (over uninvolved appendages).

generalized dermatosis; namely, lichen planus. LPLK may be a violaceous or white-gray papule on the hands, forearms, face, or chest in middle-aged individuals.[27] Clinically, this lesion is often misdiagnosed as a basal cell carcinoma or squamous cell carcinoma. The microscopic findings in LPLK include irregular acanthosis, focal hypergranulosis, hyperkeratosis, and lichenoid lymphocytic inflammation that often obscures the dermal—epidermal junction. There is also vacuolar change in the basal layer keratinocytes and numerous densely eosinophilic Civatte bodies are present (Fig. 8.7).[28] Although there are subtle microscopic differences between lichen planus-like keratosis and individual papules of lichen planus,[29] the most pragmatic way of separating these entities is to ascertain whether the lesion in question is solitary; if so, LPLK is the preferred diagnosis.

Pseudoepitheliomatous hyperplasia (PEH) is an epithelial reaction pattern that may clinically imitate a skin tumor. Microscopically, one sees marked acanthosis with bulbous downgrowths of squamous epithelium that have rounded contours.[30,31] A dermal inflammatory infiltrate may also be present, depending on the underlying cause of PEH. Although this condition may mimic squamous cell carcinoma histologically, it lacks significant nuclear atypia and mitotic activity; moreover, the tongues of proliferating epidermis in PEH penetrate to roughly the same level in the dermis and may be interconnected, unlike the image of squamous carcinoma.

Many specific causes exist for PEH, but they are generally related to chronic irritation and/or infection.[32] An association may also be seen with Spitz nevi, selected malignant melanomas, cutaneous granular cell tumors, and cutaneous T-cell lymphomas.[33]

Actinic (solar) keratosis (AK) is a flat erythematous and scaly lesion, usually <1 cm in diameter, that occurs on the sun-exposed skin of middle-aged or elderly individuals. This is a premalignant epidermal alteration that is clearly linked to solar damage. If left untreated, 8% to 20% of these lesions will gradually transform to in-situ or invasive squamous cell carcinomas.[34] One study calculated that the risk of malignant transformation of any given actinic keratosis within a particular calendar year was <1/1000.[35]

Microscopically, AK shows basal keratinocytic nuclear atypia with an associated loss of an orderly epidermal maturation pattern. Mitotic figures may be seen. Adnexal structures are often uninvolved by AKs, giving the stratum corneum over the lesion a distinctive alternating pattern of parakeratosis (over actinic epidermis) and orthokeratosis (over uninvolved appendages) (Fig. 8.8). As expected, extensive solar elastosis is present in the dermis. Some AKs exhibit only minimal basal keratinocytic atypia and these require comparison to the surrounding epidermis in order to establish the diagnosis. On the other hand, lesions with obvious epidermal atypia may border on squamous cell carcinoma in situ, and are termed 'bowenoid' actinic keratoses. Other variants of AK include *acantholytic* lesions that display a lack of cohesion between atypical keratinocytes;[36] *hypertrophic* AKs which feature acanthosis and marked hyperkeratosis;[37] *lichenoid* AKs with a superficial dermal band of lymphocytic inflammation and scattered apoptotic keratinocytes;[38,39] and *pigmented* AK, with hyperpigmentation in both the lesional keratinocytes and melanocytes of the basal epidermis.[40]

DEVELOPMENTAL CYSTS

Although not all epithelial cysts in the skin are derived from the surface epithelium or its appendages, a spectrum of these entities is considered here for the sake of convenience.

Bronchogenic cysts and *branchial cleft cysts* have in common a derivation from the embryological branchial apparatus, and, as such, are primarily limited to the head and neck. They may be superficial or deep, with rare communication to the pharynx. The microscopic image of such lesions features a wall lined by ciliated and squamous epithelium. Other distinctive findings of bronchogenic cysts include accessory bronchial glands, cartilage, and smooth muscle.[41,42] Branchial cleft cysts are exclusively located in the lateral neck and are largely lined by squamous cells and abundant lymphocytes, often with formation of germinal centers.[43]

Cutaneous ciliated cysts, which have purportedly Müllerian or eccrine differentiation,[44–46] are found on the extremities and usually occur in females. These lesions have a similar epithelial lining to that of bronchogenic cysts but are devoid of accessory bronchial tissue, as described above.[47]

Dermoid cyst (DC) is encountered most frequently in the facial midline of children and should be recognized as distinct from the more ordinary *epi*dermal inclusion cyst. DC is located more deeply in the skin and may even demonstrate connection to the central nervous system. Unlike epidermoid inclusion cysts, DCs contain adnexal structures and their epithelial lining may occasionally be glandular as well.[48]

Median raphe cyst is found between the urethral meatus and the anus and is considered to be a developmental midline closure deformity. Cilia are rarely seen in this lesion, with a pseudostratified columnar glandular lining.[49]

MALIGNANT EPITHELIAL NEOPLASMS RELATED TO THE SURFACE EPITHELIUM

Basal cell carcinoma

Basal cell carcinoma (BCC) is the most common cutaneous malignancy, with an incidence that is directly related to duration and intensity of sun exposure;[50,51] hence, elderly patients are typically affected. We, however, have encountered undeniable examples of BCC in children, some of whom have been less than 10 years of age. The overwhelming majority of these tumors occur in the head and neck where they appear as papules or nodules, often with a pearly surface or rolled edge. They may also be erythematous plaques or ulcers with surrounding induration. Uncommonly, BCC may arise in nonsolar skin areas as well, such as the genitoperineal skin or the feet.

Despite the existence of several morphologic subtypes and diverse patterns of differentiation, BCC has several constant features that allow for its pathologic recognition. The typical appearance is that of a dermal proliferation of variably sized nodules consisting of basaloid cells that are compact and polygonal, with hyperchromatic nuclei and scant amphophilic cytoplasm. Within the individual

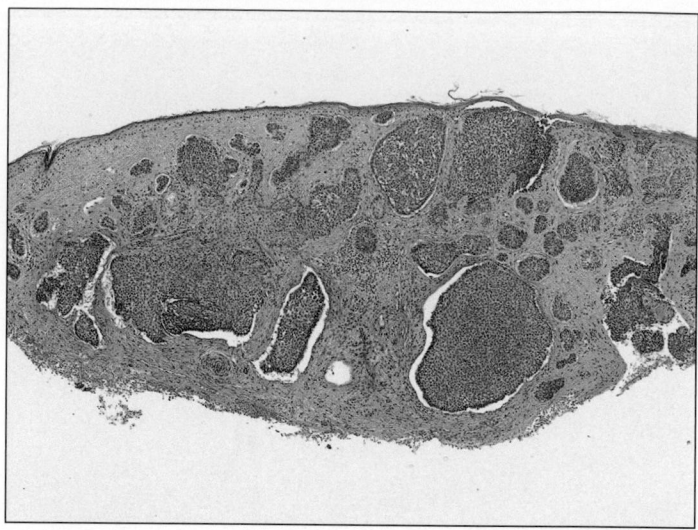

Fig. 8.9 The nodular form of basal cell carcinoma contains variably sized nodules of basophilic cells within the dermis. Note the stromal retraction around tumor islands.

nodules, palisading of nuclei is common at the periphery with blunt spindle-cell change in more central cells. Scattered apoptotic bodies are characteristically present in the centers of the cell nests. In formalin-fixed specimens, adjacent fibromyxoid stroma tends to retract from the edges of the epithelial nodules, leaving an artifactual slit-like clear space (Fig. 8.9). Small collections of stromal mucin may be present around and within the cell nests of BCC, and this finding is particularly helpful in tumor identification when other confounding features are present. Cystic change with pseudoluminal debris is a result of geographic necrosis, but this is seen in a minority of cases. Nuclear features are generally bland with inconspicuous nucleoli. A variant with nuclear anaplasia does exist but its evolution is similar to that of the common forms of BCC.[52] Mitotic activity is variable, ranging up to 10 division figures per high-power (×400) field; pathologically shaped mitoses are rare, and again do not appear to influence biological behavior.

Of the numerous subtypes of BCC only a few are associated with unusual aggressiveness. *Infiltrative* BCC, a term which is sometimes used synonymously with 'morpheaform' or 'sclerosing' BCC, is represented by small, angular nests, short cords, and single tumor cells that permeate randomly into a desmoplastic and fibromyxoid stroma (Fig. 8.10). The term *metatypical* has been used for those lesions having variable degrees of squamoid differentiation, whereas *basosquamous* is the preferred term for tumors showing truly conjoint basal and squamous differentiation in well-defined, separate regions, yielding a type of 'collision' tumor. All of these variants of BCC have an increased rate of recurrence, and basosquamous carcinoma may metastasize as well in some instances. *Superficial* basal cell carcinoma is not an aggressive subtype, but it may be difficult to eradicate because of the presence of many 'plates' of tumor cells attached to the basal epidermis (Fig. 8.11). In two dimensions, these exhibit 'skip' areas along the skin surface, producing an appearance that has been referred to as 'multifocal.' In three dimensions, all of the tumor cell nests are likely interconnected.[53] The *micronodular* variant of BCC manifests several widely scattered tiny nodules in the dermis, with a similar recalcitrance to surgical extirpation.

Histological variants whose natural histories are comparable include *nodulocystic* BCC, in which the cell islands are arranged as

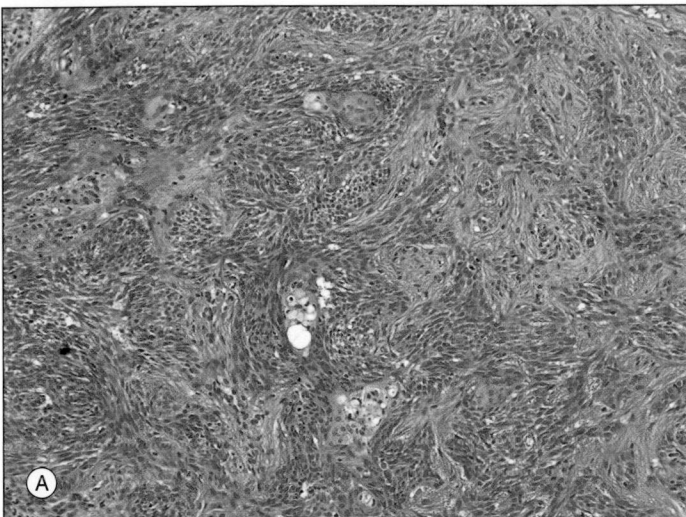

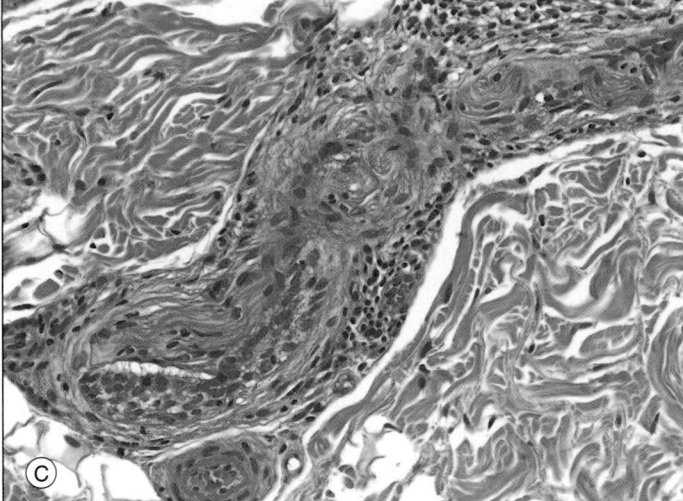

Fig. 8.10 Basal cell carcinoma **A**, Irregularly jagged-shaped nests infiltrate a sclerotic dermis with basophilic mucinous change; **B**, Some prefer the designation of morpheaform type for tumors with this densely eosinophilic stroma; **C**, Perineural invasion is an uncommon finding in the infiltrative type.

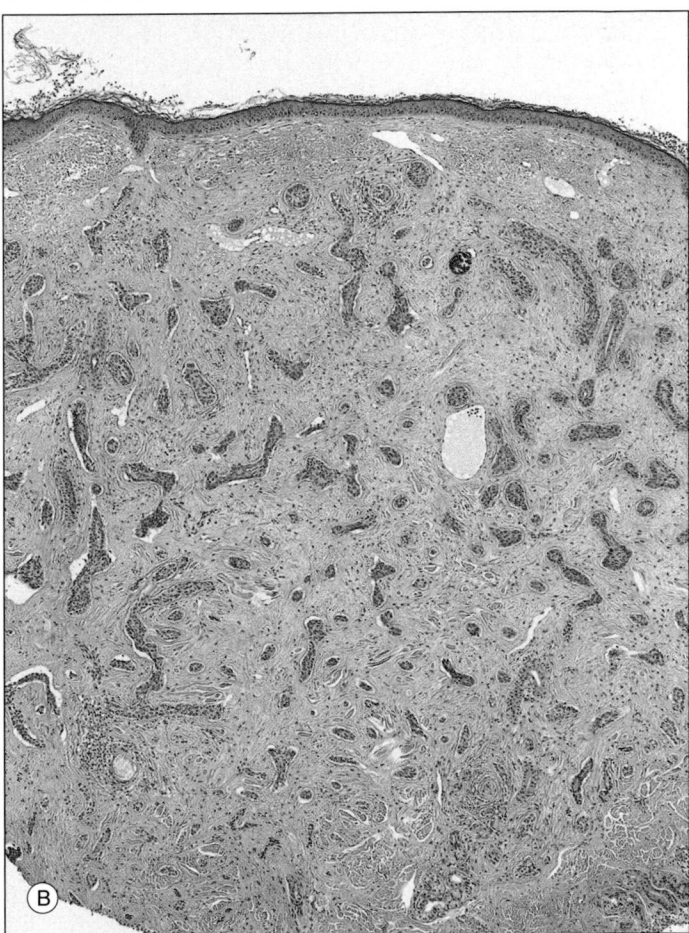

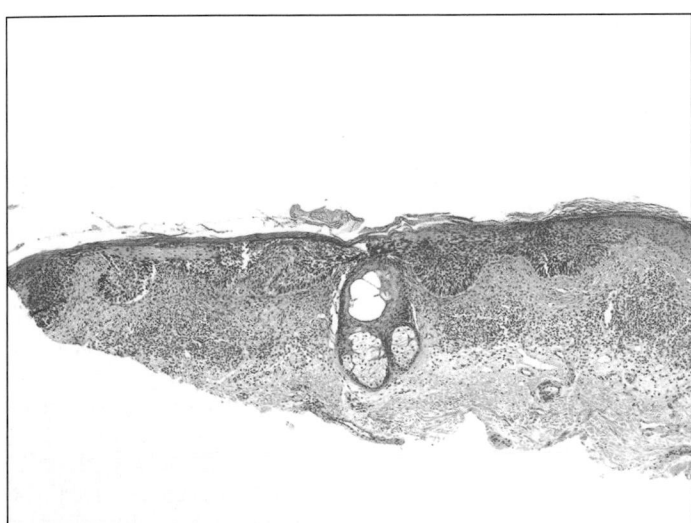

Fig. 8.11 Epidermal attachment is maintained in superficial basal cell carcinoma.

dermal nodules with limited or no epidermal attachment; *adenoid* or *pseudoglandular* BCC, with its recapitulation of glandular structures and common mucin content; *pigmented* BCC, featuring melaninization of the tumor cells, clinically imitating melanoma; *pilar* or *organotypical* BCC, showing an advanced degree of follicular differentiation; and *fibroepitheliomatous* BCC (of Pinkus), denoting a tumor with thin, interconnected strands of basaloid cells in a background of slightly hypercellular stroma.[54] Other less common forms of this tumor type include *adamantanoid*, *organoid*, *signet-ring-cell, clear cell*, and '*dedifferentiated*' (*sarcomatoid*) BCC. Among all of the entities mentioned in this paragraph, the adenoid variant is probably the most common source of diagnostic difficulty in regard to its separation from adnexal adenocarcinomas. The simplest solution to that problem is an immunostain for epithelial membrane antigen (EMA); it is expected to yield positivity in examples of adnexal carcinoma but not BCC, adenoid or otherwise. We are, of course, aware that, historically, BCC was considered to *be* a form of adnexal skin tumor. Nevertheless, from a pragmatic clinical perspective, it does not behave as such and should be clearly separated from sweat gland carcinomas diagnostically.

With regard to other differential diagnostic considerations, the striking histological similarity of BCC to *classical trichoepithelioma*

(CTE) has generated substantial debate over the possible interrelationship of those lesions.[55] In its usual form, CTE contains organoid dermal arrays of basaloid cells that demonstrate discernible pilar differentiation, with cellular formations that simulate embryonic hair buds. Small keratinous microcysts may be present,[56] but the stroma of CTE lacks the retraction artifact that is seen in basal cell carcinoma. Our approach is to follow convention and label tumors with all of the expected histological features of CTE as such. However, at a conceptual level, we believe that it is probably merely a highly differentiated version of organotypical/pilar BCC. That opinion is bolstered by the knowledge that no consistent immunophenotypic or genotypic differences have been found between BCC and CTE. *Desmoplastic trichoepithelioma* (DTE) occurs in a younger patient population than that in which BCC is usually observed, in the facial skin; the former lesion contains narrow cords of basaloid cells arranged in a confined plate-like fashion in the reticular dermis. These connect to pilar keratinous microcysts, some of which are calcified, and often are accompanied by overlying epidermal hyperplasia. DTE is easily recognized when suitable biopsies are obtained that show the base of the lesion; otherwise, one must rely on the presence or absence of stromal mucin or retraction artifact to distinguish it from morpheaform/sclerosing BCC. *Small cell squamous carcinoma* lacks fibromyxoid stroma and the nuclear palisading of BCC, and demonstrates more nuclear atypia with discernible nucleoli. *Sebaceous carcinoma with basaloid features* is likewise more anaplastic cytologically than BCC, and occasionally shows pagetoid involvement of the overlying epidermis. Cytoplasmic lipid droplets are evident in sebaceous carcinomas, at least focally, on close inspection.

In those cases of BCC that show indeterminate histologic features or multilineage differentiation, immunohistochemical studies may be helpful in diagnosis. Two antibodies of importance are those against bcl-2 protein, an inhibitor of apoptosis,[57–59] and Ber-EP4, a cell membrane glycoprotein that is present on many epithelial cells.[60] Both are expressed by BCC but not by squamous cell carcinoma or actinic keratosis.[61] On the other hand, as mentioned earlier, an opposite pattern of staining is often observed for EMA.[62] The latter maxim also holds true for CD15, S-100 protein, and carcinoembryonic antigen.[63,64] BCC routinely synthesizes low molecular weight keratins (40–46 kd),[65] making antibodies directed towards them useful in the distinction from squamous cell carcinoma.

The separation of BCC from *adnexal tumors* is somewhat more complicated because many of the latter also express Ber-EP4, but EMA usually represents a discriminating marker in that setting (see above). It is found in both sweat glandular and sebaceous neoplasms. Several proposals have been advanced regarding an immunohistochemical approach to distinguishing BCC from CTE,[66] but we believe that endeavor to be unproductive. Immunoreactivity in BCC for cellular proliferation markers – such as proliferating cell nuclear antigen and the Ki-67 antigen – and beta-2-microglobulin have been reported as indicators of aggressive behavior, but we likewise believe that those determinants have little utility.[67,68]

BCC is most commonly treated successfully by complete excision, either by traditional surgery or chemosurgery (Mohs' technique). Local recurrence may be encountered, but metastases are extraordinarily rare. Curettage, with or without electrodesiccation, is also an acceptable treatment modality for some BCCs. Recently, imiquimod, a topical immune modulator, also has been reported as effective in the treatment of superficial basal cell carcinoma.[69]

Squamous cell carcinoma

Squamous cell carcinoma in situ is known in the clinical lexicon as 'Bowen's disease,' but that synonymity is only partial. True Bowen's

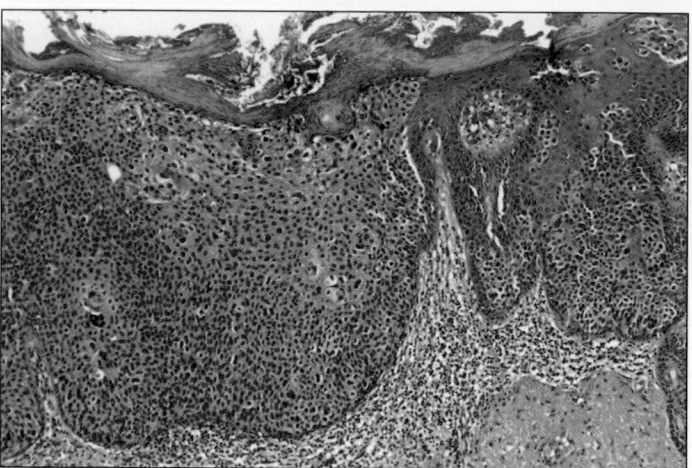

Fig. 8.12 Squamous cell carcinoma in situ. There is full-thickness keratinocyte atypia associated with disordered maturation and mitotic activity at all levels of the epidermis. Note the pagetoid spread of atypical keratinocytes in the upper right of the photomicrograph.

disease presents as a circumscribed, erythematous, slightly scaly patch, usually on the sun-exposed skin of elderly persons. The most common cause of this lesion is solar damage, but it may also be induced by human papillomavirus (HPV) infection, arsenic exposure, and psoralen-ultraviolet light (PUVA) treatment. Immunosuppression also increases the risk of that condition. Other clinical forms of squamous cell carcinoma in situ (SCCIS) are indistinguishable from actinic keratosis. Thus, our preference is to use the more generic designation of SCCIS (rather than Bowen's disease) in pathologic reports. Ordinary in situ squamous carcinoma becomes invasive in only a small percentage of cases.[70] However, when SCCIS occurs in mucosal sites such as the glans penis ('erythroplasia of Queyrat') or the vulva ('vulvar intraepithelial neoplasia, grade III') it is potentially associated with more aggressive behavior.[71] 'Bowenoid papulosis' is, at least conceptually, another histological variant of SCCIS. That condition is clearly related to HPV infection of the genitoperineal skin, but its clinical indolence – with an absence of invasion – justifies its continued designation as a separate clinicopathologic entity. Clinically, it presents as multiple pigmented papules in the anogenital region, resembling condyloma acuminata. Although the histologic appearance of Bowenoid papulosis is comparable to that of conventional SCCIS, some lesions may, in fact, regress spontaneously.[72]

Microscopically, SCCIS shows transepidermal keratinocytic atypia that is associated with disordered maturation, mitotic activity at all levels of the epidermis, acanthosis, atypical parakeratosis, dyskeratosis, and elongation of the rete ridges (Fig. 8.12). Multinucleation may also be present in the tumor cells. Although the basement membrane of the epidermis is intact, SCCIS may involve the follicular infundibula and other skin appendages. There is often a reaction beneath the lesion that may vary from scant lymphocytic infiltration to intense chronic inflammation with lichenoid features.[73]

Several histological variants of SCCIS have been described. The atrophic, psoriasiform, and verrucous variants have full-thickness keratinocyte atypia superimposed on histologic changes that are implicit in their names.[73] Rare metaplastic variants with mucinous or sebaceous differentiation have been described.[74] The pagetoid variant displays atypical keratinocytes with pale to clear cytoplasm

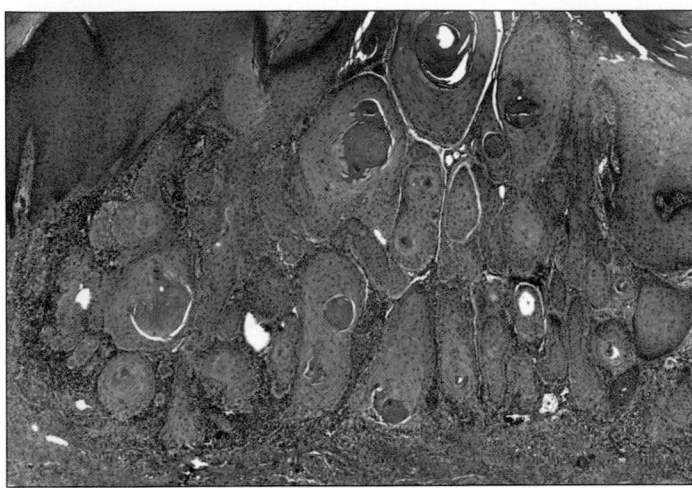

Fig. 8.13 Squamous cell carcinoma. Atypical polygonal cells with eosinophilic cytoplasm form irregular nests that invade the dermis. Deeply eosinophilic keratin pearls are seen in the centers of some of the nests.

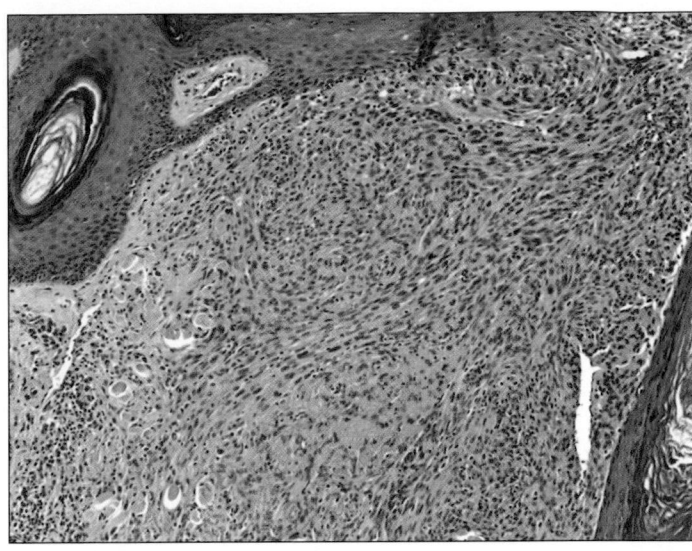

Fig. 8.14 Squamous cell carcinoma, spindle cell type. Sheets of atypical spindle cells invade the dermis.

that proliferate as nests and single cells within the epidermis. This form of squamous cell carcinoma in situ is sometimes difficult to distinguish from mammary Paget's disease, extramammary Paget's disease, or superficial spreading malignant melanoma in situ. Immunohistochemical stains may be quite helpful in differentiating these possibilities. Melanoma cells are easily detected by S-100 and both forms of Paget's disease often display carcinoembryonic antigen (CEA).[75] Cytokeratin 7 (CK7) has been considered a marker for mammary Paget's disease.[76] However, cases of pagetoid squamous cell carcinoma in situ have been reported to be positive for this marker.[77] Although most cases can be sorted out by immunohistochemistry, some cases will not allow easy definition. Reliance on clinical history may be the best recourse in this situation, e.g. proximity to breast or perineum and presence or absence of internal malignancy.

Conventional invasive cutaneous squamous cell carcinoma (SCC) usually occurs in the sun-damaged skin fields of adults over the age of 45 years. The most common locations for this tumor are the face, neck, lower lip, and dorsal hands.[78] Rarely, SCC develops in sites of chronic cutaneous inflammation and regeneration such as fistulas, sinus tracts, and chronic ulcers.[79,80] This tumor is uncommon in black people, but may indeed occur, often in the setting of a scar or an area of depigmentation.[81] Immunosuppression is again a predisposing factor for SCC, particularly in organ transplant recipients.[82] Clinically, this lesion usually takes the form of a shallow ulcer with an inflamed base and a keratinous crust, or, if originating in a precancerous lesion such as AK, SCC may be a hyperkeratotic nodule.

Histologically, SCC comprises nests of variably atypical polygonal cells with eosinophilic or amphophilic cytoplasm and vesicular nuclei (Fig. 8.13). It connects to the basal epidermis and infiltrates the corium in jagged tongues of cells.[83] In well-differentiated tumors, cells may form localized concentric whorls around a central deposit of anucleated or parakeratotic keratin – so-called keratin 'pearls.' Low-grade SCCs usually extend no more deeply than the mid-reticular dermis, and their bland cytologic attributes may make it necessary to rely on architectural atypia to make a firm diagnosis. Fibrosis and lymphoplasmacytic inflammation are typically evident at the interface between the tumor and the dermis, but necrosis is

rare. SCCs arising in sun-exposed areas often show residual changes of actinic keratosis and solar elastosis in the adjacent skin.

Moderately and poorly differentiated lesions demonstrate much less obvious keratinization and have less cytoplasm. They also manifest more nuclear hyperchromasia and mitotic activity as well as potential invasion into the subcutis or subjacent soft tissue. Necrosis may be present and invasion of dermal angiolymphatic spaces and nerve sheaths may be appreciated. Perineural lymphocytic inflammation within the confines of such tumors is often a clue to the presence of frank nerve invasion in serial tissue sections.[84]

Histologic subtypes of squamous cell carcinoma

Spindle cell SCC is an uncommon anaplastic variant that is composed of spindle cells with fusiform nuclei and scant cytoplasm (Fig. 8.14). Nuclear pleomorphism is variable but usually present, mitotic figures are numerous, and keratinization is absent. This tumor type usually arises in markedly sun-damaged or irradiated skin.[85] The presence of foci of more well-differentiated SCC or a connection between the spindle cell neoplasm and the epidermis are helpful in making the diagnosis. However, in most instances immunostaining for keratin is necessary to distinguish this tumor from sarcomatoid amelanotic malignant melanoma and atypical fibroxanthoma, both of which are keratin-negative but may simulate the morphologic image of spindle-cell SCC virtually perfectly.[86,87] As is true of other poorly differentiated SCCs, deep infiltration of the dermis, subcutis, and underlying soft tissue is potentially observed in cases of spindle cell SCC.

Adenoid (acantholytic/pseudoglandular) SCC most frequently arises in the skin of the head and neck in elderly males; there is probably also a higher incidence of this tumor variant in immuno-suppressed patients. The tumor cell nests in this lesion show marked central acantholysis whereas the peripheral cells remain cohesive, yielding the image of gland-like structures (Fig. 8.15).[88,89] The nonacantholytic cells generally have the phenotype of poorly differentiated squamous cell carcinoma, and there are often areas of tumoral connection to the epidermis that aid in diagnosis. Although these tumors are generally thought of as indolent, 19% metastasized in one study;[88] that behavior was most frequently associated with

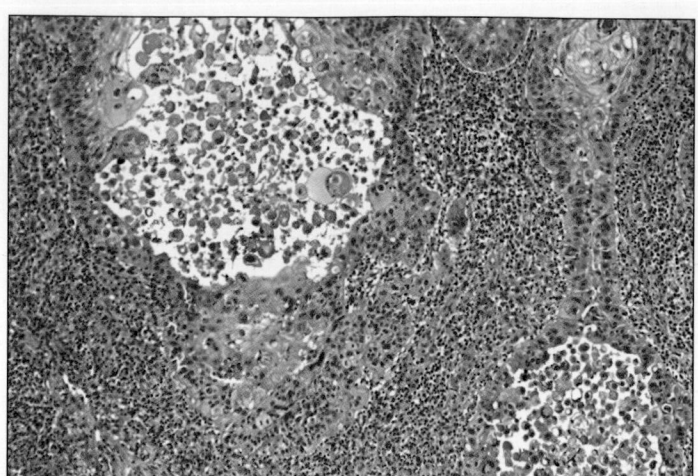

Fig. 8.15 Squamous cell carcinoma, acantholytic type. The tumor cell nests show marked central acantholysis with numerous dyskeratotic cells.

lesions that were >1.5 cm. in maximal dimension. A rare subtype of adenoid SCC is *pseudovascular squamous carcinoma*, which may be mistaken for an angiosarcoma.[90] It features marked acantholysis, with pseudovascular and interanastomosing spaces in the dermis that are lined by flattened and poorly differentiated cells. Some cases may even contain erythrocytes in the pseudovascular 'lumina.' However, the neoplastic cells in pseudovascular SCC are labeled for keratin and EMA, whereas negativity is obtained for markers of endothelial differentiation such as CD31, CD34, and von Willebrand factor.[90] This tumor type usually behaves aggressively.[91]

Verrucous carcinoma is a form of SCC that usually involves the oral cavity, larynx, or selected skin fields.[92] The plantar surfaces of the feet and the genitocrural area are favored in cutaneous cases.[93,94] Clinically, verrucous carcinomas present as large slowly growing masses that have the gross appearance of giant condylomas or warts. These tumors have had various alternative names including 'giant condyloma of Buschke and Loewenstein' in reference to penile lesions;[95] 'epithelioma cuniculatum pedis' when the plantar surface of the foot is involved;[96] and 'carcinoma cuniculatum' in other cutaneous locations.[94] All of these lesions are histologically superimposable and can be considered as a unified group.[97] Microscopically, verrucous carcinoma exhibits marked papillomatosis and acanthosis, with 'church spires' of surface keratinization. As a definitional rule, cytological atypia is minimal in this neoplasm, with scant mitotic activity and only rare foci of dyskeratosis.[98] Infiltration of the dermis takes the form of blunt irregular tongues of bland squamous epithelium, rather than the ragged profiles seen in conventional SCC.[97] Hence, an incisional or excisional biopsy will be necessary for a confident pathologic diagnosis to be made; indeed, 'shave' or punch biopsies are likely to yield a misdiagnosis of benign viral lesions or verruciform PEH. Vascular and perineural invasion are generally not seen in verrucous carcinoma,[99] and its typical clinical evolution is one of recalcitrant local growth with little if any potential for distant spread.

'Keratoacanthoma' has classically been included in pathologic discussions as a 'benign' squamous tumor. It is usually described clinically as a nodule that enlarges rapidly over a 2 to 6 week period, and is often characterized by a crater-like center that is filled with keratinous material. This lesion most commonly occurs in sun-exposed skin, especially on the face and arms of elderly adults.

Spontaneous regression often occurs over the span of several (2 to 6) months.[100] It is because of that behavioral attribute that many authors have classified keratoacanthoma as nonmalignant, with the associated assertion that it is distinct from SCC.[33] In our opinion, however, keratoacanthoma is indeed a form of low-grade squamous cell carcinoma that is uniquely capable of inducing a tumorilytic immunological host response in most (but not all) instances.[101] It may be multifocal in syndromic form; the *Grzybowski type* is characterized by eruption of hundreds of keratoacanthomas, usually in middle-aged persons.[102] In comparison, the *Ferguson-Smith type* of syndromic keratoacanthoma first appears in adolescence with the successive formation of crops of new lesions, separated in time. They typically self-heal, leaving atrophic scars.[103]

The scanning microscopic profile of keratoacanthoma resembles a volcano with a central keratin-filled crater that is surrounded by 'lips' of well-differentiated squamous epithelium. The latter structures hang over the keratinous center of the lesion, giving it a distinctly symmetrical (also known as 'buttressed') appearance. The tumor cells have a low nuclear:cytoplasmic ratio and abundant eosinophilic cytoplasm, and demonstrate only rare mitotic figures. There is usually a moderately dense mixed inflammatory infiltrate in the subjacent dermis, together with loose fibrosis.[104] Perineural invasion has, however, been observed in some examples, and there are no histologic findings which reliably assure the observer that any given keratoacanthoma will, in fact, regress on its own.[105]

When a prototypical history is obtained and the above-cited histologic image is seen, it is our practice to label the lesion as 'well-differentiated squamous cell carcinoma, with features of so-called keratoacanthoma.' This interpretation simultaneously confirms the contributing physician's clinical impression and conveys the fact that the pathologist cannot discern which keratoacanthomas will or will not regress spontaneously.

Differential diagnosis of squamous cell carcinoma

Because of its potential variability in appearance, cutaneous SCC may be confused morphologically with several other neoplasms, including spindle cell amelanotic melanoma, angiosarcoma, atypical fibroxanthoma, metatypical BCC, and sweat gland carcinoma. Despite this morphologic heterogeneity, squamous carcinomas are uniformly immunoreactive for EMA and keratin.[65] Poorly differentiated SCC may also express vimentin.[106] Amelanotic melanomas are readily distinguishable from SCCs by their strong immunoreactivity for S-100 protein, HMB-45 antigen, tyrosinase, and MART-1/melan-A, with a typical lack of staining for keratin. Rare cases of melanoma (<3%) may, in fact, demonstrate positivity for keratin, but concurrent labeling for at least 2 melanocyte-related markers would still constitute strong evidence for a nonepithelial lesion in those circumstances.[107] Angiosarcoma is separable from pseudovascular SCC by its immunoreactivity for CD34, CD31, and von Willebrand factor.[90] It must be acknowledged that squamous carcinoma may very rarely express CD31 as well, but that is clearly an anomaly.[108] Atypical fibroxanthoma is, by definition, negative for keratin and S-100 protein, but may show reactivity for CD68, factor XIIIa, or CD99.[109] Metatypical (squamoid) BCC is distinguishable from SCC because of its positivity for Ber-EP4 and bcl-2 protein, and the absence of EMA.[110]

Merkel-cell (primary cutaneous neuroendocrine) carcinoma

The Merkel cell is a normal constituent of the epidermis and is responsible for tactile sensation.[111] Primary neuroendocrine tumors

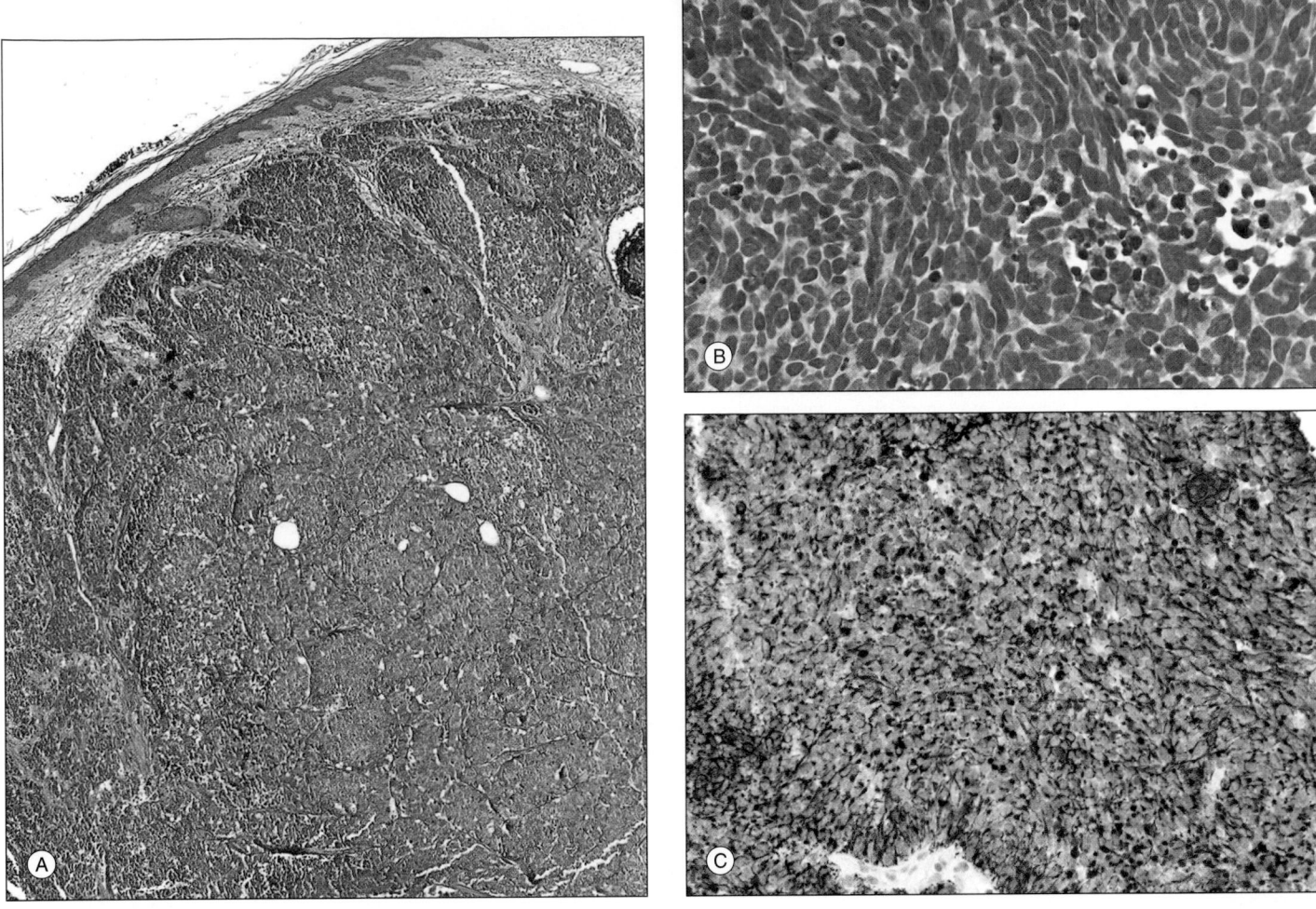

Fig. 8.16 Merkel cell carcinoma. **A,** Basophilic cells with scant cytoplasm grow as sheets within the dermis. The Grenz zone illustrated here is typical, but epidermal invasion occurs; **B,** Chromatin is finely stippled as in other neuroendocrine carcinomas; **C,** Various cytokeratins are labeled in a paranuclear dot pattern as with CAM5.2 pictured here.

of the skin that show differentiation towards this cell type have been labeled as 'Merkel cell carcinomas' (MCCs), although that nomenclature may not be fully accurate and is not universally accepted.[112] Indeed, a less contentious and alternative diagnostic label is that of 'primary cutaneous neuroendocrine carcinoma.' Sun-exposed skin fields in elderly patients are the typical setting for this tumor, which usually takes the form of an erythematous or violaceous nodule which is ulcerated in roughly 20% of cases.[113]

The originally reported series on five cases of MCC (initially termed 'trabecular carcinoma')[114] described them as having a trabecular growth pattern. Nevertheless, subsequent experience has shown that solid sheets or organoid insular nests of tumor cells are more commonly observed (Fig. 8.16A). Although the presence of a subepidermal Grenz zone is typical above this dermally based neoplasm, epidermal involvement is seen in approximately 10% of MCCs. It may simulate the junctional component of melanoma, and also can be confused with intraepithelial nests of atypical lymphocytes in cutaneous T-cell lymphomas.[112,115,116] Subcuticular infiltration is frequent in MCC, with adipocytic entrapment by tumor

cells in similarity to that seen in lymphoproliferative disorders. The cytological features of MCC are comparable to those of other small cell neuroendocrine carcinomas elsewhere in the body; they include finely stippled chromatin, high nuclear:cytoplasmic ratios, and inconspicuous nucleoli (Fig. 8.16B). Mitoses are extremely numerous in this tumor, with as many as 12 per single high-power field; apoptosis and geographic necrosis are also common. The tumoral stroma may be sclerotic, simulating the appearance of amyloid, but more often is delicately fibrovascular with arborizing small vessels. A peritumoral lymphoplasmacytic infiltrate also may be present in some examples.[117]

Morphologic variations in MCC cases include the presence of tumor giant cells, Homer-Wright-type rosettes, myxoid stroma, spindle cell foci, and divergent squamous or glandular differentiation. A purely morphological distinction from metastatic small cell neuroendocrine carcinoma of the lung may be difficult. It is aided, however, by the presence of DNA encrustation around blood vessels in metastatic tumors (the 'Azzopardi phenomenon'), which is lacking in MCC.

The potential concurrence of MCC and other cutaneous tumors such as SCC – which is the most frequent – sweat gland carcinoma,[118,119] BCC, melanoma,[120] and congenital nevi[121] has been recognized. Moreover, MCC may show multilinear differentiation in any given tumor mass towards sweat glandular structures,[119,122] squamous epithelium,[123] or even mesenchymal elements.[124,125] This fact has been cited as support for the premise that MCC arises from a pluripotent stem cell, possibly residing in the skin appendages.[122]

Cytoplasmic glycogen may be demonstrated in a minority of cases with the periodic acid–Schiff method, and stromal mucin is sometimes evident in MCC using the Alcian blue and colloidal iron staining techniques. Immunoreactivity for keratin may be diffuse throughout the cytoplasm of the tumor cells, or show more restricted labeling of the paranuclear cytoplasm with dot-like staining (Fig. 8.16C). The latter pattern is observed in the majority of cases. Cytokeratin 20 is positive in >90% of cases with a similar globular pattern.[126,127] Reactivity for chromogranin, a marker that is specific for neuroendocrine differentiation, has ranged from 33% to 100% in various reports.[128] Synaptophysin, which is also a neuroendocrine determinant, is demonstrable in 40% of MCCs.[129] Other markers that may be observed in such tumors include CD99,[130] vasoactive intestinal polypeptide, calcitonin, pancreatic polypeptide, gastrin, and somatostatin.

MCC is an aggressive neoplasm that is prone to frequent local recurrence with a high incidence of regional lymph nodal metastasis.[131] Complete surgical excision provides the best chance of cure, whereas irradiation and chemotherapy are largely palliative. Clinicopathologic indicators that suggest the need for lymph node dissection include a tumor size >2 cm, mitotic activity >10 per ten high-power fields, vascular invasion, small cell cytologic features, and palpable lymphadenopathy. Recently, the 'sentinel node' biopsy procedure has been applied to MCC as well, but its merits and impact on therapy have yet to be shown.

ADNEXAL TUMORS AND PSEUDOTUMORS OF THE SKIN

Benign pilosebaceous lesions

Nevus sebaceus of Jadassohn (NSJ; organoid nevus) is a hamartomatous proliferation that is composed of several adnexal and cutaneous elements. Clinically, this lesion presents as a plaque that ranges in size from millimeters to several centimeters in diameter, with a mamillated, hairless surface. It is usually present at birth but may become manifest early in childhood. The majority of these lesions are found on the scalp, forehead, or face.[132] The microscopic image of NSJ is variable and depends on the age of the patient. In children, immature and abnormally formed pilosebaceous units are predominant, with little alteration of the epidermis. At puberty there is enlargement of sebaceous glands in NSJ, featuring increased numbers of small lobules and abnormally placed sebaceous ducts. The sebaceous glands are abnormally superficially located in the dermis, and may connect directly to the epidermal surface (Fig. 8.17). The epidermis takes on a papillomatous and acanthotic appearance that may resemble the image of seborrheic keratosis or an epidermal nevus. In contrast, eccrine glands are reduced in number and often have dilated profiles. Hair follicles remain immature at all stages of the evolution of the lesion.[133,134] In adults, several tumors such as basal cell carcinoma, syringocystadenoma papilliferum, trichoblastoma, hidradenoma papilliferum, and nodular eccrine hidradenoma may develop in NSJ.[135] Because of that potentiality, complete excision of the lesion is the treatment of choice.

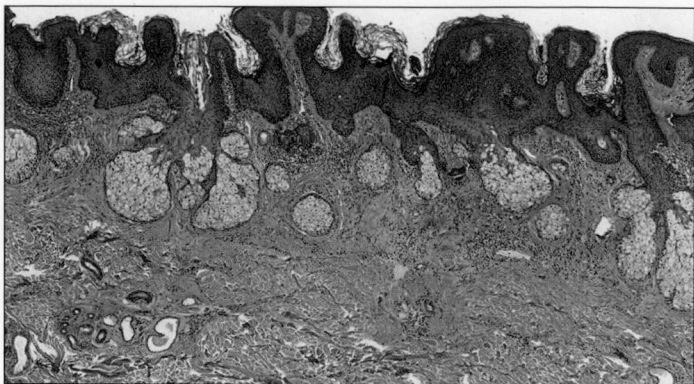

Fig. 8.17 Nevus sebaceus. The epidermis has a papillomatous and acanthotic appearance. Sebaceous glands are located abnormally high in the dermis, and often connect directly to the epidermal surface.

Sebaceous hyperplasia presents as a small, yellowish, usually umbilicated papule in the facial skin of adults. Clinically, it may be confused with basal cell carcinoma. Histologically, sebaceous hyperplasia comprises multiple enlarged sebaceous lobules, usually >3 per pilosebaceous unit, which coalesce around a centrally dilated follicle that contains debris or a vellus hair.[136] The lesion is fully mature cytologically.

Sebaceous adenoma is most commonly a solitary tan or yellowish papule in the skin of the head and neck in adult patients. The low-power microscopic image of the lesion is that of a lobulated and circumscribed mass in the upper to mid-dermis, with possible connection to the skin surface. The sebaceous lobules in sebaceous adenoma are composed of mature sebocytes with abundant finely vacuolated cytoplasm, together with a peripheral rim of smaller basaloid cells (Fig. 8.18). Occasionally, the two cell types are more intimately admixed, but mature sebocytes are always dominant. Significant nuclear atypia, mitotic activity, and necrosis are absent. Sebaceous hyperplasia differs from sebaceous adenoma in showing few if any germinative basaloid cells; moreover, hyperplasia is centered on definable hair follicles whereas adenoma is not.[137]

Any sebaceous neoplasm (including basal cell carcinoma with sebaceous differentiation) may be linked to the Muir-Torre syndrome, in which sebaceous tumors of the skin are a sign of visceral malignancy that often involves the gastrointestinal tract. Benign sebaceous lesions in the Muir-Torre syndrome sometimes have an unusual appearance, which may include proliferation of germinative elements, cyst formation, or the presence of a central debris-filled dell, yielding a configuration which resembles that of keratoacanthoma.[138]

Some benign sebaceous proliferations diverging from the prototypical image of sebaceous hyperplasia and sebaceous adenoma are difficult to classify. Another complication is a plethora of additional terms that have been used to describe such lesions. Basosebaceous epithelioma, superficial epithelioma with sebaceous differentiation, mantleoma, and sebaceoma are among them. Some authors have alternatively suggested that the designation of 'sebomatricoma' would be desirable as a unifying rubric for all benign tumors of the skin with pilosebaceous differentiation.[139,140] Histologically, lesions in this group that are nosologically challenging tend to share attributes of both sebaceous adenoma and basal cell carcinoma with sebaceous differentiation; our pragmatic approach to them has been to favor the latter of those diagnoses, to ensure that adequate surgery and follow-up are undertaken.

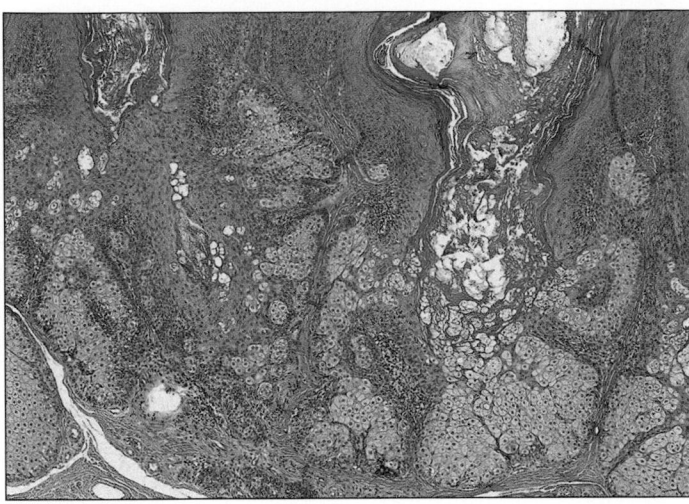

Fig. 8.18 Sebaceous adenoma. The sebaceous lobules are composed of mature sebocytes with finely vacuolated cytoplasm and a peripheral rim of smaller basaloid cells.

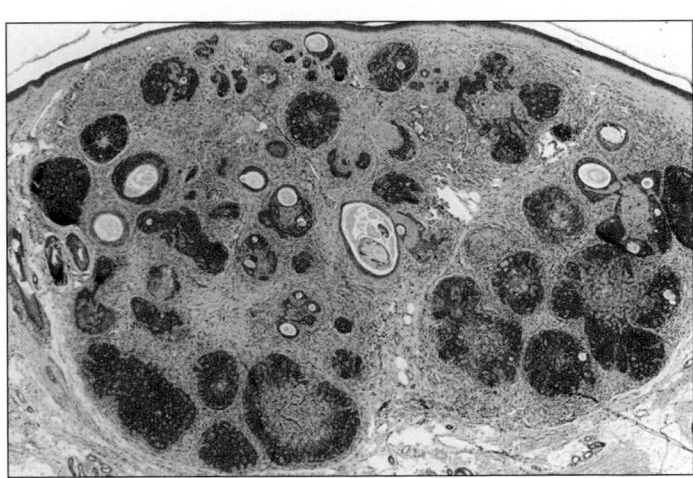

Fig. 8.20 Trichoepithelioma. Islands and cords of uniform basaloid cells contain pilar microcysts and epithelial structures resembling embryonic hair follicles with variable degrees of differentiation.

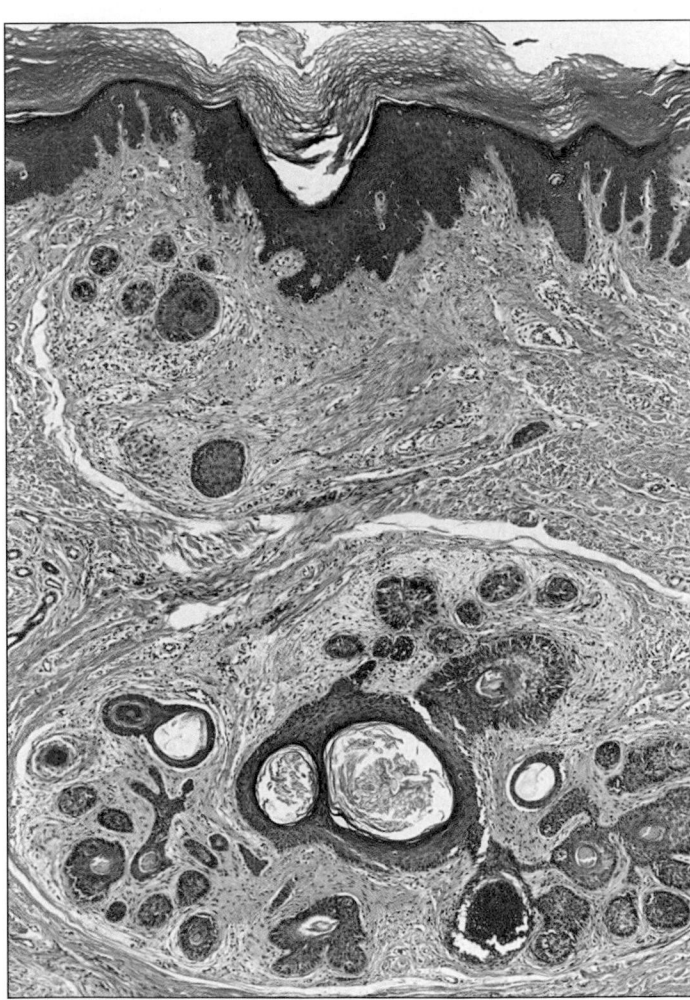

Fig. 8.19 Trichofolliculoma. Immature secondary follicles radiate from a large central dilated follicle.

Steatocystoma is considered to be a malformation of the pilosebaceous duct;[113] it most frequently presents as a multifocal nodular eruption on the chest (steatocystoma multiplex) in young individuals and has potential for autosomal dominant inheritance. However, solitary masses (steatocystoma uniplex) also may be seen. Each lesion is lined by squamous epithelium that is devoid of a granular layer. Two other distinct characteristics are an 'undulating' keratinous cyst lining and the presence of sebaceous glands in the cyst wall. Lanugo hairs and cellular debris may be present in the cyst lumen as well, but there is no lamellated keratinous accumulation as seen in ordinary epidermoid or pilar cysts.

Trichofolliculoma is a rare tumor that presents as a small, solitary, tan papule on the face. Often a tuft of fine white hair protrudes from the center of the lesion. Histologically, there is a centrally dilated follicle from which several immature secondary follicles radiate, essentially representing a caricature of the normal hair follicle (Fig. 8.19). These small follicles comprise cords of basaloid cells, vellus hairs, and, occasionally, foci of sebaceous differentiation.[141]

Trichoepithelioma is manifest as a sporadic solitary papule on the face or as multiple papules with an autosomal dominant mode of transmission (the 'epithelioma adenoides cysticum' syndrome).[142] In either eventuality the histologic features are the same. Classically, one sees a dermal mass that is composed of islands and cords of uniform basaloid cells punctuated by pilar microcysts, with some epithelial structures resembling embryonic hair follicles with variable degrees of pilar differentiation (Fig. 8.20). Some trichoepitheliomas demonstrate focal peripheral palisading of basaloid cells within cell nests and focal connection to the epidermis, engendering confusion with basal cell carcinoma. Nevertheless, trichoepitheliomas rarely demonstrate retraction artifacts between tumor cell nests and the surrounding stroma, as expected in conventional BCC. Trichoepitheliomas are also characterized by a collagenized fibrous stroma rather than the mucomyxoid stroma seen in BCC, with fewer mitotic figures and apoptotic cells.[56] A difference in proliferative capacity between the two tumors in question was demonstrated in a study showing increased immunohistochemical labeling for Ki-67 and PCNA in BCC.[143] The presence of 'papillary mesenchymal bodies' (fibrous structures representing abortive follicular papillae) in

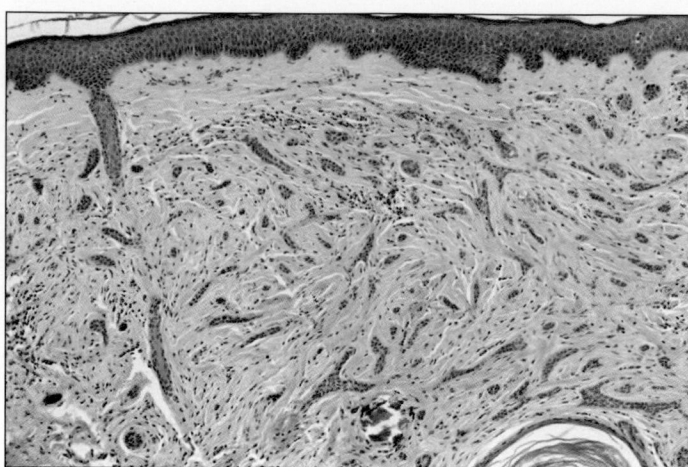

Fig. 8.21 Desmoplastic trichoepithelioma. Elongated cords and small nests of basaloid cells form a well-circumscribed 'plate-like' proliferation in the upper dermis. A keratinous horn cyst is seen in the lower right portion of the photomicrograph. The stroma is desmoplastic and hypocellular.

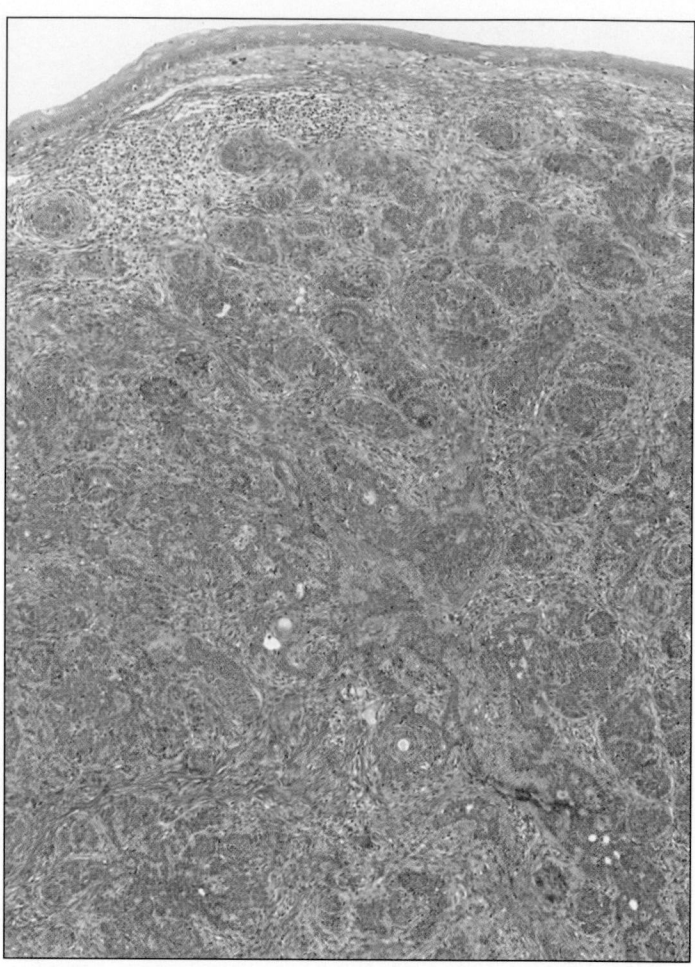

Fig. 8.22 Trichoblastoma. There are irregular nests and cords of basaloid cells that do not have a connection to the epidermis. Within the nests there is pilar differentiation in the form of primitive hair follicles.

trichoepithelioma is also said to be helpful in distinguishing it from BCC.[144]

Immunohistochemical studies have suggested that overexpression of bcl-2 protein is unique to BCC in this specific context.[59] However, more recent analyses have observed shared reactivity for that marker in trichoepithelioma as well.[66] Although trichoepithelioma and BCC have classically been regarded as distinct and unrelated tumor entities, it is probable that a continuum exists between the two. Our practice is to continue to utilize both diagnostic labels, but we advise complete excision of trichoepitheliomas whenever that intervention is clinically feasible.

Desmoplastic trichoepithelioma usually takes the form of a firm solitary nodule or plaque with central umbilication. It occurs almost exclusively in the facial skin and shows a predilection for young women. This neoplasm is composed of elongated cords and small nests of basaloid cells with scant cytoplasm, which form a well-circumscribed 'plate-like' proliferation in the upper dermis with an interlacing pattern. There are numerous small keratinous horn cysts that are connected to the cellular nests. The stroma is desmoplastic and hypocellular (Fig. 8.21). Dystrophic calcification of lesional microcysts is commonly seen as well.[145] The differential diagnosis of this lesion includes syringoma, morpheaform basal cell carcinoma, and microcystic adnexal carcinoma. Syringomas typically lack horn cysts and dystrophic calcification, and contain more tubular cell nests than those seen in desmoplastic trichoepithelioma. Moreover, syringomas are multifocal and typically affect the lower eyelids, whereas desmoplastic trichoepithelioma (DTE) is solitary and usually arises in the central facial region. Morphea-like basal cell carcinomas (MBCC) show artifactual clefts between tumor cell nests and stroma, and often contain small foci of other typical morphotypes of BCC.[146] The presence of Merkel cells, detected by immunohistochemistry, is much more common in DTE than in MBCC.[147] Microcystic adnexal carcinoma deeply invades the dermis, in contrast to DTE, and displays immunoreactivity for carcinoembryonic antigen which is not apparent in the latter lesion.[148]

Trichoblastoma is a very rare tumor that frequently affects the scalp but may involve almost any body site. It is thought to be a tumor of 'hair germ' that displays differentiation resembling both the epithelial and mesenchymal portions of the hair follicle.[149]

These tumors form a spectrum of differentiation from epithelial-predominant *trichoblastomas* to mesenchymal-predominant *trichoblastic fibromas*.[150] Another rare variant of this tumor is the *cutaneous lymphadenoma* that displays a prominent lymphoid component.[151]

Microscopically, trichoblastomas are composed of irregular nests and cords of basaloid cells that do not have a connection to the epidermis. Within the nests there is often pilar differentiation in the form of primitive hair follicles (Fig. 8.22).[142] These tumors bear a striking resemblance to basal cell carcinoma but lack the epidermal connection, mitotic activity, single-cell necrosis and clefting artifact of the latter. Trichoblastic fibromas display an intimate relationship between the basaloid nests and a dense fibrocellular stroma.[152] Cutaneous lymphadenomas contain an intense infiltrate of small lymphocytes that course through the basaloid nests. Some authors have likened this histology to that of an adamantinoma (Fig. 8.23).[153]

Trichilemmoma is usually a solitary keratotic papule on the face. Multiple lesions of this type are a cutaneous marker for *Cowden's syndrome*, a complex that has autosomal dominant inheritance and a predilection for visceral hamartomas and carcinomas of the breast and thyroid gland.[154] This syndrome is associated with a mutation in the *PTEN* gene on chromosome 10q23.[155] Microscopically, trichilemmoma is composed of squamoid cells with abundant clear

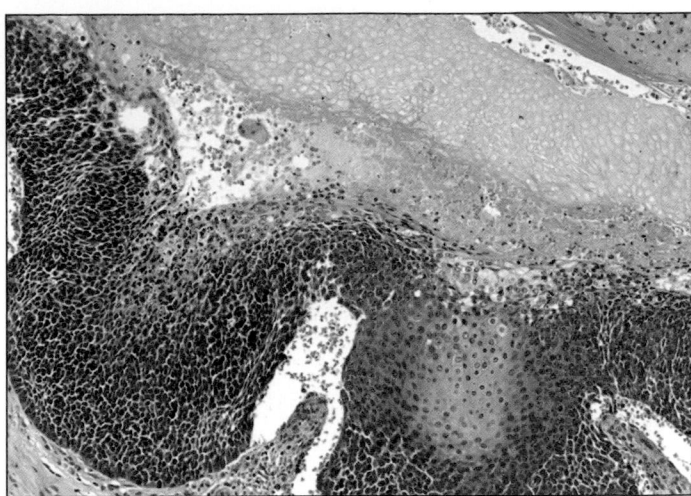

Fig. 8.25 Pilomatrixoma. Note the biphasic cell population composed of basaloid germinative cells and eosinophilic 'shadow' cells.

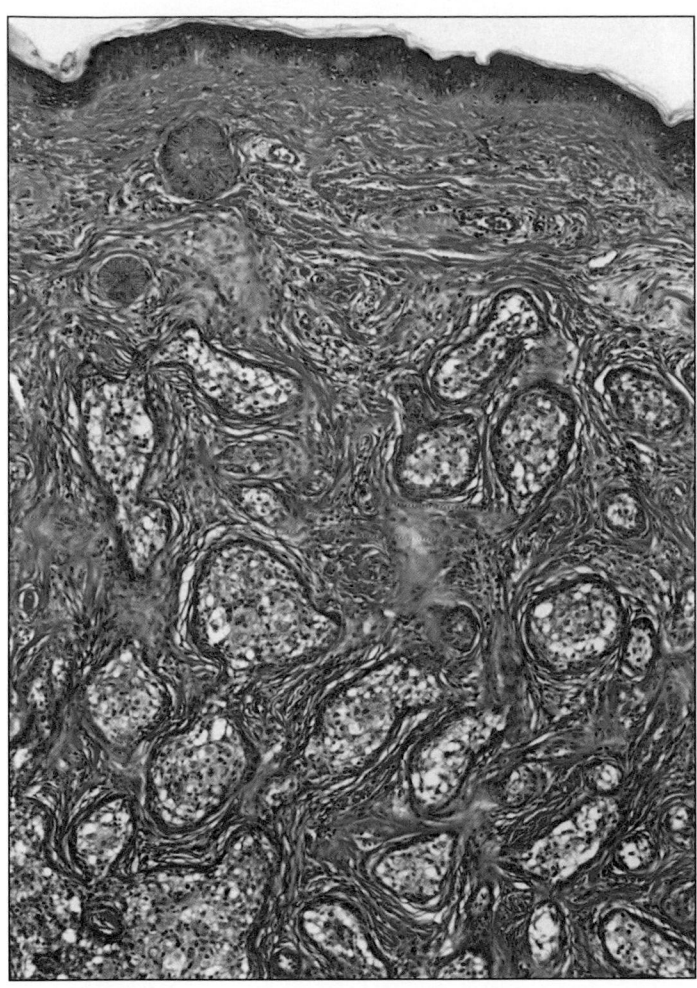

Fig. 8.23 Lymphadenoma. An infiltrate of small lymphocytes courses through the basaloid nests.

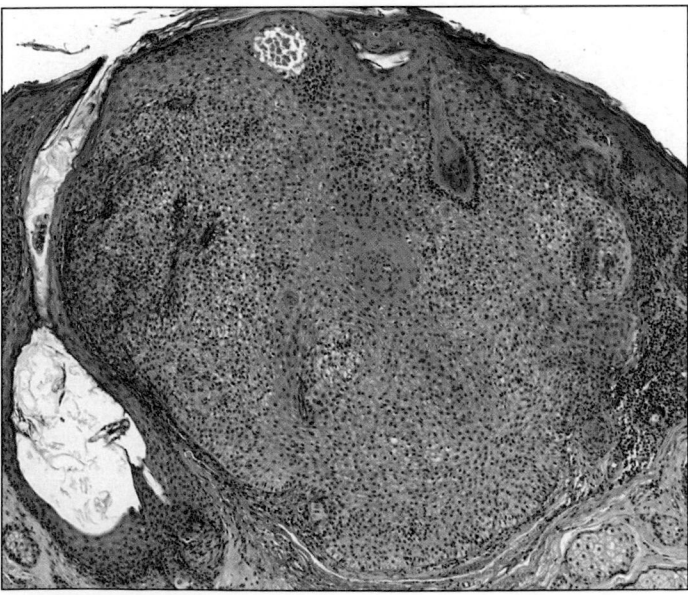

Fig. 8.24 Trichilemmoma. Squamoid cells with abundant clear cytoplasm, form a lobule that attaches to a pilosebaceous unit. There is a peripheral palisade of cells that simulates the outer root sheath of normal hair follicles.

cytoplasm, forming one or more lobules that are attached to the epithelial surface or a pilosebaceous unit (Fig. 8.24). The lobules often contain a peripheral palisade of cells that simulate the outer root sheath of normal hair follicles. A glassy eosinophilic basement membrane ('cuticle') may partially envelop the tumor cell lobules as well.[156] A desmoplastic form of trichilemmoma has also been described, in which cords and islands of tumor cells are trapped in a densely fibroblastic stroma, imitating the appearance of an invasive carcinoma. However, the overall circumscription of that tumor type and the presence of a thick eosinophilic cuticle around tumor cell islands provide clues to its benign nature.[157] Some authors have questioned the pathogenesis of trichilemmomas, suggesting that they are actually involuting folliculocentric verrucae rather than true neoplasms.[158] We continue to prefer the latter interpretation, especially given the association of this lesion with Cowden's syndrome.[159]

Pilomatrixoma (pilomatricoma; calcifying epithelioma of Malherbe) is a relatively common dermal tumor that is encountered most often in children and young adults. It is a solitary, deeply seated nodule, usually in the skin of the head and neck, with a strong female predilection.[160] Pilomatrixomas are sharply circumscribed and centered in the corium, but they often extend into the subcutis. Microscopically, there is a biphasic cell population comprising basaloid germinative cells and eosinophilic 'shadow' cells. The former of those elements contain scant cytoplasm, hyperchomatic nuclei, and numerous mitotic figures, and are usually found at the periphery of the neoplasm (Fig. 8.25). 'Shadow' cells have abundant eosinophilic cytoplasm, but demonstrate only ghost-like outlines of nuclear membranes; they are often associated with foci of dystrophic calcification or even metaplastic ossification. The number of basaloid cells decreases with the age of the lesion;[142,161] accordingly, some pilomatrixomas may be composed exclusively of shadow cells. Other findings may include the presence of foreign-body-type granulomas and lesional pigmentation, either with hemosiderin or melanin.[142,162] Although locally aggressive forms of pilomatrixoma have been described – which exhibit permeative growth into a desmoplastic stroma – ordinary versions of these tumors uncommonly recur even if they are incompletely excised. Important differential diagnostic considerations in cases of pilomatrixoma, especially in frozen section preparations, include basal cell carcinoma and squamous cell

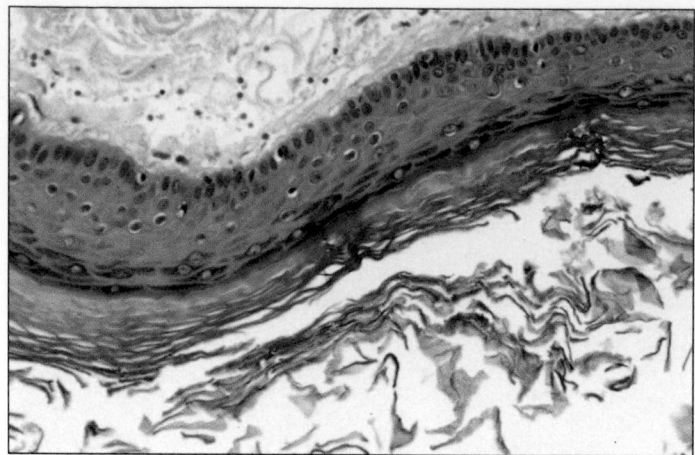

Fig. 8.26 Epidermoid cyst. The cyst wall is composed of stratified squamous epithelium with a keratohyaline-containing granular layer. 'Keratin flakes' are seen on the luminal side of the cyst.

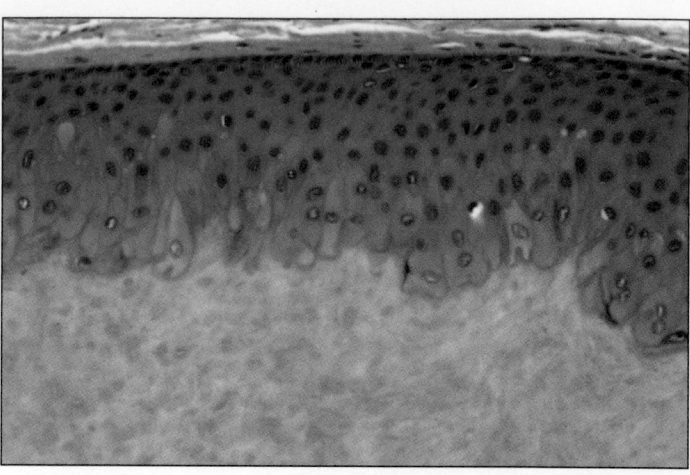

Fig. 8.27 Pilar cyst. The cyst wall consists of stratified squamous epithelium that shows 'abrupt' dense keratinization without an interposed granular layer.

carcinoma. BCC may occasionally manifest ghost-cell differentiation but has unique characteristics reflecting the interrelationship between tumor cell nests and their stroma, as described above. Squamous cell carcinoma lacks ghost cells and is not expected to occur in the age range that is usually applicable to pilomatrixoma.

Epidermoid (infundibular) cysts are thought to arise developmentally from the infundibular portion of hair follicles. However, traumatic implantation of the epidermis may also be causally responsible, especially in acral locations. The walls of the cysts are composed of stratified squamous epithelium with a keratohyaline-containing granular layer (Fig. 8.26). The rupture of epidermoid cysts will cause a local foreign body giant cell reaction, which may completely obliterate the original lesion.[33] The only remaining evidence of a cyst in that instance may be residual 'keratin flakes' within foreign-body-type giant cells. Multifocal cyst formation is sometimes associated with *Gardner's* syndrome.[163] Although malignant transformation of epidermoid cysts is extremely rare, it still seems reasonable to submit those that are excised for histological examination.[164,165]

A *milium* is a small intradermal cyst (1–2 mm) that is most commonly found on the face or cheeks. Several layers of stratified squamous epithelium line such lesions, and there is keratinous material in their centers. In essence, they are miniature epidermoid inclusion cysts. The importance of milia lies in their potential association with other cutaneous disorders such as discoid lupus erythematosus and porphyria cutanea tarda.[33]

Pilar (trichilemmal) inclusion cysts have a strong predilection for the scalp. Their walls consist of stratified squamous epithelium that shows 'abrupt' (trichilemmal) keratinization (without an interposed granular layer) (Fig. 8.27). Trichilemmal cysts also differ from epidermoid cysts in that they are rarely inflamed, with the common presence of cholesterol clefts and calcifications internally.[166] Occasionally, *hybrid cysts* with morphological features of both pilar and epidermoid cysts are encountered.[167]

Proliferating pilar (trichilemmal) tumor presents as a deep dermal to subcutaneous nodule, usually on the scalp. It is typically 2–10 cm in diameter, but may reach huge proportions. This neoplasm is 2 to 3 times more common in women and usually occurs in middle-aged to elderly individuals.[168] It usually forms a well-

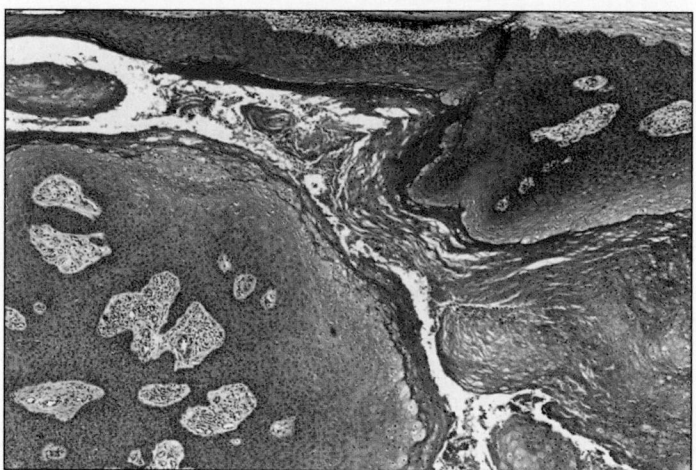

Fig. 8.28 Proliferating pilar tumor. Keratinocytes with eosinophilic cytoplasm form lobules with areas of trichilemmal keratinization. A central cystic area is present.

circumscribed multilobulated mass in the dermis that is composed of keratinocytes with densely eosinophilic cytoplasm and foci of trichilemmal keratinization (Fig. 8.28). Central cystic areas may be present, as well as foci resembling ordinary pilar inclusion cyst. In a substantial proportion of cases, one sees nuclear atypia in the proliferating cells, as well as brisk mitotic activity. Moreover, zones of spontaneous degeneration and calcification may be mistaken for necrosis.[169] These often alarming findings may lead to an erroneous diagnosis of squamous cell carcinoma.[170] However, attention to the low-power microscopic profile of the tumor, with its sharply demarcated borders and lack of stromal invasion, should yield the correct interpretation.

Tumor of the follicular infundibulum is a rare pilar neoplasm that is composed of cords of basaloid cells which form an interlocking network in the papillary and upper reticular dermis. Typically, the tumor cells bud from the bases of follicular ostia. Some of the neoplastic elements may have relatively abundant pale cytoplasm.[171]

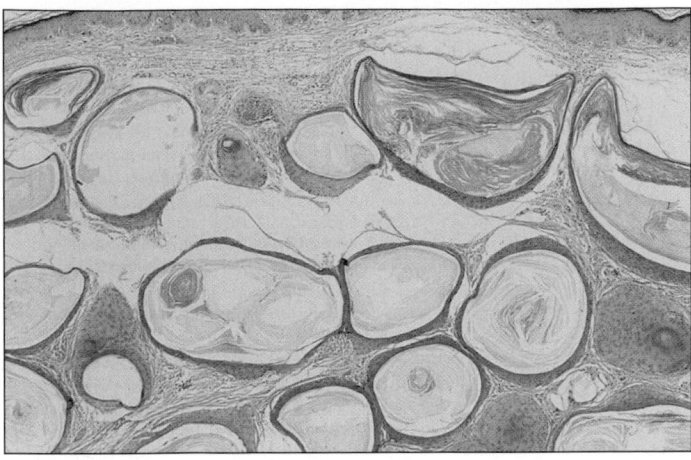

Fig. 8.29 Trichoadenoma. Microcystic epithelial structures resemble cross-sections of follicular infundibula. No hair shafts are present.

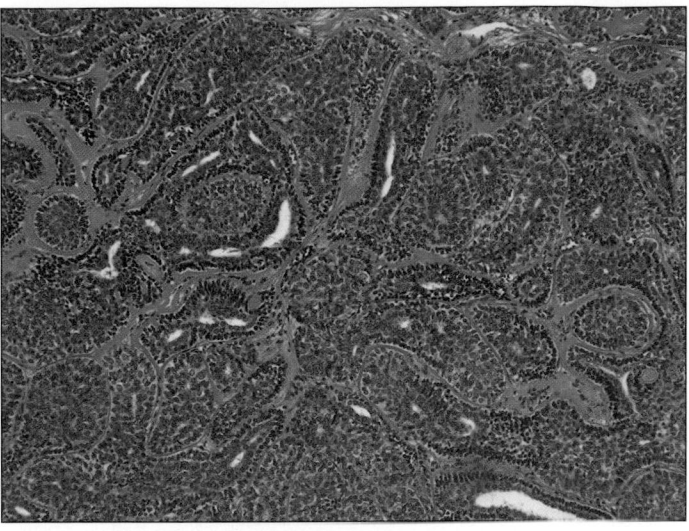

Fig. 8.31 Cylindroma. The distinctive appearance of cylindroma with its interlocking cell aggregates separated by thick eosinophilic bands is shared on occasion with spiradenoma.

Although tumor of the follicular infundibulum may be mistaken for a superficial basal cell carcinoma, it lacks the mucomyxoid stromal reaction and artifactual stromal-epithelial clefting of the latter lesion.

Trichoadenoma (of Nikolowski) is a very uncommon tumor comprising a circumscribed proliferation of microcystic epithelial structures that resemble cross-sections of follicular infundibula (Fig. 8.29). However, there are no hair shafts in this lesion.[172] Trichoadenomas are most often found on the face or buttocks.

Benign sweat gland proliferations

Hidrocystoma presents almost exclusively on the face, often in a periorbital location, as one or more cystic papules. Whether this is a true neoplasm or results from ductal obstruction is uncertain; however, by convention, it has been felt that the apocrine variant of hidrocystoma is indeed neoplastic and some have applied to it the term apocrine 'cystadenoma.'[173] Microscopically, one sees internal layers of epithelium with a basal myoepithelial component surrounding a central unilocular cyst; up to ten layers have been reported in some lesions. Luminal cells in apocrine hidrocystoma often manifest decapitation-type secretion (Fig. 8.30).[174,175]

Dermal cylindroma, or *'turban tumor,'* a term that is used for the syndromic form of that lesion,[176] is a neoplasm consisting of small nests of basaloid cells in the corium, with a pattern reminiscent of a jigsaw puzzle. Around the cell clusters there are eosinophilic hyalinized zones that are largely composed of basement membrane material containing collagen types IV and VII (Fig. 8.31).[177,178]

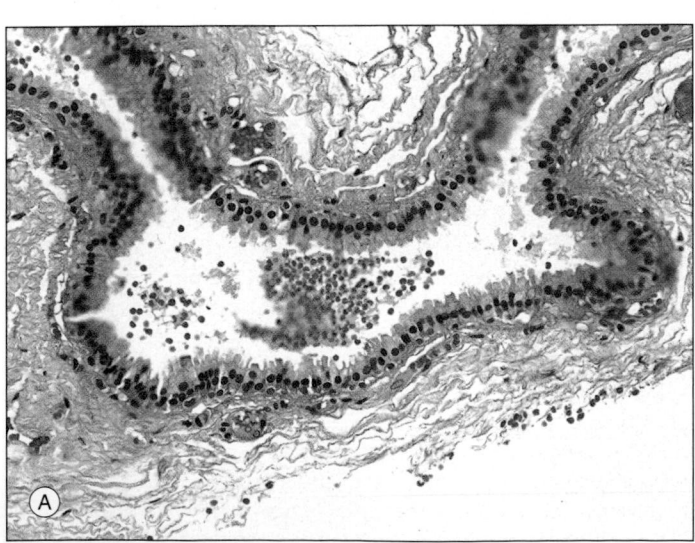

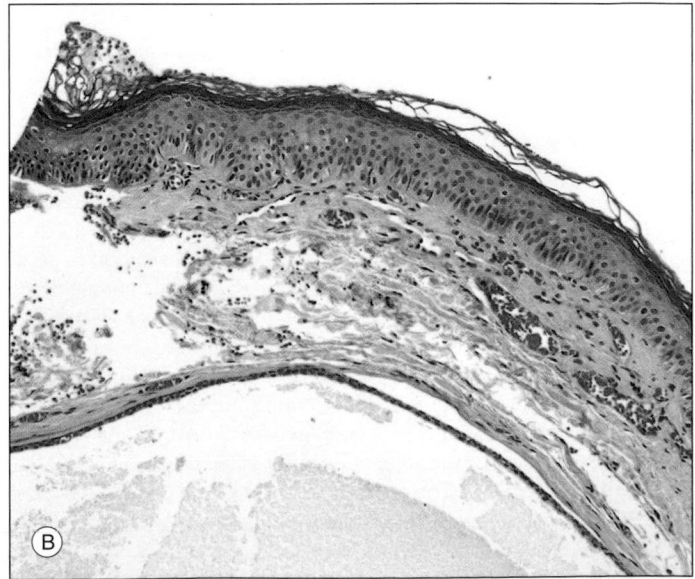

Fig. 8.30 Hidrocystoma. **A**, The apical cell decapitation of the apocrine variant distinguishes it from the eccrine with a low cuboidal, often flattened, epithelium (**B**).

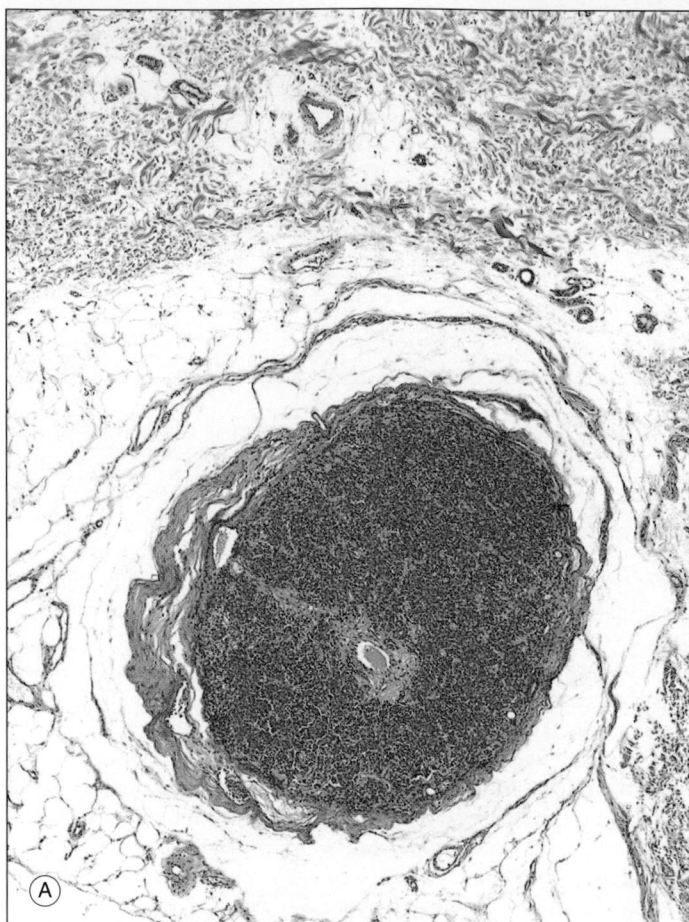

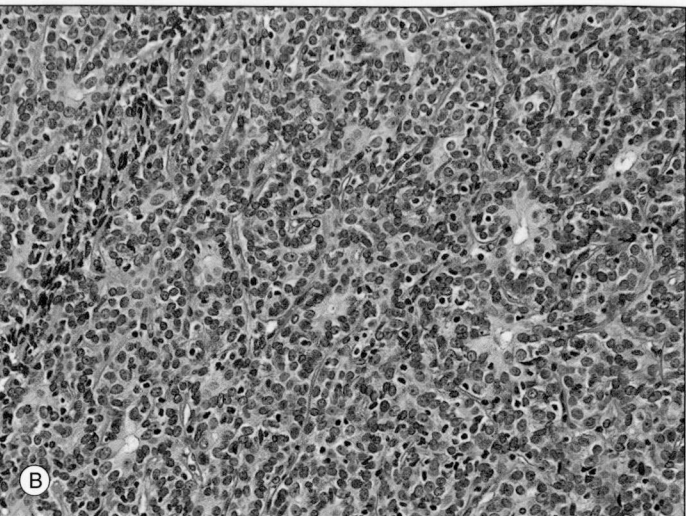

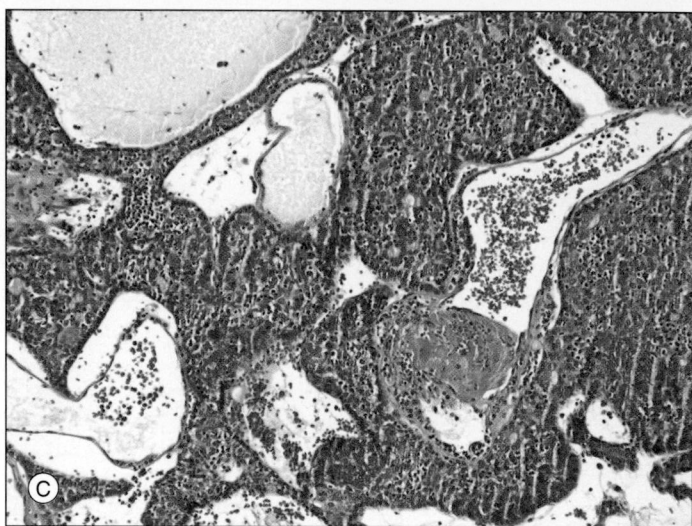

Similar matrix may be seen in the form of intercellular globules. A dual cell population can usually be appreciated in cylindroma, with small basaloid elements that are disposed at the periphery of the cell nests and a second population of more epithelioid elements in the center of the nests. Small duct-like structures may occasionally be formed by the latter component. Mitotic activity and detachment of small buds of tumor cells at the periphery of cylindromas are both common, and they are associated with no adverse behavior.

Eccrine spiradenoma is as a reddish or violaceous nodule that is usually seen in the skin of the head and neck or the trunk. This tumor is potentially painful when traumatized or palpated, but that is an inconstant finding.[179,180] Spiradenoma morphologically resembles cylindroma in many respects; its scanning microscopic appearance is that of a basophilic dermal nodule with an irregular peripheral profile (Fig. 8.32A). In comparison with cylindroma, however, the dual cell population of spiradenoma is better developed and duct-like formations are more common. Lesional basement membrane material is usually not as prominent in spiradenoma, and mature lymphocytes are consistently scattered throughout that tumor, recalling the attributes of thymic tissue (Fig. 8.32B). Dilated blood vessels are common in spiradenoma as well, both within the tumor cell nodules and in the perilesional stroma. Indeed, they may be

prominent enough to justify the diagnostic label of 'giant vascular spiradenoma' (Fig. 8.32C).

Syringoma is most commonly seen on the face of young women; like hidrocystoma, it has a predilection for a periorbital location but is typically multifocal. Similar tumors also occur in the genital skin.[173] Some 'eruptive' syringomas have been reported in familial settings, and an association with the Down syndrome is also possible.[181] These tumors are well-circumscribed, dermal collections of small, angulated tubules set in a densely collagenized stroma (Fig. 8.33). A double layer of cuboidal epithelium comprises the tubules, often mantled internally by a luminal cuticle. Mitotic activity and nuclear atypia are lacking in syringoma. Circumscription and a superficial location help to distinguish syringoma from microcystic adnexal carcinoma (see below), with which it shares several morphologic features. A reactive proliferation of eccrine ducts, variably termed *syringometaplasia* or *syringoma-like sweat duct proliferation*, has been reported in association with alopecias and inflammatory dermatoses, and represents yet another differential diagnostic consideration.[182,183] Ultimately, information on the clinical appearance of syringoma is usually sufficient to resolve these difficulties.

The *eccrine poroma/acrospiroma* category of tumors is plagued by nosological controversy, and it encompasses several pathologic

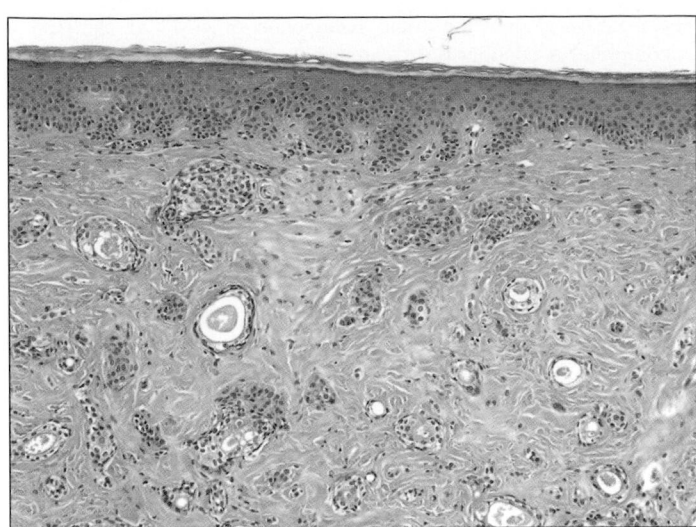

Fig. 8.33 Syringoma differentiates towards the eccrine sweat duct with a double layer of cells, sometimes with clear cytoplasm.

entities with overlapping histological features.[113,184] Typical *poroma* occurs on the extremities, particularly on the palms and soles, and is a proliferation of interconnecting cords and sheets of compact polyhedral cells that grow into the dermis from multifocal epidermal attachments and intraepidermal tumor cell 'lakes.' The overall pattern simulates that of the non-neoplastic acrosyringium.[185] Poroma cells in the surface epithelium are distinct from adjacent keratinocytes (Fig. 8.34A)[186–188] Occasional ducts may be scattered throughout the dermal component of the tumor but they may be difficult to find (Fig. 8.34B). Poroma is one of very few nonmelanocytic skin tumors that may contain melanin pigment, along with basal cell carcinoma, actinic keratosis, and seborrheic keratosis.

Several separate but related variants of poroma are recognized. *Dermal duct tumor* is similar in virtually all respects but lacks an obvious epidermal attachment;[189] conversely, *hidroacanthoma simplex* is conceptualized as an entirely intraepidermal poroma. All poroma subtypes may contain focally cellular stroma, but *syringofibroadenoma*, a tumor that is considered to be synonymous with *acrosyringeal nevus*,[190–194] shows a uniformly proliferative connective tissue component that is admixed with poroma-like epithelial elements (Fig. 8.35). The overall microscopic profile of that lesion is very similar to that of mammary fibroadenoma.

Nodular hidradenoma or *acrospiroma* is also felt by some to be a subtype of poroma.[187] Those terms denote a poroma-like neoplasm that has a wider topographic distribution and a greater tendency for local recurrence than does poroma,[113] but with microscopic attributes that are closely similar to the latter. Acrospiroma is distinguished morphologically from classical poroma by a lack of epidermal attachment and a more heterogeneous cellular constituency, including clear glycogenated cells, others with eosinophilic cytoplasm, and even squamoid elements (Fig. 8.36).[195] There is also a tendency for the tumor cells to be arranged in larger sheets and nodules. Both solid and cystic variants of acrospiroma occur and those patterns often coexist within the same lesion. Small papillae sometimes protrude into microcystic lumina in such neoplasms. In similarity to classical poroma, ducts are sparse in acrospiromas. The latter tumors are circumscribed on scanning microscopy; indeed, the presence of irregular, invasive nests at the periphery of such masses is sufficient grounds for a diagnosis of low-grade hidradenocarcinoma. Conservative but complete excision is prudent in those instances where small biopsy specimens do not allow for complete examination of the perimeter of the lesion. The diagnostic terminology attending such tumors will no doubt continue to evolve over time.[196,197]

Papillary eccrine adenoma (also known as tubulopapillary hidradenoma) occurs most commonly in African-American females on the lower extremities; some examples may, in fact, demonstrate apocrine rather than eccrine differentiation. Duct-like structures of

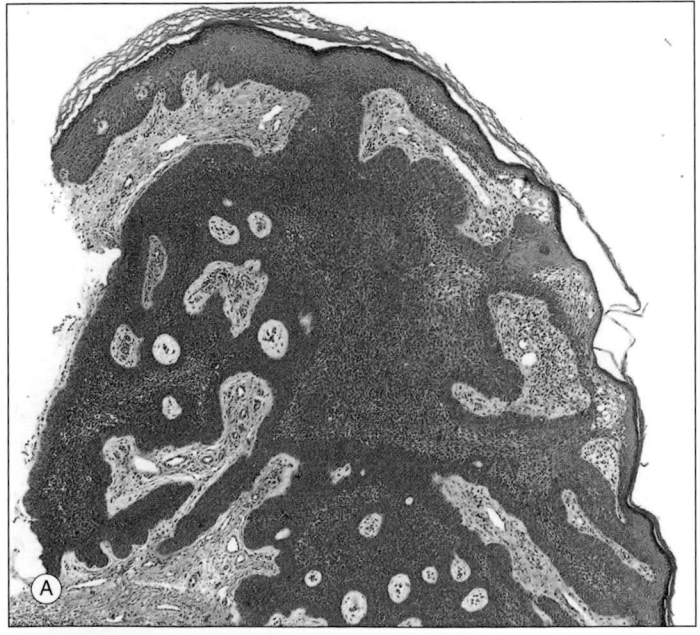

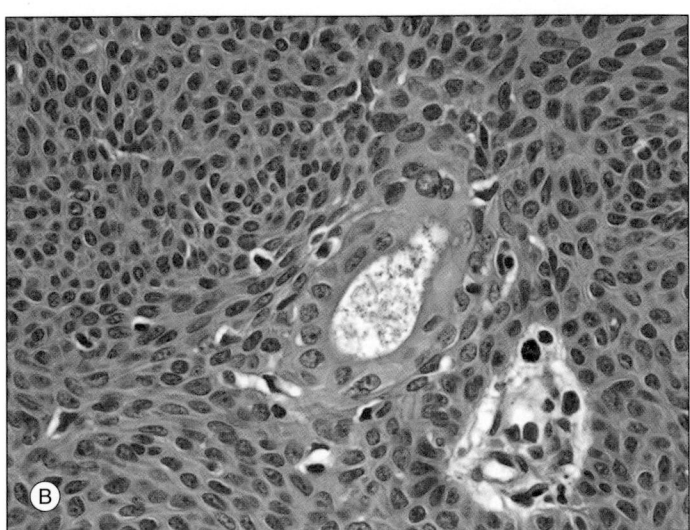

Fig. 8.34 Poroma. **A**, Basaloid cells descend from a multifocal epidermal attachment among which eccrine differentiation is evident (**B**).

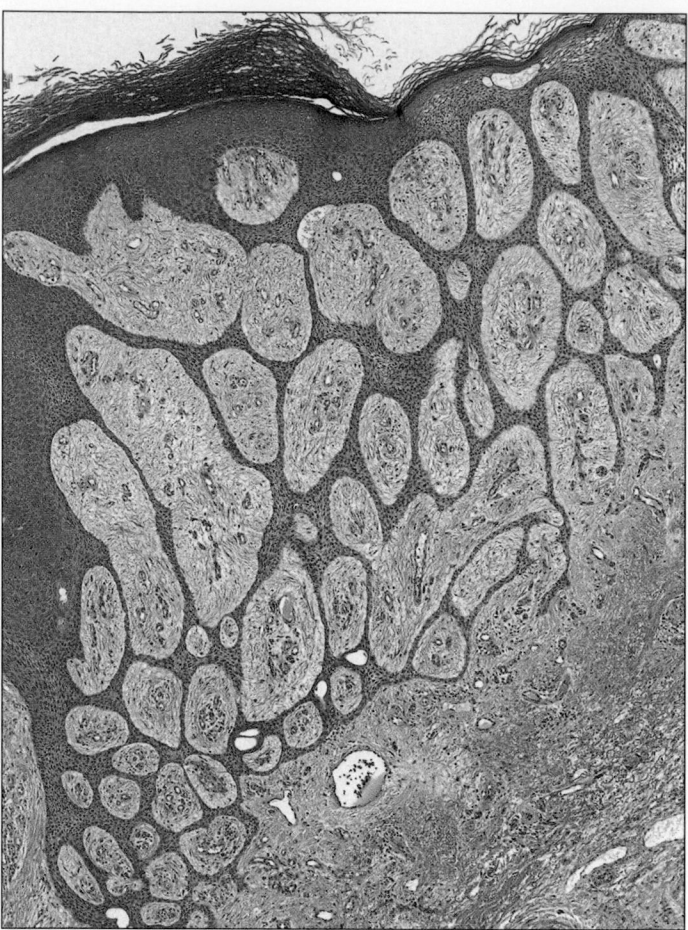

Fig. 8.35 Syringofibroadenoma differs from the related poroma by more delicate epithelial strands separated by a hypercellular, myxoid stroma, but eccrine ducts remain evident.

variable size are seen in this lesion, and they contain distinctive luminal micropapillary fronds comprising cuboidal epithelium that is two or more cell layers in thickness (Fig. 8.37).[198,199] Squamous and clear cell metaplasia is potentially seen. The configuration of this lesion is analogous to that of florid 'simple' intraductal hyperplasia in the breast. That is an important concept, because the poor circumscription of papillary eccrine adenoma and the presence of focal luminal 'pseudonecrotic' secretion may give a false impression of malignancy. Misdiagnosis of digital papillary adenocarcinoma, as described subsequently, can be avoided by attention to the lack of *macro*cysts in papillary eccrine adenoma. It is likely that a morphological continuum exists between the latter lesion and 'tubular apocrine adenoma' or 'apocrine tubulopapillary hidradenoma'; hence, eccrine-'specific' immunohistological reagents[200] have failed to label papillary 'eccrine' adenomas consistently.

Cutaneous mixed tumor (CMT; 'chondroid syringoma') is analogous in most respects to pleomorphic adenoma of the salivary glands. It usually manifests in the skin as a firm tan nodule in the scalp or on the face, in adult patients. Sometimes, the lesion may be deeply situated in the subcutis and can simulate a soft tissue tumor clinically. Microscopically, CMT shows an admixture of bland cuboidal epithelium, arranged in cords, tubules, nests, or sheets, with variably myxochondroid stroma (Fig. 8.38).[201] The lesion may demonstrate micronodular 'budding' at its periphery, and this

feature can account for local recurrence of CMT if excision is incomplete. A peculiarity of *cutaneous* mixed tumor is its capacity to demonstrate divergent and mixed differentiation. The epithelial component of this lesion may include eccrine, apocrine, squamous, sebaceous, and follicular elements, and its mesenchymal-like component can exhibit differentiation into smooth muscle, cartilage, fat, and bone.[202,203] Moreover, 'hyaline' plasmacytoid epithelial cells or myoepithelial spindle cells may dominate the histologic image. The evolution of a true carcinoma originating by clonal transformation of CMT ('carcinoma *ex* mixed tumor') is vanishingly rare in the skin.[204]

Syringocystadenoma papilliferum (SCP) is a singular neoplasm that most often arises in the skin of the scalp or the face; it may also complicate nevus sebaceus, as mentioned earlier in this discussion. It may be seen in patients of all ages as a friable reddish nodular lesion measuring up to several centimeters in diameter. SCP is typified microscopically by the presence of a micropapillary proliferation that is sharply demarcated from the surrounding epidermis and sits in a 'dell' in the superficial corium (Fig. 8.39A).[205] One to two layers of cuboidal epithelium that often demonstrate decapitation-type secretion mantle the individual papillary structures; tumoral epithelium at the lesional surface also commonly exhibits squamous metaplasia. The connective tissue cores of the micropapillae usually contain chronic inflammatory cells, particularly plasmacytes (Fig. 8.39B).[206] The morphologic profile of this tumor is distinctive enough to preclude meaningful differential diagnosis.

Hidradenoma papilliferum (HP) is an apocrine tumor that is restricted to the eyelids, axillae, and genitoperineal skin in adult patients. It takes the form of a nodular bluish-red dermal lesion, usually <3 cm in diameter. Microscopically, HP shows a circumscribed proliferation of large papillae that fill a cystic space in the dermis (Fig. 8.40).[205] The papillae arborize and interconnect, and are mantled by cuboidal to low columnar epithelial cells with obvious luminal decapitation 'snouts.' Smaller tubules may also be seen at the lesional periphery. Differential diagnosis is largely regionally determined; the most problematic alternatives include Bartholin gland tumors in the vulva, metastatic well-differentiated breast carcinoma in the axilla, and low-grade adenocarcinoma of the rectum in reference to HPs that arise at the anal verge. The characteristic morphologic features of HP should be sufficient to distinguish it from those other possibilities.

Malignant pilosebaceous neoplasms

Sebaceous carcinomas (SCs) most commonly arise in the skin of the eyelids. Clinically, these tumors may simulate inflammatory conditions such as chalazion. Extraocular SCs may arise in most any skin field, but they have a predilection for the head and neck.[207] Microscopically, SC shows a wide range of differentiation, from lesions that comprise obviously multivacuolated epithelial cells to poorly differentiated basaloid or squamoid populations with more occult cytoplasmic lipid content. The tumor cells are most commonly arranged in rounded nests in the dermis, but infiltrative cords may be observed in high-grade examples.[137,208] Approximately 50% of cases also manifest pagetoid involvement of the overlying epidermis.[209] Foci of in situ sebaceous carcinoma within the confines of neighboring pilosebaceous units may be seen surrounding invasive SCs. The nuclear features of SCs are similar to those of squamous cell carcinomas, and mitotic activity is usually easily found. However, the cytoplasm of SC is more amphophilic or basaloid in comparison to that of squamous tumors. Overt sebaceous differentiation, represented by complex, multivacuolated or 'bubbly' cytoplasm, is often best seen in the central portions of tumor cell lobules (Fig. 8.41). This is the single most useful feature in separating SC diagnostically from other

Fig. 8.36 Hidradenoma. **A**, This example has solid tumor growth within a larger cyst and contains areas of clear cell change (**B**) as well as squamous-like whorls (**C**).

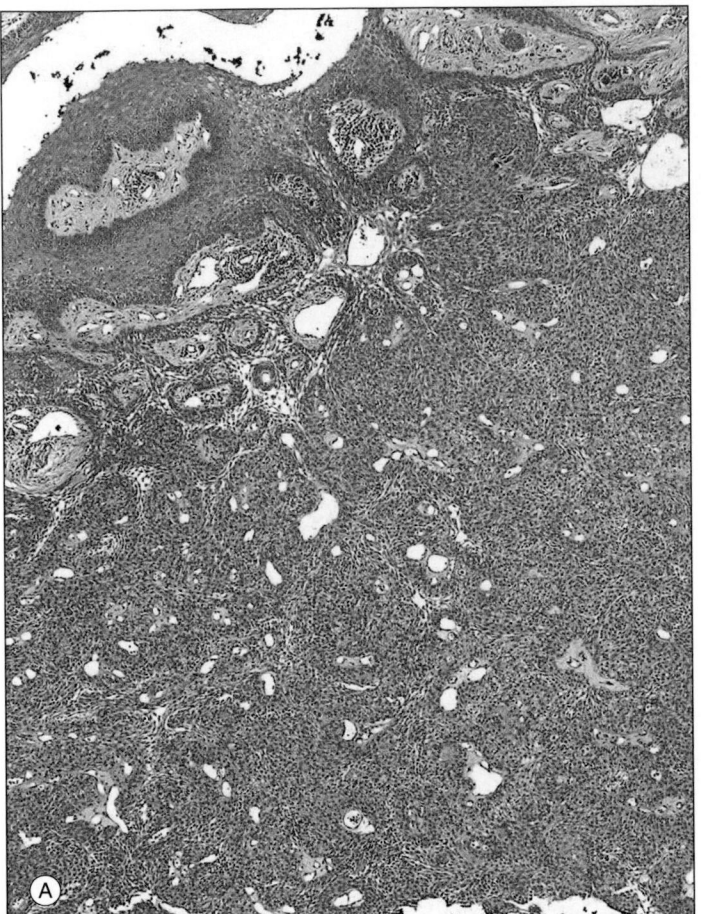

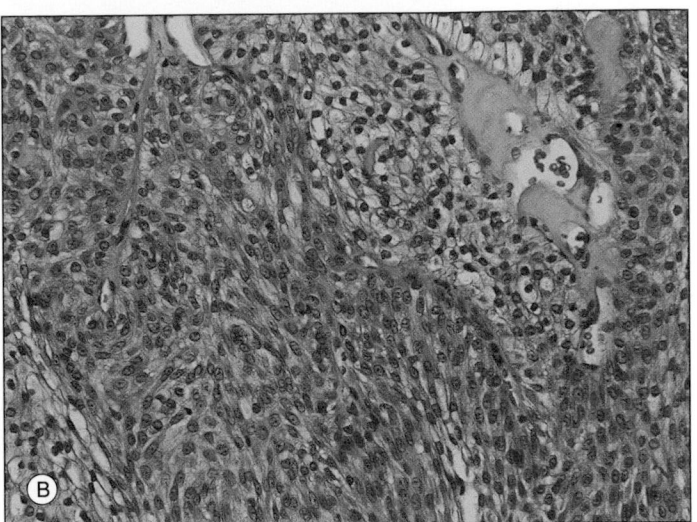

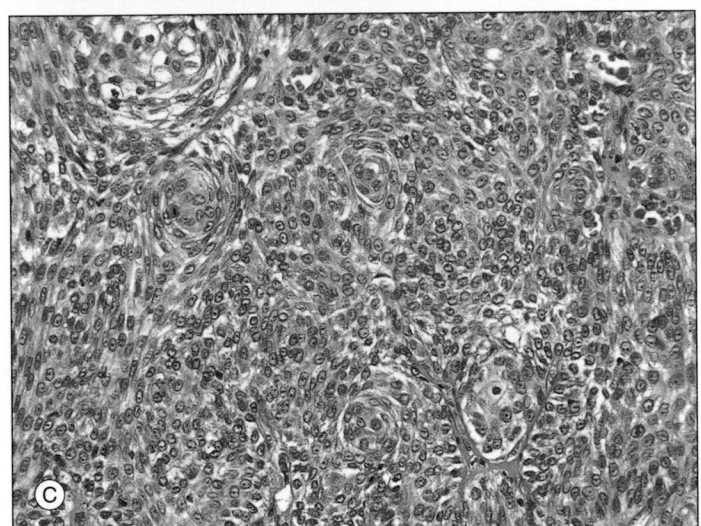

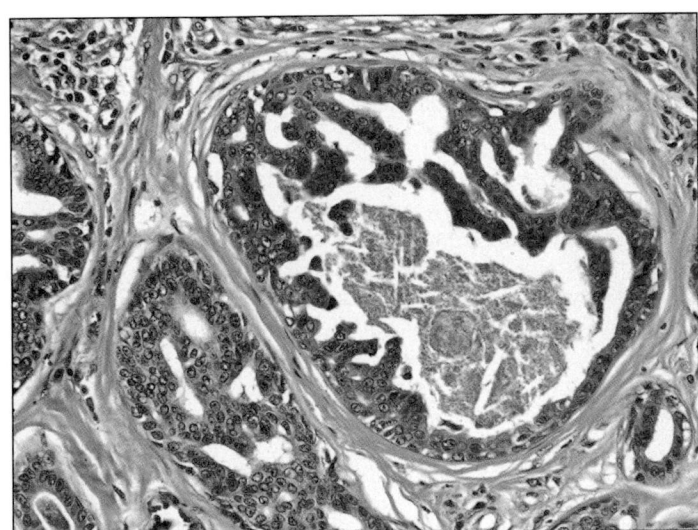

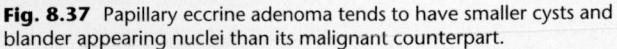

Fig. 8.37 Papillary eccrine adenoma tends to have smaller cysts and blander appearing nuclei than its malignant counterpart.

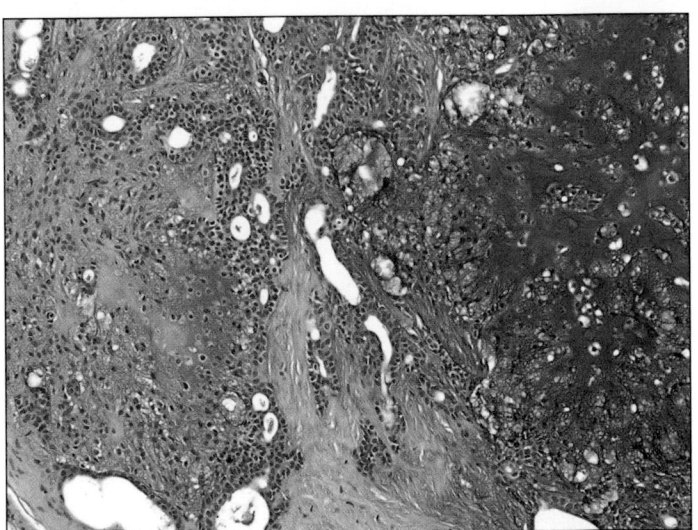

Fig. 8.38 Mixed tumor of the skin, like its analogue in the salivary gland, has a wide range of appearances in which the mesenchymal component may be sparse or compose the bulk of the tumor.

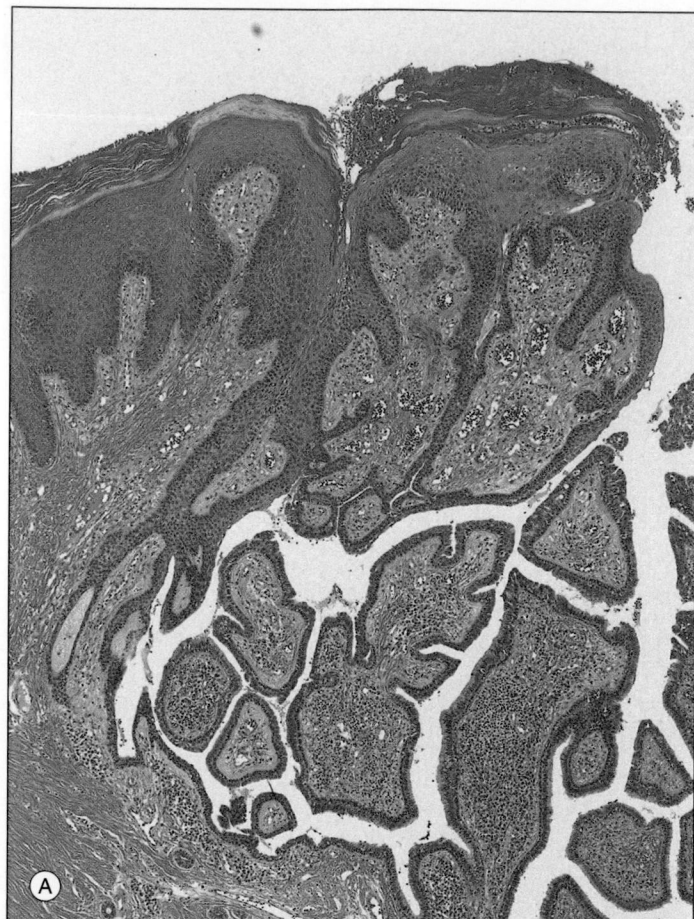

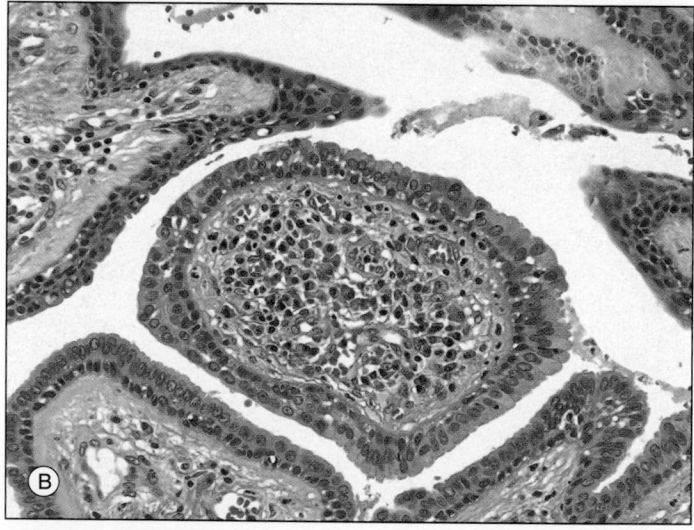

Fig. 8.39 Syringocystadenoma papilliferum often has (**A**) epidermal attachment and (**B**) numerous plasma cells. The double layer of epithelium is almost always present, but is not unique to this tumor type.

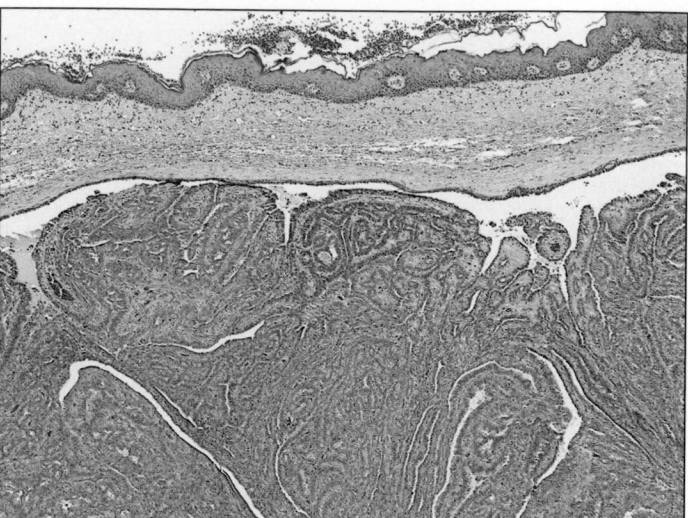

Fig. 8.40 Hidradenoma papilliferum with a large cystic space and numerous papillae lined by cuboidal epithelium with underlying myoepithelial cells.

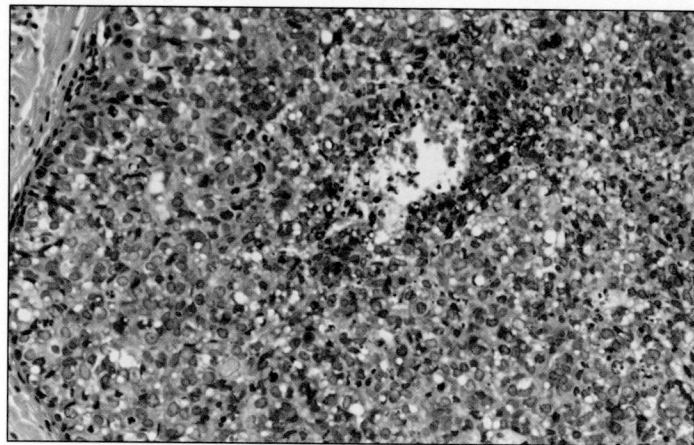

Fig. 8.41 Sebaceous carcinoma. Multivacuolated cells are indicative of sebaceous differentiation. There is a central area of necrosis.

Those two patterns may be misinterpreted as markers of adenocarcinoma or squamous carcinoma, respectively. Immunohistochemical studies demonstrate that the tumor cells of SC are reactive for androgen receptor protein. No labeling is seen with antibodies to carcinoembryonic antigen (CEA), S-100 protein, or gross cystic disease fluid protein-15 (GCDFP-15).[210]

The list of differential diagnostic possibilities for SC includes basal cell carcinoma with sebaceous differentiation, malignant clear cell acrospiroma, hydropic squamous cell carcinoma, trichilemmal carcinoma, 'balloon cell' melanoma, and metastatic visceral clear cell carcinoma, particularly from the kidneys. Application of selected immunostains and attention to histologic nuances usually allows for separation of those lesions from one another.

Trichilemmal carcinoma (TLC) was first described by Headington,[142] but, until recently, that entity received little attention. Microscopically, TLC is characterized by a lobular proliferation of atypical polyhedral cells with clear cytoplasm that partially or

clear cell neoplasms of the skin. Cytoplasmic lipid vacuoles may be highlighted with fat stains on frozen sections of SC, or by immunostaining for epithelial membrane antigen (EMA). Relatively frequently, SC demonstrates comedo-like central necrosis within tumor cell islands; keratin 'pearl' formation also may be observed.

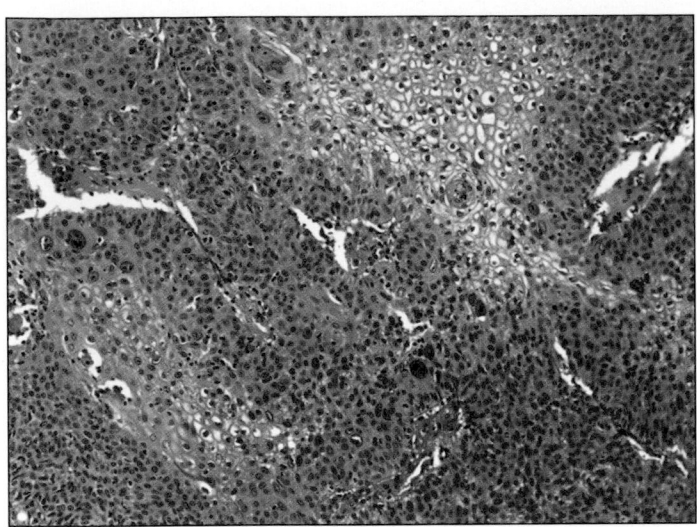

Fig. 8.42 Trichilemmal carcinoma displays clear cells, abrupt pilar type keratinization, and marked nuclear atypia.

completely replaces pilosebaceous units (Fig. 8.42). There is also frequent involvement of the interfollicular epidermis with a 'skipping' pattern. The tumor cells show marked nuclear atypia and mitotic figures are easily appreciated. This lesion commonly displays nuclear palisading at the periphery of tumor lobules and multifocal 'abrupt' pilar-type keratinization.[211,212] Superficial ulceration of these lesions may be noted. Although TLCs may be completely intraepithelial, many show infiltrative 'pushing' growth into the dermis. Clinically, the tumors may display locally aggressive growth but are generally considered to be indolent, approximating the behavior of low-grade cutaneous squamous carcinomas. One series of TLCs with long-term follow-up showed no recurrences or examples of metastasis.[213]

Pilomatrix carcinoma (PMC) is a rare tumor with a predilection for the head and neck. Although it retains a biphasic microscopic appearance, as seen in ordinary pilomatrixoma (with sheets of viable epithelial cells and shadow cells), PMC exhibits overtly malignant cytologic attributes that include atypical mitotic figures, enlarged vesicular nuclei with prominent nucleoli, and infiltrative borders.[214] Indeed, aside from its areas of ghost-cell keratinization, PMC assumes the histological image of a lymphoepithelioma-like carcinoma. The behavior of this tumor is generally limited to local aggressiveness, but distant metastases have been reported in some cases.[215]

Malignant proliferating pilar cyst/tumor may be separated from ordinary proliferating pilar tumor by its uniformly high-grade cytological appearance and, more importantly, the presence of irregular tongues of tumor cells that invade the dermis and subcutis.[216] There is usually a portion of the tumor that can be recognized as an underlying benign proliferating pilar tumor. Surgical excision with clear margins is the standard treatment for this tumor. However, both recurrences and metastasis have been reported in the literature.[217,218]

Malignant sweat gland tumors

A very diverse group of diagnostic terms has been used in the past in reference to malignant sweat gland tumors.[219] This problem relates in part to the infrequency with which such lesions are encountered; they account for approximately 0.005% of all cutaneous neoplasms. Also, occasional divergent differentiation may be seen micro-

scopically, causing further nomenclatural difficulty.[220,221] The most common form of sweat gland carcinoma in our experience is the *low-grade eccrine hidradenocarcinoma* or *malignant acrospiroma*. It shows a predilection for the face and the extremities.[222] Aggressive local behavior may be observed, with several recurrences, but metastases are not expected when the cytologic features of the lesion approximate those of ordinary acrospiroma (see above).[222,223] A lack of circumscription with irregular tongues of peripheral invasive tumor is the key to diagnosis of this entity. Similar tumors with prominent intraepidermal involvement (showing discrete 'lakes' of tumor cells in the epidermis), more basaloid cytologic features, and internal ductal structures have been regarded as representative of *porocarcinoma*;[224] however, that lesion also may demonstrate obvious nuclear anaplasia, squamoid or clear cell foci, and pathologically shaped mitotic figures. In a recent series, porocarcinomas were associated with lymph node metastasis in 15–20% of cases.[225]

Microcystic adnexal carcinoma (MAC) is a tumor with essentially no metastatic potential; it usually occurs on the face in middle-aged or elderly persons.[226–228] Despite the banal cytologic attributes of MAC, it exhibits perineural and perivascular extension along with deep infiltration of the subcutis, muscle, and even bone, and may cause death because of recalcitrant local growth into the mouth, nose, and orbits. Small angulated or tubular glands, concentric cellular arrays, and single tumor cells are widely scattered throughout the affected tissue in MAC (Fig. 8.43A), distinguishing it from syringoma, with which it may be confused in superficial ('shave') biopsies. Microcysts in MAC often contain pilar-type keratin (Fig. 8.43B). When they are inconspicuous, however, the alternative term of *sclerosing sweat duct carcinoma*[229] has been applied. Eccrine, apocrine, pilar, and sebaceous differentiation have all been observed in MAC, sometimes in the same tumor mass.

Ductal eccrine adenocarcinoma (DEA) is a sweat glandular malignancy that essentially perfectly imitates the microscopic appearance of metastatic ductal breast cancer in the skin. In distinct contrast to the latter condition, however, DEA is typically a solitary lesion that evolves over a period of >6 months.[219,230] It affects the head and neck and extremities preferentially, and although DEA has been observed in patients of all ages, it strongly favors adults. The lesion usually takes the form of a nondescript tan-pink nodule that may become ulcerated with time. Histologically, DEA shows randomly disposed, invasive cords and nests of large epithelioid cells in the dermis, sometimes with vascular and perineural infiltration. Ductal luminal differentiation may be apparent, and nuclear atypicality is typically obvious. Squamoid foci, spindle cell change, or a small cell constituency – imitating the appearance of Merkel cell carcinoma – are potential variations in the histopathologic image of DEA. Differential diagnosis with breast carcinoma is, as preceding comments suggest, best resolved by attention to clinical details. That is true because there is nothing in the microscopic profile, ultrastructural features, or immunophenotype of DEA (including analyses for expression of estrogen and progesterone receptor proteins) that differs consistently from the features of metastatic mammary tumors.

Mucinous eccrine adenocarcinoma (MEA) has also been termed 'colloid' carcinoma of the skin, in analogy to lesions that are seen more often in the breast and gastrointestinal tract.[231] This neoplasm also favors the skin of the head and neck in adults, as a nondescript but slightly fluctuant solitary tan nodule that evolves over months or years. Histologically, MEA shows clusters and cords of relatively bland epithelioid cells – with compact oval nuclei and eosinophilic or amphophilic cytoplasm – that are suspended in pools of extracellular mucin. The latter labels with the mucicarmine method

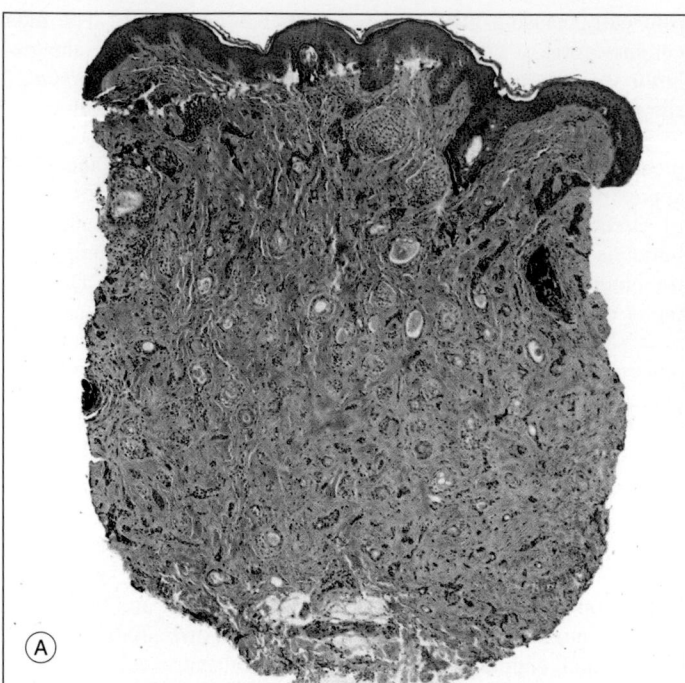

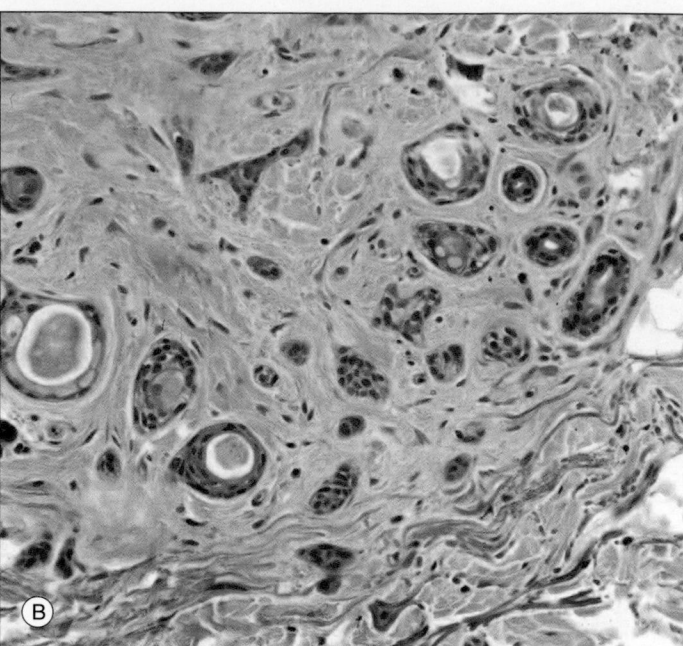

Fig. 8.43 Microcystic adnexal carcinoma. **A,** Deep, poorly circumscribed penetration with subcuticular extension is common as is cystic pilar epithelium with luminal keratin (**B**).

or the digested periodic acid–Schiff technique. Peripheral borders of MEA are vaguely infiltrative, and involvement of vascular adventitia or nerve sheaths may be appreciated. Differential diagnosis centers on metastasis to the skin from mucinous carcinomas of the viscera. Because the latter event does not occur except in the context of disseminated disease, MEA can, for practical purposes, be recognized confidently as a primary cutaneous lesion because of its distinctive microscopic image.

Clear cell eccrine adenocarcinoma (CCEA) is probably closely related conceptually to low-grade malignant acrospiroma/eccrine hidradenocarcinoma, but it demonstrates a greater degree of nuclear and architectural atypia. This tumor is potentially seen in any skin field, but favors sun-exposed areas. CCEA is observed much more often in adults than in children. It shows nests and cords of relatively large polyhedral cells in the corium, with clear cytoplasm, invasive borders, and a delicate fibrovascular stroma. Nuclei are more anaplastic than those of low-grade hidradenocarcinoma, with the consistent presence of nucleoli. Foci of spontaneous tumor necrosis, vascular invasion, and perineural infiltration also may be present. Differential diagnosis is comparable to that associated with trichilemmal carcinoma, as discussed above. In particular, a distinction must be made between CCEA and metastatic renal cell carcinoma in the skin. Again, the former of those tumors is solitary and slowly growing, in contrast to the latter. Moreover, renal cell carcinoma often contains microscopic 'blood lakes,' or hemorrhage into tumor cell tubules, whereas that feature is not seen in CCEA.

The original description of digital papillary sweat gland tumors[232,233] was made by Kao et al. in 1987, suggesting that they could be divided into benign and malignant variants. A recent series and review, however, have indicated that all of these neoplasms should be considered as malignant ab initio (*digital papillary eccrine adenocarcinoma* [DPEA]), because of their frequent recurrence and metastases in 14% of cases.[234,235] Limitation to the fingers, toes, and

adjacent acral sites is the norm for such lesions. Histologically, one sees dermal cysts of varying sizes – but consistently larger than those of papillary eccrine adenoma – which are lined by one or several layers of atypical cuboidal cells (Fig. 8.44). A distinctive feature of DPEA is the formation of macropapillae, many of which project into the cystic lumina. Cribriform architecture and spindle cell or clear cell foci also may be observed in some cases. Necrotic debris may be present within the cysts. DPEA may infiltrate deeply into underlying soft tissue and even into bone, and digital amputation is warranted in some cases to gain local control of the tumor.[232,236]

Adenoid cystic carcinoma of the skin (ACCS) has morphologic features which are identical to those of its salivary glandular and mammary counterparts, and they allow for recognition of this rare cutaneous tumor.[237] In keeping with the theme of sweat gland carcinomas in general, ACCS is a single and slowly developing lesion that has typically been present for several years. Perineural and vascular invasion are relatively frequent. Immunostaining for carcinoembryonic antigen, epithelial membrane antigen, and S-100 protein in ACCS allow for its distinction from adenoid basal cell carcinoma, which may be quite similar microscopically.

Although the clinical appearance of *extramammary Paget's disease* (EPD) – with an erythematous or eczematous plaque – is similar to that of Paget's disease of the breast, EPD differs in lacking an underlying carcinoma in most instances. Outside of the perianal skin field, <1% of such lesions are associated with invasive tumors. In the perineum and surrounding the anus, this figure increases to 80% of EPD cases, which are linked to the concurrent presence of uterine cervical, anorectal, Bartholin gland, or urinary bladder tumors.[238] EPD is conceptualized as an adnexal tumor that arises within the skin surface, from primitive stem cells that undergo glandular differentiation.[239,240] Tumor cells are scattered haphazardly throughout the epidermis; they are large with pleomorphic nuclei, which, along with cytoplasmic clearing, glandular lumen formation,

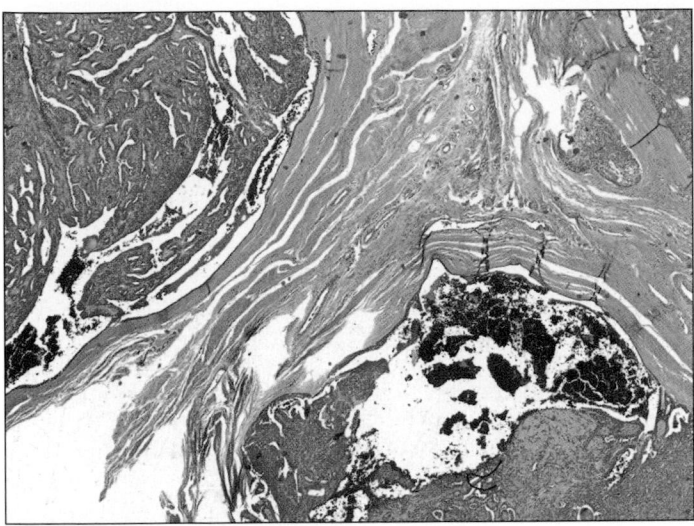

Fig. 8.44 Cellular atypia and mitoses are common, but not invariable in digital papillary adenocarcinoma. More reliable for diagnosis are large, variably sized cysts with papillary fronds.

immunoreactivity for cytokeratin 20 have been reported to show a particular linkage to regional visceral malignancies, particularly in the large intestine and anus.[76] S-100 protein is consistently absent.

Malignant cylindroma and *malignant spiradenoma* are both unique among sweat gland carcinomas because they arise from benign 'parent' tumors through clonal evolution.[219] By definition, one therefore observes obvious and usually high-grade carcinoma in juxtaposition to ordinary cylindroma or spiradenoma. Paradoxically, although such tumors are typically anaplastic histologically, their risk of distant metastasis appears to be very limited.

Other sweat gland carcinomas

Other very rare sudoriferous malignancies include various forms of apocrine adenocarcinoma,[243,244] 'malignant mixed tumor' (cutaneous 'carcinosarcoma'),[219] and 'polymorphous sweat gland carcinoma.'[245] A discussion of the details of those lesions is left to the contents of more specialized reference sources.

and vacuolization, help to distinguish them from the surrounding keratinocytes (Fig. 8.45A). Epidermal squamous hyperplasia may be present in reaction to EPD. In sharp contrast to pagetoid squamous cell carcinoma in situ (Fig. 8.45B) and pagetoid in situ malignant melanoma, which represent its principal differential diagnostic alternatives, EPD exhibits the presence of cytoplasmic mucin in the majority of cases with histochemical methods such as the Alcian blue technique at pH 2.5 and Hale's colloidal iron stain.[241,242] Immunohistochemical study is also helpful, because the tumor cells of EPD are potentially positive for cytokeratin 7, GCDFP-15, and carcinoembryonic antigen, whereas melanoma lacks all three of those markers. Those cases of perineal/perianal EPD that manifest

SELECTED MESENCHYMAL TUMORS AND PSEUDOTUMORS OF THE SKIN

Cutaneous mesenchymal neoplasms are a broad group, with several constituents that also occur in deeper soft tissue. Accordingly, only those lesions that preferentially affect the skin will be considered in the following sections. Readers are referred to the excellent chapter by Montgomery in this textbook for a broader discussion of soft tissue lesions.

Fibrohistiocytic and fibroblastic proliferations

Whereas the line of differentiation for many mesenchymal skin tumors is frequently discernible through morphologic study alone or the use of ancillary studies, the 'fibrohistiocytic' category of lesions remains enigmatic in that regard. They probably differentiate simultaneously towards several cell types that include fibroblasts, myofibroblasts, 'dermal dendrocytes,' and, perhaps, fixed phagocytic

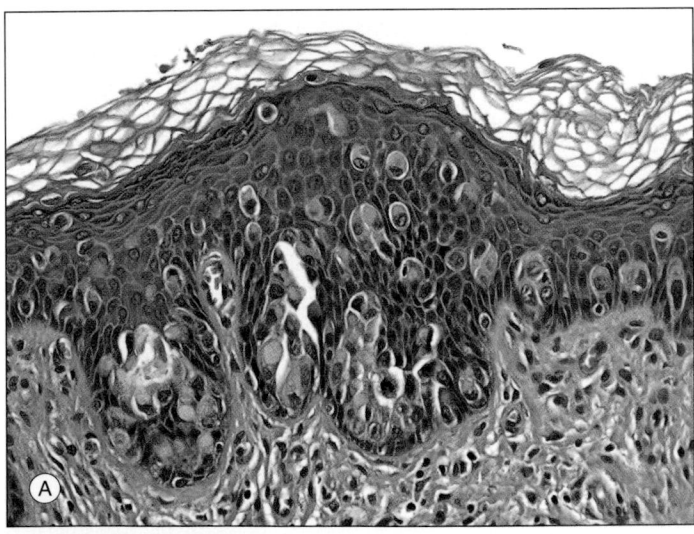

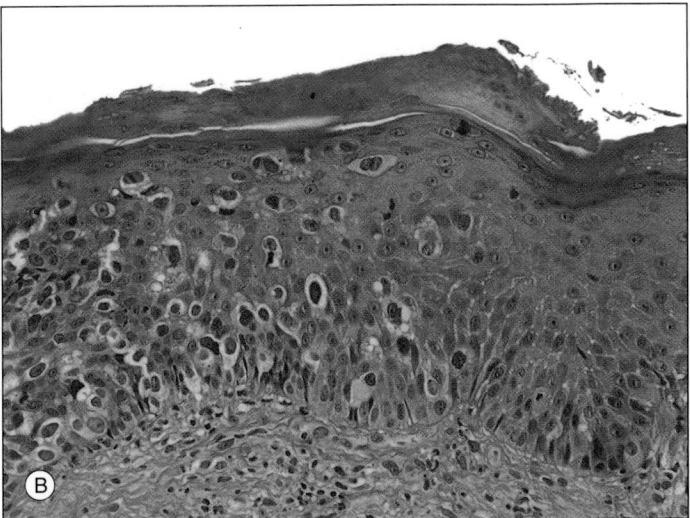

Fig. 8.45 A, Extramammary Paget's disease, a tumor of glandular epithelial differentiation, can be indistinguishable from (**B**) pagetoid squamous cell carcinoma or melanoma without ancillary studies.

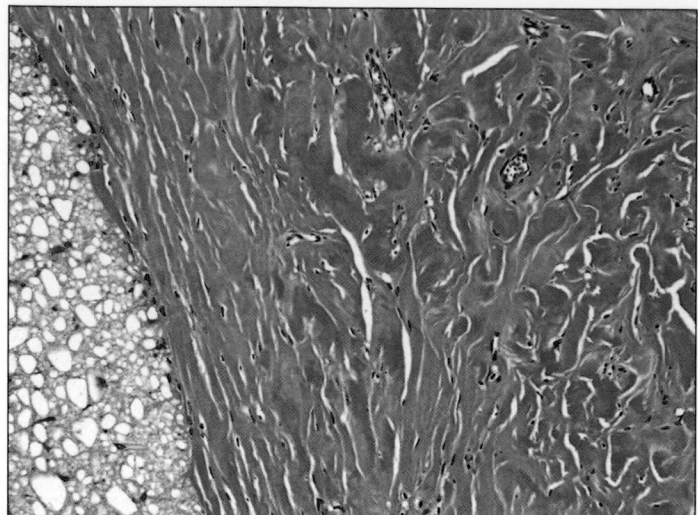

Fig. 8.46 Dense, hyalinized bands of collagen typify this keloid in which there is evidence of prior corticosteroid injection (left).

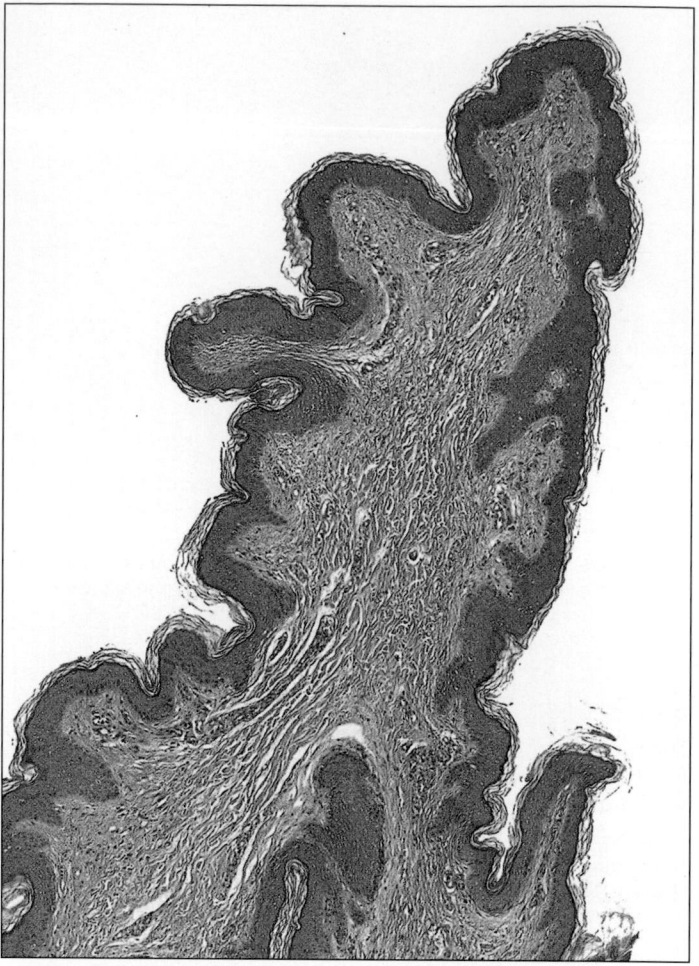

Fig. 8.47 The fibroepithelial polyp's core varies in stromal cellularity and vascular density. Torsion and trauma often result in epidermal ulceration and even polyp infarction.

cells. Myofibroblasts are recognizable through their expression of muscle specific actin and the ultrastructural presence of subplasmalemmal dense plaques. Dermal dendrocytes can be immunolabeled for factor XIIIa and CD34.[246,247] Among all proliferations of the skin that are felt to show 'fibrohistiocytic' features, only those that are encountered with any frequency in general surgical pathology practice will be considered here.

Hypertrophic scar and *keloid* are part of the same pathologic spectrum of wound repair, and they represent a clinical and histological continuum.[248–250] Both may extend outside the boundaries of the initial injury, and they also may recur after surgical excision. Classical keloids are manifest as broad bands of brightly eosinophilic hypocellular hyalinized dermal collagen (Fig. 8.46). Hypertrophic scars show a greater degree of fibroblastic proliferation, sometimes with deposition of matrical mucopolysaccharide as well, but such foci shade into keloidal areas in many cases. The proliferation is arranged parallel to the skin surface, with perpendicularly oriented capillaries. S-100 protein-containing dendritic cells may be present in hypertrophic scars and one should be wary of misusing that fact to render a diagnosis of desmoplastic melanoma.

Simple *fibroepithelial polyps of the skin* (FPS) are linked to a plethora of alternative terms, including cutaneous papilloma, soft fibroma, skin tag, and the etymologically problematic term 'acrochordon' (because the lesion in question is seldom seen on the extremities and only vaguely string-like). They need not be excised except when irritated or located in cosmetically sensitive areas of the skin.[251] The incidence of FPS increases with age, and they are often seen in the skin of the head and neck, axillae, and inframammary regions as papules, polyps, or sac-like excrescences.[252] Microscopically, a central core of loose fibrous tissue is seen along with variable numbers of small vessels (Fig. 8.47). Adipose tissue may also constitute a major portion of the tissue in some cases (so-called 'fibrolipomas').

Nevus lipomatosus represents a connective tissue nevus that takes the form of a yellowish cutaneous plaque, usually in the skin over the pelvic girdle or buttocks; it is detected in the first two decades of life. Mature lobules of adipose tissue are seen in the dermis in this lesion, and they may or may not have a subcutaneous attachment.

Other attendant mesenchymal abnormalities include thickening of collagen bundles, quantitative variation in elastic tissue content, and an increase in the number of small dermal blood vessels.[253] The 'solitary' form of nevus lipomatosus, which is a papule or nodule in adults and located anywhere on the body, is considered by many to be an adipose tissue-rich variant of fibroepithelial polyp.[253,254]

Fibrous papule is an exceedingly common lesion, usually seen on or near the nose but potentially anywhere on the face. It is best categorized as an *angiofibroma* and is clearly not a form of melanocytic nevus as originally proposed.[255–257] Syndromic facial or periungual cutaneous angiofibromas are part of tuberous sclerosis (Bourneville's disease) and the former have been incorrectly called 'adenoma sebaceum.' Associated findings in such cases include connective tissue nevi ('shagreen patches') and hypopigmented macules ('ashleaf spots').[258] Multiple endocrine neoplasia is another syndrome in which multiple angiofibromas are present. The '*pearly penile papule*' is also an angiofibroma, presenting in multiple form as ring-like papules of the penile corona or sulcus.[259] Histologically, all of these lesions show similar features, including papillary dermal fibroblastic hyperplasia, and the presence of stellate mesenchymal cells that are immunoreactive for factor XIIIa (Fig. 8.48).[260–262] Degenerative-type nuclear atypia is potentially seen in the latter cell

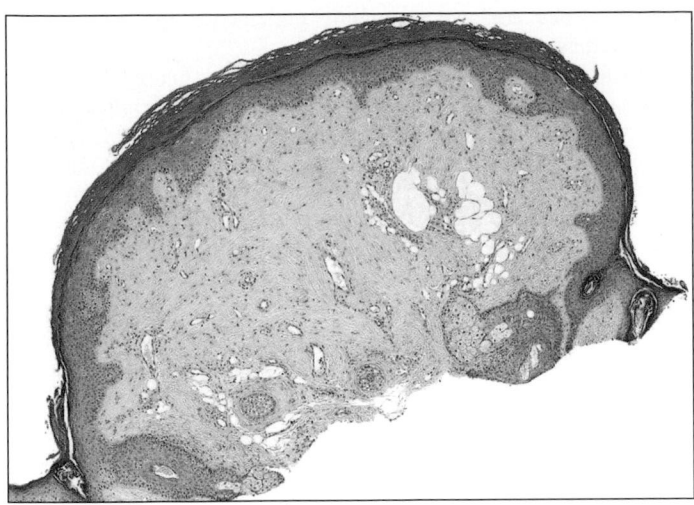

Fig. 8.48 The typical dome shape of a fibrous papule is unusually this evident, but dermal changes of stellate fibroblasts and vessel dilatation confirm its identity as an angiofibroma.

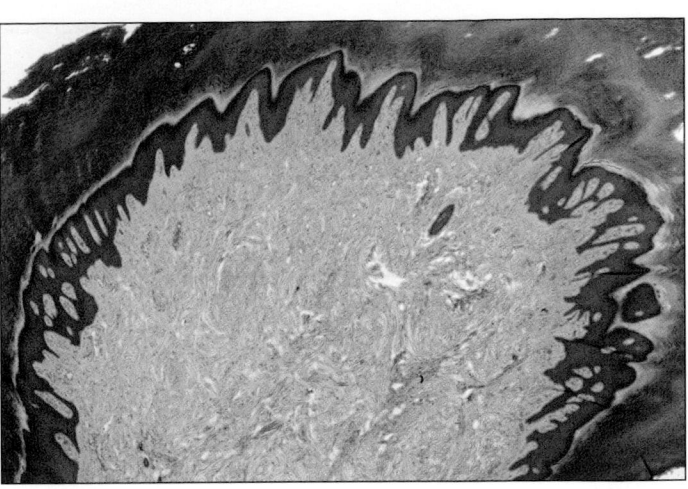

Fig. 8.49 Acral fibrokeratoma shares dermal changes with fibrous papule but differs in its more conical shape and acral-type epidermis.

type but has no clinical significance. Dilatation of small stromal vessels accompanies the spindle cell proliferation. *Acral fibrokeratoma* (Fig. 8.49), a tumor of the digits, also likely represents a form of angiofibroma.[263,264]

The relatively recently described lesion known as *pleomorphic fibroma*[265] is notable because of potentially striking atypia in its spindle cell population. The nosologic placement of that lesion is problematic; indeed, it is possible that several different tumor types may assume the image of pleomorphic fibroma as a degenerative phenomenon. These include FPS, paucivascular angiofibroma, and sclerotic dermatofibroma. No mitotic activity or necrosis is typically observed in pleomorphic fibromas, and they are sharply circumscribed. In the past, those lesions were confused with atypical fibroxanthomas (see below), which demonstrate a much higher level of cellularity with foam cell elements and atypical mitoses.

Despite its involutional appearance, *sclerotic fibroma* is a proliferative neoplasm[266] comprising storiform arrays of eosinophilic and clefted collagen bundles. Cellularity is very low with an absence of nuclear atypia.[267] An association with Cowden's disease (multiple trichilemmomas together with visceral malignancies) exists.

Dermatofibroma (DF) likely represents the most common mesenchymal tumor of the skin. The synonymous term *'fibrous histiocytoma'* is sometimes used for this lesion as well. DF is usually <1 cm in diameter and it presents on the extremities in postpubertal, often middle-aged patients. Dimpling of the skin on compression between the fingertips – the so-called 'dimple sign' – is associated with this tumor but may be seen with any lesion having deep dermal or subcutaneous attachments.[268,269] Although most DFs are easily identified by their violaceous to gray-black color and sharp circumscription, they may mimic the appearance of other tumors including malignant melanoma as well as pigmented BCC or squamous cell carcinoma. Recurrence of DF is very uncommon, even after incomplete excision. As is typical of many fibrohistiocytic tumors, DF shows a spindle cell proliferation with occasional storiform areas, usually in the superficial to mid-reticular dermis (Fig. 8.50A). There may be an admixture of vacuolated histiocytes and multinucleated or floret-type giant cells.[269,270] The tumor cells commonly splay and fragment individual collagen fibers at the periphery of the lesion, yielding rounded profiles of stromal material (Fig. 8.50B). Associated epidermal changes include acanthosis, elongation of the rete ridges, and, occasionally, a peculiar basal-cell-rich form of pseudoepitheliomatous hyperplasia that closely simulates the image of superficial BCC (Fig. 8.50C). Extension of 'deep penetrating' DFs into the subcutaneous fat occurs along pre-existing fibrous septa. This feature contrasts with broad growth into the fat and entrapment of individual adipocytes, as seen in an important differential diagnostic consideration, *dermatofibrosarcoma protuberans*. Mitotic activity in DF is variable and does not correlate with behavior. Several morphologic variants of this tumor have been described, only a few of which have any clinical importance. *Cellular and deep penetrating* DFs do appear to be more prone to recur, possibly because of larger size and involvement of the subcutis.[271] The *aneurysmal* variant of DF may be associated with systemic symptoms such as fever and may attain a size of >10 cm. Within a dense spindle cell background in that variant, one sees blood-filled cavernous spaces that are devoid of an endothelial lining.[272,273] *Atypical DF*, an entity that is arguably synonymous with *'benign recurring fibrous histiocytoma,'* has been described as a fibrohistiocytic tumor that shows focal nuclear pleomorphism and hyperchromasia, as well as micronodularity, a deeper location, and a larger size than that of banal DF. Kaddu et al. and others have demonstrated that 'atypical' DF has a tendency for recurrence.[274,275] Other DF patterns with little clinical significance include *lichenoid, myoid, palisading, clear cell, granular cell,* and *lymphocyte-rich* lesions.[276,277] The presence of factor XIIIa in these tumors is relatively non-specific. However, that finding is helpful in conjunction with CD34 negativity in distinguishing DF from dermatofibrosarcoma protuberans. It should be noted, however, that DF may indeed demonstrate CD34 positivity at its advancing edge.[278,279]

Dermatomyofibroma is felt to be distinct from DF, because it occurs as a plaque located predominantly over the shoulder girdle in young adults.[280,281] This lesion is much broader than DF, and demonstrates obvious myofibroblastic or myogenous differentiation in addition to areas that do resemble those of DF histologically. In contrast to cutaneous leiomyomas, dermatomyofibromas show only weak reactivity for alpha-isoform actin and tend to be desmin

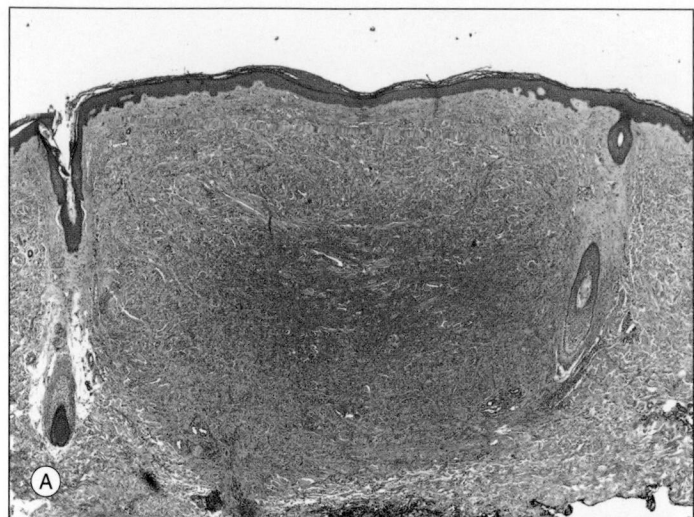

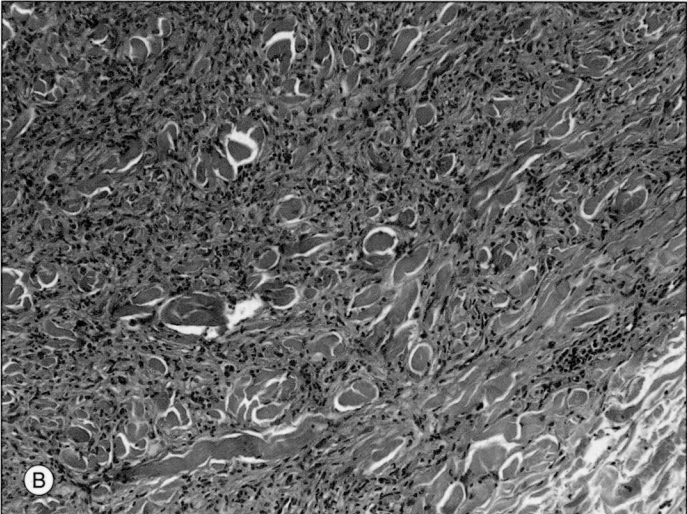

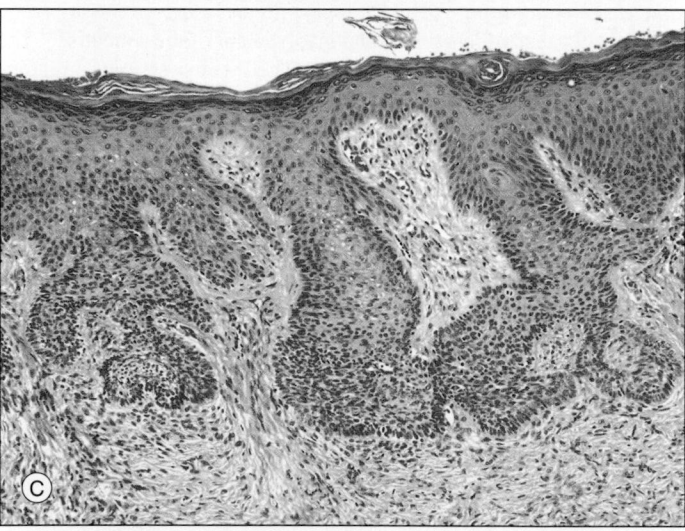

Fig. 8.50 Dermatofibroma. **A**, Relative circumscription is typical as is (**B**) encirclement of peripheral collagen bundles; **C**, Basal cell hyperplasia may rarely mimic basal cell carcinoma.

negative. They are also frequently nonreactive for factor XIIIa, unlike ordinary DF.[282]

Dermatofibrosarcoma protuberans (DFSP) is a tumor of borderline malignancy. It is most often seen in adults, but cases in childhood have been well documented. DFSP may recur in up to 50% of cases following simple excision, and, after multiple recurrences, it may even metastasize.[283,284] This tumor shows a predilection for the trunk and proximal extremities and is a violaceous nodule or plaque. A tendency for DFSP to protrude above the surrounding skin surface is reflected by its name. Subcutaneous extension is usual (Fig. 8.51A)[285,286] Microscopically, a storiform (pinwheel-like) growth pattern is prototypically represented in DFSP (Fig. 8.51B). Mitotic activity may be brisk but atypical forms are absent; significant cellular pleomorphism should be absent. In particular, foam cells, multinucleated giant cells, and hemosiderinized cells are not seen in DFSP. Some lesions of this type show areas of sharply increased cellularity with heightened nuclear atypia and a 'herringbone' growth pattern, simulating the image of fibrosarcoma. Whether or not this is associated with a worsened prognosis is a debatable point, however.[284] The pigmented variant of DFSP (Bednar's tumor) comprises only 1–5 % of all cases. A proportion of the tumor cells in that subtype contain melanin.[287] Myxoid DFSP exhibits a lower cellularity than the ordinary form and has a less well-developed storiform pattern. *Giant cell fibroblastoma* is a pediatric lesion that differs from classical DFSP histologically but is clearly related to it clinically, immuno-histologically, and cytogenetically. The former of those lesions shows a biphasic growth pattern, with a loose proliferation of spindle cells and floret-type giant cells in the superficial reticular dermis, and a deeper component that features the formation of pseudovascular ('angiectoid') spaces that are mantled by floret cells.

Occasional lesions in this group can be regarded as *fibrohistiocytic tumors of indeterminate biological potential*; these have morphologic and immunophenotypic features which straddle those of DF and DFSP.[288] As alluded to earlier, DFSP classically exhibits diffuse CD34 positivity and lacks factor XIIIa.[289,290] It represents another tumor type that can contain numerous stromal dendritic cells, which may label for S-100 protein; this finding should not be misinterpreted as support for a diagnosis of melanoma, especially in reference to Bednar tumors.

Although *atypical fibroxanthoma* (AFX) has been recognized for almost half a century[291] its classification as a superficial form of malignant fibrous histiocytoma (MFH) is still a contentious one.[292] The classic presentation of AFX is on the face of elderly patients; in the past, it was said that 25% arose on the extremities of young adults, but it is now thought that those lesions represent examples of pleomorphic fibroma rather than AFX.[283] The usual clinical appearance of AFX is that of a red-pink, variably ulcerated nodule, with an average size of 2 cm. Despite the fact that this tumor has been called a 'pseudosarcoma' and 'benign' by some authors, that is clearly untrue.[293] Cases of AFX that show vascular invasion, deep growth into the subcutis or underlying soft tissue, or repeated recurrence may metastasize to distant sites. Hence, it is more apropos to consider the lesion as a 'borderline' malignancy. Indeed, if a lesion with the morphologic attributes of AFX were larger and more deeply located, it would undoubtedly be labeled as MFH by most observers. The histologic epicenter of AFX is typically in the reticular dermis. Its borders are indistinct and prominent actinic change is apparent in the adjacent corium. In similarity to deep MFH, individual tumor cells in AFX show striking nuclear atypia, common multinucleation, and a high mitotic rate as well as abnormal division figures (Fig. 8.52). Focal necrosis and the presence of vacuolated histiocyte-like cells are also commonly seen. Some tumors may exhibit divergent differentiation with chondro-osseous, osteoclast-

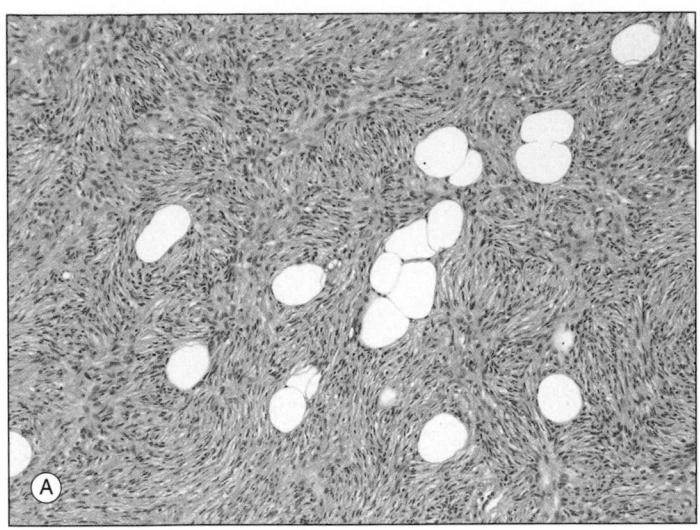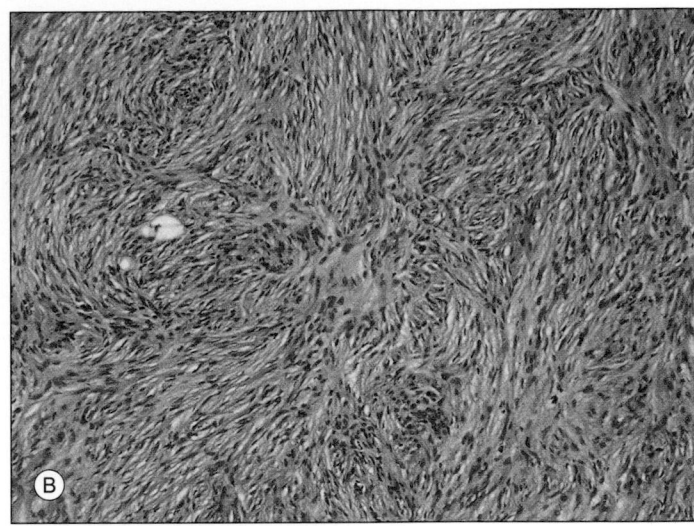

Fig. 8.51 A, Dermatofibrosarcoma protuberans often diffusely infiltrates the subcutis in contrast to dermatofibroma that grows along existing fibrous septa; **B,** Storiform growth is prototypical in this tumor.

rich, and myxoid foci.[294] A purely spindle cell variant of AFX also exists.

Two tumors with which AFX is potentially confused are spindle cell squamous carcinoma and sarcomatoid malignant melanoma. Immunohistology should be employed routinely in the diagnostic separation of those neoplastic entities; indeed, the authors' experience has shown the imprudence of failing to do so. Vimentin positivity is seen in all three of these tumor types, but AFX is not labeled for cytokeratin or S-100 protein as true of squamous carcinoma and melanoma, respectively.

Benign chondro-osseous lesions

Cutaneous ossification is not a true neoplasm, but may resemble one. It can be seen as a primary lesion (osteoma cutis) in the dermis or subcutis, corresponding to the clinical entities known as *congenital plaque-like osteomatosis, multiple osteomatosis* (Fig. 8.53), and *Albright's hereditary osteodystrophy*. All of those conditions occur principally in children and young adults.[295–299] *Secondary ossification* is more common in the skin; it is typically encountered in older individuals in association with other neoplasms, antecedent trauma, and prior infection.[300,301] Histologically, foci of ossification in the skin typically lack interposed cartilage, osteoblastic proliferation, and osteoclastic elements, as seen in conventional bone formation.[300] Primary *osteosarcoma* of the skin is extraordinarily rare and has a histological appearance that is comparable to its intraosseous counterpart.

Benign myxoid lesions

Cutaneous myxoma (superficial angiomyxoma) is a benign tumor that has a predilection for the head and neck, trunk, and lower extremities. It usually presents in middle-aged adults as single nodules or polypoid lesions that may be clinically confused with a skin tag or neurofibroma.[302] When this lesion occurs in the setting of Carney's complex (cutaneous and cardiac myxomas, spotty pigmentation, and endocrine overactivity) they are often multiple and frequently occur in the eyelid or external ear.[303] Histologically,

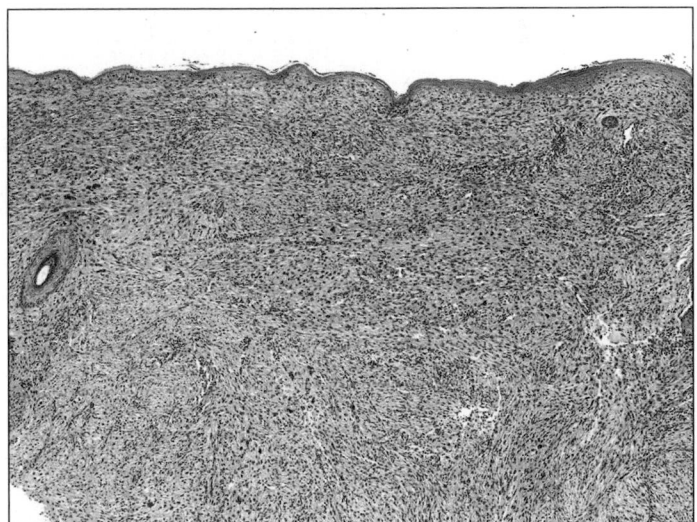

Fig. 8.52 The relationship to deep malignant fibrous histiocytoma is evident in this atypical fibroxanthoma with pleomorphic spindle cells and foamy macrophages.

this tumor has a lobular low-power appearance with a circumscribed border that involves the dermis and sometimes the subcutis. Small spindle shaped cells are set in a background of abundant myxoid stroma (Fig. 8.54). The nuclear features of these cells are bland and mitotic figures are rare. A prominent arborizing vasculature may be seen. Occasionally, there are epithelial structures within the tumor that may represent entrapped adnexal elements. By immunohistochemistry the spindle cells are positive for vimentin and negative for cytokeratins and S-100 protein.[304] Although this tumor is benign it does have a propensity for local recurrence.[302]

Superficial acral fibromyxoma is a recently described lesion with a predilection for the hands and feet, especially the periungual regions. Microscopically, there is moderate cellular proliferation of

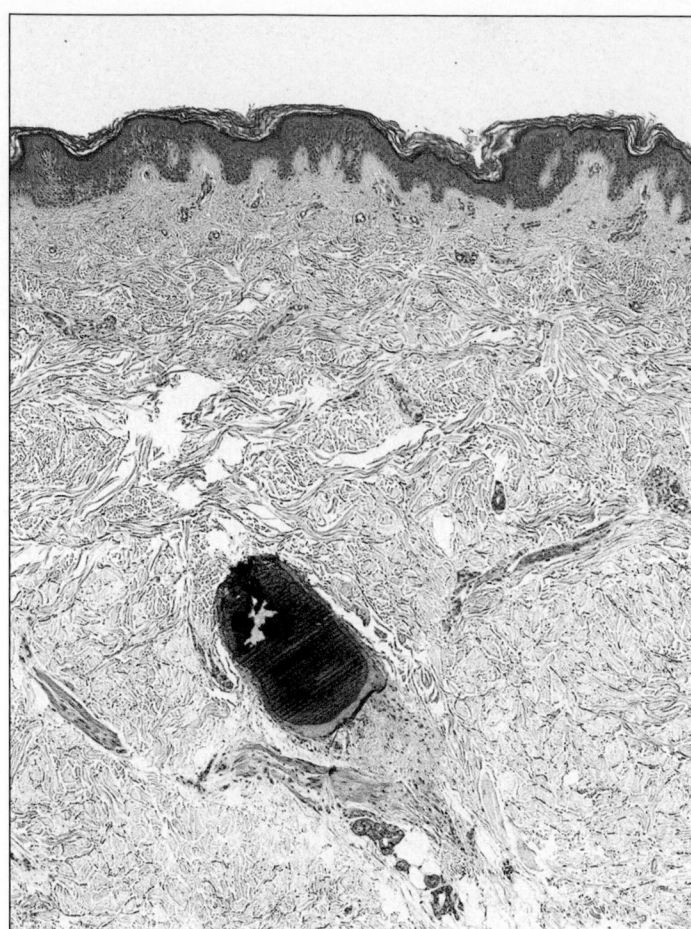

Fig. 8.53 Osteoma cutis (milium osteoma) is most often incidental, but a potential relationship with prior trauma or abnormal calcium/phosphorus metabolism should be kept in mind.

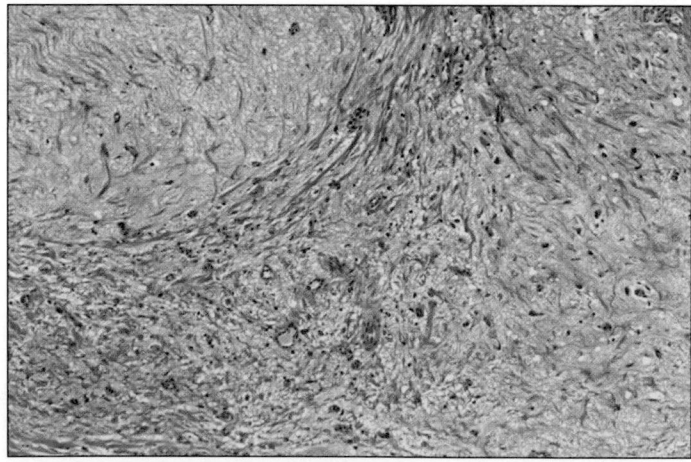

Fig. 8.54 Cutaneous myxoma. Scattered spindle cells and small vessels are imbedded in a myxoid matrix.

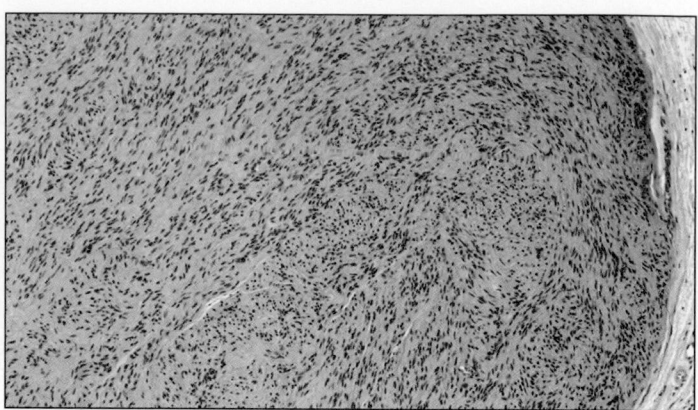

Fig. 8.55 Solitary circumscribed neuroma. There are interlacing fascicles of spindle cells that variably display nuclear palisading.

spindled to stellate fibroblast-like cells set in a myxoid or myxo-collagenous background. There is often accentuated vasculature, particularly in the examples that contain more myxoid stroma. Focal cytologic atypia and rare mitotic figures may be seen. In comparison to cutaneous myxoma this tumor tends to be much more cellular. By immunohistochemistry the spindle cells express CD34 and CD99.[305]

Benign peripheral nerve tumors

Solitary circumscribed neuroma (palisaded and encapsulated neuroma) is an uncommon slow-growing tumor that usually presents as a small papule on the face of a middle-aged individual.[306] Microscopically, there are interlacing fascicles of spindle cells that variably display nuclear palisading (Fig. 8.55). Rarely, the cells may have an epithelioid appearance.[307] This tumor is generally well circumscribed and may or may not have a thin connective tissue capsule. By immuno-histochemistry, the spindle cells are strongly S-100 positive.[308]

Benign vascular tumors of the skin

Nevus flammeus is a generic term for a vascular malformation that is commonly known as 'port-wine stain,' 'salmon patch' or 'stork bite.' Clinically, it is represented by a pink to red patch, usually on the scalp, face, or neck, but occasionally located elsewhere as well. Large lesions have a slightly raised surface and a darker red color; these are typically categorized as port-wine stains. In all lesions in this category, one sees relatively little microscopically except for ectatic thin-walled vessels in the dermis (Fig. 8.56). Therefore, clinicopathologic correlation is necessary for a correct diagnosis to be made.[309] Nevus flammeus has principal importance as a cutaneous marker of multiorgan vascular malformation syndromes. In *Sturge-Weber syndrome* a large unilateral, facial port-wine stain is associated with intracranial vascular malformations. Large port-wine stains occurring on a hypertrophied limb are seen in *Klippel-Trenaunay-Weber syndrome*.[310] Despite these associations, most examples of nevus flammeus are sporadic.

Lymphangioma circumscriptum is a superficial lymphatic malformation that makes itself apparent early in life as vesicle-like papules that resemble 'frog spawn.' Sites of predilection for these lesions include the trunk, axillae, and tongue. Histologically, lymphangioma circumscriptum comprises multiple dilated lymphatic channels that are located immediately beneath the epidermis and are filled with

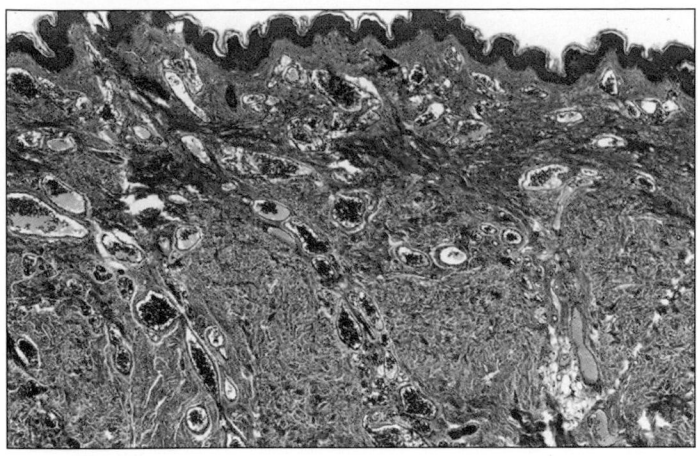

Fig. 8.56 Nevus flammeus. Note the ectatic thin-walled vessels in the dermis.

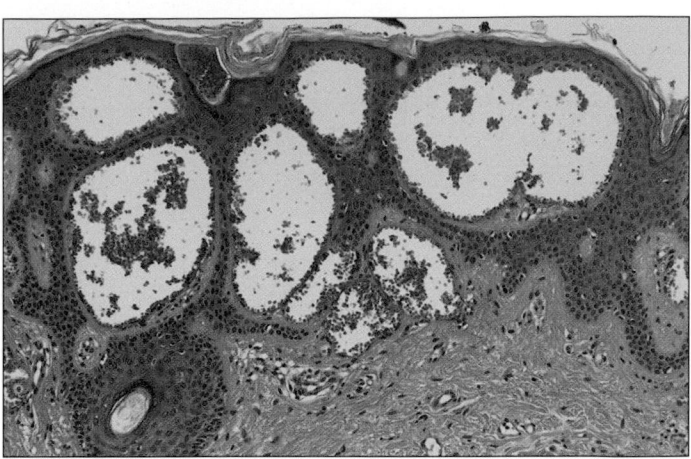

Fig. 8.58 Angiokeratoma. Dilated papillary dermal blood vessels push up on an acanthotic epidermis. Elongated rete ridges often partially or completely surround the vessels.

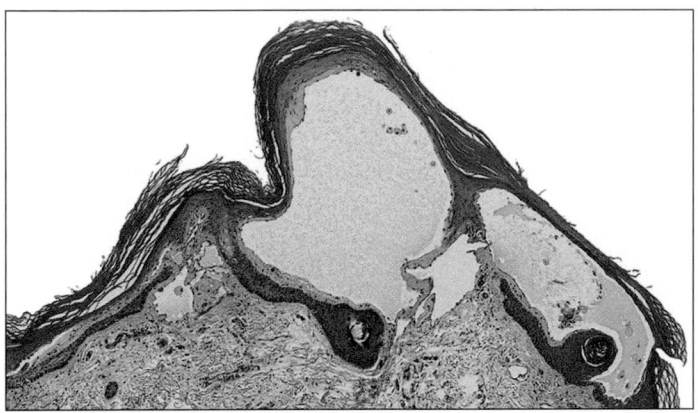

Fig. 8.57 Lymphangioma circumscriptum. Multiple dilated lymphatic channels located beneath the epidermis are filled with proteinaceous fluid.

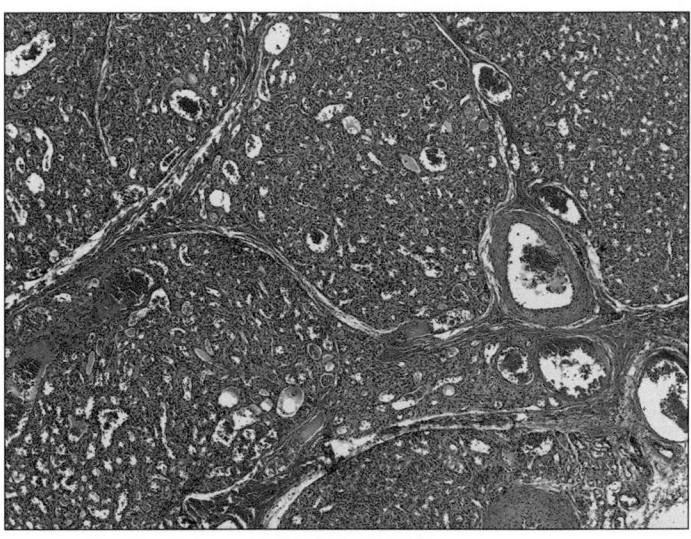

Fig. 8.59 Juvenile capillary hemangioma. There are cellular lobules composed of densely apposed capillaries with little or no lumen formation. Note the larger feeder vessels that connect to the lobules.

proteinaceous fluid (Fig. 8.57). These spaces elevate the epidermis and give it a papular raised contour. Occasionally, blood cells are found within the vascular spaces as well. Epidermal hyperplasia and lymphocytic exocytosis may also be seen.[311]

Angiokeratomas are characterized by dilated papillary dermal blood vessels that are intimately associated with irregularly acanthotic epidermis (Fig. 8.58). Elongated rete ridges often partially or completely surround the vessels in angiokeratomas. Other associated findings include hyperkeratosis and vascular thrombosis. A number of clinical variants of angiokeratoma have been described, but these all have similar histologic features. The *solitary type* occurs predominately on the lower extremities as a warty papule. The *Mibelli type* is seen in children as multiple verrucoid lesions on the hands, feet, elbows, trunk, or knees.[312] The *Fordyce type* is characterized by numerous red papules that are distributed over the scrotum or vulva in adult individuals.[313,314]

The term '*capillary hemangioma*' encompasses a number of neoplastic entities that are clinically distinct but have comparable histological appearances. These include juvenile capillary hemangioma, lobular capillary hemangioma, cherry angioma, verrucous hemangioma, and acquired tufted hemangioma. Capillary-sized vessels proliferate to form discrete lobules in the dermis in all of these tumors. Each lobule contains a central 'feeder' vessel that has a relatively large caliber, and the size of constituent vessels decreases as one moves to the periphery of the lobular array. The amount of stroma between the lobules is variable. Circumscription and a lobular architecture are the principal clues to the benign nature of these lesions.

Juvenile capillary hemangioma ('strawberry nevus') is the most common tumor of infancy. It shows a female predominance, and the head, neck, and trunk are its most common locations. This lesion is usually not seen at birth, but appears during the first few weeks of life and pursues a course marked by variable regression thereafter.[315,316] The histologic image depends on the age of the lesion when it is biopsied. Early tumors are composed of highly cellular lobules comprising densely apposed capillaries with little or no lumen formation (Fig. 8.59). Both the dermis and subcutis may be involved

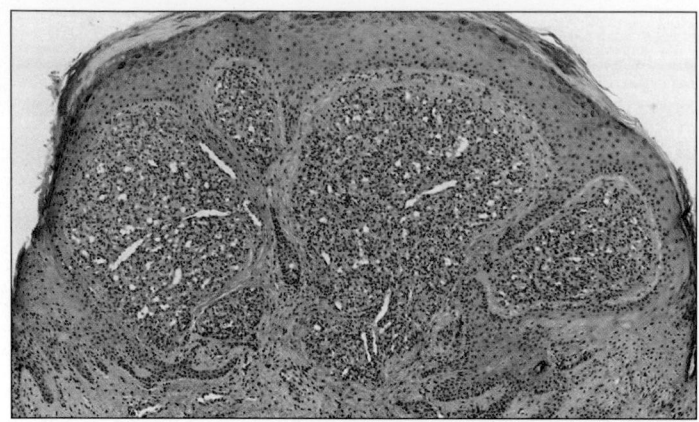

Fig. 8.60 Lobular capillary hemangiomas. This tumor has a prototypically lobular architecture with a polypoid configuration and an adjacent 'collarette' of epithelium.

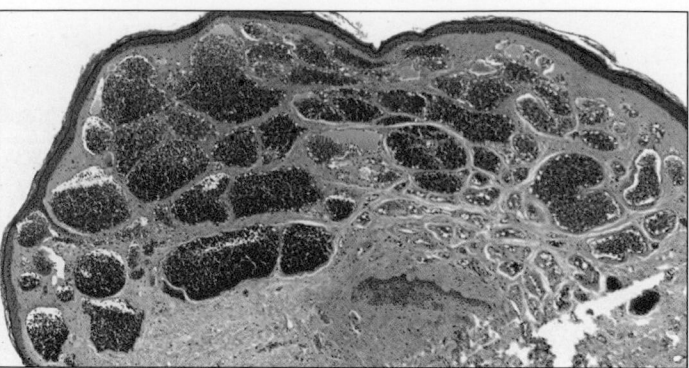

Fig. 8.61 Cherry angioma. Dilated and interconnecting capillaries fill the papillary dermis.

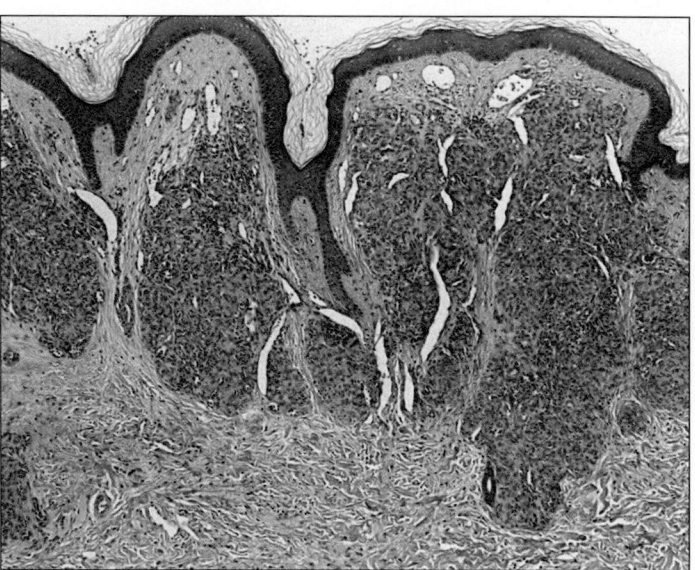

Fig. 8.62 Acquired tufted hemangioma. Lobules of capillary-sized vascular channels project into the semicircular lumina of pre-existing vessels.

and mitotic figures are usually present; hence, these features should not be accorded any negative portent. Although capillary hemangiomas are completely benign and generally do not recur, perineural infiltration may be present as well.[317] Older lesions show progressively better-defined vascular lumina and luminal dilatation, as well as stromal fibrosis.

Lobular capillary hemangiomas (LCHs; 'pyogenic granulomas') are very common vascular proliferations that clinically resemble exuberant granulation tissue. These tumors usually occur on the extremities or at sites of trauma in children.[318] There is also a peculiar predilection for the oral cavity in pregnant women ('granuloma gravidarum').[319] Very rarely, an extreme multiplicity of lesions or repeated recurrence of LCH may be encountered. Morphologically, it closely resembles juvenile capillary hemangioma but has a more prototypically lobular architecture. The former of those lesions usually has a polypoid configuration as well, with an adjacent 'collarette' of appendageal epithelium (Fig. 8.60). Surface ulceration may lead to lesional edema, stromal infiltration by neutrophils and lymphocytes, and regenerative nuclear atypia and striking mitotic activity in the proliferating endothelial cells. These changes should not be misinterpreted as those of a vascular sarcoma.[320]

Cherry angioma is another common tumor in the general adult population. It is represented by one or more small red papules with a predilection for the trunk and upper extremities. The number of lesions present on any given individual increases with age. Histologically, this tumor is composed of dilated and interconnecting capillaries that fill the papillary dermis (Fig. 8.61). A vaguely lobular architecture may be present. The tumoral vessels sometimes push against the epidermis and create a polypoid lesion,[321] but ulceration and inflammation are distinctly unusual.

Verrucous hemangioma presents as a wart-like lesion on the lower extremities, usually in children. At birth the lesion often clinically resembles a juvenile capillary hemangioma but becomes progressively verrucoid afterwards. The histologic image of this lesion features epidermal acanthosis and papillomatosis overlying a localized proliferation of dilated capillaries. 'Collarettes' may extend downward to surround the lesion, as observed in angiokeratomas. Some authors believe these lesions are vascular malformations rather than neoplasms.[322]

Acquired tufted hemangioma ('angioblastoma of Nakagawa') is a microscopically unusual vascular proliferation that is found primarily in children and young adults. It is characterized macroscopically by multiple ill-defined red macules, often with confluence. The lesions slowly expand with time and usually stop growing in adulthood.[323,324] Microscopically, this tumor demonstrates lobules of capillary-sized vascular channels that project into the lumina of pre-existing blood vessels in the dermis (Fig. 8.62). These lobules are sometimes widely dispersed. This arrangement yields a low-power pattern which has been likened to 'cannonballs' by Wilson-Jones and Orkin.[323] Individual lobules of tumor cells include spindle cells as well, a finding that may cause confusion with Kaposi's sarcoma. However, tufted angiomas lack the cellular atypia and architectural disorganization that is seen in that entity. It is likely that reports of 'intravascular pyogenic granuloma' and acquired tufted hemangioma describe comparable neoplasms.[325]

Cavernous hemangioma is typically a childhood lesion, and takes the form of an ill-defined red to blue mass in the deep dermis and subcutis. Microscopically, it is a proliferation of dilated thin-walled vessels that are lined by flattened endothelial cells (Fig. 8.63).

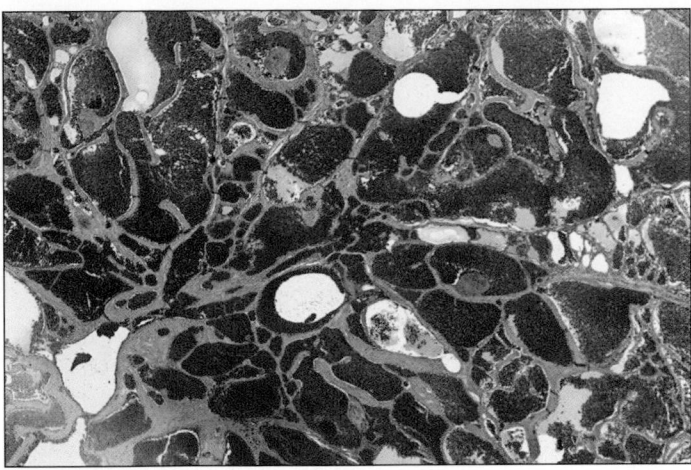

Fig. 8.63 Cavernous hemangioma. Dilated thin-walled vessels are lined by flattened endothelial cells.

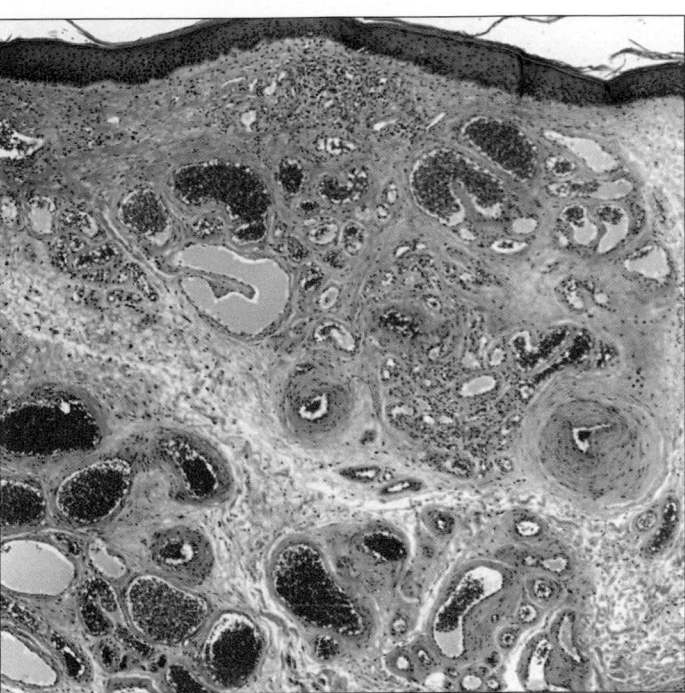

Fig. 8.64 Cutaneous arteriovenous hemangioma. There is a mixture of thin- and thick-walled vessels, with the latter predominating.

These are usually congested and may contain focal thromboses. In contrast to capillary hemangiomas, cavernous hemangiomas lack a lobular architecture.[326] In rare instances they are associated with *Kasabach-Merritt syndrome*[327] (consumption coagulopathy and thrombocytopenia), *blue rubber bleb syndrome*[328] (multiple cutaneous and gastrointestinal cavernous hemangiomas) or *Maffucci's syndrome*[329] (multiple cutaneous vascular tumors and enchondromas of long and small bones). *Sinusoidal hemangioma* is a probable variant of cavernous hemangioma that is seen in adults. That lesion exhibits thin-walled dilated vessels that anastomose to create complex sieve-like or pseudopapillary configurations in the dermis. Despite these worrisome histologic attributes, sinusoidal hemangiomas are well circumscribed and often lobulated, supporting their innocuous nature.[330]

Cutaneous arteriovenous hemangioma ('acral arteriovenous tumor') occurs in middle-aged adults on the lips, nose, and eyelids. It is a small red to blue papule that is often painful. Despite the name given to this tumor, no significant arteriovenous shunting is present in association with it. Microscopically, one observes a mixture of thin- and thick-walled vessels, with the latter predominating (Fig. 8.64). They have muscular walls, which tend to merge with those of neighboring tumor vessels. Although there are both venous and arterial forms of arteriovenous hemangioma, they have no particular clinical significance and it is usually difficult to tell them apart without the use of elastic stains. Some lesions of this type also contain small zones of proliferative capillaries that resemble those of capillary hemangiomas.[331]

True arteriovenous malformation has a completely different clinical profile. The latter lesion presents as a large deep-seated tumor in a limb or on the head and neck in children and young adults. It frequently causes arteriovenous shunting and may lead to limb hypertrophy, high-output cardiac failure, and a consumptive coagulopathy.[332]

Glomeruloid hemangioma is a rare vascular neoplasm that is composed of congeries of small dermal blood vessels that resemble renal glomeruli on scanning microscopy. It presents with numerous firm red papules on the trunk and proximal extremities. Constituent endothelial cells may be vacuolized or contain distinctive eosinophilic cytoplasmic inclusions that represent immunoglobulin deposits. The significance of this tumor lies in its potential association with the

'POEMS' syndrome, a constellation of disorders (*p*olyneuropathy, *o*rganomegaly, *e*ndocrinopathy, *M*-protein, *s*kin changes) that sometimes overlaps with the components of multicentric Castleman's disease.[333] In that regard, it should be noted some patients with POEMS syndrome have only ordinary capillary hemangiomas of the skin rather than the glomeruloid form of those tumors.

Epithelioid hemangioma ('angiolymphoid hyperplasia with eosinophilia;' 'histiocytoid hemangioma') is a benign vascular tumor represented by a pink to red papule or nodule, usually in the skin of the head and neck, in young to middle-aged adults. Multiple lesions may be present in some cases. Microscopically, one observes a vaguely lobular proliferation of thin-walled vessels that are lined by 'epithelioid' endothelial cells with abundant cytoplasm and large rounded nuclei (Fig. 8.65). Cytoplasmic vacuoles may be present in some cells. The stroma contains an inflammatory infiltrate of variable density, comprising lymphocytes and eosinophils. Lymphoid follicles also may be seen but are relatively rare. The stroma may be myxoid or fibrous. Although the etiology of epithelioid hemangioma is unknown, recent studies have suggested its constituents show a resemblance to damaged endothelial cells.[334,335] The lesion known as *Kimura's disease/tumor* was once thought to be identical to epithelioid hemangioma. However, the current literature indicates that they are two completely different conditions with only a few superficial similarities.[336–338] Kimura's tumor is limited almost exclusively to Asian individuals. It takes the form of large subcutaneous masses that are often concentrated around the ears or located adjacent to the parotid glands. Lymph node involvement is frequent and peripheral eosinophilia is often seen. Histologically, Kimura's tumor demonstrates a striking lymphoid infiltrate containing numerous reactive lymphoid follicles and abundant interspersed eosinophils; the latter may even form eosinophilic abscesses. In contrast to epithelioid hemangioma, the vascular component of Kimura's tumor is much less prominent with no epithelioid endothelial cells.

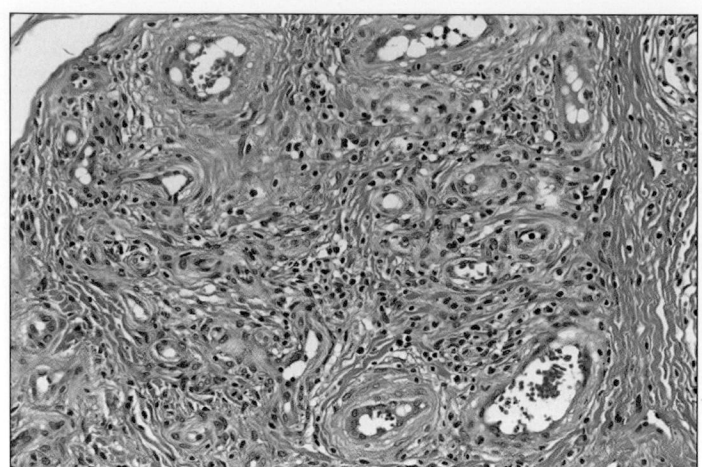

Fig. 8.65 Epithelioid hemangioma. A vaguely lobular proliferation of thin-walled vessels is lined by 'epithelioid' endothelial cells with abundant cytoplasm and large rounded nuclei. Note the cytoplasmic vacuoles in some of the endothelial cells. Eosinophils are scattered between the vessels.

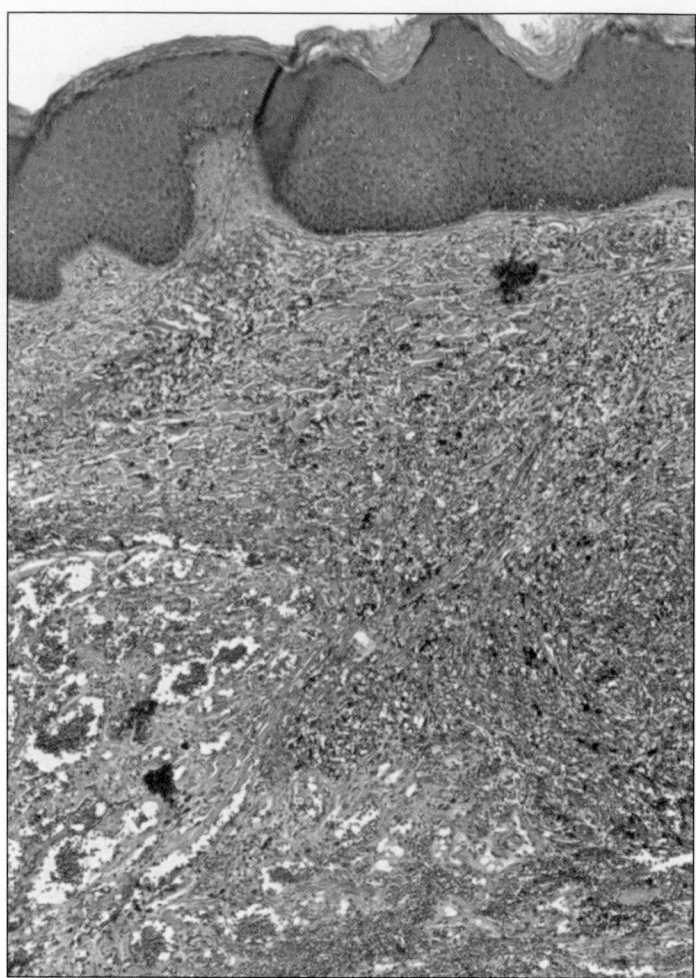

Fig. 8.66 Hobnail hemangioma. A biphasic vascular composition is seen. There are dilated vessels lined by a single layer of plump endothelial cells in the lower left portion of the micrograph. Interanastomosing slit-like vessels that dissect the dermal collegen surround this area. Stromal hemosiderin deposition and lymphocyte infiltration are prominent in this case.

Hobnail hemangioma (HH; 'targetoid hemosiderotic hemangioma;' 'atypical hemangioma') is a recently recognized benign vascular tumor represented by a violaceous papule surrounded by an ecchymotic or brown ring. This configuration gives the lesion a 'targetoid' macroscopic appearance.[339] HH usually occurs in young to middle-aged patients and may show episodic swelling, darkening, or involution. Microscopically, it has a biphasic vascular composition in well-developed form. In the papillary dermis there are dilated vessels lined by a single layer of plump endothelial cells, often likened to 'hobnails,' protruding into the luminal spaces (Fig. 8.66). Small papillary projections of bland endothelial cells also may be present. Reticular dermal tumor vessels assume an interanastomosing slit-like appearance that appears to 'dissect' through the stromal collagen.[340,341] Stromal hemosiderin deposition and scattered lymphocytes are also common in the deep corium. A lesion closely allied to hobnail hemangioma is *microvenular hemangioma*.[342,343] That tumor is composed of small tubular vessels that ramify between dermal collagen bundles. Pericytic cells partially invest the lesional vascular channels, and occasional lobules may be seen.

Spindle cell hemangioma (SCH; formerly called 'spindle cell 'hemangioendothelioma'') is a vascular tumor of the dermis and subcutis that usually presents as a single nodule on the distal extremities. Some examples may be multinodular and affect a regional skin area. Although the majority of these tumors are seen in children or young adults, they may occur at any age.[344] The microscopic appearance of SCH features a biphasic pattern including dilated cavernous vascular spaces that are admixed with solid areas of spindle cell proliferation with slit-like vascular channels, resembling those of Kaposi's sarcoma (Fig. 8.67). Intralesional thrombi may be present. The spindle cell foci also contain plumper endothelial elements with cytoplasmic vacuoles, simulating cells seen in various forms of hemangioendothelioma (see below). In general, nuclear atypia is modest and there are only rare mitotic figures.[345] Even in the recent past, SCH was considered to have low-grade malignant potential, accounting for its alternative designation of spindle cell 'hemangioendothelioma.'[346] Recent evidence suggests that this tumor entity may arise as a consequence of local vascular malformations.[347] Local 'recurrences' of SCH are

common but may actually represent the metachronous growth of multicentric lesions.[345]

Glomus tumor presents as painful bluish nodule, usually in a subungual location. Indeed, these neoplasms are most commonly found in the acral skin. Rarely, glomus tumors have arisen in visceral organs as well.[348] They are thought to resemble the glomus apparatus histologically, in that layers of glomus cells surround vascular structures and resemble non-neoplastic Sucquet-Hoyer complexes.[349] The *glomangioma* is a variant of glomus tumor that contains prominently dilated stromal blood vessels. It is typically painless and rarely affects subungual locations.[350] Multiple glomangiomas may occur with an autosomal dominant mode of inheritance.[351] Histologically, the glomus tumor is composed of solid nests of compact polyhedral cells surrounding small vessels in the dermis (Fig. 8.68). It is well circumscribed but unencapsulated, and the background stroma may be fibrous or myxoid. No nuclear pleomorphism or mitotic activity is apparent in this lesion. Glomangiomas are less well circumscribed and contain large vascular channels that are surrounded by several layers of cells like those seen in glomus tumor. In some cases, the latter are so sparse that it is difficult to distinguish the lesion from typical cavernous

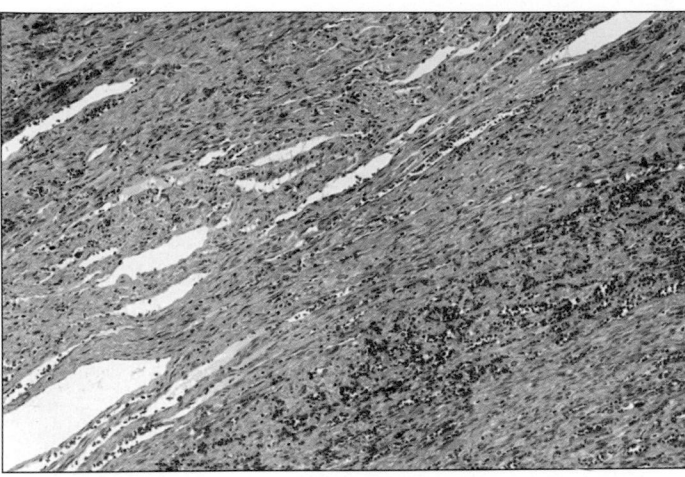

Fig. 8.67 Spindle cell hemangioma. Note the biphasic pattern. There are dilated cavernous vascular spaces admixed with solid areas of spindle cell proliferation that have slit-like vascular channels, resembling those of Kaposi's sarcoma.

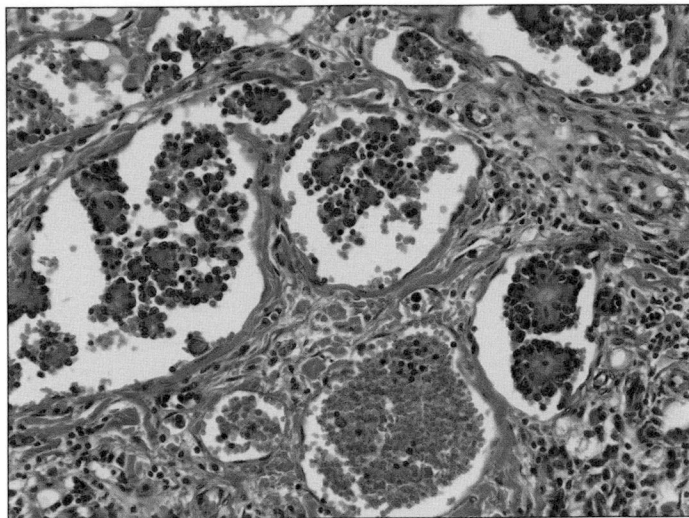

Fig. 8.69 Dabska's tumor. Papillary endothelial micropapillae project into vascular spaces. These are lined by 'hobnail' cells that surround cores of hyalinized basement membrane material.

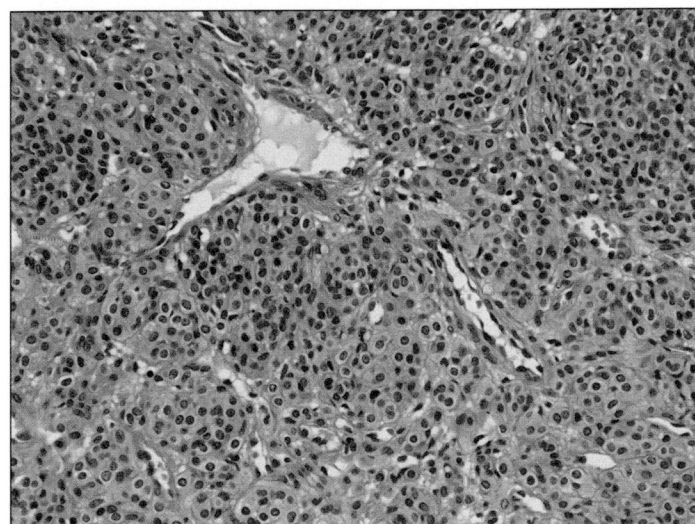

Fig. 8.68 Glomus tumor. Solid nests of compact polyhedral cells surround small vessels in the dermis.

hemangioma. Glomus tumors and glomangiomas are peculiar smooth muscle neoplasms rather than endothelial lesions, as reflected by their immunoreactivity for muscle-specific actin and alpha-isoform actin.[352] Endothelial cell markers are absent in the tumor cells.[353] 'Malignant' glomus tumors have been described, with infiltrative borders, a size >2 cm, atypical mitotic figures, and nuclear atypia. However, whether these lesions are truly aggressive biologically is a debatable point.[354]

Borderline vascular tumors of the skin

The term 'hemangioendothelioma' has been used to denote vascular tumors that have a borderline clinical behavior between that of hemangioma and Kaposi's sarcoma or angiosarcoma. The neoplasms in the former group generally have the ability to recur but metastasize

to distant sites only infrequently. *Epithelioid hemangioendothelioma*, which is uncommonly seen in the skin (see Ch. 9), has a small but significant risk of lymph nodal metastasis and may even prove fatal.[355] On the other hand, retiform hemangioendothelioma and endovascular papillary angioendothelioma, both of which show a predilection for the skin, rarely cause fatality. Spindle cell 'hemangioendothelioma' has been renamed spindle cell *hemangioma* (see above) in recent years because long-term follow-up has revealed a general lack of metastatic potential and it demonstrates an association with malformative conditions in the soft tissue.[345]

Endovascular papillary angioendothelioma was first described by Dabska in 1969[356] and subsequently has been designated using her name, as *Dabska's tumor*. This lesion presents in children and young adults as a slowly growing intradermal violaceous nodule or plaque.[357] There are rare reports of Dabska's tumor involving the spleen or deep soft tissue, but the diagnosis in such cases is questionable.[358,359] Endovascular papillary angioendothelioma should be considered as a low-grade malignancy with a generally favorable prognosis.[360] However, it does have the potential to recur and occasionally metastasizes to regional lymph nodes.[356,357]

The microscopic features of this tumor are distinctive. It shows a proliferation of well-formed, endothelial-lined vascular spaces in the dermis and has a low-power microscopic pattern recalling the image of lymphangiectasia or lymphangioma.[361] Papillary endothelial micropapillae project into the vascular spaces and are lined by 'hobnail' cells that surround cores of hyalinized basement membrane material (Fig. 8.69). The tumor cells have high nuclear-to-cytoplasmic ratios, but they lack nuclear atypia and mitotic figures are rare. Zones of densely collagenized stroma, containing lymphocyte aggregates, are seen between the vascular spaces. Some cases show intravascular lymphocytic clusters around the papillary projections; this feature has led some authors to suggest that Dabska's tumor demonstrates features of 'high' endothelial differentiation as seen in postcapillary venules.[362] Immunohistochemical studies have demonstrated the expression of vascular endothelial cell growth factor receptor 3 (VEGFR 3) in endovascular papillary angioendotheliomas; this marker labels non-neoplastic lymphatic endothelium, stimulating the suggestion that Dabska's tumor should be renamed as papillary *intralymphatic* angioendothelioma.[360] However, it should be noted that VEGFR 3 is not specific for lymphatic differentiation when applied to tumor tissue.[363] Expression of von Willebrand factor, CD31, and CD34 has also been demonstrated in Dabska's tumor.[360,364]

Retiform hemangioendothelioma (RHE) is a relatively recently documented tumor entity that is probably closely related to endovascular papillary angioendothelioma. It is seen in young adults as a slowly growing cutaneous plaque in the distal extremities. Some examples have occurred in the setting of lymphedema or within skin fields of prior radiotherapy. In contrast to endovascular papillary angioendothelioma, RHE manifests the presence of narrow slit-like vessels that infiltrate the reticular dermis and subcutis in a pattern which simulates that of the rete testis (Fig. 8.70).[365] Monomorphic, 'hobnail' endothelial cells with hyperchromatic but bland nuclei line the lesional vessels. Small focal endothelial papillae also may be observed, like those seen in Dabska's tumor. A prominent intravascular or stromal lymphoid infiltrate is also shared by RHE and endovascular papillary angioendothelioma, and their immunophenotypes are similar. Although RHE may be locally aggressive, only one case with lymph nodal metastasis has been reported.[365] Weiss & Goldblum have proposed the term *hobnail hemangioendothelioma* as a unifying diagnosis to encompass both RHE and Dabska's tumor.[366]

Kaposiform hemangioendothelioma is a rare tumor that occurs mainly in children as a rapidly expanding cutaneous red plaque or nodule or a deeply seated (often retroperitoneal) tumor. The second of those presentations is sometimes associated with a consumption coagulopathy and thrombocytopenia (Kasabach-Merritt syndrome) and a poor prognosis.[367] Histologically, one sees a poorly circumscribed dermal mass composed of irregular micronodules of tumor cells in the dermis and subcutis. Constituent lesional vessels have a slit-like configuration and may be surrounded by zones of spindle cells, yielding an image which is partially like that of Kaposi's sarcoma. Those foci are admixed with areas resembling the phenotype of capillary hemangiomas. Hemosiderin deposits and cytoplasmic hyaline globules may also be present in the spindle cell areas. However, nuclear atypia and mitotic activity are minimal.[368]

It is often difficult to distinguish Kaposiform hemangioendothelioma from Kaposi's sarcoma morphologically, in small biopsy specimens. However, Kaposi's sarcoma lacks a capillary hemangioma-like component and is extraordinary in children. A childhood 'lymphadenopathic' form of the latter neoplasm has been described in African patients[369] but is virtually unknown in Western countries. A viral association with Kaposi's sarcoma further distinguishes it from Kaposiform hemangioendothelioma. Integrated nucleic acid sequences of human herpesvirus-8 (HHV8) have not been detected in the second of those neoplasms, but they are present in virtually all examples of Kaposi's sarcoma.[370]

Malignant endothelial neoplasms of the skin

Kaposi's sarcoma (KS) is an aggressive endothelial tumor that has four distinct clinical variants. As just mentioned, all forms of this neoplasm are linked to HHV-8 infection.[371,372]

Classical (Mediterranean) Kaposi's sarcoma is an indolent form of the tumor that is seen in middle-aged to elderly men of Mediterranean or Eastern European heritage. In most instances such lesions are limited to the skin of the lower extremities; they are red or brown macules, plaques, or nodules. Lymphedema may be present in the affected skin field surrounding the tumors. Rarely, lymph nodal or visceral involvement by classical KS is encountered. Although this tumor variant typically pursues a chronic course, it seems to have little impact on life expectancy.[373,374]

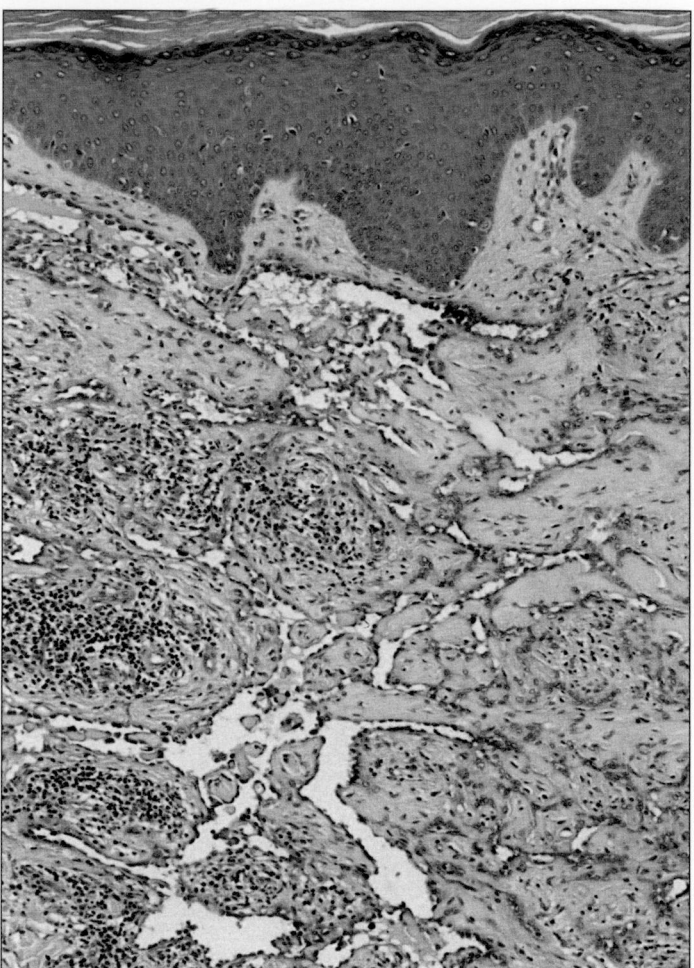

Fig. 8.70 Retiform hemangioendothelioma. Narrow slit-like vessels infiltrate the reticular dermis and subcutis in a pattern which simulates the rete testis. Monomorphic, 'hobnail' endothelial cells with hyperchromatic but bland nuclei line the lesional vessels.

African-type Kaposi's sarcoma is endemic to equatorial Africa, where it affects children and middle-aged adults that are not infected with the human immunodeficiency (HIV) virus. There are two subtypes of this neoplasm in adults. The indolent form has a presentation and course which is similar to that of classic KS.[373] The second subtype is more aggressive, with extensive cutaneous involvement and infiltration of underlying soft tissue and even bone. The 'lymphadenopathic' variant of African KS primarily affects children, as cited earlier. It shows extensive lymph nodal involvement with few if any cutaneous lesions, and is often rapidly fatal.[369]

Iatrogenic Kaposi's sarcoma is a potential complication of long-term immunosuppressive therapy in solid organ transplantation or prolonged corticosteroid treatment. This tumor variant is usually more aggressive than classical KS. However, spontaneous regression of the lesions may occur if immunosuppressive therapy is discontinued or decreased significantly.[375]

Acquired immunodeficiency syndrome (AIDS)/HIV-associated Kaposi's sarcoma is the most aggressive form of KS. The distribution of the lesions in this subtype differs from that seen in the classical type, with a preference for the skin of the arms, trunk, head, and neck. Mucosal surfaces, the lungs, the gastrointestinal tract, and lymph nodes are also frequently involved. The macroscopic characteristics of individual lesions often are dissimilar from those of classical KS as well; those in HIV-related disease commonly resemble ecchymoses or vascular nevi, at least early in their evolution. The extent of cutaneous involvement in AIDS-associated KS may not correlate well with the presence of visceral tumor. Morbidity from this variant is considerable, but, because of the many other medical problems seen in AIDS patients, they often die from opportunistic infections or other complications instead of KS.[376-378]

The histological features of KS are identical in all of its clinical forms.[376] In early or *patch-stage* lesions, one sees an irregular dermal proliferation of jagged thin-walled vascular channels that are lined by a single layer of endothelium (Fig. 8.71). These dissect through collagen and partially encircle pre-existing vessels and adnexal structures in the corium. Those structures often protrude into the lumina of the neovascular channels, yielding the so-called 'promontory sign.' Lesional endothelial cells contain scant cytoplasm and have hyperchromatic nuclei, but there is little nuclear atypia. Scattered collections of peritumoral lymphocytes and plasma cells are often present in the dermis. Extravasated erythrocytes and deposits of hemosiderin are frequently deposited around neoplastic vessels in more advanced histological forms of KS, in which spindle cells become increasingly prominent. The *plaque stage* of KS features the presence of cellular fascicles with a largely spindle cell composition; the tumor cells are relatively uniform and manifest modest nuclear atypia. Intracytoplasmic and extracellular hyaline eosinophilic globules are commonly found in this lesional variant; they are PAS-positive and represent red blood cell fragments that have been phagocytosed (Fig. 8.72).[379] The *nodular stage* of KS is characterized by a mass of fusiform neoplastic cells which form interlacing bundles. Slit-like spaces are scattered throughout the tumor, yielding a sieve-like appearance. Although the spindle cells do not manifest marked nuclear atypia, mitotic figures are easily found. Hyaline globules, extravasated red blood cells, and hemosiderin deposits are also notable at this stage.[380]

The immunohistochemical characteristics of Kaposi's sarcoma have been variable in reported series on this tumor. In general, positivity for CD34 and CD31 is demonstrable in the patch stage of KS, with lesser labeling of the spindle cells of nodular tumors.[381] Some studies have claimed to show focal labeling of KS for factor VIII-related antigen (von Willebrand factor).[382] However, that has not been our experience with this neoplasm. Indeed, more than an occasional case of spindle cell KS is completely nonreactive for all endothelial markers. A much more helpful immunohistologic diagnostic marker is represented by anti-human herpesvirus-8 latent nuclear antigen-1. It is present in virtually all examples of KS but is lacking in morphologic simulants of that tumour.[382a,382b]

Early lesions of KS are often subtle and must be separated from benign entities such as telangiectasias, pigmented purpuric dermatoses, and acroangiodermatitis. Vascular channels in patch-stage KS tend to have a more irregular and less well-formed appearance in comparison with those of benign proliferations. A plasma cell-rich inflammatory infiltrate is also much more frequently seen in KS. KS lesions with a predominant spindle cell component can imitate cutaneous smooth muscle tumors, dermatofibromas, proliferating scars, and spindle cell hemangiomas.[346,383] In general, the presence of slit-like vascular channels and hyaline globules strongly favors a diagnosis of KS in that specific context.

Cutaneous angiosarcomas comprise three distinct clinical subtypes. *Idiopathic cutaneous angiosarcoma* typically manifests itself as violaceous plaques involving the upper face or scalp in elderly patients. This lesion often has vague macroscopic borders and areas of

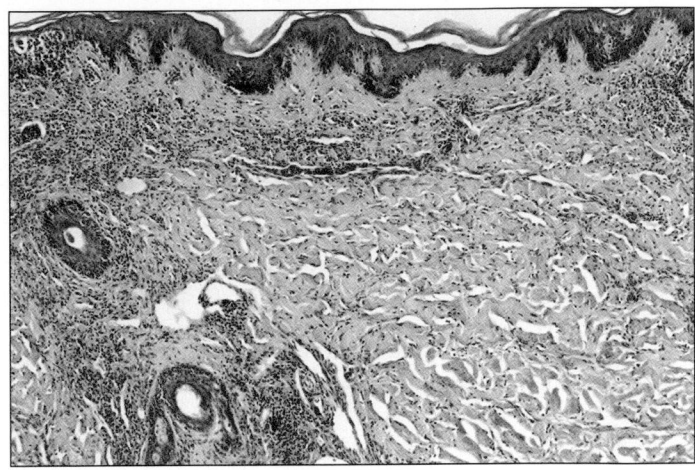

Fig. 8.71 Kaposi's sarcoma, patch stage. Jagged thin-walled vascular channels lined by a single layer of endothelium dissect through collagen and partially encircle pre-existing vessels and adnexal structures in the dermis. A single pre-existing vascular structure protrudes into the lumin of a neovascular channel (promontory sign) on the left side of the photomicrograph.

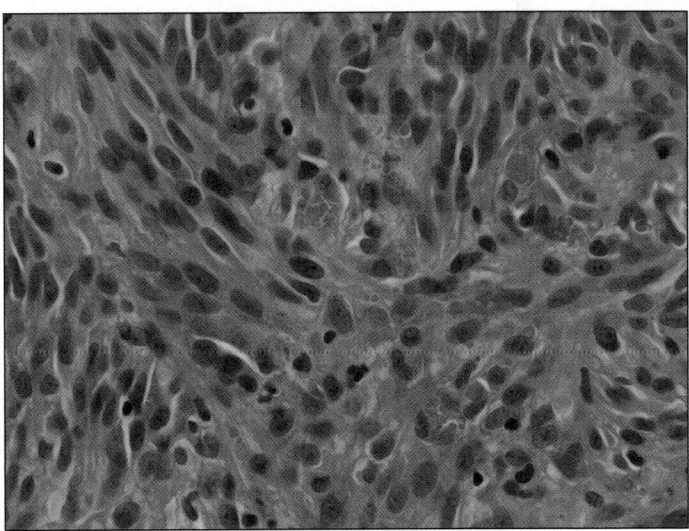

Fig. 8.72 Kaposi's sarcoma. Both plaque and nodular stages feature the presence of cellular fascicles with a largely spindle-cell composition. The tumor cells are relatively uniform and manifest modest nuclear atypia. Intracytoplasmic and extracellular hyaline globules are prominent in this case.

discontinuous cutaneous growth, making frozen section evaluation of surgical margins nearly impossible. Metastasis to regional lymph nodes or the lungs often becomes evident even if treatment has apparently eradicated the primary tumor.[384] Accordingly, long-term prognosis is poor. In one study, 50% of patients died within 15 months of presentation and only 12% survived for >5 years.[385]

Angiosarcoma arising in chronic lymphedema was first described by Stewart and Treves in 1948.[386] Their series documented a group of women who had undergone radical mastectomy and developed subsequent chronic edema in the ipsilateral arm. The development of purple macular or polypoid tumors was seen in those extremities

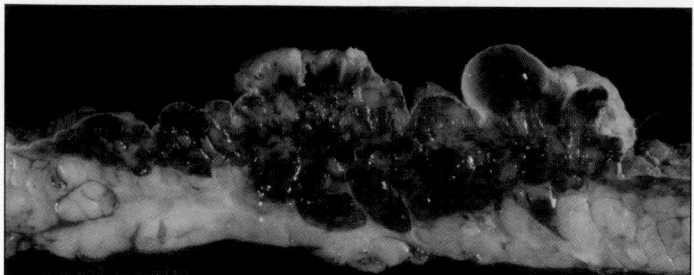

Fig. 8.73 Cutaneous angiosarcoma. This cut section surgical specimen, from an irradiated skin field, displays tumor nodules protruding above the skin surface and invading the subcutis. (Courtesy of Dr. Todd E. Abbott)

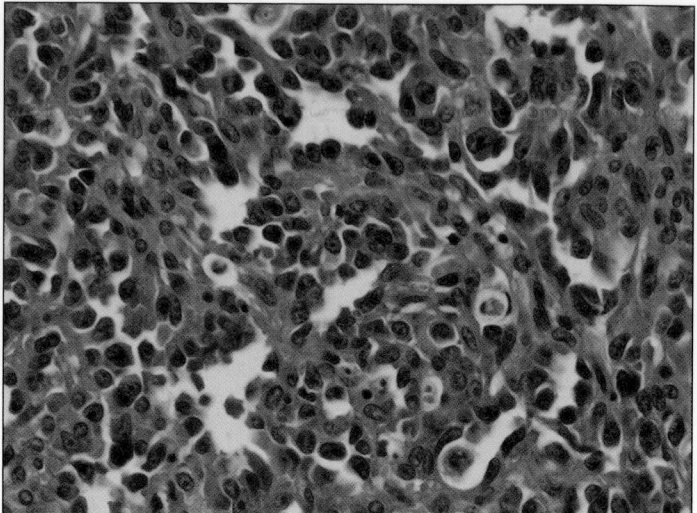

Fig. 8.75 Cutaneous angiosarcoma. Poorly differentiated angiosarcomas may display fusiform cells and a decrease in the number of obvious vascular channels. The nuclei are often pleomorphic and densely hyperchromatic.

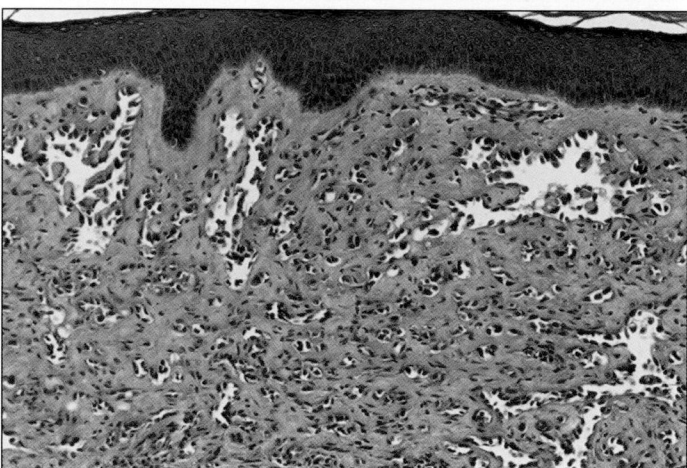

Fig. 8.74 Cutaneous angiosarcoma, well differentiated. Irregular neovascular channels dissect through the dermal collagen in a complex interanastomosing pattern.

at an average of 12.5 years after surgery. Similar angiosarcomas may occur in congenital lymphedema (Milroy's disease) and in other conditions causing long-term lymphatic stasis.[387,388] However, for unknown reasons, angiosarcoma rarely occurs in the setting of chronic filarial lymphedema.[389]

Postirradiation angiosarcomas are rare and often present after periods of 'latency' after therapy has been completed. Such lesions are most common following irradiation for malignant tumors of various types (Fig. 8.73).[390] There are also reports of angiosarcomas in a skin field that had harbored a benign hemangioma which had been irradiated. The prognosis for this tumor variant is poor, with a 5-year survival rate of 10%.[391]

Histologically, all of the aforementioned angiosarcoma subtypes are identical. Neovascular channels that dissect through the dermal collagen are common to all of them, regardless of their level of differentiation. Tumor vessels show irregular outlines and a complex interanastomosing ('racemose') pattern (Fig. 8.74). Nuclei of the neoplastic endothelial cells usually are hyperchromatic, with pleomorphism and mitotic activity. Although cytoplasm is scant in most tumor cells, some contain cytoplasmic vacuoles that probably reflect the presence of primitive vascular lumina. 'Piling up' of the neoplastic cells, with the formation of intravascular tufts or papillae, is seen more often in well-differentiated angiosarcoma than in anaplastic versions of that neoplasm. A peritumoral lymphocytic

infiltrate may also be apparent in such tumors. In poorly differentiated angiosarcomas the neoplastic cells may become fusiform, and the number of obvious vascular channels decreases. Nuclei in high-grade tumors are often pleomorphic and densely hyperchromatic (Fig. 8.75). Some angiosarcomas may be so anaplastic that they simulate such pleomorphic soft tissue tumors as malignant fibrous histiocytoma.[392] An epithelioid variant of angiosarcoma has also been well described in the skin, and it is capable of simulating carcinoma or melanoma histologically.

Immunohistochemical markers of endothelial differentiation, including CD34, CD31, factor VIII-related antigen, and *Ulex europaeus*-I lectin, have been used to distinguish angiosarcomas from their microscopic simulators.[393] The most sensitive and specific among these is CD31. However, it is wisest to utilize a panel of immunostains that includes antibodies to pankeratin and S-100 protein, as well as several endothelial determinants. In that regard, it must be remembered that a minority of angiosarcomas aberrantly expresses keratin proteins; these are usually epithelioid variants.[394] In the absence of positivity for CD31 or CD34, that immunophenotypic peculiarity could result in misdiagnosis of angiosarcoma as pseudovascular squamous cell carcinoma.

The distinction between malignant tumors with blood vessel differentiation (angiosarcoma) and lymphatic vessel differentiation (lymphangiosarcoma) is difficult given that both tumors may stain for endothelial markers CD31, CD34, and Ulex europaeus-I lectin.[108] Although some studies have shown that the immunohistochemical marker vascular endothelial growth factor receptor 3 (VEGFR 3) selectively labels tumors with lymphatic differentiation,[360] others have refuted this finding.[363] We believe it is best to consider these two tumors as part of a spectrum of malignant lesions with endothelial differentiation.

MELANOCYTIC PROLIFERATIONS

Melanocytes historically have been thought to derive embryologically from the neural crest, and they serve the primary function of pigment

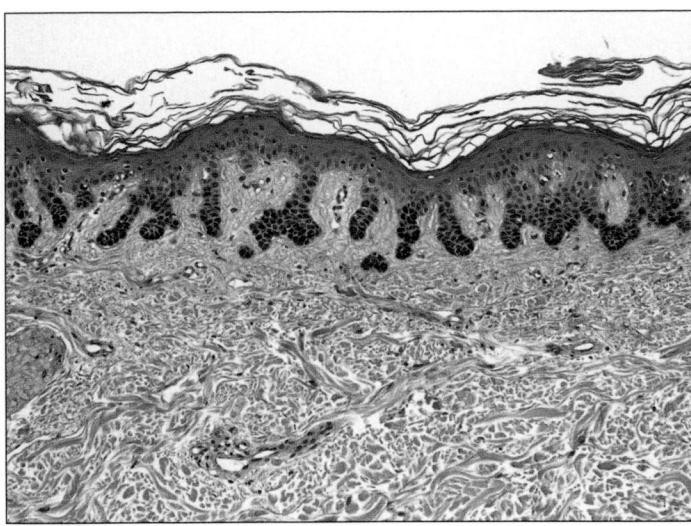

Fig. 8.76 Note the lack of nevocyte nesting in this lentigo simplex. The almost reticular retia elongation may prompt the designation of solar lentigo by some.

production in the skin via the development of cytoplasmic organelles called melanosomes. The dendritic processes of melanocytes intercalate among the epidermal keratinocytes; the former of those cells are located in the basal epidermis in a ratio of 1 melanocyte per 5 to 10 adjacent keratinocytes. Classification of melanocytic disorders includes some diseases featuring abnormal quantities of intracellular pigment, and others in which melanocytic proliferation is dominant. It is the latter of those categories that will be considered in this chapter. In the following discussion, the term 'nevus' will be used colloquially (as in common medical practice) to refer to a *melanocytic* nevus. We have made that specific qualification because the true definition of 'nevus' is much broader and includes hamartomatous proliferations of several cell types.[395]

Benign melanocytic lesions other than 'nevi'

Lentigo simplex is not congenital but usually begins its development in early childhood on sun-exposed skin surfaces. Unlike ephelides ('freckles;' macules reflecting sun-induced hypermelaninization rather than melanocytic proliferation), lentigos persist throughout life. Their clinical appearance is that of a hyperpigmented tan or brown macule, measuring up to several millimeters in diameter. Multiple lentigines may be seen in some syndromic conditions including the LEOPARD complex and Carney's syndrome. Microscopically, one observes hyperpigmentation in linear arrangements of melanocytes along the basal epidermis that are quantitatively increased over those of the normal skin. This particular constellation of findings, with no nesting of melanocytes, is what distinguishes lentigos from junctional nevi (Fig. 8.76). Associated findings include elongation of the rete ridges and slight epidermal acanthosis.

Labial and genital melanotic macules arise on the vermilion borders of the lips and the vulvar or penile skin, respectively. Conceptually, they also represent a type of clinical lentigo, but most quantitative studies have shown no clear augmentation in the number of melanocytes.[396,397] Melanotic macules are typically 1–2 mm in diameter; they remain stable for long periods of time and show no relationship to melanoma.[396,398,399] Histologically, one sees more pronounced elongation of the rete ridges than that of lentigo simplex,

but comparable basal epidermal hyperpigmentation. Melanophages in the dermis are more common in genital macules than in lesions of the lip.[397]

Solar (senile) lentigo shows a strong association with sun exposure and therefore features the regular presence of dermal elastosis. It exhibits melanocytic hyperpigmentation as well as a conjoint proliferation of both keratinocytes and melanocytes. The former of those cell types additionally manifests nuclear atypia that is similar to that of AK. Indeed, 'pigmented actinic keratosis' is regarded as a synonym for solar lentigo by many observers.

Speckled lentiginous nevus (also known as *nevus spilus*) is a flat patch of slight hyperpigmentation with superimposed punctate brown macules. Histologically, the basic lesion resembles lentigo simplex but with a superimposition of junctional or compound melanocytic nevi in those areas that represent the darker macules at a macroscopic level.[400]

Melanocytic nevi

Although lentigo technically could be considered a type of nevus, the latter term is usually restricted to those melanocytic proliferations that contain overt nests of melanocytes microscopically. The most common nevi are usually acquired in childhood, although some may be present at birth. These lesions progressively mature through junctional, compound, and intradermal stages. Nevi typically decrease in number with increasing age of the host, because of tumor involution or extrusion through the skin surface as 'pseudoacrochordons.' Their incidence is directly related to sun exposure in childhood or adolescence,[401–404] but they may occur in any skin region.

The *junctional nevus* is a flat or slightly raised brown macule with a melanocyte proliferation that is confined to the dermal—epidermal junction with a proclivity towards nesting at the tips of rete ridges (Fig. 8.77A). Individual cells are rounded with pericellular clear zones that are seen because of cytoplasmic retraction from surrounding keratinocytes. Although they are typically larger than normal melanocytes, the cells of junctional nevi show no nuclear atypia. Small nucleoli and rare mitoses, however, may be present. An association of junctional nevus with lentigo simplex is recognized in some cases, and hybrid tumors are common, with morphologic features that bridge those entities.[405] These have been called *nevoid lentigo* and *lentiginous junctional nevus*.[406]

Mechanisms of nevus cell descent *from* the epidermis or upward migration from the corium *into* the epidermis have been proposed for development of *compound nevi* (CN). In those lesions, dermal nevus cells are present in addition to a junctional component (Fig. 8.77B).[407–410] Clinical palpability and diminished pigmentation accompany the development of dermal growth. As true of their putative predecessor lesions (junctional nevi), CN are small and a diameter >5–7 mm is unusual.[410] The junctional melanocytes in CN are arranged in cords as well as small nests, and are usually dispersed in a symmetrical fashion throughout the lesion. Smaller cell size and decreased pigment content characterize the nevus cells in CN as one progresses from top to bottom in the dermis. If dermal mitoses are present at all, they should be limited to 1 or 2 in the entire nevus.

CN in selected anatomical sites often show unusual or atypical morphological features, and these may raise concern over the biological potential of such lesions. At this point, however, so many cutaneous fields have been associated with these 'privileged' nevi that their identity as distinct entities is in question. They have been recognized in the genital, acral,[411–413] flexural,[414] palmoplantar,[415,416] nail-matrical,[417] and periumbilical skin. Nevi that arise during pregnancy or adolescence have also demonstrated similar histological

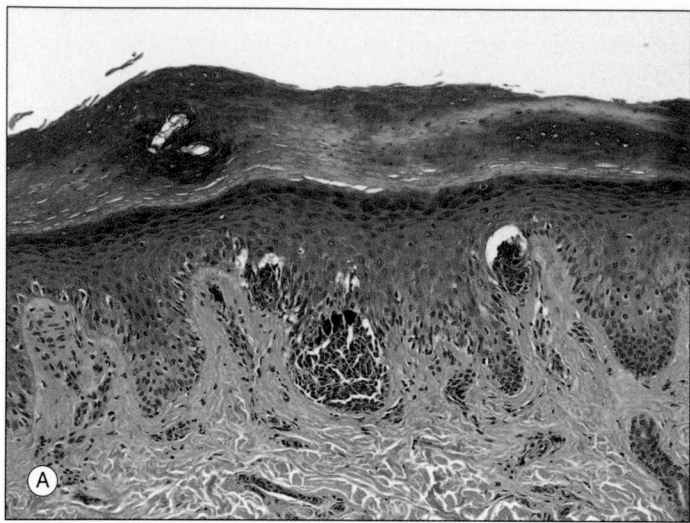
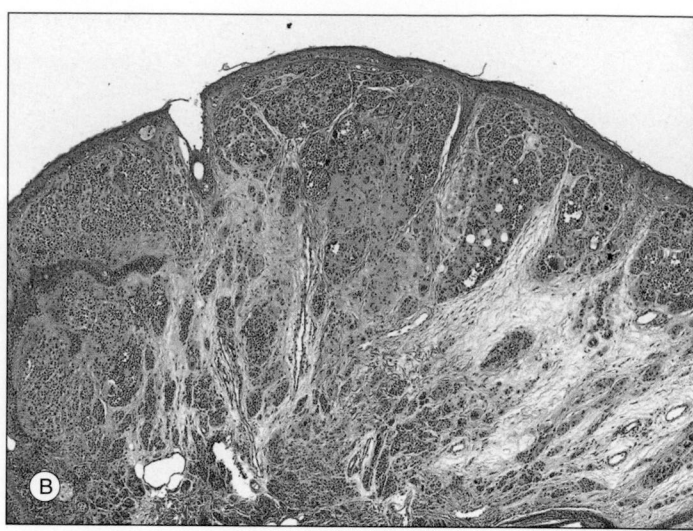

Fig. 8.77 Unlike this purely nested junctional nevus most contain a lentiginous component (**A**); a tumor combining this junctional process with an intradermal component is a compound nevus (**B**).

features.[418] Such changes include an increase in the size of individual melanocytes, irregular sizes and shapes of nevocytic nests, pagetoid spread of melanocytes within the epidermis, and limited intercellular dyshesion. Asymmetry of the lesions and fusion of junctional nests may be seen, but dermal fibroplasia is lacking in 'privileged' CN.[411]

In the *intradermal nevus* (IDN) there is a complete absence of junctional melanocytic nests. This nevus type is represented by a papule or nodule that may be pedunculated, and constituent dermal nevocytes have a banal appearance. The presence of multinucleated melanocytes in the dermis is common, and, unlike similar cells at the dermal—epidermal junction, they are reassuring of the benignancy of the lesion. Involutional changes commonly occur as an IDN ages, including neurotization[419] (metaplasia towards neural tissue), as well as dermal sclerosis and replacement of the melanocytes by fat or fibroelastic tissue.[420–422]

Congenital nevi

The entity of *congenital nevus* (CGN) deserves separate consideration because of its capacity to attain a large size and pose a cosmetic problem. Moreover, a selected subset of congenital nevi (CGN) may have an increased risk of malignant transformation. Small lesions in this category (<1.5 cm in diameter) and those of intermediate size (1.5–19.9 cm) probably have no greater incidence of melanomatous change than do ordinary nevi.[423,424] CGN with a definite risk of that eventuality are those over 20 cm in diameter or which cover at least 5% of the body surface area.[425,426] Malignant melanoma develops in approximately 4–10 % of these large or 'giant' CGN. When considering such data, however, one must be aware that benign but pseudomelanomatous proliferations may be seen in CGN as well.[427] The only completely reliable indicator of a congenital nature for any given nevus is its presence by visual inspection at birth.[428,429]

Histological indicators of CGN, however, do exist; these are principally represented by interdigitation of nevus cells with the epithelial cells of appendageal structures.[430] Involvement of neurovascular bundles and the subcutaneous tissue may also be seen, but those findings are less specific diagnostically.[429,431] Approximately 10% of CGN show atypical features that include asymmetry, growth of junctional nevocytic nests outside the confines of the dermal

melanocytic population, upward epidermal 'migration' of nevocytes, dermal fibroplasias, and cytological atypia. These should not be interpreted as evidence of malignancy.[432] Indeed, in our experience, CGN that undergo true malignant transformation evolve into highly anaplastic versions of melanoma that do not pose diagnostic problems.

Spitz (spindle-cell and epithelioid-cell) nevus

Dr. Sophie Spitz originally described *Spitz nevus* (SN) as 'juvenile melanoma' in 1948.[433] Up to that time, this lesion was often mistaken, both histologically and clinically, for malignant melanoma.[434] The term 'spindle-cell and epithelioid-cell nevus' is synonymous with Spitz nevus and is more descriptive of the entity.[434–436] SN is classically a rapidly growing, pink or tan papule on the face of a child or adolescent (Fig. 8.78A),[436] but pigmentation and a truncal location are more common in older patients.[437,438] Multiple or agminate lesions also occur.[439] After the age of 25 years, the incidence of SN decreases progressively. Accordingly, extreme caution is advised before making such a diagnosis in a patient over 60.

Overall architectural symmetry and circumscription are maintained in SN, which is usually a wedge-shaped proliferation of melanocytes with its base at the dermal—epidermal junction (Fig. 8.79A). The majority of Spitz nevi are compound, but purely junctional and intradermal forms occur. The former of those tumor types is probably equivalent to '*pigmented spindle-cell nevus of Reed*' (see below). Accompanying epidermal hyperplasia[440] often envelops nevocytic nests in SN; the keratinocytes that interface with such nests show a peculiar but reproducible tendency to pull away from them, producing artifactual clefts. One also may see basal epidermal deposits of eosinophilic basement membrane material that are known as 'Kamino bodies'[441–443] in SN (Fig. 8.79B). Although they are common, such structures are not uniformly present in Spitz nevi and may also be seen in melanomas. Individual cells in SN are either epithelioid, with abundant pale eosinophilic cytoplasm, or spindle shaped. They form nests at the dermal—epidermal junction, from which spindle cell fascicles often descend in a 'raining-down' fashion (Fig. 8.79B). Both epithelioid and fusiform cells in SN are larger than the elements of

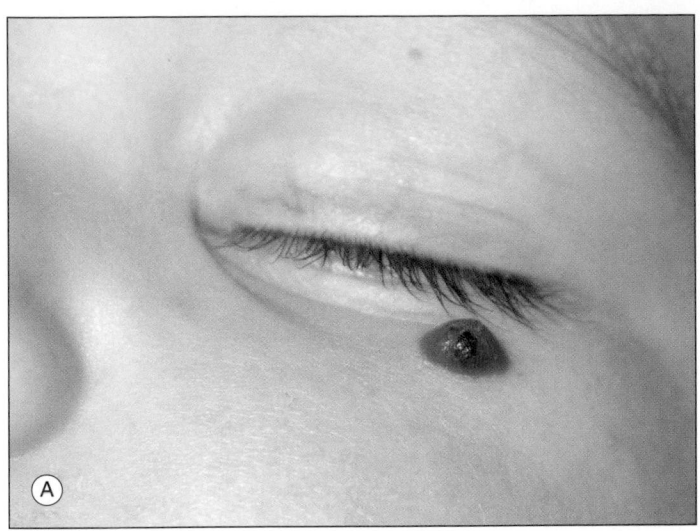
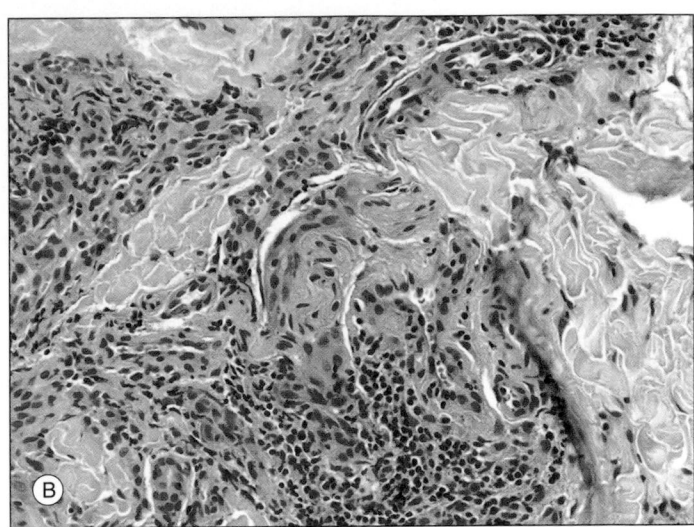

Fig. 8.78 A, Spitz nevus with ulceration in a 19-month-old female. Hemangioma was favored by the clinician; **B**, Perineural invasion was seen within the deep corium adjacent to subcuticular tumor extension.

ordinary nevi. Moreover, the dermal component in SN shows characteristic single-cell infiltration of the stromal collagen at the base of the tumor. Cells with nuclear atypia and mitoses are typically confined to the superficial aspects of Spitz nevi (Fig. 8.79C).[412,438,444] Invasion of adnexal, vascular, and neural structures by the nevocytes in this lesion is an uncommon but acceptable finding, as is multinucleation of constituent cells (see Fig. 8.79B).[445] When stromal fibrosis or hyalinization in SN is extensive, the term *sclerotic Spitz nevus* is preferred. The word 'desmoplastic' should be avoided diagnostically in that context, to avoid confusion with desmoplastic melanoma.[446,447]

Pigmented spindle cell nevus of Reed has been regarded as a distinct entity by some,[448–450] or a variant of Spitz nevus by others.[424] It is a darkly pigmented papule, usually seen on the proximal extremities of young women. Histologically, the junctional component in this tumor type comprises interconnected fascicles of spindle cells that form a broad shelf-like base. Dermal involvement, when it is present at all, is usually superficial. Dense pigmentation is distributed uniformly throughout the tumor and is a consistent feature of it. Symmetry, circumscription, possible focal cytological atypia, the potential presence of Kamino bodies, and junctional clefts with adjacent keratinocytes may be encountered in Reed's nevus as well as SN.[450,451]

In adult patients, the diagnostic separation of SN and melanoma can be extremely difficult or impossible in selected cases.[452] When melanomas exhibit Spitz-like features, particular attention must be given to asymmetry, deep mitotic activity, the presence of fine ('dusty') cytoplasmic pigment, and uniform nuclear atypia as indicators of the malignant potential of such neoplasms.[452,453] A progressive decrease in cell size as the tumor 'descends' into the dermis ('maturational descent') is variably present in 'Spitzoid' melanomas, but is certainly more typical of SN.[454,455] In those instances where one is uncertain of malignancy despite meticulous microscopic study, the diagnostic term *atypical melanocytic neoplasm with features of Spitz nevus* is recommended, in lieu of 'probable Spitz nevus' or 'atypical Spitz nevus.'[456,457] The first of those designations correctly implies that the biological potential is unknown, and that fact should be further specified in a comment in the surgical pathology report. Accordingly, excision should be done as if the tumor were indeed malignant. Another term, '*malignant Spitz nevus*,' has been used for tumors that resemble SN but which are >1 cm in diameter with more extensive cellular pleomorphism, deeper intradermal growth, and more widespread mitotic activity. These have a capacity for regional lymph node metastasis,[458] and, in our view, should more properly be regarded as outright melanomas and designated as such.

Blue nevus

Blue nevus (BN) most often occurs in childhood on the distal extremities, as a blue or black papule or macule that measures <5 mm.[459] Infrequently, multiple lesions comprise a confluent plaque or form an agminate congerie, and sizes up 24 cm have been reported.[460] The epithelioid cell variant of BN has an association with Carney's syndrome,[461,462] including ephelides, endocrine overactivity, and myxomas of the skin, heart, and soft tissue. Although conventional nevus cells are polyhedral or rounded and grow in a nesting pattern, individual cells in BN maintain a dendritic configuration and are dispersed singly or in small groups through the dermal interstitium. Long, slender cell processes with heavy pigmentation are typical of this tumor (Fig. 8.80), but recognition of BN may be more difficult in its hypopigmented forms; indeed, the differential diagnosis of dermatofibroma is often erroneously favored for such lesions in the absence of immunohistologic data.[463–465] Rarely, a junctional nevocytic component is seen over BN.[466] Progressive dermal sclerosis over time eventually may result in hypocellular fibrotic replacement of the lesional melanocytes in this tumor type.

Conversely, small areas of hypercellularity in BN[467] should not be equated with a diagnosis of '*cellular*' blue nevus. That distinctive entity most often is seen on the dorsal feet or buttocks as a multinodular mass averaging 1.8 cm in diameter; it shows greater variability in pigmentation than does typical BN.[468] Microscopically, cellular BN is lobulated or dumbbell-shaped, with deep dermal extension and bulbous encroachment into the subcutaneous fat.[460] Individual tumor cells in this neoplastic variant are plump with an epithelioid or fusiform appearance. Areas of striking cellularity may be seen, causing alarm over the possibility of malignancy. Nevertheless, only those lesions with numerous deep mitotic figures,

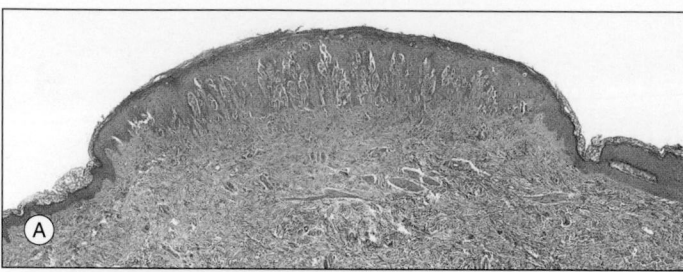

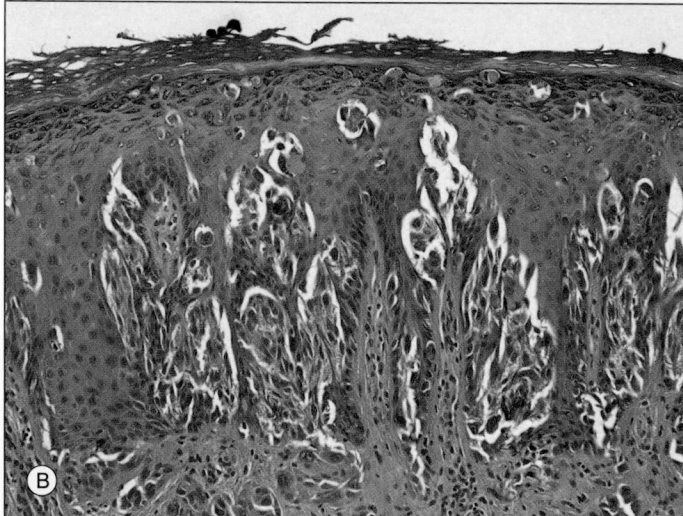

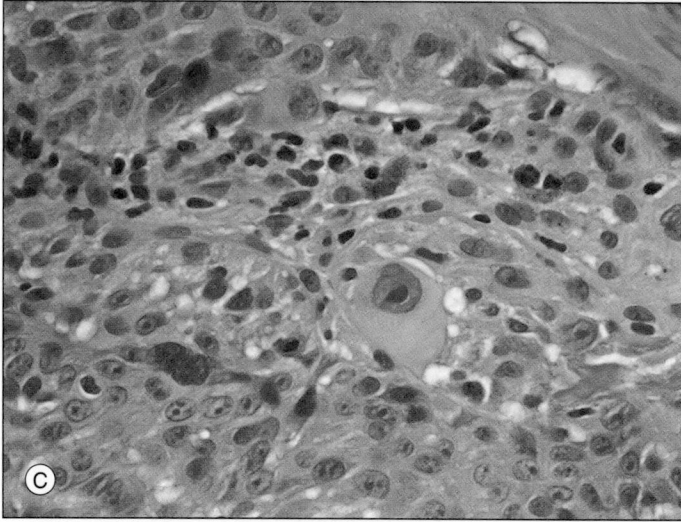

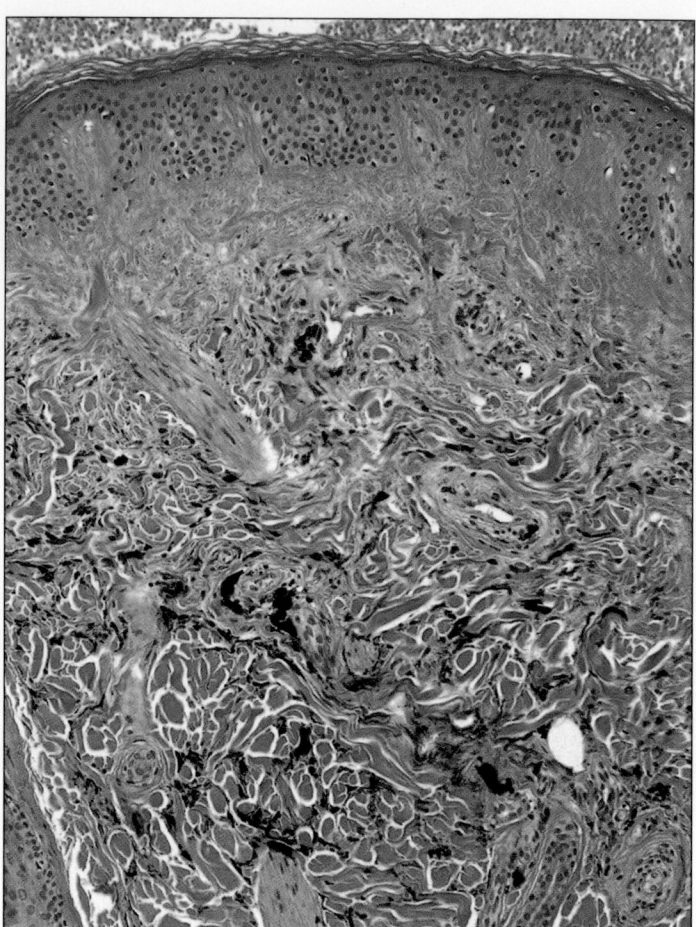

Fig. 8.79 Spitz nevus. **A**, Small size, symmetry, and circumscription are important features in distinction from melanoma; **B**, Other delineations include Kamino bodies and a raining-like descent of spindle cells; **C**, Cellular atypia may be striking.

Fig. 8.80 On first glance blue nevus may be mistaken for melanin incontinence, but the long, slender, dendritic, melanocytic processes and deep nevus extension are distinctive.

marked global nuclear atypia, or necrosis qualify for a diagnosis of *malignant blue nevus*.[469]

Atypical ('dysplastic;' architecturally-disordered) melanocytic nevus

Clark introduced the term 'dysplastic nevus' over two decades ago to denote a clinically and histologically distinct form of melanocytic lesion that occurred in patients who were felt to have an increased risk of melanoma. He described individuals with the familial

occurrence of multiple nevi as a part of the '*B-K mole syndrome*,' named after the two probands. The term '*dysplastic nevus syndrome*' has subsequently been used in reference to patients with similar lesions in both familial *and* nonfamilial settings.[470–473] Although an increased risk of melanoma in families with 'atypical moles' is generally accepted,[474,475] the chance of that malignancy developing in a patient with multiple sporadic lesions of this kind remains largely undetermined.[424,476] Similarly, little is known concerning the risk of melanoma in individuals with a *single* dysplastic nevus; reports favoring[477–480] and denying[473,481] such an association are both well represented in the pertinent literature.

Based on this controversy, and the observation that the term 'dysplasia' is used in other organs for lesions with an indisputable linkage to malignancy, a Consensus Conference convened at the US National Institutes of Health in 1992 recommended that the melanocytic lesions in question should be called 'atypical nevi' clinically and reported pathologically as 'nevi with architectural disorder,' with comments regarding the presence and significance of any cytological atypia.[482] *Clark's nevus* has been proposed as an alternative name for the lesion as well.[483,484]

Atypical nevi are usually somewhat larger than conventional nevi, and the former have irregular borders and show internal variation in color. Histologically, atypical nevi are usually compound lesions, although both junctional and intradermal variants do occur. Some investigators apply rigid criteria with requisite architectural *and* cytological atypia before rendering a diagnosis of atypical nevus.[424,485,486] Because of the significant variability of morphologic features in individual lesions of this type, we prefer a more flexible approach following the recommendations of the NIH Consensus Conference. An interpretation is made that includes the general type of nevus being studied (compound, etc.) along with a comment detailing the particular architectural and cytological changes that are present.

The assessment of architectural disorder should first include attention to lesional symmetry and peripheral circumscription. Varying degrees of nevus cell proliferation in lentiginous, nested, or spindle cell patterns are combined with extension and fusion of rete ridges (Fig. 8.81A), and bridging of melanocytic groups in the rete. There is a tendency in atypical nevi for the growth of nevus cell nests between the rete and along their lateral aspects, contrasting with the image of banal nevi in which nevocytic groups favor the tips of the rete. 'Shouldering' in architecturally disordered nevi (ADN) is represented by the extension of junctional melanocytes beyond the peripheral margins of the dermal component of the lesion, usually greater than three rete ridges away, but this is not a mandatory component of the lesion.[487,488] Dermal stromal fibroplasia is always apparent, taking the form of plate-like lamellar deposition of collagen immediately below the basal epidermis, or concentric fibrosis (Fig. 8.81B) around the tips of the rete with an eosinophilic or hyaline appearance.[489] A modest lymphocytic host response is often present in ADN. Architectural disorder may also be appreciated in their dermal components, where nevocytic nests are seen that are larger than their junctional counterparts.[490–495]

Cytological atypia principally appears as nuclear enlargement to a size over that of the nuclei in basal keratinocytes.[490] Other changes include cytomegaly in the constituent nevocytes, assumption of an epithelioid appearance, and nuclear hyperchromasia with occasionally prominent nucleoli. Scattered multinucleated nevocytes may be present in the basal epidermis, but if these are numerous, serious consideration should be given to a diagnosis of melanoma *in situ* (Fig. 8.81C). Dusty cytoplasmic pigmentation is another potentially identifying feature of ADN. Atypical cells in these lesions are usually randomly situated throughout, in contrast to their confluence in melanoma in situ. Grading of nuclear atypia in ADN has been proposed as useful in some publications, but is not generally done.[471]

In a recent survey conducted by the American Academy of Dermatologists the majority of respondents treated 'dysplastic nevi'/ADN by complete surgical removal with a <2 mm margin, although larger excisions were sometimes done depending on the presence of 'histological atypia.'[496] More comprehensive data on this point are unavailable, however, to indicate whether this approach in any way alters the risk of melanoma in patients with ADN.[497]

Other nevus variants

Recurrent or *persistent nevus* ('nevus recurrens;' 'nevus perstans') simply represents a nevocytic lesion that has been incompletely excised, usually because of the abominable, but, unfortunately, common practice of doing shave or punch biopsies of pigmented skin lesions.[498,499] The typical morphologic form of these proliferations is that of a junctional and partially confluent proliferation of atypical nevocytes that is separated by scar tissue from a blander dermal component. Similar atypical cells may also be entrapped in the scar. The overall image of nevus recurrens may be sufficiently atypical that melanoma is a real consideration.[500,501] However, dense pigmentation of the junctional component in that tumor type is a

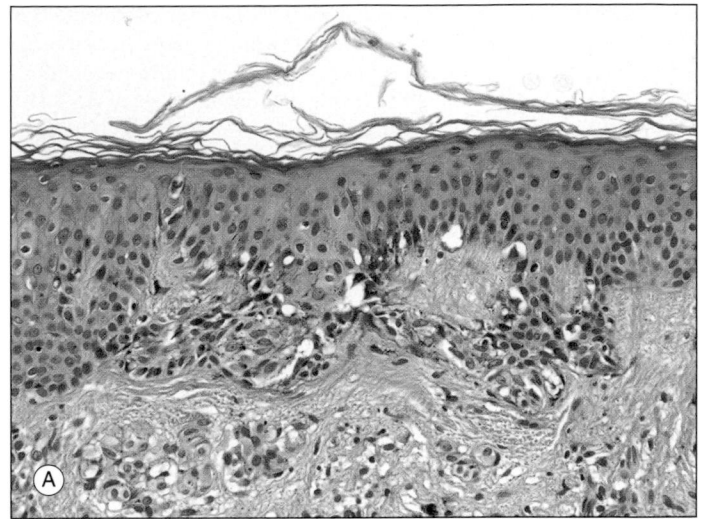

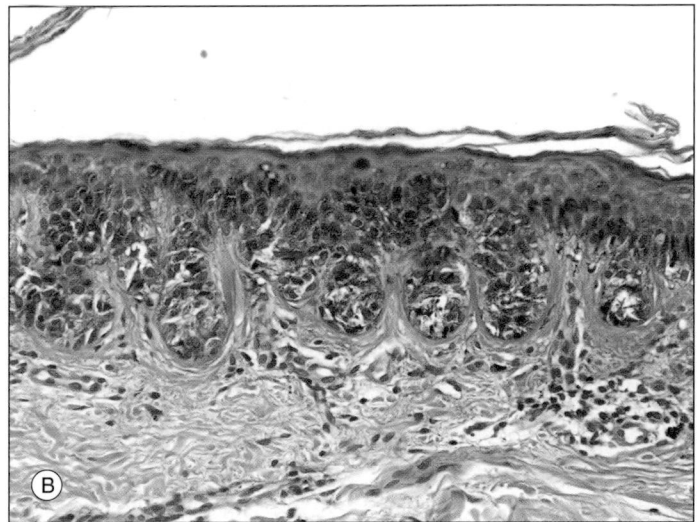

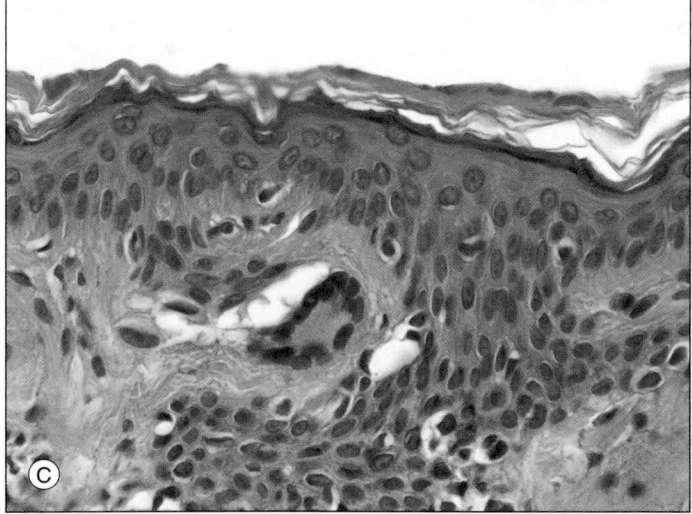

Fig. 8.81 Atypical nevi. (**A**) Retia fusion and (**B**) concentric eosinophilic fibroplasia are features of architectural disorder in these junctional and compound nevi, respectively. In addition to atypical nevi (**C**) junctional melanocytic florets may be present in malignant melanoma.

histologic clue to its proper recognition, as is strict confinement of the atypical junctional cells to the area over the dermal component of the neoplasm. Obviously, a history of surgery for a nevus at the anatomic site in question is invaluable diagnostically.

Halo nevus, which was first described by Sutton,[502] is a clinically distinct lesion that is characterized by a circumferential zone of hypopigmentation around a conventional nevus. The latter phenomenon is thought to reflect an antibody- and cell-mediated host response to the melanocytic tumor,[503,504] and, as such, represents a form of involution. Halo change may be seen around several types of melanocytic tumors, including melanoma.[505–507]

Histologically, one sees a dense band of dermal lymphocytes around the nevocytic proliferation in halo nevus, admixed with pigmented macrophages and 'incontinent' pigment in the corium. As the lesion evolves, stromal fibrosis replaces the nevus cells and inflammation subsides. The number of melanocytes in the adjacent epidermis also decreases,[508] for unknown reasons. In the absence of a clinical halo, a lymphocyte infiltrate in nevi may be designated as a *halo-like phenomenon*. As mentioned earlier, a similar host response may be present in melanomas; however, in order to avoid overdiagnosis of the latter, it should be remembered that a limited degree of melanocytic atypia is seen in halo nevi as 'reactive' change attributable to the inflammation.[506]

'Balloon'-cell nevus denotes a lesion that is dominated by cytologically bland melanocytes with abundant, lucent, sometimes-vacuolated cytoplasm. A morphologic continuum can be recognized that links conventional nevi to 'balloon'-cell nevi, reinforcing a conviction that the former of those lesions represent a peculiar form of degenerative change rather than a distinct pathologic entity.[406,509]

Deep penetrating nevus (probably synonymous with *plexiform spindle cell nevus*) may attain a size of up to 3 cm in diameter and show pigmentary variegation. Both of those attributes can lead to a mistaken clinical diagnosis of melanoma. Considerable histological overlap exists between deep penetrating nevus (DPN) and other nevus morphotypes with a dominant dermal component. These include Spitz nevus, pigmented spindle cell nevus, and blue nevus.[510–512] DPN shows a wedge-shaped configuration on scanning microscopic examination, with its base at the dermal—epidermal junction (Fig. 8.82). It has a plexiform or fascicular growth pattern and shows irregular pigmentation. Constituent cells are compactly epithelioid or bluntly fusiform. Limited pagetoid spread of melanocytes may occasionally be observed over the dermal component of DPN, but nuclear atypia in the nevocytes and deep mitotic activity are lacking.

Dermal melanocytosis comprises a number of related clinical entities.[513,514] *Nevi of Ota*[515] *and Ito*[516] are two separate congenital melanocytic proliferations that are seen in the facial region and shoulder, respectively, usually in patients of Asian descent. Macrophages and dendritic melanocytes that are similar to those seen in blue nevus are present in the upper reticular dermis in those lesions.[517] Unlike the *Mongolian spot*, a histologically similar nevus with a predilection for the sacral skin of Asian individuals, nevi of Ota and Ito generally do not regress with age.[514]

Café-au-lait spots are found both sporadically and in patients who have neurofibromatosis (von Recklinghausen's disease).[518] A histological increase in intraepidermal pigment is more readily appreciated in such lesions than is melanocytosis.

Becker's nevus is usually encountered in adolescence; it is a 'nevus' only in the sense of being a hamartoma, but does not feature the presence of melanocytic nests. This lesion is typically seen on the shoulders of male patients as a hyperpigmented patch or plaque that is associated with 'pseudourtication' when scratched. Hypertrichosis is commonly seen in Becker's nevus, in contradistinction to the clinical

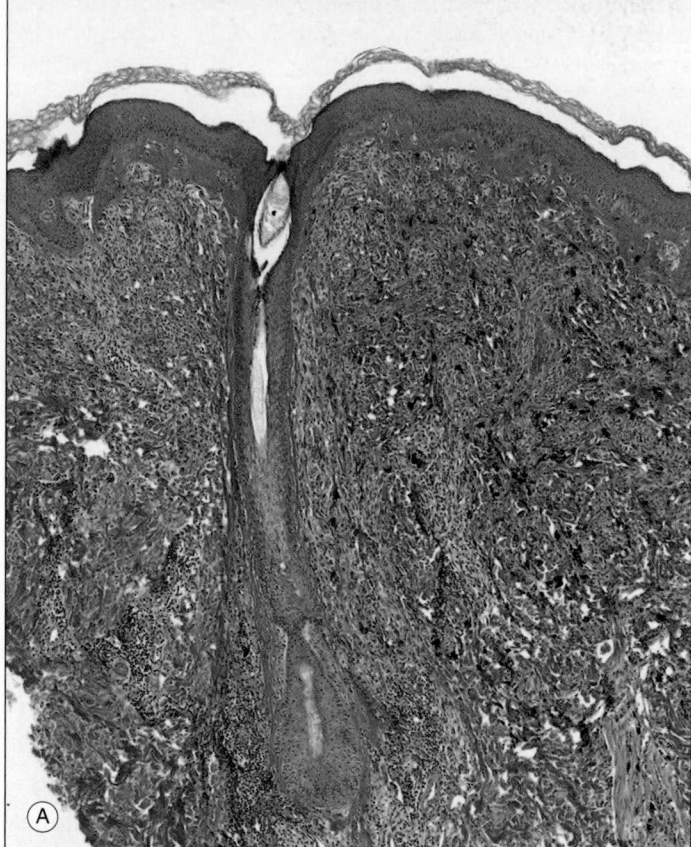

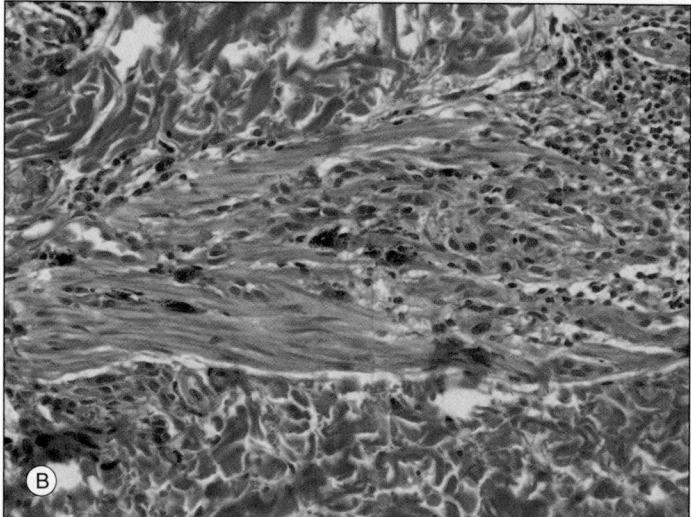

Fig. 8.82 A, Deep penetrating nevus with wedge-shaped fasicles; **B,** Adnexal involvement is common as seen here in this erector pilar muscle.

profile of congenital melanocytic nevus.[519,520] In addition, the former of those entities shows acanthosis and smooth muscle hyperplasia at a histological level.[521]

Malignant melanoma

Melanoma is a relatively infrequently seen tumor in the general population, being responsible for approximately 3% of cutaneous malignancies, but its aggressive behavior –accounting for 60% of all skin cancer-related deaths – makes it an extremely important entity.[522] The latter figure has declined somewhat in recent years, possibly relating to the earlier detection of melanoma,[523,524] but overall survival has not increased in a statistically significant manner.[525] As recently as 1994, the incidence of melanoma continued to rise worldwide. More recent analyses indicate a slight decrease, particularly among individuals in the third and fourth decades of life.[526,527] A clear relationship of melanomagenesis to sun exposure has been demonstrated, primarily in pale-skinned, light-haired persons. The number of acute episodes of sunburn is probably best associated with overall risk,[528–531] but chronic sun exposure may be contributory as well.[532–534] The association of melanoma with congenital and atypical nevi has been addressed previously in this discussion, as has the existence of families with a hereditary tendency to develop this neoplasm. The cyclin-dependent kinase inhibitor (2A-related protein) designated as 'p16,' which is encoded on chromosome 9, is structurally or functionally abnormal in a significant percentage of familial melanomas, and some sporadic tumors as well.[535–539]

Clinically, melanoma is most often a tumor of adults with an average patient age in the fourth decade. Only 0.3% to 0.9% of cases are seen in prepubescent patients.[540–542] Melanomas are characterized by *A*symmetry of the tumor, *B*order irregularity, *C*olor variegation, and *D*iameter >6 mm, commonly abbreviated as 'ABCD.'[543,544]

Melanoma in situ

There is general agreement that an atypical intraepidermal melanocytic proliferation precedes the development of invasive melanoma. Terms for this incipient stage have included *atypical melanocytic hyperplasia*, *severe melanocytic dysplasia*, *pagetoid melanocytosis*, *pagetoid melanocytic proliferation*, *precancerous melanosis*, and *dysplastic nevus*.[545,546] Today, the designation of *melanoma in situ* is preferred for intraepithelial lesions in which the degree of cytologic atypia and architectural distortion approximates that of invasive intradermal melanoma. In situ melanoma has the capacity in most cases for long-term persistence without invasion. For instance, the lifetime rate of progression of 'lentigo maligna' (see below; a particular clinical form of in situ melanoma) to invasive disease has been estimated at <5%.[547] Although controversy exists over the diagnostic criteria for melanoma in situ (MIS),[482,548–550] we make that interpretation for melanocytic proliferations that are limited to the epidermis and which show global nuclear atypia, at-least-regional cellular confluence, and areas of intercellular dyshesion.

Several patterns of cellular confluence are potentially seen in MIS. These include the fusion of adjacent melanocytic nests at the dermal—epidermal junction (DEJ), bridging of nests in adjacent rete ridges, arrays of single tumor cells extending along the DEJ and into dermal adnexae, or combinations thereof (Fig. 8.83). Another common feature is the random intraepidermal pagetoid spread of malignant cells that may reach the granular layer and stratum corneum. The presence of eosinophilic nucleoli with zones of lucency around them is also helpful in the recognition of cytologic atypia in MIS.

Lentigo maligna, originally called *Hutchinson's melanotic freckle* over 100 years ago,[551] may be conceptualized as a special type of MIS. It develops in sun-exposed skin, usually in elderly persons, and is typified by confluent basal epidermal single-cell melanocytic proliferation with little tendency towards nesting or pagetoid spread (Fig. 8.84). Multinucleated melanocytes with a 'floret'-like image are often seen at the dermal—epidermal junction, and the individual lesional melanocytes may be surprisingly bland.[552,553] Because the term 'lentigo maligna' is really a clinical one, we prefer the

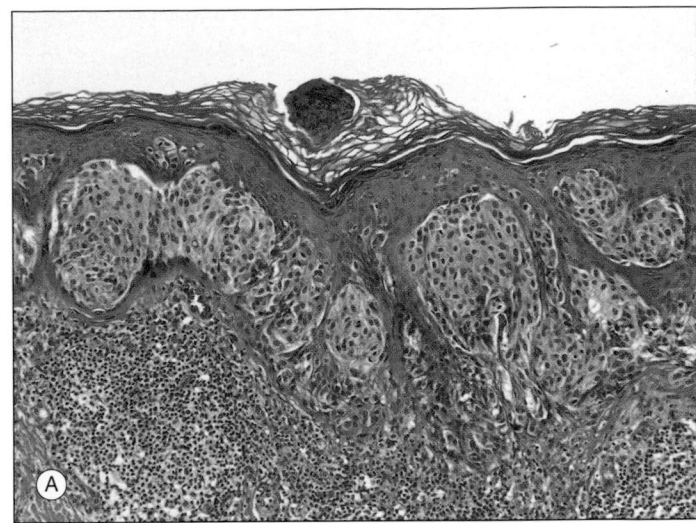

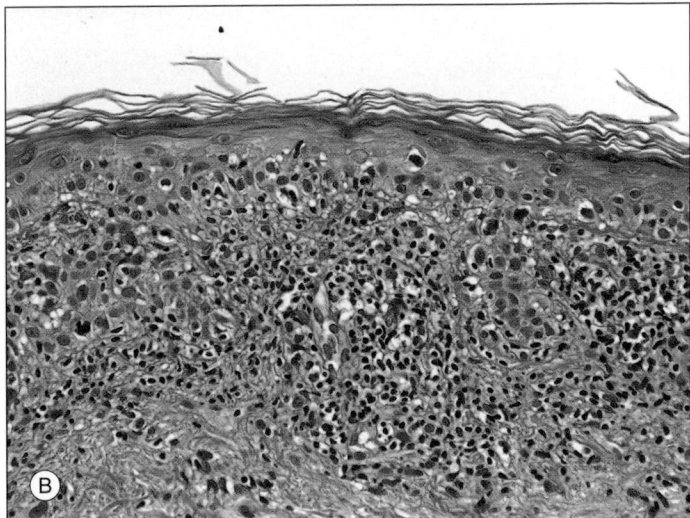

Fig. 8.83 Melanoma in situ. **A**, Nesting of malignant melanocytes is particularly prominent in this example; **B**, Close scrutiny is required to exclude invasion in the face of this lichenoid lymphocytic response.

designation of 'lentiginous MIS' to refer to tumors with the above-cited microscopic features.[554,555]

Invasive melanoma

The current classification of invasive melanoma is based on paradigms that were codified by Clark in 1969 and shortly afterwards by McGovern.[556,557] This approach relies largely on distinctions between patterns of epidermal and dermal involvement by any given tumor. In decreasing order of frequency, the major histologic types of invasive melanoma are superficial spreading, nodular, lentiginous, and acral-lentiginous. We agree with Ackerman and others that the clinical identification of these various types is difficult, if not impossible, and that similar divisions based on histopathology realistically have little if any prognostic significance.[558–561] Nevertheless, a traditional approach to this topic is used in the ensuing discussion.

Superficial spreading melanoma may present anywhere on the body at almost any age. It begins as a small, dark brown macule that may eventually attain a size of 10 cm. With enlargement, variegations in color appear that include hues of tan, red, black, blue, and even

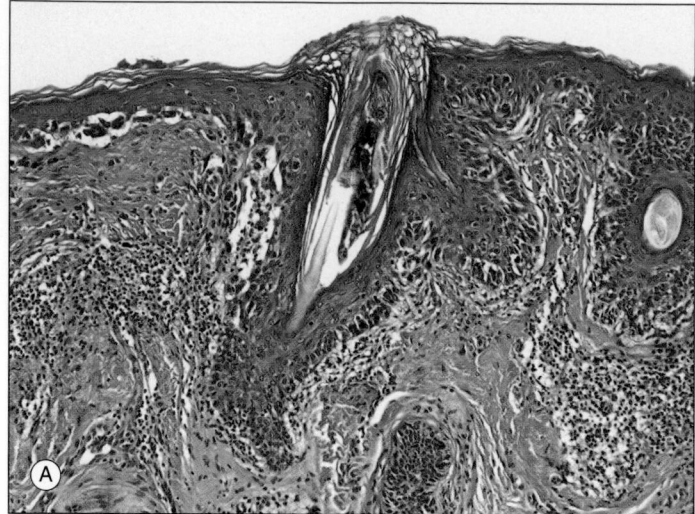

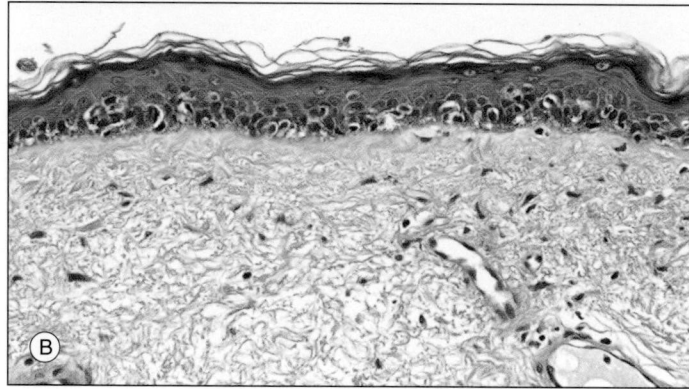

Fig. 8.84 Lentigo maligna. **A**, In diagnosis of all types of melanoma in situ confluence of tumor cells is requisite, and adnexal extension is frequent. **B**, In elderly patients cytology may be deceptively bland.

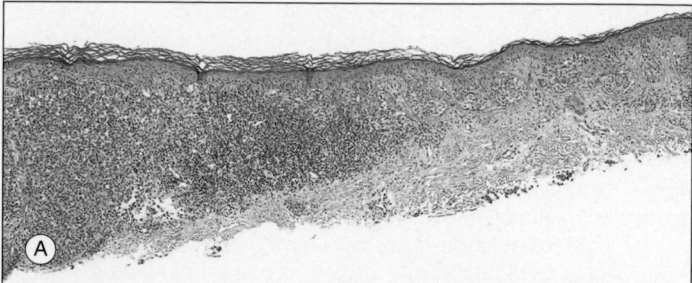

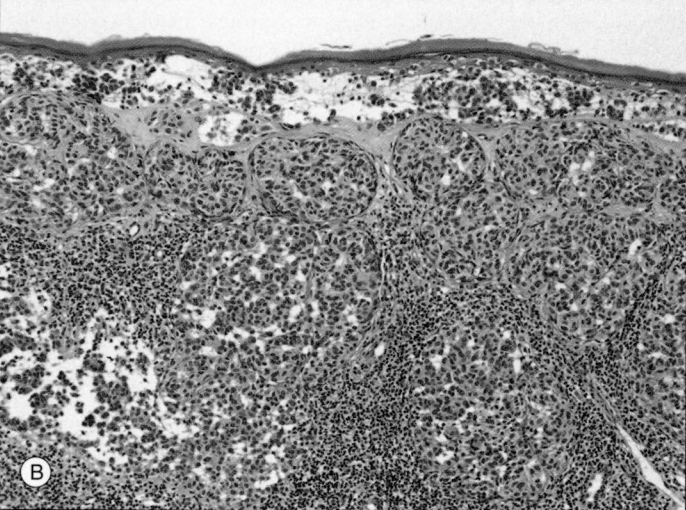

Fig. 8.85 Superficial spreading melanoma. **A**, Expansion of junctional tumor (right) beyond that in the dermis (far left) is definitional. Lymphocytes are interposed; **B**, Vertical growth phase is diagnosed here by enlargement of dermal nests and filling of the papillary dermis by tumor cells. Note the brisk lymphocytic response.

white. Irregularity of the lesional borders is common and with the development of the vertical growth phase (see below) a palpable mass appears.[453] Dermal invasion in this variant may be represented by only a few cells in the papillary dermis that are distributed singly or in very small nests, in which case there is usually no significant metastatic potential because the lesion is still in the *radial growth phase*.[562–565] The presence of this phase is definitional of the superficial spreading type and denotes the presence of centrifugally oriented tumor spread in the epidermis or superficial dermis or both (Fig. 8.85A). Cytologic features are similar to those described above for melanoma in situ. A host lymphocytic response often accompanies early invasion (Fig. 8.86).

The term *vertical growth phase* is used for those melanomas that have penetrated the corium to the level of the reticular dermis, usually equating with the attainment of metastatic capability. More generally speaking, melanomas are in vertical growth when at least one dermal tumor cell nest is larger than any single melanocytic cell group in the epidermis (see Fig. 8.85B); when dermal mitoses are present; when at least one tumor cell nest in the dermis is >10 cells in diameter; when cytologic features of dermal tumor cells are dissimilar to those of the intraepidermal component; and when a substantial lymphocytic host response surrounds the dermal tumor. In our view, entrance into the vertical growth phase is the single most

prognostically adverse finding in melanomas. Indeed, the reason the Breslow microstaging system – which is predicated on tumor depth in millimeters – is effective is that an increasing thickness in melanoma generally parallels the development of vertical growth characteristics. A roughly linear relationship exists between survival and the degree of tumor invasion, once a threshold depth of 0.76 mm has been reached. In addition, tumor location on the upper back, proximal arms, neck, or shoulders is prognostically adverse. Finally, men with melanoma tend to have worse outcomes than women with morphologically comparable tumors, for unknown reasons.

Nodular melanoma is the melanoma type that, by definition, enters vertical growth virtually concomitantly with invasion of the dermis. It includes some polypoid or pedunculated lesions.[566,567] Intraepidermal tumor does not extend laterally beyond the breadth of the intradermal component in nodular melanoma, because a radial growth phase in this lesion is thought to be absent. Rarely, epidermal tumor cells are lacking altogether.

Lentiginous invasive melanoma (formerly called 'lentigo maligna melanoma' [a confusing term that should be avoided]) is comparable behaviorally to melanomas of other morphotypes but equal depth,[568] despite past anecdotal claims to the contrary. It is typified by a prominent radial growth phase component, with well-developed intraepidermal tumor that is essentially identical histologically to

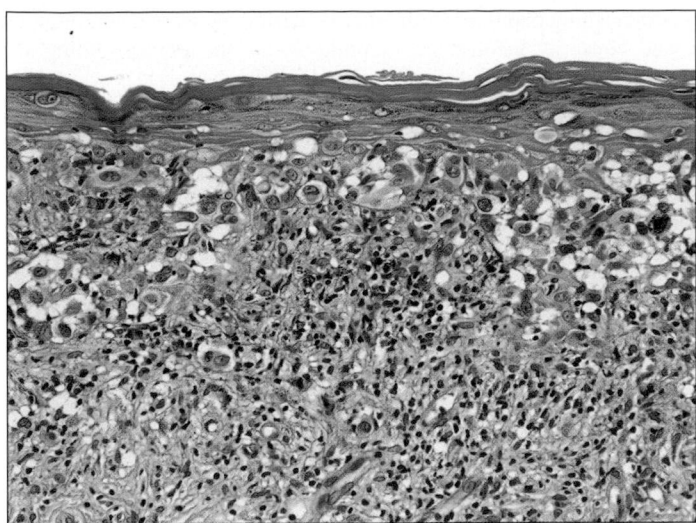

Fig. 8.86 Diffuse cellular atypia, pagetoid spread, and lymphocytic infiltrate aid in diagnosing this as invasive melanoma.

lentiginous MIS.[556,569] The intradermal element comprises epithelioid or spindle cells, with the latter of those being more common than in other forms of invasive melanoma.

Acral-lentiginous melanoma (ALM) arises on the distal extremities in palmar, plantar, or subungual locations and shows a predilection for elderly Asian and African-American individuals.[570–574] Other salient clinical features include frequent ulceration (a definitely negative prognostic feature) and deep penetration into the dermis at the time of diagnosis. Microscopic findings in ALM are hybrids of those seen in lentiginous and superficial spreading melanomas. One sees basal confluence of single tumor cells along with a limited degree of nesting and pagetoid growth.[570,572] Acanthosis, transepidermal pigment elimination, and band-like dermal lymphocytosis are often seen as well. Cytological banality of the epidermal component is relatively common, in likeness to that of lentiginous MIS.

Other variants of melanoma

Unusual variants of invasive melanoma include desmoplastic/neuroid ('neurotropic') and 'minimal-deviation/nevoid' types, among others. *Desmoplastic melanoma* often shows a relationship to pre-existing lentiginous MIS and is seen often on the head or neck in elderly patients.[575,576] It is so named because dense fibrosis surrounds and is admixed with the invasive dermal tumor, comprising fusiform, often deceptively bland cells (Fig. 8.87A). As such, desmoplastic melanoma is a subtype of *spindle-cell/sarcomatoid melanoma*. An absence of melanin in the neoplastic cells is common, a feature that may make clinical diagnosis difficult.[577] Immunohistological studies are often necessary to define the location and number of intradermal tumor cells. Antibodies to S-100 protein routinely decorate these elements, but reactivity for HMB-45, tyrosinase, melan-A, and microophthalmia transcription factor-1 is almost always absent in desmoplastic melanoma. Some studies have suggested that desmoplastic melanoma has a relatively favorable prognosis, stage for stage, but there is no consensus on that point.[577,578]

Neuroid melanoma has a tendency to invade dermal perineurial sheaths or recapitulate nerve-like structures, and is felt to be closely related conceptually to desmoplastic melanoma (Fig. 8.87B).[579] '*Minimal-deviation*' melanoma was originally described by Reed in 1978;[580] it has the overall architectural pattern of a vertical growth phase melanoma but is composed of relatively bland individual tumor cells that superficially simulate those of ordinary nevi. '*Nevoid*' melanoma is generally used as a synonym.[581–583] We do not utilize the terms 'minimal-deviation' or 'nevoid' in final diagnostic labels referring to melanomas, because there is no general agreement on criteria for doing so and no clinical data that suggest convincingly that the behavior of such lesions is unique. A resemblance to nevocytic lesions can be mentioned descriptively in such cases, along with the rationale for making a final diagnosis of melanoma, for the benefit of other pathologists who may review the lesions.

Other variant cytomorphologic patterns existing in vertical growth phase melanomas include pseudoglandular, pseudopapillary, spitzoid, myxoid, small-cell, rhabdoid, balloon-cell, hemangiopericytoid, and signet-ring-cell tumors.[584–588] Metastatic melanomas in the skin are most often dermal nodules that lack an epidermal attachment. Junctional components and pagetoid involvement of the surface

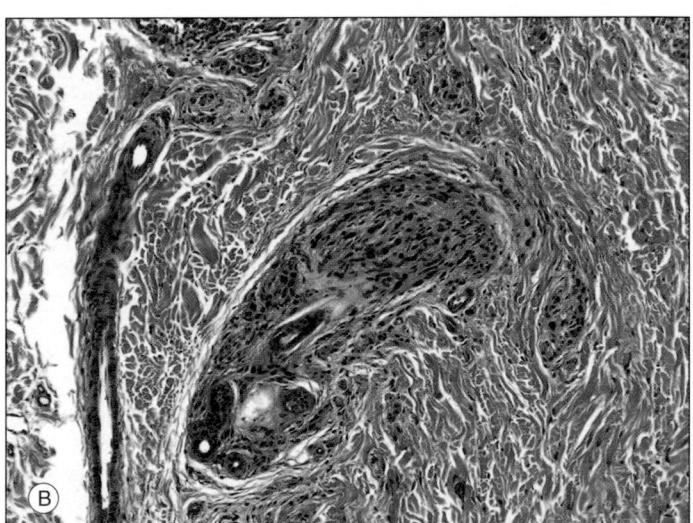

Fig. 8.87 Desmoplastic melanoma. **A,** Fortunately, junctional activity almost always allows recognition of this nondescript spindle tumor as melanocytic, but even then immunohistochemistry is often required; **B,** Neural tissue may be both invaded and morphologically mimicked.

epithelium, however, have indeed been reported in such lesions, and a confident distinction between a new primary melanoma and a metastatic deposit cannot be made in selected cases.[589]

Histochemistry and immunohistochemistry of melanocytic lesions

In the absence of a well-defined junctional component or in tumors that are amelanotic, the diagnostic recognition of melanoma may require special techniques. Histochemical stains for the identification of melanoma – such as the Fontana-Masson, Warthin-Starry, or Schmorl methods[590,591] – are currently not often employed, but they still have definite utility. The labeling of melanocyte-related proteins by immunohistochemistry is the most common means of identifying melanomas, with a sensitivity of >95% in most studies.[592–594] None of the markers used for that purpose is absolutely specific for melanoma, but that fact is not problematic if such determinants are used in the proper differential diagnostic contexts. gp100, a protein found in premelanosomes, is labeled by the monoclonal antibody known as HMB-45; it is present in both melanoma and several forms of benign melanocytic proliferation. As stated earlier, an exception to that statement is represented by desmoplastic/spindle cell melanoma.[107] Antibodies to melan-A (also known as MART-1), another gp100-related polypeptide, demonstrate a superior sensitivity to that of HMB-45 and a greater specificity in comparison with S-100 protein, a calcium flux-related protein that is shared by all melanocytes and other cell types of various lineages.[595,596] Again, however, desmoplastic melanomas are typically negative for melan-A. Tyrosinase, an enzyme involved in the catalysis of tyrosine to melanin, is limited to melanin-producing cells and may be identified by two monoclonal antibodies that are best used in combination.[597–600] It should be emphasized that there are no immunohistologic markers that can be used to separate benign and malignant melanocytic proliferations.

Microstaging and other prognostic indicators for melanoma

As true of many other malignancies, tumor stage in melanomas is the best predictor of patient survival. For example, five-year survival rates are 95% and 28% for stage I and stage IIIC tumors,[601] respectively. As stated previously, the most important histological prognostic factor in primary melanoma is its depth of invasion, expressed in millimeters as the *Breslow thickness*,[602] in recognition of the seminal work of Dr. Alexander Breslow on that topic. This is the vertical distance from the granular cell layer of the epidermis to the deepest melanoma cell in the dermis. Areas of invasion arising from adnexal structures rather than the skin surface are excluded from consideration. The Breslow thickness has largely superceded 'Clark levels' in prognostication of melanomas, but many pathologists still include both in their diagnostic reports.[603] Dr. Wallace Clark's microstaging system is based on anatomical skin compartments.[556] Level I melanomas are tumors confined to the epidermis; level II lesions are represented by those that partially fill the papillary dermis; others that fill and expand that compartment are classified as level III in the classical Clark system, but the McGovern modification of it redefined level III melanomas as lesions that invaded into the superficial reticular dermis. Level IV tumors in the original Clark paradigm included *any* that had entered the reticular dermis; however, McGovern used level IV to refer to melanomas in the *deep* reticular corium. Finally, level V neoplasms involve the subcutis or deeper soft tissue.

The highest interobserver variability in using the Clark system centers on level III and IV tumors, because of imprecision in distinguishing papillary from reticular dermis. A second confounding issue concerns inconsistent definitions for the phrase 'filling the papillary dermis' in reference to level III lesions.

The risk of metastasis from melanoma in situ is nil, and that of thinly invasive lesions is minimal; some studies show 100% 5-year survival for tumors <0.76 mm in Breslow thickness.[604] More recently, 1 mm has been suggested as the threshold for definition of 'thick' melanomas, under which consideration of regional lymph node dissection is unnecessary.[605] In fact, Reed and Martin consider melanomas <1 mm in thickness as 'borderline' or biologically 'indeterminate.'[606] In regard to the latter point, however, we return to our earlier statement that vertical growth phase characteristics are probably paramount in determining behavior. Thus, it is clearly possible for 'thin' melanomas to have entered that growth phase and attained metastatic capability, explaining why adverse outcomes in melanoma cases lie along a continuum of increasing tumor thickness.[603]

Tumor *ulceration* has clearly been shown to have independent power as a determinant of aggressiveness in melanoma cases. That fact is reflected in the American Joint Committee on Cancer (AJCC) staging criteria that divide tumors into Ta (without ulceration) or Tb (with ulceration), with the latter being associated with decreased survival.[607] A *mitotic rate* of >6/mm^2 is also an untoward prognostic indicator.[563,608] On the other hand, a *lymphocytic response* to melanomas, with intercalation of the lymphocytes among the tumor cells (a so-called 'brisk' response) has been linked to a favorable course.[563] *Microscopic 'satellitosis'* differs from clinically defined tumor satellites in the AJCC staging paradigm and is rather vaguely defined as nodules 'separated from the main body of the tumor.'[609,610] *Vascular invasion* is thought to 'guarantee' the eventual and inevitable appearance of metastasis, and is, therefore, a serious finding indeed.[611] *Regression* of melanoma, in its classic form, is defined as an area of effacement of the rete ridges with subjacent dermal fibrosis, lymphocytic infiltration, and melanophagocytosis, in which melanoma cells are absent. Persistent tumor may be seen at the borders of the area in question (Fig. 8.88). Paradoxically, *complete* regression of melanoma is associated with a relatively high risk of metastasis and adverse behavior, for reasons that are poorly understood. There is no agreement on the significance of varying degrees of subtotal regression, but we believe that involution of >75% of the dermal tumor mass most often portends an unfavorable outcome.[612,613]

Treatment of melanoma

Surgical excision of primary melanoma remains the mainstay of treatment, but the wide margins of excision that were sought even 15 years ago are no longer thought to be necessary. Current recommendations indicate that margins for MIS need be no more than 0.5 mm from the tumor, and 1 cm margins are used for invasive tumors up to 1 mm in Breslow thickness.[614,615] Margins of 2–3 cm are felt to be appropriate for lesions of greater thickness.[616,617]

The status of the 'sentinel' lymph node, the first node in any given chain draining a lesion in question, is thought to predict the status of its distal counterparts (also known as the 'nodal basin').[618,619] Discovery of metastasis in the sentinel node is followed by a completion lymphadenectomy and possibly by adjuvant therapy. We are unconvinced, however, that this approach has any benefits whatsoever on long-term survival, based on the results of many studies from the past showing no salutary effects of elective lymph node dissections for melanoma. Accordingly, sentinel lymph node biopsy is not considered to be a clinically validated practice, especially in Europe.[620,621] Despite that fact, there is a growing demand by

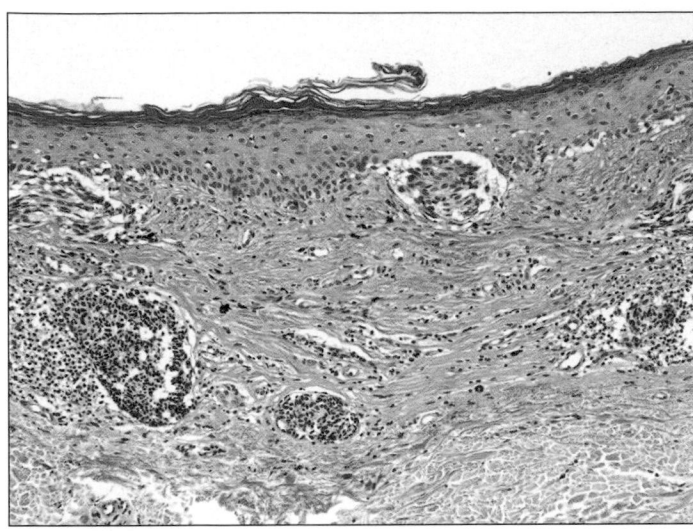

Fig. 8.88 Focal absence of melanocytes, stromal fibrosis, and melanophages indicate regression in this invasive melanoma.

surgeons for pathologists to use extensive serial sectioning of the sentinel node, immunohistochemical analysis with melanocyte-related antibodies, and the polymerase chain reaction with primer segments of the tyrosinase gene, to detect microscopic metastases of melanoma. We cannot endorse these practices (especially the latter two), because there is no objective outcome-related evidence to support their clinical value. Moreover, frozen section examination of sentinel nodes is completely unwarranted and unwise.[622–628]

HISTIOCYTIC PROLIFERATIONS

Our understanding of the cell type known as the 'histiocyte' is far from complete and continues to evolve. A recent codification by the

Histiocyte Society and the WHO Committee divides 'histiocytes' into two cell types – the *macrophage*, whose primary responsibility is that of phagocytosis, and the *dendritic cell*, an antigen-presenting cell which interacts with T- and B-lymphocytes.[629,630] The antibodies HAM-56, CD68, and CD14 identify the former of those cellular entities. Dendritic cells of the skin include dermal dendrocytes, whose expression of factor XIIIa helps to distinguish them from macrophages. Also included among the latter are Langerhans cells and the related 'indeterminate' histiocyte. Both of them express S-100 protein and CD1a; Birbeck granules can be identified ultrastructurally in Langerhans cells but are lacking in 'indeterminate' histiocytes.[629] Often, the neoplastic *versus* reactive nature of cutaneous histiocytic accumulations is unknown. Somewhat arbitrarily, we will herein consider those lesions that commonly assume a nodular or tumor-like clinical appearance, regardless of their precise biological underpinnings. Given the inconsistent identification of exact cell types in the histiocytic proliferations of the skin, these disorders are traditionally grouped according to the lipid content of the predominant cell type; 'nonxanthomatous' lesions refer to those containing few if any foamy, lipid-laden histiocytes, and 'xanthomatous' proliferations are those in which foam cells are numerous. Patients with the latter disorders usually demonstrate elevations in serum lipid levels, but that is not invariably true.[631]

Juvenile xanthogranuloma or, more generically, *solitary xanthogranuloma* (SXG) is the most commonly encountered nonxanthomatous histiocytic tumor of the skin. It presents as a solitary nodule on the head, neck, or upper trunk, usually in young children.[632] Less commonly, agminated lesions are seen or adults are affected.[633] Spontaneous involution of SXG is common, but rapidly growing facial tumors, particularly near the eyelids, may require excision. Histologically, the pathognomonic cell type in this lesion is the 'Touton' giant cell, with a wreath-like arrangement of nuclei surrounded by frothy cytoplasm. Typical mononuclear histiocytes are also numerous, some of which are also xanthomatized (Fig. 8.89). Neutrophils, plasma cells, and eosinophils may be present in SXG as well. In time, fibrotic involution of the lesion ensues. SXG shows variable immunoreactivity for CD68 and factor XIIIa; there is no labeling of the tumor cells for CD1a or S-100 protein.[634]

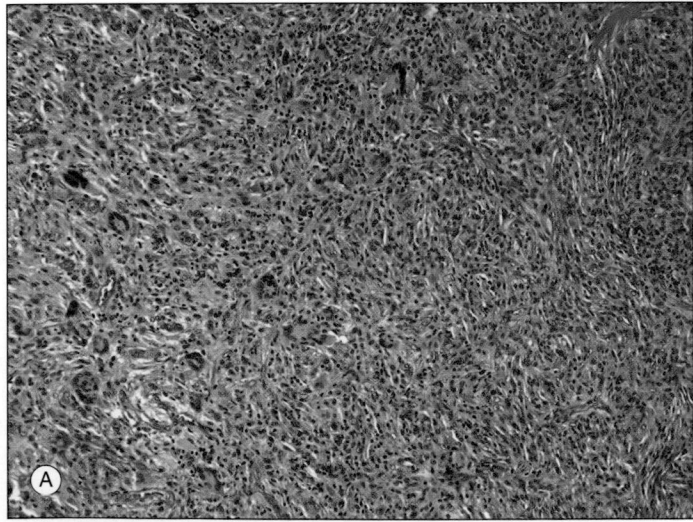

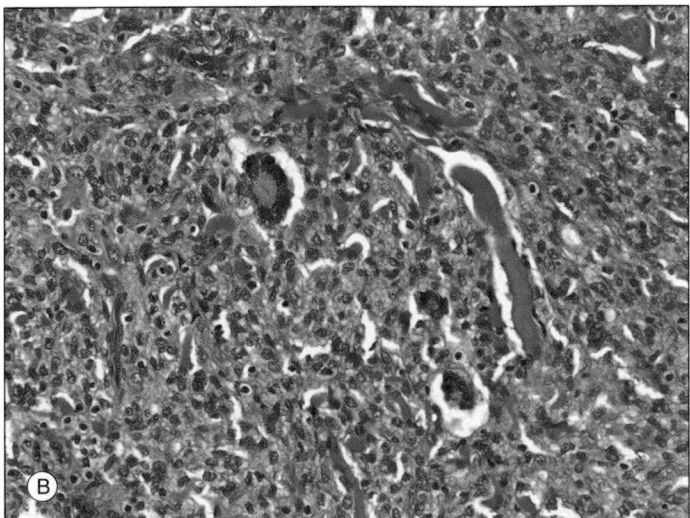

Fig. 8.89 A, The mononuclear cell infiltrate of xanthogranuloma may mimic that of dermatofibroma; **B**, A xanthomatous halo is distinctive of multinucleated cells of the Touton type.

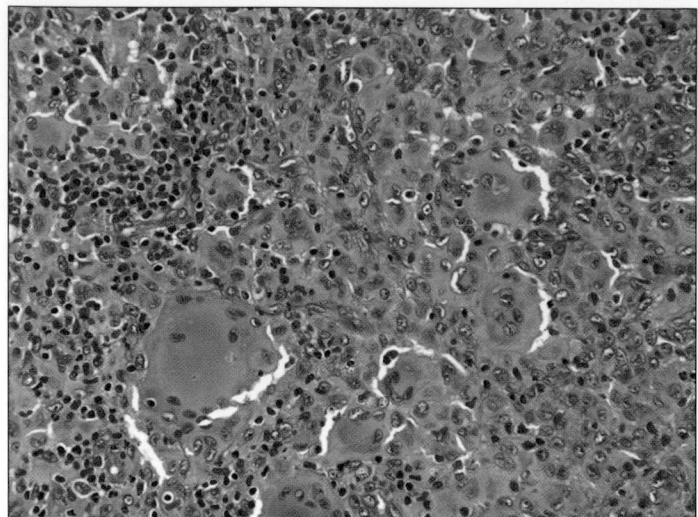

Fig. 8.90 Cytoplasmic hyalinization helps to distinguish this solitary reticulohistiocytoma from solitary xanthogranuloma.

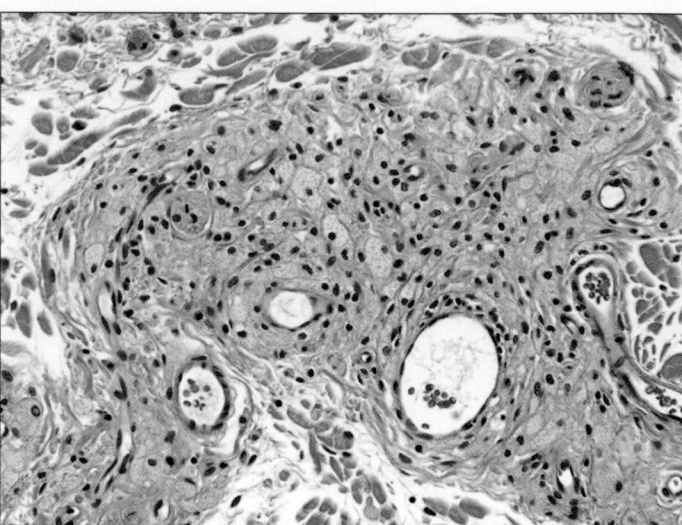

Fig. 8.91 Xanthomatous cells are perivascular in this example of xanthelasma, but diffuse papillary dermal infiltration is common.

Other rare cutaneous histiocytic proliferations that are thought to have a close relationship with SXG include *benign cephalic histiocytosis,*[635] *generalized eruptive histiocytosis,*[636,637] *progressive nodular histiocytosis,*[638] and *xanthoma disseminatum.*[639] The last of these lesions is typically seen in normolipemic patients, despite the contrary implications of its name. All of these conditions except xanthoma disseminatum feature the presence of dermal aggregates of bland mononuclear histiocytes and lack significant numbers of multinucleated cells, usually without discernible cytoplasmic vacuolization. A diagnostic distinction between them is best made with close attention to clinical information, because their histologic features are quite similar.

Multicentric reticulohistiocytosis is a systemic disorder characterized by numerous cutaneous papules and nodules on the face and the extremities, concentrated near joints. Histiocytic infiltrates are found in the skin lesions as well as the synovium of several joints, with resulting destructive arthritis.[640] Visceral and pharyngeal involvement has been reported. A similar disorder manifests itself only with skin lesions, in which case the terms *diffuse cutaneous reticulohistiocytosis* or *solitary reticulohistiocytoma* have been applied. The morphologic features of all three of these entities are comparable, with multinucleate cells and variable numbers of mononuclear histiocytes dispersed in the reticular dermis. The cells contain PAS-positive, diastase-resistant material and are immunoreactive for CD68, with or without factor XIIIa.[641] Intralesional lymphocytes and neutrophils are also present in many cases. In the solitary reticulohistiocytomas the multinucleated cells have a 'ground glass' appearance rather than the xanthomatized image seen in SXG (Fig. 8.90).

Necrobiotic xanthogranuloma is distinctive among the histiocytic tumors because of its association with paraproteinemia. These neoplasms are large yellowish plaques that favor the periorbital skin. Histologically, they contain broad zones of necrobiosis that are surrounded by mononuclear and multinucleated histiocytes, with admixed foam cells. The multinucleated elements commonly show polarization of the nuclei toward one side of the cell, with nuclear hyperchromasia and atypia. However, mitotic activity is limited.

Rosai–Dorfman disease (RDD; sinus histiocytosis with massive lymphadenopathy) is primarily a disorder of lymph nodes. Nonetheless,

it involves the skin in approximately 10% of cases,[642,643] and isolated cutaneous involvement also has been reported. Microscopic attributes of the skin lesions in RDD are similar to those of lymph nodal involvement. They include effacement of the dermis and superficial subcutis by a lymphoid infiltrate that features compartmentalizing fibrosis, with a peculiar dispersion of large mononuclear histiocytes having eosinophilic cytoplasm. The latter cells are situated in spaces that resemble nodal sinusoids. Characteristically, the lesional histiocytes in RDD exhibit a phenomenon known as 'emperipolesis,' wherein inflammatory cells (usually lymphocytes) are engulfed and contained intact in the cytoplasm. The large cells in this disorder are unusual in their immunoreactivity for S-100 protein but not CD1a, and they variably express CD68 and factor XIIIa as well.

'*Malignant reticulohistiocytosis*' is an old term for malignant histiocytosis, the existence of which is seriously questioned at the present time. Many lesions that were labeled as such in the past have proven to represent examples of CD30+ anaplastic large cell lymphoma (see below).

Xanthomatous infiltrates of the skin are considered together because they often share a common clinical configuration. Papules, nodules, and plaques are seen – potentially in almost any skin area – with a distinctive yellow cast that reflects a histological predominance of lipidized macrophages (foam cells). The presence of hyperlipidemia and lipoprotein abnormalities is inconstant in these disorders. Lesions of *eruptive xanthoma, tuberous xanthoma,* and *tendinous xanthoma* all favor the extremities but with nuances in the appearance of the respective lesions. These conditions are linked, in order of their listing above, with elevations in plasma triglyceride levels; both cholesterol and triglycerides (familial dysbetalipoproteinemia); and cholesterol alone (familial hypercholesterolemia).[634] Plaques of *xanthelasma* (Fig. 8.91), a type of *planar xanthoma,* arise on the eyelids and are also associated with hypercholesterolemia in roughly 50% of cases.[644] *Verruciform xanthoma* and *papular xanthoma* are almost never accompanied by systemic lipid abnormalities.

Histologically, all of these disorders have similar features, with dermal infiltrates of foam cells and occasional Touton-type giant cells. Eruptive xanthoma and verruciform xanthoma additionally contain neutrophils, lymphocytes, and other inflammatory cells –

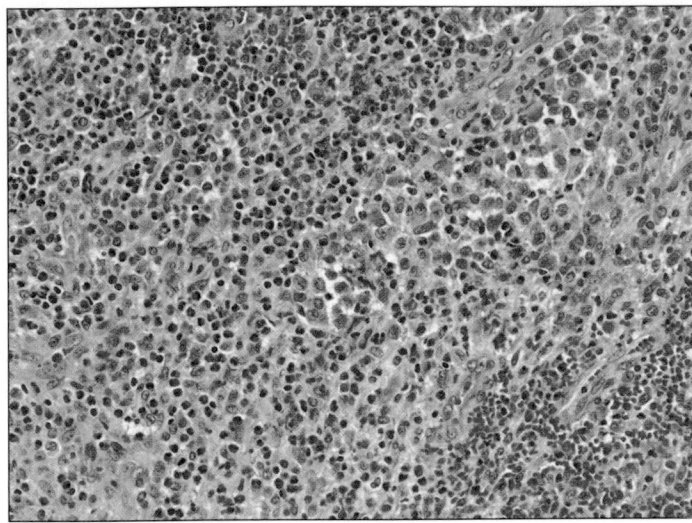

Fig. 8.92 In Langerhans histiocytosis the neoplastic cells contain nuclear convolution and linear grooving. Admixed inflammatory cells including eosinophils are common.

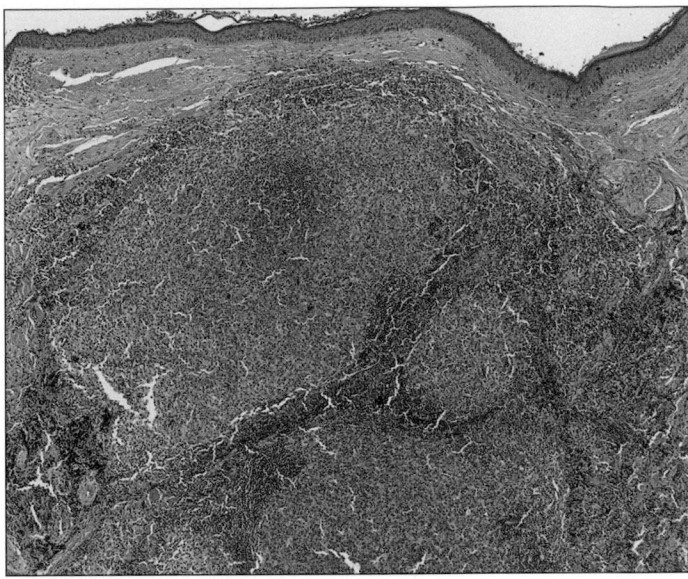

Fig. 8.93 Follicular lymphoma. There is a nodular lymphoid infiltrate in the dermis composed of neoplastic follicles that are irregularly shaped.

particularly early in their evolution – and the latter of those lesions incites the presence of marked epidermal acanthosis. Xanthelasma shows the presence of dermal foam cells that are arranged in small, scattered groups throughout the corium.

'Histiocytosis-X' is a term that is generally no longer used, referring to tumefactive proliferations of Langerhans-type histiocytes. *Langerhans-cell histiocytosis* (LCH) is now the preferred unifying designation for those conditions, and it is a potentially systemic disease that is primarily (but not exclusively) seen in children. LCH has several reproducible clinical presentations that were formerly given special names such as 'eosinophilic granuloma;' 'Hand-Schuller-Christian disease;' and 'Letterer-Siwe syndrome.' The bones, liver, spleen, bone marrow, lymph nodes, thymus, and skin may all be involved by LCH, singly or in combination. Cutaneous lesions are multifocal, papular, and variably crusted or hemorrhagic.[645] *'Congenital self-healing histiocytosis'* is also considered to be a part of the spectrum of LCH. That disease is observed in infants and often spontaneously resolves; however, some cases do progress to widespread systemic involvement.[646]

Langerhans cells in cutaneous lesions of LCH form either diffuse or nodular dermal infiltrates, with limited involvement of the epidermis and epidermal spongiosis or vesiculation. The nuclei of the lesional cells are distinctive, with an elongated or reniform shape and convoluted nuclear membranes (Fig. 8.92). These features often result in recognizable longitudinal nuclear grooves. Admixed neutrophils, eosinophils, and lymphocytes may be present in the infiltrates but should not be considered diagnostically mandatory. The cellular milieu of LCH, when combined with the presence of multinucleated cells, may falsely imitate the image of a granulomatous dermatitis; however, attention to the nuclear features of the constituent histiocytes usually allows one to recognize them successfully. A correct diagnosis is also facilitated by immunoreactivity for S-100 protein and CD1a.[647] In adults, solitary lesions of LCH may assume a modestly atypical cytological image; this characteristic, along with conjoint dermal—epidermal involvement and S-100 protein positivity, may engender a mistaken interpretation of melanoma unless additional studies are obtained.

HEMATOPOIETIC TUMORS OF THE SKIN

B-cell lymphomas

Follicular lymphoma of the skin (cutaneous follicular center-type lymphoma) is a low-grade B-cell malignancy that usually pursues an indolent course. This tumor usually involves the head and neck in adults and almost invariably remains confined to the skin for very prolonged periods. Histologically, one sees a nodular lymphoid infiltrate in the dermis and occasionally the subcutis; the epidermis is spared (Fig. 8.93). The lesional follicles are composed of a variable mixture of centrocytes (cleaved follicular cells) and centroblasts (large noncleaved follicle center cells) with incomplete or absent mantle zones. Interfollicular zones variably contain small mature lymphocytes, histiocytes, plasma cells, and occasional eosinophils.[648] The grade of follicular lymphomas can be determined by counting the number of centroblasts per single high-power microscopic field (grade 1 lesions show 0–5 centroblasts; grade 2 has 6–15 centroblasts; grade 3 is >15 centroblasts).[649] The neoplastic cells express CD10, CD19, and CD20. Unlike their nodal counterparts, cells in the central aspects of neoplastic follicles in primary skin lesions often lack bcl-2 protein expression and the t(14;18) chromosomal translocation; however, these features are thought to be more common in low-grade tumors.[650] Histologic features that help to separate follicular lymphoma from follicular hyperplasias include the presence of cytologically monotonous follicular lymphoid cells, irregularly shaped follicles with incomplete mantle zones, and a lack of tingible-body macrophages.

Extranodal marginal-zone lymphoma of the MALT type (MALToma) is the most common low-grade cutaneous B-cell malignancy. This tumor has also been called 'immunocytoma' in the EORTC classicification. However, that term has been discredited because it causes confusion with the dissimilar entity of nodal lymphoplasmacytoma/immunocytoma in the REAL paradigm for lymphomas. Cutaneous MALToma presents with red or purple nodules or plaques on the head, neck, or trunk. Although its long-term prognosis is generally good, recurrence in the skin and involvement of lymph nodes and viscera has been reported. When

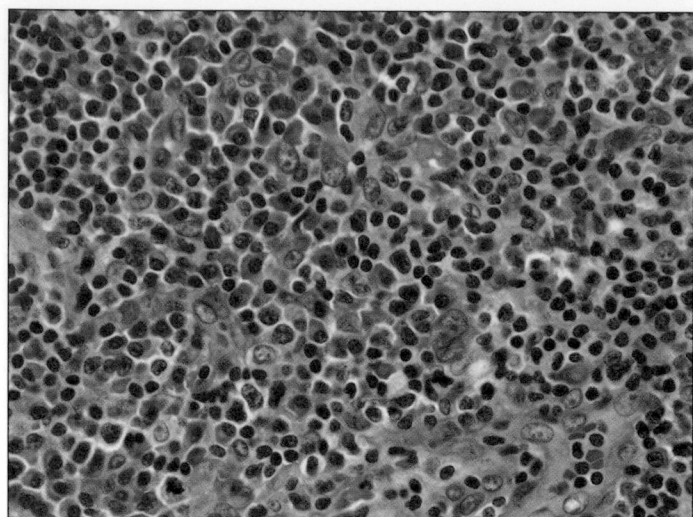

Fig. 8.94 Extranodal marginal-zone lymphoma. The dermis is infiltrated by neoplastic lymphocytes with a spectrum of cytologic phenotypes, including centrocyte-like, monocytoid B-cell-like, and small lymphocyte-like cells. Aggregates of plasma cells are a prominent feature in this case.

MALToma is present in other organs such as the stomach, it is thought to be possibly initiated by chronic antigenic stimulation owing to an infection, particularly with *Helicobacter pylori*.[651] Analogously, several studies on cutaneous lesions of this type have linked *Borrelia burgdorferi* infection to extranodal marginal zone lymphoma of the skin.[652,653] Regression of the lesions after antibiotic therapy has also been demonstrated. However, it is important to note that the great majority of cutaneous MALTomas are not caused by this pathogenetic process.

Histologically, the dermis in MALTomas is infiltrated by neoplastic lymphocytes with a spectrum of cytologic phenotypes, including centrocyte-like, monocytoid B-cell-like, and small lymphocyte-like cells (Fig. 8.94). Aggregates of plasma cells and plasmacytoid cells may be a prominent feature, often at the periphery of the infiltrate. 'Russell' bodies (cytoplasmic inclusions of immunoglobulin) are sometimes found in the plasmacytes. The overall pattern of dermal infiltration may be nodular or diffuse, and reactive lymphoid follicles may be scattered throughout the lesion.[654,655] The latter structures may be 'colonized' by neoplastic lymphocytes, but this finding should not be interpreted as diagnostic of follicular lymphoma. Although MALTomas in other sites show prominent infiltration of glandular epithelium (lymphoepithelial lesions), that attribute is rarely seen in the cutaneous adnexal structures,[656]

Immunohistochemically, the neoplastic cells of MALTomas express CD20 and CD79a. Reactivity for bcl-2 protein may also seen but the t(14;18) chromosomal translocation of follicular lymphoma is uniformly absent. A lack of CD5 and cyclin-D1 further aids in distinguishing MALToma from nodal-type mantle cell lymphoma and small lymphocytic lymphomas that may secondarily involve the skin. Similarly, a lack of staining for CD10 in cutaneous marginal zone lymphoma may help to separate it from follicular lymphoma when the latter lesion shows extensive follicular colonization.[654]

Primary diffuse large B-cell lymphoma of the skin (DLBCL) is a neoplastic proliferation of large B-cells that have a nuclear size which is at least twice that of mature lymphocytes. Although this cutaneous lymphoma morphotype may arise de novo, some cases of DLBCL represent variants of cutaneous follicular lymphoma or large-cell transformations of cutaneous MALTomas. Some observers also separately recognize *large B-cell lymphoma of the legs* that is said to have a worse prognosis than that of DLBCL in other sites, but that assertion is debatable.[657–659] A rare variant of cutaneous diffuse large B-cell lymphoma, called 'T-cell and histiocyte-rich B-cell lymphoma,' contains large numbers of reactive T cells and macrophages and a relatively small number of neoplastic B cells.[660]

DLBCLs tend to affect the skin of the head and neck, trunk, and lower legs, but not the arms. The course of this lymphoma variant is usually indolent, but extracutaneous spread does occur in some instances. The skin lesions tend to be single nodules or grouped papules, with a violaceous hue. The cytologic features of the neoplastic B cells are variable. Usually they resemble centroblasts, with large round nuclei and small peripheral nucleoli. However, other elements with an immunoblast-like image may be encountered, with oval nuclei and single prominent nucleoli. Similarly, large centrocytes (large cleaved cells) and anaplastic pleomorphic lymphoid cells resembling those of anaplastic large cell lymphomas are sometimes apparent. Biopsies of small clinical lesions of DLBCL show a periadnexal and perivascular distribution of the lesional cells in the dermis. More advanced lesions exhibit diffuse infiltration of the corium and the subcutis. There is usually a Grenz zone between the dermal infiltrate and the epidermis. The immunophenotype of DLBCL features positivity for CD20 and CD79a. Many cases also express CD10 and bcl-2 protein.[659,661]

Lymphomatoid granulomatosis (LYG) was once thought to be a quasi-malignant proliferative disorder of T lymphocytes. It is now known to be a B-cell lymphoma that is associated with the Epstein-Barr virus. LYG usually presents with pulmonary nodules but may involve other organs as well, including the brain, kidneys, liver, and gastrointestinal tract.[662] The skin is frequently involved.[663] Histologically, there is a polymorphous lymphoid infiltrate in the dermis that is primarily perivascular, periappendageal, and perineural. The infiltrate contains a mixture of small lymphocytes with a few scattered large lymphocytes that may resemble immunoblasts or, less commonly, Reed-Sternberg cells. A variable number of plasma cells and histiocytes also are seen. The lymphoid cell population may also show variable degrees of angioinvasion and angiodestruction. Cells in vessel walls are usually small lymphocytes and histiocytes (Fig. 8.95). When there is prominent fibrinoid necrosis of vascular structures, primary vasculitides such as Wegener's granulomatosis must also be considered in the differential diagnosis. Immuno-histologically, the majority of cells in LYG are CD3+ and CD4+ T lymphocytes. However, the large atypical elements are B cells, which label for CD20 and LMP1 (Epstein-Barr virus Latent Membrane Protein-1), indicating integration of nucleic acid sequences of the Epstein-Barr virus.[664,665]

Intravascular large B-cell lymphoma (intravascular lymphomatosis) is a rare form of non-Hodgkin's lymphoma that involves several organ systems, especially the central nervous system and skin. The cutaneous lesions take the form of erythematous to blue plaques. Histologically, one sees a proliferation of large dyshesive round cells within the lumina of dermal vessels. Those elements are many times larger than endothelial cells and have prominent nucleoli. Small vessels in the corium are often partially or completely occluded by the proliferation, leading to ischemic change in the surrounding tissue. In most cases the atypical cells, which label for CD45, are strictly confined to vascular lumina.[666] Some authors have suggested that this phenomenon is due to a defect in synthesis of the homing receptors β1-integrin and ICAM-1 on the neoplastic cells.[667] Although the majority of these cases are B-cell lymphomas, and are

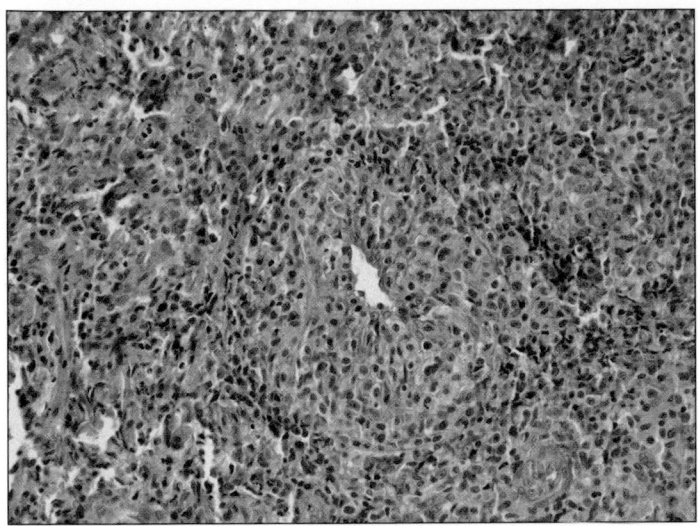

Fig. 8.95 Lymphomatoid granulomatosis. A mixture of small lymphocytes, macrophages, and immunoblast-like cells infiltrates a vessel at the center of the photomicrograph.

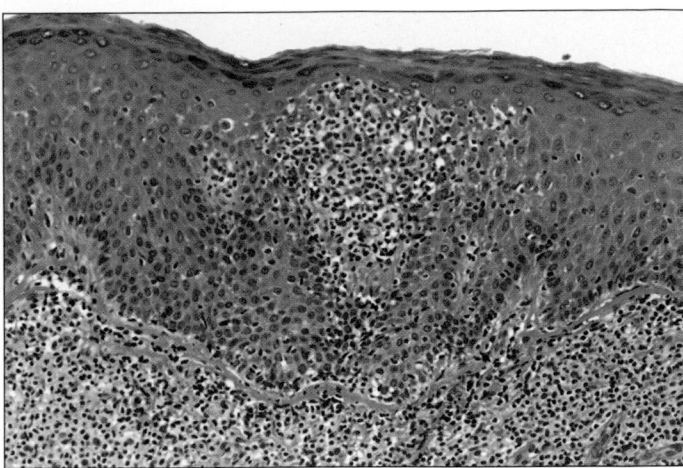

Fig. 8.96 Mycosis fungoides. A dense infiltrate of atypical lymphocytes fills the papillary dermis in a band-like fashion. There is a Grenz zone between this infiltrate and the epidermis with atypical lymphocytes lining up at the dermal-epidermal junction. Marked epidermotropism of atypical lymphocytes is seen in the center of the photomicrograph.

immunoreactive for CD20 and CD79a, rare examples with a T-cell lineage have been reported as well.[668]

Other B-cell lymphomas

Other B-cell lymphomas that are primarily nodally based may show secondary involvement of the skin. These include *mantle cell lymphoma*, *plasmacytoma*, and *small lymphocytic lymphoma/chronic lymphocytic leukemia*. As expected, cutaneous implants of these neoplasms arc similar histologically and immunohistochemically to nodal lesions.

T-cell lymphomas of the skin

Mycosis fungoides (cutaneous T-cell lymphoma; CTCL) is the most common primary lymphoma of the skin.[669] Most cases begin in middle-aged or elderly individuals but rare examples with disease onset in childhood or adolescence have also been reported.[670] The male-to-female ratio is 2:1. CTCL is considered by many dermatologists to be one of the 'great imitators;' a recent review by Zackheim & McCalmont. cited at least 25 dermatological diseases that it could simulate.[671]

Mycosis fungoides usually pursues an indolent course. Before diagnostic changes develop at a histopathologic level, many patients will have had ill-defined scaly eruptions for years that show non-specific histologic attributes like those of chronic spongiotic dermatitides. Some authors have used the term *large plaque parapsoriasis* for those precursor lesions.[672,673] The *patch stage* of CTCL is characterized by erythematous to brown patches that have a fine scale and indistinct borders. These lesions tend to be located on the lower trunk, buttocks, and thighs and may persist over many years. Development of the *plaque stage* is characterized by more well-defined lesions with an annular or arciform shape. They are erythematous to violaceous and may be slightly raised. Eventually the *tumor stage* may develop, manifested by violaceous nodules that are often ulcerated.[674] Erythroderma may develop at any stage of CTCL.[675] This manifestation in mycosis fungoides is distinguished from Sezary's syndrome by the presence of circulating neoplastic T cells (Sezary cells) in the latter but not the former condition.

The histology of CTCL varies depending on the clinical stage at which the biopsy is taken. In patch-stage lesions there is a relatively sparse papillary dermal lymphocytic infiltrate with epidermotropic lymphoid cells confined to the basal epidermis. These lymphocytes are often surrounded by a clear halo and may be aligned along the dermal–epidermal junction like a 'string of pearls.'[676] Papillary dermal fibrosis with thick bundles of 'wiry' collagen may also be present.

In plaque-stage lesions the dermal infiltrate is denser and band-like, and nuclear atypicality is apparent (Fig. 8.96). The lymphoid cells show nuclear enlargement, hyperchromasia, and a convoluted nuclear outline that is often described as 'cerebriform.' Although lymphocytes are the predominant cell type, there are also scattered eosinophils and plasma cells in the infiltrate. 'Pautrier microabscesses' are common in this phase as well; they are small dense intraepidermal collections of atypical lymphocytes (Fig. 8.97). Other epidermal changes include parakeratosis and psoriasiform hyperplasia.[667] Although the presence of spongiosis does not absolutely exclude the diagnosis of mycosis fungoides, it is an unusual finding and should lead to consideration of other diagnoses. This is especially true if spongiotic microvesicles are present.[678] Conversely, pseudo-Pautrier microabscesses may be present in spongiotic dermatoses, such as contact dermatitis, and should not be overinterpreted. They comprise monocyte-like cells, Langerhans histiocytes, and occasional lymphocytes,[679] and can be distinguished from true Pautrier micro-abscesses by their lack of nuclear atypia and greater dyshesion.

In tumoral-stage CTCL there is a dense infiltrate of atypical lymphocytes that fills the entire dermis and often extends into the subcutis. The tumor cells have a monomorphic appearance and greatly outnumber reactive lymphocytes; if they are large and pleomorphic, the term 'transformed' CTCL is appropriate. Epidermotropism and Pautrier microabscesses are unusual at this stage.[677]

Immunohistologically, the tumor cells in CTCL are reactive for CD2, CD3, and CD4, and usually negative for CD8 and CD30. Rare cases are CD8 positive and CD4 negative.[680] In many instances the tumor cells also lack CD7 expression.[681] This aberrant loss of a pan-T-cell marker is sometimes helpful in distinguishing mycosis

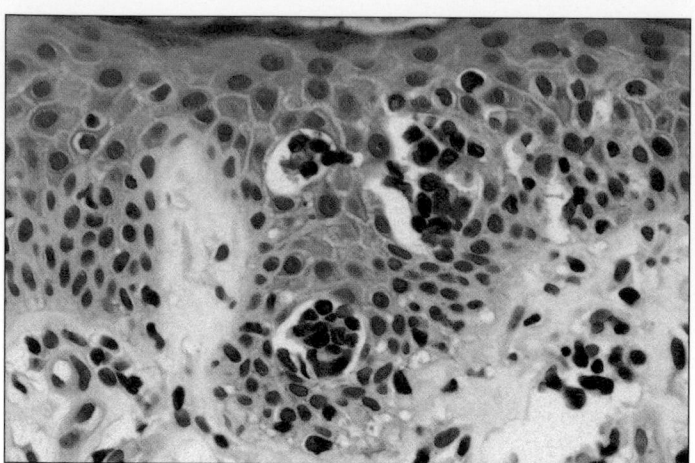

Fig. 8.97 Mycosis fungoides, Pautrier microabscesses. Small dense collections of atypical lymphocytes are seen in the epidermis.

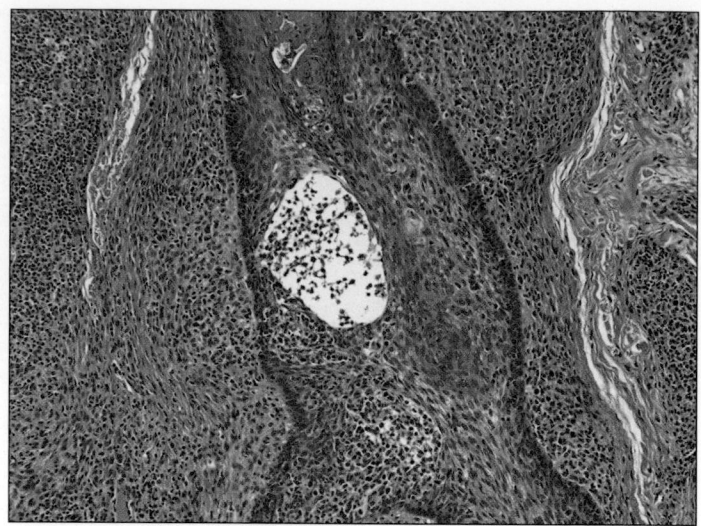

Fig. 8.98 Mycosis fungoides–associated follicular mucinosis. Hair follicles are infiltrated by atypical lymphocytes. The epidermis is uninvolved.

fungoides from its benign simulants. However, it has also been reported in some inflammatory conditions and should not be ascribed undue importance.[682]

Mycosis fungoides may sometimes progress to secondary anaplastic large cell lymphoma (ALCL), as cited above. When this occurs the neoplastic cells often acquire the CD30 (Ki-1) antigen. Transformation to ALCL is not associated with the t(2;5) chromosomal translocation, as seen in primary nodal anaplastic large cell lymphomas; transformed CTCL with these features has a poor prognosis.[683,684]

The distinction of mycosis fungoides from inflammatory dermatoses is often difficult. There is a broad spectrum of histological findings in CTCL that includes almost every major pattern seen in inflammatory skin disease.[677] However, selected key microscopic features favor CTCL in this context. These include Pautrier micro-abscesses; epidermal lymphocytes being larger than dermal lymphocytes; 'haloed' lymphocytes in the epidermis; lymphocytes aligned along the basal layer; and the presence of large convoluted nuclei.[685] Guitart et al. have attempted to standardize the diagnosis of CTCL by using specific criteria in a codified grading system.[686] In our experience, however, the most practical approach to the diagnosis is a multifactorial one, including attention to clinical information, application of histological criteria, immunophenotyping, and occasionally molecular evaluations for T-cell receptor gene rearrangements.

Variants of mycosis fungoides

Pagetoid reticulosis is a rare variant of CTCL in which the neoplastic T cells are strictly confined to the epidermis. The epidermis is usually markedly acanthotic and the distribution of atypical intraepithelial lymphocytes is reminiscent of the patterns in Paget's disease or pagetoid melanoma. The tumor cells have morphologic features that are similar to those of conventional mycosis fungoides. They may be either CD4+ or CD8+ and often express CD30 as well. There are two subtypes of pagetoid reticulosis – localized/unifocal (Woringer-Kolopp disease) and disseminated/multifocal (Ketron-Goodman syndrome). The localized form of the disease has an excellent prognosis, but Ketron-Goodman syndrome behaves comparably to conventional CTCL.[687]

Mycosis fungoides-associated follicular mucinosis is an unusual variant of mycosis fungoides that preferentially affects hair follicles.

It is characterized by papules on the head and neck that may coalesce to form plaques. Histologically, pilar units are infiltrated by atypical lymphocytes like those of classical CTCL (Fig. 8.98). There is also mucinous degeneration of the follicular epithelium with the formation of mucin pools. The epidermis is often uninvolved.[688]

Granulomatous slack skin is an exceedingly rare disease featuring pendulous folds of skin that slowly develop in pre-existing erythematous plaques. It preferentially involves the axillae or groin. Histologically, one sees permeation of the dermis and subcutis by atypical lymphocytes, and many multinucleated giant cells are evenly distributed throughout the infiltrate. The giant cells often contain phagocytosed lymphocyte nuclei and elastic fibers, and the Verhoeff-van Gieson method typically shows a complete absence of elastin in the corium. Although granulomatous slack skin is considered to be a variant of CTCL, it has also been associated with Hodgkin's lymphoma in some cases.[689]

Sezary syndrome is the leukemic form of CTCL. It presents with erythroderma, lymphadenopathy, and circulating neoplastic T cells that can be seen on blood smears or by flow cytometry of peripheral blood. The cutaneous lesions in Sezary syndrome have a histologic image which is comparable to that of mycosis fungoides, but there is usually less epidermotropism in the former condition. In some instances, skin biopsy changes are minimal, represented only by nondescript papillary dermal lymphocytic infiltrates that are concentrated around blood vessels. Lymph node biopsies in Sezary syndrome show effacement of normal nodal architecture by a paracortical or diffuse infiltrate of monotonous atypical lymphocytes, with or without superimposed changes of dermatopathic lympha-denopathy. Sezary cells in the peripheral blood have hyperchromatic and highly convoluted nuclei, a feature that is well seen by electron microscopy. They may be small ('Lutzner cells') or large (classic Sezary cells). No consensus exists on the exact number of peripheral Sezary cells required for diagnosis. This disease is more aggressive than mycosis fungoides and has a 5-year survival of only 11%.[690]

Primary cutaneous CD30+ T-cell lymphomas

Primary cutaneous ALCL predominantly affects middle-aged or elderly adults, with single or multiple nodules that are violaceous

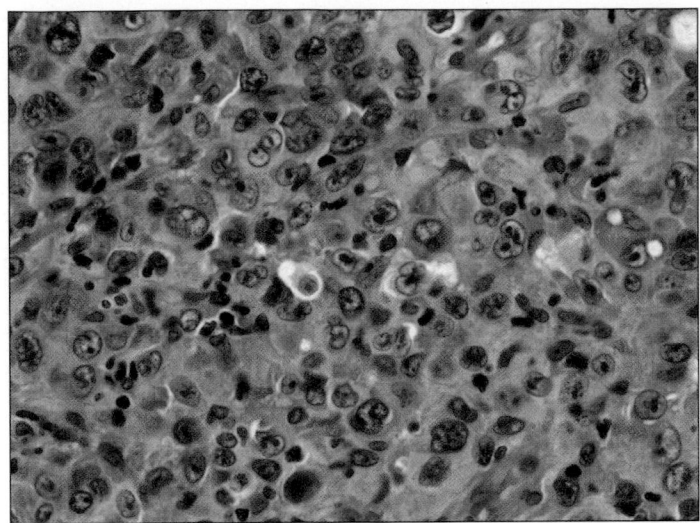

Fig. 8.99 Primary cutaneous anaplastic large cell lymphoma. The neoplastic cells are very large and have abundant pink cytoplasm. The nuclei have multiple lobes and multiple eosinophilic nucleoli.

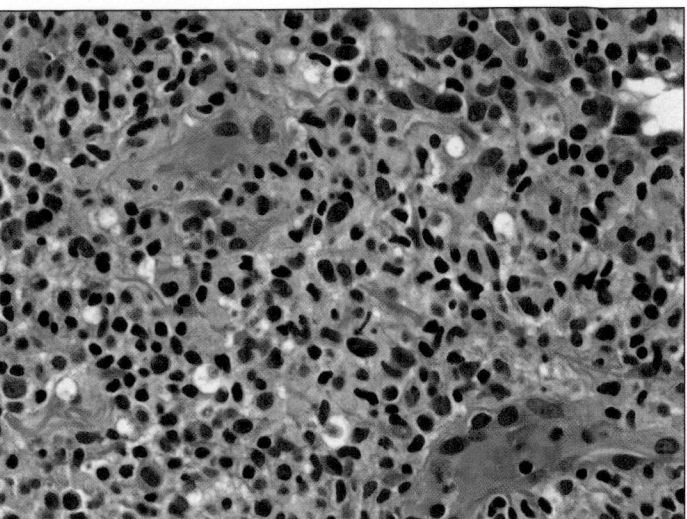

Fig. 8.100 Lymphomatoid papulosis, type A. Large atypical lymphocytes similar to those seen in anaplastic large cell lymphoma are set in a background of small lymphocytes and histocytes.

and sometimes ulcerated.[691] Local excision or cutaneous radiotherapy may be the only treatment that is necessary in some cases for prolonged periods of time. Lymph nodal involvement eventuates in a minority of cases. The prognosis is excellent with a 5-year survival of 97.5% in one series.[692] Primary ALCL of the skin is rare in children, but has indeed been reported.[693]

Histologically, this disease features the presence of atypical lymphocytes in the dermis, forming a cohesive cellular sheet that may extend into the subcutis (Fig. 8.99). The neoplastic cells are large with relatively abundant cytoplasm. Nuclei are often multilobated with several eosinophilic nuclcoli, and multinucleated cells resembling Reed-Sternberg cells may be present. The majority of the tumor cells express CD30, CD3, and CD4.[691] Most lack the anaplastic lymphoma kinase (ALK-1) fusion protein, related to the t(2;5) chromosomal aberration mentioned above. Indeed, the presence of immunohistological ALK-1 positivity in a cutaneous lesion usually indicates *secondary* involvement of the skin by a primary nodal ALCL, because the t(2;5) translocation is very rarely found in primary cutaneous disease.[694] Making that distinction is an important issue, because secondary ALCL in the skin has a relatively adverse prognosis.

Lymphomatoid papulosis (LYP) is a chronic low-grade lymphoproliferative disorder that mainly occurs in the third and fourth decades of life but may also be seen in children. It is characterized by recurrent crops of papules and nodules on the trunk and proximal limbs, which spontaneously regress over time. The lesions may ulcerate and sometimes heal, leaving atrophic scars. The course of LYP may span decades, with a variable number of lesions appearing with each new episode. The EORTC oncology study group reported 100% 5-year survival in a group of 70 patients with LYP.[690] However, some reports of transformation to systemic disease have appeared,[695,696] and it is currently felt that LYP represents a peculiar form of lymphoma that is kept in a localized cutaneous 'symbiotic' relationship with the host in most instances.

The histologic features of this disease are divided into three types. In *type A* LYP there are a variable number of large atypical lymphocytes, similar to those of ALCL, set in a background

population of small lymphocytes, eosinophils, neutrophils, and histiocytes (Fig. 8.100). The scanning image of the lesion is usually wedge-shaped, with the base of the lesion at the dermal—epidermal junction; there is no epidermotropism. *Type B* LYP shows a band-like infiltrate in the dermis comprising small to medium-sized atypical lymphocytes with cerebriform nuclei. Epidermotropism is usually apparent and there is a close resemblance to plaque-stage mycosis fungoides. *Type C* LYP lesions manifest a monotonous and dense dermal infiltrate of large atypical cells, comparable to those in primary cutaneous ALCL.[690]

Immunohistologically, the tumor cells in types A and C LYP have a profile which is similar to that of ALCL (CD30+, CD3+, CD4+/–, CD8–, ALK-1–). The cells in type B disease are phenotypically comparable to the elements of mycosis fungoides (CD3+, CD4+, CD8–).[690,697] Obviously, clinical data, histologic findings, and immunohistological information must all be considered and integrated before making a final diagnosis of LYP.

Other T-cell lymphomas

Subcutaneous panniculitis-like T-cell lymphoma (SPTL) is a rare disorder that presents with multiple tender subcutaneous nodules on the legs or the trunk. Although it affects patients of any age, most cases occur in young adults. Some may have a hemophagocytic syndrome that includes fever, pancytopenia, and hepatosplenomegaly.[698] Indeed, in the past, cases of so-called *cytophagic histocytic panniculitis* were felt to represent an inflammatory disorder, but it is now generally accepted that they are, in fact, examples of SPTL.[699] Histologically, this tumor shows an atypical lymphocytic infiltrate in the subcutaneous tissue, with a pattern that superficially resembles that of lobular panniculitis. Individual lymphocytes are small to medium-sized with irregular hyperchromatic nuclei, and atypical lymphocytes may surround individual adipocytes (Fig. 8.101). Karyorrhectic debris and foamy macrophages are interspersed throughout the infiltrate. Occasionally one also sees large histiocytes, known as 'bean-bag cells,' containing abundant cellular debris. The majority of SPTLs have a CD8+ T-cell immunophenotype with alpha-beta T-cell receptors. Rare examples alternatively show a CD8–, CD4–, CD56+,

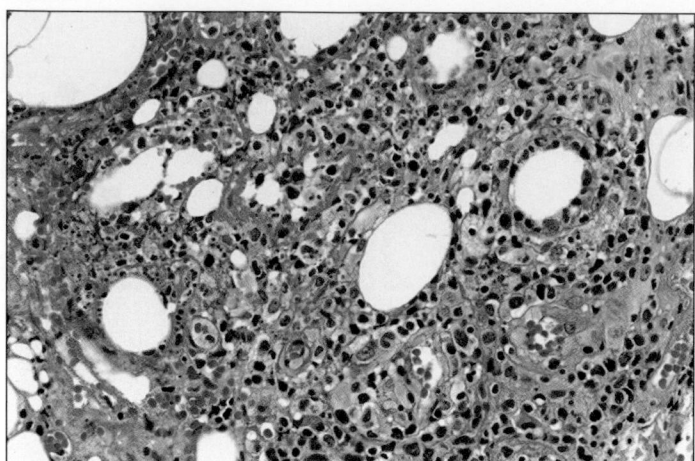

Fig. 8.101 Subcutaneous panniculitis-like T-cell lymphoma. A rim of atypical lymphocytes surrounds individual fat cells. Karyorrhectic debris and foamy macrophages are also present.

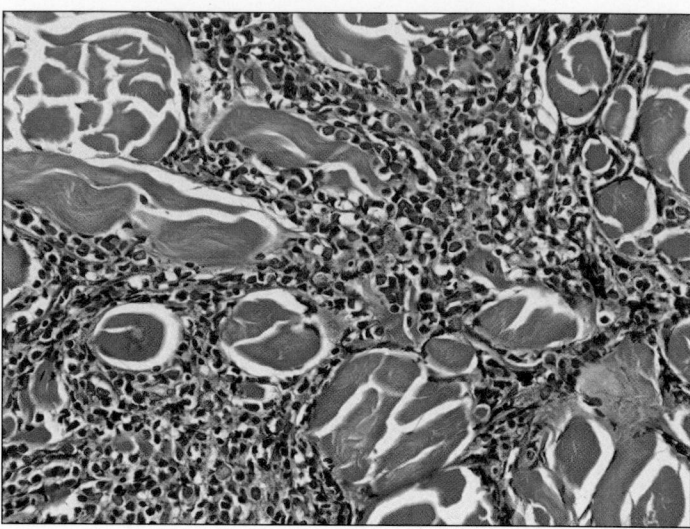

Fig. 8.102 Leukemia cutis, acute myelogenous leukemia. A dense dermal infiltrate of myeloblasts migrates between collagen bundles. This is a poorly differentiated example with few mature myeloid cells present.

and a gamma-delta T-cell receptor profile. The later cases are typically more aggressive.[700]

Peripheral T-cell lymphoma (not further specified) (PTCL) is a designation given to T-cell lymphomas that do not fit into another known clinicopathologic subtype. This category accounts for approximately 10% of all lymphomas in Western countries.[701] Although PTCL is primarily a nodal lymphoma type, it also commonly involves extranodal sites such as the skin. Microscopically, the cutaneous lesions exhibit a polymorphous cellular composition in the dermis, with medium-sized to large lymphocytes having irregular, pleomorphic nuclear contours. There is often a background of reactive cells including mature lymphocytes, eosinophils, plasma cells, and histiocytes. The general immunophenotype of these tumors is CD4+, CD8– and CD30+/–.[702,703] A rare variant of PTCL known as *Lennert's lymphoma* demonstrates the presence of clustered intralesional epithelioid histiocytes, and only uncommonly involves the skin.[704]

Adult T-cell lymphoma/leukemia (ATLL) is a peripheral T-cell lymphoproliferative disease that is associated with human T-cell lymphotropic virus type 1 (HTLV-1). This agent is endemic to Japan, the Caribbean, and parts of Central Africa. Sporadic cases of ATLL have also been reported in Europe and the United States.[705] Individuals infected with HTLV-1 carry a lifetime risk of 2–6% for the development of ATLL.[706] The course of that malignancy ranges from that of an aggressive leukemia – with lymph nodal, visceral, and osseous lesions – to a more indolent form that has no nodal involvement and few lymphomatous cells in the peripheral blood. However, cutaneous lesions may be present regardless of those nuances, usually in the form of erythematous patches or plaques or more rarely as an erythrodermatous eruption.[707]

Histologically, the lesions of ATLL may resemble those of CTCL with epidermotropism and formation of Pautrier microabscesses, but some cases show infiltrates that are confined to the superficial dermis.[708] Individual neoplastic cells are medium-sized to large and they are often pleomorphic with convoluted nuclear outlines. Tumor cells in the peripheral blood often have polylobated nuclei as well, but their morphologic profile is said to differ from that of cells in the Sezary syndrome.[709] The immunophenotype of ATLL is CD3+, CD4+, CD7– and CD8–. CD25 is also expressed in nearly all cases, helping to distinguish this disease from CTCL.[710]

Leukemia cutis

Leukemic infiltrates in the skin usually take the form of violaceous to red papules, nodules, or plaques, and are known as *leukemia cutis*. In most instances the cutaneous lesions are a late manifestation of leukemia, and may herald a rapid subsequent progression of the disease. However, in a small subset of cases leukemia cutis *precedes* overt leukemia by several months or longer ('*aleukemic leukemia cutis*').[711] Acute myeloid leukemias (AMLs) are the most common underlying conditions. Their tumefactive cutaneous manifestations have been given several special names, including *chloroma*, *granulocytic sarcoma*, and *extramedulary myeloid cell tumor*. Chronic lymphocytic leukemia (of both B-cell and T-cell types) also commonly produces infiltrates in the skin, but <10% of acute lymphoid leukemias (i.e. precursor-B-cell and T-cell lymphoblastic leukemias) are associated with cutaneous involvement.[712]

The histology of the dermal infiltrate obviously depends on the type of underlying leukemia.[713] AMLs produce a dense infiltrate of myeloblasts, with or without myelocytes, and scattered mature myeloid cells. There is typically a Grenz zone in the corium between the infiltrate and the epidermal basement membrane, and single cells often 'dissect' between dermal collagen bundles (Fig. 8.102). Chronic myelogenous leukemias may be associated with a variable mixture of granulocytic cells – including myelocytes, metamyelocytes, eosinophilic metamyelocytes, and neutrophils – or a monomorphous infiltrate of mononuclear cells.[714] Infiltrates of chronic lymphocytic leukemia comprise a monomorphous population of small round lymphocytes in the dermis with perivascular, periadnexal, nodular, band-like, or diffuse configurations. Acute lymphoblastic leukemias show cells with high nuclear-to-cytoplasmic ratios and finely dispersed chromatin; nuclear contours may also be convoluted.

Most cases of aleukemic cutaneous leukemia require intensive application of histochemical and immunohistochemical methods to determine the lineage of the disease. Myeloid leukemias commonly show histochemical positivity for chloroacetate esterase (the von Leder stain), as well as immunoreactivity for CD45, CD43, lysozyme, and myeloperoxidase.[714] Lymphoid leukemias express

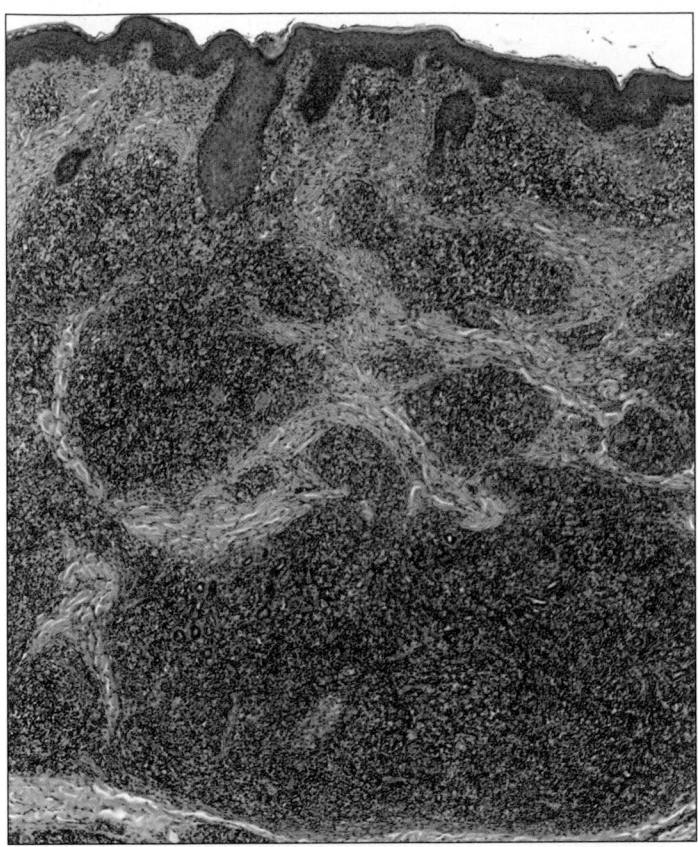

Fig. 8.103 Benign lymphoid infiltrates. There is dense infiltrate of small lymphocytes and histiocytes in the dermis. This example has a predominantly nodular configuration.

infiltration; manifestations of epidermal damage; and associated vascular proliferation.[719,720] Despite the usual configurational resemblance of CLH to a B-cell lesion, with formation of follicles, immunohistology most often demonstrates a predominance of T lymphocytes in hyperplasias. One study showed that a B-to-T-cell ratio of >3:1 was seen in 40% of low-grade B-cell lymphomas in the skin, but it excluded a diagnosis of lymphoid hyperplasia.[655] The use of molecular techniques to determine the presence of lymphoid clonality is controversial in this context, because occasional cases of CLH will demonstrate an apparent clonal IgH gene rearrangement and yet still behave in a benign fashion.[721]

Occasionally, examples of CLH have a 'T-cell pattern,' with clinical and histological features that are reminiscent of mycosis fungoides. Those lesions may be idiopathic, but they more commonly arise in the setting of chronic sun damage ('*actinic reticuloid*')[722] or as a reaction to certain medications (particularly phenytoin, phenothiazines, and carbamazepine).[723] Microscopically, one sees a band-like lymphoid infiltrate in the dermis in T-cell CLH, with or without epidermotropism. Occasional lymphocytes may have hyperchromatic and convoluted nuclei, and Pautrier microabscess-like cell groups may be present in the epidermis.[720] In 'actinic reticuloid,' immunohistochemical analysis may help in demonstrating a predominance of CD8+ T cells in the epidermis, contrasting with usual findings in mycosis fungoides.[724] The separation of idiopathic or drug-induced T-cell CLH from CTCL may require strong reliance on clinical-pathological integration, heavily utilizing historical information in conjunction with morphological and adjunctive laboratory data for successful identification of these lesions. Even after that has been done, some cases will inevitably be encountered where a diagnosis of 'CTCL' is accompanied by complete resolution of the skin lesions in question, after an offending medication has been discontinued.

Mast cell infiltrates in the skin
Mast cell infiltrates in the skin are associated with several distinct clinical manifestations, all of which have histological similarities. This group of diseases can be divided into two broad categories – cutaneous mastocytosis and systemic mastocytosis.

Cutaneous mastocytosis
Urticaria pigmentosa (UP) is the most common form of cutaneous mast cell disease. It manifests as multiple red-brown macules on the trunk and extremities in children. The lesions may be sparse and scattered or they may number in the hundreds. Most examples of UP make their appearance before 4 years of age, and they spontaneously resolve by puberty; systemic involvement is unusual in childhood cases. UP appearing for the first time in adults is often persistent and accompanied by visceral disease.[725,726] A useful clinical clue in recognizing cutaneous mastocytosis is *Darier's sign*, in which the lesion develops a wheal and flare after vigorous rubbing.[727] *Solitary mastocytomas* also occur in infants, most frequently on the trunk or wrists; they spontaneously resolve without treatment. *Diffuse cutaneous mastocytosis* is a rare disorder that is seen almost exclusively in infants. They have diffuse thickening of the skin with an erythematous or yellow-brown coloration, and secondary nodular lesions may develop therein; systemic involvement frequently supervenes.[728] *Telangiectasia macularis eruptiva perstans* or '*TMEP*' is an adult form of cutaneous mastocytosis that frequently is associated with systemic involvement. It is reflected by hundreds of small brown macules and fine telangiectasias that cover the trunk and proximal extremities.[729] Multiple myeloma has rarely been linked to TMEP.[730]

markers that reflect their level of B-cell or T-cell differentiation, including CD5, CD10, CD20, *PAX-5*, terminal deoxynucleotidyl transferase, and CD99.

Benign lymphoid infiltrates
One of the most difficult differential diagnostic problems in cutaneous pathology is the separation of exuberant lymphoid hyperplasias from forms of malignant lymphoma. Indeed, many examples of cutaneous lymphoid hyperplasia are clinically and microscopically similar to low-grade cutaneous B-cell lymphomas. Most of those lesions are idiopathic, but some have been linked etiologically to arthropod bites,[715] tattoos,[716] or *Borrelia* infections.[717] They usually present as solitary papules or nodules on the face, or, less commonly, on the trunk or extremities. Several clinical terms have been applied to benign cutaneous lymphoid infiltrates, including *lymphadenoma benigna cutis*, *lymphocytoma cutis of Spiegler-Fendt*, *benign lymphocytic infiltrate of Jessner*, and *pseudolymphoma*.[718] Practically speaking, these are arcane names that engender confusion for nondermatologists, and are best replaced generically by the designation of 'cutaneous lymphoid hyperplasia' (CLH).

Microscopically, CLH is represented by a dense dermal infiltrate of small lymphocytes and histiocytes, with either a nodular or a diffuse pattern (Fig. 8.103). Features that suggest a benign rather than a neoplastic infiltrate include cellular heterogeneity with admixed eosinophils, plasma cells, and tingible-body macrophages; formation of lymphoid follicles, with or without germinal centers; a predominant pattern of perivascular and periappendageal lymphoid

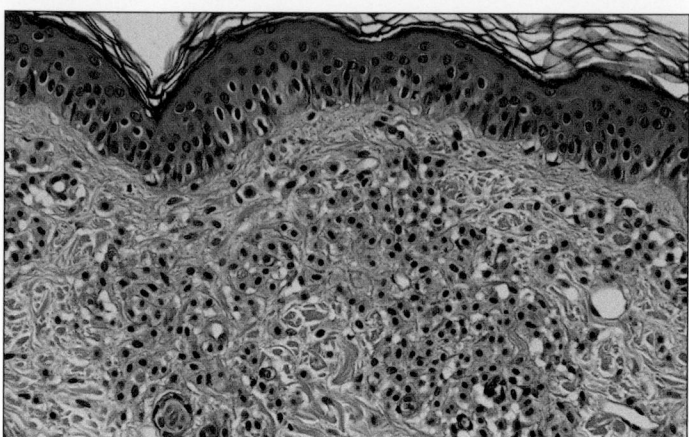

Fig. 8.104 Cutaneous mastocytosis. Aggregates of mast cells with amphophilic cytoplasm infiltrate the papillary dermis.

The histological features of cutaneous mastocytosis are similar in all of its clinical variants.[729] They are composed of aggregated polygonal or elongated mast cells that infiltrate the papillary dermis and sometimes extend into the reticular corium as well (Fig. 8.104). Their nuclei are round and compact, and cytoplasm is amphophilic and granular. Typical cytoplasmic mast cell granules are often difficult to see in hematoxylin and eosin-stained sections, and often require the use of special histochemical or immunohistochemical stains (see below). Hyperpigmentation of the basal epithelium may be present, along with scattered eosinophils and dermal edema. Some cases of UP show extremely sparse infiltrates that are primarily perivascular; individual cells in those cases are often cuboidal rather than spindle shaped. In solitary mastocytomas the cellular infiltrates are typically dense, often filling the dermis and involving the subcutis as well. TMEP shows an increase in dermal mast cells that are most concentrated around dilated dermal blood vessels. Sometimes these changes are so subtle that they require formal quantitation of mast cells and comparisons with biopsies of nonlesional skin; in one study, the number of mast cells in TMEP was at least twice that of the normal dermis.[731] In diffuse cutaneous mastocytosis, mast cell infiltrates are loosely arranged in bands in the upper corium. As mentioned earlier, histochemical and immuno-histochemical techniques are helpful in identifying mast cells. The Giemsa and toluidine blue methods both metachromatically label the cytoplasmic granules of mast cells. The von Leder stain decorates the granules with a bright red color. Immunohistochemical detection of CD117 (c-*kit*-encoded tyrosine kinase receptor protein) is also an extremely sensitive marker of mast cells.[732]

Systemic mastocytosis

In systemic mastocytosis, the bone marrow is the most frequent site of involvement, followed by the liver, spleen, gastrointestinal tract, and lymph nodes. The skin may or may not be affected.[733] Symptoms in this form of mastocytosis may include flushing, asthmatic-like attacks, nausea, vomiting, syncope, bone pain, and weight loss, and its prognosis is unpredictable.[734] Some patients develop aggressive disease including a leukemic evolution ('malignant mastocytosis');[735] others have an indolent course with little or no impact on long-term survival. An important prognostic factor in this setting appears to be the presence of skin involvement. Somewhat paradoxically, patients with cutaneous infiltrates in systemic mastocytosis usually have an indolent course, but those who lack skin disease have a more unfavorable prognosis.[736] The histological, histochemical, and immunohistologic features of cutaneous lesions in systemic mastocytosis are identical to those described above in reference to cutaneous mastocytosis.

REFERENCES

1. Hurwitz S. Epidermal nevi and tumors of epidermal origin. Pediatr Clin North Am 1983; 30(3): 483–494.

2. Su WP. Histopathologic varieties of epidermal nevus. A study of 160 cases. Am J Dermatopathol 1982; 4(2): 161–170.

3. Altman J, Mehregan AH. Inflammatory linear verrucose epidermal nevus. Arch Dermatol 1971; 104(4): 385–389.

4. Morag C, Metzker A. Inflammatory linear verrucous epidermal nevus: report of seven new cases and review of the literature. Pediatr Dermatol 1985; 3(1): 15–18.

5. Hodge SJ, Barr JM, Owen LG. Inflammatory linear verrucose epidermal nevus. Arch Dermatol 1978; 114(3): 436–438.

6. Dupre A, Christol B. Inflammatory linear verrucose epidermal nevus. A pathologic study. Arch Dermatol 1977; 113(6): 767–769.

7. Jablonska S. Wart viruses: human papillomaviruses. Semin Dermatol 1984; 3: 120–129.

8. Young R, Jolley D, Marks R. Comparison of the use of standardized diagnostic criteria and intuitive clinical diagnosis in the diagnosis of common viral warts (verrucae vulgaris). Arch Dermatol 1998; 134(12): 1586–1589.

9. Steigleder GK. Histology of benign virus induced tumors of the skin. J Cutan Pathol 1978; 5(2): 45–52.

10. Brown TJ, Yen-Moore A, Tyring SK. An overview of sexually transmitted diseases. Part II. J Am Acad Dermatol 1999; 41(5 Pt 1): 661–77; quiz 678–680.

11. Jablonska S, Orth G. Epidermodysplasia verruciformis. Clin Dermatol 1985; 3(4): 83–96.

12. Androphy EJ, Dvoretzky I, Lowy DR. X-linked inheritance of epidermodysplasia verruciformis. Genetic and virologic studies of a kindred. Arch Dermatol 1985; 121(7): 864–868.

13. Ramoz N, et al. Mutations in two adjacent novel genes are associated with epidermodysplasia verruciformis. Nat Genet 2002; 32: 579–581.

14. Majewski S, et al. Partial defects of cell-mediated immunity in patients with epidermodysplasia verruciformis. J Am Acad Dermatol 1986; 15(5 Pt 1): 966–973.

15. Glinski W, et al. T cell defect in patients with epidermodysplasia verruciformis due to human papillomavirus type 3 and 5. Dermatologica 1981; 162(3): 141–147.

16. van Voorst Vader PC, et al. Epidermodysplasia verruciformis. Skin carcinoma containing human papillomavirus type 5 DNA sequences and primary hepatocellular carcinoma associated with chronic hepatitis B virus infection in a patient. Acta Derm Venereol 1986; 66(3): 231–236.

17. Harris AJ, et al. A novel human papillomavirus identified in epidermodysplasia verruciformis. Br J Dermatol 1997; 136(4): 587–591.

18. Nuovo GJ, Ishag M. The histologic spectrum of epidermodysplasia verruciformis. Am J Surg Pathol 2000; 24(10): 1400–1406.

19. Barzegar C, et al. Epidermodysplasia verruciformis-like eruption complicating human immunodeficiency virus infection. Br J Dermatol 1998; 139(1): 122–127.

20. Yeatman JM, Kilkenny M, Marks R. The prevalence of seborrhoeic keratoses in an Australian population: does exposure to sunlight play a part in their frequency? Br J Dermatol 1997; 137(3): 411–414.

21. Sanderson KV. The structure of seborrhoeic keratoses. Br J Dermatol 1968; 80(9): 588–593.

22. Wade TR, Ackerman AB. The many faces of seborrheic keratoses. J Dermatol Surg Oncol 1979; 5(5): 378–382.

23. Farrell AM, Dawber RP. Sign of Leser-Trelat. J Am Acad Dermatol 1997; 37(1): 138–139.

24. Brownstein MH, Fernando S, Shapiro L. Clear cell acanthoma: clinicopathologic analysis of 37 new cases. Am J Clin Pathol 1973; 59(3): 306–311.

25. Tanay A, Mehregan AH. Warty dyskeratoma. Dermatologica 1969; 138(3): 155–164.

26. Szymanski F. Warty dyskeratoma. A benign cutaneous tumor resembling Darier's disease microscopically. Arch Dermatol 1957; 75: 567–572.

27. Laur WE, Posey RE, Waller JD. Lichen planus-like keratosis. A clinicohistopathologic correlation. J Am Acad Dermatol 1981; 4(3): 329–336.

28. Prieto VG, Casal M, McNutt NS. Lichen planus-like keratosis. A clinical and histological reexamination. Am J Surg Pathol 1993; 17(3): 259–263.

29. Frigy AF, Cooper PH. Benign lichenoid keratosis. Am J Clin Pathol 198; 83(4): 439–443.

30. Grunwald MH, Lee JY, Ackerman AB. Pseudocarcinomatous hyperplasia. Am J Dermatopathol 1988; 10(2): 95–103.

31. Ju DM. Pseudoepitheliomatous hyperplasia of the skin. Dermatol Int 1967; 6(2): 82–92.

32. Civatte J. Pseudo-carcinomatous hyperplasia. J Cutan Pathol 1985; 12(3–4): 214–223.

33. Weedon D. Skin pathology, 2nd edn. New York: Churchill Livingstone; 2002.

34. Pinkus H, Mehregan, AH. Premalignant skin lesions. Clin Plast Surg 1980; 7(3): 289–300.

35. Marks R, Rennie G, Selwood TS. Malignant transformation of solar keratoses to squamous cell carcinoma. Lancet 1988; 1(8589): 795–797.

36. Carapeto FJ, Garcia-Perez A. Acantholytic keratosis. Dermatologica 1974; 148(4): 233–239.

37. Billano RA, Little WP. Hypertrophic actinic keratosis. J Am Acad Dermatol 1982; 7(4): 484–489.

38. Hirsch P, Marmelzat WL. Lichenoid actinic keratosis. Dermatol Int 1967; 6(2): 101–103.

39. Tan CY, Marks R. Lichenoid solar keratosis – prevalence and immunologic findings. J Invest Dermatol 1982; 79(6):365–367.

40. James MP, Wells GC, Whimster IW. Spreading pigmented actinic keratoses. Br J Dermatol 1978; 98(4): 373–379.

41. Patterson JW, Pittman DL, Rich JD. Presternal ciliated cyst. Arch Dermatol 1984; 120(2): 240–242.

42. Kural YB, et al. Cutaneous bronchogenic cysts. Int J Dermatol 1998; 37(2): 137–140.

43. Betti R, et al. Branchial cyst of the neck. Br J Dermatol 1992; 127(2): 195.

44. al-Nafussi AI, Carder P. Cutaneous ciliated cyst: a case report and immunohistochemical comparison with fallopian tube. Histopathology 1990; 16(6): 595–598.

45. Ashton MA. Cutaneous ciliated cyst of the lower limb in a male. Histopathology 1995; 26(5): 467–469.

46. Dini M, et al. Cutaneous ciliated cyst: a case report with immunohistochemical evidence for dynein in ciliated cells. Am J Dermatopathol 2000; 22(6): 519–523.

47. Cortes-Franco R, et al. Cutaneous ciliated cyst. Int J Dermatol 1995; 34(1): 32–33.

48. Brownstein MH, Helwig EB. Subcutaneous dermoid cysts. Arch Dermatol 1973; 107(2): 237–239.

49. Nagore E, et al. Median raphe cysts of the penis: a report of five cases. Pediatr Dermatol 1998; 15(3): 191–193.

50. Long CC, Marks R. Increased risk of skin cancer: another Celtic myth? A review of Celtic ancestry and other risk factors for malignant melanoma and nonmelanoma skin cancer. J Am Acad Dermatol 1995; 33(4): 658–661.

51. Robinson JK. Risk of developing another basal cell carcinoma. A 5-year prospective study. Cancer 1987; 60(1): 118–120.

52. Okun M, Blumenthal G. Basal cell epithelioma with giant cells and nuclear atypicality. Arch Dermatol 1964; 89: 598–602.

53. Lang PG Jr, McKelvey AC, Nicholson JH. Three-dimensional reconstruction of the superficial multicentric basal cell carcinoma using serial sections and a computer. Am J Dermatopathol 1987; 9(3): 198–203.

54. Betti R, et al. Age and site prevalence of histologic subtypes of basal cell carcinomas. Int J Dermatol 1995; 34(3): 174–176.

55. Wallace ML, Smoller BR. Trichoepithelioma with an adjacent basal cell carcinoma, transformation or collision? J Am Acad Dermatol 1997; 37(2 Pt 2): 343–5.

56. Bettencourt MS, Prieto VG, Shea CR. Trichoepithelioma: a 19-year clinicopathologic re-evaluation. J Cutan Pathol 1999; 26(8): 398–404.

57. Jimenez FJ, et al. Ber-EP4 immunoreactivity in normal skin and cutaneous neoplasms. Mod Pathol 1995; 8(8): 854–858.

58. Morales-Ducret CR, et al. bcl-2 expression in primary malignancies of the skin. Arch Dermatol 1995; 131(8): 909–912.

59. Smoller BR, et al. bcl-2 expression reliably distinguishes trichoepitheliomas from basal cell carcinomas. Br J Dermatol 1994; 131(1): 28–31.

60. Tellechea O, et al. Monoclonal antibody Ber EP4 distinguishes basal-cell carcinoma from squamous-cell carcinoma of the skin. Am J Dermatopathol 1993; 15(5): 452–455.

61. Mills AE. Solar keratosis can be distinguished from superficial basal cell carcinoma by expression of bcl-2. Am J Dermatopathol 1997; 19(5): 443–445.

62. Sinard JH. Immunohistochemical distinction of ocular sebaceous carcinoma from basal cell and squamous cell carcinoma. Arch Ophthalmol 1999; 117(6): 776–783.

63. Gatter KC, et al. An immunohistological study of benign and malignant skin tumours: epithelial aspects. Histopathology 1984; 8(2): 209–227.

64. Wick M, Swanson P. Immunohistochemical findings in tumors of the skin. In: DeLellis RA, ed. Advances in immunohistochemistry. New York: Raven Press; 1988: 395–429.

65. Thomas P, et al. Profiles of keratin proteins in basal and squamous cell carcinomas of the skin. An immunohistochemical study. Lab Invest 1984; 50(1): 36–41.

66. Swanson PE, et al. Immunohistologic differential diagnosis of basal cell carcinoma, squamous cell carcinoma, and trichoepithelioma in small cutaneous biopsy specimens. J Cutan Pathol 1998; 25(3): 153–159.

67. Geary WA, Cooper PH. Proliferating cell nuclear antigen (PCNA) in common epidermal lesions. An immunohistochemical study of proliferating cell populations. J Cutan Pathol 1992; 19(6): 458–468.

68. Healy E, et al. Prognostic value of Ki67 antigen expression in basal cell carcinomas. Br J Dermatol 1995; 133(5): 737–741.

69. Geisse JK, et al. Imiquimod 5% cream for the treatment of superficial basal cell carcinoma: a double-blind, randomized, vehicle-controlled study. J Am Acad Dermatol 2002; 47(3): 390–398.

70. Kao GF. Carcinoma arising in Bowen's disease. Arch Dermatol 1986; 122(10): 1124–1126.

71. Degos R, et al. Mucocutaneous Bowen's disease. 243 clinical cases. Ann Dermatol Syphiligr (Paris) 1976; 103(1): 5–14.

72. Patterson JW, et al. Bowenoid papulosis. A clinicopathologic study with ultrastructural observations. Cancer 1986; 57(4): 823–836.

73. Strayer DS, Santa Cruz JD. Carcinoma in situ of the skin: a review of histopathology. J Cutan Pathol 1980; 7(4): 244–259.

74. Fulling KH, Strayer DS, Santa Cruz JD. Adnexal metaplasia in carcinoma in situ of the skin. J Cutan Pathol 1981; 8(2): 79–88.

75. Guldhammer Bnorgaard T. The differential diagnosis of intraepidermal malignant lesions using immunohistochemistry. Am J Dermatopathol 1986; 8(4): 295–301.

76. Ohnishi Twatanabe S. The use of cytokeratins 7 and 20 in the diagnosis of primary and secondary extramammary Paget's disease. Br J Dermatol 2000; 142(2): 243–247.

77. Williamson JD, et al. Pagetoid Bowen disease: a report of 2 cases that express cytokeratin 7. Arch Pathol Lab Med 2000; 124(3): 427–430.

78. Johnson TM, et al. Squamous cell carcinoma of the skin (excluding lip and oral mucosa). J Am Acad Dermatol 1992; 26(3 Pt 2): 467–484.

79. Barr LH, Menard JW. Marjolin's ulcer. The LSU experience. Cancer 1983; 52(1): 173–175.

80. Cruickshank AH, Miller DG. Malignancy in scars, chronic ulcers, and sinuses. J Clin Pathol 1963; 16: 573–580.

81. Mora RG, Perniciaro C. Cancer of the skin in blacks. I. A review of 163 black patients with cutaneous squamous cell carcinoma. J Am Acad Dermatol 1981; 5(5): 535–543.

82. Jensen P, et al, Skin cancer in kidney and heart transplant recipients and different long-term immunosuppressive therapy regimens. J Am Acad Dermatol 1999; 40(2 Pt 1): 177–186.

83. Broders A. Squamous cell epithelioma of the skin. Ann Surg 1921; 73: 141–160.

84. Subtil A, LeBoit PE. Lymphocytes + nerves = ? Am J Dermatopathol 2000; 22(4): 362–364.

85. Evans HL, Smith JL. Spindle cell squamous carcinomas and sarcoma-like tumors of the skin: a comparative study of 38 cases. Cancer 1980; 45(10): 2687–2697.

86. Eusebi V, et al. Spindle cell tumours of the skin of debatable origin. An immunocytochemical study. J Pathol 1984; 144(3): 189–199.

87. Argenyi ZB. Spindle cell neoplasms of the skin: a comprehensive diagnostic approach. Semin Dermatol 1989; 8(4): 283–297.

88. Nappi O, Pettinato G, Wick MR. Adenoid (acantholytic) squamous cell carcinoma of the skin. J Cutan Pathol 1989; 16(3): 114–121.

89. Johnson WC, Helwig EB. Adenoid squamous cell carcinoma (adenoacanthoma). A clinicopathologic study of 155 patients. Cancer 1966; 19(11): 1639–1650.

90. Nappi O, et al. Pseudovascular adenoid squamous cell carcinoma of the skin. A neoplasm that may be mistaken for angiosarcoma. Am J Surg Pathol 1992; 16(5): 429–438.

91. Nagore E, et al. Pseudovascular squamous cell carcinoma of the skin. Clin Exp Dermatol 2000; 25(3): 206–208.

92. Kraus FT, Perezmesa C. Verrucous carcinoma. Clinical and pathologic study of 105 cases involving oral cavity, larynx and genitalia. Cancer 1966; 19(1): 26–38.

93. McKee PH, et al. Carcinoma (epithelioma) cuniculatum: a clinico-pathological study of nineteen cases and review of the literature. Histopathology 1981; 5(4): 425–436.

94. Kao GF, Graham JH, Helwig EB. Carcinoma cuniculatum (verrucous carcinoma of the skin): a clinicopathologic study of 46 cases with ultrastructural observations. Cancer 1982; 49(11): 2395–2403.

95. Schwartz RA. Buschke-Loewenstein tumor: verrucous carcinoma of the penis. J Am Acad Dermatol 1990; 23(4 Pt 1): 723–727.

96. Reingold IM, Smith BR, Graham JH. Epithelioma cuniculatum pedis, a variant of squamous cell carcinoma. Am J Clin Pathol 1978; 69(5): 561–565.

97. Headington JT. Verrucous carcinoma. Cutis 1978; 21(2): 207–211.

98. Prioleau PG, et al. Verrucous carcinoma: a light and electron microscopic, autoradiographic, and immunofluorescence study. Cancer 1980; 45(11): 2849–2857.

99. Mills SE, Gaffey MJ, Frierson HF. Tumors of the upper aerodigestive tract, Fascicle 26. Washington DC: Armed Forces Institute of Pathology; 2000.

100. Schwartz RA. Keratoacanthoma. J Am Acad Dermatol 1994; 30(1): 1–19; quiz 20–22.

101. Hodak E, Jones RE, Ackerman AB. Solitary keratoacanthoma is a squamous-cell carcinoma: three examples with metastases. Am J Dermatopathol 1993; 15(4): 332–342; discussion 343–352.

102. Jaber PW, Cooper PH, Greer KE. Generalized eruptive keratoacanthoma of Grzybowski. J Am Acad Dermatol 1993; 29(2 Pt 2): 299–304.

103. Alexander JO, Lyell A. Multiple keratoacanthomas. J Am Acad Dermatol 1985; 12(2 Pt 1): 376–377.

104. Kern WH, McCray MK. The histopathologic differentiation of keratoacanthoma and squamous cell carcinoma of the skin. J Cutan Pathol 1980; 7(5): 318–325.

105. Lapins NA, Helwig EB. Perineural invasion by keratoacanthoma. Arch Dermatol 1980; 116(7): 791–793.

106. Smith KJ, et al. Spindle cell neoplasms coexpressing cytokeratin and vimentin (metaplastic

squamous cell carcinoma). J Cutan Pathol 1992; 19(4): 286–293.

107. Wick MR. Immunohistologic features of melanocytic neoplasms. In: Dabbs DJ, ed. Diagnostic immunohistochemistry. New York: Churchill Livingstone; 2002.

108. De Young BR, et al. CD31 immunoreactivity in carcinomas and mesotheliomas. Am J Clin Pathol 1998; 110(3): 374–377.

109. Longacre TA, Smoller BR, Rouse RV. Atypical fibroxanthoma. Multiple immunohistologic profiles. Am J Surg Pathol 1993; 17(12): 1199–1209.

110. Beer TW, Shepherd P, Theaker JM. Ber EP4 and epithelial membrane antigen aid distinction of basal cell, squamous cell and basosquamous carcinomas of the skin. Histopathology 2000; 37(3): 218–223.

111. Narisawa Y, Hashimoto K, Kohda H. Merkel cells of the terminal hair follicle of the adult human scalp. J Invest Dermatol 1994; 102(4): 506–510.

112. Rocamora A, et al. Epidermotropic primary neuroendocrine (Merkel cell) carcinoma of the skin with Pautrier-like microabscesses. Report of three cases and review of the literature. J Am Acad Dermatol 1987; 16(6): 1163–1168.

113. Weedon D. Skin pathology. 2nd edn. Philadelphia: Churchill Livingstone; 2002: 1158.

114. Toker C. Trabecular carcinoma of the skin. Arch Dermatol 1972; 105(1): 107–110.

115. Hashimoto K., et al. Pagetoid Merkel cell carcinoma: epidermal origin of the tumor. J Cutan Pathol 1998; 25(10): 572–579.

116. Traest K, De Vos R, van den Oord JJ. Pagetoid Merkel cell carcinoma: speculations on its origin and the mechanism of epidermal spread. J Cutan Pathol 1999; 26(7): 362–365.

117. Wick M, Scheithauer B. Primary neuroendocrine carcinoma of the skin. In: Wick MR, ed. Pathology of unusual malignant cutaneous tumors. New York: Marcel Dekker; 1985: 107–180.

118. Gould VE, et al. Neuroendocrine (Merkel) cells of the skin: hyperplasias, dysplasias, and neoplasms. Lab Invest 1985; 52(4): 334–353.

119. Gould E, et al. Eccrine and squamous differentiation in Merkel cell carcinoma. An immunohistochemical study. Am J Surg Pathol 1988; 12(10): 768–772.

120. Silva EG, et al. Endocrine carcinoma of the skin (Merkel cell carcinoma). Pathol Annu 1984; 19 Pt 2: 1–30.

121. Wick M. Cutaneous tumors and pseudotumors of the head and neck. In: Gnepp D, ed. Diagnostic surgical pathology of the head and neck. Philadelphia: WB.Saunders; 2001: 777–856.

122. Kroll MH, Toker C. Trabecular carcinoma of the skin: further clinicopathologic and morphologic study. Arch Pathol Lab Med 1982; 106(8): 404–408.

123. Layfield L, et al. Neuroendocrine carcinoma of the skin: an immunohistochemical study of tumor markers and neuroendocrine products. J Cutan Pathol 1986; 13(4): 268–273.

124. Eusebi V, et al. Small cell neuroendocrine carcinoma with skeletal muscle differentiation: report of three cases. Am J Surg Pathol 2000; 24(2): 223–230.

125. Rios-Martin JJ, et al. Neuroendocrine carcinoma of the skin with a lymphoepithelioma-like histological pattern. Br J Dermatol 2000; 143(2): 460–462.

126. Miettinen M. Keratin 20: immunohistochemical marker for gastrointestinal, urothelial, and Merkel cell carcinomas. Mod Pathol 1995; 8(4): 384–388.

127. Chan JK, et al. Cytokeratin 20 immunoreactivity distinguishes Merkel cell (primary cutaneous neuroendocrine) carcinomas and salivary gland small cell carcinomas from small cell carcinomas of various sites. Am J Surg Pathol 1997; 21(2): 226–234.

128. DeLellis R, Shin S. Diagnostic immunohistochemistry of endocrine tumors, In: Dabbs DJ, ed. Diagnostic immunohistochemistry. Philadelphia: Churchill Livingstone; 2002: 209–240.

129. Brinkschmidt C, et al. Immunohistochemical demonstration of chromogranin A, chromogranin B and secretoneurin in Merkel cell carcinoma of the skin: An immunohistochemical study suggesting two types of Merkel cell carcinoma. Appl Immunohistochem 1995; 3: 37–44.

130. Nicholson SA, et al. CD99 and cytokeratin-20 in small-cell and basaloid tumors of the skin. Appl Immunohistochem Mol Morphol 2000; 8(1): 37–41.

131. Goepfert H, et al. Merkel cell carcinoma (endocrine carcinoma of the skin) of the head and neck. Arch Otolaryngol 1984; 110(11): 707–712.

132. Mehregan AH. Sebaceous tumors of the skin. J Cutan Pathol 1985; 12(3–4): 196–199.

133. Alessi E, Sala F. Nevus sebaceus. A clinicopathologic study of its evolution. Am J Dermatopathol 1986; 8(1): 27–31.

134. Morioka S. The natural history of nevus sebaceus. J Cutan Pathol 1985; 12(3–4): 200–213.

135. Kaddu S, et al. Basaloid neoplasms in nevus sebaceus. J Cutan Pathol 2000; 27(7): 327–337.

136. Prioleau PG, Santa Cruz DJ. Sebaceous gland neoplasia. J Cutan Pathol 1984; 11(5): 396–414.

137. Rulon DB, Helwig EB. Cutaneous sebaceous neoplasms. Cancer 1974; 33(1): 82–102.

138. Burgdorf WH, Pitha J, Fahmy A. Muir-Torre syndrome. Histologic spectrum of sebaceous proliferations. Am J Dermatopathol 1986; 8(3): 202–208.

139. Sachez Yus E, et al. Sebomatricoma: a unifying term that encompasses all benign neoplasms with sebaceous differentiation. Am J Dermatopathol 1995; 17(3): 213–221.

140. Yus ES, Simon P. About benign neoplasms with sebaceous differentiation. Am J Dermatopathol 1999; 21(3): 298–300.

141. Mehregan AH. Hair follicle tumors of the skin. J Cutan Pathol 198; 12(3–4): 189–195.

142. Headington JT. Tumors of the hair follicle. A review. Am J Pathol 1976; 85(2): 479–514.

143. Abdelsayed RA, et al. Immunohistochemical evaluation of basal cell carcinoma and trichepithelioma using Bcl-2, Ki67, PCNA and P53. J Cutan Pathol 2000; 27(4): 169–175.

144. Brooke JD, Fitzpatrick JE, Golitz LE. Papillary mesenchymal bodies: a histologic finding useful in differentiating trichoepitheliomas from basal cell carcinomas. J Am Acad Dermatol 1989; 21(3 Pt 1): 523–528.

145. Brownstein MH, Shapiro L. Desmoplastic trichoepithelioma. Cancer 1977; 40(6): 2979–2986.

146. Takei Y, Fukushiro S, Ackerman AB. Criteria for histologic differentiation of desmoplastic trichoepithelioma (sclerosing epithelial hamartoma) from morphea-like basal-cell carcinoma. Am J Dermatopathol 1985; 7(3): 207–221.

147. Hartschuh W, Schulz T. Merkel cells are integral constituents of desmoplastic trichoepithelioma: an immunohistochemical and electron microscopic study. J Cutan Pathol 1995; 22(5): 413–421.

148. Landau-Price D, et al. The value of carcinoembryonic antigen in differentiating sclerosing epithelial hamartoma from syringoma. J Cutan Pathol 1985; 12(1): 8–12.

149. Headington JT, French AJ. Primary neoplasms of the hair follicle. Histogenesis and classification. Arch Dermatol 1962; 86: 430–441.

150. Slater DN. Trichoblastic fibroma: hair germ (trichogenic) tumours revisited. Histopathology 1987; 11(3): 327–331.

151. Santa Cruz DJ, Barr RJ, Headington JT. Cutaneous lymphadenoma. Am J Surg Pathol 1991; 15(2): 101–110.

152. Altman DA, et al. Trichoblastic fibroma. A series of 10 cases with report of a new plaque variant. Arch Dermatol 1995; 131(2): 198–201.

153. Soyer HP, Kutzner H, Jacobson M, et al. Cutaneous lymphadenoma is adamantinoid trichoblastoma. Dermatopathology: Practical & Conceptual 1996; 2: 32–38.

154. Salem OS, Steck WD. Cowden's disease (multiple hamartoma and neoplasia syndrome). A case report and review of the English literature. J Am Acad Dermatol 1983; 8(5): 686–696.

155. Bussaglia E, et al. PTEN mutations in eight Spanish families and one Brazilian family with Cowden syndrome. J Invest Dermatol 2002; 118(4): 639–644.

156. Brownstein MH, Shapiro L. Trichilemmoma. Analysis of 40 new cases. Arch Dermatol 1973; 107(6): 866–869.

157. Tellechea O, Reis JP, Baptista AP. Desmoplastic trichilemmoma. Am J Dermatopathol 1992; 14(2): 107–104.

158. Ackerman AB. Trichilemmoma. Arch Dermatol 1978; 114(2): 286.

159. Brownstein MH. Trichilemmoma. Benign follicular tumor or viral wart? Am J Dermatopathol 1980; 2(3): 229–231.

160. Marrogi AJ, Wick MR, Dehner LP. Pilomatrical neoplasms in children and young adults. Am J Dermatopathol 1992; 14(2): 87–94.

161. Booth JC, Kramer H, Taylor KB. Pilomatrixoma calcifying epithelioma (Malherbe). Pathology 1969; 1(2): 119–127.

162. Cazers JS, Okun MR, Pearson SH. Pigmented calcifying epithelioma. Review and presentation of a case with unusual features. Arch Dermatol 1974; 110(5): 773–774.

163. Leppard B, Bussey HJ. Epidermoid cysts, polyposis coli and Gardner's syndrome. Br J Surg 1975; 62(5): 387–393.

164. Wade CL, Haley JC, Hood AF. The utility of submitting epidermoid cysts for histologic examination. Int J Dermatol 2000; 39(4): 314–315.

165. Lopez-Rios F, et al. Squamous cell carcinoma arising in a cutaneous epidermal cyst: case report and literature review. Am J Dermatopathol 1999; 21(2): 174–177.

166. Leppard BJ, Sanderson KV. The natural history of trichilemmal cysts. Br J Dermatol 1976; 94(4): 379–390.

167. Brownstein MH. Hybrid cyst: a combined epidermoid and trichilemmal cyst. J Am Acad Dermatol 1983; 9(6): 872–875.

168. Poiares Baptista A, Garcia ESL, Born MC. Proliferating trichilemmal cyst. J Cutan Pathol 1983; 10(3): 178–187.

169. Sau P, Graham JH, Helwig EB. Proliferating epithelial cysts. Clinicopathological analysis of 96 cases. J Cutan Pathol 1995; 22(5): 394–406.

170. Brownstein MH, Arluk DJ. Proliferating trichilemmal cyst: a simulant of squamous cell carcinoma. Cancer 1981; 48(5): 1207–1214.

171. Mehregan AH. Infundibular tumors of the skin. J Cutan Pathol 1984; 11(5): 387–395.

172. Rahbari H, Mehregan A, Pinkus H. Trichoadenoma of Nikolowski. J Cutan Pathol 1977; 4(2): 90–98.

173. Smith JD, Chernosky ME. Apocrine hidrocystoma (cystadenoma). Arch Dermatol 1974; 109(5): 700–702.

174. Requena L, Kiryu H, Ackerman AB. Neoplasms with apocrine differentiation. Philadelphia: Lippincott-Raven and Ardor Scribendi; 1997.

175. Simon RS, Sanches Yus E. Does eccrine hidrocystoma exist? J Cutan Pathol 1998; 25(3): 182–184.

176. Crain RC, Helwig EB. Dermal cylindroma (dermal ecrine cylindroma). Am J Clin Pathol 1961; 35: 504–515.

177. Pfaltz M, Bruckner-Tuderman L, Schnyder UW. Type VII collagen is a component of cylindroma basement membrane zone. J Cutan Pathol 1989; 16(6): 388–395.

178. Bruckner-Tuderman L, Pfaltz M, Schnyder UW. Cylindroma overexpresses collagen VII, the major anchoring fibril protein. J Invest Dermatol 1991; 96(5): 729–734.

179. Mambo NC. Eccrine spiradenoma: clinical and pathologic study of 49 tumors. J Cutan Pathol 1983; 10(5): 312–320.

180. Kersting DW, Helwig EB. Eccrine spiradenoma. Arch Dermatol 1956; 73: 199–227.

181. Urban CD, Cannon JR, Cole RD. Eruptive syringomas in Down's syndrome. Arch Dermatol 198; 117(6): 374–375.

182. Mehregan AH. Proliferation of sweat ducts in certain diseases of the skin. Am J Dermatopathol 1981; 3(1): 27–31.

183. Mehregan AH, Mehregan DA. Syringoma-like sweat duct proliferation in scalp alopecias. J Cutan Pathol 1990; 17: 355–357.

184. Wilson-Jones E. Pigmented nodular hidradenoma. Arch Dermatol 1971; 104(2): 117–123.

185. Pylyser K, DeWolf-Peeters C, Marien K. The histology of eccrine poroma. Dermatologica 1983; 167: 243–249.

186. Tellechea O, et al. Tubular apocrine adenoma with eccrine and apocrine immunophenotypes or papillary tubular adenoma? Am J Dermatopathol 1995; 17(5): 499–505.

187. Johnson BL Jr, Helwig EB. Eccrine acrospiroma. A clinicopathologic study. Cancer 1969l 23(3): 641–657.

188. Helwig EB. Eccrine acrospiroma. J Cutan Pathol 1984; 11(5): 415–420.

189. Hu CH, Marques AS, Winkelmann RK. Dermal duct tumor: a histochemical and electron microscopic study. Arch Dermatol 1978; 114(11): 1659–1664.

190. Mehregan AH, Marufi M, Medenica M. Eccrine syringofibroadenoma (Mascaro). Report of two cases. J Am Acad Dermatol 1985; 13(3): 433–436.

191. Utani A, Hattori Y. A reactive acrosyringeal proliferation in a patient with ectodermal dysplasia: eccrine syringofibroadenoma-like lesion. J Dermatol 1999; 26(1): 36–43.

192. Hara K, et al. Acrosyringeal adenomatosis (eccrine syringofibroadenoma of Mascaro). A case report and review of the literature. Am J Dermatopathol 1992; 14(4): 328–339.

193. Hurt MA, Igra-Serfaty H, Stevens CS. Eccrine syringofibroadenoma (Mascaro). An acrosyringeal hamartoma. Arch Dermatol 1990; 126(7): 945–949.

194. Weedon D. Eccrine syringofibroadenoma versus acrosyringeal nevus. J Am Acad Dermatol 1987; 16(3 Pt 1): 622–623.

195. Cho S, et al. Poroid hidradenoma. Int J Dermatol 2001; 40(1): 62–64.

196. Biernat W, Pytel J. Retiform/racemiform neoplasm with features of clear cell hidradenoma. Am J Dermatopathol 1999; 21(5): 479–482.

197. Gianotti R, Alessi E. Clear cell hidradenoma associated with the folliculo-sebaceous-apocrine unit. Histologic study of five cases. Am J Dermatopathol 1997; 19(4): 351–347.

198. Rulon DB, Helwig EB. Papillary eccrine adenoma. Arch Dermatol 1977; 113(5): 596–598.

199. Cooper PH, Frierson HF. Papillary eccrine adenoma. Arch Pathol Lab Med 1984; 108(1): 55–57.

200. Ishihara M, et al. Staining of eccrine and apocrine neoplasms and metastatic adenocarcinoma with IKH-4, a monoclonal antibody specific for the eccrine gland. J Cutan Pathol 1998; 25(2): 100–105.

201. Hassab-el-Naby HM, et al. Mixed tumors of the skin. A histological and immunohistochemical study. Am J Dermatopathol 1989; 11(5): 413–428.

202. Akasaka T, Onodera H, Matsuta M. Cutaneous mixed tumor containing ossification, hair matrix, and sebaceous ductal differentiation. J Dermatol 1997; 24(2): 125–131.

203. Wong TY, et al. Benign cutaneous adnexal tumors with combined folliculosebaceous, apocrine, and eccrine differentiation. Clinicopathologic and immunohistochemical study of eight cases. Am J Dermatopathol 1996; 18(2): 124–136.

204. Bates AW, Baithun SI. Atypical mixed tumor of the skin: histologic, immunohistochemical, and ultrastructural features in three cases and a review of the criteria for malignancy. Am J Dermatopathol 1998; 20(1): 35–40.

205. Massa MC, Medenica, M. Cutaneous adnexal tumors and cysts: a review. Part II – Tumors with apocrine and eccrine glandular differentiation and miscellaneous cutaneous cysts. Pathol Annu 1987; 22 Pt 1: 225–276.

206. Vanatta PR, Bangert JL, Freeman RG. Syringocystadenoma papilliferum. A plasmacytotropic tumor. Am J Surg Pathol 1985; 9(9): 678–683.

207. Nelson BR, et al. Sebaceous carcinoma. J Am Acad Dermatol 1995; 33(1): 1–15; quiz 16–18.

208. Rao NA, et al. Sebaceous carcinomas of the ocular adnexa: A clinicopathologic study of 104 cases, with five-year follow-up data. Hum Pathol 1982; 13(2): 113–122.

209. Russell WG, et al. Sebaceous carcinoma of meibomian gland origin. The diagnostic importance of pagetoid spread of neoplastic cells. Am J Clin Pathol 1980; 73(4): 504–511.

210. Ansai S, et al. A histochemical and immunohistochemical study of extra-ocular sebaceous carcinoma. Histopathology 1993; 22(2): 127–133.

211. Boscaino A, et al. Tricholemmal carcinoma: a study of seven cases. J Cutan Pathol 1992; 19(2): 94–99.

212. Swanson PE, et al. Tricholemmal carcinoma: clinicopathologic study of 10 cases. J Cutan Pathol 1992; 19(2): 100–109.

213. Wong TY, Suster S. Tricholemmal carcinoma. A clinicopathologic study of 13 cases. Am J Dermatopathol 1994; 16(5): 463–473.

214. Manivel C, Wick MR, Mukai K. Pilomatrix carcinoma: an immunohistochemical comparison with benign pilomatrixoma and other benign cutaneous lesions of pilar origin. J Cutan Pathol 1986; 13(1): 22–29.

215. Gould E, et al. Pilomatrix carcinoma with pulmonary metastasis. Report of a case. Cancer 1984; 54(2): 370–372.

216. Mehregan AH, Lee KC. Malignant proliferating trichilemmal tumors – report of three cases. J Dermatol Surg Oncol 1987; 13(12): 1339–1342.

217. Weiss J, et al. Malignant proliferating trichilemmal cyst. J Am Acad Dermatol 1995; 32(5 Pt 2): 870–873.

218. Amaral AL, Nascimento GN, Goellner JR. Proliferating pilar (trichilemmal) cyst. Report of two cases, one with carcinomatous transformation and one with distant metastases. Arch Pathol Lab Med 1984; 108(10): 808–810.

219. Santa Cruz DJ. Sweat gland carcinomas: a comprehensive review. Semin Diagn Pathol 1987; 4(1): 38–74.

220. Wick MR, et al. Adnexal carcinomas of the skin. I. Eccrine carcinomas. Cancer 1985; 56(5): 1147–1162.

221. Nakhleh RE, Swanson PE, Wick MR. Cutaneous adnexal carcinomas with divergent differentiation. Am J Dermatopathol 1990; 12(4): 325–334.

222. Berg J, McDivitt R. Pathology of sweat gland carcinoma. Pathol Annu 1968; 3: 123–144.

223. Waxtein L, et al. Malignant nodular hidradenoma. Int J Dermatol 1998; 37(3): 225–228.

224. Mehregan AH, Hashimoto K, Rahbari H. Eccrine adenocarcinoma. A clinicopathologic study of 35 cases. Arch Dermatol 1983; 119(2): 104–114.

225. Robson D, et al. Eccrine porocarcinoma (malignant eccrine poroma): a clinicopathologic study of 69 cases. Am J Surg Pathol 2001; 25(6): 710–720.

226. Henner MS, et al. Solitary syringoma. Report of five cases and clinicopathologic comparison with microcystic adnexal carcinoma of the skin. Am J Dermatopathol 1995; 17(5): 465–470.

227. LeBoit PE, Sexton M. Microcystic adnexal carcinoma of the skin. A reappraisal of the differentiation and differential diagnosis of an underrecognized neoplasm. J Am Acad Dermatol 1993; 29(4): 609–618.

228. Goldstein DJ, Barr RJ, Santa Cruz DJ. Microcystic adnexal carcinoma: a distinct clinicopathologic entity. Cancer 1982; 50(3): 566–572.

229. Cooper PH. Sclerosing carcinomas of sweat ducts (microcystic adnexal carcinoma). Arch Dermatol 1986; 122(3): 261–264.

230. Goto M, et al. Digital syringomatous carcinoma mimicking basal cell carcinoma. Br J Dermatol 2001; 144(2): 438–439.

231. Urso C, et al. Carcinomas of sweat glands: report of 60 cases. Arch Pathol Lab Med 2001; 125(4): 498–505.

232. Singla AK, Shearin JC. Aggressive surgical treatment of digital papillary adenocarcinoma. Plast Reconstr Surg 1997; 99(7): 2058–2060.

233. Kao GF, Helwig EB, Graham JH. Aggressive digital papillary adenoma and adenocarcinoma. A clinicopathological study of 57 patients, with histochemical, immunopathological, and ultrastructural observations. J Cutan Pathol 1987; 14(3): 129–146.

234. Duke WH, Sherrod TT, Lupton GP. Aggressive digital papillary adenocarcinoma (aggressive digital papillary adenoma and adenocarcinoma revisited). Am J Surg Pathol 2000; 24(6): 775–784.

235. Jih DM, et al. Aggressive digital papillary adenocarcinoma: a case report and review of the literature. Am J Dermatopathol 2001; 23(2): 154–157.

236. Inaloz HS, Patel GK, Knight AG. An aggressive treatment for aggressive digital papillary adenocarcinoma. Cutis 2002; 69(3): 179–182; quiz 210.

237. van der Kwast TH, et al. Primary cutaneous adenoid cystic carcinoma: case report, immunohistochemistry, and review of the literature. Br J Dermatol 1988; 118(4): 567–577.

238. Merot Y, et al. Extramammary Paget's disease of the perianal and perineal regions. Evidence of apocrine derivation. Arch Dermatol 1985; 121(6): 750–752.

239. Lloyd J, Flanagan AM. Mammary and extramammary Paget's disease. J Clin Pathol 2000; 53(10): 742–749.

240. Zollo JD, Zeitouni NC. The Roswell Park Cancer Institute experience with extramammary Paget's disease. Br J Dermatol 2000; 142(1): 59–65.

241. Sitakalin C, Ackerman AB. Mammary and extramammary Paget's disease. Am J Dermatopathol 1985; 7(4): 335–340.

242. Helm KF, Goellner JR, Peters MS. Immunohistochemical stains in extramammary Paget's disease. Am J Dermatopathol 1992; 14(5): 402–407.

243. Kiyohara T, et al. Apocrine carcinoma of the vulva in a band-like arrangement with inflammatory and telangiectatic metastasis via local lymphatic channels. Int J Dermatol 2003; 42(1): 71–74.

244. Shintaku M, et al. Apocrine adenocarcinoma of the eyelid with aggressive biological behavior: report of a case. Pathol Int 2002; 52(2): 169–173.

245. Suster S, Wong TY. Polymorphous sweat gland carcinoma. Histopathology 1994; 25(1): 31–39.

246. Steinman R, Hoffman L, Pope M. Maturation and migration of cutaneous dendritic cells. J Invest Dermatol 1995; 105(1 Suppl): 2S–7S.

247. Nestle FO, Nickoloff BJ. A fresh morphological and functional look at dermal dendritic cells. J Cutan Pathol 1995; 22(5): 385–393.

248. Sahl WJ Jr, Clever H. Cutaneous scars: Part II. Int J Dermatol 1994; 33(11): 763–769.

249. Sahl WJ Jr, Clever H. Cutaneous scars: Part I. Int J Dermatol 1994; 33(10): 681–691.

250. Murray JC, Pollack SV, Pinnell SR. Keloids: a review. J Am Acad Dermatol 1981; 4(4): 461–470.

251. Eads TJ, et al. The utility of submitting fibroepithelial polyps for histological examination. Arch Dermatol 1996; 132(12): 1459–1462.

252. Banik R, Lubach D. Skin tags: localization and frequencies according to sex and age. Dermatologica 1987; 174(4): 180–183.

253. Mehregan AH, Tavafoghi V, Ghandchi A. Nevus lipomatosus cutaneus superficialis (Hoffmann-Zurhelle). J Cutan Pathol 1975; 2(6): 307–313.

254. Nogita T, et al. Pedunculated lipofibroma. A clinicopathologic study of thirty-two cases supporting a simplified nomenclature. J Am Acad Dermatol 1994; 31(2 Pt 1): 235–240.

255. McGibbon DH, Jones EW. Fibrous papule of the face (nose). Fibrosing nevocytic nevus. Am J Dermatopathol 1979; 1(4): 345–348.

256. Ragaz A, Berezowsky V. Fibrous papule of the face. A study of five cases by electron microscopy. Am J Dermatopathol 1979; 1(4): 353–356.

257. Nemeth AJ, Penneys NS, Bernstein HB. Fibrous papule: a tumor of fibrohistiocytic cells that contain factor XIIIa. J Am Acad Dermatol 1988; 19(6): 1102–1106.

258. Webb DW, et al. The cutaneous features of tuberous sclerosis: a population study. Br J Dermatol 1996; 135(1): 1–5.

259. Ackerman ABKronberg R. Pearly penile papules. Acral angiofibromas. Arch Dermatol 1973; 108(5): 673–675.

260. Bhawan J, Edelstein L. Angiofibromas in tuberous sclerosis: a light and electron microscopic study. J Cutan Pathol 1977; 4(6): 300–307.

261. Graham JH, et al. Fibrous papule of the nose: a clinicopathological study. J Invest Dermatol 1965; 45(3): 194–203.

262. Cerio R, et al. A study of factor XIIIa and MAC 387 immunolabeling in normal and pathological skin. Am J Dermatopathol 1990; 12(3): 221–233.

263. Hare PJ, Smith, PA. Acquired (digital) fibrokeratoma. Br J Dermatol 1969; 81(9): 667–670.

264. Cahn RL. Acquired periungual fibrokeratoma. A rare benign tumor previously described as the garlic-clove fibroma. Arch Dermatol 1977; 113(11): 1564–1568.

265. Kamino H, Lee JY, Berke A. Pleomorphic fibroma of the skin: a benign neoplasm with cytologic atypia. A clinicopathologic study of eight cases. Am J Surg Pathol 1989; 13(2): 107–113.

266. McCalmont TH. Sclerotic fibroma: a fossil no longer. J Cutan Pathol 1994; 21(1): 82–85.

267. Garcia-Doval I, Casas L, Toribio J. Pleomorphic fibroma of the skin, a form of sclerotic fibroma: an immunohistochemical study. Clin Exp Dermatol 1998; 23(1): 22–24.

268. Fitzpatrick TB, Gilchrest BA. Dimple sign to differentiate benign from malignant pigmented cutaneous lesions. N Engl J Med 1977; 296(26): 1518.

269. Gonzalez S, Duarte I. Benign fibrous histiocytoma of the skin. A morphologic study of 290 cases. Pathol Res Pract 1982; 174(4): 379–391.

270. Marrogi AJ, et al. Benign cutaneous histiocytic tumors in childhood and adolescence, excluding Langerhans' cell proliferations. A clinicopathologic and immunohistochemical analysis. Am J Dermatopathol 1992; 14(1): 8–18.

271. Calonje E, Mentzel T, Fletcher CD. Cellular benign fibrous histiocytoma. Clinicopathologic analysis of 74 cases of a distinctive variant of cutaneous fibrous histiocytoma with frequent recurrence. Am J Surg Pathol 1994; 18(7): 668–676.

272. Costa MJ, Weiss SW. Angiomatoid malignant fibrous histiocytoma. A follow-up study of 108 cases with evaluation of possible histologic predictors of outcome. Am J Surg Pathol 1990; 14(12): 1126–1132.

273. Calonje E, Fletcher CD. Aneurysmal benign fibrous histiocytoma: clinicopathological analysis of 40 cases of a tumour frequently misdiagnosed as a vascular neoplasm. Histopathology 1995; 26(4): 323–331.

274. Tamada S, Ackerman SB. Dermatofibroma with monster cells. Am J Dermatopathol 1987; 9(5): 380–387.

275. Kaddu S, McMenamin ME, Fletcher CD. Atypical fibrous histiocytoma of the skin: clinicopathologic analysis of 59 cases with evidence of infrequent metastasis. Am J Surg Pathol 2002; 26(1): 35–46.

276. Zelger BG, et al. Granular cell dermatofibroma. Histopathology 1997; 31(3): 258–262.

277. Soyer HP, Metze D, Kerl H. Granular cell dermatofibroma. Am J Dermatopathol 1997; 19(2): 168–173.

278. Cerio R, Spaull J, Jones EW. Histiocytoma cutis: a tumour of dermal dendrocytes (dermal dendrocytoma). Br J Dermatol 1989; 120(2): 197–206.

279. Goldblum JR, Tuthill RJ. CD34 and factor-XIIIa immunoreactivity in dermatofibrosarcoma protuberans and dermatofibroma. Am J Dermatopathol 1997; 19(2): 147–153.

280. Kamino H, et al. Dermatomyofibroma. A benign cutaneous, plaque-like proliferation of fibroblasts and myofibroblasts in young adults. J Cutan Pathol 1992; 19(2): 85–93.

281. Rose C, Brocker EB. Dermatomyofibroma: case report and review. Pediatr Dermatol 1999; 16(6): 456–459.

282. Colome MI, Sanchez RL. Dermatomyofibroma: report of two cases. J Cutan Pathol 1994; 21(4): 371–376.

283. Manivel JC, Dehner LP, MR W. Nonvascular sarcomas of the skin. In: Wick MR, ed. Pathology of unusual malignant cutaneous tumors. New York: Marcel Dekker; 1985: 211–279.

284. McPeak CJ, Cruz T, Nicastri DN. Dermatofibrosarcoma protuberans: an analysis of 86 cases – five with metastasis. Ann Surg 1967; 166(5): 803–816.

285. Kamino H, Jacobson M. Dermatofibroma extending into the subcutaneous tissue. Differential diagnosis from dermatofibrosarcoma protuberans. Am J Surg Pathol 1990; 14(12): 1156–1164.

286. Burkhardt BR, et al. Dermatofibrosarcoma protuberans. Study of fifty-six cases. Am J Surg 1966; 111(5): 638–644.

287. Dupree WB, Langloss JM, Weiss SW. Pigmented dermatofibrosarcoma protuberans (Bednar tumor). A pathologic, ultrastructural, and immunohistochemical study. Am J Surg Pathol 1985; 9(9): 630–639.

288. Horenstein MG, et al. Indeterminate fibrohistiocytic lesions of the skin: is there a spectrum between dermatofibroma and dermatofibrosarcoma protuberans? Am J Surg Pathol 2000; 24(7): 996–1003.

289. Cohen PR, Rapin R, Farhood AI. Dermatofibroma and dermatofibrosarcoma protuberans: differential expression of CD34 and factor XIIIa. Am J Dermatopathol 1994; 16(5): 573–574.

290. Aiba S, et al. Dermatofibrosarcoma protuberans is a unique fibrohistiocytic tumour expressing CD34. Br J Dermatol 1992; 127(2): 79–84.

291. Helwig EB. Atypical fibroxanthoma. Texas J Med 1963; 59: 664–697.

292. Oshiro Y, Fukuda T, Tsuneyoshi M. Atypical fibroxanthoma versus benign and malignant fibrous histiocytoma. A comparative study of their proliferative activity using MIB-1, DNA flow cytometry, and p53 immunostaining. Cancer 1995; 75(5): 1128–1134.

293. Grosso M, et al. Metastatic atypical fibroxanthoma of skin. Pathol Res Pract 1987; 182(3): 443–447.

294. Wilson PR, Strutton GM, Stewart MR. Atypical fibroxanthoma: two unusual variants. J Cutan Pathol 1989; 16(2): 93–98.

295. Touart DM, Sau P. Cutaneous deposition diseases. Part II. J Am Acad Dermatol 1998; 39(4 Pt 1): 527–544; quiz 545–546.

296. Sanmartin O, et al. Congenital platelike osteoma cutis: case report and review of the literature. Pediatr Dermatol 1993; 10(2): 182–186.

297. Gardner RJ, Yun K, Craw SM. Familial ectopic ossification. J Med Genet 1988; 25(2): 113–117.

298. Eyre WG, Reed WB. Albright's hereditary osteodystrophy with cutaneous bone formation. Arch Dermatol 1971; 104(6): 634–642.

299. Goeteyn V, De Potter CR, Naeyaert JM. Osteoma cutis in pseudohypoparathyroidism. Dermatology 1999; 198(2): 209–211.

300. Roth S, Stowell R, Helwig E. Cutaneous ossification. Arch Pathol 1963; 76: 44–54.

301. Burgdorf W, Nasemann T. Cutaneous osteomas: a clinical and histopathologic review. Arch Dermatol Res 1977; 260(2): 121–135.

302. Allen PW, Dymock RB, MacCormac LB. Superficial angiomyxomas with and without epithelial components. Report of 30 tumors in 28 patients. Am J Surg Pathol 1988; 12(7): 519–530.

303. Ferreiro JA, Carney JA. Myxomas of the external ear and their significance. Am J Surg Pathol 1994; 18(3): 274–280.

304. Calonje E, et al. Superficial angiomyxoma: clinicopathologic analysis of a series of distinctive but poorly recognized cutaneous tumors with tendency for recurrence. Am J Surg Pathol 1999; 23(8): 910–917.

305. Fetsch JF, Laskin WB, Miettinen M. Superficial acral fibromyxoma: a clinicopathologic and immunohistochemical analysis of 37 cases of a distinctive soft tissue tumor with a predilection for the fingers and toes. Hum Pathol 2001; 32(7): 704–714.

306. Megahed M. Palisaded encapsulated neuroma (solitary circumscribed neuroma). A clinicopathologic and immunohistochemical study. Am J Dermatopathol 1994; 16(2): 120–125.

307. Tsang WY Chan JK. Epithelioid variant of solitary circumscribed neuroma of the skin. Histopathology 1992; 20(5): 439–441.

308. Argenyi ZB. Immunohistochemical characterization of palisaded, encapsulated neuroma. J Cutan Pathol 1990; 17(6): 329–335.

309. Finley JL, et al. Port-wine stains. Morphologic variations and developmental lesions. Arch Dermatol 1984; 120(11): 1453–1455.

310. Requena Lsangueza OP. Cutaneous vascular anomalies. Part I. Hamartomas, malformations, and dilation of preexisting vessels. J Am Acad Dermatol 1997; 37(4): 523–549; quiz 549–552.

311. Whimster IW. The pathology of lymphangioma circumscriptum. Br J Dermatol 1976; 94(5): 473–486.

312. Imperial R, Helwig EB. Angiokeratoma. A clinicopathological study. Arch Dermatol 1967; 95(2): 166–175.

313. Imperial R, Helwig EB. Angiokeratoma of the scrotum (Fordyce type). J Urol 1967; 98(3): 379–387.

314. Imperial R, Helwig EB. Angiokeratoma of the vulva. Obstet Gynecol 1967; 29(3): 307–312.

315. MacCollum DW, Martin LW. Hemangiomas in infancy and childhood. A report based on 6470 cases. Surg Clin North Am 1956; 36: 1647–1663.

316. Bowers RE, Graham EA, Tomlinson KM. The natural history of the strawberry nevus. Arch Dermatol 1960; 82: 667–668.

317. Calonje E, Mentzel T, Fletcher CD. Pseudomalignant perineurial invasion in cellular ('infantile') capillary haemangiomas. Histopathology 1995; 26(2): 159–164.

318. Patrice SJ, Wiss K, Mulliken JB. Pyogenic granuloma (lobular capillary hemangioma): a clinicopathologic study of 178 cases. Pediatr Dermatol 1991; 8(4): 267–276.

319. Mussalli NG, Hopps RM, Johnson NW. Oral pyogenic granuloma as a complication of pregnancy and the use of hormonal contraceptives. Int J Gynaecol Obstet 1976; 14(2): 187–191.

320. Mills SE, Cooper PH, Fechner RE. Lobular capillary hemangioma: the underlying lesion of pyogenic granuloma. A study of 73 cases from the oral and nasal mucous membranes. Am J Surg Pathol 1980; 4(5): 470–479.

321. Tuder RM, et al. Adult cutaneous hemangiomas are composed of nonreplicating endothelial cells. J Invest Dermatol 1987; 89(6): 594–597.

322. Puig L, et al. Verrucous hemangioma. J Dermatol Surg Oncol 1987; 13(10): 1089–1092.

323. Jones EW, Orkin M. Tufted angioma (angioblastoma). A benign progressive angioma, not to be confused with Kaposi's sarcoma or low-grade angiosarcoma. J Am Acad Dermatol 1989; 20(2 Pt 1): 214–225.

324. Cho KH, et al. Angioblastoma (Nakagawa) – is it the same as tufted angioma? Clin Exp Dermatol 1991; 16(2): 110–113.

325. Padilla RS, Orkin M, Rosai J. Acquired 'tufted' angioma (progressive capillary hemangioma). A distinctive clinicopathologic entity related to lobular capillary hemangioma. Am J Dermatopathol 1987; 9(4): 292–300.

326. Requena L, Sangueza OP. Cutaneous vascular proliferation. Part II. Hyperplasias and benign neoplasms. J Am Acad Dermatol 1997; 37(6): 887–919; quiz 920–922.

327. Esterly NB. Kasabach-Merritt syndrome in infants. J Am Acad Dermatol 1983; 8(4): 504–513.

328. Morris SJ, et al. Blue rubber-bleb nevus syndrome. JAMA 1978; 239(18): 1887.

329. Loewinger RJ, et al. Maffucci's syndrome: amesenchymal dysplasia and multiple tumour syndrome. Br J Dermatol 1977; 96(3): 317–322.

330. Calonje E, Fletcher CD. Sinusoidal hemangioma. A distinctive benign vascular neoplasm within the group of cavernous hemangiomas. Am J Surg Pathol 1991; 15(12): 1130–1135.

331. Connelly MG, Winkelmann RK. Acral arteriovenous tumor. A clinicopathologic review. Am J Surg Pathol 1985; 9(1): 15–21.

332. Girard C, Graham JH, Johnson WC. Arteriovenous hemangioma (arteriovenous shunt). A clinicopathological and histochemical study. J Cutan Pathol 1974; 1(2): 73–87.

333. Chan JK, et al. Glomeruloid hemangioma. A distinctive cutaneous lesion of multicentric Castleman's disease associated with POEMS syndrome. Am J Surg Pathol 1990; 14(11): 1036–1046.

334. Onishi Yohara K. Angiolymphoid hyperplasia with eosinophilia associated with arteriovenous malformation: a clinicopathological correlation with angiography and serial estimation of serum levels of renin, eosinophil cationic protein and interleukin 5. Br J Dermatol 1999; 140(6): 1153–1156.

335. Vadlamudi G, Schinella R. Traumatic pseudoaneurysm: a possible early lesion in the spectrum of epithelioid hemangioma/angiolymphoid hyperplasia with eosinophilia. Am J Dermatopathol 1998; 20(2): 113–117.

336. Googe PB, Harris NL, Mihm MC Jr. Kimura's disease and angiolymphoid hyperplasia with eosinophilia: two distinct histopathological entities. J Cutan Pathol 1987; 14(5): 263–271.

337. Kung IT, Gibson JB, Bannatyne PM. Kimura's disease: a clinico-pathological study of 21 cases and its distinction from angiolymphoid hyperplasia with eosinophilia. Pathology 1984; 16(1): 39–44.

338. Urabe A, Tsuneyoshi M, Enjoji M. Epithelioid hemangioma versus Kimura's disease. A comparative clinicopathologic study. Am J Surg Pathol 1987; 11(10): 758–766.

339. Carlson JA, Daulat S, Goodheart HP. Targetoid hemosiderotic hemangioma – a dynamic vascular tumor: report of 3 cases with episodic and cyclic changes and comparison with solitary angiokeratomas. J Am Acad Dermatol 1999; 41(2 Pt 1): 215–224.

340. Santa Cruz DJ, Aronberg J. Targetoid hemosiderotic hemangioma. J Am Acad Dermatol 1988; 19(3): 550–558.

341. Guillou L, et al. Hobnail hemangioma: a pseudomalignant vascular lesion with a reappraisal of targetoid hemosiderotic hemangioma. Am J Surg Pathol 1999; 23(1): 97–105.

342. Hunt SJ, Santa Cruz DJ, Barr RJ. Microvenular hemangioma. J Cutan Pathol 1991; 18(4): 235–240.

343. Aloi F, Tomasini C, Pippione M. Microvenular hemangioma. Am J Dermatopathol 1993; 15(6): 534–538.

344. Tomasini C, et al. Spindle cell hemangioma. Dermatology 1999; 199(3): 274–276.

345. Perkins P, Weiss SW. Spindle cell hemangioendothelioma. An analysis of 78 cases with reassessment of its pathogenesis and biologic behavior. Am J Surg Pathol 1996; 20(10): 1196–1204.

346. Weiss SW, Enzinger FM. Spindle cell hemangioendothelioma. A low-grade angiosarcoma resembling a cavernous hemangioma and Kaposi's sarcoma. Am J Surg Pathol 1986; 10(8): 521–530.

347. Fletcher CD, Beham A, Schmid C. Spindle cell haemangioendothelioma: a clinicopathological and immunohistochemical study indicative of a non-neoplastic lesion. Histopathology 1991; 18(4): 291–301.

348. Appelman HD, Helwig EB. Glomus tumors of the stomach. Cancer 1969; 23(1): 203–213.

349. Goodman TF. Fine structure of the cells of the Suquet-Hoyer canal. J Invest Dermatol 1972; 59(5): 363–369.

350. Peretz E, et al. Solitary glomus tumour. Australas J Dermatol 1999; 40(4): 226–227.

351. Blume-Peytavi U, et al. Multiple familial cutaneous glomangioma: a pedigree of 4 generations and critical analysis of histologic and genetic differences of glomus tumors. J Am Acad Dermatol 2000; 42(4): 633–639.

352. Dervan PA, et al. Glomus tumours: an immunohistochemical profile of 11 cases. Histopathology 1989; 14(5): 483–491.

353. Schurch W, et al. Intermediate filament proteins and actin isoforms as markers for soft-tissue tumor differentiation and origin. III. Hemangiopericytomas and glomus tumors. Am J Pathol 1990; 136(4): 771–786.

354. Folpe AL, et al. Atypical and malignant glomus tumors: analysis of 52 cases, with a proposal for the reclassification of glomus tumors. Am J Surg Pathol 2001; 25(1): 1–12.

355. Quante M, et al. Epithelioid hemangioendothelioma presenting in the skin: a clinicopathologic study of eight cases. Am J Dermatopathol 1998; 20(6): 541–546.

356. Dabska M. Malignant endovascular papillary angioendothelioma of the skin in childhood. Clinicopathologic study of 6 cases. Cancer 1969; 24(3): 503–510.

357. Schwartz RA, Dabski C, Dabska M. The Dabska tumor: a thirty-year retrospect. Dermatology 2000; 201(1): 1–5.

358. Argani P, Athanasian E. Malignant endovascular papillary angioendothelioma (Dabska tumor) arising within a deep intramuscular hemangioma. Arch Pathol Lab Med 1997; 121(9): 992–995.

359. Katz JA, et al. Endovascular papillary angioendothelioma in the spleen. Pediatr Pathol 1988; 8(2): 185–193.

360. Fanburg-Smith JC, et al. Papillary intralymphatic angioendothelioma (PILA): a report of twelve cases of a distinctive vascular tumor with phenotypic features of lymphatic vessels. Am J Surg Pathol 1999; 23(9): 1004–1010.

361. Kempson RL, Fletcher CDM, Evans HL, et al. Tumors of the soft tissues. Third series. Atlas of tumor pathology. Vol. 30. Washington DC: Armed Forces Institute of Pathology; 2001.

362. Manivel JC, et al. Endovascular papillary angioendothelioma of childhood: a vascular lesion possibly characterized by 'high' endothelial cell differentiation. Hum Pathol 1986; 17(12): 1240–1244.

363. Partanen TA, Alitalo K, Miettinen M. Lack of lymphatic vascular specificity of vascular endothelial growth factor receptor 3 in 185 vascular tumors. Cancer 1999; 86(11): 2406–2412.

364. Folpe AL, et al. Vascular endothelial growth factor receptor-3 (VEGFR-3): a marker of vascular tumors with presumed lymphatic differentiation, including Kaposi's sarcoma, kaposiform and Dabska-type hemangioendotheliomas, and a subset of angiosarcomas. Mod Pathol 2000; 13(2): 180–185.

365. Calonje E, et al. Retiform hemangioendothelioma. A distinctive form of low-grade angiosarcoma delineated in a series of 15 cases. Am J Surg Pathol 1994; 18(2): 115–125.

366. Weiss SW, Goldblum J. Enzinger and Weiss's soft tissue tumors. 4th edition. Philadelphia: Mosby; 2001.

367. Beaubien ER, Ball NJ, Storwick GS. Kaposiform hemangioendothelioma: a locally aggressive vascular tumor. J Am Acad Dermatol 1998; 38(5 Pt 2): 799–802.

368. Zukerberg LR, Nickoloff BJ, Weiss SW. Kaposiform hemangioendothelioma of infancy and childhood. An aggressive neoplasm associated with Kasabach-Merritt syndrome and lymphangiomatosis. Am J Surg Pathol 1993; 17(4): 321–328.

369. Slavin G, et al. Kaposi's sarcoma in East African children: a report of 51 cases. J Pathol 1970; 100(3): 187–199.

370. Vin-Christian K, McCalmont TH, Frieden IJ. Kaposiform hemangioendothelioma. An aggressive, locally invasive vascular tumor that can mimic hemangioma of infancy. Arch Dermatol 1997; 133(12): 1573–1578.

371. Li N, Anderson WK, Bhawan J. Further confirmation of the association of human herpesvirus 8 with Kaposi's sarcoma. J Cutan Pathol 1998; 25(8): 413–419.

372. Antman K, Chang Y. Kaposi's sarcoma. N Engl J Med 2000; 342(14): 1027–1038.

373. Requena L, Sangueza OP. Cutaneous vascular proliferations. Part III. Malignant neoplasms, other cutaneous neoplasms with significant vascular component, and disorders erroneously considered as vascular neoplasms. J Am Acad Dermatol 1998; 38(2 Pt 1): 143–175; quiz 176–178.

374. Cottoni F, De Marco R, Montesu MA. Classical Kaposi's sarcoma in north-east Sardinia: an overview from 1977 to 1991. Br J Cancer 1996; 73(9): 1132–1133.

375. Stribling J, Weitzner S, Smith GV. Kaposi's sarcoma in renal allograft recipients. Cancer 1978; 42(2): 442–446.

376. Chor PJ, Santa Cruz DJ. Kaposi's sarcoma. A clinicopathologic review and differential diagnosis. J Cutan Pathol 1992; 19(1): 6–20.

377. Lemlich G, Schwam L, Lebwohl M. Kaposi's sarcoma and acquired immunodeficiency syndrome. Postmortem findings in twenty-four cases. J Am Acad Dermatol 1987; 16(2 Pt 1): 319–325.

378. Friedman-Kien AE, Saltzman BR. Clinical manifestations of classical, endemic African, and epidemic AIDS-associated Kaposi's sarcoma. J Am Acad Dermatol 1990; 22(6 Pt 2): 1237–1250.

379. Kao GF, Johnson FB, Sulica VI. The nature of hyaline (eosinophilic) globules and vascular slits of Kaposi's sarcoma. Am J Dermatopathol 1990; 12(3): 256–267.

380. Templeton AC. Kaposi's sarcoma. Pathol Annu 1981; 16(Pt 2): 315–336.

381. DeYoung BR, et al. CD31 immunoreactivity in mesenchymal neoplasms of the skin and subcutis: report of 145 cases and review of putative immunohistologic markers of endothelial differentiation. J Cutan Pathol 1995; 22(3): 215–222.

382. Miettinen M, Lindenmayer AE, Chaubal A. Endothelial cell markers CD31, CD34, and BNH9 antibody to H- and Y-antigens – evaluation of their specificity and sensitivity in the diagnosis of vascular tumors and comparison with von Willebrand factor. Mod Pathol 1994; 7(1): 82–90.

382a. Cheuk W, Wong KO, Wong CS, et al. Immunostaining for human herpesvirus-8 latent nuclear antigen-1 helps distinguish Kaposi sarcoma from its mimickers. Am J Clin Pathol 2004; 121: 335–342.

382b. Robin YM, Guillou L, Michels JJ, Coindre JM. Human herpesvirus-8 immunostaining: a sensitive and specific method for diagnosing Kaposi sarcoma in paraffin-embedded sections. Am J Clin Pathol 2004; 121: 330–334.

383. Blumenfeld W, Egbert BM, Sagebiel RW. Differential diagnosis of Kaposi's sarcoma. Arch Pathol Lab Med 1985; 109(2): 123–127.

384. Rosai J, et al. Angiosarcoma of the skin. A clinicopathologic and fine structural study. Hum Pathol 1976; 7(1): 83–109.

385. Holden CA, Spittle MF, Jones EW. Angiosarcoma of the face and scalp, prognosis and treatment. Cancer 1987; 59(5): 1046–1057.

386. Stewart FW, Treves N. Classics in oncology: lymphangiosarcoma in postmastectomy lymphedema: a report of six cases in elephantiasis chirurgica. CA Cancer J Clin 1981; 31(5): 284–299.

387. Offori TW, et al. Angiosarcoma in congenital hereditary lymphoedema (Milroy's disease) – diagnostic beacons and a review of the literature. Clin Exp Dermatol 1993; 18(2): 174–177.

388. Alessi E, Sala F, Berti E. Angiosarcomas in lymphedematous limbs. Am J Dermatopathol 1986; 8(5): 371–378.

389. Muller R, Hajdu SI, Brennan MF. Lymphangiosarcoma associated with chronic filarial lymphedema. Cancer 1987; 59(1): 179–183.

390. Goette DK, Detlefs RL. Postirradiation angiosarcoma. J Am Acad Dermatol 1985; 12(5 Pt 2): 922–926.

391. Caldwell JB, et al. Cutaneous angiosarcoma arising in the radiation site of a congenital hemangioma. J Am Acad Dermatol 1995; 33(5 Pt 2): 865–870.

392. Cooper PH. Angiosarcomas of the skin. Semin Diagn Pathol 1987; 4(1): 2–17.

393. Ohsawa M, et al. Use of immunohistochemical procedures in diagnosing angiosarcoma. Evaluation of 98 cases. Cancer 1995; 75(12): 2867–2874.

394. Miettinen Mfetsch JF. Distribution of keratins in normal endothelial cells and a spectrum of vascular tumors: implications in tumor diagnosis. Hum Pathol 2000; 31(9): 1062–1067.

395. Happle R. What is a nevus? A proposed definition of a common medical term. Dermatology 1995; 191(1): 1–5.

396. Gupta G, Williams RE, Mackie RM. The labial melanotic macule: a review of 79 cases. Br J Dermatol 1997; 136(5): 772–775.

397. Lenane P, et al. Genital melanotic macules: clinical, histologic, immunohistochemical, and ultrastructural features. J Am Acad Dermatol 2000; 42(4): 640–644.

398. Sexton FM, Maize CJ. Melanotic macules and melanoacanthomas of the lip. A comparative study with census of the basal melanocyte population. Am J Dermatopathol 1987; 9(5): 438–444.

399. Ho KK, et al. Labial melanotic macule: a clinical, histopathologic, and ultrastructural study. J Am Acad Dermatol 1993; 28(1): 33–39.

400. Hwang SM, et al. Nevus spilus (speckled lentiginous nevus) associated with a nodular neurotized nevus. Am J Dermatopathol 1997; 19(3): 308–311.

401. Gallagher RP, et al. Anatomic distribution of acquired melanocytic nevi in white children. A comparison with melanoma: the Vancouver Mole Study. Arch Dermatol 1990; 126(4): 466–471.

402. Pope DJ, et al. Benign pigmented nevi in children. Prevalence and associated factors: the West Midlands, United Kingdom Mole Study. Arch Dermatol 1992; 128(9): 1201–1206.

403. Richard MA, et al. Role of sun exposure on nevus. First study in age-sex phenotype-controlled populations. Arch Dermatol 1993; 129(10): 1280–1285.

404. Kelly JW, et al. Sunlight: a major factor associated with the development of melanocytic nevi in Australian schoolchildren. J Am Acad Dermatol 1994; 30(1): 40–48.

405. Maize JC, Ackerman AB. Pigmented lesions of the skin: clinicopathologic correlations. Philadelphia: Lea & Febiger; 1987.

406. Elder DE, Murphy GF. Melanocytic tumors of the skin. Atlas of tumor pathology. Sobin LH, ed. Vol. 2. Washington DC: Armed Forces Institute of Pathology; 1991: 216.

407. Yaar M, Woodley DT, Gilchrest BA. Human nevocellular nevus cells are surrounded by basement membrane components. Immunohistologic studies of human nevus cells and melanocytes in vivo and in vitro. Lab Invest 1988; 58(2): 157–162.

408. Schmoeckel C. Classification of melanocytic nevi: do nodular and flat nevi develop differently? Am J Dermatopathol 1997; 19(1): 31–34.

409. Worret WI, Burgdorf WH. Which direction do nevus cells move? Abtropfung reexamined. Am J Dermatopathol 1998; 20(2): 135–139.

410. Cramer SF. The melanocyte differentiation pathway in spitz nevi. Am J Dermatopathol 1998; 20(6): 555–570.

411. Clemente C, et al. Acral-lentiginous naevus of plantar skin. Histopathology 1995; 27(6): 549–555.

412. LeBoit PE. Simulants of malignant melanoma: a rogue's gallery of melanocytic and nonmelanocytic imposters. Pathology (Phila) 1994; 2(2): 195–258.

413. Boyd AS, Rapini RP. Acral melanocytic neoplasms: a histologic analysis of 158 lesions. J Am Acad Dermatol 1994; 31(5 Pt 1): 740–745.

414. Rongioletti F, et al. Histopathological features of flexural melanocytic nevi: a study of 40 cases. J Cutan Pathol 2000; 27(5): 215–217.

415. Signoretti S, et al. Melanocytic nevi of palms and soles: a histological study according to the plane of section. Am J Surg Pathol 1999; 23(3): 283–287.

416. Fallowfield ME, Collina G, Cook MG. Melanocytic lesions of the palm and sole. Histopathology 1994; 24(5): 463–467.

417. Tosti A, et al. Nail matrix nevi: a clinical and histopathologic study of twenty-two patients. J Am Acad Dermatol 1996; 34(5 Pt 1): 765–771.

418. Foucar E, et al. A histopathologic evaluation of nevocellular nevi in pregnancy. Arch Dermatol 1985; 121(3): 350–354.

419. Misago N. The relationship between melanocytes and peripheral nerve sheath cells (Part I): melanocytic nevus (excluding so-called 'blue nevus') with peripheral nerve sheath differentiation. Am J Dermatopathol 2000; 22(3): 217–229.

420. Weedon D. Unusual features of nevocellular nevi. J Cutan Pathol 1982; 9(5): 284–292.

421. Eng W, Cohen PR. Nevus with fat: clinical characteristics of 100 nevi containing mature adipose cells. J Am Acad Dermatol 1998; 39(5 Pt 1): 704–711.

422. Maize JC, Foster G. Age-related changes in melanocytic naevi. Clin Exp Dermatol 1979; 4(1): 49–58.

423. Sahin S, et al. Risk of melanoma in medium-sized congenital melanocytic nevi: a follow-up study. J Am Acad Dermatol 1998; 39(3): 428–433.

424. Crowson AN, Magro CM, Mihm MC. The melanocytic proliferations: A comprehensive textbook of pigmented lesions. New York: Wiley-Liss; 2001: 539.

425. Swerdlow AJ, English JS, Qiao Z. The risk of melanoma in patients with congenital nevi: a cohort study. J Am Acad Dermatol 1995; 32(4): 595–599.

426. Rhodes AR. Pigmented birthmarks and precursor melanocytic lesions of cutaneous melanoma identifiable in childhood. Pediatr Clin North Am 1983; 30(3): 435–463.

427. Mancianti ML, et al. Malignant melanoma simulants arising in congenital melanocytic nevi do not show experimental evidence for a malignant phenotype. Am J Pathol 1990; 136(4): 817–829.

428. Walton RG, Jacobs AH, Cox AJ. Pigmented lesions in newborn infants. Br J Dermatol 1976; 95(4): 389–396.

429. Cribier BJ, Santinelli F, Grosshans E. Lack of clinical-pathological correlation in the diagnosis of congenital naevi. Br J Dermatol 1999; 141(6): 1004–1009.

430. Zitelli JA, et al. Histologic patterns of congenital nevocytic nevi and implications for treatment. J Am Acad Dermatol 1984; 11(3): 402–409.

431. Mark GJ, et al. Congenital melanocytic nevi of the small and garment type. Clinical, histologic, and ultrastructural studies. Hum Pathol 1973; 4(3): 395–418.

432. Rhodes AR, et al. The malignant potential of small congenital nevocellular nevi. An estimate of association based on a histologic study of 234 primary cutaneous melanomas. J Am Acad Dermatol 1982; 6(2): 230–241.

433. Spitz S. Melanomas of childhood. Am J Pathol 1948; 24: 591–610.

434. Kernan J, Ackerman AB. Spindle cell nevi and epithelioid cell nevi (so-called juvenile melanomas in children and adults): A clinicopathological study of 27 cases. Cancer 1960; 13: 612–625.

435. Helwig EB. Seminar on skin neoplasms and dermatoses: Twentieth seminar of the American Society of Clinical Pathologists. Washington DC: American Society of Clinical Pathologists; 1954: 63–67.

436. Paniago-Pereira C, Maize JC, Ackerman AB. Nevus of large spindle and/or epithelioid cells (Spitz's nevus). Arch Dermatol 1978; 114(12): 1811–1823.

437. Dal Pozzo V, et al. Clinical review of 247 case records of Spitz nevus (epithelioid cell and/or spindle cell nevus). Dermatology 1997; 194(1): 20–25.

438. Weedon D, Little JH. Spindle and epithelioid cell nevi in children and adults. A review of 211 cases of the Spitz nevus. Cancer 1977; 40(1): 217–225.

439. Akyurek M, et al. Multiple agminated Spitz nevi of the scalp. Ann Plast Surg 1999; 43(4): 459–460.

440. Scott G, Chen KT, Rosai J. Pseudoepitheliomatous hyperplasia in Spitz nevi. A possible source of confusion with squamous cell carcinoma. Arch Pathol Lab Med 1989; 113(1): 61–63.

441. Havenith MG, et al. Basement membrane deposition in benign and malignant naevo-melanocytic lesions: an immunohistochemical study with antibodies to type IV collagen and laminin. Histopathology 1989; 15(2): 137–146.

442. Kamino H, Jagirdar J. Fibronectin in eosinophilic globules of Spitz's nevi. Am J Dermatopathol 1984; 6 Suppl: 313–316.

443. Kamino H, et al. Eosinophilic globules in Spitz's nevi. New findings and a diagnostic sign. Am J Dermatopathol 1979; 1(4): 319–324.

444. Binder SW, et al. The histology and differential diagnosis of Spitz nevus. Semin Diagn Pathol 1993; 10(1): 36–46.

445. Howat AJ, Variend S. Lymphatic invasion in Spitz nevi. Am J Surg Pathol 1985; 9(2): 125–128.

446. Barr RJ, Morales RV, Graham JH. Desmoplastic nevus: a distinct histologic variant of mixed spindle cell and epithelioid cell nevus. Cancer 1980; 46(3): 557–564.

447. Harris GR. Desmoplastic (sclerotic) nevus: an underrecognized entity that resembles dermatofibroma and desmoplastic melanoma. Am J Surg Pathol 1999; 23(7): 786–794.

448. Barnhill RL, et al. The histologic spectrum of pigmented spindle cell nevus: a review of 120 cases with emphasis on atypical variants. Hum Pathol 1991; 22(1): 52–58.

449. Smith NP. The pigmented spindle cell tumor of Reed: an underdiagnosed lesion. Semin Diagn Pathol 1987; 4(1): 75–87.

450. Sau P, Graham JH, Helwig EB. Pigmented spindle cell nevus: a clinicopathologic analysis of ninety-five cases. J Am Acad Dermatol 1993; 28(4): 565–571.

451. Wistuba I, Gonzalez S. Eosinophilic globules in pigmented spindle cell nevus. Am J Dermatopathol 1990; 12(3): 268–271.

452. Barnhill RL, et al. Atypical Spitz nevi/tumors: lack of consensus for diagnosis, discrimination from melanoma, and prediction of outcome. Hum Pathol 1999; 30(5): 513–520.

453. Perkocha LA. Classification of melanoma in adults and children. In: LeBoit PE, ed. Malignant melanoma and melanotic neoplasms. Philadelphia: Hanley & Belfus; 1994: 299–338.

454. Goovaerts G, Buyssens N. Nevus cell maturation or atrophy? Am J Dermatopathol 1988; 10(1): 20–27.

455. Ruhoy SM, et al. Malignant melanoma with paradoxical maturation. Am J Surg Pathol 2000; 24(12): 1600–1614.

456. Piepkorn M. On the nature of histologic observations: the case of the Spitz nevus. J Am Acad Dermatol 1995; 32(2 Pt 1): 248–254.

457. Weyers W. The 21st Colloquium of the International Society of Dermatopathology. Am J Dermatopathol 2001; 23(3): 232–234.

458. Barnhill RL. Childhood melanoma. Semin Diagn Pathol 1998; 15(3): 189–194.

459. Radentz WH, Vogel P. Congenital common blue nevus. Arch Dermatol 1990; 126(1): 124–125.

460. Busam KJ, et al. Large plaque-type blue nevus with subcutaneous cellular nodules. Am J Surg Pathol, 2000; 24(1): 92–99.

461. Carney JA, Ferreiro JA. The epithelioid blue nevus. A multicentric familial tumor with important associations, including cardiac myxoma and psammomatous melanotic Schwannoma. Am J Surg Pathol 1996; 20(3): 259–272.

462. Carney JA, Stratakis CA. Epithelioid blue nevus and psammomatous melanotic Schwannoma: the unusual pigmented skin tumors of the Carney complex. Semin Diagn Pathol 1998; 15(3): 216–224.

463. Carr S, et al. Hypopigmented common blue nevus. J Cutan Pathol 1997; 24(8): 494–498.

464. Bhawan J, Cao SL. Amelanotic blue nevus: a variant of blue nevus. Am J Dermatopathol 1999; 21(3): 225–228.

465. Bolognia JL, Glusac EJ. Hypopigmented common blue nevi. Arch Dermatol 1998; 134(6): 754–756.

466. Kamino H, Tam ST. Compound blue nevus: a variant of blue nevus with an additional junctional dendritic component. A clinical, histopathologic, and immunohistochemical study of six cases. Arch Dermatol 1990; 126(10): 1330–1333.

467. Harvell JD, White WL. Persistent and recurrent blue nevi. Am J Dermatopathol 1999; 21(6): 506–517.

468. Rodriguez HA, Ackerman LV. Cellular blue nevus. Clinicopathologic study of forty-five cases. Cancer 1968; 21(3): 393–405.

469. Granter SR, et al. Melanoma associated with blue nevus and melanoma mimicking cellular blue nevus: a clinicopathologic study of 10 cases on the spectrum of so-called 'malignant blue nevus'. Am J Surg Pathol 2001; 25(3): 316–323.

470. Reimer RR, et al. Precursor lesions in familial melanoma. A new genetic preneoplastic syndrome. JAMA 1978; 239(8): 744–746.

471. Sagebiel RW. The dysplastic melanocytic nevus. J Am Acad Dermatol 1989; 20(3): 496–501.

472. Clark WH Jr, et al. Origin of familial malignant melanomas from heritable melanocytic lesions. 'The B-K mole syndrome'. Arch Dermatol 1978; 114(5): 732–738.

473. Elder DE, et al. Dysplastic nevus syndrome: a phenotypic association of sporadic cutaneous melanoma. Cancer 1980; 46(8): 1787–1794.

474. Ford D, et al. Risk of cutaneous melanoma associated with a family history of the disease. The International Melanoma Analysis Group (IMAGE). Int J Cancer 1995; 62(4): 377–381.

475. Greene MH, et al. High risk of malignant melanoma in melanoma-prone families with dysplastic nevi. Ann Intern Med 1985; 102(4): 458–465.

476. Rhodes AR, et al. Dysplastic melanocytic nevi in histologic association with 234 primary cutaneous melanomas. J Am Acad Dermatol 1983; 9(4): 563–574.

477. Garbe C, Orfanos CE. [Epidemiology of malignant melanoma in West Germany in an international comparison]. Onkologie 1989; 12(6): 253–262.

478. Marchesi L, et al. Combined Clark's nevus. Am J Dermatopathol 1994; 16(4): 364–371.

479. Rigel DS, et al. Dysplastic nevi. Markers for increased risk for melanoma. Cancer 1989; 63(2): 386–389.

480. Barnhill RL. Current status of the dysplastic melanocytic nevus. J Cutan Pathol 1991; 18(3): 147–159.

481. Ahmed I, et al. Histopathologic characteristics of dysplastic nevi. Limited association of conventional histologic criteria with melanoma risk group. J Am Acad Dermatol 1990; 22(5 Pt 1): 727–733.

482. National Institutes of Health Consensus Development Conference Statement on Diagnosis and Treatment of Early Melanoma, January 27–29, 1992. Am J Dermatopathol 1993; 15(1): 34–43; discussion 46–51.

483. Ackerman AB, Milde P. Naming acquired melanocytic nevi. Common and dysplastic, normal and atypical, or Unna, Miescher, Spitz, and Clark? Am J Dermatopathol 1992; 14(5): 447–453.

484. Ackerman AB. Enough mysticism about dysplastic nevi. Dermatopathology: Practical & Conceptual 2001; 7: 86–88.

485. Clemente C, et al. Histopathologic diagnosis of dysplastic nevi: concordance among pathologists convened by the World Health Organization Melanoma Programme. Hum Pathol 1991; 22(4): 313–319.

486. Rivers JK, et al. Quantification of histologic features of dysplastic nevi. Am J Dermatopathol 1990; 12(1): 42–50.

487. Ackerman AB. What naevus is dysplastic, a syndrome and the commonest precursor of malignant melanoma? A riddle and an answer. Histopathology 1988; 13(3): 241–256.

488. Clark WH Jr, Ackerman AB. An exchange of views regarding the dysplastic nevus controversy. Semin Dermatol 1989; 8(4): 229–250.

489. Piepkorn M. A perspective on the dysplastic nevus controversy. In: LeBoit P, ed. Malignant melanoma and melanocytic neoplasms. Philadelphia: Hanley & Belfus; 1994: 259–279.

490. Steijlen PM, et al. The efficacy of histopathological criteria required for diagnosing dysplastic naevi. Histopathology 1988; 12(3): 289–300.

491. Rhodes AR, Mihm MC Jr, Weinstock MA. Dysplastic melanocytic nevi: a reproducible histologic definition emphasizing cellular morphology. Mod Pathol 1989; 2(4): 306–319.

492. Barnhill RL, Roush GC, Duray PH. Correlation of histologic architectural and cytoplasmic features with nuclear atypia in atypical (dysplastic) nevomelanocytic nevi. Hum Pathol 1990; 21(1): 51–58.

493. Elder DE, et al. The dysplastic nevus syndrome: our definition. Am J Dermatopathol 1982; 4(5): 455–460.

494. Cook MG, Fallowfield ME. Dysplastic naevi – an alternative view. Histopathology 1990; 16(1): 29–35.

495. Elder DE, et al. The early and intermediate precursor lesions of tumor progression in the melanocytic system: common acquired nevi and atypical (dysplastic) nevi. Semin Diagn Pathol 1993; 10(1): 18–35.

496. Tripp JM, et al. Management of dysplastic nevi: a survey of fellows of the American Academy of Dermatology. J Am Acad Dermatol 2002; 46(5): 674–682.

497. Kanzler MH, Mraz-Gernhard S. Primary cutaneous malignant melanoma and its precursor lesions: diagnostic and therapeutic overview. J Am Acad Dermatol 2001; 45(2): 260–276.

498. Sexton M, Sexton CW. Recurrent pigmented melanocytic nevus. A benign lesion, not to be mistaken for malignant melanoma. Arch Pathol Lab Med 1991; 115(2): 122–126.

499. Hoang MP, et al. Recurrent melanocytic nevus: a histologic and immunohistochemical evaluation. J Cutan Pathol 2001; 28(8): 400–406.

500. Park HK, et al. Recurrent melanocytic nevi: clinical and histologic review of 175 cases. J Am Acad Dermatol 1987; 17(2 Pt 1): 285–292.

501. Kornberg R, Ackerman AB. Pseudomelanoma: recurrent melanocytic nevus following partial surgical removal. Arch Dermatol 1975; 111(12): 1588–1590.

502. Sutton R. An unusual variety of vitiligo (leukoderma acquisitum centrifugum). J Cutan Dis 1916; 34: 797–800.

503. Berman B, et al. Halo giant congenital melanocytic nevus: in vitro immunologic studies. J Am Acad Dermatol 1988; 19(5 Pt 2): 954–960.

504. Baranda L, et al. Presence of activated lymphocytes in the peripheral blood of patients with halo nevi. J Am Acad Dermatol 1999; 41(4): 567–572.

505. Berman A, Herszenson S. Vascular response in halo of recent halo nevus. J Am Acad Dermatol 1981; 4(5): 537–540.

506. Mooney MA, Barr RJ, Buxton MG. Halo nevus or halo phenomenon? A study of 142 cases. J Cutan Pathol 1995; 22(4): 342–348.

507. Langer K, Konrad K. Congenital melanocytic nevi with halo phenomenon: report of two cases and a review of the literature. J Dermatol Surg Oncol 1990; 16(4): 377–380.

508. Wayte DM, Helwig EB. Halo nevi. Cancer 1968; 22(1): 69–90.

509. Schrader WA, Helwig EB. Balloon cell nevi. Cancer 1967; 20(9): 1502–1514.

510. Seab JA Jr, Graham JH, Helwig EB. Deep penetrating nevus. Am J Surg Pathol 1989; 13(1): 39–44.

511. Cooper PH. Deep penetrating (plexiform spindle cell) nevus. A frequent participant in combined nevus. J Cutan Pathol 1992; 19(3): 172–180.

512. Mehregan DA, Mehregan AH. Deep penetrating nevus. Arch Dermatol 1993; 129(3): 328–331.

513. Carmichael AJ, Tan CY, Abraham SM. Adult onset Mongolian spot. Clin Exp Dermatol 1993; 18(1): 72–74.

514. Stanford DG, Georgouras KE. Dermal melanocytosis: a clinical spectrum. Australas J Dermatol 1996; 37(1): 19–25.

515. Ota M, Tanino H. Nevus fusco-caeruleus ophthalmomaxillaris and melanosis bulbi. Tokyo Iji Shinshi 1939; 63: 1243–1245.

516. Ito M. Nevus fusco-caeruleus acromio-deltoideus. Tohoku Exp Med 1954; 60:10.

517. Mishama Y, Mevorah B. Nevus Ota and nevus Ito in American negroes. J Invest Dermatol 1961; 36: 133–154.

518. Landau M, Krafchik BR. The diagnostic value of cafe-au-lait macules. J Am Acad Dermatol 1999; 40(6 Pt 1): 877–890; quiz 891–892.

519. Picascia DD, Esterly NB. Congenital Becker's melanosis. Int J Dermatol 1989; 28(2): 127–128.

520. Jain HC, Fisher, BK. Familial Becker's nevus. Int J Dermatol 1989; 28(4): 263–264.

521. Urbanek RW, Johnson WC. Smooth muscle hamartoma associated with Becker's nevus. Arch Dermatol 1978; 114(1): 104–106.

522. Radovic-Kovacevic V, et al. [Survival analysis in patients with cutaneous malignant melanoma]. Srp Arh Celok Lek 1997; 125(5–6): 132–137.

523. Richert SM, D'Amico F, Rhodes AR. Cutaneous melanoma: patient surveillance and tumor progression. J Am Acad Dermatol 1998; 39(4 Pt 1): 571–577.

524. Storm HH, Engholm G. [Relative survival of Danish cancer patients diagnosed 1981 to 1997 and followed to 2001. A status report]. Ugeskr Laeger 2002; 164(22): 2855–2864.

525. MacKie RM. Melanoma and the dermatologist in the third millennium. Arch Dermatol 2000; 136(1): 71–73.

526. Geller AC, et al. Melanoma incidence and mortality among US whites, 1969–1999. JAMA 2002; 288(14): 1719–1720.

527. Hall HI, et al. Update on the incidence and mortality from melanoma in the United States. J Am Acad Dermatol 1999; 40(1): 35–42.

528. Beitner H, et al. Further evidence for increased light sensitivity in patients with malignant melanoma. Br J Dermatol 1981; 104(3): 289–294.

529. Beral V, et al. Cutaneous factors related to the risk of malignant melanoma. Br J Dermatol 1983; 109(2): 165–172.

530. Katsambas A, Nicolaidou E. Cutaneous malignant melanoma and sun exposure. Recent developments in epidemiology. Arch Dermatol 1996; 132(4): 444–450.

531. Whiteman DC, Green AC. Melanoma and sun exposure: where are we now? Int J Dermatol 1999; 38(7): 481–489.

532. Whiteman DC, Whiteman CA, Green AC. Childhood sun exposure as a risk factor for melanoma: a systematic review of epidemiologic studies. Cancer Causes Control 2001; 12(1): 69–82.

533. Schreiber MM, Moon TE, Bozzo PD. Chronic solar ultraviolet damage associated with malignant melanoma of the skin. J Am Acad Dermatol 1984; 10(5 Pt 1): 755–759.

534. Kopf AW, Kripke ML, Stern RS. Sun and malignant melanoma. J Am Acad Dermatol 1984; 11(4 Pt 1): 674–684.

535. Piepkorn M. The expression of p16(INK4a), the product of a tumor suppressor gene for melanoma, is upregulated in human melanocytes by UVB irradiation. J Am Acad Dermatol 2000; 42(5 Pt 1): 741–745.

536. Funk JO, et al. p16INK4a expression is frequently decreased and associated with 9p21 loss of heterozygosity in sporadic melanoma. J Cutan Pathol 1998; 25(6): 291–296.

537. Piepkorn M. Melanoma genetics: an update with focus on the CDKN2A(p16)/ARF tumor suppressors. J Am Acad Dermatol 2000; 42(5 Pt 1): 705–722; quiz 723–726.

538. Bataille V. Genetics of familial and sporadic melanoma. Clin Exp Dermatol 2000; 25(6): 464–470.

539. Zhu G, et al. A major quantitative-trait locus for mole density is linked to the familial melanoma gene CDKN2A: a maximum-likelihood combined linkage and association analysis in twins and their sibs. Am J Hum Genet 1999; 65(2): 483–492.

540. Roth ME, et al. Melanoma in children. J Am Acad Dermatol 1990; 22(2 Pt 1): 265–274.

541. Chun K, Vazquez M, Sanchez JL. Malignant melanoma in children. Int J Dermatol 1993; 32(1): 41–43.

542. Handfield-Jones SE, Smith NP. Malignant melanoma in childhood. Br J Dermatol 1996; 134(4): 607–616.

543. Guibert P, et al. Melanoma screening: report of a survey in occupational medicine. Arch Dermatol 2000; 136(2): 199–202.

544. Baade PD, et al. Community perceptions about the important signs of early melanoma. J Am Acad Dermatol 1997; 36(1): 33–39.

545. Stern JB, Haupt HM. Pagetoid melanocytosis: tease or tocsin? Semin Diagn Pathol 1998; 15(3): 225–229.

546. Schmoeckel C. How consistent are dermatopathologists in reading early malignant melanomas and lesions 'precursor' to them? An international survey. Am J Dermatopathol 1984; 6 Suppl: 13–24.

547. Weinstock MA, Sober AJ. The risk of progression of lentigo maligna to lentigo maligna melanoma. Br J Dermatol 1987; 116(3): 303–310.

548. Ackerman AB, Borghi S. 'Pagetoid melanocytic proliferation' is the latest evasion from a diagnosis of 'melanoma in situ.' Am J Dermatopathol 1991; 13(6): 583–604.

549. Ackerman AB. Histopathologists can diagnose malignant melanoma in situ correctly and consistently. Am J Dermatopathol 1984; 6 Suppl: 103–107.

550. Mihm MC Jr, Murphy GF. Malignant melanoma in situ: an oxymoron whose time has come. Hum Pathol 1998; 29(1): 6–7.

551. Hutchinson J. Notes on the cancerous process and on new growths in general. Arch Surg (Lond) 1890; 2: 83–86.

552. Cohen LM. The starburst giant cell is useful for distinguishing lentigo maligna from photodamaged skin. J Am Acad Dermatol 1996; 35(6): 962–968.

553. Katz SK, Guitart J. Starburst giant cells in benign nevomelanocytic lesions. J Am Acad Dermatol 1998; 38(2 Pt 1): 283.

554. Tannous ZS, et al. Progression to invasive melanoma from malignant melanoma in situ, lentigo maligna type. Hum Pathol 2000; 31(6): 705–708.

555. Finan MC, Perry HO. Lentigo maligna: a form of malignant melanoma in situ. Geriatrics 1982; 37(12): 113–115.

556. Clark WH Jr, et al. The histogenesis and biologic behavior of primary human malignant melanomas of the skin. Cancer Res 1969; 29(3): 705–727.

557. McGovern VJ, et al. The classification of malignant melanoma and its histologic reporting. Cancer 1973; 32(6): 1446–1457.

558. Ackerman AB, David KM. A unifying concept of malignant melanoma: biologic aspects. Hum Pathol 1986; 17(5): 438–440.

559. Flotte TJ, Mihm MC Jr. Melanoma: the art versus the science of dermatopathology. Hum Pathol 1986; 17(5): 441–442.

560. Weyers W, et al. Classification of cutaneous malignant melanoma: a reassessment of histopathologic criteria for the distinction of different types. Cancer 1999; 86(2): 288–299.

561. Sober AJ, Fitzpatrick TB, Mihm MC Jr. Primary melanoma of the skin: recognition and management. J Am Acad Dermatol 1980; 2(3): 179–197.

562. Clark WH Jr, Elder DE, Van Horn M. The biologic forms of malignant melanoma. Hum Pathol 1986; 17(5): 443–450.

563. Clark WH Jr, et al. Model predicting survival in stage I melanoma based on tumor progression. J Natl Cancer Inst 1989; 81(24): 1893–1904.

564. Guerry DT, et al. Lessons from tumor progression: the invasive radial growth phase of melanoma is common, incapable of metastasis, and indolent. J Invest Dermatol 1993; 100(3): 342S–345S.

565. Abramova L, Slingluff CL Jr, Patterson JW. Problems in the interpretation of apparent 'radial growth phase' malignant melanomas that metastasize. J Cutan Pathol 2002; 29(7): 407–414.

566. Plotnick H, Rachmaninoff N, VandenBerg HJ Jr. Polypoid melanoma: a virulent variant of nodular melanoma. Report of three cases and literature review. J Am Acad Dermatol 1990; 23(5 Pt 1): 880–884.

567. Kiene P, Petres-Dunsche C, Folster-Holst R. Pigmented pedunculated malignant melanoma. A rare variant of nodular melanoma. Br J Dermatol 1995; 133(2): 300–302.

568. Koh HK, et al. Lentigo maligna melanoma has no better prognosis than other types of melanoma. J Clin Oncol 1984; 2(9): 994–1001.

569. Cohen LM. Lentigo maligna and lentigo maligna melanoma. J Am Acad Dermatol 1995; 33(6): 923–936; quiz 937–940.

570. Kato T, et al. Clinicopathological study of acral melanoma in situ in 44 Japanese patients. Dermatology 1996; 193(3): 192–197.

571. Cho KH, Han KH, Minn KW. Superficial spreading melanoma arising in a longstanding melanocytic nevus on the sole. J Dermatol 1998; 25(5): 337–340.

572. Arrington JH 3rd, et al. Plantar lentiginous melanoma: a distinctive variant of human cutaneous malignant melanoma. Am J Surg Pathol 1977; 1(2): 131–143.

573. Levit EK, et al. The ABC rule for clinical detection of subungual melanoma. J Am Acad Dermatol 2000; 42(2 Pt 1): 269–274.

574. Banfield CC, Redburn JC, Dawber RP. The incidence and prognosis of nail apparatus melanoma. A retrospective study of 105 patients in four English regions. Br J Dermatol 1998; 139(2): 276–279.

575. Egbert B, Kempson R, Sagebiel R. Desmoplastic malignant melanoma. A clinicohistopathologic study of 25 cases. Cancer 1988; 62(9): 2033–2041.

576. Skelton HG, et al. Desmoplastic malignant melanoma. J Am Acad Dermatol 1995 32(5 Pt 1): 717–725.

577. Carlson JA, et al. Desmoplastic neurotropic melanoma. A clinicopathologic analysis of 28 cases. Cancer 1995; 75(2): 478–494.

578. Quinn MJ, et al. Desmoplastic and desmoplastic neurotropic melanoma: experience with 280 patients. Cancer 1998; 83(6): 1128–1135.

579. Reed RJ, Leonard DD. Neurotropic melanoma. A variant of desmoplastic melanoma. Am J Surg Pathol 1979; 3(4): 301–311.

580. Reed RJ. Minimal deviation malignant melanoma arising in a congenital nevus. Am J Surg Pathol 1978; 2(2): 215–220.

581. Schmoeckel C, Castro CE, Braun-Falco O. Nevoid malignant melanoma. Arch Dermatol Res 1985; 277(5): 362–369.

582. Wong TY, et al. Nevoid melanoma: a clinicopathological study of seven cases of malignant melanoma mimicking spindle and epithelioid cell nevus and verrucous dermal nevus. Hum Pathol 1995; 26(2): 171–179.

583. Banerjee SS, Harris M. Morphological and immunophenotypic variations in malignant melanoma. Histopathology 2000; 36(5): 387–402.

584. Prieto VG. et al. Primary cutaneous myxoid melanoma: immunohistologic clues to a difficult diagnosis. J Am Acad Dermatol 1994; 30(2 Pt 2): 335–339.

585. McCluggage WG, Shah V, Toner PG. Primary cutaneous myxoid malignant melanoma. Histopathology 1996; 28(2): 179–182.

586. Perniciaro C. Dermatopathologic variants of malignant melanoma. Mayo Clin Proc 1997; 72(3): 273–279.

587. Breier F, et al. Primary invasive signet-ring cell melanoma. J Cutan Pathol 1999; 26(10): 533–536.

588. House NS, et al. Malignant melanoma with clinical and histologic features of Merkel cell carcinoma. J Am Acad Dermatol 1994; 31(5 Pt 2): 839–842.

589. White WL, Hitchcock MG. Dying dogma: the pathological diagnosis of epidermotropic metastatic malignant melanoma. Semin Diagn Pathol 1998; 15(3): 176–188.

590. van Duinen SG, Ruiter DJ, Scheffer E. A staining procedure for melanin in semithin and ultrathin epoxy sections. Histopathology 1983; 7(1): 35–48.

591. Carson FL. Histotechnology: a self-instructional text. 2nd edn. Chicago: ASCP Press; 1997: 304.

592. Fernando SS, Johnson S, Bate J. Immunohistochemical analysis of cutaneous malignant melanoma: comparison of S-100 protein, HMB-45 monoclonal antibody and NKI/C3 monoclonal antibody. Pathology 1994; 26(1): 16–19.

593. Argenyi ZB, et al. S-100 protein-negative malignant melanoma: fact or fiction? A light-microscopic and immunohistochemical study. Am J Dermatopathol 1994; 16(3): 233–240.

594. Smoller BR. Immunohistochemistry in the diagnosis of melanocytic neoplasms. Pathology (Phila) 1994; 2(2): 371–383.

595. Blessing K, Sanders DS, Grant JJ. Comparison of immunohistochemical staining of the novel antibody melan-A with S100 protein and HMB-45 in malignant melanoma and melanoma variants. Histopathology 1998; 32(2): 139–146.

596. Clarkson KS, Sturdgess IC, Molyneux AJ. The usefulness of tyrosinase in the immunohistochemical assessment of melanocytic lesions: a comparison of the novel T311 antibody (anti-tyrosinase) with S-100, HMB45, and A103 (anti-melan-A). J Clin Pathol 2001; 54(3): 196–200.

597. Orchard GE. Comparison of immunohistochemical labelling of melanocyte differentiation antibodies melan-A, tyrosinase and HMB 45 with NKIC3 and S100 protein in the evaluation of benign naevi and malignant melanoma. Histochem J 2000; 32(8): 475–481.

598. Jungbluth AA, et al. T311 – an anti-tyrosinase monoclonal antibody for the detection of melanocytic lesions in paraffin embedded tissues. Pathol Res Pract 2000; 196(4): 235–242.

599. Kaufmann O, et al. Tyrosinase, melan-A, and KBA62 as markers for the immunohistochemical identification of metastatic amelanotic melanomas on paraffin sections. Mod Pathol 1998; 11(8): 740–746.

600. de Vries TJ, et al. High expression of immunotherapy candidate proteins gp100, MART-1, tyrosinase and TRP-1 in uveal melanoma. Br J Cancer 1998; 78(9): 1156–1161.

601. Melanoma of the skin. In: Greene FL, Page DL, Fleming ID, eds. American Joint Committee on Cancer, Cancer staging manual, 6th edn. New York: Springer-Verlag; 2002: 209–220.

602. Breslow A. Thickness, cross-sectional areas and depth of invasion in the prognosis of cutaneous melanoma. Ann Surg 1970; 172(5): 902–908.

603. Vollmer RT, Seigler HF. Using a continuous transformation of the Breslow thickness for prognosis in cutaneous melanoma. Am J Clin Pathol 2001; 115(2): 205–212.

604. Lemish WM, et al. Survival from preinvasive and invasive malignant melanoma in Western Australia. Cancer 1983; 52(3): 580–585.

605. Balch CM, et al. Prognostic factors analysis of 17,600 melanoma patients: validation of the American Joint Committee on Cancer melanoma staging system. J Clin Oncol 2001; 19(16): 3622–3634.

606. Reed RJ, Martin P. Variants of melanoma. Semin Cutan Med Surg 1997; 16(2): 137–158.

607. Balch CM, et al. Final version of the American Joint Committee on Cancer staging system for cutaneous melanoma. J Clin Oncol 2001; 19(16): 3635–3648.

608. Day CL Jr, et al. A prognostic model for clinical stage I melanoma of the upper extremity. The importance of anatomic subsites in predicting recurrent disease. Ann Surg 1981; 193(4): 436–440.

609. Day CL Jr, et al. Prognostic factors for patients with clinical stage I melanoma of intermediate thickness (1.51–3.39 mm). A conceptual model for tumor growth and metastasis. Ann Surg 1982; 195(1): 35–43.

610. Kelly JW, et al. The frequency of local recurrence and microsatellites as a guide to reexcision margins for cutaneous malignant melanoma. Ann Surg 1984; 200(6): 759–763.

611. Paichitrojjana A. Hemangiolymphatic invasion at the site of a primary cutaneous melanoma is virtually equivalent to metastasis. Dermatopathology: Practical & Conceptual 2001; 7: 21–27.

612. Trau H, et al. Regression in malignant melanoma. J Am Acad Dermatol 1983; 8(3): 363–368.

613. Massi D, et al. Thin cutaneous malignant melanomas (< or = 1.5 mm): identification of risk factors indicative of progression. Cancer 1999; 85(5): 1067–1076.

614. Veronesi U, et al. Thin stage I primary cutaneous malignant melanoma. Comparison of excision with margins of 1 or 3 cm. N Engl J Med 1988; 318(18): 1159–1162.

615. Heenan PJ, et al. The effects of surgical treatment on survival and local recurrence of cutaneous malignant melanoma. Cancer 1992; 69(2): 421–426.

616. Kaufmann R. Surgical management of primary melanoma. Clin Exp Dermatol 2000; 25(6): 476–481.

617. Piepkorn M, Barnhill RL. A factual, not arbitrary, basis for choice of resection margins in melanoma. Arch Dermatol 1996; 132(7): 811–814.

618. Cherpelis BS, et al. Sentinel lymph node micrometastasis and other histologic factors that predict outcome in patients with thicker melanomas. J Am Acad Dermatol 2001; 44(5): 762–766.

619. Reintgen D, Shivers S. Sentinel lymph node micrometastasis from melanoma. Proven methodology and evolving significance. Cancer 1999; 86(4): 551–552.

620. Yu, L, et al. Detection of microscopic melanoma metastases in sentinel lymph nodes. Cancer 1999; 86(4): 617–627.

621. Thomas JM, Patocskai EJ. The argument against sentinel node biopsy for malignant melanoma. Br Med J 2000; 321(7252): 3 4.

622. Messina JL, Glass LF. Pathologic examination of the sentinel lymph node. J Fla Med Assoc 1997; 84(3): 153–156.

623. Baisden BL, et al. HMB-45 immunohistochemical staining of sentinel lymph nodes: a specific method for enhancing detection of micrometastases in patients with melanoma. Am J Surg Pathol 2000; 24(8): 1140–1146.

624. Hatta N, et al. Polymerase chain reaction and immunohistochemistry frequently detect occult melanoma cells in regional lymph nodes of melanoma patients. J Clin Pathol 1998; 51(8): 597–601.

625. Cochran AJ. Surgical pathology remains pivotal in the evaluation of 'sentinel' lymph nodes. Am J Surg Pathol 1999; 23(10): 1169–1172.

626. Shivers SC, et al. The clinical relevance of molecular staging for melanoma. Recent Results Cancer Res 2001; 158: 187–199.

627. Blumenthal R, et al. Morbidity and outcome after sentinel lymph node dissection in patients with early-stage malignant cutaneous melanoma. Swiss Surg 2002; 8(5): 209–214.

628. Starz H, et al. A micromorphometry-based concept for routine classification of sentinel lymph node metastases and its clinical relevance for patients with melanoma. Cancer 2001; 91(11): 2110–2121.

629. Wright-Browne V, et al. Physiology and pathophysiology of dendritic cells. Hum Pathol 1997; 28(5): 563–579.

630. Favara BE, et al. Contemporary classification of histiocytic disorders. The WHO Committee On Histiocytic/Reticulum Cell Proliferations. Reclassification Working Group of the Histiocyte Society. Med Pediatr Oncol 1997; 29(3): 157–166.

631. Cruz PD Jr, East C, Bergstresser PR. Dermal, subcutaneous, and tendon xanthomas: diagnostic markers for specific lipoprotein disorders. J Am Acad Dermatol 1988; 19(1 Pt 1): 95–111.

632. Torok E, Daroczy J. Juvenile xanthogranuloma: an analysis of 45 cases by clinical follow-up, light- and electron microscopy. Acta Derm Venereol 1985; 65(2): 167–169.

633. Whitmore SE. Multiple xanthogranulomas in an adult: case report and literature review. Br J Dermatol 1992; 127(2): 177–181.

634. Sanguesa OP, et al. Juvenile xanthogranuloma: a clinical, histopathologic and immunohistochemical study. J Cutan Pathol 1995; 22(4): 327–335.

635. Jih DM, Salcedo SL, Jaworsky C. Benign cephalic histiocytosis: a case report and review. J Am Acad Dermatol 2002; 47(6): 908–913.

636. Marzano AV, Facchetti M, Caputo R. Guess what! Generalized eruptive histiocytosis (histiocytoma). Eur J Dermatol 2002; 12(2): 205–206.

637. Jang KA, et al. Generalized eruptive histiocytoma of childhood. Br J Dermatol 1999; 140(1): 174–176.

638. Vadoud-Seyedi J, Vadoud-Seyedi R, De Dobbeleer G. Progressive nodular histiocytomas. Br J Dermatol 2000; 143(3): 678–679.

639. Rupec RA, Schaller M. Xanthoma disseminatum. Int J Dermatol 2002; 41(12): 911–913.

640. Gorman JD, et al. Multicentric reticulohistiocytosis: case report with immunohistochemical analysis and literature review. Arthritis Rheum 2000; 43(4): 930–938.

641. Zelger B, et al. Reticulohistiocytoma and multicentric reticulohistiocytosis. Histopathologic and immunophenotypic distinct entities. Am J Dermatopathol 1994; 16(6): 577–584.

642. Brenn T, et al. Cutaneous Rosai-Dorfman disease is a distinct clinical entity. Am J Dermatopathol 2002; 24(5): 385–391.

643. Tsunemi Y, et al. Rosai-Dorfman disease presenting as large pigmented indurated plaques. Acta Derm Venereol 2003; 83(1): 57–58.

644. Bergman R. The pathogenesis and clinical significance of xanthelasma palpebrarum. J Am Acad Dermatol 1994; 30(2 Pt 1): 236–242.

645. Munn S, Chu AC. Langerhans cell histiocytosis of the skin. Hematol Oncol Clin North Am 1998; 12(2): 269–286.

646. Inuzuka M, et al. Congenital self-healing reticulohistiocytosis presenting with hemorrhagic bullae. J Am Acad Dermatol 2003; 48(5 Suppl): S75–S77.

647. Shani-Adir A, et al. A child with both Langerhans and non-Langerhans cell histiocytosis. Pediatr Dermatol 2002; 19(5): 419–422.

648. Cerroni L, et al. Primary cutaneous follicle center cell lymphoma with follicular growth pattern. Blood 2000; 95(12): 3922–3928.

649. Mann RB, Berard CW. Criteria for the cytologic subclassification of follicular lymphomas: a proposed alternative method. Hematol Oncol 1983; 1(2): 187–192.

650. Lawnicki LC, et al. The t(14;18) and bcl-2 expression are present in a subset of primary cutaneous follicular lymphoma: association with lower grade. Am J Clin Pathol 2002; 118(5): 765–772.

651. Wotherspoon AC, et al. Helicobacter pylori-associated gastritis and primary B-cell gastric lymphoma. Lancet 1991; 338(8776): 1175–1176.

652. Goodlad JR, et al. Primary cutaneous B-cell lymphoma and Borrelia burgdorferi infection in patients from the Highlands of Scotland. Am J Surg Pathol 2000; 24(9): 1279–1285.

653. Cerroni L, et al. Infection by Borrelia burgdorferi and cutaneous B-cell lymphoma. J Cutan Pathol 1997; 24(8): 457–461.

654. Cerroni L, et al. Primary cutaneous marginal zone B-cell lymphoma: a recently described entity of low-grade malignant cutaneous B-cell lymphoma. Am J Surg Pathol 1997; 21(11): 1307–1315.

655. Baldassano MF, et al. Cutaneous lymphoid hyperplasia and cutaneous marginal zone lymphoma: comparison of morphologic and immunophenotypic features. Am J Surg Pathol 1999; 23(1): 88–96.

656. Pelstring RJ, et al. Diversity of organ site involvement among malignant lymphomas of mucosa-associated tissues. Am J Clin Pathol 1991; 96(6): 738–745.

657. Vermeer MH, et al. Primary cutaneous large B-cell lymphomas of the legs. A distinct type of cutaneous B-cell lymphoma with an intermediate prognosis. Dutch Cutaneous Lymphoma Working Group. Arch Dermatol 1996; 132(11): 1304–1308.

658. Paulli M, et al. Primary cutaneous large B-cell lymphoma of the leg: histogenetic analysis of a controversial clinicopathologic entity. Hum Pathol 2002; 33(9): 937–943.

659. Fernandez-Vazquez A, et al. Primary cutaneous large B-cell lymphoma: the relation between morphology, clinical presentation, immunohistochemical markers, and survival. Am J Surg Pathol 2001; 25(3): 307–315.

660. Sander CA, et al. T-cell-rich B-cell lymphoma presenting in skin. A clinicopathologic analysis of six cases. J Cutan Pathol 1996; 23(2): 101–108.

661. Kurtin PJ, et al. Primary cutaneous large cell lymphomas. Morphologic, immunophenotypic, and clinical features of 20 cases. Am J Surg Pathol 1994; 18(12): 1183–1191.

662. Jaffe ES, Wilson WH. Lymphomatoid granulomatosis: pathogenesis, pathology and clinical implications. Cancer Surv 1997; 30: 233–248.

663. James WD, Odom RB, Katzenstein AL. Cutaneous manifestations of lymphomatoid granulomatosis. Report of 44 cases and a review of the literature. Arch Dermatol 1981; 117(4): 196–202.

664. Beaty MW, et al. Cutaneous lymphomatoid granulomatosis: correlation of clinical and biologic features. Am J Surg Pathol 2001; 25(9): 1111–1120.

665. McNiff JM, et al. Lymphomatoid granulomatosis of the skin and lung. An angiocentric T-cell-rich B-cell lymphoproliferative disorder. Arch Dermatol 1996; 132(12): 1464–1470.

666. Wick MR, Mills SE. Intravascular lymphomatosis: clinicopathologic features and differential diagnosis. Semin Diagn Pathol 1991; 8(2): 91–101.

667. Ponzoni M, et al. Lack of CD 29 (beta1 integrin) and CD 54 (ICAM-1) adhesion molecules in intravascular lymphomatosis. Hum Pathol 2000; 31(2): 220–226.

668. Sanguesa O, Hyder DM, Sanguesa P. Intravascular lymphomatosis: report of an unusual case with T cell phenotype occurring in an adolescent male. J Cutan Pathol 1992; 19(3): 226–231.

669. Zackheim HS, et al. Relative frequency of various forms of primary cutaneous lymphomas. J Am Acad Dermatol 2000; 43(5 Pt 1): 793–796.

670. Koch SE, et al. Mycosis fungoides beginning in childhood and adolescence. J Am Acad Dermatol 1987; 17(4): 563–570.

671. Zackheim HS, McCalmont TH. Mycosis fungoides: the great imitator. J Am Acad Dermatol 2002; 47(6): 914–918.

672. Lambert WC, Everett MA. The nosology of parapsoriasis. J Am Acad Dermatol 1981; 5(4): 373–395.

673. Simon M, et al. Large plaque parapsoriasis: clinical and genotypic correlations. J Cutan Pathol 2000; 27(2): 57–60.

674. Abel EA. Clinical features of cutaneous T-cell lymphoma. Dermatol Clin 1985; 3(4): 647–664.

675. Grekin DA, Zackheim HS. Mycosis fungoides. Med Clin North Am 1980; 64(5): 1005–1016.

676. Nickoloff BJ. Light-microscopic assessment of 100 patients with patch/plaque-stage mycosis fungoides. Am J Dermatopathol 1988; 10(6): 469–477.

677. Shapiro PE, Pinto FJ. The histologic spectrum of mycosis fungoides/Sezary syndrome (cutaneous T-cell lymphoma). A review of 222 biopsies, including newly described patterns and the earliest pathologic changes. Am J Surg Pathol 1994; 18(7): 645–667.

678. LeBoit PE. Variants of mycosis fungoides and related cutaneous T-cell lymphomas. Semin Diagn Pathol 1991; 8(2): 73–81.

679. Candiago E, et al. Nonlymphoid intraepidermal mononuclear cell collections (pseudo-Pautrier abscesses): a morphologic and immunophenotypical characterization. Am J Dermatopathol 2000; 22(1): 1–6.

680. Ralfkiaer E. Immunohistological markers for the diagnosis of cutaneous lymphomas. Semin Diagn Pathol 1991; 8(2): 62–72.

681. Ormsby A, et al. Evaluation of a new paraffin-reactive CD7 T-cell deletion marker and a polymerase chain reaction-based T-cell receptor gene rearrangement assay: implications for diagnosis of mycosis fungoides in community clinical practice. J Am Acad Dermatol 2001; 45(3): 405–413.

682. Harmon CB, et al. Detection of circulating T cells with CD4+CD7– immunophenotype in patients with benign and malignant lymphoproliferative dermatoses. J Am Acad Dermatol 1996; 35(3 Pt 1): 404–410.

683. Kaudewitz P, et al. Primary and secondary cutaneous Ki-1+ (CD30+) anaplastic large cell lymphomas. Morphologic, immunohistologic, and clinical characteristics. Am J Pathol 1989; 135(2): 359–367.

684. Salhany KE, et al. Transformation of cutaneous T cell lymphoma to large cell lymphoma. A clinicopathologic and immunologic study. Am J Pathol 1988; 132(2): 265–277.

685. Glusac EJ. Of cells and architecture: new approaches to old criteria in mycosis fungoides. J Cutan Pathol 2001; 28(4): 169–173.

686. Guitart J, et al. Histologic criteria for the diagnosis of mycosis fungoides: proposal for a grading system to standardize pathology reporting. J Cutan Pathol 2001; 28(4): 174–183.

687. Burns MK, Chan LS, Cooper KD. Woringer-Kolopp disease (localized pagetoid reticulosis) or unilesional mycosis fungoides? An analysis of eight cases with benign disease. Arch Dermatol 1995; 131(3): 325–329.

688. Flaig MJ, et al. Follicular mycosis fungoides. A histopathologic analysis of nine cases. J Cutan Pathol 2001; 28(10): 525–530.

689. LeBoit PE. Granulomatous slack skin. Dermatol Clin 1994; 12(2): 375–389.

690. Willemze R, et al. EORTC classification for primary cutaneous lymphomas: a proposal from the Cutaneous Lymphoma Study Group of the European Organization for Research and Treatment of Cancer. Blood 1997; 90(1): 354–371.

691. Krishnan J, Tomaszewski MM, Kao GF. Primary cutaneous CD30-positive anaplastic large cell lymphoma. Report of 27 cases. J Cutan Pathol 1993; 20(3): 193–202.

692. Vergier B, et al. Statistical evaluation of diagnostic and prognostic features of CD30+ cutaneous lymphoproliferative disorders: a clinicopathologic study of 65 cases. Am J Surg Pathol 1998; 22(10): 1192–1202.

693. Tomaszewski MM, Moad JC, Lupton GP. Primary cutaneous Ki-1(CD30) positive anaplastic large cell lymphoma in childhood. J Am Acad Dermatol 1999; 40(5 Pt 2): 857–861.

694. Herbst H, et al. Absence of anaplastic lymphoma kinase (ALK) and Epstein-Barr virus gene products in primary cutaneous anaplastic large cell lymphoma and lymphomatoid papulosis. Br J Dermatol 1997; 137(5): 680–686.

695. Harrington DS, et al. Lymphomatoid papulosis and progression to T cell lymphoma: an immunophenotypic and genotypic analysis. J Am Acad Dermatol 1989; 21(5 Pt 1): 951–957.

696. Kadin ME. Lymphomatoid papulosis and associated lymphomas. How are they related? Arch Dermatol 1993; 129(3): 351–353.

697. Willemze R. Lymphomatoid papulosis. Dermatol Clin 1985; 3(4): 735–747.

698. Romero LS, et al. Subcutaneous T-cell lymphoma with associated hemophagocytic syndrome and terminal leukemic transformation. J Am Acad Dermatol 1996; 34(5 Pt 2): 904–910.

699. Wick MR, Patterson JW. Cytophagic histiocytic panniculitis – a critical reappraisal. Arch Dermatol 2000; 136(7): 922–924.

700. Salhany KE, et al. Subcutaneous panniculitis-like T cell lymphoma: clinicopathologic, immunophenotypic, and genotypic analysis of alpha/beta and gamma/delta subtypes. Am J Surg Pathol 1998; 22(7): 881–893.

701. Lopez-Guillermo A, et al. Peripheral T-cell lymphomas: initial features, natural history, and prognostic factors in a series of 174 patients diagnosed according to the R.E.A.L. Classification. Ann Oncol 1998; 9(8): 849–855.

702. Beljaards RC, et al. Primary cutaneous T-cell lymphoma: clinicopathological features and prognostic parameters of 35 cases other than mycosis fungoides and CD30-positive large cell lymphoma. J Pathol 1994; 172(1): 53–60.

703. Weis JW, et al. Peripheral T-cell lymphomas: histologic, immunohistologic, and clinical characterization. Mayo Clin Proc 1986; 61(6): 411–426.

704. Kiesewetter F, et al. Cutaneous lymphoepithelioid lymphoma (Lennert's lymphoma). Combined immunohistological, ultrastructural, and DNA-flow-cytometric analysis. Am J Dermatopathol 1989; 11(6): 549–554.

705. Gross DJ, Kavanaugh A. HTLV-I. Int J Dermatol 1990; 29(3): 161–165.

706. Tajima K, Cartier L. Epidemiological features of HTLV-I and adult T cell leukemia. Intervirology 1995; 38(3–4): 238–246.

707. Shimoyama M. Diagnostic criteria and classification of clinical subtypes of adult T-cell leukemia-lymphoma. A report from the Lymphoma Study Group (1984-87). Br J Haematol 1991; 79(3): 428–437.

708. DiCaudo DJ, et al. Clinical and histologic spectrum of human T-cell lymphotropic virus type I-associated lymphoma involving the skin. J Am Acad Dermatol 1996; 34(1): 69–76.

709. Luca DC, August CZ, Weisenberg E. Adult T-cell leukemia/lymphoma in a peripheral blood smear. Arch Pathol Lab Med 2003; 127(5): 636.

710. Maeda K, Takahashi M. Characterization of skin infiltrating cells in adult T-cell leukaemia/lymphoma (ATLL): clinical, histological and immunohistochemical studies on eight cases. Br J Dermatol 1989; 121(5): 603–612.

711. Ohno S, et al. Aleukemic leukemia cutis. J Am Acad Dermatol 1990; 22(2 Pt 2): 374–377.

712. Aboud H, et al. An adult with common acute lymphoblastic leukaemia (C-ALL) presenting with skin infiltration. Br J Dermatol 1991; 124(1): 84–85.

713. Buechner SA, Li CY, Su WP. Leukemia cutis. A histopathologic study of 42 cases. Am J Dermatopathol 1985; 7(2): 109–119.

714. Kaddu S, et al. Specific cutaneous infiltrates in patients with myelogenous leukemia: a clinicopathologic study of 26 patients with assessment of diagnostic criteria. J Am Acad Dermatol 1999; 40(6 Pt 1): 966–978.

715. Peretz E, et al. Follicular B-cell pseudolymphoma. Australas J Dermatol 2000; 41(1): 48–49.

716. Blumental G, Okun MR, Ponitch JA. Pseudolymphomatous reaction to tattoos. Report of three cases. J Am Acad Dermatol 1982; 6(4 Pt 1): 485–488.

717. Albrecht S, et al. Lymphadenosis benigna cutis resulting from *Borrelia* infection (Borrelia lymphocytoma). J Am Acad Dermatol 1991; 24(4): 621–625.

718. Ploysangam T, Breneman DL, Mutasim DF. Cutaneous pseudolymphomas. J Am Acad Dermatol 1998; 38(6 Pt 1): 877-95; quiz 896–897.

719. Rijlaarsdam JU, Meijer CJ, Willemze R. Differentiation between lymphadenosis benigna cutis and primary cutaneous follicular center cell lymphomas. A comparative clinicopathologic study of 57 patients. Cancer 1990; 65(10): 2301–2306.

720. Smoller BR, Glusac EJ. Histologic mimics of cutaneous lymphoma. Pathol Annu 1995; 30 (Pt 1): 123–141.

721. Ceballos KM, et al. Heavy multinodular cutaneous lymphoid infiltrates: clinicopathologic features and B-cell clonality. J Cutan Pathol 2002; 29(3): 159–167.

722. Toonstra J. Actinic reticuloid. Semin Diagn Pathol 1991; 8(2): 109–116.

723. Rijlaarsdam U, et al. Mycosis fungoides-like lesions associated with phenytoin and carbamazepine therapy. J Am Acad Dermatol 1991; 24(2 Pt 1): 216–220.

724. Heller P, et al. Chronic actinic dermatitis. An immunohistochemical study of its T-cell antigenic profile, with comparison to cutaneous T-cell lymphoma. Am J Dermatopathol 1994; 16(5): 510–516.

725. Allison MA, Schmidt CP. Urticaria pigmentosa. Int J Dermatol 1997; 36(5): 321–325.

726. Azana JM, et al. Urticaria pigmentosa: a review of 67 pediatric cases Pediatr Dermatol 1994; 11(2): 102–106.

727. Odom R, James WD, Berger TG. Andrews' diseases of the skin: clinical dermatology. 9th edn. New York: WB Saunders; 2000.

728. Kanwar AJ, Dhar S. Diffuse cutaneous mastocytosis: a rare entity. Pediatr Dermatol 1993; 10(3): 301–302.

729. Mihm MC, et al. Mast cell infiltrates of the skin and the mastocytosis syndrome. Hum Pathol 1973; 4(2): 231–239.

730. Bachmeyer C, et al. Telangiectasia macularis eruptiva perstans and multiple myeloma. J Am Acad Dermatol 2000; 43(5 Pt 2): 972–974.

731. Olafsson JH, Roupe G, Enerback L. Dermal mast cells in mastocytosis: fixation, distribution and quantitation. Acta Derm Venereol 1986; 66(1): 16–22.

732. Natkunam Y, Rouse RV. Utility of paraffin section immunohistochemistry for C-KIT (CD117) in the differential diagnosis of systemic mast cell disease involving the bone marrow. Am J Surg Pathol 2000; 24(1): 81–91.

733. Brunning RD, et al. Systemic mastocytosis. Extracutaneous manifestations. Am J Surg Pathol 1983; 7(5): 425–438.

734. Longley J, Duffy TP, Kohn S. The mast cell and mast cell disease. J Am Acad Dermatol 1995; 32(4): 545–561; quiz 562–564.

735. Travis WD, et al. Mast cell leukemia: report of a case and review of the literature. Mayo Clin Proc 1986; 61(12): 957–966.

736. Travis WD, et al. Systemic mast cell disease. Analysis of 58 cases and literature review. Medicine (Baltimore) 1988; 67(6): 345–368.

Soft tissue tumors

Elizabeth Montgomery

9

INTRODUCTION

Soft tissue tumors are a heterogeneous group of benign and malignant processes, some presumed to be reactive and others clearly neoplastic. Because of their rarity, they frequently pose diagnostic problems for surgical pathologists. Accurate diagnosis of these tumors is enhanced by knowledge of the clinical features of the given lesions and, at times, by application of immunohistochemical and molecular techniques. In this chapter the lesions are described essentially in accordance with the World Health Organization (WHO) classification.[1,2] It is beyond the scope of this chapter to cover all described soft tissue entities; both detailed[3] and abbreviated[4] textbooks are also available.

GRADING AND STAGING

Grading soft tissue tumors applies only to sarcomas. Histologic grade is an important (if not the most important) prognostic parameter in soft tissue neoplasia.[5–7] Many sarcomas can be assigned a grade definitionally based on their subtype. Overall, the rarity of soft tissue tumors does not practically allow for separate grading criteria for each subtype. Therefore, general grading schemes have been devised and studied over the past several decades that correlate with prognosis, recurrence, metastasis-free survival, and overall survival. Earlier grading systems were four-tiered and correlated histologic grade nicely with risk of metastasis and survival but three-tier systems are similarly effective.[6] For example, in one early study, overall survival rates for grades 1, 2, and 3 were 97%, 67%, and 38%, respectively.[7] The National Cancer Institute (NCI) regarded tumor necrosis as the most important prognostic indicator in separating grades 2 and 3. Necrosis was predictive of survival after the first recurrence.[5] The key in the NCI histopathologic grading system is the use of more or less than 15% necrosis to separate grades 2 and 3. Many authors have found that this scheme accurately predicts prognosis in soft tissue tumors. The French Federation of Cancer Centers has used differentiation, mitosis, and necrosis in their grading system, which also provides similar prognostic information.[8] The NCI and French grading systems are presented in Tables 9.1–9.3.

A study comparing the French system and the NCI systems found a slightly better predictability of the French system over the NCI system.[9] However, when used consistently in a single institution, either system is serviceable and reproducible.

It is perhaps the ultimate goal in soft tissue tumors to select a group of patients (such as those with grade 2 tumors) who may benefit from surgery alone versus a combination of surgery with adjuvant therapy. A large number of proliferation markers have been explored for this purpose. At present, however, histologic grading remains the foundation of clinical decision making for most

Table 9.1 National Cancer Institute histopathologic grading of soft-tissue tumors

Histologic parameters
Tumor type
Necrosis
Mitoses
Grade
I – Well differentiated
II – <15% necrosis (none or minimal)
III – >15% necrosis (moderate or marked)

National Cancer Institute three-grade system

Grade I	Grade I–III
Well differentiated liposarcoma	Leiomyosarcoma*
Myxoid liposarcoma	Chondrosarcoma
Dermatofibrosarcoma protuberans	Malignant peripheral nerve sheath tumor†
	Hemangiopericytoma‡
	Fibrosarcoma*
	Myxoid chondrosarcoma§

Grade II–III	Grade III
Round cell liposarcoma	Ewing's sarcoma
Malignant fibrous histiocytoma	Osteosarcoma
Clear cell sarcoma	Alveolar soft part sarcoma
Angiosarcoma	Primitive neuroectodermal tumor
Epithelioid sarcoma	Malignant triton tumor
Malignant granular cell tumor	Mesenchymal chondrosarcoma
Fibrosarcoma	
Synovial sarcoma	
Rhabdomyosarcoma	
Pleomorphic liposarcoma	

* Grade I, absent necrosis, low mitotic activity (<6 mitoses/10 hpf)
† Grade I, appearance of neurofibroma but with mitoses (<6 mitoses/10 hpf)
‡ Grade I, <1 mitosis/10 hpf
§ Grade I, uniformly hypocellular, myxoid, devoid of mitoses
Modified from Guillou L, Coindre JM, Bonichon F, et al. Comparative study of the National Cancer Institute and French Federation of Cancer Centers Sarcoma Group grading systems in a population of 410 adult patients with soft tissue sarcoma. J Clin Oncol 1997;15(1): 350–362.

sarcomas, although genetic markers are promising in well studied pediatric sarcomas and in sarcomas with established translocations such as synovial sarcoma and alveolar rhabdomyosarcoma.

Staging of any cancer is a portrait of its anatomic location and the extent of disease at the time of initial diagnosis. The staging of soft tissue sarcomas presents a set of unique problems given that these tumors are so rare, have a wide range of histologic features and anatomic locations and, at times, unpredictable biologic behavior.

Table 9.2 French Federation of Cancer Centers (FNCLCC, Fédération nationale des centres de lutte contre le cancer) grading system

Histologic parameters
Tumor differentiation
Mitosis count
Tumor necrosis
Scores are added to assign grade

Grade
1 – Score 2–3
2 – Score 4–5
3 – Score 6–8

Scoring parameters

Score	Differentiation	Mitosis	Necrosis
0	(not used)	(not used)	No necrosis
1	Resembling normal tissue	0–9/field	<50% necrosis
2	Sarcomas for which histologic typing certain	10–19/field	>50% necrosis
3	Embryonal and undifferentiated sarcomas	>20/field	(not used)

Table 9.3 Differentiation scores

Histologic type	Tumor differentiation score
Well differentiated liposarcoma	1
Myxoid liposarcoma	2
Round cell liposarcoma	3
Pleomorphic liposarcoma	3
Dedifferentiated liposarcoma	3
Conventional fibrosarcoma	2
Poorly differentiated fibrosarcoma	3
Well differentiated malignant schwannoma	1
Conventional malignant schwannoma	2
Poorly differentiated malignant schwannoma	3
Epithelioid malignant schwannoma	3
Malignant triton tumor	3
Well differentiated hemangiopericytoma	2
Conventional malignant hemangiopericytoma	3
Myxoid malignant fibrous histiocytoma (MFH)	2
Storiform pleomorphic MFH	2
Giant cell and inflammatory MFH	3
Well differentiated leiomyosarcoma	1
Conventional leiomyosarcoma	2
Poorly diff/pleo/epithelioid leiomyosarcoma	3
Biphasic/monophasic synovial sarcoma	3
All rhabdomyosarcoma	3
Well differentiated chondrosarcoma	1
Myxoid chondrosarcoma	2
Mesenchymal chondrosarcoma	3

Modified from Guillou L, Coindre JM, Bonichon F, et al. Comparative study of the National Cancer Institute and French Federation of Cancer Centers Sarcoma Group grading systems in a population of 410 adult patients with soft tissue sarcoma. J Clin Oncol 1997;15(1): 350.

Furthermore, the controversies surrounding histologic grade directly influence the stage of disease because, unique to sarcomas, grade itself is incorporated into the staging schemes.

Staging of cancers began in 1959 with the organization of the American Joint Committee for cancer staging and end results reporting (AJC). The AJC used the TNM system for staging cancers and published its first clinical and pathologic staging system for sarcomas in 1977.[10] Over time the AJC became the American Joint Committee on Cancer (AJCC) and together with the International Union against Cancers devised a four-stage system applicable to soft tissue tumors in a variety of anatomical locations. An alternative system is the Enneking system, published in 1980.[11] In contrast to the AJCC system, this system highlights additional clinical and surgical management perspectives of extremity tumors. However the basic principles of each staging system incorporate grade, tumor size, local extent, and metastasis.

The 6th edition AJCC system[12] applies to all soft tissue sarcomas except Kaposi's sarcoma, dermatofibrosarcoma protuberans, infantile fibrosarcoma, and angiosarcoma. Sarcomas of the brain and parenchymal organs are not optimally staged by this system although gastrointestinal stromal tumors are staged using general sarcoma criteria. A key feature of the AJCC staging system is that 5 cm appears to be a prognostic 'cut-off' size. It should also be noted that, in contrast to carcinomas, lymphoid metastasis is not a typical feature of sarcomas with the following exceptions: synovial sarcoma, rhabdomyosarcoma, epithelioid sarcoma, and clear cell sarcoma. The AJCC staging system appears in Table 9.4.

CLASSIFICATION OF SOFT TISSUE TUMORS

Soft tissue tumors are classified according to the adult tissue types that the lesional cells resemble. This does not necessarily imply that the tumor arose from such cells. In the future, classification may be established on molecular grounds but presently morphologic features remain the basis of classification. Table 9.5 presents known translocations and their associated gene products.

FIBROUS TISSUE TUMORS

FIBROMA

Collagenous

Collagenous fibroma was first described by Evans using the term desmoplastic fibroblastoma. Since the latter name is potentially confusing to clinicians, later observers preferred the term collagenous fibroma. Evans initially described seven cases of this distinctive fibrous soft tissue tumor, all in adults and located in multiple sites.[13] A large Armed Forces Institute of Pathology (AFIP) study[14] confirmed that these lesions tended to occur in adults over a wide age range (16–81 years) with a wide anatomic distribution (arm, shoulder, girdle, posterior neck and upper back, feet and ankles, leg, hand, abdominal wall, and hip). The tumors were painless and slowly growing and often present for years. The AFIP series included tumors ranging in size from 1–20 cm (median 3 cm) and all behaved in a benign fashion without recurrences or metastasis despite incomplete excision in some cases. Collagenous fibromas are predominantly subcutaneous but occasionally involve fascial structures; a few have extensions into skeletal muscle. They are elongated and lobulated and typically infiltrative into fat. On microscopic examination the lesions are composed of bland

Table 9.4 Definition of TNM

Primary tumor (T)

TX	Primary tumor cannot be assessed
T0	No evidence of primary tumor
T1	Tumor 5 cm or less in greatest dimension
	T1a Superficial tumor
	T1b Deep tumor
T2	Tumor more than 5 cm in greatest dimension
	T2a Superficial tumor
	T2b Deep tumor

Regional lymph nodes (N)

NX	Regional lymph nodes cannot be assessed
N0	No regional lymph node metastasis
N1*	Regional lymph node metastasis

*Note: Presence of positive nodes (N1) is considered to be stage IV.

Distant metastasis (M)

MX	Distant metastasis cannot be assessed
M0	No distant metastasis
M1	Distant metastasis

Stage grouping

Stage I	T1a, 1b, 2a, 2b	N0	M0	G1–2	G1	Low
Stage II	T1a, 1b, 2a	N0	M0	G3–4	G2–3	High
Stage III	T2b	N0	M0	G3–4	G2–3	High
Stage IV	Any T	N1	M0	Any G	Any G	High or low
	Any T	N0	M1	Any G	Any G	High or low

Histologic grade (G)

GX	Grade cannot be assessed
G1	Well differentiated
G2	Moderately differentiated
G3	Poorly differentiated
G4	Poorly differentiated or undifferentiated (four-tiered systems only)

Source: AJCC Cancer Staging Manual, 6th edn.

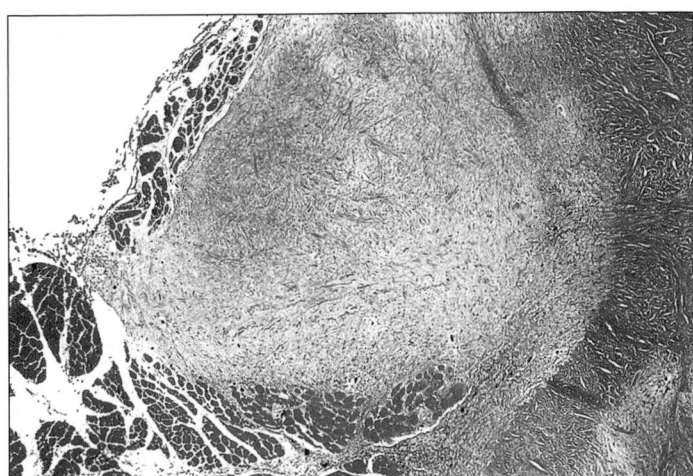

Fig. 9.1 Collagenous fibroma. This loosely circumscribed nodule is present in skeletal muscle.

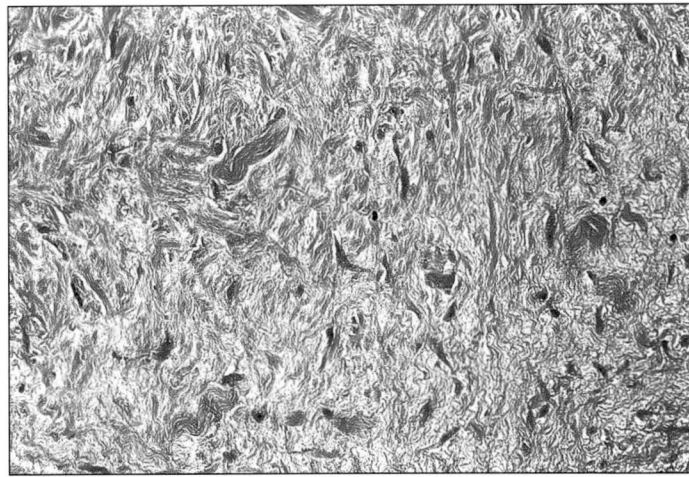

Fig. 9.2 Collagenous fibroma. Note the stellate appearance of the fibroblasts.

stellate and spindle-shaped fibroblasts set in a densely collagenized or myxocollagenous matrix, mitotic activity is absent or minimal (Figs 9.1, 9.2). In the AFIP study, some lesional cells had a myofibroblastic immunophenotype with scattered reactivity for alpha smooth muscle actin (SMA). Desmin, S100 protein and CD34 were lacking in these fibroblastic lesions. Ultrastructural studies on collagenous fibroma have yielded fibroblastic or myofibroblastic lineage[15] and they are diploid on flow cytometry. However, in one karyotyped case, an 11q12 rearrangement was found.[16] Since fibroma of tendon sheath also has rearrangements of 11q12, collagenous fibromas and fibromas of tendon sheath may be genetically linked. Reported attempts to diagnosis collagenous fibroma by cytology were nondiagnostic based on low cellularity.[17] The key point in recognizing collagenous fibromas is that their dense collagenized appearance and occasionally large size suggests that these lesions are, instead, musculoaponeurotic fibromatoses (desmoid tumors, see below). However these are substantially less cellular and lack the sweeping fascicular architecture at low magnification that is characteristic of fibromatosis. Collagenous fibromas are readily recognized as benign.

Fibroma of tendon sheath

Fibroma of tendon sheath was first well characterized by Chung and Enzinger.[18] Fibroma of tendon sheath tends to occur between the third and fifth decades and is more common in males. Most affect the tendons and tendon sheaths of the fingers, hand, and wrist and usually present as insidiously growing masses associated with mild tenderness and pain in about one third of patients. The finding of t(2;11)(q31–32;q12) in a reported case suggests that these are neoplasms rather than reactive lesions.[19] Fibroma of tendon sheath is typically well circumscribed and lobulated and measures approximately 2 cm, although the largest in the original series was 5.5 cm. On gross examination the tumors are found attached to tendons and tendon sheaths and are usually well circumscribed and sometimes appear encapsulated. They are distinctly lobulated grossly and gray to ivory or pearly white on cut surface. Most are firm with collagenous consistency. Microscopically fibroma of tendon sheath is lobulated and consists of scattered fibroblasts associated with dense fibrous stroma, similar to collagenous fibroma but better marginated (Figs 9.3, 9.4). Fibromas of tendon sheath often contain slit-like vascular channels, which bear some resemblance to entrapped

Table 9.5 Specific chromosomal translocations established cytogenetically and the corresponding gene changes mesenchymal tumors

Tumors	Translocation	Gene changes
Alveolar rhabdomyosarcoma	t(2;13)(q35;q14)	PAX3–FKHR
	t(1;13)(p36;q14)	PAX7–FKHR
Alveolar soft part sarcoma	t(X;17)(p11.2;q25)	ASPL–TFE3
Clear cell sarcoma (malignant melanoma of soft parts)	t(12;22)(q13;q12)	ATF1–EWS
Congenital fibrosarcoma and mesoblastic nephroma	t(12;15)(p13;q25)	ETV6–NTRK3
Dermatofibrosarcoma protuberans (giant cell fibroblastoma)	t(17;22)(q22;q13)	COL1A1–PDGFB
Desmoplastic small round cell tumor	t(11;22)(p13;q12)	WT1–EWS
Endometrial stromal sarcoma	t(7;17)(p15;q21)	JAZF1–JJAZ1
Ewing's sarcoma and peripheral primitive neuroectodermal tumors	t(11;22)(q24;q12)	EWS–FLI1
	t(21;22)(q22;q12)	EWS–ERG
	t(7;22)(p22;q12)	EWS–ETV1
	t(17;22)(q12;q12)	EWS–E1AF
	t(2;22)(q33;q12)	FEV–EWS
Inflammatory myofibroblastic tumor	t(2;19)(p23;p13.1)	ALK–TPM4
	t(1;2)(q22–23;p23)	TPM3–ALK
Myxoid chondrosarcoma, extraskeletal	t(9;22)(q22;q12)	EWS–CHN(TEC)
	t(9;17)(q22;q11)	RBP56–CHN(TEC)
	t(9;15)(q22;q21)	TEC/TCF12
Myxoid liposarcoma	t(12;16)(q13;p11)	TLS(FUS)–CHOP
	t(12;22)(q13;q12)	EWS–CHOP
Synovial sarcoma	t(X;18)(p11;q11)	SYT–SSX1
		SYT–SSX2
Low-grade fibromyxoid sarcoma	t(7;16)(q33;p11)	FUS–BBF2H7

Modified from Sandberg AA. Translocations in malignant tumors. Am J Pathol 2001;159:1979.

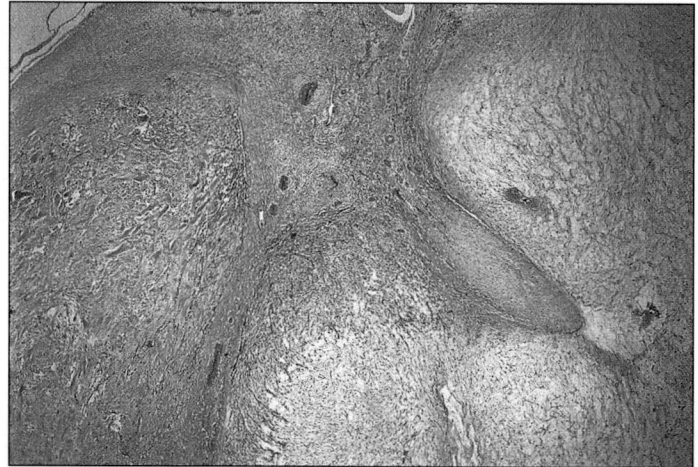

Fig. 9.3 Fibroma of tendon sheath. At low magnification, a lobulated pattern can be seen with tissue clefting.

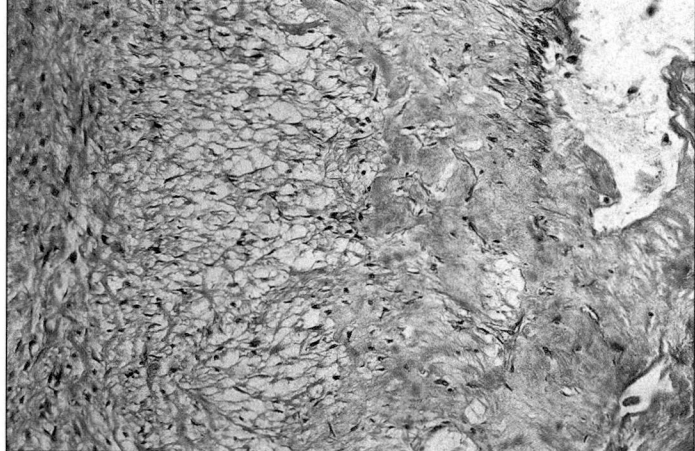

Fig. 9.4 Fibroma of tendon sheath. Bland-appearing stellate cells and myxoid change can overlap with nodular fasciitis. Heavily collagenized zones may also be found.

tenosynovial clefts. Typically the fibroblasts are spindle-shaped and the fibrous stroma markedly collagenized with zones of myxoid degeneration in which stellate fibroblasts are observed. It is important to note that in cellular (probably early) variants of fibroma of tendon sheath the spindle cells are arranged in fascicles and occasionally accompanied by mucoid matrix, extravasated erythrocytes and sprinkled mononuclear cells indistinguishable from nodular fasciitis (described below). Immunohistochemistry and ultrastructural studies of these tumors yield fibroblastic and myofibroblastic features.[20,21] Fibroma of tendon sheath may recur locally if incompletely excised but is benign.

Elastofibroma

Elastofibroma is a slowly growing fibroelastic proliferation believed to result from mechanical friction between the scapula and the chest wall. Tumors typically occur on the backs of predominantly female

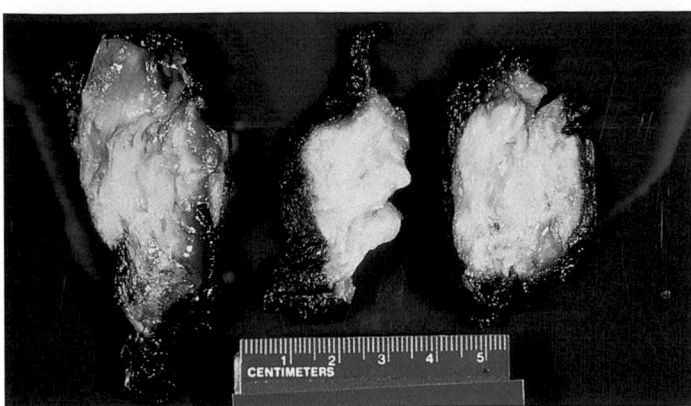

Fig. 9.5 Elastofibroma. This appears as an irregular sclerotic mass in subcutaneous fat.

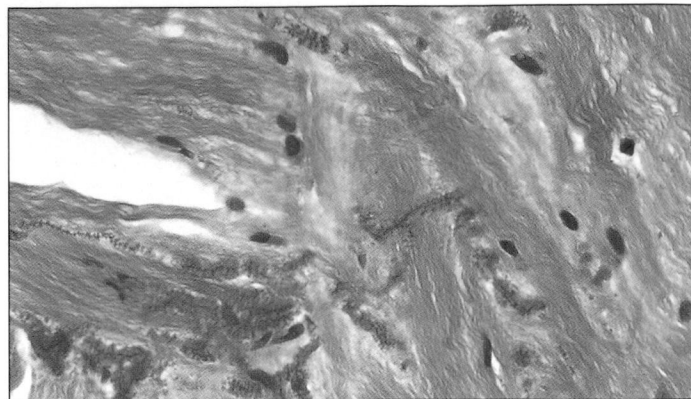

Fig. 9.6 Elastofibroma. Degenerating collagen fibers are seen on H&E sections.

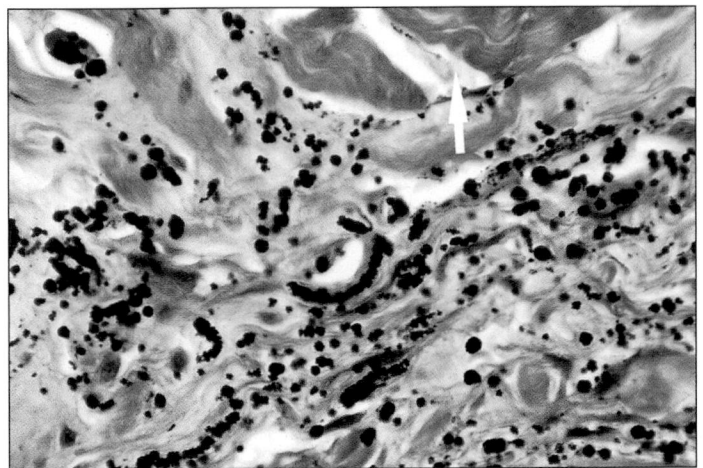

Fig. 9.7 Elastofibroma. Elastic staining highlights chenille (caterpillar) bodies.

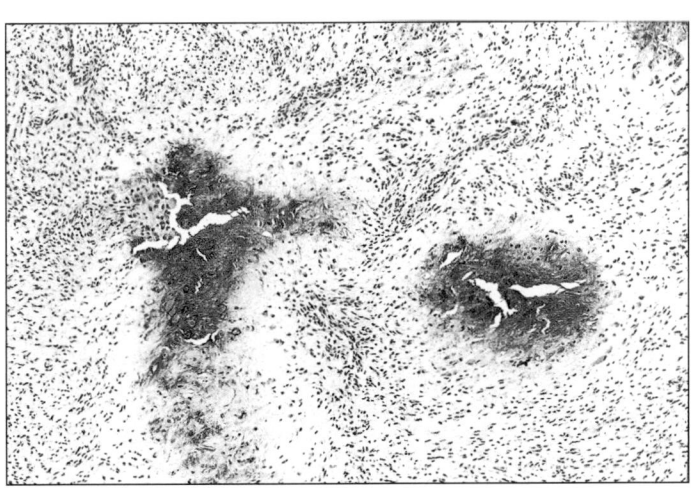

Fig. 9.8 Calcifying aponeurotic fibroma. In its classic form, lesions are punctuated by irregular calcified foci.

patients with a history of mechanical labor. Although these lesions have been presumed to be reactive in the past[22], recent studies suggest that they have a variety of chromosomal alterations and could instead be neoplasms.[23] Bilaterality is also known.[24] Grossly the excised mass is a firm ill-defined lesion with a glistening surface and foci of cystic degeneration and interspersed fatty areas (Fig. 9.5). On microscopic examination the mass consists of intertwining eosinophilic collagen and thickened serrated deeply eosinophilic elastic fibers that have a degenerated beaded appearance or are fragmented into globules (chenille, French for 'caterpillar', bodies) or flower like arrangements (Fig. 9.6). Elastic stain characteristically highlights the degenerate appearance of the elastic fibers (Fig. 9.7). Like other densely collagenized fibroblastic lesions, these do not lend themselves to accurate diagnosis by fine-needle aspiration cytology (FNA) but aspirate findings are occasionally highly suggestive of the diagnosis if the 'petaloid' structures are found on the smear.[25] Elastofibromas are benign.

Calcifying aponeurotic fibroma

Calcifying aponeurotic fibroma primarily affects the hands and feet of children between birth and 16 years.[26] As with any tumor type,

however, there are exceptions; extra-axial examples may be observed.[27] The tumor usually presents as a slow growing, poorly circumscribed mass. Calcifying aponeurotic fibroma has a tendency to local recurrence. On radiologic examination, it may have calcific stippling. Grossly it is an ill defined, gritty mass with punctate calcification. Microscopically the nodules are characterized by infiltrative fibrous growth of plump oval fibroblasts arranged in cords. There is rich cellularity and dense collagen. Not infrequently, the nodules may be attached to an aponeurosis or tendon. Focal calcification can be seen microscopically, except in cases occurring early in infants or small children. Typically band-like or serpiginous central calcification is surrounded by chondroid matrix (Fig. 9.8). Variable numbers of giant cells may also be seen. Cases with no calcification may be difficult to distinguish from infantile fibromatosis (Fig. 9.9). However, calcifying aponeurotic fibroma has plumper spindle cells, is associated with dense collagen, and occurs in the hands and feet, whereas fibromatoses tend to involve more proximal anatomic sites.

On immunohistochemical staining, calcifying aponeurotic fibroma expresses vimentin, sometimes muscle-specific actin (MSA), sometimes SMA, CD99, S100 protein, and CD68. Although calcifying

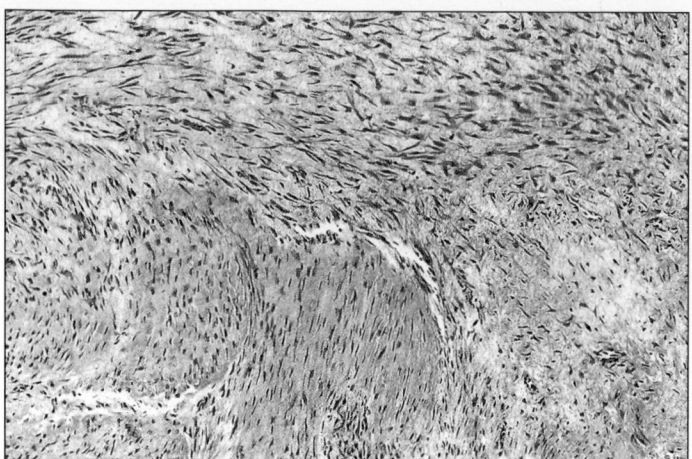

Fig. 9.9 Calcifying aponeurotic fibroma. Cellular examples can appear similar to fibromatoses. However, these tumors are typically acral whereas fibromatoses are more axial.

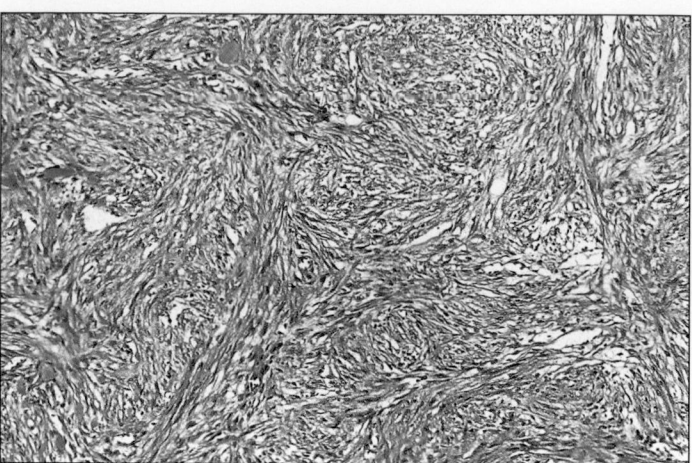

Fig. 9.10 Nodular fasciitis. At scanning magnification, most examples display a loose storiform pattern.

aponeurotic fibroma is a benign lesion, aneuploidy has been reported.[28] On aspiration cytology, it has been reported to display benign appearing spindled cells, chondroid cells, multinucleated giant cells, and calcific debris, recapitulating its histologic features.[29]

BENIGN FIBROBLASTIC/MYOFIBROBLASTIC PSEUDOSARCOMATOUS PROLIFERATIONS

Pseudosarcomatous proliferative lesions of soft tissue are fascia-based fibroblastic and myofibroblastic lesions that have the potential to be overdiagnosed as sarcoma. They are usually subtyped according to the location, depth of involvement, age at presentation, and histologic features. They are presumed to be reactive and recurrences are only rarely encountered after surgical excision. However, there are reports of cytogenetic alterations.[30,31] These lesions, including nodular fasciitis, proliferative myositis, and proliferative fasciitis, were all diploid in one flow cytometric study and cell cycle analysis did not correlate with mitotic counts.[32]

Nodular fasciitis

Nodular fasciitis, first described in the 1950s,[33] is the most frequently encountered pseudosarcomatous lesion. It is sometimes mistaken for a sarcoma because of its rapid growth, increased cellularity and high mitotic index.[34–38] Nodular fasciitis occurs mostly in the third to fourth decades as a rapidly growing solitary mass of the upper extremities. The second most common site is the head and the neck region, which is the most frequent site in infants and children. No gender predilection has been observed.

Grossly the lesion is a well circumscribed, nonencapsulated nodule, usually less than 2 cm in diameter, although lesions as large as 10 cm are known. Tumors are loosely marginated and their cut surfaces vary from fibrous to gelatinous or mucoid. Histologically, nodular fasciitis usually involves subcutaneous tissue, but intramuscular and fascial forms also occur. The nodule consists primarily of plump myofibroblasts that appear similar to those seen in tissue culture or granulation tissue. The myofibroblasts are arranged in a whorled/storiform pattern, slightly curved or S-shaped pattern or haphazardly (Fig. 9.10). The cells are bland in appearance, with pale nuclei and small nucleoli. The mitotic rate is fairly high but atypical

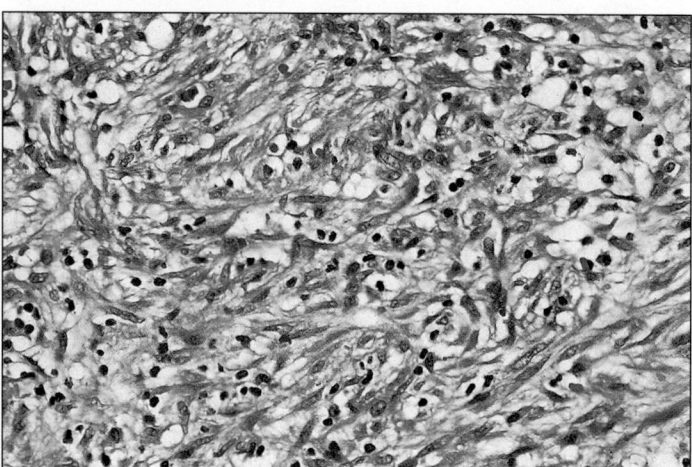

Fig. 9.11 Nodular fasciitis. Lymphocytes may be a prominent feature but plasma cells are not usually found.

mitoses are absent. Intermixed with the fibroblasts are lymphocytes (Fig. 9.11), and extravasated erythrocytes (Fig. 9.12) with variable numbers of macrophages and giant cells (Fig. 9.13). The intervening matrix is myxoid, imparting a feathery appearance, whereas cellular forms exhibit dense cellularity and have less matrix. Microcysts and or macrocysts, and areas of microhemorrhages can be seen. Lesions of short duration usually are myxoid whereas long-standing ones are more fibrotic or hyalinized with cyst formation.

Variants of nodular fasciitis merit brief description. *Ossifying fasciitis* is a nodular fasciitis-like fibroblastic proliferation with osseous metaplasia[39] similar to myositis ossificans. Related proliferations have even been described in the mesentery and also likened to myositis ossificans.[40] *Intravascular fasciitis* is a rare variant of nodular fasciitis arising from small or medium-sized vessels[41] (Fig. 9.14). The lesion presents as a soft tissue mass with focal intravascular extension or a multinodular predominantly intravascular mass. Despite the intravascular location the lesion behaves in a benign fashion with no tendency to recur or metastasize. *Cranial fasciitis* involves soft tissues of the scalp and underlying skull of infants. It usually erodes the bone but may penetrate through the

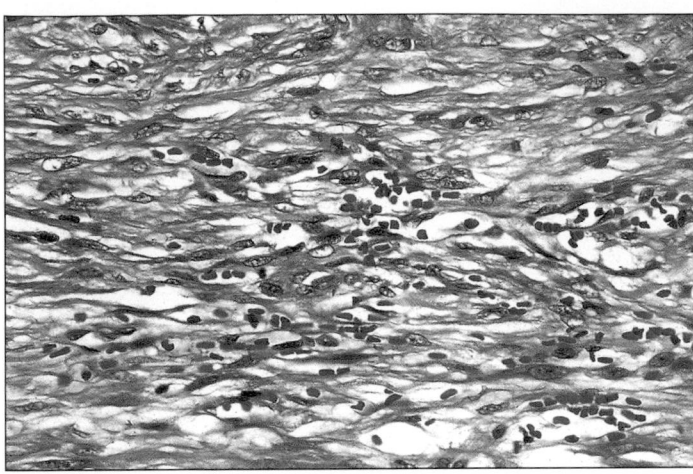

Fig. 9.12 Nodular fasciitis. Extravasated erythrocytes are constant findings. Note that there is no associated hemosiderin. The nuclei have smooth nuclear membranes and delicate nucleoli.

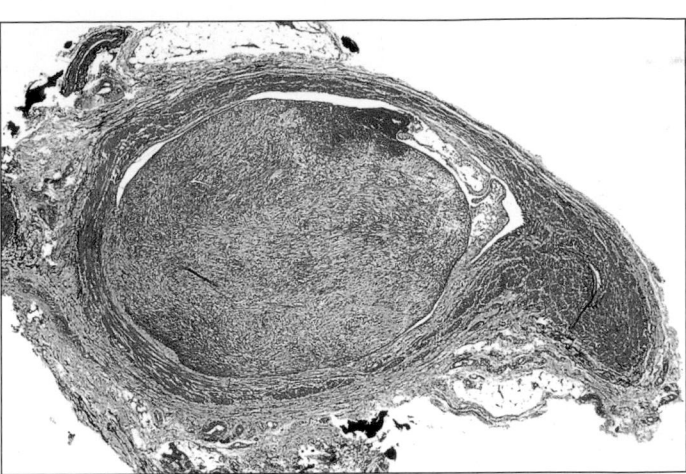

Fig. 9.14 Intravascular fasciitis. (Movat stain.)

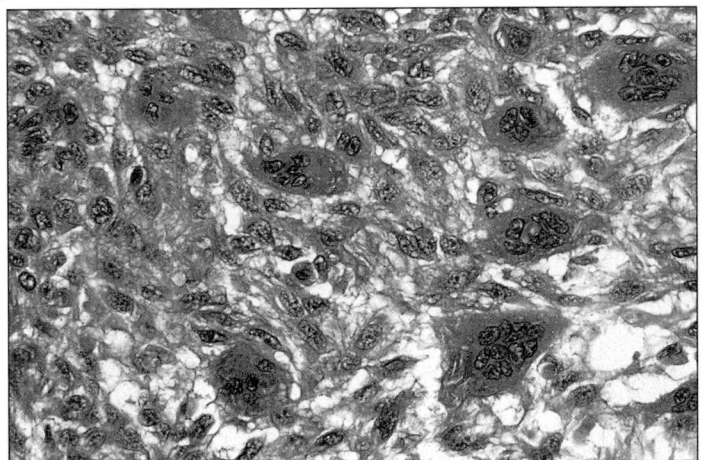

Fig. 9.13 Nodular fasciitis. Many lesions have osteoclast-like giant cells.

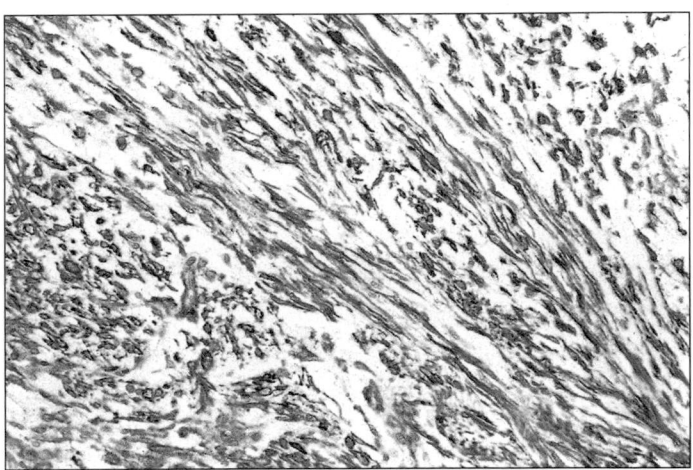

Fig. 9.15 Nodular fasciitis. This is a myofibroblastic process and, consequently, SMA is expressed. Awareness of this phenomenon can prevent overdiagnosis as leiomyosarcoma.

bone to involve the meninges. Fragments of bone may be seen at the periphery of this lesion. Birth trauma is presumed to be the inciting stimulus.[42]

If immunohistochemistry is performed, these lesions invariably express MSA, SMA (Fig. 9.15), and calponin owing to their myofibroblastic differentiation, a feature that may result in their misclassification as leiomyosarcoma. In contrast to leiomyosarcoma, nodular fasciitis typically lacks immunoreactivity for desmin and caldesmon. Nodular fasciitis also lacks S100 protein and keratin. Many admixed cells in nodular fasciitis stain with KP1 (CD68), including the osteoclast-like giant cells, which are highlighted by CD68 staining in lesions where they were initially inconspicuous.

The proliferating cells in the pseudosarcomas typically have benign-appearing nuclei and stellate cytoplasm on aspiration[43] (Figs 9.16, 9.17). They can generally be recognized as cytologically benign but have overlapping features with other myofibroblastic processes.

Proliferative fasciitis

Proliferative fasciitis is less common than nodular fasciitis.[44] It mainly occurs in adults with no gender predilection. This proliferation often presents as a palpable mobile rapidly growing subcutaneous nodule in the extremities, especially the forearm and the thigh.

Grossly it appears as poorly circumscribed elongated mass mainly involving the interlobular fibrous tissue septa of the subcutis. Histologically, in addition to stellate cells, there are ganglion-like cells (Figs 9.18, 9.19) with basophilic cytoplasm, one or two nucleoli, and occasional cytoplasmic inclusions. There is variable myxoid stroma that becomes more collagenized as lesions persist. It is the large 'ganglion-like' cells that are readily mistaken as malignant.

The differential diagnosis includes malignant fibrous histiocytoma (MFH), which has more atypia and pleomorphic giant cells (as opposed to ganglion-like cells). Ganglioneuroblastoma contains, in addition to small round cells, true ganglion cells and may resemble proliferative myositis. However, ganglion cells express neuroendocrine markers whereas the ganglion-like cells in proliferative fasciitis are modified fibroblasts, thus retaining the same staining criteria. *Rhabdomyosarcoma* also enters in the differential diagnosis as the ganglion-like cells may bear resemblance to the rhabdomyoblasts, a consideration apt to arise in pediatric examples of proliferative fasciitis.[45] Immunohistochemistry can assist in any

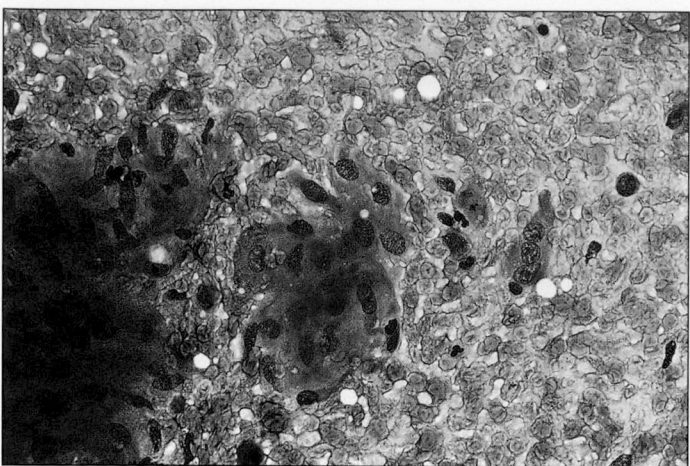

Fig. 9.16 Nodular fasciitis, fine-needle aspirate. As is typical for benign soft tissue lesions on aspiration, most cells are cohesive and a few are shed singly. The nuclei are not substantially larger than 'control' erythrocytes and inflammatory cells in the field.

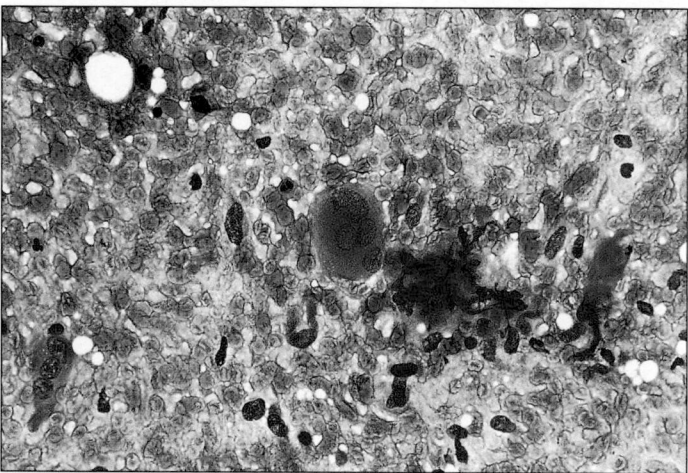

Fig. 9.17 Nodular fasciitis, fine-needle aspirate. Note the osteoclast-like giant cell.

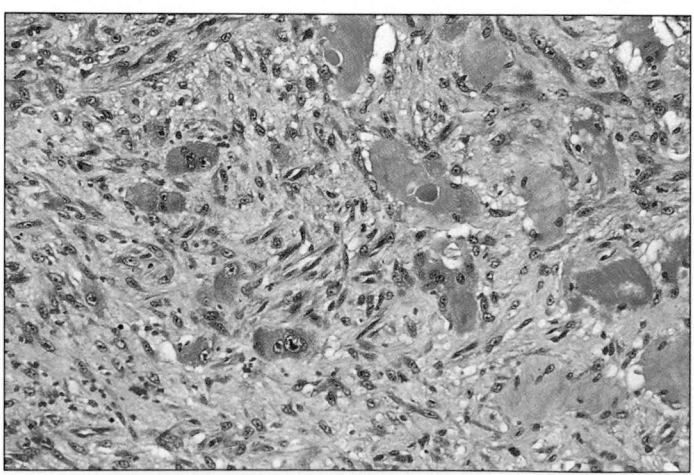

Fig. 9.18 Proliferative fasciitis. The background is that of nodular fasciitis but enlarged 'ganglion-like' fibroblasts are apparent.

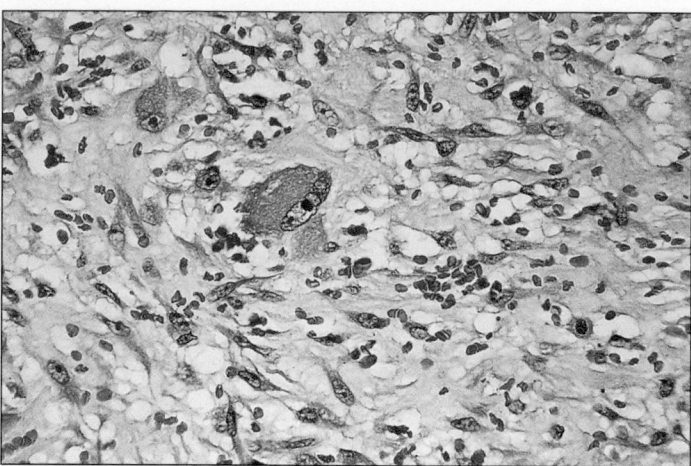

Fig. 9.19 Proliferative fasciitis. Ganglion-like fibroblasts and extravasated erythrocytes are present.

doubtful case, as rhabdomyoblasts are desmin-positive whereas ganglion-like cells of proliferative fasciitis are desmin-negative. Such errors should be a thing of the past since newer antibodies (such as MyoD1, myogenin) reliably identify rhabdomyosarcomas whereas they do not react with the fibroblastic nuclei of proliferative fasciitis.

Proliferative myositis

Proliferative myositis is the deep or intramuscular counterpart of proliferative fasciitis. It typically presents as a rapidly growing mass affecting the muscles of the trunk and the limb girdles. Grossly the tumor/nodule is poorly circumscribed, appearing as pale, scar-like induration of the muscle and overlying fascia. Histologically, it is a poorly demarcated process with fibroblastic proliferation involving the epimysium, perimysium, and endomysium with scattered large basophilic ganglion-like giant cells. At low magnification, alternating areas of proliferated fibroblasts and remnants of infiltrated muscle tissue produce a 'checkerboard' pattern. A variable amount of myxoid to collagenized stroma is present. Focal areas of ossification can be seen, although this finding is less conspicuous in proliferative myositis than in myositis ossificans.

The differential diagnosis is from proliferative fasciitis.

Atypical decubital fibroplasia/ischemic fasciitis

Atypical decubital fibroplasia,[46] also known as ischemic fasciitis,[47] was first described by Montgomery et al. It has some resemblance to proliferative fasciitis and is considered a degenerative and reparative process. It typically occurs as a mass lesion over bony prominences (e.g. sacrum or ischial tuberosities) as a result of prolonged pressure and impaired circulation, mainly in elderly debilitated, immobilized, or wheelchair-bound patients. It is essentially a unique pressure sore that results in a mass effect rather than an ulcer. Microscopically there is a lobular or zonal pattern with central fibrinous and myxoid areas rimmed by ingrowing thin-walled ectatic vascular channels (Fig. 9.20). There is proliferation of fibroblasts with scattered ganglion-like giant cells with basophilic cytoplasm, large hyperchromatic nuclei with smudged nuclear chromatin and prominent nucleoli (Fig. 9.21). These cells are intermixed with inflammatory cells, areas of hemorrhage, granulation tissue, focal fibrinoid necrosis with fibrosis, and cystic changes (seen more often in older cases).

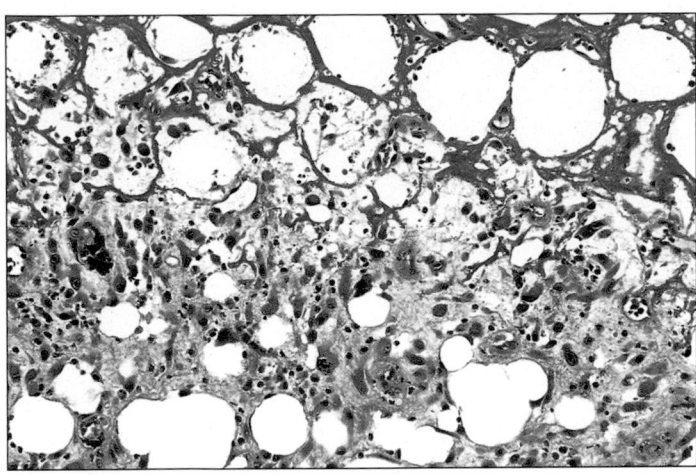

Fig. 9.20 Atypical decubital fibroplasia/ischemic fasciitis. The fat in this field shows coagulative necrosis with a fibrinoid appearance. There is ingrowth of enlarged fibroblasts.

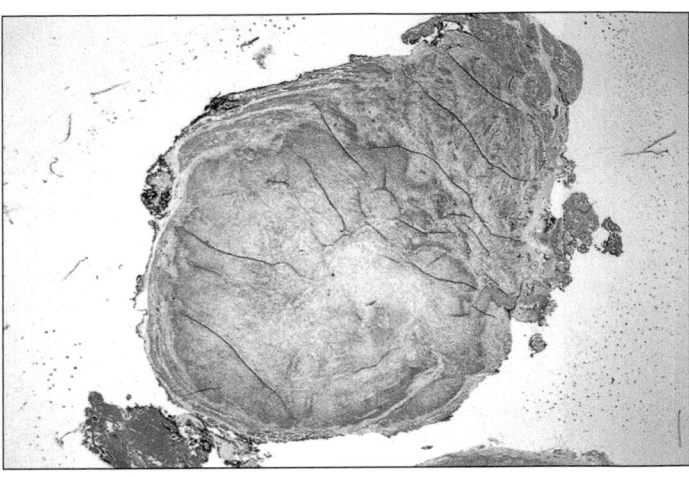

Fig. 9.22 Myofibroma. This was a solitary pediatric lesion from the neck. Note the lobulated appearance.

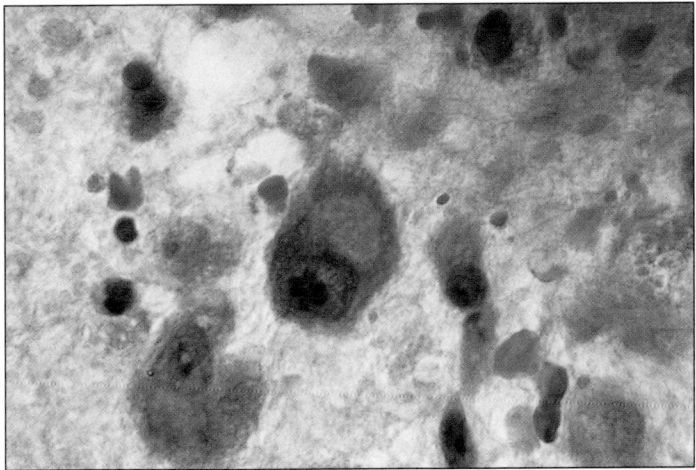

Fig. 9.21 Atypical decubital fibroplasia. Higher magnification of enlarged fibroblasts. This cell has a nucleolus similar to that in the ganglion-like cells of proliferative fasciitis but with a more 'smudged' and degenerative appearance.

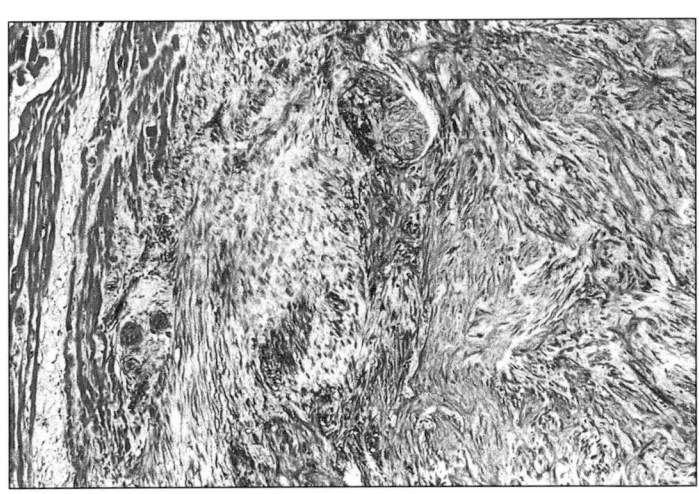

Fig. 9.23 Myofibroma, myoid area.

MYOFIBROMA AND MYOFIBROMATOSIS

In 1954, Stout introduced the term 'congenital generalized fibromatosis,'[48] which later gave way to 'infantile myofibromatosis', to describe findings in a group of infants having multifocal lesions. A comprehensive review by Chung and Enzinger concluded that such lesions were, in fact, typically solitary (74%), affecting the dermis or subcutis.[49] These tumors were subsequently recognized in adults and termed 'myofibromas.'[50] Isolated myofibromas of both children and adults have since been reported in a variety of sites. The presence of familial examples suggests that they are a neoplastic rather than reactive condition.[51] Recurrence is rare and attributable to incomplete excision.

Solitary myofibromas most commonly present in the head and neck region. Solitary myofibromas of the skeleton are quite rare, although when they do occur in bone, the head and neck region is by far the most common location. The largest series of solitary skeletal myofibromas was published by Inwards.[52] Of 14 cases found in the Mayo clinic files, eight involved the skull, five the mandible, and one the distal tibial diametaphysis.

Myofibroma is a biphasic tumor composed of lobules of myofibroblasts with intervening foci of small dark cells with hemangiopericytoma-like vessels (Figs 9.22–9.24). Although the myofibroblastic areas appear similar to smooth muscle, the biphasic nature of these lesions allows distinction from leiomyoma and leiomyosarcoma. A pitfall in diagnosis of these tumors is that they assume a more fascicular appearance when there is overlying mucosal ulceration and they can appear sarcoma-like on superficial biopsies.[53] There is limited experience with these tumors on FNA, although in one series of pediatric FNA the single myofibroma yielded insufficient material for diagnosis[54] and in another case report the diagnosis of myofibromatosis was suggested on FNA.[55] Early on, when these tumors are cellular, they can be mistaken for malignancy on FNA.

Myofibromas display ultrastructural features of myofibroblastic differentiation, namely cytoplasmic filaments with dense bodies, basal lamina, pinocytotic vesicles, and nuclear invaginations.

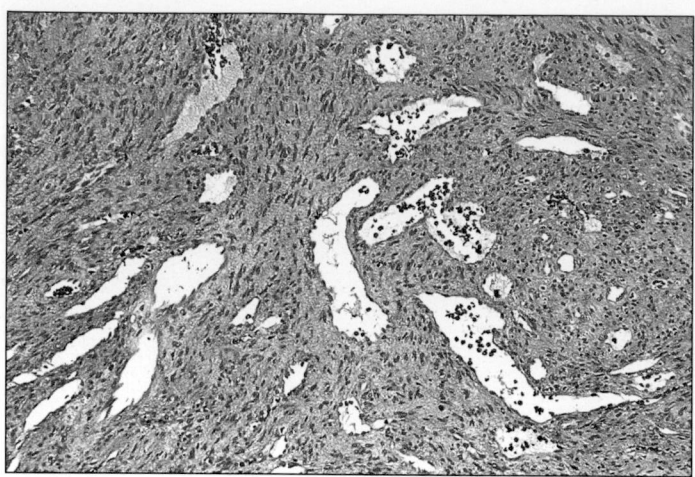

Fig. 9.24 Myofibroma, hemangiopericytoma-like area.

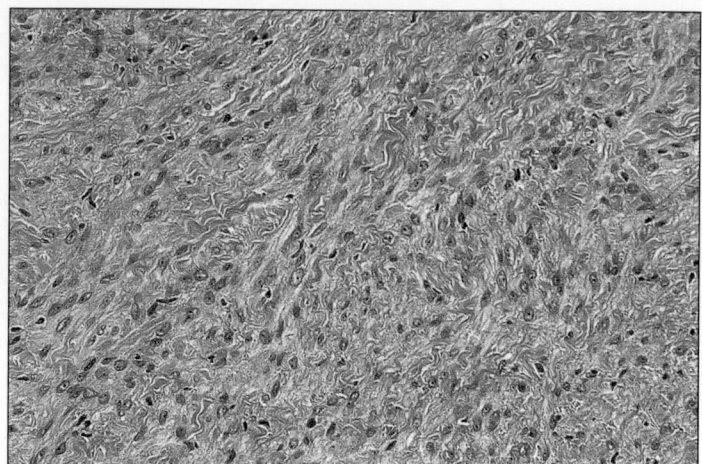

Fig. 9.25 Myofibroblastoma. This breast lesion displays bland uniform cells similar to the myofibroblasts in nodular fasciitis but arranged in alignment rather than in a storiform array. There are no secondary background changes (such as extravasated erythrocytes or inflammation).

Immunohistochemical investigation discloses a myofibroblastic profile (strongly actin- reactive, focal or negative desmin expression, nonreactive with S100 and keratin preparations).

The differential diagnosis of myofibromas includes both benign lesions and low-grade sarcomas, specifically fibromatoses and fibrosarcoma. However, myofibromas differ from both fibromatoses and fibrosarcoma by their zonation/lobulation, their myoid appearance, and their general lack of mitotic activity. This distinction is important since both fibromatoses and fibrosarcomas are prone to local recurrence and to metastases in the case of the latter, whereas myofibromas are usually cured by local and even incomplete excision. As most of these lesions present in infants and children, the differential diagnosis is usually with the infantile form of fibrosarcoma, which carries a better prognosis than the adult counterpart.

The differential diagnosis between smooth muscle lesions and solitary myofibroma can be difficult. Both leiomyoma and myofibroma express smooth muscle antigens and have myofilaments ultrastructurally but myofibromas display lobulation with zones of smaller rounded cells and cells with tapered nuclei and a hemangiopericytomatous vascular pattern, whereas leiomyomas consist of perpendicularly oriented fascicles of homogeneous cells with blunt-ended nuclei. The distinction between leiomyomas and solitary myofibromas is of no clinical consequence, although making the correct diagnosis would be critical in a patient with multiple lesions.

Myofibroblastoma (Figs 9.25, 9.26) should be noted here since this name is similar to 'myofibroma' and thus these two entities may be confused. A group of 16 breast lesions having ultrastructural characteristics of myofibroblasts was described in 1987[56] as 'myofibroblastomas,' although a number of isolated cases had been described prior to this series. Extramammary lesions have subsequently been reported in a variety of sites; the lymph nodes were the first highlighted.[57,58] Although these lesions may have a vaguely lobulated architecture, they differ from myofibromas by lacking the hemangiopericytoma-like areas between lobules and they have a divergent immunohistochemical phenotype. They express both CD34 and desmin (Figs 9.27, 9.28) in a significant number of cases, raising the possibility that they either overlap with or are tantamount to solitary fibrous tumors, which have also been reported in multiple sites.[59] However, solitary fibrous tumors do not express desmin, whereas myofibroblastomas are unusual in expressing both desmin and CD34, markers that are not typically coexpressed in myo-

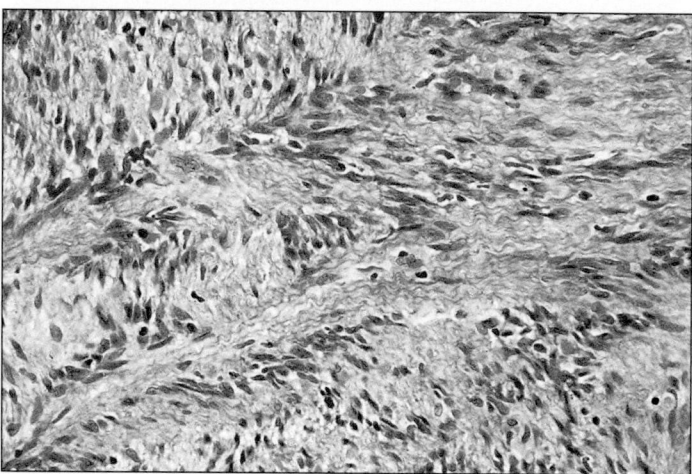

Fig. 9.26 Palisaded myofibroblastoma of lymph node. Despite the palisaded appearance, the cells are more uniform than those of schwannoma. This lesion expressed actin and lacked S100 protein.

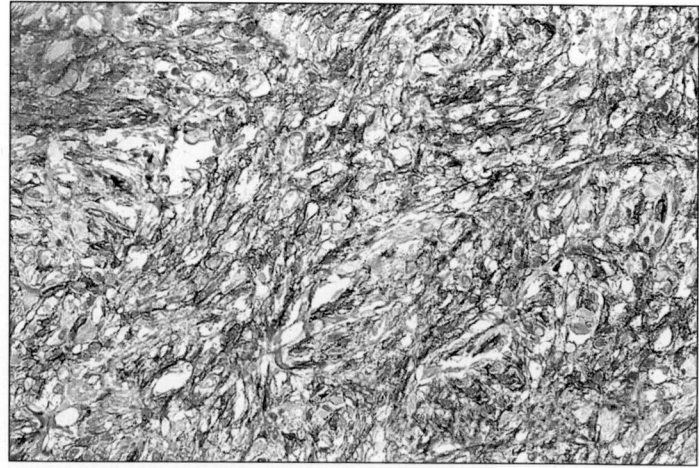

Fig. 9.27 Myofibroblastoma of breast. CD34 is strongly reactive.

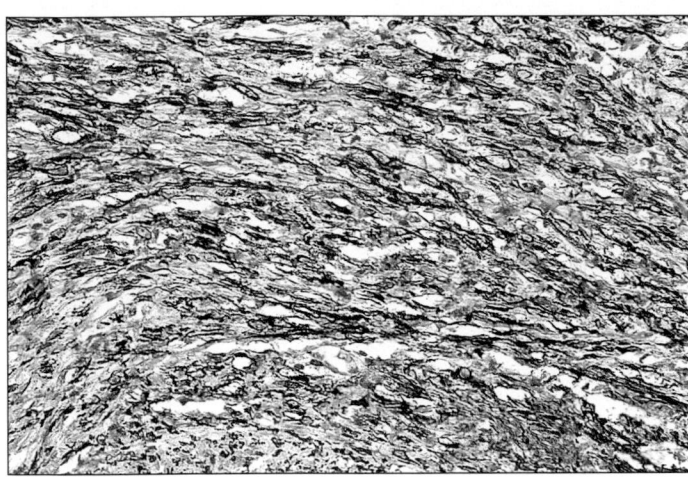

Fig. 9.28 Myofibroblastoma of breast with strong desmin expression.

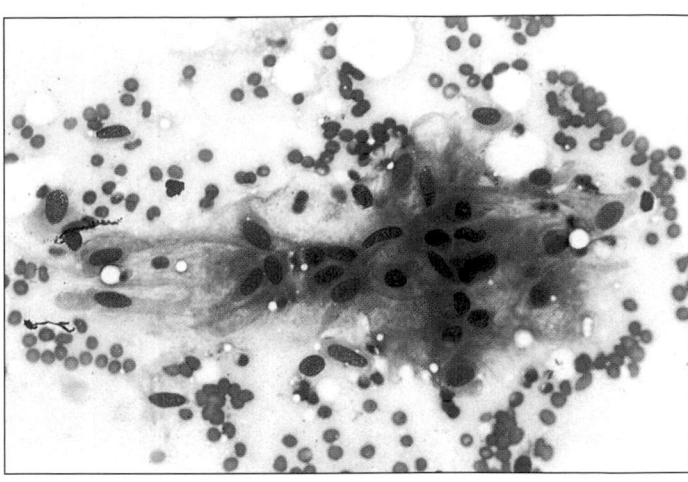

Fig. 9.30 Myofibroblastoma of breast, aspiration cytology. At higher magnification, the spindle cells have smooth nuclear contours.

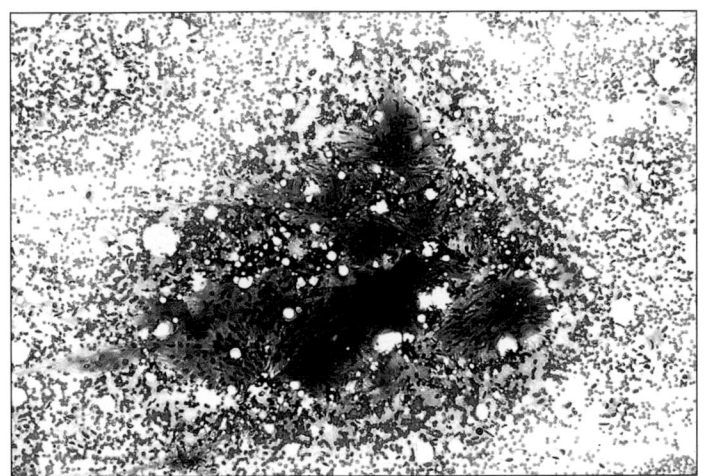

Fig. 9.29 Myofibroblastoma of breast, aspiration cytology. Most cells are cohesive, with a few 'spilling off' the aspirated clump, a feature of benignity.

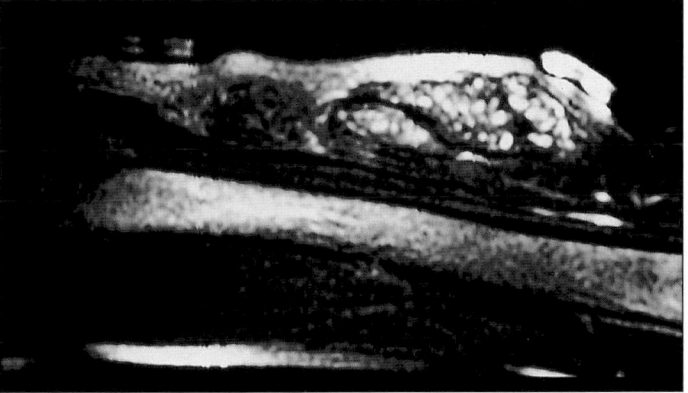

Fig. 9.31 Calcifying fibrous tumor, MRI. While these are histologically obviously benign, their clinical presentation is more alarming.

fibroblastic lesions. On aspiration cytology, these tumors appear similar to nodular fasciitis but lack osteoclast-like giant cells (Figs 9.29, 9.30).

CALCIFYING FIBROUS PSEUDOTUMOR

These tumors were originally described as 'childhood fibrous tumor with psammoma bodies.'[60] Calcifying fibrous tumor/pseudotumor is a rare benign fibrous lesion. Most soft tissue examples affect children and young adults without gender predilection[61] whereas visceral examples usually occur in adults.[62–65] These tumors were originally described in the subcutaneous and deep soft tissues (extremities, trunk, neck, and scrotum)[60,61] but have subsequently been reported all over the body, notably in the mesentery and peritoneum[64–68] and pleura (sometimes multiple).[62,63,69] Soft tissue examples present as painless masses. Visceral examples may produce site-specific symptoms.[62–64] Radiographs show well margined,

noncalcified tumors. Calcifications are apparent on computed tomography (CT) and may be thick and band-like or punctate.[69] On magnetic resonance imaging (MRI), masses appear similar to fibromatoses, with a mottled appearance and a signal closer to that of muscle than fat[61] (Fig. 9.31). Although examples have followed trauma[62,70] and occurred in association with Castleman's disease[71] and inflammatory myofibroblastic tumors,[72,73] the pathogenesis remains unknown.

Grossly these lesions are well marginated but unencapsulated, ranging in size from <1–15 cm. Some show indistinct boundaries with infiltration into surrounding tissues. On occasion, a gritty texture is noted on sectioning, which reveals a firm white lesion. Microscopically, calcifying fibrous tumor consists of well circumscribed, unencapsulated, paucicellular, hyalinized fibrosclerotic tissue with a variable inflammatory infiltrate consisting of lymphocytes and plasma cells (Fig. 9.32). Lymphoid aggregates may be present. Calcifications, both psammomatous and dystrophic, are scattered throughout (Fig. 9.33). Lesional cells express vimentin and factor XIIIa but usually lack actins, desmin, factor VIII, S100 protein, neurofilament protein, cytokeratins (CK), CD34, and CD31. The immunophenotype differs from that of inflammatory myofibro-

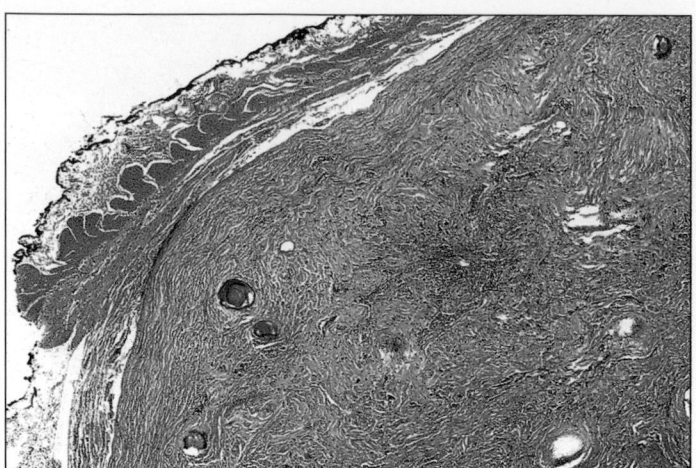

Fig. 9.32 Calcifying fibrous tumor. The lesion is well circumscribed and is paucicellular at scanning power but calcifications are apparent.

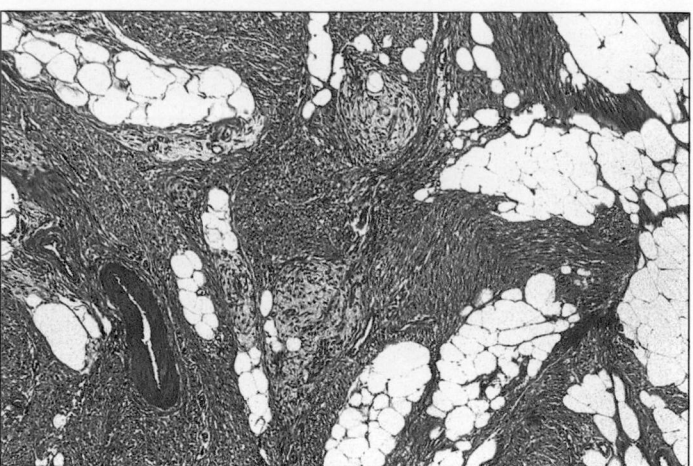

Fig. 9.34 Fibrous hamartoma of infancy. At scanning power, the three components are evident: fat, spindled fibroblastic/myofibroblastic cells, and organoid nodules of smaller cells.

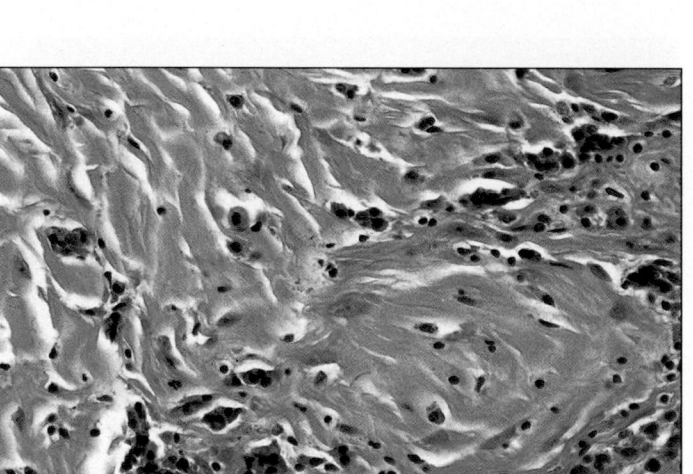

Fig. 9.33 Calcifying fibrous tumor. At high magnification, plasma cells and bland fibroblasts are evident.

blastic tumors in that most calcifying fibrous pseudotumors lack actin and anaplastic lymphoma kinase (ALK).[67,74] Occasional lesions have expressed CD34.[68,74] On electron microscopy, fibroblasts are accompanied by collagen fibrils.[62,75] Flow cytometry has revealed diploidy in one case.[76] These tumors are benign; occasional recurrences are recorded.[61,74]

FIBROUS HAMARTOMA OF INFANCY

Fibrous hamartoma of infancy is an uncommon benign fibroblastic and myofibroblastic proliferation that typically occurs in the axillary or shoulder region of males in their first 2 years of life[77,78], usually presenting as a solitary, small, rapidly growing, soft-to-firm mass. About 20% of cases are congenital. The lesion only rarely occurs on the hands and feet.

Grossly, this process is poorly circumscribed with firm gray-white tissue admixed with fat. Histologically the lesion consists of

several cell types: fibroblasts, myofibroblasts, primitive mesenchymal cells, and haphazardly distributed fat. Three tissue components are seen in varying proportions: (1) fibrous trabeculae or septae composed of spindle cells separated by collagen; (2) myxoid foci containing primitive round or stellate mesenchymal cells; and (3) interspersed mature fat (Fig. 9.34). The lesion has an organoid pattern.

Generally most pathologists recognize this entity as a benign process, however examples with predominant myofibroblastic differentiation and sparse numbers of the primitive cells may be confused with infantile fibromatosis. The latter is a locally aggressive tumor whereas fibrous hamartoma of infancy is cured by local excision and is not locally destructive. Occasionally, fibrous hamartoma of infancy can occur in the genital region,[78] where it may mimic embryonal rhabdomyosarcoma clinically, although the pathologic features are quite distinct if the pathologist is aware of this presentation. The characteristic 'organoid' pattern helps in distinguishing fibrous hamartoma of infancy from rhabdomyosarcoma and other sarcomas such as infantile fibrosarcoma. There may be a histologic resemblance to calcifying aponeurotic fibroma, especially in earlier lesions when the tumor may grow in a trabecular pattern and lack calcifications. These lesions, however, usually occur on the palms of older children.

NUCHAL FIBROMA AND NUCHAL FIBROCARTILAGINOUS TUMOR

Benign soft tissue tumors with a predilection for the head and neck region include spindle cell lipomas, pleomorphic lipomas, and nuchal fibromas. Nuchal fibroma is a rare fibrous proliferation of subcutis that mainly involves the interscapular and paraspinal regions of adult patients.[79,80] The majority are men in their fifth decade of life and more likely to have diabetes. Most examples are found in the nuchal region, followed by the back and shoulders, although other sites are infrequently involved. Occasionally, these tumors are associated with familial adenomatous polyposis (FAP)/Gardner syndrome, and they are occasionally a harbinger of this condition.[81] If incompletely excised, the lesion may recur.

The excised specimen is poorly marginated, has a hard consistency and off-white color and is typically about 3 cm. The tumor

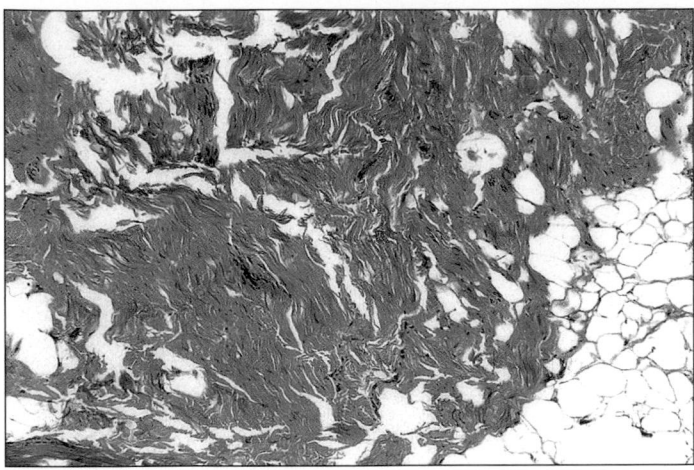

Fig. 9.35 Nuchal fibroma. This mass shows paucicellular dense collagen.

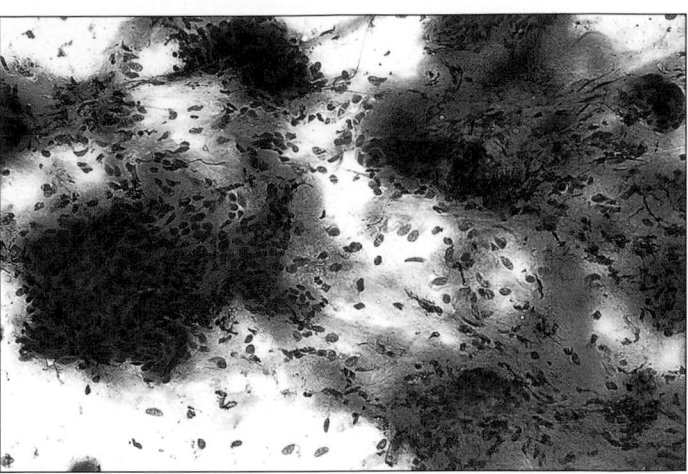

Fig. 9.36 Fibromatosis colli, fine-needle aspiration. Most cells are cohesive. Dense collagen appears magenta on Diff-Quik preparations (Courtesy of Dr William Frable).

lacks a capsule and shows paucicellular dense collagen with interspersed mature fat and entrapment of nerve fibers (Fig. 9.35). Variable amounts of calcification and, rarely, ossification may be present. If immunohistochemistry is performed, these lesions express vimentin and, peculiarly, may display CD99/O13 as well as CD34 positivity[82] but lack epithelial membrane antigen (EMA), actins, and S100 protein staining.

Nuchal fibrocartilaginous pseudotumor is a distinctive soft-tissue lesion that occurs in the posterior aspect of the base of the neck, at the junction of the nuchal ligament and the deep cervical fascia.[83] It was first believed to be a variant of nuchal fibroma, although several differences were noted. Nuchal fibroma is not confined to the midline, lacks an association with ligaments, and occurs superficial to the fascia. Nuchal fibrocartilaginous pseudotumor is associated with prior neck injury and histologically shows fibrocartilaginous metaplasia.

FIBROMATOSIS COLLI

Fibromatosis colli is a fibrous growth involving the distal portion of the sternocleidomastoid muscle. The lesion typically presents between the second to fourth week of life, is more common in males, and, for obscure reasons, affects the right side more than the left. In about half of cases, a history of a complicated delivery is elicited. It is characterized by a rapid growth phase leading to a stationary phase and eventually to regression such that, in a matter of 1–2 years, the mass is no longer palpable.

If the lesion is indeed excised it shows partial replacement of the sternocleidomastoid muscle by a bland-appearing fibrous proliferation without inflammatory cells. However, this is a situation where aspiration cytology can be helpful in reassuring the patient's family of benignity while awaiting regression of the lesion[84] (Figs 9.36, 9.37).

LIPOFIBROMATOSIS

Described by Fetsch, lipofibromatosis is a pediatric lesion with a characteristic appearance with features of lipomatosis and fibromatosis.[85] The initial report was of 45 cases involving 32 boys

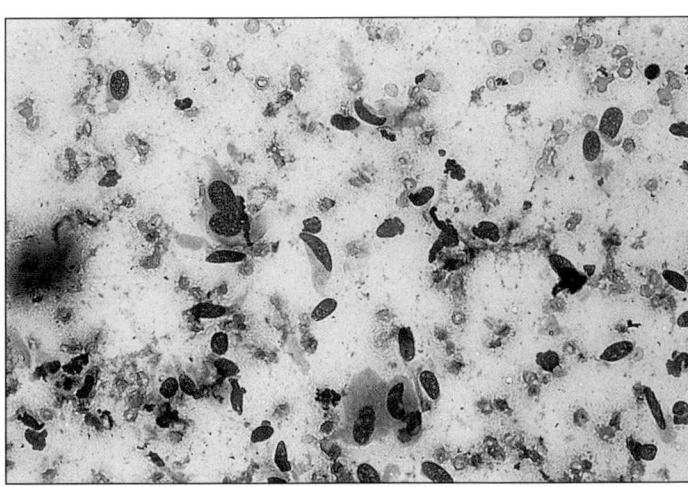

Fig. 9.37 Fibromatosis colli, fine-needle aspiration. The individual fibroblasts are uniform and have smooth nuclear membranes. They are not particularly enlarged.

and 12 girls ranging in age from 11 days to 12 years (median age, 1 year). Tumors involved the hand (18 cases, 40%), arm (8 cases), leg (7 cases), foot (6 cases), chest (3 cases), abdomen (2 cases), and head (1 case). There were eight congenital lesions. The masses were typically described as painless and slow-growing.

On excision, lesions ranged from 1–7 cm (median, 2 cm) and had a yellowish or tan–white color, often with fatty or fibrofatty tissue. Microscopically, lipofibromatosis is poorly marginated and consists of abundant fat with an accompanying fibroblastic proliferation coursing along fat septa and forming an integral component (Fig. 9.38). The tumor is variably collagenized and the proliferating fibroblasts are uniform. In areas where the fibroblasts merge with fat, univacuolated cells reminiscent of lipoblasts are identified (Fig. 9.39). The tumors lack the 'primitive cell' component of fibrous hamartoma of infancy. Mitotic activity is typically minimal. The lesion infiltrates regional structures, including vessels, nerves, skin adnexa, and skeletal muscle.

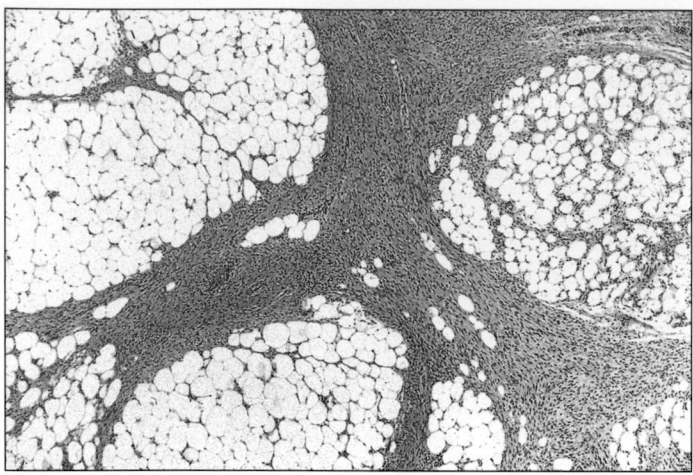

Fig. 9.38 Lipofibromatosis. Fat and sweeping fascicles of fibroblasts are intimately associated.

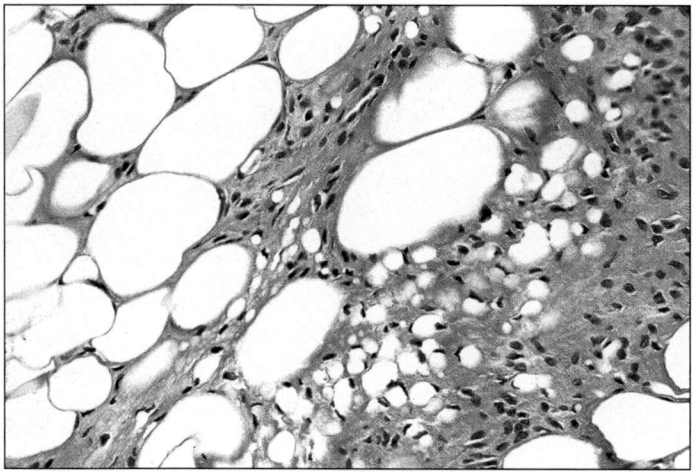

Fig. 9.39 Lipofibromatosis. Where fat and fibroblasts collide, an appearance simulating lipoblasts is produced.

With immunohistochemical staining, the spindle cell component expresses CD99, CD34, and SMA in most cases and variably expresses Bcl-2, S100 protein, MSA, and EMA. Keratin and desmin are absent.

On follow-up, the majority (72%) of reported cases recurred but there were no metastases. Recurrent tumors were more likely to be congenital, occur in boys, involve the hands and feet, be incompletely excised, and display mitotic activity.

FIBROMATOSES

The fibromatoses are classified as superficial and deep.[1,2] The superficial fibromatoses encompass small lesions of the hands (palmar fibromatoses/Dupuytren's contractures, knuckle pads, infantile digital fibromatoses), feet (plantar fibromatoses/Ledderhose's disease), and penis (penile fibromatoses/Peyronie's disease).[86] Palmar fibromatosis is the most common of these, occurring in 1–2% of the population with a male predominance, frequently

presenting bilaterally. Plantar fibromatoses occur in a younger age group and are also prone to bilaterality. As the name implies, infantile digital fibromatoses arise in the digits of infants and young children and are characterized by peculiar inclusion-like condensations of cytoplasmic actin.[87,88] Penile fibromatoses are uncommon, and tend to present in association with other superficial fibromatoses. The deep fibromatoses are also called 'aggressive fibromatoses' and desmoid tumors.

Probably the best estimates for the incidence of desmoid tumors overall come from studies of the Finnish population, where the incidence is 2.4–4.3 new cases per 1 million inhabitants per year.[89] In children, most desmoid tumors are extra-abdominal with a female predominance whereas those occurring in young adults are nearly always in the abdominal wall (of women). As patients approach their fifties, the sex ratio approaches 1:1 and most tumors continue to affect the abdominal wall. As patients age still further, the sex ratio remains 1:1 but the sites of disease vary. It is worthwhile to be aware of these trends when encountering a paucicellular fibroblastic lesion. It is more important for the treating surgeon to be aware of these trends, since the 'juvenile' type is particularly prone to recurrence (70% in one series, versus 45% for extra-abdominal and 10% for abdominal).[90] These tumors are usually large and local control can prove difficult but, despite their capacity for local aggression, deep fibromatoses do not metastasize. However, they are managed clinically in the same fashion as low-grade sarcomas.

Since fibromatoses may be a component of the Gardner syndrome (FAP)[91–93] it is not surprising that virtually all Gardner-syndrome-associated lesions harbor mutations of the adenomatous polyposis coli (*APC*) gene.[94–99] This observation has led to the study of *APC* mutations in sporadic desmoid tumors. Since one function of the *APC* gene involves regulation of the cellular level of β-catenin, the interaction between these two molecules has been explored in tandem. Although sporadic desmoid tumors may have *APC* mutations,[100–102] they are more likely to have *β-catenin* mutations.[103,104] The majority of desmoid tumors, both familial and sporadic, have mutations of one of these two genes.

Standard karyotyping analysis of a large series of superficial and deep fibromatoses has revealed clonal chromosomal aberrations in about half of the deep fibromatoses and 10% of superficial lesions.[105] Loss of 5q, which houses the *APC* gene, was detected in two of the deep fibromatoses in the latter series but not in superficial lesions. *β-catenin* and *APC* gene alterations are uniformly absent in superficial lesions and thus they are genetically distinct from deep fibromatoses.[106]

Several other cytogenetic abnormalities have been reported in desmoids, including trisomy 8, trisomy 20, and abnormalities of the Y chromosome. A specific history of trauma at the precise point of growth is often elicited. Hormonal effects and pregnancy are believed to influence the growth of this tumor. Some tumors express hormone receptors (estrogen and progesterone) and therefore tamoxifen and other hormonal modulators are among the adjuvant therapies for this tumor.[107,108]

As above, fibromatoses are divided into superficial and deep types based on their distinctive features.

1. Superficial fibromatoses (fascial)
   a. Palmar fibromatosis
   b. Plantar fibromatosis
   c. Penile fibromatosis
   d. Knuckle pads
   e. Infantile digital

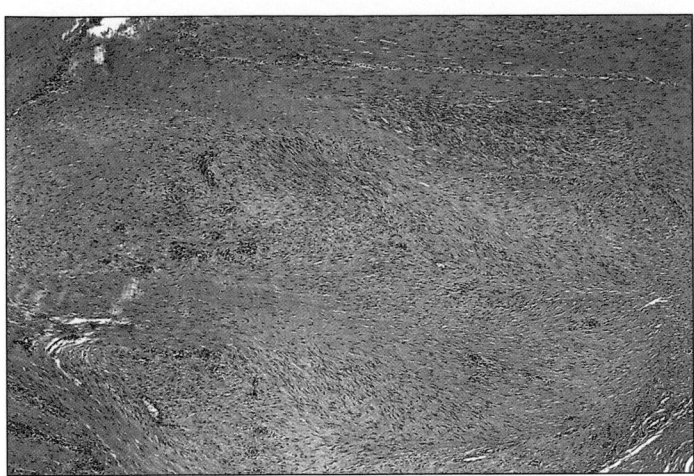

Fig. 9.40 Palmar fibromatosis. A dense uniform proliferation of fibroblasts is intimately associated with a tendon aponeurosis.

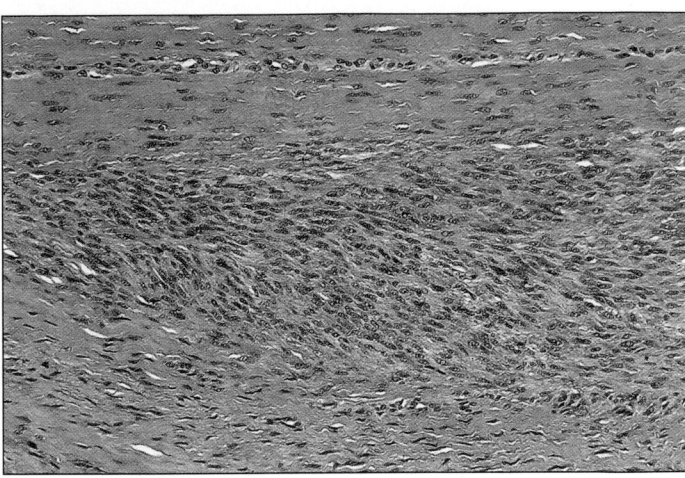

Fig. 9.41 Palmar fibromatosis, higher magnification.

2. Deep fibromatoses (musculoaponeurotic)
   a. Extraabdominal fibromatosis/desmoid
   b. Abdominal fibromatosis/desmoid
   c. Intraabdominal fibromatosis/desmoid

Superficial fibromatoses

Palmar fibromatosis (Dupuytren's contracture)

Palmar fibromatosis is probably the commonest of all fibromatoses. Its incidence is 1–2% and lesions present as slowly growing, small, subcutaneous nodules or plaques involving the dermis or underlying fascia. These nodules may lead to contractures. They may be bilateral, familial, and multiple. There is association between Dupuytren's contractures and alcoholism, epilepsy, diabetes, and chronic lung disease. There is also coexistence of palmar fibromatosis with other superficial types (plantar and penile) but not with deep fibromatoses. There is a tendency to local recurrence after surgical excision.

Grossly the lesion usually consists of a single nodule or a multi-nodular mass closely associated with thickened palmar aponeurosis. Microscopically, the palpable nodule or plaque consists of multiple tiny fibrovascular proliferations with narrow blood vessels surrounded by a thin cuff of collagen situated near the center of these nodules (Fig. 9.40). Lesions of short duration are more cellular with plump, immature-appearing fibroblasts that are uniform in appearance and contain variable numbers of mitotic figures (Fig. 9.41). Lesions of longer duration are less cellular and contain increased dense collagen. Variable amount of myxoid matrix is usually present and, rarely, long-standing lesions may develop cartilaginous or osseous metaplasia.

Plantar fibromatosis

Plantar fibromatosis, like palmar fibromatosis, is a nodular fibrous proliferation of plantar aponeurosis but is less likely to develop contractures and has a higher recurrence rate.[109] There is an increased incidence in patients with palmar or penile fibromatosis. Although the lesions may be entirely asymptomatic, they may cause mild pain, or paraesthesia if there is superficial plantar nerve entrapment.

Grossly and histologically the lesion is similar to palmar fibromatosis (Fig. 9.42), although the presence of striking cellularity and numerous mitoses can raise the possibility of malignancy, an

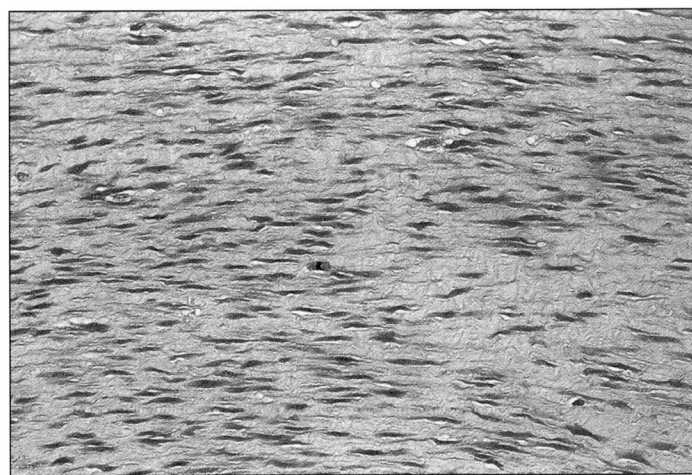

Fig. 9.42 Plantar fibromatosis. Mitoses and striking cellularity may be a feature.

interpretation avoided by attention to the clinical history. Giant cells may also be a feature of plantar fibromatosis[110]

Penile fibromatosis (Peyronie's disease/plastic induration of the penis)

Peyronie's disease is a localized fibromatosis that affects the tunica albuginea of the penis. It begins as an inflammatory disorder, subsequently leading to fibrous plaques on the dorsum of the penis causing it to curve towards the affected side. Often there is difficulty in passing urine and pain on erection and intercourse. It is much less common than palmar and plantar fibromatosis but is seen more frequently in patients with palmar or plantar fibromatosis. Multiple clonal chromosomal abnormalities have been described in Peyronie's disease.[111]

Histologically there is relatively little fibrosis with predominance of inflammatory cells in earlier lesions, as opposed to older lesions, which are more fibrotic with only scant inflammatory cells. There is patchy deposition of elastic fibers, thickened fibrous plaques, destruction of smooth muscle, and/or ossification (Fig. 9.43).

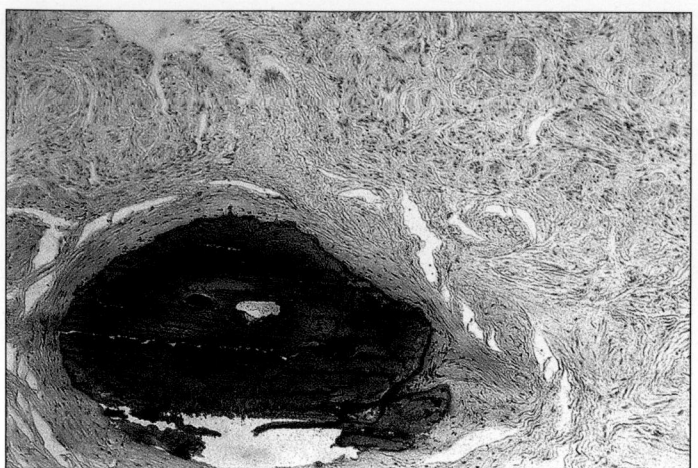

Fig. 9.43 Penile fibromatosis. This example displays focal ossification.

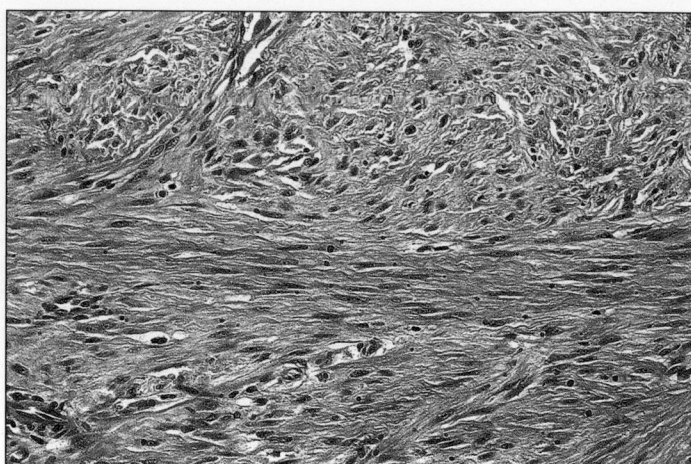

Fig. 9.44 Infantile digital fibromatosis. These lesions appear much like the other superficial fibromatoses but differ by the presence of many tiny eosinophilic cytoplasmic inclusions.

Knuckle pads

Knuckle pads are infrequent, flat or dome-shaped fibrous thickenings of the dorsal aspect of proximal interphalangeal or metacarpophalangeal joints. They are seen more frequently in patients with palmar or plantar fibromatosis. Microscopically they resemble palmar fibromatosis but there are no contractures. Knuckle pads should be distinguished from Heberden's nodes of osteoarthritis and hyperkeratosis secondary to chronic irritation or trauma.

Infantile digital fibromatosis

Infantile digital fibromatosis is a distinct tumor of the dermis and subcutis of the fingers and toes of infants. Approximately 30% of cases are congenital. The salient feature of this tumor is the presence of cytoplasmic inclusion bodies. The lesion may be single or multiple and has a tendency to recur. The ultimate prognosis is excellent and most tumors will eventually regress spontaneously after the initial growth period. These tumors are capable of causing contracture deformities.

Grossly the tumor is poorly circumscribed and is attached to the overlying skin. Microscopically, there are fascicles of bland-appearing fibroblasts that appear similar to those of other superficial fibromatoses (Fig. 9.44). The characteristic globular, eosinophilic cytoplasmic inclusion bodies can be seen on routine hematoxylin and eosin staining but appear bright red with the Masson trichrome stain (Fig. 9.45). They stain with actin antibodies immunohistochemically.[88] The inclusions are variable in number and are seen less frequently in cases with more fibrosis.

Deep fibromatoses (desmoid tumors, 'aggressive fibromatoses')

Extra-abdominal fibromatosis (desmoid)

Extra-abdominal desmoid is a relatively common lesion that has deceptively bland histomorphology but a tendency to recur locally and infiltrate the surrounding tissue, hence the name 'aggressive fibromatosis'. It arises primarily in the connective tissue of muscle and the overlying fascia or aponeurosis (musculoaponeurotic fibromatosis). Although many organs can be involved, such as breast, vulva, and spermatic cord, the most common location is the shoulder girdle, followed by chest wall and back, thigh, and head and neck[86,89,106–108,112–122] (Fig. 9.46). Although chest wall is a common

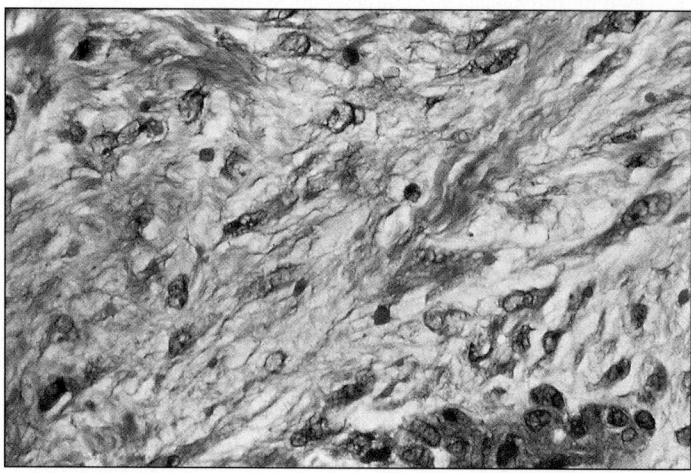

Fig. 9.45 Infantile digital fibromatosis. Trichrome staining highlights the inclusions, which are also actin-reactive.

location anyway, the tumor has rarely been associated with breast implants.[123] Fibromatosis of the head and neck is seen more commonly in children, in which case the lesions tend to be more cellular and may grow more aggressively, even encroaching on the trachea with destruction of adjacent bone and a fatal outcome. Although these tumors do not metastasize, multicentricity has been described.[124,125]

Clinically the lesions present as deep-seated, firm, nonencapsulated, slowly growing, locally invasive, painless masses. They are seen most commonly in young women, although children and even infants may be affected.

Grossly the tumor is firm with coarse white trabeculation resembling a scar and cuts with a gritty sensation (Fig. 9.47). Microscopically, the lesion is poorly defined with infiltrative margins consisting of spindled fibroblasts separated by abundant collagen (Fig. 9.48). Cells and collagen are organized in parallel arrays. Keloid-like collagen and hyalinization may be so extensive as to obscure the original pattern of the tumor. Scattered thin-walled, elongated, and compressed vessels are usually seen with focal areas

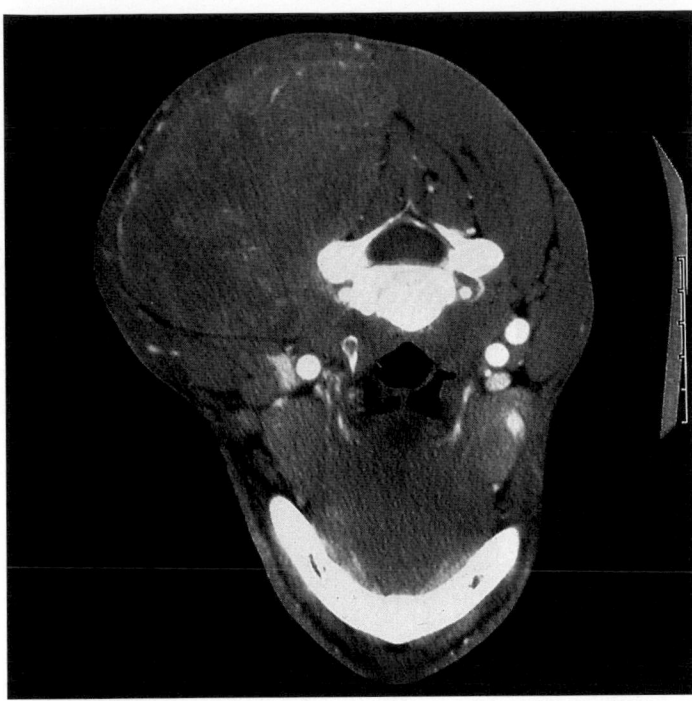

Fig. 9.46 Fibromatosis/extra-abdominal desmoid tumor. Most occur in the shoulder region, but the head and neck is also a favored site. CT.

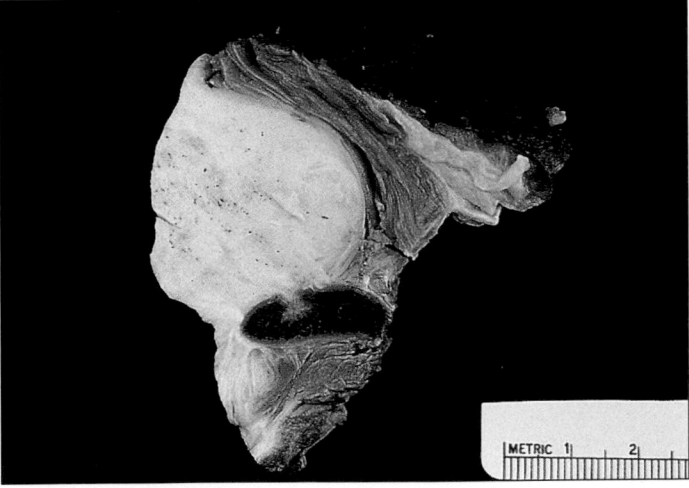

Fig. 9.47 Fibromatosis/extra-abdominal desmoid tumor. This example arose in the shoulder region of a young woman and invaded the scapula. Note the white fibrous appearance of the cut surface.

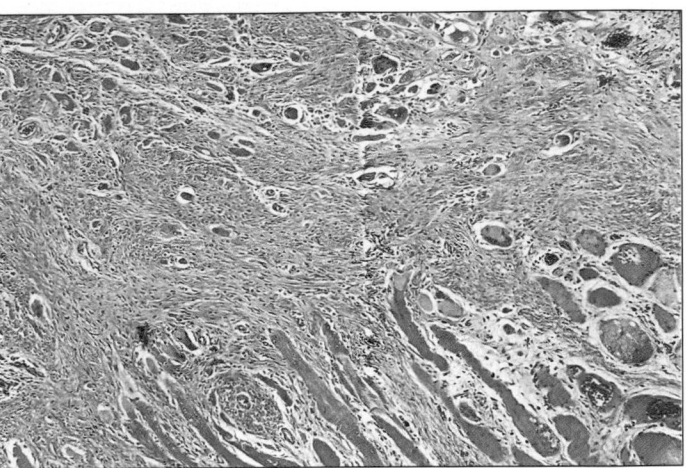

Fig. 9.48 Fibromatosis. At scanning power, there is a sweeping fascicular architecture and infiltration into skeletal muscle. Individual myocytes assume a degenerative appearance.

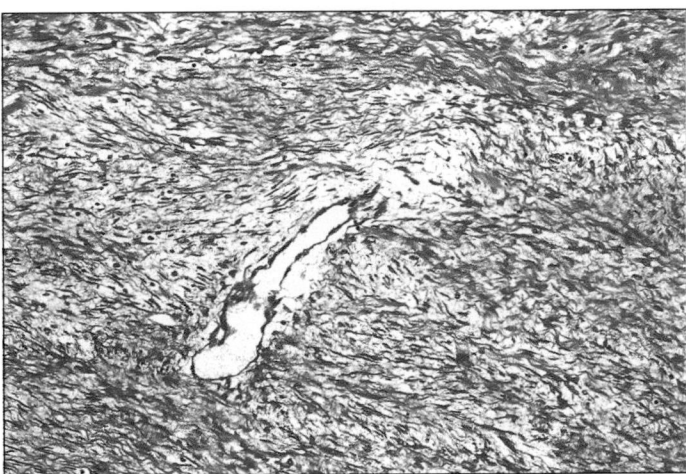

Fig. 9.49 Fibromatosis. The small vessel in the center of the field appears to be stretched open by the proliferating myo/fibroblasts.

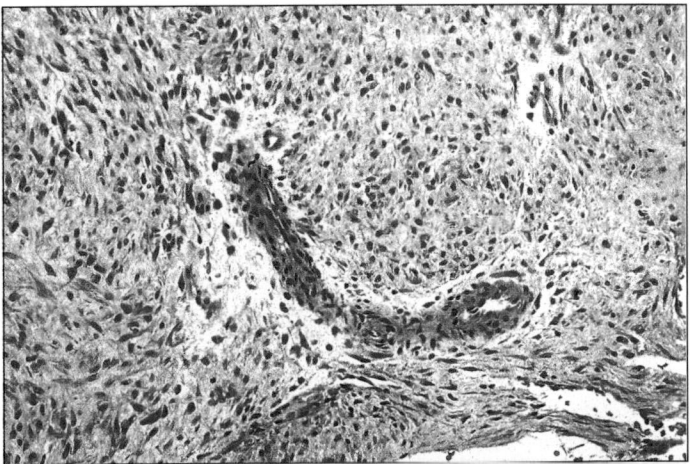

Fig. 9.50 Fibromatosis. Note the prominent appearance of the small vessel.

of hemorrhage, lymphoid aggregates, and, rarely, calcification or chondro-osseous metaplasia. Typically the vessels, though thin-walled, appear conspicuous at scanning magnification. The nuclei of the proliferating lesion are typically tinctorially lighter than those of the endothelial cells and the smooth muscle cytoplasm in vessel walls is pinker than the surrounding myofibroblastic cytoplasm of the tumor cells (Figs 9.49–9.51). Mitotic figures are infrequent. These tumors are so well collagenized that diagnosing them by FNA can be frustrating owing to difficulty in sampling. However, loosely

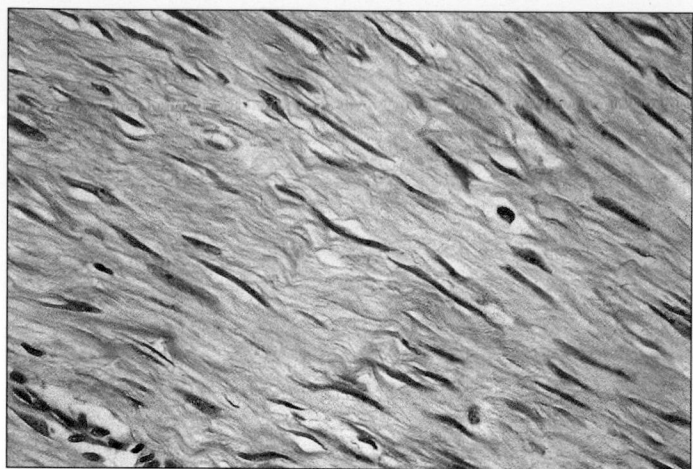

Fig. 9.51 Fibromatosis. Despite its aggressive local behavior, fibromatosis is composed of bland-appearing cells with dainty, inconspicuous nucleoli.

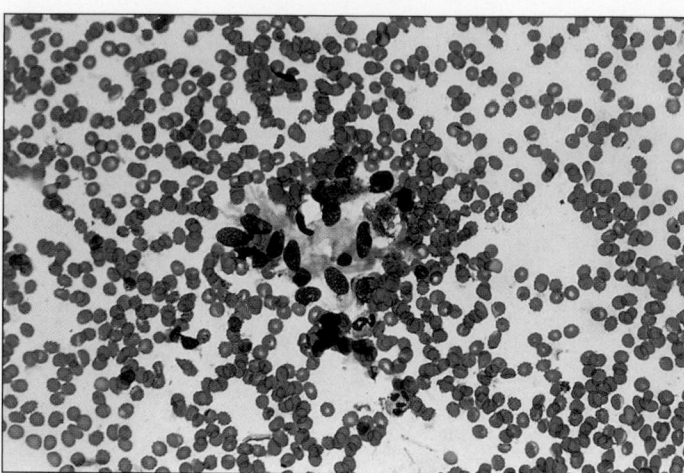

Fig. 9.53 Fibromatosis, aspiration cytology. The spindle cells are uniform and not particularly enlarged.

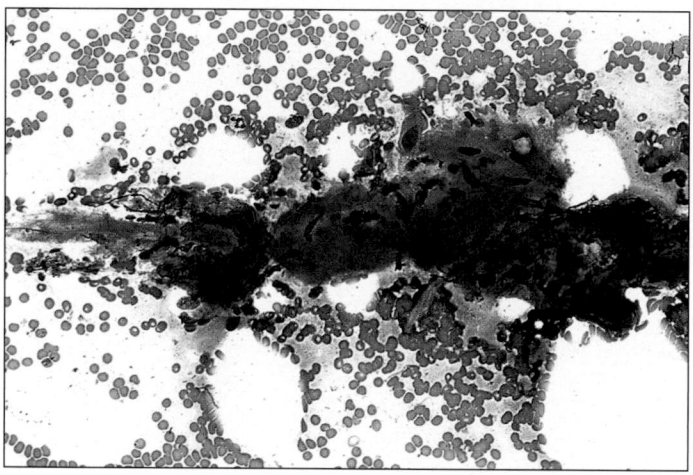

Fig. 9.52 Fibromatosis, aspiration cytology. These tumors frequently yield insufficient material for interpretation but, like other benign soft tissue tumors, may give up cohesive 'chunks' of tissue.

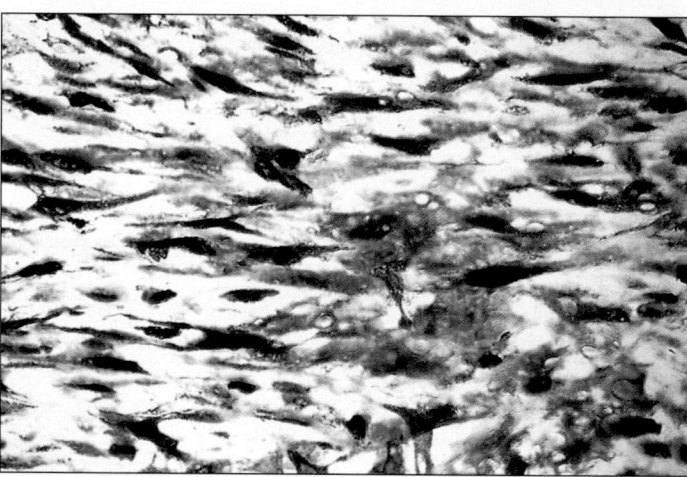

Fig. 9.54 Fibromatosis. Beta catenin over-expression is detected in most cases of deep fibromatoses (but not in superficial fibromatoses). Nuclear staining is required but cytoplasmic staining is often also present and is regarded as non-specific.

cohesive and single bland spindle cells are found if there is sufficient FNA material[126] (Figs 9.52, 9.53).

The differential diagnosis includes fibrosarcoma and benign fibroblastic proliferative lesions. Classic *fibrosarcomas* are, in general, more cellular with a herringbone pattern, have increased mitotic figures, i.e. at least one mitosis per high power field (hpf), and atypical mitoses. Both lesions have infiltrative margins, although well differentiated fibrosarcoma may appear less invasive into adjacent structures and occasionally has a tendency to form a pseudocapsule. The tumor cells and collagen of well differentiated fibrosarcoma are arranged in bundles and bands in a manner resembling fibromatoses. Mitoses are rare and the classic herringbone pattern may not be a prominent feature in the better differentiated tumors. The distinction between these two entities, which revolves around identification of subtle nuclear atypia in fibrosarcomas, may be extremely difficult, if not impossible, particularly in small biopsy specimens. A *scar* may also resemble a fibromatosis, especially in a small biopsy where the

relationship with adjacent tissue cannot be assessed. We have occasionally found the presence of nuclear β-catenin (which is seen in the majority of fibromatoses) helpful in distinction between fibromatoses and exuberant scars (Fig. 9.54).[127]

Fibromatoses are myofibroblastic lesions and, as such, frequently express smooth muscle markers by immunohistochemistry.[112] Fibromatosis may also focally exhibit a whorled/storiform pattern mimicking *nodular fasciitis* but this is never such a prominent or uniform feature as typically seen in nodular fasciitis. *Myxomas* may come into the differential as fibromatosis may have areas of myxoid degeneration. However, fibromatoses are usually more cellular and have more collagen than myxomas. *Desmoplastic fibromas* of bone are histologically indistinguishable from fibromatoses.

Abdominal fibromatosis (desmoid)

This tumor has identical morphology to the extra-abdominal desmoids but is far less prone to recurrences than desmoid tumors in other sites. It usually occurs in the abdominal wall of women of childbearing age during or after pregnancy. It typically manifests as a slow-growing progressive mass, which becomes more prominent on abdominal muscle contraction. The gross and microscopic features are identical to those of extra-abdominal fibromatosis.

Intra-abdominal fibromatosis (desmoid)

This includes several entities that have similar morphologic findings but distinct clinical presentations.[120,121] *Pelvic fibromatosis* typically involves the lower portion of the pelvis where it presents as a slowly growing mass in young females but has no relationship to gestation. *Mesenteric fibromatosis* is probably the commonest among the intra-abdominal fibromatosis group. It usually presents as a slowly growing mass that involves small bowel mesentery or retro-peritoneum where distinction may become extremely difficult from retroperitoneal fibrosis. There are cases associated with pregnancy and Crohn's disease,[128] even though the majority are considered to be secondary to trauma in individuals with the appropriate predisposition. Mesenteric fibromatosis in patients with Gardner syndrome appears to have a substantially higher recurrence rate than in patients without this syndrome.[120,121,129] Gardner syndrome is an autosomal dominant familial disease with a female predilection and consists of numerous colorectal adenomatous polyps, osteomas, cutaneous cysts, soft tissue masses, and other manifestations.[91–93] Gardner's syndrome is related to FAP, a disorder caused by germline *APC* gene mutations. It is associated with an 8–12% incidence of developing fibromatosis.

Among patients with FAP, intestinal and extraintestinal neoplasms typically arise through bi-allelic (germline then somatic) inactivation of the *APC* gene, whereas the corresponding tumors in non-FAP patients occur either through somatic bi-allelic APC inactivation or somatic mutation of a single β-catenin allele. As the various FAP-associated tumors have been studied, somatic alterations of the APC/β-catenin pathway have been initially detected in familial examples and then subsequently demonstrated in the sporadic counterparts. The first tumors studied were gastrointestinal adenomas,[130] followed by desmoid tumors,[101,103,104] medulloblastomas, childhood hepatoblastomas, gastric fundic gland polyps, and nasopharyngeal angiofibromas, all of which occur more frequently in FAP patients than in controls. It has been estimated that FAP patients in general have an 852-fold increased risk of developing desmoids, typically intra-abdominal lesions.[131] In fact, there is a unique French-Canadian kindred harboring a germline mutation of codon 2643–2644 of the *APC* gene.[132] These patients have a penetrance of desmoid tumors approaching 100% and have cutaneous cysts, but few manifest colon polyposis. Noteworthy is that, among the fibromatoses found in these specialized carriers, virtually all were axial and none were superficial. These observations of familial lesions suggest that the pathobiology of deep and superficial fibromatoses differs and that they are truly two divergent and probably biologically unrelated processes. The absence of both β-catenin and *APC* gene mutations in superficial fibromatoses in contrast to common mutations of these genes in deep fibromatoses is one of many examples wherein the existing WHO classification (based on light microscopic and clinical features) reflects a biologic distinction that has subsequently been confirmed on genetic grounds.[106]

A further point of interest and caveat concerning mesenteric fibromatosis is that these tumors frequently need to be distinguished from gastrointestinal stromal tumors (GISTs). Although their features are readily distinguishable on routine H&E-stained slides,

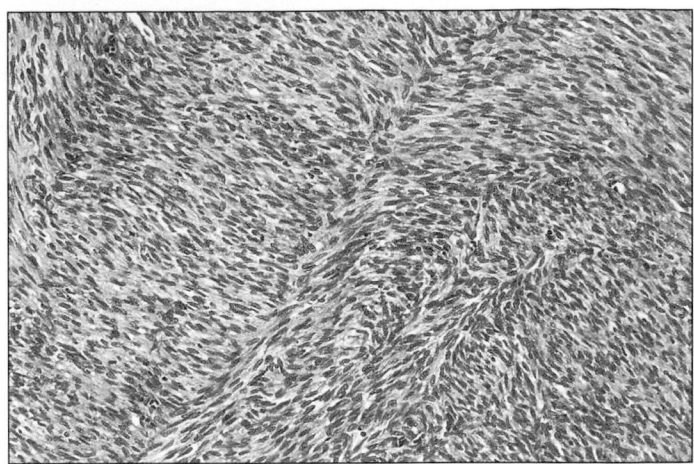

Fig. 9.55 Classic fibrosarcoma. This lesion has a 'herringbone' pattern.

since there is recent interest in performing C-kit/CD117 staining on mesenteric lesions to direct therapy, pathologists should be aware that fibromatoses may react with some commercially available CD117 antibodies.[133] Staining is typically weaker than that seen with true GISTs but in doubtful cases β-catenin staining can be helpful, since nuclear staining is only seen in desmoids[127] (Fig. 9.54).

FIBROSARCOMA

Classic adult

Once regarded as the most common type of sarcoma,[10] adult fibrosarcoma is now rarely diagnosed. It is essentially a diagnosis of exclusion, since many lesions classified as fibrosarcomas in the past are readily recognized as malignant peripheral nerve sheath tumors, synovial sarcomas, or pseudosarcomas using current criteria and modern ancillary studies. However, adult fibrosarcoma is defined, as it was at the time of its initial description, as a malignant tumor composed of fibroblasts.[134] It must be distinguished from congenital–infantile fibrosarcoma and from other specific types of fibroblastic sarcomas. It probably accounts for 1–5% of adult sarcomas.[135] Classical fibrosarcoma is most common in middle-aged and older adults with no gender predilection. Fibrosarcoma usually involves deep soft tissues of the extremities, trunk, head, and neck. Hypoglycemia has been reported and has been related to elaboration of insulin-like growth factor by the tumor cells, a phenomenon also observed in association with solitary fibrous tumors of the pleura.[136,137] Fibrosarcoma can arise in dermatofibrosarcoma protuberans (see Chapter 8).

On gross examination, tumors are circumscribed, white or tan, and firm. Hemorrhage and necrosis can be seen in high-grade tumors. This neoplasm is composed of spindle-shaped cells, characteristically arranged in sweeping fascicles that are angled in a chevron-like or herringbone pattern (Fig. 9.55). Storiform areas can be seen. The cells have tapered, darkly staining nuclei with variably prominent nucleoli and scant cytoplasm (Figs 9.56, 9.57). Mitotic activity is almost always present but variable. Higher-grade tumors have more densely staining nuclei and can display focal round cell change and multinucleated cells, but sarcomas with significant pleomorphism are currently classified as MFH. The stroma has

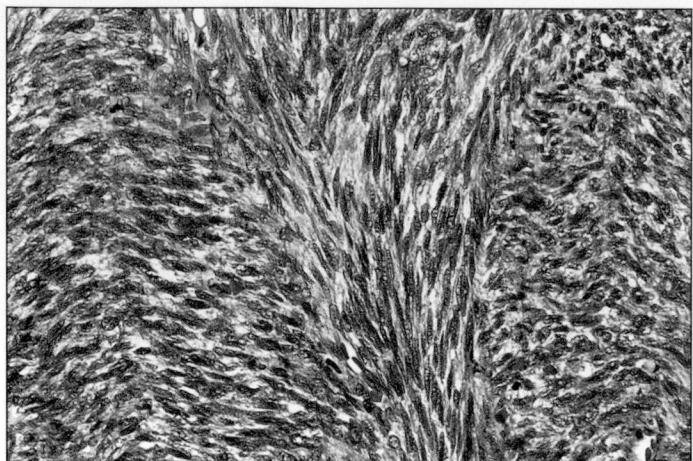

Fig. 9.56 Classic fibrosarcoma.

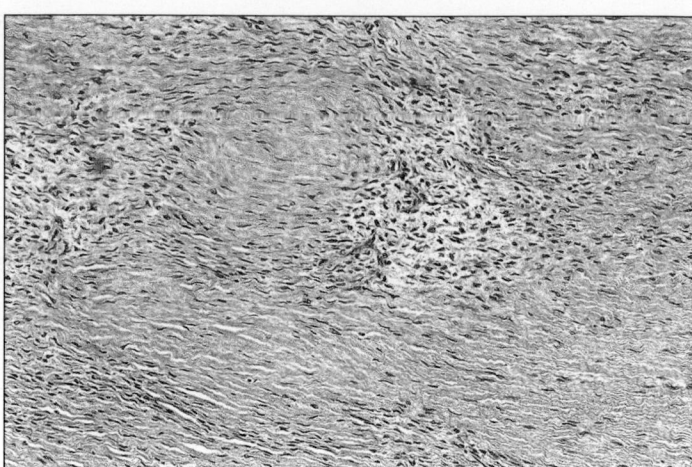

Fig. 9.58 Low-grade fibromyxoid sarcoma. This tumor appears similar to a fibromatosis but differs by having a vaguely swirled architecture and less architectural uniformity than the fibromatoses depicted in Figures 9.48–9.50.

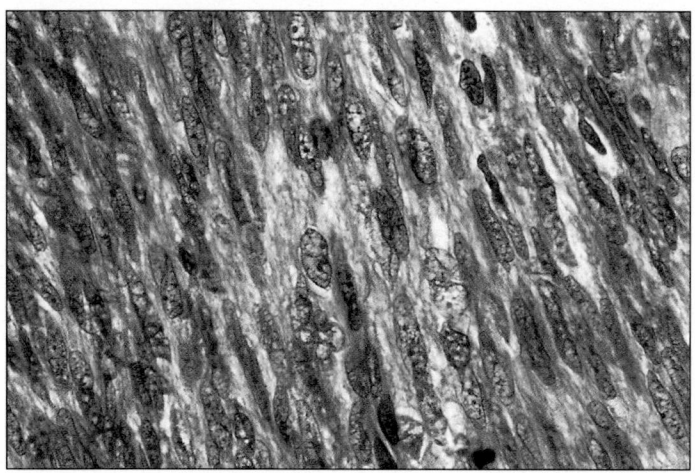

Fig. 9.57 Classic fibrosarcoma, cytologic features.

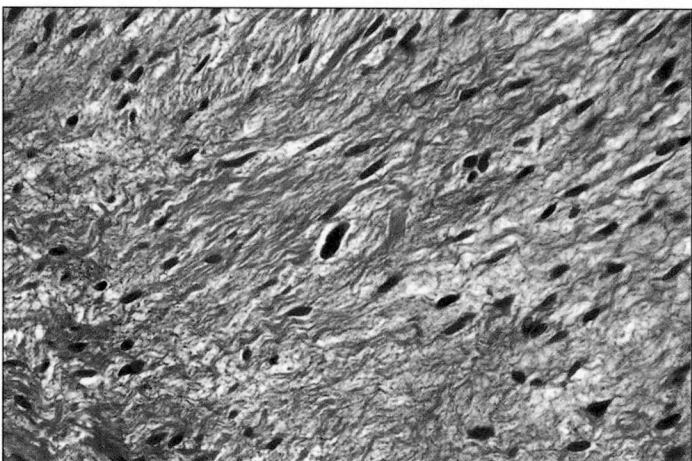

Fig. 9.59 Low-grade fibromyxoid sarcoma. Nuclear hyperchromasia is seen. Compare this field to the one depicted in Figure 9.51. These fields were photographed at the same magnification from slides prepared in the same laboratory.

variable collagen from a delicate intercellular network to pauci-cellular areas with diffuse or 'keloid-like' sclerosis or hyalinization. Myxoid change and osteochondrous metaplasia can occur. Fibrosarcomas are positive for vimentin and very focally for SMA representing myofibroblastic differentiation. Some cases arising in dermatofibrosarcoma are CD34-positive. On ultrastructural study, fibrosarcoma is composed of fibroblasts with prominent rough endoplasmic reticulum and absence of myofilaments, external lamina or intercellular junctions. An occasional cell has peripheral filament bundles suggestive of myofibroblastic differentiation but tumors in which this is a prominent feature should be classified as myofibrosarcomas.

There are no recent series of fibrosarcomas classified using modern techniques. In the older literature, behavior relates to grade and to general factors of tumor size and depth from the skin. The probability of local recurrence relates to completeness of excision.[138–140] Fibrosarcomas metastasize to lungs and bone, especially the axial skeleton, and rarely to lymph nodes in about 10–65% of patients. Five-year survival is on the order of 50%.

Low-grade fibromyxoid sarcoma (Evans) and hyalinizing spindle cell tumor with giant rosettes

Low-grade fibromyxoid sarcoma is a tumor composed of bland, fibroblast-like cells with a swirling, whorled, vaguely storiform pattern in a fibrous and focally myxoid stroma, occasionally with plexiform vasculature. These were first reported by Evans, who noted their deceptive resemblance to fibromatoses[141] (Figs 9.58, 9.59). Evans later expanded his observations and included examples that had undergone dedifferentiation to higher-grade sarcomas.[142] These tumors have little mitotic activity and minimal nuclear pleomorphism. This lesion recurs, but many cases also metastasize (e.g. to lung, Fig. 9.60). This tumor is not quite equivalent to low-grade examples of myxofibrosarcoma, as originally defined, since the latter occur in older patients, are more pleomorphic and less fibrous, and seldom metastasize when superficial. Ultrastructural

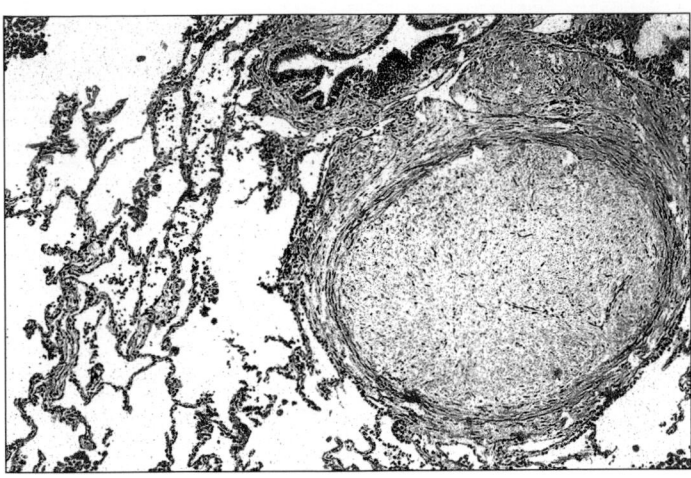

Fig. 9.60 Low-grade fibromyxoid sarcoma. Note the deceptively bland appearance of this lung metastasis.

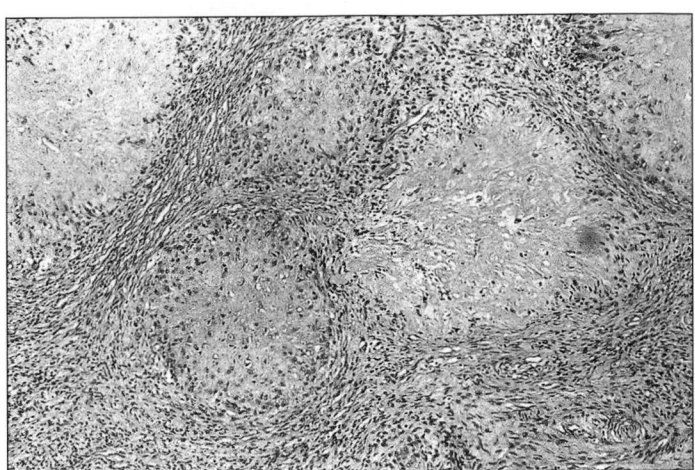

Fig. 9.61 Hyalinizing spindle cell tumor with giant rosettes. The rosettes are found in tumors that are otherwise indistinguishable from low-grade fibromyxoid sarcoma. These two tumors variants both behave as low-grade sarcomas.

reports have shown fibroblastic differentiation and this tumor is regarded as a low-grade variant of fibrosarcoma. The differential diagnosis of low-grade fibromyxoid sarcoma includes fibromatosis, which differs by having blander nuclei, no swirling architectural pattern, and a characteristic vascular pattern, and perineurioma, which displays EMA reactivity and has classic ultrastructural features.

Hyalinizing spindle cell tumor with giant rosettes is an entity closely resembling low-grade fibromyxoid sarcoma. Some 19 examples were reported by Lane et al. in 1997[143], as occurring principally as a painless, slowly growing, deeply situated mass of the proximal extremities in young to middle-aged adults (age range 14–65 years, mean 38). 13 of the cases (68%) were in males. 14 tumors were in skeletal muscle and three in subcutis. Although grossly circumscribed, the tumors had infiltrative borders microscopically and were composed of bland spindled cells situated in a hyalinized to myxoid stroma, often with 'cracking' artifact in the collagen. Characteristics were scattered large, rosette-like structures that often merged with serpiginous areas of dense hyalinization (Fig. 9.61). The rosettes consist of a central collagen core surrounded by a rim of rounded cells morphologically and immunophenotypically different from the cells of the spindled stroma. These cells express a number of antigens, including S-100 protein, neuron-specific enolase (NSE), and Leu 22, in contrast to the stroma, which usually lacks these antigens.

Of the 12 patients with available follow-up information in the original series, one patient treated with simple excision clinically developed local recurrence of the tumor 20 months later. No other recurrences were reported during the limited follow-up period, and no patient developed metastatic disease. However, the authors thought that the favorable prognosis might relate to the limited follow-up period (approximately 3 years), as well as to initial treatment by wide excision in nearly half of the patients. They regarded this entity as a distinctive type of low-grade fibroblastic tumor that with time may prove to behave similarly to low-grade fibromyxoid sarcoma and therefore represent a variant of it. Subsequently such a case was reported to metastasize by Woodruff et al.[144] and a further study showed that the Evans tumor and the hyalinizing spindle cell tumor with giant rosettes were indeed ends of a diagnostic spectrum.[145] The final component of the story has been the observation that there

is the identical characteristic translocation in both types of tumors[146] with its own fusion gene product;[147,148] t(7;16)(q33;p11) fuses the *FUS* gene to *BBF2H7*.

There are no prospective reports of diagnosis of low-grade fibromyxoid sarcoma or hyalinizing spindle cell tumor by aspiration cytology, although, given that these tumors can be subtle to diagnose on open biopsies, accurate diagnosis by aspiration cytology would seem unrealistic.

The differential diagnosis of both ends of this spectrum is primarily with fibromatosis, which, as above, differs by featuring sweeping fascicles of bland spindle cells rather than a swirled architecture punctuated by rosettes. Nuclei are pale-staining and not prominent at scanning magnification. Additionally, fibromatoses display nuclear β cantenin on immunohistochemistry whereas low grade fibromyxoid sarcomas do not. Schwannomas are not likely to have rosettes and the cells are typically not rounded as the ones in the current lesion. If S100 staining is performed, all cells are reactive rather than a subgroup. Fibroma of tendon sheath is a paucicellular lobulated lesion that lacks rosettes. In its cellular phase, it resembles nodular fasciitis and features bland hyperchromatic cells arranged in a loose storiform pattern.

Acral myxoinflammatory fibroblastic sarcoma (inflammatory myxohyaline tumor)

'Acral myxoinflammatory fibroblastic sarcoma' and 'inflammatory myxohyaline tumor' are terms used to describe the same entity.

A series of 51 cases of a unique soft tissue tumor with a proclivity for the hands and feet were initially described as inflammatory myxohyaline tumor by Montgomery et al.[149] These occurred over a wide age range (4–81 years; median 40 years) and affected the sexes equally. Most involved the hands (25, 50%) and feet (7, 14%), presenting as painless masses. The wrist/lower arm and the ankles/lower leg were also affected. Tumors were infiltrative and multinodular (Fig. 9.62), characterized histologically by dense inflammation merging with stroma varying from myxoid to hyalinized and containing sheets of epithelioid spindled cells (Figs 9.63, 9.64). Some lesions contained foamy histiocytes, giant cells, and

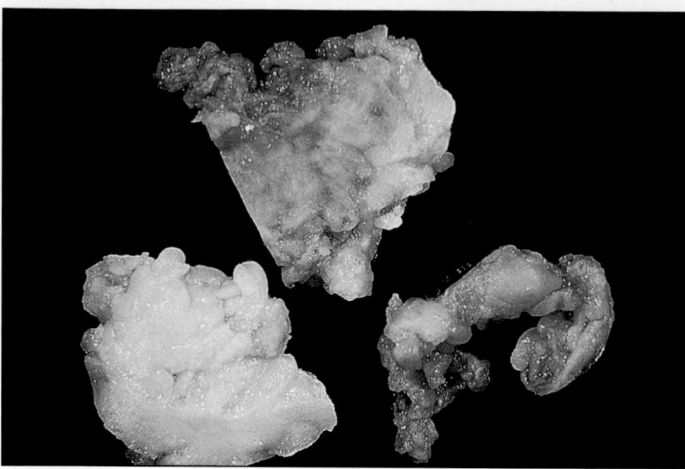

Fig. 9.62 Inflammatory myxohyaline tumor/acral low-grade fibroblastic sarcoma. It is clear from this gross photograph that these lesions are infiltrative, this one of subcutaneous fat.

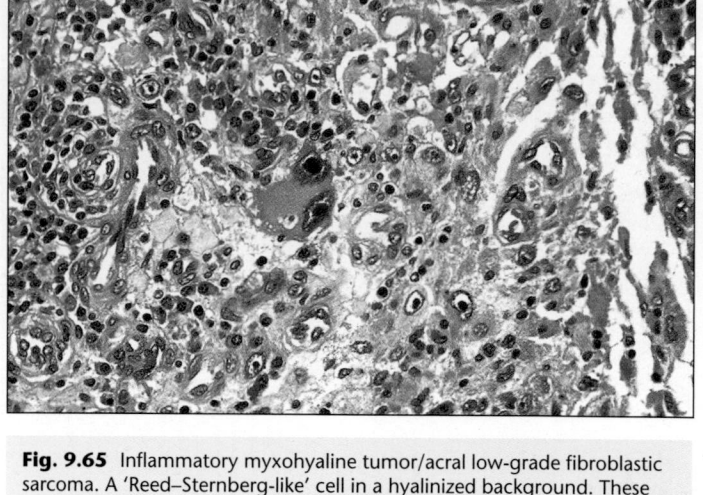

Fig. 9.65 Inflammatory myxohyaline tumor/acral low-grade fibroblastic sarcoma. A 'Reed–Sternberg-like' cell in a hyalinized background. These cells are fibroblastic ultrastructurally and do not react with CD15/CD30.

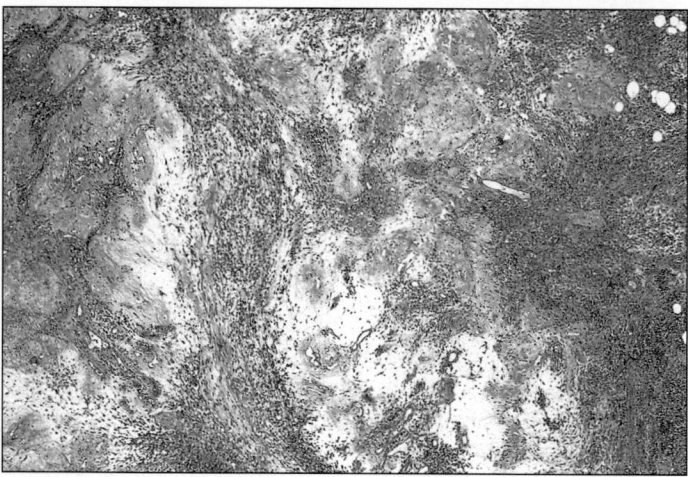

Fig. 9.63 Inflammatory myxohyaline tumor/acral low-grade fibroblastic sarcoma. At scanning power, myxoid zones are seen in an inflammatory backdrop.

hemosiderin. Amid the inflammatory backdrop, scattered bizarre cells having large vesicular nuclei and macronucleoli reminiscent of Reed–Sternberg cells (Fig. 9.65) or virocytes were present. Neither cytomegalovirus nor Epstein–Barr virus was detected. Despite the cytologic atypia, mitotic activity was minimal (mean, 1 mitotic figure per 50 high-power fields). Recurrences were noted in six of 27 patients (22%) at follow-up. Many of the patients were treated aggressively for their tumors since these cases were initially diagnosed as low-grade sarcomas.

Subsequently, a series of 44 identical tumors was reported as 'acral myxoinflammatory fibroblastic sarcoma',[150] the term currently preferred by the WHO, with confirmation of the proclivity for local recurrences and histologic documentation of metastasis in one case. Presumably the finding of metastasis in the second series was a reflection of initial diagnoses of reactive processes; the recurrence rate in this series was substantially higher as well. Ultrastructural studies in this second series demonstrated fibroblastic characteristics.

On immunohistochemical staining, inflammatory myxohyaline tumor expresses vimentin and may have focal CD68 positivity. There may be occasional keratin or CD34 positive cells[149] or CD34.[150] The tumors lack S100 protein, desmin, actin, NSE, EMA and leukocyte markers (CD15, CD30, CD45). Cytogenetics have been studied for one lesion, which displayed a complex karyotype.[151] On FNA, cytologic features are similar to 'malignant fibrous histiocytoma' in that pleomorphic fibroblastic cells are found in an inflammatory background. Rendering a specific diagnosis would be difficult, although features of one such case are depicted in Figure 9.66.

Myxofibrosarcoma (myxoid malignant fibrous histiocytoma)

Myxoid MFH as described by Weiss and Enzinger,[152] comprised 20% of all MFH and was defined as having over 50% of myxoid change, with characteristic nodularity, vascular pattern, atypical spindle cells, and a tendency to superficial location (Fig. 9.67). The myxoid nodules merged into areas of pleomorphic MFH. The likelihood of metastasis related to depth from the skin and was inversely proportional to the amount of myxoid change.

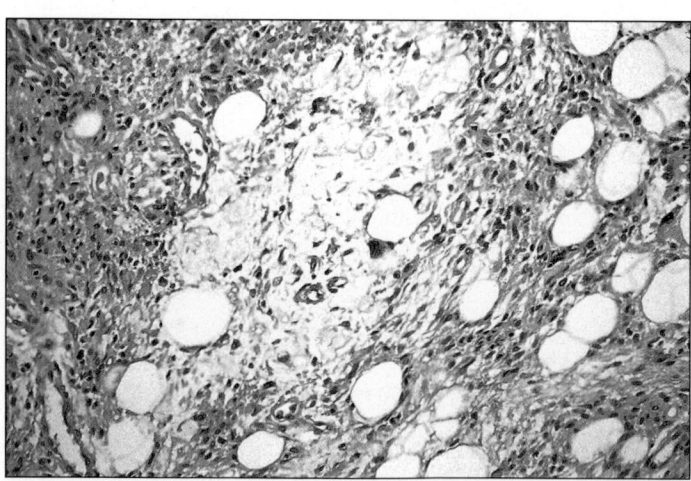

Fig. 9.64 Inflammatory myxohyaline tumor/acral low-grade fibroblastic sarcoma, myxoid zone.

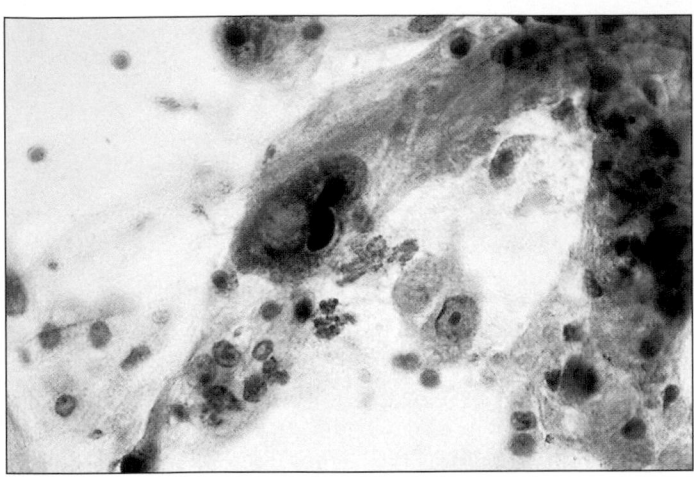

Fig. 9.66 Inflammatory myxohyaline tumor/acral low-grade fibroblastic sarcoma, aspiration cytology. The large nuclei are seen on this aspirate, although it would seem difficult to diagnose these tumors prospectively on aspiration cytology.

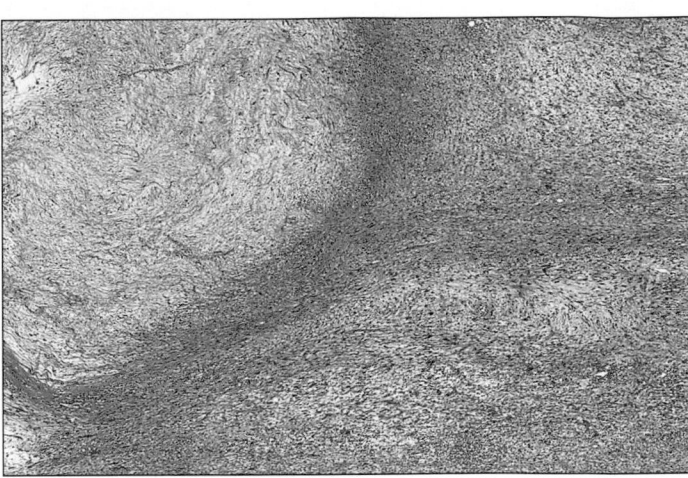

Fig. 9.68 Myxofibrosarcoma/myxoid malignant fibrous histiocytoma. This example displays a lobulated appearance at scanning magnification.

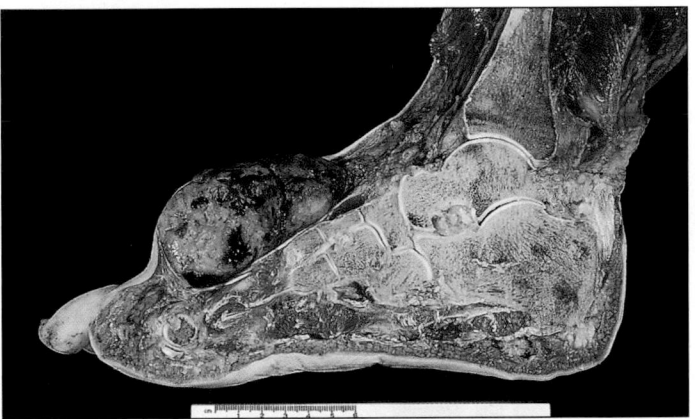

Fig. 9.67 Myxofibrosarcoma/myxoid malignant fibrous histiocytoma. Although the distal extremity is an unusual site for these tumors, the superficial location seen in this case is not. Note the gelatinous multinodular appearance of this example.

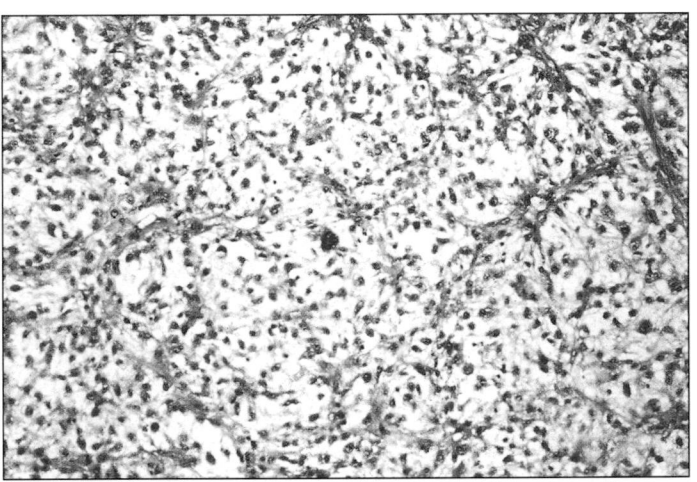

Fig. 9.69 Myxofibrosarcoma/myxoid malignant fibrous histiocytoma. Rich vascular and scattered pleomorphic cells in a myxoid background are typical of these sarcomas.

Myxofibrosarcoma was described at the same time[153] as a subcutaneous or deep multinodular tumor of older adults composed of thin tapered spindle cells in a myxoid pattern, with a prominent vascular pattern (Figs 9.68–9.70). The tumor cells are sometimes vacuolated, resembling lipoblasts, but are irregularly shaped and contain alcianophilic secretion (Fig. 9.71). Four grades were initially recognized depending on degree of cellularity and pleomorphism; higher grades were considered equivalent to myxoid MFH. Comparing grade with outcome in a large series, metastases were found in 0%, 21%, 47%, and 38% of patients with grades I–IV respectively.[154]

Another series[155] reaffirmed the morphologic findings. On follow-up in this series, in which tumors were graded using a three-tier system, 23% of patients developed metastases, all of whom had intermediate or high-grade tumors. Over half of the low-grade tumors (6/11) recurred locally. Two of the latter six tumors recurred as higher-grade lesions.

When these lesions are aspirated, there is copious myxoid background punctuated by pleomorphic cells in higher-grade tumors (Fig. 9.72). Unfortunately, it is impossible to definitively distinguish low-grade examples from benign myxoid lesions on aspiration, as doing so is based on architecture and cytologic alterations that may be subtle in low-grade tumors. As such, it may be best to avoid diagnosing 'myxoma' definitively on aspiration cytology.

Sclerosing epithelioid fibrosarcoma

Sclerosing epithelioid fibrosarcoma was first described by Meis-Kindbom et al.[156] Its primary significance is that this variant of fibrosarcoma can mimic metastatic carcinoma, particularly lobular carcinoma of the breast. 25 cases were initially reported, affecting primarily the deep musculature of adults without gender predilection. About half affected the lower limbs and limb girdles and the remainder were distributed over the trunk, upper limb girdles and neck. Most were large (median size 7 cm). These lesions display a

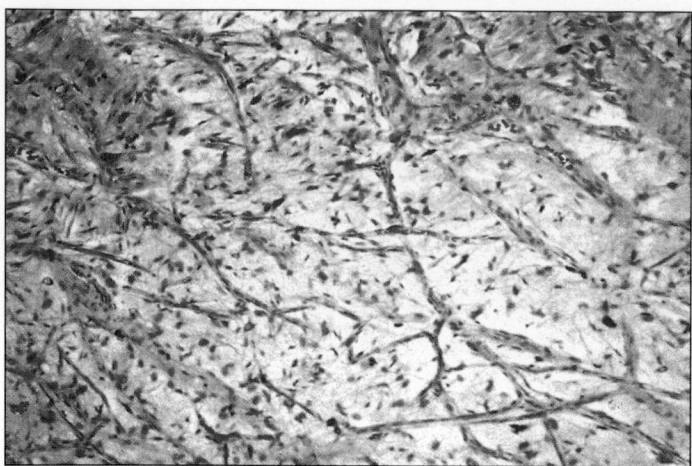

Fig. 9.70 Myxofibrosarcoma/myxoid malignant fibrous histiocytoma. This example displays a rich array of curvilinear vessels and scattered pleomorphic fibroblasts, an appearance that may be mistaken for myxoid liposarcoma. The latter has rich vascularity but lacks such large pleomorphic cells.

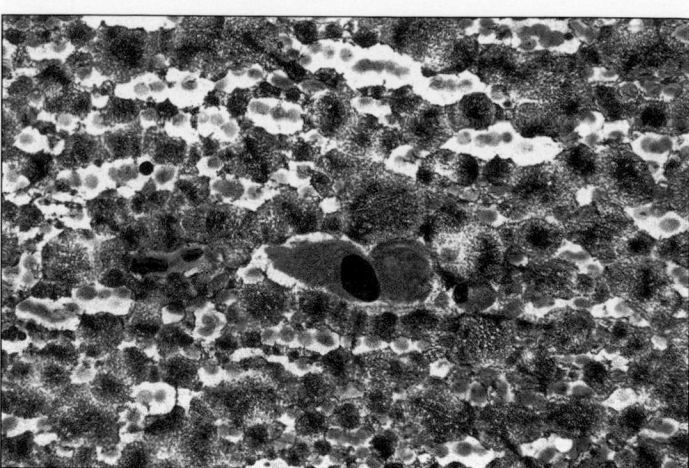

Fig. 9.72 Myxofibrosarcoma/myxoid malignant fibrous histiocytoma, aspiration cytology. A large pleomorphic cell is suspended in ample mucoid matrix. The cell in the center of the field is substantially larger than 'control' lymphocytes. Contrast this with nuclei in previously depicted benign lesions.

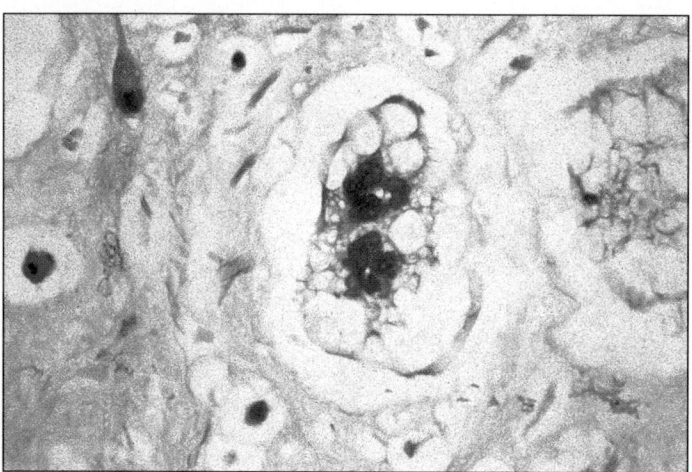

Fig. 9.71 Myxofibrosarcoma/myxoid malignant fibrous histiocytoma. Abundant mucoid material in the cytoplasm of cells with pleomorphic nuclei is reminiscent of lipoblasts. However, lipoblasts have crisply indented nuclei.

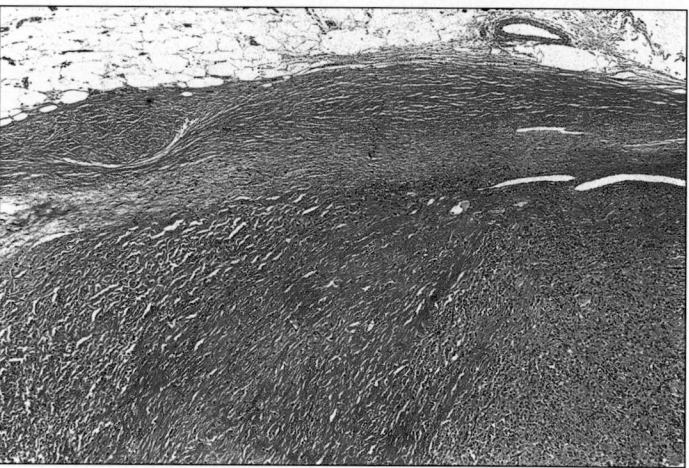

Fig. 9.73 Sclerosing epithelioid fibrosarcoma. Small epithelioid cells in a collagenized background.

white–gray cut surface characterized microscopically by a uniform population of small, slightly angulated, rounded cells with scant cytoplasm arranged in nests, cords, and sometimes in an 'Indian file' array (Figs 9.73, 9.74). There is a background of dense sclerosis, minimal inflammation and sometimes zones of cartilage and mineralization. Mitotic activity is scant. Patchy EMA, S100 protein, and patchy keratin have all been reported in these lesions, which display ultrastructural features of fibroblasts.[157] Since the histologic differential diagnosis is carcinoma, the keratin and EMA can pose diagnostic problems if attention is not paid to the patchy pattern of the reactivity. There are no reports on diagnosis of these by FNA cytology. These tumors can behave quite aggressively. In the earlier series, 53% of patients had persistent disease or local recurrence and 43% had metastases. 86% of patients in the more recent series had

metastases and over half of the reported patients had died of disease during the follow-up period.

Congenital/infantile fibrosarcoma

Infantile fibrosarcoma primarily presents during infancy. Up to 40% of cases are congenital.[158] Although the tumor closely resembles classic adult fibrosarcoma, it must be considered as a separate entity because of the marked difference in the clinical behavior.[158,159] Infantile fibrosarcoma has a much better prognosis than its adult counterpart despite its ominous histological features. Rarely, the tumor has the potential to recur and even metastasize. It is seen slightly more commonly in boys[158] and paraneoplastic behavior is possible.[160] Infantile fibrosarcomas show a significantly lower proliferative index and a higher apoptotic index when compared with adult tumors.[161] Of recent interest is the discovery in these tumors of trisomy 11, and t(12;15)(p13;q25) and the resulting gene fusion

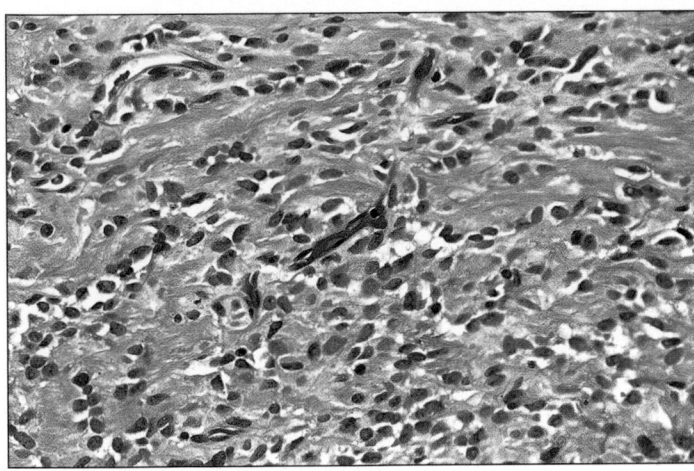

Fig. 9.74 Sclerosing epithelioid fibrosarcoma. These tumors have subtle cytologic features of malignancy and their pattern is reminiscent of metastatic lobular breast carcinoma.

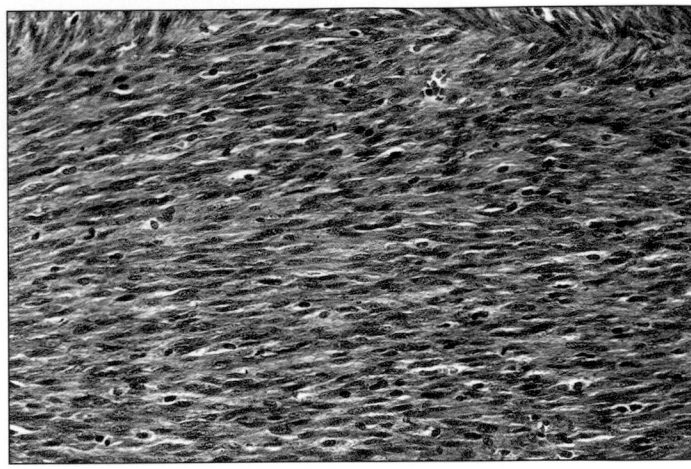

Fig. 9.76 Infantile fibrosarcoma. These tumors appear similar to classic adult fibrosarcoma. In contrast, they display a characteristic translocation, t(12;15), and behave indolently.

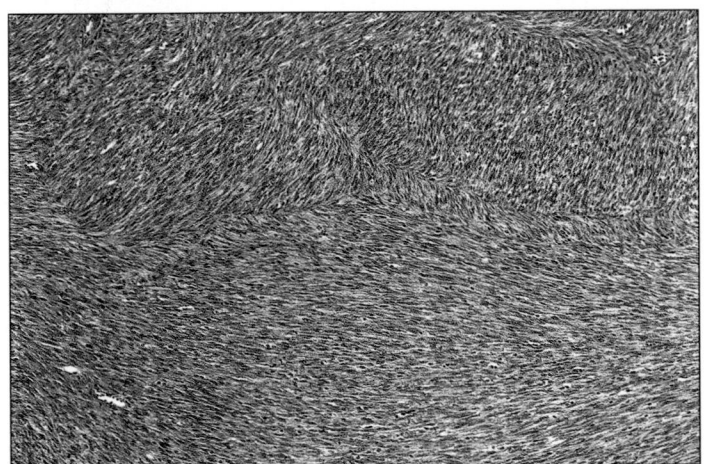

Fig. 9.75 Infantile fibrosarcoma. Note the striking cellularity.

ETV6–NTRK3 (ETS variant gene 6; neurotrophic tyrosine kinase receptor type 3). The same fusion product is detected in mesoblastic nephroma of kidney, now regarded as the same entity.[162] The gene product can be detected in paraffin-embedded material[163], although this is currently of little clinical use as these rare lesions pose little diagnostic difficulty on routine histologic sections. There is little experience in the literature with aspiration cytology of these tumors. However, tumors with characteristic translocations can often be diagnosed with a miniscule sample if molecular diagnostic capacities are available. Diagnosis of this tumor type, like that of other pediatric tumors having characteristic genetic findings, might lend itself to these techniques.

Grossly, the tumor usually consists of a large, rapidly growing, poorly circumscribed, painless mass commonly involving the distal extremities, which may even entirely replace the distal portion of the limb. Microscopically, the lesion consists of spindled to round, small, primitive fibroblasts arranged in vague fascicles or bundles that are separated by variable amounts of collagen (Figs 9.75, 9.76). Mitotic figures are common. Scattered lymphocytes are often seen. Necrosis and hemorrhage are commonly present, which often leads

to marked distortion of larger tumors. Areas of rich vascularity are also often seen. Other mesenchymal lesions can often be confused with infantile fibrosarcoma, although the solid growth pattern with spindle cells in fascicles with lack of cell differentiation are fairly characteristic. Application of a panel of immunohistochemical stains can be helpful in excluding other pediatric sarcomas.

INFLAMMATORY MYOFIBROBLASTIC TUMOR/INFLAMMATORY FIBROSARCOMA

Although these lesions were originally described as separate entities, they are now recognized as ends of a spectrum of tumors unified by a common molecular profile.[67,164–166] They are grouped together by the WHO.[1,2] Gene fusions involving anaplastic lymphoma kinase (ALK) at chromosome 2p23 have been described in these lesions.[166–169] By immunohistochemistry, ALK has been detected in about 60% of cases, a finding that can sometimes be exploited for diagnosis.[167] In a subset of cases, ALK C-terminal kinase domain is fused with tropomyosin N-terminal coiled-coil domain and other cases have shown fusion of ALK with the clathrin heavy chain.[166] The cytologic findings of these tumors are not well described.

Inflammatory fibrosarcoma

This is most common in childhood with a mean age of 8 years (range 2 months to 74 years). As described in the AFIP series,[170] this tumor arises within the abdomen, involving mesentery, omentum and retroperitoneum (over 80% of cases), with occasional cases in the mediastinum, abdominal wall and liver. Sometimes there are associated systemic symptoms. The tumor can be solitary or multinodular (30%) and up to 20 cm in diameter (Fig. 9.77). The tumors are composed of myofibroblasts and fibroblasts in fascicles or whorls, and also histiocytoid cells. Pleomorphism is moderate but mitoses are infrequently seen. There is a variable but often marked inflammatory infiltrate, predominantly plasmacytic but with some lymphocytes, and occasionally neutrophils or eosinophils as well (Fig. 9.78). Fibrosis and calcification can be seen in the stroma. Immunostaining is positive for SMA and some

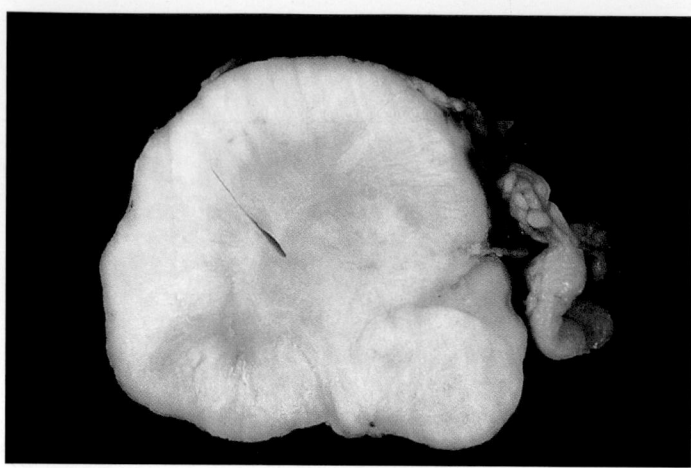

Fig. 9.77 Inflammatory fibrosarcoma/Inflammatory myofibroblastic tumor. These are classically large intra-abdominal pediatric tumors associated with systemic symptoms.

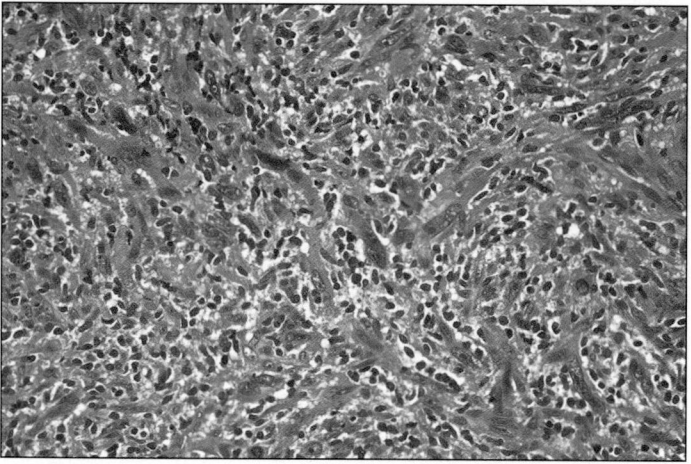

Fig. 9.78 Inflammatory fibrosarcoma/inflammatory myofibroblastic tumor. Enlarged fibroblasts and myofibroblasts in an inflammatory background.

examples express cytokeratin, especially where there is sub-mesothelial extension. The tumors invade adjacent viscera; 37% recurred and three cases (11%) metastasized. A quarter of the patients died of disease.

The differential diagnosis from inflammatory myofibroblastic tumor is subjective as these conditions are ends of a spectrum (one case was included in both the original papers describing these two conditions). Essentially, it depends on the presence of pleomorphism in cases designated as 'fibrosarcoma'. Retroperitoneal fibrosis is clinically distinctive, being more inflammatory than spindled and lacking pleomorphism. Inflammatory MFH has atypical xanthomatous cells, and inflammatory leiomyosarcoma is more myoid. Solitary fibrous tumor has CD34 positivity, and sarcomatoid mesothelioma displays epithelial marker positivity.

Inflammatory myofibroblastic tumor

Also known as inflammatory pseudotumor, this entity was first well described in the lungs and later became recognized in extrapulmonary

locations.[171] Recent cytogenetic and molecular evidence in both inflammatory myofibroblastic tumor and inflammatory fibrosarcoma supports a clonal origin, implying that this process is neoplastic. It is found in soft tissue, in omentum and retroperitoneum and involving viscera. Inflammatory myofibroblastic tumor has been reported in patients between 3 months and 46 years, but mostly in childhood (mean age 9 years) with a slight male predominance, and some cases are associated with systemic symptoms. A small number recur, especially when multinodular. They form firm, white, infiltrative masses, and histologically there are three patterns: (1) fasciitis-like, with vascular, myxoid and inflamed stroma, including plasma cells; (2) fascicular MFH- or leiomyosarcoma-like spindle cell areas with inflammation; and (3) sclerosed desmoid-like areas with calcification.

MYOFIBROSARCOMA

It has become accepted that fibrosarcomas also contain myofibro-blasts, although the problem arises of distinction from poorly differentiated smooth muscle tumors. When leiomyosarcomas become less differentiated, decreasing cytoplasmic volume and eosinophilia plus increasing nuclear atypia leads to a resemblance to fibro-sarcoma or to the spindle cells of MFH. A category composed purely or predominantly of myofibroblasts ('myofibrosarcoma') has recently received attention.

With the *electron microscope*, smooth muscle differentiation is characterized by the presence of cytoplasmic myofilament bundles with focal dense bodies. Other features include pinocytosis, cell membrane thickenings and interrupted or continuous external lamina, prominent paranuclear Golgi, and variable amounts of rough endoplasmic reticulum. These features are inconsistently developed, so that these cells may be indistinguishable from myofibroblasts. In the latter, the myofilaments form a peripheral cytoplasmic band and there is more rough endoplasmic reticulum, as well as the so-called fibronexus fibril. Both myofibroblasts and smooth muscle cells can have detectable desmin, MSA, and SMA.

Myofibroblast-like cells have been observed in several malig-nancies, although in some these probably represent reactive stromal cells. However, the concept of myofibroblastic sarcoma is somewhat controversial, because: (1) there is a close relationship between the fibroblast and myofibroblast; (2) it is difficult to recognize purely myofibroblastic differentiation without electron microscopy; and (3) even with electron microscopy, diagnostic features overlap with those of smooth muscle cells. In neoplastic cells these features are incomplete or abnormally developed and it is not always possible to define a cell type with certainty. Immunohistochemical positivity for SMA or MSA or sometimes desmin can indicate myofibroblastic differentiation. This is also found in smooth muscle and other cell types and does not always correlate with ultrastructure. Further-more, some myofibroblasts express only vimentin. It has been questioned whether sarcomas of myofibroblasts have yet been unequivocally demonstrated although recently 'myofibrosarcoma' has become accepted as an entity.[172–175]

There have been two larger series of such tumors as well as small series and isolated case reports.[172,173,175,176] Histologically, a spec-trum of myofibroblastic differentiation is described from fasciitis-like (Fig. 9.79) to sarcomatous. Most lesions include plump, focally atypical spindle cells in irregular fascicles, which can be focally myxoid, with prominent mitoses and necrosis. Occasionally, more cellular areas with polygonal cells are seen, as well as osteoclast-like giant cells. Recurrences are often more pleomorphic. Immunohisto-chemistry shows most cases express SMA, and about a third are also

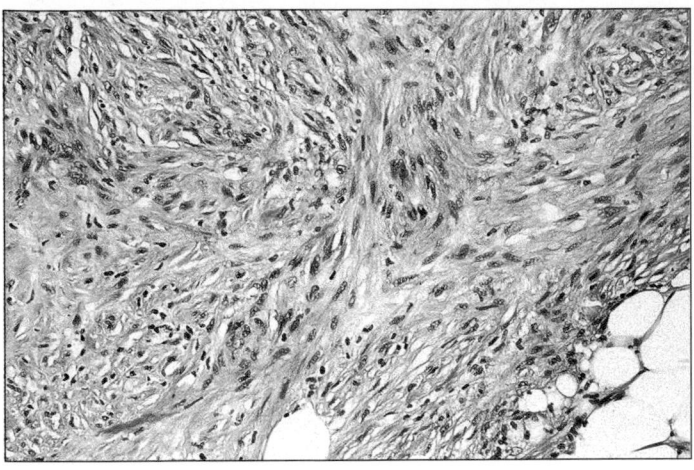

Fig. 9.79 Myofibrosarcoma. Although fasciitis-like, this neoplasm displays subtle nuclear hyperchromasia.

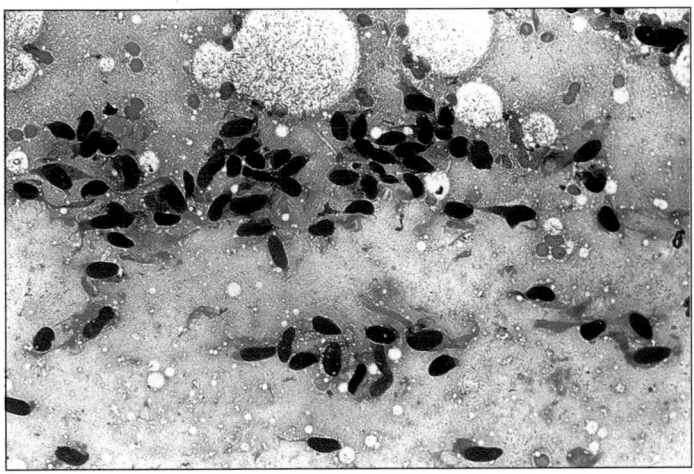

Fig. 9.80 Myofibrosarcoma, needle aspiration. It would be impossible to diagnose this lesion as such prospectively. The predominance of singly shed cells with enlarged nuclei is a clue that this aspirate is from a low-grade sarcoma.

desmin positive. Some tumors display fibronectin but not collagen IV or laminin. Electron microscopy shows myofibroblasts with variable rough endoplasmic reticulum, myofilaments, and in some cases minimal external lamina, and fibronectin fibrils and fibronexus,[172] as well as collagen secretion granules. As for many recently recognized and rare low-grade sarcoma types, there is little experience with cytology of these lesions. However, an example of one tumor is illustrated in Figure 9.80.

Clinically, low-grade myofibrosarcomas can be indolent but can relapse and metastasize even after a long period. Distinction is required from fasciitis, leiomyosarcoma, and fibrosarcoma. High-grade examples are equivalent to 'MFH'.[174]

FIBROHISTIOCYTIC TUMORS

Fibrous histiocytoma (dermatofibroma), juvenile xanthogranuloma, reticulohistiocytoma, xanthoma, angiomatoid fibrous histiocytoma, atypical fibroxanthoma (superficial malignant fibrous histiocytoma), dermatofibrosarcoma protuberans, pigmented dermatofibrosarcoma protuberans (Bednar tumor), and giant cell fibroblastoma are all discussed in Chapter 8.

MALIGNANT FIBROUS HISTIOCYTOMA

Malignant fibrous histiocytiocytoma was initially classified into storiform–pleomorphic, myxoid, giant cell, xanthomatous, and angiomatoid types. The angiomatoid type is now regarded as a 'borderline' lesion, renamed angiomatoid fibrous histiocytoma (and is covered in Chapter 8). The myxoid subtype is, for practical purposes, subsumed under myxofibrosarcoma and discussed above. This category assumes many tumors that were historically classified as fibrosarcoma, pleomorphic rhabdomyosarcoma, or undifferentiated pleomorphic sarcoma. It was the most common sarcoma diagnosis rendered in the 1980s and early 1990s but application of newer techniques has reduced the number of cases so diagnosed in more recent years, also eliminating many misdiagnosed cases of pleomorphic sarcomatoid carcinomas, melanomas, and lymphomas. It has been suggested that MFH is not an entity but a collection of poorly differentiated neoplasms better classified with comprehensive examination.[177] Certainly there may be neoplasms 'lumped' in this classification that could be better characterized, but the term MFH remains a reasonable descriptive one and this is a phenotype that can be recognized reproducibly. Masqueraders are now readily unmasked with modern immunohistochemistry.

Storiform pleomorphic

This most common variant of MFH is a tumor of older adults and usually affects the limbs and limb girdles followed by the retroperitoneum, trunk, or head and neck. Pediatric cases are uncommon but behave similarly.[178] Occasional examples have been associated with hyperlipidemia[179] and even as a component of hereditary nonpolyposis colon cancer syndrome with mismatch repair defects.[180] These neoplasms typically attain a large size with zones of hemorrhage and necrosis. Deep tumors are usually circumscribed whereas superficial ones can sometimes track along connective tissue septa and often require a wider excision than palpation would suggest.[181] There are many published studies of these tumors and behavior is similar in all of them;[174,182–184] overall survival is usually of the order of 50% and the key prognosticators are tumor grade and tumor size.

Histologically there is, at least focally, a storiform pattern (Fig. 9.81) and the tumor consists of a variable proportion of atypical pleomorphic spindle cells and polygonal cells (Fig. 9.82). There are frequently abundant pleomorphic multinucleated cells with ample eosinophilic cytoplasm. The stroma has variable amounts of collagen. Tumor cells have ultrastructural features of fibroblasts, myofibroblasts, and cells lacking differentiation.[135,174] There is no specific immunohistochemical profile for MFH. The tumor should lack specific differentiation but various intermediate filaments may be expressed. Most MFHs react with vimentin but desmin or keratin may be expressed. Tumors having desmin or keratin might be interpreted as carcinomas, pleomorphic rhabdomyosarcomas, or pleomorphic leiomyosarcomas, but such tumors can lack ultrastructural features of specific differentiation.[185,186] Expression of smooth muscle type markers (actins, desmin, calponin) may be best attributable to myofibroblastic differentiation in these tumors ('pleomorphic myofibrosarcoma').[172,174] Based on ultrastructural data, it has been suggested that these sarcomas should be regarded

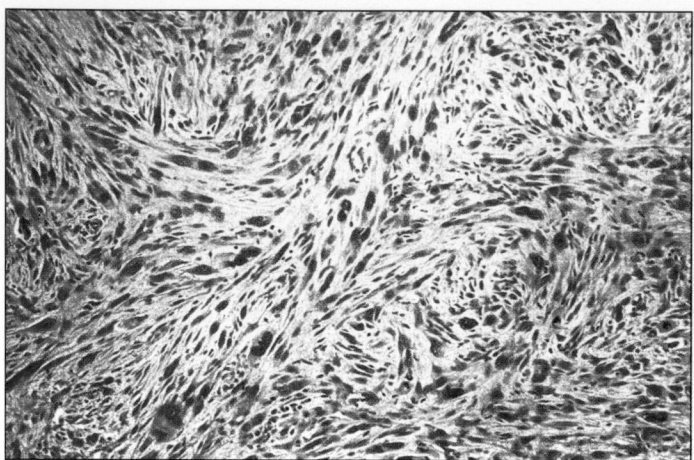

Fig. 9.81 Malignant fibrous histiocytoma showing a storiform pattern.

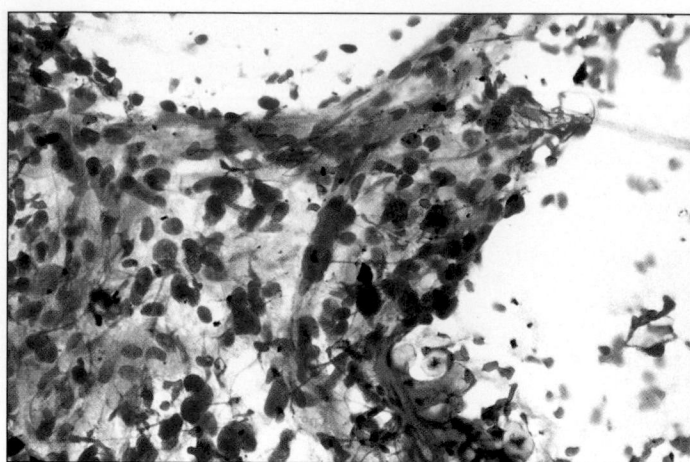

Fig. 9.83 Malignant fibrous histiocytoma. On aspiration cytology, discohesive cells are present. Note the striking nuclear enlargement.

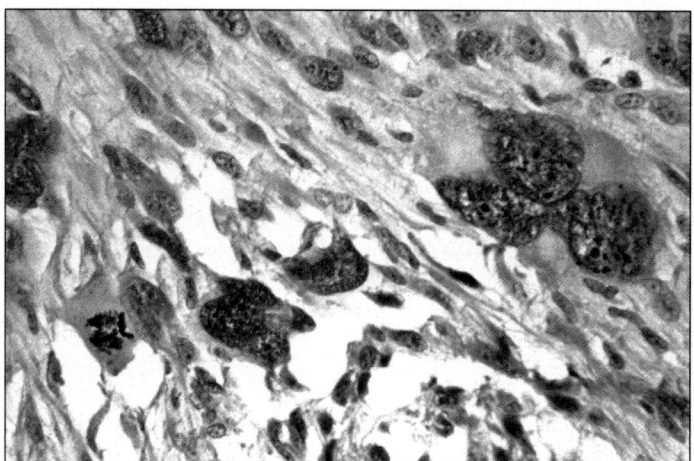

Fig. 9.82 Malignant fibrous histiocytoma with nuclear pleomorphism.

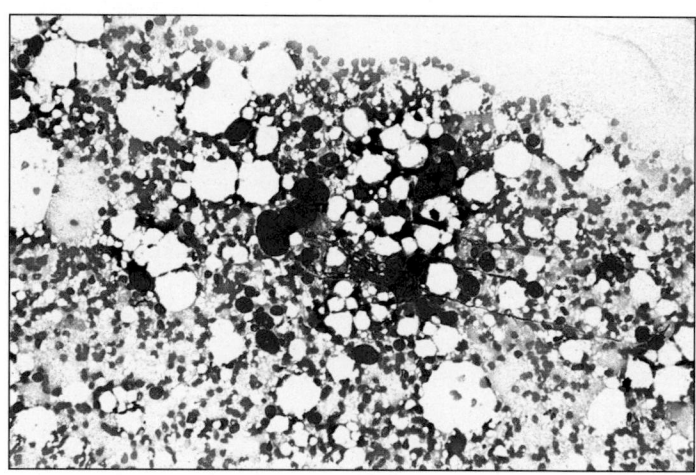

Fig. 9.84 Malignant fibrous histiocytoma, fine-needle aspiration, Diff-Kwik.

as 'pleomorphic fibrosarcomas'.[187] However, on the basis of comparative genomic hybridization data,[188] other observers have suggested that they are poorly differentiated leiomyosarcomas. Cytogenetic/molecular studies yield complex karyotypes[189] and there is no specific genetic alteration. Cytologic findings are not specific but pleomorphic multinucleation and tumor cell phagocytosis were considered helpful criteria for diagnosis[190] (Figs 9.83–9.86).

The differential diagnosis of pleomorphic spindle cell tumors includes spindled carcinomas, lymphomas, and melanomas, as well as pleomorphic sarcomas. The history and immunohistochemistry usually allow exclusion of carcinoma, lymphoma, and melanoma. Occasionally, extranodal examples of Rosai–Dorfman disease may be mistaken for MFH, but these display emperipolesis in S100-reactive histiocytic cells in a plasma-cell-rich background[191] (Figs 9.87, 9.88). Among sarcomas, pleomorphic liposarcoma, leiomyosarcoma, rhabdomyosarcoma, and dedifferentiated sarcomas, especially liposarcoma, require consideration. For these, the presence in an MFH-like pleomorphic sarcoma of even very focal differentiation is taken to be sufficient for diagnosis. For example,

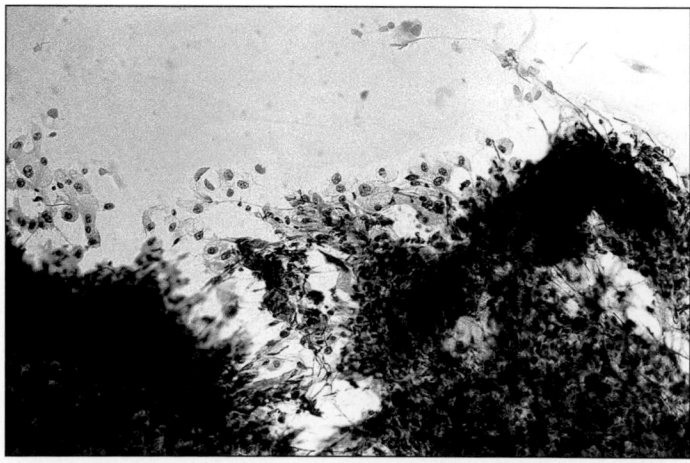

Fig. 9.85 Malignant fibrous histiocytoma, fine-needle aspiration, Papinicolaou stain. There is prominent cellularity.

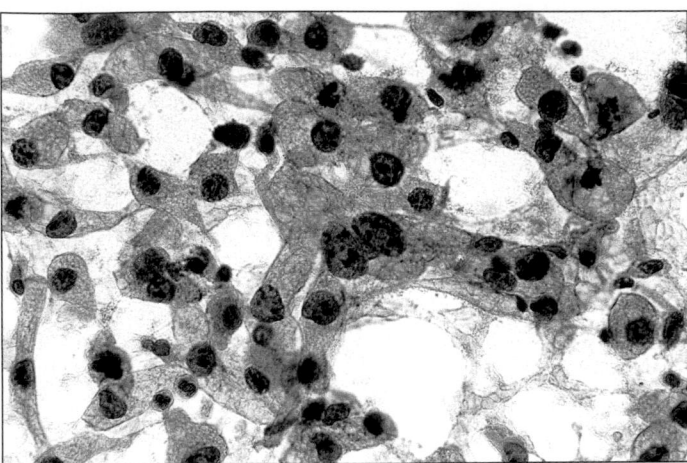

Fig. 9.86 Malignant fibrous histiocytoma, fine-needle aspiration. This lesion displays the foamy histiocytoid cytology some observers have regarded as diagnostic. Preparation of cell blocks for immunohistochemistry for primary diagnosis is recommended.

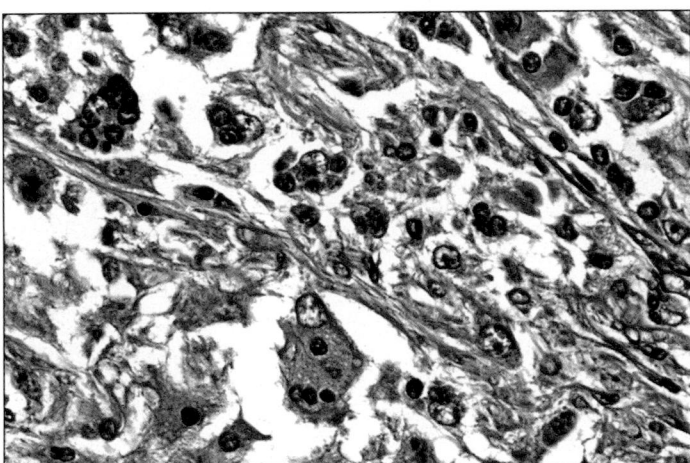

Fig. 9.87 Rosai–Dorfman disease of soft tissue. The multinucleated cells are Langerhans histiocytes displaying emperipolesis.

the WHO classification states that, in the case of pleomorphic liposarcoma, a tumor may resemble an MFH except for the presence of pleomorphic lipoblasts, which can be very scanty. Pleomorphic rhabdomyosarcomas have few or many rhabdomyoblasts, which can be demonstrated ultrastructurally or by positivity for desmin *and* nuclear MyoD1.[192–195] Thus focal specific differentiation suffices for diagnosis of various subtypes of pleomorphic sarcomas.

Pleomorphic sarcomas of various histologic types are remarkably similar clinically. The prognosis of pleomorphic sarcomas is generally poor, and about 40% of patients with high-grade MFH are dead of disease at 5 years. Data for patients with pleomorphic soft tissue leiomyosarcomas are few but, in one series, 65% of patients with pleomorphic leiomyosarcoma had died of disease.[196] The tumors in the latter series displayed marked pleomorphism but had areas with light microscopic features typical of smooth muscle differentiation (perpendicularly oriented fascicles of brightly eosinophilic spindle cells with blunt-ended nuclei and paranuclear vacuoles).

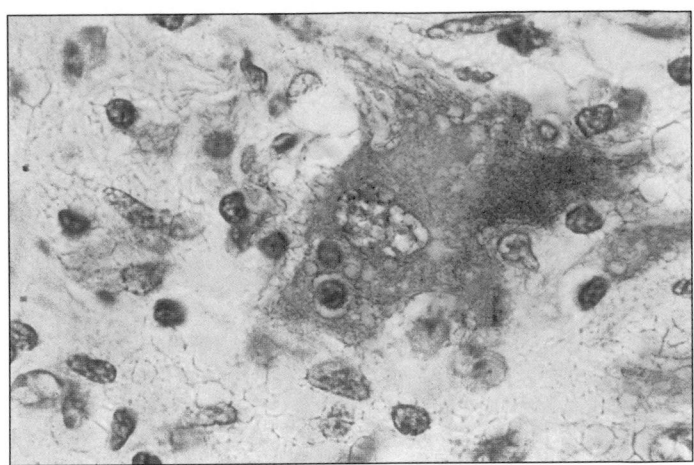

Fig. 9.88 Rosai–Dorfman disease of soft tissue. (S100 protein stain.)

The prognosis for dedifferentiated liposarcomas, which differ by typically presenting in the retroperitoneum, may be somewhat better than with other pleomorphic sarcomas; metastases were documented in four of 27 (15%) patients in one series and in 17% in a more comprehensive report.[197,198] In the latter, 28% of patients died of disease but 17% died of local effects of retroperitoneal tumors rather than of metastases. The outcome for pleomorphic rhabdomyosarcoma, however, appears to be relatively poor; in a large series[193] 70% of patients died of disease. It appears, therefore, that it may be important to identify pleomorphic rhabdomyosarcomas and dedifferentiated liposarcomas in daily practice but the specific separation of pleomorphic liposarcoma, pleomorphic leiomyosarcoma, or pleomorphic myofibrosarcoma from MFH is not clinically important at this time.

Myxoid
These neoplasms are discussed above under myxofibrosarcoma.

Giant cell
Giant cell MFH accounts for about 10% of all MFH and features numerous osteoclast-like giant cells in addition to the atypical spindle and polygonal cells (Fig. 9.89). It is typically multinodular and may be surrounded by peripheral bone formation.[199] This latter component may be metaplastic or neoplastic. Distinguishing such cases from extraskeletal osteosarcoma is difficult.

Inflammatory (xanthomatous)
This variety accounts for fewer than 5% of MFH and tends to be located in the retroperitoneum. These are aggressive tumors[200,201] composed of sheets of large histiocyte-like cells, many of which have a bland appearance also but with scattered pleomorphic tumor cells. There is often an intense background neutrophilic infiltrate and minimal collagen (Fig. 9.90). Since they are so rare, they are not well studied but most are probably, dedifferentiated liposarcomas;[202] see below.

ADIPOSE TISSUE TUMORS

Adipose tissue tumors span the spectrum from benign to malignant and a number of subtypes have been recognized over the years. Key

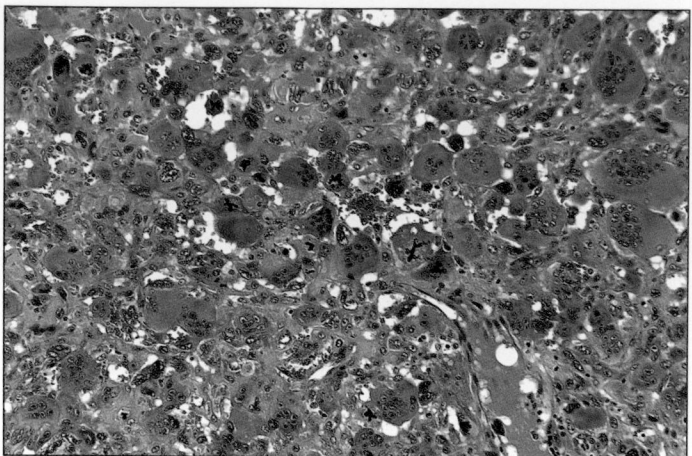

Fig. 9.89 Giant cell malignant fibrous histiocytoma (Courtesy of Dr Cyril Fisher).

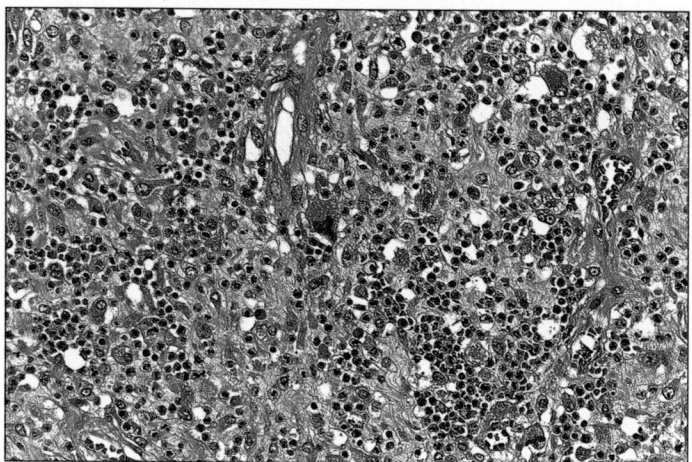

Fig. 9.90 Inflammatory malignant fibrous histiocytoma (Courtesy of Dr Cyril Fisher).

cytogenetic findings are tabulated in Table 9.6.[189,203–206] Lipomas and liposarcomas are the commonest mesenchymal neoplasms of the somatic soft tissue. As is the case for most other soft tissue neoplasms (the main exception being skeletal muscle tumors), the benign variants of adipose tumors (lipomas) greatly outnumber the malignant ones (liposarcomas). The vast majority of these neoplasms occur in adulthood and only rare specific subtypes occur in children. As with other soft tissue tumors, the cell of origin of adipose neoplasms is unknown. In this regard these neoplasms, like most other soft tissue tumors, are classified based on the resemblance of the lesional neoplastic cells to normal cells (in this case the adipocyte and its various precursor cells). Mature adipocytes are spherical cells whose cytoplasm is distended by a single lipid vacuole. The vacuole compresses the nucleus, which is seen microscopically at the periphery of the cell as a thin dark crescent. Immunohistochemically mature fat cells express vimentin and S100 protein but lack other markers. Immature fat cells contain multiple lipid vacuoles and exhibit a higher nuclear to cytoplasmic ratio. A variety of adipose neoplasms contain cells resembling these

Table 9.6 Adipose tissue tumor cytogenetics

Tumor type	Alteration
Lipomas	12q13–5;3q22
Hibernomas	11q13 breakpoints
Chondroid lipoma	t(11;16)
Angiolipoma	Consistently none
Atypical lipoma/well differentiated liposarcoma	Giant marker and ring chromosomes (q12)
Myxoid/round cell liposarcoma	T(12;16), t(12;22)
Pleomorphic liposarcoma	Complex rearrangements, extra chromosomes

precursor cells. Such multivacuolated cells are termed lipoblasts when they occur in the setting of liposarcoma and lipoblast-like cells when present in benign neoplasms or reactive conditions. The diagnostic significance of these multivacuolated cells, particularly regarding their specificity for liposarcoma, has been over-emphasized in the past. Lipoblast-like cells are present in several variants of lipoma.

BENIGN TUMORS

Lipoma

Lipomas, benign tumors composed of cells resembling mature adipocytes, are the most common soft tissue tumors of adulthood. Most arise between the ages of 40 and 60 years. They are more common in obese individuals. The tumors may arise in the subcutaneous tissue (*superficial lipoma*) or within deep soft tissues (*deep lipoma*) or even from the surfaces of bone (*parosteal lipoma*). Occasionally, lipomas can have areas of bone formation (*osteolipoma*), nodules of cartilage (*chondrolipoma*), abundant fibrous tissue (*fibrolipoma*), extensive myxoid change (*myxolipoma*) or a smooth muscle component (*myolipoma*).[207] These microscopic subtypes do not have clinical significance.

Superficial lipomas present as painless, soft, mobile masses that are generally small at the time of diagnosis (<5.0 cm). They are treated by simple excision. Recurrences are uncommon. Deep lipomas are generally larger at the time of diagnosis (>5.0 cm). They are typically painless but occasionally cause symptoms when they compress peripheral nerves. Deep-seated lipomas that arise within or between skeletal muscles are called intramuscular and intermuscular lipomas respectively. *Intramuscular lipomas* affect patients in middle to late adult life. They occur in various locations including the trunk, upper and lower extremities.[208] Intramuscular lipomas may be infiltrative or well circumscribed. This clinicopathologic distinction is important, as the infiltrative type has a tendency to recur locally following incomplete excision. The *intermuscular lipoma*, as the name implies, arises between muscles. It also affects adults and arises most often in the anterior abdominal wall. These are usually cured by local excision.

Grossly, most lipomas are well circumscribed, encapsulated and have a yellow, greasy cut surface. Intramuscular lipomas may appear as ill-defined regions of pallor within skeletal muscles. Typically they lack a capsule. Microscopically, conventional lipoma is composed of lobules of mature adipocytes (Figs 9.91, 9.92). In the infiltrative type of intramuscular lipoma the mature

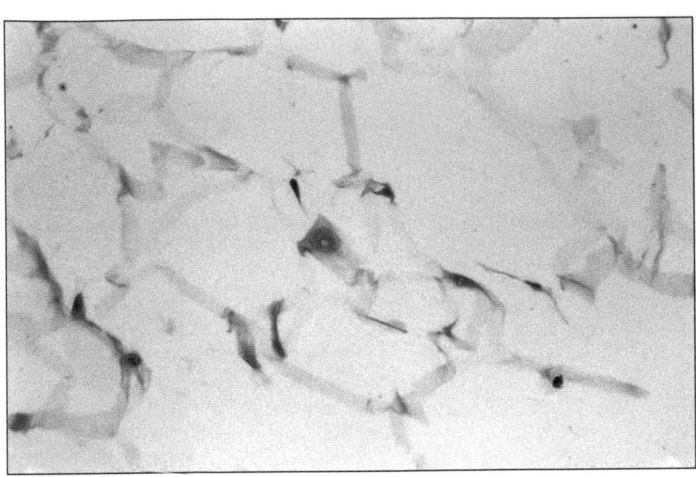

Fig. 9.91 Lipoma. This field is indistinguishable from normal fat. A cell in the center shows an intranuclear cytoplasmic invagination. This is *not* a lipoblast.

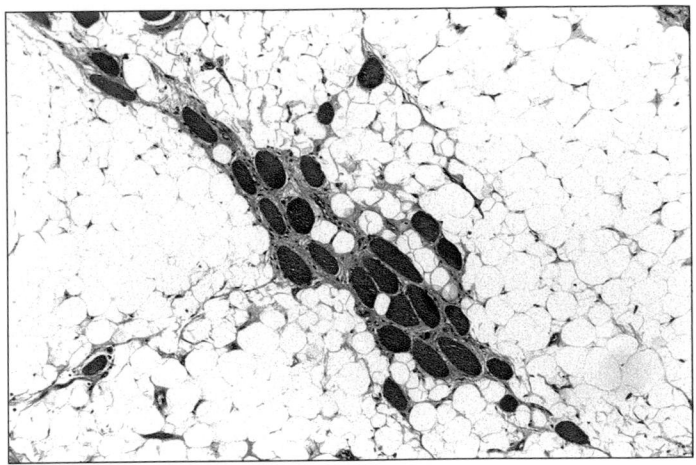

Fig. 9.93 Intramuscular lipoma. These benign tumors sometimes recur as they are infiltrative.

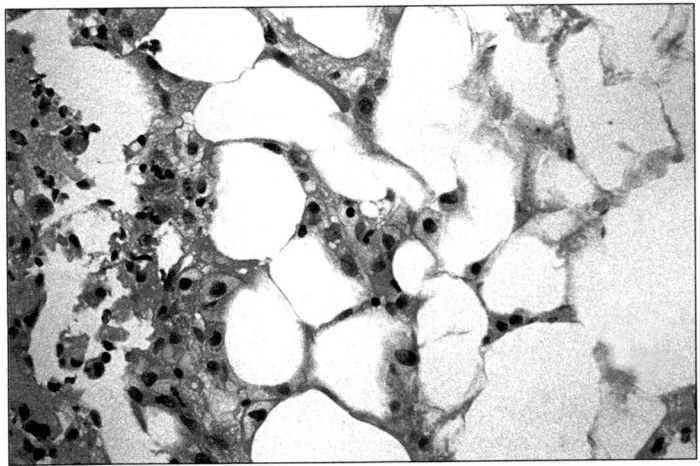

Fig. 9.92 Fat necrosis in a lipoma. The larger nuclei are histiocytic, not lipoblasts.

adipocytes are arranged between skeletal myocytes (Fig. 9.93). The majority of lipomas demonstrate karyotypic abnormalities involving 12q.

The most important pathologic differential diagnosis, especially for deep-seated lipomas, is low-grade liposarcoma. *Well differentiated liposarcoma* generally has sclerotic bands containing cells with bizarre, hyperchromatic nuclei and occasional lipoblasts, whereas deep lipomas are composed only of mature adipocytes that do not demonstrate hyperchromasia or nuclear enlargement. Intramuscular *hemangioma* can have a prominent fatty component that can simulate intramuscular lipoma. Microscopically, however, vessels are present in addition to mature adipose tissue and atrophic skeletal muscle.

Multiple lipomas/lipomatosis

Multiple lipomas are found in about 5% of patients with lipomas. Hundreds of lipomas can be present in these patients. The back, shoulder and upper arms are the most common location and men are affected more frequently than women. Familial cases of multiple lipomas have been described that seem to have a dominant inheritance pattern and to be associated with other syndromes. In lipomatosis, there is a diffuse, non-lobular proliferation of fat in the affected tissues. The subcutaneous fat of the back of the neck and shoulder are involved in nearly every individual.[209–212] Lipomatosis is thought to be secondary to a defect in lipid metabolism and patients with diffuse lipomatosis have the clinical appearance of obesity; mediastinal involvement can cause venous obstruction, with stasis and airway obstruction.[209–212]

The lipomas in these patients have the same gross and histologic features as conventional lipoma. The adipocytes have a normal appearance, except for slightly smaller size.

Lipoblastoma/lipoblastomatosis

Lipoblastoma is a benign tumor exclusively arising in infants, typically during the first 3 years of life.[213–216] The term lipoblastomatosis is used to describe poorly circumscribed masses of similar immature-appearing adipose tissue. Patients with lipoblastoma tend to be slightly older than those with lipoblastomatosis. Lipoblastoma is more common in boys. It most frequently involves the extremities and presents as a slow-growing painless mass. Other locations include the neck, trunk, retroperitoneum, groin, axilla, back, labia, flank, and mediastinum. Lipoblastoma generally involves the subcutaneous tissue but can also involve deeper tissue especially the diffuse (lipoblastomatosis) form. Lipoblastoma and lipoblastomatosis are treated by local resection. Local recurrence has been reported in 9–22% of patients; recurrences are more common in patients with the diffuse (lipoblastomatosis) form. Metastases do not occur. These tumors have alterations (rearrangements) of the long arm of chromosome 8.[217]

Grossly, lipoblastomas have a lobulated, myxoid or pale cut surface. Occasionally, they can have cystic areas filled with mucoid material. They are typically well circumscribed. Lipoblastomatosis, however, is poorly circumscribed and infiltrates the subcutaneous tissue and occasionally also underlying skeletal muscle. Most tumors are less than 5 cm in diameter but larger tumors, measuring over 20 cm, occasionally occur. Microscopically, lipoblastoma is lobular, with the individual lobules separated by fibrous connective tissue septa (Fig. 9.94). It is composed of primitive stellate and spindle-shaped cells, multivacuolated adipocytes, and univacuolated 'signet ring' cell

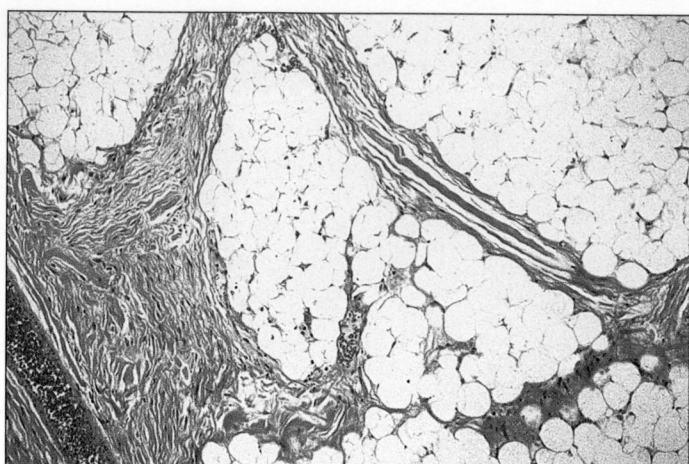

Fig. 9.94 Lipoblastoma. Note the prominent lobulations at scanning power.

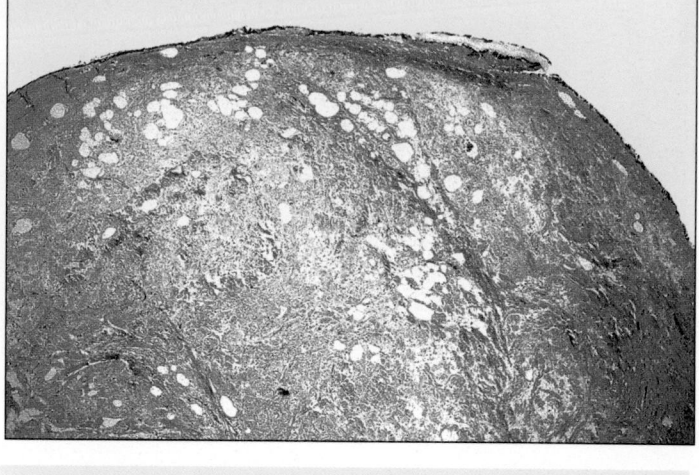

Fig. 9.96 Spindle cell lipoma. Note the sharp circumscription.

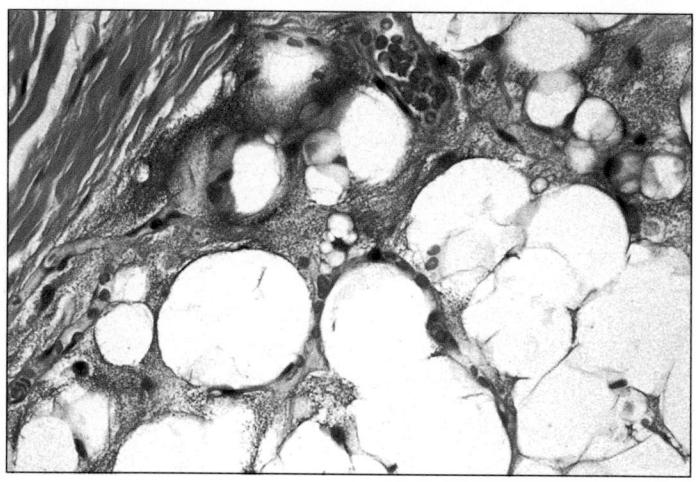

Fig. 9.95 Lipoblastoma. There is a lipoblast in the center of the field and a myxoid background, an appearance very similar to myxoid liposarcoma. These lesions typically affect children (in contrast to liposarcomas) and are lobulated so most are easily distinguishable from liposarcomas.

adipocytes (Fig. 9.95). Mitotic figures are rare and always normal in appearance. The supporting extracellular stroma is myxoid and commonly demonstrates a plexiform vascular pattern very much like the vascular pattern in myxoid liposarcoma. Sometimes these tumors mature to conventional lipomas. Aspiration cytologic findings have been described in case report form.[218]

The main differential diagnosis of lipoblastoma/lipoblastomatosis is myxoid liposarcoma. *Myxoid liposarcoma* is extremely rare in children and lacks the well formed lobular growth pattern seen in lipoblastoma. In a doubtful case, cytogenetics might be useful in this distinction.

Angiolipoma
These tumors are covered in Chapter 8.

Spindle cell lipoma
Spindle cell lipoma was first recognized by Enzinger & Harvey.[219] Although it can arise in various locations, the classic presentation is that of a painless subcutaneous mass involving the shoulder, back, or posterior neck in a middle-aged to elderly man. Most tumors are solitary but occasionally they can be multiple. In rare cases there may be a familial tendency towards multiple lesions.[220] The treatment is excision. Recurrences are rare.

Grossly, the tumors are well circumscribed and typically measure between 3 and 5 cm, although larger examples occasionally occur. On sectioning they have yellow areas, representing the mature fat, and gray-gelatinous areas representing the spindle cell component. Microscopically, spindle cell lipoma is usually well circumscribed (Fig. 9.96); however, focal infiltration into surrounding tissue can be seen, especially in those spindle cell lipomas that involve the deeper structures. Spindle cell lipoma is composed of an admixture of mature adipocytes and spindle cells embedded in myxoid matrix that contains collagen fibers (Fig. 9.97). The spindle cell component can be focal or it can involve almost the entire lesion, obscuring its lipomatous nature. The mature adipocytes have identical features to those of conventional lipoma. The spindle cells have oval to elongated uniform dark-staining nuclei and bipolar eosinophilic cytoplasm. Mitotic figures are rare. The matrix is variably myxoid and characteristically contains bright eosinophilic collagen fibers. Scattered mast cells are present (Fig. 9.98). The vascular pattern is usually inconspicuous but occasionally this tumor can have a 'pseudo-angiomatous' appearance secondary to myxoid degenerative changes. On aspiration cytology, spindle cell lipomas display a mixture of mature adipocytes, uniform spindle cells, and collagen bundles and/or fibers.[221] Immunohistochemically, the mature adipocytes, but not the spindle cells, stain for S-100 protein. In contrast, the spindle cells stain for CD34. Cytogenetic studies have shown abnormalities involving 13q and 16q.[222,223]

Pleomorphic lipoma
Pleomorphic lipoma is clinically, morphologically, and cytogenetically related to spindle cell lipoma and can be considered a pleomorphic variant of spindle cell lipoma.[222–225] Like spindle cell lipoma, pleomorphic lipoma generally occurs in males and involves the posterior neck, shoulder, and back. Patients typically present with a long-standing solitary subcutaneous mass. As is the case with spindle cell lipoma, treatment is excision and recurrences are rare.

Grossly, pleomorphic lipomas are well circumscribed with a yellow or grayish-tan cut surface. Microscopically, they closely resemble

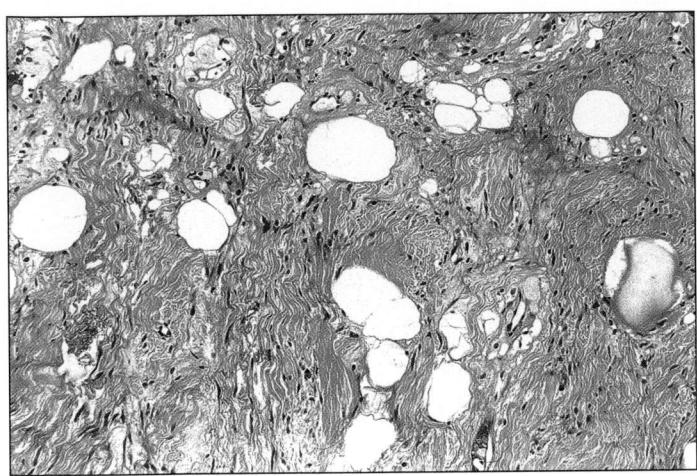

Fig. 9.97 Spindle cell lipoma. Dense collagen, fat, and spindle cells are all present.

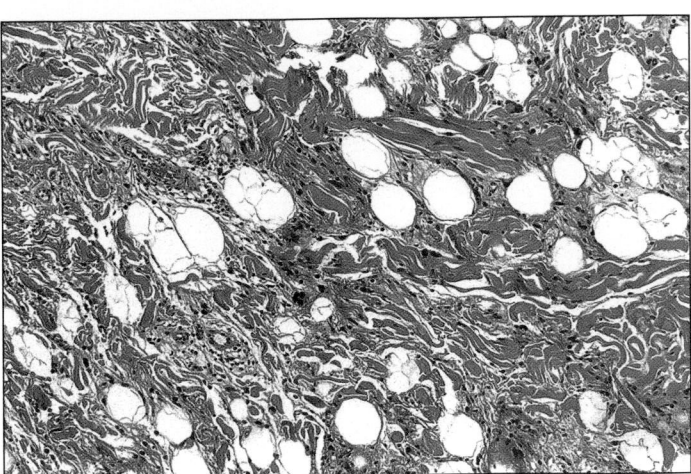

Fig. 9.99 Pleomorphic lipoma. These are otherwise similar to spindle cell lipomas but have enlarged hyperchromatic atypical cells.

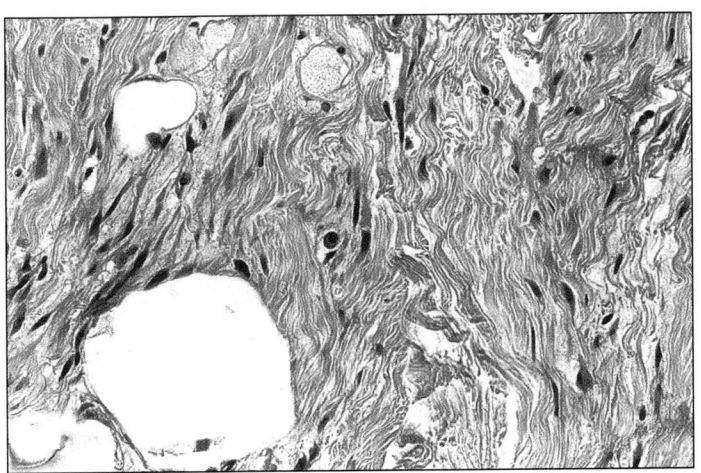

Fig. 9.98 Spindle cell lipoma. This tumor often features prominent mast cells.

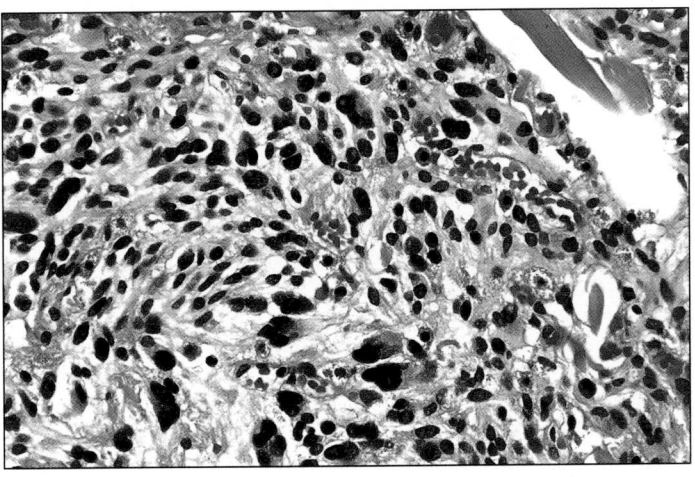

Fig. 9.100 Pleomorphic lipoma showing several 'floret' cells.

spindle cell lipomas. However, in addition, pleomorphic lipoma contains variable numbers of hyperchromatic multinucleated giant cells that frequently demonstrate a concentric or 'floret-like' arrangement of the nuclei (Figs 9.99, 9.100). These cells have eosinophilic cytoplasm with the nuclei arranged peripherally and circumferentially. The nuclei overlap and have finely dispersed or, less frequently, smudgy chromatin and small eosinophilic nucleoli. These pleomorphic cells are highly variable in number. The extracellular matrix is myxoid and contains thick eosinophilic collagen fibers. Lipoblast-like cells may be present. Because of this latter feature, these neoplasms are a real pitfall for aspiration cytology.[226,227] On cytogenetic studies, this tumor displays similar chromosomal abnormalities to those found in spindle cell lipoma.

Distinguishing pleomorphic lipoma from well differentiated sclerosing liposarcoma can be problematic, especially as lipoblast-like cells can be seen in pleomorphic lipoma. However, the clinical setting of a slow growing tumor arising in the subcutaneous tissue of the posterior neck, shoulder, or back is very characteristic for pleomorphic lipoma, whereas sclerosing liposarcoma arises in

the deep soft tissues or the retroperitoneum. Also, sclerosing liposarcoma has large areas of collagen deposition (sclerosis), more easily identified multivacuolated lipoblasts, and fewer 'floret-like' giant cells. In practical terms the diagnosis of pleomorphic lipoma should not be considered outside of the appropriate clinical setting of a superficial shoulder/neck adipose tissue tumor.

Chondroid lipoma

Chondroid lipoma was first described by Meis & Enzinger,[228] although an example of this tumor had been previously reported as 'extraskeletal chondroma with lipoblast-like cells.'[229] These tumors have a female predominance. They usually arise in the extremities but can also involve other sites. All reported examples of chondroid lipoma have behaved in a benign fashion. The treatment is excision.

Grossly, chondroid lipoma is well circumscribed and has a yellow cut surface. Microscopically, it is lobulated (Fig. 9.101) with the neoplastic cells growing in sheets, cords, or as single cells, separated by extracellular eosinophilic ('chondroid') matrix. The cells have well

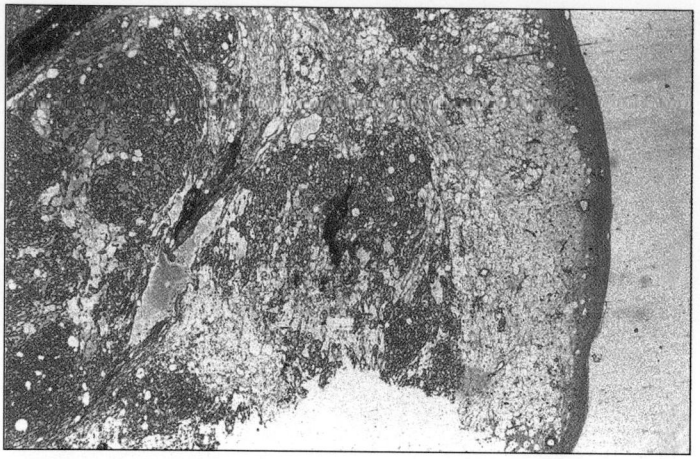

Fig. 9.101 Chondroid lipoma. This is a well circumscribed fatty tumor.

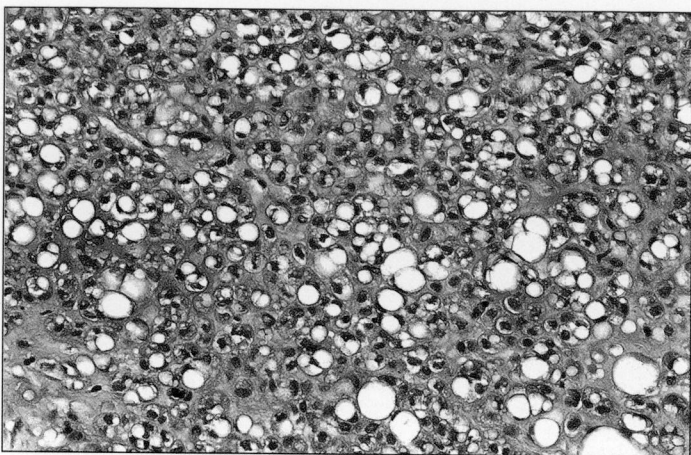

Fig. 9.102 Chondroid lipoma. The bubbly cells are reminiscent of both lipoblasts and chondrocytes.

defined cell membranes and small, dark-staining nuclei surrounded by granular eosinophilic cytoplasm. Many cells contain clear intracytoplasmic fat vacuoles indenting the nucleus, making them indistinguishable from lipoblasts (lipoblast-like cells, Fig. 9.102). However, mature adipocytes are present in all of the tumors. Immunohistochemically, the chondroid-like cells stain for vimentin and S-100 protein in a manner similar to normal adipocytes. Ultra-structural studies have shown a spectrum of differentiation with the cells showing features of prelipoblasts and chondroblasts.[230–232] Cyto-genetic analysis reveals a balanced translocation t11,16(q13;p12–13) distinct from the known translocation involving 16p11 in myxoid and round-cell liposarcoma. The 11q13 breakpoint was previously noted in hibernomas, raising the possibility of a common genetic deregulation.[233–235] On aspiration cytology, they feature clustered, variably mature, multivacuolated, hibernoma-like cells enmeshed in a capillary plexus, with a background of chondromyxoid material.[233–235]

Because of the myxoid ground substance and multivacuolated lipoblast-like cells, chondroid lipoma may simulate myxoid lipo-sarcoma. Myxoid liposarcoma, however, contains a prominent plexi-form vascular pattern and myxoid stroma instead of the eosinophilic, 'chondroid' stroma seen in chondroid lipoma.

Angiomyolipoma

The majority of these tumors appear in the kidney and the reader is directed to Chapter 32 for full coverage of this tumor type. However, these are well known to occur in the soft tissues of the retro-peritoneum and in the liver.[236–240] Other sites have been reported. Like their renal counterparts, they stain with HMB-45, MART (melanoma-type markers), and smooth muscle markers but usually lack S100 protein. Most behave in a benign fashion, but not all. Aspiration cytology is difficult unless one considers the diagnosis and performs confirmatory immunohistochemistry.

Myelolipoma

These are typically adrenal lesions, although extra-adrenal examples have been reported. Like their adrenal counterparts, this tumor dis-plays bone marrow elements admixed in an adipose tissue neoplasm.

Myolipoma

As the name implies, myolipoma is a benign-appearing tumor composed of an admixture of smooth muscle and adipose tissue[207]

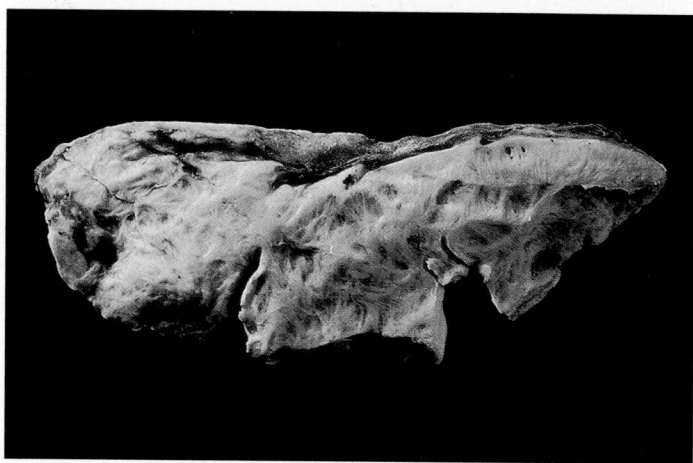

Fig. 9.103 Myolipoma. This large retroperitoneal tumor behaved in a benign fashion. The cut surface displays both fat and solid areas.

(Figs 9.103, 9.104). Only a small number of such cases are well documented and it should be noted that large, deep soft tissue masses composed of either fat or smooth muscle tend to be malig-nant. This rare tumor may be found in the retroperitoneum, where it may attain a large size (26 cm reported).

Hibernoma

Hibernoma is an uncommon benign tumor in which the lesional cells demonstrate morphological features of brown fat cells. Hibernomas generally arise in locations where brown fat is found in fetuses and infants, such as the interscapular region, neck, medi-astinum, axilla, posterior abdominal wall, and retroperitoneum adjacent to the kidney and adrenal gland.[241] They can also arise in areas that normally do not harbor brown fat, such as the thigh. Hibernoma presents as a painless, slow-growing mass. Hibernomas are benign and are treated by local excision.

Grossly, hibernomas are tan or red-brown, usually measuring 5–10 cm; tumors greater than 20 cm occasionally occur. Micro-scopically hibernoma demonstrates a lobular architecture and is composed of large polygonal cells supported by small branching

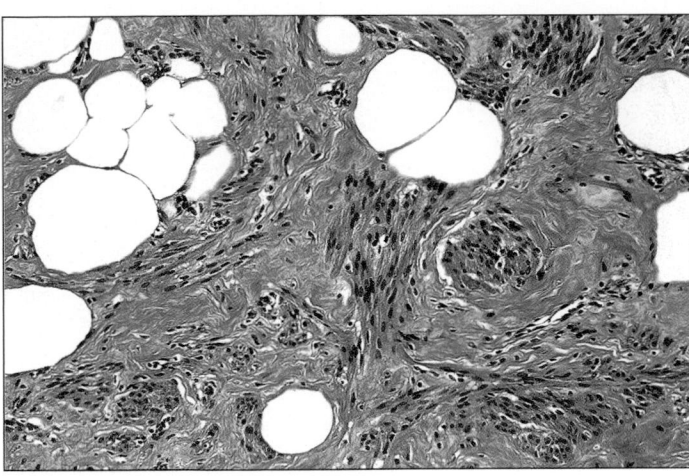

Fig. 9.104 Myolipoma featuring smooth muscle and mature fat.

capillaries. Three cell types can be identified; those with abundant mitochondria have a granular eosinophilic cytoplasm. Other cells have granular eosinophilic cytoplasm and numerous lipid vacuoles that typically indent the centrally located nucleus. The third type resembles a mature univacuolar adipocyte. Cytogenetically, hibernomas demonstrate aberrations of chromosome 11q13.[242]

MALIGNANT TUMORS

Liposarcoma
The WHO recognizes the following subtypes of liposarcoma:[1–3]

1. Well differentiated liposarcoma/dedifferentiated liposarcoma
2. Myxoid liposarcoma/round cell liposarcoma
3. Pleomorphic liposarcoma

Well differentiated liposarcoma and dedifferentiated liposarcoma are related: the latter arises from the former. Myxoid and round cell liposarcoma are two biological and clinical ends of a spectrum. Both have a single cytogenetic abnormality.

Well differentiated liposarcoma
Well differentiated liposarcoma is the commonest subtype of liposarcoma. These tumors nearly always occur in adults, with no gender predilection.[243–249] They most commonly arise in the deep soft tissues of the proximal extremities and the retroperitoneum. Occasionally, retroperitoneal liposarcomas may present as groin masses by virtue of local extension into the peritoneum-lined scrotal sac.[250] When well differentiated liposarcomas occur within the subcutaneous tissues they have been classified as 'atypical lipomas'.[243,246,251,252] Although these tumors are histologically and cytogenetically identical to their deeply located counterparts, the natural history of the superficial tumors is sufficiently different for them to be considered as a separate group. However, they are not immune to dedifferentiation to a high-grade sarcoma.[247,253]

Most patients with well differentiated liposarcomas present with painless, slow-growing soft tissue masses. Intra-abdominal tumors typically are larger than the extremity tumors and patients with abdominal tumors may present with altered abdominal girth or altered gastrointestinal tract function. Primary groin tumors commonly simulate inguinal or femoral hernias.[254] CT and MRI imaging effectively demonstrate these neoplasms, highlighting their relation-

ship to muscle, bone, and neurovascular structures. Using both these modalities, most well differentiated liposarcomas exhibit similar signal qualities to normal fat. Strands of soft tissue with signal characteristics similar to muscle are often present within these tumors. If large volumes of this intermediate signal material is present within a neoplasm that otherwise is composed predominantly of fat, this suggests the possibility of a dedifferentiated liposarcoma. In the absence of dedifferentiation, distant metastases from well differentiated liposarcomas essentially never occur and extremity tumors often recur many years after the original surgical procedure. Local recurrence in the extremities is typically not associated with destructive growth.

For these reasons well differentiated liposarcoma is managed by wide local excision, if technically possible. Local or marginal excision is preferable to ablative surgical procedures that result in major functional compromise. Retroperitoneal tumors are treated by debulking, which virtually always results in residual gross or microscopic tumor. Treated in this way well differentiated liposarcoma of the extremity demonstrates a recurrence rate of approximately 40–50%, while groin and retroperitoneal tumors nearly always recur (80–90%). The extremity tumors do not result in patient deaths but the retroperitoneal and groin tumors have a poor long-term prognosis due to uncontrolled local growth within the abdominal cavity.[243,245,246,252]

Well differentiated liposarcomas demonstrate ring chromosomes and long marker chromosomes derived from the q13–15 region of chromosome 12. These findings are present regardless of anatomic location, including tumors that arise in the superficial soft tissue.[203,204]

Well differentiated liposarcomas are usually large. Tumors in excess of 20 cm are not uncommon. They typically demonstrate a multinodular growth within and between skeletal muscles. The tumors are soft and pale yellow on cut section. The cut surface often is a paler yellow than adjacent normal fat because of the presence of excessive interstitial collagen within the tumor in comparison to the normal fat.

Three microscopic variants of well differentiated liposarcoma occur.

The most common is the *lipoma-like variant*. As its name suggests, this tumor morphologically resembles lipoma. As such, this subtype is composed predominantly of cells that resemble mature adipocytes. In contrast to lipoma there is a greater variability in adipocyte size. Additionally, there is usually an increase in interstitial collagen within the tumor, both within thickened fibrous bands that traverse the tumor and diffusely within the extracellular space. The diagnostic hallmark of lipoma-like liposarcoma is atypical hyperchromatic nuclei within the cells showing adipose differentiation in addition to non-specific spindled cells embedded within the collagenous bands and interstitial matrix. These latter nuclei are enlarged and characterized by intense hyperchromasia, coarsely clumped chromatin, and convoluted nuclear membranes (Figs 9.106, 9.107). Lipoblasts are often present in lipoma-like liposarcoma, particularly adjacent to the collagenous septa, but their identification is not a requirement for the diagnosis of well differentiated liposarcoma. Mitotic figures are typically few in pure well differentiated liposarcoma. Focal regions of fat necrosis with cystic change and a histiocytic inflammatory reaction are commonly present. Other microscopic findings that may be present include the atypical stromal cells within the muscular walls of veins in the tumor, stromal myxoid change, and focal myoid differentiation.[255–257] The last finding although rare, is more commonly present in dedifferentiated tumors.

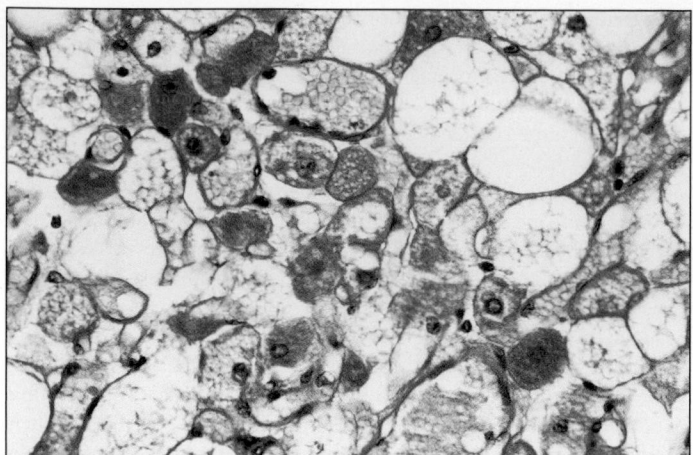

Fig. 9.105 Hibernoma. Like brown fat, these tumors have plentiful capillaries and foamy, granular appearing cells.

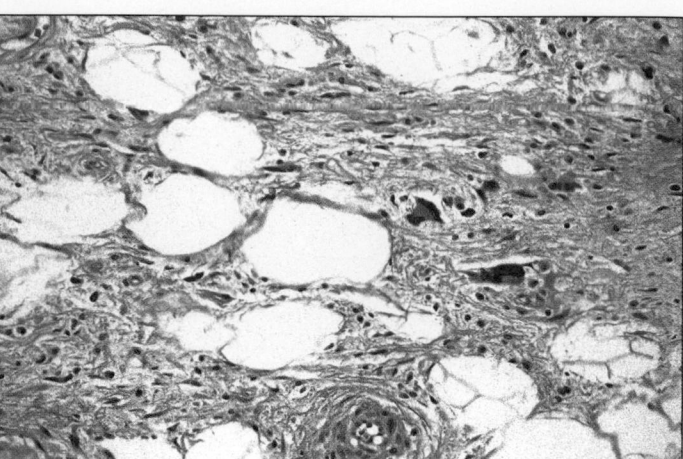

Fig. 9.107 Well differentiated liposarcoma. Usually the hyperchromatic cells are found along fibrous septa.

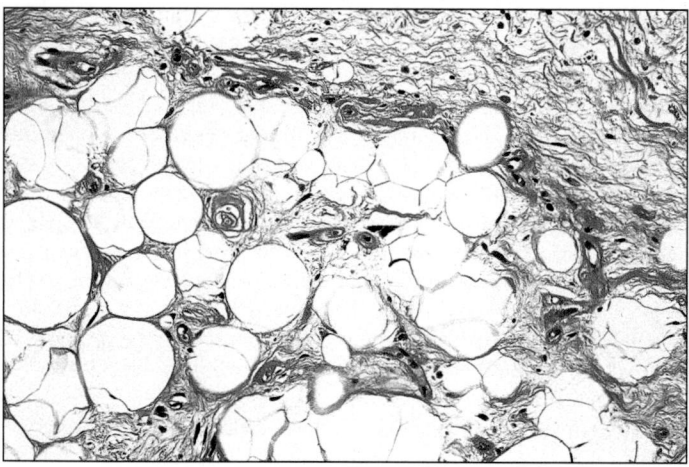

Fig. 9.106 Well differentiated liposarcoma showing enlarged hyperchromatic cells in a fatty background.

The second most common histologic variant of well differentiated liposarcoma is the so-called *sclerosing type*. When exclusively sclerosing, the radiographic and gross appearance of the neoplasm will suggest a nonfatty tumor since the degree of adipocytic differentiation present may be scant. Typically, however, there are transitions between lipoma-like and sclerosing regions within a single neoplasm. In sclerosing regions the tumor is dominated by interstitial collagen that separates the widely spaced tumor cells. Only a minority of the embedded cells will exhibit recognizable adipocytic differentiation. The majority appear as non-specific spindled cells or markedly atypical stromal cells similar to the type present within the lipoma-like variant. The extracellular collagen that separates the lesional cells varies from fibrillary to hyalinized but the cellularity remains relatively low. Hypercellularity with fascicular growth suggests dedifferentiation (see below). As with the more common lipoma-like variant, mitotic figures are infrequently found.

The least common histologic subtype of well differentiated liposarcoma is the *inflammatory type*.[258] Both lipoma-like and sclerosing well differentiated liposarcoma may rarely contain focal regions of

tumor with extensive lymphoid infiltrates. These regions may exhibit follicle formation with germinal centers, sheets and clusters of plasma cells, and even admixed neutrophils and eosinophils (Fig. 9.108). The atypical stromal cells that characterize all types of well differentiated liposarcoma are found admixed with these inflammatory cells, which may cause confusion with malignant lymphoma.

None of the histologic variants of low-grade liposarcoma are clinically or prognostically relevant.

On aspiration cytology, sheets of mature adipose are punctuated by enlarged hyperchromatic cells, often with bare nuclei (Figs 9.109, 9.110).

The term *atypical lipoma* has been applied to well differentiated liposarcomas that occur in the subcutis.[243,246,251] This is because tumors in this location have an excellent prognosis and an extremely low rate of dedifferentiation. Historically, the term atypical lipoma was applied to well differentiated liposarcomas of the deep soft tissues of the extremities but current favored terminology is as above.

Finally, the term 'atypical lipomatous tumor' has been suggested as an encompassing term for well differentiated liposarcomas regardless of their location. However, some discourage the use of this term because of its non-specificity and its application to tumors of different biologic potential, including pleomorphic lipoma. *Pleomorphic lipoma* is distinguished from well differentiated liposarcoma principally by its location and the presence of spindle cell lipoma-like regions within these tumors.

Myxoid change in well differentiated liposarcoma of the lipoma-like variant may occasionally simulate *myxoid liposarcoma*. The latter tumor may be distinguished morphologically and cytogenetically. Well differentiated liposarcoma must also be distinguished from a number of non-neoplastic inflammatory conditions, which are characterized by the infiltrates of so-called lipoblast-like histiocytes. This pattern of inflammation is often associated with the injection of lipid material or silicone implants of various types. The multivacuolated cells that form as a reaction to the foreign material may closely resemble lipoblasts. Lastly, massively obese patients may develop lymphedema-associated tumefactions that display mature fat traversed by fibrous bands containing mildly enlarged reactive fibroblasts, an overall pattern that may be mistaken for well differen-

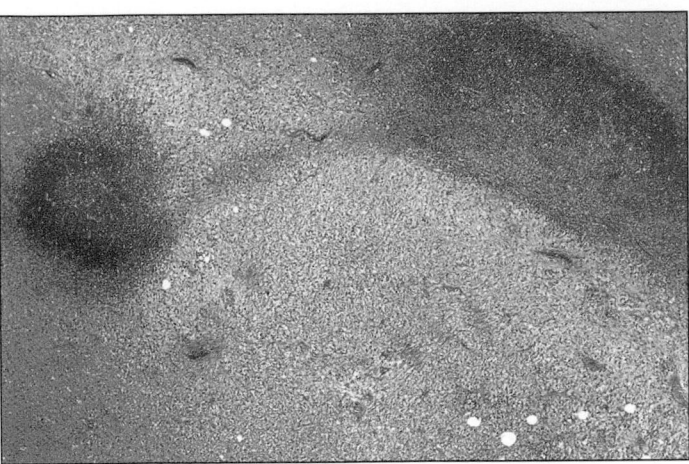

Fig. 9.108 Well differentiated liposarcoma. A rich inflammatory background may be present.

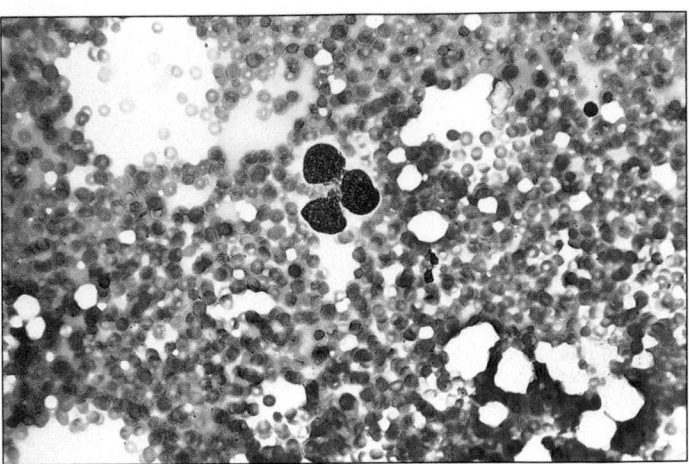

Fig. 9.110 Well differentiated liposarcoma, aspiration cytology. This focus, from the same tumor depicted in Figure 9.109, together with the imaging impression, allowed for the correct interpretation. This cell is reminiscent of the 'floret' cells in pleomorphic lipoma but, in the setting of a retroperitoneal mass, is in keeping with well differentiated liposarcoma.

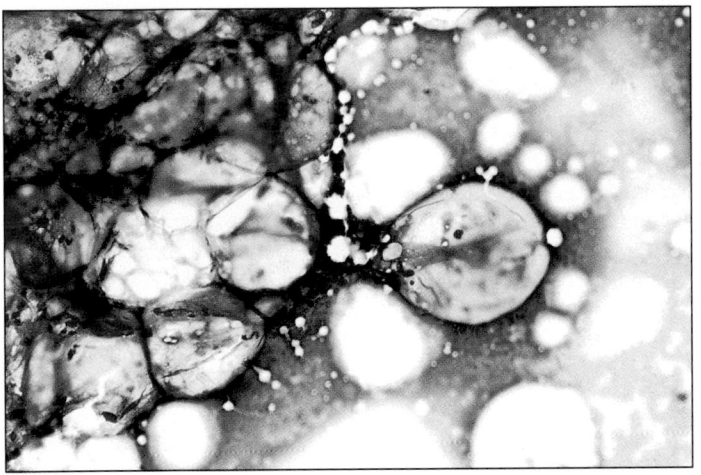

Fig. 9.109 Well differentiated liposarcoma, aspiration cytology. Sampling error can be a problem. This focus from a retroperitoneal tumor has the appearance of normal fat.

tiated liposarcoma. There is usually also prominent lymphedema displayed in the sections.[259]

Dedifferentiated liposarcoma

The term dedifferentiated liposarcoma describes a spindle cell non-lipogenic sarcoma occurring in association with a well differentiated low-grade liposarcoma.[197,198,246,247,252,253] In the majority of cases the spindle cell sarcoma and low-grade liposarcoma regions are found in the same tumor at the time of diagnosis ('primary dedifferentiated liposarcoma').[198] In a minority of cases the spindle cell sarcoma is identified at the time of a local recurrence of a previously resected low-grade liposarcoma ('secondary dedifferentiated liposarcoma').[198] In the latter situation the dedifferentiated tumor may contain a mixture of well differentiated liposarcoma and spindle cell sarcoma or be composed only of the non-lipogenic component.

Dedifferentiated liposarcoma affects the same patient population as well differentiated liposarcomas. There is no sex predilection. In the past it was suggested that dedifferentiation only occurred in the

setting of retroperitoneal low-grade liposarcoma and that this phenomenon was site-dependent but more recent experience has shown that well differentiated liposarcomas in all locations may undergo dedifferentiation (Fig. 9.111). The concept that dedifferentiation is 'time-dependent' rather than 'site-dependent' has been proposed.[198] The clinical significance of dedifferentiation is that once it occurs in a well differentiated liposarcoma then the tumor acquires the capacity for distant metastases and hence should be considered biologically high-grade. The metastatic rate for dedifferentiated liposarcoma ranges between 15% and 30%. Dedifferentiation also typically portends more aggressive local growth, an increased risk of local recurrence, and higher tumor-related mortality. Some reported dedifferentiation rates are tabulated by site (Table 9.7).

Dedifferentiated liposarcoma is cytogenetically related to low-grade liposarcoma. Although these tumors may demonstrate complex karyotypes similar to those found in undifferentiated sarcomas such as MFH, the majority of dedifferentiated liposarcomas exhibit the ring chromosomes characteristic of well differentiated liposarcoma. Dedifferentiated liposarcoma is treated by radical surgical excision, if feasible. Adjuvant radiation therapy and/or chemotherapy may also be considered, as for other high-grade soft tissue sarcomas.

Like well differentiated liposarcomas, dedifferentiated tumors are typically large (greater than 10 cm) and demonstrate multi-nodular growth. There is no minimum amount of nonlipogenic spindle cell sarcoma that must be present for a tumor to be classified as dedifferentiated. Approximately 90% of these tumors are primary dedifferentiated liposarcomas and these often show admixtures of pale, soft, yellow fat representing the well differentiated liposarcoma component and firmer, tan tissue representing the nonlipogenic spindle cell sarcoma. Secondary dedifferentiated tumors may consist only of nonlipogenic sarcoma at the time of recurrence or contain an admixture of both adipose and nonadipose components. The adipose components of the dedifferentiated tumors are histologically identical to usual well differentiated liposarcoma. In the majority of instances, the spindle cell sarcoma component is undifferentiated and histo-

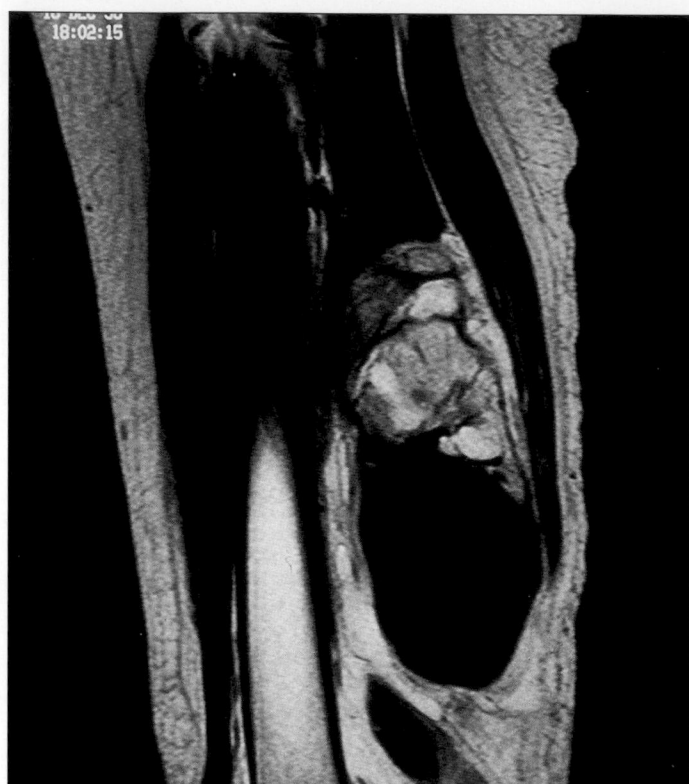

Fig. 9.111 Dedifferentiated liposarcoma. Note that much of this tumor of the thigh has the same signal as the subcutaneous fat. However, the dedifferentiated component has the same signal as muscle. This was a recurrent lesion; the initial tumor was purely fatty.

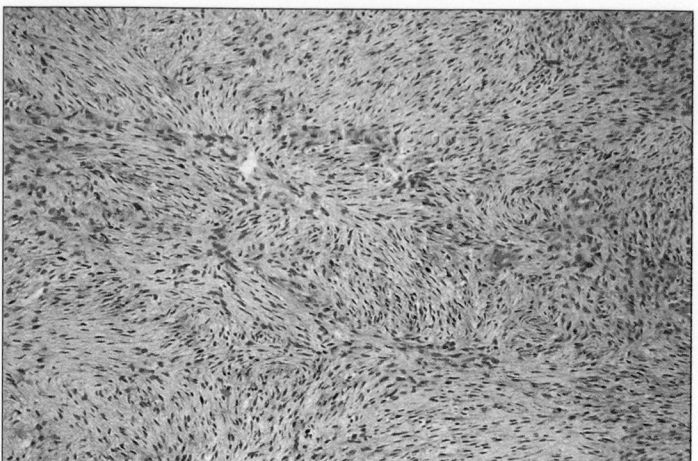

Fig. 9.112 Dedifferentiated liposarcoma. High-grade dedifferentiation is similar to a malignant fibrous histiocytoma.

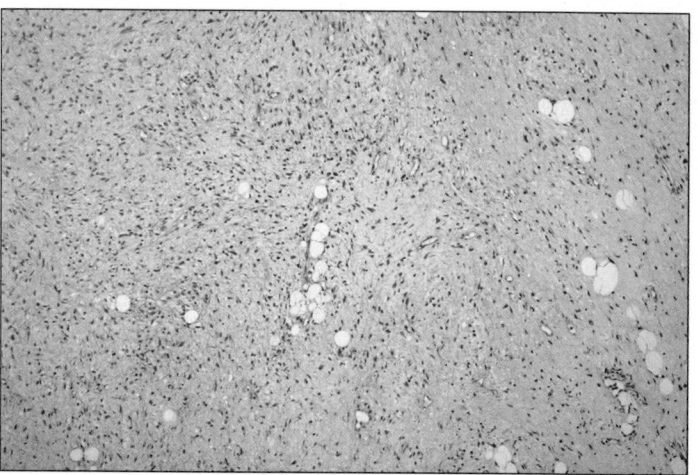

Fig. 9.113 Dedifferentiated liposarcoma. Low-grade dedifferentiation has been defined as a region devoid of lipogenic differentiation occupying at least a low-power (10× objective) microscopic field, having cellularity in excess of that encountered in sclerosing well differentiated liposarcoma and similar to that encountered in a fibromatosis or low-grade fibrosarcoma.

Table 9.7 Liposarcoma: dedifferentiation – frequency by site

Year	Author	All	Extremities	Retroperitoneum, etc.	Other
1979	Evans	–	1/4	6/12	–
1982	Hashimoto	4/14	–	–	–
1987	Azumi	5/69	0/24	5/25	0/20
1992	Weiss	11/92	3/46	8/37	0/9
1994	Lucas	10/58	2/32	7/24	1/2
Total		30/233	6/106	26/98	1/31
%		12.8	5.6	26.5	3

logically high-grade (Fig. 9.112), resembling MFH. These two components may show abrupt interfaces, gradual transitions, or a more diffuse admixture. The first of these is the most typical with the last the least common. The dedifferentiated component of the tumor characteristically demonstrates marked hypercellularity, nuclear pleomorphism, and a high mitotic rate.

A number of morphological variations of the dedifferentiated foci of the tumor have been described. It is now clear that in a minority of cases the dedifferentiated regions may appear histologically low-grade, resembling fibromatosis or low-grade fibrosarcoma[198] (Fig. 9.113). Additionally, occasionally the dedifferentiated regions may exhibit a microscopic nodularity resembling meningothelial whorls.[260,261] Finally, heterologous differentiation towards leiomyosarcoma, rhabdomyosarcoma, and/or osteosarcoma rarely occurs.[255] These histologic variants of dedifferentiation do not appear to be prognostically relevant. 'Low-grade' dedifferentiated is believed to reflect an earlier step towards high-grade dedifferentiation and is also associated with metastases.

The differential diagnosis of dedifferentiated liposarcoma includes well differentiated liposarcoma and spindle cell sarcomas. Dedifferentiated tumors with heterologous differentiation can be distinguished from the various sarcomas they resemble by the presence of the accompanying well differentiated liposarcoma.

Myxoid and round cell liposarcoma

Up to half of all liposarcomas are of myxoid/round cell type. Although these two lesions have historically been considered to be

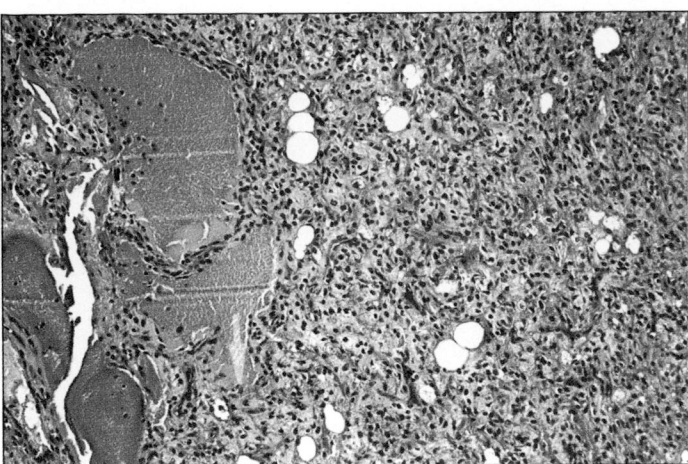

Fig. 9.114 Myxoid liposarcoma. This scanning power image shows cystic change, rich vascularity, uniform cytology, and lipoblasts, all features of myxoid liposarcoma.

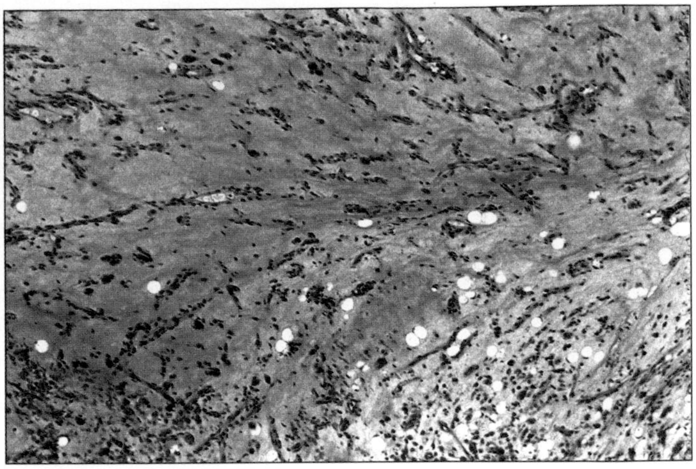

Fig. 9.115 Myxoid liposarcoma. This hypocellular tumor shows many lipoblasts 'hugging' the vasculature.

separate histologic entities it is now apparent that these two diagnostic terms describe different histologic and clinical ends of a spectrum that is genetically homogeneous.[206,262–267] Tumors with pure myxoid liposarcoma morphology demonstrate a better prognosis than those with round cell features.[246,264,267] Pure round cell morphology is extremely uncommon and most tumors classified as round cell liposarcoma are composed of mixtures of myxoid and round cell components. These tumors typically affect adults and are most common in the fifth decade. Rare myxoid/round cell liposarcomas occur in children. Males are affected more commonly than females. The deep soft tissue of the thigh is the single most common location for these neoplasms. Primary tumors also arise in the soft tissue of the arms, trunk, and retroperitoneum. The majority are deep to the fascia. Patients typically complain of a painless soft tissue mass. Myxoid/round cell liposarcoma is treated by wide surgical excision with or without radiation therapy. Approximately 30% of patients develop distant metastases. Like most other sarcomas these often involve the lungs; however, myxoid/round cell liposarcoma often metastasizes to nonpulmonary sites, including the retroperitoneum, soft tissue, and skeleton.[266] Histologic grading appears to be of value in predicting those patients at risk for metastases. Specifically, as the cellularity of the tumor increases and the degree of tumor composed of round cell liposarcoma or so-called cellular myxoid liposarcoma increases, there is an increased risk of metastasis.

Most myxoid/round cell liposarcomas demonstrate the chromosomal translocation t(12;16)(q13;p11) that results in the rearrangement of the *CHOP* and *FUS* genes.[206,262,263,268,269] This translocation appears to be specific for these tumors. A minority of myxoid/round cell liposarcomas may demonstrate variants of this translocation, which typically also involve a 12q13 breakpoint.

Grossly myxoid/round cell liposarcomas have a wide range in size although most measure more than 10 cm. They typically demonstrate a lobulated, smooth outline and may appear encapsulated. The cut surface of the tumor varies from gelatinous and tan to opaque and yellow. Focal hemorrhage is common but necrosis or gross cystic change is unusual. It is usually not possible to grossly distinguish those parts of the tumor that harbor round cell foci. As stated above, virtually all tumors in the myxoid/round cell spectrum contain myxoid regions.

Myxoid liposarcoma is composed of aggregated lobules of low to moderately cellular, uniform, small, spindled and oval tumor cells embedded in a richly myxoid ground substance (Fig. 9.114). The tumor cells are arranged as cords and clusters although individual cells are usually readily separable from adjacent ones by ground substance (Fig. 9.115). Most characteristically, an acute angle (plexiform) branching capillary vasculature is present within the ground substance. The majority of the tumor cells have scant cytoplasm and uniform dark-staining nuclei. Nucleoli or mitotic figures are typically not prominent. Tumor cells tend to aggregate closer to each other at the periphery of individual tumor lobules and adjacent to blood vessels. Univacuolar and multivacuolar lipoblasts are scattered throughout the tumor. The number and distribution of these cells varies considerably; however, they are often most prominent at the periphery of the tumor lobules.

Round cell liposarcoma is characterized by a relative increase in cellularity of the tumor such that individual tumor cells lie in direct apposition to each other without intervening matrix (Fig. 9.116). When this occurs the capillary vasculature becomes less distinct and the tumor cell nuclei often are enlarged and exhibit pale-staining nuclear chromatin with prominent nucleoli. Mitotic figures are typically more visible within these round cell regions.

One of the difficulties in precise classification of myxoid/round cell liposarcoma is that there are no universally acceptable criteria for minimum levels of cellularity and nuclear atypia that define round cell foci within these tumors. The 'cut-off' as to when a cellular myxoid liposarcoma becomes a round cell liposarcoma is imprecise, since some lesions seem to appear intermediate to these two ends of the spectrum. The term 'transitional' was coined by Smith et al.[267] to describe areas in these tumors that are more cellular than those of myxoid liposarcoma but with preservation of the vascular pattern and readily apparent myxoid matrix (Fig. 9.117). When unassociated with round cell areas, transitional morphology appears not to relate to prognosis. Like most myxoid neoplasms, diagnosis of myxoid liposarcoma from frozen sections can be perilous (Fig. 9.118). Aspiration or intraoperative cytology can be diagnostic (Figs 9.119, 9.120).

As for prognosis, although Smith and colleagues suggest that a prognostic 'cutoff' occurs at greater than 5% cellular areas,[267] other authors prefer to rely on a higher figure (25%).[252,264]

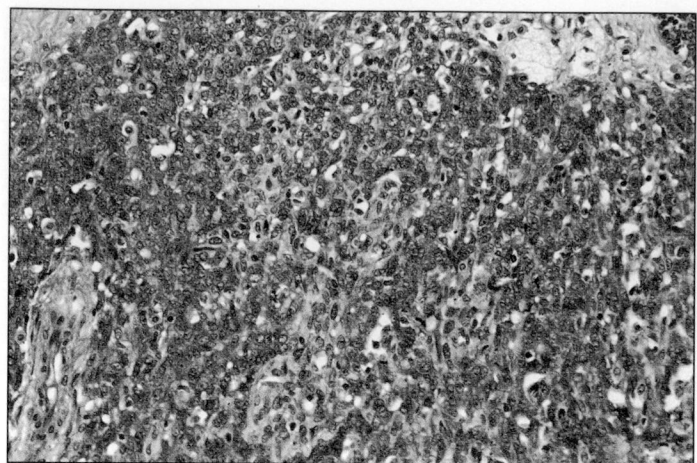

Fig. 9.116 Round cell liposarcoma. Overlapping cells and an obscured vascular pattern are seen.

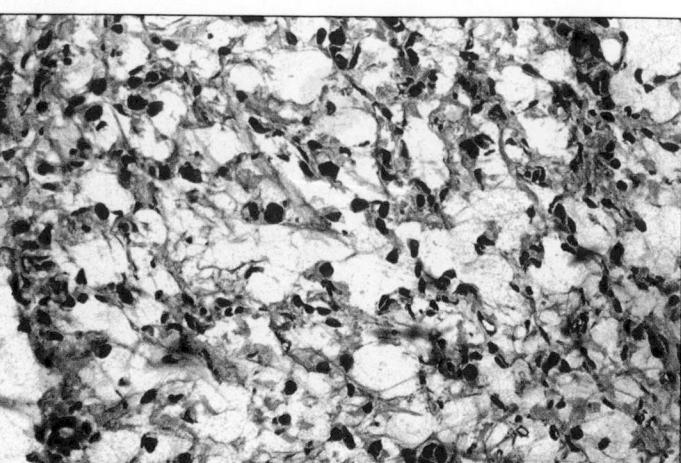

Fig. 9.118 Myxoid liposarcoma, frozen section. Diagnosing myxoid lesions on frozen sections is prone to inaccuracy.

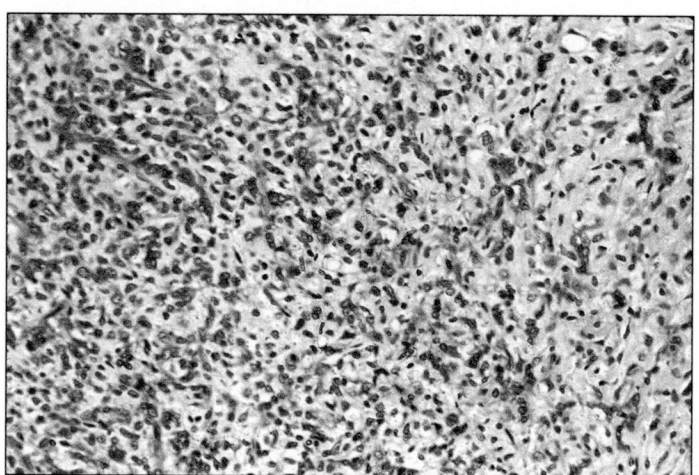

Fig. 9.117 Is this myxoid or round cell liposarcoma? Some observers have applied the term 'transitional' to lesions like this. This appearance does not impact prognosis whereas round cell pattern conveys a poor prognosis in relation to its percentage.

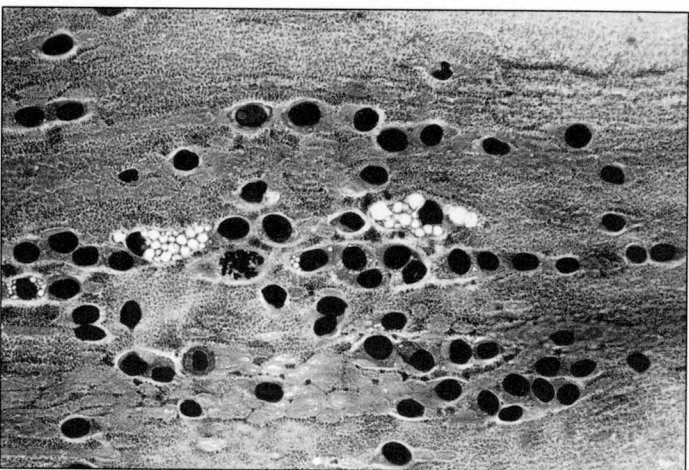

Fig. 9.119 Myxoid liposarcoma, aspiration cytology. Note the perfectly preserved lipoblasts. The cells have small uniform nuclei but the myxoid background and lipoblasts allow a diagnosis on this Diff-Quik preparation.

Pleomorphic liposarcoma

Pleomorphic liposarcoma is the rarest subtype of liposarcoma. Few series of this variant of liposarcoma have been reported and most published examples have been as small numbers of tumors included within larger series of the more common types of liposarcoma.[270–272] They typically occur in adults over the age of 50 years. Males and females are both affected. Pleomorphic liposarcoma in childhood is extremely uncommon. Most tumors arise in the deep soft tissues of the thigh, trunk, or retroperitoneum, where they produce symptoms related to a painless mass. These tumors are often large and typically exceed 10 cm. There are no consistent or specific cytogenetic abnormalities within this subgroup of liposarcoma and they display complex karyotypes.[189] Pleomorphic liposarcomas are treated by wide surgical excision with or without adjuvant radiation therapy. The role of chemotherapy remains unclear. Pleomorphic liposarcomas have a very high incidence of metastases and tumor-related mortality.

Pleomorphic liposarcomas are large multinodular tumors that typically are yellow to tan on their cut surface (Fig. 9.121). Grossly recognizable fat is usually not present but regions of hemorrhage and/or necrosis are common. There are two microscopic subtypes of pleomorphic liposarcoma. In both, clusters of markedly pleomorphic multivacuolated lipoblasts are present. In fact pleomorphic liposarcoma features the most numerous and bizarre lipoblasts of all liposarcomas types (Figs 9.122, 9.123). Mitotic figures, including atypical forms, are readily found. Lipoblasts with more than 20 separate cytoplasmic vacuoles arranged around a central atypical nucleus are not uncommon. In the more common variant of pleomorphic liposarcoma these cells comprise the majority of the tumor. In the other histologic variant, clusters of these bizarre lipoblasts are embedded in a background of otherwise undifferentiated pleomorphic spindle cell sarcoma resembling MFH. There is usually an abrupt transition between these two microscopically distinct regions. Both variants of

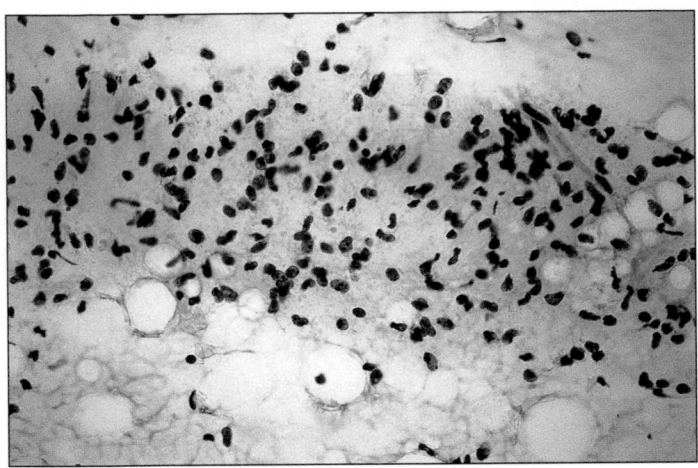

Fig. 9.120 Myxoid liposarcoma, aspiration cytology. The Papanicolaou stain does now allow for such easy recognition of lipoblasts as does the Diff-Quik. Note the striking uniformity of the cells.

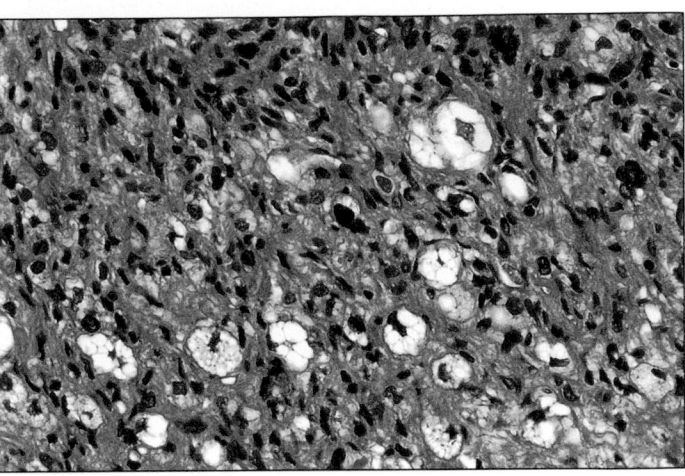

Fig. 9.122 Pleomorphic liposarcoma. Abundant lipoblasts are seen in this field.

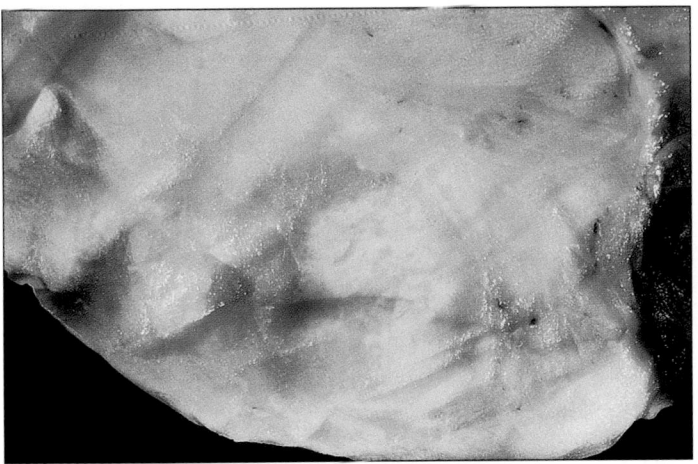

Fig. 9.121 Pleomorphic liposarcoma. The gross appearance is both fatty and like 'fish-flesh.'

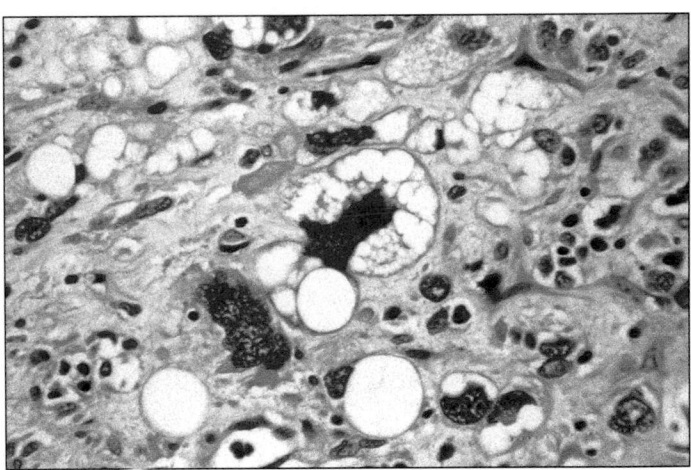

Fig. 9.123 Pleomorphic liposarcoma. These pleomorphic lipoblasts have crisp indentations of their nuclei by lipid. Compare this to the appearance of myxoid malignant fibrous histiocytoma/myxofibrosarcoma in Figure 9.71.

pleomorphic liposarcoma may exhibit a well developed capillary vascular pattern, which may appear somewhat 'plexiform'.

The differential diagnosis of pleomorphic liposarcoma includes other variants of liposarcoma and undifferentiated soft tissue sarcomas such as MFH. Pleomorphic liposarcoma may be distinguished from undifferentiated sarcomas such as MFH by the presence of pleomorphic lipoblasts. Clearly if the microscopically examined tissue lacks these cells then appropriate diagnosis is not possible. A minority of myxoid MFHs (high-grade myxofibrosarcomas) contain vacuolated oval pleomorphic tumor cells. These vacuoles, which correspond to markedly dilated rough endoplasmic reticulum, may simulate the lipid vacuoles of pleomorphic liposarcoma. Careful microscopic examination usually reveals the presence of basophilic flocculent material within the vacuole in contrast to the completely 'empty' appearance of a genuine lipid vacuole. The basophilic material is microscopically and ultrastructurally identical to the abundant extracellular matrix found in myxoid MFH.

SMOOTH MUSCLE TUMORS, INCLUDING CUTANEOUS EXAMPLES

LEIOMYOMA

Benign smooth muscle neoplasms are relatively common tumors. Most occur in the female genital tract. Less frequent sites include the gastrointestinal tract, the skin and subcutaneous tissues, the genitourinary tract, and the deep soft tissues.

Grossly, leiomyomas are typically well circumscribed nodular tumors with a firm, gray to white cut surface displaying a whorled or lobulated pattern. Degenerative changes include hemorrhage with central brownish-red softening, myxoid change with a hydropic, gelatinous appearance, and cystic change. Calcification is common. The presence of significant hemorrhage and/or necrosis within a large tumor suggests potential malignancy.

Microscopic features of smooth muscle differentiation include spindle-shaped cells arranged into interlacing bundles or fascicles, which often intersect at right angles. The nuclei are typically blunt-ended or 'cigar-shaped' and often show nuclear membrane indentations. Juxtanuclear vacuoles containing glycogen, as demonstrated by periodic acid–Schiff (PAS) staining, are commonly seen. The cytoplasm contains longitudinally arranged myofilaments that are seen as eosinophilic striations and are highlighted by their fuchsinophilia with the Masson trichrome stain. A thin outer basal lamina is present between the cells, which can be demonstrated by PAS or reticulin staining, or by immunohistochemical staining for collagen type IV.

The most characteristic microscopic pattern is that of intersecting fascicles of well differentiated spindled smooth muscle cells. However, a diversity of other cytologic and architectural patterns may be encountered. Myxoid change or extensive hyalinization may be present. Nuclear palisading, resembling the so-called Verocay bodies of benign nerve sheath tumors, is common. Long-standing tumors may show focal calcification and, less frequently, metaplastic ossification. Bizarre, enlarged, and hyperchromatic nuclei are sometimes present (symplastic change). These nuclear changes may initially appear alarming but the lack of associated mitotic activity is often a clue to the degenerative nature of such pleomorphism. Occasionally, smooth muscle tumors are comprised of cytologically round cells with an 'epithelioid' appearance (formerly designated leiomyoblastoma). Formalin fixation may cause artifactual perinuclear vacuolization.

Leiomyomas consistently express vimentin, desmin, MSA, SMA, calponin, and h-caldesmon. MSA is almost always present in leiomyomas. However, it is also expressed in skeletal and cardiac muscle as well as pericytes, myofibroblasts, myoepithelial cells, and decidual cells. Staining for more specific antibodies to alpha and gamma isoforms of SMA may also be performed. Normal smooth muscle, pericytes, myoepithelium, myofibroblasts, and most benign smooth muscle tumors also display SMAs. Calponin and h-caldesmon are both reactive with smooth muscle; h-caldesmon is more specific for smooth muscle. Calponin also stains myofibroblasts (as do MSA and SMA).[273]

Leiomyomas of the skin and subcutaneous tissue

Leiomyomas of the skin and subcutaneous tissues (leiomyoma cutis) can be divided into three distinct subtypes. These include the superficial cutaneous (pilar) leiomyoma, the genital leiomyoma (including those arising in the nipple, scrotum, and vulva), and the more deeply situated angioleiomyoma (vascular leiomyoma).

Cutaneous (pilar) leiomyoma

Superficial cutaneous leiomyomas usually present during early adulthood, occur with equal frequency in both sexes, and most commonly involve the extensor surfaces of the extremities. Other common locations include the trunk, face, and chest. Patients typically present with multiple, small, slow-growing tumor papules and nodules, which may be present individually or in groups. The grouped nodules may coalesce to form plaques in a linear or arciform distribution, often corresponding to a dermatome. More than one body site may be synchronously affected. Individual tumor nodules are small, usually less than 2–3 cm in diameter. The skin surface over the tumor nodules is often pink to red, but may appear yellow to brown. Occasionally, the nodules appear waxy, glistening, or semi-translucent. Telangiectatic vessels may be seen on the surface.

Burning, pinching, or stabbing pain that is exacerbated by fluctuations in temperature or application of pressure is frequently described.

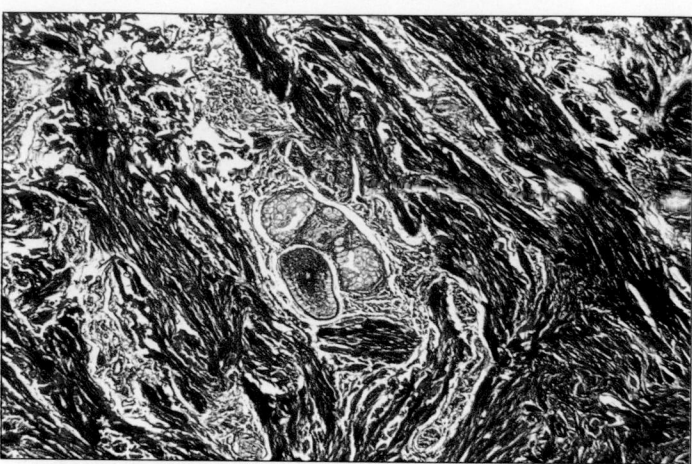

Fig. 9.124 Cutaneous leiomyoma, Masson stain. This tumor is intimately associated with the arrector pili muscle. The cytoplasm of the cells is characterized by delicate longitudinal striations.

Several reports have described a hereditary form of multiple leiomyomas of the skin. Pedigree analysis in these families suggests an autosomal dominant mode of inheritance. Familial multiple leiomyomas have also been described in association with dermatitis herpetiformis, FAP of the gastrointestinal tract (Gardner's syndrome), multiple uterine leiomyomas (Reed's syndrome), and multiple endocrine neoplasia (type 1).[274]

Multifocal cutaneous leiomyomas are thought to arise from the arrectores pilorum muscles within the dermis. This hypothesis is supported by the occasional histologic finding of an arrector pili muscle adjacent to or fused with the leiomyoma. Grossly, small, firm, nodular masses are present beneath the skin surface that display a grayish white cut surface. Microscopically, a poorly circumscribed mass, comprised of intersecting bundles of spindle-shaped cells with typical features of smooth muscle differentiation (see above) is seen within the reticular dermis. Infrequently, the tumor may encroach upon the deeper subcutaneous fat. The smooth muscle bundles commonly show interdigitation of the fibers into the adjacent collagenous dermal stroma along the peripheral edge of the tumor, while the central portion of the tumor consists of solidly packed smooth muscle bundles. Above the tumor, a grenz zone of uninvolved papillary dermis separates the tumor from an often atrophic overlying epidermis. Importantly, mitotic activity is low and should be less than 1 mitotic figure/10 hpf.[275] When the mitotic frequency equals or exceeds 1 mitotic figure/10 hpf, the possibility of leiomyosarcoma should be considered, as discussed below.

Solitary cutaneous leiomyomas occur less frequently than multifocal tumors. When they occur in nongenital sites, they are histologically similar to the multifocal lesions described above (Fig. 9.124). The microscopic differential diagnosis of cutaneous pilar leiomyomas includes fibrous histiocytoma, cutaneous smooth muscle hamartoma, and accessory nipple.

Although malignant transformation does not occur, the multifocal nature of these lesions may make them difficult to manage

Genital leiomyoma

Smooth muscle tumors classified as genital leiomyomas include those involving the nipple, the scrotum, and the vulva. Although they are often grouped together, published reports have identified distinguishing features of these tumors at the different genital sites.

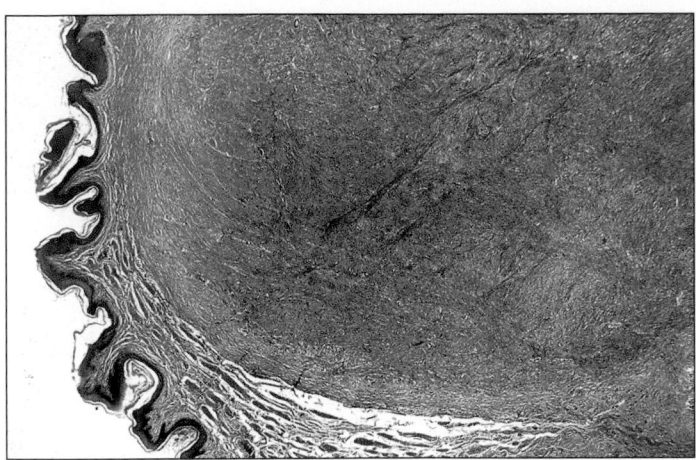

Fig. 9.125 Scrotal leiomyoma.

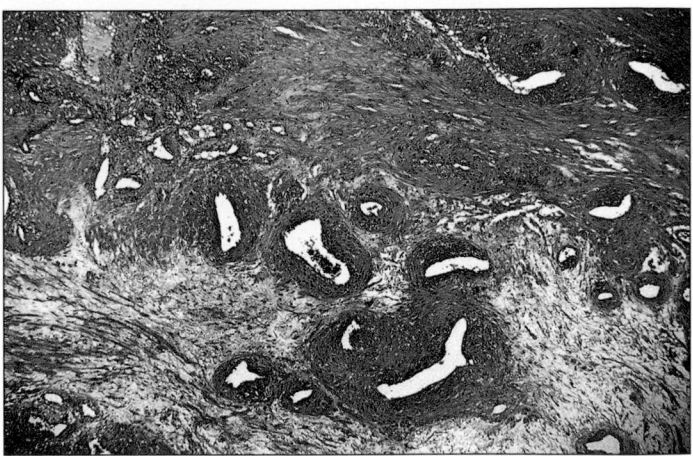

Fig. 9.126 Angiomyoma. Note that the vessels appear to merge with the surrounding lesion.

Leiomyoma of the nipple occurs in young adults and presents as a painful small nodular mass arising from the muscularis mammillae and areolae. These tumors are generally less than 1 cm in diameter. Microscopically, fascicles of well differentiated, spindled smooth muscle cells are seen in the mid to upper dermis. At the peripheral margin of the tumor, the fascicles interdigitate between the adjacent dermal collagen, creating an irregular margin. Hyperplasia of the superficial epidermis may be seen. Importantly, cytologic atypia and mitoses are not generally present. These smooth muscle tumors of the nipple are almost always benign and are considered to be analogous to cutaneous pilar leiomyomas.[276] Extremely rare cases of leiomyosarcoma of the nipple have been reported.[277,278]

Scrotal leiomyomas typically occur in middle-aged adults. These tumors are thought to arise from the dartos muscle (Fig. 9.125). They are relatively larger than other genital leiomyomas, with tumors as large as 14 cm reported in the literature. Clinically, they are usually painless lesions often mistaken for benign epidermal inclusion cysts. Microscopically, fascicles of well differentiated spindled smooth muscle cells are seen within the dermis and are surrounded by dartoic muscle fibers. As with cutaneous pilar and nipple leiomyomas, the peripheral margin typically shows an irregular interdigitating, infiltrating border. Bizarre nuclei featuring nuclear enlargement, pleomorphism, hyperchromasia, macronucleoli, and multinucleation are occasionally present.[279] These pleomorphic, bizarre nuclei are considered a degenerative phenomenon and are unassociated with mitotic activity. A grenz zone of uninvolved superficial papillary dermis is often present. Prominent lymphoid aggregates are frequently seen. The presence of mitotic figures is suggestive of malignancy.[280]

Vulvar leiomyomas occur in early to middle adulthood. Clinically, these lesions often present as a painless lump on gynecological examination and may be mistaken for a Bartholin's gland cyst. The labium majus is the most common location. Although they vary in size, as a group they are generally smaller than scrotal leiomyomas. Microscopically, these tumors are comprised of fascicles of well differentiated spindled smooth muscle cells. In contrast to the other types of genital leiomyoma, these tumors are often well circumscribed. Infiltrating margins are not frequently seen and, when present in combination with other unfavorable features, may suggest malignancy. Myxoid change (common in pregnant patients) and hyalinization may be prominent. Criteria for defining malignancy have been difficult to establish with certainty. Although no single criterion has proved reliable, features suggesting potentially malignant behavior include tumors larger than 5 cm in diameter, 5 or more mitoses per hpf, and an infiltrating margin.[281–283]

Angioleiomyoma/angiomyoma (vascular leiomyoma)

Angioleiomyoma typically presents as a clinically painful, solitary nodular mass, most frequently located in the extremities or head and neck region. This tumor often occurs in middle-aged adults and is more common in females. Tactile pressure and exposure to cold temperatures exacerbate symptomatic pain, which may relate to vascular contraction with ischemia and/or the occasional presence of intratumoral nerve fibers. The pain may worsen during pregnancy or menses. These tumors typically have been present for several years at the time of presentation and rarely recur following excision.

Grossly, these neoplasms are often small, firm, nodular, and well circumscribed masses. Most tumors measure less than 2 cm in diameter. Upon sectioning, a gray-white or brown cut surface is seen. In contrast to the cutaneous leiomyomas of pilar origin, these tumors are located more deeply in subcutaneous tissue. Microscopically, these tumors are comprised of a mixture of smooth muscle and vascular elements (Fig. 9.126). Occasionally, a small component of adipose tissue and/or nerve is present. Myxoid and hyaline changes are common. Other occasional findings include calcification, hemosiderin, and lymphocytic inflammatory infiltrates. These lesions are essentially amitotic.

Three subtypes of angioleiomyoma have been described: solid, cavernous, and venous.[284] Most tumors are of the solid type, with compact, spindled smooth muscle bundles that surround and extend tangentially outward from small, slit-like vascular channels. The venous type is second in frequency, with less compact smooth muscle bundles surrounding venous vessels with thick muscular walls. Finally, the cavernous type is comprised of a smaller amount of smooth muscle surrounding dilated vascular channels, sometimes containing luminal thrombi.

The microscopic differential diagnosis includes another painful lesion, the glomus tumor. Epithelioid, rounded cytology, a more abundant component of nerve fibers, and the classic subungual location distinguish the glomus tumor. Glomus tumors express SMA but typically lack desmin.

Leiomyoma of deep soft tissue

Benign smooth muscle neoplasms of the deep soft tissues are rare.[285–287] They may occur at any age and with equal frequency in males and females. Clinically, these tumors often present as a painless mass, which may have been present for several years. They arise in the deep subcutaneous tissues or muscles of the extremities, the abdominal cavity, or the retroperitoneum.

Grossly, these tumors are relatively large, often more than 5 cm in diameter. Their larger size, as compared with leiomyomas at other sites, may reflect a long, clinically asymptomatic growth period. They are typically well circumscribed and display a gray-white, whorled cut surface. Hemorrhage, cystic degeneration, and calcification may be present. Necrosis is notably absent.

Microscopically, these tumors are comprised of intersecting fascicles of bland, spindled smooth muscle cells with elongated, tapering eosinophilic cytoplasm. Most lack both significant nuclear pleomorphism and prominent nucleoli. However, cystic degeneration can be seen and may be associated with atypical, pleomorphic, bizarre nuclear morphology akin to that seen in the so-called 'ancient' schwannoma (symplastic change). This nuclear atypia is considered a degenerative phenomenon associated with long-standing, slow-growing tumors. Other microscopic features include nuclear palisading, myxoid change, stromal hyalinization, dystrophic calcification, metaplastic ossification, and the presence of mature adipose tissue (lipoleiomyoma or myolipoma,[207] see Figs 9.103, 9.104). Importantly, mitotic figures are notably scarce and should not be atypical. Quantitatively, they do not exceed 1 mitosis per 50 hpf and should even be absent.

Deep soft tissue leimoyomas are far exceeded by leiomyosarcomas in frequency and should therefore be diagnosed with caution. Although a specific threshold is difficult to establish, it has been suggested that when the mitotic rate exceeds 1 mitosis per 20 hpf, the potential for malignancy should be considered. Mitotic counts cannot be used as a criterion in isolation, since retroperitoneal smooth muscle tumors with extremely low mitotic activity have been known to metastasize.[288] Adequate sampling of tissue for thorough microscopic examination is required.

In females, it is also particularly important to note the precise location of tumors arising within the abdomen, as they may be detached pedunculated uterine leiomyomas. Mitotic rates in uterine tumors may be higher and this may result in an erroneous diagnosis of deep soft tissue leiomyosarcoma.[286] Tumors arising in the vicinity of the pelvis in females should also be distinguished from the broad ligament, which may microscopically simulate a leiomyoma. Lastly, there is a subset of deep leiomyomas found in the retroperitoneum and abdomen of young women that are hormone-receptor-positive and resemble uterine lesions despite extrauterine location[285]

LEIOMYOSARCOMA

Malignant smooth muscle neoplasms account for approximately 5–10% of all sarcomas. Although they may occur at any age, they are more common during adulthood and are more frequent in women. They arise at various locations and can bear a close gross resemblance to leiomyomas. Like leiomyomas, leiomyosarcomas have distinct, sharply marginated borders. They appear as firm, nodular masses with a fleshy, gray-white to beige whorled or lobulated cut surface. Cystic degeneration may be prominent. In contrast to leiomyomas, leiomyosarcomas are typically solitary, larger, and frequently display areas of hemorrhage and necrosis

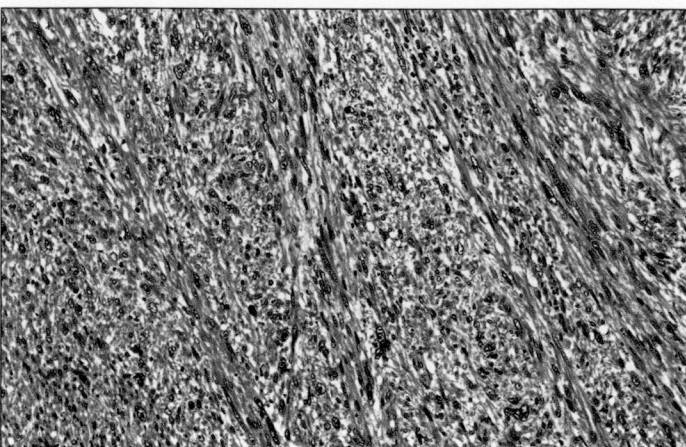

Fig. 9.127 Leiomyosarcoma. The brightly eosinophilic fascicles are perpendicularly oriented.

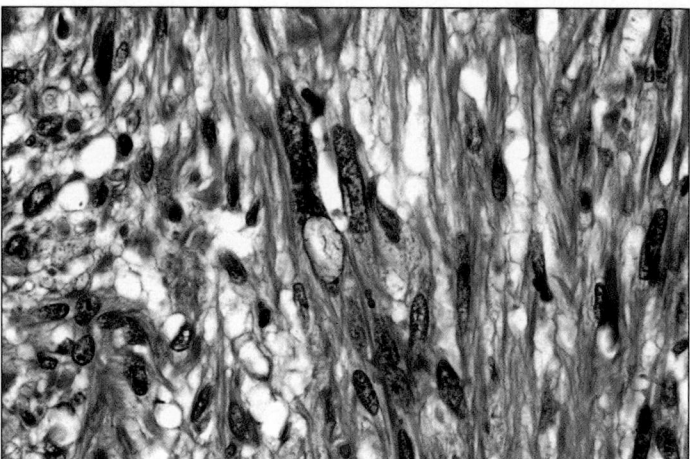

Fig. 9.128 Leiomyosarcoma. Blunt-ended nuclei, paranuclear vacuoles, and delicate eosinophilic cytoplasmic longitudinal striations are all seen in this field.

Microscopically, well differentiated leiomyosarcomas show typical features of smooth muscle differentiation similar to those described above for leiomyomas (Figs 9.127, 9.128). Increased mitotic activity is an important criterion in establishing a malignant diagnosis. With lesser degrees of differentiation, atypical cytologic features are often present. Architecturally, moderately differentiated tumors are less orderly, with a more haphazard fascicular pattern. A greater degree of nuclear hyperchromasia and pleomorphism is seen, often with conspicuous nucleoli. The poorly differentiated tumors demonstrate an even greater degree of architectural disarray and nuclear anaplasia. Bizarre, pleomorphic, or multinucleated giant cells can be seen. As is common in leiomyomas, nuclear palisading reminiscent of peripheral nerve sheath tumors may be prominent. Hemorrhage and/or necrosis are common, often corresponding to the gross appearance. A diagnostically important feature is the presence of mitotic figures. Mitotic figures are useful in establishing malignancy and are discussed below in the specific discussions of leiomyosarcoma at various sites.

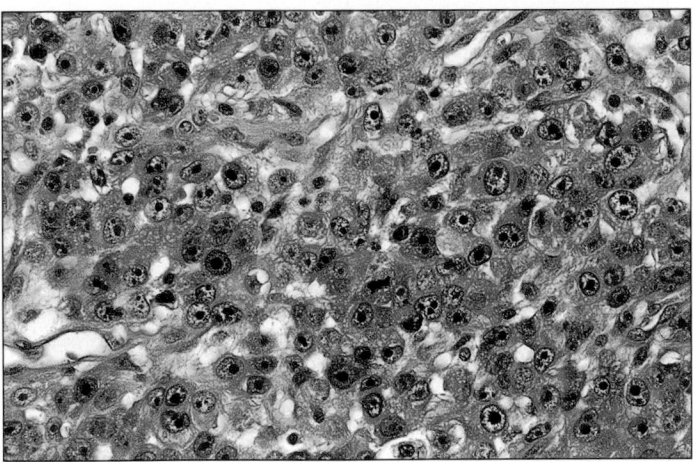

Fig. 9.129 Epithelioid leiomyosarcoma.

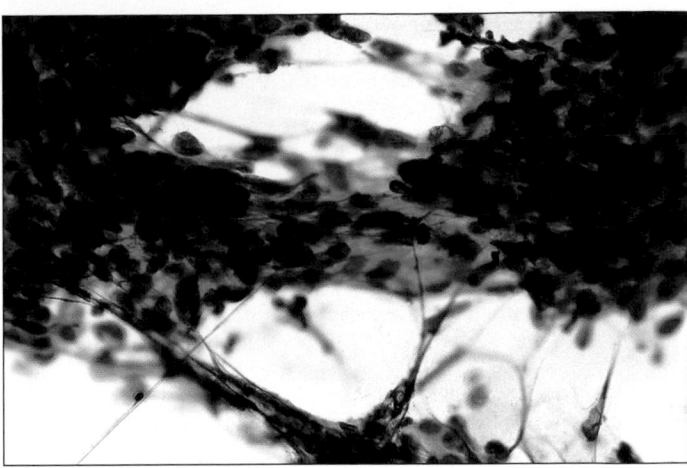

Fig. 9.131 Leiomyosarcoma, aspiration cytology. The fibrillary cytoplasm and blunt-ended nuclei are apparent on Papanicolaou stain.

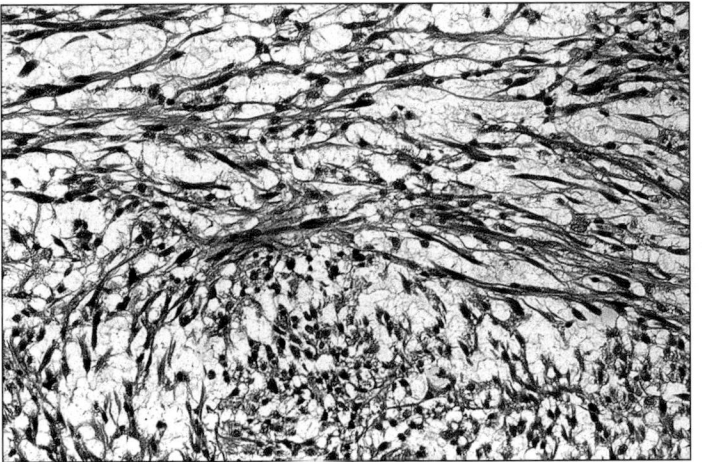

Fig. 9.130 Myxoid leiomyosarcoma.

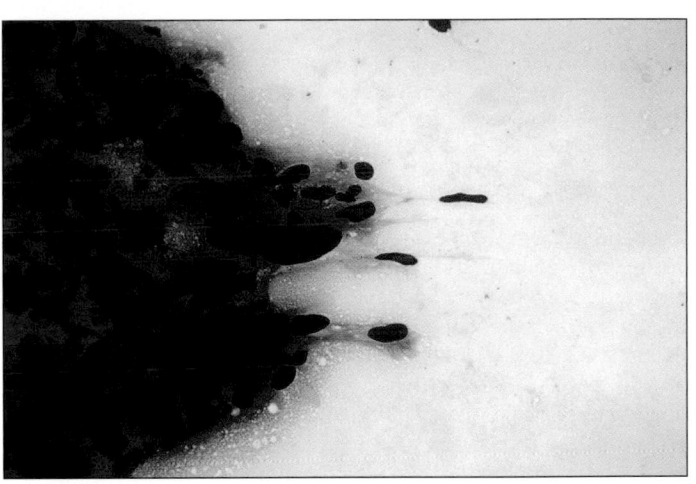

Fig. 9.132 Leiomyosarcoma, aspiration cytology. The Diff-Quik highlights the fibrillary cytoplasm.

Several microscopic variants of the usual well differentiated smooth muscle pattern exist. One common variant, the 'epithelioid' leiomyosarcoma (formerly designated leiomyoblastoma), is comprised of round, rather than spindled, cells with central nuclei and abundant eosinophilic cytoplasm, imparting an epithelioid appearance (Fig. 9.129). The cytoplasm contains fewer myofilaments than the typical well differentiated leiomyosarcoma. The epithelioid component is often admixed with a population of spindled cells showing typical features of smooth muscle differentiation. These epithelioid leiomyosarcomas commonly show artifactual cytoplasmic perinuclear clearing (vacuolar change) due to formalin fixation. This clear cell morphology can lead to difficulty in microscopically distinguishing these tumors from carcinoma, liposarcoma, and melanoma. Importantly, these clear vacuoles do not stain for mucins, fat, or glycogen. Other variant patterns include a myxoid pattern (Fig. 9.130), which may show microcystic change, a well vascularized, pericytomatous pattern, a 'storiform' pattern reminiscent of fibrohistiocytic tumors, a hyalinized and often hypocellular pattern, and a 'dedifferentiated' pattern with prominent nuclear enlargement,

hyperchromasia, and pleomorphism. Granular leiomyosarcomas have also been described.

On fine-needle aspirates, leiomyosarcomas can sometimes be recognized by their fibrillary cytoplasm and blunt-ended nuclei (Figs 9.131, 9.132).

The histologic differential diagnosis of leiomyosarcoma includes other spindle cell neoplasms, such as fibrosarcoma, malignant peripheral nerve sheath tumor, hemangiopericytoma, synovial sarcoma, and MFH. When evaluating cutaneous tumors, spindle cell melanoma, spindle cell squamous cell carcinoma, and atypical fibroxanthoma also need to be considered. Epithelioid tumors may be difficult to distinguish from carcinoma and melanoma. Clear cell (vacuolar) change may suggest a clear cell carcinoma or liposarcoma.

In contrast to leiomyoma, desmin expression in leiomyosarcoma is often only focal or even absent. One early series reported a lack of desmin expression in almost half of the leiomyosarcomas examined,[289] although more recent reports note more consistent staining.[280,290] Muscle-specific actin is expressed in many leiomyosarcomas but is not specific. It is also expressed in tumors with skeletal muscle, pericytic, and myofibroblastic differentiation. Leiomyosarcomas show variable expression of SMAs. The positive yield with SMA antibodies may reflect the degree of differentiation within the tumor.

An interesting and important immunohistochemical feature of leiomyosarcoma is the occasional expression of epithelial antigens. One early series documented both cytokeratin and EMA staining in approximately half of the reported cases.[291] This emphasizes the need for a panel approach in classifying tumors by immunohisto-chemistry. A variety of sarcomas (e.g. leiomyosarcoma, synovial sarcoma, epithelioid sarcoma, angiosarcoma) may express epithelial markers. In contrast to other spindle cell tumors, there is no characteristic cytogenetic/molecular profile for leiomyosarcomas although site-specific patterns of alterations have been described.[292]

Criteria for malignancy

Leiomyosarcomas of the soft tissues include those found within the deep soft tissues and retroperitoneum, skin and subcutaneous tissue, and blood vessels. An important concept to appreciate is that micro-scopically similar smooth muscle neoplasms arising at different sites do not always behave in the same manner. Hence, the establishment of criteria for malignancy has been difficult and has required correlation of site-specific pathological findings with patient outcome. Criteria for malignancy, including tumor location, size, and mitotic rate, are discussed below for individual soft tissue sites. Still, in some cases, it may not be possible to make a definitively malignant interpretation and the designation of a tumor as 'border-line' or 'of uncertain malignant potential' may be appropriate.

Deep soft tissue/retroperitoneal leiomyosarcomas

Malignant smooth muscle neoplasms arising in the deep soft tissues and retroperitoneum can occur at any age, but most are diagnosed during middle age, between 40 and 70 years.[288,293–297] At the time of diagnosis, these tumors have been present for a period of weeks to several years. The majority of reports have shown a female pre-dominance, especially among the retroperitoneal tumors.[294] Clinically, abdominal pain, nausea, vomiting, anorexia, weight loss, fatigue, and malaise are common presenting symptoms.[288]

Correlation between size, mitotic rate, and clinical outcome attest to the fact that all smooth muscle neoplasms arising in these locations should be regarded with caution. While the average reported size of malignant tumors in several series ranged between 5 and 7.5 cm in diameter, recurrence has been described for tumors as small as 1.5 cm. Similarly low thresholds for establishing malignancy apply when using mitotic index criteria. It has been suggested that tumors with 1–4 mitoses/10 hpf should be regarded as potentially malignant, and those with 5 or more mitoses/10 hpf as malignant. However, it is important to remain aware that malignancy has been associated with as few as 1 mitotic figure/10 hpf.[288] Truly benign leiomyomas of the deep soft tissue are exceedingly rare and such a diagnosis requires attention to mitotic index and cytologic criteria. Any smooth muscle neoplasm of the deep soft tissue with more than 1 mitotic figure per 20 hpf should be regarded as suspicious for malignancy.[286] If cytologic atypia is found, any mitoses at all are tantamount to malignancy.[297] Thus, most tumors arising at these sites are best regarded as malignant, as neither small size nor low mitotic activity necessarily predicts a benign outcome. Metastases are most commonly to lungs and liver. Less common sites include other soft tissues, skin, gastrointestinal tract, bone, and lymph nodes.

Cutaneous/subcutaneous leiomyosarcomas

Superficial leiomyosarcomas typically occur in middle-aged to elderly adults. In contrast to those in the retroperitoneum and

deep soft tissues, they are more frequent in males.[298,299] The extremities are the most common site. Patients clinically present with a raised nodular mass below the skin. Pain is reported in the majority of cases. Other symptoms include pruritus, burning, and bleeding.

These superficial tumors have been subdivided into cutaneous and subcutaneous leiomyosarcomas.[300] This distinction reflects the hypothetical smooth muscle source from which these neoplasms arise. The more superficial cutaneous tumors are thought to arise from the arrector pili muscle in the dermis or from superficial blood vessels, while the deeper subcutaneous tumors probably arise from deeper vessels. Two distinctly different growth patterns have been described. The cutaneous tumors arising from arrector pili muscle show a diffuse growth pattern, characterized by a non-encapsulated, infiltrative proliferation of well differentiated spindle cells, arranged in intersecting fascicles, extending into the adjacent collagen. They frequently display low cellularity, minimal cytologic atypia, lower mitotic rates, and a lack of tumor necrosis. In contrast, other tumors presumably of vascular origin, both cutaneous and subcutaneous, are characterized by a nodular growth pattern. These well circumscribed neoplasms are more likely to show increased cellularity, nuclear pleomorphism, multi-nucleation, numerous mitoses, necrosis, and extension into the subcutaneous tissue. Epithelioid variants have been encountered in the skin/subcutis.[301]

As with smooth muscle neoplasms arising in the peripheral soft tissue and retroperitoneum, the clinical behavior of superficial leiomyosarcomas is often difficult to predict. Hence, criteria for establishing malignancy reflect such uncertainty. While there does appear to be some correlation between large size, high mitotic counts, and recurrence or metastasis, tumors with as few as 1 mitosis/10 hpf and as small as 0.8 cm in diameter have demonstrated malignant behavior.[299,300] Perhaps more importantly, the depth of these superficial tumors within the skin and subcutaneous tissue has prognostic sig-nificance. While cutaneous smooth muscle neoplasms have been reported to recur locally in 25–50% of cases, metastases are exceedingly rare. A single case of a dermal tumor that metastasized and eventually led to the death of the patient has been reported. However, the location of the tumor in that case was described as 'deep' dermis and was specifically distinguished from the location of more superficial cutaneous tumors in that series.[302] In contrast, both recurrence (50–70% of cases) and metastases (30–40% of cases) have been reported more frequently with the deeper sub-cutaneous tumors.[303] Therefore, any subcutaneous tumor should be regarded as having potential for recurrence or metastasis, while the cutaneous tumors are only likely to recur. Large tumor size and high mitotic rates are also useful but are not reliable indicators of malig-nancy. Any tumor with 1 or more mitotic figure/10 hpf, regardless of location, should be considered potentially malignant. Metastases from these superficial leiomyosarcomas commonly involve the lungs, liver, and bone. Because both types of tumor may recur locally, wide surgical excision of these lesions is warranted and is the treatment of choice.

Vascular leiomyosarcomas

Vascular leiomyosarcomas are derived from smooth muscle cells within the medial layer of blood vessels. These tumors commonly occur within veins, most often the inferior vena cava (IVC). Other locations, in order of frequency, are the peripheral veins, the pul-monary artery, and the peripheral arterial vessels.[304] In fact, it has been suggested that most soft tissue leiomyosarcomas are of vascular origin.[297]

Leiomyosarcoma of the IVC typically presents during middle adulthood, predominantly in women. Patient symptoms vary with the location of the tumor. Those arising in the middle portion of the IVC (infrahepatic/suprarenal) are most frequent (41.7%) and often present as a palpable abdominal mass with associated abdominal pain, weight loss, and occasional lower limb swelling. Clinically, the abdominal pain is often erroneously attributed to biliary tract disease. Evidence of renal dysfunction suggests extension into or obstruction of the renal vein. Those tumors involving the lower portion of the IVC (infrarenal) are next in frequency (34%). Patients more often present with a palpable abdominal mass, flank pain, and lower extremity edema. Finally, patients with tumors of the superior portion of the IVC (suprahepatic) (24.3%) can manifest symptoms of the Budd–Chiari syndrome (hepatic vein thrombosis) with associated jaundice, ascites, and hepatomegaly. Other general signs and symptoms in all groups include dyspnea, fever, night sweats, weakness, anorexia, nausea, vomiting, and increasing abdominal girth.

Vascular leiomyosarcomas are relatively slow-growing tumors that are typically attached to the wall of the vena cava and exhibit extraluminal growth. Yet some do project into the lumen and are often associated with luminal thrombosis. Intraluminal tumor thrombi may extend into the renal veins, the hepatic vein, or even the right atrium. These tumors may also extend outward into the retroperitoneum. Reported cases range in size from 2 to 30 cm, with a mean diameter of 11 cm. Histologically, typical features of smooth muscle differentiation are present with varying degrees of cytologic atypia. Mitoses are often plentiful[305] but there is no specific mitotic threshold for determining malignancy. Surgical resection seems to offer the only chance for survival. Half of all patients develop metastases. Common sites include the lung, liver, kidney, pleura, chest wall, and bone.

Venous leiomyosarcomas of the extremities also occur in middle-aged to elderly adults but have an equal sex distribution. Peripheral veins of the lower extremities, including the iliac, femoral, popliteal, and saphenous veins, are most often involved. Clinically, the characteristic presentation is lower extremity edema. Projection into the vascular lumen with associated thrombosis is common. Reported cases vary in size, some measuring as large as 18 cm. Histologically, typical features of smooth muscle differentiation are seen, including interlacing fascicles of spindled cells, with variable mitotic rates and foci of hemorrhage and necrosis. Mitoses are generally frequent and do not appear to be useful in predicting outcome. Criteria for malignancy are not well defined. Surgical excision is the treatment of choice. Common metastatic sites include the lungs and liver.

Pulmonary artery leiomyosarcomas occur less frequently than intimal sarcomas, comprising approximately 20% of all pulmonary artery sarcomas. These tumors also arise in middle-aged adults with an approximately equal sex distribution. Clinically, symptoms include dyspnea, chest or back pain, cough, dizziness or syncope, hemoptysis, cyanosis, and evidence of right-sided heart failure. This combination of symptoms is often incorrectly attributed to pulmonary thromboembolism; the correct diagnosis is often made at autopsy. The tumors usually arise within the main pulmonary artery near the base of the heart with extension into the main pulmonary branches and sometimes into the lung. Pulmonary metastases are most frequent, but distant sites may be involved. The average survival from diagnosis is approximately 1 year.

Uterine leiomyosarcomas, leiomyomatosis peritonealis disseminata, intravenous leiomyomatosis, and benign metastasizing leiomyoma are covered in the chapter on gynecologic pathology.

IMMUNOSUPPRESSION-ASSOCIATED SMOOTH MUSCLE NEOPLASMS

Benign and malignant smooth muscle neoplasms have been described in association with immunosuppression. The typical clinical settings include both human immunodeficiency virus (HIV) infection[306–312] and post-transplantation therapeutic immunosuppression.[313] The reported HIV-associated cases predominantly involve children and young adults with a predilection for visceral organs rather than the soft tissues. Common sites include the lungs, gastrointestinal tract, and liver, but other sites are also reported, including the adrenal gland and spleen.

Several reports have demonstrated the presence of Epstein–Barr virus within these tumors by in situ hybridization. Smooth muscle tumors in non-immunocompromised patients were negative for Epstein–Barr virus viral sequences.[307]

Criteria for establishing malignancy generally reflect those applied to smooth muscle neoplasms arising at the particular site in non-immunocompromised patients. The designation of malignancy is particularly difficult in visceral organs, such as the liver, where criteria are not well defined. In such cases, a designation of smooth muscle neoplasm of undetermined malignant potential may be appropriate. While multifocality might suggest malignant behavior with metastases, the association with Epstein–Barr virus in these cases could also indicate multiple primary sites.

The differential diagnosis of these smooth muscle neoplasms includes those previously mentioned for smooth muscle tumors in general. However, in the setting of immunosuppression, this is expanded to include Kaposi's sarcoma and mycobacterial spindle cell pseudotumor. Kaposi's sarcoma is discussed below. Mycobacterial spindle cell pseudotumor is seen in immunosuppressed patients and commonly involves the lymph nodes and spleen. These lesions comprised a multinodular or diffuse proliferation of spindle cells with storiform architecture admixed with chronic inflammatory cells. The spindle cells are histiocytes and contain numerous intracytoplasmic acid-fast bacilli,[314] which are easily demonstrated by Ziehl Neelsen staining. Immunohistochemical staining should be interpreted with caution, as the histiocytic spindle cells may show desmin or CD31 positivity.

EXTRAINTESTINAL TUMORS OF THE GASTROINTESTINAL STROMAL TYPE

Gastrointestinal stromal tumors (GISTs) in general are covered in the gastrointestinal pathology section and their morphologic features are described there. Mazur and Clark introduced the term stromal tumor in 1983, after failing to find ultrastructural evidence of smooth muscle or nerve sheath differentiation in several gastric tumors.[315] Of course, most gastrointestinal wall tumors formerly classified as leiomyosarcomas prove to be GISTs using newer criteria, but true leiomyosarcomas do exist. They lack characteristic c-*kit* mutations.[316]

GISTs have undergone a conceptual revolution in the last few years, with the discovery that many of them show differentiation towards interstitial cells of Cajal, the 'pacemaker' cells of the gut.[317] This category also subsumes the ultrastructurally defined rare lesions previously known as gastrointestinal autonomic nerve tumors (GANT).[318,319] The availability of c-Kit/CD117 antibodies has facilitated diagnosis.

GISTs comprise 5–10% of all sarcomas. Approximately 25% of GISTs are malignant, representing about 1% of all gastrointestinal

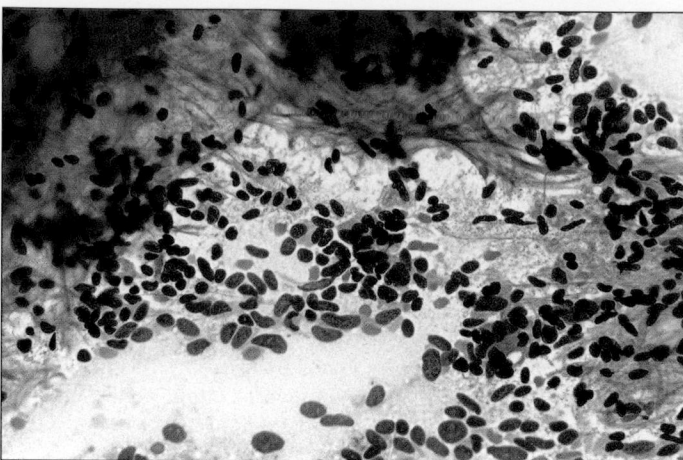

Fig. 9.133 Extragastrointestinal GIST. This aspirate is from a malignant GIST. Without performing CD117 on a cell block, it would be difficult to make a diagnosis in isolation but the striking cellularity and abundance of singly shed cells are features that suggest malignancy in aspirates.

malignancies. Extraintestinal GISTs are now known: GIST-type tumors arising in omentum,[320] peritoneum, and retroperitoneum[321] have been identified, comprising 6.7% of the large Armed Forces Institute of Pathology series of 1008 GISTs.[322] Miettinen et al.[320] described 13 omental and 10 mesenteric cases and Reith et al.[321] described 48 tumors, in 32 women and 16 men, of which 40 involved omentum or mesentery (these were not analyzed separately), and eight arose in the retroperitoneum. About 40% of the reported patients developed metastases or died of disease. In multivariate analysis, mitoses >2/50 hpf and necrosis were predictive factors of a poor outcome. It has been suggested that GISTs of omentum resemble those of stomach and that GISTs of mesentery are similar to small intestinal tumors, including a worse outcome.

The cytologic findings of a malignant retroperitoneal GIST are illustrated in Figure 9.133.

SKELETAL MUSCLE TUMORS

INTRODUCTION

When soft tissue tumors are considered in total, benign lesions outnumber malignant ones by a margin of over 100:1. The distribution is reversed, however, among skeletal muscle tumors, where rhabdomyosarcomas are 50 times more common than rhabdomyomas. Most rhabdomyosarcomas are found in children.

RHABDOMYOMAS

Rhabdomyomas have been classified as follows:

I. Cardiac rhabdomyoma
II. Extracardiac rhabdomyoma
  1. Adult rhabdomyoma
  2. Fetal rhabdomyoma
    a. Classic type
    b. Intermediate type
  3. Genital rhabdomyoma

Cardiac rhabdomyoma

Cardiac rhabdomyomas are the most common of all rhabdomyomas, presenting almost exclusively in children. These have been considered hamartomatous lesions. Between 51% and 86% of cases are associated with tuberous sclerosis.[323–328] This syndrome is characterized by a collection of hamartomatous lesions including brain malformations, epidermal nevi, facial angiofibroma, and renal angiomyolipoma. Cardiac rhabdomyomas associated with the syndrome are congenital and frequently multiple. They often regress but can cause life-threatening ventricular outflow obstruction and arrhythmias. Hence, surgery is indicated for symptomatic lesions and clinical observation for the rest.[329–331]

These lesions most commonly involve the ventricle and range from multiple microscopic lesions to large solitary tumors up to 9 cm. Microscopically, they are well demarcated and composed of uniformly vacuolated clear cells. Many contain a central vesicular nucleus, from which radiate thin strands of pink cytoplasm extending to the cell membrane, separated by large cytoplasmic vacuoles. These are called 'spider cells.' The vacuolization is created by cytoplasmic glycogen, which can be demonstrated as positivity on PAS stains that disappears with diastase pretreatment. The cells have a skeletal muscle immunophenotype, staining for desmin, actin, and myoglobin. Ultrastructurally, they demonstrate features of altered cardiac myocytes, containing myofibrils, Z-bands, and intercalated discs. Large pools of β-glycogen particles fill the cytoplasm.

Adult rhabdomyoma

Fewer than 100 cases of adult rhabdomyoma are reported in the literature.[332] Cytogenetic alterations support a neoplastic rather than a reactive condition.[333] The mean age at the time of diagnosis is approximately 50 years, with the reported age at presentation ranging from 2–82 years. The male to female ratio is approximately 4:1. Over 90% of all adult rhabdomyomas occur in the head and neck region. The most common locations are the oropharyngeal cavity (base of the tongue, palate, floor of the mouth) and the larynx.

The most common presentation of adult rhabdomyoma is that of a slow-growing unicentric mass. When tumors grow submucosally, they may obstruct the upper aerodigestive tract, leading to symptoms of hoarseness, dysphagia, foreign body sensation, or dyspnea/ stridor. Rare tumors are truly multicentric, although approximately 25% are composed of multiple grossly contiguous nodules (see below). Spontaneous regression has not been documented.

Adult rhabdomyomas are usually encapsulated, well circumscribed, unifocal lesions. Approximately 25% are grossly multinodular.[334] The median size is 3 cm. The cut surface is typically uniform, tan-brown, and rubbery. Necrosis is absent.

Histologically, these lesions have a lobular architecture and characteristically contain closely packed large polygonal cells with abundant, eosinophilic granular cytoplasm, and usually peripherally placed nuclei. The deeply eosinophilic cytoplasm of the cells reflects their prominent myofibril content. However, since the myofibrils are typically haphazardly oriented, cross-striations are only occasionally evident by light microscopy, found within scattered elongated 'strap' cells. A consistent feature is the presence of haphazardly arranged, rod-like intracytoplasmic crystals. These structures, termed 'matchstick' or 'jack-straw' crystals, actually represent clusters of randomly oriented, elongated, hypertrophic Z-bands. Both cross-striations and 'jack straw' crystals are readily highlighted with phosphotungstic

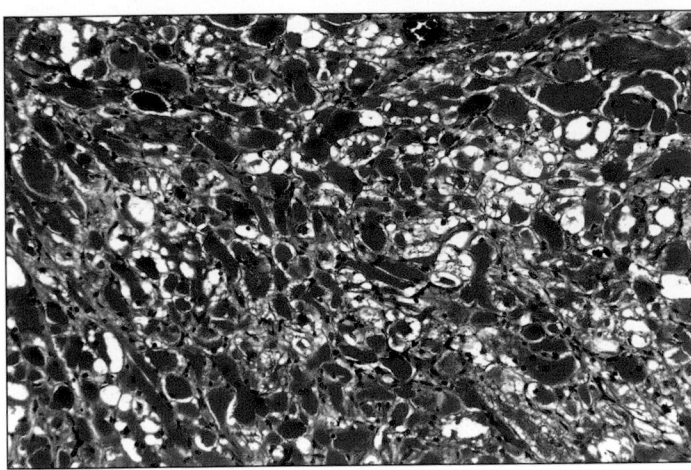

Fig. 9.134 Adult rhabdomyoma. This lesion has both striations and 'spider cells.'

acid–hematoxylin (PTAH) stain. Cytoplasmic vacuoles containing variable amounts of glycogen and lipid can be identified, although few cells have sufficient vacuolization to impart the 'spider-cell' morphology that is typical of cardiac rhabdomyomas (Fig. 9.134). Intranuclear inclusions are occasionally identified.

Immunohistochemical stains are useful for confirming myogenic differentiation. Desmin, MSA, and myoglobin stains are usually strongly positive. Cytokeratin, EMA, glial filament acid protein (GFAP), CD68, and leukocyte common antigen stains are negative. Variable results have been obtained with S-100, Leu-7, and vimentin. Of interest, several antigens that are normally restricted to fetal muscle have been detected in adult rhabdomyoma. These include fetal myosin[335] and CD56 (neural-cell adhesion molecule)[333], which is expressed strongly in fetal muscle at 18 weeks gestation but weakly at 35 weeks. These findings indicate that adult rhabdomyoma may in fact be less differentiated than their appearance would suggest.

It is remarkable that there is no record of an adult rhabdomyoma arising in the abundant skeletal musculature of the limbs. The predilection for the head and neck may relate to the fact that the skeletal muscle in this area is distinct embryologically: it is derived from the third and fourth branchial arches, unlike the peripheral musculature, which is derived from myotomes.

Adult rhabdomyomas are benign. Recurrence is common and is attributed to incomplete excision.[333,334]

The differential diagnosis for adult rhabdomyoma is granular cell tumor, alveolar soft part sarcoma, hibernoma, crystal-storing histiocytosis[334], paraganglioma, and rhabdomyosarcoma.

Fetal rhabdomyoma

Fetal rhabdomyomas are even rarer than adult rhabdomyoma. Their histopathology recapitulates the normal histology of developing fetal skeletal muscle. As such, they pose significant potential for confusion with rhabdomyosarcoma. Like adult rhabdomyomas, these tumors occur most commonly in the head and neck region. An association with the basal cell nevus syndrome (odontogenic keratocysts of the jaw, rib abnormalities, and macrocephaly, predisposition to basal cell carcinoma and other neoplasms) has been described. Fetal rhabdomyomas are often divided into two types: the classic (or myxoid) type and the intermediate (also known as cellular or juvenile) type.

Fetal rhabdomyoma, classic type

The classic fetal rhabdomyoma has a predilection for children less than 1 year of age, although it has been reported in adults. The male to female ratio is approximately 3:1. While the head and neck is the favored site, rare cases have been reported elsewhere. Within the head and neck region, fetal rhabdomyoma targets the periauricular region. The usual presentation is that of a slowly growing mass. Up to 25% are congenital.[336]

Classic fetal rhabdomyomas are unencapsulated but well demarcated, noninfiltrative lesions. The usual size range is 2–6 cm, with larger examples reported. They are almost always unifocal. Importantly, tumors are usually located superficial to the underlying musculature, often in the subcutaneous tissue or submucosa. On cut section, tumors are gray in color, often mucoid in texture, and do not show necrosis.

The histopathology of classic fetal rhabdomyoma resembles normal developing fetal musculature of 6–12 weeks gestation. The stroma is abundant and mucoid, composed of mucopolysaccharides that stain positively with Alcian blue. Two cell types are loosely arranged in this matrix. First is a population of oval to spindle-shaped primitive mesenchymal cells with indistinct cytoplasm, analogous to the primitive fibroblastic cells of developing skeletal muscle. Second is a population of immature elongated skeletal muscle fibers that resemble fetal myotubes. The latter are scattered haphazardly as single cells within the lesion, although they tend to be more abundant at its perimeter. They contain centrally placed oval nuclei with fine chromatin and inconspicuous nucleoli and tapered, thin, often bipolar cell processes. The cytoplasm is pale pink and in most cases cross-striations can be identified (although a thorough search is often required). Mitoses and pleomorphism are not present.

Fetal rhabdomyoma, intermediate type

The intermediate variant of fetal rhabdomyoma also most frequently presents in the head and neck region. In contrast to the classical variant, adults are more commonly affected. The documented age range falls between 2.5 and 60 years with a male to female preponderance of approximately 3:1. These tumors also usually present as slowly growing, asymptomatic masses. While the classical fetal rhabdomyoma tends to be superficially located, intermediate fetal rhabdomyomas are found in the deep tissues of the head and neck and often are submucosal.

Like the classic type, these tumors are well circumscribed but usually unencapsulated. Reported sizes range from 1.0–5.0 cm. The cut surface shows firm light tan to gray-white tissue without hemorrhage or necrosis.

The intermediate fetal rhabdomyoma shows a degree of rhabdomyoblastic differentiation that is greater than that of classic fetal rhabdomyoma and approaches but does not reach the level of adult rhabdomyoma. Hence, it is 'intermediate' in its level of differentiation. In contrast to the classic type of fetal rhabdomyoma, the intermediate type shows minimal to no myxoid matrix and only scattered primitive mesenchymal cells. The lesion is dominated instead by tightly packed, elongated spindled muscle fibers (hence the alternative name 'cellular'). Tumor cells are often strap-shaped and have central vesicular nuclei with variably prominent nucleoli and deeply eosinophilic cytoplasm with frequent cross-striations. They are larger than the primitive myotubes of classic fetal rhabdomyoma, and the cytoplasmic and nuclear features reflect more advanced muscular differentiation. These fibers are arranged somewhat haphazardly but often as intersecting fascicles. Occasionally, a herringbone or plexiform pattern can be appreciated. Some cells show vacuolization due to intracellular glycogen but only rare cells are large and rounded like those of adult rhabdomyoma. Some cases may display mild pleomorphism, and occasional mitoses can be present. However, abundant mitotic figures and extreme pleomorphism are not attributes of this lesion and suggest instead the diagnosis of rhabdomyosarcoma.

The immunohistochemical staining pattern of fetal rhabdomyomas of both classic and intermediate types is generally similar to that of adult rhabdomyomas. Tumors express myoglobin, desmin, and MSA. Variable staining is reported with vimentin, S100 protein, SMA, and glial fibrillary acidic protein. Cytokeratin, EMA, CD68, and Leu-7 are negative.

Fetal rhabdomyomas are postulated to be hamartomatous lesions, based upon their morphologic resemblance to developing fetal skeletal muscle.[336–338] However, cytogenetic analysis is not available on such cases to date. Their occurrence as congenital lesions supports this concept, as does their association with the malformative basal cell nevus syndrome. Their occasional association with peripheral nerves has raised the possibility of a relationship to neuromuscular hamartoma.

Fetal rhabdomyomas are usually cured by complete excision; only rare recurrences and no metastases of well characterized lesions have been reported. Their benign nature is questioned only by isolated, somewhat controversial case reports of an association with rhabdomyosarcoma.[339]

The distinction of fetal rhabdomyoma from rhabdomyosarcoma is crucial, since a misdiagnosis of rhabdomyosarcoma will trigger unnecessary and potentially harmful chemotherapy. Embryonal rhabdomyosarcoma, particularly its well differentiated spindle cell variant, is the main consideration. The intermediate type of fetal rhabdomyoma, being more cellular and having occasional mitoses and mild pleomorphism, is more likely to cause confusion. Both architectural and cytologic features can be helpful in this differential diagnosis. In contrast to fetal rhabdomyoma, rhabdomyosarcomas are usually situated deeper in the soft tissue and have an infiltrative border. While submucosal rhabdomyosarcomas may show a cambium layer, fetal rhabdomyomas do not. Cytologically, rhabdomyosarcomas show pleomorphism in the form of enlarged, hyperchromatic, angulated nuclei beyond what is acceptable in fetal rhabdomyoma. On careful examination, rhabdomyosarcomas usually show more than the scattered mitoses that are acceptable in fetal rhabdomyoma. Necrosis is often present in rhabdomyosarcoma but absent in fetal rhabdomyoma.

Genital rhabdomyoma

These tumors present as slow growing, polypoid masses in the genital tract of middle-aged women.[340] Tumors most commonly involve the vulva or vagina but rarely have arisen in the cervix. Most are asymptomatic, although some lesions cause vaginal bleeding and/or dyspareunia.[341–347] There is a single case report of tumor recurrence[341] but no recorded metastases.

Genital rhabdomyomas are polypoid lesions that usually measure less than 3 cm in diameter. They are typically covered by a smooth, intact epithelial surface. They are unencapsulated and composed of grey to pink, homogeneous, firm tissue.

The characteristic histology is that of scattered, highly mature skeletal muscle fibers set in an abundant hypocellular stroma. The fibers range from long, thin spindled cells to strap cells, with dense eosinophilic cytoplasm containing easily discernible cross-striations. Neither cytoplasmic vacuoles nor crystalline inclusions are demonstrated, and mitoses are absent. The cells usually have one central round nucleus with a prominent nucleolus, but pleomorphism is not present. Nuclei are sometimes peripherally located, as is seen in mature skeletal muscle. The stroma is variably fibrous and myxoid

and contains thin-walled blood vessels. The overlying mucosa is intact, and subepithelial condensations of cells (cambium layer) are not present.

Immunohistochemically, the tumor cells express desmin, myoglobin, actin, and myosin.

Embryonal rhabdomyosarcoma has different clinical and pathologic features. It typically occurs in younger patients: approximately 90% are less than 5 years of age. Rhabdomyosarcomas are often grossly larger than the usual genital rhabdomyoma and usually are more infiltrative. Microscopically, the cells are more primitive, mitotically active, and form subepithelial condensations (cambium layer).

Benign fibroepithelial stromal polyps of the vulva and vagina are the main clinical differential diagnosis. These can be seen at any age but also usually affect middle-aged women. The composition of their stroma is varied, ranging from nondescript bland spindle cells to pleomorphic multinucleated cells with pink cytoplasm that can simulate rhabdomyoblasts. However, true cross-striations are not identified. While the stromal cells are usually immunoreactive for desmin, curiously they are often nonimmunoreactive for actin stains. They also typically stain for estrogen and progesterone receptors, which may explain the association of these polyps with pregnancy.[348]

RHABDOMYOSARCOMA

Embryonal and alveolar rhabdomyosarcoma

Rhabdomyosarcoma is the most common pediatric soft tissue sarcoma, comprising 80–90% of reported cases. Although the name implies that these tumors arise from striated muscle, in fact a substantial percent arise from areas without it, such as the urinary bladder, prostate, common bile duct, and vagina. Thus the term reflects the tendency of the tumors to recapitulate skeletal myoblasts rather than to arise from them.

In the 1950s, rhabdomyosarcoma were subclassified into embryonal, alveolar, botryoid, and pleomorphic subtypes.[349] The histologic category of the tumor was soon found to correspond to clinical groupings, and correlation with genetic features has been subsequently demonstrated. As such, rhabdomyosarcoma encompasses a group of biologically dissimilar sarcomas that recapitulate the myogenesis pathway of embryonic tissues.

In the 1980s, it became apparent that there were additional variants that belonged in the rhabdomyosarcoma classification scheme. It was noted that the alveolar category could be expanded to encompass cytologically similar but histologically dissimilar tumors[350] (solid variant). Similarly, it was found that the embryonal category could be subdivided further into more differentiated spindle cell lesions ('spindle cell rhabdomyosarcoma') dissimilar from typical embryonal tumors[351] and might encompass neoplasms without overt myogenesis.[352] Concurrently, the development of molecular techniques has demonstrated that characteristic genetic events correlate with traditional classification schemes.[353] The existence of a large multi-institutional database and slide repository, the Intergroup Rhabdomyosarcoma Study, has been the grist for sophisticated studies that have emerged in recent years.[354–362] The current classification of rhabdomyosarcomas appears in Table 9.8.

Clinical symptomatology reflects the affected organ system. Orbital tumors present with proptosis and diplopia. Parameningeal tumors often cause neurologic defects related to spinal cord encroachment. Urinary tract tumors arising in the bladder or prostate typically present with urinary retention. Cervicovaginal tumors cause vaginal bleeding, and large masses extruding from the introitus may be evident. Painless masses are typical of extremity tumors. Biliary

Table 9.8 International classification of pediatric rhabdomyosarcoma[362]

Embryonal rhabdomyosarcoma (includes embryonal sarcoma[352])
Alveolar rhabdomyosarcoma (includes solid variants)
Botryoid rhabdomyosarcoma
Spindle cell rhabdomyosarcoma
Rhabdomyosarcoma, not otherwise classified
Undifferentiated sarcoma
Sarcoma, not classifiable

Pleomorphic rhabdomyosarcoma, although the most common form of adult rhabdomyosarcoma, is vanishingly rare in children and is not included in this pediatric classification.

Table 9.9 Rhabdomyosarcoma TNM pretreatment staging system

Stage	Sites	T	Tumor size	N	M
I	Orbit Head and neck (excluding parameningeal) Genitourinary – nonbladder/nonprostate	T1 or T2	a or b	N0 or N1 or Nx	M0
II	Bladder/prostate Extremity Head and neck parameningeal Other (including trunk, retroperitoneum, etc.)	T1 or T2	a	N0 or Nx	M0
III	Bladder/prostate Extremity Head and neck parameningeal Other (including trunk, retroperitoneum, etc.)	T1 or T2	a b	N1 N0 or N1 or Nx	M0
IV	All	T1 or T2	a or b	N0 or N1	M1

For definitions of T, N, and M, see Table 9.10

Table 9.10 Definitions of T, N, and M classifications

Classification	Description
Tumor	
T1	Confined to anatomic site of origin
A	<5 cm in diameter
B	≥5 cm in diameter
T2	Extended into or fixed in surrounding tissue
A	<5 cm in diameter
B	≥5 cm in diameter
Regional lymph nodes	
N0	Regional lymph nodes not clinically involved
N1	Regional lymph nodes clinically involved
Nx	Clinical status of regional lymph nodes unknown
Metastasis	
M0	No distant metastasis
M1	Metastasis present

tumors lead to jaundice, and nasal/paranasal lesions may cause obstructive symptoms. Of particular note is that occasional extremely aggressive rhabdomyosarcomas may present with widespread bone marrow metastases lacking an apparent primary source.[363] This presentation can mimic a hematologic malignancy, particularly as rare examples express lymphoid antigens.[364,365]

Stage, histologic type, and site of origin are the most important prognostic considerations. The TNM staging scheme for rhabdomyosarcoma is presented in Tables 9.9 and 9.10.

Histologic type is also predictive of rhabdomyosarcoma therapy response and clinical outcome,[362] independently of clinical grouping. To some degree this observation reflects the tendency of certain subtypes to manifest in particular sites and ages. As examples, embryonal rhabdomyosarcomas are most frequently head and neck and genitourinary lesions of young children, whereas alveolar rhabdomyosarcomas are most frequently extremity and parameningeal lesions of adolescents and young adults.

Over the past century, the prognosis for embryonal rhabdomyosarcomas has improved dramatically. This trend is illustrated by comparing outcomes for the large consecutive trials directed by the Intergroup Rhabdomyosarcoma Study Group (IRSG).[360] For example, outcome for group 3 embryonal rhabdomyosarcoma treated with IRSG therapy improved from an overall 5-year survival rate of 50% reported in 1988[366] to a progression-free 5-year survival rate of 65% reported in 1993.[360] Newer data appear better still at 3 years.[356]

Unfortunately, the improvements in outcome for embryonal rhabdomyosarcoma have not been mirrored by alveolar rhabdomyosarcoma, although more aggressive therapy used with the latter tumors may ameliorate some of the differences in outcome.[367]

Rhabdomyosarcomas are generally fleshy, nondescript pale gray–yellow masses with areas of necrosis and hemorrhage. They insidiously invade adjacent tissues, so that microscopic areas of marginal involvement may be apparent even with grossly resected lesions. Of particular note is the gross appearance of the botryoid variant of rhabdomyosarcoma, so named for its resemblance to a cluster of grapes (Fig. 9.135). This tumor arises exclusively along mucosa-lined surfaces such as the bladder or vagina. External examples may arise from the conjunctiva. Whether these neoplasms are embryonal rhabdomyosarcomas with mucosal involvement or a separate entity has been debated, but they are genetically identical to other embryonal rhabdomyosarcomas. Botryoid rhabdomyosarcomas have a proven superior prognosis.[361]

The primary distinguishing characteristic of rhabdomyosarcomas is their capacity for myogenesis at the microscopic level. Rhabdomyoblasts display brightly eosinophilic cytoplasm. At the more differentiated end of the spectrum, rhabdomyoblasts acquire microscopically visible cytoplasmic cross-striations that result from the submicroscopic alignment of myofilaments in register. At the less differentiated (and more common) end of the spectrum, ancillary methods of demonstrating myogenesis are often necessary for diagnostic confirmation.

Rhabdomyoblasts display a variety of odd forms such as tadpole cells, racquet cells, strap cells, spider cells, and multinucleated giant cells. Cytoplasmic glycogen is often abundant and may be manifested as clear cytoplasm, which can be demonstrated with the PAS stain (disappearing with diastase digestion). Morphologically similar

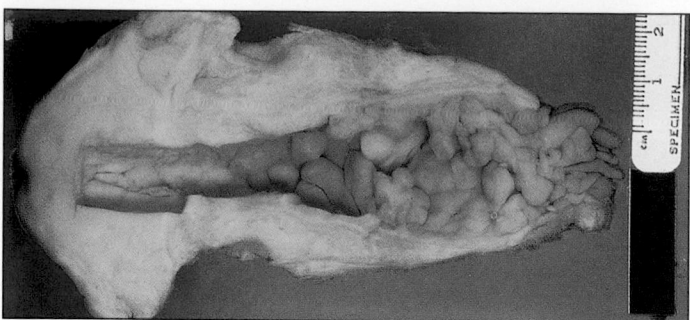

Fig. 9.135 Botryoid rhabdomyosarcoma. Note the polypoid protrusions in this infant's vagina. Such specimens are seldom seen in recent years since most tumors are biopsied and treated by chemotherapy and radiation (Courtesy of Dr Frederick Askin).

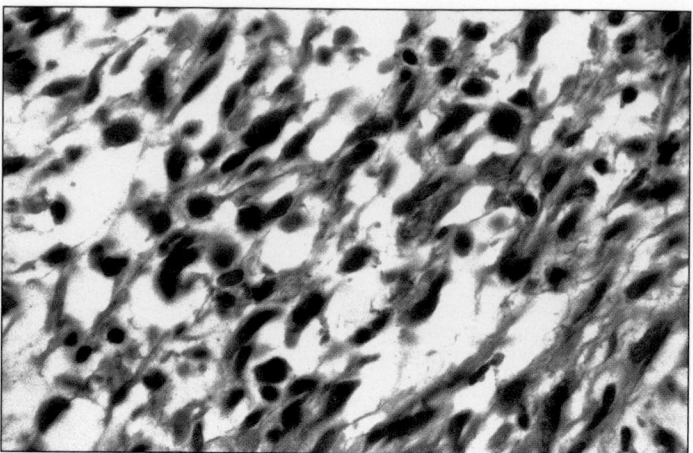

Fig. 9.137 Embryonal rhabdomyosarcoma. Rhabdomyoblasts.

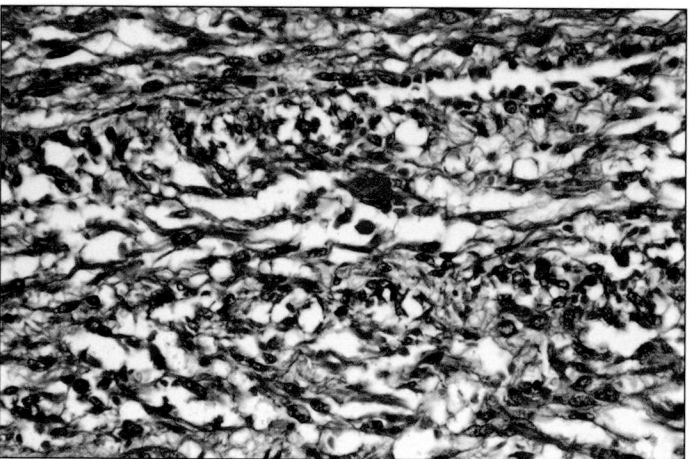

Fig. 9.136 Embryonal rhabdomyosarcoma showing a haphazard arrangement of pink rhabdomyoblasts.

neoplasms such as lymphomas and neuroblastomas generally do not contain glycogen, but exceptions occur.[368]

After finding clear evidence of myogenesis, diagnosis of rhabdomyosarcomas is a matter of subclassification, which is critical to both therapy and prognosis. Most crucial to therapy is recognition of the alveolar subtype. Although prognostically diverse, the other subtypes are currently lumped together for treatment purposes.

The most common subtype is embryonal rhabdomyosarcoma, so named for its remarkable resemblance to developing muscle in embryos and fetuses. Embryonal rhabdomyosarcoma is typified by alternating areas of cellular condensation and hypocellularity, with cells floating in mucoid ground substance. These tumors may exhibit a heterogeneous degree of differentiation, matrix, and cellularity from case to case or even within individual tumors (Figs 9.136, 9.137). Under the influence of chemical or physical agents such as oncolytic drugs, X-irradiation, cyclic adenosine monophosphate (AMP), or *cis*-retinoic acid, the cells may terminally differentiate into mature myoblasts that histologically resemble normal muscle cells.[353,369] This phenomenon can lead to difficulties in evaluating post-treatment excisions or biopsies, as tumor cells may not be separable from entrapped normal muscle.

Embryonal sarcoma is a category of soft tissue sarcoma described by the Société Internationale d'Oncologie Pédiatrique (SIOP).[352] This tumor is unrelated to embryonal sarcoma of the liver. Histologically it is characterized by a resemblance to embryonal rhabdomyosarcoma without light microscopic evidence of myogenesis. Theoretically it represents the most primitive end of the mesenchymal spectrum of embryonal rhabdomyosarcoma. Since muscle proteins may be demonstrable by immunohistochemistry, most observers regard these as embryonal rhabdomyosarcoma. It has been included in the embryonal rhabdomyosarcoma category in the International Classification and appears to have a better prognosis than classic embryonal rhabdomyosarcoma.[370]

Just as it displays a typical gross appearance that resembles a cluster of grapes, botryoid rhabdomyosarcoma also exhibits a key histologic feature, namely its cambium layer. A cambium layer consists of a subepithelial condensation of tumor cells, named for its resemblance to the more rapidly growing layer of a tree juxtaposed to its bark (Fig. 9.138). In the current international classification,[362] this feature is required for diagnosis, although it may be obscured by mucosal erosion.

Spindle cell rhabdomyosarcoma is another subtype that is associated with a better prognosis. However, spindle cell variants arise almost exclusively in the paratesticular region, a site with an independently better prognosis, so that an argument might be made that this observation is site-dependent. Grossly, spindle cell rhabdomyosarcomas have a fibrous, whorled appearance. Microscopically, these tumors are more differentiated than the usual rhabdomyosarcoma and exhibit a heavy content of muscle proteins by immunohistochemistry.[351] They histologically mimic other spindle cell sarcomas, as storiform areas may resemble fibrous histiocytoma and wavy neuroid foci may mimic nerve sheath tumors. Scattered individual round cells with larger, atypical nuclei or multinucleated giant cells with bright pink cytoplasm often punctuate these wavy and whorled bundles of spindle cells. The molecular basis for this particular variant of rhabdomyosarcoma is uncertain at present.

Alveolar rhabdomyosarcoma is a highly aggressive sarcoma. Microscopically, alveolar rhabdomyosarcomas form nests separated by a prominent framework of fibrovascular septa, thus displaying some resemblance to lung alveoli[371] (Fig. 9.139). Rows of tumor cells are suspended from these alveoli-like septa in a 'picket fence'

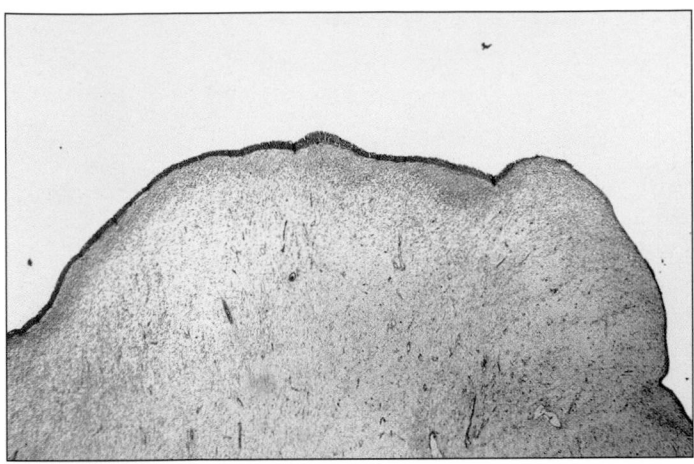

Fig. 9.138 Botryoid rhabdomyosarcoma. Note the increased cellularity just under the epithelium (cambium layer).

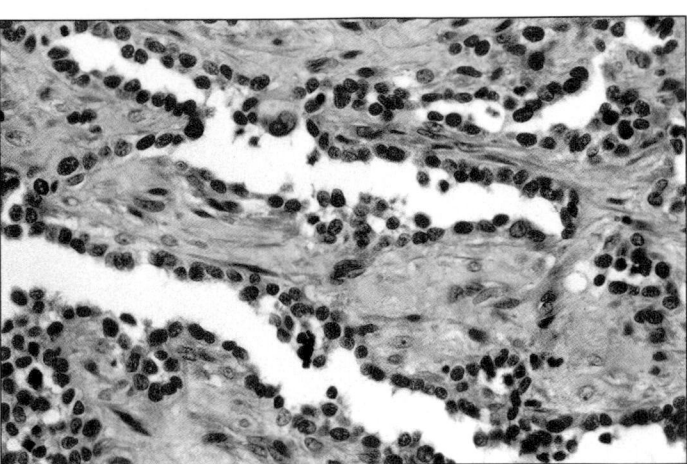

Fig. 9.140 Alveolar rhabdomyosarcoma. The rhabdomyoblasts line the alveolar-like spaces, some spilling into the space. The cells are brightly eosinophilic.

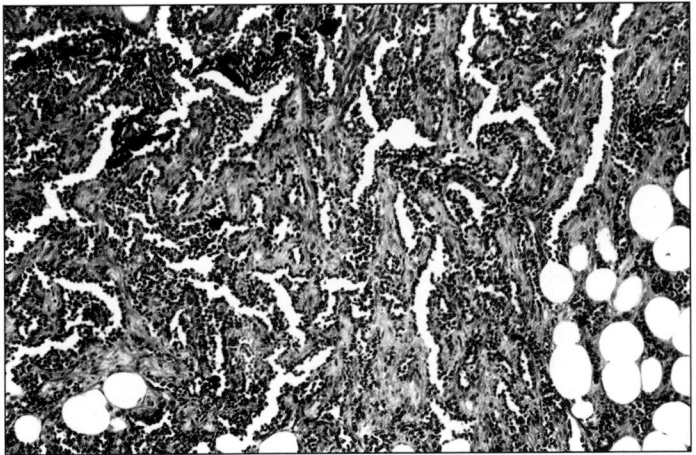

Fig. 9.139 Alveolar rhabdomyosarcoma. This tumor has a well developed alveolar pattern.

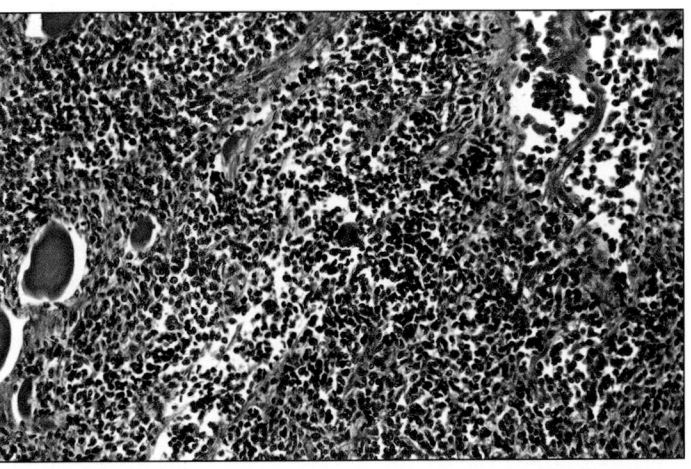

Fig. 9.141 Alveolar rhabdomyosarcoma, solid type. The proliferating cells are the same as in typical alveolar rhabdomyosarcoma but they are arranged in solid sheets.

arrangement, with loss of tumor cell cohesion at the periphery of the alveolar nests and increased cohesion in their central portions (Fig. 9.140). The majority of tumor cells are usually poorly differentiated with little cytoplasm, but scattered multinucleated tumor giant cells are common.

Sometimes the nested pattern with fibrous septa is absent. Otherwise these 'solid variants' show the crowded, highly cellular, undifferentiated round cell features of typical alveolar tumors (Figs 9.141, 9.142). Solid alveolar rhabdomyosarcomas display the same genetic alterations as the classic form.

Pleomorphic rhabdomyosarcomas are discussed below and are currently regarded as primarily neoplasms of adults. A few examples are reported in children using current criteria.[195] An overlapping concept between pleomorphic rhabdomyosarcoma and juvenile rhabdomyosarcoma is anaplastic rhabdomyosarcoma. Anaplasia may occur focally or diffusely in rhabdomyosarcoma and is defined by the present of enlarged cells with hyperchromatic nuclei and often bizarre, multipolar mitoses. These cytologic changes are sometimes seen in other pediatric tumors, such as Wilms tumor and neuroblastoma, and they may occur in any variety of rhabdo-

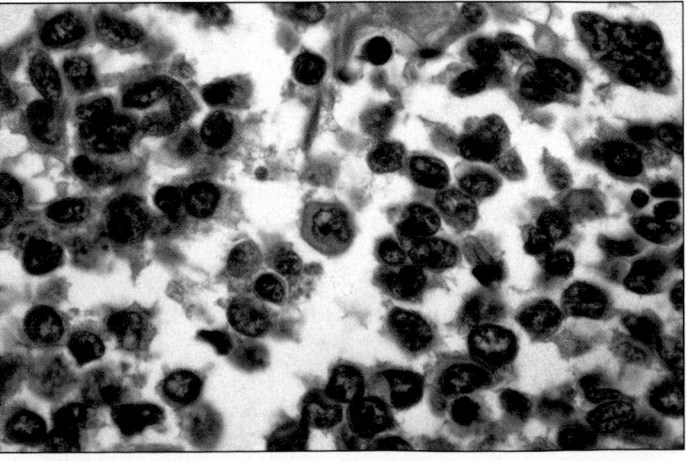

Fig. 9.142 Alveolar rhabdomyosarcoma, solid type, high magnification.

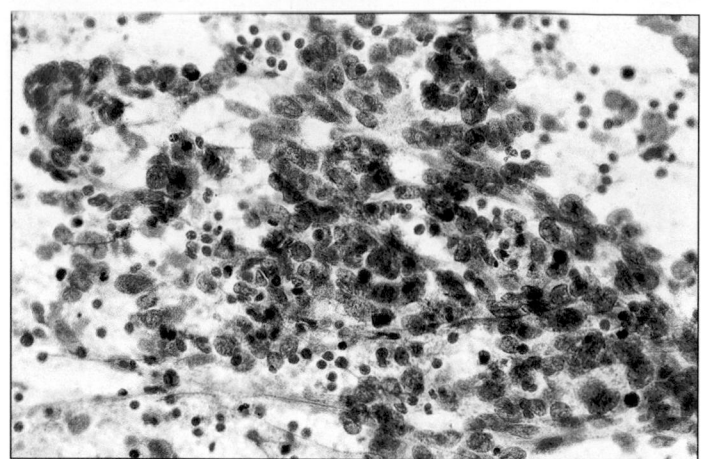

Fig. 9.143 Alveolar rhabdomyosarcoma. Aspiration cytology can be diagnostic with modern ancillary studies (immunohistochemistry and, at times, molecular studies). The aspirated cells are shed singly and have enlarged nuclei and scanty cytoplasm. Papanicolaou stain.

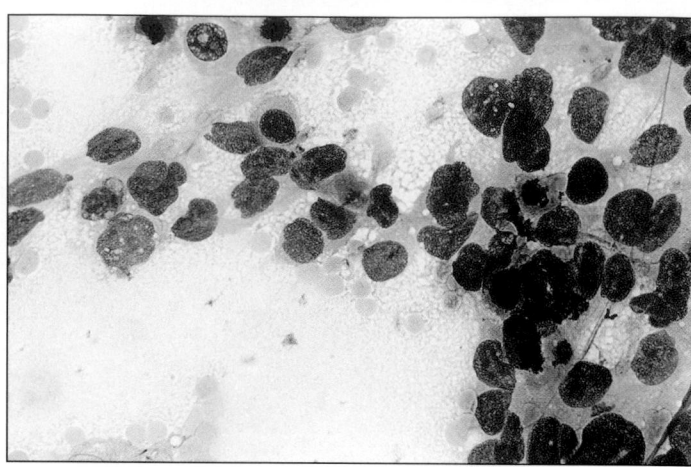

Fig. 9.144 Alveolar rhabdomyosarcoma. Aspiration cytology, Diff-Kwik stain.

myosarcoma. When anaplasia occurs diffusely, it portends a poor prognosis, whereas focal anaplasia has less significance.[192]

'Rhabdomyosarcoma not otherwise specified' refers to those biopsies that contain rhabdomyoblasts but that have limited material, precluding further characterization. Similarly, 'sarcoma not otherwise specified' refers to lesions that contain limited material without definitive rhabdomyoblasts but with cells resembling rhabdomyosarcoma. Both of these categories generally represent rhabdomyosarcomas but with biopsies having scant material or abundant artifact or cellular degeneration. The patients from these groups are placed on study but without further pathologic categorization. On the other hand, undifferentiated sarcomas generally contain adequate material but consist of primitive cells that lack sufficient differentiation for further categorization. These lesions cannot be proved to be rhabdomyosarcomas and are probably a diverse group of high-grade pediatric sarcomas with a poor outcome.

The IRSG also recognizes a group of rare and unusual lesions that express features of both muscle cells and nerve cells, ectomesenchymomas. At one end of the spectrum, these comprise spindle cell or embryonal rhabdomyosarcomas containing scattered mature ganglion cells. Conversely, primitive lesions with peripheral neuroectodermal tumor-like areas may coexist with primitive rhabdomyosarcoma, either alveolar or embryonal. Their behavior generally mirrors the histologic pattern of rhabdomyosarcoma.[372] Immunohistochemistry and electron microscopy may be used to confirm the coexistence of two cell types. Molecular biologic studies have demonstrated features of either alveolar rhabdomyosarcoma, peripheral primitive neuroectodermal tumor (see below), or both.[373]

Rhabdomyosarcomas can easily be confused by a variety of other small cell neoplasms. In previous decades, diagnosis was resolved by prolonged and often futile searches for cross-striations but, using newer immunohistochemical stains and molecular techniques, most cases can be reliably classified. Furthermore, newer techniques allow accurate diagnosis on tiny specimens, such as those afforded by aspiration cytology (Figs 9.143, 9.144).

Electron microscopy discloses bundles of 'thick' 15-nm myosin and 'thin' 6-nm actin filaments in hexagonal arrays that can occasionally be found in cells lacking microscopic cross-striations.

Earlier ultrastructural stages of myogenesis correlate with complexes of thick (myosin) filaments associated with free ribosomes.[374] On immunohistochemistry, rhabdomyosarcomas variably express MSA and desmin. More recently, a family of muscle protein transcription promoters have been discovered that includes MyoD and myogenin; these act by binding to DNA and initiating the molecular events leading to the formation of muscle-specific proteins. MyoD protein is formed early in the myogenesis pathway and myogenin is created later; these are both reliable markers of skeletal muscle differentiation. Nuclear staining is required for diagnosis. Non-specific cytoplasmic staining and decreased sensitivity result from the use of paraffin-embedded tissues rather than frozen specimens for MyoD staining, so a panel approach is best.[375–377] As a word of caution, when searching for metastatic rhabdomyosarcoma in effusions by cytologic examination, it is worthwhile to be aware that mesothelial cells are desmin-reactive. Specific staining with MyoD1 or myogenin should be sought before making a diagnosis of metastatic rhabdomyosarcoma.[378–381]

Myoglobin is found primarily in differentiated cells and so is of little utility in diagnosing primitive tumors. Muscle-specific actin also stains smooth and cardiac muscle as well as myofibroblasts and myoepithelial cells. Exploiting newer molecular techniques for diagnosis is limited to alveolar rhabdomyosarcoma, which displays a characteristic fusion between the *PAX3* gene on chromosome 2 and the *FKHR* gene on chromosome 13, visualized by standard karyotyping as the t(2;13)(q35;q14) translocation.[353,382–386] This translocation fuses two DNA-binding transcription factors and appears to cause the abnormal cell proliferation.[387,388] Another PAX gene, *PAX7*, located on chromosome 1, may also fuse with the *FKHR* gene and produce alveolar rhabdomyosarcomas containing a similar aberrant fusion gene, the t(1;13)(p36;q14). Although similar in molecular composition and in tumorigenesis, the two translocations are dissimilar in affected patient age, stage, location, and metastatic pattern, with t(1;13)(p36;q14) lesions comprising less aggressive tumors and occurring in younger children.[383]

Currently there is no genetic test for embryonal rhabdomyosarcoma, as no specific gene or mutation has been found to date. However, comparative genomic hybridization studies show that embryonal rhabdomyosarcomas may have novel genomic im-

Table 9.11 Differential diagnosis of rhabdomyosarcoma – small round blue cell tumors

Ewing's sarcoma

Primitive peripheral neuroectodermal tumor

Neuroblastoma

Pigmented neuroectodermal tumor

Esthesioneuroblastoma

Lymphoblastic lymphoma

Small noncleaved cell lymphoma

Wilms tumor

Embryonal sarcoma of liver

Pleuropulmonary blastoma

Malignant melanoma

Desmoplastic small round cell tumor

Synovial sarcoma

Malignant peripheral nerve sheath tumor

Germ cell tumors

Histiocytoses

Table 9.12 Differential diagnosis of rhabdomyosarcoma – myogenous/ pseudomyogenous tumors

Rhabdomyoma

Nerve sheath tumors, benign and malignant (Triton tumor)

Rhabdoid tumor

Inflammatory myofibroblastic tumor

Eosinophilic cystitis

Various carcinomas with heterologous muscle

Various sarcomas with heterologous muscle

Sex cord tumors with heterologous muscle

Germ cell tumors

Embryonal sarcoma of liver

Pleuropulmonary blastoma

Ectomesenchymoma (primitive neuroectodermal tumor plus rhabdomyosarcoma)

Malignant mesenchymoma (fibrosarcoma/malignant fibrous histiocytoma plus rhabdomyosarcoma and/or other heterologous elements)

balances that may be useful in directing further molecular studies for the determination of key genes.[389]

Differential diagnosis of rhabdomyosarcoma relates to two phenomena: their primitive, undifferentiated nature (Table 9.11) and their tendency to myogenesis (Table 9.12).

Pleomorphic rhabdomyosarcoma

This tumor was first described by Arthur Purdy Stout in 1946 as the classic form of rhabdomyosarcoma.[390] Pleomorphic rhabdomyosarcoma was soon after accepted as one of the more common adult pleomorphic sarcomas. Horn and Enterline included pleomorphic rhabdomyosarcoma in their early histologic classification of rhabdomyosarcoma, along with the embryonal, botryoid, and alveolar types.[349] The introduction of the concept of MFH in the 1970s and its subsequent acceptance by pathologists as the most common pleomorphic sarcoma in adults dramatically changed the view of pleomorphic rhabdomyosarcoma. Pleomorphic rhabdomyosarcoma became an extremely uncommon diagnosis but newer techniques have allowed pathologists to better recognize these tumors in recent years.

Pleomorphic rhabdomyosarcoma accounts for 5–7% of all pleomorphic adult soft tissue sarcomas. In a review by Schürch of 325 pleomorphic adult sarcomas,[391] 18 (5%) pleomorphic rhabdomyosarcomas were found; the age range of this group was 28–84 years with a mean age of 61 years. Gaffney and colleagues reported a similar (6.8%) incidence of pleomorphic rhabdomyosarcoma.[194] The age range in this series was 27–84 years with a mean age of 56 years. No cases of pediatric pleomorphic rhabdomyosarcoma were identified in either series.

Pleomorphic rhabdomyosarcoma usually arises in the large skeletal muscles of the extremities, most commonly in the thigh, although multiple other sites have been reported. Males appear to be affected more frequently than females. Patients usually present with a painless but rapidly growing soft tissue mass. Metastases to the lungs are not uncommonly present at time of diagnosis.

Pleomorphic rhabdomyosarcoma are usually unicentric, large (>10 cm) tumors that are centered within the deep skeletal muscle.

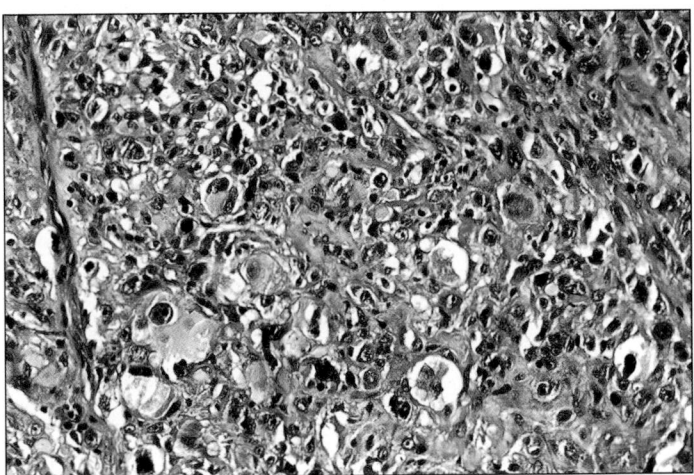

Fig. 9.145 Pleomorphic rhabdomyosarcoma. These are adult tumors. This lesion appears similar to malignant fibrous histiocytoma but the marked eosinophilia should suggest the need to perform immunohistochemistry for skeletal muscle markers.

The tumors are usually well circumscribed with a fleshy, gray-pink cut surface. Extensive necrosis is nearly universal while cystic change and focal hemorrhage is not uncommon.

Microscopically these are pleomorphic sarcomas composed of undifferentiated round to spindle cells and an admixture of polygonal cells with densely eosinophilic cytoplasm in spindle, tadpole, and racket-like contours (Figs 9.145, 9.146). Some observers have classified adult lesions into 'classic' (pleomorphic rhabdomyoblasts in sheets), 'round cell,' and 'spindle cell' patterns.[193] Cross-striations are vanishingly rare in all cases. The presence of pleomorphic polygonal rhabdomyoblasts on routine hematoxylin and eosin stains coupled with immunohistochemical evidence of at least one skeletal-muscle specific marker by immunohistochemistry is required for diagnosis.[193] Aspiration cytology has been reported to yield a

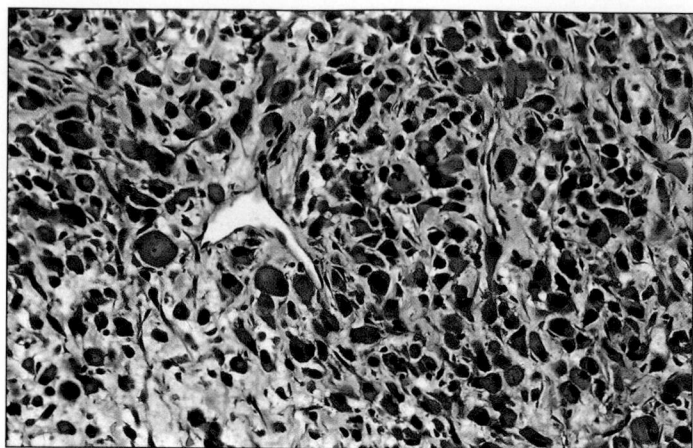

Fig. 9.146 Pleomorphic rhabdomyosarcoma.

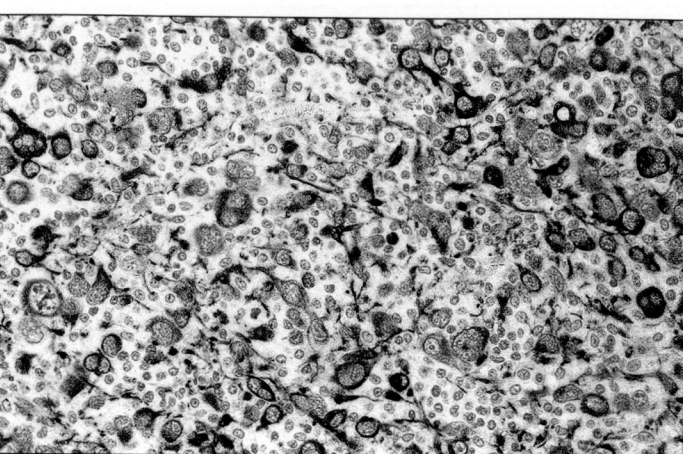

Fig. 9.147 Pleomorphic rhabdomyosarcoma, desmin stain.

pleomorphic population of clustered and single cells with hyper-chromatic nuclei; granular, pink cytoplasm; and isolated, large cells with whiplike or globoid cytoplasmic processes and occasional striations.[392]

Pleomorphic rhabdomyosarcomas, like other rhabdomyosarcoma types, express myoglobin, MyoD1, skeletal muscle myogenin, fast skeletal muscle myosin, and desmin (Fig. 9.147). Nuclear staining is required when evaluating MyoD1 or myogenin (Fig. 9.148). These sarcomas variably express MSA, SMA, and muscle-specific myogenin. They lack epithelial markers or S100 protein.

The differential diagnosis of pleomorphic rhabdomyosarcoma is extremely broad. Once mimics of neoplasia, like regenerating skeletal muscle[393] and myositis, are eliminated, the differential diagnosis comes down to that of pleomorphic malignant neoplasms. Carcinomas and melanomas are far more common than sarcomas and merit serious consideration in each case. Negativity for cytokeratins and S100 protein usually excludes these entities. The potential for anaplastic large cell lymphoma to present as a soft tissue mass requires addition of CD30 and ALK1 antibodies. Other pleomorphic sarcomas, such as MFH, pleomorphic liposarcoma, and pleomorphic leiomyosarcoma, can be virtually indistinguishable from pleomorphic rhabdomyosarcoma on light microscopy. While MFH and pleomorphic leiomyosarcoma typically feature storiform and fascicular patterns respectively, compared to the usual nondescript patterns of rhabdomyosarcoma, these features are not uniform. The presence of pleomorphic lipoblasts characterizes pleomorphic liposarcoma but non-specific vacuolization can occur in any anaplastic cell. Since the morphologic features can overlap, ancillary studies (myoglobin or MyoD1/myogenin immunostains or electron microscopy) are generally needed to confirm sarcomeric differentiation.

Once a malignant tumor has been shown to demonstrate rhabdomyoblastic differentiation, other entities must be excluded. Heterologous rhabdomyosarcomatous differentiation occurs in a broad range of neoplasms, some of which are more common than rhabdomyosarcoma. These include carcinosarcomas from a variety of sites, malignant mixed müllerian tumor of the uterus and ovary, ovarian Sertoli–Leydig cell tumor, malignant peripheral nerve sheath tumor (malignant triton tumor), malignant ectomesenchymoma (containing ganglion cells and neuroblasts), malignant mesenchymoma (containing liposarcomatous or osteoid/cartilaginous elements), and

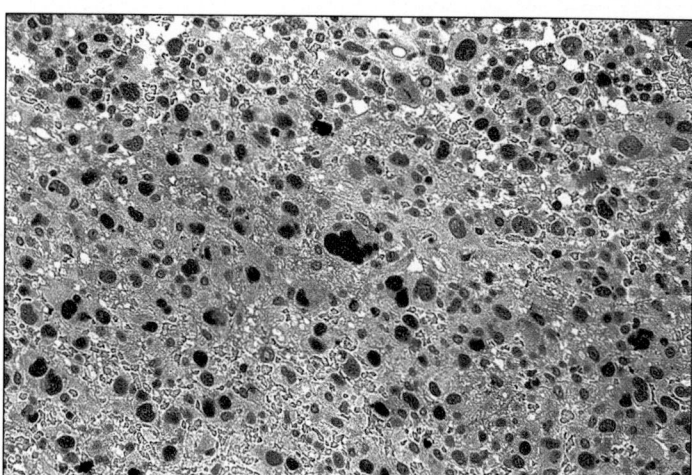

Fig. 9.148 Pleomorphic rhabdomyosarcoma, MyoD1 stain. Nuclear staining is required. These tumors are worth separating from malignant fibrous histiocytoma since their prognosis is worse.

Wilms tumor. Attention to the clinical presentation and thorough sampling will help distinguish these entities.

Preliminary cytogenetic study has yielded complex karyotypes.[189,394]

The prognosis for these tumors is poor and prognostic factors have yet to be developed. In two series with follow-up, about 75% of patients died of disease.[193,194]

VASCULAR TUMOURS

PAPILLARY ENDOTHELIAL HYPERPLASIA

This benign reactive process is an unusually exuberant form of organizing vascular thrombus and was first called 'vegetant intravascular hemangioendothelioma.' The initial example was described in the dilated vessels of thrombosed hemorrhoids and likened to a cherry.[395] Papillary endothelial hyperplasia may occur at any age and

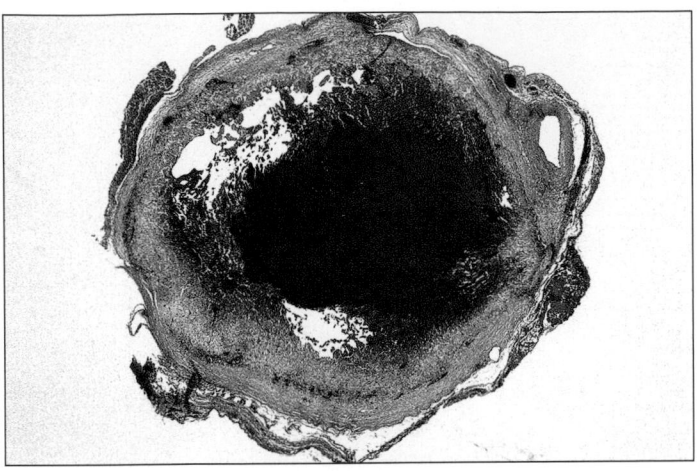

Fig. 9.149 Papillary endothelial hyperplasia. This process is confined to the lumen of a vessel.

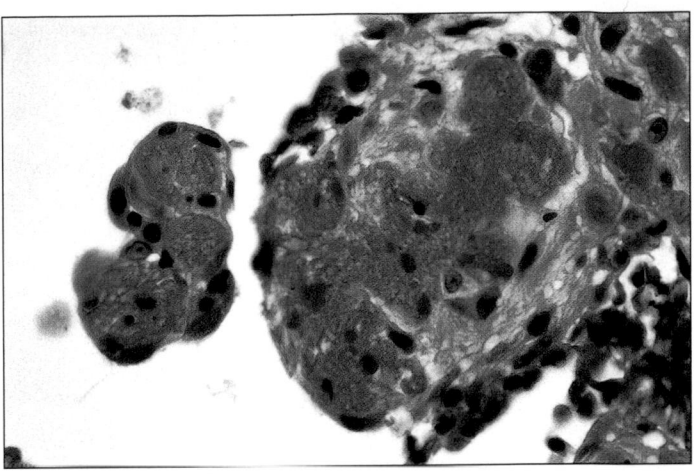

Fig. 9.151 Papillary endothelial hyperplasia. A central fibrin core is coated by endothelial cells.

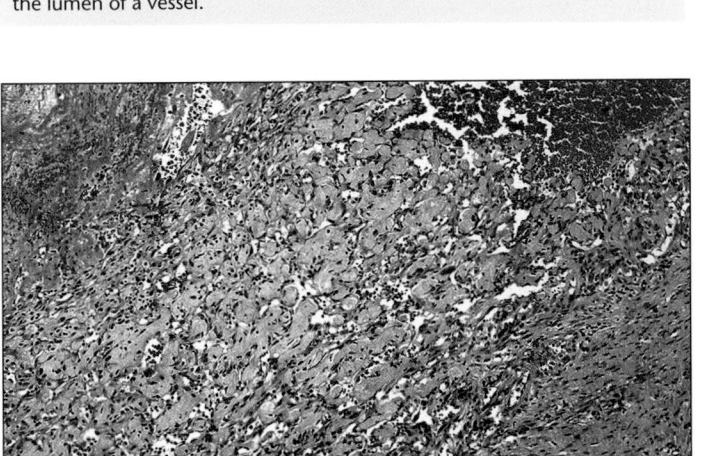

Fig. 9.150 Papillary endothelial hyperplasia. This example arose in an organizing hematoma.

involve virtually any vessel, including those of neoplastic processes and vascular malformations. However, in its 'pure' form it typically presents as a solitary, superficial, firm, bluish or erythematous mass involving the fingers, head and neck or anorectal region. Commonly, physical examination reveals limited mobility of the process about its longitudinal axis. Gross examination may reveal confinement of the process to the lumen of a dilated vessel, usually a vein.

Histologically, the lesion shows papillary fronds with a core of fibrin or hyalinized collagen lined by a single layer of endothelial cells, which may be plump or swollen but lack significant atypia or mitotic activity (Figs 9.149–9.151). Occasionally the fronds appear to be 'free-floating' within the vessel lumen. Extravascular extension may occasionally be seen, although it is usually not extensive.

The following features differentiate papillary endothelial hyperplasia from angiosarcoma, a tumor with which it has occasionally been confused: (1) the frequent confinement of the process to a vascular lumen; (2) lack of cellular pleomorphism; (3) the typical arrangement of the endothelium in a monolayer; (4) low mitotic rate; and (5) lack of cellular necrosis.

HEMANGIOMA

These lesions are discussed in Chapter 8. However, it should be noted that capillary and cavernous hemangiomas may be encountered in all sites. Large hemangiomas (as well as malignant vascular tumors) may all be associated with the Kasabach–Merritt syndrome, in which disseminated intravascular coagulation is initiated by the vast endothelial surface, a complication that can be life-threatening.[396]

ARTERIOVENOUS MALFORMATIONS

Lesions with arteriovenous anastomoses may be either acquired or congenital. The former are usually solitary and traumatic in origin. Congenital arteriovenous connections are often multiple, involving a significant portion of an extremity or the head and neck region with a female predilection. Arteriovenous malformations that have a prominent superficial component, associated with substantial shunting, present as pulsating collections of tortuous vessels and are sometimes referred to as cirsoid aneurysms, racemose aneurysms, aneurysms by anastomosis, or pulsating angiomas. Examples that contain large dilated vessels have been designated arteriovenous aneurysms.

The age at which patients come to medical attention is typically related to the conspicuousness of any surface component. The most common presenting complaint is swelling of the extremity, followed by cosmetic disfigurement and visible pulsations. Pain is less common. Superficial varicosities, increased warmth, and thrills or bruits are often present over the affected site. Systemic hemodynamic effects, such as cardiac enlargement, high output cardiac failure, and Branham's sign (bradycardia elicited by digital pressure on the afferent arterial supply), are identified only rarely in congenital arteriovenous malformations. Traumatic fistulas, however, are somewhat more likely to be associated with these findings. This difference is attributed to more extensive, tortuous, and narrower arteriovenous communications in congenital examples, which allow the peripheral resistance to be maintained.

In 1900, Klippel and Trenaunay summarized a group of patients with the following triad: (1) a lower extremity port wine stain; (2) varicose veins; and (3) skeletal and soft tissue hypertrophy of the affected site with lengthening of the limb.[397] Seven years later, Parkes Weber[398] described a similar group of cases but included two individuals who also had extensive arteriovenous malformations. Patients with all four of the above features are now said to have the Parkes Weber or Klippel–Trenaunay–Weber syndrome.

The diagnosis of arteriovenous malformation is made with greater accuracy on the basis of clinical and radiographic findings than by histologic examination. Arteriography confirms the presence of arteriovenous anastomoses and demonstrates cases where superficial varicosities are attributable to deep venous obstruction or the congenital absence of deep veins rather than an arteriovenous malformation. Excision of superficial veins in the latter case is contraindicated. Further, arteriography is also needed to assess the feasibility of surgery since arteriovenous malformations often have several feeding vessels and therefore there is a tendency for recurrence via collateral circulation if they are incompletely excised.

The histology of arteriovenous malformations may vary considerably. Foci identical to capillary or cavernous hemangiomas may even be present. The identification of direct arteriovenous anastomoses may require extensive tissue sampling. When these are not seen, the presence of juxtaposed medium-sized or larger arteries and veins and the identification of arterialized veins, characterized by prominent fibrointimal hyperplasia and medial muscular hypertrophy, aid in this diagnosis.

INTRAMUSCULAR HEMANGIOMAS

Intramuscular hemangiomas/angiomas are relatively uncommon, accounting for 0.8–4.4% of all vascular tumors in two large series.[399,400] There does not appear to be a distinct gender predilection.[399–401] The majority of cases are identified in the first three decades of life.[399–401] The lower extremity, in particular the quadriceps femoris, is the most frequent site affected. However, any muscle may be involved. Many examples are less than 5 cm in maximum dimension at the time of diagnosis, although tumors over 20 cm in size have been recorded.[401] Soft tissue swelling and pain are respectively the most frequent sign and symptom.

The recurrence rates in recent series range from a low of 18%[401] to a high of 61%.[399] Recurrent disease is attributable to incomplete excision.

The gross appearance varies widely, depending on the type and size of vessels that predominate and the extent to which supporting elements such as adipose and fibrous connective tissue are represented. Tumors composed predominantly of small capillary-sized vessels (Fig. 9.152) vary in color from whitish-tan to reddish-brown and are poorly circumscribed. Tumors dominated by a large vessel pattern (i.e. cavernous spaces, dilated venous) are much more likely to be recognized grossly as vascular anomalies. Intramuscular hemangiomas are frequently accompanied by abundant adipose tissue (Fig. 9.153). Occasionally foci of ossification may be seen. This seems to occur most frequently in lesions with a complex vascular pattern, containing an arteriovenous component.[399]

In the past, most authors have categorized benign intramuscular vascular tumors according to vessel size or type. However, it has been proposed that all these lesions, including capillary, cavernous, arteriovenous, lymphangiomatous, and complex malformation types, be regarded as intramuscular 'angiomas',[399] since (1) most examples have mixed features and (2) there is no correlation between the predominant vessel type and the clinical outcome. However, there is some correlation between vessel pattern and anatomic site:

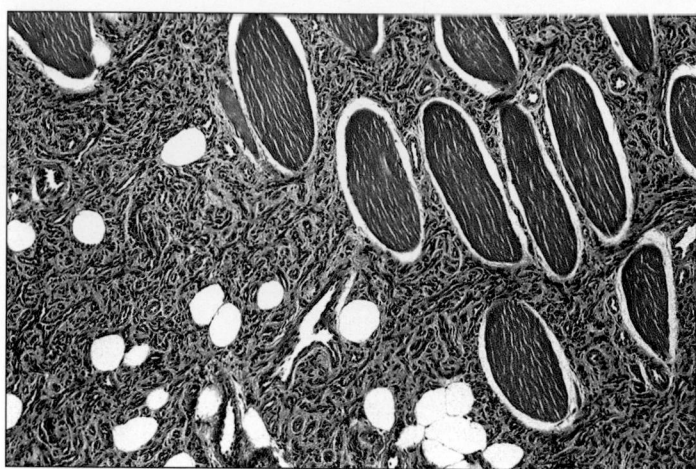

Fig. 9.152 Intramuscular hemangioma. This lesion is of the capillary type. Even this cellular example still has a minor fatty component.

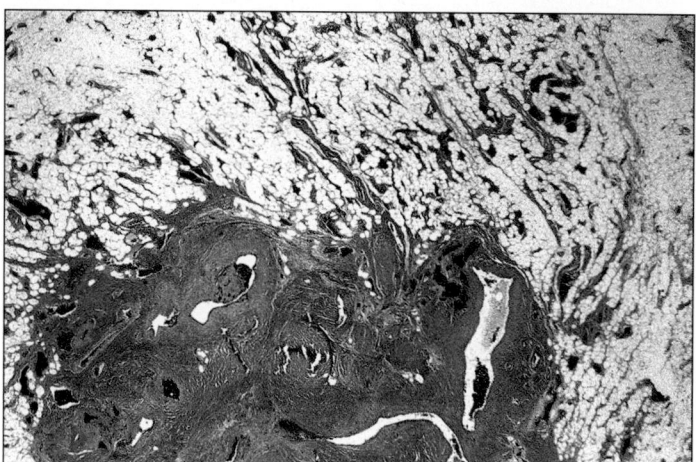

Fig. 9.153 This intramuscular hemangioma displays a large vessel pattern and striking overgrowth of fat.

intramuscular capillary hemangiomas and lymphangiomas favor the upper half of the body.

The differential diagnosis of intramuscular hemangioma/angioma includes angiomatosis, angiosarcoma and lipoma/liposarcoma. Angiomatosis is primarily a clinical diagnosis, based on extent of the process.

Angiosarcoma may be entertained when dealing with a cellular small-vessel variant of intramuscular hemangioma. However, the latter lacks an interanastomosing sinusoidal pattern, nuclear pleomorphism, and atypical mitotic activity. When considering this possibility, one should be aware of the rarity of primary angiosarcomas of skeletal muscle. The young age of many patients with intramuscular hemangioma also is against a diagnosis of angiosarcoma.

As mentioned earlier, intramuscular hemangiomas with abundant fat can be confused with lipogenic neoplasms. However, the latter rarely contain large, dilated or 'gaping' vasculature and their small-vessel pattern lacks the exuberance of that seen in hemangiomas.

ANGIOMATOSIS

Angiomatosis is a term that has been applied to a variety of processes, including papillary endothelial hyperplasia, encephalofacial vascular malformations in Sturge–Weber syndrome, and extensive multifocal benign vascular proliferations in children that may be associated with a poor prognosis due to organ compromise or hemorrhage. For the purposes of this discussion, angiomatosis is used as defined by Rao and Weiss,[402] who characterized the process as a histologically benign vascular proliferation growing contiguously in multiple tissue planes or extensively in tissues of the same type (e.g. apposed muscles). Multifocal vascular proliferations were excluded from their definition. Similar criteria were provided by Howat and Campbell.[403] The lesions tend to be based in the deep subcutaneous tissue and muscles, but more superficial tissues or underlying bone may also be involved.

Rao and Weiss's series included 31 females and 20 males. Over half of the patients were brought to medical attention prior to age 29 and of these, 11 were evaluated in the first year of life. The most common symptoms are persistent diffuse swelling, pain, and tenderness. Limb hypertrophy is present only infrequently. Vascular lesions are, in many instances, not suspected clinically since superficial discoloration is frequently absent and arteriovenous shunting is usually not apparent. The lower extremity, including the buttock, is the most frequently affected site, followed by the trunk and the upper extremity. Less commonly, the head and neck, back, pelvis, and retroperitoneum may be involved.

Angiomatosis is characterized histologically by an admixture of large irregular venous segments with disorganized muscular walls, cavernous vessels, and capillary channels, scattered diffusely throughout tissue planes and often associated with large amounts of adipose tissue (Fig. 9.154). Arteries and lymphatic channels may also be noted but are typically not seen in direct communication with the former. Features that are distinctive, though not specific, include the presence of capillary-sized vessels proliferating adjacent to, and within the walls of, the disorganized venous segments.

Angiomatosis, as defined above, is a vascular anomaly with a strong propensity for local recurrence. This can be expected in the majority of patients. Management appears to reflect a balance between complete extirpation of the lesion and obviating excessive morbidity. Malignant transformation has not been reported.

The differential diagnosis of angiomatosis includes intramuscular hemangioma and diffuse arteriovenous malformation. The former distinction is primarily clinical, based on extent of the process. Diffuse arteriovenous malformation can have a clinical appearance similar to angiomatosis but in general it is more likely to be associated with edema, phlebectasia, increased warmth, a bruit, and other features consistent with shunting. Arteriography is an invaluable aid in the diagnosis of this process. In general, arteriovenous malformation differs histologically from angiomatosis by featuring a greater abundance of thick-walled arteries and juxtaposed 'arterialized' veins.

Epithelioid hemangioma (angiolymphoid hyperplasia with eosinophilia), acquired tufted hemangioma (angioblastoma), and targetoid hemosiderotic ('hobnail') hemangioma are all discussed in Chapter 8.

'HEMANGIOENDOTHELIOMA'

This is a confusing term since it has been applied to both benign and malignant vascular lesions in the past. For example, completely

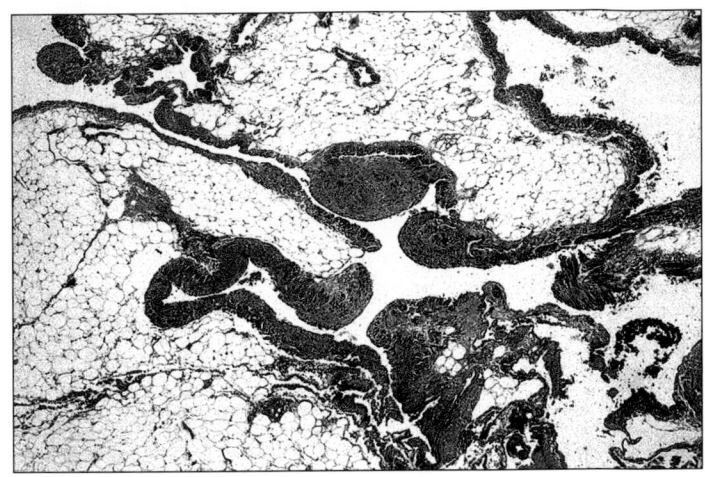

Fig. 9.154 Angiomatosis. Note the large ectatic vessels. This diagnosis is established on clinicopathologic rather than purely histologic grounds.

benign lesions now typically diagnosed as 'juvenile hemangioma' or 'cellular capillary hemangioma' were referred to as 'hemangioendothelioma' in the older literature. Papillary endothelial hyperplasia was also initially described as a type of hemangioendothelioma. In contrast, epithelioid hemangioendotheliomas are unequivocally malignant, metastasizing in a significant number of cases, but have been considered 'borderline' in the past. At present, most observers would use the term 'hemangiothelioma' to refer to malignant vascular neoplasms that are less aggressive than angiosarcomas. However, spindle cell hemangioendothelioma/hemangioma is benign and capable of multicentricity as a 'field effect,' but was initially believed to be malignant.

Spindle cell hemangioendothelioma (spindle cell hemangioma)

These lesions are depicted and discussed in more detail in Chapter 8. Briefly, spindle cell hemangioendothelioma typically presents as a superficial, slow-growing, painless mass involving the dermis and/or subcutis. It was initially believed to be a low-grade sarcoma[404] but further evidence does not support this view.[405] These lesions may develop at any age, may be single or multifocal, and most commonly involve the hands and feet. A small number of cases have been associated with other disease processes such as Maffucci syndrome, Klippel–Trenaunay syndrome and an early onset of varicose veins. The lesions tend to recur and grow in multifocal fashion (in 'crops') but do not metastasize.[405]

The histology of spindle cell hemangioendothelioma is highly characteristic, with a well marginated lesion showing two components: (1) cavernous vascular spaces, similar to those seen in a cavernous hemangioma, lined by epithelioid endothelial cells with occasional intracytoplasmic lumina, frequently associated with phleboliths; and (2) a spindle cell proliferation vaguely reminiscent of Kaposi's sarcoma.

Endovascular papillary angioendothelioma (Dabska tumor)

These lesions are also discussed in Chapter 8. This is an exceedingly rare tumor, seen chiefly in children, that is capable of regional lymph node metastasis.[406–413] The tumors tend to be superficial, primarily

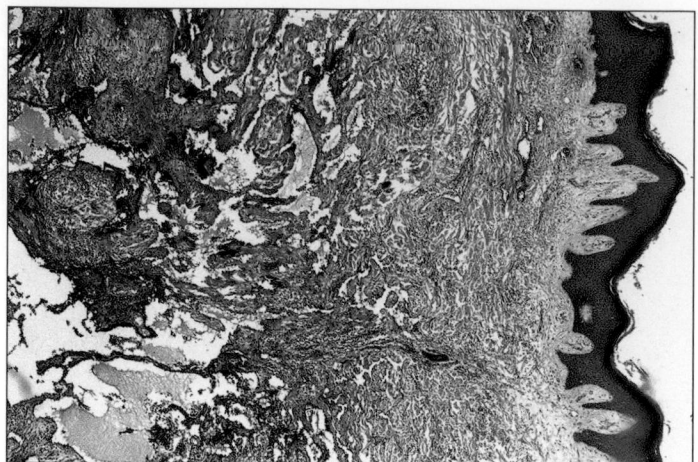

Fig. 9.155 Retiform hemangioendothelioma. These tumors are so-named for their architectural resemblance to rete testis.

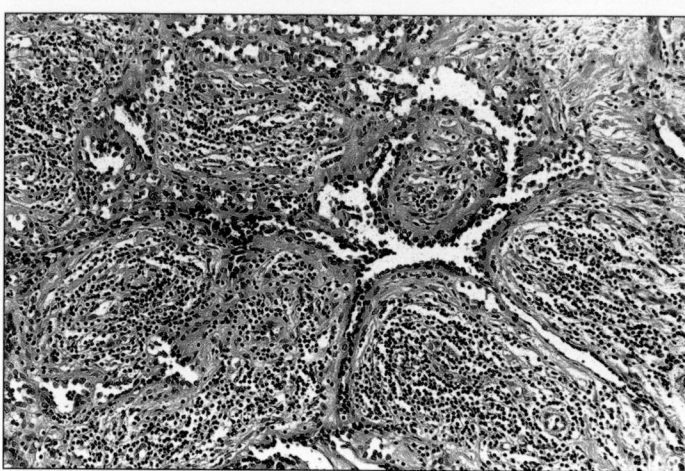

Fig. 9.156 Retiform hemangioendothelioma. Lymphocytes are closely intermingled with endothelial cells, a pattern also seen in Dabska tumor.

involving the skin and subcutis, and are composed of a proliferation of capillary-sized vessels lined by cuboidal or columnar endothelial cells occasionally forming intraluminal tufts. Lymphocytes are commonly seen intravascularly and surrounding the capillary proliferation. Epithelioid endothelial cells with intracytoplasmic lumina are often seen in Dabska tumor.

Retiform hemangioendothelioma

Retiform hemangioendothelioma is a distinctive form of low-grade angiosarcoma of the skin that recurs frequently but has a very low metastatic rate.[414–417] No tumor-related deaths have been reported so far, underscoring the importance of accurate distinction from conventional angiosarcoma. Most tumors present in the second to fourth decade with no sex predilection. The lesions are located preferentially on the lower and upper limbs, although any site can be involved. Clinically the tumor presents as a slow-growing exophytic mass or plaque-like skin nodule.

Histologically, typical features are the presence of long arborizing vessels reminiscent of normal rete testes lined by monomorphic hobnail endothelial cells, a prominent lymphocytic infiltrate, and focal intraluminal papillary projections similar to those seen in Dabska's tumor (Figs 9.155–9.157). There seems to be considerable overlap between Dabska's tumor and retiform hemangio-endothelioma and they are probably ends of a spectrum.[413] *By immunohistochemistry the endothelial cells are positive for factor-VIII-related antigen, CD31,CD34, and* Ulex europaeus I lectin. Viral sequences of herpesvirus 8 associated with Kaposi's sarcoma have been detected in one case, the significance of which is not clear.[417]

Kaposiform (infantile) hemangioendothelioma

Kaposiform hemangioendothelioma is a rare vascular tumor first described in infants and children manifesting as a large retroperitoneal mass frequently associated with consumptive coagulopathy (Kasabach–Merritt syndrome).[418–420] Subsequently, both adult[419] and superficial[418] variants have been described. The tumor is reported to have an association with lymphangiomatosis and is sometimes complicated by intestinal obstruction, jaundice and hemoperitoneum. This lesion can be lethal because of its aggressive local behavior, although distant metastases have not been reported.

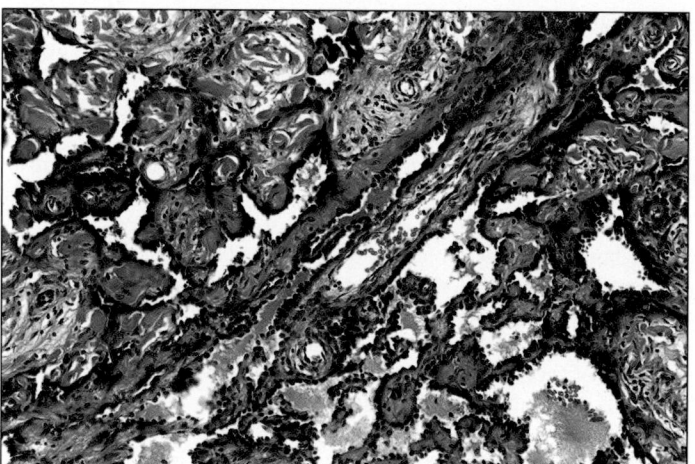

Fig. 9.157 Retiform hemangioendothelioma. Endothelial cells protrude into lumina and some have individual intracytoplasmic lumina.

The tumors are characterized histologically by infiltrative, lobular growth of well formed capillaries, sometimes containing fibrin thrombi, admixed with short fascicles of spindle cells with slit-like spaces (Figs 9.158, 9.159).

Features that distinguish kaposiform hemangioendothelioma from Kaposi's sarcoma include the usual young age of the patients, lack of an association with HIV status, confinement of the process to one general site or location, which is usually deep-seated, lobulated architecture of the vascular proliferation, less pronounced lympho-plasmacytic response, and hyaline globules, which, although documented in kaposiform hemangioendothelioma, are much less frequent than in Kaposi's sarcoma.

Epithelioid hemangioendothelioma

Epithelioid hemangioendothelioma is a low-grade vascular neoplasm that can occur at any age. There is no sex predilection. Predominant sites of involvement are the soft tissue, lungs, liver, and bones.[421–425] The tumors typically present as superficial or deep

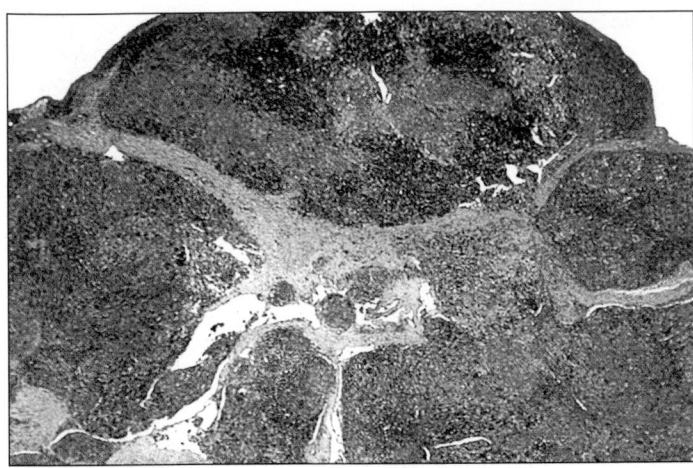

Fig. 9.158 Kaposiform hemangioendothelioma. Despite dense cellularity, this tumor maintains a lobular architecture.

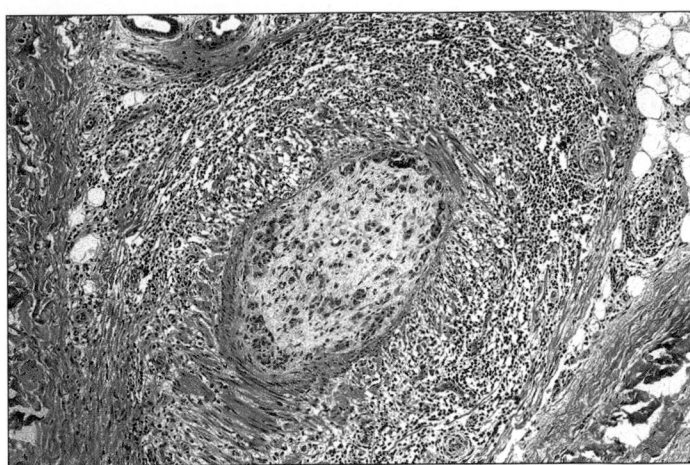

Fig. 9.160 Epithelioid hemangioendothelioma. Note the vasocentricity. This lesion has destroyed the vessel in which it arose. The center of the lesion shows a chondroid background.

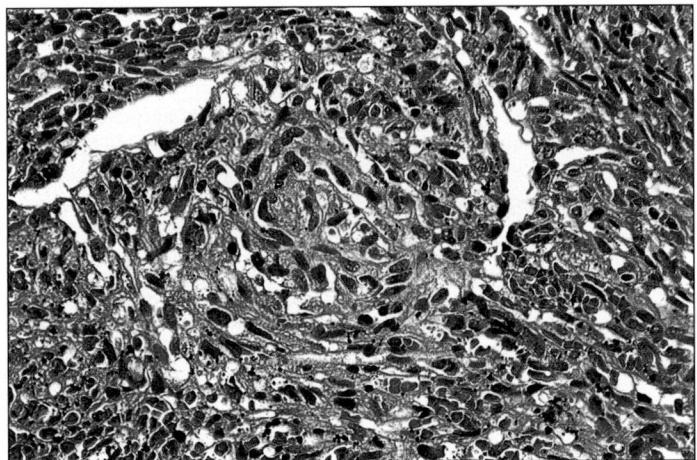

Fig. 9.159 Kaposiform hemangioendothelioma. At high magnification, the tumor is composed of spindle cells and well formed capillaries. These tumors can be lethal based on local growth and consumptive coagulopathy but they do not metastasize.

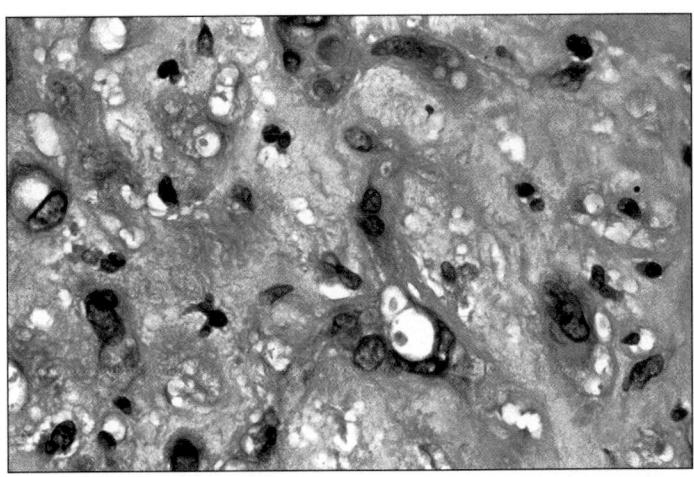

Fig. 9.161 Epithelioid hemangioendothelioma. Occasionally erythrocytes can be found in intracytoplasmic lumina.

solitary masses, or occasionally multiple masses, with a predilection for the extremities. Lesions in the soft tissue are frequently associated with a vessel, most commonly a vein. The local recurrence rate is about 15%, the metastasis rate of about 30%, mostly to regional lymph nodes, and mortality rate is about 15%. Features that were correlated (in soft tissue lesions) with more aggressive biologic behavior include mitotic counts of greater than 1 mitosis/10 hpf, spindled tumor cell morphology, the presence of necrosis, and cytologic atypia.[423,424] Specific histologic features seem to correlate poorly with outcome for liver lesions.[426] Liver and lung lesions are discussed in pertinent chapters.

Grossly the tumor, regardless of the site, is well marginated, firm, rubbery, and has a cartilaginous consistency. Calcifications may occasionally be seen. Microscopically the tumor is commonly angiocentric and composed of short cords and nests of epithelioid endothelial cells with eosinophilic cytoplasm, occasionally showing intracellular vacuole/lumen, embedded in myxohyaline matrix (Figs 9.160, 9.161). The intracytoplasmic vacuoles may contain

intraluminal erythrocytes, a sign of 'primitive' vasoformative differentiation. Epithelioid hemangioendothelioma usually expresses vascular markers (Fig. 9.162) (CD34, CD31) and may have focal keratin expression. It should be noted that CD31 antibodies are reactive with intratumoral macrophages, which can lead to an erroneous interpretation of vascular neoplasia in other types of tumors.[427] More recently, FLI1 antibodies have been shown to react with vascular lesions, despite their original utility in separating round cell tumors of childhood.[428,429]

The differential diagnosis includes adenocarcinoma, with infiltrating cells showing intracytoplasmic vacuoles or signet ring cells. However carcinoma is not vasocentric and different areas may show obvious gland formation. The vacuoles of carcinoma are also mucicarmine-positive and the neoplastic cells are positive for antibodies against cytokeratin and negative for vascular markers by immunohistochemistry. A panel approach is recommended, as occasionally epithelioid hemangioendothelioma may show some cytokeratin positivity. Melanoma also comes into the differential

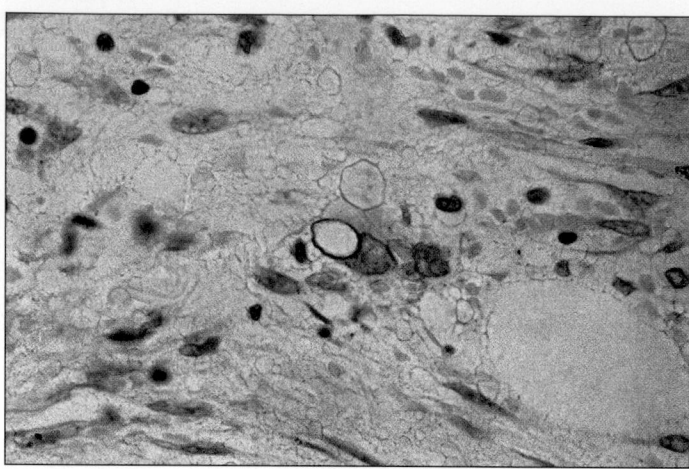

Fig. 9.162 Epithelioid hemangioendothelioma. An intracytoplasmic lumen is highlighted by CD34.

diagnosis and may appear as infiltrating epithelioid cells with eosinophilic cytoplasm. Close attention should be paid to melanin pigment, binucleation, and prominent intranuclear inclusions. By immunohistochemistry, melanoma cells are usually positive for S-100 protein and HMB-45 and negative for vascular markers and keratin. Epithelioid angiosarcoma is readily distinguished, in most instances, by its paucity of myxohyaline matrix and its tendency for more atypism, cellularity, mitotic activity, and necrosis. Interanastomosing vascular channels with prominent melanoma-like intranuclear inclusions are also more prevalent in angiosarcoma.

Features that serve to distinguish epithelioid hemangioendothelioma from epithelioid hemangioma (see Chapter 8) are infiltrative growth pattern, less pronounced inflammatory response, more primitive vascular pattern as opposed to well formed vessels, and cytologic atypia. Epithelioid sarcoma also comes into the differential diagnosis. It differs histologically by featuring a rather distinctive geographic or granulomatous growth pattern with central necrosis. Chondrosarcoma, like epithelioid hemangioendothelioma, contains sulfated acid mucins. However, in contrast to chondrosarcoma, the neoplastic cells of epithelioid hemangioendothelioma typically lack S100 protein expression. Epithelioid hemangioendothelioma exhibiting pleural or peritoneal extension can grow in an organ-encasing manner and produce a pattern reminiscent of malignant mesothelioma. Intraosseous epithelioid hemangioendothelioma, especially if multifocal, can be confused histologically with myeloma, since both tumors may feature coarsely granular nuclear chromatin and hyaline-like eosinophilic cytoplasm.

KAPOSI'S SARCOMA

Kaposi's sarcoma was first described as 'idiopathic multiple pigmented sarcoma of the skin' in 1872.[430] There are different epidemiological subgroups that are at high risk for Kaposi's sarcoma.[431]

Classic or European form

This subtype classically affects elderly males with an increased incidence in Ashkenazi Jews and people of Mediterranean descent. The disease has an indolent course with lesions involving predominantly the lower legs. Secondary malignancies have been reported in more than 30% of cases, mostly of hematopoietic origin.[432]

African or endemic form

This variant originally had its highest incidence in Zaire and Uganda.[433–435] The disease has been subsequently subdivided into two groups: young to middle-aged adults with mostly benign nodular disease, and children with fulminant lymphadenopathic disease typically fatal in a 2–3-year period.

Iatrogenic form associated with immunosuppression

This subtype is found in transplant patients. It is usually more aggressive than the classic form but regression frequently follows discontinuation of immunosuppression.[433–435]

Acquired immunodeficiency syndrome (AIDS)-associated or epidemic form

The risk of developing Kaposi's sarcoma was reported as 300 times greater in AIDS patients than other immunosuppressed patients in the 1990 following the US AIDS epidemic that began in 1981.[436] However, during the mid 1990s, the incidence of Kaposi's sarcoma declined sharply. For example, in San Francisco, where rates were about 33/100 000 in 1991, the incidence declined to 2.8/100 000 in 1998 (a tenfold reduction).[437] This reduction is probably a result of highly active antiretroviral therapy.[438] Since earlier observers noted that Kaposi's sarcoma was most frequent in homosexual men with AIDS practicing oroanal and anal intercourse, it was suspected that an infectious agent incited Kaposi's sarcoma. Many agents have been implicated but most recently, a unique human herpesvirus, now called Kaposi's sarcoma-associated herpesvirus (KSHV) or human herpesvirus 8, has been isolated from HIV-associated and non-AIDS-related Kaposi's sarcoma lesions. Furthermore, this virus is consistently present in a specific type of non-Hodgkin's lymphoma frequently although not exclusively occurring in patients with AIDS (i.e. the primary effusion lymphoma, previously called body-cavity-based lymphoma). KSHV is also present in a significant proportion of cases of AIDS- and non-AIDS-related multicentric Castleman's disease.[439–444] Additional experience with this virus will probably result in improved treatment strategies for Kaposi's sarcoma.[438,445,446]

Three clinical disease patterns of Kaposi's sarcoma have been recognized: (1) nodular; (2) aggressive; and (3) generalized. *Nodular disease* is characterized by the presence of circumscribed cutaneous or subcutaneous nodules. It usually pursues an indolent course, although internal involvement, which is frequently asymptomatic, is often present at the time of death. The *aggressive form* of Kaposi's sarcoma generally arises from a background of pre-existing nodular disease. It is characterized by extensive exophytic and ulcerative or deep infiltrative growth usually involving the extremities. Osseous and visceral involvement are commonly present but may be clinically silent. The *generalized form* of Kaposi's sarcoma includes lymphadenopathic disease with or without systemic involvement primarily occurring in children. AIDS-associated Kaposi's sarcoma may appear at any stage but usually affects those with advanced immune suppression and CD4+ T-cell counts of less than 500 cells/mm^3. In contrast to the classic form, AIDS-associated Kaposi's sarcoma lesions are often seen over the chest and face (Fig. 9.163).

Kaposi's sarcoma is a vascular/lymphatics-related process with endothelial and vascular-derived supporting cells being the key elements. Flow cytometric analyses of Kaposi's lesions show predominantly a diploid pattern (or a low level of aneuploidy).[447–450] Histologically there are no well defined differences between the four subtypes of Kaposi's sarcoma. The earliest or *patch lesions* occur in the upper dermis. The changes appear very inconspicuous and may be easily missed as an inflammatory condition (Fig. 9.164). Charac-

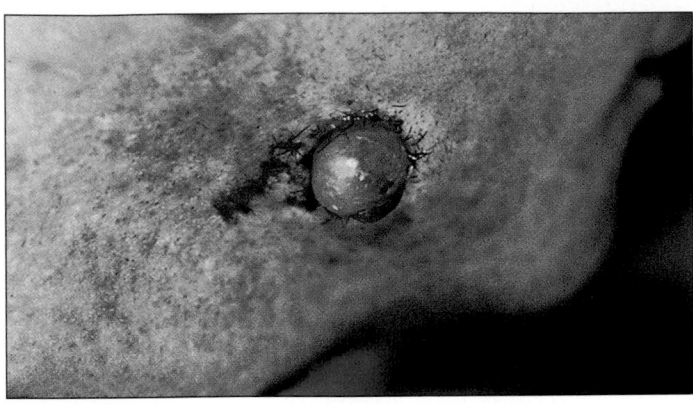

Fig. 9.163 Kaposi's sarcoma. Epidemic (AIDS-associated) lesions are often on the face.

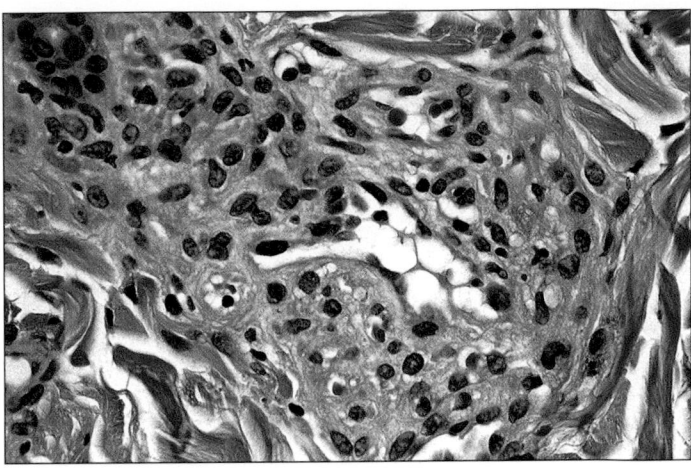

Fig. 9.165 Kaposi's sarcoma. At the patch stage, the lesion proliferates around pre-existing vessels (promontory sign).

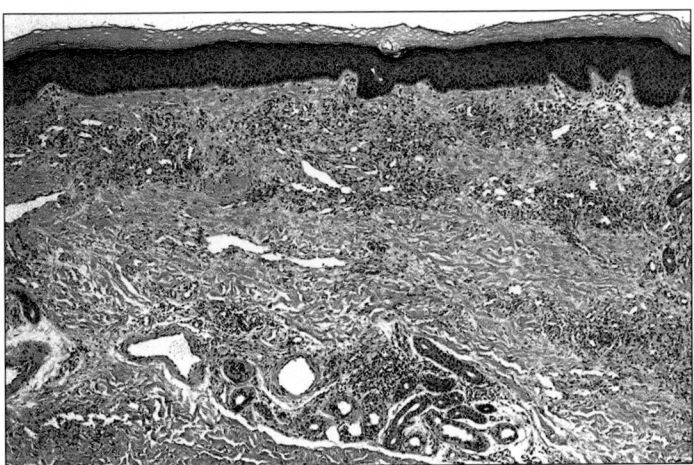

Fig. 9.164 Kaposi's sarcoma. Early (patch stage) lesions can be difficult to diagnosis. Note the subtle hypercellularity in the superficial dermis.

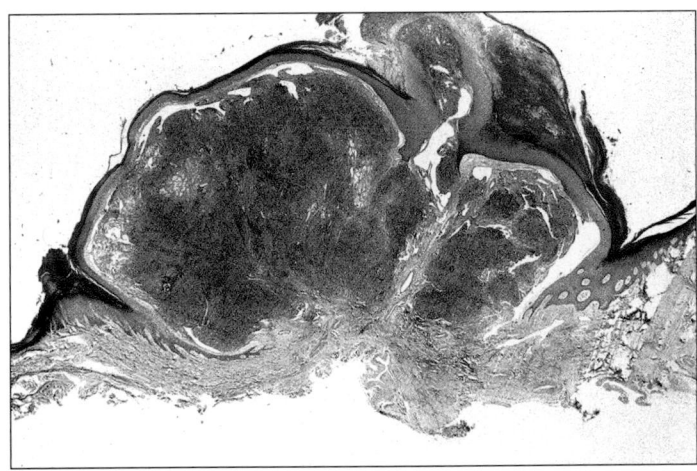

Fig. 9.166 Kaposi's sarcoma, nodular stage.

teristically there is proliferation of thin-walled, jagged capillaries around pre-existing dermal vessels and adnexa, sometimes protruding into the lumen of a pre-existing larger dermal vessel resulting in the so called 'promontory sign' (Fig. 9.165). Some endothelial cells may contain apoptotic nuclei. Variable numbers of inflammatory cells dominated by lymphocytes and plasma cells are usually seen, along with extravasated erythrocytes, hemosiderin deposition, and intracytoplasmic PAS-positive hyaline globules. As the process progresses to involve the full thickness of the dermis it becomes palpable, clinically recognized as *plaque stage*, which has a more prominent spindled cell component dispersed amongst the dermal collagen, forming slit-like spaces that frequently contain red blood cells. *Nodular lesions* of Kaposi's sarcoma (Fig. 9.166) represent further development and grossly appear as well circumscribed, violaceous, dome-shaped or polypoid masses. The spindle cells dominate forming fascicles and sheets with scattered extravasated red blood cells, hemosiderin-laden macrophages, hyaline globules, and inflammatory cells (Fig. 9.167). Although atypia is not typical it may be seen along with mitotic figures. Aspiration cytology can be diagnostic at this stage in the appropriate clinical setting (Figs 9.168, 9.169).

Rarely, a *lymphangioma-like variant* may occur.[451–456] Its clinical presentation does not appear to vary substantially from more typical cases. However, its histology differs by featuring a predominance of ectatic lymphatic-like channels that permeate the dermis. Associated inflammation is minimal but hemosiderin deposition is seen. A minor, ill-defined, spindle cell component may be present but it is not usually intermingled with the vascular clefts as in more typical Kaposi's lesions.

There are no well defined morphologic or immunohistochemical differences between the classical, endemic, iatrogenic (immunosuppressive), and AIDS-associated forms of Kaposi's sarcoma. While the histologic diagnosis of well developed nodular or plaque lesions is generally not difficult, early patch (macular) lesions may have sufficiently subtle morphology that a definite diagnosis can not be rendered. In the latter instance, little is usually lost by adopting a conservative stance, providing supportive medical management, and rebiopsying the patient at a later date when more typical lesions are present.

Pleomorphic or anaplastic change ('malignant transformation') has, on rare occasions, been reported in Kaposi's sarcoma. Lesions with this morphology are believed capable of true metastasis. In some instances, the morphology is indistinguishable from a spindled

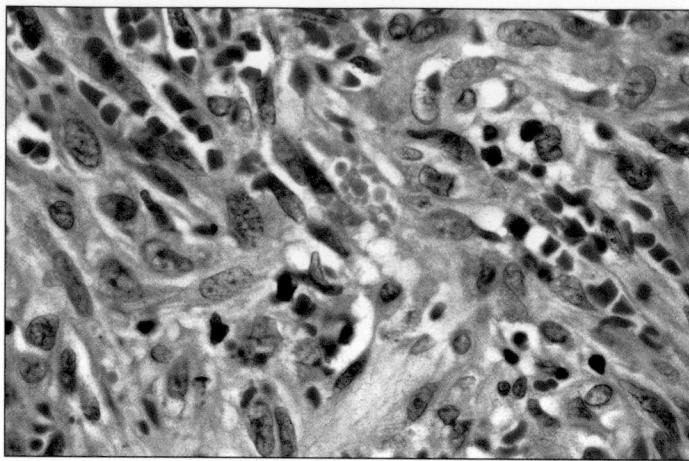

Fig. 9.167 Kaposi's sarcoma. The atypical spindle cells are accompanied by extravasated erythrocytes, hemosiderin, and hyaline globules. Plasma cells are present.

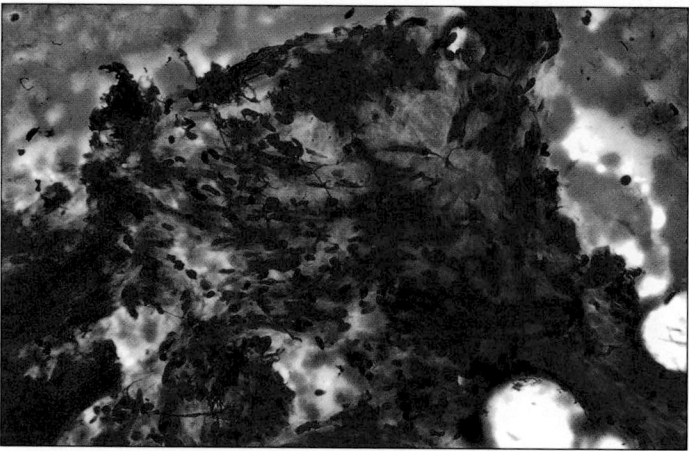

Fig. 9.168 Kaposi's sarcoma. The aspiration appearance recapitulates the histologic appearance.

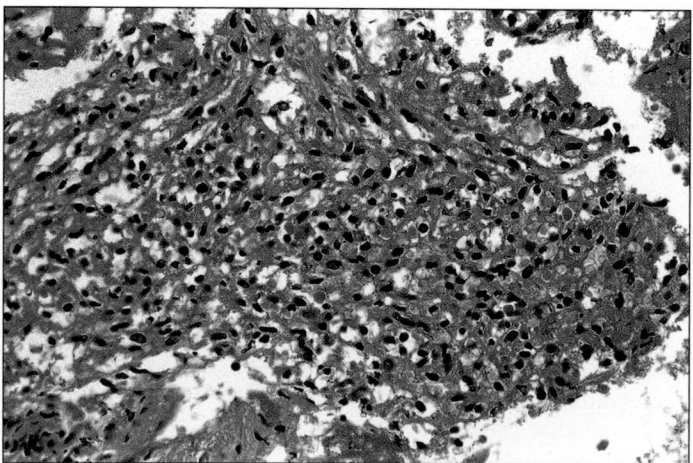

Fig. 9.169 Kaposi's sarcoma. This is the cell block from the aspirate depicted in Figure 9.170 It has a sieve-like appearance, another feature of Kaposi's sarcoma.

or poorly differentiated angiosarcoma. Other examples have been likened to fibrosarcoma or an undifferentiated malignancy.[457,458]

Kaposi's sarcoma may involve lymph nodes, either as an initial, sometimes isolated manifestation or as a later component of disseminated disease. Like cutaneous examples, it is readily recognized when the process is fully established but is difficult to characterize in its initial stages. Early changes include subcapsular sinus ectasia and intrasinusoidal vascular proliferation. Step sectioning may be required to identify a spindle cell component. Caution is advised when diagnosing early nodal Kaposi's sarcoma, especially when clinical details are not at hand, since other intranodal vascular proliferations may exhibit some morphologic overlap (i.e. vascular transformation of sinuses/nodal angiomatosis).[459,460]

The clinical differential diagnosis of Kaposi's sarcoma is quite long because of the various stages through which the disease progresses. It includes acro/angiodermatitis, bacillary angiomatosis, pyogenic granuloma, melanoma, cutaneous lymphoma, blue nevus, dermatofibroma, hemangioma, cicatrix, postinflammatory pigmentation, and a number of other conditions. The challenge lies in recognizing early stages of the disease as well as unusually aggressive examples. An accurate diagnosis in these instances is dependent on a high index of suspicion and appropriate clinicopathologic correlation.

Pseudo-Kaposi's sarcoma is an unfortunate term that includes acrodermatitis/angiodermatitis, which refers to skin lesions on lower extremities of patients with chronic venous insufficiency, and Stewart–Bluefarb syndrome, which consists of an arteriovenous malformation that clinically resembles Kaposi's sarcoma. Both types of lesion resemble Kaposi's sarcoma clinically but are quite distinct histologically. In acrodermatitis the histopathologic changes are those of stasis dermatitis with increased number of thick-walled blood vessels lined by plump endothelial cells, hemosiderin deposition, and extravasated red blood cell's. In Stewart–Bluefarb syndrome an arteriovenous shunt may be identified. *Targetoid hemosiderotic hemangioma* may mimic Kaposi's sarcoma histologically, but the clinical presentation is quite different. The lesions of targetoid hemosiderotic hemangioma have a characteristic target-like gross appearance. *Acquired progressive lymphangioma* (benign lymphangioendothelioma) has not been described in immunocompromised patients or in association with HSV 8.[461–466] This lesion presents as a solitary macule or plaque that slowly enlarges and is cured by local excision. Histologically, there are interanastomosing endothelium-lined vascular clefts lacking red blood cells, with a collagen dissecting pattern. *Bacillary angiomatosis* enters into the differential diagnosis since it has both a predilection for immunosuppressed patients and is typically a multifocal or generalized process. In fact, in the AIDS population, it is not uncommon for this disease to coexist with Kaposi's sarcoma. Its proper distinction is important since it is the result of a treatable infection that, if unmanaged, can prove fatal.

Nodular Kaposi's sarcoma features a prominent spindled component that commonly contains areas with a fascicular growth pattern. As a result, soft tissue sarcomas, including fibrosarcoma and leiomyosarcoma, may occasionally be considered in the differential diagnosis. All three tumors contain cells capable of reacting with immunohistochemical antibodies directed against MSA and SMA. Although longitudinal cytoplasmic fibrillations may also be seen in all three, they are much more prevalent and better defined in leiomyosarcoma. The latter entity differs further from the other two by featuring blunt-ended nuclei and more abundant eosinophilic cytoplasm. The plasma cell infiltrate, slit-like vascular spaces, degree of red blood cell extravasation, and hyaline globules in

Kaposi's sarcoma set it apart from both leiomyosarcoma and fibrosarcoma.

ANGIOSARCOMA

In this discussion, angiosarcoma is used to encompass fully malignant neoplasms of endothelial derivation whether originating from lymphatics (lymphangiosarcoma) or blood vessels (hemangiosarcoma). Angiosarcoma is a rare tumor, estimated to comprise fewer than 1% of all sarcomas. It can occur in a variety of clinical settings involving any site, but there is a particularly strong predilection for the skin and subcutis. In this superficial location angiosarcoma occurs in three distinct clinical settings: (1) face and scalp of the elderly;[467–471] (2) extremities of patients with chronic lymphedema;[472–479] and (3) at sites previously subjected to radiation therapy.[480–489] Angiosarcomas may develop in association with foreign bodies,[490–492] defunctionalized arteriovenous fistulas,[493–498] and also are seen with increased frequency in patients with neurofibromatosis.[499–503] Other carcinogenic agent exposures have also been implicated, particularly in hepatic tumors, e.g. thorotrast,[504–506] arsenic compounds,[506,507] and vinyl chloride.[506,508]

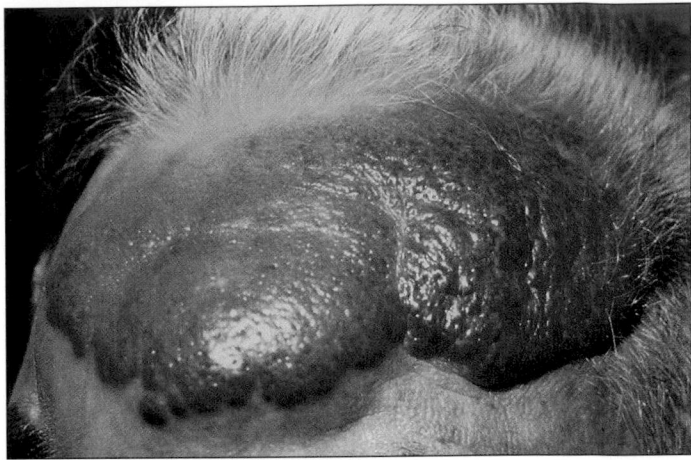

Fig. 9.170 Angiosarcoma. The scalp is a classic location for these aggressive tumors.

Angiosarcoma of the face and scalp (Wilson Jones angiosarcoma)

Cutaneous angiosarcoma of the face and scalp affects predominantly elderly patients and is usually found on the scalp and upper forehead (Fig. 9.170). It is more common in men than in women with no predisposing factors identified. Most cases show multifocality. Clinically, the lesion appears as an ill-defined, bruise-like area, occasionally starting as erythema and edema. More advanced cases appear as indurated plaques/nodules that may ulcerate, with or without small satellite nodules in the vicinity. The tumor grows slowly and centrifugally. The single most important prognostic factor is tumor size. The prognosis is poor.[468,470,471]

Lymphedema-associated angiosarcoma (Stewart–Treves syndrome)

Lymphedema-associated angiosarcoma was first described by Stewart and Treves in patients with breast carcinoma status following radical mastectomy with or without radiation developing chronic postoperative edema.[509] The average interval between the onset of postmastectomy lymphedema and the appearance of angiosarcoma is approximately 5–10 years. Later reports have described tumors in areas of lymphedema secondary to a variety of other mechanisms. Patients with congenital lymphedema tend to develop a superimposed angiosarcoma at an earlier age than their postmastectomy counterparts. Lymphedema is usually present for 20 years or more. These patients may have a somewhat longer mean survival time.[510] Gross examination typically reveals pitting, indurated skin with red or bluish purple macular, papular, polypoid, or fungating lesions. The tumors may be either solitary or multicentric, sometimes with an appearance of a dominant mass with satellite nodules. The overall prognosis of lymphedema-associated angiosarcoma is as bad as other forms of conventional angiosarcoma, if not worse.

Postirradiation angiosarcoma

Postirradiation angiosarcomas have a predilection for the skin and subcutis, although they occasionally arise in more deep-seated sites.

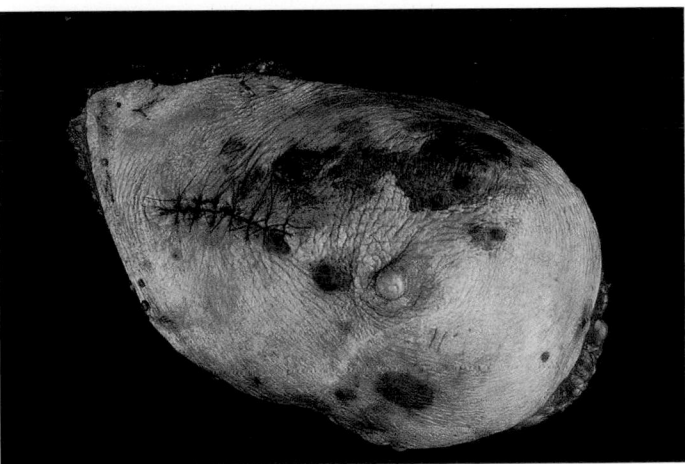

Fig. 9.171 Postradiation angiosarcoma of the breast. Note the purplish nodules.

Affected individuals can be subdivided into two groups based on whether radiotherapy was given for a benign disorder such as hemangioma or eczema, or for a malignancy such as gynecologic or breast cancers. The mean interval to angiosarcoma was shorter in the group treated for a malignancy, approximately 11 years versus 22 years for benign conditions. This difference could be due to the use of higher irradiation dosages in the malignant group. Postradiation well differentiated angiosarcoma in the breast (Fig. 9.171) must be distinguished from benign lymphangiomatous papules.[511] Such lesions were described in 1994 as 'atypical vascular lesions'[512] and consist of focal proliferation of dilated vascular spaces lined predominantly with a single layer of plump and sometimes hyperchromatic endothelial cells. Over time, these have been shown to be benign lesions and termed 'lymphangiomatous papules.'[511]

Angiosarcoma of deep soft tissue

Angiosarcoma of the deep tissue is rare and information about it is limited. Most cases involve the extremities or trunk and many are

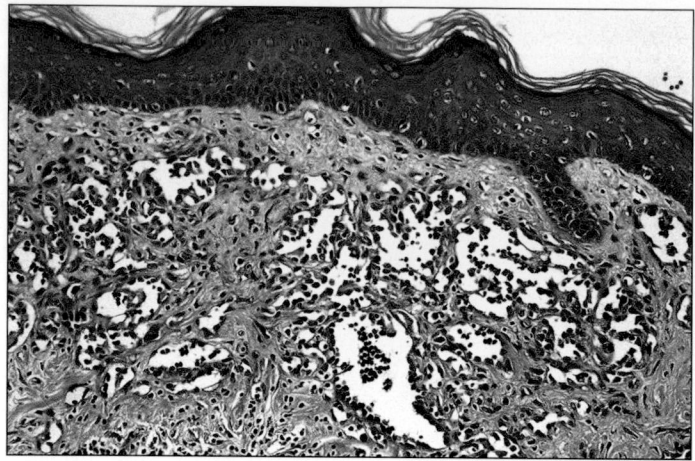

Fig. 9.172 Cutaneous angiosarcoma. Note the prominent endothelial cells, even at scanning magnification.

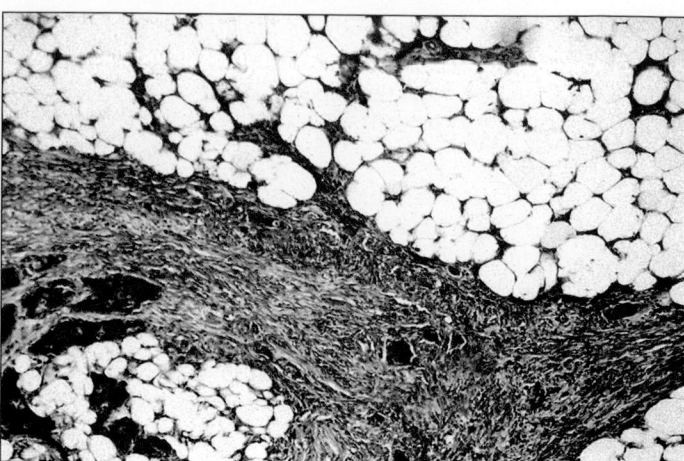

Fig. 9.174 This mesenteric angiosarcoma tracked along fat septa.

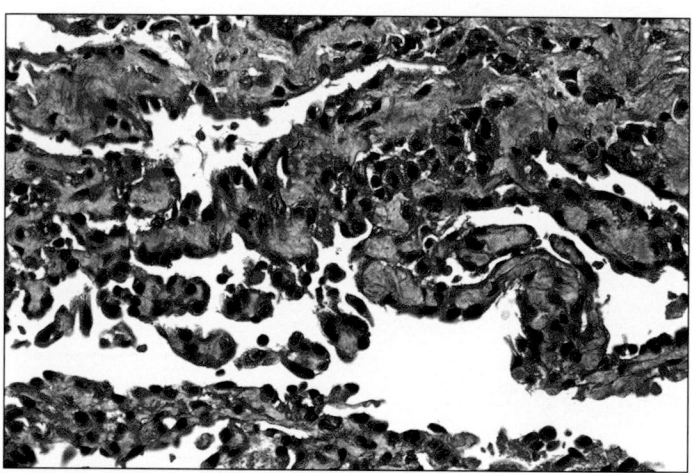

Fig. 9.173 Angiosarcoma composed of interanastomosing vasoformative channels.

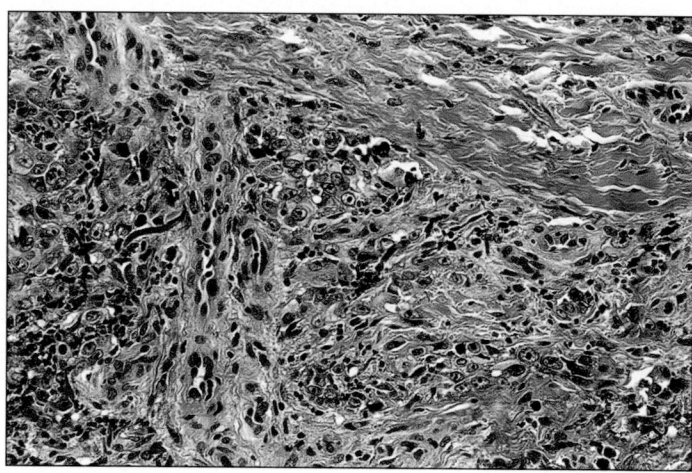

Fig. 9.175 Spindled and epithelioid angiosarcoma. Diagnosis of a lesion such as this is best made together with an immunohistochemical panel.

poorly differentiated. In general these tumors behave as high-grade sarcomas. Some deep-seated tumors appear to originate from medium to large vessels. Epithelioid morphology is well documented in this group and may lead to an erroneous diagnosis of carcinoma or melanoma.[513,514]

Angiosarcoma of the breast parenchyma

Angiosarcomas arising in the breast (de novo and unassociated with radiation or lymphedema) account for about less than 0.1% of all malignant neoplasms in the breast and are covered in Chapter 10.

Morphology of angiosarcomas

Histopathologically, angiosarcoma has a broad morphologic spectrum (Figs 9.172–9.177). At one extreme, the tumor may consist entirely of well developed hemangioma or lymphangioma-like vascular tissue in which the only clues to malignancy are the interanastomosing and infiltrative nature of the process, the presence of mild nuclear hyperchromasia, and an occasional crowding or piling up of the endothelium, sometimes forming small papillations.

The opposite end of the spectrum includes both a spindle cell pattern reminiscent of fibrosarcoma or Kaposi's sarcoma and an 'undifferentiated' pattern consisting of plump epithelioid neoplastic cells with prominent nucleoli and diffuse sheet-like growth, suggestive of carcinoma or melanoma. A high index of suspicion, knowledge of the clinical findings, and thorough tumor sampling are essential to establish the correct diagnosis at these morphologic extremes. When well developed vessels are not apparent, the presence of cytoplasmic vacuolization consistent with early lumen development and a milieu rich in red blood cells or hemosiderin may serve as important clues pointing in the direction of a vascular tumor. A reticulin stain can help to highlight tube-like vascular growth that may be inapparent in sections stained with hematoxylin and eosin.

Immunohistochemistry can prove invaluable when vasoformative architecture is minimal or absent. The endothelial cells stain positive with factor-VIII-related antigen, CD34, CD31, and *Ulex europaeus*. However, a panel approach is recommended as poorly differentiated tumors may not be positive for all the vascular markers. The epithelioid variants may stain with epithelial cell

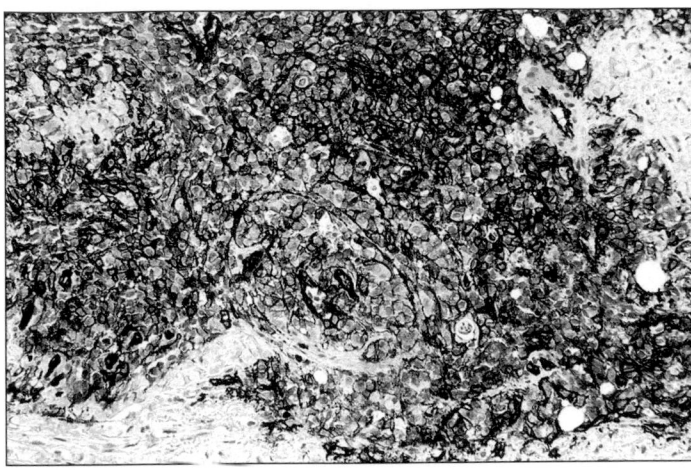

Fig. 9.176 Spindled and epithelioid angiosarcoma. This is the CD34 from the case depicted in Figure 9.175.

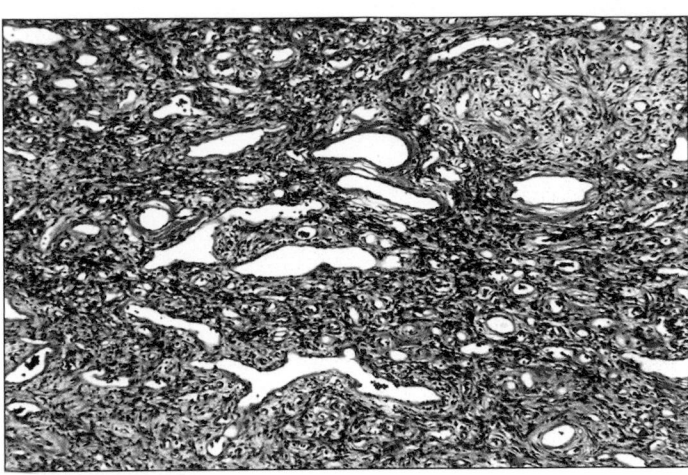

Fig. 9.178 Hemangiopericytoma, showing the classic staghorn vascular pattern.

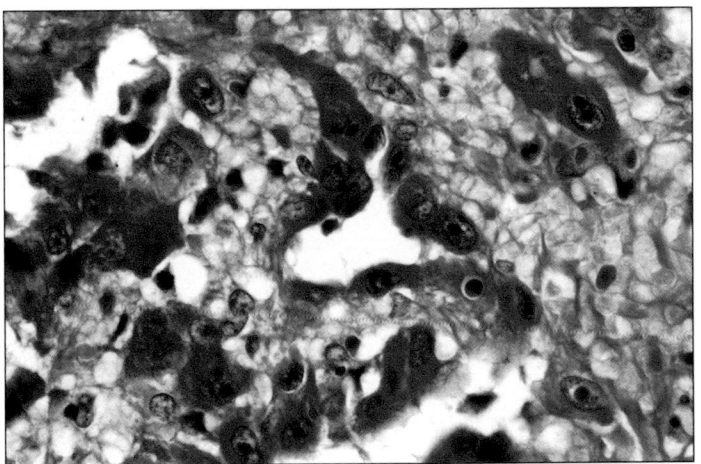

Fig. 9.177 Epithelioid angiosarcoma. This field is vasoformative but much of this tumor was not. Such cases should be subjected to a panel of immunohistochemical stains. This tumor was keratin-positive but strongly expressed vascular markers.

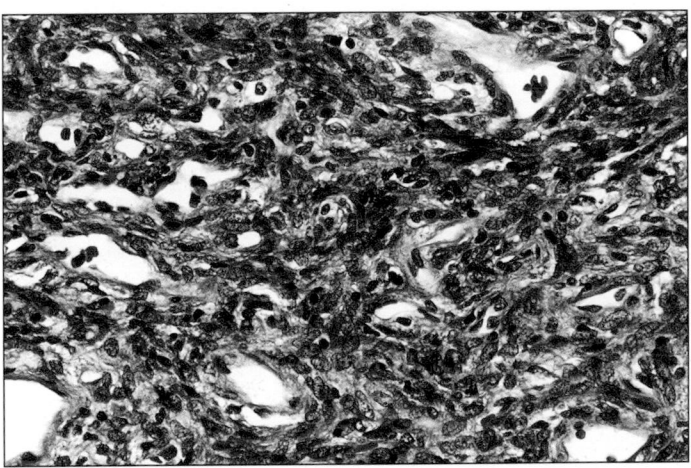

Fig. 9.179 Hemangiopericytoma. The lesional cells are angulated and immunohistochemically 'inert'.

markers such as cytokeratin. As noted previously, CD31 antibodies are reactive with intratumoral macrophages, which can lead to an erroneous interpretation of vascular neoplasia in other types of tumor.[427] Also, FLI1 antibodies have been shown to react with vascular lesions, despite their original utility in separating round small cell tumors of childhood.[428,429]

PERIVASCULAR TUMORS

HEMANGIOPERICYTOMA

Most tumors with a hemangiopericytomatous vascular pattern are not hemangiopericytomas but these masqueraders can generally be unmasked with an appropriate immunohistochemical pattern. What remains is a lesion most commonly involving the thigh or retroperitoneum of adults that weakly expresses CD34 but is otherwise

immunohistochemically 'inert'. The largest series to date remains Enzinger and Smith's, 106 cases published in 1976.[515] This series may have contained some examples of other entities, particularly solitary fibrous tumor (for example, one patient in Enzinger's series had tumor-associated hypoglycemia) but the authors carefully excluded the most important congener, synovial sarcoma, by noting the fascicular pattern of the latter. Today, this distinction is readily made with appropriate immunohistochemistry since synovial sarcomas express epithelial markers whereas hemangiopericytomas do not. These neoplasms have their classic 'staghorn' vascular pattern and small angulated cells (reticulin preparations show enclosure of every cell) (Figs 9.178–9.180). Although the diagnosis would be impossible prospectively on aspiration cytology, an aspirate from such a case is depicted in Figure 9.181.

Hemangiopericytomas can usually but not always be distinguished from solitary fibrous tumors. In general, solitary fibrous tumors have more abundant collagen than hemangiopericytoma and also strongly express CD34. Criteria for malignancy in both tumor types are similar. Solitary fibrous tumors have been shown to have a

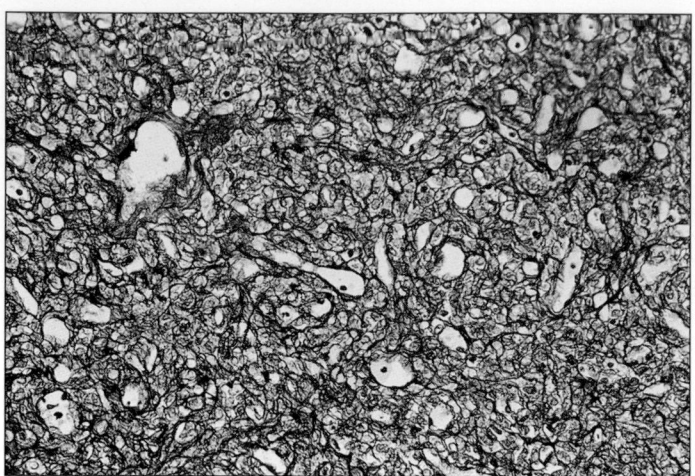

Fig. 9.180 Hemangiopericytoma. Reticulin encloses every cell.

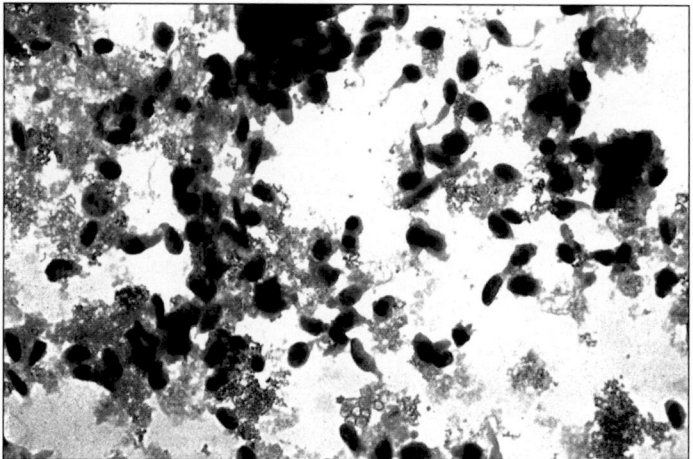

Fig. 9.181 Hemangiopericytoma, aspiration cytology. Such tumors have a low probability of accurate diagnosis on aspiration cytology.

different comparative genomic hybridization pattern than hemangio-pericytomas.[516] A group of hybrid tumors displaying fat as well as classic hemangiopericytomatous features have been recently described as 'lipomatous hemangiopericytomas'.[517–520]

GLOMUS TUMOR

These lesions are discussed in Chapter 8.

SYNOVIUM-RELATED TUMORS

TENOSYNOVIAL GIANT CELL TUMOR

Localized tenosynovial giant cell tumor (giant cell tumor of tendon sheath)

Localized or nodular tenosynovial giant cell tumor is far more common than the diffuse form and is, next to ganglion cyst, the most frequently encountered tumor affecting the hand. The lesion has a peak incidence between 30 and 50 years of age. Tumors involving the hand occur more commonly in males while an equal sex distribution has been reported for tumors arising in the toes. The tumor less frequently develops in the knee, ankle, wrist, and elbow. Polyarticular involvement by localized tenosynovial giant cell tumor occurs rarely. There has yet to be convincing evidence that this process is neoplastic and it seems to lack clonality.[521]

In the digit, localized tenosynovial giant cell tumor usually presents as a slow-growing, painless mass with discomfort or pain reported in only about 20% of tumors.[522] Tumors arising in the knee are more often associated with tenderness or a locking or snapping sensation with joint movement. On physical examination, the lesion is nonfluctuant and usually not attached to the overlying skin. However, tumors developing in the distal aspect of the finger or toe may become adherent to the skin and ulcerate. Plain radiographs of the lesion may show cortical erosion of the underlying bone, particularly in tumors involving the toes. The outcome of localized tenosynovial giant cell tumor is excellent, with only a 10–20% recurrence rate, this being attributable to incomplete excision. At surgery, a lobulated mass with a fibrous pseudocapsule and an attachment to the underlying synovium is the usual finding.

At gross examination, localized tenosynovial giant cell tumor appears as a firm, well circumscribed, lobulated mass. Tumors of the digits are small, typically measuring between 0.5 and 4 cm. Lesions arising in the wrist, ankle, and especially the knee, are generally larger and show more variability in shape. The tumor has a firm consistency and the cut surface is gray-white. The presence of yellow foci within the tumor represents aggregates of xanthoma cells, whereas brown pigment indicates hemosiderin deposition.

At low magnification, localized tenosynovial giant cell tumor is a well circumscribed, partially encapsulated mass (Fig. 9.182). It consists of an admixture of polygonal and spindled mononuclear cells, xanthoma cells, and multinucleated giant cells set in a collagenous, variably hyalinized stroma that is punctuated by rounded and cleft-like spaces. The overall cellularity and the distribution and relative proportions of these cellular elements characteristically vary throughout a given lesion. The central portion of the tumor tends to be more cellular than the well marginated periphery of the nodule where the cells become smaller, aggregates of xanthoma cells and hemosiderin-laden cells are usually in relatively greater abundance, and stroma is more densely collagenized (peripheral maturation).

The chief proliferating element is a mononuclear cell with a polygonal or short spindled shape, a scanty amount of pale to eosinophil cytoplasm, and a centrally-positioned, oval to reniform nucleus that often possesses a longitudinal groove (Figs 9.183, 9.184). These cells grow in a sheet-like configuration or within tightly aggregated nests invested by collagen. Mitotic activity is typically higher in more cellular tumors. The osteoclast-like giant cells have nuclei that appear similar to those of the surrounding mononuclear cells, suggesting that the giant cells form from fusion of the mononuclear cells. Cells containing lipid (foamy or xanthomatous cells) and hemosiderin deposits are present in the majority of cases. Touton giant cells are occasionally observed.

Cleft-like, pseudoglandular spaces are characteristic of tenosynovial giant cell tumor and are more commonly observed in tumors arising in association with larger joints, such as the knee and ankle.[522] Some of these elongated spaces are partially lined by synovium-like cells and probably represent native synovium engulfed by the advancing tumor. In time, these spaces lose their cellular lining. The spaces may contain xanthoma cells.

The amount and type of stromal collagen depends partially on the cellularity of the lesion. Tumors studied early in their evolution are generally more cellular and have relatively small quantities of delicate collagen. In older lesions, thick bands of dense collagen and extensively hyalinized collagen reminiscent of osteoid (pseudo-osteoid) prevail. There may be cartilaginous or osseous metaplasia. Inflammation is sparse but scattered collections of lymphocytes may be identified.

Immunohistochemically, both reactive synovial lining cells and the cells of the tenosynovial giant cell tumor demonstrate mono-cytic/histiocytic differentiation. Along with vimentin, the mononuclear cells express macrophage-related antigens CD68 (KP1), HAM56, and alpha-1-antichymotrypsin. Anti-vimentin, CD68 (KP1), alpha-1-antichymotrypsin, and leukocyte common antigen (LCA) stain the multinucleated giant cells. Both components variably express the dendritic fibroblast marker factor XIIIa.[523,524]

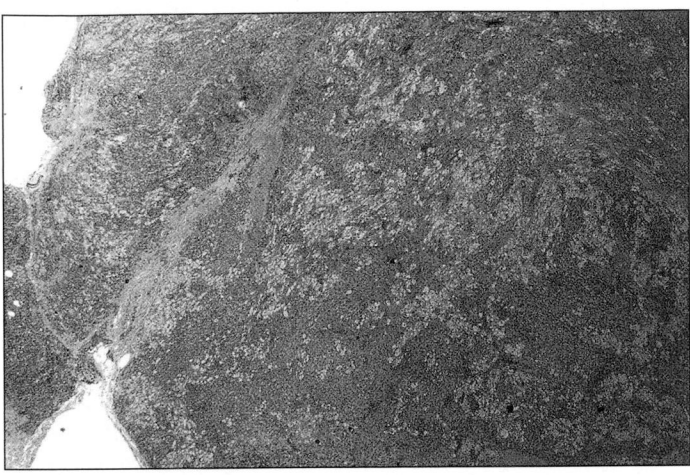

Fig. 9.182 Tenosynovial giant cell tumor, localized type (giant cell tumor of tendon sheath). At scanning power, lobulation and foamy macrophages are apparent.

Diffuse tenosynovial giant cell tumor (pigmented villonodular tenosynovitis)

Jaffe, Lichtenstein, and Sutro first coined the term, 'pigmented villonodular synovitis' (PVNS) for this family of localized and diffuse tenosynovium- and bursa-based giant cell tumors.[525] In present-day practice, this terminology is reserved for the diffuse intra-articular form of the disease. Most cases of extra-articular diffuse giant cell tumor are probably extension of PVNS outside the joint space.

The clinical features and outcome of diffuse tenosynovial giant cell tumor more closely parallel those of PVNS than localized tenosynovial giant cell tumor. In comparison to localized tenosynovial giant cell tumor, diffuse tenosynovial giant cell tumor (and PVNS) occurs in a slightly younger population with approximately 50% of the patients diagnosed prior to 40 years of age. The lesion involves females slightly more often than males. The para-articular soft tissue and intra-articular surface of the knee are the most common locations for diffuse tenosynovial giant cell tumor and PVNS respectively. The ankle, foot, and wrist are less commonly involved sites for diffuse tenosynovial giant cell tumor according to the records of the AFIP.[3] Tumors have also been reported in the hip, sacroiliac joint, vertebral column, and digits. Unlike the usual presentation for localized tenosynovial giant cell tumor, diffuse tenosynovial giant cell tumor (and PVNS) more commonly causes joint pain, functional impairment, including limitation of motion of the joint, joint effusion, and hemarthrosis. The duration of symptoms range from months to decades.

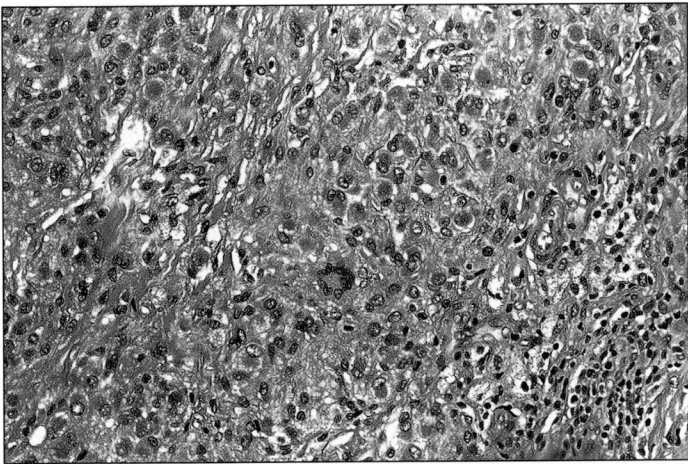

Fig. 9.183 Tenosynovial giant cell tumor, localized type (giant cell tumor of tendon sheath). Sometimes giant cells are numerous in these tumors, although this example had only a few.

The recurrence rate of diffuse tenosynovial giant cell tumor is similar to that of PVNS: 40–50% of patients develop local recurrence. The basic approach to treatment should be an attempt to remove as much of the tumor as possible while trying to maintain the function of the involved extremity.

The bulky, sheet-like, and multinodular growth pattern of diffuse tenosynovial giant cell tumor helps distinguish it from the localized variant. Unfortunately, both localized and diffuse tumors may show similar gross features early in their evolution. Diffuse tenosynovial giant cell tumor has a firm consistency with a variegated tan-yellow to red-brown cut surface. In contrast to localized tenosynovial giant cell tumor, the tumor lacks a fibrous capsule and has more prominent cleft-like invaginations. The shaggy, matted villous projections so characteristic of PVNS are not generally seen in diffuse tenosynovial giant cell tumor.

The cellular composition, fibrous stroma, and cleft-like and rounded spaces differ little from those described for localized

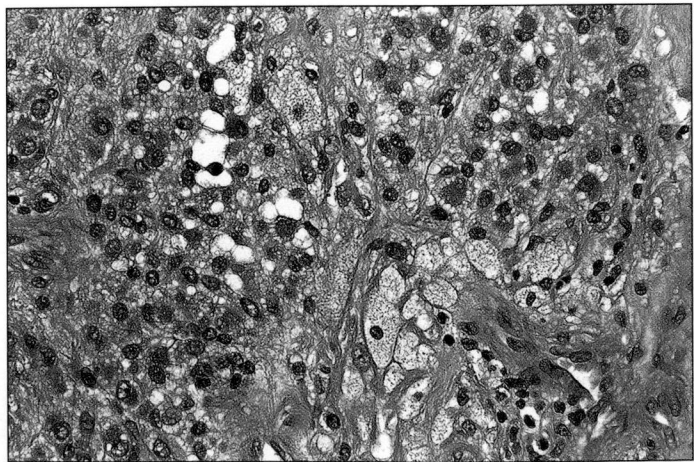

Fig. 9.184 Tenosynovial giant cell tumor, localized type (giant cell tumor of tendon sheath). These display monotonous cytologic features.

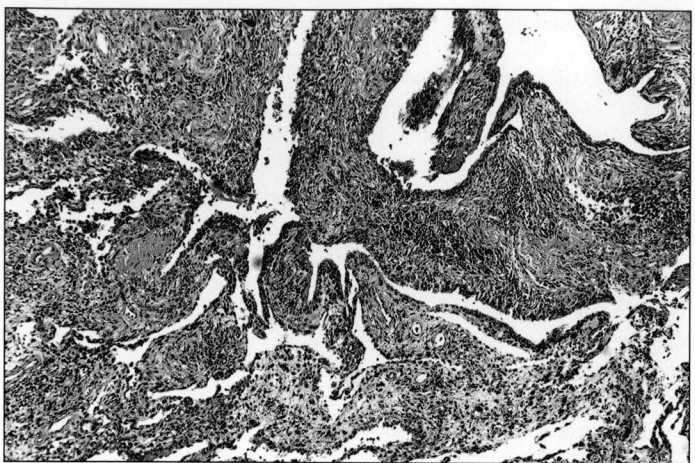

Fig. 9.185 Tenosynovial giant cell tumor, diffuse type (pigmented villonodular tenosynovitis). This lesion displays prominent hemosiderin deposition and is associated with synovium but is otherwise similar to the localized form.

tenosynovial giant cell tumor (Fig. 9.185). The tumor grows in an expansile manner and lacks a fibrous capsule. Multinucleation and xanthomatous change are less commonly observed in diffuse than in the localized variant.

Reactive synovial hyperplasias associated with hemarthrosis, degenerative and destructive joint diseases, and failed orthopedic prosthetics grossly and histologically imitate PVNS. These processes cause villous expansion of the synovium. However, unlike PVNS, this synovial proliferation is principally due to collagen deposition, an increase in the number of reactive vessels, and, in some instances, a pronounced chronic inflammatory cell infiltrate. Although the number of synovial lining cells may be modestly increased in these disorders, they do not form a tumoral mass.

The failure of the pathologist or surgeon to identify a tenosynovial or bursal origin for diffuse tenosynovial giant cell tumor, coupled with its expansile growth pattern, may lead to a consideration of sarcoma. The absence of cellular pleomorphism and atypical mitotic figures, presence of cleft-like spaces, an occasional multi-nucleated cell or cells containing fat or hemosiderin, and the appreciation of 'peripheral maturation' will help the pathologist arrive at the correct diagnosis.

Malignant tenosynovial giant cell tumor

The existence of a malignant form of tenosynovial giant cell tumor has been the subject of controversy. First, the nature of the tenosynovial giant cell tumor remains unknown; some investigators favor a reactive etiology. Furthermore, early studies of tumors categorized as malignant tenosynovial giant cell tumor included unrelated neoplasms such as giant cell MFH, clear cell sarcoma, and epithelioid sarcoma.

For the diagnosis of malignant tenosynovial giant cell tumor, the malignant lesion should either coexist with or present as a recurrence of a documented, conventional tenosynovial giant cell tumor.[3] Bertoni et al.[526] broadened the definition to include any synovium-based sarcoma with overlapping histopathologic features of a conventional PVNS. These are extremely rare lesions. The location, age range, and clinical signs and symptoms of malignant tenosynovial giant cell tumor closely parallel those of diffuse tenosynovial giant cell

tumor. Females are affected more often than males.[526] The mean age of clinical recognition is about one or two decades later (sixth to seventh decade) than for diffuse tenosynovial giant cell tumor. The majority of tumors occur in the knee, followed by the ankle and foot.[526] Commonly reported complaints include joint swelling, pain, and effusion.

The reported data on the behavior of these lesions is sparse but indicates that malignant tenosynovial giant cell tumor is a locally aggressive neoplasm with the potential for metastasis. The lung was the most common metastatic site and all patients with pulmonary metastasis died.[526]

On gross examination, the neoplasm has a bulky, multinodular appearance with an intra-articular component and extension beyond the joint space into the surrounding skeletal muscle and fat.

Malignant tenosynovial giant cell tumor grows in infiltrating nodules. Sheets of tumor cells are accompanied by sparse stroma. Necrosis is a conspicuous feature and focal hemorrhage may also be present. In contrast to diffuse tenosynovial giant cell tumor, malignant tenosynovial giant cell tumor has a more monotonous cytologic appearance as xanthoma cells and hemosiderin-laden cells are virtually absent. Mitotic activity is variable but atypical mitotic figures can be observed. Peripheral maturation is absent in malignant lesions and the cleft-like and rounded spaces are also markedly diminished in size and number.

SOLITARY FIBROUS TUMOR

In early literature, these tumors were described as pleura-based lesions believed to be the benign localized counterpart of 'fibrous' mesotheliomas, an assertion supported by tissue culture studies. Subsequent ultrastructural and early immunohistochemical studies supported a fibroblastic origin for the proliferating cells.[527] The clinical behavior of the pleura-based tumors was well delineated by England et al.,[528] who described 223 cases from AFIP archives and offered criteria for separating malignant from benign examples. These included the presence of >4 mitoses/10 hpf, prominent nucleoli, and nuclear pleomorphism in malignant lesions. These tumors were also known to elaborate insulin-like growth factors and were sometimes associated with hypoglycemia. Solitary fibrous tumors have now been described in many sites, including the soft tissues.[529–535] Criteria for malignancy are not well established but the criteria developed for the pleural tumors are serviceable.

Grossly, regardless of their location, solitary fibrous tumors are typically well marginated.

Microscopically, solitary fibrous tumors characteristically display a 'patternless pattern' of spindled fibroblast-like cells and collagen in varying proportions arranged in a disorderly fashion (Figs 9.186–9.187). The individual cells have spindled to plump, ovoid nuclei and eosinophilic cytoplasm. They may also appear hemangiopericytoma-like with closely packed cells with amphophilic cytoplasm arranged around staghorn-shaped vessels, or they may have a myxoid appearance (Fig. 9.188).

On immunohistochemical staining, solitary fibrous tumors consistently express CD34 (Fig. 9.189), regardless of their malignant potential[531,536,537] and lack muscle markers (actins and desmin), keratins, and S100 protein. The are said to retain their 'patternless pattern' on aspiration cytology, although diagnosis by aspiration biopsy can probably only be suggested in lesions with striking CD34 positivity on cell blocks. One is unlikely to be able to assess malignant potential from aspiration cytology[538,539] (Figs 9.190, 9.191).

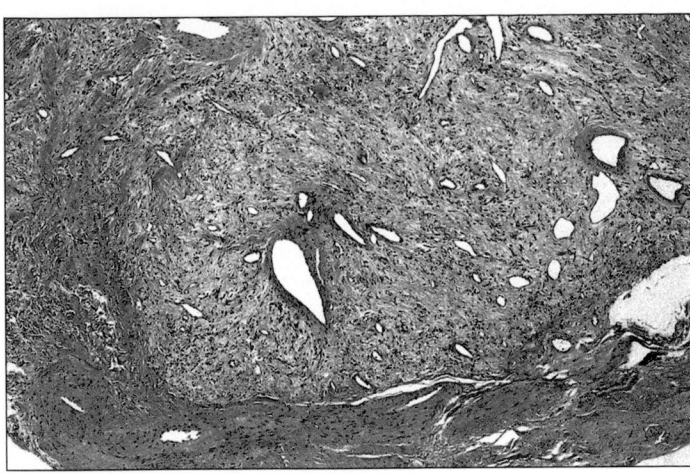

Fig. 9.186 Solitary fibrous tumor. A patternless pattern, wiry collagen, and staghorn vessels are all features of solitary fibrous tumor.

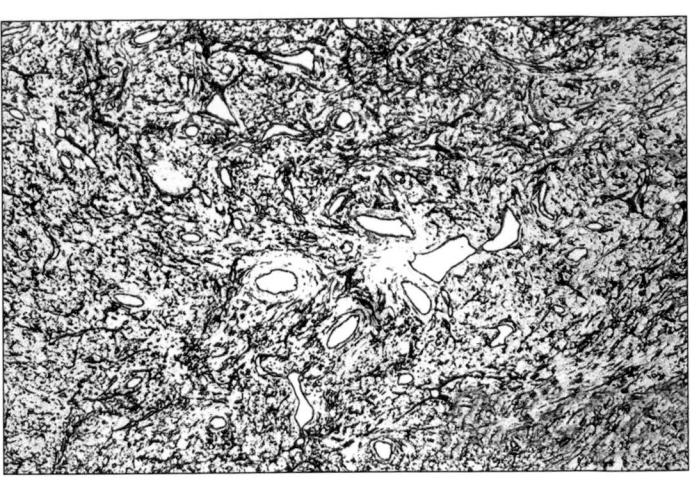

Fig. 9.189 Solitary fibrous tumor expresses CD34 consistently.

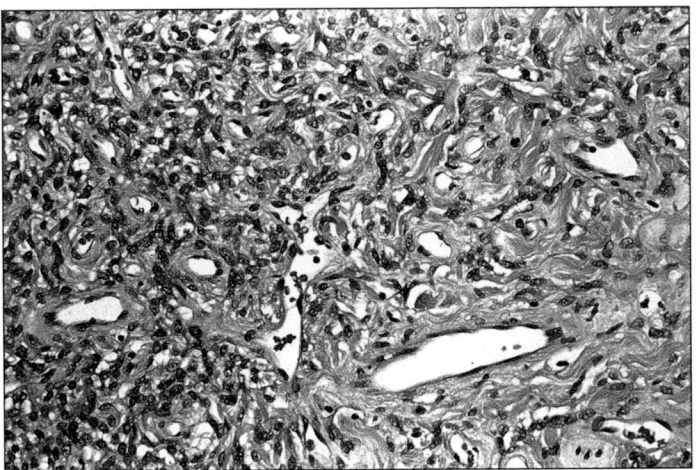

Fig. 9.187 Solitary fibrous tumor. Uniform angulated cells comprise this lesion.

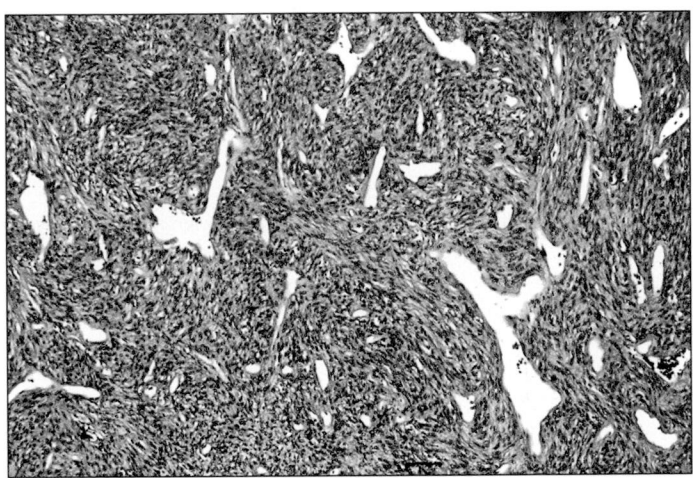

Fig. 9.190 This example of solitary fibrous tumor had abundant mitoses and behaved in a malignant fashion; note the prominent staghorn (hemangiopericytoma-like) vascular pattern and marked cellularity compared to the lesions depicted in Figures 9.188–9.190.

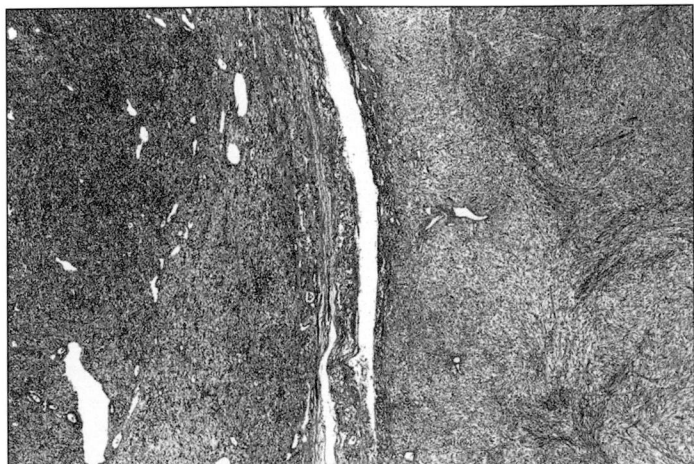

Fig. 9.188 Solitary fibrous tumor. The left side of this field shows the usual pattern, whereas the right side is quite myxoid, a feature that sometimes predominates in these tumors.

The differential diagnosis of solitary fibrous tumor revolves around fibroblastic lesions with abundant collagen and neoplasms with a hemangiopericytoma-like vascular pattern (Table 9.13). Separating them from fibromatoses is straightforward as fibromatoses seldom express CD34 and are infiltrative. Low-grade fibrosarcomas are also generally CD34-negative. This then leads to other CD34-positive lesions and hemangiopericytoma-like lesions as the principal contenders in the differential diagnosis. Myofibroblastoma (see Figs 9.25–9.30), like solitary fibrous tumor, contains wiry collagen, is well marginated grossly, and uniformly and strongly expresses CD34.[59] Some observers believe they are the same tumor.[59] Myofibroblastomas differ from solitary fibrous tumors in that malignant examples are not described and by their expression of muscle markers immunohistochemically and ultrastructural demonstration of myofibroblastic features. They have been described in the breast,[56] lymph nodes,[57,58] and a variety of other sites and are benign. One of their characteristic features is the presence of wiry collagen fibers called 'amianthoid fibers'.[58] Myofibroblastomas may also

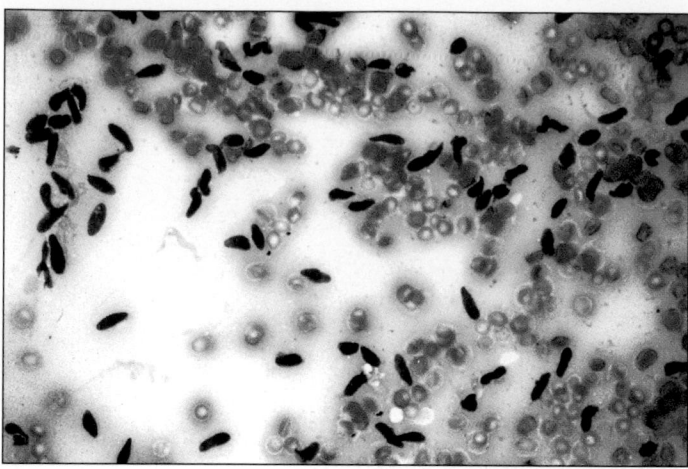

Fig. 9.191 Aspiration cytology from the tumor depicted in Figure 9.192. This would be difficult to diagnose prospectively.

show areas of typical smooth muscle differentiation,[540–542] a finding not reported in solitary fibrous tumors.

NEURAL TUMORS

TRAUMATIC NEUROMA

Traumatic neuromas are the most common reactive lesion of peripheral nerves and are the prototypic true neuromas. They are formed by disorganized growth of peripheral nerve tissue after neural disruption. Following either partial or complete severance of a peripheral nerve, axons and myelin sheaths distal to the injury site degenerate. Residual Schwann cells, with associated basement membrane, form tubules that are awaiting the extension of regenerating axons emanating from the intact proximal aspect of the nerve. If the proximal and distal portions of the nerve have been widely displaced or the path of regeneration is blocked, the proliferating proximal nerve elements cannot reach the distal nerve tubes and instead grow in an aimless and disorganized manner. This resulting disordered growth is referred to as an amputation or traumatic neuroma. The development of a traumatic neuroma takes

Table 9.13 Differential diagnosis of solitary fibrous tumor of soft tissue

Tumor type	Solitary fibrous tumor	Hemangiopericytoma	Myofibroblastoma	Myofibroma	Synovial sarcoma	Mesenchymal chondrosarcoma
Criteria for malignancy	>4 mits/10 hpf, nucleoli and pleomorphism in malignant cases	>4 mits/10 hpf, nucleoli and pleomorphism in malignant cases	Benign	Benign	Malignant	Malignant
IHC	CD34+ SMA− MSA− DES− CK− S100− CD99+ Bcl-2+	CD34− weak SMA− MSA− DES− CK− S100− CD99+	CD34+ SMA+ MSA+ DES− (variable) CK− S100− Bcl-2 +	CD34− SMA+ MSA+ DES− (variable) CK− S100−	CD34− SMA− MSA− DES− CK-focal S100-focal CD99+ Bcl-2+ EMA+ Calponin+	CD34− SMA− MSA− DES− CK− S100-focal CD99+ Bcl-2+ EMA−
Molecular/ cytogenetic	t(4, 19), t(12, 19) (not specific)	Trisomy 8 (not specific)	?	?	t(X;18) SSX1 and SSX2	No specific abnormality
Electron microscopic	Fibroblastic	Primitive cells with basal lamina, pinocytosis,	Myofibroblastic	Myofibroblastic	Scattered poorly formed desmosome-type intercellular junctions	Cartilage areas: well developed Golgi, glycogen, and rough endoplasmic reticulum (cartilaginous features). Small cells: minimal organelles (undifferentiated features)
Morphology	'Patternless pattern', wiry abundant collagen, 'amianthoid' fibers, every cell invested by reticulin	Uniform angulated cells with minimal collagen, classic staghorn vessels, every cell invested by reticulin	Similar to solitary fibrous tumor; divergent immuno-histochemistry, no malignant examples	Lobulated myoid lobules separated by primitive areas with staghorn vasculature. Reticulin invests every cell	Spindled, scant cytoplasm, biphasic and monophasic variants. Reticulin invests every cell.	Uniform 'blue cells' with inconspicuous nucleoli punctuated by islands of mature cartilage. Reticulin invests groups of cells.

several weeks and clinically the patient presents with a painful nodule at the site of prior trauma.

The histologic findings of this process are distinctive. Grossly traumatic neuromas display bulbous white tissue with an associated segment of peripheral nerves. Typically, amputation neuromas are incidental findings identified only microscopically. Histologically these consist of a haphazard tangle of peripheral nerve tissue arranged in microfasicals with abundant interspersed fibroblasts. S100 staining can highlight normal nerves and EMA staining can highlight perineurial tissue admixed in the process and outlining each small fascicle.

MORTON'S NEUROMA

Morton's neuroma is also referred to as localized interdigital neuritis. It is a degenerative change of plantar digital nerves with associated fibrosis and enlargement of the affected site. This lesion predominantly affects women as a consequence of tight, ill-fitting shoes. The classic clinical presentation is of a woman with unilateral burning pain localized to the plantar aspect of the foot and sometimes radiating into a toe, which is relieved by resting the foot or removing the shoe. The nerves most typically affected are the digital nerves of the second and third metatarsal phalangeal interspaces. Chronic compression of these nerves with vascular compromise is believed to be the cause of this disorder. Grossly the process is a nodule or fusiform soft tissue enlargement. Microscopically, all nerve layers (epineurium, perineurium, and endoneurium) are sclerosed to varying degrees. Clear-cut thickening of the perineurium is a typical finding. In addition to endoneural fibrosis, myxoid changes in the endoneurium may be found. Thickened, occluded small digital arteries are often seen. In many examples, the adjacent intermetatarsal bursa displays degenerative changes.

As a clinical pathologic entity Morton's neuroma is specific. However, microscopically these lesions are readily mistaken for other processes. For example, they may appear similar to ganglion cysts owing to adjacent degenerative bursal tissue. However, ganglion cysts do not display degenerative changes in adjacent neurovascular tissue, a characteristic of Morton's neuroma. Morton's neuroma may also be mistaken for amputation neuromas.

SCHWANNOMA

Schwannomas are discussed in Chapter 45. As a general comment, the majority of schwannomas arise in the head and neck area[543] although they can be found emanating from nerves anywhere in the body. As a note of caution, while most schwannomas are well circumscribed, when cellular examples (having a predominance of Antoni A areas) arise in the paranasal areas, they are infiltrative and mimic sarcomas.[544] However, they have strong diffuse S100 expression (in contrast to malignant nerve sheath tumors, which have weak focal S100 protein).

Neurofibroma, granular cell tumor, neurothekeoma and nerve sheath myxoma, perineurioma, and ganglioneuroma are discussed in Chapter 45.

OSSIFYING FIBROMYXOID TUMOR

In 1989 Enzinger et al.[545] described the clinicopathologic features of 59 examples of ossifying fibromyxoid tumor of soft parts (OFT).

Since this initial report, other examples have appeared in the literature as case reports and small series. Many studies have concentrated on the immunohistochemical profile or ultrastructural features of the tumor in an attempt to clarify its histogenesis. The immunoexpression of neural markers, including S100 protein in the majority of these tumors, and the presence of discontinuous runs of thick basal lamina and interdigitating cytoplasmic processes on ultrastructural examination support the view that OFT is closely related to elements of the peripheral nerve sheath.[546–555] Cytogenetic and flow-cytometric studies have not yielded consistent findings.[553,556,557]

OFT occurs over a wide age range (14–79 years of age) with a peak incidence in the fifth decade.[545] Men are affected more often than women. The tumor clinically presents as a slow-growing, asymptomatic nodule or mass within the subcutaneous tissue or, less often, skeletal muscle. Multiple lesions have been documented at presentation[546] and are usually grouped in the same general area. The shoulder, upper arm, buttock, and thigh are the preferentially involved sites of origin. The tumor arises less frequently in the head and neck region and trunk. In the initial study, duration of preoperative disease varied from less than 1 year to over 20 years.[545]

OFT appears to have low-grade malignant potential. In the original series, the local recurrence rate was 27%, with multiple recurrences documented in three patients. One patient with three recurrences developed a presumed metastasis to the opposite thigh 20 years after initial excision.[545] A subset of 'atypical and malignant' OFTs characterized by tumors exhibiting increased cellularity and mitotic activity have been reported.[551] Two of the six patients in this study developed recurrent disease and one experienced a pulmonary metastasis. Other examples of metastatic lesions have also been reported[556,558] and in a larger recent series, 8/44 patients with OFT had metastases. Surgery is presently the mainstay of therapy for OFT.

The tumors vary in size from about 1 cm to as large as 17 cm. OFT appears as either a well circumscribed, single round to oval nodule (Fig. 9.192) or as a multinodular or lobulated mass. Most lesions have a firm to hard, cartilage-like consistency. The tumor may feel gritty on sectioning because of its variably calcified or ossified pseudocapsule (Fig. 9.193).

At low-power magnification, OFT is composed of uniform-appearing, small, round to polygonal cells embedded in a myxohyalin to collagenous stromal matrix. The cells are arranged in lobules that vary in size and cellularity and are partially separated by fibrous bands. The tumor is surrounded by an incomplete fibrous pseudocapsule composed of dense fibrous and hyalinized connective tissue. Nests of tumor may be seen infiltrating through rents in this fibrous shell. Most tumors have calcified lamellar (sometimes with marrow) or woven bone within the pseudocapsule (Figs 9.194, 9.195).

The proliferating cells are small with lightly eosinophilic to clear cytoplasm and a cytologically bland-appearing, round to spindle-shaped nucleus containing a small nucleolus (Fig. 9.196). The occasional presence of a clear space around the cell mimics the appearance of chondrocytic differentiation. In zones with an abundant myxocollagenous stromal matrix, the cells interconnect to form anastomosing, thin, cord-like arrangements. A vaguely fascicular growth pattern of spindled cells occurs in the more collagenous areas of the tumor. Polygonal cells with distinct cell borders may aggregate around vessels in a manner reminiscent of a glomus tumor. In conventional examples, the mitotic activity is low. In fact, many examples of this tumor lack bone in their capsule (nonossifying variant).[559] The stromal mucin is chiefly composed of hyaluronic acid. Collagen deposition varies from delicate fibers in the myxoid

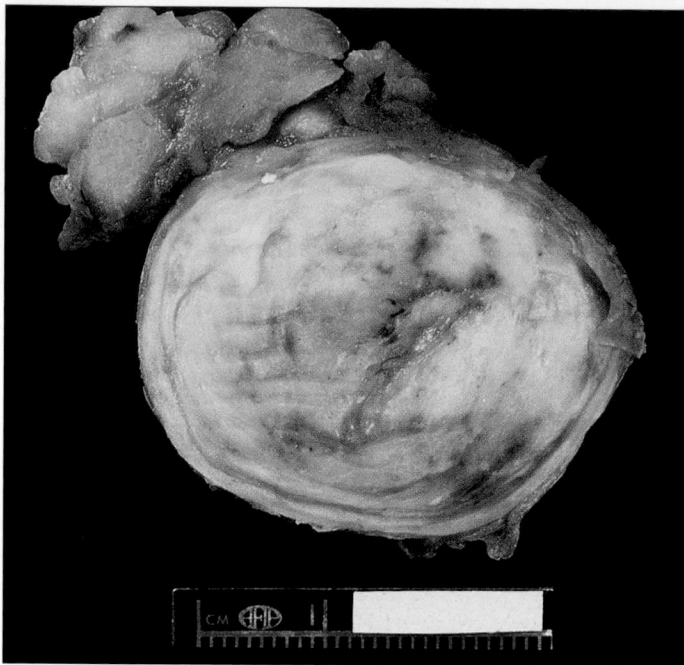

Fig. 9.192 Ossifying fibromyxoid tumor. This tumor has a prominent capsule.

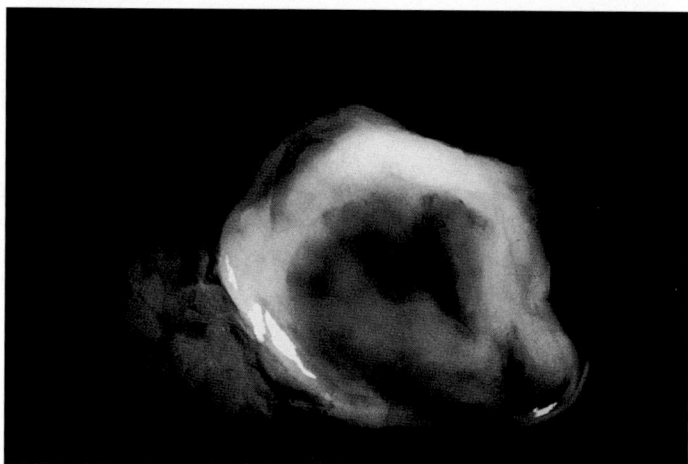

Fig. 9.193 Ossifying fibromyxoid tumor. The shell of bone is apparent on this specimen radiograph.

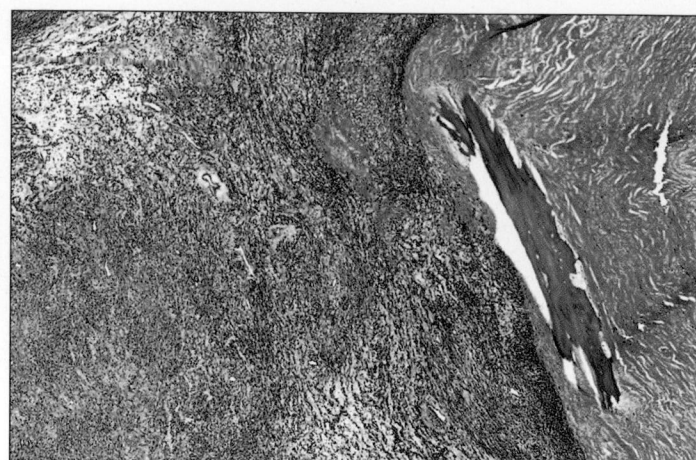

Fig. 9.194 Ossifying fibromyxoid tumor. This area shows sheets of uniform round cells. The shell of bone is seen.

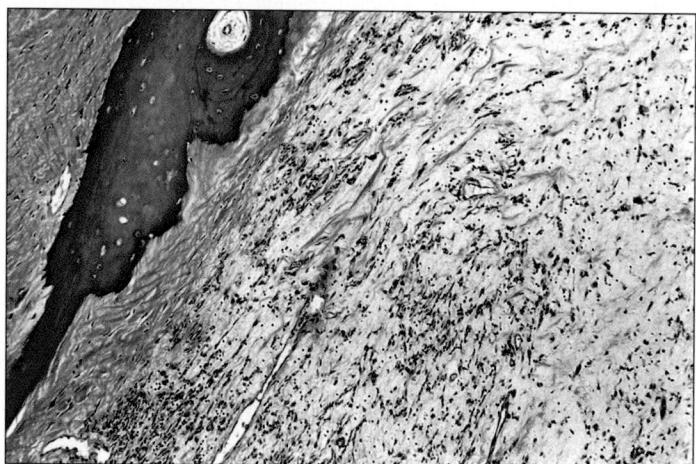

Fig. 9.195 Ossifying fibromyxoid tumor. In this field, the tumor cells are arranged in cords in a myxoid background.

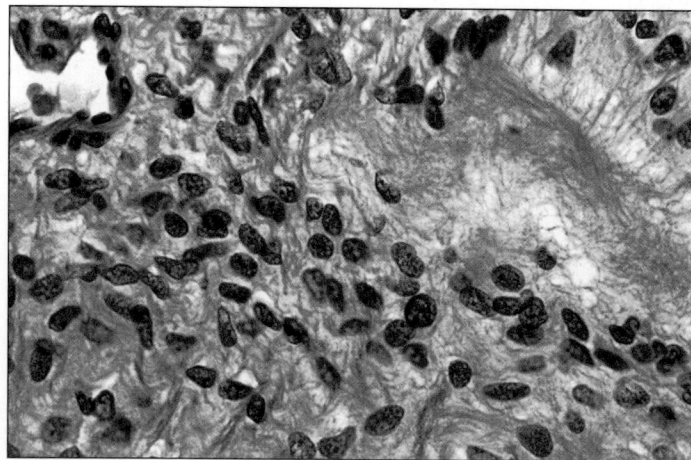

Fig. 9.196 Ossifying fibromyxoid tumor. Note the uniform cytologic features.

zones to thick bands of hyalinized collagen that occasionally contain spicules of bone or osteoid. Mature cartilage is infrequently identified in OFT. A rich network of thin-walled vessels, often showing perivascular fibrosis, is a consistent finding.

OFTs with aggressive histopathologic features have been described. Tumors reported in the literature as 'atypical' or 'malignant' OFTs show increased cellularity and are composed of a more pleomorphic cell population exhibiting nuclear hyperchromatism and increased mitotic activity (>2 mitoses/10 hpf).[551]

The immunohistochemical profile of conventional OFT includes immunoreactivity for neural and myogenic markers. Along with strong and diffuse expression of vimentin, approximately half to three quarters of tumors tested variably express S100 protein and

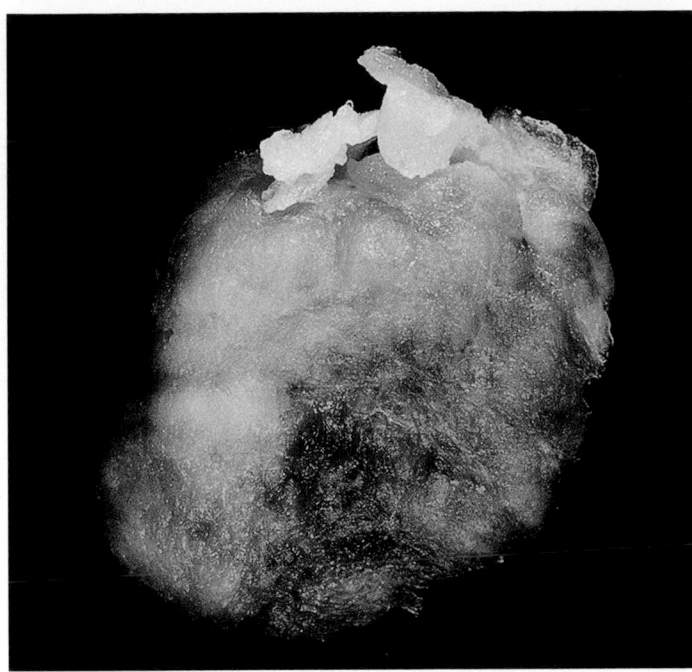

Fig. 9.197 Clear cell sarcoma. This tumor is loosely marginated but unencapsulated.

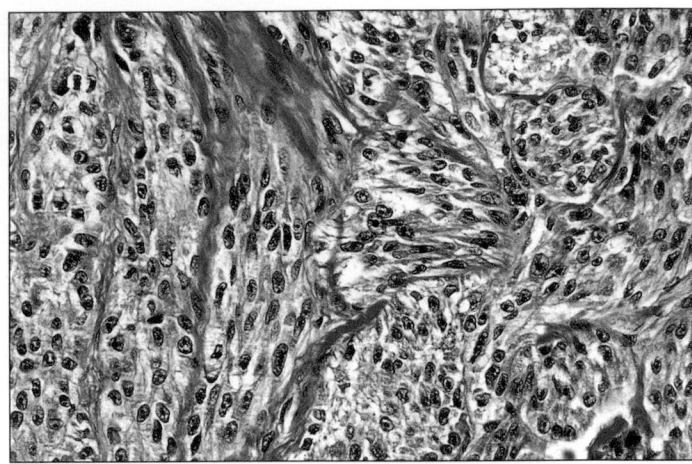

Fig. 9.198 Clear cell sarcoma. This example shows packeted fascicular nests of spindle cells with clear cytoplasm and uniform enlarged nuclei.

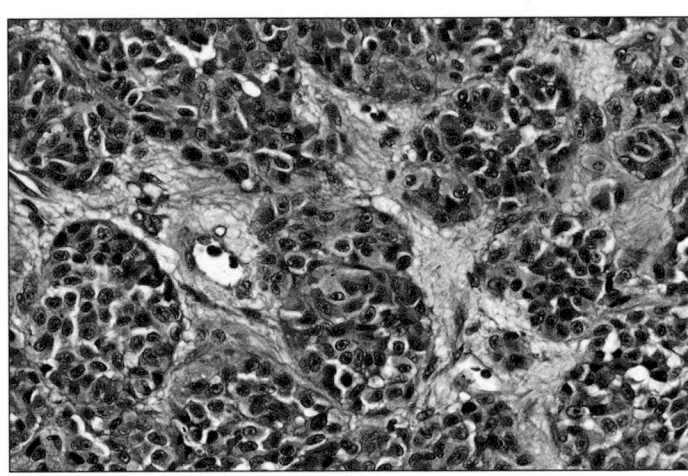

Fig. 9.199 Clear cell sarcoma displaying nests of cells with uniform nuclei, each with a prominent round nucleolus.

more than half express CD57 (Leu-7).[546,559–561] In one study,[560] 70% of tumors expressed desmin. Limited expression of NSE, GFAP, alpha-SMA, and MSA has also been documented.[546,560,561] Aspiration findings have been described in one malignant example although it seems unlikely that this diagnosis could be made prospectively.[558]

MALIGNANT PERIPHERAL NERVE SHEATH TUMOR

Malignant peripheral nerve sheath tumors (MPNST, malignant schwannoma, neurofibrosarcoma) are discussed in Chapter 48.

CLEAR CELL SARCOMA

Clear cell sarcoma (malignant melanoma of soft parts) was described by Enzinger in 1965[562] as a unique sarcoma associated with tendons and aponeuroses of the hands and feet. At the time of Enzinger's initial description, the nature of this lesion was unclear, although he raised the possibility of a melanocytic lesion. Subsequent studies reported the presence of melanosomes and the name 'melanoma of soft parts' was adopted.[563–567] These tumors mainly affect the distal extremities, particularly the feet and ankles (9/21 cases in Enzinger's initial series, 18/58[568], 7/17[569], 39/141[565] in subsequent reports), and occur in young adults.[562,565,568,570]

On gross examination, the tumors are well marginated with a smooth white firm cut surface and range in size from 0.6–15 cm[565,568] (Fig. 9.197). They consist of a packeted and fascicular arrangement of uniform round to spindled cells with clear to eosinophilic cytoplasm and often containing abundant glycogen (Figs 9.198, 9.199). The individual cells have uniform and prominent nucleoli. Tumor giant cells with a peripheral wreath-like arrangement of nuclei are found in some cases (Fig. 9.200). Melanin can

occasionally be seen. Necrosis is found in a minority of cases. The vast majority of cases are reactive with S100 protein (Fig. 9.201) and melanoma markers, both HMB-45 (Fig. 9.202)[565,568,570] and newer ones.

Some observers have speculated that these are simply melanomas of connective tissue. However, this is probably incorrect for several reasons. (1). Their histologic features are very monotonous whereas skin melanomas feature more prominent cytologic pleomorphism. (2). Their clinical behavior is also markedly different. Whereas an excellent prognosis would be expected for a 1-cm clear cell sarcoma, a nodular skin melanoma of this size would be rapidly lethal. In fact, most patients with tumors smaller than 2.5 cm fare well on follow-up[568] (although 54% of all patients were dead of disease in a Mayo clinic study[570] and 53/115 were dead in an AFIP study[565]) (3). Finally, clear cell sarcoma has a characteristic 12;22 translocation whereas skin melanomas have complex karyotypes.[571–578] The gene product afforded by this translocation, the EWS–ATF1 fusion transcript, can be detected by reverse transcriptase polymerase chain

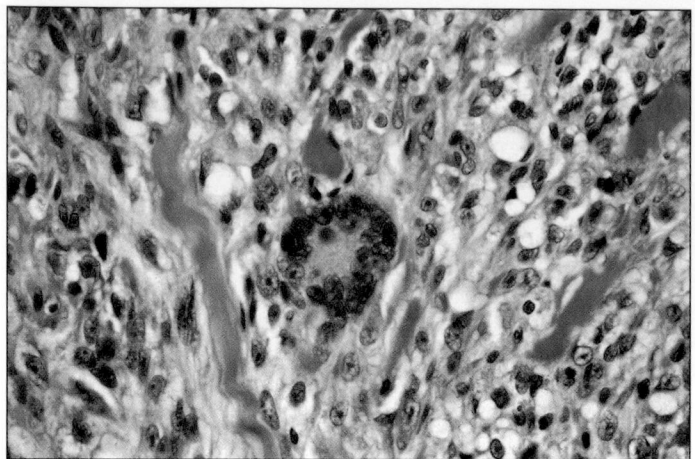

Fig. 9.200 Clear cell sarcoma. Wreath-like cells are sometimes abundant.

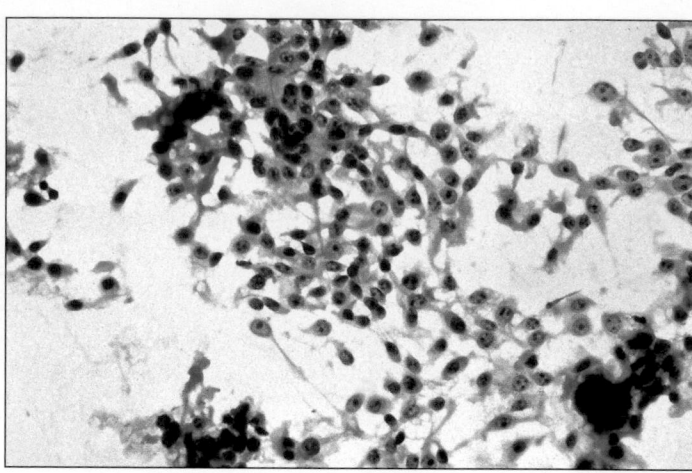

Fig. 9.203 Clear cell sarcoma. On aspirate, a cellular specimen with a spindle cell pattern is present (Courtesy of D. William Frable).

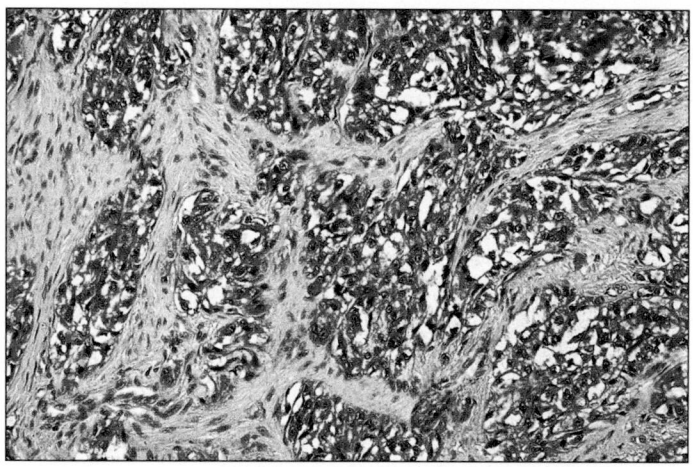

Fig. 9.201 Clear cell sarcoma. Strong S100 protein expression is a constant feature.

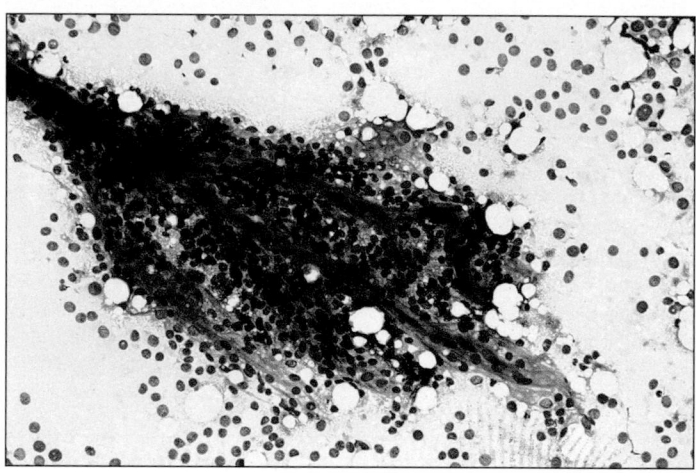

Fig. 9.204 Clear cell sarcoma, aspiration cytology. The packeted appearance is maintained in this sample.

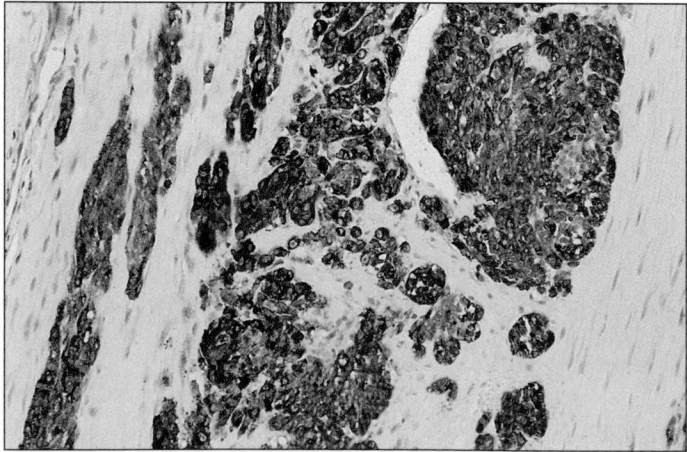

Fig. 9.202 Clear cell sarcoma. HMB-45 often stains clear cell sarcoma more intensely than S100 protein.

reaction (RT-PCR) and thus diagnosis of clear cell sarcoma can be made by molecular means, although it is usually not difficult by light microscopy.[578] Aspiration cytology could easily be diagnostic with the correct supporting evidence (Figs 9.203–9.205).

The differential diagnosis of clear cell sarcoma is primarily from monophasic synovial sarcoma, fibrosarcoma, malignant peripheral nerve sheath tumor (particularly the epithelioid variant), and cutaneous melanoma. However, occasional examples with giant cells have been mistaken for giant cell tumor of tendon sheath (easily resolved by performing S100 and HMB-45 staining) while the strong S100 staining can lead to a misinterpretation as benign schwannoma (easily resolved with HMB-45 staining).

Synovial sarcoma has long fascicles of cells rather than packets, typically lacks nucleoli, and has a hemangiopericytoma-like vascular pattern. There is also focal expression of epithelial markers and synovial sarcoma lacks HMB-45 (although it often expresses S100 protein in a patchy distribution).[579]

The distinction from epithelioid malignant peripheral nerve sheath tumor may be difficult since both clear cell sarcoma and

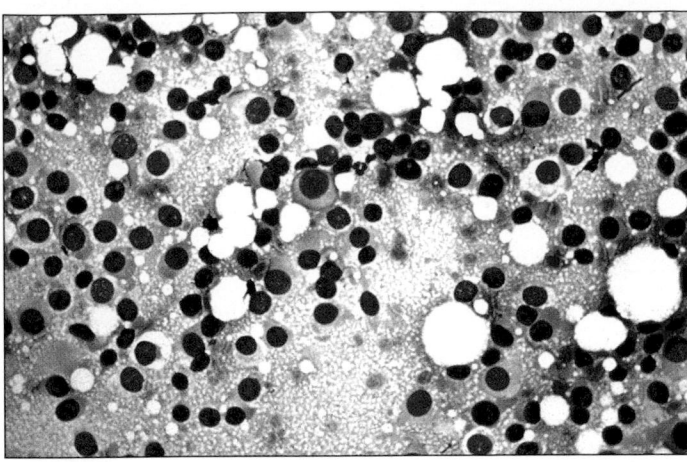

Fig. 9.205 Clear cell sarcoma, aspiration cytology. The cytologic uniformity and nucleoli are apparent.

Table 9.14 International neuroblastoma staging system (INSS)

Stage 1	Localized tumor with complete gross excision, with or without microscopic residual disease; representative ipsilateral lymph nodes negative for tumor microscopically (nodes attached to and removed with the primary tumor may be positive).
Stage 2A	Localized tumor with incomplete gross resection; representative ipsilateral non-adherent lymph nodes negative for tumor microscopically.
Stage 2B	Localized tumor with or without complete gross excision, with ipsilateral non-adherent lymph nodes positive for tumor; enlarged contralateral lymph nodes must be negative microscopically.
Stage 3	Unresectable unilateral tumor infiltrating across the midline, with or without regional lymph node involvement; or localized unilateral tumor with contralateral regional lymph node involvement; or midline tumor with bilateral extension by infiltration (unresectable) or by lymph node involvement.
Stage 4	Any primary tumor with dissemination to distant lymph nodes, bone, bone marrow, liver, skin, and/or other organs (except as defined for Stage 4S).
Stage 4S	Localized primary tumor (as defined for Stage 1, 2A or 2B) with dissemination limited to skin, liver, and/or bone marrow (limited to infants <1 year of age).

epithelioid MPNST feature strong S100 reactivity and prominent nucleoli. Epithelioid MPNST has a cord-like arrangement of cells and usually also has areas of conventional MPNST.[580] Furthermore, it lacks staining for HMB-45. Conventional MPNST typically has only patchy S100 protein positivity and also lacks nucleoli. Distinction from cutaneous melanoma may also be difficult since these tumors have an identical immunohistochemical profile. True melanomas usually have more pleomorphic nuclei than clear cell sarcomas, but overlapping features may exist and require clinicopathologic correlation. Obviously skin involvement favors melanoma. Such cases may also be resolved by molecular methods.[578]

NEUROBLASTOMA

Neuroblastic tumors are frequently confused with primitive neuro-ectodermal tumors (PNETs), although they are dissimilar lesions, affecting different age groups, metastasizing to different locations, presenting in different foci, having different differentiation potentials and biologic features, and, most importantly, requiring different therapy and staging. The key biologic difference is that neuro-blastomas are adrenergic tumors, as reflected by their predilection for the adrenal glands and sympathetic ganglia, whereas PNETs are cholinergic tumors.[581]

Neuroblastic tumors are generally classified by their differentiation capacity, reflected as the formation of mature ganglia and Schwann cells. For example, ganglioneuroma is composed of non-metastasizing mature elements and is most frequently encountered in the posterior mediastinum of young children. Neuroblastoma most commonly involves the adrenal gland and is one of the most common congenital neoplasms, frequently differentiating into mature tissues in prenatal and early life. Neuroblastomas are one of the most common malignant tumors in children, following leukemias and brain tumors. In between neuroblastoma and ganglioneuroma is ganglioneuroblastoma, a partially differentiated lesion that nevertheless has full metastatic potential because it harbors neuroblasts.

Clinically, neuroblastic tumors produce not only mass effects but also a host of systemic symptoms including watery diarrhea secondary to secretion of vasoactive intestinal polypeptide.

Neuroblastomas are potentially aggressive lesions whose clinical behavior depends on genetic, histologic, and staging factors. The bone marrow is a common site of metastatic disease and is emphasized in staging schemes. The staging system in current use by the Pediatric Oncology Group is set out in Table 9.14. Using this system, multifocal primary tumors (e.g. bilateral adrenal primary tumors) should be staged according to the greatest extent of disease. Defining the vertebral column as the midline, tumors arising unilaterally and extending past the midline must cross into the opposite side of the vertebral column. Also, metastatic disease may be present in stage 4S tumors, which paradoxically have a good outcome. Marrow involvement in Stage 4S nevertheless should be minimal, with malignant cells comprising fewer than 10% of nucleated cells. The unexpectedly excellent behavior of Stage 4S neuroblastomas has been confirmed by a number of investigators and has led to speculation concerning their biology.[582–585]

Neuroblastomas are typically fleshy masses discolored by abundant hemorrhage. As such they produce raised purplish masses when metastasizing to skin and subcutaneous soft tissues. Affected infants have been termed 'blueberry muffin babies.' Adrenal masses usually compress the normal gland into a thin cap that partially rims the fibrous capsule. Paravertebral tumors invade through the neural foramina in a dumbbell fashion that is apparent on MRI. Paravertebral lesions may also completely overrun adjacent lymph nodes but this observation does not have the significance of separate metastases. Chalky foci of calcification are typically present.

Ganglioneuromas form firm yellow-tan masses with a whorled, fibroma-like cut surface. They may appear locally invasive but they are terminally differentiated lesions by definition and usually don't grow even if incompletely excised[586] Ganglioneuroblastomas, in the composite form, comprise both firm yellow-tan ganglioneuromatous masses and nodular foci of fleshy, hemorrhagic tissue constituting

Table 9.15 Neuroblastoma grading system of Shimada

Good prognostic lesions

Stroma-rich (Schwann-cell-rich) tumors with intermixed differentiating neuroblastic elements

Stroma-poor (Schwann-cell-poor) tumors in patients <1.5 years of age, with MKI <200

Stroma-poor tumors in patients 1.5 to 5 years of age, with ganglionic differentiation and MKI >100.

Poor prognostic lesions

Stroma-rich nodular tumors (nodular ganglioneuroblastomas; see text description)

Stroma-poor tumors in patients <1.5 years of age, with MKI >200

Stroma-poor tumors in patients 1.5–5 years of age, with MKI >100

Stroma-poor tumors of all types in patients >5 years of age

MKI = mitotic karyorrhectic index, determining by counting the number of mitoses and karyolytic bodies among 5000 tumor cells.

their neuroblastomatous elements. The gross appearance of ganglioneuroblastomas reflects their relative proportions of mature schwannian and immature neuroblastic tissues.

Neuroblastic tumors histologically comprise a heterogeneous group, ranging from the primitive neuroblastoma to the terminally differentiated ganglioneuroma. The key element of neuroblastoma is the production of neuropil, a wispy, lightly eosinophilic, fibrillar material, by otherwise undifferentiated-appearing neuroblasts; these cells are characterized by their granular, 'salt and pepper' chromatin. The 'wispy' material ultrastructurally corresponds to elongate dendritic processes that interdigitate in a manner reminiscent of nervous system development. Rosettes similar to those described for PNET are commonly seen and have cores filled with neuropil. A diagnostically helpful feature is the presence of islands of dystrophic calcification, which often grow to sufficient size to be detectable radiographically and grossly.

Early cytologic differentiation into ganglionic cells is evidenced in neuroblasts that contain nuclei with prominent nucleoli and acquire an eccentric triangular rim of cytoplasm. In ganglioneuroblastomas, which are graded by their degree of differentiation,[587–589] progressive acquisition of neural features results in mature ganglion cells with pale nuclei, prominent nucleoli, and abundant cytoplasm with Nissl substance. Mature neuronal cells tend to be diffusely dispersed among the less differentiated elements, except in the more compartmentalized composite ganglioneuroblastoma.

In ganglioneuromas, scattered isolated nests of mature ganglion cells actually become overgrown by Schwann cells, which imparts a fibrous gross appearance. Ganglioneuromas also typically contain the scattered clusters of mature lymphocytes seen in more primitive lesions, so that caution is advised in interpreting FNAs to avoid overdiagnosis of benign small cell elements. Ganglioneuromatous areas frequently occur in post-treatment excisions of primary and metastatic lesions and represent therapy-induced maturation.

Histologic examination is important in neuroblastoma not only for diagnosis but also for grading, which has distinct prognostic significance. The currently used grading system is that of Shimada[589] outlined in Table 9.15. Note that, besides maturation, the age of the patient and the amount of mitosis/apoptosis are important in dividing patients into prognosis groups. The latter feature

theoretically requires counting mitotic figures and karyolytic bodies among 5000 tumor cells, although in reality estimates are used. Shimada grading is reproducible, commonly used, and prognostically significant.

In general, neuroblastomas express neural markers, namely NSE, chromogranin, synaptophysin, neurofilament protein, and microtubule-associated protein 2.[590–592] They often lack S100 protein. In contrast to Ewing's sarcoma/PNET (ES/PNET), chromogranin is more likely to be positive with neuroblastoma, while CD99/O13 appears largely restricted to tumors of the (ES/PNET) type, a helpful tool for distinguishing the two.[593] However, CD99/O13 is not entirely specific for ES/PNET tumors and newer antibodies to the protein encoded by the *EWS–FLI1* fusion transcript in ES/PNET may also be helpful in selected cases.[429] Cytogenetics itself distinguishes between neuroblastoma and PNET. Whereas *EWS–ETS* fusions are characteristic of the latter lesion, neuroblastomas are distinguished by frequent deletions in chromosome 1p, common amplifications of the N-*myc* oncogene, and resultant double minute chromosomes and homogeneously staining regions that contain the amplified oncogene segments.[594,595] This N-*myc* amplification phenomenon results in a dramatic increase in the number of DNA segments transcribing this gene and causes unrestrained growth in vitro and aggressive clinical behavior in vivo. Fluorescence in situ hybridization (FISH) can be used to directly visualize and count the number of copies per tumor cell nucleus. This technique has become the standard method of genetic testing for N-*myc* amplification.

Cytologic preparations and bone marrow aspirates are often used for primary diagnosis. However, occasional examples show minimal or no differentiation at the light microscopic level, necessitating use of the ancillary techniques described above. Essential elements to consider are the clinical settings and radiographic images, as calcified adrenal masses in infants and very young children are almost always neuroblastomas. Another important feature is urinary catecholamine secretion, whose measurement should be considered prior to excision of these tumors to avoid postexcisional decline to nondiagnostic levels. Neuroblastic tumors are also morphologically similar to PNETs but there are great treatment differences, so it is important for the pathologist to perform ancillary studies as described above if distinction is an issue. Usually this is a problem with paravertebral, thoracic, and pelvic tumors, as both entities may occur in these locations.

Other entities that may be considered include Wilms tumors, as distinction between Wilms tumors with adrenal extension and neuroblastomas with renal extension or origin can be difficult both radiographically and clinically. The pathology is generally straightforward, although Wilms tumors may contain neural elements, so that some degree of caution is advised in questionable cases. Pigmented neuroectodermal tumor (or retinal anlage tumor) is a neuroblastic lesion, unrelated to typical neuroblastoma and usually occurring in the head and neck region of young children. Because neuroblastoma may occur within the neck, there is potential clinical overlap, but pigmented neuroectodermal tumor generally does not metastasize. Distinction between the two entities is made by the presence of nests of melanocytic cells laden with dark brown pigment. This is the key diagnostic feature of pigmented neuroectodermal tumor.

Esthesioneuroblastoma (olfactory neuroblastoma), a primitive neural tumor arising from the neuroepithelium of the olfactory placode, is an invasive, aggressive neoplasm that erodes into the cribriform plate and thus into the base of the brain. It requires intensive combined therapy. Some geneticists have observed the

EWS–FLI1 fusion of PNET in these tumors, linking it to the Ewing family,[596] but others have not.[597] Esthesioneuroblastoma displays epithelial markers expected of its neuroepithelial origin and lacks CD99, which further separates it from PNET.[372]

NEUROEPITHELIOMA AND EXTRASKELETAL EWING'S SARCOMA

Ewing family of tumors (ES/PNETs)

It is only within the past couple of decades that we have realized that two histologically distinct neoplasms, Ewing's sarcoma and PNET (also referred to as peripheral neuroepithelioma), are biologically related. James Ewing described a peculiar undifferentiated round cell tumor of bone in adolescents[598] and Arthur Purdy Stout published a case report of a primitive rosette-forming neoplasm of the ulnar nerve of a young adult.[599] Ewing's sarcoma became a standard diagnosis by the 1950s, whereas PNET was largely unrecognized until Askin and colleagues described a peculiar small cell tumor of the chest wall in adolescents (Askin tumor).[600] Subsequently, based on cytogenetic, ultrastructural, and biologic studies, the commonality of these three lesions, Ewing's sarcoma, PNET, and Askin tumors, became apparent and they are presently referred to as the PNET or Ewing family of tumors.[601–606] Soft tissue examples of these neoplasms are now recognized as the second most common pediatric soft tissue sarcoma following rhabdomyosarcoma. Excellent reviews of this topic are available.[605,607]

Ewing family tumors are primarily bone lesions: only a relatively small percentage arise in soft tissue. These involve the chest wall, paravertebral region, pelvis, and proximal extremities of adolescents and young adults, although small children may be affected. Among organ systems, the kidneys are probably the most common site.[608] Because these latter tumors more typically arise in older children and adults,[608] they must be distinguished from blastema-predominant Wilms tumor and other primitive renal tumors that require different therapy. As is the case for neuroblastoma (above), FLI-1 and WT-1 immunohistochemistry appear to separate ES/PNET tumors from Wilms tumor but there is a known immunophenotypic overlap between ES/PNET and blastema-predominant Wilms tumor with regard to CD99, cytokeratin, and desmin.

Ewing family tumors are aggressive lesions that are best considered systemic rather than localized phenomena. Systemic symptoms such as fever and elevated erythrocyte sedimentation rate may occur. As with all sarcomas, metastases at presentation (typically to lungs) are indicators of poor prognosis. Because of their biologic relatedness, soft tissue lesions in this group currently are treated similarly to skeletal ones in the Intergroup Ewing's Sarcoma Study. Recent advances in chemotherapy, such as the addition of ifosfamide to the therapeutic regimen, have resulted in improvements in outcome.[609–611]

Ewing family tumors are typically fleshy, yellow-tan lesions that may contain degenerate areas of necrosis and hemorrhage. They occasionally arise from peripheral nerves. Chest wall examples may or may not arise from ribs; by definition the Askin tumor does not. This distinction is best made radiographically. After therapy, Ewing tumors often regress, leaving a fibrous scar that may contain microscopic nests of residual viable tumor. Postchemotherapy tumor regression is associated with a good prognosis.[612,613]

Homer Wright rosettes are the hallmark of primitive neuroectodermal tumors (whereas Ewing's sarcomas lack these). These microscopic structures comprise wreaths of dark, oval nuclei that circumscribe wispy, lightly pink, neurofibrillary cores. By electron microscopy, these fibrillary cores correspond with elongated, dendritic tumor cell processes that intertwine in a fashion similar to

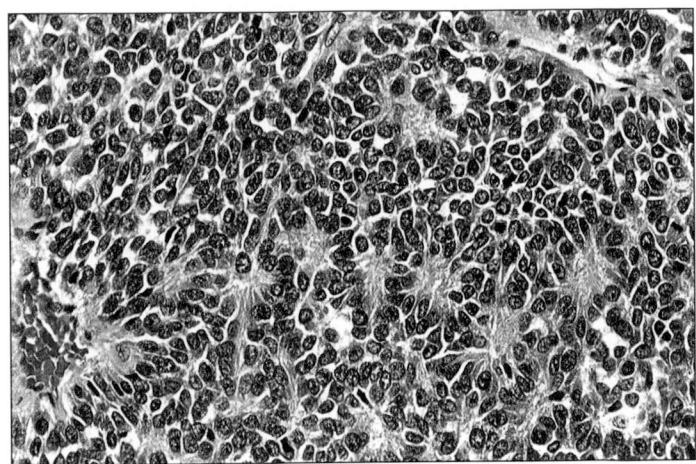

Fig. 9.206 Primitive neuroectodermal tumor. Note the rosettes (Courtesy of Dr Pedram Argani).

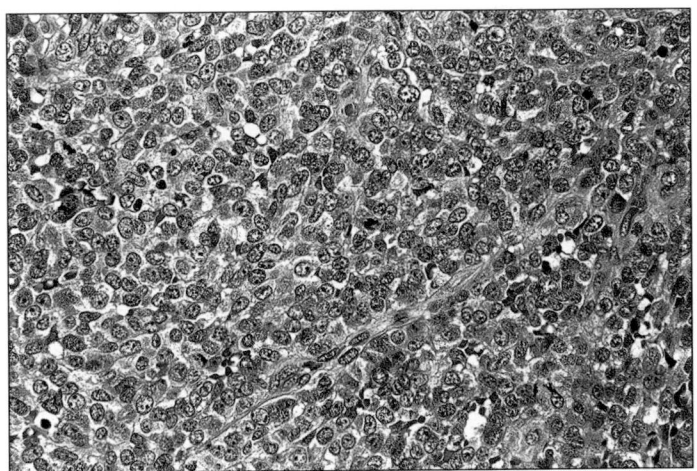

Fig. 9.207 Extraskeletal Ewing's sarcoma. Although related to primitive neuroectodermal tumor, these undifferentiated neoplasms lack rosettes.

a skein of yarn. The presence of well defined rosettes suffices to categorize a lesion histologically as PNET (Fig. 9.206).

On the other end of the differentiation spectrum lies typical Ewing's sarcoma, which by its primitive nature is the quintessential 'small, round, blue cell' tumor (Fig. 9.207). These are composed of highly compressed cellular masses that usually occur in diffuse sheets. The tumor cell nuclei typically possess round, even contours and smooth chromatin with inconspicuous nucleoli, being similar to but larger than lymphoid cells. One prominent distinction is their cytoplasm, which is often clear or bubbly because of an abundance of glycogen demonstrable by PAS stain. At first glance, this cytoplasmic vacuolization may resemble the neurofibrillary material found in rosettes but neural similarities are otherwise lacking. Another prominent feature is the presence of interspersed amorphous clusters of cells with more condensed nuclei and lightly eosinophilic cytoplasm. This creates a pattern of alternating 'light' cells and 'dark' cells. Although these are rapidly growing lesions, the mitotic index is often paradoxically low in typical Ewing's sarcoma.

In some Ewing tumors, the above typical features are distorted, so that cells are larger and display more uneven contours, irregular chromatin, and an increased mitotic index. These tumors are referred to as 'atypical Ewing's sarcomas' or 'large cell Ewing's sarcomas.'[614] Atypical Ewing's sarcomas may comprise a 'missing link' between typical Ewing's sarcomas and PNETs, as they often express a solitary neural marker such as NSE or show rudimentary neuronal features by ultrastructural examination.[615] The presence of atypia does not seem to have prognostic significance.[615]

Commonly used neural markers include synaptophysin, chromogranin, NSE, CD57 (also known as Leu-7), and S100. Each of these markers has inherent problems. For example, synaptophysin requires optimal fixation, whereas the more stable chromogranin is unfortunately rarely positive in PNET, perhaps because of the relative rarity of neurosecretory granules. Non-specificity is a problem with the other markers, particularly NSE, which is often expressed by atypical Ewing tumors.[615] S100 is present in a host of cell types, including cartilage, fat, and Schwann cells. Its presence in PNET may indicate differentiation into the latter elements. CD99 (O13), formerly known as the MIC2 antigen, is expressed in over 95% of ES/PNET cases with a distinctive diffuse membranous pattern of immunoreactivity. However, being derived from a lymphoblastic cell line, it may react with lymphoblastic tumors. Rhabdomyosarcomas occasionally may also yield positive immunostaining, although generally in a focal cytoplasmic or nuclear pattern of reactivity. Thus, as with the other markers, CD99 stains are best interpreted in the context of a diagnostic panel of immunostains. A newer antibody to the FLI1 protein product of the *EWS–FLI1* fusion gene offers improved specificity.[429,604,608]

The Ewing family of tumors is genetically characterized by a gene fusion between the *FLI1* gene on chromosome 11 and the *EWS* gene on chromosome 22. Karyotypically this is expressed by the reciprocal translocation t(11;22)(q24;q12). Unlike alveolar rhabdomyosarcoma, which has a single reproducible fusion point, a variety of fusions may occur, all of which fuse the two translated protein molecules. In this chimeric protein, a DNA transcription factor (EWS) is joined to an RNA binding factor (FLI1) causing abnormal DNA regulation and leading to tumorigenesis. The length of the resultant protein, which varies with the fusion combination, may have prognostic significance.[616] An intriguing phenomenon is that fusions of *EWS* with non-*ETS* genes, such as the *WT1* gene or the *ATF-1*[118] genes on chromosomes 11 and 12 respectively, produce dissimilar tumors, i.e. desmoplastic small cell tumor and the clear cell sarcoma. Extraskeletal myxoid chondrosarcoma is also characterized by a *EWS* gene type fusion.

The genetic aberrations of the Ewing family tumors can be exploited for diagnosis. Standard karyotyping will reveal the t(11;22)(q24;q12), and the resultant m-RNA can be probed using RT-PCR. However, additional testing is required to more completely screen for the host of fusions possible with the *EWS* gene. Using modern techniques, aspiration biopsy can be diagnostic for these tumors.

A common mimic of tumors in the Ewing's family is the solid variant of *alveolar rhabdomyosarcoma*. These two tumor entities occur in identical locations and affect identical age groups of patients, with the caveat that Ewing tumors are exceedingly rare in black children. Most cases can be resolved using immunohistochemistry. Lymphoma is less of a problem, given its usual presentation in lymph nodes, but soft tissue examples are well known. Diagnosis of lymphoma is made particularly treacherous because of its reactivity with CD99 and frequent non-reactivity with CD45, the common leukocyte antigen. Attention to cytologic detail

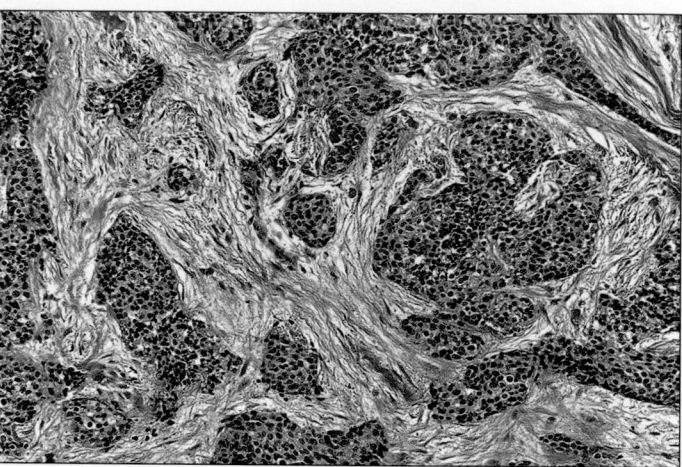

Fig. 9.208 Desmoplastic small round cell tumor. These primitive 'round blue cell tumors' are typically intra-abdominal and display nests of cells punctuating myofibroblastic stroma. They express desmin, keratin, and neural markers.

is thus important, as well as use of a panel that includes neural, muscle, and lymphoid antigens.

DESMOPLASTIC SMALL ROUND CELL TUMOR

Desmoplastic small cell tumor is a descriptively named malignancy that primarily affects adolescents and young adults and arises within the peritoneal cavity and retroperitoneum.[617] Although initially considered to originate exclusively from these sites, further reports have expanded its distribution.[618–632] Desmoplastic small cell tumor is an aggressive, highly malignant neoplasm. Its peritoneal seeding, abdominal adhesion, and omental cake formation are all reminiscent of mesothelioma and ovarian surface carcinomas. Some have considered it a primitive variety of mesothelioma. Treatment attempts have been largely unsuccessful.

In its typical intra-abdominal location, desmoplastic small cell tumor occurs as a sclerotic, locally invasive mass that may arise anywhere from the surface of the ovary to the pancreas, with frequent peritoneal spread.

Desmoplastic small cell tumor consists of nests of primitive small cells encircled by dense fibrotic tissue (Fig. 9.208). The small cell foci may contain vague rosettes or epithelioid features, and often cells have a rhabdoid appearance, raising a differential diagnosis of alveolar rhabdomyosarcoma because of their abundant pinkish cytoplasm containing hyaline inclusions.

These tumors display a range of markers by immunohistochemistry. Tumors often express desmin, vimentin, EMA, cytokeratin, NSE, S100 protein, synaptophysin, and CD57.

As might be expected from a hybrid lesion, desmoplastic small cell tumor is genetically characterized by a fusion of the *WT1* gene on chromosome 11 and the *EWS* gene on chromosome 22, karyotypically expressed by a reciprocal translocation, t(11;22)(p13;q12). It is important to note that, although similar chromosomes are involved, the breakpoint on chromosome 11 differs from that of the Ewing family of tumors. As with Ewing tumors and alveolar rhabdomyosarcomas, RT-PCR or FISH can be used to support the diagnosis by demonstration of this chimeric gene. A noteworthy feature of the *WT1* gene involvement in desmoplastic small cell tumor is that this gene is important not only for normal kidney development but also for mesothelial development. Strong expression of *WT1* by splanchnic mesoderm occurs during embryogenesis. This may link the desmoplastic small cell tumor with its predilection for mesothelial tissues.

The differential diagnosis includes Wilms tumors, Ewing family tumors, which may have a nested alveolar-like pattern, and alveolar rhabdomyosarcoma, in which this pattern is typical. The key distinguishing features are the typical clinical presentation, the polyphenotypia with combined expression of epithelial, neural, and mesenchymal markers, and the *EWS–WT1* genetic marker, which is demonstrable by the t(11;22)(p13;q12) with standard karyotyping. As noted in the section on rhabdomyosarcoma, when searching for metastatic desmoplastic small round cell tumor in effusions by cytologic examination, it is worthwhile to be aware that mesothelial cells are desmin-reactive.[618] Aspiration biopsy shows showed moderate to high cellularity with cells arranged singly and in clusters. The cells have high nuclear:cytoplasmic ratios, granular chromatin, usually inconspicuous nucleoli, smooth to irregular nuclear membranes, and frequent nuclear molding. The cytoplasm is scant to moderate, pale blue, and occasionally vacuolated. Pseudorosettes may be observed. Stromal fragments may be found in direct smears but are uncommon in liquid-based specimens.[623,629,631]

CARTILAGE AND BONE TUMORS IN SOFT TISSUE

MYOSITIS OSSIFICANS

Myositis ossificans is a non-neoplastic bone-forming reactive 'pseudotumor' occurring in soft tissue.[633,634] The term myositis ossificans is misleading since the process is not primarily inflammatory, nor exclusively confined to muscle. Histological and clinically identical forms may occur in tendons and aponeuroses.[634] Some authors recognize two distinct forms, termed 'post-traumatic' and 'pseudomalignant.'[633,634] Myositis ossificans is commonest in the second and third decades of life and without gender predilection. The masses most commonly arise within the large skeletal muscles of the proximal extremities. The quadriceps and the brachialis are affected in most cases.[635] Patients present with a short history of pain and swelling in the affected region. In early lesions (within the first 3 weeks), radiographs demonstrate only a soft tissue mass. Typically, soft tissue calcification is evident only after approximately 6 weeks.[636] Mature lesions of myositis ossificans appear as ossified soft tissue nodules. Resection results in cure. Local recurrence is extremely uncommon, even following incomplete excision.[633–635]

Since myositis ossificans is a reactive process, the histologic appearance of an individual lesion will depend on the part of the mass that is examined and the point in time at which it is excised. In general, the quantity of bone and the degree of maturity increase with time. One of the defining microscopic features of myositis ossificans is a reproducible transition from cellular sheets of spindle cells in the center of the mass to a less cellular bone-rich periphery. This phenomenon, virtually pathognomonic of myositis ossificans, is termed 'zoning'. The central aspect consists of intersecting fascicles of plump spindle cells demonstrating central elongate nuclei and visible nucleoli. Mitotic figures are readily found but marked nuclear atypia is not seen. The spindle cells gradually merge with thin trabeculae of woven bone that appear to arise directly from the stroma. As the trabeculae become more defined, prominent surface layers of osteoblasts are evident, so-called osteoblastic rimming. These intersecting trabeculae of woven bone demonstrate a gradual transition to mature lamellar bone at the periphery of the mass.

FIBRODYSPLASIA (MYOSITIS) OSSIFICANS PROGRESSIVA

Fibrodysplasia ossificans progressiva (FOP) is an extremely rare (<1 person per million affected) autosomal dominant inherited condition characterized by extensive soft tissue ossification at multiple sites without gender predilection.[637–644] The progressive nature of the process results in severe disability. Affected patients have a variety of skeletal abnormalities, particularly of the digits and cervical spine. The most common and virtually diagnostic finding is the presence of short great toes. Soft tissue ossification typically begins in the first decade of life. Trauma, either accidental or surgical, often initiates the process and the children present with painful swollen soft tissues at the affected site with progressive stiffness and loss of function of the muscles in the area. Development of soft tissue calcification and ossification ensues within 2–3 months. Any tissue site may be affected but the ossifying process is usually worse in the paraspinal region, especially within cervical musculature. Mutations in the genes encoding for bone morphogenetic protein are the most likely cause.[640,643] Surgical intervention should be avoided in this disease, since excision of a mass of heterotopic bone results in rapid recurrence with accelerated ossification.[640] Most patients with FOP do not have affected family members, suggesting that virtually all cases reflect sporadic mutations. Some relief is afforded by treatment with Accutane.[637]

Since FOP is essentially a reactive process in which there is uncontrolled inappropriate soft tissue ossification, the histologic appearance will vary depending on the time course of the disease, in a fashion similar to myositis ossificans. However, several differences between the two conditions are evident. Unlike myositis ossificans, FOP presents as a confluence of multiple nodules. The morphology of an individual lesion depends on its stage of development. Early unmineralized lesions typically show an intramuscular proliferation of uniform mitotically active spindle-shaped fibroblasts embedded within myxoid extracellular ground substance. The cells and myxoid material are seen between skeletal myocytes, an appearance closely resembling infantile fibromatosis. As lesions develop there is increasing production of cartilage and bone matrix. With time, complete maturation to lamellar bone occurs. Late lesions are composed entirely of lamellar cortical and cancellous bone and may contain bone marrow.

The most important differential diagnoses for FOP are infantile fibromatosis and soft tissue sarcoma, such as infantile fibrosarcoma or embryonal rhabdomyosarcoma. The clinical scenario is extremely important, since small biopsy samples of early lesions may closely simulate fibromatosis. Attention to clinical details, with examination of the child's feet for the characteristic short great toes, is useful. Distinction of FOP from soft tissue sarcoma is based on recognition of the bland proliferating cells in this disorder. Immunohistochemistry for myogenin and MyoD1 may assist in doubtful cases.

FIBRO-OSSEOUS PSEUDOTUMOR OF DIGITS

Fibro-osseous pseudotumor of digits,[645] also referred to as florid reactive periostitis,[646] is a non-neoplastic, reactive, bone- and

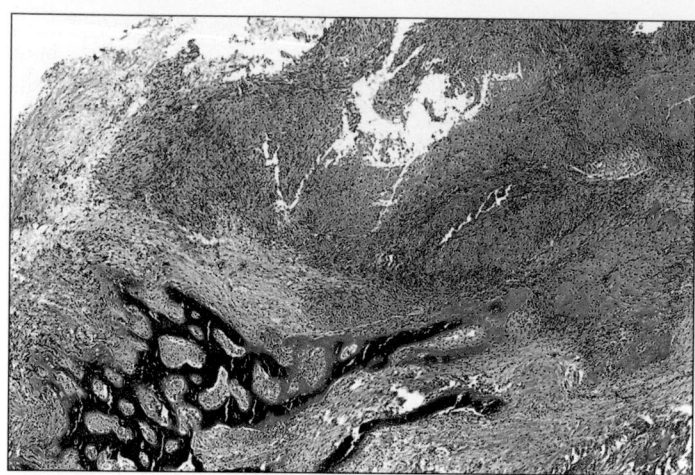

Fig. 9.209 Fibro-osseous pseudotumor of digits. This lesion is fasciitis-like but is 'zonated' and ossifies.

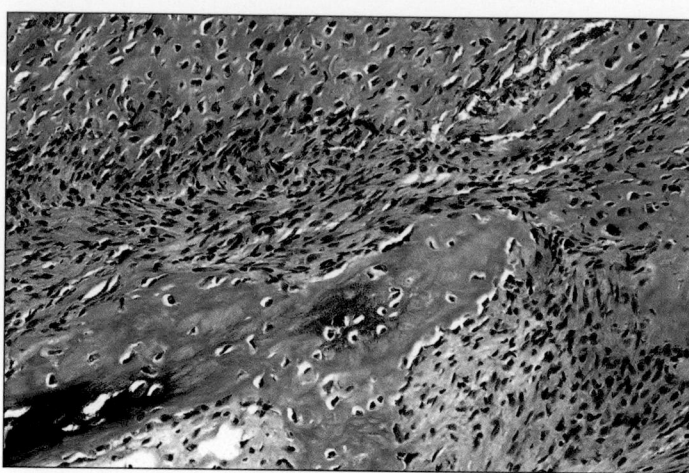

Fig. 9.210 Fibro-osseous pseudotumor of digits. At times, prominent cellularity in these lesions raises the concern of extraskeletal osteosarcoma; the acral location would be unusual for osteosarcoma.

cartilage-rich mass of the soft tissues of the distal extremities, predominantly the digits of the hands. It is essentially the distal soft tissue equivalent of myositis ossificans. This condition affects males and females equally and is most common in the second and third decade. Patients characteristically present with a short history of a painful or painless digital swelling. Fewer than half of the patients give a history of trauma to the site. In a minority there is localized erythema. Radiographs demonstrate soft tissue swelling of the affected digit and, in a minority, linear 'periosteal' bone formation on the underlying phalanx. The majority of the masses lack detectable mineralization at presentation. Most fibro-osseous pseudotumors measure less than 3.0 cm and are described as firm or rubbery at the time of excision. Local excision is curative. Recurrence is unusual despite frequent incomplete excision.[645,646]

Many of the histologic features of myositis ossificans are found in fibro-osseous pseudotumor of digits. Specifically, this condition is characterized by considerable hypercellularity, an often high mitotic rate and bone formation that varies depending on the stage at which the lesion is removed (Figs 9.209, 9.210). A transition from fascicles of spindle cells to progressively mature bone, resulting in a 'zonal' appearance similar to myositis ossificans, is found in a minority of examples.

The differential diagnosis of fibro-osseous pseudotumor includes all the previously discussed entities with the addition of soft tissue osteosarcoma, discussed below. These masses also should be distinguished from fracture callus occurring in association with phalangeal fracture. Finally, fibro-osseous pseudotumor has many similarities with bizarre parosteal osteochondromatous proliferation.[647,648] However, the latter condition demonstrates radiographically detectable attachment to the underlying phalanx and microscopically lacks the callus-like appearance of fibro-osseous pseudotumor.

SOFT TISSUE OSTEOSARCOMA

Soft tissue osteosarcomas are rare malignant neoplasms, accounting for fewer than 1% of soft tissue sarcomas.[649–653] In contrast to conventional osseous osteosarcoma, which typically affects young adults in the second and third decades, soft tissue osteosarcoma occurs in older patients, predominantly in the fifth and sixth decades. A minority of affected patients have a history of prior radiation therapy. The tumors typically arise in the proximal extremities and present as a painless or minimally tender mass. Most measure more than 5 cm. Radiographs usually show only a soft tissue mass without calcification. The underlying skeleton appears normal. Soft tissue osteosarcomas are high-grade malignant tumors. Up to 85% of patients develop metastases and ultimately die of tumor.[649–653]

The majority of soft tissue osteosarcomas are composed of pleomorphic spindle cells. All the histologic subtypes of osseous osteosarcoma occur in the soft tissues. Therefore, tumors can be classified as osteoblastic, chondroblastic, fibroblastic, small cell, telangiectatic, or resembling MFH. The latter is the most common. In these, the majority of the tumor resembles a high-grade undifferentiated pleomorphic sarcoma such as storiform pleomorphic MFH. Mitotic figures are readily found and atypical forms may be seen. Necrosis is common. The neoplastic bone matrix is minimally mineralized or unmineralized and outlines individual tumor cells in a lace-like manner. Bone matrix production is also typically patchy. Large expanses of tumor may be devoid of any recognizable bone or osteoid. This can result in diagnostic error on small biopsy samples. In chondroblastic tumors, pleomorphic chondrocytes embedded within irregular hyaline cartilage matrix are found admixed with other high-grade foci of tumor. The small cell and telangiectatic variants of osteosarcoma are the rarest subtypes to be found in the soft tissues. In the former, the tumor is composed of undifferentiated 'small blue' cells similar to those found in ES/PNET. The small cells however, are associated with lace-like neoplastic bone production in osteosarcoma, in contrast to Ewing's sarcoma. In the telangiectatic variant of soft tissue osteosarcoma blood filled spaces that lack an endothelial lining are present within the tumor.

Soft tissue osteosarcoma closely resembles other pleomorphic high-grade soft tissue sarcomas such as MFH, pleomorphic liposarcoma, and high-grade leiomyosarcoma. It is distinguished from these by the presence of neoplastic bone and osteoid matrix and the absence of other lines of differentiation. One of the most important differential diagnostic considerations is myositis ossificans. Soft tissue osteosarcoma demonstrates consistently greater cytologic atypia, and the 'zoning' phenomenon that is the histologic hallmark of myositis ossificans is not present in osteosarcoma. Myositis ossificans also affects a distinctly different age group of patients.

SOFT TISSUE CHONDROMA

Soft tissue chondromas are benign cartilage neoplasms that predominantly occur in adults in the fourth to seventh decades of life.[646,654–656] There is a slight male predominance. Soft tissue chondromas most commonly arise in the superficial soft tissues of the distal extremities, particularly on the volar aspect of the wrist, where they present as a painless soft tissue nodule. Radiographs often reveal calcification, with an arrangement of rings and arcs characteristic of hyaline cartilage. During excision, they often 'pop out.' Most soft tissue chondromas measure less than 3.0 cm. Soft tissue chondromas are treated by local resection. Recurrence develops in a minority of cases following excision.

Soft tissue chondromas are well circumscribed neoplasms composed of hyaline cartilage in the majority of instances. Within an individual tumor there are multiple compressed lobules of cartilage that are separated by collagen bands. The lobules exhibit relative hypercellularity and clusters of chondrocytes. Individual cells often demonstrate enlarged nuclei and visible nucleoli. Mitoses, however, are rare. Overall, the degree of cellularity and cytologic atypia in soft tissue chondroma equals or exceeds that found in low-grade intraosseous chondrosarcoma. This characteristic feature may result in diagnostic confusion. The hyaline cartilage matrix often undergoes calcification and ossification, accounting for the radiographic findings. The calcifications appear as purple granules that frequently outline individual chondrocytes in a lace-like manner. A minority of soft tissue chondromas are composed of myxoid cartilage as opposed to hyaline cartilage. In these tumors the chondrocytes lie within flocculent granular extra-cellular matrix and lack well developed lacunas. A cellular giant-cell-rich infiltrate may be found at the periphery of these tumors. The chondrocytes of soft tissue chondroma express S100 protein and vimentin immunohistochemically.

Soft tissue chondroma should be distinguished from soft tissue chondrosarcomas of myxoid and mesenchymal types, discussed below. Foci of cellular hyaline cartilage may be found in reactive bone-producing conditions such as myositis ossificans, FOP, and fibro-osseous pseudotumor of digits. Primary skeletal chondrosarcoma with soft tissue extension may simulate soft tissue chondroma.

EXTRASKELETAL MYXOID CHONDROSARCOMA

Extraskeletal myxoid chondrosarcomas (EMCs) are rare soft tissue sarcomas that predominantly occur in adulthood.[657–659] There is a slight male predilection. The tumors most commonly occur in the deep soft tissues of the extremities. They usually present as a painless or minimally tender, slow-growing mass. Most of the tumors are larger than 5 cm. In Enzinger's original series, this tumor was considered to be relatively low-grade, with a low incidence of metastasis and an indolent clinical course.[658] More recent experience shows that the estimated 5-, 10-, and 15-year survival rates were 90%, 70%, and 60% respectively. Older patient age, larger tumor size, and tumor location in the proximal extremity or limb girdle were adverse

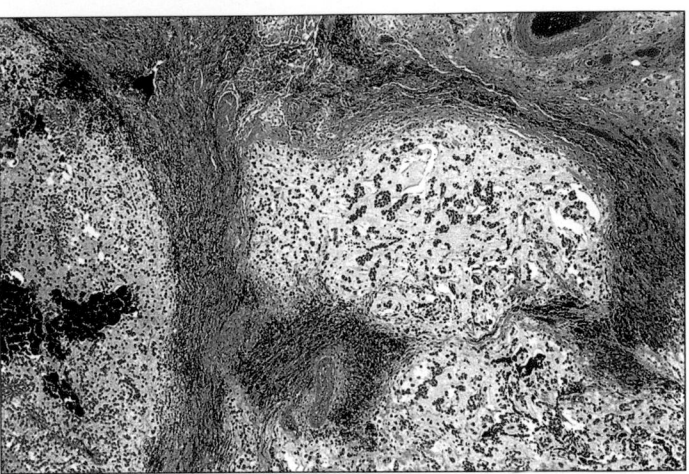

Fig. 9.211 Extraskeletal myxoid chondrosarcoma. This tumor has a prominent lobulated architecture.

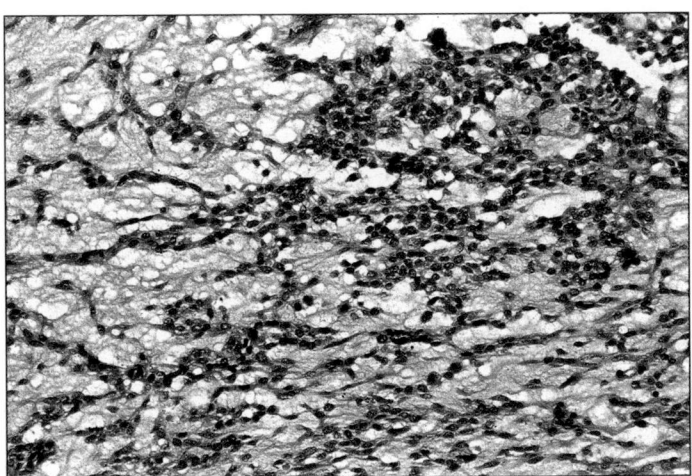

Fig. 9.212 Extraskeletal myxoid chondrosarcoma. Cords of cells are embedded in myxoid matrix.

prognostic factors identified by multivariate analysis. EMC has a unique clinical course, including a high rate of local recurrence, prolonged survival after metastasis in some cases, and eventually a high rate of death due to tumor. These features distinguish EMC from low-grade sarcomas. Histologic grading is of no prognostic value in EMC because prognosis is dictated primarily by clinical features.[657] Cytogenetic analysis of EMC demonstrates a consistent translocation between chromosomes 9 and 22, t(9;22)(q22–31;q11–12), which serves as a diagnostic marker for this neoplasm since it results in a specific fusion product.[657,660–668]

EMCs are lobulated myxoid tumors that characteristically demonstrate low cellularity (Fig. 9.211). The individual tumor cells are small, oval and have minimal amounts of eosinophilic cytoplasm surrounding the nucleus. The nuclei are central, dark-staining, and usually lack visible nucleoli. Tumor cells are arranged in linear arrays that appear as straight lines or curves (Figs 9.212, 9.213). Mitotic figures are usually inconspicuous. The tumor cells are embedded within a hypovascular basophilic flocculent matrix. A distinctly nodular/lobular growth is evident. The lobules are

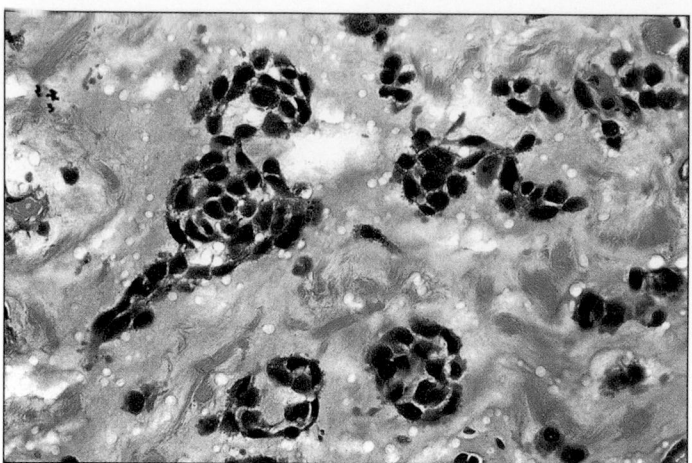

Fig. 9.213 Extraskeletal myxoid chondrosarcoma. In this example, the cells are nested.

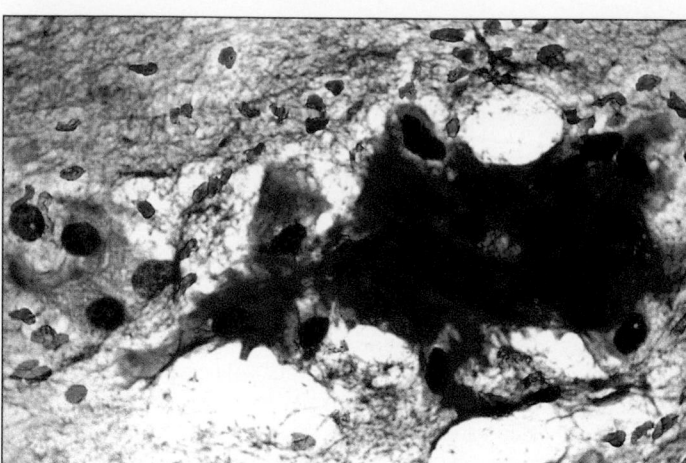

Fig. 9.215 Extraskeletal myxoid chondrosarcoma, aspiration cytology. The cells are relatively uniform and lack the bubbled appearance of chordoma.

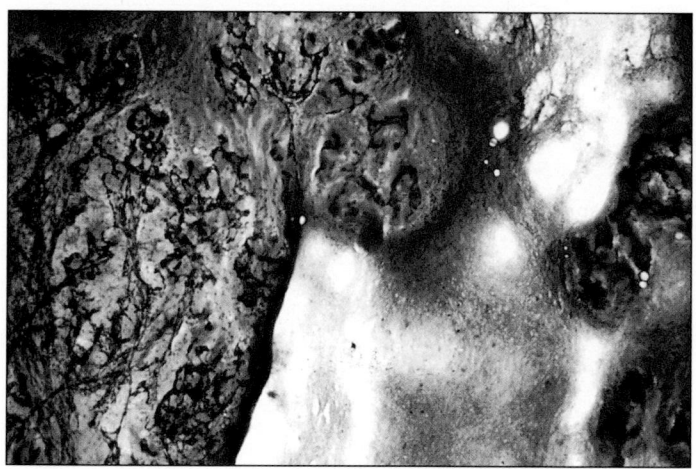

Fig. 9.214 Extraskeletal myxoid chondrosarcoma, aspiration cytology. On Diff-Kwik staining, the myxoid matrix is readily apparent (Courtesy of Dr William Frable).

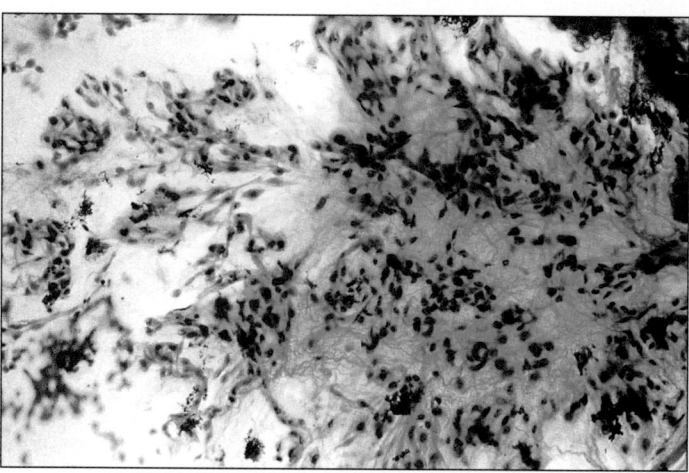

Fig. 9.216 Extraskeletal myxoid chondrosarcoma, aspiration cytology. The matrix is less apparent on Papanicolaou stain.

separated by strands of eosinophilic collagen. In low-grade tumors there is low cellularity and higher-grade tumors typically show greater cellularity with less extracellular matrix. Hyaline cartilage is not found in EMC. Rarely dedifferentiation to a high-grade sarcoma occurs in EMC.[659] Immunohistochemical stains demonstrate vimentin and S100 protein expression in the majority of cases. Aspiration cytologic features recapitulate the histologic ones and are depicted in Figures 9.214–9.217.

EMC should be distinguished from soft tissue chondroma and from myxoid liposarcoma. It is typically more myxoid than the former and lacks the vascular pattern of the latter.

EXTRASKELETAL MESENCHYMAL CHONDROSARCOMA

The largest series of these lesions has been published from the Mayo Clinic by Nakashima and colleagues.[669] About two thirds arise in

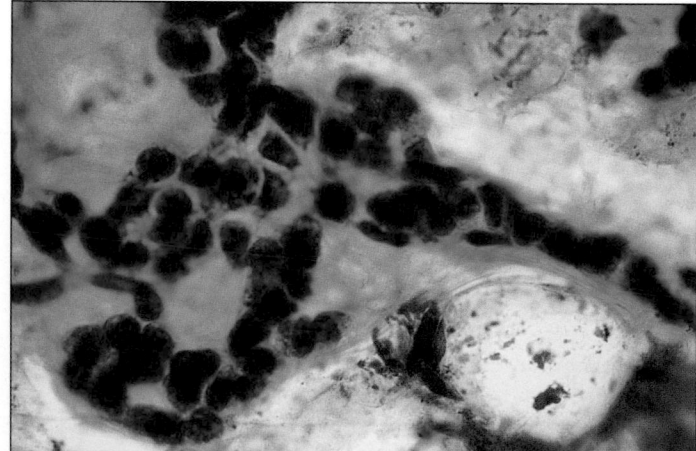

Fig. 9.217 Extraskeletal myxoid chondrosarcoma, aspiration cytology. The Papanicolaou stain shows uniform nuclear features.

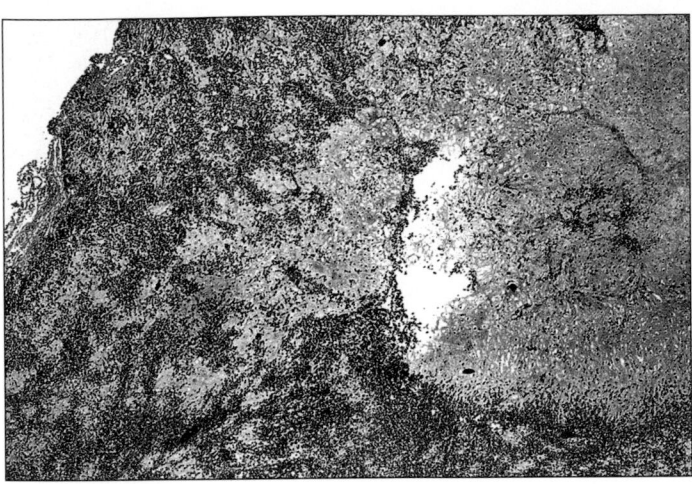

Fig. 9.218 Mesenchymal chondrosarcoma. These lesions classically display juxtaposed primitive cells and mature cartilage.

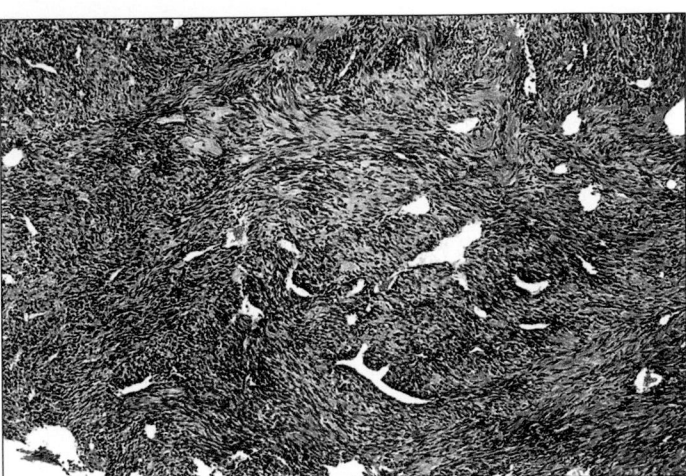

Fig. 9.220 Mesenchymal chondrosarcoma. Some lesions display a spindled appearance and abundant hemangiopericytoma-like vasculature and the mature islands of cartilage are found only after careful search.

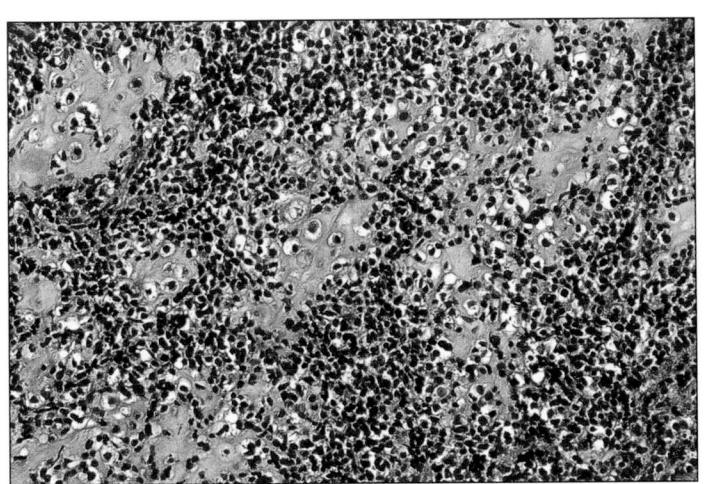

Fig. 9.219 Mesenchymal chondrosarcoma, higher magnification.

bone and the remainder in soft tissue. In skeletal sites, the mandible, rib, pelvic bones, and femur are the most common locations, whereas extraskeletal examples present in lower extremities, followed by the meninges. Most lesions present in the second and third decades of life. Central nervous system examples have been reviewed by Rushing et al.[670] Vencio has called attention to the fact that, while these are generally aggressive tumors, examples arising in the jaw bones can pursue a more indolent course.[671] Their histologic features are usually diagnostic without ancillary studies, as these tumors consist of 'small round cells' with scant cytoplasm arranged around hemangiopericytoma-like vasculature and punctuated by islands of mature-appearing cartilage (Figs 9.218, 9.219). Reticulin staining encloses small groups of cells. Ultrastructure of the cartilage areas discloses well developed Golgi, glycogen, and rough endoplasmic reticulum (features in keeping with cartilaginous differentiation), whereas the small cells show minimal organelles (undifferentiated features).[672,673] When the cartilage islands are not well represented or when the cells assume a spindled pattern,

mesenchymal chondrosarcoma can be more difficult to recognize. Immunohistochemistry can be helpful in such cases, which can bear a striking resemblance to both solitary fibrous tumor (Fig. 9.220) and poorly differentiated synovial sarcoma. These tumors are CD99(013)-positive[674] and show S100 in the zones of cartilage as well as in scattered small cells.[670] They lack actins, desmin, and EMA (synovial sarcoma usually has focal EMA). Central nervous system examples sometimes have glial fibrillary acid protein and focal keratin. Since CD99 has been found in several tumors in the differential diagnosis (poorly differentiated synovial sarcoma, solitary fibrous tumor, and hemangiopericytoma),[675] a panel approach is always warranted.

OTHER MATRIX-CONTAINING SOFT TISSUE TUMORS

ANEURYSMAL CYST OF SOFT TISSUE

Primary soft tissue tumors histologically identical to osseous aneurysmal bone cysts have been designated aneurysmal cysts of soft tissue. These are extremely rare lesions and only a handful have been reported.[676] They occur in all age groups. There is no sex predilection. Patients present with symptoms related to an enlarging soft tissue mass, usually of short duration. The underlying skeleton is normal. Local resection is curative. There have been no cases of local recurrence. Aneurysmal bone cyst had been regarded as a reactive phenomenon but cytogenetic data suggest that it is instead truly neoplastic.[677,678]

Aneurysmal cyst of soft tissue demonstrates all the histologic features of aneurysmal bone cyst (Fig. 9.221). These lesions contain blood-filled cystic spaces that lack endothelial lining. The solid components between the cysts are composed of moderately cellular spindle cell nodules, often with abundant osteoclast-like giant cells. These solid foci, in addition to the septa that divide the cysts, contain linear strands of woven bone with osteoblastic rimming. Aggregates of moderately cellular basophilic 'chondroid' material may also be present. The latter appears relatively specific for aneurysmal cysts of bone and soft tissue.

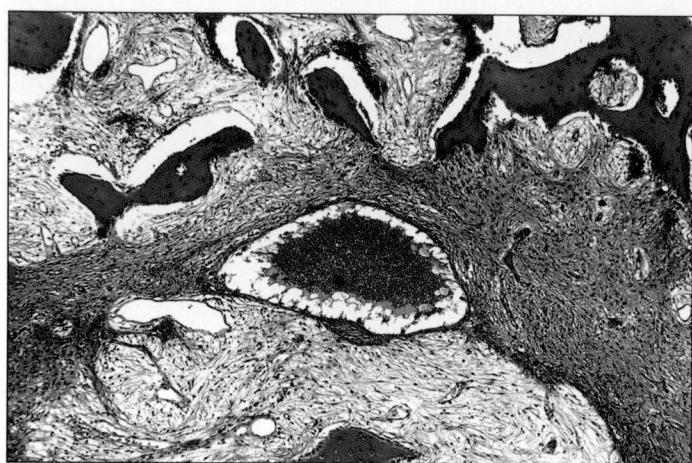

Fig. 9.221 Aneurysmal cyst of soft tissue. These tumors are identical to their skeletal counterparts.

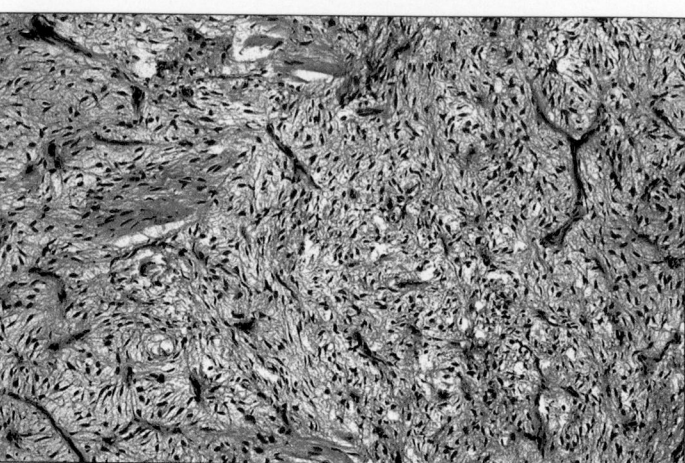

Fig. 9.223 Superficial acral fibromyxoma. Prominent vessels and bland spindled cells. These lesions express epithelial membrane antigen.

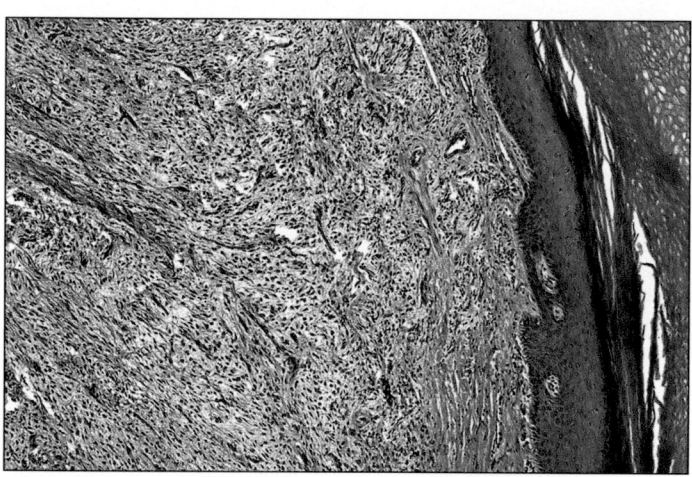

Fig. 9.222 Superficial acral fibromyxoma. Many of these tumors proliferate in the nail bed (Courtesy of Dr John Fetsch).

MISCELLANEOUS TUMOR TYPES

Superficial angiomyxoma is discussed in Chapter 8.

SUPERFICIAL ACRAL FIBROMYXOMA

Fetsch et al. described superficial acral fibromyxoma. They identified 37 cases from 25 men and 12 women ranging in age from 14–72 years. The tumors were solitary, involving a toe (20 cases), a finger (13 cases), or the palmar surface of the hand (four cases) and often (16 cases) involved the nail region. The lesions were slow-growing and typically asymptomatic (three were painful). Tumors ranged in size from <1 to 5 cm and most were well marginated grossly, although five were described as infiltrative. They were centered in the dermis (Fig. 9.222). Microscopically, tumors were moderately cellular and consisted of stellate to spindled fibroblastic cells set in myxoid to collagenous stroma. Vasculature was prominent (Fig. 9.223). Some cases displayed focal loose storiform

growth similar to fibrous histiocytoma. Scattered multinucleated cells were found in about half of cases. Only slight nuclear pleomorphism was detected and mitotic activity was present in seven of the tumors, including some with mild cytologic atypia. No atypical mitoses were found and mitoses were not numerous (highest reported, 1 mitotic figure/10 hpf). With the exception of mast cells, which were present in most of the lesions, there was minimal inflammation. The immunohistochemical profile was highly distinctive in that the vast majority of cases displayed immunoreactivity for EMA, CD34, and CD99 but lacked actins, desmin, glial fibrillary acid protein, and keratins and did not stain with HMB-45. One case had weak focal reactivity for S100 protein.

The differential diagnosis of superficial acral fibromyxoma includes fibrous histiocytoma, sclerosing perineurioma, superficial angiomyxoma, and inflammatory myxohyaline tumor. Fibrous histiocytoma is typically not myxoid and lacks CD34. The differential diagnosis of an EMA-positive lesion of the distal extremity includes sclerosing perineurioma (also described by Fetsch et al.),[679] but the latter lacks CD34 and features small, uniform, epithelioid cells arranged in cords and whorls. Superficial angiomyxoma, as its name suggests, is also superficial and myxoid, and often has a multi-nodular configuration and an entrapped epithelial component.[680,681] Superficial angiomyxoma may express CD34[682] but not EMA. Inflammatory myxohyaline tumor differs from superficial acral fibromyxoma by its infiltrative multinodular growth pattern, its inflammatory background, and the presence of bizarre fibroblasts with inclusion-like nucleoli. Inflammatory myxohyaline tumor may have CD34 reactivity, but EMA expression has not been reported.

INTRAMUSCULAR MYXOMA

Intramuscular myxoma affects individuals over an age range of 20–84 years but has a peak incidence in middle-aged adults, with a female majority.[683–686] The tumor develops in association with deep skeletal muscle. The thigh and pelvic girdle, shoulder, and upper arm are the common sites in decreasing order of frequency. The lesion usually presents as a slow-growing, painless mass with less than 25% of tumors associated with discomfort or pain. The mass is moveable when the affected muscle relaxes but becomes fixed when

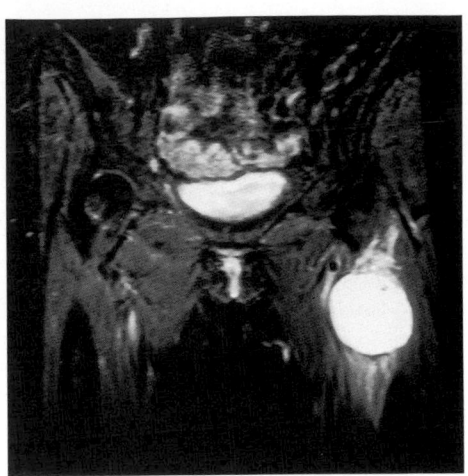

Fig. 9.224 Intramuscular myxoma. The bright signal on T2 images is in keeping with a myxoid lesion.

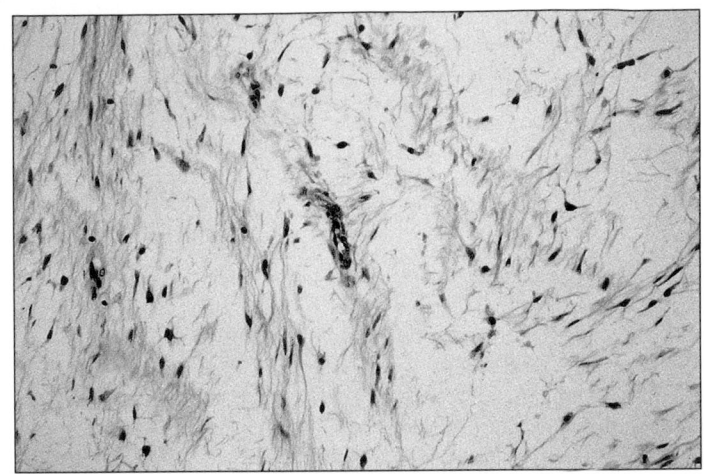

Fig. 9.226 Intramuscular myxoma. These tumors have low cellularity and vascularity and mitotic activity is essentially nil. Hypercellular forms maintain their bland cytologic features and lack mitoses.

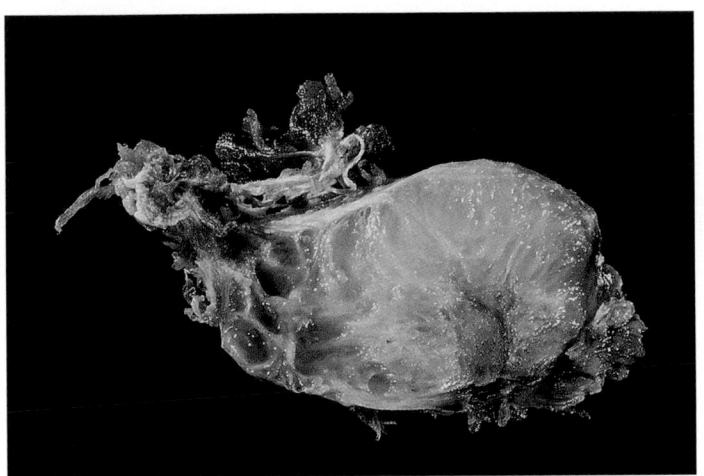

Fig. 9.225 Intramuscular myxoma. Note the gelatinous gross appearance.

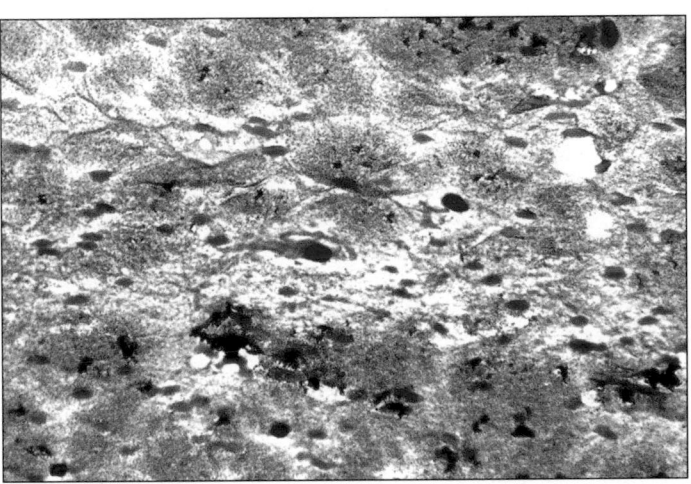

Fig. 9.227 Intramuscular myxoma, aspiration biopsy. Although this lesion displays only minimal nuclear enlargement compared with the myxoid malignant fibrous histiocytoma depicted in Figure 9.72, sampling error could easily be a factor in such cases.

the muscle contracts. The duration of signs and symptoms prior to presentation varies from months to years.

The presence of multiple lesions is a rare phenomenon and is usually associated with a coexistent fibrous dysplasia of bone.[687,688] In such cases, the manifestations of fibrous dysplasia typically appear first. In most reported cases, the fibrous dysplasia involves more than one bone (polyostotic) and, in some instances, can be associated with Albright syndrome (polyostotic fibrous dysplasia, café-au-lait spots on the skin, and endocrine abnormalities). The intramuscular myxoma typically arises in the same general vicinity as the bone(s) involved by fibrous dysplasia. Intramuscular myxoma is a benign tumor that rarely recurs and is managed with local excision.

The tumors are located within the skeletal muscle or attached to the muscular fascia. Most range in size from 5–10 cm (Fig. 9.224). On gross inspection, the tumor has an oval or lobular shape and appears well circumscribed. The cut surface has a soft, mucoid consistency and a gray-white color (Fig. 9.225) with thin, traversing fibrous trabeculae and small mucin-filled cysts. On close inspection, the process can be observed infiltrating into surrounding, edematous skeletal muscle.

On microscopic examination, intramuscular myxoma is characterized by scattered, bland, spindle-shaped and stellate cells, sparse small vessels, and numerous thin collagen fibers suspended in a richly myxoid stromal matrix (Fig. 9.226). The spindle-shaped and stellate cells have a small nucleus and a meager amount of pale, occasionally vacuolated, eosinophilic cytoplasm. The ill defined cytoplasmic processes of the lesional cells are often continuous with delicate strands of collagen that run haphazardly throughout the tumor. The mitotic activity is virtually nonexistent. The hyaluronic-acid-rich, mucinous stroma often contains small cystic spaces. Occasionally, residual atrophic skeletal muscle fibers, foamy histiocytes, and, rarely, mast cells are identified within the myxoid matrix. Simple, nonarborizing, capillary-sized vessels are scattered throughout the process. At the periphery of the lesion, skeletal muscle fibers adjacent to the tumor are atrophic and separated by edema fluid or infiltrating tumor. Fat cells are commonly interspersed in the skeletal muscle. Aspiration cytology yields mucoid matrix and bland-appearing nuclei (Fig. 9.227).

Rarely, intramuscular myxoma may have areas exhibiting increased cellularity, more abundant collagen, and an increased number of vessels. These cellular myxomas lack the mitotic activity, cytologic atypia, branching vascular network, and necrosis characteristic of a sarcoma.[686]

JUXTA-ARTICULAR MYXOMA

Juxta-articular myxoma (JAM) arises in association with large joints.[689] As this tumor may exhibit large size, poor circumscription, and focal hypercellularity, recognition of JAM as a distinct benign entity is important.

Although JAM affects patients over a wide age range (16–83 years), almost three-quarters of cases occur in men in the third to fifth decades. Most lesions develop around the lateral or medial aspect of the knee. JAM usually presents as a swelling or mass, with over 50% of patients giving a history of pain or tenderness. There is often a history of trauma.

Although JAM is a benign tumor with no potential for metastatic spread, it recurs in about a third of patients. Half of these patients experience more than one recurrence.

JAM is centered primarily within the subcutaneous tissue but can extend into the overlying dermis or the deep fibrous structures of the joint. It may abut the synovium or invade skeletal muscle. When the process involves the knee, the main tumor mass may be associated with smaller, ganglion-like structures within the lateral or medial semilunar cartilage. The tumors range in size from lesions approximating the dimensions of a ganglion to masses over 10 cm in greatest dimension. The lesion appears as a lobulated, unilocular or multilocular cyst lined by a thin fibrous membrane. The tumor has a soft, jelly-like consistency. The cut surface is myxoid, gelatinous, or slimy in appearance and has a white to tan-yellow color.

JAM is chiefly composed of bland-appearing, oval, spindled and stellate cells embedded in a relatively hypovascular, hyaluronic-acid-rich mucinous stroma through which run numerous strands of delicate collagen. Variably sized cystic spaces are identified in the majority of cases. JAM is often seen infiltrating and entrapping subcutaneous fat. Focal increased cellularity or fibrosis may be present, especially in recurrent lesions. In the cellular foci, the spindled cells maintain their benign cytologic appearance and lack increased mitotic activity.

Both ganglion and JAM exhibit cystic change and, rarely, a ganglion may show a modest cellular proliferation. However, the former entity occurs more commonly in females, is a smaller lesion, and arises chiefly in the joint capsule or tendinous tissue of the wrist. Ganglion cyst also contains less mucin than does intramuscular myxoma or JAM.

Intramuscular myxoma differs from JAM by its deep location and association with the large muscle groups of the thigh, pelvic girdle, or shoulder. Microscopically, intramuscular myxoma is better circumscribed than JAM and does not undergo as much cystic change. Foci of increased cellularity or vascularity also occur less commonly in intramuscular myxoma than in JAM.

Angiomyofibroblastoma and aggressive angiomyxoma are both discussed in Chapter 37.

JUVENILE NASAL ANGIOFIBROMA

Juvenile nasopharyngeal angiofibroma (JNA) is an uncommon vascular tumor occurring almost exclusively in adolescent males. JNAs constitute approximately 0.5% of head and neck tumors. Although histologically benign, they can recur following surgical therapy and can be locally aggressive. JNAs typically arise from the posterolateral wall of the nasal cavity and grow by erosion of bone and displacement of adjacent structures; eventually these lesions can involve the nasopharynx, paranasal sinuses, orbit, and skull base with intracranial extension. They occur more frequently in patients with FAP.[690,691] Histopathologically, JNAs are characterized by proliferating, irregular vascular channels within a fibrous stroma. The stromal compartment consists of plump cells that can be spindled or stellate in shape and give rise to varying amounts of collagen fibers. The stromal component seems to house the actual lesional cells. The occurrence of nasopharyngeal angiofibromas in the nasal region of pubescent males, their histologic similarity to erectile tissue, and their expression of multiple sex hormone receptors have remained tantalizing observations with possible implications about the origin of these neoplasms. Mutations in exon 3 of the β-catenin gene have been detected in 75% (12 of 16) sporadic JNAs from non-FAP patients.[100]

PARACHORDOMA

Parachordoma is an extremely rare soft tissue neoplasm with microscopic features that overlap with classical chordoma and, to some extent, with EMC and mixed tumor of the skin and soft tissue. Dabska[692] is credited with fully characterizing the clinicopathologic features of this unusual neoplasm in a study of 10 cases that included five examples reported earlier by Laskowski as 'chordoma periphericum.' Dabska concluded that parachordoma is histologically similar to chordoma, arises in the deep soft tissue of the extremities, and follows a benign clinical course if adequately excised. These tumors have been comprehensively reviewed by Fisher.[693]

Since Dabska's study, only scattered reports of parachordoma or chordoma periphericum have appeared in the literature. Recent investigations have focused on the ultrastructural characteristics and immunoprofile of parachordoma in an attempt to differentiate it from tumors with similar histology and to establish its histogenesis. In general, electron microscopic and immunohistochemical studies have shown that the cells of parachordoma possess features resembling those of chordoma.[694,695]

Several histogenetic origins have been proposed for parachordoma but none are universally accepted. Laskowski considered a specialized synovial cell with the capacity for chondroid differentiation as the progenitor cell.[692] At present, the term 'parachordoma' denotes a presumably benign soft tissue neoplasm with histomorphologic, immunohistochemical, and ultrastructural features similar to chordoma but taking origin in extra-axial sites.

Parachordoma arises mainly in tenosynovial and aponeurotic tissue or on the surface of bone in close relation to the periosteum. One tumor has been reported within subcutaneous tissue.[695] The tumor presents as a slow-growing mass in adolescents and adults, without sex predilection. The majority of lesions are painless, although Dabska reported that two subperiosteal tumors were painful.[692] Parachordoma can recur with inadequate excision but does not metastasize.

The neoplasm is described as an ovoid, lobulated, well circumscribed mass that is sometimes surrounded by a thin fibrous pseudocapsule. In Dabska's series, the tumors ranged from 2.5–8 cm with the majority measuring 5 cm or less.

At low magnification, the neoplasm is characterized by epithelioid-appearing cells arranged in small nests, cord-like arrays,

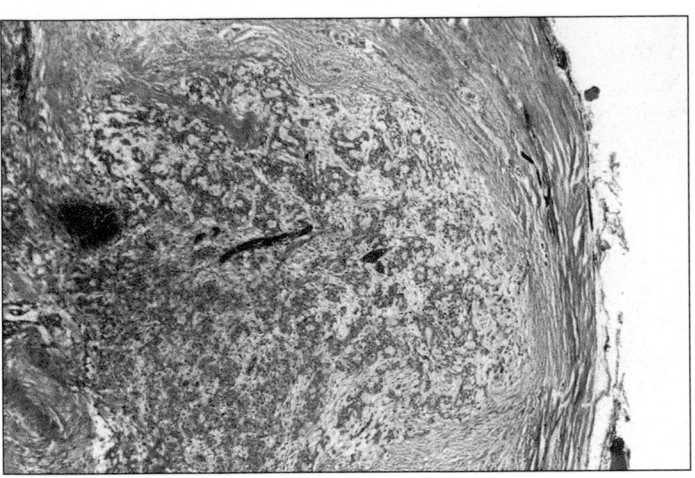

Fig. 9.228 Parachordoma. The tumor is well marginated at scanning power (Courtesy of Dr Cyril Fisher).

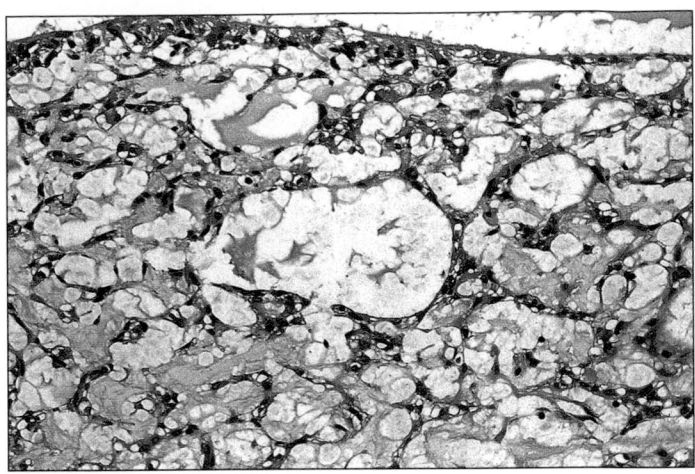

Fig. 9.230 Parachordoma. The cells are arranged in a lace-like configuration.

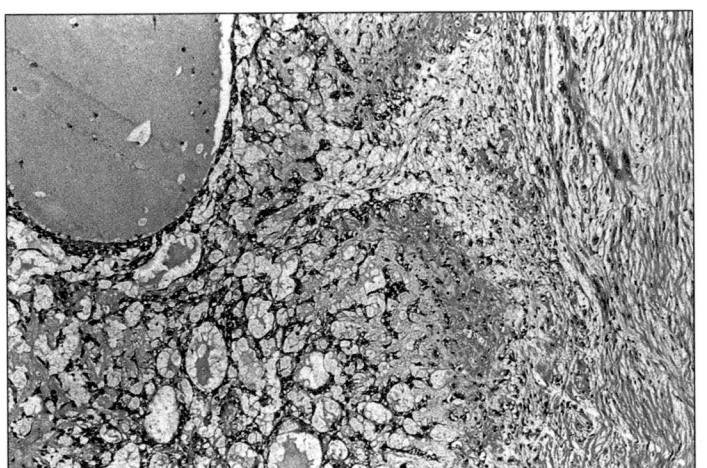

Fig. 9.229 Parachordoma. Nests, cords, and cystic spaces are all present.

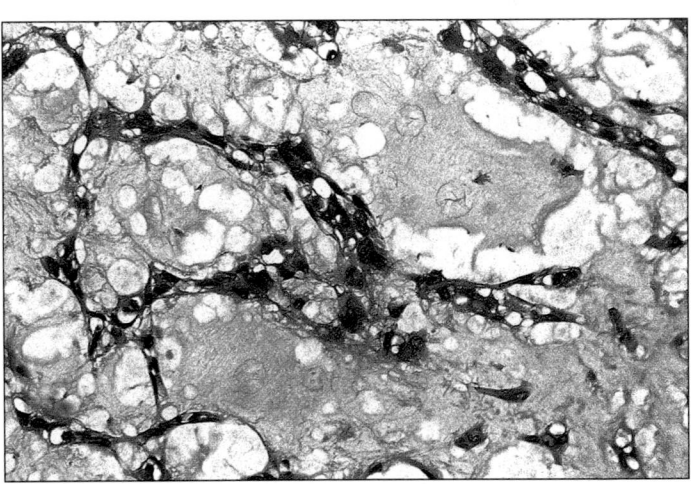

Fig. 9.231 Parachordoma. The individual cells are uniform and bland-appearing. Cytoplasmic vacuoles are present but the intensely vacuolated cells that characterize classic chordomas are lacking.

and pseudoglandular structures within a myxohyaline stroma (Figs 9.228–9.230). Irregular bands of fibrous tissue traverse the tumor, imparting a lobular architecture.

The proliferating cells have abundant clear to pale eosinophilic cytoplasm that is variably vacuolated, sometimes to the point of resembling physaliphorous cells of classical chordoma (Fig. 9.231). Myxoid material can be identified within the intracytoplasmic vacuoles (with Alcian blue stain). PAS stain demonstrates the presence of intracytoplasmic glycogen. The nuclei range in morphology from a large structure with bland, vesicular chromatin and a prominent nucleolus to a small, pyknotic form. Multinucleation is occasionally observed. Mitotic activity is minimal and lymphatic or vascular invasion is not observed. Some tumors have a minor component of short, spindle-shaped cells with scant cytoplasm and elongated, hyperchromatic nuclei arranged in cords within in a fibrous matrix. The stromal matrix of the lobules varies from a purely myxoid to a more chondroid or hyalin-like composition.

Immunohistochemical analysis of parachordoma demonstrates immunoexpression of vimentin, S100 protein, and EMA in most

tumors tested. Parachordomas are CAM5.2 (CK8 and 18) immuno-reactive but lack AE1 and CK19 expression.[694,695]

Conventional chordoma and EMC are the main contenders in the differential diagnosis of parachordoma. Their separation from the latter neoplasms is clinically important, as both of these are malignant. Parachordomas are also distinguishable from cutaneous mixed tumors, although some observers believe they fall within the spectrum of cutaneous mixed tumors.[1]

Chordomas develop exclusively in the axial skeleton, with the majority of neoplasms occurring in the sacrococcygeal region, followed by the spheno-occipital area of the cranium. In contradistinction to the relatively asymptomatic clinical presentation exhibited by most parachordomas, chordoma almost always produces symptoms related to its location within the axial skeleton. The radiograph of the latter neoplasm characteristically shows destruction of the involved bone and soft tissue spread of tumor. Histologically, the cells of chordoma generally grow in a more cord-like fashion and do not exhibit the nested and gland-like growth patterns seen in parachordoma.

EMC bears a resemblance to parachordoma due to its lobular architecture and mucopolysaccharide-rich stroma. This sarcoma, however, generally arises within deep skeletal muscle. The cells of myxoid chondrosarcoma are smaller and contain more intensely eosinophilic, less vacuolated cytoplasm than the cells of parachordoma. Moreover, they have a tendency to grow in anastomosing thin trabecula, unlike the cells within parachordoma. Although the cells of both neoplasms express S100 protein, the cells of the myxoid chondrosarcoma do not express cytokeratin or EMA. Ultrastructurally, the cells of myxoid chondrosarcoma possess microtubular aggregates within dilated rough endoplasmic reticulum and lack features of epithelial differentiation.[695] These two lesions are also cytogenetically distinct, although limited data are available on parachordoma.[694] One case of parachordoma studied cytogenetically disclosed trisomy 15, and monosomies of 1, 16, and 17 in contrast to the t(9;22) reported in EMC and the monosomies of 3, 4, 10, and 13 seen in chordoma.

Most examples of mixed tumor of the soft tissues arise in the skin (chondroid syringoma) but rare cases have been reported in deep subcutaneous and subfascial sites.[696] Tumors with a preponderance of myoepithelial cells may show histologic features reminiscent of parachordoma, including lobular arrays of rounded myoepithelial cells arranged in nests or cords within a chondromyxoid matrix. The presence of any epithelial differentiation, such as the formation of ductal structures or epithelial-lined cysts, favors a mixed tumor. As both myoepithelial cells and the cells of parachordoma express S100 protein, cytokeratin, and EMA, other discriminating immunomarkers for myoepithelial differentiation, such as alpha-SMA, glial fibrillary acidic protein, or calponin, as well as evaluation of ultrastructure, may be helpful in differentiating these lesions.

PLEOMORPHIC HYALINIZING ANGIECTATIC TUMOR

Pleomorphic hyalinizing angiectatic tumor (PHAT), described in 1996[697] is of uncertain histogenesis. This extremely rare neoplasm exhibits histologic features that overlap with both ancient schwannoma and a pleomorphic sarcoma. Unlike schwannoma and high-grade-appearing sarcomas, PHAT appears to have the potential for local recurrence but possibly not for metastatic spread.

PHAT has been described in adults (age 32–83 years).[697] The chief complaint is the presence of a slow-growing mass. Most lesions arise in subcutaneous tissue, with a few reported intramuscularly. The lower extremity is the most common site. In the series by Smith et al., four of eight patients with follow-up data experienced a recurrence and one patient had multiple recurrences over a 25-year period.[697] No metastases have been reported. One example has been diploid on flow cytometry.[698]

PHAT is described as a lobulated tumor ranging from 2–8 cm in greatest dimension. The tumors are unencapsulated and most have an infiltrative border. The cut surface of the neoplasm is white-tan with areas of hemorrhage.

Microscopically, PHAT features clusters of dilated, irregularly contoured blood vessels and an accompanying relatively cellular population of pleomorphic, plump, spindled and multinucleated cells proliferating haphazardly in a variably collagenous stroma (Figs 9.232, 9.233). In less vascularized examples, a fascicular growth pattern can be observed. The tumors usually have an infiltrative border.

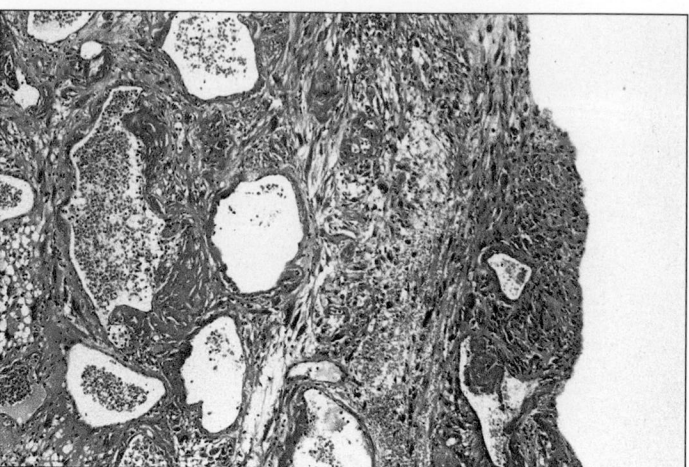

Fig. 9.232 Pleomorphic hyalinizing angiectatic tumor. Ectatic vessels are accompanied by fibrous stroma containing atypical cells.

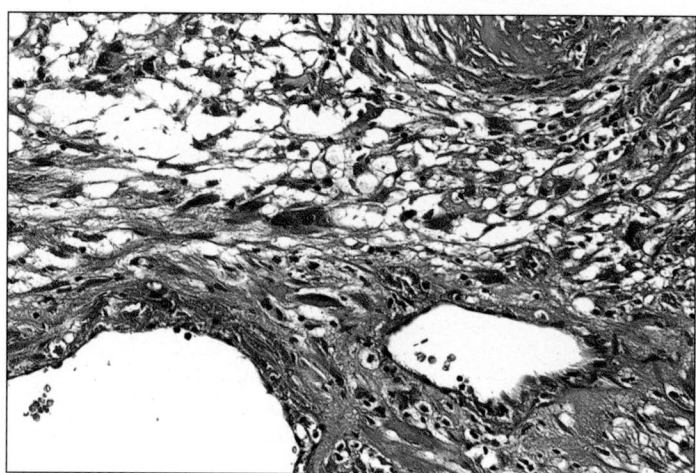

Fig. 9.233 Pleomorphic hyalinizing angiectatic tumor, higher magnification.

The ectatic vessels within the tumor show marked fibrinoid change, perivascular hyaline fibrosis, and may contain intraluminal fibrin and thrombi. Hemosiderin deposition is noted in the tumor cells adjacent to the ectatic vessels. The stroma is composed of loose collagen but focal mucin can be observed. Mast cells are commonly identified and a few tumors contain collections of lymphocytes.

The tumor cells lack immunoreactivity for S100 protein, EMA, CD31, and desmin. CD34 immunoreactivity has been demonstrated in about half the tumors tested. Immunoelectron microscopy revealed large numbers of cytoplasmic vimentin-positive filaments within the tumor cells.[697]

Dilated vessels with hyalinized walls and pleomorphic spindled cells with intranuclear pseudoinclusions are microscopic features shared by PHAT and ancient schwannoma (neurilemmoma). Unlike PHAT, neurilemmoma is generally encapsulated and noninvasive. Its cells are arranged in sharply demarcated Antoni A and Antoni B zones and they strongly express S100 protein in contrast to PHAT.

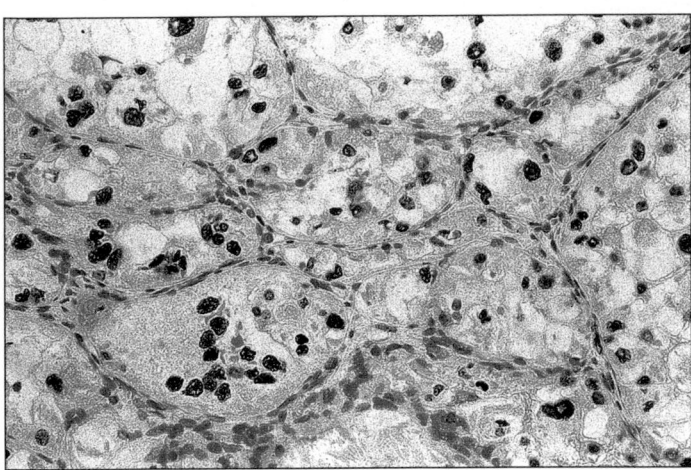

Fig. 9.234 Alveolar soft part sarcoma, immunohistochemical preparation for the TFE3 gene product (Courtesy of Dr Pedram Argani).

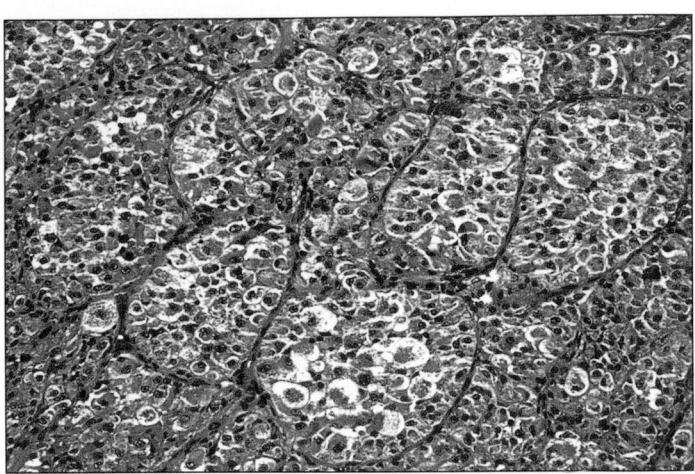

Fig. 9.235 Alveolar soft part sarcoma. This adult example displays a striking alveolar pattern and uniform granular eosinophilic cells.

ALVEOLAR SOFT PART SARCOMA

Despite the fact that alveolar soft part sarcoma (ASPS) accounts for fewer than 1% of all soft tissue sarcomas,[3] it is the grist for numerous studies attempting to establish histogenesis.[699] Early reports claimed that ASPS is a variant of paraganglioma or granular cell tumor, a neoplasm exhibiting skeletal muscle differentiation, or a neoplasm capable of producing renin.

A prevailing theory has been that ASPS differentiates along skeletal muscle lineage. This hypothesis gained initial support when investigators claimed that the intracytoplasmic, membrane-bound crystals in ASPS ultrastructurally resembled the crystalline structures detected in nemaline myopathy or adult rhabdomyoma.[700] Furthermore, a few studies have identified myogenic proteins, including the highly sensitive and specific skeletal muscle marker MyoD1, within cells of ASPS on frozen tissue.[701] However evidence for skeletal muscle differentiation has been contested, as specific ultrastructural features of muscle differentiation have not been identified within ASPS. Researchers have not been able to demonstrate nuclear expression of MyoD1 or myogenin, two key proteins in skeletal muscle differentiation, using immunohistochemistry, Western blot analysis, or molecular techniques.[702,703]

Karyotyping studies in the early 1990s[702] yielded two clonally abnormal lines. One demonstrated trisomy 47,XX+5, the other 46,XX,1p-,17q+. Subsequently, Ladanyi et al. identified the *ASPL–TFE3* fusion gene in tumors characterized by der(17)t(X;17)(p11.2;q25). This unbalanced translocation results in fusion of the *TFE3* gene on Xp11.2 to a novel gene named *ASPL*. The protein product can be detected immunohistochemically[704] (Fig. 9.234). Therefore, ASPS can also be diagnosed by molecular techniques. A group of pediatric renal neoplasms have also been described that bear a histologic resemblance to ASPS and harbor the same translocation.[705]

ASPS principally affects adolescents and young adults, with a slight female predominance,[706–711] but pediatric cases are known[712] and older adults may also be affected. The tumor arises primarily in the deep soft tissues of the lower extremity, particularly the anterior thigh and the buttock,[707] followed by the chest and abdominal wall. Unusual locations include the retroperitoneum,[707] mediastinum,[713]

and female genital tract.[714] In children, ASPS has a proclivity for the head and neck region, especially the periorbital soft tissue and tongue. ASPS clinically presents as a slow-growing, painless mass, which may be apparent for months to years before the patient seeks medical attention. Unfortunately, sometimes metastatic disease to the lung or brain heralds the presence of an occult sarcoma.

ASPS has a poor long-term survival. In a clinicopathologic study covering over 60 years, Lieberman et al.[707] documented a 5-year survival for patients presenting without metastatic disease of 60%, a 10-year survival of 38%, and a 20-year survival of only 15%. Death usually results from metastases to vital organs. The principal metastatic sites are the lung, followed by the brain and bone.[707] Children with ASPS fare better than adults; possibly earlier detection is a factor.[710,712]

ASPS varies in size from less than 5 cm to over 20 cm. The tumor is usually well circumscribed and may be partially surrounded by a fibrous pseudocapsule. Large, tortuous vessels can be identified in the surrounding normal tissue. The tumor has a firm, but friable consistency. The cut surface has an overall gray color with areas of hemorrhage and necrosis resulting in red-tan and yellow-white foci respectively. Thin fibrous septa may be observed.

At low magnification, ASPS displays a distinctive nested or organoid arrangement of large, polygonal cells with eosinophilic cytoplasm (Fig. 9.235). The nests are separated from one another by thin-walled, sinusoidal vascular channels. Protrusion of nests of tumor into these vessels and frank vascular invasion are common findings in ASPS. Loss of cellular cohesion results in intact and degenerated cells floating in the center of a tumor cell nest and imparts a pseudoalveolar appearance to the otherwise ball-like arrangement of cells. ASPS can also be composed of small, compact nests of cells without prominent vascularity, an architectural pattern seen more commonly in children (Fig. 9.236).

The neoplastic cells have a uniform, oval to polygonal shape with distinct cell borders and an ample amount of finely granular, eosinophilic cytoplasm. The cells possess one or two eccentrically positioned, uniformly round to reniform nuclei with vesicular chromatin and prominent nucleoli. Mitotic activity is characteristically low. PAS stain detects intracytoplasmic glycogen and highlights elongated and rhomboid crystalline

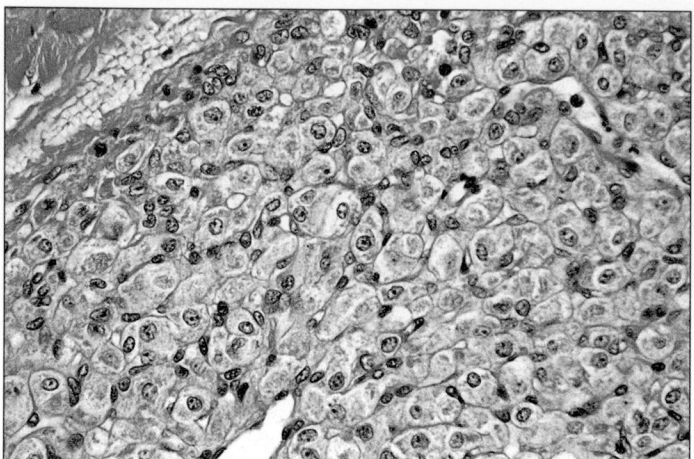

Fig. 9.236 Alveolar soft part sarcoma. This more solid example was from the tongue of a child.

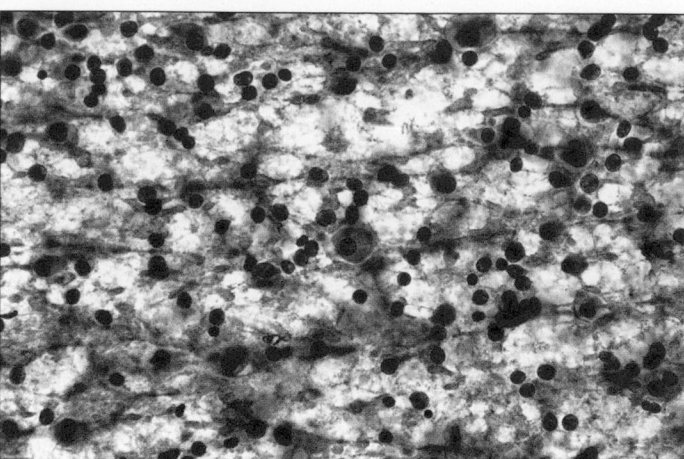

Fig. 9.238 Alveolar soft part sarcoma, aspiration cytology. The cytoplasm is fragile but well preserved cells display the characteristic prominent nucleoli.

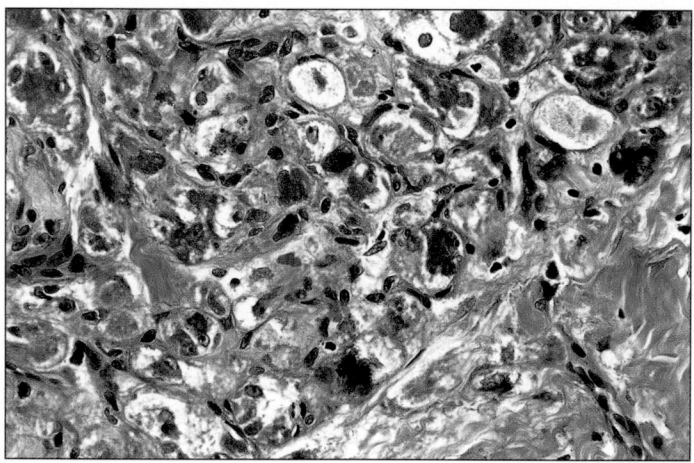

Fig. 9.237 Alveolar soft part sarcoma. The PAS stain shows 'chunky' positivity and crystalline-like structures.

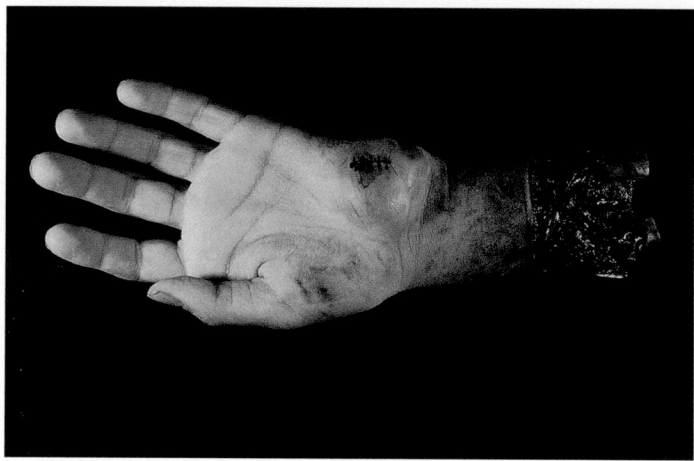

Fig. 9.239 Epithelioid sarcoma. These tumors most commonly affect the hand/wrist.

structures commonly disposed in sheaf-like aggregates within the cytoplasm (Fig. 9.237).

Unusual histomorphologic variants include a pleomorphic form of ASPS characterized by loss of the nestlike growth, cellular pleomorphism, and high mitotic activity.[708] Examples of ASPS featuring a spindle cell component[715] and psammomatous calcifications[716] have been documented in the literature.

The immunohistochemical profile of ASPS is broad and rather nonspecific. Most cases of ASPS exhibit some degree of vimentin, desmin, and MSA expression. S100 protein immunoreactivity has been observed in some tumors.[707,710,715,717]

Aspiration cytology can yield cells with a resemblance to a carcinoma. Aspirated cells display prominent nuclear pleomorphism and dissociated, large neoplastic cells with round to plasmacytoid morphology, cytoplasmic fragility, and granularity with abundant, atypical, naked nuclei[716,718] (Fig. 9.238).

The differential diagnosis of ASPS is primarily with paraganglioma, adult rhabdomyoma, granular cell tumor (GCT), rhabdomyosarcoma, and metastatic renal cell carcinoma.

EPITHELIOID SARCOMA

These tumors were first described by Laskowski in 1961.[719] Enzinger subsequently reported the clinicopathologic features of 62 cases and coined the term epithelioid sarcoma,[720] recognizing that this neoplasm was distinct from synovial sarcoma and, later, from clear cell sarcoma.

Epithelioid sarcoma is the most common primary sarcoma of the hand and wrist[3] (Fig. 9.239). The clinical and histologic features of epithelioid sarcoma can mimic those of a non-neoplastic process, so that the sarcoma may be misdiagnosed until recurrence or metastasis reveals its true nature. The histogenesis of epithelioid sarcoma remains unknown. Electron microscopy reveals a spectrum of ultrastructural differentiation ranging from epithelial-appearing cells with intercellular junctions and surface microvilli to near-totally undifferentiated, fibroblast-like cells with a paucity of organelles.[721] Genetic evaluation of epithelioid sarcoma has yet to yield a consistent event.

Epithelioid sarcoma has been reported in almost all ages but is most prevalent in patients between 10 and 39 years of age,[722] with a male predominance.[723] The flexor surfaces of the hand, fingers, and forearm are the most commonly involved sites, followed by the knee and lower leg, proximal lower and upper extremity, ankle, and the feet and toes. The trunk and head and neck regions are the least commonly involved sites. Penile and vulvar cases have been reported. A history of trauma is elicited in about 20–25% of cases.[722,723]

Epithelioid sarcoma arising in the dermis most often presents as a slow-growing, painless, usually solitary nodule or plaque. Epithelioid sarcoma situated in the subcutaneous or fascial tissue frequently presents as fixed, relatively hard nodule. Tumors of the hand and penis can clinically mimic superficial fibromatoses. Dermal and subcutaneous lesions characteristically develop a cleft of the overlying skin, which eventually ulcerates.[724] These innocuous clinical presentations not uncommonly lead the clinician to an erroneous diagnosis of a benign lesion. The neoplasm spreads proximally up the extremity producing numerous cutaneous nodules and ulcerative lesions.

In a study of 202 patients with follow-up over 10 years from the AFIP,[722] over three-quarters of patients developed at least one recurrence. Other series document recurrence rates ranging from about 35–70%.[725,726] Multiple recurrences are characteristic. Metastases were reported in 45% of patients followed over 10 years in the AFIP study.[722] Lung and regional lymph nodes are the most common metastatic sites, followed by skin, soft tissue, and central nervous system. Although the reported 5-year survival for epithelioid sarcoma is at least 60% in most studies,[723,725–728] the overall survival of patients with epithelioid sarcoma is probably quite low. Parameters that impact adversely on survival include large size, vascular invasion, lymph node metastasis, and the presence of necrosis. Proximal and deep location, male sex, older age, high mitotic activity, and presence of pulmonary metastasis have also been reported to correlate with decreased survival. Radical local excision or amputation is recommended therapy. Adjuvant radiotherapy helps to provide local control. Since lymph node involvement is more common in epithelioid sarcoma than in other types of sarcoma, regional lymph node dissection should be attempted.

Tumors located in the distal aspect of the extremity are situated in the superficial soft tissue (dermis and/or subcutaneous tissue) and appear as small (generally less than 5 cm), nonencapsulated nodules with a firm to hard consistency. The lesions may appear well circumscribed or invade surrounding tissue in a fashion similar to a squamous cell carcinoma. The cut surface of the tumor is gray-white to tan with centrally located yellow to brown foci of necrosis and/or hemorrhage.

Tumors arising in the more proximal locations tend to be large, deeply situated masses (deep fascia or tendons) with a multinodular growth pattern and an ill-defined, infiltrating margin. The nodules grow along fascial planes, surround nerves and vessels, or diffusely invade tendons and muscle.

Epithelioid sarcoma is characterized by a predominantly nodular growth pattern of epithelioid and plump, spindled cells. The center of the nodule commonly undergoes degenerative change characterized by necrosis, hemorrhage, cyst formation, focal calcification, or replacement of tumor cells by a myxohyaline stroma (Figs 9.240–9.242). At the periphery of the nodules, the epithelioid cells occasionally grow in a cord-like fashion and the spindled cells form vague fascicles as these elements mingle with dense, eosinophilic collagen. The nodules have a tendency to coalesce. When the tumor spreads along fascial planes and aponeurotic connective tissue, the confluent nodules align themselves along the length of the tissue plane, resulting in a band of tumor cells surrounding hypocellular or necrotic zones (garland-like configuration).

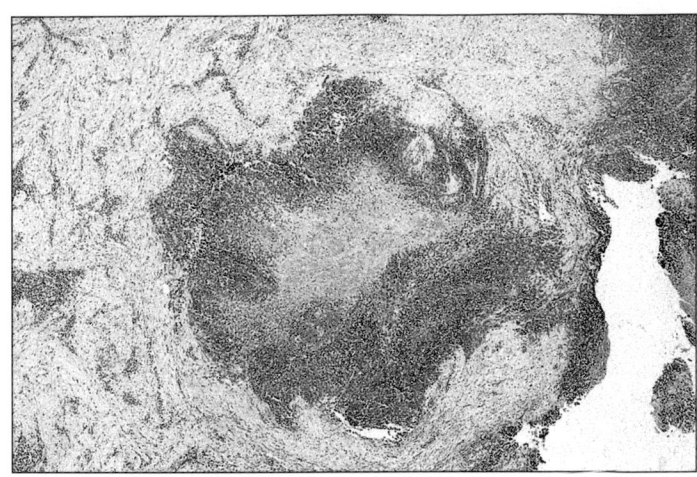

Fig. 9.240 Epithelioid sarcoma. The presence of necrosis in the center of collections of tumor cells often results in misdiagnosis of granulomatous processes.

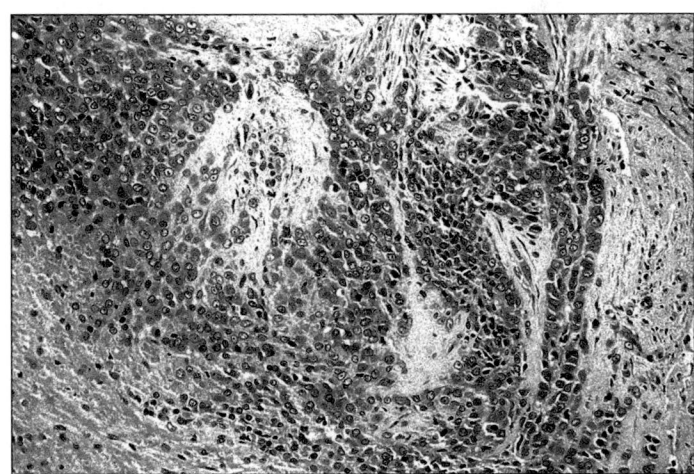

Fig. 9.241 Epithelioid sarcomas display cells with ample eosinophilic cytoplasm.

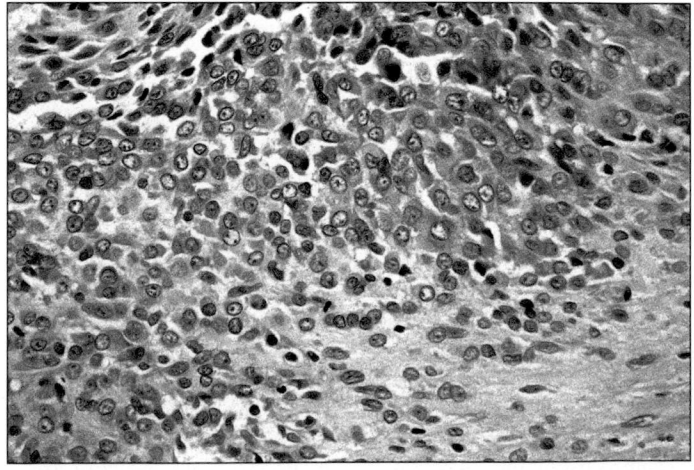

Fig. 9.242 Epithelioid sarcoma, higher magnification.

The neoplastic cells have an epithelioid or plump spindle cell morphology and usually exhibit mild to moderate pleomorphism. The cells possess eosinophilic cytoplasm with fairly well defined cell borders. The nucleus has a round to slightly irregular, ovoid contour with irregularly distributed, vesicular chromatin and a conspicuous nucleolus. Multinucleated cells can be identified as a minor component in some cases. The mitotic rate in epithelioid sarcoma varies but is usually <10 mitoses/10 hpf. Cells with an eccentrically positioned nucleus, a prominent nucleolus, and a pale eosinophilic intracytoplasmic inclusion (rhabdoid cell morphology) may be interspersed in the tumor cell population or, in some cases, represent a significant component of the tumor.

The proximal type of epithelioid sarcoma,[729] which arises primarily in axial sites as a large, generally deeply-seated mass, is composed of pleomorphic epithelioid cells, including a significant rhabdoid component. This variant has histologic overlap with both extrarenal malignant rhabdoid tumor and carcinoma. Rarely, epithelioid sarcoma consists predominantly of bland-appearing spindle cells arranged in a storiform or fascicular growth pattern with interspersed epithelioid and rhabdoid cells (fibroma-like variant).[730]

The characteristic immunoprofile of epithelioid sarcoma is the coexpression of keratin and vimentin. Cytokeratin is expressed in over 75% of cases using older immunohistochemistry techniques[731] whereas, in a more recent series,[732] nearly all epithelioid sarcomas with typical histology (94%) were positive for keratin 8 (K8), whereas 72% were positive for K19, 48% for intermediate- and high-molecular-weight keratins (34βEH12), and 22% for K7. Reactivity with the latter two antibodies was usually seen in only a minority of tumor cells. EMA is expressed in 50–96% of tumors[732–735] and its pattern of reactivity also demonstrates variability within the same lesion. CD34 is reportedly expressed in about 50% of tumors tested.[732,733,736] Carcinoembryonic antigen (CEA) immunoreactivity can be focally identified in epithelioid sarcoma. Desmin expression has been observed, mainly in the rhabdoid cell component of the proximal type of epithelioid sarcoma.[729]

Necrobiotic granulomas, including granuloma annulare and rheumatoid nodule, are reactive lesions that may histologically resemble epithelioid sarcoma. In contrast to epithelioid sarcoma, necrobiotic granulomas exhibits less cellular atypia and lower mitotic activity, and the inflammatory infiltrate is generally heavier than that of epithelioid sarcoma. Langhans giant cells may be present in necrobiotic granulomas but are not a component of epithelioid sarcoma. While the cells of necrobiotic granulomas express histiocyte/monocyte-related immunomarkers, they lack keratin, EMA, or convincing CD34 immunoreactivity.

The presence of eosinophilic, epithelioid cells attached to and ulcerating the skin may suggest the diagnosis of squamous cell carcinoma. Additionally, proximal-type epithelioid sarcoma, with its deeply located nodules of large, eosinophilic, epithelioid-appearing cells, may also masquerade as a squamous cell carcinoma. As most cases of squamous carcinoma arise in sun-damaged skin, the absence of atypical squamous epithelium in the adjacent nonulcerated epidermis is a feature against squamous carcinoma. Unlike squamous carcinoma, epithelioid sarcoma lacks intercellular bridges and keratinization. Squamous carcinoma does not express CD34[732,736] and has a different keratin profile than epithelioid sarcoma; CK5/6 is detected in squamous cell carcinoma but not in epithelioid sarcoma.[737]

Melanoma may be mistaken for epithelioid sarcoma. The cytoplasm of melanoma cells has a more amphophilic appearance than that of epithelioid sarcoma. Importantly, melanoma cells express S100 protein and HMB-45, but not EMA or keratin. Vascular tumors with epithelioid endothelial cells, including epithelioid hemangioendothelioma and epithelioid angiosarcoma, may histologically resemble epithelioid sarcoma. In contrast to the cells of epithelioid sarcoma, the cells of epithelioid hemangioendothelioma have pale cytoplasm and typically exhibit intracytoplasmic lumina containing red blood cells or their debris. They are arranged in small nests or thin trabeculae and attempt to form primitive vascular lumina. Large nodules with central necrosis are not indicative of epithelioid hemangioendothelioma. The epithelioid variant of angiosarcoma is the most common morphologic expression of high-grade angiosarcoma involving the soft tissues. The epithelioid appearance of the cells and formation of solid nests without discernible vascular differentiation mimic the histopathologic features of epithelioid sarcoma, particularly, the proximal type of epithelioid sarcoma. Careful search, however, will typically uncover vascular channels lined by the neoplastic cells or the presence of intracellular vacuoles containing red blood cells or their debris. The cells of both vascular neoplasms express CD34 and can focally express keratin and EMA. However, in contrast to epithelioid sarcoma, they also express factor-VIII-related antigen and CD31.

SYNOVIAL SARCOMA

Synovial sarcoma is the paradigm for the discovery first of a characteristic translocation and then the elucidation of key molecular events in a solid tumor. An excellent review of the pathology of this tumor by Fisher[738] is available. Synovial sarcoma is a rare but distinctive soft tissue neoplasm showing epithelial differentiation. The term synovial sarcoma has become well established, but is a misnomer. This tumor has no demonstrable relationship with synovium.

Between 5 and 10% of all soft tissue sarcomas are synovial sarcoma, with approximately 800 new cases a year in the United States.[739] Synovial sarcoma are mainly tumors of young adults with a male predominance. The tumor presents typically as an otherwise asymptomatic, deep-seated, slow-growing mass. About 90% occur on the extremities, with a third around the knee. Origin within a joint or bursa represents fewer than 5% of cases.[740,741] A distinct region of involvement is the head and neck, most commonly the paravertebral region with pharyngeal presentation.

Some tumors, especially in the lower limb, have radiologically detectable scattered calcifications. This is diagnostically useful, as they are rare in other types of sarcoma, although calcifications may be found in benign processes (e.g., calcifying fibrous pseudotumor). Tumors are typically 3–10 cm in diameter, multinodular, and infiltrating irregularly into adjacent soft tissues (Figs 9.243, 9.244). Slowly growing lesions can be circumscribed but lack a capsule, and peripheral satellite nodules are occasionally seen. The lesional tissue is pale brown or gray and often is relatively soft and friable because of the paucity of intercellular stroma. Unlike most other soft tissue sarcomas, synovial sarcoma can become multicystic; the cysts, of varying size, have a smooth lining and frequently contain blood, with hemosiderin deposition in the adjacent tumor tissue. This cystic change can be the source of false-negative diagnoses on aspiration cytology.

Biphasic synovial sarcoma has an epithelial and a spindle cell component (Figs 9.245–9.247). The epithelial cells have round to oval vesicular nuclei, abundant cytoplasm, and distinct cell borders. Classically, they form glands with lumina, or prominent papillary structures with spindle cells rather than connective tissue in the papillary core. In both there is usually a single layer of rather uni-

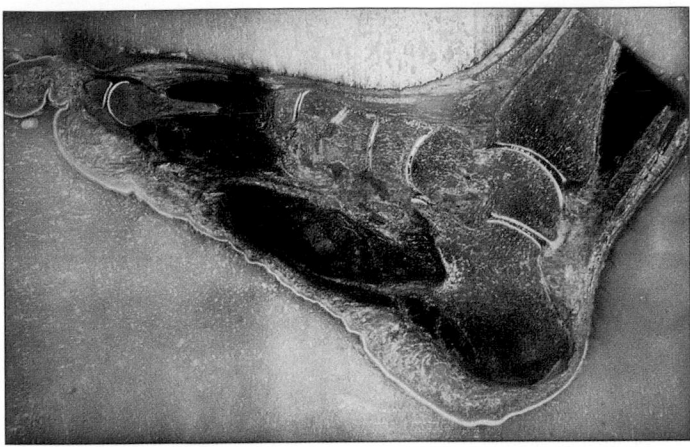

Fig. 9.243 Synovial sarcoma. This tumor is multinodular.

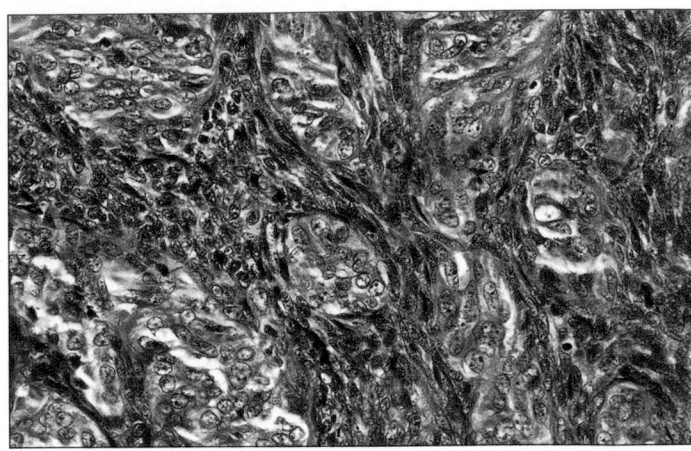

Fig. 9.246 Synovial sarcoma. In this biphasic lesion, spindle cells surround islands with a syncytial appearance.

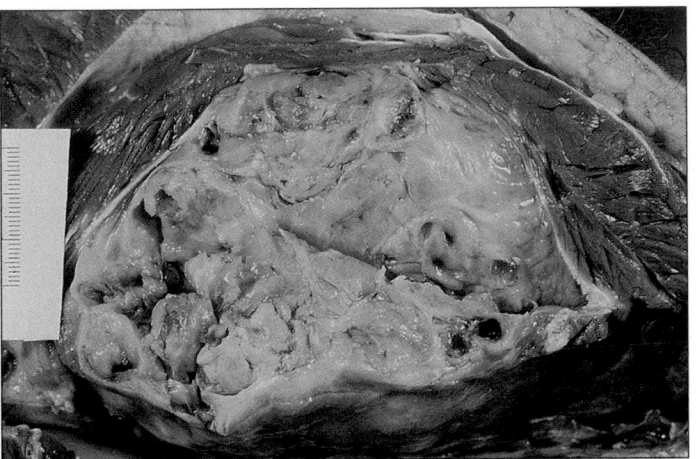

Fig. 9.244 Synovial sarcoma. This large tumor has cystic areas.

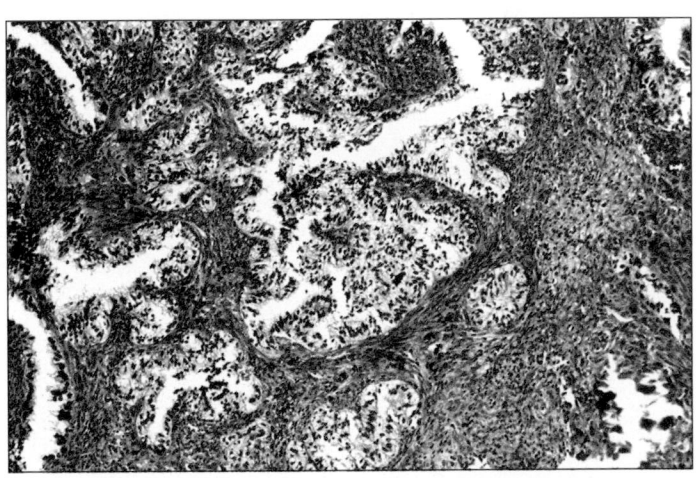

Fig. 9.247 This synovial sarcoma has overt gland formation.

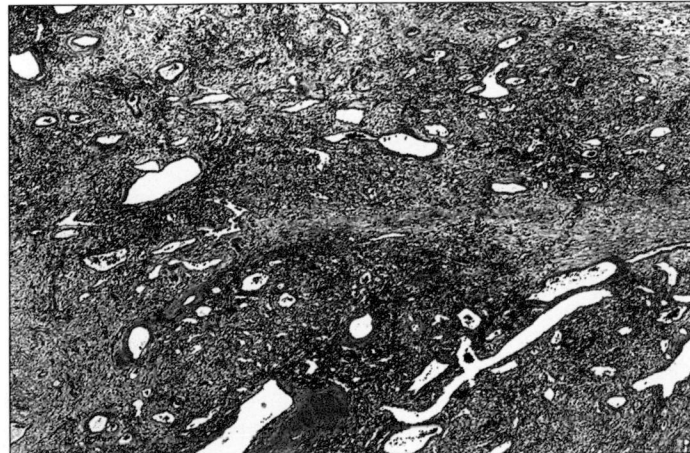

Fig. 9.245 Synovial sarcoma. At scanning power, this biphasic example has a prominent hemangiopericytoma-like vascular pattern.

form cells, but occasionally multilayering or tufting is seen, with or without pleomorphism. The glandular component can be sparse, requiring numerous blocks to be sampled for its detection, or 'overwhelming'[742] with large, closely packed glands and scant intervening spindle component. The glandular lumina contain mucin. The nuclei of the spindle cells are typically uniform, relatively small, ovoid, and pale-staining with inconspicuous nucleoli. Cytoplasm is scant and the cell membranes are indistinct, so that nuclei overlap (Figs 9.248, 9.249). Mitotic figures can be scarce despite the cellularity, but are more frequent in the poorly differentiated type.

The spindle cell component can predominate or occur alone. This was recognized from the earliest reports, but monophasic synovial sarcoma (MSS) closely resembles other spindle cell sarcomas and its distinctive features have only become appreciated and fully accepted in the last two decades. Many MSSs display, at least focally, a prominent hemangiopericytoma-like vascular architecture, with open, branching thin-walled vessels of variable caliber. An obvious epithelial component can sometimes be found by extensive sampling, but this is not necessary to make the diagnosis.

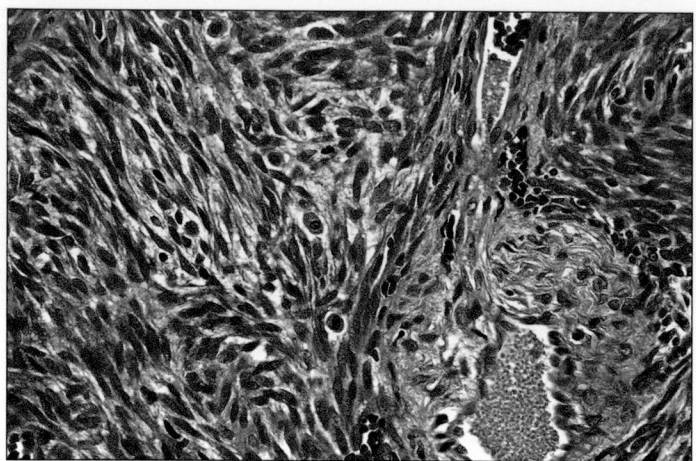

Fig. 9.248 Synovial sarcoma. Monophasic synovial sarcomas often have few mitoses and a rather uniform appearance. A diagnostic clue is that the nuclei overlap.

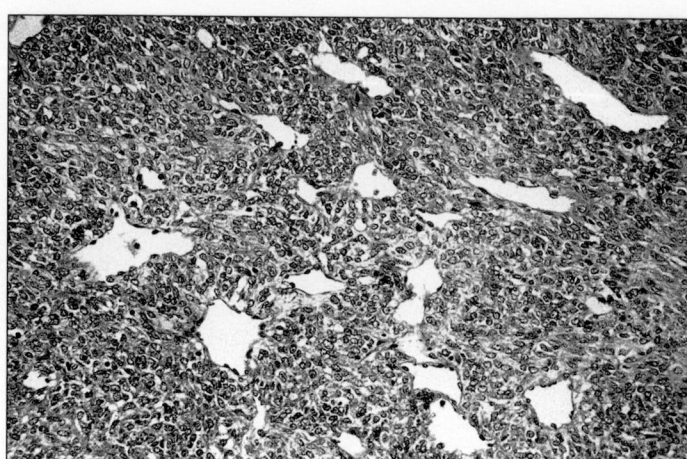

Fig. 9.250 Poorly differentiated synovial sarcoma. These tumors in many ways resemble other 'round blue cell tumors' but the hemangiopericytoma-like vascular pattern in this example suggests the correct diagnosis.

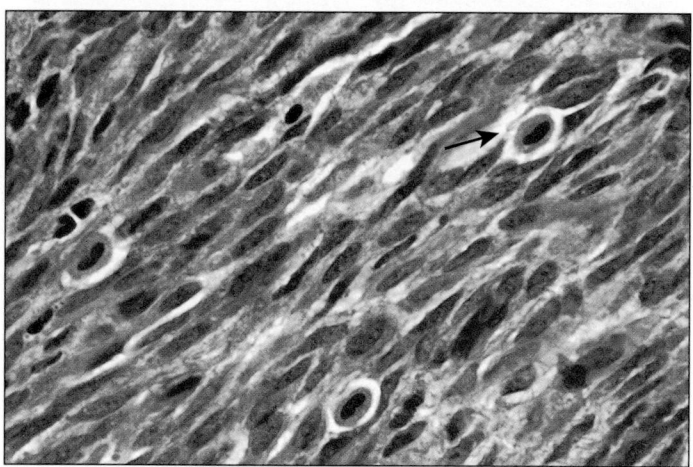

Fig. 9.249 Synovial sarcoma. This lesion has numerous mast cells (arrow).

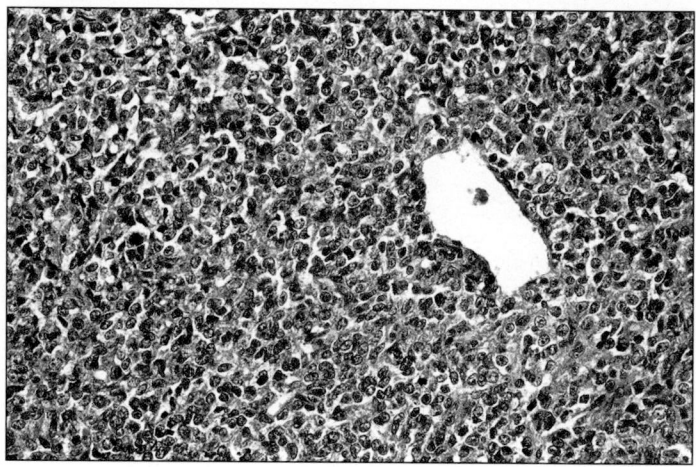

Fig. 9.251 Poorly differentiated synovial sarcoma, high magnification.

Synovial sarcoma with a very prominent glandular component, in which the spindle cells are scarce, must be distinguished from purely glandular MSS (i.e. those without any discernible spindle cell component). Such tumors theoretically exist,[743,744] but resemble adenocarcinomas and are probably best identified by cytogenetics.

About one third of synovial sarcomas have focal calcification, with or without ossification. However, in some tumors, calcification is extensive, and the improved prognosis in such cases merits their separation as a subtype. This phenomenon is more common in tumors of the lower extremities and is rarely seen in examples arising in the head and neck. The 32 calcifying synovial sarcoma described by Varela-Duran and Enzinger[745] were all biphasic, but calcifying MSS exists.

Many synovial sarcoma (biphasic and monophasic) have poorly differentiated areas characterized by high cellularity, numerous mitoses, and often necrosis. Predominantly poorly differentiated synovial sarcoma (PDSS) has a similar range of immunohistologic and ultrastructural findings, and the same cytogenetic and molecular genetic abnormalities, as typical synovial sarcoma.[746]

PDSS shows sheets of darkly staining ovoid or rounded cells, which resemble those in other small round cell tumors, especially ES/PNET (Figs 9.250, 9.251).

The majority of synovial sarcoma display positivity for cytokeratins (Fig. 9.252) and EMA (Fig. 9.253). In biphasic synovial sarcoma, the epithelial component is strongly positive, as are scattered cells in the spindle cell component. CK-positive cells can usually be found in MSS, singly, in cords or in small nests, although their detection sometimes requires examination of several blocks. Several subtypes of cytokeratin are expressed. Compared with other types of spindle cell sarcoma where CK8 and CK18 are also present, CK7 and CK19 appear to be more or less restricted to synovial sarcomas.[747]

EMA is also seen in many synovial sarcomas with a frequency similar to that of cytokeratin.[748,749] A significant number of cases are EMA-positive but CK-negative, or vice versa.[748,749] Both markers should therefore be used as they can complement each other. EMA outlines glandular lumina, and slit-like spaces in solid epithelial areas, and can appear on the surface of single cells or small nests in MSS.

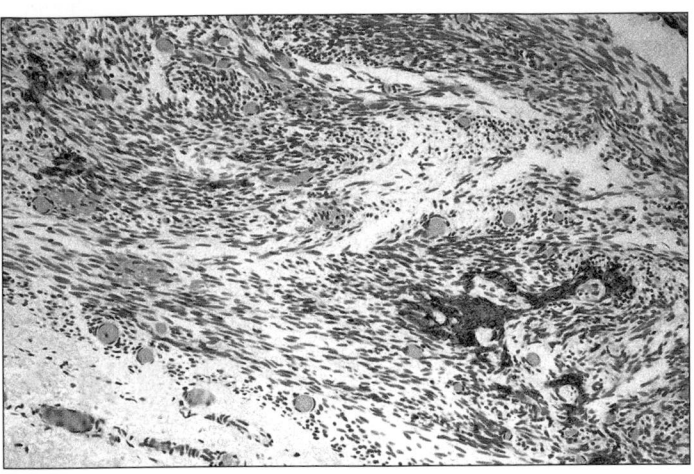

Fig. 9.252 Synovial sarcoma. Keratin stains both the glands and the spindled cells.

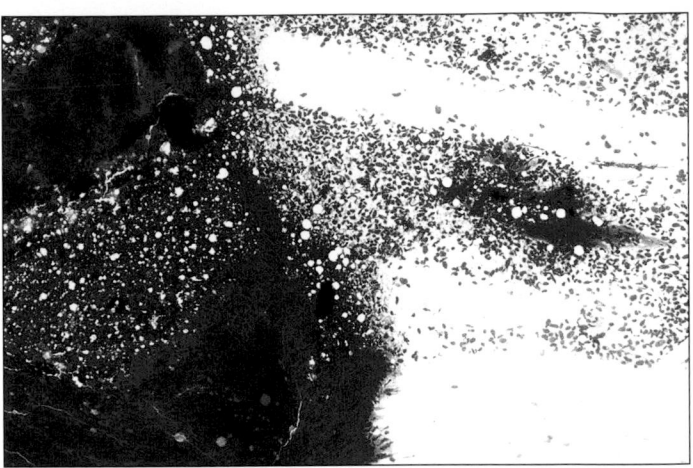

Fig. 9.254 Synovial sarcoma, aspiration cytology. These tumors yield cellular specimens with both aggregated and singly shed cells. This aspirate was from a monophasic lesion.

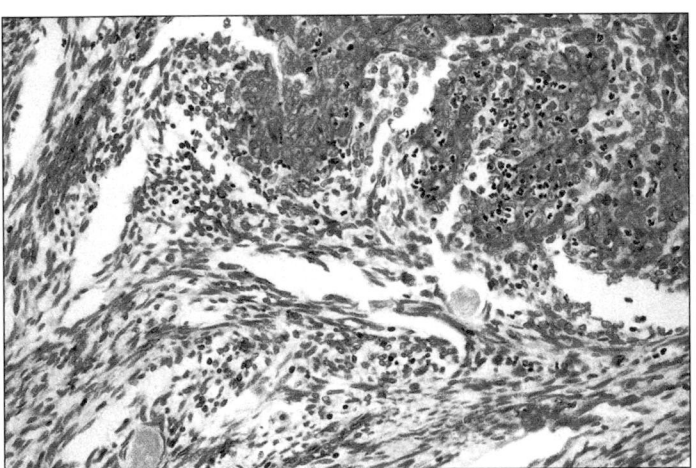

Fig. 9.253 Synovial sarcoma. Epithelial membrane antigen sometimes stains more cells than keratin in any given case. This is from the same case as the keratin in Figure 9.258.

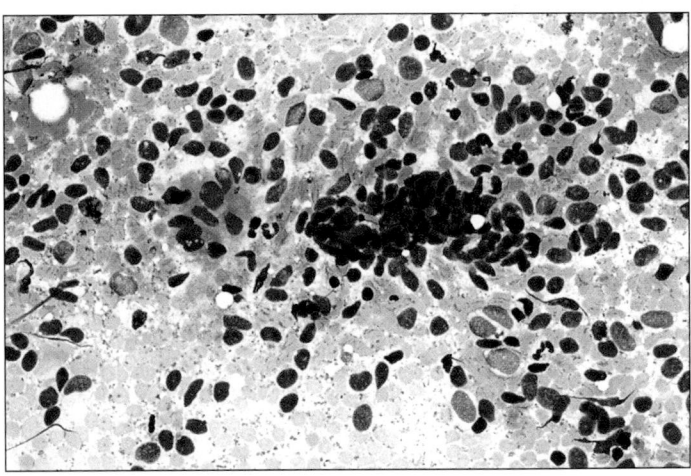

Fig. 9.255 Synovial sarcoma, aspiration cytology. Note the presence of a cluster probably corresponding to the glandular component and a spindled background.

S100 protein positivity is detectable in nearly a third of synovial sarcomas, including spindle cell MSS.[579]

CD99 (MIC2), is commonly positive in synovial sarcomas, with a membranous or cytoplasmic pattern,[675,746] raising the possibility of PNET. This is particularly relevant for the diagnosis of PDSS. Newer antibodies to FLI1 are more specific for ES/PNET[429] and can be applied for this distinction. CD34 is virtually always negative in synovial sarcoma but bcl-2 protein has been found in most synovial sarcomas in a diffuse and strongly positive fashion.[750] Demonstration of bcl-2 positivity in a spindle cell sarcoma is sometimes diagnostically useful as leiomyosarcomas and fibrosarcomas are negative and malignant peripheral nerve sheath tumors only inconsistently and focally positive.[750] As in most mesenchymal lesions, vimentin is present in the spindle cells of synovial sarcoma. Staining for desmin is usually absent, but occasionally in otherwise typical MSS there is focal positivity for both MSA (represented by the HHF35 antibody) and α-SMA. Calponin is also expressed by synovial sarcoma.[751]

Using immunohistochemistry in concert with aspiration cytology can allow accurate diagnosis of synovial sarcoma[752] (Figs 9.254–9.256).

A specific translocation involving chromosomes X and 18 has been described in synovial sarcoma.[753] This balanced reciprocal translocation, t(x;18)(p11.2;q11.2), is found in the vast majority of reported synovial sarcomas. The resultant fusion gene product, SYT–SSX chimeric RNA,[754] can be detected by RT-PCR in frozen and paraffin-embedded material.[755,756] These techniques are of diagnostic use as this translocation has not convincingly been demonstrated in any other tumor types[756] despite assertions of one group of investigators concerning SYT–SSX in nerve sheath tumors.[757]

The breakpoints of the t(X;18) involve the fusion of the *SYT* gene at 18q11 to either of two highly homologous genes at Xp11 called *SSX1* and *SSX2*. Although there appear to be exceptions, a correlation between the biphasic subtype of synovial sarcoma and involvement of the *SSX1* gene has been found. Involvement of the *SSX2* gene is associated with MSS, although around half of the

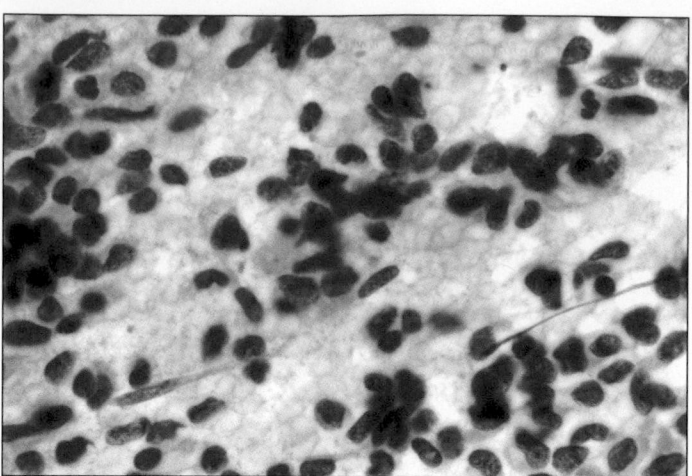

Fig. 9.256 Synovial sarcoma, aspiration cytology. Although correct diagnosis might require immunohistochemistry, the nuclear features in this lesion are malignant. These cells display clumped irregular chromatin and are quite enlarged.

monophasic variants involve *SSX1* disruption. More importantly, a significantly longer metastasis-free survival period has been associated with patients with the *SSX1* gene.[758]

There is usually no difficulty in recognizing biphasic synovial sarcoma. The major difficulties lie in the diagnosis of the MSS, which can resemble many other cell neoplasms, including fibrosarcoma, leiomyosarcoma, malignant peripheral nerve sheath tumor, angiosarcoma, hemangiopericytoma, and spindle cell carcinoma or melanoma. Furthermore, poorly differentiated synovial sarcoma can be confused with any of the small round cell tumors of childhood type, as well as carcinoma and epithelioid sarcoma, and the calcifying and ossifying variants with osteosarcoma as well as benign lesions.

Many MSS were interpreted as fibrosarcomas in the past but the classic adult-type fibrosarcoma, with the so-called 'herringbone' pattern of fascicles of long cells with slim and tapering nuclei, is now rarely diagnosed. By definition, fibrosarcomas are immunoreactive only for vimentin, although SMA is sometimes seen if there is significant myofibroblastic differentiation. An epithelial phenotype is diagnostic of synovial sarcoma but in marker-negative cases the nuclear morphology is probably the most useful histological discriminant between synovial sarcoma and fibrosarcoma.

Some synovial sarcoma contain spindle cells with eosinophilic cytoplasm, mimicking smooth muscle. In leiomyosarcoma, however, the bundles and fascicles, arranged perpendicularly, are more discrete and well defined. The nuclei are blunt-ended with paranuclear vacuoles rather than smoothly oval and well separated. Leiomyosarcomas express desmin and muscle actins, and usually lack bcl-2 protein.

Malignant peripheral nerve sheath tumor typically has a fascicular architecture displaying alternating cellularity, which can also be seen in synovial sarcoma; more specific but less common features are neuroid-type whorls, and perivascular or subintimal involvement of blood vessels by tumor. In malignant peripheral nerve sheath tumor, nuclei are often bullet- or arrowhead-shaped, with one blunt and one tapered end. Bent or buckled nuclei are also a useful finding, as are 'wavy' or serpiginous nuclei, although these are less specific. About two thirds of malignant peripheral nerve sheath tumors are S100-protein-positive (as are some synovial sarcoma) but most lack epithelial markers, whereas synovial sarcomas with S100 protein positivity also have cytokeratin and EMA.

The frequently prominent hemangiopericytomatous vascular pattern can lead to a diagnosis of benign or malignant hemangiopericytoma. This now rare entity is essentially a diagnosis of exclusion as the characteristic vascular pattern is seen in a host of benign and malignant tumors. Hemangiopericytoma has the pericytomatous appearance throughout the histologic sections and lacks immunohistochemical differentiation except for focal CD34 reactivity. In synovial sarcoma, this vascular pattern is focal and often peripheral, and CD34 is absent. A similarly distributed hemangiopericytomatous pattern is also seen in solitary fibrous tumor, which, like synovial sarcoma, is also positive for bcl-2 protein.[750] However, solitary fibrous tumor has variable cellularity with an irregular growth pattern and more collagen, and is characteristically strongly and diffusely positive for CD34.

Poorly differentiated synovial sarcoma resembles small round cell tumors including ES/PNET, neuroblastoma, rhabdomyosarcoma, and even lymphoma. In ES/PNET, rosette formations can be seen and the cells are more discrete as the nuclei, which have a somewhat clumped chromatin pattern, do not appear to overlap. The reticulin pattern is also distinctive in many cases, because in PDSS the fibers are often pericellular whereas in PNETs they enclose large reticulin-free cellular nodules.

The immunohistochemical profiles of ES/PNET and PDSS overlap. CD99 is seen in synovial sarcoma[675,746] as well as in ES/PNET, and epithelial markers can be absent in PDSS yet focally detectable in ES/PNET; however, the patterns of expression of cytokeratin subtypes differ and use of FLI1 antibodies can also be helpful,[429] although these also react with vascular lesions.[428] Positivity for neural differentiation markers such as NSE, PGP9.5, chromogranin, or synaptophysin is more in favor of ES/PNET and, when suitable tissue is available, the cytogenetic demonstration of t(11;22)(q24;q12) or of chimeric gene transcripts for *EWS–FLI1* will confirm the diagnosis. Neuroblastoma almost always occurs in a specific clinical setting in early childhood and nearly all cases lack both CD99 and cytokeratins. Rhabdomyosarcoma is readily excluded by the absence of desmin, myoglobin, and MyoD1 and lymphomas can be ruled out by the use of appropriate immunostains. Poorly differentiated synovial sarcoma is also consistently reactive with calponin antibodies whereas the other 'round, blue cell tumors' are not.[751]

There is local recurrence of tumor in up to 50% of cases of synovial sarcoma.[3] Metastases are usually blood-borne, to lungs and bone, but, perhaps reflecting the epithelial differentiation, they can involve regional lymph nodes in over 20% of cases. The usual course of synovial sarcoma is that of a high-grade sarcoma. However, the calcifying variant has a better long-term prognosis: the 5-year survival is 83%, and 66% of patients are alive after 10 years. In contrast, PDSSs generally behave more aggressively than the average and metastasize in a higher percentage of cases. In one series of patients with PDSS, 50% of patients died, with a mean survival of 33 months.[746]

EXTRARENAL RHABDOID TUMOR

Malignant rhabdoid tumor was initially characterized as a highly aggressive renal neoplasm affecting children less than 2 years of age.[759] The tumor derives its name from the early observation that the cells comprising this unique renal tumor cytologically resembled those of rhabdomyosarcoma but lacked ultrastructural evidence of myogenesis.[760]

Despite the continuing controversy that surrounds the specificity of the rhabdoid phenotype, there appears to be a subset of childhood soft tissue tumors with rhabdoid features that display significant clinico-pathologic overlap with malignant renal rhabdoid tumor and are considered a distinct clinicopathologic entity. Alterations at chromosome band 22q11.2 in a group of congenital malignant extrarenal rhabdoid tumors and in some examples of malignant rhabdoid tumor of the kidney, brain, liver, and retroperitoneum further suggest that there exists a select group of malignant rhabdoid tumors that are interrelated.[761]

The vast majority of extrarenal rhabdoid tumors occur in infants and young children, although they may rarely affect adolescents and adults. They have been described in the soft tissues of the head and neck, paravertebral region, shoulder, trunk, extremities, mediastinum, and retroperitoneum[761,762] as well as multiple other sites. The clinical course of the extrarenal rhabdoid tumor is marked by early dissemination and death.[761,762]

Nearly all the tumors arising in the soft tissues of the neck, thorax, and extremities are deep, intramuscular lesions. The masses are partially pseudoencapsulated and have a soft to firm consistency. Their cut surface is gray-tan to white with foci of necrosis.

Microscopically, the hallmark cytologic features of the rhabdoid cell are: (1) a round to polygonal shape and amphophilic to lightly basophilic cytoplasm that commonly has a weakly PAS-positive, paranuclear globoid inclusion with a pale eosinophilic, glassy appearance, and (2) a large, eccentrically positioned nucleus with a round to reniform configuration and prominent nucleoli.

The cells are generally noncohesive but may focally grow in a trabecular pattern or adhere to vessel walls or fibrous septa. Mitotic figures are easily observed but atypical mitotic figures are infrequent. The cells form bulky, ill defined sheets or large irregular nests. The stromal matrix is usually edematous but may be myxoid. Lymphatic and blood vessel invasion are frequently identified.

Extrarenal rhabdoid tumor shows rather consistent immuno-expression of vimentin and the majority of tumors display keratin and EMA. In one study, over half of tumors expressed the Ewing's marker (CD99), synaptophysin, Leu-7 (CD57), and NSE.[763] Focal immunoreactivity has been reported for desmin and MSA.

A number of neoplasms, including carcinomas, melanomas, and soft tissue sarcomas, may have foci exhibiting the cytomorphologic features of a malignant rhabdoid tumor and extrarenal rhabdoid tumor is thus a diagnosis of exclusion. Poorly differentiated foci of synovial sarcoma, malignant epithelioid schwannoma, EMC, mesothelioma, and the intra-abdominal desmoplastic small round cell tumor are some of the soft tissue sarcomas that can demonstrate rhabdoid features. However, rhabdomyosarcoma and epithelioid sarcoma are the two neoplasms that bear the closest histologic resemblance to extrarenal rhabdoid tumor.

Rhabdomyosarcoma, like extrarenal rhabdoid tumor, arises principally in the deep soft tissues and mostly affects children. Rhabdomyoblasts express desmin and MyoD1 but not keratin or EMA. Epithelioid sarcoma can also have cells with rhabdoid features. In contrast to extrarenal rhabdoid tumor, epithelioid sarcoma affects mostly adolescents and young adults and has a predilection for the hand and forearm area. The tumoral cells of epithelioid sarcoma form cohesive nodules that frequently coalesce and exhibit central necrosis. The proximal type of epithelioid sarcoma is composed of large epithelioid cells, including a significant component of rhabdoid-appearing cells arranged in large, bulky nodules. In some instances, the number of rhabdoid-appearing cells in this variant of epithelioid sarcoma may make the separation from extrarenal rhabdoid tumor almost impossible. Although coexpression of vimentin and keratin is a feature shared by both epithelioid sarcoma and extrarenal rhabdoid tumor, the former neoplasm demonstrates CD34 immunoreactivity in 50% of cases.

REFERENCES

1. Fletcher C, Unni K, Mertens FE. World Health Organization classification of tumours. Pathology and genetics of tumours of soft tissue and bone. Lyon: IACR Press; 2002.

2. Weiss S. Histological typing of soft tissue tumours. Berlin: Springer-Verlag; 1994.

3. Weiss S, Goldblum J. Enzinger and Weiss's soft tissue tumors. 4th edn. St Louis: Mosby; 2001.

4. Montgomery E, Aaron AE. Clinical pathology of soft tissue tumors. New York: Marcel Dekker; 2001.

5. Costa J, Wesley RA, Glatstein E, Rosenberg SA. The grading of soft tissue sarcomas. Results of a clinicohistopathologic correlation in a series of 163 cases. Cancer 1984; 53(3): 530–541.

6. Markhede G, Angervall L, Stener B. A multivariate analysis of the prognosis after surgical treatment of malignant soft-tissue tumors. Cancer 1982; 49(8): 1721–1733.

7. Myhre-Jensen O, Kaae S, Madsen EH, Sneppen O. Histopathological grading in soft-tissue tumours. Relation to survival in 261 surgically treated patients. Acta Pathol Microbiol Immunol Scand [A] 1983; 91(2): 145–150.

8. Trojani M, Contesso G, Coindre JM, et al. Soft-tissue sarcomas of adults; study of pathological prognostic variables and definition of a histopathological grading system. Int J Cancer 1984; 33(1): 37–42.

9. Guillou L, Coindre JM, Bonichon F, et al. Comparative study of the National Cancer Institute and French Federation of Cancer Centers Sarcoma Group grading systems in a population of 410 adult patients with soft tissue sarcoma. J Clin Oncol 1997; 15(1): 350–362.

10. Russell WO, Cohen J, Enzinger F, et al. A clinical and pathological staging system for soft tissue sarcomas. Cancer 1977; 40(4): 1562–1570.

11. Enneking WF, Spanier SS, Goodman MA. A system for the surgical staging of musculoskeletal sarcoma. Clin Orthop 1980(153): 106–120.

12. Greene F, Page D, Fleming I, et al. AJCC cancer staging manual, 6th edn. Chicago: American Joint Committee on Cancer; 2002.

13. Evans HL. Desmoplastic fibroblastoma. A report of seven cases. Am J Surg Pathol 1995; 19(9): 1077–1081.

14. Miettinen M, Fetsch JF. Collagenous fibroma (desmoplastic fibroblastoma): a clinicopathologic analysis of 63 cases of a distinctive soft tissue lesion with stellate-shaped fibroblasts. Hum Pathol 1998; 29(7): 676–682.

15. Huang HY, Sung MT, Eng HL, et al. Superficial collagenous fibroma: immunohistochemical, ultrastructural, and flow cytometric study of three cases, including one pemphigus vulgaris patient with a dermal mass. Apmis 2002; 110(4): 283–289.

16. Sciot R, Samson I, van den Berghe H, et al. Collagenous fibroma (desmoplastic fibroblastoma): genetic link with fibroma of tendon sheath? Mod Pathol 1999; 12(6): 565–856.

17. Ogose A, Hotta T, Emura I, et al. Collagenous fibroma of the arm: a report of two cases. Skeletal Radiol 2000; 29(7): 417–420.

18. Chung EB, Enzinger FM. Fibroma of tendon sheath. Cancer 1979; 44(5): 1945–5194.

19. Dal Cin P, Sciot R, De Smet L, Van den Berghe H. Translocation 2; 11 in a fibroma of tendon sheath. Histopathology 1998; 32(5): 433–435.

20. Hashimoto H, Tsuneyoshi M, Daimaru Y, et al. Fibroma of tendon sheath: a tumor of myofibroblasts. A clinicopathologic study of 18 cases. Acta Pathol Jpn 1985; 35(5): 1099–1107.

21. Lundgren LG, Kindblom LG. Fibroma of tendon sheath. A light and electron-microscopic study of 6 cases. Acta Pathol Microbiol Immunol Scand [A] 1984; 92(6): 401–409.

22. Kransdorf MJ, Meis JM, Montgomery E. Elastofibroma: MR and CT appearance with radiologic-pathologic correlation. AJR 1992; 159(3): 575–579.

23. Nishio J, Iwasaki H, Ohjimi Y, et al. Gain of Xq detected by comparative genomic hybridization in elastofibroma. Int J Mol Med 2002; 10(3): 277–280.

24. Turna A, Yilmaz MA, Urer N, et al. Bilateral elastofibroma dorsi. Ann Thorac Surg 2002; 73(2): 630–632.

25. Harigopal M, Seshan SV, DeLellis RA, et al. Aspiration cytology of elastofibroma dorsi: Case report with ultrastructural and immunohistochemical findings. Diagn Cytopathol 2002; 26(5): 310–313.

26. Keasbey L. Juvenile aponeurotic fibroma (calcifying fibroma): A distinctive tumor arising in the palms and soles of young children. Cancer 1953; 6:338–346.

27. Fetsch JF, Miettinen M. Calcifying aponeurotic fibroma: a clinicopathologic study of 22 cases arising in uncommon sites. Hum Pathol 1998; 29(12): 1504–1510.

28. Alho A, Skjeldal S, Pettersen EO, et al. Aneuploidy in benign tumors and nonneoplastic lesions of musculoskeletal tissues. Cancer 1994; 73(4): 1200–1205.

29. Tai LH, Johnston JO, Klein HZ, et al. Calcifying aponeurotic fibroma features seen on fine-needle aspiration biopsy: case report and brief review of the literature. Diagn Cytopathol 2001; 24(5): 336–339.

30. Birdsall SH, Shipley JM, Summersgill BM, et al. Cytogenetic findings in a case of nodular fasciitis of the breast. Cancer Genet Cytogenet 1995; 81(2): 166–168.

31. Weibolt VM, Buresh CJ, Roberts CA, et al. Involvement of 3q21 in nodular fasciitis. Cancer Genet Cytogenet 1998; 106(2): 177–179.

32. el-Jabbour JN, Wilson GD, Bennett MH, et alK. Flow cytometric study of nodular fasciitis, proliferative fasciitis, and proliferative myositis. Hum Pathol 1991; 22(11): 1146–1149.

33. Konwaler B, Keasbey L, Kaplan L. Subcutaneous pseudosarcomatous fibromatosis (fasciitis). Am J Clin Pathol 1955; 25:241–252.

34. Allen PW. Nodular fasciitis. Pathology 1972; 4(1): 9–26.

35. Montgomery EA, Meis JM. Nodular fasciitis. Its morphologic spectrum and immunohistochemical profile. Am J Surg Pathol 1991; 15(10): 942–948.

36. Shimizu S, Hashimoto H, Enjoji M. Nodular fasciitis: an analysis of 250 patients. Pathology 1984; 16(2): 161–166.

37. Meister P, Buckmann FW, Konrad E. Nodular fasciitis (analysis of 100 cases and review of the literature). Pathol Res Pract 1978; 162(2): 133–165.

38. Wirman JA. Nodular fasciitis, a lesion of myofibroblasts: an ultrastructural study. Cancer 1976; 38(6): 2378–2389.

39. Daroca PJ Jr, Pulitzer DR, LoCicero J III. Ossifying fasciitis. Arch Pathol Lab Med 1982; 106(13): 682–685.

40. Wilson JD, Montague CJ, Salcuni P, et al. Heterotopic mesenteric ossification ('intraabdominal myositis ossificans'): report of five cases. Am J Surg Pathol 1999; 23(12): 1464–1470.

41. Patchefsky AS, Enzinger FM. Intravascular fasciitis: a report of 17 cases. Am J Surg Pathol 1981; 5(1): 29–36.

42. Lauer DH, Enzinger FM. Cranial fasciitis of childhood. Cancer 1980; 45(2): 401–406.

43. Aydin O, Oztuna V, Polat A. Three cases of nodular fasciitis: primary diagnoses by fine needle aspiration cytology. Cytopathology 2001; 12(5): 346–347.

44. Chung EB, Enzinger FM. Proliferative fasciitis. Cancer 1975; 36(4): 1450–1458.

45. Meis JM, Enzinger FM. Proliferative fasciitis and myositis of childhood. Am J Surg Pathol 1992; 16(4): 364–372.

46. Montgomery EA, Meis JM, Mitchell MS, Enzinger FM. Atypical decubital fibroplasia. A distinctive fibroblastic pseudotumor occurring in debilitated patients. Am J Surg Pathol 1992; 16(7): 708–715.

47. Perosio PM, Weiss SW. Ischemic fasciitis: a juxta-skeletal fibroblastic proliferation with a predilection for elderly patients. Mod Pathol 1993; 6(1): 69–72.

48. Stout A. Juvenile fibromatosis. Cancer 1954; 7: 953–978.

49. Chung EB, Enzinger FM. Infantile myofibromatosis. Cancer 1981; 48(8): 1807–1818.

50. Smith KJ, Skelton HG, Barrett TL, et al. Cutaneous myofibroma. Mod Pathol 1989; 2(6): 603–609.

51. Bracko M, Cindro L, Golouh R. Familial occurrence of infantile myofibromatosis. Cancer 1992; 69(5): 1294–1299.

52. Inwards CY, Unni KK, Beabout JW, Shives TC. Solitary congenital fibromatosis (infantile myofibromatosis) of bone. Am J Surg Pathol 1991; 15(10): 935–941.

53. Montgomery E, Speight PM, Fisher C. Myofibromas presenting in the oral cavity: a series of 9 cases. Oral Surg Oral Med Oral Pathol Oral Radiol Endod 2000; 89(3): 343–348.

54. Kilpatrick SE, Ward WG, Chauvenet AR, Pettenati MJ. The role of fine-needle aspiration biopsy in the initial diagnosis of pediatric bone and soft tissue tumors: an institutional experience. Mod Pathol 1998; 11(10): 923–928.

55. Ostrowski ML, Bradshaw J, Garrison D. Infantile myofibromatosis: diagnosis suggested by fine-needle aspiration biopsy. Diagn Cytopathol 1990; 6(4): 284–288.

56. Wargotz ES, Weiss SW, Norris HJ. Myofibroblastoma of the breast. Sixteen cases of a distinctive benign mesenchymal tumor. Am J Surg Pathol 1987; 11(7): 493–502.

57. Weiss SW, Gnepp DR, Bratthauer GL. Palisaded myofibroblastoma. A benign mesenchymal tumor of lymph node. Am J Surg Pathol 1989; 13(5): 341–346.

58. Suster S, Rosai J. Intranodal hemorrhagic spindle-cell tumor with 'amianthoid' fibers. Report of six cases of a distinctive mesenchymal neoplasm of the inguinal region that simulates Kaposi's sarcoma. Am J Surg Pathol 1989; 13(5): 347–357.

59. Damiani S, Miettinen M, Peterse JL, Eusebi V. Solitary fibrous tumour (myofibroblastoma) of the breast. Virchows Arch 1994; 425(1): 89–92.

60. Rosenthal NS, Abdul-Karim FW. Childhood fibrous tumor with psammoma bodies. Clinicopathologic features in two cases. Arch Pathol Lab Med 1988; 112(8): 798–800.

61. Fetsch JF, Montgomery EA, Meis JM. Calcifying fibrous pseudotumor. Am J Surg Pathol 1993; 17(5): 502–508.

62. Pinkard NB, Wilson RW, Lawless N, et al. Calcifying fibrous pseudotumor of pleura. A report of three cases of a newly described entity involving the pleura. Am J Clin Pathol 1996; 105(2): 189–194.

63. Hainaut P, Lesage V, Weynand B, et al. Calcifying fibrous pseudotumor (CFPT): a patient presenting with multiple pleural lesions. Acta Clin Belg 1999; 54(3): 162–164.

64. Ben-Izhak O, Itin L, Feuchtwanger Z, et al. Calcifying fibrous pseudotumor of mesentery presenting with acute peritonitis: case report with immunohistochemical study and review of literature. Int J Surg Pathol 2001; 9(3): 249–253.

65. Chen K. Intraabdominal calcifying fibrous pseudotumor. Int J Surg Pathol 1996; 4(1): 9–12.

66. Kocova L, Michal M, Sulc M, Zamecnik M. Calcifying fibrous pseudotumour of visceral peritoneum. Histopathology 1997; 31(2): 182–184.

67. Sigel JE, Smith TA, Reith JD, Goldblum JR. Immunohistochemical analysis of anaplastic lymphoma kinase expression in deep soft tissue calcifying fibrous pseudotumor: evidence of a late sclerosing stage of inflammatory myofibroblastic tumor? Ann Diagn Pathol 2001; 5(1): 10–14.

68. Weynand B, Draguet AP, Bernard P, et al. Calcifying fibrous pseudotumour: first case report in the peritoneum with immunostaining for CD34. Histopathology 1999; 34(1): 86–87.

69. Erasmus JJ, McAdams HP, Patz EF Jr, et al. Calcifying fibrous pseudotumor of pleura: radiologic features in three cases. J Comput Assist Tomogr 1996; 20(5): 763–765.

70. Zamecnik M, Dorociak F, Vesely L. Calcifying fibrous pseudotumor after trauma. Pathol Int 1997; 47(11): 812.

71. Dargent JL, Delplace J, Roufosse C, et al. Development of a calcifying fibrous pseudotumour within a lesion of Castleman disease, hyaline-vascular subtype. J Clin Pathol 1999; 52(7): 547–549.

72. Van Dorpe J, Ectors N, Geboes K, et al. Is calcifying fibrous pseudotumor a late sclerosing stage of inflammatory myofibroblastic tumor? Am J Surg Pathol 1999; 23(3): 329–335.

73. Pomplun S, Goldstraw P, Davies SE, et al. Calcifying fibrous pseudotumour arising within an inflammatory pseudotumour: evidence of progression from one lesion to the other? Histopathology 2000; 37(4): 380–382.

74. Hill KA, Gonzalez-Crussi F, Chou PM. Calcifying fibrous pseudotumor versus inflammatory myofibroblastic tumor: a histological and immunohistochemical comparison. Mod Pathol 2001; 14(8): 784–790.

75. Maeda T, Hirose T, Furuya K, Kameoka K. Calcifying fibrous pseudotumor: an ultrastructural study. Ultrastruct Pathol 1999; 23(3): 189–192.

76. Fukunaga M, Kikuchi Y, Endo Y, Ushigome S. Calcifying fibrous pseudotumor. Pathol Int 1997; 47(1): 60–63.

77. Dickey GE, Sotelo-Avila C. Fibrous hamartoma of infancy: current review. Pediatr Dev Pathol 1999; 2(3): 236–243.

78. Popek EJ, Montgomery EA, Fourcroy JL. Fibrous hamartoma of infancy in the genital region: findings in 15 cases. J Urol 1994; 152(3): 990–993.

79. Balachandran K, Allen PW, MacCormac LB. Nuchal fibroma. A clinicopathological study of nine cases. Am J Surg Pathol 1995; 19(3): 313–317.

80. Michal M, Fetsch JF, Hes O, Miettinen M. Nuchal-type fibroma: a clinicopathological study of 52 cases. Cancer 1999; 85(1): 156–163.

81. Wehrli BM, Weiss SW, Yandow S, Coffin CM. Gardner-associated fibromas (GAF) in young patients: a distinct fibrous lesion that identifies unsuspected Gardner syndrome and risk for fibromatosis. Am J Surg Pathol 2001; 25(5): 645–651.

82. Zamecnik M, Michal M. Nuchal-type fibroma is positive for CD34 and CD99. Am J Surg Pathol 2001; 25(7): 970.

83. O'Connell JX, Janzen DL, Hughes TR. Nuchal fibrocartilaginous pseudotumor: a distinctive soft-tissue lesion associated with prior neck injury. Am J Surg Pathol 1997; 21(7): 836–840.

84. Wakely PE Jr, Price WG, Frable WJ. Sternomastoid tumor of infancy (fibromatosis colli): diagnosis by aspiration cytology. Mod Pathol 1989; 2(4): 378–381.

85. Fetsch JF, Miettinen M, Laskin WB, et al. A clinicopathologic study of 45 pediatric soft tissue tumors with an admixture of adipose tissue and fibroblastic elements, and a proposal for classification as lipofibromatosis. Am J Surg Pathol 2000; 24(11): 1491–1500.

86. Allen PW. The fibromatoses: a clinicopathologic classification based on 140 cases. Am J Surg Pathol 1977; 1(3): 255–270.

87. Iwasaki H, Tsuneyoshi M, Enjoji M. Infantile digital fibromatosis. Histopathological and electron microscopic study with a review of the literature. Acta Pathol Jpn 1974; 24(6): 717–732.

88. Iwasaki H, Kikuchi M, Ohtsuki I, et al. Infantile digital fibromatosis. Identification of actin filaments in cytoplasmic inclusions by heavy meromyosin binding. Cancer 1983; 52(9): 1653–1661.

89. Reitamo JJ, Hayry P, Nykyri E, Saxen E. The desmoid tumor. I. Incidence, sex-, age- and anatomical distribution in the Finnish population. Am J Clin Pathol 1982; 77(6): 665–673.

90. Reitamo JJ. The desmoid tumor. IV. Choice of treatment, results, and complications. Arch Surg 1983; 118(11): 1318–1322.

91. Gardner E. A genetic and clinical study of intestinal polyposis, a predisposing factor for carcinoma of the colon and rectum. Am J Human Genet 1951; 3:167–176.

92. Gardner E, Richards R. Multiple cutaneous and subcutaneous lesions occurring simultaneously with hereditary polyposis and osteomatosis. Am J Hum Genet 1953; 5: 139–147.

93. Gardner E. Follow-up study of a family group exhibiting dominant inheritance for a syndrome including intestinal polyps, osteomas, fibromas, and epidermal cysts. Am J Hum Genetics 1962; 14:376–390.

94. Caspari R, Olschwang S, Friedl W, et al. Familial adenomatous polyposis: desmoid tumours and lack of ophthalmic lesions (CHRPE) associated with APC mutations beyond codon 1444. Hum Mol Genet 1995; 4(3): 337–340.

95. Davies DR, Armstrong JG, Thakker N, et al. Severe Gardner syndrome in families with mutations restricted to a specific region of the APC gene. Am J Hum Genet 1995; 57(5): 1151–1158.

96. Eccles DM, van der Luijt R, Breukel C, et al. Hereditary desmoid disease due to a frameshift mutation at codon 1924 of the APC gene. Am J Hum Genet 1996; 59(6): 1193–1201.

97. Enomoto M, Konishi M, Iwama T, et al. The relationship between frequencies of extracolonic manifestations and the position of APC germline mutation in patients with familial adenomatous polyposis. Jpn J Clin Oncol 2000; 30(2): 82–88.

98. Halling KC, Lazzaro CR, Honchel R, et al. Hereditary desmoid disease in a family with a germline Alu I repeat mutation of the APC gene. Hum Hered 1999; 49(2): 97–102.

99. Scott RJ, Froggatt NJ, Trembath RC, et al. Familial infiltrative fibromatosis (desmoid tumours) (MIM135290) caused by a recurrent 3′ APC gene mutation. Hum Mol Genet 1996; 5(12): 1921–1924.

100. Abraham SC, Montgomery EA, Giardiello FM, Wu TT. Frequent beta-catenin mutations in juvenile nasopharyngeal angiofibromas. Am J Pathol 2001; 158(3): 1073–1078.

101. Alman BA, Li C, Pajerski ME, et al. Increased beta-catenin protein and somatic APC mutations in sporadic aggressive fibromatoses (desmoid tumors). Am J Pathol 1997; 151(2): 329–334.

102. Giarola M, Wells D, Mondini P, et al. Mutations of adenomatous polyposis coli (APC) gene are uncommon in sporadic desmoid tumours. Br J Cancer 1998; 78(5): 582–587.

103. Tejpar S, Nollet F, Li C, et al. Predominance of beta-catenin mutations and beta-catenin dysregulation in sporadic aggressive fibromatosis (desmoid tumor). Oncogene 1999; 18(47): 6615–6620.

104. Miyoshi Y, Iwao K, Nawa G, et al. Frequent mutations in the beta-catenin gene in desmoid tumors from patients without familial adenomatous polyposis. Oncol Res 1998; 10(11–12): 591–594.

105. De Wever I, Dal Cin P, Fletcher CD, et al. Cytogenetic, clinical, and morphologic correlations in 78 cases of fibromatosis: a report from the CHAMP Study Group. Mod Pathol 2000; 13(10): 1080–1085.

106. Montgomery E, Lee JH, Abraham SC, Wu TT. Superficial fibromatoses are genetically distinct from deep fibromatoses. Mod Pathol 2001; 14(7): 695–701.

107. Hayry P, Reitamo JJ, Totterman S, et al. The desmoid tumor. II. Analysis of factors possibly contributing to the etiology and growth behavior. Am J Clin Pathol 1982; 77(6): 674–680.

108. Hayry P, Reitamo JJ, Vihko R, et al. The desmoid tumor. III. A biochemical and genetic analysis. Am J Clin Pathol 1982; 77(6): 681–685.

109. Aluisio FV, Mair SD, Hall RL. Plantar fibromatosis: treatment of primary and recurrent lesions and factors associated with recurrence. Foot Ankle Int 1996; 17(11): 672–678.

110. Evans HL. Multinucleated giant cells in plantar fibromatosis. Am J Surg Pathol 2002; 26(2): 244–248.

111. Guerneri S, Stioui S, Mantovani F, et al. Multiple clonal chromosome abnormalities in Peyronie's disease. Cancer Genet Cytogenet 1991; 52(2): 181–185.

112. Wilson RW, Gallateau-Salle F, Moran CA. Desmoid tumors of the pleura: a clinicopathologic mimic of localized fibrous tumor. Mod Pathol 1999; 12(1): 9–14.

113. Mehrotra AK, Sheikh S, Aaron AD, et al. Fibromatoses of the extremities: clinicopathologic study of 36 cases. J Surg Oncol 2000; 74(4): 291–296.

114. Enzinger FM, Shiraki M. Musculo-aponeurotic fibromatosis of the shoulder girdle (extra-abdominal desmoid). Analysis of thirty cases followed up for ten or more years. Cancer 1967; 20(7): 1131–1140.

115. Haggitt RC, Booth JL. Bilateral fibromatosis of the breast in Gardner's syndrome. Cancer 1970; 25(1): 161–166.

116. Rosen PP, Ernsberger D. Mammary fibromatosis. A benign spindle-cell tumor with significant risk for local recurrence. Cancer 1989; 63(7): 1363–1369.

117. Naylor EW, Gardner EJ, Richards RC. Desmoid tumors and mesenteric fibromatosis in Gardner's syndrome: report of kindred 109. Arch Surg 1979; 114(10): 1181–1185.

118. Ayala AG, Ro JY, Goepfert H, et al. Desmoid fibromatosis: a clinicopathologic study of 25 children. Semin Diagn Pathol 1986; 3(2): 138–150.

119. Wargotz ES, Norris HJ, Austin RM, Enzinger FM. Fibromatosis of the breast. A clinical and pathological study of 28 cases. Am J Surg Pathol 1987; 11(1): 38–45.

120. Burke AP, Sobin LH, Shekitka KM. Mesenteric fibromatosis. A follow-up study. Arch Pathol Lab Med 1990; 114(8): 832–835.

121. Burke AP, Sobin LH, Shekitka KM, et al. Intra-abdominal fibromatosis. A pathologic analysis of 130 tumors with comparison of clinical subgroups. Am J Surg Pathol 1990; 14(4): 335–341.

122. Abraham SC, Reynolds C, Lee JH, et al. Fibromatosis of the breast and mutations involving the APC/beta-catenin pathway. Hum Pathol 2002; 33(1): 39–46.

123. Aaron AD, O'Mara JW, Legendre KE, et al. Chest wall fibromatosis associated with silicone breast implants. Surg Oncol 1996; 5(2): 93–99.

124. Zayid I. Multicentric fibromatosis of familial inheritance. Arch Pathol Lab Med 1988; 112(6): 577.

125. Zayid I, Dihmis C. Familial multicentric fibromatosis–desmoids. A report of three cases in a Jordanian family. Cancer 1969; 24(4): 786–795.

126. Raab SS, Silverman JF, McLeod DL, et al. Fine needle aspiration biopsy of fibromatoses. Acta Cytol 1993; 37(3): 323–328.

127. Montgomery E, Torbenson MS, Kaushal M, et al. beta-Catenin Immunohistochemistry Separates Mesenteric Fibromatosis From Gastrointestinal Stromal Tumor and Sclerosing Mesenteritis. Am J Surg Pathol 2002; 26(10): 1296–1301.

128. Slater G, Greenstein AJ. Mesenteric fibromatosis in Crohn's disease. J Clin Gastroenterol 1996; 22(2): 147–149.

129. Harvey JC, Quan SH, Fortner JG. Gardner's syndrome complicated by mesenteric desmoid tumors. Surgery 1979; 85(4): 475–477.

130. Herter P, Kuhnen C, Muller KM, et al. Intracellular distribution of beta-catenin in colorectal adenomas, carcinomas and Peutz–Jeghers polyps. J Cancer Res Clin Oncol 1999; 125(5): 297–304.

131. Gurbuz AK, Giardiello FM, Petersen GM, et al. Desmoid tumours in familial adenomatous polyposis. Gut 1994; 35(3): 377–381.

132. Couture J, Mitri A, Lagace R, et al. A germline mutation at the extreme 3′ end of the APC gene results in a severe desmoid phenotype and is associated with overexpression of beta-catenin in the desmoid tumor. Clin Genet 2000; 57(3): 205–212.

133. Yantiss RK, Spiro IJ, Compton CC, Rosenberg AE. Gastrointestinal stromal tumor versus intra-abdominal fibromatosis of the bowel wall: a clinically important differential diagnosis. Am J Surg Pathol 2000; 24(7): 947–957.

134. Stout A. Fibrosarcoma. The malignant tumor of fibroblasts. Cancer 1948; 1:30–63.

135. Fisher C. The value of electronmicroscopy and immunohistochemistry in the diagnosis of soft tissue sarcomas: a study of 200 cases. Histopathology 1990; 16(5): 441–454.

136. Kotani K, Tsuji M, Oki A, et al. IGF-II producing hepatic fibrosarcoma associated with hypoglycemia. Intern Med 1993; 32(12): 897–901.

137. Fukasawa Y, Takada A, Tateno M, et al. Solitary fibrous tumor of the pleura causing recurrent hypoglycemia by secretion of insulin-like growth factor II. Pathol Int 1998; 48(1): 47–52.

138. Pritchard DJ, Soule EH, Taylor WF, Ivins JC. Fibrosarcoma – a clinicopathologic and statistical study of 199 tumors of the soft tissues of the extremities and trunk. Cancer 1974; 33(3): 888–897.

139. Pritchard DJ, Sim FH, Ivins JC, et al. Fibrosarcoma of bone and soft tissues of the trunk and extremities. Orthop Clin North Am 1977; 8(4): 869–881.

140. Scott SM, Reiman HM, Pritchard DJ, Ilstrup DM. Soft tissue fibrosarcoma. A clinicopathologic study of 132 cases. Cancer 1989; 64(4): 925–931.

141. Evans HL. Low-grade fibromyxoid sarcoma. A report of two metastasizing neoplasms having a deceptively benign appearance. Am J Clin Pathol 1987; 88(5): 615–619.

142. Evans HL. Low-grade fibromyxoid sarcoma. A report of 12 cases. Am J Surg Pathol 1993; 17(6): 595–600.

143. Lane KL, Shannon RJ, Weiss SW. Hyalinizing spindle cell tumor with giant rosettes: a distinctive tumor closely resembling low-grade fibromyxoid sarcoma. Am J Surg Pathol 1997; 21(12): 1481–1488.

144. Woodruff JM, Antonescu CR, Erlandson RA, Boland PJ. Low-grade fibrosarcoma with palisaded granulomalike bodies (giant rosettes): report of a case that metastasized. Am J Surg Pathol 1999; 23(11): 1423–1428.

145. Folpe AL, Lane KL, Paull G, Weiss SW. Low-grade fibromyxoid sarcoma and hyalinizing spindle cell tumor with giant rosettes: a clinicopathologic study of 73 cases supporting their identity and assessing the impact of high-grade areas. Am J Surg Pathol 2000; 24(10): 1353–1360.

146. Reid R, de Silva MV, Paterson L, et al. Low-grade fibromyxoid sarcoma and hyalinizing spindle cell tumor with giant rosettes share a common t(7; 16)(q34; p11) translocation. Am J Surg Pathol 2003; 27(9): 1229–1236.

147. Panagopoulos I, Storlazzi CT, Fletcher CD, et al. The chimeric FUS/CREB3l2 gene is specific for low-grade fibromyxoid sarcoma. Genes Chromosomes Cancer 2004; 40(3): 218–228.

148. Storlazzi CT, Mertens F, Nascimento A, et al. Fusion of the FUS and BBF2H7 genes in low-grade fibromyxoid sarcoma. Hum Mol Genet 2003; 12(18): 2349–2358.

149. Montgomery EA, Devaney KO, Giordano TJ, Weiss SW. Inflammatory myxohyaline tumor of distal extremities with virocyte or Reed–Sternberg-like cells: a distinctive lesion with features simulating inflammatory conditions, Hodgkin's disease, and various sarcomas. Mod Pathol 1998; 11(4): 384–391.

150. Meis-Kindblom JM, Kindblom LG. Acral myxoinflammatory fibroblastic sarcoma: a low-grade tumor of the hands and feet. Am J Surg Pathol 1998; 22(8): 911–924.

151. Lambert I, Debiec-Rychter M, Guelinckx P, et al. Acral myxoinflammatory fibroblastic sarcoma with unique clonal chromosomal changes. Virchows Arch 2001; 438(5): 509–512.

152. Weiss SW, Enzinger FM. Myxoid variant of malignant fibrous histiocytoma. Cancer 1977; 39(4): 1672–1685.

153. Angervall L, Kindblom LG, Merck C. Myxofibrosarcoma. A study of 30 cases. Acta Pathol Microbiol Scand [A] 1977; 85A(2): 127–140.

154. Merck C, Angervall L, Kindblom LG, Oden A. Myxofibrosarcoma. A malignant soft tissue tumor of fibroblastic- histiocytic origin. A clinicopathologic and prognostic study of 110 cases using multivariate analysis. Acta Pathol Microbiol Immunol Scand Suppl 1983; 282:1–40.

155. Mentzel T, Calonje E, Wadden C, et al. Myxofibrosarcoma. Clinicopathologic analysis of 75 cases with emphasis on the low-grade variant. Am J Surg Pathol 1996; 20(4): 391–405.

156. Meis-Kindblom JM, Kindblom LG, Enzinger FM. Sclerosing epithelioid fibrosarcoma. A variant of fibrosarcoma simulating carcinoma. Am J Surg Pathol 1995; 19(9): 979–993.

157. Antonescu CR, Rosenblum MK, Pereira P, et al. Sclerosing epithelioid fibrosarcoma: a study of 16 cases and confirmation of a clinicopathologically distinct tumor. Am J Surg Pathol 2001; 25(6): 699–709.

158. Chung EB, Enzinger FM. Infantile fibrosarcoma. Cancer 1976; 38(2): 729–739

159. Coffin CM, Jaszcz W, O'Shea PA, Dehner LP. So-called congenital–infantile fibrosarcoma: does it exist and what is it? Pediatr Pathol 1994; 14(1): 133–150.

160. Michigami T, Yamato H, Mushiake S, et al. Hypercalcemia associated with infantile fibrosarcoma producing parathyroid hormone-related protein. J Clin Endocrinol Metab 1996; 81(3): 1090–1095.

161. Kihara S, Nehlsen-Cannarella N, Kirsch WM, et al. A comparative study of apoptosis and cell proliferation in infantile and adult fibrosarcomas. Am J Clin Pathol 1996; 106(4): 493–497.

162. Argani P, Fritsch M, Kadkol SS, et al. Detection of the ETV6–NTRK3 chimeric RNA of infantile fibrosarcoma/cellular congenital mesoblastic nephroma in paraffin-embedded tissue: application to challenging pediatric renal stromal tumors. Mod Pathol 2000; 13(1): 29–36.

163. Sheng WQ, Hisaoka M, Okamoto S, et al. Congenital-infantile fibrosarcoma. A clinicopathologic study of 10 cases and molecular detection of the ETV6–NTRK3 fusion transcripts using paraffin-embedded tissues. Am J Clin Pathol 2001; 115(3): 348–355.

164. Coffin CM, Dehner LP, Meis-Kindblom JM. Inflammatory myofibroblastic tumor, inflammatory fibrosarcoma, and related lesions: an historical review with differential diagnostic considerations. Semin Diagn Pathol 1998; 15(2): 102–110.

165. Meis-Kindblom JM, Kjellstrom C, Kindblom LG. Inflammatory fibrosarcoma: update, reappraisal, and perspective on its place in the spectrum of inflammatory myofibroblastic tumors. Semin Diagn Pathol 1998; 15(2): 133–143.

166. Bridge JA, Kanamori M, Ma Z, et al. Fusion of the ALK gene to the clathrin heavy chain gene, CLTC, in inflammatory myofibroblastic tumor. Am J Pathol 2001; 159(2): 411–415.

167. Cook JR, Dehner LP, Collins MH, et al. Anaplastic lymphoma kinase (ALK) expression in the inflammatory myofibroblastic tumor: a comparative immunohistochemical study. Am J Surg Pathol 2001; 25(11): 1364–1371.

168. Lawrence B, Perez-Atayde A, Hibbard MK, et al. TPM3–ALK and TPM4–ALK oncogenes in inflammatory myofibroblastic tumors. Am J Pathol 2000; 157(2): 377–384.

169. Sirvent N, Hawkins AL, Moeglin D, et al. ALK probe rearrangement in a t(2; 11; 2)(p23; p15; q31) translocation found in a prenatal myofibroblastic fibrous lesion: toward a molecular definition of an inflammatory myofibroblastic tumor family? Genes Chromosomes Cancer 2001; 31(1): 85–90.

170. Meis JM, Enzinger FM. Inflammatory fibrosarcoma of the mesentery and retroperitoneum. A tumor closely simulating inflammatory pseudotumor. Am J Surg Pathol 1991; 15(12): 1146–1156.

171. Coffin CM, Watterson J, Priest JR, Dehner LP. Extrapulmonary inflammatory myofibroblastic tumor (inflammatory pseudotumor). A clinicopathologic and immunohistochemical study of 84 cases. Am J Surg Pathol 1995; 19(8): 859–872.

172. Watanabe K, Ogura G. Fibronexus in 'malignant fibrous histiocytoma' of the bone: a case report of pleomorphic myofibrosarcoma. Ultrastruct Pathol 2002; 26(1): 47–51.

173. Montgomery E, Goldblum J, Fisher C. Myofibrosarcoma: a clinicopathologic study. Am J Surg Pathol 2001; 25: 219–228.

174. Montgomery E, Fisher C. Myofibroblastic differentiation in malignant fibrous histiocytoma (pleomorphic myofibrosarcoma): a clinicopathologic study. Histopathology 2001; 38(6): 499–509.

175. Mentzel T, Dry S, Katenkamp D, Fletcher CD. Low-grade myofibroblastic sarcoma: analysis of 18 cases in the spectrum of myofibroblastic tumors. Am J Surg Pathol 1998; 22(10): 1228–1238.

176. Smith DM, Mahmoud HH, Jenkins JJ III, et al. Myofibrosarcoma of the head and neck in children. Pediatr Pathol Lab Med 1995; 15(3): 403–418.

177. Fletcher CD. Pleomorphic malignant fibrous histiocytoma: fact or fiction? A critical reappraisal based on 159 tumors diagnosed as pleomorphic sarcoma. Am J Surg Pathol 1992; 16(3): 213–228.

178. Cole CH, Magee JF, Gianoulis M, Rogers PC. Malignant fibrous histiocytoma in childhood. Cancer 1993; 71(12): 4077–4083.

179. Laskin WB, Conklin RC, Enzinger FM. Malignant fibrous histiocytoma associated with hyperlipoproteinemia. Am J Surg Pathol 1988; 12(9): 727–732.

180. Sijmons R, Hofstra R, Hollema H, et al. Inclusion of malignant fibrous histiocytoma in the tumour spectrum associated with hereditary non-polyposis colorectal cancer. Genes Chromosomes Cancer 2000; 29(4): 353–355.

181. Fanburg-Smith JC, Spiro IJ, Katapuram SV, et al. Infiltrative subcutaneous malignant fibrous histiocytoma: a comparative study with deep malignant fibrous histiocytoma and an observation of biologic behavior. Ann Diagn Pathol 1999; 3(1): 1–10.

182. Weiss SW, Enzinger FM. Malignant fibrous histiocytoma: an analysis of 200 cases. Cancer 1978; 41(6): 2250–2266.

183. Pezzi CM, Rawlings MS Jr, Esgro JJ, et al. Prognostic factors in 227 patients with malignant fibrous histiocytoma. Cancer 1992; 69(8): 2098–103.

184. Le Doussal V, Coindre JM, Leroux A, et al. Prognostic factors for patients with localized primary malignant fibrous histiocytoma: a multicenter study of 216 patients with multivariate analysis. Cancer 1996; 77(9): 1823–1830.

185. Rosenberg AE, O'Connell JX, Dickersin GR, Bhan AK. Expression of epithelial markers in malignant fibrous histiocytoma of the musculoskeletal system: an immunohistochemical and electron microscopic study. Hum Pathol 1993; 24(3): 284–293.

186. Lawson CW, Fisher C, Gatter KC. An immunohistochemical study of differentiation in malignant fibrous histiocytoma. Histopathology 1987; 11(4): 375–383.

187. Kesavan S, Rosenberg A, Selig M, Nielsen G. The reclassification of MFH as fibrosarcoma: a proposal based on the analysis of the ultrastructural features of 100 cases. Mod Pathol 2001; 14: 14A (abstract 59).

188. Derre J, Lagace R, Nicolas A, et al. Leiomyosarcomas and most malignant fibrous histiocytomas share very similar comparative genomic hybridization imbalances: an analysis of a series of 27 leiomyosarcomas. Lab Invest 2001; 81(2): 211–215.

189. Mertens F, Fletcher CD, Dal Cin P, et al. Cytogenetic analysis of 46 pleomorphic soft tissue sarcomas and correlation with morphologic and clinical features: a report of the CHAMP Study Group. Chromosomes and Morphology. Genes Chromosomes Cancer 1998; 22(1): 16–25.

190. Walaas L, Angervall L, Hagmar B, Save-Soderbergh J. A correlative cytologic and histologic study of malignant fibrous histiocytoma: an analysis of 40 cases examined by fine-needle aspiration cytology. Diagn Cytopathol 1986; 2(1): 46–54.

191. Montgomery EA, Meis JM, Frizzera G. Rosai–Dorfman disease of soft tissue. Am J Surg Pathol 1992; 16(2): 122–129.

192. Kodet R, Newton WA Jr, Hamoudi AB, et al. Childhood rhabdomyosarcoma with anaplastic (pleomorphic) features. A report of the Intergroup Rhabdomyosarcoma Study. Am J Surg Pathol 1993; 17(5): 443–453.

193. Furlong MA, Mentzel T, Fanburg-Smith JC. Pleomorphic rhabdomyosarcoma in adults: a clinicopathologic study of 38 cases with emphasis on morphologic variants and recent skeletal muscle-specific markers. Mod Pathol 2001; 14(6): 595–603.

194. Gaffney EF, Dervan PA, Fletcher CD. Pleomorphic rhabdomyosarcoma in adulthood. Analysis of 11 cases with definition of diagnostic criteria. Am J Surg Pathol 1993; 17(6): 601–609.

195. Furlong MA, Fanburg-Smith JC. Pleomorphic rhabdomyosarcoma in children: four cases in the pediatric age group. Ann Diagn Pathol 2001; 5(4): 199–206.

196. Oda Y, Miyajima K, Kawaguchi K, et al. Pleomorphic leiomyosarcoma: clinicopathologic and immunohistochemical study with special emphasis on its distinction from ordinary leiomyosarcoma and malignant fibrous histiocytoma. Am J Surg Pathol 2001; 25(8): 1030–1038.

197. McCormick D, Mentzel T, Beham A, Fletcher CD. Dedifferentiated liposarcoma. Clinicopathologic analysis of 32 cases suggesting a better prognostic subgroup among pleomorphic sarcomas. Am J Surg Pathol 1994; 18(12): 1213–1223.

198. Henricks WH, Chu YC, Goldblum JR, Weiss SW. Dedifferentiated liposarcoma: a clinicopathological analysis of 155 cases with a proposal for an expanded definition of dedifferentiation. Am J Surg Pathol 1997; 21(3): 271–281.

199. Guccion JG, Enzinger FM. Malignant giant cell tumor of soft parts. An analysis of 32 cases. Cancer 1972; 29(6): 1518–1529.

200. Kyriakos M, Kempson RL. Inflammatory fibrous histiocytoma. An aggressive and lethal lesion. Cancer 1976; 37(3): 1584–1606.

201. Merino MJ, LiVolsi VA. Inflammatory malignant fibrous histiocytoma. Am J Clin Pathol 1980; 73(2): 276–281.

202. Coindre JM, Hostein I, Maire G, et al. Inflammatory malignant fibrous histiocytomas and dedifferentiated liposarcomas: histological review, genomic profile, and MDM2 and CDK4 status favour a single entity. J Pathol 2004; 203(3): 822–830.

203. Fletcher CD, Akerman M, Dal Cin P, et al. Correlation between clinicopathological features and karyotype in lipomatous tumors. A report of 178 cases from the Chromosomes and Morphology (CHAMP) Collaborative Study Group. Am J Pathol 1996; 148(2): 623–630.

204. Rosai J, Akerman M, Dal Cin P, et al. Combined morphologic and karyotypic study of 59 atypical lipomatous tumors. Evaluation of their relationship and differential diagnosis with other adipose tissue tumors (a report of the CHAMP Study Group). Am J Surg Pathol 1996; 20(10): 1182–1189.

205. Sciot R, Akerman M, Dal Cin P, et al. Cytogenetic analysis of subcutaneous angiolipoma: further evidence supporting its difference from ordinary pure lipomas: a report of the CHAMP Study Group. Am J Surg Pathol 1997; 21(4): 441–444.

206. Tallini G, Akerman M, Dal Cin P, et al. Combined morphologic and karyotypic study of 28 myxoid liposarcomas. Implications for a revised morphologic typing (a report from the CHAMP Group). Am J Surg Pathol 1996; 20(9): 1047–1055.

207. Meis JM, Enzinger FM. Myolipoma of soft tissue. Am J Surg Pathol 1991; 15(2): 121–125.

208. Kindblom LG, Angervall L, Stener B, Wickbom I. Intermuscular and intramuscular lipomas and hibernomas. A clinical, roentgenologic, histologic, and prognostic study of 46 cases. Cancer 1974; 33(3): 754–762.

209. Gamez J, Playan A, Andreu AL, et al. Familial multiple symmetric lipomatosis associated with the A8344G mutation of mitochondrial DNA. Neurology 1998; 51(1): 258–260.

210. Ronan SJ, Broderick T. Minimally invasive approach to familial multiple lipomatosis. Plast Reconstr Surg 2000; 106(4): 878–880.

211. Tsao H, Sober AJ. Multiple lipomatosis in a patient with familial atypical mole syndrome. Br J Dermatol 1998; 139(6): 1118–1119.

212. Stoll C, Alembik Y, Truttmann M. Multiple familial lipomatosis with polyneuropathy, an inherited dominant condition. Ann Genet 1996; 39(4): 193–196.

213. Hicks J, Dilley A, Patel D, et al. Lipoblastoma and lipoblastomatosis in infancy and childhood: histopathologic, ultrastructural, and cytogenetic features. Ultrastruct Pathol 2001; 25(4): 321–333.

214. Mentzel T, Calonje E, Fletcher CD. Lipoblastoma and lipoblastomatosis: a clinicopathological study of 14 cases. Histopathology 1993; 23(6): 527–533.

215. Collins MH, Chatten J. Lipoblastoma/lipoblastomatosis: a clinicopathologic study of 25 tumors. Am J Surg Pathol 1997; 21(10): 1131–1137.

216. Chung EB, Enzinger FM. Benign lipoblastomatosis. An analysis of 35 cases. Cancer 1973; 32(2): 482–492.

217. Dal Cin P, Sciot R, De Wever I, et al. New discriminative chromosomal marker in adipose tissue tumors. The chromosome 8q11–q13 region in lipoblastoma. Cancer Genet Cytogenet 1994; 78(2): 232–235.

218. Jadusingh IH. Fine needle aspiration cytology of lipoblastoma. Acta Cytol 2000; 44(1): 104–107.

219. Enzinger FM, Harvey DA. Spindle cell lipoma. Cancer 1975; 36(5): 1852–1859.

220. Fanburg-Smith JC, Devaney KO, Miettinen M, Weiss SW. Multiple spindle cell lipomas: a report of 7 familial and 11 nonfamilial cases. Am J Surg Pathol 1998; 22(1): 40–48.

221. Domanski HA, Carlen B, Jonsson K, et al. Distinct cytologic features of spindle cell lipoma. A cytologic-histologic study with clinical, radiologic, electron microscopic, and cytogenetic correlations. Cancer 2001; 93(6): 381–389.

222. Dal Cin P, Sciot R, Polito P, et al. Lesions of 13q may occur independently of deletion of 16q in spindle cell/pleomorphic lipomas. Histopathology 1997; 31(3): 222–225.

223. Mandahl N, Mertens F, Willen H, et al. A new cytogenetic subgroup in lipomas: loss of chromosome 16 material in spindle cell and pleomorphic lipomas. J Cancer Res Clin Oncol 1994; 120(12): 707–711.

224. Azzopardi JG, Iocco J, Salm R. Pleomorphic lipoma: a tumour simulating liposarcoma. Histopathology 1983; 7(4): 511–23.

225. Shmookler BM, Enzinger FM. Pleomorphic lipoma: a benign tumor simulating liposarcoma. A clinicopathologic analysis of 48 cases. Cancer 1981; 47(1): 126–33.

226. Verghese A, Smith RA, Stock D, Lewis MH. Aspiration cytology of a pleomorphic lipoma – a cautionary note. Cytopathology 1999; 10(4): 280–282.

227. Thirumala S, Desai M, Kannan V. Diagnostic pitfalls in fine needle aspiration cytology of pleomorphic lipoma. A case report. Acta Cytol 2000; 44(4): 653–656.

228. Meis JM, Enzinger FM. Chondroid lipoma. A unique tumor simulating liposarcoma and myxoid chondrosarcoma. Am J Surg Pathol 1993; 17(11): 1103–1112.

229. Chan JK, Lee KC, Saw D. Extraskeletal chondroma with lipoblast-like cells. Hum Pathol 1986; 17(12): 1285–1287.

230. Zamecnik M, Michal M, Fakan F. Ultrastructural study of so called chondroid lipoma. Hum Pathol 1998; 29(1): 98–100.

231. Nielsen GP, O'Connell JX, Dickersin GR, Rosenberg AE. Chondroid lipoma, a tumor of white fat cells. A brief report of two cases with ultrastructural analysis. Am J Surg Pathol 1995; 19(11): 1272–1276.

232. Kindblom LG, Meis-Kindblom JM. Chondroid lipoma: an ultrastructural and immunohistochemical analysis with further observations regarding its differentiation. Hum Pathol 1995; 26(7): 706–715.

233. Gisselsson D, Domanski HA, Hoglund M, et al. Unique cytological features and chromosome aberrations in chondroid lipoma: a case report based on fine-needle aspiration cytology, histopathology, electron microscopy, chromosome banding, and molecular cytogenetics. Am J Surg Pathol 1999; 23(10): 1300–1304.

234. Thomson TA, Horsman D, Bainbridge TC. Cytogenetic and cytologic features of chondroid lipoma of soft tissue. Mod Pathol 1999; 12(1): 88–91.

235. Thomson TA, Bainbridge TC, Horsman D. Unique cytologic and chromosome aberrations in chondroid lipoma. Am J Surg Pathol 2000; 24(7): 1035.

236. Ji Y, Zhu X, Xu J, et al. Hepatic angiomyolipoma: a clinicopathologic study of 10 cases. Chin Med J (Engl) 2001; 114(3): 280–285.

237. Tang P, Alhindawi R, Farmer P. Case report: primary isolated angiomyolipoma of the spleen. Ann Clin Lab Sci 2001; 31(4): 405–410.

238. Tsutsumi M, Yamauchi A, Tsukamoto S, Ishikawa S. A case of angiomyolipoma presenting as a huge retroperitoneal mass. Int J Urol 2001; 8(8): 470–471.

239. Johnson SR, Clelland CA, Ronan J, et al. The TSC-2 product tuberin is expressed in lymphangioleiomyomatosis and angiomyolipoma. Histopathology 2002; 40(5): 458–463.

240. Barnard M, Lajoie G. Angiomyolipoma: immunohistochemical and ultrastructural study of 14 cases. Ultrastruct Pathol 2001; 25(1): 21–29.

241. Furlong MA, Fanburg-Smith JC, Miettinen M. The morphologic spectrum of hibernoma: a clinicopathologic study of 170 cases. Am J Surg Pathol 2001; 25(6): 809–814.

242. Gisselsson D, Hoglund M, Mertens F, et al. Hibernomas are characterized by homozygous deletions in the multiple endocrine neoplasia type I region. Metaphase fluorescence in situ hybridization reveals complex rearrangements not detected by conventional cytogenetics. Am J Pathol 1999; 155(1): 61–66.

243. Evans HL, Soule EH, Winkelmann RK. Atypical lipoma, atypical intramuscular lipoma, and well differentiated retroperitoneal liposarcoma: a reappraisal of 30 cases formerly classified as well differentiated liposarcoma. Cancer 1979; 43(2): 574–584.

244. Elgar F, Goldblum JR. Well-differentiated liposarcoma of the retroperitoneum: a clinicopathologic analysis of 20 cases, with particular attention to the extent of low-grade dedifferentiation. Mod Pathol 1997; 10(2): 113–120.

245. Lucas DR, Nascimento AG, Sanjay BK, Rock MG. Well-differentiated liposarcoma. The Mayo Clinic experience with 58 cases. Am J Clin Pathol 1994; 102(5): 677–683.

246. Evans HL. Liposarcoma: a study of 55 cases with a reassessment of its classification. Am J Surg Pathol 1979; 3(6): 507–523.

247. Weiss SW, Rao VK. Well-differentiated liposarcoma (atypical lipoma) of deep soft tissue of the extremities, retroperitoneum, and miscellaneous sites. A follow-up study of 92 cases with analysis of the incidence of 'dedifferentiation'. Am J Surg Pathol 1992; 16(11): 1051–1058.

248. Enzinger F, Winslow D. Liposarcoma: A study of 103 cases. Virchow's Archives A Pathol Anat Histopathol 1962; 335: 367–388.

249. Shmookler BM, Enzinger FM. Liposarcoma occurring in children. An analysis of 17 cases and review of the literature. Cancer 1983; 52(3): 567–574.

250. Montgomery E, Fisher C. Paratesticular liposarcoma: a clinicopathologic study. Am J Surg Pathol 2002; 27(1): 40–47.

251. Azumi N, Curtis J, Kempson RL, Hendrickson MR. Atypical and malignant neoplasms showing lipomatous differentiation. A study of 111 cases. Am J Surg Pathol 1987; 11(3): 161–183.

252. Evans H. Liposarcomas and atypical lipomatous tumors: a study of 66 cases followed for a minimum of 10 years. Surgical Pathology 1988; 1(1): 41–54.

253. Yoshikawa H, Ueda T, Mori S, et al. Dedifferentiated liposarcoma of the subcutis. Am J Surg Pathol 1996; 20(12): 1525–1530.

254. Montgomery E, Fisher C. Paratesticular liposarcoma: a clinicopathologic study. Am J Surg Pathol 2003; 27(1): 40–47.

255. Evans HL, Khurana KK, Kemp BL, Ayala AG. Heterologous elements in the dedifferentiated component of dedifferentiated liposarcoma. Am J Surg Pathol 1994; 18(11): 1150–1157.

256. Evans HL. Smooth muscle in atypical lipomatous tumors. A report of three cases. Am J Surg Pathol 1990; 14(8): 714–718.

257. Vartanian R, O'Connell J, Holden J, et al. Primary jejunal well-differentiated liposarcoma (atypical lipomatous tumor) with leiomyosarcomatous differentiation. Int J Surg Pathol 1996; 4(1): 29–36.

258. Argani P, Facchetti F, Inghirami G, Rosai J. Lymphocyte-rich well-differentiated liposarcoma: report of nine cases. Am J Surg Pathol 1997; 21(8): 884–895.

259. Farshid G, Weiss SW. Massive localized lymphedema in the morbidly obese: a histologically distinct reactive lesion simulating liposarcoma. Am J Surg Pathol 1998; 22(10): 1277–1283.

260. Nascimento AG, Kurtin PJ, Guillou L, Fletcher CD. Dedifferentiated liposarcoma: a report of nine cases with a peculiar neural-like whorling pattern associated with metaplastic bone formation. Am J Surg Pathol 1998; 22(8): 945–955.

261. Fanburg-Smith JC, Miettinen M. Liposarcoma with meningothelial-like whorls: a study of 17 cases of a distinctive histological pattern associated with dedifferentiated liposarcoma. Histopathology 1998; 33(5): 414–424.

262. Antonescu CR, Tschernyavsky SJ, Decuseara R, et al. Prognostic impact of P53 status, TLS-CHOP fusion transcript structure, and histological grade in myxoid liposarcoma: a molecular and clinicopathologic study of 82 cases. Clin Cancer Res 2001; 7(12): 3977–3987.

263. Antonescu CR, Elahi A, Healey JH, et al. Monoclonality of multifocal myxoid liposarcoma: confirmation by analysis of TLS-CHOP or EWS-CHOP rearrangements. Clin Cancer Res 2000; 6(7): 2788–2793.

264. Kilpatrick SE, Doyon J, Choong PF, et al. The clinicopathologic spectrum of myxoid and round cell liposarcoma. A study of 95 cases. Cancer 1996; 77(8): 1450–1458.

265. Oliveira AM, Nascimento AG, Okuno SH, Lloyd RV. p27(kip1) protein expression correlates with survival in myxoid and round-cell liposarcoma. J Clin Oncol 2000; 18(15): 2888–2893.

266. Spillane AJ, Fisher C, Thomas JM. Myxoid liposarcoma–the frequency and the natural history of nonpulmonary soft tissue metastases. Ann Surg Oncol 1999; 6(4): 389–394.

267. Smith TA, Easley KA, Goldblum JR. Myxoid/round cell liposarcoma of the extremities. A clinicopathologic study of 29 cases with particular attention to extent of round cell liposarcoma. Am J Surg Pathol 1996; 20(2): 171–180.

268. Paulien S, Turc-Carel C, Dal Cin P, et al. Myxoid liposarcoma with t(12; 16) (q13; p11) contains site-specific differences in methylation patterns surrounding a zinc-finger gene mapped to the breakpoint region on chromosome 12. Cancer Res 1990; 50(24): 7902–7907.

269. Sreekantaiah C, Karakousis CP, Leong SP, Sandberg AA. Trisomy 8 as a nonrandom secondary change in myxoid liposarcoma. Cancer Genet Cytogenet 1991; 51(2): 195–205.

270. Downes KA, Goldblum JR, Montgomery EA, Fisher C. Pleomorphic liposarcoma: a clinicopathologic analysis of 19 cases. Mod Pathol 2001; 14(3): 179–184.

271. Miettinen M, Enzinger FM. Epithelioid variant of pleomorphic liposarcoma: a study of 12 cases of a distinctive variant of high-grade liposarcoma. Mod Pathol 1999; 12(7): 722–728.

272. Reddick RL, Michelitch H, Triche TJ. Malignant soft tissue tumors (malignant fibrous histiocytoma, pleomorphic liposarcoma, and pleomorphic rhabdomyosarcoma): an electron microscopic study. Hum Pathol 1979; 10(3): 327–343.

273. Miettinen MM, Sarlomo-Rikala M, Kovatich AJ, Lasota J. Calponin and h-caldesmon in soft tissue tumors: consistent h-caldesmon immunoreactivity in gastrointestinal stromal tumors indicates traits of smooth muscle differentiation. Mod Pathol 1999; 12(8): 756–762.

274. Vellanki LS, Camisa C, Steck WD. Familial leiomyomata. Cutis 1996; 58(1): 80–82.

275. Raj S, Calonje E, Kraus M, et al. Cutaneous pilar leiomyoma: clinicopathologic analysis of 53 lesions in 45 patients. Am J Dermatopathol 1997; 19(1): 2–9.

276. Nascimento AG, Karas M, Rosen PP, Caron AG. Leiomyoma of the nipple. Am J Surg Pathol 1979; 3(2): 151–154.

277. Hernandez FJ. Leiomyosarcoma of male breast originating in the nipple. Am J Surg Pathol 1978; 2(3): 299–304.

278. Lonsdale RN, Widdison A. Leiomyosarcoma of the nipple. Histopathology 1992; 20(6): 537–539.

279. Slone S, O'Connor D. Scrotal leiomyomas with bizarre nuclei: a report of three cases. Mod Pathol 1998; 11(3): 282–287.

280. Fisher C, Goldblum JR, Epstein JI, Montgomery E. Leiomyosarcoma of the paratesticular region: a clinicopathologic study. Am J Surg Pathol 2001; 25(9): 1143–1149.

281. Tavassoli FA, Norris HJ. Smooth muscle tumors of the vulva. Obstet Gynecol 1979; 53(2): 213–217.

282. Tavassoli FA, Norris HJ. Smooth muscle tumors of the vagina. Obstet Gynecol 1979; 53(6): 689–693.

283. Newman PL, Fletcher CD. Smooth muscle tumours of the external genitalia: clinicopathological analysis of a series. Histopathology 1991; 18(6): 523–529.

284. Hachisuga T, Hashimoto H, Enjoji M. Angioleiomyoma. A clinicopathologic reappraisal of 562 cases. Cancer 1984; 54(1): 126–130.

285. Billings SD, Folpe AL, Weiss SW. Do leiomyomas of deep soft tissue exist? An analysis of highly differentiated smooth muscle tumors of deep soft tissue supporting two distinct subtypes. Am J Surg Pathol 2001; 25(9): 1134–1142.

286. Kilpatrick SE, Mentzel T, Fletcher CD. Leiomyoma of deep soft tissue. Clinicopathologic analysis of a series. Am J Surg Pathol 1994; 18(6): 576–582.

287. Fletcher CD, Kilpatrick SE, Mentzel T. The difficulty in predicting behavior of smooth-muscle tumors in deep soft tissue. Am J Surg Pathol 1995; 19(1): 116–117.

288. Shmookler BM, Lauer DH. Retroperitoneal leiomyosarcoma. A clinicopathologic analysis of 36 cases. Am J Surg Pathol 1983; 7(3): 269–280.

289. Azumi N, Ben-Ezra J, Battifora H. Immunophenotypic diagnosis of leiomyosarcomas and rhabdomyosarcomas with monoclonal antibodies to muscle-specific actin and desmin in formalin-fixed tissue. Mod Pathol 1988; 1(6): 469–474.

290. Montgomery E, Goldblum JR, Fisher C. Leiomyosarcoma of the head and neck: a clinicopathological study. Histopathology 2002; 40(6): 518–525.

291. Miettinen M. Immunoreactivity for cytokeratin and epithelial membrane antigen in leiomyosarcoma. Arch Pathol Lab Med 1988; 112(6): 637–640.

292. Mandahl N, Fletcher CD, Dal Cin P, et al. Comparative cytogenetic study of spindle cell and pleomorphic leiomyosarcomas of soft tissues: a report from the CHAMP Study Group. Cancer Genet Cytogenet 2000; 116(1): 66–73.

293. Hashimoto H, Daimaru Y, Tsuneyoshi M, Enjoji M. Leiomyosarcoma of the external soft tissues. A clinicopathologic, immunohistochemical, and electron microscopic study. Cancer 1986; 57(10): 2077–2088.

294. Wile AG, Evans HL, Romsdahl MM. Leiomyosarcoma of soft tissue: a clinicopathologic study. Cancer 1981; 48(4): 1022–1032.

295. Swanson PE, Wick MR, Dehner LP. Leiomyosarcoma of somatic soft tissues in childhood: an immunohistochemical analysis of six cases with ultrastructural correlation. Hum Pathol 1991; 22(6): 569–577.

296. Rajani B, Smith TA, Reith JD, Goldblum JR. Retroperitoneal leiomyosarcomas unassociated with the gastrointestinal tract: a clinicopathologic analysis of 17 cases. Mod Pathol 1999; 12(1): 21–28.

297. Farshid G, Pradhan M, Goldblum J, Weiss SW. Leiomyosarcoma of somatic soft tissues: a tumor of vascular origin with multivariate analysis of outcome in 42 cases. Am J Surg Pathol 2002; 26(1): 14–24.

298. Kaddu S, Beham A, Cerroni L, et al. Cutaneous leiomyosarcoma. Am J Surg Pathol 1997; 21(9): 979–987.

299. Dahl I, Angervall L. Cutaneous and subcutaneous leiomyosarcoma. A clinicopathologic study of 47 patients. Pathol Eur 1974; 9(4): 307–315.

300. Fields JP, Helwig EB. Leiomyosarcoma of the skin and subcutaneous tissue. Cancer 1981; 47(1): 156–169.

301. Suster S. Epithelioid leiomyosarcoma of the skin and subcutaneous tissue. Clinicopathologic, immunohistochemical, and ultrastructural study of five cases. Am J Surg Pathol 1994; 18(3): 232–240.

302. Swanson PE, Stanley MW, Scheithauer BW, Wick MR. Primary cutaneous leiomyosarcoma. A histological and immunohistochemical study of 9 cases, with ultrastructural correlation. J Cutan Pathol 1988; 15(3): 129–141.

303. Wascher RA, Lee MY. Recurrent cutaneous leiomyosarcoma. Cancer 1992; 70(2): 490–492.

304. Kevorkian J, Cento DP. Leiomyosarcoma of large arteries and veins. Surgery 1973; 73(3): 390–400.

305. Varela-Duran J, Oliva H, Rosai J. Vascular leiomyosarcoma: the malignant counterpart of vascular leiomyoma. Cancer 1979; 44(5): 1684–1691.

306. Boman F, Gultekin H, Dickman PS. Latent Epstein–Barr virus infection demonstrated in low-grade leiomyosarcomas of adults with acquired immunodeficiency syndrome, but not in adjacent Kaposi's lesion or smooth muscle tumors in immunocompetent patients. Arch Pathol Lab Med 1997; 121(8): 834–838.

307. McClain KL, Leach CT, Jenson HB, et al. Association of Epstein–Barr virus with leiomyosarcomas in children with AIDS. N Engl J Med 1995; 332(1): 12–18.

308. Orlow SJ, Kamino H, Lawrence RL. Multiple subcutaneous leiomyosarcomas in an adolescent with AIDS. Am J Pediatr Hematol Oncol 1992; 14(3): 265–268.

309. Brown HG, Burger PC, Olivi A, et al. Intracranial leiomyosarcoma in a patient with AIDS. Neuroradiology 1999; 41(1): 35–39.

310. Bejjani GK, Stopak B, Schwartz A, Santi R. Primary dural leiomyosarcoma in a patient infected with human immunodeficiency virus: case report. Neurosurgery 1999; 44(1): 199–202.

311. Morgello S, Kotsianti A, Gumprecht JP, Moore F. Epstein–Barr virus-associated dural leiomyosarcoma in a man infected with human immunodeficiency virus. Case report. J Neurosurg 1997; 86(5): 883–887.

312. Sabatino D, Martinez S, Young R, et al. Simultaneous pulmonary leiomyosarcoma and leiomyoma in pediatric HIV infection. Pediatr Hematol Oncol 1991; 8(4): 355–359.

313. Timmons CF, Dawson DB, Richards CS, et al. Epstein–Barr virus-associated leiomyosarcomas in liver transplantation recipients. Origin from either donor or recipient tissue. Cancer 1995; 76(8): 1481–1489.

314. Suster S, Moran CA, Blanco M. Mycobacterial spindle-cell pseudotumor of the spleen. Am J Clin Pathol 1994; 101(4): 539–542.

315. Mazur MT, Clark HB. Gastric stromal tumors. Reappraisal of histogenesis. Am J Surg Pathol 1983; 7(6): 507–519.

316. Miettinen M, Sarlomo-Rikala M, Sobin LH, Lasota J. Gastrointestinal stromal tumors and leiomyosarcomas in the colon: a clinicopathologic, immunohistochemical, and molecular genetic study of 44 cases. Am J Surg Pathol 2000; 24(10): 1339–1352.

317. Kindblom LG, Remotti HE, Aldenborg F, Meis-Kindblom JM. Gastrointestinal pacemaker cell tumor (GIPACT): gastrointestinal stromal tumors show phenotypic characteristics of the interstitial cells of Cajal. Am J Pathol 1998; 152(5): 1259–1269.

318. Lauwers GY, Erlandson RA, Casper ES, et al. Gastrointestinal autonomic nerve tumors. A clinicopathological, immunohistochemical, and ultrastructural study of 12 cases. Am J Surg Pathol 1993; 17(9): 887–897.

319. Lee JR, Joshi V, Griffin JW Jr, et al. Gastrointestinal autonomic nerve tumor: immunohistochemical and molecular identity with gastrointestinal stromal tumor. Am J Surg Pathol 2001; 25(8): 979–987.

320. Miettinen M, Monihan JM, Sarlomo-Rikala M, et al. Gastrointestinal stromal tumors/smooth muscle tumors (GISTs) primary in the omentum and mesentery: clinicopathologic and immunohistochemical study of 26 cases. Am J Surg Pathol 1999; 23(9): 1109–118.

321. Reith JD, Goldblum JR, Lyles RH, Weiss SW. Extragastrointestinal (soft tissue) stromal tumors: an analysis of 48 cases with emphasis on histologic predictors of outcome. Mod Pathol 2000; 13(5): 577–585.

322. Emory TS, Sobin LH, Lukes L, et al. Prognosis of gastrointestinal smooth-muscle (stromal) tumors: dependence on anatomic site. Am J Surg Pathol 1999; 23(1): 82–87.

323. Krapp M, Baschat AA, Gembruch U, et al. Tuberous sclerosis with intracardiac rhabdomyoma in a fetus with trisomy 21: case report and review of literature. Prenat Diagn 1999; 19(7): 610–613.

324. Bosi G, Lintermans JP, Pellegrino PA, et al. The natural history of cardiac rhabdomyoma with and without tuberous sclerosis. Acta Paediatr 1996; 85(8): 928–931.

325. Nir A, Tajik AJ, Freeman WK, et al. Tuberous sclerosis and cardiac rhabdomyoma. Am J Cardiol 1995; 76(5): 419–421.

326. Bordarier C, Lellouch-Tubiana A, Robain O. Cardiac rhabdomyoma and tuberous sclerosis in three fetuses: a neuropathological study. Brain Dev 1994; 16(6): 467–471.

327. Harding CO, Pagon RA. Incidence of tuberous sclerosis in patients with cardiac rhabdomyoma. Am J Med Genet 1990; 37(4): 443–446.

328. Webb DW, Osborne JP. Incidence of tuberous sclerosis in patients with cardiac rhabdomyoma. Am J Med Genet 1992; 42(5): 754–755.

329. Wu SS, Collins MH, de Chadarevian JP. Study of the regression process in cardiac rhabdomyomas. Pediatr Dev Pathol 2002; 5(1): 29–36.

330. D'Addario V, Pinto V, Di Naro E, et al. Prenatal diagnosis and postnatal outcome of cardiac rhabdomyomas. J Perinat Med 2002; 30(2): 170–175.

331. Carrico A, Moura C, Baptista MJ, et al. Cardiac rhabdomyomas presenting in neonates. Rev Port Cardiol 2001; 20(11): 1095–1101.

332. Willis J, Abdul-Karim FW, di Sant'Agnese PA. Extracardiac rhabdomyomas. Semin Diagn Pathol 1994; 11(1): 15–25.

333. Gibas Z, Miettinen M. Recurrent parapharyngeal rhabdomyoma. Evidence of neoplastic nature of the tumor from cytogenetic study. Am J Surg Pathol 1992; 16(7): 721–728.

334. Kapadia SB, Meis JM, Frisman DM, et al. Adult rhabdomyoma of the head and neck: a clinicopathologic and immunophenotypic study. Hum Pathol 1993; 24(6): 608–617.

335. Eusebi V, Ceccarelli C, Daniele E, et al. Extracardiac rhabdomyoma: An immunocytochemical study and review of the literature. Appl Pathol 1988; 6(3): 197–207.

336. Kapadia SB, Meis JM, Frisman DM, et al. Fetal rhabdomyoma of the head and neck: a clinicopathologic and immunophenotypic study of 24 cases. Hum Pathol 1993; 24(7): 754–765.

337. Dehner LP, Enzinger FM, Font RL. Fetal rhabdomyoma. An analysis of nine cases. Cancer 1972; 30(1): 160–166.

338. Szadowska A, Giryn I, Zawadzki R. The value of electron microscopic examination of differential diagnosis of fetal rhabdomyoma and embryonal rhabdomyosarcoma of urinary bladder. Acta Med Pol 1979; 20(4): 459–460.

339. Kodet R, Fajstavr J, Kabelka Z, et al. Is fetal cellular rhabdomyoma an entity or a differentiated rhabdomyosarcoma? A study of patients with rhabdomyoma of the tongue and sarcoma of the tongue enrolled in the intergroup rhabdomyosarcoma studies I, II, and III. Cancer 1991; 67(11): 2907–2913.

340. Konrad EA, Meister P, Hubner G. Extracardiac rhabdomyoma: report of different types with light microscopic and ultrastructural studies. Cancer 1982; 49(5): 898–907.

341. Losi L, Choreutaki T, Nascetti D, Eusebi V. [Recurrence in a case of rhabdomyoma of the vagina]. Pathologica 1995; 87(6): 704–708.

342. Lopez JI, Brouard I, Eizaguirre B. Rhabdomyoma of the vagina. Eur J Obstet Gynecol Reprod Biol 1992; 45(2): 147–148.

343. Gee DC, Finckh ES. Benign vaginal rhabdomyoma. Pathology 1977; 9(3): 263–267.

344. Hanski W, Hagel E. Histological and ultraststructural studies of a case of rhabdomyoma polyposum vaginae. Ann Med Sect Pol Acad Sci 1976; 21(1–2): 47–48.

345. Gad A, Eusebi V. Rhabdomyoma of the vagina. J Pathol 1975; 115(3): 179–181.

346. Leone PG, Taylor HB. Ultrastructure of a benign polypoid rhabdomyoma of the vagina. Cancer 1973; 31(6): 1414–1417.

347. Ceremsak RJ. Benign rhabdomyoma of the vagina. Am J Clin Pathol 1969; 52(5): 604–606.

348. Nucci MR, Young RH, Fletcher CD. Cellular pseudosarcomatous fibroepithelial stromal polyps of the lower female genital tract: an underrecognized lesion often misdiagnosed as sarcoma. Am J Surg Pathol 2000; 24(2): 231–240.

349. Horn R, Enterline H. Rhabdomyosarcoma: a clinicopathologic study of 39 cases. Cancer 1958; 11: 181–199.

350. Tsokos M, Webber BL, Parham DM, et al. Rhabdomyosarcoma. A new classification scheme related to prognosis. Arch Pathol Lab Med 1992; 116(8): 847–855.

351. Cavazzana AO, Schmidt D, Ninfo V, et al. Spindle cell rhabdomyosarcoma. A prognostically favorable variant of rhabdomyosarcoma. Am J Surg Pathol 1992; 16(3): 229–235.

352. Caillaud JM, Gerard-Marchant R, Marsden HB, et al. Histopathological classification of childhood rhabdomyosarcoma: a report from the International Society of Pediatric Oncology pathology panel. Med Pediatr Oncol 1989; 17(5): 391–400.

353. Parham DM. Pathologic classification of rhabdomyosarcomas and correlations with molecular studies. Mod Pathol 2001; 14(5): 506–514.

354. Raney RB, Anderson JR, Barr FG, et al. Rhabdomyosarcoma and undifferentiated sarcoma in the first two decades of life: a selective review of intergroup rhabdomyosarcoma study group experience and rationale for Intergroup Rhabdomyosarcoma Study V. J Pediatr Hematol Oncol 2001; 23(4): 215–220.

355. Raney RB, Meza J, Anderson JR, et al. Treatment of children and adolescents with localized parameningeal sarcoma: experience of the Intergroup Rhabdomyosarcoma Study Group protocols IRS-II through -IV, 1978–1997. Med Pediatr Oncol 2002; 38(1): 22–32.

356. Crist WM, Anderson JR, Meza JL, et al. Intergroup rhabdomyosarcoma study-IV: results for patients with nonmetastatic disease. J Clin Oncol 2001; 19(12): 3091–3102.

357. Neville HL, Andrassy RJ, Lobe TE, et al. Preoperative staging, prognostic factors, and outcome for extremity rhabdomyosarcoma: a preliminary report from the Intergroup Rhabdomyosarcoma Study IV (1991–1997). J Pediatr Surg 2000; 35(2): 317–321.

358. Newton WA Jr, Webber B, Hamoudi AB, et al. Early history of pathology studies by the Intergroup Rhabdomyosarcoma Study Group. Pediatr Dev Pathol 1999; 2(3): 275–285.

359. Qualman SJ, Coffin CM, Newton WA, et al. Intergroup Rhabdomyosarcoma Study: update for pathologists. Pediatr Dev Pathol 1998; 1(6): 550–561.

360. Maurer HM, Gehan EA, Beltangady M, et al. The Intergroup Rhabdomyosarcoma Study-II. Cancer 1993; 71(5): 1904–1922.

361. Newton WA Jr, Soule EH, Hamoudi AB, et al. Histopathology of childhood sarcomas, Intergroup Rhabdomyosarcoma Studies I and II: clinicopathologic correlation. J Clin Oncol 1988; 6(1): 67–75.

362. Newton WA Jr, Gehan EA, Webber BL, et al. Classification of rhabdomyosarcomas and related sarcomas. Pathologic aspects and proposal for a new classification–an Intergroup Rhabdomyosarcoma Study. Cancer 1995; 76(6): 1073–1085.

363. Etcubanas E, Peiper S, Stass S, Green A. Rhabdomyosarcoma, presenting as disseminated malignancy from an unknown primary site: a retrospective study of ten pediatric cases. Med Pediatr Oncol 1989; 17(1): 39–44.

364. Parham DM, Pinto A, Tallini G, Novak RW. Rhabdomyosarcoma mimicking acute leukemia. Arch Pathol Lab Med 1998; 122(12): 1047.

365. Pinto A, Tallini G, Novak RW, et al. Undifferentiated rhabdomyosarcoma with lymphoid phenotype expression. Med Pediatr Oncol 1997; 28(3): 165–170.

366. Maurer HM, Beltangady M, Gehan EA, et al. The Intergroup Rhabdomyosarcoma Study-I. A final report. Cancer 1988; 61(2): 209–220.

367. Crist W, Gehan EA, Ragab AH, et al. The Third Intergroup Rhabdomyosarcoma Study. J Clin Oncol 1995; 13(3): 610–630.

368. Triche TJ, Ross WE. Glycogen-containing neuroblastoma with clinical and histopathologic features of Ewing's sarcoma. Cancer 1978; 41(4): 1425–1432.

369. Parham DM. The molecular biology of childhood rhabdomyosarcoma. Semin Diagn Pathol 1994; 11(1): 39–46.

370. Wijnaendts LC, van der Linden JC, van Unnik AJ, et al. Histopathological classification of childhood rhabdomyosarcomas: relationship with clinical parameters and prognosis. Hum Pathol 1994; 25(9): 900–907.

371. Enzinger FM, Shiraki M. Alveolar rhabdomyosarcoma. An analysis of 110 cases. Cancer 1969; 24(1): 18–31.

372. Parham D. Pediatric small-cell tumors of soft tissue. In: Montgomery E, Aaron A, eds. Clinical pathology of soft tissue tumors. New York: Marcel Dekker; 2001: 543–600.

373. Sorensen PH, Shimada H, Liu XF, et al. Biphenotypic sarcomas with myogenic and neural differentiation express the Ewing's sarcoma EWS/FLI1 fusion gene. Cancer Res 1995; 55(6): 1385–1392.

374. Erlandson RA. The ultrastructural distinction between rhabdomyosarcoma and other undifferentiated 'sarcomas'. Ultrastruct Pathol 1987; 11(2–3): 83–101.

375. Cessna M, Zhou H, Perkins S, et al. Are myogenin and MyoD1 expression specific for rhabdomyosarcoma? A study of 150 cases with emphasis on spindle cell mimics. Am J Surg Pathol 2001; 25(9): 1150–1157.

376. Dias P, Parham DM, Shapiro DN, et al. Myogenic regulatory protein (MyoD1) expression in childhood solid tumors: diagnostic utility in rhabdomyosarcoma. Am J Pathol 1990; 137(6): 1283–1291.

377. Folpe AL. MyoD1 and myogenin expression in human neoplasia: a review and update. Adv Anat Pathol 2002; 9(3): 198–203.

378. Choi YW, Heath EI, Heitmiller R, et al. Mutations in beta-catenin and APC genes are uncommon in esophageal and esophagogastric junction adenocarcinomas. Mod Pathol 2000; 13(10): 1055–1059.

379. Davidson B, Nielsen S, Christensen J, et al. The role of desmin and N-cadherin in effusion cytology: a comparative study using established markers of mesothelial and epithelial cells. Am J Surg Pathol 2001; 25(11): 1405–1412.

380. Gill SA, Meier PA, Kendall BS. Use of desmin immunohistochemistry to distinguish between mesothelial cells and carcinoma in serous fluid cell block preparations. Acta Cytol 2000; 44(6): 976–980.

381. Hurlimann J. Desmin and neural marker expression in mesothelial cells and mesotheliomas. Hum Pathol 1994; 25(8): 753–757.

382. Chen B, Dias P, Jenkins JJ III, et al. Methylation alterations of the MyoD1 upstream region are predictive of subclassification of human rhabdomyosarcomas. Am J Pathol 1998; 152(4): 1071–1079.

383. Sorensen PH, Lynch JC, Qualman SJ, et al. PAX3–FKHR and PAX7–FKHR gene fusions are prognostic indicators in alveolar rhabdomyosarcoma: a report from the children's oncology group. J Clin Oncol 2002; 20(11): 2672–2679.

384. Douglass EC, Rowe ST, Valentine M, et al. Variant translocations of chromosome 13 in alveolar rhabdomyosarcoma. Genes Chromosomes Cancer 1991; 3(6): 480–482.

385. Barr FG, Qualman SJ, Macris MH, et al. Genetic heterogeneity in the alveolar rhabdomyosarcoma subset without typical gene fusions. Cancer Res 2002; 62(16): 4704–4710.

386. Douglass EC, Shapiro DN, Valentine M, et al. Alveolar rhabdomyosarcoma with the t(2; 13): cytogenetic findings and clinicopathologic correlations. Med Pediatr Oncol 1993; 21(2): 83–87.

387. Shapiro DN, Sublett JE, Li B, et al. Fusion of PAX3 to a member of the forkhead family of transcription factors in human alveolar rhabdomyosarcoma. Cancer Res 1993; 53(21): 5108–5112.

388. Shapiro DN, Valentine MB, Sublett JE, et al. Chromosomal sublocalization of the 2; 13 translocation breakpoint in alveolar rhabdomyosarcoma. Genes Chromosomes Cancer 1992; 4(3): 241–249.

389. Bridge JA, Liu J, Weibolt V, et al. Novel genomic imbalances in embryonal rhabdomyosarcoma revealed by comparative genomic hybridization and fluorescence in situ hybridization: an intergroup rhabdomyosarcoma study. Genes Chromosomes Cancer 2000; 27(4): 337–344.

390. Stout A. Rhabdomyosarcoma of the skeletal muscle. Ann Surg Oncol 1946; 123:447–472.

391. Schurch W, Begin LR, Seemayer TA, et al. Pleomorphic soft tissue myogenic sarcomas of adulthood. A reappraisal in the mid-1990s. Am J Surg Pathol 1996; 20(2): 131–147.

392. Ali SZ, Smilari TF, Teichberg S, Hajdu SI. Pleomorphic rhabdomyosarcoma of the heart metastatic to bone. Report of a case with fine needle aspiration biopsy findings. Acta Cytol 1995; 39(3): 555–558.

393. Guillou L, Coquet M, Chaubert P, Coindre JM. Skeletal muscle regeneration mimicking rhabdomyosarcoma: a potential diagnostic pitfall. Histopathology 1998; 33(2): 136–144.

394. Sonobe H, Takeuchi T, Taguchi T, et al. A new human pleomorphic rhabdomyosarcoma cell-line, HS-RMS-1, exhibiting MyoD1 and myogenin. Int J Oncol 2000; 17(1): 119–125.

395. Masson P. Hemangioendotheliome vegetant intravasculaire. Bull Soc Anat Paris 1923; 93: 517–523.

396. Kasabach H, Merritt K. Capillary hemangioma with extensive purpura: Report of a case. Am J Dis Child 1940; 59: 1063–1070.

397. Klippel M, Trenaunay P. Du naevus variqueux osteo-hypertrophique. Arch Gen Med (Paris) 1900; 185: 641–672.

398. Parkes Weber F. Angioma formation in connection with hypertrophy of limbs and hemihypertrophy. Br J Dermatol 1907; 19: 231–235.

399. Beham A, Fletcher CD. Intramuscular angioma: a clinicopathological analysis of 74 cases. Histopathology 1991; 18(1): 53–59.

400. Watson W, McCarthy W. Blood and blood vessel tumors: 1056 cases. Surg Gynecol Obstet 1940; 71: 569–588.

401. Allen PW, Enzinger FM. Hemangioma of skeletal muscle. An analysis of 89 cases. Cancer 1972; 29(1): 8–22.

402. Rao VK, Weiss SW. Angiomatosis of soft tissue. An analysis of the histologic features and clinical outcome in 51 cases. Am J Surg Pathol 1992; 16(8): 764–771.

403. Howat AJ, Campbell PE. Angiomatosis: a vascular malformation of infancy and childhood. Report of 17 cases. Pathology 1987; 19(4): 377–382.

404. Weiss SW, Enzinger FM. Spindle cell hemangioendothelioma. A low-grade angiosarcoma resembling a cavernous hemangioma and Kaposi's sarcoma. Am J Surg Pathol 1986; 10(8): 521–530.

405. Perkins P, Weiss SW. Spindle cell hemangioendothelioma. An analysis of 78 cases with reassessment of its pathogenesis and biologic behavior. Am J Surg Pathol 1996; 20(10): 1196–204.

406. Dabska M. Malignant endovascular papillary angioendothelioma of the skin in childhood. Clinicopathologic study of 6 cases. Cancer 1969; 24(3): 503–510.

407. Quecedo E, Martinez-Escribano JA, Febrer I, et al. Dabska tumor developing within a preexisting vascular malformation. Am J Dermatopathol 1996; 18(3): 302–307.

408. Argani P, Athanasian E. Malignant endovascular papillary angioendothelioma (Dabska tumor) arising within a deep intramuscular hemangioma. Arch Pathol Lab Med 1997; 121(9): 992–5.

409. Yamada A, Uematsu K, Yasoshima H, et al. Endovascular papillary angioendothelioma (Dabska tumor) in an elderly woman. Pathol Int 1998; 48(2): 164–7.

410. Fukunaga M. Endovascular papillary angioendothelioma (Dabska tumor). Pathol Int 1998; 48(10): 840–1.

411. McCarthy EF, Lietman S, Argani P, Frassica FJ. Endovascular papillary angioendothelioma (Dabska tumor) of bone. Skeletal Radiol 1999; 28(2): 100–3.

412. Schwartz RA, Dabski C, Dabska M. The Dabska tumor: a thirty-year retrospect. Dermatology 2000; 201(1): 1–5.

413. Fanburg-Smith JC, Michal M, Partanen TA, Alitalo K, Miettinen M. Papillary intralymphatic angioendothelioma (PILA): a report of twelve cases of a distinctive vascular tumor with phenotypic features of lymphatic vessels. Am J Surg Pathol 1999; 23(9): 1004–10.

414. Calonje E, Fletcher CD, Wilson-Jones E, Rosai J. Retiform hemangioendothelioma. A distinctive form of low-grade angiosarcoma delineated in a series of 15 cases. Am J Surg Pathol 1994; 18(2): 115–125.

415. Duke D, Dvorak A, Harris TJ, Cohen LM. Multiple retiform hemangioendotheliomas. A low-grade angiosarcoma. Am J Dermatopathol 1996; 18(6): 606–610.

416. Sanz-Trelles A, Rodrigo-Fernandez I, Ayala-Carbonero A, Contreras-Rubio F. Retiform hemangioendothelioma. A new case in a child with diffuse endovascular papillary endothelial proliferation. J Cutan Pathol 1997; 24(7): 440–444.

417. Schommer M, Herbst RA, Brodersen JP, et al. Retiform hemangioendothelioma: another tumor associated with human herpesvirus type 8? J Am Acad Dermatol 2000; 42(2 Pt 1): 290–292.

418. Mac-Moune Lai F, To KF, Choi PC, et al. Kaposiform hemangioendothelioma: five patients with cutaneous lesion and long follow-up. Mod Pathol 2001; 14(11): 1087–1092.

419. Mentzel T, Mazzoleni G, Dei Tos AP, Fletcher CD. Kaposiform hemangioendothelioma in adults. Clinicopathologic and immunohistochemical analysis of three cases. Am J Clin Pathol 1997; 108(4): 450–455.

420. Zukerberg LR, Nickoloff BJ, Weiss SW. Kaposiform hemangioendothelioma of infancy and childhood. An aggressive neoplasm associated with Kasabach–Merritt syndrome and lymphangiomatosis. Am J Surg Pathol 1993; 17(4): 321–328.

421. Dail DH, Liebow AA, Gmelich JT, et al. Intravascular, bronchiolar, and alveolar tumor of the lung (IVBAT). An analysis of twenty cases of a peculiar sclerosing endothelial tumor. Cancer 1983; 51(3): 452–464.

422. Ishak KG, Sesterhenn IA, Goodman ZD, et al. Epithelioid hemangioendothelioma of the liver: a clinicopathologic and follow-up study of 32 cases. Hum Pathol 1984; 15(9): 839–852.

423. Weiss SW, Ishak KG, Dail DH, et al. Epithelioid hemangioendothelioma and related lesions. Semin Diagn Pathol 1986; 3(4): 259–287.

424. Weiss SW, Enzinger FM. Epithelioid hemangioendothelioma: a vascular tumor often mistaken for a carcinoma. Cancer 1982; 50(5): 970–981.

425. Tsuneyoshi M, Dorfman HD, Bauer TW. Epithelioid hemangioendothelioma of bone. A clinicopathologic, ultrastructural, and immunohistochemical study. Am J Surg Pathol 1986; 10(11): 754–764.

426. Makhlouf HR, Ishak KG, Goodman ZD. Epithelioid hemangioendothelioma of the liver: a clinicopathologic study of 137 cases. Cancer 1999; 85(3): 562–582.

427. McKenney JK, Weiss SW, Folpe AL. CD31 expression in intratumoral macrophages: a potential diagnostic pitfall. Am J Surg Pathol 2001; 25(9): 1167–1173.

428. Folpe AL, Chand EM, Goldblum JR, Weiss SW. Expression of Fli-1, a nuclear transcription factor, distinguishes vascular neoplasms from potential mimics. Am J Surg Pathol 2001; 25(8): 1061–1066.

429. Folpe AL, Hill CE, Parham DM, et al. Immunohistochemical detection of FLI-1 protein expression: a study of 132 round cell tumors with emphasis on CD99-positive mimics of Ewing's sarcoma/primitive neuroectodermal tumor. Am J Surg Pathol 2000; 24(12): 1657–1662.

430. Kaposi M. Idiopathic multiple pigmented sarcomas of the skin. Arch F Dermatol Syph 1872; 4: 265–273. (Translated from German in CA Cancer J Clin 1982; 32: 342–347.)

431. Krown SE. Acquired immunodeficiency syndrome-associated Kaposi's sarcoma. Biology and management. Med Clin North Am 1997; 81(2): 471–494.

432. Safai B, Mike V, Giraldo G, et al. Association of Kaposi's sarcoma with second primary malignancies: possible etiopathogenic implications. Cancer 1980; 45(6): 1472–1479.

433. Ziegler JL, Templeton AC, Vogel CL. Kaposi's sarcoma: a comparison of classical, endemic, and epidemic forms. Semin Oncol 1984; 11(1): 47–52.

434. Taylor JF, Templeton AC, Vogel CL, et al. Kaposi's sarcoma in Uganda: a clinico-pathological study. Int J Cancer 1971; 8(1): 122–135.

435. Templeton AC. Kaposi's sarcoma. Pathol Annu 1981; 16(Pt 2): 315–336.

436. Beral V, Peterman TA, Berkelman RL, Jaffe HW. Kaposi's sarcoma among persons with AIDS: a sexually transmitted infection? Lancet 1990; 335(8682): 123–128.

437. Eltom MA, Jemal A, Mbulaiteye SM, et al. Trends in Kaposi's sarcoma and non-Hodgkin's lymphoma incidence in the United States from 1973 through 1998. J Natl Cancer Inst 2002; 94(16): 1204–1210.

438. Cattelan AM, Trevenzoli M, Aversa SM. Recent advances in the treatment of AIDS-related Kaposi's sarcoma. Am J Clin Dermatol 2002; 3(7): 451–462.

439. Chang Y, Cesarman E, Pessin MS, et al. Identification of herpesvirus-like DNA sequences in AIDS-associated Kaposi's sarcoma. Science 1994; 266(5192): 1865–1869.

440. Knowles DM, Cesarman E. The Kaposi's sarcoma-associated herpesvirus (human herpesvirus-8) in Kaposi's sarcoma, malignant lymphoma, and other diseases. Ann Oncol 1997; 8 Suppl 2: 123–129.

441. Cesarman E, Knowles DM. Kaposi's sarcoma-associated herpesvirus: a lymphotropic human herpesvirus associated with Kaposi's sarcoma, primary effusion lymphoma, and multicentric Castleman's disease. Semin Diagn Pathol 1997; 14(1): 54–66.

442. Nador RG, Milligan LL, Flore O, et al. Expression of Kaposi's sarcoma-associated herpesvirus G protein-coupled receptor monocistronic and bicistronic transcripts in primary effusion lymphomas. Virology 2001; 287(1): 62–70.

443. Moore PS, Gao SJ, Dominguez G, et al. Primary characterization of a herpesvirus agent associated with Kaposi's sarcomae. J Virol 1996; 70(1): 549–558.

444. Mesri EA, Cesarman E, Arvanitakis L, et al. Human herpesvirus-8/Kaposi's sarcoma-associated herpesvirus is a new transmissible virus that infects B cells. J Exp Med 1996; 183(5): 2385–2390.

445. Boivin G, Cote S, Cloutier N, et al. Quantification of human herpesvirus 8 by real-time PCR in blood fractions of AIDS patients with Kaposi's sarcoma and multicentric Castleman's disease. J Med Virol 2002; 68(3): 399–403.

446. Hengge UR, Ruzicka T, Tyring SK, et al. Update on Kaposi's sarcoma and other HHV8 associated diseases. Part 2: pathogenesis, Castleman's disease, and pleural effusion lymphoma. Lancet Infect Dis 2002; 2(6): 344–352.

447. Reizis Z, Trattner A, Katzenelson V, et al. Flow cytometric DNA analysis of classic and steroid-induced Kaposi's sarcoma. Br J Dermatol 1995; 132(4): 548–550.

448. Eto H, Toriyama K, Tsuda N, et al. Flow cytometric DNA analysis of vascular soft tissue tumors, including African endemic-type Kaposi's sarcoma. Hum Pathol 1992; 23(9): 1055–1060.

449. Fukunaga M, Silverberg SG. Kaposi's sarcoma in patients with acquired immune deficiency syndrome. A flow cytometric DNA analysis of 26 lesions in 21 patients. Cancer 1990; 66(4): 758–764.

450. Bisceglia M, Bosman C, Quirke P. A histologic and flow cytometric study of Kaposi's sarcoma. Cancer 1992; 69(3): 793–798.

451. Davis DA, Scott DM. Lymphangioma-like Kaposi's sarcoma: etiology and literature review. J Am Acad Dermatol 2000; 43(1 Pt 1): 123–127.

452. Noel JC, de Thier F, de Dobbeleer G, Heenen M. Demonstration of herpes virus 8 in a lymphangioma-like Kaposi's sarcoma occurring in a non-immunosuppressed patient. Dermatology 1997; 194(1): 90–91.

453. Bossuyt L, Van den Oord JJ, Degreef H. Lymphangioma-like variant of AIDS-associated Kaposi's sarcoma with pronounced edema formation. Dermatology 1995; 190(4): 324–326.

454. Leibowitz MR, Dagliotti M, Smith E, Murray JF. Rapidly fatal lymphangioma-like Kaposi's sarcoma. Histopathology 1980; 4(5): 559–566.

455. Gange RW, Jones EW. Lymphangioma-like Kaposi's sarcoma. A report of three cases. Br J Dermatol 1979; 100(3): 327–334.

456. Cossu S, Satta R, Cottoni F, Massarelli G. Lymphangioma-like variant of Kaposi's sarcoma: clinicopathologic study of seven cases with review of the literature. Am J Dermatopathol 1997; 19(1): 16–22.

457. Smith KJ, Skelton HG, James WD, et al. Angiosarcoma arising in Kaposi's sarcoma (pleomorphic Kaposi's sarcoma) in a patient with human immunodeficiency virus disease. Armed Forces Retroviral Research Group. J Am Acad Dermatol 1991; 24(5 Pt 1): 790–792.

458. Steiner MC, Smith ME, Spittle MF. A patient with classical Kaposi's sarcoma and angiosarcoma: bad luck or a common aetiology? Clin Oncol 1997; 9(3): 186–188.

459. Chan JK, Warnke RA, Dorfman R. Vascular transformation of sinuses in lymph nodes. A study of its morphological spectrum and distinction from Kaposi's sarcoma. Am J Surg Pathol 1991; 15(8): 732–743.

460. Chan JK, Frizzera G, Fletcher CD, Rosai J. Primary vascular tumors of lymph nodes other than Kaposi's

sarcoma. Analysis of 39 cases and delineation of two new entities. Am J Surg Pathol 1992; 16(4): 335–350.

461. Guillou L, Fletcher CD. Benign lymphangioendothelioma (acquired progressive lymphangioma): a lesion not to be confused with well-differentiated angiosarcoma and patch stage Kaposi's sarcoma: clinicopathologic analysis of a series. Am J Surg Pathol 2000; 24(8): 1047–1057.

462. Grunwald MH, Amichai B, Avinoach I. Acquired progressive lymphangioma. J Am Acad Dermatol 1997; 37(4): 656–657.

463. Kato N, Isu K, Kikuta H. Absence of human herpesvirus 8/Kaposi's sarcoma-associated herpesvirus in a case of benign lymphangioendothelioma associated with periosteal haemangioma. Br J Dermatol 2002; 146(1): 157–159.

464. Jones EW, Winkelmann RK, Zachary CB, Reda AM. Benign lymphangioendothelioma. J Am Acad Dermatol 1990; 23(2 Pt 1): 229–235.

465. Sevila A, Botella-Estrada R, Sanmartin O, et al. Benign lymphangioendothelioma of the thigh simulating a low-grade angiosarcoma. Am J Dermatopathol 2000; 22(2): 151–154.

466. Soohoo L, Mercurio MG, Brody R, Zaim MT. An acquired vascular lesion in a child. Acquired progressive lymphangioma. Arch Dermatol 1995; 131(3): 341–345.

467. Maddox JC, Evans HL. Angiosarcoma of skin and soft tissue: a study of forty-four cases. Cancer 1981; 48(8): 1907–1921.

468. Haustein UF. Angiosarcoma of the face and scalp. Int J Dermatol 1991; 30(12): 851–856.

469. Holden CA, Wilson Jones E. Angiosarcoma of the face and scalp. J R Soc Med 1985; 78(Suppl 11): 30–31.

470. Holden CA, Spittle MF, Jones EW. Angiosarcoma of the face and scalp, prognosis and treatment. Cancer 1987; 59(5): 1046–1057.

471. Holden CA, Spaull J, Das AK, et al. The histogenesis of angiosarcoma of the face and scalp: an immunohistochemical and ultrastructural study. Histopathology 1987; 11(1): 37–51.

472. Nakazono T, Kudo S, Matsuo Y, et al. Angiosarcoma associated with chronic lymphedema (Stewart–Treves syndrome) of the leg: MR imaging. Skeletal Radiol 2000; 29(7): 413–416.

473. Trattner A, Shamai-Lubovitz O, Segal R, Zelikovski A. Stewart–Treves angiosarcoma of arm and ipsilateral breast in post-traumatic lymphedema. Lymphology 1996; 29(2): 57–59.

474. Kirchmann TT, Smoller BR, McGuire J. Cutaneous angiosarcoma as a second malignancy in a lymphedematous leg in a Hodgkin's disease survivor. J Am Acad Dermatol 1994; 31(5 Pt 2): 861–866.

475. Chen KT, Bauer V, Flam MS. Angiosarcoma in postsurgical lymphedema. An unusual occurrence in a man. Am J Dermatopathol 1991; 13(5): 488–492.

476. Schmitz-Rixen T, Horsch S, Arnold G, Peters PE. Angiosarcoma in primary lymphedema of the lower extremity – Stewart–Treves syndrome. Lymphology 1984; 17(2): 50–53.

477. McBride CM, Reeder JW, Smith JL. Angiosarcoma in the lymphedematous limb. South Med J 1969; 62(4): 378–380.

478. Shaw MB, Vycital RO. Angiosarcoma: a complication of postoperative lymphedema of the extremity. Clin Orthop 1968; 56:51–56.

479. Baes H. Angiosarcoma in a chronic lymphedematous leg. Dermatologica 1967; 134(5): 331–336.

480. Polgar C, Orosz Z, Szerdahelyi A, et al. Postirradiation angiosarcoma of the chest wall and breast: issues of radiogenic origin, diagnosis and treatment in two cases. Oncology 2001; 60(1): 31–34.

481. Yasumatsu R, Hirakawa N, Tomita K. Postradiation angiosarcoma of the tongue. Eur Arch Otorhinolaryngol 2000; 257(8): 464–465.

482. Vesoulis Z, Cunliffe C. Fine-needle aspiration biopsy of postradiation epithelioid angiosarcoma of breast. Diagn Cytopathol 2000; 22(3): 172–175.

483. Aitola P, Poutiainen A, Nordback I. Small-bowel angiosarcoma after pelvic irradiation: a report of two cases. Int J Colorectal Dis 1999; 14(6): 308–310.

484. Williams EV, Banerjee D, Dallimore N, Monypenny IJ. Angiosarcoma of the breast following radiation therapy. Eur J Surg Oncol 1999; 25(2): 221–222.

485. Edeiken S, Russo DP, Knecht J, Parry LA, Thompson RM. Angiosarcoma after tylectomy and radiation therapy for carcinoma of the breast. Cancer 1992; 70(3): 644–647.

486. Stokkel MP, Peterse HL. Angiosarcoma of the breast after lumpectomy and radiation therapy for adenocarcinoma. Cancer 1992; 69(12): 2965–2968.

487. Nanus DM, Kelsen D, Clark DG. Radiation-induced angiosarcoma. Cancer 1987; 60(4): 777–779.

488. Caldwell JB, Ryan MT, Benson PM, James WD. Cutaneous angiosarcoma arising in the radiation site of a congenital hemangioma. J Am Acad Dermatol 1995; 33(5 Pt 2): 865–870.

489. Parham DM, Fisher C. Angiosarcomas of the breast developing post radiotherapy. Histopathology 1997; 31(2): 189–195.

490. Ben-Izhak O, Kerner H, Brenner B, Lichtig C. Angiosarcoma of the colon developing in a capsule of a foreign body. Report of a case with associated hemorrhagic diathesis. Am J Clin Pathol 1992; 97(3): 416–420.

491. Jennings TA, Peterson L, Axiotis CA, et al. Angiosarcoma associated with foreign body material. A report of three cases. Cancer 1988; 62(11): 2436–2444.

492. Hayman J, Huygens H. Angiosarcoma developing around a foreign body. J Clin Pathol 1983; 36(5): 515–518.

493. Wehrli BM, Janzen DL, Shokeir O, et al. Epithelioid angiosarcoma arising in a surgically constructed arteriovenous fistula: a rare complication of chronic immunosuppression in the setting of renal transplantation. Am J Surg Pathol 1998; 22(9): 1154–1159.

494. Bessis D, Sotto A, Roubert P, et al. Endothelin-secreting angiosarcoma occurring at the site of an arteriovenous fistula for haemodialysis in a renal transplant recipient. Br J Dermatol 1998; 138(2): 361–363.

495. Byers RJ, McMahon RF, Freemont AJ, et al. Angiosarcoma at the site of a ligated arteriovenous fistula in a renal transplant recipient. Nephrol Dial Transplant 1994; 9(1): 112.

496. Keane MM, Carney DN. Angiosarcoma arising from a defunctionalized arteriovenous fistula. J Urol 1993; 149(2): 364–365.

497. Byers RJ, McMahon RF, Freemont AJ, et al. Epithelioid angiosarcoma arising in an arteriovenous fistula. Histopathology 1992; 21(1): 87–89.

498. Faggioli GL, Bertoni F, Bacchini P, et al. Angiosarcoma in a limb with arteriovenous fistulas and elephantiasis. Int Angiol 1989; 8(3): 161–170.

499. Andreu V, Elizalde I, Mallafre C, et al. Plexiform neurofibromatosis and angiosarcoma of the liver in von Recklinghausen disease. Am J Gastroenterol 1997; 92(7): 1229–1230.

500. Brown RW, Tornos C, Evans HL. Angiosarcoma arising from malignant schwannoma in a patient with neurofibromatosis. Cancer 1992; 70(5): 1141–1144.

501. Lederman SM, Martin EC, Laffey KT, Lefkowitch JH. Hepatic neurofibromatosis, malignant schwannoma, and angiosarcoma in von Recklinghausen's disease. Gastroenterology 1987; 92(1): 234–239.

502. Riccardi VM, Wheeler TM, Pickard LR, King B. The pathophysiology of neurofibromatosis. II. Angiosarcoma as a complication. Cancer Genet Cytogenet 1984; 12(3): 275–280.

503. Millstein DI, Tang CK, Campbell EW. Angiosarcoma developing in a patient with Neurofibromatosis (von Recklinghausen's disease). Cancer 1981; 47(5): 950–954.

504. Falk H, Telles NC, Ishak KG, et al. Eidemiology of thorotrast-induced hepatic angiosarcoma in the United States. Environ Res 1979; 18(1): 65–73.

505. Ito Y, Kojiro M, Nakashima T, Mori T. Pathomorphologic characteristics of 102 cases of thorotrast-related hepatocellular carcinoma, cholangiocarcinoma, and hepatic angiosarcoma. Cancer 1988; 62(6): 1153–1162.

506. Popper H, Thomas LB, Telles NC, et al. Development of hepatic angiosarcoma in man induced by vinyl chloride, thorotrast, and arsenic. Comparison with cases of unknown etiology. Am J Pathol 1978; 92(2): 349–369.

507. Falk H, Caldwell GG, Ishak KG, et al. Arsenic-related hepatic angiosarcoma. Am J Ind Med 1981; 2(1): 43–50.

508. Falk H. Vinyl chloride-induced hepatic angiosarcoma. Princess Takamatsu Symp 1987; 18:39–46.

509. Stewart F, Treves N. Lymphangiosarcoma in postmastectomy lymphedema. Cancer 1948; 1:64–81.

510. Mackenzie DH. Lymphangiosarcoma arising in chronic congenital and idiopathic lymphoedema. J Clin Pathol 1971; 24(6): 524–529.

511. Diaz-Cascajo C, Borghi S, Weyers W, et al. Benign lymphangiomatous papules of the skin following radiotherapy: a report of five new cases and review of the literature. Histopathology 1999; 35(4): 319–327.

512. Fineberg S, Rosen PP. Cutaneous angiosarcoma and atypical vascular lesions of the skin and breast after radiation therapy for breast carcinoma. Am J Clin Pathol 1994; 102(6): 757–763.

513. Fletcher CD, Beham A, Bekir S, et al. Epithelioid angiosarcoma of deep soft tissue: a distinctive tumor readily mistaken for an epithelial neoplasm. Am J Surg Pathol 1991; 15(10): 915–924.

514. Meis-Kindblom JM, Kindblom LG. Angiosarcoma of soft tissue: a study of 80 cases. Am J Surg Pathol 1998; 22(6): 683–697.

515. Enzinger FM, Smith BH. Hemangiopericytoma. An analysis of 106 cases. Hum Pathol 1976; 7(1): 61–82.

516. Miettinen MM, el-Rifai W, Sarlomo-Rikala M, et al. Tumor size-related DNA copy number changes occur in solitary fibrous tumors but not in hemangiopericytomas. Mod Pathol 1997; 10(12): 1194–1200.

517. Ceballos KM, Munk PL, Masri BA, O'Connell JX. Lipomatous hemangiopericytoma: a morphologically distinct soft tissue tumor. Arch Pathol Lab Med 1999; 123(10): 941–945.

518. Folpe AL, Devaney K, Weiss SW. Lipomatous hemangiopericytoma: a rare variant of hemangiopericytoma that may be confused with liposarcoma. Am J Surg Pathol 1999; 23(10): 1201–1207.

519. Guillou L, Gebhard S, Coindre JM. Lipomatous hemangiopericytoma: a fat-containing variant of solitary fibrous tumor? Clinicopathologic, immunohistochemical, and ultrastructural analysis of a series in favor of a unifying concept. Hum Pathol 2000; 31(9): 1108–1115.

520. Nielsen GP, Dickersin GR, Provenzal JM, Rosenberg AE. Lipomatous hemangiopericytoma. A histologic, ultrastructural and immunohistochemical study of a unique variant of hemangiopericytoma. Am J Surg Pathol 1995; 19(7): 748–756.

521. Vogrincic GS, O'Connell JX, Gilks CB. Giant cell tumor of tendon sheath is a polyclonal cellular proliferation. Hum Pathol 1997; 28(7): 815–819.

522. Ushijima M, Hashimoto H, Tsuneyoshi M, Enjoji M. Giant cell tumor of the tendon sheath (nodular tenosynovitis). A study of 207 cases to compare the large joint group with the common digit group. Cancer 1986; 57(4): 875–884.

523. O'Connell JX, Fanburg JC, Rosenberg AE. Giant cell tumor of tendon sheath and pigmented villonodular synovitis: immunophenotype suggests a synovial cell origin. Hum Pathol 1995; 26(7): 771–775.

524. Maluf HM, DeYoung BR, Swanson PE, Wick MR. Fibroma and giant cell tumor of tendon sheath: a comparative histological and immunohistological study. Mod Pathol 1995; 8(2): 155–1559.

525. Jaffee H, Lichtenstein L, Sutro C. Pigmented villonodular synovitis, bursitis, and tenosynovitis. A discussion of the synovial and bursal equivalents of the tenosynovial lesion commonly denoted as xanthoma, xanthogranuloma, giant cell tumor, or myeloplaxoma of the tendon sheath, with some consideration of this tendon sheath lesion itself. Arch Pathol 1941; 31: 731–765.

526. Bertoni F, Unni KK, Beabout JW, Sim FH. Malignant giant cell tumor of the tendon sheaths and joints (malignant pigmented villonodular synovitis). Am J Surg Pathol 1997; 21(2): 153–163.

527. Carter D, Otis CN. Three types of spindle cell tumors of the pleura. Fibroma, sarcoma, and sarcomatoid mesothelioma. Am J Surg Pathol 1988; 12(10): 747–753.

528. England DM, Hochholzer L, McCarthy MJ. Localized benign and malignant fibrous tumors of the pleura. A clinicopathologic review of 223 cases. Am J Surg Pathol 1989; 13(8): 640–658.

529. Witkin GB, Rosai J. Solitary fibrous tumor of the mediastinum. A report of 14 cases. Am J Surg Pathol 1989; 13(7): 547–557.

530. Witkin GB, Rosai J. Solitary fibrous tumor of the upper respiratory tract. A report of six cases. Am J Surg Pathol 1991; 15(9): 842–848.

531. Westra WH, Gerald WL, Rosai J. Solitary fibrous tumor. Consistent CD34 immunoreactivity and occurrence in the orbit. Am J Surg Pathol 1994; 18(10): 992–998.

532. Westra WH, Grenko RT, Epstein J. Solitary fibrous tumor of the lower urogenital tract: a report of five cases involving the seminal vesicles, urinary bladder, and prostate. Hum Pathol 2000; 31(1): 63–68.

533. Weidner N. Solitary fibrous tumor of the mediastinum. Ultrastruct Pathol 1991; 15(4–5): 489–492.

534. Zukerberg LR, Rosenberg AE, Randolph G, et al. Solitary fibrous tumor of the nasal cavity and paranasal sinuses. Am J Surg Pathol 1991; 15(2): 126–130.

535. Khalifa MA, Montgomery EA, Azumi N, et al. Solitary fibrous tumors: a series of lesions, some in unusual sites. South Med J 1997; 90(8): 793–799.

536. Van de Rijn M, Lombard CM, Rouse RV. Expression of CD34 by solitary fibrous tumors of the pleura, mediastinum, and lung. Am J Surg Pathol 1994; 18(8): 814–820.

537. Flint A, Weiss SW. CD-34 and keratin expression distinguishes solitary fibrous tumor (fibrous mesothelioma) of pleura from desmoplastic mesothelioma. Hum Pathol 1995; 26(4): 428–431.

538. Caruso RA, LaSpada F, Gaeta M, et al. Report of an intrapulmonary solitary fibrous tumor: fine-needle aspiration cytologic findings, clinicopathological, and immunohistochemical features. Diagn Cytopathol 1996; 14(1): 64–67.

539. Weynand B, Noel H, Goncette L, et al. Solitary fibrous tumor of the pleura: a report of five cases diagnosed by transthoracic cutting needle biopsy. Chest 1997; 112(5): 1424–1428.

540. Thomas TM, Myint A, Mak CK, Chan JK. Mammary myofibroblastoma with leiomyomatous differentiation. Am J Clin Pathol 1997; 107(1): 52–55.

541. Fukunaga M, Endo Y, Ushigome S. Atypical leiomyomatous features in myofibroblastoma of the breast [letter]. Histopathology 1996; 29(6): 592–593.

542. Fukunaga M, Ushigome S. Myofibroblastoma of the breast with diverse differentiations. Arch Pathol Lab Med 1997; 121(6): 599–603.

543. Das Gupta TK, Brasfield RD, Strong EW, Hajdu SI. Benign solitary Schwannomas (neurilemomas). Cancer 1969; 24(2): 355–366.

544. Hasegawa SL, Mentzel T, Fletcher CD. Schwannomas of the sinonasal tract and nasopharynx. Mod Pathol 1997; 10(8): 777–784.

545. Enzinger FM, Weiss SW, Liang CY. Ossifying fibromyxoid tumor of soft parts. A clinicopathological analysis of 59 cases. Am J Surg Pathol 1989; 13(10): 817–827.

546. Miettinen M. Ossifying fibromyxoid tumor of soft parts. Additional observations of a distinctive soft tissue tumor. Am J Clin Pathol 1991; 95(2): 142–149.

547. Hanski W, Lewicki Z. New observations on three cases of ossifying fibromyxoid tumor of soft parts. Pol J Pathol 1994; 45(3): 231–238.

548. Donner LR. Ossifying fibromyxoid tumor of soft parts: evidence supporting Schwann cell origin. Hum Pathol 1992; 23(2): 200–202.

549. Yang P, Hirose T, Hasegawa T, et al. Ossifying fibromyxoid tumor of soft parts: a morphological and immunohistochemical study. Pathol Int 1994; 44(6): 448–453.

550. Fisher C, Hedges M, Weiss SW. Ossifying fibromyxoid tumor of soft parts with stromal cyst formation and ribosome-lamella complexes. Ultrastruct Pathol 1994; 18(6): 593–600.

551. Kilpatrick SE, Ward WG, Mozes M, et al. Atypical and malignant variants of ossifying fibromyxoid tumor. Clinicopathologic analysis of six cases. Am J Surg Pathol 1995; 19(9): 1039–1046.

552. Zamecnik M, Michal M, Simpson RH, et al. Ossifying fibromyxoid tumor of soft parts: a report of 17 cases with emphasis on unusual histological features. Ann Diagn Pathol 1997; 1(2): 73–81.

553. Ekfors TO, Kulju T, Aaltonen M, Kallajoki M. Ossifying fibromyxoid tumour of soft parts: report of four cases including one mediastinal and one infantile. Apmis 1998; 106(12): 1124–1130.

554. Matsumoto K, Yamamoto T, Min W, et al. Ossifying fibromyxoid tumor of soft parts: clinicopathologic, immunohistochemical and ultrastructural study of four cases. Pathol Int 1999; 49(8): 742–746.

555. Shet T, Desai S, Kane S, Vora I. Nerve cell markers in ossifying fibromyxoid tumour of soft parts. Indian J Pathol Microbiol 2001; 44(2): 163–167.

556. Nishio J, Iwasaki H, Ohjimi Y, et al. Ossifying fibromyxoid tumor of soft parts. Cytogenetic findings. Cancer Genet Cytogenet 2002; 133(2): 124–128.

557. Sovani V, Velagaleti GV, Filipowicz E, et al. Ossifying fibromyxoid tumor of soft parts: report of a case with novel cytogenetic findings. Cancer Genet Cytogenet 2001; 127(1): 1–6.

558. Minami R, Yamamoto T, Tsukamoto R, Maeda S. Fine needle aspiration cytology of the malignant variant of ossifying fibromyxoid tumor of soft parts: a case report. Acta Cytol 2001; 45(5): 745–755.

559. Folpe A, Weiss S. Ossifying fibromyxoid tumor of soft parts: a clinicopathologic study of 66 cases with emphasis on atypical and malignant variants. Mod Pathol 2002; 15:14A (abstract 46).

560. Schofield JB, Krausz T, Stamp GW, et al. Ossifying fibromyxoid tumour of soft parts: immunohistochemical and ultrastructural analysis. Histopathology 1993; 22(2): 101–112.

561. Williams SB, Ellis GL, Meis JM, Heffner DK. Ossifying fibromyxoid tumour (of soft parts) of the head and neck: a clinicopathological and immunohistochemical study of nine cases. J Laryngol Otol 1993; 107(1): 75–80.

562. Enzinger F. Clear cell sarcoma of tendons and aponeuroses: an analysis of 21 cases. Cancer 1965; 18: 1163–1174.

563. Bearman RM, Noe J, Kempson RL. Clear cell sarcoma with melanin pigment. Cancer 1975; 36(3): 977–984.

564. Benson JD, Kraemer BB, Mackay B. Malignant melanoma of soft parts: an ultrastructural study of four cases. Ultrastruct Pathol 1985; 8(1): 57–70.

565. Chung EB, Enzinger FM. Malignant melanoma of soft parts. A reassessment of clear cell sarcoma. Am J Surg Pathol 1983; 7(5): 405–413.

566. Ekfors TO, Kujari H, Isomaki M. Clear cell sarcoma of tendons and aponeuroses (malignant melanoma of soft parts) in the duodenum: the first visceral case. Histopathology 1993; 22(3): 255–259.

567. Ekfors TO, Rantakokko V. Clear cell sarcoma of tendons and aponeuroses: malignant melanoma of soft tissues? Report of four cases. Pathol Res Pract 1979; 165(4): 422–428.

568. Montgomery E, Meis J, Ramos A, et al. Clear cell sarcoma of tendons and aponeuroses. A clinicopathologic study of 58 cases with analysis of prognostic factors. Int J Surg Pathol 1993; 1: 89–100.

569. Sara AS, Evans HL, Benjamin RS. Malignant melanoma of soft parts (clear cell sarcoma). A study of 17 cases, with emphasis on prognostic factors. Cancer 1990; 65(2): 367–374.

570. Lucas DR, Nascimento AG, Sim FH. Clear cell sarcoma of soft tissues. Mayo Clinic experience with 35 cases. Am J Surg Pathol 1992; 16(12): 1197–1204.

571. Reeves BR, Fletcher CD, Gusterson BA. Translocation t(12; 22)(q13; q13) is a nonrandom rearrangement in clear cell sarcoma. Cancer Genet Cytogenet 1992; 64(2): 101–103.

572. Bridge JA, Sreekantaiah C, Neff JR, Sandberg AA. Cytogenetic findings in clear cell sarcoma of tendons and aponeuroses. Malignant melanoma of soft parts. Cancer Genet Cytogenet 1991; 52(1): 101–106.

573. Fujimura Y, Ohno T, Siddique H, et al. The *EWS-ATF-1* gene involved in malignant melanoma of soft parts with t(12; 22) chromosome translocation, encodes a constitutive transcriptional activator. Oncogene 1996; 12(1): 159–167.

574. Langezaal SM, Graadt van Roggen JF, Cleton-Jansen AM, et al. Malignant melanoma is genetically distinct from clear cell sarcoma of tendons and aponeurosis (malignant melanoma of soft parts). Br J Cancer 2001; 84(4): 535–538.

575. Mrozek K, Karakousis CP, Perez-Mesa C, Bloomfield CD. Translocation t(12; 22)(q13; q12.2–12.3) in a clear cell sarcoma of tendons and aponeuroses. Genes Chromosomes Cancer 1993; 6(4): 249–252.

576. Nedoszytko B, Mrozek K, Roszkiewicz A, et al. Clear cell sarcoma of tendons and aponeuroses with t(12; 22) (q13; q12) diagnosed initially as malignant melanoma. Cancer Genet Cytogenet 1996; 91(1): 37–39.

577. Zucman J, Delattre O, Desmaze C, et al. *EWS* and *ATF-1* gene fusion induced by t(12; 22) translocation in malignant melanoma of soft parts. Nat Genet 1993; 4(4): 341–345.

578. Antonescu CR, Tschernyavsky SJ, Woodruff JM, et al. Molecular diagnosis of clear cell sarcoma: detection of EWS-ATF1 and MITF-M transcripts and histopathological and ultrastructural analysis of 12 cases. J Mol Diagn 2002; 4(1): 44–52.

579. Fisher C, Schofield JB. S-100 protein positive synovial sarcoma. Histopathology 1991; 19(4): 375–377.

580. Laskin WB, Weiss SW, Bratthauer GL. Epithelioid variant of malignant peripheral nerve sheath tumor (malignant epithelioid schwannoma). Am J Surg Pathol 1991; 15(12): 1136–1145.

581. Thiele CJ, McKeon C, Triche TJ, et al. Differential protooncogene expression characterizes histopathologically indistinguishable tumors of the peripheral nervous system. J Clin Invest 1987; 80(3): 804–811.

582. Nickerson HJ, Matthay KK, Seeger RC, et al. Favorable biology and outcome of stage IV-S neuroblastoma with supportive care or minimal therapy: a Children's Cancer Group study. J Clin Oncol 2000; 18(3): 477–486.

583. Etoh T, Takahashi H, Ohnuma N, et al. Kinetics of cytotoxic T lymphocytes in stage IV-S neuroblastoma. J Pediatr Surg 1987; 22(4): 356–359.

584. Evans AE, Baum E, Chard R. Do infants with stage IV-S neuroblastoma need treatment? Arch Dis Child 1981; 56(4): 271–274.

585. Stevens MM. Stage IV-S neuroblastoma: disseminated malignancy with a favourable prognosis. Three case reports. Aust Paediatr J 1979; 15(1): 39–43.

586. Hayes FA, Green AA, Rao BN. Clinical manifestations of ganglioneuroma. Cancer 1989; 63(6): 1211–1214.

587. Umehara S, Nakagawa A, Matthay KK, et al. Histopathology defines prognostic subsets of ganglioneuroblastoma, nodular. Cancer 2000; 89(5): 1150–1161.

588. Aoyama C, Qualman SJ, Regan M, Shimada H. Histopathologic features of composite ganglioneuroblastoma. Immunohistochemical distinction of the stromal component is related to prognosis. Cancer 1990; 65(2): 255–264.

589. Shimada H, Chatten J, Newton WA Jr, et al. Histopathologic prognostic factors in neuroblastic tumors: definition of subtypes of ganglioneuroblastoma and an age-linked classification of neuroblastomas. J Natl Cancer Inst 1984; 73(2): 405–416.

590. Franquemont DW, Mills SE, Lack EE. Immunohistochemical detection of neuroblastomatous foci in composite adrenal pheochromocytoma-neuroblastoma. Am J Clin Pathol 1994; 102(2): 163–170.

591. Triche TJ, Tsokos M, Linnoila RI, et al. NSE in neuroblastoma and other round cell tumors of childhood. Prog Clin Biol Res 1985; 175: 295–317.

592. Tsokos M, Linnoila RI, Chandra RS, Triche TJ. Neuron-specific enolase in the diagnosis of neuroblastoma and other small, round-cell tumors in children. Hum Pathol 1984; 15(6): 575–584.

593. Pappo AS, Douglass EC, Meyer WH, et al. Use of HBA 71 and anti-beta 2-microglobulin to distinguish peripheral neuroepithelioma from neuroblastoma. Hum Pathol 1993; 24(8): 880–885.

594. Schwab M, Ellison J, Busch M, et al. Enhanced expression of the human gene N-myc consequent to amplification of DNA may contribute to malignant progression of neuroblastoma. Proc Natl Acad Sci USA 1984; 81(15): 4940–4944.

595. Rosen N, Reynolds CP, Thiele CJ, et al. Increased N-myc expression following progressive growth of human neuroblastoma. Cancer Res 1986; 46(8): 4139–4142.

596. Sorensen PH, Wu JK, Berean KW, et al. Olfactory neuroblastoma is a peripheral primitive neuroectodermal tumor related to Ewing sarcoma. Proc Natl Acad Sci USA 1996; 93(3): 1038–1043.

597. Argani P, Perez-Ordonez B, Xiao H, et al. Olfactory neuroblastoma is not related to the Ewing family of tumors: absence of EWS/FLI1 gene fusion and MIC2 expression. Am J Surg Pathol 1998; 22(4): 391–398.

598. Ewing J. Diffuse endothelioma of bone. Proc NY Pathol Soc 1921; 21:17–24.

599. Stout A. A tumor of the ulnar nerve. Proc NY Pathol Soc 1918; 18: 2–22.

600. Askin FB, Rosai J, Sibley RK, et al. Malignant small cell tumor of the thoracopulmonary region in childhood: a distinctive clinicopathologic entity of uncertain histogenesis. Cancer 1979; 43(6): 2438–2451.

601. Douglass EC, Rowe ST, Valentine M, et al. A second nonrandom translocation, der(16)t(1; 16)(q21; q13), in Ewing sarcoma and peripheral neuroectodermal tumor. Cytogenet Cell Genet 1990; 53(2–3): 87–90.

602. Downing JR, Head DR, Parham DM, et al. Detection of the (11; 22)(q24; q12) translocation of Ewing's sarcoma and peripheral neuroectodermal tumor by reverse transcription polymerase chain reaction. Am J Pathol 1993; 143(5): 1294–1300.

603. Sorensen PH, Lessnick SL, Lopez-Terrada D, et al. A second Ewing's sarcoma translocation, t(21; 22), fuses the EWS gene to another ETS-family transcription factor, ERG. Nat Genet 1994; 6(2): 146–151.

604. Weidner N, Tjoe J. Immunohistochemical profile of monoclonal antibody O13: antibody that recognizes glycoprotein p30/32MIC2 and is useful in diagnosing Ewing's sarcoma and peripheral neuroepithelioma. Am J Surg Pathol 1994; 18(5): 486–494.

605. Yunis EJ. Ewing's sarcoma and related small round cell neoplasms in children. Am J Surg Pathol 1986; 10 Suppl 1: 54–62.

606. Delattre O, Zucman J, Melot T, et al. The Ewing family of tumors – a subgroup of small-round-cell tumors defined by specific chimeric transcripts. N Engl J Med 1994; 331(5): 294–299.

607. Dehner LP. Primitive neuroectodermal tumor and Ewing's sarcoma. Am J Surg Pathol 1993; 17(1): 1–13.

608. Jimenez RE, Folpe AL, Lapham RL, et al. Primary Ewing's sarcoma/primitive neuroectodermal tumor of the kidney: a clinicopathologic and immunohistochemical analysis of 11 cases. Am J Surg Pathol 2002; 26(3): 320–327.

609. Raney RB, Asmar L, Newton WA Jr, et al. Ewing's sarcoma of soft tissues in childhood: a report from the Intergroup Rhabdomyosarcoma Study, 1972 to 1991. J Clin Oncol 1997; 15(2): 574–582.

610. Wexler LH, DeLaney TF, Tsokos M, et al. Ifosfamide and etoposide plus vincristine, doxorubicin, and cyclophosphamide for newly diagnosed Ewing's sarcoma family of tumors. Cancer 1996; 78(4): 901–911.

611. Gururangan S, Marina NM, Luo X, et al. Treatment of children with peripheral primitive neuroectodermal tumor or extraosseous Ewing's tumor with Ewing's-directed therapy. J Pediatr Hematol Oncol 1998; 20(1): 55–61.

612. Picci P, Bohling T, Bacci G, et al. Chemotherapy-induced tumor necrosis as a prognostic factor in localized Ewing's sarcoma of the extremities. J Clin Oncol 1997; 15(4): 1553–1559.

613. Bacci G, Ferrari S, Bertoni F, et al. Prognostic factors in nonmetastatic Ewing's sarcoma of bone treated with adjuvant chemotherapy: analysis of 359 patients at the Istituto Ortopedico Rizzoli. J Clin Oncol 2000; 18(1): 4–11.

614. Soule EH, Newton W Jr, Moon TE, Tefft M. Extraskeletal Ewing's sarcoma: a preliminary review of 26 cases encountered in the Intergroup Rhabdomyosarcoma Study. Cancer 1978; 42(1): 259–264.

615. Pinto A, Grant LH, Hayes FA, et al. Immunohistochemical expression of neuron-specific enolase and Leu 7 in Ewing's sarcoma of bone. Cancer 1989; 64(6): 1266–1273.

616. De Alava E, Kawai A, Healey JH, et al. EWS–FLI1 fusion transcript structure is an independent determinant of prognosis in Ewing's sarcoma. J Clin Oncol 1998; 16(4): 1248–1255.

617. Gerald WL, Miller HK, Battifora H, et al. Intra-abdominal desmoplastic small round-cell tumor. Report of 19 cases of a distinctive type of high-grade polyphenotypic malignancy affecting young individuals. Am J Surg Pathol 1991; 15(6): 499–513.

618. Choi JK, van Hoeven K, Brooks JJ, Gupta PK. Desmoplastic small round cell tumor presenting in pleural fluid and accompanied by desmin-positive mesothelial cells. Acta Cytol 1995; 39(2): 377–378.

619. Ohno T, Ouchida M, Lee L, et al. The EWS gene, involved in Ewing family of tumors, malignant melanoma of soft parts and desmoplastic small round cell tumors, codes for an RNA binding protein with novel regulatory domains. Oncogene 1994; 9(10): 3087–3097.

620. Prat J, Matias-Guiu X, Algaba F. Desmoplastic small round-cell tumor. Am J Surg Pathol 1992; 16(3): 306–307.

621. Sawyer JR, Tryka AF, Lewis JM. A novel reciprocal chromosome translocation t(11; 22)(p13; q12) in an intraabdominal desmoplastic small round-cell tumor. Am J Surg Pathol 1992; 16(4): 411–416.

622. Setrakian S, Gupta PK, Heald J, Brooks JJ. Intraabdominal desmoplastic small round cell tumor. Report of a case diagnosed by fine needle aspiration cytology. Acta Cytol 1992; 36(3): 373–376.

623. Bian Y, Jordan AG, Rupp M, et al. Effusion cytology of desmoplastic small round cell tumor of the pleura. A case report. Acta Cytol 1993; 37(1): 77–82.

624. Ladanyi M, Gerald W. Fusion of the EWS and WT1 genes in the desmoplastic small round cell tumor. Cancer Res 1994; 54(11): 2837–2840.

625. Parkash V, Gerald WL, Parma A, et al. Desmoplastic small round cell tumor of the pleura. Am J Surg Pathol 1995; 19(6): 659–665.

626. Ordonez NG. Desmoplastic small round cell tumor: I: a histopathologic study of 39 cases with emphasis on unusual histological patterns. Am J Surg Pathol 1998; 22(11): 1303–1313.

627. Perez RP, Zhang PJ. Detection of EWS–WT1 fusion mRNA in ascites of a patient with desmoplastic small round cell tumor by RT-PCR. Hum Pathol 1999; 30(2): 239–242.

628. Wolf AN, Ladanyi M, Paull G, et al. The expanding clinical spectrum of desmoplastic small round-cell tumor: a report of two cases with molecular confirmation. Hum Pathol 1999; 30(4): 430–435.

629. Insabato L, Di Vizio D, Lambertini M, et al. Fine needle aspiration cytology of desmoplastic small round cell tumor. A case report. Acta Cytol 1999; 43(4): 641–646.

630. Kawano N, Inayama Y, Nagashima Y, et al. Desmoplastic small round-cell tumor of the paratesticular region: report of an adult case with demonstration of EWS and WT1 gene fusion using paraffin-embedded tissue. Mod Pathol 1999; 12(7): 729–734.

631. Crapanzano JP, Cardillo M, Lin O, Zakowski MF. Cytology of desmoplastic small round cell tumor. Cancer 2002; 96(1): 21–31.

632. Finke NM, Lae ME, Lloyd RV, et al. Sinonasal desmoplastic small round cell tumor: a case report. Am J Surg Pathol 2002; 26(6): 799–803.

633. Angervall L, Stener B, Stener I, Ahren C. Pseudomalignant osseous tumour of soft tissue. A clinical, radiological and pathological study of five cases. J Bone Joint Surg Br 1969; 51(4): 654–663.

634. Lagier R, Cox JN. Pseudomalignant myositis ossificans. A pathological study of eight cases. Hum Pathol 1975; 6(6): 653–665.

635. Ogilvie-Harris DJ, Fornasier VL. Pseudomalignant myositis ossificans: heterotopic new-bone formation without a history of trauma. J Bone Joint Surg Am 1980; 62(8): 1274–1283.

636. Kransdorf MJ, Meis JM, Jelinek JS. Myositis ossificans: MR appearance with radiologic-pathologic correlation. AJR Am J Roentgenol 1991; 157(6): 1243–1248.

637. Jones G, Rocke DM. Multivariate survival analysis with doubly-censored data: application to the assessment of Accutane treatment for fibrodysplasia ossificans progressiva. Stat Med 2002; 21(17): 2547–2562.

638. Kocyigit H, Hizli N, Memis A, Sabah D. A severely disabling disorder: fibrodysplasia ossificans progressiva. Clin Rheumatol 2001; 20(4): 273–275.

639. Smith R, Athanasou NA, Vipond SE. Fibrodysplasia (myositis) ossificans progressiva: clinicopathological features and natural history. Q J Med 1996; 89(6): 445–446.

640. Bridges AJ, Hsu KC, Singh A, et al. Fibrodysplasia (myositis) ossificans progressiva. Semin Arthritis Rheum 1994; 24(3): 155–164.

641. Heidelberger KP, DiPietro M. Fibrodysplasia ossificans progressiva. Pediatr Pathol 1987; 7(1): 105–109.

642. Cramer SF, Ruehl A, Mandel MA. Fibrodysplasia ossificans progressiva: a distinctive bone-forming lesion of the soft tissue. Cancer 1981; 48(4): 1016–1021.

643. Kaplan FS, McCluskey W, Hahn G, et al. Genetic transmission of fibrodysplasia ossificans progressiva. Report of a family. J Bone Joint Surg Am 1993; 75(8): 1214–1220.

644. Maxwell WA, Spicer SS, Miller RL, et al. Histochemical and ultrastructural studies in fibrodysplasia ossificans progressiva (myositis ossificans progressiva). Am J Pathol 1977; 87(3): 483–498.

645. Dupree WB, Enzinger FM. Fibro-osseous pseudotumor of the digits. Cancer 1986; 58(9): 2103–2109.

646. Spjut HJ, Dorfman HD. Florid reactive periostitis of the tubular bones of the hands and feet. A benign lesion which may simulate osteosarcoma. Am J Surg Pathol 1981; 5(5): 423–433.

647. Nora FE, Dahlin DC, Beabout JW. Bizarre parosteal osteochondromatous proliferations of the hands and feet. Am J Surg Pathol 1983; 7(3): 245–250.

648. Meneses MF, Unni KK, Swee RG. Bizarre parosteal osteochondromatous proliferation of bone (Nora's lesion). Am J Surg Pathol 1993; 17(7): 691–697.

649. Bane BL, Evans HL, Ro JY, et al. Extraskeletal osteosarcoma. A clinicopathologic review of 26 cases. Cancer 1990; 65(12): 2762–2770.

650. Chung EB, Enzinger FM. Extraskeletal osteosarcoma. Cancer 1987; 60(5): 1132–1142.

651. Lee JS, Fetsch JF, Wasdhal DA, et al. A review of 40 patients with extraskeletal osteosarcoma. Cancer 1995; 76(11): 2253–2259.

652. Lidang Jensen M, Schumacher B, Myhre Jensen O, et al. Extraskeletal osteosarcomas: a clinicopathologic study of 25 cases. Am J Surg Pathol 1998; 22(5): 588–594.

653. Sordillo PP, Hajdu SI, Magill GB, Golbey RB. Extraosseous osteogenic sarcoma. A review of 48 patients. Cancer 1983; 51(4): 727–734.

654. Chung EB, Enzinger FM. Chondroma of soft parts. Cancer 1978; 41(4): 1414–1424.

655. Dahlin DC, Salvador AH. Cartilaginous tumors of the soft tissues of the hands and feet. Mayo Clin Proc 1974; 49(10): 721–726.

656. Humphreys S, Pambakian H, McKee PH, Fletcher CD. Soft tissue chondroma–a study of 15 tumours. Histopathology 1986; 10(2): 147–159.

657. Meis-Kindblom JM, Bergh P, Gunterberg B, Kindblom LG. Extraskeletal myxoid chondrosarcoma: a reappraisal of its morphologic spectrum and prognostic factors based on 117 cases. Am J Surg Pathol 1999; 23(6): 636–650.

658. Enzinger FM, Shiraki M. Extraskeletal myxoid chondrosarcoma. An analysis of 34 cases. Hum Pathol 1972; 3(3): 421–435.

659. Antonescu CR, Argani P, Erlandson RA, et al. Skeletal and extraskeletal myxoid chondrosarcoma: a comparative clinicopathologic, ultrastructural, and molecular study. Cancer 1998; 83(8): 1504–1521.

660. Turc-Carel C, Dal Cin P, Rao U, et al. Recurrent breakpoints at 9q31 and 22q12.2 in extraskeletal myxoid chondrosarcoma. Cancer Genet Cytogenet 1988; 30(1): 145–150.

661. Turc-Carel C, Dal Cin P, Sandberg AA. Nonrandom translocation in extraskeletal myxoid chondrosarcoma. Cancer Genet Cytogenet 1987; 26(2): 377.

662. Stenman G, Andersson H, Mandahl N, et al. Translocation t(9; 22)(q22; q12) is a primary cytogenetic abnormality in extraskeletal myxoid chondrosarcoma. Int J Cancer 1995; 62(4): 398–402.

663. Sciot R, Dal Cin P, Fletcher C, et al. t(9; 22)(q22–31; q11–12) is a consistent marker of extraskeletal myxoid chondrosarcoma: evaluation of three cases. Mod Pathol 1995; 8(7): 765–768.

664. Sjogren H, Meis-Kindblom J, Kindblom LG, et al. Fusion of the EWS-related gene TAF2N to TEC in extraskeletal myxoid chondrosarcoma. Cancer Res 1999; 59(20): 5064–5067.

665. Sjogren H, Wedell B, Kindblom JM, et al. Fusion of the NH2-terminal domain of the basic helix-loop-helix protein TCF12 to TEC in extraskeletal myxoid chondrosarcoma with translocation t(9; 15)(q22; q21). Cancer Res 2000; 60(24): 6832–6835.

666. Brody RI, Ueda T, Hamelin A, et al. Molecular analysis of the fusion of EWS to an orphan nuclear receptor gene in extraskeletal myxoid chondrosarcoma. Am J Pathol 1997; 150(3): 1049–1058.

667. Day SJ, Nelson M, Rosenthal H, et al. Der(16)t(1; 16)(q21; q13) as a secondary structural aberration in yet a third sarcoma, extraskeletal myxoid chondrosarcoma. Genes Chromosomes Cancer 1997; 20(4): 425–427.

668. Hirabayashi Y, Ishida T, Yoshida MA, et al. Translocation (9; 22)(q22; q12). A recurrent chromosome abnormality in extraskeletal myxoid chondrosarcoma. Cancer Genet Cytogenet 1995; 81(1): 33–37.

669. Nakashima Y, Unni KK, Shives TC, et al. Mesenchymal chondrosarcoma of bone and soft

tissue. A review of 111 cases. Cancer 1986; 57(12): 2444–2453.

670. Rushing EJ, Armonda RA, Ansari Q, Mena H. Mesenchymal chondrosarcoma: a clinicopathologic and flow cytometric study of 13 cases presenting in the central nervous system. Cancer 1996; 77(9): 1884–1891.

671. Vencio EF, Reeve CM, Unni KK, Nascimento AG. Mesenchymal chondrosarcoma of the jaw bones: clinicopathologic study of 19 cases. Cancer 1998; 82(12): 2350–2355.

672. Bertoni F, Picci P, Bacchini P, et al. Mesenchymal chondrosarcoma of bone and soft tissues. Cancer 1983; 52(3): 533–541.

673. Steiner GC, Mirra JM, Bullough PG. Mesenchymal chondrosarcoma. A study of the ultrastructure. Cancer 1973; 32(4): 926–939.

674. Granter SR, Renshaw AA, Fletcher CD, et al. CD99 reactivity in mesenchymal chondrosarcoma. Hum Pathol 1996; 27(12): 1273–1276.

675. Renshaw A. O13 (CD99) in spindle cell tumors. Reactivity with hemangiopericytoma, solitary fibrous tumor, synovial sarcoma and meningioma but rarely with sarcomatoid mesothelioma. Appl Immunohistochem 1995; 3:250–256.

676. Nielsen GP, Fletcher CD, Smith MA, et al. Soft tissue aneurysmal bone cyst: a clinicopathologic study of five cases. Am J Surg Pathol 2002; 26(1): 64–69.

677. Winnepenninckx V, Debiec-Rychter M, Jorissen M, et al. Aneurysmal bone cyst of the nose with 17p13 involvement. Virchows Arch 2001; 439(5): 636–639.

678. Sciot R, Dorfman H, Brys P, et al. Cytogenetic-morphologic correlations in aneurysmal bone cyst, giant cell tumor of bone and combined lesions. A report from the CHAMP study group. Mod Pathol 2000; 13(11): 1206–1210.

679. Fetsch JF, Miettinen M. Sclerosing perineurioma: a clinicopathologic study of 19 cases of a distinctive soft tissue lesion with a predilection for the fingers and palms of young adults. Am J Surg Pathol 1997; 21(12): 1433–1442.

680. Allen PW, Dymock RB, MacCormac LB. Superficial angiomyxomas with and without epithelial components. Report of 30 tumors in 28 patients. Am J Surg Pathol 1988; 12(7): 519–530.

681. Calonje E, Guerin D, McCormick D, Fletcher CD. Superficial angiomyxoma: clinicopathologic analysis of a series of distinctive but poorly recognized cutaneous tumors with tendency for recurrence. Am J Surg Pathol 1999; 23(8): 910–917.

682. Fetsch JF, Laskin WB, Tavassoli FA. Superficial angiomyxoma (cutaneous myxoma): a clinicopathologic study of 17 cases arising in the genital region. Int J Gynecol Pathol 1997; 16(4): 325–334.

683. Caraway NP, Staerkel GA, Fanning CV, et al. Diagnosing intramuscular myxoma by fine-needle aspiration: a multidisciplinary approach. Diagn Cytopathol 1994; 11(3): 255–261.

684. Kindblom LG, Stener B, Angervall L. Intramuscular myxoma. Cancer 1974; 34(5): 1737–1744.

685. Logel RJ. Recurrent intramuscular myxoma associated with Albright's syndrome. J Bone Joint Surg Am 1976; 58(4): 565–568.

686. Nielsen GP, O'Connell JX, Rosenberg AE. Intramuscular myxoma: a clinicopathologic study of 51 cases with emphasis on hypercellular and hypervascular variants. Am J Surg Pathol 1998; 22(10): 1222–1227.

687. Ireland DC, Soule EH, Ivins JC. Myxoma of somatic soft tissues. A report of 58 patients, 3 with multiple tumors and fibrous dysplasia of bone. Mayo Clin Proc 1973; 48(6): 401–410.

688. Wirth WA, Leavitt D, Enzinger FM. Multiple intramuscular myxomas. Another extraskeletal manifestation of fibrous dysplasia. Cancer 1971; 27(5): 1167–1173.

689. Meis JM, Enzinger FM. Juxta-articular myxoma: a clinical and pathologic study of 65 cases. Hum Pathol 1992; 23(6): 639–646.

690. Giardiello FM, Hamilton SR, Krush AJ, et al. Nasopharyngeal angiofibroma in patients with familial adenomatous polyposis. Gastroenterology 1993; 105(5): 1550–1552.

691. Guertl B, Beham A, Zechner R, et al. Nasopharyngeal angiofibroma: An APC-gene-associated tumor? Hum Pathol 2000; 31(11): 1411–1413.

692. Dabska M. Parachordoma: a new clinicopathologic entity. Cancer 1977; 40(4): 1586–1592.

693. Fisher C. Parachordoma exists–but what is it? Adv Anat Pathol 2000; 7(3): 141–148.

694. Folpe AL, Agoff SN, Willis J, Weiss SW. Parachordoma is immunohistochemically and cytogenetically distinct from axial chordoma and extraskeletal myxoid chondrosarcoma. Am J Surg Pathol 1999; 23(9): 1059–1067.

695. Fisher C, Miettinen M. Parachordoma: a clinicopathologic and immunohistochemical study of four cases of an unusual soft tissue neoplasm. Ann Diagn Pathol 1997; 1(1): 3–10.

696. Kilpatrick SE, Hitchcock MG, Kraus MD, et al. Mixed tumors and myoepitheliomas of soft tissue: a clinicopathologic study of 19 cases with a unifying concept. Am J Surg Pathol 1997; 21(1): 13–22.

697. Smith ME, Fisher C, Weiss SW. Pleomorphic hyalinizing angiectatic tumor of soft parts. A low-grade neoplasm resembling neurilemoma. Am J Surg Pathol 1996; 20(1): 21–29.

698. Groisman GM, Bejar J, Amar M, Ben-Izhak O. Pleomorphic hyalinizing angiectatic tumor of soft parts: immunohistochemical study including the expression of vascular endothelial growth factor. Arch Pathol Lab Med 2000; 124(3): 423–426.

699. Weiss SW. Alveolar soft part sarcoma: are we at the end or just the beginning of our quest? Am J Pathol 2002; 160(4): 1197–1199.

700. Fisher ER, Reidbord H. Electron microscopic evidence suggesting the myogenous derivation of the so-called alveolar soft part sarcoma. Cancer 1971; 27(1): 150–159.

701. Rosai J, Dias P, Parham DM, et al. MyoD1 protein expression in alveolar soft part sarcoma as confirmatory evidence of its skeletal muscle nature. Am J Surg Pathol 1991; 15(10): 974–981.

702. Cullinane C, Thorner PS, Greenberg ML, et al. Molecular genetic, cytogenetic, and immunohistochemical characterization of alveolar soft-part sarcoma. Implications for cell of origin. Cancer 1992; 70(10): 2444–2450.

703. Wang NP, Bacchi CE, Jiang JJ, et al. Does alveolar soft-part sarcoma exhibit skeletal muscle differentiation? An immunocytochemical and biochemical study of myogenic regulatory protein expression. Mod Pathol 1996; 9(5): 496–506.

704. Argani P, Lal P, Hutchinson B, et al. Aberrant nuclear immunoreactivity for TFE3 in neoplasms with TFE3 gene fusions. Am J Surg Pathol 2003; 27(6): 750–761.

705. Argani P, Antonescu CR, Illei PB, et al. Primary renal neoplasms with the *ASPL–TFE3* gene fusion of alveolar soft part sarcoma: a distinctive tumor entity previously included among renal cell carcinomas of children and adolescents. Am J Pathol 2001; 159(1): 179–192.

706. Van Ruth S, van Coevorden F, Peterse JL, Kroon BB. Alveolar soft part sarcoma: a report of 15 cases. Eur J Cancer 2002; 38(10): 1324–1328.

707. Lieberman PH, Brennan MF, Kimmel M, et al. Alveolar soft-part sarcoma. A clinico-pathologic study of half a century. Cancer 1989; 63(1): 1–13.

708. Evans HL. Alveolar soft-part sarcoma. A study of 13 typical examples and one with a histologically atypical component. Cancer 1985; 55(4): 912–917.

709. Portera CA Jr, Ho V, Patel SR, et al. Alveolar soft part sarcoma: clinical course and patterns of metastasis in 70 patients treated at a single institution. Cancer 2001; 91(3): 585–591.

710. Matsuno Y, Mukai K, Itabashi M, et al. Alveolar soft part sarcoma. A clinicopathologic and immunohistochemical study of 12 cases. Acta Pathol Jpn 1990; 40(3): 199–205.

711. Auerbach HE, Brooks JJ. Alveolar soft part sarcoma. A clinicopathologic and immunohistochemical study. Cancer 1987; 60(1): 66–73.

712. Pappo AS, Parham DM, Cain A, et al. Alveolar soft part sarcoma in children and adolescents: clinical features and outcome of 11 patients. Med Pediatr Oncol 1996; 26(2): 81–84.

713. Flieder DB, Moran CA, Suster S. Primary alveolar soft-part sarcoma of the mediastinum: a clinicopathological and immunohistochemical study of two cases. Histopathology 1997; 31(5): 469–473.

714. Nielsen GP, Oliva E, Young RH, et al. Alveolar soft-part sarcoma of the female genital tract: a report of nine cases and review of the literature. Int J Gynecol Pathol 1995; 14(4): 283–292.

715. Jong R, Kandel R, Fornasier V, et al. Alveolar soft part sarcoma: review of nine cases including two cases with unusual histology. Histopathology 1998; 32(1): 63–68.

716. Persson S, Willems JS, Kindblom LG, Angervall L. Alveolar soft part sarcoma. An immunohistochemical, cytologic and electron-microscopic study and a quantitative DNA analysis. Virchows Arch A Pathol Anat Histopathol 1988; 412(6): 499–513.

717. Miettinen M, Ekfors T. Alveolar soft part sarcoma. Immunohistochemical evidence for muscle cell differentiation. Am J Clin Pathol 1990; 93(1): 32–38.

718. Lopez-Ferrer P, Jimenez-Heffernan JA, Vicandi B, et al. Cytologic features of alveolar soft part sarcoma: Report of three cases. Diagn Cytopathol 2002; 27(2): 115–119.

719. Laskowski J. Sarcoma aponeuroticum. Nowotwory 1961; 11: 61–67.

720. Enzinger F. Epithelioid sarcoma. A sarcoma simulating a granuloma or a carcinoma. Cancer 1970; 26: 1029–1041.

721. Fisher C. Epithelioid sarcoma: the spectrum of ultrastructural differentiation in seven immunohistochemically defined cases. Hum Pathol 1988; 19(3): 265–275.

722. Chase DR, Enzinger FM. Epithelioid sarcoma. Diagnosis, prognostic indicators, and treatment. Am J Surg Pathol 1985; 9(4): 241–263.

723. Prat J, Woodruff JM, Marcove RC. Epithelioid sarcoma: an analysis of 22 cases indicating the prognostic significance of vascular invasion and regional lymph node metastasis. Cancer 1978; 41(4): 1472–1487.

724. Dabska M, Koszarowski T. Clinical and pathologic study of aponeurotic (epithelioid) sarcoma. Pathol Annu 1982; 17(1): 129–153.

725. Halling AC, Wollan PC, Pritchard DJ, et al. Epithelioid sarcoma: a clinicopathologic review of 55 cases. Mayo Clin Proc 1996; 71(7): 636–642.

726. Ross HM, Lewis JJ, Woodruff JM, Brennan MF. Epithelioid sarcoma: clinical behavior and prognostic factors of survival. Ann Surg Oncol 1997; 4(6): 491–495.

727. Bos GD, Pritchard DJ, Reiman HM, et al. Epithelioid sarcoma. An analysis of fifty-one cases. J Bone Joint Surg Am 1988; 70(6): 862–870.

728. Evans HL, Baer SC. Epithelioid sarcoma: a clinicopathologic and prognostic study of 26 cases. Semin Diagn Pathol 1993; 10(4): 286–291.

729. Guillou L, Wadden C, Coindre JM, et al. 'Proximal-type' epithelioid sarcoma, a distinctive aggressive neoplasm showing rhabdoid features. Clinicopathologic, immunohistochemical, and ultrastructural study of a series. Am J Surg Pathol 1997; 21(2): 130–146.

730. Mirra JM, Kessler S, Bhuta S, Eckardt J. The fibroma-like variant of epithelioid sarcoma. A fibrohistiocytic/myoid cell lesion often confused with benign and malignant spindle cell tumors. Cancer 1992; 69(6): 1382–1395.

731. Chase DR, Enzinger FM, Weiss SW, Langloss JM. Keratin in epithelioid sarcoma. An immunohistochemical study. Am J Surg Pathol 1984; 8(6): 435–441.

732. Miettinen M, Fanburg-Smith JC, Virolainen M, et al. Epithelioid sarcoma: an immunohistochemical analysis of 112 classical and variant cases and a discussion of the differential diagnosis. Hum Pathol 1999; 30(8): 934–942.

733. Daimaru Y, Hashimoto H, Tsuneyoshi M, Enjoji M. Epithelial profile of epithelioid sarcoma. An immunohistochemical analysis of eight cases. Cancer 1987; 59(1): 134–141.

734. Wick MR, Manivel JC. Epithelioid sarcoma and isolated necrobiotic granuloma: a comparative immunocytochemical study. J Cutan Pathol 1986; 13(4): 253–260.

735. Wick MR, Manivel JC. Epithelioid sarcoma and epithelioid hemangioendothelioma: an immunocytochemical and lectin-histochemical comparison. Virchows Arch A Pathol Anat Histopathol 1987; 410(4): 309–316.

736. Arber DA, Kandalaft PL, Mehta P, Battifora H. Vimentin-negative epithelioid sarcoma. The value of an immunohistochemical panel that includes CD34. Am J Surg Pathol 1993; 17(3): 302–307.

737. Lin L, Montgomery E, Bergfeld W, et al. The utility of cytokeratin 5/6 in distinguishing superficial epithelioid sarcoma from cutaneous spindled squamous cell carcinoma. Mod Pathol 2002; 15:101A (abstract 413).

738. Fisher C. Synovial sarcoma. Ann Diagn Pathol 1998; 2(6): 401–421.

739. Kransdorf MJ. Malignant soft-tissue tumors in a large referral population: distribution of diagnoses by age, sex, and location. AJR 1995; 164(1): 129–134.

740. Dardick I, O'Brien PK, Jeans MT, Massiah KA. Synovial sarcoma arising in an anatomical bursa. Virchows Arch A Pathol Anat Histol 1982; 397(1): 93–101.

741. McKinney CD, Mills SE, Fechner RE. Intraarticular synovial sarcoma. Am J Surg Pathol 1992; 16(10): 1017–1020.

742. Majeste RM, Beckman EN. Synovial sarcoma with an overwhelming epithelial component. Cancer 1988; 61(12): 2527–2531.

743. Farris KB, Reed RJ. Monophasic, glandular, synovial sarcomas and carcinomas of the soft tissues. Arch Pathol Lab Med 1982; 106(3): 129–132.

744. Weidner N, Goldman R, Johnston J. Epithelioid monophasic synovial sarcoma. Ultrastruct Pathol 1993; 17(3–4): 287–294.

745. Varela-Duran J, Enzinger FM. Calcifying synovial sarcoma. Cancer 1982; 50(2): 345–352.

746. Van de Rijn M, Barr FG, Xiong QB, et al. Poorly differentiated synovial sarcoma: an analysis of clinical, pathologic, and molecular genetic features. Am J Surg Pathol 1999; 23(1): 106–112.

747. Smith TA, Machen SK, Fisher C, Goldblum JR. Usefulness of cytokeratin subsets for distinguishing monophasic synovial sarcoma from malignant peripheral nerve sheath tumor. Am J Clin Pathol 1999; 112(5): 641–648.

748. Abenoza P, Manivel JC, Swanson PE, Wick MR. Synovial sarcoma: ultrastructural study and immunohistochemical analysis by a combined peroxidase-antiperoxidase/avidin-biotin-peroxidase complex procedure. Hum Pathol 1986; 17(11): 1107–1115.

749. Fisher C. Synovial sarcoma: ultrastructural and immunohistochemical features of epithelial differentiation in monophasic and biphasic tumors. Hum Pathol 1986; 17(10): 996–1008.

750. Suster S, Fisher C, Moran CA. Expression of bcl-2 oncoprotein in benign and malignant spindle cell tumors of soft tissue, skin, serosal surfaces, and gastrointestinal tract. Am J Surg Pathol 1998; 22(7): 863–872.

751. Healy V, Fisher C. Calponin and h-caldesmon expression in synovial sarcoma. Mod Pathol 2002; 15:16A (abstract 51).

752. Kilpatrick SE, Teot LA, Stanley MW, et al. Fine-needle aspiration biopsy of synovial sarcoma. A cytomorphologic analysis of primary, recurrent, and metastatic tumors. Am J Clin Pathol 1996; 106(6): 769–775.

753. Smith S, Reeves BR, Wong L, Fisher C. A consistent chromosome translocation in synovial sarcoma [letter]. Cancer Genet Cytogenet 1987; 26(1): 179–180.

754. Clark J, Rocques PJ, Crew AJ, et al. Identification of novel genes, SYT and SSX, involved in the t(X;18)(p11.2; q11.2) translocation found in human synovial sarcoma. Nat Genet 1994; 7(4): 502–508.

755. Coindre JM, Hostein I, Benhattar J, et al. Malignant peripheral nerve sheath tumors are t(X; 18)-negative sarcomas. Molecular analysis of 25 cases occurring in neurofibromatosis type 1 patients, using two different RT-PCR-based methods of detection. Mod Pathol 2002; 15(6): 589–592.

756. Van de Rijn M, Barr FG, Collins MH, et al. Absence of SYT-SSX fusion products in soft tissue tumors other than synovial sarcoma. Am J Clin Pathol 1999; 112(1): 43–49.

757. O'Sullivan MJ, Kyriakos M, Zhu X, et al. Malignant peripheral nerve sheath tumors with t(X; 18). A pathologic and molecular genetic study. Mod Pathol 2000; 13(12): 1336–1346.

758. Kawai A, Woodruff J, Healey JH, et al. SYT–SSX gene fusion as a determinant of morphology and prognosis in synovial sarcoma. N Engl J Med 1998; 338(3): 153–160.

759. Weeks DA, Beckwith JB, Mierau GW, Luckey DW. Rhabdoid tumor of kidney. A report of 111 cases from the National Wilms' Tumor Study Pathology Center. Am J Surg Pathol 1989; 13(6): 439–458.

760. Haas JE, Palmer NF, Weinberg AG, Beckwith JB. Ultrastructure of malignant rhabdoid tumor of the kidney. A distinctive renal tumor of children. Hum Pathol 1981; 12(7): 646–657.

761. White FV, Dehner LP, Belchis DA, et al. Congenital disseminated malignant rhabdoid tumor: a distinct clinicopathologic entity demonstrating abnormalities of chromosome 22q11. Am J Surg Pathol 1999; 23(3): 249–256.

762. Kodet R, Newton WA Jr, Sachs N, et al. Rhabdoid tumors of soft tissues: a clinicopathologic study of 26 cases enrolled on the Intergroup Rhabdomyosarcoma Study. Hum Pathol 1991; 22(7): 674–684.

763. Fanburg-Smith JC, Hengge M, Hengge UR, et al. Extrarenal rhabdoid tumors of soft tissue: a clinicopathologic and immunohistochemical study of 18 cases. Ann Diagn Pathol 1998; 2(6): 351–362.

The breast

10

James L. Connolly   Timothy W. Jacobs

INTRODUCTION

Lesions of the breast are among the most common surgical pathology specimens in general practice. With the advent of modern screening and advanced imaging, smaller lesions are being identified and biopsied. Fine-needle aspiration (FNA) and core needle biopsy (CNB) are less intrusive than open biopsy but require clinical and imaging correlation.

The pathologist must not only be able to distinguish benign from malignant lesions but also know the biologic potential of the various lesions. Among benign lesions the pathologist must distinguish between lesions associated with varying risk. With in situ and invasive cancers the pathologist must know the traditional and newer prognostic factors in order to order appropriate tests and report necessary histopathologic findings. Management of patients with breast lesions is very much a team effort. The pathologist must cooperate with the breast imager, surgeon, radiation oncologist, and medical oncologist. The pathologist should be aware of the clinical and imaging findings and ensure they are in concert with the pathologic findings.

EMBRYOLOGY AND HISTOLOGY

The understanding and correct interpretation of the morphologic lesions of mammary tissue require a knowledge of the normal histologic structures and their embryological origins.

The early embryo produces a ventral, linear, ectodermal thickening extending from the axillary region to the inguinal region along both sides of the midsagittal plane. These thickenings are the milk ridges. By the ninth week of embryonic development, these ridges persist only in the pectoral region, where the ectoderm undergoes further thickening and produces solid cords of cells that burrow into the underlying mesenchyme[1] (Fig. 10.1).

Near the end of the embryonic period, these cords become hollow and thus constitute the future mammary gland parenchyma: the lactiferous sinus, the lactiferous ducts, and the secretory alveoli.[2] The stroma of the future mammary gland includes tissue situated around the lobar glandular formations and constitutes is the intralobar connective tissue. Beyond the limits of the intralobar connective tissue, the stroma is denser and constitutes the interlobar connective tissue. The resting gland consists of approximately 15–25 lobes separated by the dense interlobar fibrous septa. Each lobe is subdivided into lobules that represent the functional units of the mammary parenchyma. A surface ectodermal thickening, pushed anteriorly by the mesenchyme, constitutes the nipple, which is surrounded by a pigmented ectodermal zone called the areola. Ultrastructurally, the walls of the glandular system consist of a basal lamina, a discontinuous layer of myoepithelial cells, and two layers

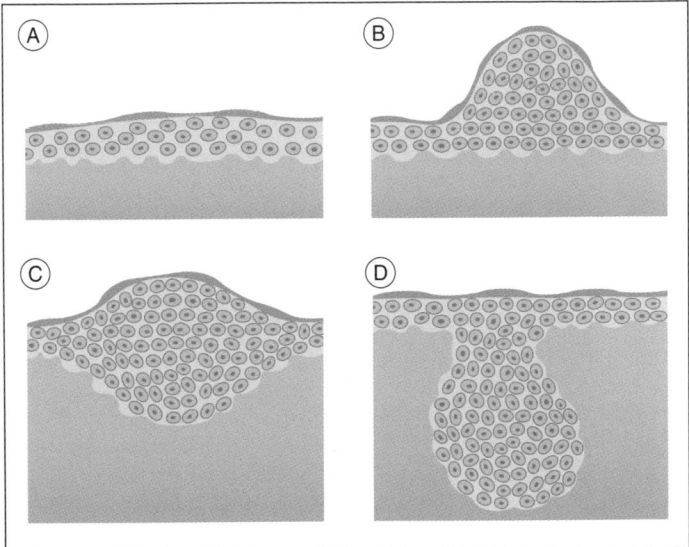

Fig. 10.1 Embryonic development of the mammary gland. **(A)** Ectoderm. **(B, C)** Thickening of ectoderm. **(D)** Solid ectodermal cord invading the underlying mesenchyme.

of columnar cells. The columnar cells possess numerous microvilli on the luminal surface as well as between the cells, and the myoepithelial cells are characterized by an abundant contractile fibrillar cytoplasmic apparatus.[3]

During gestation, the fetal mammary gland undergoes hormonal stimulation of maternal origin, producing signs of secretory activity that regress at birth.[4] At puberty, under the influence of hormones, the female mammary gland acquires its ultimate maturation: the development of the lactiferous duct system and the process of lobulation occur simultaneously with a proliferation of the surrounding connective and adipose tissues (Fig.10.2).

In a mature woman, the mammary gland reacts to the influences of the hormonal cycle and the glandular system thus undergoes a cellular proliferation during the estrogenic phase, followed by discrete secretory activity at the end of the cycle.[5] Concomitant with these changes, the intralobular connective tissue increases its capacity to bind water, particularly near the end of the cycle. This phenomenon explains the impression of heaviness and fullness experienced by many women in the premenstrual period.

During periods of lactation, under the action of different hormones (estrogens, progesterone, prolactin, and others such as cortisol and insulin), the acinar cells undergo a marked secretory differentiation and the lobules become enlarged and crowded (Fig. 10.3). The interlobular septa are markedly thinned. Colostrum production and

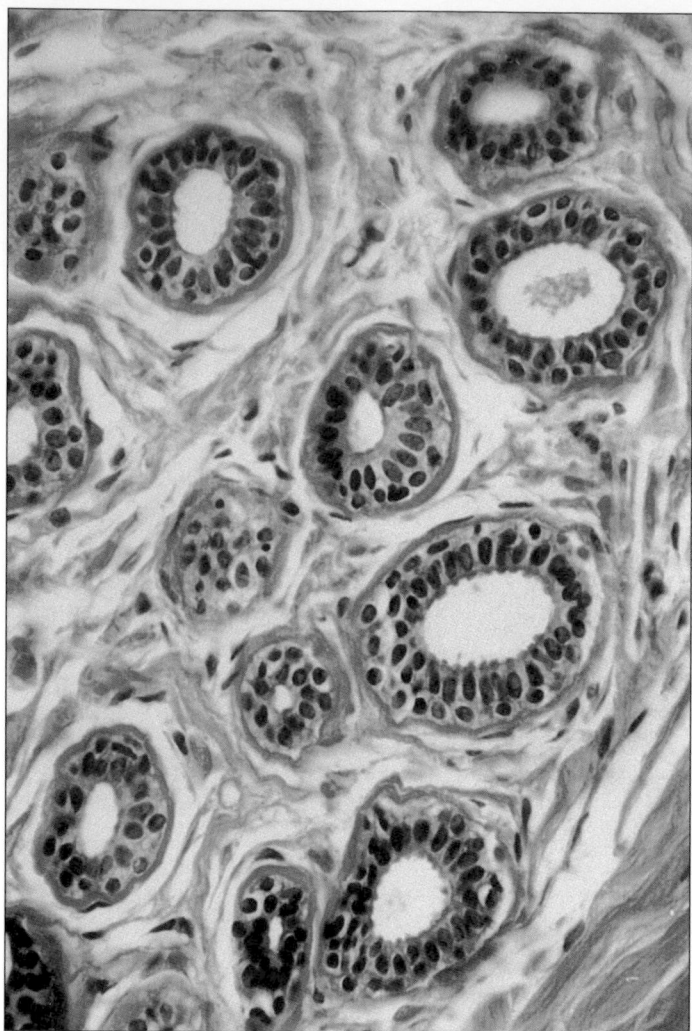

Fig. 10.2 Normal mammary gland. Lactiferous ducts and the surrounding connective tissue are shown.

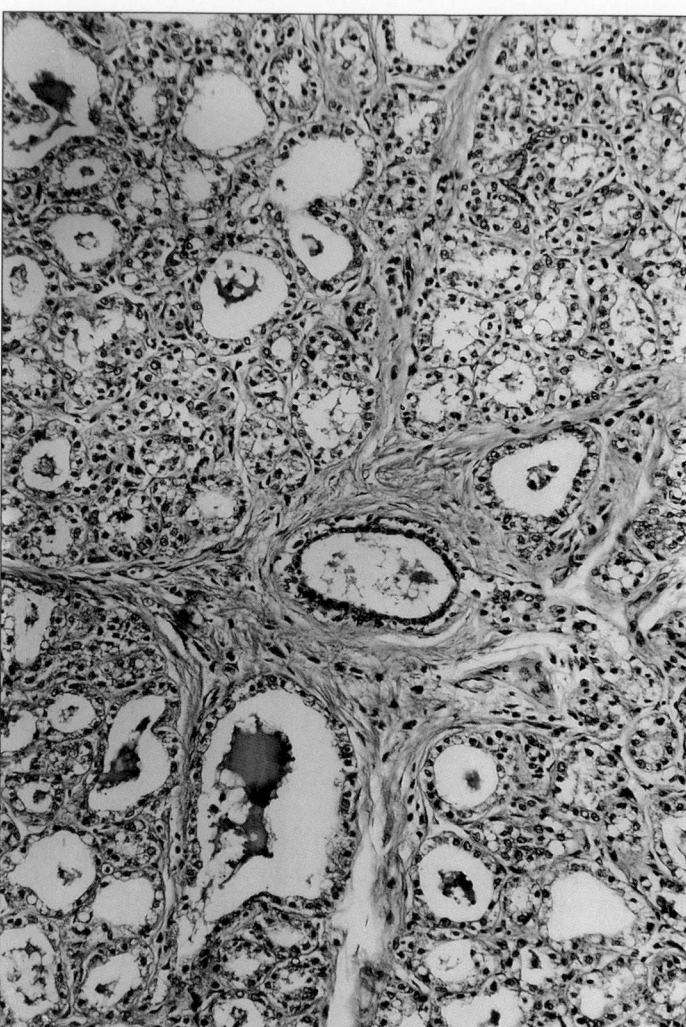

Fig. 10.3 Lactating mammary gland, secretory differentiation of acinar cells. Note the structural difference between the secretory acini and the lactiferous ducts.

subsequently milk production occur at the distal part of the glandular system, the cellular activities of which thus comprise protein and lipid synthesis. Once secreted, ejection of the milk requires sucking, oxytocin secretion, and myoepithelial cell contraction. After menopause, the lobules become atrophic and the excretory ducts undergo cystic degenerative dilatation. The surrounding stroma manifests a loss of cellularity accompanied by fibrosis.[6]

MACROSCOPIC ANATOMY

The breast is a glandular system surrounded by fibroadipose tissue that rests on a musculoconnective tissue bed. The gland is covered by the epidermis. Centrally located is the nipple, which is surrounded by a circular, pigmented area called the areola; the tubercles of Montgomery[7] are specialized sebaceous glands of the areola that enlarge during pregnancy and lactation. The arteries of the mammary gland are branches of the internal mammary, external mammary, and intercostal arteries. The veins are the axillary, internal mammary, and intercostal veins.

The structure of the lymphatic system has a direct influence on the mode of dissemination of tumors (Fig.10.4). The cutaneous lymphatics and some of the perilobular, perialveolar, and ductal lymphatic pathways drain into the areolar plexus.[8] Three main lymphatic groups arise from the plexus: the external, internal, and inferior groups. Most of the deep lymphatics bypass the areolar plexus and drain into these groups. The external mammary lymphatics terminate in the external mammary nodes. These nodes are in continuity with the different axillary groups: the scapular nodes, the central nodes, the axillary vein nodes, and the subclavicular nodes. From there, large lymphatic trunks drain into the jugular–subclavian venous system. The interpectoral nodes (Rotter's) are usually not dissected unless the pectoralis major muscle is removed. The internal mammary lymphatics drain into the internal mammary nodes between the costal cartilages. These nodes surround the internal mammary vessels and are usually small. They receive some drainage from the lateral half of the breast. Connecting lymphatics between the left and right lymphatic chains exist at the level of the first costal interspace. The inferior mammary lymphatics empty into the anterior pectoral, axillary, and subclavicular nodes. When the lymphatic drainage is

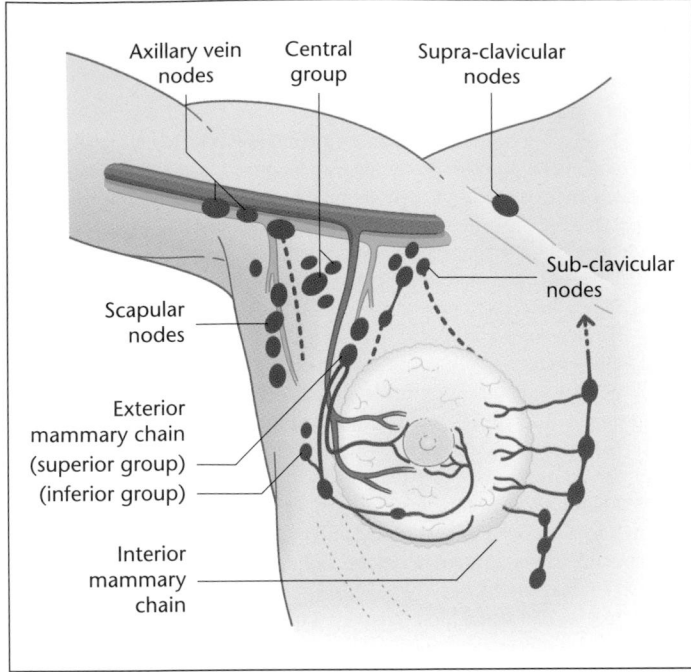

Fig. 10.4 Structure of the lymphatic system of the mammary gland.

blocked by metastases, retrograde lymphatic spread may develop. Intramammary lymph nodes are frequently aspirated or removed as mammographically detected masses.[9]

CONGENITAL ABNORMALITIES

Like other organs, the mammary glands can present congenital anomalies resulting from improper embryonic development:

- *Athelia:* lack of nipple; generally occurs with amastia, both rare
- *Amastia:* absence of the mammary gland; can be uni- or bilateral
- *Polythelia:* the presence of supernumerary nipples
- *Polymastia:* presence of supernumerary mammary glands (polymastia and polythelia result from the persistence of portions of the milk ridge that normally undergo involution).

NEUROENDOCRINE ABNORMALITIES

The normal development of the mammary gland is under the influence of the neuroendocrine system. When this stimulation is absent or disturbed, abnormalities occur:

- *Precocious development* of the breast occurs as part of the clinical presentation of premature – although normal – adolescence. Rarely, it is associated with estrogen-producing ovarian tumors, lutein cysts, or tumors of the adrenal cortex.
- *Micromastia* is insufficient development of the gland at puberty. Failure of development can be due to ovarian insufficiency or congenital adrenal hyperplasia, or the development may simply be delayed because of late menarche.
- *Macromastia* is hypertrophy of the mammary gland.[10] When it occurs, it is generally at puberty and may result in markedly voluminous breasts. This hypertrophy is due to an abnormal

sensitivity to estrogenic hormones and may be symmetric. The microscopic structure reveals a remarkable growth of the connective and adipose tissues. A few cases of massive breast hypertrophy have been reported during pregnancy.

- *Gynecomastia* is the unilateral or bilateral development of the mammary gland in the male. When it occurs, it is usually at puberty or in old age. This anomaly is discussed in detail later in the section on pathologic conditions of the male breast.

PATHOLOGIC EVALUATION OF BREAST SPECIMENS

Several diagnostic and therapeutic procedures are available, yielding a variety of types of breast specimens for interpretation by the pathologist. In order to obtain maximum clinically relevant information from these specimens, the pathologist requires an understanding of their strengths, limitations and unique features to allow appropriate processing and interpretation.

CYTOLOGY SPECIMENS

The use of cytology for the diagnosis of breast lesions in the US dates back to the early 1930s, when Martin and Ellis first reported their experience with FNA at the Memorial Hospital for Cancer and Allied Diseases in New York.[11] The popularity of breast FNA has steadily increased since then; however, in the latter part of the 20th century this modality was challenged by CNB of the breast.[12] More recently, breast ductal lavage has emerged as a new cytologic technique for both diagnosing breast lesions and possible risk assessment.[13,14] This introductory cytology section will cover our approach to the diagnosis of breast cytology specimens. Cytologic features unique to specific disease entities will be incorporated in the sections which follow, as appropriate.

Fine needle aspiration (FNA)

Specimen adequacy

How best to define breast FNA specimen adequacy has been a matter of much debate among cytopathologists.[15–19] Authorities have varied in their definitions, with some applying strict quantitative criteria, such as those based on the number and/or type of cells present on the smear,[15–17,19–21] number of slides with epithelial cells required,[22] and number of needle passes needed.[23] Others have advocated a more qualitative, clinically oriented approach, taking into account the impression of the aspirator in conjunction with imaging and cytologic findings.[24–27]

Most authorities who define a numerical cut-off for cellularity have required at least six epithelial cell groups for adequacy (usually with five to ten cells per group).[15,16,21] Others have included bipolar nuclei in their criteria, either as an alternative to[16] or in addition to[20] the epithelial cell requirement. Some studies have found false-negative results to be more common in hypocellular smears,[16] making a minimal cell count requirement for adequacy intuitively attractive. However, there are drawbacks to this approach. It fails to take into account the inherent variability of breast lesions aspirated, with many benign lesions, because of their histomorphologic nature, yielding an aspirate of low cellularity with a low epithelial cell count regardless of the accuracy of lesion targeting or the experience of the operator. Lesions such as fat necrosis, hyalinized fibroadenoma, or nonproliferative fibrocystic changes may yield specimens of low cellularity, which may still be diagnostic.[28,29] For example, a hypo-cellular FNA sample of fat necrosis containing rare epithelial cells with scattered foam cells, stromal cells, and a few giant cells is diagnostic of this entity but would be categorized as nondiagnostic if a specific epithelial cell count is used as a cut-off. Categorizing such a lesion as nondiagnostic limits a clinician's management options. It has also been suggested that a specific cell count cut-off may be more appropriate for benign or negative aspirates to avoid the problem of false-negative results.[30] In contrast, a cut-off may not be needed if any atypical or suspicious cells are found on an aspirate, as this finding would prompt further investigation of the lesion (such as repeat FNA or excision) irrespective of cellularity or how definitive the cytologic diagnosis is.[30]

As a corollary to these numerical cut-off criteria, a 'diagnostic' specimen with 'adequate' cellularity does not necessarily ensure accuracy of diagnosis for the particular lesion targeted. In other words, despite an 'adequate' smear, the diagnosis rendered may still be false-negative if the lesion of interest is missed.[17] An adequate FNA specimen is not merely a function of the cellularity of the cytology specimen obtained but is dependent on the lesion of clinical interest being adequately sampled. Furthermore, FNA samples should only be interpreted in the appropriate clinical context. To this end, correlation of clinical, imaging and FNA cytology findings is essential to accurate diagnosis.[24–26] This 'triple test' as originally described by Hermansen and colleagues[24] relies on complete concordance between these three modalities for an adequate diagnosis. Discordance among any of these parameters requires further investigation, such as re-aspiration, core biopsy, or excision as clinically indicated. For example, a lesion that is suspicious both clinically and mammographically but with moderately cellular 'benign' cytology requires investigation to exclude a malignant lesion. Butler et al.[25] applied the triple test prospectively to breast FNA specimens with excision follow-up. These authors found a correct diagnosis of carcinoma in 97% of patients and of benign in 100% of patients when all three tests (cytology, clinical examination, and radiology) were concordant.

The National Cancer Institute (NCI) sponsored a multidisciplinary consensus conference on breast FNA in 1996, which included recommendations for specimen adequacy[31] (Table 10.1). Rather than exact epithelial cell counts, the recommendations are for the pathologist interpreting the smear to comment primarily on the quality of the cytologic preparations, such as clarity, preservation, and stain quality of the material on the slide. A qualitative description can also be provided as to the cellularity of the specimen (few, moderate, or abundant epithelial cells present). Of note, there is no national standard for a specific cell count defining adequacy and, according to the NCI consensus conference, this requirement should be at the discretion of the individual cytology laboratory. Rather, the adequacy should ideally be determined by a combination of the pathologist's judgment of interpretability of the slides and the aspirator's clinical impression (correlating the cytologic diagnosis and clinical findings and adequacy of sampling).

In our cytology practice, we endorse the approach of the 1996 NCI consensus conference[31] and do not have a threshold for adequate versus inadequate specimens. We provide a qualitative indication of the level of cellularity at the beginning of the report (i.e. cellular, moderately cellular, or low cellularity). In the case of a smear with particularly low cellularity, we alert the clinician that the sample may not be representative of the lesion sampled, with qualifiers such as 'suboptimal hypocellular specimen' at the beginning of a descriptive report. In a similar fashion, Abele and co-workers[27] have suggested a nonjudgmental approach to reporting FNA specimens

Table 10.1 Recommendations for specimen adequacy of FNA samples: 1996 National Cancer Institute (NCI)-sponsored consensus conference

---

Adequacy of FNA samples of solid nodules

A. An adequate specimen obtained by aspiration is one that leads to resolution of a problem presented by a lesion in a particular patient's breast. There is no specific requirement for a minimum number of ductal cells to be present for specimen adequacy.

B. Adequacy is determined by two judgments:
   1. Opinion of the aspirator that the cytologic findings based on the report are consistent with the clinical findings and that the lesion was adequately sampled
   2. Opinion of the pathologist examining the smears that the slides do not have significant distortion or artifacts and can be interpreted.

C. Specimen description should include quantity of epithelial cells:
   1. Few (occasional clusters)
   2. Moderate (clusters easy to find)
   3. Abundant (epithelial cells in almost every field).

D. Other cellular components should also be in the specimen description.

E. Laboratories may choose to require a specific cell count as one of their own criteria for adequacy.

F. There is no national standard requiring that a given number of cells be present for specimen adequacy.

Adequacy of FNA sample from cyst

A. Adequacy of a benign cyst:
   1. When contents consist of thin, watery, green-gray fluid and there is no residual mass palpable following evacuation of the cyst contents, the fluid from such a lesion may be examined or discarded at the discretion of an experienced aspirator
   2. Any residual, clinically significant mass requires further evaluation (FNA, biopsy)
   3. Any brown or red discoloration in the aspirate not considered to be traumatic warrants careful clinical and cytologic evaluation.

Source: with permission from The uniform approach to breast fine-needle aspiration biopsy. National Cancer Institute Fine-Needle Aspiration of Breast Workshop Subcommittees. Diagn Cytopathol 1997; 16(4): 295–311.

of low cellularity, using phrases such as 'acellular aspirate sample' or 'benign breast cells,' with a note recommending clinical and radiologic correlation and mentioning the false-negative rates of such samples (3–5%). It is crucial for clinicians to understand that the absence of malignant cells on a cytology smear does not necessarily mean the absence of malignancy in the lesion targeted.

Related to adequacy is the issue of specimen processing. Most cytologists are probably more comfortable interpreting direct smears. However, the preparation of an adequate direct smear, free of air-drying and other artifacts, requires that the individual smearing the slide be appropriately trained in the technique.[32] This might not always be feasible in a busy clinical or radiologic practice without cytology support. In this situation, liquid-based samples (such as ThinPrep, TriPath, Cytospin preparations) are appropriate, transferring the responsibility of preparation to the cytology laboratory. Other advantages of thin-layer techniques include excellent cellular preservation, more even distribution of cells, cleaner, less bloody background, and availability of material for ancillary studies (e.g. hormone receptor immunohistochemistry, fluorescence in situ hybridization (FISH) for oncogenes). Detractors cite alteration of architecture and some loss of background material on thin-layer preparations as possibly contributing to suboptimal diagnosis. However, recent data has shown that liquid-based, thin-layer techniques are as accurate as direct smears in the interpretation of breast FNA.[33] Most importantly, the cytopathologist should be comfortable when interpreting a particular type of cytologic specimen. When faced with an unfamiliar cytology preparation, a conservative and cautious approach to diagnosis is advisable.

The probabilistic approach to diagnosis of breast cytology

FNA of the breast is far more sensitive and specific for diagnosing malignant neoplasms than for borderline or benign lesions. Furthermore, attempts at precisely correlating breast cytology findings with histologic features of a particular lesion may in many cases prove unrewarding and frustrating. A diagnostic approach based on the probability of identifying malignancy in a breast sampled by FNA is therefore more clinically appropriate and would draw on the strengths of the FNA technique in identifying carcinoma. Predicting the chance of malignancy in a particular lesion rather than accurately and precisely predicting the corresponding histology of the lesion is more important in optimizing further patient management. This has been termed the *probabilistic approach* to the diagnosis of carcinoma. Wang and Ducatman[34] were the first to report this probabilistic diagnostic approach with validation in a large cohort of patients who had prospectively undergone breast FNA with biopsy or surgical follow-up. The diagnostic categories used by these investigators were essentially similar to those sanctioned by the 1996 NCI-sponsored consensus conference on breast FNA[31] and supported by other authorities.[15,35,36]

The aim of the probabilistic approach is to identify malignancy, the diagnostic categories are defined from the perspective of what constitutes a definitive diagnosis of malignancy (i.e. positive for carcinoma). Five categories are defined, with: '(1) Positive for carcinoma' corresponding to the highest probability of malignancy (i.e. 100%), followed by a decreasing likelihood of malignancy through the other four categories; '(2) Suspicious for carcinoma;' '(3) Epithelial proliferative lesion with atypia;' '(4) Epithelial proliferative lesion without atypia;' and '(5) Unremarkable':[34]

(1) Positive for carcinoma

For a definitive diagnosis of carcinoma, all four of the following criteria must be met: hypercellularity, cellular dyshesion, cytologic atypia, and one cellular population (Fig. 10.5).

- *Cellular dyshesion* refers to the presence of abundant single epithelial cells or loosely cohesive groups of epithelial cells present. (This excludes single bipolar or stromal cells.)
- *Cytologic atypia* may be variable but should at least include increased nuclear:cytoplasmic ratios and markedly eccentrically located nuclei (sometimes described as 'protuberant', or leading to a 'comet-shaped' cell). Other useful features, which may or may not be present depending on the level of pleomorphism, include nuclear membrane irregularities, coarse and clumped chromatin, and multiple and irregular nucleoli.
- *One cell population* refers to one population of atypical epithelial cells, as opposed to a mixed population of atypical and benign-appearing epithelial cells or atypical epithelial cells and stromal cells.
- *Hypercellularity* refers to the atypical epithelial cell population only, rather than increased cellularity due to another component such as inflammatory or stromal cells. This is the most subjective of the criteria to apply, with the most interobserver variability.

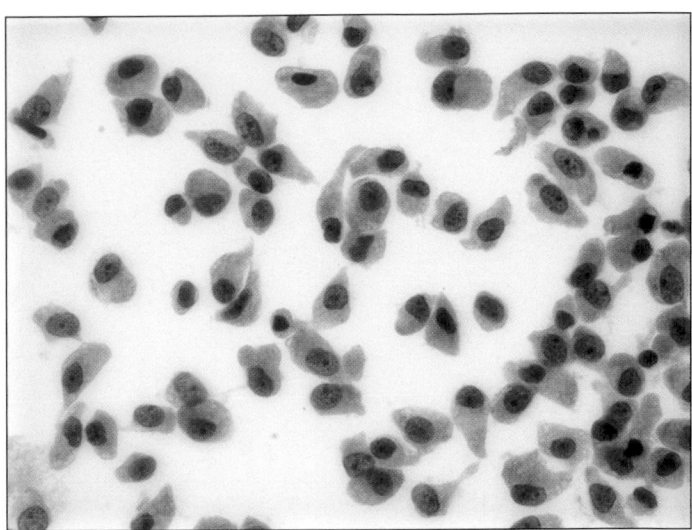

Fig. 10.5 Example of positive cytology, showing a cellular specimen with many single, atypical cells, exhibiting high nuclear:cytoplasmic ratios, with eccentric pleomorphic nuclei that are hyperchromatic with coarse chromatin. (ThinPrep, Papanicolaou stain, ×600.)

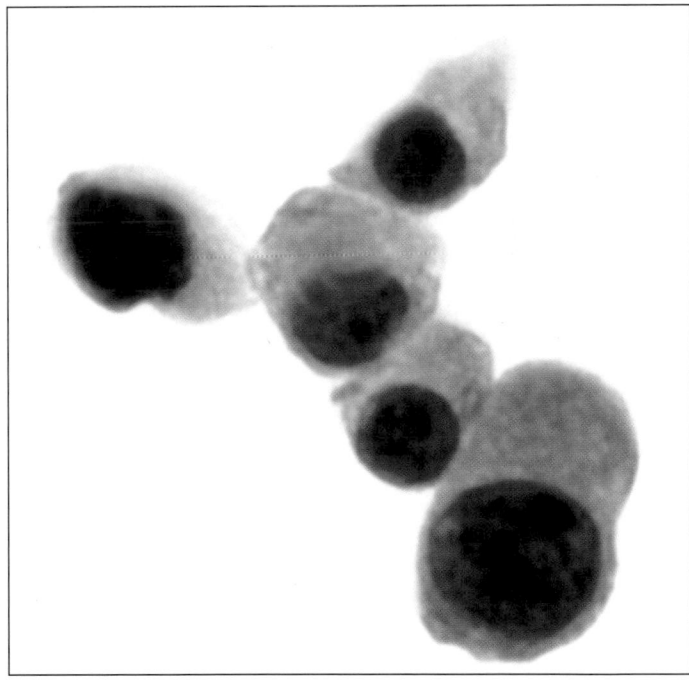

Fig. 10.6 Cytology of a suspicious ductal lesion. Example of *suspicious* cytology, showing few highly atypical cells present in a loosely cohesive cluster, in a specimen which lacked hypercellularity. (ThinPrep, Papanicolaou stain, ×600.)

(2) Suspicious for carcinoma

When any three of the above four features for malignancy are present, a suspicious diagnosis is rendered (Fig. 10.6).

(3) Epithelial proliferative lesion with atypia

This diagnosis is rendered when the specimen is cellular with many epithelial cells and when the epithelial cells present in groups and

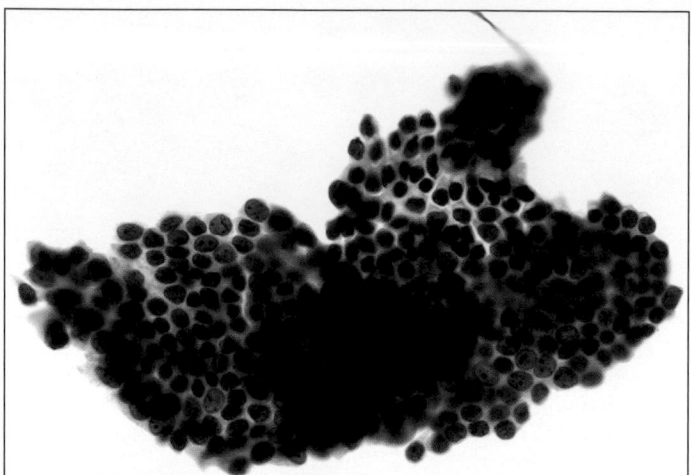

Fig. 10.7 Cytology of an atypical proliferative ductal lesion. Example of an *epithelial proliferative lesion with atypia* cytology, showing cohesive group of ductal epithelial cells with crowding and overlapping, but with mild cytologic atypia. (ThinPrep, Papanicolaou stain, ×400.)

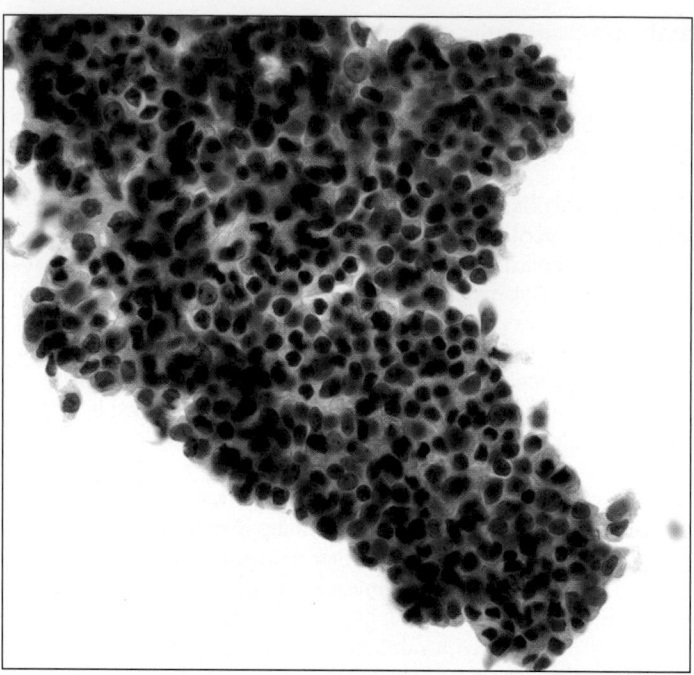

Fig. 10.8 Cytology of a proliferative lesion. Example of an *epithelial proliferative lesion without atypia* showing cohesive group cells exhibiting mild crowding and overlapping, but no appreciable cytologic atypia. Note the admixed myoepithelial cells (with darker staining, smaller nuclei). (ThinPrep, Papanicolaou stain, ×400.)

show significant crowding and overlapping and/or the specimen shows one other feature of malignancy (i.e. cellular dyshesion, cytologic atypia, or one cell population) (Fig. 10.7). It is important to note that the term 'atypia' in this context is not equivalent to that used in the histologic sense, such as 'atypical ductal hyperplasia' (ADH). Rather, atypia is used here to denote a small but finite probability that the aspirated lesion might be malignant. As noted above, the cytologic–histologic correlation of ADH is poor, in part because the diagnosis of ADH is based on a combination of cytological and architectural features.[37]

(4) Epithelial proliferative lesion without atypia

This category is used when a specimen is cellular with many epithelial cells and the epithelial cells in groups show no or mild crowding and overlapping, with obvious myoepithelial cells present and no other features of carcinoma (Fig. 10.8). Although the ability to discriminate among various benign proliferative lesions is very difficult on cytology, most fibroadenomas tend to fall into this category.

(5) Unremarkable

When none of the four features of malignancy is present, the specimen is categorized as unremarkable. The cytologic findings should be described, such as benign-appearing ductal cells, apocrine metaplastic cells, bipolar cells, foam cells, etc. (Fig. 10.9). We do not use the term 'negative for malignant cells' because clinical and radiologic correlation are crucial in this situation (see the triple test, above). Many samples in this category tend to be hypocellular, and a descriptive diagnosis is rather provided, with the onus upon the clinician to judge whether the particular sample is representative of the lesion targeted. If appropriate, we might add a statement such as 'the findings are consistent with cyst contents' if the clinical and radiologic findings concur with the cytologic findings (e.g. apocrine metaplastic cells, benign ductal cells, and numerous foam cells).

Using this probabilistic approach, Wang and Ducatman[34] found excellent concordance between their cytologic diagnoses and pathologic categories of excised lesions. Based on the findings of their study, in conjunction with the clinicians' actions following the

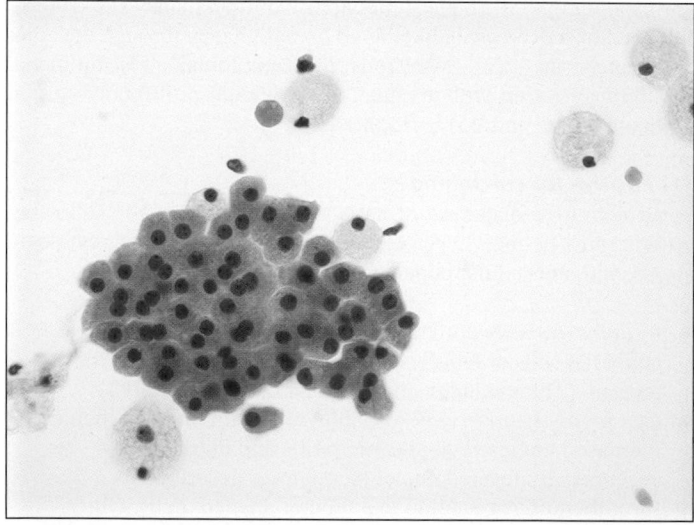

Fig. 10.9 Cytology of a cyst aspirate. Aspirate of cyst, showing cluster of apocrine metaplastic cells and foam cells present singly. This lesion would be classified as *unremarkable*. (ThinPrep, Papanicolaou stain, ×400)

cytologic diagnoses, these authors have proposed management recommendations for each diagnostic category (Table 10.2). The validity of the probabilistic approach has been further highlighted by a recent study that demonstrated excellent accuracy and interobserver reproducibility irrespective of the level of experience of the pathologist participating.[38]

Table 10.2 Recommendations for management by category of cytologic diagnosis using the probabilistic approach

Cytologic category	Management recommendation
Positive for carcinoma	Definitive surgery*. If DCIS is a possibility based on clinical and/or imaging findings, a preceding frozen section confirmation of invasive carcinoma is necessary
Suspicious for carcinoma	Excisional biopsy or definitive surgery preceded by frozen section confirmation
Epithelial proliferative lesion with atypia	Excisional or core biopsy
Epithelial proliferative lesion without atypia	Follow-up if clinical and imaging findings concur with cytology and are not suspicious. Otherwise biopsy
Unremarkable	Follow-up if clinical and imaging findings concur with cytology and are not suspicious. Otherwise re-aspirate or biopsy

* Definitive surgery: mastectomy or lumpectomy and axillary lymph node dissection/sampling. Source: adapted from Wang & Ducatman.[34]

Nipple discharge and nipple sampling techniques

In the majority of women presenting with nipple discharge, the underlying lesion is benign; however, the appearance of nipple discharge is often a cause of significant anxiety for patients. In contrast to a physiologic nipple discharge, one that is pathologic is usually spontaneous, arises from a single duct, is persistent, and is blood-stained (or positive for occult blood on testing). However, fewer than 10% of women with a bloody discharge actually have an underlying malignancy.[39] In contrast, male patients with nipple discharge have a much higher incidence of malignancy.[40]

The use of exfoliative cytology to detect carcinoma cells from nipple discharge was first described by Papanicolaou and colleagues.[41,42] Although this technique has a good specificity for malignancy, the sensitivity is low (less than 50%).[40,43] Obtaining more fluid by use of a suction device similar to a modified breast milk pump has improved cellular yield.[44–47] Installation of fluid via catheter, followed by breast massage and fluid aspiration, further improved specimen yield.[13,48] More recently, ductal lavage, which uses an improved microcatheter design to irrigate the ductal system, has emerged as a technique to further increase the cellular yield of nipple ducts sampled.[14,49,50] In addition to sampling techniques involving the nipple ducts, direct scrape preparations may be prepared of the nipple surface, particularly in patients suspected of having Paget's disease of the nipple.[51,52]

Smears of spontaneous nipple discharge

Most smears prepared from spontaneous nipple discharges are acellular or hypocellular.[40] The commonest cells found are foam cells, which contain abundant finely vacuolated cytoplasm and exhibit an eccentrically placed, small nucleus.[53] These cells are akin to histiocytes, with recent evidence supporting a monocyte.[54] Apocrine metaplastic cells may also be present, and are characterized by finely granular cytoplasm with a single small, uniform, round nucleus containing a small but prominent nucleolus. Inflammatory cells may also be present depending on the etiology of the discharge, with benign squamous cells and/or acellular squames often also present. These benign cellular components (foam cells, apocrine metaplastic cells, inflammatory cells, squamous elements) constitute an unremarkable smear. However, because of the low sensitivity of this test, a 'negative' smear does not exclude malignancy in the patient's breast. Therefore, we do not use the word 'negative' but rather provide a descriptive diagnosis for such smears, with the responsibility of the clinician to correlate the findings. The presence of *any* ductal epithelial cells (even if benign-appearing) on a smear from a spontaneous nipple discharge is abnormal and we categorize these smears as 'atypical'. In addition, if ductal cells are present in papillary or three-dimensional clusters, these are also classified as atypical or suspicious, depending on the degree of cellularity and/or cytologic atypia present. Overtly malignant smears are classified as positive, using the same criteria as applied in the probabilistic approach to FNA (see above).

Ductal lavage

In contrast to nipple aspiration (which uses a device similar to a breast milk pump), ductal lavage uses a microcatheter device to infuse a selected nipple duct system with saline, followed by collection of that fluid for cytologic analysis. A recent multicenter study found the cellular yield of duct lavage to be high, with a median of 13 500 epithelial cells obtained per duct and an insufficiency rate of 22%.[50] In contrast, nipple aspiration yielded a median of 120 cells per breast with an insufficiency rate of 73%.[50] Other advantages of ductal lavage compared to nipple aspiration include better preservation of cytologic material and the ability to target a specific duct system. In addition to cytologic examination, the lavaged fluid obtained may be used for ancillary or molecular diagnostic studies. Because of the high yield and relatively good cellular preservation, ductal lavage material may be interpreted in a similar fashion to that of breast FNA. Five diagnostic categories have been proposed by investigators in this field[50] and are as follows: (a) inadequate for diagnosis (<10 epithelial cells per sample or poor technical quality); (b) benign; (c) mild atypia; (d) marked atypia (equivalent to suspicious); and (e) malignant. An initial multicenter study has shown that this procedure is safe and well tolerated by patients.[50] Of particular interest are the potential of ductal lavage as a screening test for women at high risk for breast carcinoma[14] and the potential use of ductal lavage fluid for molecular analysis as a screening test for women at risk of breast carcinoma. For example, a recent study demonstrated the feasibility of performing methylation-specific polymerase chain reaction (PCR) on ductal lavage fluid, showing a high concordance between methylated markers, atypical cytology, and the presence of carcinoma.[49]

Nipple scrape cytology

This technique is of use if the superficial surface of the nipple is clinically diseased, and is particularly helpful in the diagnosis of Paget's disease of the nipple. Paget's disease presents as an eczematous, scaly nipple lesion, and the area of interest may be directly sampled by scraping the nipple and preparing a cytology slide. The characteristic 'Paget' cells are large with abundant dense cytoplasm, which may be vacuolated and contain nuclei with prominent nucleoli. These cells are shed singly or in clusters and may be found in a background of squamous and keratinaceous material.[51,52] Because of the presence of squamous elements (predominantly from the nipple skin), squamous carcinoma often enters into the differential diagnosis. Useful features for differentiating Paget's disease from squamous carcinoma include the presence of three-dimensional groups of malignant cells, occasional glandular type acini, eccentric nuclei, or the presence of cytoplasmic vacuoles. A mucin stain may also be useful, which is usually positive in Paget cells.[52]

Limitations of FNA

One disadvantage of FNA is that the distinction of invasive from in situ carcinoma is not practically possible. Several studies have examined a variety of cytologic features in an attempt to identify invasion on FNA; however, no features have been found to be entirely specific or frequent enough to be reliably applicable[55–61]

Although FNA specimens of breast are highly sensitive and specific at detecting poorly differentiated malignant tumors, they are more problematic for borderline, atypical, or benign lesions. Specifically, FNA is limited in the ability to discriminate among nonproliferative lesions, proliferative lesions without atypia, atypical hyperplasia, and low-grade ductal carcinoma in situ (DCIS).[58,62–68]

In an attempt to further refine benign FNA diagnoses, some authorities have proposed criteria for distinguishing these lesions on cytology.[58,69] However the criteria proposed did not appear to be generally applicable. A study under the auspices of the Papanicolaou Society of Cytopathology evaluated these published cytologic criteria[58,69] for the categorization of proliferative breast disease.[66] FNA specimens of biopsy-proven nonproliferative lesions, proliferative lesions without atypia, atypical hyperplasia, and low-grade DCIS were evaluated by six expert breast cytopathologists. Cytologic–histologic concordance was achieved in 36% of cases overall. When the cases were divided into two categories of 'low risk' (nonproliferative and proliferative without atypia) and 'high risk' (atypical hyperplasia and DCIS), the interobserver agreement and cytohistologic correlation improved markedly. Based on these findings, we suggest using fewer diagnostic categories for proliferative lesions and employing a terminology that is more clinically applicable and oriented to patient management.[66]

There are high insufficiency rates for the FNA technique when applied to nonpalpable lesions. In a large multicenter study (the Radiologic Diagnostic Oncology Group 5 Study), the overall insufficiency rate among the 18 participating institutions for image-guided FNA of nonpalpable lesions ranged from 3–80% (mean 34%).[70,71] The rate of sample insufficiency varied by the type of lesion targeted, with calcified lesions yielding insufficient samples more often than masses (46% vs 29% respectively). The insufficiency rate was higher for benign than for malignant samples. The insufficiency rate was influenced by the guidance system used, with overall adequacy for ultrasound superior to those FNAs obtained via stereotactic guidance (8% vs 40% insufficiency respectively). Lastly, the type of institution and expertise varied widely, with no special training for FNA technique or specimen preparation required. FNA adequacy is known to be highly operator-dependent, with better specimen acquisition by those aspirators with more training in FNA technique, a higher volume of cases performed, and a higher level of interest in FNA.[72,73]

In contrast, insufficiency rates for palpable breast masses have been consistently lower (<10%), and the presence of an on-site cytopathologist at the time of aspiration significantly improves sufficiency rates.[74,75]

Core needle biopsy

Core needle biopsy yields tissue fragments suitable for routine histologic examination. CNB has been used for many years for the evaluation of palpable breast lesions. More recently, CNB using image-directed guidance methods (i.e. stereotactic mammography and ultrasound) has become widely used for the initial evaluation of clinically occult breast lesions and represent a practical alternative to open surgical biopsy for many patients.[76–78]

CNB was developed with two goals in mind: (1) to eliminate the need for open biopsy in patients with benign lesions and (2) to provide a nonsurgical means to definitively diagnose breast cancer. CNB also increases likelihood of negative margins at surgical excision performed for carcinoma.[79–81] CNB specimens are also suitable for immunohistochemical studies of markers of potential therapeutic or prognostic importance, including hormone receptors, proliferation markers, oncoproteins (e.g. HER2/neu), and others.[82]

There is excellent correlation between the findings on CNB and those on open biopsy. The level of diagnostic agreement among pathologists in the interpretation of CNB specimens is extremely high. In one study, over 2000 CNB specimens were initially diagnosed by multiple pathologists at 22 hospitals around the US and then sent for central review by one of three reference pathologists. The initial diagnosis and the central review diagnosis were concordant in 96% of the cases. This level of agreement was comparable to that observed among over 550 open surgical biopsies obtained from the patients in that study.[83]

Core needle biopsy techniques

CNB procedures employ computer-assisted stereotactic mammography or ultrasound for localization of the target lesion and an automated spring-loaded biopsy gun equipped with a large core (preferably 14-gauge) cutting needle. Of note, the sensitivity of this automated biopsy gun is in large part related to the size of the needle.[84]

Directional vacuum-assisted biopsy devices (VABD) employ vacuum assistance to draw the tissue into the needle and permit the use of larger needles (e.g. 11-gauge), thus resulting in larger specimens. One of the major advantages of VABDs over the automated biopsy gun is the procurement of larger and longer tissue specimens with the former, even when using needles of similar gauge.[85,86] VABDs allow multiple, contiguous specimens to be obtained with a single needle insertion. Furthermore, a higher calcification retrieval rate is possible, with more complete sampling of the target lesion.[87,88] The likelihood of completely removing the mammographic lesion is higher with VABDs than with the automated biopsy gun[89] and smaller diameters of microcalcifications can be sampled by CNB when using a VABD compared to the automated biopsy gun.[90] A significant advantage of VABDs is that a clip can be placed at the biopsy site to mark the area should subsequent wire localization excision be necessary. This is particularly important if the visible findings are completely removed.

Other types of devices are available or in development.

Pathologic–radiologic concordance

Similar to the 'triple test' in breast cytology (see above), mammographic–pathologic concordance is essential with any CNB technique. The pathologist should be provided with the essential clinical information in order to judge if his diagnosis is concordant with the clinical/imaging findings. Discordant diagnoses must be reconciled and repeat CNB or surgical excision may be required. In addition, if the CNB is performed because of the presence of mammographic microcalcifications without a soft tissue density, specimen radiography is essential to confirm the presence of calcifications within the specimens. The likelihood that the pathologist will be able to render a specific diagnosis on such a specimen is significantly greater when calcifications are identified on the specimen radiograph than when they are not.[91,92] Furthermore, the calcifications should be identified by the pathologist microscopically and their location indicated in the final pathology report.

Diagnostic and management problems on CNB

There are a number of recurring diagnostic problems encountered in CNB specimens. These are generally similar to those encountered in open surgical excision specimens such as distinguishing ADH from low-grade DCIS, identifying foci of stromal invasion in cases of DCIS, distinguishing between tubular carcinoma and benign sclerosing lesions such as sclerosing adenosis and radial scars, distinguishing among benign papillomas, atypical papillomas, and papillary forms of DICS, distinguishing mucocele-like lesions from mucinous carcinomas, and distinguishing low-grade phyllodes tumors from cellular fibroadenomas. The most prudent approach for the pathologist in the face of any of these diagnostic uncertainties is to provide enough of a diagnosis to prompt a surgical excision if clinically indicated without overdiagnosing the lesion.

Certain nonmalignant lesions pose dilemmas with regard to the most appropriate clinical management subsequent to CNB (i.e. surgical excision versus clinical and radiologic follow-up). Many of these lesions are encountered relatively infrequently so that few data are available on which to base rational management decisions, but they occur frequently enough to create continual discussion and debate regarding their appropriate post-CNB management.[93] These lesions include ADH, lobular neoplasia (atypical lobular hyperplasia (ALH) and lobular carcinoma in situ(LCIS)), papillary lesions, radial scars, fibroepithelial lesions, mucocele-like lesions, and columnar cell lesions. The management of these lesions on CNB will be briefly covered in the sections that follow. For a detailed review of this topic see Jacobs et al.[94]

Processing of CNB specimens

CNB specimens should be submitted for microscopic evaluation in their entirety and drying and distortion of the specimens should be avoided. It is generally acknowledged that levels should be cut from each paraffin block to ensure adequate sampling; however the optimal number of levels required is not well defined.[95] Immuno-histochemical evaluation of hormone receptors and a wide variety of other biological markers can be readily performed on CNB specimens. Immediate diagnosis is rarely needed and the use of frozen sections is discouraged because of the small size of these specimens. If, however, there is a need for an immediate evaluation, touch imprint cytology can provide highly accurate results without compromising the specimen.[96]

Limitations of CNB

A diagnosis of DCIS on CNB does not exclude a coexistent invasive carcinoma.

The diagnosis of ADH on CNB is also not definitive and represents an underdiagnosis in many cases, with DCIS or invasive carcinoma found in up to 33–87% of patients who go on to have an excision.[97-101] For these reasons, surgical excision is still recommended in all cases with a diagnosis of ADH on CNB.[102] Similar management uncertainty exists for other specific nonmalignant diagnoses on CNB, such as lobular neoplasia, radial scar, and papillary lesions (for review, see Jacobs et al.[94]).

The most important thing to keep in mind when evaluating CNBs is that they are a sampling technique. The pathologic diagnosis must be concordant with the imaging/clinical findings. When the findings are discordant there is a substantial incidence of a missed cancer.[99]

Incisional biopsies

Most incisional biopsies should be submitted completely for histopathologic examination. As for CNB specimens, these specimens are suitable for the evaluation of hormone receptor status and other biological markers.

Excisional biopsy (lumpectomy, partial mastectomy) performed for a palpable mass

Careful macroscopic examination of excisional biopsy specimens is an essential component of their evaluation. Every breast excision should be measured; if a palpable tumor is present, it should also be measured and its relationship to overlying skin or underlying fascia or skeletal muscle, if present, should be noted. The distance of any macroscopically evident tumor from the margins of excision should also be recorded.

Numerous studies have now demonstrated that the presence of carcinoma at the final microscopic margins of breast excision specimens is a significant and independent risk factor for local recurrence in patients with invasive breast cancer treated with conservative surgery and radiation therapy.[103-108] Therefore, the status of the microscopic margins is one of the major factors taken into consideration in determining patient suitability for this treatment approach.

Methods of margin evaluation

There are a number of ways to evaluate margins. If margins are not separately submitted by the surgeon, accurate assessment of the microscopic margins requires that the specimen be presented to the pathologist as a single intact tissue fragment. It may be difficult or impossible to evaluate the margins of specimens that have been previously incised or that are in more than one fragment. Ideally, the intact specimen should be oriented by the surgeon by means of sutures, clips, or a diagram. Specimen orientation is useful in directing further surgery to a particular area of margin involvement rather than re-excising the entire biopsy site. In addition, if the positive margin is deep or at skin, further surgery may not be required.

There are a number of methods available for microscopic margin evaluation.[109] In the method most commonly employed, the specimen surface is dried, then painted with an insoluble ink or dye prior to sectioning. Adherence of the ink may be improved by dipping the specimen in alcohol or acetic acid after applying the ink.

If the specimen is oriented, different colors of ink may be used to denote specific margins in oriented specimens. The specimen is then sectioned through the equatorial plane ('breadloafed'), with sections perpendicular to the inked tissue edges submitted for microscopic evaluation. Using this method, the precise distance between the carcinoma and the inked margin can be determined histologically. When reporting the margin status the presence of DCIS and invasive carcinoma should be reported separately. In addition, an attempt should be made to quantify the extent of involvement.

To overcome the limitations of the inked margin method, some authors have proposed peeling or shaving some or all of the surface of the specimen and submitting these tangentially obtained (en face) sections for histological examination.[110,111] Using this method, a margin is considered positive when cancer cells are present anywhere on the histologic sections of these margins. The advantage of this method is that it permits examination of a large proportion of the specimen's surface with relatively few sections. However this method may overestimate margin positivity.[111]

A third method of margin evaluation consists of the surgeon removing arcs of additional tissue from the medial, lateral, inferior, superior, and deep walls of the biopsy cavity immediately after the surgical specimen has been excised. These are then submitted to the pathologist as separate specimens and processed individually.[112] As when the pathologist shaves margins, this technique has the potential to overestimate margin positivity.

It should be noted that virtually all the clinical studies in which margin status has been related to local recurrence risk are based on margins evaluated with sections taken perpendicular to the inked surfaces. It may not be appropriate to generalize these results to patients who have margins evaluated in a different manner. Therefore, it is essential that clinicians formulating therapeutic options for patients with breast cancer understand how the margins from that patient were evaluated, particularly if the patient had her surgery at another institution.

Intraoperative evaluation of margins

With rare exceptions, we do not recommend frozen sections or cytologic techniques for intraoperative margin evaluation.

Needle localization breast biopsies for nonpalpable lesions

With the increasing use of mammographic screening, a growing number of breast biopsies are performed because of an abnormality detected by mammography in the absence of a palpable mass. These lesions may be sampled by image-directed core biopsy or FNA. In many cases, the needle localization technique is used to guide the surgeon to the area of mammographic abnormality. Communication among the radiologist, surgeon, and pathologist is essential to ensure proper processing and evaluation of such specimens.[109]

The most frequent mammographic abnormalities prompting biopsy are microcalcifications, a soft tissue density, or a combination of the two. Specimen radiography is a crucial component in the evaluation of these specimens in order to both document the presence of the lesion detected by mammography and localize the suspicious area for histologic examination. Specimen radiology is of limited value in assessing margins.[113,114]

Several aspects of specimen radiography merit comment. Magnification views frequently permit the identification of mammographic abnormalities (particularly microcalcifications) that are not well demonstrated using standard nonmagnified radiographs. Second, many radiologists consider specimen compression an essential component of specimen radiography, since this enhances image resolution. With or without specimen compression there is an artificial decrease in margin width due to specimen flattening after removal.[115] Finally, specimen radiographs should always be compared with the preoperative mammograms to be certain that the lesion of concern has been excised. It should be noted, however, that, if the biopsy has been performed for a soft tissue density without calcifications, the lesion may be difficult or impossible to detect on the specimen radiograph unless it has a well defined configuration (i.e. a stellate mass or a sharply circumscribed nodule).

After radiography of the intact specimen has demonstrated that the lesion of interest is present within the specimen, this area must be identified by the pathologist. Some specimens will contain a grossly evident tumor. If there is no grossly evident lesion, a number of methods can be used to identify the lesion within the specimen. One simple method consists of comparing the gross specimen with the specimen radiograph and placing a pin or needle into the specimen at the site of the mammographic lesion to permit the identification of its location by the prosector. Another method consists of performing the initial specimen radiograph after placing the tissue in a specimen holder that incorporates a grid that is visible on the radiograph. The holder containing the specimen and the specimen radiograph are then compared to precisely locate the target lesion using the X and Y coordinates of the grid.

The method we prefer involves slicing the specimen, after inking, at 2–3-mm intervals and obtaining a radiograph of the sliced specimen. The slices on the radiograph can then be marked and the corresponding tissue slices placed in labeled tissue cassettes to permit correlation between the histologic sections and the radiograph of the sliced specimen.

Beyond submitting the breast tissue containing the mammographically detected lesion, the extent to which the remaining breast tissue is sampled for microscopic evaluation varies among different institutions. Our preference for calcifications is to submit the slices with calcifications and the adjacent slices as a first pass. All of our slices are cassetted sequentially in disposable cassettes so that if the first sections reveal DCIS we can go back and submit more while keeping the orientation.

In some cases, the initial histologic sections of breast specimens containing radiographic calcifications fail to reveal microscopic calcifications, even when the specimen radiograph clearly indicated that the calcifications are contained within the specimen. There are several possible explanations for this. First, the calcifications may be composed of calcium oxalate (weddellite) rather than the usual calcium phosphate.[116] Both types of calcium deposit produce the mammographic appearance of microcalcifications but they appear different histologically. The basophilic nature of calcium phosphate deposits are well known and easily recognized by pathologists. In contrast, calcium oxalate deposits on hematoxylin–eosin sections are pale and refractile and may be difficult to identify using routine microscopy. Examination of such specimens under polarized light, however, readily demonstrates this type of calcification. If, after examination under polarized light, there is still no microscopic evidence of calcifications, other possibilities must be considered. For example, the paraffin blocks may not have been cut deeply enough to provide histologic sections that demonstrate the calcifications. To investigate this possibility, the blocks may themselves be radiographed; any blocks containing radiographic calcifications should be cut more deeply until the calcifications are microscopically identified. Finally, in some cases, larger calcifications may shatter out of the block during sectioning and will, therefore, not be demonstrable on histologic sections. In cases such as this the large calcification may tear its way through the section. This tear is a clue that this may have happened and examination of the edges of the tear may reveal fragments of calcium. It should be emphasized that it is incumbent upon the pathologist to make every effort to identify histologically the lesion for which the surgical excision was performed.

There are several potential pitfalls in the histologic examination of needle localization breast biopsies. While some authors have reported that frozen section diagnosis can be performed on nonpalpable breast lesions with a high degree of accuracy,[117,118] the routine use of frozen sections to examine such lesions should be discouraged.[119] Many of these lesions are small and it may not be possible to both perform a frozen section and to retain a sufficient amount of lesional tissue for permanent sections. Moreover, artifacts resulting from freezing the specimen may make it extremely difficult or impossible to accurately evaluate the permanent sections. Finally, at many institutions, the results of the frozen section will not alter the immediate management of the patient. For these reasons, nonpalpable breast lesions are usually best evaluated on permanent sections only.

Calcifications are commonly identified in histologic sections of breast tissue, even in breast biopsies performed for indications other than mammographic microcalcifications. Therefore, in order to ensure accurate mammographic–pathologic correlation, the calcifications identified histologically should correspond to the mammographic calcifications.

Needling procedures such as FNA, CNB, and wire localization can induce a number of artifacts in subsequent breast excision specimens, including displacement of benign ductal epithelium or DCIS cells into the stroma or into vascular spaces.[120–124] This can result in an erroneous diagnosis of invasive or intralymphatic/intravascular cancer in a patient with benign disease or DCIS.

Re-excision specimens

Re-excision specimens are in general handled the same as excision specimens.

There are only limited data addressing the most cost-effective method to sample re-excision specimens, which are often large and rarely exhibit grossly identifiable areas of carcinoma. One study suggested that, for grossly benign re-excisions, submitting two tissue blocks for each centimeter of the largest specimen diameter is sufficient for providing the clinically essential information needed from these specimens in most cases.[125]

Mastectomy specimens

The methods used for examination of a mastectomy specimen as well as the extent of sampling depend, in part, upon the type of surgical procedure and the reasons for which the procedure was performed. Nonetheless, several aspects of the examination apply to all mastectomy specimens. Ideally, the specimen should be oriented for the pathologist by the surgeon, particularly for mastectomy specimens that do not have a contiguous axillary tail. The following features should be recorded before any mastectomy specimen is incised: the specimen weight; the overall dimensions; descriptions and measurements of the skin, areola, nipple, and any incisions or scars; composition of the deep margin (i.e. presence of fascia or muscle); description of the axillary tail (if present); and the location and size of any palpable tumor, with careful attention paid to its relationship to the overlying skin and deep margin.

Prior to incising the specimen, the deep margin should be painted with ink to facilitate its identification on histologic sections. Superficial margins in general should not be inked since there are no clinical studies that have evaluated the significance of tumor involvement of these surfaces of the specimen. Further examination of the specimen is best performed by placing the specimen skin side down and making multiple parallel incisions through the deep aspect 1–2 cm apart, leaving the skin intact. The cut surfaces of each slice should be examined carefully for the presence of grossly evident tumor and/or biopsy site.

Sampling for histologic examination should include sections of any grossly apparent tumor and/or biopsy site, the deep margin, the overlying skin (including scars), the nipple, and random sections (approximately two) of the grossly unremarkable quadrants of breast tissue. If the specimen is a radical mastectomy the interpectoral fascia should be examined for the presence of Rotter's node(s).

In a number of situations, more extensive examination of a mastectomy specimen may be required. In patients with DCIS, particularly those with larger lesions, many sections may be required to determine the presence of stromal invasion. Similarly, extensive sampling may be required to identify a carcinoma in the breast in patients with Paget's disease of the nipple and in patients who present with metastatic carcinoma in an axillary lymph node and an 'occult' primary tumor. In these situations, radiography of the mastectomy specimen (either intact or after it has been sectioned) may be of value in directing histologic sampling to areas with calcifications, mass lesions, or architectural distortion. Some patients with operable breast cancer and locally advanced breast cancer undergo neoadjuvant chemotherapy prior to mastectomy. It is important for the pathologist to carefully examine the mastectomy specimen in such cases to assess the therapeutic response and to document the morphologic effects of treatment on the tumor.[126–129]

Axillary lymph nodes

Pathologic evaluation of axillary lymph nodes is used to assess prognosis and to determine the need for adjuvant systemic therapy. For any axillary specimen, initial pathologic examination should include gross inspection and palpation for lymph nodes. The adipose tissue should then be carefully dissected in the fresh state to retrieve excised lymph nodes. The number, size range, and gross appearance of the identified nodes should be recorded. Although we advocate dissection of larger axillary dissections in the fresh state, a variety of other methods are available for further examination of these specimens. Special techniques such as radiographic imaging of the axillary specimen[130,131] or clearing of the specimen[132] increase the number of lymph nodes identified; however, the additional information obtained is of questionable clinical value.[133]

Sentinel lymph nodes

More recently, sentinel lymph node biopsy has emerged as an alternative surgical technique to a more extensive axillary dissection.[134–139] By definition, the sentinel node is the first lymph node or nodes that receive lymphatic drainage from the tumor. To this end, colored dye (usually blue) and/or radioactive tracer are injected into or in the vicinity of the tumor or in the dermis over the tumor in order to facilitate the identification of the sentinel node. The sentinel lymph node is usually an axillary node; however, it may rarely be intramammary, interpectoral (Rotter's) or internal mammary in location. For sentinel node biopsy procedures, the smaller tissue sample usually has limited associated adipose tissue, and therefore retrieval of lymph nodes is easier.

Extent of lymph node sampling for microscopic evaluation

The extent to which axillary lymph nodes are sampled for microscopic evaluation has long been a subject of debate, but this subject has received more attention recently with the advent of the sentinel lymph node biopsy technique. It is of interest to note that, despite the acknowledged importance of the axillary lymph node status in patients with breast cancer, there is wide variation among pathologists with regard to the extent of lymph node examination. Although a number of studies have clearly shown that more thorough gross and microscopic sampling results in an increase in the detection of positive lymph nodes and a change in the lymph node status from negative to positive in some patients,[140–142] the optimal means for the routine pathologic examination of axillary lymph nodes, particularly sentinel is still largely undecided.[143,144]

For full axillary dissections as well as for sentinel node biopsy, lymph nodes grossly uninvolved by tumor should be submitted for histologic examination in their entirety. However, representative sections of grossly positive lymph nodes are sufficient. Small lymph nodes may be submitted intact, whereas larger lymph nodes should be sectioned at 2–3-mm intervals. The College of American Pathologists suggested that examination of one microscopic slide for each tissue block is sufficient either for sentinel lymph nodes or those from full axillary dissections.[145] However, most experts believe that sentinel lymph nodes require more extensive examination than this, and a recent consensus conference recommended that each paraffin block of sentinel lymph nodes be cut at three levels.[146]

Numerous studies have shown that microscopic deposits of tumor cells may be found in up to 20% of lymph nodes classified as negative on hematoxylin and eosin (H&E) staining with the use of immunohistochemistry or molecular techniques such as the polymerase chain reaction (PCR).[139,140,147–149] However, the clinical significance of such occult micrometastases is uncertain and controversial.[147,148,150–153] In particular, the appropriate management of patients with lymph nodes containing single cells detected by immunohistochemistry for cytokeratins is not known.[140,147,148,153] The 6th edition of the AJCC staging manual considers patients with tumor deposits detected by any method that measure 0.2 mm or less as node negative.[154] At the present time therefore, there are insufficient data to justify the routine use of cytokeratin immunohistochemistry or PCR to detect occult metastases both in either sentinel or nonsentinel lymph nodes. Cytokeratin immunostains may however be utilized to confirm the presence of metastases in specific areas of concern on H&E-stained sections. In addition to noting the total number of lymph nodes examined and number of involved nodes, the size of the largest metastatic deposit should be included in the pathology report as well as a comment as to the presence of extranodal extension.

Surgeons may elect to do a complete axillary dissection on patients who have a positive sentinel lymph node, and in these cases intraoperative assessment may be helpful to avoid a second procedure. In these circumstances, intraoperative gross examination and touch imprint cytology[155–157] is preferable to frozen section analysis, which may cause unnecessary loss of lymph node tissue.[145]

Benign breast disorders

It has been known for many years that some benign breast lesions are more highly associated with breast cancer than others.[158,159]

More recent studies have evaluated the subsequent risk of developing breast cancer in patients who have had a benign breast biopsy and for whom long-term follow-up is available.[160–171] In these studies, the benign biopsies were reviewed and the types of benign lesion present were recorded and related to the risk of breast cancer. The findings of these studies have indicated that terms such as 'fibrocystic disease,' 'chronic cystic mastitis,' and 'mammary dysplasia' are not clinically meaningful since they encompass a heterogeneous group of processes, some physiologic and some pathologic, with widely varying cancer risks.[172–174]

The seminal study evaluating benign breast disease and cancer risk is the retrospective cohort study of Dupont and co-workers.[161,175] In this study, the slides of benign breast biopsies from over 3000 women in Nashville, TN, were reviewed, and the histologic lesions present were categorized using strictly defined criteria[37,161,175] into one of three categories: nonproliferative lesions, proliferative lesions without atypia, and atypical hyperplasias (Table 10.3). The risk of developing breast cancer was then determined for each of these groups. This system provides a pragmatic, clinically relevant approach to benign

Table 10.3 Categorization of benign breast lesions according to the criteria of Dupont, Page, and Rogers[37,161,175]

Nonproliferative
Cysts
Papillary apocrine change
Epithelial-related calcifications
Mild hyperplasia of the usual type
Proliferative lesions without atypia
Moderate or florid ductal hyperplasia of the usual type (usual ductal hyperplasia)
Intraductal papilloma
Sclerosing adenosis
Fibroadenoma
Atypical hyperplasia
Atypical ductal hyperplasia
Atypical lobular hyperplasia

breast lesions. Studies from other groups have largely confirmed the initial observations of the Nashville group and have extended these findings by providing important new information regarding benign breast disease and breast cancer risk[164,165,168,170,171] (Table 10.4).

Nonproliferative lesions

Nonproliferative lesions, as defined by Dupont and Page,[161] include cysts, papillary apocrine change, epithelium-related calcifications, and mild hyperplasia of the usual type.

Cysts are fluid-filled round to ovoid structures that vary in size from microscopic to grossly evident (Fig. 10.10). 'Gross cysts,' as defined by Haagensen, are those that are large enough to produce palpable masses.[176] Cysts are derived from the terminal duct lobular unit. The epithelium usually consists of two layers: an inner (luminal) epithelial layer and an outer myoepithelial layer. In some cysts, the epithelium is markedly attenuated or absent; in others, the lining epithelium shows apocrine metaplasia, characterized by granular eosinophilic cytoplasm and apical cytoplasmic protrusions ('snouts').

Papillary apocrine change is characterized by a proliferation of ductal epithelial cells in which all of the cells show apocrine features as described above. *Epithelium-related calcifications* are frequently observed in breast tissue and may be seen in normal ducts and lobules or in virtually any pathologic condition in the breast. Calcifications may also be seen in the breast stroma as well as in blood vessel walls. *Mild hyperplasia of the usual type* is defined as an increase in the number of epithelial cells within a duct that is less

Table 10.4 Relative risk of breast cancer according to histologic category of benign breast disease in studies using the criteria of Dupont, Page, and Rogers[164,165,168,170,171]

Study	Study design	Nonproliferative	Proliferative without atypia	Atypical hyperplasia
Nashville[161]	Retrospective cohort	1	1.9 (1.0–2.3)	5.3 (3.1–8.8)
Nurses' Health Study[165]	Case-control	1	1.6 (1.2–2.2)	3.9 (2.6–5.9)
Breast Cancer Detection and Demonstration Project[168]	Case-control	1	1.3 (0.77–2.2)	4.3 (1.7–11.0)
Florence, Italy[164]	Case-control	1	1.3 (0.5–3.5)	13.0 (4.1–41.7)

Numbers in parentheses represent 95% confidence intervals

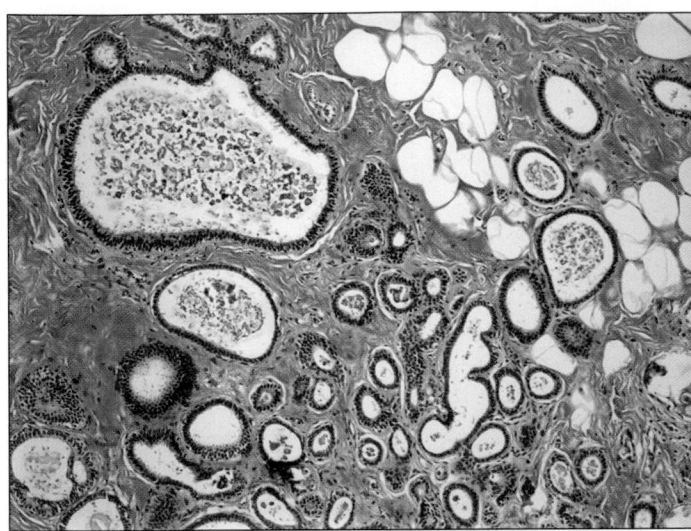

Fig. 10.10 Microcyst. Dilated lobule with microcyst formation (×100.)

than four epithelial cells in depth. In this type of hyperplasia, the epithelial cells do not cross the lumen of the involved space. Patients in this category are not at increased risk.

FNA specimens of *nonproliferative lesions* are usually of low cellularity; however, they may be difficult to distinguish from *proliferative lesions without atypia* (see introductory cytology section above). Depending on the lesion aspirated, the smear may be composed of apocrine metaplastic cells (in sheets, clusters, and singly), cohesive clusters of benign epithelial cells, and/or foam cells. Cyst fluid characteristically contains abundant foam cells, accompanied by varying proportions of apocrine metaplastic cells, benign ductal epithelial cells, and inflammatory cells in a background of proteinaceous debris.

Proliferative lesions without atypia

Included within the group of proliferative lesions without atypia are *moderate or florid hyperplasias of the usual type, intraductal papillomas, sclerosing adenosis, radial scars and fibroadenomas*.[161,177,178] As noted, women who have had a benign breast biopsy showing proliferative lesions without atypia, as defined above, have a mildly elevated breast cancer risk, approximately 1.5–2.0 times that of the reference population (*intraductal papillomas, radial scars,* and *fibroadenomas* are discussed elsewhere in this chapter).

Moderate or florid hyperplasias of the usual type, also known as usual ductal hyperplasias, are intraductal epithelial proliferations more than four epithelial cells in depth. They are characterized by a tendency to bridge and often distend the involved space. The proliferation may have a solid, fenestrated or papillary architecture. If spaces remain within the duct lumen, they are irregular and variable in shape. These spaces are often slit-like and arranged around the periphery of the proliferation, with their long axes parallel to the basement membrane. The cells comprising this type of proliferation are cytologically benign and variable in size, shape, and orientation, and typically are arranged in a 'swirling' pattern. It is often possible to discern two distinct cell populations: epithelial cells and myoepithelial cells. A fibrovascular stroma is sometimes present (Figs 10.11–10.14).

Sclerosing adenosis is usually an incidental finding but may present as a mammographic abnormality, microcalcifications,

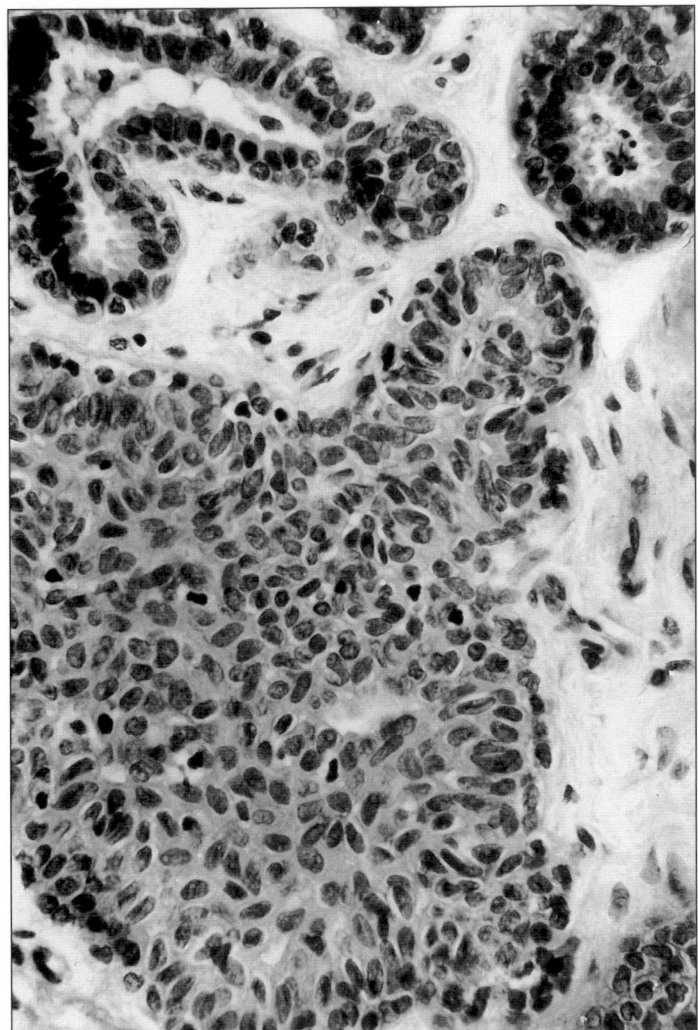

Fig. 10.11 Ductal hyperplasia. Note the solid cellular growth without marked cellular atypia; partial obliteration of the ductular lumen by cellular proliferation; and absence of cellular atypia and mitoses (high magnification).

distorted architecture, or a mass lesion, also known as 'nodular adenosis' or 'adenosis tumor'.[179] This lesion is composed of distorted epithelial, myoepithelial, and sclerotic stromal elements arising in association with the terminal duct lobular unit. This 'lobulocentric' pattern is key to the correct diagnosis of sclerosing adenosis and its variants, and is best appreciated at low-power microscopic examination (Figs 10.15–10.17). The epithelium in sclerosing adenosis may undergo apocrine metaplasia, when it is also known as 'apocrine adenosis.'[180,181] The apocrine metaplastic cells may show cytologic atypia, raising the differential diagnosis of invasive carcinoma if the lesion is examined at high microscopic power without accounting for lobulocentric architecture appreciated at low power.[182] Sclerosing adenosis may also be involved by ALH and/or LCIS, ADH, or DCIS.[183–186] Perineural 'pseudoinvasion' may be present in approximately 2% of sclerosing adenosis cases and should not be confused with invasive carcinoma.[187] Because of the distorted glandular pattern of sclerosing adenosis, this lesion may be confused with a low-grade invasive carcinoma, particularly tubular carcinoma. Importantly, as opposed to tubular carcinoma, sclerosing

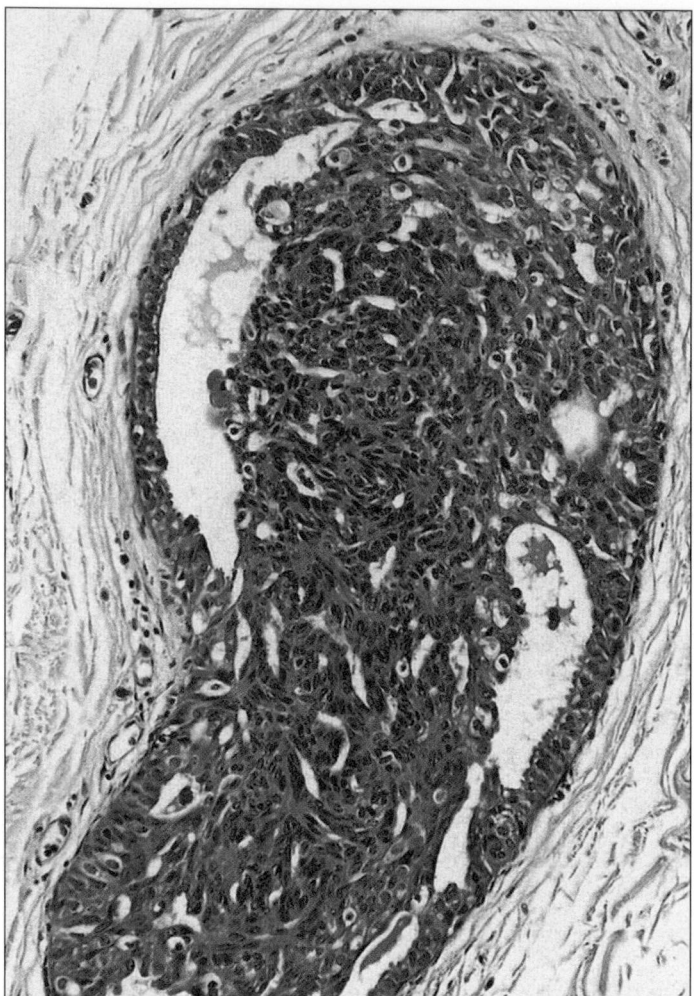

Fig. 10.12 Ductal hyperplasia without atypia. Irregularity in size and shape of lumina within the intraductal proliferation is emphasized here, as are cell streaming and lack of nuclear atypia.

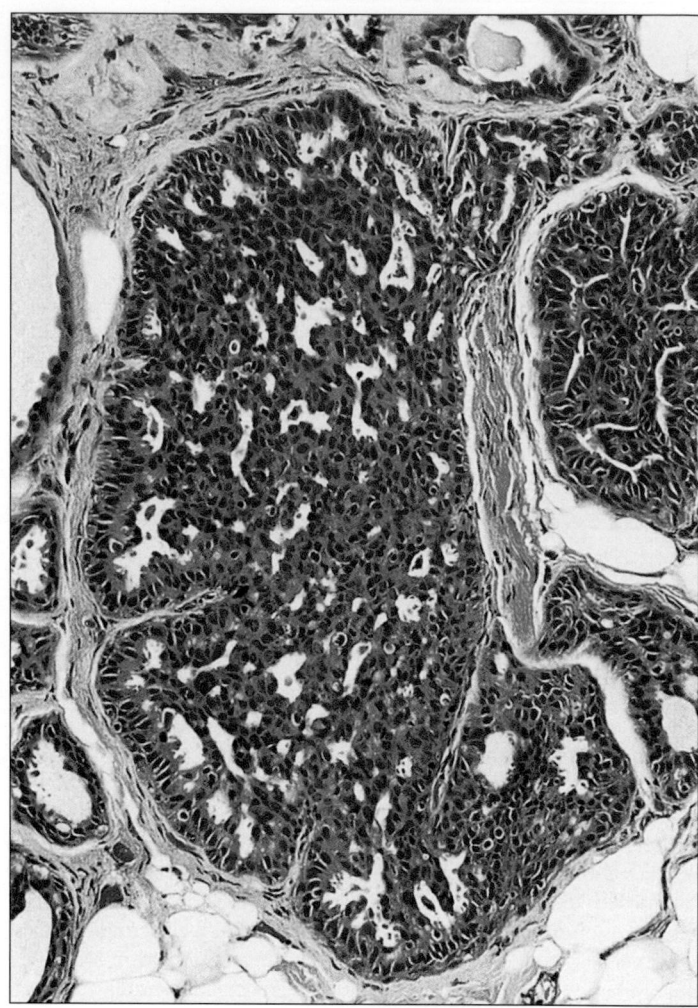

Fig. 10.13 Ductal hyperplasia without atypia. Note bimorphic cell population, lack of nuclear atypia, and irregularly sized and shaped intraluminal spaces.

adenosis contains myoepithelial cells, which may be highlighted by immunohistochemistry.

Atypical hyperplasia

Atypical hyperplasias have been defined as proliferative lesions of the breast that possess some but not all of the features of carcinoma in situ and are classified as either ductal or lobular type.[37,161] *Atypical ductal hyperplasias* are lesions that have some of the architectural and cytologic features of low-grade DCIS, such as nuclear monomorphism, regular cell placement, and round regular spaces, in at least part of the involved space. The cells may form tufts, micropapillations, arcades, bridges, solid, and cribriform patterns.[188] A second cell population which has similar features to those seen in usual ductal hyperplasia is also typically present (Fig. 10.18).

Atypical lobular hyperplasia is composed of cells identical to those found in LCIS. These cells are monomorphic, evenly spaced, and dyshesive, with round or oval, usually eccentric nuclei and pale cytoplasm, often with intracytoplasmic vacuoles. Although criteria for the distinction between ALH and LCIS differ among experts, we use the criteria proposed by Page and Anderson and diagnose ALH

when the characteristic cells are present but less than one half of the acini of a lobular unit are filled, distorted, or distended[189] (Fig. 10.19). In addition to involving lobular units, the cells of ALH may also involve ducts.[190]

The likelihood of finding atypical hyperplasia varies with the reason for the biopsy. Biopsies performed for a palpable mass reveal atypical hyperplasia is in 2–4% of cases.[161,191] In contrast, atypical hyperplasia is identified in 12–17% of biopsies performed because of mammographic microcalcifications.[192,193]

Women who have had a benign breast biopsy that demonstrates atypical hyperplasia are at a substantially increased risk for developing breast cancer, approximately 3.5–5.0 times that of the reference population. In the two largest studies,[170,175,190] the risk associated with ALH was greater than that associated with ADH. These studies have shown that the risk of the subsequent breast cancer in patients with atypical lobular hyperplasia is greater in the ipsilateral than the contralateral breast; however, the risk for women with ADH is bilateral.[170,194]

The cytologic diagnosis of 'atypia' is not equivalent to that used in the histologic sense (i.e. ADH or ALH). Because the histologic criteria for atypical hyperplasia are in large part dependent on

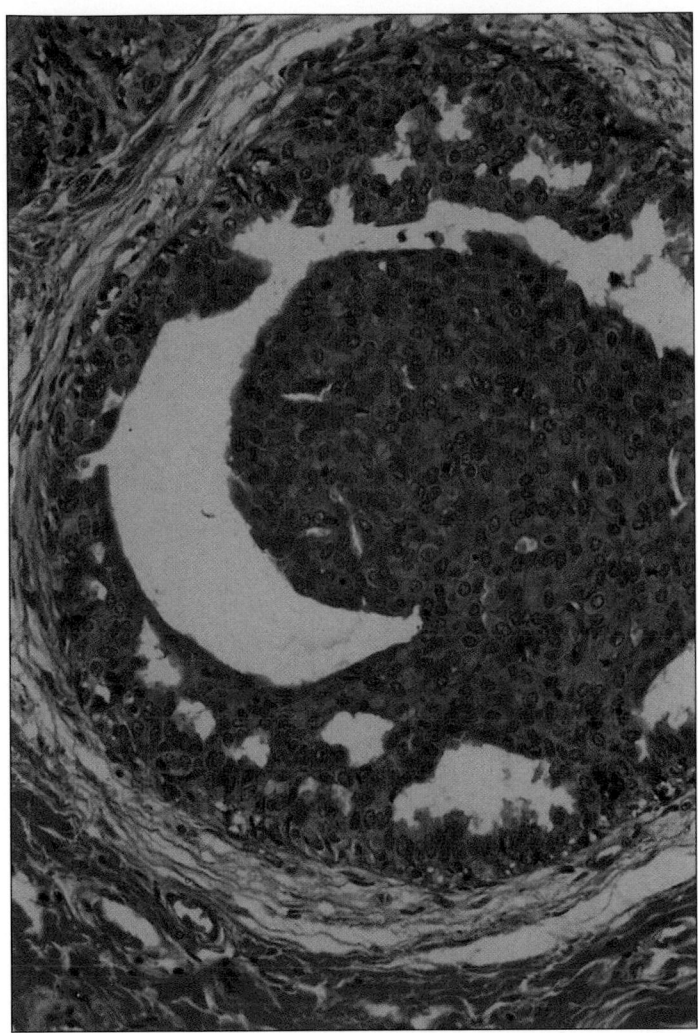

Fig. 10.14 Ductal hyperplasia without atypia. Solid proliferation extending into lumen shows prominent swirling of uniform cells with somewhat ovoid nuclei.

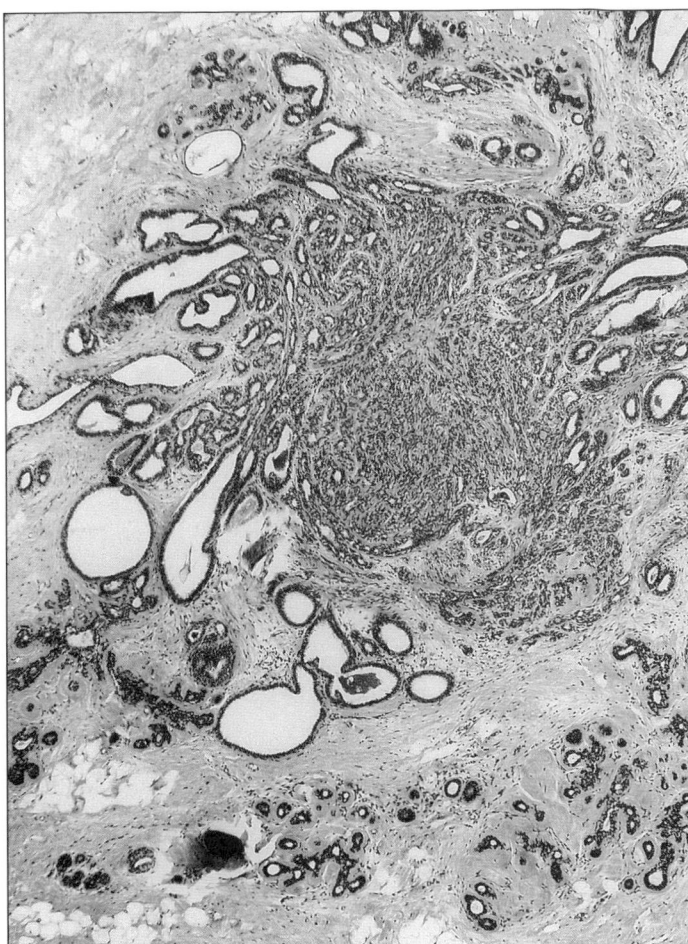

Fig. 10.15 Sclerosing adenosis. Note the dense cellular area composed of epithelial structures modified by the stromal proliferation. This should not be misinterpreted as a malignant proliferation. Retained lobular configuration and peripheral dilatation are characteristic and useful findings, as are lack of cytologic atypia and mitotic activity.

architectural features, the cytologic–histologic correlation of atypical hyperplasia (particularly ADH) is poor. Atypia, particularly in the context of the probabilistic approach to cytologic diagnosis, should rather be used to denote a small but finite chance that the aspirated lesion might be malignant.

Factors modifying breast cancer risk in women with biopsy-proven benign breast disease

There are a number of factors that appear to modify the breast cancer risk associated with biopsy-proven benign breast disease, including a family history of breast cancer, which increases the risk to some extent, and being premenopausal, which increases the risk relative to being postmenopausal.[161,168,170,175]

Some authors have suggested that quantitative criteria should also be used to aid in the distinction between ADH and DCIS. For example, Page and co-workers require that all of the features of low-grade DCIS be uniformly present throughout at least two separate spaces before DCIS is diagnosed.[175] Lesions that have the qualitative features of low-grade DCIS that do not fulfill this quantitative criterion are categorized as atypical hyperplasias. Tavassoli and Norris classify lesions that fulfill the qualitative criteria for low-

grade DCIS but that are 2 mm in size or smaller as atypical intraductal hyperplasias.[163] However, in contrast to studies using the Page criteria, the risk is greater in the ipsilateral breast when using the 2-mm criteria. In our experience ADHs are usually limited to part of one space. Therefore we do not use size criteria for that diagnosis.

To overcome some of the limitations of morphology, studies have attempted to identify biological or genetic markers that may be useful adjuncts to histopathology in distinguishing among these various proliferative lesions. Unfortunately at this time there are no reliable markers to routinely separate these lesions.

SPECIFIC BENIGN LESIONS

BENIGN NEOPLASMS AND PROLIFERATIVE LESIONS

Fibroadenomas

On gross examination, fibroadenomas are pseudoencapsulated and are sharply delimited from the surrounding breast tissue. They are

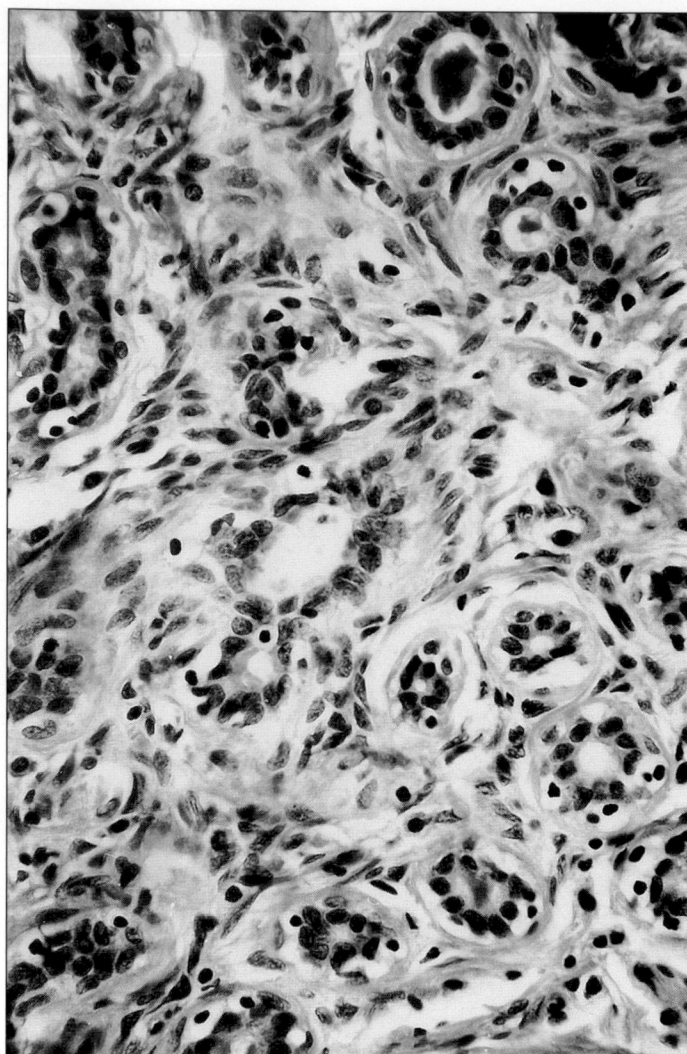

Fig. 10.16 Sclerosing adenosis. Detail showing bimorphic appearance and lack of atypia.

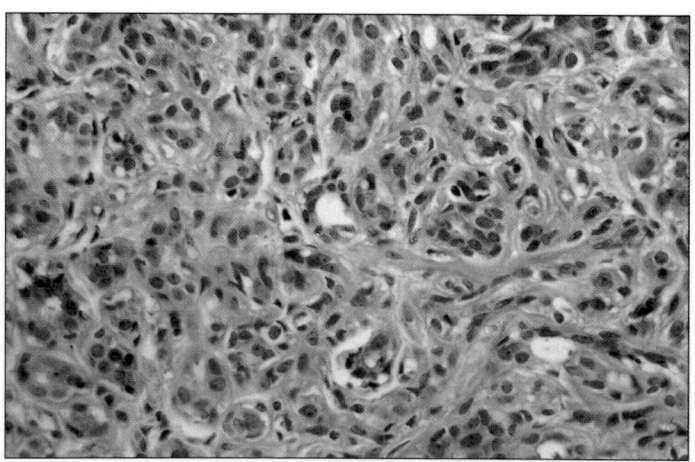

Fig. 10.17 Sclerosing adenosis. Distortion of the epithelial structures by interstitial fibrosis is seen.

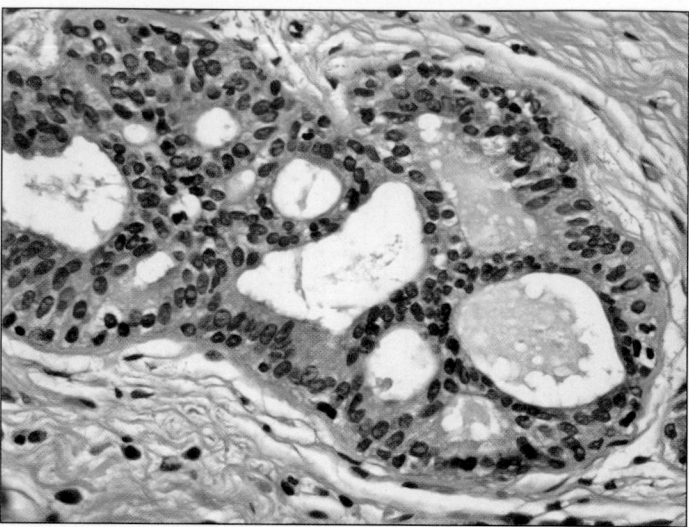

Fig. 10.18 Atypical ductal hyperplasia. A ductal proliferation with 'rigid bars' and central cellular monomorphism.

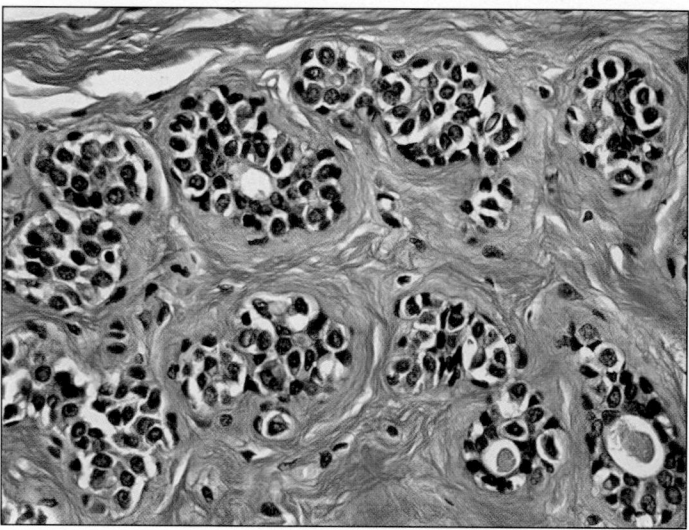

Fig. 10.19 Atypical lobular hyperplasia: Proliferation of small monomorphic cells that lack cohesion.

usually spherical or ovoid but may be multilobular. When cut, the tumor bulges above the level of the surrounding breast tissue. The cut surface is most typically grey-white and small, punctate, yellow to pink soft areas and slit-like spaces are commonly observed. Occasionally, the tumor has a gelatinous, mucoid consistency.

Microscopically, fibroadenomas have both an epithelial and stromal component. The histologic pattern depends upon which of these components predominates. In general, the epithelial component consists of well defined, gland-like, and duct-like spaces lined by cuboidal or columnar cells with uniform nuclei. Varying degrees of epithelial hyperplasia are frequently observed. The stromal component consists of connective tissue that has a variable content of acid mucopolysaccharides and collagen (Figs 10.20–10.22). In older lesions and in postmenopausal patients, the stroma may become hyalinized, calcified, or even ossified (ancient fibroadenoma). On rare occasions, mature adipose tissue or smooth muscle may comprise a

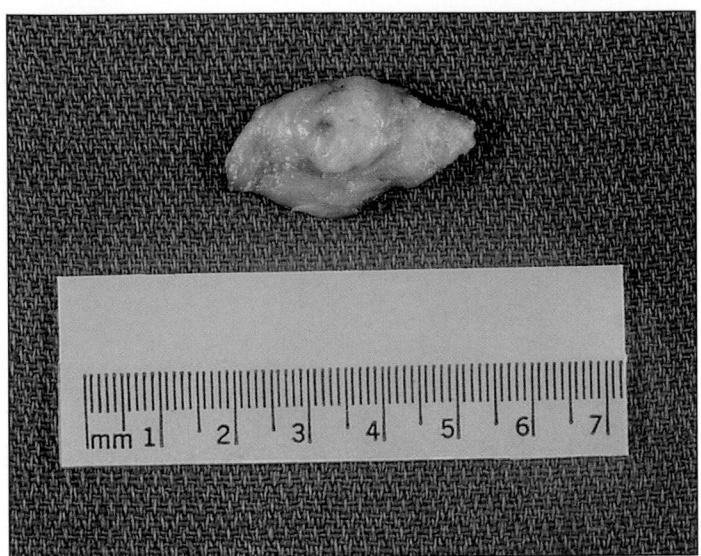

Fig. 10.20 Fibroadenoma, gross appearance.

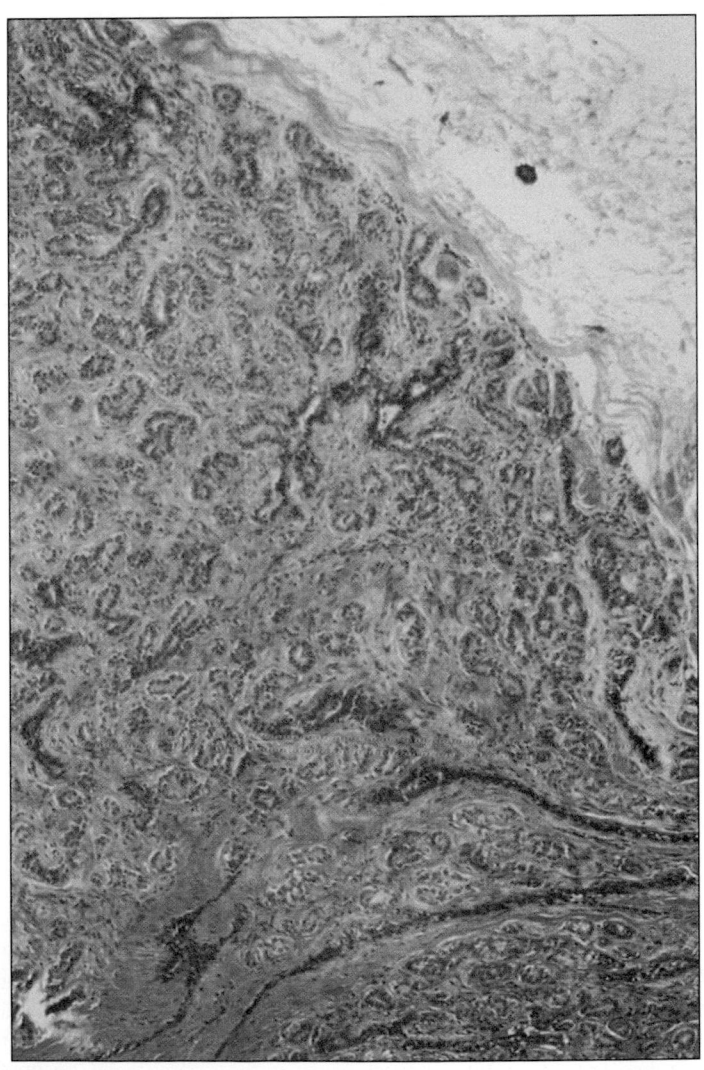

Fig. 10.21 Fibroadenoma, pericanalicular type.

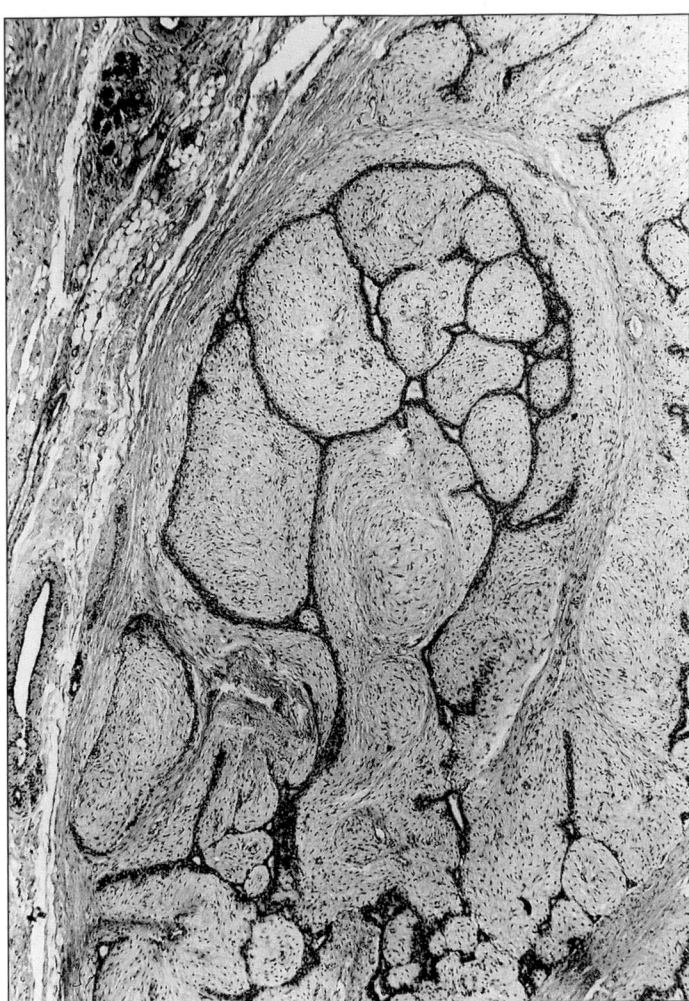

Fig. 10.22 Fibroadenoma, intracanalicular type.

portion of the stroma.[195,196] The term 'intracanalicular' has been used to describe tumors in which the stromal component compresses the glands into slit-like spaces, whereas 'pericanalicular' tumors are those in which the rounded configuration of the glandular structures is maintained. In fact, these two patterns often coexist in the same lesion, and this distinction has no clinical significance.

Juvenile fibroadenomas

Most fibroadenomas in adolescents and younger women are of the usual type seen in older patients. A minority present a different clinical and pathologic picture and are termed juvenile fibroadenomas.[197–200] Unfortunately, this term has been used by different authors to describe different lesions. Some authors use the term to refer to fibroadenomatous lesions that grow rapidly and may show venous dilatation in the overlying skin. Such lesions may clinically resemble virginal hypertrophy, and only surgical exploration will reveal a circumscribed tumor.[197–199] Microscopically, these lesions are more floridly glandular and have greater stromal cellularity than the more common adult-type fibroadenoma. Mies and Rosen use the term 'juvenile fibroadenomas' to refer to fibroadenomatous lesions that demonstrate severe epithelial hyperplasia, which may border on carcinoma in situ.[200] Nevertheless, these lesions behave in a clinically benign fashion.

Giant fibroadenomas

Some tumors that are histologically typical fibroadenomas may attain great size. Unfortunately, several authors have used the terms 'giant fibroadenoma' and 'benign cystosarcoma phyllodes' synonymously and have created considerable confusion regarding these entities. A lesion that has the microscopic appearance of a conventional fibroadenoma but that is large should still be classified as a fibroadenoma and may be treated adequately by enucleation. The major feature that distinguishes a phyllodes tumor from a giant fibroadenoma is the cellularity of the stromal component in the former.[195] It must be noted, however, that the distinction between these two entities may be extremely difficult in some cases. Because juvenile fibroadenomas may attain great sizes, some authors consider them to be variants of giant fibroadenomas.[199]

Infarction

Fibroadenomas may undergo partial, subtotal, or total infarction. Pregnancy and lactation are the most common predisposing factors. It has been postulated that a relative vascular insufficiency in the face of increased metabolic activity in the breast underlies this phenomenon.[195]

Involvement of fibroadenomas by atypical hyperplasia

Atypical hyperplasia of both ductal and lobular types may occasionally be found within a fibroadenoma. In a study of almost 2000 fibroadenomas, atypical hyperplasia was found in 0.81% of the cases.[201] Of note in that study, the presence of atypia in a fibroadenoma did not predict for the presence of atypical hyperplasia in the surrounding breast tissue nor was it associated with a significant increase in the risk of subsequent breast cancer.

Involvement of fibroadenomas by carcinoma

This subject has been reviewed by Azzopardi[195] and by Pick and Iossifides.[202] Infrequently, carcinoma may occur in association with a fibroadenoma. The most frequent type of carcinoma involving fibroadenomas is LCIS. Infiltrating carcinomas of various types and DCIS can also occur within fibroadenomas. In almost half the reported cases, the malignant tumor also involves the surrounding breast tissue. Given this and the fact that the epithelial component of a fibroadenoma may communicate with the surrounding ducts, re-excision of the surrounding tissue is advisable when DCIS or invasive carcinoma is present in a fibroadenoma. The prognosis of carcinoma limited to a fibroadenoma is excellent.

Phyllodes tumors

Phyllodes tumors are uncommon tumors. In one community-based study compared to breast cancer patients, they had a frequency of 0.5%.[203] Patients generally are over the age of 40 and the lesions may be quite large, although at the present time the average size is approximately 5 cm[203,204] (Fig. 10.23). Grossly, the lesions are usually well circumscribed and one may see the characteristic leaf-like pattern in large lesions. Microscopically, these are biphasic lesions with epithelial and stromal proliferation. The stroma is more cellular than that of a fibroadenoma and, in contrast to a fibroadenoma, the stromal cellularity is greater around epithelial elements than elsewhere in the lesion. The characteristic leaf-like pattern is helpful but may also be seen in fibroadenomas and is not seen in every phyllodes tumor. The main criteria separating a phyllodes tumor from a fibroadenoma is increased stromal cellularity. If one sees what appears to be a sarcoma in the breast, one should carefully sample a lesion for the presence of phyllodes tumor since the prognosis of a phyllodes tumor is better than other lesions that may be sarcomatous.

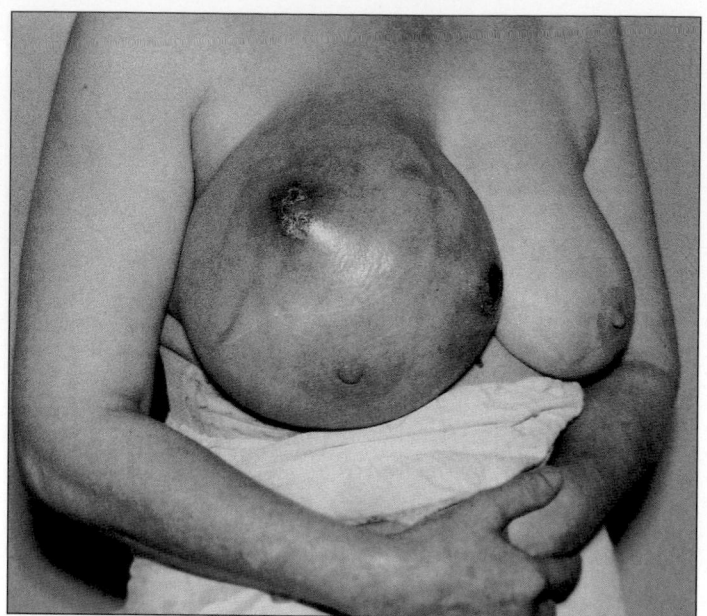

Fig. 10.23 Phyllodes tumor in a 52-year-old woman.

The prognosis of a phyllodes tumor depends upon whether it is benign, borderline, or malignant. The definition of benign, borderline and malignant, however, is not universally agreed upon. The most reliable criteria for predicting malignant behavior in a phyllodes tumor is the presence of heterologous sarcomatous elements, i.e. liposarcoma, rhabdomyosarcoma, osteosarcoma, etc.[204–207] Other than that, factors that may help predict for malignant behavior include an infiltrative border, cellular overgrowth (which is defined as a 4× low-power field with only stromal elements),[208] moderate to marked stromal atypia, and a high mitotic count. Generally, a high mitotic count is considered to be 10 or more mitoses per 10 high power fields (hpf). Lesions with pushing margins, minimal cellular atypia, and fewer than 4 mitoses/10 hpf are generally felt to be benign and lesions with characteristics in between fall into a borderline category[209] (Figs 10.24, 10.25).

In a series of articles summarized in references 209–215,[210] when lesions were divided into benign, borderline, and malignant in a series of 467 total cases, lesions classified as benign had an 18% local recurrence rate (generally attributed to lack of adequate initial excision) but no metastases or deaths. A series of 36 cases classified as borderline had a 33% risk of local recurrence but only a 6% risk of metastasis or death, and 131 cases classified as malignant had a 15% risk of local recurrence but only an 8% chance of metastasis or death. These figures are in sharp contrast to a number of series that have been reported from cancer hospitals or sarcoma units in which, in a highly selected population of patients, the risk of death is up to 27%.[211]

Therefore, it seems wise to consider most phyllodes tumors as benign lesions that require adequate excision. Even tumors that histologically appear malignant have a very low risk (8%) of metastasis or death.

Cytology of fibroadenoma

Most fibroadenomas fall into the category of 'epithelial proliferative lesion without atypia' on cytology (see probabilistic approach

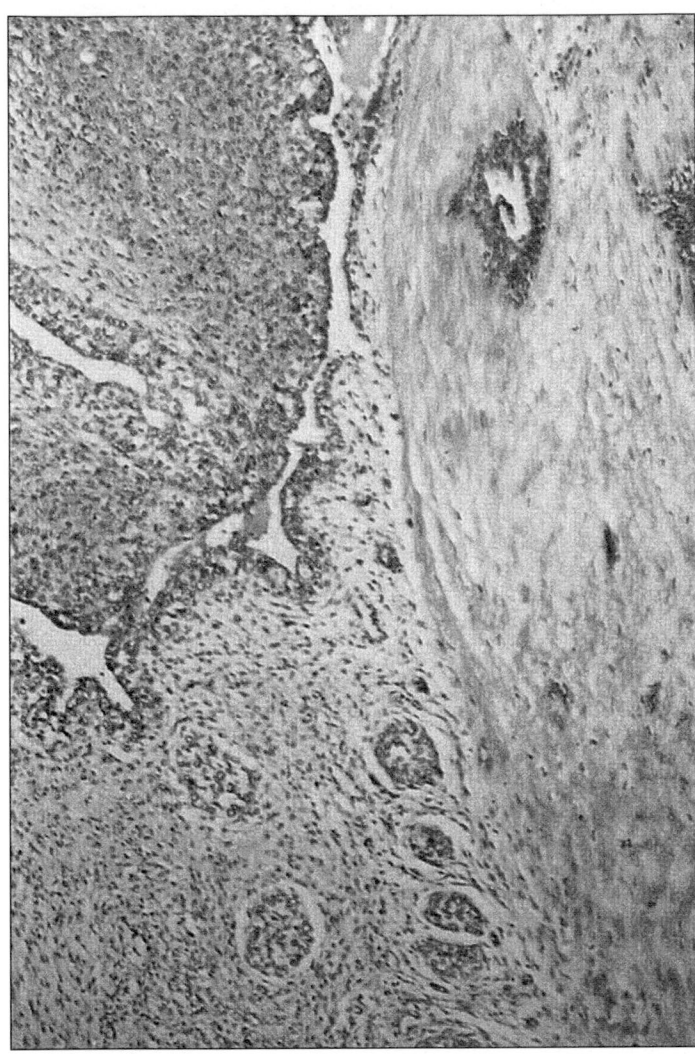

Fig. 10.24 Phyllodes tumor. Low-grade phyllodes tumor, note hypercellular periductal stroma with minimal atypia, and well demarcated tumor border.

above). Aspirates are usually cellular but some may have low cellularity, depending upon the degree of sclerosis of the lesion (particularly in older patients). Classically, smears of fibroadenoma are composed of cohesive sheets and clusters of ductal epithelial cells in a background of bipolar cells and stromal fragments.[28,216,217] Characteristically, the epithelial cell sheets show branching patterns, giving rise to 'staghorn' arrangements (Fig. 10.26). These staghorn arrangements, when present, are the most specific feature of fibroadenoma; however, they may not be seen in all cases and therefore have low sensitivity. Bipolar cells exhibit oval to elongated, spindle-shaped, bland nuclei with absent or inconspicuous nucleoli. The cytoplasm is usually scant and is often absent, giving rise to 'naked' nuclei (Fig. 10.27). A proportion of bipolar cells are of myoepithelial origin, with the remainder of stromal origin. Although abundantly present in fibroadenomas, bipolar cells may be as numerous in other proliferative lesions and are therefore not discriminatory in the diagnosis. Although stromal fragments are found in fibroadenoma, they tend to be more prominent in phyllodes tumor[218–221] (Fig. 10.28).

Confusion of fibroadenoma with carcinoma on FNA cytology is a well known diagnostic pitfall.[222–225] The epithelial cells of fibro-

adenoma may show nuclear atypia with crowding, small prominent nuclei, and clumped chromatin. These features may be particularly troublesome when there are fewer bipolar cells or stromal fragments in the background. In these cases, a diagnosis of 'proliferative lesion with atypia' may be rendered, and in rarer circumstances the diagnosis may be 'suspicious'. The absence of many single epithelial cells and the presence of some stromal or bipolar component should prevent a diagnosis of carcinoma. The clinical and imaging findings of a well circumscribed mass lesion used as part of the 'triple test' (see above) should assist in preventing overdiagnosis of cancer.

Adenoma

Adenomas of the breast are well circumscribed tumors composed of benign epithelial elements with sparse, inconspicuous stroma.[226] The last feature differentiates these lesions from fibroadenomas, in which the stroma is an integral part of the tumor. For practical purposes, adenomas may be divided into two major groups: tubular adenomas and lactating adenomas.

Tubular adenomas

Tubular adenomas present in young women as well defined, freely movable nodules which clinically resemble fibroadenomas.[226] Gross examination reveals a well circumscribed, tan-yellow, firm tumor. On microscopic examination, tubular adenomas are separated from the adjacent breast tissue by a pseudocapsule, and are composed of a proliferation of uniform, small tubular structures with a scant amount of intervening stroma. The tubules are composed of an inner epithelial layer and an outer myoepithelial layer, and resemble normal breast acini both at the light and ultrastructural level. The tubular lumens often contain eosinophilic material. In some cases, this pattern is admixed with that of a fibroadenoma, suggesting a relationship between the two tumors.

On cytologic examination, tubular adenoma may mimic carcinoma.[227] The smears are often cellular, with abundant small, cohesive, gland-like clusters of uniform epithelial cells. Myoepithelial cells and/or bipolar cells are usually scant (Fig. 10.29). The distinction from low-grade or tubular carcinomas may be particularly difficult, and atypical or even suspicious diagnoses are not uncommon in these circumstances.

Lactating adenomas (nodular lactational hyperplasia)

Lactating adenomas present as one or more freely movable masses during pregnancy or the postpartum period.[226] They are grossly well circumscribed and lobular, and on cut section appear tan and softer than tubular adenomas. On microscopic examination, these lesions have lobulated borders and are composed of glands lined by cuboidal cells with secretory activity, identical to the lactational changes normally observed in breast tissue during pregnancy and the puerperium (Fig. 10.30). Although some authors believe that these lesions are the result of lactational changes superimposed on a pre-existing tubular adenoma, others have suggested that they represent de novo lesions and are merely nodular foci of hyperplasia in the lactating breast.

Cytologically, aspirates of lactating breasts are usually cellular, with numerous single epithelial cells present in a background of proteinaceous debris. Variable proportions of inflammatory cells may be present, depending on the clinical context. The epithelial cells characteristically have wispy, delicate, foamy cytoplasm, which is most often stripped, resulting in numerous naked nuclei. The epithelial nuclei are enlarged and hyperchromatic but are uniform in size, with an accentuated smooth nuclear membrane. A single prominent nucleolus is found, which is mostly centrally located

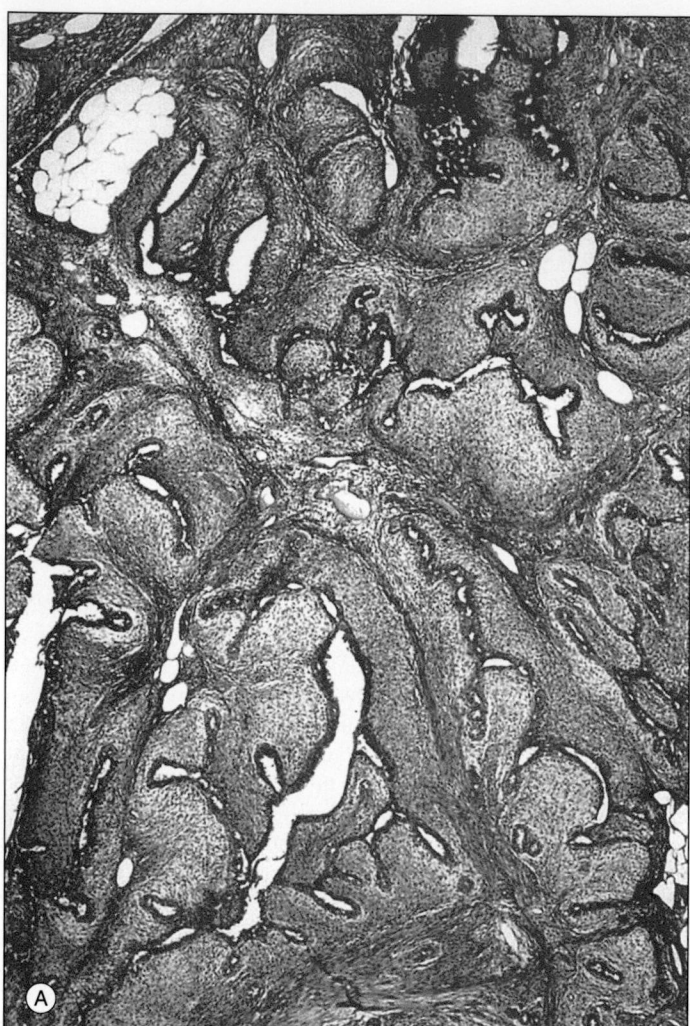

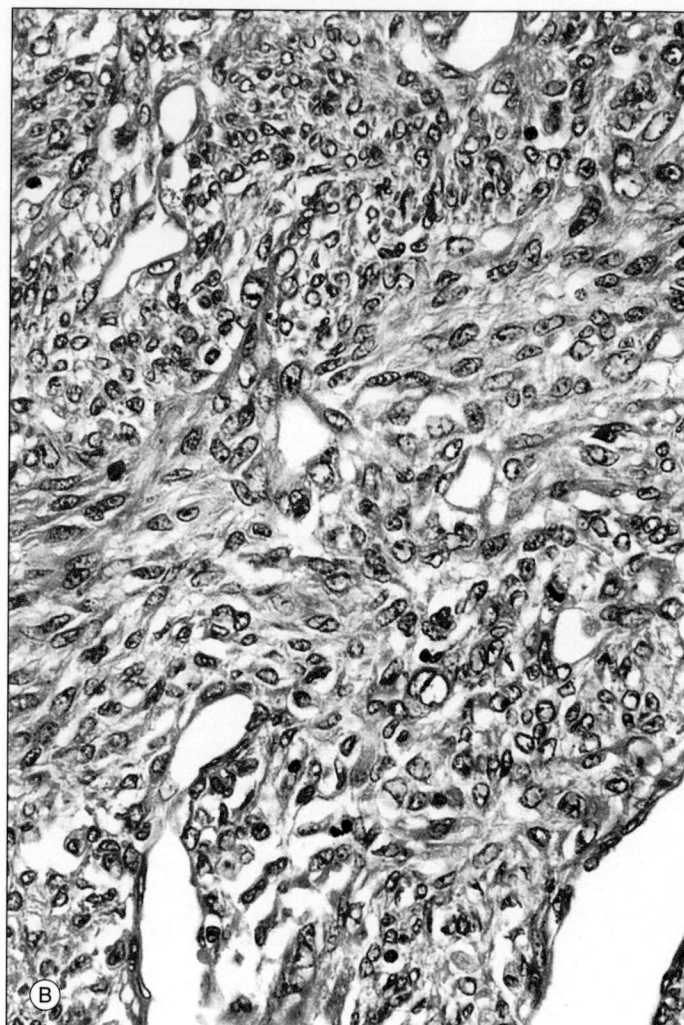

Fig. 10.25 Phyllodes tumor. High-grade phyllodes tumor. **(A)** Slit like ductal spaces cuffed by hypercellular stroma. **(B)** Focus of stromal overgrowth with atypia and increased mitotic activity.

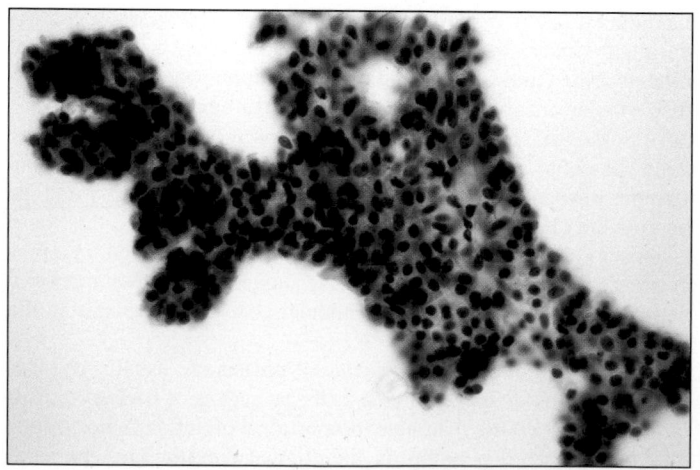

Fig. 10.26 Cytology of a fibroadenoma. Aspirate of fibroadenoma showing cohesive flat sheet of ductal epithelial cells with papillations in 'stag-horn' configuration. (ThinPrep, Papanicolaou stain, ×400.) (Courtesy of Dr Helen Wang, Beth Israel Deaconess Medical Center, Boston, MA.)

within the nucleus (Fig. 10.31).[228] This is in contrast to carcinoma, where the nucleus is usually eccentrically placed, with pleomorphism, irregular nuclear membranes, and variable, often multiple haphazardly placed nucleoli. Because of their high cellularity, abundance of single cells, and perceived nuclear atypia, lactating adenomas may easily be confused with carcinoma. However, if the characteristic cytologic features are considered and the smear is interpreted in the clinical context, an appropriate diagnosis is possible.

Carcinoma of the breast may occur during pregnancy and lactation, and these cases may be particularly challenging to diagnose on cytology. Nonetheless, the nuclear features of carcinoma such as nuclear membrane irregularities, angulated, and pleomorphic nuclei may be distinguished from lactation. Other helpful features in favor of carcinoma in the presence of lactation include crowding and overlapping of nuclei, coarse chromatin, and mitoses.[229]

Rarely, adenomatous tumors resembling dermal sweat gland neoplasms are observed as primary lesions in the breast parenchyma (e.g. clear cell hidradenoma and eccrine spiradenoma)[202,230] or nipple (e.g. syringomatous adenoma).[231,232] Pleomorphic adenomas histologically identical to those seen in the salivary glands and skin have also been described in the breast.[233–236] While some of these

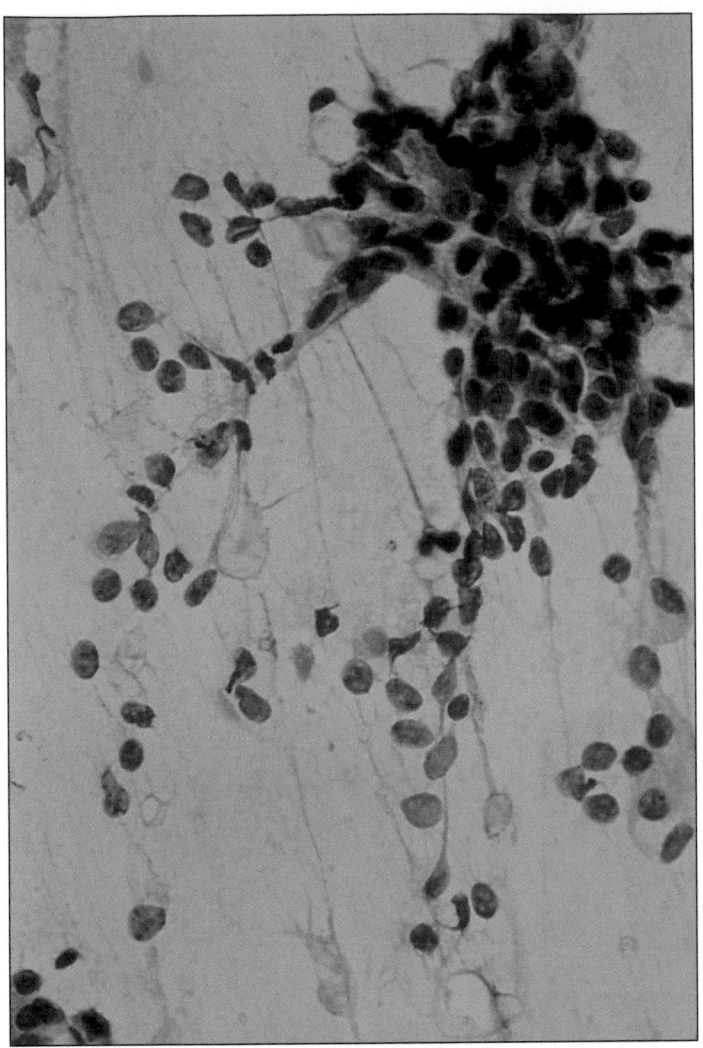

Fig. 10.27 Cytology of a fibroadenoma. Aspirate of fibroadenoma displaying naked nuclei in the background and spindled myoepithelial cells within the cluster of epithelial cells. (Papanicolaou stain, ×200.)

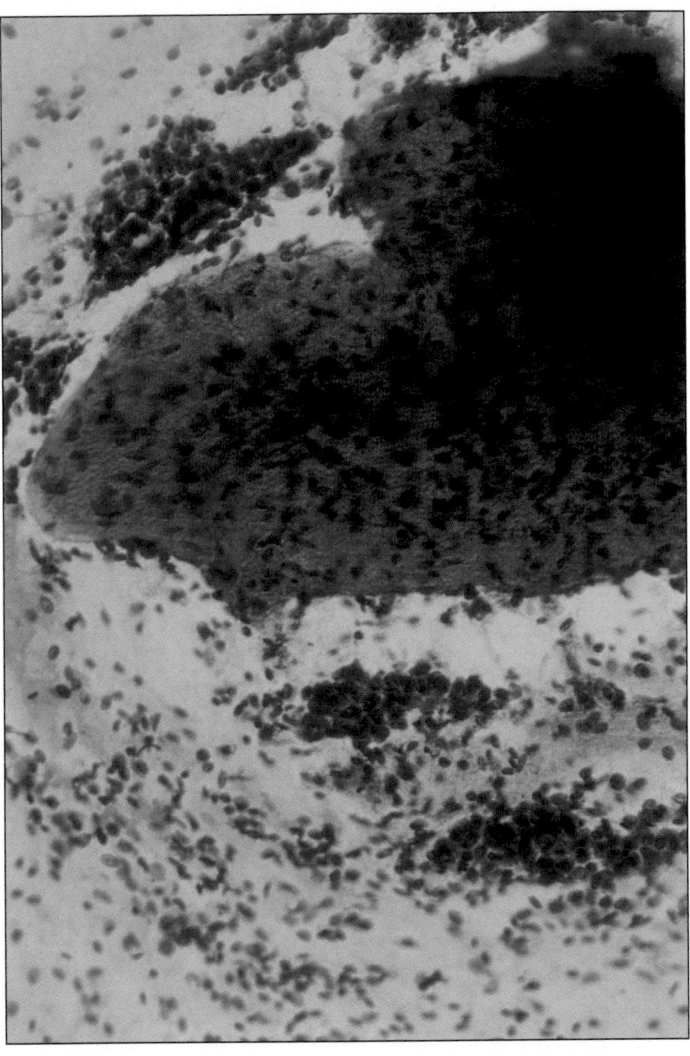

Fig. 10.28 Cytology of a phyllodes tumor. Biphasic pattern seen in an aspirate of low-grade phyllodes tumor, similar to features seen in fibroadenomas. (Papanicolaou stain, ×200.)

lesions appear to arise from the breast tissue de novo, others appear to represent variants of intraductal papillomas.[236]

Adenomas of the nipple

Adenoma of the nipple has been described under a variety of names, including florid papillomatosis of the nipple ducts,[237] subareolar duct papillomatosis,[195] papillary adenoma of the nipple,[238] and erosive adenomatosis of the nipple.[239]

On macroscopic examination, some adenomas of the nipple appear as solid, grey-tan, poorly demarcated tumors in the nipple and subareolar region; in other cases, no gross lesion is evident. Microscopically, the dominant feature is a proliferation of small, gland-like structures. Solid and papillary proliferation of ductal epithelium is also usually evident; however, the papillary pattern may be inconspicuous or totally absent. In advanced lesions, glandular epithelium extends out on to the surface of the nipple. It is this phenomenon that results in the clinically apparent reddish, granular appearance that clinically mimics Paget's disease. Squamous epithelium frequently extends into the superficial regions of the involved ducts, sometimes with the formation of keratinaceous cysts. The

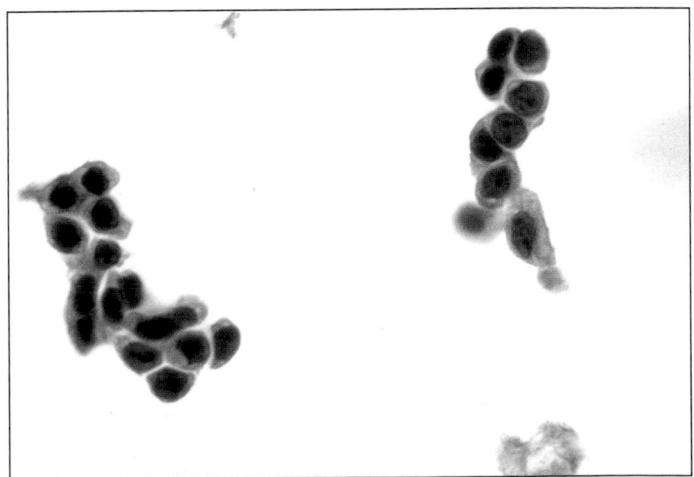

Fig. 10.29 Cytology of a tubular adenoma. Fine-needle aspiration cytology of tubular adenoma, showing small, loosely cohesive clusters of atypical ductal epithelial cells. (ThinPrep, Papanicolaou stain, ×400.)

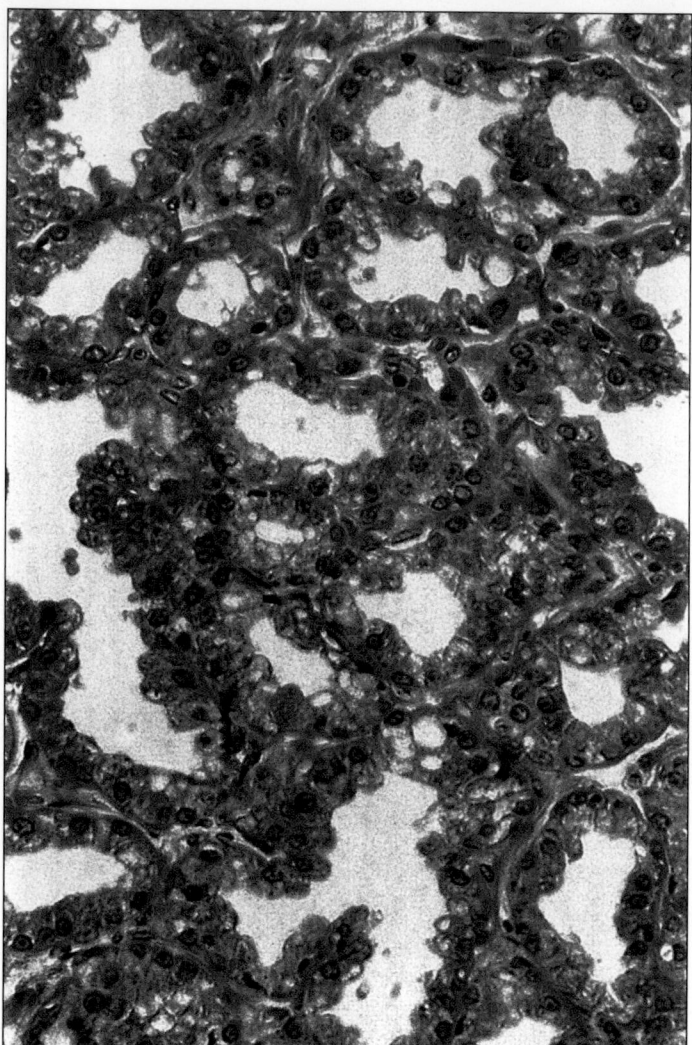

Fig. 10.30 Lactating adenoma. Note bubbly vacuolated cytoplasm.

lesions usually show considerable stromal fibrosis. This connective tissue may distort and entrap the epithelial elements, resulting in a pattern mimicking invasive carcinoma. The lesion is distinguishable from carcinoma by the preservation of the myoepithelial layer, minimal nuclear atypicality, usual absence of necrosis, and the overall low-power configuration (Fig. 10.32). In problematic cases, immunohistochemical stains for myoepithelial cells may be of value in distinguishing a nipple adenoma from invasive carcinoma.

A few cases of carcinoma associated with adenomas of the nipple have been reported.[240] However, in the majority of cases the lesion is entirely benign. Reports of recurrence most probably represent cases in which the initial resection failed to remove the lesion completely.

Syringomatous adenoma of the nipple
Syringomatous adenoma of the nipple is an uncommon benign breast lesion that is similar in histologic appearance to eccrine syringoma of the skin. The usual clinical presentation is as a mass lesion in the region of the nipple–areola complex. Microscopic examination reveals an infiltrative pattern of epithelial islands that are angulated or comma shaped as well as tubular or solid in configuration. The glandular lumens are small or obliterated. Squamous metaplasia is usually present within a variable proportion of epithelial islands, which have an inconspicuous or absent outer myoepithelial layer (Fig. 10.33). The epithelial elements infiltrate between normal structures, mimicking invasive carcinoma.[231] Perineural invasion is common.

It is important to distinguish syringomatous adenoma from the malignant lesions, tubular carcinoma and low-grade adenosquamous carcinoma. The glandular structures of tubular carcinoma are mostly angular, with open lumens, compared to the epithelial islands of syringomatous adenoma, which have smaller or absent lumens and often have characteristic 'comma' or 'tadpole' shapes. In addition, the glands of tubular carcinoma are composed of a single cell population as opposed to those of syringomatous adenoma, which have a variable amount of squamous metaplasia. Unlike syringomatous adenoma, tubular carcinoma often has associated DCIS. Low-grade adenosquamous carcinoma is virtually indistinguishable from syringomatous adenoma but usually involves the deeper parenchyma of the breast. If low-grade adenosquamous carcinoma involves the nipple–areola complex, the lesion may be impossible to distinguish from syringomatous adenoma.

Papillary lesions
A variety of lesions in the breast are characterized by a papillary configuration grossly and/or microscopically. These include solitary intraductal papillomas, multiple (peripheral) papillomas and papillomatosis. *Solitary intraductal papilloma* represents a distinct clinicopathologic entity, as described below. *Papillomatosis* is a term used to describe microscopic foci of intraductal hyperplasia that have a papillary architecture. *Multiple (peripheral) papillomas* are lesions that are less uniformly recognized. While some authors include these in the category of papillomatosis, others recognize a clinicopathologic entity characterized clinically by an indistinct mass with or without nipple discharge and pathologically by multiple small, but grossly evident papillary lesions.[176]

Solitary intraductal papillomas
Solitary intraductal papillomas are tumors of the major lactiferous ducts, most frequently observed in women 30–50 years of age. These lesions often present with unilateral nipple discharge. These lesions are generally less than 1 cm in diameter, usually measuring 3–4 mm. Occasionally, they may be as large as 4–5 cm. On gross examination, intraductal papillomas are tan-pink, friable tumors within a dilated duct or cyst. A frankly papillary configuration may or may not be apparent. The tumor is usually attached to the wall of the involved duct by a delicate stalk but it may be sessile.

Benign papillary lesions have fibrovascular stalks with both an epithelial and a myoepithelial layer. Microscopically, these tumors are composed of multiple, branching, and interanastomosing papillae, each with a central fibrovascular core and a covering layer of cuboidal to columnar epithelial cells (Figs 10.34, 10.35). In some areas, the complex growth pattern of the papillae results in the formation of gland-like spaces. Variable amounts of fibrosis may result in the entrapment of epithelial elements, producing a pseudo-infiltrative pattern. Many lesions, designated by some authors as 'ductal adenomas,' appear to represent extensively sclerotic intraductal papillomas.[241,242] In addition, florid epithelial proliferation is sometimes observed in intraductal papillomas. At times, the epithelial cell hyperplasia or fibrosis (or both) and the architectural distortion make it extremely difficult to distinguish between benign papilloma and papillary DCIS (or intracystic papillary carcinoma). Features helpful in making this distinction have been elucidated by Kraus and Neubecker[243] and by Azzopardi[195] (Table 10.5).

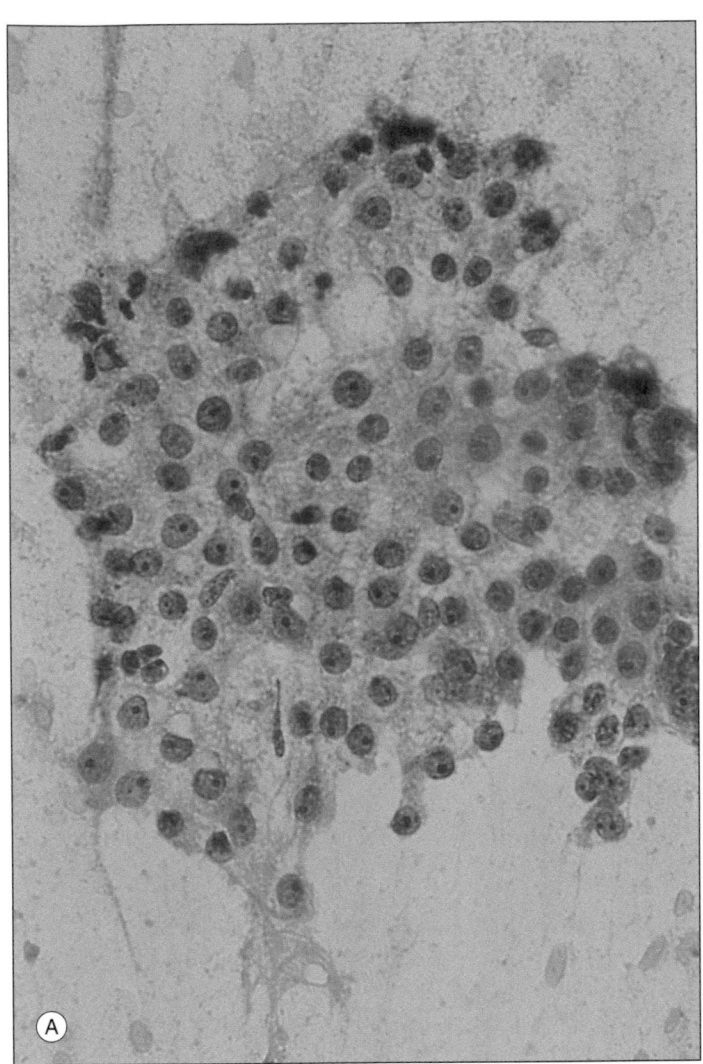
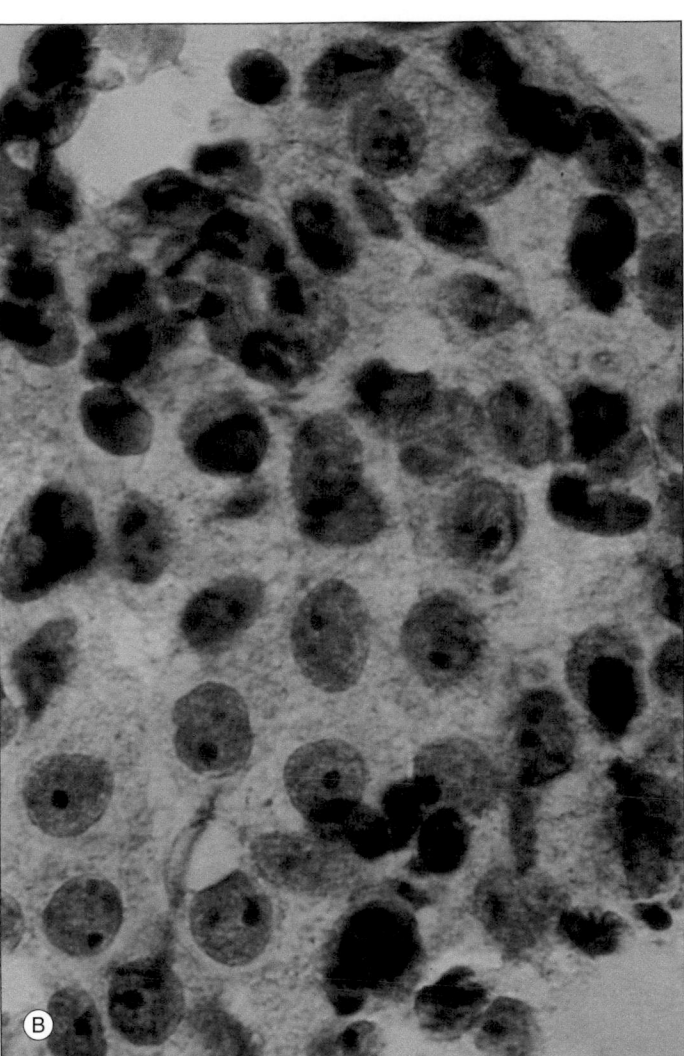

Fig. 10.31 **(A)** Direct smear from a lactating adenoma showing loosely cohesive clusters of epithelial cells in the proteinaceous background. (Papanicolaou stain ×200.) **(B)** Higher magnification of the same case featuring reactive epithelial changes with prominent nucleoli and abundant cytoplasm with ill-defined borders. (Papanicolaou stain, ×400.)

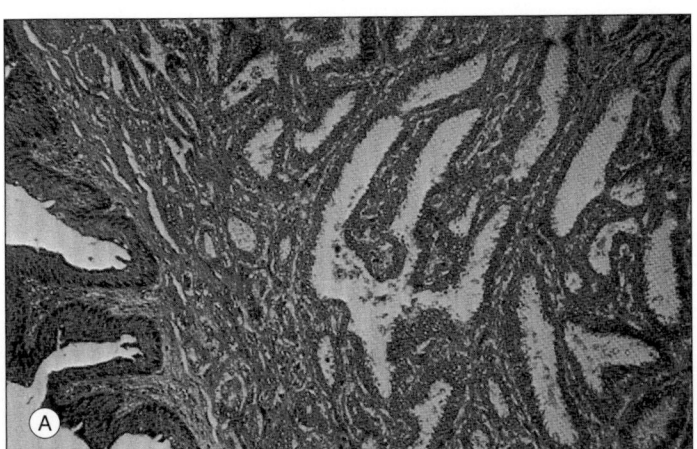
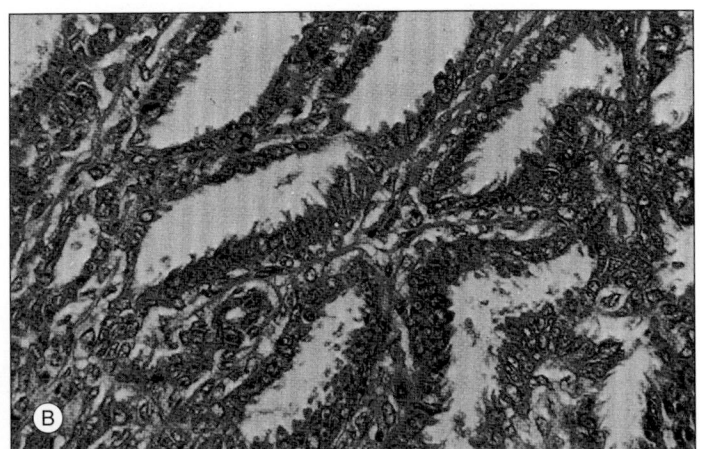

Fig. 10.32 Nipple adenoma. **(A)** Low magnification. Ductal proliferation is localized beneath the mammary skin (seen at left). **(B)** High magnification. The glandular structures are lined by columnar epithelium underlain by myoepithelium. The nuclei are regular and mitoses are absent.

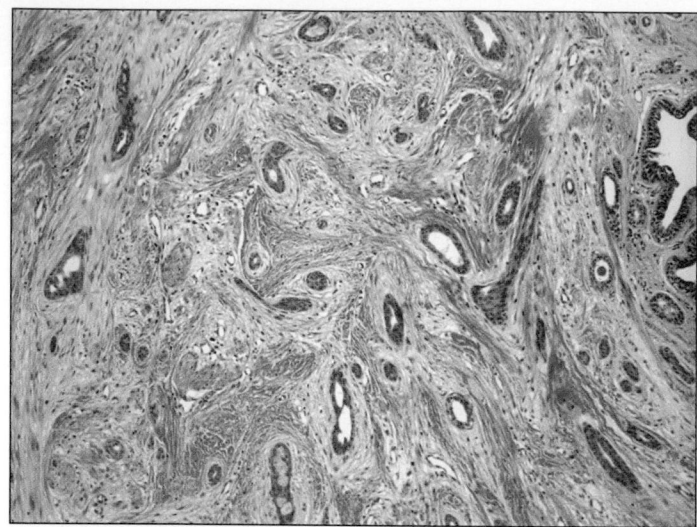

Fig. 10.33 Syringomatous adenoma of the nipple. Infiltrative comma-shaped small ducts without a stromal response.

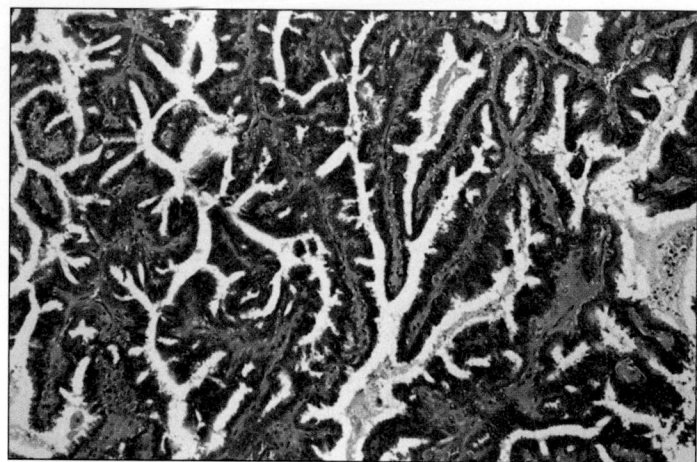

Fig. 10.35 Intraductal papilloma. High power of an intraductal papilloma showing fibrovascular cores.

Table 10.5 Histologic criteria for distinguishing benign intraductal papilloma from papillary ductal carcinoma in situ (DCIS)

Histologic feature	Intraductal papilloma	Papillary DCIS
Cell types	Epithelial, myoepithelial	Epithelial
Cell orientation	Haphazard	Perpendicular to fibrovascular stalk, uniform
Nuclei	Normochromatic	Hyperchromatic
Apocrine metaplasia	Present	Absent
Glandular pattern	Complex	Uniform
Stroma	Prominent, fibrosis	Delicate or absent
Associated epithelial proliferation	Hyperplasia	DCIS
Adjacent epithelial proliferation	Hyperplasia	DCIS

Source: adapted from Kraus and Neubecker[243]

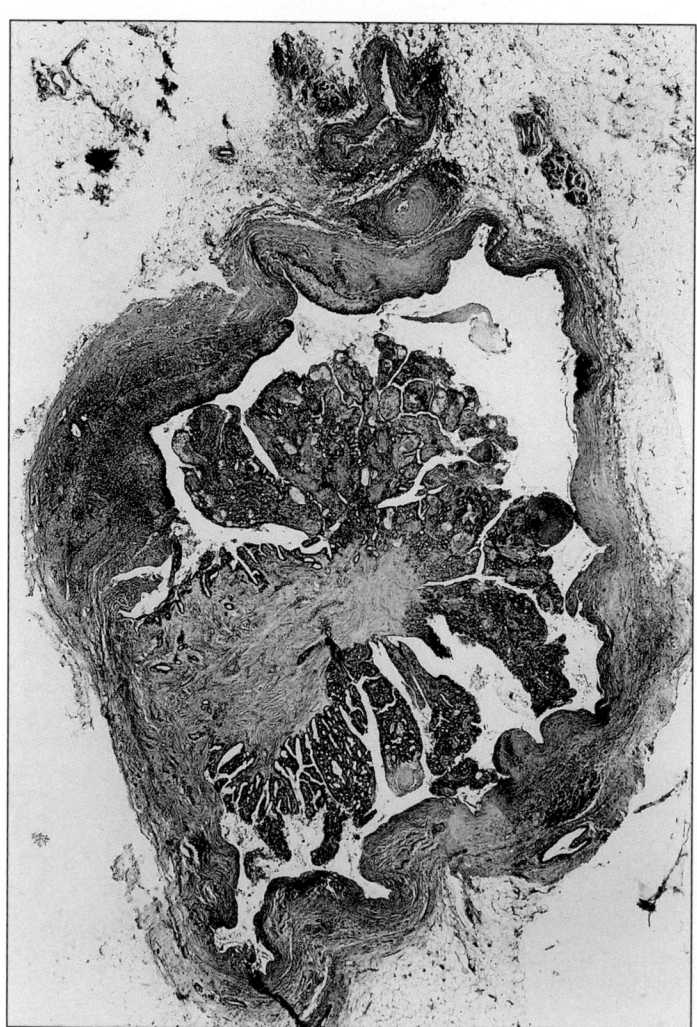

Fig. 10.34 Intraductal papilloma.

The cardinal feature of papillomas (compared to papillary DCIS) is the presence of a layer of myoepithelial cells between the epithelial cells and the fibrovascular cores they cover. At low power, the papillary/glandular pattern of benign papilloma is 'disorganized' and complex compared to the orderly fine and uniform pattern observed in papillary DCIS. The fibrovascular cores of papilloma are prominent, often with fibrosis, compared to those of papillary DCIS, which are delicate or minimally present. As opposed to the neoplastic epithelial cells in papillary DCIS, which are uniform and mostly oriented perpendicular to the fibrovascular cores, those of benign papilloma have a haphazard 'windswept' arrangement. The epithelial cell nuclei of benign papillomas are also normochromatic compared to the hyperchromatic nuclei of papillary DCIS. A useful feature, if present, in favor of an intraductal papilloma is the presence of apocrine metaplasia. Lastly, the epithelial proliferation within and adjacent to benign papillomas is characteristically usual-type ductal hyperplasia, while that in and adjacent to papillary DCIS may be DCIS.

The presence of myoepithelial cells beneath the epithelium covering the fibrovascular cores in benign papillomas (and their absence in papillary DCIS) may be demonstrated by immuno-histochemistry for myoepithelial markers.[244] Because of the fine fibrovascular cores present in papillary carcinoma, immunostaining of blood vessels may be misinterpreted as positively stained myoepithelial cells; p63 immunostaining is often easiest to interpret because it is more specific for myoepithelial cells and does not stain vasculature.

A study has suggested that the epithelial cells of benign intraductal papillomas are monoclonal in origin.[245] It should be apparent from the foregoing description that careful evaluation of intraductal papillomas can only be accomplished with paraffin-embedded sections. Therefore, frozen-section evaluation of papillary lesions of the breast is strongly discouraged.

Papillomas may undergo partial or total infarction, often accompanied by distortion of the adjacent, viable epithelium and production of a pattern that may simulate invasive carcinoma. Squamous metaplasia is common with or without infarction. This phenomenon may also result in a disturbing growth pattern that may be confused with carcinoma.[246]

Papillomas with atypia

Intraductal papillomas exhibit areas of atypia that range from foci resembling ADH to areas qualitatively similar to low-grade DCIS. The decision to classify a papilloma as atypical versus having DCIS within it varies among authors. Some authors classify a papilloma as atypical if low-grade DCIS is limited to one-third of the lesion (Tavassoli). In a study by Page and coworkers, the subsequent breast cancer risk associated with the presence of ADH or limited (<3 mm) low-grade DCIS within a papilloma was similar to that of patients with atypical hyperplasia in the breast parenchyma (four- to fivefold relative risk). In contrast to the risk seen with ADH in ducts, the breast cancer risk in these patients was largely confined to the ipsilateral breast in the area of the original papilloma.[247] If a papilloma has areas that would qualify as DCIS if they were in breast parenchyma we would diagnose DCIS in the papilloma and advise treating appropriately. Given the continuity of the ductal system with the papilloma, we advocate examination of tissue adjacent to papillomas with atypia (no matter what definition is used) to exclude DCIS.

Multiple (peripheral) intraductal papillomas

Compared to solitary intraductal papillomas, multiple intraductal papillomas tend to occur in younger patients, are less often associated with nipple discharge, are more frequently peripheral, and are more often bilateral. Most importantly, these lesions are associated with the development of carcinoma.[176] A study in which specimens from patients with multiple peripheral papillomas were examined with three-dimensional reconstruction confirms these observations.[248] All the multiple papillomas in the series were found to originate in the terminal duct–lobular unit, the most peripheral portion of the duct system. Carcinoma was found to be associated with these multiple peripheral papillomas in over one third of the cases. In contrast, no cases of carcinoma were found to be associated with solitary papillomas involving the large ducts. These findings support the observation that peripheral papillomas, in contrast to solitary central papillomas, have a higher association with carcinoma. The associated carcinomas are usually well differentiated DCIS. Infiltrating carcinomas are unusual.[249]

Cytology of papillary lesions

Papillary lesions may be sampled for cytologic examination from nipple discharge (a common presentation), duct lavage, or FNA. Cytologically, intraductal papillomas classically consist of epithelial cells arranged in three-dimensional papillary clusters, often with

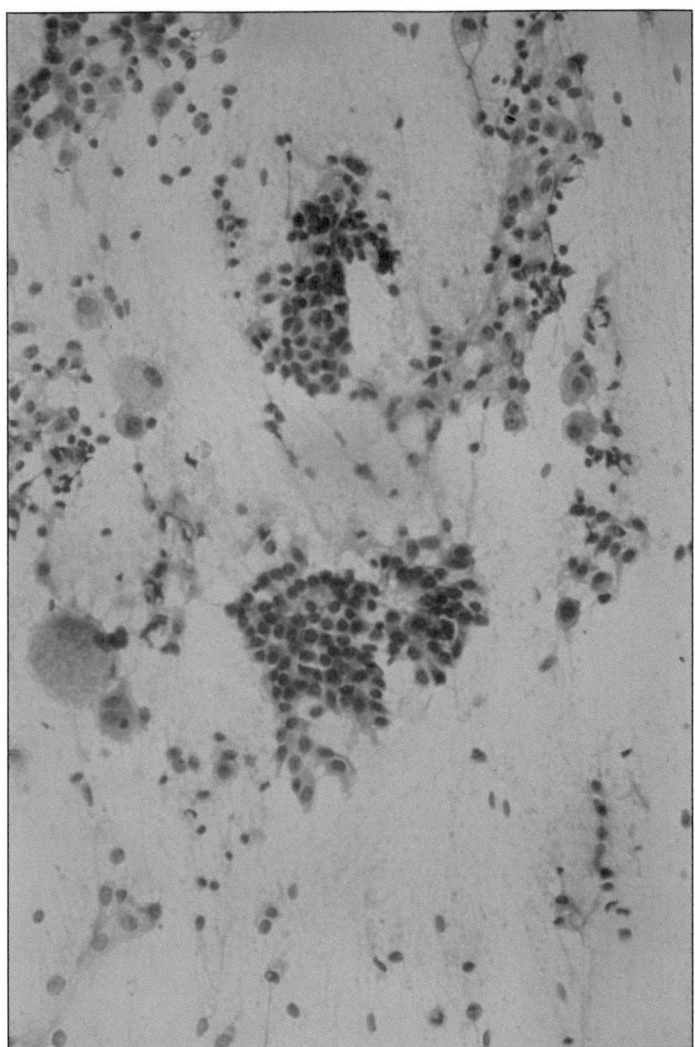

Fig. 10.36 A cellular aspirate obtained from an intraductal papilloma, showing crowded clusters of epithelial cells, macrophages, and columnar cells in a proteinaceous background. (Papanicolaou stain, × 200.)

associated foam cells, apocrine cells, in a background of debris and/or blood (Figs 10.36, 10.37).[250,251] In contrast, papillary DCIS is more often characterized by taller columnar cells, hyperchromatic nuclei with numerous mitotic figures present, and cellular dyshesion in a background of old blood.[252–256] However, for practical purposes, the distinction between intraductal papilloma and papillary DCIS on cytology is particularly challenging and may be impossible in some circumstances.[250] For this reason, a conservative diagnostic approach is prudent unless overt features of malignancy are present. A tentative diagnosis, such as 'papillary neoplasm, recommend surgical excision' is most appropriate in these circumstances.

Juvenile papillomatosis (Swiss cheese disease)

This lesion occurs most commonly in adolescents and young women (mean age of 23, range 12–48 years).[257] Patients typically present with a painless mass, which, on physical examination, is circumscribed, easily movable, and often mistaken for a fibroadenoma.

On gross pathologic examination, the lesions range in size from 1–8 cm. Multiple cysts up to 1 cm in diameter are generally apparent,

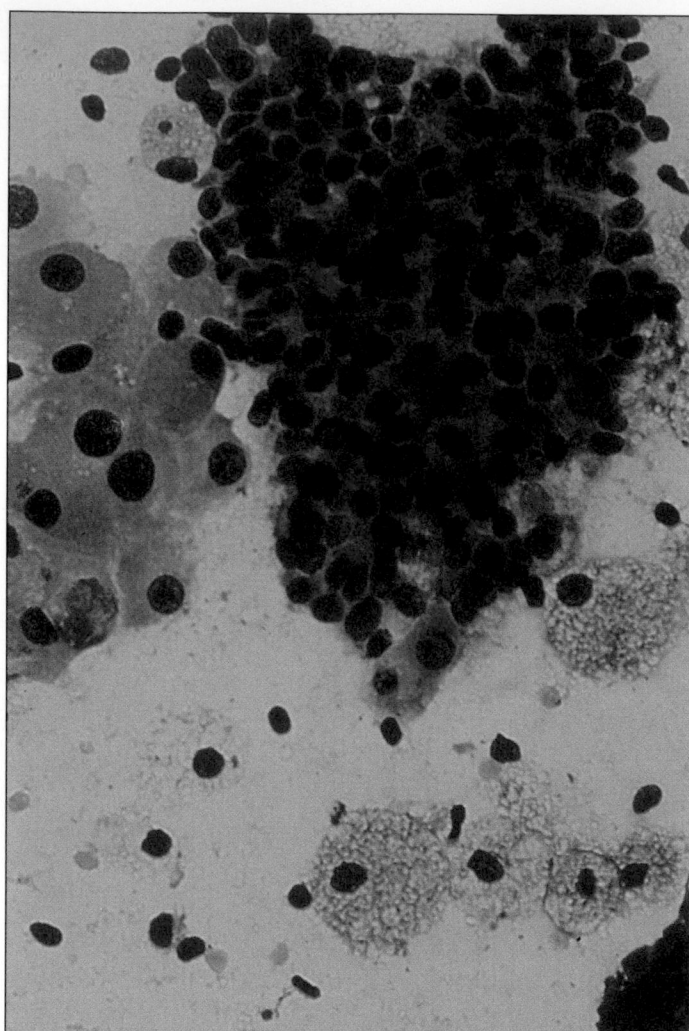

Fig. 10.37 Higher magnification of the same case as in Fig. 10.36 showing apocrine cells, epithelial cells, and foamy macrophages (Diff-Quik, ×400.)

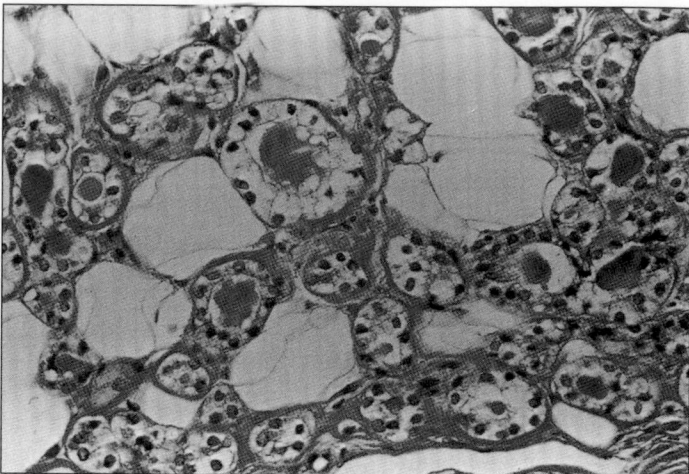

Fig. 10.38 Microglandular adenosis. Uniform small, round glands extended through mammary fat without a stromal response. Glands are lined by a single layer of clear cells and contain intraluminal dense eosinophilic material.

hence the term 'Swiss cheese disease'. The microscopic features of juvenile papillomatosis are not unique to this entity. The constellation of histologic features, however, form a characteristic complex. These lesions appear to be well circumscribed but not encapsulated, and are characterized by the following elements: duct papillomatosis, apocrine and nonapocrine cysts, papillary apocrine hyperplasia, sclerosing adenosis, and ductal hyperplasia. There may be areas of necrosis and the epithelial proliferation in these lesions is usually quite pronounced.

Follow-up studies have suggested that juvenile papillomatosis is associated with a higher incidence of breast cancer in the patient's female relatives, and that the patient herself may be at increased risk for developing carcinoma, particularly if the lesion is bilateral and the patient has a family history of breast cancer.[258–261]

Microglandular adenosis

Microglandular adenosis (MGA) is an uncommon lesion, of uncertain malignant potential, that may be found incidentally in breast tissue excised for other lesions, or it may present as a mass lesion.[262–264] Most women in whom this lesion has been reported are older than 40 years of age, but patients as young as 28 years and as old

as 82 years have been reported to have MGA.[265] The importance of this lesion is twofold: first it may be mistaken for a well differentiated (tubular) carcinoma on histological examination, and second it may be associated with carcinoma.

On gross examination, MGA has generally been described as an ill-defined area of firm, rubbery tissue. Microscopically, the lesion is characterized by a poorly circumscribed, haphazard proliferation of small, round glands in the breast stroma and adipose tissue. Unlike sclerosing adenosis, MGA does not have a lobulocentric, organoid configuration. Like tubular carcinoma, the glands are composed of a single cell layer and lack an outer myoepithelial layer. However, in contrast to tubular carcinoma, the glands are round (not angular). The single layer of cuboidal epithelial cells have clear to slightly eosinophilic cytoplasm and small, regular nuclei, but unlike tubular carcinoma, they lack apical secretory snouts. The cells stain strongly for S100 protein and not for estrogen receptors. The glands are surrounded by basement membrane material.[266,267] Dense, periodic acid–Schiff (PAS)-positive, eosinophilic secretions are frequently present within the glandular lumina. As opposed to the desmoplastic stroma associated with tubular carcinoma, the stroma in MGA is typically composed of dense, relatively acellular collagen, which usually demarcates the lesion from the adjacent parenchyma. In some areas, the stroma is minimal and the proliferating glands lie exposed in adipose tissue. A large proportion of tubular carcinomas have associated DCIS, which is uniformly absent in MGA (Fig. 10.38).

The relationship between MGA and cancer has been addressed in several studies. The incidence of simultaneous or subsequent carcinoma ranges from 0–31% depending on the study.[263–269] Atypical MGA may represent a transitional form between typical MGA and carcinomas arising in this setting.[270] At the present time, the recommended approach to the management of patients with MGA is complete, local excision of the lesion and careful follow-up. If found on CNB, excision is warranted.

Radial scars

Radial scars were first recognized by Semb in 1928.[271] Linell et al.[272] proposed the name 'radial scar' in 1980, which was a translation of Hamperl's 'strahlige Narben' introduced in 1975.[273] They have been described in the literature by a variety of other names, including sclerosing papillary proliferation, non-encapsulated sclerosing lesion, indurative mastopathy, and radial sclerosing lesion.[236,274–277] The term 'complex sclerosing lesion' is sometimes used for similar lesions that are larger than 1 cm in size or for those lesions with several fibroelastotic areas in close contiguity.[189] The importance of these lesions is twofold. First, they may, on mammographic, gross, and microscopic examination, simulate breast carcinomas. Second, although the relationship between the presence of radial scars and subsequent breast cancer has long been a matter of controversy, recent evidence suggests that the presence of a radial scar is associated with an increased risk of subsequent breast cancer.[278]

Radial scars are most often incidental microscopic findings in breast biopsies performed for other indications.[275,278,279] However, some are large enough to be detected mammographically, on which they appear as spiculated masses that cannot be reliably distinguished from carcinomas.[280] The reported incidence of radial scars varies from 4–28%.[275,281,282] In a recent nested case-control study, radial scars were identified in 7% of benign breast biopsies reviewed.[278] Several studies have found radial scars to have a high incidence of bilaterality and multicentricity.[279,282,283] They are often multiple, with as many as 31 lesions having been observed in a single breast.[281]

On gross examination, radial scars are irregular, grey-white, and indurated with central retraction – an appearance identical to that of scirrhous carcinoma. On microscopic examination, radial scars are characterized by a central zone of fibroelastosis from which ducts and lobules radiate, exhibiting various benign alterations such as microcysts, apocrine metaplasia, and proliferative changes, such as florid hyperplasia and papillomas. Within the central area of fibro-elastostotic stroma, smaller entrapped ducts are present, which are often distorted or angular in appearance. These ducts are lined by one or more layers of epithelium and an outer myoepithelial cell layer (Figs 10.39, 10.40). The presence of these myoepithelial cells may be confirmed immunohistochemcally. Radial scars may be involved by atypical hyperplasia (either ductal or lobular) and LCIS, DCIS, or invasive carcinoma may rarely be present. Of note, atypical hyperplasia and carcinoma are more common in larger lesions and in radial scars in women over 50 years of age.[280]

Tubular carcinoma may be confused with radial scars microscopically for several reasons. First, on low-power examination, radial scars and tubular carcinomas may have a similar stellate configuration. Second, at higher magnification, the entrapped, distorted glands within the fibroelastotic center of a radial scar may be confused with invasive carcinoma. However, the entrapped glands within the radial scar fibroelastotic core are surrounded at least in part by myoepithelial cells, which are absent in tubular carcinoma. The stroma of radial scars is characteristically composed of hyalinized collagen and elastic tissue and is present only in the center of the lesion. In contrast, the stroma of tubular carcinoma tends to be more cellular and is typically present throughout the lesion. Other evidence in support of a benign diagnosis is the presence of cysts and/or proliferative changes, which increase in magnitude peripherally in a radial fashion from the central core. This configuration is usually not present in tubular carcinoma. In addition, tubular carcinoma is often associated with low-grade DCIS (usually cribriform and/or micropapillary patterns).

Granular cell tumor

Granular cell tumors are uncommonly found in the breast but, when present, simulate carcinoma on clinical, mammographic, and pathologic examination.[284] Microscopically, these lesions are identical to granular cell tumors in other sites.

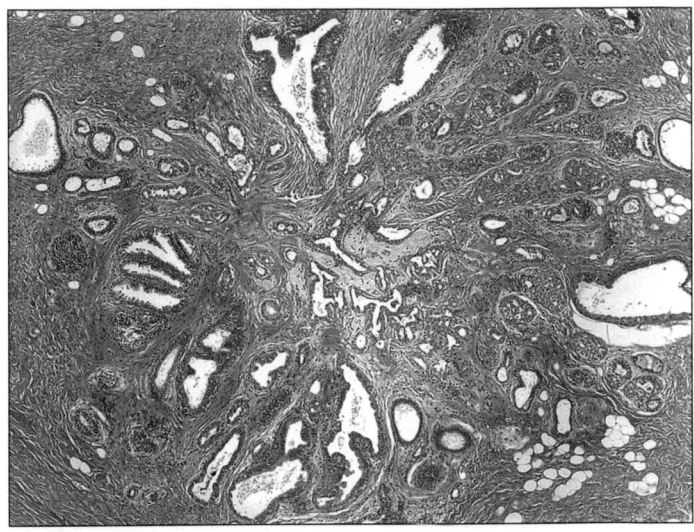

Fig. 10.39 Radial scar with a central core and radiating intraductal proliferation.

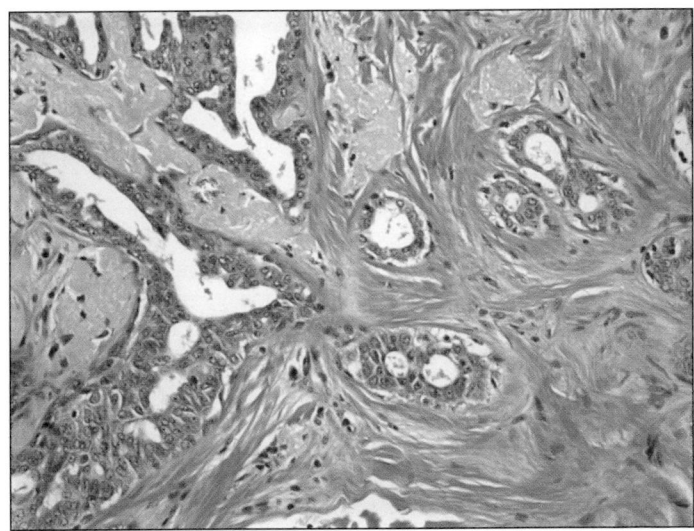

Fig. 10.40 Higher power of the radial scar showing elastosis and entrapped epithelium.

Fibromatosis

Fibromatosis of the breast is analogous to fibromatosis in other sites and is characterized by a locally invasive, non-encapsulated proliferation of well differentiated spindle cells.[285,286] These tumors have the capacity to recur locally if inadequately excised, but they do not metastasize. One of the main concerns is to distinguish these lesions from well differentiated 'fibromatosis like' metaplastic carcinomas (see section on metaplastic carcinomas).

Miscellaneous benign lesions

Lipomas

Lipomas consist of encapsulated nodules of mature adipose tissue. Although true lipomas occur in the breast, many lesions designated 'lipoma' probably represent foci of fatty breast tissue without a true

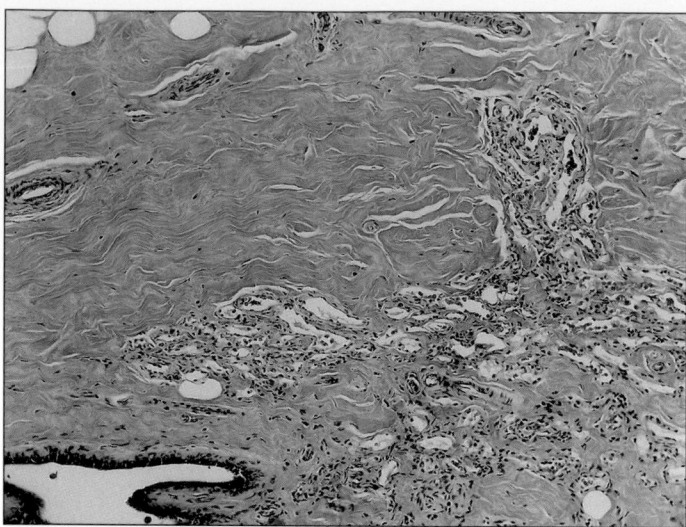

Fig. 10.41 Perilobular hemangioma.

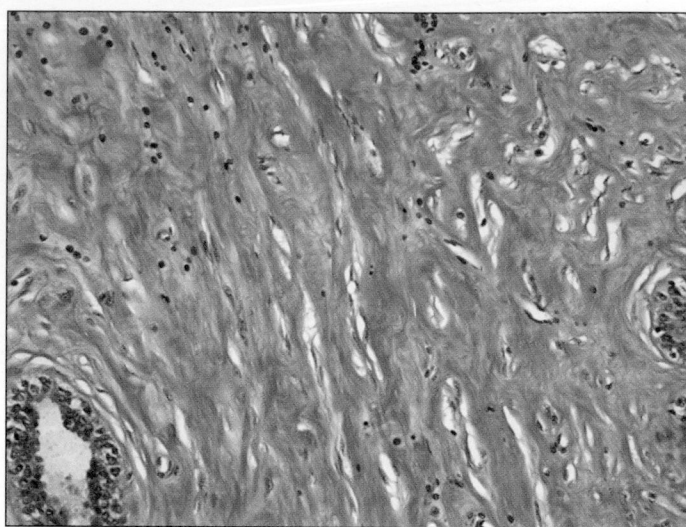

Fig. 10.42 Pseudoangiomatous stromal hyperplasia: the slit like spaces are not lined by endothelial cells.

capsule. 'Adenolipoma' is a term applied to a benign fatty tumor of the breast containing entrapped lobular epithelial elements;[195] however, the distinction between this lesion and breast tissue with prominent stromal adipose tissue is often unclear.

Vascular lesions

Benign vascular lesions of the breast parenchyma are relatively uncommon and most often represent incidental microscopic findings. In a series of 550 mastectomy specimens from patients with breast carcinoma, the incidence of benign hemangiomas was 1.2%.[287] Benign vascular lesions of the breast may be divided into four major categories: *perilobular hemangiomas, angiomatoses, venous hemangiomas, and hemangiomas involving the mammary subcutaneous tissue.*[288–291] The major significance of these lesions is that they must be distinguished from angiosarcomas.[292] Benign angiomatous lesions are almost always microscopic in size and lack interanastomosing channels, endothelial proliferation, and atypia. Benign angiomatous lesions usually respect breast parenchyma and do not 'invade' lobules. The one exception is the perilobular hemangiomas, which may involve lobules. The perilobular hemangiomas is always small (usually less than 4 mm) and lacks atypia (Fig. 10.41). Complete excision is recommended for all vascular lesions of the breast. Recently, atypical vascular lesions have been described in the skin of the breast and the mammary parenchyma in women who have been treated with conservative surgery and radiation therapy for breast cancer.[293]

Pseudoangiomatous stromal hyperplasia

Pseudoangiomatous hyperplasia of the mammary stroma is a benign stromal proliferation that simulates a vascular lesion.[294] The lesion is often seen as an incidental microscopic finding but may present as a palpable mass. Microscopic examination reveals complex interanastomosing spaces, some of which have spindle-shaped stromal cells at their margins simulating endothelial cells (Fig. 10.42). However, ultrastructural examinations and immunocytochemical studies have demonstrated that the spaces are not vascular and that the associated spindle cells are fibroblasts. The significance of this lesion is that it must be distinguished from angiosarcoma.

Chondromatous lesions

Chondromatous lesions of the breast are uncommon. Chondromatous metaplasia is most often seen in breast carcinomas and sarcomas. Rarely chondroid metaplasia may be seen in fibroadenomas and intraductal papillomas and lipomas.

Leiomyoma

Leiomyomas of the breast are most often seen in the areolar region and rarely occur in the breast parenchyma.[195] The histologic characteristics are the same as those of leiomyomas in other tissue.

Neural lesions

Neurofibromas and neurilemomas (schwannomas) are most frequently seen in the breast in patients with neurofibromatosis and are most common in the areolar area.[295]

Adenomyoepithelioma

The term adenomyoepithelioma has been used to describe a variety of lesions. Some of these lesions are well recognized but occasionally have a more prominent myoepithelial component than usual. Examples include papillomas, ductal adenomas, and sclerosing adenosis. They usually present as palpable masses that are grossly circumscribed. Microscopically these lesions are usually nodular or multinodular and are composed of a combination of epithelial and myoepithelial elements. The myoepithelial cells may be polygonal or spindle-shaped (Fig. 10.43). The biologic behavior of these lesions is difficult to predict; most are adequately treated by complete local excision but some recur locally.[296,297] Lesions composed exclusively of myoepithelial cells (*myoepitheliomas*) have also been described.[297]

An unusual entity has been described that is characterized by having two components. The first component has glandular elements lined by epithelial cells, usually with apocrine features, surrounded by myoepithelial cells. The second component has solid nests of myoepithelial cells, usually with clear cytoplasm, with only occasional glands. The behavior of these lesions is also hard to predict.[298]

Malignant myoepithelial lesions are rarely encountered. The malignant component can be epithelial, myoepithelial, or both. Some metaplastic carcinomas, including low-grade adenosquamous

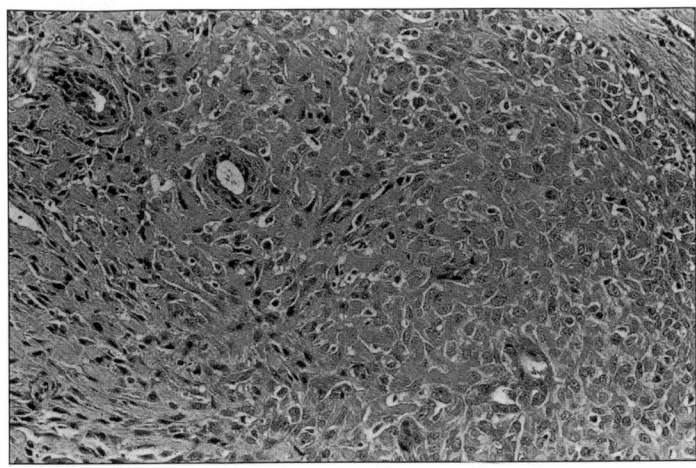

Fig. 10.43 Adenomyoepithelioma. Locally recurrent tumor contains small ductal structures engulfed by polygonal myoepithelial cells becoming spindled at periphery of nodule.

carcinomas, may be myoepithelial in origin.[299–304] Tumors with only myoepithelial characteristics have been described.[297]

Hamartoma

Hamartoma is a term used to describe an entity that has a characteristic well demarcated mammographic appearance but is histologically nondescript. Microscopically, these lesions are composed of an admixture of ducts, lobules, fibrous stroma, and adipose tissue in varying proportions (Fig. 10.44).[305] Occasional lesions also contain smooth muscle (*myoid hamartomas*). These lesions frequently go unrecognized by the pathologist, since they histologically resemble other benign or physiologic changes in the breast.

Myofibroblastoma

Myofibroblastomas are uncommon benign mesenchymal tumors occurring more often in males than females. These lesions are typically well circumscribed and are composed of a proliferation of haphazardly arranged but uniform-appearing spindle cells in a densely collagenized stroma. The cells comprising the tumor show features of myofibroblasts on ultrastructural and immunohistochemical examination.[306] FNA cytology yields non-specific findings, with bland, loosely cohesive groups of spindle cells present.[307]

Mucocele-like lesion

Mucocele-like lesions are composed of mucin-containing cysts, which often rupture, with resultant extravasation of mucin into surrounding stroma.[308] The mucoid character of these lesions is usually evident on gross examination. The epithelium lining these cysts may range from benign (including flat or cuboidal epithelium and hyperplasia, including papillary) to ADH to DCIS[309] (Fig. 10.45). The distinction between mucocele-like lesion and mucinous (colloid) carcinoma may be difficult, particularly if there are epithelial cells floating within the mucin. Therefore, these lesions must be completely excised and carefully examined histologically (with multiple sections if necessary) in order to rule out the possibility of an invasive mucinous carcinoma.[308–312]

The distinction between mucocele-like lesion and mucinous carcinoma may be impossible in the limited, fragmented material obtained with CNB. The problem of sampling error on CNB is further complicated by the possibility that mucocele-like lesions,

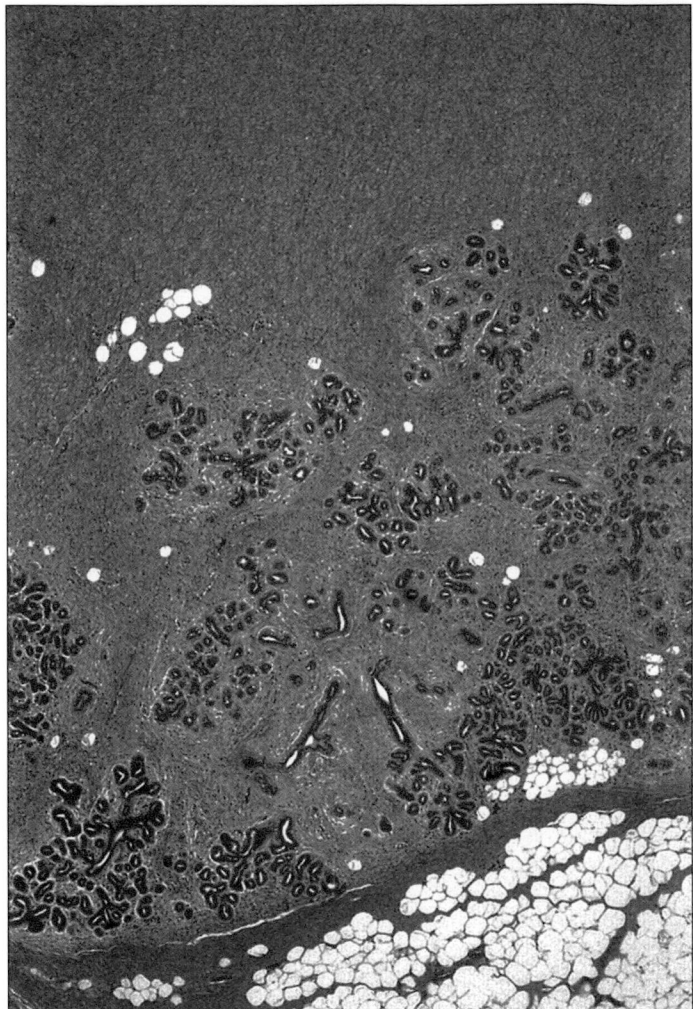

Fig. 10.44 Mammary hamartoma. Circumscribed mass of irregularly distributed mammary ducts, lobules, and stroma including adipose tissue.

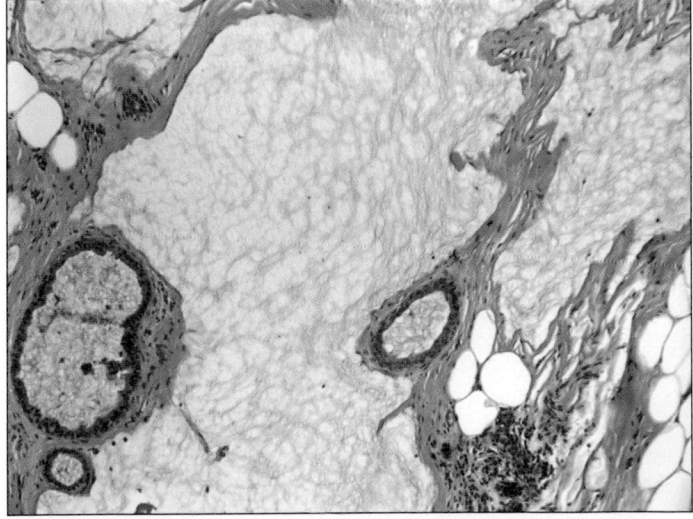

Fig. 10.45 Mucocele-like lesion. Mucin is free in the stroma with no epithelial cells present.

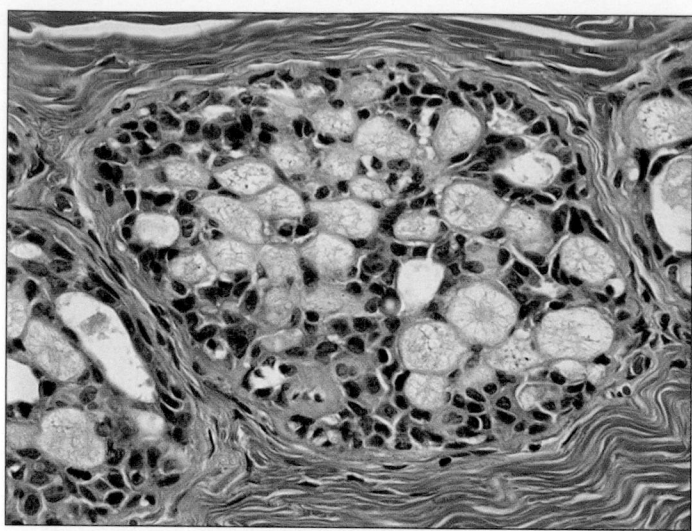

Fig. 10.46 Collagenous spherulosis. A duct contains acellular hyaline spherules surrounded by small regular cells.

mucinous DCIS and mucinous carcinoma may represent a pathologic continuum and that this spectrum of mucinous features may coexist in the breast.[310–314] For these reasons, it is strongly advised that the presence of either a mucocele-like lesion or of stromal mucin pools on CNB should prompt an excision to rule out mucinous DCIS or an invasive mucinous carcinoma.

On FNA cytology, mucocele-like lesions yield abundant mucus.[315] However, as with CNB, sampling issues may not allow mucinous carcinoma to be excluded with certainty. Therefore, the presence of mucin on FNA cytology requires further investigation to rule out a mucinous carcinoma in the patient's breast.

Collagenous spherulosis

Collagenous spherulosis is most often an incidental microscopic finding in breast tissue removed for another abnormality. This lesion appears to be more frequent in breasts containing sclerosing lesions, such as radial scars or sclerosed papillomas. Occasionally collagenous spherulosis may calcify and present as mammographic microcalcifications. This lesion is characterized by a lobulocentric aggregates of eosinophilic fibrillar and/or hyaline spherules which are surrounded by an inner myoepithelial layer and outer epithelial layers.[316] This arrangement gives rise to an appearance of a fenestrated or 'cribriform' proliferation at low-power microscopic examination (Fig. 10.46). The spherules are composed of variable amounts of basement-membrane-like material and type IV collagen and are positive for PAS and Alcian blue.

Occasionally the spherules of collagenous spherulosis may be present on FNA cytology. These are seen as hyaline spherules or globules on Papanicolaou-stained smears and appear metachromatic on air-dried Diff-Quick stains, surrounded by benign-appearing ductal and bipolar cells.[317–319]

This lesion must be distinguished from cribriform DCIS and adenoid cystic carcinoma.[316] At low-power microscopic view, both cribriform DCIS and collagenous spherulosis appear fenestrated. However, the pseudolumens of collagenous spherulosis contain the characteristic eosinophilic spherules, which are hyaline or fibrillar as opposed to cribriform DCIS true lumens, which may be empty or contain calcifications, debris, or necrotic material. Importantly, the

spherules of collagenous spherulosis are lined by a layer of myoepithelial cells, whereas the myoepithelial cells associated with DCIS are adjacent to the basement membrane and do not line the lumens. Collagenous spherulosis may mimic cribriform DCIS if it is involved by ALH or LCIS.[320]

Collagenous spherulosis similar to adenoid cystic carcinoma has cylindromatous areas comprised of pseudolumens, containing basement-membrane-type material, surrounded by myoepithelial cells. Adenoid cystic carcinoma usually presents as a mass lesion, whereas collagenous spherulosis is most often an incidental finding. In addition, the growth pattern of adenoid cystic carcinoma is infiltrative as opposed to the lobulocentric pattern of collagenous spherulosis. The secretions in adenoid cystic carcinoma are either PAS- and Diastase-positive in the ductlike structures or Alcian-blue-positive in the pseudolumens (cylindromatous areas), whereas in collagenous spherulosis the staining pattern is more variable, often with dual staining in the same spherule.[321]

Reactive/inflammatory lesions

Mammary duct ectasia (periductal mastitis)

Mammary duct ectasia occurs primarily in perimenopausal and postmenopausal women and is characterized by dilatation of the subareolar ducts.[176] Considerable controversy exists regarding the most appropriate name for this condition. This controversy has arisen from the fact that some authors consider ductal dilatation to be the primary event whereas others consider the ectatic ducts to be the consequence of prior periductal inflammation.

Duct ectasia is a frequent pathologic finding in breast tissue obtained at autopsy and in surgically excised material. It has been observed on microscopic examination in 30–40% of women older than 50 years of age. Clinically evident disease, however, occurs much less frequently.[322]

A wide spectrum of pathologic changes is observed in this condition. Cut section of the gross specimen often reveals dilated, thick-walled ducts that contain pasty, yellow-brown secretions. The intervening stroma may be fibrotic. On microscopic examination, some cases show prominent inspissation of lipid-rich material within ducts, accompanied by periductal inflammation. Rupture or leakage of these ducts results in release of this material into the adjacent stroma, with subsequent inflammation and fat necrosis. Plasma cells may be a prominent component of the periductal and stromal inflammatory infiltrate. It should be noted that many cases previously designated as plasma cell mastitis probably represent a stage in the evolution of duct ectasia. In other cases, the histologic picture is dominated by periductal fibrosis and ductal dilatation with minimal inflammation (Fig. 10.47).

The pathogenesis of this condition has not been fully established. Dixon and associates originally suggested that the primary event was periductal inflammation and that duct ectasia was the ultimate outcome of this disorder.[322] Thus, their postulated sequence of events in the evolution of this disease was that periductal inflammation leads to periductal fibrosis, which subsequently results in ductal dilatation. However, in a more recent study, this group of investigators has suggested that periductal mastitis and duct ectasia should be considered two separate entities, based on differences between women with these two disorders with regard to age, clinical history, and smoking history.[323]

Fat necrosis

Fat necrosis may closely simulate carcinoma both clinically and on mammographic examination.[176,324]

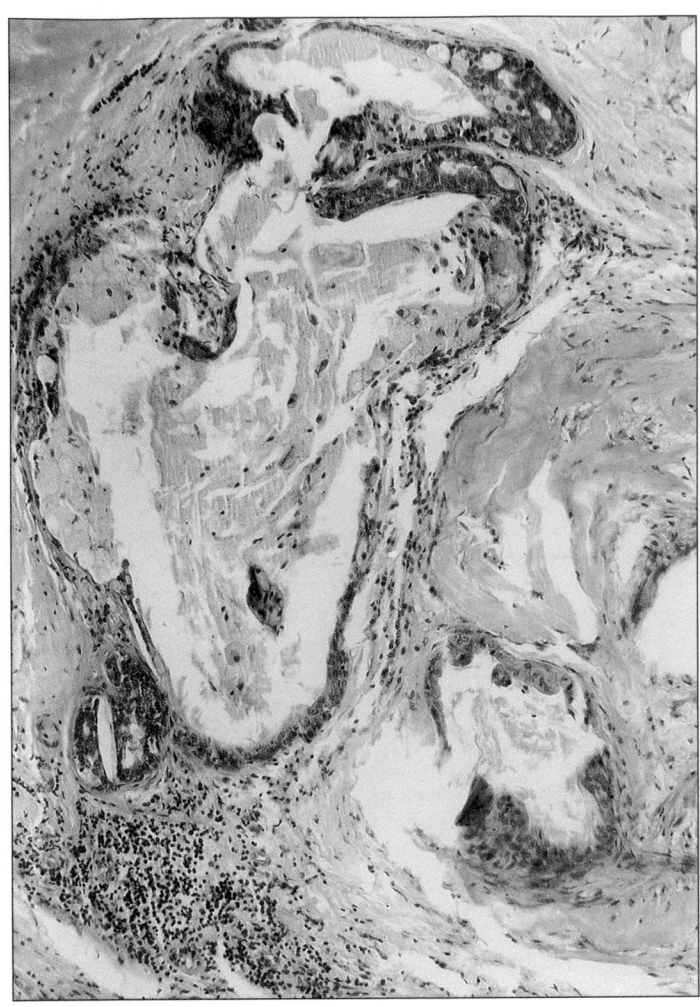

Fig. 10.47 Plasma cell mastitis. Dilated lactiferous ducts with inflammatory infiltrate and giant cell granulomas around cellular debris and lipids.

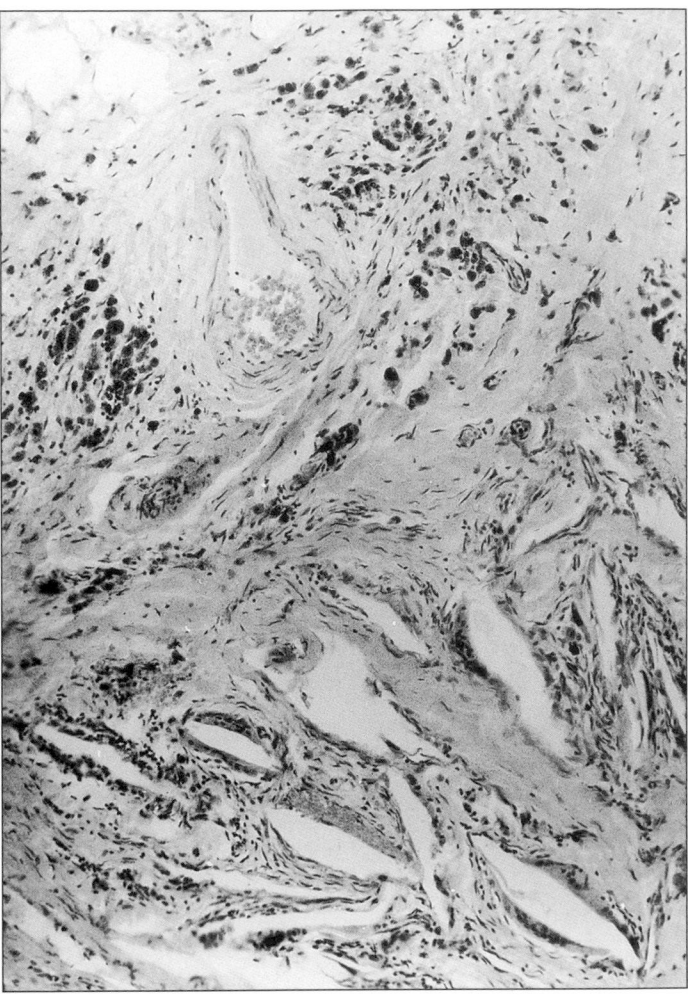

Fig. 10.48 Fat necrosis. Inflammatory granuloma with areas of fibrosis and lipid crystals surrounded by multinucleated giant cells.

The macroscopic appearance of fat necrosis depends on its age. In early lesions, there is hemorrhage and indurated fat. With time, a rounded, firm lesion is formed. The cut surface of the lesion at this stage has a variegated, yellow-grey appearance with focal hemorrhage. Cavitation may subsequently occur, owing to liquefactive necrosis. The lesion may eventually be converted to a dense, fibrous scar or may remain a cystic cavity with calcification of its walls.

On microscopic examination, early lesions show cystic spaces surrounded by lipid-laden macrophages and foreign-body-type giant cells with foamy cytoplasm. A variable, acute inflammatory cell infiltrate may be present, and there may be focal hemorrhage. With time, there is fibroblastic proliferation with deposition of collagen. Scattered, chronic inflammatory cells are usually present, and focal hemosiderin deposition may be observed. Even in older lesions, scattered, foamy histiocytes and foreign body giant cells are usually discernible (Fig. 10.48). A similar pathologic appearance may be seen after surgical trauma to the breast and after radiation therapy for carcinoma (see the section on pathologic changes associated with radiation therapy, below).

FNA of fat necrosis usually yields a hypocellular specimen with scant (or absent) epithelial cells, comprised predominantly of foam cells, with variable proportions of inflammatory cells and foreign body giant cells, depending on the age of the lesion (Fig. 10.49). In the appropriate clinical setting (e.g. following trauma), it is important to not categorize such cases as 'inadequate' or 'insufficient' merely because of lack of epithelial cells or hypocellularity. A descriptive diagnosis is best, with the recommendation that clinical and radiologic correlation be made.

Reactions to foreign material

Foreign-body-type granulomatous inflammation has been described following injection within the breast of a variety of substances, including paraffin and silicone. Clinically, these lesions generally appear as firm nodules, which may be tender.[324]

A variety of tissue reactions has been reported in association with mammary implants.[325,326] Histological examination of the capsular tissue shows varying degrees of fibrosis, chronic inflammation, fat necrosis, granulation tissue, fibrin deposition, and histiocytes and foreign body giant cells, often with demonstrable silicone or polyurethane when it has been used as part of the implant shell. In some cases the capsule surrounding breast implants develops a cellular lining that resembles normal synovium or synovium with papillary hyperplasia.[327]

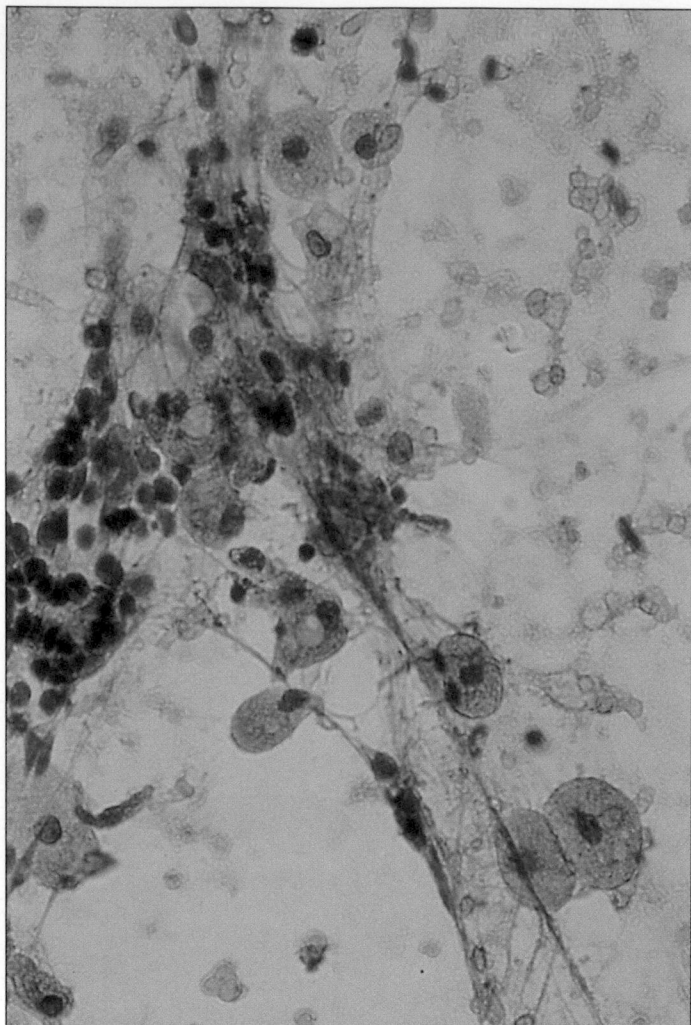

Fig. 10.49 Cellular debris, inflammatory cells, small vessels, and lipid-laden macrophages in an aspirate of fat necrosis. (Papanicolaou stain, ×400.)

FNA cytology of silicone-augmented breast tissue yields histiocytes and foreign body giant cells containing numerous perfectly round, empty-appearing cytoplasmic vacuoles. The silicone is often present within these vacuoles and appears as refractile (but not birefringent) homogeneous globules of pale blue or yellow foreign semitransparent material (Fig. 10.50). The cellularity is variable, as is the accompanying inflammatory infiltrate. On air-dried Diff-Quick smears, silicone appears as a thick, amorphous material, present both intra- and extracellularly.[328] Occasionally, silicone may migrate to the axillary lymph nodes, presenting as an enlarged lymph node. FNA will yield characteristic silicone-laden macrophages and giant cells.[329]

Mondor's disease (phlebitis of the thoracoepigastric vein)

Mondor's disease is phlebitis of the thoracoepigastric vein. On pathologic examination, there is phlebitis and periphlebitis. The obliterative endophlebitis is associated with varying degrees of thrombosis, and the adventitia and media may be completely destroyed in advanced cases.[330,331]

Pathologic changes associated with radiation therapy for carcinoma

The effects of therapeutic doses of ionizing radiation on the skin of the breast have been well described and are identical to the radiation-induced alterations occurring in skin from any irradiated site.[332] Fat necrosis may occur in the breast following local excision and radiation therapy for carcinoma. These lesions may be indistinguishable from carcinoma by clinical and radiographic examination, requiring complete histologic examination for accurate diagnosis.[333] The most characteristic pathologic finding in breast tissue excised following primary radiation therapy for carcinoma is epithelial cell atypicality in the terminal duct–lobular unit, usually associated with varying degrees of lobular sclerosis and atrophy[334] (Fig. 10.51). These changes may be distinguished from carcinoma involving the terminal duct–lobular unit by the focality of the change, the preservation of polarity and cohesion, and the absence of cellular proliferation and distention of the involved terminal duct–lobular unit in areas of radiation-induced change. Similar epithelial changes have been described in patients treated with chemotherapy prior to tumor excision.[335] Less frequently, epithelial atypia in large (extralobular) ducts, atypical fibroblasts in the stroma, and radiation-related vascular changes may be observed. Interestingly, stromal fibrosis, a characteristic feature of radiation effect in other organs, is so variable among both irradiated patients and non-irradiated control subjects that it is not by itself a reliable marker for radiation-induced injury in the breast.

FNA cytology specimens of radiation effect are usually hypocellular with scattered atypical cells present. The atypical cells may show marked nuclear pleomorphism but with smudged rather than coarse chromatin. The cytoplasm is usually abundant, often with vacuolization, and nuclear:cytoplasmic ratios are low (in contrast to carcinoma). As opposed to benign radiation change, aspirates of carcinoma are usually more cellular, with increased cellular dyshesion (Fig. 10.52).[336–339] Squamous metaplasia following radiation may be markedly atypical and easily mistaken for carcinoma.[340]

Sarcoidosis

Involvement of the breast by sarcoidosis is rare but, when present, may clinically simulate a neoplasm.[341,342] Histologically, the lesions consist of typical, noncaseating granulomas with varying numbers of giant cells, which are present in the interlobular and intralobular connective tissue. A diagnosis of sarcoidosis should be made only after the exclusion of other causes of granulomatous inflammation, such as mycobacterial, fungal, and parasitic infections or reactions to foreign materials. Sarcoidosis should also be distinguished from 'granulomatous mastitis,' a lesion in which the granulomas are associated with microabscesses and which may respond to corticosteroid therapy.[343,344]

Diabetic and lymphocytic mastopathy

These may represent the same entity or a spectrum of histologically similar changes of various etiologies. This condition affects young to middle-aged women and is associated with insulin-dependent diabetes or other autoimmune conditions.[345–347] These women develop painful breast masses that may be multiple, bilateral, palpable, or simply a mammographic finding.[348,349] These include dense fibrosis and lymphocytic infiltrates in association with ducts and lobules. Over time, lobular atrophy and sclerosis develop with resolution of the inflammatory component (Fig. 10.53). Epithelioid stromal cells may be prominent and may mimic infiltrating carcinoma.[347] These epithelioid cells are probably myoepithelial in origin since they are cytokeratin-negative and smooth muscle actin-

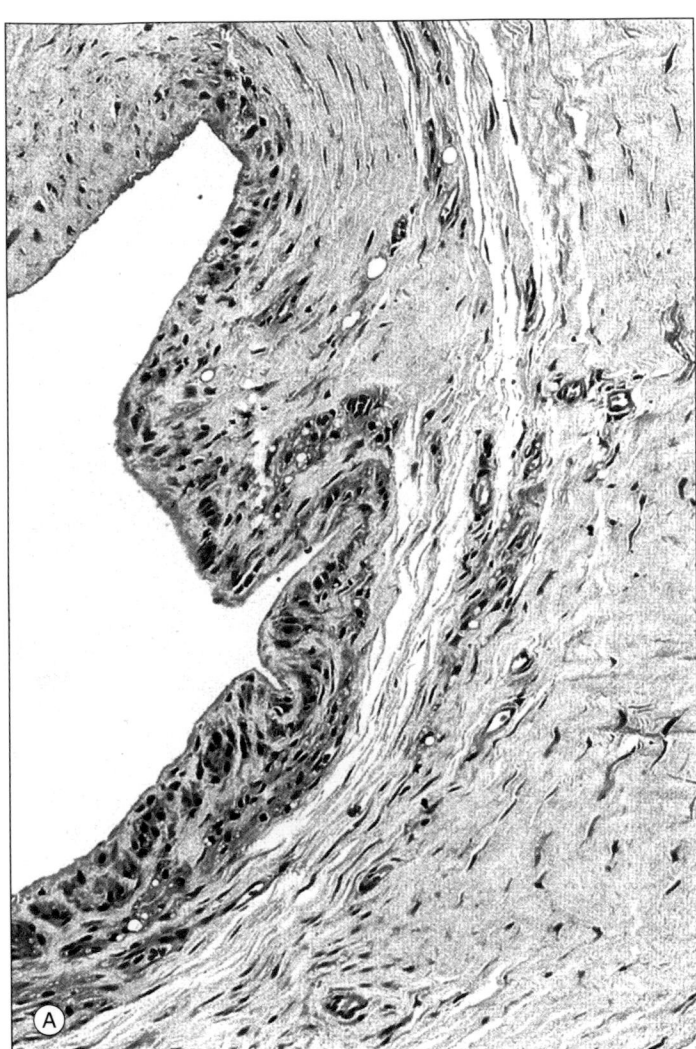

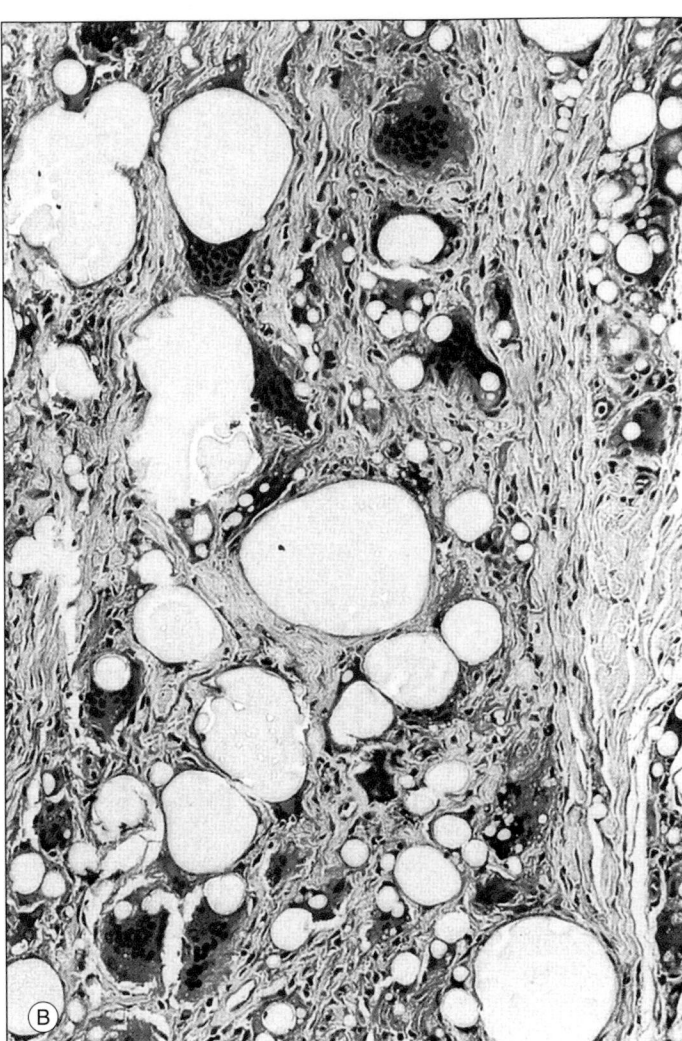

Fig. 10.50 **(A)** Capsule of silicone implant, with synovial metaplasia. **(B)** Underlying foreign body reaction with large spaces, some containing silicon particles.

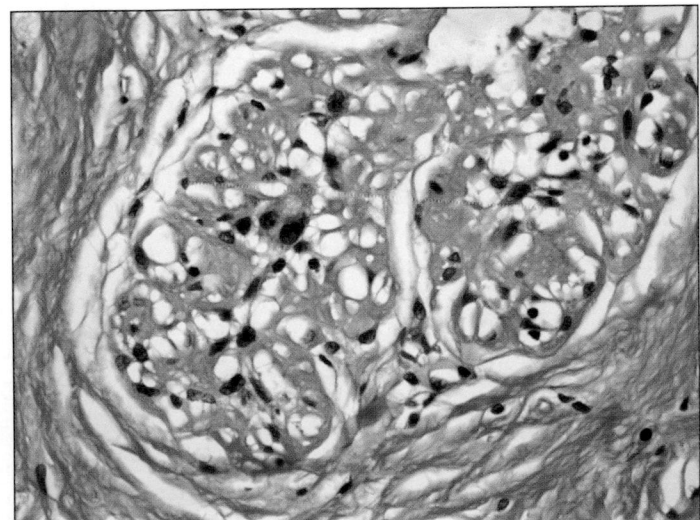

Fig. 10.51 Radiation change. A sclerotic lobule with atypical cells. Note the lack of proliferation and vacuolated cytoplasm.

positive.[347] These patients often have circulating antibodies associated with HLA types DR3, 4 or 5, supporting an autoimmune etiology for these disorders.[345,346]

Gynecomastia

Enlargement of the male breast can occur at any time during life. During adolescence, such enlargements are generally bilateral and temporary. This temporary hypertrophy may be due to some hormonal stimulation, which usually regresses spontaneously after a few months.

In adults, gynecomastia is usually idiopathic; however, it may be due to a variety of conditions associated with hormone imbalance or secondary to various drugs.[350-352] The process may be localized, generalized, unilateral, or bilateral. A unilateral presentation is most common. The histologic appearance varies. Microscopically, gynecomastia consists of varying proportions of stroma and ducts. Early the stroma surrounding the proliferating ducts is loose, with a bluish coloration, later it may be densely fibrotic. The stroma may contain varying numbers of plasma cells and lymphocytes. The epithelial proliferation within the ducts may be minimal or multilayered, with those layers at the luminal surface demonstrating tufting. These tufts have pointed tips containing small hyper-

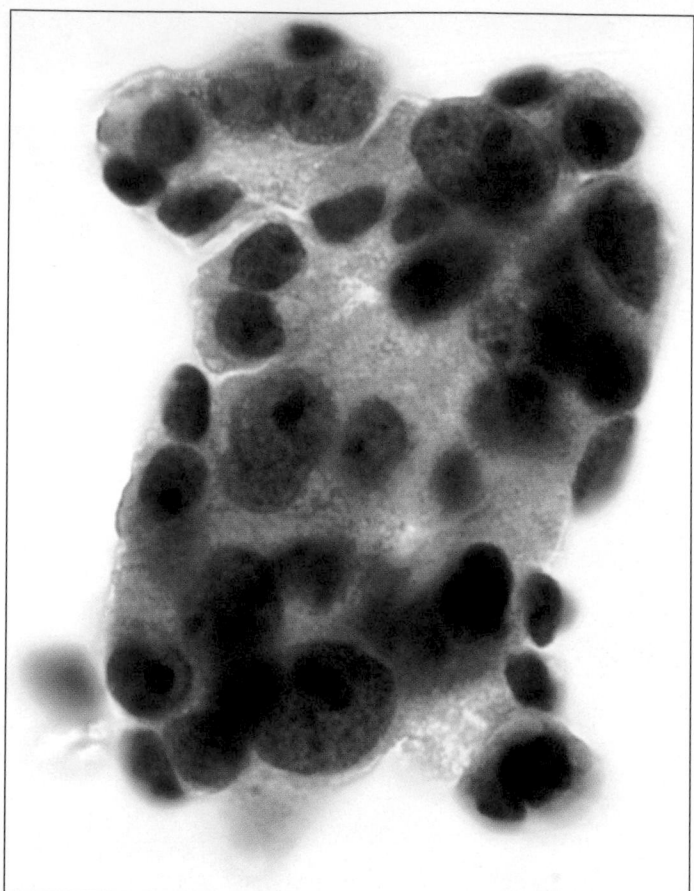

Fig. 10.52 Cytology of radiation change, showing a cohesive cluster of ductal epithelial cells with focal markedly atypical nuclei but normal nuclear:cytoplasmic ratios. (ThinPrep, Papanicolaou stain, ×1000)

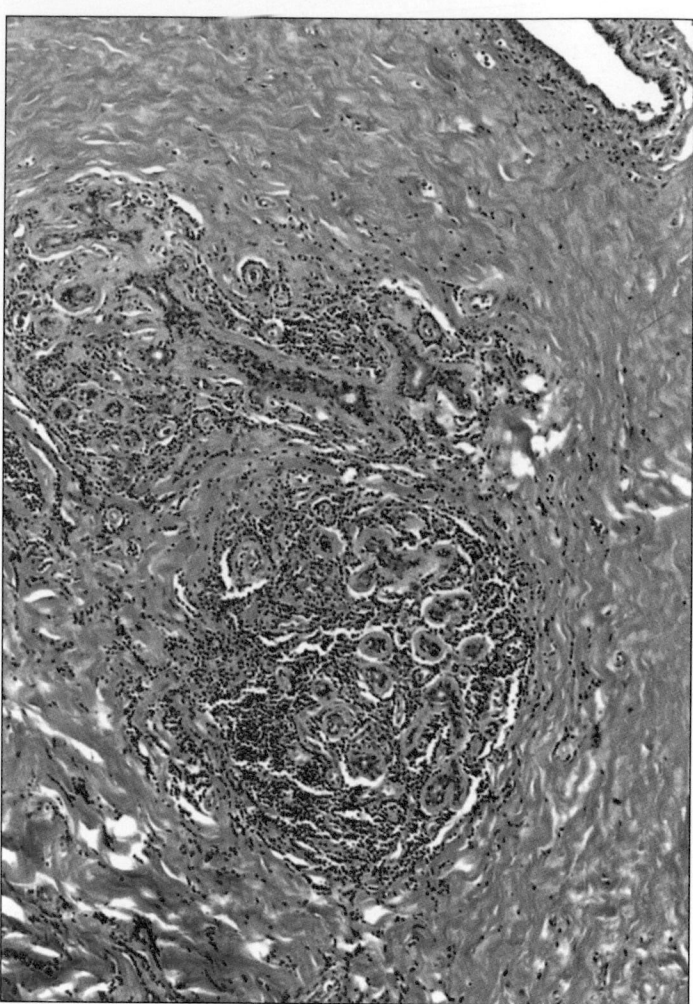

Fig. 10.53 Lymphocytic mastopathy. Note lymphocytic infiltrate cuffing atrophic ducts and lobules, and surrounding keloid-like dense fibrosis.

chromatic cells This appearance is worrisome but should not be interpreted as atypical or a DCIS (Fig. 10.54).[353]

FNA smears of gynecomastia vary in cellularity. Characteristically tightly cohesive clusters of ductal cells are found, which may exhibit crowding and overlapping. The nuclei are usually uniform with inconspicuous nucleoli. Single epithelial cells are rarely found, and bipolar cells are usually present in the background (Fig. 10.55).[354,355] Cytologic atypia is not uncommon in gynecomastia, manifesting as crowded clusters, focal cellular dyshesion, nuclear variability, and occasionally single columnar cells. These findings may pose diagnostic difficulty, particularly in conjunction with a cellular smear. However, overt features of malignancy are usually not present and the correct diagnosis can be rendered if the appropriate clinical context is taken into consideration.[354,355]

DUCTAL CARCINOMA IN SITU

CLASSIFICATION

The term ductal carcinoma in situ (DCIS) encompasses a pathologically heterogeneous group of lesions that differ in their growth pattern and cytological features. While the diversity of DCIS lesions is well recognized, at present there is no universal agreement as to how best to subclassify these lesions. Proposed classification

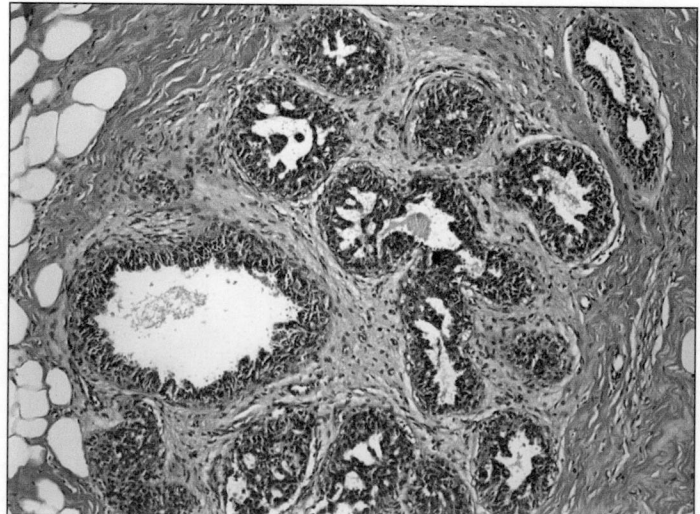

Fig. 10.54 Gynecomastia. The stroma is edematous and the ductal proliferation is tufting.

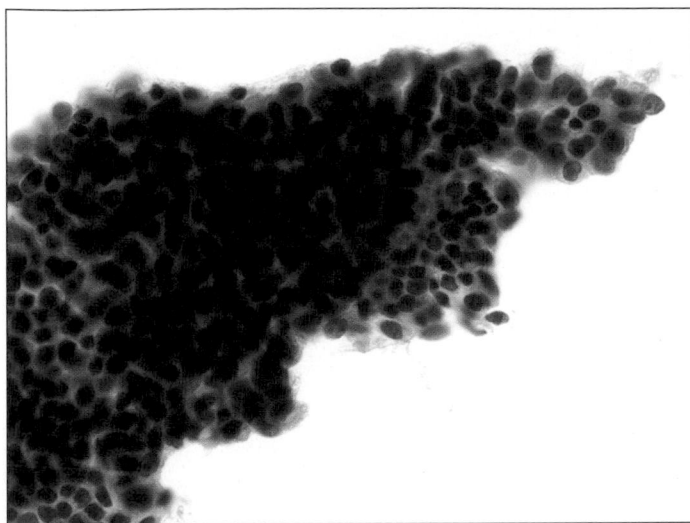

Fig. 10.55 Fine-needle aspirate of gynecomastia, showing a group of ductal epithelial cells with crowding and overlapping. Myoepithelial cells are also evident (with darker and smaller nuclei). (ThinPrep, Papanicolaou stain, ×600).

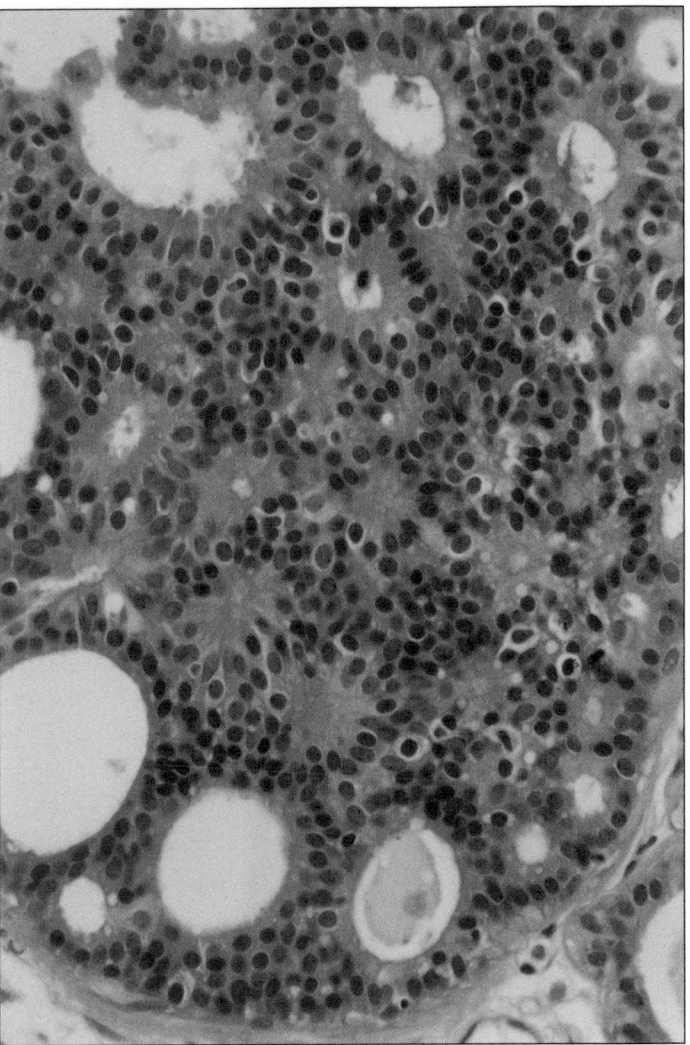

Fig. 10.56 Cribriform pattern ductal carcinoma in situ. The cells comprising this lesion grow in a fenestrated, sieve-like pattern. This example has low-grade nuclei.

schemes for DCIS have variously emphasized architectural features or growth pattern of the neoplastic cells within the ductal-lobular system, cytologic features of the neoplastic cells, and cellular necrosis, singly and in combination.[356]

Traditionally, DCIS has been classified by growth pattern into five main architectural subtypes: cribriform, micropapillary, papillary, solid, and comedo.[189,236,357] Cribriform DCIS is composed of uniform, small to intermediate-sized cells arranged in a fenestrated pattern (Fig. 10.56). Micropapillary DCIS is also composed of small to intermediate-sized tumor cells, but these grow in club-shaped tufts, usually with bulbous ends, oriented perpendicular to the basement membrane and projecting toward the duct lumen (Figs 10.57, 10.58). As opposed to the micropapillary pattern, papillary DCIS is composed of fibrovascular cores around which the neoplastic cells are arranged (Fig. 10.59). In one variant of papillary DCIS, the tumor cells are primarily or exclusively present in a single cystically dilated space (intracystic or encysted papillary carcinoma).[358–360] In solid DCIS, the tumor cells fill the duct space and lack fenestrations, necrosis, or other papillations. The neoplastic cells may be small or large (Fig. 10.60). The comedo pattern has prominent central necrosis with or without calcifications. The central necrotic area is surrounded by viable ductal neoplastic cells, which are most often pleomorphic with high nuclear grade, often with conspicuous mitotic figures (Figs 10.61, 10.62).

The criteria for classifying DCIS using this traditional approach are not well defined and are subjective, and there is considerable interobserver variability. Furthermore, there is considerable variability in the architectural appearance of a single lesion from area to area.[361,362] Although the architectural classification scheme was perfectly acceptable in the era when all cases of DCIS were treated by mastectomy, there is a pressing clinical need to develop a classification system that has prognostic significance in patients considered for treatment with breast conservation.

A number of alternative classification schemes for DCIS have recently been proposed in an attempt to overcome the limitations of the traditional, primarily architectural classification system.[363–365] These newer classification systems stratify DCIS lesions primarily on the basis of nuclear grade and/or necrosis, with architectural pattern given secondary or no consideration (Fig. 10.63).[366–371] Other classification systems have been proposed by other authors as well.[363,364,372–374] To attain widespread clinical use, any classification system must be not only clinically relevant but also reproducibly applicable by different observers.

In 1997, a consensus conference was convened in an attempt to reach agreement on the classification of DCIS.[112] While the panel did not endorse any one system of classification, there was agreement that certain features should be routinely documented in pathology reports of DCIS lesions. These include nuclear grade (low, intermediate, or high grade), the presence of necrosis (comedo or punctate), cell polarization, and architectural pattern(s). In fact, if these individual features are recorded, there will be sufficient information available to permit the categorization of a DCIS lesion according to virtually all the newly proposed classification schemes. Information derived from ongoing genetic and molecular studies of DCIS will probably provide important new insights into these lesions and may ultimately provide the basis for a biologically-based classification system.[375–377]

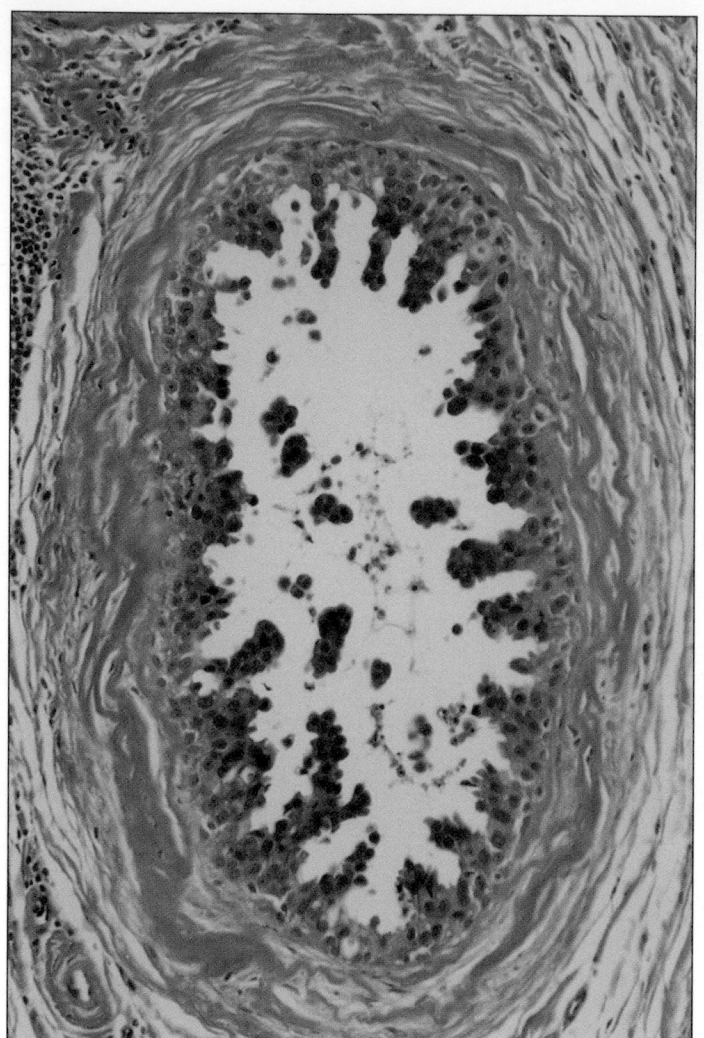

Fig. 10.57 Ductal carcinoma in situ, micropapillary type. Papillae have no connective tissue cores and are lined by cells with modest atypia.

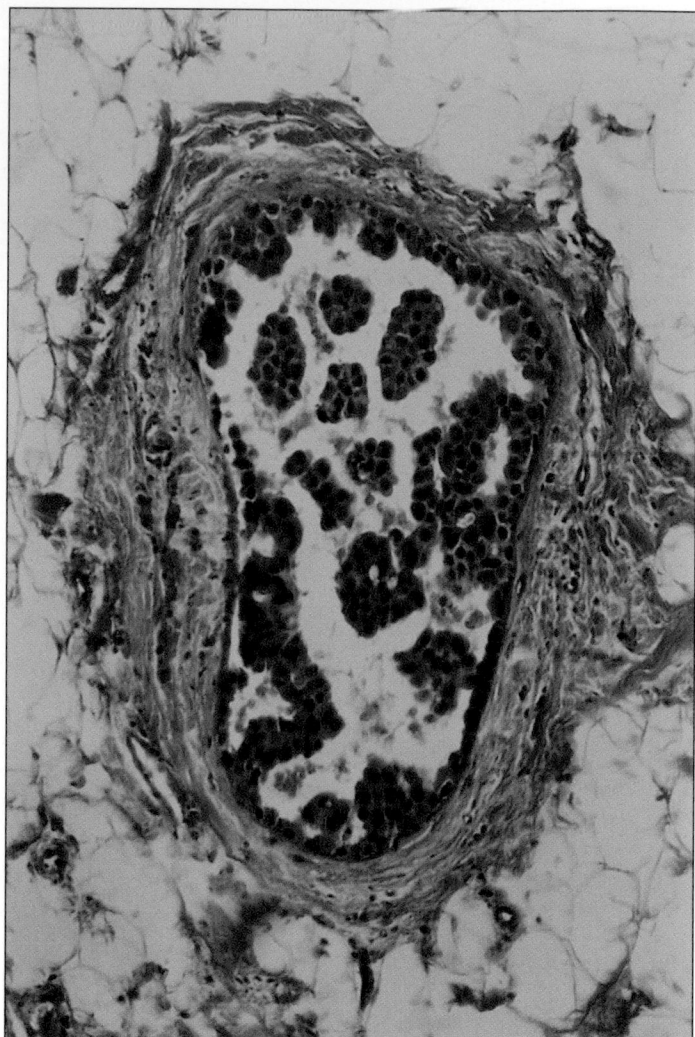

Fig. 10.58 Ductal carcinoma in situ, micropapillary type. Another case with somewhat more atypia than seen in Fig. 10.57.

BIOLOGICAL MARKERS

There has been considerable interest in the study of tumor markers in DCIS in order to provide a better understanding of the biology of these lesions and to aid in their classification. Although the results of studies of these markers are somewhat difficult to compare because of differences in the classification used for the DCIS, patient populations, and methodology, a number of trends have emerged. These studies have generally shown that high-grade DCIS more often than low-grade DCIS exhibits a profile of biological markers that has been associated with aggressive clinical behavior in invasive cancers. For example, high-grade lesions more frequently than low-grade lesions lack estrogen and progesterone receptors,[378–382] have a high proliferative rate,[380–384] and exhibit aneuploidy,[385] over-expression of the *HER2/neu* oncogene,[379–383,386–388] mutations of the p53 tumor suppressor gene with accumulation of its protein product,[379–383,389–391] and angiogenesis in the surrounding stroma.[392,393]

In addition, recent genetic studies have indicated that the number and type of chromosomal alterations differ according to DCIS pattern and grade.[375,394,395] For example, using comparative genomic hybridization analysis, high-grade DCIS has been shown to exhibit

more numerous chromosomal losses and gains than low-grade lesions.[375] Furthermore, the particular chromosomal loci that are altered appear to differ among different grades of DCIS, with losses of material on chromosomes 17p and 16q particularly common in low-grade DCIS, gains of 1q and losses of 11q common in inter-mediate grade DCIS, and gains of 17q and 11q common in high-grade DCIS.[375,376] It is hoped that further understanding of the genetic and molecular alterations in these lesions will lead to a biologically-based classification system of DCIS.

OTHER IMPORTANT FEATURES

High-grade DCIS is more malignant cytologically[189,236,357] and is more often associated with microinvasion[361,396,397] than are the other DCIS types. Another difference reported for these two groups is in regard to the relationship between the extent of microcalcifications on the mammogram and the histologic extent of the lesion. Using standard two-view mammography, the histologic extent of high-grade (comedo-type) DCIS is highly correlated with the extent of the calcifications on the mammogram in most cases. In contrast, the

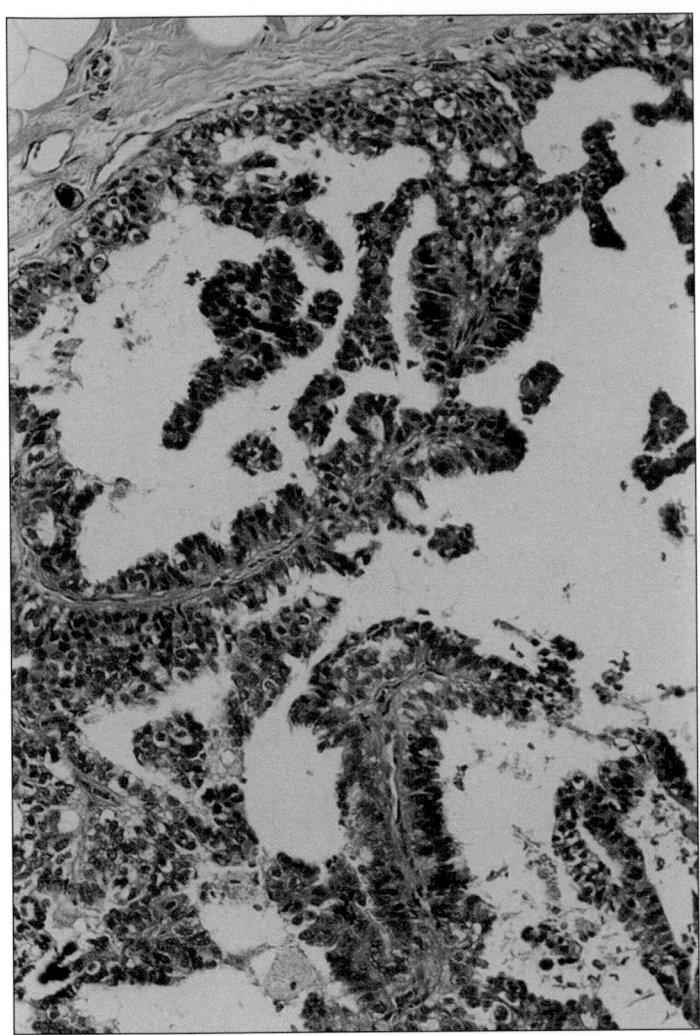

Fig. 10.59 Ductal carcinoma in situ, papillary stratified spindle cell type. The papillae are larger than in the micropapillary type and have connective tissue cores (compare with Figs 10.57 and 10.58). Stratification, lack of myoepithelial cells, and nuclear atypia distinguish this from intraductal papilloma.

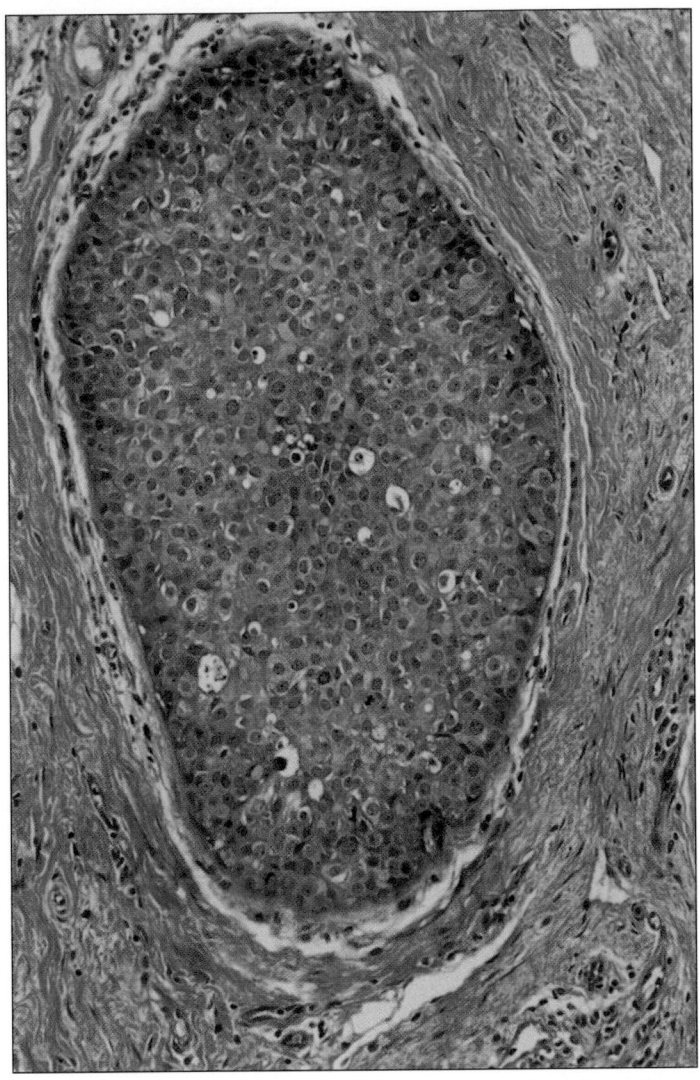

Fig. 10.60 Ductal carcinoma in situ, solid type. The marked atypia noted in comedocarcinoma (see Figs 10.61 and 10.62) is not present.

mammographic extent of the calcifications associated with low-grade (noncomedo) DCIS frequently underestimates the pathologic extent of the lesion.[398] With magnification views there is a much better correlation between the extent of mammographic calcifications and the histologic extent of the lesion[399]

The reported incidence of 'multicentricity' in mastectomy specimens from patients with DCIS varies considerably and has ranged from 0–47%.[400] Older studies found that the rates of multicentricity increased with large lesions (5 cm or greater) or with a greater number of involved ducts, and with micropapillary histology.[361,373,396,401] More recent studies suggest that, in most cases, true multicentricity in DCIS is rare. Holland and Hendriks studied 119 mastectomy specimens containing DCIS by a subgross pathologic–mammographic technique.[399] In all but one case, the tumor was confined to a single 'segment' of the breast. There was clear-cut multicentric distribution (defined in this study as foci of DCIS separated by 4 cm or more of uninvolved breast tissue) in only one patient. In another study using stereomicroscopic three-dimensional analysis to define the growth pattern of DCIS within the

mammary duct system, Faverly et al. studied 60 mastectomy specimens containing DCIS.[402] They found that, within the segment of breast involved by DCIS, growth was continuous in some cases and discontinuous in others. Overall, 50% of cases showed a continuous growth pattern and 50% showed a discontinuous pattern, characterized by uninvolved breast tissue between foci of DCIS ('gaps'). In most instances, these gaps were small (<5 mm in 82% of cases) and the likelihood of finding such gaps was related to the histologic type of the lesion. Whereas 90% of the cases of poorly differentiated DCIS grew in a continuous manner without gaps, only 30% of well differentiated lesions and 45% of intermediately differentiated lesions were continuous. The 'gaps' in low- and intermediate-grade DCIS are likely to be 'diagnostic' rather than biologic. This is due to the necessity to define architectural alterations to make the diagnosis of low-grade DCIS. The findings in these two studies indicate that in most cases DCIS involves the breast in a segmental distribution and that truly multicentric disease is uncommon. However, in some cases, the segment involved by DCIS may be quite large. A study of clonality in DCIS supports the contention that most DCIS is unifocal, at least

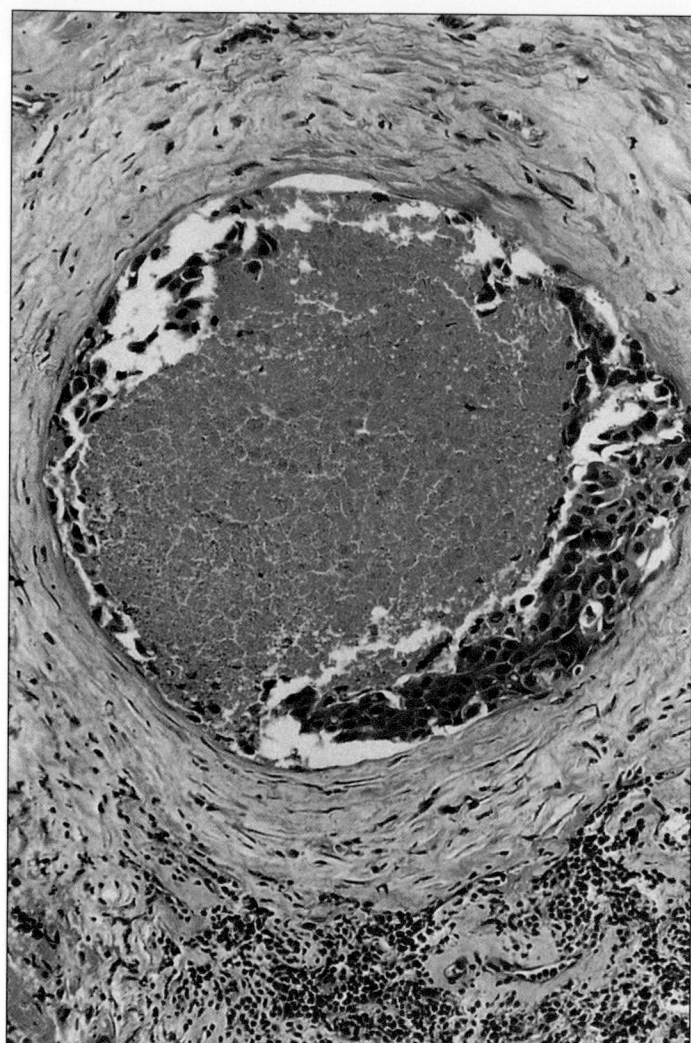

Fig. 10.61 Ductal carcinoma in situ, comedo type. Solid growth pattern, central necrosis, and marked nuclear atypia are characteristic. The surrounding sclerosing and lymphoid reaction is typical in this type of DCIS but may be absent and is often present in other types.

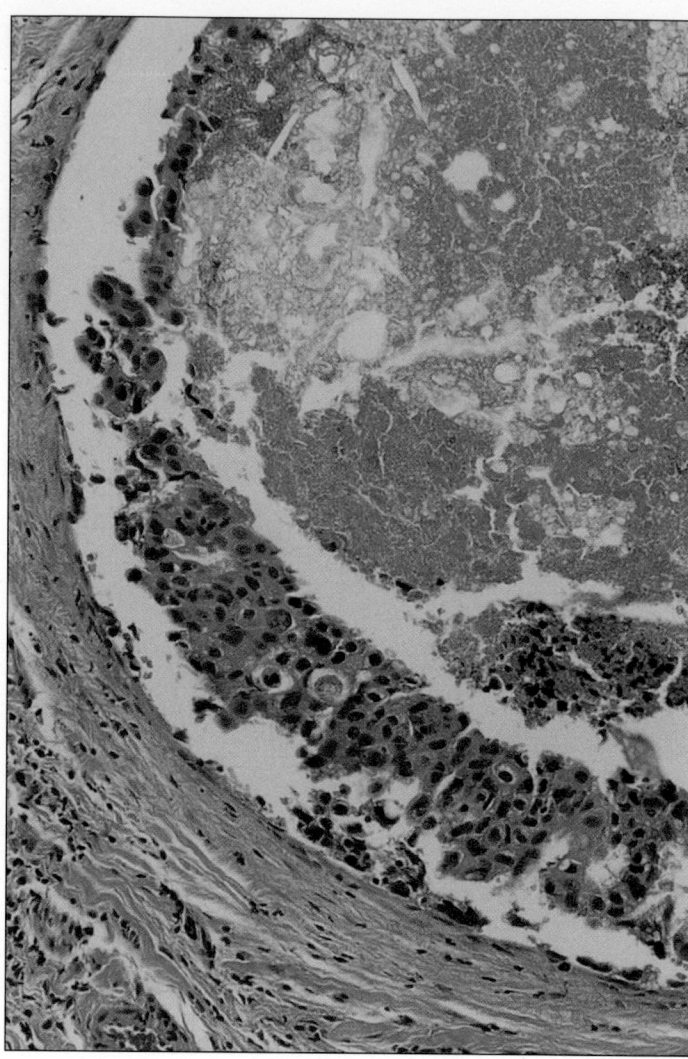

Fig. 10.62 Ductal carcinoma in situ, comedo type. High magnification of another case to show marked (grade 3) nuclear atypia.

with regard to comedo lesions.[403] In that study, clonality was assessed in widely separated sites of comedo-type DCIS in the same breast. These widely separated sites were each found to be monoclonal.

The incidence of occult invasion, either near the primary tumor or in other parts of the breast, has also examined in mastectomy series. The reported incidence of occult invasion ranges from 0–26%.[400] The likelihood of finding occult invasion appears to be related to the size of the index lesion. In one series, patients with lesions larger than 2.5 cm were more likely to have occult invasion.[401] The frequency of occult invasion is also related to the method of detection of the DCIS. DCIS that presents as a palpable mass is more likely to be associated with occult invasion than lesions detected mammographically.[404,405] The incidence of occult invasion also appears to be correlated with the histologic type of DCIS, being much more common in high-grade (comedo) lesions.[361]

Incidence rates reported for axillary nodal involvement in patients given the diagnosis of DCIS range from 0–7%,[357] with the higher rates noted in studies performed in the premammographic era when most patients with DCIS presented with a palpable mass. In

such cases, invasion is undoubtedly present but is either not recognized by the pathologist or is undetected due to sampling error. Axillary lymph node involvement in patients with mammographically detected DCIS is a rare event. In a series of 189 patients with DCIS, most of whose tumors were detected by mammography alone, none showed metastases on axillary dissection.[406]

PAGET'S DISEASE

Paget's disease is a form of DCIS characterized by involvement of the nipple epidermis (Figs 10.64, 10.65). The DCIS is almost always of high grade. The clinical manifestation includes crusting and erosion of the nipple, pruritus, and bloody discharge. Paget's disease is seen in 1–2% of all breast cancers; it rarely occurs in men.[407] Microscopically, the nipple epidermis is infiltrated by large, ovoid or round cells with a round nucleus and abundant clear cytoplasm (Fig. 10.65). These cells (Paget cells) may exhibit hyperchromatic irregular nuclei and mitoses. They are isolated or constitute small

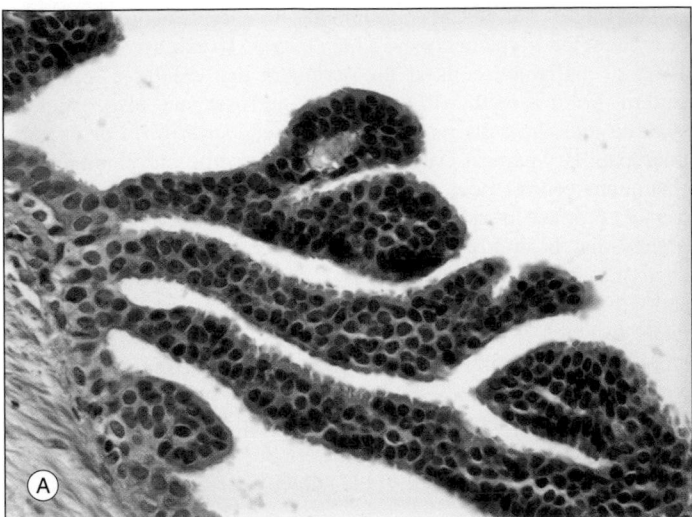

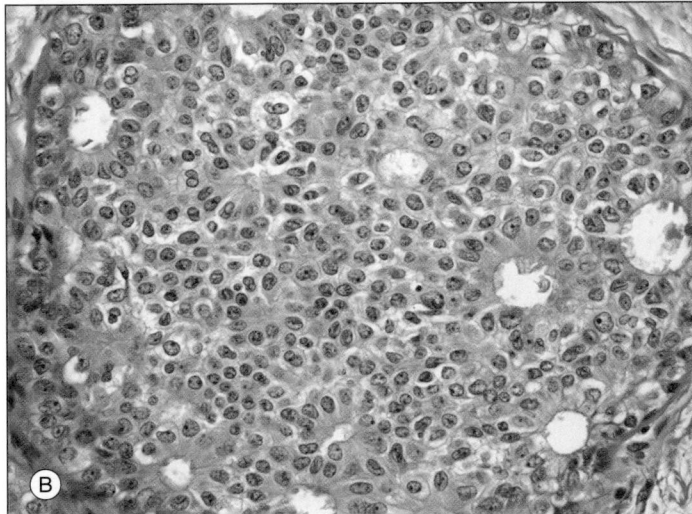

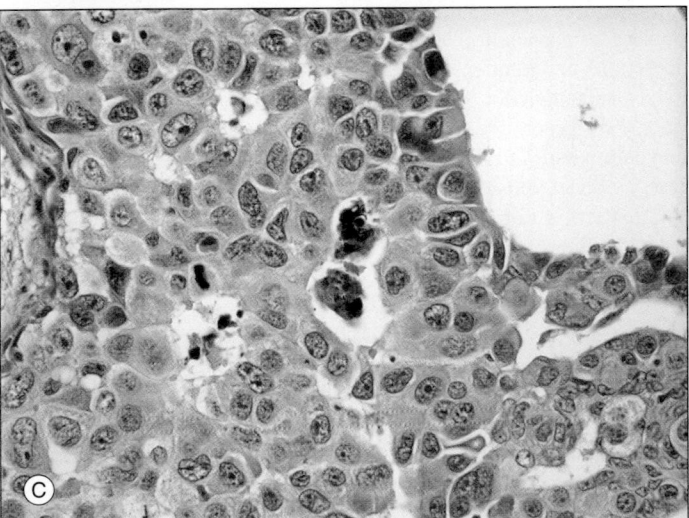

Fig. 10.63 Nuclear grading in ductal carcinoma in situ. **(A)** Low nuclear grade. **(B)** Intermediate nuclear grade. **(C)** High nuclear grade.

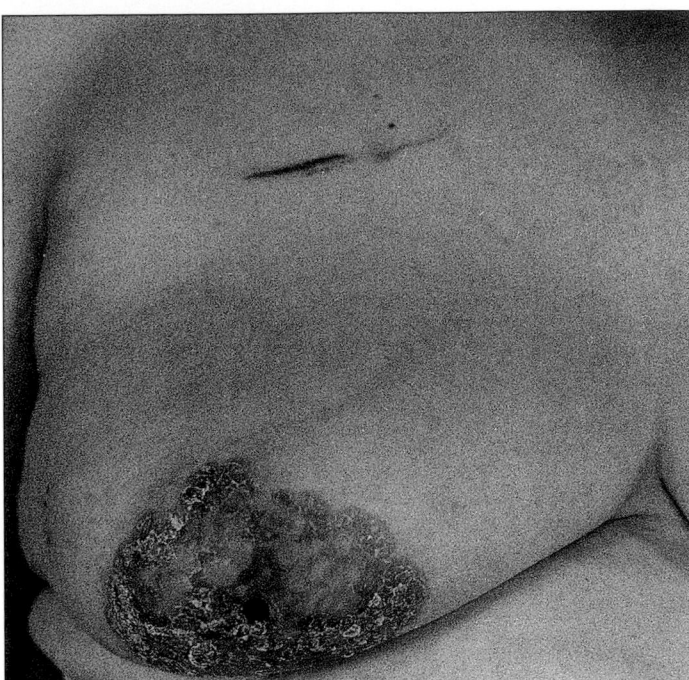

Fig. 10.64 Paget's disease, clinical appearance.

masses or clumps and rarely small glands, usually located in the deeper layers of the epithelium. When the cells occur in nests, this arrangement may recall the junctional component of an amelanotic melanoma; compounding the difficulty is the fact that Paget cells may occasionally contain melanin granules.[408] However, melanoma of the nipple virtually never occurs. A form of Paget's disease in which the cells largely replace the normal squamous cells of the nipple epidermis (so-called anaplastic Paget's disease)[409] occasionally occurs; in this situation the differential diagnosis is with in situ squamous carcinoma (Bowen's disease). Again, as with melanoma, Bowen's disease of the nipple is exceedingly rare. If the diagnosis is in doubt, mucin staining (PAS with diastase digestion) and immunoreactivity for cytokeratin CAM5.2 and *HER2/neu*[410,411] are characteristic of Paget cells. All of these findings should be negative in melanoma and Bowen's disease. Immunostaining for human milk fat globulin and carcinoembryonic antigen (CEA), although generally positive, has not been as reliable.[412]

Clear cells with small regular nuclei normally occur in the epidermis of the nipple (Toker cells) and should not be mistaken for Paget cells. The distinction should also be made from direct invasion from an underlying invasive carcinoma.

Cytologically, Paget's disease is characterized by a pleomorphic population of neoplastic epithelial cells. The cells are large with centrally located nuclei and abundant clear cytoplasm. Tumor cells are seen in a background of keratinous debris, inflammatory cells, and squamous cells. The differential diagnosis (because of the location of the lesion) includes subareolar abscess and periareolar duct hyperplasias. In these cases, although some degree of atypia may be seen in epithelial cells, the clustering of cohesive aggregates of epithelial cells favors the benign nature of these lesions. Malignant melanoma, although extremely rare, may cytologically present with features similar to Paget's disease. Distinction from malignant melanoma is possible by immunocytochemistry, as discussed above.

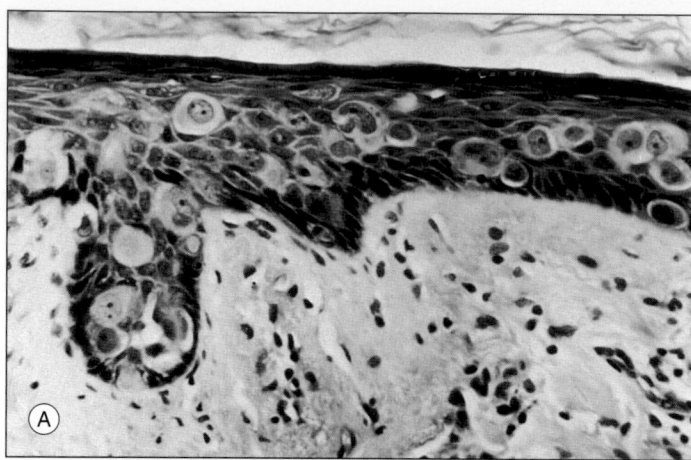

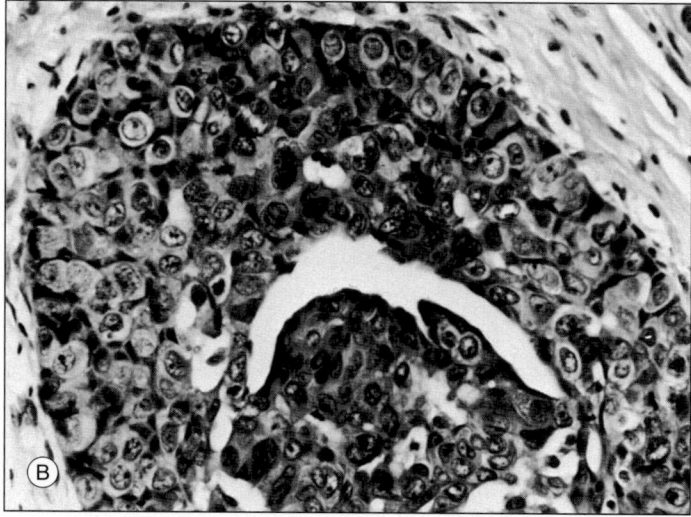

Fig. 10.65 Paget's disease. **(A)** The nipple epidermis is infiltrated by large round cells with a round nucleus and abundant clear cytoplasm. **(B)** An underlying lactiferous duct is infiltrated by the same type of neoplastic cells.

The histogenesis of the disease has been controversial, but immunohistochemical studies have confirmed their glandular epithelial phenotype.[413] Thus, there is thought to be an extension of the malignant cells upward in the duct system with final infiltration of the overlying cutaneous epithelium. In rare instances, underlying DCIS is not found. In these cases the Paget cells may have arisen from a very localized DCIS in the lactiferous sinus or from epidermally located mammary ductal epithelial cells.

The prognosis depends on the underlying mammary tumor. Treatment is directed at the intraductal and/or infiltrating duct carcinoma. Primary carcinoma of the nipple is a rarity and should not be misinterpreted as Paget's disease; both basal cell and squamous carcinoma of the nipple epithelium have been described.[414]

CHARACTERISTICS OF DUCTAL CARCINOMA IN SITU BY TYPE

High-grade ductal carcinoma in situ
High-grade DCIS (poorly differentiated DCIS, comedo DCIS) is usually not a diagnostic problem because the nuclei are overtly malignant. Cell polarization or architectural differentiation, as defined by

Holland et al.,[370] is absent or minimal. These lesions commonly have central comedo-type necrosis, which may be so extensive as to leave a rim of malignant cells at the periphery that creates a 'clinging' pattern. Solid growth without central necrosis may also occur. In some lesions the cells may grow in a pseudocribriform or pseudo-micropapillary pattern. Autophagocytosis is common. When there is prominent central necrosis the calcifications are amorphous and usually produce a typical branching, linear pattern on mammography that is highly suspicious for malignancy.[399] The involved ducts may be very distended. This type of DCIS is rapid-growing and is often quite large at presentation. This type of DCIS is more likely to result in a palpable abnormality in the breast than other types of DCIS. This is partly because of the surrounding stromal reaction, which is usually more evident in this pattern of DCIS than in others. Involvement of lobules (cancerization) is frequent. Paget's disease of the nipple is almost invariably associated with DCIS composed of cells with high-grade nuclei.

Low-grade ductal carcinoma in situ
Low-grade or well differentiated DCIS, composed of cells of low nuclear grade, is sometimes difficult to differentiate from florid ductal hyperplasia. The most striking feature is the monotonous appearance of the cells. The growth pattern of most lesions of this group is true cribriform, micropapillary, or solid. Architectural differentiation (cell polarization) is prominent. In the cribriform pattern, intercellular lumina between the proliferating cells are rigid, rounded and usually evenly distributed within the cell masses. The cells within the center of the proliferating strands forming the bridges and arcades are arranged regularly or lie at right angles to the plane of the cellular strands. In the micropapillary pattern, proliferating cells extend into the lumen of the glandular structure but without a fibrovascular stalk. The papillae frequently have a club-like appearance with even distribution of the cells within the papillae. The cells between papillae are also atypical but often have more cytoplasm than the cells in the papillae. Occasionally, true papillae with fibrovascular cores are present, together with the micropapillae. When the growth pattern is solid, necrosis is rarely present in association with cells of low nuclear grade. However, secretions are frequently present within the duct lumen and should not be mistaken for necrosis. Calcification is not as frequent as in poorly differentiated DCIS and, when present, is usually rounded and laminated and deposited within the secretions. Such calcification produces clusters of granular particles on mammography and this pattern is not as distinctive as that of the calcification seen in poorly differentiated, high-grade DCIS, since similar patterns may also occur in benign lesions.[399] Some patterns of well differentiated DCIS are difficult to distinguish from LCIS. Furthermore, some in situ carcinomas may show mixed ductal and lobular features.

Intermediate-grade ductal carcinoma in situ
The third type of DCIS shows features in between those of the high-grade, poorly differentiated and low-grade, well differentiated types. The presence of cell polarization is not as prominent and uniform as in the well differentiated type.[370] The growth pattern varies and may be solid, cribriform, micropapillary, or clinging. Necrosis may or may not be present. Calcification, when present, may be laminated or amorphous.[399]

Clinging ductal carcinoma in situ
The terms *clinging DCIS* and *clinging carcinoma* have been applied to two histologically distinct lesions, both of which are characterized by the presence of one or two cell layers adjacent to the basement

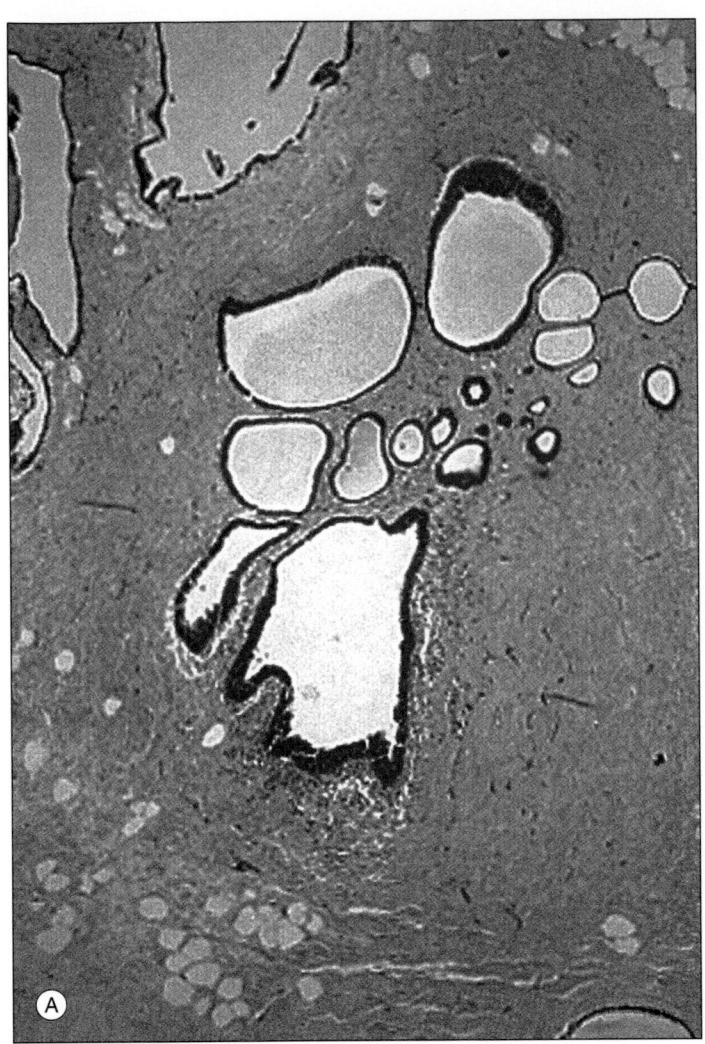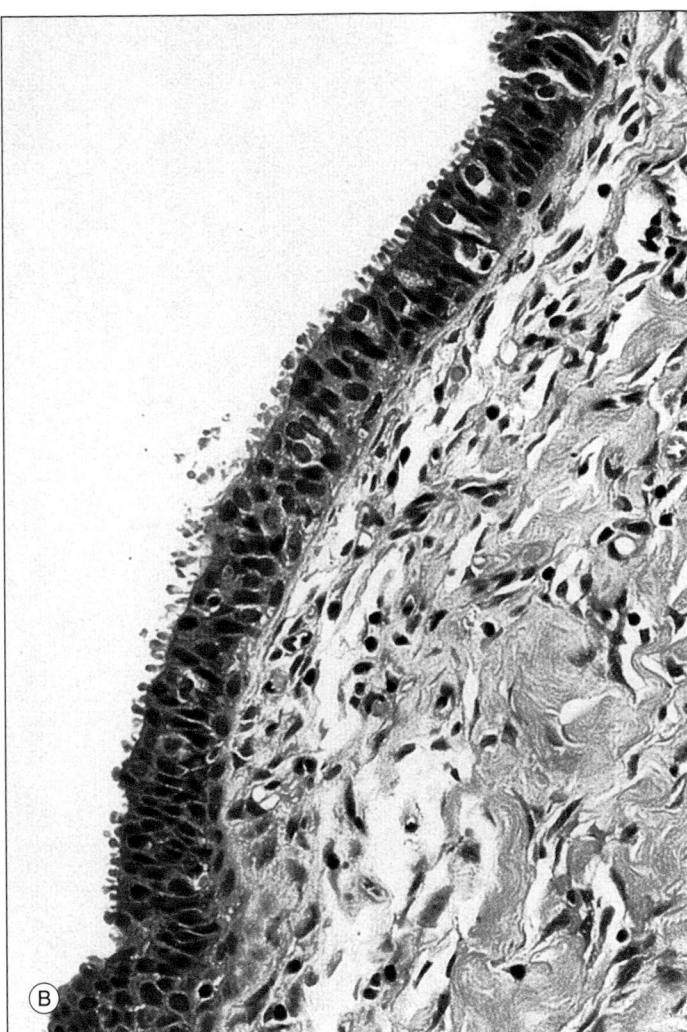

Fig. 10.66 Columnar cell hyperplasia with atypia. This lesion has been variously categorized as 'clinging carcinoma,' atypical ductal hyperplasia, or columnar cell hyperplasia with atypia. **(A)** Low power view. **(B)** Detail.

membrane. The most common lesions in this group are composed of small uniform cells with low-grade nuclei, characteristic of well differentiated DCIS.[195,415] In many such lesions, the cells are columnar. When lesions of this type are seen in conjunction with low-grade DCIS with cribriform or micropapillary patterns one can be confident that they are part of the readily diagnosable DCIS. However they are being encountered with increasing frequency as isolated lesions in breast biopsies performed because of mammographic microcalcifications. In isolation, this pattern is not universally recognized as representing fully developed DCIS and, indeed, some consider it to be part of the spectrum of ADH[416] or columnar cell hyperplasia with atypia (Fig. 10.66).[417] In fact, such lesions do not appear to be associated with as high a risk of breast cancer as fully developed forms of low-grade DCIS.[415,418] In the second form of clinging DCIS the cells lining the involved spaces have high-grade nuclei. In these cases, there may be evidence of central necrosis, and these lesions represent examples of poorly differentiated DCIS.[195,415]

Rarely, clinging DCIS is composed of one or two layers of very atypical cells. This is a variant of a high-grade DCIS or comedo type carried to the extreme. It is best classified as such to prevent confusion.

Apocrine ductal carcinoma in situ

Apocrine proliferations within the breast represent a spectrum of changes ranging from usual apocrine metaplasia at the benign end to overt apocrine DCIS at the malignant end. In between these two easily identifiable entities are a range of atypical apocrine lesions that are often difficult to categorize accurately. Because usual benign apocrine metaplasia is characterized by a uniform population of cells, most often with well formed architectural structures (bridges, micropapillae, etc.), the threshold for diagnosing DCIS or ADH is raised. The classification and management of atypical apocrine lesions is therefore a controversial topic with few studies and limited clinical outcome data available.

O'Malley et al.[419] categorized atypical apocrine lesions based on their level of nuclear atypia (none, moderate, or marked) combined with the size of the area involved (<4 mm, 4–8 mm, and >8 mm). Moderate nuclear atypia included cells showing nuclei '2–3 times the size of usual apocrine nuclei with slightly irregular nuclear membranes and 2–3 small nucleoli in some cells.' Marked nuclear atypia (noncomedo DCIS) showed 'irregular nuclear membranes, coarse chromatin pattern and multiple nucleoli.' These authors formulated several categories based on the combination of atypicality

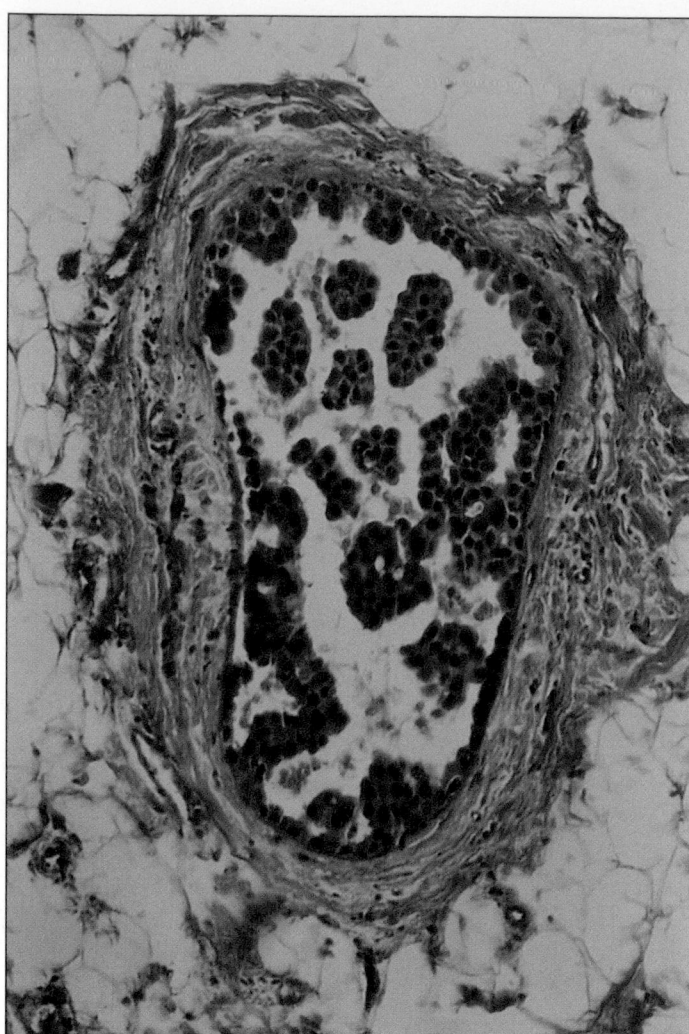

Fig. 10.67 Ductal carcinoma in situ, apocrine type. Note bizarre cells with apocrine cytoplasm.

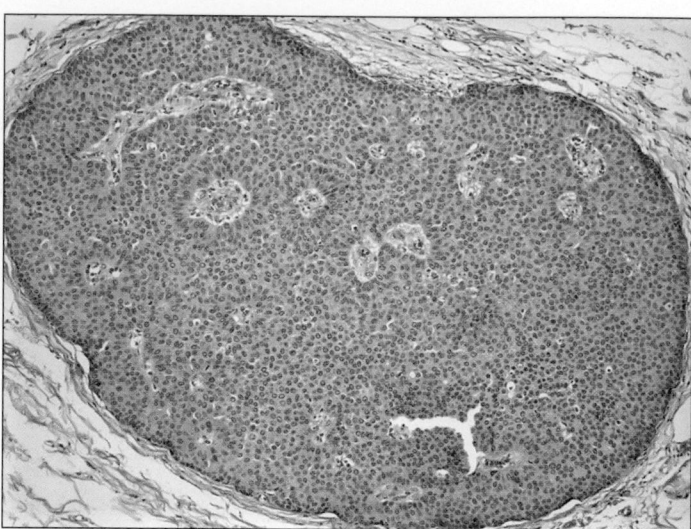

Fig. 10.68 Solid papillary DCIS. This variant is usually seen in older women and usually stains for neuroendocrine markers.

and size criteria. Overt apocrine DCIS was diagnosed if the cells had marked nuclear atypia or if the lesion was larger than 8 mm with moderate atypia (Fig. 10.67). Further categories of borderline apocrine DCIS and apocrine atypia were also defined. Unfortunately, no outcome data were reported in this study. In another study, Tavassoli and Norris[420] divided their atypical apocrine lesions into three categories: atypical apocrine metaplasia, atypical apocrine hyperplasia, and apocrine DCIS. Most of their apocrine DCIS cases were of high nuclear grade. These authors advised caution in diagnosing apocrine DCIS in the absence of marked nuclear atypia and necrosis.

In the absence of substantive outcome data, it is prudent to apply a cautious and conservative approach to the diagnosis of apocrine DCIS. For a diagnosis of overt apocrine DCIS we require either of the following:

- *Marked nuclear atypia*, characterized by irregular nuclear membranes, marked pleomorphism, coarse chromatin, and multiple nucleoli[419]
- *Perfect architectural pattern* (e.g. cribriform, micropapillary, necrosis) in the presence of moderate nuclear atypia (2–3 times

the size of usual apocrine nuclei with slightly irregular nuclear membranes and 2–3 small nucleoli in some cells).[419]

Apocrine lesions that do not meet these criteria should be considered on a case-by-case basis, and are probably best categorized as atypical.

Endocrine (argyrophilic) ductal carcinoma in situ (solid papillary ductal carcinoma in situ)

A solid pattern of DCIS with neuroendocrine histologic features has also been recognized.[421–424]

Such lesions are usually seen in elderly patients and often present with a bloodstained nipple discharge. The involved glandular elements are often markedly distended. The proliferating cells have a polygonal, oval, or spindle morphologic appearance and granular eosinophilic cytoplasm with intervening fibrovascular cores and septae (Fig. 10.68). Rosettes and ribboning may be evident, as may mucin production and microglandular spaces.[424] In some examples, the component cells are a mixture of spindle cell and argyrophilic signet ring cells (see Figs 10.33, 10.34)[422] Because of the frequent lack of overt cytologic atypia, this type of DCIS can easily be misdiagnosed as benign.[424] Small foci of invasive carcinoma are present in a significant number of cases and, in one series, 20 of 34 examples of endocrine DCIS had associated invasion. In another 18 examples there were nearby papillomas colonized by endocrine DCIS.[422] 'Solid papillary carcinoma'[423] of the breast would appear to be related to, if not identical with, neuroendocrine DCIS.

Signet ring cell ductal carcinoma in situ

While signet ring cell formation is more commonly seen in in situ lobular carcinomas, DCIS consisting predominantly of signet ring cells has been described.[425]

Cystic hypersecretory ductal carcinoma in situ

In this uncommon type of DCIS the gross appearance is characteristic, consisting of cysts filled with viscid material. Microscopic examination reveals multiple cystlike structures containing homogeneous eosinophilic material that resembles thyroid colloid.[426]

Some are lined by histologically benign, flat, or columnar epithelium. In others the lining epithelium shows various degrees of hyperplasia, with foci of low-grade DCIS. The lining cells may show evidence of secretory activity with features reminiscent of the lactating breast. Stains for mucin show focal positivity within the epithelial cells, with the majority of the cyst contents being negative. Rarely, the same pattern is seen without fully developed carcinoma in situ. Such lesions are termed *cystic hypersecretory hyperplasia*.[427]

Ductal carcinoma in situ involving lobules (cancerization of lobules)

When DCIS is extensive it causes involved lobules to expand or unfold. This causes the lobule to lose its characteristic low-power appearance and the lobule appears as a group of expanded ducts involved by DCIS. When DCIS is seen within obviously lobular structures, the term *cancerization of lobules* has been used to describe this finding. It is nearly always associated with one of the typical patterns of DCIS described above, but very occasionally occurs alone. The appearance should not be misinterpreted as invasive carcinoma, a possibility that is enhanced when the process is further complicated by the presence of sclerosing adenosis. Differentiation from invasive carcinoma, as well as differentiation of lobular cancerization by DCIS from LCIS, is discussed later.

DIFFERENTIAL DIAGNOSIS OF DUCTAL CARCINOMA IN SITU

From ductal hyperplasia

In most cases of DCIS, there is no diagnostic problem; however, on occasion, differentiation from intraductal hyperplasia can be difficult. The features suggestive of DCIS at low power are an even distribution of cells, geometric intercellular spaces, and bridges that appear well defined or rigid. Necrosis can occur in many benign lesions but its presence raises the suspicion of DCIS.

At a higher magnification there is only one cell type (monomorphism). The nuclei of cells forming bridges or lining spaces are either randomly arranged or lie perpendicular to bridges or radially around spaces. The nuclei do not show streaming. Unless it is apocrine DCIS, areas of apocrine metaplasia are not seen (see above). While in low-grade, DCIS nuclear pleomorphism may be minimal, the cells are usually hyperchromatic and have at least one prominent nucleolus and an increased nuclear/cytoplasmic ratio. Mitotic figures are difficult to find in well differentiated, low-grade DCIS.

Use of the term *atypical ductal hyperplasia* should be reserved for cases showing some of the aforementioned features but not showing the full picture of DCIS.

From other lesions

See specific sections, such as on papillary lesions, apocrine lesions, LCIS.

LOBULAR CARCINOMA IN SITU

Lobular carcinoma in situ (LCIS) is not detectable on macroscopic examination and is therefore an incidental microscopic finding in breast tissue removed for another reason. In contrast to DCIS, which is highly heterogeneous in its histologic appearance, the histologic features of LCIS show little variation and are usually easily recognized.[189,236,357,428] LCIS is most often characterized by a solid proliferation of small cells with small, uniform, round to oval nuclei,

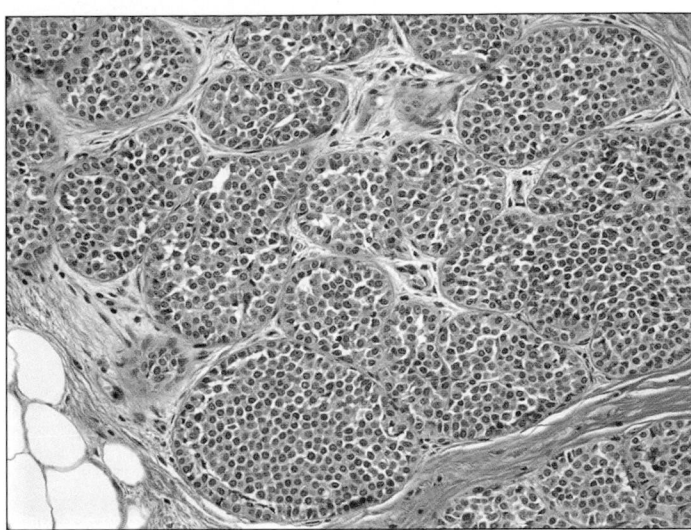

Fig. 10.69 LCIS. Enlarged acini are filled with uniform cells lacking pleomorphism or mitotic activity.

and variably distinct cell borders (Fig. 10.69). The cells often show loss of cohesion. Loss of cohesion is a hallmark of these lesions and is best demonstrated in well fixed preparations. The cytoplasm is clear to lightly eosinophilic; occasionally, the cells contain intracytoplasmic vacuoles that may be large enough to produce signet ring cell forms. This description refers to the type of LCIS described by Haagensen as type A, or classical type.[429] Some cases of LCIS are, however, characterized by larger cells with larger nuclei that show minimal pleomorphism, referred to by Haagensen as type B cells[429] (see Fig. 10.2). LCIS is typically present in the terminal duct–lobular units and distends and distorts the involved spaces. In some instances, LCIS cells involve extralobular ducts. The growth within these ducts may be either solid or pagetoid (i.e. the LCIS cells are insinuated between the duct basement membrane and the native ductal epithelial cells). Although some authors previously recognized a cribriform pattern of involvement of extralobular ducts by LCIS,[430] in situ lesions with a cribriform pattern are best categorized as DCIS.

Cell kinetic studies have shown that LCIS has a low proliferative rate.[381,382] The cells of LCIS are also typically estrogen-receptor-positive,[381,382] and rarely show overexpression of the *HER2/neu* oncogene[381,382] or accumulation of the p53 protein.[381,382] In addition, studies have indicated that the cells of LCIS are characterized by loss of expression of the adhesion molecule E-cadherin (Fig. 10.70).[431]

DIFFERENTIAL DIAGNOSIS

Atypical lobular hyperplasia

The cells composing atypical lobular hyperplasia (ALH) are the same as in LCIS but in ALH the degree of involvement of the terminal ducts and lobules is less extensive (see Fig. 10.19). Unfortunately, there is no sharp dividing line between ALH and LCIS and diagnostic criteria for this distinction vary among experts. Some authors require that at least 50% of the spaces in a given lobule be filled with and distended by the characteristic cells to warrant a diagnosis of LCIS[189] whereas others do not consider lobular distension and enlargement an essential feature for the diagnosis of LCIS.[236] The most important

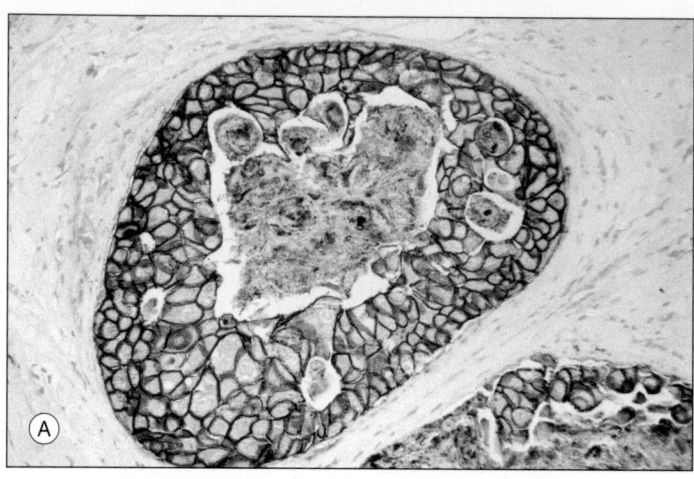
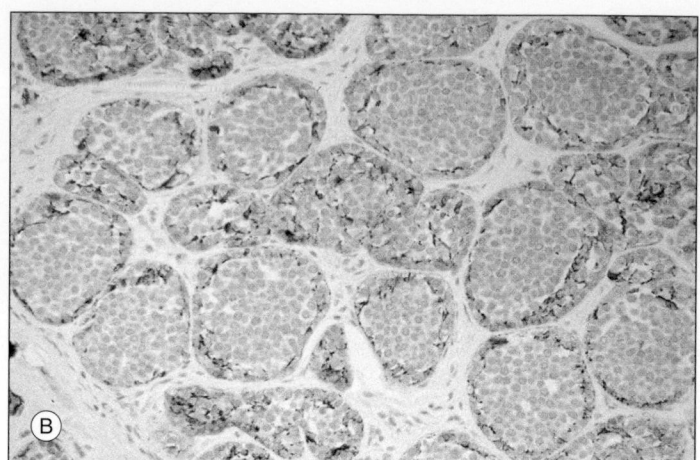

Fig. 10.70 **(A)** High-grade DCIS with typical E-cadherin membrane staining. **(B)** LCIS with the characteristic lack of E-cadherin membrane staining.

factor is to recognize the lesion as an atypical lobular lesion (LCIS, ALH, lobular neoplasia). All of these lesions are associated with a substantially elevated risk for the subsequent development of cancer.[161,165] In addition, patients with ALH or LCIS may benefit from chemopreventive therapy.[432,433]

Lobular carcinoma in situ involving pre-existing benign lesions

In some patients, LCIS may involve areas of breast tissue that have pre-existing benign alterations; for example, LCIS may involve foci of sclerosing adenosis and produce a pattern that mimics invasive carcinoma.[183] However, low-power examination in such specimens usually reveals the lobulocentric configuration characteristic of adenosis. When LCIS involves collagenous spherulosis the pattern mimics low-grade DCIS, cribriform pattern.

Lobular carcinoma in situ versus ductal carcinoma in situ

Although the distinction between DCIS and LCIS is usually not difficult to make, there are areas of overlap between these two lesions:

- DCIS may extend into recognizable lobules and be confused with LCIS[434] and LCIS may involve extralobular ducts,[430] mimicking DCIS. It is important to note that the classification of in situ lesions (whether ductal or lobular) is based on their specific cytologic and architectural features within the space involved, rather than the site involved (i.e. lobule vs extralobular duct). Therefore, irrespective of the site involved, the cells of DCIS will remain more cohesive and maintain their characteristic cytologic features, in contrast to those of LCIS, the cells of which are relatively smaller, more uniform, and dyshesive.
- DCIS and LCIS may coexist in the same breast and even in the same ductal-lobular unit.[435]
- In some in situ carcinomas, the cytologic and/or architectural features deviate from the usual patterns, making it difficult to determine if the proliferation is ductal or lobular in nature (see following section).

CARCINOMAS IN SITU WITH INDETERMINATE FEATURES

There has been no general agreement as how best to classify such in situ lesions with indeterminate features (CIS-IF) between DCIS and LCIS. Some authors have proposed a combined or mixed ductal and lobular category[436,437] and others have favored categorization of these lesions as either DCIS or LCIS.[189,438–441] E-cadherin immunostaining may be of use in classifying these indeterminate in situ lesions.[442]

A number of studies have shown E-cadherin protein expression to be lost in invasive lobular carcinoma[443,444] and in LCIS,[443,444] but not in invasive ductal carcinoma[443,444] or DCIS[443,444] (Fig. 10.70). In at least some studies, loss of E-cadherin expression in lobular carcinomas is due to a mutation of the E-cadherin gene, predominantly in the part that encodes the extracellular domain.[445–448]

Cases of in situ carcinoma with cytologic atypia that show a lack of cell-to-cell cohesion are classified by some as in situ carcinomas with mixed ductal and lobular features and by others as pleomorphic LCIS[438,439] (Fig. 10.71). These cases are typically negative for E-cadherin immunostaining, suggesting a lobular phenotype.

E-cadherin immunohistochemistry therefore appears to be a valuable adjunct in the categorization of carcinoma in situ lesions with indeterminate features. However, until clinical outcome data are available to determine the true behavior of these lesions, E-cadherin immunostaining of CIS-IF lesions should be interpreted with caution and be assessed on a case-by-case basis. In particular, all histologically ambiguous in situ carcinomas found on CNB specimens should undergo surgical excision irrespective of their E-cadherin immunostaining pattern. In our opinion, pleomorphic in situ carcinomas, whether or not they show loss of E-cadherin staining, should at the present time be treated as one would DCIS.

INVASIVE BREAST CANCER

Invasive breast cancers are a very varied group of lesions with regard to their presentation and biologic potential. The classification of invasive breast cancers used in this chapter (with minor modifications), is that of the World Health Organization (2nd edition)[449]

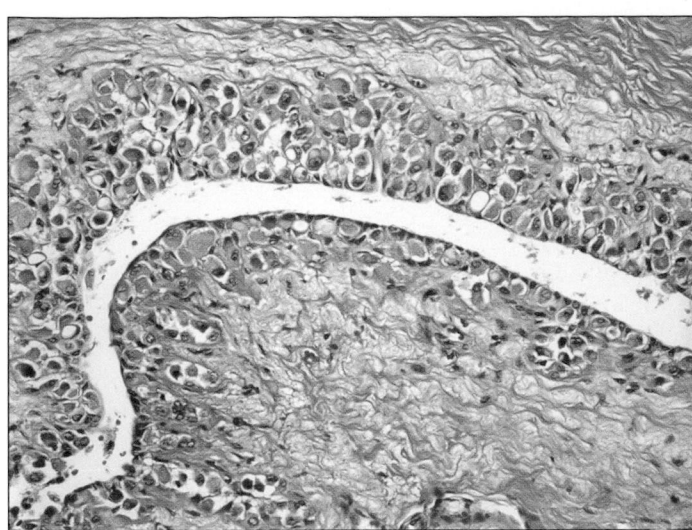

Fig. 10.71 Pleomorphic LCIS. In this example of lobular carcinoma in situ, the lesion is composed of larger tumor cells that show more atypical nuclei than the usual LCIS.

Table 10.6 World Health Organization. Classification of Carcinomas of the Breast

Noninvasive
Intraductal carcinoma
    With Paget's disease
Lobular carcinoma in situ
Invasive
Invasive ductal carcinoma
    With Paget's disease
Invasive ductal carcinoma with a predominant intraductal component
Invasive lobular carcinoma
Medullary carcinoma
Mucinous carcinoma
Invasive papillary carcinoma
Tubular carcinoma
Adenoid cystic carcinoma
Secretory (juvenile) carcinoma
Apocrine carcinoma
Carcinoma with metaplasia
Inflammatory carcinoma (unusual clinical presentation)

Source: World Health Organization. Classification of Tumors. Tumors of the Breast and Female Genital Organs. Geneva: World Health Organization; 2003.

(Table 10.6). Most invasive breast cancers arise in the terminal duct lobular unit, regardless of histologic type.[159] Therefore the terms 'ductal' and 'lobular' imply typical cytologic and histologic growth patterns and not histogenesis.

The most common type of invasive breast cancer is infiltrating (invasive) ductal carcinoma.[189,450,451] To distinguish these tumors from invasive breast cancers with specific histological features (such as invasive lobular, tubular, mucinous, medullary, and other rare types), some authorities prefer the term infiltrating ductal carcinoma not otherwise specified (IDC-NOS)[450] or infiltrating carcinoma of no special type (IC-NST).[189] In fact, the diagnosis of invasive ductal carcinoma is a diagnosis by default, since this tumor type is defined as a type of cancer 'not classified into any of the other categories of invasive mammary carcinoma.'[449] In this chapter, the terms invasive ductal carcinoma, infiltrating ductal carcinoma, and infiltrating or invasive carcinoma of no special type are synonymous.

Depending upon authors definition and patient population the percentages of special types varies. In order to qualify as a special type cancer at least 90% of a tumor should demonstrate the defining histological characteristics of a special type cancer to be designated as that histological type.[189,452] With these criteria 20–30% of invasive carcinomas will qualify as special types.

Mammography has resulted in a change in the distribution of the histological features of the invasive breast cancers detected. In particular, special type cancers (particularly tubular carcinomas)[453,454] and cancers of lower histological grade[455–457] have been more frequently observed in mammographically screened populations than in patients who present with a palpable mass, particularly in the prevalent round of screening.[458]

Invasive carcinomas derive from the in situ component. This is based on the frequent coexistence of the two lesions, on the histological similarities between the invasive and in situ components within the same lesion, and on the fact that coexisting invasive and in situ carcinomas often share the same immunophenotype and genetic alterations.[230] For example, a number of studies have clearly documented that low-grade invasive cancers are most often associated with low-grade DCIS and high-grade invasive cancers with high-grade in situ lesions.[459–461]

INVASIVE (INFILTRATING) DUCTAL CARCINOMA

As noted above, invasive ductal carcinomas represent the single largest group of invasive breast cancers. Although these tumors are most commonly encountered in pure form, a substantial minority exhibit admixed foci of other histologic types. In one series of 1000 invasive breast cancers, such combinations of invasive ductal carcinoma and other types were seen in 28% of cases.[450] The classification of tumors composed primarily of invasive ductal carcinoma with a minor component consisting of one or more other histological types is problematic. Some authorities categorize such lesions as invasive ductal carcinomas (or invasive carcinomas of no special type) and simply note the presence of the other types,[189] whereas others classify them as 'mixed.'[452]

Clinical presentation
Invasive ductal carcinomas most often present as a palpable mass and/or mammographic abnormality. There are no clinical or mammographic characteristics that distinguish invasive ductal carcinomas from other histologic types of invasive cancer. Rarely, these lesions present with Paget's disease of the nipple.

Gross pathology
The classical macroscopic appearance of invasive ductal carcinoma is that of a scirrhous carcinoma, characterized by a firm, sometimes rock-hard mass that on cut section has a grey-white, gritty surface (Fig. 10.72). This consistency and appearance is due to the desmoplastic tumor stroma and not to the neoplastic cells themselves. Some invasive ductal carcinomas are composed primarily of tumor cells with little desmoplastic stromal reaction, and such lesions are grossly tan and soft. Although most invasive ductal cancers have a stellate or spiculated contour with irregular peripheral margins, some lesions have rounded, pushing margins and are grossly well

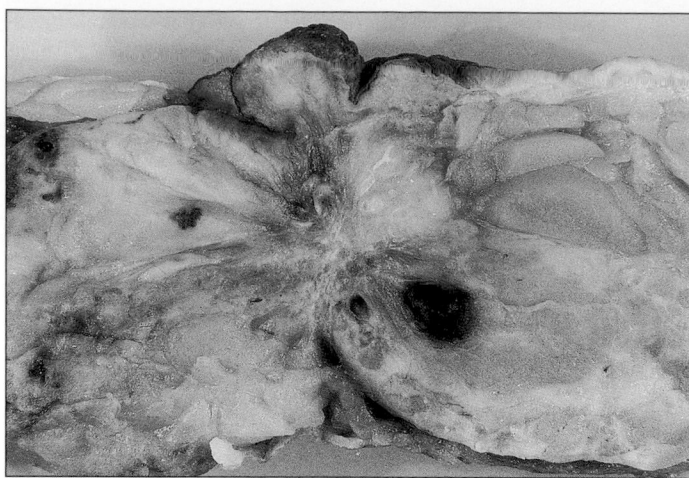

Fig. 10.72 Infiltrating duct carcinoma. Typical gross appearance of a firm, stellate, scar-like process.

circumscribed, and rarely they lack a significant tumor stroma and are indistinct.

Histopathology

The microscopic appearance of invasive ductal carcinomas is highly heterogeneous with regard to growth pattern, cytologic features, mitotic activity, stromal desmoplasia, extent of the associated DCIS, and contour. Variability in histologic features may even be seen within a single case. The tumor cells may be arranged as glandular structures, as nests, cords, or trabeculae of various sizes, or as solid sheets. Foci of necrosis are evident in some cases and may be extensive. Cytologically, the tumor cells range from those that show little deviation from normal breast epithelial cells to those exhibiting marked cellular pleomorphism and nuclear atypia. Mitotic activity can range from imperceptible to marked. Stromal desmoplasia is prominent in some cases and minimal in others. At the other end of the spectrum, some tumors show such prominent stromal desmoplasia that the tumor cells constitute only a minor component of the lesion. Similarly, some invasive ductal carcinomas have no identifiable component of DCIS, whereas in others the in situ carcinoma is the predominant component of the tumor. Finally, the microscopic margins of these cancers may be infiltrating, pushing, circumscribed or mixed (Figs 10.73, 10.74).

Recognizing that invasive ductal carcinomas are a histologically diverse group of lesions, many investigators have attempted to stratify them on the basis of certain microscopic features. The most common method of subclassifying invasive ductal carcinomas is grading. Grading in some systems is based solely on nuclear features (nuclear grading). The nuclear grading system that was most commonly employed was that of Black et al.[462,463] The most commonly used and recommended grading systems use a combination of architectural and nuclear characteristics (histologic grading). In histologic grading, breast carcinomas are categorized based on the evaluation of three features: tubule formation, nuclear pleomorphism, and mitotic activity. The histologic grading system currently in most widespread use is the Nottingham system. This system is a modification by Elston and Ellis[464] of the grading system proposed by Bloom and Richardson, but provides strictly defined criteria that are lacking in the original description. Tubule formation, nuclear pleomorphism, and mitotic activity are each scored on a 1–3 scale.

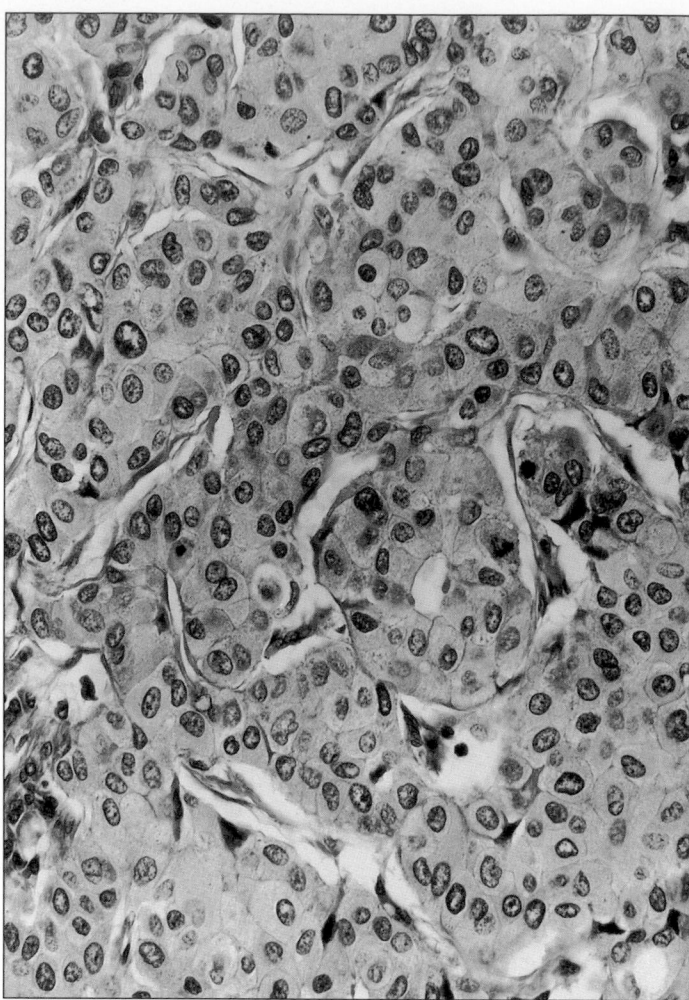

Fig. 10.73 Infiltrating duct carcinoma. Numerous glandular formations lined by large cells with hyperchromatic but relatively uniform nuclei are seen. Minimal stroma is present.

The sum of the scores for these three parameters provides the overall histologic grade, such that tumors in which the sum of the scores is 3–5 are designated grade 1 (well differentiated), those with score sums of 6 and 7 are designated grade 2 (moderately differentiated), and those with score sums of 8 and 9 are designated grade 3 (poorly differentiated) (Table 10.7). Attempts at correlating cytologic findings with the Elston–Ellis histologic grading system have not been successful. As could be expected, the parameter that correlates best is usually nuclear pleomorphism.[465] When done properly, histologic grading is highly predictive of outcome (see Prognostic factors, below).

The expression of biologic markers, such as estrogen and progesterone receptors, growth factors, oncogene and tumor suppressor gene products, and other markers is highly variable in invasive ductal carcinomas as might be anticipated from their histologic heterogeneity.

Clinical course and prognosis

Although invasive ductal carcinomas have among the poorest prognosis of all invasive breast cancers, even within this group prognostically favorable subsets can be identified, as discussed in the section on Prognostic Factors below.

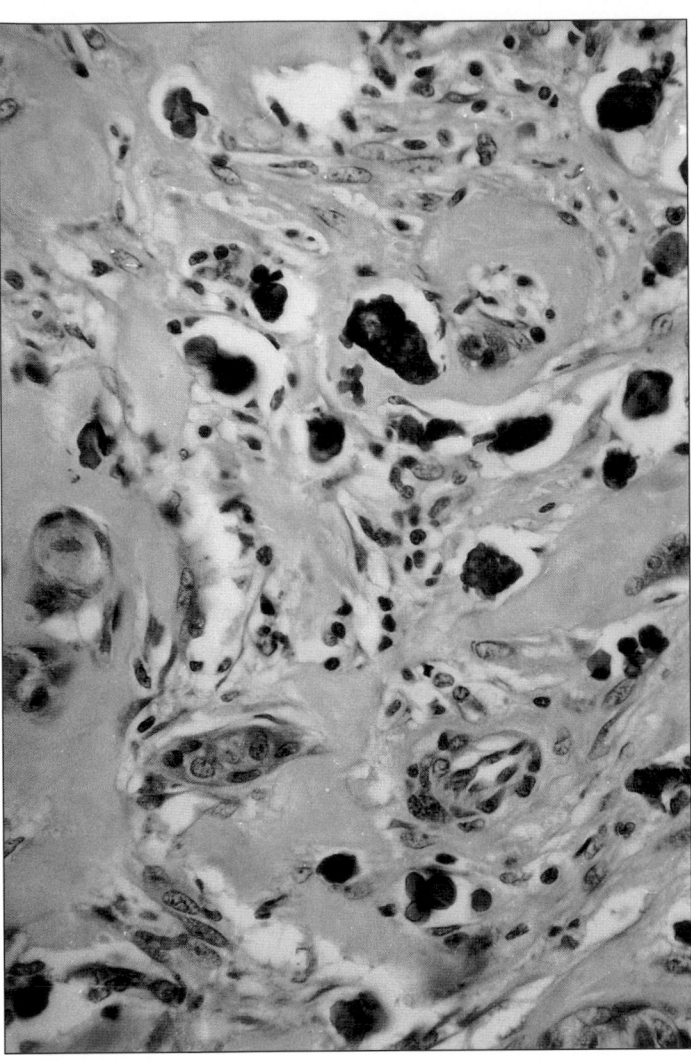

Fig. 10.74 Infiltrating duct carcinoma. Note the presence of diffuse fibrosis and numerous microcalcifications.

Table 10.7 Histologic grading system for invasive breast cancers – Elston and Ellis modification of Bloom and Richardson grading system

Components of grade	Score
Tubules	
>75% of tumor composed of tubules	1 point
10–75% of tumor composed of tubules	2 points
<10% of tumor composed of tubules	3 points
Nuclear grade	
Nuclei small and uniform	1 point
Moderate variation in nuclear size/shape	2 points
Marked nuclear pleomorphism	3 points
Mitotic rate	
Dependent on microscope field area*	1–3 points
Histologic grade	**Total points**
1 (well differentiated)	3–5
2 (moderately differentiated)	6–7
3 (poorly differentiated)	8–9

It is very important to measure the diameter of the high-power field used and correct for the mitotic count. For a typical 44 mm field diameter a mitotic count of 0–5/hpf is 1 point, 6–10 is 2 points and >11 is 3 points. Larger fields will proportionately require higher mitotic counts per point.
Source: from Elston CW, Ellis IO. Assessment of histologic grade. In: Elston CW, Ellis IO (eds) The breast. Edinburgh: Churchill Livingstone; 1998: 365–384.

prominent sclerosis in the tumor. This is best exemplified in scirrhous-type infiltrating duct carcinoma, which yields hypocellular aspirates and may contain few neoplastic cells. Thus, attempts should be made to perform multiple aspirations of the lesion and remain sensitive to the adequacy of the specimen. The presence of benign epithelial cells and stromal components does not exclude the possibility of an infiltrating duct carcinoma. These elements may be introduced during aspiration via accidental sampling of surrounding breast tissue.

INVASIVE (INFILTRATING) LOBULAR CARCINOMA

Invasive lobular carcinomas constitute the second most frequent type of invasive breast cancer. The reported incidence of this tumor type has ranged from less than 1% to as high as 20%.[466] In most series, these tumors account for approximately 5–10% of invasive breast carcinomas.[189,450,451,467] Some of this difference may be related to differences in patient populations. However, much of this variability appears to be related to differences in diagnostic criteria. In addition, a recent study suggested that the increase in the frequency of infiltrating lobular carcinoma may be in part related to the use of postmenopausal hormone replacement therapy.[468]

Invasive lobular carcinomas are characterized by apparent multi-focality in the ipsilateral breast and appear to be more often bilateral than other types of invasive breast cancer, although the reported range of bilaterality has been broad (6–47%).[450,469–473] In two recent clinical follow-up studies of patients with invasive lobular carcinoma, however, the incidence of subsequent contralateral breast cancer among patients with invasive lobular carcinoma was similar to that of patients with invasive ductal carcinoma.[474,475]

Lobular carcinoma in situ coexists with invasive lobular carcinoma in the majority of cases. Overall, approximately 70–80% of cases of invasive lobular carcinoma contain foci of LCIS.[195]

Cytologic features

The cellularity of IDC-NOS is variable and, depending on the degree of fibrous response, aspirates may be quite hypocellular. However, in most cases, infiltrating duct carcinomas are rich in cellularity and the aspirated smears show tumor cells in a dispersed cell pattern displaying various degrees of polymorphism. Scattered individual cells and aggregates of tumor cells as three-dimensional clusters, syncytial groupings, or occasionally gland-like arrangements characterize the neoplasm (Figs 10.75, 10.76). The background contains cellular debris, microcalcific particles, and red blood cells. Cell size varies and ranges from relatively uniform small cells to large and markedly bizarre forms. However, the tumor cells are often pleomorphic with hyperchromatic nuclei and prominent nucleoli. Anisonucleosis is conspicuous and mitoses may also occasionally be seen. Nuclear molding and overriding and crowding of the nuclei are also common. Poorly differentiated infiltrating duct cell carcinoma can form multinucleated giant cells, often seen intermingled with mononuclear neoplastic epithelial cells.

Overall, the frequency of false-negative diagnosis of infiltrating duct carcinoma is relatively low. False-negative diagnosis may be due either to poor aspiration biopsy technique or to the presence of

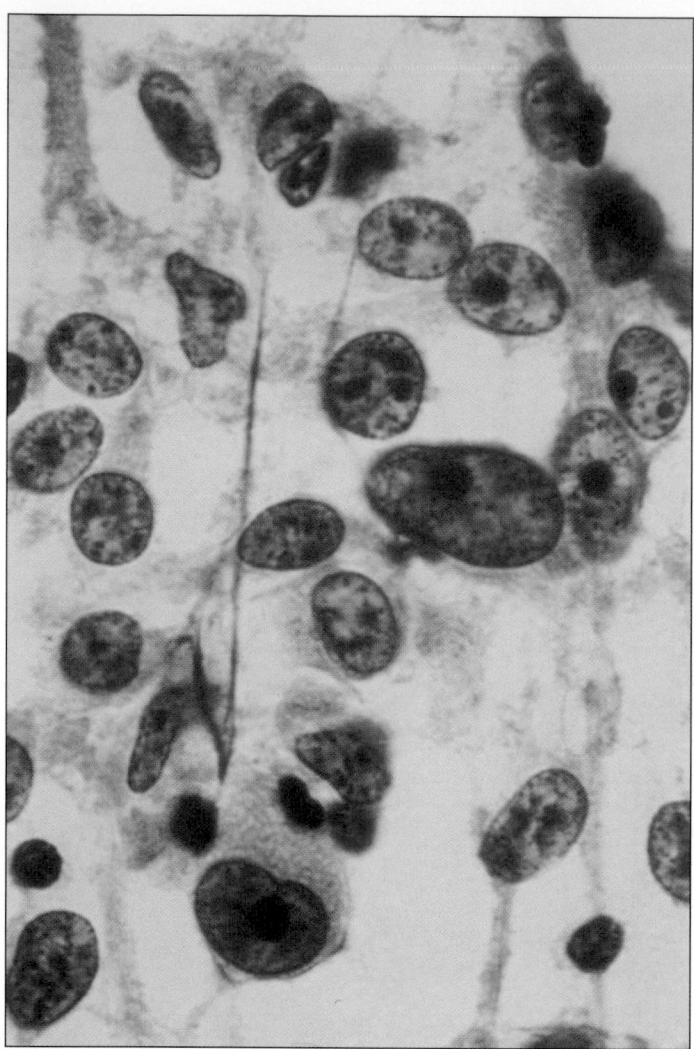

Fig. 10.75 Aspirate of an infiltrating duct carcinoma shows a dispersed cell pattern with conspicuous anisonucleosis and nuclear atypia. (Papanicolaou stain, ×1000.)

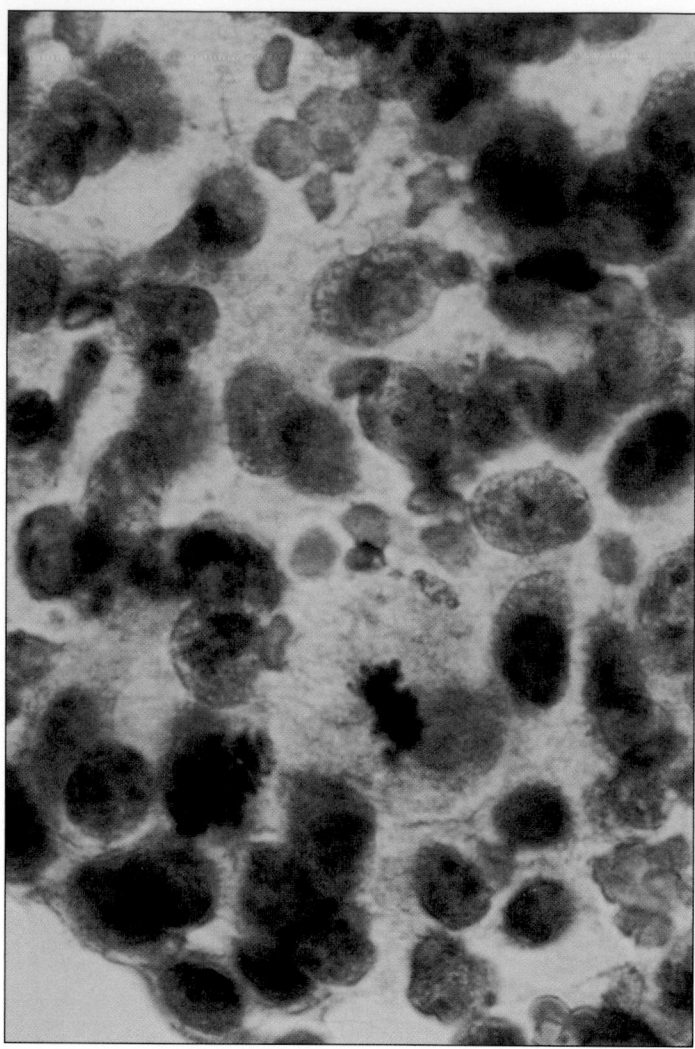

Fig. 10.76 Another view of the same case featuring a mitotic figure. (Papanicolaou stain, ×1000.)

Clinical presentation

While invasive lobular carcinoma may present as a palpable mass or a mammographic abnormality with characteristics similar to those of invasive ductal carcinomas, the findings on physical examination and the mammographic appearance of invasive lobular carcinomas are often quite subtle because of a lack of tumor stroma and a diffuse infiltrative pattern. On physical examination, there may be no findings or only a vague area of thickening or induration, without definable margins. Mammographic findings may be equally subtle, with many invasive lobular carcinomas appearing as poorly defined areas of asymmetric density with architectural distortion, and others revealing no mammographic abnormalities, even in the presence of a palpable mass.[476–481] In fact, the extent of the tumor is often substantially underestimated by both physical examination and mammography.

Gross pathology

In many cases, no mass is grossly evident and the breast tissue may have only a rubbery consistency. In still other cases, no abnormality is evident on visual inspection or upon palpation of the involved breast tissue and the presence of carcinoma is revealed only upon microscopic examination. Finally some invasive lobular carcinomas appear as firm, gritty, grey-white masses, indistinguishable from invasive ductal carcinomas.

Histopathology

Invasive lobular carcinomas as a group show distinctive cytologic features and patterns of tumor cell infiltration of the stroma. The *classical form* is characterized by small, relatively uniform neoplastic cells that invade the stroma singly and in a single-file pattern, which results in the formation of linear strands (Fig. 10.77).[449,467,482–485] These cells frequently encircle mammary ducts in a targetoid manner. Furthermore, the tumor cells may infiltrate the breast stroma and adipose tissue in an insidious fashion, invoking little or no desmoplastic stromal reaction. This feature accounts for the difficulty in detecting some invasive lobular carcinomas on physical examination, mammography and gross pathologic examination. The nuclei of the neoplastic cells are small, show little variation in size, and are often eccentric. Mitotic figures are infrequent. The cells may contain intracytoplasmic lumina, which, in some, may be large enough to

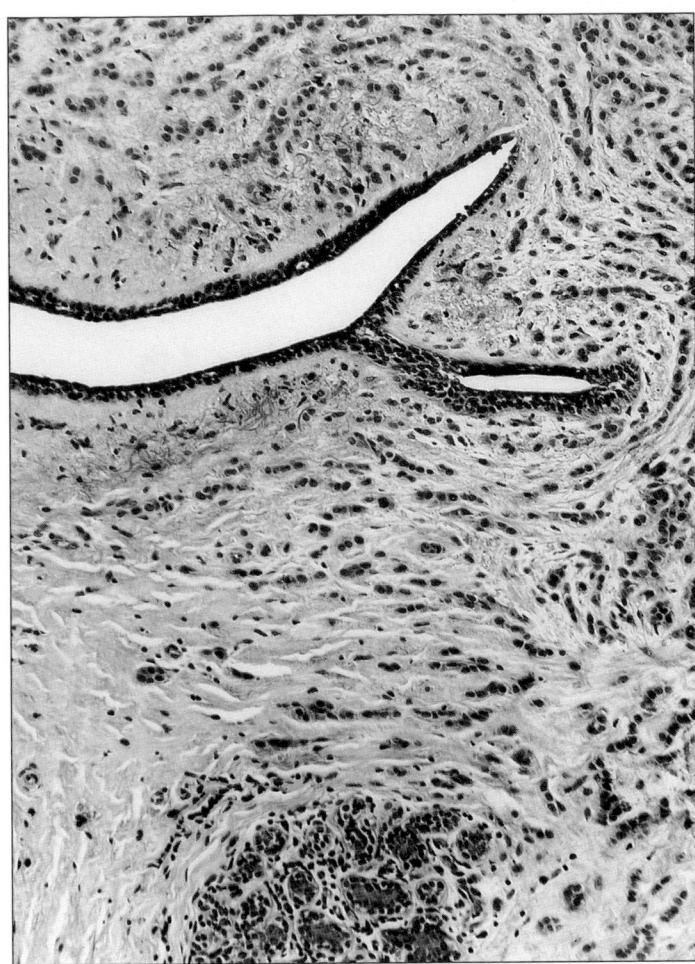

Fig. 10.77 Infiltrating lobular carcinoma. Note the single-file arrangement and swirling around normal duct.

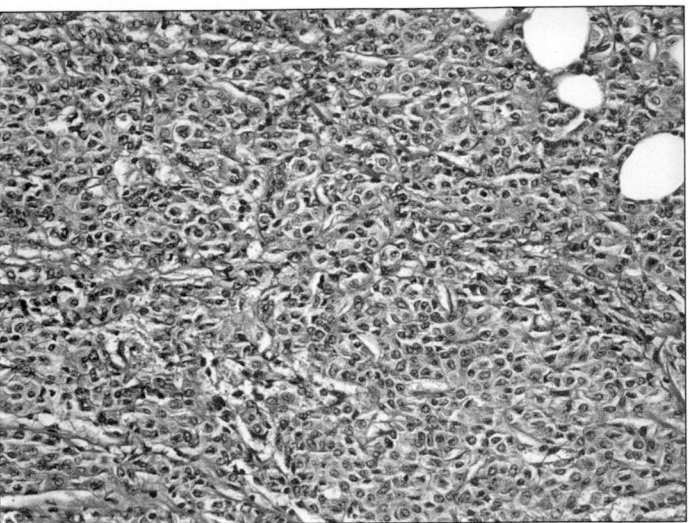

Fig. 10.78 Solid infiltrating lobular carcinoma. Irregular solid nests of small tumor cells.

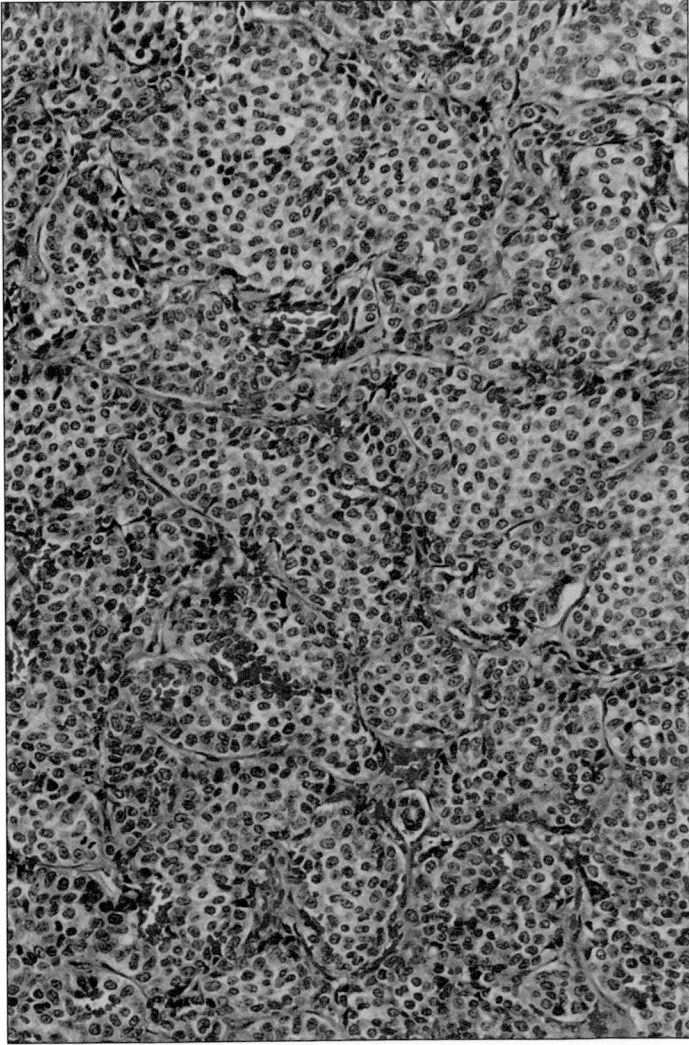

Fig. 10.79 Infiltrating lobular carcinoma, alveolar type. This infiltrating tumor forms round aggregates of uniform small cells, reminiscent of lobular carcinoma in situ.

impart a signet ring cell appearance. However, in the classical form of invasive lobular carcinoma, cells with a signet ring configuration comprise only a small proportion of the tumor cell population. Many examples of invasive lobular carcinoma (as well as LCIS) are characterized histologically by tumor cells that are loosely cohesive. This phenotype may at least be partially related to the fact that both in situ and invasive lobular carcinomas typically show loss of expression of the adhesion molecule E-cadherin,[443,444] in many cases as a result of mutations in the gene encoding this protein.[447] This feature distinguishes lobular carcinomas from ductal-type carcinomas, which characteristically exhibit E-cadherin protein expression, albeit to a variable degree.[443,444]

Variant forms of invasive lobular carcinoma differ from the classical form with regard to architectural and/or cytologic features. In the solid, alveolar and tubulolobular variants, the cells comprising the lesion have features characteristic of the classical form of invasive lobular carcinoma but differ from the classical form with regard to the growth pattern of the tumor cells.[467,485–489] In the *solid form*, the neoplastic cells grow in large confluent sheets with little intervening stroma (Fig. 10.78).[467,484–486,490] The *alveolar form* is characterized by tumor cells that grow in groups of 20 or more cells. These cellular aggregates are separated from one another by a delicate fibrovascular stroma (Fig. 10.79).[467,484–486,490] Although a *trabecular variant* has also been described,[467] there is considerable

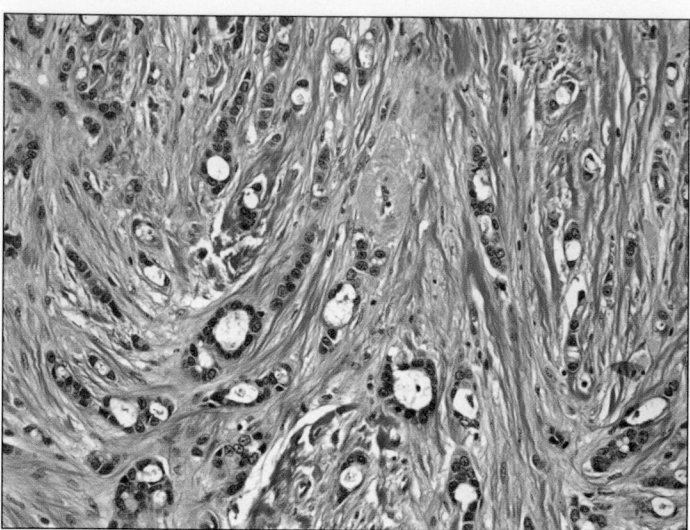

Fig. 10.80 Tubulolobular variant. Uniform small cells invade in a discohesive and tubular fashion.

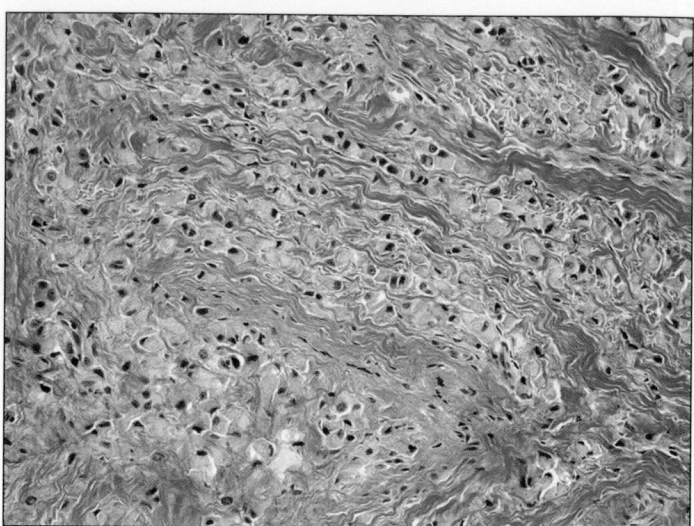

Fig. 10.82 Histiocytoid carcinoma. An apocrine variant of invasive lobular carcinoma where the tumor cells have a histiocyte-like appearance with abundant, foamy, pale, eosinophilic cytoplasm and mild nuclear atypia.

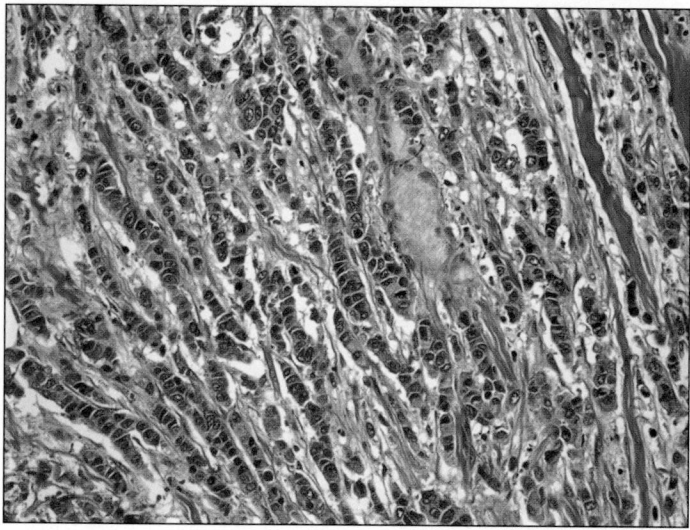

Fig. 10.81 Pleomorphic invasive lobular carcinoma. A classic invasive lobular pattern but with pleomorphic mitotically active cells.

overlap between this pattern and that seen in the classical form of invasive lobular carcinoma. In the *tubulolobular variant*, some of the tumor cells invade in the linear strands characteristic of the classical form of invasive lobular carcinoma whereas others form small tubules, which tend to have rounded to ovoid contours[487,489] (Fig. 10.80). These tubules are smaller and less angular than those seen in tubular carcinoma. Since the tumor forms tubules it may not represent a true lobular variant. In other variants, the invasive pattern is similar to that seen in the classical form of invasive lobular carcinoma but the cytologic features differ. In the *pleomorphic variant* the neoplastic cells are larger and exhibit more nuclear variation than is seen in the classical form of invasive lobular carcinoma (Fig. 10.81).[439,484,491–495] Although signet ring cell forms can be seen in the classical type of invasive lobular carcinoma as

well as in some examples of invasive ductal carcinoma,[496,497] tumors that are composed of a prominent component of signet ring cells that otherwise have the characteristic features of invasive lobular carcinoma are considered to represent the *signet ring cell variant* of invasive lobular carcinoma.[496,498–501] *Histiocytoid carcinoma* is an apocrine variant of invasive lobular carcinoma where the tumor cells have a histiocyte-like appearance with abundant foamy pale eosinophilic cytoplasm and mild nuclear atypia (Fig. 10.82). The cells are PAS- and Diastase-positive and stain for gross cystic disease fluid protein (GCDFP) by immunohistochemistry.[502–505] Several authors have recognized a 'mixed' category of invasive lobular carcinomas. This term is generally used to designate lesions in which no single pattern comprises more than 80–85% of the lesion.[189,490,506] However, Dixon et al. also included in their 'mixed' group the pleomorphic variant.[473]

The relative frequency of these various lobular subtypes is difficult to discern since not all subtypes have been recognized in all series and criteria for categorization of the subtypes varied from study to study. The classic variant is the most common (30–77%) with the mixed next.[452,473,490] The pleomorphic variant is uncommon.[439]

Classical invasive lobular carcinomas typically show expression of estrogen and progesterone receptors and rarely show expression of the HER2/Neu oncoprotein[507] or accumulation of the p53 gene product.[508] Gross cystic disease fluid protein is seen in about one third of all invasive lobular carcinomas but is present in the vast majority of lesions that show prominent signet ring cell features.[509] While pleomorphic lobular carcinomas are also frequently estrogen-receptor- and progesterone-receptor-positive, they also frequently show HER2 protein overexpression and p53 protein accumulation.[494,495]

Cytopathology

Infiltrating lobular carcinoma is a diagnostic pitfall on FNA cytology. Smears are usually moderately cellular but often hypocellular, and this, coupled with the low nuclear pleomorphism of the neoplastic cells, may lead to false-negative diagnoses.[510–512]

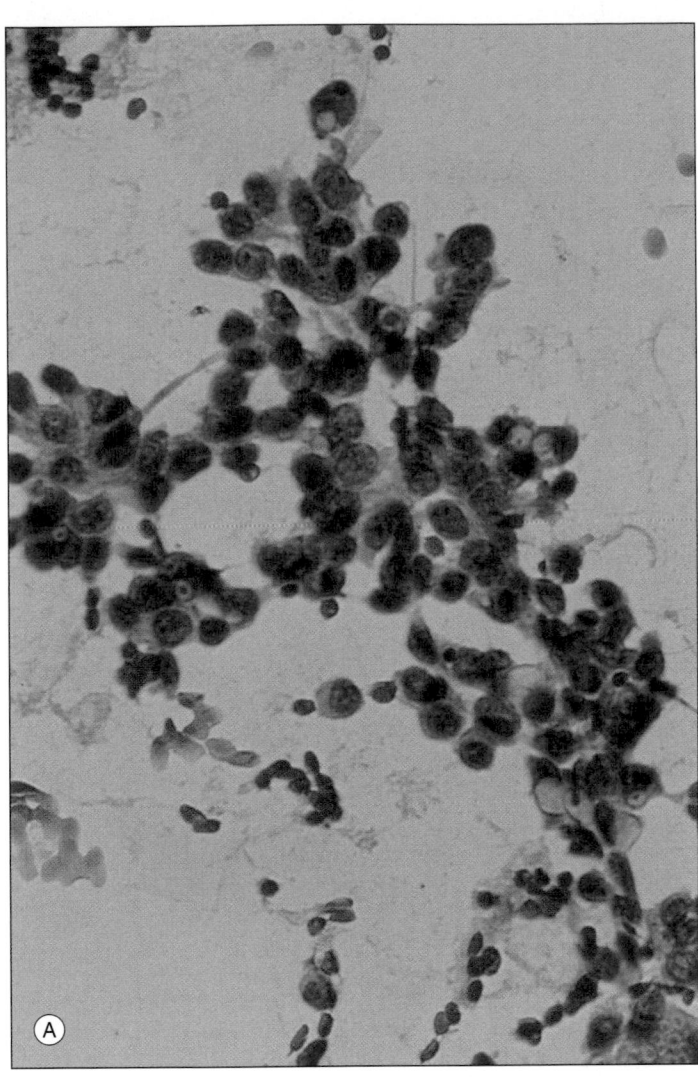 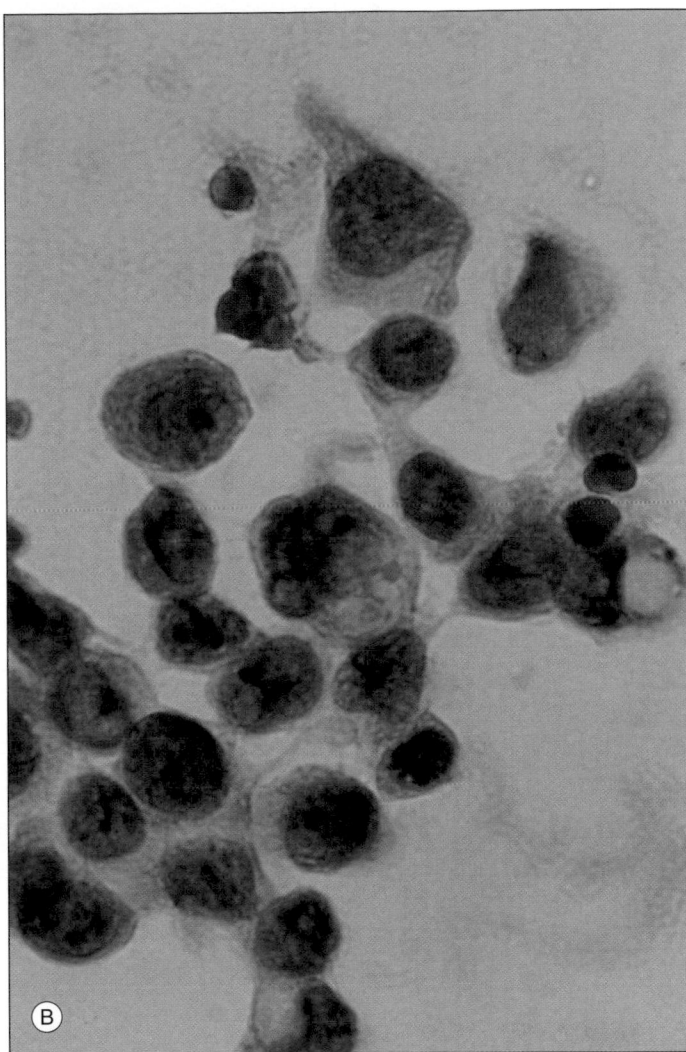

Fig. 10.83 (A) Aspirate of an infiltrating lobular carcinoma with small uniform cells and a few signet ring cells. (Papanicolaou stain, ×200.) **(B)** High magnification of the same case displaying a few signet rings. (Papanicolaou stain, ×400.)

Characteristically, infiltrating lobular carcinoma yields monomorphic dyshesive cells, mostly present singly. The cells often have scant cytoplasm with intracytoplasmic vacuoles (often with signet ring forms) and uniform, vesicular, occasionally grooved nuclei containing inconspicuous nucleoli[510,513–515] (Fig. 10.83). Although nuclear molding, 'single filing,' and signet ring cells are characteristic of lobular carcinoma, these features may also be found in infiltrating ductal carcinoma and are therefore not entirely discriminatory.[515] FNA of LCIS may also yield single neoplastic cells indistinguishable from those found in invasive lobular carcinoma.[516] This may result in a false-positive result, especially if the LCIS is extensive.[34]

As with histologic sections, histiocytoid carcinoma may mimic macrophages on FNA cytology and therefore may also be a cause for false-negative diagnoses.[517,518] These cells may be particularly deceptive without the benefit of architectural pattern found on histopathology. As expected from the degree of cellular atypia, pleomorphic infiltrating lobular carcinoma usually does not cause diagnostic problems on cytology regarding categorization as malignant, in contrast to the classic or other variants or infiltrating lobular carcinoma.[519]

Clinical course and prognosis

There are several aspects of the clinical course of invasive lobular carcinomas that merit consideration. First, a number of studies have noted differences in the pattern of metastatic spread between invasive lobular and invasive ductal carcinomas. In particular, metastases to the lungs, liver, and brain parenchyma appear to be less common in patients with lobular than ductal cancers.[520–523] Some authors have also noted bone metastases to be more frequent in patients with invasive lobular carcinoma.[520] In contrast, lobular carcinomas have a greater propensity to metastasize to the leptomeninges, peritoneal surfaces, retroperitoneum, gastrointestinal tract, and reproductive organs. In fact, the majority of cases of carcinomatous meningitis in patients with metastatic breast cancer occur in patients with lobular cancers.[520,521,523–525] Peritoneal metastases may appear as numerous small nodules studding the peritoneal surfaces in a manner similar to that seen in ovarian carcinoma.[496,520,521,523] Metastases to the stomach can produce an appearance that simulates an infiltrative (linitis plastica) type of primary gastric carcinoma.[526,527] Involvement of the uterus may result in vaginal bleeding,[528] whereas metastatic tumor in the ovary may produce ovarian enlargement and the appearance of a Krukenberg tumor.

Whether or not invasive lobular carcinomas differ in overall prognosis from invasive ductal carcinomas is difficult to determine, largely because of variations in the application of histologic criteria for the diagnosis of invasive lobular carcinoma. However, the prognosis of patients with invasive lobular carcinoma as a group has not consistently been shown to different from that of patients with invasive ductal carcinoma.[437] Several studies have suggested that the prognosis for the classical form of invasive lobular carcinoma is better than that of the solid variant[452,473,490] and that the tubulo-lobular variant has a particularly favorable prognosis.[452] However, attempts to assess prognostic differences between classical and variant forms of invasive lobular carcinoma have been limited by the small numbers of patients in the variant subgroups in virtually all the published series as well as failure in some series to stratify patients by stage, and the results across studies have been inconsistent. Some studies have suggested that the classical form of invasive lobular carcinoma is associated with a more favorable prognosis than invasive ductal carcinoma.[452,490,529] However, in the study of DiCostanzo et al., a prognostic advantage for invasive lobular carcinomas over invasive ductal cancers was seen only among patients with stage I disease.[490] Available evidence suggests that the pleomorphic variant[439,491,492] and the signet ring cell variant (when defined as lesions in which more than 10% of the neoplastic cells are of the signet ring cell type)[501] appear to be associated with a particularly poor clinical outcome. While in the past, invasive lobular carcinomas were typed but not graded it is now recommended that they be graded using the Nottingham system.[530]

Numerous clinical follow-up studies have indicated that patients with invasive lobular carcinoma can be adequately treated with conservative surgery and radiation therapy following a complete gross excision of the tumor, with local recurrence rates comparable to those seen in patients with invasive ductal carcinoma (reviewed in reference[531]).

INVASIVE CARCINOMAS WITH DUCTAL AND LOBULAR FEATURES

A small proportion of invasive breast cancers are not readily classifiable as either ductal or lobular. This was acknowledged by Azzopardi, who noted that 'infiltrating ductal and infiltrating lobular carcinoma cannot be separated quite as easily as is implied by much of the literature.' Such tumors account for between 2.2% and 4.7% of invasive breast cancers.[452,474,528,532] However the biologic behavior of these lesions is not unique: in three large series, lesions designated as having both ductal and lobular features were not distinctive in their rate of local recurrence or distant failure when compared with patients with invasive ductal or invasive lobular carcinomas.[195,474,532]

TUBULAR CARCINOMA

Tubular carcinoma is a special type of cancer that is typically associated with limited metastatic potential and an excellent prognosis. The reported incidence of tubular carcinoma varies depending upon the histologic definition and the method of cancer detection. In most studies performed prior to the widespread use of screening mammography, tubular carcinomas accounted for less than 1–4% of all breast cancers.[450,533] However, these tumors account for a much higher proportion of cancers detected in mammographically screened populations, with incidence rates ranging from 7.7–27%.[534–536]

Clinical presentation

The mean age at presentation for patients with tubular carcinoma is in the early sixth decade (range 23–89 years).[537 539]

Mammographic abnormalities have been reported in the majority (80%) of patients with tubular carcinomas, most often in the absence of palpable abnormalities. However, mammographically occult tubular carcinomas are not infrequent.[540] When a mammographic abnormality is present, it is usually a mass lesion, most commonly with spiculated margins, is only occasionally associated with micro-calcifications, and cannot be distinguished radiologically from infiltrating ductal carcinomas.

Gross pathology

Pure tubular carcinomas are typically small, with an average diameter <1.0 cm in most series.[537–539,541] Tubular carcinomas detected by screening mammography are typically smaller than palpable lesions.[542,543] Grossly, tubular carcinomas are firm, spiculated lesions that are indistinguishable from infiltrating ductal carcinomas.

Histopathology

Tubular carcinomas are characterized by a proliferation of well formed glands or tubules formed by a single layer of epithelial cells without a myoepithelial cell component. These tubules tend to be ovoid in shape and have sharply angular contours with tapering ends and open lumens. The cells comprising these tubules are characterized by low-grade nuclear features and are usually polarized toward the lumen, often exhibiting apical cytoplasmic 'snouting' (Figs 10.84, 10.85). To qualify as a tubular carcinoma there is now general agreement that 90% of the tumor must have these features[189,452] and tumors with less than 90% tubular elements are generally referred to as 'mixed' tubular carcinomas. However, the proportion required for this diagnosis in published studies has varied from 75–100%. Tubular carcinomas should not be confused with invasive ductal carcinomas with gland-like structures in which the cells are typically less well differentiated.[449] The stroma of tubular carcinomas usually has desmoplastic features, and prominent elastosis may be present in some cases.[544]

The majority of tubular carcinomas have an associated component of DCIS.[533,543,545–548] The DCIS seen in association with tubular carcinoma is usually of low nuclear grade, with cribriform, micropapillary, papillary, or solid patterns, and does not typically comprise a large proportion of the tumor mass. In addition, atypical columnar cell lesions that do not fulfill the diagnostic criteria for DCIS (i.e. columnar cell change with atypia and columnar cell hyperplasia with atypia) are often found in the vicinity of tubular carcinomas.[417] LCIS is also observed in association with tubular carcinoma but only in a minority of cases.[542,543,546,548–550] There is a higher incidence of reported multifocality and multicentricity in tubular carcinoma than for infiltrating ductal carcinomas.[542] The incidence of contralateral breast cancers in patients with tubular carcinomas ranges from 4.5–38%.[533,537,542,545,546,548,551–553]

The expression of various biologic markers in tubular carcinomas generally reflects the well differentiated nature and good prognosis associated with these lesions. Estrogen receptor positivity has been reported in 70–100% of tubular carcinomas and progesterone receptor positivity in 60–83%.[533,537,538,554–557] In addition, these lesions are almost always diploid, have a low proliferative rate, and rarely show HER2 overexpression or p53 protein accumulation.[557–560] In addition, when compared to invasive carcinomas of no special type, tubular carcinomas exhibit fewer overall chromosomal changes, more often show losses of 16q, and less often show losses of 17p.[561]

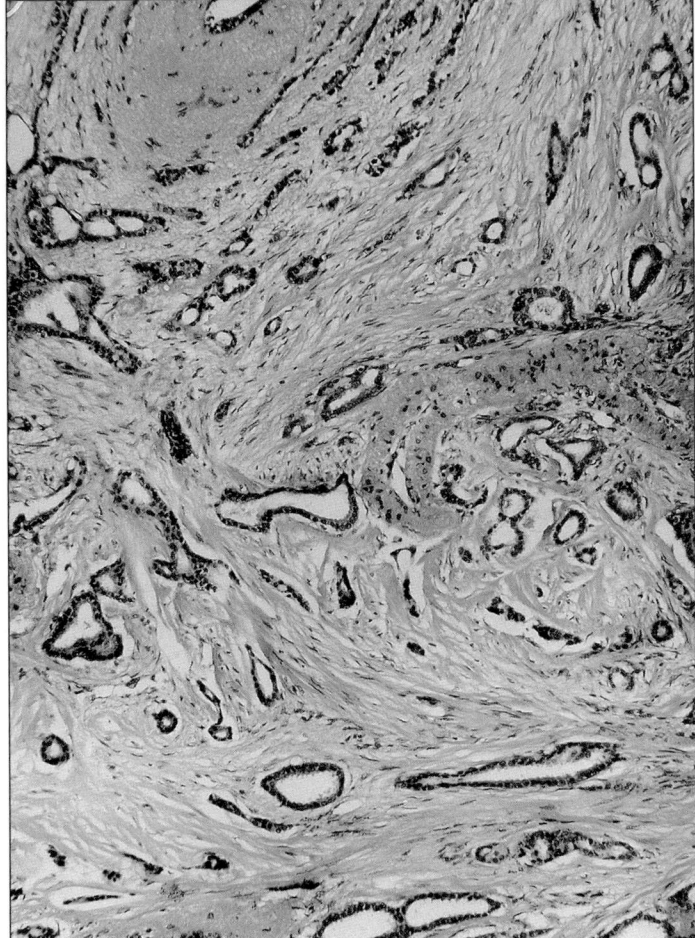

Fig. 10.84 Tubular carcinoma. Widely separated tubules lined by a single layer of small uniform cells.

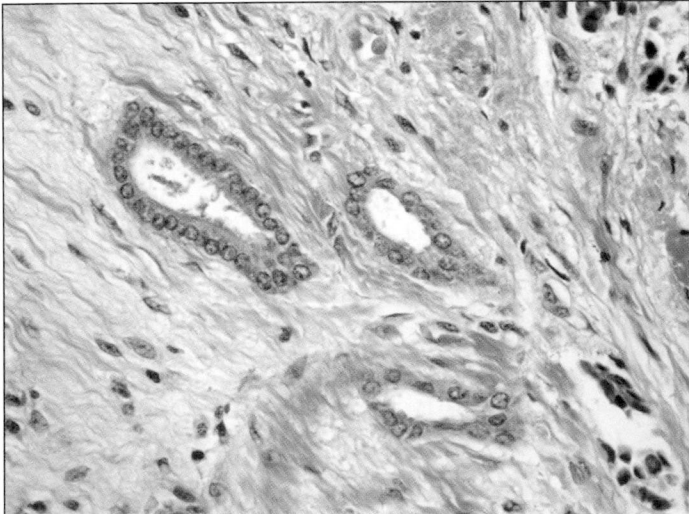

Fig. 10.85 Tubular carcinoma. Higher power illustrating fibrotic stroma, angulated glands, apical snouting, and well differentiated nuclei.

Because these lesions are extremely well differentiated, several benign entities such as sclerosing adenosis, radial scars, complex sclerosing lesions, and microglandular adenosis may enter into the differential diagnosis. In such cases, the use of adjunctive immuno-histochemical stains may be necessary in order to arrive at the correct diagnosis.[562–565] Although stains for myoepithelial cells are useful for distinguishing between tubular carcinomas and benign sclerosing lesions (i.e. sclerosing adenosis, radial scars and complex sclerosing lesions), they do not permit a distinction between tubular carcinoma and microglandular adenosis.

Cytopathology

As with infiltrating lobular carcinoma, FNA cytology of tubular carcinoma may result in a false-negative diagnosis.[62,566,567] In addition to having minimal cytologic atypia, the neoplastic cells of tubular carcinoma lack dyshesion and are characteristically present in tightly cohesive groups, features not usually associated with carcinoma.

Smears are usually moderately cellular and are characterized by cohesive groups of epithelial cells with few single epithelial cells present. In their analysis of tubular carcinoma on FNA, Bondeson and Lindholm[568] found prominent cellular dissociation in only two-thirds of cases. The tumor cells are monomorphic and usually show minimal to absent pleomorphism, with finely dispersed chromatin and small inconspicuous nucleoli. The cellular groups are characteristically present as three-dimensional angular configurations or tubular structures. The borders of these structures are notably straight and rigid, with absent myoepithelial cells. Bipolar cells are also characteristically scant or absent in the background but their presence does not exclude a diagnosis of tubular carcinoma[62,568–572] (Fig. 10.86).

Even considering the above classic features, the definitive diagnosis of malignancy may be particularly difficult in any individual case, and an atypical or suspicious diagnosis is often rendered. In fact, Bondeson and Lindholm[568] found the classic three-dimensional cohesive clusters present in only 56% of cases of tubular carcinoma. Furthermore, Rogers and Lee[566] found that no combination of features accurately separated all benign and malignant lesions in their cytologic analysis of borderline lesions. However, these authors did find that if easily discernible small nucleoli were present, as well as many single bipolar nuclei in the background, a benign lesion was more likely. In contrast, nuclear hyperchromasia usually indicated a malignant diagnosis. Immunocytochemistry for myoepithelial markers such as smooth muscle actin may be helpful, with absent immuno-staining of epithelial clusters in cases of tubular carcinoma.[569]

Clinical course and prognosis

The reported incidence of axillary lymph node metastases in patients with tubular carcinomas has a vide range. Patients with 'pure' tubular carcinomas have nodal metastases in up to 15% of cases.[537]

With regard to survival, all studies suggest that patients with tubular carcinoma have a good prognosis.[452,533,534,537–543,545–553,573–580]

When tubular carcinoma does metastasize to axillary lymph nodes, usually one and seldom more than three level I nodes are involved.[533,537,542,543,547,550] The presence of nodal disease in patients with tubular carcinoma does not seem to affect disease-free and/or overall survival in these patients.[537,549]

In patients treated with conservative surgery and radiation therapy there are no significant differences in local recurrence rates when patients with tubular carcinomas are compared to patients with invasive ductal carcinoma.[532,579]

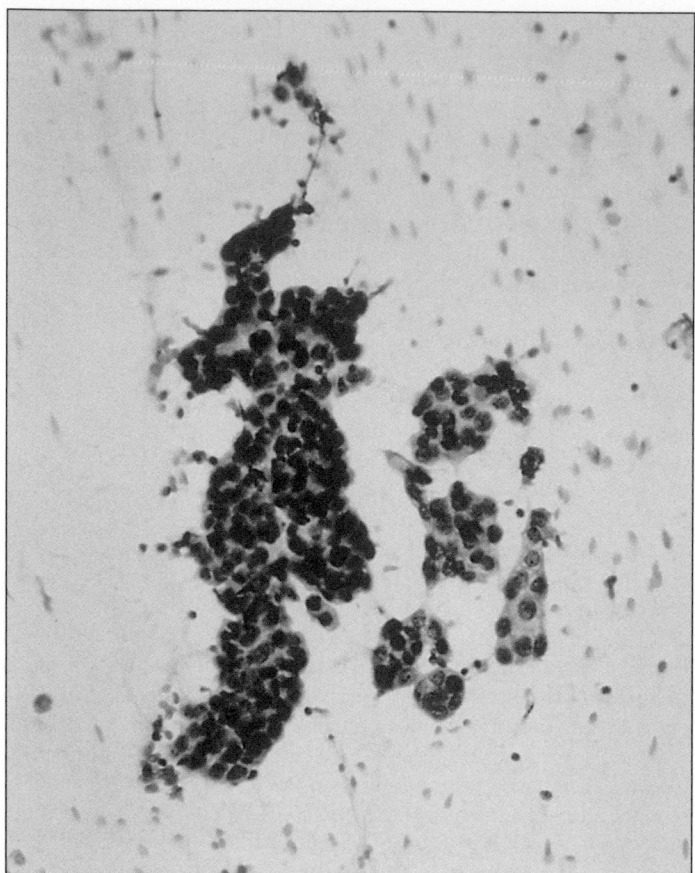

Fig. 10.86 Smear of an aspirate from a tubular carcinoma. Uniform small tumor cells are forming tubules. (Papanicolaou stain, × 200.)

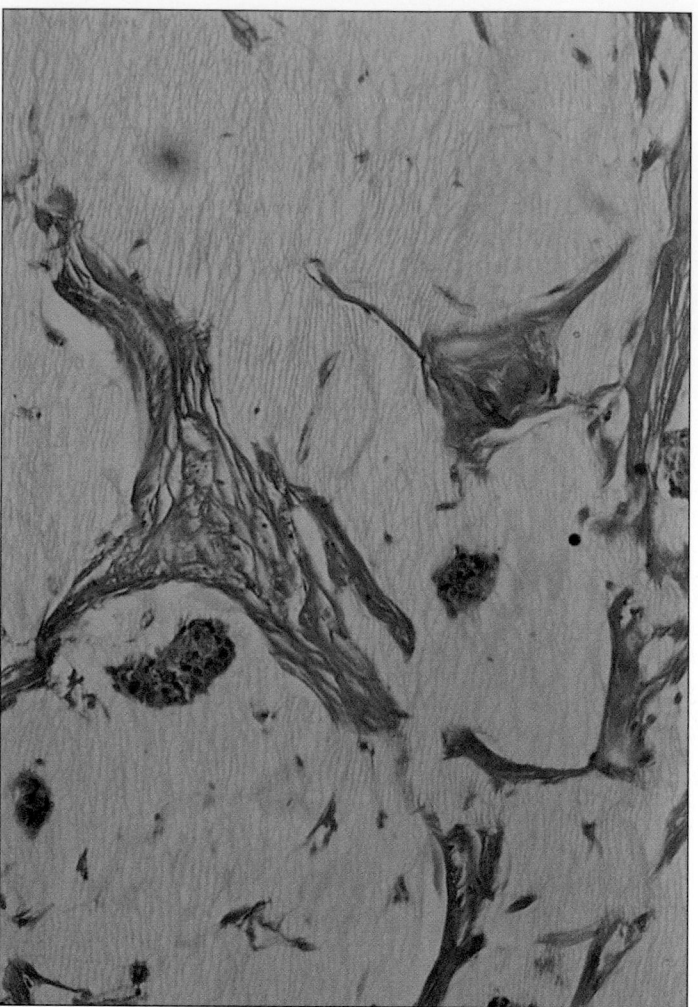

Fig. 10.87 Mucinous carcinoma. Well differentiated tumor cells in pools of extracellular mucin.

MUCINOUS CARCINOMA

Mucinous carcinoma (also known as colloid carcinoma) is another special type of cancer that is associated with a relatively favorable prognosis. The reported incidence of mucinous carcinoma varies depending on the histologic criteria. Most studies have indicated that less than 5% of invasive breast carcinomas have a mucinous component and of these less than half represent pure mucinous carcinomas.[581–583]

Clinical presentation

The mean age at presentation for patients with mucinous carcinoma is in the seventh decade in most studies (range 21–94 years), greater than that for patients with breast cancers of no special type.[581,582,584–591] Most patients in the past presented with palpable tumors. However, more recent reports suggest that a substantial proportion of patients with mucinous carcinoma (30–70%) present with nonpalpable mammographic abnormalities.[592,593]

Mammographically, mucinous carcinomas are most often poorly defined or lobular mass lesions that are rarely associated with calcification.[592–595] On ultrasound examination, mucinous carcinomas are typically hypoechoic mass lesions.[595]

Gross pathology

Mucinous carcinomas average approximately 3 cm in size, with a wide range reported in the literature.[236] In some studies, tumors composed exclusively of mucinous features are smaller, on average, than mixed tumors.[589,592] Mucinous carcinomas have a distinctive gross appearance. These lesions are typically circumscribed and have a variably soft, gelatinous consistency and a glistening cut surface. However, lesions with a greater amount of fibrous stroma may have a firmer consistency.

Histopathology

The hallmark of mucinous carcinomas is extracellular mucin production. However, the extent of extracellular mucin varies from tumor to tumor. Typically, tumor cells in small clusters, sheets, or papillary configurations are dispersed within pools of extracellular mucin (Fig. 10.87). This characteristic histology should comprise at least 90% of the tumor[452] to qualify for the diagnosis of mucinous carcinoma. Mucinous neoplasms intermixed with other nonmucinous histologic are classified as the other type but with mucinous areas. The cellularity of mucinous carcinomas is variable and some tumors are relatively paucicellular; in these cases the differential diagnosis includes mucocele-type tumors, which are benign lesions characterized by cystically dilated ducts associated with rupture and extravasation of mucin into the stroma.[308,309] The cells comprising mucinous carcinomas are usually of low or intermediate nuclear grade. Many studies have documented endocrine differentiation in a significant subset of lesions, although this finding does not appear to be clinically meaningful.[583] Mucinous carcinomas are often accompanied by a DCIS component. which may have a papillary, micropapillary, cribriform, or even a comedo pattern. In some cases, the DCIS may also exhibit prominent extracellular mucin production.[236]

The expression of various biological markers in mucinous carcinomas generally reflects the good prognosis associated with these lesions. Estrogen receptor positivity has been reported in 86–92% of tumors[554,556,590] and progesterone receptor positivity in 63–68%.[555–557] In addition, mucinous carcinomas do not usually overexpress the HER2/Neu oncoprotein (0–4% of cases) or show p53 protein accumulation (18% of cases).[557–560] DNA studies of 26 pure mucinous carcinomas revealed that 25 (96%) were diploid compared to only eight of 19 mixed tumors (42%). The rate of diploidy among the mixed tumors was comparable to that seen in breast cancers of no special type.[596] Mucinous carcinomas show substantially fewer chromosomal abnormalities than invasive carcinomas of no special type.[597]

Cytopathology

FNA smears of mucinous carcinoma characteristically contain abundant extracellular mucin. Although mucin is seen with Papanicolaou-stained direct and liquid-based smears, it is best seen on air-dried Diff-Quick preparations, where it appears metachromatic. Dispersed within the mucin are relatively small three-dimensional clusters or 'balls' of cells. The neoplastic cells within these clusters are bland-appearing and relatively uniform in size but have increased nuclear:cytoplasmic ratios and often contain cytoplasmic vacuoles (Fig. 10.88).[598–600]

As noted previously in the discussion of mucocele-like lesions, if mucus is obtained on breast FNA without epithelial cells, a diagnosis of mucinous carcinoma cannot be excluded and will require excision for definitive diagnosis.[315] Fibroadenomas may yield mucinous-type stroma and, particularly if there is accompanying epithelial atypia, these lesions may mimic mucinous carcinoma.[601]

Clinical course and prognosis

The incidence of axillary lymph node metastases in pure mucinous carcinomas, although variable (range 4–39%, average 15%), is significantly less than the incidence of node positivity seen in mixed mucinous tumors (38–59%) or breast cancers of no special type (43–63%).[581,582,584–590] In contrast to patients with tubular carcinoma, patients with mucinous carcinoma with nodal metastases do not have as good a prognosis as those without nodal metastases.

Pure mucinous carcinomas have a much better prognosis than tumors with mixed histologic features and infiltrating ductal carcinomas.[452,578–590,602] Data from the SEER study reported that the patients with mucinous carcinoma present with localized disease more commonly than patients with invasive ductal carcinoma (78.1% vs 53.1%). In addition, even after prolonged follow-up, only 25.1% of patients with mucinous carcinoma died as a consequence breast cancer, compared to 58.3% of patients with invasive ductal carcinoma.[591]

Three studies have examined the use of conservative surgery and radiation therapy in patients with mucinous carcinoma and report no significant differences in local recurrence rates compared to patients with invasive ductal carcinoma.[532,579,603]

Several studies have noted that a significant number of late recurrences are seen in patients with mucinous carcinoma,[587,604] with one report documenting a recurrence 30 years after initial treatment.[604]

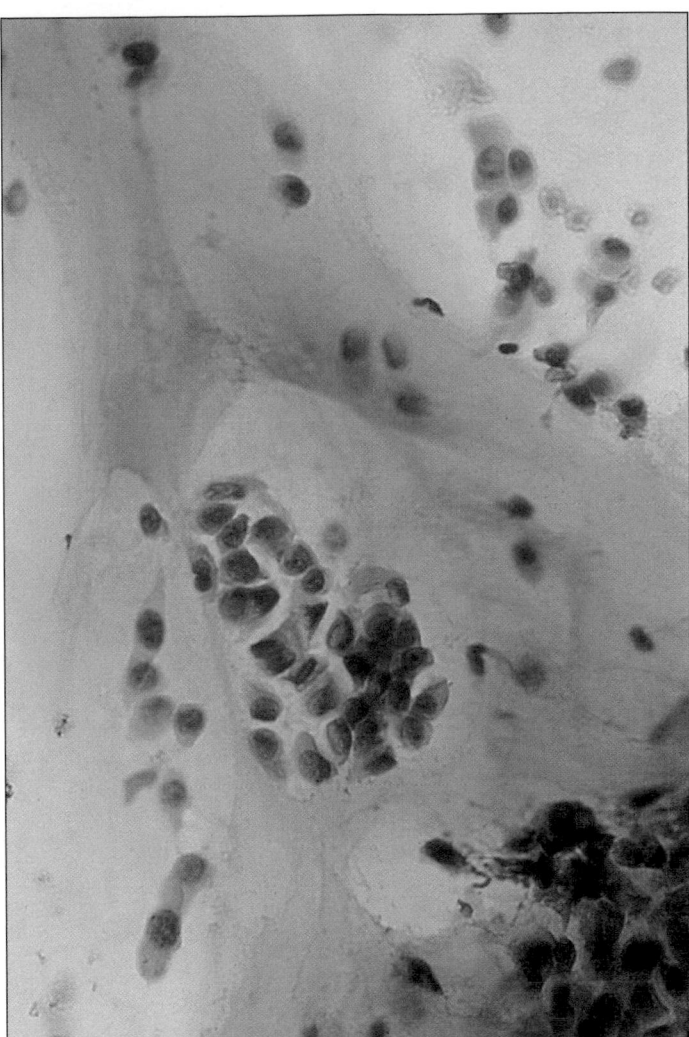

Fig. 10.88 Direct smear from an aspirate of mucinous carcinoma. The epithelial cells are seen singly and in clusters in mucoid background. (Papanicolaou stain, ×400.)

MEDULLARY CARCINOMA

Medullary carcinomas account for less than 5–7% of all invasive breast cancers.[236] Some studies have indicated that this type of breast cancer has a favorable prognosis, despite its aggressive histologic appearance.[605–612] However, there is considerable controversy regarding the appropriate histologic definition of medullary carcinoma, as well as the reproducibility of this diagnosis among pathologists. As a result, the prognostic implications of this diagnosis are uncertain.[605–619]

Clinical presentation

Patients with medullary carcinoma usually present at a relatively younger age than patients with other breast cancers: the mean age at presentation is in the late fifth and early sixth decade, with a wide age range reported.[605–612] The majority of patients with medullary carcinoma present with a palpable mass.[612] Rare examples of medullary carcinoma have been reported in males.[608] A number of studies have found an association between mutations in the *BRCA1* breast cancer susceptibility gene and the occurrence of medullary

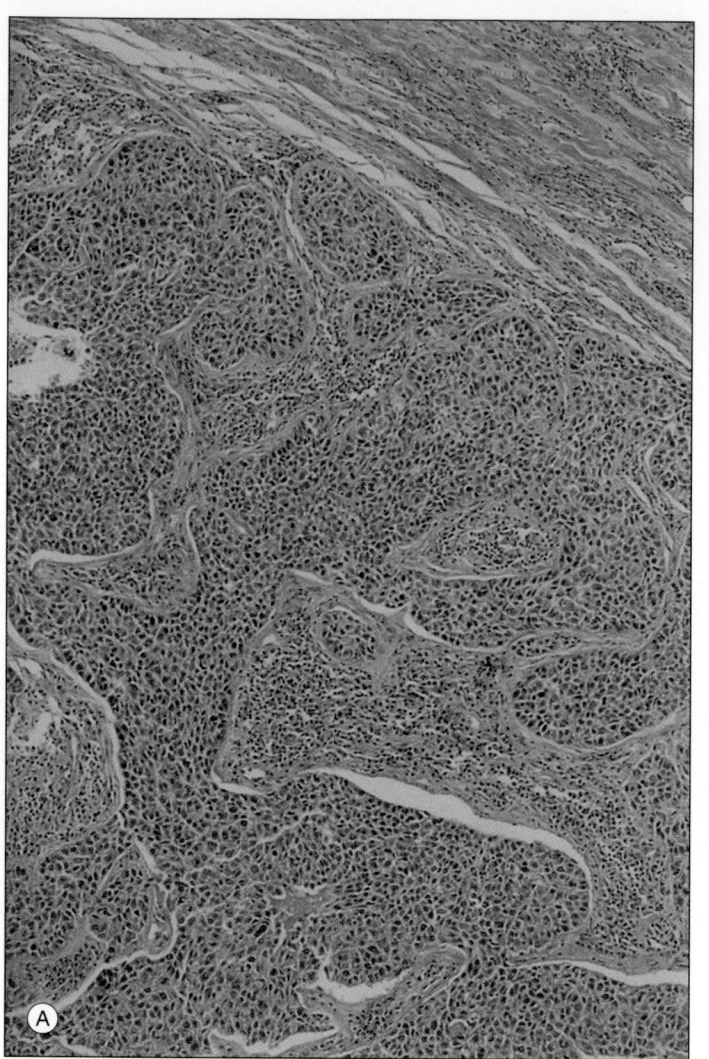

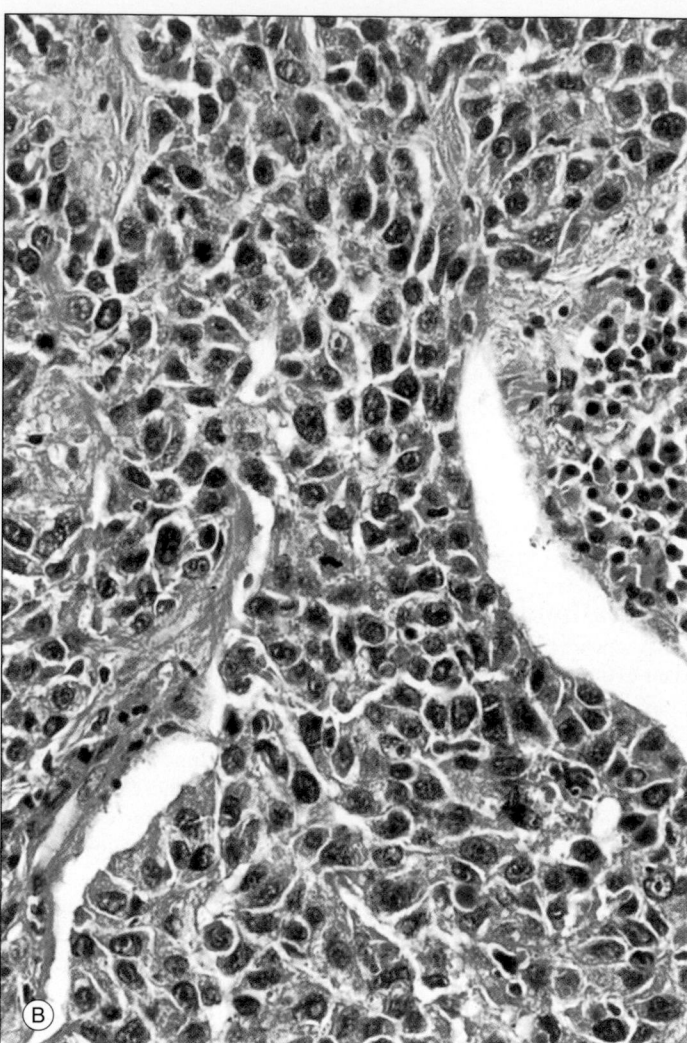

Fig. 10.89 Medullary carcinoma. **(A)** Low-power photomicrograph shows pushing tumor border, 'syncytial' growth pattern, and prominent lymphoid infiltration. **(B)** Detail of large pleomorphic tumor cells and lymphoplasmacytic infiltrate.

carcinomas and invasive ductal carcinomas with medullary features.[620]

To some degree, the mammographic features of medullary carcinoma reflect the pathologic features, although they are not specific. Most lesions are associated with a moderately well defined mass unassociated with calcifications.[621,622] On ultrasound examination, medullary carcinomas are generally well circumscribed, frequently lobular, and hypoechoic.[622,623]

Gross pathology

The mean size of medullary carcinomas is similar to that of breast cancers of no special type.[236] Grossly, these lesions are well circumscribed, soft, tan-brown to gray tumors that bulge above the cut surface of the specimen. A multinodular appearance may be appreciated in some cases. Areas of hemorrhage, necrosis, or cystic degeneration may be present in tumors of any size, but prominent necrosis is usually seen in larger tumors.

Histopathology

Three similar but distinct classification systems for the histologic diagnosis of medullary carcinomas have been proposed by

Ridolfi,[607] Wargotz,[610] and Pedersen.[611] All three classification schemes recognize the following attributes of medullary carcinomas, but the relative importance and the mandatory nature of each are stressed to a different degree: (1) syncytial growth pattern of the tumor cells in more than 75% of the tumor; (2) admixed lymphoplasmacytic infiltrate; (3) microscopic circumscription; (4) grade 2 or 3 nuclei; and (5) absence of glandular differentiation (Fig. 10.89). Tumors that lack a variable number of these characteristics (depending on the system used) are classified as either invasive ductal carcinoma or 'atypical medullary carcinoma.' Regardless of the classification system used, however, medullary carcinoma is frequently overdiagnosed.[617,624]

In addition to the histologic features listed above, medullary carcinomas may be associated with a DCIS component (usually comprised of cells that are morphologically similar to the invasive component), hemorrhage, tumor necrosis, cystic degeneration, and various types of metaplasia of the tumor cells, most often squamous metaplasia.[236] There does not appear to be an increased incidence of multicentricity or contralateral cancers in patients with medullary carcinoma.[609]

The expression of various biological markers in medullary carcinomas is reflective of the poorly differentiated histologic features

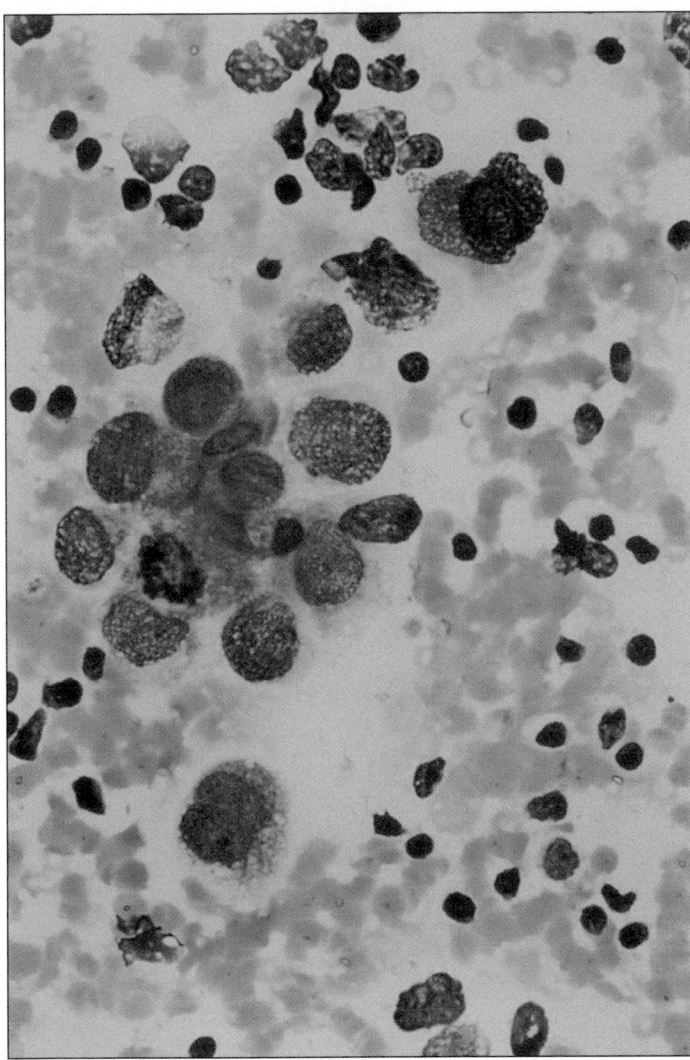

Fig. 10.90 Aspirate of medullary carcinoma. The neoplastic epithelial cells are large and pleomorphic and are surrounded by lymphocytes. (Diff-Quick, ×400.)

of these tumors. Estrogen receptor positivity has been reported in only 0–33% of medullary carcinomas[554–556,612,615] and progesterone receptor positivity in 0–36%.[554–556,612] DNA studies indicate that most tumors are aneuploid.[615] In addition, medullary carcinomas are associated with p53 protein accumulation in the majority of cases,[560] while *HER2/neu* overexpression is uncommon.[558,559]

Cytopathology

FNA biopsies of medullary carcinoma yield cellular smears with a dual population of highly atypical epithelial cells present singly and in sheets, admixed with polymorphous benign-appearing lymphocytes and plasma cells (Fig. 10.90).[513] These cytologic features will only be suggestive of a diagnosis of medullary carcinoma because definitive categorization requires fulfillment of criteria only possible on histologic examination. Depending on the predominance of carcinoma cells or lymphoid cells, the differential diagnosis will include poorly differentiated infiltrating ductal carcinoma at one end of the spectrum and a benign inflammatory infiltrate or intramammary lymph node at the other. In addition, high-grade DCIS may be accompanied by a marked lymphocytic infiltrate, further complicating the differential

diagnosis. Lymphoproliferative disorders may also enter the differential, depending on the atypia or monomorphism and relative abundance of the lymphoid population.

Clinical course and prognosis

Although studies have differed in the histologic criteria employed, most studies indicate that the incidence of axillary lymph node metastases is lower in patients with medullary carcinomas (19–46%) than in those with atypical medullary carcinomas (30–52%) or invasive ductal carcinomas (29–65%).[607–610,612]

Data regarding survival rates in patients with medullary carcinoma vary depending on the histologic criteria used for diagnosis and the investigators. Many studies report a better survival than atypical medullary carcinoma or infiltrating ductal carcinomas.[607,609,610] However, several other reports have found little difference in prognosis or proposed different classification systems.[452,611,612,614,615]

In addition to the clinical follow-up studies that question a favorable prognosis for medullary carcinoma, several studies have also questioned the practical applicability of the diagnostic criteria.[613,616,617]

In summary, although there may be patients with medullary carcinoma who have improved survival compared to patients with breast cancers of no special type, the ability of pathologists to reliably and reproducibly identify this subset of patients is suboptimal. It is essential that clinicians are aware of these limitations when confronted with a pathology report suggesting the diagnosis of medullary carcinoma. Given the difficulty in diagnosing these lesions, it could be argued that treatment decisions, particularly those related to the use of adjuvant chemotherapy, should not rest solely on assumptions regarding the prognostic implications of medullary carcinoma.

The results of the use of breast-conserving therapy in patients with medullary carcinoma have been reported in three studies. In all three studies there were no significant differences in local recurrence rates among patients with medullary carcinoma compared to patients with invasive ductal carcinoma. Thus, the available limited data suggest that conservative surgery and radiation therapy is appropriate local treatment for patients with medullary carcinoma.[532,579,603]

INVASIVE CRIBRIFORM CARCINOMA

Invasive cribriform carcinoma is a well differentiated cancer that shares some morphologic features with tubular carcinoma and is also associated with a favorable prognosis. Approximately 5–6% of invasive breast cancers show at least a partial invasive cribriform component.[625,626]

Clinical presentation

The majority of patients with invasive cribriform carcinoma present in the sixth decade (range 19–86 years).[625,626] A significant proportion of invasive cribriform carcinomas were mammographically occult.[627] The remaining lesions showed non-specific mammographic findings, usually spiculated masses with or without calcification.[627]

Gross pathology

No distinctive gross features of invasive cribriform carcinoma have been described.

Histopathology

Invasive cribriform carcinomas are characterized by tumor cells that invade the stroma in a cribriform, or fenestrated growth pattern

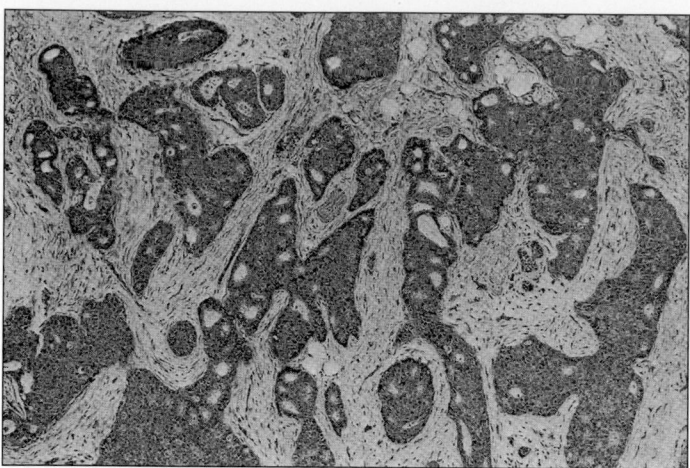

Fig. 10.91 Infiltrating cribriform carcinoma. Irregular nests of infiltrating carcinoma are punctuated by uniform punched-out spaces lined by well differentiated tumor cells.

similar to that seen in the cribriform pattern of DCIS (Fig. 10.91). These tumors often show admixtures of other histologic patterns of invasive breast cancer, particularly tubular carcinoma, which is seen in 17–23% of cases. The 'classic' variant of invasive cribriform carcinoma[625] is defined as a tumor composed of an exclusively invasive cribriform pattern or a tumor with more than 50% invasive cribriform features in which the remainder of the tumor exhibits features of tubular carcinoma. The cribriform component of these lesions is associated with low or intermediate grade nuclear features. Significant nuclear pleomorphism is generally not present. In both studies, most invasive cribriform carcinomas were associated with DCIS, usually of the cribriform type. The average size of these tumors was relatively large, and varied from 3.1 cm (range 1–14 cm) for the classical variant of cribriform carcinoma to 4.2 cm (range 2–9 cm) for tumors of mixed histology.[625]

The tumors are generally estrogen- and progesterone-receptor-positive and HER2/Neu-negative.[558,626]

The main lesion to distinguish from invasive cribriform carcinoma is the cribriform pattern of DCIS. It is clearly important to not confuse a purely in situ carcinoma from one that is invasive. However, the proportion of invasive and in situ cribriform components within a tumor is also important with regard to accurately sizing the invasive component and determining whether the invasive tumor has an extensive intraductal component.[628] Invasive cribriform carcinoma ignores normal breast architecture and infiltrates between ducts and lobules, in contrast to DCIS, which maintains the normal ductal and lobular architecture. In contrast to cribriform DCIS, where the involved spaces have smooth, rounded contours, the infiltrating glands of invasive cribriform carcinoma have irregular, sharp, and angular borders. As mentioned above, invasive cribriform carcinoma is frequently associated with foci of classic tubular carcinoma, which is helpful if attempting to distinguish a lesion composed of only DCIS. The stroma in invasive cribriform carcinoma tends to be desmoplastic compared to that associated with cribriform DCIS. Lastly, the main distinguishing feature is the lack of myoepithelial cells surrounding the glandular islands of invasive cribriform carcinoma, in contrast to their presence in cribriform DCIS. The presence of myoepithelial cells may be confirmed with immuno-histochemical markers.

Clinical course and prognosis

Patients with pure cribriform carcinomas or those mixed only with tubular carcinoma have an excellent prognosis, rarely result in distant metastasis, and have a significantly better overall survival compared to control groups including patients with tumors without a cribriform component.[452,625,626]

INVASIVE PAPILLARY CARCINOMA

Invasive papillary carcinomas comprise from <1% to 2% of invasive breast cancers and are characterized by a relatively good prognosis.[629,630]

Clinical presentation

Invasive papillary carcinomas are diagnosed predominantly in postmenopausal patients. Fisher et al. noted a disproportionate number of cases in non-Caucasian women.[629]

Mammographically, invasive papillary carcinoma is usually characterized by nodular densities, which may be multiple and are frequently lobular.[630–632] These lesions are often hypoechoic on ultrasound.[632] One study noted the difficulty in distinguishing between intracystic papillary carcinoma, intracystic papillary carcinoma with invasion, and invasive papillary carcinoma.[632]

Gross pathology

Fisher et al. reported that invasive papillary carcinoma is grossly circumscribed in two thirds of cases.[629] Other invasive papillary carcinomas are grossly indistinguishable from invasive breast cancers of no special type.

Histopathology

Microscopically, invasive papillary carcinomas are characteristically circumscribed, show delicate or blunt papillae, and show focal solid areas of tumor growth. The cells typically show amphophilic cytoplasm but may have apocrine features and also may exhibit apical 'snouting' of cytoplasm similar to tubular carcinoma. The nuclei of tumor cells are typically intermediate-grade, and most tumors are histologic grade 2.[629] Tumor stroma is not abundant in most cases and occasional cases show prominent extracellular mucin production. Calcifications, although not usually mammographically evident, are commonly seen histologically but are usually present in associated DCIS. DCIS is present in more than 75% of cases and usually but not exclusively has a papillary pattern. In some lesions in which both the invasive and in situ components have papillary features, it may be difficult to determine the relative proportion of each.[629]

Estrogen and progesterone receptor positivity is common.[554] Invasive papillary carcinomas are not usually associated with p53 protein accumulation or HER2/Neu oncoprotein overexpression.[558,560]

Clinical course and prognosis

While there are only limited data on the prognostic significance of invasive papillary carcinoma,[580,629,633] these patients appear to have a good prognosis.

INVASIVE MICROPAPILLARY CARCINOMA

Invasive micropapillary carcinoma is an entity that, unlike invasive papillary carcinoma, appears to be associated with a poor prognosis.[634–639] Tumors with pure micropapillary carcinoma comprised 1.7% of cases in one study[637] and 2.7% in another.[635]

Clinical presentation

The mean age at presentation for patients with invasive micropapillary carcinoma is 54–62 years (range 36–92 years).[634,635,638,639] Most cases present with a palpable mass.[634]

The mammographic features of this tumor type have not been well defined.

Gross pathology

No distinguishing gross features have been described. The median size varies and may be significantly larger than invasive carcinomas of no special type.[635]

Histopathology

In most reported cases, invasive micropapillary carcinomas have been admixed to a variable degree with invasive carcinomas of no special type or, in a minority of cases, with mucinous carcinoma. However, unlike other special-type carcinomas, the prognostic implications appear to be the same whether the micropapillary component is present focally or diffusely within the tumor.[635,639] The lesions are characterized by clusters of cells in a micropapillary or tubular–alveolar arrangement that appear to be suspended in a clear space or in some cases a mucinous or aqueous fluid. These micropapillary clusters, unlike 'true' papillary lesions, lack fibro-vascular cores. The cells clusters appear to have an 'inside-out' arrangement, with the apical surface polarized to the outside (Fig. 10.92). The overall appearance of invasive micropapillary carcinoma may mimic serous papillary carcinomas of the ovary, or may simulate lymphatic/vascular space invasion.[634] True lymphatic/vascular space invasion has been reported in 33–67% of cases, and may be extensive.[634,635,638] Cytologically, the cells comprising the invasive micropapillary carcinoma have variable-grade nuclei. The majority of tumors (67–70%) are associated with a DCIS component with micropapillary and cribriform patterns.[634,635] A minority of cases (33%) have shown calcifications histologically.[634]

In a large analysis, an invasive micropapillary component was found in 6% of all breast carcinomas.[639] However, this component usually made up a small proportion of the overall tumor, involving less than 20% of the tumor mass in 53% of these cases.[639]

Cytopathology

Cytologic features parallel those found on histology and have recently been described.[640–642] The smears consist of clusters of cells with hyperchromatic, irregular, crowded nuclei. The cytoplasm is characteristically peripherally located, consistent with an 'inside-out' orientation, with a scalloped edge to the clusters.

Immunohistochemical studies of invasive micropapillary carcinoma have reported that 72–75% were positive for estrogen receptor and 45% were positive for progesterone receptor. HER2/Neu overexpression was observed in 36% of cases and p53 protein accumulation was seen in 12% of cases, with 66% bcl-2 positive.[643,644]

Clinical course and prognosis

Invasive micropapillary carcinomas are more likely to have positive lymph nodes and multiple positive lymph nodes than invasive ductal carcinomas.[635,638,639] There appears to be no significant difference in lymph node status, ER status, tumor size, tumor grade, or lymphatic vascular invasion between tumors with predominant versus focal invasive micropapillary components. While most studies report a worse prognosis for this subtype in one large study, the clinical outcome of tumors with invasive micropapillary histology did not differ from infiltrating ductal carcinomas of similar stage (i.e. nodal status).[639]

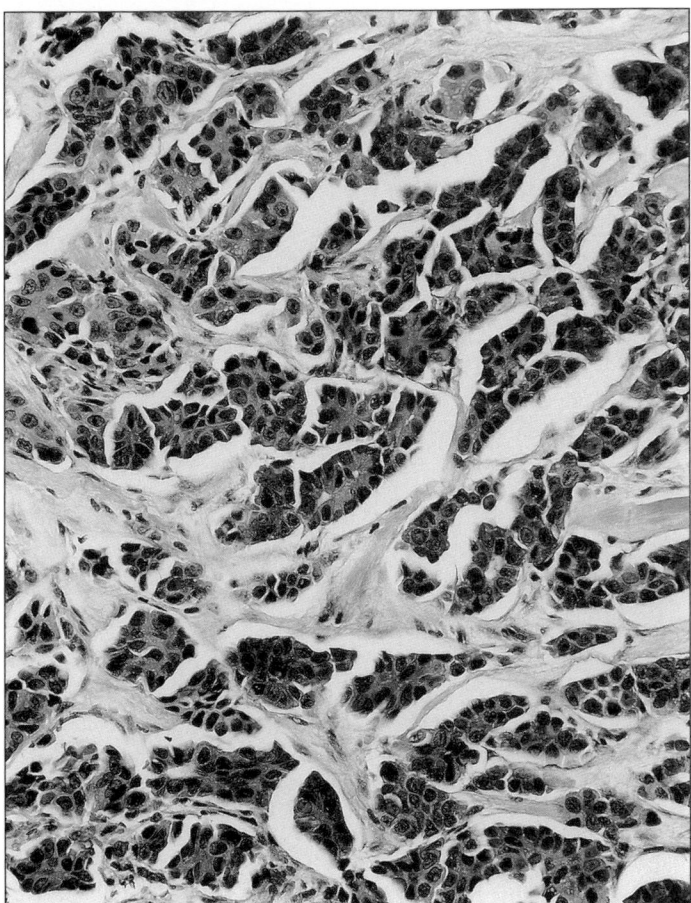

Fig. 10.92 Infiltrating micropapillary carcinoma. Note resemblance to ovarian serous carcinoma.

METAPLASTIC CARCINOMA

Metaplastic carcinomas represent a morphologically heterogeneous group of invasive breast cancers in which a variable portion of the glandular epithelial cells comprising the tumor have undergone transformation into an alternate cell type – either a nonglandular epithelial cell type (e.g. squamous cell) or a mesenchymal cell type (spindle cell, chondroid, osseous, myoid, etc.). There are numerous published reports describing various aspects of metaplastic carcinomas, and numerous appellations have been applied to the various tumors comprising this group.[299–304,645–659] However, there is no uniformly agreed-upon classification scheme for these tumors. Metaplastic carcinomas are uncommon lesions, representing less than 5% of all of breast cancers. The prognostic implications of metaplastic carcinomas are difficult to define, and relate to the type of metaplasia present, as discussed below.

Clinical presentation

Patients with metaplastic carcinoma are similar to patients with IC-NST with regard to their age at presentation, the manner in which their tumors are detected, and the location within the breast in which these tumors arise.[650,660] Most patients present with a single palpable lesion that is often associated with rapid growth.[650]

The mammographic appearance of metaplastic carcinoma is not specific. Most are fairly circumscribed, noncalcified lesions that in

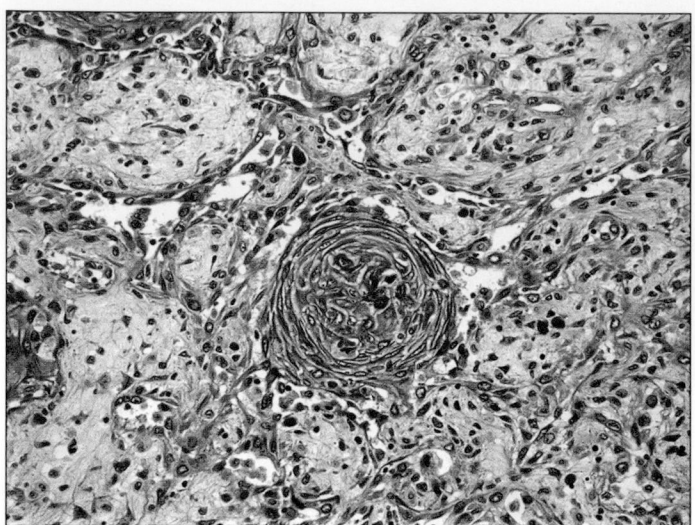

Fig. 10.93 Metaplastic carcinoma. All elements are malignant. Note the spindle cell and squamous areas.

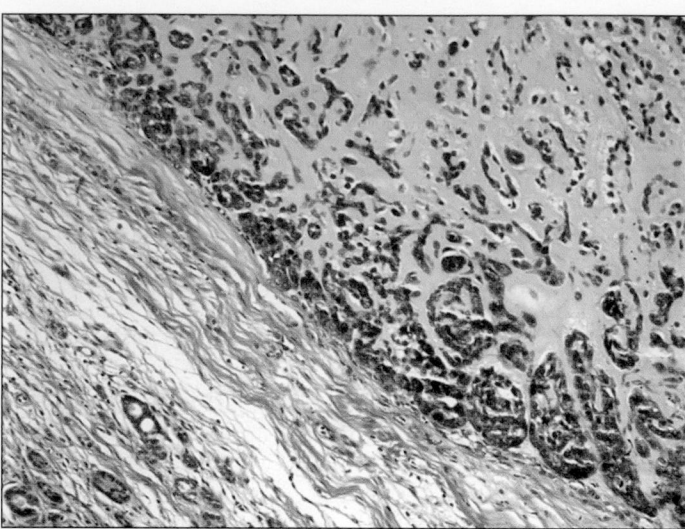

Fig. 10.94 Metaplastic carcinoma. A metaplastic carcinoma with chondroid differentiation.

some cases appear benign.[654] Some show both a circumscribed portion and a spiculated portion, which in one study correlated with the metaplastic and invasive epithelial components respectively.[654,655] Foci of osseous metaplasia may be detected mammographically in a subset of cases.

Gross pathology

The gross appearance of metaplastic carcinomas is not distinctive and these tumors can either be well circumscribed or show an indistinct or irregular border. Cystic degenerative changes are not infrequent, particularly in lesions with squamous differentiation. In general, metaplastic carcinomas tend to be relatively large tumors, compared to IC-NST.

Histopathology

Microscopically, metaplastic carcinomas are highly distinctive but vary in the types and extent of metaplastic changes. Most reports divide metaplastic carcinomas into two broad categories: those that show squamous differentiation[302,646] and those that feature heterologous elements, such as cartilage, bone, muscle, adipose tissue, vascular elements, and even melanocytes, among others.[300,301,303,649–654,659–661] Investigators at the Armed Forces Institute of Pathology categorize metaplastic carcinomas into five categories: squamous cell carcinomas,[302] spindle cell carcinomas,[299] carcinosarcomas,[301] matrix-producing carcinomas,[300] and carcinomas with osteoclast-like giant cells,[303] although others consider this last group to be a separate entity.

Squamous differentiation can range from well to poorly differentiated. In some tumors composed primarily of squamous cells, there is prominent cystic degeneration. In such cases, parts of the tumor may be composed of squamous epithelium-lined cysts resembling benign epidermal inclusion cysts. Spindle-cell differentiation is common in metaplastic carcinomas, and is frequently seen in association with squamous differentiation (Fig. 10.93). A low-grade metaplastic breast tumor composed of spindle cells that resemble those seen in fibromatosis has been described.[662,663]

The most common heterologous types of metaplastic carcinoma show chondroid and/or osseous differentiation (Fig. 10.94). In these tumors, the cartilage and bone may appear histologically benign or

frankly malignant, resembling chondrosarcoma and osteosarcoma respectively. If the heterologous metaplastic component of a particular tumor predominates, the differential diagnosis must include a sarcoma, either primary or metastatic. Metaplastic carcinomas resembling sarcomas are far more common than primary or metastatic sarcomas to the breast. The correct diagnosis in such cases may require extensive tissue sampling in order to demonstrate epithelial elements and immunohistochemical staining for epithelial markers, such as keratin, may be required for proper diagnosis (Figs 10.95, 10.96). While this is often helpful in tumors with spindle cell differentiation, not all metaplastic carcinomas show expression of epithelial markers, particularly those with heterologous differentiation. The results of immunohistochemical staining for other markers have been even more variable and this subject has been reviewed in detail.[437]

Low-grade adenosquamous carcinoma, an unusual subtype of metaplastic carcinoma, appears to represent a distinct clinico-pathologic entity.[304,657,658] These tumors are typically smaller than other metaplastic carcinomas, with a median size between 2 and 2.8 cm (range 0.5–8.6 cm).[304,657] They exhibit a firm, yellow cut surface with irregular borders. Histologically, these tumors are well differentiated and show epidermoid differentiation and a peculiar collagenized, lamellated stroma. Areas of squamous differentiation are present in most tumors and are admixed with areas of glandular differentiation. The glands often show elongated, compressed lumens, which may suggest syringomatous differentiation. Other than location, the histology is very similar to syringomatous adenoma of the nipple (see Fig. 10.33). Microcysts filled with keratinaceous material may be present. DCIS is usually not seen.

The differential diagnosis of low-grade adenosquamous carcinoma includes syringomatous adenoma of the nipple, reactive squamous metaplasia and tubular carcinoma.

These lesions may be locally aggressive but have a relatively good prognosis when compared with other metaplastic carcinomas.[304,657,658]

The frequency of DCIS seen in association with metaplastic carcinoma varies among published reports. In lesions characterized by a prominent mesenchymal component in which a true sarcoma is

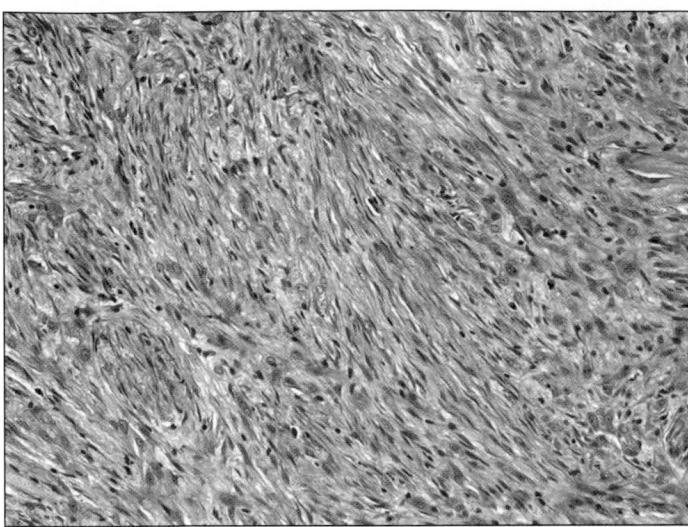

Fig. 10.95 Metaplastic carcinoma. A pure spindle cell metaplastic carcinoma. These lesions can be difficult to differentiate from benign and malignant stromal lesions.

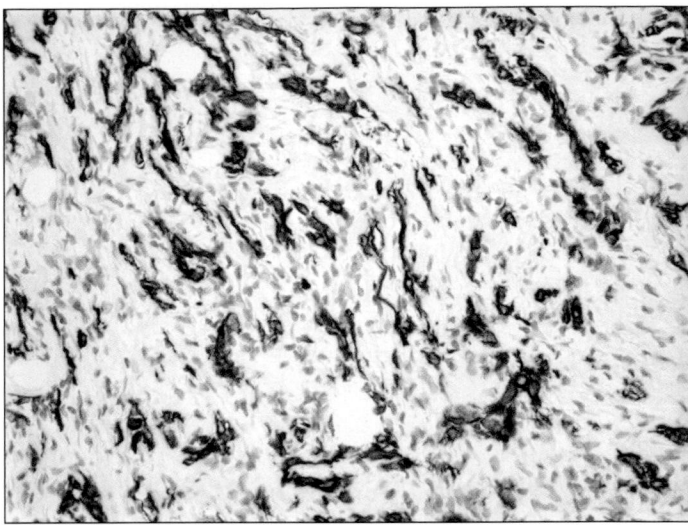

Fig. 10.96 Metaplastic carcinoma. The same spindle cell metaplastic carcinoma as in Fig. 10.94 immunostained for keratin.

in the differential diagnosis, the presence of DCIS or ADH argues in favor of metaplastic carcinoma.

Estrogen and progesterone receptor studies in metaplastic carcinomas are typically negative, regardless of the histologic subtype examined.[299–302,648,650,651,653,658,661,664] Metaplastic carcinomas are typically aneuploid or tetraploid.[651,655]

A small study of metaplastic carcinomas demonstrated identical clonality of the epithelial and mesenchymal components. The conclusion was that the mesenchymal component of these lesions arose from mutation of the epithelial component.[656] 'Fibromatosis-like' metaplastic carcinoma is a well differentiated variant of monophasic (sarcomatoid) metaplastic carcinoma. Similar to fibromatosis, these lesions are composed of a monotonous proliferation of bland, elongated spindle cells with an infiltrative pattern of growth and an invasive edge. The neoplastic cells have mild (or no) nuclear pleomorphism, variable (but low) mitoses and are disposed within a collagenous stroma. Focal biphasic (epithelial), heterologous (e.g. cartilage, bone) and/or in situ areas may be found in metaplastic carcinoma, which will not be present in fibromatosis. Therefore, multiple sections of a low-grade spindle cell lesion such as this should be submitted for microscopic examination. Furthermore, immunohistochemistry for cytokeratins and epithelial membrane antigen (EMA) are very useful if positive, as fibromatosis is negative for these markers whereas metaplastic carcinoma usually stains positively. Immunostaining may be focal in metaplastic carcinoma and therefore a negative result still does not rule out the diagnosis.

Cytopathology

Because metaplastic carcinomas are a heterogeneous group of lesions, the findings on FNA cytology are variable and are highly dependent on the proportion of cell types (i.e. spindle versus epithelial), the presence of heterologous elements, and the cellularity of the lesion being aspirated. As a consequence, reports of metaplastic carcinomas in the literature have ranged from those with bland spindle cells to overtly malignant including sarcomatoid, biphasic and/or squamous proliferations. In addition, the smear cellularity and background is also variable[665–676] (Fig. 10.97).

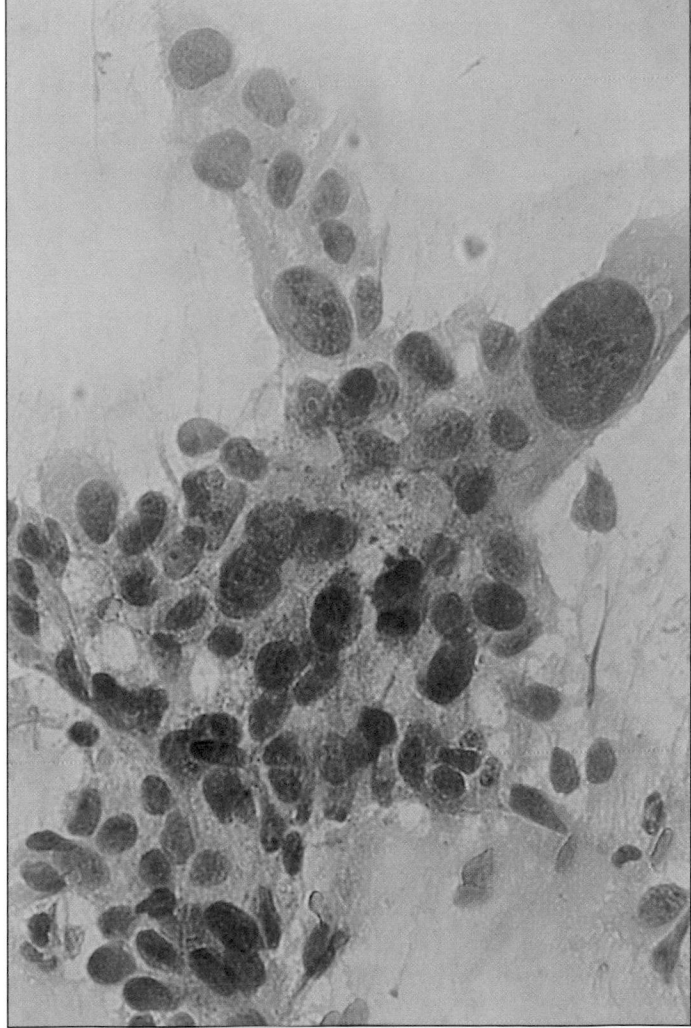

Fig. 10.97 Sinus catarrh-like pattern of lymph node metastasis in metaplastic carcinoma.

It is extremely important to consider metaplastic carcinoma in the differential diagnosis of any spindle cell lesion found on FNA cytology, even if the cells lack significant pleomorphism or the smear is not very cellular. Even in biphasic tumors, the epithelial component may be absent or difficult to appreciate on FNA smears.[669] Lesions such as fibromatosis, myofibroblastoma, adenomyoepithelioma, the stromal component of phyllodes tumor, and frank sarcomas enter into this differential diagnosis.[665,669,676,677] In addition, if the epithelial component of a biphasic metaplastic carcinoma is disproportionately present on the smear, distinction from ductal carcinoma NOS may not be feasible.

Clinical course and prognosis

The reported frequency of axillary lymph node metastases in patients with squamous or spindle cell carcinomas ranges from 6–54% of cases.[299,302,650,678] In patients with metaplastic carcinoma with heterologous elements, lymph node metastases have been noted in 6–31% of cases.[300,650,651,653,660,678]

In most cases, the routes of metastatic dissemination in metaplastic carcinomas are similar to those seen in breast cancers of no special type, including lymphatic spread to axillary lymph nodes, rather than the hematogenous spread characteristic of mammary sarcoma. Metastatic lesions may either demonstrate an epithelial phenotype, the metaplastic phenotype, or both. Tumors in which the sarcomatous elements predominate are more likely to have metastatic spread similar to a sarcoma.

Survival data reported in various studies are difficult to compare because of the relatively small numbers of patients included in the studies, differences in tumor types, differences in treatment and follow-up intervals, and differences in the use of appropriate control groups. Overall survival seems to be similar to that of grade- and stage-matched patients with infiltrating ductal carcinoma.[299,300,302,650,651,653,660,678]

In summary, the available data suggest that the prognosis for patients with metaplastic carcinoma is not appreciably different from that of invasive carcinomas of no special type when tumor size and stage are taken into consideration. The one exception among the variants of metaplastic carcinoma that does appear to have prognostic implications is low-grade adenosquamous carcinoma, which only rarely develops metastatic spread.[304,657] The use of conservative surgery and radiation therapy for patients with metaplastic carcinoma should follow the same guidelines used for patients with conventional types of invasive breast cancer.

INVASIVE CARCINOMA WITH NEUROENDOCRINE DIFFERENTIATION

Some invasive breast cancers show evidence of neuroendocrine differentiation at the morphologic level, histochemical level, immunohistochemical level, or some combination of these. In addition, in rare instances, breast carcinomas can secrete hormonal products that cause clinical symptoms.

Clinical presentation

With the exception of the very rare functioning neuro-endocrine tumor, which results in clinical manifestations due to hormone production and secretion,[679–682] carcinomas with neuro-endocrine differentiation do not demonstrate unique clinical manifestations.[683–688] Most of these tumors have been diagnosed in females but neuroendocrine tumors have also been reported in males[689] and some types may be proportionally more common in males than

females.[683] In most studies, the median age of patients and the location in the breast in which these tumors arise are similar to those seen in invasive cancers of no special type.

Distinctive mammographic or ultrasound characteristics of invasive carcinomas with neuroendocrine differentiation have not been reported.

Gross pathology

Invasive carcinomas with neuroendocrine differentiation are not associated with distinctive gross characteristics and the reported mean size in most studies is similar to invasive cancers of no special type.

Histopathology

Carcinomas with neuroendocrine differentiation represent a heterogeneous group of neoplasms[690] and, as discussed in a prior section, this feature is common in mucinous carcinomas. A study from Nottingham, UK, evaluated neuroendocrine differentiation in a series of breast carcinomas using modern immunohistochemical techniques for neuron-specific enolase, chromogranin A, and synaptophysin.[688] These authors found immunopositivity for more than one neuro-endocrine marker in 11% of cases. There was no significant association between neuroendocrine differentiation and tumor size, grade, or stage. In addition, overall or disease-free survival did not differ among patients with tumors with or without neuroendocrine differentiation.[688] This has led some authorities to propose separating breast carcinomas with neuroendocrine differentiation into cases with focal endocrine differentiation and those with overwhelming endocrine differentiation.[691] The latter tumors usually have distinct clinicopathologic features, are usually found in older patients, and show differentiation typical of neuroendocrine tumors at other sites.

With regard to tumors that show histologic evidence of neuroendocrine differentiation by routine light microscopy, several distinct morphologic subtypes have been recognized. Although there is debate regarding the histogenesis of such lesions, primary tumors that are morphologically indistinguishable from carcinoid tumors occurring elsewhere in the body can arise in the breast, and these tumors comprise less than 1% of all breast cancers.[684] These tumors must be distinguished from metastatic carcinoids,[692–697] which may even initially present as breast masses.[696] If present, DCIS in the region of the tumor can assist with this differential diagnosis. In equivocal cases, a search for an alternate primary site may be required.

At the other end of the neuroendocrine spectrum are primary breast carcinomas, which are indistinguishable from small cell neuroendocrine (oat cell) carcinomas in other sites.[698–705] These tumors must be distinguished from metastatic small cell neuroendocrine carcinoma involving the breast.[706,707]

The percentages of cases positive for estrogen and progesterone receptors is similar to tumors of no special type.[422,708–710]

Clinical course and prognosis

The available data do not point to any difference in prognosis from that of patients with invasive cancers of no special type. The exception, as may be expected, is small cell carcinoma: most[694,696,698] but not all[697,705] reports indicate an aggressive clinical course in patients with primary small cell carcinoma of the breast.

The use of breast-conserving treatment for patients with neuroendocrine carcinomas is too limited to draw any conclusions from.[709,705] At this time it seems that patients with invasive breast cancers with neuroendocrine differentiation should be treated in a manner appropriate for the size and stage of the lesion.

ADENOID CYSTIC CARCINOMA

Adenoid cystic carcinoma is a rare and morphologically distinct form of invasive carcinoma.[711–738] These tumors comprise 0.1% of all breast cancers,[716,721] and are associated with an excellent prognosis.

Clinical presentation

The age range, physical and mammographic findings are similar to those of tumors of no special type.[623,734] The majority of lesions are discovered in the subareolar or central region of the breast.[714,716,731,736] Skin involvement is uncommon.[720] These lesions are rarely multicentric and the incidence of contralateral breast cancers does not appear to be increased. Rarely, this tumor has been reported in males.[718,724,727,736]

Gross pathology

The reported size range of adenoid cystic carcinomas is broad. In one recent study, the mean size was 1.8 cm.[736] Grossly, these tumors are usually circumscribed and nodular; however, the microscopic extent of the lesion may be appreciably greater than the grossly evident lesion in 50–65% of cases.[723–725,732,734–736]

Histopathology

Histologically, these tumors are similar to adenoid cystic carcinomas, which arise in the salivary glands and are composed of epithelial cells with variable degrees of glandular, squamous, and sebaceous differentiation, myoepithelial cells, and characteristic collections of acellular basement membrane material (Fig. 10.98).[733,734] The epithelial component can assume variable architectural patterns, including solid, cribriform, tubular, and trabecular configurations. A solid variant of adenoid cystic carcinoma in which the cells display prominent basaloid features has been described.[739] Immunohistochemical studies have documented the presence of true lumens in the glandular component, lined by cytokeratin-positive cells with intact polarity, as well as pseudolumens surrounded by cells immunohistochemically consistent with myoepithelial cells.[735] Associated DCIS is seen in a minority of cases. Perineural invasion is also seen in some cases and may be prominent. Lymphatic vessel invasion is only rarely identified.[734]

Because of the fenestrated appearance found in adenoid cystic carcinoma, this lesion may mimic collagenous spherulosis, invasive cribriform carcinoma, and cribriform DCIS.[316,721,740] In contrast to the infiltrative pattern of adenoid cystic carcinoma, DCIS maintains the normal architectural relationship of ducts and lobules. Compared to the characteristic secretions present in the lumens of adenoid cystic carcinoma, the cribriform spaces of DCIS are either empty or contain calcifications, necrotic debris, or mucin. DCIS has an outer peripheral myoepithelial layer, whereas the adenoid cystic carcinoma has no outer myoepithelial layer, with only the pseudolumens lined by cells that immunostain as myoepithelial cells.

The tumors are usually estrogen- and progesterone-receptor-negative.[554,722,723,725,729,734,737] However, estrogen receptor positivity rates of up to 46%[736,738] have been reported in other series. Most cases are diploid[725,738] and have a low proliferative rate.[738]

Cytopathology

FNA smears of adenoid cystic carcinoma are characteristically cellular with uniform, small, hyperchromatic cells present singly and in loosely cohesive clusters. The cells have scant cytoplasm and naked nuclei may be present in the smear. The nuclei may have small

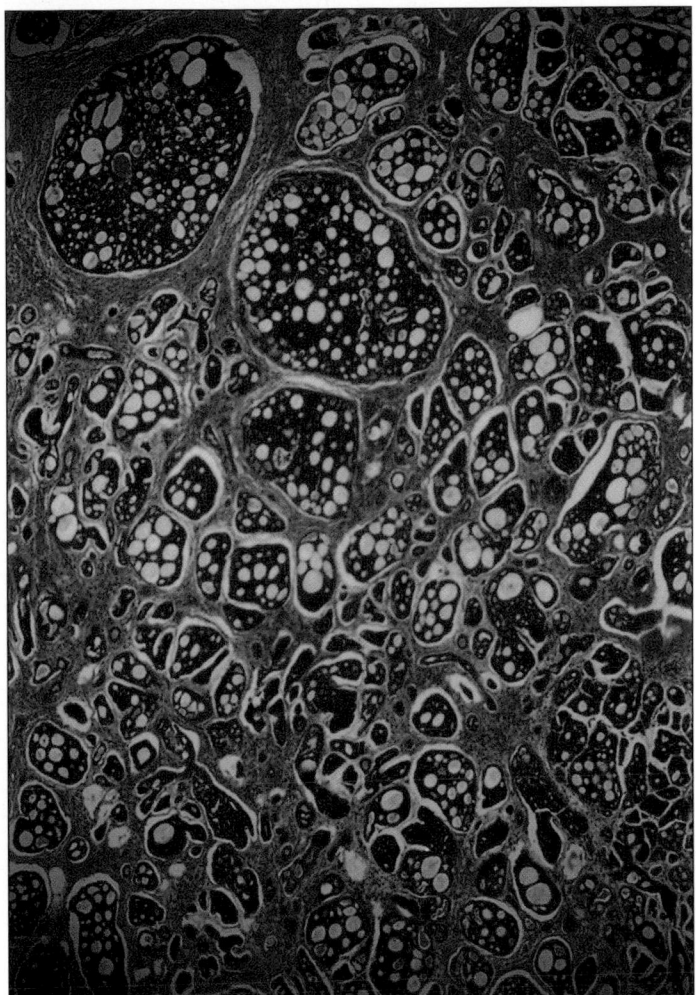

Fig. 10.98 Adenoid cystic carcinoma. Typical cylindromatous pattern.

but inconspicuous nucleoli. As with the salivary gland counterpart, the tumor cells surround cores and balls of acellular, homogeneous material, which appears translucent on Papanicolaou stain but pink-metachromatic on Diff-Quick stain (Fig. 10.99).[722,729,741–743] The differential diagnosis on cytology includes lesions with small hyperchromatic dyshesive cells such as lobular carcinoma, lymphoma, neuroendocrine tumors, and small cell carcinoma. Rarely, the basement-membrane-type spherular material may be mistaken for extracellular mucin, and mucinous carcinoma would then enter the differential diagnosis. In this respect, a recent study has reported utility of immunostaining for type IV collagen on FNA specimens of adenoid cystic carcinoma.[744]

Clinical course and prognosis

Patients with adenoid cystic carcinoma usually have an excellent prognosis with rare axillary lymph node metastases[725–727,731] or distant metastases.[711,728–732,738,739] Death due to adenoid cystic carcinoma is exceedingly rare.[731]

There are only sporadic reports of breast-conserving treatment for patients with adenoid cystic carcinoma. While local recurrences following excision alone have been described,[713,717,719,728,731,736] details regarding microscopic margin status are rarely provided. At the present time treatment of patients with adenoid cystic carcinoma

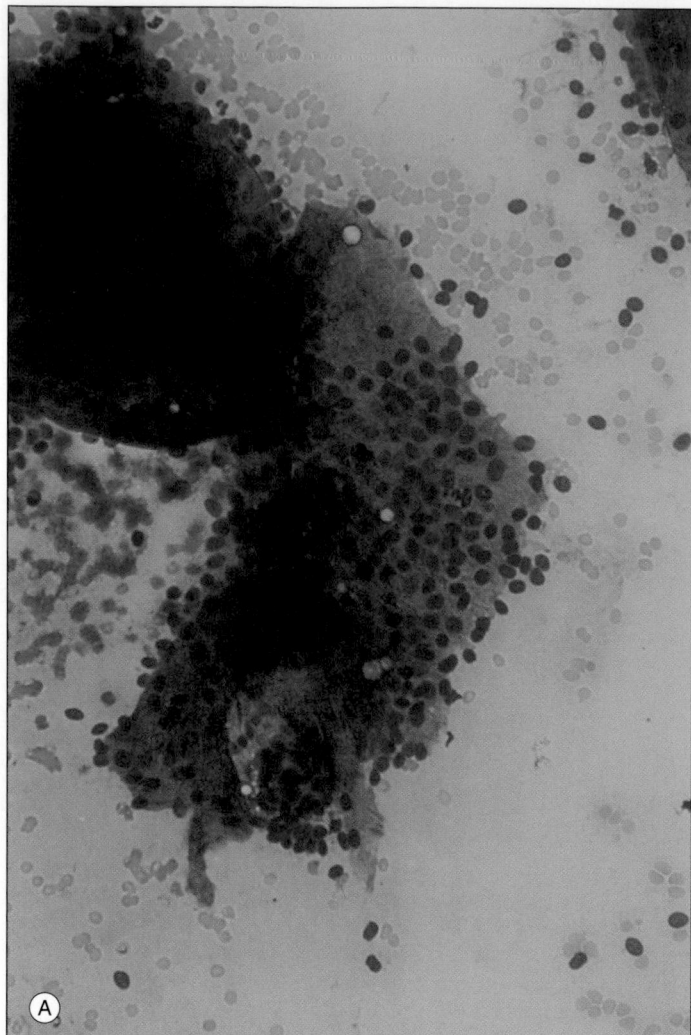
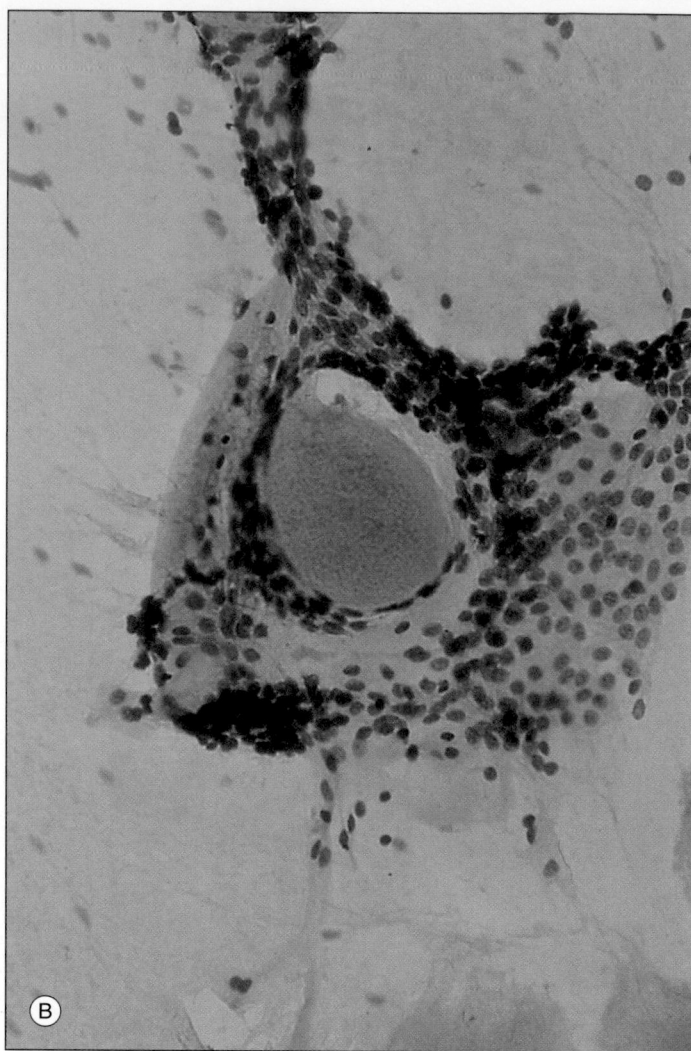

Fig. 10.99 (A) Diff-Quick-stained smear from an aspirate of adenoid cystic carcinoma. The cells are small and uniform and surround acellular homogeneous material. **(B)** Papanicolaou-stained smear of the same case displaying similar features. (×400.)

should follow the same guidelines as for other invasive breast cancers.

INVASIVE APOCRINE CARCINOMA

Although many invasive breast cancers of various types show some evidence of apocrine differentiation, fewer than 1% of invasive breast carcinomas demonstrate pure apocrine features (i.e. exhibit cytologic characteristics that resemble apocrine sweat glands).[745] While the morphologic features of these tumors are distinctive, available evidence suggests that patients with these tumors have the same prognosis as patients with invasive breast cancers of no special type. The clinical presentation, mammographic features, and gross findings are the same as for tumors of no special type.

Histopathology

In contrast, the histologic features of apocrine carcinoma are highly distinctive.[505,745–754] The invasive patterns are usually those seen in carcinomas of no special type, but in some cases lesions with apocrine

cytology can exhibit a pattern of invasion more characteristic of invasive lobular carcinoma.[754] One variant with a distinctive dyshesive and diffusely infiltrative pattern has been designated as having 'myoblastoid' or 'histiocytoid' features[505] and in some cases this lesion may mimic a granular cell tumor. Cytologically, the tumor cells have cytoplasm that is abundant and eosinophilic, with obvious granularity in some cases. The nuclei vary in grade, but typically show prominent nucleoli (Fig. 10.100). There is frequently associated DCIS, which may have apocrine features.

Apocrine carcinomas characteristically show immunostaining for GCDFP.[509]

Clinical course and prognosis

The clinical course and prognosis is the same as for carcinomas of no special type.

SECRETORY CARCINOMA

Secretory carcinoma is an exceedingly rare form of invasive breast carcinoma that accounts for <0.01% of all breast cancers.[755]

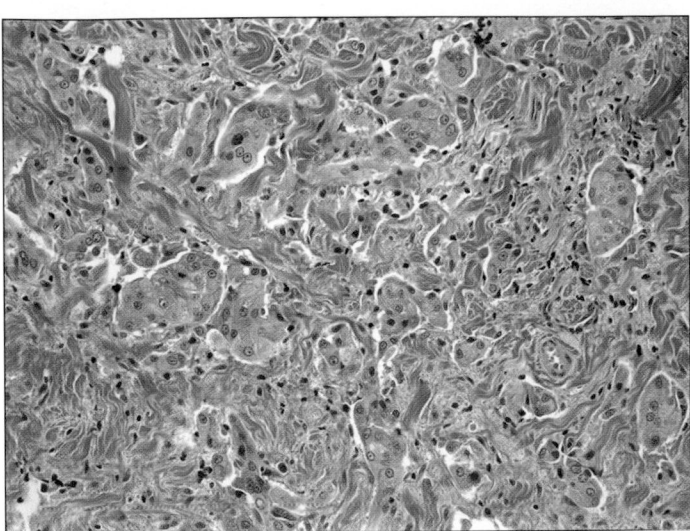

Fig. 10.100 Apocrine carcinoma. Invasive apocrine carcinoma has the invasive pattern of an NST tumor with apocrine type cells.

Sporadic reports regarding hormone receptor status in secretory carcinoma indicate that approximately one third of cases are estrogen-receptor-positive and three-quarters are progesterone-receptor-positive.[755,765,766,770,772] In addition, DNA studies indicate that virtually all secretory carcinomas are diploid or near diploid.[755,772,773]

Clinical course and prognosis

The majority of patients with secretory carcinoma have stage I disease and an indolent clinical course. Nevertheless, approximately one-quarter to one-third of the reported cases of secretory carcinomas have been associated with axillary lymph node metastases in both younger and older age groups,[755,758,760,762,763,768,774] usually to three lymph nodes or fewer. Information on recurrence rates of patients with secretory carcinoma is limited. Local recurrence in the breast[756,757,759,760,762,768] and chest wall[772] is recorded and the time to recurrence can be quite prolonged.

Distant metastases are very uncommon and have resulted in patient deaths in rare instances.[760,768] Neither the efficacy of conservative surgery and radiation therapy nor the role of adjuvant chemotherapy in patients with secretory carcinoma have been defined.

Although secretory carcinomas occur over a wide age range, they account for a substantial number of primary breast cancers diagnosed in childhood and have therefore also been referred to as 'juvenile' carcinomas. In most cases, secretory carcinomas are associated with an indolent clinical course.

Clinical presentation

Secretory carcinomas present over a wide age range (3–73 years) with a median age in the third decade.[755–775] The majority of reported cases have been in females but rare cases have occurred in males.[755,767,768,773,774] Most lesions are detected as palpable masses, and these can arise anywhere in the breast, with no obvious site predilection. No association has been documented with underlying medical conditions or hormonal abnormalities. In addition, no increased incidence of a positive family history of breast cancer has been reported in patients with secretory carcinoma. Only rare cases have been reported to be multicentric[769] and there does not appear to be an increased incidence of contralateral breast cancer in these patients.

Mammographic abnormalities associated with secretory carcinoma in adults have not been described in detail. On ultrasound examination, these lesions sometimes appear as hypoechoic lesions with heterogeneous internal echo texture and posterior acoustic enhancement, similar to a fibroadenoma.[623]

Gross pathology

Secretory carcinomas are typically grossly circumscribed. A broad size range has been reported, with a median size of 3 cm noted in one relatively large series.[760]

Histopathology

Histologically, these lesions are characterized by a proliferation of relatively low-grade tumor cells that form glandular structures and microcystic spaces filled with a vacuolated, lightly eosinophilic secretion. The tumor cells have abundant eosinophilic or clear cytoplasm. DCIS is frequently present in association with the invasive component and can be of the solid, cribriform, or papillary patterns, most often with low-grade nuclear features.

MISCELLANEOUS RARE INVASIVE BREAST CANCERS

Invasive carcinoma with osteoclast-like giant cells

Invasive carcinoma with osteoclast-like giant cells is characterized by an invasive epithelial component with admixed giant cells that morphologically resemble osteoclasts and have the phenotypic features of histiocytes on immunohistochemical and ultrastructural analysis.[776–787] The clinical features of patients with these tumors and their location within the breast are similar to patients with invasive carcinomas of no special type. Invasive carcinoma with osteoclast-like giant cells is associated with a benign appearance both mammographically[779,786] and grossly, because of the presence of circumscribed borders. On macroscopic examination, these lesions are typically circumscribed, fleshy and brown in color as a result of recent and remote hemorrhage and benign vascular proliferation. The epithelial component of the tumor is usually moderately to poorly differentiated carcinoma of no special type, but osteoclast-like giant cells have been reported in invasive lobular carcinomas and most other special-type cancers (Fig. 10.101).[778,780,782,783,787,788] The giant cell component can be but is not invariably present in metastatic lesions.[783] Available evidence suggests that these tumors do not appear to be any more or less aggressive than carcinomas of no special type.

Invasive carcinoma with choriocarcinomatous features

Invasive carcinoma with choriocarcinomatous features is an exceedingly rare form of breast cancer. Only two reports have described the presence of choriocarcinomatous elements (i.e. trophoblastic differentiation) admixed with conventional breast carcinomas.[789,790] The choriocarcinomatous component was associated with a carcinoma of no special type in one case[789] and metastatic mucinous carcinoma in the second.[790] The choriocarcinomatous elements in these tumors produce human chorionic gonadotropin.[789] If choriocarcinomatous features are encountered in a breast tumor, the differential diagnosis should include choriocarcinoma metastatic to the breast, as several such cases have been reported.[791]

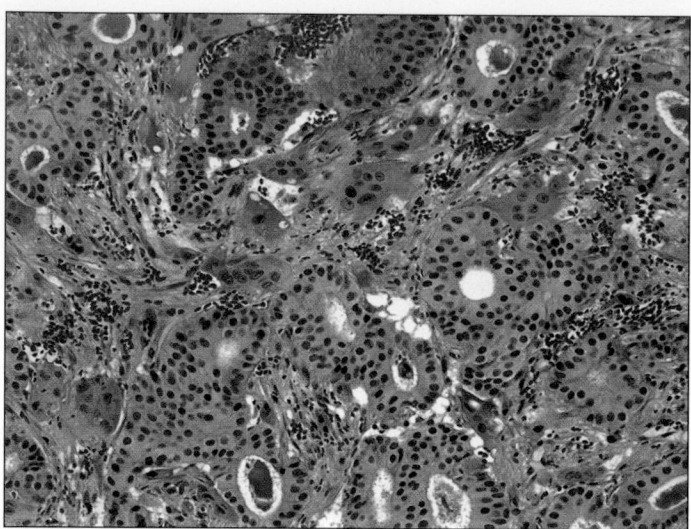

Fig. 10.101 Invasive carcinoma with osteoclast-like giant cells. The tumor has an NST pattern with osteoclast like giant cells.

Lipid-rich carcinoma

Lipid-rich carcinoma is a rare type of invasive breast carcinoma that is characterized by tumor cells that contain abundant lipid within their cytoplasm.[792–796] On routine light microscopy the tumor cells comprising these lesions show vacuolated, clear cell cytoplasmic features due to the fact that the lipid is dissolved during tissue processing. The importance of recognizing this tumor lies in the fact that it may mimic other forms of malignancy that may have metastasized to the breast, such as renal cell carcinoma. The prognostic significance of lipid-rich carcinoma is currently not known.

Glycogen-rich carcinoma

Glycogen-rich carcinoma is a rare variant of invasive breast carcinoma characterized by tumor cells that contain abundant glycogen within their cytoplasm.[796–803] As with lipid-rich carcinoma, the intracytoplasmic glycogen is often dissolved during specimen processing, imparting a vacuolated or 'clear cell' appearance to the tumor cells. Although relatively few cases have been reported, some have suggested that these tumors are associated with a more aggressive clinical course than invasive carcinomas of no special type.[803]

Mucinous cystadenocarcinoma

Mucinous cystadenocarcinoma is a variant of invasive breast carcinoma that is morphologically indistinguishable from mucinous cystadenocarcinoma of the ovary or pancreas and has 'ovarian type stroma.'[804] Although these tumors may be associated with the extravasation of mucin, they are otherwise morphologically distinct from conventional mucinous carcinoma of the breast and are therefore considered separately. The importance of recognizing these tumors is that they must be distinguished from metastatic lesions in the breast, particularly those of ovarian origin.[805] The prognostic significance of primary mucinous cystadenocarcinoma of the breast is currently unknown.

CARCINOMA OF THE MALE BREAST

Rare in those under 30 years of age, carcinoma of the breast in men arises at a later age than in women and is approximately 100 times less frequent than carcinoma of the female breast. It is more frequent in certain parts of the world, such as Egypt, where it is related to chronic liver disease secondary to schistosomiasis. Hormonal factors play a probable causal role in fewer cases than in women, and radiation exposure and genetic factors may therefore be more important.[806–808] An association has also been noted with Klinefelter syndrome,[809] gynecomastia,[810] and prostate cancer. The last of these associations is difficult to evaluate because of both the use of estrogens to treat prostate cancer[811] and the likelihood of prostate cancer to metastasize to the breast, where it may be confused with primary breast cancer.[812,813] Familial cases have been reported.[814]

Grossly, the tumor infiltrates the small mammary gland and may involve skin and the pectoral fascia. Ulceration of the overlying skin is common. Infiltrating carcinoma of no special type is the most common histologic type, but all types of carcinoma have been reported. Their cytologic appearance is as expected.[815,816] The prognosis is poorer than in women.[817] HER2 positivity has been reported to be related to prognosis[817] but ploidy and receptor status may not be.[817,818] Estrogen and progesterone receptors are present in an even higher percentage than in female patients.[817,819]

EXTRAMAMMARY MALIGNANCIES METASTATIC TO THE BREAST

There are numerous reports of metastatic tumors involving the breast. Secondary tumor deposits in the breast may emanate from the contralateral breast[820] or from virtually any nonmammary site. In one series, metastases to the breast from nonmammary malignancies comprised 1.2% of all malignancies diagnosed in the breast.[707] Because many nonmammary malignancies can mimic the features of usual or unusual types of primary breast tumor, it can be very difficult to distinguish between the two in a subset of cases, particularly when there is no history of a prior nonmammary malignancy. Nevertheless, this distinction is critical for appropriate patient management.

Metastatic lesions involving the breast almost never occur in the absence of metastases to other sites, even when the breast metastasis is the first clinically detected site. When metastases are detected in the breast, a solitary unilateral lesion is present in 85% of cases; multiple lesions are present in 10% of cases, and diffuse involvement of the breast occurs in 5% of cases.[821]

Although metastatic lesions in the breast can mimic the mammographic appearance of primary breast cancers, they are more likely to be multiple, bilateral, and exhibit well defined margins without evidence of spiculation.[623,805,821]

Metastatic tumors to the breast have a variable gross appearance, depending on the type of metastasis. In general, however, these lesions may be single or multiple and are generally well demarcated from the surrounding breast parenchyma. The histologic and cytologic appearance of these neoplasms is related to the site of origin of the primary tumor. Metastatic lesions most frequently described in the breast include malignant melanoma,[707,820–825] lung carcinoma,[706,707,821,826–828] prostate carcinoma,[813,829–834] and carcinoid tumors from a variety of primary sites.[692–697,835–840] Any carcinoma, sarcoma, or hematopoietic malignancy can involve the breast.

To a variable degree, many metastases may mimic unusual primary breast carcinomas. Therefore it is imperative that the pathologist considers the possibility of metastasis, particularly in a case associated with unusual clinical, mammographic, or pathologic features. It is also imperative that relevant information (such as a history of prior malignancy or simultaneous unexplained masses occurring elsewhere) is relayed to the pathologist. If a tumor displays unusual histologic findings that raise the possibility of metastases, the pathologist may opt to additionally sample the tumor to look for areas more typical of primary breast carcinoma, as well as associated DCIS. In addition, immunohistochemical stains for a variety of markers may be helpful to provide adjunctive evidence of mammary or nonmammary derivation in a subset of cases.

PATHOLOGIC FEATURES OF BREAST CANCER IN PATIENTS WITH *BRCA1* AND *BRCA2* MUTATIONS

There has been general agreement that *BRCA1*-related cancers are more frequently medullary carcinomas, atypical medullary carcinomas, and high-grade invasive ductal carcinomas than are cancers in patients without this genetic alteration. Cancers associated with *BRCA1* mutations have a significantly higher mitotic rate, more lymphocytic infiltration, and a larger proportion of the tumor with a continuous pushing margin, than sporadic breast cancers. In addition, *BRCA1*-related cancers are less often estrogen- and progesterone-receptor-positive, are more often aneuploid, more often have a high S-phase fraction, and more often show accumulation of the p53 protein than sporadic breast cancers and surprisingly, given the other tumor parameters, are less often HER2-positive.[620,841–853] It should be noted, however, that none of these features, singly or in combination, uniquely identifies a cancer as being related to *BRCA1* mutation.[854] Despite this constellation of adverse features, most studies have indicated that the clinical outcome of patients with *BRCA1*-related cancers is similar to that of patients with sporadic breast cancer.[841,843,845,846,851,855,856]

The histologic features reported in *BRCA2*-related breast cancers have been less consistent. One study noted a significantly higher proportion of tubular–lobular group cancers (including tubular, lobular, tubulolobular, and invasive cribriform carcinomas) than in other patients.[841,851] However, another group found tubular carcinomas to be less common in *BRCA2* mutation carriers.[842] In another small study, the pleomorphic variant of invasive lobular carcinoma was related to *BRCA2* mutation.[850] Some investigators have reported that *BRCA2*-related cancers tend to be of high histologic grade,[842,857] whereas others have not noted a significant difference in histologic grade when *BRCA2*-related cancers are compared with controls.[858]

SARCOMAS

Sarcomas are very uncommon cancers of the breast, representing about 0.5% of mammary tumors.[859] They include all tumors originating in the mesenchymal stroma of the mammary gland. Most lesions that resemble sarcomas are in fact metaplastic carcinomas. Therefore metaplastic carcinomas should first be excluded before one diagnoses a mammary sarcoma. The most important sarcoma that occurs primarily in the breast is angiosarcoma. Sarcomas also develop in the context of phyllodes tumors. For a discussion of all other sarcomas refer to the appropriate chapters.

ANGIOSARCOMA

Angiosarcoma is an infrequent tumor that manifests as a rapidly growing breast mass with a blue-red discoloration of the overlying skin. It may appear in women of all ages. Microscopically, it consists of numerous irregular blood vessels in which the endothelial cells show nuclear and cytoplasmic anomalies, often separated by spindle cells. Immunohistochemical staining confirm the endothelial location and nature of the neoplastic elements. Thrombi as well as necrotic and hemorrhagic zones are common. Hematogenous metastases are the rule. The prognosis is very poor in the high-grade sarcomas but may be more favorable in the better differentiated ones[139] (Fig. 10.102). Mammary angiosarcoma should not be mistaken for highly vascular or acantholytic carcinoma, or for benign or malignant vascular tumors of the skin of the breast. Angiosarcomas primarily of the skin of the breast but also of the breast itself are increased after radiotherapy for breast carcinoma.[860] Although deceptively benign-appearing angiosarcomas do occur, so do truly benign hemangiomas. Other than microscopic perilobular hemangiomas, benign vascular lesions respect breast parenchyma and do not 'invade lobules.' The presence of a palpable mass and of communicating vascular channels favor low-grade angiosarcoma over these benign lesions.

CYTOPATHOLOGY OF MAMMARY SARCOMAS

As with other breast lesions, sarcomas of the breast can be diagnosed by FNA biopsy.[665]

Although they are rare, there are sufficient numbers of reports in the literature that define the cytomorphology of various types. Cytologically, aspirates from sarcomas are rich in cellularity and demonstrate a population of pleomorphic spindle cells with conspicuous numbers of mitoses and evidence of necrosis. Multinucleation, cytoplasmic vacuolation, and phagocytosis are common. To differentiate sarcomas of the breast from metaplastic carcinoma and carcinoma with giant cells, it is essential to use immunocytochemistry. The cytopathology of sarcomas of the breast is essentially identical to that of their more common soft tissue counterparts, and is discussed in more detail in the appropriate chapters of this text.

LYMPHOMAS AND LEUKEMIAS

Different types of lymphomas and leukemic infiltrates may be observed as primary tumors of the breast. Most cases, however, represent part of the spectrum of a disseminated disease. Primary localizations manifest as a single nodule or as a diffuse infiltrative process. Microscopically, the infiltrating cells extend around the ducts and lobules and infiltrate the adjacent stroma and fatty tissue.

Lymphoid and hematopoietic tumors must also be distinguished from infiltrating lobular carcinomas, which can also infiltrate as noncohesive small round cells. Signet ring cells with intracellular lumina are a useful marker of lobular carcinoma. If there is any doubt, immunohistochemical staining for epithelial and leukocytic/lymphoid markers will provide the answer.

Cytologically, FNA from malignant lymphoma of the breast, whether primary or secondary, present with a cellular sample. The tumor cells appear in a dispersed pattern and lymphoglandular bodies are seen in the background. The cytomorphology of breast lymphoma varies according to the histologic subtype of the lesion. It ranges from a uniform monotonous cell population to a pleomorphic population of atypical lymphoid cells.

An incorrect diagnosis of carcinoma may result in unnecessary surgery, since the treatment of lymphoma is chemotherapy and/or radiotherapy. By contrast, a false-negative diagnosis of chronic

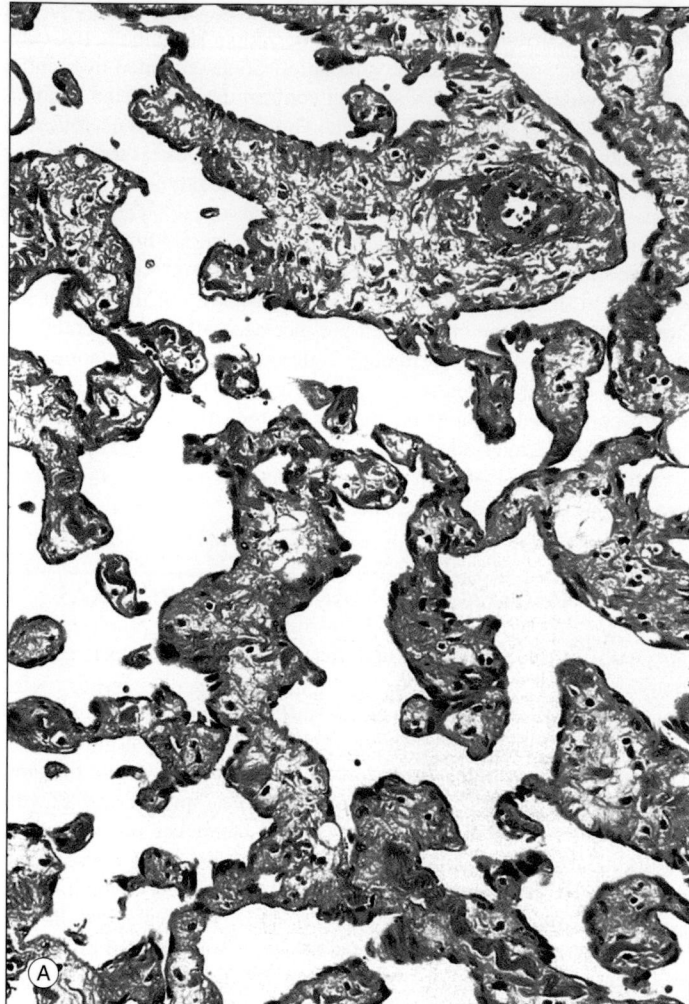
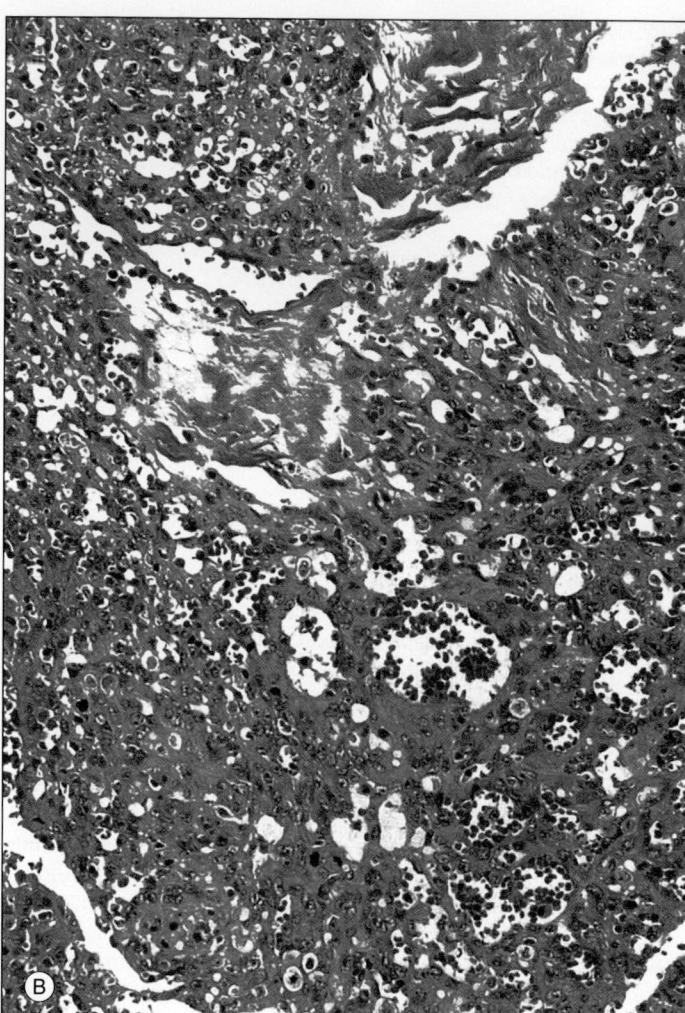

Fig. 10.102 Angiosarcoma. **(A)** Low-grade focus with complex papillary architecture as the major clue to a malignant tumor; endothelial cells are increased in number but small and flat. **(B)** High-grade focus in same tumor with solid nests of anaplastic tumor cells with numerous mitotic figures.

mastitis or fat necrosis may delay appropriate treatment. In the absence of a clinical history of a generalized lymphoma, the presence of lymphoid cells in breast aspirates may be misinterpreted as chronic mastitis, fat necrosis, medullary carcinoma, duct cell carcinoma with lymphocytic infiltration, carcinoid tumor, or primary or metastatic small cell carcinoma. Reactive processes, as well as unremarkable intramammary lymph nodes, can also yield a cellular aspirate consisting of lymphoid cells. The diagnosis of malignant lymphoma is therefore usually established by immunocytochemistry and/or flow cytometry.

GROWTH RATES OF BREAST CANCERS

It has been estimated from observing breast cancer growth in women that the 'average' breast cancer takes at least 8 years to reach 1 cm.[861] It is clear that there is a wide variation in growth rates depending on both tumor and host factors. The histologic type, grade, multifocality, proliferative index, associated biological markers, and patient age are all associated with growth rate.[862–867] Some investigators feel that the growth rate is very predictable and can be applied to individual patients.[868]

PATHOLOGIC FACTORS USEFUL IN ASSESSING PROGNOSIS

There is currently considerable interest in identifying biological, molecular, and genetic markers that may useful to help assess the prognosis of patients with invasive breast cancer. However a considerable amount of useful prognostic information can be obtained from routine pathologic examination of specimens containing breast cancer without the need for special diagnostic procedures, equipment, or reagents. Clinical follow-up studies have repeatedly demonstrated that features such as axillary lymph node status, histologic grade, histologic type, and lymphatic vessel invasion represent powerful and independent prognostic indicators. Tumor size is a much weaker independent factor but is strongly tied to other factors such as lymph node status and grade. Other factors have also been shown to provide important prognostic information in many studies.[869–871] In fact, these traditional prognostic factors should be considered to be the standard against which any new prognostic factors are measured.

Axillary lymph node status

There is uniform agreement that the status of the axillary lymph nodes is the single most important prognostic factor for patients with breast cancer and that disease-free and overall survival decrease as the number of positive lymph nodes increases. Evaluation of lymph nodes and sentinel lymph nodes is discussed above in the section on tissue processing.

Tumor size

After lymph node status, tumor size, primarily because it correlates with nodal status, represents the next most important prognostic factor for patients with breast cancer. Even among patients with breast cancers 1 cm and smaller (T1a and T1b), size represents an important prognostic factor for axillary lymph node involvement and outcome.[872] It should be noted, however, that the manner in which the pathologic tumor size is reported has not yet been standardized, with some pathologists reporting the size of the macroscopically identified tumor, some reporting a microscopic size that includes both the invasive and in situ components, and still others reporting the microscopic size of the invasive component only. Prior studies have shown that, particularly for small breast cancers, there is often a poor correlation between the tumor size determined by gross pathologic examination and the size of the invasive component of the tumor as determined by measurement from the histologic sections.[873] Moreover, it is the size of the invasive component that is the most clinically significant determinant of outcome. In fact, the sixth edition of the American Joint Committee on Cancer (AJCC) cancer staging manual indicates that 'the pathologic tumor size for the T classification is a measurement of *only the invasive component.*'[154] Therefore, when there is a discrepancy between the gross tumor size and the microscopic size of the invasive component, particularly of small breast cancers, it is the microscopic size that takes precedence. The gross size must be correlated with the microscopic size and appearance of the invasive component of the tumor. For example, if a tumor grossly 3 cm in greatest dimension is verified microscopically to be primarily invasive, then that is the size to report for staging purposes. However if a 3-cm gross tumor is primarily DCIS and the invasive component verified microscopically is 6 mm, then that is the size to report for staging purposes.

Histologic type

Some histologic types of breast cancer are associated with a particularly favorable clinical outcome.[452,578] Special types of tumor that have consistently been shown to have an excellent prognosis include tubular, invasive cribriform, mucinous, and adenoid cystic carcinomas. Moreover, Rosen et al. have shown that the 20-year recurrence-free survival of special-type tumors 1.1–3.0 cm in size is similar to that of invasive ductal carcinomas 1 cm and smaller (87% and 86% respectively).[578] However, strict diagnostic criteria must be employed in order to observe the favorable outcome reported for these lesions. For a tumor to be classified as a special type at least 90% of the tumor should be of that type.

Histologic grade

The importance of tumor grading as a prognostic factor in patients with breast cancer has been clearly demonstrated in numerous clinical outcome studies. These studies have repeatedly shown higher rates of distant metastasis and poorer survival in patients with higher-grade (poorly differentiated) tumors, independent of lymph node status and tumor size.[145,455,580,869–871,874–883]

In fact, tumor grading has been shown to be of prognostic value even in patients with breast cancers 1 cm and smaller.[872] Although a variety of methods of nuclear and histologic grading have been used in these studies, the grading method in most widespread clinical use at the present time is the Nottingham, UK, modification of the Scarff–Bloom–Richardson histologic grading system by Elston and Ellis[880] (see Table 10.7). These authors advocate the use of histologic grading for all types of invasive breast cancer, acknowledging, however, that histologic grade partially defines some of these histologic types (for example, tubular carcinomas are by definition grade 1 and medullary carcinomas are grade 3 lesions). However, these authors have also pointed out that the combination of histologic type and grade provides a more accurate assessment of prognosis than does histologic type alone.[530]

Some studies have suggested that histologic grade may provide useful information with regard to response to chemotherapy and may therefore be of value as a predictive factor as well as a prognostic indicator. The results of several studies have suggested that the presence of high histologic grade is associated with a better response to certain chemotherapy regimens than low histologic grade.[884,885]

A frequent criticism of the use of histologic grading is that this assessment is subjective and, as a consequence, prone to considerable interobserver variability.[886–888] Most of the studies that have suggested this have used grading systems that lack precisely defined criteria and/or did not attempt to educate the participating pathologists in the use of the system evaluated. Studies have indicated using the Elston and Ellis grading system[889] that the use of strict criteria and guidelines for histologic grading can result in acceptable levels of interobserver agreement.

Lymphatic vessel invasion

Lymphatic vessel invasion has been shown in numerous studies to be an important and independent prognostic factor. Its major clinical value at this time is in identifying node-negative patients at increased risk for axillary lymph node involvement[890–897] and adverse outcome.[879,892,893,898,899] The identification of lymphatic vessel invasion may be of particular importance in patients with T1 node-negative breast cancers, since this finding may permit the identification of a subset of patients at increased risk for axillary lymph node involvement and distant metastasis in this otherwise favorable group.[872] In a study of 461 patients with T1 node-negative breast cancer, patients with tumors lacking lymphatic vessel invasion had a 20-year survival rate of 81% compared with 64% for those whose tumors exhibited lymphatic vessel invasion.[578] Similar findings have been reported by others,[900–902] even when the analysis is restricted to the subset of T1 breast cancers that are 1 cm and smaller.[899,900]

As with histologic grade, the ability of pathologists to reproducibly identify lymphatic vessel invasion has been challenged.[903] However, a higher level of interobserver agreement has been noted in other studies.[890–893,902] The use of strict criteria for the identification of lymphatic vessel invasion is therefore imperative. The following are our suggestions. To avoid overdiagnosing lymphatic invasion it should be evaluated outside the invasive tumor. It is most common at the periphery of the invasive tumor. Lymphatics are found in vascular bundles as well as around ducts and lobules. Endothelial cells are difficult to distinguish from myofibroblasts but when present are helpful. In contrast to retraction artifact, tumor in lymphatics does not usually have the same shape as the outline of the space it is in. Nests of tumor cells with a targetoid appearance around a duct commonly represent lymphatic invasion. It is not important to distinguish a lymphatic space from a small blood vessel.

A number of investigators have evaluated the use of immunohistochemical stains for endothelial cells (including stains for factor VIII related antigen, CD34, *Ulex europaeus* agglutinin I, and blood group isoantigens) and basement membrane components as an aid in the identification of lymphatic vessel invasion.[904–911] However, these stains have been of limited value in this context. Therefore, at the present time, lymphatic vessel invasion is best assessed on routine H&E-stained sections using strict diagnostic criteria.

Other factors

A number of other histologic factors have been reported to have prognostic value in patients with invasive breast cancer. The presence of *blood vessel invasion* (i.e. invasion of veins and arteries) has been reported to have an adverse effect on clinical outcome.[450,894,901,902,912–916] Blood vessel invasion is highly correlated with lymphatic invasion. It is rare to see invasion of large arteries and veins. Elastic stains are of no use since large ducts often acquire an elastic layer and DCIS may be mistaken for vascular invasion. At the present time we report all small vessel invasion as lymphatic–small vessel invasion.

The prognostic significance of *tumor necrosis* has also been investigated in a number of studies.[902,917–920] In most studies, the presence of necrosis has been associated with an adverse effect on clinical outcome,[917–920] although in one of these studies necrosis was associated with a worse prognosis only within the first 2 years after diagnosis.[919] The presence of necrosis is highly correlated with other features associated with a poor prognosis such as larger tumor size and high histologic grade,[882,917] and it is not clear if the adverse prognostic influence of necrosis is independent of these other factors.

The relationship between clinical outcome and the extent of *mononuclear inflammatory cell infiltrate* in association with invasive breast cancers has also been investigated. The presence of a prominent mononuclear cell infiltrate has been correlated in some studies with high histologic grade.[882] However the prognostic significance of this finding is controversial, with some studies noting an adverse effect of a prominent mononuclear cell infiltrate on clinical outcome[463,921–924] and others observing either no significant effect or a beneficial effect.[878,901,921,925]

The presence of *perineural invasion* is sometimes observed in invasive breast cancers. This phenomenon is often seen in association with lymphatic vessel invasion but it has not been shown to be an independent prognostic factor.[437]

The *extent of ductal carcinoma* in situ associated with invasive cancers has also been studied as a potential prognostic factor. Numerous investigators have shown that the presence of an extensive intraductal component is a prognostic factor for local recurrence in the breast in patients treated with conservative surgery and radiation therapy when the status of the excision margins is unknown. An extensive ductal component (EIC) has been defined in a number of ways. The authors define it as an infiltrating carcinoma with prominent DCIS (often referred to as 25%) within the confines of the invasive tumor and any adjacent to it or cases of DCIS with foci of invasion. However, more recent studies have indicated that this factor is not an independent predictor of local recurrence following conservative surgery and radiation therapy when the microscopic margin status is taken into consideration (reviewed in Schnitt[531]). The issue is complicated by the fact that some studies have shown that even in patients with negative margins the amount of DCIS near margins was predictive of breast recurrence.[926,927] Silverberg and Chitale reported an inverse relationship between the amount of DCIS and both the risk of axillary lymph node metastasis and the 5-year survival rate in a series of patients with invasive ductal carcinoma treated by mastectomy.[928] However, in another series of 573 patients with invasive ductal carcinoma treated by mastectomy there was no significant relationship between the extent of intraductal involvement and either recurrence or survival.[929]

Similarly, among 533 patients with invasive carcinoma treated with conservative surgery and radiation therapy the presence of an extensive intraductal component was not associated with the risk of distant metastasis in a multiple logistic regression analysis.[930] Therefore, while the extent of associated DCIS is a consideration in the local management of patients treated with breast-conserving therapy, it does not appear to be a significant prognostic factor with regard to distant metastasis or survival.

Combining prognostic factors

Although a variety of prognostic factors have been reported for patients with invasive breast cancer, how best to integrate these factors to assess patient outcome and formulate therapeutic decisions is an unresolved issue.[931] Several authors have developed prognostic indices for this purpose that take into account various combinations of factors. One of these, the Nottingham Prognostic Index, takes into consideration tumor size, lymph node status, and histologic grade. The three factors in the index are tumor size, grade, and lymph node status. The numerical scores are assigned as follows: Tumor size in cm is multiplied by 0.2 + Grade (1–3) + nodal stage (1–3). Nodal stage is as follows: Stage 1, no nodal involvement. Stage 2, involvement of one to three low axillary nodes or an internal mammary node. Stage 3, involvement of four or more low axillary nodes and/or the apical node or any axillary node and internal mammary node simultaneously. There are then four prognostic groups assigned: a Good Prognostic Group (score 2.1≤3.4), a Moderate Prognostic Group (score 3.41–5.4) and a Poor Prognostic Group (score >5.41).[932] This index has been used to stratify patients with breast cancer into good, moderate, and poor prognostic groups with 15-year survival rates of 80%, 42%, and 13% with age-matched controls of 83%. In addition, within the Prognostic Group score a subset with an excellent prognosis was identified with survival the same as for age-matched controls. Another group of investigators has proposed a prognostic index that combines tumor size, lymph node status, and mitotic index (morphometric prognostic index).[933] This index has been shown to be a useful prognostic discriminator for premenopausal patients with both node-negative and node-positive disease. Prognostic indices represent important attempts to refine prognostication in patients with invasive breast cancer.

Biological markers

Hormone receptor status

The presence of steroid hormone receptors (estrogen receptor, progesterone receptor) represents a relatively weak prognostic factor for patients with breast cancer but these receptors are the strongest predictive factors for response to hormonal therapy.[145,869–871,874,875] In recent years, immunohistochemical staining has replaced the ligand binding biochemical assay for assessment of ER and PR status. In fact, the immunohistochemical method is easier to perform and has recently been shown to be equivalent or better than the biochemical assay in predicting the response to adjuvant endocrine therapy.[934] While a number of methods for scoring receptor positivity have been proposed, patients respond to therapy if there is any staining and therefore reporting tumors as positive or negative should be sufficient in most cases.

Newer factors

Numerous biological and molecular markers have been reported to have prognostic and/or predictive value in patients with breast cancer, including DNA content (ploidy), proliferative rate, apoptosis, oncogenes, suppressor genes, proteases, adhesion molecules, and angiogenesis, among others.[145,869–871] Some of the factors initially reported to be significant, independent prognostic markers have subsequently been shown to have little or no independent prognostic value (e.g. ploidy, cathepsin D). Among most of the other reported factors, variations in study design, methodology, and statistical analysis have led to conflicting and contradictory data.[935] A comprehensive review of biological and molecular prognostic and predictive factors is beyond the scope of this chapter. However, one of these factors, HER2/neu, has been the subject of much recent discussion and controversy and merits detailed consideration.

The analysis of breast cancer specimens for alterations in the HER2/neu (c-erbB-2) gene or its protein product has now become common practice in surgical pathology laboratories. Although some clinicians use the information derived from these assays in assessing patient prognosis and in evaluating the likelihood of response to various chemotherapeutic agents and to tamoxifen, currently the major clinical role of assessment of HER2 status is to help determine patient suitability for treatment with trastuzumab, a monoclonal antibody targeted to the HER2 protein.[936,937]

Although there are a variety of methods available to assess HER2 status in clinical breast cancer specimens, assessment of protein overexpression using immunohistochemistry and evaluation of gene amplification using FISH are the methods most commonly employed in clinical practice today.[938,939]

While the clinical value of assessing HER2 status in human breast cancers to help determine suitability for trastuzumab therapy is indisputable, the manner in which the test should be performed and the results evaluated and reported is a matter of heated debate and controversy.[940] The College of American Pathologists recently issued recommendations regarding HER2 testing for patients with breast cancer.[145] However, these recommendations largely reflect the current lack of consensus with regard to how best to evaluate HER2 status.

CURRENT STATUS OF PROGNOSTIC AND PREDICTIVE FACTORS

At the 1990 NIH Consensus Development Conference on the treatment of early-stage breast cancer, tumor size, histologic type, nuclear grade, proliferative rate, and hormone receptors were considered the major useful prognostic factors in patients with node-negative breast cancer.[874] At the 1998 St Gallen Conference on Adjuvant Therapy of Primary Breast Cancer, nodal status was recognized as the most important breast cancer prognostic factor. Among patients with node-negative disease, tumor size, histologic or nuclear grade, hormone receptor status, and lymphatic vessel invasion were considered to be the most relevant prognostic factors.[875] More recently, at a 1999 Consensus Conference held under the auspices of the College of American Pathologists (CAP), a multidisciplinary group of pathologists, clinicians, and statisticians reviewed breast cancer prognostic and predictive factors and categorized them into three groups based on the strength of the published data[145]:

- Category I: Well supported by the literature; generally used in patient management (nodal status, size, histologic type, histologic grade, mitotic figure count, hormone receptor status).
- Category II: Extensively studied biologically and/or clinically
  - A. Tested in clinical trials
  - B. Biological and correlative studies done, few clinical outcome studies (HER2, p53, lymphatic vessel invasion, other proliferation markers such as MIB-1)

- Category III: Currently does not meet criteria for category I or category II (ploidy, cathepsin D, angiogenesis, and others).

Of note, the factors considered most relevant at the 1999 CAP Consensus Conference (category I) are virtually identical to those considered most important at the 1990 NIH Consensus Development Conference

The American Joint Committee on Cancer (AJCC) and the International Union Against Cancer (UICC) have developed criteria to assess the value of putative prognostic and predictive factors.[935] The criteria include clinical importance (the factor is a powerful predictor that can be used in patient management), independence (the factor retains its prognostic or predictive value when other factors are combined with it), and significance (the prognostic or predictive accuracy of the factor rarely occurs by chance). In addition, there must be standardization with regard to methods, interpretation and reporting. It is hoped that the recognition and widespread adoption of these criteria will result in greater clarity of the value of the newer putative prognostic and predictive factors.

Finally, while the evaluation of individual prognostic and predictive factors has value, there is a pressing clinical need to develop a comprehensive profile of the biological and molecular characteristics of a tumor that may aid in the assessment of prognosis and the prediction of response to various therapeutic modalities. The tools of modern molecular biology, such as microarray technology, may ultimately provide such an assessment by permitting high throughput, parallel analysis of hundreds or thousands of parameters.[941]

CONTENTS OF THE FINAL SURGICAL PATHOLOGY REPORT

The final surgical pathology report for specimens containing invasive breast cancer should include, in addition to the diagnosis, information needed for staging and therapeutic decision-making.[942,943] The information used by clinicians in determining treatment options varies among different institutions. However, at a minimum, every surgical pathology report for specimens containing an invasive breast cancer should include the type of specimen submitted, laterality, specimen size, tumor size, histologic type, histologic grade, presence or absence of lymphatic vessel invasion, presence or absence of an extensive intraductal component (EIC), the status of the microscopic margins, and lymph node status (if applicable). In addition, for specimens removed because of the presence of a mammographically detected microcalcifications, it is important to note the location of the calcifications (i.e. in association with invasive cancer, carcinoma in situ, benign breast ducts and lobules, stroma, or blood vessels). If ancillary studies are in progress (hormone receptor assays, prognostic markers, etc.), this should also be documented in the final report. The use of a standardized, synoptic-type report, either in addition to or in place of a narrative report, should also be considered.[942,943] The Association of Directors of Anatomic and Surgical Pathology (ADASP) and the College of American Pathologists (CAP) have both posted guidelines and synoptic report forms on their websites. Both of these formats will satisfy the American College of Surgery for cancer center approval.

ACKNOWLEDGMENT

We would like to thank Dr Stuart Schnitt for help and advice with the manuscript and Drs Silverberg and Masood for our use of text and illustrations from the last edition.

REFERENCES

1. Propper A. Etude experimentale des premiers stades de la morphogenese mammaire. [Experimental study of the first stages of mammary morphogenesis]. Annee Biol 1970; 9(5): 267–275.

2. Page DL, Anderson TJ. Stages of breast development. In: Page DL, Anderson TJ (eds) Diagnostic histopathology of the breast. Edinburgh: Churchill Livingstone; 1987: 11–29.

3. Ozzello L. Ultrastructure of the human mammary gland. Pathol Annu 1971; 6: 1–59.

4. Forsyth IA. The mammary gland. Baillières Clin Endocrinol Metab 1991; 5(4): 809–832.

5. Vogel PM, Georgiade NG, Fetter BF, et al. The correlation of histologic changes in the human breast with the menstrual cycle. Am J Pathol 1981; 104(1): 23–34.

6. Kramer WM, Rush BF Jr. Mammary duct proliferation in the elderly. A histopathologic study. Cancer 1973; 31(1): 130–137.

7. Smith DM Jr, Peters TG, Donegan WL. Montgomery's areolar tubercle. A light microscopic study. Arch Pathol Lab Med 1982; 106(2): 60–63.

8. Halsell JT, Smith JR, Bentlage CR, et al. Lymphatic drainage of the breast demonstrated by vital dye staining and radiography. Ann Surg 1965; 162: 221–226.

9. Egan RL, McSweeney MB. Intramammary lymph nodes. Cancer 1983; 51(10): 1838–1842.

10. Strombeck JO. Macromastia in women and its surgical treatment. A clinical study based on 1042 cases. Acta Chir Scand Suppl 1964; 341: 1–129.

11. Martin HE, Ellis EB. Biopsy needle puncture and aspiration. Ann Surg 1930; 92: 169–181.

12. Tabbara SO, Frost AR, Stoler MH, et al. Changing trends in breast fine-needle aspiration: results of the Papanicolaou Society of Cytopathology Survey. Diagn Cytopathol 2000; 22(2): 126–30.

13. Sartorius OW, Smith HS, Morris P, et al. Cytologic evaluation of breast fluid in the detection of breast disease. J Natl Cancer Inst 1977; 59(4): 1073–1080.

14. O'Shaughnessy JA, Ljung BM, Dooley WC, et al. Ductal lavage and the clinical management of women at high risk for breast carcinoma: a commentary. Cancer 2002; 94(2): 292–298.

15. Sneige N, Staerkel GA, Caraway NP, et al. A plea for uniform terminology and reporting of breast fine needle aspirates. MD Anderson Cancer Center proposal. Acta Cytol 1994; 38(6): 971–972.

16. Layfield LJ, Mooney EE, Glasgow B, et al. What constitutes an adequate smear in fine-needle aspiration cytology of the breast? Cancer Cytopathol 1997; 81(1): 16–21.

17. Rubenchik I, Sneige N, Edeiken B, et al. In search of specimen adequacy in fine-needle aspirates of nonpalpable breast lesions. Should specimen adequacy be determined by the opinion of the aspirator or by the cells on the slides? [editorial; comment]. Am J Clin Pathol 1997; 108(1): 13–18.

18. Abati A. To count or not to count? A review of the issue of adequacy in breast FNA. Diagn Cytopathol 1999; 21(2): 142–147.

19. Eckert R, Howell LP. Number, size, and composition of cell clusters as related to breast FNA adequacy. Diagn Cytopathol 1999; 21(2): 105–111.

20. Stanley MW, Abele J, Kline T, et al. What constitutes adequate sampling of palpable breast lesions that appear benign by clinical and mammographic criteria? Diagn Cytopathol 1995; 13(5): 473–482.

21. Kline TS. Adequacy and aspirates from the breast: a philosophical approach. Diagn Cytopathol 1995; 13(5): 470–472.

22. Scopa CD, Koukouras D, Androulakis J, Bonikos D. Sources of diagnostic discrepancies in fine-needle aspiration of the breast. Diagn Cytopathol 1991; 7(5): 546–548.

23. Pennes DR, Naylor B, Rebner M. Fine needle aspiration biopsy of the breast. Influence of the number of passes and the sample size on the diagnostic yield. Acta Cytol 1990; 34(5): 673–676.

24. Hermansen C, Skovgaard Poulsen H, Jensen J, et al. Diagnostic reliability of combined physical examination, mammography, and fine-needle puncture ('triple-test') in breast tumors. A prospective study. Cancer 1987; 60(8): 1866–1871.

25. Butler JA, Vargas HI, Worthen N, Wilson SE. Accuracy of combined clinical-mammographic-cytologic diagnosis of dominant breast masses. A prospective study. Arch Surg 1990; 125(7): 893–5; discussion 896.

26. Negri S, Bonetti F, Capitanio A, Bonzanini M. Preoperative diagnostic accuracy of fine-needle aspiration in the management of breast lesions: comparison of specificity and sensitivity with clinical examination, mammography, echography, and thermography in 249 patients. Diagn Cytopathol 1994; 11(1): 4–8.

27. Abele J, Stanley MW, Rollins SD, Miller TR. What constitutes an adequate smear in fine-needle aspiration cytology of the breast? [letter; comment]. Cancer 1998; 84(1): 57–61.

28. Linsk J, Kreuzer G, Zajicek J. Cytologic diagnosis of mammary tumors from aspiration biopsy smears. II. Studies on 210 fibroadenomas and 210 cases of benign dysplasia. Acta Cytol 1972; 16(2): 130–138.

29. Abele JS, Miller TR, Goodson WH III, et al. Fine-needle aspiration of palpable breast masses. A program for staged implementation. Arch Surg 1983; 118(7): 859–863.

30. Sneige N. Should specimen adequacy be determined by the opinion of the aspirator or by the cells on the slides? Cancer Cytopathol 1997; 81(1): 3–5.

31. The uniform approach to breast fine-needle aspiration biopsy. National Cancer Institute Fine-Needle Aspiration of Breast Workshop Subcommittees. Diagn Cytopathol 1997; 16(4): 295–311.

32. Crystal BS, Wang HH, Ducatman BS. Comparison of different preparation techniques for fine needle aspiration specimens. A semiquantitative and statistical analysis. Acta Cytol 1993; 37(1): 24–28.

33. Bedard YC, Pollett AF. Breast fine-needle aspiration. A comparison of ThinPrep and conventional smears. Am J Clin Pathol 1999; 111(4): 523–527.

34. Wang HH, Ducatman BS. Fine needle aspiration of the breast. A probabilistic approach to diagnosis of carcinoma. Acta Cytol 1998; 42(2): 285–289.

35. Page DL, Johnson JE, Dupont WD. Probabilistic approach to the reporting of fine-needle aspiration cytology of the breast. Cancer 1997; 81(1): 6–9.

36. Logrono R, Kurtycz DF, Inhorn SL. Criteria for reporting fine needle aspiration on palpable and nonpalpable masses of the breast [editorial]. Acta Cytol 1997; 41(3): 623–627.

37. Page DL, Rogers LW. Combined histologic and cytologic criteria for the diagnosis of mammary atypical ductal hyperplasia. Hum Pathol 1992; 23(10): 1095–1097.

38. Ayata G, Abu-Jawdeh G, Fraser J, et al. Accuracy and reproducibility of a probabilistic approach to reporting breast fine needle aspiration (FNA) (meeting abstract). Mod Pathol 2001; 14(1): 49A.

39. Dixon JM, Bundred NJ. Management of disorders of the ductal system and infections. In: Harris JR, Lippman ME, Morrow M, Osborne CK (eds) Diseases of the breast. 2nd edn. Philadelphia, PA: Lippincott Williams & Wilkins; 2000.

40. Johnson TL, Kini SR. Cytologic and clinicopathologic features of abnormal nipple secretions: 225 cases. Diagn Cytopathol 1991; 7(1): 17–22.

41. Papanicolaou GN, Bader GM, Holmquist DG, et al. Cytologic evaluation of breast secretions. Ann NY Acad Sci 1956; 63: 1409–1421.

42. Papanicolaou GN, Holmquist DG, Bader GM, et al. Exfoliative cytology of the human mammary gland and its value in the diagnosis of cancer and other diseases of the breast. Cancer 1958; 11: 377–409.

43. Groves AM, Carr M, Wadhera V, Lennard TWJ. An audit of cytology in the evaluation of nipple discharge: a retrospective study of 10 years' experience. Breast 1996; 5: 96.

44. Buehring GC. Screening for breast atypias using exfoliative cytology. Cancer 1979; 43(5): 1788–1799.

45. Leif RC, Bobbitt D, Railey C, et al. Centrifugal cytology of nipple aspirate cells. Acta Cytol 1980; 24(3): 255–261.

46. Wrensch MR, Petrakis NL, King EB, et al. Breast cancer incidence in women with abnormal cytology in nipple aspirates of breast fluid. Am J Epidemiol 1992; 135(2): 130–141.

47. Sauter ER, Ross E, Daly M, et al. Nipple aspirate fluid: a promising non-invasive method to identify cellular markers of breast cancer risk. Br J Cancer 1997; 76(4): 494–501.

48. Hou M, Tsai K, Lin H, et al. A simple intraductal aspiration method for cytodiagnosis in nipple discharge. Acta Cytol 2000; 44(6): 1029–1034.

49. Evron E, Dooley WC, Umbricht CB, et al. Detection of breast cancer cells in ductal lavage fluid by methylation-specific PCR. Lancet 2001; 357(9265): 1335–1336.

50. Dooley WC, Ljung BM, Veronesi U, et al. Ductal lavage for detection of cellular atypia in women at high risk for breast cancer. J Natl Cancer Inst 2001; 93(21): 1624–1632.

51. Masukawa T, Kuzma JF, Straumfjord JV. Cytologic detection of early Paget's disease of breast with improved cellular collection method. Acta Cytol 1975; 19(3): 274–278.

52. Samarasinghe D, Frost F, Sterrett G, et al. Cytological diagnosis of Paget's disease of the nipple by scrape smears: a report of five cases. Diagn Cytopathol 1993; 9(3): 291–295.

53. DeMay RM. The art and science of cytopathology. Chicago: ASCP Press; 1996.

54. Dabbs DJ. Mammary ductal foam cells: macrophage immunophenotype. Hum Pathol 1993; 24(9): 977–981.

55. Wang HH, Ducatman BS, Eick D. Comparative features of ductal carcinoma in situ and infiltrating ductal carcinoma of the breast on fine-needle aspiration biopsy. Am J Clin Pathol 1989; 92(6): 736–740.

56. Sneige N, White VA, Katz RL, et al. Ductal carcinoma-in-situ of the breast: fine-needle aspiration cytology of 12 cases. Diagn Cytopathol 1989; 5(4): 371–377.

57. Silverman JF, Masood S, Ducatman BS, et al. Can FNA biopsy separate atypical hyperplasia, carcinoma in situ, and invasive carcinoma of the breast? Cytomorphologic criteria and limitations in diagnosis. Diagn Cytopathol 1993; 9(6): 713–728.

58. Sneige N, Staerkel GA. Fine-needle aspiration cytology of ductal hyperplasia with and without atypia and ductal carcinoma in situ. Hum Pathol 1994; 25(5): 485–492.

59. Venegas R, Rutgers JL, Cameron BL, et al. Fine needle aspiration cytology of breast ductal carcinoma in situ. Acta Cytol 1994; 38(2): 136–143.

60. Maygarden SJ, Brock MS, Novotny DB. Are epithelial cells in fat or connective tissue a reliable indicator of tumor invasion in fine-needle aspiration of the breast? Diagn Cytopathol 1997; 16(2): 137–142.

61. Shin HJ, Sneige N. Is a diagnosis of infiltrating versus in situ ductal carcinoma of the breast possible in fine-needle aspiration specimens? Cancer 1998; 84(3): 186–191.

62. Al-Kaisi N. The spectrum of the 'gray zone' in breast cytology. A review of 186 cases of atypical and suspicious cytology. Acta Cytol 1994; 38(6): 898–908.

63. Thomas PA, Raab SS, Cohen MB. Is the fine-needle aspiration biopsy diagnosis of proliferative breast disease feasible? Diagn Cytopathol 1994; 11(3): 301–306.

64. Frost AR, Aksu A, Kurstin R, Sidawy MK. Can nonproliferative breast disease and proliferative breast disease without atypia be distinguished by fine-needle aspiration cytology? Cancer Cytopathol 1997; 81(1): 22–28.

65. Lee WY, Wang HH. Fine-needle aspiration is limited in the classification of benign breast diseases. Diagn Cytopathol 1998; 18(1): 56–61.

66. Sidawy MK, Stoler MH, Frable WJ, et al. Interobserver variability in the classification of proliferative breast lesions by fine-needle aspiration: results of the Papanicolaou Society of Cytopathology Study. Diagn Cytopathol 1998; 18(2): 150–165.

67. Frost AR, Tabbara SO, Poprocky LA, et al. Cytologic features of proliferative breast disease: a study designed to minimize sampling error. Cancer 2000; 90(1): 33–40.

68. Sidawy MK, Tabbara SO, Bryan JA, et al. The spectrum of cytologic features in nonproliferative breast lesions. Cancer 2001; 93(2): 140–145.

69. Masood S, Frykberg ER, McLellan GL, et al. Cytologic differentiation between proliferative and nonproliferative breast disease in mammographically guided fine-needle aspirates. Diagn Cytopathol 1991; 7(6): 581–590.

70. Pisano ED, Fajardo LL, Tsimikas J, et al. Rate of insufficient samples for fine-needle aspiration for nonpalpable breast lesions in a multicenter clinical trial: The Radiologic Diagnostic Oncology Group 5 Study. The RDOG5 investigators. Cancer 1998; 82(4): 679–688.

71. Pisano ED, Fajardo LL, Caudry DJ, et al. Fine-needle aspiration biopsy of nonpalpable breast lesions in a multicenter clinical trial: results from the radiologic diagnostic oncology group V. Radiology 2001; 219(3): 785–792.

72. Hayes MK, DeBruhl ND, Hirschowitz S, et al. Mammographically guided fine-needle aspiration cytology of the breast: reducing the rate of insufficient specimens. AJR 1996; 167(2): 381–384.

73. Giard RW, Hermans J. The value of aspiration cytologic examination of the breast. A statistical review of the medical literature. Cancer 1992; 69(8): 2104–2110.

74. Lannin DR, Silverman JF, Walker C, Pories WJ. Cost-effectiveness of fine needle biopsy of the breast. Ann Surg 1986; 203(5): 474–480.

75. Silverman JF, Lannin DR, O'Brien K, Norris HT. The triage role of fine needle aspiration biopsy of palpable breast masses. Diagnostic accuracy and cost-effectiveness. Acta Cytol 1987; 31(6): 731–736.

76. Dershaw DD, Liberman L. Stereotactic breast biopsy: indications and results. Oncology (Huntingt) 1998; 12(6): 907–922.

77. Meyer JE, Smith DN, Lester SC, et al. Large-core needle biopsy of nonpalpable breast lesions. JAMA 1999; 281(17): 1638–1641.

78. Liberman L. Centennial dissertation. Percutaneous imaging-guided core breast biopsy: state of the art at the millennium. AJR 2000; 174(5): 1191–1199.

79. Liberman L, LaTrenta LR, Dershaw DD, et al. Impact of core biopsy on the surgical management of impalpable breast cancer. AJR 1997; 168(2): 495–499.

80. Smith DN, Christian R, Meyer JE. Large-core needle biopsy of nonpalpable breast cancers. The impact on subsequent surgical excisions. Arch Surg 1997; 132(3): 256–259; discussion 260.

81. Liberman L. Cost-effectiveness of percutaneous image-guided core breast biopsy. Semin Breast Dis 2001; 4: 68–77.

82. Jacobs TW, Siziopikou KP, Prioleau JE, et al. Do prognostic marker studies on core needle biopsy specimens of breast carcinoma accurately reflect the marker status of the tumor? Mod Pathol 1998; 11(3): 259–264.

83. Collins L, Connolly JL, Page D, et al. Diagnostic agreement in breast core needle biopsies: results from a randomized clinical trial. (Meeting Abstract). Mod Pathol 2000; 13: 19A.

84. Nath ME, Robinson TM, Tobon H, et al. Automated large-core needle biopsy of surgically removed breast lesions: comparison of samples obtained with 14-, 16-, and 18-gauge needles. Radiology 1995; 197(3): 739–742.

85. Berg WA, Krebs TL, Campassi C, et al. Evaluation of 14- and 11-gauge directional, vacuum-assisted biopsy probes and 14-gauge biopsy guns in a breast parenchymal model. Radiology 1997; 205(1): 203–208.

86. Burbank F, Parker SH, Fogarty TJ. Stereotactic breast biopsy: improved tissue harvesting with the Mammotome. Am Surg 1996; 62(9): 738–744.

87. Meyer JE, Smith DN, DiPiro PJ, et al. Stereotactic breast biopsy of clustered microcalcifications with a directional, vacuum-assisted device. Radiology 1997; 204(2): 575–576.

88. Liberman L, Smolkin JH, Dershaw DD, et al. Calcification retrieval at stereotactic, 11-gauge, directional, vacuum-assisted breast biopsy. Radiology 1998; 208(1): 251–260.

89. Jackman RJ, Marzoni FA Jr, Nowels KW. Percutaneous removal of benign mammographic lesions: comparison of automated large-core and directional vacuum-assisted stereotactic biopsy techniques. AJR 1998; 171(5): 1325–1330.

90. Meyer JE, Smith DN, Lester SC, et al. Large-needle core biopsy: nonmalignant breast abnormalities evaluated with surgical excision or repeat core biopsy. Radiology 1998; 206(3): 717–720.

91. Liberman L, Evans WP III, Dershaw DD, et al. Radiography of microcalcifications in stereotaxic mammary core biopsy specimens. Radiology 1994; 190(1): 223–225.

92. Mainiero MB, Philpotts LE, Lee CH, et al. Stereotaxic core needle biopsy of breast microcalcifications: correlation of target accuracy and diagnosis with lesion size. Radiology 1996; 198(3): 665–669.

93. Reynolds HE. Core needle biopsy of challenging benign breast conditions: a comprehensive literature review. AJR 2000; 174(5): 1245–1250.

94. Jacobs TW, Connolly JL, Schnitt SJ. Non-malignant lesions in breast core needle biopsies: to excise or not to excise? Am J Surg Pathol 2002; 26(9): 1095–1110.

95. Renshaw AA. Adequate histologic sampling of breast core needle biopsies. Arch Pathol Lab Med 2001; 125(8): 1055–1057.

96. Jacobs TW, Silverman JF, Schroeder B, et al. Accuracy of touch imprint cytology of image-directed breast core needle biopsies. Acta Cytol 1999; 43(2): 169–714.

97. Jackman RJ, Nowels KW, Shepard MJ, et al. Stereotaxic large-core needle biopsy of 450 nonpalpable breast lesions with surgical correlation in lesions with cancer or atypical hyperplasia. Radiology 1994; 193(1): 91–95.

98. Liberman L, Cohen MA, Dershaw DD, et al. Atypical ductal hyperplasia diagnosed at stereotaxic core biopsy of breast lesions: an indication for surgical biopsy. AJR 1995; 164(5): 1111–1113.

99. Dahlstrom JE, Sutton S, Jain S. Histological precision of stereotactic core biopsy in diagnosis of malignant and premalignant breast lesions. Histopathology 1996; 28(6): 537–541.

100. Moore MM, Hargett CW III, Hanks JB, et al. Association of breast cancer with the finding of atypical ductal hyperplasia at core breast biopsy. Ann Surg 1997; 225(6): 726–731; discussion 731–733.

101. Jackman RJ, Nowels KW, Rodriguez-Soto J, et al. Stereotactic, automated, large-core needle biopsy of nonpalpable breast lesions: false-negative and histologic underestimation rates after long-term follow-up. Radiology 1999; 210(3): 799–805.

102. Bassett L, Winchester DP, Caplan RB, et al. Stereotactic core-needle biopsy of the breast: a report of the Joint Task Force of the American College of Radiology, American College of Surgeons, and College of American Pathologists. CA Cancer J Clin 1997; 47(3): 171–190.

103. Schnitt SJ, Abner A, Gelman R, et al. The relationship between microscopic margins of resection and the risk of local recurrence in patients with breast cancer treated with breast-conserving surgery and radiation therapy. Cancer 1994; 74(6): 1746–1751.

104. Gage I, Schnitt SJ, Nixon AJ, et al. Pathologic margin involvement and the risk of recurrence in patients treated with breast-conserving therapy. Cancer 1996; 78(9): 1921–1928.

105. Smitt MC, Nowels KW, Zdeblick MJ, et al. The importance of the lumpectomy surgical margin status in long-term results of breast conservation. Cancer 1995; 76(2): 259–267.

106. Solin LJ, Fowble BL, Schultz DJ, Goodman RL. The significance of the pathology margins of the tumor excision on the outcome of patients treated with definitive irradiation for early stage breast cancer. Int J Radiat Oncol Biol Phys 1991; 21(2): 279–287.

107. Wazer DE, Schmidt-Ullrich RK, Ruthazer R, et al. Factors determining outcome for breast-conserving irradiation with margin-directed dose escalation to the tumor bed. Int J Radiat Oncol Biol Phys 1998; 40(4): 851–858.

108. Park CC, Mitsumori M, Nixon A, et al. Outcome at 8 years after breast-conserving surgery and radiation therapy for invasive breast cancer: influence of margin status and systemic therapy on local recurrence. J Clin Oncol 2000; 18(8): 1668–1675.

109. Schnitt SJ, Connolly JL. Processing and evaluation of breast excision specimens. A clinically oriented approach. Am J Clin Pathol 1992; 98(1): 125–137.

110. Carter D. Margins of 'lumpectomy' for breast cancer. Hum Pathol 1986; 17(4): 330–332.

111. Guidi AJ, Connolly JL, Harris JR, Schnitt SJ. The relationship between shaved margin and inked margin status in breast excision specimens. Cancer 1997; 79(8): 1568–1573.

112. Consensus Conference on the classification of ductal carcinoma in situ. The Consensus Conference Committee. Cancer 1997; 80(9): 1798–1802.

113. Graham RA, Homer MJ, Sigler CJ, et al. The efficacy of specimen radiography in evaluating the surgical margins of impalpable breast carcinoma. AJR 1994; 162(1): 33–36.

114. Lee CH, Carter D. Detecting residual tumor after excisional biopsy of impalpable breast carcinoma: efficacy of comparing preoperative mammograms with radiographs of the biopsy specimen. AJR 1995; 164(1): 81–86.

115. Graham RA, Homer MJ, Katz J, et al. The pancake phenomenon contributes to the inaccuracy of margin assessment in patients with breast cancer. Am J Surg 2002; 184(2): 89–93.

116. Radi MJ. Calcium oxalate crystals in breast biopsies. An overlooked form of microcalcification associated with benign breast disease. Arch Pathol Lab Med 1989; 113(12): 1367–1369.

117. Bianchi S, Palli D, Ciatto S, et al. Accuracy and reliability of frozen section diagnosis in a series of 672 nonpalpable breast lesions. Am J Clin Pathol 1995; 103(2): 199–205.

118. Ferreiro JA, Gisvold JJ, Bostwick DG. Accuracy of frozen-section diagnosis of mammographically directed breast biopsies. Results of 1,490 consecutive cases. Am J Surg Pathol 1995; 19(11): 1267–1271.

119. Connolly JL, Fechner RE, Page DL, Silverberg SG. Immediate management of mammographically detected breast lesions. Association of Directors of Anatomic and Surgical Pathology. Am J Surg Pathol 1993; 17(8): 850–851.

120. Lee KC, Chan JK, Ho LC. Histologic changes in the breast after fine-needle aspiration. Am J Surg Pathol 1994; 18(10): 1039–1047.

121. Youngson BJ, Cranor M, Rosen PP. Epithelial displacement in surgical breast specimens following needling procedures. Am J Surg Pathol 1994; 18(9): 896–903.

122. Youngson BJ, Liberman L, Rosen PP. Displacement of carcinomatous epithelium in surgical breast

123. Tavassoli FA, Pestaner JP. Pseudoinvasion in intraductal carcinoma. Mod Pathol 1995; 8(4): 380–383.

124. Diaz LK, Wiley EL, Venta LA. Are malignant cells displaced by large-gauge needle core biopsy of the breast? AJR 1999; 173(5): 1303–1313.

125. Abraham SC, Fox K, Fraker D, et al. Sampling of grossly benign breast reexcisions: a multidisciplinary approach to assessing adequacy. Am J Surg Pathol 1999; 23(3): 316–322.

126. Honkoop AH, Pinedo HM, De Jong JS, et al. Effects of chemotherapy on pathologic and biologic characteristics of locally advanced breast cancer. Am J Clin Pathol 1997; 107(2): 211–218.

127. Bonadonna G, Valagussa P, Brambilla C, et al. Primary chemotherapy in operable breast cancer: eight-year experience at the Milan Cancer Institute. J Clin Oncol 1998; 16(1): 93–100.

128. Kuerer HM, Newman LA, Smith TL, et al. Clinical course of breast cancer patients with complete pathologic primary tumor and axillary lymph node response to doxorubicin-based neoadjuvant chemotherapy. J Clin Oncol 1999; 17(2): 460–469.

129. Fisher ER, Wang J, Bryant J, et al. Pathobiology of preoperative chemotherapy: findings from the National Surgical Adjuvant Breast and Bowel (NSABP) protocol B-18.Cancer 2002; 95(4): 681–695.

130. Andersen J, Jensen J. Lymph node identification. Specimen radiography of tissue predominated by fat. Am J Clin Pathol 1977; 68(4): 511–512.

131. Groote AD, Oosterhuis JW, Molenaar WM, et al. Radiographic imaging of lymph nodes in lymph node dissection specimens. Lab Invest 1985; 52(3): 326–329.

132. Durkin K, Haagensen CD. An improved technique for the study of lymph nodes in surgical specimens. Ann Surg 1980; 191(4): 419–429.

133. Morrow M, Evans J, Rosen PP, Kinne DW. Does clearing of axillary lymph nodes contribute to accurate staging of breast carcinoma? Cancer 1984; 53(6): 1329–1332.

134. Krag DN, Weaver DL, Alex JC, Fairbank JT. Surgical resection and radiolocalization of the sentinel lymph node in breast cancer using a gamma probe. Surg Oncol 1993; 2(6): 335–339; discussion 340.

135. Giuliano AE, Kirgan DM, Guenther JM, Morton DL. Lymphatic mapping and sentinel lymphadenectomy for breast cancer. Ann Surg 1994; 220(3): 391–398; discussion 398–401.

136. Albertini JJ, Lyman GH, Cox C, et al. Lymphatic mapping and sentinel node biopsy in the patient with breast cancer. Jama 1996; 276(22): 1818–1822.

137. Veronesi U, Paganelli G, Galimberti V, et al. Sentinel-node biopsy to avoid axillary dissection in breast cancer with clinically negative lymph-nodes. Lancet 1997; 349(9069): 1864–1867.

138. Krag D, Weaver D, Ashikaga T, et al. The sentinel node in breast cancer – a multicenter validation study. N Engl J Med 1998; 339(14): 941–946.

139. Rosen PP, Kimmel M, Ernsberger D. Mammary angiosarcoma. The prognostic significance of tumor differentiation. Cancer 1988; 62(10): 2145–2151.

140. De Mascarel I, Bonichon F, Coindre JM, Trojani M. Prognostic significance of breast cancer axillary lymph node micrometastases assessed by two special techniques: reevaluation with longer follow-up. Br J Cancer 1992; 66(3): 523–527.

141. Niemann TH, Yilmaz AG, Marsh WL Jr, Lucas JG. A half a node or a whole node: a comparison of methods for submitting lymph nodes. Am J Clin Pathol 1998; 109(5): 571–576.

142. Zhang PJ, Reisner RM, Nangia R, et al. Effectiveness of multiple-level sectioning in detecting axillary nodal micrometastasis in breast cancer: a retrospective study with immunohistochemical analysis. Arch Pathol Lab Med 1998; 122(8): 687–690.

143. Lucci A Jr, Kelemen PR, Miller C III, et al. National practice patterns of sentinel lymph node dissection for breast carcinoma. J Am Coll Surg 2001; 192(4): 453–458

144. Turner R. Histopathologic processing of the sentinel lymph node. Semin Breast Dis 2002; 5: 35–40.

145. Fitzgibbons PL, Page DL, Weaver D, et al. Prognostic factors in breast cancer. College of American Pathologists Consensus Statement 1999. Arch Pathol Lab Med 2000; 124(7): 966–978.

146. Schwartz GF, Giuliano AE, Veronesi U. Proceedings of the consensus conference on the role of sentinel lymph node biopsy in carcinoma of the breast, April 19–22, 2001, Philadelphia, Pennsylvania. Cancer 2002; 94(10): 2542–2551.

147. Trojani M, de Mascarel I, Bonichon F, et al. Micrometastases to axillary lymph nodes from carcinoma of breast: detection by immunohistochemistry and prognostic significance. Br J Cancer 1987; 55(3): 303–306.

148. Sedmak DD, Meineke TA, Knechtges DS, Anderson J. Prognostic significance of cytokeratin-positive breast cancer metastases. Mod Pathol 1989; 2(5): 516–520.

149. Noguchi S, Aihara T, Nakamori S, et al. The detection of breast carcinoma micrometastases in axillary lymph nodes by means of reverse transcriptase-polymerase chain reaction. Cancer 1994; 74(5): 1595–1600.

150. Huvos AG, Hutter RV, Berg JW. Significance of axillary macrometastases and micrometastases in mammary cancer. Ann Surg 1971; 173(1): 44–46.

151. Clayton F, Hopkins CL. Pathologic correlates of prognosis in lymph node-positive breast carcinomas. Cancer 1993; 71(5): 1780–1790.

152. Rosen PP, Saigo PE, Braun DW Jr, et al. Occult axillary lymph node metastases from breast cancers with intramammary lymphatic tumor emboli. Am J Surg Pathol 1982; 6(7): 639–641.

153. Carter BA, Simpson JF, Jensen RA, Page DL. Significance of and redefinition of types of micrometastases in the sentinel node. Semin Breast Dis 2002; 5: 41–46.

154. AJCC Cancer Staging Manual. 6th ed. New York: Springer; 2002.

155. Rubio IT, Korourian S, Cowan C, et al. Use of touch preps for intraoperative diagnosis of sentinel lymph node metastases in breast cancer. Ann Surg Oncol 1998; 5(8): 689–694.

156. Kane RA III, Edge SB, Winston JS, et al. Intraoperative pathologic evaluation of a breast cancer sentinel lymph node biopsy as a determinant for synchronous axillary lymph node dissection. Ann Surg Oncol 2001; 8(4): 361–367.

157. Lee A, Krishnamurthy MD, Sahin A, et al. Intraoperative touch imprint of sentinel lymph nodes in breast carcinoma patients. Cancer 2002; 25;96(4): 225–231.

158. Page DL, Dupont WD. Anatomic indicators (histologic and cytologic) of increased breast cancer risk. Breast Cancer Res Treat 1993; 28(2): 157–166.

159. Wellings SR, Jensen HM, Marcum RG. An atlas of subgross pathology of the human breast with special reference to possible precancerous lesions. J Natl Cancer Inst 1975; 55(2): 231–273.

160. Kodlin D, Winger EE, Morgenstern NL, Chen U. Chronic mastopathy and breast cancer. A follow-up study. Cancer 1977; 39(6): 2603–2607.

161. Dupont WD, Page DL. Risk factors for breast cancer in women with proliferative breast disease. N Engl J Med 1985; 312(3): 146–151.

162. Carter CL, Corle DK, Micozzi MS, et al. A prospective study of the development of breast cancer in 16,692 women with benign breast disease. Am J Epidemiol 1988; 128(3): 467–477.

163. Tavassoli FA, Norris HJ. A comparison of the results of long-term follow-up for atypical intraductal hyperplasia and intraductal hyperplasia of the breast. Cancer 1990; 65(3): 518–529.

164. Palli D, Rosselli del Turco M, Simoncini R, Bianchi S. Benign breast disease and breast cancer: a case-control study in a cohort in Italy. Int J Cancer 1991; 47(5): 703–706.

165. London SJ, Connolly JL, Schnitt SJ, Colditz GA. A prospective study of benign breast disease and the risk of breast cancer. JAMA 1992; 267(7): 941–944.

166. Krieger N, Hiatt RA. Risk of breast cancer after benign breast diseases. Variation by histologic type, degree of atypia, age at biopsy, and length of follow-up. Am J Epidemiol 1992; 135(6): 619–631.

167. McDivitt RW, Stevens JA, Lee NC, et al. Histologic types of benign breast disease and the risk for breast cancer. The Cancer and Steroid Hormone Study Group. Cancer 1992; 69(6): 1408–1414.

168. Dupont WD, Parl FF, Hartmann WH, et al. Breast cancer risk associated with proliferative breast disease and atypical hyperplasia. Cancer 1993; 71(4): 1258–1265.

169. Bodian CA, Perzin KH, Lattes R, et al. Prognostic significance of benign proliferative breast disease. Cancer 1993; 71(12): 3896–3907.

170. Marshall LM, Hunter DJ, Connolly JL, et al. Risk of breast cancer associated with atypical hyperplasia of lobular and ductal types. Cancer Epidemiol Biomarkers Prev 1997; 6(5): 297–301.

171. Shaaban AM, Sloane JP, West CR, et al. Histopathologic types of benign breast lesions and the risk of breast cancer: case-control study. Am J Surg Pathol 2002; 26(4): 421–430.

172. Love SM, Gelman RS, Silen W. Sounding board. Fibrocystic 'disease' of the breast–a nondisease? N Engl J Med 1982; 307(16): 1010–1014.

173. Hutter RV. Goodbye to 'fibrocystic disease' [editorial]. N Engl J Med 1985; 312(3): 179–181.

174. Hughes LE, Mansel RE, Webster DJ. Aberrations of normal development and involution (ANDI): a new perspective on pathogenesis and nomenclature of benign breast disorders. Lancet 1987; 2(8571): 1316–1319.

175. Page DL, Dupont WD, Rogers LW, Rados MS. Atypical hyperplastic lesions of the female breast. A long-term follow-up study. Cancer 1985; 55(11): 2698–2708.

176. Haagensen CD. Diseases of the breast, 3rd ed. Philadelphia, PA: WB Saunders; 1986.

177. Jensen RA, Page DL, Dupont WD, Rogers LW. Invasive breast cancer risk in women with sclerosing adenosis. Cancer 1989; 64(10): 1977–1983.

178. Dupont WD, Page DL, Parl FF, et al. Long-term risk of breast cancer in women with fibroadenoma. N Engl J Med 1994; 331(1): 10–15.

179. Nielsen BB. Adenosis tumour of the breast–a clinicopathological investigation of 27 cases. Histopathology 1987; 11(12): 1259–1275.

180. Seidman JD, Ashton M, Lefkowitz M. Atypical apocrine adenosis of the breast: a clinicopathologic study of 37 patients with 8.7-year follow-up. Cancer 1996; 77(12): 2529–2537.

181. Eusebi V, Damiani S, Losi L, Millis RR. Apocrine differentiation in breast epithelium. Adv Anat pathol 1997; 4: 139.

182. Carter DJ, Rosen PP. Atypical apocrine metaplasia in sclerosing lesions of the breast: a study of 51 patients. Mod Pathol 1991; 4(1): 1–5.

183. Fechner RE. Lobular carcinoma in situ in sclerosing adenosis. A potential source of confusion with invasive carcinoma. Am J Surg Pathol 1981; 5(3): 233–239.

184. Chan JK, Ng WF. Sclerosing adenosis cancerized by intraductal carcinoma. Pathology 1987; 19(4): 425–428.

185. Eusebi V, Collina G, Bussolati G. Carcinoma in situ in sclerosing adenosis of the breast: an immunocytochemical study. Semin Diagn Pathol 1989; 6(2): 146–152.

186. Fechner RE. Carcinoma in situ involving sclerosing adenosis. Histopathology 1996; 28(6): 570.

187. Taylor HB, Norris HJ. Epithelial invasion of nerves in benign diseases of the breast. Cancer 1967; 20(12): 2245–2249.

188. Jensen RA, Dupont WD, Page DL. Diagnostic criteria and cancer risk of proliferative breast lesions. J Cell Biochem Suppl 1993; 17G:59–64.

189. Page DL, Anderson TJ. Diagnostic histopathology of the breast. Edinburgh: Churchill Livingstone; 1987.

190. Page DL, Dupont WD, Rogers LW. Ductal involvement by cells of atypical lobular hyperplasia in the breast: a long-term follow-up study of cancer risk. Hum Pathol 1988; 19(2): 201–207.

191. Schnitt SJ, Wang HH. Histologic sampling of grossly benign breast biopsies. How much is enough? Am J Surg Pathol 1989; 13(6): 505–512.

192. Owings DV, Hann L, Schnitt SJ. How thoroughly should needle localization breast biopsies be sampled for microscopic examination? A prospective mammographic/pathologic correlative study. Am J Surg Pathol 1990; 14(6): 578–583.

193. Rubin E, Visscher DW, Alexander RW, et al. Proliferative disease and atypia in biopsies performed for nonpalpable lesions detected mammographically. Cancer 1988; 61(10): 2077–2082.

194. Page DL, Schuyler PA, Dupont WD, et al. Atypical lobular hyperplasia as a unilateral predictor of breast cancer risk: a retrospective cohort study. Lancet 2003; 361(9352): 125–129.

195. Azzopardi JG. Problems in breast pathology. Philadelphia, PA: WB Saunders; 1979.

196. Goodman ZD, Taxy JB. Fibroadenomas of the breast with prominent smooth muscle. Am J Surg Pathol 1981; 5(1): 99–101.

197. Oberman HA. Breast lesions in the adolescent female. In: Sommers SC, Rosen PP (eds) Pathology annual, part 1. Norwalk, CT: Appleton-Century-Crofts; 1979.

198. Nambiar R, Kutty MK. Giant fibro-adenoma (cystosarcoma phyllodes) in adolescent females – a clinicopathological study. Br J Surg 1974; 61(2): 113–117.

199. Ashikari R, Farrow JH, O'Hara J. Fibroadenomas in the breast of juveniles. Surg Gynecol Obstet 1971; 132(2): 259–262.

200. Mies C, Rosen PP. Juvenile fibroadenoma with atypical epithelial hyperplasia. Am J Surg Pathol 1987; 11(3): 184–190.

201. Carter BA, Page DL, Schuyler P, et al. No elevation in long-term breast carcinoma risk for women with fibroadenomas that contain atypical hyperplasia. Cancer 2001; 92(1): 30–3.

202. Pick PW, Iossifides IA. Occurrence of breast carcinoma within a fibroadenoma. A review. Arch Pathol Lab Med 1984; 108(7): 590–594.

203. Moffat CJ, Pinder SE, Dixon AR, et al. Phyllodes tumours of the breast: a clinicopathological review of thirty-two cases. Histopathology 1995; 27(3): 205–218.

204. Hawkins RE, Schofield JB, Fisher C, et al. The clinical and histologic criteria that predict metastases from cystosarcoma phyllodes. Cancer 1992; 69(1): 141–147.

205. Norris HJ, Taylor HB. Relationship of histologic features to behavior of cystosarcoma phyllodes. Analysis of ninety-four cases. Cancer 1967; 20(12): 2090–2099.

206. Qizilbash AH. Cystosarcoma phyllodes with liposarcomatous stroma. Am J Clin Pathol 1976; 65(3): 321–327.

207. Cohn-Cedermark G, Rutqvist LE, Rosendahl I, Silfversward C. Prognostic factors in cystosarcoma phyllodes. A clinicopathologic study of 77 patients. Cancer 1991; 68(9): 2017–2022.

208. Ward RM, Evans HL. Cystosarcoma phyllodes. A clinicopathological study of 26 cases. Cancer 1986; 58(10): 2282–2289.

209. Elston CE, Ellis IO. The breast. Edinburgh: Churchill Livingstone; 1998.

210. Hajdu SI, Espinosa MH, Robbins GF. Recurrent cystosarcoma phyllodes: a clinicopathologic study of 32 cases. Cancer 1976; 38(3): 1402–1406.

211. McDivitt RW, Urban JA, Farrow JH. Cystosarcoma phyllodes. Johns Hopkins Med J 1967; 120(1): 33–45.

212. Pietruszka M, Barnes L. Cystosarcoma phyllodes: a clinicopathologic analysis of 42 cases. Cancer 1978; 41(5): 1974–1983.

213. Hart WR, Bauer RC, Oberman HA. Cystosarcoma phyllodes. A clinicopathologic study of twenty-six hypercellular periductal stromal tumors of the breast. Am J Clin Pathol 1978; 70(2): 211–216.

214. Hines JR, Murad TM, Beal JM. Prognostic indicators in cystosarcoma phylloides. Am J Surg 1987; 153(3): 276–280.

215. Salvadori B, Cusumano F, Del Bo R, et al. Surgical treatment of phyllodes tumors of the breast. Cancer 1989; 63(12): 2532–2536.

216. Bottles K, Chan JS, Holly EA, et al. Cytologic criteria for fibroadenoma. A step-wise logistic regression analysis. Am J Clin Pathol 1988; 89(6): 707–713.

217. Dejmek A, Lindholm K. Frequency of cytologic features in fine needle aspirates from histologically and cytologically diagnosed fibroadenomas. Acta Cytol 1991; 35(6): 695–699.

218. Stanley MW, Tani EM, Rutqvist LE, Skoog L. Cystosarcoma phyllodes of the breast: a cytologic and clinicopathologic study of 23 cases. Diagn Cytopathol 1989; 5(1): 29–34.

219. Dusenbery D, Frable WJ. Fine needle aspiration cytology of phyllodes tumor. Potential diagnostic pitfalls. Acta Cytol 1992; 36(2): 215–221.

220. Shimizu K, Masawa N, Yamada T, et al. Cytologic evaluation of phyllodes tumors as compared to fibroadenomas of the breast. Acta Cytol 1994; 38(6): 891–897.

221. Krishnamurthy S, Ashfaq R, Shin HJ, Sneige N. Distinction of phyllodes tumor from fibroadenoma: a reappraisal of an old problem. Cancer 2000; 90(6): 342–349.

222. Kline TS. Masquerades of malignancy: a review of 4,241 aspirates from the breast. Acta Cytol 1981; 25(3): 263–266.

223. Stanley MW, Tani EM, Skoog L. Fine-needle aspiration of fibroadenomas of the breast with atypia: a spectrum including cases that cytologically mimic carcinoma. Diagn Cytopathol 1990; 6(6): 375–382.

224. Benoit JL, Kara R, McGregor SE, Duggan MA. Fibroadenoma of the breast: diagnostic pitfalls of fine-needle aspiration. Diagn Cytopathol 1992; 8(6): 643–647; discussion 647–648.

225. Simsir A, Waisman J, Cangiarella J. Fibroadenomas with atypia: causes of under- and overdiagnosis by aspiration biopsy. Diagn Cytopathol 2001; 25(5): 278–284.

226. Hertel BF, Zaloudek C, Kempson RL. Breast adenomas. Cancer 1976; 37(6): 2891–2905.

227. Mulvany N, Lowhagen T, Skoog L. Fine needle aspiration cytology of tubular adenoma of the breast. A report of two cases. Acta Cytol 1994; 38(6): 961–964.

228. Novotny DB, Maygarden SJ, Shermer RW, Frable WJ. Fine needle aspiration of benign and malignant breast masses associated with pregnancy. Acta Cytol 1991; 35(6): 676–686.

229. Mitre BK, Kanbour AI, Mauser N. Fine needle aspiration biopsy of breast carcinoma in pregnancy and lactation. Acta Cytol 1997; 41(4): 1121–1130.

230. O'Connell P, Pekkel V, Fuqua SA, et al. Analysis of loss of heterozygosity in 399 premalignant breast lesions at 15 genetic loci. J Natl Cancer Inst 1998; 90(9): 697–703.

231. Rosen PP. Syringomatous adenoma of the nipple. Am J Surg Pathol 1983; 7(8): 739–745.

232. Jones MW, Norris HJ, Snyder RC. Infiltrating syringomatous adenoma of the nipple. A clinical and pathological study of 11 cases. Am J Surg Pathol 1989; 13(3): 197–201.

233. Chen KT. Pleomorphic adenoma of the breast. Am J Clin Pathol 1990; 93(6): 792–794.

234. Moran CA, Suster S, Carter D. Benign mixed tumors (pleomorphic adenomas) of the breast. Am J Surg Pathol 1990; 14(10): 913–921.

235. Ballance WA, Ro JY, el-Naggar AK, et al. Pleomorphic adenoma (benign mixed tumor) of the breast. An immunohistochemical, flow cytometric, and ultrastructural study and review of the literature. Am J Clin Pathol 1990; 93(6): 795–801.

236. Rosen PP, Oberman HA. Tumors of the mammary gland. Washington, DC: Armed Forces Institute of Pathology; 1993.

237. Jones DB. Florid papillomatosis of the nipple ducts. Cancer 1955; 8: 315.

238. Perzin KH, Lattes R. Papillary adenoma of the nipple (florid papillomatosis, adenoma, adenomatosis). A clinicopathologic study. Cancer 1972; 29(4): 996–1009.

239. Smith EJ, Kron SD, Gross PR. Erosive adenomatosis of the nipple. Arch Dermatol 1970; 102(3): 330–332.

240. Rosen PP, Caicco JA. Florid papillomatosis of the nipple. A study of 51 patients, including nine with mammary carcinoma. Am J Surg Pathol 1986; 10(2): 87–101.

241. Azzopardi JG, Salm R. Ductal adenoma of the breast: a lesion which can mimic carcinoma. J Pathol 1984; 144(1): 15–23.

242. Lammie GA, Millis RR. Ductal adenoma of the breast – a review of fifteen cases. Hum Pathol 1989; 20(9): 903–908.

243. Kraus FT, Neubecker RD. The differential diagnosis of papillary tumors of the breast. Cancer 1962; 15: 444–455.

244. Yaziji H, Gown AM, Sneige N. Detection of stromal invasion in breast cancer: the myoepithelial markers. Adv Anat Pathol 2000; 7(2): 100–109.

245. Noguchi S, Motomura K, Inaji H, et al. Clonal analysis of solitary intraductal papilloma of the breast by means of polymerase chain reaction. Am J Pathol 1994; 144(6): 1320–1325.

246. Flint A, Oberman HA. Infarction and squamous metaplasia of intraductal papilloma: a benign breast lesion that may simulate carcinoma. Hum Pathol 1984; 15(8): 764–767.

247. Page DL, Salhany KE, Jensen RA, Dupont WD. Subsequent breast carcinoma risk after biopsy with atypia in a breast papilloma. Cancer 1996; 78(2): 258–266.

248. Ohuchi N, Abe R, Kasai M. Possible cancerous change of intraductal papillomas of the breast. A 3-D reconstruction study of 25 cases. Cancer 1984; 54(4): 605–611.

249. Papotti M, Gugliotta P, Ghiringhello B, Bussolati G. Association of breast carcinoma and multiple intraductal papillomas: an histological and immunohistochemical investigation. Histopathology 1984; 8(6): 963–975.

250. Jeffrey PB, Ljung BM. Benign and malignant papillary lesions of the breast. A cytomorphologic study. Am J Clin Pathol 1994; 101(4): 500–507.

251. Bardales RH, Suhrland MJ, Stanley MW. Papillary neoplasms of the breast: fine-needle aspiration findings in cystic and solid cases. Diagn Cytopathol 1994; 10(4): 336–341.

252. Kline TS, Kannan V. Papillary carcinoma of the breast. A cytomorphologic analysis. Arch Pathol Lab Med 1986; 110(3): 189–191.

253. Naran S, Simpson J, Gupta RK. Cytologic diagnosis of papillary carcinoma of the breast in needle aspirates. Diagn Cytopathol 1988; 4(1): 33–37.

254. Corkill ME, Sneige N, Fanning T, el-Naggar A. Fine-needle aspiration cytology and flow cytometry of intracystic papillary carcinoma of breast. Am J Clin Pathol 1990; 94(6): 673–680.

255. Nguyen GK, Redburn J. Aspiration biopsy cytology of papillary carcinoma of the breast. Diagn Cytopathol 1992; 8(5): 511–516.

256. Dei Tos AP, Della Giustina D, Bittesini L. Aspiration biopsy cytology of malignant papillary breast neoplasms. Diagn Cytopathol 1992; 8(6): 580–584.

257. Rosen PP, Cantrell B, Mullen DL, DePalo A. Juvenile papillomatosis (Swiss cheese disease) of the breast. Am J Surg Pathol 1980; 4(1): 3–12.

258. Rosen PP, Lyngholm B, Kinne DW, Beattie EJ Jr. Juvenile papillomatosis of the breast and family history of breast carcinoma. Cancer 1982; 49(12): 2591–2595.

259. Rosen PP, Holmes G, Lesser ML, et al. Juvenile papillomatosis and breast carcinoma. Cancer 1985; 55(6): 1345–1352.

260. Bazzocchi F, Santini D, Martinelli G, et al. Juvenile papillomatosis (epitheliosis) of the breast. A clinical and pathologic study of 13 cases. Am J Clin Pathol 1986; 86(6): 745–748.

261. Rosen PP, Kimmel M. Juvenile papillomatosis of the breast. A follow-up study of 41 patients having biopsies before 1979. Am J Clin Pathol 1990; 93(5): 599–603.

262. Clement PB, Azzopardi JG. Microglandular adenosis of the breast–a lesion simulating tubular carcinoma. Histopathology 1983; 7(2): 169–180.

263. Rosen PP. Microglandular adenosis. A benign lesion simulating invasive mammary carcinoma. Am J Surg Pathol 1983; 7(2): 137–144.

264. Tavassoli FA, Norris HJ. Microglandular adenosis of the breast. A clinicopathologic study of 11 cases with ultrastructural observations. Am J Surg Pathol 1983; 7(8): 731–737.

265. Millis RR. Microglandular adenosis of the breast. Adv Anat Pathol 1995; 2: 10.

266. Diaz NM, McDivitt RW, Wick MR. Microglandular adenosis of the breast. An immunohistochemical comparison with tubular carcinoma. Arch Pathol Lab Med 1991; 115(6): 578–582.

267. Tavassoli FA, Bratthauer GL. Immunohistochemical profile and differential diagnosis of microglandular adenosis. Mod Pathol 1993; 6(3): 318–322.

268. Rosenblum MK, Purrazzella R, Rosen PP. Is microglandular adenosis a precancerous disease? A study of carcinoma arising in microglandular adenosis. Lab Invest 1985; 52: 57A.

269. James BA, Cranor ML, Rosen PP. Carcinoma of the breast arising in microglandular adenosis. Am J Clin Pathol 1993; 100(5): 507–513.

270. Koenig C, Dadmanesh F, Bratthauer GL, Tavassoli FA. Carcinoma arising in microglandular adenosis: an immunohistochemical analysis of 20 intraepithelial and invasive neoplasms. Int J Surg Pathol 2000; 8(4): 303–315.

271. Semb C. Pathologico-anatomical and clinical investigations of fibro-adenomatosis cystica mammae and its relation to other pathological conditions in the mamma, especially cancer. Acta Chir Scand (Suppl) 1928; 64: 1–484.

272. Linell F, Ljungberg O, Anderson I. Breast carcinoma. Aspects of early stages, progression and related problems. Acta Pathol Microbiol Scand Suppl 1980(272): 1–233.

273. Hamperl H. Strahlige Narben und obliterierende Mastopathie. Beitrage zur pathologischen Histologie der Mamma. XI. Virchows Arch A Pathol Anat Histol 1975; 369(1): 55–68.

274. Fenoglio C, Lattes R. Sclerosing papillary proliferations in the female breast. A benign lesion often mistaken for carcinoma. Cancer 1974; 33(3): 691–700.

275. Fisher ER, Palekar AS, Kotwal N, Lipana N. A nonencapsulated sclerosing lesion of the breast. Am J Clin Pathol 1979; 71(3): 240–246.

276. Rickert RR, Kalisher L, Hutter RV. Indurative mastopathy: a benign sclerosing lesion of breast with elastosis which may simulate carcinoma. Cancer 1981; 47(3): 561–571.

277. Andersen JA, Gram JB. Radial scar in the female breast. A long-term follow-up study of 32 cases. Cancer 1984; 53(11): 2557–2560.

278. Jacobs TW, Byrne C, Colditz G, et al. Radial scars in benign breast-biopsy specimens and the risk of breast cancer. N Engl J Med 1999; 340(6): 430–436.

279. Anderson TJ, Battersby S. Radial scars of benign and malignant breasts: comparative features and significance. J Pathol 1985; 147(1): 23–32.

280. Sloane JP, Mayers MM. Carcinoma and atypical hyperplasia in radial scars and complex sclerosing lesions: importance of lesion size and patient age. Histopathology 1993; 23(3): 225–231.

281. Wellings SR, Alpers CE. Subgross pathologic features and incidence of radial scars in the breast. Hum Pathol 1984; 15(5): 475–479.

282. Nielsen M, Jensen J, Andersen JA. An autopsy study of radial scar in the female breast. Histopathology 1985; 9(3): 287–295.

283. Nielsen M, Christensen L, Andersen J. Radial scars in women with breast cancer. Cancer 1987; 59(5): 1019–1025.

284. Damiani S, Koerner FC, Dickersin GR, et al. Granular cell tumour of the breast. Virchows Arch A Pathol Anat Histopathol 1992; 420(3): 219–226.

285. Wargotz ES, Norris HJ, Austin RM, Enzinger FM. Fibromatosis of the breast. A clinical and pathological study of 28 cases. Am J Surg Pathol 1987; 11(1): 38–45.

286. Rosen PP, Ernsberger D. Mammary fibromatosis. A benign spindle-cell tumor with significant risk for local recurrence. Cancer 1989; 63(7): 1363–1369.

287. Rosen PP, Ridolfi RL. The perilobular hemangioma. A benign microscopic vascular lesion of the breast. Am J Clin Pathol 1977; 68(1): 21–23.

288. Jozefczyk MA, Rosen PP. Vascular tumors of the breast. II. Perilobular hemangiomas and hemangiomas. Am J Surg Pathol 1985; 9(7): 491–503.

289. Rosen PP. Vascular tumors of the breast. III. Angiomatosis. Am J Surg Pathol 1985; 9(9): 652–658.

290. Rosen PP, Jozefczyk MA, Boram LH. Vascular tumors of the breast. IV. The venous hemangioma. Am J Surg Pathol 1985; 9(9): 659–665.

291. Rosen PP. Vascular tumors of the breast. V. Nonparenchymal hemangiomas of mammary subcutaneous tissues. Am J Surg Pathol 1985; 9(10): 723–729.

292. Donnell RM, Rosen PP, Lieberman PH, et al. Angiosarcoma and other vascular tumors of the breast. Am J Surg Pathol 1981; 5(7): 629–642.

293. Fineberg S, Rosen PP. Cutaneous angiosarcoma and atypical vascular lesions of the skin and breast after radiation therapy for breast carcinoma. Am J Clin Pathol 1994; 102(6): 757–763.

294. Vuitch MF, Rosen PP, Erlandson RA. Pseudoangiomatous hyperplasia of mammary stroma. Hum Pathol 1986; 17(2): 185–191.

295. Cohen MB, Fisher PE. Schwann cell tumors of the breast and mammary region. Surg Pathol 1991; 4: 47–56.

296. Rosen PP. Adenomyoepithelioma of the breast. Hum Pathol 1987; 18(12): 1232–1237.

297. Tavassoli FA. Myoepithelial lesions of the breast. Myoepitheliosis, adenomyoepithelioma, and myoepithelial carcinoma. Am J Surg Pathol 1991; 15(6): 554–568.

298. Eusebi V, Casadei GP, Bussolati G, Azzopardi JG. Adenomyoepithelioma of the breast with a distinctive type of apocrine adenosis. Histopathology 1987; 11(3): 305–315.

299. Wargotz ES, Deos PH, Norris HJ. Metaplastic carcinomas of the breast. II. Spindle cell carcinoma. Hum Pathol 1989; 20(8): 732–740.

300. Wargotz ES, Norris HJ. Metaplastic carcinomas of the breast. I. Matrix-producing carcinoma. Hum Pathol 1989; 20(7): 628–635.

301. Wargotz ES, Norris HJ. Metaplastic carcinomas of the breast. III. Carcinosarcoma. Cancer 1989; 64(7): 1490–1499.

302. Wargotz ES, Norris HJ. Metaplastic carcinomas of the breast. IV. Squamous cell carcinoma of ductal origin. Cancer 1990; 65(2): 272–276.

303. Wargotz ES, Norris HJ. Metaplastic carcinomas of the breast: V. Metaplastic carcinoma with osteoclastic giant cells. Hum Pathol 1990; 21(11): 1142–1150.

304. Rosen PP, Ernsberger D. Low-grade adenosquamous carcinoma. A variant of metaplastic mammary carcinoma. Am J Surg Pathol 1987; 11(5): 351–358.

305. Oberman HA. Hamartomas and hamartoma variants of the breast. Semin Diagn Pathol 1989; 6(2): 135–145.

306. Wargotz ES, Weiss SW, Norris HJ. Myofibroblastoma of the breast. Sixteen cases of a distinctive benign mesenchymal tumor. Am J Surg Pathol 1987; 11(7): 493–502.

307. Amin MB, Gottlieb CA, Fitzmaurice M, et al. Fine-needle aspiration cytologic study of myofibroblastoma of the breast. Immunohistochemical and ultrastructural findings. Am J Clin Pathol 1993; 99(5): 593–597.

308. Rosen PP. Mucocele-like tumors of the breast. Am J Surg Pathol 1986; 10(7): 464–469.

309. Ro JY, Sneige N, Sahin AA, et al. Mucocelelike tumor of the breast associated with atypical ductal hyperplasia or mucinous carcinoma. A clinicopathologic study of seven cases. Arch Pathol Lab Med 1991; 115(2): 137–140.

310. Weaver MG, Abdul-Karim FW, al-Kaisi N. Mucinous lesions of the breast. A pathological continuum. Pathol Res Pract 1993; 189(8): 873–876.

311. Fisher ER, Palekar AS, Stoner F, Costantino J. Mucocele-like lesions and mucinous carcinoma of the breast. Int J Surg Pathol 1994; 1: 213.

312. Hamele-Bena D, Cranor ML, Rosen PP. Mammary mucocele-like lesions. Benign and malignant. Am J Surg Pathol 1996; 20(9): 1081–1085.

313. Fisher CJ, Millis RR. A mucocele-like tumour of the breast associated with both atypical ductal hyperplasia and mucoid carcinoma. Histopathology 1992; 21(1): 69–71.

314. Kulka J, Davies JD. Mucocoele-like tumours: more associations and possibly ductal carcinoma in situ? Histopathology 1993; 22(5): 511–512.

315. Bhargava V, Miller TR, Cohen MB. Mucocele-like tumors of the breast. Cytologic findings in two cases. Am J Clin Pathol 1991; 95(6): 875–877.

316. Clement PB, Young RH, Azzopardi JG. Collagenous spherulosis of the breast. Am J Surg Pathol 1987; 11(6): 411–417.

317. Tyler X, Coghill SB. Fine needle aspiration cytology of collagenous spherulosis of the breast. Cytopathology 1991; 2(3): 159–162.

318. Johnson TL, Kini SR. Cytologic features of collagenous spherulosis of the breast. Diagn Cytopathol 1991; 7(4): 417–419.

319. Highland KE, Finley JL, Neill JS, Silverman JF. Collagenous spherulosis. Report of a case with diagnosis by fine needle aspiration biopsy with immunocytochemical and ultrastructural observations. Acta Cytol 1993; 37(1): 3–9.

320. Sgroi D, Koerner FC. Involvement of collagenous spherulosis by lobular carcinoma in situ. Potential confusion with cribriform ductal carcinoma in situ. Am J Surg Pathol 1995; 19(12): 1366–1370.

321. Ellis IO, Elston CW, Goulding H, Pinder SE. Miscellaneous benign lesions. In: Elston CW, Ellis, I. O (eds) The breast. Edinburgh: Churchill Livingstone; 1998.

322. Dixon JM, Anderson TJ, Lumsden AB, et al. Mammary duct ectasia. Br J Surg 1983; 70(10): 601–603.

323. Dixon JM, Ravisekar O, Chetty U, Anderson TJ. Periductal mastitis and duct ectasia: different conditions with different aetiologies. Br J Surg 1996; 83(6): 820–822.

324. Symmers W. The breasts. In: Symmers W (ed.). Systemic pathology. Edinburgh: Churchill Livingstone; 1978.

325. Bridges AJ, Vasey FB. Silicone breast implants. History, safety, and potential complications. Arch Intern Med 1993; 153(23): 2638–2644.

326. Noone RB. A review of the possible health implications of silicone breast implants. Cancer 1997; 79(9): 1747–1756.

327. Raso DS, Crymes LW, Metcalf JS. Histological assessment of fifty breast capsules from smooth and textured augmentation and reconstruction mammoplasty prostheses with emphasis on the role of synovial metaplasia. Mod Pathol 1994; 7(3): 310–316.

328. Dodd LG, Sneige N, Reece GP, Fornage B. Fine-needle aspiration cytology of silicone granulomas in

the augmented breast. Diagn Cytopathol 1993; 9(5): 498–502.

329. Tabatowski K, Elson CE, Johnston WW. Silicone lymphadenopathy in a patient with a mammary prosthesis. Fine needle aspiration cytology, histology and analytical electron microscopy. Acta Cytol 1990; 34(1): 10–14.

330. Honig C, Rado R. Mondor's disease – superficial phlebitis of the chest wall: a review of seven cases. Ann Surg 1961; 153: 589.

331. Tabar L, Dean PB. Mondor's disease: Clinical, mammographic, and pathologic features. Breast 1981; 7: 18.

332. Fajardo LJ. Pathology of radiation injury. New York: Masson Publishing; 1982.

333. Clarke D, Curtis JL, Martinez A, et al. Fat necrosis of the breast simulating recurrent carcinoma after primary radiotherapy in the management of early stage breast carcinoma. Cancer 1983; 52(3): 442–445.

334. Schnitt SJ, Connolly JL, Harris JR, Cohen RB. Radiation-induced changes in the breast. Hum Pathol 1984; 15(6): 545–550.

335. Kennedy SM, Merino MJ. Histologic evaluation of the effects of chemotherapy and hormonal therapy in residual and tumoral breast tissues: their significance in diagnoses. Lab Invest 1988; 58: 47A.

336. Bondeson L. Aspiration cytology of radiation-induced changes of normal breast epithelium. Acta Cytol 1987; 31(3): 309–310.

337. Pedio G, Landolt U, Zobeli L. Irradiated benign cells of the breast: a potential diagnostic pitfall in fine needle aspiration cytology. Acta Cytol 1988; 32(1): 127–128.

338. Peterse JL, Thunnissen FB, van Heerde P. Fine needle aspiration cytology of radiation-induced changes in nonneoplastic breast lesions. Possible pitfalls in cytodiagnosis. Acta Cytol 1989; 33(2): 176–180.

339. Gupta RK. Radiation-induced cellular changes in the breast: a potential diagnostic pitfall in fine needle aspiration cytology. Acta Cytol 1989; 33(1): 141–142.

340. Saad RS, Silverman JF, Julian T, et al. Atypical squamous metaplasia of seromas in breast needle aspirates from irradiated lumpectomy sites: a potential pitfall for false-positive diagnoses of carcinoma. Diagn Cytopathol 2002; 26(2): 104–108.

341. Gansler TS, Wheeler JE. Mammary sarcoidosis. Two cases and literature review. Arch Pathol Lab Med 1984; 108(8): 673–675.

342. Fitzgibbons PL, Smiley DF, Kern WH. Sarcoidosis presenting initially as breast mass: report of two cases. Hum Pathol 1985; 16(8): 851–852.

343. Kessler E, Wolloch Y. Granulomatous mastitis: a lesion clinically simulating carcinoma. Am J Clin Pathol 1972; 58(6): 642–646.

344. Kessler EI, Katzav JA. Lobular granulomatous mastitis. Surg Pathol 1990; 3: 115–120.

345. Schwartz IS, Strauchen JA. Lymphocytic mastopathy. An autoimmune disease of the breast? Am J Clin Pathol 1990; 93(6): 725–730.

346. Lammie GA, Bobrow LG, Staunton MD, et al. Sclerosing lymphocytic lobulitis of the breast–evidence for an autoimmune pathogenesis. Histopathology 1991; 19(1): 13–20.

347. Ashton MA, Lefkowitz M, Tavassoli FA. Epithelioid stromal cells in lymphocytic mastitis–a source of confusion with invasive carcinoma. Mod Pathol 1994; 7(1): 49–54.

348. Tomaszewski JE, Brooks JS, Hicks D, Livolsi VA. Diabetic mastopathy: a distinctive clinicopathologic entity. Hum Pathol 1992; 23(7): 780–786.

349. Seidman JD, Schnaper LA, Phillips LE. Mastopathy in insulin-requiring diabetes mellitus. Hum Pathol 1994; 25(8): 819–824.

350. Williams MJ. Gynecomastia. Its incidence, recognition and host characterization in 447 autopsy cases. Am J Med 1963; 34: 103–112.

351. Bannayan GA, Hajdu SI. Gynecomastia: clinicopathologic study of 351 cases. Am J Clin Pathol 1972; 57(4): 431–437.

352. Carlson HE. Gynecomastia. N Engl J Med 1980; 303(14): 795–799.

353. Nicolis GL, Modlinger RS, Gabrilove JL. A study of the histopathology of human gynecomastia. J Clin Endocrinol Metab 1971; 32(2): 173–178.

354. Russin VL, Lachowicz C, Kline TS. Male breast lesions: gynecomastia and its distinction from carcinoma by aspiration biopsy cytology. Diagn Cytopathol 1989; 5(3): 243–247.

355. Amrikachi M, Green LK, Rone R, Ramzy I. Gynecomastia: cytologic features and diagnostic pitfalls in fine needle aspirates. Acta Cytol 2001; 45(6): 948–952.

356. Jacobs TW, Connolly JL. Current status of classifications schemes for ductal carcinoma in situ. Semin Breast Dis 2000; 3: 200–208.

357. Azzopardi JG. Problems in breast pathology. Philadelphia, PA: WB Saunders; 1983.

358. Carter D, Orr SL, Merino MJ. Intracystic papillary carcinoma of the breast. After mastectomy, radiotherapy or excisional biopsy alone. Cancer 1983; 52(1): 14–19.

359. Lefkowitz M, Lefkowitz W, Wargotz ES. Intraductal (intracystic) papillary carcinoma of the breast and its variants: a clinicopathological study of 77 cases. Hum Pathol 1994; 25(8): 802–809.

360. Leal C, Costa I, Fonseca D, et al. Intracystic (encysted) papillary carcinoma of the breast: a clinical, pathological, and immunohistochemical study. Hum Pathol 1998; 29(10): 1097–1104.

361. Patchefsky AS, Schwartz GF, Finkelstein SD, et al. Heterogeneity of intraductal carcinoma of the breast. Cancer 1989; 63(4): 731–741.

362. Lennington WJ, Jensen RA, Dalton LW, Page DL. Ductal carcinoma in situ of the breast. Heterogeneity of individual lesions. Cancer 1994; 73(1): 118–124.

363. Millis RR. Classification of ductal carcinoma in situ. Adv Anat Pathol 1996; 3: 114–129.

364. Schnitt SJ, Connolly JL. Classification of ductal carcinoma in situ: striving for clinical relevance in the era of breast conserving therapy [editorial; comment]. Hum Pathol 1997; 28(8): 877–880.

365. Shoker BS, Sloane JP. DCIS grading schemes and clinical implications. Histopathology 1999; 35(5): 393–400.

366. Lagios MD, Margolin FR, Westdahl PR, Rose MR. Mammographically detected duct carcinoma in situ. Frequency of local recurrence following tylectomy and prognostic effect of nuclear grade on local recurrence. Cancer 1989; 63(4): 618–624.

367. Scott MA, Lagios MD, Axelsson K, et al. Ductal carcinoma in situ of the breast: reproducibility of histological subtype analysis. Hum Pathol 1997; 28(8): 967–973.

368. Poller DN, Silverstein MJ, Galea M, et al. Ideas in pathology. Ductal carcinoma in situ of the breast: a proposal for a new simplified histological classification association between cellular proliferation and c-erbB-2 protein expression. Mod Pathol 1994; 7(2): 257–262.

369. Silverstein MJ, Poller DN, Waisman JR, et al. Prognostic classification of breast ductal carcinoma-in-situ. Lancet 1995; 345(8958): 1154–1157.

370. Holland R, Peterse JL, Millis RR, et al. Ductal carcinoma in situ: a proposal for a new classification. Semin Diagn Pathol 1994; 11(3): 167–180.

371. Pathology ECWGoBS. Consistency achieved by 23 European pathologists in categorizing ductal carcinoma in situ of the breast using five classifications. European Commission Working Group on Breast Screening Pathology. Hum Pathol 1998; 29(10): 1056–1062.

372. Ottesen GL, Graversen HP, Blichert-Toft M, et al. Ductal carcinoma in situ of the female breast. Short-term results of a prospective nationwide study. The Danish Breast Cancer Cooperative Group. Am J Surg Pathol 1992; 16(12): 1183–1196.

373. Bellamy CO, McDonald C, Salter DM, et al. Noninvasive ductal carcinoma of the breast: the relevance of histologic categorization. Hum Pathol 1993; 24(1): 16–23.

374. Tavassoli FA, Man Y. Morphofunctional features of intraductal hyperplasia, atypical intraductal hyperplasia, and various grades of intraductal carcinoma. Breast J 1995; 1: 155–162.

375. Buerger H, Otterbach F, Simon R, et al. Comparative genomic hybridization of ductal carcinoma in situ of the breast—evidence of multiple genetic pathways. J Pathol 1999; 187(4): 396–402.

376. Van Diest PJ. Ductal carcinoma in situ in breast carcinogenesis. J Pathol 1999; 187(4): 383–384.

377. Adeyinka A, Emberley E, Niu Y, et al. Analysis of gene expression in ductal carcinoma in situ of the breast. Clin Cancer Res 2002; 8(12): 3788–3795.

378. Bur ME, Zimarowski MJ, Schnitt SJ, et al. Estrogen receptor immunohistochemistry in carcinoma in situ of the breast. Cancer 1992; 69(5): 1174–1181.

379. Bose S, Lesser ML, Norton L, Rosen PP. Immunophenotype of intraductal carcinoma. Arch Pathol Lab Med 1996; 120(1): 81–85.

380. Bobrow LG, Happerfield LC, Gregory WM, et al. The classification of ductal carcinoma in situ and its association with biological markers. Semin Diagn Pathol 1994; 11(3): 199–207.

381. Albonico G, Querzoli P, Ferretti S, et al. Biological profile of in situ breast cancer investigated by immunohistochemical technique. Cancer Detect Prev 1998; 22(4): 313–318.

382. Rudas M, Neumayer R, Gnant MF, et al. p53 protein expression, cell proliferation and steroid hormone receptors in ductal and lobular in situ carcinomas of the breast. Eur J Cancer 1997; 33(1): 39–44.

383. Mack L, Kerkvliet N, Doig G, O'Malley FP. Relationship of a new histological categorization of ductal carcinoma in situ of the breast with size and the immunohistochemical expression of p53, c-erb B2, bcl-2, and ki-67. Hum Pathol 1997; 28(8): 974–979.

384. Meyer JS. Cell kinetics of histologic variants of in situ breast carcinoma. Breast Cancer Res Treat 1986; 7(3): 171–180.

385. Killeen JL, Namiki H. DNA analysis of ductal carcinoma in situ of the breast. A comparison with histologic features. Cancer 1991; 68(12): 2602–2607.

386. Van de Vijver MJ, Peterse JL, Mooi WJ, et al. Neu-protein overexpression in breast cancer. Association with comedo- type ductal carcinoma in situ and limited prognostic value in stage II breast cancer. N Engl J Med 1988; 319(19): 1239–1245.

387. Bartkova J, Barnes DM, Millis RR, Gullick WJ. Immunohistochemical demonstration of c-erbB-2 protein in mammary ductal carcinoma in situ. Hum Pathol 1990; 21(11): 1164–1167.

388. Lodato RF, Maguire HC Jr, Greene MI, et al. Immunohistochemical evaluation of c-erbB-2 oncogene expression in ductal carcinoma in situ and atypical ductal hyperplasia of the breast. Mod Pathol 1990; 3(4): 449–454.

389. Poller DN, Roberts EC, Bell JA, et al. p53 protein expression in mammary ductal carcinoma in situ: relationship to immunohistochemical expression of estrogen receptor and c-erbB-2 protein. Hum Pathol 1993; 24(5): 463–468.

390. O'Malley FP, Vnencak-Jones CL, Dupont WD, et al. p53 mutations are confined to the comedo type ductal carcinoma in situ of the breast. Immunohistochemical and sequencing data. Lab Invest 1994; 71(1): 67–72.

391. Done SJ, Eskandarian S, Bull S, et al. p53 missense mutations in microdissected high-grade ductal carcinoma in situ of the breast. J Natl Cancer Inst 2001; 93(9): 700–704.

392. Guidi AJ, Fischer L, Harris JR, Schnitt SJ. Microvessel density and distribution in ductal carcinoma in situ of the breast. J Natl Cancer Inst 1994; 86(8): 614–619.

393. Engels K, Fox SB, Whitehouse RM, et al. Distinct angiogenic patterns are associated with high-grade in situ ductal carcinomas of the breast. J Pathol 1997; 181(2): 207–212.

394. Tsuda H, Fukutomi T, Hirohashi S. Pattern of gene alterations in intraductal breast neoplasms associated

with histological type and grade. Clin Cancer Res 1995; 1(3): 261–267.

395. Lakhani SR. The transition from hyperplasia to invasive carcinoma of the breast. J Pathol 1999; 187(3): 272–278.

396. Schwartz GF, Patchefsky AS, Finklestein SD, et al. Nonpalpable in situ ductal carcinoma of the breast. Predictors of multicentricity and microinvasion and implications for treatment. Arch Surg 1989; 124(1): 29–32.

397. Silverstein MJ, Waisman JR, Gamagami P, et al. Intraductal carcinoma of the breast (208 cases). Clinical factors influencing treatment choice. Cancer 1990; 66(1): 102–108.

398. Holland R, Hendriks JH, Vebeek AL, et al. Extent, distribution, and mammographic/histological correlations of breast ductal carcinoma in situ. Lancet 1990; 335(8688): 519–522.

399. Holland R, Hendriks JH. Microcalcifications associated with ductal carcinoma in situ: mammographic-pathologic correlation. Semin Diagn Pathol 1994; 11(3): 181–192.

400. Fowble B. In situ breast cancer. In: Fowble B, Goodman RL, Glick JH, Rosato EF (eds) Breast cancer treatment. A comprehensive guide to management. St. Louis, MO: Mosby Year-Book; 1991.

401. Lagios MD, Westdahl PR, Margolin FR, Rose MR. Duct carcinoma in situ. Relationship of extent of noninvasive disease to the frequency of occult invasion, multicentricity, lymph node metastases, and short-term treatment failures. Cancer 1982; 50(7): 1309–1314.

402. Faverly DR, Burgers L, Bult P, Holland R. Three dimensional imaging of mammary ductal carcinoma in situ: clinical implications. Semin Diagn Pathol 1994; 11(3): 193–198.

403. Noguchi S, Motomura K, Inaji H, et al. Clonal analysis of predominantly intraductal carcinoma and precancerous lesions of the breast by means of polymerase chain reaction. Cancer Res 1994; 54(7): 1849–1853.

404. Gump FE, Jicha DL, Ozello L. Ductal carcinoma in situ (DCIS): a revised concept. Surgery 1987; 102(5): 790–795.

405. Fentiman IS, Fagg N, Millis RR, Hayward JL. In situ ductal carcinoma of the breast: implications of disease pattern and treatment. Eur J Surg Oncol 1986; 12(3): 261–266.

406. Silverstein MJ, Gierson ED, Waisman JR, et al. Axillary lymph node dissection for T1a breast carcinoma. Is it indicated? Cancer 1994; 73(3): 664–667.

407. Lancer HA, Moschella SL. Paget's disease of the male breast. J Am Acad Dermatol 1982; 7(3): 393–396.

408. Neubecker RD, Bradshaw RP. Mucin, melanin, and glycogen in Paget's disease of the breast. Am J Clin Pathol 1961; 36: 49–53.

409. Rayne SC, Santa Cruz DJ. Anaplastic Paget's disease. Am J Surg Pathol 1992; 16(11): 1085–1091.

410. Kaya H, Ragazzini T, Aribal E, et al. Her-2/neu gene amplification compared with HER-2/neu protein overexpression on ultrasound guided core-needle biopsy specimens of breast carcinoma. Pathol Oncol Res 2001; 7(4): 279–283.

411. Anderson JM, Ariga R, Govil H, et al. Assessment of Her-2/Neu status by immunohistochemistry and fluorescence in situ hybridization in mammary Paget disease and underlying carcinoma. Appl Immunohistochem Mol Morphol 2003; 11(2): 120–124.

412. Hitchcock A, Topham S, Bell J, et al. Routine diagnosis of mammary Paget's disease. A modern approach. Am J Surg Pathol 1992; 16(1): 58–61.

413. Chaudary MA, Millis RR, Lane EB, Miller NA. Paget's disease of the nipple: a ten-year review including clinical, pathological, and immunohistochemical findings. Breast Cancer Res Treat 1986; 8(2): 139–146.

414. Shertz WT, Balogh K. Metastasizing basal cell carcinoma of the nipple. Arch Pathol Lab Med 1986; 110(8): 761–762.

415. Eusebi V, Feudale E, Foschini MP, et al. Long term follow-up of in situ carcinoma of the breast. Semin Diagn Pathol 1994; 11(3): 223–235.

416. Page DL, Dupont WD. Anatomic markers of human premalignancy and risk of breast cancer. Cancer 1990; 66(6 Suppl): 1326–1335.

417. Schnitt SJ, Vincent-Salomon A. Columnar cell lesions of the breast. Adv Anat Pathol 2003; 10(3): 113–124.

418. Bijker N, Peterse JL, Duchateau L, et al. Risk factors for recurrence and metastasis after breast-conserving therapy for ductal carcinoma-in-situ: analysis of European Organization for Research and Treatment of Cancer Trial 10853. J Clin Oncol 2001; 19(8): 2263–2271.

419. O'Malley FP, Page DL, Nelson EH, Dupont WD. Ductal carcinoma in situ of the breast with apocrine cytology: definition of a borderline category. Hum Pathol 1994; 25(2): 164–168.

420. Tavassoli FA, Norris HJ. Intraductal apocrine carcinoma: a clinicopathologic study of 37 cases. Mod Pathol 1994; 7(8): 813–818.

421. Cross AS, Azzopardi JG, Krausz T, et al. A morphological and immunocytochemical study of a distinctive variant of ductal carcinoma in-situ of the breast. Histopathology 1985; 9(1): 21–37.

422. Maluf HM, Zukerberg LR, Dickersin GR, Koerner FC. Spindle-cell argyrophilic mucin-producing carcinoma of the breast. Histological, ultrastructural, and immunohistochemical studies of two cases. Am J Surg Pathol 1991; 15(7): 677–686.

423. Maluf HM, Koerner FC. Solid papillary carcinoma of the breast. A form of intraductal carcinoma with endocrine differentiation frequently associated with mucinous carcinoma. Am J Surg Pathol 1995; 19(11): 1237–1244.

424. Tsang WY, Chan JK. Endocrine ductal carcinoma in situ (E-DCIS) of the breast: a form of low-grade DCIS with distinctive clinicopathologic and biologic characteristics. Am J Surg Pathol 1996; 20(8): 921–943.

425. Fisher ER, Brown R. Intraductal signet ring carcinoma. A hitherto undescribed form of intraductal carcinoma of the breast. Cancer 1985; 55(11): 2533–2537.

426. Rosen PP, Scott M. Cystic hypersecretory duct carcinoma of the breast. Am J Surg Pathol 1984; 8(1): 31–41.

427. Guerry P, Erlandson RA, Rosen PP. Cystic hypersecretory hyperplasia and cystic hypersecretory duct carcinoma of the breast. Pathology, therapy, and follow-up of 39 patients. Cancer 1988; 61(8): 1611–1620.

428. Wheeler JE, Enterline HT, Roseman JM, et al. Lobular carcinoma in situ of the breast. Long-term followup. Cancer 1974; 34(3): 554–563.

429. Haagensen CD, Lane N, Lattes R, Bodian C. Lobular neoplasia (so-called lobular carcinoma in situ) of the breast. Cancer 1978; 42(2): 737–769.

430. Fechner RE. Epithelial alterations in the extralobular ducts of breasts with lobular carcinoma. Arch Pathol 1972; 93(2): 164–171.

431. Vos CB, Cleton-Jansen AM, Berx G, et al. E-cadherin inactivation in lobular carcinoma in situ of the breast: an early event in tumorigenesis. Br J Cancer 1997; 76(9): 1131–1133.

432. Wickerham DL. Tamoxifen's impact as a preventive agent in clinical practice and an update on the STAR trial. Recent Results Cancer Res 2003; 163: 87–95; discussion 264–266.

433. Smith RE, Good BC. Chemoprevention of breast cancer and the trials of the National Surgical Adjuvant Breast and Bowel Project and others. Endocr Relat Cancer 2003; 10(3): 347–357.

434. Fechner RE. Ductal carcinoma involving the lobule of the breast. A source of confusion with lobular carcinoma in situ. Cancer 1971; 28(2): 274–281.

435. Rosen PP. Coexistent lobular carcinoma in situ and intraductal carcinoma in a single lobular-duct unit. Am J Surg Pathol 1980; 4(3): 241–246.

436. Fisher ER, Costantino J, Fisher B, et al. Pathologic findings from the National Surgical Adjuvant Breast Project (NSABP) Protocol B-17. Five-year observations concerning lobular carcinoma in situ. Cancer 1996; 78(7): 1403–1416.

437. Rosen PP. Rosen's breast pathology. 2nd edn. Philadelphia, PA: Lippincott-Raven; 2001.

438. Frost AR, Tsangaris TN, Silverberg SG. Pleomorphic lobular carcinoma in situ. Pathol Case Rev 1996; 1: 27.

439. Bentz JS, Yassa N, Clayton F. Pleomorphic lobular carcinoma of the breast: clinicopathologic features of 12 cases. Mod Pathol 1998; 11(9): 814–822.

440. Tavassoli FA. Pathology of the breast. 2nd edn. Stamford, CT: Appleton & Lange; 1999.

441. Koerner F, Maluf H. Uncommon morphologic patterns of lobular neoplasia. Ann Diagn Pathol 1999; 3(4): 249–259.

442. Jacobs TW, Pliss N, Kouria G, Schnitt SJ. Carcinomas in situ of the breast with indeterminate features: role of E-cadherin staining in categorization. Am J Surg Pathol 2001; 25(2): 229–236.

443. Moll R, Mitze M, Frixen UH, Birchmeier W. Differential loss of E-cadherin expression in infiltrating ductal and lobular breast carcinomas. Am J Pathol 1993; 143(6): 1731–1742.

444. Rasbridge SA, Gillett CE, Sampson SA, et al. Epithelial (E-) and placental (P-) cadherin cell adhesion molecule expression in breast carcinoma. J Pathol 1993; 169(2): 245–250.

445. Kanai Y, Oda T, Tsuda H, et al. Point mutation of the E-cadherin gene in invasive lobular carcinoma of the breast. Jpn J Cancer Res 1994; 85(10): 1035–1039.

446. Berx G, Cleton-Jansen AM, Nollet F, et al. E-cadherin is a tumour/invasion suppressor gene mutated in human lobular breast cancers. Embo J 1995; 14(24): 6107–6115.

447. Berx G, Cleton-Jansen AM, Strumane K, et al. E-cadherin is inactivated in a majority of invasive human lobular breast cancers by truncation mutations throughout its extracellular domain. Oncogene 1996; 13(9): 1919–1925.

448. De Leeuw WJ, Berx G, Vos CB, et al. Simultaneous loss of E-cadherin and catenins in invasive lobular breast cancer and lobular carcinoma in situ. J Pathol 1997; 183(4): 404–411.

449. The World Health Organization histological typing of breast tumors – second edition. Am J Clin Pathol 1982; 78(6): 806–816.

450. Fisher ER, Gregorio RM, Fisher B, et al. The pathology of invasive breast cancer. A syllabus derived from findings of the National Surgical Adjuvant Breast Project (protocol no. 4). Cancer 1975; 36(1): 1–85.

451. Rosen PP. The pathological classification of human mammary carcinoma: past, present and future. Ann Clin Lab Sci 1979; 9(2): 144–156.

452. Ellis IO, Galea M, Broughton N, et al. Pathological prognostic factors in breast cancer. II. Histological type. Relationship with survival in a large study with long-term follow-up. Histopathology 1992; 20(6): 479–489.

453. Cowan WK, Kelly P, Sawan A, et al. The pathological and biological nature of screen-detected breast carcinomas: a morphological and immunohistochemical study. J Pathol 1997; 182(1): 29–35.

454. Mustafa IA, Cole B, Wanebo HJ, et al. The impact of histopathology on nodal metastases in minimal breast cancer. Arch Surg 1997; 132(4): 384–390; discussion 390–391.

455. Henson DE, Ries L, Freedman LS, Carriaga M. Relationship among outcome, stage of disease, and histologic grade for 22,616 cases of breast cancer. The basis for a prognostic index. Cancer 1991; 68(10): 2142–2149.

456. Rosner D, Lane WW. Should all patients with node-negative breast cancer receive adjuvant therapy? Identifying additional subsets of low-risk patients who are highly curable by surgery alone. Cancer 1991; 68(7): 1482–1494.

457. Tabar L, Fagerberg G, Duffy SW, et al. Update of the Swedish two-county program of mammographic screening for breast cancer. Radiol Clin North Am 1992; 30(1): 187–210.

458. Anderson TJ, Lamb J, Donnan P, et al. Comparative pathology of breast cancer in a randomised trial of screening. Br J Cancer 1991; 64(1): 108–113.

459. Lampejo OT, Barnes DM, Smith P, Millis RR. Evaluation of infiltrating ductal carcinomas with a DCIS component: correlation of the histologic type of the in situ component with grade of the infiltrating component. Semin Diagn Pathol 1994; 11(3): 215–222.

460. Moriya T, Silverberg SG. Intraductal carcinoma (ductal carcinoma in situ) of the breast. A comparison of pure noninvasive tumors with those including different proportions of infiltrating carcinoma. Cancer 1994; 74(11): 2972–2978.

461. Gupta SK, Douglas-Jones AG, Fenn N, et al. The clinical behavior of breast carcinoma is probably determined at the preinvasive stage (ductal carcinoma in situ). Cancer 1997; 80(9): 1740–1745.

462. Black MM, Speer FD. Nuclear structure in cancer tissues. Surg Gynecol Obstet 1957; 105: 97.

463. Cutler SJ, Black MM, Mork T, et al. Further observations on prognostic factors in cancer of the female breast. Cancer 1969; 24(4): 653–667.

464. Elston CW, Ellis IO. Assessment of histologic grade. In: Elston CW, Ellis IO (eds) The breast. Edinburgh: Churchill Livingstone; 1998: 365–384.

465. Ducatman BS, Emery ST, Wang HH. Correlation of histologic grade of breast carcinoma with cytologic features on fine-needle aspiration of the breast. Mod Pathol 1993; 6(5): 539–543.

466. Simpson JF. Predictive utility of the histopathologic analysis of carcinoma of the breast. Adv Pathol Lab Med 1994; 7: 107.

467. Martinez V, Azzopardi JG. Invasive lobular carcinoma of the breast: incidence and variants. Histopathology 1979; 3(6): 467–488.

468. Chen CL, Weiss NS, Newcomb P, et al. Hormone replacement therapy in relation to breast cancer. JAMA 2002; 287(6): 734–741.

469. Ashikari R, Huvos AG, Urban JA, Robbins GF. Infiltrating lobular carcinoma of the breast. Cancer 1973; 31(1): 110–116.

470. Lesser ML, Rosen PP, Kinne DW. Multicentricity and bilaterality in invasive breast carcinoma. Surgery 1982; 91(2): 234–240.

471. Tinnemans JG, Wobbes T, van der Sluis RF, et al. Multicentricity in nonpalpable breast carcinoma and its implications for treatment. Am J Surg 1986; 151(3): 334–338.

472. Gump FE, Shikora S, Habif DV, et al. The extent and distribution of cancer in breasts with palpable primary tumors. Ann Surg 1986; 204(4): 384–390.

473. Dixon JM, Anderson TJ, Page DL, et al. Infiltrating lobular carcinoma of the breast: an evaluation of the incidence and consequence of bilateral disease. Br J Surg 1983; 70(9): 513–516.

474. Sastre-Garau X, Jouve M, Asselain B, et al. Infiltrating lobular carcinoma of the breast. Clinicopathologic analysis of 975 cases with reference to data on conservative therapy and metastatic patterns. Cancer 1996; 77(1): 113–120.

475. Peiro G, Bornstein BA, Connolly JL, et al. The influence of infiltrating lobular carcinoma on the outcome of patients treated with breast-conserving surgery and radiation therapy. Breast Cancer Res Treat 2000; 59(1): 49–54.

476. Mendelson EB, Harris KM, Doshi N, Tobon H. Infiltrating lobular carcinoma: mammographic patterns with pathologic correlation. AJR 1989; 153(2): 265–271.

477. Hilleren DJ, Andersson IT, Lindholm K, Linnell FS. Invasive lobular carcinoma: mammographic findings in a 10-year experience. Radiology 1991; 178(1): 149–154.

478. Le Gal M, Ollivier L, Asselain B, et al. Mammographic features of 455 invasive lobular carcinomas. Radiology 1992; 185(3): 705–708.

479. Helvie MA, Paramagul C, Oberman HA, Adler DD. Invasive lobular carcinoma. Imaging features and clinical detection. Invest Radiol 1993; 28(3): 202–207.

480. Krecke KN, Gisvold JJ. Invasive lobular carcinoma of the breast: mammographic findings and extent of disease at diagnosis in 184 patients. AJR 1993; 161(5): 957–960.

481. White JR, Gustafson GS, Wimbish K, et al. Conservative surgery and radiation therapy for infiltrating lobular carcinoma of the breast. The role of preoperative mammograms in guiding treatment. Cancer 1994; 74(2): 640–647.

482. Wheeler JE, Enterline HT. Lobular carcinoma of the breast in situ and infiltrating. Pathol Annu 1976; 11: 161–188.

483. Foote FW Jr, Foote FW. A histologic classification of carcinoma of the breast. Surgery 1946; 19: 74.

484. Dixon JM, Anderson TJ, Page DL, et al. Infiltrating lobular carcinoma of the breast. Histopathology 1982; 6(2): 149–161.

485. Du Toit RS, Locker AP, Ellis IO, et al. Invasive lobular carcinoma of the breast–the prognosis of histopathological subtypes. Br J Cancer 1989; 60(4): 605–609.

486. Fechner RE. Histologic variants of infiltrating lobular carcinoma of the breast. Hum Pathol 1975; 6(3): 373–378.

487. Fisher ER, Gregorio RM, Redmond C, Fisher B. Tubulolobular invasive breast cancer: a variant of lobular invasive cancer. Hum Pathol 1977; 8(6): 679–683.

488. Van Bogaert LJ, Maldague P. Infiltrating lobular carcinoma of the female breast. Deviations from the usual histopathologic appearance. Cancer 1980; 45(5): 979–984.

489. Green I, McCormick B, Cranor M, Rosen PP. A comparative study of pure tubular and tubulolobular carcinoma of the breast. Am J Surg Pathol 1997; 21(6): 653–657.

490. DiCostanzo D, Rosen PP, Gareen I, et al. Prognosis in infiltrating lobular carcinoma. An analysis of 'classical' and variant tumors. Am J Surg Pathol 1990; 14(1): 12–23.

491. Eusebi V, Magalhaes F, Azzopardi JG. Pleomorphic lobular carcinoma of the breast: an aggressive tumor showing apocrine differentiation. Hum Pathol 1992; 23(6): 655–662.

492. Weidner N, Semple JP. Pleomorphic variant of invasive lobular carcinoma of the breast. Hum Pathol 1992; 23(10): 1167–1171.

493. Frolik D, Caduff R, Varga Z. Pleomorphic lobular carcinoma of the breast: its cell kinetics, expression of oncogenes and tumour suppressor genes compared with invasive ductal carcinomas and classical infiltrating lobular carcinomas. Histopathology 2001; 39(5): 503–513.

494. Radhi JM. Immunohistochemical analysis of pleomorphic lobular carcinoma: higher expression of p53 and chromogranin and lower expression of ER and PgR. Histopathology 2000; 36(2): 156–160.

495. Middleton LP, Palacios DM, Bryant BR, et al. Pleomorphic lobular carcinoma: morphology, immunohistochemistry, and molecular analysis. Am J Surg Pathol 2000; 24(12): 1650–1656.

496. Merino MJ, Livolsi VA. Signet ring carcinoma of the female breast: a clinicopathologic analysis of 24 cases. Cancer 1981; 48(8): 1830–1837.

497. Hull MT, Seo IS, Battersby JS, Csicsko JF. Signet-ring cell carcinoma of the breast: a clinicopathologic study of 24 cases. Am J Clin Pathol 1980; 73(1): 31–35.

498. Steinbrecher JS, Silverberg SG. Signet-ring cell carcinoma of the breast. The mucinous variant of infiltrating lobular carcinoma? Cancer 1976; 37(2): 828–840.

499. Raju U, Ma CK, Shaw A. Signet ring variant of lobular carcinoma of the breast: a clinicopathologic and immunohistochemical study. Mod Pathol 1993; 6(5): 516–520.

500. Eltorky M, Hall JC, Osborne PT, el Zeky F. Signet-ring cell variant of invasive lobular carcinoma of the breast. A clinicopathologic study of 11 cases. Arch Pathol Lab Med 1994; 118(3): 245–248.

501. Frost AR, Terahata S, Yeh IT, et al. The significance of signet ring cells in infiltrating lobular carcinoma of the breast. Arch Pathol Lab Med 1995; 119(1): 64–68.

502. Eusebi V, Betts C, Haagensen DE Jr, et al. Apocrine differentiation in lobular carcinoma of the breast: a morphologic, immunologic, and ultrastructural study. Hum Pathol 1984; 15(2): 134–140.

503. Allenby PA, Chowdhury LN. Histiocytic appearance of metastatic lobular breast carcinoma. Arch Pathol Lab Med 1986; 110(8): 759–760.

504. Walford N, ten Velden J. Histiocytoid breast carcinoma: an apocrine variant of lobular carcinoma. Histopathology 1989; 14(5): 515–522.

505. Eusebi V, Foschini MP, Bussolati G, Rosen PP. Myoblastomatoid (histiocytoid) carcinoma of the breast. A type of apocrine carcinoma. Am J Surg Pathol 1995; 19(5): 553–562.

506. Pinder SE, Elston CW, Ellis IO. Invasive carcinoma – usual histological types. In: Elston CW, Ellis IO (eds) The breast. Edinburgh: Churchill Livingstone; 1998: 283–337.

507. Porter PL, Garcia R, Moe R, et al. C-erbB-2 oncogene protein in in situ and invasive lobular breast neoplasia. Cancer 1991; 68(2): 331–334.

508. Domagala W, Markiewski M, Kubiak R, et al. Immunohistochemical profile of invasive lobular carcinoma of the breast: predominantly vimentin and p53 protein negative, cathepsin D and oestrogen receptor positive. Virchows Arch A Pathol Anat Histopathol 1993; 423(6): 497–502.

509. Mazoujian G, Bodian C, Haagensen DE Jr, Haagensen CD. Expression of GCDFP-15 in breast carcinomas. Relationship to pathologic and clinical factors. Cancer 1989; 63(11): 2156–2161.

510. Joshi A, Kumar N, Verma K. Diagnostic challenge of lobular carcinoma on aspiration cytology. Diagn Cytopathol 1998; 18(3): 179–183.

511. Abdulla M, Hombal S, al-Juwaiser A, et al. Cellularity of lobular carcinoma and its relationship to false negative fine needle aspiration results. Acta Cytol 2000; 44(4): 625–632.

512. Lerma E, Fumanal V, Carreras A, et al. Undetected invasive lobular carcinoma of the breast: review of false-negative smears. Diagn Cytopathol 2000; 23(5): 303–307.

513. Kline TS, Kannan V, Kline IK. Appraisal and cytomorphologic analysis of common carcinomas of the breast. Diagn Cytopathol 1985; 1(3): 188–193.

514. Leach C, Howell LP. Cytodiagnosis of classic lobular carcinoma and its variants. Acta Cytol 1992; 36(2): 199–202.

515. Greeley CF, Frost AR. Cytologic features of ductal and lobular carcinoma in fine needle aspirates of the breast. Acta Cytol 1997; 41(2): 333–340.

516. Salhany KE, Page DL. Fine-needle aspiration of mammary lobular carcinoma in situ and atypical lobular hyperplasia. Am J Clin Pathol 1989; 92(1): 22–26.

517. Cohen H, Szvalb S, Bickel A, et al. Myoblastomatoid carcinoma of the breast: an unusual variant of apocrine carcinoma: report of a case with fine-needle aspiration cytology and immunohistochemical study. Diagn Cytopathol 1997; 16(2): 145–148.

518. Cangiarella J, O'Connell Mazzei E, Weg N, et al. Aspiration biopsy in a case of apocrine adenocarcinoma with foam cells (myoblastomatoid or histiocytoid adenocarcinoma). Diagn Cytopathol 2002; 26(5): 320–323.

519. Auger M, Huttner I. Fine-needle aspiration cytology of pleomorphic lobular carcinoma of the breast. Comparison with the classic type. Cancer 1997; 81(1): 29–32.

520. Harris M, Howell A, Chrissohou M, et al. A comparison of the metastatic pattern of infiltrating lobular carcinoma and infiltrating duct carcinoma of the breast. Br J Cancer 1984; 50(1): 23–30.

521. Lamovec J, Bracko M. Metastatic pattern of infiltrating lobular carcinoma of the breast: an autopsy study. J Surg Oncol 1991; 48(1): 28–33.

522. Borst MJ, Ingold JA. Metastatic patterns of invasive lobular versus invasive ductal carcinoma of the breast. Surgery 1993; 114(4): 637–641; discussion 641–642.

523. Dixon AR, Ellis IO, Elston CW, Blamey RW. A comparison of the clinical metastatic patterns of invasive lobular and ductal carcinomas of the breast. Br J Cancer 1991; 63(4): 634–635.

524. Smith DB, Howell A, Harris M, et al. Carcinomatous meningitis associated with infiltrating lobular carcinoma of the breast. Eur J Surg Oncol 1985; 11(1): 33–36.

525. Lamovec J, Zidar A. Association of leptomeningeal carcinomatosis in carcinoma of the breast with infiltrating lobular carcinoma. An autopsy study. Arch Pathol Lab Med 1991; 115(5): 507–510.

526. Cormier WJ, Gaffey TA, Welch TA, et al. Linitis plastica caused by metastatic lobular carcinoma of the breast. Mayo Clinic Proc 1980; 55: 747.

527. Battifora H. Metastatic breast carcinoma to the stomach simulating linitis plastica. Appl Immunohistochem 1994; 2: 225.

528. Kumar NB, Hart WR. Metastases to the uterine corpus from extragenital cancers. A clinicopathologic study of 63 cases. Cancer 1982; 50(10): 2163–2169.

529. Silverstein MJ, Lewinsky BS, Waisman JR, et al. Infiltrating lobular carcinoma. Is it different from infiltrating duct carcinoma? Cancer 1994; 73(6): 1673–1677.

530. Pereira H, Pinder SE, Sibbering DM, et al. Pathological prognostic factors in breast cancer. IV: Should you be a typer or a grader? A comparative study of two histological prognostic features in operable breast carcinoma. Histopathology 1995; 27(3): 219–226.

531. Schnitt S. Morphologic risk factors for local recurrence in patients with invasive breast cancer treated with conservative surgery and radiation therapy. Breast J 1997; 3: 261.

532. Weiss MC, Fowble BL, Solin LJ, et al. Outcome of conservative therapy for invasive breast cancer by histologic subtype. Int J Radiat Oncol Biol Phys 1992; 23(5): 941–947.

533. McBoyle MF, Razek HA, Carter JL, Helmer SD. Tubular carcinoma of the breast: an institutional review. Am Surg 1997; 63(7): 639–644; discussion 644–645.

534. Patchefsky AS, Shaber GS, Schwartz GF, et al. The pathology of breast cancer detected by mass population screening. Cancer 1977; 40(4): 1659–1670.

535. Report of the Working Group to Review the National Cancer Institute-American Cancer Society Breast Cancer Detection Demonstration Projects. J Natl Cancer Inst 1979; 62(3): 639–709.

536. Feig SA, Shaber GS, Patchefsky A, et al. Analysis of clinically occult and mammographically occult breast tumors. AJR 1977; 128(3): 403–408.

537. Winchester DJ, Sahin AA, Tucker SL, Singletary SE. Tubular carcinoma of the breast. Predicting axillary nodal metastases and recurrence. Ann Surg 1996; 223(3): 342–347.

538. Berger AC, Miller SM, Harris MN, et al. Axillary dissection for tubular carcinoma of the breast. Breast J 1996; 2: 204.

539. Feig SA, Shaver GS, Patchefsky AS. Tubular carcinoma of the breast: mode of presentation, mammographic appearance and pathologic correlation. Diagn Radiol 1993; 129: 311.

540. Elson BC, Helvie MA, Frank TS, et al. Tubular carcinoma of the breast: mode of presentation, mammographic appearance, and frequency of nodal metastases. AJR 1993; 161(6): 1173–1176.

541. Eusebi V, Betts CM, Bussolati G. Tubular carcinoma: a variant of secretory breast carcinoma. Histopathology 1979; 3(5): 407–419.

542. Lagios MD, Rose MR, Margolin FR. Tubular carcinoma of the breast: association with multicentricity, bilaterality, and family history of mammary carcinoma. Am J Clin Pathol 1980; 73(1): 25–30.

543. Leibman AJ, Lewis M, Kruse B. Tubular carcinoma of the breast: mammographic appearance. AJR 1993; 160(2): 263–265.

544. Tremblay G. Elastosis in tubular carcinoma of the breast. Arch Pathol 1974; 98(5): 302–307.

545. Carstens PH, Huvos AG, Foote FW Jr, Ashikari R. Tubular carcinoma of the breast: a clinicopathologic study of 35 cases. Am J Clin Pathol 1972; 58(3): 231–238.

546. Oberman HA, Fidler WJ Jr. Tubular carcinoma of the breast. Am J Surg Pathol 1979; 3(5): 387–35.

547. McDivitt RW, Boyce W, Gersell D. Tubular carcinoma of the breast. Clinical and pathological observations concerning 135 cases. Am J Surg Pathol 1982; 6(5): 401–411.

548. Deos PH, Norris HJ. Well-differentiated (tubular) carcinoma of the breast. A clinicopathologic study of 145 pure and mixed cases. Am J Clin Pathol 1982; 78(1): 1–7.

549. Cooper HS, Patchefsky AS, Krall RA. Tubular carcinoma of the breast. Cancer 1978; 42(5): 2334–2342.

550. Parl FF, Richardson LD. The histologic and biologic spectrum of tubular carcinoma of the breast. Hum Pathol 1983; 14(8): 694–698.

551. Carstens PH. Tubular carcinoma of the breast. A study of frequency. Am J Clin Pathol 1978; 70(2): 204–210.

552. Taylor HB, Norris HJ. Well-differentiated carcinoma of the breast. Cancer 1970; 25(3): 687–692.

553. Peters GN, Wolff M, Haagensen CD. Tubular carcinoma of the breast. Clinical pathologic correlations based on 100 cases. Ann Surg 1981; 193(2): 138–149.

554. Reiner A, Reiner G, Spona J, et al. Histopathologic characterization of human breast cancer in correlation with estrogen receptor status. A comparison of immunocytochemical and biochemical analysis. Cancer 1988; 61(6): 1149–1154.

555. Helin HJ, Helle MJ, Kallioniemi OP, Isola JJ. Immunohistochemical determination of estrogen and progesterone receptors in human breast carcinoma. Correlation with histopathology and DNA flow cytometry. Cancer 1989; 63(9): 1761–1767.

556. Stierer M, Rosen H, Weber R, et al. Immunohistochemical and biochemical measurement of estrogen and progesterone receptors in primary breast cancer. Correlation of histopathology and prognostic factors. Ann Surg 1993; 218(1): 13–21.

557. Diab SG, Clark GM, Osborne CK, et al. Tumor characteristics and clinical outcome of tubular and mucinous breast carcinomas. J Clin Oncol 1999; 17(5): 1442–1448.

558. Soomro S, Shousha S, Taylor P, et al. c-erbB-2 expression in different histological types of invasive breast carcinoma. J Clin Pathol 1991; 44(3): 211–214.

559. Somerville JE, Clarke LA, Biggart JD. c-erbB-2 overexpression and histological type of in situ and invasive breast carcinoma. J Clin Pathol 1992; 45(1): 16–20.

560. Rosen PP, Lesser ML, Arroyo CD, et al. p53 in node-negative breast carcinoma: an immunohistochemical study of epidemiologic risk factors, histologic features, and prognosis. J Clin Oncol 1995; 13(4): 821–830.

561. Waldman FM, Hwang ES, Etzell J, et al. Genomic alterations in tubular breast carcinomas. Hum Pathol 2001; 32(2): 222–226.

562. Flotte TJ, Bell DA, Greco MA. Tubular carcinoma and sclerosing adenosis: the use of basal lamina as a differential feature. Am J Surg Pathol 1980; 4(1): 75–77.

563. Ekblom P, Miettinen M, Forsman L, Andersson LC. Basement membrane and apocrine epithelial antigens in differential diagnosis between tubular carcinoma and sclerosing adenosis of the breast. J Clin Pathol 1984; 37(4): 357–363.

564. O'Leary TJ, Mikel UV, Becker RL. Computer-assisted image interpretation: use of a neural network to differentiate tubular carcinoma from sclerosing adenosis. Mod Pathol 1992; 5(4): 402–405.

565. Eusebi V, Foschini MP, Betts CM, et al. Microglandular adenosis, apocrine adenosis, and tubular carcinoma of the breast. An immunohistochemical comparison. Am J Surg Pathol 1993; 17(2): 99–109.

566. Rogers LA, Lee KR. Breast carcinoma simulating fibroadenoma or fibrocystic change by fine-needle aspiration. A study of 16 cases. Am J Clin Pathol 1992; 98(2): 155–160.

567. Layfield LJ, Dodd LG. Cytologically low grade malignancies: an important interpretative pitfall responsible for false negative diagnoses in fine-needle aspiration of the breast. Diagn Cytopathol 1996; 15(3): 250–259.

568. Bondeson L, Lindholm K. Aspiration cytology of tubular breast carcinoma. Acta Cytol 1990; 34(1): 15–20.

569. Fischler DF, Sneige N, Ordonez NG, Fornage BD. Tubular carcinoma of the breast: cytologic features in fine-needle aspirations and application of monoclonal anti-alpha-smooth muscle actin in diagnosis. Diagn Cytopathol 1994; 10(2): 120–125.

570. Dei Tos AP, Della Giustina D, De Martin V, et al. Aspiration biopsy cytology of tubular carcinoma of the breast. Diagn Cytopathol 1994; 11(2): 146–150.

571. Dawson AE, Logan-Young W, Mulford DK. Aspiration cytology of tubular carcinoma. Diagnostic features with mammographic correlation. Am J Clin Pathol 1994; 101(4): 488–492.

572. Cangiarella J, Waisman J, Shapiro RL, Simsir A. Cytologic features of tubular adenocarcinoma of the breast by aspiration biopsy. Diagn Cytopathol 2001; 25(5): 311–315.

573. Tobon H, Salazar H. Tubular carcinoma of the breast. Clinical, histological, and ultrastructural observations. Arch Pathol Lab Med 1977; 101(6): 310–316.

574. Kouchoukos NT, Ackerman LV, Butcher HR Jr. Prediction of axillary nodal metastases from the morphology of primary mammary carcinomas. Guide to operative therapy. Cancer 1967; 20(6): 948–960.

575. Van Bogaert LJ. Clinicopathologic hallmarks of mammary tubular carcinoma. Hum Pathol 1982; 13(6): 558–562.

576. Carstens PH, Greenberg RA, Francis D, Lyon H. Tubular carcinoma of the breast. A long term follow-up. Histopathology 1985; 9(3): 271–280.

577. Gadaleanu V, Galatar N, Tzortzi E. Tubular carcinoma of the breast. Morphol Embryol (Bucur) 1985; 31(3): 197–204.

578. Rosen PP, Groshen S, Kinne DW, Norton L. Factors influencing prognosis in node-negative breast carcinoma: analysis of 767 T1N0M0/T2N0M0 patients with long-term follow-up. J Clin Oncol 1993; 11(11): 2090–2100.

579. Haffty BG, Perrotta PL, Ward BE, et al. Conservatively treated breast cancer: Outcome by histologic subtype. Breast J 1997; 3: 7.

580. Fisher ER, Anderson S, Redmond C, Fisher B. Pathologic findings from the National Surgical Adjuvant Breast Project protocol B-06. 10-year pathologic and clinical prognostic discriminants. Cancer 1993; 71(8): 2507–2514.

581. Norris HJ, Taylor HB. Prognosis of mucinous (gelatinous) carcinoma of the breast. Cancer 1965; 18: 879.

582. Silverberg SG, Kay S, Chitale AR, Levitt SH. Colloid carcinoma of the breast. Am J Clin Pathol 1971; 55(3): 355–363.

583. Rasmussen BB. Human mucinous breast carcinomas and their lymph node metastases. A histological review of 247 cases. Pathol Res Pract 1985; 180(3): 377–382.

584. Clayton F. Pure mucinous carcinomas of breast: morphologic features and prognostic correlates. Hum Pathol 1986; 17(1): 34–38.

585. Rasmussen BB, Rose C, Christensen IB. Prognostic factors in primary mucinous breast carcinoma. Am J Clin Pathol 1987; 87(2): 155–160.

586. Komaki K, Sakamoto G, Sugano H, et al. Mucinous carcinoma of the breast in Japan. A prognostic

587. Toikkanen S, Kujari H. Pure and mixed mucinous carcinomas of the breast: a clinicopathologic analysis of 61 cases with long-term follow-up. Hum Pathol 1989; 20(8): 758–764.

588. Andre S, Cunha F, Bernardo M, et al. Mucinous carcinoma of the breast: a pathologic study of 82 cases. J Surg Oncol 1995; 58(3): 162–167.

589. Fentiman IS, Millis RR, Smith P, et al. Mucoid breast carcinomas: histology and prognosis. Br J Cancer 1997; 75(7): 1061–1065.

590. Avisar E, Khan MA, Axelrod D, Oza K. Pure mucinous carcinoma of the breast: a clinicopathologic correlation study. Ann Surg Oncol 1998; 5(5): 447–451.

591. Northridge ME, Rhoads GG, Wartenberg D, Koffman D. The importance of histologic type on breast cancer survival. J Clin Epidemiol 1997; 50(3): 283–290.

592. Wilson TE, Helvie MA, Oberman HA, Joynt LK. Pure and mixed mucinous carcinoma of the breast: pathologic basis for differences in mammographic appearance. AJR 1995; 165(2): 285–289.

593. Cardenosa G, Doudna C, Eklund GW. Mucinous (colloid) breast cancer: clinical and mammographic findings in 10 patients. AJR 1994; 162(5): 1077–1079.

594. Goodman DN, Boutross-Tadross O, Jong RA. Mammographic features of pure mucinous carcinoma of the breast with pathological correlation. Can Assoc Radiol J 1995; 46(4): 296–301.

595. Chopra S, Evans AJ, Pinder SE, et al. Pure mucinous breast cancer-mammographic and ultrasound findings. Clin Radiol 1996; 51(6): 421–424.

596. Toikkanen S, Eerola E, Ekfors TO. Pure and mixed mucinous breast carcinomas: DNA stemline and prognosis. J Clin Pathol 1988; 41(3): 300–303.

597. Fujii H, Anbazhagan R, Bornman DM, et al. Mucinous cancers have fewer genomic alterations than more common classes of breast cancer. Breast Cancer Res Treat 2002; 76(3): 255–260.

598. Duane GB, Kanter MH, Branigan T, Chang C. A morphologic and morphometric study of cells from colloid carcinoma of the breast obtained by fine needle aspiration. Distinction from other breast lesions. Acta Cytol 1987; 31(6): 742–750.

599. Stanley MW, Tani EM, Skoog L. Mucinous breast carcinoma and mixed mucinous-infiltrating ductal carcinoma: a comparative cytologic study. Diagn Cytopathol 1989; 5(2): 134–138.

600. Gupta RK, McHutchison AG, Simpson JS, Dowle CS. Value of fine needle aspiration cytology of the breast, with an emphasis on the cytodiagnosis of colloid carcinoma. Acta Cytol 1991; 35(6): 703–709.

601. Simsir A, Tsang P, Greenebaum E. Additional mimics of mucinous mammary carcinoma: fibroepithelial lesions. Am J Clin Pathol 1998; 109(2): 169–172.

602. Scopsi L, Andreola S, Pilotti S, et al. Mucinous carcinoma of the breast. A clinicopathologic, histochemical, and immunocytochemical study with special reference to neuroendocrine differentiation. Am J Surg Pathol 1994; 18(7): 702–711.

603. Kurtz JM, Jacquemier J, Torhorst J, et al. Conservation therapy for breast cancers other than infiltrating ductal carcinoma. Cancer 1989; 63(8): 1630–1635.

604. Sharnhorst D, Huntrakoon M. Mucinous carcinoma of the breast: recurrence 30 years after mastectomy. Southern Med J 1988; 81(656).

605. Richardson WW. Medullary carcinoma of the breast. A distinctive tumor type with a relatively good prognosis following radical mastectomy. Br J Cancer 1956; 10: 415.

606. Bloom HJ, Richardson WW, Field JR. Host resistance and survival in carcinoma of breast: a study of 104 cases of medullary carcinoma in a series of 1,411 cases of breast cancer followed for 20 years. Br Med J 1970; 3(716): 181–188.

607. Ridolfi RL, Rosen PP, Port A, et al. Medullary carcinoma of the breast: a clinicopathologic study

608. Maier WP, Rosemond GP, Goldman LI, et al. A ten year study of medullary carcinoma of the breast. Surg Gynecol Obstet 1977; 144(5): 695–698.

609. Rapin V, Contesso G, Mouriesse H, et al. Medullary breast carcinoma. A reevaluation of 95 cases of breast cancer with inflammatory stroma. Cancer 1988; 61(12): 2503–2510.

610. Wargotz ES, Silverberg SG. Medullary carcinoma of the breast: a clinicopathologic study with appraisal of current diagnostic criteria. Hum Pathol 1988; 19(11): 1340–1346.

611. Pedersen L, Holck S, Schiodt T, et al. Medullary carcinoma of the breast, prognostic importance of characteristic histopathological features evaluated in a multivariate Cox analysis. Eur J Cancer 1994; 30A(12): 1792–1797.

612. Pedersen L, Zedeler K, Holck S, et al. Medullary carcinoma of the breast. Prevalence and prognostic importance of classical risk factors in breast cancer. Eur J Cancer 1995; 31A(13–14). 2289–2295.

613. Pedersen L, Holck S, Schiodt T, et al. Inter- and intraobserver variability in the histopathological diagnosis of medullary carcinoma of the breast, and its prognostic implications. Breast Cancer Res Treat 1989; 14(1): 91–99.

614. Pedersen L, Zedeler K, Holck S, et al. Medullary carcinoma of the breast, proposal for a new simplified histopathological definition. Based on prognostic observations and observations on inter- and intraobserver variability of 11 histopathological characteristics in 131 breast carcinomas with medullary features. Br J Cancer 1991; 63(4): 591–595.

615. Fisher ER, Kenny JP, Sass R, et al. Medullary cancer of the breast revisited. Breast Cancer Res Treat 1990; 16(3): 215–229.

616. Rigaud C, Theobald S, Noel P, et al. Medullary carcinoma of the breast. A multicenter study of its diagnostic consistency. Arch Pathol Lab Med 1993; 117(10): 1005–1008.

617. Gaffey MJ, Mills SE, Frierson HF Jr, et al. Medullary carcinoma of the breast: interobserver variability in histopathologic diagnosis. Mod Pathol 1995; 8(1): 31–38.

618. Crotty TB. Medullary carcinoma: is it a reproducible and prognostically significant type of mammary carcinoma? Adv Anat Pathol 1996; 3: 179.

619. Jensen ML, Kiaer H, Andersen J, et al. Prognostic comparison of three classifications for medullary carcinomas of the breast. Histopathology 1997; 30(6): 523–532.

620. Shousha S. Medullary carcinoma of the breast and BRCA1 mutation. Histopathology 2000; 37(2): 182–185.

621. Neuman ML, Homer MJ. Association of medullary carcinoma with reactive axillary adenopathy. AJR 1996; 167(1): 185–186.

622. Meyer JE, Amin E, Lindfors KK, et al. Medullary carcinoma of the breast: mammographic and US appearance. Radiology 1989; 170(1 Pt 1): 79–82.

623. Kopans DB. Breast imaging. 2nd ed. Philadelphia, PA: Lippincott-Raven; 1997.

624. Rubens JR, Lewandrowski KB, Kopans DB, et al. Medullary carcinoma of the breast. Overdiagnosis of a prognostically favorable neoplasm. Arch Surg 1990; 125(5): 601–604.

625. Page DL, Dixon JM, Anderson TJ, et al. Invasive cribriform carcinoma of the breast. Histopathology 1983; 7(4): 525–536.

626. Venable JG, Schwartz AM, Silverberg SG. Infiltrating cribriform carcinoma of the breast: a distinctive clinicopathologic entity. Hum Pathol 1990; 21(3): 333–338.

627. Stutz JA, Evans AJ, Pinder S, et al. The radiological appearances of invasive cribriform carcinoma of the breast. Nottingham Breast Team. Clin Radiol 1994; 49(10): 693–695.

628. Boyages J, Recht A, Connolly JL, et al. Early breast cancer: predictors of breast recurrence for patients

treated with conservative surgery and radiation therapy. Radiother Oncol 1990; 19(1): 29–41.

629. Fisher ER, Palekar AS, Redmond C, et al. Pathologic findings from the National Surgical Adjuvant Breast Project (protocol no. 4). VI. Invasive papillary cancer. Am J Clin Pathol 1980; 73(3): 313–322.

630. Schneider JA. Invasive papillary breast carcinoma: mammographic and sonographic appearance. Radiology 1989; 171(2): 377–379.

631. Mitnick JS, Vazquez MF, Harris MN, et al. Invasive papillary carcinoma of the breast: mammographic appearance. Radiology 1990; 177(3): 803–806.

632. McCulloch GL, Evans AJ, Yeoman L, et al. Radiological features of papillary carcinoma of the breast. Clin Radiol 1997; 52(11): 865–868.

633. Fisher ER, Costantino J, Fisher B, Redmond C. Pathologic findings from the National Surgical Adjuvant Breast Project (Protocol 4). Discriminants for 15-year survival. National Surgical Adjuvant Breast and Bowel Project Investigators. Cancer 1993; 71(6 Suppl): 2141–2150.

634. Siriaunkgul S, Tavassoli FA. Invasive micropapillary carcinoma of the breast. Mod Pathol 1993; 6(6): 660–662.

635. Luna-More S, Gonzalez B, Acedo C, et al. Invasive micropapillary carcinoma of the breast. A new special type of invasive mammary carcinoma. Pathol Res Pract 1994; 190(7): 668–674.

636. Middleton LP, Tressera F, Sobel ME, et al. Infiltrating micropapillary carcinoma of the breast. Mod Pathol 1999; 12(5): 499–504.

637. Paterakos M, Watkin WG, Edgerton SM, et al. Invasive micropapillary carcinoma of the breast: a prognostic study. Hum Pathol 1999; 30(12): 1459–1463.

638. Walsh MM, Bleiweiss IJ. Invasive micropapillary carcinoma of the breast: eighty cases of an underrecognized entity. Hum Pathol 2001; 32(6): 583–589.

639. Nassar H, Wallis T, Andea A, et al. Clinicopathologic analysis of invasive micropapillary differentiation in breast carcinoma. Mod Pathol 2001; 14(9): 836–841.

640. Khurana KK, Wilbur D, Dawson AE. Fine needle aspiration cytology of invasive micropapillary carcinoma of the breast. A report of two cases. Acta Cytol 1997; 41(4 Suppl): 1394–1398.

641. Wong SI, Cheung H, Tse GM. Fine needle aspiration cytology of invasive micropapillary carcinoma of the breast. A case report. Acta Cytol 2000; 44(6): 1085–1089.

642. Ng WK, Poon CS, Kong JH. Fine needle aspiration cytology of invasive micropapillary carcinoma of the breast: review of cases in a three-year period. Acta Cytol 2001; 45(6): 973–979.

643. Luna-More S, de los Santos F, Breton JJ, Canadas MA. Estrogen and progesterone receptors, c-erbB-2, p53, and Bcl-2 in thirty-three invasive micropapillary breast carcinomas. Pathol Res Pract 1996; 192(1): 27–32.

644. Luna-More S, Casquero S, Perez-Mellado A, et al. Importance of estrogen receptors for the behavior of invasive micropapillary carcinoma of the breast. Review of 68 cases with follow-up of 54. Pathol Res Pract 2000; 196(1): 35–39.

645. Cornog JL, Mobini J, Steiger E, Enterline HT. Squamous carcinoma of the breast. Am J Clin Pathol 1971; 55(4): 410–417.

646. Eusebi V, Lamovec J, Cattani MG, et al. Acantholytic variant of squamous-cell carcinoma of the breast. Am J Surg Pathol 1986; 10(12): 855–861.

647. Gersell DJ, Katzenstein AL. Spindle cell carcinoma of the breast. A clinicopathologic and ultrastructural study. Hum Pathol 1981; 12(6): 550–561.

648. Merino MJ, LiVolsi VA, Kennedy S, et al. Spindle-cell carcinoma of teh breast: A clinicopathologic, ultrastructural and immunohistochemical study of eight cases. Surg Pathol 1988; 1: 193.

649. Kahn LB, Uys CJ, Dale J, Rutherford S. Carcinoma of the breast with metaplasia to chondrosarcoma: a light and electron microscopic study. Histopathology 1978; 2(2): 93–106.

650. Oberman HA. Metaplastic carcinoma of the breast. A clinicopathologic study of 29 patients. Am J Surg Pathol 1987; 11(12): 918–929.

651. Pitts WC, Rojas VA, Gaffey MJ, et al. Carcinomas with metaplasia and sarcomas of the breast. Am J Clin Pathol 1991; 95(5): 623–632.

652. Foschini MP, Dina RE, Eusebi V. Sarcomatoid neoplasms of the breast: proposed definitions for biphasic and monophasic sarcomatoid mammary carcinomas. Semin Diagn Pathol 1993; 10(2): 128–136.

653. Chhieng C, Cranor M, Lesser ME, Rosen PP. Metaplastic carcinoma of the breast with osteocartilaginous heterologous elements. Am J Surg Pathol 1998; 22(2): 188–194.

654. Patterson SK, Tworek JA, Roubidoux MA, et al. Metaplastic carcinoma of the breast: mammographic appearance with pathologic correlation. AJR 1997; 169(3): 709–712.

655. Flint A, Oberman HA, Davenport RD. Cytophotometric measurements of metaplastic carcinoma of the breast: correlation with pathologic features and clinical behavior. Mod Pathol 1988; 1(3): 193–197.

656. Zhuang Z, Lininger RA, Man YG, et al. Identical clonality of both components of mammary carcinosarcoma with differential loss of heterozygosity. Mod Pathol 1997; 10(4): 354–362.

657. Van Hoeven KH, Drudis T, Cranor ML, et al. Low-grade adenosquamous carcinoma of the breast. A clinocopathologic study of 32 cases with ultrastructural analysis. Am J Surg Pathol 1993; 17(3): 248–258.

658. Drudis T, Arroyo C, Van Hoeven KH, et al. The pathology of low grade adenosquamous carcinoma of the breast. An immunohistochemical study. Pathol Annu 1994; part 2.

659. Ruffolo EF, Koerner FC, Maluf HM. Metaplastic carcinoma of the breast with melanocytic differentiation. Mod Pathol 1997; 10(6): 592–596.

660. Kaufman MW, Marti JR, Gallager HS, Hoehn JL. Carcinoma of the breast with pseudosarcomatous metaplasia. Cancer 1984; 53(9): 1908–1917.

661. Brenner RJ, Turner RR, Schiller V, et al. Metaplastic carcinoma of the breast: report of three cases. Cancer 1998; 82(6): 1082–1087.

662. Gobbi H, Simpson JF, Borowsky A, et al. Metaplastic breast tumors with a dominant fibromatosis-like phenotype have a high risk of local recurrence. Cancer 1999; 85(10): 2170–2182.

663. Sneige N, Yaziji H, Mandavilli SR, et al. Low-grade (fibromatosis-like) spindle cell carcinoma of the breast. Am J Surg Pathol 2001; 25(8): 1009–1016.

664. Bauer TW, Rostock RA, Eggleston JC, Baral E. Spindle cell carcinoma of the breast: four cases and review of the literature. Hum Pathol 1984; 15(2): 147–152.

665. Silverman JF, Geisinger KR, Frable WJ. Fine-needle aspiration cytology of mesenchymal tumors of the breast. Diagn Cytopathol 1988; 4(1): 50–58.

666. Boccato P, Briani G, d'Atri C, et al. Spindle cell and cartilaginous metaplasia in a breast carcinoma with osteoclastlike stromal cells. A difficult fine needle aspiration diagnosis. Acta Cytol 1988; 32(1): 75–78.

667. Stanley MW, Tani EM, Skoog L. Metaplastic carcinoma of the breast: fine-needle aspiration cytology of seven cases. Diagn Cytopathol 1989; 5(1): 22–28.

668. Kline TS, Kline IK. Metaplastic carcinoma of the breast–diagnosis by aspiration biopsy cytology: report of two cases and literature review. Diagn Cytopathol 1990; 6(1): 63–67.

669. Jebsen PW, Hagmar BM, Nesland JM. Metaplastic breast carcinoma. A diagnostic problem in fine needle aspiration biopsy. Acta Cytol 1991; 35(4): 396–402.

670. Castella E, Gomez-Plaza MC, Urban A, Llatjos M. Fine-needle aspiration biopsy of metaplastic carcinoma of the breast: report of a case with abundant myxoid ground substance. Diagn Cytopathol 1996; 14(4): 325–327.

671. Straathof D, Yakimets WW, Mourad WA. Fine-needle aspiration cytology of sarcomatoid carcinoma of the breast: a cytologically overlooked neoplasm. Diagn Cytopathol 1997; 16(3): 242–246.

672. Nogueira M, Andre S, Mendonca E. Metaplastic carcinomas of the breast–fine needle aspiration (FNA) cytology findings. Cytopathology 1998; 9(5): 291–300.

673. Gupta RK. Cytodiagnostic patterns of metaplastic breast carcinoma in aspiration samples: a study of 14 cases. Diagn Cytopathol 1999; 20(1): 10–12.

674. Ferrara G, Nappi O, Wick MR. Fine-needle aspiration cytology and immunohistology of low-grade adenosquamous carcinoma of the breast. Diagn Cytopathol 1999; 20(1): 13–18.

675. Yen H, Florentine B, Kelly LK, et al. Fine-needle aspiration of a metaplastic breast carcinoma with extensive melanocytic differentiation: a case report. Diagn Cytopathol 2000; 23(1): 46–50.

676. Ribeiro-Silva A, Luzzatto F, Chang D, Zucoloto S. Limitations of fine-needle aspiration cytology to diagnose metaplastic carcinoma of the breast. Pathol Oncol Res 2001; 7(4): 298–300.

677. Chhieng DC, Cangiarella JF, Waisman J, et al. Fine-needle aspiration cytology of spindle cell lesions of the breast. Cancer 1999; 87(6): 359–371.

678. Huvos AG, Lucas JC Jr, Foote FW Jr. Metaplastic breast carcinoma. Rare form of mammary cancer. NY State J Med 1973; 73(9): 1078–1082.

679. Mavligit GM, Cohen JL, Sherwood LM. Ectopic production of parathyroid hormone by carcinoma of the breast. N Engl J Med 1971; 285(3): 154–156.

680. Kaneko H, Hojo H, Ishikawa S, et al. Norepinephrine-producing tumors of bilateral breasts: a case report. Cancer 1978; 41(5): 2002–2007.

681. Cohle SD, Tschen JA, Smith FE, et al. ACTH-secreting carcinoma of the breast. Cancer 1979; 43(6): 2370–2376.

682. Woodard BH, Eisenbarth G, Wallace NR, et al. Adrenocorticotropin production by a mammary carcinoma. Cancer 1981; 47(7): 1823–1827.

683. Scopsi L, Andreola S, Pilotti S, et al. Argyrophilia and granin (chromogranin/secretogranin) expression in female breast carcinomas. Their relationship to survival and other disease parameters. Am J Surg Pathol 1992; 16(6): 561–576.

684. Fisher ER, Palekar AS. Solid and mucinous varieties of so-called mammary carcinoid tumors. Am J Clin Pathol 1979; 72(6): 909–916.

685. Taxy JB, Tischler AS, Insalaco SJ, Battifora H. 'Carcinoid' tumor of the breast. A variant of conventional breast cancer? Hum Pathol 1981; 12(2): 170–179.

686. Azzopardi JG, Muretto P, Goddeeris P, et al. 'Carcinoid' tumours of the breast: the morphological spectrum of argyrophil carcinomas. Histopathology 1982; 6(5): 549–569.

687. Bussolati G, Gugliotta P, Sapino A, et al. Chromogranin-reactive endocrine cells in argyrophilic carcinomas ('carcinoids') and normal tissue of the breast. Am J Pathol 1985; 120(2): 186–192.

688. Miremadi A, Pinder SE, Lee AH, et al. Neuroendocrine differentiation and prognosis in breast adenocarcinoma. Histopathology 2002; 40(3): 215–222.

689. Feczko JD, Rosales RN, Cramer HM, et al. Fine needle aspiration cytology of a male breast carcinoma exhibiting neuroendocrine differentiation. Report of a case with immunohistochemical, flow cytometric and ultrastructural analysis. Acta Cytol 1995; 39(4): 803–808.

690. Fetissof F, Dubois MP, Arbeille-Brassart B, et al. Argyrophilic cells in mammary carcinoma. Hum Pathol 1983; 14(2): 127–134.

691. Sapino A, Bussolati G. Is detection of endocrine cells in breast adenocarcinoma of diagnostic and clinical significance? Histopathology 2002; 40(3): 211–214.

692. Kashlan RB, Powell RW, Nolting SF. Carcinoid and other tumors metastatic to the breast. J Surg Oncol 1982; 20(1): 25–30.

693. Ordonez NG, Manning JT Jr, Raymond AK. Argentaffin endocrine carcinoma (carcinoid) of the pancreas with concomitant breast metastasis: an immunohistochemical and electron microscopic study. Hum Pathol 1985; 16(7): 746–751.

694. Fishman A, Kim HS, Girtanner RE, Kaplan AL. Solitary breast metastasis as first manifestation of ovarian carcinoid tumor. Gynecol Oncol 1994; 54(2): 222–226.

695. Moreno A, Gonzalo MA, Sarasa JL, Herrera-Pombo JL. Bilateral breast metastases as the first manifestation of an occult ileocecal carcinoid. Med Clin (Barcelona) 1995; 104(13): 515–516.

696. Wozniak TC, Naunheim KS. Bronchial carcinoid tumor metastatic to the breast. Ann Thorac Surg 1998; 65(4): 1148–1149.

697. Rubio IT, Korourian S, Brown H, et al. Carcinoid tumor metastatic to the breast. Arch Surg 1998; 133(10): 1117–1119.

698. Toyoshima S. Mammary carcinoma with argyrophil cells. Cancer 1983; 52(11): 2129–2138.

699. Yogore MG III, Sahgal S. Small cell carcinoma of the male breast: report of a case. Cancer 1977; 39(4): 1748–1751.

700. Wade PM Jr, Mills SE, Read M, et al. Small cell neuroendocrine (oat cell) carcinoma of the breast. Cancer 1983; 52(1): 121–125.

701. Jundt G, Schulz A, Heitz PU, Osborn M. Small cell neuroendocrine (oat cell) carcinoma of the male breast. Immunocytochemical and ultrastructural investigations. Virchows Arch A Pathol Anat Histopathol 1984; 404(2): 213–221.

702. Papotti M, Gherardi G, Eusebi V, et al. Primary oat cell (neuroendocrine) carcinoma of the breast. Report of four cases. Virchows Arch A Pathol Anat Histopathol 1992; 420(1): 103–108.

703. Francois A, Chatikhine VA, Chevallier B, et al. Neuroendocrine primary small cell carcinoma of the breast. Report of a case and review of the literature. Am J Clin Oncol 1995; 18(2): 133–138.

704. Carlson HJ, Trujillo YP, Taxy JB. Prolonged survival in a case of small cell carcinoma of the breast. Breast J 1996; 2: 160.

705. Shin SJ, DeLellis RA, Ying L, Rosen PP. Small cell carcinoma of the breast: a clinicopathologic and immunohistochemical study of nine patients. Am J Surg Pathol 2000; 24(9): 1231–1238.

706. Deeley TJ. Secondary deposits in the breast. Br J Cancer 1965; 19(4): 738–743.

707. Hajdu SI, Urban JA. Cancers metastatic to the breast. Cancer 1972; 29(6): 1691–1696.

708. Clayton F, Sibley RK, Ordonez NG, Hanssen G. Argyrophilic breast carcinomas: evidence of lactational differentiation. Am J Surg Pathol 1982; 6(4): 323–333.

709. Jablon LK, Somers RG, Kim PY. Carcinoid tumor of the breast: treatment with breast conservation in three patients. Ann Surg Oncol 1998; 5(3): 261–264.

710. Birsak CA, Janssen PJ, van Vroonhoven CC, et al. Sex steroid receptor expression in 'carcinoid' tumours of the breast. Breast Cancer Res Treat 1996; 40(3): 243–249.

711. Nayer HR. Cylindroma of the breast with pulmonary metastases. Dis Chest 1957; 31: 324.

712. Wilson WB, Spell JP. Adenoid cystic carcinoma of breast: a case with recurrence and regional metastasis. Ann Surg 1967; 166(5): 861–864.

713. Cavanzo FJ, Taylor HB. Adenoid cystic carcinoma of the breast. An analysis of 21 cases. Cancer 1969; 24(4): 740–745.

714. Friedman BA, Oberman HA. Adenoid cystic carcinoma of the breast. Am J Clin Pathol 1970; 54(1): 1–14.

715. Eisner B. Adenoid cystic carcinoma of the breast. Pathol Euro 1970; 3: 357.

716. Anthony PP, James PD. Adenoid cystic carcinoma of the breast: prevalence, diagnostic criteria, and histogenesis. J Clin Pathol 1975; 28(5): 647–655.

717. Qizilbash AH, Patterson MC, Oliveira KF. Adenoid cystic carcinoma of the breast. Light and electron

microscopy and a brief review of the literature. Arch Pathol Lab Med 1977; 101(6): 302–306.

718. Hjorth S, Magnusson PH, Blomquist P. Adenoid cystic carcinoma of the breast. Report of a case in a male and review of the literature. Acta Chir Scand 1977; 143(3): 155–158.

719. Peters GN, Wolff M. Adenoid cystic carcinoma of the breast. Report of 11 new cases: review of the literature and discussion of biological behavior. Cancer 1983; 52(4): 680–686.

720. Wells CA, Nicoll S, Ferguson DJ. Adenoid cystic carcinoma of the breast: a case with axillary lymph node metastasis. Histopathology 1986; 10(4): 415–424.

721. Sumpio BE, Jennings TA, Merino MJ, Sullivan PD. Adenoid cystic carcinoma of the breast. Data from the Connecticut Tumor Registry and a review of the literature. Ann Surg 1987; 205(3): 295–301.

722. Lamovec J, Us-Krasovec M, Zidar A, Kljun A. Adenoid cystic carcinoma of the breast: a histologic, cytologic, and immunohistochemical study. Semin Diagn Pathol 1989; 6(2): 153–164.

723. Due W, Herbst WD, Loy V, Stein H. Characterisation of adenoid cystic carcinoma of the breast by immunohistology. J Clin Pathol 1989; 42(5): 470–476.

724. Miliauskas JR, Leong AS. Adenoid cystic carcinoma in a juvenile male breast. Pathology 1991; 23(4): 298–301.

725. Pastolero G, Hanna W, Zbieranowski I, Kahn HJ. Proliferative activity and p53 expression in adenoid cystic carcinoma of the breast. Mod Pathol 1996; 9(3): 215–219.

726. Lusted D. Structural and growth patterns of adenoid cystic carcinoma of breast. Am J Clin Pathol 1970; 54(3): 419–425.

727. Verani RR, Van der Bel-Kahn J. Mammary adenoid cystic carcinoma with unusual features. Am J Clin Pathol 1973; 59(5): 653–658.

728. Lim SK, Kovi J, Warner OG. Adenoid cystic carcinoma of breast with metastasis: a case report and review of the literature. J Natl Med Assoc 1979; 71(4): 329–330.

729. Zaloudek C, Oertel YC, Orenstein JM. Adenoid cystic carcinoma of the breast. Am J Clin Pathol 1984; 81(3): 297–307.

730. Koller M, Ram Z, Findler G, Lipshitz M. Brain metastasis: a rare manifestation of adenoid cystic carcinoma of the breast. Surg Neurol 1986; 26(5): 470–472.

731. Ro JY, Silva EG, Gallager HS. Adenoid cystic carcinoma of the breast. Hum Pathol 1987; 18(12): 1276–1281.

732. Herzberg AJ, Bossen EH, Walther PJ. Adenoid cystic carcinoma of the breast metastatic to the kidney. A clinically symptomatic lesion requiring surgical management. Cancer 1991; 68(5): 1015–1020.

733. Tavassoli FA, Norris HJ. Mammary adenoid cystic carcinoma with sebaceous differentiation. A morphologic study of the cell types. Arch Pathol Lab Med 1986; 110(11): 1045–1053.

734. Rosen PP. Adenoid cystic carcinoma of the breast. A morphologically heterogeneous neoplasm. Pathol Annu 1989; 24(2): 237–254.

735. Kasami M, Olson SJ, Simpson JF, Page DL. Maintenance of polarity and a dual cell population in adenoid cystic carcinoma of the breast: an immunohistochemical study. Histopathology 1998; 32(3): 232–238.

736. Kleer CG, Oberman HA. Adenoid cystic carcinoma of the breast: value of histologic grading and proliferative activity. Am J Surg Pathol 1998; 22(5): 569–575.

737. Trendell-Smith NJ, Peston D, Shousha S. Adenoid cystic carcinoma of the breast: a tumour commonly devoid of oestrogen receptors and related proteins. Histopathology 1999; 35(3): 241–248.

738. Arpino G, Clark GM, Mohsin S, et al. Adenoid cystic carcinoma of the breast: molecular markers, treatment, and clinical outcome. Cancer 2002; 94(8): 2119–2127.

739. Shin SJ, Rosen PP. Solid variant of mammary adenoid cystic carcinoma with basaloid features: a study of nine cases. Am J Surg Pathol 2002; 26(4): 413–420.

740. Harris M. Pseudoadenoid cystic carcinoma of the breast. Arch Pathol Lab Med 1977; 101(6): 307–309.

741. Galed-Placed I, Garcia-Ureta E. Fine needle aspiration biopsy diagnosis of adenoid cystic carcinoma of the breast. A case report. Acta Cytol 1992; 36(3): 364–366.

742. Stanley MW, Tani EM, Rutquist LE, Skoog L. Adenoid cystic carcinoma of the breast: diagnosis by fine-needle aspiration. Diagn Cytopathol 1993; 9(2): 184–187.

743. Culubret M, Roig I. Fine-needle aspiration biopsy of adenoid cystic carcinoma of the breast: a case report. Diagn Cytopathol 1996; 15(5): 431–434.

744. Quinodoz IS, Berger SD, Schafer P, Remadi S. Adenoid cystic carcinoma of the breast: utility of immunocytochemical study with collagen IV on fine-needle aspiration. Diagn Cytopathol 1997; 16(5): 442–445.

745. Mossler JA, Barton TK, Brinkhous AD, et al. Apocrine differentiation in human mammary carcinoma. Cancer 1980; 46(11): 2463–2471.

746. D'Amore ES, Terrier-Lacombe MJ, Travagli JP, et al. Invasive apocrine carcinoma of the breast: a long term follow-up study of 34 cases. Breast Cancer Res Treat 1988; 12(1): 37–44.

747. Bryant J. Male breast cancer: a case of apocrine carcinoma with psammoma bodies. Hum Pathol 1981; 12(8): 751–753.

748. Abati AD, Kimmel M, Rosen PP. Apocrine mammary carcinoma. A clinicopathologic study of 72 cases. Am J Clin Pathol 1990; 94(4): 371–377.

749. Gilles R, Lesnik A, Guinebretiere JM, et al. Apocrine carcinoma: clinical and mammographic features. Radiology 1994; 190(2): 495–497.

750. Frable WJ, Kay S. Carcinoma of the breast. Histologic and clinical features of apocrine tumors. Cancer 1968; 21(4): 756–763.

751. Yates AJ, Ahmed A. Apocrine carcinoma and apocrine metaplasia. Histopathology 1988; 13(2): 228–231.

752. Lee BJ, Pack GT, I. S. Sweat gland cancer of the breast. Surg Gynecol Obstet 1933; 54: 975.

753. Eusebi V, Millis RR, Cattani MG, et al. Apocrine carcinoma of the breast. A morphologic and immunocytochemical study. Am J Pathol 1986; 123(3): 532–541.

754. Raju U, Zarbo RJ, Kubus J, Schultz DS. The histologic spectrum of apocrine breast proliferations: a comparative study of morphology and DNA content by image analysis. Hum Pathol 1993; 24(2): 173–181.

755. Lamovec J, Bracko M. Secretory carcinoma of the breast: light microscopical, immunohistochemical and flow cytometric study. Mod Pathol 1994; 7(4): 475–479.

756. McDivitt RW, Stewart FW. Breast carcinoma in children. JAMA 1966; 195(5): 388–390.

757. Oberman HA, Stephens PJ. Carcinoma of the breast in childhood. Cancer 1972; 30(2): 470–474.

758. Byrne MP, Fahey MM, Gooselaw JG. Breast cancer with axillary metastasis in an eight and one-half-year-old girl. Cancer 1973; 31(3): 726–728.

759. Sullivan JJ, Magee HR, Donald KJ. Secretory (juvenile) carcinoma of the breast. Pathology 1977; 9(4): 341–346.

760. Tavassoli FA, Norris HJ. Secretory carcinoma of the breast. Cancer 1980; 45(9): 2404–2413.

761. Masse SR, Rioux A, Beauchesne C. Juvenile carcinoma of the breast. Hum Pathol 1981; 12(11): 1044–1046.

762. Botta G, Fessia L, Ghiringhello B. Juvenile milk protein secreting carcinoma. Virchows Arch A Pathol Anat Histol 1982; 395(2): 145–152.

763. Karl SR, Ballantine TV, Zaino R. Juvenile secretory carcinoma of the breast. J Pediatr Surg 1985; 20(4): 368–371.

764. d'Amore ES, Maisto L, Gatteschi MB, et al. Secretory carcinoma of the breast. Report of a case with fine needle aspiration biopsy. Acta Cytol 1986; 30(3): 309–312.

765. Abe R, Masuda T. Secretory carcinoma of the breast in a Japanese woman. Jpn J Surg 1986; 16(1): 52–55.

766. Ferguson TB Jr, McCarty KS Jr, Filston HC. Juvenile secretory carcinoma and juvenile papillomatosis: diagnosis and treatment. J Pediatr Surg 1987; 22(7): 637–639.

767. Roth JA, Discafani C, O'Malley M. Secretory breast carcinoma in a man. Am J Surg Pathol 1988; 12(2): 150–154.

768. Krausz T, Jenkins D, Grontoft O, et al. Secretory carcinoma of the breast in adults: emphasis on late recurrence and metastasis. Histopathology 1989; 14(1): 25–36.

769. Richard G, Hawk JC III, Baker AS Jr, Austin RM. Multicentric adult secretory breast carcinoma: DNA flow cytometric findings, prognostic features, and review of the world literature. J Surg Oncol 1990; 44(4): 238–244.

770. Dominguez F, Riera JR, Junco P, Sampedro A. Secretory carcinoma of the breast. Report of a case with diagnosis by fine needle aspiration. Acta Cytol 1992; 36(4): 507–510.

771. Serour F, Gilad A, Kopolovic J, Krispin M. Secretory breast cancer in childhood and adolescence: report of a case and review of the literature. Med Pediatr Oncol 1992; 20(4): 341–344.

772. Mies C. Recurrent secretory carcinoma in residual mammary tissue after mastectomy. Am J Surg Pathol 1993; 17(7): 715–721.

773. Pohar-Marinsek Z, Golouh R. Secretory breast carcinoma in a man diagnosed by fine needle aspiration biopsy. A case report. Acta Cytol 1994; 38(3): 446–450.

774. Kuwabara H, Yamane M, Okada S. Secretory breast carcinoma in a 66-year-old man. J Clin Pathol 1998; 51(7): 545–547.

775. Furugaki K, Nagai E, Shinohara M, et al. Secretory carcinoma of the breast in an elderly woman: report of a case. Surg Today 1998; 28(2): 219–222.

776. Factor SM, Biempica L, Ratner I, et al. Carcinoma of the breast with multinucleated reactive stromal giant cells. A light and electron microscopic study of two cases. Virchows Arch A Pathol Anat Histol 1977; 374(1): 1–12.

777. Sugano I, Nagao K, Kondo Y, et al. Cytologic and ultrastructural studies of a rare breast carcinoma with osteoclast-like giant cells. Cancer 1983; 52(1): 74–78.

778. Fisher ER, Palekar AS, Gregorio RM, Paulson JD. Mucoepidermoid and squamous cell carcinomas of breast with reference to squamous metaplasia and giant cell tumors. Am J Surg Pathol 1983; 7(1): 15–27.

779. Holland R, van Haelst UJ. Mammary carcinoma with osteoclast-like giant cells. Additional observations on six cases. Cancer 1984; 53(9): 1963–1973.

780. Nielsen BB, Kiaer HW. Carcinoma of the breast with stromal multinucleated giant cells. Histopathology 1985; 9(2): 183–193.

781. McMahon RF, Ahmed A, Connolly CE. Breast carcinoma with stromal multinucleated giant cells–a light microscopic, histochemical and ultrastructural study. J Pathol 1986; 150(3): 175–179.

782. Ichijima K, Kobashi Y, Ueda Y, Matsuo S. Breast cancer with reactive multinucleated giant cells: report of three cases. Acta Pathol Jpn 1986; 36(3): 449–457.

783. Tavassoli FA, Norris HJ. Breast carcinoma with osteoclastlike giant cells. Arch Pathol Lab Med 1986; 110(7): 636–639.

784. Athanasou NA, Wells CA, Quinn J, et al. The origin and nature of stromal osteoclast-like multinucleated giant cells in breast carcinoma: implications for tumour osteolysis and macrophage biology. Br J Cancer 1989; 59(4): 491–498.

785. Phillipson J, Ostrzega N. Fine needle aspiration of invasive cribriform carcinoma with benign osteoclast-like giant cells of histiocytic origin. A case report. Acta Cytol 1994; 38(3): 479–482.

786. Viacava P, Naccarato AG, Nardini V, Bevilacqua G. Breast carcinoma with osteoclast-like giant cells: immunohistochemical and ultrastructural study of a case and review of the literature. Tumori 1995; 81(2): 135–141.

787. Takahashi T, Moriki T, Hiroi M, Nakayama H. Invasive lobular carcinoma of the breast with osteoclastlike giant cells. A case report. Acta Cytol 1998; 42(3): 734–741.

788. Agnantis NT, Rosen PP. Mammary carcinoma with osteoclast-like giant cells. A study of eight cases with follow-up data. Am J Clin Pathol 1979; 72(3): 383–389.

789. Saigo PE, Rosen PP. Mammary carcinoma with 'choriocarcinomatous' features. Am J Surg Pathol 1981; 5(8): 773–778.

790. Green DM. Mucoid carcinoma of the breast with choriocarcinoma in its metastases. Histopathology 1990; 16(5): 504–506.

791. Alvarez RD, Gleason BP, Gore H, Partridge EE. Coexisting intraductal breast carcinoma and metastatic choriocarcinoma presenting as a breast mass. Gynecol Oncol 1991; 43(3): 295–299.

792. Aboumrad MH, Horn RC, Fine G. Lipid-secreting mammary carcinoma: report of a case associated with Paget's disease of the nipple. Cancer 1963; 16: 521.

793. Ramos CV, Taylor HB. Lipid-rich carcinoma of the breast. A clinicopathologic analysis of 13 examples. Cancer 1974; 33(3): 812–819.

794. Van Bogaert LJ, Maldague P. Histologic variants of lipid-secreting carcinoma of the breast. Virchows Arch A Pathol Anat Histol 1977; 375(4): 345–353.

795. Lapey JD. Lipid-rich mammary carcinoma–diagnosis by cytology. Case report. Acta Cytol 1977; 21(1): 120–122.

796. Dina R, Eusebi V. Clear cell tumors of the breast. Semin Diagn Pathol 1997; 14(3): 175–182.

797. Hull MT, Priest JB, Broadie TA, et al. Glycogen-rich clear cell carcinoma of the breast: a light and electron microscopic study. Cancer 1981; 48(9): 2003–2009.

798. Benisch B, Peison B, Newman R, et al. Solid glycogen-rich clear cell carcinoma of the breast (a light and ultrastructural study). Am J Clin Pathol 1983; 79(2): 243–245.

799. Fisher ER, Tavares J, Bulatao IS, et al. Glycogen-rich, clear cell breast cancer: with comments concerning other clear cell variants. Hum Pathol 1985; 16(11): 1085–1090.

800. Hull MT, Warfel KA. Glycogen-rich clear cell carcinomas of the breast. A clinicopathologic and ultrastructural study. Am J Surg Pathol 1986; 10(8): 553–559.

801. Sorensen FB, Paulsen SM. Glycogen-rich clear cell carcinoma of the breast: a solid variant with mucus. A light microscopic, immunohistochemical and ultrastructural study of a case. Histopathology 1987; 11(8): 857–869.

802. Toikkanen S, Joensuu H. Glycogen-rich clear-cell carcinoma of the breast: a clinicopathologic and flow cytometric study. Hum Pathol 1991; 22(1): 81–83.

803. Hayes MM, Seidman JD, Ashton MA. Glycogen-rich clear cell carcinoma of the breast. A clinicopathologic study of 21 cases. Am J Surg Pathol 1995; 19(8): 904–911.

804. Koenig C, Tavassoli FA. Mucinous cystadenocarcinoma of the breast. Am J Surg Pathol 1998; 22(6): 698–703.

805. Bohman LG, Bassett LW, Gold RH, Voet R. Breast metastases from extramammary malignancies. Radiology 1982; 144(2): 309–312.

806. Mabuchi K, Bross DS, Kessler, II. Risk factors for male breast cancer. J Natl Cancer Inst 1985; 74(2): 371–375.

807. Casagrande JT, Hanisch R, Pike MC, et al. A case-control study of male breast cancer. Cancer Res 1988; 48(5): 1326–1330.

808. Wolman SR, Sanford J, Ratner S, Dawson PJ. Breast cancer in males: DNA content and sex chromosome constitution. Mod Pathol 1995; 8(3): 239–243.

809. Evans DB, Crichlow RW. Carcinoma of the male breast and Klinefelter's syndrome: is there an association? CA Cancer J Clin 1987; 37(4): 246–251.

810. Heller KS, Rosen PP, Schottenfeld D, et al. Male breast cancer: a clinicopathologic study of 97 cases. Ann Surg 1978; 188(1): 60–65.

811. Schlappack OK, Braun O, Maier U. Report of two cases of male breast cancer after prolonged estrogen treatment for prostatic carcinoma. Cancer Detect Prev 1986; 9(3–4): 319–322.

812. Sobin LH, Sherif M. Relation between male breast cancer and prostate cancer. Br J Cancer 1980; 42(5): 787–790.

813. Yan Z, Hummel P, Waisman J, et al. Prostatic adenocarcinoma metastatic to the breasts: report of a case with diagnosis by fine needle aspiration biopsy. Urology 2000; 55(4): 590.

814. Kozak FK, Hall JG, Baird PA. Familial breast cancer in males. A case report and review of the literature. Cancer 1986; 58(12): 2736–2739.

815. Sneige N, Holder PD, Katz RL, et al. Fine-needle aspiration cytology of the male breast in a cancer center. Diagn Cytopathol 1993; 9(6): 691–697.

816. Das DK, Junaid TA, Mathews SB, et al. Fine needle aspiration cytology diagnosis of male breast lesions. A study of 185 cases. Acta Cytol 1995; 39(5): 870–876.

817. Joshi MG, Lee AK, Loda M, et al. Male breast carcinoma: an evaluation of prognostic factors contributing to a poorer outcome. Cancer 1996; 77(3): 490–498.

818. Gattuso P, Reddy VB, Green L, et al. Prognostic significance of DNA ploidy in male breast carcinoma. A retrospective analysis of 32 cases. Cancer 1992; 70(4): 777–780.

819. Pegoraro RJ, Nirmul D, Joubert SM. Cytoplasmic and nuclear estrogen and progesterone receptors in male breast cancer. Cancer Res 1982; 42(11): 4812–4814.

820. Sandison. Metastatic tumors in the breast. Br J Surg 1959; 47: 54.

821. Toombs BD, Kalisher L. Metastatic disease to the breast: clinical, pathologic, and radiographic features. AJR 1977; 129(4): 673–676.

822. Pressman PI. Malignant melanoma and the breast. Cancer 1973; 31(4): 784–792.

823. Silverman JF, Feldman PS, Covell JL, Frable WJ. Fine needle aspiration cytology of neoplasms metastatic to the breast. Acta Cytol 1987; 31(3): 291–300.

824. Sneige N, Zachariah S, Fanning TV, et al. Fine-needle aspiration cytology of metastatic neoplasms in the breast. Am J Clin Pathol 1989; 92(1): 27–35.

825. Cangiarella J, Symmans WF, Cohen JM, et al. Malignant melanoma metastatic to the breast: a report of seven cases diagnosed by fine-needle aspiration cytology. Cancer 1998; 84(3): 160–162.

826. Kelly C, Henderson D, Corris P. Breast lumps: rare presentation of oat cell carcinoma of lung. J Clin Pathol 1988; 41(2): 171–172.

827. McCrea ES, Johnston C, Haney PJ. Metastases to the breast. AJR 1983; 141(4): 685–690.

828. Nielsen M, Andersen JA, Henriksen FW, et al. Metastases to the breast from extramammary carcinomas. Acta Pathol Microbiol Scand [A] 1981; 89(4): 251–256.

829. Salyer WR, Salyer DC. Metastases of prostatic carcinoma to the breast. J Urol 1973; 109(4): 671–675.

830. Hartley LC, Little JH. Bilateral mammary metastases from carcinoma of the prostate during oestrogen therapy. Med J Aust 1971; 1(8): 434–436.

831. Scott J, Robb-Smith AH, Burns I. Bilateral breast metastases from carcinoma of the prostate. Br J Urol 1974; 46(2): 209–214.

832. Benson WR. Carcinoma of the prostate with metastases to the breast and testes. Cancer 1957; 10: 1235.

833. Malek GH, Madsen PO. Carcinoma of the prostate with unusual metastases. Cancer 1969; 24(1): 194–197.

834. Wilson SE, Hutchinson WB. Breast masses in males with carcinoma of the prostate. J Surg Oncol 1976; 8(2): 105–112.

835. Harrist TJ, Kalisher L. Breast metastasis: an unusual manifestation of a malignant carcinoid tumor. Cancer 1977; 40(6): 3102–3106.

836. Turner M, Gallager HS. Occult appendiceal carcinoid. Report of a case with fatal metastases. Arch Pathol 1969; 88(2): 188–190.

837. Schurch W, Lamoureux E, Lefebvre R, Fauteux JP. Solitary breast metastasis: first manifestation of an occult carcinoid of the ileum. Virchows Arch A Pathol Anat Histol 1980; 386(1): 117–124.

838. Hawley PR. A case of secondary carcinoid tumours in both breasts following excision of primary carcinoid tumour of the duodenum. Br J Surg 1966; 53(9): 818–820.

839. Landon G, Sneige N, Ordonez NG, Mackay B. Carcinoid metastatic to breast diagnosed by fine-needle aspiration biopsy. Diagn Cytopathol 1987; 3(3): 230–233.

840. Lozowski MS, Faegenburg D, Mishriki Y, Lundy J. Carcinoid tumor metastatic to breast diagnosed by fine needle aspiration. Case report and literature review. Acta Cytol 1989; 33(2): 191–194.

841. Marcus JN, Watson P, Page DL, et al. Hereditary breast cancer: pathobiology, prognosis, and *BRCA1* and *BRCA2* gene linkage. Cancer 1996; 77(4): 697–709.

842. Breast Cancer Linkage Consortium. Pathology of familial breast cancer: differences between breast cancers in carriers of *BRCA1* or *BRCA2* mutations and sporadic cases. Lancet 1997; 349(9064): 1505–1510.

843. Robson M, Gilewski T, Haas B, et al. *BRCA*-associated breast cancer in young women. J Clin Oncol 1998; 16(5): 1642–1649.

844. Karp SE, Tonin PN, Begin LR, et al. Influence of *BRCA1* mutations on nuclear grade and estrogen receptor status of breast carcinoma in Ashkenazi Jewish women. Cancer 1997; 80(3): 435–441.

845. Verhoog LC, Brekelmans CT, Seynaeve C, et al. Survival and tumour characteristics of breast-cancer patients with germline mutations of BRCA1. Lancet 1998; 351(9099): 316–321.

846. Johannsson OT, Idvall I, Anderson C, et al. Tumour biological features of *BRCA1*-induced breast and ovarian cancer. Eur J Cancer 1997; 33(3): 362–371.

847. Eisinger F, Stoppa-Lyonnet D, Longy M, et al. Germ line mutation at BRCA1 affects the histoprognostic grade in hereditary breast cancer. Cancer Res 1996; 56(3): 471–474.

848. Lynch BJ, Holden JA, Buys SS, et al. Pathobiologic characteristics of hereditary breast cancer. Hum Pathol 1998; 29(10): 1140–1144.

849. Lakhani SR, Jacquemier J, Sloane JP, et al. Multifactorial analysis of differences between sporadic breast cancers and cancers involving *BRCA1* and *BRCA2* mutations. J Natl Cancer Inst 1998; 90(15): 1138–1145.

850. Armes JE, Egan AJ, Southey MC, et al. The histologic phenotypes of breast carcinoma occurring before age 40 years in women with and without *BRCA1* or *BRCA2* germline mutations: a population-based study. Cancer 1998; 83(11): 2335–2345.

851. Marcus JN, Page DL, Watson P, et al. *BRCA1* and *BRCA2* hereditary breast carcinoma phenotypes. Cancer 1997; 80(3): 543–556.

852. Lakhani SR, Van De Vijver MJ, Jacquemier J, et al. The pathology of familial breast cancer: predictive value of immunohistochemical markers estrogen receptor, progesterone receptor, HER-2, and p53 in patients with mutations in *BRCA1* and *BRCA2*. J Clin Oncol 2002; 20(9): 2310–2318.

853. Quenneville LA, Phillips KA, Ozcelik H, et al. HER-2/neu status and tumor morphology of invasive breast carcinomas in Ashkenazi women with known BRCA1 mutation status in the Ontario Familial Breast Cancer Registry. Cancer 2002; 95(10): 2068–2075.

854. Henderson IC, Patek AJ. Are breast cancers in young women qualitatively distinct? Lancet 1997; 349(9064): 1488–1489.

855. Lynch HT, Watson P. BRCA1, pathology, and survival. J Clin Oncol 1998; 16(2): 395–396.

856. Watson P, Marcus JN, Lynch HT. Prognosis of BRCA1 hereditary breast cancer. Lancet 1998; 351(9099): 304–305.

857. Agnarsson BA, Jonasson JG, Bjornsdottir IB, et al. Inherited BRCA2 mutation associated with high grade breast cancer. Breast Cancer Res Treat 1998; 47(2): 121–127.

858. Marcus JN, Watson P, Page DL, et al. BRCA2 hereditary breast cancer pathophenotype. Breast Cancer Res Treat 1997; 44(3): 275–277.

859. Norris HJ, Taylor HB. Sarcomas and related mesenchymal tumors of the breast. Cancer 1968; 22(1): 22–28.

860. Buatti JM, Harari PM, Leigh BR, Cassady JR. Radiation-induced angiosarcoma of the breast. Case report and review of the literature. Am J Clin Oncol 1994; 17(5): 444–447.

861. Collins V LR, Tivey H. Observations in the growth rate of human tumors. 1956; 76: 988.

862. Von Fournier D, Weber E, Hoeffken W, et al. Growth rate of 147 mammary carcinomas. Cancer 1980; 45(8): 2198–2207.

863. Kusama S, Spratt JS Jr, Donegan WL, et al. The gross rates of growth of human mammary carcinoma. Cancer 1972; 30(2): 594–599.

864. Moskowitz M. Breast cancer: age-specific growth rates and screening strategies. Radiology 1986; 161(1): 37–41.

865. Spratt JA, von Fournier D, Spratt JS, Weber EE. Mammographic assessment of human breast cancer growth and duration. Cancer 1993; 71(6): 2020–2026.

866. Spratt JS, Heuser L, Kuhns JG, et al. Association between the actual doubling times of primary breast cancer and histopathologic characteristics and Wolfe's parenchymal mammographic patterns. Cancer 1981; 47(9): 2265–2268.

867. Taylor GW. Inflammatory carcinoma of the breast. AM J Cancer 1938; 33: 33.

868. Friberg S, Mattson S. On the growth rates of human malignant tumors: implications for medical decision making. J Surg Oncol 1997; 65(4): 284–297.

869. Mansour EG, Ravdin PM, Dressler L. Prognostic factors in early breast carcinoma. Cancer 1994; 74(1 Suppl): 381–400.

870. Weidner N, Cady B, Goodson WH III. Pathologic prognostic factors for patients with breast carcinoma. Which factors are important. Surg Oncol Clin North Am 1997; 6(3): 415–462.

871. Donegan WL. Tumor-related prognostic factors for breast cancer. CA Cancer J Clin 1997; 47(1): 28–51.

872. Chen YY, Schnitt SJ. Prognostic factors for patients with breast cancers 1cm and smaller. Breast Cancer Res Treat 1998; 51(3): 209–225.

873. Abner AL, Collins L, Peiro G, et al. Correlation of tumor size and axillary lymph node involvement with prognosis in patients with T1 breast carcinoma. Cancer 1998; 83(12): 2502–2508.

874. NIH Consensus Conference. Treatment of early-stage breast cancer. J Am Med Assoc 1990; 265: 391–395.

875. Goldhirsch A, Glick JH, Gelber RD, Senn HJ. Meeting highlights: International Consensus Panel on the Treatment of Primary Breast Cancer. J Natl Cancer Inst 1998; 90(21): 1601–1608.

876. Davis BW, Gelber RD, Goldhirsch A, et al. Prognostic significance of tumor grade in clinical trials of adjuvant therapy for breast cancer with axillary lymph node metastasis. Cancer 1986; 58(12): 2662–2670.

877. Contesso G, Mouriesse H, Friedman S, et al. The importance of histologic grade in long-term prognosis of breast cancer: a study of 1,010 patients, uniformly treated at the Institut Gustave-Roussy. J Clin Oncol 1987; 5(9): 1378–1386.

878. Le Doussal V, Tubiana-Hulin M, Friedman S, et al. Prognostic value of histologic grade nuclear components of Scarff–Bloom–Richardson (SBR). An improved score modification based on a multivariate analysis of 1262 invasive ductal breast carcinomas. Cancer 1989; 64(9): 1914–1921.

879. Rosen PP, Groshen S, Saigo PE, et al. Pathological prognostic factors in stage I (T1N0M0) and stage II (T1N1M0) breast carcinoma: a study of 644 patients with median follow-up of 18 years. J Clin Oncol 1989; 7(9): 1239–1251.

880. Elston CW, Ellis IO. Pathological prognostic factors in breast cancer. I. The value of histological grade in breast cancer: experience from a large study with long-term follow-up. Histopathology 1991; 19(5): 403–410.

881. Page DL. Prognosis and breast cancer. Recognition of lethal and favorable prognostic types. Am J Surg Pathol 1991; 15(4): 334–349.

882. Nixon AJ, Schnitt SJ, Gelman R, et al. Relationship of tumor grade to other pathologic features and to treatment outcome of patients with early stage breast carcinoma treated with breast-conserving therapy. Cancer 1996; 78(7): 1426–1431.

883. Roberti NE. The role of histologic grading in the prognosis of patients with carcinoma of the breast: is this a neglected opportunity? Cancer 1997; 80(9): 1708–1716.

884. Pinder SE, Murray S, Ellis IO, et al. The importance of the histologic grade of invasive breast carcinoma and response to chemotherapy. Cancer 1998; 83(8): 1529–1539.

885. Fisher ER, Redmond C, Fisher B. Pathologic findings from the National Surgical Adjuvant Breast Project. VIII. Relationship of chemotherapeutic responsiveness to tumor differentiation. Cancer 1983; 51(2): 181–191.

886. Stenkvist B, Westman-Naeser S, Vegelius J, et al. Analysis of reproducibility of subjective grading systems for breast carcinoma. J Clin Pathol 1979; 32(10): 979–985.

887. Delides GS, Garas G, Georgouli G, et al. Intralaboratory variations in the grading of breast carcinoma. Arch Pathol Lab Med 1982; 106(3): 126–128.

888. Harvey JM, de Klerk NH, Sterrett GF. Histological grading in breast cancer: interobserver agreement, and relation to other prognostic factors including ploidy. Pathology 1992; 24(2): 63–68.

889. Frierson HF Jr, Wolber RA, Berean KW, et al. Interobserver reproducibility of the Nottingham modification of the Bloom and Richardson histologic grading scheme for infiltrating ductal carcinoma. Am J Clin Pathol 1995; 103(2): 195–198.

890. Pinder SE, Ellis IO, Galea M, et al. Pathological prognostic factors in breast cancer. III. Vascular invasion: relationship with recurrence and survival in a large study with long-term follow-up. Histopathology 1994; 24(1): 41–47.

891. Orbo A, Stalsberg H, Kunde D. Topographic criteria in the diagnosis of tumor emboli in intramammary lymphatics. Cancer 1990; 66(5): 972–977.

892. Rosen PP. Tumor emboli in intramammary lymphatics in breast carcinoma: pathologic criteria for diagnosis and clinical significance. Pathol Annu 1983; 18(2): 215–232.

893. Davis BW, Gelber R, Goldhirsch A, et al. Prognostic significance of peritumoral vessel invasion in clinical trials of adjuvant therapy for breast cancer with axillary lymph node metastasis. Hum Pathol 1985; 16(12): 1212–1218.

894. Lauria R, Perrone F, Carlomagno C, et al. The prognostic value of lymphatic and blood vessel invasion in operable breast cancer. Cancer 1995; 76(10): 1772–1778.

895. Chen YY, Connolly JL, Harris J, Schnitt S. Predictors of axillary lymph node metastases (ALNM) in patients with breast cancers 1 cm or smaller (T1a, b): Implications for axillary dissection (Meeting Abstract). Mod Pathol 1998; 78: 17A.

896. Fein DA, Fowble BL, Hanlon AL, et al. Identification of women with T1-T2 breast cancer at low risk of positive axillary nodes. J Surg Oncol 1997; 65(1): 34–39.

897. Chadha M, Chabon AB, Friedmann P, Vikram B. Predictors of axillary lymph node metastases in patients with T1 breast cancer. A multivariate analysis. Cancer 1994; 73(2): 350–353.

898. Nealon TF Jr, Nkongho A, Grossi C, Gillooley J. Pathologic identification of poor prognosis stage I (T1N0M0) cancer of the breast. Ann Surg 1979; 190(2): 129–132.

899. Leitner SP, Swern AS, Weinberger D, Duncan LJ, Hutter RV. Predictors of recurrence for patients with small (one centimeter or less) localized breast cancer (T1a,b N0 M0). Cancer 1995; 76(11): 2266–74.

900. Lee AK, Loda M, Mackarem G, et al. Lymph node negative invasive breast carcinoma 1 centimeter or less in size (T1a,bN0M0): clinicopathologic features and outcome. Cancer 1997; 79(4): 761–771.

901. Rosen PP, Saigo PE, Braun DW Jr, et al. Predictors of recurrence in stage I (T1N0M0) breast carcinoma. Ann Surg 1981; 193(1): 15–25.

902. Roses DF, Bell DA, Flotte TJ, et al. Pathologic predictors of recurrence in stage 1 (T1N0M0) breast cancer. Am J Clin Pathol 1982; 78(6): 817–820.

903. Gilchrist KW, Gould VE, Hirschl S, et al. Interobserver variation in the identification of breast carcinoma in intramammary lymphatics. Hum Pathol 1982; 13(2): 170–172.

904. Lee AK, DeLellis RA, Silverman ML, Wolfe HJ. Lymphatic and blood vessel invasion in breast carcinoma: a useful prognostic indicator? Hum Pathol 1986; 17(10): 984–987.

905. Bettelheim R, Mitchell D, Gusterson BA. Immunocytochemistry in the identification of vascular invasion in breast cancer. J Clin Pathol 1984; 37(4): 364–366.

906. Lee AK, DeLellis RA, Rosen PP, et al. ABH blood group isoantigen expression in breast carcinomas–an immunohistochemical evaluation using monoclonal antibodies. Am J Clin Pathol 1985; 83(3): 308–319.

907. Lee AK, DeLellis RA, Wolfe HJ. Intramammary lymphatic invasion in breast carcinomas. Evaluation using ABH isoantigens as endothelial markers. Am J Surg Pathol 1986; 10(9): 589–594.

908. Martin SA, Perez-Reyes N, Mendelsohn G. Angioinvasion in breast carcinoma. An immunohistochemical study of factor VIII-related antigen. Cancer 1987; 59(11): 1918–1922.

909. Saigo PE, Rosen PP. The application of immunohistochemical stains to identify endothelial-lined channels in mammary carcinoma. Cancer 1987; 59(1): 51–54.

910. Ordonez NG, Brooks T, Thompson S, Batsakis JG. Use of Ulex europaeus agglutinin I in the identification of lymphatic and blood vessel invasion in previously stained microscopic slides. Am J Surg Pathol 1987; 11(7): 543–550.

911. Hanau CA, Machera H, Meittinen M. Immunohistochemical evaluation of vascular invasion in carcinomas with five different markers. Appl Immunohistochem 1993; 1: 46.

912. Rosen PP, Saigo PE, Braun DW, et al. Prognosis in stage II (T1N1M0) breast cancer. Ann Surg 1981; 194(5): 576–584.

913. Bell JR, Friedell GH, Goldenberg IS. Prognostic significance of pathologic findings in human breast carcinoma. Surg Gynecol Obstet 1969; 129(2): 258–262.

914. Kister SJ, Sommers SC, Haagensen CD, Cooley E. Re-evaluation of blood-vessel invasion as a prognostic factor in carcinoma of the breast. Cancer 1966; 19(9): 1213–1216.

915. Sampat MB, Sirsat MV, Gangadharan P. Prognostic significance of blood vessel invasion in carcinoma of the breast in women. J Surg Oncol 1977; 9(6): 623–632.

916. Weigand RA, Isenberg WM, Russo J, et al. Blood vessel invasion and axillary lymph node involvement as prognostic indicators for human breast cancer. Cancer 1982; 50(5): 962–969.

917. Fisher ER, Palekar AS, Gregorio RM, et al. Pathological findings from the national surgical

adjuvant breast project (Protocol No. 4). IV. Significance of tumor necrosis. Hum Pathol 1978; 9(5): 523–530.

918. Carter D, Pipkin RD, Shepard RH, et al. Relationship of necrosis and tumor border to lymph node metastases and 10-year survival in carcinoma of the breast. Am J Surg Pathol 1978; 2(1): 39–46.

919. Gilchrist KW, Gray R, Fowble B, et al. Tumor necrosis is a prognostic predictor for early recurrence and death in lymph node-positive breast cancer: a 10-year follow-up study of 728 Eastern Cooperative Oncology Group patients. J Clin Oncol 1993; 11(10): 1929–1935.

920. Parham DM, Hagen N, Brown RA. Simplified method of grading primary carcinomas of the breast. J Clin Pathol 1992; 45(6): 517–520.

921. Stenkvist B, Bengtsson E, Dahlqvist B, et al. Predicting breast cancer recurrence. Cancer 1982; 50(12): 2884–2893.

922. Black MM, Barclay TH, Hankey BF. Prognosis in breast cancer utilizing histologic characteristics of the primary tumor. Cancer 1975; 36(6): 2048–2055.

923. Alderson MR, Hamlin I, Staunton MD. The relative significance of prognostic factors in breast carcinoma. Br J Cancer 1971; 25(4): 646–656.

924. Berg JW. Morphological evidence for immune response to breast cancer. An historical review. Cancer 1971; 28(6): 1453–1456.

925. Dawson PJ, Ferguson DJ, Karrison T. The pathological findings of breast cancer in patients surviving 25 years after radical mastectomy. Cancer 1982; 50(10): 2131–2138.

926. Vicini FA, Goldstein NS, Pass H, Kestin LL. Use of pathologic factors to assist in establishing adequacy of excision before radiotherapy in patients treated with breast-conserving therapy. Int J Radiat Oncol Biol Phys 2004; 60(1): 86–94.

927. Crombie N, Rampaul RS, Pinder SE, et al. Extent of ductal carcinoma in situ within and surrounding invasive primary breast carcinoma. Br J Surg 2001; 88(10): 1324–1329.

928. Silverberg SG, Chitale AR. Assessment of significance of proportions of intraductal and infiltrating tumor growth in ductal carcinoma of the breast. Cancer 1973; 32(4): 830–837.

929. Rosen PP, Kinne DW, Lesser M, Hellman S. Are prognostic factors for local control of breast cancer treated by primary radiotherapy significant for patients treated by mastectomy? Cancer 1986; 57(7): 1415–1420.

930. Park C, Misumori M, Recht A, et al. The relationship between pathologic margin status and outcome after breast conserving therapy. Int J Radiat Oncol Biol Phys 1998; 42 (suppl): 125.

931. McGuire WL, Clark GM. Prognostic factors and treatment decisions in axillary-node-negative breast cancer. N Engl J Med 1992; 326(26): 1756–1761.

932. Galea MH, Blamey RW, Elston CE, Ellis IO. The Nottingham Prognostic Index in primary breast cancer. Breast Cancer Res Treat 1992; 22(3): 207–219.

933. Van Diest PJ, Baak JP. The morphometric prognostic index is the strongest prognosticator in premenopausal lymph node-negative and lymph node-positive breast cancer patients. Hum Pathol 1991; 22(4): 326–330.

934. Harvey JM, Clark GM, Osborne CK, Allred DC. Estrogen receptor status by immunohistochemistry is superior to the ligand-binding assay for predicting response to adjuvant endocrine therapy in breast cancer. J Clin Oncol 1999; 17(5): 1474–1481.

935. Hammond ME, Fitzgibbons PL, Compton CC, et al. College of American Pathologists Conference XXXV: solid tumor prognostic factors-which, how and so what? Summary document and recommendations for implementation. Cancer Committee and Conference Participants. Arch Pathol Lab Med 2000; 124(7): 958–965.

936. Yamauchi H, Stearns V, Hayes DF. When is a tumor marker ready for prime time? A case study of c-erbB-2 as a predictive factor in breast cancer. J Clin Oncol 2001; 19(8): 2334–2356.

937. Slamon DJ, Leyland-Jones B, Shak S, et al. Use of chemotherapy plus a monoclonal antibody against HER2 for metastatic breast cancer that overexpresses HER2. N Engl J Med 2001; 344(11): 783–792.

938. Jacobs TW, Gown AM, Yaziji H, et al. Comparison of fluorescence in situ hybridization and immunohistochemistry for the evaluation of HER-2/neu in breast cancer. J Clin Oncol 1999; 17(7): 1974–1982.

939. Hanna W, Kahn HJ, Trudeau M. Evaluation of HER-2/neu (erbB-2) status in breast cancer: from bench to bedside. Mod Pathol 1999; 12(8): 827–834.

940. Schnitt SJ, Jacobs TW. Current status of HER2 testing: caught between a rock and a hard place. Am J Clin Pathol 2001; 116(6): 806–810.

941. Lichter P. New tools in molecular pathology. J Mol Diagn 2000; 2(4): 171–173.

942. Association of Directors of Anatomic and Surgical Pathology. Recommendations for the reporting of breast carcinoma. Am J Clin Pathol 1995; 104(6): 614–619.

943. Henson DE, Oberman HA, Hutter RV. Practice protocol for the examination of specimens removed from patients with cancer of the breast: a publication of the Cancer Committee, College of American Pathologists. Members of the Cancer Committee, College of American Pathologists, and the Task Force for Protocols on the Examination of Specimens from Patients with Breast Cancer. Arch Pathol Lab Med 1997; 121(1): 27–33.

Hematopoietic system

Lymph nodes and spleen

Karen L. Chang   Daniel A. Arber   Karl K. Gaal   Lawrence M. Weiss

11

PATHOLOGIC EVALUATION OF THE LYMPH NODE

The practicing surgical pathologist commonly encounters lymph node biopsies in daily practice. Not only are enlarged peripheral lymph nodes readily accessible to the surgeon or radiologist, the lymph nodes may yield a host of varied information about systemic and localized diseases, ranging from benign, infectious, and metabolic disorders, as well as to metastatic and primary tumors.

Major advances in diagnostic technology serve the field of lymph node and spleen pathology well, helping to immunologically and phenotypically characterize pathologic processes. Yet the sine qua non of diagnostic pathology remains the clinical history, which guides the pathologist to a narrow list of differential diagnoses. Relevant history is especially important in cases where the amount of evaluable tissue is small, such as in fine needle aspirate smears or radiologically guided needle biopsies.

EXCISIONAL LYMPH NODE BIOPSY

An excised lymph node biopsy should be received fresh (and not in fixative), intact, preferably sterile, and always with complete clinical information. Placing the specimen on a dry towel or sponge will introduce artifacts. If a long period must elapse before receipt by the pathologist, the node may be placed in sterile saline, although this may introduce undesirable artifacts into subsequent frozen section studies. One should first harvest tissue for sterile studies, which may include microbiologic cultures and cytogenetic studies, if indicated. Fresh tissue for possible frozen section immunohistochemical, flow cytometric, and molecular studies should also be taken at this time. If a metastatic tumor is a possibility, a small piece should also be appropriately fixed for electron microscopy. Rapid frozen section evaluation may be quite helpful for determining adequacy of the tissue, establishing a tentative diagnosis, and determining which special studies may be particularly useful to obtain at once. Only a small piece of tissue should be frozen and, if necessary, this piece may be kept frozen for possible future frozen section immunohistochemical studies or molecular studies. Contrary to historic belief, we find frozen section diagnosis of hematolymphoid disorders to be reliable, as long as the limitations of the technique are recognized. Cytologic characteristics are often not well appreciated in frozen sections, but touch or rapidly fixed scrape preparations (we prefer the latter) may demonstrate cytologic features as well as or even better than in paraffin sections. Distinctions that can usually be made in frozen sections include benign versus malignant, hematolymphoid versus nonhematolymphoid, Hodgkin's versus non-Hodgkin's lymphoma, and low-grade versus high-grade non-Hodgkin's lymphoma. We try to provide as much of a diagnosis as necessary for immediate clinical decisions and avoid making distinctions that are not needed rapidly. Of course, the diagnosis should always be deferred in cases in which significant doubt exists.

Prompt and proper tissue fixation is more important than choice of fixative in the preparation of good histologic sections. The sections should be thinly cut and not underfixed, as this will hinder morphologic interpretation, or overfixed, as this may hinder immunohistochemical studies. If formalin is used as the primary fixative, it should be freshly prepared and at the proper pH. Some pathologists use a second fixative, usually a metal-based fixative such as B5, for fixation of lymph nodes. Sections should be cut thinly, to better evaluate nuclear features. Hematoxylin and eosin (H&E)-stained sections are usually adequate for morphologic interpretation, but some pathologists supplement this with reticulin-van Gieson (to evaluate the architecture), Giemsa (to better visualize the nuclear features), and methyl green-pyronine stains (to obtain a rough estimate of the RNA content of the cytoplasm).

NEEDLE CORE BIOPSIES

Using a variety of radiographic techniques, the surgeon or radiologist may obtain a percutaneous or invasive fiber-optic biopsy, with or without the support of CT or MRI technology, or ultrasound.[1] The amount of tissue obtained from these procedures is often small and thus, should be preserved for light microscopy. Paraffin immunohistochemistry is often available, but the quantity of tissue may be too low to allow the use of other ancillary techniques, such as flow cytometry analysis, cytogenetics, or molecular studies.

FINE NEEDLE ASPIRATION BIOPSY

Fine needle aspiration biopsy is also used for the evaluation of lymphadenopathy.[2] This technique may be used to determine whether a suspected enlarged lymph node is indeed lymphoid tissue, to obtain material for special studies (including culture, immunophenotyping studies, and molecular studies), to diagnose metastatic tumors, to diagnose reactive hyperplasia or infectious lymphadenitis, to diagnose and stage Hodgkin's disease and non-Hodgkin's lymphomas, to identify residual recurrent lymphoma, and to diagnose transformation of lymphoma. The efficacy varies with the clinical situation. It is probably best applied in cases in which reactive hyperplasia is suspected and least effective in cases in which the initial diagnosis of a non-Hodgkin's lymphoma is the primary clinical consideration. In our experience, the amount of tissue obtained by fine needle aspiration biopsy is insufficient for flow cytometry analysis.

SPECIAL STUDIES

In diagnostically difficult cases, H&E-stained sections are usually supplemented with a panel of *paraffin section immunohistochemical studies*, with the particular selected panel components dependent on the differential diagnosis suggested by the morphologic features. A listing of many of the important leukocyte antigens easily detectable in paraffin sections is presented in Table 11.1. Some suggested panels are given in Table 11.2. Immunostains are helpful by providing an indication as to the immunoarchitecture and cell lineage, and by providing an assessment of cancer in some cases. Immunostains can demonstrate the B- and T-cell areas or show that architecture has been altered or effaced. Stains for follicular dendritic cells can indicate the presence of follicles and other structures, while antibodies such as

Table 11.1 Selected useful major leukocyte antigens detectable in paraffin sections

Antibody	Predominant hematolymphoid cell expression
bcl-1	Mantle cell lymphoma
bcl-2	Nongerminal center B cells, most T cells, most follicular lymphomas, many low-grade and some higher-grade B-cell lymphomas
bcl-6	Diffuse large B cell lymphoma, subset of follicular lymphoma, Burkittlymphoma, nodular lymphocyte predominance Hodgkin's disease; not chronic lymphocytic leukemia, hairy cell leukemia, mantle cell or marginal zone-derived lymphomas
CD1	Thymocytes and some T-lymphoblastic lymphomas, Langerhans cells, and Langerhans cell histiocytosis
CD2	T cells and T-cell lymphomas
CD3	T cells and many T-cell lymphomas
CD4	Histiocytes and histiocytic neoplasms, T-helper cells and many T-cell lymphomas
CD5	T cells and many T-cell lymphomas, many B small lymphocytic lymphomas/chronic lymphocytic leukemia, mantle cell lymphoma
CD7	Most T cells and T-cell lymphomas, some myeloid leukemias
CD8	T cytotoxic/suppressor cells, some T-cell lymphomas
CD10 (CALLA)	Precursor B cells and B-lymphoblastic neoplasms, many follicular lymphomas
CD15	Myeloid cells, Hodgkin's disease, some non-Hodgkin's lymphomas
CD20	B cells and B-cell lymphomas, nodular L&H lymphocyte predominance
CD21	Follicular dendritic cells, mantle and marginal zone B cells and neoplasms
CD23	Mantle zone B cells and most B small lymphocytic lymphomas/chronic lymphocytic leukemia
CD25 (TAC)	Activated lymphoid cells, adult T-cell lymphoma/leukemia, hairy cell leukemia, most anaplastic large cell lymphomas, most Hodgkin's disease, subset of other B- and T-cell lymphomas
CD30	Activated lymphoid cells, Hodgkin's disease, anaplastic large cell lymphoma
CD34	Progenitor cells, some myeloid leukemias, some lymphoblastic neoplasms
CD35	Follicular dendritic cells, macrophages, monocytes, neutrophils
CD38	Plasma cells and plasma cell neoplasms, B and T precursor cells and lymphoblastic neoplasms
CD43	T cells, myeloid cells, mast cells, T-cell lymphomas, some B-cell lymphomas, myeloid leukemia, mast cell neoplasms
CD45/CD45RB	Hematolymphoid cells
CD45RA	B cells and subset of T cells, B-cell lymphomas, nodular L&H lymphocyte predominance
CD45RO	Most T cells, histiocytes, myeloid cells, T-cell lymphomas
CD56	Natural killer cells and subset of T-cell/natural killer lymphomas
CD57	Subset of T cells and natural killer cells, subset of T-cell lymphomas
CD61	Megakaryocytes
CD68	Histiocytes, myeloid cells, mast cells and neoplasms, some non-Hodgkin's lymphomas
CD79a	Immature and mature B cells and lymphomas, plasma cells and plasma cell neoplasms
CD99	Broadly expressed on all hematoprietic cells, especially lymphoblastic neoplasms
CD117	Immature myeloid cells including promyelocytes (normal 1–4% in bone marrow)
CD138	Plasma cells
CD163	Macrophages, (does not stain dendritic cells, interdigitating reticulum cells, or Langerhans cells)
Epithelial membrane antigen	Plasma cells and plasma cell neoplasms, many nodular L&H lymphocyte predominance, anaplastic large cell lymphoma, and T-cell rich B-cell lymphoma
EBV latent membrane protein	Some EBV-infected cells (most notably EBV-positive Hodgkin's cells, post-transplant lymphoproliferations, and EBV-associated infectious mononucleosis)
Granzyme B	T/NK cell malignancies except hepatosplenic T-cell lymphoma
Immunoglobulin light and heavy chains	Plasma cells, plasma cell and plasmacytoid neoplasms, some follicular lymphomas

Table 11.1 Selected useful major leukocyte antigens detectable in paraffin sections (*cont'd*)

Antibody	Predominant hematolymphoid cell expression
Ki-67 (mib-1)	Proliferating cells
KSHV	Cells infected with Kaposi sarcoma herpes virus
Lysozyme	Histiocytes, myeloid cells, histiocytic neoplasms, and myeloid leukemia
Myeloperoxidase	Myeloid cells and myeloid leukemia
Perforin	T/NK cell malignancies except hepatosplenic T-cell lymphoma
TdT	Thymic lymphoid cells and lymphoblastic neoplasms
TIA-1	Anaplastic large cell lymphoma; cytotoxic T/NK neoplasms
Tryptase	Mast cells and mast cell tumors
ZAP-70	Expression in chronic lymphocytic leukemia correlates with I_gV_H mutational status, disease progression, and survival; also seen in minority of other low grade B-cell neoplasms

TdT, terminal deoxynucleotidyl transferase; L&H, lymphocytic and histiocytic; EBV, Epstein-Barr virus.
Modified from Weiss et al.[912]

Table 11.2 Suggested paraffin immunohistochemistry panels for unknown primary malignant neoplasms

Differentiation of neoplasms	Suggested panels
Hematolymphoid vs. nonhematolymphoid	Keratin, S-100, CD45/CD45RB (initial) CD20, CD30, and CD43 (second line)
Carcinoma, unknown primary	Keratin 7, keratin 20, (CAM 5.2/AE1), canalicular CEA, (CDX2), (GCDFP-15), (GFAP), (hepatocyte),(PSA/PacP), (RCC), (TTF-1), (other keratin subsets)
Is this breast carcinoma?	ER/PR, GCDFP-15, bcl-2, S-100, (keratin 7, keratin 20)
Metastatic breast carcinoma vs. metastatic lung carcinoma	ER, TTF-1, GCDFP-15, bcl-2, (S-100) (in general, not CEA, vimentin, keratin 7, keratin 20), WT-1
Metastatic breast carcinoma vs. nonmucinous ovarian carcinoma	GCDFP-15 (in general, not ER, S-100, CEA, vimentin, keratin 7, keratin 20)
Small cell carcinoma of lung vs. Merkel cell carcinoma	Keratin 8/18, keratin 20, TTF-1
Carcinoid of gastrointestinal tract vs. carcinoid of lung	Keratin 7, keratin 8/18, keratin 19, TTF-1
Neuroendocrine carcinoma	Chromogranin, synaptophysin, neuron-specific enolase, (keratin 7, keratin 20)
Mesothelioma vs. carcinoma	CEA, CD15, Ber-EP4, B72.3, calretinin, keratin 5/6, thrombomodulin, TTF-1, WT-1
Is this melanoma?	S-100, vimentin, HMB-45, Melan-A
Spindled cutaneous neoplasm	Vimentin, keratin, S-100, (smooth muscle actin, collagen IV, factor XIII)
Sarcoma, unknown type	Vimentin, keratin, desmin, actin, smooth muscle actin, collagen IV, (CD-31), (CD34), (CD/17), (vWF), (Ulex)
Is this small round blue cell tumor of childhood?	CD99, CD45/RB, vimentin, neurofilament, chromogranin, synaptophysin, desmin, actin, TdT
Germ cell tumor	Placental alkaline phosphatase, keratin (hCG, AFP, EMA, CD30)
Neural vs. meningioma	GFAP, S-100, EMA (CD57), (neurofilament)

Table 11.3 Selected useful major leukocyte antigens detectable only in suspensions or frozen sections

Antibody	Predominant hematolymphoid expression
CD11c	Histiocytes and histiocytic neoplasms, M4 and M5 myeloid leukemia, hairy cell leukemia, marginal cell lymphoma
CD16	Natural killer cells and neoplasms
CD19	B cells and B-cell lymphomas
CD22	B cells and B-cell lymphomas
CD38	Plasma cells and plasma cell neoplasms, B and T precursor cells and lymphoblastic neoplasms

Modified from Weiss et al.[912]

Ki-67 can provide a measure of cell proliferation of various compartments or cell populations. Cell lineage studies that can be performed in paraffin sections help one decide between hematolymphoid versus nonhematolymphoid, and B versus T versus other lineages. Examples of immunostudies that strongly favor a diagnosis of hematolymphoid malignant tumor in paraffin sections include the demonstration of immunoglobulin light chain restriction in B-cell lymphomas (usually in plasmacytoid neoplasms, but occasionally in follicular lymphomas), reactivity of follicular B cells with bcl-2 protein (in follicular lymphoma), the aberrant coexpression of CD43 (or less commonly CD5 or CD45RO) with B-lineage markers (in diffuse B-cell lymphomas), and expression of *alk*-protein in CD30-positive anaplastic lymphoid cells (in anaplastic large cell lymphoma). The aberrant coexpression of CD43 may also be used to help in subclassification due to its differential expression in different subtypes of B-cell lymphoma.[3]

Additional antibodies can be used in *cell suspension studies* or acetone-fixed *frozen sections*[4,5] (Table 11.3). However, innovations in *paraffin section immunohistochemistry* and monoclonal antibody technology have allowed many antibodies formerly available only in frozen sections to be widely available in paraffin immunohistochemistry.[6,7,8]

Flow cytometry studies are of particular use in quantifying immunoglobulin light chain ratios and in the performance of double-labeling studies.[9] Flow cytometry studies are also used by some to determine cell proliferation and DNA content.[10–12] Studies of both have shown correlation with the grade of the lymphomas as well as specific prognosis. Another advantage of flow cytometry is its applicability to fluid specimens such as aspiration biopsies, although immunocytochemical studies can be performed on cell smears. Disadvantages of flow cytometry include the difficulty in obtaining adequate numbers of cells in fibrotic tissues (particularly in extranodal sites), the inability to visualize the individual staining cells (although one can 'gate' on certain populations by differential cell size and granularity), and the inability to relate the flow cytometric results to specific architectural compartments. Frozen section immuno-histochemical studies have the advantage of allowing correlation of staining with architecture. However, morphology is less than optimal and therefore it is difficult to assign accurate staining profiles to rare cell populations such as Reed-Sternberg cells, particularly when there is staining of adjacent cells. With the numerous monoclonal antibodies reacting in cell suspension, frozen sections, and paraffin-embedded tissues, one can apply additional criteria for malignant tumors.[4] These include aberrant absence of immunoglobulin (common in diffuse large B-cell lymphoma) or other B-lineage antigens (uncommon in B-cell lymphoma), and the aberrant absence of T-lineage antigens in peripheral T-cell lymphoma. In addition, these studies may be useful in the subclassification of lymphomas. For example, the low-grade B-cell lymphomas may be more easily subclassified by their differential expression of CD5, CD10, and CD23.[13,14]

Molecular studies may be helpful in selected cases. The detection of clonal immunoglobulin light and heavy chain gene and T-cell receptor gene rearrangements is a very useful tool in hematopathology.[15–20] Although the identification of a monoclonal population is not completely synonymous with cancer, these studies may be very helpful in difficult cases. Antigen receptor gene rearrangements may be detected by Southern blot hybridization with a sensitivity of approximately 1–5%, but it generally requires frozen tissue and takes about 2 weeks to complete. Sufficient DNA may be obtained by fine needle aspiration biopsy.[21] Alternatively, one may also use the polymerase chain reaction (PCR) technique, which may not detect all gene rearrangements but has a shorter turnaround time of less than 1 week and can usually be performed in tissue taken from paraffin blocks. In cases with detectable gene rearrangements, the sensitivity of PCR for the detection of lymphoma cells may be very high, but there is also a potential for false-positive results as a result of contamination during the analysis. Both Southern blot hybridization and PCR can be used to accurately stage patients with known lymphoma and to identify recurrent or residual disease, with PCR having a higher potential sensitivity.[19] In situ hybridization uses a molecular probe to hybridize to messenger RNA or DNA directly in the histologic or cytologic material. It is useful for the assessment of light chain restriction in lymphomas and detection of microorganisms such as Epstein-Barr virus (EBV) and Kaposi's sarcoma herpesvirus/human herpesvirus-8 (KSHV/HHV-8).[22–24] DNA microarray technology holds great promise in lymphoma and leukemia therapeutic and prognostic information and is discussed in greater detail in the individual entities. Briefly, different gene expression patterns may be used to identify various subtypes of leukemia, predict response to therapy, and predict risk of drug-induced therapies.[25] Other laboratory methods for molecular pathology, such as in situ PCR, laser capture microdissection, microsatellite analysis, and assessment of telomerase, are not yet readily available or well characterized for diagnostic hematopathology.

Cytogenetics may be useful in diagnosis and classification of lymphoproliferations in some instances. Certain lymphomas are associated with characteristic cytogenetic abnormalities, usually translocations (see section on non-Hodgkin's lymphomas).[26] Cytogenetic abnormalities may be detected by classic metaphase analysis after brief cell culture, by fluorescence in situ hybridization (FISH) on cells in interphase, by Southern blotting, or by PCR. Classic cytogenetics requires fresh, sterile tissue but does not require foreknowledge of the translocation being sought. FISH can be performed on paraffin sections, but one can only examine the section for one translocation at a time.[27] Both Southern blot hybridization and PCR require knowledge of the specific translocation. In the case of Southern blot hybridization, a specific probe that hybridizes to the area of the genome just adjacent to the translocation must be available and in the case of PCR, the sequence of DNA flanking both sides of the translocation must be known. Although classic cytogenetics may reveal a characteristic translocation, the actual breakpoint may occur in widely varying locations in the genome at the molecular level. Therefore, there is a potential for false-negative results by Southern blot hybridization and PCR methodologies, depending on the specific translocation. Although chromosomal translocations are specific for neoplasia when they are detected by classic cytogenetics, FISH, and Southern blotting, this may not be the case when the translocation is detected by the highly sensitive PCR technique. For example, the t(14;18) has been detected by PCR in tissues with reactive follicular hyperplasia from patients without a history of lymphoma.[28]

NONHEMATOPOIETIC LESIONS IN LYMPH NODES

The following is a list of the various nonhematopoietic lesions that may be encountered in lymph nodes:

Metastatic tumors
    Carcinoma
    Germ cell tumor
    Malignant melanoma
    Sarcoma
    Childhood tumors
    Unknown primary site
Congenital rests and inclusions
    Epithelial
        Salivary gland
        Breast
        Thyroid
        Müllerian
        Squamous
        Mesothelial
    Stromal
        Müllerian
    Nevomelanocytic
        Ordinary nevus
        Blue nevus
Primary mesenchymal lesions
    Lipomatosis
    Vascular
        Vascular transformation of sinuses
        Bacillary angiomatosis
        Kaposi's sarcoma
        Intranodal hemangioma and variants
        Lymphangioma
        Hemangioendothelioma and variants
        Angiosarcoma

Smooth muscle
    Smooth muscle proliferation of the nodal hilum
    Intranodal leiomyoma
    Angiomyomatous hamartoma
    Leiomyomatosis
    Lymphangiomyomatosis
    Angiomyolipoma
  Myofibroblast
    Inflammatory pseudotumor
    Mycobacterial pseudotumor
    Palisaded myofibroblastoma
    Reactive mediastinal spindle cell pseudotumor
Protein Deposition
  Proteinaceous lymphadenopathy
  Amyloid

METASTATIC TUMORS[29]

Metastatic tumors are the most frequent and most important nonhematopoietic lesions encountered in lymph nodes. Carcinoma, germ cell tumor, malignant melanoma, and sarcoma may all involve lymph nodes, often in the local lymph node regions, but not infrequently in distant sites. In any lymph node dissection, all lymph nodes should be grossly identified and submitted for microscopic examination. The number of involved nodes, as well as the total number of lymph nodes examined, should be specified. In many cases, this information should be given by the specific node group. If only one lymph node is involved, it is often useful to comment on whether the metastasis is macroscopic or microscopic (<3 mm). If the anatomic area may be treated with irradiation, one should comment on the presence of any significant extranodal soft tissue extension.[29] Whether immunohistochemical stains should be performed to facilitate detection of histologically unapparent metastases is a subject of debate.[30] It is our opinion that these studies are not usually necessary in the absence of specific clinical protocols, because many studies have not demonstrated that the detection of these micrometastases has a significant impact on prognosis.

Sentinel lymph node dissection is a well-accepted surgical technique for staging of breast cancer in patients without palpable lymphadenopathy.[31] The technique is based on the hypothesis that the histology of the first draining lymph node accurately predicts the histological character of the rest of the axillary lymph nodes. Careful morphologic and keratin immunohistochemical examination of the sentinel lymph node is required. For cases that are negative at the time of frozen section examination, the pathologist should examine each half of a bisected sentinel lymph node with one section each of H&E and cytokeratin stains from at least two levels, 40 μm apart, of the paraffin block (total of eight sections).[32,33] These parameters allow for optimal histological sensitivity, with no undue financial or labor burden to the laboratory. The technique of sentinel lymph node dissection is also used in patients with micrometastatic malignant melanoma.[34]

A lymph node biopsy may show an undifferentiated malignant tumor that cannot be classified by histologic examination. Application of a limited panel of immunohistochemical markers will resolve most cases (see Table 11.2). A panel of antibodies is needed because tumors frequently may have overlapping antibody reactivities. Most undifferentiated tumors presenting in lymph nodes comprise non-Hodgkin's lymphomas. Because CD45/45RB (leukocyte common antigen) stains about 90% of cases of non-Hodgkin's lymphoma, this antibody is an excellent initial screening tool for these neoplasms. The category of non-Hodgkin's lymphoma most likely to be

CD45/45RB negative is anaplastic large cell lymphoma; these cases may be identified by use of CD30 antibodies.[35,36] CD43 is also useful for identifying CD45/45RB-negative hematolymphoid neoplasms such as some T-cell lymphomas, histiocytic sarcoma, and granulocytic sarcoma.[3] Embryonal carcinoma may be positive for CD30, but that tumor should also be strongly positive for keratin.[35] Malignant lymphomas may rarely express keratin, but the staining is usually focal, globular, and paranuclear. After malignant lymphoma, carcinoma represents the next most common neoplasm to present as an undifferentiated tumor in the lymph node. In particular, undifferentiated nasopharyngeal carcinoma may closely mimic immunoblastic lymphoma. In addition to keratin stains, in situ hybridization for EBV is usually positive in this tumor.[37]

Carcinoma presents in lymph nodes without a known primary in about 3% of cases, so-called carcinoma of unknown origin.[38] Breast, lung, and renal carcinomas are the most common carcinomas to present in this fashion. The anatomic site of the lymph node may suggest the primary site. A neck presentation should suggest carcinoma of the upper aerodigestive tract or thyroid.[39] Even extensive head and neck examination may not reveal the primary site. An axillary presentation should suggest ipsilateral breast carcinoma; mammography may sometimes be necessary to reveal the primary lesion. However, carcinomas from the lung, skin, stomach, or pharynx may all present in an axillary node.[40] A supraclavicular presentation should suggest a lung, gastrointestinal tract, or genitourinary tract primary (particularly the ovary, in a woman).[41] An inguinal presentation should suggest carcinoma of the skin, genitourinary tract, and lower gastrointestinal tract. Immunohistochemical studies may help to identify the primary site. For example, thyroglobulin is specific for thyroid carcinoma, prostatic specific antigen and prostatic acid phosphatase are specific for prostate carcinoma, whereas estrogen receptor is positive in a restricted set of neoplasms, including breast carcinoma, carcinomas of the female genital tract, and some thyroid neoplasms. Antibodies with high specificity for hepatocytes, renal cell carcinoma, and colon carcinoma are also available.[42–46] Although the mere expression of keratin is sufficient to diagnose carcinoma, the pattern of positivity may yield a clue as to the nature of the carcinoma. Carcinomas with neuroendocrine differentiation may show dot-like positivity. The expression of keratin subsets in tumors mimics their expression in the corresponding normal tissue counterparts and thus the cytokeratin profile of a carcinoma may be useful in determining the primary site of origin (Table 11.4).[47] Also, the cytokeratin profile of a primary tumor is typically preserved in a metastasis or recurrence.

Malignant melanoma may present in lymph nodes, particularly in the axillary and inguinal groups, and may be distinguished by reactivity for S-100, Melan-A, and HMB-45, with the caveat that none of those three antibodies, in and of themselves, is absolutely specific. Occasionally, small round blue cell tumors of childhood may present in lymph nodes; immunohistochemical studies, electron microscopy, and possibly specialized molecular studies may all be helpful in arriving at the correct diagnosis.

Fine needle aspiration biopsy is a highly effective method for diagnosing metastatic neoplasms in lymph nodes. Key features in the identification of carcinoma include cohesive cell groupings, common cell borders, cytoplasmic differentiation (such as mucin vacuoles or squamous features), and nuclear molding. Key features in the identification of melanoma by fine needle aspiration biopsy include abundant cytoplasm, the presence of melanin pigment, rounded or oblong nuclei, intranuclear cytoplasmic invaginations, and prominent nucleoli. Material obtained by fine needle aspiration may be subjected to immunocytochemical studies, including keratin and S-100 stains for confirmation.

Table 11.4 Differential cytokeratin 7 and cytokeratin 20 expression of selected carcinomas*

Cytokeratin 7 positive Cytokeratin 20 positive	Cytokeratin 7 positive Cytokeratin 20 negative	Cytokeratin 7 negative Cytokeratin 20 positive	Cytokeratin 7 negative Cytokeratin 20 negative
Ovarian mucinous carcinoma	Breast carcinoma	Colorectal adenocarcinoma	Hepatocellular carcinoma
Pancreatic adenocarcinoma	Endometrial carcinoma		Prostatic adenocarcinoma
Transitional cell carcinoma	Epithelial mesothelioma		Renal cell carcinoma
	Lung adenocarcinoma		Small cell neuroendocrine carcinoma
	Ovarian serous adenocarcinoma		Squamous cell carcinoma
	Thymoma		

*This general guide to cytokeratin expression should not be considered absolute because a subset of each malignant neoplasm may not show the most common differential keratin expression.

CONGENITAL RESTS AND INCLUSIONS

Not all epithelial elements found in lymph nodes represent metastatic carcinoma. Inclusions of salivary gland, breast, thyroid, and Müllerian epithelium have all been described. *Inclusions of salivary gland tissue* are commonly found in adjacent lymph nodes, usually within the lymph node parenchyma. Most often, ducts alone are encountered but acini may also be seen. These inclusions may become clinically evident when they are cystically dilated, as frequently occurs in human immunodeficiency virus (HIV)-infected patients, forming so-called benign lymphoepithelial cysts.[48] These cysts may be confused with cystic variants of metastatic squamous cell carcinoma; the key feature is the cytologic atypia present in the lining cells in the latter. The salivary gland inclusions may give rise to neoplasms, the most common example being Warthin tumor.

Inclusions of breast epithelium have been rarely reported in axillary lymph nodes, most often in the intracapsular or subcapsular regions.[49] These inclusions may undergo the same changes as normal breast epithelium, including atypical hyperplasia, carcinoma in situ, and, rarely, primary carcinoma. *Thyroid inclusions* have also been reported in lateral cervical lymph nodes, usually in subcapsular regions. To accept a thyroid inclusion as ectopic and not metastatic, one should see completely follicular architecture with no papillary structures, psammoma bodies, or atypical nuclear features, i.e. no suggestion of the cytology of papillary carcinoma.[50]

Inclusions of Müllerian epithelium are seen within the capsule and parenchyma in 5–40% of intra-abdominal lymph nodes of females (and rarely in males), according to a large autopsy and surgical study (Fig. 11.1).[51] Occasionally, inclusions may be found within germinal centers or the sinuses. Müllerian epithelial inclusions seem to be more common in patients with epithelial tumors of the ovary, particularly borderline serous tumors. They usually consist of tubuloglandular structures lined by a single layer of epithelial cells with a distinct basement membrane. Occasionally, papillary structures can be found. Müllerian inclusions have bland nuclear features with basal orientation, differentiated cytoplasm – with the frequent presence of cilia, the lack of a stromal response, and the presence of a basement membrane, which are not features of metastases. When unaccompanied by endometrial stroma, the inclusions are sometimes termed *endosalpingiosis*; when endometrial stroma is present, the term *endometriosis* should be applied.[52] Occasionally, only stroma is present; this is most commonly seen when deciduosis is identified in pregnant women.[53]

Benign intranodal squamous inclusions may be difficult to distinguish from metastatic carcinoma in patients undergoing

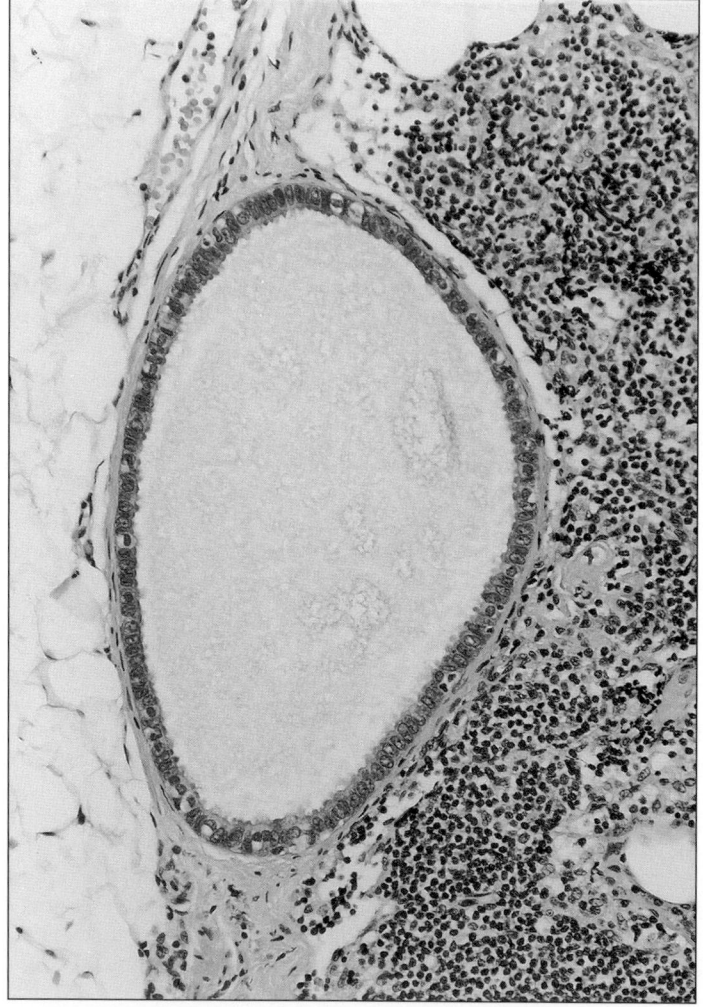

Fig. 11.1 Müllerian inclusion in a lymph node. Note the bland nuclear features and the presence of cilia.

nephrectomy for Wilms' tumor or other renal malignant neoplasm. These cells are thought to originate from metaplastic calyceal urothelium.[54]

Benign mesothelial inclusions in lymph nodes are extremely rare but have been reported in mediastinal, pelvic, and abdominal lymph

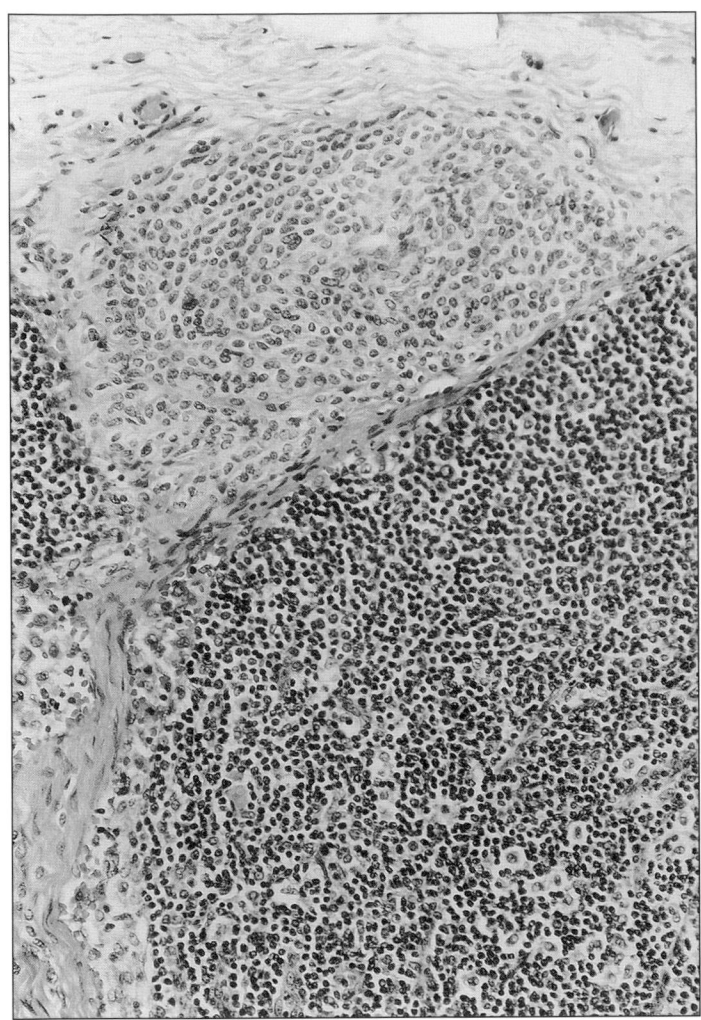

Fig. 11.2 Nevus cell inclusion. There is a nest of nevus cells in the lymph node capsule.

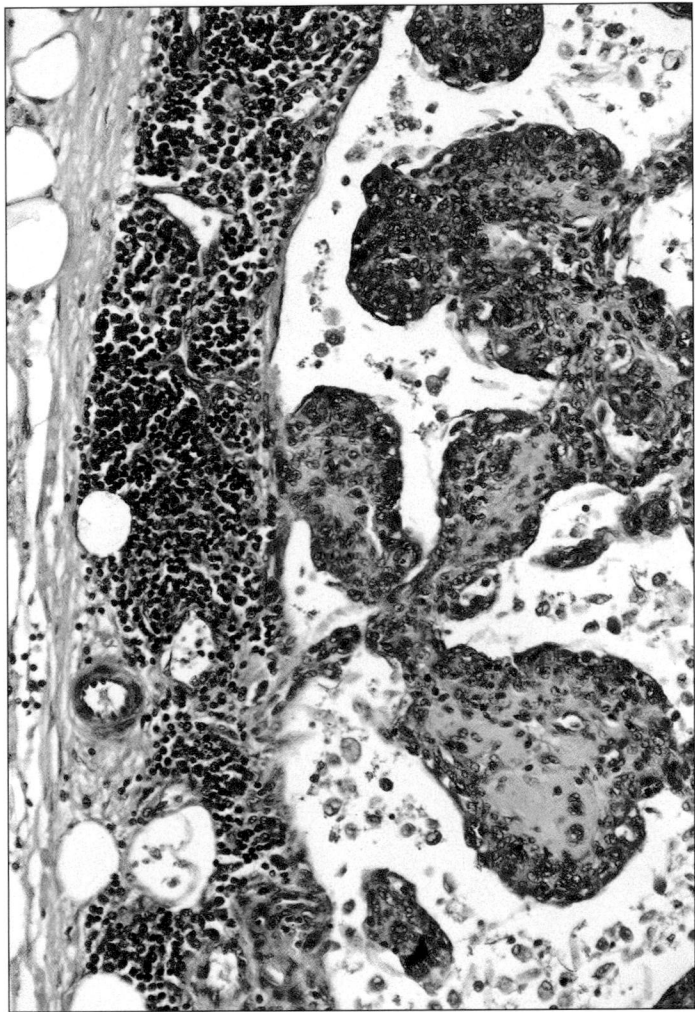

Fig. 11.3 Vascular transformation of lymph node sinuses, nodular spindle cell variant. The cells lining the spaces do not stain with epithelial markers.

nodes.[54–58] Immunohistochemistry is useful to distinguish these inclusions from metastatic carcinoma, mesothelioma, or melanoma.

Nevus cell inclusions are also relatively common, seen in about 3% of axillary node dissections by light microscopic examination, and about 5% of cases when S-100 staining is used (Fig. 11.2).[59] They have also been reported in inguinal and cervical lymph nodes. The inclusions are composed of cells resembling the cells of benign intradermal nevi, but inclusions resembling blue nevus have also been reported.[60] The keys to the distinction from metastatic tumor are the nevus cell inclusion's bland cytologic features, nesting architecture, and presence in the lymph node capsule in contrast to the subcapsular sinus, as more typically seen in carcinoma. Occasionally, the subcapsular sinus is involved by nevus cell inclusions, but there is virtually always more extensive involvement of the adjacent capsule.

MESENCHYMAL LESIONS

Lipomatosis, or fatty replacement of the lymph node, is a relatively common occurrence.[61] The fatty replacement begins in the lymph node hilum, leaving a rim of normal lymphoid tissue at the outer cortex. It is usually clinically insignificant, but may be a cause of lymphadenopathy, particularly in obese individuals.

Vascular transformation of lymph node sinuses is a reactive proliferation of blood vessels in the lymph node sinuses, probably as a result of venous obstruction.[62] It is most often observed in intra-abdominal lymph nodes removed in lymphoma staging procedures and in axillary lymph nodes removed after radical mastectomy.[62] The vessels range from endothelial-lined small dilated vascular channels through well-formed blood vessels, and are generally associated with fibrosis. There is also a *nodular spindle cell variant of vascular transformation*, characterized by a proliferation of spindle cells forming irregular interlacing bundles and cuffs around endothelium-lined vascular channels, most often seen in retroperitoneal lymph nodes draining carcinomas (Fig. 11.3).[63] Vascular transformation of lymph node sinuses is usually an incidental finding but occasionally may present as lymphadenopathy. Its significance lies in not confusing it with other more clinically important vascular lesions of lymph nodes, such as Kaposi's sarcoma. The nodular spindle cell variant must not be mistaken for lymph node involvement by metastatic carcinoma.

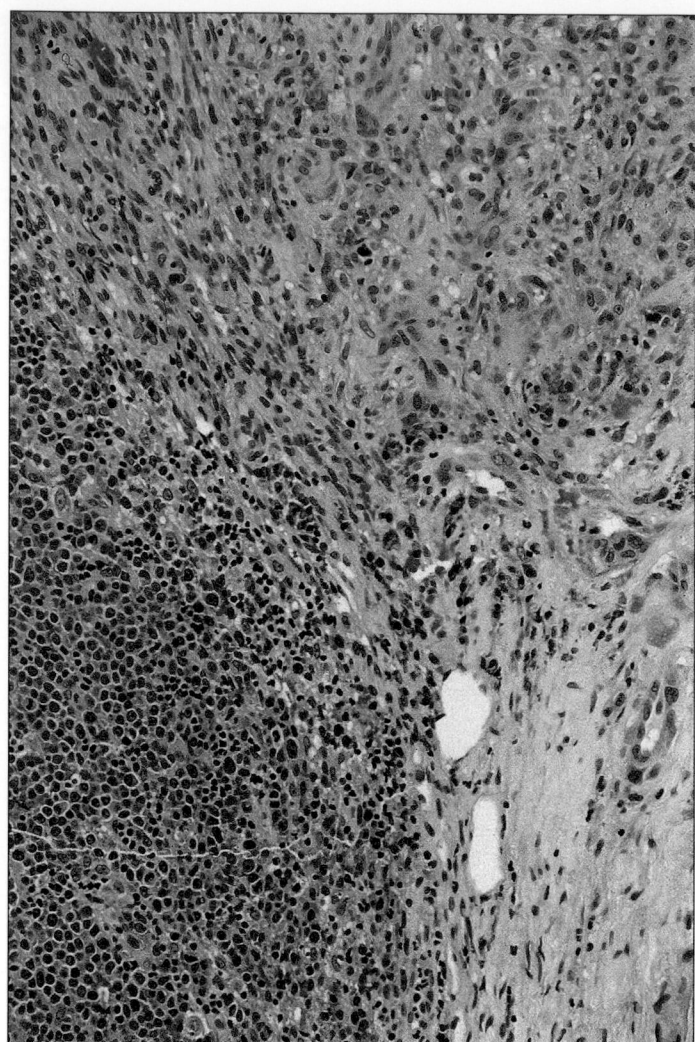

Fig. 11.4 Kaposi's sarcoma. Capsular involvement is seen in this case.

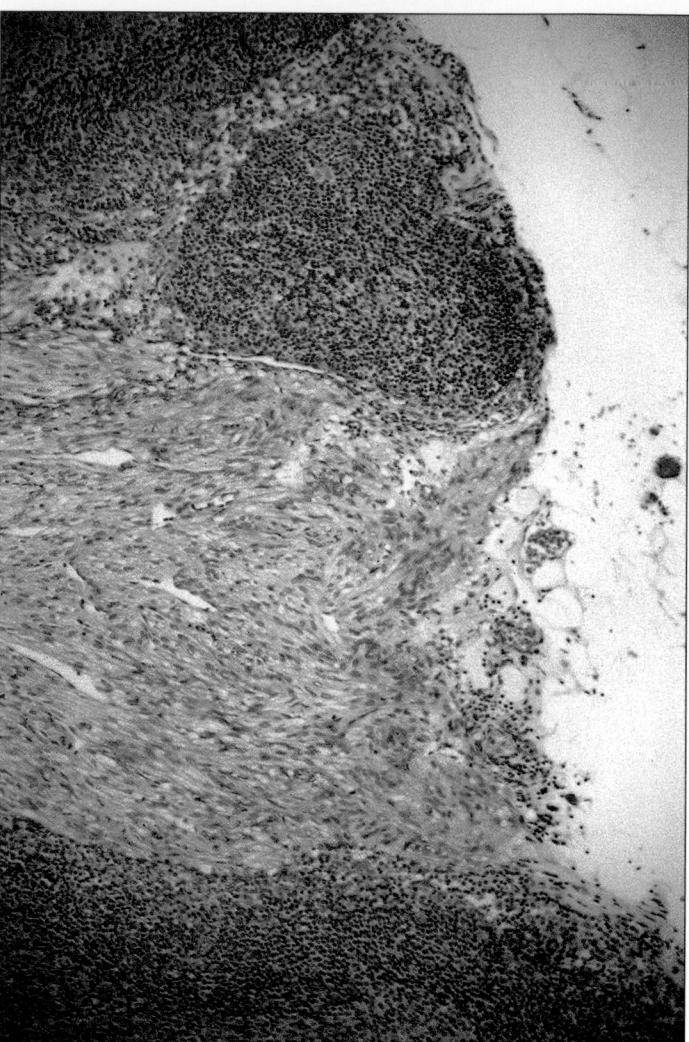

Fig. 11.5 Lymphangiomyomatosis. The spindle cells stained for smooth muscle actin and HMB-45.

Bacillary angiomatosis is another reactive proliferation of blood vessels that may involve lymph nodes.[64] It is a pseudoneoplastic vascular proliferation caused by the *Bartonella* species.[65] Although more common in skin, involved lymph nodes show patchy involvement by coalescent nodules of proliferating blood vessels lined by reactive endothelial cells. Admixed are scattered neutrophils and an eosinophilic material, which can be shown to represent bacilli on Warthin-Starry stain. There is no reported association with KSHV/HHV-8.

Kaposi's sarcoma is the most common primary vascular tumor of lymph nodes. In the USA it is usually seen as a complication of HIV infection, particularly in homosexual men but is also seen as a lymphadenopathic form in children and young adults in Africa.[66] It is also rarely present in nodal form as a complication of classic Kaposi's sarcoma occurring in Mediterranean populations or as a complication of organ transplantation.[67,68] All forms of Kaposi's sarcoma are associated with KSHV/HHV-8.[69–74] Lymph nodes involved by Kaposi's sarcoma may show complete effacement of architecture, one or several nodules, or subtle subcapsular involvement (Fig. 11.4). Uninvolved lymph node parenchyma may show non-specific reactive hyperplasia or Castleman's-like features. In fact,

Kaposi's sarcoma may be seen in patients with multicentric Castleman's disease.[75] Histologically, Kaposi's sarcoma involving lymph nodes is identical to that involving other organs.

Other primary vascular neoplasms of lymph nodes are rare and include intranodal hemangioma, epithelioid hemangioma, lymphangioma, epithelioid hemangioendothelioma, spindle and epithelioid (histiocytoid) hemangioendothelioma, polymorphous hemangioendothelioma, and angiosarcoma.[76–78] There are many rare *smooth muscle proliferations* that may involve the lymph node.[61] Lymphangiomyomatosis (related to vascular leiomyomatosis), a proliferation of smooth muscle and lymphatics, and angiomyolipoma, a proliferation of smooth muscle, adipose tissue, and thick-walled blood vessels, are associated with tuberous sclerosis, and share HMB-45 positivity (Fig. 11.5).[79] Smooth muscle proliferation of the nodal hilum is an irregular proliferation of smooth muscle cells, accompanied by fibrosis, limited to the hilum, and is usually found in inguinal lymph nodes.[80] Angiomyomatous hamartoma is an irregular proliferation of smooth muscle cells associated with blood vessels that also has a predilection for inguinal lymph nodes; however, it can involve all parts of the lymph node.[77] Leiomyomatosis of the lymph node consists of a proliferation of bland smooth muscle cells in the

An atypical mycobacterial infection known as *mycobacterial pseudotumor* can closely simulate inflammatory pseudotumor.[87,88] The clinical setting (HIV positivity) may suggest atypical mycobacterial infection; acid-fast stains will resolve any dubious cases and S-100 and CD68 staining of the spindle cells of mycobacterial pseudotumor also differentiates this from Kaposi's sarcoma, which does not have S-100-positive or CD68-positive spindle cells.

Palisaded myofibroblastoma (hemorrhagic spindle cell tumor with amianthoid fibers) is a distinctive benign neoplasm showing myofibroblastic differentiation that is almost always found in inguinal lymph nodes.[89–91] It consists of a proliferation of spindle cells with bland, spindled nuclei. The cytoplasm occasionally shows intracytoplasmic globules of actin filaments. The most characteristic feature of this neoplasm is the presence of stellate areas of extracellular collagen deposition, termed *amianthoid fibers*. The spindle cells stain for vimentin, muscle-specific actin, and myosin, whereas the amianthoid fibers may stain uniformly for type IV collagen and peripherally for type II collagen. Metaplastic bone formation may be present.[92,93]

A rare lesion known as *reactive mediastinal spindle cell pseudotumor* has also been described in lymph nodes.[94] They are associated with anthracosis and anthracosilicosis, most likely due to their location. This shows a prominent storiform pattern of spindled cells, which may involve the surrounding soft tissues or nerves. Polarizable material and nodular hyaline scars are also present. This entity has a benign clinical course.

PROTEIN DEPOSITION

Proteinaceous lymphadenopathy, also known as angiocentric sclerosing lymphadenopathy, is a rare disease of unknown etiology.[95,96] It is thought to be an unusual variant of plasma cell dyscrasia. Patients have been reported to present with generalized lymphadenopathy and polyclonal hypergammaglobulinemia. Involved lymph nodes show obliteration of the normal architecture by deposition of a nonamyloid material, which appears to be composed of bundles of fine reticulin fibers. Typically, this material lines vessel walls. Lymphocytes and plasma cells are very rarely seen. The lack of light chain predominance, the paucicellularity, and the global angiosclerotic changes of proteinaceous lymphadenopathy are morphologic features not found in light chain deposition disease or multiple myeloma.

Amyloid deposits are frequently seen in the lymph nodes of patients with systemic amyloidosis.[97] Less commonly, amyloid may be identified in the lymph nodes of patients with plasmacytoma, lymphoplasmacytic lymphoma, or Castleman's disease.[98] Amyloid lymphadenopathy in the absence of systemic amyloidosis or lymphoproliferative disease is extremely rare. The morphologic features of amyloid in lymph nodes are consistent, despite the clinical presentation. The deposits may involve the walls of the lymph node vessels, may partially or completely replace the lymph node follicles, or may be diffusely present throughout the lymph node parenchyma (Fig 11.7). Congo red cytochemical staining shows the amorphous eosinophilic amyloid material to have a unique characteristic apple-green birefringence. Proteinaceous lymphadenopathy can easily be distinguished from amyloid lymphadenopathy, because of the typical onion skinning on reticulin stain and lack of Congo red birefringent staining in the globular deposits of the former entity. *Para-amyloid* refers to a periodic acid–schiff (PAS)-positive, Congo red nonbirefringent inflammatory or abnormal immunoreaction product seen in lymph nodes with angioimmunoblastic lymphadenopathy or Hodgkin's

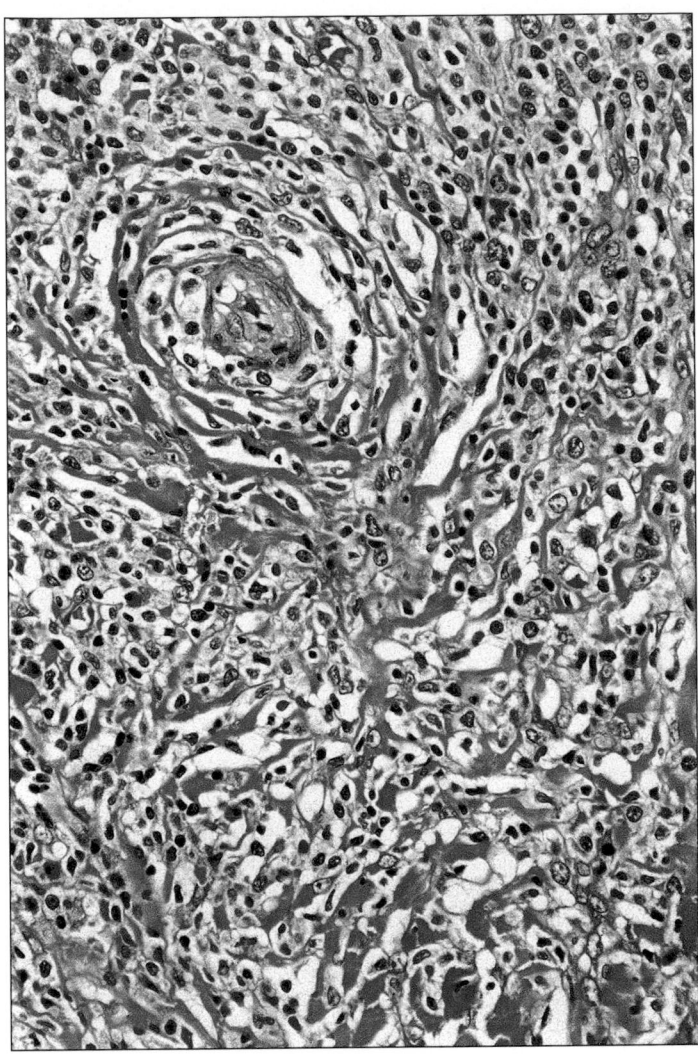

Fig. 11.6 Inflammatory pseudotumor. The capsule is fibrotic and contains a reactive lymphoid infiltrate.

intra-abdominal lymph nodes of women.[81] Patients usually have coexisting uterine leiomyomas, although this is not always the case.

Inflammatory pseudotumor is a reactive proliferation of myofibroblasts and inflammatory cells.[82–84] It usually occurs in young adults with an equal male/female ratio. Patients present with one or several moderately enlarged lymph nodes that may be matted together into larger masses up to 10 cm. There are often systemic symptoms such as fever and night sweats. The lesion is benign, but may recur. Histologically, there is infiltration of the lymph node capsule and hilum by spindled and inflammatory cells with an edematous to fibrous background (Fig. 11.6). The spindled cells consist of myofibroblasts and fibroblasts, whereas the inflammatory cells are small lymphocytes, plasma cells, immunoblasts, eosinophils, neutrophils, and histiocytes. There is also a proliferation of small blood vessels. The remaining lymph node parenchyma is unremarkable and generally nonreactive. This most likely represents the end stage of a variety of inflammatory lesions that may affect the lymph node. Some cases harbor EBV.[85] No heavy chain or T-cell receptor gene rearrangements are present.[82,86] The differential diagnosis includes Kaposi's sarcoma and the spindle cell variant of atypical mycobacterial infection. Kaposi's sarcoma generally has a greater degree of cellularity, with slit-like spaces and hemorrhage.

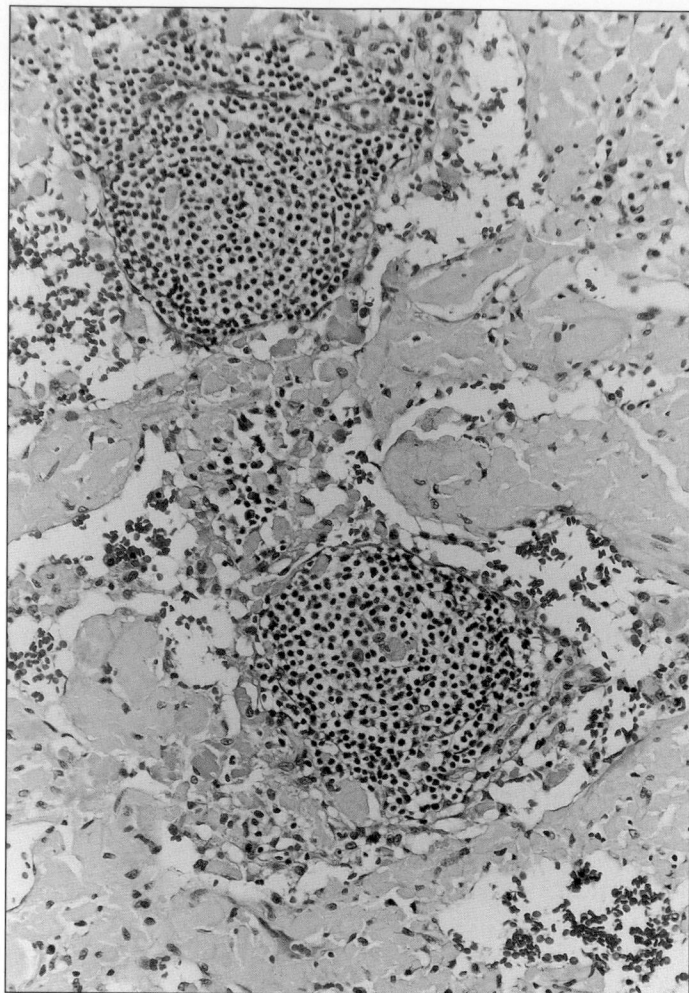

Fig. 11.7 Amyloidosis. Preferential paracortical involvement is seen in this case. The amorphous material showed apple-green birefringence on Congo red stain.

disease, or due to iatrogenic causes. The sclerosis commonly seen in inguinal and pelvic lymph nodes stains for collagen and does not show Congo red birefringence, distinguishing it from amyloid lymphadenopathy.

REACTIVE LYMPHADENOPATHY

The lymph node may undergo a variety of changes in response to reactive conditions. Broadly, these changes can be divided into two groups: lymphadenitis and lymphoid hyperplasia. The term *lymphadenitis* is used when an infectious agent is highly probable, whereas the term *lymphoid hyperplasia* is applied when it is presumed that the lymph node changes have occurred in response to antigenic stimulation without actual infectious involvement of the node. Several different patterns can be seen in lymphoid hyperplasia, including reactive follicular hyperplasia, caused by preferential stimulation of the B-cell compartment of the node; reactive paracortical hyperplasia, caused by preferential stimulation of the T-cell compartment; and reactive histiocytic hyperplasia, caused by preferential stimulation of the histiocytic compartment. Often,

combinations of these patterns are observed, as it is unusual for one compartment to be stimulated without some involvement of the others. Nonetheless, it is useful to classify the various lymphadenopathies according to their predominant pattern of involvement. In some diseases, necrosis is the predominant histologic pattern. Granulomatous disorders are considered separately.

The following is a list of reactive lymphadenopathies:

Follicular
    Non-specific reactive follicular hyperplasia
    Rheumatoid arthritis
    Sjögren syndrome
    Kimura disease
    Toxoplasmosis
    Syphilis
    Castleman's disease
    HIV-associated lymphadenopathy
    Progressive transformation of germinal centers
Paracortical
    Non-specific reactive paracortical hyperplasia
    Viral
        Epstein-Barr virus
        Cytomegalovirus
        Herpesvirus
    Drug-induced/postvaccinial
    Dermatopathic lymphadenitis
Sinusoidal
    Sinus histiocytosis
    Monocytoid B-cell hyperplasia
    Hemophagocytic syndrome
    Sinus histiocytosis with massive lymphadenopathy
    Whipple's disease
    Exogenous lipids
Extensive necrosis
    Complete necrosis/infarction
    Kikuchi histiocytic necrotizing lymphadenitis
    Systemic lupus erythematosus
    Kawasaki disease
Granulomatous
    Noninfectious
        Hodgkin's-associated and non-Hodgkin's-associated
        Sarcoidosis
    Infectious
        Nonsuppurative
            Tuberculosis
            Atypical mycobacterium
            Leprosy
            Fungal infections
            Pneumocystis carinii
        Suppurative
            Cat-scratch disease
            Lymphogranuloma venereum
            Yersinia

Fine needle aspiration biopsy is an effective method for the evaluation of reactive lymphadenopathy, both by ruling out carcinoma and by suggesting a specific etiology to a reactive condition. Material may also be obtained for appropriate microbiologic studies. The diagnosis of reactive lymphoid hyperplasia should only be made in a setting in which adequate clinical follow-up is available. If adenopathy persists or further enlargement occurs after a reactive diagnosis has been rendered based on a fine needle aspiration biopsy, one must either repeat the aspiration biopsy or perform an open biopsy.

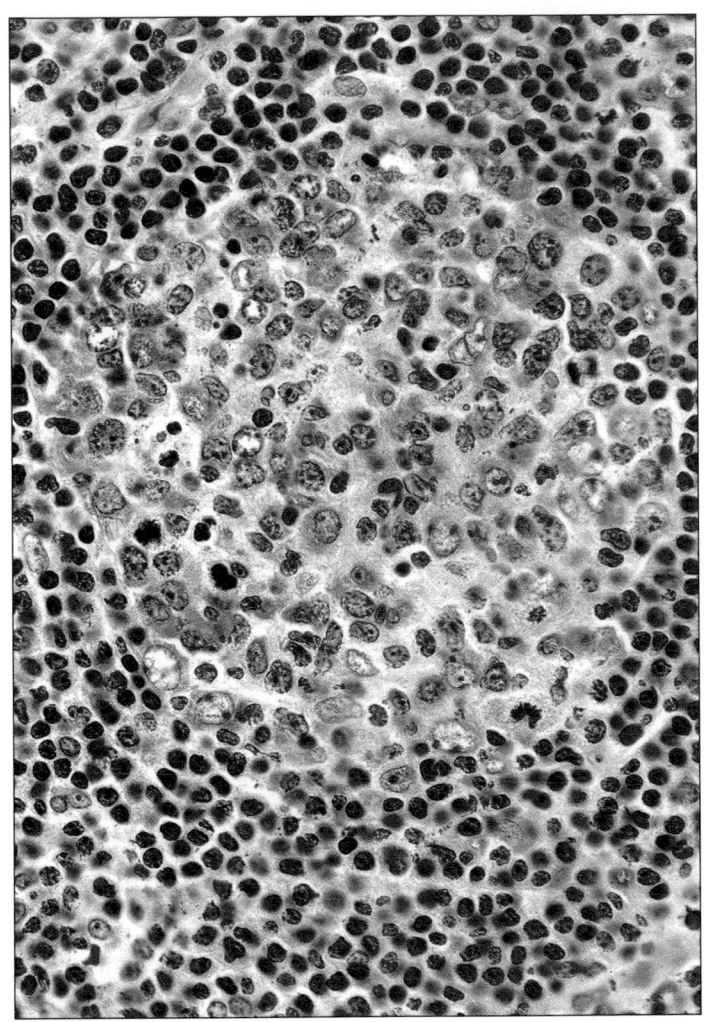

Fig. 11.8 Reactive germinal center. Note the differences in cell types at the left versus the right; this phenomenon has been called polarization.

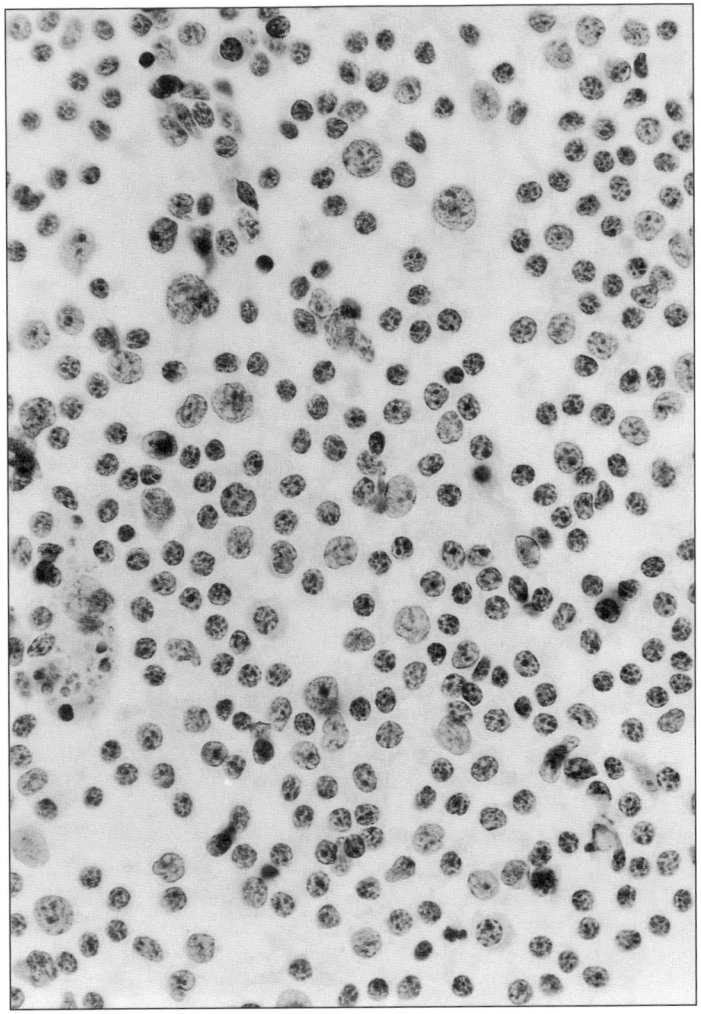

Fig. 11.9 Reactive follicular hyperplasia, fine needle aspiration. Note the mixture of lymphoid cells, with a tingible body macrophage present at the edge of the field.

REACTIVE FOLLICULAR HYPERPLASIA

The follicles represent the B-cell compartment of the lymph node. Unstimulated follicles are termed *primary follicles*. They consist of small B-lineage lymphocytes (CD20+) that are easily seen, embedded in a network of dendritic reticulum cells that are not easily appreciated morphologically, but can always be demonstrated by appropriate immunohistochemical studies for these cells (CD21 or CD35). With the appropriate stimulation, *secondary follicles* are formed. The most prominent feature of the secondary follicle is the germinal center. Germinal centers are composed of a mixture of small and large cleaved and noncleaved follicular center cells – a polytypic mixture of kappa- and lambda-bearing cells – with admixed small T lymphocytes (CD4+/CD57+), tingible body macrophages (CD68+), and occasionally polyclonal plasma cells, all embedded in a network of dendritic reticulum cells. In highly reactive follicles, polarization is seen, with one axis of the germinal center composed primarily of large noncleaved cells and tingible body macrophages (the dark zone), and the other axis composed primarily of small cleaved cells (the pale zone) (Fig. 11.8). Surrounding the germinal center is a mantle of small B lymphocytes, which share morphologic and immunologic features with the cells that are found in the centers of primary follicles. In the spleen and occasionally in abdominal lymph nodes, there is an outer layer of marginal B cells, which have slightly irregular nuclei, a moderate rim of pale to clear cytoplasm, and occasional plasmacytoid features. The follicles are surrounded by a paracortical region that is often expanded.

Follicular hyperplasia refers to an increased number and/or size of the reactive follicles, which may show great variation in shape. Adjacent germinal centers may fuse and assume large, bizarre geographic shapes. As the germinal centers expand, the surrounding mantle zones may correspondingly thin out. The germinal centers contain numerous mitotic figures, which impart a 'starry-sky' appearance, and the proliferative rate of the germinal centers is extremely high. CD21 and CD35 paraffin immunohistochemical stains highlight a greatly expanded dendritic network.

Reactive follicular hyperplasia may be recognized in fine needle aspiration specimens by the presence of small cellular aggregates at low magnification and the presence of a polymorphous population of lymphoid cells at high magnification (Fig. 11.9). Tingible body macrophages are also present.

Table 11.5 Histologic features useful in the distinction of reactive follicular hyperplasia vs. follicular lymphoma

Reactive follicular hyperplasia	Follicular lymphoma
Follicles limited to cortical region	Follicles present throughout the node
Follicles do not extend beyond capsule	Follicles extend beyond capsule
Low density of follicles	High density of follicles
Abundant interfollicular areas	Compressed interfollicular areas
No areas of diffuse effacement	Areas of diffuse effacement or architecture
Follicles of uneven size and shape	Follicles of similar size and shape
Mantle zone distinct	Mantle zone indistinct or absent
Mixture of cell types in germinal center	Monomorphic or polymorphic population
Tingible body macrophages present	Tingible body macrophages usually absent
Low to high mitotic rate	Low to moderate mitotic rate
Cell polarization often evident	Cell polarization absent

Table 11.6 Immunohistochemical and molecular features useful in the distinction of reactive follicular hyperplasia vs. follicular lymphoma

Reactive follicular hyperplasia	Follicular lymphoma
bcl-2 protein negative in follicles	bcl-2 protein often positive in follicles
CD10 weak to negative and confined to follicles	CD10 often strong in follicles and interfollicular lymphoma cells
MT2 positive in follicles	MT2 sometimes negative in follicles
Polytypic immunoglobulins in follicles, often detectable in paraffin sections	Monotypic or absent immunoglobulins in follicles, usually detectable only in frozen sections
Polytypic immunoglobulin in mRNA in follicles, often detectable in paraffin sections	Monotypic or absent immunoglobulin mRNA in follicles
Germline immunoglobulin gene	Monoclonal rearrangements of immunoglobulin genes
Germline *bcl-2* genes by Southern blot	Rearranged *bcl-2* gene in most cases
t(14;18) not detectable by classic cytogenetics	t(14;18) usually detectable by classic cytogenetics
t(14;18) usually not detectable by PCR	t(14;18) usually detectable by PCR

The major differential diagnosis of reactive follicular hyperplasia is follicular lymphoma. Numerous histologic criteria have been proposed for the distinction (Table 11.5),[99,100] but one must keep in mind that no one criterion is diagnostic. In practice, one must assess many features in combination, also considering clinical factors such as the relative rarity of follicular lymphoma in patients under the age of 40 years. Particularly helpful histologic features include the greater density and size uniformity of follicles and uniformity of cellular composition in follicular lymphoma as opposed to reactive follicular hyperplasia. The interfollicular areas of follicular lymphoma also contain the neoplastic cells, in contrast to the interfollicular areas of follicular hyperplasia, which may be broad and contain a mixture of reactive cells. The presence of a mantle zone, polarity, tingible body macrophages, and numerous mitotic figures all favor a reactive follicular hyperplasia. In difficult cases, immunohistochemical and molecular studies may be helpful in determining the correct diagnosis (Table 11.6). Bcl-2 protein expression in neoplastic as opposed to reactive follicles is usually very useful, with the caveat that bcl-2 protein may be absent in some follicular lymphomas, particularly follicular large cell lymphomas.[101–105] In addition, bcl-2 protein may be expressed by the T-helper cells in reactive follicles; comparison of bcl-2 stains with B- and T-lineage stains will prevent mistaking bcl-2 reactivity of T cells for bcl-2 reactivity in follicular lymphoma. At least 90% of follicular lymphomas have the structural cytogenetic t(14;18), which is absent in reactive tissues.[106] Under some conditions, the t(14;18) may be detected by PCR in reactive tissues,[28] but this is generally not a problem in protocols generally used for routine diagnosis.[107] CD10 expression, as detected by paraffin immunohistochemistry and flow cytometry, is often strong in follicular lymphoma, as opposed to follicular hyperplasia.[108,109]

Other neoplasms that should be considered in the differential diagnosis include the nodular variant of mantle cell lymphoma and interfollicular Hodgkin's disease. In the former, the lymphoid follicles become entirely replaced by neoplastic mantle cells, mimicking primary follicles. However, in contrast to reactive primary follicles, the follicles of mantle cell lymphoma are larger and the cells comprising the neoplastic nodules usually have a greater degree of nuclear atypia

than those of primary follicles. Paraffin section immunohistochemical studies often demonstrate aberrant coexpression of CD20 and CD43 in the cells of mantle cell lymphoma, as well as bcl-1 positivity.[3,110–112] The interfollicular variant of Hodgkin's disease can closely mimic reactive follicular hyperplasia, in that both may show highly reactive germinal centers. Examination of the interfollicular areas in the former will demonstrate Reed-Sternberg cells and variants in the appropriate milieu.[113] Immunohistochemical studies will usually demonstrate positivity for CD15 and negativity for CD45 in the Hodgkin cells of most cases of Hodgkin's disease; however, stains for CD30 may not be of use, as scattered CD30+ cells may be found in both disorders: CD30+ Reed-Sternberg cells and variants in Hodgkin's disease and CD30+ immunoblasts in reactive follicular hyperplasia.

Once a diagnosis of reactive follicular hyperplasia is established, one should attempt to identify a specific etiology. This may be possible in only a minority of cases. Nonetheless, many diseases showing reactive follicular hyperplasia have distinctive features that either allow their identification or suggest their diagnosis, prompting the appropriate confirmatory studies. Non-specific reactive follicular hyperplasia is common in the younger age groups, and generally resolves spontaneously without further consequences for the patient.[114] By contrast, non-specific reactive follicular hyperplasia occurring in the elderly often involves multiple lymph nodes and has been associated with concurrent or subsequent malignant lymphoma in a significant subset of cases.[115]

RHEUMATOID LYMPHADENOPATHY

Patients with rheumatoid arthritis commonly have lymphadenopathy, but biopsies are usually performed only if the lymph node reaches an unusually large size or grows at an unusually fast rate. The characteristic features of rheumatoid lymphadenopathy include a marked generalized reactive follicular hyperplasia with a paracortical polyclonal plasmacytosis.[116,117] The reactive changes are often present throughout the lymph node and may occur outside the capsule as well. Occasionally, there is a sinusoidal hyperplasia containing numerous neutrophils. The differential diagnosis includes secondary syphilis, the plasma cell variant of Castleman's disease, and other collagen vascular diseases, particularly Sjögren disease. In some cases, a paracortical proliferation may predominate, mimicking a peripheral T-cell lymphoma.

SJÖGREN LYMPHADENOPATHY

The lymph node findings in Sjögren disease may be indistinguishable from rheumatoid lymphadenopathy.[118] However, the former often contains a proliferation of monocytoid B cells in the sinusoidal or paracortical regions. When extensive, these proliferations may be indistinguishable from or may actually represent early low-grade B-cell lymphoma of mucosa-associated lymphoid tissue (MALT). Because these proliferations often show lymphoplasmacytoid features, staining for immunoglobulin light chains may be helpful in the differential diagnosis. Evidence of aberrant coexpression of CD20 and CD43 or the identification of significant monoclonal populations on molecular analysis of the immunoglobulin genes would favor the diagnosis of lymphoma. The significance of small clonal B-cell populations is not yet clear.

KIMURA LYMPHADENOPATHY

Kimura disease is a benign chronic inflammatory disease of probable allergic etiology. It predominantly affects Asians of young to middle age, but may occasionally affect other ethnic groups and other ages. Patients usually present with subcutaneous or soft tissue masses of the head and neck, often with infiltration of the salivary gland and involvement of regional lymph nodes. However, patients may occasionally present with isolated lymphadenopathy. Laboratory studies characteristically reveal eosinophilia with increased levels of IgE.

Involved lymph nodes usually show a characteristic triad of florid reactive follicular hyperplasia, increased vascularity, and marked eosinophilia of the paracortical regions[119–121] (Fig. 11.10). The reactive follicles frequently contain a proteinaceous material and many show prominent vascularization. Those that are highly vascularized usually show eosinophilia, which can be intense enough to form eosinophilic microabscesses. The germinal centers may also contain polykaryocytes of the Warthin-Finkeldey type. Occasionally, focal necrosis of the germinal centers can be seen. Immunohistochemical studies show large amounts of IgE on the processes of the follicular dendritic cells. The paracortical regions are also highly vascularized with numerous postcapillary venules. The most characteristic finding is marked eosinophilic infiltration, sometimes with the formation of eosinophilic abscesses. Scattered plasma cells and mast cells are also present. The sinuses also show marked eosinophilia. Other lymph node findings include the presence of polykaryocytes and focal sclerosis.

The differential diagnosis of Kimura lymphadenopathy includes many diseases with eosinophilia, such as drug-induced lymphadenopathy, parasitic infestation, Langerhans cell histiocytosis, Hodgkin's disease, and non-Hodgkin's lymphoma with eosinophilia. In drug-induced lymphadenopathy, the primary changes are in the paracortex, which contains a mixed population including immunoblasts and plasma cells, as well as eosinophils. Parasitic infestation can usually be suggested from the history; the lymph node may show direct evidence of the organism. Langerhans cell histiocytosis preferentially involves the sinuses and does not contain Warthin-

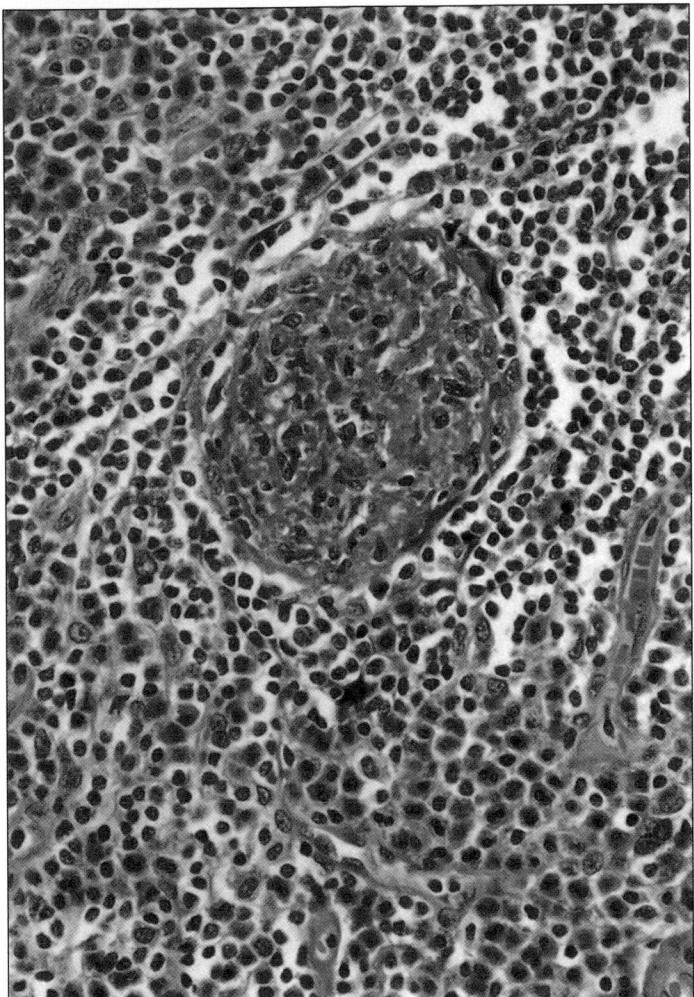

Fig. 11.10 Kimura's disease. The germinal center shows deposition of a proteinaceous material, while the paracortical area shows intense eosinophilia.

Finkeldey-type giant cells. Hodgkin's disease and non-Hodgkin's lymphoma with eosinophilia, particularly interfollicular variants, may be confused with Kimura disease, but attention to the identification of atypical cytology should allow easy distinction. Kimura disease should not be confused with *angiolymphoid hyperplasia with eosinophilia (epithelioid hemangioma)* in any way except the name.[120,121] The latter is a primary vascular proliferation characterized by an epithelioid appearance of the lining endothelial cells. Although there is often eosinophilia, the clinical picture and, most important, the histologic appearance, are otherwise markedly different.

TOXOPLASMIC LYMPHADENITIS

The symptoms of toxoplasmic lymphadenitis, caused by infection with the protozoon *Toxoplasma gondii*, may range from enlargement of a solitary node, usually posterior cervical, to a generalized lymphadenopathy with fever, resembling acute infectious mononucleosis. A characteristic triad of findings is seen, including 1) florid reactive follicular hyperplasia, 2) clusters of epithelioid histiocytes, and 3) reactive monocytoid B-cell proliferation in sinuses (Fig. 11.11).[122,123] This triad of findings is often found in close spatial relationship to one another. The epithelioid histiocytes are

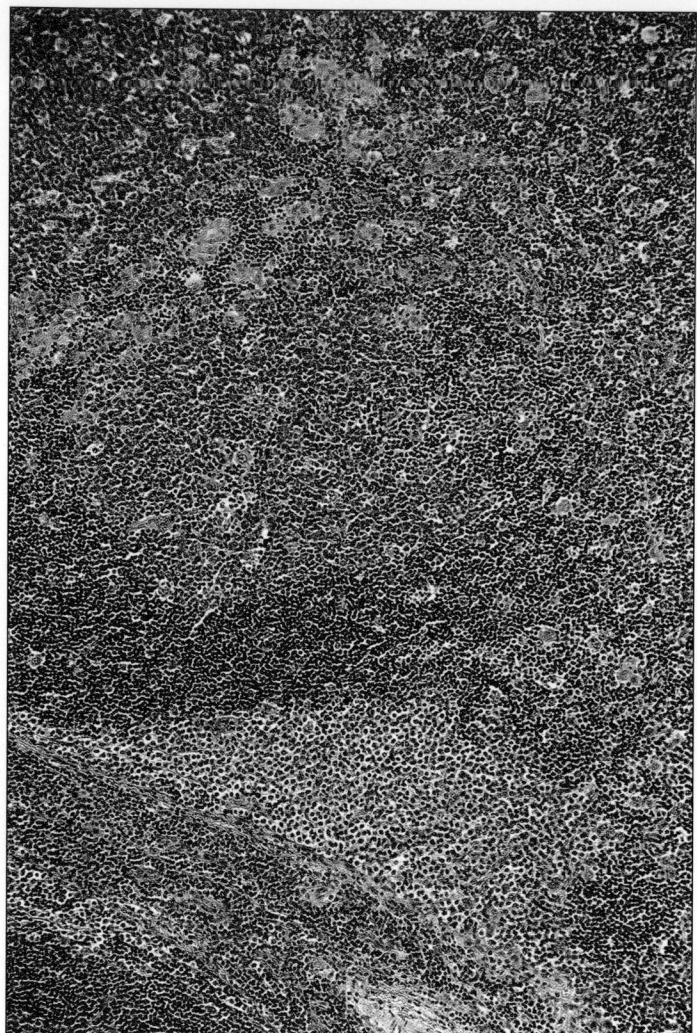

Fig. 11.11 Toxoplasmic lymphadenitis. This field shows the characteristic triad of reactive follicular hyperplasia, clusters of epithelioid histiocytes, and a reactive monocytoid B-cell proliferation.

can usually be identified if the histiocytes are carefully examined. The appropriate serologic studies for toxoplasmosis should be performed to confirm a diagnosis of toxoplasmic lymphadenitis.

SYPHILITIC LYMPHADENITIS

Enlargement of lymph nodes occurs in primary and secondary syphilis. Follicular hyperplasia and extensive paracortical plasmacytosis are common histologic features.[125] Frequently, the capsule is fibrotic, and contains an obliterative endarteritis with a perivascular lymphoplasmacytosis. In addition, aggregates of epithelioid histiocytes or small noncaseating granulomas may be present. Spirochetes are usually identified by Warthin-Starry silver stain or by immunohistochemical studies in the walls of postcapillary venules, in areas of necrosis, or occasionally within germinal centers. In recent years, the surgical pathologist is more likely than in the past to observe this disease, as the incidence of syphilitic or luetic lymphadenitis is on the rise. Inguinal lymph nodes are the most frequently biopsied site.

PROGRESSIVE TRANSFORMATION OF GERMINAL CENTERS

Progressive transformation of germinal centers is a variant of nonspecific reactive follicular hyperplasia in which some follicles undergo a marked enlargement up to four times normal size (Fig. 11.12).[126–128] The enlarged follicles consist of numerous small lymphocytes, often admixed with residual germinal center cells, the latter sometimes forming clusters. The progressively transformed germinal centers are found in a background of smaller, typical-appearing secondary lymphoid follicles, with transitional follicles usually present. Immunohistochemical studies of the small lymphocytes show the typical phenotype of polyclonal mantle zone B cells, with an expanded network of follicular dendritic cells forming the framework of the nodule.

Progressive transformation of germinal centers is more common in males and occurs in all age groups, although there is a predilection for the young. The most frequent presentation is that of an asymptomatic, solitary, enlarged lymph node, usually in the neck or inguinal region. The disease may recur in a significant subset of patients, but is otherwise not generally clinically significant. Progressive transformation of germinal centers has been reported to coexist with lymphocytic and histiocytic (L&H) lymphocyte predominance Hodgkin's disease.[129] In addition, patients with progressive transformation of germinal centers may develop the latter lymphoma, but only in a very low percentage of cases.[130]

L&H lymphocyte predominance Hodgkin's disease represents the most important entity to be distinguished from progressive transformation of germinal centers; this differential diagnosis is discussed in the section on L&H lymphocyte predominance Hodgkin's disease. Progressive transformation of germinal centers must also be distinguished from follicular lymphoma, particularly the floral variant. The progressively transformed germinal centers are generally larger than the follicles of follicular lymphoma. In addition, the background of reactive follicular hyperplasia in progressive transformation of germinal centers is different than that of follicular lymphoma, in which all the follicles are generally neoplastic. In difficult cases, immunohistochemical or molecular studies may be necessary. Occasional cases of mantle cell lymphoma may be difficult to distinguish from progressive transformation of germinal centers. The cells of mantle cell lymphoma usually have more irregular

not organized into well-formed granulomas, giant cells are rare if at all present, and eosinophils and necrosis are not seen. Rather, ill-defined aggregates of epithelioid histiocytes are seen in paracortical areas, in the mantle zones (impinging on the germinal centers), and occasionally present within germinal centers. In addition to the characteristic triad, there is often a plasmacytosis. Only rarely can the organism be identified morphologically as intracellular trophozoites or cysts. The lymph node findings most likely represent a reaction to antigens associated with the organism rather than the organism itself, since PCR studies for *T. gondii* are usually negative in toxoplasmic lymphadenitis.[124]

The characteristic histologic triad is both a sensitive and a relatively specific marker of toxoplasmic lymphadenitis, and the diagnosis should be suggested if these findings are encountered. HIV-associated lymphadenopathy, including florid reactive follicular hyperplasia and sinusoidal-parafollicular monocytoid B-cell proliferation, usually does not contain clusters of epithelioid histiocytes, and has follicular lysis and hemorrhage, which are usually not seen in toxoplasmosis. In addition, leishmaniasis can cause very similar histologic findings to toxoplasmosis, although the characteristic intracellular organisms

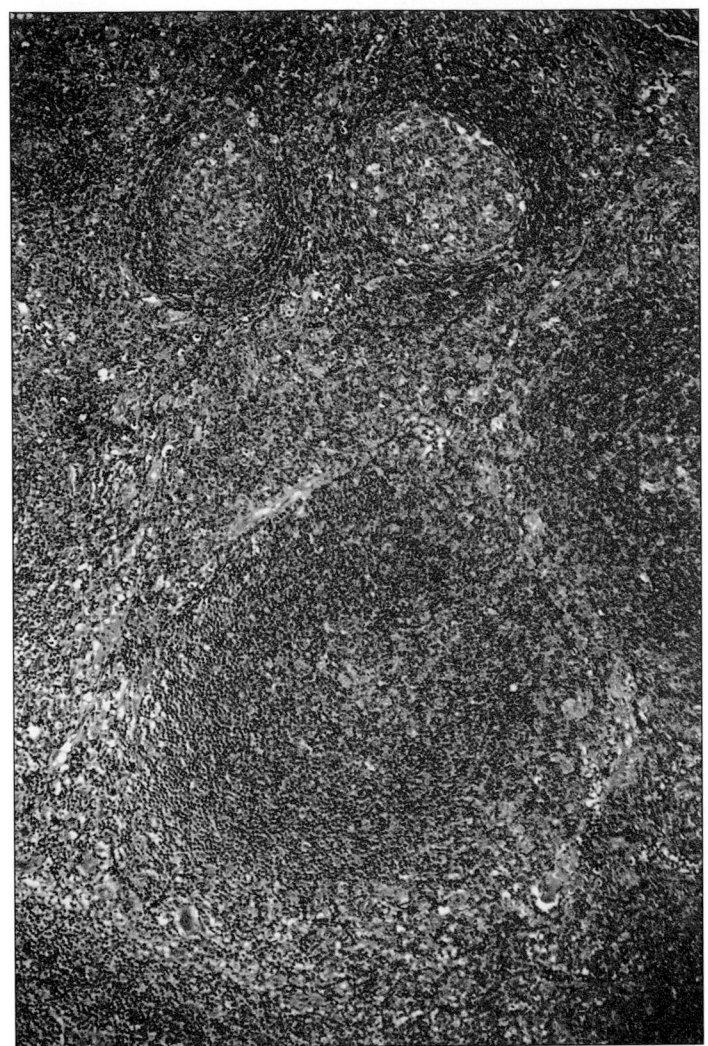

Fig. 11.12 Progressive transformation of germinal centers. Two reactive follicles are seen at top, while a progressively transformed germinal center is seen at bottom.

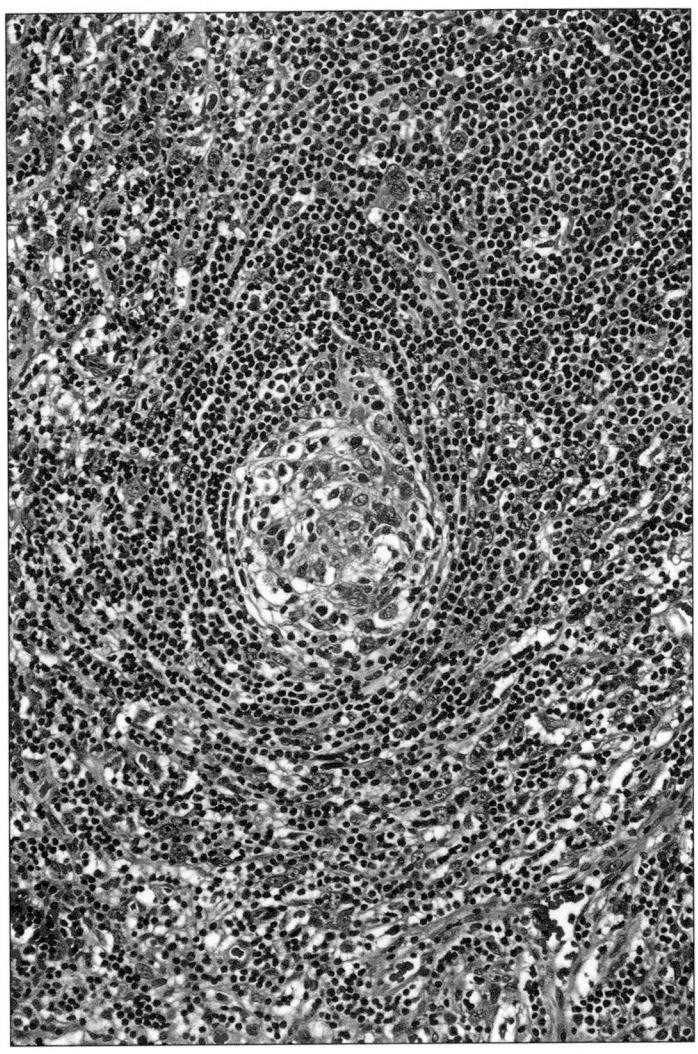

Fig. 11.13 Castleman's disease. A hyaline-vascular follicle is shown.

nuclear contours than the round lymphocytes in progressive transformation of germinal centers.

CASTLEMAN'S DISEASE

Castleman's disease, also known as angiofollicular lymph node hyperplasia or giant lymph node hyperplasia, may be localized or multicentric.[131] Localized Castleman's disease can be divided into hyaline-vascular, plasma cell, transitional, and stromal rich types.[132–134] In the hyaline-vascular type of localized Castleman's disease, there is no age or sex predilection. Patients generally present with a mass that is usually asymptomatic, except when the mass impinges on adjacent structures. The mediastinum is the most common site of involvement, followed by the abdomen, lung, skeletal muscle, and axillary and cervical soft tissue. The lesion is cured by surgical excision. Some cases are associated with a vascular or follicular dendritic cell neoplasm or an angiolipomatous hamartoma.[135–137]

Histologically, the hyaline vascular type of *localized Castleman's disease* shows numerous regressively transformed germinal centers

(Fig. 11.13). The mantle zones are expanded and usually have an 'onion-skin' appearance. The germinal centers are typically small, hypervascular, and occasionally multiple. One may see small germinal centers within a larger germinal center. They usually show lymphocyte depletion, with a hyalinized appearance. Penetrating vessels may sometimes be seen entering the follicle from the interfollicular region. The interfollicular region is hypervascular and is composed of a mixture of small lymphocytes, plasmacytoid monocytes, and plasma cells.[138] Occasionally, cells with large, hyperchromatic nuclei are present. In rare cases, the interfollicular areas may be markedly expanded, with increased numbers of spindled cells; this is more frequently present in abdominal cases. The so-called lymphoid variant of the hyaline vascular type refers to those cases in which the atrophic germinal centers are nearly completely obscured by small mantle zone lymphoctyes. The sinuses are usually obliterated and there is often a thickened capsule, with extension of the fibrosis around blood vessels. Immunohistochemical studies for CD21, CD35, and fascin demonstrate that the follicles are composed predominantly of follicular dendritic cells with scattered polyclonal B cells.[7] The interfollicular areas are composed mostly of T cells, with polyclonal plasma cells.

Molecular studies show a germline configuration of lymphocyte antigen receptor genes, and no viruses have been identified.[139]

Hyaline-vascular follicles have been reported in other types of reactive follicular hyperplasia, including HIV-associated lymphadenopathy.[131] However, the interfollicular regions in HIV-associated lymphadenopathy tend to be more polymorphous, with greater numbers of plasma cells and immunoblasts and generally lack the intense vascularity of Castleman's disease. In hyaline-vascular Castleman's disease, capsular fibrosis is more prominent and the lymph node is usually much larger in overall size. The expanded mantle zones in hyaline-vascular Castleman's disease may also mimic mantle cell lymphoma, but the cells in the reactive mantle zones lack the cytologic atypia commonly seen in the lymphoma; immunologic studies may also be helpful in making this distinction.

The plasma cell type of localized Castleman's disease is about one-tenth as common as the hyaline-vascular type; it also does not have an age or sex predilection.[133] However, patients frequently have systemic symptoms that resolve after surgical removal of the lesion. They include fever with a raised erythrocyte sedimentation rate (ESR), sweating, and fatigue; hematologic abnormalities, including thrombocytopenia and anemia;[140] and immunologic disorders, including hyperglobulinemia and rarely myasthenia gravis. Almost all patients have increased levels of serum interleukin-6.[141,142] In contrast to the hyaline-vascular type, the abdomen (particularly the small intestinal mesentery) is the most common site involved by the plasma cell type.

In the plasma cell type, the clinical mass is usually a collection of discrete, enlarged lymph nodes. The most striking histologic finding is the presence of sheets of mature plasma cells in the interfollicular regions. Other cells are few, except for occasional immunoblasts. There is no increase in vascularity. The follicles usually contain large germinal centers with mitotic figures, nuclear debris, and histiocytes. No central blood vessel is seen, and there is no hyalinization, although some follicles may be of the hyaline-vascular type. The nodal architecture is usually at least partially preserved, with patent sinuses. Immunohistochemical studies reveal the interfollicular plasma cells to be monotypic in about one-half of cases.[143] Interleukin-6 is found in the germinal center cells and immunoblasts.[144]

The differential diagnosis of the plasma cell type of Castleman's disease includes rheumatoid disease, syphilis, HIV-associated lymphadenopathy, and lymph nodes involved by or adjacent to other neoplasms (particularly Kaposi's sarcoma and Hodgkin's disease). Studies to rule out these other diseases should be performed before making a diagnosis of the plasma cell type of Castleman's disease.

Rare cases transitional between the hyaline-vascular and plasma cell types of localized Castleman's disease have been reported.[132] The clinical features more closely resemble the hyaline-vascular type. Histologically, the follicles are mostly of the hyaline-vascular type, although hyperplastic follicles may also be present. The interfollicular regions show both marked vascularity and extensive polyclonal plasmacytosis.

A stromal-rich variant of Castleman's disease has been described.[134,145] The lesions tend to be large and are usually found in the abdomen or retroperitoneal soft tissue. Histologically, the interfollicular zones are enlarged in size, so that they comprise greater than 75% of the size of the mass. These areas are rich in spindle cells, mostly endothelial cells, histiocytes, follicular dendritic cells, and fibroblastic reticulum cells.

Multicentric Castleman's disease usually occurs in older patients and is associated with systemic manifestations.[146,147] There is multicentric lymph node enlargement and splenomegaly is common. Patients are usually anemic and have polyclonal hypergamma-globulinemia. As a rule, there is evidence of multisystem disease, such as involvement of the liver, kidney, skin, and central nervous system. The bone marrow often shows plasmacytosis. Some patients may present with POEMS syndrome (polyneuropathy, organomegaly, endocrinopathy, M-protein, and skin symptoms).[148] To distinguish this from neuropathy associated with monoclonal gammopathy of uncertain significance, some authors have suggested additional criteria for diagnosing a patient with POEMS syndrome: a bone lesion, Castleman's disease, organomegaly (or lymphadenopathy), endocrinopathy, edema (peripheral edema, ascites, or effusions), and skin changes.[149] In many POEMS patients, the disease has an aggressive course with a fatal outcome.

Histologically, the nodes resemble the plasma cell type of Castleman's disease, although some hyaline-vascular follicles may be present.[147,150] Immunohistochemical studies reveal the interfollicular plasma cells to be monotypic or polytypic. Molecular studies may show a germline configuration of the lymphocyte antigen receptor genes or may demonstrate small clonal populations of T or B cells.[151] Evidence of EBV or KSHV/HHV-8 has been found in many cases.[151–156] KSHV has been shown to infect monotypic but polyclonal naive B cells of multicentric Castleman's disease. These infected cells (plasmablasts) are associated with a range of lymphoproliferative disorders from polyclonal isolated plasmablasts and microlymphomas to monoclonal microlymphoma and frank plasmablastic lymphomas in multicentric Castleman's disease patients.[157]

Histologic changes indistinguishable from multicentric Castleman's disease may be found in Kaposi's sarcoma and acquired immunodeficiency syndrome (AIDS). In addition, multicentric Castleman's disease may be complicated by malignant lymphoma.[158] Therefore, studies should be done to exclude these possibilities in any patient for whom a diagnosis of multicentric Castleman's disease is being considered.

HIV-ASSOCIATED LYMPHADENOPATHY

HIV-associated lymphadenopathy is included in the section on reactive follicular hyperplasia because patients usually show some type of follicular hyperplasia at the time of lymph node biopsy. Nonetheless, it must be acknowledged that follicular involution and lymphoid depletion may sometimes be the dominant findings, although usually at a late stage in the disease course and more commonly at autopsy than in surgical specimens. Lymphadenopathy is common in HIV-infected patients. Biopsies are generally performed in this population to rule out infection or a neoplasm such as malignant lymphoma or Kaposi's sarcoma. However, persistent generalized lymphadenopathy is a part of the spectrum of HIV-associated disease, defined by the Centers for Disease Control and Prevention as lymph node enlargement of at least 3 months' duration, absence of any illness or drug use known to cause lymph node enlargement, and histologic evidence of reactive follicular hyperplasia.[159] HIV-related lymphadenopathy is often associated with a heterogeneous EBV population.[160,161]

Three to four main stages of lymph node changes have been described.[162–166] 'Explosive' reactive follicular hyperplasia represents the earliest and most common histologic finding (Fig. 11.14). In explosive reactive follicular hyperplasia, there are numerous secondary follicles distributed throughout the lymph node, with highly irregular sizes and shapes. The germinal centers frequently show polarization and contain a mixture of germinal center B cells and numerous tingible body macrophages. Typically, the mantle zones are thinned and may be entirely absent, simulating malignant lymphoma. In some follicles, the phenomenon of follicle lysis may be

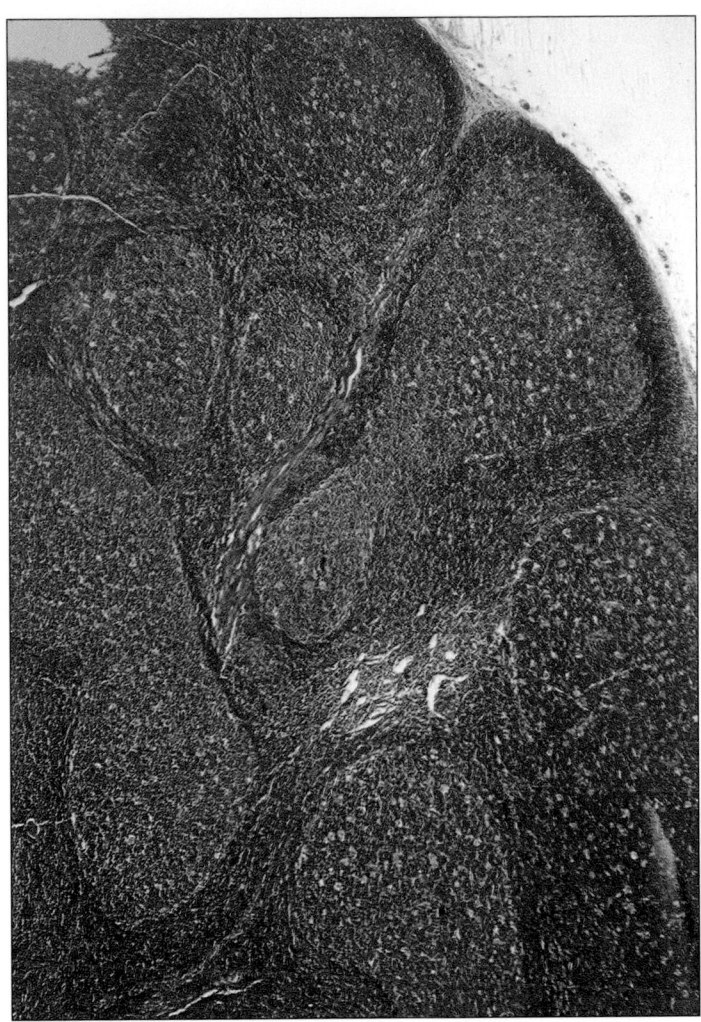

Fig. 11.14 HIV-associated lymphadenopathy. 'Explosive' reactive follicular hyperplasia is seen.

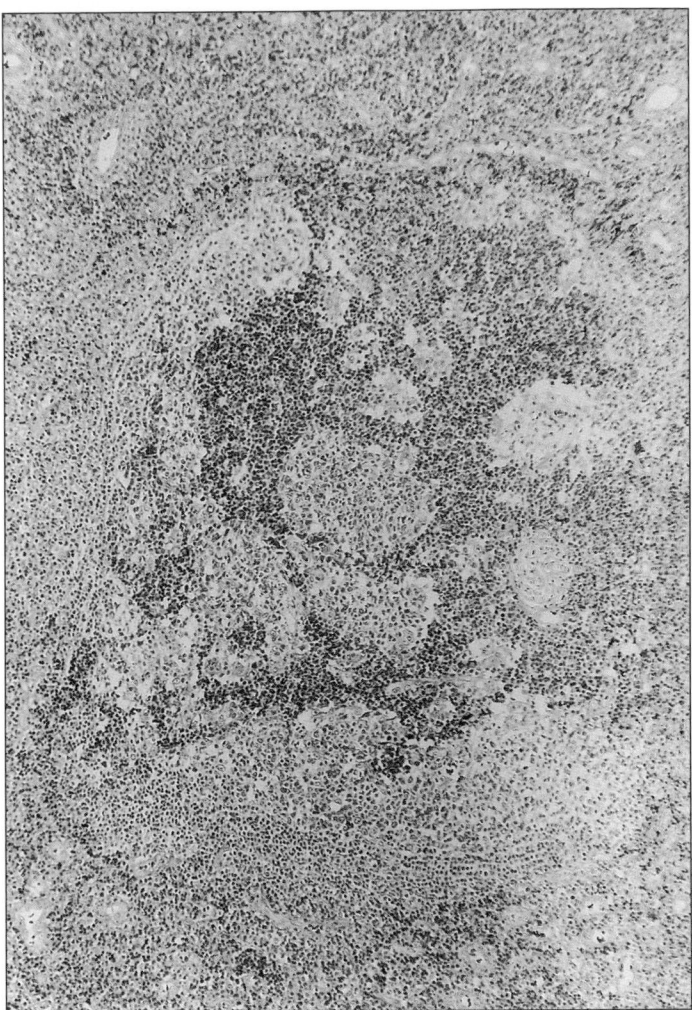

Fig. 11.15 HIV-associated lymphadenopathy. This follicle is undergoing follicle lysis.

seen (Fig. 11.15). In follicle lysis, there is invagination of small lymphocytes into the germinal center, with separation of the clusters of germinal center cells into irregular clusters. In contrast to progressive transformation of germinal centers, the affected follicles are of normal size. This is often accompanied by follicular hemorrhage. The paracortical lymphoid tissue is often reduced in size, but is usually hypervascular and contains a mixed infiltrate including plasma cells and sometimes immunoblasts, eosinophils, and epithelioid histiocytes. Other characteristic features include a proliferation of monocytoid B cells in paracortical regions, focal dermatopathic changes, and Warthin-Finkeldey-type giant cells (in follicles or the paracortical regions).[167]

Over time, floridly reactive follicles are found admixed with hyaline-vascular follicles (follicular involution) that closely resemble the characteristic follicles of the hyaline-vascular Castleman's disease. Early on, the paracortical region is diminished in size but over time, the paracortical areas become expanded with hypervascularity and numerous plasma cells, forming a picture that closely mimics the plasma cell variant of Castleman's disease. Finally, in lymphocyte depletion, there is a generalized loss of lymphoid cells in both the follicles and paracortical regions (Fig. 11.16). The germinal centers are entirely absent or reduced to skeletons of follicular dendritic cells, endothelial cells, and histiocytes. The paracortical region is also

greatly diminished in size and consists of histiocytes and plasma cells, but only scattered lymphoid cells. There may be a granulomatous appearance imparted by the numerous histiocytes, a finding that should prompt appropriate special stains for *Mycobacteria avium-intracellulare* or other organisms. Due to diminution of the follicular and paracortical areas, the sinusoidal areas often appear prominent. Lymph nodes with lymphocyte depletion are generally smaller, not larger, than usual, and therefore usually not seen in surgical specimens, but are often obtained at autopsy.

In explosive reactive follicular hyperplasia, HIV can be demonstrated in the follicular dendritic cells by electron microscopy, immunohistochemical studies, or in situ hybridization; these cells represent a major reservoir of HIV in the latent phase prior to the development of AIDS.[168] In follicle lysis, a disrupted network of follicular dendritic cells can be demonstrated by immunohistochemical studies.[169,170] The paracortical areas have a decreased CD4/CD8 ratio, similar to that seen in the peripheral blood in these patients.

Patients with explosive reactive follicular hyperplasia or mixed reactive follicular hyperplasia with hyaline-vascular follicles are generally in the pre-AIDS state with a relatively good prognosis. Patients without follicular hyperplasia – those with follicular involution or lymphocyte depletion – have a poor prognosis and

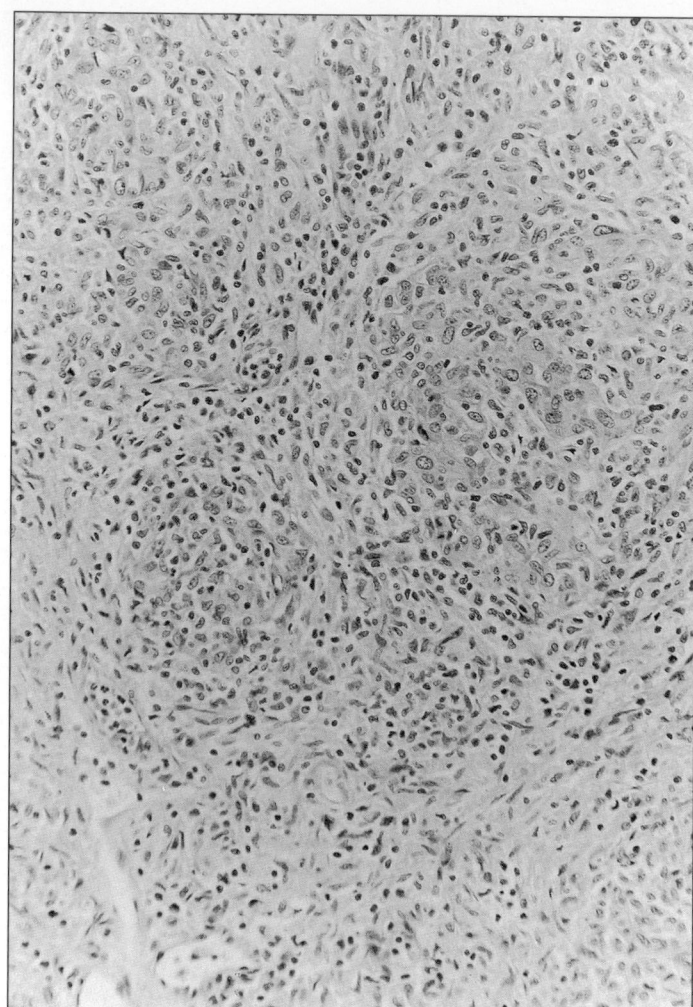

Fig. 11.16 HIV-associated lymphadenopathy. Marked lymphocyte depletion is present.

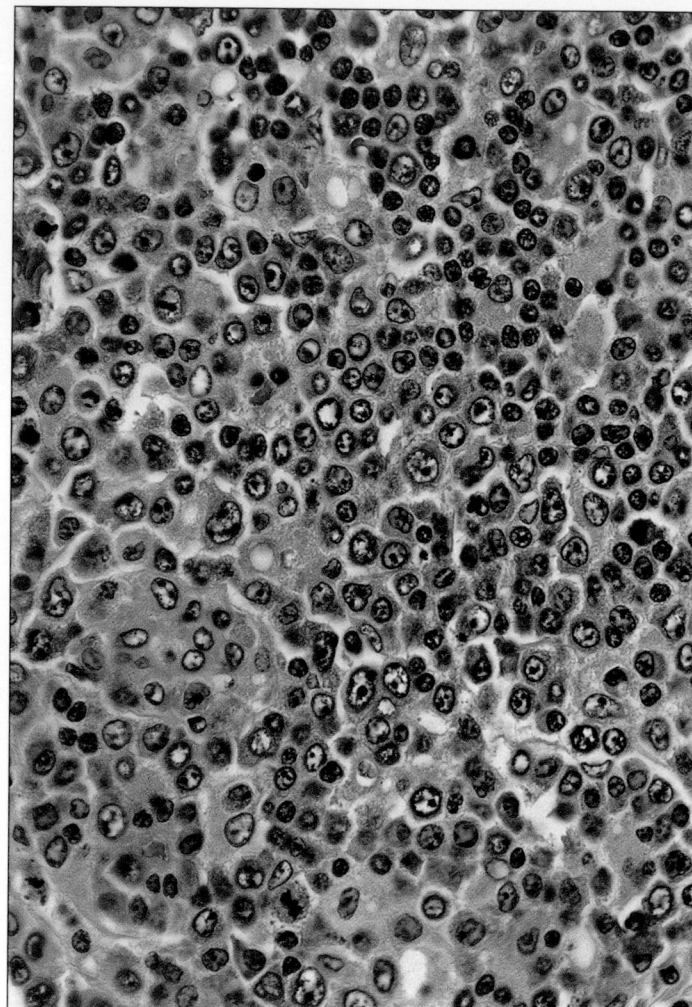

Fig. 11.17 Reactive paracortical hyperplasia. A spectrum of lymphoid differentiation, including numerous immunoblasts, is seen. This case was EBV-associated acute infectious mononucleosis.

usually have clinical AIDS.

None of the above described changes is diagnostic of HIV-associated lymphadenopathy. Nonetheless, the identification of this constellation of findings should at least prompt the suggestion of this diagnosis, particularly in the appropriate clinical settings. Several phases of this disorder can show a close resemblance to the several types of Castleman's disease. If a diagnosis of HIV-associated lymphadenopathy is suspected, one should also carefully scrutinize the lymph node for concurrent infection as well as malignant neoplasms. In particular, Kaposi's sarcoma may be present as a very focal finding in the capsule of the lymph node, particularly in cases showing hyaline-vascular follicles with Castleman's-like features or lymphocyte depletion. In addition, areas of concomitant non-Hodgkin's lymphoma should not be overlooked.

REACTIVE PARACORTICAL HYPERPLASIA

The paracortex represents the T-cell zone of the lymph node. It contains numerous T cells (with CD4+ cells generally outnumbering CD8+ cells); scattered B cells and plasma cells; histiocytes; occasional interdigitating dendritic cells (S-100+; no Birbeck granules) and Langerhans cells (S-100+; Birbeck granules); and fibroblastic reticulum cells (Fig. 11.17). In addition, there are high endothelial venules. In the unstimulated state, almost all of the lymphoid cells are small with a condensed chromatin pattern. On immune stimulation, the paracortex becomes expanded, with greater numbers of small and large B and T cells and plasma cells, giving rise to an overall mottled appearance. Many of the large cells have features of classic immunoblasts – cells with large nuclei with vesicular chromatin and prominent nucleoli. There is also a proliferation of high endothelial venules. Benign paracortical hyperplasia is virtually always accompanied by some degree of reactive follicular hyperplasia and often reactive sinus hyperplasia. Most of the time, a specific etiology cannot be determined, but some disorders are associated with characteristic or occasionally diagnostic features. Fine needle aspiration biopsy of reactive paracortical hyperplasia reveals a polymorphous population of lymphoid cells, including small, medium, and large lymphoid cells with scattered plasma cells.

VIRAL LYMPHADENITIS

Viral lymphadenitis represents a common cause of reactive paracortical hyperplasia. Although florid reactive follicular hyperplasia may be a prominent histologic finding in early lesions, reactive paracortical hyperplasia soon becomes the dominant feature and, in some cases, overruns the follicles and leads to diffuse effacement of nodal architecture. In florid cases, focal necrosis may be present in either the follicles or the paracortical region. The sinuses may show histiocytic hyperplasia, occasionally with hemophagocytosis; a range of plasmacytoid cells, including immunoblasts; or a proliferation of monocytoid B cells. The monocytoid B cells may extend into the paracortical areas.

The differential diagnosis includes several types of malignant lymphoma. Sheets of immunoblasts may be focally present, leading to potential confusion with large cell non-Hodgkin's lymphoma. In some cases, Reed-Sternberg-like cells may be found, leading to potential confusion with Hodgkin's disease. In both situations, attention should be given to identifying overall retention of architecture (when present) and a spectrum of identifiable cell types in reactive paracortical hyperplasia. Typically, one can identify small lymphocytes, plasma cells, and plasmacytoid immunoblasts in varying numbers. In difficult cases, immunohistochemical studies may be of value, with a mixture of B and T cells with polyclonal plasmacytoid lymphocytes and plasma cells in reactive paracortical hyperplasia. By contrast, non-Hodgkin's lymphoma generally shows sheets of B cells or T cells in B-cell and T-cell lymphomas, respectively, with monotypic plasmacytoid cells or plasma cells in lymphoplasmacytic lymphomas. The immunoblasts in reactive paracortical hyperplasia usually have basophilic cytoplasm, sometimes with a paranuclear hof, basophilic nucleoli, and are CD45+ and CD15−, whereas Hodgkin cells have amphophilic to eosinophilic cytoplasm lacking a hof, eosinophilic nucleoli, and are CD45− and CD15+. In addition, Hodgkin cells are found in their characteristic milieu, which usually includes eosinophils and lacks a spectrum of plasmacytoid cells.

Epstein-Barr virus (EBV)-associated acute infectious mononucleosis represents a prototype of reactive paracortical hyperplasia[171–173] (see Fig. 11.17). The specific diagnosis may be suggested by clinical studies, including a lymphocytosis with atypical lymphocytes and a positive monospot test or other EBV serologic studies. Immunohistochemical studies for EBV latent membrane protein (LMP) or in situ hybridization for Epstein-Barr early RNA (EBER) may be useful in identifying specific evidence of EBV, although one must keep in mind that other lymphoproliferations such as Hodgkin's disease and some non-Hodgkin's lymphomas may be EBV-associated and that EBV-seropositive individuals may have rare EBV-positive cells (EBER+, but LMP−) in benign lymphoid tissues.

Cytomegalovirus (CMV) in both immunocompetent and immunocompromised hosts may show features of reactive paracortical hyperplasia similar to EBV-associated infectious mononucleosis.[174] Although the characteristic CMV inclusions are generally easy to find in immunocompromised patients, they are usually very rare and require careful search. The infected cells are mostly T cells of both helper and suppressor phenotype. In addition to reactive paracortical hyperplasia, CMV lymphadenitis usually shows a florid reactive follicular hyperplasia with a proliferation of monocytoid B cells in sinuses that extends into the paracortex. The differential diagnosis of CMV lymphadenitis includes other causes of reactive immunoblastic hyperplasia as well as Hodgkin's disease, due to the superficial resemblance of CMV-infected cells to Reed-Sternberg cells. In

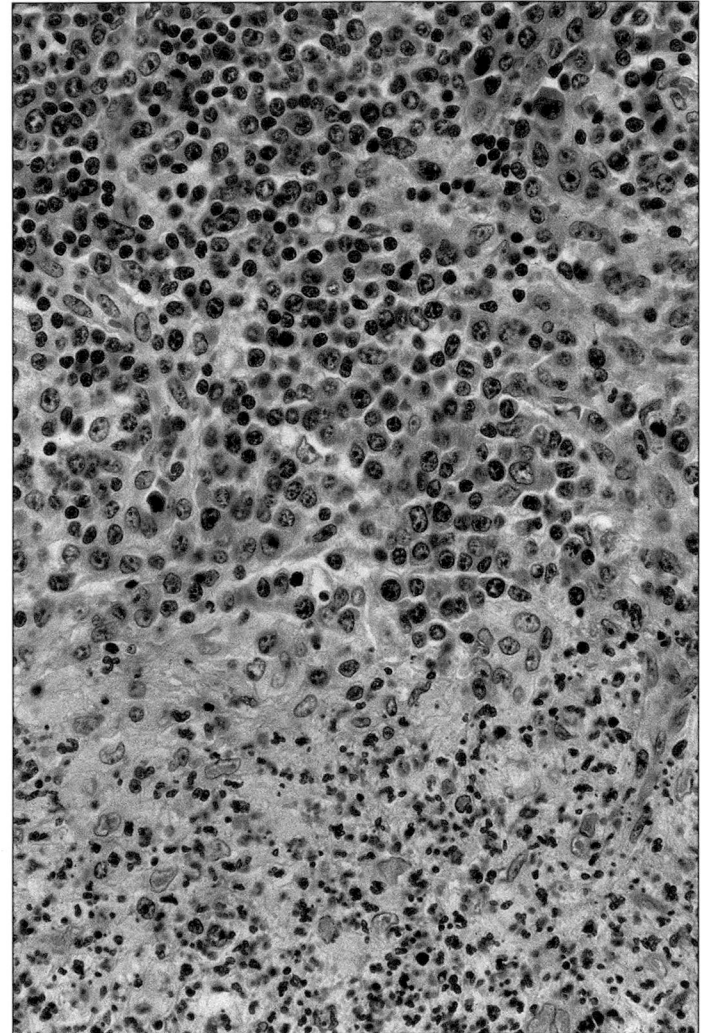

Fig. 11.18 Herpes lymphadenitis. A reactive infiltrate is seen at top, while necrosis with herpetic inclusions is seen at bottom.

addition, CMV-infected cells may be CD15+, similar to Reed-Sternberg cells.[175] Immunohistochemical studies for CMV antigens or in situ hybridization studies for CMV DNA should resolve any problematic cases.[176,177]

Herpes simplex lymphadenitis is common in patients with clinically evident skin lesions, and also rarely occurs as isolated lymph node enlargement.[178,179] The histologic appearance can be indistinguishable from non-specific reactive paracortical hyperplasia. However, there is often necrosis, which may be extensive and accompanied by neutrophils and granulation tissue (Fig. 11.18). The characteristic inclusions of herpes simplex are typically found within the areas of necrosis or in the viable lymphoid tissue at the edge of the necrosis. In situ hybridization for herpes simplex DNA can provide confirmation of the diagnosis.

DRUG-INDUCED LYMPHADENOPATHY

A wide variety of drugs, most notably diphenylhydantoin (Dilantin), can cause lymph node enlargement.[180–182] The lymphadenopathy

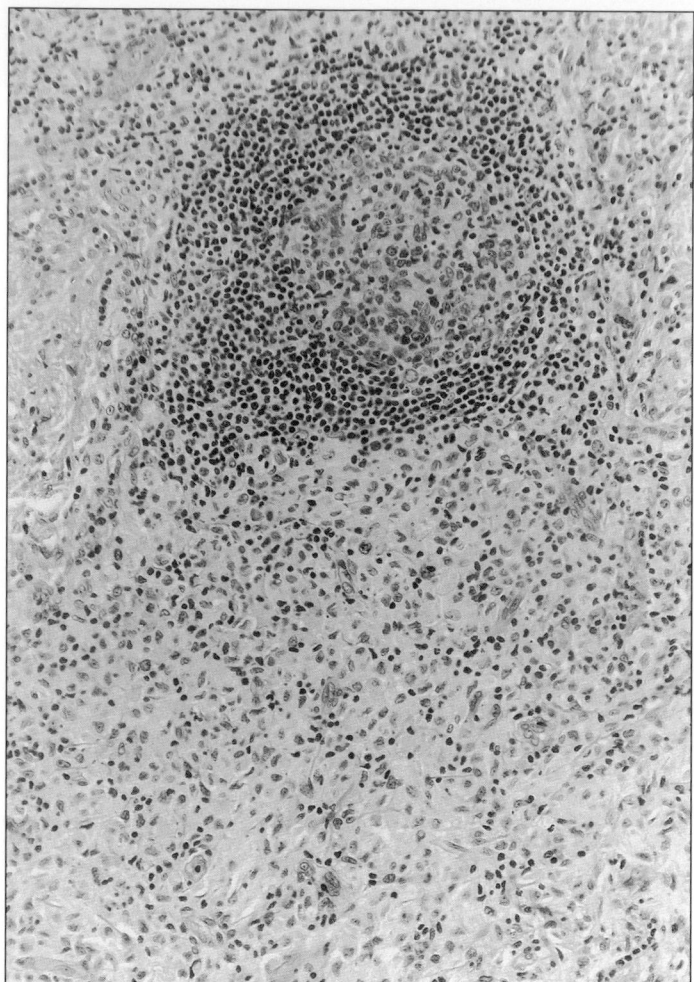

Fig. 11.19 Dermatopathic lymphadenopathy. The paracortical region is pale, due to a proliferation of cytoplasm-rich dendritic cells and macrophages.

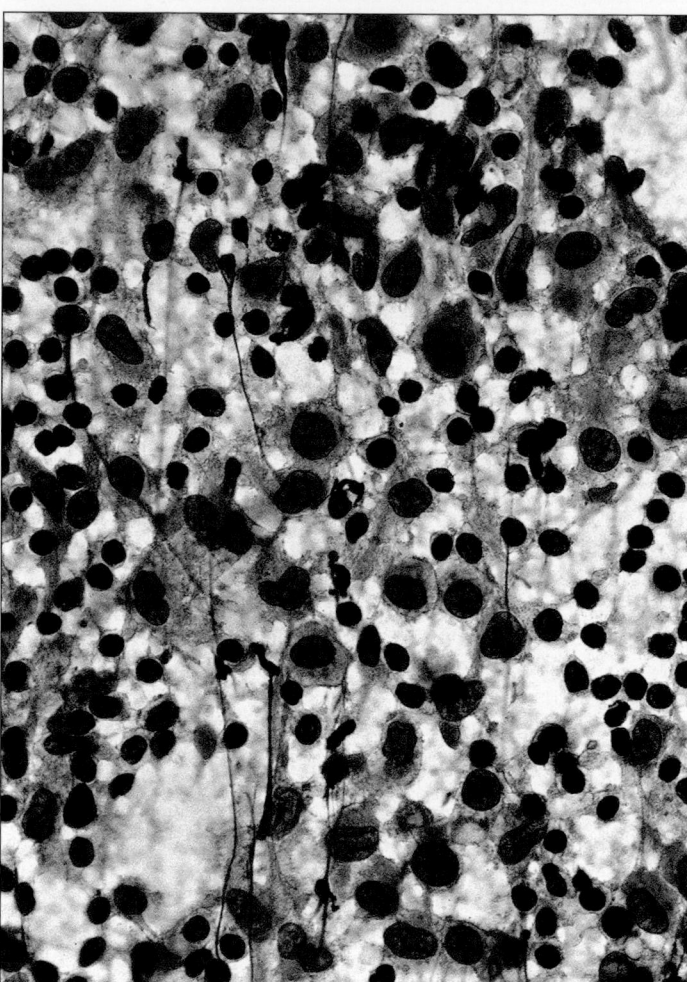

Fig. 11.20 Dermatopathic lymphadenopathy, fine needle aspiration. The characteristic grooved nuclei of interdigitating cells and Langerhans cells are easy to recognize in smear preparations.

usually occurs within several weeks after therapy is begun, and resolves within several weeks after the medication is stopped. Typically, reactive paracortical hyperplasia is seen, usually accompanied by eosinophils. Even in the absence of the appropriate history, the presence of these two features in combination should prompt a suggestion of drug-induced lymphadenopathy. However, the histologic findings may not be completely specific, and the findings may be indistinguishable from viral lymphadenitis or even angioimmunoblastic lymphadenopathy. Similar to viral lymphadenitis, a reactive follicular hyperplasia is often found in the early stages of drug-induced lymphadenopathy.

The differential diagnosis of drug-induced lymphadenopathy includes angioimmunoblastic lymphadenopathy, peripheral T-cell lymphoma, and Hodgkin's disease, diseases that commonly have a reactive component that includes eosinophils. In contrast to these other diseases, the overall lymph node architecture is usually retained in drug-induced lymphadenopathy. In addition, the spectrum of lymphoid atypia seen in peripheral T-cell lymphoma is absent in drug-induced lymphadenopathy, and the presence of numerous immunoblasts and plasma cells is unusual for Hodgkin's disease. The lymph node findings in *postvaccinial lymphadenopathy* may be indistinguishable from drug-induced lymphadenopathy. This disorder is rare now that smallpox vaccinations have been discontinued, but can be encountered following tetanus inoculations.

DERMATOPATHIC LYMPHADENOPATHY

Dermatopathic lymphadenopathy is a special form of paracortical hyperplasia in which the predominant hyperplastic elements are the dendritic cells (Fig. 11.19).[183–186] This disorder is associated with a variety of skin disorders, particularly those that lead to disruption of the skin barrier, but interestingly has been reported in patients without clinically evident skin lesions. In dermatopathic lymphadenopathy, there is a proliferation of interdigitating dendritic cells, Langerhans cells, histiocytes, eosinophils, as well as a range of lymphoid cells, imparting a mottled appearance at low magnification. The interdigitating dendritic cells and Langerhans cells, usually not morphologically identifiable in normal lymph nodes, are easy to recognize in dermatopathic lymphadenopathy, because of their characteristic grooved nuclei. The histiocytes often (but not always) contain visible melanin pigment. The dendritic cells and melanin-laden macrophages may be easily recognized in fine needle aspiration biopsy specimens (Fig. 11.20).[187] The lymphoid cells vary from small, round lymphocytes to small lymphocytes with irregular nuclear contours to immunoblasts. Confirmation of the diagnosis can be achieved with an S-100 stain, which should label both the interdigitating dendritic cells and Langerhans cells.

The diagnosis of dermatopathic lymphadenopathy is usually very straightforward. Although proliferating Langerhans cells are also seen in Langerhans cell histiocytosis, that disorder primarily affects the sinuses with secondary extension into the paracortical areas. The most difficult point in the differential diagnosis is the evaluation of dermatopathic nodes in patients with known or suspected mycosis fungoides, a topic covered in the section on mycosis fungoides later in this chapter.

SINUS HYPERPLASIA

Non-specific sinus histiocytosis

Sinus histiocytosis is often seen in lymph nodes that drain the extremities and the mesentery, and in lymph nodes that drain sites of malignant tumors or of prosthesis placement.[188–190] It is often idiopathic. Morphologically, one sees uniformly sized histiocytes with cytologically bland nuclei and abundant cytoplasm that fill and distend subcapsular and trabecular lymph node sinuses. Rarely, there may be histiocytes with prominent erythrophagocytosis, particularly in the axillary lymph nodes of patients with breast cancer.[191] A rare signet-ring variant of sinus histiocytosis may occur, also in the axillary lymph nodes of patients with breast cancer.[192,193]

Monocytoid B-cell hyperplasia

Monocytoid B-cell hyperplasia is seen in the sinuses or parasinusoidal areas in about 10% of reactive lymph nodes (Fig. 11.21).[194] It is almost invariably seen in toxoplasmosis,[123] and is also commonly found in HIV-associated benign lymphadenopathy, suppurative granulomatous lymphadenitis, and viral lymphadenitis.[195,196] Monocytoid B cells are medium-sized cells with small nuclei, irregular nuclear outlines, and a bland chromatin pattern. There is a moderate rim of pale to clear cytoplasm that forms distinct cell borders with adjacent cells. Usually, there are admixed neutrophils and plasma cells, and occasionally, immunoblasts can be seen. Monocytoid B cells stain for CD20 but not for bcl-2 protein, and polytypic cytoplasmic immunoglobulins can occasionally be demonstrated.

Monocytoid B-cell hyperplasia may be easily confused with marginal zone B-cell lymphoma, which was formerly known as monocytoid B-cell lymphoma.[197] Features favoring lymphoma include the proliferation comprising more than 50% of the lymph node with confluent extension into the paracortical areas, a greater degree of nuclear atypia and a higher mitotic rate, and the presence of a component of another lymphoma, such as follicular lymphoma or a malignant lymphoplasmacytic proliferation. Staining for immunoglobulin light chains and bcl-2 protein may be of value in this situation.[7,104] Marginal zone B-cell lymphoma has monotypic light chains and is usually bcl-2 protein positive, whereas monocytoid B-cell hyperplasia has polytypic light chains and is bcl-2 protein negative.

Infection-associated hemophagocytic syndrome

Infection-associated hemophagocytic syndrome is a non-neoplastic, systemic proliferation of benign-appearing histiocytes.[198–200] It may be caused by almost any infectious agent. Most patients have a documented primary or iatrogenic (e.g. organ transplant-related) immunodeficiency. Patients usually have fever and other consti-

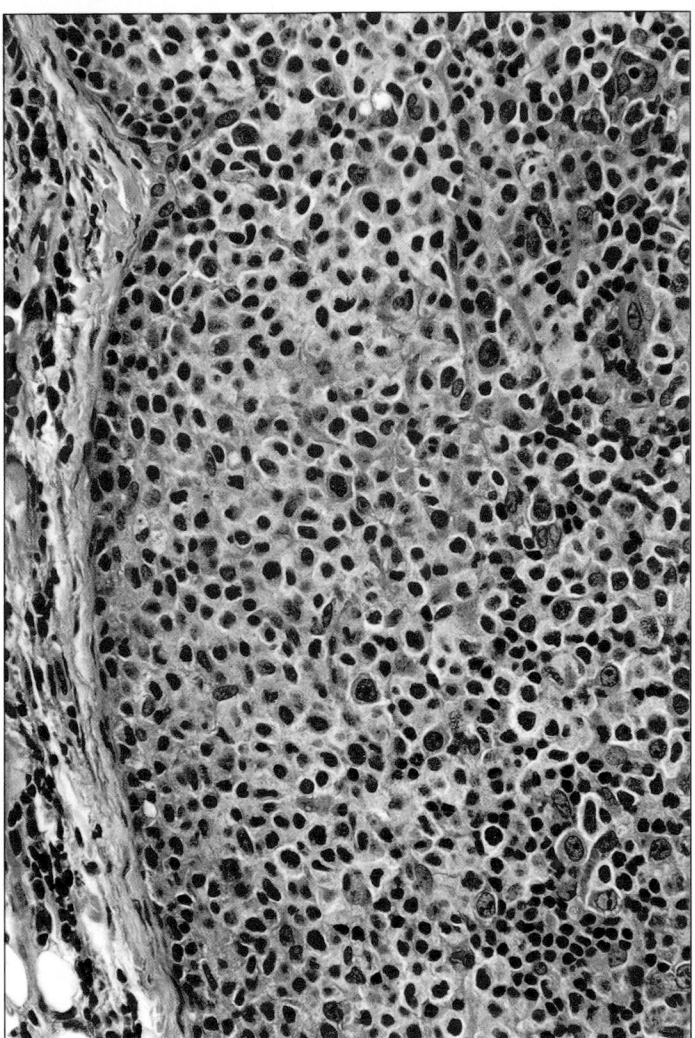

Fig. 11.21 Monocytoid B-cell hyperplasia. The sinuses and parasinusoidal regions are expanded by medium-sized cells with small bland nuclei and abundant clear cytoplasm.

tutional symptoms, hepatosplenomegaly, and generalized lymphadenopathy, and less often a skin rash and bilateral pulmonary infiltrates. Laboratory evaluation usually reveals pancytopenia and liver function abnormalities. Infection-associated hemophagocytic syndrome is a benign, self-limiting condition. However, affected patients may die during the acute disease episode due to multisystem failure or later due to infectious complications exacerbated by their underlying immunodeficiency.[198] In addition, EBV-associated hemophagocytic syndrome appears to be a particularly virulent form of this syndrome, affecting young children and leading rapidly to death.[201–203]

The pathologic features vary with the time that biopsies are performed. Early in the disease, lymph nodes are only partially involved by a small number of histiocytes and a marked immunoblastic proliferation. Later in the disease, one sees massive sinusoidal infiltration by benign-appearing histiocytes (Fig. 11.22). The histiocytes may show prominent hemophagocytosis and platelet phagocytosis. Germinal centers, if present, are inconspicuous.

The differential diagnosis of infection-associated hemophagocytic syndrome includes malignant lymphomas associated with benign

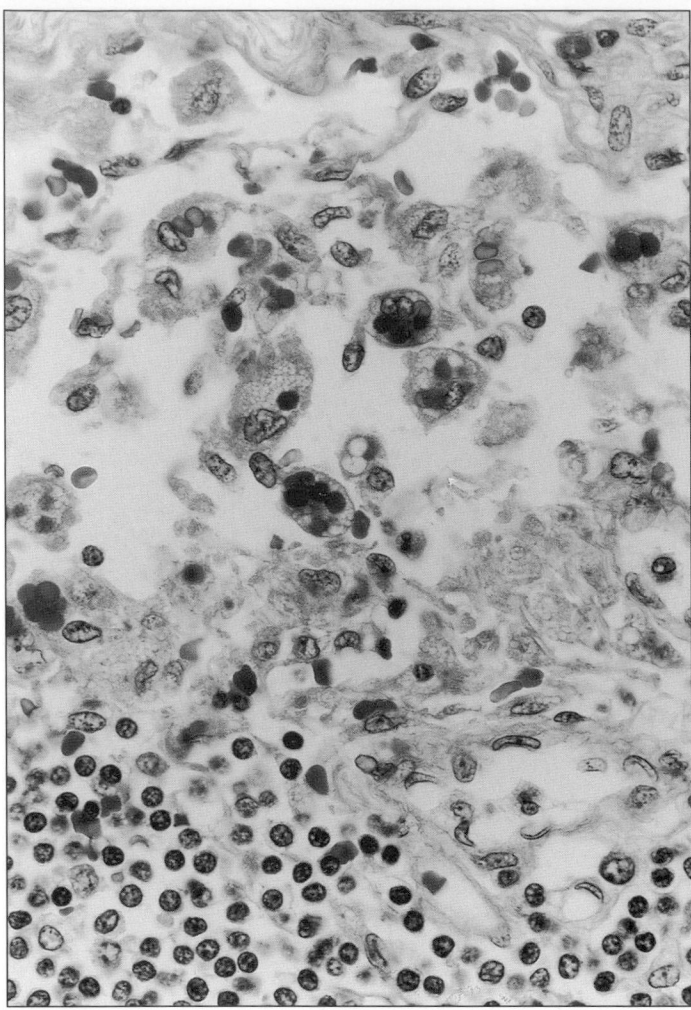

Fig. 11.22 Infection-associated hemophagocytic syndrome. The sinuses contain numerous histiocytes exhibiting erythrophagocytosis.

hemophagocytosis and familial hemophagocytic lymphohistiocytosis, both of which are discussed below.

Familial hemophagocytic lymphohistiocytosis

Familial hemophagocytic lymphohistiocytosis is a rare and usually fatal disease that is characterized by marked lymphohistiocytic infiltration in multiple organs.[198,204–206] Most patients are less than 1 year old. Approximately three-fourths of cases are familial, with an autosomal recessive mode of inheritance. The infants usually present with fevers, hepatosplenomegaly, pulmonary effusions, and a skin rash. Laboratory findings include pancytopenia and a severe hypofibrinogenemia without abnormalities of other clotting factors. Impaired cellular and humoral immunity are features of this disorder.[207] The disease is usually rapidly fatal (within weeks), with death due to sepsis or bleeding. Rare patients have survived several months to years.

The lymph nodes and bone marrow are the most frequently involved organs, followed by the spleen, liver, and the central nervous system. Lymph nodes in patients with familial hemophagocytic lymphohistiocytosis are partially to completely effaced by a sinusoidal infiltrate of benign-appearing histiocytes, lymphocytes, and plasma cells. The histiocytosis is quite pronounced and is accompanied by prominent erythrophagocytosis as well as phagocytosis of lymph-

cytes and other cellular debris. Other organs of the reticuloendothelial system may also contain large numbers of hemophagocytic histiocytes.

Familial hemophagocytic lymphohistiocytosis and infection-associated hemophagocytic syndrome may be clinically and morphologically similar. In fact, they may represent the same disease, with familial hemophagocytic lymphohistiocytosis presenting as infection-associated hemophagocytic syndrome in individuals with familial immunodeficiencies.

Malignant lymphoma with benign erythrophagocytosis

Malignant lymphoma with benign erythrophagocytosis refers to a condition in which lymphoma is associated with a reactive hemophagocytic disorder.[208,209] T-cell lymphomas and less often other lymphomas may induce a marked hyperplasia of cytologically benign hemophagocytosing histiocytes.[209,210] Malignant lymphoma with benign erythrophagocytosis may present in two different ways. In the first presentation, patients with known (usually disseminated) lymphoma develop a syndrome mimicking infection-associated hemophagocytic syndrome.[209,210] Most patients do not also have a systemic infection, although in one study approximately 20% of such patients had active infections, predominantly of viral origin.[211] Morphologically, the lymph node sinuses are filled with abundant cytologically benign histiocytes that show erythrophagocytosis as well as phagocytosis of leukocytes and platelets.[209,210] Malignant lymphoma cells are found at anatomic sites without the histiocytic proliferation. The occurrence of erythrophagocytosis is usually a terminal event in a patient with advanced-stage lymphoma.[211] In the second clinical presentation, the hemophagocytic syndrome occurs in the absence of any previously diagnosed cancer and usually prompts a search for a malignant tumor.[208] In this setting, benign hemophagocytizing histiocytes are intimately interspersed with lymphoma cells. Paraffin and frozen section immunophenotyping studies usually demonstrate a T-cell lineage. The prognosis is extremely poor in most patients.

Malignant lymphoma with benign erythrophagocytosis may be confused with infection-associated hemophagocytic syndrome.[209,211] Identification of the lymphoma cells distinguishes the malignant tumor from infection-associated hemophagocytic syndrome. Also, the lymphomas are usually not associated with a systemic infection, as is infection-associated hemophagocytic syndrome. Biopsies of other organs may be needed for cases in which this distinction may be difficult.

Sinus histiocytosis with massive lymphadenopathy

Sinus histiocytosis with massive lymphadenopathy (Rosai-Dorfman disease) is a rare idiopathic disease of proliferating histiocytes.[212,213] The disorder is most commonly seen in children, but the disease affects all age groups.[214] Approximately 90% of patients present with massive bilateral and painless cervical lymphadenopathy. Axillary, inguinal, para-aortic, and mediastinal lymph nodes may also be involved, with or without concomitant cervical disease. Solitary lymph node involvement is unusual. Extranodal sites are involved in approximately 40% of cases.[214–216] Constitutional symptoms are common, but hepatosplenomegaly is rare. Most afflicted patients undergo spontaneous remission, with disease manifestations gradually subsiding over several months to years.[214,217] Sinus histiocytosis with massive lymphadenopathy may cause or significantly contribute to death in a small number of patients.[214,217]

The lymph nodes are markedly enlarged and often matted together; the cut surface is a dull yellow-white. Microscopically, one

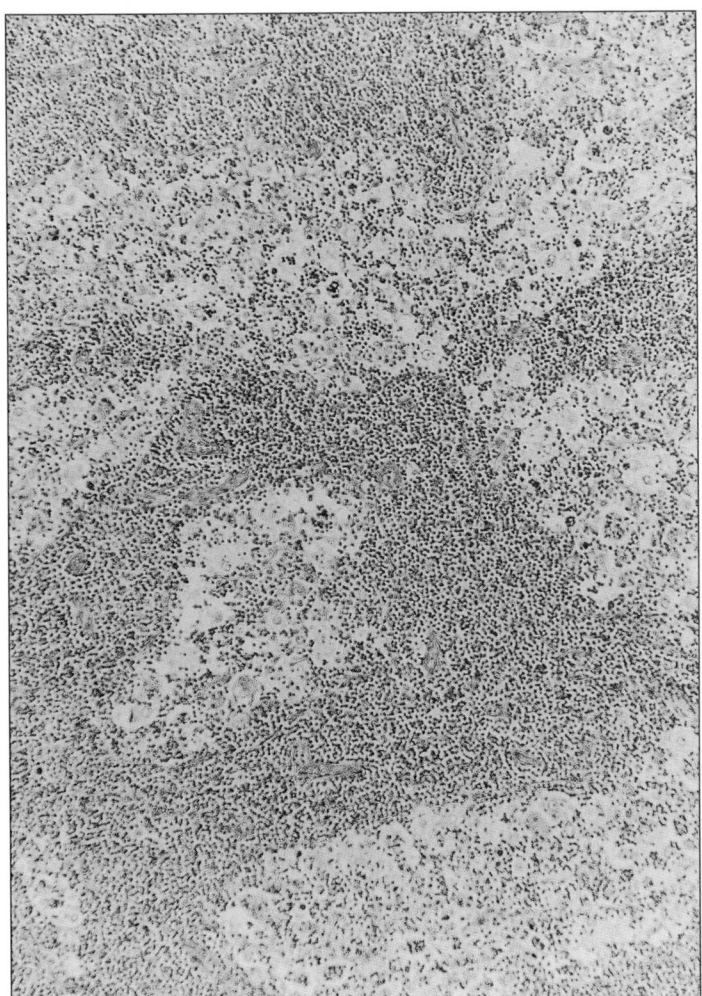

Fig. 11.23 Sinus histiocytosis with massive lymphadenopathy. An exquisitely sinusoidal pattern is seen at low magnification.

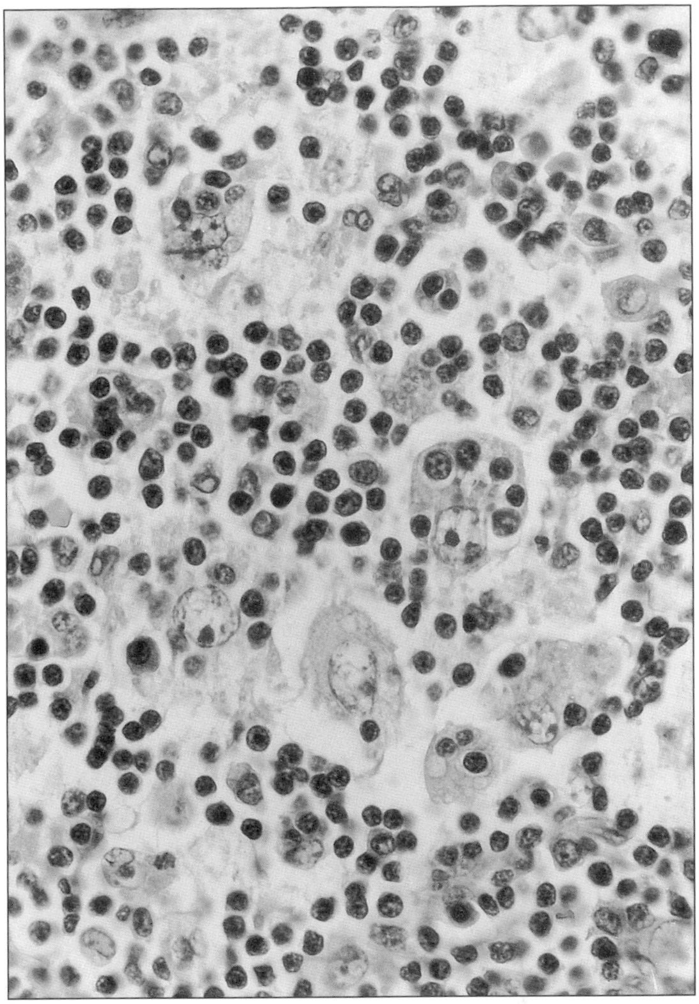

Fig. 11.24 Sinus histiocytosis with massive lymphadenopathy. Histiocytic cells with a vesicular nucleus and abundant cytoplasm exhibiting lymphophagocytosis is characteristic of this disease.

sees extensive fibrosis limited to the capsule. The normal lymph node architecture is partially or completely effaced due to massively dilated sinuses, which are filled with numerous characteristic histiocytes (Fig. 11.23). The nuclei of these unique histiocytes are intermediately sized, have a vesicular chromatin pattern, and contain one to several nucleoli (Fig. 11.24). The nuclear membranes are well delineated and delicate. Cytologic atypia is unusual. The cytoplasm is abundant, amphophilic in H&E stains, and contains intact lymphocytes (termed *lymphophagocytosis* or *emperipolesis*). Less often, the histiocytes may phagocytose plasma cells, neutrophils, or red blood cells. Plasma cells are easily found in the sinuses and intrasinusal tissues. Eosinophils are not seen.

Ultrastructurally, the proliferating histiocytes contain lipid vacuoles, numerous complex filopodia, and varying numbers of lysosomes, and lack Birbeck granules. Immunohistochemical studies show that the cells express S-100 protein and other markers associated with macrophages.[218] The cells do not express the CD1 antigen found on Langerhans cells, and also lack expression of R4/23, a monoclonal antibody with high specificity for follicular dendritic cells.[219–221] Molecular studies show a germline configuration for both the immunoglobulin heavy chain gene and the beta-T cell receptor gene.[221] Some investigators have detected late-phase HHV-6 antigens, suggesting possible pathogenetic involvement of HHV-6 in some cases of Rosai-Dorfman disease.[222]

The differential diagnosis includes reactive sinus histiocytosis and Langerhans cell histiocytosis (histiocytosis X), both of which may have low-power appearances similar to sinus histiocytosis with massive lymphadenopathy. However, the sinuses are far more distended than in the former two disorders. Also, the histiocytes of reactive sinus histiocytosis differ cytologically from the characteristic cells of sinus histiocytosis with massive lymphadenopathy and do not uniformly express S-100 protein. Likewise, the cytologic characteristics of Langerhans cells and the presence of eosinophils help to separate Langerhans cell histiocytosis from sinus histiocytosis with massive lymphadenopathy. CD1 expression, the presence of Birbeck granules, and lack of emperipolesis in Langerhans cell histiocytosis also help differentiate Langerhans cell histiocytosis from sinus histiocytosis with massive lymphadenopathy. The differential diagnosis of sinus histiocytosis with massive lymphadenopathy in a lymph node also includes sinusoidal involvement by metastatic carcinoma, malignant melanoma, and sinusoidal malignant lymphoma. Careful attention to the cytologic features of the proliferating cells and differing immunohistochemical profiles will distinguish sinus histiocytosis with massive lymphadenopathy from the malignant tumors. Rarely, patients with sinus histiocytosis with massive lymphadenopathy also have malignant lymphoma, usually involving anatomic sites different from those involved by sinus histiocytosis with massive lymphadenopathy.[223]

Whipple's disease

Whipple's disease is a bacterial infection involving the small intestine caused by *Tropheryma whipplei*.[224] Typically, Whipple's disease is seen in adult men who have symptoms of malabsorption.[225] Regional lymph nodes are frequently involved and peripheral lymphadenopathy may be seen in approximately one-half of cases. Microscopically, the lymph node sinuses are dilated and filled with enlarged histiocytes and large round empty spaces. The cytoplasm of the histiocytes contains copious amounts of diastase-resistant PAS-positive rod-shaped forms that correspond to the causative bacillus.[225–227] The vacuoles are formed by loss of lipid materials during tissue processing. These features are similar to lymphadenopathy due to the deposition of exogenous lipid substances. *Mycobacterium avium-intracellulare* infection of the lymph node, which may be seen in patients with AIDS, may be mistaken for Whipple's disease involving the lymph node, because the histiocytes of both entities contain PAS-positive material. An acid-fast stain reveals that histiocytes are stuffed with acid-fast bacilli in the mycobacterial infection, allowing easy distinction from Whipple's disease, which is acid-fast negative.

Lymphadenopathy due to deposition of exogenous lipids

Exogenous lipid substances may be deposited in lymph nodes and be responsible for lymphadenopathy in several settings, including lymphangiography dye and silicone, polyvinylpyrrolidone, and prosthetic materials. Lymphangiography dye contains an oily base that reaches the lymph nodes via the lymphatics. The material collects in the sinuses, and a foreign body giant cell reaction ensues.[228] During routine tissue processing, the injected medium dissolves, leaving behind sinuses with large empty vacuoles up to 100 μm in diameter. Silicone lymphadenopathy usually involves lymph nodes draining the site of silicone implants, usually from breast or joints. The histologic findings resemble lymphangiography changes, but since the process has usually been around for a longer period, there are usually more foamy histiocytes (Fig. 11.25).[229] Silicone is usually not completely removed during processing, so that refractile, nonbirefringent material can often be demonstrated in the spaces.

The deposition of exogenous lipids in lymph nodes must be distinguished from endogenous lipid deposition. *Lipogranulomatosis* refers to the reaction in lymph node (or spleen) to any lipid material arising from such endogenous sources as hematomas, tumors, cholesterol deposits, xanthomatous lesions, fat embolism, and fat necrosis.[230] Lymph nodes in the porta hepatis and celiac axis are most frequently involved. The lipid accumulation manifests as vacuolization of sinus histiocytes, eventually with the formation of small lipid granulomas with multinucleated giant cells. The vacuoles are much smaller than those seen with lymphangiography effect or silicone.

BENIGN LYMPHADENOPATHY WITH PROMINENT NECROSIS

Any benign lymphadenopathy or lymphadenitis may have focal areas of necrosis, including both primary follicular or paracortical hyperplasias.[231] However, in some diseases, extensive necrosis is the

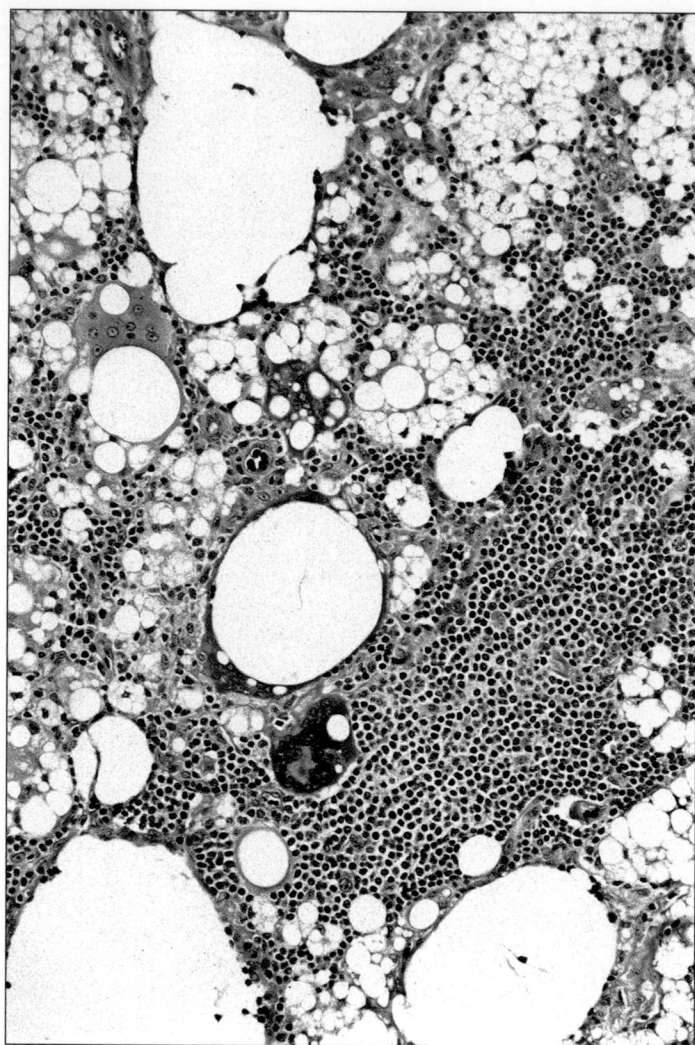

Fig. 11.25 Silicone lymphadenopathy. There are large spaces lined by attenuated foreign body giant cells and numerous foamy macrophages.

primary or most characteristic finding. The lymph node necrosis may be complete or subtotal.

Complete lymph node necrosis

Complete lymph node necrosis is seen within two main settings. In the first, there is liquefactive necrosis, consisting of karyorrhectic debris and fragments of neutrophils, often with abscess formation.[231] This is more commonly seen at autopsy than in surgical specimens, but may be seen in the setting of AIDS, either due to fungi such as histoplasmosis or a wide variety of bacteria.

In the second type of complete necrosis, coagulative necrosis is seen as a result of vascular compromise (Fig. 11.26). The areas of necrosis often show ghosts of lymphoid cells and generally lack inflammatory cells. The rim of the lymph node may be partially viable, whereas the perinodal soft tissue usually contains granulation tissue, and there may be venous thrombosis. The most important cause of coagulative necrosis is malignant lymphoma, usually a non-Hodgkin's lymphoma of diffuse large cell type.[232] Occasionally, the lymphoma may be identified in a rim of viable lymph node parenchyma. More often, immunostains will identify a diffuse infiltrate of ghosts of B cells in the infarcted area, as the membrane antigens remain viable

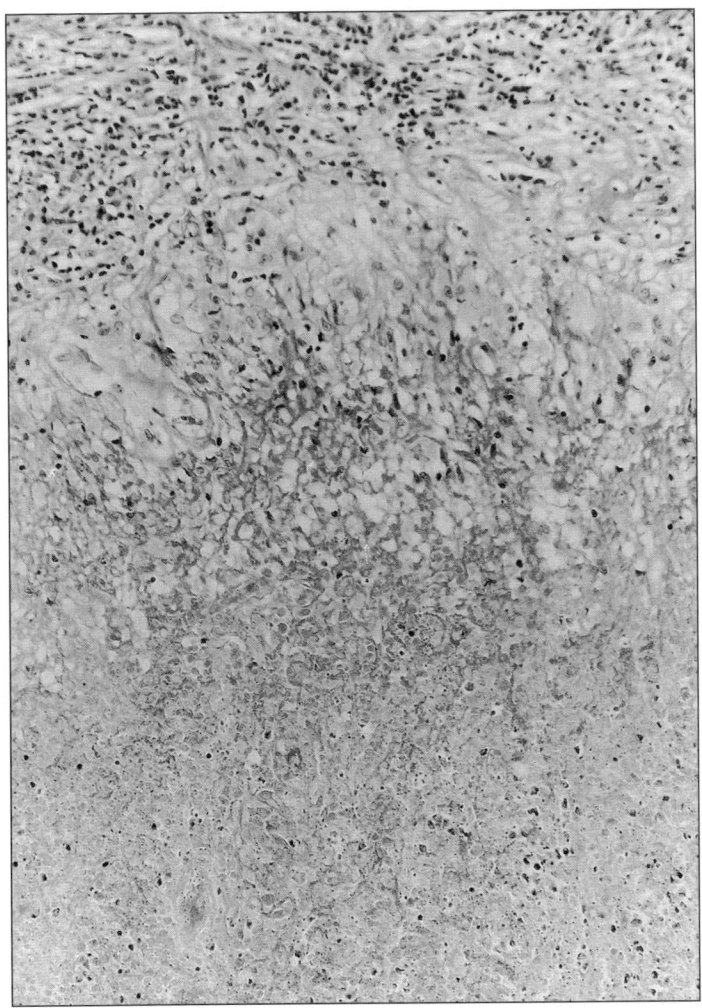

Fig. 11.26 Complete lymph node infarction. The infarcted area is rimmed by granulation tissue.

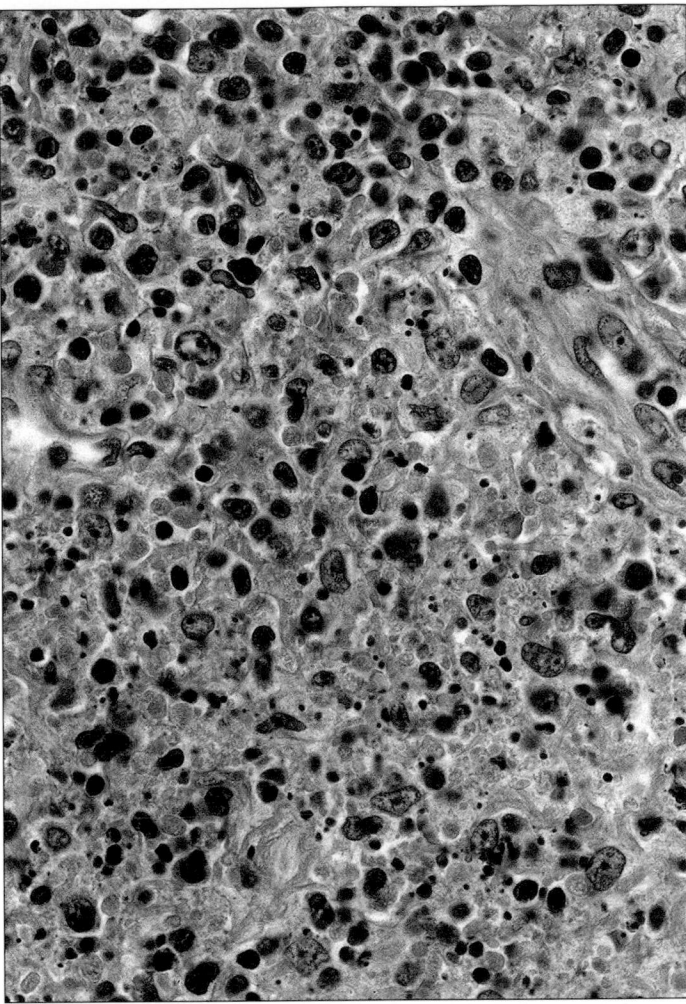

Fig. 11.27 Kikuchi's histiocytic necrotizing lymphadenitis. There is abundant necrosis with karyorrhectic debris and histiocytes with twisted nuclei.

for a time after the cells have histologically undergone complete necrosis.[233] Rebiopsy, either immediately or within 6 months, will often reveal more definitive evidence of malignant lymphoma.

Kikuchi histiocytic necrotizing lymphadenitis

Histiocytic necrotizing lymphadenitis (of Kikuchi and Fujimoto) is a self-limiting, well-defined clinicopathologic disorder of unknown etiology that most commonly affects young Asian women, although both sexes and all ages and ethnic groups may be afflicted.[234–237] Patients usually present with isolated cervical or posterior cervical lymphadenopathy, which may be tender to palpation. Lymphadenopathy of several months' duration is the only symptom in most patients. However, reported symptomatology may also include a mild fever associated with upper respiratory symptoms and constitutional symptoms. The prognosis for the large majority of patients with histiocytic necrotizing lymphadenitis is excellent, with spontaneous resolution of the disease usually occurring within 1 to 4 months.

Microscopically, the lymph node architecture is only partially effaced, and the uninvolved lymphoid tissue is usually normal, with dormant nonhyperplastic follicles.[238] Scattered throughout the paracortex, and less often the cortex, are discrete foci of large deposits of eosinophilic amorphous material, abundant karyorrhectic debris, and viable cells (Fig. 11.27). The latter consist of histiocytes that exhibit phagocytosis and occasionally contain foamy cytoplasm, reactive immunoblasts, and plasmacytoid monocytes. The absence of intact neutrophils, plasma cells, and eosinophils in the areas of extensive necrosis is a very useful diagnostic feature. Immediately adjacent to the well-circumscribed necrotic areas, one generally sees a proliferation of reactive immunoblasts. The sinuses may be focally distended by monocytoid B lymphocytes, but this is not a usual finding. The lymph node capsule may be thickened adjacent to the necrotic foci.

Immunohistochemical studies show a predominance of T cells and macrophages within involved areas of the lymph node. In lesions detected and biopsied early, helper/inducer T cells may predominate, whereas the majority of biopsies taken late after presentation appear to contain cytotoxic/suppressor T cells. There is some evidence that the karyorrhectic debris may be derived from T-lineage-associated plasmacytoid cells.[239] Other authors have detected myeloperoxidase expression in the nonphagocytosing mononuclear cells and phagocytosing histiocytes of Kikuchi lymphadenitis, an observation not made in non-necrotizing lymphadenitidies or accessory cell neoplasms.[240] Molecular studies show no monoclonal T-cell populations.[241] The etiology of this disease is not yet known, but investigators have hypothesized a role for HHV-6, as well as KSHV/HHV-8, even in the absence of HIV infection or other immunosuppression.[242]

Eliciting the characteristic clinical history of histiocytic necrotizing lymphadenitis is extremely useful in distinguishing it from non-Hodgkin's lymphoma.[238] The abundant karyorrhectic debris and sheets of macrophages seen in histiocytic necrotizing lymphadenitis may impart a superficial appearance of a high-grade lymphoma. However, one must keep in mind that the only lymphomas to have a large amount of karyorrhexis are Burkitt-type and large cell immunoblastic lymphoma. The monotonous and malignant cells of these lymphomas are not present in lymph nodes with histiocytic necrotizing lymphadenitis. In node-based non-Hodgkin's lymphoma, the infarcted areas are generally rimmed by granulation tissue and may contain the 'ghosts' of the malignant cells. The differential diagnosis of histiocytic necrotizing lymphadenitis also includes Hodgkin's disease and lymph nodes with manifestations of infectious agents such as *Yersinia* enterocolitis or the cat-scratch organism, because they all are associated with stellate areas of necrosis (stellate microabscesses). In the latter entities, the presence of neutrophils in and around the necrotic foci allow easy separation from histiocytic necrotizing lymphadenitis. The differentiation of histiocytic necrotizing lymphadenitis from systemic lupus erythematosus and Kawasaki disease is discussed below.

Systemic lupus erythematosus lymphadenopathy

Lymph nodes involved by systemic lupus erythematosus share morphologic features with lymph nodes involved by histiocytic necrotizing lymphadenitis, particularly the presence of discrete necrotic foci and eosinophilic deposits.[243] Histologic features that favor systemic lupus erythematosus are the presence of basophilic necrotic material that is often deposited in vessel walls and sometimes forms hematoxyphilic bodies, and the presence of more than occasional plasma cells. However, distinguishing between histiocytic necrotizing lymphadenitis and lupus may be impossible on a purely morphologic basis, so clinical investigation should be undertaken. Some investigators hypothesize that histiocytic necrotizing lymphadenitis represents a self-limited autoimmune condition resembling systemic lupus erythematosus.

Kawasaki disease lymphadenopathy

Kawasaki disease (mucocutaneous lymph node syndrome) is an acute febrile disease of uncertain etiology, usually occurring in young children.[244,245] Five of the following six clinical criteria must be present to establish the diagnosis: fever, congestion of the conjunctiva, oral mucous membrane lesions, distal extremity lesions, polymorphous exanthem, and acute cervical adenopathy. The disease may be life threatening when coronary arteritis is present. Lymph node biopsies from patients with Kawasaki disease show necrotizing lesions, with fibrin, karyorrhectic debris, and neutrophils in association with the areas of necrosis (Fig. 11.28).[246] In addition, fibrin thrombi in small vessels is usually a prominent feature, and an arteritis with fibrinoid necrosis may be present. Fibrin thrombi may also occur in thrombocytopenic purpura and rickettsial infection. Histiocytic necrotizing lymphadenitis may have fibrin thrombi, but they are not usually a prominent feature; the presence of neutrophils should also suggest Kawasaki disease. Rare cases of malignant lymphoma following Kawasaki disease have been reported.[247]

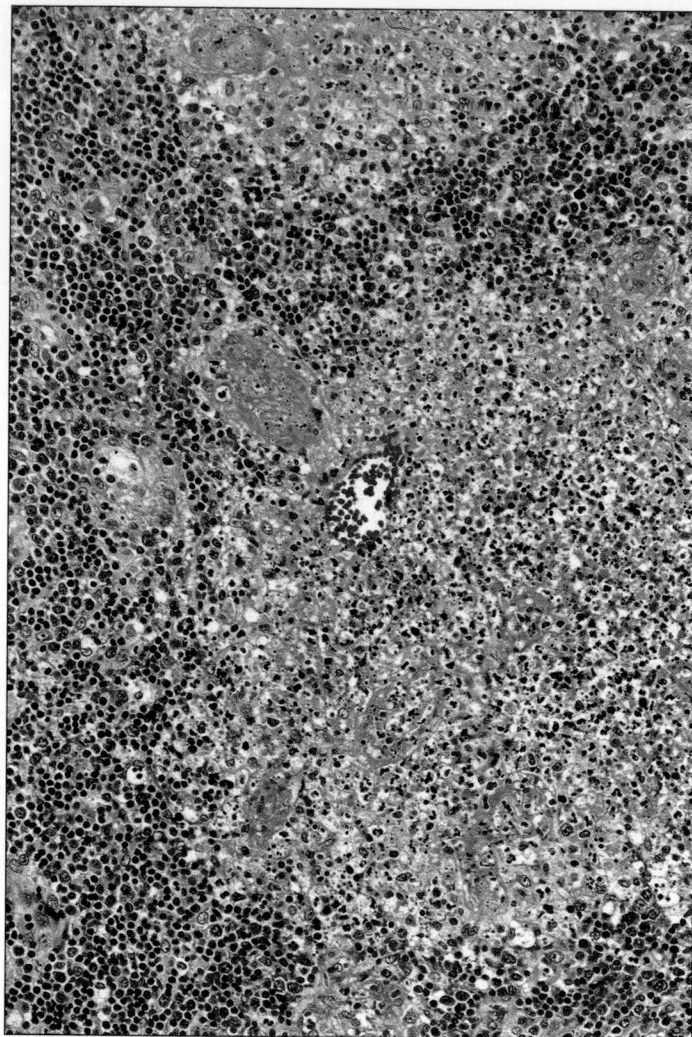

Fig. 11.28 Kawasaki disease. There are numerous fibrin thrombi in small vessels in and adjacent to areas of necrosis.

GRANULOMATOUS DISORDERS

Noninfectious granulomatous lymphadenopathy

Granulomatous lymphadenopathy may be noninfectious or infectious. Noninfectious causes of granulomatous lymphadenopathy include berylliosis, Hodgkin's disease, non-Hodgkin's lymphomas, lymph nodes draining neoplasms, lymph nodes draining Crohn's disease, and sarcoidosis.[248,249] Granulomas may be found in the lymph nodes of Hodgkin's disease and non-Hodgkin's lymphoma under two circumstances. First, they may be seen in conjunction with involvement of the lymph node by neoplasm. In Hodgkin's disease, the granulomas may be so numerous as to easily obscure the Reed-Sternberg cells and variants. The phenomenon is less common in non-Hodgkin's lymphomas, but has been reported in a variety of types, including Burkitt's lymphoma.[250] Similar to Hodgkin's disease, some cases have such an exuberant granulomatous response that the lymphoma may be obscured.[251] Second, noncaseating granulomas may be seen in uninvolved lymph nodes in patients with Hodgkin's disease, non-Hodgkin's lymphomas, as well as carcinoma and other neoplasms. In Hodgkin's disease, the presence of noncaseating granulomas may be associated with a slightly better prognosis within a given stage.[252]

Sarcoidosis is a systemic disease of unknown etiology that affects adults most commonly between the ages of 20 and 40 years.[248] The male/female ratio is 2:1 and blacks are affected approximately 10 times more frequently than whites. Multiorgan involvement is the rule, particularly lymph nodes, lungs, eyes, and skin. Mediastinal and hilar lymph nodes are most frequently involved, but there may be generalized lymphadenopathy. The lymph node architecture is partially or wholly replaced by well-formed noncaseating granulomas. The granulomas contain numerous epithelioid histiocytes, Langerhans-type multinucleated giant cells, and scattered lymphocytes. Occasional granulomas may show central foci of fibrinoid necrosis, but foci of classic caseating necrosis should be absent. Birefringent crystals (3–10 μm) of calcium oxalate are common and should not be mistaken for foreign body material. In addition, Schaumann bodies (large concentrically laminated basophilic bodies consisting of protein containing calcium carbonate and iron), asteroid bodies (acidophilic star-shaped inclusions), and Hamazaki-Wesenberg bodies (PAS-positive intracellular and extracellular inclusions that represent giant lysosomes) may also be present, but have no diagnostic significance. Supporting laboratory data such as a positive skin test (Kveim test) and an elevated serum angiotensin-converting enzyme level may support the diagnosis, but are not specific to sarcoidosis. Despite long-standing intensive research, the etiology of sarcoidosis is still not known. However, researchers hypothesize that the etiology of systemic sarcoidosis is linked to a genetically determined enhanced T-helper type immune response to a limited number of microbial pathogens.[253]

The differential diagnosis of sarcoidosis includes infectious granulomatous lymphadenitis as well as all of the other causes of noninfectious granulomatous lymphadenitis. Special stains for organisms are generally not of use unless some necrosis is present. However, appropriate cultures for acid-fast, fungal, and bacterial organisms should be performed on any case in which an infectious etiology is being considered.

Infectious granulomatous lymphadenitis

Two types of infectious granulomatous lymphadenitis have been recently delineated. In the classic type (as exemplified by tuberculosis), nonsuppurative, hypersensitivity-type granulomas are found.[254] Immunohistochemical studies demonstrate a predominance of histiocytes with lesser numbers of T cells and dendritic cells. Small, round mantle B cells are found at the periphery of the granulomas, but no B cells are present within the granulomas. In the second type (as exemplified by cat-scratch disease), suppurative granulomas containing numerous neutrophils and monocytoid B cells are found.[255] Immunohistochemical studies also demonstrate a predominance of histiocytes, but show variable numbers of B cells either at the periphery or in the center of suppurative granulomas in addition to T cells and dendritic cells. It has been suggested that the monocytoid B cells are recruited by the development of a T-cell-independent, macrophage-mediated immune response against antigens. Furthermore, the monocytoid B cells may have a role in the recruitment of neutrophils and in the development of the necrosis. Alternatively, the presence of aggregates of monocytoid B cells may be the primary event, followed by necrosis and infiltration by neutrophils, followed finally by the formation of granulomatous inflammation at the periphery.

Tuberculosis, once thought to be under control, has undergone a dramatic resurgence in the number of cases, due to complacency and the growing number of drug-resistant strains. Involvement of lymph nodes is usually accompanied by pulmonary involvement, but lymphadenopathy, usually cervical, accounts for about 40% of nonrespiratory infections. Tuberculous lymphadenopathy may be histologically indistinguishable from sarcoidosis, although the former usually contains caseating granulomas or areas of caseation with a rim of granulomatous reaction. When necrosis is prominent, there is sometimes a draining sinus to the skin. Organisms are most easily demonstrated by PCR or appropriate culture. When organisms are demonstrable by acid-fast stains, it is usually in the necrotic areas.

Atypical mycobacterial infections are an even more common cause of isolated granulomatous lymphadenitis than tuberculosis. Again, cervical lymph nodes are most commonly involved. The histologic changes may be similar to tuberculosis or may show less granulomatous changes and a greater degree of acute inflammation with abscess formation.[256] In immunocompromised patients such as AIDS patients, different features may be seen. There is often foamy histiocytic infiltration beginning in the superficial paracortex and extending to involve the entire parenchyma. An acid-fast stain reveals tremendous numbers of acid-fast bacilli in the histiocytes. Alternatively, there may be a more spindled proliferation of fibroblasts and histiocytes mimicking inflammatory pseudotumor.[87] Special stains demonstrate the presence of numerous bacilli within the spindled histiocytes.

A variety of histologic appearances may also be seen in *lepromatous lymphadenitis*, depending on the status of the patient's immunity. In patients with relatively intact cellular immunity, the tuberculoid form of leprosy is seen. Generally, lymph nodes are uninvolved by leprosy but may be enlarged due to reactive paracortical hyperplasia. In patients with borderline leprosy, numerous noncaseating granulomas are found in the paracortex; acid-fast organisms may or may not be identified by Fite stains. In patients with defective cellular immunity, the lepromatous form of leprosy is seen. In this form, generalized lymphadenopathy is often present. There are numerous foamy macrophages containing numerous organisms present in the paracortical areas, and there may also be reactive follicular hyperplasia with abundant plasma cells. The macrophages may coalesce into syncytial clumps and giant cells may be seen, but true granulomas are not present.

Fungal infections seldom present initially in lymph nodes but rather usually involve lymph nodes as part of a systemic fungal infection. A wide variety of fungi may cause lymphadenitis, but histoplasmosis most commonly causes isolated lymphadenitis. Histologically, a granulomatous reaction is usually seen, although one may also see acute inflammation with abscess formation. Organisms are most easily demonstrated by appropriate fungal cultures although fungal organisms may often be demonstrated by PAS, Gridley, or Grocott-methenamine-silver stains.

Pneumocystis carinii is a protozoal organism that is seen most commonly in patients with AIDS. Lymph nodes are rarely involved, but cases of lymphadenitis with granulomatous lesions containing the organism have been reported.[257]

Cat-scratch lymphadenitis is the most common cause of suppurative granulomas in lymph nodes.[258] It is a benign infectious illness caused by a bacterium introduced through the skin following a scratch by a cat or, less commonly, by a dog. A skin lesion may or may not be present. This is followed in several weeks by regional lymphadenopathy, usually in the axillary, inguinal, or cervical regions. The disease usually affects children and young adults, with an equal male/female ratio. It has been demonstrated that cat-scratch disease is caused by *Bartonella henselae* (formerly known as *Rochalimaea henselae*).[259]

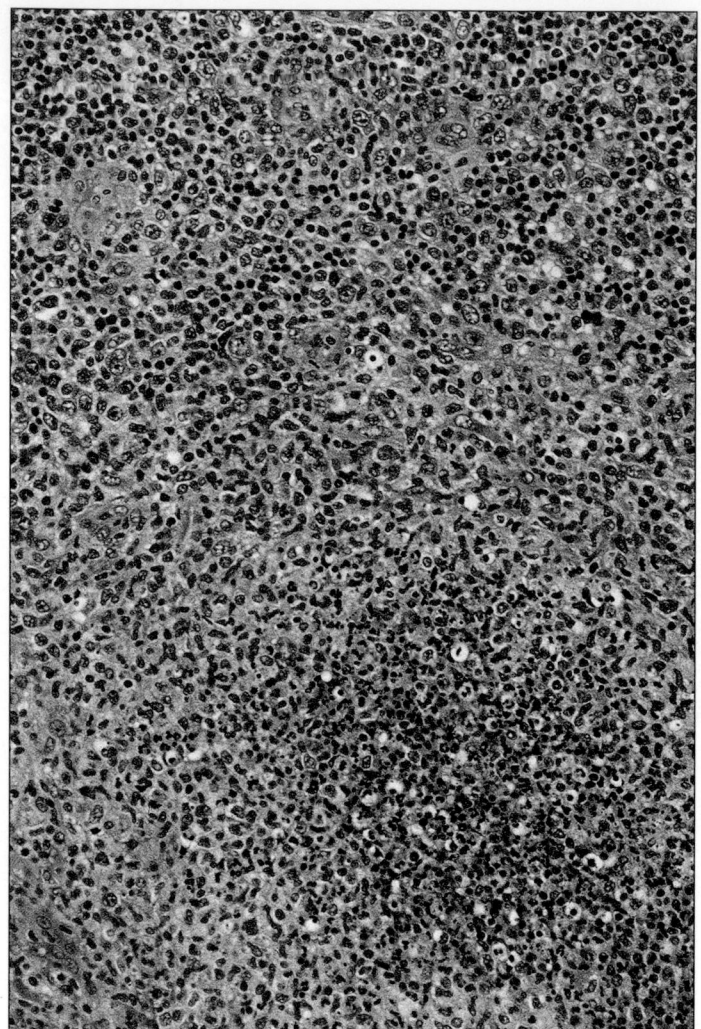

Fig. 11.29 Cat-scratch disease. A suppurative granuloma is seen.

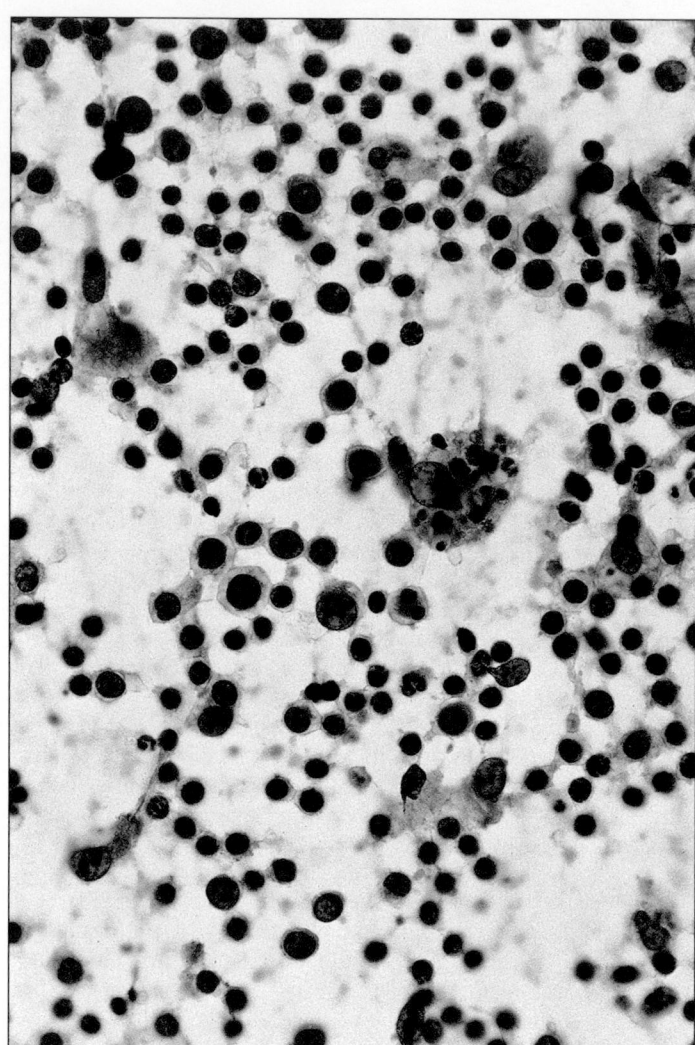

Fig. 11.30 Cat-scratch disease, fine needle aspiration. A mixture of lymphoid cells, with scattered tingible body macrophages and neutrophils, is seen.

Lymph nodes of cat-scratch disease initially show florid reactive follicular hyperplasia with a monocytoid B-cell proliferation in the sinuses and paracortical areas.[260] Subsequently, there are small suppurative granulomas located adjacent to or within the monocytoid B cells composed of histiocytes with central aggregates of neutrophils (Figs. 11.29 and 11.30). In the final stages, there are discrete stellate microabscesses composed of neutrophils and necrotic or fibrinoid material, with a rim of palisading epithelioid histiocytes. Langerhans-type giant cells are generally not frequent, but numerous mature plasma cells and occasional immunoblasts may be present at the periphery of some of the granulomas and in the paracortical areas. The lymph node capsule is often fibrotic or acutely inflamed.

In cat-scratch disease, Warthin-Starry silver impregnation stain performed at a pH of 3.8 to 4.0 may show delicate pleomorphic bacilli; the Gram stain is usually negative.[261] The bacilli are commonly observed in the walls of capillaries, in macrophages lining sinuses or near germinal centers, and in areas of necrosis; they may occur singly, in chains, or in clumps. The *Chlamydia* of lymphogranuloma venereum are not highlighted by the Warthin-Starry stain. Detection

of antibodies to *B. henselae* and amplification of *B. henselae* DNA in affected tissue specimens are useful in the diagnosis and therapeutic evaluation of cat-scratch disease.[262–265]

The differential diagnosis of cat-scratch disease includes the other bacterial causes of suppurative granulomatous lymphadenitis discussed below as well as some of the fungal and mycobacterial organisms discussed previously. The clinical setting can usually differentiate among the different infectious possibilities. In questionable cases, an indirect fluorescent-antibody test is available and serology, culture, and PCR tests may also be used to specifically identify the organism. The differential diagnosis also includes causes of nonsuppurative granulomatous lymphadenitis; these can be distinguished histologically by the absence of stellate microabscesses or large numbers of B cells (including monocytoid B cells) and the more frequent occurrence of Langhans giant cells in the latter. Hodgkin's disease, in particular the syncytial variant of nodular sclerosing type, may also be difficult to distinguish from cat-scratch disease. Close examination of the cells at the edge of the necrosis will disclose numerous Reed-Sternberg cells and variants in this type of Hodgkin's disease.

Lymphogranuloma venereum is a sexually transmitted disease caused by *Chlamydia*.[266] It almost always affects inguinal lymph nodes. Because this lesion often presents at a later stage, there is often more matting of adjacent nodes than typically seen in cat-scratch disease. Histologically, the changes are very similar to that seen in cat-scratch disease. However, early lesions are less often seen, and at the time of biopsy there are usually multiple stellate abscesses within the nodal parenchyma, sometimes with coalescence and often with extension outside the fibrotic capsule into the adjacent perinodal soft tissues. Giemsa staining may show inclusion bodies. The diagnosis can be confirmed by serologic testing.

Yersinial lymphadenitis is caused by the bacteria *Yersinia enterocolitica* or *pseudotuberculosis*.[267] It usually occurs in children or young adults who present with symptoms of acute appendicitis. However, laparoscopy reveals a grossly normal appendix, but markedly enlarged mesenteric lymph nodes draining the ileocecal region. Histologically, the lymph nodes initially show florid reactive hyperplasia. Later, there are suppurative granulomas identical to those seen in cat-scratch disease. However, the suppurative granulomas may commonly involve the germinal centers. Gram-negative, acid-fast diplobacilli may be identified in the lesions. Similar changes may be noted in the appendix when it is removed.

ANGIOIMMUNOBLASTIC LYMPHADENOPATHY

The category of abnormal immune responses of lymph nodes includes two closely related entities, angioimmunoblastic lymphadenopathy with dysproteinemia (AILD) and immunoblastic lymphadenopathy (IBL), which were originally described as benign lymphoproliferative disorders occurring in older men (Fig. 11.31).[268–270] The clinical behavior was highly unpredictable, varying from some patients having an indolent course and others having a rapidly progressive one. Response to therapy, including chemotherapy and steroids, was also unpredictable. Many patients succumbed to severe infections. The presence of clonal T-cell receptor gene rearrangements and clonal cytogenetic abnormalities, as well as evolution to malignant lymphoma in a high number of cases, led to the belief that those AILD-IBL cases were most likely lymphomas at the onset rather than abnormal immune reactions.[271–275] This is discussed in greater detail in the section on AILD-like T-cell lymphomas.

CLASSICAL HODGKIN'S DISEASE

Hodgkin's disease is a neoplastic proliferation of Reed-Sternberg cells and variants (Hodgkin cells). Lukes and Butler recognized six categories of Hodgkin's disease, including nodular and diffuse lymphocytic and histiocytic (L&H), nodular sclerosis, mixed cellularity, diffuse fibrosis, and reticular.[276] In the subsequent 1996 Rye modification, the categories of nodular and diffuse L&H were combined into a new category of lymphocyte predominance, whereas diffuse fibrosis and reticular were combined into lymphocyte depletion.[277] The nodular lymphocyte predominance form of Hodgkin's disease was subsequently found to represent a distinct clinicopathological entity separate from the other categories of Hodgkin's disease.[278–280] Thus, in the 2001 World Health Organization (WHO) Classification, *nodular lymphocyte predominance Hodgkin's disease* was placed in a separate category and the other categories were lumped into a new category of *classical Hodgkin's disease*. The other forms of lymphocyte predominance are in the category of

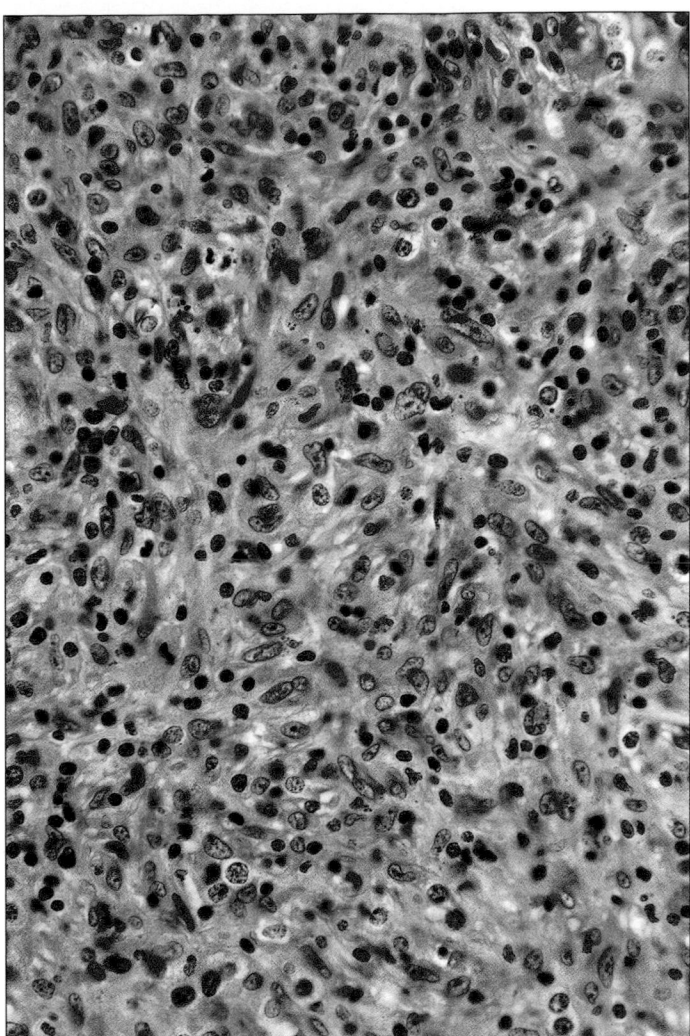

Fig. 11.31 Angioimmunoblastic lymphadenopathy. There is lymphoid depletion with marked hypervascularity. A mixture of lymphoid cells is seen, without striking atypia.

lymphocyte-rich within the category of classical Hodgkin's disease. Although the WHO Classification advocates the term *Hodgkin lymphoma*, the authors retain the old-fashioned term of '*Hodgkin's disease*' in this chapter and in daily use.

Hodgkin's disease accounts for about 15% of all cases of malignant lymphoma, with about 8000 new cases per year.[281] Classical Hodgkin's disease accounts for approximately 95% of new Hodgkin's disease cases. The overall male/female ratio is 1.5:1, although the male predominance is not seen in cases of nodular sclerosis.[282] In the United States, there is a peak of incidence in young adults with a second slow rise of incidence in older adults.[283] About 40% to 50% of cases have been associated with EBV in the neoplastic cells, although a clear etiologic role has not yet been identified.[284,285] Cases of mixed cellularity and lymphocyte depletion, particularly occurring in children or older adults, are most likely to be associated with EBV. Antecedent infectious mononucleosis has been identified as a statistically significant event in predisposition to Hodgkin's disease.[286] There may be a genetic component to Hodgkin's disease, particularly in cases of nodular sclerosis occurring in young adulthood.[287] Some other environmental/genetic factors that have been implicated include

Table 11.7 The Cotswolds staging classification of Hodgkin's disease

Classification	Description
Stage I	Involvement of a single lymph node region or lymphoid structure
Stage II	Involvement of two or more lymph node regions on the same side of the diaphragm (the mediastinum is considered a single site, whereas hilar lymph nodes are considered bilaterally)
Stage III	Involvement of lymph node regions or structures on both sides of the diaphragm
Stage III-1	With or without involvement of splenic hilar, celiac, or portal nodes
Stage III-2	With involvement of para-aortic, iliac, and mesenteric nodes
Stage IV	Involvement of one or more extranodal sites in addition to a site for which the designation 'E' has been used
Designations applicable to any disease stage:	
A	No symptoms
B	Fever (temperature >38°C), drenching night sweats, unexplained loss of >10% of body weight within the preceding 6 months
X	Bulky disease (a widening of the mediastinum by more than one-third or the presence of a nodal mass with a maximal dimension >10 cm)
E	Involvement of a single extranodal site that is contiguous or proximal to the known nodal site
CS	Clinical stage
PS	Pathologic stage (as determined by laparotomy)

Data from Lister et al.[295,296]

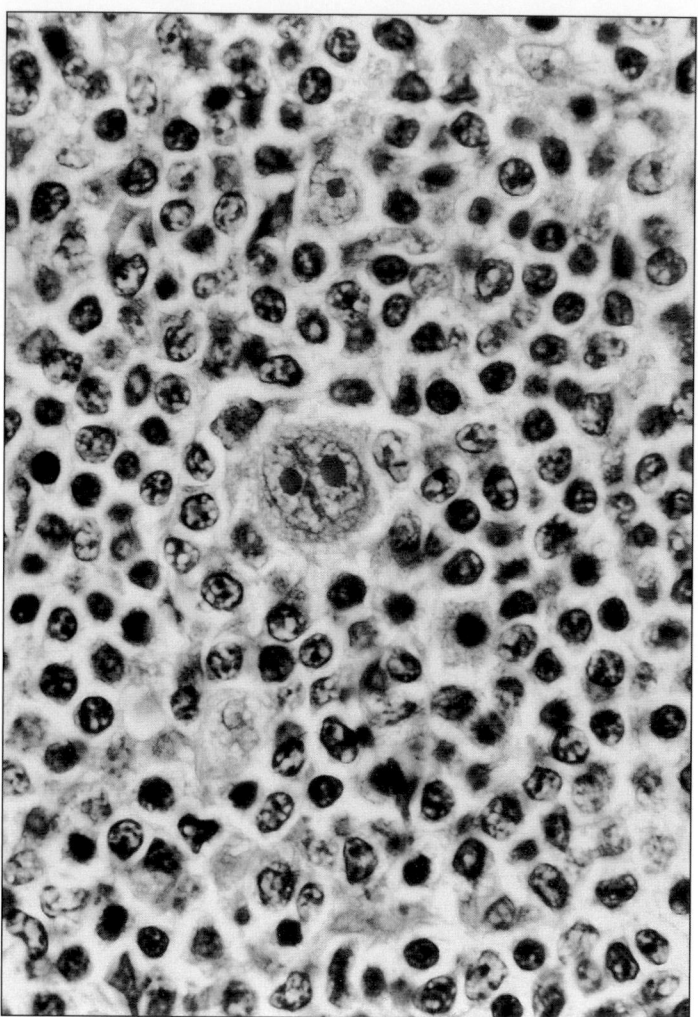

Fig. 11.32 Hodgkin's disease. A so-called diagnostic Reed-Sternberg cell is present.

higher social class, employment in wood-related industries, and certain HLA types.[288–292]

Patients with Hodgkin's disease usually present with slowly growing, enlarged lymph nodes, most often in the cervical or axillary regions, or a mediastinal mass.[293] Low neck or mediastinal presentations are particularly common in females with nodular sclerosis. About one-quarter of patients have constitutional symptoms (so-called B symptoms), including unexplained fever (>38°C) during the previous months, recurrent drenching night sweats during the previous month, and unexplained weight loss (>10% of body weight) during the previous six months. Pruritus or pain after alcohol ingestion may also occur. Laboratory studies can usually document a deficiency in cellular immunity.

Hodgkin's disease spreads in a predictable fashion, usually from one contiguous lymph node group to another; therefore, staging is generally of great use in determining the optimal treatment.[293,294] The Cotswolds staging classification, a minor modification of the Ann Arbor classification, is outlined in Table 11.7.[295,296] Clinical staging includes history, physical examination, plain chest radiograph, and computed tomography of chest and abdomen.[297] Additional studies that are commonly performed in many institutions include lymphangiography, magnetic resonance imaging, and gallium scanning. Routine pathologic staging procedures include bilateral bone marrow trephine biopsies (and not bone marrow aspirate smears).[298] Staging laparotomy is no longer routinely performed in many institutions due to long-term increase in the risk of acute leukemia and infections,

but still may be performed when detection of disease might alter therapy.[297]

HISTOPATHOLOGIC DIAGNOSIS

The diagnosis of Hodgkin's disease is established by the definitive identification of Reed-Sternberg cells and variants (Hodgkin cells). Their identification is facilitated by recognition of the characteristic cellular milieu in which these cells are usually found. Thus, attention to both the atypical cells as well as the background cells is important to the histologic diagnosis of Hodgkin's disease. Reed and Sternberg described the classic Reed-Sternberg cell as a large cell with multilobed nucleus, often 'owl's-eye' with two mirror-image nuclei, each containing a single large inclusion-like eosinophilic nucleolus; the cytoplasm is abundant and eosinophilic (Fig. 11.32). Mononuclear variants are similar to the classic Reed-Sternberg cells, but have a single nucleus and large eosinophilic nucleoli (Fig. 11.33). Formalin-fixed cases of nodular sclerosis contain many lacunar cells, which are mononuclear cells with abundant clear cytoplasm, and relatively less conspicuous nucleoli (Fig. 11.34). In all types of classical Hodgkin's disease, one can see apoptotic Hodgkin cells ('mummified' cells), with

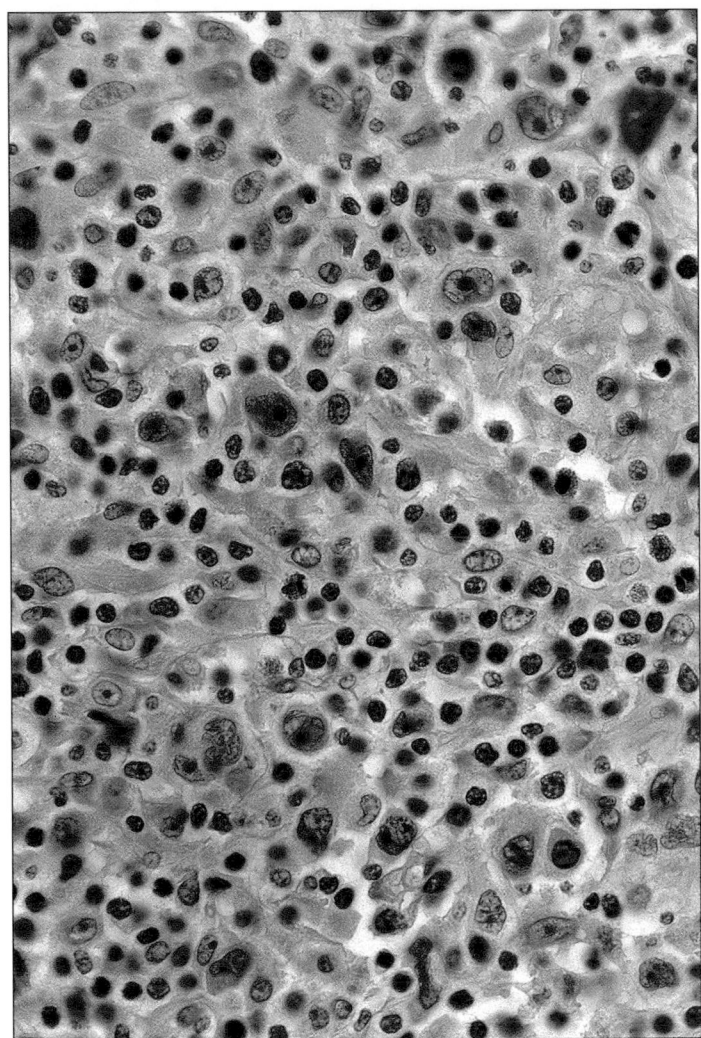

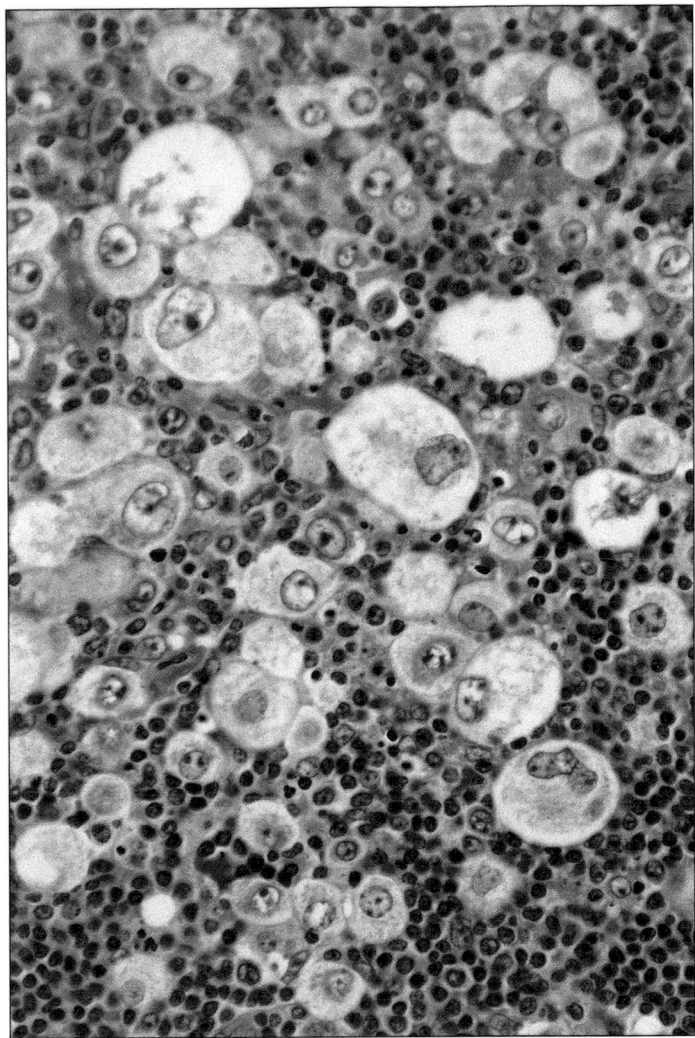

Fig. 11.33 Hodgkin's disease, mixed cellularity type. Several mononuclear Hodgkin cells are present. Note also the background cells, including small round lymphocytes, histiocytes, eosinophils, and plasma cells.

Fig. 11.34 Hodgkin's disease, nodular sclerosing type. Several lacunar cells are seen.

degenerated nuclei and shrunken, highly eosinophilic cytoplasm. Although most hematopathologists require the presence of at least one classic Reed-Sternberg cell to establish a definitive diagnosis of Hodgkin's disease, we disagree and merely require that one is confident in the identification of Hodgkin cells, either by histopathologic examination or by confirmation with immunohistochemical stains. At the time of surgery, touch or scrape preparations may be more useful than the actual frozen section for the recognition of Hodgkin cells.

Hodgkin cells generally comprise <1% of the cellular elements of the involved tissue. The background cells usually consist of varying numbers of small, round lymphocytes, histiocytes, eosinophils, neutrophils, plasma cells, and fibroblasts. Occasional immunoblasts may be present, but a spectrum of lymphoid size and atypia should raise consideration of diagnoses other than Hodgkin's disease. The histiocytes may be epithelioid in appearance, and occasionally well-formed granulomas may be found. On rare occasions, foamy histiocytes may predominate. Eosinophils may vary in number from few to many, with the formation of eosinophilic abscesses. Tissue eosinophilia may be a strong adverse prognostic factor.[299,300] Neutrophils are usually not abundant in number, and tend to be most

often found in patients with 'B' symptoms. Plasma cells are usually scattered throughout the tissue and when found in sheets should raise doubt about the diagnosis of Hodgkin's disease. Fibroblasts are usually few in number, but may occasionally be so numerous as to simulate a sarcoma such as malignant fibrous histiocytoma.

As discussed above, the Rye classification of Hodgkin's disease recognized nodular sclerosis, lymphocyte predominance, mixed cellularity, and lymphocyte depletion types.[276] In the WHO classification, the term lymphocyte-rich classical Hodgkin's disease is included to recognize those cases of lymphocyte predominance that are not of the L&H type.[14,301] Nodular sclerosis is the most frequently diagnosed subtype of Hodgkin's disease, comprising about 70% of cases in Western populations, and is defined by the presence of at least focal fibrous bands (Fig. 11.35).[276] These bands usually extend from a thickened capsule to separate the lymphoid parenchyma into nodules, but may be extremely focal, with the remainder of the lymph node showing diffuse effacement or rarely an interfollicular pattern of infiltration. The bands are composed of dense collagen with interspersed small lymphocytes and usually incorporate blood vessels radiating from the capsule. The nodules

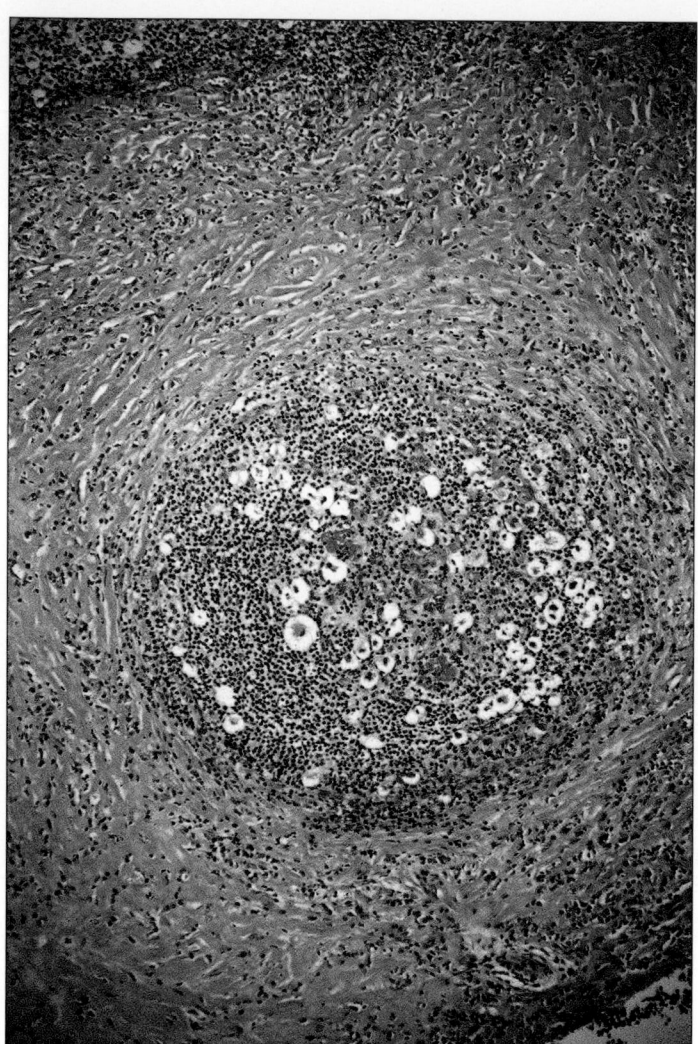

Fig. 11.35 Hodgkin's disease, nodular sclerosing type. A nodule is delineated by broad fibrous bands.

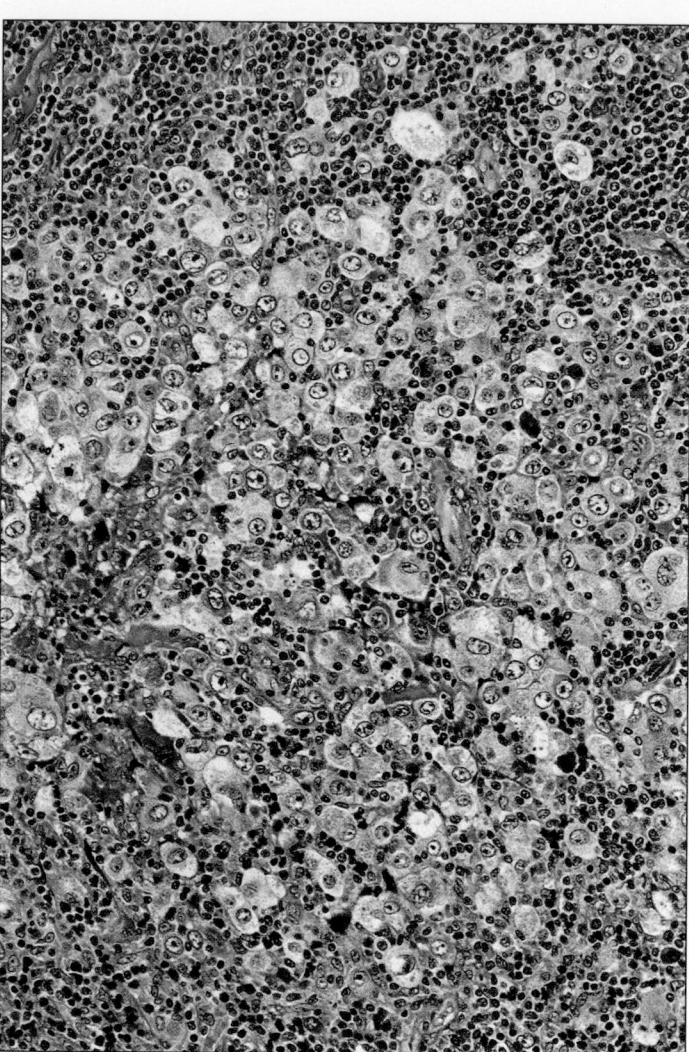

Fig. 11.36 Hodgkin's disease, nodular sclerosing type, syncytial type. Sheets of lacunar cells are seen, adjacent to an area of necrosis.

are usually composed of lacunar cells, which may be few in number or quite numerous, the latter termed the *syncytial variant* of nodular sclerosis (Fig. 11.36).[302] Eosinophils are generally abundant.

The WHO Classification has subdivided cases of nodular sclerosis into two grades based on the British National Lymphoma Investigation group; in some series, these two grades have prognostic value.[303–306] Cases are classified as grade 2 if 1) more than 25% of the nodules show reticular or pleomorphic lymphocyte depletion; 2) greater than 25% of the nodules show fibrohistiocytic lymphocyte depletion; or 3) more than 25% of the nodules contain numerous bizarre and highly anaplastic-appearing Hodgkin cells with lymphocyte depletion (syncytial variant).[306] All other cases are classified as grade 1.

Lymphocyte-rich classical Hodgkin's disease (5% of classical Hodgkin's disease), mixed cellularity (20% of classical Hodgkin's disease), and lymphocyte depletion (<5% of classical Hodgkin's disease) represent a spectrum of the remainder of cases not of the nodular sclerosis subtype. Generally, diffuse effacement of architecture is present, although a vague nodularity is characteristic at low magnification. In rare cases, however, an interfollicular pattern of involvement is present;[113] even more rarely, Hodgkin's disease may have a follicular pattern.[307,308] The capsule is usually intact, without extension of the lymphoid proliferation into the surrounding soft tissues. Varying amounts of interstitial fibrosis may be seen, particularly in lymphocyte depletion in which individual cells are often surrounded by thin wisps of collagen. The presence of any discrete, thick bands would exclude any of these subtypes and warrant classification as nodular sclerosis. There are no quantitative cutoffs between lymphocyte-rich classic Hodgkin's disease, mixed cellularity, and lymphocyte depletion, although in practice, almost all cases not of nodular sclerosing type represent mixed cellularity.

Determination of the subtype of Hodgkin's disease is best made on the initial biopsy, and preferably in a lymph node. Recurrences of Hodgkin's disease in untreated sites usually resemble the initial specimen, but Hodgkin's recurrences in treated sites generally show an increase in the number and atypia of the Hodgkin cells.[309] Hodgkin's disease at autopsy may show a striking degree of Hodgkin cell proliferation and atypia.[310] Biopsies performed in successfully treated cases of Hodgkin's disease often show hypocellular or

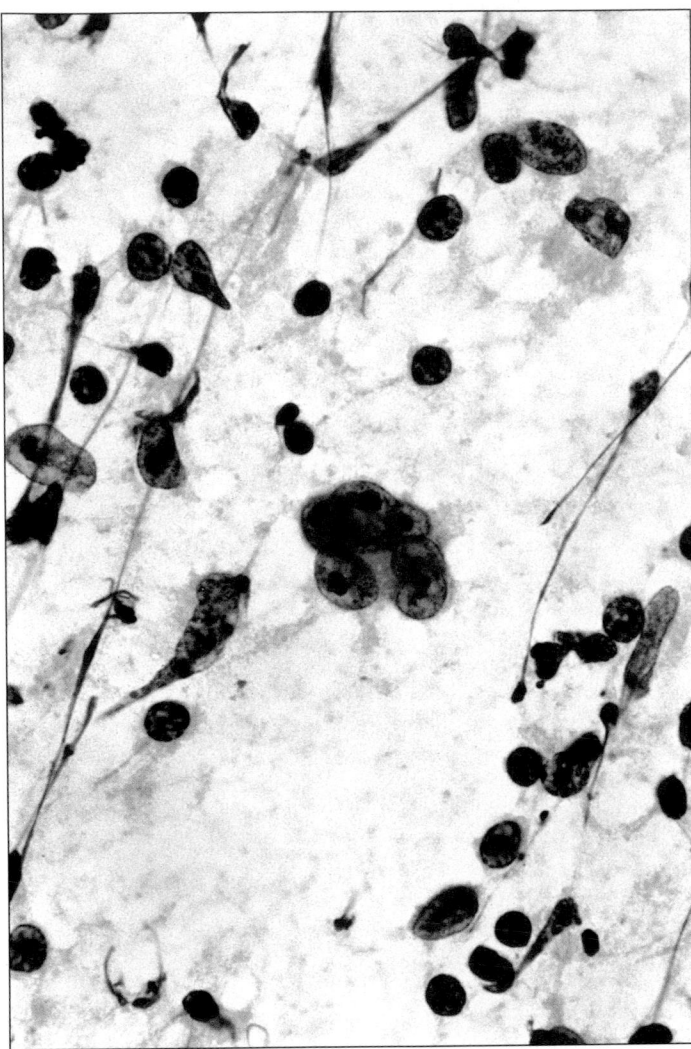

Fig. 11.37 Hodgkin's disease, fine needle aspiration. Hodgkin cells are usually easily appreciated in smear preparations.

Table 11.8 Paraffin section immunophenotype of Hodgkin cells vs. L&H cells vs. non-Hodgkin lymphoma cells

	Hodgkin cells (%)	L&H cells (%)	B-cell lymphoma cells (%)	T-cell lymphoma cells (%)
CD45	10	90	>95	90
CD30	90	40	5	40
CD15	90	10[a]	<5	20
CD20	25	90	94	0
CD3	5	0	<1	>99
CD43	5	0	25	100
EMA	0	40	<10	0

EMA, epithelial membrane antigen; L&H, lymphocytic and histiocytic.
[a] Without neuraminidase predigestion.

acellular fibrous scars. These scars may present as mass-occupying lesions that necessitate biopsy to rule out residual or recurrent disease.

FINE NEEDLE ASPIRATION CYTOPATHOLOGY

Fine needle aspiration biopsy may be a means of diagnosing and staging Hodgkin's disease; in one study, the accuracy for diagnosing Hodgkin's disease was over 90%.[311] On low magnification, the aspirate smears usually show a dispersed population of lymphoid cells in which scattered large cells are evident (Fig. 11.37). At high magnification, these latter cells have bilobed or polylobated nuclei with prominent nucleoli and moderately abundant cytoplasm. Immunohistochemical studies may be helpful for confirmation. Fine needle aspiration studies are of less use in subclassifying Hodgkin's disease, although one study reported an accuracy of 58%.[311] Fine needle aspiration may be of great use in the diagnosis of recurrence of Hodgkin's disease, as Hodgkin cells are sometimes more easily identified in this instance.

ADJUNCTIVE STUDIES

Immunohistochemical studies have become an essential adjunct to the diagnosis of Hodgkin's disease.[312,313] Paraffin section studies are better than frozen sections for the assessment of Hodgkin cells, because morphology is much better preserved. Flow cytometry studies in Hodgkin's disease are not generally of use and may even be misleading. Typically, the latter merely demonstrate a polyclonal population of B cells and a mixture of helper and suppressor T cells; the phenotype of the Hodgkin cells is not demonstrated, even with attempts to gate on the large cell population, due to the infrequency of these cells. In paraffin sections, Hodgkin cells have a characteristic phenotype: positive for CD30 and CD15, and negative for CD45, CD3, and CD43 (Table 11.8 and Fig. 11.38).[3,35,36,314,315] CD20 is positive in approximately 20–25% of cases of classical Hodgkin's disease, with the number of positive cells and the strength of staining slightly less than seen in B-cell non-Hodgkin's lymphomas. As Table 11.8 indicates, exceptions are seen with all stains and therefore one needs to assess the overall staining pattern. In addition to case-to-case variation, the phenotype may vary from biopsy to biopsy, a factor to consider when evaluating possible recurrences.[316,317] Fascin is usually positive, but approximately 60% of cases of anaplastic large cell lymphoma are also positive.[318] Immunohistochemical detection of bcl-6 in classical Hodgkin's disease is not seen.[319] Cases of EBV-associated Hodgkin's disease will show positivity for the EBV latent membrane protein.[285] Approximately 60% of cases of classical Hodgkin's disease contain bcl-2-positive Reed-Sternberg cells. In one large clinical study, bcl-2 expression predicted a statistically significant poorer prognosis in patients treated with adriamycin, bleomycin, vinblastine, and dacarbazine (ABVD) or equivalent regimens.[320]

Molecular studies are not generally of practical use in Hodgkin's disease with the exception that a positive characteristic gene rearrangement may establish a diagnosis of non-Hodgkin's lymphoma.[321] Southern blotting studies of classical Hodgkin's disease usually demonstrate a germline configuration for the immunoglobulin and beta-T-cell receptor genes, although some cases, particularly those that have large numbers of Hodgkin cells, have demonstrated clonal rearrangements (most often of the immunoglobulin genes).[322–324] Similarly, highly sensitive PCR studies have identified small monoclonal immunoglobulin gene rearrangements, particularly in cases expressing B-lineage antigens such as CD20.[325] Cytogenetic studies are generally not useful in the routine diagnosis of Hodgkin's disease due to the scarcity of Hodgkin cells and their slow growth in

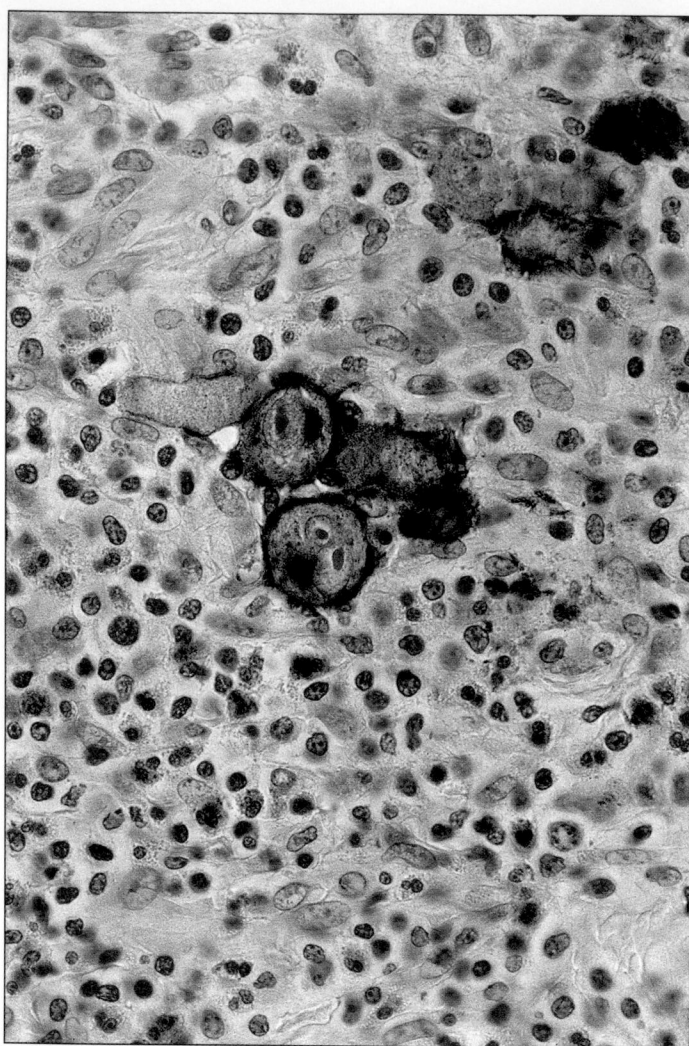

Fig. 11.38 Hodgkin's disease, CD15 stain. Membrane and paranuclear staining of Hodgkin cells is present.

cell culture. Successful studies usually show complex hyperdiploid karyotypes without consistent structural abnormalities.[326] EBV EBER in situ hybridization is a reliable test to identify this virus in EBV-associated cases.[23,327,328]

Despite years of investigation, the cell of origin of Hodgkin's disease has not been definitively established; however, a lymphoid origin is favored by most investigators.[329] Lymphoid antigens, particularly B-lineage antigens, can be identified in many cases when an extensive battery of paraffin and frozen section studies is performed, and the immunoglobulin-associated heterodimer has been identified in Reed-Sternberg cells.[322,323] In addition, the presence of clonal lymphoid antigen receptor genes in some cases strongly supports a lymphoid origin. Furthermore, molecular studies have established their derivation from germinal center B cells.[330] Gene microarray technology in Hodgkin's disease has helped identify decreased mRNA levels for nearly all established B-lineage-specific genes, but no mutations. Researchers hypothesize that the lost B-lineage identity in Reed-Sternberg cells may explain their survival without B-cell receptor expression and reflect a fundamental defect in maintaining the B-cell differentiation state in Reed-Sternberg cells, which is likely caused by a novel, yet unknown,

pathogenic mechanism.[331] However, other possibilities are considered by some investigators, particularly a follicular dendritic cell lineage.[332] Although *bcl-2* gene rearrangements have been identified in Hodgkin tissues by PCR,[333] it is likely that they derived from the reactive population and not the Reed-Sternberg cells.[321] The t(2;5), a translocation typically found in T-cell/null-cell anaplastic large cell lymphoma, is not found in Hodgkin's disease.[334,335]

The nature of the accompanying infiltrate in Hodgkin's disease has also been the focus of intense interest. It is likely that much of the reactive lymphoid infiltrate represents an immune response to the neoplastic element. However, it has been demonstrated that Hodgkin cells express a wide range of cytokines, including various interleukins, tumor necrosis factor, and transforming growth factor-β.[336] Production of one or more of these factors may explain some of the characteristic features of individual cases. For example, the production of interleukin-5 has been correlated with tissue and blood eosinophilia,[337] and the expression of TGR-β? may account for the fibrosis.[338]

DIFFERENTIAL DIAGNOSIS

The differential diagnosis of Hodgkin's disease is wide and includes carcinoma, malignant melanoma, germ cell tumor, sarcoma, reactive lymphoid hyperplasia, and malignant lymphoma. Cases of nodular sclerosing Hodgkin's disease with numerous Reed-Sternberg cells (the syncytial variant) can easily be misdiagnosed as a carcinoma, malignant melanoma, or a germ cell tumor. The localization of the neoplastic cells adjacent to areas of necrosis, the presence of admixed inflammatory cells (particularly eosinophils), and subtotal lymph node involvement may suggest the possibility of Hodgkin's disease. In difficult cases, immunohistochemical studies may be of great use, with the demonstration of keratin positivity in carcinoma, S-100 positivity in malignant melanoma, and placental alkaline phosphatase and/or keratin positivity in germ cell tumors. The latter stain is particularly important because embryonal carcinoma may be CD30 positive, but is always keratin positive. Hodgkin's disease is CD30 positive but keratin negative. As mentioned above, Hodgkin's disease may sometimes be confused with sarcoma, particularly in cases with an exuberant fibroblastic proliferation. Attention should be given to the cells possessing cytologic atypia. In sarcomas, the spindle cell elements will show significant atypia, while in Hodgkin's disease the spindled cells have bland nuclei and the atypical cells have rounded features.

Reactive immunoblastic proliferations may be easily confused with Hodgkin's disease, particularly interfollicular variants. In reactive immunoblastic proliferations, numerous immunoblasts with large nuclei and prominent nucleoli are found in expanded paracortical areas; occasionally, architectural effacement may be present. Cells resembling diagnostic Reed-Sternberg cells may even be found. The immunoblasts tend to be evenly dispersed in reactive conditions, whereas clustering of the atypical cells is typical of Hodgkin's disease. In addition, there is usually a background of numerous plasma cells and lymphoplasmacytoid cells in reactive immunoblastic proliferations, whereas only scattered plasma cells without lymphoplasmacytoid cells are found in Hodgkin's disease. Immunohistochemical studies may be of great use, as reactive immunoblasts are usually CD45+ and CD15−, while Hodgkin cells are CD45− and CD15+; both are usually CD30+. In addition, the immunoblasts as well as the lympho-plasmacytic elements may show polyclonal staining for cytoplasmic immunoglobulins.

Necrotizing granulomatous lymphadenitis may also be difficult to distinguish from Hodgkin's disease, which may show patchy areas of necrosis. In these cases, it is important to examine the areas adjacent to the necrosis. In Hodgkin's disease, Hodgkin cells will almost always be found adjacent to the necrosis, while in necrotizing granulomatous lymphadenitis, the lining cells will be bland histiocytes, often with epithelioid features.

Non-Hodgkin's lymphomas may be even more difficult to distinguish from Hodgkin's disease. Cases of small lymphocytic lymphoma may be confused with cases of lymphocyte-rich classic Hodgkin's disease. Large cells with prominent nucleoli are typically found as part of the proliferating element in small lymphocytic lymphoma; attention should be given to the background proliferation of small, regular lymphoid cells and the lack of eosinophils and other inflammatory elements. Immunohistochemical studies demonstrate a predominant B-cell proliferation (often with coexpression of CD43) in small lymphocytic lymphoma and a predominant T-cell proliferation in Hodgkin's disease. The small lymphocytes of lymphocyte-rich Hodgkin's disease are CD20+, but do not coexpress CD43 or CD5. CD15 and CD30 also highlight the Reed-Sternberg cells, which are not present in small lymphocytic lymphoma.

Rare cases of small lymphocytic lymphoma may have Reed-Sternberg-like cells or even true Reed-Sternberg cells.[339] The biology of these cases has yet to be fully clarified, but they may represent true composite lymphoma, as some of these patients, particularly those in which the atypical cells have the typical immunophenotype of Hodgkin cells, eventually developed disseminated Hodgkin's disease. Most of these cases may be identified by EBV in situ hybridization, as the Reed-Sternberg-like cells (and not the small lymphocytes) are EBV-positive in almost all cases.

Peripheral T-cell lymphoma may be easily mistaken for Hodgkin's disease, because both diseases commonly feature a mixed proliferation of cells with an inflammatory component including eosinophils, histiocytes (including epithelioid histiocytes), and plasma cells. A range of cytologic atypia is usually found in peripheral T-cell lymphoma, with atypical small, medium, and large-sized cells. Immunohistochemical studies will demonstrate a T-cell prominence in both neoplasms, and CD30+ and even CD15+ cells may be present in both. The identification of CD45 and T-lineage or T-associated antigens such as CD3 and CD43 on the atypical cells favors peripheral T-cell lymphoma. Immunohistochemical studies will demonstrate an aberrant T-cell phenotype in the majority of cases of peripheral T-cell lymphoma. Occasionally, gene rearrangement studies may be necessary; the identification of a sizeable monoclonal beta-T-cell receptor gene rearrangement would favor T-cell lymphoma over Hodgkin's disease. T-cell-rich B-cell lymphoma may be difficult to distinguish from cases of lymphocyte-rich or mixed cellularity Hodgkin's disease, as the neoplastic B cells in T-cell-rich lymphoma may very closely simulate Hodgkin cells. Hodgkin's disease may also be confused with diffuse large B-cell lymphoma, particularly in cases in which the Hodgkin cells form sheets, such as in the syncytial variant of nodular sclerosis Hodgkin's disease. Large-cell B-cell lymphoma may show significant amounts of sclerosis, particularly in the mediastinum, the site where the syncytial variant of nodular sclerosis most commonly occurs. The demonstration of CD45 negativity and CD15 positivity strongly favors Hodgkin's disease over these B-cell lymphomas; one must keep in mind that CD20 is positive in 10–20% percent of cases of Hodgkin's disease. Rarely, Hodgkin's disease and B-cell lymphoma may coexist in the same patient, either simultaneously in the same site (composite lymphoma), or simultaneously at different sites (discordant lymphoma).[340] Non-Hodgkin's lymphomas may arise in patients successfully treated for Hodgkin's disease,[341] and conversely, Hodgkin's disease may occur in patients with a history of non-Hodgkin's lymphoma.[342]

Finally, anaplastic large cell lymphoma may be extremely difficult to distinguish from Hodgkin's disease, because both neoplasms contain a proliferation of large, highly atypical cells with prominent nucleoli. Clinical features may be of use, as anaplastic large cell lymphoma frequently involves the skin, an infrequent site of solitary occurrence of Hodgkin's disease, and is more common in children. A preferential localization to sinuses would favor anaplastic large cell lymphoma over Hodgkin's disease, because Hodgkin's disease usually does not involve sinuses until there is extensive involvement of the paracortical region. The presence of abundant neutrophils and plasma cells would also favor anaplastic large cell lymphoma over Hodgkin's disease, which usually has more numerous eosinophils. Both neoplasms are CD30+, and CD45 may be negative in up to one-third of cases of anaplastic large cell lymphoma.[35] The expression of epithelial membrane antigen or T-lineage-associated antigens such as CD43 would favor anaplastic large cell lymphoma, and the expression of CD15 would favor Hodgkin's disease. Molecular studies are helpful, as the presence of a sizeable monoclonal beta-T-cell receptor gene rearrangement or the demonstration of a t(2;5) establishes the diagnosis of anaplastic large cell lymphoma and excludes Hodgkin's disease. The *alk*-1 protein, the product overexpressed in the t(2;5), correlates well with t(2;5) and is expressed in a large percentage of cases of anaplastic large cell lymphoma and not in Hodgkin's disease.[343–346]

LYMPHOCYTE PREDOMINANCE HODGKIN'S DISEASE

As discussed above, Lukes and Butler recognized nodular and diffuse L&H categories of Hodgkin's disease.[276] In the latter portion of the 21st century, a plethora of evidence established that the L&H variants of Hodgkin's disease represented a clinicopathologic entity distinct from classic Hodgkin's disease and thus the WHO Classification included them as a separate category of *nodular lymphocyte predominance Hodgkin's disease*.[278] Nodular lymphocyte predominance Hodgkin's disease is defined as a neoplastic proliferation of L&H cells, cells morphologically and immunologically distinct from the Reed-Sternberg cells and variants found in classical Hodgkin's disease. It is also known as nodular paragranuloma in the European literature.[127]

Lymphocyte predominance comprises approximately 4% of cases of Hodgkin's disease.[279,347] There is a male/female ratio of about 2.5:1, and the disease occurs in all age groups, with a median age of about 35 years.[348,349] It is not associated with EBV,[350] and there are no known predisposing factors, although rare patients have a history of progressive transformation of germinal centers.[127,129] Patients usually present with isolated lymphadenopathy of greater than 3 months' duration, usually involving cervical, axillary, or inguinal lymph nodes.[348,349] About one-half of patients present in Ann Arbor stage I, and 'B' symptoms are uncommon. Liver and spleen involvement occur in about 10% to 15% of cases, but bone marrow and other visceral organ involvement is very uncommon. In one study of nodular lymphocyte predominance, the disease tended to recur independently of time and treatment, suggesting a clinical course distinct from classical Hodgkin's disease,[351] although not all other studies have confirmed this finding. The optimal treatment of lymphocyte predominance is still not clear.[279] The overall prognosis is excellent and similar to that of the general population,

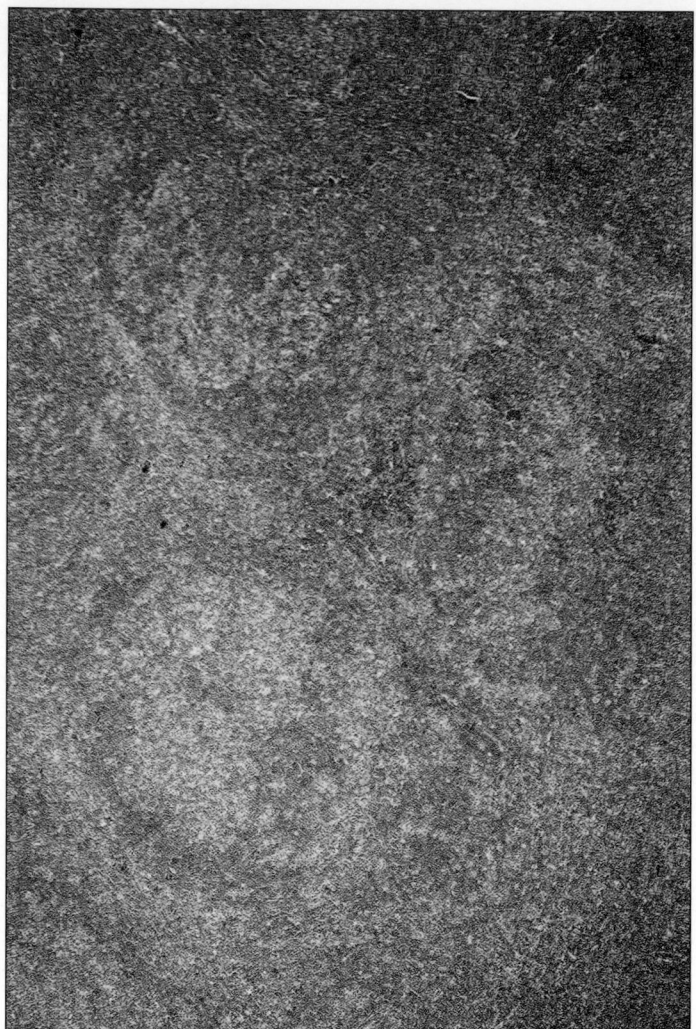

Fig. 11.39 L&H lymphocyte predominance Hodgkin's disease. At low magnification, large nodules are almost always present.

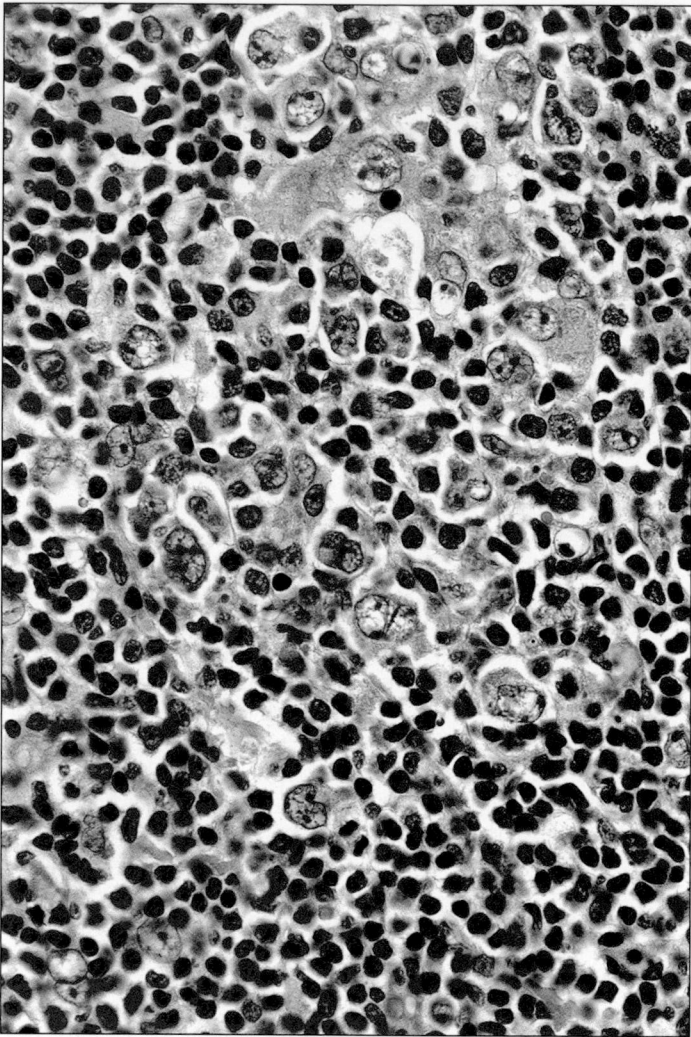

Fig. 11.40 L&H lymphocyte predominance Hodgkin's disease. Several L&H cells are seen, including a polylobated one in the center.

particularly in patients with low-stage disease. Patients with stage III disease with splenic involvement and stage IV disease have only about a 60% survival, with death usually occurring within the first year.[349]

At low magnification, lymphocyte predominance usually shows a nodular architecture, with the nodules larger than the follicles of follicular lymphoma (Fig. 11.39). Occasionally, the nodules are highlighted by a rim of epithelioid histiocytes. Often, there is a rim of uninvolved lymph node that may show reactive follicular hyperplasia or progressive transformation of germinal centers. The nodules are composed of numerous small, round lymphocytes and scattered epithelioid histiocytes and L&H cells. L&H cells are large cells with large nuclei and scant cytoplasm (Fig. 11.40). The nuclear outlines are usually highly irregular ('popcorn' or 'elephant foot' cells), but may be round. The chromatin is usually vesicular. There are one to several moderately sized nucleoli that are usually less eosinophilic and smaller in size than in the Reed-Sternberg cells of classical Hodgkin's disease. Although rare cells closely resembling classic Reed-Sternberg cells may be found, these are not a requisite for the diagnosis. The internodular areas are usually compressed and

are composed of small, round lymphocytes and scattered plasma cells. Eosinophils are generally sparse in both the nodular and internodular areas.

Whether a purely diffuse form of lymphocyte predominance exists has not been firmly established. One should avoid making the diagnosis of diffuse lymphocyte predominance on small biopsy specimens or without immunohistochemistry stains. If no nodular areas are seen when the entire node is excised, one should give consideration to the diagnoses of T-cell rich large B-cell lymphoma, diffuse large B-cell lymphoma (not otherwise specified), or lymphocyte-rich classical Hodgkin's disease.

L&H cells show a B-lineage immunophenotype distinct from the Reed-Sternberg cells of classical Hodgkin's disease. The cells typically stain for CD45 and CD20, and not for CD15. Staining with CD30 is infrequent and epithelial membrane antigen may or may not be present.[312,352–355] J chain, a protein associated with immunoglobulin synthesis, has been found in the cytoplasm of L&H cells,[356] but the expression of immunoglobulins is controversial. In some studies, a polyclonal staining pattern is seen,[355] in other studies no expression is seen,[349,353, 356,357] while in one study kappa light chain restriction was found in most cases.[358] The large cells also express bcl-6.[359] Most of the small lymphocytes in the nodules are polyclonal B lymphocytes, although there are also significant numbers of T cells.[355] Many of these T cells express the natural killer (NK) marker CD57, and a ring of CD57+ cells may sometimes be found around the L&H cells.[360] A network of dendritic reticulum cells is found in the nodules.[361]

The true nature of the L&H cells is still not clear. Immunophenotyping studies have indicated that they are of germinal center cell-derived origin, but whether they are polyclonal or monoclonal has not been resolved.[319] As mentioned above, the results of immunoglobulin protein studies have been controversial. The results of in situ hybridization studies for immunoglobulin mRNA have been equally confusing and have paralleled the immunohistochemical studies, with some studies demonstrating a lack of immunoglobulin mRNA,[357] other studies demonstrating a polyclonal pattern, and still other studies finding monotypic kappa mRNA restriction.[350] One PCR study employing single-cell dissection found a polyclonal pattern of light chain mRNA expression.[362]

DIFFERENTIAL DIAGNOSIS

The differential diagnosis of lymphocyte predominance is wide and includes progressive transformation of germinal centers, classical Hodgkin's disease, and non-Hodgkin's lymphomas, including follicular lymphoma, T-cell-rich/histiocyte-rich B-cell lymphoma, and diffuse large B-cell lymphoma. Progressive transformation generally does not show the architectural effacement seen in lymphocyte predominance; rather, the progressively transformed germinal centers are found in the context of reactive follicular hyperplasia.[129] However, the most important differentiating feature is the presence of L&H cells in lymphocyte predominance and their absence in progressive transformation. Immunostains for CD20 may be very useful in highlighting the L&H cells, although it must be remembered that CD20+ immunoblasts may be present in progressive transformation. Stains for epithelial membrane antigen are positive in a subset of cases of lymphocyte predominance but always negative in immunoblasts.[312,363] In addition, CD57 staining of small lymphocytes in lymphocyte predominance may also be helpful, particularly when there is ringing of CD57+ cells around the L&H cells.[360]

Lymphocyte-rich cases of classical Hodgkin's disease may be difficult to distinguish from lymphocyte predominance, particularly diffuse variants of lymphocyte predominance.[301] It is likely that both were included in the Rye category of lymphocyte predominance Hodgkin's disease. Although a distinctly nodular architecture would favor lymphocyte predominance, the crucial difference rests in the character of the large atypical cells, L&H cells versus other Hodgkin cells. L&H cells tend to have more delicate and more irregular nuclear membranes and less prominent nucleoli than classic Hodgkin cells. In difficult cases, immunohistochemical studies may be of great use (see Table 11.8).

Follicular lymphoma, particularly the floral variant, may be difficult to distinguish from nodular forms of lymphocyte predominance.[364] The nodules in lymphocyte predominance are almost always larger than seen in follicular lymphoma, and there is usually not the compression between adjacent follicles seen in the latter. Cytologically, lymphocyte predominance does not contain the small and large cleaved cells that compose the neoplastic element of follicular lymphoma. The distinction between T-cell-rich/histiocyte-rich B-cell lymphoma and lymphocyte predominance may be extremely difficult. A significant degree of nodularity would favor lymphocyte predominance, whereas clustering of the large atypical cells into small sheets of cells would favor B-cell lymphoma. Immunohistochemical studies may not be helpful, since the B-lineage phenotype with possible expression of epithelial membrane antigen may be identical. In fact, some have speculated that histiocyte-rich B-cell lymphoma and diffuse lymphocyte predominance represent the same disease, although it is stated that the histiocytes are epithelioid and nonepithelioid in lymphocyte predominance, but nonepithelioid in histiocyte-rich B-cell lymphoma.[365] However, molecular studies have shown some differences in the number and distribution of genomic imbalances in the two entities.[366]

Some cases of lymphocyte predominance contain large numbers of L&H cells, raising consideration of large cell lymphoma, a complication that has been reported in about 5% of cases.[367] We diagnose large cell transformation when sheets of large cells are present in the internodular areas. The large cell lymphomas complicating lymphocyte predominance are usually (but not always) of B lineage, and lack EBV or bcl-2 gene rearrangements.[368] Studies have demonstrated that the same B-cell clone was found in the B-cell lymphomas associated with lymphocyte predominance Hodgkin's disease.[369–371]

NON-HODGKIN'S LYMPHOMA

Non-Hodgkin's lymphoma is defined by what it is not; that is, it includes all neoplasms of lymphoid origin other than Hodgkin's disease. It occurs five times more frequently than Hodgkin's disease, with about 50 000 new cases each year. The rate increased in the latter half of the 20th century by a rate of 3–4% per year but has stabilized in the last few years.[372–374] Some of the increase is due to the increase in number of HIV-associated cases.[375] Environmental exposures, such as exposure to hair dyes, herbicides, and organic chemicals, may account for an additional part of the increase.[376–378] A subset of cases is associated with human T-cell leukemia virus (HTLV)-1,[379] and other subsets of cases are associated with EBV.[285] Non-Hodgkin's lymphoma occurs in both children and adults, with an overall male/female ratio of 1.3:1. Although more common in adults, it accounts for a relatively high percentage of cancer occurring in children.

Non-Hodgkin's lymphoma usually presents as painless, localized, or generalized enlargement of lymph nodes with or without hepatosplenomegaly. However, it may present as a tonsillar, mediastinal, or abdominal mass, or as localized or generalized lesions involving every organ or organ system. 'B' symptoms may occur, but are less commonly seen than in Hodgkin's disease. The signs and symptoms may occur acutely or may have been present for a long period of time, occasionally years. Although progression does not occur in as orderly a fashion as in Hodgkin's disease, the Ann Arbor system has been used for the staging of non-Hodgkin's lymphoma.[380]

Non-Hodgkin's lymphomas represent a heterogeneous mixture of neoplasms of different cell lineages frozen at different stages of development. Eighty percent to 90% represent B-lineage neoplasms, most often related to cells of the germinal center.[381,382] Other B-cell lymphomas may be related to cells of the B-cell mantle or marginal zone or B-cell populations native to extranodal tissues. A minority of cases comprise T-lineage neoplasms, including neoplasms of immature (thymic) as well as mature T-cell phenotype (post-thymic or peripheral). Some cases may be of NK cell lineage or indeterminate lineage, the latter usually referred to as null cell type. Some

Table 11.9 Non-Hodgkin's lymphomas and frequency of monoclonal gene rearrangements

	Ig Heavy (%)	Ig Light (%)	T-Beta (%)
Most B-cell lymphomas	100	100	5–10
B lymphoblastic	100	40	20–30
Peripheral T-cell lymphoma	5–10	<1	90
T lymphoblastic	20–30	1	90

Ig, immunoglobulin.
Modified from Weiss et al.[912]

Table 11.10 Common chromosomal translocations found in non-Hodgkin's lymphomas

Translocation	Lymphoma	Antigen receptor gene	Oncogene
t(11;14)(q13;q32)	Mantle cell	IgH	PRAD1/cyclin/CCND1/bcl-1
t(14;18)(q32;q21)	Follicular; some diffuse large cell	IgH	bcl-2
t(3;v)(q27;v)	Diffuse large cell lymphoma	Variable	bcl-6/laz-3
t(2;5)(p23;q35)	Anaplastic large cell lymphoma	Not involved (npm gene)	alk
t(8;14)(q24;q32)	Burkitt's; some diffuse large cell	IgH	c-myc
t(2;8)(p12;q24)	Burkitt's; some diffuse large cell	Kappa	c-myc
t(8;22)(q24;q11)	Burkitt's; some diffuse large cell	Lambda	c-myc
t(9;14)(p13;q32)	Lymphoplasmacytic lymphoma	IgH	PAX5
t(11;18)(q21;q21)	Low-grade B-cell lymphoma of MALT type	API2	MLT
i(7)(q10),+8	Hepatosplenic γ/δ T-cell lymphoma		
t(3;v)(q27;v)	Diffuse large B-cell lymphoma		BCL6/LAZ3
der(3)(q27)	Diffuse large B-cell lymphoma	variable	BCL6

Modified from Weiss et al.[912]

investigators include neoplasms of true histiocytic lineage among the malignant lymphomas, because of clinical and morphologic similarities.

In general, non-Hodgkin's lymphomas are monoclonal proliferations.[18] Thus, B-cell lymphomas expressing immunoglobulin will generally show only one of the light chains, so-called light chain restriction. Monoclonal immunoglobulin gene rearrangements are usually detectable, and aberrant clonal rearrangements of the β-T-cell receptor gene are also detectable in a minority of cases, particularly in the immature lymphoblastic neoplasms (Table 11.9). There is no good marker for monoclonality analogous to analysis of light chains for T-cell lymphomas, although many T-cell lymphomas may show aberrant loss of one or more T-lineage antigens.[383] Monoclonal β-T-cell receptor gene rearrangements are found in most, but not all, T-cell lymphomas, and similar to B-cell lymphomas, aberrant monoclonal immunoglobulin heavy chain gene rearrangements are also detectable in a minority of cases, again particularly in the immature lymphoblastic neoplasms. Many types of non-Hodgkin's lymphomas are associated with characteristic cytogenetic abnormalities, usually balanced translocations (Table 11.10).[384,385] Typically, a cellular oncogene is translocated to adjacent to one of the antigen receptor genes.

The WHO Classification of hematopoietic neoplasms is the most widely accepted classification scheme for non-Hodgkin's lymphomas (Table 11.11). All previous classifications were based primarily on morphology, with increasingly sophisticated classifications that paralleled developments in immunology, ontogeny, or molecular genetics. The WHO Classification, which is based on the Revised European-American Lymphoma (REAL) classification (Table 11.12),[14] recognizes about 25 separate categories of lymphoma thought to represent well-established clinicopathologic entities as defined by combined morphologic, immunologic, ontogenic, and molecular genetic features. The REAL Classification itself was based on the 1982 Working Formulation (Table 11.13),[386] (which in turn was based on the 1966 Rappaport classification,[99] and was used primary in the United States for nearly two decades) and the Updated Kiel classification of 1988 (Table 11.14)[387] (used primarily in Europe). The earlier classification schemes divided lymphomas into two or three categories of prognostic interest.

Complicating the difficulty in classification of non-Hodgkin's lymphomas is the recognition that a minority of lymphomas may have different histologic appearances in different sites; these lymphomas are termed *discordant lymphomas*. Rarely, lymphomas may have two or more distinctly different histologic appearances at the same site (including coexisting non-Hodgkin's lymphoma and Hodgkin's disease); these lymphomas are termed *composite lymphoma*.[340,388–390] In addition, it is not uncommon for a low-grade lymphoma to transform over time to a lymphoma of higher grade.

Finally, some lymphomas show close overlap with leukemic counterparts, and it is likely that both represent the same biologic entity with different clinical manifestations.

Fine needle aspiration biopsy has been used for the primary diagnosis of non-Hodgkin's lymphoma, but there are limitations due to the difficulties involved in both the diagnosis as well as classification.[391,392] The key to the recognition of most non-Hodgkin's lymphomas on fine needle aspiration is the identification of a monotonous lymphoid cell population. The monotony is reflected not so much in the nuclear size, but in the essentially uniform cell-to-cell appearance of the chromatin pattern. Lymphomas composed of a heterogeneous mixture of neoplastic cells (e.g. peripheral T-cell lymphoma) may be very difficult to recognize by fine needle aspiration, unless highly bizarre or pleomorphic cells are identified. The efficacy of fine needle aspiration biopsy in the primary diagnosis of non-Hodgkin's lymphoma can be dramatically improved when supplemented with immunohistochemical and molecular studies. Precise classification may still be quite difficult to perform; however, the distinction between low-grade and high-grade lymphomas can usually be made. In one series, about 90% of non-Hodgkin's lymphomas were correctly diagnosed, with the correct assignment of grade in virtually all cases.[393] The specific diagnosis of low-grade lymphomas is more difficult to make than with high-grade lymphomas. Fine needle aspiration biopsy is more easily applied to the staging of non-Hodgkin's lymphoma, allowing easy, widespread sampling of different sites. It may also

Table 11.11 WHO classification of tumors of lymphoid tissues

I **B-cell neoplasms**
  A **Precursor B-cell neoplasm**
    1. Precursor B-lymphoblastic leukemia/lymphoma
  B **Mature B-cell neoplasms**
    1. Chronic lymphocytic leukemia/small lymphocytic lymphoma
    2. B-cell prolymphocytic leukemia
    3. Lymphoplasmacytic lymphoma
    4. Splenic marginal zone lymphoma
    5. Hairy cell leukemia
    6. Plasma cell myeloma
    7. Solitary plasmacytoma of bone
    8. Extraosseous plasmacytoma
    9. Extranodal marginal zone B-cell lymphoma of mucosa-associated lymphoid tissue (MALT-lymphoma)
    10. Nodal marginal zone B-cell lymphoma
    11. Follicular lymphoma
    12. Mantle cell lymphoma
    13. Diffuse large B-cell lymphoma
    14. Mediastinal (thymic) large B-cell lymphoma
    15. Intravascular large B-cell lymphoma
    16. Primary effusion lymphoma
    17. Burkitt's lymphoma/leukemia
  C **B-cell proliferations of uncertain malignant potential**
    1. Lymphomatoid granulomatosis
    2. Post-transplant lymphoproliferative disorder, polymorphic

II **T-cell and NK-cell neoplasms**
  A **Precursor T-cell neoplasms**
    1. Precursor T-lymphoblastic leukemia/lymphoma
    2. Blastic NK cell lymphoma
  B **Mature T-cell and NK-cell neoplasms**
    1. T-cell prolymphocytic leukemia
    2. T-cell large granular lymphocytic leukemia
    3. Aggressive NK cell leukemia
    4. Adult T-cell leukemia/lymphoma
    5. Extranodal NK/T cell lymphoma, nasal type
    6. Enteropathy-type T-cell lymphoma
    7. Hepatosplenic T-cell lymphoma
    8. Subcutaneous panniculitis-like T-cell lymphoma
    9. Mycosis fungoides
    10. Sezary syndrome
    11. Primary cutaneous anaplastic large cell lymphoma
    12. Peripheral T-cell lymphoma, unspecified
    13. Angioimmunoblastic T-cell lymphoma
    14. Anaplastic large cell lymphoma
  C **T-cell proliferation of uncertain malignant potential**
    1. Lymphomatoid papulosis

III **Hodgkin's disease (Hodgkin's lymphoma)**
  A **Nodular lymphocyte predominant Hodgkin's lymphoma**
  B **Classical Hodgkin's lymphoma**
  C **Nodular sclerosis classical Hodgkin's lymphoma**
  D **Lymphocyte-rich classical Hodgkin's lymphoma**
  E **Mixed cellularity classical Hodgkin's lymphoma**
  F **Lymphocyte-depleted classical Hodgkin's lymphoma**

IV **Histiocytic and dendritic-cell neoplasms**
  A **Macrophage/histiocytic neoplasm**
    1. Histiocytic sarcoma
  B **Dendritic cell neoplasms**
    1. Langerhans cell histiocytosis
    2. Langerhans cell sarcoma
    3. Interdigitating dendritic cell sarcoma/tumor
    4. Follicular dendritic cell sarcoma/tumor
    5. Dendritic cell sarcoma, not otherwise specified

Table 11.11 WHO classification of tumors of lymphoid tissues *(cont'd)*

V **Mastocytosis**
  A **Cutaneous mastocytosis**
  B **Indolent systemic mastocytosis**
  C **Systemic mastocytosis with associated clonal, hematological non-mast cell lineage disease**
  D **Aggressive systemic mastocytosis**
  E **Mast cell leukemia**
  F **Mast cell sarcoma**
  G **Extracutaneous mastocytoma**

be used to diagnose recurrent or residual disease, or to identify large cell transformation in a patient with a history of low-grade lymphoma.

An International Prognostic Index has been developed for aggressive non-Hodgkin's lymphoma patients, based on age, stage, number of extranodal sites of disease, performance status, and serum lactate dehydrogenase levels (Table 11.15).[394] This index may also be applicable to other types of non-Hodgkin's lymphoma.[395] Other clinical factors such as sex, size of tumor, and beta-2-microglobulin have been found to affect prognosis.[396–402]

Histologic grade also affects prognosis. In addition, a variety of factors may be of importance in determining prognosis, including proliferative rate, cytotoxic T-cell response, loss of molecules of immune recognition, loss of cell adhesion antigens, gain of drug resistance molecules, acquisition of aneuploidy, gain of specific oncogenes, or loss of specific tumor suppressor genes, and genomic imbalances.[395,403–406]

FOLLICULAR LYMPHOMA

Follicular lymphoma is defined as a neoplasm of follicle center B-cell derivation showing some component of follicular architecture. In the WHO Classification, it is divided into three cytologic grades.[407]

Follicular lymphoma is a relatively common type of non-Hodgkin's lymphoma, representing about 35% of such cases in the United States and 22% worldwide, with a slightly lower incidence in Europe, Asia, and underdeveloped countries.[408,409] The mean age of occurrence is 55 years, with only rare cases reported in childhood, and few under the age of 40 years.[410–412] Roughly equal numbers of cases occur in males and females. Patients usually present with one or several enlarged lymph nodes, often of long duration. Only one-third of patients are Stage I or II at the time of diagnosis.[408] The vast majority of cases are already in stage IV, with bone marrow, liver, and spleen involvement common. Involvement of peripheral blood also occurs frequently, either at presentation or during the course of disease.

Follicular lymphoma is usually an indolent lymphoma, with occasional spontaneous regressions, slow progression, and numerous relapses occurring over time, seemingly independent of treatment.[413,414] Because of this, most cases of follicular lymphoma are not treated aggressively, although the large-cell variant is often treated with standard anthracyclin-based chemotherapy with curative intent.[395] In about 40–50% of cases, transformation to a diffuse large cell lymphoma occurs. With this event, survival is usually less than one year, although some patients undergo remissions with aggressive chemotherapy. The transformation of follicular lymphoma to

Table 11.12 List of lymphoid neoplasms recognized by the International Lymphoma Study Group

B-cell neoplasms
  I **Precursor B-cell neoplasm: B-precursor lymphoblastic leukemia/lymphoma**
  II **Peripheral B-cell neoplasms**
    1. B-cell chronic lymphocytic leukemia/prolymphocytic leukemia/small lymphocytic lymphoma
    2. Lymphoplasmacytoid lymphoma/immunocytoma
    3. Mantle cell lymphoma
    4. Follicle center lymphoma, follicular
       Provisional cytologic grades: I (small cell), II (mixed small and large cell), III (large cell)
       Provisional subtype: diffuse, predominantly small cell type
    5. Marginal zone B-cell lymphoma
       Extranodal (MALT type ± monocytoid B cells)
       Provisional category: nodal (± monocytoid B cells)
    6. Provisional category: splenic marginal zone lymphoma (± villous lymphocytes)
    7. Hairy cell leukemia
    8. Plasmacytoma/plasma cell myeloma
    9. Diffuse large B-cell lymphoma
       Subtype: primary mediastinal (thymic) B-cell lymphoma
    10. Burkitt's lymphoma
    11. Provisional category: high-grade B-cell lymphoma, Burkitt's-like

T-cell and putative NK cell neoplasms
  I **Precursor T-cell neoplasm: T-precursor lymphoblastic lymphoma/leukemia**
  II **Peripheral T-cell and NK-cell neoplasms**
    1. T-cell chronic lymphocytic leukemia/prolymphocytic leukemia
    2. Large granular lymphocyte leukemia (LGL)
    3. Mycosis fungoides/Sezary syndrome
    4. Peripheral T-cell lymphoma, unspecified
       Provisional cytologic categories: subtypes: medium-sized cell, mixed medium and large cell, large cell, lymphoepithelioid cell
       Provisional subtype: hepatosplenic gamma/delta T-cell lymphoma
       Provisional subtype: subcutaneous panniculitic T-cell lymphoma
    5. Angioimmunoblastic T-cell lymphoma (AILD)
    6. Angiocentric lymphoma
    7. Intestinal T-cell lymphoma (± enteropathy associated)
    8. Adult T-cell lymphoma/leukemia (ATL/L)
    9. Anaplastic large cell lymphoma (ALCL), CD30+, T and null cell types
    10. Provisional subtype: anaplastic large cell lymphoma, Hodgkin's-like

Hodgkin's disease
  I **Lymphocyte predominance**
  II **Nodular sclerosis**
  III **Mixed cellularity**
  IV **Lymphocyte depletion**
  V **Provisional entity: lymphocyte-rich classic Hodgkin's disease**

From Harris et al.[14]

Table 11.13 Working Formulation of non-Hodgkin's lymphomas for clinical usage

Low grade
  A **Small lymphocytic**
     Consistent with CLL; plasmacytoid
  B **Follicular predominantly small cleaved cell**
     Diffuse areas, sclerosis
  C **Follicular mixed small cleaved and large cell**
     Diffuse areas, sclerosis
Intermediate grade
  D **Follicular predominantly large cell**
     Diffuse areas, sclerosis
  E **Diffuse small cleaved cell**
     Sclerosis
  F **Diffuse mixed, small and large cell**
     Sclerosis, epithelioid cell component
  G **Diffuse large cell**
     Cleaved cell, noncleaved cell, sclerosis
High grade
  H **Large cell, immunoblastic**
     Plasmacytoid, clear cell, polymorphous, epithelioid cell component
  I **Lymphoblastic**
     Convoluted, nonconvoluted
  J **Small noncleaved cell**
     Burkitt's, follicular areas
Miscellaneous
     Composite, mycosis fungoides, histiocytic, extramedullary plasmacytoma, unclassifiable, other

Modified from Non-Hodgkin's Lymphoma Pathologic Classification Project.[386]

Table 11.14 Updated Kiel classification of non-Hodgkin's lymphomas

	B cell	T cell
Low grade	Lymphocytic – chronic lymphocytic and prolymphocytic leukemia; hairy cell leukemia	Lymphocytic, chronic lymphocytic, and prolymphocytic leukemia
	Lymphoplasmacytic/cytoid	Lymphoepithelioid
	Plasmacytic	Angioimmunoblastic
	Centroblastic/centrocytic	T zone
	Centrocytic	Pleomorphic, small cell
High grade	Centroblastic	Pleomorphic, medium and large cell
	Immunoblastic	Immunoblastic
	Large cell anaplastic	Large cell anaplastic
	Burkitt's lymphoma	Lymphoblastic
	Lymphoblastic	Rare types

Rare types From Stansfeld et al.[387]

diffuse large cell lymphoma has been shown to be associated with the acquisition of a wide variety of genomic imbalances affecting recurrent chromosomal areas.[415]

The hallmark of follicular lymphoma is the presence of a true follicular architecture, at least focally within the tumor (Fig. 11.41). In most cases, the follicles are evenly dispersed throughout the entire lymph node parenchyma, often with extension into the

Table 11.15 International prognostic index for aggressive lymphomas

Risk factors	
Age >60 years	
Stage III or IV	
Number of extranodal sites of disease >1	
Performance status <2	
Serum lactate dehydrogenase level greater than normal	
Low risk (73% 5 year survival)	0 or 1 of above risk factors
Low intermediate risk (51% 5 year survival)	2 of above risk factors
High intermediate risk (43% 5 year survival)	3 of above risk factors
High risk (26% 5 year survival)	4 or 5 of above risk factors

Data from The International Non-Hodgkin's Lymphoma Prognostic Factors Project.[394]

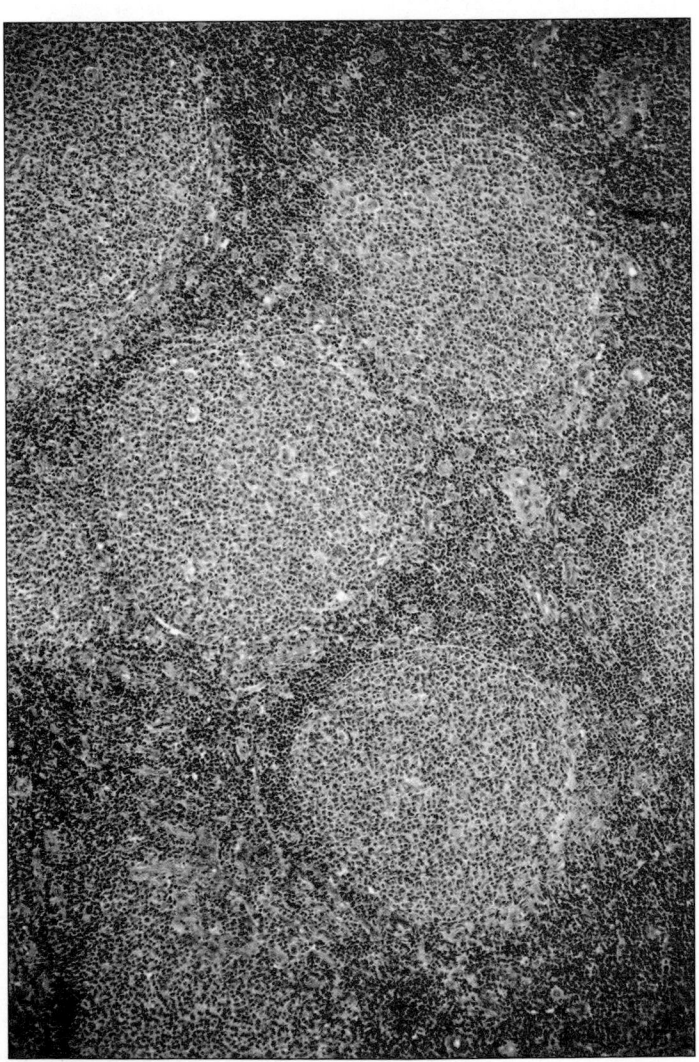

Fig. 11.41 Follicular lymphoma. Numerous follicles are present, with only a small amount of intervening interfollicular areas.

perinodal adipose tissue. In some cases, there are areas of follicular and diffuse effacement of architecture (most often seen in Grade 3). Occasionally, the follicular areas may only be focally appreciated; usually the remainder of the lymph node shows diffuse effacement of architecture, although rarely there is normal architecture. In the latter case, adjacent lymph nodes may show a greater degree of involvement. According to the WHO scheme, the pattern is reported as follicular (>75% follicular), follicular and diffuse (25–75% follicular), or minimally follicular (<25% follicular). The presence of diffuse areas may adversely affect prognosis, particularly in the mixed and large-cell variants.[395,416] The follicles are classically round and relatively homogeneously sized; occasionally however, the follicles are highly irregular, with varied size and shape. The mantles are usually absent, but when present are a thin rim or of normal thickness. Rarely, small mantle cells may invaginate between and separate small clusters of follicular lymphoma cells, expanding the neoplastic follicles in the process; these unusual cases have been termed the *floral variant of follicular lymphoma*.[364,417] In most cases, the interfollicular regions are compressed, and often there is a back-to-back arrangement of the follicles. In some cases, the follicles coalesce into one another. However, in some cases the interfollicular areas may be of normal size, and the follicles clearly distinct. In rare cases, the marginal zones (the areas just outside of the mantle zone) may be expanded by a proliferation of monocytoid cells forming a pale collar around the neoplastic follicles; in these cases, the proliferating monocytoid cells are part of the lymphomatous process.[418,419] Sclerosis is common in follicular lymphoma and usually consists of broad collagenous bands. Deposition of an amorphous extracellular material may be found within the follicles, but is not specific for neoplastic follicles.

The cytologic features are as important as the architectural features in establishing a morphologic diagnosis of follicular lymphoma. The cells in the follicles are varying mixtures of centrocytes (or cleaved follicle center cells) and centroblasts (or noncleaved follicle center cells) (Figs. 11.42 and 11.43). These correspond roughly to small cleaved cell and large cleaved cell types of the Working Formulation. Centrocytes are slightly larger than small, mature lymphocytes and have relatively condensed chromatin without prominent nucleoli. The most distinctive feature is the highly irregular nuclear outlines, which are contorted and twisted. One may also see slightly larger centrocytes with similar nuclear chromatin and shape, but with nuclei about two to three times the size of regular centrocytes. Centroblasts are slightly larger in size and have rounded nuclear outlines, a vesicular chromatin pattern, and one to several moderately sized nucleoli, often apposed to the nuclear membrane. A moderate amount of amphophilic or slightly basophilic cytoplasm is typically present.

The WHO Classification divides follicular lymphoma into 3 grades. Cases are usually classified as Grade 1 when there are greater than 75% centrocytes or 0 to 5 centroblasts per high-power field (×10 eyepiece and ×40 objective).[61,420,421] Cases are usually classified as Grade 2 when there are between 25% and 50% centrocytes or 6 to 15 centroblasts per high-power field. Cases are usually classified as Grade 3 when there are greater than 50% centroblasts or greater than 15 centroblasts per high-power field. In practice, the distinction is often arbitrary, perhaps at least partially explaining the poor reproducibility even among experienced hematopathologists. Approximately two-thirds of cases of follicular lymphoma are Grade 1, about 25% of cases are diagnosed as Grade 2, and about 10% are classified as Grade 3. Tingible body macrophages are rare in Grade 1 or Grade 2 follicular lymphoma, but may be a feature of Grade 3. Similarly, the mitotic rate is usually low in Grades 1 and 2, but may be brisk in Grade 3. Grade 3 is further subdivided into grades 3a

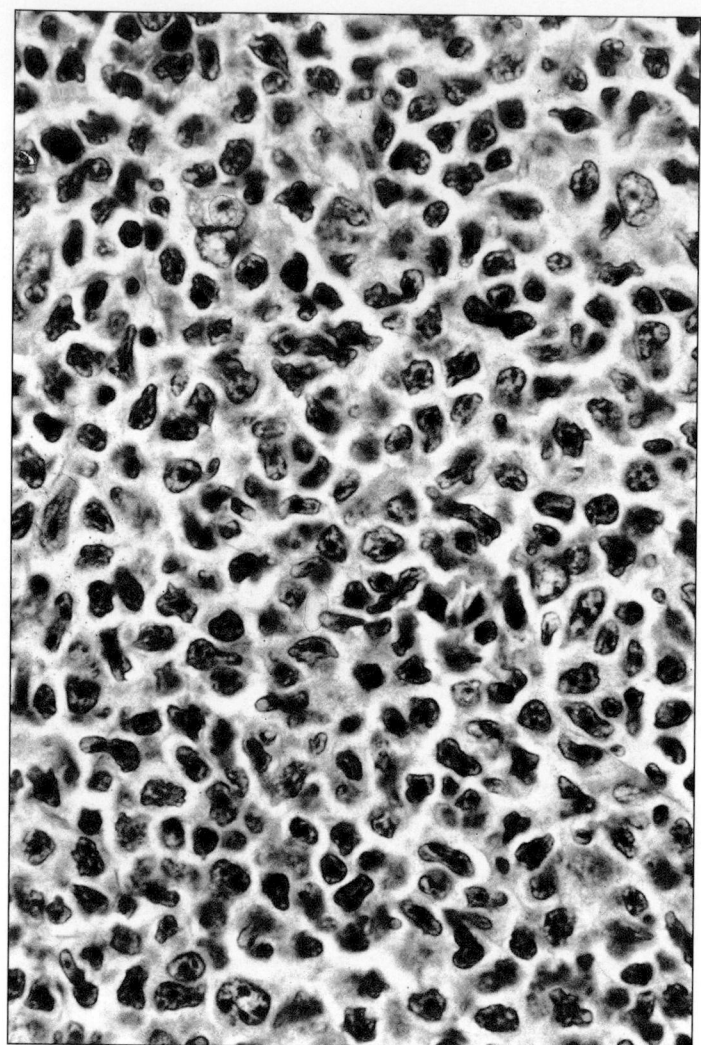

Fig. 11.42 Follicular lymphoma, predominantly small cleaved cell type. Most of the cells are small and have contorted nuclear outlines, but occasional larger cells are also present.

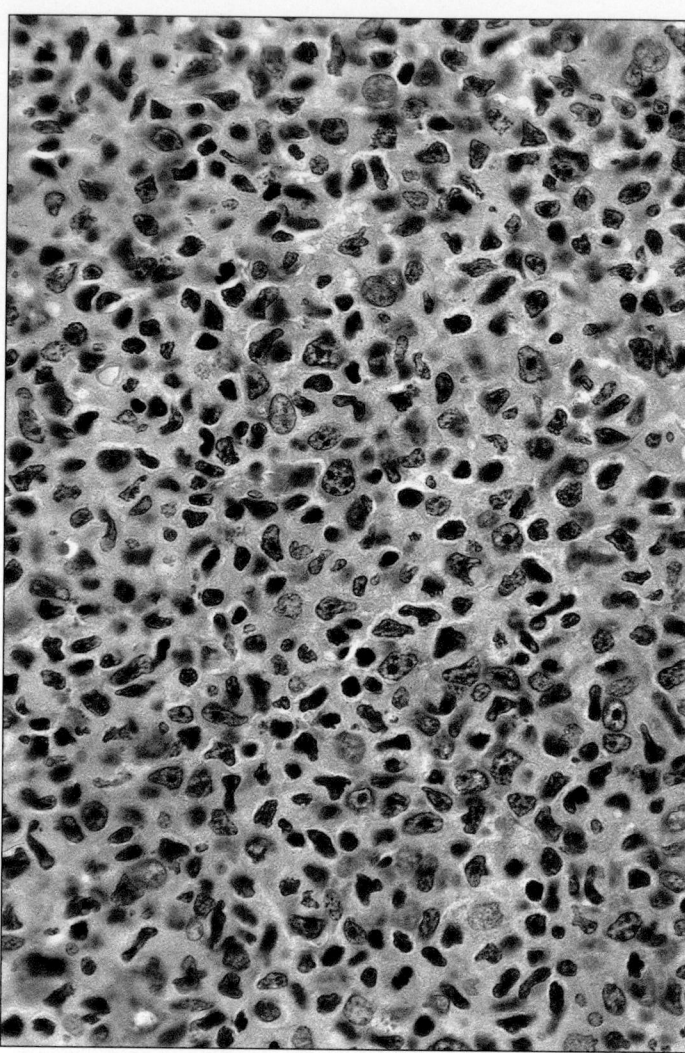

Fig. 11.43 Follicular lymphoma, mixed small cleaved cell and large cell type. A mixture of atypical cells is seen. Both large cleaved and large noncleaved cells are present.

(centrocytes present) and 3b (sheets of centroblasts). The subtypes of Grade 3 have uncertain clinical importantance.[422,423]

In addition to the floral variant of follicular lymphoma, other rare cytologic variants of follicular lymphoma have been reported. These include the presence of clear or eosinophilic cytoplasmic inclusions, the so-called signet-ring cell variant of follicular lymphoma (Fig. 11.44).[424] In addition, the tumor cells may rarely have small round nuclei (termed *follicular small lymphocytic lymphoma*),[425] cerebriform nuclei reminiscent of the cells of mycosis fungoides,[426] multilobated nuclei,[427] plasmacytoid nuclear and cytoplasmic features,[428] immunoblastic features,[429] blastic nuclei resembling the nuclei of lymphoblastic leukemia,[430] or intracytoplasmic light chain crystals.[431] Another rare variant termed 'in situ localization of follicular lymphoma' has also been described. This unusual 'lymphoma in situ' contains focal germinal centers with strong bcl-2 positivity, with most of the remaining lymph node showing bcl-2-negative follicular hyperplasia. This most likely represents follicular lymphoma at the earliest stage of development or a preneoplastic event, requiring a second hit for neoplastic transformation.[432]

Fine needle aspiration biopsy smears of follicular lymphoma often show vague nodular aggregates, imparting a nodular pattern at low magnification.[433,434] Centrocytes appear as small hyperchromatic cells with a wrinkled or indented nuclear outline (Fig. 11.45). Centroblasts typically have rounded or cleaved vesicular nuclei with irregularly thick and thin nuclear membranes. The recognition of Grade 2 follicular lymphoma may be extremely difficult cytologically, but immunohistochemical and molecular studies may be helpful in establishing a diagnosis of follicular lymphoma.

Immunophenotypic studies demonstrate that all follicular lymphomas are of B lineage, expressing multiple B-lineage antigens in both paraffin and frozen sections, and flow cytometry (Table 11.16).[315,435–439] Approximately 90% express surface immunoglobulins by flow cytometry/immunohistochemistry, usually IgM, and sometimes with a second isotype.[439] The large-cell subtype is most likely to be immunoglobulin negative. Monotypic immunoglobulin may also be detected in paraffin sections in a significant proportion of cases, but this procedure is less dependable than frozen section studies. The bcl-2 oncoprotein is expressed by

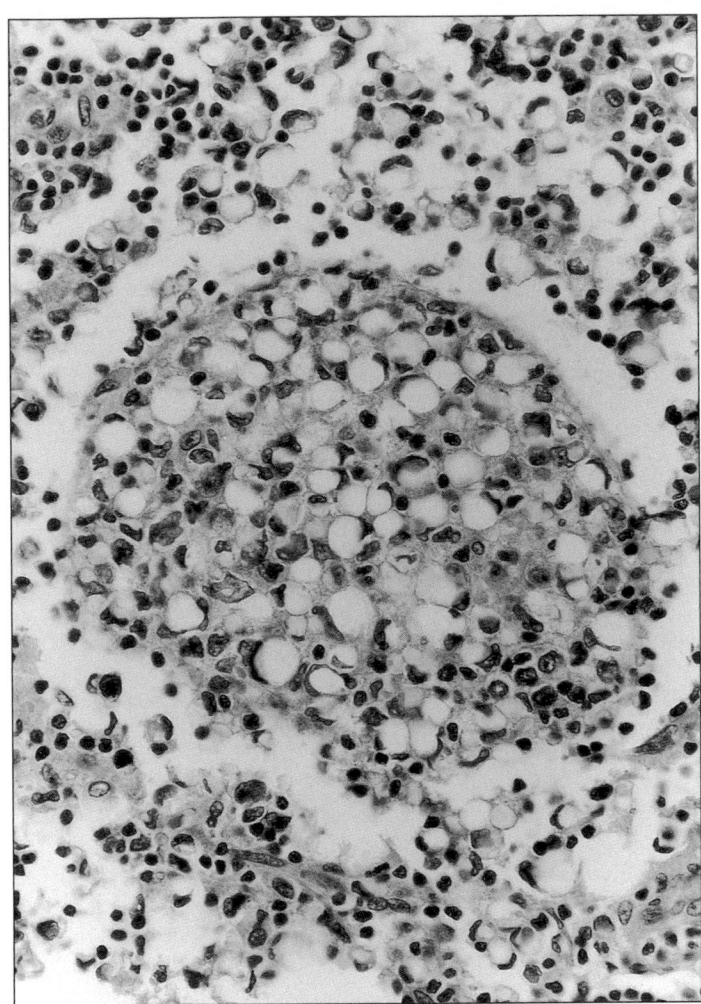

Fig. 11.44 Follicular lymphoma, signet-ring cell type. Striking cytoplasmic vacuolization is seen in this unusual variant of follicular lymphoma.

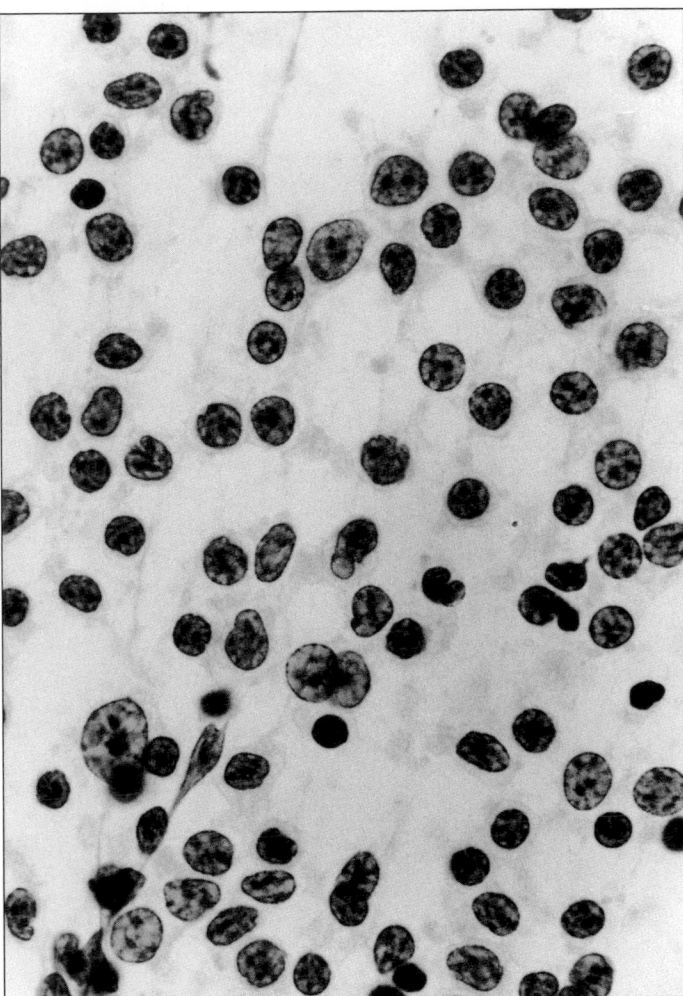

Fig. 11.45 Follicular lymphoma, fine needle aspiration. Many of the small lymphoid cells have irregular nuclear contours. This feature is often difficult to appreciate in smear preparations, unless the cells are carefully examined.

the neoplastic cells in about 80–90% of adult cases (Fig. 11.46); again, the large-cell subtype is most likely to be bcl-2 protein-negative.[104,106,440] Pediatric follicular lymphoma is also likely to be bcl-2 negative (confirmed by lack of bcl-2 gene rearrangements); when present, bcl-2 is considered an adverse prognostic marker.[411] The neoplastic cells express CD10 in about 50–60% of cases, are usually negative for CD23, and are almost always negative for CD5.[109,441] Again, the subtype most likely to be CD10 negative is Grade 3 follicular lymphoma. Therefore, lack of CD10 and bcl-2 expression on small specimens, such as from needle core biopsy or fine-needle aspiration, does not preclude the possibility of a diagnosis of follicular lymphoma. Also, lack of CD10 or bcl-2 expression in diffuse large B-cell lymphoma does not exclude the possibility of follicle center cell origin.[442] Flow cytometric detection of CD10+ cells with high bcl-2 expression is highly specific for follicular lymphoma over reactive follicular hyperplasia.[443,444] Bcl-6 immunohistochemical staining is common in follicular lymphomas.[445,446] Bcl-6 expression may be independent of chromosome 3q27 rearrangements.[447] T-lineage antibodies rarely, if ever, stain the neoplastic cells, but demonstrate a significant population of T cells within the neoplastic follicles.[3,113,448] A subset

Table 11.16 Summary of immunophenotypes of low- to intermediate-grade B-cell lymphomas

	Follicular	SLL/CLL	Marginal	Lym-Plas	Mantle
Ig	90%	98%	98%	98%	98%
Heavy	IgM, G	IgM ± IgD	IgM, D, A	IgM	IgM + IgD
K/L	2:1	2:1	2:1	2:1	1:1
CD20	100%	98%	98%	98%	99%
CD43	2%	85%	50%	60%	60%
CD5	1%	90%	10%	25%	80%
CD10	60%	10%	10%	10%	25%
CD23	5%	90%	15%	30%	15%

SLL/CLL, small lymphocytic lymphoma/chronic lymphocytic leukemia; Lym-Plas, lymphoplasmacytic; Ig, immunoglobulin; heavy, common heavy chain(s); K, kappa; L, lambda.

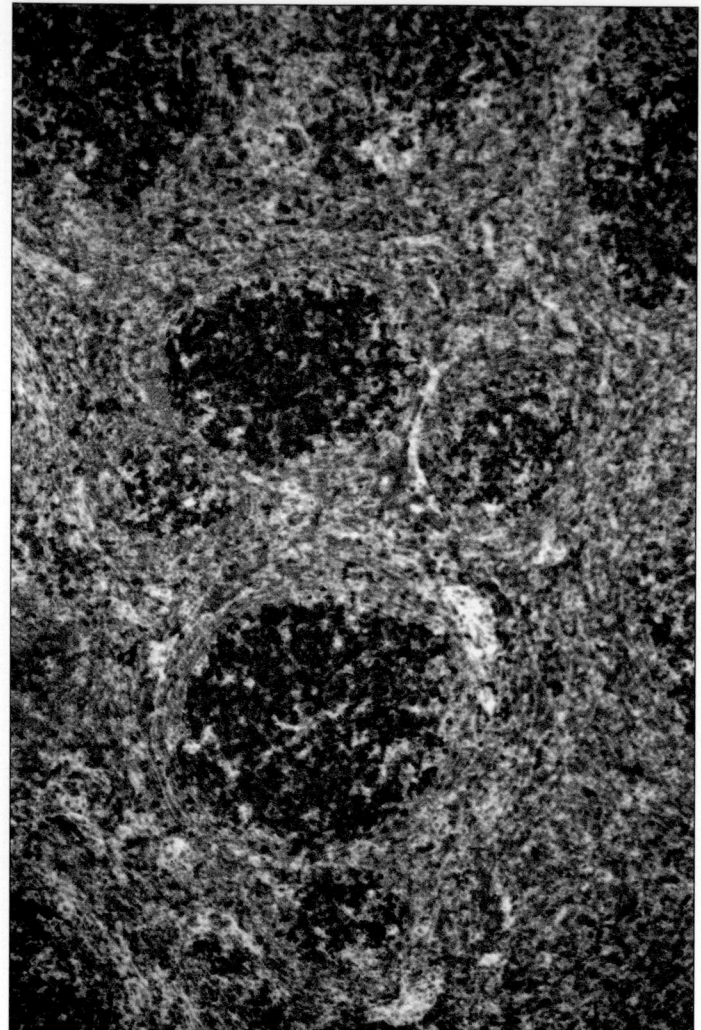

Fig. 11.46 Follicular lymphoma, bcl-2 stain. The follicles are strongly labeled for bcl-2, consistent with a follicular lymphoma.

of these T cells express the NK marker CD57. Stains such as CD23 and CD35 demonstrate a rich network of follicular dendritic cells, similar to that seen in non-neoplastic follicles.

Clonal immunoglobulin heavy and light chain gene rearrangements are detectable in virtually all cases of follicular lymphoma.[307,449,450] Almost all cases of follicular lymphoma have a cytogenetic abnormality.[451] In addition, evidence of the t(14;18) can be found by a variety of techniques in about 90% of cases.[21,384,452–455] The t(14;18) at the molecular level involves translocation of the *bcl-2* gene on chromosome 18 into the immunoglobulin heavy chain gene, leading to its deregulation and overexpression.[456] Evidence of the t(14;18) can also be detected by sensitive molecular techniques in a high proportion of peripheral blood and bone marrow specimens from these patients, consistent with the disseminated nature of the disease.[457] The chromosome 3q27 region (location of the *bcl-6* gene) is also commonly involved in follicular lymphoma, and appears to be mutually exclusive with t(14;18), at least in the subset of Grade 3 follicular lymphomas.[458] The presence of other cytogenetic abnormalities, such as abnormalities involving chromosome regions 1p21-22, 6q23-26, and the short arm of chromosome 17 may be

associated with adverse prognosis.[451] Mutations of the tumor suppressor gene p53 have been identified in a subset of cases of large-cell transformation.[459,460]

The differential diagnosis of follicular lymphoma versus reactive follicular hyperplasia has already been discussed in the section on reactive follicular hyperplasia. The differential diagnosis with nodular L&H lymphocyte predominance Hodgkin's disease has been discussed in the section on that disease. Follicular lymphoma may also be confused with mantle cell lymphoma and marginal cell lymphoma. Mantle cell lymphoma may have nodular variants in which the germinal centers as well as the mantle zone regions become replaced by neoplastic mantle cells. Cytologically, mantle cell lymphomas are characterized by a homogeneous population of small atypical cells without admixed large cleaved and noncleaved cells. Immunohistochemical studies may be very helpful, as the cells of mantle cell lymphoma often show aberrant coexpression of CD5 or CD43, as well as bcl-1, very rare findings in follicular lymphoma. Marginal zone lymphomas may mimic follicular lymphoma by virtue of colonization of reactive germinal centers by neoplastic cells. The identification of typical areas of marginal zone lymphoma is helpful on low-power magnification. The identification of moderate to abundant pale cytoplasm and the lack of truly cleaved nuclei are helpful features on high-power magnification. Bcl-2 oncoprotein may be immunohistochemically positive in follicles colonized by marginal cell lymphoma, but evidence of a t(14;18) is lacking.

SMALL LYMPHOCYTIC LYMPHOMA

The WHO recognizes the definition of small lymphocytic lymphoma as the lymph node equivalent of classic B-cell chronic lymphocytic leukemia. According to the WHO definition, the diagnosis of small lymphocytic lymphoma (but not chronic lymphocytic leukemia) can be made only in the absence of bone marrow or blood involvement, as chronic lymphocytic leukemia also infiltrates lymph nodes, liver, and spleen, and perhaps even extranodal sites such as skin, breast, and ocular adnexae. One group has recommended designating cases as chronic lymphocytic leukemia if patients have greater than 5000/mm³ circulating lymphocytes and greater than 30% lymphocytes in the marrow but the distinction is arbitrary.[461]

In the past, the equivalent Working Formulation morphologic category of low-grade small lymphocytic lymphoma included other clinicopathologic entities characterized by diffuse proliferation of relatively small lymphoid cells, including marginal zone B-cell lymphoma (particularly the extranodal variants) and lymphoplasmacytic lymphoma/immunocytoma. These other entities are now recognized in the WHO Classification as separate categories of B-cell lymphoma.[14]

Small lymphocytic lymphoma is almost always seen in adults over age 40 years, with a peak in the seventh decade.[462–465] Most patients present with generalized lymphadenopathy. Many of these patients have or will develop involvement of the peripheral blood at some point in their course. Regardless of the clinical symptoms, the patients are usually in a high stage at diagnosis, with frequent bone marrow, liver, and spleen involvement. Similar to low-grade follicular lymphoma, the clinical course is indolent, with occasional spontaneous regressions, slow progression, and numerous relapses occurring over time, seemingly independent of treatment. In about 10–20% of patients, transformation to large cell lymphoma occurs (Richter's syndrome).[466] As discussed above, rare cases may transform to a lymphoma with a Hodgkin-like histologic appearance or even true Hodgkin's disease.[339,467] Combinations of purine

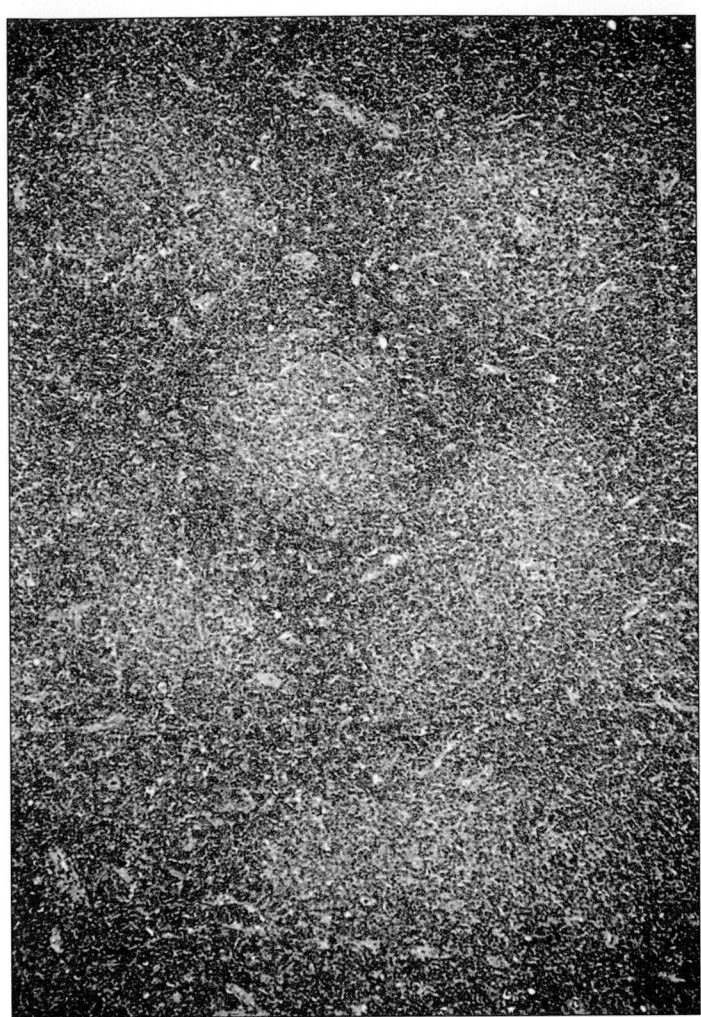

Fig. 11.47 Small lymphocytic lymphoma. The pale areas are termed proliferation centers.

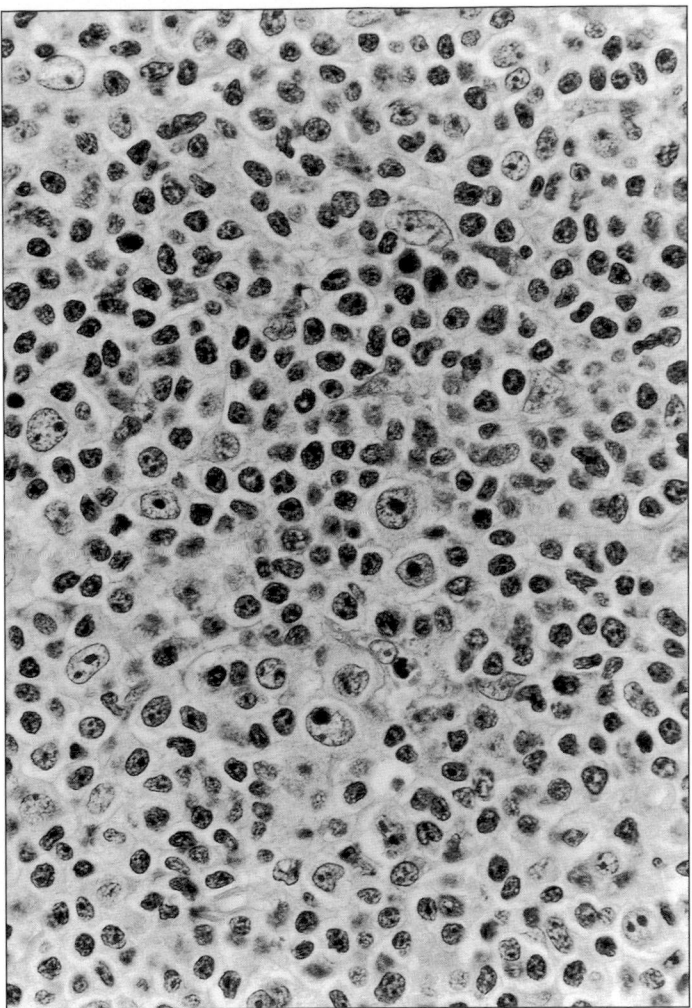

Fig. 11.48 Small lymphocytic lymphoma. Although most of the cells are small lymphocytes with round nuclear contours, a population of larger cells with prominent nucleoli is also characteristic of this lymphoma.

analogs, such as fludarabine or 2-chlorodeoxyadenosine, with alkylating agents are emerging as treatments. Also seen has been the emergence of two monoclonal antibodies, rituximab and anti-CD52, as therapy.[467] The presence of immunoglobulin heavy chain gene mutation and ZAP-70 protein in small lymphocytic lymphoma cells have been associated with more aggressive disease.[468]

At low magnification, diffuse effacement of lymph node architecture is usually seen, although occasionally germinal centers are still present.[469] There is often infiltration of the perinodal adipose tissues. In many cases, particularly cases associated with a peripheral blood lymphocytosis, pale areas can be discerned, representing proliferation centers (also called pseudofollicles) (Fig. 11.47).[470] The mitotic rate is generally low, but higher numbers may be found in the proliferation centers. At high magnification, the predominant cell type is a small lymphocyte with condensed chromatin (Fig. 11.48). Although the cells are usually round, a mild degree of irregularity may be present.[14] Nucleoli are generally small, but may be moderate in size in some cases. Cytoplasm is generally scant, although some cases may have cells with somewhat plasmacytoid features. In addition to these small cells, a population of larger cells is always present. These cells may be medium sized, termed *prolymphocytes*

or *paraimmunoblasts* or large sized, termed *immunoblasts*. Both have round nuclei with a vesicular chromatin pattern and medium-to large-sized nucleoli. It is the presence of these cells in aggregates that give rise to the proliferation centers appreciated at low magnification. Large numbers of other cells, including eosinophils, neutrophils, and histiocytes, are not found. Rarely, paraimmunoblasts can predominate, termed the *paraimmunoblastic variant of small lymphocytic lymphoma*; these cases have a worse prognosis than other cases of small lymphocytic lymphoma, but still better than cases of de novo diffuse large cell lymphoma.[471] However, when immunoblasts predominate and form sheets, the prognosis is significantly worse, indicating transformation to a higher-grade lymphoma. In rare cases, the tumor cells may be confined solely to a marginal zone, perifollicular, or interfollicular distribution.[472] Fine needle aspiration biopsy smears show a preponderance of small lymphoid cells with round, regular nuclear membranes and clumped chromatin, with occasional admixed cells of similar size with an open chromatin pattern and a prominent nucleolus, representing prolymphocytes (Fig. 11.49).

By definition, small lymphocytic lymphoma is a neoplasm of B cell lineage, expressing CD20 in both paraffin and frozen sections (Fig. 11.50; see Table 11.16). Immunoglobulin expression with light

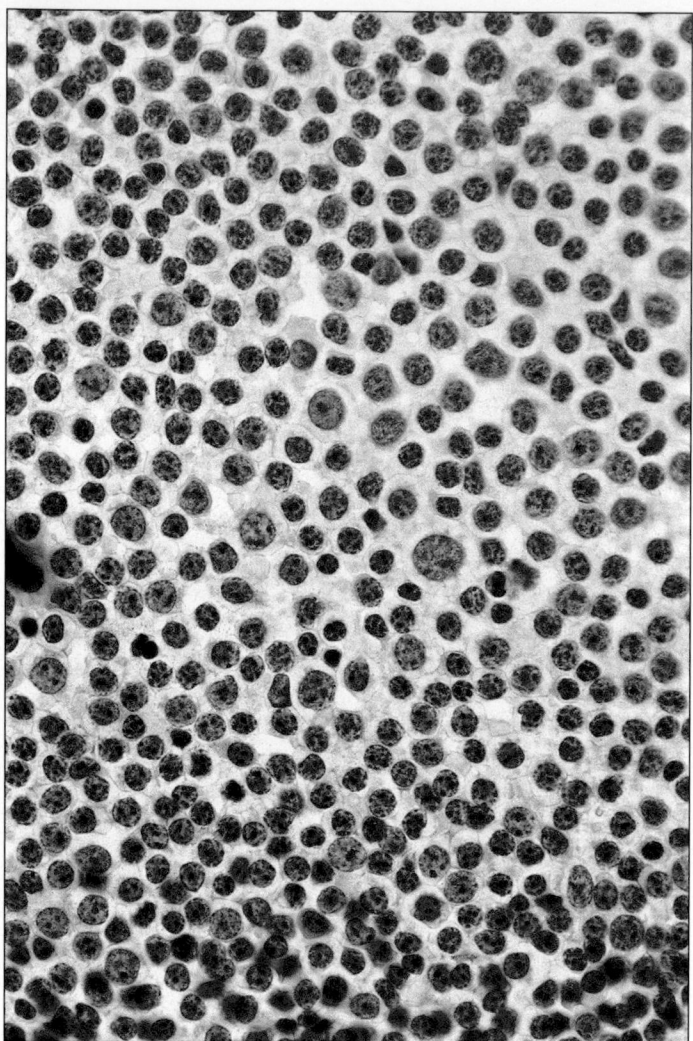

Fig. 11.49 Small lymphocytic lymphoma, fine needle aspiration. Similar to histologic sections, the cells consist mainly of small lymphocytes with round nuclear contours, with a minority population of larger cells with evident nucleoli.

found in about 20–30% of cases.[481–483] Deletions at 13q14 occur in approximately 50% of cases. Deletions at 11q22-q23, 6p21, or 17p13 (p53 locus) occur in approximately 20%, 5%, and 10% of cases, respectively.[484–486] The chromosomal abnormalities del(17)(p13.1) or del(11)(q22-q23) are associated with aggressive clinical course and inferior survival time and may predict poor response to rituximab therapy.[487,488]

The differential diagnosis of small lymphocytic lymphoma is wide and includes reactive lymphoid proliferations, follicular lymphoma, and other low- to intermediate-grade diffuse small cell B-cell lymphomas. Small lymphocytic lymphoma can usually be distinguished from reactive lymphoid proliferations by its monotonous cellular population. In difficult cases, paraffin section immunohistochemical stains are of great use, demonstrating a diffuse B-cell infiltrate, most often with aberrant coexpression of CD43 and CD5. Flow cytometry shows light chain restriction and aberrant CD5 expression. If proliferation centers are prominent, one may mistake small lymphocytic lymphoma for follicular lymphoma. However, the proliferation centers are always more poorly defined than neoplastic follicles and lack small cleaved cells. They may contain follicular dendritic cells by immunohistochemistry, but the network is never as well developed as seen in follicular lymphoma. Small lymphocytic lymphoma may be very difficult to distinguish from other low- to intermediate-grade diffuse small cell B-cell lymphomas. The presence of proliferation centers or CD23 positivity would favor small lymphocytic lymphoma over the other neoplasms. The presence of scattered larger cells also distinguishes small lymphocytic lymphoma from mantle cell lymphoma, whereas the identification of a t(11;14) would favor mantle cell lymphoma. The cells of marginal zone B-cell lymphoma generally have more abundant cytoplasm than small lymphocytic lymphoma, and the former disease commonly has extranodal sites of involvement. Although small lymphocytic lymphoma may show somewhat plasmacytoid features, the presence of marked plasmacytic differentiation with Dutcher bodies and Russell bodies is more consistent with lymphoplasmacytic lymphoma. Clinically, patients with lymphoplasmacytic lymphoma often have large M protein spikes or even symptoms of Waldenström macroglobulinemia. The presence of Reed-Sternberg cells in rare cases of small lymphocytic lymphoma may cause confusion with classical Hodgkin's disease, as previously discussed.

chain restriction is seen in virtually all cases by flow cytometry/frozen section studies. Characteristically, both mu and delta heavy chains are present. Flow cytometry studies demonstrate that the level of immunoglobulin expression is typically low. When plasmacytoid features are seen histologically, immunoglobulin light chain restriction can also be demonstrated in paraffin sections. Aberrant expression of the paraffin T/myeloid marker CD43 is found in about 80% of cases (see Fig. 11.50) and aberrant expression of the flow cytometry/frozen section T-cell marker CD5 is found in about 80–90% of cases.[4,101,473,474] In contrast to most other low-grade B-cell lymphomas, CD23 is usually positive (unlike mantle cell lymphoma), and CD10 is usually negative (unlike follicular lymphoma).[13,14,475,476] Monoclonal rearrangement of the immunoglobulin heavy and light chain genes is seen in virtually all cases. The mutational status of the immunoglobulin VH genes appears to define two prognostically distinct types of small lymphocytic lymphoma/chronic lymphocytic leukemia: one group is consistent with naive B cells, while the other group appears to be derived from postgerminal center B cells.[477–480] Trisomy of chromosome 12 is

NODAL MARGINAL ZONE B-CELL LYMPHOMA

The normal marginal zone is the area just peripheral to the mantle zone of a secondary follicle. It is best seen in the spleen and is not easy to appreciate in normal lymph nodes outside of the abdominal region. Nodal marginal zone B-cell lymphoma is a low-grade lymphoma theoretically showing differentiation similar to normal marginal zone B cells, cells that may differentiate into either monocytoid B cells or plasma cells. It represents the entity of monocytoid B-cell lymphoma of the lymph node and is the nodal counterpart to splenic or extranodal marginal zone B-cell lymphoma.[489–494] Extranodal marginal zone B-cell lymphoma is also known colloquially as lymphoma of mucosa-associated lymphoid tissues (MALToma),[197,489,491,495] a term that may not be the most appropriate because this lymphoma may occur in extranodal sites that are not usually thought of as mucosa-associated. In the Working Formulation, all variants of marginal zone B-cell lymphoma were probably classified as low grade, small lymphocytic, with or without plasmacytoid differentiation.[386]

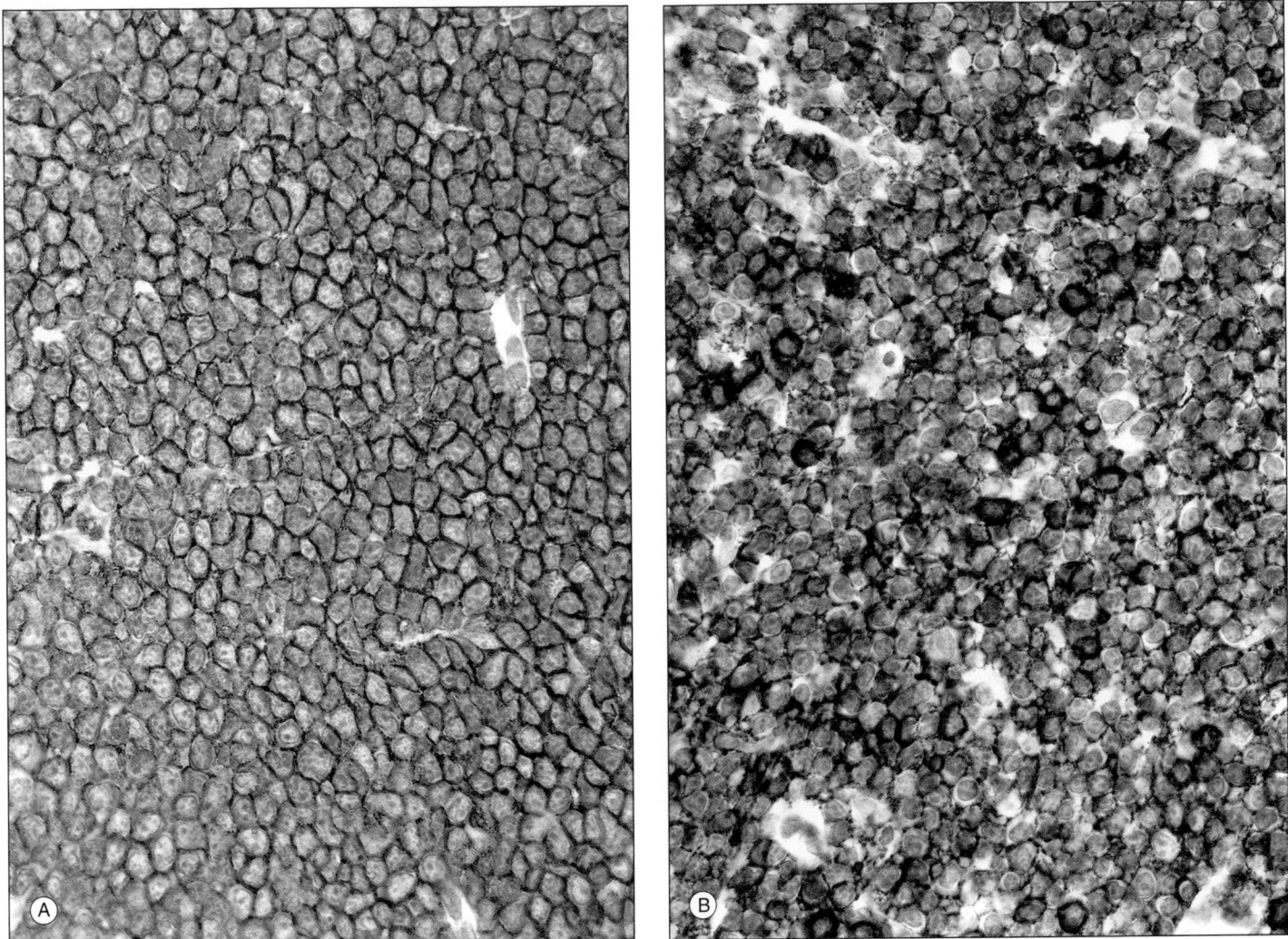

Fig. 11.50 Small lymphocytic lymphoma. **A,** CD20 stain. Diffuse positivity is present, consistent with a B-cell lymphoma. **B,** CD43 stain. Diffuse positivity is also present, consistent with aberrant coexpression in a B-cell lymphoma. The most strongly stained cells probably represent reactive T cells.

Nodal marginal zone B-cell lymphoma is most often a disease of the elderly, with a median age of about 60 years; the male/female ratio is about 1:2.[408,496–498] Rare cases have been reported in children and young adults.[499] It accounts for <2% of lymphomas. Patients usually present with isolated or generalized lymphadenopathy. Bone marrow involvement occurs in 40%, splenomegaly in 20%, hepatomegaly in 15%, and involvement of the peripheral blood occurs in 5%. The presence of bone marrow or peripheral blood involvement adversely affects prognosis.[500] Nodal marginal zone B-cell lymphoma is an indolent lymphoma, but transformation to large cell lymphoma occurs in about 10% of cases and is another poor prognostic sign.[497] MALTomas typically occur in patients with a long history of autoimmune disease or antigenic stimulation, such as Sjögren syndrome, Hashimoto thyroiditis, or *Helicobacter* gastritis.[491,501–503] Many different extranodal organs may be affected, particularly the gastrointestinal tract, salivary glands, and conjunctiva.[489,491,501,502,504] Even organs without true mucosa, such as thyroid, soft tissue, and skin, may be affected. Patients with MALToma tend to have recurrences in other extranodal sites. If lymph nodes are involved, they tend to be regional nodes draining an area affected by MALToma.

At low magnification, involved lymph nodes may have partial or complete effacement of architecture.[197] Partial involvement preferentially affects the areas adjacent to the follicular mantle, the so-called marginal zone. In some cases, lymph nodes contain another lymphoma, usually follicular type.[497] At high magnification, the typical neoplastic monocytoid B cell has a small to medium-sized nucleus with round to slightly irregular nuclear outlines (Fig. 11.51). The chromatin is usually condensed and nucleoli are indistinct. A very characteristic feature is the presence of moderately abundant clear to pale cytoplasm. The cell membranes are often distinct and highlighted when two cells with clear or pale cytoplasm abut one another. Immunoblasts are often scattered among the monocytoid B cells. Lymphoid cells with plasmacytoid features (including Dutcher bodies) and mature plasma cells may also be present, either admixed with the other cells, or segregated apart, often next to the capsule or trabeculae. In some cases, one can see scattered neutrophils, similar to what may be seen in reactive monocytoid proliferations.

All marginal zone B-cell lymphomas are of B lineage and almost all cases express surface immunoglobulin (see Table 11.16). About one-half of cases also express cytoplasmic immunoglobulin

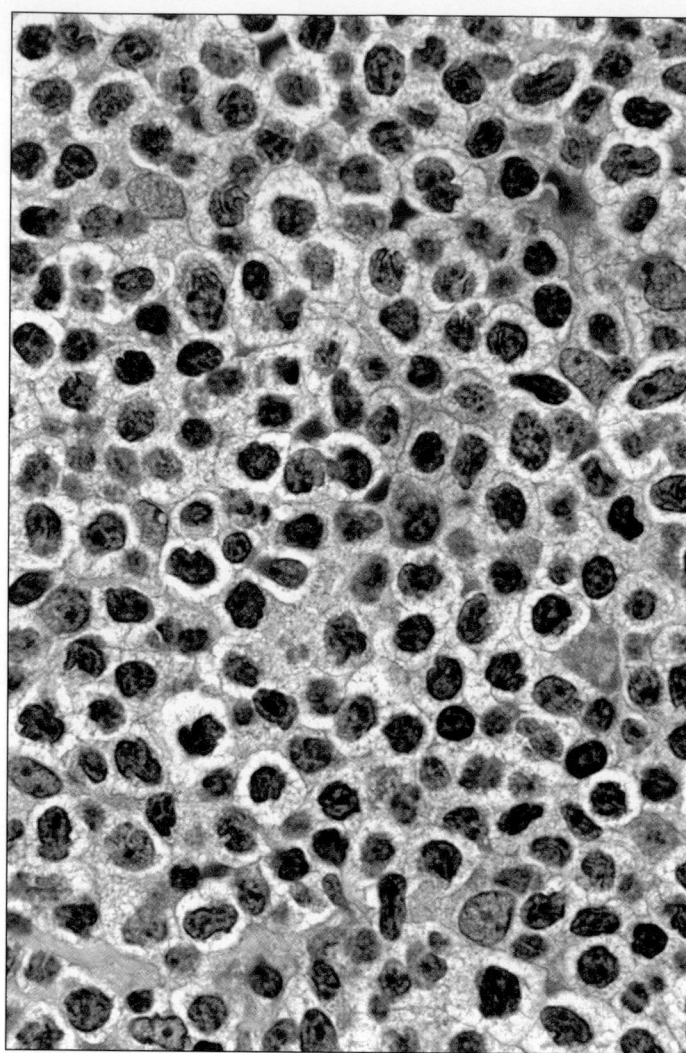

Fig. 11.51 Marginal zone B-cell lymphoma. Medium-sized cells with small bland nuclei and abundant clear cytoplasm are present.

detectable in paraffin sections, particularly cases with plasmacytoid differentiation.[505] About one-half of cases show aberrant coexpression of CD43, a helpful feature also demonstrable in paraffin sections.[506] CD5, CD10, and CD23 are usually negative.[7,109] Bcl-2 immunohistochemistry is usually positive. Monoclonal immunoglobulin heavy and light chain gene rearrangements are usually detectable, but *bcl-1* and *bcl-2* genes are germline.[507,508] Trisomy 3 has been detected in a majority of cases of both nodal and extranodal cases, and numeric abnormalities of chromosomes 12 and 18 have also been found.[508–516]

The differential diagnosis of marginal zone B-cell lymphoma includes the other low to intermediate grade B-cell lymphomas. The cells of marginal zone B-cell lymphoma generally have more abundant pale cytoplasm than the cells of small lymphocytic lymphoma, and proliferation centers are not seen. Coexpression of CD5 is usually seen in small lymphocytic lymphoma, but is present in only 10% of cases of marginal zone B-cell lymphoma.[517] Marginal zone B-cell lymphoma may be difficult to distinguish from lymphoplasmacytic lymphoma, because both may have areas with marked plasmacytoid differentiation, including Dutcher bodies. The presence of cells with

more abundant pale cytoplasm would exclude lymphoplasmacytic lymphoma. Mantle cell lymphoma contains a more homogeneous population of cells and lacks large transformed cells, and the cells have a greater degree of nuclear irregularities. Coexpression of CD5 is usually seen, distinct from marginal zone B-cell lymphoma.[517] Occasionally, marginal zone B-cell lymphoma is difficult to distinguish from follicular lymphoma because the cells of marginal zone B-cell lymphoma may colonize reactive germinal centers. Attention should be given to the cytologic features of cells, both within and outside the germinal centers. Truly small cleaved cells are absent within the germinal centers, whereas typical marginal zone B cells are found both within and outside the germinal centers. One must keep in mind, however, that true follicular lymphoma may also be found composite with marginal zone B-cell lymphoma.[497] Marginal zone B-cell lymphoma may be very difficult to distinguish histologically from lymph node involvement by hairy cell leukemia. However, the clinical circumstances are very different, as lymph node involvement by hairy cell leukemia never occurs without marked splenomegaly and obvious changes in the blood or bone marrow.

LYMPHOPLASMACYTIC LYMPHOMA/WALDENSTRÖM MACROGLOBULINEMIA

In the WHO Classification, lymphoplasmacytic lymphoma/ Waldenström macroglobulinemia are considered together as a low-grade lymphoma of small lymphocytes, plasma cells, and transitional forms between the two. It was known as lymphoplasmacytoid lymphoma in the REAL classification, small lymphocytic with plasmacytoid differentiation in the Working Formulation, and lymphoplasmacytic immunocytoma in the Updated Kiel classification.[14,386,387] It is an uncommon lymphoma, comprising about 1–2% of non-Hodgkin's lymphomas in the United States, and remains a diagnosis of exclusion.[518] It is a disease of the elderly. Some patients present with symptoms of Waldenström macroglobulinemia, with high amounts of a monoclonal serum paraprotein of IgM type, often with symptoms of hyperviscosity, whereas others present with symptoms resembling small lymphocytic lymphoma, with generalized lymphadenopathy with or without splenomegaly, and without paraproteinemia.[463] At least a portion of Waldenström macroglobulinemia cases are familial.[519] Dermal and neurologic complications may occur as a results of IgM deposits.[520] The clinical course is generally indolent, but transformation to large cell lymphoma, usually an immunoblastic lymphoma with plasmacytoid features, may occur in 5–10% of cases and indicates a poor prognosis.

Histologically, there is diffuse architectural effacement. Proliferation centers are not present, but in occasional cases the germinal centers are still present. At high magnification, there is a mixed population of small lymphocytes, plasmacytoid lymphocytes, and plasma cells (Fig. 11.52). Scattered plasmacytoid immunoblasts are also often found. In occasional cases, numerous plasmacytoid immunoblasts may be present (polymorphous immunocytoma); these cases may be classified as diffuse mixed small and large cell with plasmacytoid differentiation in the Working Formulation, since they may be more aggressive. Dutcher bodies are usually frequently and easily identified and Russell bodies may also be present. Scattered epithelioid histiocytes may be present and occasionally marked infiltration may be seen, masking the lymphoma or simulating T-cell lymphoma.[521] Mast cells may also be numerous. Rare cases may contain numerous histiocytes containing crystals of monotypic immunoglobulin.[522,523]

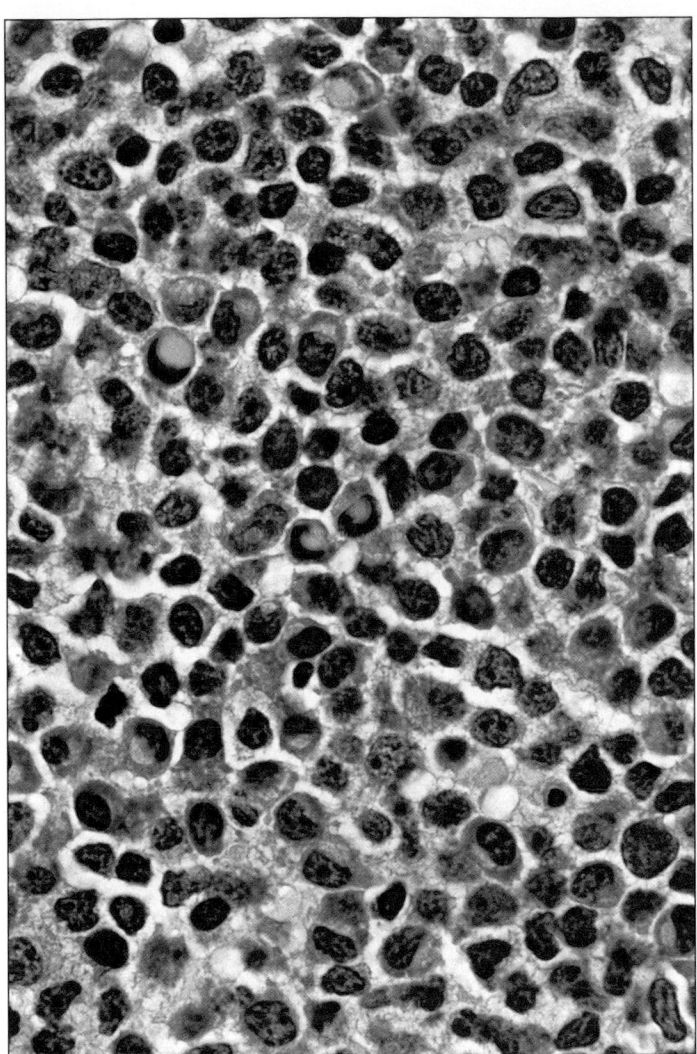

Fig. 11.52 Lymphoplasmacytic lymphoma. There is a range of lymphoplasmacytic differentiation. Note the numerous Dutcher bodies in this field.

which it is categorized.[529] In contrast to lymphoplasmacytic lymphomas unassociated with paraproteinemia and with frequent t(9;14)(p13;q32) translocations, IgH translocations are not found in Waldenström macroglobulinemia. However, Waldenström macroglobulinemia tumor cells often have deletions of 6q21.[520]

The differential diagnosis of lymphoplasmacytic lymphoma includes reactive lymphoplasmacytic proliferations, other low to intermediate grade B-cell lymphomas, Hodgkin's disease, and T-cell lymphoma. The presence of more than rare numbers of Dutcher bodies would favor lymphoplasmacytic lymphoma over a reactive lymphoplasmacytic proliferation, but the distinction is perhaps most reliably accomplished by paraffin section staining for cytoplasmic immunoglobulin: polytypic in reactive proliferations and monotypic in lymphoplasmacytic lymphoma. All other low to intermediate grade B-cell lymphomas may have lymphoplasmacytic differentiation. The diagnosis of lymphoplasmacytic differentiation is almost a diagnosis of exclusion – the lymphoma must lack evidence of other types of lymphomas. The presence of proliferation centers indicates a diagnosis of small lymphocytic lymphoma rather than lymphoplasmacytic lymphoma, despite the presence of lymphoplasmacytic features. Similarly, the presence of areas of neoplastic monocytoid B cells indicates a diagnosis of marginal zone B-cell lymphoma. The presence of a homogeneous population of lymphoplasmacytoid cells with irregular nuclei favors mantle cell lymphoma, a diagnosis that may be supported by immunophenotypic studies demonstrating CD5 positivity. Even follicular lymphoma may rarely show lymphoplasmacytic features with numerous Dutcher bodies. Hodgkin's disease and peripheral T-cell lymphoma may have scattered plasma cells and epithelioid histiocytes, which can simulate lymphoplasmacytic lymphoma. However, the plasma cells are polyclonal and both neoplasms feature neoplastic elements (Reed-Sternberg cells in Hodgkin's disease and a spectrum of atypical lymphoid cells in peripheral T-cell lymphoma) not present in lymphoplasmacytic lymphoma.

MANTLE CELL LYMPHOMA

Mantle cell lymphoma has morphologic, immunologic, biologic, and molecular/genetic features distinct from other non-Hodgkin's B-cell lymphomas and has emerged in the past two decades as one of the better-defined and more easily recognizable entities in the WHO classification. Mantle cell lymphoma was previously recognized in the 1970s as 'centrocytic lymphoma' by Lennert in the Kiel classification and 'intermediate differentiated lymphocytic lymphoma' by Berard.[532–534] In the Working Formulation, most mantle cell lymphomas were categorized as intermediate grade 'diffuse small cleaved cell' lymphomas. Improved and new immunologic techniques and molecular/genetic studies subsequently led to the prevailing concept that these tumors likely originate from cells of the mantle zone, and not germinal center cells, resulting in the now favored terminology 'mantle cell lymphoma.'[110]

Mantle cell lymphoma is relatively common, comprising up to 10% of lymphomas in the United States. It occurs most commonly in elderly adults, and is rare in children. The male/female ratio is at least 2:1. Patients often present in advanced stage with generalized lymphadenopathy and frequent involvement of spleen and bone marrow. Peripheral blood involvement is also quite common (25–30%), usually occurring with widely disseminated disease, but occasionally presenting as a primarily leukemic picture without prominent lymphadenopathy. Other commonly involved extranodal sites include Waldeyer's ring and the gastrointestinal tract, the latter

The immunophenotypic hallmark of this lymphoma is the uniform presence of monotypic cytoplasmic and surface immunoglobulin of IgM type, usually easily demonstrated in paraffin sections (see Table 11.16). As expected, these neoplasms usually express B-lineage markers and often show aberrant coexpression of CD43 in paraffin sections.[524] The neoplastic cells usually do not stain for CD5, CD10, or CD23 in frozen sections or flow cytometric studies, but exceptions occur. Approximately 50% of lymphoplasmacytic lymphoma cases may have a t(9;14)(p13;q32), del(7)(32), or rearrangement of the PAX-5 gene.[525–528] These genetic abnormalities are not specific to lymphoplasmacytic lymphoma, but are seen in other lymphomas with plasmacytic differentiation and are usually not associated with paraproteinemia.[465,520,529–531] Monoclonal gene rearrangements of the immunoglobulin heavy and light chain genes are detected in virtually all cases of lymphoplasmacytic lymphomas. The genetic makeup of the plasma cells in Waldenström macroglobulinemia appears to be different than other lymphomas associated with plasma cells, including the lymphoplasmacytic lymphomas with

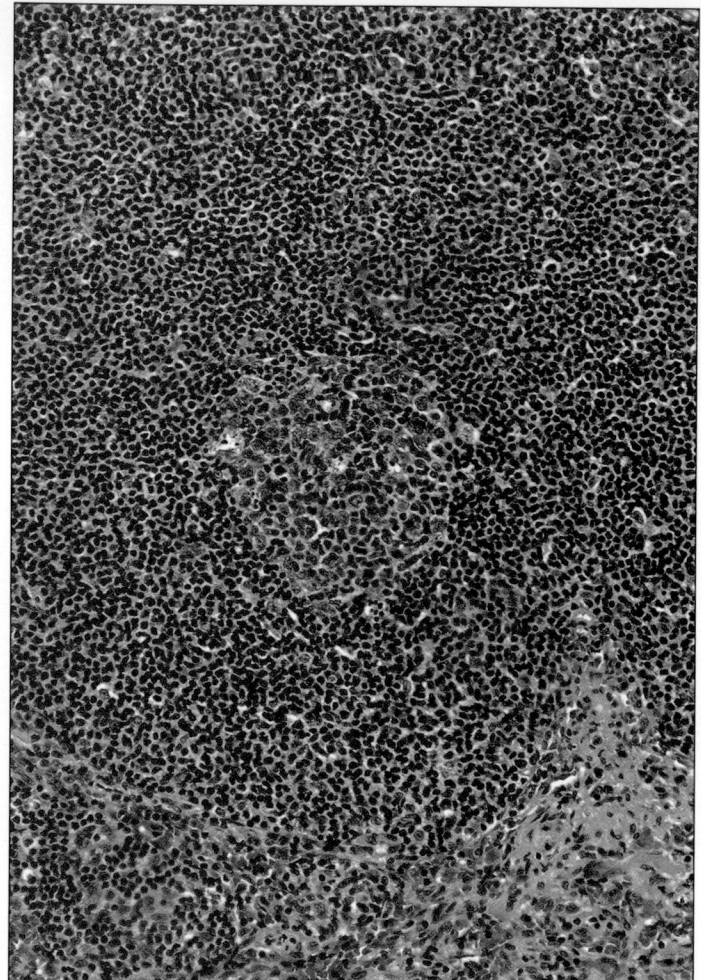

Fig. 11.53 Mantle cell lymphoma. A mantle zone architecture is present, with expanded mantle zones, with a small reactive germinal center.

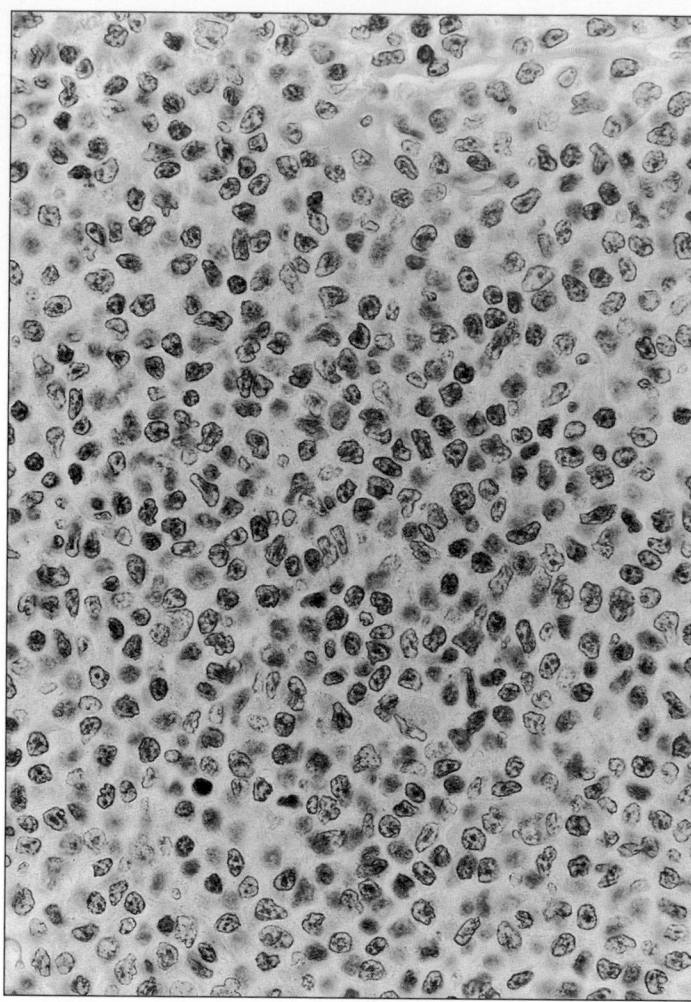

Fig. 11.54 Mantle cell lymphoma. A homogeneous population of small lymphoid cells with irregular nuclear contours is seen.

characteristically displaying multiple polypoid masses (multiple lymphomatous polyposis).[535]

Mantle cell lymphoma is more aggressive than indolent low-grade B-cell lymphomas, with a median survival measured at 3–5 years.[536] However, similar to the low-grade lymphomas, there is no plateau in survival (patients are incurable) and relapses occur independently of time.[466,537,538] Unlike other B-cell lymphomas, transformation to large cell lymphoma is rare, if it occurs at all; but transformation to a more aggressive 'blastoid' variant is not uncommon and portends a poor prognosis.[13,537,538]

Architecturally, three patterns may be seen. Most often, there is diffuse effacement of architecture. Occasionally, the neoplastic infiltrate replaces the mantle zone of reactive follicles, leaving naked germinal centers surrounded by thickened cuffs (Fig. 11.53); this 'mantle zone' pattern may be a focal finding or may be present throughout the biopsy.[539] In a subset of cases, the germinal centers may also become replaced by the neoplastic infiltrate, leaving large nodules of mantle cell lymphoma. Cytologically, there is usually a highly monomorphic population of small- to medium-sized lymphocytes with condensed chromatin, inconspicuous nucleoli, and irregular nuclear outlines (Fig. 11.54). The nuclear irregularities are often marked, with abrupt deep indentations. Large transformed

lymphoid cells, commonly scattered about in other low-grade B-cell lymphomas (including CLL/SLL and follicular lymphomas), are noticeably rare or absent in mantle cell lymphoma. The cellular monotony and lack of transformed cells provides a valuable histologic clue to the diagnosis. It is important, however, not to confuse residual germinal centers overrun by tumor, which may appear as loose clusters of large cells, for 'proliferation centers' of transformed tumor cells. Scattered epithelioid histiocytes are also commonly seen in mantle cell lymphoma and can be helpful in suggesting the diagnosis. Fine needle aspiration biopsy smears of mantle cell lymphoma show small lymphoid cells with irregular nuclear contours. The chromatin pattern is usually less clumped or coarse than that seen in small lymphocytic or follicular small cleaved cell lymphoma.[540]

Mantle cell lymphoma has several cytologic variants, which otherwise share immunologic and molecular features with more typical mantle cell lymphoma. The blastoid variants have a high mitotic rate and carry a worse prognosis. The classic blastoid variant resembles lymphoblastic lymphoma in its uniform population with finely dispersed chromatin.[537] The pleomorphic blastoid or anaplastic variant shows a more heterogeneous population with variable numbers of larger cells having large irregular nuclei and prominent nucleoli.[387,541,542] Small round lymphocytes resembling small lymphocytic lymphoma, or rarely, cells with more abundant cytoplasm resembling marginal zone lymphoma may be seen but are not likely of any clinical significance.[541,542]

The immunophenotype of mantle cell lymphoma by flow cytometry or immunohistochemistry usually permits distinction from other B-cell lymphomas, or at least suggests the correct diagnosis (see Table 11.16). Immunophenotypic studies show monotypic B lineage with coexpression of T-cell associated antigen CD5. CD5 may be negative in a small minority of cases.[543] Most cases are CD23 and CD10 negative. FMC7, CD22, and CD79b are typically positive. Interestingly, there is an unexplained slight predilection for lambda as opposed to kappa light chain restriction. Aberrant coexpression of CD43 is also seen in about 60% of cases.

The t(11;14)(q13;q32) translocation is characteristic of mantle cell lymphoma and is diagnostically useful, but not entirely specific. Fluorescent in situ hybridization (FISH) is the most sensitive technique for demonstrating the translocation.[544] Direct PCR and Southern blot techniques are less useful due to variability of breakpoints, necessitating multiple probes and resulting in lower sensitivity. The translocation results in overexpression of the *cyclin D1 (BCL-1, PRAD1, CCND1)* gene by juxtaposition of the *bcl-1* locus on the long arm of chromosome 11 with an immunoglobulin heavy chain gene enhancer sequence on chromosome 14.[541,545-549] Cyclin D1 overexpression may be detected by quantitative reverse transcription PCR, Northern blot (both detecting mRNA), or immunohistochemistry for the *bcl-1* protein.[545,550] Paraffin section immunohistochemistry for cyclin D1 is the most widely available method and when optimally performed provides a very sensitive test for confirming a diagnosis of mantle cell lymphoma.[551] Positive cyclin D1 staining is nuclear. About 10% of cases of mantle cell lymphoma may truly be negative for cyclin D1.[551,552] Some cases of myeloma and hairy cell leukemia are also cyclin D1 positive by immunohistochemistry, but are easily distinguished by other features.[553,554]

The differential diagnosis of mantle cell lymphoma includes other diffuse or occasionally nodular, low- to intermediate-grade B-cell lymphomas. Morphologically, the very monotonous cellular population and lack of proliferation centers or larger transformed cells help distinguish mantle cell lymphoma from small lymphocytic lymphoma, with which it is most often confused. Other low-grade lymphomas, including marginal zone lymphoma and lympho-plasmacytoid lymphoma, also usually show scattered transformed cells or have other distinguishing features (e.g. monocytoid cells, plasmacytoid differentiation) not found in typical mantle cell lymphoma. Mantle cell lymphoma typically, but not exclusively, has greater nuclear irregularities than low-grade B-cell lymphomas. Although both typically coexpress CD5 and CD43, helpful immunophenotypic differences exist between small lymphocytic lymphoma (dim sIg, CD23+, CD79b–, FMC7–) and mantle cell lymphoma (strong sIg, CD23–, CD79b+, FMC7+). As in most of hematopathology, patterns of immunoreactivity are most useful and reliance on a single marker is discouraged. Evidence of cyclin D1 protein overexpression or t(11;14) would strongly favor mantle cell lymphoma.

When mantle cell lymphoma has a mantle zone or nodular pattern, there may be confusion with follicular lymphoma. In the mantle zone pattern, the germinal centers are reactive and not neoplastic, and have the architectural and cytologic characteristics of reactive germinal centers. In the nodular pattern, the nodules are generally somewhat larger than the follicles of follicular lymphoma (because they encompass both the region of the germinal center and the mantle zone). In addition, the follicles of follicular lymphoma virtually always include at least some large cells, whereas the cells

of mantle cell lymphoma are usually more homogeneous, without large cells. Follicular lymphoma is negative for *bcl-1* and CD43 whereas mantle cell lymphoma is positive for *bcl-1* and usually shows CD43 coexpression.

The classic blastic variant of mantle cell lymphoma may be very difficult to distinguish from lymphoblastic lymphoma. A history of mantle cell lymphoma or the presence of areas of typical mantle cell lymphoma within the same specimen would favor mantle cell lymphoma. In addition, the cells of mantle cell lymphoma are terminal deoxynucleotidyl transferase (TdT) negative and *bcl-1* positive, whereas TdT is almost always positive and *bcl-1* negative in lymphoblastic lymphoma. Of note, CD10 may occasionally be expressed in blastic mantle cell lymphoma, similar to lymphoblastic lymphoma.

DIFFUSE LARGE B-CELL LYMPHOMAS

Diffuse large B-cell lymphomas constitute a heterogeneous group of diffuse aggressive lymphomas with a significant component of large B-lineage lymphoid cells. The WHO[555] classification and its immediate predecessor REAL[14] schemes combine most diffuse proliferations of large B cells into the single entity known as 'diffuse large B-cell lymphoma.' The category specifically excludes Burkitt's and lymphoblastic lymphomas. The category of diffuse large B-cell lymphoma encompasses diffuse mixed small and large cell, diffuse large cell, and large cell immunoblastic lymphomas of the Working Formulation[386] and centroblastic and B-immunoblastic lymphomas of the Updated Kiel classification.[387] While acknowledging that this "lumping" results in a rather heterogeneous group, the lack of well-defined, clinically relevant subtypes and poor reproducibility of histologic subtyping among even expert hematopathologists provided the rationale for the "lumpers".[14,353,386,408,556-558] This concept has been generally accepted by most researchers, although some investigators maintain immunoblastic lymphomas do more poorly than other large B-cell lymphomas and can be distinguished by high-quality sections.[559] The WHO recognizes a few variants of diffuse large B-cell lymphoma with unique clinicopathologic and histologic features, namely mediastinal large B-cell lymphoma, intravascular large B-cell lymphoma and primary effusion lymphoma (the latter will be discussed later under immunodeficiency related lymphomas).

Diffuse large B-cell lymphomas comprise about one-third of all non-Hodgkin's lymphomas and occur in all age groups, with a median age at presentation of about 60 years.[386] The male/female ratio is about 1.2:1. Most patients present with a single mass, either an enlarged lymph node (two-thirds of cases) or at an extranodal site (one-third of cases). Diffuse large B-cell lymphomas may occur de novo or may represent transformations of various low-grade B-cell lymphomas, including follicular lymphoma, small lymphocytic lymphoma, marginal zone B-cell lymphoma and lymphoplasma-cytoid lymphoma. Various immunodeficiency related large B-cell lymphomas also occur and are discussed later.[556] The International Prognostic Index for Aggressive Lymphomas was designed for large cell lymphoma and works well to stratify patients into clinically important prognostic groups.[394] These lymphomas are generally treated with multidrug chemotherapy, with response rates above 80%, and survival rates of about 60%.[560-562] Relapses generally occur early, with a plateau in survival seen after a few years. Clinical studies combining anti-CD20 monoclonal antibody with chemotherapy have demonstrated improved overall survival in diffuse large cell lymphoma.[563] Mediastinal large B-cell lymphoma occurs as a localized mediastinal mass in younger adults, with a male/female ratio

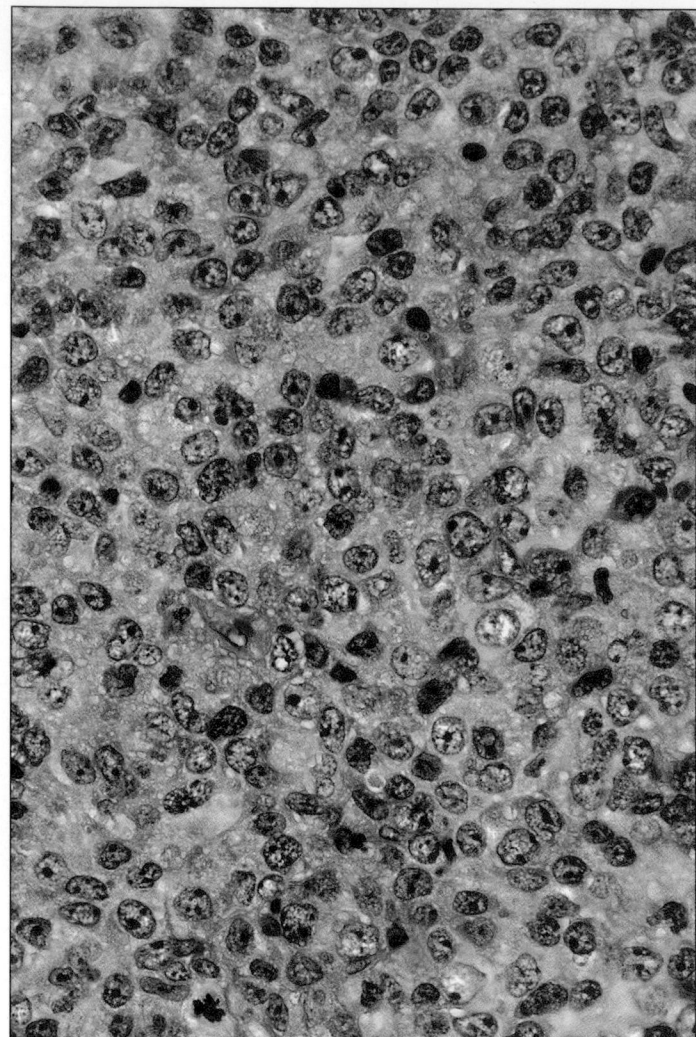

Fig. 11.55 Diffuse large B-cell lymphoma. A mixture of large cleaved and large noncleaved cells is present.

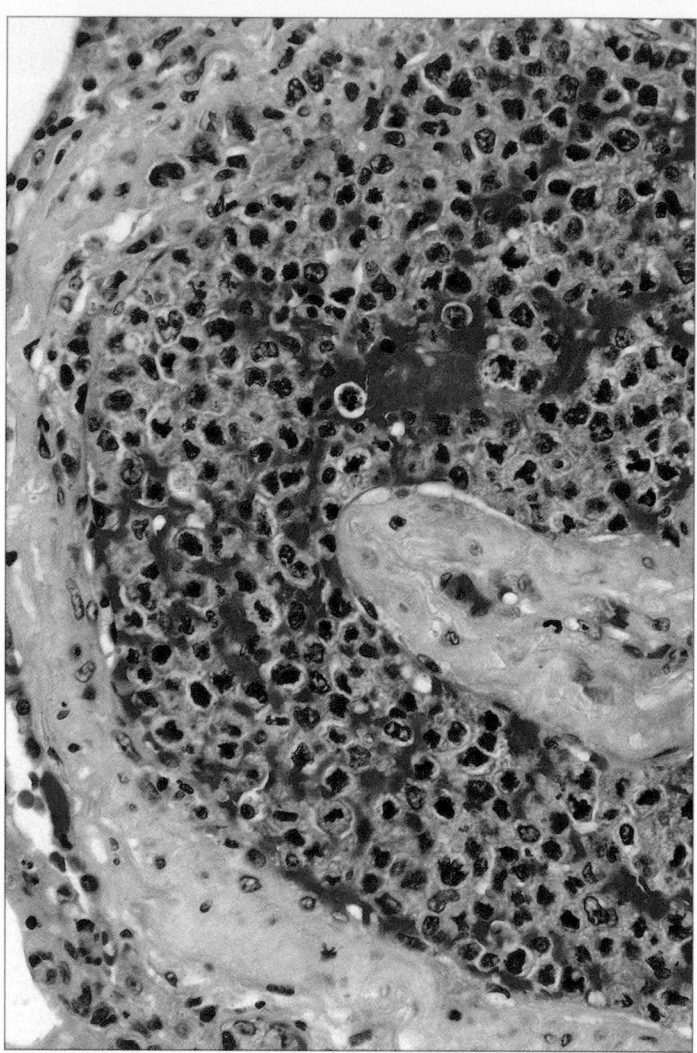

Fig. 11.56 Diffuse large B cell lymphoma, intravascular pattern. The small vessels of the lung are packed with large cell lymphoma cells in this case.

of about 1:1.5 and may be locally aggressive.[557,564–567] Intravascular large B-cell lymphoma is a very aggressive variant with highly variable presentation, including frequent skin involvement.[568]

By definition, these lymphomas have a diffuse architecture (Fig. 11.55). Focal follicular areas may be seen in a minority of cases, representing an antecedent follicular lymphoma that has transformed. Similarly, in a subset of cases, one may recognize areas of other low-grade lymphomas, from which the diffuse large cell lymphoma has transformed. Complete lymph node effacement is common, although partial involvement may be seen. An exclusive or predominant intravascular pattern defines intravascular large B-cell lymphoma (Fig. 11.56).[568] Sclerosis occurs in up to one-half of cases and may consist of broad bands surrounding large areas of tumor, a fine sclerosis enveloping single cells, or a compartmentalizing fibrosis enclosing clusters of cells. The latter pattern is particularly common in mediastinal large B-cell lymphoma (Fig. 11.57).[567] Rarely, large cell lymphomas may form rosette-like structures (Fig. 11.58) or have myxoid or fibrillary stroma.[569,570]

All of these lymphomas have a significant component of large cells, which varies widely in number from scattered large cells to confluent sheets (see Fig. 11.55). Morphologic subtypes that are recognized by the WHO but are not considered separate clinicopathologic entities include centroblastic, immunoblastic, T-cell/histiocyte-rich and anaplastic variants. Centroblasts are large lymphoid cells that have generally round or oval nuclei with vesicular chromatin and 2–3 membrane-bound nucleoli, and usually scant cytoplasm. Nuclear irregularity, however, is quite variable within the centroblastic subtype. Immunoblasts show noncleaved nuclei with a vesicular chromatin pattern and a single prominent central nucleolus and more abundant basophilic cytoplasm, which may demonstrate plasmacytoid differentiation. The immunoblastic variant should have >90% immunoblasts (Fig. 11.59); any lesser number of immunoblasts is categorized as centroblastic variant. The large cells of T-cell/histiocyte-rich variant are not distinctive; rather, this histologic variant is defined by the associated predominant non-neoplastic infiltrate and scarcity of large tumor cells.[365,571–574] In the anaplastic variant, the cells resemble those of poorly differentiated carcinoma, or the cells of anaplastic large cell lymphoma of T-cell lineage. They have large pleomorphic nuclei and often abundant cytoplasm, which may grow in a cohesive pattern or in a sinusoidal

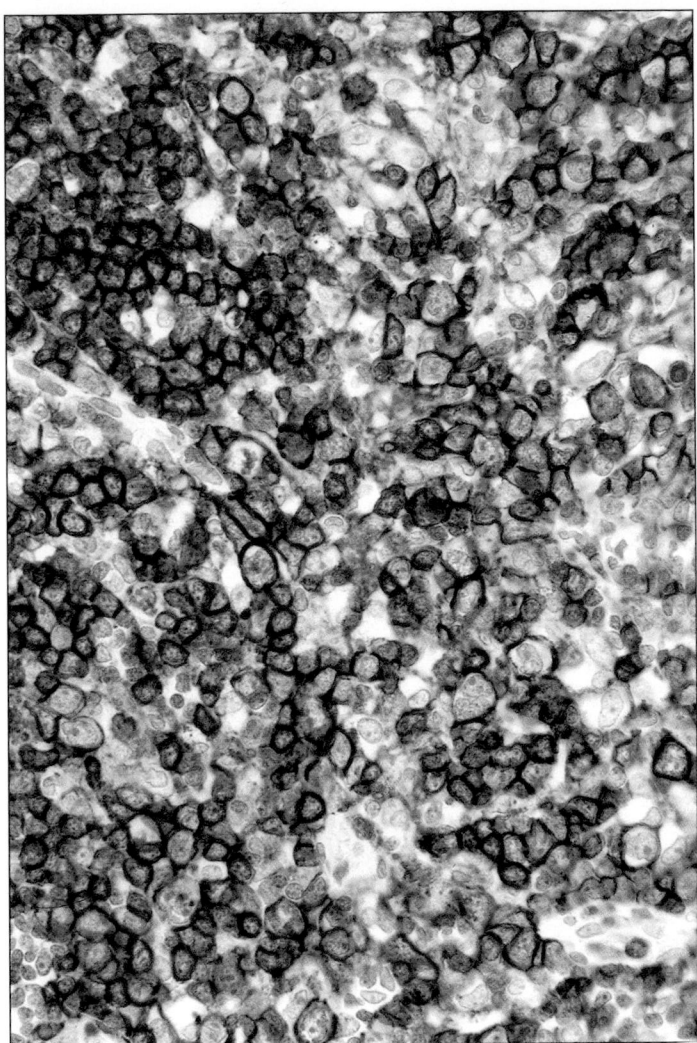

Fig. 11.63 Peripheral T-cell lymphoma, CD45RO stain. The atypical lymphoid cells are labeled with this T-lineage marker. The CD20 stain was negative.

a reactive proliferation. As mentioned above, the histologic distinction between B- and T-cell lymphoma is very difficult, even for experienced hematopathologists. A diffuse proliferation of atypical lymphoid cells, the presence of a spectrum of lymphoid atypia, the presence of more than occasional eosinophils, or a paracortical distribution should all raise the possibility of a T-cell lymphoma. Nonetheless, any histologic suspicions should always be confirmed by immunohistochemical or molecular studies. The presence of CD3+ atypical cells is a good indication of a T-cell lymphoma, but staining for CD45RO or CD43 alone should not be used as definitive evidence for a T-cell lymphoma, because both may stain some B-cell lymphomas. However, positivity for CD45RO or CD43 in the absence of staining for the reliable B-lineage markers CD20 and CD79a is strong presumptive evidence for T-cell lymphoma.

Anaplastic large cell lymphoma (ALCL) is a neoplasm of highly pleomorphic lymphoid cells that show membrane staining of CD30 antigen.[597–599] There is no true equivalent in the Working Formulation, but cases were most likely classified as high-grade, immunoblastic, polymorphous type.[386] The WHO classification recognizes only the T-cell and null-cell types of ALCL, with the B-cell type of ALCL (Updated Kiel classification) no longer recognized as a distinct entity.[14,387] Any lymphomas with morphologic features of ALCL but of B-lineage phenotype should be included within the category of diffuse large B-cell lymphoma in the WHO classification.

Anaplastic large cell lymphoma comprises less than 5% of all non-Hodgkin's lymphomas, but comprises approximately 10–30% of the lymphomas in the pediatric age group.[598,600,601] Most cases of ALCL are positive for the anaplastic large cell lymphoma kinase (ALK) protein, but cases of ALK-negative ALCL are also seen. The WHO classification includes two subtypes of ALCL: primary systemic type and primary cutaneous type. Primary systemic cases of ALK-positive ALCL involve lymph nodes and extranodal sites, which include skin, bone, soft tissue, lung, and liver, and rarely the digestive tract and central nervous system.[602] This lymphomatous presentation is the most common mode of presentation and has a bimodal age distribution, with one peak in childhood and the second in the fifth decade. Patients usually present with advanced stage III to IV disease and show 'B' symptoms, especially high fever. The clinical course in these cases is aggressive, similar to other large cell non-Hodgkin's lymphomas and with a similar response to multidrug chemotherapy. ALK-negative cases less frequently involve extranodal sites.[598] In the second type of presentation, which occurs primarily in adults, there are one to multiple skin papules and nodules without extracutaneous involvement, similar to lymphomatoid papulosis; in fact, there is probably a clinical, histologic, and biologic continuum between this type of ALCL and lymphomatoid papulosis.[603–605] This ALCL type is very indolent, does not require systemic therapy, and waxes and wanes over time, although systemic dissemination may occur eventually, heralding a more aggressive course. Another type of presentation is of patients with a history of another type of lymphoma, including both non-Hodgkin's lymphoma and Hodgkin's disease, transforming to ALCL. The prognosis in these cases is usually poor.

Involved lymph nodes may show complete architectural effacement, but partial involvement is more common. Characteristically, there is preferential infiltration of the sinuses (Fig. 11.64), although extension to the paracortical regions is very common. Often there is capsular fibrosis, with focal extension into the lymph node parenchyma. The mitotic rate is high and a starry-sky pattern may be present. The most common morphologic variant (so-called '*common*' *variant*), which accounts for approximately 70% of cases, contains numerous highly anaplastic cells, often with multilobation or multinucleation (Fig. 11.65).[606,607] Cells with doughnut-shaped nuclei (so-called 'hallmark' cells) and Reed-Sternberg-like cells can be identified. Monomorphic tumor cells with large round to oval nuclei, no multinucleation, and fairly abundant basophilic cytoplasm without a paranuclear hof, may also be present. Usually accompanying the neoplastic population are a mixed population of host reactive cells, including small lymphocytes, histiocytes, plasma cells, eosinophils, and neutrophils. Several variants of ALCL have been recognized. The *lymphohistiocytic variant* accounts for approximately 10% of cases. It contains numerous benign histiocytes, which are present in such quantities as to obscure the tumor cells, which may be smaller than seen in the common variant.[608] The *small cell variant* (5–10% of cases) contains tumor cells that are small with highly irregular nuclear outlines, with scattered anaplastic large cells present singly or in small groups.[609] The relationship to ALCL is inferred by the characteristic immunohistochemical profile as well as progression in some cases to typical ALCL. Other histologic patterns are seen, including *sarcomatoid type*,[610] *signet-ring-like subtype*, and a *Hodgkin-like variant*, featuring Reed-Sternberg-like cells.[611] The Hodgkin-like variant is particularly common in the

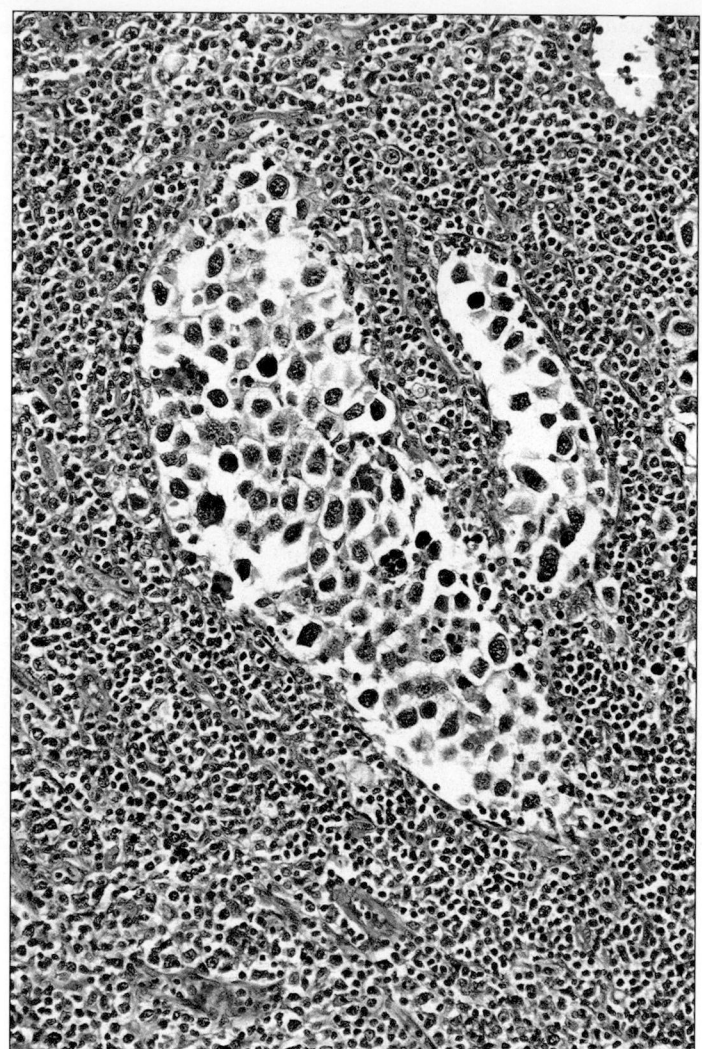

Fig. 11.64 Anaplastic large cell lymphoma. A striking sinusoidal pattern of infiltration is seen.

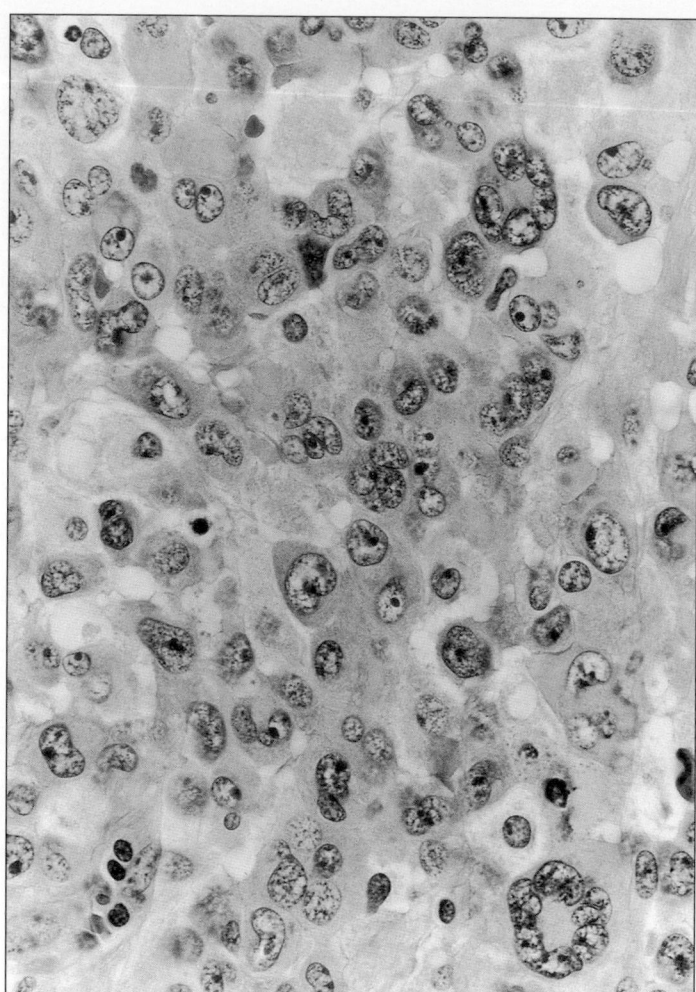

Fig. 11.65 Anaplastic large cell lymphoma. Large pleomorphic cells are seen, including two 'doughnut' cells.

mediastinum and may actually represent an anaplastic variant of nodular sclerosing Hodgkin's disease.

The immunohistochemical hallmark of ALCL is the universal expression of CD30 (Fig. 11.66).[597,598] Typically, all or nearly all of the neoplastic cells show membrane and cytoplasmic (Golgi) positivity for CD30. This is in contrast to CD30 expression when it occurs in most other non-Hodgkin's lymphomas, in which the staining is usually focal. CD45 is positive in only two-thirds of cases, the lowest rate of positivity of any of the major categories of non-Hodgkin's lymphoma.[36] Most cases are of T lineage, expressing CD43, CD3, and CD45RO and showing aberrant T-cell phenotypes in frozen section studies.[597,598] A significant minority are of null cell lineage, although CD43 is still usually positive. Epithelial membrane antigen is usually positive in systemic cases,[612] whereas the cutaneous lymphocyte antigen HECA-452 is usually positive in the cutaneous cases.[603] Occasional cases may be CD15+,[613] and rare cases may be keratin positive.[614] EBV-LMP is absent.

About 90% of ALCL cases have detectable monoclonal gene rearrangements of the beta-T-cell receptor gene, regardless of T-cell antigen expression.[615,616] About one-half of cases of systemic ALCL possess a translocation involving the *Alk* gene on chromosome 2p23.[346,617–619] This is usually a t(2;5) involving the *npm* gene on chromosome 5q35, but may involve the tropomyosin 3 gene on chromosome 1, the *Trk* fusion gene on chromosome 3, the *ATIC* gene on chromosome 2 (manifesting as an (inv)2), or the clathrin heavy chain gene on chromosome 17.[620–624] The incidence of a translocation involving *Alk* is higher in neoplasms from children than from adults, in systemic cases compared to cutaneous cases, and in T-cell or null-cell cases compared to B-cell cases. The *alk-npm* gene product may be detected by paraffin section immunohistochemistry.[625] The staining is usually nuclear, cytoplasmic, and nucleolar when a t(2;5) occurs, and cytoplasmic when the other translocations are involved.[346,622,624,626]

The *differential diagnosis* of ALCL includes metastatic carcinoma and malignant melanomas (covered in the section on metastatic neoplasms), classical Hodgkin's disease (covered in the section on Hodgkin's disease), other large cell lymphomas, and malignant histiocytosis. Anaplastic large cell lymphoma is distinguished from other large cell lymphomas by the combination of its characteristic anaplastic histologic appearance and diffuse positivity for CD30. Most non-Hodgkin's lymphomas usually show negative or focal staining for CD30, with only occasional cases exhibiting diffuse

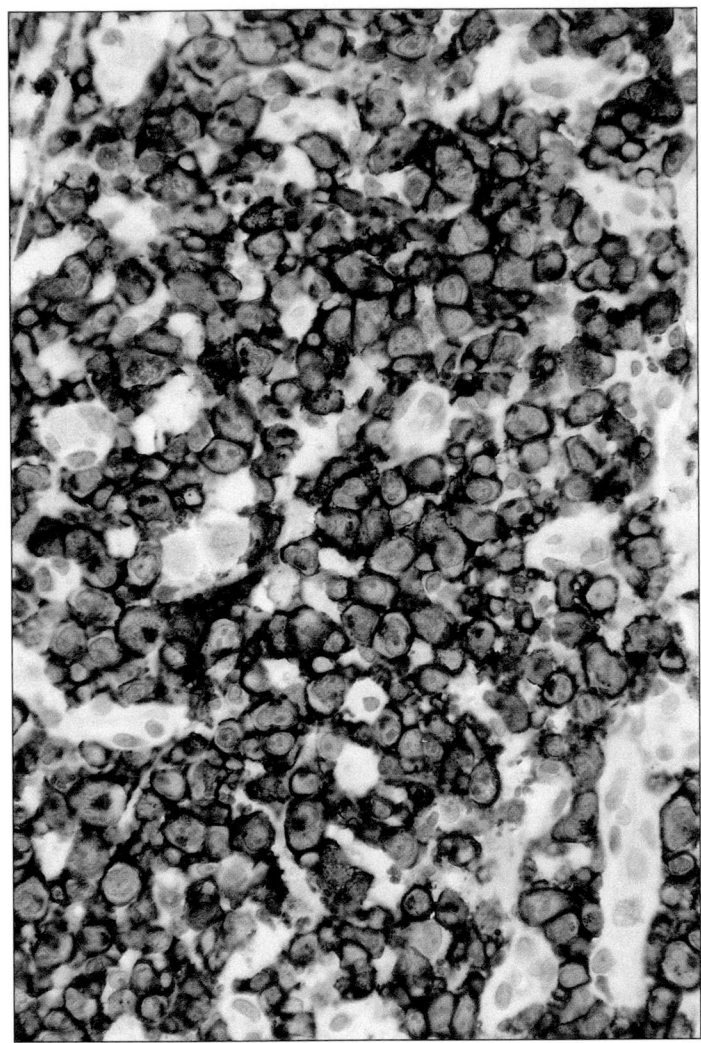

Fig. 11.66 Anaplastic large cell lymphoma, CD30 stain. Diffuse strong reactivity is seen on the tumor cell membranes.

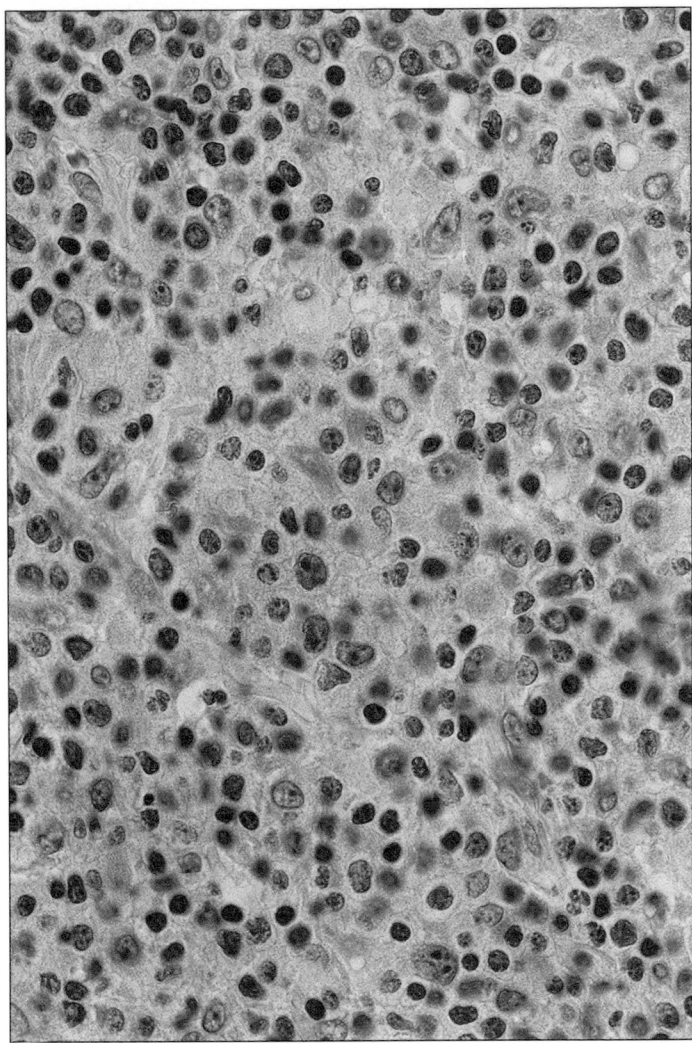

Fig. 11.67 Lymphoepithelioid T-cell (Lennert's) lymphoma. The sheets of epithelioid histiocytes masked the tumor cell population.

positivity. As discussed above, the WHO classification excludes a diagnosis of ALCL in any B-lineage neoplasm, despite the presence of *Alk* rearrangements in rare B-cell lymphomas.[627]

Malignant histiocytosis was described as a sinusoidal neoplasm of histiocytic derivation, but many of the cases previously diagnosed as malignant histiocytosis have been found to be ALCL when studied using modern techniques.[628] Complete immunophenotyping should be performed in any case suspected to be of histiocytic derivation to rule out the possibility of ALCL.

Two other nodal-based T/NK-type lymphomas are lympho-epithelioid lymphoma and angioimmunoblastic T-cell lymphoma. *Lymphoepithelioid T-cell lymphoma (Lennert's lymphoma)* is not so much a specific clinicopathologic entity as it is a peripheral T-cell lymphoma (not otherwise specified) with distinctive histologic features. The characteristic finding is the presence of numerous epithelioid histiocytes throughout the lymph node, as single cells or small clusters, but not forming discrete granulomas (Fig. 11.67).[629] The neoplastic component may be overshadowed by the epithelioid histiocytes unless the biopsy is carefully examined. One should keep in mind that lymphoplasmacytic lymphoma may occasionally have extensive infiltrates of epithelioid histiocytes. The absence of well-

formed granulomata and necrosis makes granulomatous lymphadenitis an unlikely diagnosis.

Angioimmunoblastic T-cell lymphoma (also known as angio-immunoblastic lymphadenopathy (AILD)-like T-cell lymphoma) is a peripheral T-cell lymphoma with clinical and histologic features similar to AILD.[271,272] As discussed in the section on AILD, some hematopathologists consider all cases of AILD to represent AILD-like lymphoma ab initio, whereas other hematopathologists still regard AILD as a possible polyclonal or preneoplastic T-cell disorder. Lymphoma should be suspected when there are clusters and small sheets of atypical lymphoid cells (Fig. 11.68), particularly around vessels, and should be diagnosed when there are large sheets of atypical lymphoid cells, immunohistochemical evidence of an aberrant T-cell immunophenotype, or molecular evidence of a sizeable (>1–5%) monoclonal T-cell population.[274] The neoplastic cell express pan-T-cell antigens and show unique coexpression of *bcl-6* and CD10.[275,630] Most cases are EBV-positive. T-cell receptor gene rearrangements are found in approximately 75% of cases, and immunoglobulin gene rearrangements have been identified in approximately 10% of cases.

Extranodal subtypes of T/NK cell neoplasms include the following.

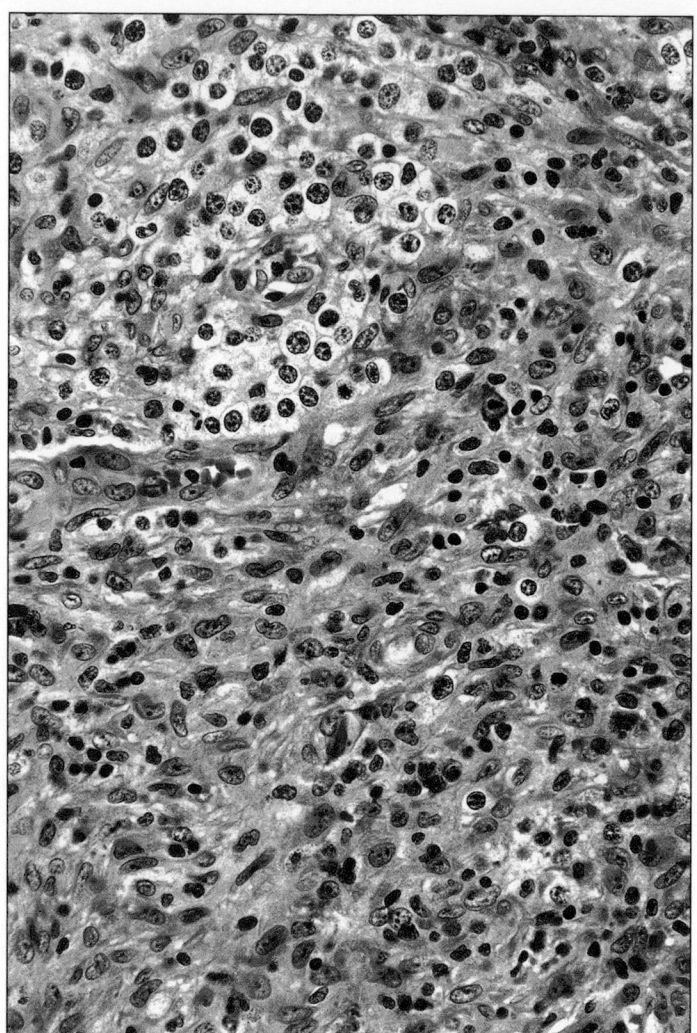

Fig. 11.68 Angioimmunoblastic lymphadenopathy-like peripheral T-cell lymphoma. Although the overall features resemble angioimmunoblastic lymphadenopathy, there are small sheets of atypical cells with clear cytoplasm.

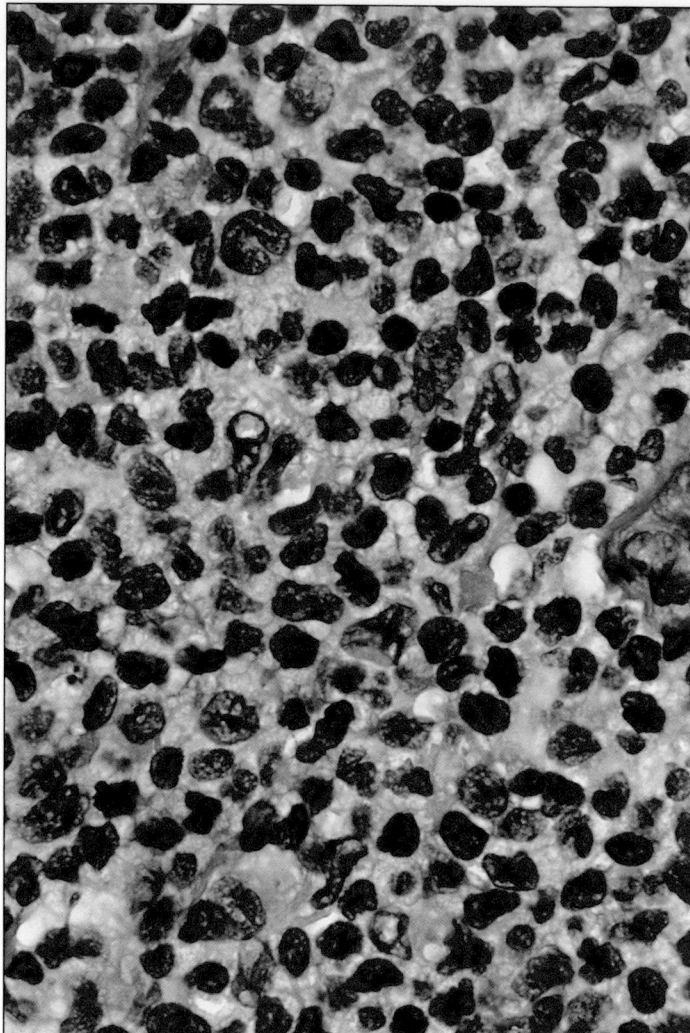

Fig. 11.69 Mycosis fungoides. Sheets of atypical small lymphoid cells are present in this case.

Mycosis fungoides is a peripheral T-cell lymphoma of CD4+ helper T-cells arising in skin or rarely, another epithelial site. It is an indolent disease, characterized by a neoplastic proliferation of small cerebriform cells. Patients with mycosis fungoides often have lymph node enlargement due to dermatopathic lymphadenitis, but lymph node involvement by mycosis fungoides may also commonly occur.[631] Lymph node involvement begins as very subtle infiltrates of atypical cells among the dendritic cells and macrophages within the areas of dermatopathic change. The diagnosis of mycosis fungoides can generally be established histologically only when aggregates of cerebriform cells of 15 or more cells are found in the paracortical areas or when architectural effacement is present (Fig. 11.69). Determining histologic grades from multiple lymph nodes may allow a more accurate stage and prognosis to be assigned to mycosis fungoides patients.[632]

Transformation to large cell lymphoma may occur, and confers a poor prognosis.[633,634] Molecular studies to detect beta-T-cell gene rearrangements are usually a more sensitive indicator of involvement by mycosis fungoides than light microscopy or immunohistochemistry in this setting.[635]

Adult T cell leukemia/lymphoma (ATLL) is a specific clinicopathologic variant caused by the human T-cell leukemia virus (HTLV)-1.[636,637] The virus is endemic in southwestern Japan,[638] but can occur in other areas.[639] About 3–5% of HTLV-1-infected individuals generally develop ATLL after a 40–60 year period of clinical latency. Patients usually present with widespread disease, including generalized lymphadenopathy. The patients are often hypercalcemic. Characteristic atypical lymphoid cells with cloverleaf nuclei are usually seen in the peripheral blood. Less commonly, lymphomatous, chronic, and smoldering forms may occur.[640] Involved lymph nodes show histologic features similar to that described for peripheral T-cell lymphoma, although marked pleomorphism may be seen.[379] Tumor cells usually express CD3, CD4, CD5, and CD25 and not CD7 and CD8.[641] Molecular studies show clonal integration of HTLV-1 in the tumor cells.[637]

Extranodal NK/T cell lymphoma, nasal type (angiocentric T-cell lymphoma in the REAL classification) is found in extranodal sites such as the upper respiratory tract, particularly the nose.[642–645]

Secondary nodal involvement may be present. A subset of cases of lymphomatoid granulomatosis may also represent extranodal T/NK-cell lymphoma but in general is more properly classified as an EBV-positive T-cell rich B-cell lymphoproliferation.[646] Nasal type extranodal T/NK-cell lymphomas occur more commonly in Asian, Central American, and South American populations but also occur sporadically in the United States. Histologically, there is an angiocentric and angiodestructive atypical infiltrate in the wall of blood vessels, usually leading to extensive necrosis of the surrounding tissues. There is large cytologic variation, from small to large and possibly anaplastic. Chromatin is granular and nucleoli are not prominent. Cytoplasm is pale and moderate in amount. Mitotic activity is high. Most of these tumors express CD2, cytoplasmic CD3, and the NK-associated antigen CD56, but lack surface CD3 and other pan-T-cell antigens.[647] The presence of markers of cytotoxic granules (granzyme B, perforin, and TIA-1) and EBV expression are essential to distinguish nasal-type extranodal T/NK-cell lymphomas[285,643–645,648–650] from peripheral T-cell lymphomas, which may be CD56+ but generally lack EBV and do not express granzyme B, perforin, or TIA-1.[643–645] Many of these cases lack multiple T-cell antigens and beta-T-cell receptor gene rearrangements.[651] The differential diagnosis includes blastic or monomorphic NK cell lymphoma/leukemia, CD56-positive peripheral T-cell lymphoma, and enteropathy-associated T-cell lymphoma.[652]

Hepatosplenic T cell lymphoma is a rare lymphoma of gamma/delta T cells, as opposed to the usual alpha/beta T cells.[653] Patients present with hepatosplenomegaly. Histologic involvement of the splenic red pulp and the hepatic sinusoids is seen. The tumor cells exhibit an aberrant T-cell phenotype and have detectable rearrangements of the delta- and gamma-T-cell receptor gene, whereas the beta-T-cell receptor gene is germline. The neoplasm is discussed further in the section on lymphomas in the spleen.

Enteropathy-type T cell lymphoma (ulcerative jejunitis or intestinal-type T-cell lymphoma) is a rare lymphoma derived from the intestinal intraepithelial T cells.[654,655] It usually occurs in patients with a history of celiac sprue. Patients often present with an acute abdomen and ulcers are often found in the jejunum or less commonly the ileum. The base of the ulcer contains an infiltrate of atypical lymphoid cells and atypical cells are often found in the adjacent nonulcerated mucosa. The tumor is often deeply invasive. An aberrant T-cell phenotype is usually present, expressing pan-T-cell antigens and not expressing CD4 or CD5. CD103 is usually expressed; this is a marker of normal mucosal-associated T lymphocytes.[656] T-cell beta and gamma genes show clonal rearrangements.[657]

Subcutaneous panniculitis-like T-cell lymphoma is a rare cytotoxic T-cell lymphoma that occurs preferentially within the interstitium of subcutaneous fat lobules.[658–661] The disease mimics lobular panniculitis. Patients usually have multiple subcutaneous tumors or plaques involving the extremities or trunk but no other sites of disease. Patients may develop systemic hemophagocytic syndrome and related constitutional symptoms. The epidermis and dermis are uninvolved but the subcutaneous adipose tissue contains neoplastic small cells, which have slightly irregular nuclear shapes and a moderate amount of pale-staining cytoplasm, such that there is widening of the intralobular septa. Large-cell transformation is infrequent. There is often an admixture of histiocytes, which sometimes form noncaseating granulomas. Karyorrhectic debris and fat necrosis with foamy macrophages are often seen. Hemophagocytosis by benign histiocytes may be present. The tumors show a characteristic staining pattern of CD8+ suppressor T cells rimming the non-neoplastic adipocytes. By paraffin immunohistochemistry, the cells

stain with markers of cytotoxic granules, including TIA-1 and perforin.[659] Clonal T-cell gene rearrangements are frequently found. Epstein-Barr virus has not been identified in cases of subcutaneous panniculitis-like T-cell lymphoma. Most cases are derived from alpha/beta cells and approximately 25% are of gamma/delta phenotype. The latter cases are usually CD4–/CD8–and carry a poorer prognosis than those of the alpha/beta phenotype, which are more indolent.

The differential diagnosis includes another CD8+ primary cutaneous lymphoma, which is the rare epidermotropic cytotoxic T-cell lymphoma. The latter, which has a tendency for metastases, affects the epidermis with variable degrees of spongiosis, intra-epidermal blistering, and necrosis.[662]

Blastic NK cell lymphomas are a rare type of lymphoma with NK-cell lineage, often involving the skin and possibly multiple other sites, including lymph nodes, soft tissues, and bone marrow.[626,642,645,651,663,664] The cytologic features are similar to those of lymphoblasts, with medium-sized nuclei with fine delicate chromatin. Rarely, Homer-Wright rosette-like cells may be seen. Necrosis and angiocentric/angiodestructive infiltrates are usually not seen. The cells are positive for cytoplasmic CD3 and CD56, and negative for surface CD3, myeloperoxidase and CD33. Positivity for TdT and/or CD34 has been described. T-cell receptor gene rearrangements and EBV are not found.[665]

LYMPHOBLASTIC LYMPHOMA

Lymphoblastic lymphoma is a neoplasm of cells frozen at the level of immature lymphoid cells, either T-lineage thymocytes or immature B-lineage bone marrow lymphoid cells. In the WHO classification, it is separated into B-cell and T-cell types and is called precursor lymphoblastic lymphoma/lymphoblastic leukemia. This nomenclature underscores the fact that the cells of lymphoblastic lymphoma are equivalent to the neoplastic cells of acute lymphoblastic leukemia. When greater than 10% circulating blasts are found in the peripheral blood or greater than 25% bone marrow involvement is seen, many clinicians prefer using the designation acute lymphoblastic leukemia over acute lymphoblastic lymphoma, but the cutoff between the two entities is arbitrary.[666,667]

Lymphoblastic lymphoma has a median age of incidence of 17 years and a male/female ratio of 2:1.[666–669] Accounting for about one-third of non-Hodgkin's lymphomas in childhood, it nonetheless occurs in all age groups. Patients usually present with a symptomatic mediastinal mass, often associated with pleural or pericardial effusions, or supradiaphragmatic lymphadenopathy. Mediastinal presentation is a strong predictor for a T-cell phenotype, although rare cases of B-lineage mediastinal lymphoblastic lymphoma have been reported. Skin involvement is relatively common in cases of B lineage.[670] Lymphoblastic lymphoma shows rapid progression, often with involvement of the peripheral blood and bone marrow, central nervous system, and gonads. It responds well to multidrug chemotherapeutic regimens similar or identical to those given for acute lymphoblastic leukemia. Adverse prognostic factors include high stage, involvement of the central nervous system, and a high serum lactate dehydrogenase.[666]

Histologically, lymphoblastic lymphoma shows diffuse effacement of normal nodal architecture. In fact, lymphoblastic lymphoma often effaces the entire lymph node structure, with capsular destruction and extensive infiltration of the adjacent soft tissues. In the soft tissues and in the adventitia of blood vessels, single-file cell infiltration is often seen. The mitotic rate is generally high and a starry-sky pattern may be focally present. It is a monomorphous lymphoma, composed

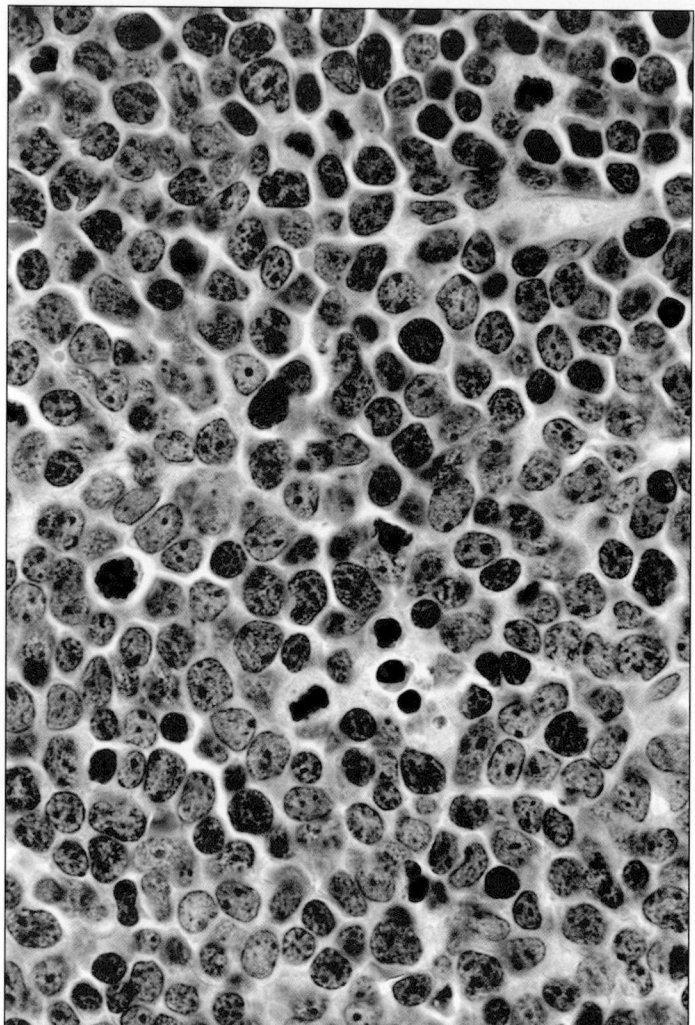

Fig. 11.70 Lymphoblastic lymphoma. A diffuse proliferation of medium-sized cells with a fine chromatin pattern is present. Note the high mitotic rate.

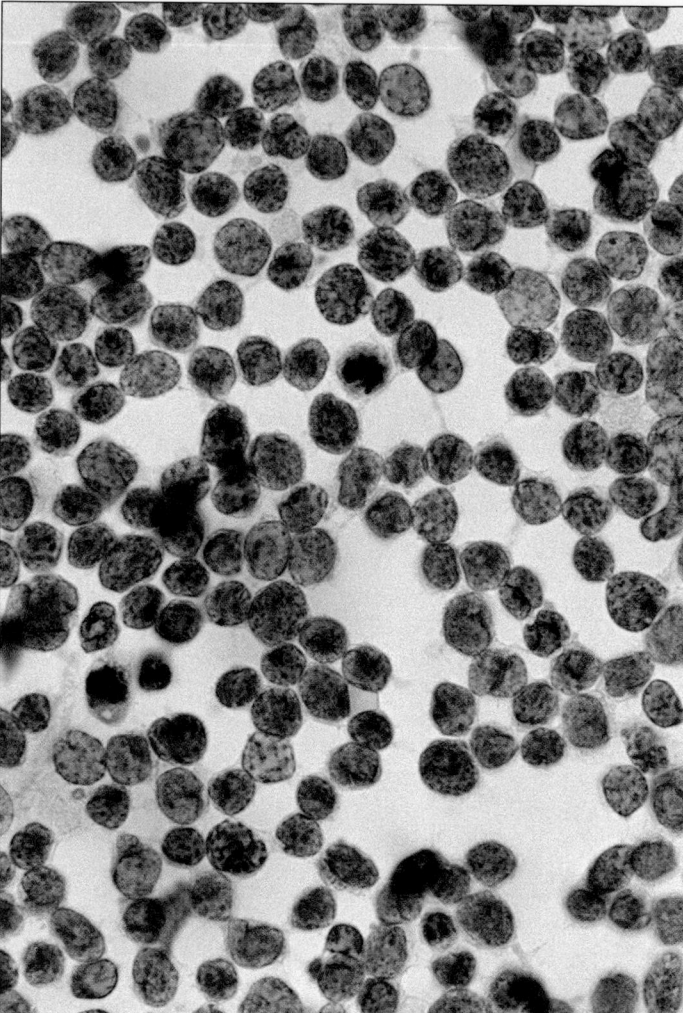

Fig. 11.71 Lymphoblastic lymphoma, fine needle aspiration. The nuclei have a very fine chromatin pattern without discernible nucleoli. Several mitotic figures are present in this field.

of a uniform population of small to medium-sized cells (Fig. 11.70). These cells have a very fine chromatin pattern with inconspicuous nucleoli and only a small amount of cytoplasm. In many cases, the nuclear outlines are highly irregular and convoluted (convoluted variant), whereas in other cases the nuclear outlines appear rounded or oval (nonconvoluted variant). In about 10% of cases, the cells may be slightly larger than usual and may possess larger nuclei that may contain one or two small but distinct nucleoli.[671] There are usually very few host cells, although occasional cases may have scattered plasma cells or eosinophils. Fine needle aspiration smears of lymphoblastic lymphoma show a monomorphous population of medium-sized lymphoid cells with a very fine chromatin pattern and very inconspicuous nucleoli (Fig. 11.71). The cytologic appearance is identical to acute lymphoblastic leukemia in bone marrow aspirate or peripheral blood smears.

Virtually all lymphoblastic lymphomas express TdT, a marker that can be applied in frozen and paraffin sections, and by flow cytometry.[672,673] CD45 is positive in about 80% of cases, a rate of positivity lower than all non-Hodgkin's lymphoma except anaplastic large cell lymphoma.[36] About 85–90% of lymphoblastic lymphomas

Table 11.17 Stages of T-cell maturation

Prethymic	CD7+	CD2–	cCD3±					
Stage I	CD7+	CD2+	cCD3+	CD1–	CD4–	CD8+		
Stage II	CD7+	CD2+	cCD3+	CD1+	CD4–	CD8–	or CD4+	CD8+
Stage III	CD7+	CD2+	sCD3+	CD1–	CD4+	CD8–	or CD4–	CD8+

c, cytoplasmic; s, surface.

are T-lineage neoplasms, almost always expressing CD43, CD7, and cytoplasmic or surface CD3.[674,675] These cases express phenotypes consistent with the different stages of intrathymic T-cell maturation (Table 11.17),[676] including early, thymic (cortical), and mature subtypes. Some studies indicate that patients with a thymic subtype have a better clinical outcome than the other immunologic subtypes.[677] About 20% of these cases may also show strong positivity for the NK markers CD16 and CD57; in one study, these latter cases occurred more often in females and had a more aggressive course.[678,679] About 15% of cases of lymphoblastic lymphoma are of B lineage.[674,675] Due to their immaturity, only about one-half of cases express CD20, but all B-lineage cases will express the B-lineage markers CD19, cytoplasmic CD22, PAX-5 and CD79a (flow cytometry or paraffin/frozen immunohistochemistry) and most cases express the CALLA antigen CD10 (common or intermediate or precursor B stage).[680,681] Cytoplasmic immunoglobulin may be positive (mature precursor B) and surface immunoglobulin is only rarely positive.[682,683] In fact, some cases reported as precursor B-cell lymphoblastic leukemia with light chain expression in fact represent circulating blastic mantle cell lymphoma.[683] CD13 and CD33 may be positive in either T- or B-lineage lymphoblastic neoplasms and do not by themselves imply a biphenotypic malignancy.

Hyperdiploidy between 51 and 65 chromosomes or the presence of t(12;21) are each associated with a good prognosis.[684–686] Cases with a pre-B (or early precursor B) phenotype (CD10 negative) are characterized by a high proportion of t(4;11). The t(1;19) is present in approximately 25% of cases with cytoplasmic mu expression. Cases with a common precursor B phenotype show a high incidence of positivity for the Philadelphia chromosome/BCR-ABL. The t(4;11), t(1;19) and Ph cytogenetic abnormalities, as well as hypodiploidy, are each associated with an inferior outcome. The prognostic impact of other aberrations (+8, 7 abnormalities) is less clear. Various cytogenetic changes associated with T-lymphoblastic neoplasms are also known, although their effect on clinical outcome does not appear to be significant. About 90% of T-lineage lymphoblastic lymphomas have detectable monoclonal beta-T-cell receptor gene rearrangements; in addition, immunoglobulin heavy chain gene rearrangements may be present in about 25% of cases.[687,688] Virtually all B-lineage lymphoblastic lymphomas have detectable monoclonal immunoglobulin heavy chain gene rearrangements, but light chain gene rearrangements are detectable in only about 40% of cases. Similar to the presence of immunoglobulin heavy chain gene rearrangements in T-lineage lymphoblastic lymphoma, beta-T-cell receptor gene rearrangements may be present in 25% of cases of B-lineage lymphoblastic lymphoma.[687,689]

The differential diagnosis of lymphoblastic lymphoma includes other types of non-Hodgkin's lymphoma, myeloid sarcoma, thymoma, and small cell undifferentiated carcinoma. TdT is an extremely useful marker in the differential diagnosis of lymphoblastic lymphoma versus other non-Hodgkin's lymphomas, as it is positive in virtually all cases of lymphoblastic lymphoma, but negative in all other types of non-Hodgkin's lymphoma.[673] Morphologically, lymphoblastic lymphoma can be easily confused with Burkitt's-type lymphoma and the blastic variant of mantle cell lymphoma. The cells of lymphoblastic lymphoma have a finer chromatin pattern than those of Burkitt's-type lymphoma, whereas the latter have more distinct nucleoli and a greater amount of cytoplasm that tends to square off on adjacent cells. The blastic variant of mantle cell lymphoma may be morphologically indistinguishable from lymphoblastic lymphoma. Areas of more typical mantle cell lymphoma or a past history of that lymphoma can be helpful, but immunohistochemical studies may be necessary. Besides TdT (negative in mantle cell lymphoma) and bcl-1 (negative in lymphoblastic lymphoma), lineage determination may be of use, because most cases of lymphoblastic lymphoma are of T lineage.

Lymphoblastic lymphoma may also be very difficult to distinguish from a myeloid sarcoma (extramedullary myeloid tumor), because both can show a single-file pattern of infiltration in fibrous tissue and both feature a fine chromatin pattern. The presence of eosinophils or cells with more than scant cytoplasm should suggest the diagnosis of myeloid sarcoma. Occasional cases of myeloid sarcoma may be TdT-positive. Myeloperoxidase is a relatively sensitive marker for myeloid sarcoma, but rare cases may be negative. Peripheral blood and bone marrow examination are recommended in any questionable cases. The proliferating thymocytes of thymoma may have close morphologic and immunohistochemical similarities to the cells of lymphoblastic lymphoma.[690] Attention should be given to the presence of the epithelial cells of thymoma, which are scattered larger cells with vesicular chromatin. Confirmation can be obtained using keratin stains, which demonstrate a network of epithelial cells throughout thymoma, keeping in mind that occasional residual thymic epithelial cells can be seen in mediastinal masses of lymphoblastic lymphoma. The confusion between the thymocytes of thymoma and the cells of lymphoblastic lymphoma can be greatest when examining flow cytometric data, which may demonstrate an immature thymic phenotype in thymoma and not detect the epithelial population. Finally, small cell undifferentiated carcinoma can be confused with lymphoblastic lymphoma, particularly in suboptimal preparations. Immunohistochemical studies including keratin should be performed in any questionable case.

BURKITT'S LYMPHOMA

Burkitt's lymphoma is an extremely aggressive B-lineage lymphoma associated with a MYC gene translocation. It often presents in extranodal sites or as an acute leukemia. Criteria for making the diagnosis of Burkitt's lymphoma are more restrictive in the WHO classification compared to previous classification schemes.

There are three clinical forms of Burkitt's lymphoma: 1) endemic, 2) sporadic, and 3) immunodeficiency-associated. The endemic form, which occurs in primarily in equatorial Africa and less frequently in Papua New Guinea, affects children (particularly males) who present with jaw tumors or other extranodal masses.[691] Sporadic Burkitt's lymphoma occurs throughout the world, including North and South America, Western Europe, and Northern Africa and has peaks of incidence in both childhood and adults, with abdominal presentations most common.[692–695] Immunodeficiency-associated Burkitt's lymphoma is commonly associated with HIV infection, but has been described in other immunodeficiency states.[696] Bone marrow and lymph node involvement are common in the HIV-associated cases.

The WHO classification recognizes three morphologic variants: 1) classical, which corresponds to small noncleaved Burkitt's lymphoma in the Working Formulation, 2) atypical/Burkitt's-like types, which corresponds to the small noncleaved, non-Burkitt's type of lymphoma in the Working Formulation, and 3) showing plasmacytoid differentiation. Burkitt's lymphoma with plasmacytoid differentiation is usually seen in immunodeficiency states, although it also is seen in children.

At low magnification, Burkitt's lymphoma usually shows diffuse effacement of architecture, although rare cases show focal involvement of germinal centers.[697] A striking finding is the presence of a 'starry-sky' pattern, imparted by a high mitotic rate, numerous apoptotic cells, and evenly dispersed tingible body macrophages (Fig. 11.72); this pattern is invariably present in the classic subtype and almost always present in the other two subtypes. At high magnification, Burkitt's lymphoma is composed of a very homogeneous population of medium-sized cells with round nuclei, a vesicular chromatin pattern, several moderately sized nucleoli, and a moderate rim of basophilic cytoplasm that tends to square off as it

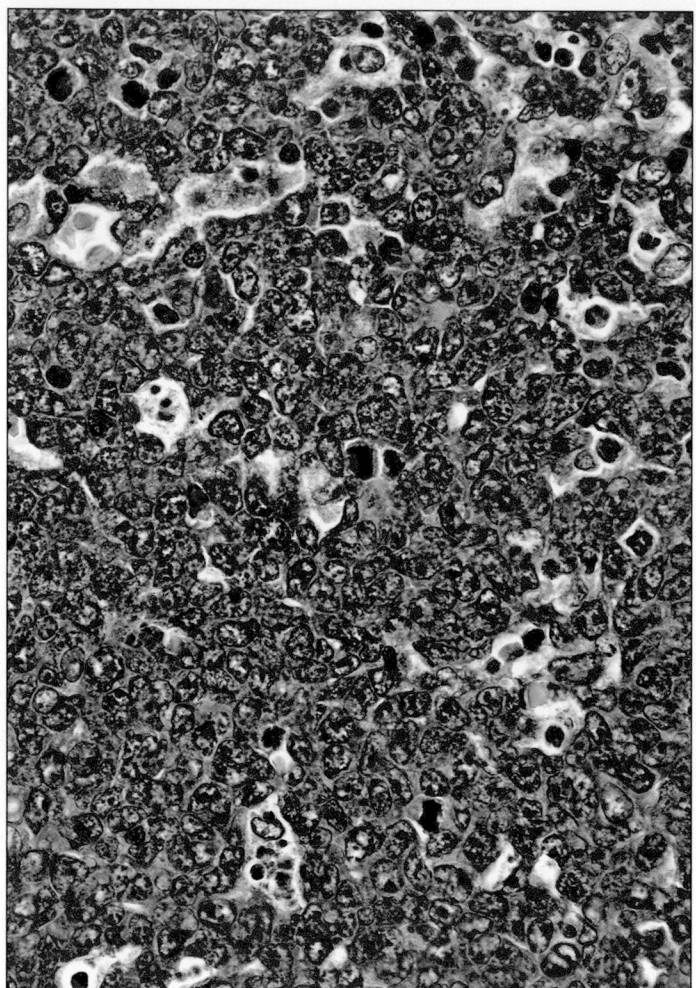

Fig. 11.72 Small noncleaved lymphoma, Burkitt's type. A starry-sky pattern is present. The tumor cells are very homogeneous.

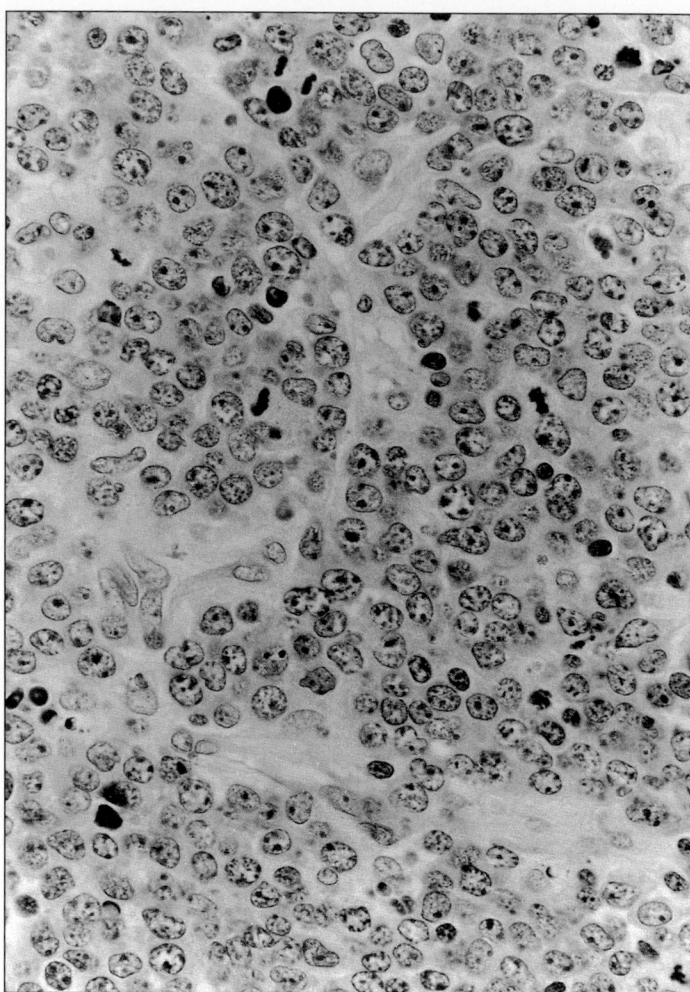

Fig. 11.73 Small noncleaved lymphoma, non-Burkitt's type. The mitotic rate is very high. Although the cells are somewhat monomorphous, some variability is present.

abuts adjacent cells (see Fig. 11.72). In the atypical/non-Burkitt's subtype, more cell-size and shape heterogeneity is seen, and nucleoli tend to be fewer in number, but more prominent (Fig. 11.73). The plasmacytoid variant also has morphologic features similar to classic Burkitt's lymphoma, with the exception of some plasmacytoid tumor cells exhibiting eccentric basophilic cytoplasm (corresponding to monotypic immunoglobulin), a small degree of pleomorphism in nuclear size and shape, and only a single central nucleolus. Fine needle aspirate smears of Burkitt's lymphoma show a homogeneous population of medium-sized cells with round nuclei, a coarsely reticulated chromatin pattern, and several nucleoli. The cytoplasm is relatively abundant, basophilic, and usually shows small vacuoles on air-dried smears. The atypical/Burkitt's-like type contains similarly sized rounded nuclei with a finer chromatin pattern and usually one conspicuous nucleolus.

All cases of Burkitt's lymphoma are mature B-lineage neoplasms, expressing CD20, CD19, CD22, and CD79a, and almost always expressing monotypic immunoglobulins. Aberrant coexpression of CD43 is seen in a significant subset of cases. CD10 and *bcl-6* are usually positive, but CD5, CD23, and TdT are negative. *Bcl-2* expression is variable.[104] The proliferative rate as measured by Ki-67

is extremely high, approaching 100%. Virtually all cases have detectable immunoglobulin heavy and light chain gene rearrangements. In addition, all Burkitt's subtypes have a translocation involving the *MYC* gene on chromosome 8 band q24 – either a t(8;14) involving the immunoglobulin heavy chain gene, found in 85% of cases, a t(2;8) involving the kappa gene, found in 10% of cases, or a t(8;22) involving the lambda gene, found in 5% of cases.[698,699]

The differential diagnosis of Burkitt's lymphoma includes lymphoblastic lymphoma and diffuse large B-cell lymphomas, particularly those with a large number of immunoblasts. Burkitt's lymphoma is generally more homogeneous than diffuse large B-cell lymphoma, lacking host cells other than histiocytes, and more consistently has a starry-sky appearance. Although one would expect that size could be used as a criterion in the discrimination between Burkitt's lymphoma and the large cell lymphomas, in practice there is a gradation of nuclear sizes for each, without distinct differences in many cases. In questionable cases, Ki-67 (mib-1) stains to assess the proliferative index may be helpful, with the highest rates present in Burkitt's lymphoma.[700] TdT positivity also helps to distinguish lymphoblastic lymphoma from Burkitt's lymphoma, which is TdT negative.

LYMPHOPROLIFERATIONS IN IMMUNODEFICIENT INDIVIDUALS

Patients with immunodeficiencies are at increased risk of developing lymphoproliferative disorders, most often EBV-associated non-Hodgkin's lymphomas. The incidence and specific types of lymphoproliferative disorders vary with the specific type of immunodeficiency. The WHO classification scheme divides these immunodeficiency-associated lymphoproliferative disorders into four broad clinical settings: 1) primary immunodeficiency syndromes and other primary immune disorders; 2) infection by the human immunodeficiency virus (HIV); 3) iatrogenic immunosuppression in patients who have received solid organ or bone marrow allografts; and 4) iatrogenic immunosuppression associated with methotrexate treatment, most commonly for autoimmune disease. As expected, the large variety of underlying immune disorders results in a heterogeneous group of lymphoproliferative disorders.

The primary immunodeficiencies most often associated with lymphoproliferative disorders are X-linked lymphoproliferative syndrome, ataxia-telangiectasia, common variable immunodeficiency, Wiskott-Aldrich syndrome, and severe combined immunodeficiency.[701] Nijmegen breakage syndrome, hyper-IgM syndrome, and autoimmune lymphoproliferative syndrome are other primary immune disorders associated with the development of lymphoproliferative disorders. B-lineage proliferations occur much more frequently than T-cell disorders. The development of a lymphoproliferative disorder may be preceded by lymphoid hyperplasia, particularly in patients with Wiskott-Aldrich syndrome and autoimmune lymphoproliferative syndrome. Patients with common variable immunodeficiency more often have lymphadenopathy that reveals chronic granulomatous inflammation, reactive hyperplasia, or atypical lymphoid hyperplasia.[702] Patients with X-linked lymphoproliferative disorder and severe combined immunodeficiency may develop fatal infectious mononucleosis, which has similar morphology to the previously described nonfatal cases of infectious mononucleosis, with the addition of hemophagocytosis in some patients. About 65% of patients with X-linked lymphoproliferative syndrome, 15% of patients with Wiskott-Aldrich syndrome, 5% of patients with common variable immunodeficiency syndrome, and variable numbers of patients with common variable immunodeficiency and Nijmegen breakage syndrome develop diffuse large B-cell lymphoma, which may be extranodal. About 10% of patients with ataxia-telangiectasia and 3% of patients with severe combined immunodeficiency develop lymphoid neoplasia, including both non-Hodgkin's lymphoma and Hodgkin's disease. Ataxia-telangiectasia patients are more likely to develop T-cell lymphomas than B-cell neoplasms. In terms of T-cell proliferations, patients with primary immune disorders more often have benign T-cell expansions of CD4−/CD8− alpha/beta T cells than they develop T-cell lymphomas.

Secondary immunodeficiencies associated with lymphoproliferative disorders include HIV infection and iatrogenic causes, usually as a result of immunosuppression after organ transplantation, but occasionally after treatment for a collagen vascular disease. The benign lymphadenopathies associated with HIV infection have already been discussed. About 3% of HIV-infected patients develop non-Hodgkin's lymphoma, roughly accounting for about 10% of cases of non-Hodgkin's lymphoma currently diagnosed in the United States.[375] These lymphomas are usually B lineage, and include lymphoma types that occur in immunocompetent patients (primarily diffuse large B-cell lymphoma or Burkitt's lymphoma) and lesions that occur specially in HIV-positive patients (*primary effusion lymphoma* and *plasmablastic lymphoma* of the oral cavity).

HIV-positive patients may also develop lesions resembling polymorphic B-cell post-transplant lymphoproliferative disorders and have a higher incidence of classical Hodgkin's disease.[703] HIV-infected patients occasionally develop other types of malignant lymphoma, including Hodgkin's disease and T-cell lymphomas.[704] Rare HIV-infected patients have developed MALT lymphoma, peripheral T-cell lymphomas, and natural killer cell lymphomas. Diffuse large B-cell lymphoma and classical type Burkitt's lymphoma account for 25% and 30%, respectively, of HIV-associated lymphomas. The HIV-associated Burkitt's lymphomas may also have plasmacytoid differentiation, as described in the section on Burkitt's lymphomas, and account for approximately 20% of lymphomas in HIV-infected patients. Primary effusion lymphomas are B-lineage lymphoma involving the body cavities, most often the pleural or peritoneal spaces.[705,706] Rarely, primary effusion lymphoma may present as a solid tumor mass. The primary effusion lymphomas contain the Kaposi's sarcoma-associated herpesvirus (HHV-8) and are also associated with multicentric Castleman's disease. The cells are highly pleomorphic and may be admixed with a few small lymphocytes. The nuclei are large and irregular and contain prominent nucleoli. The cytoplasm is variable in amount and may show plasmacytoid differentiation. Gene expression profile analysis shows plasmablastic derivation, with features of both immunoblasts and plasma cells.[707] Plasmablastic lymphoma is a rare HIV-related non-Hodgkin's lymphoma that is generally limited to the oral cavity and jaw at the time of diagnosis, although extension to distant sites may occur at a later stage.[708–711] The tumor cells have vesicular nuclear chromatin, prominent nucleoli, and abundant plasmacytoid cytoplasm. Immunohistochemistry shows the cells are negative for CD45/45RB and CD20, but they are positive for the plasma cell-reactive antibody VS38c and CD138, and they are usually positive for CD79a antibody. There is moderate association with EBV and no known association with HHV-8. Most cases have cytoplasmic immunoglobulin and approximately one-half show monoclonal immunoglobulin heavy chain gene rearrangement.[712]

Patients who receive immunosuppression after organ transplantation are at greatly increased risk of developing post-transplantation lymphoproliferative disorders (PTLDs), with the specific risk dependent on age, the type of organ transplant, and the drug regimen used. The WHO divides these lesions into four categories: 1) early lesions, 2) polymorphic PTLDs, 3) monomorphic PTLDs, and 4) Hodgkin's disease and Hodgkin's disease-like PTLD.[407,713] The early lesions comprise reactive plasmacytic hyperplasia and infectious mononucleosis-like lesions.[713] Plasmacytic hyperplasia is characterized by an expansion of the paracortical areas predominantly by plasmacytoid lymphocytes and plasma cells. Plasmacytoid immunoblasts and cytologic atypia are usually not seen. Follicles may be hyperplastic, regressive, or absent. Plasmacytic hyperplasia is polyclonal and one generally sees regression of the lesion with reduction in immunosuppression. The polymorphic PTLDs are characterized by disruption of the normal nodal architecture, with the presence of the entire range of B-lymphocyte forms, including small lymphocytes, plasma cells, small lymphoplasmacytoid forms, plasmacytoid immunoblasts, and small and large cleaved and noncleaved lymphoid cells (Fig. 11.74). Necrosis and cytologic atypia may also be seen. The clinical course varies greatly, from partial to complete regression following immunosuppression reduction to progression despite therapy. Disease progression appears to correlate with *bcl-6* gene mutation.[714] The monomorphic PTLDs are subtyped by the specific histologic type of lymphoma. Most of them are diffuse large B-cell lymphomas, with most of the remainder as plasma cell myeloma and rare cases of plasmacytoma-like PTLD.[713] Rare cases

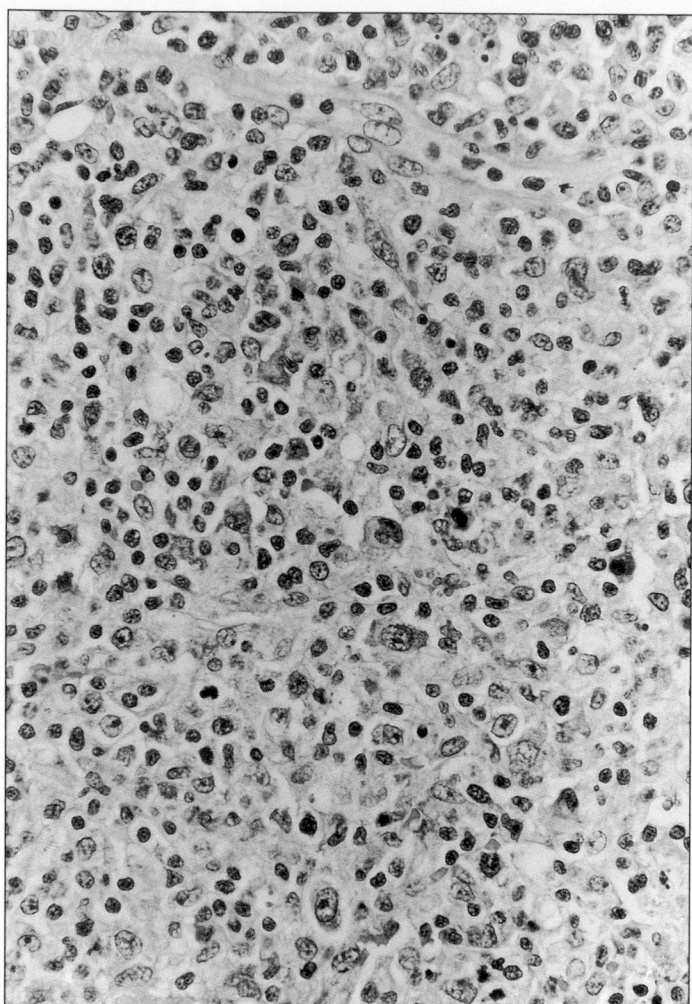

Fig. 11.74 Post-transplantation lymphoproliferative disorder, polymorphous hyperplasia type. A mixed population of lymphoid cells is seen, without striking atypia.

modulatory therapy, including cyclosporin, corticosteroids, and azathioprine.[696] Some of these lymphomas have undergone regression upon withdrawal of the drug.

The rare entity of 'senile EBV-positive B-cell lymphoproliferative disorder' has morphologic and immunohistochemical features analogous to those of immunodeficiency-associated B-cell lymphoproliferative disorder but none of the elderly patients (median age 75.5 years) had evidence of underlying immunodeficiency-related diseases.[719]

OTHER NEOPLASMS

LANGERHANS CELL HISTIOCYTOSIS (HISTIOCYTOSIS X)

Langerhans cell histiocytosis, also known as histiocytosis X and Langerhans cell granulomatosis, is a tumorous proliferation of specialized dendritic cells resembling the normal antigen-presenting Langerhans cells primarily found in skin. Historically, three main and sometimes overlapping clinical syndromes have been recognized: solitary eosinophilic granuloma, Hand-Schüller-Christian syndrome (triad of bony lesions, exophthalmos, and diabetes insipidus), and Letterer-Siwe syndrome (aggressive, disseminated histiocytosis in young children).[720] These and other presentations are believed to all represent manifestations of one entity, Langerhans cell histiocytosis. Subclassification is based on whether the lesion is single or multiple (unifocal versus multifocal), and whether one or multiple organ systems are involved (unisystem versus multisystem). The pattern of organ involvement has prognostic significance.[721] Lymph nodes may be the site of unifocal disease or multifocal unisystem disease, or as part of multifocal multisystem disease. Isolated lymph node involvement (usually cervical or inguinal region) is most often found in children or young adults who are typically afebrile and may have painful lymphadenopathy.[722,723] However, bone and skin are much more commonly involved sites than lymph nodes in both unifocal or multifocal disease. Of note, pulmonary Langerhans cell histiocytosis in adults may represent a clinicopathologic entity distinct from the others, showing features suggesting an unusual reactive proliferation, including being found almost exclusively in smokers and having a tendency for spontaneous remission.[724] Occasionally, Langerhans cell histiocytosis may be associated with other malignancies.[722,725,726]

Involved lymph nodes in disseminated and localized forms of Langerhans cell histiocytosis show similar histology with a sinusoidal pattern of involvement (Fig. 11.75). Affected lymph nodes may be small and only focally involved. Most cases have intact lymph node architecture. One may see extensive disease with marked sinusoidal distention or even architectural effacement in very advanced cases. The Langerhans cells are accompanied by mononuclear and multinucleated histiocytes, eosinophils, neutrophils, and small lymphocytes; plasma cells are rare or absent. Clusters of eosinophils may be associated with necrosis, forming so-called eosinophilic microabscesses. Dermatopathic changes may also be seen.

Cytologically, Langerhans cells have characteristic folded or grooved nuclei ('coffee-bean' appearance), inconspicuous nucleoli, and abundant eosinophilic cytoplasm (Fig. 11.76). The nuclei appear bland. Mitotic activity varies widely from lesion to lesion, but is generally low. Rare cases with frankly malignant cytologic features and high mitotic rates have been called malignant histiocytosis X or Langerhans cell sarcoma.[727,728] These cases may arise de novo or may follow pre-existing Langerhans cell proliferations.

of Burkitt's-type or Burkitt's-like lymphomas have been reported in post-transplant recipients.[696] Molecular studies demonstrate that almost all the polymorphic B-cell lesions and all of the monomorphic lesions harbor monoclonal B-cell populations and are almost all EBV associated.[713] T-cell lymphomas arising after organ transplant are rare and tend to occur much later after transplant than their B-cell counterparts. Most are EBV negative. The T-cell lesions include lymphoblastic lymphoma, peripheral T-cell lymphoma, and anaplastic large cell lymphoma. Hodgkin's disease and Hodgkin's disease-like lesions have also been reported in patients receiving organ transplant, particularly allogeneic bone marrow transplantation.[715] They are almost always associated with EBV.

Patients with autoimmune disease who are treated with methotrexate may develop a lymphoproliferative disorder, including diffuse large B-cell lymphoma, Hodgkin's disease, and polymorphous PTLD.[716–718] Other subtypes of lymphoma as well as lymphoplasmacytic infiltrates also occur. The lymphomas are classified according to their specific histologic subtype. They are usually EBV negative and many cases occur in extranodal sites. Nontransplantation iatrogenically-induced lymphoproliferative disorders have also been described in association with patients receiving other immuno-

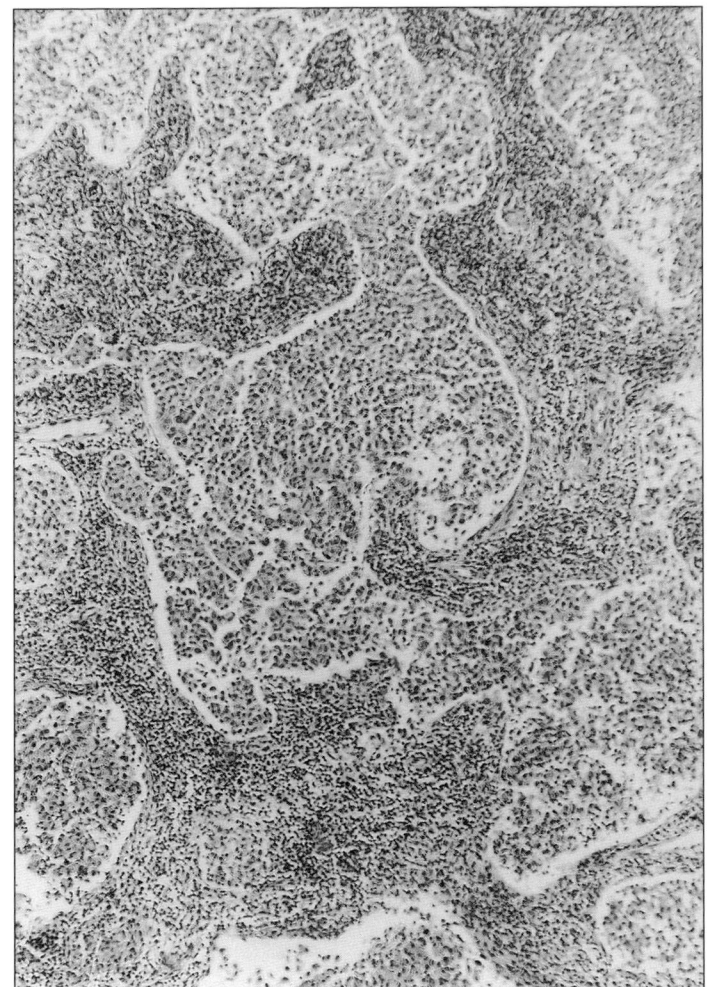

Fig. 11.75 Langerhans cell histiocytosis. A sinusoidal pattern of infiltration is present.

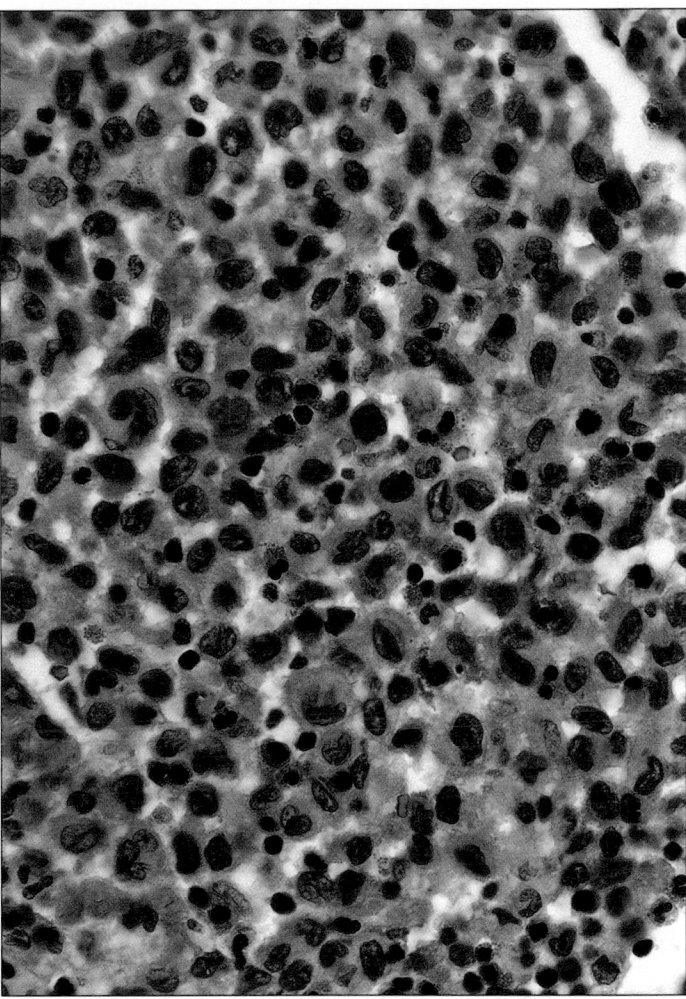

Fig. 11.76 Langerhans cell histiocytosis. Langerhans cells, with their characteristic grooved nuclei, are seen admixed with eosinophils.

Neoplastic Langerhans cells resemble their normal counterparts by immunohistochemistry and virtually always express S-100 protein and CD1a. [728–731] CD68 and fascin are often expressed, but lysozyme is only weakly expressed in a subset of tumor cells. [728,732] CD1a expression is not found in other histiocytic and dendritic cells, and is very useful in differential diagnosis. [733] Ultrastructurally, one should see characteristic Birbeck granules, which are racket-shaped organelles approximately 200–400 nm long, 33 nm wide, with an osmiophilic core and a double outer sheath. [734] By studying the patterns of X-chromosome inactivation in the X-linked human androgen-receptor gene, researchers have demonstrated that Langerhans cell histiocytosis is a monoclonal proliferation. [735] Molecular studies show a germline configuration for the immunoglobulin heavy chain and T-cell receptor genes. [736]

Lymph node involvement by Langerhans cell histiocytosis must be distinguished from other diseases with sinusoidal distribution, including reactive sinus hyperplasia, sinus histiocytosis with massive lymphadenopathy, metastatic neoplasms, and sinusoidal malignant lymphoma. The characteristic cytologic features of Langerhans cells and abundant eosinophils seen in Langerhans cell histiocytosis are not features of benign sinusoidal hyperplasia. The histiocytes of sinus histiocytosis with massive lymphadenopathy show rounded nuclei with vesicular chromatin and prominent nucleoli, differing from the folded, grooved nuclei of Langerhans cell histiocytosis. Also, in contrast to Langerhans cell histiocytosis, sinus histiocytosis with massive lymphadenopathy lymph nodes shows phagocytosis and high numbers of plasma cells. If necessary, immunostaining for CD1a will separate Langerhans cells from all other types of histiocytes/dendritic cells. Malignant cytologic features differentiate metastatic malignancies and sinusoidal malignant lymphoma from most cases of Langerhans cell histiocytosis, except for the rare Langerhans cell sarcoma. Immunohistochemistry is necessary to resolve morphologically atypical cases. Large numbers of non-neoplastic Langerhans cells (S-100+ and CD1a+) are present in dermatopathic lymphadenitis, but differ in distribution, involving the paracortex and not the sinuses, as in Langerhans cell histiocytosis. Melanin pigment may also be found in dermatopathic lymphadenitis. [184]

DENDRITIC CELL NEOPLASMS

Dendritic cell neoplasms are rare tumors derived from specialized antigen-presenting dendritic cells and are composed primarily of two entities in the WHO classification: follicular dendritic cell

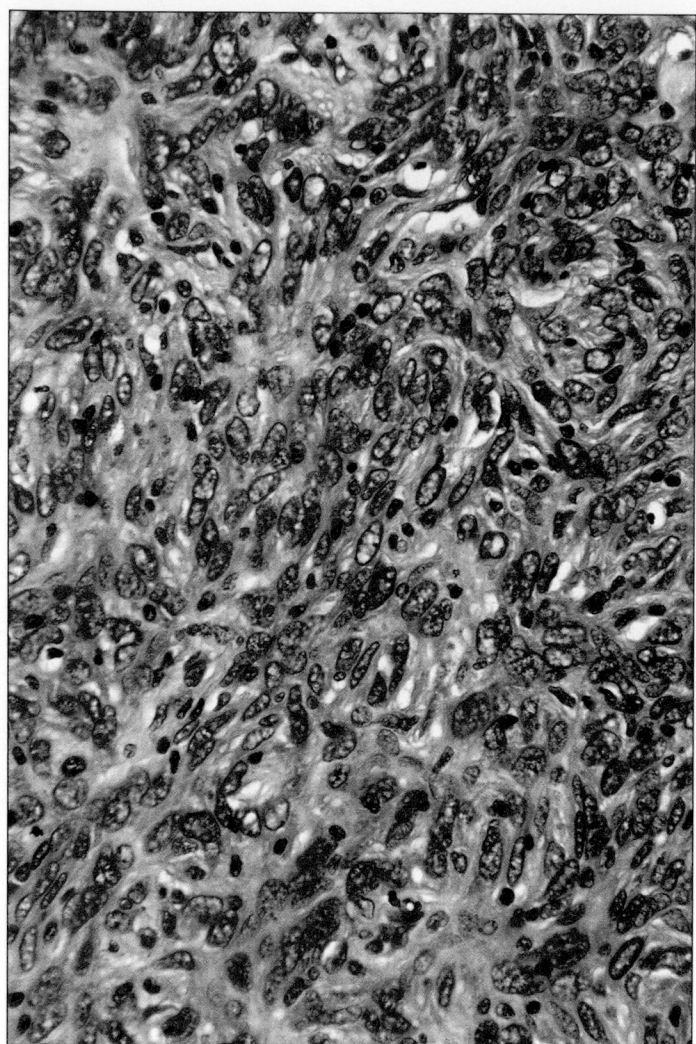

Fig. 11.77 Follicular dendritic cell tumor. A spindle cell proliferation is seen. Note the admixed small lymphocytes.

formed desmosomes.

Immunohistochemistry is essential for diagnosing dendritic tumors.[728] Follicular dendritic cell sarcoma/tumor expresses CD21 and/or CD35, antigens detectable in paraffin sections. Interdigitating dendritic cell sarcoma/tumor is negative for both CD21 and CD35, but positive for S-100 protein (CD1a negative). Both tumors are negative for B- and T-lineage antigens and show no B-cell or T-cell gene rearrangements.

The category of 'dendritic cell sarcoma, not otherwise specified' encompasses the entity formerly known as indeterminate cell neoplasms (also known as indeterminate cell histiocytosis).[728] These are rare lesions that show differentiation toward indeterminate cells, which are normal cells with morphologic and immunologic similarities to normal Langerhans cells, but without Birbeck granules by electron microscopy. These are usually dermal-based tumors, occasionally with epidermal extension, and only rarely found in lymph nodes. The cells are large with highly irregularly shaped nuclei and abundant cytoplasm. Multinucleated and foam cells may be present. Other electron microscopic findings include numerous interdigitating dendritic processes. Vimentin, CD45, CD1, S-100, fascin, and macrophage-associated antigens are usually positive. Because of its specific defining features of lack of Birbeck granules and CD1 positivity, both ultrastructural and immunohistochemical studies are required for establishing a firm diagnosis.

The differential diagnosis of dendritic cell neoplasms includes any spindle-cell lesion occurring in lymph nodes, including thymoma, melanoma, spindled carcinoma, and sarcoma. Immunohistochemistry can exclude these other entities, and is necessary to prove dendritic cell phenotype. The differentiation between follicular dendritic cell sarcoma/tumor and interdigitating dendritic cell sarcoma/tumor also rests on immunohistochemistry.

HISTIOCYTIC SARCOMA/TRUE HISTIOCYTIC LYMPHOMA

Histiocytic sarcoma, true histiocytic lymphoma, and malignant histiocytosis are terms for a rare neoplasm in which the malignant cells demonstrate lineage consistent with histiocytes.[745,746] Historically, the diagnosis of malignant histiocytosis was more frequently made when the morphologic and cytochemical features of the tumor cells were considered those of histiocytes.[747] Unfortunately, neither the appearance nor the cytochemistry was unique for histiocytic lineage. With the use of more recently available study techniques that have high specificity, the majority of cases of malignant histiocytosis studied in earlier reports are now known to be lymphoid in origin.[748–751]

Histiocytic sarcoma accounts for approximately 0.5% of all hematolymphoid neoplasms and occurs most commonly in adults.[752] Cases have been roughly equally distributed among lymph nodes, skin, and other extranodal sites.[747,753] Some cases have been associated with or subsequent to a non-Hodgkin's lymphoma.[754,755] Patients generally present with fever, fatigue, and weakness, and may have weight loss, lymphadenopathy, skin lesions, or splenomegaly. The clinical course is very aggressive and most patients die from progressive disease.

Involved lymph nodes may be partially or completely effaced by a proliferation of cytologically malignant cells with some resemblance to histiocytes (Fig. 11.78). The malignant cells vary in size and have a large, eccentrically placed, oval nucleus with a prominent irregular nucleolus and abundant eosinophilic cytoplasm. Multinucleated tumor cells with bizarre nuclei and multiple nucleoli are often present. Despite histiocytic origin, hemophagocytosis occurs only occasionally. Mitotic activity is quite brisk.

sarcoma/tumor and interdigitating dendritic cell sarcoma/tumor.[61,737–741] The terminology 'sarcoma/tumor' used in WHO classification reflects variable clinical behavior and lack of predictability based on histology. Both dendritic tumor types are predominantly nodal, but may be extranodal. Follicular dendritic cell neoplasms have a tendency to recur, either locally or at multiple sites, although the prognosis has generally been good. Approximately 10–20% of cases are associated with Castleman's disease, mostly of the hyaline vascular type but also rarely with the plasma cell variant.[741–743] Interdigitating dendritic cell neoplasms seem to be more aggressive, with approximately one-half of patients dying of their disease.

Follicular dendritic cell sarcoma/tumors are composed of spindle cells containing oval to spindled nuclei with bland nuclear features, exhibiting a whorled, fascicular, or storiform pattern (Fig. 11.77).[744] Admixed small lymphocytes are often found between the tumor cells and in perivascular spaces. By electron microscopy, long cytoplasmic processes are evident, connecting to one another by numerous desmosomes. *Interdigitating dendritic cell sarcoma/tumors* also show spindled to ovoid cells, in paracortical distribution, with whorls or fascicles. Electron microscopy of interdigitating dendritic cell tumors reveals interdigitating cell processes without well-

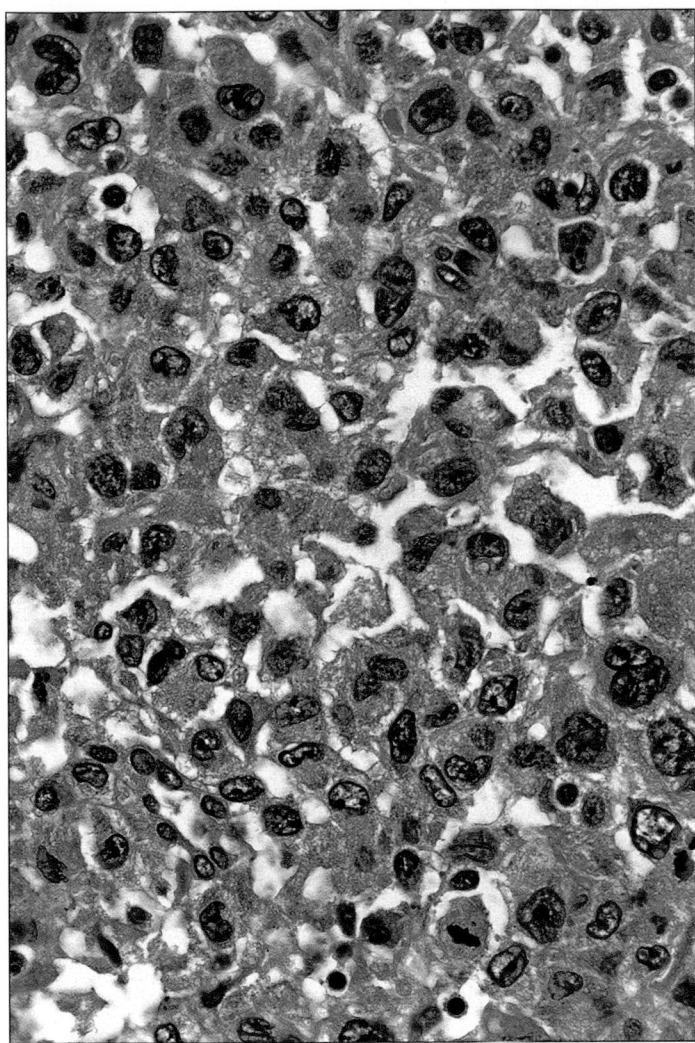

Fig. 11.78 True histiocytic tumor. This case was proved to be a true histiocytic lymphoma after a large panel of immunohistochemical and molecular studies. The cells have pleomorphic nuclei and abundant cytoplasm.

Diagnosis of this rare entity requires exhaustive exclusion of other more common entities by various immunophenotypic and molecular studies. One must have strong immunologic evidence of histiocytic lineage, accompanied by absence of specific T- and B-lineage markers, lack of T-cell receptor and immunoglobulin genes rearrangement by molecular studies.[4,616,747,748] Histiocytic lineage may be demonstrated with expression of CD68, CD163, and lysozyme. Of note, some histiocytic sarcomas may also be S-100 positive.[728] Rare cases are CD56 positive.[663] They should not stain with CD30, any B-lineage or T-lineage-specific antibodies, dendritic cell markers (CD21, CD35), CD1a, CD34, any of the anti-keratin antibodies, or HMB45.[728,745,751,752]

The differential diagnosis of true histiocytic sarcoma includes a variety of tumors with anaplastic morphology, including anaplastic large cell lymphoma, B- or T-cell large cell lymphomas, anaplastic carcinomas, follicular dendritic cell neoplasms, and melanoma. Strict attention to the immunophenotypic and molecular criteria of true histiocytic sarcoma, along with clinical presentation, will help exclude these other more common anaplastic tumors.[211,747,756,757]

Extramedullary acute monoblastic leukemias have smaller, more monomorphic, tumor cells, and may express the immature marker CD34.[728] Reactive histiocytic proliferations, including hemophagocytic syndromes and storage diseases, can generally be excluded because of lack of malignant cytologic features.[756,757]

MYELOID SARCOMA (EXTRAMEDULLARY MYELOID TUMOR)

When acute myeloid leukemia involves extramedullary sites, it is known as myeloid or granulocytic sarcoma, extramedullary myeloid tumor, or chloroma.[758] Lymph node involvement has several modes of presentation.[759,760] It may occur at presentation or as relapse in patients with known acute myeloid leukemia, as the first sign of blastic transformation in a patient with a known myeloproliferative or myelodysplastic disorder, or by itself in a patient with no known hematopoietic malignancy.

Histologically, acute leukemia may involve the sinusoidal, interfollicular, or perinodal spaces of a lymph node or diffusely efface the normal lymph node architecture. Sheets of monotonous malignant cells are often accompanied by eosinophilic myelocytes (Fig. 11.79). The malignant cells have intermediately sized round or lobated nuclei, with fine delicate or vesicular chromatin and small to prominent nucleoli. The cytoplasm is scant or moderate and may contain granules. The tumor usually has a high mitotic rate and a starry-sky pattern may be seen, owing to interspersed tingible body macrophages. Touch imprints or frozen sections, if available, can be examined cytochemically for myeloperoxidase or Sudan black B.[758,761] In tissues, the Leder stain (chloroacetate esterase reaction) will be positive in approximately 75% of cases, but the number of positive blasts can be very low. Immunohistochemistry is extremely useful, with antimyeloperoxidase, CD43, CD68, and antilysozyme, each positive in a high percentage of cases.[762] The immature marker CD34 may also be positive, although less frequently in cases with monocytic differentiation. Flow cytometry may also demonstrate an immature myelomonocytic phenotype (e.g. CD34, CD33, CD13, CD117).

The differential diagnosis generally includes high-grade lymphomas (lymphoblastic, large cell, Burkitt's, blastoid mantle cell) and, in children, other small round blue cell tumors. A history of a previous or concurrent acute leukemia, chronic myeloproliferative disorder, or myelodysplasia should alert one to the possibility of an extramedullary myeloid tumor. The larger size and more prominent nucleoli of myelomonocytic cells compared to lymphoblasts and the finer chromatin pattern compared to cells of large cell lymphoma may help distinguish between these entities. Identifying admixed eosinophilic myelocytes or cytoplasmic granules in touch preparations also should suggest the diagnosis. Immunologic (flow cytometric and/or immunohistochemical) and cytochemical studies to demonstrate a myelomonocytic phenotype are particularly helpful in establishing a definitive diagnosis and excluding other entities.

MISCELLANEOUS NEOPLASMS

Hairy cell leukemia may involve the lymph nodes, but rarely without concomitant involvement of the bone marrow and spleen.[763] The outer cortex of the lymph node is preferentially involved and the morphology and immunologic profile are the same as those of hairy cell leukemia involving other sites. Regional lymph nodes near a site of solitary plasmacytoma may be involved by plasmacytoma.[764] *Primary plasmacytoma* of lymph node is extremely rare. Rare cases of

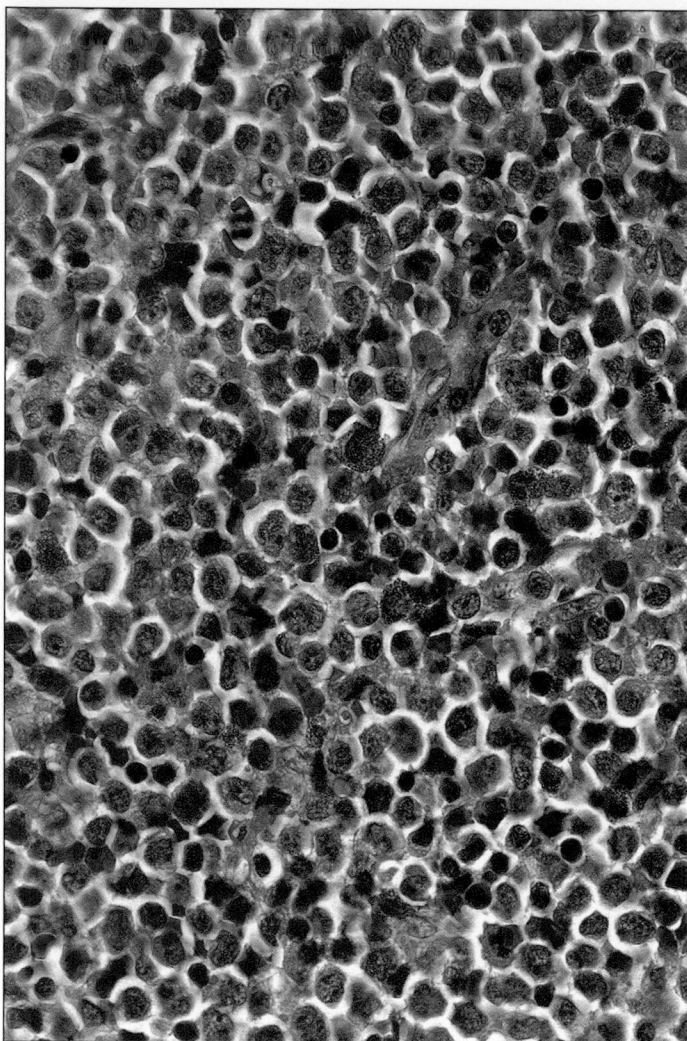

Fig. 11.79 Extramedullary myeloid tumor. A relatively monomorphous population of cells with a fine chromatin pattern is seen. Note the occasional eosinophilic myelocytes.

plasmacytoma of lymph node are associated with amyloidosis.[765,766] Lymph nodes may be involved in cases of *systemic mastocytosis*.[767,768] The mast cell infiltrate is found predominantly in the medullary cords and perivascular areas and is composed of bland cells, with small or indented nuclei, fine chromatin, and a moderate or pale cytoplasm. Eosinophils and sclerosis typically accompany the mast cell clusters. Histochemical stains, Giemsa, chloracetate esterase, and toluidine blue stains can identify mast cell granules; however, immunohistochemistry for tryptase is the most sensitive approach to diagnosis.[768] Mast cell disease is discussed more thoroughly below in the section on splenic mastocytosis.

THE SPLEEN

While the most common spleen specimen received in most laboratories is the result of splenectomy, an increasing number of splenic fine needle aspirations, ultrasound or computed tomography-guided biopsies, and laparoscopic biopsies or total splenectomies are now performed. These procedures have been accurately used to diagnose metastatic disease, splenic involvement by malignant lymphoma, primary splenic tumors, as well as infectious diseases, with very little morbidity.[769-773] While laparoscopic splenectomies are fragmented, which limits gross pattern evaluation of tumors, they usually yield diagnostically useful material. Fine needle aspiration is best for evaluating for metastatic tumors, but may also be used to evaluate for a primary hematologic malignancy. Because of the high frequency of hematologic neoplasms in the spleen, causing either diffuse or focal tumor lesions, flow cytometric immunophenotyping should be considered with most splenic fine needle aspirations. The cytologic features of the individual hematologic tumors studied by fine needle aspiration are usually similar to those in lymph nodes and will not be described in detail.

A wide range of clinical events may result in a patient undergoing a splenectomy or splenic biopsy. While a spleen removed due to traumatic injury, either preoperatively or intraoperatively, generally offers little difficulty to the surgical pathologist, most other causes for splenectomy are diagnostically challenging. A variety of reactive, metabolic, autoimmune, and neoplastic processes can result in splenic enlargement,[774,775] and the clinical indication for splenectomy must be adequately communicated to the pathologist examining the specimen. Although splenic enlargement is often related to a systemic disease process, the splenectomy specimen may be the first opportunity for diagnosis.[776] Adequate sampling, fixation, and processing are all vital to identify many of these disease processes, which may be histologically subtle.

Whenever possible, the spleen should be examined, weighed, and sectioned prior to fixation. One-centimeter-thick sections can be easily made through a fresh specimen, although thinner sectioning may be desired when the splenectomy is performed as a staging procedure. Each breadloafed section should be carefully examined and accentuations of the white pulp should be sampled. The sections submitted for tissue processing and microscopic examination should be thin (2 mm or less in thickness) and adequately fixed prior to processing. We routinely fix one specimen in B5 and place the remaining sections in formalin. If B5 is not available, formalin fixation alone is generally adequate. The tissue, however, must be fixed adequately in the formalin and should be fixed overnight prior to processing if the specimen is received late in the day. The number of required sections will vary greatly by the clinical indication for the procedure. Touch preparations of the fresh spleen should also be made for Wright-Giemsa staining. The cut surface of the spleen should be dried with towels to reduce the amount of blood prior to making the impressions. The touch preparations should be made from areas that include areas of accentuated white pulp, if present.

Additional tissue may also be collected from the fresh specimen. A portion of tissue should be snap frozen if there is any possibility of an hematopoietic neoplasm. This tissue should be stored for possible gene rearrangement studies. Also, if available, fresh tissue should be collected for possible flow cytometric immunophenotyping and cytogenetic study if a hematopoietic neoplasm is in the differential diagnosis.

We find hematoxylin and eosin-stained sections to be adequate for evaluation of most spleen sections, although others have advocated the routine use of silver stains and the PAS stain. Reticulin staining and iron stains may be useful in selected cases.

NORMAL HISTOLOGY

The normal anatomy and histology of the spleen are described in more detail elsewhere.[777,778] The simplest approach to spleen

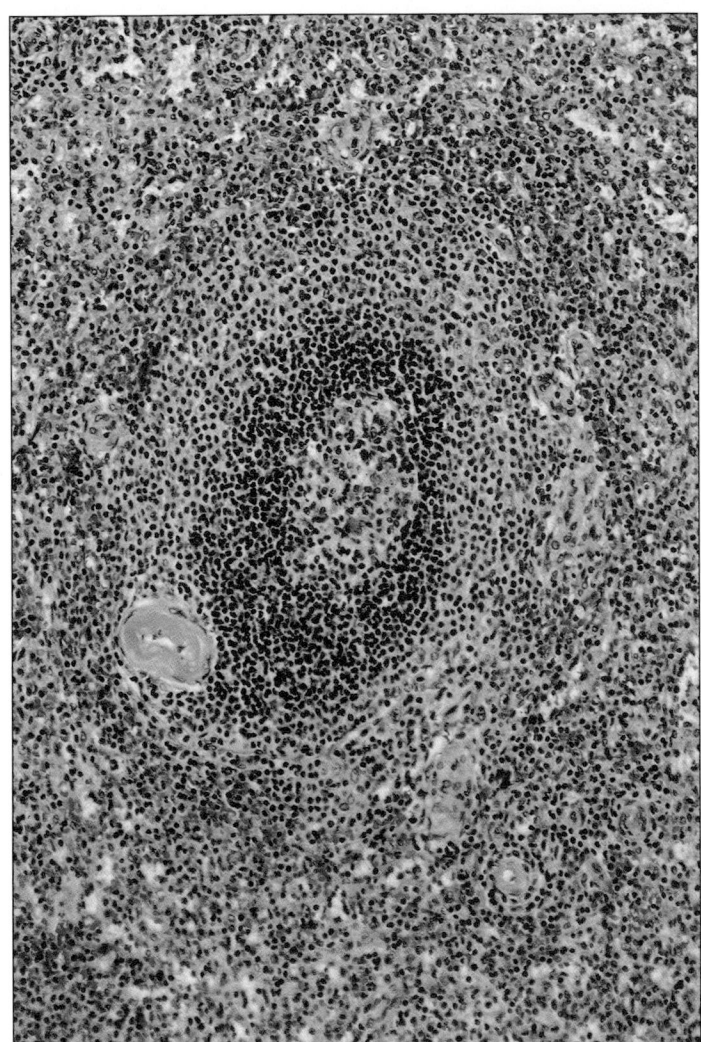

Fig. 11.80 Splenic white pulp in an antigenically stimulated adult. Note the central germinal center, the surrounding, darkly stained mantle zone, and the outer, more pale-staining splenic marginal zone.

histology is to divide the cellular constituents into the white and red pulp. The red pulp is the larger of the two components and is involved in the filtering function of the spleen. It is primarily composed of the open sinuses lined by flattened endothelium and is surrounded by the splenic cords (of Billroth). The lymphoid component of the normal red pulp is minimal, with only rare scattered lymphocytes and plasma cells identified by immunohistochemical studies. The white pulp contains the major lymphoid component of the spleen, with a fairly high proportion of B lymphocytes. The Malpighian corpuscles vary in their appearance with age, with prominent germinal center formation present in children and in antigenically stimulated adults (Fig. 11.80). Adults that are not antigenically stimulated have more involuted white pulp without germinal center formation.

In the child, three distinct white pulp zones of lymphocytes are seen. The central germinal center and surrounding mantle zone are B-cell regions that are similar to the primary follicle of the lymph node. A third distinct lymphocyte zone is also normally present in the splenic white pulp. This splenic marginal zone is composed predominantly of B lymphocytes with slightly more open nuclear chromatin than the mantle zone cells and with moderately abundant, clear cytoplasm. These cells are morphologically similar to the monocytoid B lymphocytes seen in some reactive lymph nodes. The region analogous to the normal splenic marginal zone, however, is not present routinely in lymph nodes. T lymphocytes are scattered within the germinal centers, similar to lymph node follicles, as well as admixed around white pulp follicles with the marginal-zone cells. In addition, periarterial lymphatic sheaths without follicle formation and small red pulp arterioles are surrounded by T lymphocytes.

SPLENOSIS AND ACCESSORY SPLEEN

Splenosis is the term for autotransplantation of the spleen following surgery or trauma that results in multiple small, dark red nodules attached to the abdominal mesentery.[779,780] Microscopically, most cases show a diffuse red pulp proliferation; however, lymphoid nodules with or without germinal centers (white pulp elements) may be seen. The capsule of splenosis is often thinner than the usual splenic capsule. Accessory spleens are present in 16%–19% of individuals and may have similar morphologic features to a nodule of splenosis with both red and white pulp elements.[774,781] Most accessory spleens are solitary, in contrast to the multiple nodules usually found with splenosis.[774,781] The distinction between these two processes may not be possible solely on morphologic grounds, and may depend on the clinical and operative findings.

SPLENIC RUPTURE

Examination of the ruptured spleen following major trauma is of value primarily to document the gross pathologic findings. Microscopic examination of the spleen when it is ruptured in relation to minor or no trauma is important since this unusual occurrence is usually related to an underlying disease process involving the spleen. A variety of infectious disease processes are associated with splenic rupture; most notable of these are infectious mononucleosis and malaria. In addition, patients with splenic involvement by lymphoma, acute leukemia, or metastatic malignancies may rarely present with spontaneous splenic rupture.[782,783] Splenic rupture may be the initial manifestation of the disease process in these patients. Even in the absence of a specific disease, ruptured spleens are more likely than controls to have white pulp germinal centers and hyperplasia, suggesting prior immunologic stimulation.[784,785]

INFECTIOUS DISEASES

Splenomegaly may be caused by a variety of infectious diseases. *Splenic abscesses* are rare, but may be treated by splenectomy.[786,787] They may be single or multiple, and may occur following trauma, and in patients with bacterial endocarditis (especially intravenous drug users), sepsis, and sickle cell disease.[786,788,789] The abscess is usually well circumscribed with a fibrous wall and may be accompanied by white pulp hyperplasia of the surrounding splenic tissue. Bacterial and fungal cultures should be taken in all cases, since many different organisms have been implicated in abscess formation,[790] although *Salmonella* is the most common organism in patients with sickle cell disease.[789] Rarely, patients with splenic abscess have presented with splenic rupture.[786]

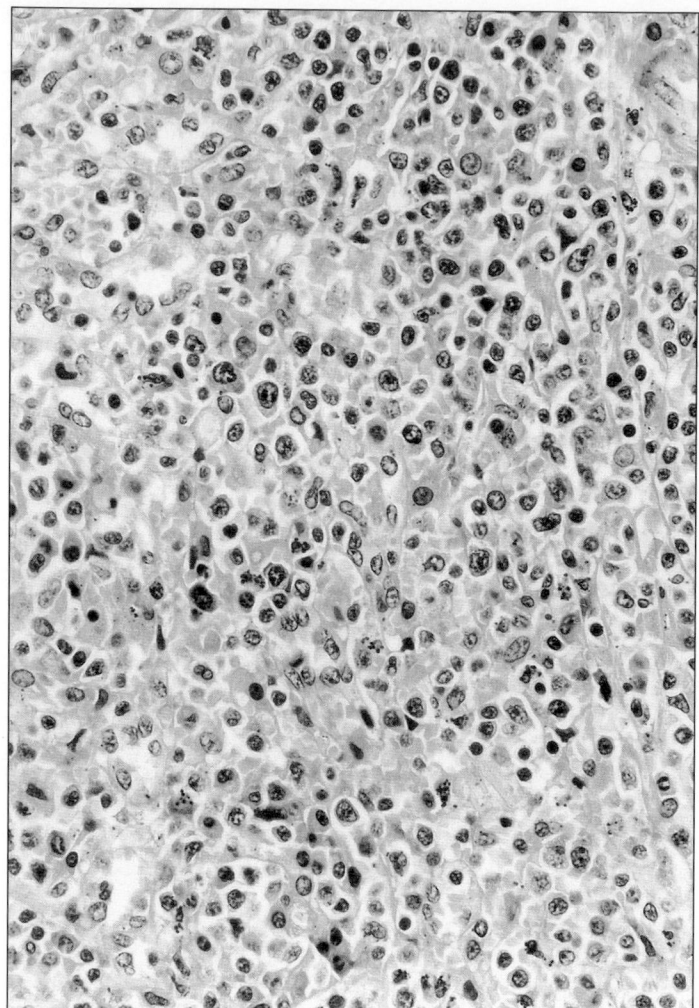

Fig. 11.81 Infectious mononucleosis involving the spleen showing a spectrum of lymphocytes, including plasmacytoid immunoblasts.

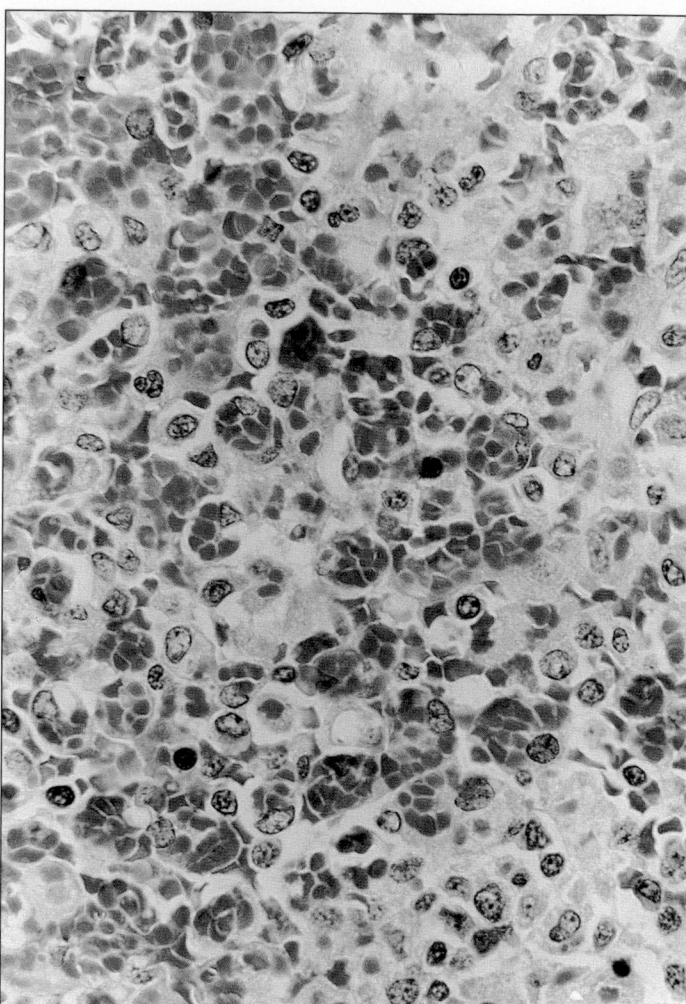

Fig. 11.82 Infection-associated hemophagocytosis showing marked erythrophagocytosis within the splenic red pulp.

More than half of patients of patients with *infectious mononucleosis* have associated splenomegaly. Although many different infectious diseases are associated with an increased risk of rupture, only recurrent malaria infection is associated with more splenic ruptures than Epstein-Barr virus infection.[791] The majority of cases of splenic rupture in infectious mononucleosis are associated with trauma, often minor, although rare cases of spontaneous rupture have been documented.[786,792,793] The morphologic features of infectious mononucleosis in the spleen may be confused with malignant lymphoma. The white pulp may be expanded or depleted with a wide spectrum of cell types (Fig. 11.81) ranging from small lymphocytes and plasma cells to plasmacytoid immunoblasts and cells simulating Reed-Sternberg cells. Such cells may also be seen in increased numbers in the red pulp cords and are generally of T lineage with a suppressor cell phenotype. Areas of individual cell necrosis may be present as well as larger areas of necrosis. Epithelioid granulomas may also be seen. The striking polymorphism of the cellular infiltrate is helpful for excluding a malignant process. In addition, discrete nodules as typically seen in Hodgkin's disease are not usually present in infectious mononucleosis.

Infection-associated, familial, and *secondary hemophagocytoses* (Fig. 11.82) also frequently result in splenomegaly and are often associated with Epstein-Barr virus infection, although other infectious agents may cause identical finding.[794] Two morphologic patterns may be seen with the infection-associated and the familial disorders. The most common is one of white pulp atrophy which is usually accompanied by lymphocyte depletion of lymph nodes. This may be accompanied by red pulp fibrosis.[795] A second pattern of white pulp expansion with cellular polymorphism is similar to that seen in infectious mononucleosis. Both patterns also exhibit a marked expansion of the red pulp by histiocytes showing marked hemophagocytosis.[794] Secondary hemophagocytosis occurs in patients with T-cell lymphomas,[794,796] and evidence of hemophagocytosis may be present in organs that are not involved by lymphoma. Many of these T-cell lymphomas are Epstein-Barr virus-related, and admixed pleomorphic large lymphoid cells may be seen within the splenic red pulp along with the non-neoplastic hemophagocytic histiocytes.

Granulomas are commonly seen in the spleen and may be associated with infectious diseases as well as with malignancies. Tuberculosis, fungal diseases, infectious mononucleosis, and brucellosis, among others, all may cause extensive necrotizing granuloma formation in the spleen, similar to the those seen in lymph nodes. Granulomas of the spleen, however, are not always infection-related and may also be seen in patients with Hodgkin's disease, non-Hodgkin's lymphomas, sarcoidosis, chronic uremia, and selective IgA deficiency.[797] In Hodgkin's disease, granulomas may be present in an otherwise uninvolved spleen and care must be taken to not overinterpret such granulomas as representing disease involvement. The presence of epithelioid granulomas in Hodgkin's disease has been reported to be a favorable prognostic sign.[252,798] Lipogranulomas (follicular lipidosis or mineral oil lipidosis) of the spleen are common in North America, present in approximately half of autopsy specimens, while virtually nonexistent in other geographic areas.[799,800] This difference is presumed to be due to differences in dietary intake or food packaging. Aggregates of vacuolated histiocytes are present, surrounded by lymphocytes and plasma cells. They differ from lymphangiography-associated changes by the lack of epithelioid, foreign body type histiocytes that are commonly seen in tissues following the radiographic procedure. Reactive histiocyte proliferations without granuloma formation may be seen adjacent to splenic trabeculae in patients that have undergone hip or knee replacements.[801]

SPLENIC-GONADAL FUSION

Splenic-gonadal fusion is a congenital disorder that primarily affects males, almost always involving the left testicle. Putschar and Manion[802] described two forms. *Continuous* splenic-gonadal fusion has a direct cord-like attachment of splenic and fibrous tissue between the gonad and the spleen, while the *discontinuous* type represents a fusion between an accessory spleen and the gonad. A subset of cases are associated with congenital defects of the extremities and mandible.[803]

METABOLIC DISEASES

A variety of congenital enzyme deficiencies cause the red pulp accumulation of histiocytes in the spleen with resultant splenomegaly.[804,805] The lysosomal storage diseases are the major group that result in splenomegaly. These disorders generally present in infants and children, although adults are affected by some of these storage diseases, such as type 1 Gaucher disease. The enlarged spleen generally demonstrates a firm mottled to homogeneous cut surface. The red pulp cords are expanded by large aggregates of histiocytes with abundant cytoplasm. The morphologic detail of the histiocytes is best visualized on touch imprints where the tissue-paper character of the Gaucher cell cytoplasm (Fig. 11.83) can more easily be distinguished from the multivacuolated cytoplasm seen with Niemann-Pick disease. Heavily vacuolated balloon cells may be seen with both the gangliosidoses, including Tay-Sach's disease, and the mucopolysaccharidoses, including Hunter's and Hurler's syndromes. Less descript foamy-appearing histiocytes are seen in several disorders, including Fabry's disease, Wolman's disease and von Gierke's disease, while ceroid-containing histiocytes (sea blue histiocytes) with granular cytoplasm may be seen in familial Hermansky-Pudlak syndrome. The presence of ceroid histiocytes, however, is non-specific and they may be seen in other storage diseases as well as in chronic myelogenous leukemia, red blood cell disorders, and autoimmune disorders.[777]

Tangier's disease (familial high protein lipoprotein deficiency) may also result in splenomegaly. The red pulp histiocytes seen in

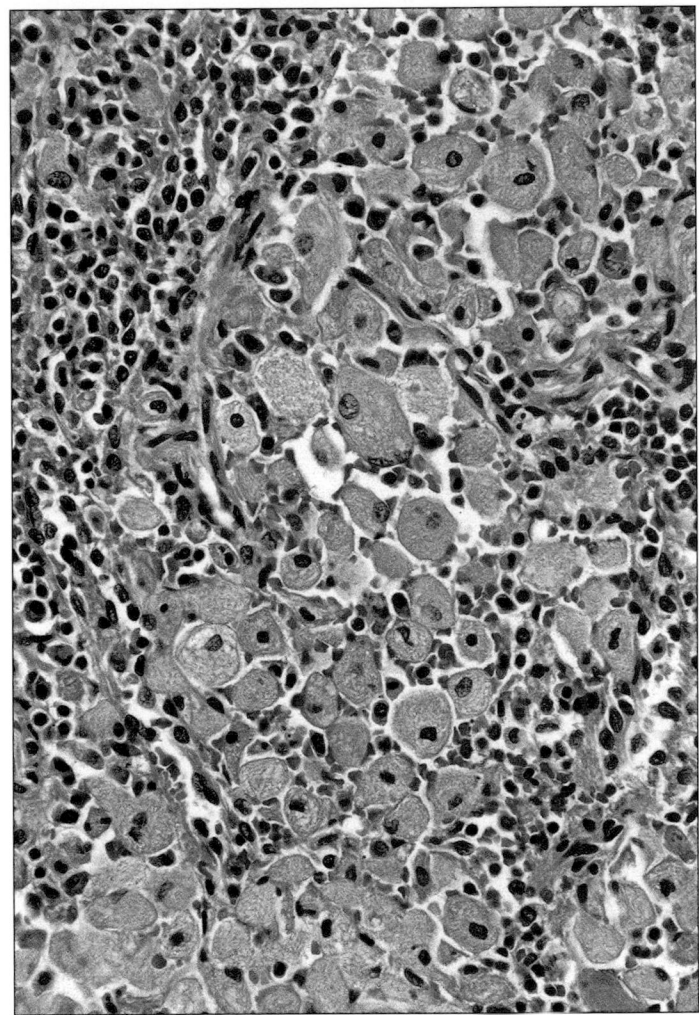

Fig. 11.83 Gaucher's disease. Aggregates of Gaucher's cells expand the splenic red pulp.

these patients contain intracytoplasmic lipid droplets as well as identifiable cholesterol crystals.[804]

The wide morphologic overlap in these diseases makes a definite diagnosis difficult by H&E alone, and differences in cytochemical staining patterns may be useful to differentiate some of these processes. Gaucher cells and ceroid histiocytes contain strongly diastase-resistant, PAS-positive material, in comparison to the cells of Niemann-Pick disease which are only weakly PAS positive. In addition, Niemann-Pick cells contain neutral fat that can be demonstrated in unfixed tissue with an oil red O or other fat stain. In addition to being PAS positive, ceroid histiocytes are positive for acid-fast stains. Specific ultrastructural changes are also described for certain storage diseases, and fresh tissue might be collected for electron microscopy in certain cases. This requires communication between the clinician and pathologist prior to examination and fixation of the specimen. Biochemical evaluation to determine the enzymatic defect is essential for the precise classification of the various storage diseases. Many of the genes involved in these disorders have now been cloned and molecular studies will continue to gain diagnostic importance in these diseases as well. The pathologist must correlate the molecular and enzymatic ancillary test results with the morphologic findings to properly diagnose these cases.

RED BLOOD CELL DISORDERS

Splenomegaly may result from abnormalities of red blood cells. Hereditary spherocytosis is probably the best example of this phenomenon. The red cells in this usually autosomal dominant disorder have abnormalities of the surface protein spectrin or other related proteins. These defects result in a loss of red cell pliability, which is needed for the cells to pass through the cords of Billroth into the splenic sinuses. The sequestration of red blood cells that subsequently occurs results in splenomegaly and anemia. The initial diagnosis is generally made prior to surgery, and splenectomy for this disease is a therapeutic procedure. The morphologic features consist of an expanded red pulp with red blood cell engorgement of the cords and relatively clear sinuses.

Sickle cell anemia is another disorder of red blood cells that the surgical pathologist may encounter. While autosplenectomy frequently occurs in late childhood, splenomegaly is more common in infants and young children with sickle cell anemia. Again, the loss of pliability of the sickled red blood cells within the spleen leads to splenic sequestration and splenomegaly. The morphologic features of such a spleen are similar to those of hereditary spherocytosis, with engorged cords and fairly clear sinuses. With good histologic preservation, sickled red blood cells can be identified within the cords. Other less common red blood cell disorders, including hemoglobin C disease and hemoglobin SC disease, may also result in splenomegaly with similar features. Both α and β thalassemia are also associated with progressive splenomegaly, although such spleens are not commonly received as surgical pathology specimens.

IDIOPATHIC THROMBOCYTOPENIC PURPURA

The surgical pathologist frequently receives splenectomy specimens for idiopathic thrombocytopenic purpura (ITP). The diagnosis is usually well established prior to surgery. Gross examination of these specimens is often only remarkable for slight accentuation of the white pulp. The most common microscopic findings are white pulp hyperplasia with secondary follicle formation and focal red pulp lymphoplasmacytic aggregates. In addition, phagocytosed platelets and extramedullary hematopoiesis may be seen in the red pulp. Foamy, lipid-laden macrophages are also commonly present, containing the degenerated by-products of phagocytosed platelets.[806,807] The plasmacytosis and white pulp hyperplasia, which is also seen with Felty's syndrome,[808] may be absent in ITP patients treated with corticosteroids prior to splenectomy. The platelet-filled red pulp foamy macrophages, however, are usually still present after steroid therapy.[809] The microscopic examination of the spleen in these cases is most important to exclude other causes of hypersplenism, particularly splenic involvement by malignant lymphoma or chronic lymphocytic leukemia. The morphologic features of these latter disorders will be described subsequently.

Rarely, multiple myeloma will involve the spleen with aggregates of red pulp plasma cells, morphologically mimicking ITP. The clinical presentation of these two disorders is usually quite different and can aid in this differential diagnosis. If necessary, immunohistochemical studies on paraffin sections will usually identify a monotypic plasma cell population in multiple myeloma in contrast to the polytypic plasma cells of ITP.

Table 11.18 Splenic cysts

Type	Characteristic features
Primary (true) cyst	
Parasitic	Entirely or partially epithelial lined, parasite scolices identified
Nonparasitic	Entirely or partially epithelial lined, no scolices identified
Secondary (false) cyst	No epithelial lining identified on examination of multiple histologic sections, ± calcification

CYSTS

Cysts of the spleen are found in less than 1% of splenectomy specimens.[810] These rare lesions most frequently occur in young adults in the third decade, but may be seen at any age, and a male predominance has been reported. An abdominal mass is the most common presenting symptom, although abdominal pain and other gastrointestinal tract disturbances may be present or the patient may be asymptomatic. In one large series,[811] the average size of splenic cysts was 10 cm.

Fairly elaborate classification systems have been proposed for the different cyst types;[810,812–814] however, we prefer the simple classification[811] of primary (or true) cysts and secondary (or false) cysts (Table 11.18). Most cysts of either type are unilocular. Primary cysts have a firm but slightly roughened to trabecular internal surface that has been likened to the endocardial surface of the heart. The cyst wall is composed of thick fibrous tissue that is at least partially surfaced by mesothelium, squamous epithelium, or a mixture of both (Fig. 11.84). Subdivision of these cysts based on the type of lining probably does not accurately reflect a difference in pathogenesis.[815] Primary cysts may be parasitic or nonparasitic. There are geographic differences in the frequency of primary parasitic (echinococcal) cysts. Garvin and King[811] found parasitic cysts to represent less than 2% of all splenic cysts accessioned at the Armed Forces Institute of Pathology. The nonparasitic, primary cysts are felt to arise from congenital inclusions.

Secondary cysts are approximately four times as common as primary cysts and are frequently associated with a history of significant trauma. Their gross appearance is similar to the primary cyst, except the lining is generally smoother. Microscopically, the cyst wall is composed of dense fibrous tissue without any lining and approximately 25% of cases will have areas of calcification within the cyst wall. Iron may be demonstrated within the cyst wall, probably reflecting previous hemorrhage related to trauma. Since the major difference in the two cyst types is based on the presence or absence of cyst lining cells, multiple sections of the cyst wall should be submitted to identify the possibly incomplete epithelial lining of primary cysts.

Mucinous cysts in the spleen are usually not an isolated finding and are associated with mucinous tumors of other sites.[816] Therefore, the finding of such a cyst should prompt investigation for an underlying mucinous tumor. Small, incidental, multiloculated and subcapsular cystic lesions that were originally considered subcapsular splenic lymphangiomas are now recognized to be incidental mesothelial cysts in the spleen.[817] Such cysts are usually of little clinical significance.

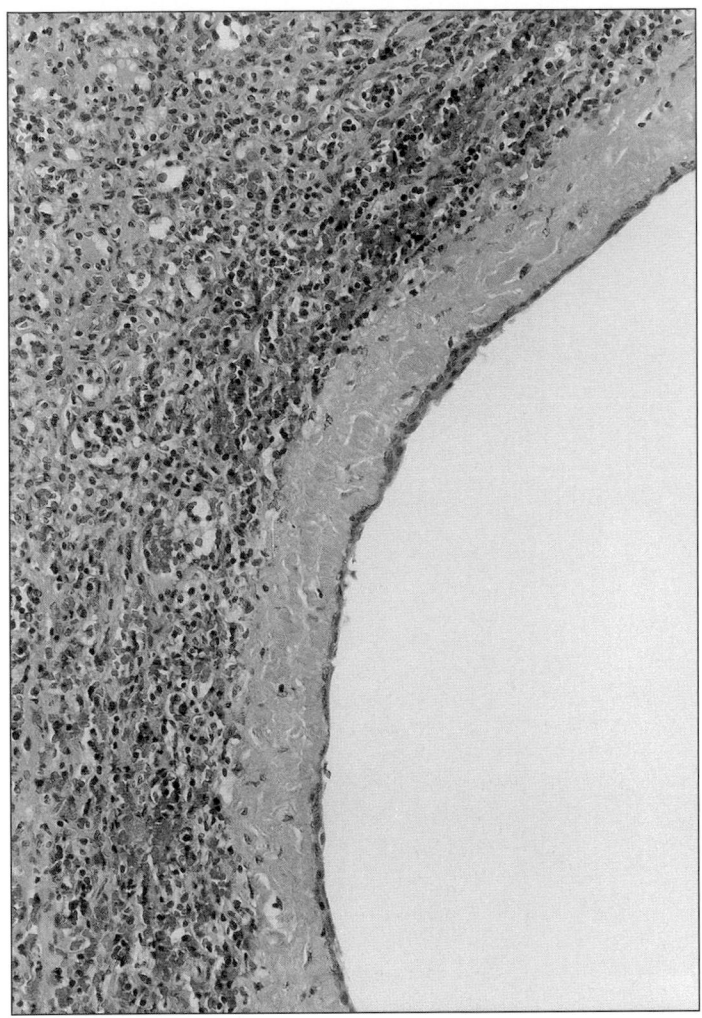

Fig. 11.84 Primary or true splenic cyst. Note that the cyst is lined by a thin layer of flattened epithelium.

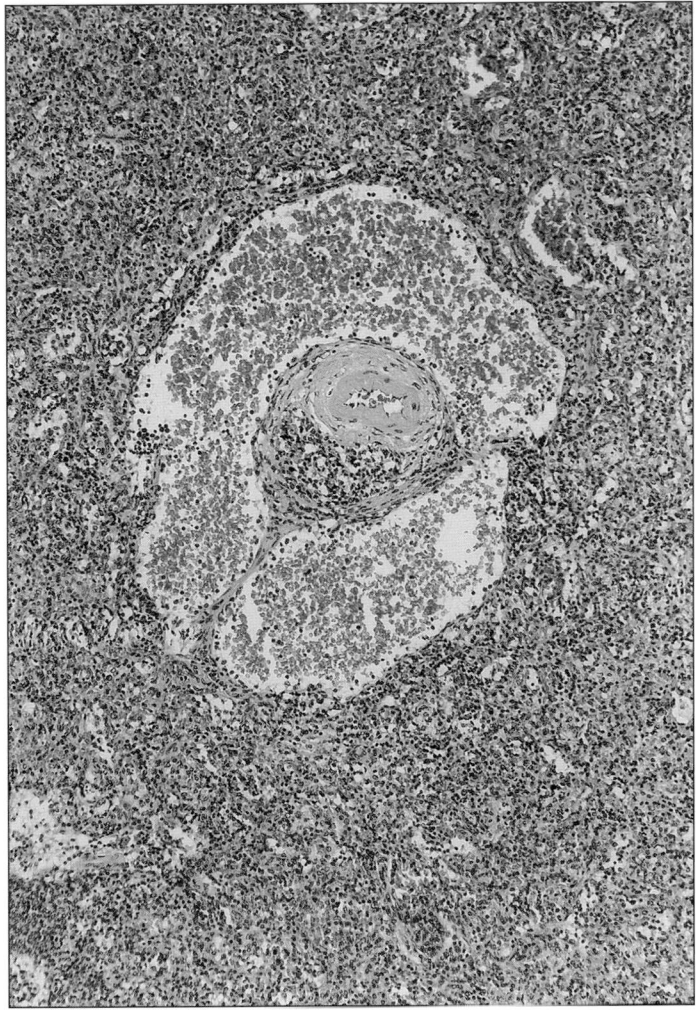

Fig. 11.85 Peliosis of the spleen. Oval blood-filled spaces are present throughout the splenic parenchyma.

BENIGN TUMORS AND PROLIFERATIONS

Vascular and lymphatic proliferations

Hemangiomas are the most common primary tumors of the spleen. Similar to splenic cysts, these lesions are seen most often in young adults.[811,818] They are often asymptomatic, but may present as abdominal masses, with abdominal discomfort or hypersplenism. The spleen is usually only slightly enlarged (300–400 g) with an average size of the lesion reported as 5–8 cm.[811] The lesion generally has a cystic and bloody gross appearance. The morphologic features are similar to hemangiomas at other sites and usually have a cavernous component. Hemangiomas may undergo infarction with resultant fibrosis and possible cystic change.

A subset of hemangiomas in the spleen may be unique. These were recently described as *sclerosing angiomatoid nodular transformation*.[819] This grossly nodular tumor has a multinodular microscopic appearance composed of plump, spindled cells with slit-like vascular spaces. The nodules are surrounded by fibrosis and the spindled cells show no cytologic atypia, mitotic activity, or necrosis. This tumor does not appear to recur, and probably includes some cases that were considered to be epithelioid and spindled heman-

gioendotheliomas. Cases that appear to be similar to this proliferation have been described as having myoid and angioendotheliomatous features.[820]

Peliosis of the spleen is a rare, diffuse vascular proliferation, primarily of adults, which is infrequently associated with splenomegaly. It is usually an incidental finding, although rare cases have been associated with splenic rupture.[821,822] Although it is usually found in conjunction with peliosis of the liver, approximately 17% of cases of peliosis involve only the spleen.[823] Peliosis of the spleen is most often associated with anabolic steroid use, malignancy, tuberculosis, and aplastic anemia. It has also been reported in association with splenic involvement by chronic myelomonocytic leukemia.[874] The process is usually evident grossly with diffuse, dilated vascular spaces of up to 1 mm.[823,825] Microscopically, round to oval blood-filled spaces are lined by a single layer of cells without cordal fibrosis (Fig. 11.85).

Patients with *lymphangiomas* may be asymptomatic or present with abdominal pain. The cystic nature of the gross lesions may suggest a primary or secondary cyst in some cases, and 10% of cystic spleen lesions described by Fowler[813] were considered lymphangiomas. Smaller lymphangiomas may be less cystic in appearance and multiple splenic lymphangiomas may also occur.[826] These proliferations are most often found in children and young adults and have a reported predilection for a subcapsular location,[811] compared to hemangiomas which occur in no specific splenic location. However, these small, incidental subcapsular lesions were recently shown to actually represent small mesothelial cystic proliferations, mimicking lymphangiomas.[817] These lesions are lined by bland, plump cells that are keratin positive. Microscopically, true lymphangiomas consist of a single layer of endothelium surrounding the variably sized cystic spaces containing proteinaceous material. The lining cells immunoreact for Factor VIII-related antigen as well as CD31, while negative for CD68 and keratin. *Lymphangiomatosis* is a rare condition associated with lymphangiomas of multiple sites, including the spleen as well as other organs, including bone.[827]

Littoral cell angioma of the spleen is an endothelial-lined proliferation of the spleen that differs both morphologically and immunohistochemically from hemangiomas and lymphangiomas.[818] The tumor may occur at any age. Patients most commonly presented with splenomegaly in the report of Falk et al.,[828] although the tumors in that series varied greatly in size, from 0.2 to 9 cm. Littoral cell angiomas are grossly nodular dark spongy lesions that are frequently multiple and may be cystic. Microscopically, they contain tall endothelial cells with small nucleoli, a low mitotic rate, and no nuclear pleomorphism although the cells may be large with abundant cytoplasm and enlarged nuclei (Fig. 11.86). The endothelial cells commonly form papillary projections that are often accompanied by endothelial cell sloughing into the lumina of the lesion. The intraluminal cells may show evidence of hemophagocytosis. Littoral cell angioma may be confused with other benign vascular lesions or with angiosarcoma, although mitoses are not increased and nuclear atypia is not prominent. Immunohistochemically, the lining cells of littoral cell angioma stain for Factor VIII-related antigen as well as for CD21, CD31, and CD68.[818,828] The expression of CD68 presumably reflects a pattern of dual differentiation in this lesion of both vascular and histiocytic origin. Unlike normal sinus lining cells, the lining cells of littoral angioma do not express CD8. The expression of CD21 is a useful feature in excluding other vascular lesions.

Littoral cell angioma is generally a benign proliferation, but a case has been reported to recur many years after splenectomy.[829] This so-called littoral cell hemangioendothelioma showed morphologic and immunophenotypic features of littoral cell angioma, as well as focal areas of necrosis, which is not a typical finding in littoral cell angioma. Therefore, necrotic foci in a tumor that is otherwise typical for littoral cell angioma may be a feature to suggest the possibility of low-grade malignancy in this tumor.

Tumors described as littoral cell angiosarcoma have been reported based on expression of CD68 and CD8 on the tumor cells.[830–832] This immunophenotype, however, may be seen in other angiosarcomas,[818] and does not appear to be specific for a sinus lining cell-derived tumor.

Hamartoma

Splenic hamartoma, also termed splenoma or 'spleen in spleen' syndrome, is a rare, generally asymptomatic lesion with only three such lesions found in almost 200 000 surgical spleen specimens in one series.[833] Since most lesions are incidental autopsy findings, they have been found most commonly in elderly patients with no apparent sex predilection. Hamartomas, however, may occur at any age, and may be seen in spleens removed for other causes. In addition, rare cases may present with splenomegaly, hypersplenism or splenic rupture.[834,835]

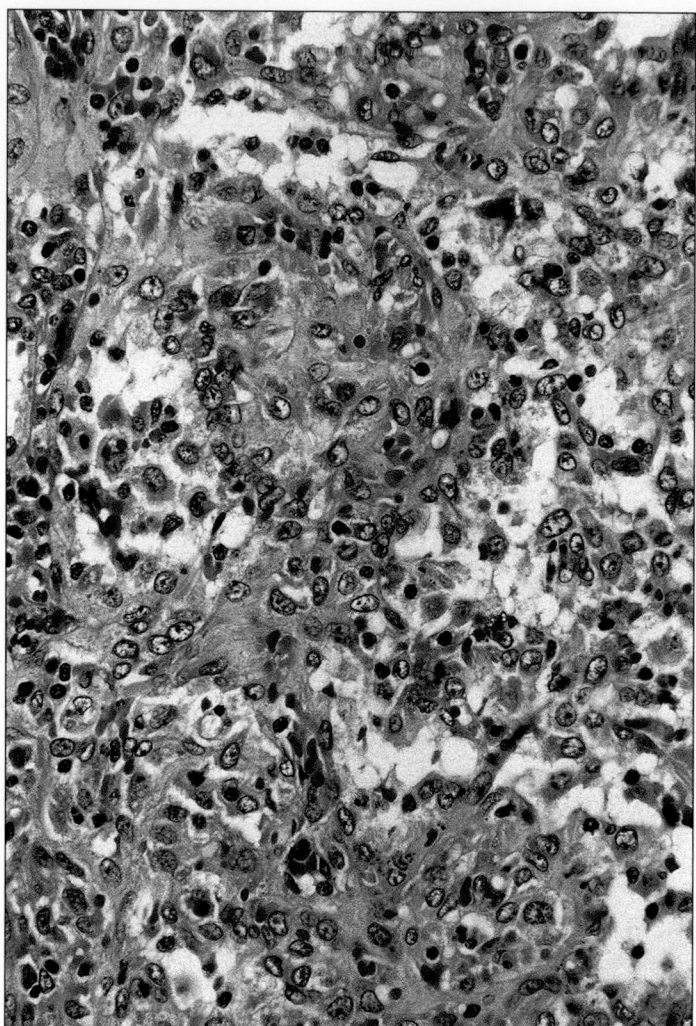

Fig. 11.86 Littoral cell angioma. Papillary projections are present with sloughing of endothelial cells into the lumina. Although there is enlargement of the endothelial cells, no nuclear atypia is seen.

Grossly, hamartomas appear well-circumscribed and have a characteristic bulging cut surface. Other than the bulging surface, they frequently have a similar gross appearance to the surrounding splenic parenchyma. Microscopically, they are not encapsulated, but compress the surrounding normal splenic tissue. The hamartoma is composed of a homogeneous proliferation of splenic sinuses and cords similar to the surrounding red pulp without Malpighian corpuscles or periarterial lymphoid sheaths. An increase in B and T lymphocytes as well as plasma cells has been seen in some cases.[836] While some reports have described white pulp elements with hamartomas,[837] they are characteristically absent. This can be confirmed by a lack of CD21-positive dendritic cells in areas of lymphocytes within the hamartoma, as compared to the normal dendritic cell network in the white pulp nodules outside of the hamartoma.[836]

Hemangioma is the major splenic tumor to be considered in the differential diagnosis of hamartoma. Because hamartomas are proliferations of normal red pulp cells, CD8-positive sinus lining cells are present in splenic hamartoma but the vascular cells of

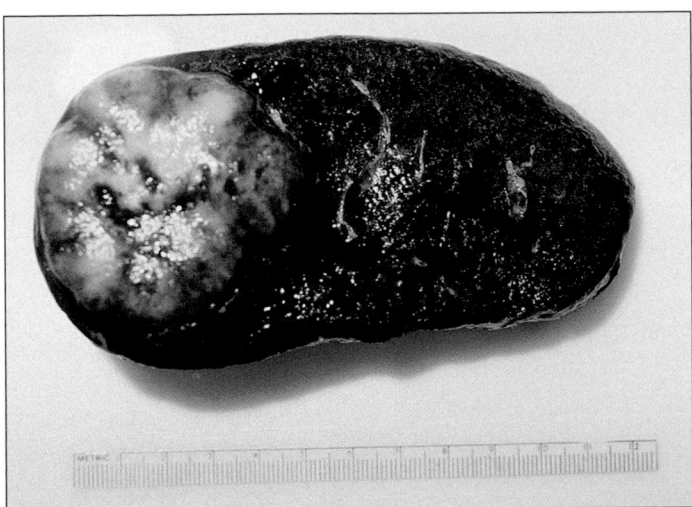

Fig. 11.87 Inflammatory pseudotumor of the spleen forming a large, well-circumscribed nodule, simulating a malignant neoplasm.

hemangiomas are usually CD8 negative.[818,838] Morphologically, the absence of a cavernous component associated with the vascular channels is a helpful finding in excluding hemangioma.

Inflammatory pseudotumor

Inflammatory pseudotumor (also known as inflammatory myofibroblastic tumor) of the spleen is now well described,[839–841] and may be seen in a wide age range, from young adulthood to the elderly. The patients may be asymptomatic or may present with abdominal pain or an abdominal mass. Some patients present with anemia, weight loss, malaise, and fever, suggestive of an infectious disease. The lesions may or may not be associated with splenomegaly and are usually solitary, although occasional multifocal lesions are seen. Inflammatory pseudotumors are characteristically well circumscribed, but not encapsulated, with a white or yellow cut surface that may contain areas of necrosis (Fig. 11.87). They can vary greatly in size, from 1.5 cm to over 12 cm. Microscopically, they are composed of an admixture of cells. Lymphocytes and plasma cells are present at least focally, and foci of neutrophils and occasional eosinophils may also be present. Clusters of histiocytes, often foamy, are present in some tumors. Fibrosis, sclerosis, plump spindled cells and often vascular proliferation are other characteristic features of these tumors (Fig. 11.88). Foci of necrosis are present in some cases. Although the etiology of most cases of inflammatory pseudotumor at any site is not known, the tumors of the liver and spleen are often associated with evidence of the Epstein-Barr virus.[842] In particular, the spindle cells of these tumors have been shown to contain this virus. These spindle cells also express CD21, leading some authors to suggest that they represent unusual types of follicular dendritic cell tumors.[85,843] Cases of inflammatory pseudotumor have recurred as follicular dendritic cell tumors, but the detection of the Epstein-Barr virus in follicular dendritic cell tumors is extremely unusual at other sites, suggesting that these proliferations are unique to the liver and spleen.

The gross appearance of these tumors may simulate a metastatic lesion, and the morphologic features may superficially mimic those of Hodgkin's disease. The lack of identifiable Reed-Sternberg cells or their mononuclear variants excludes such a neoplastic process.

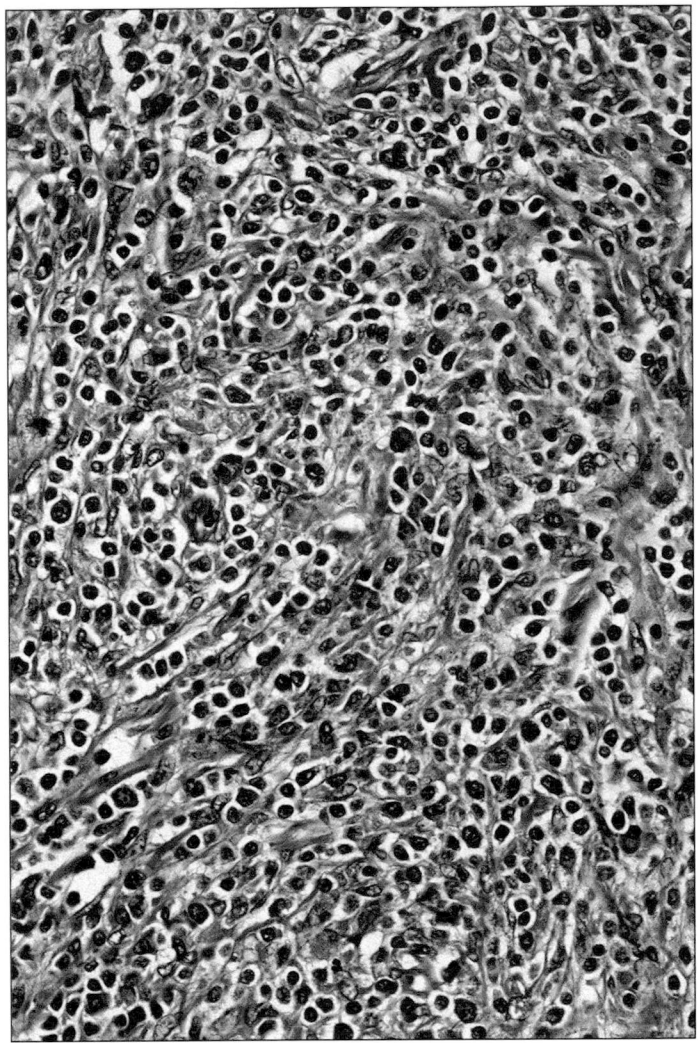

Fig. 11.88 Inflammatory pseudotumor of the spleen. An admixture of stromal cells, lymphocytes, and plasma cells is present.

Localized reactive lymphoid hyperplasia

Small localized hyperplastic foci of the spleen have been reported, usually in spleens of normal weight, which may grossly mimic malignancy.[844] Similar to inflammatory pseudotumors, these foci are well-circumscribed, but are not encapsulated. They are smaller than inflammatory pseudotumors, usually 0.1–1.0 cm, and contain prominent reactive follicular hyperplasia. Some cases may have accompanying sclerosis and a plasma cell infiltrate. The surrounding splenic white pulp in these cases frequently shows evidence of reactive hyperplasia. These lesions offer a similar differential diagnosis to inflammatory pseudotumors, and caution must be used in diagnosing localized reactive lymphoid hyperplasia in the setting of Hodgkin's disease. In these cases, it is advisable to examine multiple tissue levels for the presence of neoplastic cells.

The relationship between these lesions and inflammatory pseudotumor is not clear since there is some overlap in the morphologic features of the two proliferations in the spleen. Small size and the presence of abundant lymphoid hyperplasia would favor a diagnosis of localized reactive lymphoid hyperplasia.

Systemic mast cell disease

Systemic mast cell disease, or mastocytosis, is a rare multi-organ proliferation of mast cells that may be subclassified into benign and malignant categories. Patients with malignant mastocytosis have an associated malignancy, usually a myeloproliferative disorder or myelodysplasia, and usually do not have the cutaneous involvement seen in benign mast cell disease. Over two-thirds of patients with systemic mast cell disease have splenomegaly,[845] and a splenectomy specimen may be the first diagnostic specimen received in such a patient. The spleen may vary widely in weight, from a normal weight to over 2000 grams.[767,845] The largest spleens are seen in patients with malignant mastocytosis, although pathologic examination of the spleen alone cannot conclusively distinguish between the benign and malignant forms of mast cell disease. The splenic capsule usually shows fibrous thickening, and the cut surface demonstrates an expanded red pulp without prominent white pulp. In spleens of near normal weight, no other gross lesions may be identifiable. Nodules of 1–2 mm may be identified throughout the cut surface in the more enlarged specimens.

Microscopically, the grossly identified nodules represent multiple areas of fibrosis, usually radiating from blood vessels, or nodular collections of mast cells. The mast cells have central, dark staining, round to irregular nuclei, and abundant, often clear, cytoplasm or they may have a more spindled cell appearance admixed with a surrounding fibrous stroma (Fig. 11.89). Only rare, more typical mast cells with basophilic or granular cytoplasm may be present, and eosinophils may be more obvious than the mast cells in many cases. Despite the pattern, the fibrous areas of the spleen are almost pathognomonic of mast cell disease, forming multiple areas of stellate fibrosis. Both a diffuse red pulp and focal white pulp pattern of splenic involvement by mastocytosis have been described;[845] however, the multifocal fibrotic pattern is the most common one seen. These fibrous areas are often so prominent that the underlying mast cells are easily missed. Identification of the pattern of fibrosis as well as the scattered eosinophils should increase the surgical pathologist's index of suspicion of a mast cell proliferation. In addition to the multiple aggregates of mast cells or the stellate areas of fibrosis, the splenic red pulp may be expanded in patients with mast cell disorders. Extramedullary hematopoiesis is frequently present. Mast cells are generally positive with chloracetate esterase, Giemsa and toluidine blue stains, although the demonstration of neoplastic mast cells with cytochemical stains is frequently pH dependent.[846] Mast cells may also express the CD43, CD45, and CD68 antigens.[847] Although all of these antigens can be detected in paraffin sections, they are also relatively non-specific. Mast cells, however, show very high expression of CD117 and are tryptase positive,[768] and these two markers are useful in the immunohistochemical evaluation of this disease.

Malignant mast cell disease is associated with several malignancies.[848] In the spleen, these patients may have acute or chronic myeloproliferative disorders or myelodysplastic syndromes that infiltrate the splenic red pulp. Careful attention, therefore, must be placed on the identification of a second process in these patients. Solid tumors, in organs other than the spleen, may also be present in patients with mast cell disease.

MALIGNANCIES INVOLVING THE SPLEEN

Leukemias

Acute leukemias may secondarily involve the spleen with resultant splenomegaly. Both acute myeloid and lymphoblastic leukemia

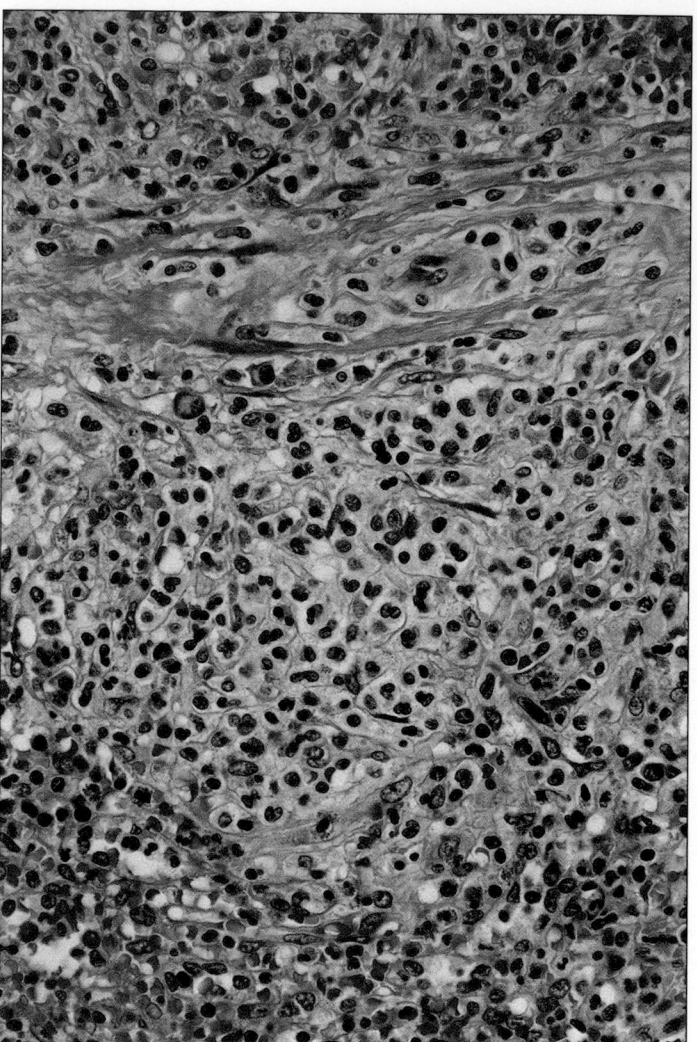

Fig. 11.89 Systemic mast cell disease of the spleen. An aggregate of mast cells with abundant clear cytoplasm is present with adjacent fibrosis.

predominantly involve the splenic red pulp. Blast cells are identifiable in both the splenic cords and sinuses as a relatively monotonous cell composition with fine nuclear chromatin and a high mitotic rate. Lymphoblasts may be difficult to distinguish from small lymphocytes if the cytologic details are not well-preserved. Paraffin section immunohistochemistry may be helpful in determining the lineage of the cellular infiltrate as well as confirming the immature nature of lymphoid cells. Myeloperoxidase staining will identify the majority of cells of myeloid derivation. Precursor-B lymphoblasts may be identified by staining for both the B-cell antigen CD79a and TdT. CD3 antigen and TdT expression may be detected in many cases of acute lymphoblastic leukemia of T lineage. An even more detailed phenotypic analysis may be performed if fresh tissue is submitted for flow cytometric evaluation.

The chronic myeloproliferative disorders all generally cause splenomegaly to varying degrees. Splenectomy may be performed for some of these disorders, most notably for *myelosclerosis with myeloid metaplasia* (agnogenic myeloid metaplasia).[849] In myelosclerosis with myeloid metaplasia, the spleen is almost always significantly enlarged, averaging approximately 2000 grams.[850,851] The splenic capsule is often thickened with patchy fibrosis, and the spleen has a

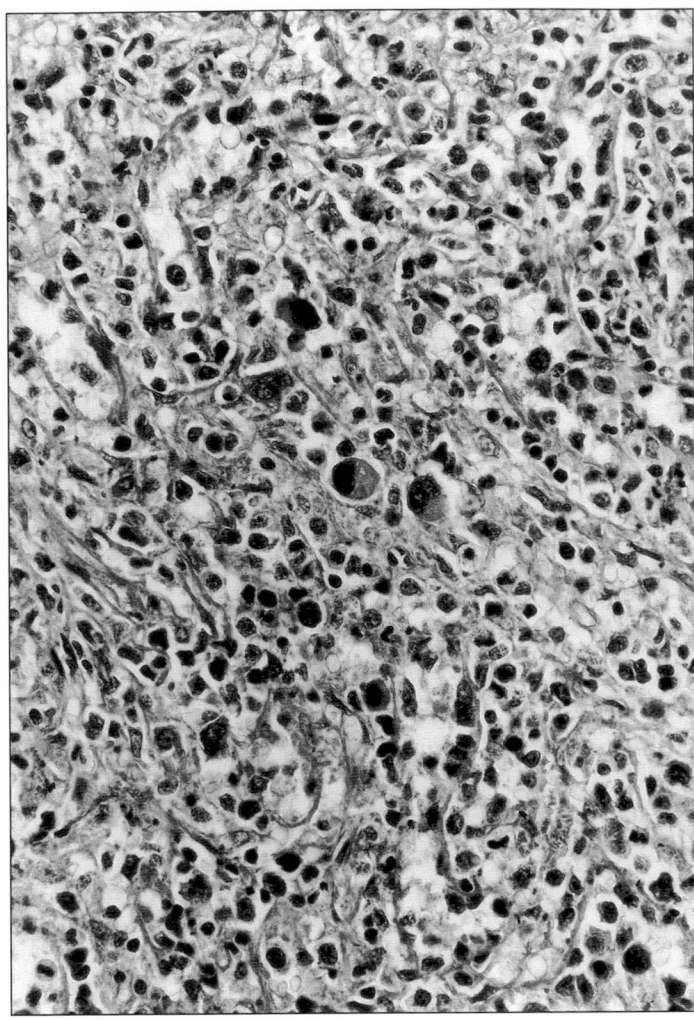

Fig. 11.90 Myelosclerosis with myeloid metaplasia. Extramedullary hematopoiesis is present in the splenic red pulp. Megakaryocytes are the cell type most easily identified.

homogeneous red to brown cut surface with indistinct Malpighian corpuscles. Areas of infarction may be present, especially in the larger spleens. Gross nodules corresponding to areas of hematopoiesis are occasionally seen. Microscopically, the white pulp is decreased or absent with little or no germinal center formation. The red pulp is congested with prominent areas of extramedullary hematopoiesis present in both the cords and sinuses, but primarily within the splenic cords (Fig. 11.90). Of the maturing hematopoietic elements, the megakaryocytes are the most morphologically striking, showing dysplastic features with smaller cells and pleomorphic nuclei as well as the presence of immature megakaryocytes.[851,852] Some cases may show a predominance of immature, or left-shifted, granulocytes. Fibrosis of the red pulp cords may be prominent, especially in the larger spleens. The etiology of this fibrosis appears to differ from the bone marrow fibrosis seen in these patients and does not appear to be related to the megakaryocytic proliferation. Instead, the splenic fibrosis appears to be secondary to splenic congestion, similar to the red pulp fibrosis found in patients with portal hypertension. Additional cases may demonstrate a red pulp plasmacytosis, and others may contain areas of hemorrhage and scarring. The morphologic findings of the spleen in myelosclerosis with myeloid metaplasia are not

pathognomonic, and similar findings may be found in the other chronic myeloproliferative disorders, especially chronic myelogenous leukemia. Correlation with clinical, cytogenetic, peripheral blood, and bone marrow findings are all essential for the proper classification of these disorders. The identification of a predominance of immature granulocytes or microscopic evidence of infarction are associated with decreased post-splenectomy survival.[853]

In *chronic myelogenous leukemia*, the red that pulp infiltrate of the spleen may show more numerous maturing myeloid cells and a lesser degree of extramedullary hematopoiesis than that seen in myelosclerosis with myeloid metaplasia. Varying numbers of blast cells may also be present, and blast crisis of CML may present with a rapidly enlarging spleen. In *essential thrombocythemia*, the spleen may be small and atrophic or enlarged.[812] When enlarged, the red pulp is congested and contains numerous platelet-filled histiocytes. Occasional megakaryocytes may be present, but other evidence of extramedullary hematopoiesis is not prominent. In *polycythemia vera*, there are two different patterns of splenomegaly.[854] In the erythrocytotic phase of polycythemia vera, the white pulp is decreased and there is marked congestion of the red pulp by red blood cells. This congestion is presumably secondary to the elevated red blood cell mass in these patients. Extramedullary hematopoiesis is minimal, and the average splenic weight is 800–900 grams. In the spent phase of polycythemia vera, the spleen is even larger, averaging over 2000 grams. Marked extramedullary hematopoiesis is present in the splenic cords and sinuses with all three bone marrow cell lines evident. Immature precursor cells become more evident as the spleen enlarges.

Patients receiving growth factors, especially granulocyte colony stimulating factor (G-CSF), may have myeloid proliferations of the spleen that mimic involvement by a chronic myeloproliferative disorder.[855] Therefore, correlation with the clinical medication history is suggested before interpreting a spleen as being involved by a myeloproliferative disorder.

The chronic lymphoid leukemias also frequently involve the spleen. *Chronic lymphocytic leukemia* and *prolymphocytic leukemia* primarily involve the splenic white pulp with secondary involvement of the red pulp. This distribution will be discussed in more detail below with small lymphocytic lymphoma. *Hairy cell leukemia* is a rare chronic lymphoid leukemia of B lineage that frequently presents in elderly patients with pancytopenia and splenomegaly.[763] The spleen in this disorder is massively enlarged, usually over 1000 grams, although splenic involvement by hairy cell leukemia without splenomegaly has been reported.[856] The spleen has a homogeneous cut surface with diminished Malpighian bodies. Unlike the majority of chronic lymphoproliferative disorders of B lineage, hairy cell leukemia primarily involves the splenic red pulp. A diffuse red pulp proliferation, with or without residual white pulp follicles, is present, composed of small, relatively homogeneous lymphoid cells with ovoid nuclei and abundant clear to pink-staining cytoplasm (Fig. 11.91). Dilated, blood-filled sinuses, also known as red cell lakes, may be present, but are not pathognomonic. Paraffin section immunohistochemistry for CD20 may be useful to identify the marked increase of B-lineage cells within the red pulp. In addition, the cells characteristically express the CD103 antigen. Immunophenotyping will identify a monoclonal B-cell population that is CD5-negative and usually CD10-negative while commonly expressing CD11c and CD25. Imprint preparations will more clearly demonstrate the cytologic features of the tumor cells than can be appreciated on H&E sections. The cells have slightly indented nuclei with abundant cytoplasm and irregular (hairy) cytoplasmic borders. Cytochemical studies may be performed on imprint preparations to demonstrate

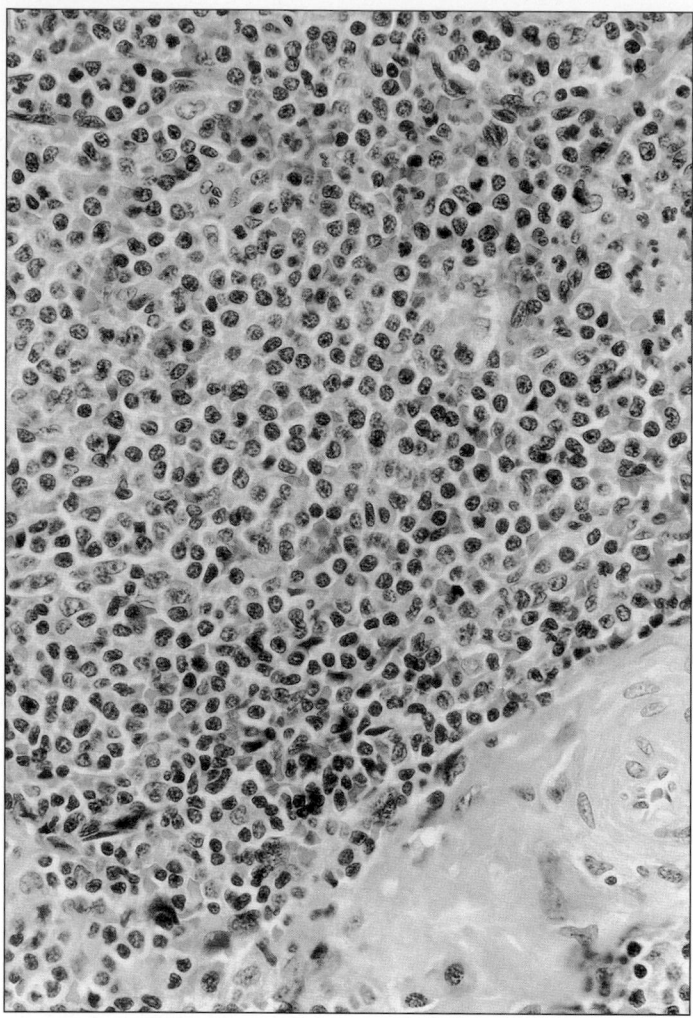

Fig. 11.91 Hairy cell leukemia. A monotonous population of small lymphoid cells with moderately abundant cytoplasm diffusely replace the splenic red pulp.

Table 11.19 Common patterns of splenic involvement by hematopoietic malignant tumors

Predominantly white pulp disease
  Chronic lymphocytic leukemia/small lymphocytic lymphoma
  Prolymphocytic leukemia
  Follicular center lymphoma[a]
  Mantle cell lymphoma
  Splenic marginal zone lymphoma/marginal zone B-cell lymphoma
  Lymphoplasmacytic lymphoma[a]
  Early involvement by B-lineage large cell and immunoblastic lymphoma[a]

Predominantly red pulp disease
  Acute myeloid leukemia
  Acute lymphoblastic leukemia/lymphoblastic lymphoma
  Chronic myeloproliferative disorders
  Hairy cell leukemia
  Lymphoplasmacytic lymphoma[a]
  Hepatosplenic T-cell lymphoma
  Large granular lymphocytosis
  Some T-cell lymphomas[a]
  Rare B-lineage large cell lymphomas[a]

Predominantly nodular disease
  Most large cell and immunoblastic lymphomas, B or T lineage[a]
  Some follicular center lymphomas[a]
  Hodgkin's disease

[a] More than one pattern may be seen with these tumor types.

the characteristic tartrate resistant acid phosphatase (TRAP) positivity of the hairy cells, but a commercially available TRAP antibody is now available for paraffin section immunohistochemistry and this methodology has replaced the cytochemical study in most laboratories.

Large granular lymphocytosis is a T-cell or natural killer cell proliferation that is associated with neutropenia and an increased risk of infections. Splenectomy has been reported to reduce the degree of neutropenia in these patients.[857] Grossly, the spleen is enlarged, weighing from 450 to 1650 grams with no gross lesions.[857,858] Microscopically, the white pulp may be expanded, but is uninvolved by the neoplastic proliferation while the red pulp is expanded by the tumor cells. On H&E sections, the infiltrate has the appearance of small lymphocytes and may be confused with hairy cell leukemia. Well-fixed sections, however, will show that the cells lack the abundant clear cytoplasm of hairy cells. Imprint preparations show the characteristic large cytoplasmic granules that are associated with the NK/T cell phenotype of this proliferation. Immunohistochemical studies will also exclude a B-cell proliferation such as hairy cell leukemia. The large granular lymphocytes are often CD3 positive or mark for the less specific T-lineage associated antigen CD43. Many cases also express CD8, CD57 (Leu 7), TIA-1 or granzyme B, which

can also be detected by paraffin section immunohistochemistry. Correlation with the peripheral blood and clinical findings is helpful in the differential diagnosis with other T-cell proliferations, especially hepatosplenic T-cell lymphoma.

Malignant lymphoma secondarily involving the spleen

Malignant lymphoma of the spleen usually represents secondary involvement. Any of the malignant lymphomas previously described can secondarily involve the spleen with morphologic features similar to lymph node involvement. A great deal has been written concerning the pattern of splenic involvement by various malignancies, especially lymphoma.[859–863] Traditionally, malignant lymphomas of B lineage and chronic lymphocytic leukemia are described as involving primarily the white pulp while acute leukemias, chronic myeloproliferative disorders, histiocytic malignancies, and T-cell lymphomas reportedly primarily involve the splenic red pulp. These generalizations hold true for the leukemias, but are fairly inconsistent for the malignant lymphomas. Immunophenotyping studies demonstrate that some T-lineage neoplasms involve the white pulp primarily and many B-lineage lymphomas may primarily involve the red pulp.

Table 11.19 shows the overlap of pattern of splenic lymphomas. Most low-grade B-cell lymphomas diffusely involve the splenic white pulp and often cause gross accentuation of the Malpighian bodies. The spleen may be massively enlarged in these patients. In chronic lymphocytic leukemia and small lymphocytic lymphoma, the markedly expanded white pulp nodules fuse to form large dumbbell-shaped aggregates of tumor. In addition, small lymphoid cells of B lineage spill over into the surrounding red pulp (Fig. 11.92). This secondary red pulp infiltration is a helpful feature in distinguishing

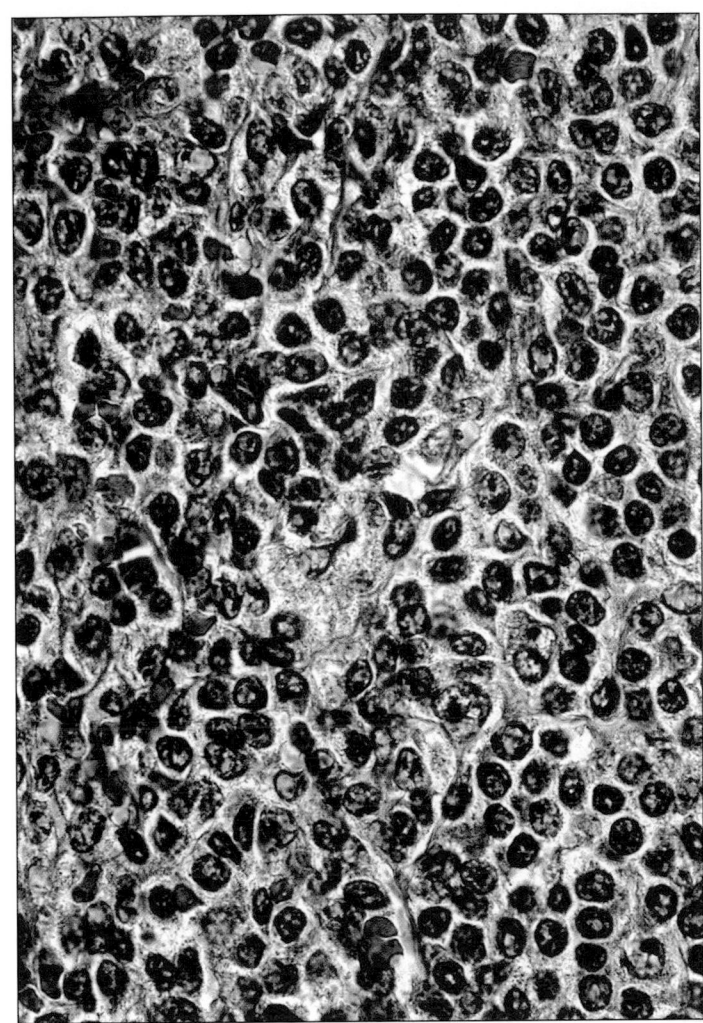

Fig. 11.92 Small lymphocytic lymphoma/chronic lymphocytic leukemia. Small lymphocytes with scattered larger prolymphocytes expand the splenic white pulp and secondarily infiltrate the red pulp. This red pulp involvement, demonstrated in the figure, is a helpful clue in the diagnosis of splenic involvement by lymphoma.

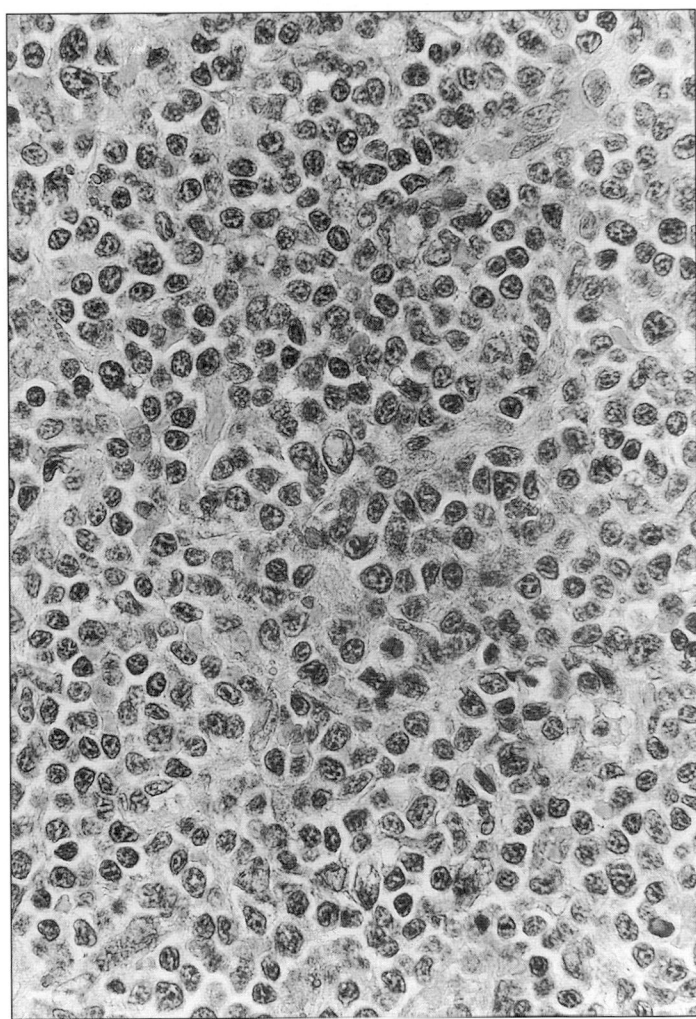

Fig. 11.93 Lymphoplasmacytic lymphoma. The entire splenic parenchyma may be replaced by plasmacytoid cells. The identification of intranuclear inclusions (Dutcher bodies) is a useful diagnostic feature.

large reactive white pulp hyperplasia from splenic lymphoma since this differential diagnosis may be problematic in patients who undergo splenectomy for presumed immune thrombocytopenic purpura (ITP) that is actually related to low-grade lymphoma. Early involvement of the spleen by lymphoma may be morphologically similar to the expanded white pulp of an ITP patient and immunohistochemical studies are useful to demonstrate an abnormal increase in red pulp B lymphocytes in involved spleens. Prolymphocytoid transformation of small lymphocytic lymphoma and prolymphocytic leukemia may show a zone of transformed cells at the periphery of the expanded white pulp, adjacent to the red pulp.[864]

Lymphoplasmacytic lymphomas, which may cause massive splenomegaly in clinical Waldenström macroglobulinemia, may have the white pulp pattern of small lymphocytic lymphomas or may diffusely infiltrate the splenic red pulp (Fig. 11.93). The frequent presence of intranuclear inclusions, or Dutcher bodies, is helpful in distinguishing this type of lymphoma from leukemic infiltrates, including hairy cell leukemia. Monotypic light chain expression of

the plasmacytoid cells is often identifiable with paraffin section immunohistochemistry in these cases.

Mantle cell lymphoma of the spleen shows a similar pattern of splenic involvement to small lymphocytic lymphoma, but does not contain the larger prolymphocytes seen in small lymphocytic lymphoma (Fig. 11.94). Clusters of epithelioid histiocytes may be present in cases of mantle cell lymphoma and may obscure the neoplastic infiltrate in rare cases. Some patients with mantle cell lymphoma will present with splenomegaly and peripheral blood involvement without lymphadenopathy.[865]

Follicular lymphomas also primarily involve the splenic white pulp. They generally involve the central portion of the Malpighian body with surrounding residual nonlymphomatous white pulp elements. With extensive splenic involvement, follicular nodules may become evident within a markedly expanded white pulp nodule. Rare cases may also show follicular proliferation attached to the capsule. Some follicular lymphomas of the spleen will show typical features in the central white pulp, but will have expanded marginal zones of clonal B cells. Such cases appear to represent marginal

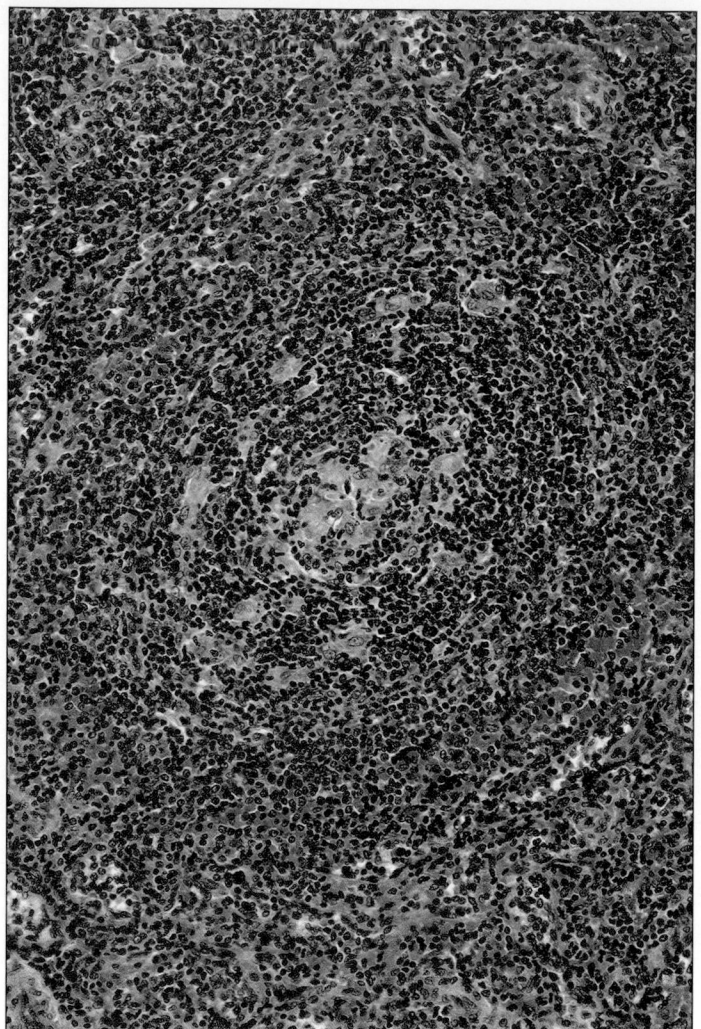

Fig. 11.94 Mantle cell lymphoma. A distinct mantle zone pattern may not be obvious in all cases. The lack of prolymphocytes is useful in distinguishing this lymphoma type from small lymphocytic lymphoma.

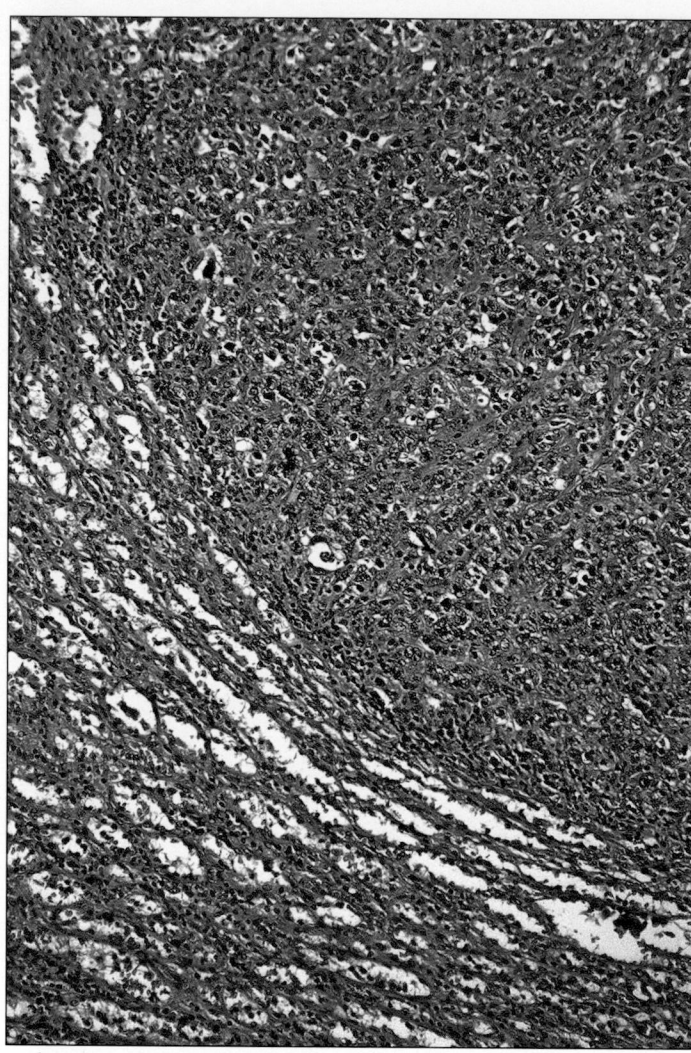

Fig. 11.95 Large cell lymphoma forming a large tumor aggregate within the spleen.

zone differentiation of the follicular lymphoma, rather than a composite lymphoma.[866]

Large cell lymphomas of either T or B lineage frequently form tumor nodules that are grossly apparent.[863,867] Such nodules are presumably overgrowths of the white pulp. These firm tan-white nodules are grossly similar to splenic involvement by metastatic carcinoma or Hodgkin's disease (Fig. 11.95). Case of T-cell/histiocyte-rich large B-cell lymphoma presenting in the spleen may be particularly challenging. These tumors may form only microscopic nodules of tumor.[868] Similar to its nodal counterpart, this lymphoma is composed of large numbers of small T cells with smaller numbers of admixed histiocytes and large atypical B cells. Some T-cell lymphomas will not form nodules and will primarily involve the splenic red pulp. Many such cases in the past were considered examples of malignant histiocytosis. Rarely, large cell lymphomas of B lineage will primarily involve the splenic red pulp (Fig. 11.96), and immunohistochemical studies may be necessary to differentiate these tumors from T-cell lymphomas or leukemic infiltrates. These red pulp large B-cell lymphomas may represent a splenic presentation of angiotropic B-cell lymphoma.[852] Because of the great variability in the

pattern of splenic involvement by malignant lymphoma, it is ill-advised to presume lineage of a process without immunophenotypic studies.

Hodgkin's disease characteristically forms grossly obvious tumor nodules that are similar to the nodules of large cell lymphoma and metastatic carcinoma (Fig. 11.97). Very early involvement of the spleen by Hodgkin's disease may only demonstrate a small tan-white nodule and may grossly mimic an area of accentuated white pulp. The spleen should be carefully examined for such minute nodules in any patient with a history of Hodgkin's disease. As discussed previously, however, the presence of granulomatous inflammation is not sufficient for a diagnosis of splenic involvement by Hodgkin's disease. Reed-Sternberg cells or their mononuclear variants must be identified for such a diagnosis. Nodular lymphocyte predominance Hodgkin's disease only rarely involves extranodal sites, but when present it also generally forms tumor nodules in the spleen.[869]

Primary splenic lymphomas

Any type of malignant lymphoma may on rare occasion present as a primary splenic lymphoma,[863,870–872] although most cases that present

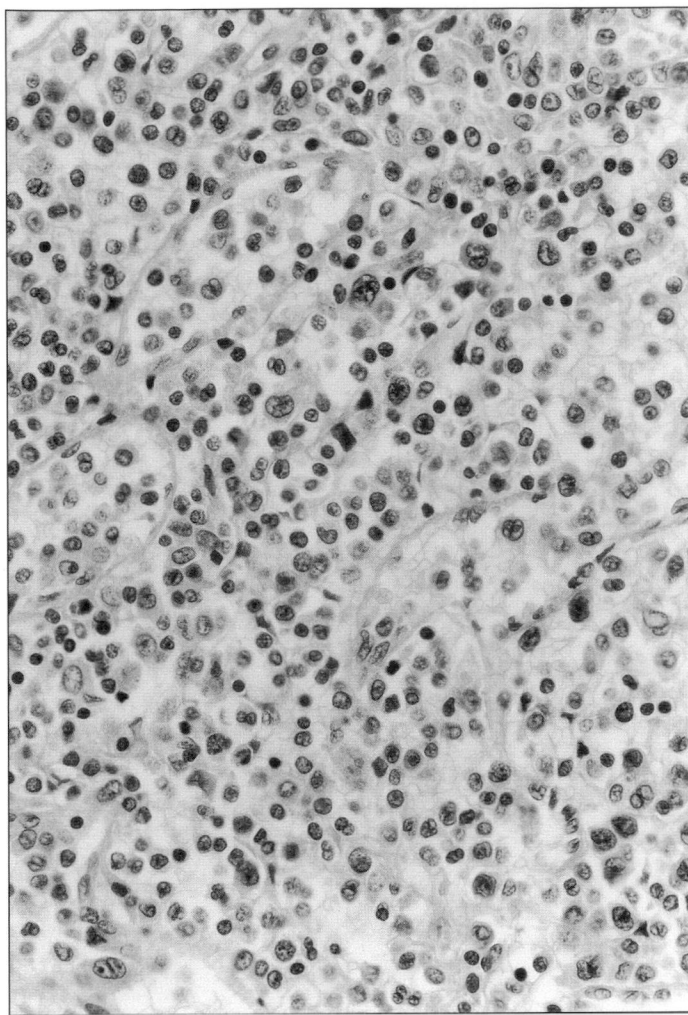

Fig. 11.96 Large cell lymphoma primarily involving the splenic red pulp. This relatively unusual pattern of splenic involvement by large cell lymphoma can easily be mistaken for splenic involvement by acute leukemia.

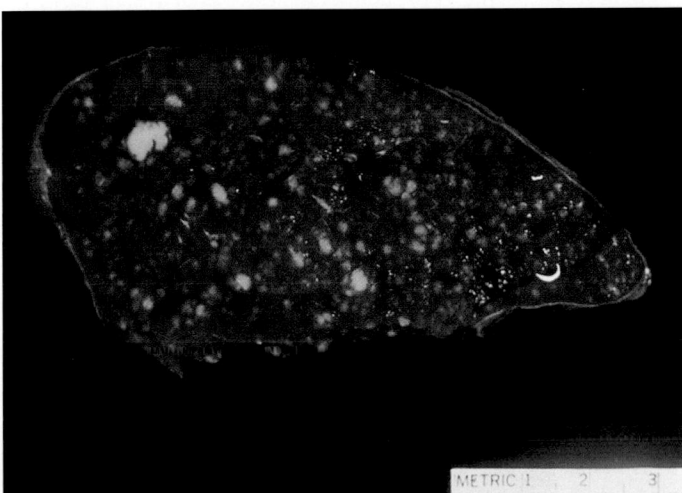

Fig. 11.97 Hodgkin's disease. A similar gross pattern of splenic involvement may be seen with large cell lymphoma.

with splenomegaly have evidence of disease elsewhere at the time of splenectomy. For this reason, it is not clear if these cases actually represent primary splenic lymphomas, and some authors have used the term malignant lymphoma with prominent splenomegaly rather than primary splenic lymphoma.[873] Three other described disorders appear to be unique to the spleen and will be discussed in more detail.

Splenic marginal zone lymphoma

Splenic marginal zone lymphoma is a unique form of B-cell lymphoma that involves the central portion and the marginal zone of the splenic white pulp.[874,875,876] The tumor is distinct from nodal marginal zone lymphomas, including monocytoid B-cell lymphoma and low-grade B-cell lymphoma of mucosa associated lymphoid tissue.[877] This entity was originally described by Neiman et al.[874] in 1979 as a malignant lymphoma that simulated hairy cell leukemia, and was latter described as splenic marginal zone lymphoma.[875]

In most cases, the spleen is massively enlarged, weighing 1000 grams or more. Rarely, involved spleens are normal in weight or only slightly enlarged, apparently representing an early phase of the disease.[878] The cut splenic surface of the cases with splenomegaly shows a miliary pattern similar to the gross pattern of involvement by other low-grade lymphomas. On microscopic examination, the white pulp is markedly expanded. This expansion is due to a biphasic cell population that includes a clonal population of small lymphocytes in the central white pulp and an expansion of cytologically different cells in the surrounding marginal zone (Fig. 11.98). The marginal zone cells are small to medium-sized lymphocytes with moderately abundant cytoplasm and little to no nuclear pleomorphism. In addition to the expanded marginal zones, aggregates of lymphoma cells form small nodules within the splenic red pulp. The neoplastic B cells are characteristically CD20 positive, CD5 negative, CD10 and CD43 negative. The t(11;18), present in a subset of extranodal marginal zone lymphomas, is not detected in the splenic form of the disease. Other cytogenetic aberrations, particularly loss of 7q31 and gain of 3q, have been reported in splenic marginal zone lymphoma.[879,880]

The differential diagnosis of splenic marginal zone lymphoma includes hairy cell leukemia and reactive marginal zone cell hyperplasia. The diffuse red pulp involvement of hairy cell leukemia, sparing the residual white pulp, is not seen in marginal zone lymphoma. In addition, the neoplastic marginal zone cells differ from hairy cells by being TRAP-1 negative and usually negative for the antigens CD11c and CD103. An expanded marginal zone may also be seen in reactive conditions and in other lymphomas involving the spleen[881] and care must be taken not to overdiagnose marginal zone lymphoma in these cases. The lack of a red pulp component is helpful in suggesting a reactive process. Immunophenotyping or molecular studies for clonality are useful for this differential diagnosis, especially in cases that are not accompanied by massive splenic enlargement. Unlike reactive marginal zone (monocytoid) B cells in other sites, however, reactive splenic marginal zone lymphocytes express bcl-2 protein, and this feature is not useful in the differential diagnosis of splenic marginal zone hyperplasia and lymphoma.[104,882]

Although splenic marginal zone lymphoma is generally an indolent disease,[883] 13% of cases are reported to relapse as, or transform to, large B-cell lymphoma.[884]

Splenic lymphoma with circulating villous lymphocytes

Splenic lymphoma with circulating villous lymphocytes (SLVL) is a rare clinicopathologic disorder that is most common in elderly males and is characterized by splenomegaly, a mild lymphocytosis and circulating lymphocytes with unipolar villous cytoplasmic

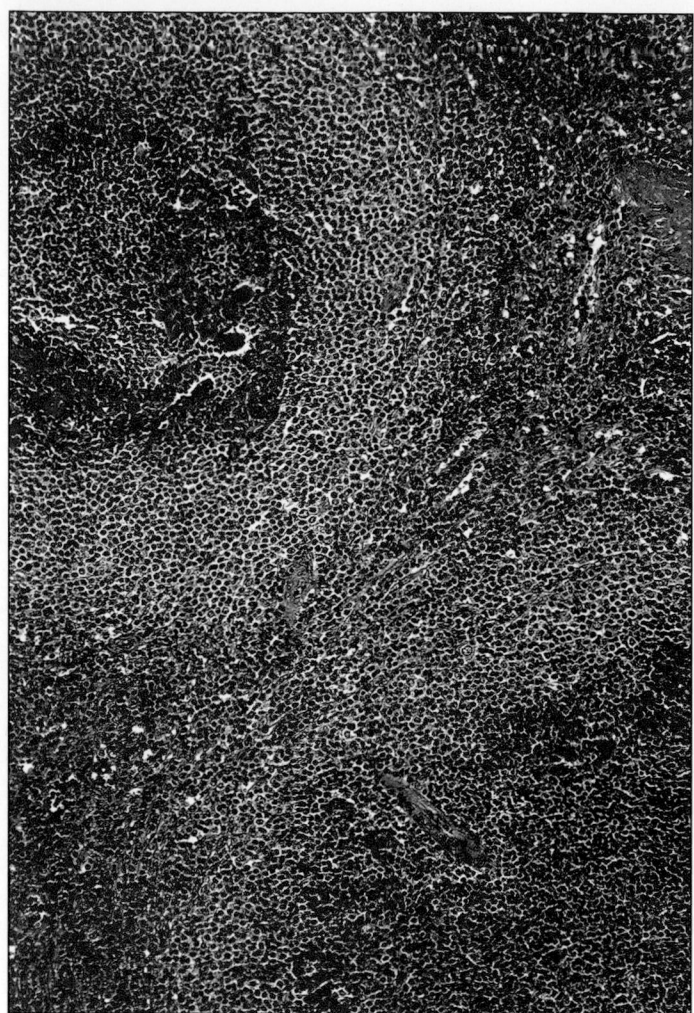

Fig. 11.98 Splenic marginal zone lymphoma. The marginal zone is expanded by cells with pale-staining cytoplasm. Small aggregates of similar cells are usually also seen within the splenic red pulp.

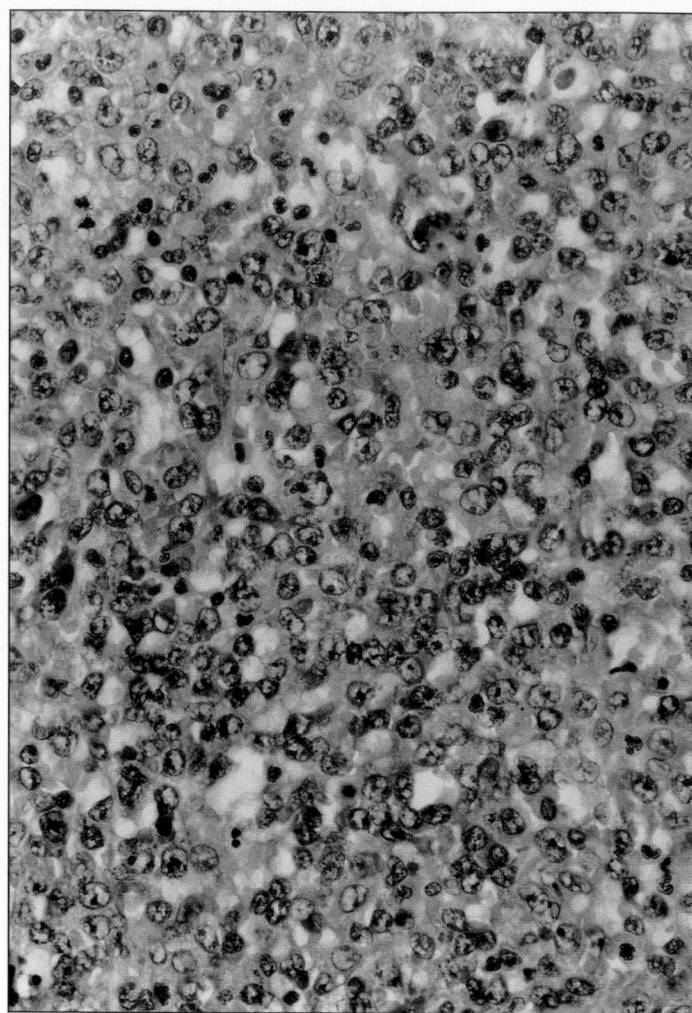

Fig. 11.99 Hepatosplenic T-cell lymphoma. The splenic red pulp is expanded by a mixture of medium-sized and large lymphoid cells.

projections.[885] Clinically, the disorder is most likely to mimic hairy cell leukemia; however, the gross appearance of the enlarged spleen in SLVL shows the miliary pattern more characteristic of a low-grade lymphoma. Most cases of SLVL represent peripheral blood involvement by splenic marginal zone lymphoma.[886] Rarely, other lymphoma types may mimic this presentation.[885,887,888] We favor the concept that a variety of malignant lymphomas can cause the clinical syndrome of SLVL, and we prefer to classify the underlying splenic lymphoma based on the morphologic, immunologic, and molecular characteristics of the tumor. Therefore, we do not use the term 'splenic lymphoma with circulating villous lymphocytes' diagnostically. Splenic marginal zone lymphoma may also involve the blood with cells with abundant cytoplasm and no villous projections.

Hepatosplenic T-cell lymphoma

This rare type of aggressive lymphoma is also known as hepatosplenic γδ T-cell lymphoma and probably includes cases originally described as erythrophagocytic Tγ lymphoma.[653,889–894] It is a neoplastic proliferation of T lymphocytes, which are most commonly γδ T lymphocytes. While the majority of normal circulating T lymphocytes are αβ T cells, approximately 4% of T cells carry the γδ T-cell antigen receptor. In the normal spleen, these γδ cells are over-represented, accounting for approximately 17% of all splenic T lymphocytes, and are localized to the splenic red pulp.[895]

Patients with hepatosplenic T-cell lymphoma are usually adolescents or young men who present with hepatosplenomegaly and no adenopathy, but this disease may also occur after solid organ transplantation.[896,897] The patients may also have anemia and/or thrombocytopenia and subtle bone marrow involvement by the disease at the time of diagnosis. Grossly, the spleen is usually massively enlarged, often weighing several thousand grams, with a diffuse pattern of involvement. On microscopic examination, the red pulp cords and sinuses are extensively infiltrated by medium to large lymphoid cells with open nuclear chromatin and slightly irregular nuclear contours (Fig. 11.99). The cells may have moderately abundant cytoplasm, imparting a low-power impression of splenic involvement by hairy cell leukemia. Rare cases of hepatosplenic T-cell lymphoma are associated with prominent erythrophagocytosis, presumably mimicking malignant histiocytosis, but this feature is not pronounced in most cases. Involvement of the hepatic sinuses by identical neoplastic T cells exists at the time of splenectomy.

Immunophenotyping easily excludes hairy cell leukemia from the differential diagnosis by the failure to identify evidence of B lineage. On paraffin sections, the neoplastic cells are usually positive for the T-lineage and T-lineage associated antigens CD2, CD3, CD5, CD43, and CD45RO. The cells differ from αβ T cells by being characteristically CD4 and CD8 negative. Some cases express natural killer cell associated antigens, including CD16 and CD56, as well as TIA. The neoplastic cells usually fail to immunoreact with the βF1 antibody that detects the β chain of αβ T cells, while they generally react with the TCR-δ1 antibody or other antibodies for the T-cell δ or γ chains. T-cell receptor γ chain gene rearrangements are detectable in these patients while β chain rearrangements may or may not be detectable. The cytogenetic abnormalities isochrome 7q and trisomy 8 are consistently associated with this disease.[812,898,899] Several cases of an essentially identical proliferation arising from αβ T cells have now been described,[900] and subclassification based on the T-cell type is probably of no significance.

In addition to hairy cell leukemia, the morphologic findings of hepatosplenic T-cell lymphoma overlap with splenic involvement by large granular lymphocytosis (LGL). A morphologic distinction between these two diseases may not be possible and the clinical setting must be considered. In LGL, the patients are older, have a more indolent clinical course and frequently have an autoimmune disease. In addition, many LGL cases have CD57-positive lymphocytes, an antigen that is not commonly expressed by hepatosplenic T-cell lymphoma cells.

Vascular malignancies

Angiosarcoma is the most common primary nonhematopoietic malignancy of the spleen.[811,901] In a series of 40 primary angiosarcomas of the spleen, Falk et al. found this tumor to occur at a median age of 59 years with no sex predilection.[902] Unlike angiosarcoma of the liver, there is no apparent relationship between splenic tumors and exposure to arsenic, vinyl chloride, or Thorotrast. Most patients present with splenomegaly and abdominal pain and have a short survival, often dying within a year of diagnosis. Thirteen percent to 18% of patients will present with spontaneous splenic rupture, and the disease is often associated with peripheral blood cytopenias and coagulation disorders.

Grossly, the spleen is enlarged, usually weighing over 500 grams.[902] The cut splenic surface characteristically demonstrates multiple nodules, some of which may have a diffuse, infiltrating pattern or hemorrhagic cystic spaces. Areas of hemorrhage are present in over half of cases and approximately one-quarter of cases will have associated areas of infarction. Microscopically, angiosarcoma of the spleen may demonstrate great morphologic variation (Fig. 11.100). Solid areas of sarcomatous proliferation may be difficult to distinguish from malignant fibrous histiocytoma or fibrosarcoma on H&E-stained sections alone. More vascular areas, however, are invariably present in other areas of the tumor, forming irregular vascular channels with atypical endothelial cells. Papillary and spindle cell patterns may also be seen. Hobnail cells with enlarged, atypical nuclei may be present, even in the absence of an obvious increase in mitotic figures. Immunohistochemical studies demonstrate vascular antigen expression in the tumor cells, which are characteristically von Willebrand factor, CD31, and CD34 positive.[818] These tumors may also express CD68 and CD8, and we do not find these markers useful in determining whether an angiosarcoma is primary to the spleen or represents secondary involvement of this organ.

Epithelioid hemangioendothelioma and *epithelioid and spindle-cell hemangioendothelioma* are low-grade angiosarcomas that have more abundant epithelioid cells and small signet-ring-like vascular

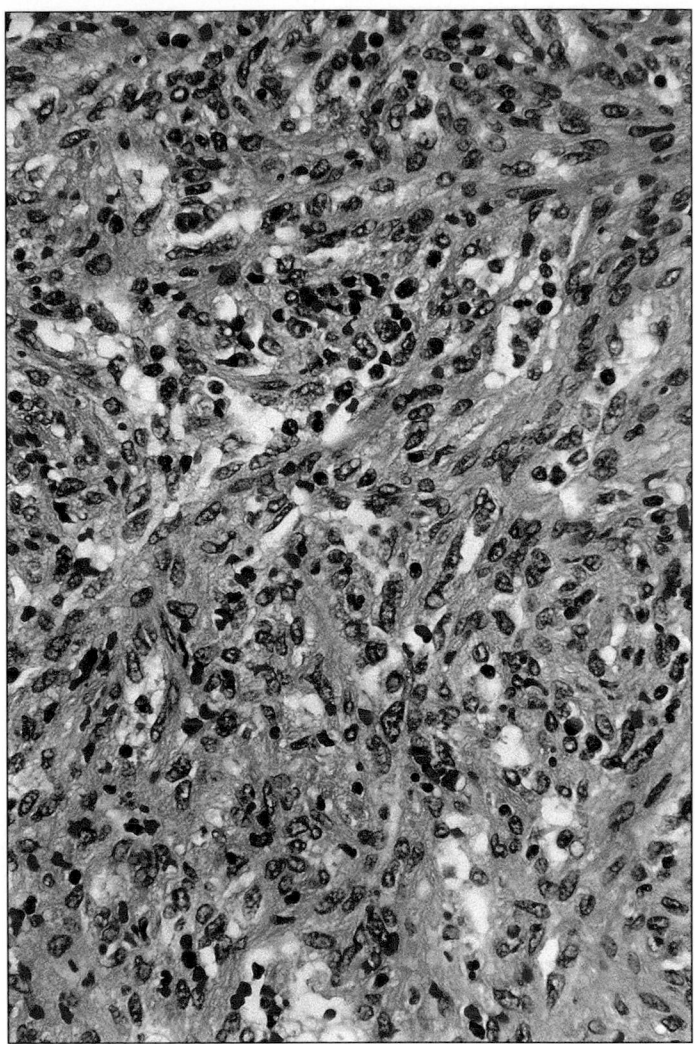

Fig. 11.100 Angiosarcoma of the spleen. Solid areas of spindled cells may mimic other types of sarcoma.

tumor cells. These tumors have a similar clinical presentation and gross appearance to high-grade angiosarcomas, but several reports suggest a better survival than with typical angiosarcomas of the spleen.[903–905]

The differential diagnosis of angiosarcoma includes both benign and malignant proliferations. Benign vascular proliferations, such as hemangiomas and peliosis, do not demonstrate the nuclear atypia of angiosarcoma. In addition, the lack of an infiltrating gross and microscopic pattern into the surrounding red pulp is useful for the diagnosis of hemangioma. Some tumors previously reported as splenic hemangioendotheliomas may actually represent the recently described *splenic multinodular hemangioma* (see above).[819] These proliferations would differ from true hemangioendotheliomas by their lack of cytologic atypia, necrosis, or mitotic activity. Littoral cell angiomas do have nuclear enlargement of lining cells, but not the nuclear atypia of angiosarcoma. Rare cases of *littoral cell angiosarcoma* and *littoral cell hemangioendothelioma* have been reported[830–832] in which cytologic atypia was present as well as an infiltrating gross appearance and immunohistochemical evidence of both vascular and histiocytic antigen expression. Despite these reports, most of this type of antigen expression is fairly non-specific, and we would not consider a case in this category unless it expressed CD21 in a manner similar to traditional littoral cell angiomas.

Kaposi's sarcoma may also rarely involve the spleen.[902,906,907] When present, Kaposi's sarcoma usually forms small tumor nodules without associated hemorrhage, in contrast to the more characteristic massive splenic involvement with hemorrhage of angiosarcoma. Numerous hyaline globules are also frequently present in Kaposi's sarcoma, as are areas of collagenous fibrosis. These features are uncommon in angiosarcoma.

The distinction of angiosarcoma from other sarcomas, especially malignant fibrous histiocytoma and fibrosarcoma, can be difficult in tumors that have extensive solid sarcomatous areas. Even when this pattern predominates, foci of irregular vascular channels lined by atypical tumor cells are usually present; therefore, extensive tumor sampling is essential. The immunohistochemical detection of vascular-associated antigens, such as von Willebrand factor, *Ulex europaeus* lectin, CD31, and CD34, is also helpful in excluding other types of sarcomas.

OTHER SARCOMAS AND METASTATIC TUMORS

Other primary sarcomas of the spleen are extremely rare, with reports of malignant fibrous histiocytoma, fibrosarcoma, and leiomyosarcoma primarily involving the spleen.[811,901] Careful sampling and immunohistochemical studies help to exclude an angiosarcoma mimicking one of these rare tumors.

Metastatic tumors involving the spleen are also quite rare and are usually discovered on autopsy. Solitary metastases may present with splenomegaly and may be treated with splenectomy.[908] Rare cases of splenic rupture have also been reported due to metastatic tumors.[909,910] In one autopsy series, one-third of patients with splenic metastases had no gross evidence of splenic tumor. When grossly seen, the majority of tumors formed large nodules, often with areas of necrosis. Lung and breast carcinomas are the most common primary tumors to metastasize to the spleen, although virtually any tumor may secondarily involve the spleen on rare occasions. [105,911,912]

REFERENCES

1. Zinzani PL, Colecchia A, Festi D, et al. Ultrasound-guided core-needle biopsy is effective in the initial diagnosis of lymphoma patients. Haematologica 1998; 83: 989–992.

2. Weiss LM, Pitts WC. The role of fine needle aspiration biopsy in diagnosis and management of hematopoietic neoplasms. In: Knowles DM, ed. Neoplastic hematopathology. 2nd edn. Philadelphia: Lippincott Williams & Wilkins; 2001: 483–505.

3. Arber DA, Weiss LM. CD43: A review. Appl Immunohistochem 1993; 1:88–96.

4. Picker LJ, Weiss LM, Medeiros LJ, et al. Immunophenotypic criteria for the diagnosis of non-Hodgkin's lymphoma. Am J Pathol 1987; 128: 181–201.

5. Stein H, Lennert K, Feller AC, et al. Immunohistological analysis of human lymphoma: correlation of histological and immunological categories. Adv Cancer Res 1984; 42: 67–147.

6. Cattoretti G, Pileri S, Parravicini C, et al. Antigen unmasking on formalin-fixed, paraffin embedded tissue sections. J Pathol 1993; 171: 83–98.

7. Chu PG, Chang KL, Arber DA, et al. Practical applications of immunohistochemistry for hematolymphoid disorders: An updated review. Ann Diagn Pathol 1999; 3: 104–133.

8. Shi SR, Cote RJ, Taylor CR. Antigen retrieval immunohistochemistry: past, present and future. J Histochem Cytochem 1997; 45: 327–343.

9. Borowitz MJ, Bray R, Gascoyne R, et al. U.S.-Canadian consensus recommendations on the immunophenotypic analysis of hematologic neoplasia by flow cytometry: data analysis and interpretation. Cytometry 1997; 30: 236–244.

10. Braylan RC, Benson NA, Nourse VA. Cellular DNA of human neoplastic B-cells measured by flow cytometry. Cancer Res 1984; 44: 5010–5016.

11. Shackney SE, Skramstad KS, Cunningham RE, et al. Dual parameter flow cytometry studies in human lymphomas. J Clin Invest 1980; 66: 1281–1294.

12. Costa A, Mazzini G, Delbino G, et al. DNA content and kinetic characteristics of non-Hodgkin's lymphoma: Determined by flow cytometry and autoradiography. Cytometry 1981; 2: 185–188.

13. Zukerberg LR, Medeiros LJ, Ferry JA, et al. Diffuse low-grade B-cell lymphomas: four clinically distinct subtypes defined by a combination of morphologic and immunophenotypic features. Am J Clin Pathol 1993; 100: 373–385.

14. Harris NL, Jaffe ES, Stein H, et al. A revised European-American classification of lymphoid neoplasms. A proposal from the International Lymphoma Study Group. Blood 1994; 84: 1361–1392.

15. Cossman J, Aehnbauer B, Garrett CT, et al. Gene rearrangements in the diagnosis of lymphoma/leukemia: guidelines for use based on a multiinstitutional study. Am J Clin Pathol 1991; 95: 347–354.

16. Cossman J, Uppenkamp M, Sundeen J, et al. Molecular genetics and the diagnosis of lymphoma. Arch Pathol Lab Med 1988; 134: 117–127.

17. Davis RE, Warnke RA, Dorfman RF, et al. Utility of molecular genetic analysis for the diagnosis of neoplasia in morphologically and immunophenotypically equivocal hematolymphoid lesions. Cancer 1991; 67: 2890–2899.

18. Sklar J, Weiss LM. Applications of antigen receptor gene rearrangements to the diagnosis and characterization of lymphoid neoplasms. Ann Rev Med 1988; 39: 315–334.

19. Weiss LM, Spagnolo DV. Assessment of clonality in lymphoid proliferations. Am J Pathol 1993; 142: 1679–1682.

20. Stevenson GT, Cragg MS. Molecular markers of B-cell lymphoma. Semin Cancer Biol 1999; 9: 139–147.

21. Hu E, Horning S, Flynn S, et al. Diagnosis of B cell lymphoma by analysis of immunoglobulin gene rearrangements in biopsy specimens obtained by fine needle aspiration. J Clin Oncol 1986; 4: 278–283.

22. Weiss LM, Movahed LA, Chen Y-Y, et al. Detection of immunoglobulin light-chain mRNA in lymphoid tissues using a practical in situ hybridization method. Am J Pathol 1990; 137: 979–988.

23. Chang KL, Chen Y-Y, Shibata D, et al. Description of an in situ hybridization methodology for detection of Epstein-Barr virus RNA in paraffin-embedded tissues, with a survey of normal and neoplastic tissues. Diagn Mol Pathol 1992; 1: 246–255.

24. Du M, Diss TC, Liu H, et al. KSHV-and EBV-associated germinotropic lymphoproliferative disorder. Blood 2002; 100: 3415–3418.

25. Yeoh E, Ross M, Shurtleff S, et al. Classification, subtype discovery, and prediction of outcome in pediatric acute lymphoblastic leukemia by gene expression profiling. Cancer Cell 2002; 1:133–143.

26. Schlegelberger B, Zwingers T, Harder L, et al. Clinicopathogenetic significance of chromosomal abnormalities in patients with blastic peripheral B-cell lymphoma. Blood 1999; 94: 3114–3120.

27. Anastasi J. Interphase cytogenetic analysis in the diagnosis and study of neoplastic disorders. Am J Clin Pathol (suppl) 1991; 95: S22–S28.

28. Aster JC, Kobayashi Y, Shiota M, et al. Detection of the t(14;18) at similar frequencies in hyperplastic lymphoid tissues from American and Japanese patients. Am J Pathol 1992; 141: 291–299.

29. Fisher ER, Gregorio RM, Redmond C, et al. Pathologic findings from the National Surgical Adjuvant Breast Project (Protocol No. 4). III The significance of extranodal extension of axillary metastases. Am J Clin Pathol 1976; 65: 439–444.

30. Wells CA, Heryet A, Brochier J, et al. The immunocytochemical detection of axillary micrometastases in breast cancer. Br J Cancer 1984; 50: 193–197.

31. Rubio IT, Korourian S, Cowan C, et al. Sentinel lymph node biopsy for staging breast cancer. Am J Surg 1998; 176: 532–537.

32. Turner RR, Ollila DW, Krasne DL, et al. Histopathologic validation of the sentinel lymph node hypothesis for breast carcinoma. Ann Surg 1997; 226: 271–276.

33. Turner RR, Ollila DW, Stern S, et al. Optimal histopathologic examination of the sentinel lymph node for breast carcinoma staging. Am J Surg Pathol 1999; 23: 263–267.

34. Gershenwald JE, Thompson W, Mansfield PF, et al. Multi-institutional melanoma lymphatic mapping experience: the prognostic value of sentinel lymph node status in 612 stage I or II melanoma patients. J Clin Oncol 1999; 17: 976–983.

35. Chang KL, Arber DA, Weiss LM. CD30: A review. Appl Immunohistochem 1993; 1: 244–255.

36. Weiss LM, Arber DA, Chang KL. CD45: a review. Appl Immunohistochem 1993; 1: 166–181.

37. Weiss LM, Movahed LA, Butler AE, et al. Analysis of lymphoepithelioma and lymphoepithelioma-like carcinomas for Epstein-Barr viral genomes by in situ hybridization. Am J Surg Pathol 1989; 13: 625–631.

38. Robert NJ, Garnick MB, Frei E. Cancers of unknown origin: current approaches and future perspectives. Semin Oncol 1983; 9: 526–531.

39. Jesse RH, Perez CA, Fletcher G. Cervical lymph node metastasis; unknown primary cancer. Cancer 1973; 31: 854–859.

40. Copeland EM, McBride CM. Axillary metastasis from an unknown primary site. Ann Surg 1973; 178: 25–27.

41. Molinari R, Cantu G, Chiesa F, et al. A statistical approach to detection of the primary cancer based on the site of neck lymph node metastases. Tumori 1977; 63: 267–282.

42. Avery AK, Beckstead J, Renshaw AA, et al. Use of antibodies to RCC and CD10 in the differential

diagnosis of renal neoplasms. Am J Surg Pathol 2000; 24: 203–210.

43. Wieczorek TJ, Pinkus JL, Glickman JN, et al. Comparison of thyroid transcription factor-1 and hepatocyte antigen immunohistochemical analysis in the differential diagnosis of hepatocellular carcinoma, metastatic adenocarcinoma, renal cell carcinoma, and adrenal cortical carcinoma. Am J Clin Pathol 2002; 118: 911–921.

44. Almeida R, Silva E, Santos-Silva F, et al. Expression of intestine-specific transcription factors, CDX1 and VDX2, in intestinal metaplasia and gastric carcinomas. J Pathol 2003; 199: 36–40.

45. Moskaluk CA, Zhang H, Powell SM, et al. Cdx2 protein expression in normal and malignant human tissues: an immunohistochemical survey using tissue microarrays. Mod Pathol 2003; 16: 913–919.

46. Werling RW, Yazigi H, Bacchi CE, et al. CDX2, a highly sensitive and specific marker of adenocarcinomas of intestinal origin: an immunohistochemical survey of 476 primary and metastatic carcinomas. Am J Surg Pathol 2003; 27: 303–310.

47. Chu PG, Weiss LM. Keratin expression in human tissues and neoplasms. Histopathology 2002; 40: 403–439.

48. Ryan JR, Ioachim HL, Marmer J, et al. Acquired immune deficiency syndrome-related lymphadenopathies presenting in the salivary gland lymph nodes. Arch Otolaryngol 1985; 111: 554–556.

49. Holdsworth PJ, Hopkinson JM, Leveson SH. Benign axillary epithelial lymph node inclusions – a histological pitfall. Histopathology 1988; 13: 226–228.

50. Rosai J, Carcangiu, ML, DeLellis RA. Thyroid tissue in abnormal locations. In: Atlas of tumor pathology: tumors of the thyroid gland. 3rd edn, vol. 5. Washington DC: Armed Forces Institute of Pathology; 1992: 323.

51. Karp LA, Czernobilsky B. Glandular inclusions in pelvic and abdominal paraaortic lymph nodes, a study of autopsy and surgical material in males and females. Am J Clin Pathol 1969; 52: 212–218.

52. Clement PB. Pathology of endometriosis. Pathol Annu 1990; 25: 245–295.

53. Mills SE. Decidua and squamous metaplasia in abdomino-pelvic lymph nodes. Int J Gynecol Pathol 1983; 2: 209–215.

54. Weeks DA, Beckwith JB, Mierau GW. Benign nodal lesions mimicking metastases from pediatric renal neoplasms: a report of the National Wilms' Tumor Study Pathology Center. Hum Pathol 1990; 21: 1239–1244.

55. Rutty GN, Lauder I. Mesothelial cell inclusions within mediastinal lymph nodes. Histopathology 1994; 25: 483–487.

56. Cohn DE, Folpe AL, Gown AM, et al. Mesothelial pelvic lymph node inclusions mimicking metastatic thyroid carcinoma. Gynecol Oncol 1998; 68: 210–213.

57. Suarez VD, Izquierdo Garcia FM. Embolization of mesothelial cells in lymphatics: the route to mesothelial inclusions in lymph nodes? Histopathology 1998; 33: 570–575.

58. Parkash V, Vidwans M, Carter D. Benign mesothelial cells in mediastinal lymph nodes. Am J Surg Pathol 1999; 23: 1264–1269.

59. Bautista NC, Cohen S, Anders KH. Benign melanocytic nevus cells in axillary lymph nodes. A prospective incidence and immunohistochemical study with literature review. Am J Clin Pathol 1994; 102: 102–108.

60. Epstein JI, Erlandson RA, Rosen PP. Nodal blue nevi. A study of three cases. Am J Surg Pathol 1984; 8: 907–915.

61. Warnke RA, Weiss LM, Chan JKC, et al. Tumors of the lymph nodes and spleen. 3rd edn, volume 14, Washington DC: Armed Forces Institute of Pathology; 1995.

62. Chan JKC, Warnke RA, Dorfman RF. Vascular transformation of sinuses in lymph nodes: a study of

its morphologic spectrum and distinction from Kaposi's sarcoma. Am J Surg Pathol 1991; 15: 732–743.

63. Cook PD, Czerniak B, Chan JKC, et al. Nodular spindle cell vascular transformation of lymph nodes: a benign process occurring predominantly in retroperitoneal lymph nodes draining carcinomas that can simulate Kaposi's sarcoma or metastatic tumor. Am J Surg Pathol 1995; 19: 1010–1020.

64. Chan JKC, Lewin KJ, Lombard CD, et al. The histopathology of bacillary angiomatosis of lymph nodes. Am J Surg Pathol 1991; 14: 430–437.

65. Koehler JE, Sanchez MA, Garrido CS, et al. Molecular epidemiology of Bartonella infections in patients with bacillary angiomatosis-peliosis. N Eng J Med 1997; 337: 1876–1883.

66. Finkbeiner WE, Egbert BM, Groundwater JR, et al. Kaposi's sarcoma in young homosexual men, a histopathologic study with particular reference to lymph node involvement. Arch Pathol Lab Med 1982; 106: 261–264.

67. Yokois NU, Perlman ER, Colombani P, et al. Kaposi's sarcoma presenting as a protracted multisystem illness in an adolescent liver transplant recipient. Liver Transpl Surg 1997; 3: 541–544.

68. Wang AY, Li PK, To KF, et al. Coexistence of Kaposi's sarcoma and tuberculosis in a renal transplant recipient. Transplantation 1998; 66: 115–118.

69. Chang Y, Cesarman E, Pessin MS, et al. Identification of herpesvirus-like DNA sequences in AIDS-associated Kaposi's sarcoma. Science 1994; 266: 1865–1869.

70. Chang Y, Moore PS. Kaposi's sarcoma (KS)-associated herpesvirus and its role in KS. Infect Agents Dis 1996; 5: 215–222.

71. Moore PS, Kingsley LA, Holmberg SD, et al. Kaposi's sarcoma-associated herpesvirus infection prior to onset of Kaposi's sarcoma. AIDS 1996; 10: 175–180.

72. Kennedy MM, Cooper K, Howells DD, et al. Identification of HHV8 in early Kaposi's sarcoma: implications of Kaposi's sarcoma pathogenesis. Mol Pathol 1998; 51: 14–20.

73. Dupin N, Fisher C, Kellam P, et al. Distribution of human herpesvirus-8 latently infected cells in Kaposi's sarcoma, multicentric Castleman's disease, and primary effusion lymphoma. Proc Natl Acad Sci USA 1999; 96: 4546–4551.

74. Cesarman E, Knowles DM. Kaposi's sarcoma-associated herpesvirus: a lymphotropic human herpesvirus associated with Kaposi's sarcoma, primary effusion lymphoma, and multicentric Castleman's disease. Semin Diagn Pathol 1997; 14: 54–66.

75. Chen KTK. Multicentric Castleman's disease and Kaposi's sarcoma. Am J Surg Pathol 1984; 8: 287–293.

76. Tsang WYW, Chan JKC, Dorfman RF, et al. Vasoproliferative lesions of lymph nodes. Pathol Annu 1994; 29 (Pt 1): 63–133.

77. Chan JK, Frizzera G, Fletcher CD, et al. Primary vascular tumors of lymph nodes other than Kaposi's sarcoma: analysis of 39 cases and delineation of two new entities. Am J Surg Pathol 1992; 16: 335–350.

78. Cho NH, Yang WI, Lee WJ. Spindle and epithelioid haemangioendothelioma of the inguinal lymph nodes. Histopathology 1997; 30: 595–598.

79. Chan JK, Tsang WY, Pau MY, et al. Lymphangiomyomatosis and angiomyolipoma: closely related entities characterized by hamartomatous proliferation of HMB-45-positive smooth muscle. Histopathology 1993; 22: 445–455.

80. Channer JL, Davies JD. Smooth muscle proliferation in the hilum of superficial lymph nodes. Virchow Arch [A] 1985; 406: 261–270.

81. Abell MR, Littler ER. Benign metastasizing uterine leiomyoma: multiple lymph node metastasis. Cancer 1975; 36: 2206–2213.

82. Davis RE, Warnke RA, Dorfman RF. Inflammatory pseudotumor of lymph nodes. Additional

observations and evidence for an inflammatory etiology. Am J Surg Pathol 1991; 15: 744–756.

83. Perrone T, De Wolf-Peeters C, Frizzera G. Inflammatory pseudotumor of lymph nodes. A distinctive pattern of nodal reaction. Am J Surg Pathol 1988; 12: 351–361.

84. Coffin CM, Dehner LP, Meis-Kindblom JM. Inflammatory myofibroblastic tumor, inflammatory fibrosarcoma, and related lesions: An historical review with differential diagnostic considerations. Semin Diagn Pathol 1998; 15: 102–110.

85. Arber DA, Weiss LM, Chang KL. Detection of Epstein-Barr virus in inflammatory pseudotumor. Semin Diagn Pathol 1998; 15: 155–160.

86. Menke DM, Griesser H, Araujo I, et al. Inflammatory pseudotumors of lymph node origin show macrophage-derived spindle cells and lymphocyte-derived cytokine transcripts without evidence of T-cell receptor gene rearrangements. Implications for pathogenesis and classification as an idiopathic retroperitoneal fibrosis-like sclerosing immune reaction. Am J Clin Pathol 1996; 105: 430–439.

87. Chen KTK. Mycobacterial spindle cell pseudotumor of lymph nodes. Am J Surg Pathol 1992; 16: 276–281.

88. Logani S, Lucas DR, Cheng JD, et al. Spindle cell tumors associated with mycobacteria in lymph nodes of HIV-positive patients: 'Kaposi sarcoma with mycobacteria' and 'mycobacterial pseudotumor'. Am J Surg Pathol 1999; 23: 656–661.

89. Suster S, Rosai J. Intranodal hemorrhagic spindle cell tumor with "amianthoid" fibers. Report of six cases of a distinctive mesenchymal neoplasm of the inguinal region that simulates Kaposi's sarcoma. Am J Surg Pathol 1989; 13: 347–357.

90. Weiss SW, Gnepp DR, Bratthauer GL. Palisaded myofibroblastoma. A benign mesenchymal tumor of lymph node. Am J Surg Pathol 1989; 13: 341–346.

91. Fletcher CD, Stirling RW. Intranodal myofibroblastoma presenting in the submandibular region: evidence of a broader clinical and histological spectrum. Histopathology 1990; 16: 287–293.

92. Creager AJ, Garwacki CP. Recurrent intranodal palisaded myofibroblastoma with metaplastic bone formation. Arch Pathol Lab Med 1999; 123: 433–436.

93. Rossi A, Bulgarini A, Rondanelli E, et al. Intranodal palisaded myofibroblastoma: report of three new cases. Tumori 1995; 81: 464–468.

94. Argani P, Ghossein R, Rosai J. Anthracotic and anthracosilicotic spindle cell pseudotumors of mediastinal lymph nodes: report of five cases of a reactive lesion that simulates malignancy. Hum Pathol 1998; 29: 851–855.

95. Michaeli J, Niesvizky R, Siegel D, et al. Proteinaceous (angiocentric sclerosing) lymphadenopathy: a polyclonal systemic, nonamyloid deposition disorder. Blood 1995; 86: 1159–1162.

96. Osborne BM, Butler JJ, MacKay B. Proteinaceous lymphadenopathy with hypergammaglobulinaemia. Am J Surg Pathol 1979; 3: 137–145.

97. MacKenzie DH. Amyloidosis presenting as lymphadenopathy. Br Med J 1963; 2: 1449–1450.

98. Ordi J, Grau JM, Junque A, et al. Secondary (AA) amyloidosis associated with Castleman's disease. Report of two cases and review of the literature. Am J Clin Pathol 1993; 100: 393–397,

99. Rappaport H. Tumors of the hematopoietic system. 1st edn. Washington DC: Armed Forces Institute of Pathology; 1966.

100. Nathwani BN, Winberg CD, Diamond LW, et al. Morphologic criteria for the differentiation of follicular lymphoma from florid reactive follicular hyperplasia: a study of 80 cases. Cancer 1981; 48: 1794–1806.

101. Ngan BY, Picker LJ, Medeiros LJ, et al. Immunophenotypic diagnosis of non-Hodgkin's lymphoma in paraffin sections. Co-expression of L60(Leu-22) and L26 antigens correlates with

malignant histologic findings. Am J Clin Pathol 1989; 91: 579–583

102. Wood BL, Bacchi MM, Bacchi CE, et al. Immunocytochemical differentiation of reactive hyperplasia from follicular lymphoma using monoclonal antibodies to cell surface and proliferation-related markers. Appl Immunohistochem 1994; 2: 48–53.

103. Utz GL, Swerdlow SH. Distinction of follicular hyperplasia from follicular lymphoma in B5-fixed tissues: comparison of MT2 and bcl-2 antibodies. Hum Pathol 1993; 24: 1155–1158.

104. Lai R, Arber DA, Chang KL, et al. Frequency of bcl-2 expression in non-Hodgkin's lymphoma. A study of 798 cases with comparison of marginal zone lymphoma and monocytoid B cell hyperplasia. Mod Pathol 1998; 11: 864–869.

105. Fakan F, Michal M. Nodular transformation of splenic red pulp due to carcinomatous infiltration. A diagnostic pitfall. Histopathology 1994; 25: 175–178.

106. Ngan B, Chen-Levy Z, Weiss LM, et al. Expression in non-Hodgkin's lymphoma of the bcl-2 protein associated with the t(14;18) chromosomal translocation. N Engl J Med 1988; 318: 1638–1644.

107. Segal GH, Scott M, Jorgensen T, et al. Standard polymerase chain reaction analysis does not detect t(14;18) in reactive lymphoid hyperplasia. Arch Pathol Lab Med 1994; 118: 791–794.

108. Almasri NM, Iturraspe JA, Braylan RC. CD10 expression in follicular lymphoma and large cell lymphoma is different from that of reactive lymph node follicles. Arch Pathol Lab Med 1998; 122: 539–544.

109. Arber DA, Weiss LM. CD10: A review. Appl Immunohistochem 1997; 5: 125–140.

110. Banks PM, Chan J, Cleary ML, et al. Mantle cell lymphoma. A proposal for unification of morphologic, immunologic, and molecular data. Am J Surg Pathol 1992; 16: 637–640.

111. Kurtin PJ. Mantle cell lymphoma. Adv Anat Pathol 1998; 5: 376–398.

112. Campo E, Raffeld M, Jaffe ES. Mantle-cell lymphoma. Semin Hematol 1999; 36: 115–127.

113. Doggett RS, Colby TV, Dorfman RF. Interfollicular Hodgkin's disease. Am J Med 1983; 78: 22–28.

114. Segal GH, Perkins SL, Kjeldsberg CR. Benign lymphadenopathies in children and adolescents. Semin Diagn Pathol 1995; 12: 288–302.

115. Osborne BM, Butler JJ. Clinical implications of nodal reactive follicular hyperplasia in elderly patients with enlarged lymph nodes. Mod Pathol 1991; 4: 24–30.

116. Kondratowicz GM, Symmons DP, Bacon PA, et al. Rheumatoid lymphadenopathy: A morphological and immunohistochemical study. J Clin Pathol 1990; 43: 106–113.

117. Nosanchuk JS, Schnitzer B. Follicular hyperplasia in lymph nodes from patients with rheumatoid arthritis. Cancer 1969; 24: 243–254.

118. McCurley TJ, Collins D, Ball E, et al. Nodal and extranodal lymphoproliferative disorders in Sjogren's syndrome: A clinical and immunopathologic study. Hum Pathol 1990; 21: 482–492.

119. Hui PK, Chan JKC, Ng CS, et al. Lymphadenopathy of Kimura's disease. Am J Surg Pathol 1989; 13: 177–186.

120. Kuo TT, Shih LY, Chan HL. Kimura's disease. Involvement of regional lymph nodes and distinction from angiolymphoid hyperplasia with eosinophilia. Am J Surg Pathol 1988; 12: 843–854.

121. Chan JKC, Hui PK, Ng CS, et al. Epithelioid hemangioma (angiolymphoid hyperplasia with eosinophilia) and Kimura's disease in Chinese. Histopathology 1989; 15: 557–574.

122. Stansfeld AG. The histologic diagnosis of toxoplasmic lymphadenitis. J Clin Pathol 1961; 14: 565–573.

123. Dorfman RF, Remington JS. Value of lymph node biopsy in the diagnosis of toxoplasmosis. N Engl J Med 1973; 289: 878–881.

124. Weiss LM, Chen YY, Berry GJ, et al. Infrequent detection of toxoplasma gondii genome in toxoplasmic lymphadenitis. a polymerase chain reaction study. Hum Pathol 1992; 23: 154–158.

125. Hartsock RJ, Halling LW, King FM. Luetic lymphadenitis: A clinical and histologic study of 20 cases. Am J Clin Pathol 1970; 53: 304–314.

126. Hansmann ML, Fellbaum C, Hui PK, et al. Progressive transformation of germinal centers with and without association to Hodgkin's disease. Am J Clin Pathol 1990; 93: 219–226.

127. Poppema S, Kaiserling E, Lennert K. Hodgkin's disease with lymphocyte predominance, nodular type (nodular paragranuloma) and progressively transformed germinal centers: a cytohistologic study. Histopathology 1979; 3: 295–302.

128. Wilson CS, Chang KL, Weiss LM. Malignant lymphomas that mimic benign lymphoid lesions: A review of four lymphomas. Sem Diagn Pathol 1995; 12: 77–86.

129. Burns BF, Colby TV, Dorfman RF. Differential diagnostic features of nodular L&H Hodgkin's disease, including progressive transformation of germinal centers. Am J Surg Pathol 1984; 8: 253–261.

130. Osborne BM, Butler JJ. Clinical implications of progressive transformation of germinal centers. Am J Surg Pathol 1984; 8: 725–733.

131. Frizzera G. Castleman's disease and related disorders. Semin Diagn Pathol 1988; 5: 346–364.

132. Flendrig JA. Benign giant lymphoma: clinicopathologic correlation study. In: Clark RL, Curnley RW, eds. The year book of cancer. Chicago: Yearbook Medical Publishers; 1970: 296–299.

133. Keller AR, Hochholzer L, Castleman B. Hyaline-vascular and plasma-cell types of giant lymph node hyperplasia of mediastinum and other locations. Cancer 1972; 29: 670–683.

134. Danon AD, Krishnan J, Frizzera G. Morpho-immunophenotypic diversity of Castleman's disease, hyaline-vascular type: with emphasis on a stroma-rich variant and a new pathogenetic hypothesis. Virchows Arch [A] 1993; 423: 369–382.

135. Gerald W, Kostianovsky M, Rosai J. Development of vascular neoplasia in Castleman's disease. Am J Surg Pathol 1990; 14: 603–614.

136. Chan JKC, Tsang WYW, Ng CS. Follicular dendritic cell tumor and vascular neoplasm complicating hyaline-vascular Castleman's disease. Am J Surg Pathol 1994; 18: 517–525.

137. Madero S, Onate JM, Garzon A. Giant lymph node hyperplasia in an angiolipomatous mediastinal mass. Arch Pathol Lab Med 1986; 110: 853–855.

138. Harris NL, Bhan AK. Plasmacytoid T cells in Castleman's disease: Immunohistologic phenotype. Am J Surg Pathol 1987; 11: 109–113.

139. Soulier J, Grollet L, Oksenhendler E, et al. Molecular analysis of clonality in Castleman's disease. Blood 1995; 86: 1131–1138.

140. Kahn LB, Ranchod M, Stables DP, et al. Giant lymph node hyperplasia with haematological abnormalities. S Afr Med J 1973; 47: 811–816.

141. Beck JT, Hsu SM, Wijdenes J, et al. Alleviation of systemic manifestations of Castleman's disease by monoclonal interleukin-6 antibody. N Engl J Med 1994; 330: 602–605.

142. Leger-Ravet MB, Peuchmaur M, Devergne O, et al. Interleukin-6 gene expression in Castleman's disease. Blood 1991; 78: 2923–2930.

143. Radaszkiewicz T, Hansmann ML, Lennert K. Monoclonality and polyclonality of plasma cells in Castleman's disease of the plasma cell variant. Histopathology 1989; 14: 11–24.

144. Hsu SM, Waldron JA, Xie SS, et al. Expression of interleukin-6 in Castleman's disease. Hum Pathol 1993; 24: 833–839.

145. Lin O, Frizzera G. Angiomyoid and follicular dendritic cell proliferative lesions in Castleman's disease of hyaline-vascular type: a study of 10 cases. Am J Surg Pathol 1997; 21: 1295–1306.

146. Frizzera G, Peterson BA, Bayrd ED, et al. A systemic lymphoproliferative disorder with morphologic features of Castleman's disease: clinical findings and clinicopathologic correlations in 15 patients. J Clin Oncol 1985; 3: 1202–1216.

147. Weisenburger DD, Nathwani BN, Winberg CD, et al. Multicentric angiofollicular lymph node hyperplasia: a clinicopathologic study of 16 cases. Hum Pathol 1985; 16: 162–172.

148. Bitter MA, Komaiko W, Franklin WA. Giant lymph node hyperplasia with osteoblastic bone lesions and the POEMS (Takatsuki's) syndrome. Cancer 1985; 56: 188–194.

149. Dispenzieri A, Kyle R, Lacy M, et al. POEMS syndrome: definitions and long-term outcome. Blood 2003; 101: 2496–2506.

150. Frizzera G, Massarelli G, Banks PM, et al. A systemic lymphoproliferative disorder with morphologic features of Castleman's disease: pathological findings in 15 patients. Am J Surg Pathol 1983; 7: 211–231.

151. Hanson CA, Frizzera G, Patton DF, et al. Clonal rearrangement for immunoglobulin and T-cell receptor genes in systemic Castleman's disease: association with Epstein-Barr virus. Am J Pathol 1988; 131: 84–91.

152. Soulier J, Grollet L, Oksenhendler E, et al. Kaposi's sarcoma-associated herpesvirus-like DNA sequences in multicentric Castleman's disease. Blood 1995; 86: 1276–1280.

153. Menke DM, Chadburn A, Cesarman E, et al. Analysis of the human herpesvirus 8 (HHV-8) genome and HHV-8 vIL-6 expression in archival cases of Castleman disease at low risk for HIV infection. Am J Clin Pathol 2002; 117: 268–275.

154. Teruya-Feldstein J, Zauber P, Setsuda JE, et al. Expression of human herpesvirus-8 oncogene and cytokine homologues in an HIV-seronegative patient with multicentric Castleman's disease and primary effusion lymphoma. Lab Invest 1998; 78: 1637–1642.

155. Chadburn A, Cesarman E, Nador RG, et al. Kaposi's sarcoma-associated herpesvirus sequences in benign lymphoid proliferations not associated with human immunodeficiency virus. Cancer 1997; 80: 788–797.

156. Cesarman E, Knowles DM. The role of Kaposi sarcoma-associated herpesvirus (KSHV/HHV-8) in lymphoproliferative diseases. Semin Cancer Biol 1999; 3: 165–174.

157. Du M, Liu H, Diss TC, et al. Kaposi sarcoma-associated herpesvirus infects monotypic (IgM lambda) but polyclonal naïve B cells in Castleman disease and associated lymphoproliferative disorders. Blood 2001; 97: 2130–2136.

158. Oksenhendler E, Boulanger E, Galicier L, et al. High incidence of Kaposi sarcoma associated herpesvirus-related non-Hodgkin lymphoma in patients with HIV infection and multicentric Castleman disease. Blood 2002; 99: 2331–2336.

159. Centers for Disease Control. Persistent, generalized lymphadenopathy among homosexual males. MMWR 1982; 31: 249–251.

160. Ometto L, Menen C, Masiero S, et al. Molecular profile of Epstein-Barr virus in human immunodeficiency virus type 1-related lymphadenopathies and lymphomas. Blood 1997; 90: 313–322.

161. Shibata D, Weiss LM, Hernandez AM, et al. Epstein-Barr virus-associated non-Hodgkin's lymphoma in patients infected with the human immunodeficiency virus. Blood 1993; 81: 2102–2109.

162. Brynes RK, Chan WC, Spira TJ, et al. Value of lymph node biopsy in unexplained lymphadenopathy in homosexual men. JAMA 1983; 250: 1313–1317.

163. Chadburn A, Metroka C, Mouradian J. Progressive lymph node histology and its prognostic value in patients with acquired immunodeficiency syndrome and AIDS-related complex. Hum Pathol 1989; 20: 579–587.

164. Ioachim HL, Cronin W, Roy M, et al. Persistent lymphadenopathies in people at high risk for HIV

infection. Clinicopathologic correlations and long-term follow-up in 79 cases. Am J Clin Pathol 1990; 93: 208–218.

165. Pileri S, Rivano MT, Raise E, et al. The value of lymph node biopsy in patients with acquired immunodeficiency syndrome (AIDS) and the AIDS-related complex (ARC): a morphological and immunohistochemical study of 90 cases. Histopathology 1986; 10: 1107–1129.

166. Said JW. Human immunodeficiency virus-related lymphoid proliferations. Semin Diagn Pathol 1997; 14: 48–53.

167. Burns BF, Wood GS, Dorfman RF. The varied histopathology of lymphadenopathy in the homosexual male. Am J Surg Pathol 1985; 9: 287–297.

168. Biberfeld P, Chayt KJ, Marselle LM, et al. HTLV-III expression in infected lymph nodes and relevance to pathogenesis of lymphadenopathy. Am J Pathol 1986; 125: 436–442.

169. Wood GS, Garcia CF, Dorfman RF, et al. The immunohistology of follicle lysis in lymph node biopsies from homosexual men. Blood 1985; 66: 1092–1097.

170. Said JW, Pinkus JL, Yamashita J, et al. The role of follicular and interdigitating dendritic cells in HIV-related lymphoid hyperplasia: localization of fascin. Mod Pathol 1997; 10: 421–427.

171. Childs CC, Parham DM, Berard CW. Infectious mononucleosis: the spectrum of morphologic changes simulating lymphoma in lymph nodes and tonsils. Am J Clin Pathol 1987; 53: 304–314.

172. Shin SS, Berry GJ, Weiss LM. Infectious mononucleosis: Diagnosis by in situ hybridization in two cases with atypical features. Am J Surg Pathol 1991; 15: 625–631.

173. Strickler JG, Fedeli F, Horwitz CA, et al. Infectious mononucleosis in lymphoid tissue. Histopathology, in situ hybridization, and differential diagnosis. Arch Pathol Lab Med 1993; 117: 269–278.

174. Younes M, Podesta A, Helie M, et al. Infection of T but not B lymphocytes by cytomegalovirus in lymph nodes. An immunophenotypic study. Am J Surg Pathol 1991; 15: 75–80.

175. Rushin JM, Riordan GP, Hagton RB, et al. Cytomegalovirus-infected cells express LeuM1 antigen. A potential source of diagnostic error. Am J Pathol 1990; 136: 989–995.

176. Malik UR, Oleksowicz L, Dutcher JP, et al. Atypical clonal T-cell proliferation in infectious mononucleosis. Med Oncol 1996; 13: 207–213.

177. Spector SA, Hsia K, Denaro F, et al. Use of molecular probes to detect human cytomegalovirus and human immunodeficiency virus. Clin Chem 1999; 35: 1581–1587.

178. Gaffey MJ, Ben-Ezra J, Weiss LM. Herpes simplex lymphadenitis. Am J Clin Pathol 1991; 95: 709–714.

179. Tamaru JI, Mikata A, Horie H, et al. Herpes simplex lymphadenitis. Report of two cases with review of the literature. Am J Surg Pathol 1990; 14: 571–577.

180. Gams RA, Neal JA, Conrad FG. Hydantoin-induced pseudolymphoma. Ann Intern Med 1968; 69: 557–568.

181. Saltzstein SL, Ackerman LV. Lymphadenopathy induced by anticonvulsant drugs clinically and pathologically mimicking malignant lymphomas. Cancer 1959; 12: 164–182.

182. Abbondanzo SL, Irye NS, Frizzera G. Dilantin-associated lymphadenopathy: spectrum of histopathologic patterns. Am J Surg Pathol 1995; 19: 675–686.

183. Burke JS, Colby TV. Dermatopathic lymphadenopathy. Comparison of cases associated and unassociated with mycosis fungoides. Am J Surg Pathol 1981; 5: 343–352.

184. Gould E, Porto R, Albores-Saavedra J, et al. Dermatopathic lymphadenitis. The spectrum and significance of its morphologic features. Arch Pathol Lab Med 1988; 112: 1145–1150.

185. Rausch E, Kaiserling E, Goos M. Langerhans cells and interdigitating reticulum cells in the thymus-dependent region in human dermatopathic lymphadenitis. Virchows Arch B (Cell Pathol) 1977; 25: 327–343.

186. Weiss LM, Beckstead JH, Warnke RA, et al. Leu 6 expressing lymph node cells are dendritic cells and closely related to interdigitating cells. Hum Pathol 1986; 17: 179–184.

187. Sudilovsky D, Cha I. Fine needle aspiration cytology of dermatopathic lymphadenitis. Acta Cytol 1998; 42: 1341–1346.

188. Black MM, Speer F. Sinus histiocytosis of lymph node in cancer. Surg Gynecol Obstet 1958; 106: 163–175.

189. Albores-Saavedra J, Vuitch F, Delgado R, et al. Sinus histiocytosis of pelvic lymph nodes after hip replacement. A histiocytic proliferation induced by cobalt-chromium and titanium. Am J Surg Pathol 1994; 18: 83–90.

190. Vaamonde R, Cabrera JM, Vaamonde-Martin RJ, et al. Silicone granulomatous lymphadenopathy and siliconomas of the breast. Histol Histopathol 1997; 12: 1003–1011.

191. Listinsky CM. Common reactive erythrophagocytosis in axillary lymph nodes. Hum Pathol 1988; 89: 189–192.

192. Gould E, Perez J, Albores-Saavedra J, et al. Signet ring cell sinus histiocytosis: a previously unrecognized histologic condition mimicking metastatic adenocarcinoma in lymph nodes. Am J Clin Pathol 1989; 92: 509–512.

193. Frost AR, Shek YH, Lack EE. Signet ring sinus histiocytosis mimicking metastic adenocarcinoma: report of two cases wtih immunohistochemical and ultrastructural study. Mod Pathol 1992; 5: 497–500.

194. Plank L, Hansmann ML, Fischer R. The cytological spectrum of the monocytoid B-cell reaction: recognition of its large cell type. Histopathology 1993; 23: 425–431.

195. Sheibani K, Fritz RM, Winberg CD, et al. Monocytoid cells in reactive follicular hyperplasia with and without multifocal histiocytic reactions: An immunohistochemical study of 21 cases including suspected cases of toxoplasmosis lymphadenitis. Am J Clin Pathol 1984; 81: 453–458.

196. Sohn CC, Sheibani K, Winberg CD, et al. Monocytoid B lymphocytes: their relation to the patterns of the acquired immunodeficiency syndrome (AIDS) and AIDS-related lymphadenopathy. Hum Pathol 1985; 16: 979–985.

197. Nathwani BN, Mohrmann RS, Brynes RK, et al. Monocytoid B-cell lymphomas: An assessment of diagnostic criteria and a perspective on histogenesis. Hum Pathol 1992; 23: 1061–1071.

198. Favara BE. Hemophagocytic lymphohistiocytosis: a hemophagocytic syndrome. Semin Diagn Pathol 1992; 9: 63–74.

199. McKenna RW, Risdall RJ, Brunning RD. Virus associated hemophagocytic syndrome. Hum Pathol 1981; 12: 395–398.

200. Risdall RJ, McKenna RW, Nesbitt ME, et al. Virus associated hemophagocytic syndrome. A benign histiocytic proliferation distinct from malignant histiocytosis. Cancer 1979; 44: 993–1002.

201. Chen R-L, Su I-J, Lin K-H, et al. Fulminant childhood hemophagocytic syndrome mimicking histiocytic medullary reticulosis. An atypical form of Epstein-Barr virus infection. Am J Clin Pathol 1991; 96: 171–176.

202. Kikuta H, Sakiyama T, Matsumoto S, et al. Fatal Epstein-Barr virus-associated hemophagocytic syndrome. Blood 1993; 82: 3259–3264.

203. Wong KF, Chan JK, Lo ES, et al. A study of the possible etiologic association of Epstein-Barr virus with reactive hemophagocytic syndrome in Hong Kong Chinese. Hum Pathol 1996; 27: 1239–1242.

204. Farquhar JW, Claireaux AF. Familial hemophagocytic reticulosis. Arch Dis Child 1952; 27: 519–525.

205. Arico M, Janka G, Fischer A, et al. Hemophagocytic lymphohistiocytosis. Report of 122 children from the International Registry. Leukemia 1998; 10: 197–203.

206. Ost A, Nilsson-Ardnor S, Henter J-I. Autopsy findings in 27 children with haemophagocytic lymphohistiocytosis. Histopathology 1998; 32: 310–316.

207. Ladisch S, Holiman B, Poplack DG, et al. Immunodeficiency in familial erythrophagocytic lymphohistiocytosis. Lancet 1978; 1: 581–583.

208. Falini B, Pileri S, DeSolas I, et al. Peripheral T-cell lymphoma associated with hemophagocytic syndrome. Blood 1990; 75: 434–444.

209. Jaffe ES, Costa J, Fauci AS, et al. Malignant lymphoma and erythrophagocytosis simulating malignant histiocytosis. Am J Med 1983; 75: 741–749.

210. Wong KF, Chan JK. Reactive hemophagocytic syndrome – a clinicopathologic study of 40 patients in an Oriental population. Am J Med 1992; 93: 177–180.

211. Chang C-S, Wang C-H, Su I-J, et al. Hematophagic histiocytosis: a clinicopathologic analysis of 23 cases with special reference to the association with peripheral T-cell lymphoma. J Formos Med Assoc 1994; 93: 421–428.

212. Rosai J, Dorfman RF. Sinus histiocytosis with massive lymphadenopathy: A newly recognized benign clinicopathological entity. Arch Pathol 1969; 87: 63–70.

213. Rosai J, Dorfman RF. Sinus histiocytosis with massive lymphadenopathy: A pseudolymphomatous benign disorder. Analysis of 34 cases. Cancer 1972; 1174–1188.

214. Foucar E, Rosai J, Dorfman RF. Sinus histiocytosis with massive lymphadenopathy (Rosai-Dorfman disease). Review of the entity. Semin Diagn Pathol 1990; 7: 19–73.

215. Montgomery EA, Meis JM, Frizzera G. Rosai-Dorfman disease of soft tissue. Am J Surg Pathol 1992; 16: 122–129.

216. Leighton SEJ, Gallimore AP. Extranodal sinus histiocytosis with massive lymphadenopathy affecting the subglottis and trachea. Histopathology 1994; 24: 393–394.

217. Komp DM. The treatment of sinus histiocytosis with massive lymphadenopathy (Rosai-Dorfman disease). Sem Diagn Pathol 1990; 7: 83–86.

218. Eisen RN, Buckley PJ, Rosai J. Immunophenotypic characterization of sinus histiocytosis with massive lymphadenopathy (Rosai-Dorfman disease). Semin Diagn Pathol 1990; 7: 74–82.

219. Naiem M, Gerdes J, Abdulaziz A, et al. Production of a monoclonal antibody reactive with human dendritic cells and its use in the immunohistological analysis of lymphoid tissue. J Clin Pathol 1983; 36: 167–175.

220. Parwaresch MR, Radzun HJ, Hansmann M-L, et al. Monoclonal antibody Ki-M4 specifically recognizes human dendritic cells (follicular dendritic cells) and their possible precursors in blood. Blood 1983; 62: 585–590.

221. Bonetti F, Chilosi M, Menestrina F, et al. Immunohistological analysis of Rosai-Dorfman histiocytosis. A disease of S-100+CD1– histiocytes. Virchows Arch 1987; 411: 129–135.

222. Luppi M, Barozzi P, Garber R, et al. Expression of human herpesvirus-6 antigens in benign and malignant lymphoproliferative diseases. Am J Pathol 1998; 153: 815–823.

223. Lu D, Estalilla OC, Manning JTJ, et al. Sinus histiocytosis with massive lymphadenopathy and malignant lymphoma involving the same lymph node: a report of four cases and review of the literature. Mod Pathol 2000; 13: 414–419.

224. Relman DA, Schmidt TM, McDermott RP, et al. Identification of the uncultured bacillus of Whipple's disease. N Engl J Med 1992; 327: 293–301.

225. Fleming JL, Wiesner RH, Shorter RG. Whipple's disease: Clinical, biochemical, and histopathologic features and assessment of treatment in 29 patients. Mayo Clin Proc 1988; 63: 539–551.

226. Rotterdam H. Tissue diagnosis of selected AIDS-related opportunistic infections. Am J Surg Pathol 1987; 11 Suppl 1: 13–15.

227. Sieracki JC, Fine G. Whipple's disease – Observations on systemic involvement: II. Gross and histologic observations. Arch Pathol 1959; 67: 81–93.

228. Ravel R. Histopathology of lymph nodes after lymphangiography. Am J Clin Pathol 1966; 46: 335–340.

229. Truong LD, Cartwright J, Goodman D, et al. Silicone lymphadenopathy associated with augmentation mammoplasty: morphologic features of nine cases. Am J Surg Pathol 1988; 12: 484–491.

230. Warner NE, Friedman NB. Lipogranulomatous pseudosarcoid. Ann Intern Med 1956; 45: 662–673.

231. Strickler JG, Warnke RA, Weiss LM. Necrosis in lymph nodes. Pathol Annu 1987; (Pt 2) 22: 253–282.

232. Cleary KR, Osborne BM, Butler JJ. Lymph node infarction foreshadowing malignant lymphoma. Am J Surg Pathol 1982; 6: 435–442.

233. Norton AJ, Ramsey AD, Isaacson PG. Antigen preservation in infarcted lymphoid tissue: a novel approach to the infarcted lymph node using monoclonal antibodies effective in routinely processed tissues. Am J Surg Pathol 1988; 12: 759–767.

234. Pileri S, Kikuchi M, Helbron D, et al. Histiocytic necrotizing lymphadenitis without granulocytic infiltration. Virchows Arch (Pathol Anat) 1982; 395: 257–271.

235. Dorfman RF, Berry GJ. Kikuchi's histiocytic necrotizing lymphadenitis: An analysis of 108 cases with emphasis on differential diagnosis. Semin Diagn Pathol 1988; 5: 329–345.

236. Fujimoto Y, Kozima Y, Yamaguchi K. Cervical subacute necrotizing lymphadenitis. A new clinicopathologic entity. Naika 1972; 20: 920–927.

237. Kikuchi M. Lymphadenitis showing focal reticulum cell hyperplasia with nuclear debris and phagocytes: a clinico-pathological study [in Japanese]. Nippon Ketsueki Gakkai Zasshi 1972; 35: 379–380.

238. Menasce LP, Banerjee SS, Edmondson D, et al. Histiocytic necrotizing lymphadenitis (Kikuchi-Fujimoto disease): continuing diagnostic difficulties. Histopathology 1998; 33: 248–254.

239. Feller AC, Lennert K, Stein H, et al. Immunohistology and aetiology of histiocytic necrotizing lymphadenitis: report of three instructive cases. Histopathology 1983; 7: 825–829.

240. Pileri SA, Facchetti F, Ascani S, et al. Myeloperoxidase expression by histiocytes in Kikuchi's and Kikuchi-like lymphadenopathy. Am J Pathol 2001; 159: 915–924.

241. Lin CW, Chang CL, Li CC, et al. Spontaneous regression of Kikuchi lymphadenopathy with oligoclonal T-cell populations favors a benign immune reaction over a T-cell lymphoma. Am J Clin Pathol 2002; 117: 627–635.

242. Huh J, Kang GH, Gong G, et al. Kaposi's sarcoma-associated herpesvirus in Kikuchi's disease. Hum Pathol 1998; 29: 1091–1096.

243. Medeiros LJ, Kaynor B, Harris NL. Lupus lymphadenitis: report of a case with immunohistologic studies on frozen sections. Hum Pathol 1989; 20: 295–299.

244. Goldsmith RW, Gribetz D, Strauss L. Mucocutaneous lymph node syndrome (MLNS) in the continental United States. Pediatrics 1976; 57: 431–435.

245. Rowley AH, Eckerley CA, Jack HM, et al. IgA plasma cells in vascular tissue of patients with Kawasaki syndrome. J Immunol 1997; 159: 5946–5955.

246. Giesker DW, Pastuszak WT, Forouhar FA, et al. Lymph node biopsy for early diagnosis in Kawasaki disease. Am J Surg Pathol 1982; 6: 493–501.

247. Murray JC, Bomgaars LR, Carcamo B, et al. Lymphoid malignancies following Kawasaki disease. Am J Hematol 1995; 50: 299–300.

248. Bascom R, Johns CJ. The natural history and management of sarcoidosis. Adv Intern Med 1986; 31: 213–241.

249. Cook MG. The size and histological appearances of mesenteric lymph nodes in Crohn's disease. Gut 1972; 13: 970–972.

250. Hollingsworth HC, Longo DL, Jaffe ES. Small noncleaved cell lymphoma associated with florid epithelioid granulomatous response: a clinicopathologic study of seven patients. Am J Surg Pathol 1993; 17: 51–59.

251. Braylan RC, Long JC, Jaffe ES, et al. Malignant lymphoma obscured by concomitant extensive epithelioid granulomas: report of three cases with similar clinicopathologic features. Cancer 1977; 39: 1146–1155.

252. Sacks EL, Donaldson SS, Gordon J, et al. Epithelioid granulomas associated with Hodgkin's disease: clinical correlations in 55 previously untreated patients. Cancer 1978; 41: 562–567.

253. Moller DR, Chen ES. What causes sarcoidosis? Current Opinion in Pulmonary Medicine 2002; 8: 429–434.

254. van den Oord JJ, de Woolf-Peeters C, Facchetti F, et al. Cellular composition of hypersensitivity-type granulomas. Immunohistochemical analysis of tuberculous and sarcoidal lymphadenitis. Hum Pathol 1984; 15: 559–565.

255. Facchetti F, Agostini C, Chilosi M, et al. Suppurative granulomatous lymphadenitis. Immunohistochemical evidence for a B-cell-associated granuloma. Am J Surg Pathol 1992; 16: 955–961.

256. Reid JD, Wolinsky E. Histopathology of lymphadenitis caused by atypical mycobacteria. Am Rev Respir Dis 1969; 99: 8–12.

257. Barnett RN, Hull JG, Vortel V. *Pneumocystis carinii* in lymph nodes and spleen. Arch Pathol Lab Med 1969; 88: 175–180.

258. Korbi S, Toccanier MF, Leyvraz G, et al. Use of silver staining (Dieterle's stain) in the diagnosis of cat scratch disease. Histopathology 1986; 10: 1015–1021.

259. Maurin M, Birtles R, Raoult D. Current knowledge of *Bartonella* species. Eur J Clin Microbiol 1997; 16: 487–506.

260. Naji AF, Carbonell F, Barker HJ. Cat scratch disease, a report of three new cases, review of the literature, and classification of the pathologic changes in the lymph nodes during various stages of the disease. Am J Clin Pathol 1962; 38: 513–521.

261. Wear DJ, Margileth AM, Hadfield TL, et al. Cat-scratch disease: a bacterial infection. Science 1983; 221: 1403–1405.

262. Zangwill KM, Hamilton DH, Perkins BA, et al. Cat scratch disease in Connecticut: Epidemiology, risk factors, and evaluation of a new diagnostic test. N Engl J Med 1993; 329: 8–13.

263. Not T, Canciani M, Buratti E, et al. Serologic response to *Bartonella henselae* in patients with cat scratch disease and in sick and healthy children. Acta Paediatr 1999; 88: 284–289.

264. Sander A, Posselt M, Bohm N, et al. Detection of *Bartonella henselae* DNA by two different PCR assays and determination of the genotypes of strains involved in histologically defined cat scratch disease. J Clin Microbiol 1999; 37: 993–997.

265. Litwin CM, Martins TB, Hill HR. Immunologic response to *Bartonella henselae* as determined by enzyme immunoassay and Western blot analysis. Am J Clin Pathol 1997; 108: 202–209.

266. Walzer PD, Armstrong D. Lymphogranuloma venereum presenting as supraclavicular and inguinal lymphadenopathy. Sex Transm Dis 1977; 4: 12–14.

267. Schapers RFM, Reif R, Lennert K, et al. Mesenteric lymphadenitis due to *Yersinia enterocolitica*. Virchows Arch A (Pathol Anat Histol) 1981; 390: 127–138.

268. Frizzera G, Moran EM, Rappaport H. Angio-immunoblastic lymphadenopathy with dysproteinemia. Lancet 1974; 1: 1070–1073.

269. Frizzera G, Moran EM, Rappaport H. Angioimmunoblastic lymphadenopathy: diagnosis and clinical course. Am J Med 1975; 59: 803–818.

270. Lukes RJ, Tindle BH. Immunoblastic lymphadenopathy: A hyperimmune entity resembling Hodgkin's disease. N Engl J Med 1975; 292: 1–8.

271. Nathwani BN, Rappaport H, Moran EM, et al. Malignant lymphoma arising in angioimmunoblastic lymphadenopathy. Cancer 1978; 41: 578–606.

272. Shimoyama M, Minato K, Saito H, et al. Immunoblastic lymphadenopathy (IBL)-like T-cell lymphoma. Jpn Clin Oncol 1979; 9(suppl): 347–356.

273. Watanabe S, Sato Y, Shimoyama M, et al. Immunoblastic lymphadenopathy, angioimmunoblastic lymphadenopathy, and IBL-like T-cell lymphoma. A spectrum of T-cell neoplasia. Cancer 1986; 58: 2224–2232.

274. Weiss LM, Strickler JG, Dorfman RF, et al. Clonal T-cell populations in angioimmunoblastic lymphadenopathy and angioimmunoblastic lymphadenopathy-like lymphoma. Am J Pathol 1986; 122: 392–397.

275. Ferry JA. Angioimmunoblastic T-cell lymphoma. Adv Anat Pathol 2002; 273–279.

276. Lukes RJ, Butler JJ. The pathology and nomenclature of Hodgkin's disease. Cancer Res 1966; 26: 1063–1083.

277. Lukes RJ, Craver LF, Hall TC, et al. Report of the nomenclature committee. Cancer Res 1966; 26: 1311.

278. Mason DY, Banks PM, Chan J, et al. Nodular lymphocyte predominance Hodgkin's disease: a distinct clinico-pathological entity. Am J Surg Pathol 1994; 18: 528–530.

279. Diehl V, Sextro M, Fanklin J, et al. Clinical presentation, course, and prognostic factors in lymphocyte-predominant Hodgkin's disease and lymphocyte-rich classical Hodgkin's disease: report from the European Task Force on Lymphoma Project on Lymphocyte-Predominant Hodgkin's Disease. J Clin Oncol 1999; 17: 776–783.

280. Orlandi E, Lazzarino M, Brusamolino E, et al. Nodular lymphocyte predominance Hodgkin's disease: long-term observation reveals a continuous pattern of recurrence. Leuk Lymphoma 1997; 26: 359–368.

281. Ries LAG, Kosary CL, Hankey BF, et al. SEER cancer statistics review: 1973–1994. NIH publ Bethesda: National Cancer Institute 1997; 97: 2789

282. MacMahon B. Epidemiology of Hodgkin's disease. Cancer Res 1966; 26: 1189–1201.

283. Chen YZ, Zheng T, Chou MC, et al. The increase of Hodgkin's disease incidence among young adults. Experience in Connecticut. Cancer 1997; 79: 2209–2218.

284. Weiss LM, Chen Y-Y, Liu X-F, et al. Epstein-Barr virus and Hodgkin's disease: a correlative in situ hybridization and polymerase chain reaction study. Am J Pathol 1991; 139: 1259–1265.

285. Weiss LM, Chang KL. Association of the Epstein-Barr virus with hematolymphoid neoplasia. Adv Anat Pathol 1996; 3: 1–15.

286. Mueller NC, Grufferman S. The epidemiology of Hodgkin's disease. In: Mauch P, Armitage J, Diehl V, et al., eds. Hodgkin's disease. Philadelphia: Lippincott, Williams, & Wilkins; 1999: 61–77.

287. Mack TM, Cozen W, Shibata DK, et al. Concordance in identical twins suggests genetic susceptibility to young adult Hodgkin's disease. N Engl J Med 1995; 332: 413–418.

288. Gutensohn N, Cole P. Epidemiology of Hodgkin's disease in the young. Int J Cancer 1977; 19: 595–604.

289. Gutensohn N, Cole P. Childhood social environment and Hodgkin's disease. N Engl J Med 1981; 304: 135–140.

290. Grufferman S, Delzell E. Epidemiology of Hodgkin's disease. Epidemiol Rev 1984; 6: 76–106.

291. Gutensohn N, Cole P. Epidemiology of Hodgkin's disease. Semin Oncol 1980; 7: 92–102.

292. Prazak J, Hermanska Z. Study of HLA antigens in patients with Hodgkin's disease. Eur J Haematol 1989; 43: 50–53.

293. Kaplan HS. Hodgkin's disease. 2nd edn. Cambridge, MA: Harvard University Press; 1980.

294. Mauch PM, Kalish LA. Patterns of presentation of Hodgkin's disease. Implications for etiology and pathogenesis. Cancer 1993; 71: 2062–2071.

295. Lister TA, Crowther D, Sutcliffe SB, et al. Report of a committee convened to discuss the evaluation and staging of patients with Hodgkin's disease: Cotswolds meeting. J Clin Oncol 1989; 7: 1630–1636.

296. Lister TA, Crowther D. Staging for Hodgkin's disease. Semin Oncol 1990; 17: 696–703.

297. Urba WJ, Longo DL. Hodgkin's disease. N Engl J Med 1992; 326: 678–687.

298. Howell SJ, Grey M, Chang J, et al. The value of bone marrow examination in the staging of Hodgkin's lymphoma: a review of 955 cases seen in a regional cancer centre. Br J Haematol 2002; 119: 408–411.

299. von Wasielewski R, Seth S, Franklin J, et al. Tissue eosinophilia correlates strongly with poor prognosis in nodular sclerosing Hodgkin's disease, allowing for known prognostic factors. Blood 2000; 95: 1207–1213.

300. von Wasielewski S, Franklin J, Fischer R, et al. Nodular sclerosing Hodgkin disease: new grading predicts prognosis in intermediate and advanced stages. Blood 2003; 101: 4063–4069.

301. Anagnostopoulos I, Hansmann ML, Franssila K, et al. European Task Force on Lymphoma project on lymphocyte predominance Hodgkin's disease: histologic and immunohistological analysis of submitted cases reveals 2 types of Hodgkin disease with a nodular growth and abundant lymphocytes. Blood 2000; 96: 1889–1899.

302. Strickler JG, Michie SA, Warnke RA, et al. The "syncytial variant" of nodular sclerosing Hodgkin's disease. Am J Surg Pathol 1986; 10: 470–477.

303. Ferry JA, Linggood RM, Convery KM, et al. Hodgkin's disease, nodular sclerosis type: implications of histologic subclassification. Cancer 1993; 71: 457–463.

304. Wijlhuizen TJ, Vrints LW, Jairam R, et al. Grades of nodular sclerosis (NSI-NSII) in Hodgkin's disease: are they of independent prognostic value? Cancer 1989; 63: 1150–1153.

305. Georgii A, Fischer R, Hubner K, et al. Classification of Hodgkin's disease biopsies by a panel of four histopathologists. Report of 1,140 patients from the German National Trial. Leuk Lymphoma 1993; 9: 365–370.

306. MacLennan KA, Bennett MH, Tu A, et al. Relationship of histopathologic features to survival and relapse in nodular sclerosing Hodgkin's disease: a study of 1,659 patients. Cancer 1989; 64: 1686–1693.

307. Ashton-Key M, Thorpe PA, Allen JP, et al. Follicular Hodgkin's disease. Am J Surg Pathol 1995; 19: 1294–1299.

308. Kansal R, Singleton TP, Ross CW, et al. Follicular Hodgkin lymphoma: a histopathologic study. Am J Clin Pathol 2002; 117: 29–35.

309. Colby TV, Warnke RA. The histology of the initial relapse of Hodgkin's disease. Cancer 1980; 45: 289–292.

310. Colby TV, Hoppe RT, Warnke RA. Hodgkin's disease at autopsy: 1972–1977. Cancer 1981; 47: 1852–1862.

311. Das DK, Gupta SK, Datta BM, et al. Fine needle aspiration cytodiagnosis of Hodgkin's disease and its subtypes. I. Scope and limitations. Acta Cytol 1989; 34: 329–336.

312. Chittal SM, Caveriviere P, Schwarting R, et al. Monoclonal antibodies in the diagnosis of Hodgkin's disease: the search for a rational panel. Am J Surg Pathol 1988; 12: 9–21.

313. Taylor CR, Riley CR. Molecular morphology of Hodgkin lymphoma. Applied Immunohistochemistry & Molecular Morphology 2001; 9: 187–202.

314. Arber DA, Weiss LM. CD15: A review. Appl Immunohistochem 1993; 1: 17–30.

315. Chang KL, Arber DA, Weiss LM. CD20: A review. Appl Immunohistochem 1996; 4: 1–15.

316. Chu WS, Abbondanzo SL, Frizzera G. Inconsistency of the immunophenotype of Reed-Sternberg cells in simultaneous and consecutive specimens from the same patients. A paraffin section evaluation in 56 patients. Am J Pathol 1992; 141: 11–17.

317. Vasef MA, Alsabeh R, Medeiros LJ, et al. Immunophenotype of Reed-Sternberg and Hodgkin's cells in sequential biopsy specimens of Hodgkin's disease. A HIER-based study. Am J Clin Pathol 1997; 108: 54–59.

318. Fan G, Kotylo P, Neiman RS, et al. Comparison of fascin expression in anaplastic large cell lymphoma and Hodgkin disease. Am J Clin Pathol 2003; 119: 199–204.

319. Wlodarska I, Nooyen P, Maes B, et al. Frequent occurrence of BCL6 rearrangements in nodular lymphocyte predominance Hodgkin lymphoma but not in classical Hodgkin lymphoma. Blood 2003; 101: 706–710.

320. Rassidakis GZ, Medeiros LJ, Vassilakopoulos TP, et al. BCL-2 expression in Hodgkin and Reed-Sternberg cells of classical Hodgkin disease predicts a poorer prognosis in patients treated with ABVD or equivalent regimens. Blood 2002; 100: 3935–3941.

321. Weiss LM, Chang KL. Molecular biologic studies of Hodgkin's disease. Semin Diagn Pathol 1992; 9: 272–278.

322. Schmid C, Pan L, Diss T, et al. Expression of B-cell antigens by Hodgkin's and Reed-Sternberg cells. Am J Pathol 1991; 139: 701–707.

323. Kuzu I, Delsol G, Jones M, et al. Expression of the Ig-associated heterodimer (mb-1 and B29) in Hodgkin's disease. Histopathology 1993; 22: 141–144.

324. Weiss LM, Strickler JG, Hu E, et al. Immunoglobulin gene rearrangements in Hodgkin's disease. Hum Pathol 1986; 17: 1009–1014.

325. Tamaru J, Hummel M, Zemlin M, et al. Hodgkin's disease with a B-cell phenotype often shows a VDJ rearrangement and somatic mutations in the V_H genes. Blood 1994; 84: 708–715.

326. Cabanillas F. A review and interpretation of cytogenetic abnormalities identified in Hodgkin's disease. Hematol Oncol 1988; 6: 271–274.

327. Weiss LM, Strickler JG, Warnke RA, et al. Epstein-Barr viral DNA in tissues of Hodgkin's disease. Am J Pathol 1987; 129: 86–91.

328. Wu TC, Mann RB, Charache P, et al. Detection of EBV gene expression in Reed-Sternberg cells of Hodgkin's disease. Int J Cancer 1990; 46: 801–804.

329. Chan WC. The Reed-Sternberg cell in classical Hodgkin's disease. Hematol Oncol 2001; 19: 1–17.

330. Kuppers R. Molecular biology of Hodgkin's lymphoma. Adv Cancer Res 2002; 84: 277–312.

331. Schwering I, Brauninger A, Klein U, et al. Loss of the B-lineage-specific gene expression program in Hodgkin and Reed-Sternberg cells of Hodgkin lymphoma. Blood 2003; 101: 1505–1512.

332. Delsol G, Meggetto F, Brousset P, et al. Relation of follicular dendritic reticulum cells to Reed-Sternberg cells of Hodgkin's disease with emphasis on the expression of CD21 antigen. Am J Pathol 1993; 142: 1729–1738.

333. Stetler-Stevenson MA, Crush-Stanton S, Cossman J. Involvement of the bcl-2 gene in Hodgkin's disease. J Natl Cancer Inst 1990; 82: 855–858.

334. Weiss LM, Lopategui JR, Sun L-H, et al. Absence of the t(2;5) in Hodgkin's disease. Blood 1995; 85: 2845–2847.

335. Ladanyi M, Cavalchire G, Morris SW, et al. Reverse transcriptase polymerase chain reaction for the Ki-1 anaplastic large cell lymphoma-associated t(2;5) translocation in Hodgkin's disease. Am J Pathol 1994; 145: 1296–1300.

336. Hsu S-M, Waldron Jr JW, Hus P-L, et al. Cytokines in malignant lymphomas: review and prospective evaluation. Hum Pathol 1993; 24: 1040–1057.

337. Samoszuk M, Nansen L. Detection of interleukin-5 messenger RNA in Reed-Sternberg cells of Hodgkin's disease with eosinophilia. Blood 1990; 75: 13–16.

338. Kadin ME, Agnarsson BA, Ellingsworth LR, et al. Immunohistochemical evidence of a role for transforming growth factor beta in the pathogenesis of nodular sclerosing Hodgkin's disease. Am J Pathol 1990; 136: 1209–1214.

339. Momose H, Jaffe ES, Shin SS, et al. Chronic lymphocytic leukemia/small lymphocytic lymphoma with Reed-Sternberg-like cells and possible transformation to Hodgkin's disease. Mediation by Epstein-Barr virus. Am J Surg Pathol 1992; 16: 859–867.

340. Gonzalez CL, Medeiros LJ, Jaffe ES. Composite lymphoma. A clinicopathologic analysis of nine patients with Hodgkin's disease and B-cell non-Hodgkin's lymphoma. Am J Clin Pathol 1991; 96: 81–89.

341. Zarate-Osorno A., Medeiros LJ, Longo DL, et al. Non-Hodgkin's lymphomas arising in patients successfully treated for Hodgkin's disease. A clinical, histologic, and immunophenotypic study of 14 cases. Am J Surg Pathol 1992; 16: 885–895.

342. Zarate-Osorno A, Medeiros LJ, Kingma DW, et al. Hodgkin's disease following non-Hodgkin's lymphoma. A clinicopathologic and immunophenotypic study of nine cases. Am J Surg Pathol 1993; 17: 123–132.

343. Pittaluga S, Wiodarska I, Pulford K, et al. The monoclonal antibody ALK1 identifies a distinct morphological subtype of anaplastic large cell lymphoma associated with 2p23/ALK rearrangements. Am J Pathol 1997; 151: 343–351.

344. Pulford K, Lamant L, Morris SW, et al. Detection of anaplastic lymphoma kinase (ALK) and nucleolar protein nucleophosmin (NPM)-ALK proteins in normal and neoplastic cells with the monoclonal antibody ALK1. Blood 1997; 89: 1394–1404.

345. Cataldo KA, Jalal SM, Law ME, et al. Detection of t(2;5) in anaplastic large cell lymphoma: comparison of immunohistochemical studies, FISH, and RT-PCR in paraffin-embedded tissue. Am J Surg Pathol 1999; 23: 1386–1392.

346. Lamant L, Meggetto F, Al Saati T, et al. High incidence of the t(2;5)(p23;q35) translocation in anaplastic large cell lymphoma and its lack of detection in Hodgkin's disease. Comparison of cytogenetic analysis, reverse transcriptase chain reaction, and P-80 immunostaining. Blood 1996; 87: 284–291.

347. Lukes RJ, Butler JJ, Hicks EB. Natural history of Hodgkin's disease as related to its pathologic picture. Cancer 1966; 19: 317–344.

348. Poppema S, Kaiserling E, Lennert K. Epidemiology of nodular paragranuloma (Hodgkin's disease with lymphocytic predominance, nodular). J Cancer Res & Clin Oncol 1979; 95: 57–63.

349. Hansmann ML, Zwingers T, Boske A, et al. Clinical features of nodular paragranuloma (Hodgkin's disease, lymphocyte predominance type, nodular). J Cancer Res & Clin Oncol 1984; 108: 321–330.

350. Stoler MH, Nichols GE, Symbula M, et al. Nodular L&H lymphocyte predominance Hodgkin's disease: evidence for a kappa light chain-restricted monotypic B cell neoplasm. Am J Pathol 1995; 146: 812–818.

351. Regula DP, Hoppe RT, Weiss LM. Nodular and diffuse types of lymphocyte predominance Hodgkin's disease. N Engl J Med 1988; 318: 214–219.

352. Dorfman RF, Gatter KC, Pulford KAF, et al. An evaluation of the utility of anti-granulocyte and anti-leukocyte monoclonal antibodies in the diagnosis of Hodgkin's disease. Am J Pathol 1986; 123: 508–519.

353. Pinkus GS, Said JW. Hodgkin's disease, lymphocyte predominance type, nodular – a distinct entity? Unique staining profile of L&H variants of Reed-Sternberg cells defined by monoclonal antibodies to leukocyte common antigen, granulocyte specific antigen, and B-cell specific antigen. Am J Pathol 1985; 116: 1–6.

354. Pinkus GS, Said JW. Hodgkin's disease, lymphocyte predominance type, nodular – further evidence for a B cell derivation: L&H variants of Reed-Sternberg cells express L26, a pan B cell marker. Am J Pathol 1988; 133: 211–217.

355. Timmens W, Visser L, Poppema S. Nodular lymphocyte predominance type of Hodgkin's disease

is a germinal center lymphoma. Lab Invest 1986; 54: 457–461.

356. Stein H, Hansmann ML, Lennert K, et al. Reed-Sternberg and Hodgkin's cells in lymphocyte-predominant Hodgkin's disease of nodular subtype contain J chain. Am J Clin Pathol 1986; 86: 292–297.

357. Momose H, Chen YY, Ben-Ezra J, et al. Nodular, lymphocyte predominant Hodgkin's disease: study of immunoglobulin light chain protein and mRNA expression. Hum Pathol 1992; 23: 1115–1119.

358. Schmid C, Sargent C, Isaacson PG. L and H cells of nodular lymphocyte predominant Hodgkin's disease show immunoglobulin light-chain restriction. Am J Pathol 1991; 139: 1281–1289.

359. Kraus MD, Haley J. Lymphocyte predominance Hodgkin's disease: the use of bcl-6 and CD57 in diagnosis and differential diagnosis. Am J Surg Pathol 2000; 24: 1068–1078.

360. Kamel OW, Gelb AB, Shibuya RB, et al. Leu7 (CD57) reactivity distinguishes nodular lymphocyte predominance Hodgkin's disease, T cell rich B cell lymphoma and follicular lymphoma. Am J Pathol 1993; 142: 541–546.

361. Alavaikko JF, Hansmann ML, Nebendahl C, et al. Follicular dendritic cells in Hodgkin's disease. Am J Clin Pathol 1991; 95: 194–200.

362. Delabie J, Tierens A, Wu G, et al. Lymphocyte predominance Hodgkin's disease: lineage and clonality determination using a single-cell assay. Blood 1994; 84: 3291–3298.

363. Nguyen P, Ferry J, Harris NL. Progressive transformation of germinal centers and nodular lymphocyte predominance Hodgkin's disease: a comparative immunohistochemical study. Am J Surg Pathol 1999; 22: 27–33.

364. Goates JJ, Kamel OW, LeBrun DP, et al. Floral variant of follicular lymphoma. Immunological and molecular studies support a neoplastic process. Am J Surg Pathol 1994; 18: 37–47.

365. Delabie J, Vandenberghe E, Kennes C, et al. Histiocyte-rich B-cell lymphoma. A distinct clinicopathologic entity possibly related to lymphocyte predominant Hodgkin's disease, paragranuloma subtype. Am J Surg Pathol 1992; 16: 37–48.

366. Franke S, Wlodarska I, Maes B, et al. Comparative genomic hybridization pattern distinguishes T-cell/histiocyte-rich B-cell lymphoma from nodular lymphocyte predominance Hodgkin's lymphoma. Am J Pathol 2002; 161: 1861–1867.

367. Miettinen M, Franssila KO, Saxen E. Hodgkin's disease, lymphocytic predominance nodular: increased risk for subsequent non-Hodgkin's lymphomas. Cancer 1983; 51: 2293–2300.

368. Hansmann ML, Shibata D, Lorenzen J, et al. Incidence of Epstein-Barr virus, bcl-2 expression and chromosomal translocation t(14;18) in large cell lymphoma associated with paragranuloma (lymphocyte-predominant Hodgkin's disease). Hum Pathol 1994; 25: 240–243.

369. Parrens M, Vergier B, Fitoussi O, et al. Sequential development of Hodgkin's disease and CD30+ diffuse large B-cell lymphoma in a patient with MALT-type lymphoma: evidence of different clonal origin of single microdissected Reed-Sternberg cells. Am J Surg Pathol 2002; 26: 1634–1642.

370. Wickert RS, Weisenburger DD, Tierens A, et al. Clonal relationship between lymphocyte predominance Hodgkin's disease and concurrent or subsequent large-cell lymphoma of B lineage. Blood 1995; 86: 2312–2320.

371. Ohno T, Huang J, Wu G, et al. The tumor cells in nodular lymphocyte-predominant Hodgkin disease are clonally related to the large cell lymphoma occurring in the same individual. Direct demonstration by single cell analysis. Am J Clin Pathol 2001; 506–511.

372. Boring CC, Squires TS, Tong T. Cancer Statistics. Cancer J Clin 1993; 43: 7–26.

373. Devesa SS, Fears T. Non-Hodgkin's lymphoma time trends: United States and International Data. Cancer Res 1992; 52: 5432–5440.

374. Ries LAG, Eisner MP, Kosary CL, et al. SEER Cancer Statistics Review. Bethesda, MD: National Cancer Institute; 2003.

375. Gail MH, Pluda JM, Rabkin CS, et al. Projections of the incidence of non-Hodgkin's lymphoma related to acquired immunodeficiency syndrome. JNCI 1991; 83: 695–701.

376. Cantor KP, Blair A, Everett G, et al. Hair dye use and risk of leukemia and lymphoma. Am J Public Health 1988; 78: 570–571.

377. Hoar SK, Blair A, Holmes FF, et al. Agricultural herbicide and risk of lymphoma and soft tissue sarcoma. JAMA 1986; 256: 1141–1147.

378. Scherr PA, Hutchison GB, Neiman RS. Non-Hodgkin's lymphoma and occupational exposure. Cancer Res 1992; 52: 5503–5509.

379. Jaffe ES, Blattner WA, Blayney DW. The pathologic spectrum of adult T-cell leukemia/lymphoma in the United States. Human T-cell leukemia/lymphoma virus-associated lymphoid malignancies. Am J Surg Pathol 1984; 8: 263–275.

380. Rosenberg SA. Validity of the Ann Arbor Staging Classification for the non-Hodgkin's lymphomas. Cancer Treat Rep 1977; 61: 1023–1027.

381. Lukes RJ, Collins RD. Immunologic characterization of human malignant lymphomas. Cancer 1974; 34: 1488–1503.

382. Oeschger S, Brauninger A, Kuppers R, et al. Tumor cell dissemination in follicular lymphoma. Blood 2004; 99: 2192–2198.

383. Weiss LM, Crabtree GS, Rouse RV, et al. Morphologic and immunologic characterization of 50 peripheral T-cell lymphomas. Am J Pathol 1985; 118: 316–324.

384. Fan YS, Rizkalla K. Comprehensive cytogenetic analysis including multicolor spectral karyotyping and interphase fluorescence in situ hybridization in lymphoma diagnosis. A summary of 154 cases. Cancer Genet Cytogenet 2003; 143: 73–79.

385. Godon A, Moreau A, Talmant P, et al. Is t(14;18)(q32;q21) a constant finding in follicular lymphoma? An interphase FISH study on 63 patients. Leukemia 2003; 17: 255–259.

386. National Cancer Institute sponsored study of classifications of non-Hodgkin's lymphomas: summary and description of a working formulation for clinical usage. The Non-Hodgkin's Lymphoma Pathologic Classification Project. Cancer 1982; 49: 2112–2135.

387. Stansfeld AG, Diebold J, Kapanci Y, et al. Updated Kiel classification for lymphomas (letter). Lancet 1988; 292–293.

388. Fend F, Quintanilla-Martinez L, Kumar S, et al. Composite low grade B-cell lymphomas with two immunophenotypically distinct cell populations are true biclonal lymphomas. A molecular analysis using laser capture microdissection. Am J Surg Pathol 1999; 154: 1857–1866.

389. Kim H, Hendrickson MR, Dorfman RF. Composite lymphoma. Cancer 1977; 40: 959–976.

390. Delabie J, Greiner TC, Chan WC, et al. Concurrent lymphocyte predominance Hodgkin's disease and T-cell lymphoma. A report of three cases. Am J Surg Pathol 1996; 20: 355–362.

391. Stewart CJ, Duncan JA, Farquharson M, et al. Fine needle aspiration cytology diagnosis of malignant lymphoma and reactive lymphoid hyperplasia. J Clin Pathol 1998; 51: 197–203.

392. Young NA, Al-Saleem T, Ehya H, et al. Utilization of fine-needle aspiration cytology and flow cytometry in the diagnosis and subclassificaiton of primary and recurrent lymphoma. Cancer 1998; 25: 252–261.

393. Russell J, Skinner J, Orell S, et al. Fine needle aspiration cytology in the management of lymphoma. Aust NZ J Med 1983; 13: 365–368.

394. The International Non-Hodgkin's Lymphoma Prognostic Factors Project. A predictive model for aggressive non-Hodgkin's lymphoma. N Engl J Med 1993; 329: 987–994.

395. Bartlett NL, Rizeq M, Dorfman RF, et al. Follicular large-cell lymphoma: intermediate or low grade? J Clin Oncol 1994; 12: 1349–1357.

396. Coiffier B, Gisselbrecht C, Vose JM, et al. Prognostic factors in aggressive malignant lymphomas: description and validation of a prognostic index that could identify patients requiring a more intensive therapy. J Clin Oncol 1991; 9: 211–219.

397. Velasquez WS, Jagannath S, Tucker SL, et al. Risk classification as the basis for clinical staging of diffuse large-cell lymphoma derived from 10-year survival data. Blood 1989; 74: 551–557.

398. Hoskins PJ, Ng V, Spinelli JJ, et al. Prognostic variables in patients with diffuse large-cell lymphoma treated with MACOP-B. J Clin Oncol 1991; 9: 220–226.

399. Dixon DO, Neilan B, Jones SE, et al. Effect of age on therapeutic outcome in advanced diffuse histiocytic lymphoma: the Southwest Oncology Group experience. J Clin Oncol 1986; 4: 295–305.

400. Shipp MA, Yeap BY, Harrington DP, et al. The M-BACOD combination chemotherapy regimen in large-cell lymphoma: analysis of the completed trial and comparison with the M-BACOD regimen. J Clin Oncol 1990; 8: 84–93.

401. Mok TS, Steinberg J, Chan AT, et al. Application of the International Prognostic Index in a study of Chinese patients with non-Hodgkin's lymphoma and a high incidence of primary extranodal lymphoma. Cancer 1998; 82: 2439–2448.

402. Maartense E, Le Cessie S, Kluin-Nelemans H, et al. Age-related differences among patients with follicular lymphoma and the importance of prognostic scoring systems: analysis from a population-based non-Hodgkin's lymphoma registry. Ann Oncol 2002; 1275–1284.

403. Grogan TM, Lippman SM, Spier CM, et al. Independent prognostic significance of a nuclear proliferation antigen in diffuse large cell lymphomas as determined by the monoclonal antibody Ki-67. Blood 1988; 71: 1157–1160.

404. Grogan TM, Spier CM, Richter LC, Rangel CS. Immunologic approaches to the classification of non-Hodgkin's lymphomas. In: Bennett JM, Foon KA, eds. Immunologic approaches to the classification and management of lymphomas and leukemias. Boston: Kluwer Academic; 1988: 31–148.

405. Grogan TM. Immunobiologic correlates of prognosis in lymphoma. Semin Oncol 1993; 5: 58–74.

406. Viardot A, Moller P, Hogel J, et al. Clinicopathologic correlations of genomic gains and losses in follicular lymphoma. J Clin Oncol 2002; 4523–4530.

407. Harris NL, Jaffe ES, Diebold J, et al. World Health Organization classification of neoplastic diseases of the hematopoietic and lymphoid tissues: Report of the clinical advisory committee meeting – Airlie House, Virginia, November 1997. J Clin Oncol 1999; 17: 3835–3849.

408. The Non-Hodgkin's Lymphoma Classification Project. A clinical evaluation of the International Lymphoma Study Group classification of non-Hodgkin's lymphoma. Blood 1997; 89: 3909–3918.

409. Anderson JR, Armitage JO, Weisenburger DD. Epidemiology of the non-Hodgkin's lymphomas: distributions of the major subtypes differ by geographic locations. Non-Hodgkin's Lymphoma Classification Project. Ann Oncol 1998; 9: 717–720.

410. Pinto A, Hutchison RE, Grant LH, et al. Follicular lymphomas in pediatric patients. Mod Pathol 1990; 3: 308–313.

411. Lorsbach RB, Shay-Seymore D, Moore J, et al. Clinicopathologic analysis of follicular lymphoma occurring in children. Blood 2002; 99: 1959–1964.

412. Winberg CD, Nathwani BN, Bearman RM, et al. Follicular (nodular) lymphoma during the first two decades of life: a clinicopathologic study of 12 patients. Cancer 1981; 48: 2223–2235.

413. Horning SJ, Rosenberg SA. The natural history of initially untreated low-grade non-Hodgkin's lymphomas. N Engl J Med 1984; 311: 1471–1475.

414. Rosenberg SA. The low-grade non-Hodgkin's lymphomas: Challenges and opportunities. J Clin Oncol 1985; 3: 299–310.

415. Martinez-Climent JA, Alizadeh AA, Seagraves R, et al. Transformation of follicular lymphoma to diffuse large cell lymphoma is associated with a heterogeneous set of DNA copy number and gene expression alterations. Blood 2003; 101: 3109–3117.

416. Hu E, Weiss LM, Hoppe RT, et al. Follicular and diffuse mixed small cleaved and large cell lymphoma – a clinicopathologic study. J Clin Oncol 1985; 3: 1183–1187.

417. Osborne BM, Butler JJ. Follicular lymphoma mimicking progressive transformation of germinal centers. Am J Clin Pathol 1987; 88: 264–269.

418. Slovak ML, Weiss LM, Nathwani BN, et al. Cytogenetic studies of composite lymphomas: monocytoid B-cell lymphoma and other non-Hodgkin's lymphomas. Hum Pathol 1993; 24: 1086–1094.

419. Nathwani BN, Anderson JR, Armitage JO, et al. Clinical significance of follicular lymphoma with monocytoid B cells. Hum Pathol 1999; 30: 263–268.

420. Mann RB, Berard CW. Criteria for the cytologic subclassification of follicular lymphomas: a proposed alternative method. Hematol Oncol 1982; 1: 187–192.

421. Harris NL, Ferry JA. Follicular lymphoma. In: Knowles DM, ed. Neoplastic hematopathology. Philadelphia: Lippincott, Williams,& Wilkins; 2001: 823-853.

422. Hans CP, Weisenburger DD, Vose JM, et al. A significant diffuse component predicts for inferior survival in grade 3 follicular lymphoma, but cytologic subtypes do not predict survival. Blood 2003; 101: 2363–2367.

423. Ott G, Katzenberger T, Lohr A, et al. Cytomorphologic, immunohistochemical, and cytogenetic profiles of follicular lymphoma: 2 types of follicular lymphoma grade 3. Blood 2002; 99: 3806–3812.

424. Kim H, Dorfman RF, Rappaport H. Signet-ring lymphoma: a rare morphologic and functional expression of nodular (follicular) lymphoma. Am J Surg Pathol 1978; 2: 119–132.

425. Chang KL, Arber DA, Shibata D, et al. Follicular small lymphocytic lymphoma: a rare but distinct clinicopathologic entity. Am J Surg Pathol 1994; 18: 999–1009.

426. Nathwani BN, Sheibani K, Winberg CD, et al. Neoplastic B cells with cerebriform nuclei in follicular lymphomas. Hum Pathol 1985; 16: 173–180.

427. van der Putte SC, Schuurman HJ, Rademakers LH, et al. Malignant lymphoma of follicular center cell with marked nuclear lobation. Virchows Arch [Cell Pathol] 1984; 46: 93–107.

428. Vago JF, Hurtubise PE, Redden-Borowski MN, et al. Follicular center-cell lymphoma with plasmacytic differentiation, monoclonal paraprotein, and peripheral blood involvement. Recapitulation of normal B-cell development. Am J Surg Pathol 1985; 9: 764–770.

429. Chan JK, Hui PK, Ng CS. Follicular immunoblastic lymphoma: neoplastic counterpart of the intrafollicular immunoblast? Pathology 1990; 22: 103–105.

430. Come SE, Jaffe ES, Andersen JC, et al. Non-Hodgkin's lymphomas in leukemic phase: clinicopathologic correlations. Am J Med 1980; 69: 667–674.

431. Wada R, Ebina Y, Kurotaki H, et al. Intracytoplasmic immunoglobulin crystals in follicular lymphoma. Hum Pathol 2002; 33: 1141–1144.

432. Cong P, Raffeld M, Teruya-Feldstein J, et al. In situ localization of follicular lymphoma: description and analysis by laser capture microdissection. Blood 2002; 99: 3376–3382.

433. Gong JZ, Williams DC Jr, Liu K, et al. Fine-needle aspiration in non-Hodgkin's lymphoma: evaluation of cell size by cytomorphology and flow cytometry. Am J Clin Pathol 2002; 117: 880–888.

434. Saikia UN, Dey P, Saidia B, et al. Fine-needle aspiration biopsy in diagnosis of follicular lymphoma: cytomorphologic and immunohistochemical analysis. Diagn Cytopathol 2002; 26: 251–256.

435. Kurtin PJ, Hobday KS, Ziesmer S, et al. Demonstration of distinct antigenic profiles of small B-cell lymphomas by paraffin section immunohistochemistry. Am J Clin Pathol 1999; 112: 319–329.

436. Garcia CF, Warnke RA, Weiss LM. Follicular large cell lymphoma. An immunophenotype study. Am J Pathol 1986; 123: 425–431.

437. Swerdlow SH. Small B-cell lymphomas of the lymph nodes and spleen: practical insghts to diagnosis and pathogenesis. Mod Pathol 1999; 12: 125–140.

438. DiGiuseppe JA, Borowitz MJ. Clinical utility of flow cytometry in the chronic lymphoid leukemias. Semin Oncol 1998; 25: 6–10.

439. Warnke R, Levy R. The immunopathology of follicular lymphomas: a model of B-lymphocyte homing. New Engl J Med 1978; 298: 481–486.

440. Pezzella F, Tse AG, Cordell JL, et al. Expression of the bcl-2 oncogene protein is not specific for the 14;18 chromosomal translocation. Am J Pathol 1990; 137: 225–232.

441. de Leon ED, Alkan S, Huang JC, et al. Usefulness of an immunohistochemical panel in paraffin-embedded tissues for the differentiation of B-cell non-Hodgkin's lymphomas of small lymphocytes. Mod Pathol 1998; 11: 1046–1051.

442. Eshoa C, Perkins S, Kampalath B, et al. Decreased CD10 expression in grade III and in interfollicular infiltrates of follicular lymphomas. Am J Clin Pathol 2001; 115: 862–867.

443. Xu Y, McKenna RW, Kroft SH. Assessment of CD10 in the diagnosis of small B-cell lymphomas: a multiparameter flow cytometric study. Am J Clin Pathol 2002; 117: 291–300.

444. Cook JR, Craig FE, Swerdlow SH. bcl-2 expression by multicolor flow cytometric analysis assists in the diagnosis of follicular lymphoma in lymph node and bone marrow. Am J Clin Pathol 2003; 119: 145–151.

445. Capello D, Vitolo D, Pasqualucci L, et al. Distribution and pattern of BCL-6 mutations throughout the spectrum of B-cell neoplasia. Blood 2000; 95: 651–659.

446. Dunphy CH, Polski JM, Lance Evans H, et al. Paraffin immunoreactivity of CD10, CDw75, and bcl-6 in follicle center cell lymphoma. Leuk Lymphoma 2001; 41: 585–592.

447. Jardin F, Buchonnet G, Parmentier F, et al. Follicle center lymphoma is associated with significantly elevated levels of BCL-6 expression among lymphoma subtypes, independent of chromosome 3q27 rearrangements. Leukemia 2002; 16: 2318–2325.

448. Barry TS, Jaffe ES, Kingma DW, et al. CD5+ follicular lymphoma: a clinicopathologic study of three cases. Am J Clin Pathol 2002; 118: 589–598.

449. Segal GH, Jorgensen T, Scott M, et al. Optimal primer selection for clonality assessment by polymerase chain reaction analysis: II. Follicular lymphomas. Hum Pathol 1994; 25: 1276–1282.

450. Abdel-Reheim FA, Edwards E, Arber DA. Utility of a rapid polymerase chain reaction panel for the detection of molecular changes in B-cell lymphoma. Arch Pathol Lab Med 1996; 120: 357–363.

451. Tilly H, Rossi A, Stamatoullas A, et al. Prognostic value of chromosomal abnormalities in follicular lymphoma. Blood 1994; 84: 1043–1049.

452. Yunis JJ, Mayer MG, Amesen MA. bcl-2 and other genomic alterations in the prognosis of large-cell lymphoma. N Engl J Med 1989; 320: 1047–1054.

453. Weiss LM, Warnke RA, Sklar J, et al. Molecular analysis of the t(14;18) chromosomal translocation in malignant lymphomas. N Engl J Med 1987; 317: 1185–1189.

454. Yunis JJ, Oken MM, Kaplan ME, et al. Distinctive chromosomal abnormalities in histologic subtypes of non-Hodgkin's lymphoma. N Engl J Med 1982; 307: 1231–1236.

455. Horsman DE, Gascoyne RD, Coupland RW, et al. Comparison of cytogenetic analysis, Southern analysis, and polymerase chain reaction for the detection of t(14;18) in follicular lymphoma. Am J Clin Pathol 1995; 103: 472–478.

456. Tsujimoto T, Cossman J, Jaffe E, et al. Involvement of the bcl-2 gene in human follicular lymphoma. Science 1985; 288: 1440–1443.

457. Berinstein NL, Reis MD, Ngan BY, et al. Detection of occult lymphoma in peripheral blood and bone marrow of patients with untreated early-stage and advanced-stage follicular lymphoma. J Clin Oncol 1993; 11: 1344–1352.

458. Bosga-Bouwer AG, van Imhoff GW, Boonstra R, et al. Follicular lymphoma grade 3B includes 3 cytogenetically defined subgroups with primary t(14;18), 3q27, or other translocations: t(14;18) and 3q27 are mutually exclusive. Blood 2003; 101: 1149–1154.

459. Sander CA, Yano T, Clark HM, et al. p53 mutation is associated with progression in follicular lymphoma. Blood 1993; 82: 1994–2004.

460. LoCoco F, Gaidano G, Louie DC, et al. p53 mutations are associated with histologic transformation of follicular lymphoma. Blood 1994; 92: 2289–2295.

461. Cheson BD, Bennett JM, Rai KR, et al. Guidelines for clinical protocols for chronic lymphocytic leukemia: recommendations of the National Cancer Institute-sponsored working group. Am J Hematol 1988; 29: 152–163.

462. Morrison WH, Hoppe RT, Weiss LM, et al. Small lymphocytic lymphoma. J Clin Oncol 1989; 7: 598–606.

463. Pangalis GA, Boussiotis VA, Kittas C. Malignant disorders of small lymphocytes. Small lymphocytic lymphoma, lymphoplasmacytic lymphoma, and chronic lymphocytic leukemia: their clinical and laboratory relationship. Am J Clin Pathol 1993; 99: 402–408.

464. Coiffier B, Thieblemont C, Felman P, et al. Indolent nonfollicular lymphomas: characteristics, treatment, and outcome. Semin Hematol 1999; 36: 198–208.

465. Pangalis GA, Angelopoulou MK, Vassilakopoulos TP, et al. B-chronic lymphocytic leukemia, small lymphocytic lymphoma, and lymphoplasmacytic lymphoma, including Waldenstrom's macroglobulinemia: a clinical, morphologic, and biologic spectrum of similar disorders. Semin Hematol 1999; 36: 104–114.

466. Berger F, Felman P, Sonet A, et al. Nonfollicular small B-cell lymphomas: a heterogeneous group of patients with distinct clinical features and outcome. Blood 1994; 83: 2829–2835.

467. Keating MJ. Chronic lymphocytic leukemia. Semin Oncol 1999; 26(Suppl 14): 107–114.

468. Rassenti LZ, Huynh L, Toy TL, et al. ZAP-70 compared with immunoglobulin heavy-chain gene mutation status as a predictor of disease progression in chronic lymphocytic leukemia. N Engl J Med 2004; 351: 893–901.

469. Ben-Ezra J, Burke JS, Swartz WG, et al. Small lymphocytic lymphoma: a clinicopathologic analysis of 268 cases. Blood 1989; 73: 579–587.

470. Dick FR, Maca RD. The lymph node in chronic lymphocytic leukemia. Cancer 1978; 41: 283–292.

471. Pugh WC, Manning JT, Butler JJ. Paraimmunoblastic variant of small lymphocytic lymphoma/leukemia. Am J Surg Pathol 1988; 12: 907–917.

472. Gupta D, Lim MS, Medeiros LJ, et al. Small lymphocytic lymphoma with perifollicular, marginal

zone, or interfollicular distribution. Mod Pathol 2000; 11: 1161–1166.

473. Contos MJ, Kornstein MJ, Innes DJ, et al. The utility of CD20 and CD43 in subclassification of low-grade B-cell lymphoma on paraffin sections. Mod Pathol 1992; 5: 631–633.

474. Chen CC, Raikow RB, Sonmez-Alpan E, et al. Classification of small B-cell lymphoid neoplasms using a paraffin section immunohistochemical panel. Appl Immunohistochem Mol Morphol 2000; 8: 1–11.

475. Dorfman DM, Pinkus GS. Distinction between small lymphocytic and mantle cell lymphoma by immunoreactivity for CD23. Mod Pathol 1994; 7: 326–331.

476. Benattar L, Flandrin G. Morphometric and colorimetric analysis of peripheral blood smears of lymphocytes in B-cell disorders: proposal for a scoring system. Leuk Lymphoma 2001; 42: 29–40.

477. Damle RN, Wasil T, Fais F, et al. IgV gene mutation status and CD38 expression as novel prognostic indicators in chronic lymphocytic leukemia. Blood 1999; 94: 1840–1847.

478. Hamblin TJ, Davis Z, Gardiner A, et al. Unmutated Ig V(H) genes are associated with a more aggressive form of chronic lymphocytic leukemia. Blood 1999; 94: 1848–1854.

479. Oscier DG, Thompsett A, Zhu D, et al. Differential rates of somatic hypermutation in V(H) genes among subsets of chronic lymphocytic leukemia defined by chromosomal abnormalities. Blood 1997; 89: 4153–4160.

480. Bahler DW, Aguilera NS, Chen CC, et al. Histological and immunoglobulin VH gene analysis of interfollicular small lymphocytic lymphoma provides evidence for two types. Am J Pathol 2000; 157: 1063–1070.

481. Knuutila S, Elonen E, Teerenhovi L, et al. Trisomy 12 in B cells of patients with B-cell chronic lymphocytic leukemia. N Engl J Med 1986; 314: 865–869.

482. Döhner H, Stilgenbauer S, Fischer K, et al. Cytogenetic and molecular cytogenetic analusis of B cell chronic lymphocytic leukemia: specific chromosome aberrations identify prognostic subgroups of patients and point to loci of candidate genes. Leukemia 1997; 11: S19–S24.

483. Matutes E, Oscier D, Garcia-Marco J, et al. Trisomy 12 defines a group of CLL with atypical morphology: correlation between cytogenetic, clinical and laboratory features in 544 patients. Br J Haematol 1996; 92: 382–388.

484. Döhner H, Stilgenbauer S, James MR, et al. 11q deletions identify a new subset of B-cell chronic lymphocytic leukemia characterized by extensive nodal involvement and inferior prognosis. Blood 1997; 89: 2516–2522.

485. Döhner H, Fischer K, Bentz M, et al. p53 gene deletion predicts for poor survival and non-response to therapy with purine analogs in chronic B-cell leukemias. Blood 1995; 1580–1589.

486. Döhner H, Stilgenbauer S, Dohner K, et al. Chromosome aberrations in B-cell chronic lymphocytic leukemia: reassessment based on molecular cytogenetic analysis. J Mol Med 1999; 77: 266–281.

487. Byrd JC, Smith L, Hackbarth ML, et al. Interphase cytogenetic abnormalities in chronic lymphocytic leukemia may predict response to rituximab. Cancer Res 2003; 63: 36–38.

488. Oscier DG. Cytogenetics and molecular genetics of chronic lymphocytic leukaemia. Haematologica 1999; 84: 88–91.

489. Isaacson PG, Wright DH. Malignant lymphoma of mucosa associated lymphoid tissue. A distinctive B cell lymphoma. Cancer 1983; 52: 1410–1416.

490. Sheibani K, Burke JS, Swartz WG, et al. Monocytoid B cell lymphoma. Clinicopathologic study of 21 cases of a unique type of low grade lymphoma. Cancer 1988; 62: 1531–1538.

491. Isaacson PG. Lymphomas of mucosa-associated lymphoid tissue (MALT). Histopathology 1990; 16: 617–619.

492. Campo E, Miquel R, Krenacs L, et al. Primary nodal marginal zone lymphomas of splenic and MALT type. Am J Surg Pathol 1999; 23: 59–68.

493. Mollejo M, Lloret E, Marguez J, et al. Lymph node involvement by splenic marginal zone lymphoma: morphological and immunohistochemical features. Am J Surg Pathol 1997; 21: 772–780.

494. Nathwani BN, Drachenberg MR, Hernandez AM, et al. Nodal monocytoid B-cell lymphoma (nodal marginal-zone B-cell lymphoma). Semin Hematol 1999; 36: 128–138.

495. Isaacson PG, Spencer J. Malignant lymphoma of mucosa-associated lymphoid tissue. Histopathol 1987; 11: 445–462.4p1

496. Shin SS, Sheibani K. Monocytoid B-cell lymphoma. Am J Clin Pathol 1993; 99: 421–425.

497. Ngan BY, Warnke RA, Wilson M, et al. Monocytoid B-cell lymphoma: a study of 36 cases. Hum Pathol 1991; 22: 409–421.

498. Armitage JO, Weisenburger DD. New approach to classifying non-Hodgkin's lymphomas: clinical features of the major histologic subtypes. Non-Hodgkin's Lymphoma Classification Project. J Clin Oncol 1998; 16: 2780–2795.

499. Taddesse-Heath L, Pittaluga S, Sorbara L, et al. Marginal zone B-cell lymphoma in children and young adults. Am J Surg Pathol 2003; 27: 522–531.

500. Traweek ST, Sheibani K. Monocytoid B-cell lymphoma. The biologic and clinical implications of peripheral blood involvement. Am J Clin Pathol 1992; 97: 591–598.

501. Shin SS, Sheibani K, Fishleder A, et al. Monocytoid B-cell lymphoma in patients with Sjogren's syndrome: a clinicopathologic study of 13 patients. Hum Pathol 1991; 22: 422–430.

502. Parsonnet J, Hansen S, Rodriguez L, et al. *Helicobacter pylori* infection and gastric lymphoma. N Engl J Med 1994; 330:1267–1271.

503. Royer B, Cazals-Hatem D, Sibilia J, et al. Lymphomas in patients with Sjogren's syndrome are marginal zone B-cell neoplasms, arise in diverse extranodal and nodal sites, and are not associated with viruses. Blood 1997; 90: 766–775.

504. Pelstring RJ, Essell JH, Kurtin PJ, et al. Diversity of organ site involvement among malignant lymphomas of mucosa-associated tissues. Am J Clin Pathol 1991; 96: 738–745.

505. Chan JKC. Antibiotic-responsive gastric lymphoma? Adv Anat Pathol 1994; 1: 33–37.

506. Lai R, Weiss LM, Chang KL, et al. Frequency of CD43 expression in non-Hodgkin's lymphoma. A survey of 742 cases and further characterization of rare CD43+ follicular lymphomas. Am J Clin Pathol 1999; 111: 488–494.

507. Camacho FI, Algara P, Mollejo M, et al. Nodal marginal zone lymphoma: a heterogeneous tumor: a comprehensive analysis of a series of 27 cases. Am J Surg Pathol 2003; 27: 762–771.

508. Muller-Hermelink HK. Genetic and molecular genetic studies in the diagnosis of B-cell lymphomas: marginal zone lymphomas. Hum Pathol 2003; 34: 336–340.

509. Brynes RK, Almaguer PD, Leathery KE, et al. Numerical cytogenetic abnormalities of chromosomes 3, 7, and 12 in marginal zone B-cell lymphoma. Mod Pathol 1996; 10: 995–1000.

510. Wotherspoon AC, Finn TM, Isaacson PG. Trisomy 3 in low-grade primary B-cell lymphomas of mucosa-associated lymphoid tissue (MALT). Blood 1995; 85: 2000–2004.

511. Dierlamm J, Rosenberg C, Stul M, et al. Characteristic pattern of chromosomal gains and losses in marginal zone B cell lymphoma detected by comparative genomic hybridization. Leukemia 1997; 11:747–758.

512. Auer IA, Gascoyne RD, Connors JM, et al. t(11;18)(q21;q21) is the most common translocation in MALT lymphoma. Ann Oncol 1997; 8: 979–985.

513. Rosenwald A, Ott G, Stilgenbauer S, et al. Exclusive detection of the t(11;18)(q21;q21) in extranodal marginal zone B cell lymphomas (MZBL) of MALT type in contrast to other MZBL and extranodal large B cell lymphomas. Am J Surg Pathol 1999; 155: 1817–1821.

514. Bertoni F, Cotter FE, Zucca E. Molecular genetics of extranodal marginal zone (MALT-type) B-cell lymphoma. Leuk Lymphoma 1999; 35: 57–68.

515. Dierlamm J, Baens M, Wlodarska I, et al. The apoptosis inhibitor gene *AP12* and a novel 18q gene, *MLT*, are recurrently rearranged in the t(11;18)(q21;q21) associated with mucosa-associated lymphoid tissue lymphomas. Blood 1999; 93: 3601–3609.

516. Ott G, Katzenberger T, Greiner A, et al. The t(11;18)(q21;q21) chromosome translocation is a frequent and specific aberration in low-grade but not high-grade malignant non-Hodgkin's lymphomas of the mucosa-associated lymphoid tissue (MALT)-type. Cancer Res 1997; 57: 3944–3948.

517. Arber DA, Weiss LM. CD5: A review. Appl Immunohistochem 1995; 3: 1–22.

518. Andriko JA, Swerdlow SH, Aguilera NS, et al. Is lymphoplasmacytic lymphoma/immunocytoma a distinct entity? A clinicopathologic study of 20 cases. Am J Surg Pathol 2001; 25: 742–751.

519. McMaster ML. Familial Waldenstrom's macroglobulinemia. Semin Oncol 2003; 30: 146–152.

520. Schop RF, Kuehl WM, Van Wier SA, et al. Waldenstrom macroglobulinemia neoplastic cells lack immunoglobulin heavy chain locus translocations but have frequent 6q deletions. Blood 2002; 199: 2996–3001.

521. Patsouris E, Noël H, Lennert K. Lymphoplasmacytic/lymphoplasmacytoid immunocytoma with a high content of epithelioid cells: histologic and immunohistochemical findings. Am J Surg Pathol 1990; 14: 660–670.

522. Lebeau A, Zeindl-Eberhart E, Muller EC, et al. Generalized crystal-storing histiocytosis associated with monoclonal gammopathy: molecular analysis of a disorder with rapid clinical course and review of the literature. Blood 2002; 100: 1817–1827.

523. Harada M, Shimada M, Fukayama M, et al. Crystal-storing histiocytosis associated with lymphoplasmacytic lymphoma mimicking Weber-Christian disease: immunohistochemical, ultrastructural, and gene-rearrangement studies. Histopathology 1998; 33: 459–464.

524. San Miguel JF, Vidriales MB, Ocio E, et al. Immunophenotypic analysis of Waldenstrom's macroglobulinemia. Semin Oncol 2003; 30: 187–195.

525. Offit K, Parsa NZ, Filippa D, et al. t(9;14)(p13;q32) denotes a subset of low-grade non-Hodgkin's lymphoma with plasmacytoid differentiation. Blood 1992; 80: 2594–2599.

526. Offit K, Louie DC, Parsa NZ, et al. del (7)(32) is associated with a subset of small lymphocytic lymphoma with plasmacytoid features. Blood 1995; 86: 2365–2370.

527. Iida S, Rao PH, Nallasivam P, et al. The t(9;14)(p13;q32) chromosomal translocation associated with lymphoplasmacytoid lymphoma involves the PAX-5 gene. Blood 1996; 88: 4110–4117.

528. Iida S, Rao PH, Ueda R, et al. Chromosomal rearrangement of the PAX-5 locus in lymphoplasmacytic lymphoma with t(9;14)(p13;q32). Leuk Lymphoma 1999; 34: 25–33.

529. Schop RF, Fonseca R. Genetics and cytogenetics of Waldenstrom's macroglobulinemia. Semin Oncol 2003; 39: 142–145.

530. Torlakovic E, Torlakovic G, Nguyen PL, et al. The value of anti-pax-5 immunostaining in routinely fixed and paraffin-embedded sections: a novel pan pre-B and B-cell marker. Am J Surg Pathol 2002; 26: 104–114.

531. Amakawa R, Ohno H, Fukuhara S. t(9;14)(p13;Q32) involving the PAX-5 gene: a unique subtype of 14q32 translocation in B cell non-Hodgkin's lymphoma. Int J Hematol 1999; 69: 65–69.

532. Gerard-Marchant R, Hamlin I, Lennert K, et al. Classification of non-Hodgkin's lymphomas. Lancet 1974; 2: 406–408.

533. Berard CW, Dorfman RF. Histopathology of malignant lymphomas. Clin Haematol 1974; 3: 39–76.

534. Swerdlow SH, Williams ME. From centrocytic to mantle cell lymphoma: a clinicopathologic and molecular review of 3 decades. Hum Pathol 2002; 33: 7–20.

535. O'Briain DS, Kennedy MJ, Daly PA, et al. Multiple lymphomatous polyposis of the gastrointestinal tract: a clinicopathologically distinctive form of non-Hodgkin's lymphoma of centrocytic type. Am J Surg Pathol 1989; 13: 691–699.

536. Weisenburger DD, Armitage JO. Mantle cell lymphoma – an entity comes of age. Blood 1996; 87: 4483–4494.

537. Lardelli P, Bookman MA, Sundeen J, et al. Lymphocytic lymphoma of intermediate differentiation. Morphologic and immunophenotypic spectrum and clinical correlations. Am J Surg Pathol 1990; 14: 752–763.

538. Fisher RI, Dahlberg S, Nathwani BN, et al. A clinical analysis of two indolent lymphoma entities: mantle cell lymphoma and marginal zone lymphoma (including the mucosa-associated lymphoid tissue and monocytoid B-cell categories): A Southwest Oncology Group study. Blood 1995; 85: 1075–1082.

539. Weisenburger DD, Kim H, Rappaport H. Mantle zone lymphoma. A follicular variant of intermediate lymphocytic lymphoma. Cancer 1982; 49: 1429–1438.

540. Koo CH, Rappaport H, Sheibani K, et al. Imprint cytology of non-Hodgkin's lymphomas. Based on a study of 212 immunologically characterized cases. Hum Pathol 1989; 20 (suppl): 1–137.

541. Ott MM, Ott G, Kuse R, et al. The anaplastic variant of centrocytic lymphoma is marked by frequent rearrangements of the bcl-1 gene and high proliferation indices. Histopathology 1994; 24: 329–334.

542. Lennert K, Stein H, Mohri N, et al. Malignant lymphomas other than Hodgkin's disease, histology, cytology, ultrastructure, immunology. New York: Springer-Verlag; 1978.

543. Liu Z, Dong HY, Gorczyca W, et al. CD5- mantle cell lymphoma. Am J Clin Pathol 2002; 118: 216–224.

544. Li JY, Gaillard F, Moreau A, et al. Detection of translocation t(11;14)(q13;q32) in mantle cell lymphoma by fluorescence in situ hybridization. Am J Pathol 1999; 154: 1449–1452.

545. Raffeld M, Jaffe ES. bcl-1, t(11;14), and mantle cell-derived lymphomas. Blood 1991; 78: 259–263.

546. Rimokh R, Berger F, Delsol G, et al. Rearrangement and overexpression of the BCL-1/PRAD-1 gene in intermediate lymphocytic lymphomas and in t(11q13)-bearing leukemias. Blood 1993; 81: 3063–3067.

547. Rimokh R, Berger F, Delsol G, et al. Detection of the chromosomal translocation t(11;14) by polymerase chain reaction in mantle cell lymphomas. Blood 1994; 83: 1871–1875.

548. Williams ME, Swerdlow SH, Rosenberg CL, et al. Chromosome 11 translocation breakpoints at the PRAD1/Cyclin D1 gene locus in centrocytic lymphoma. Leukemia 1993; 7: 241–245.

549. Leroux D, LeMarc'hadour F, Gressin R, et al. Non-Hodgkin's lymphomas with t(11;14)(q13;q32): a subset of mantle zone/intermediate lymphocytic lymphoma? Br J Haematol 1991; 77: 346–353.

550. DeBoer CH, VanKrieken JH, Luin-Nelemans HC, et al. Cyclin D1 messenger RNA overexpression as a marker for mantle cell lymphoma. Oncogene 1995; 10: 1833–1840.

551. Zukerberg LR, Yang W-I, Arnold A, et al. Cyclin D1 expression in non-Hodgkin's lymphomas. Detection by immunohistochemistry. Am J Clin Pathol 1995; 103: 756–760.

552. Swerdlow SH, Yang WI, Zukerberg LR, et al. Expression of cyclin D1 protein in centrocytic/mantle cell lymphomas with and without rearrangement of the BCL1/cyclin D1 gene. Hum Pathol 1995; 26: 999–1004.

553. Sawyer JR, Waldron JA, Jagannath S, et al. Cytogenetic findings in 200 patients with multiple myeloma. Cancer Genet Cytogenet 1995; 82: 41–49.

554. Bosch F, Campo E, Jares P, et al. Increased expression of the PRAD-1/CCND1 gene in hairy cell leukemia. Br J Haematol 1995; 91: 1025–1030.

555. Banks PM, Warnke RA. Pathology and genetics: tumor of haematopoietic and lymphoid tissues. In: Jaffe ES, Harris NL, Stein H, et al., eds. WHO classification of tumors. Lyon: IARC Press; 2001: 179–180.

556. Kwak LW, Wilson M, Weiss LM, et al. Clinical significance of morphologic subdivision in diffuse large cell lymphoma. Cancer 1991; 68: 1988–1993.

557. Davis RE, Dorfman RF, Warnke RA. Primary large cell lymphoma of the thymus: a diffuse B-cell neoplasm presenting as primary mediastinal lymphoma. Hum Pathol 1990; 21: 1262–1268.

558. Diebold J, Anderson JR, Armitage JO, et al. Diffuse large B-cell lymphoma: A clinicopathologic analysis of 444 cases classified according to the updated Kiel Classification. Leukemia & Lymphoma 2002; 43: 97–104.

559. Engelhard M, Brittinger G, Huhn D, et al. Subclassification of diffuse large B-cell lymphomas according to the Kiel Classification: Distinction of centroblastic and immunoblastic lymphomas is a significant prognostic risk factor. Blood 1997; 89: 2291–2297.

560. Jacobson JO, Aisenberg AC, Lamarre L, et al. Mediastinal large cell lymphoma: an uncommon subset of adult lymphoma curable with combined modality therapy. Cancer 1988; 62: 1893–1898.

561. Urba WJ, Duffey PL, Longo DL. Treatment of patients with aggressive lymphomas: an overview. JNCI Monogr 1990; 10: 29–37.

562. Armitage JO. Treatment of non-Hodgkin's lymphoma. N Engl J Med 1993; 328: 1023–1030.

563. Blum KA, Bartlett NL. Antibodies for the treatment of diffuse large cell lymphoma. Semin Oncol 2003; 30: 448–456.

564. Lamarre L, Jacobson JO, Aisenberg AC, et al. Primary large cell lymphoma of the mediastinum. Am J Surg Pathol 1989; 13: 730–739.

565. Addis BJ, Isaacson PG. Large cell lymphoma of the mediastinum: a B-cell tumour of probable thymic origin. Histopathology 1986; 10: 379–390.

566. Yousem SA, Weiss LM, Warnke RA. Primary mediastinal non-Hodgkin's lymphomas: a morphologic and immunologic study of 19 cases. Am J Clin Pathol 1985; 83: 676–680.

567. Perrone T, Frizzera G, Rosai J. Mediastinal diffuse large-cell lymphoma with sclerosis: a clinicopathologic study of 60 cases. Am J Surg Pathol 1986; 10: 176–191.

568. Sheibani K, Battifora H, Winberg CD, et al. Further evidence that "malignant angioendotheliomatosis" is an angiotropic large-cell lymphoma. N Engl J Med 1986; 314: 943–948.

569. Tsang WY, Chan JK, Tang SK, et al. Large cell lymphoma with fibrillary matrix. Histopathology 1992; 20: 80–82.

570. Dardick I, Srinivasan R, Al-Jabi M. Signet ring cell variant of large cell lymphoma. Ultrastruct Pathol 1983; 5: 195–200.

571. Ramsay AP, Smith WJ, Isaacson PG. T-cell-rich B-cell lymphoma. Am J Surg Pathol 1988; 12: 433–443.

572. Chittal SM, Brousset P, Voigt JJ, et al. Large B-cell lymphoma rich in T-cells and simulating Hodgkin's disease. Histopathology 1991; 19: 211–220.

573. Macon WR, Williams ME, Greer JP, et al. T-cell-rich B-cell lymphomas. A clinicopathologic study of 19 cases. Am J Surg Pathol 1992; 16: 351–363.

574. Krishnan J, Wallberg K, Frizzera G. T-cell-rich large B-cell lymphoma. A study of 30 cases, supporting its histologic heterogeneity and lack of clinical distinctiveness. Am J Surg Pathol 1994; 18: 455–465.

575. Moller P, Lammler B, Erberlein-Gonska M. Primary mediastinal clear cell lymphoma of B-cell type. Virchows Arch 1986; 409: 79–92.

576. Kinney MC, Glick AD, Stein H, et al. Comparison of anaplastic large cell Ki-1 lymphomas and microvillous lymphomas in their immunologic and ultrastructural features. Am J Surg Pathol 1990; 14: 1047–1060.

577. Doggett RS, Wood GS, Horning S, et al. The immunologic characterization of 95 nodal and extranodal diffuse large cell lymphomas in 89 patients. Am J Pathol 1984; 115: 245–252.

578. Piris M, Brown DC, Gatter KC, et al. CD30 expression in non-Hodgkin's lymphoma. Histopathology 1990; 17: 211–218.

579. Cleary ML, Trela MJ, Weiss LM, et al. Most null large-cell lymphomas are B cell neoplasms. Lab Invest 1985; 53: 521–525.

580. Offit K, LoCoco F, Louie DC, et al. Rearrangement of the bcl-6 gene as a prognostic marker in diffuse large-cell lymphoma. N Engl J Med 1994; 331: 74–80.

581. Tsang P, Cesarman E, Chadburn A, et al. Molecular characterization of primary mediastinal B cell lymphoma. Am J Pathol 1996; 148: 2017–2025.

582. Joos S, Otano-Joos MI, Ziegler S, et al. Primary mediastinal (thymic) B-cell lymphoma is characterized by gains of chromosomal material including 9p and amplification of the REL gene. Blood 1996; 87: 1571–1578.

583. Onciu M, Behm FG, Downing JR, et al. ALK-positive plasmablastic B-cell lymphoma with expression of the NPM-ALK fusion transcript: report of 2 cases. Blood 2003; 102: 2642–2644.

584. Adam P, Katzenberger T, Seeberger H, et al. A case of a diffuse large B-cell lymphoma of plasmablastic type associated with the t(2;5)(p23;q35) chromosome translocation. Am J Surg Pathol 2003; 27: 1473–1476.

585. Kramer MHH, Hermans J, Wijburg E, et al. Clinical relevance of BCL2, BCL6 and MYC rearrangements in diffuse large B-cell lymphoma. Blood 1998; 92: 3152–3162.

586. Alizadeh AA, Eisen MB, Davis RE, et al. Distinct types of diffuse large B-cell lymphoma identified by gene expression profiling. Nature 2000; 403: 503–511.

587. Greer JP, York JC, Cousar JB, et al. Peripheral T-cell lymphoma: a clinicopathologic study of 42 cases. J Clin Oncol 1984; 2: 788–798.

588. Horning SJ, Weiss LM, Crabtree GS, et al. Clinical and phenotypic diversity of T cell lymphomas. Blood 1986; 67: 1578–1582.

589. Weis JW, Winter MW, Phyliky RL, et al. Peripheral T-cell lymphomas: histologic, immunohistologic, and clinical characterization. Mayo Clin Proc 1986; 61: 411–426.

590. Kwak LW, Wilson M, Weiss LM, et al. Similar outcome of treatment of B-cell and T-cell diffuse large-cell lymphomas: the Stanford experience. J Clin Oncol 1991; 9: 1426–1431.

591. Lippman SM, Miller TP, Spier CM, et al. The prognostic significance of the immunotype in diffuse large-cell lymphoma: a comparative study of the T-cell and B-cell phenotype. Blood 1988; 72: 436–441.

592. Jaffe ES, Strauchen JA, Berard CW. Predictability of immunologic phenotype by morphologic criteria in diffuse aggressive non-Hodgkin's lymphomas. Am J Clin Pathol 1982; 77: 46–49.

593. Borowitz M, Reichert TA, Brynes RK, et al. The phenotypic diversity of peripheral T-cell lymphomas. The Southeastern Cancer Study Group experience. Hum Pathol 1986; 17: 567–574.

594. Kern WF, Spier CM, Hanneman EH, et al. Neural cell adhesion molecule-positive peripheral T-cell lymphoma: a rare variant with a propensity for unusual sites of involvement. Blood 1992; 79: 2432–2437.

595. Wong KF, Chan JK, Ng CS, et al. CD56 (NKH1)-positive hematolymphoid malignancies: an aggressive neoplasm featuring frequent cutaneous/mucosal involvement, cytoplasmic azurophilic granules, and angiocentricity. Hum Pathol 1992; 23: 798–804.

596. Weiss LM, Picker LJ, Grogan TM, et al. Absence of clonal beta and gamma T-cell receptor gene rearrangements in a subset of peripheral T-cell lymphomas [published erratum appears in Am J Pathol 1988;131: 604]. Am J Pathol 1988; 130: 436–443.

597. Kadin M, Sako D, Berliner N, et al. Childhood Ki-1 lymphoma presenting with skin lesions and peripheral lymphadenopathy. Blood 1986; 68: 1042–1049.

598. Stein H, Mason DY, Gerdes J, et al. The expression of the Hodgkin's disease associated antigen Ki-1 in reactive and neoplastic lymphoid tissue: evidence that Reed-Sternberg cells and histiocytic malignancies are derived from activated lymphoid cells. Blood 1985; 66: 848–858.

599. Stein H, Foss HD, Durkop H, et al. CD30 (+) anaplastic large cell lymphoma: a review of its histopathologic, genetic, and clinical features. Blood 2000; 96: 3681–3695.

600. Sandlund JT, Pui CH, Santana VM, et al. Clinical features and treatment outcome for children with CD30+ large-cell non-Hodgkin's lymphoma. J Clin Oncol 1994; 12: 895–898.

601. Reiter A, Schrappe M, Tiemann M, et al. A successful treatment strategy for Ki-1 anaplastic large cell lymphoma of childhood. A prospective analysis of 62 patients enrolled in three consecutive BFM group studies. J Clin Oncol 1994; 12: 899–908.

602. Greer JP, Kinney MC, Collins RD, et al. Clinical features of 31 patients with Ki-1 anaplastic large-cell lymphoma. J Clin Oncol 1991; 9: 539–547.

603. deBruin PC, Beljaards RC, VanHeerde P, et al. Differences in clinical behaviour and immunophenotype between primary cutaneous and primary nodal anaplastic large cell lymphoma of T-cell or null cell phenotype. Histopathology 1993; 23: 127–135.

604. Beljaards RC, Meijer CJLM, Scheffer E, et al. Prognostic significance of CD30 (Ki-1/Ber-H2) expression in primary cutaneous large-cell lymphomas of T-cell origin. A clinicopathologic and immunohistochemical study in 20 patients. Am J Pathol 1989; 135: 1169–1178.

605. Krishnan J, Tomaszewski MM, Kao GF. Primary cutaneous CD30+ anaplastic large cell lymphoma. Report of 27 cases. J Cutan Pathol 1993; 20: 193–202.

606. Chan JKC, Ng CS, Hui PK, et al. Anaplastic large cell Ki-1 lymphoma. Delineation of two morphological types. Histopathology 1989; 15: 11–34.

607. Chott A, Kaserer K, Augustin I, et al. Ki-1 positive large cell lymphoma. A clinicopathologic study of 41 cases. Am J Surg Pathol 1990; 14: 439–448.

608. Pileri S, Falini B, Delsol G, et al. Lymphohistiocytic T-cell lymphoma (anaplastic large cell lymphoma CD30+/Ki-1+) with a high content of reactive histiocytes. Histopathology 1990; 16: 383–391.

609. Kinney M, Collins RD, Greer JP, et al. A small-cell-predominant variant of primary Ki-1 (CD30)+ T-cell lymphoma. Am J Surg Pathol 1993; 17: 859–868.

610. Chan JKC, Buchanan R, Fletcher CDM. Sarcomatoid variant of anaplastic large cell Ki-1 lymphoma. J Clin Oncol 1991; 9: 539–547.

611. Pileri S, Bocchia M, Baroni CD, et al. Anaplastic large cell lymphoma (CD30+/Ki-1+): results of a prospective clinicopathologic study of 69 cases. Br J Haematol 1994; 86: 513–523.

612. Delsol G, Al-Saati T, Gatter KC, et al. Coexpression of epithelial membrane antigen (EMA), Ki-1, and interleukin-2 receptor by anaplastic large cell lymphomas. Diagnostic value in so-called malignant histiocytosis. Am J Pathol 1988; 130: 59–70.

613. Penny RJ, Blaustein JC, Longtine JA, et al. Ki-1 positive large cell lymphomas, a heterogenous group of neoplasms. Morphologic, immunophenotypic, genotypic, and clinical features of 24 cases. Cancer 1991; 68: 362–373.

614. Frierson HF, Bellafiore FJ, Gaffey MJ, et al. Cytokeratin in anaplastic large cell lymphoma. Mod Pathol 1994; 7: 317–321.

615. O'Connor NTJ, Stein H, Gatter KC, et al. Genotypic analysis of large cell lymphomas which express the Ki-1 antigen. Histopathology 1987; 11: 733–730.

616. Weiss LM, Picker LJ, Copenhaver CM, et al. Large-cell hematolymphoid neoplasms of uncertain lineage. Hum Pathol 1988; 19: 967–973.

617. Benz-Lemoine E. Malignant histiocytosis: a specific t(2;5) (p23;q35) translocation? Review of the literature. Blood 1988; 72: 1045–1047.

618. Wellmann A, Otsuki T, Vogelbruch M, et al. Analysis of the t(2;5)(p23;q35) by RT-PCR in CD30+ anaplastic large cell lymphomas, in other non-Hodgkin's lymphomas of T-cell phenotype, and in Hodgkin's disease. Blood 1995; 86: 2321–2328.

619. Lopategui JR, Sun L-H, Chan JKC, et al. Low frequency association of the t(2;5)(p23;q35) chromosomal translocation with CD30+ lymphomas from American and Asian patients. A reverse transcriptase-polymerase chain reaction study. Am J Pathol 1995; 146: 323–328.

620. Falini B, Pulford K, Pucciarini A, et al. Lymphomas expressing ALK fusion protein(s) other than NPM-ALK. Blood 1999; 94: 3509–3515.

621. Hernandez L, Pinyol M, Hernandez S, et al. TRK-fused gene (TFG) is a new partner of ALK in anaplastic large cell lymphoma producing two structurally different TFG-ALK translocations. Blood 1999; 94: 3265–3268.

622. Lamant L, Dastugue N, Pulford K, et al. A new fusion gene TPM3-ALK in anaplastic large cell lymphoma created by a (1;2)(q25;p23) translocation. Blood 1999; 93: 3088–3095.

623. Rosenwald A, Ott G, Pulford K, et al. t(1;2)(q21;p23) and t(2;3)(p23;q21): two novel variant translocations of the t(2;5)(p23;q35) in anaplastic large cell lymphoma. Blood 1999; 94: 362–364.

624. Touriol C, Greenland C, Lamant L, et al. Further demonstration of the diversity of chromosomal changes involving 2p23 in ALK-positive lymphoma: 2 cases expressing ALK kinase fused to CLTCL (clathrin chain polypeptide-like). Blood 2000; 95: 3204–3207.

625. Shiota M, Nakamura S, Ichinohasama R, et al. Anaplastic large cell lymphomas expressing the novel chimeric protein p80NPM/ALK: a distinct clinicopathologic entity. Blood 1995; 86: 1954–1960.

626. Bayerl MG, Rakozy CK, Mohamed AN, et al. Blastic natural killer cell lymphoma/leukemia: a report of seven cases. Am J Clin Pathol 2003; 117: 41–50.

627. Gascoyne RD, Lamant L, Martin-Subero JI, et al. ALK-positive diffuse large B-cell lymphoma is associated with clathrin-ALK rearrangements: report of 6 cases. Blood 2003; 102: 2568–2573.

628. Wilson MS, Weiss LM, Gatter KC, et al. Malignant histiocytosis: a reassessment of cases previously reported in 1975 based upon paraffin section immunophenotyping studies. Cancer 1990; 66: 530–536.

629. Patsouris E, Noel H, Lennert K. Histological and immunohistological findings in lymphoepithelioid cell lymphoma (Lennert's lymphoma). Am J Surg Pathol 1988; 12: 341–350.

630. Attygalle A, Al-Jehani R, Diss TC, et al. Neoplastic T cells in angioimmunoblastic T-cell lymphoma express CD10. Blood 2002; 99: 627–633.

631. Colby T, Burke J, Hoppe RT. Lymph node biopsy in mycosis fungoides. Cancer 1981; 47: 351–359.

632. Breneman DL, Raju US, Breneman JC, et al. Lymph node grading for staging of mycosis fungoides may benefit from examination of multiple excised lymph nodes. J Am Acad Dermatol 2003; 48: 702–706.

633. Salhany KE, Cousar JB, Greer JP, et al. Transformation of cutaneous T cell lymphoma to large cell lymphoma. A clinicopathologic and immunologic study. Am J Pathol 1988; 132: 265–277.

634. Vonderheid EC, Diamond LW, Lai SM, et al. Lymph node histopathologic findings in cutaneous T-cell lymphoma. A prognostic classification system based on morphologic assessment. Am J Clin Pathol 1992; 97: 121–129.

635. Weiss LM, Hu E, Wood GS, et al. Clonal rearrangements of the T cell receptor gene in mycosis fungoides and dermatopathic lymphadenopathy. N Engl J Med 1985; 313: 539–544.

636. Bunn PA, Schecter GP, Jaffe ES, et al. Clinical course of retrovirus-associated adult T-cell lymphoma in the United States. N Engl J Med 1983; 309: 257–264.

637. Mortreux F, Gabet AS, Wattel E. Molecular and cellular aspects of HTLV-1 associated leukemogenesis in vivo. Leukemia 2003; 17: 26–38.

638. Tokunaga M, Sato E. Non-Hodgkin's lymphomas in a southern prefecture in Japan: an analysis of 715 cases. Cancer 1980; 46: 1231–1239.

639. Swerdlow SH, Habeshaw JA, Rohatiner AZS, et al. Caribbean T-cell lymphoma/leukemia. Cancer 1984; 54: 687–696.

640. Kikuchi M, Mitsui T, Takeshita M, et al. Virus associated adult T-cell leukemia (ATL) in Japan: clinical, histological and immunological studies. Hematol Oncol 1986; 4: 67–91.

641. Dahmoush L, Hijazi Y, Barnes E, et al. Adult T-cell leukemia/lymphoma: a cytopathologic, immunocytochemical, and flow cytometric study. Cancer 2002; 96: 110–116.

642. Lipford EH, Margolich JB, Longo DL, et al. Angiocentric immunoproliferative lesions: a clinicopathologic spectrum of post-thymic T cell proliferations. Blood 1988; 5: 1674–1681.

643. Arber DA, Weiss LM, Albujar PF, et al. Nasal lymphomas in Peru: high incidence of T-cell immunophenotype and Epstein-Barr virus infection. Am J Surg Pathol 1993; 17: 392–399.

644. Strickler JG, Meneses M, Habermann TM, et al. Polymorphic reticulosis: a reappraisal. Hum Pathol 1994; 25: 659–665.

645. Weiss LM, Arber DA, Strickler JG. Nasal T cell lymphoma. Ann Oncol 1994; 5: 39–42.

646. Jaffe ES. Nasal/nasal type NK/T cell lymphoma (angiocentric lymphoma) and lymphomatoid granulomatosis. In: Mason DY, Harris NL, eds. Human lymphoma: clinical implications of the REAL classification. London: Springer; 1999: 32.1–32.6.

647. Yamashita Y, Yatabe Y, Tsuzuki T, et al. Perforin and granzyme expression in cytotoxic T-cell lymphomas. Mod Pathol 1998; 11: 313–333.

648. Kanavaros P, Briere J, Emile JF, et al. Epstein-Barr virus in T and natural killer (NK) cell non-Hodgkin's lymphomas. Leukemia 1996; 10: S84–S87.

649. Chan AC, Ho JW, Chiang AK, et al. Phenotypic and cytotoxic characteristics of peripheral T-cell and NK-cell lymphomas in relation to Epstein-Barr virus association. Histopathology 1999; 34: 16–24.

650. Cuadra-Garcia I, Proulx GM, Wu CL, et al. Sinonasal lymphoma: a clinicopathologic analysis of 58 cases from the Massachusetts General Hospital. Am J Surg Pathol 1999; 23: 1356–1369.

651. Nakamura S, Suchi T, Koshikawa T, et al. Clinicopathologic study of CD56 (NCAM)-positive angiocentric lymphoma occurring in sites other than the upper and lower respiratory tract. Am J Surg Pathol 1995; 19: 284–296.

652. Jaffe ES, Krenacs L, Kumar S, et al. Extranodal peripheral T-cell and NK-cell neoplasms. Am J Clin Pathol 1999; 111: S46–S55.

653. Farcet JP, Gaulard P, Marolleau JP, et al. Hepatosplenic T-cell lymphoma: sinusal/sinusoidal localization of malignant cells expressing the T-cell receptor γδ. Blood 1990; 75: 2213–2219.

654. Isaacson PG, Spencer J, Connolly CE, et al. Malignant histiocytosis of the intestine: a T-cell lymphoma. Lancet 1985; ii: 688–691.

655. Chott A, Dragosics B, Radaszkiewicz T. Peripheral T-cell lymphomas of the intestine. Am J Pathol 1992; 141: 1361–1371.

656. Spencer J, Cerf-Bensussan N, Jarry A, et al. Enteropathy-associated T-cell lymphoma is recognized by a monoclonal antibody (HML-1) that defines a membrane molecule on human mucosal lymphocytes. Am J Pathol 1988; 132: 1–5.

657. Murray A, Cuevas EC, Jones DB, et al. Study of the immunohistochemistry and T cell clonality of enteropathy-associated T cell lymphoma. Am J Pathol 1995; 146: 509–519.

658. Gonzalez CL, Medeiros LJ, Braziel RM, et al. T-cell lymphoma involving subcutaneous tissue: a clinicopathologic entity commonly associated with hemophagocytic syndrome. Am J Surg Pathol 1991; 15: 17–27.

659. Salhany KE, Macon WR, Choi JK, et al. Subcutaneous panniculitis-like T-cell lymphoma: clinicopathologic, immunophenotypic, and genotypic analysis of alpha/beta and gamma/delta subtypes. Am J Surg Pathol 1998; 22: 881–893.

660. Dargent JL, Roufosse C, Delville JP, et al. Subcutaneous panniculitis-like T-cell lymphoma: further evidence for a distinct neoplasm originating from large granular lymphocytes of T/NK phenotype. J Cutan Pathol 1998; 25: 394–400.

661. Hoque SR, Child FJ, Whittaker SJ, et al. Subcutaneous panniculitis-like T-cell lymphoma: a clinicopathological, immunophenotypic and molecular analysis of six patients. Br J Dermatol 2003; 148: 516–525.

662. Berti E, Tomasini D, Vermeer MH, et al. Primary cutaneous CD8-positive epidermotropic cytotoxic T cell lymphomas. A distinct clinicopathological entity with an aggressive clinical behavior. Am J Pathol 1999; 155: 483–492.

663. Chan JK, Sin VC, Wong KF, et al. Nonnasal lymphoma expressing the natural killer cell marker CD56: a clinicopathologic study of 49 cases of an uncommon aggressive neoplasm. Blood 1997; 89: 4501–4513.

664. Chan JK. Natural killer cell neoplasms. Adv Anat Pathol 1998; 3: 77–145.

665. DiGiuseppe JA, Louie DC, Williams JE, et al. Blastic natural killer cell leukemia/lymphoma: a clinicopathologic study. Am J Surg Pathol 1997; 21: 1223–1230.

666. Coleman CN, Picozzi VJ, Cox RS, et al. Treatment of lymphoblastic lymphoma in adults. J Clin Oncol 1986; 4: 1628–1637.

667. Murphy SB. Current concepts in cancer. Childhood non-Hodgkin's lymphoma. N Engl J Med 1978; 299: 1446–1448.

668. Nathwani BN, Kim H, Rappaport H. Malignant lymphoma, lymphoblastic. Cancer 1976; 38: 964–983.

669. Nathwani BN, Diamond LW, Winberg CD, et al. Lymphoblastic lymphoma: a clinicopathologic study of 95 patients. Cancer 1981; 48: 2347–2357.

670. Sander CA, Medeiros LJ, Abruzzo LV, et al. Lymphoblastic lymphoma presenting in cutaneous sites. A clinicopathologic analysis of six cases. J Am Acad Dermatol 1991; 25: 1023–1031.

671. Griffith RC, Kelly DR, Nathwani BN, et al. A morphologic study of childhood lymphoma of the lymphoblastic type. The Pediatric Oncology Group experience. Cancer 1987; 59: 1126–1131.

672. Orazi A, Cattoretti G, John K, et al. Terminal deoxynucleotidyl transferase staining of malignant lymphomas in paraffin sections. Mod Pathol 1994; 7: 582–586.

673. Braziel RM, Keneklis T, Donlon JA, et al. Terminal deoxynucleotidyl transferase in non-Hodgkin's lymphoma. Am J Clin Pathol 1983; 80: 655–659.

674. Weiss LM, Bindl JM, Picozzi VJ, et al. Lymphoblastic lymphoma: an immunophenotype study of 26 cases with comparison to T cell acute lymphoblastic leukemia. Blood 1986; 67: 474–478.

675. Cossman J, Chused TM, Fisher RI, et al. Diversity of immunological phenotypes of lymphoblastic lymphoma. Cancer Res 1983; 43: 4486–4490.

676. Bernard A, Boumsell L, Reinherz L, et al. Cell surface characterization of malignant T cells from lymphoblastic lymphoma using monoclonal antibodies: evidence for phenotypic differences between malignant T cells from patients with acute lymphoblastic leukemia and lymphoblastic lymphoma. Blood 1981; 57: 1105–1110.

677. Hoelzer D, Gokbuget N, Ottmann O, et al. Acute lymphoblastic leukemia. Hematology (Am Soc Hematol Educ Program) 2002; 162–192.

678. Sheibani K, Winberg CD, Burke JS, et al. Lymphoblastic lymphoma expressing natural killer cell-associated antigens: a clinicopathologic study of six cases. Leuk Res 1987; 11: 371–377.

679. Sheibani K, Nathwani BN, Winberg CD. Antigenically defined subgroups of lymphoblastic lymphoma: relationship to clinical presentation and biological behavior. Cancer 1987; 60: 183–190.

680. Mason DY, Cordell JL, Tse AG, et al. The IgM-associated protein mb-1 as a marker of normal and neoplastic B cells. J Immunol 1991; 147: 2474–2482.

681. Mason DY, vanNoesel C, Cordell JL, et al. The B29 and mb-1 polypeptides are differentially expressed during human B cell differentiation. Eur J Immunol 1992; 22: 2753–2756.

682. Navid F, Mosijczuk AD, Head DR, et al. Acute lymphoblastic leukemia with the (8;14)(q24;q32) translocation and FAB L3 morphology associated with a B-precursor immunophenotype: the Pediatric Oncology Group experience. Leukemia 1999; 13: 135–141.

683. Kansal R, Deeb G, Barcos M et al. Precursor B lymphoblastic leukemia with surface light chain immunoglobulin restriction: a report of 15 patients. Am J Clin Pathol 2004; 121: 512–525.

684. Williams DL, Tsiatis A, Brodeur GM, et al. Prognostic importance of chromosome number in 136 untreated children with acute lymphoblastic leukemia. Blood 1982; 60: 864–871.

685. Secker-Walker LM, Swansbury GJ, Hardisty RM, et al. Cytogenetics of acute lymphoblastic leukaemia in children as a factor in the prediction of long-term survival. Br J Haematol 1982; 52: 389–399.

686. Trueworthy R, Shuster J, Look T, et al. Ploidy of lymphoblasts is the strongest predictor of treatment outcome in B-progenitor cell acute lymphoblastic leukemia of childhood: A Pediatric Oncology Group study. J Clin Oncol 1992; 10: 606–613.

687. Korsmeyer SJ, Arnold A, Bakhshi A, et al. Immunoglobulin gene rearrangement and cell surface antigen expression in acute lymphocytic leukemias of T-cell and B-cell precursor origins. J Clin Invest 1983; 71: 301–313.

688. Kitchingman GR, Robigatti U, Mauer AM, et al. Rearrangement of immunoglobulin heavy chain genes in T cell acute lymphoblastic leukemia. Blood 1985; 65: 725–729.

689. Felix CA, Poplack DG, Reaman GH. Characterization of immunoglobulin and T-cell receptor gene patterns in B-cell precursor acute lymphoblastic leukemia of childhood. J Clin Oncol 1990; 8: 431–442.

690. Rouse RV, Weiss LM. Human thymomas: evidence of immunologically defined normal and abnormal microenvironmental differentiation. Cell Immunol 1988; 111: 94–106.

691. Burkitt DP. A sarcoma involving the jaws in African children. Br J Surg 1958; 197: 218–223.

692. Grogan TM, Warnke RA, Kaplan HS. A comparative study of Burkitt's and non-Burkitt's "undifferentiated" malignant lymphoma: immunologic, cytochemical, ultrastructural, cytologic, histopathologic, clinical and cell culture features. Cancer 1982; 49: 1817–1828.

693. Aine R. Small non-cleaved follicular center cell lymphoma: clinicopathologic comparison of Burkitt and non-Burkitt variants in Finnish material. Eur J Cancer Clin Oncol 1985; 21: 1179–1185.

694. Levine AM, Pavlova Z, Pockros AW, et al. Small noncleaved follicular center cell (FCC) lymphoma: Burkitt and non-Burkitt variants in the United States. I. Clinical features. Cancer 1983; 52: 1073–1079.

695. Miliauskas JR, Berard CW, Young RC, et al. Undifferentiated non-Hodgkin's lymphomas (Burkitt's and non-Burkitt's types). The relevance of making this histologic distinction. Cancer 1982; 50: 2115–2121.

696. Knowles DM. Immunodeficiency-associated lymphoproliferative disorders. Mod Pathol 1999; 12: 200–217.

697. Mann RB, Jaffe ES, Braylan RC, et al. Non-endemic Burkitt's lymphoma. A B-cell tumor related to germinal centers. N Engl J Med 1976; 295:685–691.

698. Leder P, Battey J, Lenoir G, et al. Translocations among antibody genes in human cancer. Science 1983; 222: 765–771.

699. Magrath I. The pathogenesis of Burkitt's lymphoma. Adv Cancer Res 1990; 53: 133–270.

700. Weiss LM, Strickler JG, Medeiros LJ, et al. Proliferative rates of non-Hodgkin's lymphomas as assessed by Ki-67 antibody. Hum Pathol 1987; 18: 1155–1159.

701. Filipovich AH, Mathus A, Kamat D, et al. Primary immunodeficiencies: genetic risk factors for lymphoma. Cancer Res 1992; 52: 5465s–5467s.

702. Sander CA, Medeiros LM, Weiss LM, et al. Lymphoproliferative lesions in patients with common variable immunodeficiency syndrome. Am J Surg Pathol 1992; 16: 1170–1182.

703. Nador RG, Chadburn A, Gundappa G, et al. Human immunodeficiency virus (HIV)-associated polymorphic lymphoproliferative disorders. Am J Surg Pathol 2003; 27: 293–302.

704. Schoeppel SL, Hoppe RT, Dorfman RF, et al. Hodgkin's disease in homosexual men with generalized lymphadenopathy. Ann Intern Med 1985; 102: 68–70.

705. Ansari MQ, Dawson DB, Nador R, et al. Primary body cavity-based AIDS-related lymphomas. Am J Clin Pathol 1996; 105: 221–229.

706. Cesarman E, Nador RG, Aozasa K, et al. Kaposi's sarcoma-associated herpesvirus in non-AIDS related lymphomas occurring in body cavities. Blood 1996; 88: 645–656.

707. Klein U, Gloghini A, Gaidano G, et al. Gene expression profile analysis of AIDS-related primary effusion lymphoma (PEL) suggests a plasmablastic derivation and identifies PEL-specific transcripts. Blood 2003; 101: 3115–4121.

708. Brown RS, Campbell C, Lishman SC, et al. Plasmablastic lymphoma: a new subcategory of human immunodeficiency virus-related non-Hodgkin's lymphoma. Clin Oncol (R Coll Radiol) 1998; 10: 327–329.

709. Carbone A, Gaidano G, Gloghini A, et al. AIDS-related plasmablastic lymphomas of the oral cavity and jaws: a diagnostic dilemma. Ann Otol Rhinol Laryngol 1999; 108: 95–99.

710. Delecluse HJ, Anagnostopoulos I, Dallenbach F, et al. Plasmablastic lymphomas of the oral cavity: a new entity associated with the human immunodeficiency virus infection. Blood 1997; 89: 1413–1420.

711. Raphael M, Gentilhomme O, Tulliez M, et al. Histopathologic features of high-grade non-Hodgkin's lymphomas in acquired immunodeficiency syndrome. Arch Pathol Lab Med 1991; 115: 15–20.

712. Gaidano G, Cerri M, Capello D, et al. Molecular histogenesis of plasmablastic lymphoma of the oral cavity. Br J Haematol 2002; 119: 622–628.

713. Knowles DN, Cesarman E, Chadburn A, et al. Correlative morphologic and molecular genetic analysis demonstrates three distinct categories of posttransplantation lymphoproliferative disorders. Blood 1995; 85: 552–565.

714. Cesarman E, Chadburn A, Liu YF, et al. bcl-6 gene mutations in posttransplantation lymphoproliferative disorders predict response to therapy and clinical outcome. Blood 1998; 92: 2294–2302.

715. Rowlings PA, Curtin RE, Passweg JR, et al. Increased incidence of Hodgkin's disease after allogeneic bone marrow transplantation. J Clin Oncol 1999; 17: 3122–3127.

716. Kamel OW, vandeRijn M, LeBrun DP, et al. Lymphoproliferative lesions in patients with rheumatoid arthritis and dermatomyositis: Frequency of Epstein-Barr virus and other features associated with immunosuppression. Hum Pathol 1994; 25: 638–643.

717. Kamel OW, van de Rijn M, Colby TV, et al. Hodgkin's disease in patients receiving long-term, low-dose methotrexate therapy. Am J Surg Pathol 1996; 20: 1279–1287.

718. Kamel OW. Iatrogenic lymphoproliferative disorders in nontransplantation settings. Sem Diagn Pathol 1997; 14: 27–34.

719. Oyama T, Ichimura K, Suzuki R, et al. Senile EBV + B-cell lymphoproliferative disorders: a clinicopathologic study of 22 patients. Am J Surg Pathol 2003; 27: 16–26.

720. Lichtenstein L. Histiocytosis X: integration of eosinophilic granuloma of bone, Letterer-Siwe disease and Schüller-Christian disease as related manifestations of a single nosologic entity. Arch Pathol 1953; 56: 84–102.

721. Lahey ME. Prognostic factors in histiocytosis X. Am J Pediatr Hematol Oncol 1981; 3: 57–60.

722. Motoi M, Helbron D, Kaiserling E, et al. Eosinophilic granuloma of lymph nodes: A variant of histiocytosis X. Histopathol 1980; 4: 585–606.

723. Williams JW, Dorfman RF. Lymphadenopathy as the initial manifestation of histiocytosis X. Am J Surg Pathol 1979; 3: 405–421.

724. Vassalo R, Ryu JH, Colby TV, et al. Pulmonary Langerhan's-cell histiocytosis. N Eng J Med 2000; 342: 1969–1978.

725. Burns BF, Colby TV, Dorfman RF. Langerhans' cell granulomatosis (histiocytosis X) associated with malignant lymphomas. Am J Surg Pathol 1983; 7: 529–533.

726. Egeler RA, Neglia JP, Puccetti DM, et al. Association of Langerhans cell histiocytosis with malignant neoplasms. Cancer 1993; 71: 865–873.

727. Ben-Ezra J, Bailey A, Azumi N, et al. Malignant histiocytosis X. A distinct clinicopathologic entity. Cancer 1991; 68: 1050–1060.

728. Pileri SA, Grogan TM, Banks P, et al. Tumors of histiocytes and accessory dendritic cells: an immunohistochemical approach to classification from the International Lymphoma Study Group based on 61 cases. Histopathology 2002; 41: 1–29.

729. Azumi N, Sheibani K, Swartz WG, et al. Antigenic phenotype of Langerhans cell histiocytosis. An immunohistochemical study demonstrating the value of LN-2, LN-3 and vimentin. Hum Pathol 1988; 19: 1376–1382.

730. Hage C, Willman CL, Favara BE, et al. Langerhans' cell histiocytosis (histiocytosis X): immunophenotype and growth fraction. Hum Pathol 1993; 24: 840–845.

731. Ruco LP, Pulford KAF, Mason D. Expression of macrophage-associated antigens in tissues involved by Langerhans' cell histiocytosis (histiocytosis X). Am J Clin Pathol 1989; 92: 273–279.

732. Pinkus GS, Lones MA, Matsumura F, et al. Langerhans cell histiocytosis immunohistochemical expression of fascin, a dendritic cell marker. Am J Clin Pathol 2002; 118: 335–343.

733. Krenacs L, Tiszlavicz L, Krenacs T, et al. Immunohistochemical detection of CD1a antigen in formalin-fixed and paraffin-embedded tissue sections with monoclonal antibody O10. J Pathol 1993; 171: 99–104.

734. Mierau GW, Favara BE, Brenman JM. Electron microscopy in histiocytosis X. Ultrastr Pathol 1982; 3: 137–142.

735. Willman CL, Busque L, Griffith BB, et al. Langerhans'-cell histiocytosis (histiocytosis X) – a clonal proliferative disease. N Engl J Med 1994; 331: 154–160.

736. Yu RC, Chu AC. Lack of T-cell receptor gene rearrangements in cells involved in Langerhans cell histiocytosis. Cancer 1995; 75: 1162–1166.

737. Monda L, Warnke R, Rosai J. A primary lymph node malignancy with features suggestive of dendritic reticulum cell differentiation. A report of 4 cases. Am J Surg Pathol 1986; 122: 562–572.

738. Vasef MA, Zaatari GS, Chan WC, et al. Dendritic cell tumors associated with low-grade B-cell malignancies. Report of three cases. Am J Clin Pathol 1995; 104: 696–701.

739. Nakamura S, Hara K, Suchi T, et al. Interdigitating cell sarcoma. A morphologic, immunohistologic, and enzyme-histochemical study. Cancer 1988; 61: 562–568.

740. Weiss LM, Berry GJ, Dorfman RF, et.al. Spindle cell neoplasms of lymph nodes of probable reticulum cell lineage. True reticulum cell sarcoma? Am J Surg Pathol 1990; 14: 405–414.

741. Fonseca R, Yamakawa M, Nakamura S. Follicular dendritic cell sarcoma and interdigitating reticulum cell sarcoma: a review. Am J Hematol 1998; 59: 161–167.

742. Perez-Ordonez B, Erlandson RA, Rosai J. Follicular dendritic cell tumor. Report of 13 additional cases of a distinctive entity. Am J Surg Pathol 1996; 20: 944–955.

743. Luk IS, Shek TW, Tang VW, et al. Interdigitating dendritic cell tumor of the testis: a novel testicular spindle cell neoplasm. Am J Surgical Pathol 1999; 23: 1141–1148.

744. Perez-Ordonez B, Rosai J. Follicular dendritic cell tumor: review of the entity. Semin Diag Pathol 1998; 15: 144–154.

745. Hanson CA, Jaszcz W, Kersey JH, et al. True histiocytic lymphoma: histopathologic, immunophenotypic and genotypic analysis. Br J Haematol 1989; 73: 187–198.

746. Kamel OW, Gocke CD, Kell DL, et al. True histiocytic lymphoma: a study of 12 cases based on current definition. Leuk Lymphoma 1995; 18: 81–86.

747. Copie-Bergman C, Wotherspoon AC, Norton AJ, et al. True histiocytic lymphoma. A morphologic, immunohistochemical and molecular genetic study of 13 cases. Am J Surg Pathol 1998; 22: 1386–1392.

748. Weiss LM, Trela MJ, Cleary M, et al. Frequent immunoglobulin and T cell receptor gene rearrangement in "histiocytic" neoplasms. Am J Pathol 1985; 121: 369–373.

749. Isaacson P, Wright DH, Jones DB. Malignant lymphoma of true histiocytic (monocyte-macrophage) origin. Cancer 1983; 51: 80–91.

750. Ornvold K, Carstensen H, Junge J, et al. Tumours classified as "malignant histiocytosis" in children are T-cell neoplasms. APMIS 1992; 100: 558–566.

751. Salter DM, Krajewski AS, Dewar AE. Immunophenotype analysis of malignant histiocytosis of the intestine. J Clin Pathol 1986; 39: 8–15.

752. Ralfkiaer E, Delsol G, O'Connor NTJ, et al. Malignant lymphomas of true histiocytic origin. A clinical, histological, immunophenotypic and genotypic study. J Pathol 1990; 160: 9–17.

753. Arai E, Su WPD, Roche PC, et al. Cutaneous histiocytic malignancy. Immunohistochemical re-examination of cases previously diagnosed as cutaneous "histiocytic lymphoma" and "malignant histiocytosis." J Cutan Pathol 1993; 20: 115–120.

754. Alvaro T, Bosch R, Salvado MT, et al. True histiocytic lymphoma of the stomach associated with low-grade B-cell mucosa-associated lymphoid tissue (MALT)-type lymphoma. Am J Surg Pathol 1996; 20: 1406–1411.

755. Martin-Rodilla C, Fernandez-Acenero J, Pena-Mayor L, et al. True histiocytic lymphoma as a second neoplasm in a follicular centroblastic-centrocytic lymphoma. Pathol Res Pract 1997; 193: 319–322.

756. Okada Y, Nakanishi I, Nomura H, et al. Angiotropic B-cell lymphoma with hemophagocytic syndrome. Pathol Res Pract 1994; 190: 718–727.

757. Bucksy P, Favara B, Feller AC. Malignant histiocytosis and large cell anaplastic (Ki-1) lymphoma in childhood: guidelines for differential diagnosis – report of the Histiocyte Society. Med Ped Oncol 1994; 22: 200–203.

758. Neiman RS, Barcos M, Berard C, et al. Granulocytic sarcoma: a clinicopathologic study of 61 biopsied cases. Cancer 1981; 48: 1426–1437.

759. Meis JM, Butler JJ, Osborne BM, et al. Granulocytic sarcoma in nonleukemic patients. Cancer 1986; 58: 2697–2709.

760. Muller S, Sangster G, Crocker J, et al. An immunohistochemical and clinicopathological study of granulocytic sarcoma (chloroma). Hematol Oncol 1986; 4: 101–112.

761. Roth MJ, Medeiros LJ, Elenitoba-Johnson K, et al. Extramedullary myeloid cell tumors. An immunohistochemical study of 29 cases using routinely fixed and processed paraffin-embedded tissue sections. Arch Pathol Lab Med 1995; 119: 790–798.

762. Traweek ST, Arber DA, Rappaport H, et al. Extramedullary myeloid cell tumors. An immunohistochemical and morphologic study of 28 cases. Am J Surg Pathol 1993; 17: 1011–1019.

763. Chang KL, Stroup R, Weiss LM. Hairy cell leukemia. Current status. Am J Clin Pathol 1992; 97: 719–738.

764. Addis BJ, Isaacson P, Billings JA. Plasmacytosis of lymph nodes. Cancer 1980; 46: 340–346.

765. Kahn H, Strauchen JA, Gilbert HS, et al. Immunoglobulin-related amyloidosis presenting as recurrent isolated lymph node involvement. Arch Pathol Lab Med 1991; 115: 948–950.

766. Lin BT, Weiss LM. Primary plasmacytoma of lymph nodes. Hum Pathol 1997; 28: 1083–1090.

767. Travis WD, Li CY. Pathology of the lymph node and spleen in systemic mast cell disease. Mod Pathol 1988; 1: 4–14.

768. Yang F, Tran T-A, Carlson JA, et al. Paraffin section immunophenotype of cutaneous and extracutaneous mast cell disease: Comparison to other hematopoietic neoplasms. Am J Surg Pathol 2000; 24: 703–709.

769. Bernard T, Rhodes M, Turner GE, et al. Laparoscopic splenectomy: single-centre experience of a district general hospital. Br J Haematol 1999; 106: 1065–1067.

770. Venkataramu NK, Gupta S, Sood BP, et al. Ultrasound guided fine needle aspiration biopsy of splenic lesions. Br J Radiol 1999; 72: 953–956.

771. Szold A, Schwartz J, Abu-Abeid S, et al. Laparoscopic splenectomies for idiopathic thrombocytopenic purpura: experience of sixty cases. Am J Hematol 2000; 63: 7–10.

772. Civardi G, Vallisa D, Berte R, et al. Ultrasound-guided fine needle biopsy of the spleen: high clinical efficacy and low risk in a multicenter Italian study. Am J Hematol 2001; 67: 93–99.

773. Zeppa P, Picardi M, Marino G, et al. Fine-needle aspiration biopsy and flow cytometry immunophenotyping of lymphoid and myeloproliferative disorders of the spleen. Cancer 2003; 99: 118–127.

774. Eraklis AJ, Filler RM. Splenectomy in childhood: A review of 1,413 cases. J Pediatr Surg 1972; 7: 382–388.

775. Swaroop J, O'Reilly RA. Splenomegaly at a university hospital compared to a nearby county hospital in 317 patients. Acta Haematol 1999; 102: 83–88.

776. Kraus MD, Fleming MD, Vonderheide RH. The spleen as a diagnostic specimen: a review of 10 years' experience at two tertiary care institutions. Cancer 2001; 91: 2001–2009.

777. Neiman RS, Orazi A.Embryology and anatomy. disorders of the spleen. Philadelphia: WB Saunders; 1999.

778. Chadburn A. The spleen: anatomy and anatomical function. Semin Hematol 2000; 37: 13–21.

779. Carr NJ, Turk EP. The histological features of splenosis. Histopathology 1992; 21: 549–553.

780. Fleming CR, Dickson ER, Harrison EG Jr. Splenosis: Autotransplantation of splenic tissue. Am J Med 1976; 61: 414–419.

781. Wadham BM, Adams PB, Johnson MA. Incidence and location of accessory spleens. N Engl J Med 1981; 304: 1111.

782. Bauer TW, Haskins GE, Armitage JO. Splenic rupture in patients with hematologic malignancies. Cancer 1981; 48: 2729–2733.

783. Athale UH, Kaste SC, Bodner SM, et al. Splenic rupture in children with hematologic malignancies. Cancer 2000; 88: 480–490.

784. Farhi DC, Ashfaq R. Splenic pathology after traumatic injury. Am J Clin Pathol 1996; 105: 474–478.

785. Barnard H, Dreef EJ, van Krieken JHJM. The ruptured spleen. A histological, morphometrical and immunohistochemical study. Histol Histopath 1990; 5: 299–304.

786. Chun CH, Raff MJ, Contreras L, et al. Splenic abscess. Medicine 1980; 59: 50–65.

787. Paris S, Weiss SM, Ayers WH Jr., et al. Splenic abscess. The American Surgeon 1994; 60: 358–361.

788. Gadacz T, Way LW, Dunphy JE. Changing clinical spectrum of splenic abscess. Am J Surg 1974; 128: 182–187.

789. Al-Salem AH, Qaisaruddin S, Al Jam'a AA, et al. Splenic abscess and sickle cell disease. Am J Hematol 1998; 58: 100–104.

790. Brook I, Frazier EH. Microbiology of liver and spleen abscesses. J Med Microbiol 1998; 47: 1075–1080.

791. Smithe EB, Custer RP. Rupture of the spleen in infectious mononucleosis. A clinicopathologic report of seven cases. Blood 1946; 1: 317–333.

792. Rutkow IM. Rupture of the spleen in infectious mononucleosis. A critical review. Arch Surg 1978; 113: 718–720.

793. Farley DR, Zietlow SP, Bannon MP, et al. Spontaneous rupture of the spleen due to infectious mononucleosis. Mayo Clin Proc 1992; 67: 846–853.

794. Gaffey MJ, Frierson HF Jr, Medeiros LJ, et al. The relationship of Epstein-Barr virus to infection-related and familial hemophagocytic syndrome and lymphoma-related hemophagocytosis: an in situ hybridization study. Hum Pathol 1993; 24: 657–667.

795. Imashuku S, Obayashi M, Hosoi G, et al. Splenectomy in haemophagocytic lymphohistiocytosis: report of histopathological changes with CD19+ B-cell depletion and therapeutic results. Br J Haematol 2000; 108: 505–510.

796. Su IJ, Hsu YH, Lin MT, et al. Epstein-Barr containing T cell lymphoma presents with hemophagocytic syndrome mimicking malignant histiocytosis. Cancer 1993; 72: 2019–2027.

797. Neiman RS. Incidence and importance of splenic sarcoid-like granulomas. Arch Pathol Lab Med 1977; 101: 518–521.

798. O'Connell MJ, Schimpff SC, Kirschner RH, et al. Epithelioid granulomas in Hodgkin's disease. A favorable prognostic sign? JAMA 1975; 233: 886–889.

799. Cruickshank B. Follicular (mineral oil) lipidosis: I. Epidemiologic studies of involvement of the spleen. Hum Pathol 1984; 15: 724–730.

800. Cruickshank B, Thomas MJ. Mineral oil (follicular) lipidosis: II. Histologic studies of spleen, liver, lymph nodes, and bone marrow. Hum Pathol 1984; 15: 731–737.

801. Urban RM, Jacobs JJ, Tomlinson MJ, et al. Dissemination of wear particles to the liver, spleen, and abdominal lymph nodes of patients with hip or knee replacement. J Bone Joint Surg Am 2000; 82: 457–476.

802. Putschar W, Manion W. Splenic-gonadal fusion. Am J Pathol 1956; 15–33.

803. Bonneau D, Roume J, Gonzalez M, et al. Splenogonadal fusion limb defect syndrome: report of five new cases and review. Am J Med Genet 1999; 86: 347–358.

804. Scriver CR, Beaudet AL, Sly WS, Valle D. In: Stanbury JB, Wyngaarden JB, Fredrickson DS, eds. The metabolic and molecular bases of inherited disease. New York: McGraw-Hill; 1995.

805. Neiman RS, Orazi A, eds. Disorders of the monocyte-macrophage system. In: Disorders of the spleen. Philadelphia: WB Saunders; 1999: 167–191.

806. Firkin BG, Wright R, Miller S, et al. Splenic macrophages in thrombocytopenia. Blood 1969; 33: 240–245.

807. Jiang DY, Li CY. Immunohistochemical study of the spleen in chronic immune thrombocytopenic purpura. With special reference to hyperplastic follicles and foamy macrophages. Arch Pathol Lab Med 1995; 119: 533–537.

808. Laszlo J, Jones R, Silberman H, et al. Splenectomy for Felty's syndrome. Clinicopathological study of 27 patients. Arch Intern Med 1978; 138: 597–602.

809. Hassan NMR, Neiman RS. The pathology of the spleen in steroid-treated immune thrombocytopenic purpura. Am J Clin Pathol 1985; 84: 433–438.

810. McClure RD, Altemeier WA. Cysts of the spleen. Ann Surg 1942; 116: 98–102.

811. Garvin DF, King FM. Cysts and nonlymphomatous tumors of the spleen. Pathol Annu 1981; 16: 61–80.

812. Burrig KF. Epithelial (true) splenic cysts. Pathogenesis of the mesothelial and so-called epidermoid cyst of the spleen. Am J Surg Pathol 1988; 12: 275–281.

813. Fowler RH. Nonparasitic benign cystic tumors of the spleen. International Abstracts of Surgery 1953; 96: 209–227.

814. Morgenstern L. Nonparasitic splenic cysts: pathogenesis, classification, and treatment. J Am Coll Surg 2002; 194: 306–314.

815. Bürrig K. Epithelial (true) splenic cysts. Pathogenesis of the mesothelial and so-called epidermoid cyst of the spleen. Am J Surg Pathol 1988; 12: 275–281.

816. Du Plessis DG, Louw JA, Wranz PA. Mucinous epithelial cysts of the spleen associated with pseudomyxoma peritonei. Histopathology 1999; 35: 551–557.

817. Arber DA, Strickler JG, Weiss LM. Splenic mesothelial cysts mimicking lymphangiomas. Am J Surg Pathol 1997; 21: 334–338.

818. Arber DA, Strickler JG, Chen YY, et al. Splenic vascular tumors. A histologic immunophenotypic and virologic study. Am J Surg Pathol 1997; 21: 827–835.

819. Martel M, Cheuk W, Lombardi L, et al. Sclerosing angiomatoid nodular transforming (SANT): report of 25 cases of a distinctive benign splenic lesion. Am J Surg Pathol 2004; 28: 1268–1279.

820. Kraus MD, Dehner LP. Benign vascular neoplasms of the spleen with myoid and angioendotheliomatous features. Histopathology 1999; 35: 328–335.

821. Garcia RL, Khan MK, Berlin RB. Peliosis of the spleen with rupture. Hum Pathol 1982; 13: 177–179.

822. Kohr RM, Haendiges M, Taube RR. Peliosis of the spleen: A rare cause of spontaneous splenic rupture with surgical implications. The American Surgeon 1993; 59: 197–199.

823. Tada T, Wakabayashi T, Kishimoto H. Peliosis of the spleen. Am J Clin Pathol 1983; 79: 708–713.

824. Diebold J, Audouin J. Peliosis of the spleen. Report of a case associated with chronic myelomonocytic leukemia, presenting with spontaneous splenic rupture. Am J Surg Pathol 1983; 7: 197–204.

825. Taxy JB. Peliosis: A morphologic curiosity becomes an iatrogenic problem. Hum Pathol 1978; 9: 331–340.

826. Chan KW, Saw D. Distinctive, multiple lymphangiomas of spleen. J Pathology 1980; 131: 75–81.

827. Ramani P, Shah A. Lymphangiomatosis. Histologic and immunohistochemical analysis of four cases. Am J Surg Pathol 1993; 17: 329–335.

828. Falk S, Stutte HJ, Frizzera G. Littoral cell angioma. A novel splenic vascular lesion demonstrating histiocytic differentiation. Am J Surg Pathol 1991; 15: 1023–1033.

829. Ben Izhak O, Bejar J, Ben Eliezer S, et al. Splenic littoral cell haemangioendothelioma: a new low-grade variant of malignant littoral cell tumour. Histopathology 2001; 39: 469–475.

830. Rosso R, Paulli M, Gianelli E, et al. Littoral cell angiosarcoma of the spleen – Case report with immunohistochemical and ultrastructural analysis. Am J Surg Pathol 1995; 19: 1203–1208.

831. Meybehm J, Fischer HP. Littoralzellangiosarkom der Milz. Morphologische, immunohistochemische Befunde und Uberlegungen zur Histogenese eines seltenen Milztumors. Pathologe 1997; 18: 401–405.

832. Rosso R, Gianelli U, Chan JKC. Further evidence supporting the sinus lining cell nature of splenic littoral cell angiosarcoma (letter). Am J Surg Pathol 1996; 20: 1531.

833. Silverman ML, LiVolsi VA. Splenic hamartoma. Am J Clin Pathol 1978; 70: 224–229.

834. Morgenstern L, McCafferty L, Rosenberg J, et al. Hamartomas of the spleen. Arch Surg 1984; 119: 1291–1293.

835. Beham A, Hermann W, Schmid C. Hamartoma of the spleen with haematological symptoms. Virchows Archiv A Pathol Anat 1989; 414: 535–539.

836. Falk S, Stutte HJ. Hamartomas of the spleen: A study of 20 biopsy cases. Histopathology 1989; 14: 603–612.

837. Steinberg JJ, Suhrland M, Valensi Q. The spleen in the spleen syndrome: The association of splenoma with hematopoietic and neoplastic disease – compendium of cases since 1864. J Surg Oncol 1991; 47: 193–202.

838. Zukerberg LR, Kaynor BL, Silverman ML, et al. Splenic hamartoma and capillary hemangioma are distinct entities. Immunohistochemical analysis of CD8 expression by endothelial cells. Hum Pathol 1991; 22: 1258–1261.

839. Cotelingam JD, Jaffe ES. Inflammatory pseudotumor of the spleen. Am J Surg Pathol 1984; 8: 375–380.

840. Thomas RM, Jaffe ES, Zarate-Osorno A, et al. Inflammatory pseudotumor of the spleen. A clinicopathologic and immunophenotypic study of eight cases. Arch Pathol Lab Med 1993; 117: 921–926.

841. Sheahan K, Wolf BC, Neiman RS. Inflammatory pseudotumor of the spleen: A clinicopathologic study of three cases. Hum Pathol 1988; 19: 1024–1029.

842. Arber DA, Kamel OW, van de Rijn M, et al. Frequent presence of the Epstein-Barr virus in inflammatory pseudotumor. Hum Pathol 1995; 26: 1093–1098.

843. Cheuk W, Chan JK, Shek TW, et al. Inflammatory pseudotumor-like follicular dendritic cell tumor: a distinctive low-grade malignant intra-abdominal neoplasm with consistent Epstein-Barr virus association. Am J Surg Pathol 2001; 25: 721–731.

844. Burke JS, Osborne BM. Localized reactive lymphoid hyperplasia of the spleen simulating malignant lymphoma: a report of seven cases. Am J Surg Pathol 1983; 7: 373–380.

845. Horny H, Ruck MT, Kaiserling E. Spleen findings in generalized mastocytosis. A clinicopathologic study. Cancer 1992; 70: 459–468.

846. Klatt EC, Lukes RJ, Meyer PR. Benign and malignant mast cell proliferations. Diagnosis and

separation using a pH-dependent toluidine blue stain in tissue section. Cancer 1983; 51: 1119–1124.

847. Horny H, Schaumburg-Lever G, Kaiserling E. Use of monoclonal antibody KP1 for identifying normal and neoplastic human mast cells [see comments]. J Clin Pathol 1990; 43: 719–722.

848. Travis WD, Li C, Bergsthral EJ. Solid and hematologic malignancies in 60 patients with systemic mast cell disease. Arch Pathol Lab Med 1989; 113: 365–368.

849. Barosi G, Ambrosetti A, Buratti A, et al. Splenectomy for patients with myelofibrosis with myeloid metaplasia: Pretreatment variables and outcome prediction. Leukemia 1993; 7: 200–206.

850. Pitcock JA, Reinhard EH, Justus BW, et al. A clinical and pathological study of seventy cases of myelofibrosis. Ann Intern Med 1962; 57: 73–84.

851. Falk S, Mix D, Stutte H. The spleen in osteomyelofibrosis. A morphologic and immunohistochemical study of 30 cases. Virchows Archiv A Pathol Anat 1990; 416: 437–442.

852. Kobrich U, Falk S, Karhoff M, et al. Primary large cell lymphoma of the splenic sinuses: a variant of angiotropic B-cell lymphoma (neoplastic angioendotheliomatosis)? Hum Pathol 1992; 23: 1184–1187.

853. Mesa RA, Li CY, Schroeder G, et al. Clinical correlates of splenic histopathology and splenic karyotype in myelofibrosis with myeloid metaplasia. Blood 2001; 97: 3665–3667.

854. Wolf BC, Banks PM, Mann RB, et al. Splenic hematopoiesis in polycythemia vera. A morphologic and immunohistochemical study. Am J Clin Pathol 1988; 89: 69–75.

855. Vasef MA, Neiman RS, Meletiou SD, et al. Marked granulocytic proliferation induced by granulocyte colony-stimulating factor in the spleen simulating a myeloid leukemic infiltrate. Mod Pathol 1998; 10: 1138–1141.

856. Burke JS, Sheibani K, Winberg CD, et al. Recognition of hairy cell leukemia in a spleen of normal weight. The contribution of immunohistologic studies. Am J Clin Pathol 1987; 87: 276–281.

857. Loughran TP Jr., Starkebaum G, Clark E, et al. Evaluation of splenectomy in large granular lymphocytic leukaemia. Br J Haematol 1987; 67: 135–140.

858. Griffiths DFR, Jasani B, Standen GR. Pathology of the spleen in large granular lymphocytic leukaemia. J Clin Pathol 1989; 42: 885.

859. van Krieken JHJM, Feller AC, TeVelde J. The distribution of non-Hodgkin's lymphoma in the lymphoid compartments of the human spleen. Am J Surg Pathol 1989; 13: 757–765.

860. Butler JJ. Pathology of the spleen in benign and malignant conditions. Histopathology 1983; 7: 453–474.

861. Audouin J, Diebold J, Schvartz H, et al. Malignant lymphoplasmacytic lymphoma with prominent splenomegaly (primary lymphoma of the spleen). J Pathology 1988; 155: 17–33.

862. Burke JS. Surgical pathology of the spleen: An approach to the differential diagnosis of splenic lymphomas and leukemias. Part I. Diseases of the white pulp. Am J Surg Pathol 1981; 5: 551–563.

863. Arber DA, Rappaport H, Weiss LM. Non-Hodgkin's lymphoproliferative disorders involving the spleen. Mod Pathol 1997; 10: 18–32.

864. Lampert I, Catovsky D, Marsh GW, et al. The histopathology of prolymphocytic leukaemia with particular reference to the spleen: a comparison with chronic lymphocytic leukaemia. Histopathology 1980; 4: 3–19.

865. Angelopoulou M, Siakantaris M, Vassilakopoulos T, et al. The splenic form of mantle cell lymphoma. Eur J Haematol 2002; 68: 12–21.

866. Alkan S, Ross CW, Hanson CA, et al. Follicular lymphoma with involvement of the splenic marginal zone: a pitfall in the differential diagnosis of splenic

marginal zone cell lymphoma. Hum Pathol 1996; 27: 503–506.

867. Mollejo M, Algara P, Mateo MS, et al. Large B-cell lymphoma presenting in the spleen – Identification of different clincopathologic conditions. Am J Surg Pathol 1996; 27: 895–902.

868. Dogan A, Burke JS, Goteri G, et al. Micronodular T-cell/histiocyte-rich large B-cell lymphoma of the spleen – Histology, immunophenotype and differential diagnosis. Am J Surg Pathol 2003; 27: 903–911.

869. Chang KL, Kamel OW, Arber DA, et al. Pathologic features of nodular lymphocyte predominance Hodgkin's disease involving extranodal sites. Am J Surg Pathol 1995; 19: 1313–1324.

870. Falk S, Stutte HJ. Primary malignant lymphomas of the spleen. A morphologic and immunohistochemical analysis of 17 cases. Cancer 1990; 66: 2612–2619.

871. Spier CM, Kjeldsberg CR, Eyre HJ, et al. Malignant lymphoma with primary presentation in the spleen. A study of 20 patients. Arch Pathol Lab Med 1985; 109: 1076–1080.

872. Kraemer BB, Osborne BM, Butler JJ. Primary splenic presentation of malignant lymphoma and related disorders. A study of 49 cases. Cancer 1984; 54: 1606–1619.

873. Narang S, Wolf BC, Neiman RS. Malignant lymphoma presenting with prominent splenomegaly. A clinicopathologic study with special reference to intermediate cell lymphoma. Cancer 1985; 55: 1948–1957.

874. Neiman RS, Sullivan AL, Jaffe R. Malignant lymphoma simulating leukaemic reticuloendotheliosis: a clinicopathologic study of ten cases. Cancer 1979; 43: 329–342.

875. Schmid C, Kirkham N, Diss T, et al. Splenic marginal zone cell lymphoma. Am J Surg Pathol 1992; 16: 455–466.

876. Mollejo J, Menárguez J, Lloret E, et al. Splenic marginal zone lymphoma. A distinctive type of low-grade B-cell lymphoma – A clinicopathological study of 13 cases. Am J Surg Pathol 1995; 19: 1146–1157.

877. Sol Mateo M, Mollejo M, Villuendas R, et al. Analysis of the frequency of microsatellite instability and *p53* gene mutation in splenic marginal zone and MALT lymphomas. J Clin Pathol: Mol Pathol 1998; 51: 262–267.

878. Rosso R, Neiman RS, Paulli M, et al. Splenic marginal zone cell lymphoma: Report of an indolent variant without massive splenomegaly presumably representing an early phase of the disease. Hum Pathol 1995; 26: 39–46.

879. Sole F, Salido M, Espinet B, et al. Splenic marginal zone B-cell lymphomas: two cytogenetic subtypes, one with gain of 3q and the other with loss of 7q. Haematologica 2001; 86: 71–77.

880. Algara P, Mateo MS, Sanchez-Beato M, et al. Analysis of the IgV(H) somatic mutations in splenic marginal zone lymphoma defines a group of unmutated cases with frequent 7q deletion and adverse clinical course. Blood 2002; 99: 1299–1304.

881. Piris MA, Mollejo M, Campo E, et al. A marginal zone pattern may be found in different varieties of non-Hodgkin's lymphoma: the morphology and immunohistology of splenic involvement by B-cell lymphomas simulating splenic marginal zone lymphoma. Histopathology 1998; 33: 230–239.

882. Meda BA, Frost M, Newell J, et al. BCL-2 is consistently expressed in hyperplastic marginal zones of the spleen, abdominal lymph nodes, and real lymphoid tissue. Am J Surg Pathol 2003; 27: 888–894.

883. Chacon JI, Mollejo M, Munoz E, et al. Splenic marginal zone lymphoma: clinical characteristics and prognostic factors in a series of 60 patients. Blood 2002; 100: 1648–1654.

884. Canacho FI, Mollejo M, Mateo MS, et al. Progression to large B-cell lymphoma in splenic

marginal zone lymphoma – A description of a series of 12 cases. Am J Surg Pathol 2001; 25: 1268–1276.

885. Melo JV, Hegde U, Parreira A, et al. Splenic B cell lymphoma with circulating villous lymphocytes: differential diagnosis of B cell leukaemias with large spleens. J Clin Pathol 1987; 40: 642–651.

886. Isaacson PG, Matutes E, Burke M, et al. The histopathology of splenic lymphoma with villous lymphocytes. Blood 1994; 84: 3828–3834.

887. Imbing F, Kumar D, Kumar S, et al. Splenic lymphoma with circulating villous lymphocytes. J Clin Pathol 1995; 584–587.

888. Jadayel D, Matutes E, Dyer M, et al. Splenic lymphoma with villous lymphocytes: Analysis of BCL-1 rearrangements and expression of the cyclin D1 gene. Blood 1994; 3664–3671.

889. Kadin ME, Kamoun M, Lamberg J. Erythrophagocytic Tγ lymphoma. A clinicopathologic entity resembling malignant histiocytosis. N Engl J Med 1981; 304: 648–653.

890. Wong KF, Chan JKC, Matutes E, et al. Hepatosplenic γδ T-cell lymphoma. A distinct aggressive lymphoma type. Am J Surg Pathol 1995; 19: 718–726.

891. Cooke CB, Krenacs L, Stetler-Stevenson M, et al. Hepatosplenic T-cell lymphoma: a distinct clinicopathologic entity of cytotoxic γδ T-cell origin. Blood 1996; 88: 4265–4274.

892. Chang KL, Arber DA. Hepatosplenic γδ T-cell lymphoma – not just alphabet soup. Adv Anat Pathol 1998; 5: 21–29.

893. Salhany KE, Feldman M, Kahn MJ, et al. Hepatosplenic gamma delta T-cell lymphoma: ultrastructural, immunophenotypic, and functional evidence for cytotoxic T lymphocyte differentiation. Hum Pathol 1997; 28: 674–685.

894. Weidmann E. Hepatosplenic T cell lymphoma. A review of 45 cases since the first report describing the disease as a distinct lymphoma entity in 1990. Leukemia 2000; 14: 991–997.

895. Bordessoule D, Gaulard P, Mason DY. Preferential localization of human lymphocytes bearing γδ T cell receptors to the red pulp of the spleen. J Clin Pathol 1990; 43: 461–464.

896. Ross CW, Schnitzer B, Sheldon S, et al. Gamma/delta T-cell posttransplantation lymphoproliferative disorder primarily in the spleen. Am J Clin Patholod 1994; 102: 310–315.

897. Kraus MD, Crawford DF, Kaleem Z, et al. T γ/δ hepatosplenic lymphoma in a heart transplant patient after an Epstein-Barr positive lymphoproliferative disorder. Cancer 1998; 82: 983–992.

898. Wang C-C, Tien H-F, Lin M-T, et al. Consistent presence of isochromosome 7q in hepatosplenic T γ/δ lymphoma: a new cytogenetic-clinicopathologic entity. Genes Chromosom Cancer 1995; 12:161–164.

899. Yao M, Tien H-F, Lin M-T, et al. Clinical and hematological characteristics of hepatosplenic T γ/δ lymphoma with isochromosome for long arm of chromosome 7. Leuk Lymphoma 1996; 22:495–500.

899a. Jonveaux P, Daniel MT, Martel V, et al. Isochromosome 7q and trisomy 8 are consistent primary, non-random chromosomal abnormalities associated with hepatosplenic Tγ/δ? lymphoma. Leukemia 1996; 10: 1453–1455.

900. Macon WR, Levy NB, Kurtin PJ, et al. Hepatosplenic alpha beta T-cell lymphomas – A report of 14 cases and comparison with hepatosplenic gamma delta T-cell lymphomas. Am J Surg Pathol 2001; 25: 285–296.

901. Wick MR, Smith SL, Scheithauer BW, et al. Primary nonlymphoreticular malignant neoplasms of the spleen. Am J Surg Pathol 1982; 6: 229–242.

902. Falk S, Krishnan J, Meis JM. Primary angiosarcoma of the spleen. A clinicopathologic study of 40 cases. Am J Surg Pathol 1993; 17: 959–970.

903. Suster S. Epithelioid and spindle-cell hemangioendothelioma of the spleen. Report of a distinctive splenic vascular neoplasm of childhood. Am J Surg Pathol 1992; 16: 785–792.

904. Kaw YT, Duwaji MS, Kinsley RE, et al. Hemangioendothelioma of the spleen. Arch Pathol Lab Med 1992; 116: 1079–1082.

905. Budke HL, Breitfeld PP, Neiman RS. Functional hyposplenism due to a primary epithelioid hemangioendothelioma of the spleen. Arch Pathol Lab Med 1995; 119: 755–757.

906. Falk S, Muller H, Stutte H-J. The spleen in acquired immunodeficiency syndrome (AIDS). Path Res Pract 1988; 183: 425–433.

907. Sarode VR, Datta BN, Savitri K, et al. Kaposi's sarcoma of the spleen with unusual clinical and histologic features. Arch Pathol Lab Med 1991; 115: 1042–1044.

908. Klein B, Stein M, Kuten A, et al. Splenomegaly and solitary spleen metastasis in solid tumors. Cancer 1987; 60: 100–102.

909. Gupta PB, Harvey L. Spontaneous rupture of the spleen secondary to metastatic carcinoma. Br J Surg 1993; 80: 613.

910. Karakousis CP, Elias EG. Spontaneous (pathologic) rupture of spleen in malignancies. Surgery 1974; 76: 674–677.

911. Marymont JH, Gross S. Patterns of metastatic cancer in the spleen. Am J Clin Pathol 1963; 40: 58–66.

912. Weiss LM, Chan WC, Schnitzer B. Lymph nodes. In: Damjanov I, Linder J, eds. Anderson's pathology. St. Louis: Mosby-Yearbook. 1996: 1115–1120.

Bone marrow

12

Nora C. J. Sun   Jun Wang   Eric F. Glassy

Bone marrow examination is a well established procedure in the study of hematologic disorders, in the work-up of fever of unknown origin, in the evaluation of other systemic diseases, and for the staging of malignant lymphoma. It is also used to monitor therapy and for the assessment of minimal residual disease or recurrent neoplastic disease. Sections of bone biopsy provide added advantages of being able to evaluate bony architecture and marrow cellular distribution; to identify stromal disorders (such as marrow fibrosis or serous degeneration of the marrow) or bone disease (such as Paget's disease or osteoporosis); to detect infiltrative processes (such as granuloma, lymphoma, storage disease, or metastatic tumors); to follow the course of leukemias; and to supplement the information gained from the study of aspiration smears of the bone marrow. Bone marrow biopsy sections are particularly useful whenever there is a 'dry tap' (an inability to aspirate bone marrow) regardless of whether it is caused by packed leukemic cells, bone marrow necrosis, or fibrosis.[1–8]

HANDLING AND PROCESSING OF SPECIMENS

The conventional approach to the study of bone marrow includes: (1) a pertinent clinical history and physical examination; (2) complete blood cell and white cell differential counts; (3) peripheral blood smears; (4) sections of bone marrow aspiration (clot) and/or bone marrow biopsy; (5) smears of bone marrow aspirations and/or touch preparations of bone marrow biopsy; and (6) other tests.[3] These tests include cytochemistry, immunocytochemistry, flow cytometry, cytogenetics, molecular analysis, immunohistochemistry, and electron microscopy (discussed later). Bilateral or multiple bone marrow biopsies have been advocated[9–11] in the staging of malignant lymphomas and in the search for other malignant tumors or granulomas. A recent retrospective study comparing morphologic, flow cytometric, cytogenetic and molecular studies on bilateral bone marrow biopsy specimens (1864 samples) concluded that bilateral morphologic evaluation is useful in the assessment of patients with non-Hodgkin's lymphoma, Hodgkin's lymphoma, carcinoma, and sarcoma, but pooled specimens from right and left side aspirations are more cost-effective for special studies.[11] Serial sections or step sections may be required in some instances to identify focal lesions, such as granulomas or malignant lymphoma.

The choice of a site for bone marrow aspiration and/or biopsy depends on the age of the patient, a previous history of irradiation, local skin conditions, and the preference of the examiner. In general, anterior or posterior iliac crest is the choice for adults and anterior tibia is the choice for children. The density and content of hematopoietic elements, fat, and bony trabeculae vary in different parts of the bone. If care is taken to use different entry sites, either bone marrow aspiration or biopsy can be performed first. For that approach, a generous area of periosteum should be anesthetized. A Jamshidi biopsy needle is generally used.[4] Sometimes, two different needles may be used, one for aspiration and one for biopsy, to minimize the chance of specimen clotting. A bone biopsy should never be performed with a sternal puncture. A Salah or Klima marrow-puncture needle that has an adjustable guard should be used for sternal puncture and bone marrow aspiration. A detailed description of bone marrow procedures is available in any major textbook of hematology and is not repeated here.[1–2]

Proper selection of marrow particles for smears or electron microscopic study is an art learned by practice and experience. Sections of bone marrow biopsies provide additional information to aspiration smears, as discussed earlier.[1,8,12,13] They are especially useful for the study of focal intramedullary lesions. Touch preparations should be made from the bone biopsy, especially when there is a 'dry tap.' The air-dried smears and touch preparations may be used for Romanowsky's stain, special cytochemical stains, and immunocytochemical stains for the detection of cell antigens. A recent study comparing touch preparations with aspirate smears from 173 patients with treated or untreated neoplastic hematologic disease and 87 patients without hematologic abnormality found that there was no significant difference in the differential counts from touch preparations and aspirate smears of normocellular bone marrow and that touch preparations were as reliable as aspirate smears for making diagnosis from patients with neoplastic hematologic disease involving the bone marrow.[14] If the aspirate is a 'dry tap' and a diagnosis of leukemia is entertained, an additional bone biopsy may be obtained. The marrow may be teased out under a dissecting microscope. The particles can then be submitted for cytogenetic and/or flow cytometry study.

Cytologic study is most useful in classifying leukemia and myelodysplastic syndrome (MDS), and in identifying dyspoiesis by examining the Romanowsky-stained smears. It is a valuable adjunct to the study of histologic sections. The aspirated material should be submitted for flow cytometric study, cytogenetic, or molecular analysis if the diagnosis of leukemia/lymphoma or MDS is suspected. The specimen should be placed in an anticoagulant with or without tissue culture media. The collected particles or the biopsy specimen may be submitted for immunohistochemistry or electron microscopic study if such a study is indicated. We prefer to fix the bone marrow clot in 10% buffered formalin and the bone biopsy in Zenkers or B5 solutions. Specimens that have been well fixed in 10% buffered formalin and properly processed can give satisfactory preparations for interpretation.

Decalcification of bone biopsy specimens frequently causes leaching of iron from the tissue, resulting in inaccurate assessment of body iron stores.[15] Iron stain should be performed on the section of bone marrow clot or the smear of bone marrow aspiration. Routine stains for bone marrow biopsy include hematoxylin and eosin (H&E) and periodic acid–Schiff (PAS) stains. The latter highlights myeloid cells and megakaryocytes because these cells contain glycogen. Reticulin stain is particularly helpful in the study of myelofibrosis caused by a variety of diseases and for delineation of the marrow meshwork. The specific (naphthol AS-D chloroacetate) esterase (Leder) stain may be used on formalin-fixed, paraffin-embedded sections, and is a useful marker for neutrophils and tissue mast cells.[16] This stain is ineffective on tissues fixed in mercury-based fixatives.

Recent studies indicate that enzyme cytochemistry, immunocytochemistry, flow cytometry, immunohistochemistry, molecular study, and cytogenetic examinations are invaluable tools in diagnosing and classifying hematopoietic and lymphoreticular malignancies, in predicting the prognosis for these patients, in monitoring therapy, such as detecting minimal residual disease, evaluating the success of hematopoietic stem cell transplant, and in designing and/or applying targeted therapy, such as Rituximab (anti-CD20 antibody) for B-cell lymphoma, and Gleevec (a bcr/abl tyrosine kinase inhibitor) for chronic myeloid leukemia in chronic phase, accelerated phase, and blastic crisis, as well as for Philadelphia-chromosome-positive acute leukemia.[17–47]

Cytochemistry has played an important role in the diagnosis and classification of hematologic malignancies.[2,3,16,29–30,48–50] Myeloperoxidase and/or Sudan black B stains are often used to differentiate myeloid from lymphoid leukemias, although some minimally differentiated acute myeloid leukemia or monoblastic leukemia may be negative. In addition, blasts in pure erythroid leukemia and megakaryoblastic leukemia are also negative for these cytochemical stains. The combined esterase, naphthol AS-D chloroacetate (chloroacetate esterase or CAE), and naphthol ASD acetate (non-specific esterase or NSE) esterase stain is used to differentiate cells of myeloid (CAE-positive) from monocytic (NSE strongly positive) lineages. Addition of sodium fluoride into NSE substrate can completely block the esterase reaction in monocytic cells. Alpha-naphthyl butyrate esterase stain (with or without the addition of sodium fluoride) remains one of the best methods to identify monocytic cells. B-lymphoblasts (Burkitt's lymphoma/leukemia cells) frequently contain oil-red-O-positive vacuoles. Lymphoblasts in some acute lymphoblastic leukemia contain coarse PAS-positive granules but there is no correlation of this finding with morphology (L1 or L2), immunophenotyping, or cytogenetic abnormalities. Erythroblasts in erythroleukemia (M6) also contain PAS-positive granules or have a diffusely staining cytoplasm. Acid phosphatase with or without tartaric acid inhibition may be used for the diagnosis of hairy cell leukemia, but this test has been largely replaced by immunophenotyping.

Immunophenotypic studies, especially flow cytometry, are essential for the proper diagnosis and classification of lymphoid malignancies and are also helpful in the classification of acute myeloid leukemia.[17,20,22–25] It is useful to diagnose minimally differentiated acute myeloid leukemia (AML-M0), and to identify acute biphenotypic leukemia.[35–37,51–54] The advantages and disadvantages of flow cytometric analysis are as follows: it is highly sensitive and allows for rapid analysis of multiple antigens, for quantitation of antigen expression, and for the possibility of multiple labeling. However, the equipment is expensive and requires a highly trained professional to select appropriate antibodies, to perform, and to interpret the tests. Also, the cells have to be viable; and fluorochrome intensity and epitope density may influence the results. With the newer antigen retrieval technique and the availability of an automated immunostainer, immunohistochemistry has been widely used in surgical

pathology to correlate with morphology. It has the advantage of being able to provide additional information whenever there is a 'dry tap'. Also, it allows retrospective analysis and has proved to be cost-effective. Good correlation is generally observed by using flow cytometry or immunohistochemistry.[23,24]

Cytogenetic study and molecular analysis provide powerful tools in predicting prognosis and in identifying minimal residual disease.[26,27,30–34,38] They are also helpful in the diagnosis, classification, and management of patients with hematologic malignancies. Conventional karyotype is generally the preferred first-line assay in a newly diagnosed acute leukemia and MDS. Southern blot, polymerase chain reaction (PCR) (including reverse transcriptase (RT)-PCR and competitive PCR), and in situ hybridization (ISH) for specific gene fragment(s) are frequently used molecular analyses that supplement a cytogenetic study in certain circumstances.

In summary, all these methods complement each other and provide invaluable information in appropriate clinical settings. For instance, it has been demonstrated that immunologic techniques or electron microscopy is more sensitive in detecting myeloperoxidase than enzyme cytochemistry.[24,28,35] Indeed, myeloperoxidase may be present in CD13 and CD33 antigen-negative acute leukemia.[29,30] In addition to applying ultrastructural cytochemistry for the demonstration of myeloperoxidase granules, electron microscopy may be used to diagnose acute megakaryoblastic leukemia,[50] to identify Birbeck granules[55] (Fig. 12.1), and to differentiate malignant lymphoma from solid tumors, among others. However, some of these techniques require special and expensive equipment and trained and experienced operators. If collaborative studies can be arranged, fresh specimens should be collected in tissue culture media for transportation. In most surgical pathology daily practice, a panel of polyclonal and monoclonal antibodies may be applied to formalin-fixed or B5-fixed, paraffin-embedded sections by using an immunoperoxidase or an immunoalkaline phosphatase technique for identification and classification of hematologic disorders (Table 12.1).

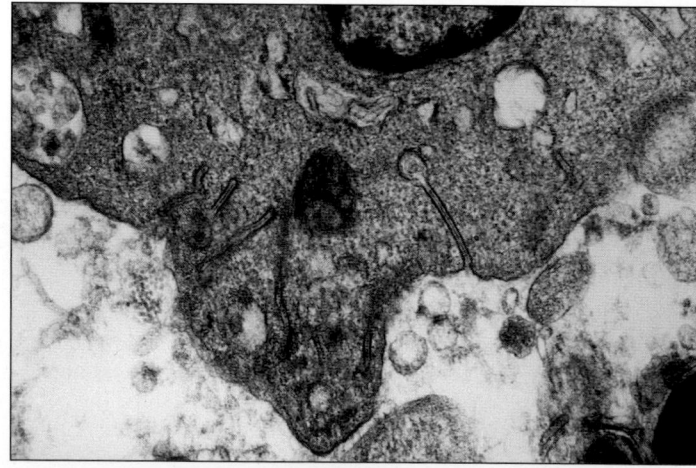

Fig. 12.1 Langerhans cell granulomatosis. This electron photomicrograph depicts several Langerhans granules or Birbeck granules, characterized by rod-shaped membranous structures having a zipper-like periodic core. They are often continuous with the plasmalemma and are probably derived from this membrane. Some of these granules have a terminal enlargement resembling a tennis racket. (×55 000.)

Table 12.1 Common markers used for antigen detection in hematologic disorders in bone marrow

Antibodies	Reactive cell lineages
Myeloid	
CD11c	Monocytes/macrophages, granulocytes, NK cells, subsets of T/B cells, HCL
CD13	Granulocytes and monocytes
CD15*	Granulocytes, monocytes, some R-S cells
CD33	Myeloid precursors, granulocytes, monocytes
CD65	Myeloid cells and monocytes
CD117* (c-Kit, SCF receptor)	Hematopoietic progenitor cells, mast cells
Myeloperoxidase*	Granulocytes, including myeloblasts, some monocytes
Tryptase**	Mast cells, basophils
Myelomonocytic	
CD14	Monocytes, some granulocytes
CD36	Monocytes, platelets, early erythroid cells
CD64	Monocytes, macrophages, dendritic cells, activated granulocytes
CD68**	Monocytes/histiocytes/macrophages, some granulocytes
Lysozyme**	Granulocytes and monocytes/histiocytes
Megakaryocytic	
CD41*	Platelets and megakaryocytes
CD61*	Platelets and megakaryocytes
Factor VIII**	Platelets, megakaryocytes, and endothelial cells
Erythroid	
HbA**	Most NRBCs and RBCs
HbF**	Minority of NRBCs and RBCs
Glycophorin A*	Most NRBCs and RBCs
T lineage	
CD1(CD1a)**	Langerhans cells, cortical thymocytes
CD2*	T cells, subset of NK cells, thymocytes
CD3 (cytoplasmic* or membranous)	Pan T cells, thymocytes
CD5*	T cells, thymocytes, subsets of B cells
CD7*	Pan T cells, thymocytes, NK subsets
CD4*	Helper/inducer T cells, subsets of thymocytes, monocytes
CD8*	Cytotoxic/suppressor T cells, subsets of thymocytes, NK subsets
CD43**	Leukocytes, except resting B cells
TIA-1**	Large granular lymphocytes
B lineage	
CD10*	Precursor B cells, B cells, and granulocytes
CD19	Precursor B cells and pan B cells
CD22*	Pan B cells
CD20*	B cells
CD79a*	Pan B cells and plasma cells
Kappa/Lambda*	Pan B cells, plasma cells
CD138*	Plasma cells, some pre B cells
Others	
CD45 (leukocyte common antigen)*	Leukocytes (except plasma cells)
CD34*	Progenitor cells, endothelial cells
HLA-DR*	B-cells, monocytes/histiocytes, activated T cells
CD56*	NK cells, activated T cells, some myeloid cells
TdT*	Lymphoid precursor cells, early B or T cells and cortical thymocytes
TRAP**	HCL
CD103	Intraepithelial (intestinal) lymphocytes, lymphocyte subset, HCL
CD30*	Activated lymphocytes and R-S cells

*Antibodies frequently used by both flow cytometry and paraffin immunohistochemistry
** Antibodies frequently used on paraffin immunohistochemistry
Those antibodies without asterisk frequently used by flow cytometry
Abbreviations: HCL, hairy cell leukemia; NRBCs, nucleated red blood cells; R-S cells, Reed–Sternberg cells;
TRAP, tartrate-resistant acid phosphatase.

NORMAL BONE MARROW

The marrow is traversed by bony trabeculae, consists of stromal cells and hematopoietic compartments, and is organized about blood vessels. The vascular sinuses play an important role in many of the marrow's functions. The adventitial reticular cells of the vascular sinuses are capable of becoming voluminous, forming gelatinous or fat cells. If such change is extensive, the marrow may become grossly gelatinous or fatty. The proportion of fatty to hematopoietic marrow varies in different bones and in different age groups under normal conditions, although the relationship in a given age group and anatomic site is usually quite constant. Hartsock and associates,[56] on the basis of a study of bone marrow from the anterior iliac crest, concluded that the amount of hematopoietic tissue in the first decade was 80%, which diminished to about 50% at the age of 30 and remained relatively constant until the age of 70, at which time the mean value became 30%. Similar trends may be seen in bone marrow obtained from the ribs, sternum, and vertebrae. It is also important to remember that marrow cavities directly adjacent to cortical bone are frequently fatty in elderly individuals and are not representative of the cellularity in the rest of the marrow. Schmid and Isaacson[57] advocate that a bone biopsy should contain at least five well preserved marrow spaces before one considers it to be an adequate specimen. The reticular cells synthesize reticular (argentophilic, reticulin) fibers that, along with their cytoplasmic processes, extend into the hematopoietic compartments and form a meshwork on which hematopoietic cells rest.

The lymphohematopoietic elements include erythrocytes, granulocytes, megakaryocytes, lymphocytes, plasma cells, macrophages, mast cells, and their precursors. They are located in the marrow spaces in the extravascular compartments in a certain topographic distribution.[58] Erythropoietic islands and megakaryocytes are associated with the sinusoids in the central regions of the marrow cavities. Early myeloid precursors lie close to the endosteal surfaces and to the arterioles. As the myeloid cells mature, they are found in the central part of the marrow cavity. The myeloid/erythroid ratio is usually 3:1 or 4:1 but may range from 2:1–6:1 under physiologic conditions. A marked derangement in myeloid/erythroid ratio indicates hematologic disorders. The histopathology of normal bone marrow has been reviewed.[13,58–60]

It is believed that a pluripotent stem cell gives rise to a series of progenitor cells for hematopoietic (erythrocytic, myeloid, and megakaryocytic) cells and to common lymphoid stem cells after a number of cell divisions and differentiation steps. These pluripotent stem cells possess the capacity of self-renewal and multilinear differentiation, whereas the progenitor cells (committed stem cells) are lineage-committed. Progenitor cells may lack self-renewal capabilities. The stromal cells consist of macrophages, fibroblasts, endothelial cells, fat cells, and reticular cells. These stromal cells and a microvascular network constitute the microenvironment that is essential for the growth and development of stem cells. The extracellular matrix is composed of a variety of substances, such as fibronectin (binds erythroid precursors), hemonectin (binds granulocytic precursors), laminin, collagen, and proteoglycans (acid mucopolysaccharides). Lymphohematopoietic growth factors (cytokines, glycoprotein hormones) regulate the proliferation and differentiation of lymphohemopoietic progenitor cells and functions of mature blood cells. They serve as either inducers or inhibitors of lymphohematopoiesis. They are produced by many types of cell and usually affect more than one lineage. These cytokines are active at very low concentrations and generally act on the malignant counterpart of their normal target cells.

Most information about lymphohematopoietic regulators is obtained from in-vitro culture systems and animal studies. Some cytokines, such as stem cell factor (SCF), interleukin (IL)-1, IL-3, IL-6, IL-11, and granulocyte–macrophage colony-stimulating factor (GM-CSF), are considered to be early-acting growth factors. Others, such as macrophage colony-stimulating factor (M-CSF), granulocyte colony-stimulating factor (G-CSF), IL-5, erythropoietin (EPO), and thrombopoietin (TP) are considered to be lineage-specific hematopoietic growth factors. Other interleukins such as IL-2, IL-4, IL-7, IL-8, IL-9, and IL-10 also participate in the regulation of hematopoiesis. Although the precise pattern of colony formation stimulated by each purified regulator is quite distinctive, there is substantial overlap in function and synergism of these regulatory factors.[61] The availability of recombinant human hematopoietic growth factors provides the basis for clinical trials. They have been used to correct iatrogenic myelosuppression secondary to chemotherapy or radiotherapy, to stimulate hematopoiesis in primary bone marrow failure (such as aplastic anemia), and to activate effector cell functions in patients with leukocyte function disorders, acquired immunodeficiency syndrome (AIDS), or other toxic conditions. They have also been used as differentiation/maturation agents for the treatment of acute myelogenous leukemias and myelodysplastic syndromes. A detailed discussion of cytokines and their inhibitors is beyond the scope of this chapter.

ERYTHROPOIESIS

Islands of erythropoiesis are easily identified on histologic sections or smears. They are characterized by perfectly round nuclei, evenly distributed chromatin, and a moderate amount of cytoplasm, which is often intensely basophilic in proerythroblasts and basophilic normoblasts by the Giemsa stain and bright red with the methyl green pyronine stain. The more mature forms (polychromatophilic and orthochromatophilic normoblasts) have more condensed or pyknotic nuclei (Fig. 12.2). The former have a clear cytoplasm and the latter have eosinophilic cytoplasm with H&E stain as hemoglobinization of the cytoplasm becomes more evident. The nucleated red blood cells (NRBCs) may be easily differentiated from myeloid precursors by their PAS-negative cytoplasm (except in erythroleukemia and a few disease entities in which the cytoplasm of erythroblasts may contain PAS-positive granules or may be diffusely stained by the PAS method). Lymphocytes or lymphoid aggregates may at times be confused with NRBCs. However, foci of erythropoiesis usually contain a spectrum of NRBCs, indicating successive maturation, whereas small lymphocytes in lymphoid aggregates tend to be monomorphic. In addition, the nuclei of lymphoid cells are usually slightly irregular, the nuclear membranes are thickened, and the chromatin is more clumped. Plasma cells, blood vessels, transformed cells, and mast cells are often found in lymphoid aggregates. Erythropoiesis tends to be present in the vicinity of sinusoids. Hemosiderin-laden macrophages, which are found in the center of an *erythroblastic island*, may be easily identified by a Prussian blue (iron) stain. These macrophages are usually surrounded by a ring of erythroblasts.

Body iron stores are best assessed by an iron (Prussian blue) stain on the bone marrow smear or clot section. Although serum ferritin correlates well with the bone marrow iron stain under normal conditions, an increased serum ferritin concentration may be found in a variety of pathologic conditions unrelated to body iron stores.[62] Normally, iron is present in the histiocytes. A few (up to four) Prussian blue-positive (siderotic) granules may be normally seen in erythroid precursors (sideroblasts). Under pathologic conditions the NRBCs contain iron-laden mitochondria (sideromitochondria),

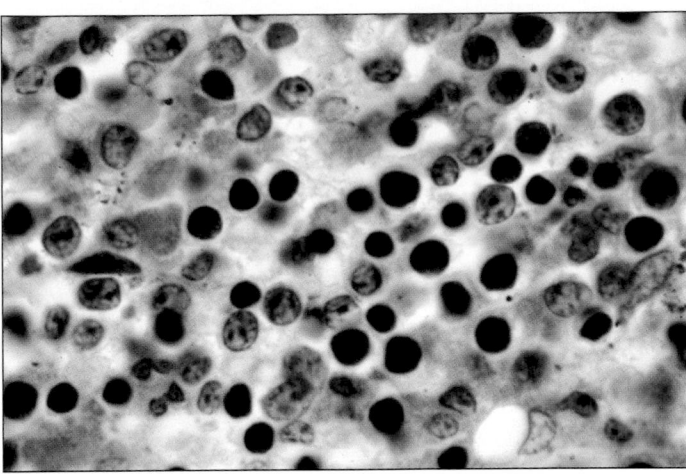

Fig. 12.2 Erythropoiesis. The early erythroid precursors have a round nucleus, evenly distributed chromatin and two or more nucleoli. The more mature erythrons have a darkly stained round nucleus. All normal erythrons have PAS-negative cytoplasm in contrast to myeloid cells or megakaryocytes, which are often PAS-positive. (PAS stain, ×630.)

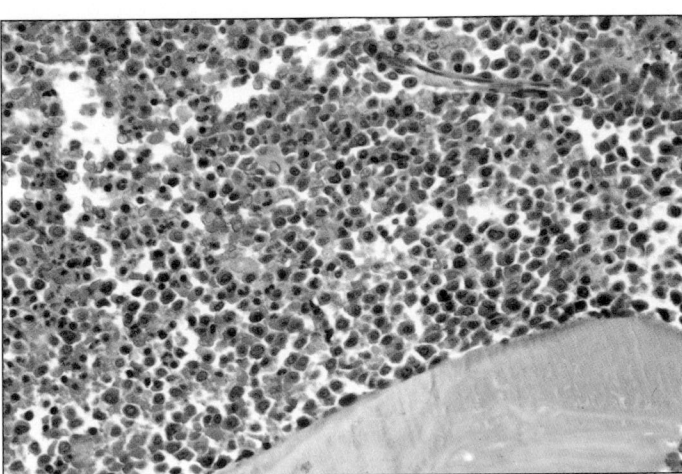

Fig. 12.3 Myelopoiesis. This bone marrow biopsy is from a patient with systemic infection. Note that the normal myelopoiesis starting at the endosteum and around the arteries. As the cells become more mature, they are pushing toward the center of the marrow cavity. (H&E stain, ×250.)

which are distributed perinuclearly in humans, thus appearing as 'ring sideroblasts' by iron stain.

MYELOPOIESIS

The earlier myeloid precursors, myeloblasts and promyelocytes, have an oval vesicular nucleus, small but distinct nucleoli, and a moderate amount of eosinophilic cytoplasm (Figs 12.3, 12.4). Primary (azurophilic) granules are synthesized in the promyelocytes, which appear as purplish granules on Romanowsky-stained smears, but are usually unidentifiable on H&E-stained sections. As the cells become more mature, the nuclear/cytoplasmic ratio decreases and specific (neutrophilic, basophilic, and eosinophilic) granules, which are synthesized by myelocytes, appear in the cytoplasm. However, neutrophilic granules are often difficult to see on H&E-stained sections, and basophilic granules dissolve during tissue processing. As mentioned earlier, PAS and specific esterase (Leder) stains are helpful in recognizing neutrophilic granulocytes, and the Leder stain will highlight mast cells. Frequently, a PAS-positive dot-like globule may be observed in the Golgi region in the promyelocytes.

MEGAKARYOPOIESIS

The more primitive cells – megakaryoblasts and promegakaryocytes – are difficult to identify on H&E-stained sections, although they are readily recognizable on Romanowsky-stained smears. Their number is increased in acute megakaryoblastic leukemia (M7), some chronic myeloproliferative disorders, and reactive conditions. Electron microscopic examination or specific monoclonal antibodies (such as *Ulex europaeus* agglutinin (UEA), von Willebrand factor (VWF), and CD61) are used to confirm their presence.[63] In our experience, antibody against CD41 gives satisfactory results. It identifies younger megakaryocytes than anti-VWF. Following subsequent maturation, the cells enlarge, the nuclei become lobulated, and the cytoplasm is voluminous and contains numerous granules on Romanowsky-stained smears or PAS-positive cytoplasm on histologic sections. Margination

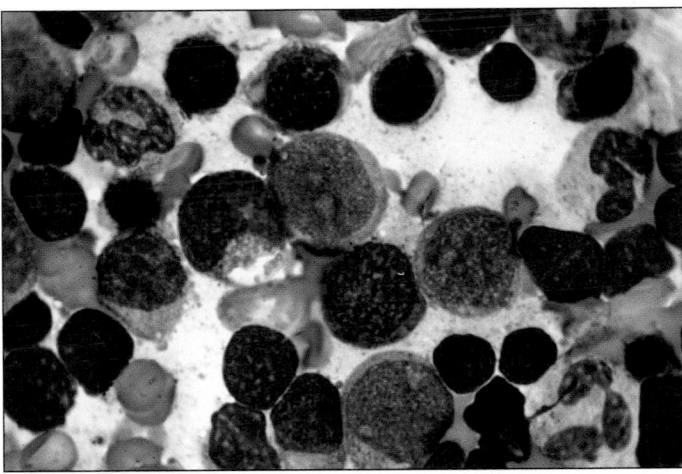

Fig. 12.4 Hematopoiesis. Note the difference in nuclear configuration, chromatin pattern, and RNA content in myeloblasts and erythroid precursors as well as lymphoid cells. (Romanowsky stain, ×630.)

of intensely PAS-positive granules may be seen on sections, which indicates platelet production. Occasionally, polymorphonuclear leukocytes or red cells are seen in the cytoplasm of megakaryocytes (emperipolesis).[64]

Megakaryocytes are easily differentiated from osteoclasts. The latter are multinucleated cells in which each nucleus is identical, with an evenly distributed chromatin pattern and a small nucleolus. Osteoclasts are present along the bony trabeculae and are considered to be generated from the same hematopoietic stem cell as monocytes. They are important in bone remodeling.[58]

OTHER CELLS

Monocytes originate from the same stem cells as myeloblasts but are difficult to find in normal bone marrow under normal conditions.

Histiocytes with phagocytosis (phagocytes, macrophages), epithelioid cells, foamy cells, or other variations are seen in normal or pathologic conditions. *Lymphocytes* are present in an appreciable number in very young and very old individuals. Lymphoid precursors (hematogones) are usually increased in young children, especially infants.[65] They may also be increased in patients who have a recent history of bone marrow suppression whether it is due to infection (such as hepatitis), chemotherapy, or other conditions.[66] Morphologically and immuno-phenotypically, they can be differentiated from leukemic blasts.[65–67] Aggregates of lymphocytes in association with capillaries, histiocytes, plasma cells, and mast cells are seen in increased frequency in elderly individuals.[68,69] Very few *plasma cells* (<2%) are normally seen in the bone marrow;[70] they are usually scattered in the marrow cavity. A perivascular cuffing of plasma cells is observed in alcoholic liver disease, cirrhosis, collagen vascular disease, and other chronic conditions (Fig. 12.5). *Osteoblasts*, cells that produce bone matrix, should be differentiated from plasma cells on bone marrow smears. These cells are often in clusters, with each cell containing one eccentrically placed oval nucleus, evenly distributed smooth chromatin, and one small nucleolus. A hof is present away from the nucleus. Osteoblasts frequently line bone trabeculae in young children or in conditions associated with bone destruction and/or remodeling, such as metastatic tumor. *Osteoclasts* absorb bone and are frequently found on the trabecular bone surface. They are multinucleated giant cells and were described earlier. *Mast cells* lie adjacent to the endothelial cells of sinusoids, at the endosteal surface of the trabecular bone, and frequently at the edges of lymphoid nodules or aggregates. They are difficult to recognize in H&E-stained sections of bone marrow but are readily identifiable by PAS or Leder stains. Antibody against tryptase is a useful marker for the diagnosis of mast cell disease (Table 12.1). Increased numbers of lymphocytes, plasma cells, and mast cells are frequently noted in hypoplastic or aplastic bone marrow.

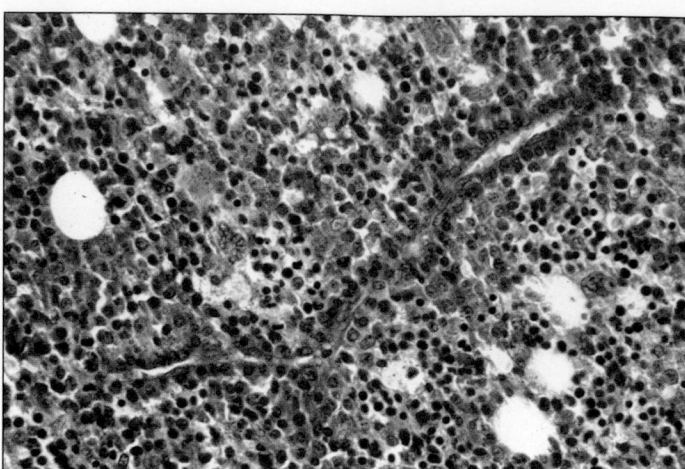

Fig. 12.5 This bone marrow biopsy is taken from a patient with HIV-infection. Note that the marrow is hypercellular, with active hematopoiesis. A prominent perivascular plasma cell cuffing is often seen in these patients. (PAS stain, ×250.)

PRACTICAL APPROACH TO BONE MARROW EXAMINATION

As stated earlier, knowledge of the clinical history, the peripheral blood cell count, the white cell differential count, and other important laboratory test results (such as serum and urine protein studies, serum levels of lactate dehydrogenase, serum iron, etc.) is essential in certain cases prior to the examination and interpretation of peripheral blood smears, bone marrow biopsy and clot sections, and bone marrow smears. A bone marrow report includes all the above information plus description, diagnosis, and comment. A checklist is included (Table 12.2).[71–72] Needless to say, all pertinent findings should be described. A systematic approach is always helpful. For example, the report can start with a short clinical history followed by the examination of the peripheral blood smear, bone marrow biopsy, bone marrow clot section, bone marrow smear and/or touch preparation, and the results of other special studies. It is important to know the patient's age (bone remodeling and cellularity), sex (especially in considering anemia), and ethnic background (e.g. hemoglobinopathy is more common in certain ethnic groups). Sometimes a definitive diagnosis cannot be made; in this case a

Table 12.2 A checklist for the preparation of bone marrow report

I.	Clinical information
II.	Pertinent laboratory data: including complete blood count and other related laboratory tests
III.	Peripheral blood smear examination:

    A. Red blood cells (RBCs)

      1. Cell size and hemoglobin content (e.g. marked anisopoikilocytosis is seen in megaloblastic anemia; spherocytosis is associated with hemolytic anemia)

      2. Presence or absence of polychromasia and nucleated red blood cells

      3. Rouleaux formation or red cell agglutination

      4. Any inclusions (Howell–Jolly bodies, hemoglobin crystal, etc.)

      5. Infectious agents (malaria, *Babesia* and *Bartonella*)

    B. White blood cells (WBCs)

      1. Increased or decreased number involving certain lineage of WBCs

      2. Cytoplasmic changes, such as toxic granules, vacuoles and Dohle bodies; or abnormal granules seen in Chédiak–Higashi syndrome

      3. Nuclear changes: Pelger–Hüet anomaly, hypersegmented neutrophils, etc.

      4. Abnormal maturation with or without dysplastic changes (such as hypogranulation, hypolobulation or apoptotic nuclei) and the presence of blasts

      5. Infectious agent (such as *Ehrlichia*, meningococci, etc.)

Table 12.2 A checklist for the preparation of bone marrow report *(cont'd)*

C. Thrombocytes (platelets)
  1. Increased or decreased number
  2. Abnormal forms: giant platelets or hypogranular platelets associated with early release from the marrow or hereditary disorders, such as Bernard–Soulier syndrome, gray platelet syndrome or May–Hegglin anomaly)
  3. Megakaryocyte nucleus or micromegakaryocytes

IV. Bone marrow biopsy section
  A. Quality of the specimen
  B. Bony architecture and content (e.g. osteoporosis, osteosclerosis)
  C. Marrow space
   1. Hematopoietic elements
     a. Cellularity (in consideration of patient's age)
     b. Fat to cell ratio
     c. Topographic distribution of hematopoiesis
     d. Erythropoiesis and maturation sequence
     e. Granulopoiesis and maturation sequence (indicate if there is abnormality in each of the cell lines)
     f. Myeloid to erythroid ratio
     g. Megakaryopoiesis and maturation sequence
     h. Dyspoiesis
     i. Marrow necrosis
   2. Stroma
     a. Fat: gelatinous or mucinous degeneration, necrosis or lipid granuloma
     b. Blood vessels: vasculitis, arteriosclerosis, amyloid deposition, intravascular fibrin or platelet thrombi, intravascular tumor, vascular proliferation, dilatation of sinuses, intrasinusoidal hematopoiesis
     c. Reticulin meshwork: fibrosis (reticulin or collagen fibrosis), collapsed reticulin meshwork
     d. Histiocytes/macrophages: foamy cells, epithelioid cells, giant cells, granulomas, abnormal histiocytes
   3. Other cells
     a. Lymphocytes: morphology and number; pattern of lymphoid aggregate distribution, interstitial, nodular, paratrabecular or diffuse; lymphoid follicle formation
     b. Plasma cells: morphology and number; perivascular, focal or diffuse infiltration
     c. Mast cells: morphology, number and location
     d. Metastatic tumor
     e. Blasts or lymphoma

V. Bone marrow aspiration smears or touch preparations of bone biopsy:
  A. Erythropoiesis and maturation sequence (normoblastic, megaloblastic, megaloblastoid; orderly maturation or left shift)
   1. Marrow polychromasia
  B. Granulopoiesis and maturation sequence (note any abnormal maturation, increased eosinophils or basophils, dysplastic changes, blasts)
  C. Megakaryopoiesis and maturation sequence (note relative number and dysplastic changes)
  D. Other cell types: increased number of lymphocytes, plasma cells, and histiocytes and their morphology; erythroblastic island, hemophagocytosis, abnormal histiocytes associated with hereditary disorders (e.g. Gaucher's disease, cystinosis), blasts, foreign cells
  E. Marrow necrosis
  F. Differential count may be indicated in some situations.

VI. Special stains:
  A. Iron stain: routinely performed on sections of bone marrow clot or smears
  B. Other stains: cytochemical, immunocytochemical and immunohistochemical stains may be performed if indicated

VII. Special studies:
  A. Flow cytometry is usually performed whenever there is a diagnosis of leukemia and non-Hodgkin's lymphoma involvement of the marrow
  B. Cytogenetic study is always undertaken whenever there is a diagnosis of leukemia
  C. In-situ hybridization: fluorescence in situ hybridization (FISH) is usually done for follow-up to detect minimal residual disease or whenever the known chromosomal abnormality is associated with cryptic gene rearrangement
  D. Other molecular analyses: Southern blot analysis or PCR may be indicated in certain circumstances

VIII. Comments and diagnosis:
  Comments and diagnosis are usually made based on clinical and laboratory information as well as morphologic examination. The classification system for hematologic malignancy is usually indicated. Also, the results of flow cytometry study are incorporated in the report. The results of other special studies, such as cytogenetic study, are usually submitted later in an addendum or as a supplementary report.

summation of pertinent findings is listed, followed by comments, which include a list of differential diagnoses and, frequently, suggestions for additional studies.

PATHOLOGY OF BONE MARROW

The pathology of bone marrow can be classified according to etiology (e.g. infectious disease, iron deficiency anemia),[73,74] type of cell involved (e.g. red cell disorders, white cell disorders, etc.), and pathologic changes. We have chosen to discuss the marrow abnormalities according to the predominant pathologic changes in the following order: (1) cellularity; (2) fibrosis; (3) lymphocytic infiltrates; (4) histiocytic proliferative disorders; (5) granulomatous changes; (6) metastatic tumors; (7) bone marrow necrosis and infarction; and (8) vascular lesions in bone marrow.

CELLULARITY

The hematopoietic elements may become hypocellular or hypercellular in normal or pathologic conditions. A hypocellular bone marrow is often associated with peripheral cytopenia, whereas hypercellular bone marrow may be manifested as polycythemia, leukocytosis, thrombocytosis, or one or more cytopenias in the peripheral blood.

Normal or hypocellular bone marrow

Hypocellular bone marrow is defined by a decrease in volume of hematopoietic elements in relation to fat (or to marrow space in postchemotherapy marrow), with the patient's age taken into consideration. The cellular components of a hypocellular marrow must be studied carefully, because the different cell series may not be affected to the same degree and because an increased number of blasts (acute leukemia) may be observed (discussed below). Lymphocytes, plasma cells, histiocytes, and mast cells are usually quite prominent in such specimens. The common causes or clinical conditions associated with hypocellular bone marrow are listed in Table 12.3. Intramedullary hemorrhage following bone marrow aspiration should not be confused with hypocellular marrow. Likewise, the marrow cavities in the subcortical region are usually more hypoplastic (especially in old age) and should not be relied on for diagnosis. Selective hypoplasia in the iliac crest has also been observed in certain conditions, such as autoimmune states.[75] Growth factors, such as IL-3 (or multi-CSF), or M-CSF, EPO, GM-CSF, and G-CSF may be selectively used to correct specific lineage hypoplasia.

Serous (mucinous, gelatinous) degeneration of the marrow

Serous degeneration of the marrow is characterized by multifocal gelatinous transformation of the nonhematopoietic marrow and is associated with malnutrition, emaciation, anorexia nervosa, and a variety of chronic disorders, including malignant disease, AIDS, tuberculosis, and chronic renal disease.[76–78] Microscopic examination reveals the fat cells to be decreased in size, with pink amorphous material in the interstitium (Fig. 12.6). They have a granular or fibrillary appearance on higher magnification and stain pale pink with the PAS stain. Histochemical studies show that the extracellular substance consists primarily of hyaluronic acid[77] and/or a large amount of sulfated glycosaminoglycan.[78] The adjacent marrow is usually hypoplastic but the total amount of hematopoietic material is

Table 12.3 Common causes or clinical conditions associated with hypocellular bone marrow

Normal aging process
Nutritional (anorexia nervosa)
Infectious (e.g. viral hepatitis or miliary tuberculosis)
Marrow toxicity (drugs, chemicals, or ionizing radiation) Some leukemias
Some myelodysplastic syndromes Paroxysmal nocturnal hemoglobinuria
Congenital (Fanconi syndrome or constitutional hypoplastic anemia) Idiopathic (aplastic anemia)

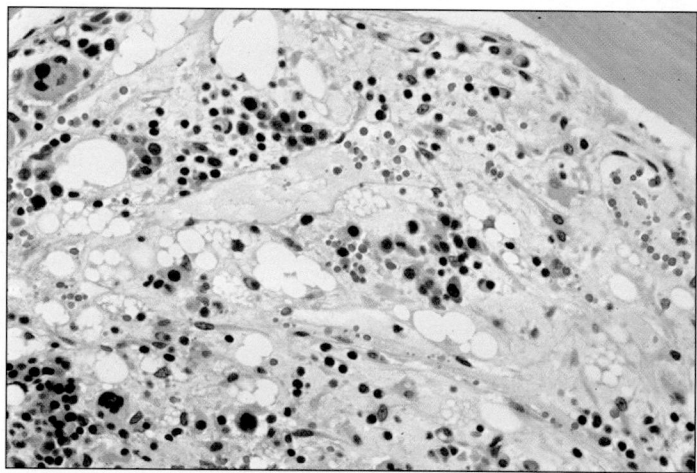

Fig. 12.6 Postchemotherapeutic effect. Note the marrow is hypocellular with marked dilatation of the sinuses, edema and deposition of eosinophilic material in the interstitium. Several adipocytes and histiocytes contain vacuoles. (H&E stain, ×250.)

usually not decreased. Serous atrophy may be found in the adipose tissue in other parts of the body.

Aplastic anemia

Aplastic anemia is defined as a nonmalignant hematopoietic disorder characterized by peripheral pancytopenia and marrow hypoplasia. Aplastic anemia can be classified as congenital/inherited or acquired.[79] Isolated single cell-line deficiency may also occur. The congenital form, such as Fanconi's anemia, is uncommon. The acquired form is frequently related to drugs, chemicals, ionizing radiation, or viral infections. Recently, an autoimmune mechanism has been proposed.[80] Sometimes the aplastic episode may be transient, and the marrow may recover after removal of the insulting agent(s). The underlying cause in most patients with acquired aplastic anemia is deficient and defective hematopoietic stem cells with normal functioning stroma,[79,81] because the stem cells are unable to respond to very high levels of hematopoietic growth factors in the colony assay study.[81,82] It has been suggested that long term use of G-CSF in nonresponders to immunosuppressive therapy may be related to secondary MDS.[83] Patients with aplastic anemia may develop MDS, paroxysmal nocturnal hemoglobinuria, or acute myeloid leukemia.[81,84,85] Peripheral bicytopenia or pancytopenia is observed.[86] Bone marrow examination reveals moderately hypocellular (hypoplastic) or severely hypocellular (aplastic) marrow with an increased amount of adipose tissue (>75% of marrow space, age-adjusted) with scattered lymphocytes, plasma cells, mast cells, and hemosiderin-laden macrophages. Small collections of erythroid, myeloid, or megakaryocytic precursors may be observed in hypoplastic anemia. There may be areas of normocellularity despite overall hypocellularity and lymphoid follicles may be prominent. Bone marrow transplantation is a treatment of choice in selected patients. Immunosuppressive therapy also results in improvement in about 70% of patients.[85] This disease must be differentiated from other causes of pancytopenia, such as hypocellular acute leukemia, hypoplastic MDS, and hairy cell leukemia, lymphomas, viral infections, mycobacterial infections, and prolonged starvation or anorexia nervosa.[86]

Pure red cell aplasia

Pure red cell aplasia may be congenital (Diamond–Blackfan anemia) or acquired (associated with spindle cell thymoma or various types of malignancy, infections, drugs, aplastic crisis in hemolytic anemia, or other conditions).[87,88] Parvovirus B19 causes a wide spectrum of diseases, including asymptomatic infection, erythema infectiosum (fifth disease), aplastic crisis in patients with underlying hemolytic disease and pure red cell aplasia in AIDS patients, among others.[89]

Bone marrow examination of parvovirus-B19-infected patients with pure red cell aplasia reveals markedly decreased or absent erythroid precursors, scattered giant proerythroblasts and intranuclear inclusions (Fig. 12.7). The diagnosis may be confirmed by immunohistochemical or molecular studies. Transient erythroblastopenia of childhood has recently been linked to human herpesvirus type 6, variant B, although the etiology of this disease in most cases is still unknown.[90] Vacuolated erythroblasts are seen in chloramphenicol-associated aplasia, erythroleukemia, and alcoholism.

Agranulocytosis

Agranulocytosis or severe neutropenia is defined as an absolute neutrophil count (ANC) less than $0.5 \times 10^9/l$ lasting for months or years. Neutropenia may be caused by decreased production, excessive destruction, or abnormal distribution of neutrophils. Thus, although granulocytic hypoplasia in the bone marrow is always associated with neutropenia in the peripheral blood, not all neutropenias are associated with granulocytic hypoplasia in the marrow. Chronic severe neutropenia may be classified as congenital and acquired.[91] Congenital abnormalities of granulopoiesis are rare.[91,92] Acquired neutropenias are usually associated with underlying diseases, such as autoimmune diseases, viral infections, hematologic disorders, or hypersplenism. Acquired neutropenias may also be drug-related or idiopathic[91,93,94] Congenital, cyclic and idiopathic neutropenia may be effectively treated with long-term G-CSF, although a cumulative risk of 13% of developing MDS and AML has been reported in patients with congenital neutropenia after 8 years of G-CSF treatment.[95]

Megakaryocytic hypoplasia

Isolated or selective megakaryocytic hypoplasia or aplasia is very rare.[96,97] Most of these cases are acquired, secondary to marrow aplasia as in aplastic anemia, radiation or chemotherapy, marrow infiltration, hematopoietic malignancies, drugs, and humoral and cellular suppression of megakaryocytic differentiation. Congenital amegakaryocytic thrombocytopenia is even rarer.[97,98] One of the examples is TAR (thrombocytopenia with absent radius). Thrombocytopenia is quite common clinically. Several thrombocytopenias, such as immune thrombocytopenic purpura (ITP) or thrombotic thrombocytopenic purpura (TTP), are associated with megakaryo-

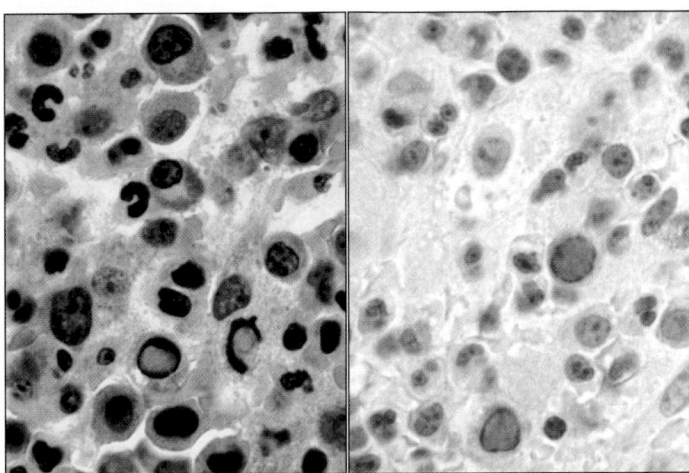

Fig. 12.7 Parvovirus infection. This composite photomicrograph illustrates several intranuclear inclusions from a patient with parvovirus B19 infection, which is confirmed by immunohistochemical technique. (H&E stain and immunoperoxidase stain, ×600.)

cytic hyperplasia, although their pathogenetic mechanisms are different. ITP is mediated by autoantibodies, whereas many patients with TTP have a deficiency of ADAMTS 13 or an inhibitor to ADAMTS 13.[99,100] TTP is a life-threatening disease characterized by fever, thrombocytopenia, microangiopathic hemolytic anemia, neurologic abnormalities, and renal dysfunctions. Wide spread hyaline/platelet thrombi are present in the small blood vessels. Concurrence of ITP and TTP has been described.[101] Refractory thrombocytopenia may be a manifestation of MDS.[102] Megakaryocytes may be quantitatively normal, increased, or decreased. However, dysmegakaryopoiesis is seen in all cases and dyspoiesis involving erythroid and/or granulocytic series is noted in some cases.[102]

Paroxysmal nocturnal hemoglobinuria

Paroxysmal nocturnal hemoglobinuria is an acquired hematopoietic stem cell disorder caused by a somatic mutation of the X-linked *PIG-A* (phosphatidyl inositol glycan class A) gene located on the $X_{p22.1}$ chromosome, which leads to reduced or absent membrane glycosyl phosphatidylinositol (GPI)- linked proteins.[81,103] Two of the GPI-linked proteins, CD55 and CD59, are important in complement regulation.[81,103] The condition is characterized by chronic recurrent intravascular complement-mediated hemolysis, pancytopenia, nocturnal exacerbations, and a tendency to thrombosis. Sucrose hemolysis and Ham acid hemolysis have been used as diagnostic tests in the past, but they have now been replaced by more sensitivity flow cytometric study, which employs monoclonal antibodies against CD55 and CD59 to the patient's granulocytes and monocytes.[81,103] Recently, Brodsky and colleagues recommended using a fluorescently labeled inactive variant of the protein aerolysin (FLAER) and flow cytometry to improve sensitivity for the diagnosis[104] The marrow cellularity is quite variable. Paroxysmal nocturnal hemoglobinuria has been associated with aplastic anemia, MDS, and acute leukemia.[81,103,105]

Hypoplastic myelodysplastic syndrome

Hypoplastic myelodysplastic syndrome (HMDS) is a well recognized disorder characterized by pancytopenia and marrow hypoplasia (<30% cellularity regardless of age).[106,107] The clinical findings and the morphologic features of the marrow may be difficult to distinguish from those associated with aplastic anemia, although cytogenetic abnormalities, dyspoiesis and abnormal localization of immature myeloid precursors (ALIP) are usually absent in aplastic anemia.[85] Orazi and associates, using monoclonal antibodies against CD34 and PCNA performed on the sections of bone marrow biopsies, were able to differentiate these two disease entities.[107] They found that CD34- and PCNA-positive cells are much higher in number in HMDS than in aplastic anemia. Cytogenetic abnormalities are detected in 33% of patients with HMDS.[106] The natural history of HMDS appears to be similar to that of normocellular and hypercellular MDS.[106]

Hypoplastic (hypocellular) acute leukemia

Hypocellular acute leukemia (HAL) is an uncommon but distinct clinicopathologic entity. It affects elderly individuals with a slight male predominance. It is characterized by severe granulocytopenia and/or variable degrees of pancytopenia with relative lymphocytosis, and hypocellular bone marrow (≤40% on bone biopsy).[108,109] Tuzuner and associates found that more than 50% of their patients had histories of antecedent hematologic disorders. Most cases of HAL are classified as FAB M1 or M2 type, and most blasts are agranular (type I). These blasts have low myeloperoxidase activity, and immunophenotypic study is needed in some cases to make the diagnosis of AML. Trilineage dysplasia is seen in more than one-third of cases,[108] and a variable degree of dysplasia involving at least one hematopoietic cell line is seen in nearly all cases. Karyotyping reveals nonrandom chromosomal abnormalities in 30% of cases analyzed.[109] Nevertheless, core biopsy of marrow supplemented by immunohistochemistry is essential for an accurate diagnosis, because the bone marrow aspiration may give a 'dry tap' (Fig. 12.8). Approximately two-thirds of patients achieved complete remission using conventional chemotherapy for acute leukemias.[108,109] HAL should be differentiated from HMDS and aplastic anemia.

Postchemotherapy bone marrow aplasia

Sequential evaluation of bone marrow changes following administration of chemotherapeutic agents for acute leukemias frequently reveals marrow necrosis and aplasia in the immediate post-therapy stage, with deposition of eosinophilic amorphous material in the interstitium, edema, and marked dilation of sinuses (see Fig. 12.6). Foamy macrophages, macrophages containing cellular debris, lymphocytes, plasma cells, mast cells, fibroblasts, and fibrocytes are increased, and loose reticulin fibrosis are frequently observed. By 7-days post-therapy, hematopoietic regeneration is usually evident in successfully treated patients. Erythroid cell regeneration usually appears first, followed by the megakaryocytic and granulocytic precursors. These regenerative foci may be present in the center of marrow cavities or along the bony trabeculae.[110–112] A similar process is observed following bone marrow necrosis of other etiologies. It should be emphasized that cytokine therapy will augment the chemotherapeutic effects on bone marrow. Special precaution should be taken when one interprets such a specimen (discussed later). Small clusters of leukemic cells are often scattered among a normocellular or hypocellular bone marrow in relapse of leukemia or in unsuccessfully treated patients with residual leukemia. Flow cytometry study and/or molecular analysis may be able to differentiate cytokine effect from residual leukemic cells.[26,27]

Bone marrow changes in transplant recipients

The sequence of changes in recipients' bone marrow following bone marrow transplant or bone marrow and peripheral blood stem cell transplants are similar to bone marrow following chemotherapy.[112] The bone marrow is usually markedly hypocellular with evidence of 'damaged' marrow (such as necrosis, edema, and an increased number

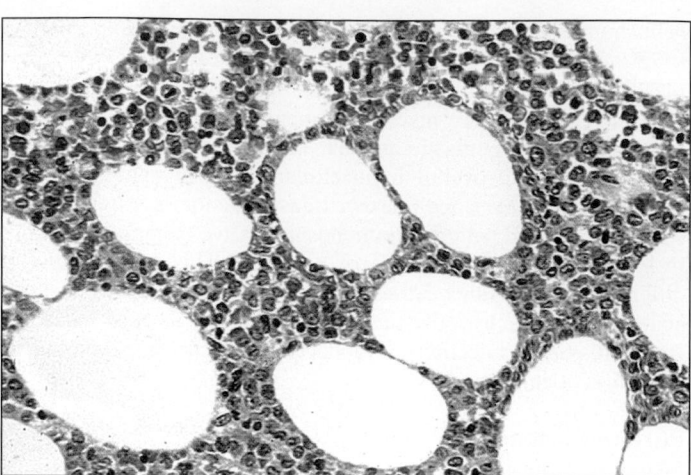

Fig. 12.8 Hypocellular acute leukemia (M1). Note that the vast majority of cells are immature with little differentiation. (H&E stain, ×250.)

of histiocytes, especially foamy macrophages, scattered lymphocytes, and plasma cells) during the first week after transplantation. The engrafted bone marrow contains isolated, small clusters of erythroid and granulocytic cells at 1–3 weeks after transplantation. However, erythropoiesis often predominates and megakaryocytes are difficult to find. By day 28, all cell lines are engrafted. Large hematopoietic islands containing mixed-lineage cell lines are evident. Dysplastic changes are minimal. Maturation proceeds normally. Once engraftment is complete, the patients may be monitored by peripheral blood cell count. Recently, peripheral blood count and morphologic examination of blood smears as well as flow cytometry assessment of blasts have replaced bone marrow examinations. Bone marrow examination should only take place when the above tests are abnormal.[112] Declining blood counts 4 weeks after transplant suggest infection or graft rejection. In the case of graft rejection, erythroid precursors decrease first, followed by other hematopoietic elements and finally by marrow aplasia. Patients with graft-versus-host disease may have an increased number of lymphocytes, plasma cells, and eosinophils in their marrow. Lymphoid aggregates and granulomas have been found in some cases. Detection of relapse or residual acute leukemia in transplant recipients by morphology alone is difficult, because lymphocytosis is common in children and regenerated left-shifted myelopoiesis may be confused with myelogenous leukemic cells in adults.

Hematogones, B lineage lymphoid precursor cells, are small to medium-sized lymphoid cells with a uniform or intermediate degree of chromatin condensation, nuclear irregularity, indistinct nucleoli, and scant agranular basophilic cytoplasm. An increased number of hematogones may be observed in regenerating bone marrow in children and in a variety of clinical conditions in adults.[65–67] Flow cytometry and cytogenetic and molecular studies may help to differentiate benign from neoplastic cells in difficult situations. Sometimes it is best to follow these cases with serial bone marrow examinations before reaching a conclusion.

Hypercellular bone marrow

Hypercellular bone marrow may be broadly classified as non-neoplastic or neoplastic hyperplasia (Table 12.4).

Non-neoplastic hyperplasia

Reactive hyperplasia is a compensatory mechanism responding to peripheral destruction or utilization of blood elements; the production

Table 12.4 Common causes or clinical conditions associated with hypercellular bone marrow

Non-neoplastic conditions
Newborn
Compensatory increase in hematopoiesis
Erythroid hyperplasia in hemoglobinopathies, hereditary red cell membrane defects, or enzymopathies, hemolytic anemia, pernicious anemia, hypoxia, and other conditions
Leukemoid reaction to infections, drug reactions, neoplasia, or others
Megakaryocytic hyperplasia in immune thrombocytopenic purpura
Panhyperplasia in hypersplenism
Congenital dyserythropoietic anemia
Multilineage or single cell line hyperplasia following cytokine (growth factor) therapy
Storage disorders, such as Gaucher's disease, Niemann–Pick disease and others
Neoplastic conditions
Leukemias, myelodysplastic syndromes, and chronic myeloproliferative disorders
Chronic lymphoproliferative disorders and plasma dyscrasias
Lymphomatous involvement
Malignant histiocytosis and true histiocytic lymphoma
Metastatic tumors

and maturation of these elements are usually normal. Sometimes non-neoplastic hyperplasia may occur under nonphysiologic conditions, such as erythroid hyperplasia following ineffective hematopoiesis associated with megaloblastic anemia, or myeloid hyperplasia following cytokine (G-CSF) therapy, or panhyperplasia in patients with hypersplenism (massive splenomegaly).

Erythroid hyperplasia   Erythroid hyperplasia may be normoblastic, megaloblastic, or megaloblastoid.

Normoblastic hyperplasia   Normoblastic hyperplasia may be manifested as peripheral erythrocytosis or anemia. Erythrocytosis (secondary polycythemia) results from increased erythropoiesis due to increased production of erythropoietin. Chronic tissue hypoxia of various etiologies (such as living at high altitude or cardiopulmonary disease resulting in a right-to-left cardiac shunt) and hemoglobinopathy with increased oxygen affinity are more common than inappropriate secretion of erythropoietin by a tumor (such as hypernephroma or cerebellar hemangioblastoma). The bone marrow shows erythroid hyperplasia without accompanying myeloid or megakaryocytic hyperplasia. Anemia of hereditary red cell abnormalities (red cell membrane defect, enzymopathy, or hemoglobinopathy) or of acquired disorders (nutritional deficiency anemia, hemolytic anemia, some forms of refractory anemias, or some forms of sideroblastic anemias) is often associated with erythroid hyperplasia. Erythroid hyperplasia also is observed a few days after acute massive hemorrhage or bleeding and in some patients with congenital dyserythropoietic anemia.[113]

Hypochromic anemia, the most common form of anemia, is characterized by normocytic or microcytic, hypochromic red cell morphology. It includes a variety of clinical conditions (such as iron deficiency anemia, thalassemia, sideroblastic anemia, and anemia of chronic disease), all of which are related to impaired hemoglobin synthesis. Of the disease entities listed above, all but iron-deficiency anemia are associated with iron overload.

Iron is stored equally as ferritin (ferric hydroxyphosphate micelles attached to apoferritin, a globulin) and hemosiderin (aggregates of ferritin particles) in the reticuloendothelial cells of the liver, spleen, and bone marrow and the parenchymal cells of the liver. Ferritin is finely dispersed within the cytoplasm, is water-soluble, and is invisible with the light microscope, although it is readily seen with the electron microscope. Hemosiderin is visible as yellow to brown granules on H&E-stained sections by light microscopy but is best demonstrated by the Prussian blue stain. The iron not utilized for the red cell pool is shifted to the stores. Prolonged intravascular hemolysis is associated with hemosiderinuria and depletion of iron stores. In extravascular hemolytic processes, including ineffective erythropoiesis (as in thalassemia), and also in patients who have received multiple blood transfusions for chronic anemias, increased hemosiderin is seen in the phagocytic histiocytes of the reticuloendothelial system (hemosiderosis). Sideroblasts are detected in normal bone marrow. Ring sideroblasts may be found in megaloblastic anemia, thalassemia, alcoholism, lead intoxication, drug reactions (to chloramphenicol or isoniazid), certain hereditary anemias, and in MDS.

Megaloblastic hyperplasia   Megaloblastic anemia includes a group of disorders characterized by one or more peripheral cytopenias, oval macrocytosis, iron overload, and megaloblastic erythroid hyperplasia. It is commonly caused by a vitamin B_{12} or folate deficiency resulting in impairment of DNA synthesis.[114] A megaloblastic erythroid cell is larger than a corresponding normoblastic cell, with a large nucleus (dyssynchrony in nuclear/cytoplasmic maturation) and an open, lacy chromatin pattern. Multinuclearity, nuclear fragments or Howell–Jolly bodies (dyserythropoiesis), and mitoses are seen. Megaloblastic change affects all dividing cells. Giant bands, monocytoid bands, hypersegmented neutrophils, and hyperlobulated megakaryocytes are all present. Ineffective erythropoiesis (premature death of erythroid cells during the maturation sequence in the marrow) is increased. Megaloblastic hyperplasia may be so florid as to be confused with acute leukemia (Fig. 12.9). Identification of intracytoplasmic HbA or HbF by an immunoperoxidase method may be helpful in recognizing that these immature cells are megaloblastic erythroblasts. Megaloblastic change is most evident on bone marrow smears.

Pernicious anemia is a form of megaloblastic anemia caused by atrophic gastritis with circulating antiparietal cell and/or intrinsic factor antibody in the blood, resulting in vitamin B_{12} deficiency.[115] The most significant clinical manifestations are neurologic symptoms due to subacute combined degeneration of the spinal cord. It primarily affects middle-aged or elderly women with a familial and racial disposition. A juvenile form has also been recognized.

Megaloblastoid hyperplasia   Megaloblastoid erythropoiesis displays morphologic features intermediate between those of megaloblastic and normoblastic erythropoiesis. A megaloblastoid erythroid cell is larger than the corresponding erythrons of the normoblastic series, with evidence of dissociation in nuclear/cytoplasmic maturation. However, the chromatin pattern is punctate and clumped, and the chromatin strands are coarser than in megaloblastic or normoblastic maturation. Thus, there are more parachromatin spaces. Multinuclearity and nuclear fragmentation are common. Both megaloblastic and megaloblastoid erythropoiesis are dyserythropoietic but the megaloblastoid change is more common clinically. It may be observed in acute and chronic myeloproliferative disorders (CMPDs), MDS, pregnancy, alcoholic

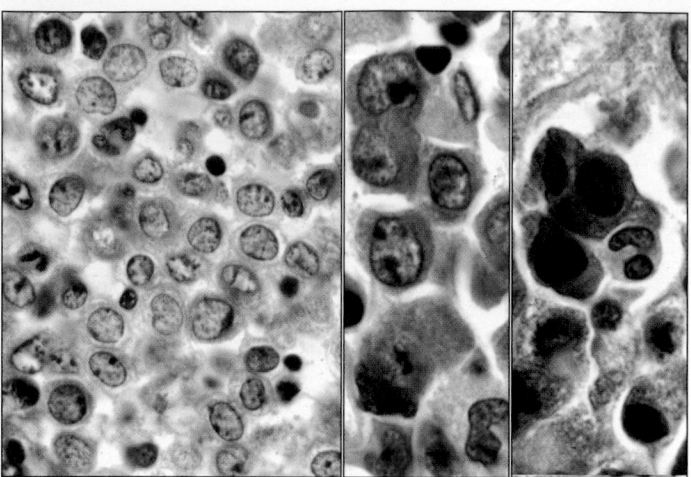

Fig. 12.9 Megaloblastic anemia. This composite picture illustrates marked megaloblastic erythroid hyperplasia. The erythroid precursors have an open chromatin pattern with nuclear to cytoplasmic dyssynchrony. The immunoperoxidase stain is used to demonstrate that these immature cells are indeed erythroid in origin, expressing hemoglobin F (middle) and hemoglobin A (right), respectively, with a normal HbA to HbF ratio. (PAS stain, ×630; and immunoperoxidase stains, ×1000.)

liver disease, and patients undergoing chemotherapy, especially those treated with antimetabolites.

Myeloid hyperplasia

Myeloid hyperplasia with peripheral leukocytosis (in excess of 20×10^9 leukocytes/l) is often seen in leukemoid reaction. Leukemoid reaction may be elicited by bacterial (neutrophilic), viral (lymphoid), allergic (eosinophilic), or inflammatory diseases, necrosis, burns, drugs, toxins, and neoplasms. Reactive myeloid hyperplasia secondary to severe sepsis may occasionally be associated with leukopenia. Myeloid hyperplasia or granulocytic hyperplasia may display normal maturation with a marked increase in the myeloid:erythroid ratio. It can also exhibit a 'shift to the left' (an increased number of the more immature granulocytic cells). The term *maturation arrest of the granulocytic series* is used to describe granulocytic hyperplasia with a shift to the left and very rare segmented neutrophils and bands. It may be associated with leukemia or it may reflect granulocytic hyperplasia associated with an increased delivery of more mature granulocytes to the peripheral blood. Histologic differentiation between a leukemoid reaction and chronic myeloid leukemia (CML) in the marrow may not be possible, but the following guidelines may be helpful:

- Granulocytic proliferation in CML is most evident along the paratrabecular region, consisting of *broad* paratrabecular and perivascular seams of immature myeloid precursors and mature granulocytes in the central regions
- Increased eosinophils and basophils are more commonly seen with CML
- Megakaryocytic hyperplasia with abnormal forms (micromegakaryocytes or dwarf megakaryocytes) is common in CML
- Increased reticulin fibers are more frequently seen in CML
- The marrow fat cells are relatively well preserved in leukemoid reaction but not in CML
- The presence of Philadelphia chromosome t(9;22)(q34;q11) confirms the diagnosis of CML.

Hematologic changes after cytokine therapy Recombinant growth factors such as EPO, G-CSF, and GM-CSF have been used to treat patients with anemia or leukopenia. These cytokines bind to specific surface receptors of lineage-specific progenitor cells and maturing cells and stimulate proliferation, differentiation, maturation, and activation of some mature cell functions. The major findings in the blood following GM-CSF or G-CSF treatment are similar to those observed in a marked inflammatory reaction, such as neutrophilia with increased azurophilic granulation (toxic granules) and prominent Döhle bodies (some of which may be seen in the eosinophils) and left-shifted myeloid cells, including myeloblasts.[116] Bone marrow examination at 2–4 days after cytokine therapy reveals marked myeloid hyperplasia with an increase in promyelocytes and myelocytes.[116,117] Both promyelocytes and myelocytes appear larger than normal. Even distribution of coarse azurophilic granules and a prominent Golgi zone are characteristic findings of abnormal promyelocytes, whereas increased azurophilic granules and cytoplasmic basophilia are common features in myelocytes. It is at times difficult to differentiate a promyelocyte from a myelocyte. Bone marrow findings at 10–15 days after cytokine therapy include a normal myeloid/erythroid ratio, although toxic granules and Döhle bodies are still visible in myelocytes, metamyelocytes, and segmented neutrophils. The differential diagnosis for a leukemic patient status post-chemotherapy includes residual leukemic cells (in the early stage of therapy) and infection. Close clinicopathologic correlations and sequential bone marrow examinations may lead to resolution of the problem.

Megakaryocytic hyperplasia Increased numbers of megakaryocytes with normal morphology are typically seen in ITP or other clinical conditions associated with increased destruction of platelets (TTP, consumption coagulopathy, and so forth) or with peripheral thrombocytosis. Increased megakaryocytes with abnormal morphology are sometimes seen in AIDS, and are also characteristically found in some CMPDs, MDS, and sometimes in acute leukemia (M7).

Neoplastic hyperplasia

Included as forms of neoplastic hyperplasia are a group of acute leukemias, CMPDs, and MDS. Chronic lymphocytic leukemia, non-Hodgkin's lymphoma, and Hodgkin's disease are discussed under the section on lymphocytic infiltrate.

Acute leukemia Acute leukemia is defined as uncontrolled clonal proliferation of immature blood cells in the blood-forming organs, which principally affects the bone marrow and eventually replaces the normal hematopoietic cell lines, resulting in peripheral cytopenias. The classification of acute leukemia is based on morphologic examination of Romanowsky-stained peripheral blood and bone marrow smears or touch preparations, supplemented by a few cytochemical stains and immunophenotyping. Cytogenetic studies have increasingly played an important role. According to the criteria proposed by the French–American–British (FAB) Cooperative Group, acute leukemia may be broadly classified into acute myeloid leukemia (AML) and acute lymphoblastic leukemia (ALL) based on the presence (AML) or absence (ALL) of 3% or more blasts containing myeloperoxidase or Sudan black B-positive granules.[48,49] It should be pointed out that blasts in M7 (megakaryoblasts) do not contain myeloperoxidase or Sudan black B-positive granules, therefore, other studies such as electron microscopy or immunocytochemistry should be performed to confirm the diagnosis.[50] Likewise, the diagnosis of minimally differentiated acute leukemia (AML-M0) has to depend on immunophenotypic study.[51]

Table 12.5 French-American-British (FAB) classification of acute myeloid leukemia

FAB subtype	Morphologic and other characteristics	Frequency (%) Adults	Children
M0	Acute myeloid leukemia, minimally differentiated (AML): ≥30% blasts; <3% blasts reactive for MPO, SBB, or NSE; blasts express CD13 and/or CD33, and may be TdT-positive	2–3	2
M1	Acute myeloblastic leukemia without maturation (AML): ≥30% blasts; ≥3% blasts reactive for MPO or SBB; blasts express CD13 and CD33; 3% may be Philadelphia-chromosome-positive	20	13
M2	Acute myeloblastic leukemia with maturation (AML): ≥30% blasts; ≥3% blasts reactive for MPO or SBB; >10% promyelocytes and maturing myeloid cells; <20% monocytic cells; blasts express CD13, CD33, CD11 and CD15; 12% have t(8;21); aberrant CD19+ and CD56+ in some cases	25–30	28
M3	Acute promyelocytic leukemia (APL): ≥30% blasts and abnormal promyelocytes; often contain bundles of Auer rods (faggot cells); hypergranular (M3) or microgranular (hypogranular, M3 variant, M3v) forms; intense MPO and SBB reactivity; blasts express CD13, CD33, CD11, and CD15; most are HLA-DR-; >90% have t(15;17); aberrant CD2+ and CD56+ in some cases	10	6
M4	Acute myelomonocytic leukemia (AMMoL): ≥30% myeloblasts, monoblasts, and promonocytes; ≥20% abnormal monocytic cells in marrow (or ≥5 × 10⁹/l monocytic cells in blood) and ≥20% myeloblasts/promyelocytes in marrow; monocytic cells reactive for NSE; monocytic cells express CD14 and CD36; ≥5% abnormal eosinophils (containing single, unsegmented nucleus and large basophilic granules) may be seen in M4Eo and associated with chromosome 16 abnormalities; aberrant CD2+ in some cases	20–25	19
M5	Acute monocytic leukemia (AMoL): ≥80% monocytic cells; MLL (11q23) abnormalities are frequently detected M5a: poorly differentiated (monoblasts ≥80% monocytic cells; NSE(+), MPO and SBB(–) or (±)) M5b: differentiated (monoblasts <80% of monocytic cells; NSE(+); MPO and SBB(±))	10–15	21
M6	Acute erythroleukemia (AEL): ≥50% erythroblasts; myeloblasts, ≥30% of NEC; abnormal multinucleated erythroblasts are usually PAS-positive and express glycophorin A and transferrin receptor	5	1
M7	Acute megakaryoblastic leukemia: ≥30% megakaryoblasts; blasts are reactive to platelet peroxidase by electron microscopy and express CD41 and CD61; myelofibrosis is common; some cases associated with t(1;22)(p13;q13)	<5	10

(+), positive; (±), weakly positive or few scattered positive granules; (–), negative; CD, cluster designation; MPO, myeloperoxidase; NEC, non-erythroid cells; NSE, nonspecific esterase; PAS, periodic acid–Schiff; SBB, Sudan black B; TdT, terminal deoxynucleotidyl transferase.
(Data from Bennett, JM et al [48–50], Pui[125], Cline[126] and Brunning et al[108, 120, 123])

The diagnosis of acute leukemia is based on the percentage of blasts in the marrow. According to the FAB classification, acute leukemia is diagnosed when there are 30% or more blasts in the peripheral blood or bone marrow. Although abnormal promyelocytes in acute promyelocytic leukemia (M3), and megakaryoblasts in acute megakaryoblastic leukemia (M7) are considered to be equivalent to myeloblasts or monoblasts,[48,49] in the newly proposed World Health Organization (WHO) classification of tumors, the requisite blast percentage for a diagnosis of acute myeloid leukemia is ≥20 myeloblasts in the blood or marrow,[118] and a precursor B- or a precursor T-lymphoblastic leukemia is diagnosed when there are more than 25% lymphoblasts in the marrow.[119] This WHO classification of acute myeloid leukemia is based on the FAB classification (Table 12.5)[48–50,118,120–126] with emphasis on cytogenetic abnormalities, effects of chemotherapy and multilineage dysplasia (Table 12.6).[118] Although cytogenetic studies and molecular analysis are important for the diagnosis, treatment (in some cases), prognosis, and detection of minimal residual diseases, the diagnosis of most cases of acute leukemia is still based on morphology supplemented by cytochemistry and immunophenotyping, of which FAB classification forms the basis for discussion.

Acute myeloid leukemias The FAB group proposes to establish the percentage of erythroblasts as the first step in classifying AMLs (Fig. 12.10).[49] If erythroblasts comprise fewer than 50% of all nucleated bone marrow cells (ANC) and there are 30% or more blasts of ANC, then the leukemia may be classified as M1 to M5, and M7. If erythroblasts account for more than 50% of ANC and blasts represent 30% or more of non-erythroid cells (NEC), a diagnosis of erythroleukemia (M6) may be made. If erythroblasts account for more than 50% of ANC but blasts account for less than 30% of NEC, a diagnosis of MDS may be considered. The WHO classification basically follows the same guideline, except that the definition of acute leukemia is based on ≥20% of blasts. In addition, pure erythroid leukemia (a subtype of M6) requires >80% of marrow cells being immature erythroid cells, and in acute megakaryoblastic leukemia ≥50% of the blasts are of megakaryocyte lineage.[120]

Acute myeloid leukemia not otherwise categorized Many of the subgroups under the heading of acute myeloid leukemia not otherwise categorized correspond to FAB subgroups (Table 12.6).[118] The application of cytochemical and immunologic studies in the modified FAB classification is illustrated in Figure 12.11.[21,127,128]

Most forms of AML exhibit a hypercellular marrow with few fat cells seen; however, hypocellular AML has been recognized and discussed earlier (see Fig. 12.8). Megakaryocytes and erythroid precursors are generally sparse, with the exception of M7 and M6 respectively. The blasts are usually large, with increased nuclear: cytoplasmic ratio, round to oval or folded nuclei, finely dispersed chromatin, and small but distinct nucleoli. Three types of blast have been described. The type I blasts resemble myeloblasts without azurophilic granules as described above. Type II blasts have identical

Table 12.6 WHO classification of acute myeloid leukemia

Acute myeloid leukemia with recurrent genetic abnormalities

Acute myeloid leukemia with t(8,21)(q22;q22); (AML1/ETO)

Acute myeloid leukemia with abnormal bone marrow eosinophils inv(16)(p13q22) or t(16;16)(p13;q22); (CBFβ/MYH11)

Acute promyelocytic leukemia [(AML with t(15:17)(q22;q12); (PML/RARα) and variants]

Acute myeloid leukemia with 11q23 (*MLL*) abnormalities

Acute myeloid leukemia with multilineage dysplasia

Following a myelodysplastic syndrome or myelodysplastic syndrome/myeloproliferative disorder

Without antecedent myelodysplastic syndrome

Acute myeloid leukemia and myelodysplastic syndromes, therapy-related

Alkylating agent related

Topoisomerase type II inhibitor related (some may be lymphoid)

Other types

Acute myeloid leukemia not otherwise categorized

Acute myeloid leukemia minimally differentiated (FAB M0)

Acute myeloid leukemia without maturation (FAB M1)

Acute myeloid leukemia with maturation (FAB M2)

Acute myelomonocytic leukemia (FAB M4)

Acute monoblastic and monocytic leukemia (FAB M5a, M5b)

Acute erythroid leukemia (FAB M6*)

Acute megakaryoblastic leukemia (FAB M7†)

Acute basophilic leukemia

Acute panmyelosis with myelofibrosis

Myeloid sarcoma

---

* A new subtype, pure erythroid leukemia in which >80% of marrow cells are immature erythroid cells has been added.

† In this entity ≥50% of blasts are of megakaryocytic lineage.

Modified from Brunning et al.[118]

---

features to type I blasts, but contain up to 20 delicate azurophilic granules in the cytoplasm. The type III blasts resemble type II blasts but have more than 20 fine azurophilic granules.[49,129] Type II and type III blasts should be differentiated from promyelocytes (Fig. 12.12). Auer rods, which appear as eosinophilic rod-like structures, may be identified (Fig. 12.13). They are composed of

primary granules and are stained by myeloperoxidase, PAS, and chloroacetate esterase (Leder) stains. They give a negative image with Sudan black B stain. A combination of chloroacetate esterase (CAE) stain, myeloperoxdase stain and immunocytochemical stain for lysozyme (muramidase) can differentiate a myelocytic component (positive with all three listed stains) from a monocytic component (negative with CAE and weakly positive with myeloperoxidase stains). Maturing granulocytic cells may be seen interspersed among blasts, in contrast to ALL, in which CAE-positive maturing granulocytes are decreased and pushed aside to the periphery of the leukemic foci. Reticulin fibers are often slightly increased.

The incidence of various subgroups is somewhat different from report to report, and is different between adults and children (see Table 12.5). However, children with Down syndrome who have had transient myeloproliferative disorder (TMPD) as newborns have a high incidence of developing M7.[130–134] Approximately 30% of infants with Down syndrome and TMPD develop M7 within 3 years. Further, the blasts in TMPD are morphologically indistinguishable from those observed in M7.[130–132] Mutations of the gene encoding the hematopoietic transcription factor *GATA1* are closely associated with M7 in Down syndrome.[132,133] It has been shown that *GATA1* is mutated in the TMPD blasts from every infant,[132] and that *GATA1* mutation is identical in sequential samples collected from a patient during TMPD and subsequent M7.[133]

Translocation – t(1;22)(p13;q13) – has been found in infants with M7 but without Down syndrome.[134–136] These children do not have antecedent history of TMPD or MDS. Organomegaly, thrombocytopenia, myelofibrosis and fibrosis of other organs are prominent features. The complete remission and median survival rates are comparable to other M7 cases, unlike children with Down syndrome with M7 who tend to have a better prognosis.[135] M7 also occurs in adults and its prognosis is poor. M6 should be differentiated from megaloblastic anemia and AML with dyserythropoiesis. Although dyserythropoiesis is seen in all three conditions, vacuolated proerythroblasts and giant erythroblasts with multinucleation are only seen in erythroleukemia (M6). Intracytoplasmic PAS-positive granules and PAS-positive cytoplasm are also characteristically seen in erythroleukemia. The erythroblasts in M6 are stained by non-specific esterase or chloroacetate esterase.[137] In addition, a therapeutic trial of vitamin B_{12} and folic acid or blood transfusion often corrects the morphologic abnormalities in megaloblastic anemia and AML with dyserythropoiesis. Clonal chromosomal abnormalities were found in 77% of patients with M6.[138] Most of these patients had

Fig. 12.10 Differentiation of acute myeloid leukemia (AML) from myelodysplastic syndrome (MDS) according to FAB classification. ANC, all nucleated cells; NEC, nonerythroid cells. Blasts, type I, type II, and type III myeloblasts. (Modified from Bennett et al.[49])

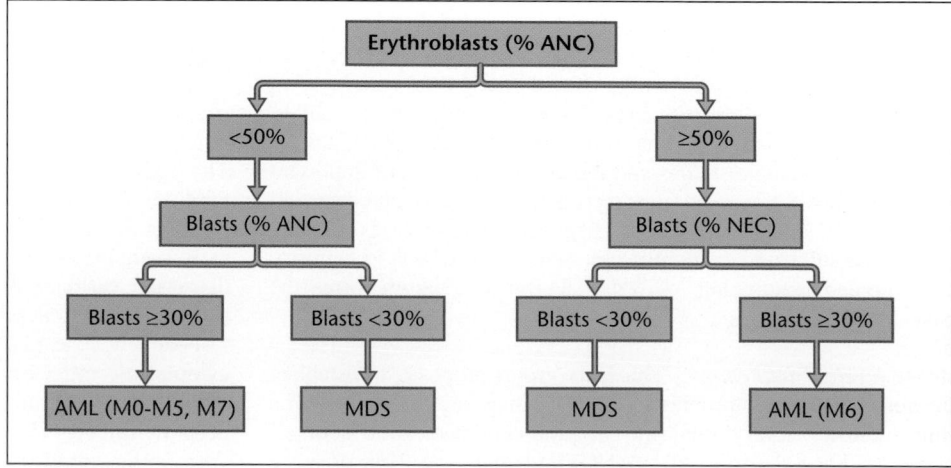

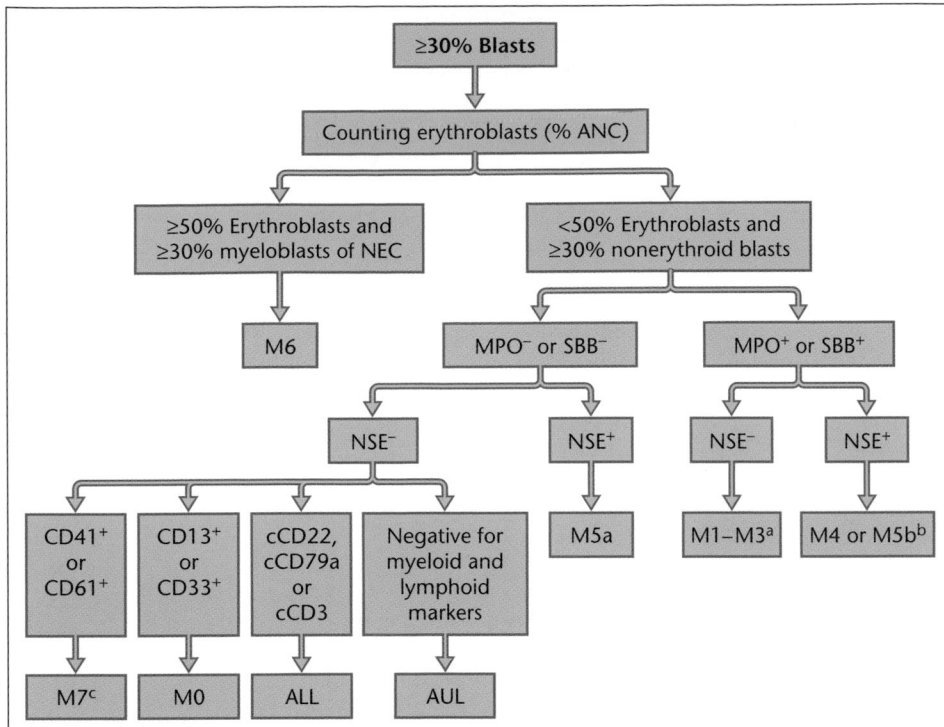

Fig. 12.11 Diagnosing acute leukemias based on cytochemical and immunologic studies according to FAB classification. ALL, acute lymphoid leukemia; ANC, all nucleated cells; AUL, acute undifferentiated leukemia; MPO myeloperoxidase; NEC, nonerythroid cells; NSE, nonspecific esterase; SBB, Sudan black B; [a]M3 may stain moderately with NSE. [b]May be NSE-negative; [c]May be ANAE-positive. (Modified from Stewart et al.[21] Franzman and Bennett,[127] and Bene et al.,[128])

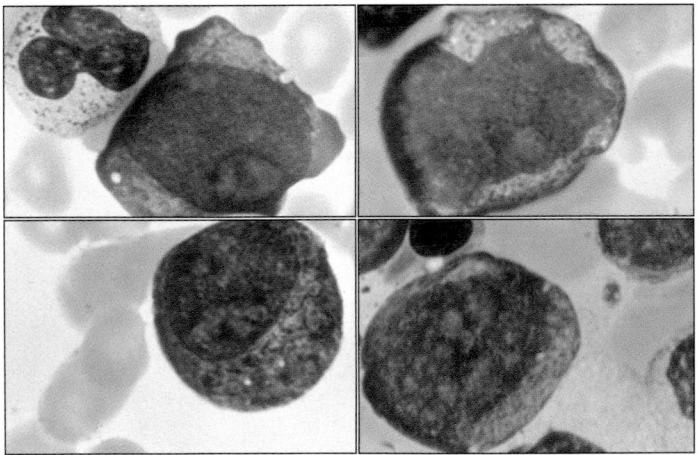

Fig. 12.12 Composite picture to compare blast types I (right lower corner), III (right upper corner), II (left upper corner), and promyelocytes (left lower corner). See text for a description of each cell type. (Romanowsky stain, ×1000.)

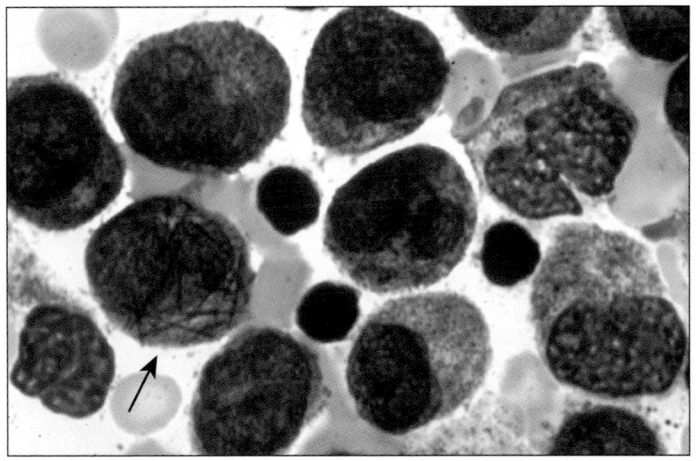

Fig. 12.13 Acute promyelocytic leukemia (M3 according to FAB classification). One of the leukemic cells contains bundles of Auer rods (faggot cell) (arrow). Leukemic cells may contain one or multiple Auer rods in their cytoplasm. (Romanowsky stain, ×1000.)

abnormalities of chromosome 5 and/or 7, similar to the incidence observed in patients with therapy-related AML.[138]

Minimally differentiated acute myeloid leukemia or AML-M0 is characterized by <3% of blasts expressing myeloperoxidase or Sudan black B, presence of at least one of the myeloid-associated antigens CD33 or CD13, and absence of B- and T-lineage-specific markers, although myeloperoxidase may be demonstrated by immunocytochemistry or immunohistochemistry and electron microscopy.[51–54] Cytoplasmic myeloperoxidase (cMPO) is considered to be lineage-specific for AML with the exception of M0, M4, or subgroups of M5 and M6, and M7, whereas cytoplasmic CD79a (cCD79a) and cytoplasmic CD22 (cCD22) are considered to be B-lineage-specific and cytoplasmic CD3 (cCD3) is T-lineage specific.[128] Flow cytometry study is essential to differentiate M0 from M7 and ALL. AML-M0s frequently express CD34, CD117, and HLA-DR; they may also be positive for TdT and CD7.[17,128,139,140] Clonal abnormalities are detected in a majority of cases.[140,141] Many of them have complex chromosomal abnormalities, −5/5q− or −7/7q−, similar to those observed in MDS or therapy-related AMLs.

Acute basophilic leukemia (ABL) is an uncommon acute leukemia with heterogeneous clinical presentations, morphologic findings and cytogenetic abnormalities.[120,142,143] Of the 16 cases reviewed by Duchayne and associates, the median age is 27 years, with four of these patients less than 1 year old.[143] Some patients presented with urticaria or gastrointestinal symptoms related to hyperhistaminemia, but the clinical presentations and morphology of the blasts in most cases are indistinguishable from others with acute leukemia.[142,143] Recognition of coarse basophilic granules in the cytoplasm of the blasts is usually the first clue in the diagnosis of this rare entity. However, the blasts in many cases are agranular. The basophilic granules are metachromatic, strongly positive for acid phosphatase and chloroacetate esterase but negative for myeloperoxidase. Immunophenotypic study reveals characteristic expressions of CD9 and CD17 in addition to myeloid markers and some activation markers (such as CD25 and CD38).[143] Identification of immature basophilic granules and theta granules in the blasts by transmission electron microscopy is diagnostic for this disease. In some cases, immature mast cell granules are also present in the blasts.[142] Chromosomal abnormalities have been associated with mature basophilic proliferations, such as the Philadelphia chromosome, t(6;9)(p23;q14), or 12p abnormality, but it appears that none of them are pathognomonic for ABL. The clinical outcomes are quite variable.[143] Duchayne and associates suggested that there were two types of ABL: (1) a pure monophenotypic ABL, with or without basophil maturation, and (2) more frequently, a mixture of blasts from different lineages and variable participation of mature or immature basophils. They speculated that the c-*myb* gene at 6q23 may be involved in the leukemogenesis in the former, whereas ABL in the latter situation may arise from a multipotent progenitor cell and is frequently associated with the Philadelphia chromosome.

Acute panmyelosis with myelofibrosis or acute malignant myelosclerosis (AMF) is a rare but rapidly fatal disease, characterized by pancytopenia and minimal or no splenomegaly.[144] Teardrop cells, characteristically seen in agnogenic myeloid metaplasia or myelosclerosis with myeloid metaplasia, are rare in AMF, and there is little anisopoikilocytosis on the peripheral blood smear. The bone marrow examination often yields a 'dry tap'. Histologic examination of bone marrow biopsy specimens shows hypercellular bone marrow with replacement of normal hematopoietic elements and fat by fibrous tissue (reticulin fibrosis) interspersed with sheets of blasts, dysplastic megakaryocytes, and residual dyspoietic hematopoietic cells. Karyotypic polymorphism was found in these patients, which supports the concept that AMF is a primary malignant tumor of hematopoietic cells associated with secondary non-neoplastic fibrosis.[145] Chemotherapy is ineffective, but marrow transplantation may offer a cure.[146] Some patients terminate in acute leukemia.[147] Some investigators found the blasts to be megakaryoblasts, indicating that these cases were variants of AML and should be classified as M7, according to FAB classifications.[147,148] Others using immunophenotypic studies found that the blasts may express myeloid, erythroid, or megakaryocytic antigens.[120] Cytogenetic studies showed changes similar to secondary AML, i.e. complex abnormalities or those involving chromosome 5 or 7.[118]

Myeloid sarcoma or extramedullary myeloid cell tumor (EMCT) The term EMCT was first introduced by Davey and associates[149] to designate malignant neoplasms of myeloid lineage that occur in a variety of anatomic sites other than the bone marrow, although *chloroma* and *granulocytic sarcoma* are better known synonyms for these neoplasms. It may develop prior to, concurrently with, or following the onset of classic AML. The tumor may occur anywhere in the body with peritoneum, soft tissue, bone, lymph node, nasal fossa, and skin as the most common sites.[150,151] Histopathologically, EMCT has been classified into: (1) well differentiated (differentiated), when numerous eosinophilic myelocytes are seen in any section of a given case; (2) poorly differentiated (immature), when only occasional eosinophilic myelocytes can be found; and (3) blastic, if there is no evidence of granulocytic differentiation.[150] The neoplastic cells in EMCT often have oval or reniform nuclei with delicate nuclear membranes, a 'dusty' or 'salt-and-pepper' chromatin pattern, and multiple small but distinct nucleoli. Commonly used special stains include Leder stain and immunoperoxidase stain for lysozyme. Traweek and associates found that 100% of their 28 cases were CD43+ and 75% were CD45+.[152] Roth and colleagues[118] concluded that CD43, lysozyme, and myeloperoxidase were all very sensitive for these tumors. In nonleukemic patients and patients with CMPDs, the occurrence of EMCT was a harbinger of AML or blast crisis. However, if patients with EMCT were appropriately treated, they might undergo complete remission, and a few might be cured;[151] thus, accurate and timely diagnosis of EMCT is important. EMCT is more frequently observed in cases with M2 (associated with t(8;21)(q22;q22)), M4Eo (inv(16)(p13;q22) or t(16;16)(p13;q22)) and M4 or M5 (associated with chromosome 11q23 abnormalities).

Acute myeloid leukemia and myelodysplastic syndromes, therapy related A greater proportion of AMLs secondary to chemotherapy and/or radiotherapy were unclassifiable according to the FAB system in comparison with de novo AMLs. These cases will be classified under AML and MDS, therapy-related under the WHO Classification (Table 12.6).[121] These patients usually present with one or more cytopenias and dyspoiesis simulating MDS (Table 12.7).[153,154] Based on whether it is alkylating agent/radiation-related or topoisomerase-II-inhibitor-related, the clinical presentations and cytogenetic abnormalities are different. The former group typically presents after a latency period of 5 years or more after receiving the treatment. They usually have refractory anemia with excess blasts or evolving AML, M2 M4, or M6 subtypes. Clonal cytogenetic abnormalities are frequently detected, such as −5/5q or −7/7q, abnormalities of 11q, inv(3) and complex or multiple abnormalities.[155–158] These types of cytogenetic abnormality are similar to de novo AML arising in the elderly.[155] Patients with topoisomerase-II-inhibitor-related AML usually develop AML in 2–3 years, and without prior manifestations of MDS.[153,154] The *MLL* gene in the 11q23 is frequently involved.[153,154] These patients tend to have monocytic leukemia, such as chronic myelomonocytic leukemia, M4 or M5. Orazi and associates[159] found that the presence of ALIP, marrow fibrosis, and augmented CD34 expression in bone marrow biopsies were ominous prognostic factors. Therapy-related MDS generally has a more aggressive clinical course than primary MDS.[159]

Acute myeloid leukemia with multilineage dysplasia as defined by WHO classification is an acute leukemia with ≥20% blasts in blood or marrow, and dysplasia (in ≥50% of the cells) in two or more hematopoietic cell lines.[122,160] This disorder usually occurs in the elderly with or without a prior history of MDS, or following a myelodysplastic/myeloproliferative disorder. The blasts usually express CD34, CD13, and CD33. There is frequent aberrant expression of CD56 and/or CD7. An increased incidence of multidrug resistant glycoprotein (MDR-1) expression on the blast cells is noted.[122]

Acute myeloid leukemia with recurrent genetic abnormalities Included in this group are recurrent cytogenetic abnormalities

Table 12.7 Morphologic abnormalities seen in myelodysplastic syndrome

Peripheral blood

Anemia with oval macrocytosis; dimorphic red cell population; anisopoikilocytosis; reticulocytopenia

Less common findings include leukoerythroblastic picture and the following:

Neutropenia or neutrophilia with qualitative granulopathy: Pelger–Hüet-like anomaly, hypersegmented neutrophils, coarse granulation, abnormal granulation (pseudo-Chédiak–Higashi), degranulation, abnormally small or large forms, mirror image of segmented nucleus or band nucleus, 'doughnut nucleus', or other nuclear abnormalities

Thrombocytopenia with bizarre platelet size and shape, abnormal granulations

Monocytosis or atypical monocytoid cells

Circulating blasts (type I, type II, or type III blasts)

Bone marrow

Erythroid hyperplasia or hypoplasia with megaloblastoid changes: dyssynchrony in nuclear/cytoplasmic maturation, multinucleation, nuclear lobulation, nuclear fragmentation, gigantic erythroblasts with abnormal nuclei, karyorrhexis, impaired hemoglobinization, ± ring sideroblasts, maturation arrest

Myeloid hyperplasia or hypoplasia with dyspoietic features described above; abnormal granulation (pseudo-Chédiak–Higashi anomaly); abnormal eosinophils with dimorphic (containing both eosinophilic and basophilic) granules; ring or rodent nuclei (doughnut-shaped nuclei); increased number of type I, II, and III blasts (but less than 20%)*; abnormal localization of immature precursors (ALIP) on sections

Megakaryocytic hyperplasia with dyspoiesis: micromegakaryocytes, polynucleated megakaryocytes, large mononucleated megakaryocytes, megakaryocytes with odd-numbered lobes; degranulated, abnormally granulated, or vacuolated cytoplasm

Increased monoblasts, promonocytes, and monocytes with dyspoiesis, reactive with naphthol-ASD-chloroacetate esterase

* Less than 20% blasts is defined by WHO classification;[118] blasts are less than 30% according to FAB classification.[48,49]

primarily caused by reciprocal chromosome translocation(s) or inversion(s) that then creates a fusion gene encoding a chimeric protein. This results in the functional inactivation or repression of the transcription factor(s) that is(are) essential for the normal regulation of hematopoiesis.[155] Most of these chromosomal abnormalities are observed in de novo AML and in adolescents and adults less than 45 years old, and are associated with favorable prognosis, except some cases of 11q23 abnormalities.[123,155] On the other hand, cytogenetic abnormalities in AML of the elderly are similar to AML that arises from antecedent MDS or therapy-related AML. These cases usually have complex patterns of chromosome gain and loss and are thought to be secondary alterations resulting from DNA damage, genome instability, defective DNA repair, or perturbations in cell signal transduction pathways.[155]

Acute myeloid leukemia with t(8;21)(q22;q22) (AML1/ETO) This chromosomal abnormality is the single most common structural rearrangement seen in AML and is most often associated with M2 morphology with large prominent Auer rods or pseudo-Chédiak–Higashi anomaly.[161] The marrow frequently has an increased number of eosinophils, with blasts containing homogeneous salmon-colored granules, large cytoplasmic globules and vacuoles (Fig. 12.14). In addition to CD13, CD33, and HLA-DR, some cases are CD15+ and CD34+. Aberrant expression of CD19 and CD56 have been observed.[17,161] Also, Arber and associates reported four cases of t(8;21) whose leukemic cells were found to be myeloperoxidase-positive but CD13− and CD33−.[30] t(8;21) commonly affects young males. Extramedullary myeloid cell tumor may be the initial clinical presentation. It is associated with a most favorable prognosis in adults but a much less favorable response to therapy in children.[161] The *AML1* gene (21q22) is also implicated in therapy-related MDS/AML.[32,158]

Acute myeloid leukemia with t(15;17)(q22;q11–22)(PML/RARα) and variants Acute promyelocytic leukemia (APL) is an uncommon AML characterized by malignant proliferation of abnormal promyelocytes in the bone marrow and is associated with a specific chromosomal abnormality, t(15;17)(q22;q11–22), in most cases.[123] This balanced translocation involves the *RARα* (17q12–22)

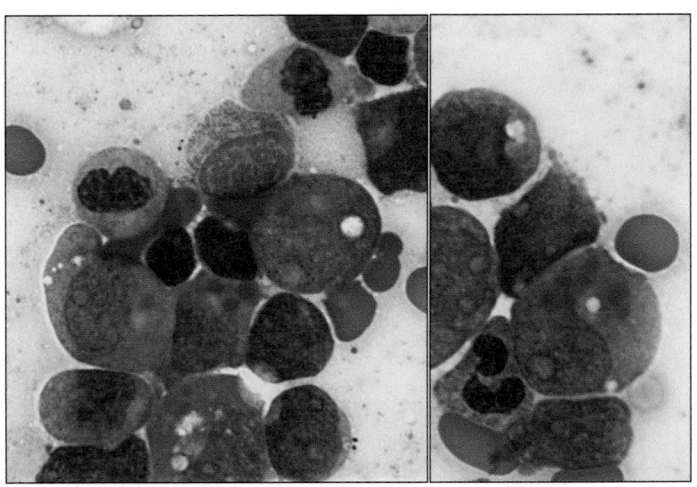

Fig. 12.14 Acute myeloid leukemia with maturation (M2 according to FAB classification). This composite photomicrograph illustrates a few leukemic cells containing several large eosinophilic or pink granules (pseudo-Chediak–Higashi granules) which may be seen in some of the M2 leukemias, especially those associated with t(8;21). (Romanowsky stain, ×1000.)

gene fused to the *PML* (15q22) gene. Cryptic *PML/RARα* fusion gene may be present in some cases, which requires RT-PCR or fluorescence in situ hybridization (FISH) for its detection.[158,162] Although the PML/RARα fusion product is characteristic for APL, it has been observed in other FAB types of AML.[163] Several variants of translocations involving *RARα* with another partner gene, such as promyelocytic leukemia zinc finger gene (*PLZF* at 11q23), nucleolar phosphoprotein nucleophosmin gene (*NPM* at 5q32–35) or nuclear mitotic apparatus protein gene (*NuMA* at 11q13), have been described.[158,162] Both hypergranular promyelocytic leukemia (M3) and microgranular promyelocytic leukemia (M3v) will have this t(15;17). Most AML-M3s display hypergranular morphology. The hypergranular promyelocytes are characterized by irregular nuclear configuration with the cytoplasm packed by coarse azurophilic granules or bundles of Auer rods ('faggot' cell) (see Fig. 12.13). Some of the promyelocytes may contain large Auer rods. Abnormal promyelocytes in the microgranular variant (M3v) are characterized by reniform or bilobed nucleus and absence or paucity of primary granules. Myeloperoxidase, Sudan black B, CAE and PAS all display strong positivity in abnormal promyelocytes. Cases that have t(5;17) show atypical morphology and lack of Auer rods. Cases with t(11;17)(q23;q21) will have increased Pelger–Hüet-like cells and blasts with regular nuclear contour, heavily granulated cytoplasm but no Auer rods.[123] Flow cytometry study of APL reveals bright CD33$^+$ and variable CD13$^+$ cells with co-expression of CD2 in some cases.[17] CD34 and HLA-DR are usually absent.[17] Cases with t(11;17)(q23;q21) may have CD56 expression.[164] APL usually affects young or middle-aged adults. Disseminated intravascular coagulation may be the initial presenting sign or soon develops after the initiation of conventional therapy. The leukemic cells can be induced to differentiate into mature granulocytes following exposure to differentiating agents such as all-*trans*-retinoic acid (ATRA). However, hyperleukocytosis develops because of a rapid increase in the number of mature leukemic cells in the blood. A *retinoic acid syndrome* may occur in some patients. These patients have hyperleukocytosis, fever, respiratory distress, episodic hypotension and acute renal failure. Pleural and pericardial effusions and peripheral edema may also develop.[165] It should be pointed out that patients with t(11;17)(q23;q21) are usually resistant to ATRA. However, when the patients are treated with a combination of ATRA and G-CSF or concurrently with ATRA and chemotherapy, remission may be attained.[162] Further, early induction of cytotoxic chemotherapy prevents onset of retinoic acid syndrome. If remission is attained, these patients tend to have a long remission duration and survival compared to other forms of AML.

Acute myeloid leukemia with inversion (16)(p13;q22) or t(16;16)(p13;q22) (CBFβ/MYH11) A subgroup of AML M4 that is characterized by bone marrow eosinophilia with atypical eosinophilic precursors is associated with inversion or translocation of chromosome 16p13q22 (Fig. 12.15).[123] These abnormalities result in fusion of the core binding factor beta gene (*CBFβ*, also known as *PEBP2β* or AML1 DNA binding factor beta) on chromosome 16q22 to the smooth muscle myosin heavy chain (*MYH11*) gene on 16p13.[158,166,167] Inversion of 16(p13;q22) have been occasionally identified in other myeloid malignancies, including AML M2, M4 without eosinophilia, M5, M7, MDS, ALL, and blast crisis of chronic myeloid leukemia.[166,167] More significantly, cryptic gene products may be detected in those patients without karyotypic abnormalities.[167] Consequently, additional screening by either RT-PCR or FISH in all AML M4 has been advocated.[167] In M4Eo, 5% or more of the non-erythroid bone marrow cells have a mixture of eosinophilic and basophilic granules. These cells are positive for CAE and PAS (coarse granules) stains. Immunophenotypic study shows that AML-M4 blasts express CD13, CD33, HLA-DR, CD14 and CD15.[17] The presence of CD2 is correlated with M4Eo.[17] This M4Eo subtype has a higher frequency of central nervous system (CNS) involvement but has a more favorable prognosis and a higher remission rate than the M4 subtype in general.

Acute myeloid leukemia with 11q23 (MLL) abnormalities The mixed-lineage leukemia gene (*MLL*, also known as *ALL-1*, *HRX* and *htrx-1*) on chromosome 11q23 may fuse with more than 20 different chromosome partners to create chimeric proteins that alter gene expression.[125,155,158,168] Translocations involving 11q23 occur in 7–10% of ALL, with the (4;11) and (11;19) translocations predominating, and 5–6% of AMLs, with the (6;11), (9;11), (10;11),

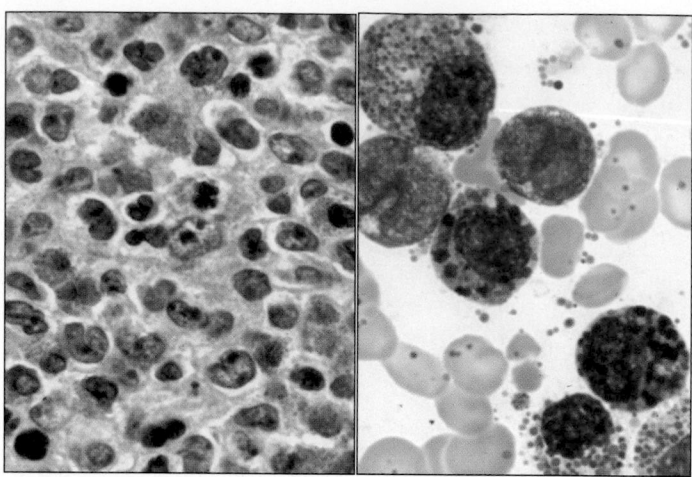

Fig. 12.15 Acute myelomonocytic leukemia (M4 according to FAB classification). This composite photomicrograph illustrates a subtype of M4, so-called M4Eo, which is frequently associated with chromosome 16 abnormality. (Note the dimorphic eosinophilic and basophilic granules in abnormal myeloid cells.) (H&E stained, ×600; Romanowsky stained, ×1000.)

and (11;19) translocations being the most common.[168,169] The 11q23 breakpoints are molecularly identical in both myeloid and lymphoblastic leukemias, suggesting that the involved gene has an important regulatory function in both differentiation pathways.[125] Chromosomal rearrangements involving MLL are the most frequent cytogenetic abnormalities in AML and ALL in infants and young children.[155] Patients who have t(9;11)(p22;q23) (MLL/AF9) tend to be young (median age 2.1 years), with low leukocyte counts at the time of diagnosis, and are more likely to have FAB M5 AML than other types. They have a favorable prognosis.[169] Patients whose leukemic cells contain t(10;11)(p12;q23) (MLL/AF10) are more likely to have FAB M5a AML, to be younger, and to have a better outcome than patients whose leukemic cells have other 11q23 abnormalities.[169] However, other investigators have found 11q23 abnormalities to be associated with a poor prognosis. Most cases of secondary AML that are induced by topoisomerase II inhibitor also have 11q23 rearrangements and AML-M5. These patients have a poor prognosis. It should be pointed out that some patients with therapy-related MDS or therapy-related AML have t(3;21)(q26;q22) abnormality.[161,170] The prior treatment includes topoisomerase II inhibitors[161] or alkylating agents and radiotherapy.[170] However, t(3;21) may be observed in CML in chronic phase, blast crisis, and MDS progressing to AML.[161,170] Abnormalities in 11q23 may not be detected by conventional karyotype. RT-PCR, Southern blot analysis, and FISH are required to identify cryptic gene rearrangement.[171]

Classification of the acute and chronic leukemias and MDS has been largely based on the criteria proposed by the FAB group based on morphology, supplemented by cytochemistry and immunophenotypic analysis. Recent progress in cytogenetic study and molecular analysis led to the new WHO classification.[172] Arber proposed a new classification that divides AML into de novo AML and AML, myelodysplasia-associated (Table 12.8).[173] The initial diagnosis is based on morphology, cytochemistry, and immunophenotype. Cytogenetic information may be added when available. It appears that this 'realistic pathologic classification' is practical, easy to remember, and includes most categories of AML. However, it remains to be seen if this classification will withstand the test of time as our understanding in pathology and molecular biology improves.

Table 12.8 Realistic pathologic classification of acute myeloid leukemia

Acute myeloid leukemia, de novo
Acute myeloid leukemia (with or without monocytic features), not otherwise specified (FAB M0, M1, M2, M4, M5)
Acute myeloid leukemia with changes suggestive of t(8;21)(q22;q22) (FAB M2)
   CD56+
   CD56−
Acute promyelocytic leukemia (FAB M3;M3v)
Variant: acute promyelocytic leukemia with features suggestive of t(11;17)(q23;q21)
Acute myeloid leukemia with abnormal eosinophils suggestive of inv (16)(p13q22) or t(16;16)(p13;q11) (FAB M4Eo)
Acute megakaryoblastic leukemia (FAB M7)

Acute myeloid leukemia, myelodysplasia-associated
Acute myeloid leukemia, treatment-related
Acute myeloid leukemia arising from myelodysplasia
Acute myeloid leukemia with associated myelodysplasia (including some FAB M6)

Adapted and modified from Arber.[173]

Acute lymphoblastic leukemia Acute lymphoblastic leukemia is more common in children than in adults. The FAB group classifies this entity into three morphologic groups: L1, L2, and L3.[48] The L1 subgroup is characterized by a homogeneous population of small cells having up to twice the diameter of a small lymphocyte. The nucleus is large and round, with occasional clefting or indentation. The amount of cytoplasm is scanty, with slight or moderate basophilia. The nucleoli are invisible or small and inconspicuous. L2 cells are large with considerable heterogeneity in size. Nuclear clefting, indentation, and folding are characteristics. Nucleoli are always present, and often large. The amount of cytoplasm varies but is often abundant. Cytoplasmic basophilia may be marked. L3 cells are large and characteristically homogeneous. The nucleus is oval to round and regular. The chromatin is finely stippled. One or more prominent vesicular nucleoli are seen in most cells. The cytoplasm is voluminous and intensely basophilic. Prominent cytoplasmic vacuolization is often present (Fig. 12.16).

With the exception of L3 (Burkitt's lymphoma/leukemia), there is no correlation between morphology and immunologic classifications. L2, which is more common in adults, has to be differentiated from AML (M0 or M1). Scattered rare azurophilic granules may be seen in L2 but these granules do not react with myeloperoxidase. The FAB group claims that the presence of up to 3% myeloperoxidase-positive blasts is still considered compatible with L2.[48] Using polyclonal antibody against myeloperoxidase and immunohisto-chemistry, Arber and associates found that blasts from 19/82 (23%) patients with adult ALL expressed polyclonal myeloperoxidase (pMPO).[174] 42% (8/19) of the pMPO+ ALL cases had Philadelphia chromosome by either karyotype or PCR. All these cases are precursor B-cell lineage, and many of them express CD13 or CD15.[174]

L3 cells carry membrane surface immunoglobulin or intracyto-plasmic immunoglobin (frequently IgM) and are B cells. The vacuoles in blasts react with oil red O or Sudan IV (neutral lipid) (Fig. 12.16). Recently, ALL with L1 or L2 morphology expressing surface immunoglobulin light chain in addition to TdT, CD19, CD20, with or without HLA-DR, or CD10 has been reported.[175] Immunologic classification of ALL is shown in Table 12.9.[17,125,176]

The WHO classification groups ALL into precursor B-lympho-blastic leukemia/lymphoblastic lymphoma and precursor T-lym-phoblastic leukemia/lymphoblastic lymphoma.[119] Unlike AML, in which tissue infiltration (myeloid sarcoma, EMCT) is uncommon, ALL frequently presents with lymphadenopathy and/or hepato-splenomegaly with neoplastic infiltrate (lymphoma) into extranodal sites. When there is extensive marrow and blood involvement, the case is classified as ALL; if the patient presents with a mass lesion and ≤25% lymphoblasts in the marrow, the term lymphoblastic lymphoma is applied. The L1 or L1/L2 ALL is frequently associated with a T-lymphoblastic lymphoma (convoluted cell lymphoma), less common with a precursor-B-lymphoblastic lymphoma, and the L3 ALL is associated with Burkitt's lymphoma. Histologic examination of ALL in bone marrow is almost identical to that of the corres-

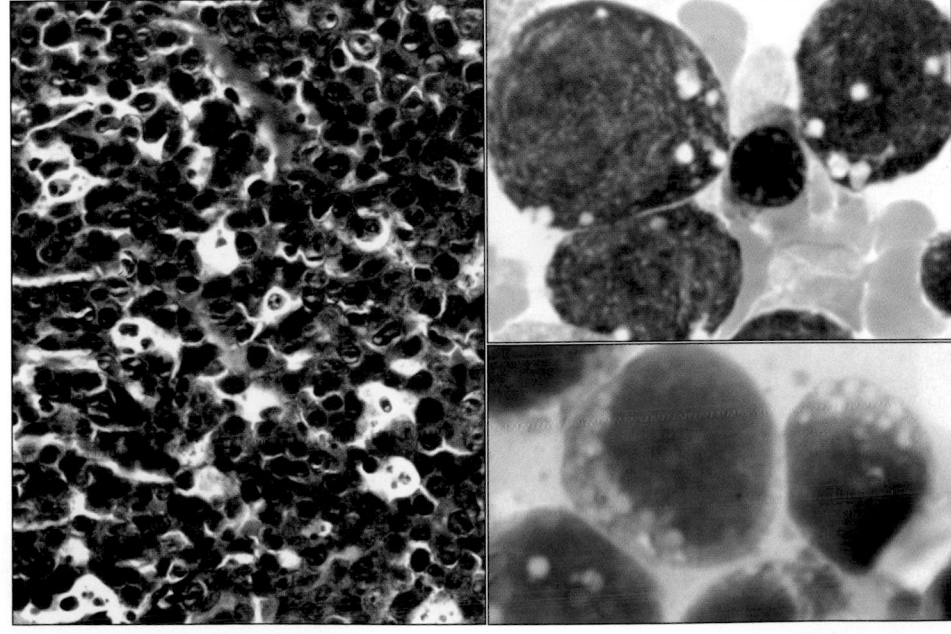

Fig. 12.16 Burkitt's lymphoma. Note the starry-sky pattern due to numerous tingible body macrophages engulfing cellular debris. The neoplastic cells are intermediate to large in size with the nucleus equal to the nucleus of a phagocytic histiocyte. They have a round or slightly oval nucleus with two or more nucleoli and moderate amount of deeply basophilic cytoplasm. The morphology of these malignant cells is indistinguishable from L3 of the FAB classification on Romanowsky-stained smear, which clearly displays prominent cytoplasmic vacuoles containing neutral lipid (lower right). (H&E stain, ×200; Romanowsky stain and oil red O stain, ×1000.)

Table 12.9 Immunologic classification of acute lymphoblastic leukemia

Immunology subtypes	Common phenotypes	Incidence (%) Children	Adults	FAB morphology	Comments
B-lineage (HLA-DR+, CD19+, cCD22+, cCD79a+)					
B-precursor ALL		70	50	L1,L2	t(12;21) in 20–25%
CALLA*-negative ALL	CD34⁺, TdT⁺				11q23 abnormalities; t(4;11) in infants
CALLA* – positive ALL	CD34⁺/⁻, TdT⁺, CD10⁺				t(9;22)
Pre-B ALL	TdT⁺/⁻, CD10⁺, cIgM⁺, CD20⁺/⁻	25	<5	L1,L2	t(1;19)
B-ALL	CD20⁺, CD10⁺/⁻, SIg⁺	2	2–5	L3	t(8;14);t(2;8);t(8;22)
T-lineage	CD7⁺, TdT⁺, cCD3⁺/⁻ (with variable expression of CD1, CD2, sCD3, CD5, CD4, CD8)	15	25	L1,L2	t(11;14);t(1;14); t(10;14);t(8;14)

*CALLA, common ALL antigen (CD10).
Data adapted from references 17, 125, 176, 187–189.

ponding non-Hodgkin's lymphoma in lymph nodes or other tissues. The marrow is markedly hypercellular with an absence of fat cells. Hematopoietic elements are markedly depleted. A few lymphocytes and plasma cells may be present, and mitoses may be numerous. Necrosis is not uncommon, but fibrosis is rarer than in AML. It should be pointed out that Burkitt's lymphoma/leukemia is classified under mature B-cell neoplasms in the WHO classification.[119]

Lymphoblastic lymphoma of T-cell type is more common than B-lymphoblastic lymphoma, comprising 85–90% of all cases; whereas T-ALL accounts for about 15% of childhood ALL and 25% of adult ALL.[124] Lymphoblastic lymphoma of T-cell type characteristically involves adolescent boys. These patients frequently present with a mediastinal mass and/or supradiaphragmatic lymphadenopathy. CNS involvement is not uncommon. Many patients also have bone marrow involvement. These patients tend to have a higher peripheral white cell count and blast count, with blasts displaying L1 (in the majority of cases) or L2 morphology. The blasts are TdT⁺, exhibiting focal globular paranuclear acid phosphatase positivity, and expressing CD7 or other T-cell markers. Most neoplastic cells in these cases express early T-precursor cell or cortical T cell antigens. A characteristic of T-cell malignancy is the loss of one or more specific T-cell antigens or the presence of aberrant combinations. Although these patients may initially respond to chemotherapy, remission duration is short, and testicular or CNS relapse is common.[177,178] Onciu and associates recently reported 26 adults with T-cell ALL and noted that patients older than 60 years had a low incidence of tissue infiltrate, with an initial WBC count less than 30 000/μl, abnormalities in chromosome 2 (especially 2q31), clonal T-cell receptor gamma (TCRγ) rearrangement, a pre-T or cortical T-cell phenotype with frequent CD34, CD13, and CD33 expression, and complete response to chemotherapy.[179] Precursor B-cell lymphoblastic lymphoma also affects young people, with 64% of patients less than 18 years old. Skin, lymph nodes, and bone are common sites of involvement; about 5% of cases present with a mediastinal mass.[180] Malignant cells express CD19, CD79a, CD10, and some of them are positive for CD20, TdT, and CD34. It is important to note that CD45 is present in 62% of cases, and 75% of cases express CD99.[180] Precursor B-ALL is common in children. Based on immunologic studies, precursor B-ALL may be subclassified into early preB-ALL(cCD79a⁺, cCD22⁺, TdT⁺, and CD19⁺), common ALL (in addition to the markers listed above, the blasts also express CD10), and preB-ALL (blasts possess all above listed antigen, also express cytoplasmic mu chain) (Table 12.9).

The WHO classification places Burkitt's lymphomas (BL) into mature B-cell neoplasms, and subgroups them into endemic BL, sporadic BL, and immunodeficiency-associated BL based on epidemiology study.[181] Morphologically, BL is classified into classical BL with a monomorphic population of medium-sized lymphoblasts, atypical Burkitt/Burkitt-like with greater pleomorphism in nuclear size and shape, and BL with plasmacytoid differentiation (more commonly seen in immunodeficiency states).[181] The endemic and sporadic BLs affect boys and young men with extranodal presentation. Over 90% of the patients with sporadic form have abdominal disease, particularly in the terminal ileum. Other sites, including bone marrow, ovary, testis, pleura, CNS, and peripheral lymph node, may also be involved. The malignant cells have a mature B-cell phenotype (Table 12.9). When it becomes leukemic, leukemic blasts display L3 morphology. Mature B-ALL constituted 2% (5/210) of pediatric and adult ALLs in a retrospective study.[182] Bone marrow involvement was found in 34% of patients in an European study of 65 adults with small noncleaved cell lymphoma and leukemia.[183] Rearrangement of c-*myc* oncogene (8q24) is frequently demonstrated.

Acute leukemias in infants   Infants less than 1 year of age account for 2.5–5% of all childhood ALL and 6–14% of all childhood AML.[184] Rearrangements of the *MLL* gene on chromosome 11q23 are the most common abnormalities, occurring in 70–80% of ALL and about 60% of AML, and are associated with an unfavorable prognosis. Translocation involving the *AF4* and *MLL* (t(4;11)) genes is most commonly seen in infants with ALL. These patients typically present with hyperleukocytosis, massive organomegaly, CNS involvement, CD10⁻ B-lineage phenotype and myeloid antigen (CD15) expression. A recent report from the MRC Childhood Leukaemia Working Party confirmed many of the above observations.[185] 11q23 rearrangement is closely linked to the monoblastic or myelomonoblastic phenotype and hyperleukocytosis.[184] The t(1;22)(p13;q13) occurs almost exclusively in infants with M7 and is associated with a low initial white cell count, bone marrow fibrosis, and organomegaly. The prognosis is poor.[135,136,184] 30–40% of reported cases with juvenile chronic myeloid leukemia occur in infants. Infants with this condition have a much better prognosis.[184] Congenital leukemia diagnosed within the first month of life is extremely uncommon. Both AML and ALL have been observed and are associated with poor prognosis.[184] Tsao and colleagues called to attention a group of patients characterized by infantile B-ALL with non-L3 morphology, expressing a mature

Table 12.10 Common nonrandom chromosomal abnormalities in acute leukemias

Disease entity	FAB classification	Chromosomal abnormalities	Genetic alterations	Frequency (%)* Adult	Children	Prognosis
AML						
	M2	t(8;21)(q22;q22)	AML1-ETO	5–10	5–10	Favorable
	M3	t(15;17)(q22;q11–22)	PML-RARα	5–10	5–10	Favorable
	M4Eo	inv(16) or t(16;16)(p13;q22)	CBFβ-MYH11	5–10	5–10	Favorable
	M4,M5	t(9;11)(p21–22;q23)	MLL-AF9	1–5	5–10	Favorable
	(M0),M1	t(9;22)(q34;q11)	bcr/abl	1–3	<1	Unfavorable
	M2,M4 marrow basophilia	t(6;9)(q23;q34)	DEK-CAN	<1	<1	Unfavorable
	M7 (infancy)	t(1;22)(p13;q13)	OTT-MAL	<1	2–3	Unfavorable
ALL						
B-lineage	L2	t(9;22)(q34;q11)	bcr/abl	25–40	4–6	Unfavorable
	L1,L2	t(1;19)(q23;p13.3)	E2A-PBX-1	2–3	5–6	Unfavorable in pre-B
	L1,L2	t(12;21)(p13;q22)	TEL-AML-1 (ETV6-CBFα2)	50	70	Favorable
	L1,L2	t(4;11)(q21;q23)	MLL-AF4	5	2	Unfavorable
	L3	t(8;14)(q24;q32.3)	MYC-IgH	4–5	1–2	Unfavorable
T-lineage	L1,L2	t(11;14)(p13;q11)	(RHOM2-TCRδ) (TTG2-TCRδ)	5–10	5–10	Unfavorable
	L1,L2	1p32	TAL-1 deletion	10–30	20–30	Some favorable

*The frequency within AML, B-lineage or T-lineage disease group.
Data from references 17, 26, 125, and 189.

B-cell phenotype (λSIg^+, $CD19^+$, $CD10^-$, $TdT^{-/+}$, and $CD34^{-/+}$), and showing MLL rearrangement with the majority being t(9;11).[186]

Clonal chromosomal abnormalities Nonrandom chromosomal changes have been frequently identified in subgroups of acute leukemia (Table 12.10).[17,26,125,187–194] Molecular studies link these structural changes to genetic alterations.[33,34] Although the mechanisms of leukemogenesis of the proto-oncogenes or tumor suppressor genes in leukemias and lymphomas are quite variable, they usually involve loss or gain of one or more entire chromosomes (hypodiploid or hyperdiploid) or long (q) or short (p) arms of a specific chromosome; other structural changes (translocations, inversions, or insertions) may also occur. Molecular studies have demonstrated that many of these structural chromosomal rearrangements create a fusion gene encoding a chimeric protein product binding to specific DNA sequences near target genes and altering the expression and/or structure of cellular gene products in hematopoietic cells. These changes result either directly or indirectly in functional activation that contributes to the promotion of leukemogenesis or inhibition of cell differentiation. These recurring (or nonrandom) chromosomal changes correlate with a particular subgroup of acute leukemias with characteristic morphologic and clinical findings. They provide important information regarding response to therapy and overall prognosis. Some of these changes, such as t(8;21); t(15;17) t(16;16) or inv(16) and 11q23 abnormalities, have been discussed earlier. The other important groups are listed below.

t(9;22) (q34;q11) (bcr/abl) The Philadelphia chromosome and its gene products first observed in >95% of patients with chronic myeloid leukemia (CML) may be detected in 3–5% of adults with de novo AML. When seen, it is most often associated with the FAB M0/M1 subtype.[190] The blasts from a number of these patients express B (CD19, CD24, CD20) and T (CD7) cell markers and CD10.[190] It is also found in 5% of children and 20–30% of adults with ALL. The c-*abl* oncogene on chromosome 9(q34) is juxtaposed to the *bcr* gene located on chromosome 22q11. Most ALL cells have a breakpoint within the *bcr* gene that differs from the breakpoint in CML. The

protein product of the fusion gene on chromosome 22 in ALL is smaller (p190) than that in CML (p210) but it also has abnormally modulated tyrosine kinase activity.[126] Philadelphia-chromosome-positive ALL is an aggressive disease both in children or adults. It frequently affects older children (median 9.6 years), with a high leukocyte count, FAB L2 morphology, and a pseudodiploid karyotype. 42 of the 56 (75%) cases with pediatric ALL are phenotyped as early pre-B, 9/56 cases as pre-B and 5/56 as T-cells.[191] In adult ALL cases, the leukemic blasts display L2 morphology, immature B-cell phenotype, with expression of CD10, and myeloid antigen (CD13 and CD33).[189] Molecular techniques or FISH are required to detect the gene rearrangement in some cases.

t(1;19)(q23;p13)(E2A/PBX-1) This chromosomal abnormality occurs quite frequently (25% in children and less than 5% in adults) in pre-B and less commonly (1%) in B-precursor ALL, AML, and T-ALL cases.[125,187,189] It is the most common translocation in childhood ALL. The presence of the t(1;19) correlates significantly with several recognized adverse prognostic indicators: high leukocyte counts, high serum lactate dehydrogenase levels, nonwhite race, DNA indexes of less than 1.6, and an increased incidence of CNS disease.[187,189] An association of pre-B-immunophenotype with t(1;19) denotes a poor prognosis and requires intensified chemotherapy. Pre-B-ALL without t(1;19) and B-precursor ALL with t(1;19) are not associated with a poor prognosis.[125]

t(4;11)(q21;q23)(AF4/MLL) Approximately 5% of all children, 70% of infants and 3–6% of adults with ALL have 11q23 rearrangements, primarily t(4;11)(q21;q23).[125,189] This chromosomal abnormality is associated with markedly elevated leukocyte count, splenomegaly, and a very poor prognosis.[192] Most cases have a B-precursor phenotype, usually CD10⁻. However, many have either features of myeloid leukemias or of mixed phenotype leukemias defined by cytochemical, immunophenotypic, or ultrastructural studies. Undifferentiated and, rarely, T cell or B cell ALL with t(4;11) have been reported. Coagulopathy and CNS involvement are characteristic of this type of leukemia.[125] RT-PCR or FISH is required to detect the genetic abnormality in some cases. Complete remission may be achieved after high-dose induction and consolidation chemotherapy.[192]

t(12;21)(p13;q22)(TEL/AML1) or (ETV6/CBFα2) Using molecular or FISH techniques, the t(12;21) is found in 25% of pediatric and 3–4% of adults with precursor-B ALL.[17,189] The t(12;21) defines a subgroup of ALL patients that are between 1 and 10 years of age (usually 3–5 years of age), with nonhyperdiploid DNA content, or B-lineage phenotype (HLA-DR⁺, CD19⁺, and CD10⁺), frequent expression (50% of cases) of myeloid-associated antigens (CD13 or CD33 or both) and an excellent prognosis.[17,18]

t(8;14)(q24;q32.3) (Myc/IGH) Reciprocal translocations involving the c-*myc* oncogene (8q24) with an immunoglobulin gene (14q32.3) are associated with FAB L3 morphology, and B cell phenotype (SIg⁺). It is found in 1–3% of cases of ALL. Less common translocations involving light chain genes ([kappa at 2p12, or lambda at 22q11 resulting in t(2;8)(p12;q24) and t(8;22)(q24;q11)]) have also been reported. Many of these patients may also have a malignant lymphoma, small noncleaved, Burkitt's type (discussed earlier). There is a high rate of CNS involvement. The prognosis is poor.

t(11;14)(p13;q11) (T-ALL/TCRα/δ)or (TTG2/TCRδ) This chromosomal abnormality is the most common form seen in childhood T-ALL.[187,193] In this condition, the *TCRα/δ* on chromosome 14q11 is spliced to a proto-oncogene (*T-ALL* on 11p13) and then serves as the driving force in dysregulated oncogene expression. A high percentage of T-cell ALL cases lack detectable cytogenetic abnormalities. Approximately 30–40% of the abnormal karyotypes in T-cell leukemias have nonrandom breakpoints within the 14q11 (*TCRα/δ*), 7q34-q36(*TCRβ*) or 7p35(*TCRγ*) region.[187,193] These T-cell receptor genes frequently form partners with one of the following genes leading to the over expression of specific genes and ultimately to leukemic transformation. Those genes that are involved in the pathogenesis of T-cell ALL include *MYC* (8q24), *TAL-1* (1p23), *TAL-2* (9q32), *LYL-1* (19p13), *LMO-1* (TTG-1, RBTN1, 11p15), *LMO-2* (RBTN2, 11p13), *HOX-11* (10q24), *LCK* (1p34) and *TAN-1* (9q34.3).[126,187,189,193]

Prognostic factors in acute leukemias As discussed above, certain nonrandomized chromosomal abnormalities have been associated with a better or worse clinical course. Currently, the overall complete remission rate for precursor B-ALL is approximately 95% in the pediatric age group and 60–85% in adults.[119] In general, about 70–80% of ALL and about 50% of AML in children is curable.[194] The results are not nearly as dramatic in adults.[195] The differing prognosis in adults and children has been attributed to differences in disease biology and in treatment tolerance. Tables 12.11 and 12.12 list the favorable and unfavorable prognostic factors in AML and ALL respectively.[118–126,135,196,197,198] Recently, *FLT3* mutations have been found to be common in acute leukemias, especially AML of M3 types.[199] Further, *FLT3* mutations are associated with young patients, higher peripheral blood blast count, normal karyotype, a higher relapse rate, and a significantly shorter event-free survival.[200]

At the present time, complete remission is defined by <5% of blasts in bone marrow examined by morphology. It is anticipated that a better estimate of the total body burden of leukemic cells would improve clinical management and cure rate. A variety of tools, such as PCR, flow cytometry combined with FISH, quantitative PCR, cell culture technique, or microarray analysis have been used to detect

Table 12.11 Prognostic factors in acute myeloid leukemias

Favorable	Intermediate	Unfavorable
t(8;21)(q22;q22)	Abnormal 11q23	Old age (>60)
t(15;17)(q22;q11)	+8	Complex chromosomal
Rearrangement of 16q22	+21	abnormalities
(inv(16) or t(16;16))	+22	t(9;22)(q34;q11)
	del (9q)	–7/7q– or –5/5q–
	del (7q)	t(1;22)(p13;q13) (infant)
	Normal karyotype	t(6;9)(p23;q34)
		Multilineage dysplasia
		Abnormal 3q
		p53 mutation
		Decreased Rb protein

Data from references 125, 126, 135,197, and 198.

Table 12.12 Prognostic factors in acute lymphoblastic leukemia

Favorable	Unfavorable
Hyperdiploid (>50 chromosomes)	Age <1 and >9
B-precursor ALL	High white blood cell count (>50×10⁹/l)
t(12;21)(p13;q22)	B- or T-cell phenotype
	Hypodiploid (<46 chromosomes)
	t(9;22)(q34;q11)
	Rearrangement of 8q24
	Rearrangement of 11q23
	t(4;11)(q21;q23)
	Pre-B-ALL with t(1;19)(q23;p13)

Data from references 119, 125, 126, and 196.

minimal residual disease (MRD).[26,31,201–203] Both the presence and the level of MRD correlate with survival.[26,31,204] It is recommended that patients who are not in 'molecular' or 'immunologic' remission, defined as fewer than one leukemic cell in 10 000 mononucleated bone marrow cells after induction therapy, should receive intensified therapy during morphologic remission.[204] Some AML-associated rearrangements continue to be positive with PCR analysis even while remission is achieved; therefore, the molecular detection of MRD, such as *AML/ETO* fusion gene, does not necessarily predict an increased risk of relapse.[205] Multidrug resistance protein (MDR-1) also known as P-glycoprotein (PgP) are detected by flow cytometry or molecular method, along with cytogenetic profile and clinical presentations, correlates with response to therapy in elderly AML patients.[17] It is obvious that large cooperative studies are needed in this area.

Acute leukemia of ambiguous lineage Truly undifferentiated acute leukemia that cannot be classified by morphology, cytochemistry, and immunophenotyping is uncommon, accounting for 1% of acute leukemias.[17] These leukemic cells express CD34 and HLA-DR but lack lineage-specific antigens. However, ALLs that co-express one or more myeloid-associated antigens or AMLs that co-express one or more lymphoid antigens are not uncommon. Thalhammer-Scherrer and associates reported an incidence of 18% and 23%, respectively, in the study of 325 adults with acute leukemias.[139] Five of 48 (9%) B-lineage ALLs and six of 14 (43%) T-lineage ALLs co-expressed myeloid markers.[139] Cruczman and

Table 12.13 Scoring system for markers proposed by the European Group for the Immunologic Classification of Leukaemia

Score	B-lymphoid	T-lymphoid	Myeloid
2	CytCD79a*†	CD3(m/cyt)†	MPO‡
	Cyt IgM	TCR α/β	
	CytCD22	TCR γ/δ	
1	CD19	CD2	CD117 (c-kit)
	CD20	CD5	CD13
	CD10	CD8	CD33
		CD10	CD65
0.5	TdT	TdT	CD14
	CD24	CD7	CD15
		CD1a	CD64

* cCD79a may also be expressed in some cases of precursor T lymphoblastic leukaemia/lymphoma.[36]
†cCD79a and cCD3 have been observed in AML.[139]
‡ MPO demonstrated by cytochemical or immunological method.
Biphenotypic acute leukaemia is defined when scores are over 2 for the myeloid and one of the lymphoid lineages.
Data adapted from references 36 and 208, with modifications.

colleagues studied 259 patients with adult ALLs and found that one-third of B-lineage ALLs and one-quarter of T-lineage ALLs co-expressed myeloid antigens.[206] In another study, Pui and co-workers found that 25 of 410 (6.1%) newly diagnosed childhood ALLs co-expressed two or more myeloid-associated antigens (My+ALL) and 16 of 95 (16.8%) newly diagnosed AMLs co-expressed two or more lymphoid associated antigens (Ly+AML).[207] These My+ALLs usually display L2 morphology, azurophilic cytoplasmic granules, acid alpha-naphthyl acetate esterase positivity, and unusual morphology (monocytoid features and cytoplasmic blebs).[207] In Ly+AML, dual populations of large and small blasts are often observed. Myeloperoxidase positivity is demonstrated in the large blasts only, but hand-mirror morphology is noted in small blasts.[207] CD2 is expressed in almost half of the cases of FAB M3, especially in microgranular variants; CD4 is expressed in two-thirds of cases of M4 or M5 leukemia; CD19 is found in three-quarters of cases of AML with t(8;21), and CD15 is expressed in two-thirds of ALL cases with t(4;11).[176] Clinically, mixed (hybrid) leukemias may be classified as biphenotypic leukemia (the individual leukemic blasts express both myeloid and lymphoid antigens), bilineal leukemia (in which the leukemic cells are heterogeneous and display either lymphoid or myeloid antigens but they originate from the same neoplastic clone), or biclonal leukemia (in which the heterogeneous leukemic cells are derived from two separate clones). Biphenotypic leukemia is probably the most common. Most investigators think that My+ALL and Ly+AML are not biphenotypic acute leukemia.[208] This term should be reserved for cases in which there is ambiguity of lineage assignment because of the presence of multiple antigens associated with more than one lineage.[208] A score system has been proposed by the European group.[209] Only when a score is more than 2 points involving the myeloid and one of the lymphoid lineages is the case classified as biphenotypic leukemia (Table 12.13).[209] Acute biphenotypic leukemias constitute 5% of all acute leukemias.[37,128] The prognosis is poor in this group of patients.[37] In addition, co-expression of CD79a and CD3 by lymphoblastic lymphoma has been reported.[210]

Myeloproliferative disorders

Chronic myeloproliferative disorders (CMPDs) are clonal disorders of the hemopoietic stem cells characterized by excessive proliferation of one or more hemopoietic cell lines with relatively normal differentiation and effective hematopoiesis, resulting in an increase in the quantities of one or more hematopoietic elements (cytosis) in the peripheral blood. Hepatomegaly and splenomegaly due to blood cell sequestration, extramedullary hematopoiesis, or leukemic infiltrate are common findings. They usually affect middle-aged or elderly individuals. CMPDs consist of four well defined clinical entities: polycythemia vera (PV), essential thrombocythemia (ET), chronic myeloid leukemia (CML), and agnogenic myeloid metaplasia (AMM, or chronic idiopathic myelofibrosis (myelofibrosis/osteomyelosclerosis)). Although the WHO classifies CMPDs into seven groups, adding chronic neutrophilic leukemia, chronic eosinophilic leukemia, and CMPD, unclassifiable,[211] we will limit the discussions to the four groups listed above.

Histologic recognition and classification of CMPDs depend on (1) the predominant proliferative cell line; (2) the degree of its differentiation; and (3) the fibrotic reaction. It should be emphasized that subgroups of CMPDs often overlap. Myelofibrosis may develop in PV, CML, and ET. Also, PV, AMM, and CML may evolve into acute leukemia. Chronic myelomonocytic leukemia (CMML) and juvenile CML share the characteristics of myeloproliferative disorder and MDS, and are discussed under MDS.

Polycythemia vera Polycythemia vera is a slowly progressive clonal stem cell disorder, characterized by an absolute erythrocytosis, hypervolemia and panhyperplasia of the bone marrow, with variable excess production of leukocytes and platelets.[212] Serum erythropoietin levels are usually low and hypersensitivity to several cytokines, including erythropoietin, insulin-like growth factor, and others in the in-vitro system has been demonstrated.[213] Bleeding and arterial and venous thrombosis are common complications that contribute to the mortality and morbidity of these patients.[214] Clinically, PV usually has an insidious onset followed by a proliferative phase and the 'spent' or postpolycythemic phase in which cytopenias are associated with ineffective hematopoiesis, bone marrow fibrosis, and extramedullary hematopoiesis. Splenomegaly is common. Some patients may develop MDS, acute leukemia, or solid tumors.[214]

The original diagnostic criteria proposed by the Polycythemia Vera Study Group have been revised as follows:

- *Category A*

1. Red cell mass >25% above mean normal predicted value (or packed cell volume (hematocrit) >0.60 for males and >0.56 for females))
2. Absence of causes of secondary erythrocytosis
3. Palpable splenomegaly
4. Clonality marker, i.e. acquired abnormal marrow karyotype

- *Category B*

1. Platelet count >400 × 10⁹/l
2. Neutrophil count >10 × 10⁹/l (in smokers >12.5 × 10⁹/l)
3. Splenomegaly demonstrated by ultrasound scanning
4. Characteristic BFU-E growth or reduced serum erythropoietin.

A diagnosis of PV is established if the following combinations are present: A1 + A2 + A3 or A4, or A1 + A2 + two of the items in category B.[212] Also, bone marrow histopathology has been proposed to be included in the diagnosis.

The peripheral blood smear usually reveals normocytic–normochromic or microcytic–hypochromic red blood cells with mild neutrophilia, eosinophilia, basophilia, and thrombocytosis at

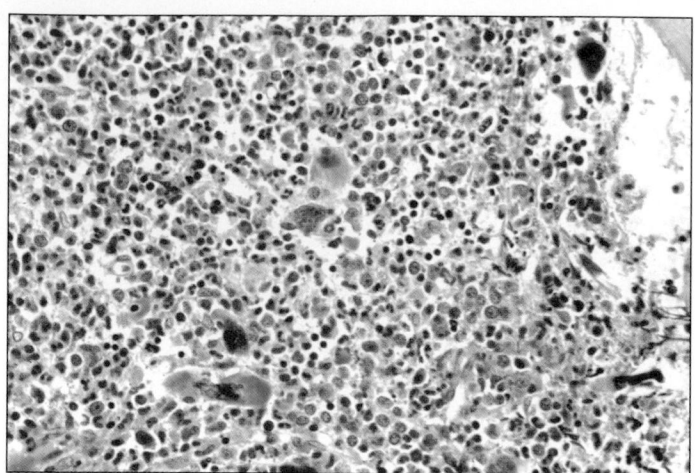

Fig. 12.17 Spent phase of polycythemia vera. Panmyelosis involving all hematopoietic cell lines with aggregates of abnormal-looking megakaryocytes. (H&E stain, ×250.)

the early stage. The bone marrow biopsy shows panhyperplasia. Megakaryocytic hyperplasia may be striking, with abnormal (dysplastic) forms present (variably sized and shaped nuclei and variable cytoplasmic density). In addition, megakaryocytes frequently form clusters. Increased reticulin fibers may be demonstrated by special stains. Irregularly dilated and expanded sinusoids may be seen, some of which contain islands of nucleated red cells and megakaryocytes. It should be pointed out that increased reticulin fibrosis and dilatation of sinusoids are more prominent in the late stage ('spent' phase) of the disease. Also, those patients with marked megakaryocytic hyperplasia on bone marrow biopsies tend to develop myelofibrosis, which may be related to the production of cytokine (such as transforming growth factor-beta, TGFβ) by these cells[213,215] (Fig. 12.17). Absent iron stores are characteristic, which may be due to increased consumption in response to erythroid hyperplasia or may be secondary to repeated phlebotomies.

Among those patients who lived more than 8 years, about 10–25% developed postpolycythemic myeloid metaplasia and another 5–10% developed AML.[216] It appears that patients who received alkylating agents had an increased incidence of malignancies, whereas those who received phlebotomy had an increased risk of thrombosis and myelofibrosis.[214]

Chromosomal abnormalities have been demonstrated in 25–50% of patients. The most common abnormalities included +8, +9, and 20q–.[217] Frequently, +8 and +9 are observed together in the same clone.[218] Recently, an association between del(13)(q12q14) in patients with PV and myelofibrosis with myeloid metaplasia has been suggested.[218] Patients who have abnormal clones at diagnosis appear to have a shorter survival than those patients who do not have them. Abnormal clones emerge with progression of the disease.

The differential diagnosis includes (1) secondary erythrocytosis, in which megakaryocytes are normal in number and in morphology, with preservation of fat cells and reticulin structure. In addition, over expression of mRNA of polycythemia rubra vera 1 (PRV-1) in mature peripheral blood granulocytes, and decreased, unevenly stained c-Mpl megakaryocytes by immunohistochemistry in bone marrow of PV patients may be used to differentiate these two entities;[219] (2) CML (in which the erythroid precursors are usually decreased in number and Philadelphia chromosome or bcr/abl is demonstrated);

and (3) AMM. However, AMM cannot be differentiated from postpolycythemic myeloid metaplasia without appropriate history.

Essential thrombocythemia Essential thrombocythemia is considered to be a clonal CMPD, characterized by persistent thrombocytosis with recurrent episodes of thrombosis (mainly arterial thrombosis) and hemorrhage. Cytogenetic studies fail to demonstrate consistent chromosomal abnormalities.[218] Clonal assessment using X-chromosome inactivation patterns reveal that, while 43% of evaluable samples display clonal hematopoiesis, the rest are polyclonal.[220] The diagnosis of ET is largely made by excluding other disorders manifested by thrombocytosis, such as reactive thrombocytosis, hereditary (familial) thrombocytosis, other CMPD or some MDS.[221,222] The updated diagnostic criteria are as follows: (1) platelet count $>600 \times 10^9/l$; (2) hematocrit <40, or normal RBC mass (males <36 ml/kg, females $<32 \times 10^9/lml/kg$); (3) stainable iron in marrow or normal ferritin or normal RBC mean corpuscular volume; (4) no Philadelphia chromosome or bcr/abl gene rearrangement; (5) collagen fibrosis of marrow (a) absent or (b) less than one-third biopsy area without both marked splenomegaly and leukoerythroblastic reaction; (6) no cytogenetic or morphologic evidence for an MDS; and (7) no cause for reactive thrombocytosis.[223,224]

ET is largely a disease of elderly patients with a male to female ratio of 0.69. At the time of diagnosis, approximately one-third of patients are asymptomatic and two-thirds of patients have symptoms and signs related to elevated platelet count and abnormal platelet functions.[225] Only one of those 147 patients followed by Fenaux and associates developed acute leukemia, 95 months after diagnosis.[225] ET is associated with a prolonged survival and about 80% are alive 5–8 years after diagnosis. Sterkers and colleagues found that 4.5% of their 357 patients progressed to acute myeloid leukemia or MDS after a median interval of 84 months between diagnosis of ET and diagnosis of AML or MDS.[226] Most patients received a variety of cytoreduction therapies. These investigators noticed an association of 17p deletion (so called 17p– syndrome) and hydroxyurea therapy. Those patient with 17p– syndrome have typical dysgranulopoiesis including pseudo-Pelger–Hüet, hypolobulation and small vacuoles in >5% neutrophils, and p53 mutation.[226] Apparently, leukemic evolution is rare in untreated ET.

The peripheral blood smear reveals thrombocytosis with platelet anisocytosis, giant platelets, bizarre shape, and pseudopods. Basophilia is absent. The bone marrow is usually hypercellular (but may be normo- or hypocellular), with moderate to marked increase in megakaryocytes. These megakaryocytes are mature with highly lobulated or polypoid nuclei (Fig. 12.18). They usually form clusters. An unevenly and decreased megakaryocyte c-Mpl staining pattern has been described in patients with ET.[219] An increase in reticulin fibers is often noted.[222] ET may progress into myelofibrosis or rarely MDS and acute leukemia.

Chronic myeloid leukemia Chronic myeloid leukemia is a clonal disorder due to malignant transformation of a primitive cell, probably involving the pluripotent hematopoietic stem cell. The Philadelphia chromosome,[227] originally described as shortening of the long arm of chromosome 22 and its fusion protein product, is identified in more than 95% of CML, 20–30% of adult ALL, and <5% of adult AML, as well as 5% of childhood ALL.[125,126] This marker chromosome, Philadelphia, has been found in erythroid, granulocytic, monocytic, and megakaryocytic lineages, as well as in B and some T cells from patients with CML. The Philadelphia (Ph) chromosome translocation activates the cellular Abelson (c-abl)

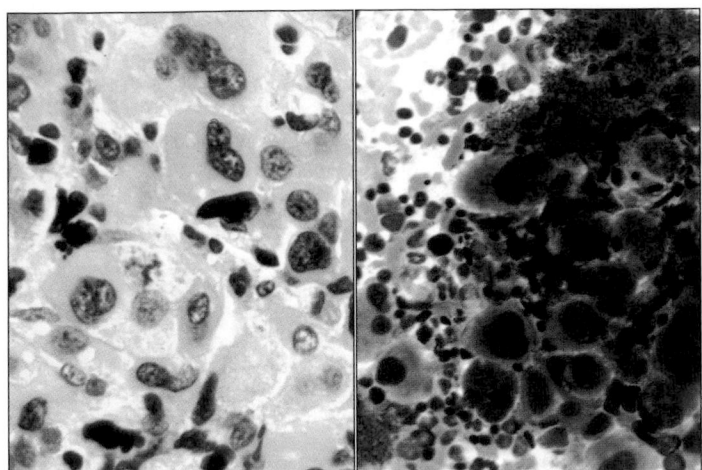

Fig. 12.18 Essential thrombocythemia. Aggregates of megakaryocytes with dysplastic features and clumps of platelets are dominant findings. (H&E stain, and Romanowsky stain, ×400.)

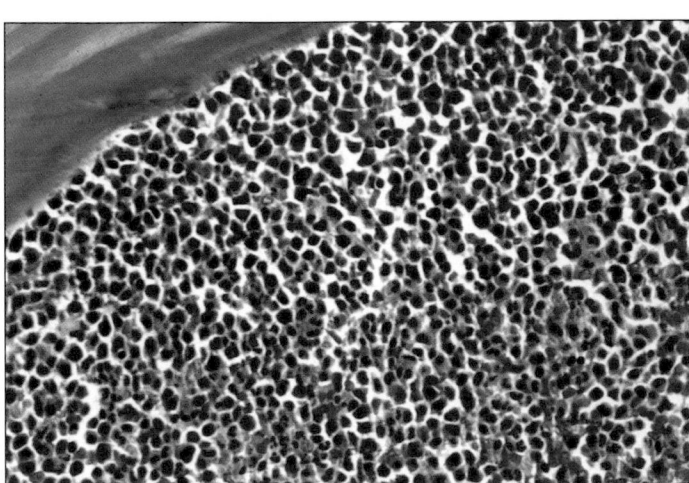

Fig. 12.19 Chronic myeloid leukemia. Note myeloid hyperplasia with 10–15 layers of immature myeloid cells present along the bony trabeculae in comparison to normal or reactive condition which has three to five layers of immature cells (see Fig. 12.3). (H&E stain, ×250.)

proto-oncogene on chromosome 9q34 by joining 3′ *abl* coding sequences with the 5′ coding sequences of the 'breakpoint cluster region' (*bcr*) gene on chromosome 22q11. The fusion proteins *bcr/abl* of CML, ALL, and AML have increased tyrosine kinase activity and show a transforming potential in vitro and in animal models. The effects of this kinase activation may include prolonged and growth-factor-independent proliferation of myeloid progenitor cells, defective adherence of CML progenitors to marrow stromal elements, and reduced apoptosis of hematopoietic cells.[228,229]

Several different breakpoints may occur on chromosome 22, resulting in at least three different *bcr/abl* chimeric proteins: m-*bcr* (p210$^{bcr/abl}$) seen in 95% or more of CML, m-*bcr* (p190$^{bcr/abl}$) in 50% of adults and 80% of children with Ph$^+$ ALL and in rare cases of CML, and μ-*bcr* (p230$^{bcr/abl}$).[228] The expression of p190$^{bcr/abl}$ in CML may be associated with monocytosis, and the expression of p230$^{bcr/abl}$ may be associated with the chronic neutrophilic variant of CML with thrombocytosis.[228] It is of note that the transforming ability of p190 is greater than that of p210 in vitro. Additional chromosomal abnormalities are often identified in CML in blast crisis, such as +8, i(17q), +19, and extra Philadelphia chromosomes.[218] About 15% of patients with CML in blast crisis have −7, −17, +17, +21, −Y or t(3;21)(q26;q22).[218]

CML is primarily a disease of middle-aged adults but may occur at any age, including infancy. The most common symptoms relate to anemia, splenomegaly, and an increased metabolic rate. The leukocyte count is usually in excess of 50×10^9/l but may be less. Signs of leukostasis may be seen in patients with excessive leukocytosis. Neutrophilia with left shift (so-called 'myelocyte bulge'), eosinophilia, basophilia, and thrombocytosis are common findings. The leukocyte alkaline phosphatase (LAP) level is decreased in most patients unless the patient has concurrent infection, in which case the LAP level may be normal or even elevated. The bone marrow is extremely hypercellular with marked granulocytic hyperplasia evidenced by broad paratrabecular and perivascular seams of immature myeloid precursors (5–10 cells in thickness compared to 1–2 cells in thickness under normal conditions) and mature granulocytes in the central regions of the marrow cavity. Although granulopoiesis appears to be normal in maturation, there is a marked increase in eosinophils and basophils.

Blasts and promyelocytes are usually less than 10% of all nucleated cells. Mast cells are usually normal. Erythropoiesis is appreciably decreased, with a myeloid to erythroid ratio of 10:1–15:1 (Fig. 12.19). The number of megakaryocytes varies even within different marrow spaces in a single biopsy; they are frequently small and hypolobulated. They may form clusters or are dispersed throughout the marrow cavities. Histiocytes containing crystalloid structures (Gaucher-like cells) or sea-blue histiocytes (usually seen on bone marrow smears) are present. Reticulin fibers may be increased.[222]

Some CML patients will develop progressive marrow failure with increasing anemia and thrombocytopenia, increasing spleen size, and increasing leukocyte count, which are unresponsive to treatment. These patients have undergone a transformation of CML from a chronic phase to an accelerated phase.[219,230,231] This condition may be recognized when one or more of the followings are present: (1) blasts 10–19%; (2) peripheral blood basophilia (>20%); (3) persistent thrombocytopenia ($<100 \times 10^9$/l) unrelated to therapy, or persistent thrombocytosis ($>1000 \times 10^9$/l) unresponsive to therapy; (4) increasing spleen size and increasing white cell count unresponsive to therapy; and (5) cytogenetic or molecular evidence of clonal evolution.[219,231] The duration for this accelerated phase is unpredictable. Progression to a blast crisis phase may occur.

Blastic transformation of CML is generally defined as 30% (20% according to WHO classification) or more blasts in the blood or bone marrow smears or a focus of blasts in a marrow biopsy or extramedullary site.[219,231] The blasts may show myeloid (about 70% of cases), lymphoid (about 30%), or mixed differentiation morphologically and immunophenotypically.[232,233] Most lymphoid blast crisis cases are of precursor B-cell linage, but rare T-cell blast crisis cases have been reported.[233] Khalidi and associates showed that it was often difficult to classify these cases of CML in blast transformation precisely based on morphology and flow cytometry studies.[232] Six cases (85.7%) with a precursor-B immunophenotype expressed two to four myeloid antigens, including myeloperoxidase (in 2/6 cases).[232] Four of the six cases fulfilled proposed criteria for biphenotypic leukemia.[36,232] Of the 13 cases that were classified as AML, 69% expressed the megakaryocyte-associated antigen CD61 and 53.8% expressed T-cell-associated antigen, CD4 and CD7.[232] It is of interest to note while p210$^{bcr/abl}$ product was detected in all

Table 12.14 Comparison of laboratory findings in chronic myeloid leukemia (CML), atypical CML (aCML), and chronic myelomonocytic leukemia (CMMoL)

	CML	aCML	CMMoL
Leukocytosis	Marked	Moderate	Mild to moderate
Monocytosis	Usually no	Variable	Yes
Absolute basophilia	Yes	No	No
Granulocytic dysplasia	–	++	+
Immature granulocytes in blood (%)	>20	10–20	≤10
Blasts (%)	≤2	>2	<2
Ph chromosome, *bcr/abl*	+	–	–
Bone marrow erythroblasts (%)	<10	≤15	>15

Data adapted from references 222, 234, 235, and 236

cases, none of them had p190$^{bcr/abl}$ product. The Ph fusion proteins, p190$^{bcr/abl}$ and p210$^{bcr/abl}$, may be used as markers to differentiate Ph$^+$ ALL from CML in blast crisis. The histopathology of the bone marrow may be indistinguishable from that of acute leukemias, except that an increase of eosinophils and basophils is more common in CML in blast crisis than in acute leukemias.

The differential diagnosis of CML includes other chronic MPD, atypical CML (aCML) and chronic myelomonocytic leukemia (CMMoL).[222,231,234,235] As stated earlier, the Philadelphia chromosome and its *bcr/abl* fusion protein are detected in more than 95% of cases with CML, and there is no difference in clinical presentations, evolution of the disease, and response to therapy in molecular Ph$^+$ but karyotypic Ph$^+$ or Ph$^-$ cases. The *bcr/abl$^-$* CML cases are heterogeneous. The major differences among CML, aCML, and CMMoL are listed in Table 12.14.[222,234–236] aCML and CMMoL will be discussed later in detail.

Much progress has been made in the treatment of CML.[237] During the chronic phase of CML, cytoreductive therapy such as hydroxyurea or busulfan leads to hematologic remissions in 90% of patients.[237] It has been reported that 70% of patients who received allogeneic bone marrow or stem cell transplant survived 10 years. For those patients who are not eligible for allogeneic bone marrow transplant, interferon alfa can induce hematologic and cytogenetic remission in patients with CML in chronic phase.[237] Thiele and associates studied sequential bone marrow biopsies on patients with Ph$^+$ CML who received busulfan, hydroxyurea, or interferon alfa.[238] They found a significant increase in the number of megakaryocytes and myelofibrosis in patients who have been treated with interferon alfa and less so with busulfan and hydroxyurea, although a complete hematologic response was noted in many patients. Hochhaus and co-workers used RT-PCR to quantify levels of *bcr/abl* transcripts in case of Ph$^+$ chronic CML who had been treated with interferon alfa, finding that molecular evidence of disease was rarely if ever eliminated even in patients with complete hematology response.[239] Recently, a tyrosine kinase inhibitor, STI571 (Gleevec, imatinib mesylate) has been introduced to treat patients with CML or CML in blast crisis.[39,40] The initial results are promising. Hematologic and morphologic responses were seen in most patients, although only one-third of patients had some degree of cytogenetic response.[229] Cytogenetic responses occurred more frequently in patients treated in the chronic phase than in patients treated in the accelerated phase or blast phase.[229] More study is needed in these areas.

Chronic idiopathic myelofibrosis Chronic idiopathic myelofibrosis (CIMF) or AMM is a clonal disorder of hematopoietic cells with reactive fibrosis. It is characterized by marked poikilocytosis with dacrocytes and a leukoerythroblastic blood picture, panmyelosis, bone marrow fibrosis, and extramedullary hematopoiesis. Patients usually present with symptoms of anemia, hepatosplenomegaly, and hyperuricemia. Atypical, large and hypogranular platelets and abnormal megakaryocyte nuclei are circulating in the blood. Blasts may be present in the blood. A basophilia is also noted. Radiographic evidence of osteosclerosis has been reported in 30–70% of patients. Bone marrow aspiration is usually unsuccessful (dry tap). Bone biopsy is necessary for diagnosis. The following histologic patterns have been described.[240]

- *Panhyperplasia:* the marrow is hypercellular with effacement of normal architecture and compartmentalization of hematopoiesis. Aggregates of dysplastic megakaryocytes are frequently surrounded by reticulin fibers. The sinusoids are irregular in shape, often dilated, with sclerosis of sinusoidal walls. Intrasinusoidal hematopoiesis is evident. This pathology is often seen in the early or prefibrotic stage of CIMF.
- *Myeloid atrophy and fibrosis:* alternating areas of fibrosis and hematopoiesis are seen. All hematopoietic cell lines are usually present but megakaryocytes predominate.
- *Myelofibrosis and osteosclerosis:* this is characterized by replacement of the marrow cavity with broad, irregular, twisted trabeculae (without the regular lamellar appearance) and fibrotic marrow. Normal hematopoietic elements are markedly decreased. The hematopoietic cells present are primarily megakaryocytes.

These different patterns may be found simultaneously in different parts of the skeleton or even of the same section, although most investigators consider that there is an early cellular phase and a late fibro-osteosclerotic stage.[219,222,233,240,241] However, as the disease progresses, reticulin fibrosis is often replaced with collagen fibrosis. It should be pointed out that myelofibrosis may be associated with a variety of benign and malignant disorders and reticulin fibrosis may not be evident in the early or cellular phase of CIMF without a reticulin stain. Likewise, extramedullary hematopoiesis or myeloid metaplasia is not pathognomonic of CIMF. A constellation of clinical and pathological characteristics is necessary to reach a correct diagnosis.[242,243]

The pathogenetic mechanisms for CIMF are not clear, although an abnormal clone has been detected in 35–60% of patients with CIMF.[218,244] The most common abnormalities are del(13q), del(20q), and partial trisomy 1q. Other findings include trisomy 8, del(7q), isochromosome long arm 17, or trisomy 9.[218,244] It should be pointed out that del(13)(q12q14) is often associated with marrow fibrosis, such as CIMF, or myelofibrosis with PV, CML, and ET.[245] A similar deletion has been found in chronic lymphocytic leukemia (CLL) and multiple myeloma (MM) patients in whom myelofibrosis was not detected.[218] It has been postulated that the stromal reaction (myelofibrosis) of the bone marrow in patients with CIMF is a reactive process mediated by cytokines that are produced by the neoplastic megakaryocytes and monocytes.[242] These cytokines may augment fibroblast proliferation (platelet-derived growth factor and calmodulin), collagen synthesis (TGFβ), angiogenesis (vascular endothelial growth factor and basic fibroblast growth factor) and osteogenesis (TGFβ and basic fibroblast growth factor).[242,243]

The differential diagnosis includes secondary myelofibrosis following other CMPDs, metastatic tumors, leukemias, Hodgkin's lymphoma, and non-Hodgkin's lymphoma. The characteristics of subgroups of CMPD are summarized in Table 12.15. Myelofibrosis

Table 12.15 Comparison of important characteristics of chronic myeloproliferative disorders

	Polycythemia vera	Chronic myeloid leukemia	Essential thrombocythemia	Chronic idiopathic myelofibrosis
Peripheral blood				
RBC count	↑↑↑	N or ↓	N or ↑	N or ↓
WBC count	N	↑ to ↑↑↑	N	N or ↑
Platelet count	↑↑	N to ↑↑↑	↑↑↑	N or ↑↑
NRBCs	Rare	Occasional	Rare	Many
Anisopoikilocytosis	0 to +	0 to +	0 to +	0 to +++
Bone marrow				
Cellularity	Panyhyperplasia, ↓ iron store	Marked myeloid hyperplasia, megakaryocytic hyperplasia ±	Marked megakaryocytic hyperplasia	Variable; with dysplastic megakaryocytes; or 'dry tap'; fibrosis
Reticulin fibers				
Early stage	Focal, mild	N to ↑	N	↑ to ↑↑
Late stage	↑↑↑*	↑ ↑ to ↑↑↑*	N to ↑↑↑*	↑↑↑
Cytogenetic abnormalities	+8, +9, 20q–, or others	Ph chromosome or *bcr/abl* fusion products	No consistent findings	13q–, 20q–, partial trisomy 1q
Frequency (% patients)	20–40	>95	5	40–60
Prognosis	Relatively good	Fair to poor	Relatively good	Poor

* Myelofibrosis may develop in 40% of patients with polycythemia vera, 20–40% with chronic myeloid leukemia, 5% or so with essential thrombocythemia.

may occur in response to other stimuli, such as toxins, drugs, radiotherapy, and bone disease.

The prognosis for patients with CIMF is poor, with a median survival of 3.5–5.5 years. Several scoring systems have been developed.[241,242,244,246] The following are considered to be the most important poor prognostic indicators: advanced age, anemia, leukopenia or leukocytosis, and abnormal karyotypes. Fibrosis of the bone marrow is discussed further in a later section. Please refer to standard hematology textbooks for other uncommon CMPDs.

Myelodysplastic syndromes Myelodysplastic syndromes encompass a group of clinically well recognized, heterogenous acquired clonal stem cell disorders characterized by qualitative and quantitative changes within one or more hematopoietic cell lines, resulting in progressive marrow failure. These disorders are refractory to treatment – most patients die of complications of bone marrow dysfunction or hematopoietic neoplasia. About 15–25% of the patients having the disease eventually develop acute leukemia. MDSs occur as primary diseases or therapy-related disorders. Therapy-related MDSs occur in patients who have been exposed to chemotherapy and radiotherapy, and have been discussed earlier. Most of the following discussions are focused on primary MDS.

Adult patients with MDSs are usually in their sixth or seventh decade. The diseases start with an insidious onset and run a slowly progressive course. Cytopenias with refractory anemia and dyspoiesis of circulating nucleated cells and of marrow cell lines are pertinent laboratory findings. The qualitative abnormalities involving hematopoiesis seen in MDSs are listed in Table 12.7. The FAB Cooperative Group subclassifies the MDSs into five groups: (1) refractory anemia (RA); (2) RA with ring sideroblasts (RARS); (3) RA with excess of blasts (RAEB); (4) chronic myelomonocytic leukemia (CMML); and (5) RAEB in transformation (RAEB-T).[247] The FAB classification is based on the presence of dyspoietic features with quantification of erythrocytic precursors (see Fig. 12.10) and the number of type I, type II and type III blasts in the bone marrow smears (see Fig. 12.12). The characteristics of the various subtypes are listed in Table

12.16.[247] The FAB states that, when the percentage of blasts present in the bone marrow is 30% or more, a diagnosis of acute leukemia is made. The number of blasts present in the bone marrow of patients with MDS can range from normal to less than 30% (see Fig. 12.10). Recognition of these subtypes may be difficult in a core biopsy specimen and immunohistochemical study may be needed to distinguish different cell lines.[248]

It should be noted that not all patients who have dysplastic changes, especially megaloblastoid erythropoiesis, have MDS. Deficiencies of vitamin B_{12} and folate, viral infections, such as infection with human immunodeficiency virus (HIV), exposure to chemotherapeutic agents, alcohol, or other chemicals can induce dysplastic changes.[249] The demonstration of a clonal chromosomal abnormality in a patient with a suspected MDS lends strong support to the diagnosis. A normal karyotype, however, does not exclude the diagnosis.

The cellularity of the bone marrow may be variable, although hypercellular marrow is most common. All hematopoietic cell lines may exhibit dysplastic changes, with increased precursors (Fig. 12.20, Table 12.16). In addition, the normal topographic distribution of erythropoiesis, myelopoiesis, and megakaryopoiesis may be disrupted. Clustered myeloblasts may be present in the central part of the marrow (abnormal localization of immature precursors) prior to the increased blast count by aspiration (Fig. 12.21). Abnormal localization of immature precursors (ALIP) is defined as the presence of three or more myeloblasts or promyelocytes clustering centrally in the marrow. There must be more than three ALIPs per section before they can be considered to be of diagnostic importance.[248,250] It should be pointed out that ALIP is not specific for MDS. Similar changes may be observed in regenerating marrows in patients who were treated for acute leukemias. They are also seen in patients with AIDS with dyspoiesis. Further, it is important to recognize that aggregates of immature erythroid and megakaryocytic cells, as demonstrated by immunohistochemistry, may also mimic the appearance of an ALIP (pseudo-ALIP).[248] The core biopsy is very useful for the detection of reticulin fibrosis (an uncommon form of MDS – MDS with

Table 12.16 Comparison of morphology features in subgroups of myelodysplastic syndrome according to FAB classification

Subgroups	Peripheral blood findings		Bone marrow findings		Others
	Blasts (%)	Abnormalities	Blasts (%)	Abnormalities	
RA	<1	Anemia; dyserythropoiesis	<5	Erythroid hyperplasia and dysplasia	–
RARS	<1	Same as above; dimorphic RBCs	<5	Same as above; ≥15% ring sideroblasts	–
RAEB	<5	Bicytopenia or pancytopenia; dyserythropoiesis and dysgranulopoiesis	5–20	Multilineage or unilineage dysplasia	No Auer rods
CMML	<5	Absolute monocytosis (>1 × 10^9/l); dysgranulopoiesis ±	<20	Same as above	Increased promonocytes
RAEB-T	>5	Bicytopenia or pancytopenia	21–29	Same as above	Auer rods +

CMML, chronic myelomonocytic leukemia; RA, refractory anemia; RAEB, refractory anemia with excess of blasts; RAEB-T, refractory anemia with excess blasts in transformation; RARS, refractory anemia with ring sideroblasts.
Data adapted from reference 247.

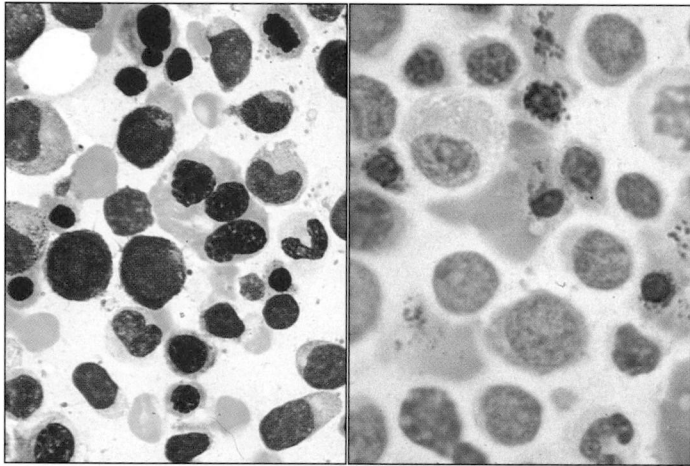

Fig. 12.20 Refractory anemia with ring sideroblasts. Note megaloblastic and megaloblastoid erythropoiesis with erythrons containing multiple nuclei. Ring sideroblasts are evident. (Romanowsky stain, ×630; Prussian blue stain, ×1000.)

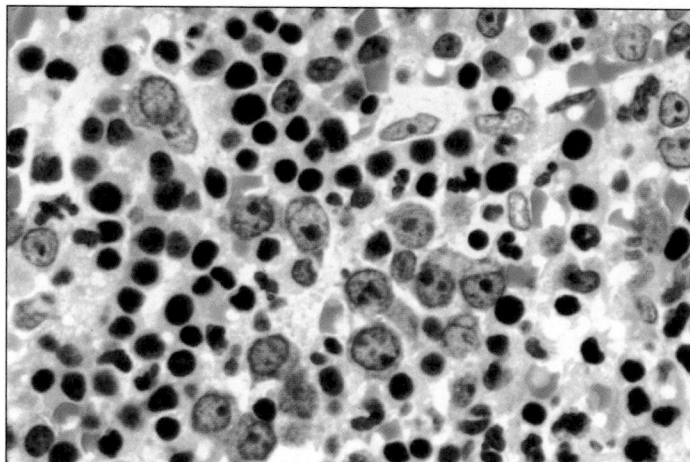

Fig. 12.21 Abnormal localization of immature myeloid precursors. Clusters of immature myeloid cells are present in the center of the marrow cavity, admixed with erythropoietic islands. Note that immature myeloid cells have an oval or round slightly eccentrically placed nucleus, evenly distributed lacy chromatin, one or more nucleoli, and a moderate amount of cytoplasm, with or without a prominent Golgi apparatus. (H&E stain, ×600.)

myelofibrosis), for the accurate diagnosis of the rare hypoplastic variant of MDS and for the identification of a uniform population of monolobulated micromegakaryocytes in 5q– syndrome.[251] Patients with *MDS with myelofibrosis* often have pancytopenia or bicytopenia, a hypercellular bone marrow with marked fibrosis, trilineage dysplasia, atypical megakaryocytic proliferation with many micromegakaryocytes, or megakaryocytes with hypolobated nuclei. Hepatosplenomegaly at diagnosis is usually minimal or absent.[252] This entity has to be differentiated from acute panmyelosis with myelofibrosis and agnogenic myelofibrosis and myelometaplasia (chronic idiopathic myelofibrosis). Hypoplastic MDS has been discussed above. *5q- syndrome* is the term used to describe those patients who have isolated deletion of 5q. Most afflicted patients are elderly females who have macrocytic anemia that is resistant to conventional therapy (refractory anemia), normal or elevated platelet count, erythroid hypoplasia, and unilobulated megakaryocytes in the marrow (Fig. 12.22).[251] The clinical course is usually mild, with infrequent progress to acute leukemia at which time additional chromosomal abnormalities are often identified.

Cytogenetic abnormalities Clonal abnormalities are found in 30–50% of de novo MDS and 80% of therapy-related MDS.[253] However, none of these cytogenetic abnormalities is specific to MDS. Unlike cases in acute leukemias, cytogenetic changes in MDS are characterized by total or partial chromosomal losses (such as 5q–, 20q–, 11q– and 7q– or –7 and –y), a relatively high incidence of chromosome gains (such as +8, +11, and acquired +21), and the rarity of translocations (except in therapy-related MDS). The unbalanced translocations generally involve chromosomes 1, 3, 5, 7, and 17. Complex cytogenetic abnormalities (involving three or more chromosomes) occur in about 15% of MDS and about 50% of therapy-related MDS. Many of these cases involve chromosomes 7 and 5.[253] Verhoef and Boogaerts found that certain chromosomal changes were more common in certain subgroups of MDS.[254] For instance, 5q–, +8 and –7 were common in RA whereas +8, 5q– and structural changes of 11q– were more frequently observed in RARS. In CMML, 5q–, –7, +8 and

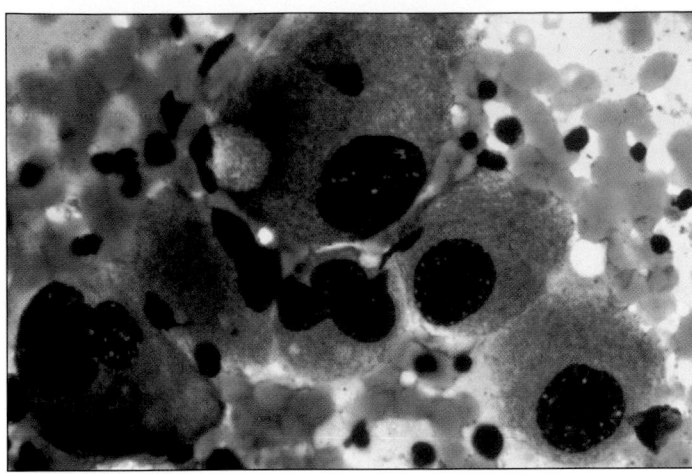

Fig. 12.22 5q– syndrome. Note an aggregate of mononucleated or hypolobated megakaryocytes. (Romanowsky stain, ×400.)

Table 12.17 International Prognostic Scoring System for myelodysplastic syndrome (survival and evolution to acute myeloid leukemia)

Prognostic variables	Score value				
	0	0.5	1.0	1.5	2.0
Bone marrow blasts (%)	<5	5–10	–	11–20	21–30
Karyotype	Good	Intermediate	Poor		
Cytopenias*	0/1	2/3			

*Cytopenias were defined as a hemoglobin level <10 g/dl, an absolute neutrophils count <1800/μl, and a platelet count <100 000/μl
From Greenberg et al.[255]

translocation or deletion of the short arm of chromosome 12 were found, but patients with RAEB or RAEB-T have more complex karyotypic abnormalities.[254]

Prognostic factors Several groups of investigators attempted to develop scoring systems using different indicators, such as hemoglobin, platelet count, blast count, cytogenetic abnormalities, etc. The most widely accepted one is the International Prognostic Scoring System (IPSS) proposed by Greenberg and associates.[255] In this scoring system, four risk groups are identified: low (score 0), intermediate 1 (0.5–1), intermediate 2 (1.5–2), and high (≥2.5). They further assigned karyotypes into good (normal karyotype, missing Y-chromosome, del(5q), del(20q)), poor (complex (≥3

abnormalities) or chromosome 7 anomalies), and intermediate (all other abnormalities). The IPSS for MDS (survival and AML evolution) is then listed as shown in Table 12.17.

By applying this scoring system to retrospectively analyze 816 patients, it was found that median survival for low, intermediate 1, intermediate 2, and high risk groups was 5.7, 3.5, 1.2, and 0.4 years respectively. The risks for 25% of patients to undergo evolution to AML were 9.4, 3.3, 1.1, and 0.2 years respectively for low, intermediate 1, intermediate 2, and high risk groups.[255]

Recently, the WHO classification for MDS has modified the FAB classification in the following ways: (1) the threshold was changed from 30% to 20% for the distinction of acute leukemia from MDS; (2) RA, RARS, and RAEB was each divided into subgroups; (3) MDS unclassified and MDS-associated with isolated del (5q) were added; (4) The RAEB-T subgroup was eliminated; and (5) a new group of disorders was created – myelodysplasia/myeloproliferative diseases.[219,256,257] The WHO classification of MDS is listed in Table 12.18. Germing and associates retrospectively studied 1600 patients with MDS using the WHO classification and found that there is (1) a significant difference in prognosis between RAEB-1 and

Table 12.18 WHO classification of myelodysplastic syndrome

Disease	Blood findings Blasts (%)	Abnormalities	Blasts (%)	Bone marrow findings Abnormalities	FAB classification
RA	Zero or <1	Anemia	<5	Erythroid dysplasia	RA
RCMD	Zero or <1	Bi- or pancytopenia	<5	Dysplasia in ≥10% of the cells of two or more myeloid cell lines	
RARS	Zero	Anemia	<5	≥15% ring sideroblasts; erythroid dysplasia	RARS
RCMD-RS	Zero or <1	Bi- or pancytopenia	<5	Dysplasia in ≥10% of the cells in two or more myeloid cell lines	
RAEB-1	<5	Cytopenias	5–9	Unilineage or multilineage dysplasia; no Auer rods	
RAEB-2	5–19; Auer rods ±	Cytopenias	10–19	Unilineage or multilineage dysplasia; Auer rods ±	RAEB
MDS-U	Zero or <1	Cytopenias	<5	Unilineage dysplasia: one myeloid cell line	
MDS with isolated del (5q)	<5	Anemia; normal or increased platelets	<5	Normal to increased megakaryocytes with hypolobated nuclei (micromegakaryocytes); isolated 5q–; no Auer rods	

Data adapted and modified from reference 256.
MDS, myelodysplastic syndrome; MDS-U, myelodysplastic syndrome, unclassified; RA, refractory anemia; RARS, refractory anemia with ringed sideroblasts; RAEB-1, refractory anemia with excess blasts –1; RAEB-2, refractory anemia with excess blasts-2; RCMD, refractory cytopenia with multilineage dysplasia; RCMD-RS, refractory cytopenia with multilineage dysplasia and ringed sideroblasts.

RAEB-2; (2) similarly, a difference in outcome between refractory anemia and refractory anemia with multilineage dysplasia; and a difference between refractory anemia with ringed sideroblasts and refractory anemia with multilineage dysplasia and ring sideroblasts.[258] They also noticed that good prognosis associated with sole 5q– anomaly only holds when the medullary blast cont is less than 5%.[258]

Myelodysplastic syndromes/chronic myeloproliferative disorders

According to the FAB classification, *chronic myelomonocytic leukemia (CMML)* possesses MDS and CMPD characteristics. These patients present with peripheral blood monocytosis ($>1 \times 10^9$/l), normocellular or hypercellular bone marrow accompanied by dysgranulopoiesis, dyserythropoiesis, or dysmegakaryopoiesis. The percentage of blasts is less than 5% in the peripheral blood and less than 20% in the bone marrow, with absent Auer rods. Although erythropoiesis and megakaryopoiesis may be ineffective, granulopoiesis is usually effective and is often associated with extreme leukocytosis. Splenomegaly and hepatomegaly are common. About 20–30% of CMML patients transform to AML, most commonly M2 or M4. Chromosomal abnormalities are found in 30–50% of patients and there are no specific clonal abnormalities that can differentiate CMML from other MDS.

The FAB group suggested that CMML might be subdivided into two groups based on an arbitrary blood leukocyte count of 13 000/µl: a myelodysplastic type (MDS-CMML) (≤13 000/µl) and a myeloproliferative type (MPD-CMML) (>13 000/µl).[234] Germing and associates retrospectively studied 158 patients with CMML using the above criterion. They found a significant difference in these two groups among the following parameters: splenomegaly, hepatomegaly, leukocytosis, neutrophilia, monocytosis, serum lactate dehydrogenase (LDH) level, and thymidine kinase level. These parameters are all more prominent or higher in MPD-CMML compared to MDS-CMML.[259] Further, immature granulocytes and nucleated red cell precursors are also commonly found in peripheral blood in MPD-CMML. The probability of transformation to AML was higher in MDS-CMML, but this difference did not reach statistical significance.[259] Onida and co-workers studied 213 patients with CMML retrospectively and found that subdivision into 'dysplastic' and 'proliferative' subgroups as defined above provided no additional benefit to prognostic stratification.[260] Instead, hemoglobin level below 12 g/dl, presence of circulating immature myeloid cells, absolute lymphocyte count above 2500/µl and marrow blasts 10% or more were independently associated with shorter survival and were used to generate a prognostic score system.[260]

Investigators using the WHO classification include chronic myelomonocytic leukemia (CMML), atypical chronic myeloid leukemia (aCML), juvenile myelomonocytic leukemia (JMML), and myelodysplasia/myeloproliferative disease, unclassifiable, into the category of myelodysplastic/myeloproliferative diseases.[257] Their criteria for the diagnosis of CMML are similar to FAB, except that they recommend dividing CMML into two subcategories, depending on the number of blasts found in the peripheral blood or bone marrow: (1) CMML-1: Blasts <5% in the blood, and <10% in the bone marrow; (2) CMML-2: Blasts 5–19% in the blood or 10–19% in the bone marrow, or when Auer rods are present and the blast count is less than 20% in the blood or the marrow. When there are 20% or more blasts in the blood and/or the marrow, the case is classified as AML.[261]

Atypical chronic myeloid leukemia (aCML) is characterized by marked myeloid hyperplasia and dysplasia, with or without relative monocytosis, circulating immature granulocytes, absence of *bcr/abl* by cytogenetic or molecular methods, and aggressive clinical course.[234,235] Multilineage dysplasia is common. Table 12.14 lists distinguishing characteristics of CML, aCML, and CMML.

Myelodysplastic syndrome in children

Myelodysplastic syndrome and MPD are uncommon in children.[262,263] However, almost all forms of MDS that affect adults also occur in children, except that RARS is rarely reported in childhood whereas CMML is more common, especially in children under the age of 5.[262,264] A number of clinical conditions have been recognized as predisposing factors for childhood MDS or MPD. These are Down syndrome, Kostmann syndrome, Fanconi's anemia, neurofibromatosis, Schwachman syndrome and others.[262]

Two types of CML in childhood have been described in the literature: the adult-type CML (or Philadelphia chromosome (*bcr/abl*)-positive CML) and juvenile CML. Most investigators now prefer the term juvenile myelomonocytic leukemia (JMML) rather than juvenile CML and consider that so called 'monosomy 7 syndrome' or 'infantile monosomy 7' and JMML probably represents a spectrum of the same disease.[262] Hasle and colleagues modified the WHO classification for childhood MDS and MPD, and proposed retaining RAEB in transformation (RAEB-T), in which peripheral blood or bone marrow blasts count 20–29%.[263]

Patients with *juvenile myelomonocytic leukemia* are usually boys less than 2 years of age.[265] Common clinical presentations include pallor, fever, infection, marked hepatosplenomegaly, generalized lymphadenopathy and skin changes (rashes, café au lait spots, xanthoma, etc.), moderate leukocytosis with monocytosis and circulating immature granulocytes, anemia with or without thrombocytopenia, frequently elevated fetal hemoglobin (>10%, age-adjusted), and hypergammoglobulinemia. Abnormal karyotype may be detected in about 40–60% of the patients, which includes monosomy 7 (most common), trisomy 8, and other complex chromosomal abnormalities.[262–265] Loss of *NF-1* gene function or *ras* gene mutations has also been observed in these patients.[262,265] Patients with infantile monosomy 7 or monosomy 7 syndrome share many of the same clinical, laboratory and pathological features of JMML except that these patients appear to have a lower level of fetal hemoglobin and a higher rate of transformation to AML in comparison to JMML.[262] It should be pointed out that monosomy 7 as a cytogenetic finding is seen in children with all forms of MDS classified according to FAB, JMML, and AML.

The diagnostic criteria for JMML as defined by the International JMML Working Group and the European Working Group on childhood MDS are as follows: (A) suggestive clinical features (hepatosplenomegaly, lymphadenopathy, pallor, fever, skin rash); (B) Minimal laboratory criteria (all three fulfilled: no Philadelphia chromosome or no *bcr/abl* rearrangement, peripheral blood monocyte count $>1 \times 10^9$/l, and bone marrow blasts <20%; (C) Criteria requested for a definitive diagnosis (at least two of the following: increased hemoglobin F for age, myeloid precursors on peripheral blood smear, white blood cell count $>10 \times 10^9$/l, clonal abnormalities, including monosomy 7, GM-CSF hypersensitivity of myeloid progenitors in vitro).[262]

The treatment of choice is bone marrow transplant. Various factors influence prognosis in JMML. The most significant determining features appear to be platelet count, hemoglobin F level, and age. Patients who are older than 2, with a low platelet count and a high hemoglobin F level, have a worse prognosis than those who do not have these characteristics.

FIBROSIS

Fibrosis of the bone marrow, or myelofibrosis, may be primary (idiopathic) or secondary. The peripheral blood in both chronic idiopathic myelofibrosis/AMM and secondary myelofibrosis is characterized by a leukoerythroblastic picture (presence of immature myeloid and erythroid series in the peripheral blood, accompanied by giant and bizarre thrombocytes) with circulating teardrop erythrocytes. The number of circulating nucleated RBCs is often excessive compared with the degree of anemia. Reticulocytosis is not seen in most cases. This peripheral blood picture is specific for myelophthisic anemia (a normocytic, normochromic anemia with leukoerythroblastosis due to replacement of normal bone marrow by nonmarrow elements). The bone marrow shows reticulin (demonstrated by silver impregnated reticulin stain) fibrosis in the early stage, and collagen fibrosis later. Clusterings of megakaryocytes with abnormal morphology are usually seen in primary myelofibrosis and myelofibrosis associated with CMPDs. These phenomena are uncommonly seen in secondary myelofibrosis.[266] Myelofibrosis is associated with a variety of benign or neoplastic clinical conditions (Table 12.19).[267,268]

Primary myelofibrosis

The clinical presentation of primary myelofibrosis may be acute or chronic. Acute myelosclerosis or acute myelofibrosis is uncommon. Patients present with rapidly developing pancytopenia without accompanying organomegaly, minimal morphologic changes in peripheral blood, panmyelosis, with dysgranulopoiesis and dysmegakaryopoiesis. Abnormal megakaryocytes, clusters of blasts, and marrow fibrosis are common features. Chronic idiopathic myelofibrosis, or agnogenic myeloid metaplasia, is a form of CMPD. Both entities have been discussed above.[144–148,240–246]

Secondary myelofibrosis

Secondary myelofibrosis may be caused by chemicals, radiation exposure, occlusive vascular disease, metastatic carcinomas, leukemias, malignant lymphomas, and other conditions (Figs 12.23, 12.24, see Table 12.19). It is also common in CMPDs, such as chronic myelogenous leukemia or polycythemia vera, and in MDS.[269,270] Focal myelofibrosis may be seen in areas of inflammatory reaction to an infectious agent (such as tuberculosis) or sarcoidosis, or in areas adjacent to bone marrow necrosis and fracture of bone.[267,268] The hematopoietic elements are normal or decreased in most of these disorders and the morphology of megakaryocytes is normal (with the exception of fibrosis associated with CMPDs and leukemias). The primary cause of fibrosis (such as metastatic carcinoma) may be identified on the same bone marrow section or on deeper sections. It is interesting to note that bone marrow fibrosis in childhood ALL is associated with common ALL antigen – CALLA-positive (CD10[+]) – and B cell markers.[271] Islam and colleagues found that at least some increase in fiber content is present in 35% of the patients with AML at presentation.[272] There is no correlation between subgroups of FAB classification and the presence or absence or the degree of marrow fibrosis. Bone marrow fibrosis regresses after effective chemotherapy. They conclude that an increase in marrow fiber content at diagnosis does not affect hematopoietic regeneration after treatment and achievement of complete remission.

Primary osseous, renal, or endocrine diseases, such as osteitis fibrosa cystica, fibrous dysplasia, and osteopetrosis, are also associated with marrow fibrosis and osteosclerosis. Microcystic resorption of

Table 12.19 Clinical conditions associated with bone marrow fibrosis

Hematopoietic disorders
Primary idiopathic myelofibrosis
  Acute myelosclerosis (acute panmyelosis with myelofibrosis)
  Chronic idiopathic myelofibrosis (CIMF)
Chronic myeloproliferative disorders
  Postpolycythemic myelofibrosis
  Transitional myeloproliferative disorder
  Chronic myeloid leukemia
  Essential thrombocythemia
Acute leukemias
Chronic lymphocytic leukemia, hairy cell leukemia, Waldenström's
  macroglobulinemia, and multiple myeloma, T-cell lymphoma/leukemia
  (e.g. adult T-cell leukemia/lymphoma)
Malignant lymphomas
Myelodysplastic syndrome
Aplastic anemia
Malignant histiocytosis
Paroxysmal nocturnal hemoglobinuria
Mast cell disease
Gray platelet syndrome

Metastatic tumors
Inflammatory and reparative processes
Infection, e.g. tuberculosis
Autoimmune diseases
Granulomatous diseases
Osteomyelitis
Previous bone marrow biopsy site
Following bone marrow necrosis or infarction
Following bone marrow radiation
Exposure to toxins, e.g. thorium dioxide or benzene

Storage diseases
Metabolic disorders
Renal osteodystrophy
Osteopetrosis
Vitamin D deficiency
Hypoparathyroidism
Hyperparathyroidism
Paget's disease of bone

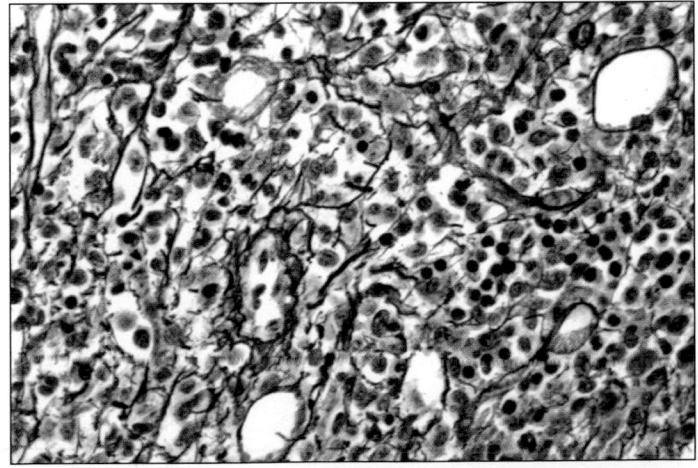

Fig. 12.23 Chronic myelomonocytic leukemia. This reticulin stain illustrates increased reticulin fibrosis in a patient with CMML. (Gridley's reticulin stain, ×400.)

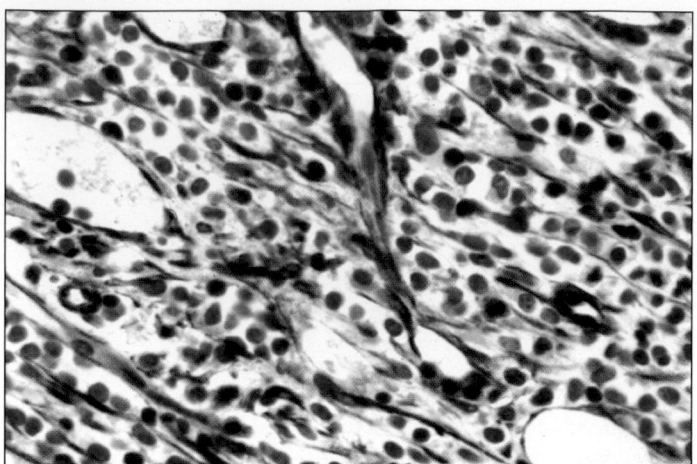

Fig. 12.24 Acute myeloid leukemia, minimally differentiated. Increased fibroblasts and fibrocytes may be seen in patients with acute leukemia. (Immunoperoxidase stain with anti-vimentin antibody, ×400.)

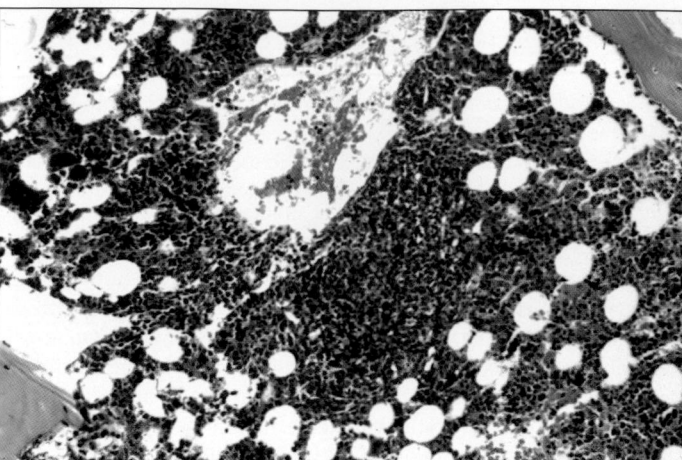

Fig. 12.25 Lymphoid aggregate. A large lymphoid aggregate, consisting of a predominance of small lymphocytes admixed with a few transformed cells, plasma cells, and histiocytes, is present close to a sinus from a patient with HIV infection. (H&E stain, ×100.)

bone, marrow fibrosis, and increased osteoclastic activity are seen in the adult T cell leukemia/lymphoma (discussed below).

LYMPHOCYTIC INFILTRATION

Lymphocytic infiltrates may be broadly separated into (1) benign lymphocytic infiltrates, which may be physiologic (in young children) or reactive (associated with drugs, infections such as infectious lymphocytosis, infectious mononucleosis, tuberculosis, etc., systemic autoimmune disorders, or chronic myeloproliferative disorders, among others); and (2) malignant lymphoproliferative disorders, including chronic lymphocytic leukemia and related disorders, bone marrow involvement by non-Hodgkin's lymphoma with or without a leukemic picture, multiple myeloma and related disorders, Hodgkin's lymphoma and some non-Hodgkin's lymphomas in which granulomatous change is part of the pathology.

Non-neoplastic lymphocytic infiltration

Lymphocytes, a normal component of the bone marrow, may constitute up to 50% of all nucleated cells in marrow in a child up to one year of age and older. Some of these lymphocytes have morphologic and immunophenotypic characteristics of hematogones.[65–67] *Hematogones* are immature B-cells. They are small to medium in size with a round to irregular nucleus nearly occupying the entire cell. They have dense homogeneous chromatin and multiple small inconspicuous nucleoli. They are CD10+ and CD19+; some may also express CD20, surface immunoglobulin, TdT or CD34.[65–67] They usually are dispersed throughout the marrow cavities in contrast to ALL cells which frequently form aggregates. *Lymphoid nodules or lymphoid aggregates* are a relatively common finding in routine bone marrow examination. These nodules are usually seen in older women and are frequently present around the blood vessels, associated with plasmacytosis and lipid granulomas. They are composed of small lymphocytes, a few plasma cells, histiocytes, and occasionally eosinophils and mast cells, organized around a capillary or arteriole within a reticulin fiber network.[68,69]

Three different types of reactive lymphoid lesions have been described: (1) reactive lymphocyte aggregates; (2) lymphoid follicles with germinal centers; and (3) reactive lymphohistiocytic infiltrate.[273] *Reactive lymphocyte aggregates* are most common. Their frequency increases with age. They have also been associated with chronic inflammatory and autoimmune diseases, malignant lymphomas or chronic myeloproliferative disorders. These aggregates are usually present in the marrow cavities away from the bony trabeculae and are usually organized around the capillaries, venous sinuses, or arterioles (Fig. 12.25). They are usually well-circumscribed and well-demarcated from the surrounding hematopoietic cells. Immunologic study reveals that they are composed of a mixture of B and T cells in variable proportions.

Lymphoid follicles with germinal centers typically are well circumscribed nodules containing tingible body macrophages surrounded by mantle zone lymphocytes. They possess the same morphologic and immunologic characteristics as those germinal centers observed in other organs. The oncoprotein *bcl-2* is negative in the germinal center cells but is expressed by mantle cells and some T-cells. These lymphoid follicles may be observed in the same clinical conditions as those associated with reactive lymphocyte aggregates.

Reactive lymphohistiocytic infiltrates are larger lesions than the reactive lymphoid aggregates with ill-defined borders. They consist of small lymphocytes with round or irregular nuclei, activated lymphocytes, immunoblasts, plasma cells, histiocytes, mast cells, and eosinophils. Epithelioid histiocytes, sometimes forming epithelioid granulomas, may also be present. These lesions contain dense reticulin network and capillaries with hypertrophic endothelial cells. Immunohistochemical study reveals a mixed population of B and T cells as well as polyclonal plasma cells. These lesions are most commonly seen in HIV-infected patients, but may also be found in other viral infections.[273] It appears that morphologically benign lymphoid aggregates should not be ignored in iliac crest biopsy specimens from patients who do not have a lymphoproliferative disorder, because Faulkner-Jones and associates[274] found that 37% of such patients eventually developed confirmed or suspected lymphoproliferative disorder.

The differential diagnosis between benign (reactive) lymphoid lesions and malignant lymphomatous involvement of marrow, especially in a patient with a history of non-Hodgkin's lymphoma,

Table 12.20 Comparison of benign (reactive) llymphocytic infiltrates and malignant lymphocytic lesions (leukemia or lymphoma) in bone marrow sections

Benign	Malignant
Randomly distributed	Frequently paratrabecular or around a large sinus
Small, well circumscribed	Large, irregularly shaped, with ill-defined borders
Polymorphic, consisting of small lymphocytes, immunoblasts and histiocytes, often organized around a capillary or blood vessel, within a delicate network of reticulin fibers	Usually monomorphic: cytology of neoplastic infiltrate depends on the type of malignant cells involved (cytologic atypia common)
Germinal centers may be present. A mixture of T and B cells by immunohistochemical study	Germinal centers are absent. Most commonly B cells with atypical morphology; aberrant T cell phenotypes in T cell lymphoproliferative disorder

Table 12.21 Chronic lymphoproliferative disorders involving bone marrow

B cells	NK/T cells
Primary leukemia	
Chronic lymphocytic leukemia (CLL)	Large granular lymphocytic leukemia
Prolymphocytic leukemia (PLL)	PLL/chronic lymphocytic leukemia
Hairy cell leukemia (HCL)	Aggressive NK-cell leukemia
Plasma cell leukemia* (PCL)	
Leukemic phase of non-Hodgkin's lymphoma	
Small lymphocytic lymphoma	Sézary syndrome
Mantle cell lymphoma	Adult T-cell leukemia/lymphoma
Follicular lymphoma	(ATLL)
Lymphoplasmacytic lymphoma	Blastic NK-cell lymphoma/leukemia
Splenic lymphoma with villous lymphocytes (marginal zone lymphoma)	Peripheral T-cell lymphoma, unspecified
Large cell lymphoma	
Pure lymphomatous infiltration†	

*Plasma cell leukemia will be discussed under plasma cell dyscrasia
† See text. Some subtypes of T-cell lymphoma (e.g. hepatosplenic T-cell lymphoma, peripheral T-cell lymphoma, unspecified, and anaplastic large cell lymphoma) frequently involve bone marrow.
Adapted and modified from references 276–279.

may be difficult. Irregularity, asymmetry, great variability in size and shape, tendency to fragmentation of the nodules, and abnormal cytology with increased number of large 'blastic' lymphocytes are criteria for malignant lymphoma. Table 12.20 lists some of the parameters that can be used to differentiate benign from malignant lymphoid lesions. However, immunohistochemical and flow cytometric study are useful to support the morphologic diagnosis.[275]

Lymphoproliferative disorders

Acute lymphocytic leukemia has been discussed earlier. Based on clinical presentations, chronic lymphoproliferative disorders may involve the bone marrow in the following ways: (1) primary leukemias; (2) leukemic phase of non-Hodgkin's lymphoma; and (3) pure lymphomatous infiltration (Table 12.21).[276–279] The FAB Cooperative Group proposed the following classifications for the chronic B and T lymphoid leukemias: the B-LPD (lymphoproliferative disorders) include CLL, PLL (prolymphocytic leukemia), HCL (hairy cell leukemia), SLVL (splenic lymphoma with villous lymphocytes), leukemic phase of non-Hodgkin's lymphoma, Waldenström's macroglobulinemia, and plasma cell leukemia. The T-LPD include CLL, PLL, ATLL (adult T cell leukemia/lymphoma), and Sézary syndrome.[280] The World Health Organization classified mature B-cell neoplasms and mature T-cell and natural killer (NK)-cell neoplasms into many subgroups.[281] Readers are referred to the chapter on malignant lymphoma (Chapter 11).

B-chronic lymphocytic leukemia and related disorders

B-chronic lymphocytic leukemia (B-CLL) is a disease of elderly men. It is the most common form of leukemia in Western countries.[276,282] The clinical manifestations are variable. For diagnosis, the National Cancer Institute-sponsored working group requires an absolute lymphocyte count of more than 5×10^9/l in the blood with mature-appearing morphology.[283] Others use mature lymphocytosis of $>3 \times 10^9$/l and $\geq 30\%$ lymphocytes in the bone marrow aspirate as diagnostic criteria.[276] Morphologically, CLL can be classified as (1) typical CLL, and (2) mixed or atypical CLL.[276,280]

The vast majority (>90%) of cells in *typical CLL* are composed of relatively uniform, small to medium sized (9–11 μm)

lymphocytes. These cells have regular cytoplasmic and nuclear outline, clumped chromatin with discernible parachromatin spaces, and scanty amount of cytoplasm. The nucleoli, if visible, are usually inconspicuous (Fig. 12.26). A small proportion (<10%) of larger cells (≥15 μm) may be present. These cells have a less condensed chromatin, prominent nucleolus, and abundant cytoplasm. They are designated as prolymphocytoid or prolymphocyte-like cells. These cells should be differentiated from large lymphocytes, which have round nuclei, clumped chromatin, no distinct nucleoli, and a moderate amount of cytoplasm. Approximately 15% of CLL cases have mixed cell types.

Two *mixed CLL* types have been described: (1) atypical CLL in which a spectrum of small to large lymphocytes (>15%) including cells with lymphoplasmacytic differentiation and/or cells with cleaved nuclei may be present. Occasional (<10%) prolymphocytes may be observed, and (2) a mixture of small lymphocytes and prolymphocytes (with prolymphocytes constituting >10% to <55%) designated CLL/PL (Fig. 12.27).[276,280] CLL/PL may be apparent at the time of diagnosis or may develop during the course of the disease.

Immunologic study shows that most of the neoplastic small lymphocytes possess weak monoclonal surface immunoglobulins (SIgM and SIgD) on their cell membrane and are monoclonal for kappa or lambda light chain. They also carry weak complement and Fc receptors as well as receptors for mouse erythrocytes. CLL cells express the following antigens: CD19, CD20, CD24, HLA-DR, CD5, CD23, and CD43. 'Deviation' from the typical CLL phenotype is seen in cases of CLL with mixed cell types, in which strong expression of SIg and reactivity with FMC7/CD22 may be seen.[280] Some CLL cells express myelomonocytic markers (such as CD11b, CD11c, CD13, and CD14),[276] although the incidence and clinical significance are uncertain. Matutes and colleagues used CD5+, CD23+, FMC-, and negative or weak membrane CD22 or CD79b expression that are characteristic for CLL to develop a score system which is used to differentiate CLL from other B-LPD. Each point

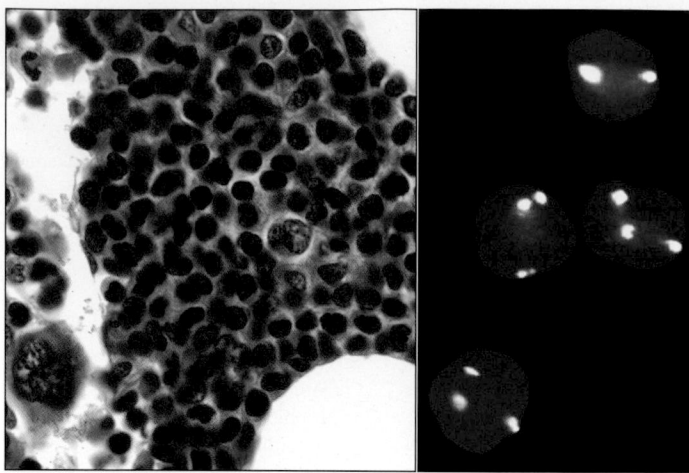

Fig. 12.26 Chronic lymphocytic leukemia. Note the interstitial pattern of infiltration from a patient with CLL. Three of the four leukemic cells from a patient with mixed CLL/PLL have trisomy 12. (H&E stain, ×603; fluorescence in-situ hybridization, ×1000.) (Courtesy of Dr Russell Brynes.)

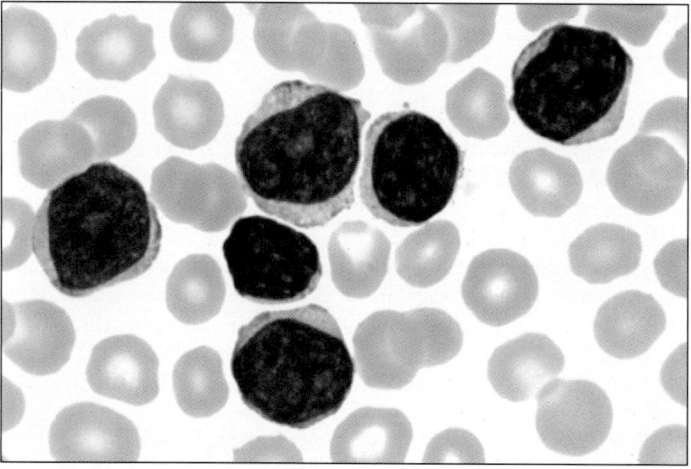

Fig. 12.27 CLL/PLL. Note that the CLL cells have a round nucleus, coarse clumped chromatin, and a minimal amount of cytoplasm, whereas the prolymphocytes are larger with a round, oval, or slightly irregular nucleus containing one large prominent nucleolus and a moderate to abundant amount of cytoplasm. (Romanowsky stain, ×1000.)

(CD5[+], CD23[+], FMC[−], SIg weak, CD22/CD79b weak/negative) scores 1. Most CLL cases score 4 or 5 and rarely 3, whereas other B-LPD score 0–2.[276] These investigators further emphasize that if the morphology is that of atypical CLL and the immunologic score is under 3 in spite of CD5[+], FISH analysis should be undertaken for the detection of trisomy 12 and t (11;14). Atypical CLL are usually trisomy 12 positive and t (11;14) negative, in contrast to mantle cell lymphoma (MCL) in leukemic phase where trisomy 12 is negative and t (11;14) is positive.[276]

A clinical staging system for CLL was introduced by Rai and colleagues[284] to assess the tumor burden. Later, Binet and associates[285] proposed a new system consisting of three stages. Both staging systems are based on the degree of peripheral lymphocytosis, thrombocytopenia, anemia, and the presence of organomegaly (liver, spleen,

cervical, axillary, and inguinal lymph nodes). For instance, Rai's 'Stage 0' is defined by lymphocytosis (>15 × 10⁹/l alone); 'stage I,' lymphocytosis and lymphadenopathy; 'stage II,' lymphocytosis, spleen or liver enlargement, or both; 'stage III,' lymphocytosis and anemia (hemoglobin <10 g/dl); 'stage IV,' lymphocytosis and thrombocytopenia (platelet count <100 × 10⁹/l). The Rai classification has now been condensed to three stages that differ with respect to survival: good prognosis (equivalent to original Rai stage 0); intermediate prognosis (Rai stage I or II); and poor prognosis (Rai stage III or IV).[283,286] The Binet staging system includes the cervical, axillary, and inguinal lymph nodes (either unilateral or bilateral), the spleen, and the liver into its consideration. In the most advanced stage, stage C, patients have anemia (hemoglobin <10 g/dl) and thrombocytopenia (platelet count <100×10⁹/l); those patients in stage A and stage B do not have evidence of impaired marrow function but have fewer than three (stage A) or three or more areas of lymph node or organ enlargement (stage B), respectively. Several studies indicate that clinical stages, bone marrow histopathologic findings, blood lymphocyte counts, lymphocyte doubling time, and cytogenetic abnormalities are good predictors of survival.[286]

Four different histologic patterns have been recognized: (1) interstitial lymphoid infiltration without displacement of fat cells; (2) nodular (abnormal lymphoid nodule without interstitial infiltration); (3) mixed (combination of interstitial and nodular patterns); and (4) diffuse (replacement of both hematopoietic cells and fat cells by lymphoid infiltration). Cytologically the neoplastic lymphocytes are small and contain round or slightly irregular nuclei, clumped chromatin, and an indiscernible amount of cytoplasm. A small nucleolus may be observed in some cells. Some intermediate lymphocytes may also be present. These transformed lymphocytes resemble those seen in proliferation centers in lymph nodes from patients with CLL. The reticulin framework is moderately accentuated in most cases. The pattern of bone marrow histology (diffuse or nondiffuse) in B-chronic lymphocytic leukemia (B-CLL) patients has been proved to be one of the best prognostic parameters.[287]

Based on the data from the Second International Working Party on Chromosomes in CLL, 311 out of 604 (51%) cases had clonal chromosome aberrations with the most common abnormality being trisomy 12 (19%), followed by structural aberrations of chromosomes 13 (10%), 14 (8%), 11 (8%), 6 (6%), and 17 (4%).[288] With the improvement in technologies and the application of fluorescence in situ hybridization, comparative genomic hybridization or other molecular methods, chromosomal aberrations were detected in 268 out of 325 (82%) cases.[289] The most frequent changes were a deletion in 13q (55%), followed by a deletion in 11q (18%), trisomy of 12q (16%), a deletion in 17p (17%) and a deletion in 6q (6%).[289] In multivariate analysis, these investigators found that the presence of a 17p deletion or an 11q deletion, age, Binet stage, the serum lactate dehydrogenase level, and the white cell count gave significant prognostic information. The median survival for 17p deletion, 11q deletion, trisomy 12q, normal karyotype, and 13q deletion was 32 months, 79 months, 114 months, 111 months and 133 months, respectively.[289]

Extensive investigations have been undertaken to identify the suppressor gene at 13q chromosome. It was found that the *RB1* (retinoblastoma) gene at 13q14 was not involved in CLL, although losses of the *BRCA2* gene in band 13q12 were reported in 80% of CLL.[288] As stated earlier, CLL patients with 13q deletion as a sole abnormality have a better survival. However, whole or partial loss of chromosome 13 in multiple myeloma patients is associated with an adverse prognosis.[288,290] Deletions of 13q14 have also been described in 25% of centroblastic–centrocytic non-Hodgkin's lymphomas,

10–28% of pre-B-ALLs, and 70% of mantle cell lymphoma (MCL) patients.[290] The 11q22–q23 deletion in CLL may be related to *ATM* (the ataxia-telangiectasia gene), which may function as a tumor suppressor gene in some CLL patients.[288,290] Patients with 11q deletion are younger (<55 years) and have more extensive lymphadenopathy with bulky masses and advanced clinical stages.[288,290] Further, these young CLL patients with the 11q deletion were associated with shorter medium survival, while there was no significant difference in older CLL patients with this chromosomal abnormality.[288,290] Trisomy 12 correlates with advanced clinical stage and atypical CLL morphology.[288,290] In univariate analysis, trisomy 12 is associated with shorter survival but its significance is lost in the multivariate analysis.[290] 6q deletion in CLL usually involves 6q21. It has been stated that patients with 6q deletions had higher white cell counts and more pronounced lymphadenopathy than patients without 6q deletion.[288] However, this chromosomal abnormality did not influence overall survival or treatment-free interval.[288]

Although deletion of 17p13 (*p53*) is not common in CLL, it is the strongest prognostic factor for survival in multivariate analysis.[288] This genetic abnormality also appears to link to treatment failure with purine analogs. Aberrations at loci involving the immunoglobulin heavy chain gene (14q32), *bcl-1* (11q13), *bcl-2* (18q21), or *bcl-3* (19q13.1) genes are uncommon in CLL, although over expression of Bcl-2 protein is observed in CLL.[288,290]

B-CLL probably arises from CD5$^+$ mantle zone lymphocytes that produce autoantibodies. Recent studies have shown that CLL may originate from a 'naive' pregerminal center cell with unmutated IgV$_H$ genes or from a committed memory postgerminal center cell having point mutations in the IgV$_H$ gene.[276,282] These studies also revealed that atypical CLLs, including CLL/PLs, are associated with no mutation (germ line configuration) of the V$_H$ region of the Ig genes, therefore derived from pregerminal center cells.[276,282] Typical CLLs, on the other hand, are derived from post-germinal-center cells with heavy mutation. Those cases express the well defined CLL immunophenotype and usually present at an early clinical stage, have chromosomal 13q14 deletions and a better prognosis.[276,282,291] Atypical CLLs usually occur in younger patients (<55 years) and present at a more advanced clinical stage. They have abnormal immunophenotype (strong SIg staining, FMC7, CD38, CD11a, CD11c, CD72 and CD21 expression), a higher incidence of cytogenetic abnormalities (61% vs 30% anomalies in typical CLL), trisomy 12, *p53* mutation, t(14;19)(q32.3;q13.2), and a poor prognosis.[276,282,291]

Recently, it has been claimed that expression of CD38 or ZAP-70 by CLL cells is associated with aggressive clinical course.[292] ZAP-70, a CD3-receptor-associated protein tyrosin kinase of T-lymphocytes, may be used to separate B-CLL into those having unmutated IgV$_H$ genes (high ZAP-70 expression) from those having mutated IgV$_H$ genes (no detectable amount of ZAP-70 proteins) in most cases.[293,294] The prognostic significance of CD38 is however not as clear as ZAP-70.[294] It appears that the flow cytometry method for CD38 has to be standardized in order to achieve reproducible results.[294] Patients with MUM1/IRF4 expression are more likely to have limited disease and a more favorable clinical course.[295]

Differential diagnosis The differential diagnosis includes a variety of chronic B cell leukemias such as prolymphocytic leukemia, hairy cell leukemia, splenic lymphoma with villous lymphocytes, leukemic phase of non-Hodgkin's lymphoma, Waldenström's macroglobulinemia, and plasma cell leukemia. The clinical presentations and morphologies of neoplastic cells in these

Table 12.22 Comparison of B-chronic lymphoproliferative disorders

	CLL	PLL	MCL	FCCL	MZL	HCL	SLVL	PCL
SIg	Weak	+	+	+	+	+	+	–
CIg	–	–/+	–	–	–/+	+/–	+/–	+
Pan B	+	+	+	+	+	+	+	
CD10	–	–	–/+	+	–	–	–	–/+
CD23	+	–/+	–	–/+	–	–	–	–
CD5	+	–/+	+	–	–	–	–/+	–
CD43	+	–/+	+	–	–/+	–	–	–
CD11c	–/+	–	–	–	–/+	+	+/–	–
CD25	–/+	–	–	–	–	+	–	–
FMC7/CD22	–/+	+	+	+	+/–	+	+	–
CD38	–/+	–/+	–	–/+	–	–/+	+	+
Bcl–1 (R)	–/+	–	+/–	–	–	–	–/+	–/+
Bcl–2 (R)	–	–	–	+	–	–	–	–

CIg, cytoplasmic immunoglobulin; CLL/SLL, chronic lymphocytic leukemia/small lymphocytic lymphoma; FCCL, follicular center cell lymphoma, small cleaved cell; HCL, hairy cell leukemia; MCL, mantle cell lymphoma; MZL, marginal zone lymphoma, including monocytoid B-cell lymphoma; PCL, plasma cell leukemia; PLL, prolymphocytic leukemia; (R), rearrangement; SIg, membrane surface immunoglobulin; SLVL, splenic lymphoma with villous lymphocytes.

entities are different from CLLs and will be discussed later. The immunophenotypic characteristics of these entities are listed in Table 12.22. It should be pointed out that rare examples of biclonal B-CLL have been reported.[296] Also, one should differentiate persistent polyclonal B-cell lymphocytosis from B-CLL.[297] *Persistent polyclonal B-cell lymphocytosis* preferentially affects middle-aged females, who are usually smokers. It is characterized by a mild to moderate polyclonal, CD5$^-$ B lymphocytosis (up to 30×10^9/l).[276,297] These circulating lymphocytes are usually medium to large in size and have a bilobed or indented nucleus, clumped chromatin, and abundant cytoplasm. These cells express CD19 and SIgM, with a normal kappa to lambda ratio. *Bcl-2* and Ig gene rearrangements have not been detected. These patients usually have HLA-DR7 phenotype and there is a suggestion of a familial occurrence.

Transformation of chronic lymphocytic leukemia In some cases of CLL there is clinical and morphologic evolution to an aggressive phase of the disease. The two most common forms of disease transformation are prolymphocytoid transformation and Richter syndrome (mostly large cell lymphoma). Acute leukemia, MDS or multiple myeloma occurring concurrently with or following CLL is very uncommon.[286]

Prolymphocytoid transformation may represent an accelerated phase of CLL in which the disease undergoes an insidious, although aggressive, change in character, with increasing refractoriness to treatment. These patients not only have a previous history of CLL but also have a double population of lymphocytes (prolymphocytes and 'mature' small lymphocytes) that retain most of the marker characteristics of B-CLL. The prolymphocytes are large cells with moderately abundant cytoplasm and a round or oval nucleus containing condensed nuclear chromatin and a large centrally located nucleolus. Bone marrow examination shows marked hypercellularity with replacement of normal marrow by a mixed infiltrate of small lymphocytes and prolymphocytes. Melo and associates divided chronic lymphocytic leukemia and prolymphocytic leukemia into three groups: (1) typical CLL group (prolymphocytes ≤10%); (2) CLL/PL group (prolymphocytes 11–55%), and (3) PLL (prolymphocytes >55%).[298,299] Patients who fell into the second group were found to have intermediate features between CLL and PLL. The degree of splenomegaly was disproportionate to the lymph node enlargement. This group includes at least two types of CLL, one with increased proportions of prolymphocytes but otherwise similar to typical CLL (absolute prolymphocytes ≤15 × 10^9/l), and another in prolymphocytoid transformation (prolymphocytes >15 × 10^9/l).[299] Those cases with absolute prolymphocytes greater than 15 × 10^9/l usually have had a clinical course similar to PLL. The third group has clinical and laboratory features characteristic of PLL. The percentage of prolymphocytes is defined as the proportion of prolymphocytes among the peripheral blood lymphoid population.[298] It was found that absolute prolymphocyte count and spleen size have prognostic significance.[299] Recently, Schlette and associates studied 20 cases of mature B-cell leukemia with more than 55% prolymphocytes in the peripheral blood or bone marrow.[300] They classified these patients into three groups: (1) de novo PLL; (2) PLL occurring in patients with a previous well-established diagnosis of CLL (PLL-Hx CLL); and (3) t(11;14)(q13;q32)-positive neoplasms. The neoplastic cells from the last group of patients were positive for CD5 and cyclin D1 and negative for CD23. These investigators classified them as MCL. Cytogenetic study showed that abnormalities of chromosome 7 were most frequent in de novo PLL, whereas trisomy 12, add 12(p), and chromosome 13 abnormalities were frequently observed in the PLL-Hx CLL group.[300]

Richter syndrome is characterized by fever, weight loss, localized lymphadenopathy, dysglobulinemia, and a pleomorphic malignant lymphoma occurring terminally in patients with a previous history of CLL.[301,302] Immunohistopathologic study has revealed that the malignant lymphoma is a large B-cell lymphoma in most instances. The incidence ranges from 1–10% of CLL patients with most reports indicating 3%. Some 33% of 39 cases studied presented with extranodal involvement.[302] The median interval between diagnosis of CLL and large cell lymphoma (Richter syndrome) was 48 months.[302] Clonality analysis suggested that Richter syndrome was most commonly a true transformational event.[302] Kroft and colleagues, after studying seven cases of large cell transformation of CLL/small lymphocytic lymphoma (CLL/SLL), concluded that the vast majority of diffuse large B-cell lymphomas retained the major immunophenotypic features of CLL/SLL, specifically expression of CD5 and CD23 with no or dim expression of FMC7.[303] Ohno and associates also found that, in some cases of Hodgkin's transformation of CLL, the Hodgkin's and Reed–Sternberg cells and the CLL cells shared the same clonality.[304] It is interesting to note that, in another study, trisomy 12 was detected in cells of Richter transformation of CLL by FISH but only in one of five cases from the original CLL specimen.[305] It is not clear whether this discrepancy is due to technical difficulty (it is likely that the original specimens were quite old) or due to the fact that trisomy 12 in Richter syndrome is an acquired abnormality.

B-cell prolymphocytic leukemia　Prolymphocytic leukemia (PLL), as first described by Galton and associates,[306] is uncommon. Patients are often elderly men, without a prior history of CLL, with massive splenomegaly, absent or minimal lymphadenopathy, striking lymphocytosis (average lymphocyte count 355 × 10^9/l), resistance to conventional therapy for CLL, and a poor prognosis.[306,307] Histo-

logically, four different patterns have been described: interstitial, mixed (interstitial-nodular), mixed (interstitial-diffuse), and diffuse.[308] Unlike CLL, the pure nodular pattern is not seen in PLL, whereas the mixed (interstitial-diffuse) pattern is observed only in PLL. Cytologically, PLL may be differentiated from CLL by the characteristic morphology of the neoplastic cells (a larger cell than CLL, with a relatively immature-appearing round nucleus containing one prominent nucleolus and an abundant amount of cytoplasm).[307] A minor population of small lymphocytes with clumped chromatin is commonly present. Phenotypically the neoplastic cells mark as B cells with bright monoclonal immunoglobulin light chain and FMC expressions. Some cases may also be CD5$^+$ (Table 12.22). Abnormalities of p53 have been reported in 75% of cases, which have been interpreted as a possible cause for the frequent resistance to therapy of this disease.[309]

It should be pointed out that in the de novo PLL group studied by Schlette and associates, the median white cell count at the time of referral to their institution was 76.5 × 10^9/l and the median percentage of prolymphocytes was 79%.[300] Further, the nuclei of prolymphocytes in some cases were located eccentrically with basophilic cytoplasm, suggestive of plasmacytoid differentiation; the nuclear contours in other cases were slightly irregular or folded; and binucleated forms were present in most cases. Many of their studied cases expressed CD5, CD23, and FMC-7 in addition to pan B-cell markers.[300] Complex cytogenetic abnormalities were found in all six cases classified as de novo PLL.[300] Four out of these six cases (67%) had abnormalities of chromosome 7 and another patient had add (12p).[300]

B-PLL should be differentiated from T-PLL, prolymphocytoid transformation of CLL, blood and bone marrow involvement by MCL, large cell lymphoma, splenic marginal zone B-cell lymphoma with or without villous lymphocytes, and hairy cell leukemia variant. Many of these entities will be discussed later. Readers are also referred to Table 12.22.

Hairy cell leukemia　Hairy cell leukemia is a chronic lymphoproliferative disorder, primarily affecting middle-aged men with a median age of 50 years at the onset of the disease. The classical triad includes bi(pan)-cytopenia and splenomegaly in the absence of lymphadenopathy, abnormal 'hairy' cells in the blood and a dry tap on bone marrow aspiration. The neoplastic cell is mononuclear and of intermediate to large size. The centrally or eccentrically located nucleus often contains lacy chromatin and a small and inconspicuous nucleolus. The light blue cytoplasm displays typical fine filamentous ('hairy') projections on peripheral blood smear. Hairy cells generally express pan B cell antigens CD19 and CD20, and monoclonal mSIg. They are also positive for PCA-1, CD11c, CD103, FMC7, CD22, and CD25[17,310,311] (Fig. 12.28, Table 12.22). Rare cases of T-cell HCL have been reported.[310] The leukemic cells are characteristically stained with acid phosphatase (multiple paranuclear granules), and this positive reaction is resistant to tartaric acid inhibition. One or more ribosome-lamellar complexes may be demonstrated intracytoplasmically by electron microscopy. They appear as rod-shaped inclusions with a pale center in the cytoplasm of the hairy cells by Romanowsky stain with light microscopic examination. However, none of these characteristics are pathognomonic, and hairy cell leukemia may simulate a variety of myeloid and lymphoid proliferative disorders.[310]

In a typical case the disease is characterized by an insidious onset, marked splenomegaly, pancytopenia, and circulating hairy cells, with minimal peripheral lymphadenopathy. The bone marrow aspiration often yields a dry tap due to reticulin fibrosis. The marrow cellularity is variable in biopsy specimen. The neoplastic infiltrate

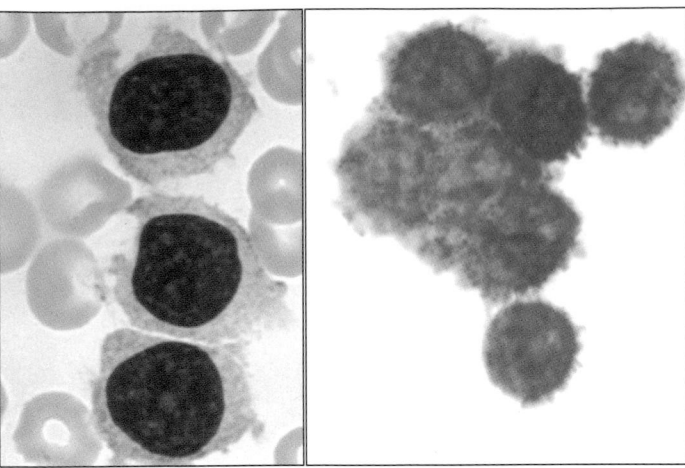

Fig. 12.28 Hairy cell leukemia. This composite picture depicts the characteristics of hairy cells. Note the typical evenly distributed nuclear chromatin and hairy cytoplasmic projection. Leukemic cells express CD11c. (Romanowsky stain and immunoalkaline phosphatase stain, ×1000.)

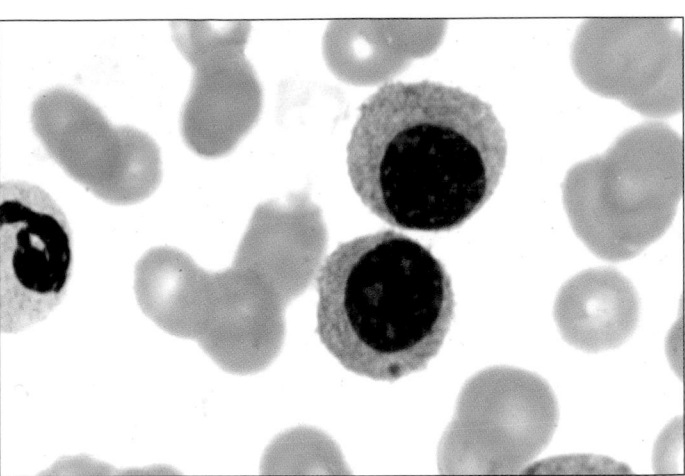

Fig. 12.30 Hairy cell leukemia variant. These leukemic cells resemble prolymphocytes characterized by a large prominent nucleolus. However, they are distinct from prolymphocytes by light blue cytoplasm with or without hairy projections. (Romanowsky stain, ×1000.)

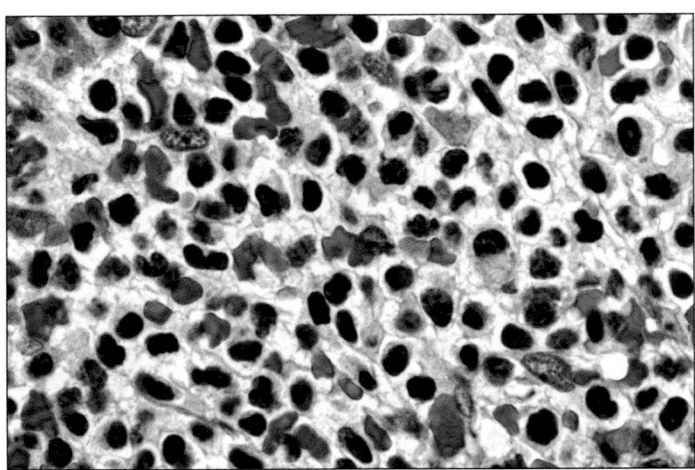

Fig. 12.29 Hairy cell leukemia. Diffuse infiltration of bone marrow. Note that each leukemia cell has a distinct cell border and clear cytoplasm. (H&E stain, ×600.)

may be focal, patchy, interstitial, or diffuse and is composed of uniform mononuclear cells with a distinct cell border, giving a 'mosaic' pattern or a 'honeycomb' or 'sponge' appearance (Fig. 12.29). The nucleus may be round, oval, indented, or coffee-bean shaped, surrounded by a 'halo' or pale cytoplasm imparting a 'fried egg' appearance; the nuclear chromatin is finely stippled and the nucleolus is indistinct. Mitoses and nuclear pleomorphism are usually absent. This loose network of monomorphic cells is in contrast to the tightly packed, paratrabecular arrangement of lymphomatous involvement of the marrow. Increased reticulin fibers are seen in the infiltrated areas.

The changes in the spleen are characteristic.[310] It is usually moderately to massively enlarged and appears congested on gross examination. Microscopically, the red pulp cords and sinuses are infiltrated by the neoplastic hairy cells, whereas the white pulp appears atrophic or totally replaced by the tumor. Blood lakes,

resulting from collections of pooled red blood cells surrounded by infiltrating hairy cells, may be observed. Involvement of liver is typically sinusoidal.

Nonrandomized chromosomal abnormalities have been reported in more than 50% of cases of HCL.[312] Clonal aberrations in chromosome 5 manifested as trisomy 5, pericentric inversions, or interstitial deletions involving band 5q13 have been demonstrated in 12 of 30 patients (40%).[312] Other important findings include pericentric inversions and deletions of chromosome 2, and structural abnormalities of band 1q42.[312] Recently, Sambani and associates found that 44% of cytogenetically evaluable HCL cases had clonal chromosome abnormalities.[313] Numerical aberrations (mostly trisomies) or structural anomalies involving many different chromosomes (chromosome 14 being most frequently affected) have been detected.[313]

Several variants of HCL (HCL-V) have been described.[310] One such variant is characterized by splenomegaly, moderate anemia, and thrombocytopenia with leukocytosis-containing neoplastic lymphoid cells.[314] Monocytopenia, which is common in typical HCL, is absent in these patients with HCL-V. The neoplastic cells are slightly smaller than typical hairy cells, with a higher nuclear to cytoplasmic ratio. They possess the morphologic characteristics between HCL and PLL. Their nucleus is round, deeply cleaved, or irregular and contains moderately condensed heterochromatin and a prominent nucleolus (Fig. 12.30). The cytoplasm is more basophilic than in HCL, with villous projections. The tartrate-resistant acid phosphatase reaction is negative. The leukemic cells from a majority of patients express CD19, CD20, CD22, FMC-7, HLA-DR, and CD11c; they are negative for CD25 and HC-2. The bone marrow is usually easily aspirated with less reticulin fibrosis than HCL. Bone marrow examination shows interstitial infiltration by neoplastic cells, which often contain condensed chromatin and visible nucleoli, are packed together, and are surrounded by a moderate amount of reticulin. The splenic infiltration is also found in the red pulp but blood lakes are uncommon. It is important to differentiate HCL from HCL-V because the latter does not respond to splenectomy nor to interferon-alfa therapy.[314]

The differential diagnosis includes splenic lymphoma with villous lymphocytes, monocytoid B cell lymphoma (marginal zone lymphoma), follicular center cell lymphoma, chronic lymphocytic leukemia, prolymphocytic leukemia, and mast cell disease. These entities are discussed elsewhere in this text.

The prognosis and long-term survival for patients with HCL have improved over the years.[315,316] These improvement may be due to early recognition of the disease, or advancement of therapy, especially interferon-alfa and purine analogs, such as deoxycoformycin and 2-chlorodeoxyadenosine.

NK-cell and T-cell leukemias

T-chronic lymphocytic leukemia and T-prolymphocytic leukemia

T-chronic lymphocytic leukemia is uncommon. Most cases that were previously referred to as T-CLL are now reclassified as large granular lymphocyte leukemia or the 'small cell variant' of T-PLL.[280,317–319] A diagnosis of T-CLL may be made if T lymphocytosis of greater than $5 \times 10^9/l$ persists for over 6 months and consists of a relatively uniform population of lymphocytes.[280] As described earlier, prolymphocytic leukemia as initially introduced by Galton is a well defined clinical and morphologic entity.[306] These patients are typically elderly male, and present with massive splenomegaly, inconspicuous or absent lymphadenopathy, marked lymphocytosis, and an aggressive clinical course. The circulating malignant cells are large, with a round nucleus, slightly condensed nuclear chromatin, a large prominent nucleolus, and a moderate amount of basophilic cytoplasm. Immunophenotypic studies showed that three out of the four cases marked as B-cells and one as a T-cell.[306]

Matutes and associates[320] collected data on 78 cases of *T-prolymphocytic leukemia*. The median age for this group of patients was 69 years, with a male:female ratio of 1.3:1. 73% of these patients presented with splenomegaly. Lymphadenopathy (53%) and hepatomegaly (40%) were also common; skin lesions were seen in 27% of patients. Most patients had leukocytosis ($>100 \times 10^9/l$) with circulating prolymphocytes (cells containing a large prominent nucleolus). A small prolymphocyte variant was described that comprised 19% of cases. The neoplastic cells expressed mature T cell phenotype with CD4$^+$, CD8$^-$ being the most common subset. The expression of CD7 was a consistent finding, in contrast to ATLL, large granular lymphocyte leukemia, and Sézary syndromes, in which CD7 was often negative. Chromosomal abnormalities involving 14q11 (inv(14)(q11;q32)), trisomy 8, and occasional cases with t(11;14) (q13;q32) have been reported.[320] An association of the *ATM* gene at 11q22.3 with T-PLL, and even B-CLL and MCL, has been recognized recently.[321] Allelic ATM inactivations by large deletions or mutations were found in approximately two-thirds of T-PLL.[322] The clinical course was progressive, with a median survival of 7.5 months. Interestingly, a subpopulation of patients with T-PLL, including many with ataxia telangiectasia, have an initial indolent disease course that eventually transforms into the more aggressive disease.[323]

The inclusion of a small cell variant is troublesome to some investigators.[324,325] These cells had irregular nuclear contours, a high nuclear to cytoplasmic ratio, and the nucleolus was not readily apparent by light microscopy but visible by electron microscopy. Hoyer and colleagues classified these cases as true T-cell CLL.[325] In their study of 25 cases, they found the median age to be 57 years, with 56% of patients having lymphadenopathy, 40% having mild to moderate splenomegaly, and 16% having erythematous skin lesions at presentation. The median lymphocyte count was lower than typical PLL at $36.3 \times 10^9/l$. The neoplastic lymphocytes were small, with a high nuclear to cytoplasmic ratio, a wide spectrum of nuclear

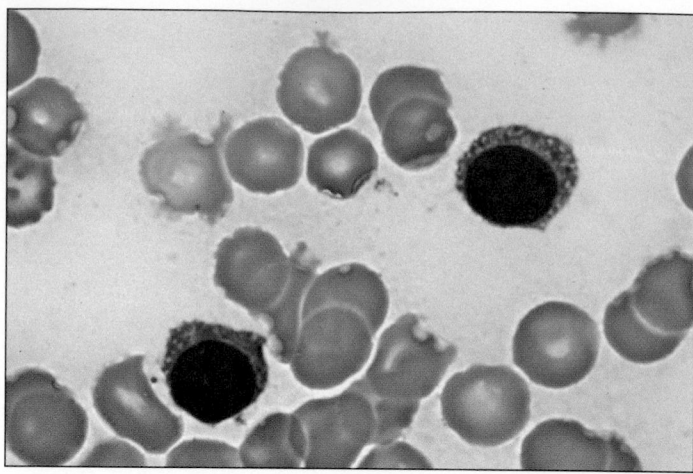

Fig. 12.31 Large granular lymphocyte leukemia. These large granular lymphocytes are abnormal with increased nuclear to cytoplasmic ratio, evenly distributed chromatin, and a small amount of deeply basophilic vacuolated cytoplasm containing many large azurophilic granules. (Romanowsky stain, ×1000.)

outlines and absent or small nucleolus. Bone marrow histopathology showed an interstitial pattern of infiltration. Immunologic studies revealed mature T-cell phenotype with a predominance of CD4 expression. Recurring structural abnormalities involving bands 14q11 (*TCRα/δ* gene locus) and 14q32 (14q32.1 is *TCL-1* locus) were the most common findings. Others involved chromosomes 7p15 (*TCRγ* region) and the long arm of chromosome 8. These patients also ran an aggressive clinical course and were refractory to conventional therapy.[325]

Large granular lymphocytosis and large granular lymphocyte leukemia

Large granular lymphocytes (LGLs) are large, and have an oval, round, or slightly folded nucleus with an abundant amount of pale blue cytoplasm that contains fine or coarse azurophilic granules. LGLs comprise 10–15% of normal blood mononuclear cells and may be of either CD3$^-$ (NK cells) or CD3$^+$ (T-cell) lineage. Deviation from normal morphology may be seen in LGL leukemia (Fig. 12.31).

T-LGL leukemia

is defined as a clonal proliferation of CD3$^+$ LGL and is found in 80% of cases with LGL leukemia. Most of these cases run a chronic clinical course and have a CD3$^+$, CD4$^-$, CD8$^+$, CD16$^+$, CD56$^-$, CD57$^+$, and often HLA-DR$^+$ phenotype. Rarely, T-LGL leukemia may be CD4$^+$ or CD4$^+$,CD8$^+$. *TCRα/β* or *TCRγ/δ* gene rearrangement is often demonstrated. Patients with T-LGL leukemia are usually old, with a median age of 60 years and an equal male to female ratio.[318] About one-third of patients are asymptomatic. Others present with severe neutropenia, anemia, or red cell aplasia. Recurrent infections, rheumatoid arthritis, and other autoimmune phenomena (such as autoantibodies) have also been observed. Hepatosplenomegaly is common; lymphadenopathy and cutaneous lesions are unusual.[318]

Bone marrow examination shows a diffuse as well as interstitial or nodular pattern of involvement by T-LGL. Immunohistochemistry demonstrated perforin, granzyme B, and T cell intracellular antigen (TIA)-1 in both NK cells and cytotoxic cells.[326] The prognosis of T-LGL leukemia is variable, but generally runs a chronic protracted

Table 12.23 Comparison of NK, NK/T and post-thymic T-cell malignancies

	CD2	sCD3*	CD5	CD7	CD4	CD8	CP†	CD16	CD56	CD57	EBV	Cell type
T-LGL	+	+	+	+/−	−	−	+	+	−	+	−	Tαβ
T-PLL	+	+	+	+	+	−	−	−	−	−	−	Tαβ
ANKL	+	−	−	−	−	−	+	+	+	−/+	+	NK
ATLL	+	+	+	−	+	−	−	−	−	−	−	Tαβ
CTCL	+	+	+	+/−	+	−	−	−	−	−	−	Tαβ
N,NTL	+	−	−	−/+	−	−/+	+	−	+	−	+	NK
BNKLL	−/+	−	−	−/+	+	−	−/+	−	+	−	−	NK
HSTCL	+	+	−/+	+/−	−	−	+	−	+	−	−	Tγδ
SPTCL	NA	+	NA	NA	−	+	+	NA	−/+	NA	−	Tαβ
ETTCL	NA	+	−	+	−	−/+	+	NA	−/+	NA	−/+	Tαβ/γδ
PTCL,US	+	−/+	+	+	−/+	−/+	−	−	−	−	−	T
ALCL	+	−/+	−	−	+	−	+	−	−/(+)	−	−	T,null

ALCL, anaplastic large cell lymphoma; ANKL, aggressive NK-cell leukemia; ATLL, adult T-cell leukemia/lymphoma; BNKLL, blastic NK-cell lymphoma/leukemia; CTCL, cutaneous T-cell lymphoma; ETTCL, enteropathy-type T-cell lymphoma, PTCL,US, peripheral T-cell lymphoma, unspecified; HSTCL, hepatosplenic (γδ) T-cell lymphoma; N,NTL, nasal or nasal-type NK/T-cell lymphoma; SPTCL, subcutaneous panniculitis-like T-cell lymphoma; T-LGL, T-large granular lymphocyte leukemia; T-PLL, T-prolymphocytic leukemia.
* sCD3, surface CD3; cells that are surface CD3− may be positive for CD3ε (cytoplasmic CD3 or cCD3).
† CP, cytoxic proteins, which include TIA-1, perforin, granzyme B.

course.[319] It should be pointed out that rare cases of T-LGL expressing CD56 have a more aggressive clinical course.[327].

NK-LGL proliferative disorders
CD3–LGL or NK-LGL proliferative disorders may be classified into chronic NK cell lymphocytosis and NK-LGL leukemia.[318,328]

Chronic NK cell lymphocytosis is very uncommon. The median age for chronic NK cell lymphocytosis is 58 years in one study,[318] and 60.5 years in another.[328] There is a definite male predominance with a male to female ratio of 3.2[318] or 7,[328] reported by two different studies. About 50% of patients are asymptomatic at presentation. Vasculitic skin lesions, non-neutropenic fever, cyclic neutropenia, pure red cell aplasia, and peripheral neuropathy have been reported. Lymphadenopathy, splenomegaly, or hepatomegaly is uncommon. The median absolute NK cell count was $4 \times 10^9/l$ in one study,[328] and $2.3 \times 10^9/l$ in another.[318] The usual phenotype is CD2+, CD3−, CD4−, CD8−, CD16+, and CD56+.[318] Bone marrow examinations showed granuloma or lymphoid aggregates.[328] The clinical features of these patients are similar to those of CD3+ LGL (or T-LGL) leukemia, except that rheumatoid arthritis is uncommon in these patients. The disease usually runs a chronic, indolent clinical course. Its status as a reactive or neoplastic disease is still uncertain.[318,328]

NK-LGL leukemias or aggressive NK-cell leukemias are more common in Asia than in Western countries. It is a disease of younger adults than T-LGL leukemia; the median age is 40 years. Patients often present with B-symptoms, pancytopenia, hepatosplenomegaly, and lymphadenopathy.[278,318,329] Some patients may have gastrointestinal involvement, neoplastic infiltration into body cavities, including cerebrospinal fluid. This disease has an aggressive course. Most patients die of multiorgan failure with or without hemophagocytosis and coagulopathy. The neoplastic cells can display a spectrum of morphology from mature, large granular lymphocytes (similar to normal large granular lymphocytes) to cells with increased nuclear/cytoplasmic ratio, open chromatin and distinct nucleoli.[329] The usual phenotype is CD3−, CD4−, CD8+, CD16+, CD56+,

TCRαβ−, TCRγδ− (Table 12.23). Expression of CD57 is variable. In paraffin sections, the neoplastic cells show reactivity with the polyclonal CD3ε antibody. Also, EBER-1 is positive in the tumor cells by in situ hybridization. Bone marrow involvement is often patchy or subtle, sometimes with marrow fibrosis. Deletions of 6q, 11q, and 17p have been reported.[330]

Two different types of precursor NK cell leukemia have also been described.[331,332] The leukemic cells in those cases described by Scott and associates have fine azurophilic granules,[331] whereas those cases reported by Suzuki and co-workers have agranular blasts that morphologically resemble L2 cells of FAB classification. These cases should be differentiated from acute myeloid leukemia with CD56 expression.

Bone marrow involvement in non-Hodgkin's lymphoma

Bone marrow involvement is quite common in non-Hodgkin's lymphoma (NHL). However, the incidence varies among different series of studies, different histologic types, and different methods of obtaining the specimens. As a rule, histologic examination of a bone marrow clot section or biopsy specimen is better than that of Wright-Giemsa-stained bone marrow smears, bilateral bone marrow biopsies are better than unilateral biopsy, and open bone marrow biopsy is better than needle biopsy. However, bilateral needle biopsies are adequate for staging purposes.[333] Bone marrow involvement was found in 89% of multiple myeloma, 64% of non-Hodgkin's lymphoma, and 8% of Hodgkin's lymphoma (HL) by Bartl and associates after studying 3229 patients with lymphoproliferative disorders.[334] Schmid and Isaacson[57] found a similar prevalence involved bone marrow: 90% (141 of 157 patients) of multiple myeloma, 64% (311 of 490) of low-grade NHL; 15% (30 of 199) of high-grade NHL, and 9% of HL. Recently, Wang and associates studied the diagnostic utility of bilateral bone marrow examinations in patients with malignant diseases and found that 29.6% of 883 specimens with a clinical diagnosis of NHL, 9.9% of 362 specimens with HL, and 77%

of 56 specimens with multiple myeloma were positive for tumor.[11] Bone marrow involvement was most common in patients with SLL/CLL (92%), followed by MCL (58%), follicular lymphoma (44.4%), marginal zone lymphoma (MZL) (29%), lymphoblastic lymphoma (25%), peripheral T-cell lymphoma (PTCL) (25%), large cell lymphoma (16.5%), and Burkitt's lymphoma (9%).[11] The clinical symptoms vary with the type of NHL. The classifications of malignant lymphomas and their clinical, histologic, immunophenotypic, and genotypic characteristics are discussed in detail in Chapter 11. The terminologies used in the International Working Formulation[335] will be used interchangeably with the new World Health Organization classification of tumor[281] in this chapter for discussion.

Bone marrow involvement is more frequently seen in patients with lymphomas of small lymphocytes (low-grade) than in those with large-cell lymphomas, high-grade NHLs, and peripheral T cell lymphoma,[334] although lymphocytic lymphomas of small lymphocytic cells and small cleaved cells (centrocytes) often have a more indolent clinical course. However, there are exceptions for the subtypes of B- and T-cell lymphomas.[336] Bone marrow examination frequently changes clinical staging from a more localized form of disease (stage I or II) to a disseminated form (stage IV). A positive bone marrow examination is frequently obtained in patients with a normal complete blood cell count and without evidence of a leukoerythroblastic picture. The absolute blood lymphocyte count is considered to be an important diagnostic criterion in differentiating malignant lymphomas from leukemic infiltration of the bone marrow; that is, when the blood lymphocyte count is $10 \times 10^9/l$ or greater, lymphocytic leukemia is the preferred diagnosis.[280]

Histopathologic examination of a bone marrow biopsy reveals the following patterns: interstitial, nodular, paratrabecular, or packed marrow (diffuse infiltration). Combinations of one or more of these patterns are also observed. The neoplastic lymphocytes are seen infiltrating between fat cells and replacing normal hematopoietic elements in the interstitial pattern. The focal or nodular involvement in small cleaved cell follicular lymphoma is characterized by a paratrabecular distribution (Fig. 12.32). Bone marrow involvement in small lymphocytic lymphomas is usually randomly focal, whereas small noncleaved cell (Burkitt's or Burkitt-like lymphomas) and lymphoblastic lymphomas generally display an interstitial or diffuse pattern of infiltration.[336] When the marrow is involved, the type of lymphoma, the pattern of infiltration, and the degree of involvement (in the form of percentage of all nucleated cells or of marrow cellularity) should all be stated in the bone marrow report. Cytologically, lymphomatous infiltration in the marrow generally shows morphologic features similar to those observed in lymph node biopsies from the same patients, with the exceptions noted below. Extensive blood involvement was noted most frequently in follicular lymphoma and MCL (Fig. 12.33). Touch imprints of bone marrow biopsy usually identify neoplastic infiltrate more easily than bone marrow aspirate smears when the infiltration is focal or patchy. Flow cytometry study and cytogenetic study may then initiate and further delineate the type of neoplastic lymphocytes and provide information for the prognosis.

Morphologic discordance between the lymph node and bone marrow

When comparative histologic examinations of malignant lymphomas in lymph node and bone marrow were made, a discordance between these two anatomic sites was noted in 22–60% of cases.[337,338] Divergent histology is common in large cell lymphomas, and in follicular and diffuse, mixed small and large cell types.[338–340] The

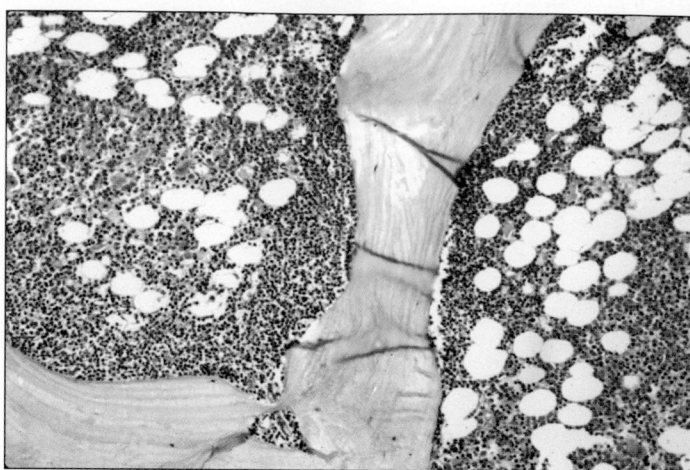

Fig. 12.32 Follicular lymphoma. Paratrabecular infiltrate is quite characteristic of small cleaved cell (centrocytic) lymphoma. (H&E stain, ×100.)

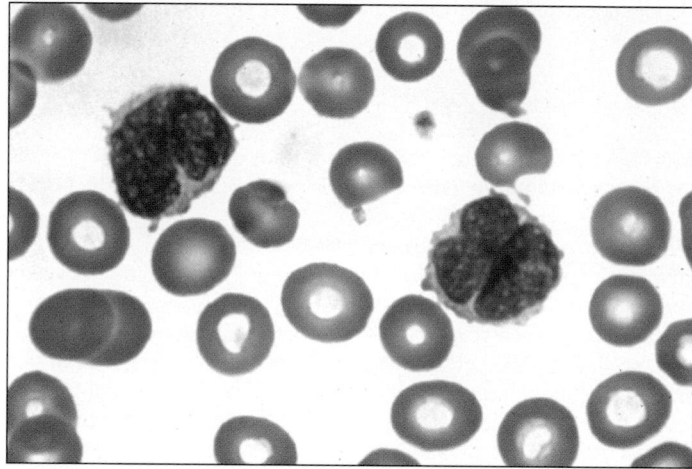

Fig. 12.33 Leukemic phase of non-Hodgkin's lymphoma. Note that neoplastic lymphocytes have deeply clefted or indented nuclei and coarse clumped chromatin. (Romanowsky stain, ×1000.)

more aggressive subtype is usually found in the lymph node. The typical discordant pattern shows large cell or immunoblastic lymphoma in the lymph node, but mixed small and large cell, small cleaved cell or small lymphocytic histology in the bone marrow.[338–340] Of the lymphomas that were immunophenotyped and had bone marrow involvement, 52% of the B-cell lymphomas and 38% of the T-cell lymphomas showed discordant histology between lymph node and bone marrow.[340]

Isolated bone marrow NHL without systemic involvement is relatively rare.[341] Three of the four cases reported by Ponzoni and Li[341] were T-cell lymphoma. They may create diagnostic difficulty. Flow cytometry, immunohistochemistry and molecular techniques may be used to detect clonal disorders.[342] Bone marrow examination is important in pathologic staging of clinical stage I or II disease and in following patients with advanced disease for response to therapy. Its significance for patients with advanced clinical stages is uncertain.

B-cell lymphomas

Small lymphocytic lymphoma Small lymphocytic lymphoma and B-chronic lymphocytic leukemia are closely related disorders with neoplastic lymphocytes displaying similar morphologic, immunophenotypic, and genotypic findings.[343] A higher CD11a/CD18 expression in SLL in comparison to B-CLL has been reported.[343] Lymphomatous involvement of the marrow is seen in nearly 90% of cases.[11,333]

Lymphoplasmacytic lymphoma Lymphoplasmacytic lymphoma is an uncommon low-grade lymphoma, although bone marrow involvement is seen in 85% of cases at the time of initial diagnosis.[334] The pattern of infiltration is nodular or interstitial/nodular. The subtype, Waldenström's macroglobulinemia, is a lymphoproliferative disorder of B-cells with variable plasmacytoid differentiation and is associated with monoclonal IgM production.[344] Clinically, these are elderly patients who may present with hyperviscosity syndrome, neuropathies, coagulopathies, cryoglobulinemia, generalized lymphadenopathy, and splenomegaly. Bone marrow is nearly 100% involved by neoplastic small lymphocytes, plasmacytoid lymphocytes, or plasma cells in a diffuse, interstitial, nodular, and paratrabecular pattern. Intranuclear or intracytoplasmic PAS-positive inclusions (Dutcher bodies) may be identified. These inclusions are usually composed of M (monoclonal) protein. Immunophenotypically, these cells are mSIg+, CD19+, CD20+, CD5-, CD10-, and CD23-. They may express CD38 or CD138. About one-third of patients who had cytogenetic studies had an abnormal karyotype. 67% of those with abnormal karyotypes had complex cytogenetic abnormalities.[345] The most common numeric abnormalities were +5 and −8; the most common structural abnormality was del(6q). A translocation involving chromosomes 9 and 14 (t(9;14)(p13;q32)) in which the *PAX5* gene at 9p13 is fused to the *IgH* gene on 14q32 has been associated with lymphoplasmacytic lymphoma.[345] Deletion of 7q32 has also been reported.[343] A post germinal center marginal zone memory B-cell origin has been proposed.[344]

Mantle cell lymphoma Mantle cell lymphoma is a disease of elderly men, characterized by generalized lymphadenopathy and liver and bone marrow involvement.[346] Other extranodal sites may also be involved. Actually, in 10–15% of cases, the clinical presentation may be an extranodal site. Bone marrow infiltration, independent of peripheral blood involvement, occurs in 50–82% of patients.[346] The pattern of infiltration may be nodular, interstitial, paratrabecular, or mixed.

Two cytologic variants of MCL have been recognized. The cells in typical (classical) MCLs are composed of a monotonous population of small to medium-sized lymphocytes with scant cytoplasm, variably irregular nuclei, evenly distributed coarse chromatin, and inconspicuous nucleoli. The morphology of malignant cells in blastic MCL is quite variable, ranging from cells resembling lymphoblasts to those large pleomorphic cells.[346] Nucleolated variants mimicking prolymphocytes have also been described.[347] Mantle cells typically express CD19, CD20, CD22, CD79a, and mSIg (usually co-expressing IgM and IgD) with aberrant expression of CD5. They are CD10- and CD23-, but they overexpress cyclin D1. Translocation involving the *IgH* gene at 14q32 and the *bcl-1* (cyclin D1, *PRAD-1*) gene at 11q13 (t(11;14)(q13;q32)) is considered to be characteristic for MCL, although this translocation has occasionally been found in other lymphomas, including multiple myeloma. Other cytogenetic abnormalities have also been described.[290,348]

Marginal zone B-cell lymphoma Marginal zone B-cell lymphoma (monocytoid B-cell lymphoma, low-grade B-cell lymphoma of MALT type) is a low-grade lymphoma and primarily involves lymph nodes or extranodal sites (mucosa-associated lymphoid tissue, MALT). Splenomegaly, bone marrow involvement, and leukemic conversion are uncommon. An incidence of 2% is cited in one report[349] and 46–53% in another.[350] Bone marrow involvement is more common in nodal type (28%) than extranodal type (15%).[351] It has been said that marrow involvement is usually more extensive and consistent in splenic MZL than the other two types.[336] In nodal MZL, the neoplastic cells are CD19+, CD20+, and often CD21+ and CD35+, but negative for CD5, CD10, CD23, and cyclin D1. Bcl-2 is positive in most cases and CD43 is positive in about 20% of cases.[351] Trisomy 3, trisomy 18, and structural abnormalities of chromosome 1 are the most common cytogenetic abnormalities described in MZL.[351] Translocation of *MLT* at 18q12 and *API* at 11q21 (t(11;18)(q21;q21)), and translocation of *bcl-10* at 1p22 and *IgH* at 14q32 (t(1;14)(p22;q32)) are significantly associated with advanced cases of MALT lymphoma.[352] These molecular abnormalities may be detected using RT-PCR, FISH, or even immunohistochemistry.[352] Recently, this lymphoma and some cases of lymphoplasmacytic lymphoma have been linked to hepatitis C virus (HCV) infection.[351]

Splenic marginal zone lymphoma/splenic lymphoma with villous lymphocytes is a low grade B cell lymphoma that is histologically indistinguishable from splenic MZL. This disease primarily afflicts elderly men or women with a median age of 66 years.[353] These patients present with anemia, thrombocytopenia, leukocytosis with circulating neoplastic cells, monoclonal gammopathy, and splenomegaly.[354] The circulating cells are slightly larger than a small lymphocyte, have a round or oval nucleus containing condensed nuclear chromatin and a small nucleolus, and exhibit short and thin cytoplasmic villi. Sometimes the cytoplasmic projections are localized to one pole or two opposite poles of the cell. The nuclear:cytoplasmic ratio is higher than in hairy cells of HCL and HCL-V. A few cells showing lymphoplasmacytic features are often present. The usual immunophenotypic findings are mSIg+, CD79b+, FMC-7+, CD22+, CD11c+, CD25−/+, CD103−/+, HC2−, CD5− and CD23− (see Table 12.22).[355] The histopathology of the spleen shows infiltration of white pulp in a marginal zone pattern or complete replacement of follicles in the white pulp, although the red pulp may show a variable degree of involvement.[355] The bone marrow is not infiltrated in half of the cases; in others there is moderate to pronounced diffuse or nodular infiltration.[280] Both bone marrow aspirate smears and trephine core biopsy are needed for the study.[355] A nodular, paratrabecular or intrasinusoidal pattern of infiltration has been described.[355] Cytogenetic abnormalities have been demonstrated in some patients especially when using FISH. These include t(11;14)(q13;q32), trisomy 3, interstitial deletion of 3q14, and trisomy 12.[355] A recent study using interferon-alfa and treating some patients with ribavirin for SLVL and HCV infection led to a partial or complete remission of SLVL in nine cases but none of the six HCV-negative patients had a response to interferon therapy.[356]

Follicular lymphoma Approximately 50% of the follicular lymphomas of predominantly small cleaved cell and follicular mixed small cleaved and large cell lymphomas involve bone marrow.[11] These types of lesions frequently display a focal and paratrabecular pattern (see Fig. 12.32). The neoplastic cells usually consist of a predominance of small cleaved cells regardless of the lymph node histology. They can be differentiated from CLL by lack of CD5 and CD23, from MCL by lack of CD5 and cyclin D1 (Bcl-1) and by its own characteristic expression of CD10, Bcl-6, and pan B (CD19, CD20) antigens using immunohistochemical techniques (Table 12.22). Although the neoplastic cells usually have t(14;18)(q32;q21), overexpression of Bcl-2 protein may be observed in normal mantle cells and some T-cells, as well as in the neoplastic cells of CLL and MCL. It should be pointed out that CD5[+] follicular lymphoma has been reported.[357] Interestingly, CD5[−] MCLs have also been described.[358] Therefore, multiparameter studies should be undertaken in the classification of NHL. A high incidence of discordant histologic types between the bone marrow and the lymph node has been observed in this group of lymphomas, as discussed earlier.[336–340]

Diffuse large cell lymphoma

Diffuse large cell lymphomas (DLCL) include a morphologic spectrum of B- and T-cell lymphomas. The overall incidence of marrow involvement for this group varies from 8–35%.[359] A discordant histology between lymph node and bone marrow is observed in this morphologic category and is more common in B cell lymphomas, especially those lymphomas of follicular origin.[338,340] *Intravascular lymphoma* is an uncommon variant of large cell lymphoma; 78% are of B-cell origin and 8% of T-cell origin.[360] Earlier reports stated that bone marrow involvement is uncommon. With the application of immunohistochemical techniques, intravascular lymphoma is found in the bone marrow of 15% of cases.[361] Another uncommon DLCL is *T-cell-rich B-cell lymphoma*. These neoplastic large B cells are often scattered among numerous T cells (>50% of all cells) and/or histiocytes. They also infiltrate bone marrow, with an incidence of 62% in one study[362] but 38% in another.[363] Again, immunohistochemistry is crucial in making the diagnosis because the lesion may resemble peripheral T-cell lymphoma and HL.

Lymphoblastic lymphoma of T- and B-cell types

Lymphoblastic lymphoma of T- and B-cell types has been discussed under ALL. The incidence of bone marrow involvement is 40–60%.[359] The histologic and cytologic features of lymphoblastic lymphoma are identical to those of ALL. The distinction is based on the percentage of neoplastic cells in the marrow. If lymphoblasts constitute more than 25% of all nucleated cells in the marrow, a diagnosis of ALL is made. The pattern of infiltration in the marrow is nearly always interstitial or diffuse. A 'starry-sky pattern' may be observed in some cases, due to the presence of tingible body macrophages. The neoplastic cells range from the size of a small lymphocyte to three or four times larger than a small lymphocyte. Nuclear irregularity, fine chromatin pattern, and a high mitotic rate are frequently observed. Immunophenotypic study shows about 70% of cases express T-cell markers and 30% of cases type as pre-B cells.

Burkitt's lymphoma

Bone marrow involvement is seen in about 20–35% of patients with Burkitt's lymphoma.[359] The pattern may be diffuse, interstitial, or focal. Focal or large areas of necrosis may be seen. The size of the neoplastic nucleus approximates that of a histiocyte. The nuclei are round or oval with coarse but evenly distributed chromatin and two to four small, distinct nucleoli. The neoplastic cells have a moderate amount of vacuolated pyroninophilic cytoplasm. Mitotic figures are numerous. Proliferation index (Ki-67) may reach 100%. Cytologic variants may be encountered in 'Burkitt-like' lymphoma.[364]

Post-thymic T- and NK-cell proliferations

Sézary syndrome

Sézary syndrome is characterized by generalized erythroderma, pruritus, peripheral lymphadenopathy,

hepatomegaly, and the presence of Sézary cells in the skin and peripheral blood. Lutzner and associates[365] proposed the term cutaneous T-cell lymphoma (CTCL) to include both Sézary syndrome and mycosis fungoides. The neoplastic cells of both diseases possess similar morphologic findings (cerebriform nuclei), express T-cell (helper cell) markers (CD2[+], CD3[+], CD4[+], and CD5[+]; TdT[−], HLA-DR[−], and CD7[−]), and have a predilection for the skin. The neoplastic cells express IL-2 receptor (CD25) in approximately 50% of patients with mycosis fungoides.[319] Circulating atypical lymphoid (Sézary) cells are classically present in Sézary syndrome but much rarer in mycosis fungoides.

Two cell types have been recognized. The large cells range from 12–25 μm in diameter and characteristically have a cerebriform nucleus. The cytoplasm is clear to slightly basophilic and may contain vacuoles. The small cells vary from 8–11 μm in diameter and may resemble normal small lymphocytes with folded nuclei. However, they contain a moderate amount of vacuolated, basophilic cytoplasm. These vacuoles are PAS-positive and form a 'necklace' around the nucleus. About 20% of patients with CTCL have marrow involvement at the time of diagnosis, and usually have peripheral blood involvement.[366] Histopathologic examination of bone marrow biopsy samples reveals that CTCL involvement is usually quite subtle and may depend on cytology or immunohistochemistry for its recognition.[366] The marrow cellularity is usually normal. The hematopoietic elements are not decreased, although the neoplastic cells may infiltrate the interstitium or form small aggregates. These cells have a very high nuclear/cytoplasmic ratio and contain a hyperchromatic nucleus with irregular nuclear contours. Nuclear indentations or convolutions may be appreciated under oil immersion with fine adjustment.

A Sézary cell leukemia has been described.[317,367] These patients have generalized lymphadenopathy, splenomegaly, lymphocytosis, and bone marrow infiltration by abnormal lymphocytes with cerebriform nuclei without skin involvement. Ultrastructurally, these lymphocytes resemble Sézary cells. Phenotypically, they are TdT[−], CD2[+/−], CD3[+]. CD5[+], and may be CD4[−]CD8[+], CD4[+]CD8[+], or CD4[−]CD8[−]. The clinical course is aggressive with a poor response to chemotherapy.

Adult T-cell leukemia/lymphoma

Adult T-cell leukemia/lymphoma is linked to human T-cell leukemia virus (HTLV-1).[368,369] This disorder was found in an endemic area in southwest Japan, the West Indies and Africa and in African-Americans in the southeastern United States.[317] The disease usually affects middle-aged men with a male to female ratio of 1.4:1. Patients may present with one of the four forms: acute leukemia (50–60% of cases), chronic leukemia (3–20%), smoldering leukemia (5–8%), and NHL with minimal or no peripheral blood involvement (20–25%).[317,369] The most common clinical manifestations are fever, lymphadenopathy, hepatosplenomegaly, lytic lesions in bones, hypercalcemia, and cutaneous lesions. The malignant cell is a small to intermediate T-cell, with a markedly irregular ('knobby') nucleus (Fig. 12.34). Polymorphism is characteristic of ATLL but there are diverse morphologies.[370] It has been said that CLL-like morphology with round nuclei is more frequent in the chronic variant and is associated with a better prognosis than those with unusual morphology.[370] These cells frequently mark as T-helper/inducer cells (CD2[+], CD3[+], CD4[+], CD5[+], and CD25[+]; and TdT[−], CD7[−], and CD8[−]), but they generally do not have detectable helper function.

Bone marrow biopsies show microcystic resorption with focal fibrosis and increased osteoclastic activity in some patients. Of those patients who had lymphomatous involvement in the marrow, the

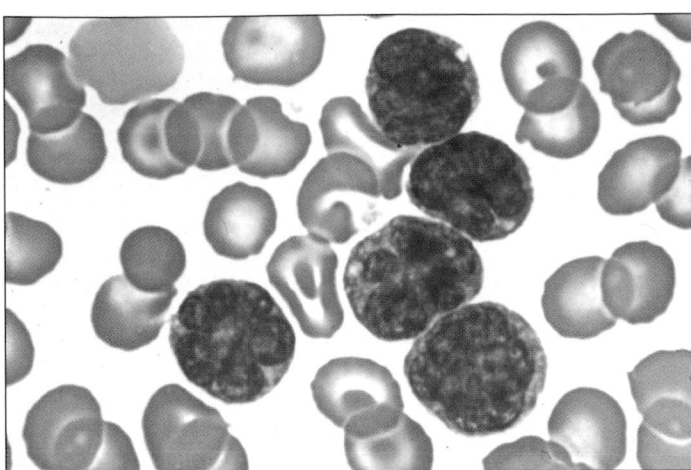

Fig. 12.34 Adult T-cell leukemia/lymphoma. Note the 'flower-like' or 'knobby' nuclei that are characteristic of this type of leukemic cells. (Romanowsky stain, ×1000.)

degree of marrow replacement was not prominent. The infiltrate is patchy or interstitial but not paratrabecular. Some patients who had circulating leukemic cells did not have evidence of bone marrow involvement.[368] Cytogenetic abnormalities including multiple trisomies, deletions of 6q and translocations involving 14q have been described.[371]

NK-cell, NK/T-cell and T-cell lymphomas NK-cell or NK/T-cell lymphomas encompass a heterogenous group of malignant lymphoproliferative disorders characterized by the expression of CD56 by malignant cells with (NK/T-cells) or without (NK-cells) T-cell receptor (*TCR*) gene rearrangement. The afflicted patients are generally younger than other patients with NHL and have extranodal clinical presentations, an aggressive clinical course, and poor prognosis.[372] CD56, an isoform of the neural cell adhesion molecule, is a sensitive marker for NK cells and is expressed on most of them. Other NK cell markers include CD11b, CD16, and CD57. Cytotoxic proteins, such as TIA-1 (resting and activated NK-cells), perforin and granzyme B (activated NK cells) may be demonstrated in these cells using an immunohistochemical method on paraffin sections. The most common NHL in this group is nasal NK/T-cell lymphoma. Chan and associates collected 49 cases of non-nasal lymphomas and classified them into: (1) nasal-type NK/T-cell lymphomas; (2) aggressive NK cell leukemia/lymphoma; (3) blastoid NK-cell lymphoma; and (4) other specific lymphoma types with CD56 expression.[329] The last category encompasses a variety of NHL including T-CLL, T-PLL, T- and B-lymphoblastic lymphoma, respectively, and true histiocytic lymphoma, among others; all exhibit CD56 expression on the malignant cells.[329] Bone marrow involvement at the time of presentation is uncommon by nasal NK-cell and nasal-type NK/T-cell lymphomas at the incidence of 2/25 (8%) and 4/34 (11.8%), respectively.[329,373] Several other types of NK-cell or NK/T-cell lymphoma have been recognized[326,374,375] and it appears that some of them involve bone marrow, which will be discussed below.

Blastic NK-cell lymphoma/leukemia With the exception of those cases reported by DiGiuseppe and associates,[376] blastic NK-cell lymphoma/leukemia affects mostly middle-aged men with a median age of 35 years in one study and 52 years in another.[277,377] These patients usually present with cutaneous lesions, lymphadenopathy

and infiltrative process in tonsils, sinuses, and cerebrospinal fluid. Bone marrow involvement is observed in more than 50% of the patients.

Suzuki and Nakamura classified malignancies of NK precursors into myeloid/NK-cell precursor acute leukemia and blastic NK-cell lymphoma/leukemia.[277] The former characteristically involves bone marrow and lymph node, and is CD34+, CD13+ and CD33+; while the latter affects skin/subcutis and is CD4+. Indeed, the neoplastic cells in blastic NK-cell lymphoma/leukemia have the characteristic sCD3−, CD4+, CD56+ phenotype (Table 12.23), and exhibit an immature (blastic) morphology. Azurophilic granules were identified in the cytoplasm on the touch imprints or bone marrow smears in some cases[277] but not in others.[376,377] Abnormal karyotypes are frequently detected[277,376,377] but no recurrent abnormalities have been found. *TCRβ* gene rearrangement was identified in 2/7 cases studied,[277] but the gene rearrangement was not found in the six cases studied by Bayerl and colleagues.[377] Epstein–Barr virus (EBV) was negative both using immunohistochemistry (LMP-1) and in situ hybridization (EBER-1).[277,376,377] The clinical outcomes in these patients were quite variable; some patients responded to chemotherapy for NHL while others died of complications or relapsed.

Feuillard and associates collected 23 cases characterized by frequent skin lesions with dissemination to other organs, bone marrow infiltrations by CD4+, CD56+ blastic cells and rapid aggressive courses.[378] The neoplastic cells have vacuolated cytoplasm but are devoid of granules. They are negative for sCD3, cCD3, CD5, CD13, CD33, myeloperoxidase, CD19, and CD20, but are frequently positive for CD68, CD36, CD38, CD71, CD7, and CD123. Based on the immunophenotype, a type 2 dendritic cell (DC2 cell) or plasmacytoid DC in origin of these tumor cells has been proposed.[378] Further, a proto-oncogene, *TCL-1*, has been detected in 83% of these blastic tumors.[379] A recent review by Bene and colleagues compared DC2 cells with NK cells[380] Readers are referred to the original article for a detailed discussion.

It is important to recognize this entity and to differentiate it from other cutaneous lymphomas, myeloid/NK cell precursor acute leukemia and aggressive NK-cell leukemia.

Hepatosplenic (g/d) T-cell lymphoma This uncommon NHL usually affects young adults with a male predominance. Patients present with cytopenias, hepatosplenomegaly with minimal or absent lymphadenopathy, with or without a leukemic blood picture.[381,382] The neoplastic cells are homogeneous, medium-sized lymphocytes with partially dispersed chromatin, inconspicuous nucleoli and a moderate amount of cytoplasm that may contain azurophilic granules. The bone marrow is nearly always involved but the sinusoidal or interstitial pattern of infiltration is very subtle and is difficult to diagnose without the aid of immunohistochemistry. The neoplastic cells also infiltrate sinusoids of the liver and the red pulp of the spleen. They have the following phenotype: CD2+, CD3+, CD4−, CD5−/(+), CD7+/(−), CD8−/(+), CD16+, CD56+, CD57−, TCRγ/δ+, TCRαβ−, TIA-1(+), and EBER-1(−) (Table 12.23). Isochromosome 7q is characteristic, although other cytogenetic abnormalities have been reported.[382,383] The prognosis is poor. Complete remission is uncommon. Of those patients with an initial response, relapses were frequent.

S-100-positive T-cell lymphoproliferative disorder This is extremely uncommon. It shares some of the same clinical characteristics of hepatosplenic T-cell lymphoma, i.e. hepatosplenomegaly with or without lymphadenopathy and sinusoidal infiltration in liver, bone marrow, and lymph node. Also, only red pulp is involved in the spleen. The neoplastic lymphocytes show heterogeneous morphology, ranging from small to intermediate size, round or irregular nuclei, coarsely clumped chromatin, small and inconspicuous nucleoli, and an abundant amount of cytoplasm without azurophilic granules. Cerebrospinal fluid involvement was observed in three of four patients reported by Hanson and associates.[384] The malignant lymphocytes possess the following phenotype: CD2$^+$, CD3$^+$, CD4$^-$, CD5$^{+/-}$, CD7$^+$, CD8$^-$, CD16$^+$, CD56$^+$ and CD57$^-$. These investigators also found clonal TCR gene rearrangements with TCRβ, γ, and δ in the two cases studied, but only TCRα and TCRβ RNA transcripts were detected by Northern blot analysis.[384] In addition, EBV was not found by molecular methods. The prognosis is very poor.

Bone marrow involvement is uncommon in *subcutaneous panniculitis-like T-cell lymphoma* and *enteropathy-type T-cell lymphoma*.[385] Readers are referred to Chapter 11 for a detailed discussion.

Peripheral T-cell lymphoma, unspecified

This term is applied to those PTCL cases that do not belong to any of the better defined entities in the WHO classification.[386] Most of the afflicted patients are adults, with a near-equal male to female ratio. They usually presented with lymphadenopathy, constitutional symptoms, disseminated disease, histopathologic diversity, and an aggressive clinical course. Paraneoplastic features, such as eosinophilia, pruritus, or hemophagocytic syndrome, may be observed. The normal architecture of the lymph node is nearly totally effaced and replaced by medium-sized or large lymphocytes with pleomorphic or irregular nuclei and clear cytoplasm. Reed–Sternberg-like cells and mitotic figures are often present. Several variants may be seen, including T-zone variant and lymphoepithelioid variant. Bone marrow involvement has been described in 32% of cases in one study[387] and 41% in another.[390]

The pattern of bone marrow infiltration may be diffuse or randomly focal. In the mixed and large cell types, the lesions are usually composed of a spectrum of lymphoid cells with variable size and configuration among a heterogeneous population of eosinophils, plasma cells, neutrophils, histiocytes, epithelioid histiocytes, and capillaries. Prominent vascularity and reticulin fibrosis are often observed. The epithelioid cells are often found in clusters and may impart a granulomatous appearance. The histopathology of PTCL in the bone marrow corresponds to that observed in lymph nodes.

Anaplastic large cell lymphoma

Anaplastic large cell lymphoma (ALCL) is a large cell lymphoma that may be confused with malignant histiocytosis or metastatic carcinoma to the lymph node because of its typical sinusoidal infiltration. The neoplastic cells express Ki-1 (CD30) antigen, epithelial membrane antigen (EMA), and CD45 (Table 12.23). However, CD30 is an activation antigen and could be expressed on T-cells, B-cells, activated histiocytes and on the prototype cells of a variety of lymphoproliferative disorders. The identification of t(2;5)(p23;q35) (a nucleophosmin (*NPM*) gene at 5q35 fuses with a gene at 2p23 encoding the receptor tyrosine kinase anaplastic lymphoma kinase (ALK)) led to the production of monoclonal antibody ALK-1. Based on the ALK expression, ALCL may be classified into ALK$^+$ systemic ALCL, ALK$^-$ systemic ALCL, and primary cutaneous ALCL that is also ALK$^-$. The ALK$^+$ ALCL occurs in children, adolescents, and young adults, and has a male predominance. These patients frequently present with B-symptoms and advanced stage disease. Extranodal involvements, especially skin, bone and soft tissue are common.[388] 17% of 42 patients with ALCL were found to have bone marrow involvement at diagnosis by

morphologic examination.[389] However, occult malignant cells were detected in 23% of the patients with negative bone marrow biopsy on routine histology after immunohistochemical stains using CD30 and EMA as markers.[389] Therefore, immunohistochemical study is crucial in the bone marrow examination of ALCL.

Angioimmunoblastic T-cell lymphoma

This condition primarily affects the middle-aged to elderly with a near-equal male to female ratio. These patients frequently present with B symptoms, skin rash with pruritus, generalized lymphadenopathy, polyclonal gammopathy, arthritis, or other stigmata of autoimmune disorders. Bone marrow involvement has been documented in 32% of cases.[390] EBV is frequently demonstrated in B cells, and perhaps T cells as well. Immunophenotypic studies are usually not that helpful. TCR genes are rearranged in a majority of cases. The most frequent cytogenetic abnormalities are trisomy 3, trisomy 5, and an additional chromosome X.[391] The disease usually runs an aggressive course.

Hodgkin's lymphoma (Hodgkin's disease)

Hodgkin's lymphoma is a lymphoreticular malignant disease, primarily affecting lymph nodes and characterized by a neoplastic proliferation of malignant cells (Reed–Sternberg cells) associated with an impaired host immune response. Identification of the classic Reed–Sternberg cells is necessary for the diagnosis of HL, although the mere presence of such a cell is not sufficient for this diagnosis. A classic Reed–Sternberg cell is binucleated or multinucleated and has a bilobed and occasionally multilobed nucleus or multiple nuclei. Each lobe or individual nucleus contains a large, homogeneous, eosinophilic, inclusion-like nucleolus, which often reaches the size of a red cell or the nucleus of a small lymphocyte. The cytoplasm contains a large quantity of ribonucleic acid and is strongly pyroninophilic when stained by methyl green pyronine (Fig. 12.35). Several types of Reed–Sternberg variant have been described and are very useful in the subclassification of the disease. These include lymphocytic and histiocytic (L&H) variants (or 'popcorn cells'), lacunar cells and pleomorphic variants.

The classification of HL has evolved throughout the years. Current classifications include two major categories: nodular lymphocyte-predominant Hodgkin's lymphoma (NLPHL), and classical Hodgkin's lymphoma.[392] The latter is further classified into nodular sclerosis, mixed cellularity, lymphocyte-rich classical HL, lymphocyte depletion, and unclassifiable classical HL.

Immunohistochemical studies are useful in the diagnosis and differential diagnosis of HL. The L&H variants that are characteristic for NLPHL are large cells having a polyploid, vesicular, multilobulated nucleus with each lobe containing a small but distinct nucleolus and scant cytoplasm. These cells usually express CD45, CD20, CD79a, Bcl-6, J chain, and CDw75. They may also be positive for EMA. The classical Reed–Sternberg cells, lacunar cells or pleomorphic variants, on the other hand, are CD45$^-$ (although some of them may be CD20$^+$). They are usually positive for CD30 and CD15 (Table 12.24). HL is considered to be a B-cell lymphoproliferative disorder in >95% of cases.[392,393]

Bone marrow involvement is not uncommon in certain subtypes of HL, although the overall frequency of bone marrow involvement reported in the literature ranges from 5–10%.[11,57,334,394] The most frequent type of HL involving bone marrow is the diffuse fibrosis of the lymphocytic depletion type, with a reported incidence varying from 40–79%.[395–397] Bone marrow involvement also occurs in patients with other types of HL. It is more commonly seen in older men who have constitutional symptoms, advanced clinical stages, and unfavorable histologic subtypes of HL.[394] The results of the

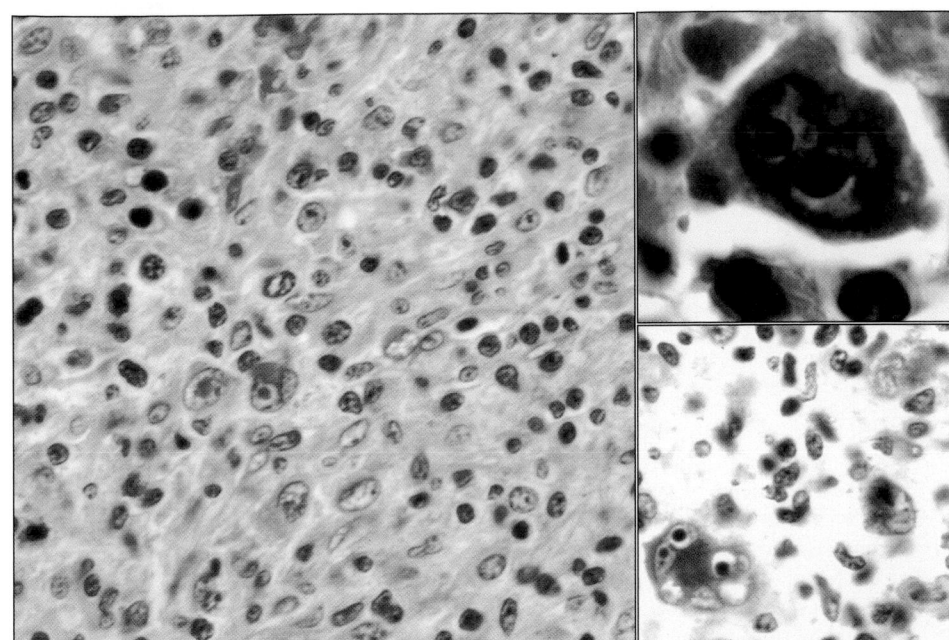

Fig. 12.35 Hodgkin's lymphoma. A mixed or polymorphic population of cells including large atypical or bizarre cells resembling Reed–Sternberg cells or Reed–Sternberg variants is frequently observed. The classical Reed–Sternberg cell is a bilobed or binucleated cell with each lobe or nucleus containing a large prominent nucleolus surrounded by perinucleolar halo, and a moderate amount of cytoplasm. These cells express CD30 or CD15 in a focal or membranous staining. (H&E stain, ×250 and ×630; immunoperoxidase stain with anti-CD15 antibody, ×250.)

Table 12.24 Differential diagnosis of Hodgkin's lymphoma

Markers	NLPHL	T/H-RBCL	CHL	PTCL	ALCL
CD45	+	+	−	+	+/−
CD20	+	+	−/(+)	−	−
CD30	−/(+)	−	+	−	+
CD15	−	−	+	−	−
CD3	−	−	−	+	+/−
CD43	−	−	−	+	+/−
EMA	+/−	−/(+)	−	−	+/−
ALK–1	−	−	−	−	+/−
λ or κ*	+	+	−/+	−	−

* Monoclonal λ or κ is usually detected in T/H-RBCL and NLPHL. The RS cells and their variants in CHL are usually double-stained by λ and κ light chains because of the presence of Fc receptor on these cells.
ALCL, anaplastic large cell lymphoma; CHL, classical Hodgkin's lymphoma; NLPHL, nodular lymphocyte predominance Hodgkin's lymphoma; PTCL, peripheral T-cell lymphoma; T/H-RBCL, T-cell/histiocyte-rich B-cell lymphoma.

German Hodgkin's Lymphoma Study Group indicated that a significant number of positive bone biopsies were detected in early stages (stage IB). These patients usually had elevated erythrocyte sedimentation rate, LDH, and alkaline phosphatase levels as well as bi- or pancytopenia.[394] It appears that bone marrow involvement does not have an adverse effect on the patient's response to treatment, ability to achieve complete remission, or overall prognosis.

The histopathologic diagnosis of HL of the marrow is not difficult to make when the normal marrow architecture is disrupted and is focally or diffusely replaced by a polymorphic cellular infiltrate consisting of lymphocytes, plasma cells, eosinophils, histiocytes, and classic Reed–Sternberg cells, especially when the diagnosis of HL has been previously established by a lymph node biopsy (Fig. 12.35). The general rule of thumb is that, if a tissue diagnosis has not been established by a previous lymph node biopsy, the criteria should be more rigid, and diagnostic or classic Reed–Sternberg cells must be identified in the lesion; otherwise, polyploid cells that contain at least one huge nucleolus or Reed–Sternberg variants in a proper cellular background are adequate for the diagnosis of Hodgkin's disease involving the marrow.[398,399] Whenever there is any double, multiple step sections or serial sections should be made to identify the diagnostic lesions. The frequency of HL involvement of marrow apparently depends on the size or volume of the specimen, the method of examination, and the histologic type.[400,401] In general, histopathologic examination of bilateral core biopsies is better than bone marrow aspiration, although touch imprints have the advantage of giving earlier results when diagnostic or classical Reed–Sternberg cell(s) is(are) found in some cases. It is not advisable to subclassify HL based on bone marrow biopsy alone. HL should be differentiated from T-cell/histiocyte-rich B-cell lymphoma (T/HRBCL), peripheral T-cell lymphoma, angioimmunoblastic lymphadenopathy, and anaplastic large cell lymphoma (Table 12.24). Immunohistochemical stains and molecular genetic analysis can usually assist in reaching a definitive diagnosis.

Sarcoid-like granulomas may be found in the bone marrow of patients with HL[402] and should not be confused with the specific lesions of this disease. It has been said, however, that survival and relapse-free survival are significantly more favorable for those patients who have noncaseating granulomas in the material obtained at initial staging procedures than for those who do not.[402] Benign lymphoid aggregates are also occasionally seen in involved or uninvolved marrow from patients with Hodgkin's disease.

PLASMA CELL DYSCRASIA AND RELATED DISORDERS

The plasma cell is an end cell of B cell lineage, and a small number of plasma cells are normally present in the marrow. Plasmacytic disorders may be divided into non-neoplastic disease, monoclonal gammopathy of undetermined significance (MGUS) and neoplastic diseases. A mixed proliferation of lymphocytes and plasma cells is sometimes seen.

Non-neoplastic plasma cell disorders

Reactive plasmacytosis is a common feature of several clinical disorders, including carcinomatosis, chronic granulomatous infections, HIV infections, hepatic diseases, and autoimmune disorders. The prevalence of plasmacytosis (defined as 2% or more of plasma cells in the differential count of the bone marrow cells) was found to be 29% in a series of consecutive studies of 1000 bone marrow aspirates.[70] The morphology of plasma cells is often mature, and they cluster around blood vessels (cuffing) on histologic sections (see Fig. 12.5). Reactive plasmacytosis should be differentiated from plasma cell myeloma. Plasma cells in the latter situation usually form aggregates or solitary lesions in the marrow and displace and/or replace normal hematopoietic elements.

Monoclonal gammopathy of undetermined significance

Bone marrow examination in patients with monoclonal gammopathy of undetermined significance (MGUS) often reveals a normal marrow, although a mild or moderate degree of plasmacytosis may be observed. These patients lack other clinical and/or laboratory findings seen in multiple myeloma, Waldenström's macroglobulinemia, heavy chain disease, or other lymphoproliferative disorders. The M-protein is usually discovered unexpectedly during serum protein electrophoresis study. The serum M-protein level is usually less than 3 g/dl, and there is no or only small amounts of M-protein in the urine. Plasma cells usually constitute less than 10% of all nucleated cells in marrow and they are normal in morphology. In addition, plasma cells are usually evenly distributed or concentrated around the blood vessels. However, continuous follow-up should be undertaken because progression to a malignant lymphoplasmacytic disorder was observed in 26% of 241 patients who had been followed at Mayo Clinic for 24–38 years.[403] The actual rate of development of these diseases was 16% at 10 years and 40% at 25 years. 68% of these patients developed multiple myeloma, 11% Waldenström's macroglobulinemia, 13% amyloidosis, and 8% lymphoma and CLL. No single factor, including measurement of serum and urine protein, magnetic resonance imaging (MRI), morphology, topographic distribution, percentage of plasma cells in bone marrow, cell marker study, cytogenetic analysis, plasma cell labeling index, and others, can differentiate patients with MGUS from those in whom a malignant plasma cell disorder will eventually develop, although the plasma cell labeling index and the presence of circulating plasma cells in the peripheral blood suggest active disease.[403]

Neoplastic proliferation of plasma cells

Neoplastic proliferation of plasma cells may be classified as follows:

I. Plasmacytomas
   A. Solitary plasmacytoma of bone
   B. Extramedullary plasmacytoma
II. Systemic tumorous plasma cell proliferation
   A. Multiple myeloma
   B. Smoldering myeloma
   C. Indolent myeloma
   D. Nonsecretory myeloma
   E. Light chain myeloma
   F. Multiple myeloma with osteosclerotic lesions.

III. Plasma cell leukemia
IV. Primary amyloidosis and monoclonal immunoglobulin deposition disease
V. Heavy chain diseases.

All these entities are associated with monoclonal gammopathies, although some of them may be difficult to detect. The closely related disorder lymphoplasmacytic lymphoma/Waldenström's macroglobulinemia was discussed earlier under the section on B-cell lymphoma.

Plasmacytoma

Plasmacytomas are clonal proliferations of plasma cells that occur as a localized osseous or extraosseous (extramedullary) tumorous growth.[404]

Solitary plasmacytoma of bone is a localized plasma cell tumor characterized by a single symptomatic area of bony destruction that is caused by a monoclonal plasma cell infiltrate without evidence of lytic lesions or bone marrow plasmacytosis in other areas. It commonly involves the spine, pelvis, and femur. Anemia, azotemia, or hypercalcemia is absent. Serum and/or urine monoclonal protein concentrations are usually low and uninvolved immunoglobulins are present in normal amounts. These patients are often a decade younger than patients with classic multiple myeloma, and they are more often male.[405] The most common symptoms at presentation are pain or pathologic fractures. Others may present with peripheral neuropathy or with features consistent with POEMS (polyneuropathy, organomegaly, endocrinopathy, monoclonal gammopathy, and skin changes). Local treatment is radiotherapy. About 5% of patients with multiple myeloma initially present with a solitary plasmacytoma. About 55% develop plasma cell myeloma after 10 years.[404]

Extramedullary plasmacytoma Solitary extramedullary plasmacytomas most often involve the mucous membranes or soft tissue of the upper respiratory tract but they may occur in other sites, such as the gastrointestinal tract, thyroid, lung, breast, testis, parotid gland, urinary bladder, central nervous system, etc. Recent studies suggest that some cases of extramedullary plasmacytoma, especially those that arise in the gastrointestinal tract, may represent marginal zone B-cell lymphomas with extensive plasmacytic differentiation.[405] Extramedullary plasmacytoma rarely evolves into multiple myeloma.

Systemic tumorous plasma cell proliferation

Multiple myeloma Multiple myeloma (plasma cell myeloma) is a multifocal, neoplastic proliferation of plasma cells in the bone marrow; it accounts for slightly more than 10% of hematologic malignant tumors. The disease commonly affects elderly men and is more frequent in blacks than other ethnicities. A recent study indicated that 2% of 1027 patients were younger than 40 years and 38% were 70 years or older.[406] The usual presentation includes bone pain, anemia, renal insufficiency, and hypercalcemia. Multiple osteolytic lesions in the bone marrow, serum monoclonal paraprotein (M-protein), and/or Bence–Jones proteinuria are frequent laboratory findings. The diagnosis is based on a combination of clinical, radiologic, laboratory, and histopathologic findings and characteristics.

The histologic pattern of myelomatous involvement of the bone marrow is variable, ranging from nodular or patchy to diffuse.[407,408] In most instances solid sheets of plasma cells infiltrate the fat and replace the normal elements of the marrow; occasionally an interstitial or a paratrabecular pattern may be observed, with preservation of fat cells but with replacement of the normal hematopoietic elements. The cytology of myeloma cells may be poorly differentiated, so called 'plasmablastic', or may be well differentiated, displaying characteristics of normal plasma cells with little cellular pleomorphism or atypism. The plasmablast has a large nucleus (>10 μm), with a large nucleolus (>2 μm), fine reticulate chromatin, and a small to moderate amount of cytoplasm that comprises less than one half the nuclear area. About 10% of patients with plasma cell myeloma display plasmablastic morphology, which is associated with a poor prognosis.[409] Binucleated, trinucleated, or tetranucleated mature-appearing (well differentiated) plasma cells, and plasma cells with intracytoplasmic inclusions, including crystalline rods, grape-like accumulations (Mott cells), and cherry-red refractive round bodies (Russell bodies), may all be observed in reactive states as well as in multiple myeloma. On the other hand, pleomorphism, irregular nuclear configuration, multinuclearity, prominent nucleoli, and nucleocytoplasmic asynchronism are helpful hints pointing to a malignant tumor. However, atypical features are not uncommon in plasma cells associated with MGUS.[410]

There is no agreement on the minimum percentage of plasma cells in the marrow that is necessary to make a diagnosis of myeloma. Recent publication by the WHO suggests that the volume of marrow occupied by plasma cells can be estimated.[404] Consequently, these investigators recommend that, when 30% of the marrow volume is comprised of plasma cells, a diagnosis of plasma cell myeloma is likely. They also established three major criteria and four minor criteria; a diagnosis of myeloma requires a minimum of one major and one minor criterion or three minor criteria, which must include (1) and (2).[404] These criteria must manifest in a symptomatic patient with progressive disease:

A. Major criteria
   1. Marrow plasmacytosis (>30%)
   2. Plasmacytoma on biopsy
   3. M-component:
      Serum: IgG >3.5 g/dl, IgA >2 g/dl
      Urine: >1 g/24 hour of Bence–Jones protein
B. Minor criteria
   1. Marrow plasmacytosis (10–30%)
   2. M-component: present but less than above
   3. Lytic bone lesions
   4. Reduced normal immunoglobulins (<50% normal levels).

The well-differentiated plasma cells do not divide and possess the following phenotype: CD38^{bright}, Syndecan-1 (CD138)^{bright}, CD19$^+$, CD45$^-$ and CD56^{weak} or CD56$^-$, SIg$^-$ and CIg$^+$. The normal plasma cells are also CD79a$^+$, PAX-5$^+$, and MUM1/IRF4$^+$. The myeloma cells are usually CD19, CD56^{bright}, CD38^{bright}, CD138^{bright}, CD20$^-$, CD126$^+$, PAX5$^-$, and CD79$^+$. They are also SIg$^-$ but CIg$^+$, and MUM1/IRF4$^+$.[404,411–413] CD138 is a very useful marker that may be applied to formalin-fixed decalcified paraffin-embedded routine trephine bone marrow biopsy. Normal and neoplastic plasma cells express clear-cut membrane immunostaining, whereas neoplastic cells from all other lymphoproliferative disorders do not.[414]

Myeloma cells are usually aneuploid. Several recurrent cytogenetic abnormalities have been demonstrated using improved techniques.[415] These include numerical abnormalities of chromosomes 1, 3, 7, 9, 11 and 15, deletion of 13q and/or 17q, trisomy 6, 7, or 9, t(11;14)(q13;q32) and others. Based on molecular cytogenetic studies, three prognostic groups have been identified: (1) poor prognosis: t(4;14)(p16;q32), t(14;16)(q32;q23), and −17p13. (2) intermediate prognosis: (−13q14), and (3) good prognosis: all others, with median survivals of 24.7, 42.3, and 50.5 months, respectively (P<0.001).[416] In addition to cytogenetic abnormalities or plasmablastic morphology, serum beta 2-microglobulin (β_2M), bone marrow and peripheral blood plasma cell labeling index (PCLI), serum levels of IL-6 and soluble IL-6 receptor (sIL-6R), increased levels of serum lactate dehydrogenase (LDH), performance status, extent of bone marrow involvement and many other tests all provide useful prognostic information.[409] A combination of independent prognostic factors provides greater prognostic information than any one prognostic factor alone. Several novel therapies have been developed which will ultimately improve morbidity and mortality.[417,418]

Smoldering myeloma   Smoldering myeloma was defined by Kyle and Greipp[419] as a group of asymptomatic patients who did not have lytic bone lesions or other features of myeloma but had 10% or more plasma cells in the bone marrow and an M-protein peak of at least 3 g/dl in the serum and remained stable without specific therapy for many years. Rosinol and colleagues followed 53 such patients for a long time and found that those patients who had progressively increased serum M protein, a previously recognized MGUS, or a significant higher proportion of IgA type developed symptomatic multiple myeloma earlier than those patients who did not have the above characteristics.[420] Most hematologists advocate no specific therapy for these patients. These cases resemble MGUS clinically.

Indolent myeloma   Patients who have systemic but asymptomatic myeloma with a low-tumor burden and slow progression are classified as having indolent myeloma.[421] These patients usually have few bone lesions without compression fractures and the M-component levels are lower (IgG <7 g/dl, IgA <5 g/dl) than overt myeloma. These patients have an intermediate survival rate between that of solitary myeloma of bone and overt myeloma.

Nonsecretory myeloma   This variant of multiple myeloma is rare (1–5% of all myelomas) and requires immunohistochemical stains or electron microscopic examination to demonstrate that the cells are capable of producing immunoglobulin. These individuals may present with typical or atypical clinical features of myeloma. M-protein cannot be detected in serum or urine. Response to therapy and survival rates vary in different series.[422] Despite bone marrow plasmacytosis greater than 20% and radiologic bone lesions, these patients have significantly longer median survival time than patients with M-protein.[423]

Light chain myeloma   The reported incidence of multiple myeloma associated with only monoclonal light chains varies from 9–26% in the literature.[424–426] Patients usually have atypical presentations, such as 'idiopathic' renal failure, 'solitary' tumor of the bone, primary amyloidosis, or leukemia. Some of the patients have light chain deposition disease which will be discussed under the section of primary amyloidosis. Serum protein study often reveals hypogammaglobulinemia and an absence of monoclonal spike. Urine protein electrophoresis may reveal an M-protein. They usually run a more aggressive clinical course with a short survival.[425,426]

Multiple myeloma with osteosclerotic lesions   Osteosclerotic lesions may appear as the only skeletal manifestation of multiple myeloma in occasional patients; in others, both osteosclerotic and osteolytic lesions coexist. Driedger and Pruzanski collected data on 68 such cases.[427] They and others found that this group of patients appears to be younger than the general group with multiple myeloma, and that peripheral neuropathy, organomegaly due to extraosseous myelomatous infiltration, endocrinopathy, monoclonal gammopathy, and skin lesions (POEMS) are common.[427,428] The monoclonal protein level is quantitatively low and usually consists of lambda light chain coupled with IgG or IgA. On radiographic examination the lesions should be differentiated from metastatic carcinoma or myelofibrosis and myeloid metaplasia. An association with Kaposi's sarcoma herpes virus/human herpes virus 8

(KSHV/HHV8) and multicentric Castleman's disease has recently been proposed.[428,429]

Plasma cell leukemia

Plasma cell leukemia (PCL) occurs rarely (2–4%) in plasma cell myeloma and is defined as circulating plasma cells that are greater than 20% of the total leukocytes or an absolute plasma cell count exceeding 2.0×10^9/l in the blood.[430] This condition may present at the time of diagnosis (primary PCL) or occurs as a terminal event in a patient with a previous diagnosis of multiple myeloma (secondary PCL). The bone marrow is hypercellular and diffusely infiltrated by neoplastic plasma cells. The cytologic characteristics of the neoplastic plasma cells vary from small, mature plasma cells resembling plasmacytoid lymphocytes to those resembling pleomorphic blastic cells (Fig. 12.36). The neoplastic cells may secrete IgG, light chains, IgA, or IgE. Patients with plasma cell leukemia are younger, have more aggressive disease with a higher frequency of extramedullary involvement (liver, spleen, and lymph node enlargement), bicytopenia, hypercalcemia, and renal function impairment in comparison with multiple myeloma. They have a poorer response to therapy and a significantly shorter survival time than patients with more typical myeloma.[430]

Primary amyloidosis and monoclonal immunoglobulin deposition disease

Both amyloidosis and monoclonal immunoglobulin deposition disease are plasma cell proliferative disorders that secrete abnormal immunoglobulins which deposit in tissue causing organ dysfunction. However, most of these patients do not present as plasma cell myeloma or lymphoplasmacytic lymphoma. Serum and urine immunoelectrophoresis and immunofixation are frequently required to identify the M-proteins. The abnormal proteins may deposit in any organs, but heart and kidneys are most commonly involved.[431,432]

Primary amyloidosis

Amyloidosis is a term used to describe a spectrum of diseases characterized by the deposition of a 'waxy' protein, amyloid, in various organs and tissues. Based on the clinical and/or chemical composition of the amyloid protein, amyloidosis may be classified as follows: (1) Primary amyloidosis (AL or AH protein); (2) secondary amyloidosis (AA protein or amyloid A protein) usually associated with chronic infections, collagen vascular disease, malignancies, etc.; (3) familial (hereditary) amyloidosis (transthyretin, fibrinogen A α-chain, lysozyme, or apolipoprotein A-1); and (4) other, such as dialysis-associated amyloidosis ($A\beta_2M$, β_2-microglobulin), Alzheimer's disease ($A\beta$, amyloid β protein precursor), and senile systemic amyloidosis (ATTR, transthyretin).[431,433,434]

Primary amyloidosis is considered to be a clonal plasma cell proliferative disorder resulting in deposition of amyloid protein in the walls of blood vessels and interstitium of visceral organs (Fig. 12.37). Amyloid protein seems to be homogeneous and amorphous by light microscopy, and is stained by Congo red, producing apple-green birefringence when viewed with polarized light. The amorphous, hyaline-like substance consists of rigid, nonbranching, aggregated fibrils 7.5–10 nm wide and of indefinite length. The fibrils consist of the N-terminal amino acid residues of the variable portion of a monoclonal light chain.[434] Primary amyloidosis may be divided into (1) primary amyloid and (2) primary amyloid associated with multiple myeloma. However, both disorders are plasma cell proliferative processes with much overlap. Of the 474 cases of

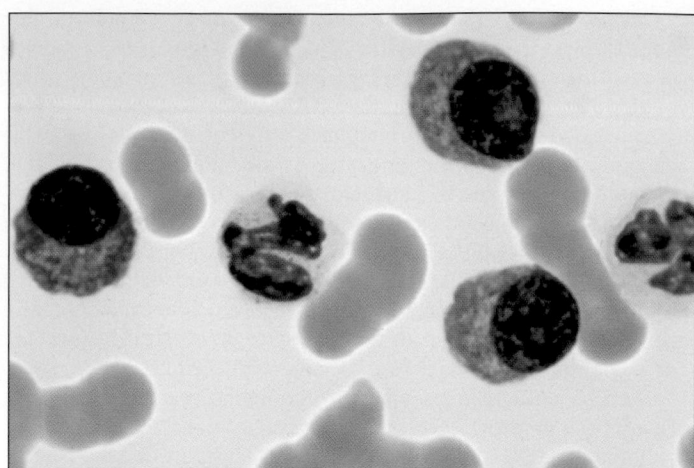

Fig. 12.36 Plasma cell leukemia. Circulating neoplastic plasma cells may be well differentiated, moderately well differentiated (as in this case), or poorly differentiated. (Romanowsky stain, ×1000.)

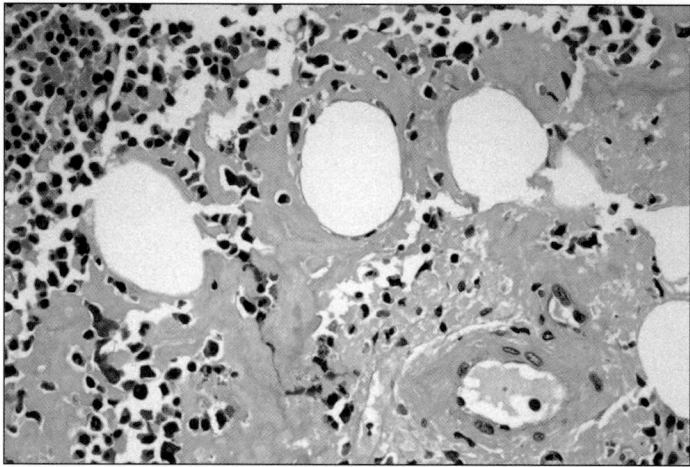

Fig. 12.37 Amyloidosis. Note the deposition of eosinophilic amorphous material within the wall of the blood vessels as well as in the interstitium. This material may be stained by PAS but should be stained by Congo red with apple-green birefringence seen under polarized light. (H&E stain, ×250.)

primary amyloidosis studied at the Mayo Clinic, 35% of patients were found to have plasma cell proliferative disorders at the time of diagnosis: 16% had monoclonal gammopathy of undetermined significance, 15% had multiple myeloma, 3% had smoldering multiple myeloma, 1% had macroglobulinemia, and 0.5% had solitary plasmacytoma of the bone.[434] The clinical symptoms and signs are often non-specific, although purpura, especially periorbital purpura, hepatomegaly, peripheral neuropathy, coagulopathy, macroglossia and hyposplenia may raise suspicions for the diagnosis.[431]

Although bone marrow aspiration and biopsy should be performed in all cases that are suspected of having primary amyloidosis, histologic sections or aspiration smears of the marrow range from having no identifiable pathologic changes to extensive replacement of the hematopoietic elements by amyloid or overt myeloma. Kyle and Gertz reported that 56% of their patients showed a positive stain for amyloid in the bone marrow biopsy, and virtually all patients had an M-protein in the serum or urine or a monoclonal population of plasma cells in the marrow.[434] Interestingly, lambda chains, especially λVI subclass of light chain, predominate in patients with amyloidosis in contrast to patients with multiple myeloma in whom kappa light chains are common.[431,434]

Patients with primary amyloidosis are frequently treated with chemotherapy. This form of treatment is contraindicated in some other forms of amyloidosis, especially the hereditary form.[433] Therefore, a correct diagnosis is most important in these patients.

Monoclonal immunoglobulin deposition diseases

This group of diseases are different from amyloid in that light chain, or less often heavy chain, or both, deposit in the tissue, appearing as amorphous substances with conventional histologic methods. These depositions do not form amyloid beta-pleated sheet and do not bind Congo red.[432] Clinical manifestations are correlated with abnormal protein deposition resulting in organ dysfunctions. These include nephrotic syndrome, acute or chronic renal failure, arthritis, congestive heart failure, coagulopathy, etc.[404,432] Serum and urine immunoelectrophoresis and immunofixation are useful to demonstrate the M-protein. However, absence of detectable M-protein has been reported in as many as 30% of patients. Biopsy of the involved organ is needed in these instances.

Heavy chain diseases

Heavy chain diseases consist of a group of lymphoproliferative disorders of B-cells characterized by the production of monoclonal defective immunoglobulins (i.e. composed of incomplete heavy chains with light chain deletions).[435] *Gamma heavy chain disease* has diverse clinical and pathologic features, and may resemble a nodal or extranodal lymphoma, CLL or even plasma cell leukemia.[404,435] The bone marrow, lymph nodes, and spleen are infiltrated by lymphoplasmacytic cells or plasma cells. Occasionally, the histopathology may mimic HL or angioimmunoblastic lymphadenopathy.[435] About 25% of patients have concurrent autoimmune diseases. The clinical outcome is variable. *Alpha chain disease* typically affects small bowel but the entire gastrointestinal tract and mesenteric lymph nodes may also be involved. There is also a respiratory variant. Those patients with the intestinal variant frequently present with chronic diarrhea, abdominal pain, and evidence of malabsorption. They are typically young males in developing countries associated with low socioeconomic status and poor hygiene. Three grades may be identified histopathologically.[435] The early lesion (grade A) is characterized by lymphoplasmacytic infiltrate in the lamina propria with or without villous atrophy and is reversible with antibiotic therapy. The highest grade (grade C) resembles a large B-cell lymphoma. Grade B is intermediate between grade A and grade C. The lesion consists of abnormal-looking plasma cells and immunoblast-like cells infiltrating into the submucosa. Some investigators consider that alpha chain disease is a variant of extranodal marginal zone B-cell lymphoma (or MALT lymphoma). Others call it Mediterranean abdominal lymphoma or immunoproliferative small intestinal disease.[435,436] Treatment and outcome are based on histopathological findings. The bone marrow is usually normal but alpha-chain-secreting plasma cells may be identified.[436] *Mu chain disease* is characterized by the presence of vacuolated plasma cells, small lymphocytes, and plasmacytoid lymphocytes in the bone marrow, with a prolonged antecedent history of CLL.[404,435] Clinically, this affects elderly patients who present with hepato-splenomegaly with minimal or absent lymphadenopathy. Cases may also mimic CLL, or multiple myeloma; others may present as systemic lupus erythematosus, hepatic cirrhosis, or myelodysplasia. Serum protein study reveals hypogammaglobulinemia with the presence of a μ chain. Light chain (especially kappa) may be detected in the urine in 50% of patients. The clinical course is quite variable.

HISTIOCYTIC PROLIFERATIVE DISORDERS

The concept and understanding of histiocytic proliferative disorders have progressed in the last 10 years with the availability of many monoclonal antibodies, molecular biologic techniques, and cytogenetic analysis. Histiocytes, originating from bone marrow CD34+ stem cells, may be divided into two functionally different systems: antigen-presenting cells, and antigen-processing cells. The former include Langerhans cells, interdigitating dendritic cells and follicular dendritic cells (FDC). Fibroblastic reticular cells (FRC) are involved in transport of cytokines and other mediators. It has been proposed that FRC and some FDC may be mesenchymal in origin.[437,438] Although tumors of FRC may arise in lymph nodes with these cells expressing vimentin, smooth muscle actin, desmin, and factor XIII,[438] they will not be discussed here; nor will some tumors of histiocytic origin that rarely involve the bone marrow. These lesions are covered in Chapter 11. The antigen-processing cells consist of monocytes and histiocytes in various organs (such as alveolar macrophages in the lung, Küpffer cells in the liver, cordal macrophages in the spleen, microglial cells in the brain, and osteoclasts in the bone).[437,439]

Several classifications have been proposed for the histiocytic proliferative disorders.[437,439] Those that involve bone marrow include reactive histiocytic proliferations (such as storage diseases, granulomatous reaction to infection, and hemophagocytic syndromes), and malignant diseases, such as acute monocytic leukemia and chronic myelomonocytic leukemia. Most of these involve monocytes–histiocytes. Acute leukemias of dendritic cell origin are exceedingly rare.[440,441] Readers are referred to the literature.[440,441] Langerhans cell histiocytosis can also involve the bone marrow and will be discussed briefly here.

All these cells have their specific cell markers and enzyme activities.[438,439] Langerhans cells and interdigitating dendritic cells are ATPase-positive. They also express CD45, HLA-DR and S100 protein. Only Langerhans cells are CD1a+ and contain Birbeck granules in the cytoplasm (see Fig. 12.1). FDCs are CD45−, but express CD21 and CD35 with variable expression of S100 protein. The antigen-processing cells (monocytes–histiocytes–phagocytes) express HLA-DR, CD45, CD11a, CD25, CD4, CD68, MAC387, CD11b, CD11c, CD14, and CD15, with variable expression of CD13 and CD33. They are also positive for lysozyme, acid phosphatase, and alpha-naphthyl esterase, and react with alpha-1-antitrypsin and alpha-1-antichymotrypsin antibodies. They contain secondary lysosomes (phagosomes) and lysosomal granules on electron microscopic examination.

Reactive histiocytic proliferation

Reactive histiocytic proliferation is usually transient and is caused by an infectious process or is associated with increased cell death, such as during chemotherapy. Granulomatous lesions, described later, are examples of histiocytic reactions. Storage diseases and some hemophagocytic syndromes are other forms of reactive histiocytic proliferation.

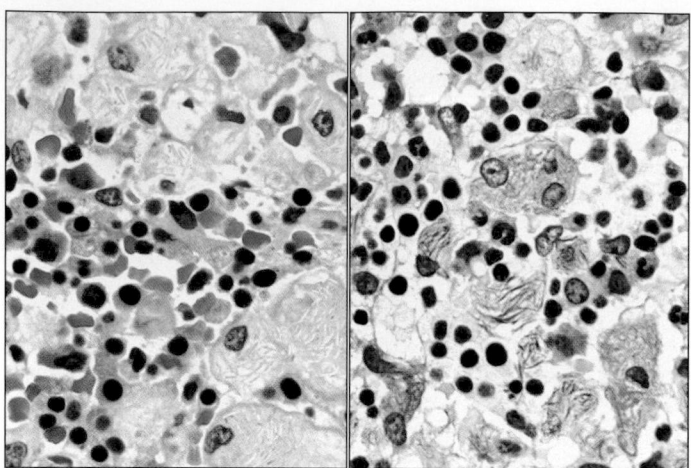

Fig. 12.38 Gaucher's disease. Note that these foamy histiocytes contain crystalloid structures in their cytoplasm characteristic of Gaucher's cells. (H&E stain and PAS stain, ×400.)

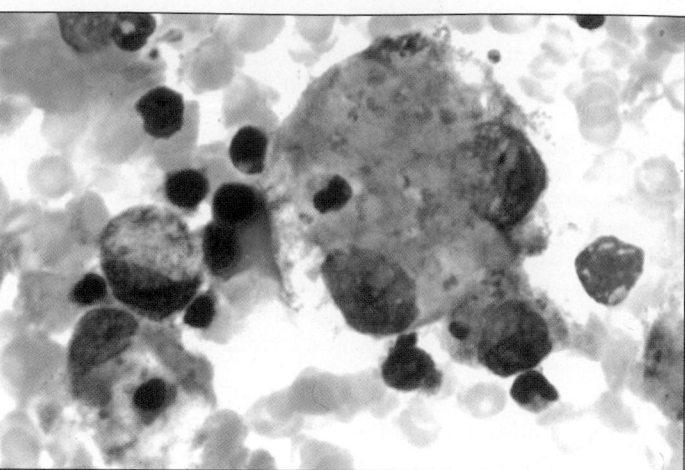

Fig. 12.39 Hemophagocytic syndrome. This photomicrograph depicts three benign-appearing histiocytes phagocytizing red blood cells, white blood cells, even platelets. This particular patient has EBV-associated T-cell lymphoma with marked hemophagocytosis in the bone marrow. (Romanowsky stain, ×600.)

Storage diseases

This group of diseases is usually caused by an enzyme defect in a normal degradative or catabolic pathway that leads to intracellular accumulation of biologic products in histiocytes. It is important to recognize that enzymatically normal macrophages can sometimes be overwhelmed by excessive tissue breakdown, such as in chronic hemolytic anemia, chronic myelogenous leukemia, or idiopathic thrombocytopenic purpura, resulting in the appearance of the cells found in the storage diseases, such as Gaucher's cells or sea-blue histiocytes. However, storage cells are much fewer in number in these conditions compared to the numbers found in genetic disorders. In addition, the underlying hematologic disorders often coexist.

Gaucher's disease is the most common storage disease and is usually readily diagnosed by bone marrow examination. Gaucher cells are large histiocytes, 20–100 μm in diameter, with one or more small, often eccentrically placed nuclei and a characteristic 'reticular', 'striated', 'fibrillary', or 'wrinkled tissue paper' appearance of the cytoplasm (Fig. 12.38). They are usually present in aggregates or sheets, focally or completely replacing the normal marrow. Characteristic storage cells can also be found in other metabolic disorders such as Niemann–Pick disease and sea-blue histiocyte syndrome. The histiocytes in Niemann–Pick disease are also large with a single, small nucleus and an abundant vacuolated cytoplasm. The sea-blue histiocytes measure up to 20 μm in diameter and are filled with sea-blue granules.

Hemophagocytic syndromes or hemophagocytic histiocytosis

Hemophagocytic syndrome (HPS) is characterized by marked systemic hemophagocytosis, associated with fever, hepatosplenomegaly, cytopenia, abnormal liver function tests, hypertriglyceridemia, elevated LDH, and coagulopathy. An infectious etiology can be detected in most cases.[442,443] A familial form (familial hemophagocytic syndrome) has also been described.[444–446] Finally, hemophagocytosis may be observed in a variety of malignant disorders in which either malignant cells phagocytize hematopoietic cells or there is hemophagocytosis by benign histiocytes as a manifestation of underlying malignant diseases.[447–452] It should be noted that hemophagocytosis by itself is not diagnostic of any disease. It indicates a stimulated (activated) monocyte–macrophage system and may be observed in a variety of clinical conditions, as described above. The pathogenesis is unclear but is probably related to defects in the immune system.

Infection-associated hemophagocytic syndrome

Infection-associated HPS (IAHS) is a systemic disorder characterized by widespread reactive proliferation of phagocytic histiocytes in response to a variety of infections. The incriminating agents include viruses (e.g. EBV, CMV, and herpes simplex virus), bacteria (*Brucella*, *Salmonella*, *Mycobacterium*), fungi (*Candida*, *Actinomyces*, *Histoplasma*), protozoa (*Leishmania*, *Babesia*), *Mycoplasma*, and others. It is considered to be a systemic reactive proliferation of phagocytic histiocytes in response to infections. Some of these patients are in immunodeficient states and others are under immunosuppressive therapy. The bone marrow shows cellular destruction with deposition of eosinophilic granular material and a decrease in density of cells. Both erythropoiesis and myelopoiesis are decreased. Megakaryopoiesis may be normal or increased. Histiocytes phagocytizing red cells, nucleated red cells, leukocytes, and platelets are diffusely scattered throughout the marrow. These histiocytes have a slightly oval nucleus, minimally condensed chromatin, and indistinct nucleoli. The voluminous cytoplasm contains hematopoietic cells or their degradation products or vacuoles (Fig. 12.39). Lymphocytes and plasma cells may be increased in number. Lymphoid aggregates and granulomas are uncommon findings. Hemophagocytosis may be observed in other organs. Some patients may respond to antimicrobial treatment, others may die during the acute phase from multisystem failure or later from infectious complications exacerbated by their underlying immunodeficiency.[453]

Familial hemophagocytic syndrome

Familial histiocytosis or familial erythrophagocytic lymphohistiocytosis is a disease of neonates and infants, although occurrence in older children has been reported.[444] It affects males and females equally and is transmitted as an autosomal recessive inheritance.

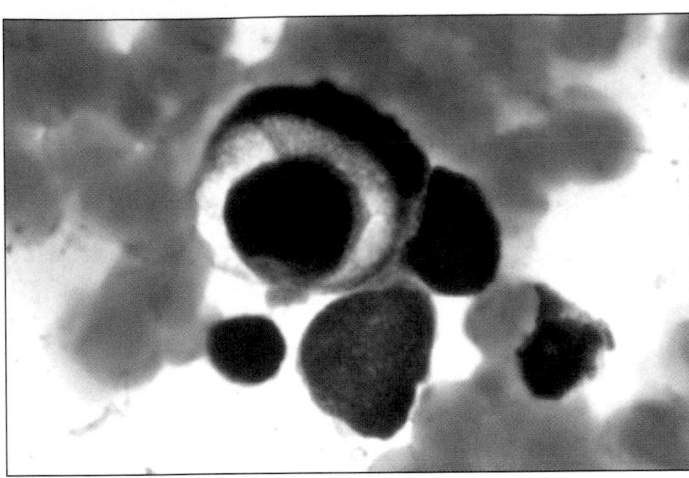

Fig. 12.40 Malignancy-associated hemophagocytosis. Note a carcinoma cell engulfs another neoplastic cell from a patient with metastatic oat cell carcinoma. There is a close resemblance of carcinoma cells to lymphoblasts. However, the carcinoma cells are very cohesive. (Romanowsky stain, ×1000)

Fever, anorexia, vomiting, irritability, and hepatosplenomegaly are common clinical presentations. The laboratory findings are similar to IAHS, except that elevated serum triglyceride is a constant feature in familial hemophagocytic syndrome (FHS). Parental consanguinity or a history of affected siblings may be helpful in making the diagnosis. Marked histiocytosis with erythrophagocytosis is seen in spleen, lymph nodes, and liver. Impairment of the immune system with defective T-cell function, T-cell and monocyte hyperactivation and hypercytokinemia is believed to be the basic pathogenetic mechanism.[445,446] Low or absent NK-cell activity as well as T-cell cytotoxicity has been reported.[445] Recently, mutation of a gene at 9q21.3–22 and 10q21–22 (perforin gene) has been linked to FHS.[454] Chemotherapy with epipodophyllotoxin and immunotherapy have limited success. Bone marrow transplant may restore NK- or T-cell function in some patients. The illness may be triggered by viral or other infectious agents.

It should be pointed out that several other well described genetic immunodeficiency syndromes, such as Chediak–Higashi syndrome, Griscelli syndrome, and X-linked lymphoproliferative syndrome can exhibit the clinical pictures of FHS.[455] In addition, children with autoimmune disease, such as rheumatic fever, may develop so called 'macrophage activation syndrome', which simulates FHS clinically.[455]

Malignancy-associated hemophagocytosis

Malignancy-associated hemophagocytosis includes a variety of hematopoietic or nonhematopoietic malignancies in which phagocytic cells may be benign histiocytes or malignant cells (Fig. 12.40). Histiocytic medullary reticulosis, originally described by Scott and Robb-Smith[456] and later renamed malignant histiocytosis (MH) by Rappaport,[457] is characterized by fever, weight loss, profound pancytopenia, skin lesions, hepatosplenomegaly, and lymphadenopathy. Widespread tissue infiltration by neoplastic ('histiocytic') cells with prominent erythrophagocytosis is a diagnostic feature. Some of these phagocytic cells are benign histiocytes; others are malignant cells. Recent studies have revealed that MH is not a single entity. It includes NK, NK/T, and PTCL, anaplastic large cell lymphoma, MH-like T-cell lymphoma, and probably truly malignant histiocytic proliferation.[438,449,450,452,458]

Patients with T-cell lymphomas, including anaplastic large cell lymphoma, may present with, or terminate in a syndrome mimicking MH. These T-cell lymphomas are nodal or extranodal (subcutaneous tissue, nose and lung) in origin, and were discussed earlier. EBV has been identified in malignant cells in some of these cases.[450,459] However, the phagocytic cells may be benign histiocytes that are present as indicators of significant underlying disease. The differential diagnoses of MH-like T-cell lymphoma from IAHS are based upon: (1) distortion of normal architecture with neoplastic proliferation of atypical cells; (2) demonstration of EBV genomes in malignant cells by in situ hybridization and clonality of EBV by Southern blot from tumor tissue; (3) rearrangement of T-cell receptor gene(s); and (4) presence of marker chromosomes. The bone marrow is usually hypocellular in IAHS, but is hypercellular with or without malignant cell infiltration in malignancy-associated hemophagocytosis. It is important to note that malignant T-cells may not be present in close proximity to benign phagocytic histiocytes in MH-like T-cell lymphoma. In that case, multiple biopsies may be required to reach an accurate diagnosis. Erythrophagocytosis in other malignancies, such as multiple myeloma, carcinoma, or acute leukemias, is usually manifested as an incidental finding in which malignant nonhematopoietic cells or hematopoietic cells display erythrophagocytosis. Antibiotic or antiviral treatment as well as immunotherapy should be instituted should infections such as EBV be a triggering agent. Of course, the malignant tumor should be treated as well. The prognosis is usually very poor.

Langerhans cell histiocytosis

The term *Langerhans cell histiocytosis* (LCH) is currently used to replace the term *histiocytosis X*, which was proposed by Lichtenstein in 1953.[460] LCH can be divided into unifocal or multifocal *eosinophilic granuloma* (the latter has also been referred to as *Hand–Schüller–Christian disease* when the classic triad of calvarial lesions, exophthalmos, and diabetes insipidus is present), and disseminated LCH (progressive LCH or *Letterer–Siwe disease*). The clinical presentation of LCH is variable depending on the type of the disease, the age of the patient, and the organ involved. However, all LCH is caused by proliferation of Langerhans histiocytes that express CD1a antigen and S-100 protein and contain Birbeck granules. In addition, they also express CD11c and CD14, which are not present in the normal Langerhans cells but are associated with phagocytic histiocytes.[460] They are positive for vimentin, CD45, CD4, CD2, HLA-DR, IL-2R, CD44, CD54 and CD58.[461] They also express fascin, although normal Langerhans cells are negative for fascin.[462] Occasionally, focal proliferation of Langerhans cells may be observed in HL and various types of lymphoma and leukemia.[461] It should be pointed out that the identification of clusters of Langerhans cells is not in itself a sufficient criterion for a diagnosis of LCH.

Eosinophilic granuloma

Unifocal eosinophilic granuloma, the most common form of LCH, seldom involves the iliac crest, although bone marrow involvement may be seen in *multifocal eosinophilic granuloma*. Both entities are characterized by chronicity and granulomatous-like lesions with or without necrosis. The Langerhans cells have an indented or grooved nucleus that contains delicate chromatin and inconspicuous nucleoli ('coffee-bean'-like nuclei). The cytoplasm is eosinophilic. Multinucleated giant cells, plasma cells, eosinophils, lymphocytes, neutrophils, and foamy histiocytes may be identified (Fig. 12.41).

Letterer–Siwe disease is commonly seen in children with visceral and hematopoietic involvement. Massive lymphadenopathy, hepatosplenomegaly, characteristic scaly brown-red eczematoid or seborrheic

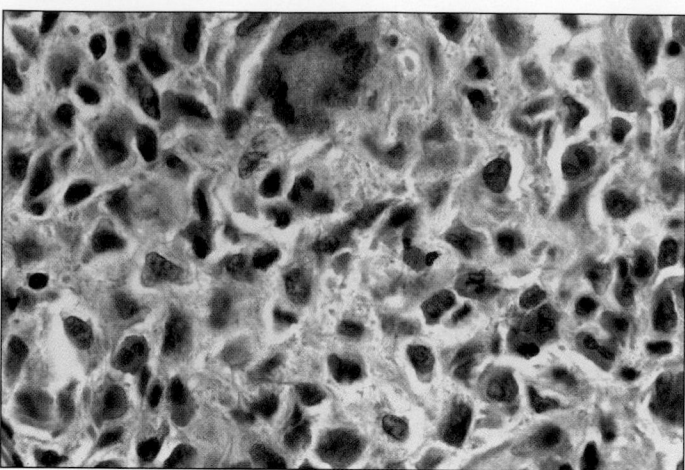

Fig. 12.41 Langerhans cell histiocytosis. In this case of unifocal eosinophilic granuloma, a mixed infiltration of Langerhans cell histiocytes and eosinophils, as well as a multinucleated Langerhans histiocyte, is present. (H&E stain, ×600.)

Table 12.25 Possible causes of granulomatous lesions in the marrow

Nonspecific
Lipid granuloma

Infectious
Mycobacteria: tuberculosis, leprosy, and atypical mycobacteria
Fungi: coccidioidomycosis, histoplasmosis, cryptococcosis, and others
Viruses: infectious mononucleosis, cytomegalovirus, hepatitis B virus, and others
Bacteria: typhoid fever, brucellosis, tularemia, and others
Rickettsial disease: Q fever, Rocky Mountain spotted fever
Spirochetes: syphilis (secondary or tertiary stage)
Others: toxoplasmosis, leishmaniasis, *Pneumocystis carinii*, mycoplasma pneumonia

Associated with neoplastic disorders
Specific lesions: Hodgkin's lymphoma, non-Hodgkin's lymphoma including peripheral T cell lymphoma, Langerhans cell histiocytosis
Non-specific lesions: sarcoid-like granuloma associated with Hodgkin's lymphoma, non-Hodgkin's lymphoma including mycosis fungoides, multiple myeloma, acute and chronic leukemia, chronic NK cell lymphocytosis, myelodysplastic syndrome, and carcinomatosis

Lesions resembling granuloma
Systemic mastocytosis, metastatic carcinoma

Miscellaneous
Sarcoidosis, angioimmunoblastic lymphadenopathy, foreign body granuloma, drug reactions, allergic/autoimmune disorders, and others

Unknown

Modified from references 273, 468–470, and 484.

cutaneous eruptions, and numerous osseous defects of the skull, ribs, and femur are common findings. Other organs involved may include thymus, bone marrow, kidney, gastrointestinal tract, muscle, lungs, and pituitary.[463,464] The proliferating cells in the bony and visceral lesions have the morphologic and phenotypic characteristics of Langerhans cells. The bone marrow may be focally or diffusely involved by the polymorphic infiltrate described above. It should be noted that there is poor correlation between the histologic appearance of the lesions and the clinical behavior of the disease.[465] All forms of Langerhans cell histiocytoses are clonal.[453] Unifocal eosinophilic granulomas, especially those in the lung that are often seen in smokers, may represent an early lesion.

Malignant histiocytic proliferative disorders

Neoplastic histiocytic proliferation includes clonal proliferation of antigen-presenting cells (which are very uncommon, with the exception of LCH; see Chapter 11) and antigen-processing cells (monocytes–phagocytes).

Acute monocytic leukemia and chronic myelomonocytic leukemia

These disorders were discussed earlier and will not be repeated here.

Malignant histiocytosis

As discussed earlier, true malignant proliferation of histiocytes, including histiocytic sarcoma, is exceedingly rare (see Chapter 11).[438,458] Nezelof and associates considered that anaplastic large cell lymphoma of childhood was actually a form of malignant histiocytosis.[466] However, this concept has not been widely accepted. The neoplastic cells in malignant histiocytes are cytologically malignant, possess monocyte–histiocyte markers, and lack of B- or T-cell gene rearrangements by molecular studies. In the aspirate smear, the malignant cells may be up to 50 μm in diameter with an increased nuclear/cytoplasmic ratio. The nucleus is large, with an irregular contour and contains reticular chromatin and a large prominent nucleolus. The cytoplasm is deeply basophilic and vacuolated. Phagocytosis may or may not be observed in the malignant histiocytes. Immunohistochemical and cytochemical studies

are essential to demonstrate the histiocytic (phagocytic) nature of the neoplastic cells. When the lesion consists of 'well differentiated' or 'reactive' histiocytes, with or without hemophagocytosis, caution should be exercised to rule out infection-associated hemophagocytic syndromes.

Malignant histiocytosis may overlap with true histiocytic sarcoma (when the disease is localized), and acute monocytic leukemia. It should be pointed out that some cases that were diagnosed as malignant histiocytosis or histiocytic medullary reticulosis are currently classified as infection-associated HPS or a variety of NHL, including PTCL and anaplastic large cell lymphoma, as discussed earlier. True histiocytic sarcomas are very uncommon and seldom involve the bone marrow.[467]

GRANULOMATOUS CHANGES AND GRANULOMA-LIKE LESIONS

A granuloma is defined as a host chronic inflammatory reaction with a predominance of cells of the macrophage series admixed with inflammatory cells, such as lymphocytes and plasma cells, with or without eosinophils. Giant cells of Langhans type or foreign body type may be present. A granulomatous reaction may be elicited by a wide variety of stimuli mediated by immunologic or chemical mechanisms, but the etiology may be difficult to establish from a tissue examination alone. A list of possible causes that may produce a granulomatous response in the bone marrow is presented in Table 12.25.[273,468–470] The reason for including some lymphoproliferative disorders under the heading of 'granulomatous changes'

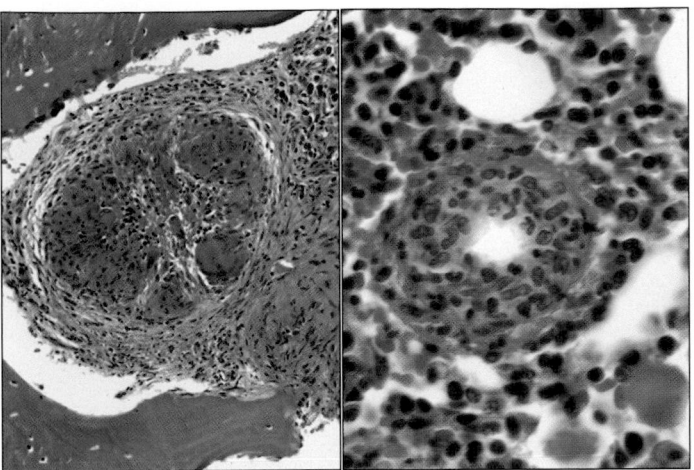

Fig. 12.42 Granulomatous diseases. This composite photomicrograph illustrates a patient with sarcoidosis with a proliferative granuloma on the left and a patient with Q fever with donut granuloma on the right. (H&E stain, ×100 on the left and ×250 on the right.)

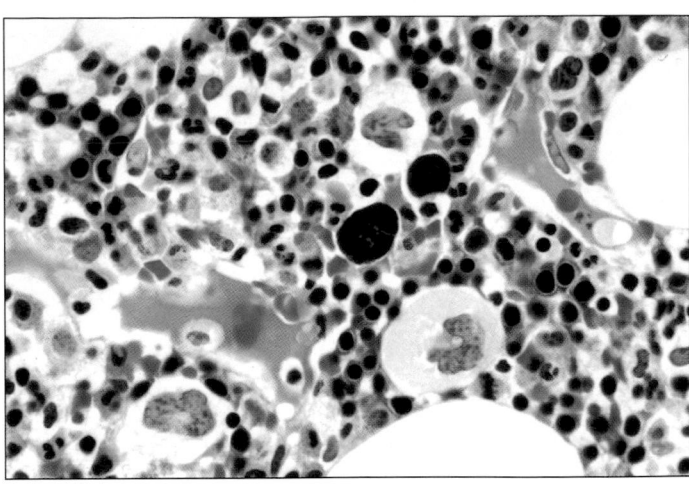

Fig. 12.43 HIV infection. This photomicrograph depicts two abnormal megakaryocytes characterized by hyperchromatic, somewhat necrotic, nuclei frequently seen in patients with HIV infection. (H&E stain, ×400.)

is to emphasize that histiocytic proliferation and granuloma formation are integral features of their pathology. Mast cell disease produces lesions mimicking granulomas and is also discussed here. Langerhans cell histiocytosis was discussed earlier.

A granulomatous lesion may be classified as proliferative, necrotic, or suppurative. The latter two types are most commonly seen in infectious disease as a form of systemic reaction. Proliferative granuloma (epithelioid granuloma) is characterized by a focal aggregation of epithelioid cells with or without Langhans giant cells and may be seen in a variety of conditions, including sarcoidosis, infectious mononucleosis, tuberculosis, HL, NHL, multiple myeloma, liver disease, and drug reactions (Fig. 12.42). It has been speculated that proliferative granuloma may be a manifestation of host immune response to overload of antigens or of defective lymphocyte-macrophage function to an infectious agent. A large study disclosed that the most common cause of granulomatous lesions in bone marrow is infection (38%), followed by malignancy (21%), drug reaction (12%), allergic or autoimmune disease (9%), and sarcoidosis (7%).[470] However, the etiology of granulomatous disease in marrow was unknown in 13% of patients in the same study. It should be pointed out that bone marrow granuloma is considered to be an uncommon finding with an incidence of 0.5–1.23% in the pre-AIDS era[470] but granulomatous change in bone marrow is very common now in HIV-infected patients, ranging from 13–24%.[471,472] A variety of microorganisms may be identified by special stains or bone marrow cultures, including *Pneumocystis carinii*.[473]

Benign nonhematologic conditions

Infectious granulomata and acquired immunodeficiency syndrome

The morphology of the granulomas in some infectious diseases is quite characteristic and is similar to that in other parts of the body. Microorganisms may be demonstrated on H&E-stained or special-stained sections. Serial sections or step sections are sometimes needed to localize the granuloma or to identify the Reed–Sternberg cells in the case of HL. A 'doughnut' granuloma, which is characterized by a central empty space surrounded by polymorphonuclear leukocytes, with or without fibrinoid material (fibrin ring), epithelioid cells, and/or eosinophils, has been observed in Q fever[474] (Fig. 12.42). Similar lesions have been described in typhoid fever and HL.[468]

Acquired immunodeficiency syndrome (AIDS) is an infectious disease caused by a retrovirus, human immunodeficiency virus. Most patients develop one or more cytopenias during the course of the disease.[471,472,475,476] Some may present with ITP- or TTP-like syndromes, and concurrence of ITP and TTP in occasional individuals has also been described.[101,475] Bone marrow examinations often reveal normocellular or hypercellular bone marrow at the early stage of the disease. With the progression of HIV infection, serous or mucinous degeneration of fat cells may be observed in the late stage of the disease, and the density of hematopoietic cells is often decreased, with deposition of eosinophilic granular or fibrillar material in the interstitium. This material may or may not be stained by PAS and is usually unstained by reticulin. Mehta and associates[78] found that the gelatinous material in AIDS patients was composed exclusively of glycosaminoglycans. They hypothesized that the damaged microenvironment leads to failure of hematopoiesis in some of these patients. In most cases, the myeloid/erythroid ratio is usually increased, with a normal or increased number of mega-karyocytes. Some megakaryocytes display dysplastic features, such as bizarre nuclear shapes, naked nuclei, hyperchromatic nuclei, and nuclear hypolobulations (Fig. 12.43).[472,475,477] Dyserythropoiesis and dysmyelopoiesis are also frequently observed; however, true MDS and acute leukemia are uncommon.[472,475] Marrow plasma cells and lymphocytes (including immunoblasts and transformed lymphocytes) are increased, with cuffing of plasma cells around the blood vessels. Lymphocytic aggregates were identified in 35% of biopsied specimens from patients with AIDS.[472] Lymphoid infiltrates may also be present. Increased iron stores are usually demonstrable by Prussian blue stain, and focal increase in reticulin fibers is also noted with the reticulin stain. A recent study showed that 49% of AIDS patients had decreased iron stores in their marrow.[478] This finding suggests that iron deficiency might be an important cause of anemia in some AIDS patients.

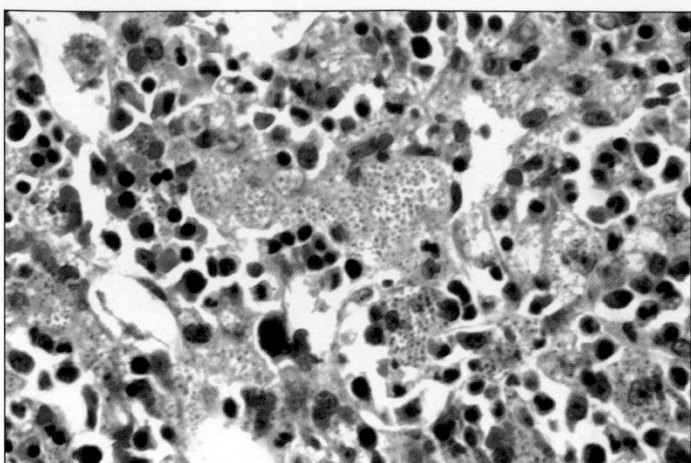

Fig. 12.44 Histoplasmosis. This photomicrograph is taken from an AIDS patient with systemic histoplasmosis. No granulomas are identified. However, numerous foamy histiocytes containing histoplasma microorganisms are observed. (H&E stain, ×400.)

Table 12.26 Clinical conditions with foamy cells in the marrow

Common conditions
Lipophages associated with alcoholic liver disease or diabetes mellitus
Fat necrosis secondary to bony fracture, infarction, pancreatitis, and status postchemotherapy for acute leukemias and other malignant tumors
Less common conditions
Infections: such as leprosy, Whipple's disease, *M. avium–intracellulare*, leishmaniasis, histoplasmosis, and others
Metastatic tumors: metastatic renal cell carcinoma and others
Storage diseases: Niemann–Pick disease, Gaucher's disease, Fabry's disease, Farber's disease, Wolman's disease, some mucopolysaccharidoses, mucolipidoses, glycogen storage disease, and others
Langerhans cell histiocytosis

Granulomas (usually small, epithelioid, and without necrosis) may be present, and special stains are required to demonstrate the microorganisms within them. Special stains for mycobacteria and fungi should be used in bone marrow specimens whenever there is clinical suspicion of systemic infection. In some severely immunosuppressed patients, no granulomas may be identified, although an increase in histiocytes with or without microorganisms (such as histoplasma) may be seen (Fig. 12.44). In addition, foamy cells in the marrow of AIDS patients should alert the observers to the possibility of *Mycobacterium avium–intracellulare* infection. Red cell hypoplasia or aplasia with gigantic or abnormal proerythroblasts with or without intranuclear inclusions should raise the suspicion of parvovirus B19 infection (Fig. 12.7).[89,475,478] Further, a variety of protozoa, such as *Leishmania*, *Toxoplasma*, and even *Pneumocystis carinii*, may be detected in the bone marrow of these patients.[475]

The mechanisms of peripheral cytopenias in an AIDS patient with normal or hypercellular marrow are probably multifactorial.[472,475,476] Hypotheses include: (1) peripheral destruction secondary to hypersplenism; (2) immune-complex-mediated autoimmune phenomenon; (3) side effects to drugs against HIV or other infectious agents or chemotherapy for neoplastic diseases; (4) stimulation of the reticuloendothelial system due to multiple viral infections; (5) damaged microenvironment; and (6) primary infection of hematopoietic stem cells by HIV. Recent studies indicate that stem cells are rarely if ever infected by HIV but endothelial cells, macrophages and other stromal cells in the bone marrow are highly permissive of HIV infection.[472,475,476] These virus-infected cells are dysfunctional, resulting in abnormal cytokine secretions which in turn create a microenvironment unsuitable for regeneration of hematopoietic cells.[476]

An increased incidence of NHL and HL in AIDS patients is well recognized.[475,476,478,479–481] Bone marrow may be involved in 20–25%, and up to 42% of patients.[478] Although the occurrence of Kaposi's sarcoma is common in HIV-infected homosexual men, its involvement of the bone marrow is very unusual.[471,482]

AIDS-related lymphoma (ARL) is usually manifested at the late stage of disease. ARL is characterized b y xtranodal presentations, wide disseminations, aggressive clinical behaviors, unfavorable histologic subtypes, frequent CNS involvement, and poor prognosis.[475,476,479–481] Some cases are associated with EBV infection, with demonstrable gene rearrangement or mutations.[475,476] It is interesting to note that bone marrow involvement in AIDS-related NHL correlates with small noncleaved pathology, thrombocytopenia ($<100\times10^9$/l), high LDH and leptomeningeal lymphoma with demonstrable malignant cells in cerebrospinal fluid.[481] The bone marrow trephine biopsy may be the initial or only diagnostic material in AIDS patients with HL.[483] However, Reed–Sternberg cells may be very few in number, and there may be granulomas with or without necrosis. Thus, step sections or immunohistochemical stains are needed to reach a correct diagnosis.

Lipid granuloma

Lipid granuloma is a relatively common finding in elderly patients and it is usually considered insignificant clinically. The morphology is similar to that found in the liver or spleen. Lipid granuloma consists of a collection of macrophages containing vacuoles of various sizes, which are, however, always smaller than the single vacuole in normal fat cells. Plasma cells, lymphocytes, and sometimes eosinophils and mast cells are all seen in the lipid granuloma. Microcysts lined by compressed histiocytes and multinucleated giant cells may also be present. Lipid granulomas associated with hyperlipidemia often contain foam cells and Touton type giant cells. Foamy cells may be seen in a variety of clinical conditions[468] (Table 12.26). It is important to differentiate the non-specific lesion of lipid granuloma from other granulomatous lesions.

Granulomatous changes associated with hematologic disorders

Lymphomas or lymphoma-like lesions may contain granulomas or display granulomatous changes.[468] These include HL, peripheral T cell lymphoma, and angioimmunoblastic lymphadenopathy. Other lesions, such as systemic mastocytosis and LCH, may produce lesions simulating granulomas. LCH and malignant lymphomas have been discussed earlier. The diagnostic criteria for these lesions in the bone marrow are the same as those in other parts of the body. Tefferi and Li reported two cases of bone marrow granuloma associated with chronic NK-cell lymphocytosis.[484] In addition to the loose aggregates of epithelioid histiocytes, there were many scattered, large mononuclear histiocytes morphologically resembling megakaryocytes.

Angioimmunoblastic (immunoblastic) lymphadenopathy

Angioimmunoblastic lymphadenopathy is a rare but distinct clinico-pathologic entity characterized by an acute clinical onset with fever, night sweats, weight loss, and generalized lymphadenopathy. Skin rash, pruritus, hepatosplenomegaly, hypergammaglobulinemia and Coombs-positive hemolytic anemia are other common features. A history of hypersensitivity reaction to drugs or other substances immediately preceding the onset of symptoms may be obtained in some patients. The disease is generally considered to be an abnormal immune response involving a deficiency of T cell regulatory function or an exaggeration of lymphocyte transformation of the B-cell system.[485,486] However, recent studies indicate that the majority of cases of angioimmunoblastic lymphadenopathy are clonal T-cell disorders.[487]

Bone marrow involvement occurred in approximately 40–70% of patients who underwent bone marrow examination.[485,488] The lesions are usually hypocellular, focal, and rarely paratrabecular in distribution. Diffuse infiltration with replacement of normal hematopoietic elements has been described.[489] Cells with fibroblast-like spindle-shaped nuclei are often prominent. In addition, lymphocytes, transformed lymphocytes, immunoblasts, histiocytes, plasma cells, and eosinophils are present in the lesion. Increased numbers of reticulin fibers that arrange in a whorled pattern are frequently demonstrated. Proliferation and arborization of small blood vessels with deposition of eosinophilic amorphous material in the interstitium are also evident. The involvement of bone marrow did not correlate with the clinical course and prognosis in one study[488] but was associated with unfavorable outcome in another.[489] The lesion should be differentiated from HL, granulomas in other disorders, and peripheral T-cell lymphomas. Transformation to malignant lymphomas has been described.[487,489]

Mast cell disease

Mast cells are derived from hematopoietic stem cells and are normally found in the bone marrow, skin, lungs, and mucosa and submucosa of other organs. Mast cell disease or mastocytosis is a proliferation of mast cells locally or systemically. *Reactive masto-cytosis* may be observed in a variety of hematopoietic or lympho-reticular disorders, chronic liver disease, chronic renal disease, and osteoporosis. Several classifications of mast cell neoplasms have been proposed.[490–492] Mast cell disease may be generally classified as cutaneous mastocytosis, systemic mastocytosis, mast cell sarcoma, and extracutaneous mastocytoma.[492] The last two entities are exceedingly rare and are beyond the scope of discussion here. Cutaneous mastocytosis is more common in children than adults. Some lesions are localized, other are disseminated in which bone marrow involvement may be observed. The term 'urticaria pigmentosa' describes the clinical features of urticaria and hyper-pigmentation and has been used as a general term for all forms of cutaneous mastocytosis.[492] Urticaria pigmentosa of children and infants is usually limited to the skin and frequently regresses at puberty. However, urticaria pigmentosa in adults usually develops into *systemic mastocytosis* (systemic mast cell disease, SMCD). Bone marrow involvement is observed in 60% of cases in one study[493] but there is no correlation of bone marrow involvement with clinical presentation, course, or associated hematologic disorders.[493] A pathologic increase of mast cells in extracutaneous tissues that is not attributable to a reactive process is the diagnostic criterion for SMCD.

SMCD may be manifested clinically in two ways: (1) an infiltra-tive process characterized by osteoporosis or osteosclerosis, hepato-

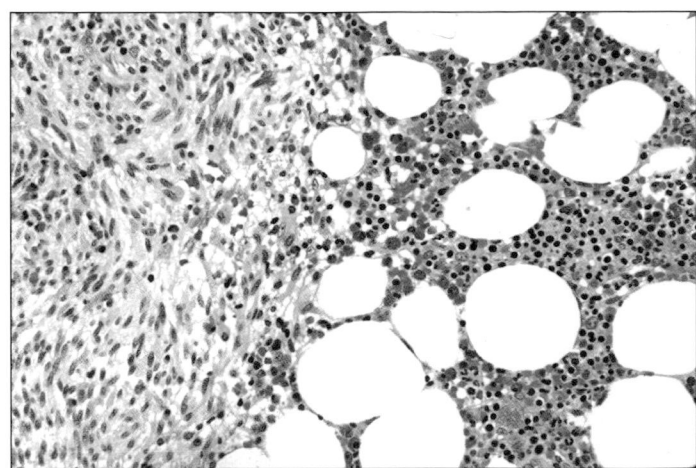

Fig. 12.45 Systemic mast cell disease. A well circumscribed lesion composed of spindle cells with elongated vesicular nuclei and abundant eosinophilic cytoplasm admixed with some hematopoietic cells, especially eosinophils, is seen in the bone marrow. (H&E stain, ×250.)

splenomegaly, lymphadenopathy, and/or mast cell infiltration in the skin (urticaria pigmentosa), bone marrow, gastrointestinal tract, heart, and lungs, and (2) pharmacologic effects secondary to release of chemicals following degranulation of mast cells. These are characterized by flushing, pounding headache, bronchospasm, hypotension, diarrhea, rhinorrhea, urticaria, palpitation, dyspnea, peptic ulcer, and gastrointestinal bleeding. Various combinations and clinical syndromes are seen.[490]

Travis and associates[494,495] classified SMCD into indolent SMCD, SMCD with associated hematologic disorders, mast cell leukemia, and aggressive SMCD (nonleukemic), based on clinical manifestations and outcomes. Urticaria pigmentosa is common in indolent SMCD but uncommon in other groups of patients, whereas patients with other groups of SMCD have constitutional symptoms and hepatosplenomegaly. Bone marrow involvement is seen in all groups.[494] Histopathologic examination of bone marrow biopsy shows patchy or focal infiltration by spindle-shaped mast cells, usually in perivascular or paratrabecular regions, with concomitant fibrosis and osteosclerosis in the vast majority of cases of SMCD (Fig. 12.45). An increased number of eosinophils, lymphocytes, and histiocytes is noted within the lesion or at the periphery. These foci often exhibit a granulomatous appearance and are sharply demarcated from the adjacent tissue. In indolent SMCD, lymphoid aggregates may be observed surrounding a collection of mast cells.[496] These lymphocytes are polyclonal, consisting of a mixture of B- and T-cells.

Although an association of SMCD with lymphoproliferative disorders is rare, it has been reported in ALL, hairy cell leukemia, or lymphoma.[496] In contrast, SMCD is more frequently associated with myeloid disorders, including MDS, MPD, and acute leukemia.[490,497] Dyspoietic features are also encountered in SMCD.[497]

The neoplastic mast cells in SMCD may be present singly or in clusters, usually at the trail of the bone marrow aspiration smears. These abnormal mast cells may resemble abnormal basophils. They may be round or spindle-shaped and have lobulated nuclei, evenly distributed fine chromatin, nucleoli, and hypogranularity with an uneven distribution of granules.[490,497] Like basophils, mast cells show metachromatic staining with Giemsa, Alcian blue or toluidine blue. Unlike basophils, they are also positive for chloroacetate esterase, epsilon aminocaproate esterase and tartrate resistant acid phosphatase.[490] Immunologically, mast cells express CD45, CD43, CD44, CD13, CD33, CD117, CD11c, CD68 and mast cell tryptase.[490] The last is specific for mast cells and may be applied to formalin-fixed, paraffin-embedded tissue sections.[490] Interestingly, bone marrow mast cells from patients with SMCD express CD2, CD25 and CD35 but are negative for CD71. These findings differ from normal mast cells.[490,498] Ultrastructurally, mast cells contain the characteristic whorls or scrolls or a crystalline structure within granules.[490] Mutations of c-*kit* (a proto-oncogene that encodes a receptor tyrosine kinase (Kit) that is the receptor for stem cell factor (SCF, also known as mast cell growth factor)) have been demonstrated in several different types of mastocytosis.[490,491] Clonal cytogenetic abnormalities including complex abnormalities or other changes, such as 5q−, del(7), monosomy 7, trisomy 8, del(11), trisomy 13, and del(20) have been reported.[490]

Diffuse marrow infiltration is seen in patients with mast cell leukemia. These patients have at least 10% atypical mast cells circulating in the peripheral blood.[494,495] The diagnosis of mast cell leukemia may be difficult because it may resemble basophilic leukemia, acute promyelocytic leukemia, or a blastic variant of hairy cell leukemia. The nuclei of many of the atypical mast cells are indented, multilobated, and multinucleated. As stated earlier, histochemical, immunohistochemical stains and ultrastructural study are useful for the identification of mast cells in mast cell disease. When mast cells account for 20% or more of the cells on the bone marrow aspirate, a diagnosis of mast cell leukemia can be suspected.[492] Readers are referred to the WHO book for detailed descriptions of diagnostic criteria of each entity.[492]

METASTATIC TUMORS

The incidence of metastatic lesions in bone marrow varies from series to series, depending on the purpose of the study, the histopathologic type of tumor, the stage of the disease, and the method of bone marrow examination. Recently, 6.8% of 381 specimens taken from patients with a diagnosis of carcinoma were found to have bone marrow metastasis.[11] Generally, both biopsy and aspiration should be performed when evaluating metastatic disease of the marrow. Trephine biopsy appears to be superior to an aspiration smear because of frequently associated fibrosis and necrosis with metastatic tumors.[499] Immunohistochemical stains increase the yield of detection.[500] Although other ancillary tests, such as flow cytometry, molecular methods, or tissue culture techniques may also be employed, immunohistochemical and immunocytochemical methods have the added advantage of being able to visualize the positive cells directly.[500–504] A cocktail of antibodies or a panel of antibodies may be used to further classify the tumors or to predict the likely primary sites.[503,504] Cautions should be exercised when an interpretation is made.[502] Also, strict quality controls should be applied during the immunohistochemical staining procedure.

The most common metastatic tumors in bone marrow are carcinomas of the lung, breast, and prostate in adults, and neuroblastomas in children. Metastatic tumor focally or diffusely infiltrates the marrow and is associated with necrosis, fibrosis, increased osteoblastic activity (most notably in carcinomas of the prostate and breast but also in other tumors), osteoclastic activity (as in metastatic oat cell carcinoma of the lung or metastatic carcinoma of the colon), or a combination of both (most common form of bone

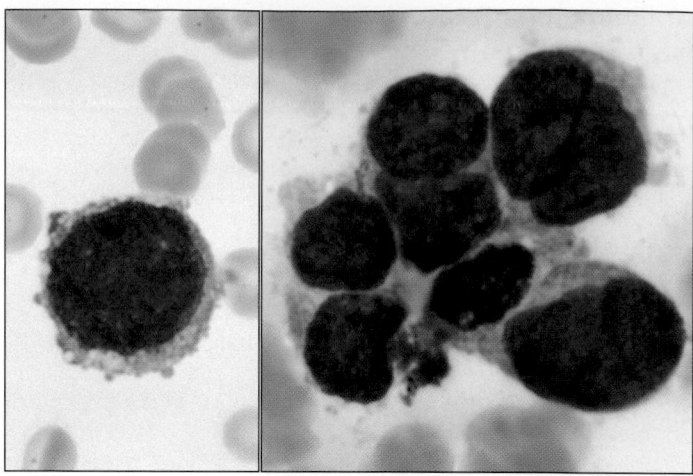

Fig. 12.46 Metastatic carcinoma and carcinocythemia. Circulating carcinoma cells may be occasionally found in the blood (carcinocythemia) (left), which is usually seen in patients with disseminated carcinomatosis. Indeed, a group of oat cell carcinoma cells is found in the bone marrow aspiration smear (right). Note the cohesiveness of the tumor cells with nuclear molding and bizarre nuclear configuration. (Romanowsky stain, ×1000.)

reaction). Oat cell carcinoma and neuroblastoma may produce a picture simulating malignant lymphoma, but metastatic tumor cells are often larger than lymphoma cells, the neoplastic cells are more cohesive than lymphoma cells, and immunohistochemical technique or electron microscopic study can differentiate these entities in a majority of difficult cases. The surrounding hematopoietic elements may show dyspoiesis and hypercellularity. In addition, increased numbers of plasma cells, eosinophils, and lymphocytes are seen. It is interesting to note that bone marrow necrosis in children with malignant disease does not appear to confer a poor prognosis,[505] and bone marrow fibrosis associated with metastatic tumor often regresses after successful treatment for malignant disease.[499]

Although the bone marrow aspiration smears are often of poor quality, isolated clusters of metastatic tumor are often found at the periphery of the smear. The neoplastic cells usually form cohesive three-dimensional structures, with considerable variability in nuclear size, shape, and staining characteristics. The nuclear/cytoplasmic ratio is variable, depending on the type of primary tumor; nevertheless, these tumor cells are usually two to five times larger than the hematopoietic cells. Nuclear molding at the cell border is often visible. The nuclear chromatin is usually hyperchromatic, with irregular condensation or a smudged appearance. The volume of cytoplasm is also variable. It may be deeply basophilic and contain vacuoles (Fig. 12.46). Rosette-like structures may be seen in metastatic neuroblastoma.

The peripheral blood findings range from mild anemia to a leukoerythroblastic picture to carcinocythemia.[499,506,507] It appears that leukoerythroblastic reaction is correlated with the extent of marrow infiltration by metastatic carcinoma. Carcinocythemia indicates a terminal event and an ominous prognosis (Fig. 12.46).[506] However, one patient who survived more than 20 months and was well and working has been reported.[507] Also, circulating malignant cells of nonhematopoietic origin may create a clinical picture simulating acute leukemia.[508]

Recent research efforts have focused on the detection of micrometastases in patients with breast cancer. Bone marrow examination

Table 12.27 Clinical conditions associated with bone marrow necrosis

Benign	Malignant
Sickle cell diseases and certain sickle cell trait	Acute or chronic myelogenous leukemia
Severe bacterial infections and septicemia	Acute or chronic lymphocytic leukemia
Tuberculosis and mycotic disease	Malignant lymphoma
Eclampsia	Multiple myeloma
Alcohol abuse	Hairy cell leukemia
Chronic renal failure	Primary thrombocythemia
Caisson disease	Metastatic carcinoma
Systemic lupus erythematosus	Metastatic neuroblastoma
Disseminated intravascular coagulation	Status post-chemotherapy or radiotherapy
Idiopathic	
Anorexia nervosa	
Antiphospholipid syndrome	

Adapted and modified from references 505, 509–511.

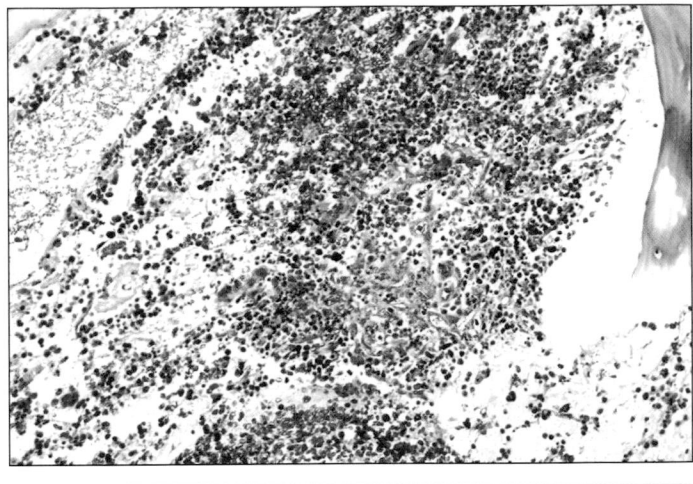

Fig. 12.47 Bone marrow necrosis. Extensive bone marrow necrosis may be observed in a variety of clinical conditions. This particular patient had a large cell lymphoma involving the bone marrow, with large areas of necrosis. (H&E stain, ×100.)

is important in identifying early recurrence, in studying hormonal receptors in patients who have not had the determination done on the primary tumor, and in the practice of autologous marrow transplants.[499,501] It also has prognostic implications.[500]

BONE MARROW NECROSIS AND INFARCTION

Bone marrow necrosis is very uncommon, with a prevalence ranging from 0.15–7% in antemortem studies.[509] The most commonly associated clinical conditions are sickle cell disease, myeloproliferative disorders, acute leukemia, malignant lymphoma, and metastatic carcinomas. Bone marrow necrosis may also occur in patients with sepsis, vasculitis, or disseminated intravascular coagulation (Table 12.27).[505,509–511] The frequency of bone marrow necrosis in an autopsy series may be as high as 15% among patients who died of acute leukemias.[509] A serious and even fatal complication is fat or bone marrow embolization.

Patients with bone marrow necrosis frequently present with bone pain, fever, pancytopenia, and leukoerythroblastic picture. Bone marrow necrosis is often a diffuse process affecting multiple foci. Frequently, the necrotic marrow cannot be aspirated, resulting in a 'dry tap' or very scant material for diagnosis. Histopathologic examination may reveal a spectrum of morphologies ranging from total necrosis and infarction to individual cell necrosis (Fig. 12.47). In foci of bone marrow necrosis, the fatty and hematopoietic marrow is replaced by granular eosinophilic debris. Ghost cells and cells with poorly defined cytoplasmic borders and pyknotic nuclei may be observed. It is important to identify the underlying disease, such as acute leukemia or metastatic carcinoma. Deep sections or step sections may be needed to search for viable cells or tissues. Occasionally, repeat biopsy is indicated.

Fat necrosis of bone marrow is identical with that seen in other adipose tissues. The causes include fracture of bone and infarction. During the healing process, lipophages (foamy cells) and lipid granulomas may be seen.

The pathogenesis of bone marrow necrosis is unclear. It may be due to vascular obstruction caused by tumor emboli or by extrinsic compression by rapidly dividing neoplastic cells. Bone marrow

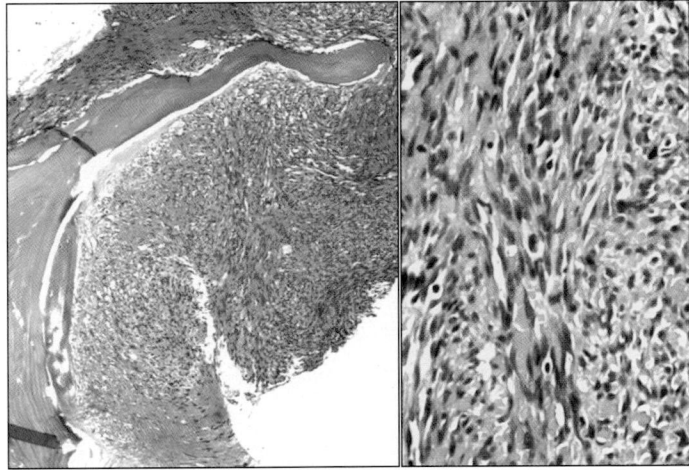

Fig. 12.48 Kaposi's sarcoma. Kaposi's sarcoma infrequently involves the bone marrow. Note the interlacing spindle cells, which form slits and spaces containing red blood cells. Mitotic figures are noted. (H&E stain, ×40, and ×100.) (Courtesy of Dr Richard Conran and associates).

necrosis may also occur after induction therapy in leukemias or malignant lymphomas.[511,512] Rapid lysis of tumor cells following effective chemotherapy may be the underlying cause of some cases. The prognosis of bone marrow necrosis associated with a malignant neoplasm is still controversial. Although some investigators believe that bone marrow necrosis in these patients is an ominous finding,[509,511] other researchers, particularly those who deal with children with acute lymphocytic leukemia and neuroblastoma, experienced a more optimistic picture.[505] Antiphospholipid syndrome is a relatively recently recognized entity characterized by antibodies directed against the phospholipid substrate. This substrate is widely distributed on cell walls and is involved in the coagulation cascade. Patients who have the syndrome often present with diverse clinical manifestations such as venous or arterial thrombosis, recurrent fetal loss, thrombocytopenia, and neurological disorders.[513] Coombs-positive hemolytic anemia, elevated levels of anticardiolipin antibody, positive anti-DNA and anti-nuclear antibodies, positive anti-SM antibody and lupus anticoagulant may be detected. It is important to include this entity in the differential diagnosis of bone marrow necrosis.

VASCULAR LESIONS IN MARROW

Vascular lesions, either localized in the marrow such as angioma or systemic lesions (whenever a pathologic process affects the blood vessels, such as arteriosclerosis, thrombosis, vasculitis, thrombotic thrombocytopenic purpura, systemic lupus erythematosus, Kaposi's sarcoma or amyloidosis), may be diagnosed on histologic sections of bone marrow.[100,434,481,514] Cholesterol emboli can be recognized with ease and may be a manifestation of a multisystem illness.[515] Kaposi's sarcoma is very uncommon in the bone marrow even in this era of the worldwide spread of AIDS; the lesion should be differentiated from a variety of disorders associated with primary or secondary myelofibrosis and vascular proliferation (Fig. 12.48). Occasionally, intravascular tumor thromboemboli, including intravascular lymphoma, may be detected in the bone marrow biopsy.[360]

REFERENCES

1. Frisch B, Bartl R. Biopsy of bone and bone marrow. In: Frisch B, Bartl R (eds). Biopsy interpretation of bone and bone marrow. Histology and immunohistology in paraffin and plastic, 2nd ed. London: Edward Arnold; 1999: 1–11.

2. Foucar K. Bone marrow examination: indications and techniques. In: Foucar K. Bone marrow pathology, 2nd ed. Chicago: ASCP Press; 2001: 30–49.

3. Naeim F. Bone marrow examination: special procedures. In: Naeim F. Pathology of bone marrow, 2nd ed. Baltimore: Williams & Wilkins; 1998: 37–81.

4. Jamshidi K, Swaim WR. Bone marrow biopsy with unaltered architecture: a new biopsy device. J Lab Clin Med 1971; 77: 335–342.

5. Islam A. A new bone marrow biopsy needle with core securing device. J Clin Pathol 1982; 35: 359–364.

6. Westerman MP. Bone marrow needle biopsy: an evaluation and critique. Semin Hematol 1981; 18: 293–300.

7. Hyun BH, Gulati GL, Ashton K. Bone marrow examination: techniques and interpretation. Hematol Oncol Clin North Am 1988; 2: 513–523.

8. Cotelingam JD. Bone marrow biopsy: interpretive guidelines for the surgical pathologist. Adv Anat Pathol 2003; 10: 8–26.

9. Ellman L. Bone marrow biopsy in the evaluation of lymphoma, carcinoma and granulomatous disorders (Review). Am J Med 1976; 60: 1–7.

10. Brunning RD, Bloomfield CD, McKenna RW, et al. Bilateral trephine bone marrow biopsies in lymphoma and other neoplastic diseases. Ann Intern Med 1975; 82: 365–366.

11. Wang J, Weiss LM, Chang KL, et al. Diagnostic utility of bilateral bone marrow examination: significance of morphologic and ancillary technique study in malignancy. Cancer 2002; 94: 1522–1531.

12. Gruber HE, Stauffer ME, Thompson ER, et al. Diagnosis of bone disease by core biopsies. Semin Hematol 1981; 18: 258–278.

13. Brown DC, Gatter KC. The bone marrow trephine biopsy: a review of normal histology. Histopathology 1993; 22: 411–422.

14. Aboul-Nasr R, Estey EH, Kantarjian HM, et al. Comparison of touch imprints with aspirate smears for evaluating bone marrow specimens. Am J Clin Pathol 1999; 111: 733–758.

15. Fong TP, Okafor LA, Thomas W Jr, et al. Stainable iron in aspirated and needle-biopsy specimens of marrow: a source of error. Am J Hematol 1977; 2: 47–51.

16. Sun NCJ. Hematologic tests and laboratory methods. In: Sun NCJ. Hematology. An atlas and diagnostic guide. Philadelphia: WB Saunders; 1983: 23–49.

17. Jennings CD, Foon KA. Recent advances in flow cytometry: application to the diagnosis of hematologic malignancy. Blood 1997; 90: 2863–2892.

18. Gozzetti A, LeBeau MM. Fluorescence in situ hybridization: uses and limitations. Semin Hematol 2000; 37: 320–333

19. Echeverri C, Fisher S, King D, et al. Immunophenotypic variability of B-cell non-Hodgkin's lymphoma. A retrospective study of cases analyzed by flow cytometry. Am J Clin Pathol 2002; 117: 615–620.

20. Todd WM. Acute myeloid leukemia and related conditions. Hematol Oncol Clin North Am 2002; 16: 301–319

21. Riley RS, Massey D, Jackson-Cook C, et al. Immunophenotypic analysis of acute lymphocytic leukemia. Hematol Oncol Clin North Am 2002; 16: 245–299

22. Chetty R, O'Leary JJ, Gatter KC. Immunocytochemistry as a diagnostic tool. Curr Diagn Pathol 1995; 2: 38–45.

23. Arber DA, Jenkins KA. Paraffin section immunophenotyping of acute leukemias in bone marrow specimens. Am J Clin Pathol 1996; 106: 462–468.

24. Manaloor EJ, Neiman RS, Heilman DK, et al. Immunohistochemistry can be use to subtype acute myeloid leukemia in routinely processed bone marrow biopsy specimens. Am J Clin Pathol 2000; 113: 814–822.

25. Hanson CA, Kurtin PJ, Katzmann JA, et al. Immunophenotypic analysis of peripheral blood and bone marrow in the staging of B-cell malignant lymphoma. Blood 1999; 94: 3889–3896.

26. Campana D, Pui C-H. (Review) Detection of minimal residual disease in acute leukemia: methodologic advances and clinical significance. Blood 1995; 85: 1416–1434.

27. Dunphy CH. Application of flow cytometry and immunohistochemistry to diagnostic hematopathology (Review). Arch Pathol Lab Med 2004; 128: 1004–1022.

28. Nguyen PL, Olszak I, Harris NL, et al. Myeloperoxidase detection by three-color flow cytometry and by enzyme cytochemistry in the classification of acute leukemia. Am J Clin Pathol 1998; 110: 163–169.

29. Kraguljac, N, Marisavljevic D, Jankovic G, et al. characterization of CD13 and CD33 surface antigen-negative acute myeloid leukemia. Am J Clin Pathol 2000; 114: 29–34.

30. Arber DA, Glackin C, Lowe G, et al. Presence of t(8; 21)(q22; q22) in myeloperoxidase-positive, myeloid surface antigen-negative acute myeloid leukemia. Am J Clin Pathol 1997; 107: 68–73.

31. Cave H, van der Werff ten Bosch J, Suciu S, et al. Clinical significance of minimal residual disease in childhood acute lymphoblastic leukemia. N Engl J Med 1998; 339: 591–598.

32. Kwong YL, Chan V, Wong KF, et al. Use of the polymerase chain reaction in the detection of AML1/ETO fusion transcript in t(8; 21). Cancer 1995; 75: 821–825.

33. Hubank M. Gene expression profiling and its application in studies of haematological malignancy. Br J Haematol 2004; 124: 577–594.

34. Bagg A, Kallakury VS. Molecular pathology of leukemia and lymphoma. Am J Clin Pathol 1999; 112(suppl.1): S76–S92.

35. Catovsky D, Matutes E, Buccheri V, et al. A classification of acute leukaemia for the 1990s. Ann Hematol 1991; 62: 16–21.

36. Bene MC, Castoldi G, Knapp W, et al. Proposals for the immunological classification of acute leukemias. Leukemia 1995; 9: 1783–1786.

37. Matutes E, Morilla R, Farahat N, et al. Definition of acute biphenotypic leukemia. Haematologica 1997; 82: 64–66.

38. Second MIC Cooperative Study Group: Morphologic, immunologic and cytogenetic (MIC) working classification of acute myeloid leukemias. Cancer Genet Cytogenet 1988; 30: 1–15.

39. Druker BJ, Sawyers CL, Kantarjian H, et al. Activity of a specific inhibitor of the BCR-ABL tyrosine kinase in the blast crisis of chronic myeloid leukemia and acute lymphoblastic leukemia with the Philadelphia chromosome. N Engl J Med 2001; 344: 1038–1042.

40. Druker BJ, Talpaz M Resta D, et al. Efficacy and safety of a specific inhibitor of the BCR-ABL tyrosine kinase in chronic myeloid leukemia. N Engl J Med 2001; 344: 1031–1037.

41. McLaughlin P, Grillo-Lopez AJ, Link BK, et al. Rituximab chimeric anti-CD20 monoclonal antibody therapy for relapsed indolent lymphoma: half of patients respond to a four-dose treatment program. J Clin Oncol 1998; 16: 2825–2833.

42. Davis TA, Grillo-Lopez AJ, White CA, et al. Rituximab anti-CD20 monoclonal antibody therapy in non-Hodgkin's lymphoma: safety and efficacy of re-treatment. J Clin Oncol 2000; 18: 3135–3143.

43. Coiffier B, Haioun C, Ketterer N, et al. Rituximab (anti-CD20 monoclonal antibody) for the treatment of patients with relapsing or refractory aggressive lymphoma: a multicenter phase II study. Blood 1998; 92: 1927–1932.

44. Foran JM, Cunningham D, Coiffier B, et al. Treatment of mantle-cell lymphoma with rituximab (chimeric monoclonal anti-CD20 antibody): analysis of factors associated with response. Ann Oncol 2000; 11(suppl. 1): 117–121.

45. Milpied M, Vasseur B, Parquet N, et al. Humanized anti-CD20 monoclonal antibody (Rituximab) in post transplant B-lymphoproliferative disorder: a retrospective analysis on 32 patients. Ann Oncol 2000; 11(suppl.1): 113–116.

46. Bain NT, Pickett JP. Glycol methacrylate for routine, special stains, histochemistry, enzyme histochemistry and immunohisto-chemistry. A simplified method for surgical biopsy tissue. J Histotechnol 1979; 2: 125–130.

47. Beckstead JH, Bainton DF. Enzyme histochemistry on bone marrow biopsies: reactions useful in the differential diagnosis of leukemia and lymphoma applied to 2-micron plastic sections. Blood 1980; 55: 386–394.

48. Bennett JM, Catovsky D, Daniel M-T, et al. Proposals for the classification of the acute leukaemias. French-American-British (FAB) Cooperative Group. Br J Haematol 1976; 33: 451–458.

49. Bennett JM, Catovsky D, Daniel M-T, et al. Proposed revised criteria for the classification of acute myeloid leukemia. A report of the French-American-British Cooperative Group. Ann Intern Med 1985; 103: 626–629.

50. Bennett JM, Catovsky D, Daniel M-T, et al. Criteria for the diagnosis of acute leukemia of megakaryocytic lineage (M7). A report of the French-American-British Cooperative Group. Ann Intern Med 1985; 103: 460–462.

51. Bennett JM, Catovsky D, Daniel M-T, et al. Proposal for the recognition of minimally differentiated acute myeloid leukaemia (AML-M0). Br J Haematol 1991; 78: 325–329.

52. Kaleem Z, White G. Diagnostic criteria for minimally differentiated acute myeloid leukemia (AML-M0). Am J Clin Pathol 2001; 115: 876–884.

53. Cohen PL, Hoyer JD, Kurtin PJ, et al. Acute myeloid leukemia with minimal differentiation. A multiple parameter study. Am J Clin Pathol 1998; 109: 32–38.

54. Bene M-C, Bernier M, Cassanovas RO, et al. Acute leukemia M0: haematological, immunophenotypic and cytogenetic characteristics and their prognostic significance: an analysis in 241 patients. Br J Haematol 2001; 113: 737–745.

55. Nezelof C, Basset F, Rousseau MF. Histiocytosis X. Histogenetic arguments for a Langerhans cell origin. Biomedicine 1973; 18: 365–371.

56. Hartsock RJ, Smith EB, Petty CS. Normal variations with aging of the amount of hematopoietic tissue in bone marrow from the anterior iliac crest. A study made from 177 cases of sudden death examined by necropsy. Am J Clin Pathol 1965; 43: 326–331.

57. Schmid C, Isaacson PG. Bone marrow trephine biopsy in lymphoproliferative disease. J Clin Pathol 1992; 45: 745–750.

58. Frisch B, Bartl R. Normal bone marrow. In: Frisch B, Bartl R. Biopsy interpretation of bone and bone marrow. Histology and immunohistology in paraffin and plastic, 2nd ed. London: Edward Arnold; 1999: 38–54.

59. Wilkins BS. Histology of normal haemopoiesis: bone marrow histology I. J Clin Pathol 1992; 45: 645–649.

60. Gulati GL, Ashton JK, Hyun BH. Structure and function of the bone marrow and hematopoiesis. Hematol Oncol Clin North Am 1988; 2: 495–511.

61. Metcalf D. Hematopoietic regulators: redundancy or subtlety? (Review) Blood 1993; 82: 3515–3523.

62. Brittenham GM, Danish EH, Harris JW. Assessment of bone marrow and body iron stores: old techniques and new technologies. Semin Hematol 1981; 18: 194–221.

63. Chuang S-S, Yung Y-C, Li C-Y. Von Willebrand factor is the most reliable immunohistochemical marker for megakaryocytes of myelodysplastic syndrome and chronic myeloproliferative disorders. Am J Clin Pathol 2000; 113: 506–511.

64. Larsen TE. Emperipolesis of granular leukocytes within megakaryocytes in human hematopoietic bone marrow. Am J Clin Pathol 1970; 53: 485–489.

65. Longacre TA, Foucar K, Crago S, et al. Hematogones: a multiparameter analysis of bone marrow precursor cells. Blood 1989; 73: 543–552.

66. Vandersteenhoven AM, Williams JE, Borowitz MJ. Marrow B-cell precursors are increased in lymphomas or systemic diseases associated with B-cell dysfunction. Am J Clin Pathol 1993; 100: 60–66.

67. Rimsza LM, Larson RS, Winter SS, et al. Benign hematogone-rich lymphoid proliferations can be distinguished from B-lineage acute lymphoblastic leukemia by integration of morphology, immunophenotype, adhesion molecule expression, and architectural features. Am J Clin Pathol 2000; 114: 66–75.

68. Thiele J, Zirbes TK, Kvasnicka HM, et al. Focal lymphoid aggregates (nodules) in bone marrow biopsies: differentiation between benign hyperplasia and malignant lymphoma – a practical guideline. J Clin Pathol 1999; 52: 294–300.

69. Fahri DC. Germinal centers in the bone marrow. Hematol Pathol 1989; 3: 133–136.

70. Hyun BH, Kwa D, Gabaldon H, et al. Reactive plasmacytic lesions of the bone marrow. Am J Clin Pathol 1976; 65: 921–928.

71. Sun NCJ. Leukocytic inclusions. In: Sun NCJ. Hematology. An atlas and diagnostic guide. Philadelphia: WB Saunders; 1983: 451–474.

72. Peterson LC, Agosti SJ, Hoyer JD, et al. Protocol for the examination of specimens from patients with hematopoietic neoplasms of the bone marrow. A basis for checklists. Arch Pathol Lab Med 2002; 126: 1050–1056.

73. Persing DH, Herwaldt BL, Glaser C, et al. Infection with a Babesia-like organism in Northern California. N Engl J Med 1995; 332: 298–303.

74. Caldwell CW, Everett D, McDonald G, et al. Lymphocytosis of γ/δ T cells in human ehrlichiosis. Am J Clin Pathol 1995; 103: 761–766.

75. Farrant A, Rodham J, Cordier A, et al. Selective hypoplasia of pelvic bone marrow. Scand J Haematol 1980; 25: 12–18.

76. Seaman JP, Kjeldsberg CR, Linker A. Gelatinous transformation of the bone marrow. Hum Pathol 1978; 9: 685–692.

77. Bohm J. Gelatinous transformation of the bone marrow: the spectrum of underlying diseases. Am J Surg Pathol 2000; 24: 56–65.

78. Mehta K, Gascon P, Robboy S. The gelatinous bone marrow (serous atrophy) in patients with acquired immunodeficiency syndrome. Evidence of excess sulfated glycosaminoglycan. Arch Pathol Lab Med 1992; 116: 504–508.

79. Guinan EC. Clinical aspects of aplastic anemia. Hematol Oncol Clin North Am 1997; 11: 1025–1044.

80. Young NS. Hematopoietic cell destruction by immune mechanisms in acquired aplastic anemia. Semin Hematol 2000; 37: 3–14.

81. Tooze JA, Marsh JCW, Gordon-Smith EC. Clonal evolution of aplastic anaemia to myelodysplasia/acute myeloid leukaemia and paroxysmal nocturnal haemoglobinuria. Leuk Lymphoma 1999; 33: 231–241

82. Baciagalupo A, Piaggio G, Figari O, et al. Response of CFU-GM to increasing doses of rhGM-CSF in patients with aplastic anemia. Exp Hematol 1991; 19: 829–832.

83. Kojima S, Ohara A, Tsuchida M, et al. Risk factors for evlution of acquired aplastic anemia into myelodysplastic syndrome and acute myeloid leukemia after immunosuppressive therapy in children. Blood 2002; 100: 786–790.

84. Narayanan MN, Geary CG, Freemont AJ, et al. Long term follow-up of aplastic anemia. Br J Haematol 1994; 86: 837–843.

85. Barrett J, Saunthararajah Y, Molldren J. Myelodysplastic syndrome and aplastic anemia: distinct entities or diseases linked by common pathophysiology? Semin Hematol 2000; 37: 15–29.

86. Marsh JC, Ball SE, Darbyshire P, et al. Guidelines for the diagnosis and management of acquired aplastic anemia. Br J Haematol 2003; 123: 782–801

87. Krijanovski OI, Sieff CA. Diamond–Blackfan anemia. Hematol Oncol Clin North Am 1997; 11: 1061–1077.

88. Erslev AJ, Soltan AJ. Pure red-cell aplasia: a review. Blood Rev 1996; 10: 20–28.

89. Vadlamudi G, Rezuke WN, Ross JW, et al. The use of monoclonal antibody R92F6 and polymerase chain reaction to confirm the presence of parvovirus B19 in bone marrow specimens of patients with acquired immunodeficiency syndrome. Arch Pathol Lab Med 1999; 123: 768–773.

90. Penchansky L, Jordan JA. Transient erythroblastopenia of childhood associated with human herpesvirus type 6, variant B. Am J Clin Pathol 1997; 108: 127–132.

91. Papadaki HA, Eliopoulos GD. An overview on the diagnosis, classification and differential diagnosis of chronic neutropenias. Haema 2002; 5: 39–49

92. Zeidler C, Schwinzer B, Welte K. Congenital neutropenias. Rev Clin Exp Hematol 2003; 7: 72–83.

93. Young NS. Agranulocytosis. JAMA 1994; 271: 935–938.

94. Welte K, Box LA. Severe chronic neutropenia: pathophysiology and therapy. Semin Hematol 1997; 34: 267–278.

95. Dale DC, Cottle TE, Fier CJ, et al. Severe chronic neutropenia: treatment and follow-up of patients in the severe Chronic Neutropenia International Registry. Am J Hematol 2003; 72: 82–93.

96. Hoffman R. Acquired pure amegaryocytic thrombocytopenic purpura. Semin Hematol 1991; 28: 303–312.

97. Ballmaier M, Germeshausen M, Schulze H, et al. c-mpl mutations are the cause of congenital amegakaryocytic thrombocytopenia. Blood 2001; 97: 139–146.

98. Geddis AE, Kaushansky K. Inherited thrombocytopenias: toward a molecular understanding of disorders of platelet production. Curr Opin Pediatr 2004; 16: 15–22.

99. Cine DB, Blanchette VS. Immune thrombocytopenic purpura (Review). N Engl J Med 2002; 346: 995–1008.

100. Moake JL. Thrombotic microangiopathies (Review). N Engl J Med 2002; 347: 589–622.

101. Yospur LS, Sun NCJ, Figueroa P, et al. Concurrent thrombotic thrombocytopenic purpura and immune thrombocytopenic purpura in an HIV-positive patient: case report and review of the literature. Am J Hematol 1996; 50: 73–78.

102. Menke DM, Colon-Otero G, Cockerill KJ, et al. Refractory thrombocytopenia: a myelodysplastic syndrome that may mimic immune thrombocytopenic purpura. Am J Clin Pathol 1992; 98: 502–510.

103. Bessler N, Hillmen P. Somatic mutation and clonal selection in the pathogenesis and in the control of paroxysmal nocturnal hemaglobinuria. Semin Hematol 1998; 35: 149–167.

104. Brodsky RA, Mukhina GL, Li S, et al. Improved detection and characterization of paroxysmal nocturnal hemoglobinuria using fluorescent aerolysin. Am J Clin Pathol 2000; 114: 459–466.

105. Dunn DE, Tanawattanacharoen P, Boccuni P, et al. Paroxysmal nocturnal hemoglobinuria cells in patients with bone marrow failure syndromes. Ann Intern Med 1999; 131: 401–408.

106. Tozuner N, Cox C, Rowe JM, et al. Hypocellular myelodysplastic syndromes (MDS): new proposals. Br J Haematol 1995; 91: 612–617.

107. Orazi A, Albitar M, Heerema NA, et al : Hypoplastic myelodysplastic syndromes can be distinguished from acquired aplastic anemia by CD34 and PCNA immunostaining of bone marrow biopsy specimens. Am J Clin Pathol 1997; 107: 268–274.

108. Tozuner N, Cox C, Rowe JM, et al. Hypocellular acute myeloid leukemia: the Rochester (New York) experience. Hematol Pathol 1995; 9: 195–203.

109. Nagai K, Kohno T, Chen Y-X, et al. Diagnostic criteria for hypocellular acute leukemia: a clinical entity distinct from overt acute leukemia and myelodysplastic syndrome. Leuk Res 1996; 20: 563–574.

110. Wittels B. Bone marrow biopsy change following chemotherapy for acute leukemia. Am J Surg Pathol 1980; 4: 135–142.

111. Dick FR, Burns CP, Weiner GJ, et al. Bone marrow morphology during induction phase of therapy for acute myeloid leukemia (AML). Hematol Pathol 1995; 9: 95–106.

112. Foucar K. Effects of therapy and transplantation, and detection of minimal residual disease. In: Foucar K. Bone marrow pathology, 2nd ed. Chicago: ASCP Press; 2001: 654–681.

113. Wickramasinghe SN. Dyserythropoiesis and congenital dyserythropoietic anemias. Br J Haematol 1997; 98: 785–797.

114. Hoffbrand AV, Herbert V. Nutritional anemias. Semin Hematol 1999; 36(suppl. 7): 13–23.

115. Toh B-H, van Driel IR, Gleeson PA. Pernicious anemia (Review). N Engl J Med 1997; 337: 1441–1448.

116. Schmitz LA, McClure JS, Litz CE, et al. Morphologic and quantitative changes in blood and marrow cells following growth factor therapy. Am J Clin Pathol 1994; 101: 67–75.

117. Harris AC, Todd WM, Hackney H, et al. Bone marrow changes associated with recombinant granulocyte-macrophage and granulocyte colony-stimulating factors. Discrimination of granulocytic regeneration. Arch Pathol Lab Med 1994; 118: 624–629.

118. Brunning RD, Vardiman J, Matutes E, et al. Acute myeloid leukaemia: introduction. In: Jaffe ES, Harris NL, Stein H, et al, eds. World Health Organization classification of tumours. Pathology and genetics of tumours of haematopoietic and lymphoid tissues. Lyon: IARC Press; 2001: 77–80.

119. Brunning RD, Flandrin G, Borowitz M, et al. Precursor B- and T-cell neoplasms. In: Jaffe ES, Harris NL, Stein H, et al, eds. World Health Organization classification of tumours. Pathology and genetics of tumours of haematopoietic and lymphoid tissues. Lyon: IARC Press; 2001: 109–117.

120. Brunning RD, Bennett J, Matutes E, et al. Acute myeloid leukaemia not otherwise categorised. In: Jaffe ES, Harris NL, Stein H, et al, eds. World Health Organization classification of tumours. Pathology and genetics of tumours of haematopoietic and lymphoid tissues. Lyon: IARC Press; 2001: 91–105.

121. Brunning RD, Bennett J, Matutes E, et al. Acute myeloid leukaemias and myelodysplastic syndromes, therapy related. In: Jaffe ES, Harris NL, Stein H, et al, eds. World Health Organization classification of tumours. Pathology and genetics of tumours of haematopoietic and lymphoid tissues. Lyon: IARC Press; 2001: 89–91.

122. Brunning RD, Vardiman J, Matutes E, et al. Acute myeloid leukaemia with multilineage dysplasia. In: Jaffe ES, Harris NL, Stein H, et al, eds. World Health Organization classification of tumours. Pathology and genetics of tumours of haematopoietic and lymphoid tissues. Lyon: IARC Press; 2001: 88–89.

123. Brunning RD, Bennett J, Matutes E, et al. Acute myeloid leukaemia with recurrent genetic abnormalities. In: Jaffe ES, Harris NL, Stein H, et al, eds. World Health Organization classification of tumours. Pathology and genetics of tumours of haematopoietic and lymphoid tissues. Lyon: IARC Press; 2001: 81–87.

124. Brunning RD. Classification of acute leukemias. Semin Diag Pathol 2003; 20: 142–153.

125. Pui C-H. Childhood leukemias, review. N Engl J Med 1995; 332: 1618–1630.

126. Cline JM. The molecular basis of leukemia, review. N Engl J Med 1994; 330: 328–336.

127. Franzman C, Bennett JM. Classification of acute leukemias. Contemp Oncol 1992; 2: 46–54.

128. Bene MC, Bernier M, Castoldi G, et al. Impact of immunophenotyping on management of acute leukemias. Haematologica 1999; 84: 1024–1034.

129. Goasguen J-E, Bennett JM, Cox C, et al. Prognostic implication and characterization of the blast cell population in the myelodysplastic syndrome. Leuk Res 1991; 15: 1159–1165.

130. Lange B. The management of neoplasstic disorders of haematopoiesis in children with Down's syndrome. Br J Haematol 2000; 110: 512–524

131. Zipursky A, Poon A, Doyle J. Leukemia in Down syndrome: a review. Pediatr Hematol Oncol 1992; 9: 139–149.

132. Mundschau G Gurbuxani S, Gamis AS, et al. Mutagenesis of GATA1 is an initiating event in Down syndrome leukemogenesis. Blood 2002; 101: 4298–4300.

133. Hitzler JK, Cheung J, Li Y, et al. GATA1 mutations in transient leukemia and acute megakaryoblastic leukemia of Down syndrome. Blood 2003; 4301–4304.

134. Lu G, Altman AJ, Benn PA. Review of the cytogenetic changes in acute megakaryoblastic leukemia: one disease or several? Cancer Genet Cytogenet 1993; 67: 81–89.

135. Bernstein J, Dastugue N, Haas OA, et al. Nineteen cases of the t(1; 22)(p13; q13) acute megakaryoblastic leukemia of infants/children and a review of 39 cases: report from a t(1; 22) study group. Leukemia 2000; 14: 216–218.

136. Mercher T, Busson-Le Coniat M, Khac FN, et al. Recurrence of OTT-MAL fusion in t(1; 22) of infant AML-M7. Genes, Chromosomes and Cancer 2002; 33: 22–28.

137. Sun NCJ. Severe Anemia with circulating blasts. In: Sun NCJ. Hematology. An atlas and diagnostic guide. Philadelphia: WB Saunders; 1983: 173–185.

138. Olopade OI, Thangavelu M, Larson RA, et al. Clinical, morphologic, and cytogenetic characteristics of 26 patients with acute erythroblastic leukemia. Blood 1992; 11: 2873–2882.

139. Thalhammer-Scherrer R, Mitterbauer G, Simonitsch I, et al. The immunophenotype of 325 adult acute leukemias. Am J Clin Pathol 2002; 117: 380–389.

140. Stasi R, Amadori S. AML-M0: a review of laboratory features and proposal of new diagnostic criteria. Blood Cells, Mol Dis 1999; 25: 120–129.

141. Cuneo A, Ferrant A, Michaux JL, et al. Cytogenetic profile of minimally differentiated (FAB M0) acute myeloid leukemia: correlation with clinicobiologic findings. Blood 1995; 85: 3688–3694.

142. Peterson LC, Parkin JL, Arthur DC, et al. Acute basophilic leukemia. A clinical, morphologic, and cytochemical study of eight cases. Am J Clin Pathol 1991; 96: 160–170.

143. Duchayne E, Demur C, Rubie H, et al. Diagnosis of acute basophilic leukemia. Leuk Lymphoma 1999; 32: 269–278.

144. Bearman RM, Pangalis GA, Rappaport H. Acute (malignant) myelosclerosis. Cancer 1979; 43: 279–293.

145. Shah I, Mayeda K, Koppitch F, et al. Karyotypic polymorphism in acute myelofibrosis. Blood 1982; 60: 841–844.

146. Rozman C, Granena A, Hernandez-Nieto M, et al. Bone marrow transplantation for acute myelofibrosis. Lancet 1982; 1: 618.

147. Truong LD, Saleem A, Schwartz MR. Acute myelofibrosis. A report of four cases and review of the literature. Medicine (Baltimore) 1984; 63: 182–187.

148. Cuneo A, Mecucci C, Kerim S, et al. Multiple stem cell involvement in megakaryoblastic leukemia. Cytologic and cytogenetic evidence in 15 patients. Blood 1989; 74: 1781–1790.

149. Davey FR, Olson S, Kurec AS, et al. The immunophenotyping of extramedullary myeloid cell tumors in paraffin-embedded tissue sections. Am J Surg Pathol 1988; 12: 699–707.

150. Neiman RS, Barcos M, Berard C, et al. Granulocytic sarcoma: a clinicopathologic study of 61 biopsies cases. Cancer 1981; 48: 1426–1437.

151. Roth MJ, Medeiros J, Elenitoba-Johnson K, et al. Extramedullary myeloid cell tumors. An immunohistochemical study of 29 cases using routinely fixed and processed paraffin-embedded tissue sections. Arch Pathol Lab Med 1995; 119: 790–798.

152. Traweek ST, Arber DA, Rappaport H, et al. Extramedullary myeloid cell tumor: an immunohistochemical and morphologic study of 28 cases. Am J Surg Pathol 1993; 17: 1011–1019.

153. Ellis M, Ravid M, Lishner M. A comparative analysis of alkylating agent and epipidophyllotoxin-related leukemias. Leuk Lymphoma 1993; 11: 9–13.

154. Thirman M, Larson RA. Therapy related myeloid leukemia. Hematol Oncol Clin North Am 1996; 10: 293–320.

155. Willman C. Molecular evaluation of acute myeloid leukemia. Semin Hematol 1999; 36: 390–400.

156. Pedersen-Bjergaard J, Andersen MK, Christiansen DH, et al. Genetic pathways in therapy-related myelodysplasia and acute myeloid leukemia. Blood 2002; 99: 1909–1912.

157. Karp JE, Sarkodee-Adoo CB. Therapy-related acute leukemia. Clin Lab Med 2000; 20: 71–79.

158. Mecucci C, Rosati R, La Starza R. Genetic profile of acute myeloid leukemia. Rev Clin Exp Hematol 2002; 6: 3–25.

159. Orazi A, Cattoretti G, Soligo D, et al. Therapy-related myelodysplastic syndromes: FAB classification, bone marrow histology, and immunohistology in the prognostic assessment. Leukemia 1993; 6: 838–847.

160. Vardiman J, Harris NL, Brunning RD. The World Health Organization (WHO) classification of the myeloid neoplasms (Review). Blood 2003; 100: 2292–2302.

161. Nucifora G, Rowley JD. AML1 and the 8; 21 and 3; 21 translocations in acute and chronic myeloid leukemia (Review article). Blood 1995; 86: 1–14.

162. Melnick A, Licht JD. Deconstructing a disease: RARα, its fusion partners, and their roles in the pathogenesis of acute promyelocytic leukemia. Blood 1999; 93: 3167–3215.

163. Virchis A, Massey E, Butler T, et al. Acute myeloblastic leukaemias of FAB type M6 and M4, with cryptic PML/RARα fusion gene formation, relapsing as acute promyelocytic leukemia M3. Br J Haematol 2001; 114: 551–556.

164. Sainty D, Liso V, Cantu-Rajnoldi A, et al. A new morphologic classification system for acute promyelocytic leukemia distinguishes cases with underlying PLZF/RARA gene rearrangements. Blood 2000; 96: 1287–1296.

165. Tallman MS, Andersen JW, Schiffer CA, et al. Clinical description of 44 patients with acute promyelocytic leukemia who developed the retinoic acid syndrome. Blood 2000; 95: 90–95.

166. Liu PP, Hajra A, Wijmenga C, et al. Molecular pathogenesis of the chromosome 16 inversion in the M4Eo subtype of acute myeloid leukemia (Review). Blood 1995; 85: 2289–2302.

167. Poirel H, Radford-Weiss I, Rack K, et al. Detection of the chromosome 16 CBFβ-MYH11 fusion transcript in myelomonocytic leukemias. Blood 1995; 85: 1313–1322.

168. Thirman MJ, Gill HJ, Burnett RC, et al. Rearrangement of the MLL gene in acute lymphoblastic and acute myeloid leukemia with 11q23 chromosomal translocation. N Engl J Med 1993; 329: 909–914.

169. Rubnitz JE, Raimondi SC, Tong X, et al. Favorable impact of the t(9; 11) in childhood acute myeloid leukemia. J Clin Oncol 2002; 20: 2302–2309.

170. Rubin CM, Larson RA, Anastasi J, et al. t(3; 21)(q26; q22): a recurring chromosomal abnormality in therapy-related myelodysplastic syndrome and acute myeloid leukemia. Blood 1990; 76: 2594–2598.

171. Ibrahim S. Estey EH, Pierce S, et al. 11q23 abnormalities in patients with acute myelogeneous leukemia and myelodysplastic syndrome as detected by molecular and cytogenetic analysis. Am J Clin Pathol 2000; 114: 793–797.

172. Bennett JM. World Health Organization classification of the acute leukemias and myelodysplastic syndrome. Int J Hematol 2000; 72: 131–133.

173. Arber DA. Realistic pathologic classification of acute myeloid leukemias. Am J Clin Pathol 2001; 115: 552–560.

174. Arber DA, Snyder DS, Fine M, et al. Myeloperoxidase immunoreactivity in adult acute lymphoblastic leukemia. Am J Clin Pathol 2001; 116: 25–33.

175. Vasef MA, Brynes RK, Murata-Collins JL, et al. Surface immunoglobulin light chain-positive acute lymphocytic leukemia of FAB L1 or L2 type. A report of 6 cases in adults. Am J Clin Pathol 1998; 110: 143–149.

176. Pui C-H, Behm FG, Crist WM. Clinical and biologic relevance of immunologic marker studies in childhood acute lymphoblastic leukemia. (Review). Blood 1993; 82: 343–362.

177. Picozzi VJ, Coleman CN. Lymphoblastic lymphoma. Semin Oncol 1990; 17: 96–103.

178. Pui CH, Behm FG, Singh B, et al. Heterogeneity of presenting features and their relation to treatment outcome in 120 children with T-cell acute lymphoblastic leukemia. Blood 1990; 75: 174–179.

179. Onciu M, Lai R, Vega F, et al. Precursor T-cell acute lymphoblastic leukemia in adults. Am J Clin Pathol 2002; 117: 252–258.

180. Maitra A, McKenna RW, Weinberg AG, et al. Precursor B-cell lymphoblastic lymphoma. A study of nine cases lacking blood and bone marrow involvement and review of the literature. Am J Clin Pathol 2001; 115: 868–875.

181. Diebold J, Jaffe E, Raphael M, et al. Burkitt lymphoma. In: Jaffe ES, Harris NL, Stein H, et al, eds. World Health Organization classification of tumours. Pathology and genetics of tumours of haematopoietic and lymphoid tissues. Lyon: IARC Press; 2001: 181–184.

182. Khalidi HS, Chang KL, Medeiros LJ, et al. Acute lymphoblastic leukemia. Survey of immunophenotype, French-American-British classification, frequency of myeloid antigen expression, and karyotypic abnormalities in 210 pediatric and adult cases. Am J Clin Pathol 1999; 111: 467–476.

183. Soussain C, Patte C, Ostronoff M, et al. Small noncleaved cell lymphoma and leukemia in adults. A retrospective study of 65 adults treated with the LMB pediatric protocols. Blood 1995; 85: 664–674.

184. Pui CH, Kane JR, Crist WM. Biology and treatment of infant leukemias (Review) Leukemia 1995; 9: 762–769.

185. Chessells JM, Harrison CJ, Kempski H, et al. Clinical features, cytogenetics and outcome in acute lymphoblastic and myeloid leukaemia of infancy: report from the MRC Childhood Leukaemia Working Party. Leukemia 2002; 16: 776–784.

186. Tsao L, Draoua HY, Osunkwo I, et al. Mature B-cell acute lymphoblastic leukemia with t(9; 11) translocation: a distinct subset of B-cell acute lymphoblastic leukemia. Mod Pathol 2004; 17: 832–839.

187. Raimondi SC. Current Status of cytogenetic research in childhood acute lymphoblastic leukemia (Review). Blood 1993; 81: 2237–2251.

188. Okuda T, Fisher R, Downing JR. Molecular diagnostics in pediatric acute leukemia (Review). Molecular Diag 1996; 1: 139–151.

189. Fernando AA, Look AT. Clinical implications of recurring chromosomal and associated molecular abnormalities in acute lymphoblastic leukemia. Semin Hematol 2000; 37: 381–395.

190. Paietta E, Racevskis J, Bennett JM, et al. Biologic heterogeneity in Philadelphia chromosome-positive acute lymphoblastic leukemia with myeloid morphology: the Eastern Cooperative Oncology Group experience. Leukemia 1998; 12: 1881–1885.

191. Crist W, Carroll A, Shuster J, et al. Philadelphia chromosome positive childhood acute lymphoblastic leukemia: clinical and cytogenetic characteristics and treatment outcome. A Pediatric Oncology Group Study. Blood 1990; 76: 489–494.

192. Cimino G, Elia L, Rapanotti MC, et al. a prospective study of residual-disease monitoring of the ALL1/AF4-transcript in patients with t(4; 11) acute lymphoblastic leukemia. Blood 2000; 95: 96–101.

193. Pui CH, Crist WM, Look AT. Biology and clinical significance of cytogenetic abnormalities in childhood acute lymphoblastic leukemia. (Review). Blood 1990; 76: 1449–1463.

194. Gaynon PS. Acute leukemia in children. Curr Opin Hematol 1995; 2: 240–246.

195. Crump M, Keating A. Acute leukemia in adults. Curr Opin Hematol 1995; 2: 247–254.

196. Pui CH, Evans WE. Acute lymphoblastic leukemia. N Engl J Med 1998; 339: 605–615

197. Grimwade D, Walker H, Oliver F, et al. The importance of diagnostic cytogenetics on outcome in AML. analysis of 1,612 patients entered into the MRC AML 10 trail. Blood 1998; 92: 2322–2333.

198. Byrd JC, Mrozek K, Dodge RK, et al. Pretreatment cytogenetic abnormalities are predictive of induction success, cumulative incidence of relapse, and overall survival in adult patients with de novo acute myeloid leukemia: result from Cancer and Leukemia Group B (CALGB 8461). Blood 2002; 100: 4325–4336.

199. Kottaridis PD, Gale RE, Linch DC. FLT3 mutations and leukemia (Review). Br J Haematol 2003; 122: 523–528.

200. Schnittger S, Schoch C, Dugas M, et al. Analysis of FLT3 length mutations in 1003 patients with acute myeloid leukemia: correlation to cytogenetics, FAB subtype, and prognosis in the AMLCG study and useful as a marker for the detection of minimal residual disease. Blood 2002; 100: 59–66.

201. Szczepanski T, Willemse MJ, Brinkhof B, et al. Comparative analysis of Ig and TCR gene rearrangements at diagnosis and at relapse of childhood precursor-B-ALL provides improved strategies for selection of stable PCR targets for monitoring of minimal residual disease. Blood 2002; 99: 2315–2323.

202. Shimada H, Ichikawa H, Ohki M. Potential involvement of AML1-MTG8 fusion protein in the granulocytic maturation of characteristic of the t(8; 21) acute myelogenous leukemia revealed by microarray analysis. Leukemia 2002; 16: 874–885.

203. Dworzak MN, Panzer-Grumayer ER. Flow cytometric detection of minimal residual disease in acute lymphoblastic leukemia. Leuk Lymphoma 2003; 44: 1445–1455.

204. Rubnitz JE, Pui CH. Molecular diagnostics in the treatment of leukemia. Curr Opin Hematol 1999; 6: 229–235.

205. Jurlander J, Caligiuri MA, Ruutu T, et al. Persistence of the AML1/ETO fusion transcript in patients treated with allogeneic bone marrow transplantation for t(8; 21) leukemia. Blood 1996; 88: 2183–2191.

206. Cruczman MS, Dodge RK, Stewart CC, et al. Value of immunophenotype in intensively treated adult acute lymphoblastic leukemia: Cancer and Leukemia Group B study 8364. Blood 1999; 93: 3931–3939.

207. Pui CH, Raimondi SC, Head DR, et al. Characterization of childhood acute leukemia with multiple myeloid and lymphoid markers at diagnosis and at relapse. Blood 1991; 78: 1327–1337.

208. Brunning RD, Head D, Matutes E, et al. Acute leukaemias of ambiguous lineage. In: Jaffe ES, Harris NL, Stein H, et al, eds. World Health Organization classification of tumours. Pathology and genetics of tumours of haematopoietic and lymphoid tissues. Lyon: IARC Press; 2001: 106–107.

209. European Group for the Immunological Classification of Leukemias: The value of c-kit in the diagnosis of biphenotypic acute leukemia. Leukemia 1998; 12: 2038.

210. Pilozzi E, Pulford K, Jones M, et al. Co-expression of CD79a (JCB117) and CD3 by lymphoblastic lymphoma. J Pathol 1998; 186: 140–143.

211. Vardiman JW, Brunning RD, Harris NL. Chronic myeloproliferative diseases: introduction. In: Jaffe ES, Harris NL, Stein H, et al, eds. World Health Organization classification of tumours. Pathology and genetics of tumours of haematopoietic and lymphoid tissues. Lyon: IARC Press; 2001: 15–19.

212. Pearson TC. Evaluation of diagnostic criteria in polycythemia vera. Semin Hematol 2001; 38(suppl. 2): 21–24.

213. Tefferi A. Pathogenetic mechanisms in chronic myeloproliferative disorders: polycythemia vera, essential thrombocythemia, agnogenic myeloid metaplasia, and chronic myelogeneous leukemia. Semin Hematol 1999; 36(suppl. 2): 3–8.

214. Gruppo Italiano Studio Policitemia: Polycythemia vera: the normal history of 1213 patients followed for 20 years. Ann Intern Med 1995; 123: 656–664.

215. Martyre MC, Romquin N, Bousse-Kerdiles MC, et al. Transforming growth factor-beta and megakaryocytes in the pathogenesis of idiopathic myelofibrosis. Br J Haematol 1994; 88: 9–16.

216. Ellis JT, Peterson P, Geller SA, et al. Studies of the bone marrow in polycythemia vera and the evolution of myelofibrosis and secondary hematologic malignancies. Semin Hematol 1986; 23: 144–155.

217. Diez-Martin JL, Graham DL, Petitt RM, et al. Chromosome studies in 104 patients with polycythemia vera. Mayo Clin Proc 1991; 66: 287–299.

218. Dewald GW, Wright PI. Chromosome abnormalities in the myeloproliferative disorders. Semin Oncol 1995; 22: 341–354.

219. Vardiman JW. Myelodysplastic syndromes, chronic myeloproliferative diseases, and myelodysplastic/myeloproliferative diseases. Semin Diag Pathol 2003; 20: 154–179.

220. Harrison CN, Gale RE, Machin SJ, et al. A large portion of patients with a diagnosis of essential thrombocythemia do not have a clonal disorder and may be at lower risk of thrombotic complications. Blood 1999; 93: 417–424.

221. Nimer SD. Essential thrombocythemia: another 'heterogeneous disease' better understood? Blood 1999; 93: 415–416.

222. Dickstein JI, Vardiman JW. Hematopathologic findings in the myeloproliferative disorders. Semin Oncol 1995; 22: 355–373.

223. Murphy S, Peterson P, Iland H, et al. Experience of the polycythemia vera study group with essential thrombocythemia: a final report on diagnostic criteria, survival and leukemia transition by treatment. Semin Hematol 1997; 34: 29–39.

224. Harrison CN, Green AR. Esssential thrombocythemia. Hematol Oncol Clin North Am 2003; 17: 1175–1190.

225. Fenaux P, Simon M, Caulier MT, et al. Clinical course of essential thrombocythemia in 147 cases. Cancer 1990; 66: 549–556.

226. Sterkers Y, Preudhomme C, Lai J-L, et al. Acute myeloid leukemia and myelodysplastic syndromes following essential thrombocythemia treated with hydroxyurea: high proportion of cases with 17p deletion. Blood 1998; 91: 616–622.

227. Nowell PC, Hungerford DA. Chromosome studies in human leukemia. II. Chronic granulocytic leukemia. J Natl Cancer Inst 1961; 27: 1013–1021.

228. Faderl S, Talpaz M, Estrov Z, et al. The biology of chronic myeloid leukemia. N Engl J Med 1999; 341: 164–172.

229. Hasserjian R, Boecklin F, Parker S, et al. STI571 (Imatinib mesylate) reduces bone marrow cellularity and normalizes morphologic features irrespective of cytogenetic response. Am J Clin Pathol 2002; 117: 360–367.

230. Silver RT. Chronic myeloid leukemia. Hematol Oncol Clin North Am 2003; 17: 1159–1173.

231. Vardiman JW, Imbert M, Pierre R, et al. Chronic myelogeneous leukemia. In: Jaffe ES, Harris NL, Stein H, et al, eds. World Health Organization classification of tumours. Pathology and genetics of tumours of haematopoietic and lymphoid tissues. Lyon: IARC Press; 2001: 20–26.

232. Khalidi HS, Brynes RK, Medeiros LJ, et al. The immunophenotype of blast transformation of chronic myelogenous leukemia: a high frequency of mixed lineage phenotype in 'lymphoid' blasts and a comparison of morphologic, immunophenotypic, and molecular findings. Mod Pathol 1998; 11: 1211–1221.

233. George TI, Arber DA. Pathology of the myeloproliferative diseases. Hematol Oncol Clin North Am 2003; 17: 1101–1127.

234. Bennett JM, Catovsky D, Daniel MT, et al. The chronic myeloid leukaemias: guidelines for distinguishing chronic granulocytic, atypical chronic myeloid, and chronic myelomonocytic leukaemia. Proposal by the French-American-British Cooperative Leukaemia Group. Br J Haematol 1994; 87: 746–754.

235. Oscier D. Atypical chronic myeloid leukemias. Pathol Biol 1997; 45: 587–593.

236. Martiat P, Michaux JL, Rodhain J, et al. Philadelphia-negative (Ph⁻) chronic myeloid leukemia (CML): comparison with Ph⁺ CML and chronic myelomonocytic leukemia. Blood 1991; 78: 205–211.

237. Sawyers CL. Chronic myeloid leukemia. N Engl J Med 1999; 340: 1330–1340.

238. Thiele J, Kvasnicka HM, Schmitt-Graeff A, et al. Effects of chemotherapy (busulfan–hydroxyurea) and interferon-alfa on bone marrow morphologic features in chronic myelogenous leukemia. Am J Clin Pathol 2000; 114: 57–65.

239. Hochhaus A, Reiter A, SauBele S, et al. Molecular heterogeneity in complete cytogenetic responders after interferon-α therapy for chronic myelogenous leukemia: low levels of minimal residual disease are associated with continuing remission. Blood 2000; 95: 62–66.

240. Ward HP, Block MH. The natural history of agnogenic myeloid metaplasia (AMM)) and a critical evaluation of its relationship with the myeloproliferative syndrome. Medicine (Baltimore) 1971; 50: 357–420.

241. Thiele J, Kvasnicka H-M, Werden C, et al. Idiopathic primary osteo-myelofibrosis: a clinico-pathological study on 208 patients with special emphasis on evolution of disease features, differentiation from essential thrombocythemia and variables of prognostic impact. Leuk Lymphoma 1996; 22: 303–317.

242. Tefferi A. Myelofibrosis with myeloid metaplasia (Review). N Engl J Med 2000; 342: 1255–1265.

243. Manoharan A. Idiopathic myelofibrosis: a clinical review (Review article). Int J Hematol 1998; 68: 355–362.

244. Reilly JT, Snowden JA, Spearing RL, et al. Cytogenetic abnormalities and their prognostic significance in idiopathic myelofibrosis: a study of 106 cases. Br J Haematol 1997; 98: 96–102.

245. Adeyinka A, Dewald GW. Cytogenetics of chronic myeloproliferative disorders and related myelodysplastic syndromes. Hematol Oncol Clin North Am 2003; 17: 1129–1149.

246. Dupriez B, Morel P, Demory JL, et al. Prognostic factors in agnogenic myeloid metaplasia: a report on 195 cases with a new scoring system. Blood 1996; 88: 1013–1018.

247. Bennett JM, Catovsky D, Daniel MT, et al. Proposals for the classification of the myelodysplastic syndromes. Br J Haematol 1982; 51: 189–199.

248. Mangi MH, Mufti GJ. Primary myelodysplastic syndromes: diagnostic and prognostic significance of immunohistochemical assessment of bone marrow biopsies. Blood 1992; 79: 198–205.

249. Heaney ML, Golde DW. Myelodysplasia (Review article). N Engl J Med 1999; 340: 1649–1660.

250. Tricot G, De Wolf-Peeters C, Vlietinck R, et al. Bone marrow histology in myelodysplastic syndromes. II. Prognostic value of abnormal localization of immature precursors in MDS. Br J Haematol 1984; 58: 217–225.

251. Boultwood J, Lewis S, Wainscoat JS. The 5q-syndrome (Review). Blood 1994; 84: 3253–3260.

252. Kampmeier P, Anastasi J and Vardiman JW. Issues in the pathology of the myelodysplastic syndromes. Hematol Oncol Clin North Am 1992; 6: 501–522.

253. Fenaux P, Morel P, Lai JL. Cytogenetics of myelodysplastic syndromes. Semin Hematol 1996; 33: 127–128.

254. Verhoef GEG, Boogaerts MA. Cytogenetics and its prognostic value in myelodysplastic syndromes. Acta Haematol 1996; 95: 95–101.

255. Greenberg P, Cox C, LeBeau MM, et al. International Scoring System for evaluating prognosis in myelodysplastic syndromes. Blood 1997; 89: 2079–2088. (Erratum: Blood 1998; 91: 1100)

256. Brunning RD, Head D, Bennett JM, et al. Myelodysplastic syndromes. In: Jaffe ES, Harris NL, Stein H, et al, eds. World Health Organization classification of tumours. Pathology and genetics of tumours of haematopoietic and lymphoid tissues. Lyon: IARC Press; 2001: 61–73.

257. Vardiman JW. Myelodysplastic/myeloproliferative diseases: introduction. In: Jaffe ES, Harris NL, Stein H, et al, eds. World Health Organization classification of tumours. Pathology and genetics of tumours of haematopoietic and lymphoid tissues. Lyon: IARC Press; 2001: 45–48.

258. Germing U, Gattermann N, Strupp C, et al. Validation of the WHO proposals for a new classification of primary myelodysplastic syndromes: a retrospective analysis of 1600 patients. Leuk Res 2000; 24: 983–992.

259. Germing U, Gattermann N, Minning H. Problems in the classification of CMML-dysplastic versus proliferative type. Leuk Res 1998; 22: 871–878.

260. Onida F, Kantarjian HM, Smith TL, et al. Prognostic factors and scoring systems in chronic myelomonocytic leukemia: a retrospective analysis of 213 patients. Blood 2002; 99: 840–849.

261. Vardiman JW, Imbert M, Pierre R, et al. Chronic myelomonocytic leukaemia. In: Jaffe ES, Harris NL, Stein H, et al, eds. World Health Organization classification of tumours. Pathology and genetics of tumours of haematopoietic and lymphoid tissues. Lyon: IARC Press; 2001: 49–52.

262. Emanuel PD. Myelodysplasia and myeloproliferative disorders in childhood: an update (Review). Br J Haematol 1999; 105: 852–863.

263. Hasle H, Niemeyer CM, Chessells JM, et al. A pediatric approach to the WHO Classification of myelodysplastic and myeloproliferative diseases (Review). Leukemia 2003; 17: 277–282.

264. Hasle H, Arica M, Basso G, et al. Myelodysplastic syndrome, juvenile myelomonocytic leukemia, and acute myeloid leukemia associated with complete or partial monosomy 7. Leukemia 1999; 13: 376–385.

265. Niemeyer CM, Arico M, Basso G, et al. Chronic myelomonocytic leukemia in childhood: a retrospective analysis of 110 cases. Blood 1997; 89: 3534–3543.

266. Bass RD, Pullarkat V, Feinstein DI, et al. Pathology of autoimmune myelofibrosis. A report of three cases and a review of the literature. Am J Clin Pathol 2001; 116: 211–216.

267. McCarthy DM. Fibrosis of the bone marrow: content and causes (annotation). Br J Haematol 1985; 59: 1–7.

268. Smith RE, Chelmowski MK, Szabo EJ. Myelofibrosis: a concise review of clinical and pathological features and treatment. Am J Hematol 1988; 29: 174–180.

269. Maschek H, Georgii A, Kaloutsi V, et al. Myelofibrosis in primary myelodysplastic syndromes: a retrospective study of 352 patients. Eur J Haematol 1992; 48: 208–214.

270. Steensma DP, Hanson CA, Letendre L, et al. Myelodysplasia with fibrosis: a distinct entity? (Invited review). Leuk Res 2001; 25: 829–838.

271. Wallis JP, Reid MM. Bone marrow fibrosis in childhood acute lymphoblastic leukaemia. J Clin Pathol 1989; 42: 1253–1254.

272. Islam A, Catovsky D, Goldman JM, et al. Bone marrow fiber content in acute myeloid leukaemia before and after treatment. Clin Pathol 1984; 37: 1259–1263.

273. Diebold J, Molina T, Camilleri-Broët S, et al. Bone marrow manifestations of infectious and systemic diseases observed in bone marrow trephine biopsy (Review). Histopathology 2000; 37: 199–211.

274. Faulkner-Jones BE, Howne AJ, Boughton BJ, et al. Lymphoid aggregates in bone marrow: study of eventual outcome. J Clin Pathol 1988; 41: 768–775.

275. Douglas VK, Gordon LI, Goolsby CL, et al. Lymphoid aggregates in bone marrow mimic residual lymphoma after Rituximab therapy for non-Hodgkin's lymphoma. Am J Clin Pathol 1999; 112: 844–853.

276. Matutes E, Polliack A. Morphological and immunophenotypic features of chronic lymphocytic leukemia. Rev Clin Exp Hematol 2000; 4: 22–47.

277. Suzuki R, Nakamura S. Malignancies of nature killer (NK) cell precursor: myeloid/NK cell precursor acute leukemia and blastic NK cell lymphoma/leukemia. Leuk Res 1999; 23: 615–624.

278. Chan JKC, Wong KF, Jaffe ES, et al. Aggressive NK-cell leukemia. In: Jaffe ES, Harris NL, Stein H, et al, eds. World Health Organization classification of tumours. Pathology and genetics of tumours of haematopoietic and lymphoid tissues. Lyon: IARC Press; 2001: 138–200.

279. Ralfkiaer E, Müller-Hermelink HK, Jaffe ES. Peripheral T-cell lymphoma, unspecified. In: Jaffe ES, Harris NL, Stein H, et al, eds. World Health Organization classification of tumours. Pathology and genetics of tumours of haematopoietic and lymphoid tissues. Lyon: IARC Press; 2001: 227–229.

280. Bennett JM, Catovsky D, Daniel M-T, et al. Proposals for the classification of chronic (mature) B and T lymphoid leukaemias. French-American-British (FAB) Cooperative Group. J Clin Pathol 1989; 42: 567–584.

281. Harris NL, Jaffe ES, Diebold J, et al. World Health Organization Classification of neoplastic diseases of the hematopoietic and lymphoid tissues: report of the Clinical Advisory Committee meeting – Airlie House, Virginia, November, 1997. J Clin Oncol 1999; 17: 3835–3839.

282. Caligaris-Cappio F, Hamblin TJ. B-cell chronic lymphocytic leukemia: a bird of a different feather (Review article). J Clin Oncol 1999; 17: 399–408.

283. Cheson BD, Bennett JM, Grever M, et al. National Cancer Institute – sponsored working group guidelines for chronic lymphocytic leukemia: revised guidelines for diagnosis and treatment. Blood 1996; 87: 4990–4997.

284. Rai KR, Sawitsky A, Cronkite EP, et al. Clinical staging of chronic lymphocytic leukemia. Blood 1975; 46: 219–234.

285. Binet J, Auquier A, Dighiero G, et al. A new prognostic classification of chronic lymphocytic leukemia derived from a multivariate analysis. Cancer 1981; 48: 198–206.

286. Rozman C, Montserrat E. Chronic lymphocytic leukemia (Review). N Engl J Med 1995; 333: 1052–1057.

287. Rozman C, Montserrat E, Rodriguez-Fernandez JM, et al. Bone marrow histologic pattern – the best single prognostic parameter in chronic lymphocytic leukemia: a multivariate survival analysis of 329 cases. Blood 1984; 64: 642–648.

288. Stilgenbauer S, Lichler P, Döhner H. Genetic features of B-cell chronic lymphocytic leukemia. Rev Clin Exp Hematol 2000; 4: 48–72.

289. Döhner H, Stilgenbauer S, Benner A, et al. Genomic aberrations and survival in chronic lymphocytic leukemia. N Engl J Med 2000; 343: 1910–1916.

290. Panayiotidis P, Kotsi P. Genetics of small lymphocyte disorders. Semin Hematol 1999; 36: 171–177.

291. Criel A, Verhoef G, Vlietinck R, et al. Further characterization of morphologically defined typical and atypical CLL: a clinical, Immunophenotypic, cytogenetic and prognostic study on 390 cases. Br J Haematol 1997; 97: 383–391.

292. Rai KR, Chiorazzi N. Determining the clinical course and outcome in chronic lymphocytic leukemia (Editorial). N Engl J Med 2003; 348: 1797–1799.

293. Orchard JA, Ibbotson RE, David Z, et al. ZAP-70 expression and prognosis in chronic lymphocytic leukaemia. Lancet 2004; 363: 105–111.

294. Kipps TJ. Immunobiology of chronic lymphocytic leukemia. Curr Opin Hematol 2003; 10: 312–318.

295. Chang C-C, Lorek J, Sabath DE, et al. Expression of MUM1/IRF4 correlates with clinical outcome in patients with B-cell chronic lymphocytic leukemia. Blood 2002; 100: 4671–4675.

296. Hsi ED, Hoeltge G, Tubbs RR. Biclonal chronic lymphocytic leukemia. Am J Clin Pathol 2000; 113: 798–804.

297. Delage R, Jacques L, Massinga-Loembe M, et al. Persistent polyclonal B-cell lymphocytosis: further evidence for a genetic disorder associated with B-cell abnormalities. Br J Haematol 2001; 114: 666–670.

298. Melo JV, Catovsky D, Galton DAG. The relationship between chronic lymphocytic leukemia and

prolymphocytic leukemia. I. Clinical and laboratory features of 300 patients and characterizations of an intermediate group. Br J Haematol 1986; 63: 377–387.

299. Melo JV, Catovsky D, Gregory WM, et al. The relationship between chronic lymphocytic leukemia and prolymphocytic leukemia. IV. Analysis of survival and prognostic features. Br J Haematol 1987; 65: 23–29.

300. Schlette E, Bueso-Ramos C, Giles F, et al. Mature B-cell leukemias with more than 55% prolymphocytes. A heterogeneous group that includes an unusual variant of mantle cell lymphoma. Am J Clin Pathol 2001; 115: 571–581.

301. Richter MN. Generalized reticular cell sarcoma of lymph nodes associated with lymphocytic leukemia. Am J Pathol 1928; 4: 285–292.

302. Robertson LE, Pugh W, O'Brien S, et al. Richter's syndrome: a report on 39 patients. J Clin Oncol 1993; 11: 1985–1989.

303. Kroft SH, Dawson B, McKenna RW. Large cell lymphoma transformation of chronic lymphocytic leukemia/small lymphocytic lymphoma. A flow cytometric analysis of seven cases. Am J Clin Pathol 2001; 115: 385–395.

304. Ohno T, Smir BN, Weisenburger DD, et al. Origin of the Hodgkin/Reed–Sternberg cells in chronic lymphocytic leukemia with 'Hodgkin's transformation'. Blood 1998; 91: 1757–1761.

305. Brynes RK, McCourty A, Sun NCJ, et al. Trisomy 12 in Richter's transformation of chronic lymphocytic leukemia. Am J Clin Pathol 1995; 104: 199–203.

306. Galton DAG, Goldman JM, Wiltshaw E, et al. Prolymphocytic leukemia. Br J Haematol 1974; 27: 7–23.

307. Stone RM. Prolymphocytic leukemia. Hematol Oncol Clin North Am 1990; 4: 457–471.

308. Nieto LH, Lampert IA, Catovsky D. Bone marrow histological patterns in B-cell and T-cell prolymphocytic leukemia. Hematol Pathol 1989; 3: 79–84.

309. Lens D, De Schouwer PJ, Hamoudi RA, et al. p53 abnormalities in B-cell prolymphocytic leukemia. Blood 1997; 89: 2015–2023.

310. Chang KL, Stroup R, Weiss LM. Hairy cell leukemia. Current status. Am J Clin Pathol 1992; 97: 719–735.

311. Robbins BA, Ellison DJ, Spinosa JC, et al. Diagnostic application of two-color flow cytometry in 161 cases of hairy cell leukemia. Blood 1993; 82: 1277–1287.

312. Haglund U, Juliusson G, Stellan B, et al. Hairy cell leukemia is characterized by clonal chromosome abnormalities clustered to specific regions. Blood 1994; 83: 2637–2645.

313. Sambani C, Trafalis DTP, Mitsoulis-Mentzikoff C, et al. Clonal chromosome rearrangements in hairy cell leukemia: personal experience and review of literature. Cancer Genet Cytogenet 2001; 129: 138–144.

314. Sainati L, Matutes E, Mulligan S, et al. A variant form of hairy cell leukemia resistant to α-interferon: clinical and phenotypic characteristics of 17 patients. Blood 1990; 76: 157–162.

315. Goodman GR, Bethel KJ, Saven A. Hairy cell leukemia: an update. Curr Opin Hematol 2003; 10: 258–266

316. Polliack A. Hairy cell leukemia and allied chronic lymphoid leukemias: current knowledge and new therapeutic options. Leuk Lymphoma 1997; 26(suppl. 1): 41–51.

317. Matutes E, Catovsky D. Mature T-cell leukemias and leukemia/lymphoma syndromes. Review of our experience in 175 cases. Leuk Lymphoma 1991; 4: 81–91.

318. Lamy T, Loughran TP, Jr. Current concepts: large granular lymphocyte leukemia. Blood Rev 1999; 13: 230–240.

319. Bartlett NL, Longo DL. T-small lymphocyte disorders. Semin Hematol 1999; 36: 164–170.

320. Matutes E, Brito-Babapulle V, Swansbury J, et al. Clinical and laboratory features of 78 cases of T-prolymphocytic leukemia. Blood 1991; 78: 3269–3274.

321. Boultwood J. Ataxia telangiectasia gene mutations in leukaemia and lymphoma. J Clin Pathol 2001; 54: 512–516.

322. Stoppa-Lyonnet D, Soulier J, Laugé A, et al. Inactivation of the ATM gene in T-cell prolymphocytic leukemias. Blood 1998; 91: 3920–3926.

323. Garand R, Goasguen J, Brizard A, et al. Indolent course as a relatively frequent presentation in T-prolymphocytic leukaemia. Groupe Francais d'Hematologie Cellulaire. Br J Haematol 1998; 103: 488–494.

324. Brunning RD. T-prolymphocytic leukemia (editorial). Blood 1991; 78: 3111–3113.

325. Hoyer JD, Ross CW, Li C-Y, et al. True T-cell chronic lymphocytic leukemia: a morphologic and immunophenotypic study of 25 cases. Blood 1995; 86: 1163–1169.

326. Jaffe ES, Ralfkiaer E. Mature T-cell and NK-cell neoplasms: Introduction. In: Jaffe ES, Harris NL, Stein H, et al, eds. World Health Organization classification of tumours. Pathology and genetics of tumours of haematopoietic and lymphoid tissues. Lyon: IARC Press; 2001: 191–194.

327. Macon WR, Williams ME, Greer JP, et al. Natural killer-like-T-cell lymphomas: aggressive lymphomas of T-large granular lymphocytes. Blood 1996; 87: 1474–1483.

328. Rabbani GR, Phyliky RL, Teffri A. A long term study of patients with chronic natural killer cell lymphocytosis. Br J Haematol 1999; 106: 960–966.

329. Chan JKC, Sin VC, Wong KF, et al. Nonnasal lymphoma expressing the natural killer cell marker CD56: a clinicopathologic study of 49 cases of an uncommon aggressive neoplasm. Blood 1997; 89: 4501–4513.

330. Siu LLP, Wong KF, Chan JKC, et al. Comparative genomic hybridization analysis of natural killer cell lymphoma/leukemia. Recognition of consistent patterns of genetic alterations. Am J Pathol 1999; 155: 1419–1425.

331. Scott AA, Head DR, Kopecky KJ, et al. HLA-DR-, CD33+, CD56+, CD16- myeloid/natural killer cell acute leukemia: a previously unrecognized form of acute leukemia potentially misdiagnosed as French-American-British acute myeloid leukemia-M3. Blood 1994; 84: 244–255.

332. Suzuki R, Yamamoto K, Seto M, et al. CD7+ and CD56+ myeloid/natural killer cell precursor acute leukemia: a distinct hematolymphoid disease entity. Blood 1997; 90: 2417–2428.

333. Juneja SK, Wolf MM, Cooper IA. Value of bilateral bone marrow biopsy specimens in non-Hodgkin's lymphoma. J Clin Pathol 1990; 43: 630–632.

334. Bartl R, Frisch B, Burkhardt R, et al. Lymphoproliferations in the bone marrow: identification and evolution, classification and staging. J Clin Pathol 1984; 37: 233–254.

335. National Cancer Institute sponsored study of classifications of non-Hodgkin's lymphoma: summary and description of a working formulation for clinical usage. The Non-Hodgkin's Lymphoma Pathology Classification Project. Cancer 1982; 49: 2112–2135.

336. Viswanatha D, Foucar K. Hodgkin and non-Hodgkin's lymphoma involving bone marrow. Semin Diag Pathol 2003; 20: 196–210

337. Bartl R, Hansmann M-L, Frisch B, et al. Comparative histology of malignant lymphomas in lymph node and bone marrow. Br J Haematol 1988; 69: 229–237.

338. Fisher DE, Jacobson JO, Ault KA, et al. Diffuse large cell lymphoma with discordant bone marrow histology. Clinical features and biological implications. Cancer 1989; 64: 1879–1887.

339. Robertson LE, Redman JR, Butler JJ, et al. Discordant bone marrow involvement in diffuse large-cell lymphoma: a distinct clinical-pathologic entity associated with a continuous risk of relapse. J Clin Oncol 1991; 9: 236–242.

340. Conlan MG, Bast M, Armitage JO, et al. Bone marrow involvement by non-Hodgkin's lymphoma: the clinical significance of morphologic discordance between the lymph node and bone marrow. J Clin Oncol 1990; 8: 1163–1172.

341. Ponzoni M, Li C-Y. Isolated bone marrow non-Hodgkin's lymphoma: a clinicopathologic study. Mayo Clin Proc 1994; 69: 37–43.

342. Crotty PL, Smith BR, Tallini G. Morphologic, Immunophenotypic and molecular evaluation of bone marrow involvement in non-Hodgkin's lymphoma. Diag Mol Pathol 1998; 7: 90–95.

343. Pangalis GA, Angelopoulou MK, Vassilakopoulos TP, et al. B-chronic lymphocytic leukemia, small lymphocytic lymphoma, and lymphoplasmacytic lymphoma, including Waldenström's macroglobulinemia: a clinical, morphologic, and biologic spectrum of similar disorders. Semin Hematol 1999; 36: 104–114.

344. Owen RG, Barrans SL, Richards SJ, et al. Waldenström macroglobulinemia. Development of diagnosis criteria and identification of prognostic factors. Am J Clin Pathol 2001; 116: 420–428.

345. Mansoor A, Medeiros LJ, Weber DM, et al. Cytogenetic findings in lymphoplasmacytic lymphoma/Waldenström macroglobulinemia. Chromosomal abnormalities are associated with the polymorphous subtype and an aggressive clinical course. Am J Clin Pathol 2001; 116: 543–549.

346. Campo E, Raffeld M, Jaffe ES. Mantle cell lymphoma. Semin Hematol 1999; 36: 115–127.

347. Wong K-F, So C-C, Chan JKC. Nucleolated variant of mantle cell lymphoma with leukemic manifestations mimicking prolymphocytic leukemia. Am J Clin Pathol 2002; 117: 246–251.

348. Onciu M, Schlette E, Medeiros LJ, et al. Cytogenetic findings in mantle cell lymphoma. Cases with a high level of peripheral blood involvement have a distinct pattern of abnormalities. Am J Clin Pathol 2001; 116: 886–892.

349. Traweek ST, Sheibani K. Monocytoid B-cell lymphoma. The biologic and clinical implications of peripheral blood involvement. Am J Clin Pathol 1992; 97: 591–598.

350. Fisher RI, Dahlberg S, Nathwani BN, et al. A clinical analysis of two indolent lymphoma entities: mantle cell lymphoma and marginal zone lymphoma (including the mucosa-associated lymphoid tissue and monocytoid B-cell subcategories): a Southwest Oncology Group Study. Blood 1995; 85: 1075–1082.

351. Nathwani BN, Drachenberg MR, Hernandez AM, et al. Nodal monocytoid B-cell lymphoma (nodal marginal-zone B-cell lymphoma). Semin Hematol 1999; 36:128–138.

352. Ye H, Chuang S-S, Dogan A, et al. t(1;14) and t(11;18) in the differential diagnosis of Waldernstrom's macroglobulinemia. Mod Pathol 2004; 17: 1150–1154.

353. Isaacson PG, Matutes E, Burke M, et al. The histopathology of splenic lymphoma with villous lymphocytes. Blood 1994; 84: 3828–3834.

354. Melo JV, Robinson DSF, Gregory C, et al. Splenic B-cell lymphoma with 'villous' lymphocytes in the peripheral blood: a disorder distinct from hairy cell leukemia. Leukemia 1987; 1: 294–298.

355. Catovsky D, Matutes E. Splenic lymphoma with circulating villous lymphocytes/splenic marginal-zone lymphoma. Semin Hematol 1999; 36: 148–154.

356. Hermine O, Lefrere F, Bronowicki J-P, et al. Regression of splenic lymphoma with villous lymphocytes after treatment of hepatitis C virus infection. N Engl J Med 2002; 347: 89–94.

357. Tiesinga JJ, Wu CD, Inghirami G. CD5+ follicle center lymphoma. Immunophenotyping detects a unique subset of 'floral' follicular lymphoma. Am J Clin Pathol 2000; 114: 912–921.

358. Liu Z, Dong HY, Gorczyca W, et al. CD5- mantle cell lymphoma. Am J Clin Pathol 2002; 118: 216–224.

359. Foucar K. Non-Hodgkin lymphoma and Hodgkin lymphoma (disease) in bone marrow. In: Foucar K. Bone marrow pathology, 2nd ed. Chicago: ASCP Press; 2001: 438–483.

360. Estalilla OC, Koo CH, Brynes RK, et al. Intravascular large B-cell lymphoma. A report of five cases initially diagnosed by bone marrow biopsy. Am J Clin Pathol 1999; 112: 248–255.

361. Tucker TJ, Bardales RH, Miranda RN. Intravascular lymphomatosis with bone marrow involvement. A case report and review of the literature. Arch Pathol Lab Med 1999; 123: 952–956.

362. Skinnider BF, Connors JM, Gascoyne RD. Bone marrow involvement in T-cell-rich B-cell lymphoma. Am J Clin Pathol 1997; 108: 570–578.

363. Aki H, Tuzuner N, Ongoren S, et al. T-cell-rich B-cell lymphoma: a clinicopathologic study of 21 cases and comparison with 43 cases of diffuse large B-cell lymphoma. Leuk Res 2004; 28: 229–236.

364. Braziel R, Arber D, Slovak M, et al. The Burkitt-like lymphomas: a Southwest Oncology Group Study delineating phenotypic, genotypic, and clinical features. Blood 2001; 97: 3713–3720.

365. Lutzner M, Edelson R, Schein P, et al. Cutaneous T-cell lymphoma: the Sézary syndrome, mycosis fungoides, and related disorders. Ann Intern Med 1975; 83: 534–552.

366. Salhany KE, Greer JP, Cousar JP, et al. Marrow involvement in cutaneous T-cell lymphoma. A clinicopathologic study of 60 cases. Am J Clin Pathol 1989; 92–747–754.

367. Pawson R, Matutes E, Brito-Babapulle V, et al. Sézary cell leukemia: a distinct T-cell disorder or a variant form of T-prolymphocytic leukemia? Leukemia 1997; 11: 1009–1013.

368. Broder S (moderator). T-cell lymphoproliferative syndrome associated with human T-cell leukemia/lymphoma virus. Ann Intern Med 1984; 100:543–557.

369. Uchiyama T. Human T cell leukemia virus type I (HTLV-1) and human disease. Annu Rev Immunol 1997; 15: 15–37.

370. Tsukasaki K, Imaizumi Y, Tawara M, et al. Diversity of leukaemic cell morphology in ATL correlates with prognostic factors, aberrant phenotype and defective HTLV-1 genotype. Br J Haematol 1999; 105: 369–375.

371. Kamada N, Sakurai M, Miyamoto K, et al. Chromosome abnormalities in adult T-cell leukemia/lymphoma: a karyotype review committee report. Cancer Res 1992; 52: 1481–1493.

372. Nakamura S, Koshikawa T, Koike K, et al. Clinicopathologic study of CD56 (NCAM)-positive angiocentric lymphoma occurring in sites other than the upper and lower respiratory tract. Am J Surg Pathol 1995; 19: 284–296.

373. Wong K-F, Chan JKC, Cheung MMC, et al. Bone marrow involvement by nasal NK cell lymphoma at diagnosis is uncommon. Am J Clin Pathol 2001; 115: 266–270.

374. Kinney MC. The role of morphologic features, phenotype, genotype and anatomic site in defining extranodal T-cell or NK-cell neoplasms. Am J Clin Pathol 1999; 111(suppl.):S104–S118.

375. Jaffe ES, Krenacs L, Kumar SK, et al. Extranodal peripheral T-cell and NK-cell neoplasms. Am J Clin Pathol 1999; 111(suppl.): S46–S55.

376. DiGiuseppe JA, Louie DC, Williams JE, et al. Blastic natural killer cell leukemia/lymphoma: a clinicopathologic study. Am J Surg Pathol 1997; 21: 1223–1230.

377. Bayerl MG, Rakozy CK, Mohamed AN, et al. Blastic natural killer cell lymphoma/leukemia. A report of seven cases. Am J Clin Pathol 2002; 117: 41–50.

378. Feuillard J, Jacob M-C, Valensi F, et al. Clinical and biologic features of CD4+CD56+ malignancies. Blood 2002; 99: 1556–1563.

379. Herling M, Teitell MA, Shen RR, et al. TCL1 expression in plasmacytoid dendritic cells (DC2s) and the related CD4+CD56+ blastic tumors of skin. Blood 2003; 101: 5007–5009.

380. Bene MC, Feuillard J, Jacob MC, et al. Plasmacytoid dendritic cells: from the plasmacytoid T-cell to type 2 dendritic cells CD4+CD56+ malignancies. Semin Hematol 2003; 40: 257–266.

381. Weidman E. Hepatosplenic T cell lymphoma. A review of 45 cases since the first report describing the disease as a distinct lymphoma entity in 1990. Leukemia 2000; 14: 991–997.

382. Vega F, Medeiros LJ, Bueso-Ramos C, et al. Hepatosplenic gamma/delta T-cell lymphoma in bone marrow. A sinusoidal neoplasm with blastic cytologic features. Am J Clin Pathol 2001; 116: 410–419.

383. Alonsozana EL, Stamberg J, Kumar D, et al. Isochromosome 7q: the primary cytogenetic abnormality in hepatoplenic gamma/delta T-cell lymphoma. Leukemia 1997; 11: 1367–1372.

384. Hanson CA, Bockenstedt PL, Schnitzer B, et al. S100-positive, T-cell chronic lymphoproliferative disease: an aggressive disorder of an uncommon T-cell subset. Blood 1991; 78: 1803–1813.

385. Jaffe ES, Krenacs L, Raffeld M. Classification of cytotoxic T-cell and natural killer cell lymphomas. Semin Hematol 2003; 40: 175–184.

386. Ralfkiaer E, Muller-Hermelink HK, Jaffe ES. Peripheral T-cell lymphoma, unspecified. In: Jaffe ES, Harris NL, Stein H, et al, eds. World Health Organization classification of tumours. Pathology and genetics of tumours of haematopoietic and lymphoid tissues. Lyon: IARC Press; 2001: 227–229.

387. Gallamini A, Stelitano C, Calvi R, et al. Peripheral T-cell lymphoma unspecified (PTCL-U): a new prognostic model from a retrospective multicentric clinical study. Blood 2004; 103: 2474–2479.

388. Stein H, Foss H-D, Dürkop H, et al. CD30+ anaplastic large cell lymphoma: a review of its histopathologic, genetic and clinical features (Review). Blood 2000; 96: 3681–3695.

389. Fraga M, Brousset P, Schlaifer D, et al. Bone marrow involvement in anaplastic large cell lymphoma. Immunohistochemical detection of minimal disease and its prognostic significance. Am J Clin Pathol 1995; 103: 82–89.

390. Lopez-Guillermo A, Cid J, Salar A, et al. Peripheral T-cell lymphomas: initial features, natural history, and prognostic factors in a series of 174 patients diagnosed according to the REAL classification. Ann Oncol 1998; 9: 849–855.

391. Jaffe ES, Ralfkiaer E. Angioimmunoblastic T-cell lymphoma. In: Jaffe ES, Harris NL, Stein H, et al, eds. World Health Organization classification of tumours. Pathology and genetics of tumours of haematopoietic and lymphoid tissues. Lyon: IARC Press; 2001: 225–226.

392. Harris NL. Hodgkin's lymphomas: classification, diagnosis and grading. Semin Hematol 1999; 36: 220–232.

393. Maratioti T, Hummel M, Foss H-D, et al. Hodgkin and Reed–Sternberg cells represent an expansion of a single clone originating from a germinal center B-cell with functional immunoglobulin gene rearrangements by defective immunoglobulin transcription. Blood 2000; 95: 1443–1450.

394. Munker R, Hasenclever D, Brostenau O, et al. Bone marrow involvement in Hodgkin's disease: an analysis of 135 consecutive cases. J Clin Oncol 1995; 13: 403–409.

395. Kinney NC, Greer JP, Stein RS, et al. Lymphocyte-depletion Hodgkin's disease. Histopathologic diagnosis of marrow involvement. Am J Surg Pathol 1986; 10: 219–226.

396. Bearman RM, Pangalis GA, Rappaport H. Hodgkin's disease, lymphocytic depletion type. A clinicopathologic study of 39 patients. Cancer 1978; 41: 293–302.

397. Neiman RS, Rosen PJ, Lukes RJ. Lymphocyte depletion Hodgkin's disease: a clinicopathologic entity. N Engl J Med 1973; 288: 751–754.

398. Lukes RJ. Criteria for involvement of lymph node, bone marrow, spleen and liver in Hodgkin's disease. Cancer Res 1971; 31: 1755–1767.

399. Rappaport H, Berard CW, Butler JJ, et al. Report of the committee on histopathological criteria contributing to staging of Hodgkin's disease. Cancer Res 1971; 31: 1864–1865.

400. Chang KL, Kamel OW, Arber DA, et al. Pathologic features of nodular lymphocyte predominance Hodgkin's disease in extranodal sites. Am J Surg Pathol 1995; 19: 1313–1324.

401. Berekman CL, Fair KP, Cotelingam JD. Comparative utility of diagnostic bone-marrow components: a ten-year study. Am J Hematol 1997; 56: 37–41.

402. Sacks EL, Donaldson SS, Gordon J, et al. Epithelioid granulomas associated with Hodgkin's disease: clinical correlations in 55 previously untreated patients. Cancer 1978; 41: 562–567.

403. Kyle RA, Rajkumar SV. Monoclonal gammopathies of undetermined significance. Hematol Oncol Clin North Am 1999; 13: 1181–1202.

404. Grogan TM, Müller-Hermelink HK, Van Camp B, et al. Plasma cell neoplasms. In: Jaffe ES, Harris NL, Stein H, et al, eds. World Health Organization classification of tumours. Pathology and genetics of tumours of haematopoietic and lymphoid tissues. Lyon: IARC Press; 2001: 142–156.

405. Dimopoulos MA, Kiamouris C, Moulopoulos LA. Solitary plasmacytoma of bone and extramedullary plasmacytoma. Hematol Oncol Clin North Am 1999; 13: 1249–1257.

406. Kyle RA, Gertz MA, Witzig TE, et al. Review of 1027 patients with newly diagnosed multiple myeloma. Mayo Clin Proc 2003; 78: 21–33.

407. Bartl R, Frisch B. Clinical significance of bone marrow biopsy and plasma cell morphology in MM and MGUS. Pathol Biol (Paris) 1999; 47: 158–168.

408. Sukpanichnant S, Cousar JB, Leelasiri A, et al. Diagnostic criteria and histologic grading in multiple myeloma: histologic and immunohistologic analysis of 176 cases with clinical correlation. Hum Pathol 1994; 25: 308–318.

409. Rajkumar SV, Greipp PR. Prognostic factors in multiple myeloma. Hematol Oncol Clin North Am 1999; 13: 1295–1314.

410. Millá F, Oriol A, Aguilar JL, et al. Usefulness and reproducibility of cytomorphologic evaluations to differentiate myeloma from monoclonal gammopathies of unknown significance. Am J Clin Pathol 2001; 115: 127–135.

411. Grogan TM. Plasma cell myeloma marrow diagnosis including morphologic and phenotypic features. Semin Diag Pathol 2003; 20: 211–225.

412. Falini B, Fizzotti M, Pucciarini A, et al. A monoclonal antibody (MUM1p) detects expression of the MUM1/IRF4 protein in a subset of germinal center B cells, plasma cells, and activated T cells. Blood 2000; 95: 2084–2092.

413. Mahmoud MS, Huang N, Nobuyoshi M, et al: altered expression of PAX5 gene in human myeloma cells Blood 1996; 87: 4311–4315

414. Chilosi M, Adami F, Lestani M, et al. CD138/Syndecan-1: a useful immunohistochemical marker of normal and neoplastic plasma cells on routine trephine bone marrow biopsies. Mod Pathol 1999; 12: 1101–1106.

415. Fonseca R, Coignet JA, Dewald GW. Cytogenetic abnormalities in multiple myeloma. Hematol Oncol Clin North Am 1999; 13: 1169–1180.

416. Fonseca R, Blood E, Rue M, et al. Clinical and biologic implications of recurrent genomic aberrations in myeloma. Blood 2003; 101: 4569–4575.

417. Kyle RA. Diagnostic challenges and standard therapy. Semin Hematol 2001; 38: 11–14.

418. Anderson KC. Advances in disease biology: therapeutic implications. Semin Hematol 2001; 38: 6–10.

419. Kyle RA, Greipp PR. Smoldering multiple myeloma. N Engl J Med 1980; 302: 1347–1349.

420. Rosinol L, Blade J, Esteve J, et al. Smoldering multiple myeloma: natural history and recognition of an evolving type. Br J Haematol 2003; 123: 631–636.

421. Alexanian R. Localized and indolent myeloma. Blood 1980; 56: 521–525.

422. Bladé J, Kyle RA. Nonsecretory myeloma, immunoglobulin D myeloma, and plasma cell leukemia. Hematol Oncol Clin North Am 1999; 13: 1259–1272.

423. Dreicer R, Alexanian R. Nonsecretory multiple myeloma. Am J Hematol 1982; 13: 313–318.

424. Kyle RA. Multiple myeloma. Review of 869 cases. Mayo Clin Proc 1975; 50: 29–40.

425. Stone MJ, Frenkel EP. The clinical spectrum of light chain myeloma. A study of 35 patients with special reference to the occurrence of amyloidosis. Am J Med 1975; 58: 601–619.

426. Shustik C, Bergsagel DE, Pruzanski W. κ and λ light chain disease: survival rates and clinical manifestations. Blood 1976; 48: 41–51.

427. Driedger H, Pruzanski W. Plasma cell neoplasia with osteosclerotic lesions. A study of five cases and a review of the literature. Arch Intern Med 1979; 139: 892–896.

428. Miralles GD, O'Fallon JR, Talley NJ. Plasma cell dyscrasia with polyneuropathy. The spectrum of POEMS syndrome. N Engl J Med 1992; 327: 1919–1923.

429. Belec L, Mohamed AS, Authier FJ, et al. Human herpesvirus 8 infection in patients with POEMS syndrome-associated multicentric Castleman's disease. Blood 1999; 93: 3643–3653.

430. Costello R, Sainty D, Bouabdallah R, et al. Primary plasma cell leukaemia: a report of 18 cases. Leuk Res 2001; 25: 103–107.

431. Gertz MA, Lacy MQ, Dispenzieri A. Amyloidosis. Hematol Oncol Clin North Am 1999; 13: 1211–1233.

432. Buxbaum J, Gallo G. Nonamyloidotic monoclonal immunoglobulin deposition disease. Light-chain, heavy-chain, and light- and heavy-chain deposition disease. Hematol Oncol Clin North Am 1999; 13: 1235–1249.

433. Lachmann HJ, Booth DR, Booth SE, et al. Misdiagnosis of hereditary amyloidosis as AL (primary amyloidosis). N Engl J Med 2002; 346: 1786–1791.

434. Kyle RA, Gertz MA. Primary systemic amyloidosis: clinical and laboratory features in 474 cases. Semin Hematol 1995; 32: 45–59.

435. Fermand J-P, Brout J-C. Heavy chain diseases. Hematol Oncol Clin North Am 1999; 13: 1281–1294.

436. Price SK. Immunoproliferative small intestinal disease: a study of 13 cases with alpha heavy-chain disease. Histopathology 1990; 17: 7–17.

437. Favara BE, Feller AC with members of the WHO Committee on Histiocytic/Reticulum Cell Proliferations: Contemporary classification of histiocytic disorders. Med Pediatr Oncol 1997; 29: 157–166.

438. Jaffe ES. Histiocytic and dendritic cell neoplasms: Introduction. In: Jaffe ES, Harris NL, Stein H, et al, eds. World Health Organization classification of tumours. Pathology and genetics of tumours of haematopoietic and lymphoid tissues. Lyon: IARC Press; 2001: 275–277.

439. Cline MJ. Histiocytes and histiocytosis, review. Blood 1994; 84: 2840–2853.

440. Srivastava BIS, Srivastava A, Srivastava MD. Phenotype, genotype and cytokine production in acute leukemia involving progenitors of dendritic Langerhans' cells. Leuk Res 1994; 18: 499–511.

441. Santiago-Schwarz F, Coppock DL, Hindenburg AA, et al. Identification of malignant counterpart of the monocyte-dendritic cell progenitor in acute myeloid leukemia. Blood 1994; 84: 3054–3062.

442. Risdall RJ, McKenna RW, Nesbit ME, et al. Virus-associated hemophagocytic syndrome: a benign histiocytic proliferation distinct from malignant histiocytosis. Cancer 1979; 44: 993–1002.

443. Reiner AP, Spivak JL. Hematophagic histiocytosis. A report of 23 new patients and a review of the literature. Medicine 1988; 67: 369–388.

444. Arica M, Janka G, Fischer A, et al. Hemophagocytic lymphohistiocytosis. Report of 122 children from the International Registry (Clinical review). Leukemia 1996; 10: 197–203.

445. Henter JI, Arica M, Elinder G, et al. Familial hemophagocytic lymphohistiocytosis. Primary hemophagocytic lymphohistiocytosis. Hematol Oncol Clin North Am 1998; 12: 417–433.

446. Öst À, Nilsson-Ardnor A, Henter J-I. Autopsy findings in 27 children with hemophagocytic lymphohistiocytosis. Histopathology 1998; 32: 310–316.

447. Colon-Orero G, Li C-Y, Dewald GW, et al. Erythrophagocytic acute lymphocytic leukemia with B-cell markers and with a 20q- chromsome abnormality. Mayo Clin Proc 1984; 59: 678–682.

448. Molad Y, Stark P, Prokocimer M, et al. Hemophagocytosis by small cell lung carcinoma. Am J Hematol 1991; 36: 154–156.

449. Kadin ME, Kamoun M, Lamberg J. Erythrophagocytic T-gamma lymphoma: a clinicopathologic entity resembling malignant histiocytosis. N Engl J Med 1981; 304: 648–653.

450. Su I-J, Hsu Y-H, Lin M-T, et al. Epstein-Barr virus containing T-cell lymphoma presents with hemophagocytic syndrome mimicking malignant histiocytosis. Cancer 1993; 72: 2019–2027.

451. Nezelof C, Barbey S, Gogusev J, et al. Malignant histiocytosis in childhood: a distinctive CD30-positive clinicopathological entity associated with a chromosomal translocation involving 5q35. Semin Diagn Pathol 1992; 9: 75–89.

452. Jaffe ES, Costa J, Fauci AS, et al. Malignant lymphoma and erythrophagocytosis simulating malignant histiocytosis. Am J Med 1983; 75: 741–749.

453. Chang KL, Gaal KK, Huang Q, et al. Histiocytic lesions ivolving the bone marrow. Semin Diag Pathol 2003; 20: 226–236.

454. Case Records of the Massachusetts General Hospital (Case 28–2004). Newborn twins with thrombocytopenia, coagulation defects, and hepatosplenomegaly. N Engl J Med 2004; 351: 1120–1130.

455. Janka GE, Schneider EM. Modern management of children with hemophagocytic lymphohistiocytosis. Br J Haematol 2004; 124: 4–14.

456. Scott RB, Robb-Smith AH. Histiocytic medullary reticulosis. Lancet 1939; 2: 194–198.

457. Rappaport H. Tumors of the hematopoietic system. In: Atlas of tumor pathology, section III, fascicle 8. Washington, DC: Armed Forces Institute of Pathology; 1966: 49–63.

458. Mongkonsritragoon W, Li CY, Phyliky, RL. True malignant histiocytosis. Mayo Clin Proc 1998; 73: 520–528.

459. Quintanilla-Martinez L, Kumar S, Fend F, et al. Fulminant EBV⁺ T-cell lymphoproliferative disorder following acute/chronic EBV infection: a distinct clinicopathologic syndrome. Blood 2000; 96: 443–451.

460. Lichentein L. Histiocytosis X, integration of eosinophilic granulomas of bone. 'Letterer–Siwe disease' and 'Schuller–Christian disease' as related manifestations of a single nosologic entity. Arch Pathol 1953; 56: 84–102.

461. Nazelof C, Basset F. Langerhans cell histiocytosis research. Past, present and future. Hematol Oncol Clin North Am 1998; 12: 385–406.

462. Pinkus GS, Lones MA, Matsumura F, et al. Langerhans cell histiocytosis. Immunohistochemical expression of fascin, a dendritic cell marker. Am J Clin Pathol 2002; 118: 335–343.

463. Dehner LP. Morphologic findings in the histiocytic syndromes. Semin Oncol 1991; 18: 3–7.

464. Schmitz L, Favara BE. Nosology and pathology of Langerhans cell histiocytosis. Hematol Oncol Clin North Am 1998; 12: 221–246.

465. Ben-Ezra J, Bailey A, Azumi N, et al. Malignant histiocytosis X. A distinct clinicopathologic entity. Cancer 1991; 68:1050–1060.

466. Gogusev J, Nezelof C. Malignant histiocytosis. Histologic, cytochemical, chromosomal, and molecular data with a nosologic discussion. Hematol Oncol Clin North Am 1998; 12: 445–463.

467. Weiss LM, Dura T, Grogan TM, et al. Histiocytic sarcoma. In: Jaffe ES, Harris NL, Stein H, et al, eds. World Health Organization classification of tumours. Pathology and genetics of tumours of haematopoietic and lymphoid tissues. Lyon: IARC Press; 2001: 278–279.

468. Sun NCJ. Spiking fever and multiple granulomas in the bone marrow. In: Sun NCJ. Hematology. An atlas and diagnostic guide. Philadelphia: WB Saunders; 1983: 398–425.

469. Bhargava V, Farhi DC. Bone marrow granulomas: clinicopathologic findings in 72 cases and review of the literature. Hematol Pathol 1988; 2: 43–50.

470. Bodem CR, Hamory BH, Taylor HM, et al. Granulomatous bone marrow diseaes. A review of the literature and clinicopathologic analysis of 58 cases. Medicine (Baltimore) 1983; 62: 372–383.

471. Karcher DS, Frost AR. The bone marrow in human immunodeficiency virus (HIV)-related disease. Morphology and clinical correlation. Am J Clin Pathol 1991; 95: 63–71.

472. Sun NCJ, Shapshak P, Lachant NA, et al. Bone marrow examination in patients with AIDS and AIDS-related complex (ARC). Morphologic and in situ hybridization studies. Am J Clin Pathol 1989; 92: 589–594.

473. Hevman MR, Rasmussen P. Pneumocystis carinii involvement of bone marrow in acquired immunodeficiency syndrome. Am J Clin Pathol 1987; 87: 780–783.

474. Eid A, Carion W, Nystrom JS. Differential diagnosis of bone marrow granuloma. West J Med 1996; 164: 510–515.

475. Bain BJ. The haematological features of HIV infection (Review). Br J Haematol 1997; 99: 1–8.

476. Moses A, Nelson J, Bagby GC, Jr. The influence of human immunodeficiency virus-1 on hematopoiesis (Review article). Blood 1998; 91: 1479–1495.

477. Gordon S, Lee S. Naked megakaryocyte nuclei in bone marrows of patients with acquired immunodeficiency syndrome: a somewhat specific finding. Mod Pathol 1994; 7: 166–168.

478. Zhao X, Sun NCJ, Witt MD, et al. Changing pattern of AIDS. A bone marrow study. Am J Clin Pathol 2004; 121: 393–401.

479. Levine AM. HIV-associated Hodgkin's disease: biologic and clinical aspects. Hematol Oncol Clin North Am 1996; 10: 1135–1148.

480. Dolcetti R, Boiocchi M, Gloghini A, et al. Pathogenetic and histogenetic features of HIV-associated Hodgkin's disease. Eur J Cancer 2001; 37: 1276–1287.

481. Seneviratne L, Espina BM, Nathwani BN, et al. Clinical, immunologic, and pathologic correlates of bone marrow involvement in 291 patients with acquired immunodeficiency syndrome-related lymphoma. Blood 2001; 98: 2358–2363.

482. Conran RM, Granger E, Reddy VB. Kaposi's sarcoma of the bone marrow. Arch Pathol Lab Med 1986; 110: 1083–1085.

483. Spina M Berretta M, Tiaelli U. Hodgkin's disease in HIV. Hematol Oncol Clin North Am 2003; 17: 843–858.

484. Tefferi A, Li C-Y. Bone marrow granulomas associated with chronic natural killer cell lymphocytosis. Am J Hematol 1997; 54: 258–262.

485. Lukes RJ, Tindle BH. Immunoblastic lymphadenopathy. A hyperimmune entity resembling Hodgkin's disease. N Engl J Med 1975; 292: 1–8.

486. Frizzera G, Moran EM, Rappaport H. Angioimmunoblastic lymphadenopathy: diagnosis and clinical course. Am J Med 1975; 59: 803–818.

487. Sallah S, Gagnon GA. Angioimmunoblastic lymphadenopathy with dysproteinemia: emphasis on pathogenesis and treatment. Acta Hematol 1998; 99: 57–64.

488. Pangalis GA, Moran EM, Rappaport H. Blood and bone marrow findings in angioimmunoblastic lymphadenopathy. Blood 1978; 51: 71–83.

489. Schnaidt U, Vykoupil KF, Thiele J, et al. Angioimmunoblastic lymphadenopathy. Histopathology of bone marrow involvement. Virchows Arch A Pathol Anat Histol 1980; 389: 369–380.

490. Bain BJ. Systemic mastocytosis and other mast cell neoplasms (Review). Br J Haematol 1999; 106: 9–17.

491. Longley BJ, Metcalfe DD. A proposed classification of mastocytosis incorporating molecular genetics. Hematol Oncol North Am 2000; 14: 697–701.

492. Valent P, Metcalfe DD, Horny H-P, et al. Mastocytosis. In: Jaffe ES, Harris NL, Stein H, et al, eds. World Health Organization classification of tumours. Pathology and genetics of tumours of haematopoietic and lymphoid tissues. Lyon: IARC Press; 2001: 293–302.

493. Topar G, Staudacher C, Geisen F, et al. Urticaria pigmentosa. A clinical, hematopathologic, and serologic study of 30 adults. Am J Clin Pathol 1998; 109: 279–285.

494. Travis WD, Li-C-Y, Hoagland HC, et al. Mast cell leukemia: report of a case and review of the literature. Mayo Clin Proc 1986; 61: 957–966.

495. Travis WD, Li-C-Y, Bergstralh EJ, et al. Systemic mast cell disease. Analysis of 58 cases and literature review. Medicine (Baltimore) 1988; 345–368.

496. Akin C, Jaffe ES, Raffeld M, et al. An immunohistochemical study of the bone marrow lesions of systemic mastocytosis. Expression of stem cell factor by lesional mast cells. Am J Clin Pathol 2002; 118: 242–247.

497. Stevens EC, Rosenthal NS. Bone marrow mast cell morphologic features and hematopoietic dyspoiesis in systemic mast cell disease. Am J Clin Pathol 2001; 116: 177–182.

498. Escribano L, Orfao A, Diaz-Agustin B, et al. Indolent systemic mast cell disease in adults: immunophenotypic characterization of bone marrow mast cells and its diagnostic implications. Blood 1998; 91: 2731–2736.

499. Papac RJ. Bone marrow metastases. A review. Cancer 1994; 74: 2403–2413.

500. Moss TJ, Reynolds P, Sather HN, et al. Prognostic value of immunocytologic detection of bone marrow metastases in neuroblastoma. N Engl J Med 1991; 324: 219–226.

501. Shpall EJ, Gee AP, Hogan C, et al. Bone marrow metastases. Hematol Oncol Clin North Am 1996; 10: 321–343.

502. Lagrange M, Ferrero JM, Lagrange JL, et al. Non-specifically labeled cells that simulate bone marrow metastases in patients with non-metastatic breast cancer. J Clin Pathol 1997; 50: 206–211.

503. Iochim HL, Pambuccian SE, Hekimgil M, et al. Lymphoid monoclonal antibodies reactive with lung tumors. Diagnostic Applications. Am J Surg Pathol 1996; 20: 64–71.

504. Brown RW, Campagna LB, Dunn JK, et al. Immunohistochemical identification of tumor markers in metastatic adenocarcinoma. A diagnostic adjunct in the determination of primary site. Am J Clin Pathol 1997; 107: 12–19.

505. Pui C-H, Stass S, Green A. Bone marrow necrosis in children with malignant disease. Cancer 1985; 56: 1522–1525.

506. Sile CC, Perry DJ, Nam L. Small cell carcinocythemia. Arch Pathol Lab Med 1999; 123: 426–428.

507. Nasr F, Corti C, Carde P, et al. Carcinoma cell leukemia. Blood 1996; 88: 2355–2357.

508. Morandi S, Manna A, Sabattini E, et al. Rhabdomyosarcoma presenting as acute leukemia. J Pediatr Hematol Oncol 1996; 18: 305–307.

509. Mehta K, Pawel BR, Gadol C. Bone marrow necrosis in leukemic phase follicular lymphoma. Arch Pathol Lab Med 1991; 115: 89–92.

510. Markovic SN, Phyliky RL, Li C-Y. Pancytopenia due to bone marrow necrosis in acute myelogenous leukemia: role of reactive CD8 cells. Am J Hematol 1998; 59: 74–78.

511. Cassileth PA, Brooks JSJ. The prognostic significance of myelonecrosis after inductor therapy in acute leukemia. Cancer 1987; 60: 2363–2365.

512. Dann EJ, Gillis S, Polliack A, et al. Tumor lysis syndrome following treatment with 2-chlorodeoxyadenosine for refractory chronic lymphocytic leukemia. N Engl J Med 1993; 329: 1547–1548.

513. Paydas S, Kocak R, Zorludemir S, et al. Bone marrow necrosis in antiphospholipid syndrome. J Clin Pathol 1997; 50: 261–262.

514. Gordon LI, Kwaan HC. Cancer- and drug-associated thrombotic thrombocytopenic purpura and hemolytic uremic syndrome. Semin Hematol 1997; 34: 140–147.

515. Pierce JR, Wren MV, Cousar JB. Cholesterol embolism: diagnosis antemortem by bone marrow biopsy. Ann Intern Med 1978; 89: 937–938.

Skeletal system

Non-neoplastic diseases of bones and joints

13

Peter G. Bullough

This chapter discusses both the special problems that relate to the interpretation of bone lesions and, briefly, the more common orthopedic diseases that may come across the surgical pathologist's desk.

METHODS OF EXAMINATION

A major problem in dealing with bone specimens is the preparation of reasonable histologic sections. In many laboratories bone tissue is either overdecalcified or the acid is inadequately removed; in both cases poor staining results. In our laboratory, after sectioning of the bone into slices 3–5 mm thick and adequate fixation with buffered formalin, decalcification is achieved with 5% nitric acid. The volume of acid should be at least 10 times that of the tissue, and because the acid is neutralized as the calcium is removed from the tissue, the acid must be changed twice a day. To ensure access of the acid to the tissue, gentle agitation is provided by means of a shaker. By using this technique, most bones are decalcified in 1 or 2 days. After decalcification, adequate washing is essential; otherwise, good differentiation of the hematoxylin and eosin (H&E) stain is not possible. We have found that better sections of bone are obtained after vacuum embedding.

GROSS

Bone specimens received by the surgical pathologist often consist only of fragments, the anatomic site of which cannot be recognized. However, when a larger piece of bone is submitted, anatomic landmarks should be carefully sought. Large specimens should be cut into parallel slices 4–5 mm thick with a band saw, so the interior appearance of the bone may be examined.

On occasion, the color of the bone may be particularly helpful; for example, necrotic bone is an opaque yellow, in contrast to the rather translucent and pink appearance of living bone. A generalized or localized increase in porosity or sclerosis should also be looked for. When multiple pieces are received, the pieces chosen for embedding should preferably be those that appear to show the most departure from normal.

A particularly useful adjunct to gross examination is the preparation of radiographs of the surgical specimens with low voltage X-rays (Faxitron X-ray machine) and industrial film (Kodalith Ortho film, type 3). These radiographs not only help in choosing the areas to section but also are frequently helpful in the interpretation of histologic material, for example, in bone-forming tumors, finding a nidus in osteoid osteoma, or defining an infarct (Fig. 13.1).

Because bone and cartilage are somewhat translucent, it is frequently difficult to get acceptable black and white photographs. This problem can be overcome by using a monochromatic shortwave light source, such as ultraviolet.[1]

MICROSCOPIC

The microscopist uses various staining techniques to demonstrate the components of the matrix.

The collagen may be demonstrated by a trichrome stain or van Gieson's stain and also by the use of polarized light. This latter technique is particularly useful because it not only clearly shows the collagen fibers but also allows us to determine the orientation of the collagen and to study the microarchitecture of the tissue.[2–4]

The proteoglycans can be demonstrated by the use of safranin O or Alcian blue stains and less specifically by toluidine blue and periodic acid–Schiff (PAS) stains.[5,6]

Undecalcified sections are particularly important in the assessment of metabolic disturbances. Mineral component of the matrix can only be demonstrated in undemineralized tissue. This is possible, by embedding the tissue in plastic and using specially hardened knives, to cut histologic sections that still contain the minerals made within the bone matrix. The mineral may be stained by two techniques: alizarin red, which will stain the calcium components of the hydroxyapatite, and the von Kossa method, which will stain the phosphate component black. The distribution of mineral in the tissue may also be studied by the technique of microradiology.[7] By using low kilovoltage X-rays from an X-ray tube with a very fine focal spot, radiographs are made from thin slices of bone, cut with a diamond saw at approximately 100 mm.

It cannot be overemphasized that an essential component in interpretation of bone and joint histology is careful correlation with the clinical radiographs and history.

BONES AND BONE TISSUE

BONES

Bone structure[8,9] may be briefly summarized as follows. Each bone has a delimiting shell or cortex, which varies in thickness from bone to bone and from area to area within a given bone. The interior of a bone is occupied by a varying amount of porous, cancellous bone tissue. The proportion of cortical to cancellous bone reflects the mechanical requirements of the bone as a whole. In the spaces between the plates and rods of cancellous bone are blood vessels, nerve fibers, fat, and hematopoietic tissue.

In the adult, most of the hematopoietic tissue is confined to the axial skeleton (spine, pelvis, and shoulder girdles). However, occasionally hematopoietic tissue may be seen in the femoral head or humeral head. By contrast, in the infant the entire skeleton contains hematopoietic tissue. During growth the hematopoietic tissue in the appendicular skeleton (arms and legs) is slowly replaced by fat advancing proximally until the adult state is reached.

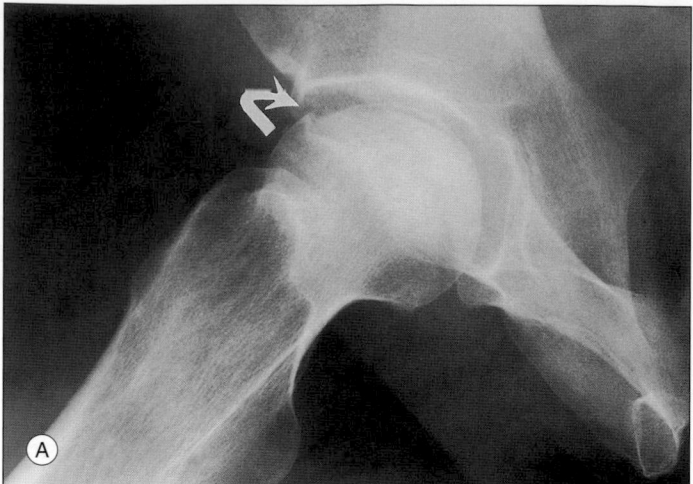

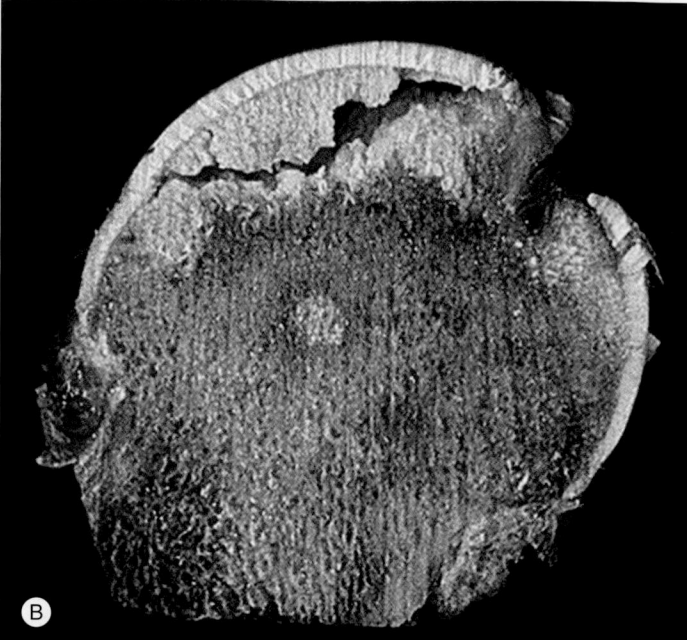

Fig. 13.1 A, Radiograph of the hip of a young person with sickle cell disease. There is segmental infarction of the superior portion of the femoral head recognized radiologically by increased density at the margin of the infarct, the presence of a small step-fracture at the lateral margin of the femoral head (arrow), and a radiolucent crescent on the superior surface of the femoral head just beneath the articular surface.
B, Photograph of a frontal section through a femoral head resected because of pain. The infarcted area is clearly differentiated from the surrounding bone by its opaque yellow-white appearance. At the margin of the infarct there is hyperemia, and there is a fracture extending from the articular surface through the infarcted bone. **C**, Radiograph of the specimen shown in **B** demonstrates that the margin of the infarct is sclerotic. This sclerosis is the result of reparative bone formation. (See also Figs 13.11 and 13.12.) (From Paget S, Bullough PG. Synovium and synovial fluid. In: Owen R, Goodfellow JW, Bullough PG, eds. Scientific foundation of orthopaedics; and traumatology. Philadelphia: Saunders, 1980: 18–22, with permission.)

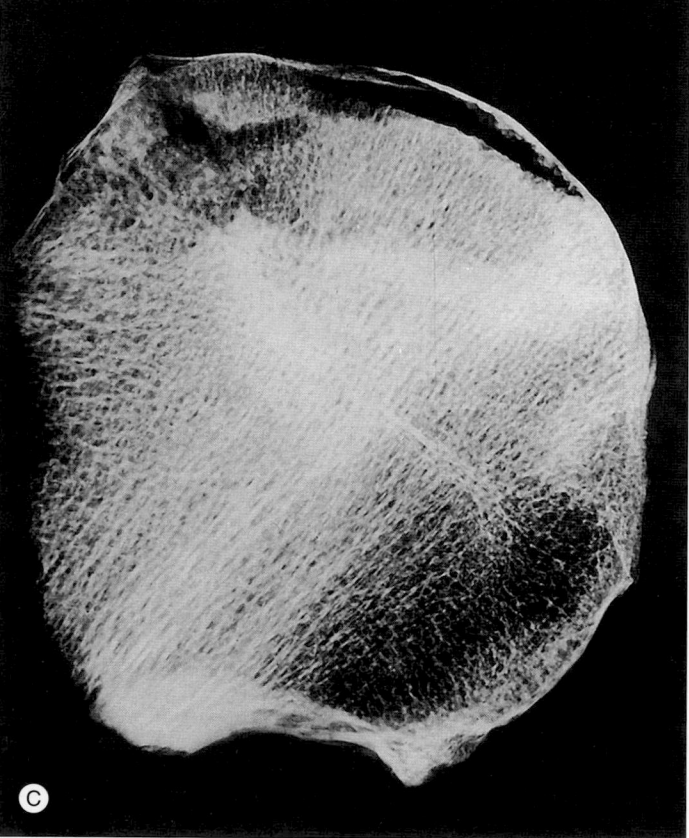

Except for the insertion of the tendons and the articular ends of the bone, the cortex is covered by a thin layer of dense fibrous tissue, the periosteum. The periosteal layer adjacent to the bone, the cambium layer, has bone-forming potential. This potential becomes apparent after trauma and infection and in association with certain tumors. In the child, the periosteum is only loosely attached to the underlying bone, whereas in the adult it is firmly attached; this accounts for the more extensive periosteal reaction that may be seen in children as compared with adults.

The terms *epiphysis, metaphysis*, and *diaphysis* are used to designate regions of bones. The epiphysis is the portion of the bone that lies between the joint and the site of the growth plate; the metaphysis is the region of bone adjacent to the growing side of the growth plate; and the diaphysis is the portion of the bone between the growth plates.

BONE TISSUE

In studying and interpreting connective tissues,[10,11] it is important to realize that unlike parenchymal organs, the bulk of which is formed of cells, the bulk of connective tissue is made up largely of an extracellular matrix, and the cells represent only a small percentage of the tissue bulk. Bone, cartilage, and fibrous tissues differ not only grossly and microscopically but also in their mechanical properties. This variation reflects the different composition of their extracellular matrices; for example, tendons, whose function is to resist tension, are formed mainly of well-oriented parallel bundles of collagen. By contrast, cartilage and bone, which are subject to compression, have in addition to collagen either large molecules of proteoglycan (cartilage) or hydroxyapatite crystals (bone). These substances, restrained by the collagen running between them, resist compressive forces and provide rigidity to the tissue.

Microscopic examination reveals two possible appearances of bone tissue, lamellar and woven. In lamellar bone, the type found normally, the collagen is in sheets of parallel fibers, stacked one upon

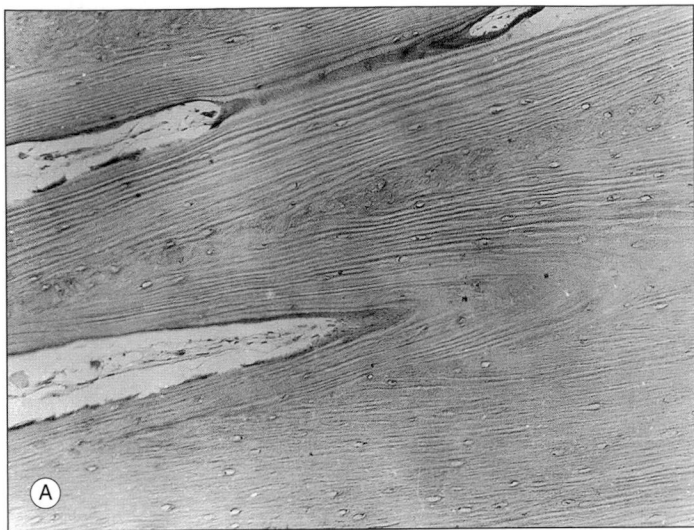

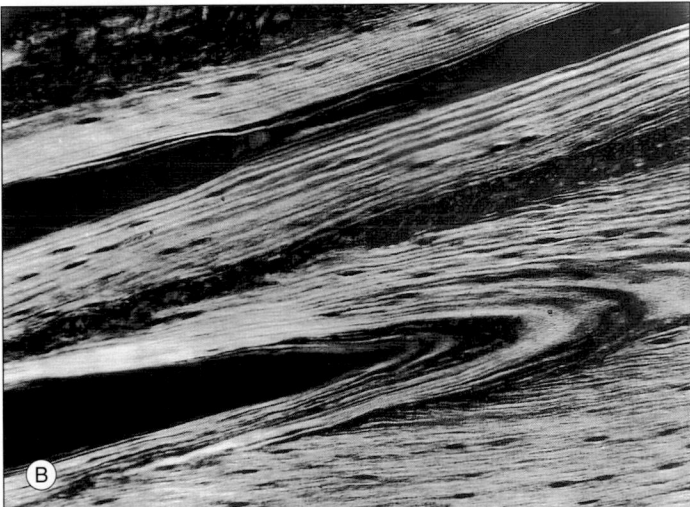

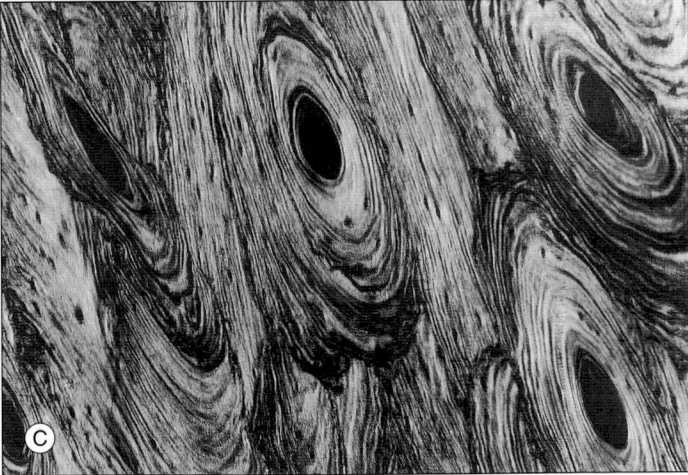

Fig. 13.2 A, Photomicrograph of lamellar bone. Note the distribution of the osteocytes in the orientation of the lamellae. **B,** Same field as in **A** but examined under polarized light. **C,** Cortical bone in transverse section to demonstrate the osteons. (Polarized light microscopy.)

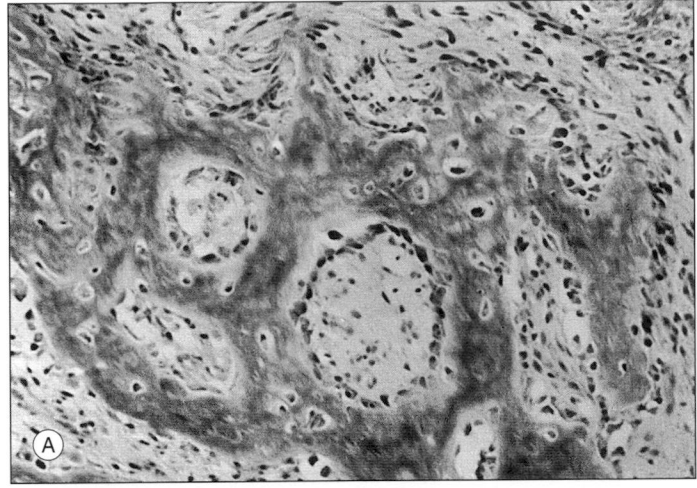

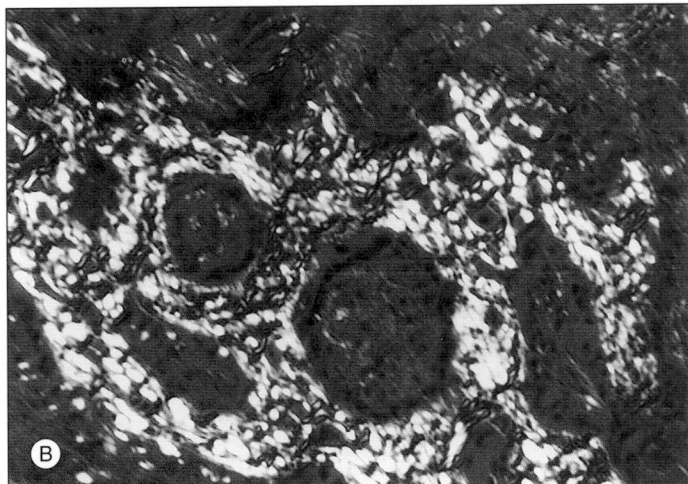

Fig. 13.3 Photomicrograph of a section taken from fracture callus to demonstrate the appearance of woven bone. Note the irregularity of the bone trabeculae that are being formed, the prominent osteoblasts and osteocytes, and the collagen fibers arranged in a basket weave pattern. **A,** Transmitted light; **B,** Polarized light. (H&E.)

another, giving rise in cross-section to a striped appearance, which is heightened by the use of polarized microscopy. The bone cells (osteocytes) are widely separated from each other, and the osteocytic lacunae are flattened (Fig. 13.2).

In the fetus and in conditions in which the metabolism of the skeleton is accelerated, such as fracture repair, Paget's disease, parathyroid dysfunction, and tumors, the collagen is arranged haphazardly, again made more apparent by examination with polarized light. The osteocytes are more closely packed together, and the lacunae are larger and rounder than those seen in lamellar bone. This type of bone is called woven bone, fiber bone, or immature bone (Fig. 13.3). (It is incorrect to refer to this type of bone as osteoid, as is often done.)

In the interpretation of bone disease recognition of these two types of bone tissue is very important to the surgical pathologist.

It is also important to look for other alterations in the intercellular matrix resulting from trauma or metabolic disturbances such as disruption of the collagen fibers, either with or without repair, metaplastic changes in the type of matrix being produced, microcystic changes, and so on; here again examination with polarized light is extremely helpful.

BONE CELLS

The skeleton is not merely an inanimate structure serving a mechanical need; it is composed of living, constantly changing tissue involved in both skeletal (structural) homeostasis (with the capability of both growth, mechanical adaptation and repair) and mineral homeostasis. These processes are affected through the bone cells, which include the osteoblasts, the osteocytes, and the osteoclasts.[10,11]

Osteoblasts

Osteoblasts are the cells responsible for the synthesis of bone matrix. They form a continuous covering over the bone tissue, and at any particular location they may be either actively forming bone matrix or dormant. The active cells are plump and crowded along the bone surface, whereas inactive osteoblasts are flat and inconspicuous. In those areas where bone is actively being made, the cells lie on a thin, smooth layer of unmineralized bone matrix called osteoid. The junction between the mineralized bone and the unmineralized osteoid at the surface is often marked in H&E-stained sections by a basophilic line indicating the mineralization front.

Osteocytes

Osteoblasts, when they have been incorporated into the bone after the process of matrix formation, are called osteocytes. The osteocytes are connected to one another and also with the surface of the bone by an intricate network of canals, the osteocytic canaliculi. Through these canaliculi cytoplasmic processes extend from osteocyte to osteocyte and also to the osteoblasts on the surface, making tight junctions with one another. The elaborate structure of the osteocytic network strongly suggests a metabolic function, probably relating to mineral homeostasis, as well as structural homeostasis.

Osteoclasts

Those portions of the bone surface which are undergoing or have undergone resorption have an irregular, gnawed-out appearance. Covering the actively resorbing surfaces are mononuclear and sometimes multinucleate osteoclasts. By electron microscopy these cells are seen to have ruffled borders on the surface facing the bone, as well as numerous cytoplasmic vesicles, lysosomal bodies, and mitochondria but, unlike osteoblasts, little endoplasmic reticulum. In sections of normal bone, multinucleate osteoclasts are rarely seen, although irregular resorbing surfaces are apparent over about 7–20% of the total bone surface. The absence of multinucleate osteoclasts from normal bone may simply reflect the fact that giant cells are obvious only when resorption is proceeding at an extraordinary or pathologic rate.

BONE PHYSIOLOGY

As already indicated, the bones have two quite different basic functions: (1) mechanical, providing for movement and protection, and (2) maintenance of the 'milieu interieur,' especially with respect to plasma calcium, phosphorus, and magnesium. As a consequence, the bone and bone tissue are a compromise in both form and structure.

The formation and resorption of bone continue throughout life, and in normal bone these processes are more or less in balance. Microscopic examination will often show one surface of a trabeculum to be smooth with a layer of active osteoblasts, while the other shows irregular resorption (Fig. 13.4). In this way, spatial reorganization of the cancellous and cortical bone to accommodate the mechanical requirements is constantly taking place. Resorbing surfaces that have become inactive later become the site for active bone deposition,

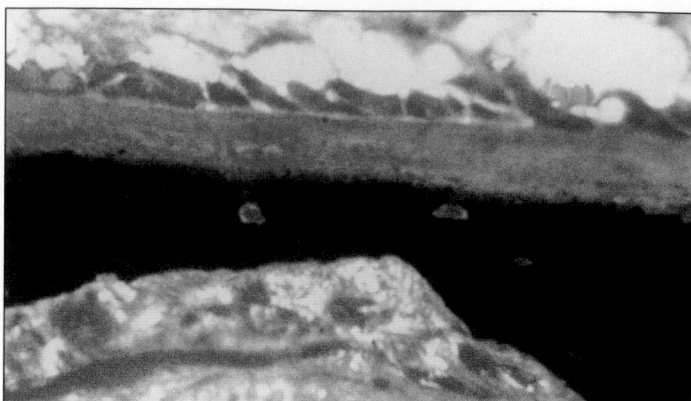

Fig. 13.4 Photomicrograph of an individual trabeculum from a patient with a metabolic disturbance, showing on the upper surface bone formation with active osteoblasts and on the lower surface the irregular gnawed-out appearance of resorption. This section of undecalcified bone was stained by the von Kossa stain. Mineralized bone is black, whereas the unmineralized osteoid is a smooth gray zone between the osteoblastic cell layer on the surface and the fully mineralized bone beneath.

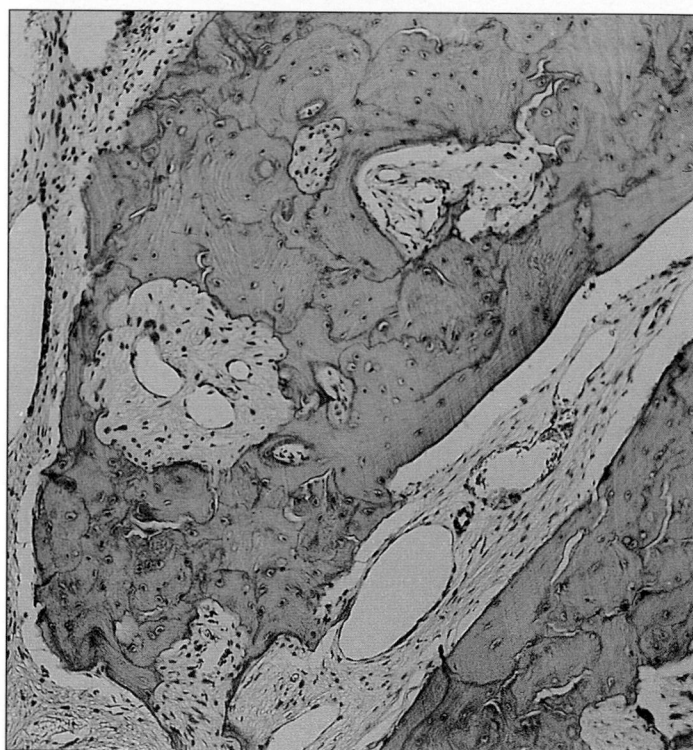

Fig. 13.5 Photomicrograph of a section taken from pagetoid bone. The cement lines are seen as irregular wavy gray lines coursing through the matrix of the bone. In many areas clefts are seen in the region of these lines. These clefts represent a cracking artifact at the time of sectioning. However, they also indicate the ease with which this bone will fracture. The marrow spaces are fibrotic, and large dilated vessels are present.

and evidence of this process is seen in the form of cement lines (reversal lines), dense basophilic lines separating distinct areas of bone matrix. The chemical composition of the cement line is not known, but examination by polarized light will show that no collagen fibers cross it.[12] In processes in which there is accelerated remodeling

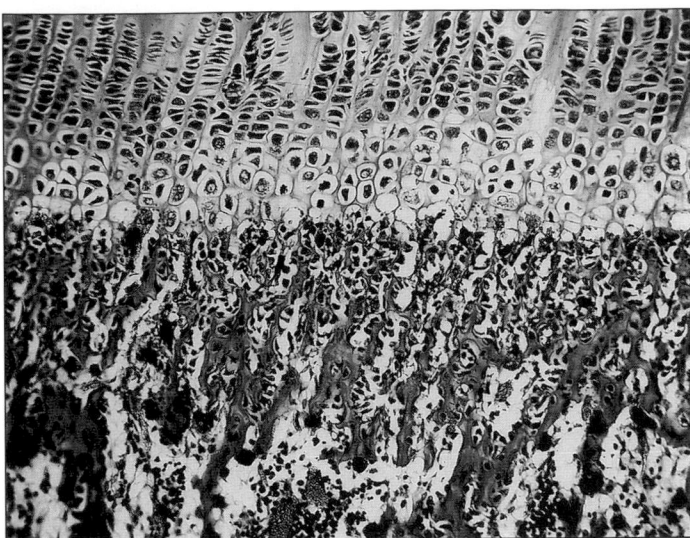

Fig. 13.6 Photomicrograph of the growth plate in a 2-month-old pig. In the upper part of the photograph one can see the columnar arrangement of the hypertrophic zone of the growth plate, which then goes into the degenerative and calcified zone of the growth plate. The calcified zone is invaded by capillaries, which deposit the first bone onto the surface of calcified cartilage matrix. The bone trabeculae of the metaphysis are therefore characterized by a central core of calcified cartilage and a thin layer of bone matrix on the surface. This bone is called the *primary spongiosa*.

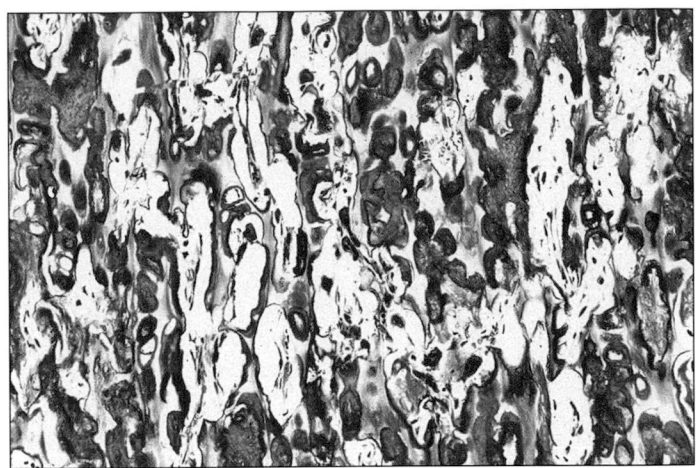

Fig. 13.7 Photomicrograph of a section of the cancellous bone from a patient with osteopetrosis. Note the increased amount of bone, the loss of the normal trabecular architecture, and the residual calcified cartilage within the bone. In this condition the osteoclasts, although present, do not appear to resorb the bone.

of bone (e.g. Paget's disease), the cement lines become more numerous (Fig. 13.5). Since fractures propagate along cement lines, an increased number of cement lines will weaken the bone.

The density of the bone in healthy people depends on several factors, including race, sex, and occupation. On the whole, blacks have heavier and denser bones than whites, men have denser bones than women, and manual workers have denser bones than sedentary workers. With advancing age, there is a steady loss of bone tissue, which occurs in everyone but is more likely to give rise to clinical problems (e.g. osteoporosis) in a white woman than in a black man, because the white woman starts with so much less bone.[13] (Osteoporosis is a clinical term which indicates an absolute loss of bone tissue sufficient to lead to fracture, whereas osteopenia indicates a decrease in bone mass and is often used by radiologists to indicate a decrease in radiodensity. Although such a decrease in radiodensity may be due to osteoporosis, it may also result from a decrease in the amount of mineralized bone tissue, as in rickets or osteomalacia, because it is only the mineralized bone that is visualized on a radiograph.)

SKELETAL DEVELOPMENT

Developmental disease is rarely seen by the surgical pathologist, with the exception of certain hamartomatous malformations, such as bone islands or fibrous dysplasia, and developmental aberrations, such as the common osteochondroma, all of which are described in Chapter 14. However, the surgical pathologist should have an understanding of the basics of bone growth and development because they are helpful to the understanding of bone disease in general.

In the fetus most bones are preformed in cartilage, which, in the course of development, undergoes central calcification followed by

vascular invasion and the laying down of osseous tissue on the remnants of calcified cartilage matrix. This process is known as endochondral ossification. The viable cartilage continues to grow and subsequently calcifies, thus providing for the growth of the skeletal elements. During most of childhood the principal source of cartilage growth and subsequent endochondral ossification is found in the growth plate. Disturbances in cell maturation in the growth plate, such as those that occur in achondroplasia and may also occur in hormonal disturbances such as hypothyroidism or hypopituitarism, result in decreased cartilage proliferation and decreased endochondral ossification; the ultimate effect is dwarfing of the child.

Hyperpituitarism in children results in gigantism and in adults acromegaly. These effects are the result of stimulation of cartilage growth and subsequently increased endochondral ossification. (Interpretation of the changes in the growth plate require familiarity with the appearance of the normal growth plate at the various stages of growth up to adolescence, as well as the molecular biology of cartilage, and such considerations are outside the scope of this chapter.)

The bone that is first laid down on the calcified cartilage is referred to as the primary spongiosa (Fig. 13.6). This mixture of bone and calcified cartilage is remodeled by osteoclastic activity and eventually the bone trabeculae are formed only of bone tissue, referred to as the secondary spongiosa. A rare disease results from a failure of the osteoclasts to effect the normal remodeling of primary to secondary spongiosa. In this condition, osteopetrosis,[14] most of the skeletal tissue is formed of primary spongiosa. In osteopetrosis the bone is extremely dense, and pieces of bone from osteopetrotic subjects will be found to be unduly heavy and difficult both to decalcify and to section (Fig. 13.7).

SKELETAL DISEASE

The clinical symptoms of disease in the skeletal tissues, whether of bones or joints, are most likely to result from mechanical failure.

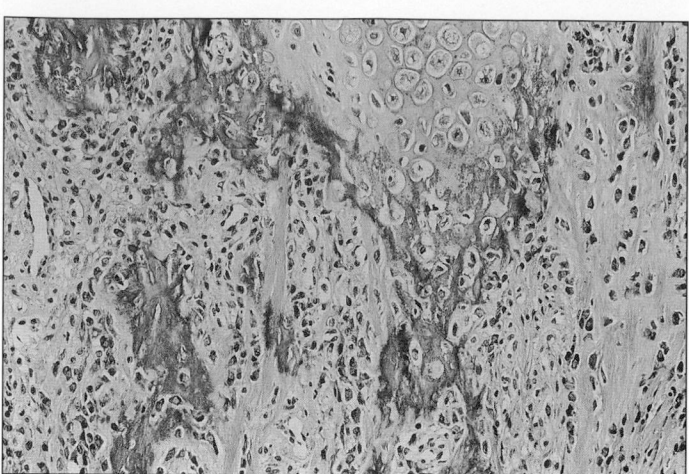

Fig. 13.8 Photomicrograph of a section taken from a fracture approximately 10 days old. The irregularity of the bone and cartilage being formed, together with the crowded and varying appearance of the stromal cells, imparts a pseudosarcomatous appearance.

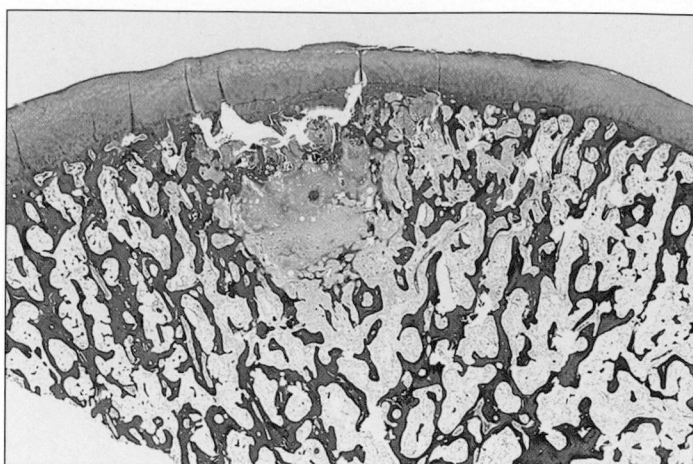

Fig. 13.9 Photomicrograph to demonstrate an area of subchondral fracture in the femoral head of an elderly female complaining of the sudden onset of hip pain.

FRACTURE HEALING

A fracture results from either a violent force to the bone or significant weakening of the bone (pathologic fracture). The latter may occur because of either a localized replacement by tumor or a generalized disturbance (e.g. senile osteoporosis, osteomalacia, Paget's disease, osteogenesis imperfecta).

The reparative response[15] depends to some extent on the site of injury and the bone involved; in general, it corresponds to the richness of the vascular bed. For example, a fracture through the midshaft of the tibia in a poorly vascularized area is notorious for both delayed healing and nonunion.[16]

A fracture inevitably results in some degree of necrosis. We tend to speak of bone necrosis, but only cells can necrose; the extracellular matrix is nonviable to begin with. However, the extracellular matrix may undergo enzymatic degradation. An example of this is the so-called hyalinization of the collagen. In favorable circumstances, the necrosis of the cellular elements (i.e. bone cells and bone marrow cells) extends for only a short distance on each side of the fracture line, but, depending on local factors, large fragments may become necrotic and significantly interfere with the healing process. (In the process of bone healing the necrotic bone will be resorbed by osteoclasts.)

The periosteum is an extremely important source of repair tissue (callus) following fracture. At the time of the initial injury the periosteum may be elevated from the underlying bone by hemorrhage, and the osteogenic cells of the cambium layer may rapidly become activated and begin to lay down woven bone. This immature subperiosteal bone eventually bridges the fracture site and thereby renders the fractured bone stable. In the medullary cavity, the osteoblasts lining the trabeculae on either side of the fracture site also become active and lay down new bone on the existing bone trabeculae.

In the face of extensive soft tissue damage, a large amount of callus may be seen in the surrounding soft tissues. This takes the form of irregular trabeculae of woven bone, and in fractures that are particularly unstable, this extraosseous callus may contain a high proportion of cellular cartilage, giving rise to a pseudosarcomatous appearance (Fig. 13.8).

After stabilization of the fracture, remodeling takes place, with restoration of anatomy similar to that present before fracture.

Stabilization of the fracture usually takes place in 4 to 8 weeks, but anatomic restitution takes many months or even years. Because the callus serves to immobilize the fracture, it should be obvious that the amount of callus is in general proportional to the stability of the fracture; therefore, in a fracture that has been immobilized surgically by internal fixation, little or no callus may form.

It is important for the surgical pathologist to know that fracture can occur in a bone without the patient being aware of it. These fractures classically occur in healthy young athletic adults and are termed *stress fractures*; they are common in the metatarsals and tibia. In such a case the patient may complain of pain and swelling over a bone, and radiographs may show localized exuberant new bone. Biopsy will show a very proliferative osseous and cartilaginous tissue, which, because of its deranged pattern and cellularity, may be mistaken for osteogenic sarcoma (see Fig. 13.8). Obviously, this is a most important differential diagnosis and requires careful correlation of the clinical history, radiographs, and pathologic findings.

Recently, clinical reports of primary subchondral insufficiency fractures (SIF) in the femoral head of renal transplant recipients and, most commonly, in our experience, elderly osteoporotic women, have stressed the importance of its differentiation from osteonecrosis (vide infra), especially when using MR imaging.[17] Many of the clinically reported cases of SIF have resolved after conservative therapy without progressing to collapse or surgery. However, in our experience, histologic evidence of subchondral fracture as the etiology of acute onset of hip pain in elderly woman has become increasingly commonplace. In the published cases of insufficiency fracture, shortly after the onset of hip pain, radiographic changes were reported unremarkable (which would seem inappropriate to the severity of the reported pain in these patients). However, MR imaging has shown a bone marrow edema pattern. Histopathologically, the most characteristics finding in the cases reported was the presence of fracture callus and granulation tissue along both edges of the fracture line.

First reported in the literature by Postel and Kerboull in 1970[18,19] (Fig. 13.9), *rapidly destructive arthrosis* (RDA) of the hip joint is a relatively uncommon form of arthritis that is seen mostly in elderly women. RDA is characterized by rapid joint destruction within 6–12 months, and disappearance of the joint space is the typical

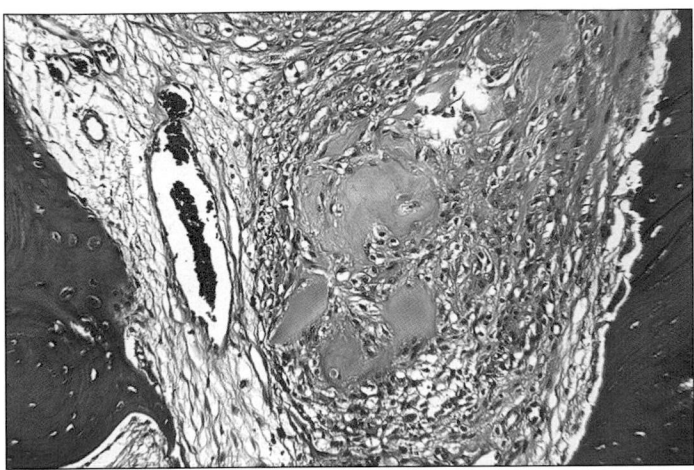

Fig. 13.10 Photomicrograph of an area of subchondral bone in the femoral head of a patient with clinical and radiographic evidence of rapid disappearance of the joint space and femoral head following the severe onset of pain in the hip. Grossly, approximately a third of the femoral head was absent. Within the marrow spaces microscopically there was bone and cartilage detritus with a surrounding histiocytic response as demonstrated in this field.

initial finding on radiographs, followed by rapid disappearance of the femoral head.

Since we became aware of SIF, we have come to realize that some cases of SIF go on to show rapid disappearance of the hip joint space. Microscopically, in the superficial portion of the marrow space in such cases of RDA, round-to-oval foci of granulomatous tissue are usually observed, in which small fragments of bone and articular cartilage embedded in amorphous eosinophilic debris are found surrounded by aggregated epithelioid histiocytes and giant cells[20] (Fig. 13.10).

BONE INFARCTION (OSTEONECROSIS)

Localized bone and bone marrow death (osteonecrosis)[21] is a common complication of osteomyelitis and conditions in which the bone marrow is replaced by massive cellular infiltrates, such as Gaucher's disease, lymphoma, or primary or metastatic tumor. Osteonecrosis may also occur as a result of the 'bends' in deep-sea divers or hemoglobinopathies such as sickle cell disease and is frequently seen in association with cortisone therapy and alcoholism. In clinical practice, osteonecrosis is most commonly seen in the juxta-articular area, usually the hip, and gives rise to articular symptoms, as described below.

Grossly, dead bone is generally yellow and chalky in appearance (see Fig. 13.1B). The recognition of dead bone microscopically is not difficult: the marrow cells are necrotic and ghost-like, the walls of the fat cells break down to form irregular fat cysts, and sometimes calcification of the fat occurs. The bone matrix is usually palely stained and the osteocytic lacunae enlarged and empty. As occurs with infarcts in other organs, the necrotic tissue is invaded at its margins by granulation tissue, removed, and replaced by scar. However, in the case of bone, the scar tissue is organized as osseous tissue (Fig. 13.11).

In revascularized necrotic bone, the bone marrow space is filled with fibrous granulation tissue, and it is common to see a layer of new living bone being deposited on a core of dead bone tissue, a process that is often referred to as 'creeping substitution' (Fig. 13.12).

Clinically, infarction is usually seen adjacent to a joint, particularly the femoral head, although it may occur in other joints. In the femoral head it commonly complicates fracture[22] but is also frequently seen without fracture, in which case there is frequently a clinical history of either cortisone therapy or alcoholism. In alcoholics and following corticosteroid therapy the systemic nature of the disease is apparent by the presence of multiple bone infarcts in almost 50% of patients.

The radiologic features of infarction of the femoral head are increased bone density and a change in joint contour. The increased density is the result of reparative new bone and trabecular thickening at the edge of the infarct. The change in the contour of the articular surface is due to a failure of repair and central collapse of the infarcted area with the overlying articular cartilage. MRI is now commonly employed for early diagnosis of osteonecrosis; however, as discussed in the section on fractures, it may be difficult for the radiologist to distinguish between infarction of the femoral head and a subchondral insufficiency fracture.

Gross examination of the femoral head resected because of early-stage osteonecrosis is likely to reveal fairly intact articular cartilage, although there will probably be wrinkling of the surface marking the edge of the necrotic area (see Fig. 13.1). On vertical sectioning, the infarcted zone exhibits a characteristic bright yellow, opaque appearance. At its margin there is a hyperemic zone or a band of fibrous scar tissue. In the later stages of the disease, the articular

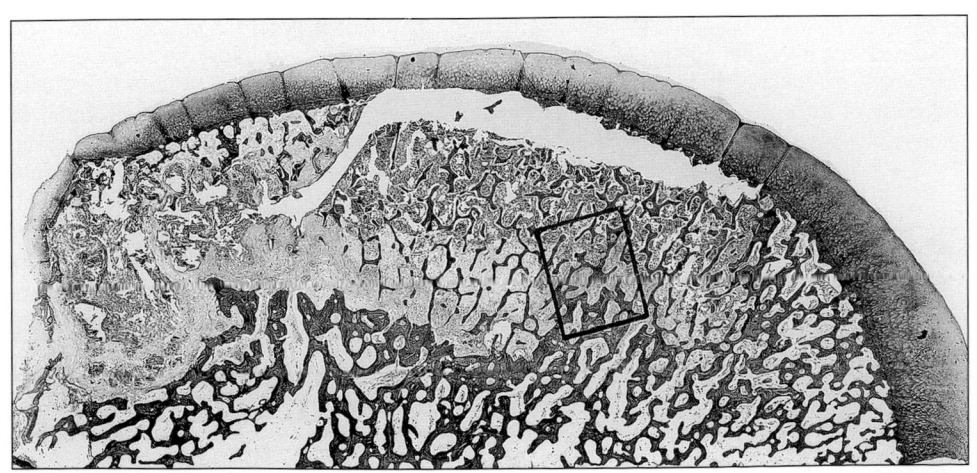

Fig. 13.11 Photomicrograph of a histologic preparation of the specimen shown in Figure 13.1. An enlarged view of the outlined area is shown in Fig. 13.12.

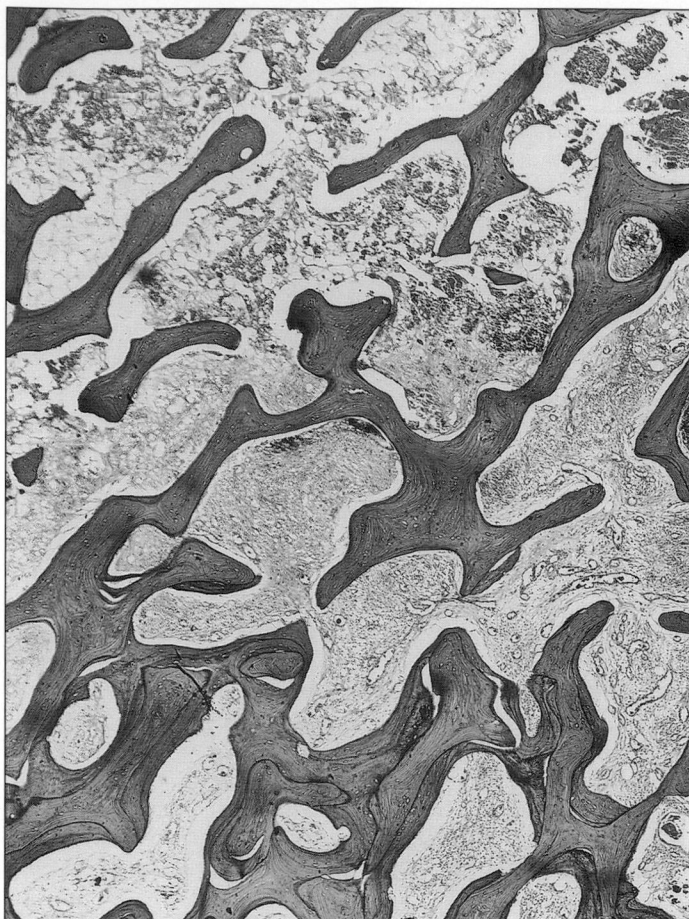

Fig. 13.12 Photomicrograph of area outlined in Fig. 13.11. In the upper part, the fatty marrow is necrotic. The amorphous granular material seen within the fat is calcium soap. In this area the bone trabeculae have a normal outline, but a close view would show that the osteocytic lacunae are empty. In the lower part of the picture, a layer of new bone is seen covering the original bone trabeculae. This is evidence of healing and is known as creeping substitution. The bone marrow in this area is hyperemic and, together with the new bone formation, represents the repairing margin of the infarct.

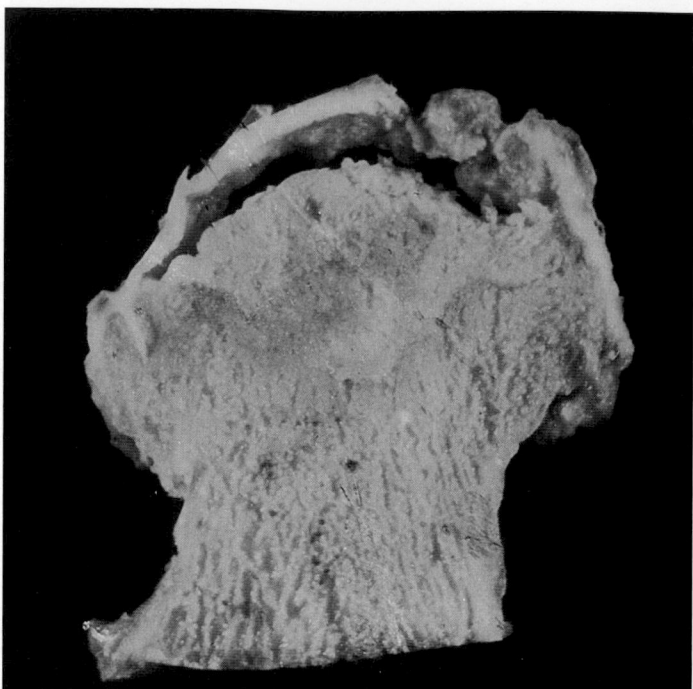

Fig. 13.13 Photograph of a coronal section through the femoral head of a patient with more advanced osteonecrosis than that shown in Figure 13.1. The articular cartilage is almost entirely detached. Once the cartilage detaches, the necrotic bone beneath will rapidly be eroded away, and secondary osteoarthritis will ensue.

cartilage becomes detached over the infarcted area, the underlying bone gradually fragments and erodes, and secondary osteoarthritis ensues (Fig. 13.13).

Infarcts in the shafts of long bones are likely to be asymptomatic.[23] They may be found as an incidental finding on radiographic films, in which case they are frequently misinterpreted as tumors, particularly cartilaginous tumors. There have been several reports of sarcomas, usually malignant fibrous histiocytoma, developing as a complication of long-standing infarcts in long bones.[24]

HETEROTOPIC CALCIFICATION AND BONE FORMATION

The distinction between calcification in soft tissue and ossification in soft tissue is an important one. Extensive calcification of soft tissue may result from disturbed calcium metabolism, as in hyperparathyroidism, metastatic carcinoma, myeloma, and hypervitaminosis D, or may complicate systemic connective tissue diseases such as scleroderma.

Localized diffuse calcification may be seen in fat necrosis, old tuberculous cavities, phlebolithiasis, or synovioma (Fig. 13.14).

The most common sites of heterotopic bone are in calcified laryngeal or tracheal cartilage and in the media of calcified arteries. In these situations bone is formed by vascular invasion of calcified tissue, similar to endochondral ossification of the growth plate (see above). However, any tissue that has calcified may later ossify.

Myositis ossificans

Two entirely separate conditions are included under the diagnosis of myositis ossificans. The first, myositis ossificans progressiva, is a very rare congenital progressive disease in which groups of tendons and muscle, usually around major joints, become progressively calcified and ossified, producing severe functional disability.[25] Microscopic examination will reveal poorly organized bone, both lamellar and woven, and dense fibrous scar tissue. Occasionally, one may observe islands of poorly formed cartilage.

The second condition is myositis ossificans circumscripta, in which the patient usually has a lump in a muscle, which has been present for some weeks and may have been somewhat painful.[26] A history of trauma can usually be elicited but is often of a trivial nature and occasionally may be absent. A radiograph taken soon after the onset of symptoms may not show an opacity, but within 1 or 2 weeks a poorly defined shadow will appear, and over the following weeks the periphery will become increasingly well delineated from the surrounding soft tissue.

On gross examination, a focus of myositis ossificans circumscripta present for a few months shows a shell of bony tissue with a more or less soft red-brown central area. It is usually 2–5 cm in diameter and adherent to the surrounding muscle.

Microscopic examination reveals, in the central part of the lesion, an irregular mass of active mesenchymal cells with foci of interstitial microhemorrhage that are rarely extensive (Fig. 13.15A). Occasionally, hemosiderin-filled macrophages and degenerative muscle fibers are encountered. The whole lesion is intensely vascular, the vessels being dilated channels lined by endothelium but without any formed media or adventitia. At some distance from the center of the lesion, depending on the age of the lesion in question, one finds small foci of osteoid production and, rarely, even cartilage production; this tissue may be disorganized and hypercellular. As one approaches the periphery there are more and more clearly defined trabeculae (see Fig. 13.15B). The bone is usually of the primitive woven type with large, round, and crowded osteocytes; however, in cases of long standing the bone is mature and has a lamellar pattern.

Histologically, it may be difficult to differentiate a focus of myositis, especially in its acute and active stage, from a sarcoma. A careful correlation of the clinical and radiographic findings is therefore essential. An important distinction that must be emphasized is that whereas myositis ossifcans is most mature at its periphery and least mature at its center (see Fig. 13.15C), the opposite is true of a soft tissue osteosarcoma. Post-traumatic reactive lesions similar to myositis ossifcans are sometimes seen on the small bones of the hand where they are often referred to as reactive periostitis.

METABOLIC DISEASE

Skeletal disease secondary to disturbed metabolism can be considered under four headings of disturbance or disease, which are discussed below.

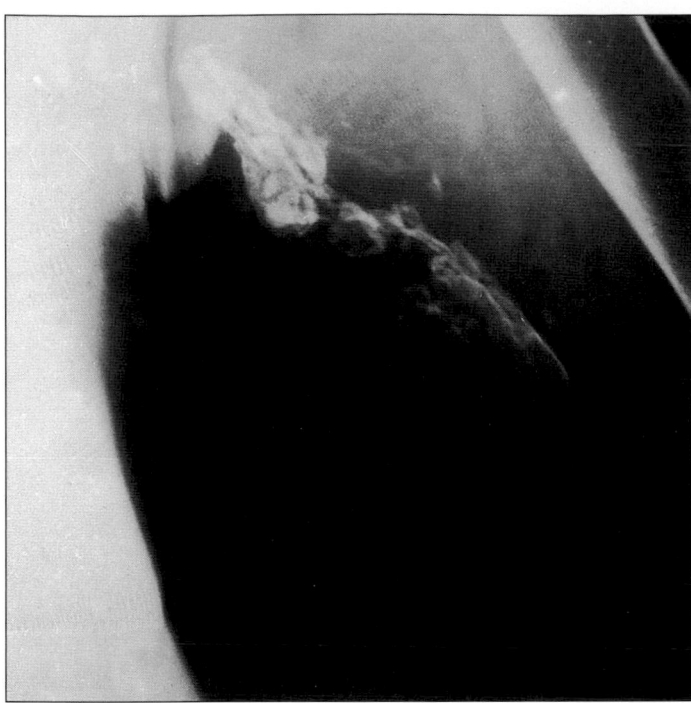

Fig. 13.14 Radiograph of the upper arm of a 50-year-old man complaining of a swelling on the inner aspect of the left arm. A heavily calcified mass is apparent which, following removal, was found to be a calcified lipoma.

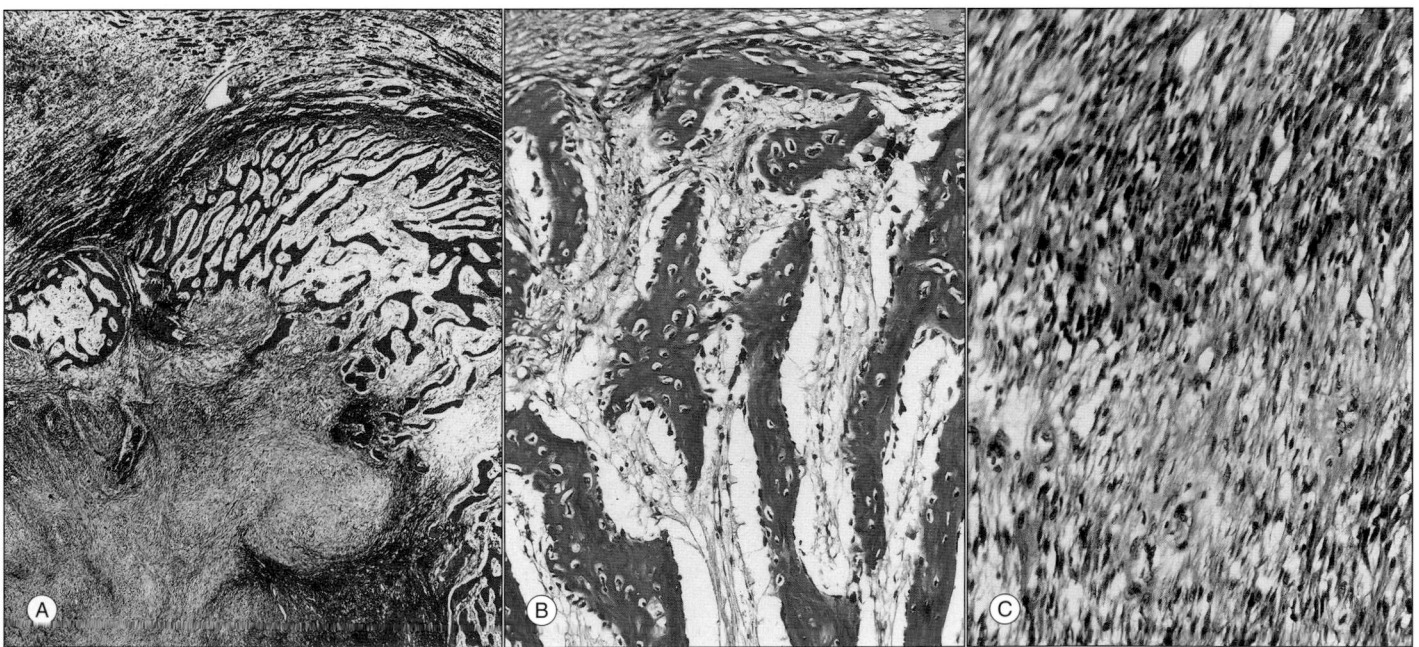

Fig. 13.15 A, Photomicrograph showing a portion of a specimen of myositis ossificans circumscripta. In the upper part of the photograph, there is scar tissue with compressed muscle fibers. The lesion itself shows trabecular bone at the periphery and at the center a cellular tissue.
B, Photomicrograph showing detail of periphery of lesion shown in A. Note the trabeculae of woven bone with crowded osteocytes and prominent osteoblasts on the surface of the trabeculae. Between the trabeculae there is innocuous fibrous tissue. **C,** Photomicrograph showing detail of center of lesion in A. Note the crowded spindle cells, which give a pseudosarcomatous appearance to the lesion.

Diseases resulting from disturbances in the formation of matrix components

Skeletal disease due to matrix component disturbances may involve the collagen, proteoglycan, or mineral components of the matrix.

Collagen

An abnormality in collagen synthesis may result from an inborn error such as occurs with osteogenesis imperfecta or the Ehlers-Danlos syndrome (diseases characterized histologically by severe osteoporosis, often a hypercellular immature bone tissue, and deficient fibrous connective tissue throughout the body)[27,28] or from extrinsic disturbances such as vitamin C deficiency and lathyrism, in which the intracellular formation of the collagen molecule is disturbed.

Proteoglycan

Most disturbances of proteoglycan metabolism are the result of overproduction of one or another type of glycosaminoglycan (mucopolysaccharide), most commonly dermatan sulfate and heparan sulfate. Accumulation of glycosaminoglycan occurs within the reticuloendothelial cells of many organs, and this may or may not be associated with excess excretion in the urine of these substances. These disorders, which are collectively known as the mucopolysaccharidoses, may exhibit marked skeletal abnormalities.[29] One of these diseases, Morquio's disease, probably specifically involves a defect in the proteoglycan metabolism of cartilage.

Minerals

Disturbances in the mineral component of the matrix may result from inborn errors in metabolism in which there is either a relative absence or excess of the enzyme alkaline phosphatase. Hypophosphatasemia[30] is characterized by an extremely osteopenic skeleton, which radiologically mimics rickets. Microscopically, the bone tissue is disorganized and poorly mineralized, with an excess of unmineralized osteoid tissue. Hyperphosphatasemia,[31] by contrast, results in a dense and irregularly formed skeleton. Histologically, the bone tissue resembles that of Paget's disease, and the condition is often referred to as juvenile Paget's disease.

A number of metallic elements may also deposit in the bone, resulting in interference with the normal process of mineralization. These include lead, iron, and aluminum. Aluminum toxicity has been recognized as a major complication of the administration of phosphate bindings in the management of renal dialysis patients. Not only does aluminum result in an encephalopathy, eventually leading to an irreversible psychosis, but it also deposits at the mineralization fronts in the bone, effectively blocking further mineralization and leading to an osteomalacia-like picture. In undecalcified sections the aluminum in the bone can be demonstrated by using the aurintricarboxylic acid stain, which stains the aluminum red.[32] Fluoride in excessive amounts, either endemic or iatrogenic, results in increased bone formation, the matrix of the newly formed bone showing a patchy and abnormal mineralization.[33]

Diseases resulting from disturbances in calcium homeostasis

Disturbances in calcium homeostasis result in osteitis fibrosa (hyperparathyroidism) and/or osteomalacia (rickets).

Hyperparathyroidism

Hyperparathyroidism may be either primary, due to a functioning adenoma, primary hyperplasia, or, rarely, a carcinoma of the

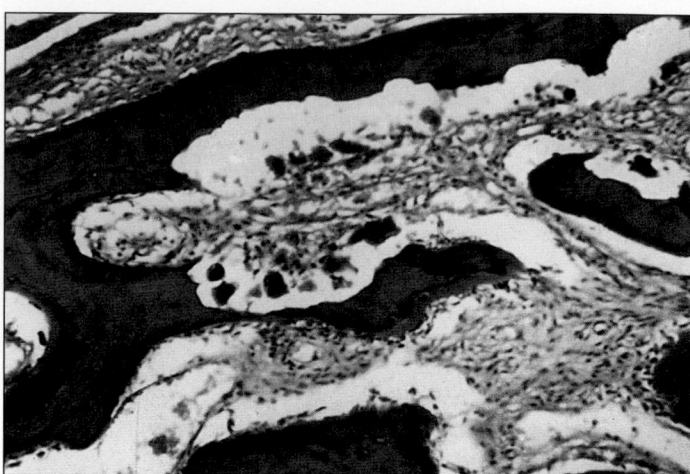

Fig. 13.16 Photomicrograph of section taken from a patient with hyperparathyroidism. Note the way the resorbing surfaces dissect into the bone trabeculae, resulting in a tunneling effect characteristic of the disease.

parathyroid glands[34] or secondary, due to renal disease.[35] With the advent of renal dialysis the latter form of disease (secondary hyperparathyroidism) has become much more frequent. In hyperparathyroid bone disease the characteristic microscopic change is localized osteoclastic resorption of the bone tissue, which characteristically and frequently shows a dissecting pattern (Fig. 13.16). Associated with the foci of osteoclastic resorption, localized fibrosis of the marrow adjacent to the bone is seen. (The localization of the fibrosis against the bone trabeculae distinguishes this type of fibrosis from that seen in myelofibrosis.) The increased bone resorption results in a secondary increase in bone formation, and the result is an increased turnover rate that is generalized throughout the skeleton, although it is more apparent in sections of cancellous bone than in sections of dense cortical bone.

Occasionally, the proliferation of osteoclasts and fibrous tissue is associated with hemorrhage and a giant cell reaction. This results in the so-called brown tumor of hyperparathyroidism, which may be confused with a giant cell tumor. This error may be avoided by careful correlation of the microscopic appearance with the clinical chemistry findings and radiographs.

Osteomalacia

Although childhood rickets is now an uncommon condition, this is not the case with adult rickets, or osteomalacia. Osteomalacia may result from malabsorption syndrome, after intestinal surgery or poor diet, or from a disturbance in vitamin D metabolism.[36] One recent cause of disturbance in vitamin D metabolism is treatment with anticonvulsive drugs such as diphenylhydantoin (Dilantin). However, whatever the cause of the disturbance in vitamin D metabolism or calcium absorption, the effects are similar. The bone that is laid down fails to be calcified. As a result the osteoblasts tend to be overactive, laying down even more bone, which in turn remains unmineralized. It is not possible to appreciate the extent of unmineralized bone tissue unless undecalcified sections are prepared (Fig. 13.17). When this is done, most of the bone trabeculae are covered by a prominent layer of unmineralized bone or osteoid, and this can be best appreciated by the use of the von Kossa stain. In osteomalacia not only is upward of 40% of the bone unmineralized, but it will also be apparent that the mineralization front is very irregular and fuzzy in appearance.

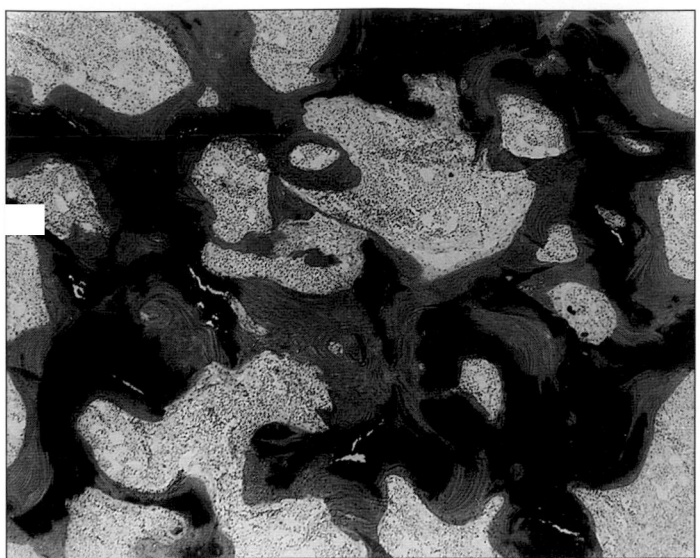

Fig. 13.17 Photomicrograph of a section taken from a patient with osteomalacia. The section has been prepared from undecalcified bone and stained by the von Kossa method. The area stained black represents mineralized bone. On the surface, there is a thick layer of nonmineralized bone matrix (osteoid). This osteoid seam, which is characteristic of osteomalacia, cannot be appreciated on decalcified sections.

Diseases resulting from disturbances in cell linkage

Skeletal tissues are in a continuous state of formation and breakdown. If the amount of tissue is to remain the same then it is necessary that the rate of tissue formation must be balanced by that of tissue breakdown. A disturbance of this linkage will give rise either to osteosclerosis or to osteopenia. Senile osteoporosis is the commonest example of the latter and Paget's disease the commonest example of the former.

Osteoporosis

Osteoporosis is a decrease in mass of normally mineralized bone, which often leads to fracture. It results in thinning of the bone cortices and in thin, widely spaced trabeculae in the cancellous bone (Fig. 13.18). It is the result of a relative decrease in osteoblastic (bone-forming) activity as compared with osteoclastic (bone-resorbing) activity, usually with an increase in osteoclastic activity.

Osteoporosis may be localized or generalized. Localized osteoporosis occurs after immobilization, for example, in a plaster cast. It may also be seen in the region of a joint associated with localized pain and hyperemia (Sudeck's atrophy). This type of localized patchy osteoporosis occasionally seems to involve several joints, usually in the lower limbs, in a transient fashion – so-called idiopathic transient osteoporosis.[37] In one form of localized osteoporosis, disappearing bone disease, the bone may eventually entirely disappear on the radiograph.[38] In all these forms of localized osteoporosis, no specific microscopic appearance other than the obvious loss of bone tissue and some increase in osteoclastic activity has been identified, although it has been suggested that there is an increased vascularity of the bone.

Clinical osteoporosis as a result of age is most common in white women for the reasons discussed earlier. It may also occur in a severe form after menopause, presumably as a result of endocrine imbalance, and it also complicates hypercortisonism.

Proper evaluation of osteoporosis, as of the other metabolic disturbances of bone, requires quantitative histology; the parameters to measure are the percentage of tissue occupied by bone tissue as opposed to marrow, and the percentage of the bone surface that is actively laying down bone or that is actually resorbing bone as compared with the inactive surfaces. (For a full discussion, see Coe and Favus.[39]) Clinical history and thorough biochemical studies are essential to determine etiology and treatment.

Paget's disease

Paget's disease[40] is a localized disturbance in bone cell activity, the cause of which is unknown, although there have been reports of viral inclusions in the osteoclasts.[41] It is a fairly common disease, occurring in about 4% of the northern European male population over the age of 40. However, in most instances the disease is not clinically significant, usually being confined to only one vertebral body or one other focus in the skeleton. Generalized clinical Paget's disease is much less common.

The microscopic appearance of Paget's disease is variable and depends on the state of activity. In active disease, the histologic

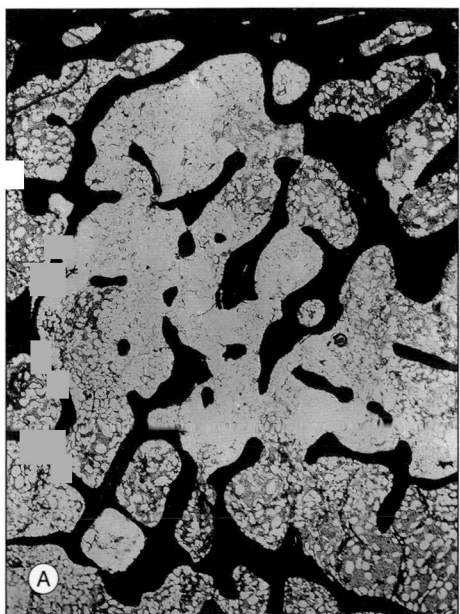

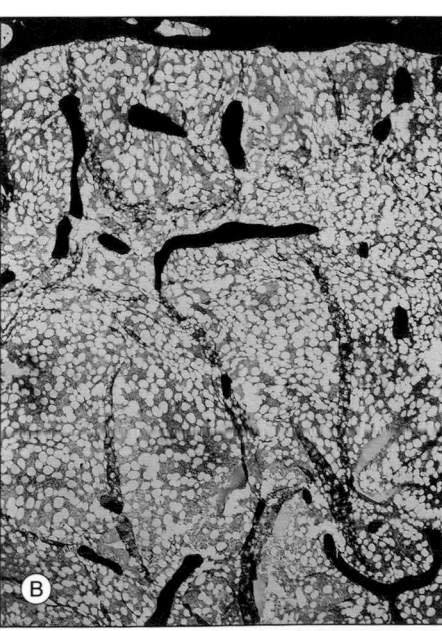

Fig. 13.18 A, Photomicrograph of a core biopsy specimen of the iliac crest in a normal 35-year-old woman. Note that for the most part the trabeculae are connected with one another and to the cortex, a portion of which is seen in the upper part of the picture. Compare this appearance with that in **B**, which is from an osteoporotic 65-year-old woman. In **B**, not only are the trabeculae much thinner and sparser, but they are not connected with one another or with the cortical bone at the surface.

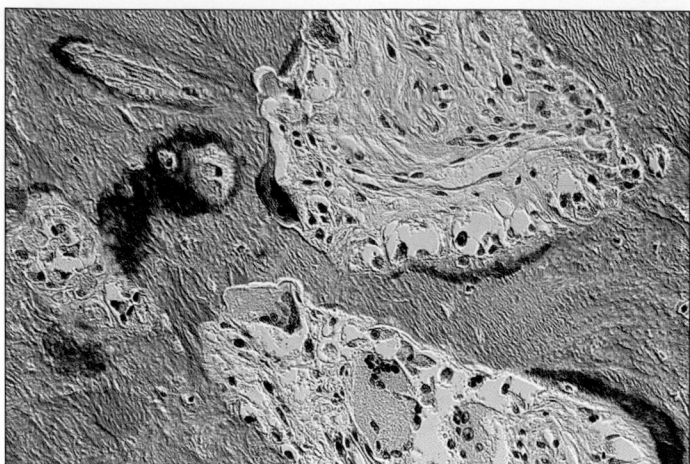

Fig. 13.19 Photomicrograph of a section taken from a patient with active Paget's disease. At the surface of the bone there is considerable osteoclastic activity. Some of these osteoclasts have many nuclei. Giant osteoclasts tend to be characteristic of Paget's disease. In other areas, abundant osteoblastic activity can be discerned, marked by the red osteoid seams (Goldner stain).

appearance is difficult to distinguish from that of hyperparathyroidism (Fig. 13.19). There is very active osteoclastic resorption and, associated with this, increased osteoblastic activity. These changes result in an increased number of reversal lines (cement lines), which are apparent even in the early or active stage of the disease. The marrow spaces are fibrosed, but the dissecting type of resorption, which typifies hyperparathyroidism, is not usually seen. In the later, quiescent stages of the disease, the bone becomes very dense, and the previous overactivity is represented by multiple cement lines, giving rise to the descriptive mosaic appearance (see Fig. 13.5). The bone marrow will be noted to have many dilated vascular channels, which is consistent with the clinical observation that these patients frequently have a high output type of failure. In a small percentage of patients sarcoma may develop[42] (see Chapter 14).

Diseases resulting from deposition of abnormal extrinsic metabolic products

The last group of metabolic disturbances commonly seen by the surgical pathologist are the conditions in which an abnormal extrinsic metabolic product is deposited in the skeleton. Such conditions include the so-called lipid histiocytoses (Gaucher's, Niemann-Pick, and Tay-Sachs diseases), ochronosis,[43,44] cystinosis, and oxalosis,[45] but the two most common diseases are calcium pyrophosphate dihydrate crystal deposition disease and gout.

Calcium pyrophosphate dihydrate deposition disease (pseudogout)

Calcium pyrophosphate dihydrate is a chalky white material often found in the synovial membrane, articular cartilage, and/or fibrocartilaginous menisci of elderly people, and it does not usually result in clinically significant disease.[46] However, some cases of inflammatory joint disease and secondary osteoarthritis may be the result of deposition of calcium pyrophosphate, and occasional patients are seen who develop clinically significant pseudogout before the age of 35. These individuals have an autosomal dominant pattern of inheritance.

The histologic appearance of these deposits, as well as the clinical presentation in some cases, is similar enough to that of gout to have given rise to the term *pseudogout* to describe the clinical syndrome. In histologic sections the material is usually crystalline, the crystals being small and rectangular and exhibiting a weak positive birefringence. On occasion, noncrystalline deposits that do not polarize may also be seen. These crystalline deposits are sometimes surrounded by giant cells and occasional histiocytes and chronic inflammatory cells (Fig. 13.20).

Gout

Gout[47] results from the precipitation of monosodium urate monohydrate in the synovial fluid and other tissues after prolonged

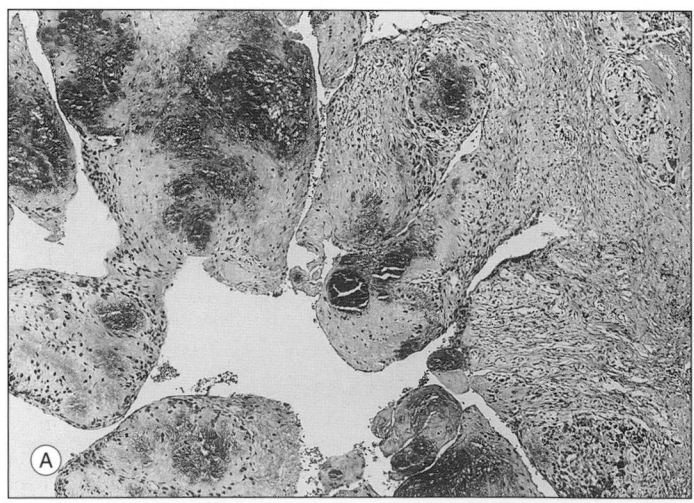

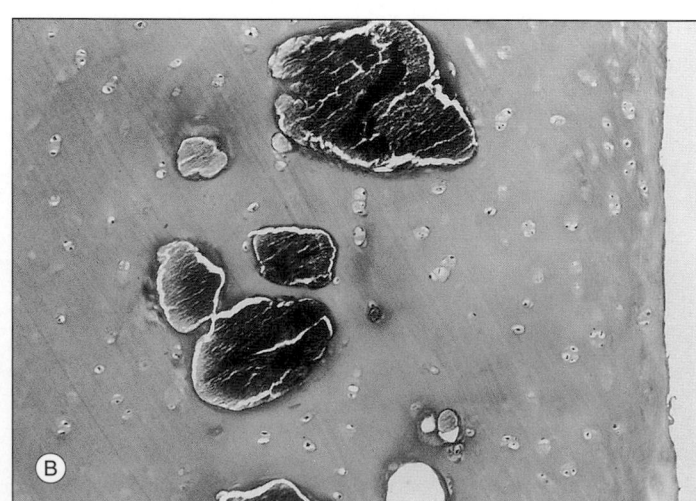

Fig. 13.20 A, Photomicrograph of a section of synovium taken from a patient with calcium pyrophosphate dihydrate deposition disease. The deposits of calcium pyrophosphate are crystalline and surrounded in some areas by histiocytes, giant cells, and a mild chronic inflammatory infiltrate. **B**, Photomicrograph of section of articular cartilage from the same case demonstrated in **A**. Large irregular noncrystalline deposits of calcified material are present. Undecalcified frozen section stained by the von Kossa method.

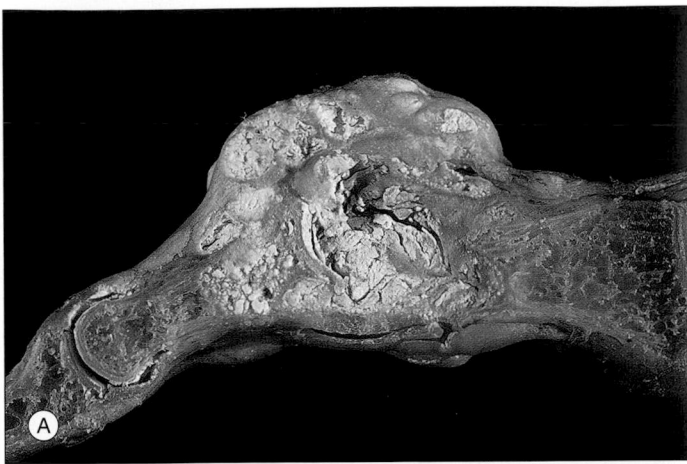

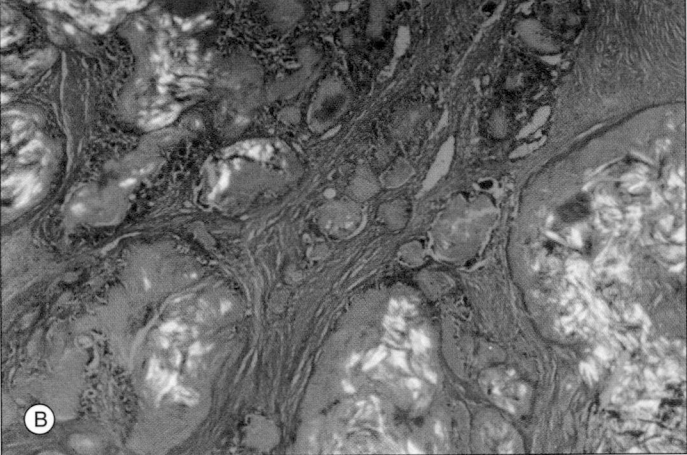

Fig. 13.21 A, Photograph of a sagittal section through a metatarsophalangeal joint affected by tophaceous gout. **B,** Photomicrograph of the sodium urate deposits with surrounding giant cell, histiocytic, and fibroblastic response in a case of tophaceous gout. As seen in this photograph the urate crystals are refractile when examined with polarized light.

hyperuricemia. It is most commonly seen in the kidney and the large joints, especially the first metatarsophalangeal joint. There are three stages of involvement to the joint by gout: (1) acute gouty synovitis; (2) the deposition of sodium urate in the form of chalky concretions or tophi in the synovium, bone, bursae, and subcutaneous tissues; and (3) chronic gouty arthritis. In patients with acute gouty arthritis, the synovial fluid invariably contains crystals that are usually needle-shaped and when examined with polarized light demonstrate strong negative birefringence. The crystals may be free in the synovial fluid or may be engulfed within polymorphonuclear leukocytes. The ingested crystals result in the release of lysosomal enzymes, which in turn perpetuate the acute inflammatory reaction. After a number of years, chalky deposits of sodium urate, known as tophi, may develop in the articular and periarticular tissues. These deposits are surrounded by chronic inflammatory cells, foreign body giant cells, and dense fibrous scar. Destruction of the bone and capsular tissues results in chronic arthritis with disabling deformities (Fig. 13.21).

Gaucher's disease

Gaucher's disease[48] is a lipid histiocytosis resulting from an accumulation of glucocerebrosides within the histiocytes of the reticuloendothelial system, particularly in bones and spleen. It is mostly seen in Ashkenazic Jews and is transmitted as an autosomal recessive trait. The bone marrow shows more or less replacement by sheets of large pale cells, with a distinctive crumpled appearance to the cytoplasm. Because the disease is inherited, the bone marrow replacement may result in developmental deformities in the more rapidly growing parts of the skeleton, that is, the lower end of the femur, the upper tibia, and the upper end of the humerus. This takes the form of widening of the metaphyseal portion of bone, resulting in a deformity known as the 'Erlenmeyer flask deformity.' Radiographically, the affected bones are frequently osteoporotic and may show a lytic or soap-bubble appearance. The extending mass of lipid-laden histiocytes may interfere with the blood supply to the bone and cause infarction. Unilateral or bilateral avascular necrosis of the femoral head is a common complication of Gaucher's disease and may be the presenting clinical sign. Because of the relative ischemia of the affected bone, biopsy is attended by a high incidence of secondary infection.

INFECTION

Before the advent of antibiotics, infection[49,50] was among the most common indications for inpatient treatment in orthopedic hospitals, and in developing countries bone infection is still the most common cause of bone and joint disease. In the United States, however, it is now rare and for this reason may give rise to problems in differential diagnosis.

Infection of the bones and joints may result from either hematogenous spread or direct implantation. In the latter case, the infection usually complicates either a compound fracture or surgery, nowadays particularly prosthetic replacement of joints.

Hematogenous osteomyelitis is most commonly seen in children and is usually due to *Staphylococcus aureus* infection. Bacteremia alone is probably not sufficient to cause osteomyelitis, and generally a history of trauma will be elicited from the patient, the trauma presumably giving rise to local blood stasis or thrombosis, thereby providing a site for bacterial growth. Infection is most commonly seen in children in the metaphyseal region of long bones and particularly around the knee joint. Usually, the patient has a high fever, pain, and local tenderness, and during the first week or so of the disease radiographs will not show any bony change. (Nowadays, because patients with fever are frequently treated with antibiotics without further diagnosis, osteomyelitis in children may present as a chronic problem.)

In adults, hematogenous osteomyelitis is less common. When it is seen, it is more common in the vertebral column. It is seen in drug addicts and may also complicate urinary tract infection, presumably via Batson's plexus. An unusual form of osteomyelitis is the multiple bony involvement seen in patients with sickle cell disease, in which the causative organism is often *Salmonella*.

In osteomyelitis, the inflammatory exudate usually results in widespread bone and bone marrow necrosis. This results from the increased pressure within the closed cavity of the cancellous bone, which rapidly leads to vascular occlusion. The inflammatory exudate tracks through the Haversian systems of the cortex to elevate the overlying periosteum, which in turn is activated to form a sleeve of new bone (the involucrum) around the necrotic infected bone (the sequestrum) beneath. This classic sequence is aborted by the use of adequate antibiotic therapy. However, unless the disease is treated with adequate doses of antibiotics, it may become chronic, and in this case is likely to continue for many years with recurrent episodes of local infection, which may be accompanied by sinus formation. Rare long-term complications of osteomyelitis include secondary amyloidosis and the formation of squamous cell carcinoma in the sinus tract.[51,52]

Occasional adult patients with hematogenous osteomyelitis may present without significant systemic signs. As likely as not, the radiologic diagnosis on these patients will be that of a tumor, possibly a malignant round cell tumor. A biopsy specimen revealing small, round inflammatory cells may also be misinterpreted by the pathologist as a round cell tumor, and on occasion this differential diagnosis may be problematic. In this regard it also should be noted that occasional children with Ewing's tumor may have an elevated temperature, increased sedimentation rate, and leukocytosis and as a consequence may initially be misdiagnosed as osteomyelitis.

Granulomatous infection is usually due to *Mycobacterium tuberculosis*, but occasionally to blastomycosis, cryptococcosis, coccidioidomycosis, or sporotrichosis; rarely, it results from sarcoidosis. These infections are most commonly seen either in the spine or in the large joints (the hip and the knee). Histologically, typical granulomas with giant cells, epithelioid cells, and chronic inflammatory cells are seen. Organisms may be difficult to demonstrate in bony tissue. Often, granulomatous infection, because of its rarity, is not suspected clinically, and the diagnosis does not become apparent until the pathologist has examined the tissue. For this reason cultures may not have been taken, and the causative organism may be difficult to establish.

THE HISTIOCYTOSES

The histiocytoses are characterized by the proliferation of histiocytes in the bone and/or soft tissues.[53] Depending on the presentation, they have been classified as eosinophilic granuloma, Hand-Schüller-Christian disease, or Letterer-Siwe disease. Nowadays, these lesions are usually all included under the rubric of eosinophilic granuloma or Langerhans granulomatosis.

In the skeleton, eosinophilic granuloma is usually unifocal but occasionally may be multifocal. Most patients are under age 10. It may occur anywhere in any bones, but the most common sites are the skull, the shafts of the long bones (particularly the femur and tibia), and the ilium. The patient usually has localized aching pain and, less commonly, a low-grade fever and an elevated erythrocyte sedimentation rate. In radiographs the lesions are osteolytic and generally round to oval, but they may show considerable periosteal reaction and a ragged appearance suggestive of infection or a malignant tumor. Involvement of the vertebral body frequently leads to collapse and flattening (so-called Calvé's disease). On gross examination, the curetted material is usually scant and pinkish-gray. Microscopic examination will reveal masses of histiocytes (Langerhans cells) and focal or diffuse collections of eosinophils (Fig. 13.22). On electron microscopic examination, the Langerhans cell displays characteristic racket-shaped inclusion bodies in the cytoplasm (Birbeck granules). Occasionally, lymphocytes and plasma cells may also be present. During the healing phase, scar tissue and lipid-laden macrophages may become predominant.

Overdecalcification of the tissue may result in the eosinophilic granules not being apparent, and the lesion may be mistaken for osteomyelitis. The numerous histiocytes, occasionally with large nuclei and even occasionally binucleate forms, can lead to the erroneous impression of Hodgkin's disease.

The term *Hand-Schüller-Christian syndrome*, which originally referred to a classic triad of skull defects, exophthalmos, and diabetes

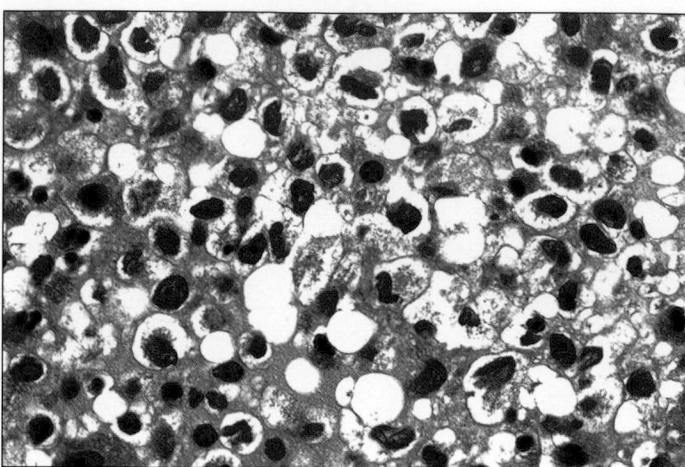

Fig. 13.22 Photomicrograph of a histologic section from a patient with eosinophilic granuloma. The lesion is composed of large histiocytes with abundant loose cytoplasm. A few eosinophils and lymphocytes are also present.

insipidus, is now used to include instances of more chronic evolution, occurring generally in children older than 3 years, with multiple cranial and other bony lesions and sometimes involvement of other systems or with one of the other classic symptoms (exophthalmos or diabetes insipidus). However, the complete triad has been rarely noted in the reported cases.

Letterer-Siwe disease is a rare condition affecting infants less than 2 years of age and is characterized by an acute onset of hepatosplenomegaly, lymphadenopathy, and sometimes bone lesions. In the past, this has been considered a form of histiocytosis, but Lieberman et al.[53] have suggested that the cases can be separated into two groups. In one group anaplastic histiocytes predominate, and this lesion would appear to be a form of malignant lymphoma. In the other group the histiocytes have a benign cytology, and this lesion may well be an infantile form of multifocal eosinophilic granuloma.

JOINT TISSUES

The joints[54] provide for motion and stability. These functions are achieved through the anatomy of the joint – its shape, the mechanical properties of the cartilage and bone of which it is made – and through the neuromuscular control of the joint. Dysfunction of the joint, which is generally called arthritis, occurs because of an alteration in the anatomy or its neuromuscular control. Obviously, such changes may result from congenital disease, metabolic disturbances, infection, or mechanical trauma.

The diarthrodial joints are composed of the articulating cartilages, synovial membrane, bone ends, and surrounding ligaments, tendons, and muscles.[55] Disease may begin in any of these structures, but by the time it comes to the attention of a physician, most or all of them are involved.

The synovial membrane, which lines the inner surface of the joint capsule and all other intra-articular structures with the exception of the articular cartilage, is composed of a smooth moist intimal layer and either a fibrous or a fatty subsynovial (or subintimal) supportive or backing layer. Microscopic examination shows at the surface a layer of closely packed cells with elliptical nuclei and abundant cytoplasm.

Table 13.1 Examination of synovial fluid

		Condition		
	Normal	Noninflammatory	Chronic inflammatory	Septic
Clinical example		Osteoarthritis	Rheumatoid arthritis	Bacterial infection
Cartilage debris	0	+	0	0
Volume (ml) (knee)	<3.5	>3.5	>3.5	>3.5
Color	Clear	Clear yellow	Opalescent yellow	Turbid yellow to green
Viscosity	High	High	Low	Low
White blood cells/mm³	200	200–2000	2000–100 000	>100 000
Polymorphonuclear leukocytes (%)	<25	<25	50% or more	90% or more
Culture	Negative	Negative	Negative	Positive
Mucin clot	Firm	Firm	Friable	Friable
Fibrin clot	None	Small	Large	Large
Glucose (% blood glucose)	≈50–100	≈50–100	≈20–75	≈1–5
Total protein		Equal to normal joint	Elevated	Elevated

From Paget S, Bullough PG. Synovium and synovial fluid. In: Owen R, Goodfellow JW, Bullough PG, eds. Scientific foundation of orthopaedics and traumatology. Philadelphia: Saunders; 1980:18–22, with permission.

The articular cartilage is largely composed of collagen, proteoglycan, and water, and it distributes the load through the joint onto the underlying subchondral bone. To achieve this, the collagen fibers are distributed in a very precise way, as is the proteoglycan.[11] The cells on the surface of the cartilage are flat with their long axes parallel to the surface. The cells that are lower down in the cartilage are rounded and lie in well-defined lacunae.

Other forms of cartilage tissue in the body (epiphyseal cartilage, fibrocartilage, and elastic cartilage) do not function in the same way as articular cartilage and therefore have a different chemical composition and a different organization of the extracellular matrix.[56]

CYTOPATHOLOGY OF SYNOVIAL FLUID

Normal synovial fluid, a dialysate of plasma to which hyaluronic acid produced by the 'B' cells of the synovial lining is added, is viscous, pale yellow, and clear. Even in large joints the volume is small.

Examination of synovial fluid may be extremely helpful in the diagnosis of arthritis for determining both the etiology and severity of the disease.[57] Whatever the cause of arthritis, the synovial fluid is altered (Table 13.1).

In cases of inflammatory arthritis, there is an increased volume of synovial fluid with large numbers of neutrophils in the fluid and some free synovial cells. The amount of hyaluronic acid is markedly diminished and this leads to a typical decrease in viscosity. However, in degenerate forms of arthritis, the amount of hyaluronic acid is increased, resulting in an extremely viscous fluid.

An important diagnostic procedure for the clinical diagnosis of crystal synovitis is examination of synovial fluid for crystals and identification of these crystals by polarized light microscopy. This examination requires a polarizing microscope with a compensating first-order red filter. With the compensating filter in position, the crystals in the synovial fluid should be aligned so that their long axis is parallel to the line that is drawn on the compensating filter, which is the axis of slow vibration.

Sodium urate crystals are usually needle-shaped and exhibit strong negative birefringence; that is, they appear bright yellow when aligned parallel with the line on the compensating filter. Calcium pyrophosphate dihydrate crystals are usually rhomboidal and they exhibit weakly positive birefringence (i.e. when their long axis is aligned with the line on the compensating filter, they appear blue and much less bright than urate crystals).

JOINT DISEASE

The most important therapeutic advance since the 1960s has been the development of artificial articulations to replace joints affected by various disease. On most orthopedic services, endoprosthetic replacements probably account for about one-third of all operations. For the surgical pathologist this means a considerable increase in the amount of orthopedically related tissue to be studied and reported on.

The most common pathologic diagnoses made in patients having total hip replacement in our experience are osteoarthritis (about 65%), avascular necrosis (about 15%), rheumatoid arthritis (about 15%), and subchondral insufficiency fractures (about 5–10%). (It should be emphasized that these diagnoses are not completely objective and that end-stage hip disease, like end-stage kidney disease or end-stage liver disease, looks very much the same regardless of its etiology.)

The arthritides that are the result of metabolic disturbances and infection have been referred to earlier and are not further discussed here.

OSTEOARTHRITIS

Osteoarthritis[58] (degenerative joint disease, osteoarthrosis) is generally regarded as a noninflammatory condition that begins as a disruption of the bearing surfaces of the articular cartilage and ends with disintegration of joint function. In about one-fifth of the cases, an antecedent condition causally related to the osteoarthritis is

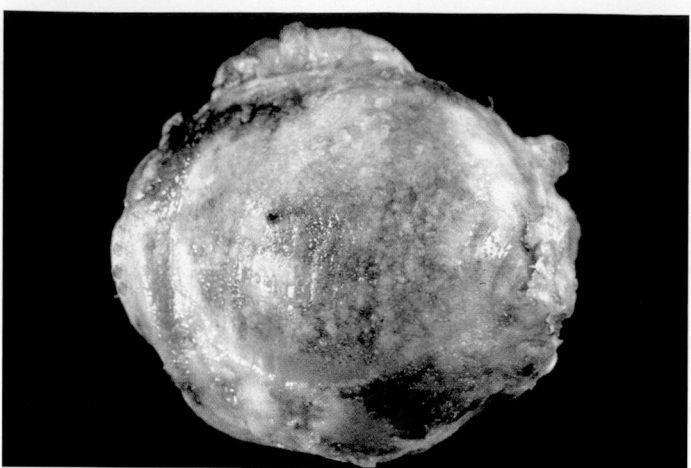

Fig. 13.23 Photograph of a femoral head removed from a patient with osteoarthritis of the hip joint. The superior articular surface has a shiny appearance where the articular cartilage has been worn away and the underlying bone exposed and polished. The cartilage that remains around the periphery is irregular and roughened.

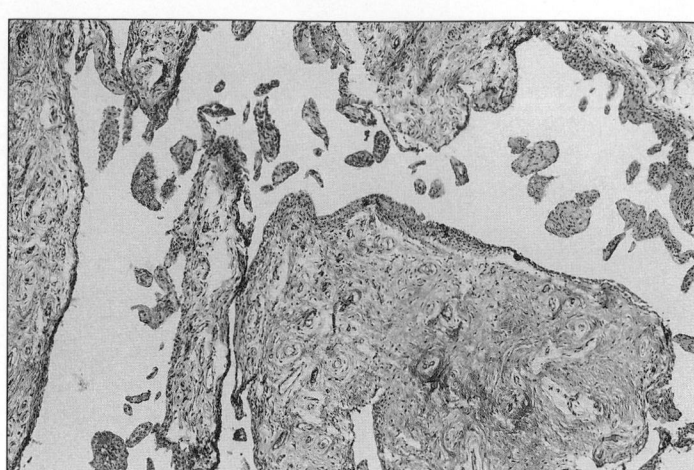

Fig. 13.25 Photomicrograph of a section of synovium taken from a patient with osteoarthritis of the hip joint. The synovial membrane is hypertrophied, hyperplastic, and thrown up into a fine villous structure. In the subsynovial tissue there is a mild chronic inflammatory infiltrate.

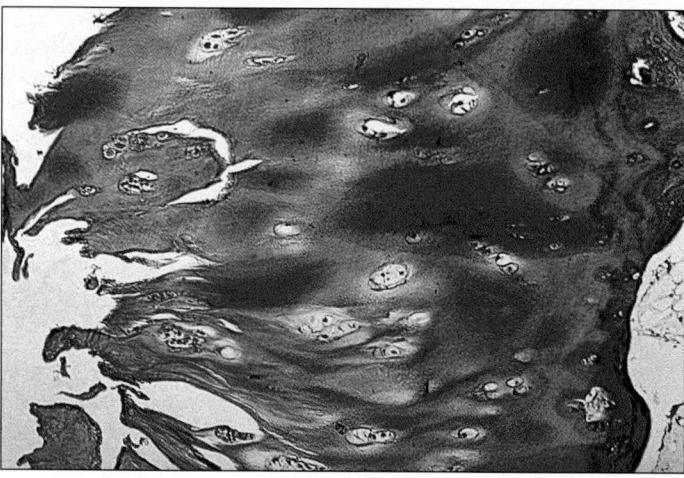

Fig. 13.24 Photomicrograph of a section of fibrillated cartilage from a patient with osteoarthritis. Note the proliferating nests of chondrocytes particularly evident towards the surface.

evident to the clinician. These conditions include Perthes disease, slipped epiphysis, previous infection, and osteonecrosis.

A patient with clinical osteoarthritis usually complains of pain and disability. Movement of the affected joint may be very limited. Examination of a joint removed at surgery or autopsy shows the most obvious features of an osteoarthritic joint to be a change in the shape of the articular surfaces and damage of the cartilage. In the weight-bearing areas of a joint, the cartilage may be entirely absent, and the exposed subchondral bone has a dense polished appearance like marble (eburnation) (Fig. 13.23). In these areas of absent cartilage, the bone trabeculae are markedly thickened (sclerotic), and, adjacent to the surface in the subchondral bone there may be cystic defects filled by loose fibromyxoid tissue or sometimes by a thick fluid. In the eburnated areas the superficial bone may be necrotic, presumably from the excessive pressure. In some specimens the

weight-bearing surface may be covered by few or many tufts of fibrocartilage, and this seems to be a reparative phenomenon. In the areas of the joint that are not weight bearing and around the margins, there are bony and cartilaginous overgrowths (osteophytes or exostoses), which on the medial and inferior aspect of the femoral head may be in the form of large, flat plaques of bone and cartilage.

The cartilage that remains on the joint surface may have many clefts in its substance, most, but by no means all, being vertical in disposition. The cartilage cells may show considerable proliferation, with the formation of prominent cell nests (Fig. 13.24). Generally, basophilic staining of the matrix with hematoxylin stain will be found to be diminished. The synovial membrane shows some villous proliferation and mild hyperplasia of the intima. There may be a mild chronic inflammation (Fig. 13.25). Small osteochondral loose bodies are not unusual both in the synovium and also free in the joint. In Charcot joints, which are very severe examples of osteoarthritis, the synovium is generally full of bone and cartilage fragments, and there are many loose bodies.

On the basis of anatomic features, Nichols and Richardson[59] in 1909 distinguished the two forms of chronic arthritis that we would call, respectively, inflammatory arthritis and degenerative arthritis – most of the former comprising the clinical syndrome of rheumatoid arthritis and the latter that of osteoarthritis.

How well are we able to distinguish rheumatoid arthritis and osteoarthritis of the hip using histopathologic criteria? This is a summary of my own experience:

1. Histologically, there is more inflammation in association with the clinical diagnosis of rheumatoid arthritis than with the clinical diagnosis of degenerative joint disease. However, there is considerable overlap, and in about 40% of the cases no clear distinction can be made on the basis of the inflammatory infiltrate.
2. Pannus, a fibrous or inflammatory covering of the cartilage, often regarded as a hallmark of rheumatoid arthritis, is not uncommon in osteoarthritis.
3. The principal difference rests in the production of osteophytes and dense sclerosis in the bony joint surfaces of osteoarthritis

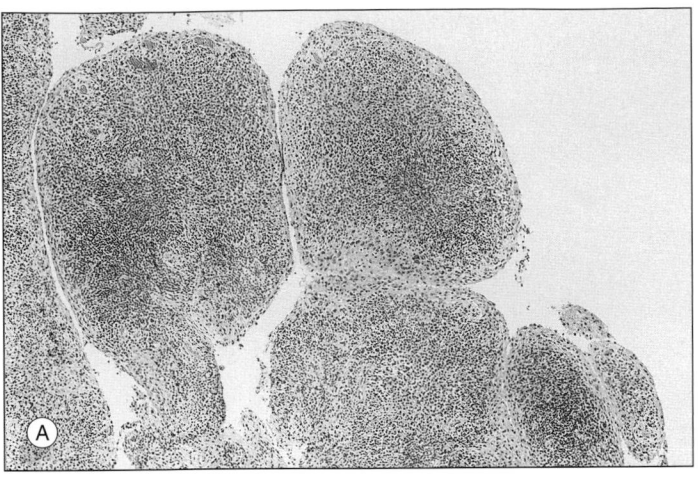 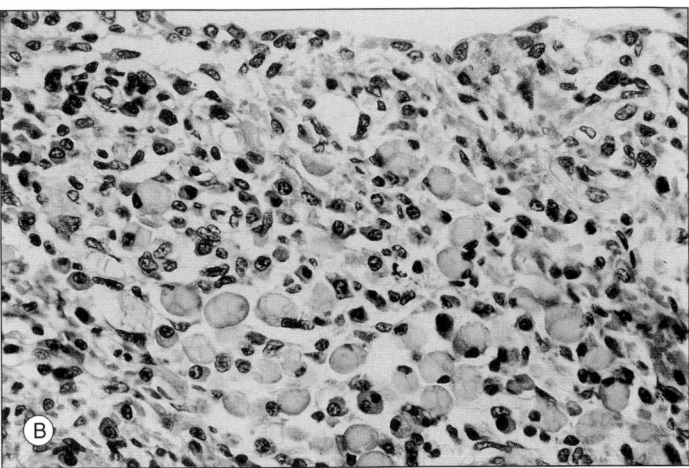

Fig. 13.26 **A**, Photomicrograph of a histologic section of synovium from a patient with rheumatoid arthritis. There is prominent villous proliferation, with a heavy subsynovial inflammatory infiltrate and marked hyperplasia of the synovial lining cells. **B**, High-power view of this synovium showing the plasma cell and lymphocyte infiltrate. Many of the plasma cells contain cytoplasmic inclusions (Russell bodies).

versus the destructive and nonproductive qualities of rheumatoid arthritis.

Haynes et al.[60] have reported on the phenotypic characterization of inflammatory cells from synovial tissue obtained from patients undergoing total hip replacement for osteoarthritis. Among patients with degenerative hip disease, two groups could be identified. In the first, there were high enzyme levels and high histologic scores. In the rest, low enzyme levels were accompanied by low histologic scores. It would seem, therefore, that there are a significant number of patients who have an inflammatory arthritis by all pathologic criteria even though clinically they have been diagnosed as having osteoarthritis.

Some patients with osteoarthritis have a spontaneous tendency to improve symptomatically and radiologically.[61] This may be explained by the histologic finding that in advanced stages of disease, eburnated areas tend to resurface with fibrocartilage. It suggests that osteoarthritis is not necessarily a progressive and continually degenerative process, but rather that there are two opposing processes occurring in a joint, namely breakdown and repair.

RHEUMATOID ARTHRITIS

Rheumatoid arthritis[62] is a chronic systemic disease frequently involving peripheral joints, two to three times more common in females, and characterized by spontaneous remission and exacerbation.[63] Of all affected patients, the majority have histocompatibility antigen HLA-DR4, which implies a strong hereditary component.[64] Family studies indicate that the disease has a dominant mode of inheritance.

Clinically, the acutely affected joint is hot, swollen, and tender. The synovial effusion is milky and turbid and contains 20 000 to 50 000 inflammatory cells, about 50% of which are polymorphonuclear leukocytes (compared with septic arthritis, in which the count is in excess of 100 000 with 75% polymorphonuclear leukocytes). No causative organism has been identified.

The principal morphologic feature of rheumatoid disease is joint destruction. Unlike osteoarthritis, there is little reparative activity, and osteophytes and new bone formation are not prominent.

The earliest histologic finding (Fig. 13.26) is a nonsuppurative chronic inflammation of the synovium characterized by:

1. Hypertrophy and hyperplasia of the synovial cells, resulting in a papillary and villous pattern at the surface of the synovium;
2. An infiltrate of lymphocytes and plasma cells, the latter often containing eosinophilic inclusions (Russell bodies, evidence of gamma globulin production); neutrophils are common in the synovial exudate but much less so in the synovial membrane;
3. Lymphoid follicles (Allison-Ghormley bodies); and
4. Fibrinous exudation both at the surface of the synovium and within the synovial tissue.

Although these histologic changes are very typical of rheumatoid arthritis, similar changes may also be seen in patients with systemic lupus erythematosus, psoriasis, Lyme disease, and other inflammatory arthritides. For this reason a definitive diagnosis of rheumatoid arthritis cannot be made on histologic examination of the synovium alone.

The hypertrophied, inflamed synovium often extends over the articular surface (pannus) and destroys the underlying cartilage by enzymatic degradation of the matrix (Fig. 13.27). The end result of this inflammatory destruction of the articular surfaces may be fusion of the joint (ankylosis), either by fibrous granulation tissue or by bone. (Note: ankylosis is not a feature of osteoarthritis.)

As well as destroying the cartilaginous surfaces of the joint, the rheumatoid synovium may invade the bone at the articular margin, the joint capsule, and other periarticular supportive tissues, resulting in marked instability of the joint and, frequently, subluxation or complete dislocation. Extra-articular synovitis may lead to carpal tunnel syndrome in which there is compression of the median nerve, or trigger finger, and on occasion these clinical syndromes may be heralds of rheumatoid arthritis.

One common histologic feature that is not usually commented on is considerable chronic inflammation and lymphoid follicle formation in the subchondral bone. In some cases this inflammatory tissue may destroy the articular cartilage from below.

Radiographs of affected joints will usually show osteopenia of the juxta-articular bone ends. This may be due either to the inflammation of the subchondral bone or to the hyperemia which is secondary to inflammation of the synovium.

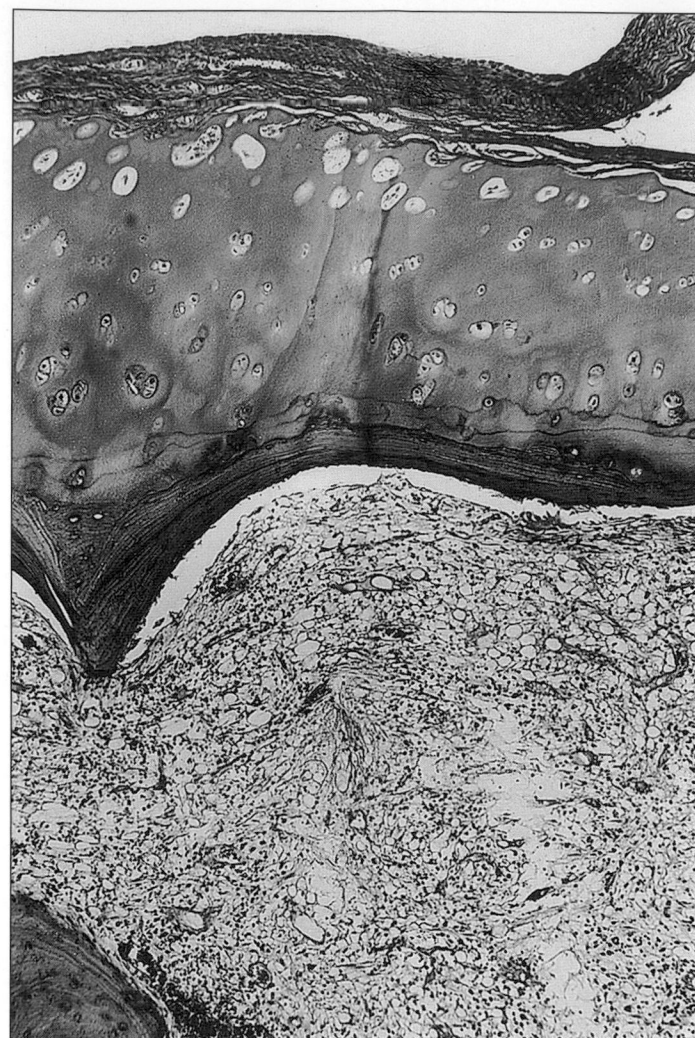

Fig. 13.27 Photomicrograph of a section of the articular surface of a joint involved by rheumatoid arthritis. Covering the articular cartilage is a layer of inflamed synovium (pannus). Underlying the pannus the chondrocytic lacunae are markedly enlarged (Weichselbaum). A heavy inflammatory infiltrate is also seen in the subchondral bone.

About 25% of patients with rheumatoid arthritis have subcutaneous nodules, most commonly over the extensor surfaces of the elbow and forearm. The nodules may also occur in synovial membrane as well as in the gastrointestinal tract, lung, and heart. The nodules may be present before any other sign of rheumatoid disease. The rheumatoid nodule is characterized histologically by an irregular shape and a central zone of necrotic fibrinoid material surrounded by histiocytes and some chronic inflammatory cells. The long axes of these histiocytes are frequently radially disposed or palisaded. Generalized vasculitis is much more common in patients with rheumatoid nodules, which is consistent with the belief that the nodules result from vascular damage (Fig. 13.28).[65]

Although the ultimate cause of rheumatoid disease is unknown, there are two important contributory factors: an immunologic reaction and increased degradative enzymes. Patients with rheumatoid arthritis have a number of immunoglobulins in their serum and synovial fluid, most commonly IgM. These immunoglobulins are known as rheumatoid factors and, as can be demonstrated by immuno-fluorescence, are made by plasma cells in the synovium and lymphoid

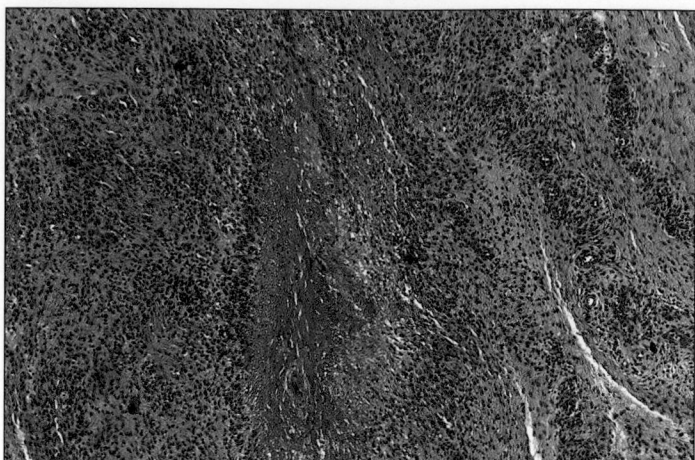

Fig. 13.28 Photomicrograph of a portion of a rheumatoid nodule. Note the geographic central fibrinoid necrosis with the surrounding palisaded histiocytes with fibrosis and chronic inflammation.

system. They can be seen microscopically in H&E-stained sections, both intracellularly and extracellularly, as dense homogeneous eosinophilic globules (Russell bodies).

As already noted, in the late stages of rheumatoid arthritis the affected joint may show very little in the way of inflammation and may be anatomically indistinguishable from osteoarthritis.

TRAUMATIC AND HEMORRHAGIC ARTHROPATHY

Severe acute or chronic trauma to a joint that results in bleeding into the joint frequently results in hemosiderotic synovitis and sometimes even green-black discoloration of the articular cartilage. As an end result, secondary osteoarthritis is not uncommon.

Hemorrhage into a joint space, resulting in a hot, painful, and swollen joint, is also one of the commonly observed clinical complications of hemophilia or other bleeding diatheses. These bloody joint effusions can be precipitated by even minor trauma and typically involve the knees, elbows, and ankles. Chronic, bloody effusions into the joint spaces may lead to a destructive arthropathy characterized on radiographic studies by a narrow joint space, cartilage destruction, bone erosion, multiple juxta-articular cysts, and, if the lesion has progressed over a long period, osteophytes. Radiographs may also reveal a juxtaepiphyseal osteoporosis. On the basis of gross examination of the hemosiderotic synovium of hemophilia and other forms of chronic bleeding into the joint, the differential diagnosis includes rheumatoid arthritis and pigmented villonodular synovitis. However, microscopic examination of the synovium in hemophilia-related destructive joint disease does not reveal the striking lymphoplasmacytic infiltrate that characterizes rheumatoid arthritis, nor is there the nodular proliferation of mononuclear and giant cells characteristic of pigmented villonodular synovitis.

SYNOVITIS AND OTHER TISSUE RESPONSES TO IMPLANTED ARTIFICIAL JOINTS

A small percentage of total joint replacements fail either because of mechanical loosening or breakage, or, less commonly, because of infection. In failed cases the prosthesis is usually removed.[66]

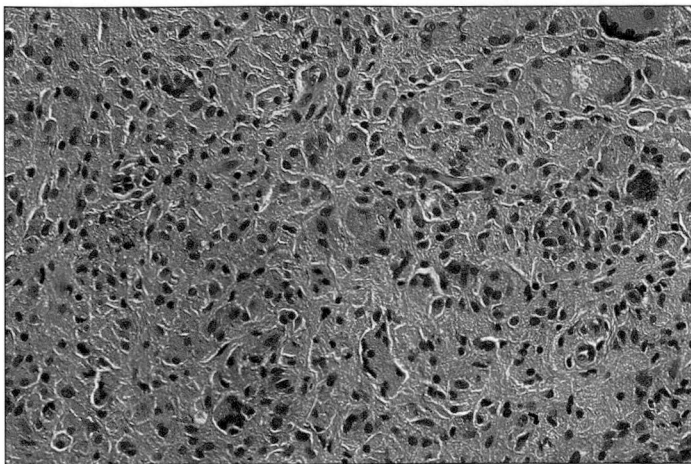

Fig. 13.29 Photomicrograph of a histologic section taken from the synovium of a patient with a failed total knee replacement. There is a marked histiocytic and giant cell reactive process. Irregular fragments of plastic can be demonstrated in these giant cells by polarized light. Proliferative synovium such as this may result in periarticular erosion of the bone.

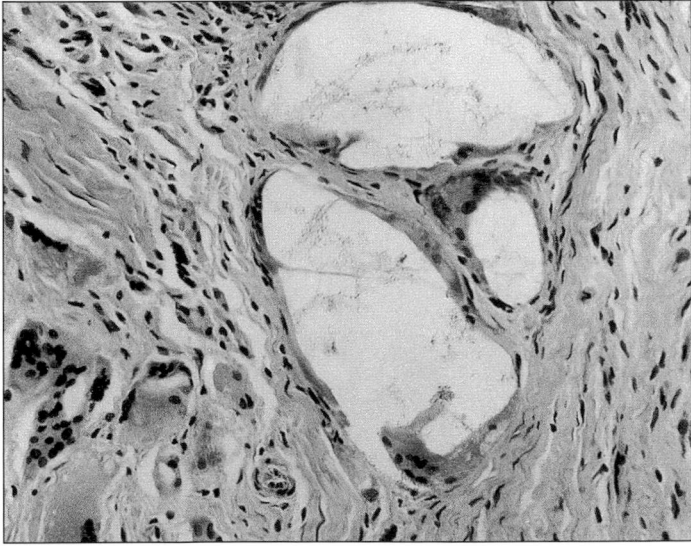

Fig. 13.30 Photomicrograph of a section of synovial tissue taken from a patient with a failed knee prosthesis. The large irregular spaces surrounded by flattened giant cells originally contained methyl methacrylate cement, dissolved out during processing. The finely granular material seen in these spaces is barium sulfate, which is used as a clinical radiopaque marker.

In patients who have had a prosthesis in which metal articulates on metal, it is not uncommon to see a distinct gray-black discoloration at the synovial surface.[66] Microscopic examination of removed tissue shows irregular metal fragments measuring between 1 mm and 3 mm, mostly within histiocytes. The metallic nature of these particles has been confirmed by various techniques.[67] In those prostheses manufactured from titanium the metallic debris may be abundant.

Wear particles from the plastic, polyethylene components of artificial joints are only visible when the tissue is examined by polarized light. Mostly, they are intracellular and thread-like and measure about 1 mm across and 4–10 mm in length. A severe histiocytic response in the synovium is frequently observed, and foreign body giant cells are common. Occasionally, the fragments of polyethylene result in a tumor-like mass developing in the joint capsular tissue, and occasionally erosion of the periarticular bone has been observed (Fig. 13.29).

Both the polyethylene and the metallic components of the artificial joint are usually keyed to the underlying bone by an interposed layer of methyl methacrylate cement.

Abraded particles of cement produce in the capsular tissues a foreign body giant cell reaction. Often the particles are fairly small (10–30 mm), in which case they are surrounded by recognizable giant cells. Sometimes the pieces are very large (≥100 mm), and in this case histologic sections reveal large irregular spaces surrounded by flattened giant cells (Fig. 13.30). In the routine preparation of histologic sections, any cement in the tissue will be dissolved out by the solvents used in the processing, and microscopic examination will reveal only spaces where the cement was. However, it usually leaves behind a marker in the form of the insoluble barium sulfate that is put into the cement to render it radiopaque.

In all the removed prostheses we have examined, wear debris from one or all of these three sources was present histologically. This debris may be found also in draining lymph nodes. The long-term effects on the body are not known.

PIGMENTED VILLONODULAR SYNOVITIS AND TENOSYNOVITIS

Pigmented villonodular synovitis (PVNS) and tenosynovitis[68,69] is characterized by a nodular or diffuse proliferation of mononuclear cells, resembling synoviocytes, in the synovium of a tendon sheath or a joint. Frequently, these cells coalesce to form multinucleate giant cells, and for this reason the lesion is sometimes called a giant cell tumor of tendon sheath. In addition to the mononuclear histiocytic-type cells, one may also see some admixed chronic inflammatory cells (Fig. 13.31). A varying degree of collagen will be observed in the lesion; this may be minimal in amount or may be so extensive as to obliterate most of the cellular elements. The more cellular the tumor, the more likely one is to see mitotic figures and occasional bizarre cells.

Although grossly these lesions most often show some brown-tan staining, despite the name pigmented villonodular synovitis hemosiderin pigment is not abundant microscopically. It is probably secondary to post-traumatic hemorrhage rather than being an etiologic factor.

PVNS is most commonly seen in the fingers, where it has been called by various names, including giant cell tumor of tendon sheath, benign synovioma, and fibroxanthoma. It usually occurs in the flexor tendon sheath and is rarely seen on the extensor surface of the finger. In most instances of major joint involvement, it is the knee that is involved, although occasionally one may see involvement of the hip or other joints. In rare instances, multiple sites may be involved in the form of multiple nodules or a diffuse involvement of the synovium. In the latter case total removal may be impossible. Often the bone underlying the lesion is eroded, which may give rise to the erroneous impression on a radiograph that one is dealing with an osseous tumor that has broken out of the bone into the soft tissue. In such a case, multiple giant cells could lead to the incorrect diagnosis of a giant cell tumor of bone.

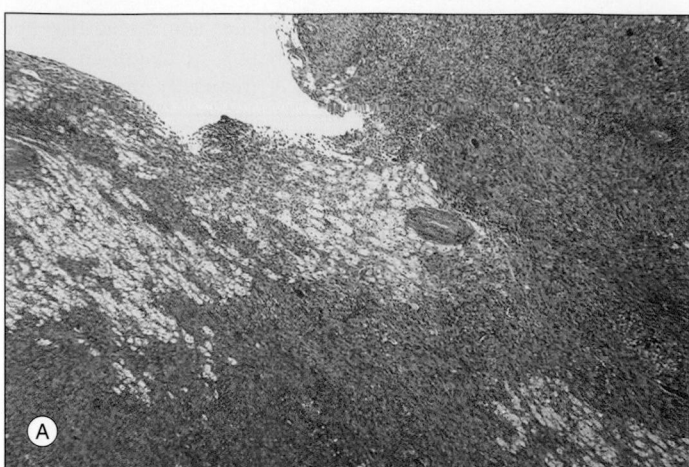

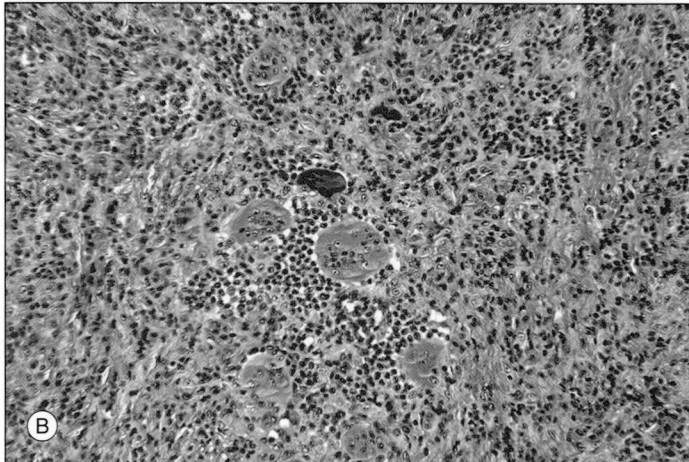

Fig. 13.31 A, Low-power view of a section taken from a patient with pigmented villonodular synovitis shows a cellular tumor with foci of foamy macrophages. **B,** Higher power shows that the tissue is composed of sheets of mononuclear cells, some of which are forming multinucleate giant cells. An admixture of chronic inflammatory cells is also present.

Although most patients with pigmented villonodular synovitis are middle-aged at the time the disease manifests, it may occur at any age. There is a high rate of local recurrence after surgery, particularly when the lesion involves a large joint.

SYNOVIAL CHONDROMATOSIS

Foci of metaplastic cartilage within the synovial tissues are not an uncommon finding in patients with various types of underlying arthritis, and often the cartilaginous nodules in the synovium may become detached and grow independently within the synovial fluid, where they may attain very large sizes.[70] In most instances, synovial cartilaginous loose bodies are secondary to some underlying joint condition, and frequently one can find at the centers of the loose bodies small fragments of bone or necrotic articular cartilage or fibrin that acted as seeds on which the cartilaginous loose body grew, rather like pearl formation inside an oyster. When such a loose body is sectioned, one will find evenly spaced chondrocytes of uniform size, although the cartilage may be excessively cellular

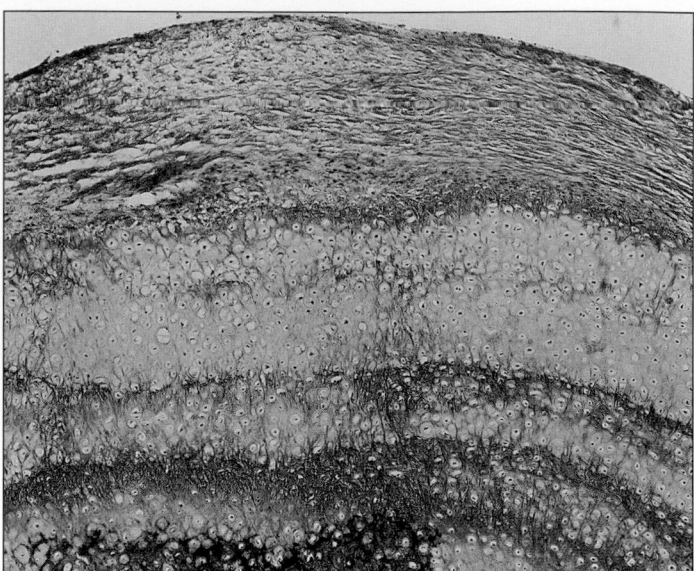

Fig. 13.32 Photomicrograph of a portion of loose body that formed secondary to a detached portion of the articular surface of a knee. The proliferating cartilage is very cellular but with regularly spaced chondrocytes. Concentric rings of calcification are apparent. Compare this photograph with Fig. 13.33.

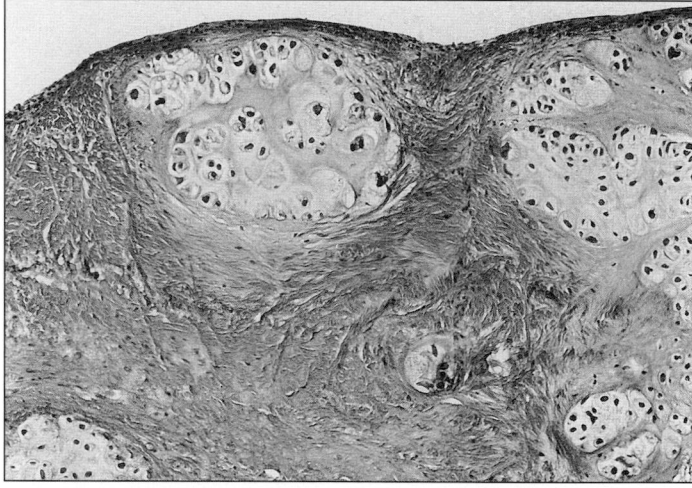

Fig. 13.33 Photomicrograph of a section taken from the synovium of a patient with primary synovial chondromatosis. The islands of cartilage, which form metaplastically within the synovium, are very irregular. The chondrocytes are crowded and vary considerably in size and shape.

(Fig. 13.32). When the cartilage nodules are in the form of loose bodies, they will undergo recurrent calcification as they get larger, leaving rings of calcium rather like the rings in a tree trunk. If the cartilage nodule is within the synovial membrane, then it may become invaded by blood vessels and endochondral ossification may occur.

Primary synovial chondromatosis, by contrast, is a very uncommon disease and is not preceded by any recognizable underlying arthritis.

Histologically, the lesions in primary synovial chondromatosis or chondrometaplasia are much more bizarre. The chondrocytes are cloned into very cellular atypical nests of chondrocytes, calcification occurs in a haphazard and diffuse manner, and the lesional tissue could easily be mistaken for chondrosarcoma (Fig. 13.33). After excision, the rate of recurrence is high. The lesions may occur both in large joints and also in the synovial sheaths of tendons, particularly in the fingers. Rare cases of malignant degeneration have been described.

TORN MENISCUS

A very common orthopedic lesion that frequently follows trauma is a tear of one or another of the menisci of the knee.[71] The tear is usually in the posterior horn and usually runs for some distance within the substance of the meniscus before turning medially to extend onto the medial edge, consequently giving rise to a tag or, on occasion, a 'bucket handle' type of tear. If these lesions have been present for a long time, the edges become very rounded, and occasionally a tag of the posterior meniscus may become detached into the joint, giving rise to a fibrocartilaginous loose body. Histologically, the meniscus is formed of a relatively avascular, highly collagenized tissue, in which the blood vessels are confined to the outer third. For this reason fibrous repair is not commonly seen; however, cystic degeneration with mucoid-filled microcysts is fairly common. Occasionally, large cysts may form, particularly in the lateral meniscus.

MISCELLANEOUS DISEASES OF CONNECTIVE TISSUE

GANGLION

A ganglion is a fibrous, walled cyst filled by clear mucinous fluid and usually without a recognizable cyst lining. Ganglia occur in the soft tissues, usually around the hands and feet, and particularly on the extensor surfaces near joints. They may arise as herniations of the synovium or from mucinous degeneration within dense fibrous connective tissue, possibly secondary to trauma. On occasion, they may erode the adjacent bone and even become totally intraosseous; the most common site for such an intraosseous ganglion is the medial malleolus of the tibia.[72]

BURSITIS

Acute or chronic bursitis is clinically characterized by pain, redness, and/or swelling of one of the many synovium-lined bursae that lie between muscles, tendons, and bone prominences, especially around the joints. Bursitis is usually caused by chronic trauma. It often occurs in the shoulders of professional athletes and in the prepatellar and infrapatellar bursae of those who frequently kneel. Bursitis is sometimes observed as a complication of rheumatoid arthritis or infection. In cases of rheumatoid arthritis, a cyst may occur, particularly in the popliteal area (where it is known as a Baker's cyst) and may extend far into the calf. In the past, bursitis from infection was frequently due to tuberculosis. The bursa may also be involved in other conditions that commonly affect the synovial membrane

(e.g. gout, synovial chondromatosis, or pigmented villonodular synovitis). Sometimes, extensive calcification may complicate a chronically inflamed bursa, which renders it visible on radiologic examination.

On gross examination of an inflamed bursa, the wall of the bursal sac is usually markedly thickened and the lining often appears injected and shaggy owing to fibrinous exudation into the cavity. The microscopic findings depend on the etiology, and the various diseases that might affect the synovium, including infection, should be carefully sought; however, most cases are post-traumatic in origin, and scarring and chronic inflammation predominate.

Treatment depends on the etiology and the extent of the lesion.

TRIGGER FINGER, DE QUERVAIN'S DISEASE, AND CARPAL TUNNEL SYNDROME

In both trigger finger and de Quervain's disease,[73] a thickening of the tendon sheath gives rise to clinical problems with movement of the tendon through the sheath. In carpal tunnel syndrome[73] there is compression of the median nerve by thickening of the tissue forming the transverse carpal ligament. These conditions may precede or accompany some systemic disease of the connective tissues such as rheumatoid arthritis. Histologic examination of the resected thickened tendon sheath will generally show a rather clear-cut cartilaginous or fibrocartilaginous metaplasia of the otherwise delicate tendon sheath (Fig. 13.34). In some cases of carpal tunnel syndrome, amyloid deposits have been recognized as the causative agent.[74]

MORTON'S NEUROMA

Morton's neuroma[75] is a lesion characterized by thickening of the interdigital nerve as it runs between the third and fourth metatarsal heads. Clinically, the patient, who is usually a woman, experiences sharp shooting pains in the sole of the foot extending onto the extensor surface. The resected specimen usually includes the neurovascular bundle and its bifurcation to the third and fourth toe. Just proximal to the bifurcation a fusiform thickening of the neurovascular bundle can usually be observed. Histologic sections will generally show two characteristic features: (1) an occlusion of the digital artery, and (2) extensive fibrosis both around and within the nerve, giving rise to a marked depletion of axons within the digital nerve (Fig. 13.35). The term neuroma is a misnomer, because there is no evidence in the vast majority of cases of either a traumatic type of neuroma or a neurilemmoma.

PROLAPSED INTERVERTEBRAL DISC

Curettage of prolapsed intervertebral disc tissue[76,77] is an operation commonly undertaken by either orthopedic surgeons or neuro-surgeons. It usually provides multiple gelatinous pieces of tissue, which on histologic examination will be seen to be composed of portions of fibrous tissue, fibrocartilage, and cartilaginous tissue, the latter with a considerable amount of myxoid material in the matrix. Often, the chondrocytes are necrotic, but in other areas the chondrocytes may be seen to be proliferating, and large clones of

Fig. 13.34 Photomicrograph of a section taken from a patient with a trigger finger. The wall of the tendon sheath, which is normally a very delicate structure, shows a localized thickening by densely collagenized tissue with cells resembling cartilage cells (i.e. fibrocartilage).

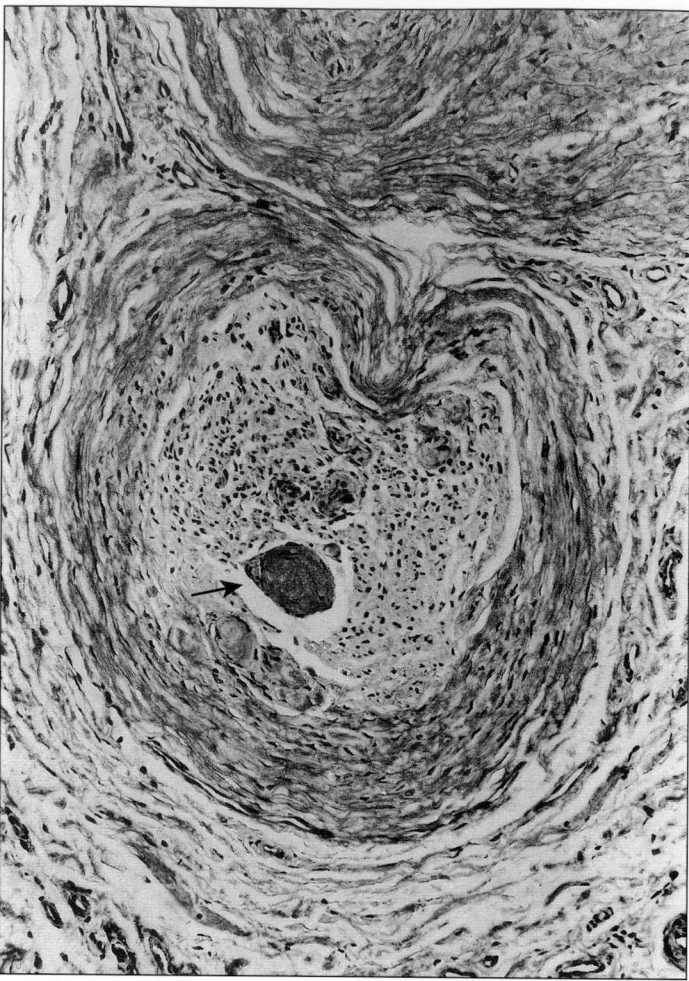

Fig. 13.35 Photomicrograph of a histologic section taken from a patient with Morton's neuroma. The nerve bundles show considerable fibrous proliferation and collagen deposition in the perineurium, as well as within the endoneurium. There is a marked diminution in the number of axons present, and on occasion focal deposits of homogeneous pink material (Renaut bodies, arrow.)

cells may be observed. Just as cartilage loose in the joint may give rise to cartilage proliferation and loose bodies, it is entirely possible that prolapsed intervertebral disc tissue may also, when removed from the constraints of the annulus fibrosa, undergo cellular proliferation and growth and result in secondary nerve root compression.

ACKNOWLEDGMENT

I am extremely grateful to Dr. E. DiCarlo and Dr. Philip Rusli for their help in the preparation of this chapter.

REFERENCES

1. Drury DJ, Bullough PG. Improved photographic reproduction of bone and cartilage specimens using ultraviolet illumination. Med Biol Illus 1970; 20:57–58.

2. Bullough P, Goodfellow J. The significance of the fine structure of articular cartilage. J Bone Joint Surg Br 1968; 50:852–857.

3. Hyttinen MM, Arokoski JP, Parkkinen JJ, et al. Age matters: collagen birefringence of superficial articular cartilage is increased in young guinea-pigs but decreased in older animals after identical physiological type of joint loading. Osteoarthritis Cartilage 2001; 9:694–701.

4. Minns RJ, Steven FS. The collagen fibril organization in human articular cartilage. J Anat 1977; 123: 37–457.

5. Scott JE. The histochemistry of cartilage proteoglycans in light and electron microscopy. In: Ali SY, Elves MW, Leaback DH, eds. Normal and osteoarthrotic articular cartilage. London: Institute of Orthopaedics (University of London); 1974: 19–32.

6. Knudson CB, Knudson W. Cartilage proteoglycans. Semin Cell Dev Biol 2001;12: 69–78.

7. Jowsey J. The bone biopsy. New York: Plenum Medical Book Co.; 1977.

8. Enlow DH. Principles of bone remodeling. An account of postnatal growth and remodeling processes in long bones and the mandible. Springfield, IL: Charles C Thomas; 1963.

9. Jaffe HL. Metabolic, degenerative, and inflammatory diseases of bones and joints. Philadelphia: Lea & Febiger; 1972.

10. Ghokaley JA, Robey PG, Boskey AL. The biochemistry of bone. In: Marcus R, Feldman D, Kelsey J, eds. Osteoporosis. San Diego: Academic Press; 2001:107–188.

11. Cormack DH. Bone. In: Cormack DH, ed. Ham's histology. Philadelphia: Lippincott-Raven; 1987.

12. Sokoloff L. Note on the histology of cement lines. In: Kenedi RM, ed. Perspectives in biomedical engineering. London: MacMillan; 1973:135.

13. Riggs BL, Melton LJ. Osteoporosis: etiology, diagnosis, and management. Philadelphia: Lippincott-Raven Publishers; 1995.

14. Johnston CC Jr, Lavy N, Lord T, et al. Osteopetrosis. A clinical, genetic, metabolic, and morphologic study of the dominantly inherited, benign form. Medicine (Baltimore) 1968; 47:149–167.

15. Ham AW, Harris WR. Repair and transplantation of bone. In: Bourne GH, ed. Biochemistry and physiology of bone. New York: Academic Press; 1971.

16. Cruess R, Dumont J. Healing of bone, tendon and ligament. In: Rockwood CA Jr, Green DP, eds. Fractures. Philadelphia: Lippincott; 1975:97.

17. Yamamoto T, Bullough PG. Subchondral insufficiency fracture of the femoral head: a differential diagnosis in acute onset of coxarthrosis in the elderly. Arthritis Rheum 1999; 42:2719–2723.

18. Postel M, Kerboull M. Total prosthetic replacement in rapidly destructive arthrosis of the hip joint. Clin Orthop 1970; 72:138–144.

19. Yamamoto T, Schneider R, Bullough PG. Insufficiency subchondral fracture of the femoral head. Am J Surg Pathol 2000; 24:464–468.

20. Yamamoto T, Bullough PG. The role of subchondral insufficiency fracture in rapid destruction of the hip joint: a preliminary report. Arthritis Rheum 2000; 43:2423–2427.

21. Urbaniak JR, Jones JP. Osteonecrosis: etiology, diagnosis, and treatment. Rosemont, IL: American Academy of Orthopaedic Surgeons; 1997.

22. Catto M. A histological study of avascular necrosis of the femoral head after transcervical fracture. J Bone Joint Surg Br 1965; 47:749–776.

23. Bullough PG, Kambolis CP, Marcove RC, et al. Bone infarctions not associated with caisson disease. J Bone Joint Surg Am 1965; 47:477–491.

24. Mirra JM, Bullough PG, Marcove RC, et al. Malignant fibrous histiocytoma and osteosarcoma in association with bone infarcts; report of four cases, two in caisson workers. J Bone Joint Surg Am 1974; 56:932–940.

25. Smith R. Fibrodysplasia (myositis) ossificans progressiva. Clinical lessons from a rare disease. Clin Orthop 1998; 346:7–14.

26. Paterson DC. Myositis ossificans circumscripta. Report of four cases without history of injury. J Bone Joint Surg Br 1970; 52:296–301.

27. Trelstad RL, Rubin D, Gross J. Osteogenesis imperfecta congenita: evidence for a generalized molecular disorder of collagen. Lab Invest 1977; 36:501–508.

28. Byers PH. Disorders of collagen biosynthesis and structure. In: Scriver CR, Beaudet AL, Sly W, Valle D, eds. The metabolic and molecular bases of inherited disease. New York: McGraw-Hill; 2001:5241–5286.

29. Neufeld EF, Muenzer J. The mucopolysaccharidoses. In: Scriver CR, Beaudet AL, Sly W, Valle D, eds. The metabolic and molecular bases of inherited disease. New York: McGraw-Hill; 2001:3421–3452.

30. Teitelbaum SL, Rosenberg EM, Bates M, Avioli LV. The effects of phosphate and vitamin D therapy on osteopenic, hypophosphatemic osteomalacia of childhood. Clin Orthop 1976; 116:38–47.

31. Whalen JP, Horwith M, Krook L, et al. Calcitonin treatment in hereditary bone dysplasia with hyperphosphatasemia: a radiographic and histologic study of bone. Am J Roentgenol 1977; 129:29–35.

32. Malluche HH, Faugere MC, Smith AJ Jr, Friedler RM. Aluminum intoxication of bone in renal failure – fact or fiction? Kidney Int Suppl 1986; 18:S70–S73.

33. Epker BN. A quantitative histologic study of the effects of fluoride on resorption and formation in animal and human bone. Clin Orthop 1966; 49:77–87.

34. Wilde CD, Jaworski ZF, Villanueva AR, Frost HM. Quantitative histological measurements of bone turnover in primary hyperparathyroidism. Calcif Tissue Res 1973; 12:137–142.

35. Teitelbaum SL, Bullough PG. The pathophysiology of bone and joint disease. Am J Pathol 1979; 96:282–354.

36. Anderson PH, O'Loughlin PD, et al. Determinants of circulating 1,25 –dihydroxyvitamin D3 levels: the role of renal synthesis and catabolism of vitamin D. J Steroid Biochem Mol Biol 2004; 89–90: 111–3.

37. Lakhanpal S, Ginsburg WW, Luthra HS, Hunder GG. Transient regional osteoporosis. A study of 56 cases and review of the literature. Ann Intern Med 1987; 106:444–450.

38. Bullough PG. Massive osteolysis. N Y State J Med 1971; 71:2267–2278.

39. Coe FL, Favus MJ. Disorders of bone and mineral metabolism. Philadelphia: Lippincott Williams & Wilkins; 2002.

40. Barry H. Paget's disease of bone. Edinburgh: Livingstone; 1969.

41. Rebel A, Malkani K, Basle M, Bregeon C. Osteoclast ultrastructure in Paget's disease. Calcif Tissue Res 1976; 2:187–199.

42. Price CH, Goldie W. Paget's sarcoma of bone. A study of eighty cases from the Bristol and the Leeds bone tumour registries. J Bone Joint Surg Br 1969; 51:205–224.

43. Gaines JJ Jr. The pathology of alkaptonuric ochronosis. Hum Pathol 1989; 20:40–46.

44. O'Brien WM, Banfield WG, Sokoloff L. Studies on the pathogenesis of ochronotic arthropathy. Arthritis Rheum 1961; 4:137–152.

45. Kinnett JG, Bullough PG. Identification of calcium oxalate deposits in bone by electron diffraction. Arch Pathol Lab Med 1976; 100:656–658.

46. McCarty DJ. Calcium pyrophosphate dihydrate crystal deposition disease. Br J Rheumatol 1993; 32:177–179.

47. Becker MA. Clinical gout and the pathogenesis of hyperuricemia. In: Koopman WJ, ed. Arthritis and allied conditions: a textbook of rheumatology. Philadelphia: Lippincott Williams & Wilkins; 2001:2281–2313.

48. Beutler E, Grabowski GA. Gaucher disease. In: Scriver CR, Beaudet AL, Sly W, Valle D, eds. The metabolic and molecular bases of inherited disease. New York: McGraw-Hill; 2001:3635–3668.

49. Lazzarini L, Mader JT, et al. Osteomyelitis in long bones. J Bone Joint Surg Am 2004; 86A: 2305–18.

50. Green NE, Edwards K. Bone and joint infections in children. Orthop Clin North Am 1987; 18:555–576.

51. Fechner RE, Mills SE. Tumors of the bones and joints. Washington, DC: Armed Forces Institute of Pathology; 1993.

52. Dorfman HD, Czerniak B. Bone tumors. St. Louis: Mosby; 1998.

53. Lieberman PH, Jones CR, Steinman RM, et al. Langerhans cell (eosinophilic) granulomatosis. A clinicopathologic study encompassing 50 years. Am J Surg Pathol 1996; 20:519–552.

54. Bullough PG. Joints. In: Sternberg SS, ed. Histology for pathologists. Philadelphia: Lippincott-Raven;1997: 107–26.

55. Hamerman D, Rosenberg LC, Schubert M. Diarthrodial joints revisited. J Bone Joint Surg Am 1970; 52:725–774.

56. Hardingham TE. Articular cartilage. In: Isenberg DA, et al., eds. Oxford textbook of rheumatology. Oxford, Oxford University Press; 2004: 325–33.

57. Paget S, Bullough PG. Synovium and synovial fluid. In: Owen R, Goodfellow JW, Bullough PG, eds. Scientific foundation of orthopaedics and traumatology. Philadelphia: Saunders; 1980:18–22.

58. Meisel AD, Bullough PG, Twersky J. Atlas of osteoarthritis. Philadelphia: Lea & Febiger; 1984.

59. Nichols EH, Richardson FL. Arthritis deformans. J Med Res 1909; 21:149–221.

60. Haynes MK, Hume EL, Smith JB. Phenotypic characterization of inflammatory cells from osteoarthritic synovium and synovial fluids. Clin Immunol 2002; 105:315–325.

61. Perry GH, Smith MJ, Whiteside CG. Spontaneous recovery of the joint space in degenerative hip disease. Ann Rheum Dis 1972; 31:440–448.

62. Firestein GS. Rheumatoid synovitis and pannus. In: Hochberg MC, Silman AJ, Smolen JS, et al., eds. Rheumatology. Edinburgh: Mosby; 2003:855–884.

63. Klippel JH, Weyand CM, Crofford LJ, Stone JH. Primer on the rheumatic diseases. Atlanta, GA: Arthritis Foundation; 2001.

64. Nepom B, King RA. Rheumatoid arthritis. In: King RA, Rotter JI, Motulsky AG, eds. The genetic basis of common diseases. Oxford, Oxford University Press; 2002: 587–603.

65. Sokoloff S. Pathophysiology of peripheral blood vessels in collagen diseases. In: Orbison JL, Smith DE, eds. The peripheral blood vessels. Baltimore: Williams & Wilkins; 1963.

66. DiCarlo EF, Bullough PG. The biologic responses to orthopedic implants and their wear debris. Clin Mater 1992; 9:235–260.

67. Willert HG, Semlitsch M. Tissue reactions to plastic and metallic wear products of joint endoprostheses. Clin Orthop 1996; 333:4–14.

68. Byers PD, Cotton RE, Deacon OW, et al. The diagnosis and treatment of pigmented villonodular synovitis. J Bone Joint Surg Br 1968; 50:290–305.

69. Schwartz HS, Unni KK, Pritchard DJ. Pigmented villonodular synovitis. A retrospective review of affected large joints. Clin Orthop 1989; 247:243–255.

70. Villacin AB, Brigham LN, Bullough PG. Primary and secondary synovial chondrometaplasia: histopathologic and clinicoradiologic differences. Hum Pathol 1979; 10:439–451.

71. Smillie IS. Injuries of the knee joint. London: Churchill Livingstone; 1978.

72. Kambolis C, Bullough PG, Jaffe HI. Ganglionic cystic defects of bone. J Bone Joint Surg Am 1973; 55:496–505.

73. Phalen GS. The birth of a syndrome, or carpal tunnel revisited. J Hand Surg [Am] 1981; 6:109–110.

74. Massachussetts General Hospital. Case records. Weekly clinicopathological exercises. Case 10. N Engl J Med 1972; 286:534–539.

75. Asbury AK, Johnson PC. Pathology of peripheral nerve. Philadelphia: Saunders; 1978.

76. Schmorl G. The displacement of intervertebral disc tissue in the human spine. In: Junghanns H, Besemann EF, eds. Health and disease. Orlando, FL: Grune & Stratton; 1971:158–184.

77. Bullough PG, Boachie-Adjei O. Atlas of spinal diseases. New York: Gower Medical Publishing; 1988.

Neoplastic and tumor-like lesions of bone

14

G. Petur Nielsen   Lester J. Layfield   Andrew E. Rosenberg

BONE TUMORS

INTRODUCTION

Neoplastic and non-neoplastic tumors of bone often pose diagnostic challenges to surgical pathologists. This is not surprising, as bone tumors have a broad spectrum of findings and are infrequently encountered in routine surgical pathology. The key to their accurate recognition is the utilization of an integrated approach that assesses and correlates the clinical, radiographic, morphologic, and biologic behavior of these lesions.

In most instances, this is best accomplished when the pathologist is a participatory member of a multidisciplinary group that includes orthopaedic surgeons, radiologists, and clinicians who specialize in the treatment of patients with these tumors. This team of physicians works together to diagnose the lesion and design an optimal treatment strategy that incorporates the stage of the tumor and the prognosis of the patient. Diagnosing bone tumors in isolation without pertinent information is inappropriate and predisposes to diagnostic errors that may have dire consequences for the patient.

EPIDEMIOLOGY

Tumors of the skeleton develop in all age groups, affect any bone in the body and can be benign or malignant. In many instances, however, there is a relationship between the age of the patient and the specific location and type of tumor (Tables 14.1, 14.2). The overall frequency of bone tumors is unknown, as most benign tumors are asymptomatic and only detected as incidental findings. Some benign tumors are quite common. For example, fibrous cortical defect develops in 50% of boys and 20% of girls older than 2 years of age, and hemangiomas of the spine can be identified in 10% of the population, indicating that benign tumors and tumor-like lesions of bone affect millions of individuals.[1-4] Based on this information, it is estimated that benign tumors and tumor-like lesions outnumber their malignant counterparts by at least 10 000:1. Bone sarcomas as these data infer are rare; only approximately 2500 new cases are diagnosed annually (0.8 cases per 100 000 persons per year) in the US, where they account for merely 0.2% of invasive cancers.[5,6] Unlike benign tumors, the majority of which occur during the first three decades of life, bone sarcomas have a bimodal age distribution; the first peak occurs in patients 10–20 years old and the second develops during the seventh decade of life. The risk of developing a bone sarcoma is equal in both of these age groups but in absolute numbers more bone sarcomas are diagnosed during the second decade of life.[7] Statistically, the younger the patient the more likely a bone tumor is to be benign, since benign tumors outnumber sarcomas, commonly occur in childhood, and their frequency diminishes with age.

Table 14.1 Association between age and type of common bone tumors

Age	Benign tumors	Malignant tumors
Infant	Myofibroma, chest wall hamartoma Langerhans cell histiocytosis	Metastatic neuroblastoma and rhabdomyosarcoma
Child	Fibrous cortical defect	Ewing's sarcoma
Adolescent	Non-ossifying fibroma Osteochondroma Unicameral bone cyst Aneurysmal bone cyst	Ewing's sarcoma Osteosarcoma
Young adult	Enchondroma Fibrous dysplasia	Osteosarcoma
Middle-aged adult	Enchondroma Giant cell tumor	Chondrosarcoma Malignant fibrous histiocytoma
Older adult	Enchondroma	Chondrosarcoma Metastatic carcinoma —-Multiple myeloma

Table 14.2 Location of primary bone tumors

Site	Benign (%)	Malignant (%)
Femur	29.5	26
Tibia	16.5	10
Humerus	11	9
Hand	7	‹1
Vertebra	6	8.9
Innominate	5.7	13

Source: modified from data from the Mayo Clinic.[4]

There is a paucity of information available regarding the distribution of benign bone tumors in relation to patient gender, which reflects the fact that most benign tumors are asymptomatic and do not undergo diagnostic evaluation. Existing estimates suggest, however, that benign tumors occur more frequently in males, although there is no clear understanding of this association. In contrast, data concerning bone sarcomas are more comprehensive and reveal that males and females are affected at a ratio of 1:0.7.[8]

Although primary tumors develop in all parts of the skeleton, most demonstrate a predilection for the long tubular bones (see Table 14.2). Benign tumors tend to arise in the appendicular skeleton, with approximately 45% developing in the femur and tibia, usually about the knee. In comparison to benign tumors, bone sarcomas more frequently involve the pelvis and axial skeleton and rarely affect the small bones of the hands and feet.

ETIOLOGY

Although it is believed that chromosomal mutations in mesenchymal stem cells are responsible for neoplastic transformation, proliferation, and, ultimately, bone tumor formation, genetic mutations specific to particular bone tumor type are infrequently identified. Benign and malignant bone tumors are, however, components of a variety of genetic syndromes including Ollier's disease, Maffucci syndrome, multiple hereditary osteochondromas, bilateral retinoblastoma, Li–Fraumeni syndrome, Gardner syndrome, Mazabraud syndrome, McCune–Albright syndrome, neurofibromatosis, and diaphyseal medullary stenosis.

A variety of diseases create conditions within bone that facilitate the development of neoplasms, especially sarcomas. The most important of these are Paget's disease, radiation injury, bone infarction, and chronic osteomyelitis. Pre-existing benign tumors undergo malignant transformation infrequently and those that do so are most commonly enchondroma and osteochondroma; rarely does it occur with fibrous dysplasia or a simple bone cyst.

Recently, reports have documented the development of sarcomas adjacent to orthopaedic implants. The incidence of this dreaded complication appears, however, to be exceedingly small, and the carcinogenic properties of the chemical components of the implants in humans are thought to be minimal. Nonetheless, this phenomenon deserves further investigation and monitoring.[9,10]

CLASSIFICATION

Primary bone tumors are classified according to the normal cell or tissue type that they recapitulate and whether they are benign or malignant (Table 14.3). The vast majority differentiates along the cell lines or tissue types that compose the skeletal system; only a small number have consistent and distinctive clinicopathologic features but lack a normal tissue counterpart. Further subclassification of bone tumors is based on their specific histological characteristics, their relationship to the underlying bone, and the presence of pre-existing conditions.

Importantly, different disease processes can produce bony changes that may mimic or simulate a bone neoplasm. Some of these more common reactive processes are listed in Table 14.4.

CLINICAL PRESENTATION

The clinical presentation of bone tumors is highly variable and generally non-specific. The vast majority of benign tumors are asymptomatic; however, larger ones may produce a palpable or visually obvious mass or deformity. Symptoms associated with benign or malignant tumors are usually localized to the affected site and include pain, swelling, and mechanical disorders. The pain may be intermittent, constant, progressive, and radiating. Rarely, its pattern is suggestive of a particular tumor, such as in osteoid osteoma, where patients typically present with night pain that is exquisitely sensitive to aspirin or nonsteroidal anti-inflammatory analgesics. Swelling of long duration is usually associated with benign lesions, whereas rapid

Table 14.3 Classification of primary bone tumors

Cartilage tumors
Cartilaginous hamartoma
Osteochondromyxoid hamartoma
Chondroma
Enchondroma
Juxtacortical
Chondroblastoma
Chondromyxoid fibroma
    Chondrosarcoma
    Conventional
        Intramedullary
        Juxtacortical
    Dedifferentiated
    Mesenchymal
    Clear cell

Bone-forming tumors
Osteoma
Enostosis (bone island)
Osteoid osteoma
Osteoblastoma
Osteosarcoma
    Intramedullary
        Conventional
            Osteoblastic
            Chondroblastic
            Fibroblastic
        Telangiectatic
        Small cell
        Well differentiated
    Juxtacortical
        Parosteal
        Periosteal
        Surface high-grade

Fibroblastic tumors
Myofibroma
Fibrous cortical defect
Non-ossifying fibroma
Benign fibrous histiocytoma
Desmoplastic fibroma
Fibrosarcoma
Malignant fibrous histiocytoma

Neuroectodermal tumors
Ewing's sarcoma/primitive neuroectodermal tumor
Pigmented neuroectodermal tumor of infancy

Notochordal tumors
Benign notochordal tumor
Chordoma

Vascular tumors
Hemangioma
Epithelioid hemangioendothelioma
Angiosarcoma

Fatty tumors
Lipoma
Liposarcoma

Smooth muscle tumors
Leiomyoma
Leiomyosarcoma

Nerve sheath tumors
Neurofibroma
Schwannoma
Malignant peripheral nerve sheath tumor

Table 14.3 Classification of primary bone tumors (*cont'd*)

Hematopoietic tumors
Malignant lymphoma
Plasmacytoma/multiple myeloma

Miscellaneous
Fibrous dysplasia
Osteofibrous dysplasia
Adamantinoma
Unicameral bone cyst
Aneurysmal bone cyst
Giant cell tumor
Giant cell reparative granuloma
Erdheim–Chester disease
Langerhans cell histiocytosis

Table 14.4 Classification of reactive lesions that simulate neoplasms

Infection

Fracture callus

Brown tumor

Subungual exostosis

Florid reactive periostitis

Bizarre parosteal osteochondromatous proliferation (BPOP)

Table 14.5 AJCC staging system of bone sarcomas

Primary tumor (T)

TX:	Primary tumor cannot be assessed
T0:	No evidence of primary tumor
T1:	Tumor ≤8 cm in greatest dimension
T2:	Tumor >8 cm in greatest dimension
T3:	Discontinuous tumors in primary bone site

Regional lymph nodes (N)

NX:	Regional lymph nodes cannot be assessed
N0:	No regional lymph node metastases
N1:	Regional lymph node metastasis

Distant metastasis (M)

MX:	Distant metastasis cannot be assessed
M0:	No distant metastasis
M1:	Distant metastasis
M1a:	Lung
M1b:	Other distant sites

Histopathologic grading (G)

TNM two-grade system	Three-grade system	Four-grade system
Low-grade	Grade 1	Grades 1 or 2
High-grade	Grades 2 or 3	Grades 3 or 4

Stages

Stage	T	N	M	Grade
Stage 1A	T1	N0,NX	M0	Low-grade
Stage 1B	T2	N0,NX	M0	Low-grade
Stage IIA	T1	N0,NX	M0	High-grade
Stage IIB	T2	N0,NX	M0	High-grade
Stage III	T3	N0,NX	M0	Any grade
Stage IVA	Any T	N0,NX	M1a	Any grade
Stage IVB	Any T	N1	Any M	Any grade
	Any T	Any N	M1b	Any grade

Source: With permission from AJCC Cancer Staging Manual, 6th edn. New York: Springer; 2002.

swelling in conjunction with skin changes, such as red-violaceous discoloration and the development of prominent blood vessels, is commonly a manifestation of malignancies. Mechanical dysfunction is usually in the form of restricted movement and may result from tumor bulk or synovitis caused by a periarticular mass. Systemic symptoms of fever, fatigue, and weight loss are usually associated with malignant bone neoplasms and are frequently indicative of advanced disease.

A minority of bone tumors are complicated by a pathologic fracture. The fracture may be the heralding event for both benign and malignant neoplasms and results from an enlarging tumor that destroys the underlying bone. Eventually, minimal trauma causes the bone to fail and break, producing sudden excruciating pain, swelling, and hemorrhage.

GRADING AND STAGING BONE SARCOMAS

The histologic grading of bone sarcomas is the pathologist's attempt to predict their biological behavior. Grading systems similar to the National Cancer Institute (NCI) and FNCC schemes devised for soft tissue sarcomas have not been developed and universally applied to bone sarcomas.[11,12] There are, however, grading schemes that some investigators have proposed for specific types of sarcomas, especially chondrosarcoma.[13] Regardless, all bone sarcomas, exclusive of Ewing's sarcoma/primitive neuroectodermal tumor and chordoma, are typically graded. The two-, three-, or four-tiered grading systems currently used are based on the assessment of standard morphologic criteria, including the degree of differentiation, cytologic atypia, mitotic activity, and necrosis. The goal of the different tiered systems is to distinguish sarcomas associated with a low probability

of dissemination (low-grade; <25% chance of metastasis) from those that are aggressive and have a high risk of systemic spread (high-grade; >25% chance of metastasis). Accordingly, in the three-tiered system, grade 1 sarcomas are low-grade and are usually hypocellular to moderately cellular. The tumor cells demonstrate mild cytologic atypia, closely resemble their normal tissue counterparts, and have few if any mitoses and minimal necrosis. For treatment purposes, grade 2 and 3 sarcomas are considered high-grade and are moderately to densely cellular. The cells are moderately to severely pleomorphic and hyperchromatic, are mitotically active with atypical forms, and the tumor contains areas of necrosis. In a similar fashion, in the four-tiered system, grade 1 and 2 sarcomas are treated as low-grade and grade 3 and 4 sarcomas are viewed as high-grade. Generally, the focus of treatment of low-grade sarcomas is local control, whereas systemic therapy combined with local control is used to attempt to cure patients with high-grade sarcomas.

Bone sarcomas are staged to help provide important prognostic information and offer guidelines for effective treatment. The two major staging systems used are those endorsed by the American Joint Commission on Cancer (AJCC) and the Musculoskeletal Tumor Society.[14,15] The AJCC system incorporates tumor grade, size, and status and location of metastases (Table 14.5). In contrast, the Musculoskeletal Tumor Society staging scheme is geared more towards surgical staging and is based on tumor grade, anatomic extent, and presence of metastases (Table 14.6).

Table 14.6 Musculoskeletal Tumor Society staging of bone sarcomas

Stage	Criteria
1A	Low-grade, intracompartmental
1B	Low-grade, extracompartmental
IIA	High-grade, intracompartmental
IIB	High-grade, extracompartmental
III	Any grade, metastasis

RADIOGRAPHIC IMAGING

Radiographic imaging permits assessment of the in vivo gross characteristics of bone tumors and the skeletal responses to them. This information is important in determining the type and aggressiveness of the lesion, which in turn are critical to the complete interpretation of histologic specimens.

Plain X-ray, the traditional technique for imaging, helps delineate the location, size, and radiodensity of the tumor and also demonstrates the type of margin, as well as the nature of the periosteal reaction, if present.[16] Tumors that are small and well circumscribed with sclerotic margins are usually benign. In contrast, neoplasms that are large and destructive with poorly defined or permeative margins are malignant until proven otherwise. Since bone tumors tend to affect certain age groups, arise in particular regions of specific bones, and have distinctive radiographic features, plain films are important in generating an appropriate differential diagnosis.

Computed tomography (CT) scans provide additional detailed information of tumors. This includes their tissue density and mineral content, their relationship to the medullary cavity, cortex, and soft tissue, the extent of periosteal reaction, and the location of the tumor with regard to important neighboring structures.[16]

Magnetic resonance imaging (MRI) is the technique of choice for assessing the composition of the tumor, the extent of involvement of the underlying bone, and the proximity of the tumor to important anatomic structures.[16] The limits of the tumor, as determined by MRI, are frequently used to map out the lines of excision required to achieve complete en bloc resection with negative margins.

Bone scintigraphy with technetium-99m-labeled diphosphonate is one of the most sensitive screening methods to evaluate the entire skeleton for many pathologic conditions. As regards bone tumors, these scans are particularly useful for identifying polyostotic disease (fibrous dysplasia, enchondromatosis, etc.) and the presence of osseous metastases. Avidity for technetium-99 correlates with the degree of vascularity and amount of cell activity within a tumor. Not surprisingly, most bone tumors are positive on these scans; however, Langerhans cell histiocytosis and malignant plasma cell tumors (plasmacytoma) are some of the few lesions that are frequently negative.

Positron emission tomography (PET scan) is a recently introduced technique that can be used for staging and assessing treatment effect in musculoskeletal malignancies.[17] Viable tumor deposits, either primary or metastatic, are usually positive on PET scan; however, PET scan turns negative once the tumor has undergone necrosis following successful treatment with either radiation and/or chemotherapy. In this manner, the effectiveness of therapy as well as the progression or recurrence of the tumor can be monitored.

BONE TUMOR SPECIMENS

Tissue from bone tumors is retrieved to make a primary diagnosis, eradicate the neoplasm, document recurrence or metastasis, and assess treatment effect. The tissue is usually obtained in the form of fine-needle aspiration cytology (FNA), needle cores, open curettage (which yields multiple, irregular fragments of tissue), or an en bloc resection. In many instances, frozen section analysis can be performed to facilitate diagnosis.

Fine-needle aspiration

Cytologic evaluation has been reliably and successfully used for many years in the investigation and diagnosis of metastases to skeletal structures. FNA of primary bone tumors, however, presents additional challenges because of the morphologic heterogeneity of the tumors and their relative rarity.[18,19] Knowledge of the cytologic appearance of primary bone tumors is important because of the speed and low cost of diagnosing them by FNA and because they may be inadvertently aspirated during the work-up of suspected metastatic disease, from which they must be distinguished.

The utility of FNA in the evaluation of skeletal lesions has been demonstrated by a favorable comparison of its accuracy rate to that achieved by other available biopsy techniques. Additionally, studies have substantiated that bone sarcomas sampled by FNA can be graded with a high degree of success.[20–22] FNA diagnosis of primary bone tumors has been reported to have an accuracy rate of 70–90% when the goal is distinguishing benign from malignant lesions.[23] Cytopathology is significantly less accurate, however, when precise subclassification of tumors is required.[23] Furthermore, not all lesions primary within the skeletal system are amenable to diagnosis by FNA. For instance, predominantly cystic lesions such as a simple bone cyst or an aneurysmal bone cyst may yield specimens of insufficient cellularity to allow diagnosis. Some bone-forming tumors, including osteoma and osteoid osteoma, produce substantial amounts of ossified matrix that precludes sampling by fine-caliber needles.

FNA evaluation is most successful when Romanowsky-stained preparations are used in conjunction with hematoxylin and eosin (H&E)-stained cell block material. The Romanowsky-based stains are superior to other methods for demonstrating cartilaginous and osseous matrix, while cell block specimens facilitate the assessment of architecture and provide tissue for special studies including immunohistochemistry, fluorescence in situ hybridization (FISH), and molecular analysis. Some authors have even suggested using FNA in conjunction with core biopsy to optimize diagnostic accuracy. Diagnosis of bone tumors by CT-directed FNA is most successful when intraoperative review is performed by a cytotechnologist or cytopathologist who is an expert in musculoskeletal lesions. Such an approach minimizes the number of passes during CT biopsy and allows optimal triage of tissue for special studies.

Needle core biopsy

If a tumor is being diagnosed via needle biopsy, which is usually performed with CT guidance, we recommend that three cores of tumor-bearing tissue be obtained. In most instances, a frozen section can be performed on one core to confirm that diagnostic tissue has been received, provide provisional diagnostic information, and facilitate triage of the remaining tissue. This core can be kept frozen for immunohistochemical and molecular studies if needed. The second core should be fixed in formalin and processed routinely for the production of standard H&E-stained slides. Portions of the third core can be submitted for electron microscopy, cytogenetics, or molecular analysis, if such ancillary techniques are warranted.

Curettage

Open biopsy for primary diagnosis typically generates specimens that are amenable to frozen section analysis. The tissue, including bone (except for pieces of cortex), can be frozen to construct a working diagnosis and allow for the appropriate triage of tissue. If curettage is going to be immediately followed by a definitive procedure during the same operation, then all the tissue submitted for initial diagnosis should undergo frozen section analysis so that errors based on sampling can be avoided. Definitive curettage specimens should be fixed, decalcified, and thoroughly sampled (minimum of ten cassettes if enough tissue is present).

En bloc resections

En bloc resections are usually performed for malignancies but occasionally a benign tumor, in an expendable bone such as the fibula or rib, will be resected intact. After orienting the specimen, the soft tissue and bone margins should be carefully assessed grossly. The margins can then be inked and the specimen transected with a bone saw through the plane that includes the greatest dimension of the tumor and its relationship to the closest soft tissue and bone margins. If needed, fresh tumor can be frozen for both diagnostic purposes and tissue triage. Subsequently, in most instances, a longitudinal slab 0.5–1 cm thick can be cut from the center of the specimen. The remaining two hemispheres of tissue can then be 'breadloafed' at 0.5–1-cm intervals in the plane perpendicular to the cut surface of the slab. Sections demonstrating the proximity of the tumor to the closest soft tissue and bone margins should be submitted and the tumor should be carefully dissected and sampled. This usually requires processing a minimum of one cassette per centimeter of tumor. The relationship between the tumor and the surrounding cancellous bone, cortex, and neighboring soft tissues should be illustrated in some of these sections.

Resected tumors that have been treated with preoperative chemotherapy (osteosarcoma, Ewing's sarcoma/primitive neuro-ectodermal tumor, dedifferentiated chondrosarcoma, mesenchymal chondrosarcoma, and high-grade malignant fibrous histiocytoma and fibrosarcoma) require determination of the percentage of tumor necrosis. To accomplish this, the central slab of tissue can be photocopied and the tumor mapped and blocked out in its entirety (Fig. 14.1). A section of tumor per centimeter (as determined by its greatest dimension) should be processed from each of the remaining two hemispheres of the specimen. During histologic review, the amount of tumor necrosis on each slide can be estimated and these scores can then be averaged to calculate the overall percentage of tumor necrosis. The location of the areas of viable and necrotic tumor can then be located on the map of the slab section, if necessary.

HISTOLOGIC DISTINCTION OF BENIGN FROM MALIGNANT TUMORS

Conventional histologic features such as degree of cellularity, mitotic activity, and necrosis are not very helpful in separating benign from malignant bone tumors. This is because benign tumors such as chondroblastoma, osteoblastoma, giant cell tumor, and solid aneurysmal bone cyst can be densely cellular, demonstrate many mitoses, and have large areas of necrosis, whereas variants of osteosarcoma, chondrosarcoma, and fibrosarcoma may be relatively hypocellular and have few mitoses and little or no necrosis. Significant pleomorphism and atypia is a telltale sign of malignancy when accompanied by concurrent cellularity and mitotic activity. The absence of these features, however, should be interpreted with

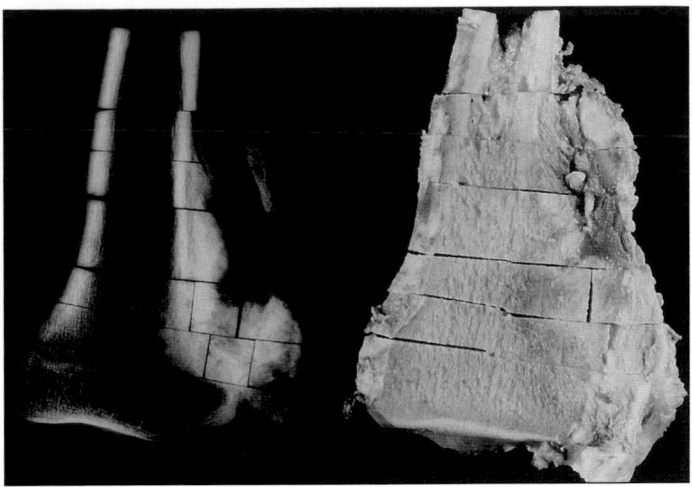

Fig. 14.1 Gross specimen and specimen X-ray of previously treated and resected osteosarcoma showing blocks on cut slab to be submitted.

caution, as degenerative nuclear atypia, similar to that seen in ancient schwannoma, may be present infrequently in a variety of benign neoplasms.

Probably the most important morphologic feature indicative of malignancy is an infiltrative growth pattern in which the tumor replaces the marrow elements, encases pre-existing bony trabeculae and percolates within haversian systems. When present, this finding is strongly suspicious of malignancy, especially for bone- and cartilage-forming neoplasms. The only benign tumor that routinely infiltrates the marrow cavity is hemangioma, although infiltration may also be seen infrequently in desmoplastic fibroma. Other processes that can cause confusion with infiltration are fracture callus and a tangential plane of section through an undulating interface between tumor and surrounding bone. The converse is also important, in that most benign tumors have well circumscribed margins and it is uncommon for bone sarcomas to be well delineated along their entire margin.

CLINICAL REPORTING OF BONE TUMOR SPECIMENS

The surgical pathology report should include a variety of information. For benign tumors, the tumor type and any unusual histologic features or underlying conditions should be noted. If resection margins are relevant then they should be noted. Results of ancillary studies including electron microscopy, immunohistochemistry, cytogenetics, and molecular analysis should also be documented.

Most sarcomas should be subtyped and graded and, if pretreated with cytotoxic therapy, the percentage of tumor necrosis should be indicated. The presence of precursor lesions or other conditions should be identified. The relationship of the tumor to important anatomic structures such as large neurovascular bundles, articular surfaces, synovium, cruciate ligaments, etc. should be commented upon. The status of the closest soft tissue and bone margins and the distances of the tumor to these surfaces need to be carefully identified, measured, assessed, and recorded. If special histochemical stains, immunohistochemistry, electron microscopy, flow cytometry, cytogenetics or molecular analyses have been performed, then their results should be integrated into the report.

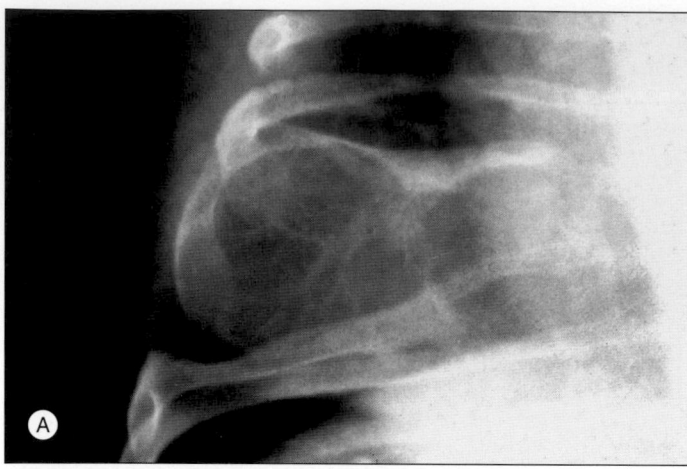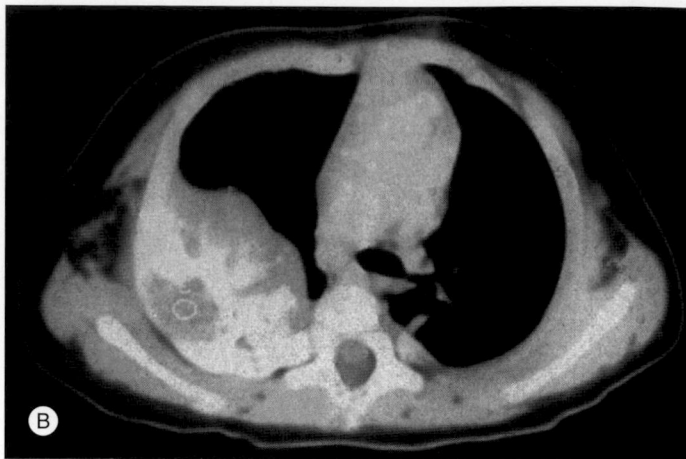

Fig. 14.2 (A) Chest X-ray showing an expansile mass in the rib. **(B)** Axial CT demonstrating the extent of the tumor.

CARTILAGE FORMING TUMORS

Neoplasms of cartilage account for a significant percentage of primary bone tumors that require surgical intervention and pathologic examination. Cartilage neoplasms exhibit a broad spectrum of biological activity ranging from an asymptomatic, indolent and slow growing mass to one that is painful, rapidly enlarging, destructive, and capable of producing metastases. Cartilage tumors recapitulate their normal tissue counterpart (hyaline, fibrous, and elastic cartilage); however the overwhelming majority, regardless of whether they are benign or malignant, produce hyaline cartilage. A small minority may contain some fibrocartilage and virtually none produce elastic cartilage. Myxoid cartilage, a more primitive form of hyaline cartilage, is generally found only in cartilage tumors and its presence should raise the suspicion for malignancy. Overall, benign cartilage tumors are much more prevalent than their malignant counterparts, and of these osteochondroma and enchondroma are the most common.

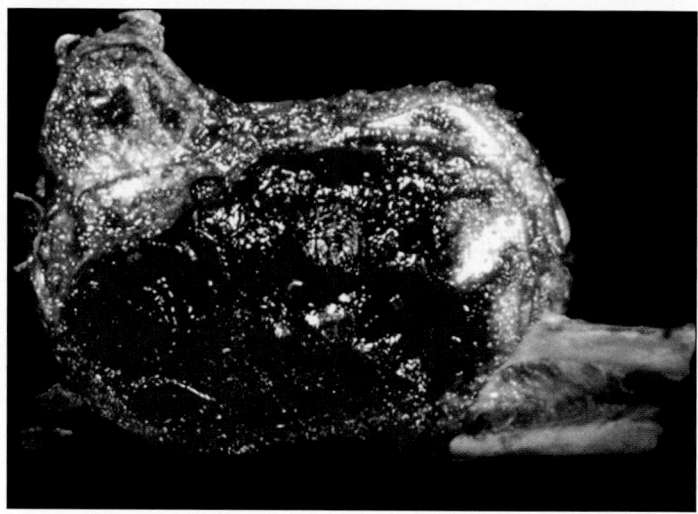

Fig. 14.3 Gross specimen of resected tumor showing a well circumscribed hemorrhagic mass.

CHEST WALL HAMARTOMA

Chest wall hamartoma, also known as vascular-cartilaginous hamartoma, vascular hamartoma of infancy, and mesenchymal hamartoma of the chest wall, is a rare mesenchymal tumor that usually develops during fetal life or the first year of infancy. Rare cases have been reported in adults.[24] The tumor arises from one or multiple ribs and may be asymptomatic or cause chest wall deformities or respiratory distress.[25] These lesions are not limited to the ribs, as we have seen several cases originate in the vertebral column. Lesions described as nasal chondromesenchymal hamartoma and osteochondromyxoma of bone may also be variants of this lesion.[26,27] Interestingly, some of the patients with osteochondromyxoma of bone also have Carney's complex, a familial lentiginous and multiorgan tumor syndrome.

Chest wall hamartoma appears on X-rays as a large expansile mass that is partially cystic and contains areas of mineralization (Fig. 14.2). Some cases may extend into adjacent soft tissues, raising concern for a more aggressive lesion.[28]

The tumors are well circumscribed and consist of an admixture of firm, gray-white, glistening, focally gritty, solid areas and numerous blood-filled cystic spaces (Fig. 14.3). They are composed of a collage of tissues including nodules of hyaline cartilage surrounded by proliferating fibrovascular tissue, newly deposited bone, and variably sized cysts (Fig. 14.4). The islands of cartilage resemble disorganized growth plate and frequently undergo endochondral ossification. The fibrovascular component is often hypercellular and mitotically active but the cells are cytologically banal. The blood vessels may be numerous and usually consist of small-caliber capillaries with scattered larger dilated vascular channels. The cystic spaces resemble those of aneurysmal bone cyst and may dominate the lesion.[29]

The treatment of choice is complete en bloc resection. Spontaneous regression is an uncommon occurrence.[30]

OSTEOCHONDROMA (EXOSTOSIS)

Osteochondroma, also known as exostosis, is a benign cartilage-capped tumor that originates on the surface of bones and enlarges

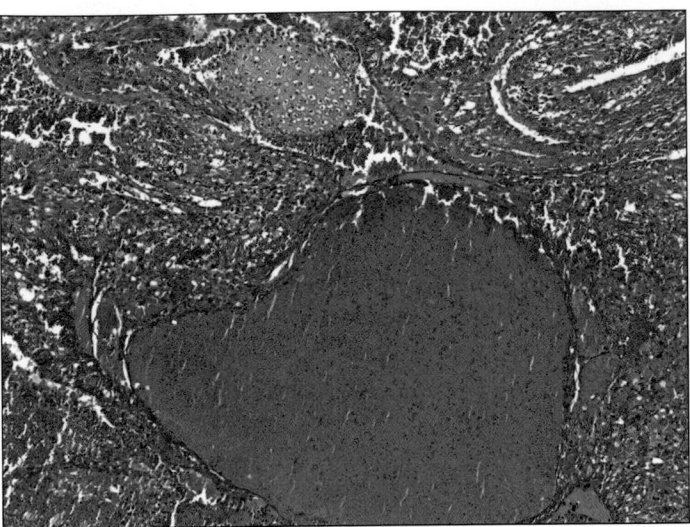

Fig. 14.4 Hemorrhagic cystic spaces with adjacent spindle cell stroma and nodules of cellular hyaline cartilage.

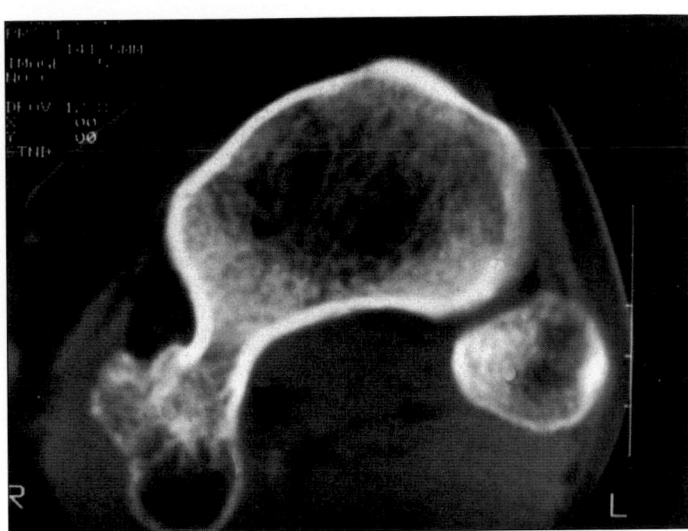

Fig. 14.5 Axial CT of osteochondroma showing continuity of the mass with the underlying cortex and medullary cavity of the tibia.

via endochondral ossification. It is one of the more common clinically significant tumors of the skeleton and in the Mayo Clinic series of surgically treated tumors it accounted for 36–50% of benign tumors and 8.5–15% of all primary bone neoplasms. In fact, some investigators estimate that 0.5% of the population may require surgical excision of an osteochondroma some time between childhood and early adulthood.[4,31]

Osteochondroma presents as a solitary lesion in slightly more than 80% of cases. Most patients are in their second decade of life at the time of diagnosis and there is a male preponderance with a male to female ratio of 1.5–2:1. Multiple osteochondromas, which are frequently polyostotic, are a manifestation of hereditary multiple exostoses, an autosomal dominant genetic disorder. This syndrome has a prevalence of 1 per 50 000 in the general population, making it one of the more common inherited skeletal diseases.[32] Patients with hereditary multiple exostoses come to medical attention at a younger age, usually during the first decade, because they have more severe skeletal deformities. In addition to the osteochondromas, patients develop modeling abnormalities in the metaphyses, including shortening, widening, and the formation of trumpet shaped bones.[33]

Osteochondromas arise in bones derived from endochondral ossification, especially long tubular bones such as the distal femur, proximal tibia, and proximal humerus. They originate from metaphyseal cortical surfaces and grow diagonally to the long axis of the bone, in the direction opposite to the nearby physeal plate. Rarely, they arise in the epiphysis, where they are known as Trevor's disease or dysplasia epiphysealis hemimelica. Osteochondromas exhibit their greatest amount of growth while the physeal plates are open and as they close the rate of enlargement diminishes and eventually ceases.[34]

Initially, it was thought that osteochondromas were caused by lateral displacement of the growth plate or defects in the surrounding periosteal cuff of bone.[35] Recent studies, however, have shown that the chondrocytes in the cartilage cap of either solitary or multiple osteochondromas have inactivating mutations involving the genes *EXT1* and *EXT2* on chromosome 8q24.[31,36,37] This indicates that the chondrocytes are derived from a monoclonal cellular proliferation and strongly suggests that the neoplastic component of

osteochondromas resides in the cartilage cap. Interestingly, osteochondromas have also been reported to be a part of other syndromes that have defects in chromosome 8q24. Additionally, a minority of osteochondromas are radiation-induced. Radiation-induced variants usually develop in children younger than 5 years of age, may be multiple, and have an indolent natural history.[38]

Many osteochondromas are asymptomatic and are only discovered as an incidental finding on X-rays. Some are first detected as a slowly enlarging, firm mass, while others produce symptoms by impinging upon adjacent neurovascular structures, fracturing, or causing an overlying inflammatory bursitis.[39,40]

Radiographically, osteochondromas are bulbous lesions with a narrow or broad (sessile) osseous radiodense stalk that is attached to the underlying bone. The cortex of the host bone merges with that of the stalk such that the medullary cavity of the bone and center of the lesion are in continuity (Fig. 14.5). The bulbous end of the osteochondroma is composed of a cartilage cap that may demonstrate variable degrees of mineralization, which is either in the form of irregular stipples or ring-like calcifications. The base of the cartilage cap merges with areas that have the appearance of cancellous bone.[41–43]

Grossly, osteochondromas range in size from 1 cm to greater than 20 cm in greatest dimension. On average, they are 3–6 cm in size and are shaped like a mushroom. The outer layer consists of a thin sheath of fibrous tissue that overlies a pearly gray-white cartilaginous cap of variable thickness, which may contain gritty areas of calcification or cystification (Fig. 14.6). The surface of the cap is smooth and lobular and the base has a sharp but undulating margin with the underlying cancellous bone. The cancellous bone frequently forms the bulk of the lesion and contains red or yellow marrow.

Histologically, the outer layer is the perichondrium, which is composed of dense fibrous tissue that overlies the hyaline cartilage cap. The cartilage cap varies in thickness and may even be several centimeters thick at its maximum. Its overall architecture recapitulates that of a disorganized growth plate (Fig. 14.7). Generally, the peripheral portion of the cap is the least cellular, with individual chondrocytes surrounded by abundant hyaline cartilage matrix. In the deeper layers, the cellularity of the cartilage increases, the chondrocytes become

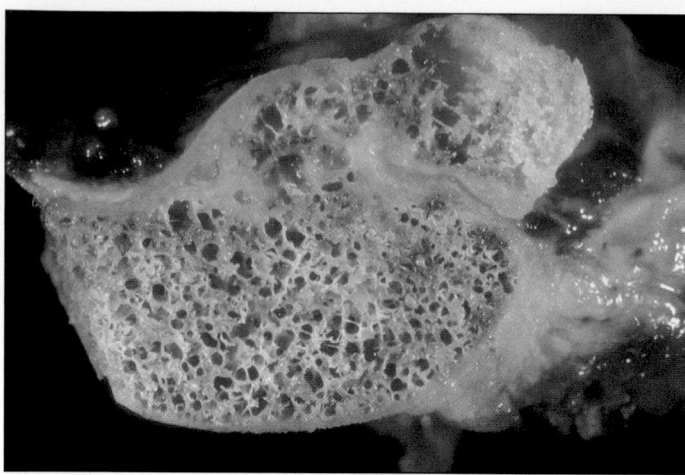

Fig. 14.6 A resected osteochondroma with attached underlying bone. Note thin cartilaginous cap and cancellous bone filling the stalk of the lesion.

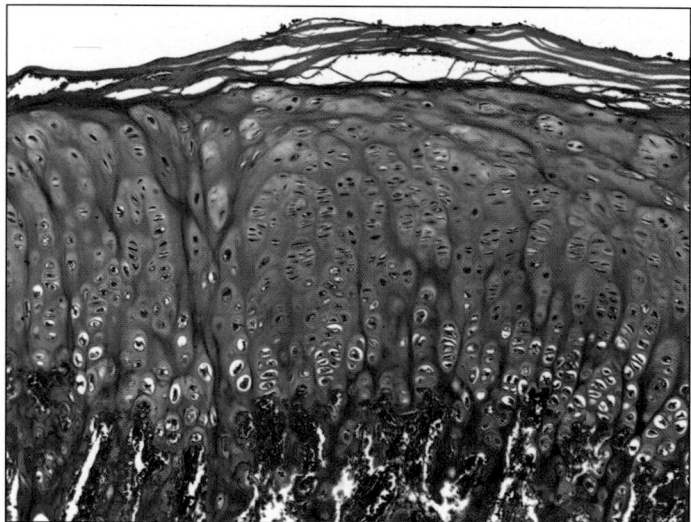

Fig. 14.7 Perichondrium overlying cartilaginous cap of an osteochondroma. The cap resembles a growth plate and is undergoing endochondral ossification.

arranged in vague columns, and their cytoplasmic volume enlarges. The chondrocytes exhibit minimal cytologic atypia and no mitotic activity; however, scattered binucleate cells may be present. At the base of the cap the matrix calcifies, the chondrocytes undergo necrosis and portions of the mineralized cartilage are resorbed by osteoclasts, leaving behind struts of matrix that act as a template for bone deposition. Eventually, the mature trabeculae formed from this process comprise the majority of the bulbous end of the lesion and are surrounded by fatty or hematopoietic marrow.

Aspirates of osteochondromas will preferentially sample the cartilaginous cap component and hence yield aspirates cytologically identical to chondromas.[23] When chondrosarcomatous dedifferentiation has occurred, the cytologic appearance will be that of a chondrosarcoma.

It is important to note that some investigators believe that, if the cap is greater than 1 cm in thickness, then by definition it is malignant and has evolved into chondrosarcoma.[41] This has no real scientific basis and other criteria, such as the cytology and the growth pattern (infiltrative versus well circumscribed) of the cartilage, should be used to make this determination.

Osteochondromas can be observed if they are small and asymptomatic. Simple excision is usually adequate for those that need to be removed. If a portion of the perichondrium or cartilage cap is left behind, then the lesion may recur. Malignant degeneration of a solitary osteochondroma is a very uncommon event (see secondary chondrosarcoma, later in this chapter).[44] This biological progression tends to develop in osteochondromas of the flat bones, particularly of the pelvis, and occurs more frequently in the setting of hereditary multiple exostoses, where, in some series, 15% of the patients eventually develop this complication. The sarcomas that arise in this setting are usually conventional well differentiated chondrosarcomas. The development of a dedifferentiated component such as a high-grade osteosarcoma or pleomorphic spindle cell sarcoma is rare.[45,46]

CHONDROMA

Chondromas are benign cartilage tumors, which may develop within or on the surfaces of bones. Most chondromas of bone are solitary, composed of hyaline cartilage, and arise within the medullary cavity. Biologically, they tend to have a limited capacity for growth and infrequently undergo malignant degeneration.

Enchondroma

Enchondromas are benign hyaline cartilage neoplasms that arise within the medullary cavity. They are relatively common, second in frequency to osteochondroma, and account for approximately 12–24% of benign primary bone tumors and 3–10% of all bone tumors.[47] The precursors of enchondromas are thought to be persistent rests of hyaline cartilage derived from the growth plate that subsequently proliferate and form tumors in the metaphysis and diaphysis.[48] Cytogenetic studies of enchondromas have identified abnormalities involving chromosomes 5, 6, 7, 12, and 17; none of these changes, however, are specific.[49]

Almost 90% of enchondromas are solitary. The remainder are multiple and occur in the setting of Ollier's disease and Maffucci syndrome.[47] They usually present during the third and fourth decades of life and have an equal gender distribution. Almost 60% develop in the bones of the hand, where they represent the most common primary tumor of bone.[47] Other frequent sites of involvement include the tubular bones of the feet, femur, tibia, humerus, fibula, and rib. As a general rule, enchondromas predominate in the distal appendicular skeleton, whereas chondrosarcomas are most common in the axial skeleton.

Enchondromas are typically asymptomatic and are identified as an incidental finding. Some, however, produce visible deformities, predispose to a pathologic fracture, or cause pain. This latter feature, especially if of long standing and progressive in nature, has been emphasized as a warning sign of malignancy. Enchondromas, however, may produce pain directly through the generation of microfractures. It is also relatively common for the pain associated with other abnormalities such as a torn meniscus or rotator cuff to be erroneously attributed to an enchondroma in a nearby bone.

The radiographic hallmarks of enchondroma are a circular or oblong lucent lesion that has well defined margins and no periosteal

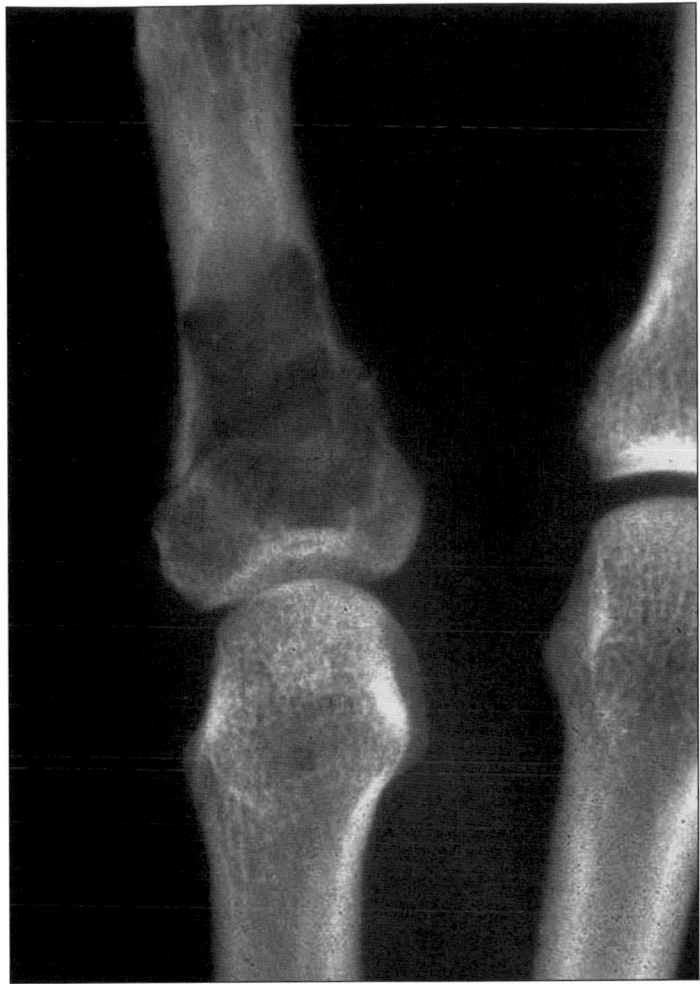

Fig. 14.8 Enchondroma of finger with pathologic fracture. The lesion is well circumscribed and lytic and has scalloped borders.

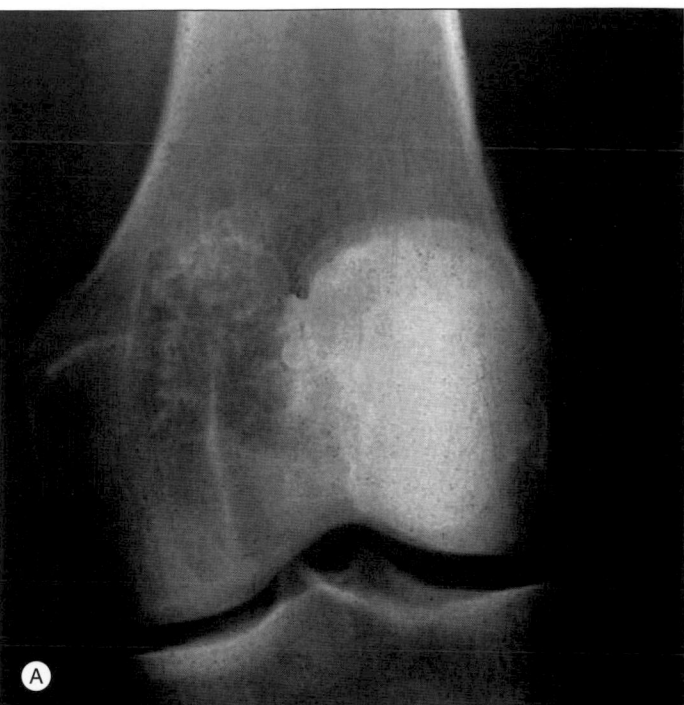

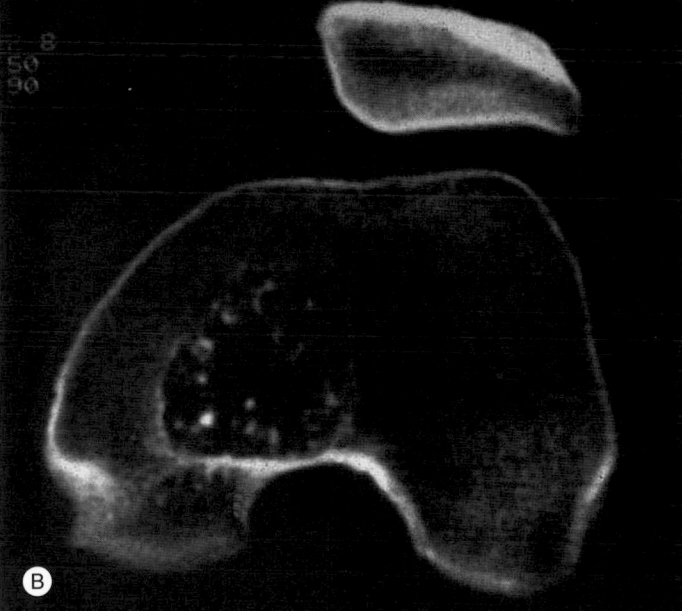

Fig. 14.9 Plain film (**A**) and axial CT (**B**) of enchondroma. The tumor has a well circumscribed and sclerotic margins and contains dense speckled and ring like radiodensities.

reaction[43] (Fig. 14.8). The extent of radiographic mineralization varies considerably; many tumors contain scattered, dense, stippled opacities that represent irregular calcification of the cartilaginous matrix and 'O'- or 'C'-ring-like mineralized structures that correlate with the presence of a thin rim of reactive bone surrounding individual nodules of lucent cartilage[50] (Fig. 14.9). In some older tumors the mineral coalesces, forming a solid, stone-like intraosseous density. The nonmineralized cartilage on MRI shows low intensity on T1-weighted images and appears bright on T2-weighted images. Enchondromas located adjacent to the cortex can produce endosteal scalloping and in small bones can even result in marked thinning of the cortex and expansion of the bone.[49] Marked bone expansion caused by an enchondroma rarely occurs in other skeletal sites. When it does, the lesion has been designated enchondroma protuberans.[51] However, cortical thinning, bone expansion, and a periosteal reaction are harbingers of malignancy when associated with cartilage tumors in flat bones and large tubular bones such as the femur, tibia, and humerus.

Grossly, enchondromas range in size from 3–5 cm and appear as coalescing nodules of firm to hard, sometimes gritty, pearly white or gray, glistening tissue that is well demarcated from the surrounding bone (Fig. 14.10). Microscopically, they are composed of nodules of cartilage that are well circumscribed and have a sharp margin with

the encompassing bone (Fig. 14.11). The cartilage is hypocellular to moderately cellular and contains chondrocytes that have uniform, small, round, hyperchromatic nuclei (Fig. 14.12). Occasional cells are binucleate. The matrix is hyaline and is the most prominent component of the lesion. Myxoid matrix is uncommon and should raise suspicion for chondrosarcoma. The hyaline matrix frequently calcifies and in these areas the chondrocytes undergo necrosis. In the absence of mineralized matrix, the finding of necrotic chondrocytes should also arouse suspicion of chondrosarcoma. The periphery of

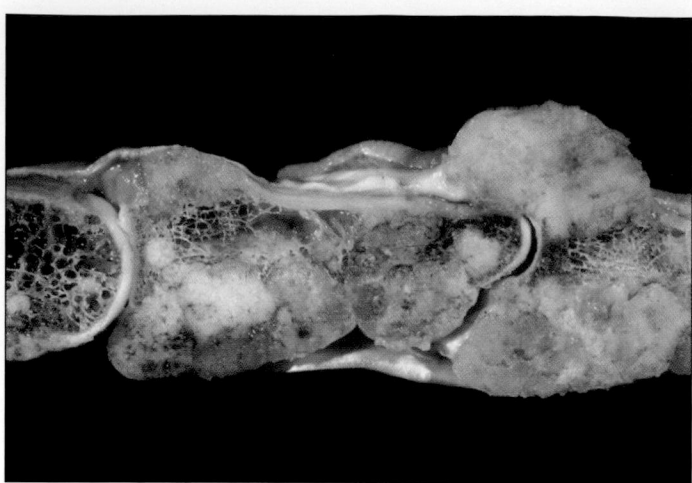

Fig. 14.10 Resected finger from a patient with Ollier's disease. Multiple enchondromas arising within and on the surfaces of the bones. The tumors are nodular, gray-white, and glistening.

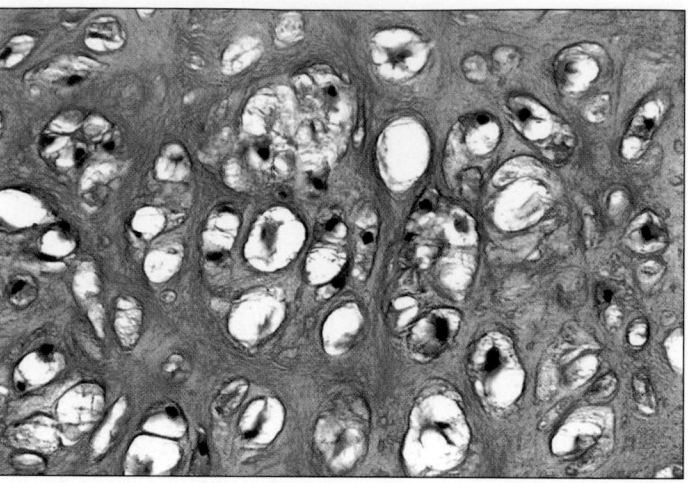

Fig. 14.12 Enchondroma composed of hyaline matrix containing bland-appearing chondrocytes.

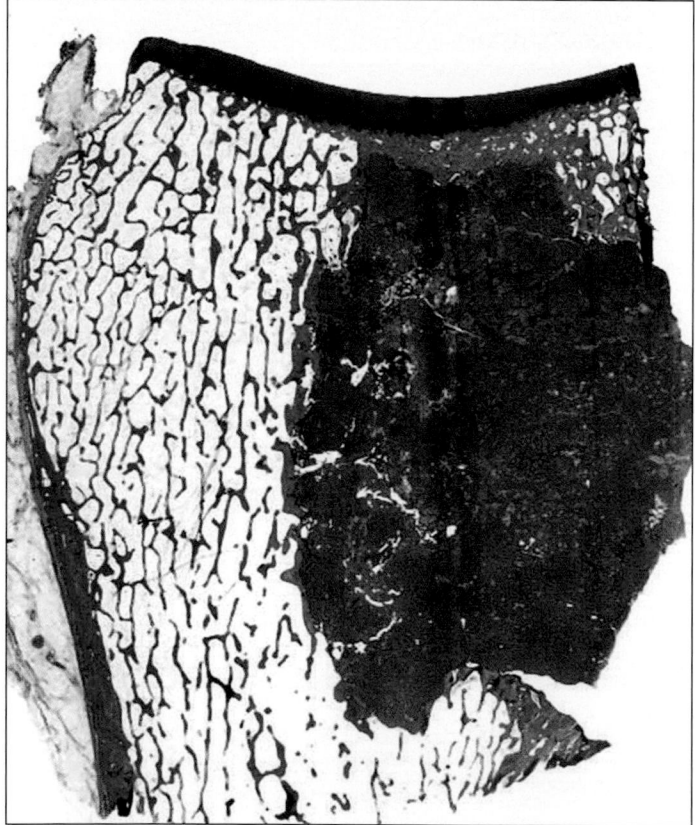

Fig. 14.11 A whole mount section stained with Goldner trichrome. Enchondroma is located in the head of the fibula. The red-staining tumor is well demarcated and surrounded by a rim of reactive sclerotic bone.

the nodules often undergoes endochondral ossification, producing a rim of bone that surrounds the nodules of cartilage. Importantly, the cartilage does not grow in an infiltrative pattern and encase pre-existing trabecular bone, which is a feature of chondrosarcoma. Enchondromas arising in digits are frequently hypercellular and

demonstrate mild cytologic atypia. Similarly, enchondromas in Ollier's disease and Maffucci syndrome may not only be cellular and exhibit cytologic abnormalities but their matrix may be focally myxoid as well.

Cytologic smears of enchondroma are dominated by a cartilaginous matrix, which on Romanowsky stain has an intensely metachromatic appearance and is often present in large, sheet-like fragments or clumps (Fig. 14.13A). Cartilage matrix may have an opaque, filmy, or glassy appearance.[52,53] The aggregates of matrix contain lacunar spaces, usually occupied by a single round cell with a nearly central, round, bland nucleus (Fig. 14.13B). At times, the cartilaginous matrix obscures cellular detail. Nucleoli are almost invariably absent from benign chondrocytes. Binucleate cells are rare and multinucleate cells and mitotic figures are absent. Within the lacunae, the cells are usually single, although rare double-nucleate chondrocytes or two closely opposed cells may be seen. When more than occasional doublets are seen, the diagnosis of chondrosarcoma should be considered. A small number of individual bland chondrocytes may be seen in the background. Enchondromas associated with Ollier's disease and Maffucci syndrome may show greater degrees of cellularity and nuclear atypia without indicating the presence of low-grade chondrosarcoma. The presence of significant myxoid change or necrosis should suggest the possibility of a chondrosarcoma.

Enchondromas have limited biologic growth potential. Most grow slowly and do not reach large size; malignant transformation is a rare event. The treatment depends on the clinical circumstances. Tumors that are asymptomatic and show no worrisome radiographic features can be followed, whereas those that are painful or have questionable radiographic findings should be biopsied or curetted.[54] The local recurrence rate following curettage is approximately 3–4%.[55,56] En bloc excision for tumors in expendable portions of bone, such as the proximal fibula, is sometimes performed.

Enchondromatosis

Multiple enchondromas occur in two clinical settings: 90% are associated with Ollier's disease and 10% are seen in Maffucci syndrome. No underlying specific genetic abnormality has been identified in these disorders.

Ollier's disease, first described by Ollier in 1900, is defined as two or more enchondromas.[57] The disease has an equal gender

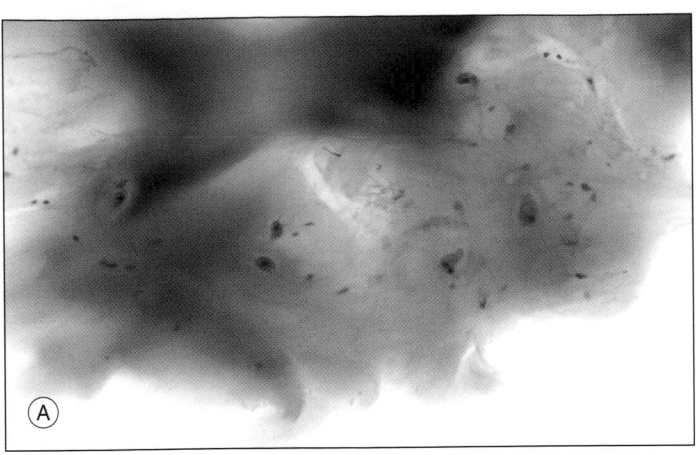
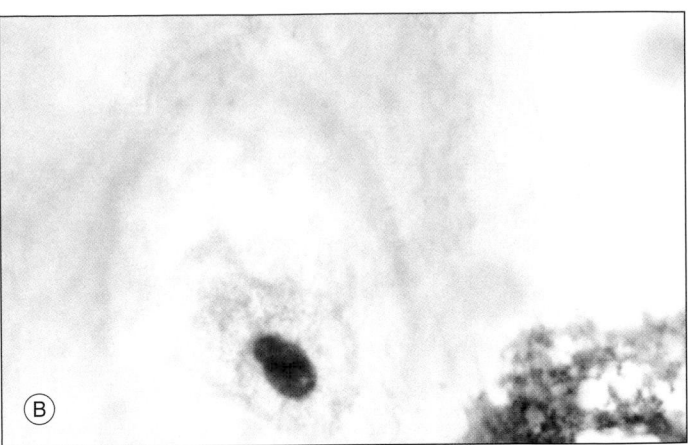

Fig. 14.13 **(A)** Large sheets of hyaline cartilage entrapping a small number of round to oval chondrocytes. The lacunar spaces contain single round cells with bland nuclei. (H&E stain.) **(B)** Chondroid matrix with a lacunar space surrounding a chondrocyte with single nucleus. The nucleus is bland with a dense even chromatin pattern. (Papanicolaou stain.)

distribution and tends to be unilateral or to affect one side of the body more severely than the other. The enchondromas are frequently first noted during childhood and the symptomatology is variable. Patients may have anything from two to hundreds of tumors, which may be asymptomatic or cause severe mechanical and cosmetic problems. The enchondromas are usually metaphyseal–diaphyseal in location and frequently affect the short tubular bones of the hands, followed by those of the feet and the long tubular bones, including the femur, tibia, and humerus. Tumors may also develop in the flat bones of the pelvis and trunk but involvement of the spinal column or skull is rare.

Taken as a whole, the radiographic features of Ollier's disease are diagnostic. The tumors are multiple, frequently eccentric, and arise in the medullary cavity, cortex, or surfaces of the bone (Fig. 14.14). In the long bones there are linear radiolucencies that extend from the metaphysis into the diaphysis and are caused by persistent columns of dysplastic cartilage that originate in the growth plate. Severely affected bones are shortened and deformed. Individual tumors have the features of a solitary chondroma and can be lucent or contain stippled calcifications.

Grossly, the tumors may consist of multiple nodules of gray, glistening cartilage, which may coalesce into large masses. The tumors are located in the medullary cavity, in the cortex, beneath the periosteum, and can even span joints (see Fig. 14.10). The chondromas of Ollier's disease are histologically similar to those of sporadic solitary tumors. However, they frequently demonstrate a greater degree of cellularity and cytologic atypia, and may contain myxoid matrix. All these features can cause confusion with chondrosarcoma.

The clinical behavior of Ollier's disease is unpredictable and there is no specialized treatment. The cartilage tumors may stabilize in size soon after puberty or continue to grow. Painful lesions may have to be removed and other forms of corrective surgery, including amputation, may be necessary for severe deformities. The most dreaded complication is malignant transformation of an enchondroma. This occurs in 25–30% of affected patients. Those patients most prone have severe forms of skeletal involvement.[58,59] The sarcomas that develop are usually low-grade conventional chondrosarcomas; however, dedifferentiated chondrosarcomas and osteosarcomas have been reported.[58,60] Accordingly, patients with Ollier's disease must have lifetime monitoring of their tumors.

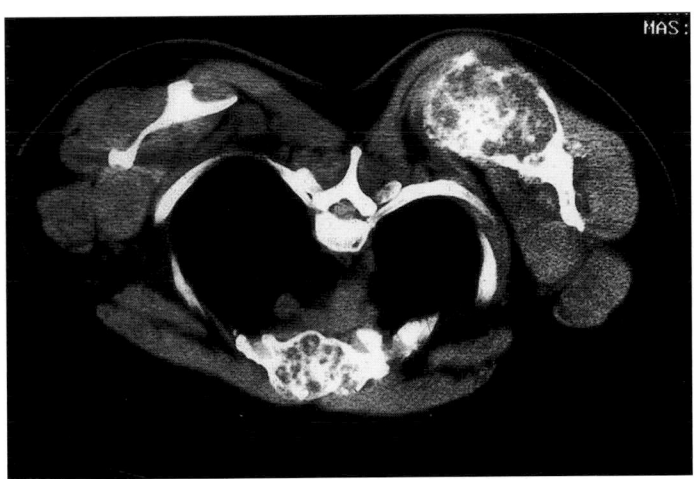

Fig. 14.14 Axial CT scan of a patient with Ollier's disease, showing multiple enchondromas associated with chondrosarcoma in the sternum and scapula.

Maffucci syndrome is defined as two or more enchondromas associated with hemangiomas, which are usually located in the skin or soft tissue but may be centered in the viscera. Originally classified as cavernous hemangiomas or arteriovenous malformations, more recent studies have shown that most of these vascular tumors are spindle cell hemangiomas.[61] The enchondromas are clinically, radiographically, grossly, and histologically similar to those seen in Ollier's disease.

An important aspect of Maffucci syndrome is the development of malignancies within the viscera as well as in the enchondromas. Carcinomas of the pancreas and malignancies of the ovaries, brain, and skeleton are commonplace. In fact, it is estimated that all patients with Maffucci syndrome will develop a malignancy, sometime during their lifetime.[59]

Juxtacortical or subperiosteal chondroma

Juxtacortical or subperiosteal chondroma is a relatively uncommon benign cartilage tumor that arises on the cortex beneath the periosteum. Less than 1% of all chondromas arise in this anatomic site.[50] Its first detailed description was by Lichtenstein and Hall in 1952, and subsequently more than 100 cases have been reported.[62–66] The tumor develops in all age groups, although most patients are in their second or third decade of life, and males are affected more frequently than females.[63]

The surface of tubular bones, particularly the metaphyseal or diaphyseal region of the humerus and femur and the short tubular bones of the hand, are characteristic sites of origin. Patients present complaining of a mass, swelling, and pain. The pain may be caused by alteration of a tendinous insertion by the tumor.

The tumor is predominately radiolucent, may contain punctuate calcifications, and has well defined margins.[62–66] The underlying cortex is eroded, occasionally scalloped, and sclerotic but is not transgressed. The periphery of the tumor is delineated by a thick, mature, buttress of reactive periosteal bone. CT scan shows that the lesion is round or oval and, in conjunction with MRI, clearly identifies the extent of the tumor and the lack of involvement of the medullary cavity.

A solid mass of glistening, gray-white cartilage that is focally gritty or mucinous is the typical gross appearance of subperiosteal chondroma. A layer of firm connective tissue, the periosteum, covers the tumor and its base is smooth or undulating and sharply demarcated from the underlying excavated cortex. The medullary cavity may be impinged upon by reactive endosteal bone but is otherwise uninvolved. The neoplastic matrix is hypocellular to moderately cellular and the chondrocytes are bland or may demonstrate mild to moderate atypia in the form of nuclear enlargement, prominent nucleoli, and binucleation. The matrix is composed of hyaline cartilage and may be focally myxoid. Some of these morphologic attributes raise the possibility of chondrosarcoma, which can be distinguished by the absence of an infiltrative growth pattern.

The treatment of juxtacortical chondroma is excision of the cartilaginous mass and the overlying periosteum. Recurrences are uncommon and malignant transformation is not of concern.

Intracortical chondroma

Intracortical chondroma is the rarest type of cartilage tumor of the skeleton. Only a few cases have been published and they have been in the form of case reports.[66,67] These tumors affect children and adults and frequently cause pain. They are small, round, and lucent on X-ray and CT, and frequently elicit a periosteal reaction.[67] Their radiographic appearance can mimic that of an osteoid osteoma. Histologically, they are composed of hypocellular, cytologically banal, hyaline cartilage. They have been successfully treated by radioablation and curettage.[67]

CHONDROBLASTOMA

Chondroblastoma, originally known as calcifying giant cell tumor, Codman's tumor, or epiphyseal chondromatous giant cell tumor, is an uncommon benign cartilage neoplasm.[68] It accounts for approximately 1% of primary bone tumors and less than 3% of benign bone tumors.[69,70]

Chondroblastoma most frequently arises in the epiphysis or apophysis of long bones. Affected individuals are typically males, skeletally immature, and usually between the ages of 10 and 25 years.

Chondroblastoma can arise in any bone that develops from endochondral ossification but most develop in the epiphyses of the distal and proximal femur, followed by the proximal tibia and proximal humerus.[70,71] Apophyseal origin is less frequent and, when

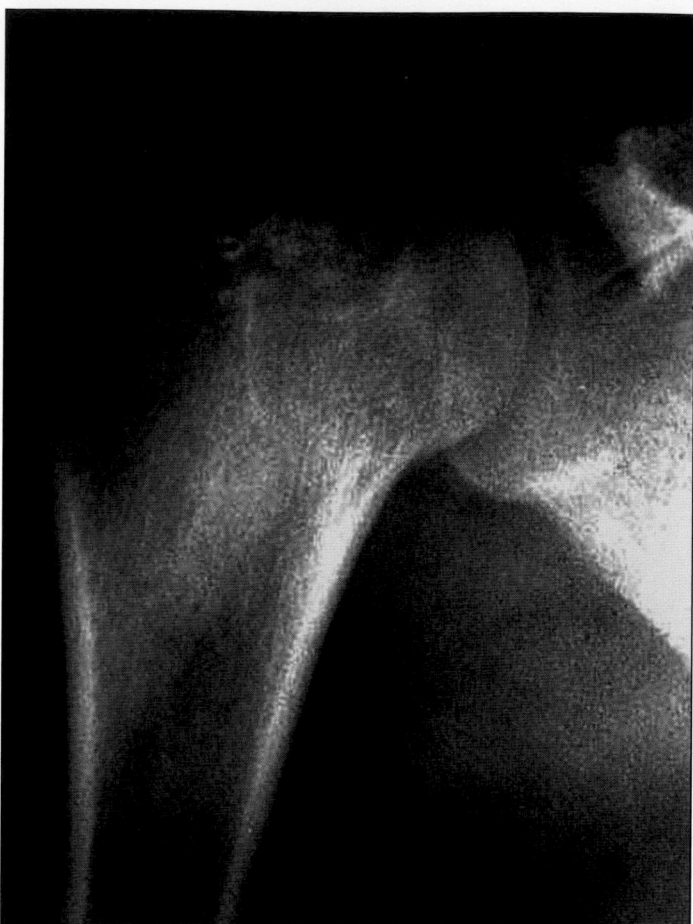

Fig. 14.15 X-ray of chondroblastoma in the humeral head. The lesion is centered in the epiphysis, is well circumscribed, and contains scattered dense calcifications.

it occurs, it usually involves the greater trochanter of the femur and the greater tuberosity of the humerus. Patients with tumors arising in the flat bones, vertebrae, and short tubular bones tend to be older and skeletally mature.[72,73] Clinically, patients with chondroblastoma usually present with pain that can be quite severe, swelling, limitation of motion of the adjacent joint, and limping.[70,74] Cytogenetic studies have shown clonal abnormalities, especially involving chromosomes 5 and 8.[75,76]

Radiographically, chondroblastoma manifests as an eccentric, intramedullary, well defined tumor that has scalloped borders and a sclerotic rim. The tumor is radiolucent but frequently contains scattered punctate calcifications[77] (Fig. 14.15). Secondary aneurysmal-bone-cyst-like changes may cause bubbly expansion of the bone and a periosteal reaction, which can mimic a more aggressive neoplasm.[77]

Grossly, chondroblastoma is gritty and grayish white with areas of hemorrhage. Hemorrhagic cystic areas are common. Histologically, chondroblastoma is densely cellular and is composed of an admixture of mononuclear chondroblasts and multinucleate osteoclast-type giant cells. The chondroblasts grow in sheets and have eosinophilic cytoplasm, delineated by well defined cell borders, and eccentrically placed reniform or coffee-bean-shaped nuclei similar to the nuclei found in Langerhans cells (Fig. 14.16). Mitotic activity and regional necrosis are commonplace. Well formed hyaline cartilage is uncommon. The matrix generally consists of poorly formed hyaline

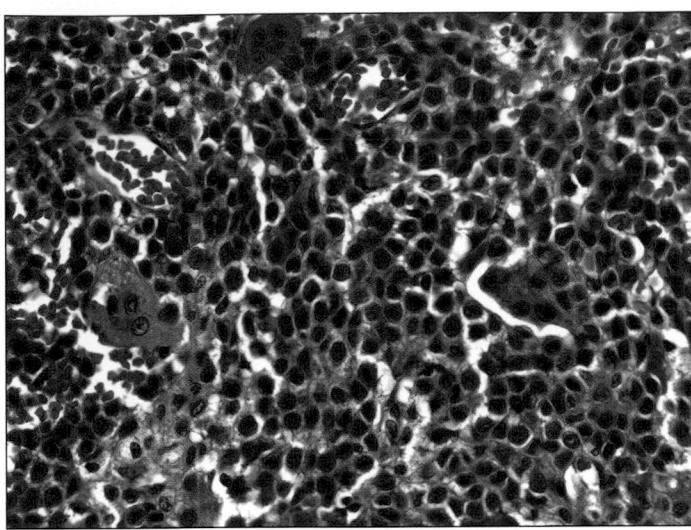

Fig. 14.16 Chondroblastoma composed of sheets of chondroblasts containing cleaved nuclei. Note scattered osteoclast type giant cells.

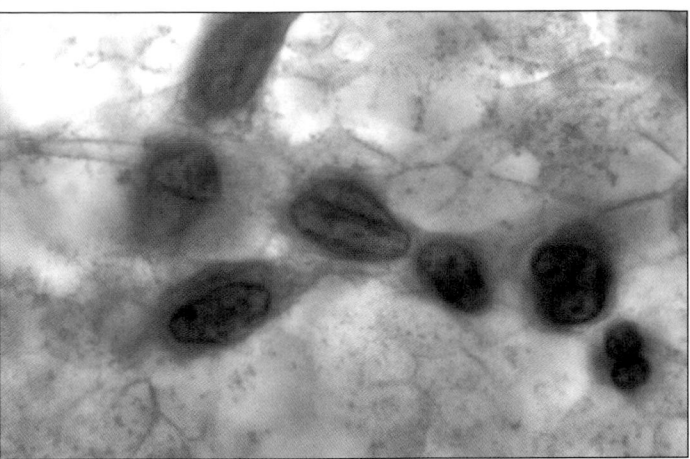

Fig. 14.18 Mononuclear cells obtained from chondroblastoma show ovoid nuclei frequently with prominent nuclear grooves. The chromatin pattern is open with small but distinct chromocenters. (Romanowsky stain.)

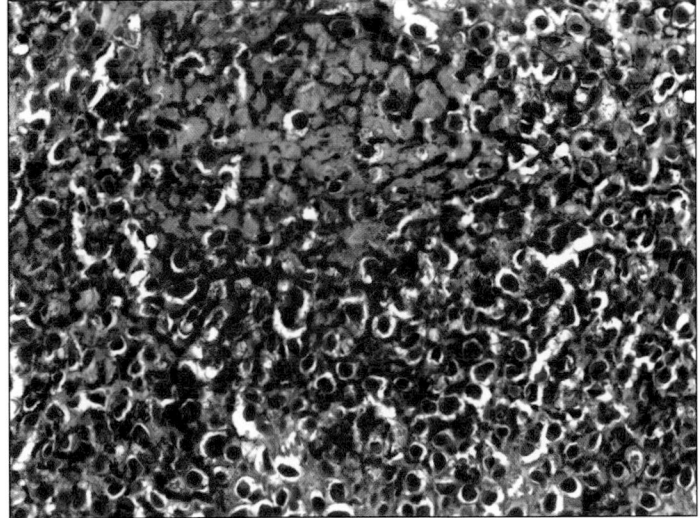

Fig. 14.17 Chicken-wire pattern of mineralization characteristic of chondroblastoma with areas of necrosis.

cartilage that is focal in distribution and deposited in small amounts outlining the neoplastic cells. Consequently, mineralization of the matrix surrounding individual cells imparts a 'chicken-wire' or 'plexiform' pattern[71] (Fig. 14.17). Areas of pink chondroid matrix that mimics bone can be identified in most tumors.[71] In fact, a recent study has actually suggested that chondroblastoma is a bone-forming and not a cartilaginous neoplasm.[78] Osteoclast-type giant cells are scattered throughout the tumor but are most numerous in areas of matrix production and hemorrhage. RANKL, a stimulator of osteoclast production and activity, is expressed by the tumor cells. It is by this mechanism that osteoclasts are recruited into the tumor and produce resorption of the underlying bone.[79] Cystic changes mimicking aneurysmal bone cyst are frequent and sometimes the cysts dominate, with only small clusters of tumor cells within their walls. An unusual finding, but one that is common in craniofacial chondroblastoma, is the presence of abundant hemosiderin in the cytoplasm of the chondroblasts.

FNA smears derived from chondroblastomas are of moderate to high cellularity[21,80,81] and contain a prominent number of multinucleate, osteoclast-like giant cells.[46] The cells lie both singly and in aggregates (see Fig. 14.12). The cell aggregates are composed of round to slightly ovoid chondroblasts surrounding multinucleate giant cells. The mononuclear chondroblasts often lie embedded in a myxoid matrix.[81] The nuclei of the mononuclear cells are round, ovoid, or reniform and lie peripherally within the cell cytoplasm. The chromatin of the chondroblasts is finely granular and small nucleoli are often present. Nuclear membrane irregularities, as exemplified by longitudinal grooves or deep convolutions, are frequent (Fig. 14.18). The cytoplasm of the chondroblasts may have a vacuolated appearance on Romanowsky staining. Cellular aggregates, in which the matrix surrounds individual cells with a chicken wire pattern of calcification, may be present and are essentially diagnostic of chondroblastoma. Such aggregates, however, are infrequent.

Immunohistochemically, the chondroblasts express S-100 protein and may also stain for muscle actin, keratin, and epithelial membrane antigen.[82,83]

The treatment of chondroblastoma usually consists of curettage and packing with bone graft.[74] Percutaneous radiofrequency heat ablation has been used in a few patients.[84] Overall, the local recurrence rate is 14–18% and seems to be higher in tumors arising in the temporal bone and ribs.[70,77] Local recurrences usually develop within the first 3 years following curettage, although they may be detected after a much longer time interval.[70,85] Pulmonary metastases from histologically benign chondroblastomas are a well recognized phenomenon. The metastases are slowly progressive, maintain the histologic appearance of benign chondroblastoma, are rarely fatal, and can be treated by resection.[86–89] The concept of 'malignant' chondroblastoma is controversial and some authors believe that most of these tumors represent either a misdiagnosis or a radiation-induced sarcoma.[70]

CHONDROMYXOID FIBROMA

Chondromyxoid fibroma is one of the least common neoplasms of bone and accounts for less than 1% of all primary bone tumors.[90] In

1948, Jaffe and Lichtenstein were the first to recognize it as a distinct entity during their review of cases previously diagnosed as chondrosarcoma.[91] Chondromyxoid fibroma still causes diagnostic difficulties, however, because of its rarity and unusual morphology.

Chondromyxoid fibroma usually arises in patients in the second to third decades of life, although it has been reported in all age groups. Males are affected slightly more frequently than females. Approximately one half of cases involve the long tubular bones (usually around the knee region: proximal tibia > distal femur), one-third arise in the flat bones (mainly the ilium) and one-fifth develop in the bones of the feet (especially the metatarsals).[90] Less common locations include the ribs, the vertebrae, and the bones of the skull and hands. Patients usually present with pain, which may be present for years, and swelling. Some tumors, however, are initially detected as incidental findings on X-rays.[92] Cytogenetic studies have demonstrated clonal rearrangement of chromosome 6, involving bands q13 and q25, suggesting a specific oncogenic transformation.[93]

Radiographically, chondromyxoid fibroma appears as an eccentric, radiolucent, multiloculated lesion in the metaphysis and ranges in size from 1–10 cm. The long axis of the tumor parallels the long axis of the bone and occasionally the mass may extend into the diaphysis or epiphysis, particularly in small tubular bones. The margins of the lesion are sharp and frequently have a sclerotic rim (Fig. 14.19). Rarely, the tumor destroys the cortex and extends into the soft tissue.

Grossly, chondromyxoid fibroma is well circumscribed, pink-tan, and glistening. Histologically, it is well defined, lobular, and composed of hypocellular chondroid or chondromyxoid tissue that is more cellular peripherally (Fig. 14.20). In the chondroid areas, the cells are oval and reside within lacunae surrounded by a poorly formed hyaline matrix. Well developed hyaline cartilage is present in only 19% of tumors and is most prominent in lesions of the small bones of the hand and feet.[90] Coarse deposits of mineral within the chondroid matrix, which may be detected radiographically, are present in approximately 20% of cases. The myxoid areas are composed of stellate cells enmeshed in a frothy basophilic matrix. Hypercellular peripheral regions may contain scattered, multinucleate, osteoclast-type giant cells and sheets of polyhedral cells resembling the cells of chondroblastoma.[94] Rarely present are so-called pseudomalignant cells, which are mitotically inactive but have enlarged, pleomorphic, and hyperchromatic nuclei similar to those present in ancient schwannoma.[90,95] The fibrous component consists of septae that subcompartmentalize the tumor into lobules. Chondromyxoid fibroma, unlike many cartilaginous tumors, frequently contains thin-walled vessels that have a hemangiopericytoma-like growth pattern.

Aspirate smears obtained from chondromyxoid fibromas are usually of low to moderate cellularity and contain a polymorphous population of round, chondroblast-like cells, stellate cells, and spindle cells lying in a fibrillar chondroid or myxoid background.[96] The chondroblast-like cells generally lie singly and are entrapped within the matrix. The majority of these cells are uninucleate but a lesser number may be bi- or multinucleate.[96] The nuclear chromatin of the chondroblast-like cells is smudgy and condensed (see Fig. 14.11) and is associated with an abundant foamy or granular cytoplasm. A small number of benign, osteoclast-like giant cells are intermingled with the other cell types.

Immunohistochemically, the cells in the cartilaginous areas stain for S-100 protein, whereas the cells in the peripheral cellular regions express muscle specific and smooth muscle actin but not S-100 protein. Ultrastructurally, the cells in the central regions have the features of chondrocytes but the cells in the peripheral regions show myofibroblastic and myochondroblastic differentiation.[97] The matrix

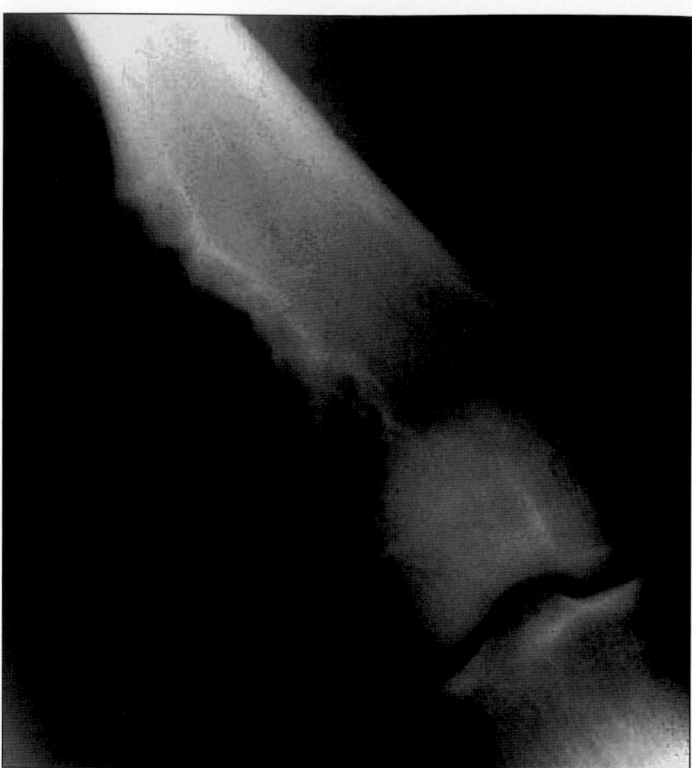

Fig. 14.19 Plain X-ray of chondromyxoid fibroma in distal femur. The tumor is eccentric, well circumscribed and radiolucent.

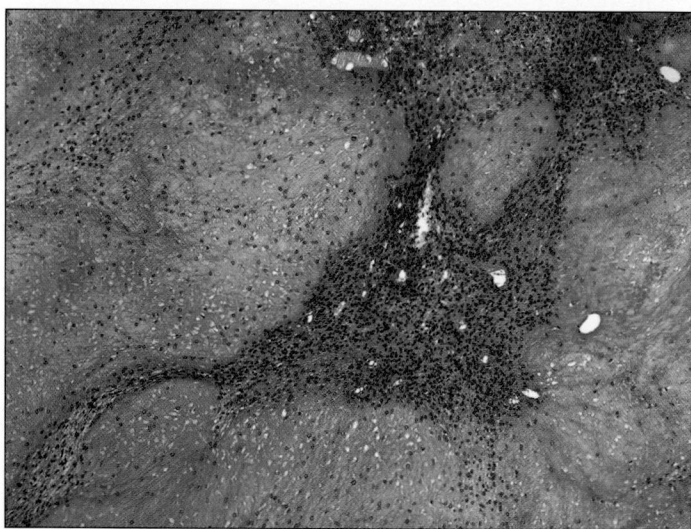

Fig. 14.20 Chondromyxoid fibroma composed of lobules of chondroid tissue separated by cellular spindle cell areas with prominent vessels.

of chondromyxoid fibroma contains collagen types I, II, III, and VI as well as hydrated proteoglycans. This composition seems to be specific for chondromyxoid fibroma and has not been found in other cartilaginous tumors such as chondroblastoma, osteochondroma, enchondroma, or chondrosarcoma.[98]

The treatment of chondromyxoid fibroma is curettage or en bloc resection, depending on the location of the tumor. The local recurrence rate is approximately 20% and predominantly complicates tumors treated by curettage. Rare examples of malignant chondromyxoid fibroma and sarcomatous transformation have been reported. Some of these cases have followed radiation therapy.[92] It is unclear, however, whether malignant chondromyxoid fibroma actually exists or whether it represents another type of sarcoma that has been misdiagnosed.

CHONDROSARCOMA

Skeletal chondrosarcoma is defined as a sarcoma that arises in bone, has a cartilaginous phenotype, and lacks osteoblastic (osteosarcomatous) differentiation. It follows osteosarcoma as the second most common sarcoma of bone and accounts for approximately 10–25% of bone sarcomas.[4,8] Chondrosarcoma is classified into different clinicopathologic types that have a wide spectrum of biologic behavior ranging from indolent tumors with minimal metastatic potential to those that are very aggressive and frequently fatal. The majority of chondrosarcomas (86%) develop de novo, while the remainder arise in association with a pre-existing condition such as osteochondroma and are known as secondary chondrosarcomas.[4] Light microscopy is adequate for diagnosis of most chondrosarcomas; however, in certain situations, additional studies including immunohistochemistry, electron microscopy, and molecular analysis are needed to definitively subclassify the neoplasm. Recently, extraskeletal myxoid chondrosarcoma has been reported to arise in bone; however, this tumor is extraordinarily rare in the skeleton and has not been shown to be of true cartilaginous differentiation. Therefore, it is not included in this section.[99]

Conventional chondrosarcoma

Conventional chondrosarcoma is defined morphologically as being composed entirely of neoplastic hyaline and/or myxoid cartilage. It accounts for more than 90% of all chondrosarcomas and the overwhelming majority of affected patients do not have Ollier's disease, Maffucci syndrome, or Multiple hereditary exostoses (syndromes associated with the development of chondrosarcoma). Chondrosarcoma usually develops in adults in the late fifth to seventh decades of life, and males are affected slightly more frequently than females.[8] It is rare in children and a diagnosis of chondrosarcoma should raise the suspicion of chondroblastic osteosarcoma, a tumor that is much more common in this age group. Chondrosarcomas can arise in any bone derived from endochondral ossification. Most originate in the pelvis, especially the ilium, followed by the proximal femur, proximal humerus, distal femur, and ribs.[4,100–102] Chondrosarcoma infrequently develops in phalanges, despite the fact that enchondroma commonly affects these bones.[103] In the skull base, an unusual location for bone tumors, chondrosarcoma follows chordoma as the most common primary bone malignancy.[104] Pain and an enlarging mass are common presenting symptoms of chondrosarcoma, with tumors centered in the skull base frequently causing headache, diplopia, and cranial nerve palsies.

Cytogenetic studies on chondrosarcoma have found different karyotypic abnormalities that lack specificity and vary in their complexity.[37] Chromosomal changes include regional deletions and mutations of tumor suppressor genes and oncogenes.[37]

The radiographic hallmark of conventional chondrosarcoma is a large, destructive, intramedullary, radiolucent mass with scattered punctate radiodensities.[43,50,77] Low-grade tumors have significant areas of mineralization and produce bone expansion, endosteal scalloping, and thickening of the cortex (Fig. 14.21). In contrast, high-grade tumors have large radiolucent areas, moth-eaten margins,

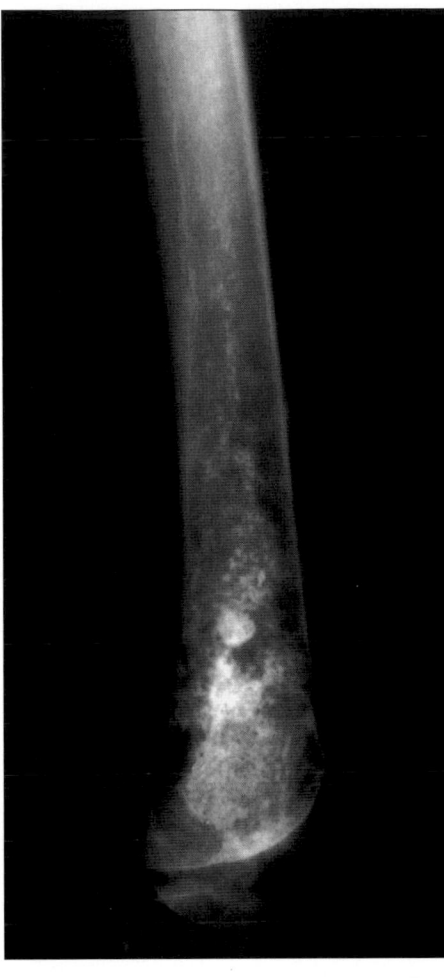

Fig. 14.21 Plain X-ray of a low-grade chondrosarcoma involving the entire distal half of the femur. Some of the dense mineralization represents an underlying enchondroma.

and cortical destruction with a significant soft tissue mass. Some chondrosarcomas contain a heavily mineralized intramedullary component, which may represent a pre-existing solitary enchondroma.[43] This finding is controversial, however, as some investigators report that it is an extremely rare event while others indicate that it is present in at least 50% of chondrosarcomas. MRI and CT are indispensable in determining the anatomic extent of the tumor and the nature of its margins. On MRI, the cartilage is dark on T1-weighted and bright on T2-weighted images. The unmineralized and mineralized components of the tumor are clearly delineated on CT scans.[43,50,77] On technetium bone scans chondrosarcomas show avid uptake.

Grossly, conventional chondrosarcomas are large, bulky tumors that are frequently 10 cm or greater in size. Low-grade tumors fill the medullary cavity, expand the bone, scallop the endosteal surface, and produce cortical thickening (Fig. 14.22). High-grade tumors destroy the cortex and form a soft tissue mass that is frequently well delineated by the raised periosteum. The neoplastic hyaline cartilage is gray, tan, and glistening and has a lobular architecture that may be accentuated by thin fibrous septa. Mineralized portions of the matrix appear as scattered, punctate, chalk-like deposits, while regions of prominent endochondral ossification are seen as hard, ivory areas of bone formation. Myxoid matrix is translucent, gray, and mucinous or watery. Large tumors have a propensity to undergo cystic degeneration.

Most chondrosarcomas grow in an infiltrative manner (Fig. 14.23). The tumor percolates through haversian systems, replaces marrow spaces and encases individual bony trabeculae. The neoplastic

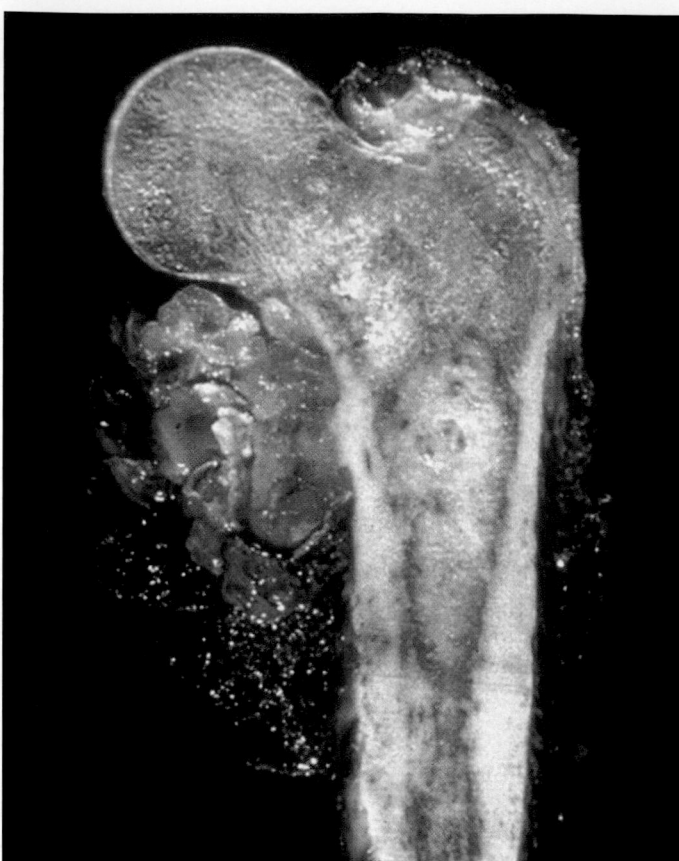

Fig. 14.22 Resected conventional chondrosarcoma of the proximal femur. The nodules of gray, glistening tumor fill the medullary cavity and extend into adjacent soft tissues.

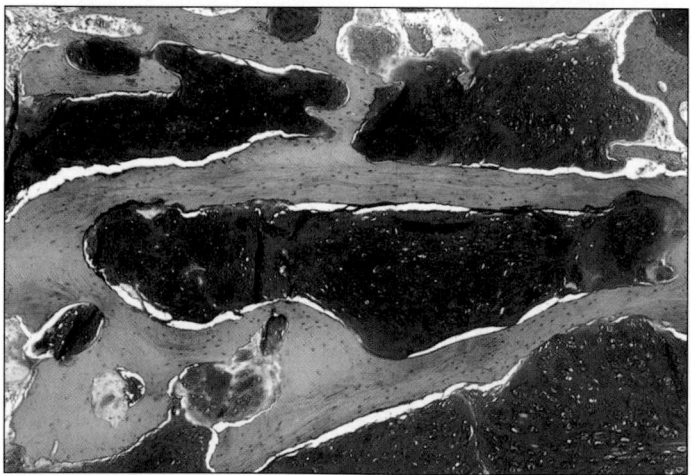

Fig. 14.23 Grade 1/3 chondrosarcoma infiltrating marrow and encasing pre-existing cancellous bone.

matrix is either hyaline or myxoid and their proportion varies greatly within individual tumors. Hyaline matrix is solid and usually basophilic, although occasionally it may be pink. Myxoid matrix is frothy or bubbly and is almost always basophilic. Both types of matrices may mineralize (which appears as amorphous purple

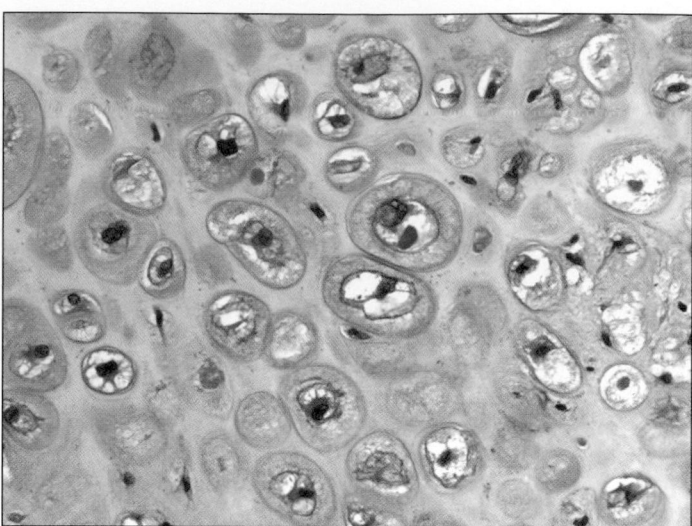

Fig. 14.24 Grade 1/3 hyaline chondrosarcoma. The cells have large nuclei with open chromatin pattern

granules) or undergo focal endochondral ossification. The neoplastic chondrocytes vary in size and have moderate amounts of eosinophilic cytoplasm that is occasionally vacuolated. The tumor cells in hyaline cartilage are round to oval and are confined to lacunar spaces. In contrast, the tumor cells in myxoid areas are bipolar or stellate and are arranged singly or in cords and strands. The cytoplasmic processes of neighboring cells come in close or direct contact with one another and form a complex cellular network. Importantly, the tumor cells are not arranged in tight cohesive nests or clusters, an architectural pattern characteristic of chordoma and carcinoma.

Conventional chondrosarcomas demonstrate varying degrees of cytologic atypia, which is determined by an assessment of the nuclear characteristics of the tumor cells and the extent of multinucleation. Aspects such as overall cell size are generally considered to be irrelevant. The combined features of cytologic atypia, cellularity, and mitotic activity have been integrated into different histological grading systems, none of which have been uniformly accepted.[13,105–107] Nonetheless, chondrosarcomas are usually graded on a three-tier system. Low-grade or grade 1 chondrosarcomas are hypocellular to moderately cellular and the chondrocyte nuclei are small, round, and dark or may be mildly enlarged with fine chromatin and small nucleoli. Occasional binucleate cells are present and mitoses are virtually absent (Fig. 14.24). Grade 1 chondrosarcomas can be very difficult, if not impossible, to distinguish from enchondromas on small biopsy specimens because of significant overlap in the cellularity and cytologic features of these tumors. Accordingly, accurate diagnosis requires careful assessment of the growth pattern (infiltrative versus well circumscribed margins) and evaluation of the radiographic findings. Intermediate grade or grade 2 chondrosarcomas are moderately cellular and the chondrocyte nuclei are roughly twice the size of those of nonneoplastic chondrocytes and are either hyperchromatic or have an open chromatin pattern and irregular contours. Binucleate cells are easily identified, trinucleate cells are uncommon, and mitotic figures are rare (Fig. 14.25). High-grade or grade 3 chondrosarcomas are densely cellular and contain many bizarre multinucleate cells that demonstrate severe pleomorphism and hyperchromasia. Mitoses, including structurally abnormal forms, are numerous (Fig. 14.26). Approximately 60% of conventional chondrosarcomas are grade 1, 35% are grade 2, and 5% are grade 3.[100–102,108,109]

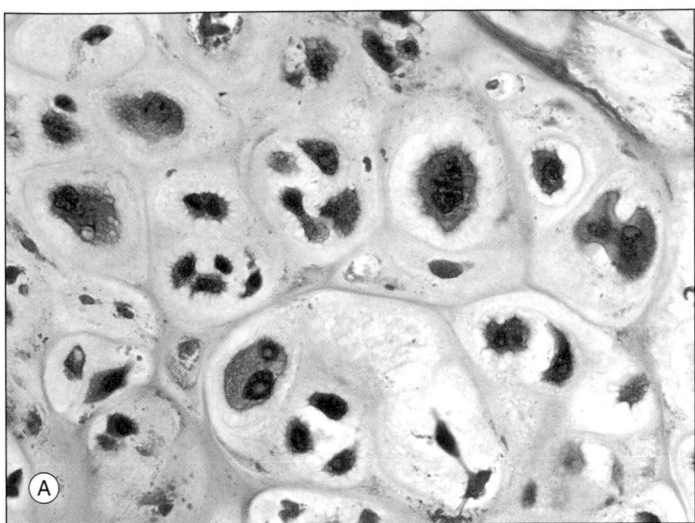 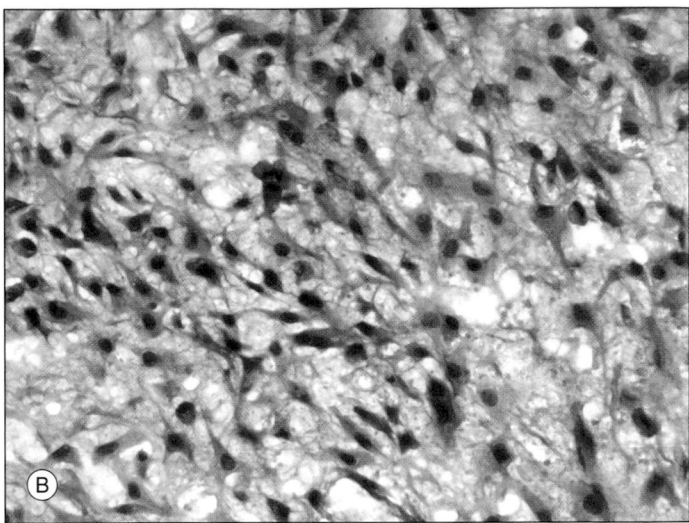

Fig. 14.25 (A) Grade 2/3 hyaline chondrosarcoma demonstrating significant cytologic atypia. **(B)** Grade 2/3 myxoid chondrosarcoma with stellate cells surrounded by a frothy basophilic matrix. Note mitotic figure in the center.

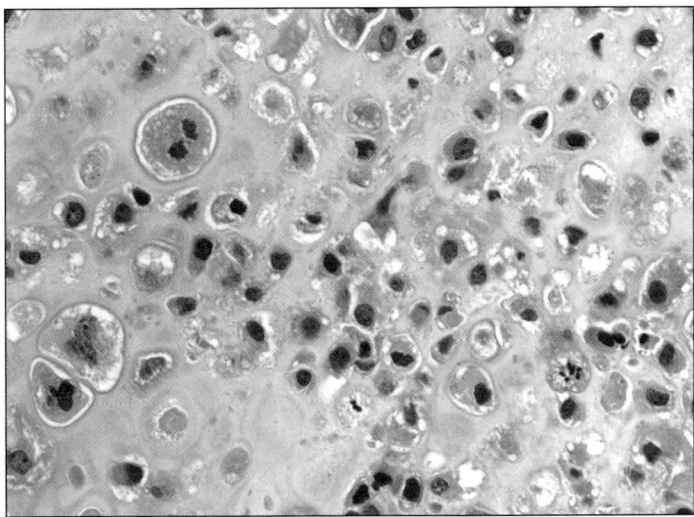 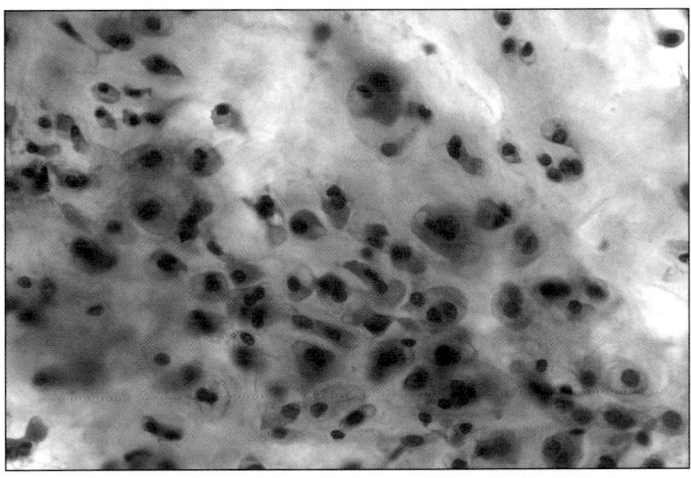

Fig. 14.27 Fragment of hyaline to myxoid chondroid stroma obtained from a grade 2 chondrosarcoma. Note the high cellularity with numerous binucleate chondrocytes. The chondrocytes show significant nuclear enlargement, hyperchromasia, and irregularity. (H&E stain.)

Fig. 14.26 Grade 3/3 hyaline chondrosarcoma. The hypercellular tumor demonstrates severe cytologic atypia and multinucleation.

Smear cellularity and matrix composition of conventional chondrosarcoma depends on the grade of the tumor.[110] Grade 1 chondrosarcomas are essentially cytologically indistinguishable from enchondromas. They contain large chunks of chondroid matrix surrounding lacunae containing one or two chondrocytes, as well as individual chondrocytes unassociated with matrix. Binucleate chondrocytes and lacunae containing two or more cells are more frequently seen in low-grade chondrosarcomas than in enchondromas; however, they are uncommon and do not permit definitive distinction between these two tumors. The nuclei of the chondrocytes are round or ovoid, may show slight degrees of nuclear enlargement and hyperchromasia, and the cytoplasm is abundant and vacuolated or finely granular.[111]

Grade 2 and 3 chondrosarcomas are associated with smears of higher cellularity, diminished amounts of hyaline cartilage, and greater quantities of myxoid–chondroid matrix.[52,53,112,113] In many grade 2 and 3 chondrosarcomas the myxoid–chondroid matrix is so abundant that it obscures the associated neoplastic chondrocytes. Significant nuclear atypia is present in at least a percentage of neoplastic chondrocytes. The nuclei are enlarged and have an open chromatin pattern, irregular contour, and prominent nucleoli (Fig. 14.27). Grade 3 chondrosarcomas demonstrate significant nuclear anaplasia, and mitotic figures, including atypical forms, are commonplace. In some cases, the chondroid matrix is very scant or absent.

The treatment of conventional chondrosarcoma has traditionally been wide surgical resection. Radiation has been used to treat tumors that are unresectable or have been incompletely excised. More recently, some investigators have advocated aggressive curettage for low-grade chondrosarcomas, especially if they are located in the appendicular skeleton. The overall local recurrence rate of conventional chondrosarcomas is approximately 20%.[100–102,108,109] Poor prognostic findings include location of the tumor in the pelvis and spine, size greater than 10 cm, and high histologic grade. The metastatic rate of conventional chondrosarcoma is approximately 14%, of which only 3% are grade 1 tumors. Conventional chondrosarcoma has an overall survival rate that ranges from 70–87% and is related to the grade of the tumor.[100–102,108,109,114] In one large series, the 5-year survival rate was 88.5% for grade 1 chondrosarcoma and 57.1% for combined grade 2 and 3 tumors.[109]

Periosteal chondrosarcoma

Conventional chondrosarcoma arising on the surface of a bone is known as periosteal or juxtacortical chondrosarcoma. This variant of conventional chondrosarcoma is rare and is approximately one-fifth as frequent as its uncommon benign counterpart periosteal chondroma.

Periosteal chondrosarcoma usually develops in adults, most frequently in the fourth decade of life. Males are affected more often than females, in a ratio as high as 5:1 according to some series.[115] Patients usually present with a painful, progressively enlarging mass that has been noted for several months to years prior to diagnosis. The tumor arises on the cortex in the metaphyseal or diaphyseal regions of the long bones, including the femur, humerus, and tibia, and the flat bones of the pelvis.[63,116]

Radiographs of periosteal chondrosarcoma show a large, cortically based tumor of soft tissue density that extends into the neighboring tissues. In many instances the soft tissue component contains scattered, irregular, spiculated calcifications.[115] The underlying cortex is frequently thickened but also contains scalloped erosions. Reactive subperiosteal bone may buttress the cortex at the proximal and distal margins of the tumor. CT and MRI reveal a lobular mass with scattered foci of mineralization. These techniques help determine the extent of the tumor and the presence of invasion into the medullary cavity, which is an uncommon occurrence.[115,117]

Macroscopically, periosteal chondrosarcoma is frequently 10 cm in dimension or larger and appears as a well circumscribed, solid, glistening, gray-tan, lobular mass. Gritty, chalk-like deposits of mineral may be scattered in the mass and ivory hard regions of endochondral ossification may also be present. The tumor is immediately adjacent to the underlying thickened cortex, which has an undulating surface caused by tumor erosion. A thin layer of periosteum separates the mass from the nearby soft tissues.

The tumor is composed of neoplastic hyaline cartilage that has the morphologic features of grade 1 or grade 2 conventional chondrosarcoma. Evidence of a higher-grade tumor should raise the possibility of juxtacortical chondroblastic osteosarcoma. The tumor extends into the soft tissues, with broad, pushing margins.

The treatment of periosteal chondrosarcoma is wide excision with a local recurrence rate of 10–20%. Metastases are very uncommon.[115,116]

Secondary chondrosarcoma

Secondary chondrosarcoma is a conventional chondrosarcoma that arises in a bone affected by a pre-existing condition or benign neoplasm. In contrast to osteosarcoma, chondrosarcoma rarely develops in irradiated bone or bone involved by Paget's disease.[118,119] Most secondary chondrosarcomas are derived from malignant transformation of a pre-existing enchondroma or osteochondroma. As discussed previously (see Conventional chondrosarcoma, above), the frequency of chondrosarcoma arising in association with a pre-existing enchondroma is controversial, but in our experience it is a common occurrence.

The true incidence of conventional chondrosarcoma developing in association with an osteochondroma (peripheral chondrosarcoma) is unknown because most osteochondromas are asymptomatic and are never detected. Additionally, the criteria for diagnosing chondrosarcoma in this setting are inadequately defined as the literature concerning this issue is based solely on surgical series, which are inherently influenced by selection bias. Consequently, the 1–2% reported risk of malignant transformation of solitary osteochondroma and the 15–25% transformation risk in multiple hereditary exostoses are significant overestimations. Supporting this view are recent analyses of kindreds with multiple hereditary exostoses that document the incidence of malignant transformation to be less than 1–3%.[33,120,121]

The absolute number of chondrosarcomas arising in solitary and multiple osteochondromas is approximately equal.[44,122] The patients are usually 10–20 years younger that those with primary chondrosarcoma and there is a male predominance. The tumors tend to develop on the surfaces of the flat and long tubular bones of the skeleton. Patients frequently complain of recent and sometimes rapid and painful enlargement of a pre-existing mass or known osteochondroma.

Chondrosarcoma arising in osteochondroma appears radiographically as a large mass that has the features inherent to osteochondroma. The cartilaginous component, however, is prominent, has irregular margins, contains considerable areas of radiolucency, and enlarges over time, developing new separate soft tissue elements that may or may not be mineralized.[44,122] Important telltale signs of malignancy are destruction of the stalk of the osteochondroma and invasion into the medullary cavity of the underlying bone.

Peripheral chondrosarcomas are well circumscribed, large, cauliflower-like masses composed of prominent lobules of gray, glistening hyaline cartilage that may contain cystic and mucinous areas and form the thickened 'cap' of the tumor. The periphery is demarcated from the surrounding soft tissues by a thin layer of fibrous tissue. Within the cap are chalky white areas of calcification, as well as ivory-colored, hard foci of endochondral ossification. Histologically, the cartilage shows the degree of cellularity and cytologic atypia associated with grade 1 or grade 2 conventional chondrosarcoma. The malignant cartilage is divided into large lobules by fibrous septae and has a pushing margin with the adjacent soft tissues. In a minority of cases the sarcoma permeates the underlying stalk and infiltrates into the marrow cavity of the host bone. Portions of the residual benign hyaline cartilage cap of the osteochondroma can be found with careful search.

The treatment of peripheral chondrosarcoma is usually excision with negative margins.[44,122] Adjuvant radiation may be used in cases in which complete surgical resection is not feasible or the margins of resection are inadequate. In the largest reported series, the 5-year and 10-year local recurrence rates were 15.9% and 17.5% respectively, and 5- and 10-year mortality rates were 1.6% and 4.8% for patients having initial treatment at the authors' institution.[44] Metastases develop in approximately 5% of cases and are discovered most frequently within the lung.[44,122] Fatal outcomes are usually caused by problems associated with local recurrence.

Dedifferentiated chondrosarcoma

Dedifferentiated chondrosarcoma is a high-grade malignant neoplasm that is composed of two components: a well differentiated cartilaginous tumor, usually a low-grade conventional chondrosarcoma or, less frequently, an enchondroma or osteochondroma, juxtaposed to a high-grade sarcoma. Whether both of these components are derived from a common precursor cell remains to be proved.[123] The presence

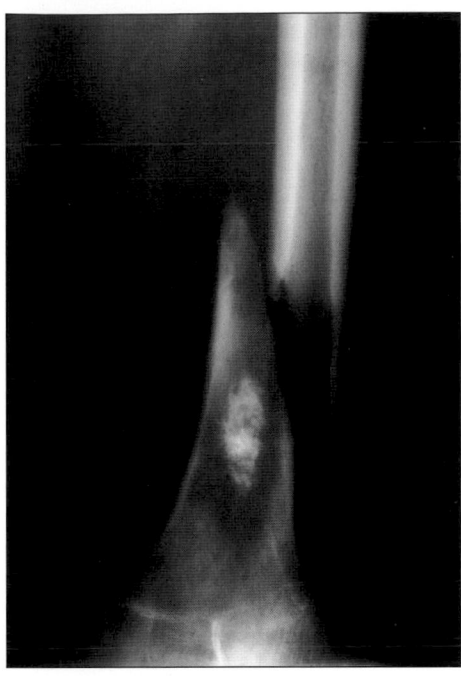

Fig. 14.28 Pathologic fracture through a destructive, lytic, dedifferentiated chondrosarcoma. The central heavily mineralized region represents an underlying enchondroma and low-grade chondrosarcoma.

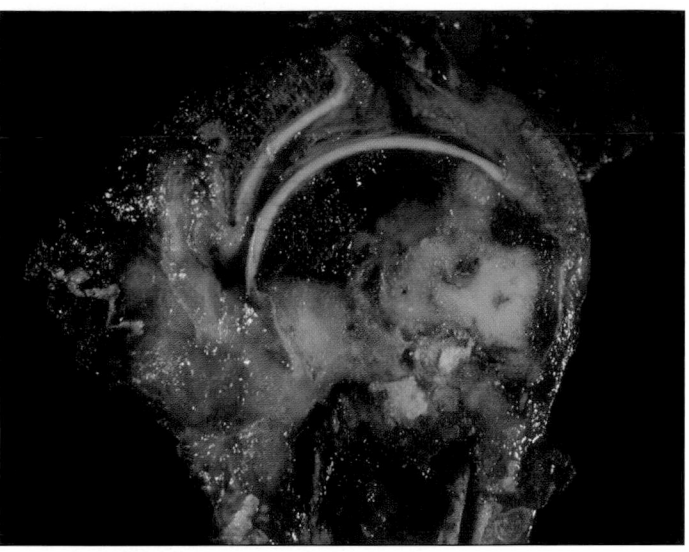

Fig. 14.29 Dedifferentiated chondrosarcoma of the proximal humerus. The central gray nodules represent the underlying low-grade chondrosarcoma. The pink-tan areas extending into the soft tissues represent the dedifferentiated component.

of identical somatic mutations and p53 overexpression in both components, however, suggests that they originate from a single progenitor cell.[123]

Dedifferentiation occurs in approximately 10% of conventional chondrosarcomas. These tumors are usually diagnosed in adults 50–70 years old. Males are affected more frequently than females.[4] Similarly to conventional chondrosarcoma, they usually develop in the pelvis, femur, or humerus. Clinically, patients present with pain, swelling, and commonly pathologic fractures.

Intramedullary dedifferentiated chondrosarcoma has two distinct radiographic components (Fig. 14.28). The low-grade element manifests as a mineralized area with rings and arches, typical of enchondroma or low-grade conventional chondrosarcoma, adjacent to a lytic permeative aggressive component that destroys the surrounding bone and frequently extends into the adjacent soft tissues. This correlates with the gross features, in which gray, glistening nodules of cartilage are adjacent to or surrounded by a pink-tan, fleshy tissue that represents the high-grade sarcoma (Fig. 14.29). Sometimes, the chondroid areas can be very small and a thorough examination is necessary to identify them. The chondroid component is well differentiated and usually has the features of a cellular enchondroma or low-grade conventional chondrosarcoma. The high-grade sarcoma is usually a pleomorphic spindle cell sarcoma with the features of malignant fibrous histiocytoma, although a variety of other phenotypes may be encountered, such as osteosarcoma, fibrosarcoma, rhabdomyosarcoma, or leiomyosarcoma[124–128] (Fig. 14.30). Rarely, the dedifferentiated component resembles a giant cell tumor.[129] The immunohistochemical and ultrastructural features of the dedifferentiated component reflects its phenotype. Occasionally, however, the dedifferentiated pleomorphic spindle cell areas may express keratin, which raises the possibility of metastatic sarcomatoid carcinoma.[130]

Dedifferentiated chondrosarcoma is a very aggressive neoplasm that requires wide excision and systemic therapy. Unfortunately, many patients are elderly and have medical conditions that limit their tolerance of necessary forms of therapy. Accordingly, the prognosis is poor and most patients die within 2 years of diagnosis.

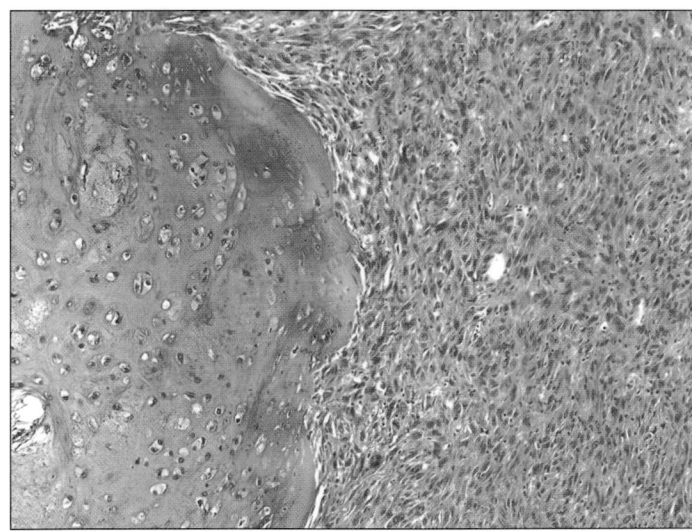

Fig. 14.30 Dedifferentiated chondrosarcoma composed of low-grade chondrosarcoma juxtaposed to a pleomorphic spindle cell sarcoma.

Mesenchymal chondrosarcoma

Mesenchymal chondrosarcoma is a rare subtype of chondrosarcoma, arising in bone and less commonly soft tissue. It was first described in 1959 by Lichtenstein and Bernstein, who encountered it in the thoracic vertebrae and parietal bone, respectively, in two young patients.[131] Mesenchymal chondrosarcoma typically occurs during the second or third decades of life and is slightly more common in females.[132,133] It has a propensity to arise in the maxilla and mandible, followed by the vertebrae, ribs, pelvis, and humerus. When it arises in the long bones, mesenchymal chondrosarcoma tends to be diaphyseal in location.[133,134] Presenting symptoms vary somewhat according to the site of origin but many are first detected as an enlarging mass, which is sometimes painful.

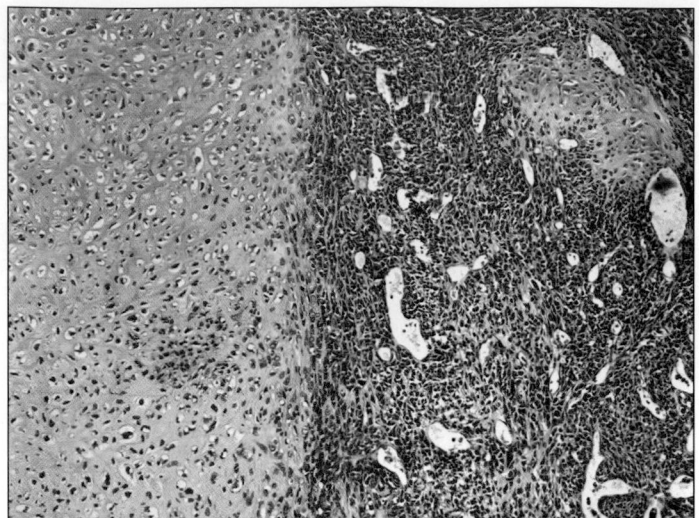

Fig. 14.31 Mesenchymal chondrosarcoma. The tumor is composed of nodules of cartilage with adjacent small round cell component. Note the prominent hemangiopericytoma-like vascular pattern.

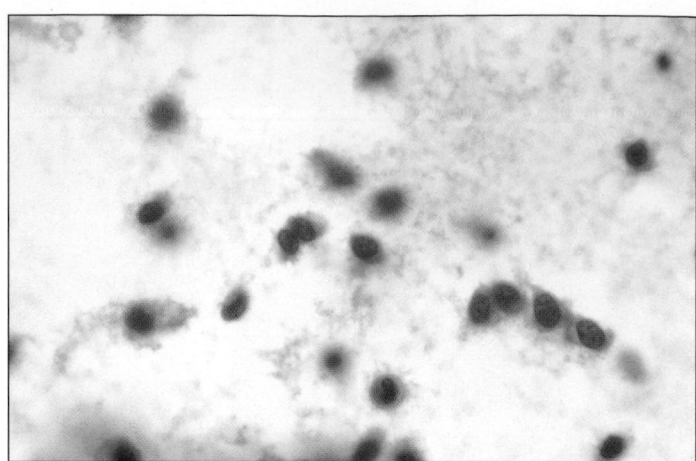

Fig. 14.32 Small round to ovoid cells with scanty cytoplasm and hyperchromatic nuclei characterize mesenchymal chondrosarcomas. The background contains granular to watery material consistent with myxoid–chondroid ground substance. (H&E stain.)

Mesenchymal chondrosarcoma is gray and fleshy with scattered areas of white calcification. Microscopically, it is composed of sheets of small, round, ovoid or spindle-shaped cells that have hyperchromatic nuclei and scant cytoplasm. Scattered throughout the tumor are nodules of mildly to moderately cellular cartilage that is hyaline or fibrous in appearance (Fig. 14.31). The matrix may be well demarcated or blend imperceptibly with the surrounding small cell component. The cartilage frequently mineralizes or undergoes endochondral ossification, which produces the radiodensities present on X-rays. In many cases, individual cells are surrounded by extracellular eosinophilic matrix resembling bone, and its presence raises the possibility that the lesion may represent a variant of osteosarcoma. The supportive stroma frequently contains a vascular tree that has a hemangiopericytoma-like pattern.

FNA of mesenchymal chondrosarcoma yields highly cellular smears in which the predominant cell type is a small round cell lying singly or in loosely cohesive clusters (Fig. 14.32).[112] The small round neoplastic cells have scant to modest amounts of granular cytoplasm with distinct borders. The central round to oval nuclei have coarsely granular chromatin and small nucleoli. The nuclear membranes are generally smooth but occasionally demonstrate longitudinal nuclear grooves. A small amount of chondroid matrix is usually present but may be exceedingly scant or altogether absent.

The cells in the cartilaginous areas stain immunohistochemically for vimentin and S-100 protein. The small blue cells stain with vimentin, CD99, Leu-7, and neuron-specific enolase. A recent study has also shown that they express SOX9 (transcription factor involved in chondrogenesis), which might be helpful in distinguishing mesenchymal chondrosarcoma from other malignant small round cell tumors,[135] especially in small biopsy specimens that lack neoplastic cartilage. Ultrastructurally, the cells in the chondroid areas have the features of chondrocytes, whereas the round cells are primitive and have large nuclei with little cytoplasm and scattered organelles. Cytogenetic studies have shown that both skeletal and extraskeletal mesenchymal chondrosarcomas have a robertsonian translocation.[136]

Mesenchymal chondrosarcoma is treated with radical surgery in conjunction with adjuvant chemotherapy and radiation therapy. The clinical course maybe protracted, and the overall 5- and 10-year survivals are approximately 55% and 27% respectively.[133] The prognosis associated with tumors arising in the jaw bones is better, with 5- and 10-year survival rates of 82% and 56% respectively.[137]

Clear cell chondrosarcoma

Clear cell chondrosarcoma is the least common variant of chondrosarcoma, accounting for 2% of all chondrosarcomas. It was initially described by Unni et al. in 1976 and behaves as a low-grade malignancy.[138,139] It arises in all age groups, with a peak incidence during the third and fourth decades of life[140] and a higher incidence in males than females. Clear cell chondrosarcoma typically arises in the epiphysis of long tubular bones, especially the proximal femur. Patients present complaining of pain that has sometimes been present for years.

Radiographically, clear cell chondrosarcoma is usually well defined, lytic, contains punctate calcifications, and may cause expansion of the bone[140] (Fig. 14.33).

The tumors range in size from 5–10 cm and are well circumscribed, solid, firm, and tan-white. They are centered in the epiphysis or apophysis. As they grow, they may destroy the cortex and extend, with pushing margins, into the adjacent soft tissues. Microscopically, clear cell chondrosarcoma has a lobular growth pattern and is composed of sheets of large cells with abundant clear or pink cytoplasm that is rich in glycogen and delineated by well defined cell borders (Fig. 14.34). Osteoclasts and trabeculae of woven bone rimmed by non-neoplastic osteoblasts are scattered throughout these tumors. Clear cell chondrosarcomas also contain areas of conventional low-grade, hyaline-type chondrosarcoma. Rare cases of dedifferentiated clear cell chondrosarcoma have been reported.[141]

Cytologic preparations from clear cell chondrosarcomas demonstrate moderate to high cellularity. The majority of cells are round to ovoid with moderate to abundant amounts of clear, frequently vacuolated cytoplasm (Fig. 14.35). The nuclei of the neoplastic cells are enlarged with a moderately to coarsely granular chromatin and large distinct nucleoli. The background has a watery, myxoid appearance

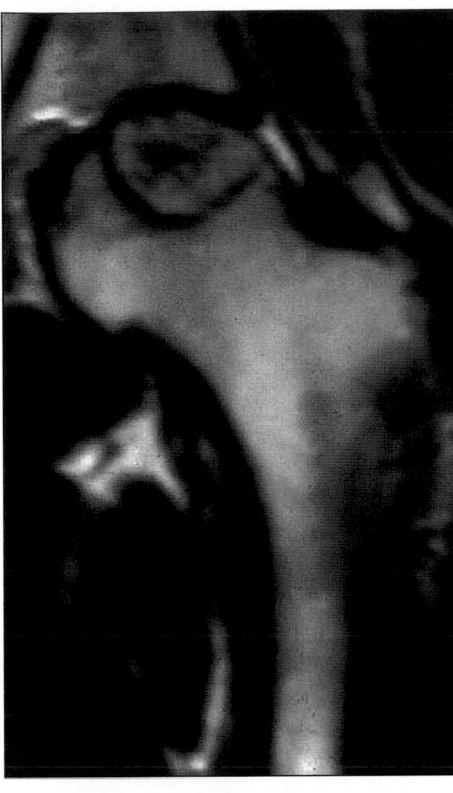

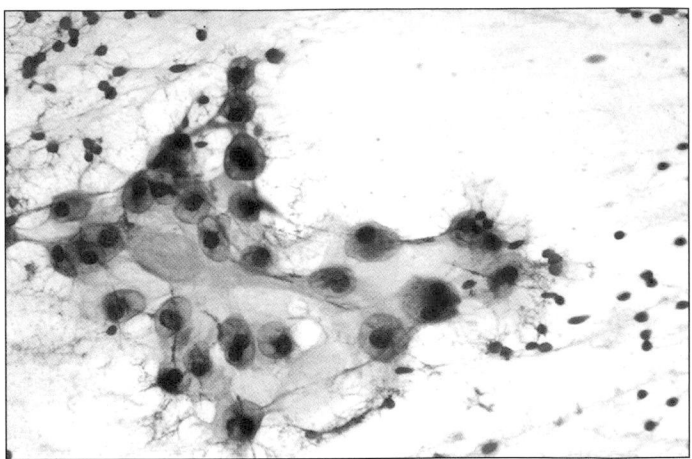

Fig. 14.33 MRI of a clear cell chondrosarcoma of proximal femur. The tumor is located within the epiphysis and has a heterogeneous pattern.

Fig. 14.35 Small fragment of chondroid stroma associated with round or polygonal cells with moderate amounts of pale to clear cytoplasm is characteristic of clear cell chondrosarcomas. The nuclei are enlarged, hyperchromatic, and possess irregular nuclear membranes. (H&E stain.)

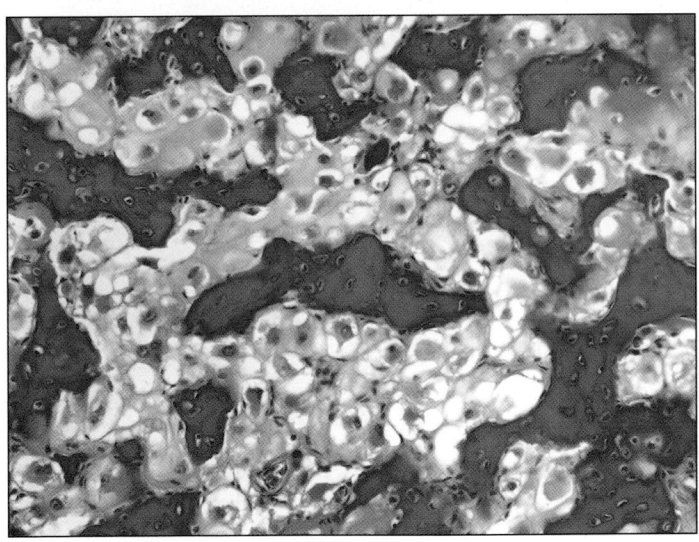

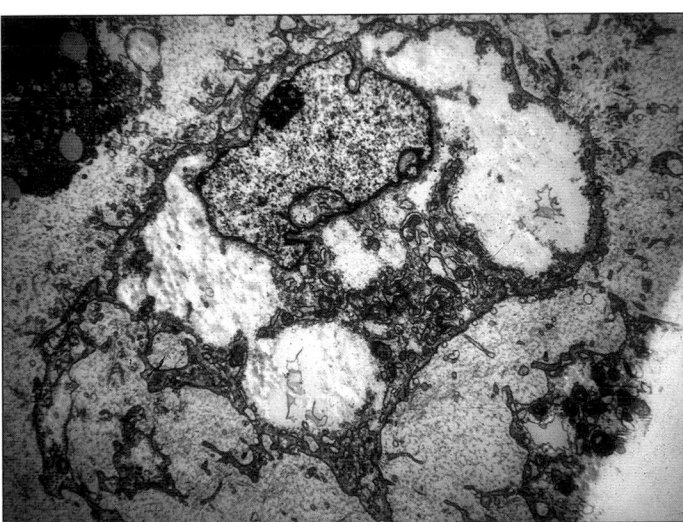

Fig. 14.34 Clear cell chondrosarcoma. Sheets of large neoplastic chondrocytes with abundant clear or pink cytoplasm admixed with metaplastic trabeculae of woven bone. Flattened osteoblasts line the surfaces of bone.

Fig. 14.36 Ultrastructurally the neoplastic cells in clear cell chondrosarcoma contain large pockets of glycogen.

consistent with myxoid–chondroid stroma. A minor component of multinucleate osteoclast-like giant cells may be present.

Immunohistochemically, the neoplastic cells express S-100 protein and type II collagen. Ultrastructurally, the neoplastic cells contain abundant intracytoplasmic glycogen, as demonstrated by a periodic acid–Schiff stain (Fig. 14.36).[142,143]

Clear cell chondrosarcoma behaves as a low-grade sarcoma and may have a prolonged clinical course. Treatment consists of wide resection, as both curettage and marginal excision are associated with a high rate of local recurrence and subsequent metastasis.[140] Overall, the local recurrence rate is approximately 16%, with 10% of patients eventually dying of their disease.[140] All three of the patients reported with dedifferentiated clear cell chondrosarcoma died of metastatic disease.[141]

BONE-FORMING TUMORS

Common to all these neoplasms is the production of bone by the neoplastic cells. The tumor bone can be deposited as cortical or cancellous, and the collagen can be arranged in a woven or lamellar pattern. In benign tumors, the bone consists of relatively well formed trabeculae of woven bone, whereas in osteosarcoma it frequently has a coarse, lace-like pattern. Lamellar cortical-type bone is only present in osteoma and enostosis, and rarely in well differentiated osteosarcoma.

BONE ISLAND

Bone island, also known as enostosis, is a benign bone-forming tumor composed of cortical-type bone that develops within the medullary cavity. Its true frequency is unknown because it is usually detected as an incidental radiographic finding. Its prevalence in pelvic bones and ribs has been reported to be 1.08% and 0.43% respectively.[144] Bone islands have been identified in all age groups, are uncommon in children, and occur equally in males and females. The pelvis, proximal femur, and ribs are the most frequently involved sites. When present in tubular bones, bone islands are usually located in the epiphyses.[145] Clinically, bone islands are asymptomatic, with only exceptional cases causing pain.

Bone islands have characteristic radiographic features.[144–148] On plain films they appear as small, round, single or multiple, homogeneously radiodense lesions with spiculated margins that merge with the surrounding cancellous bone (Fig. 14.37A). The lesions, especially larger variants, may abut or be based on the endosteal surface; however, they do not involve the cortex and do not elicit a periosteal reaction.[145–147] On CT scans, bone islands have the same characteristics as cortical bone. On MRI, they are dark; on bone scan, they are cold.

Bone islands arise in the medullary cavity, are generally not much larger than 1 cm in diameter, and are hard, solid, and tan-white. Their periphery blends into the surrounding cancellous trabeculae (Fig. 14.37B). They consist of cortical-type bone that is predominately lamellar, but may be focally woven, and contains haversian-like canals (Fig. 14.38). The osteoblasts lining the surfaces are flat and quiescent and the osteocytes are small and cytologically banal.

Osteopoikilosis is a syndrome that may be inherited in an autosomal dominant fashion and is characterized by the presence of innumerable bone islands. The enostoses are bilateral and symmetrical in distribution and are most numerous in the metaphyseal and epiphyseal regions of tubular bones, carpal and tarsal bones, and the flat bones of the proximal limb girdles (Fig. 14.39).[149] Macroscopically and histologically they are identical to sporadic, solitary bone islands.

Bone islands usually do not need any type of treatment. Occasional cases, particularly larger variants, may require a biopsy to exclude more aggressive lesions such as well differentiated osteosarcoma and sclerotic metastases.

OSTEOMA

Osteoma is a benign bone-forming tumor. Most are composed primarily of mature dense compact or cancellous bone; however, rare osteomas consist entirely of cancellous bone. Osteoma usually affects the craniofacial skeleton, where it develops on the bones forming the paranasal and frontal sinuses and the orbit (Fig. 14.40).[150] Extracranial variants are rare and most develop on the surfaces of long tubular bones (Fig. 14.41).[151] Osteoma is usually solitary but may be multiple in patients with Gardner syndrome.[152]

Craniofacial osteomas are commonly asymptomatic and are detected as an incidental radiographic finding. Larger tumors may be symptomatic and cause swelling, facial asymmetry, and symptoms secondary to sinus obstruction, including discharge and mucocele

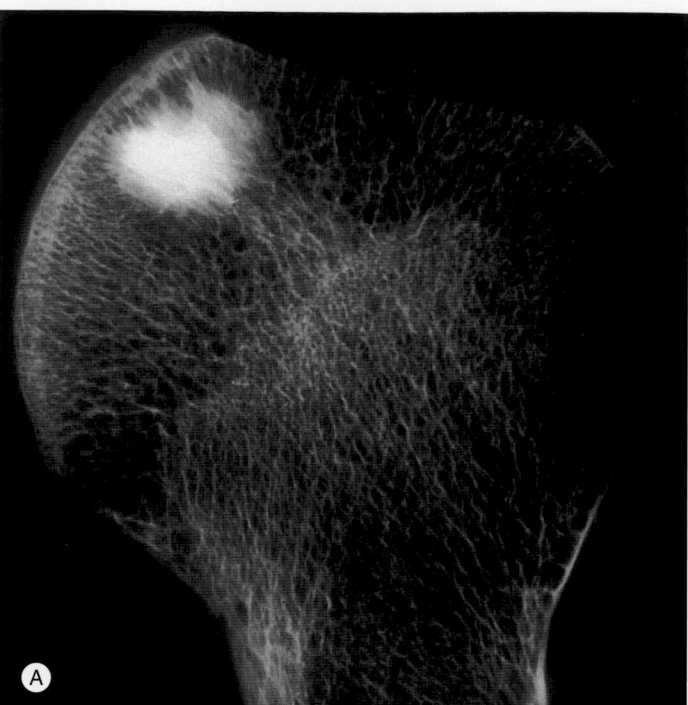

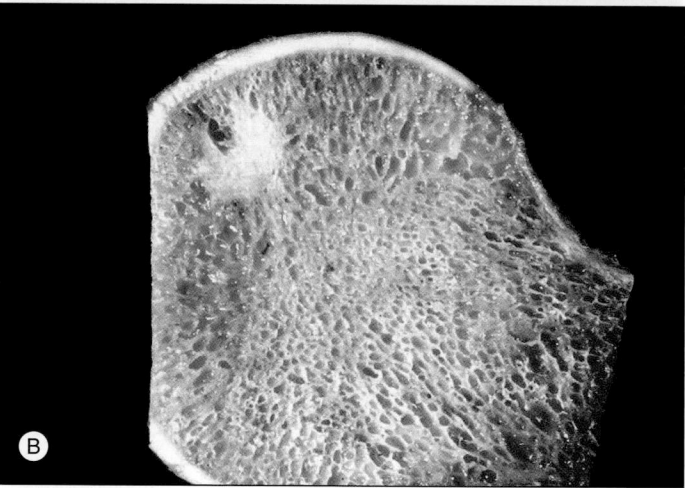

Fig. 14.37 Specimen X-ray **(A)** and gross specimen **(B)** of a bone island showing a round, homogenously mineralized, radiodense mass that merges with the surrounding cancellous bone. The tumor is hard and tan-white.

formation.[153–156] Orbital osteomas can produce a variety of ocular abnormalities.[155,157]

Radiographically, osteomas are uniformly radiodense, ovoid to mushroom-shaped lesions that are well demarcated from the surrounding soft tissues but merge with the underlying cortex. The trabecular variant is surfaced by a thin rim of compact bone that surrounds tissue with the radiodensity of cancellous bone. Grossly, osteomas are ovoid, hard, and tan-white and resemble the cortical bone with which they merge. Histologically, osteomas usually consist of lamellar bone or an admixture of lamellar and woven bone with haversian systems. The rare cancellous variant has a trabecular pattern. Only symptomatic lesions need to be treated by simple excision.

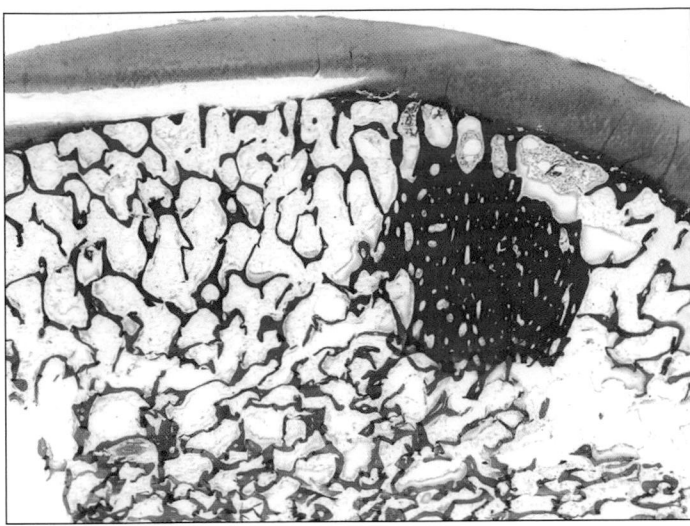

Fig. 14.38 Bone island composed of cortical-type bone merging with the surrounding cancellous bone.

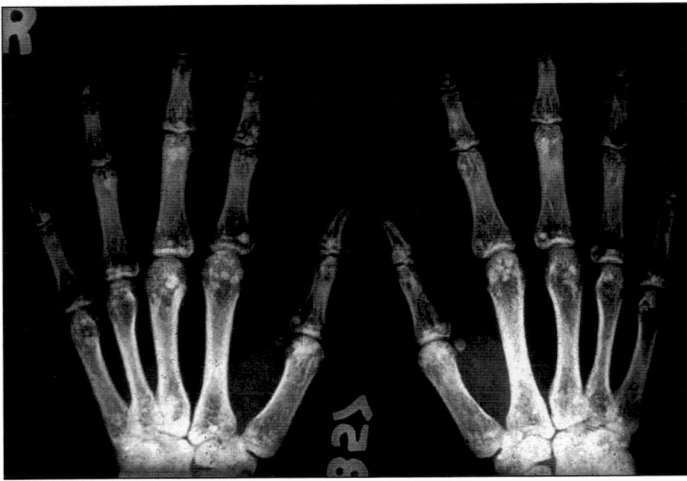

Fig. 14.39 X-ray of patient with osteopoikilosis. Numerous bone islands are scattered throughout the bones of the hand.

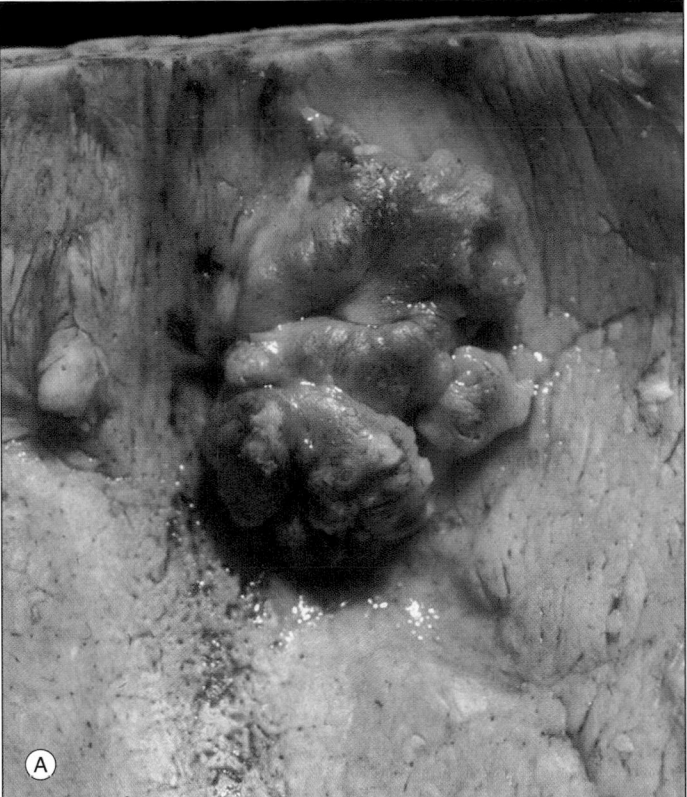

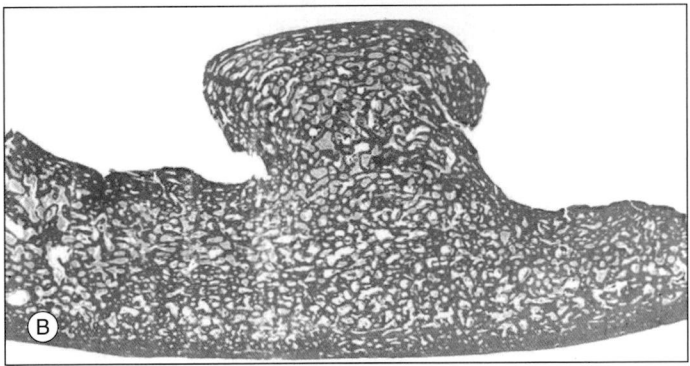

Fig. 14.40 Gross **(A)** and whole mount **(B)** specimen of an osteoma attached to the inner table of the skull. Much of the bone in this case is trabecular.

Because osteomas are composed of densely mineralized osteoid, the small diameter needles characteristically used for cytologic sampling cannot penetrate them, and material cannot be obtained for cytologic analysis. We are unaware of any published descriptions of the cytologic findings in osteomas sampled either by FNA, intraoperative scrapings, or imprint preparations.

OSTEOID OSTEOMA

Osteoid osteoma is a benign bone-forming tumor characterized by its small size, limited growth potential, and classic pattern of pain. Osteoid osteoma accounts for approximately 12% of benign bone tumors and, like osteoblastoma, most frequently develops in young adults and has a male predominance.[155,158–161] Patients typically complain of severe localized pain that is often worse at night and is relieved by aspirin or other nonsteroidal antiinflammatory medications.[155,158–161] It can involve virtually any bone in the body but is most common in the diaphysis of long bones, especially the femur. Patients with lesions located close to or within joints can present with joint pain, swelling, and effusions.[162] Tumors located in the vertebral column (usually the posterior elements) can cause painful scoliosis secondary to spasm of paravertebral muscles, while lesions of the small bones of the hand and feet may produce marked soft tissue swelling, mimicking infection.

By definition, osteoid osteoma is 1–2 cm in diameter. By convention, morphologically similar tumors larger than 2 cm are classified as osteoblastomas. Radiographically, osteoid osteoma is round and radiolucent with frequent patchy mineralization located centrally. The lesion or nidus has well defined margins and is surrounded by a zone of subperiosteal or medullary sclerosis (reactive zone), which may be so extensive that it obscures the underlying lesion and even simulates an aggressive tumor. Grossly,

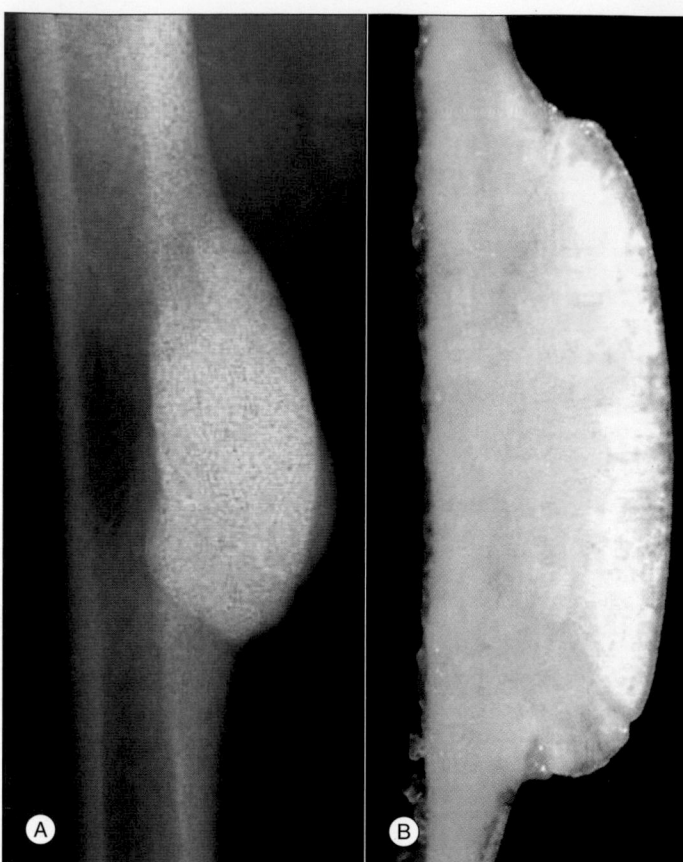

Fig. 14.41 Plain X-ray **(A)** and gross specimen **(B)** of a large osteoma of the femur. The oblong radiodense tumor merges with the underlying cortex and is hard and tan-white in appearance.

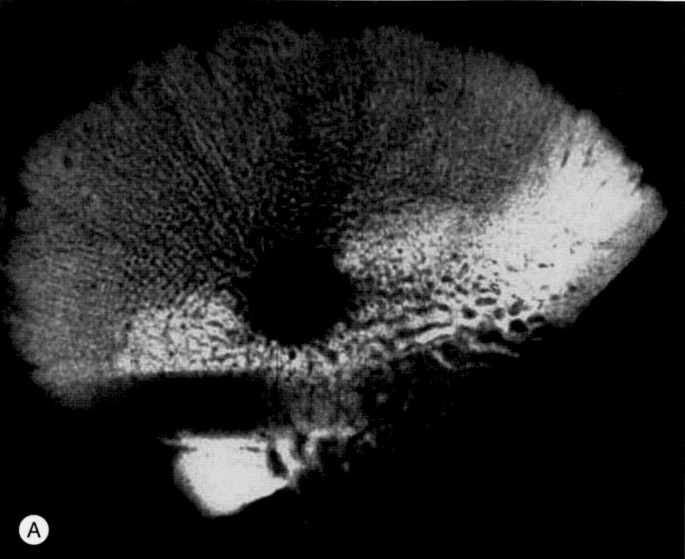

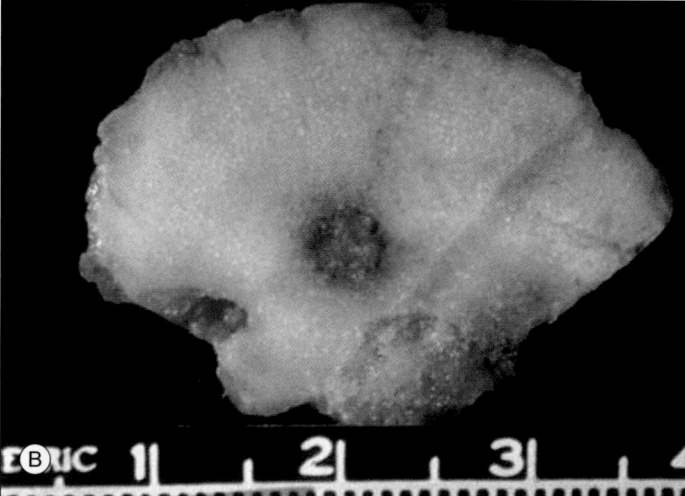

Fig. 14.42 Specimen X-ray **(A)** and resected gross specimen **(B)** of an intracortical osteoid osteoma. The pink-tan-white tumor is surrounded by abundant subperiosteal and intramedullary reactive bone. The nidus is radiolucent with central delicate calcifications.

the nidus is dark red with tan-white speckled mineralization, appears gritty, and is surrounded by dense sclerotic bone (Fig. 14.42). Histologically, it is composed of haphazard, interanastomosing trabeculae of woven bone prominently rimmed by osteoblasts. Scattered osteoclasts are also commonly present on the bony surfaces. The intervening stroma consists of richly vascularized loose connective tissue containing plump fibroblasts and thin-walled vessels with variable numbers of inflammatory cells (Fig. 14.43). In our experience, chondroid areas are very rarely seen and, when present, should raise the possibility of other types of tumor. Juxtaarticular tumors may produce a chronic synovitis with lymphoid follicles resembling rheumatoid arthritis.[163]

Osteoid osteomas, to our knowledge, have not been successfully sampled by FNA because of their intracortical location and extensive rim of sclerosis. Intraoperative scrape or touch preparations disclose a small number of plump osteoblasts, multinucleate osteoclast-like giant cells, and rare bland spindle cells. The background is rich in red blood cells, with no demonstrable osteoid. While the cytologic features are helpful in excluding metastatic disease, bone abscess, or high-grade sarcoma, they are not in themselves diagnostic. Correlation with the radiographic features is fundamental in accurately interpreting these lesions.

Immunohistochemical stains demonstrate nerve fibers within the tumor and the surrounding reactive zone. High levels of prostaglandin E_2 and prostacyclins have also been identified within the nidus,[164]

which may be related to COX-2 overexpression by osteoblasts.[165,166] Both these findings are probably responsible for the characteristic aspirin-sensitive pain.

The neoplastic potential of osteoid osteoma has been questioned because of its limited growth potential. Cytogenetic studies have shown involvement of chromosome 22q, however, suggesting that osteoid osteoma is probably a neoplasm.[167] In the past, the treatment of osteoid osteoma was frequently curettage or en bloc resection; however, in recent years radiofrequency ablation has become the treatment of choice.[168–173] The local recurrence rate following ablation is approximately 5%.

OSTEOBLASTOMA

Osteoblastoma is a rare, benign bone-forming tumor first described by Jaffe and Lichtenstein in 1956, and accounts for approximately 1% of primary bone tumors.[174,175] It usually arises in the medullary

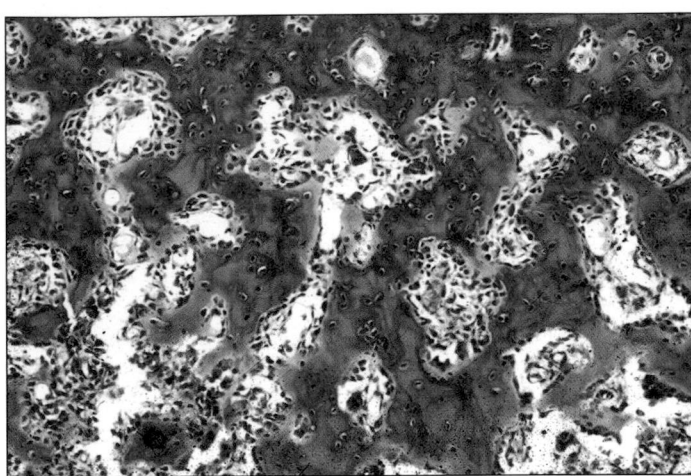

Fig. 14.43 Osteoid osteoma composed of interconnecting trabeculae of woven bone lined by prominent osteoblasts.

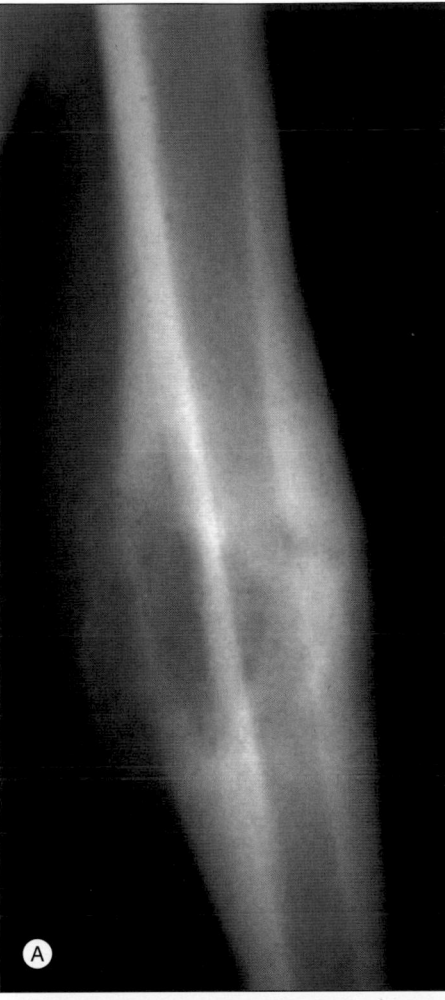

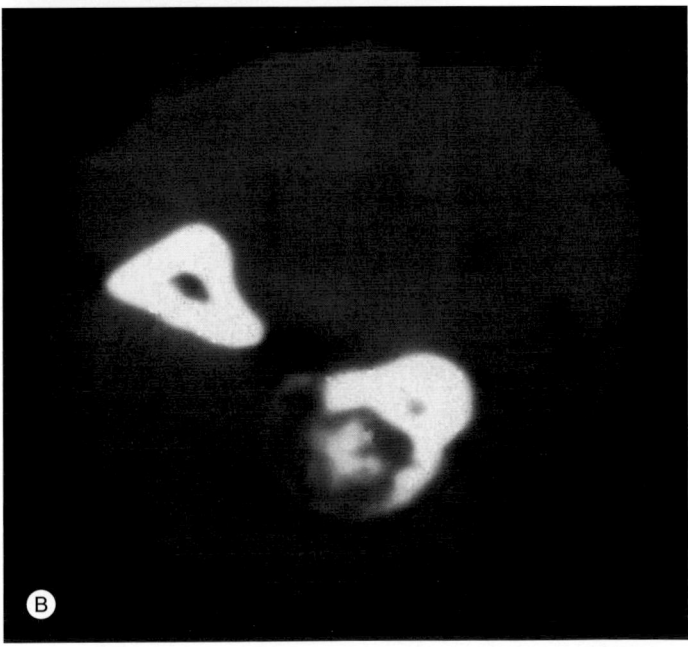

Fig. 14.44 Plain X-ray (**A**) and axial CT scan (**B**) of a subperiosteal osteoblastoma. The tumor has well circumscribed margins and contains central mineralization.

canal but may also be juxtacortical in location. In tubular bones, osteoblastomas are frequently centered in the metadiaphyseal region. In the largest series, 32% involved the spinal column, 12% the femur, 10% the tibia, and 9% the bones of the foot and ankle.[174] Osteoblastoma is usually diagnosed in young adults in the second to fourth decades of life, and males are affected approximately twice as frequently as females.[158,174–176]

Radiographically, osteoblastoma presents as a well defined, mixed lytic and blastic mass with sclerotic margins, and may expand the bone (Fig. 14.44).[174–176] Osteoblastoma is dark red because of its rich vasculature, as well as tan-white and gritty. In most cases, the tumor measures 2–5 cm in diameter (Fig. 14.45). Cystic changes (aneurysmal-bone-cyst-like changes) are seen in approximately 10% of tumors. Microscopically, osteoblastoma is well demarcated from the surrounding bone and is composed of haphazardly deposited trabeculae of woven bone rimmed by osteoblasts and scattered osteoclasts within a richly vascular stroma (Fig. 14.46). In some cases, the bone is deposited in sheets, and in 5–10% of cases a cartilaginous matrix may be present.[177] The osteoblasts in conventional tumors are ovoid or round with eccentric nuclei and moderate amounts of eosinophilic or purple cytoplasm. Mitoses are uncommon and necrosis is usually absent, unless there has been a pathologic fracture. In 10–15% of tumors, the osteoblasts are epithelioid and two to three times larger than conventional osteoblasts, and have abundant eosinophilic cytoplasm with vesicular nuclei and prominent nucleoli (Fig. 14.47). These tumors have been designated 'aggressive osteoblastoma' and have been reported to behave in a more aggressive manner than conventional tumors. The factors associated with aggressive clinical outcome have included secondary aneurysmal-bone-cyst-like changes, tumor location, and incomplete removal.[174] In the Mayo Clinic series the clinical course of 'aggressive osteoblastoma' was similar to that of conventional osteoblastoma.

Approximately 15% of osteoblastomas have several 'nidi' separated by cancellous bone that may simulate an infiltrative growth pattern. A similar number of cases may contain cells with bizarre, degenerative nuclei (pseudomalignant osteoblastoma). This finding has no clinical significance except that it may cause confusion with osteosarcoma. Rarely, osteoblastomas contain cartilage and its presence may also raise the possibility of osteosarcoma.

The size and expansile nature of osteoblastomas is such that the surrounding cortex is frequently thinned to a narrow rim of bony

sclerosis penetrable by needles traditionally used for FNA. Smears are characterized by a background rich in red blood cells and a moderately cellular, polymorphous population composed of plump osteoblasts, multinucleate osteoclasts, and bland spindle cells. The

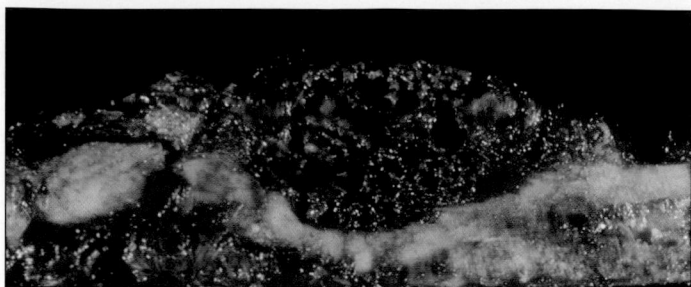

Fig. 14.45 Well circumscribed hemorrhagic osteoblastoma attached to the underlying cortex.

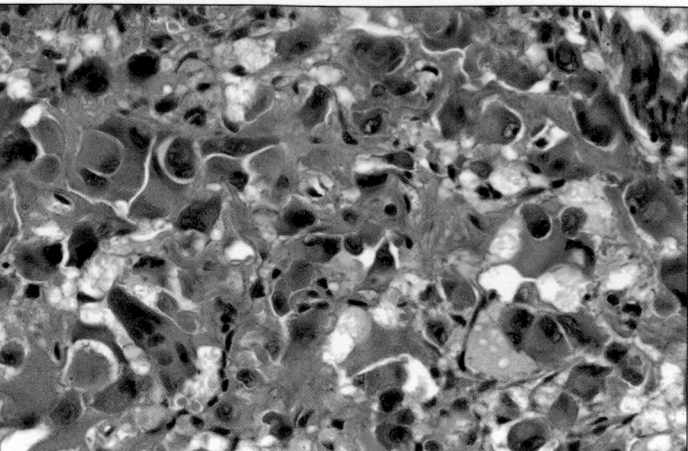

Fig. 14.47 Aggressive osteoblastoma composed of large epithelioid osteoblasts.

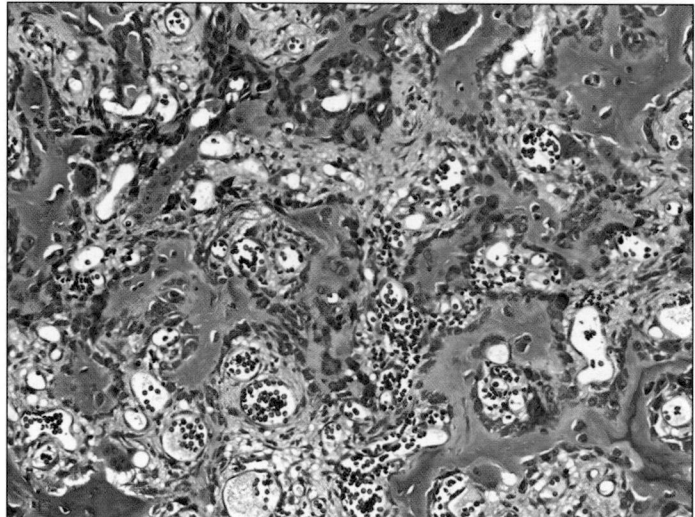

Fig. 14.46 Osteoblastoma with large osteoblasts lining anastomosing trabecular of woven bone. The intertrabecular stroma is composed of loose connective tissue with numerous blood vessels. Osteoclasts are also present.

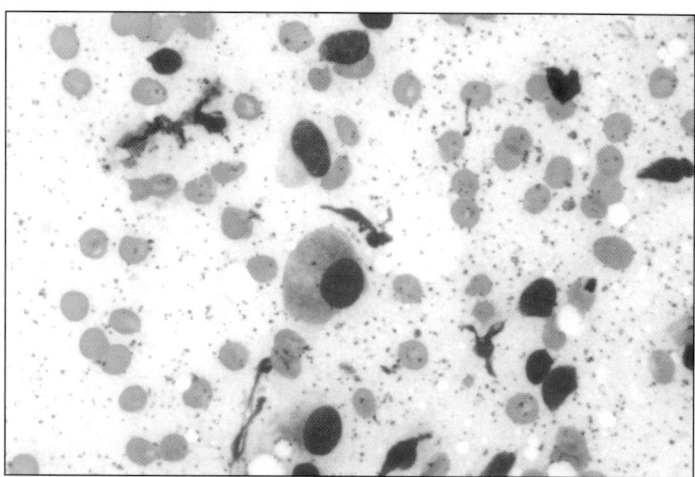

Fig. 14.48 Benign osteoblasts obtained by FNA from an osteoblastoma. The individual cells are plump with eccentric round nuclei and plasmacytoid morphology. (Romanowsky stain.)

osteoblasts may surround small fragments of osteoid or mineralized bone but more frequently are scattered as single cells in the background. They are typically large and plump and have a plasmacytoid appearance with eccentric, round nuclei that seem to protrude out of the cell. The nuclei have evenly dispersed chromatin and a single nucleolus, which may be prominent (Fig. 14.48).[18] The spindle cell component is characterized by small, bland fibroblasts and endothelial cells.[18,53]

The treatment of osteoblastoma is en bloc resection, which is usually curative. Curettage is associated with local recurrence in approximately 20% of cases.[174,176,178] Malignant transformation in osteoblastoma is exceptionally rare. In the Mayo Clinic series of 306 osteoblastomas, only two became malignant.[174]

OSTEOSARCOMA

Osteosarcoma of the skeleton is defined as a primary mesenchymal malignancy of bone in which the neoplastic cells synthesize and secrete the organic components of bone matrix, which may or may not be mineralized. There is no minimal amount of bone matrix required to classify the tumor as osteosarcoma, so the presence of any neoplastic bone, even if only microscopic in amounts, justifies categorizing the tumor as an osteosarcoma.

Classification

The classification of osteosarcoma (Table 14.7) is based on a variety of characteristics including its histologic features, biologic potential (grade), relationship to bone of origin (surface or intramedullary), multiplicity (solitary and multifocal), and the pre-existing state of underlying bone (primary or secondary).[179–183] The vast majority of osteosarcomas can be categorized into three important groups: (1) conventional osteosarcoma and its histologic subtypes; (2) intramedullary well differentiated osteosarcoma; and (3) surface osteosarcomas. Conventional osteosarcoma–garden-variety osteosarcoma–is solitary, arises in the medullary cavity of an otherwise normal bone, is high-grade, and produces neoplastic bone with or without cartilaginous or fibroblastic components. Approximately 75–80% of osteosarcomas are conventional type,

Table 14.7 Classification of osteosarcoma

Histologic features
Osteoblastic
Chondroblastic
Fibroblastic
Telangiectatic
Small cell
Giant-cell-rich
Epithelioid
Biologic potential
Low grade
Intermediate grade
High grade
Relationship to bone of origin
Intramedullary
Juxtacortical or surface
   Parosteal, periosteal, high-grade surface
Intracortical
Multiplicity
Solitary
Multifocal
   Synchronous
   Metachronous
State of underlying bone
Primary (bone normal)
Secondary (bone abnormal)
   Radiation, Paget's disease, infarction, osteomyelitis, prosthesis, preexisting benign neoplasm

5–10% are juxtacortical in origin, 10% are secondary and arise in a diseased bone, and 1% are intramedullary and well differentiated.

Grading

Grading osteosarcoma is subjective and reflects the pathologists' assessment of the biologic potential of the tumor.[181] It is founded on the relationship between clinical behavior and morphology, with the latter resting on the evaluation of histologic features such as degree of cellularity, cytologic atypia, mitotic atypia, and necrosis. As with other bone sarcomas, there is no standardized, uniform grading system for osteosarcoma that incorporates qualitative and quantitative features. Currently, the important goal is to distinguish low-grade or well differentiated osteosarcomas from high-grade tumors, as the latter require chemotherapy for adequate treatment.

Epidemiology

Osteosarcoma has been recognized for almost two centuries and is the most common primary nonhematopoietic malignancy of the skeletal system. It accounts for approximately 20% of all primary malignant bone tumors and its incidence in the United States is 4–5 per million individuals with 1000–1500 new cases diagnosed annually.[179] Osteosarcoma has a bimodal age distribution and a propensity to develop in adolescents and young adults, with 60% of tumors occurring in patients younger than 25 years and only 13–30% in persons older than 40 years.[37,118,180–224] Males are affected more frequently than females at a ratio of 1.3–1.6:1, with equal distribution among races. Osteosarcoma can arise in any bone of the body but the vast majority originate in the long bones of the appendicular skeleton, especially the distal femur, followed by the proximal tibia and proximal humerus–sites containing the most proliferative growth plates. In the long bones, the tumor is most frequently centered in the metaphysis (90%), infrequently in the diaphysis (9%), and rarely in the epiphysis.[7]

Surface osteosarcomas account for approximately 5–10% (parosteal 3–5%, periosteal 2–4%, and high-grade surface 1%) of all osteosarcomas.[202–209] Juxtacortical, well differentiated osteosarcoma (*parosteal* osteosarcoma) usually arises during the third decade of life, whereas juxtacortical, intermediate-grade, chondroblastic osteosarcoma (*periosteal* osteosarcoma) and high-grade, osteoblastic osteosarcoma (*high-grade surface* osteosarcoma) commonly develop in the second decade. Parosteal and periosteal osteosarcomas have a predilection for females, whereas high-grade surface osteosarcomas more frequently affect males. Parosteal osteosarcoma is most commonly based on the posterior femoral cortex in the metaphyseal–diaphyseal area of the popliteal region, followed by the metaphyseal–diaphyseal zone of the proximal tibia. Periosteal osteosarcoma originates from the cortex of the diaphysis or metaphysis of the tibia, followed in frequency by the femur. High-grade surface osteosarcoma arises on the metaphyseal surface of long bones in a distribution similar to conventional osteosarcoma and most frequently involves the distal femur or proximal humerus.

Intramedullary well differentiated osteosarcoma is very uncommon and represents only 1% of all osteosarcomas. Most develop during the second to fifth decades of life, and almost 50% of affected individuals are in their twenties at the time of diagnosis.[210–213]

Etiology

The etiology of osteosarcoma is unknown, but a variety of agents and disease states are associated with its development. The best-known etiologic association with osteosarcoma is radiation. Its causal relationship was first documented in luminous watch-dial painters. The painters, who were mostly women, put the tips of their brushes in their mouths to facilitate placing a fine point of radium on the watch dials.[186] After a minimum of several years, many of the women developed a skeletal osteosarcoma. Since that time, numerous studies have evaluated the minimum dosage, the accumulated dosage, and the rate of delivery of the dosage of radiation necessary to induce an osteosarcoma.[185,187] Radiation-induced osteosarcoma following therapeutic irradiation is an uncommon complication and usually develops approximately 15 (range 3–55) years following an average dosage of radiation of 6100 cGy.[118,188]

Osteosarcoma is associated with genetic syndromes including the Rothmund–Thomson syndrome (mutation of chromosome 8q24.3 encoding a DNA helicase), Bloom syndrome (mutation of chromosome 15q26.1 encoding a DNA helicase), Werner syndrome (mutation of chromosome 8p11 encoding a DNA helicase), Li–Fraumeni syndrome (mutation of chromosome 17p13 encoding p53, a tumor suppressor gene), and retinoblastoma gene (mutation of chromosome 13q14 encoding a transcription regulator). Information derived from these relationships has provided insight into the molecular pathogenesis of sporadic osteosarcoma, which appears to result from a complex accrual of a variety of genetic alterations, usually involving the inactivation of tumor suppressor genes and the overexpression of oncogenes (Table 14.8).[185]

Cytogenetic abnormalities are found in approximately 70% of osteosarcomas and are frequently complex.[185] Unfortunately, they have proved to be of little importance in diagnosing, predicting prognosis, and understanding the molecular pathogenesis of these tumors.[184] Aneuploidy is common in osteosarcoma, with DNA content ranging from near haploid to near hexaploid. Some of the more frequent numeric chromosomal abnormalities involve gain of

Table 14.8 Molecular genetic alterations implicated in the development of sporadic osteosarcoma

Tumor suppressor genes	Oncogenes
RB1	c-myc
Tp53	fos
p16	ERBB2
CDK4	met/HGF
Cyclin D1	
MDM2	
p14	

chromosome 1 and losses of genetic material on chromosomes 6, 9, 10, 13, and 17. Recurring structural rearrangements are often found in regions of chromosome 1p11–13, 1q11–12, 1q21–22, 11p14–15, 14p11–13, 15p1–13, 17p, and 19q13.[184,191,192] Comparative genomic hybridization studies have shown DNA sequence copy-number changes involving 1q21, 3q26, 6p, 8q, 12q12–13, 14q24–qter, 17p11.2–12, and 19q12–13.[37,184] Amplification of genes in the form of ring chromosomes, double minutes, and homogeneously staining regions are commonplace in osteosarcoma. Tumors with chromosomal abnormalities limited mainly to ring chromosomes, however, are almost always parosteal osteosarcomas (low-grade surface osteosarcomas) and the ring chromosomes are composed of amplified regions of 12q13–15.[193] Similar ring chromosomes, as well as abnormalities in chromosome 6p, are present in low-grade intramedullary osteosarcomas.[191]

In some populations, Paget's disease of the skeleton occurs in approximately 3–5% of adults older than 40 years. Estimates reveal that 1% of these affected individuals eventually develop osteosarcoma in an involved bone, which reflects a several thousand-fold increase in the risk of developing osteosarcoma compared to the general population.[194] Genetic predisposition to the development of Paget's disease, including its familiar form, is linked to a region on chromosome 18q.[195] Loss of heterozygosity in this locus is present in both sporadic and pagetic high-grade osteosarcomas, suggesting that this chromosomal region harbors a tumor suppressor gene important in the genesis of both diseases.

Osteosarcoma may also arise in areas of previous bone infarction, chronic osteomyelitis, pre-existing primary benign bone tumors (osteochondroma, enchondroma, fibrous dysplasia, giant cell tumor, osteoblastoma, aneurysmal bone cyst, and unicameral bone cyst), and adjacent to metallic implants. As a group, these secondary osteosarcomas account for only a very small percentage of osteosarcomas and their pathogenesis is probably related to the associated underlying disease states.

Clinical presentation

Conventional osteosarcoma typically manifests as a progressively enlarging, painful mass. The pain is deep seated, boring in nature, and frequently noted months prior to diagnosis. The pain usually increases in intensity over time, eventually producing unremitting discomfort. The overlying skin may be warm, erythematous, edematous, and cartographed by prominent engorged veins. Large tumors may restrict range of motion, decrease musculoskeletal function, produce joint effusions, and, in far advanced cases, result in weight loss and cachexia. In 5–10% of cases, the heralding event is a sudden, devastating, pathologic fracture through the destructive mass.

The *surface* osteosarcomas may or may not be associated with pain but usually present as an enlarging, fixed mass. The low-grade variants are slow growing, may be painless, and are frequently of long duration.

Well differentiated intramedullary osteosarcomas frequently cause pain that persists for months to years prior to diagnosis. In some instances, the tumor may first be detected as an enlarging palpable mass. We have also seen cases in which the neoplasm is discovered incidentally.

Laboratory studies are usually unhelpful in assessing osteosarcoma. However, the serum alkaline phosphatase level is elevated in many cases and extremely high levels are associated with the presence of metastatic disease.[196]

Radiographic manifestations

The radiographic appearance of osteosarcoma is extremely variable. Conventional tumors typically present as a large, destructive, poorly defined, mixed lytic and blastic mass that transgresses the cortex and forms a large soft tissue tumor. In some cases, the tumor is entirely lytic, which is often seen in the telangiectatic variant; while in others it is diffusely mineralized, producing a densely sclerotic mass. The periphery of the lesion is usually the least mineralized, and soft tissue components may have a fine, 'cloud-like' pattern of radiodensity. Osteosarcoma is frequently situated eccentrically within the medullary cavity and its largest dimension parallels the long axis of the underlying bone. As the enlarging mass destroys and permeates the cortex, it mechanically elevates the periosteum, producing reactive bone in the form of Codman's triangle at the proximal and distal extent of the tumor, as well as a sunburst or onion-skin-like pattern of periosteal bone formation along the bulk of its length. Conventional osteosarcoma is heterogeneous on CT and MRI, and these modalities provide valuable information regarding the overall dimensions of the tumor, its extent within the medullary cavity and soft tissue, and its relationship to important neighboring anatomic structures (Fig. 14.49). This information is vital to planning successful limb salvage surgical resection.

Surface osteosarcomas have a broad base of attachment to the underlying cortex. *Parosteal* tumors may be circumferential or mushroom-shaped and are usually densely mineralized. They may have radiolucent areas or a lobular contour with little or no periosteal reaction (Fig. 14.50). A radiolucent line separating the base of the tumor from the adjacent cortex is sometimes present.[202–204] *Periosteal* osteosarcomas are fusiform, predominately lucent, and frequently associated with a periosteal reaction in the form of Codman's triangle and perpendicular linear striae that radiate from the underlying bone (Fig. 14.51).[202,205–207] *High-grade surface* osteosarcoma is similar in appearance to periosteal osteosarcoma but, in addition, tends to have fine, cloud-like areas of radiopaucity.[208,209] CT is helpful in assessing invasion of the cortex and medullary canal. MRI facilitates the identification of cartilage, which may be in the form of a peripheral cap in parosteal osteosarcoma or scattered throughout the mass in cases of periosteal or high-grade surface osteosarcoma.

Intramedullary, well differentiated osteosarcomas have heterogeneous radiographic findings, including lytic and densely mineralized regions (Fig. 14.52). The tumors have poorly demarcated margins, may cause expansion of the underlying bone with little periosteal reaction, and, if present, have a soft tissue mass that is relatively small compared to the extent of intramedullary involvement.[210–213]

Gross morphology

Conventional osteosarcoma presents as a large, metaphyseal, intramedullary, and tan-gray-white, gritty mass (Fig. 14.53). Tumors

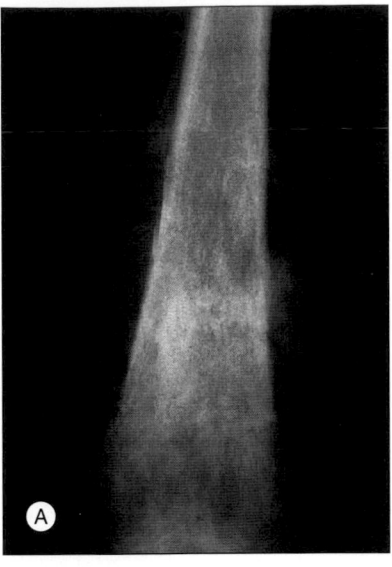

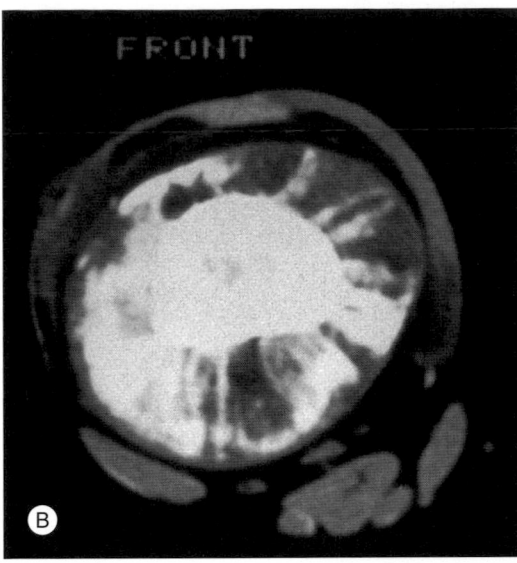

Fig. 14.49 (A) and **(B)** Plain X-ray and axial CT of a conventional osteosarcoma, showing a large destructive osteosarcoma of the distal femur. The tumor is centered in the medullary cavity and is mixed lytic and blastic. It forms a large circumferential soft tissue mass and a Codman's triangle, best seen proximally.

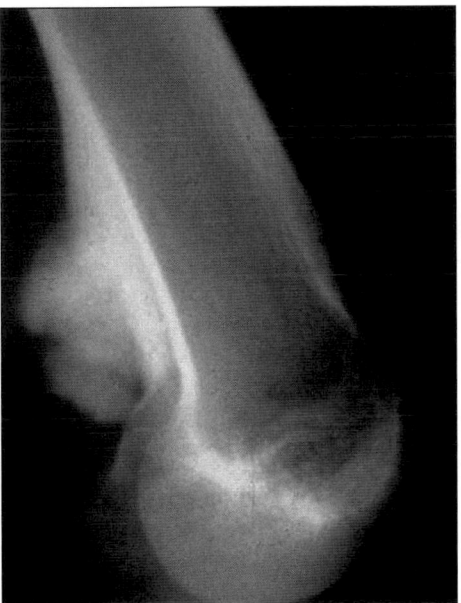

Fig. 14.50 Parosteal osteosarcoma producing a large radiodense mass arising from the posterior distal aspect of the femur.

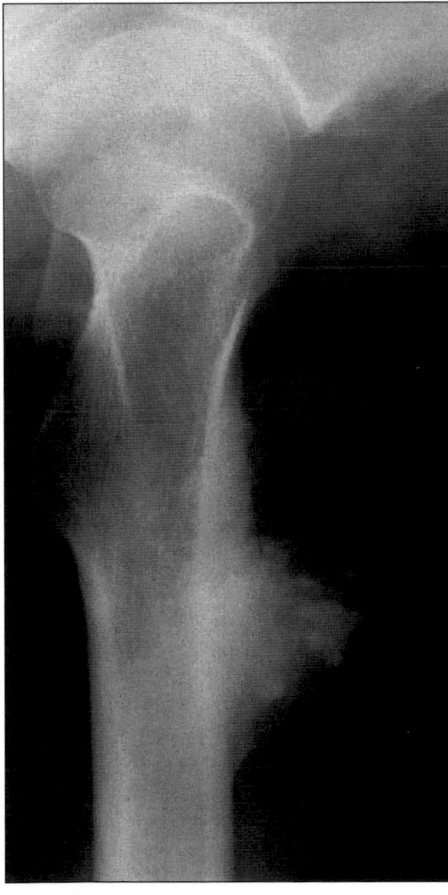

Fig. 14.51 Periosteal osteosarcoma appears as a mixed lytic and blastic mass on the proximal femoral cortex.

containing abundant mineralized bone are tan-white and hard, whereas nonmineralized cartilaginous components are glistening, gray, and may be mucinous if the matrix is myxoid or more rubbery if it is hyaline in nature (Fig. 14.54). Areas of hemorrhage and cystic change are commonplace and, when extensive, produce a friable, bloody, and spongy mass (telangiectatic osteosarcoma) (Fig. 14.55). Intramedullary involvement is often considerable, and the tumor usually destroys the overlying cortex and forms an eccentric or circumferential soft tissue component that displaces the periosteum peripherally. The dislodged periosteum becomes a sharp interface between the mass and the bordering skeletal muscle and fat. Additionally, in the proximal and distal regions, where the periosteum is first lifted from the cortex, it deposits a layer of reactive bone (Codman's triangle). Growth into the joint space, which in some cases may be associated with the tumor coating peripheral portions of the articular cartilage, follows pathways offering least resistance to

spread—beneath the synovium via extension along the cortical surface, or through tendoligamentous and joint capsule insertion sites. Open growth plates often function as effective barriers to advancing tumors; however, penetration of the physis and invasion through the epiphysis to the base of the articular surface occurs in some cases. Skip metastases, solitary or multiple, appear as intramedullary, firm, ovoid, tan-white nodules located adjacent to or far distant from the main mass.

Fig. 14.52 Intramedullary well differentiated osteosarcoma. The tumor is sclerotic and poorly delineated. A small periosteal reaction is seen.

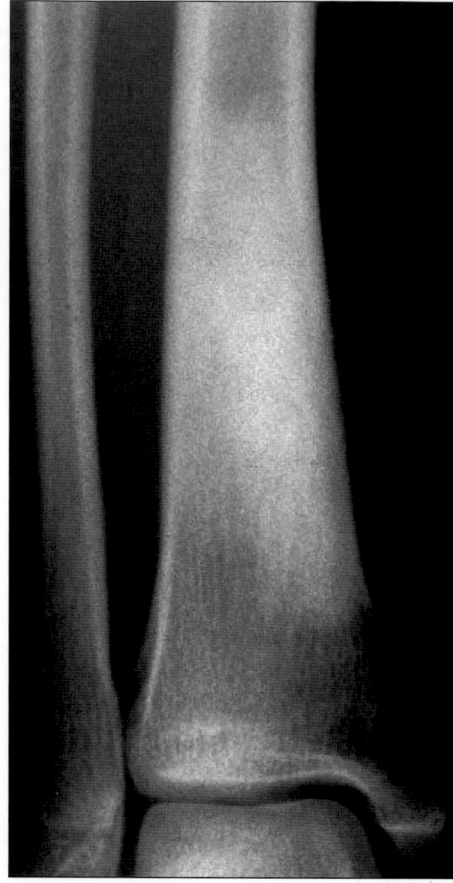

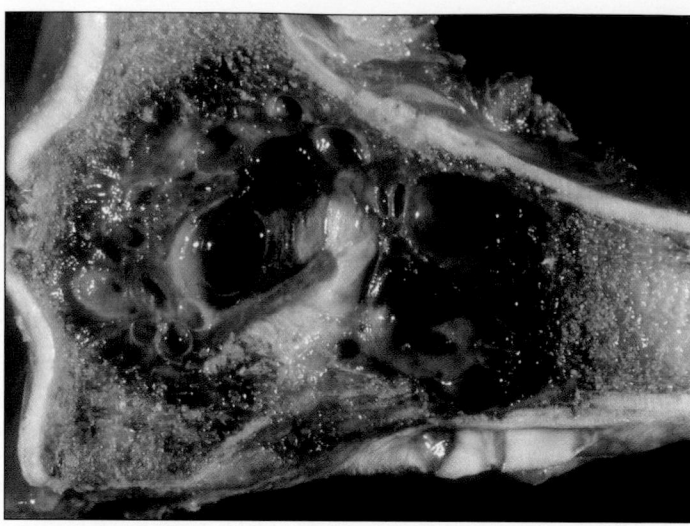

Fig. 14.55 Telangiectatic osteosarcoma with prominent hemorrhagic cysts.

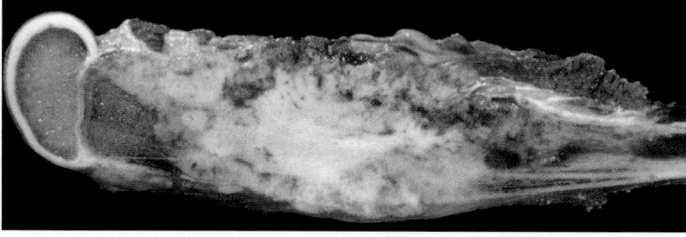

Fig. 14.53 Gross specimen of conventional osteosarcoma. The tumor is hard and tan-white. It obliterates the medullary cavity, destroys the cortex and extends into the soft tissues. The raised periosteum seen proximally and distally produces the Codman's triangle seen radiographically. The open growth plate is not transgressed by the tumor.

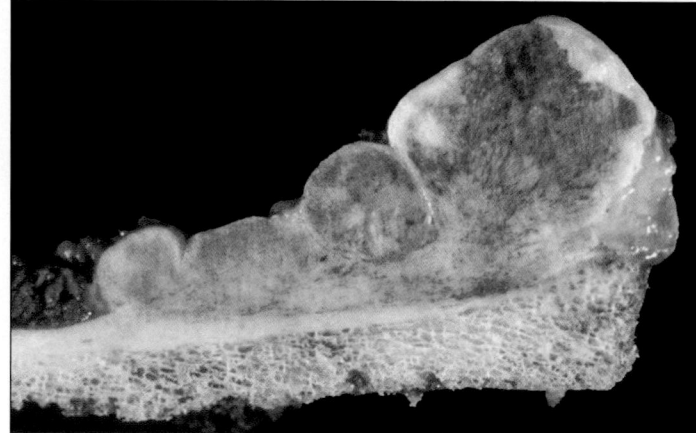

Fig. 14.56 Large bosselated parosteal osteosarcoma firmly attached to the underlying cortex. The distal surface of the tumor has a cartilaginous cap.

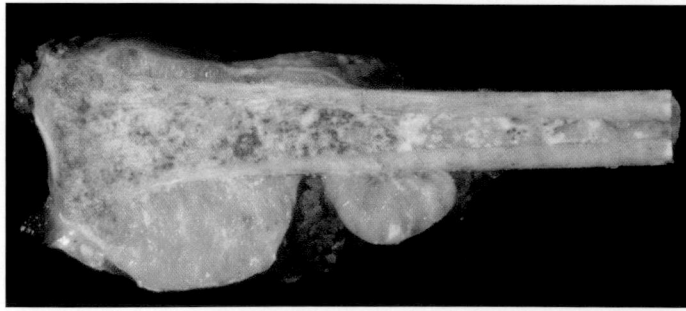

Fig. 14.54 Chondroblastic osteosarcoma composed of large nodules of gray, glistening cartilage.

Surface osteosarcomas are broad-based, rigidly attached to the underlying cortex, and usually well demarcated from the neighboring soft tissues. Well differentiated juxtacortical tumors (*parosteal osteosarcoma*) are solid, tan-white, hard, and gritty and may have a gray firm, glistening, hyaline cartilage cap or areas that are softer and fish-flesh-like, representing fibrosarcomatous elements (Fig. 14.56). High-grade juxtacortical osteosarcomas (*periosteal* and *high-grade surface*) may be dominated by cartilaginous tissue or be composed of hard, tan-white areas admixed with fish-flesh-like regions (Fig. 14.57). Destruction of the underlying cortex and invasion into the medullary canal is usually absent and, when present, is usually only focal. If extensive, it is difficult, if not impossible, to distinguish an intramedullary tumor with an eccentric soft tissue component from a surface neoplasm with extensive invasion of the medullary canal.

Intramedullary well differentiated osteosarcoma is typically centered in the medullary cavity of the metaphysis or metaphyseal–diaphyseal region. The tumor is hard, gritty, and tan-white and has

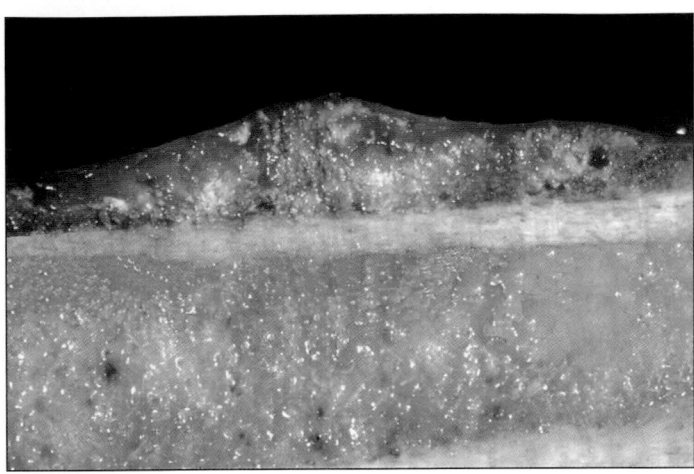

Fig. 14.57 Periosteal osteosarcoma composed of gray, glistening cartilage arising beneath the periosteum and elevating it.

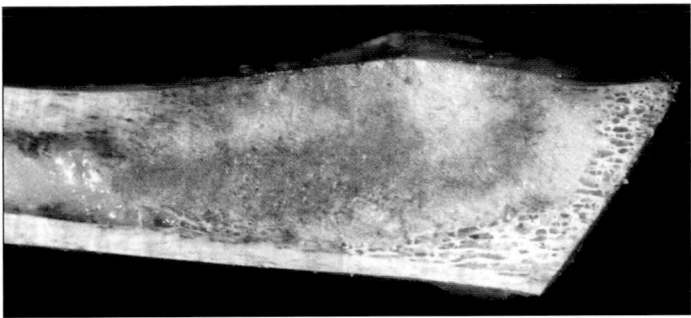

Fig. 14.58 Intramedullary well differentiated osteosarcoma composed of a solid mass of pink-tan bone (same as Fig. 14.52).

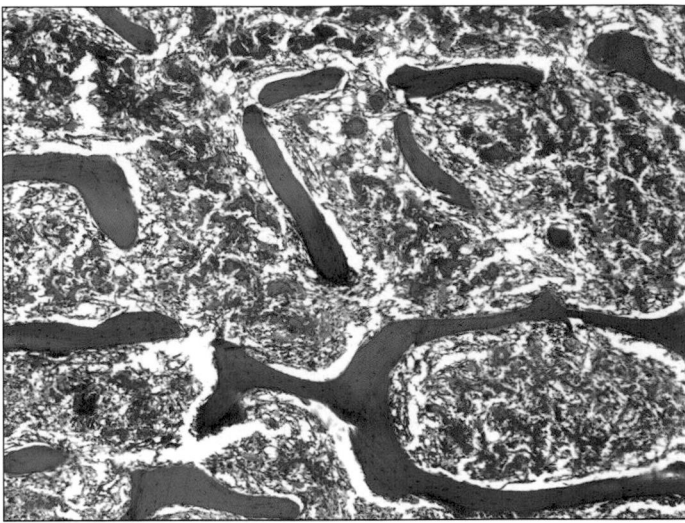

Fig. 14.59 Conventional osteoblastic osteosarcoma replacing the marrow and surrounding cancellous bone.

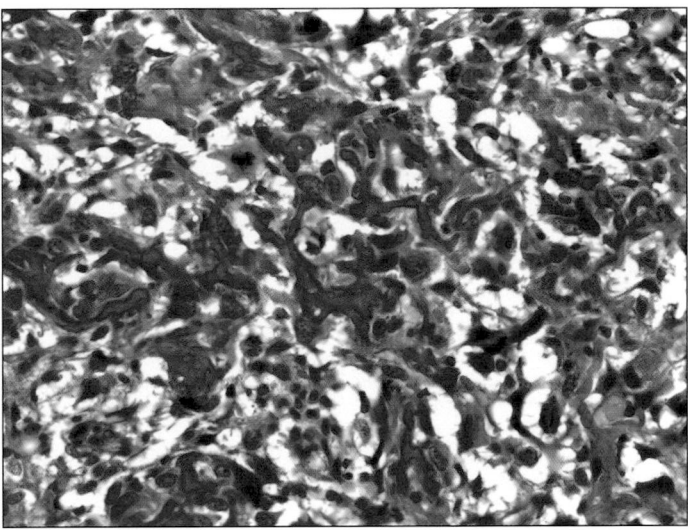

Fig. 14.60 High-grade osteoblastic osteosarcoma containing coarse, lace-like neoplastic bone. The neoplastic cells are cytologically malignant and mitotically active.

poorly defined margins (Fig. 14.58). Cortical destruction and an associated soft tissue mass may be present.

Microscopic morphology

Microscopically, high-grade osteosarcoma grows with a permeative pattern, replacing the marrow space, surrounding and eroding pre-existing bony trabeculae, and filling and expanding haversian systems (Fig. 14.59). The conventional type has been subclassified into *osteoblastic*, *chondroblastic*, *fibroblastic*, and *mixed* types, depending on the predominance of the neoplastic component (Figs 14.60–14.62). In osteoblastic foci, the malignant cells have an osteoblastic phenotype and are large, pleomorphic, and polyhedral or spindle-shaped. The nuclei are hyperchromatic, are central or eccentric in position, and may contain prominent nucleoli. The cytoplasm is eosinophilic with a volume correlating with cell size. The tumor cells are intimately related to the surface of the neoplastic bone. As they become surrounded and imprisoned by the matrix, the cells are smaller and appear less atypical. The neoplastic bone is woven in architecture, varies in quantity, and is deposited as primitive, disorganized trabeculae that produce a coarse, lace-like pattern or large, broad sheets fashioned by coalescing trabeculae as seen in the sclerosing variant. Depending on its state of mineralization, the bone is eosinophilic or basophilic and may have a pagetoid appearance caused by haphazardly deposited cement lines. Neoplastic cartilage, when

present, is usually hyaline but may be predominately myxoid, particularly in tumors arising in jaw bones. The malignant chondrocytes demonstrate severe cytologic atypia and reside in lacunar spaces in hyaline matrix, or float singly or in cords in myxoid matrix. Fibroblastic foci manifest as cytologically malignant spindle cells arranged in a herringbone of storiform pattern. The degree of atypia is variable, but is frequently severe. Mitoses are numerous and structurally abnormal forms are common.

Telangiectatic osteosarcomas are high-grade tumors that contain numerous blood-filled cystic spaces comprising the majority of the tumor.[214–216] The cyst walls contain and are lined by malignant cells that produce variable amounts of neoplastic matrix (Fig. 14.63). In *small cell* osteosarcoma, the neoplastic cells are uniform, small, round, or spindle shaped and contain little cytoplasm (Fig. 14.64).[217–220] Non-

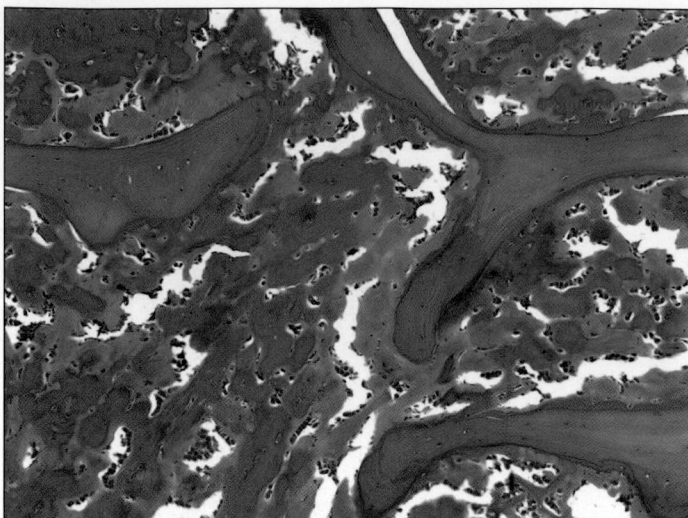

Fig. 14.61 Sclerosing variant of osteoblastic osteosarcoma.

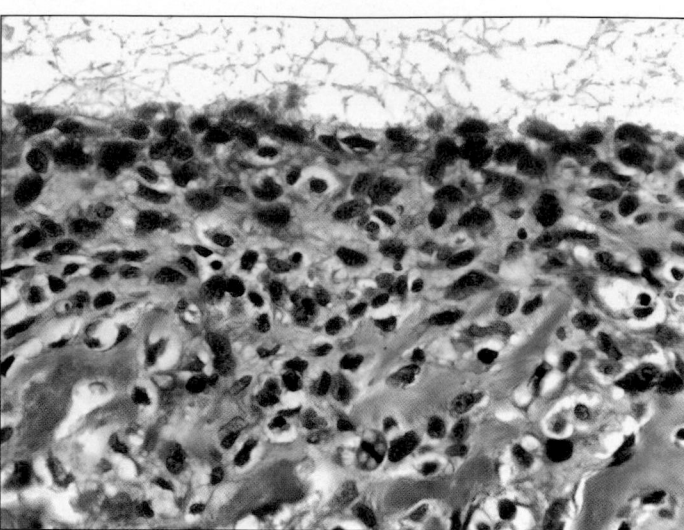

Fig. 14.63 Telangiectatic osteosarcoma. Malignant cells and tumor bone are present in the cyst wall.

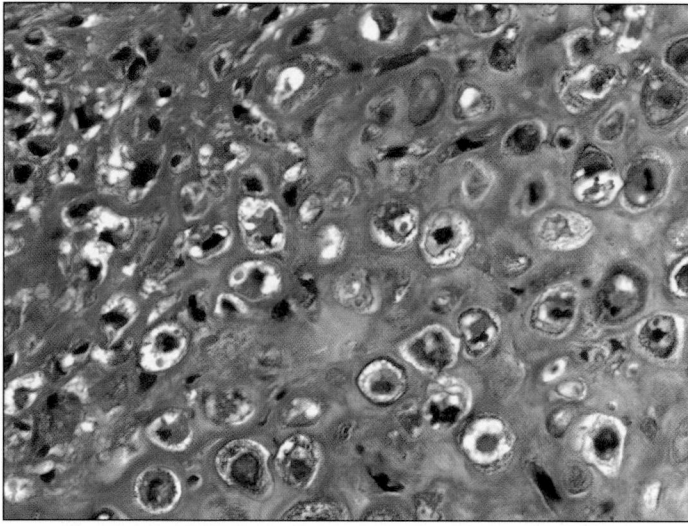

Fig. 14.62 High-grade chondroblastic osteosarcoma with malignant cartilage adjacent to lace-like neoplastic bone.

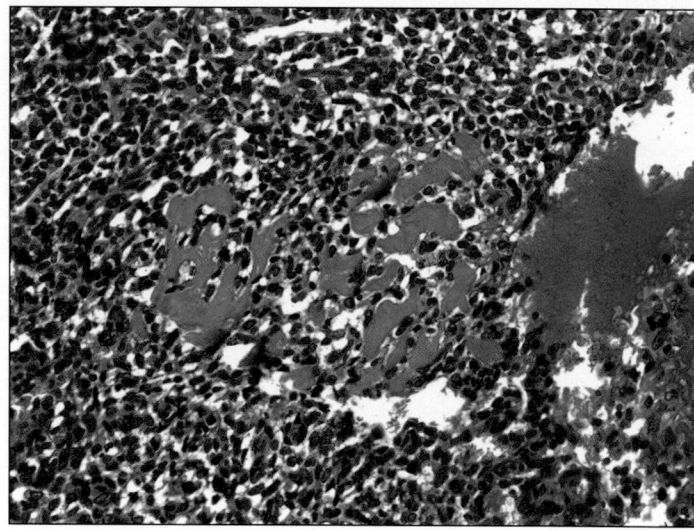

Fig. 14.64 Small cell osteosarcoma with neoplastic bone surrounded by sheets of small cells.

neoplastic, osteoclast-type giant cells scattered throughout the tumor are the hallmark of the *giant-cell-rich* variant, while large polyhedral tumor cells characterize the *epithelioid* variant.[221–223] In the *osteoblastoma-like* variant, the tumor cells may be deceptively banal and rim the neoplastic bony trabeculae in a fashion that mimics osteoblastoma. Features that permit their distinction are the permeative growth pattern and solid cellular intertrabecular tissue that are found in osteosarcoma.[225,226]

The hallmark of *parosteal* osteosarcoma is the presence of relatively well formed trabeculae of woven bone, surrounded by a mildly to moderately cellular spindle cell proliferation enmeshed in a collagenous stroma (Fig. 14.65). The spindle cells have elongate nuclei with pointed ends and demonstrate varying degrees of cytologic atypia. In the deceptively bland-appearing cases, the nuclei have finely stippled chromatin, small nucleoli, poorly defined eosinophilic cytoplasm, and few mitoses, thus resembling fibromatosis. In higher-grade tumors, the nuclei contain coarsened chromatin and demonstrate a greater degree of mitotic activity. It is not uncommon for the tumor cells in higher-grade neoplasms to be arranged in a herringbone pattern. Malignant cartilage is sometimes a component of parosteal osteosarcoma and, when present, has a hyaline matrix, contains mildly to moderately atypical chondrocytes, and grows as a cap covering the periphery of the tumor. This latter configuration can cause confusion with osteochondroma. Rarely, parosteal osteosarcoma contains foci of pleomorphic spindle cell sarcoma or even high-grade osteosarcoma. In this instance, the term *dedifferentiated parosteal* osteosarcoma is used to denote these lesions.[227–229]

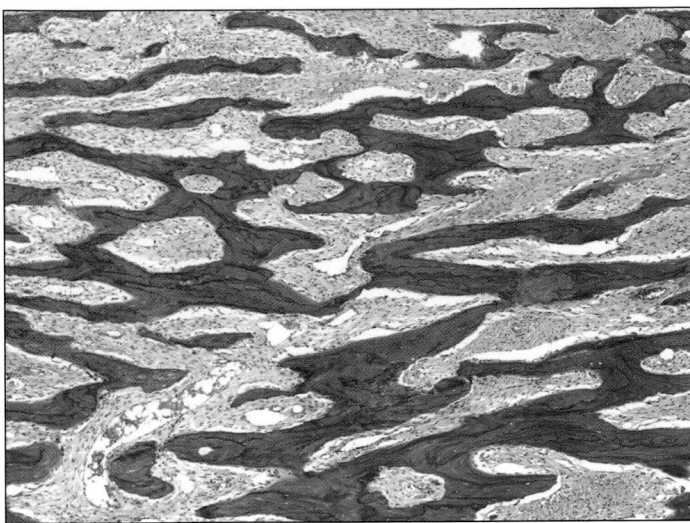

Fig. 14.65 Parosteal osteosarcoma. Long trabeculae of bone having a pagetoid appearance surrounded by moderately cellular, bland neoplastic cells.

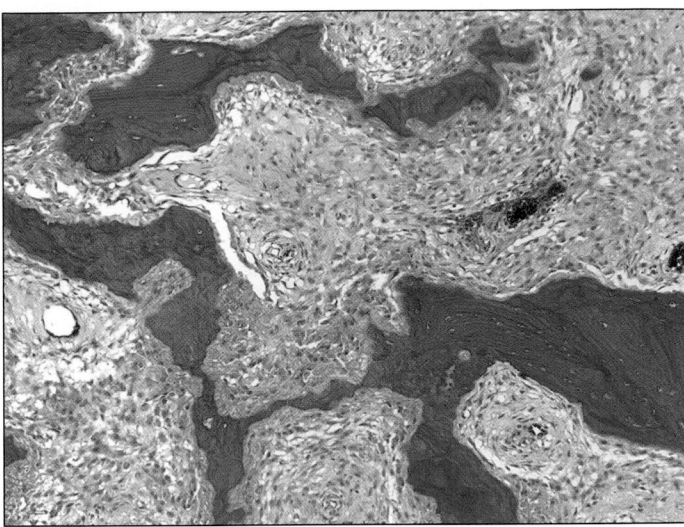

Fig. 14.66 Intramedullary well differentiated osteosarcoma. The tumor bone is deposited on the surfaces of pre-existing lamellar cancellous bone. The neoplastic cells show minimal cytologic atypia.

Periosteal osteosarcoma is a grade 2/3 chondroblastic osteosarcoma. Therefore, lobules of neoplastic cartilage, frequently hyaline, predominate, with the chondrocytes showing moderate to severe cytologic atypia as well as mitotic activity. The neoplastic bone that qualifies the tumor as an osteosarcoma usually has a coarse, lace-like pattern and either merges with or is surrounded by the cartilage, or arises in the background of significantly atypical proliferating spindle-shaped or polyhedral tumor cells.

High-grade surface osteosarcoma is essentially a high-grade osteoblastic osteosarcoma that arises on the external surface of the cortex. The tumor cells show pronounced cytologic atypia, mitotic activity, and areas of necrosis. As in all high-grade osteosarcomas, neoplastic cartilage and fibroblastic components may be present.

Intramedullary well differentiated osteosarcoma, like its juxtacortical variant, is composed of a mild to moderately cellular cytologically bland spindle cell component that is intimately associated with long trabeculae or round islands of woven bone, which may have a pagetoid appearance (Fig. 14.66). Unlike fibrous dysplasia, which it may resemble, the tumor grows with an infiltrative pattern, replacing the marrow space and surrounding pre-existing bony trabeculae, which may serve as scaffolding for the deposition of tumor bone.

Cytology

The majority of osteosarcomas can be successfully sampled by FNA because of the destructive character of these neoplasms and their proclivity for invading the surrounding soft tissues. Each subtype of osteosarcoma is associated with a rather characteristic cytologic pattern. Osteosarcomas are characterized by direct osteoid production by the neoplastic cell population. Osteoid may not always be present in smear preparations, and the diagnosis of these sarcomas depends on the recognition of a malignant osteoblastic population combined with the appropriate radiographic features of a matrix-forming sarcoma.

Smears from conventional osteosarcomas are of moderate cellularity with a background rich in red blood cells. The amount of osteoid present in the smears is variable. Its presence, when in close association with malignant osteoblasts or spindle cells, is diagnostic of

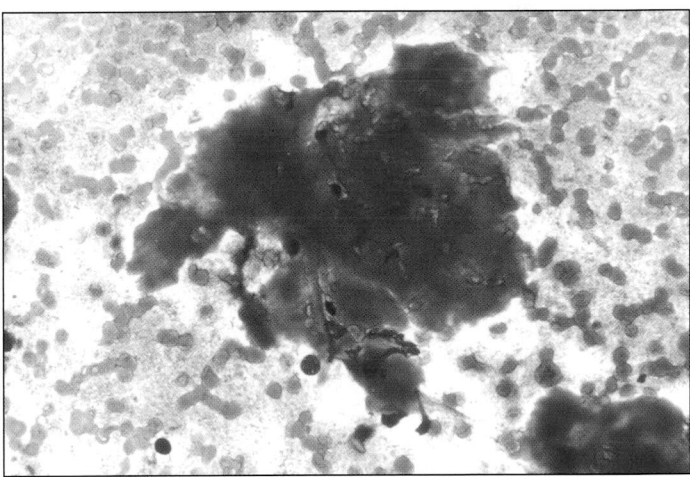

Fig. 14.67 Osteoid with a dense magenta appearance entrapping a small number of bland, oval cells. (Romanowsky stain.)

osteosarcoma in the appropriate radiographic setting. The cellular component of osteosarcomas can be quite variable in appearance, and White et al. subclassified the FNA findings of osteosarcomas into five categories: (1) pleomorphic; (2) epithelioid; (3) chondroblastic; (4) small cell; and (5) mixed.[230] In the experience of White et al. the pleomorphic pattern is the most common.[230] We have found recognition of a sixth pattern in which osteoclast-like giant cells dominate the smears.

When present, osteoid is best seen in Romanowsky-stained preparations where it forms streamers, small dense aggregates, or lace-like structures entrapping or abutting neoplastic osteoblasts (Fig. 14.67). FNA smears from osteosarcomas usually contain a prominent population of large pleomorphic cells. These cells may be mono- or multinuclear. Nuclear atypia is marked with irregular nuclear membranes and substantial variation in nuclear size and shape (Fig. 14.68). Nucleoli are prominent and mitotic figures, while

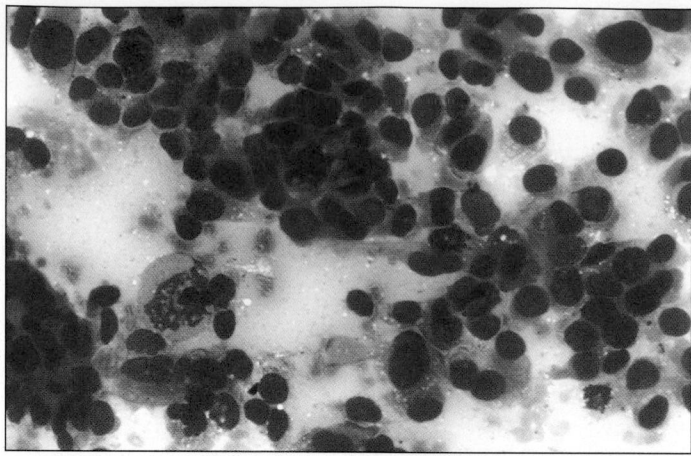

Fig. 14.68 Cellular smear material obtained from an osteosarcoma. The individual malignant osteoblasts have a plasmacytoid to plump 'spindle' shape. Moderate to abundant cytoplasm is often associated with a hyperchromatic enlarged eccentrically located nucleus. Variation in nuclear size is marked. Occasional mitotic figures are seen. (Romanowsky stain.)

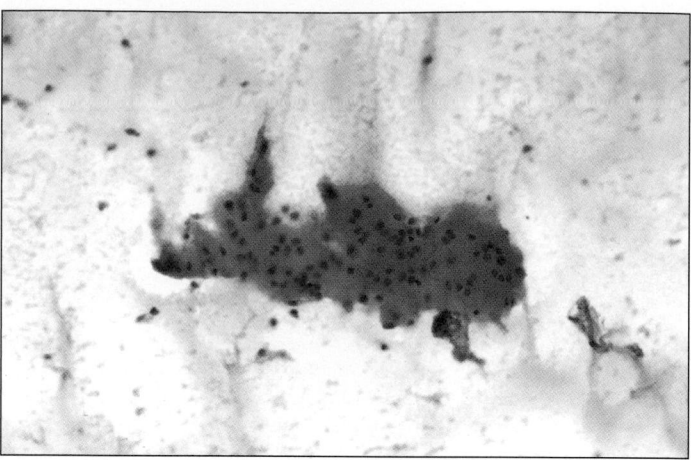

Fig. 14.70 Chondroblastic osteosarcoma. The tissue fragment has a homogeneous chondroid matrix surrounded and entrapping neoplastic round to oval cells. (H&E stain.)

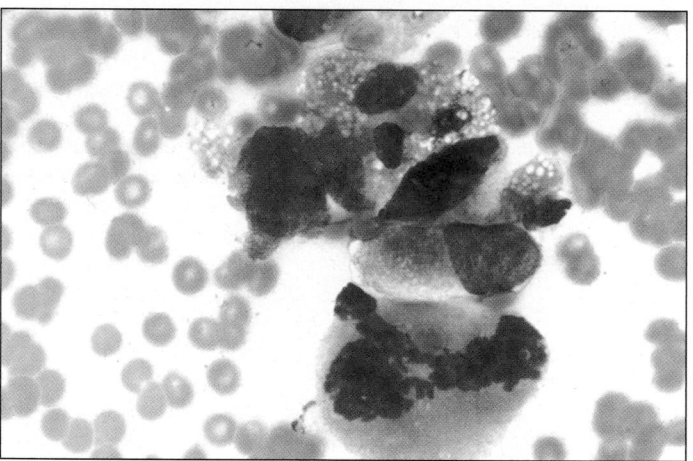

Fig. 14.69 Malignant osteoblasts obtained from an osteosarcoma. Note the atypical mitotic figure (lower right hand corner). Several of the neoplastic cells have cytoplasmic vacuoles or peripheral red granules. (Romanowsky stain.)

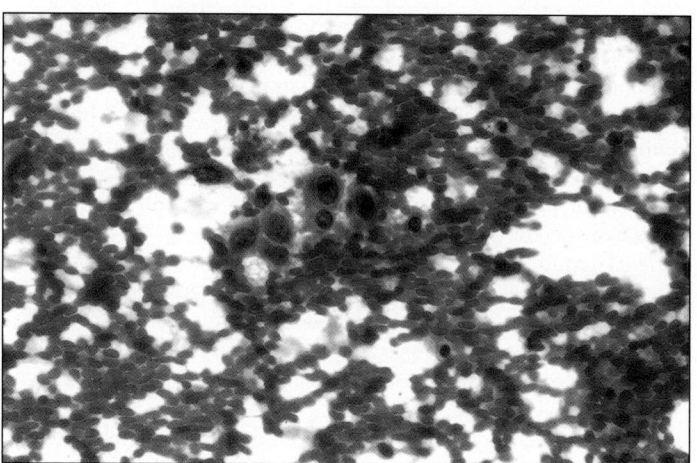

Fig. 14.71 Telangiectatic osteosarcoma. Note the bloody background which surrounds a relatively small number of enlarged round to ovoid cells with hyperchromatic nuclei. Nuclear membranes show irregularity. (H&E stain.)

infrequent, are generally identifiable and may be of atypical form. Admixed with these pleomorphic cells are a prominent number of malignant osteoblasts, which have a plasmacytoid appearance. The nuclei are eccentrically located and often appear to bulge outside the cytoplasmic membrane. These malignant osteoblasts are often associated with aggregates and streamers of osteoid. When the plasmacytoid osteoblasts dominate, the epithelioid pattern of White et al. is present.[230] Romanowsky-stained smears demonstrate vacuoles and purple-red granules in the cytoplasm of the neoplastic osteoblasts[231,232] (Fig. 14.69).

The chondroblastic pattern of osteosarcoma contains the cell types described above, as well as rounded chondroblasts with fragments of chondroid matrix (Fig. 14.70). This matrix is identical to that seen in high-grade chondrosarcomas and may have a myxoid or waxy appearance best seen with Romanowsky-stained smears.[230,233]

Fragments of chondroid matrix with well formed lacunae may be found in smears from chondroblastic osteosarcomas.

Smears obtained for telangiectatic osteosarcomas are characterized by a bloody background in which are dispersed a variable but usually small number of anaplastic cells with a plasmacytoid, spindle cell, or anaplastic giant cell morphology similar to those seen in conventional intramedullary osteosarcoma (Fig. 14.71). The large volume of blood and the characteristic radiographic appearance separates telangiectatic osteosarcoma from conventional high-grade intramedullary osteosarcoma.

In a small percentage of conventional osteosarcomas, a prominent number of benign-appearing, multinucleate, osteoclast-like giant cells are present. While these cells may suggest the differential diagnoses of chondroblastoma and conventional giant tumor of bone, the presence in the background of clearly anaplastic cells associated with fragments

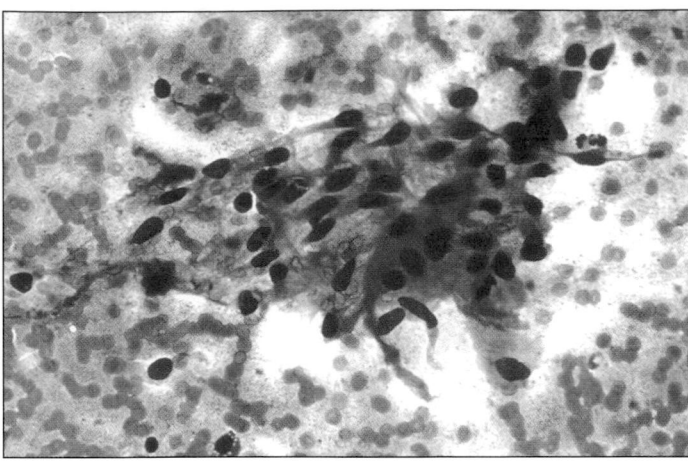

Fig. 14.72 Parosteal osteosarcoma. The smear is of relatively low cellularity with the predominant cell type being spindle-shaped and possessing relatively bland nuclei. Small streamers of magenta osteoid are intimately admixed with the cellular component. (Romanowsky stain.)

of osteoid, or the appropriate radiographic findings, establishes the diagnosis of osteosarcoma.

Cytologic smears from small cell osteosarcomas closely resemble those obtained from Ewing's sarcoma or lymphoma but lack lymphoglandular bodies and may contain small streamers of osteoid intimately associated with the small cell component.

Parosteal osteosarcoma smears are characterized by low cellularity in which the predominant cell type is a relatively bland spindle cell (Fig. 14.72). Admixed with the spindle cell element are occasional atypical oval, round or plasmacytoid cells representing neoplastic osteoblasts. Streamers of lace-like osteoid associated with entrapped osteoblasts are found in some smears.

Aspirates from periosteal and high-grade surface osteosarcomas are indistinguishable from intramedullary chondroblastic and osteoblastic osteosarcomas respectively.

Ultrastructure and immunohistochemistry

Osteosarcomas are usually diagnosed on the basis of their morphologic features, with electron microscopy and immunohistochemistry having a limited role in their evaluation.

In problematic cases, however, electron microscopic evaluation may be helpful. Osteosarcoma cells have the features of mesenchymal cells with abundant, dilated rough endoplasmic reticulum. The matrix contains collagen fibers, which may show calcium hydroxyapatite crystal deposition. These findings can be helpful in excluding Ewing's sarcoma/primitive neuroectodermal tumor, metastatic carcinoma, and melanoma, as well as lymphoma.

Osteosarcoma has a broad immunoprofile that lacks diagnostic specificity. Commonly expressed antigens include vimentin, osteocalcin, osteonectin, S-100 protein, actin, smooth muscle actin, neuron-specific enolase, and CD99.[234,235] Importantly, some tumors also stain with antibodies to keratin and epithelial membrane antigen.[236] Biopsy specimens that lack neoplastic bone can be problematic, as this staining pattern can generate a broad list of differential diagnoses that includes Ewing's sarcoma/ primitive neuroectodermal tumor, metastatic carcinoma and melanoma, leiomyosarcoma, and malignant peripheral nerve sheath tumor. It is worthy to note that osteosarcoma usually does not stain with antibodies to factor VIII, CD31, and leukocyte common antigen (LCA).

Treatment

The treatment of osteosarcoma is tailored to the age of the patient and the location, size, grade, and stage of the tumor. The goal of therapy is eradication of the primary tumor and the elimination of any metastases.[237] Local therapy is usually limb salvage, wide surgical resection with negative margins for appendicular tumors, and surgical excision in combination with radiation for tumors that are not resectable in their entirety (as is the case for neoplasms involving the axial skeleton). Adjuvant chemotherapy (methotrexate, cisplatin, doxorubicin, ifosfamide) is usually employed in the preoperative setting for all high-grade (grade 2/3, 3/3, 3/4, and 4/4) intramedullary and surface osteosarcomas, and continues after the surgical resection has been completed and wound healing has begun.[238] The integration of aggressive polychemotherapy into treatment protocols for high-grade osteosarcomas has had a dramatic impact on an otherwise fatal disease.[239] Intramedullary well differentiated osteosarcoma and parosteal osteosarcoma are usually treated by surgery alone, as they are associated with a low risk of dissemination.

Prognosis

The prognosis of patients with osteosarcoma is dependent upon a number of factors. Variables shown in some studies to have prognostic impact include patient age, gender, tumor size, location, stage, response to chemotherapy, multidrug resistance status, loss of heterozygosity of the *RB* gene, and *HER2/erbB-2* expression.[239] Of all patients with osteosarcoma who die of disease, approximately 90% result from unrelenting disease progression, while the remainder succumb to treatment-related complications (cardiomyopathy, pancytopenia, or the development of secondary malignancies).[239] Important independent prognostic factors associated with a poor outcome include proximal location in an extremity or in the axial skeleton, large tumor size, clinically detectable metastases at the time of initial diagnosis, and poor response of the tumor to preoperative chemotherapy.[239] The histologic response of the tumor to preoperative chemotherapy is felt to be one of the most important prognostic features for localized high-grade osteosarcoma of the extremities (the vast majority of the tumors): good response is 90% or greater necrosis; poor response is less than 90% necrosis. The histologic assessment of tumor necrosis requires extensive sampling and evaluation of the treated neoplasm (Fig. 14.73).[200,240,241]

Relapse-free survival rates for patients with localized conventional high-grade osteosarcoma of the extremity have been reported to vary from 50–80%.[239] Actuarial 10-year survival rates for patients with axial tumors are approximately 27% for patients presenting with metastatic disease, 53% for patients with large tumors (more than one-third length of involved bone), 47% for patients with tumors with a poor response, and 73% for patients with tumors with a good response.[239] Of conventional osteosarcoma subtypes, the chondroblastic variant has been shown to be associated with a poor preoperative chemotherapy response and, in some studies, has a worse prognosis than other variants.[238,242] Paget's osteosarcoma has a dismal prognosis, with a survival rate of approximately 10%. Radiation-induced sarcomas are also biologically aggressive and are associated with a long-term survival of 30–35%.[189,224,243]

Parosteal osteosarcoma has an excellent prognosis, with survival rates ranging from 91–100%.[203,244] Periosteal osteosarcoma has a survival rate of approximately 75%, although a recent study utilizing chemotherapy achieved a 10-year metastasis-free survival rate of 100%. High-grade surface osteosarcoma has a prognosis similar to conventional intramedullary osteosarcoma.[204–209]

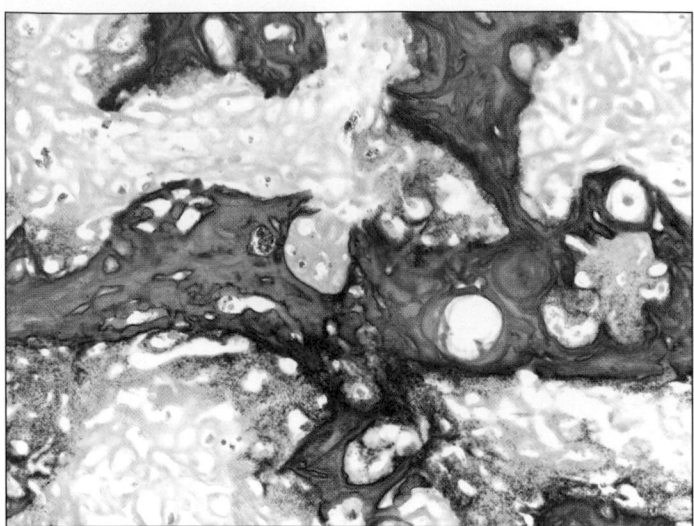

Fig. 14.73 Treated osteosarcoma with 100% necrosis. Residual neoplastic bone persists.

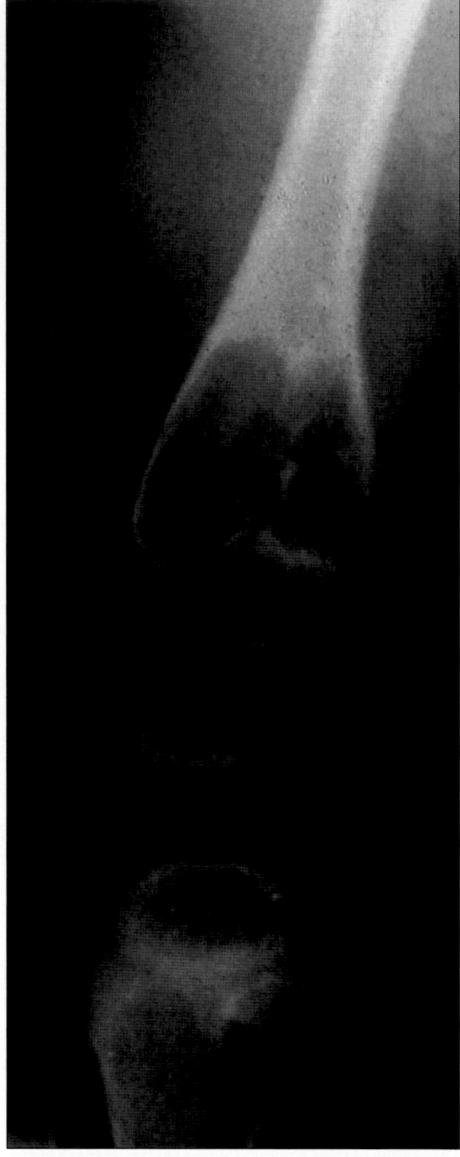

Fig. 14.74 Plain X-ray of infantile myofibroma. The intramedullary tumor is lytic and well circumscribed.

Intramedullary well differentiated osteosarcoma is an indolent tumor and is associated with a metastatic rate of approximately 15%.[210–213] Many of the metastases originate from tumors that have undergone dedifferentiation.

FIBROUS TUMORS OF BONE

Fibrous tumors of bone are defined by their composition of fibroblasts, myofibroblasts, and collagen. The benign fibrous tumors are much more common than the malignant variants. In fact, some of the benign variants are the most common tumors of the skeleton.

MYOFIBROMA OF BONE

Myofibroma is an uncommon myofibroblastic lesion that usually presents at birth, during infancy, or in early childhood. It manifests as single or multiple nodules that may involve a variety of anatomic structures including the skin, soft tissue, viscera, and skeleton.[245] Solitary tumors, which may be rapidly growing, are the most common form of presentation and frequently involve the soft tissues of the head and neck and trunk, as well as the craniofacial bones.[245] The etiology of myofibroma is unknown.

Myofibroma of bone affects very young children and many patients first develop lesions in utero. There is a male predominance and the tumors commonly involve the skull, jaw, ribs, and pelvis.[246–249] Lesions of the appendicular skeleton are less frequent and are usually located in the metaphyses of long bones. The tumors may be asymptomatic, produce a palpable mass, or cause pain and even a pathologic fracture.

Myofibromas have benign-appearing radiographic findings. They are oval or elongate and lucent, with well circumscribed, sclerotic margins, and may expand the bone (Fig. 14.74).[246–250]

Excised tumors are firm, tan-white, and well delineated. The central regions are usually densely cellular and composed of sheets of small round cells with a prominent vascular tree that has a hemangiopericytoma-like pattern (Fig. 14.75). Mitotic activity, necrosis, and dystrophic calcification are common findings. This region merges peripherally with a component composed of intersecting fascicles of plump spindle cells that have blunt-ended nuclei and conspicuous eosinophilic cytoplasm, causing them to resemble smooth muscle cells. These spindle cells have the ultrastructural and immunohistochemical characteristics of myofibroblasts.[251]

The prognosis of infantile myofibroma depends on whether there is one or multiple lesions and, importantly, whether there is visceral involvement. The prognosis of bone lesions is excellent and simple excision is usually curative. Patients with multiple visceral lesions, especially those with involvement of the gastrointestinal tract, may have a fatal outcome from severe hemorrhage.

The differential diagnosis includes cranial fasciitis, non-ossifying fibroma, rhabdomyosarcoma, Ewing's sarcoma/primitive neuroectodermal tumor, desmoplastic fibroma, and infantile or congenital fibrosarcoma. The clinical setting and unique morphologic features help distinguish myofibroma from these other tumors.

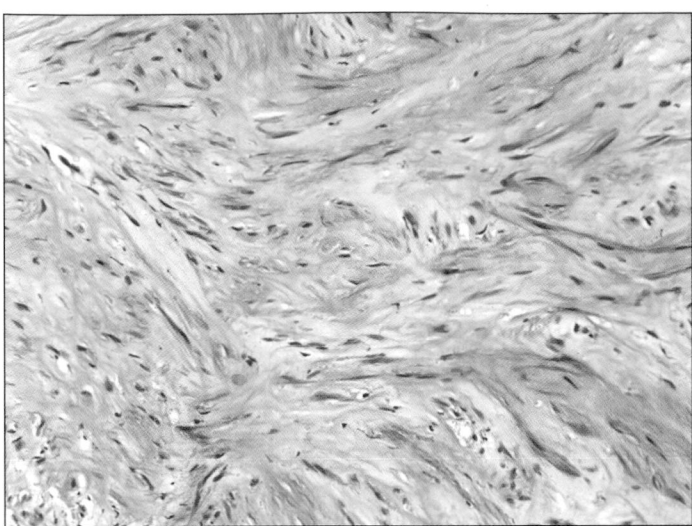

Fig. 14.75 Infantile myofibroma. The proliferating spindle cells have a distinct eosinophilic cytoplasm, typical of myofibroblasts.

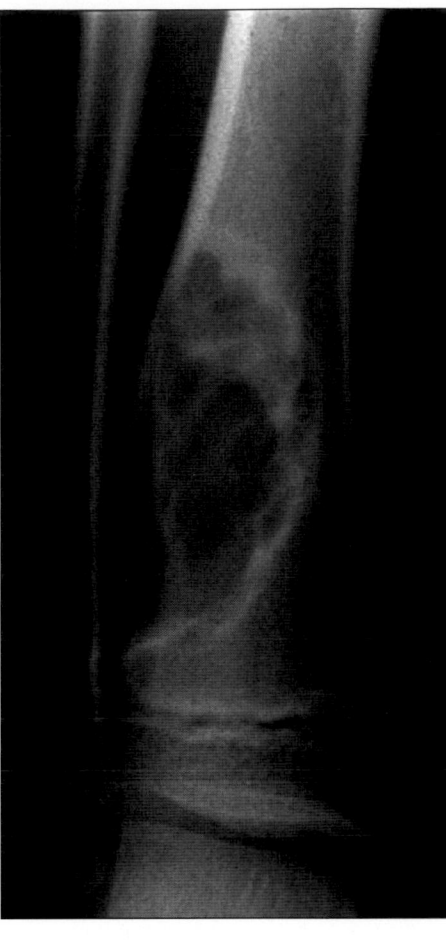

Fig. 14.76 Non-ossifying fibroma. The lesion is eccentric, metaphyseal, well circumscribed with internal trabeculations.

FIBROUS CORTICAL DEFECT AND NON-OSSIFYING FIBROMA

Non-ossifying fibroma, also known as metaphyseal fibrous defect, is considered to be a non-neoplastic process, possibly related to a defect in ossification. It classically involves the metaphysis (the growing portion of long tubular bones) in skeletally immature individuals. The term fibrous cortical defect can be applied to the lesion when it is confined to the cortex. If the lesion enlarges, however, and extends into the adjacent medullary cavity, the term non-ossifying fibroma is more appropriate.[252] Radiologic studies have shown that non-ossifying fibromas are present in 30–40% of skeletally immature individuals.[4,252] The rarity of non-ossifying fibromas among adults suggests that these lesions eventually undergo spontaneous resolution in most patients.[253] This concept is supported by the study by Sontag et al., which analyzed serial radiographs of 200 children over a defined time span.[2] The results showed that 54% of boys and 22% of girls, at an average age of 4 years, had a lesion involving the cortex. The lesions regressed spontaneously over a time of approximately 2.5 years.

Patients with non-ossifying fibroma are usually in their second decade of life at the time of diagnosis. The distal femur, proximal tibia, and distal tibia are most frequently affected; the flat or short tubular bones are rarely involved.[4] Most non-ossifying fibromas are asymptomatic and are discovered incidentally on X-rays performed for other reasons. Larger lesions can cause pain, which is probably secondary to microfractures or obvious pathologic fracture.[253,254] The vast majority of non-ossifying fibromas are single, although some may be multiple. Multiple non-ossifying fibromas may be associated with syndromes such as neurofibromatosis (von Recklinghausen's disease) and Jaffe–Campanacci syndrome.

Classic non-ossifying fibroma manifests radiographically as an eccentric, lytic lesion centered within the metaphyseal cortex and adjacent medullary cavity of long tubular bones. It is well demarcated, with sclerotic margins, and frequently contains internal trabeculations. The trabeculations are incomplete and are the result of scalloping of the affected cortex (Fig. 14.76). As the patient grows, the lesion becomes incorporated into the diaphysis. Eventually, most tumors undergo spontaneous necrosis, regression, and replacement by sclerotic bone that remodels over time, so that ultimately no abnormality is evident. The radiographic features of non-ossifying fibroma are so characteristic that in most instances a biopsy is not indicated.

Macroscopically, non-ossifying fibroma is eccentric and well circumscribed, and has sclerotic borders. The overlying cortex is attenuated and may be completely eroded. The lesion is tan-brown and frequently has areas of yellow discoloration (Fig. 14.77). Cystic changes (aneurysmal-bone-cyst-like areas) may be present and extensive areas of hemorrhage and necrosis result from pathologic fracture. The most prominent cell type in non-ossifying fibroma is spindle fibroblasts, which are arranged in a storiform pattern. The spindle cells have cytologically banal nuclei that have pointed ends and indistinct eosinophilic cytoplasm. Mitoses are few in number. Osteoclast-type giant cells are frequently scattered throughout the lesion. Other secondary findings include hemosiderin deposits and collections of foamy macrophages.

Fine-needle aspirates obtained from non-ossifying fibromas and fibrous cortical defects are identical cytologically and usually of low cellularity. Cytologic preparations demonstrate an admixture of ovoid and fusiform mononuclear stromal cells admixed with occasional osteoclast-like giant cells.[255] The mononuclear component has a spindle morphology, and the nuclei are more elongate than the nuclei of the osteoclast-like giant cells (Fig. 14.78). There is no evidence of nuclear anaplasia, and mitotic figures are not seen (Fig. 14.79).

Non-ossifying fibromas that are asymptomatic do not usually need surgical excision. Larger lesions that are painful or have an

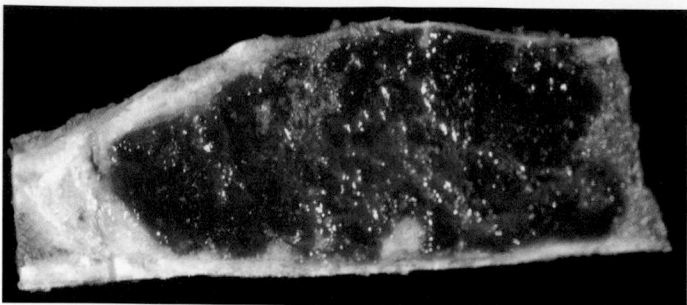

Fig. 14.77 Non-ossifying fibroma, expanding the fibula. The tumor is well circumscribed and red brown.

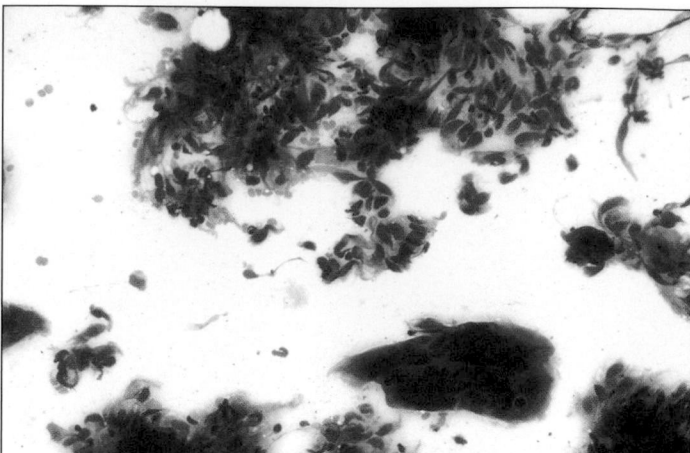

Fig. 14.79 Sheets of short spindle-shaped cells associated with multinucleate osteoclast-type giant cells are found in smears obtained from non-ossifying fibroma. The spindle cells have bland, markedly elongated nuclei. Nuclear pleomorphism is absent, with the nuclei being bland and uniform in appearance. (Romanowsky stain.)

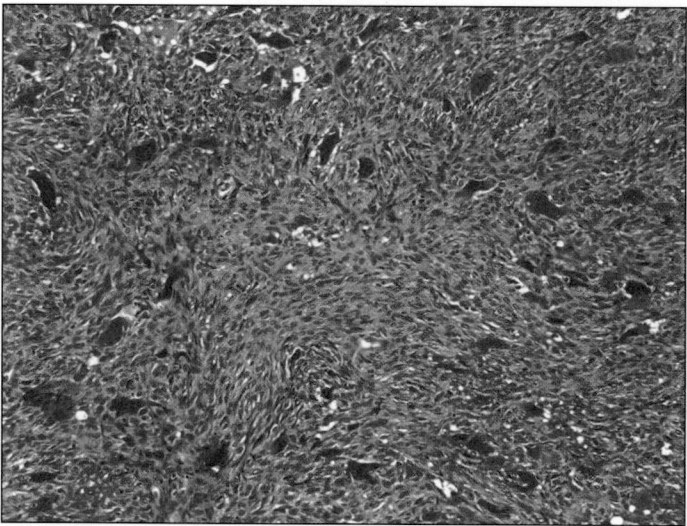

Fig. 14.78 Non-ossifying fibroma. Hypercellular spindle cells arranged in a storiform growth pattern, osteoclast type giant cells, and foci of hemorrhage.

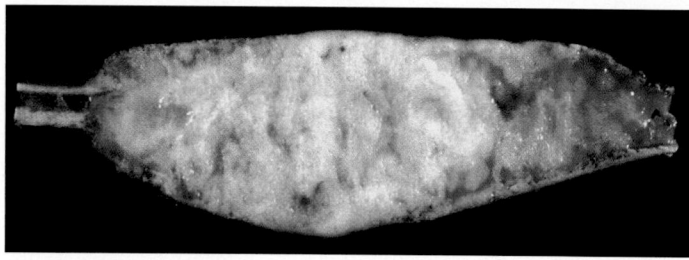

Fig. 14.80 Desmoplastic fibroma expanding the fibula and consisting of solid, white, leathery tissue.

impending or established pathologic fracture are adequately treated by curettage.

The histologic differential diagnosis of non-ossifying fibroma includes several entities. The diagnosis, however, is usually easily rendered when the patient's age and radiographic findings are correlated with the histologic findings of the tumor. Confusion may arise with non-ossifying fibromas that contain numerous osteoclastic-type giant cells. These tumors may resemble giant cell tumor of bone but their clinical and radiographic findings are distinctively different. Furthermore, in the diagnostic areas of giant cell tumor, the morphology of the nuclei in the giant cells is identical to that of the mononuclear stromal cells, a finding not present in non-ossifying fibroma.

DESMOPLASTIC FIBROMA

Desmoplastic fibroma is believed to be the intraosseous counterpart of deep-seated soft tissue fibromatosis. It is generally considered a locally aggressive tumor that does not have the capacity to metastasize. Desmoplastic fibroma is rare and accounts for only 0.1% of primary bone tumors. It affects a wide age range, including

children, but most often develops during the second or third decade of life.[256] The tumor arises in a variety of bones but most frequently develops in the metaphyses of long bones and the mandible.[257–260] It is slow growing, painful, and produces gradual enlargement of the bone. In the craniofacial skeleton, desmoplastic fibroma can cause symptoms such as headache, recurrent otitis, and hearing loss.

Desmoplastic fibroma appears as a unilocular or multilocular lucent mass that often has a honeycomb or trabeculated appearance on plain X-rays. Rarely, the tumor has a more aggressive appearance, with permeative margins.[257,261]

The tumor ranges in size from 5–10 cm and is oblong, well circumscribed, leathery or rubbery, and tan-white in appearance (Fig. 14.80). Histologically, it is similar to soft tissue fibromatosis, with variable cellularity and regions of abundant collagen (Fig. 14.81). The neoplastic cells are spindle fibroblasts arranged in broad sweeping fascicles. The tumor cells are uniform, cytologically bland, and surrounded by a collagenous matrix that contains scattered groups of extravasated red blood cells and small-caliber blood vessels. Cellular atypia and pleomorphism are absent and mitoses are inconspicuous. At the periphery of the tumor, focal infiltration of the cancellous bone may be present; however, extensive infiltration should raise concern for fibrosarcoma or low-grade osteosarcoma.[262] Desmoplastic fibroma can extend through the cortex and infiltrate adjacent soft tissue in a manner similar to soft tissue fibromatosis.

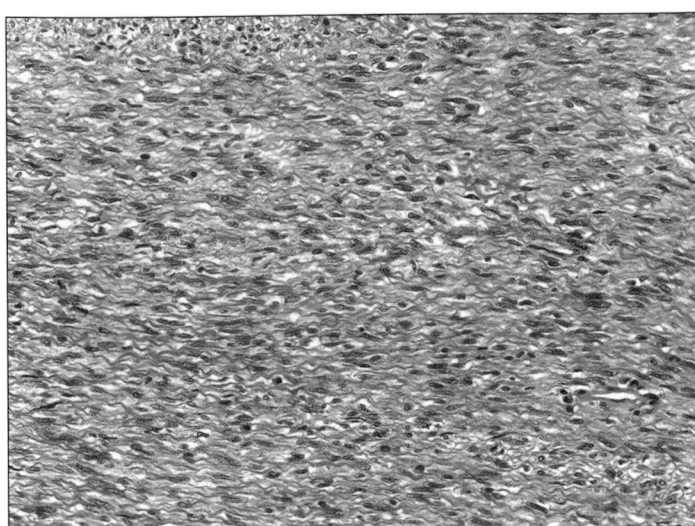

Fig. 14.81 Desmoplastic fibroma composed of uniform spindle cells growing in long fascicles and separated by eosinophilic collagen fibers.

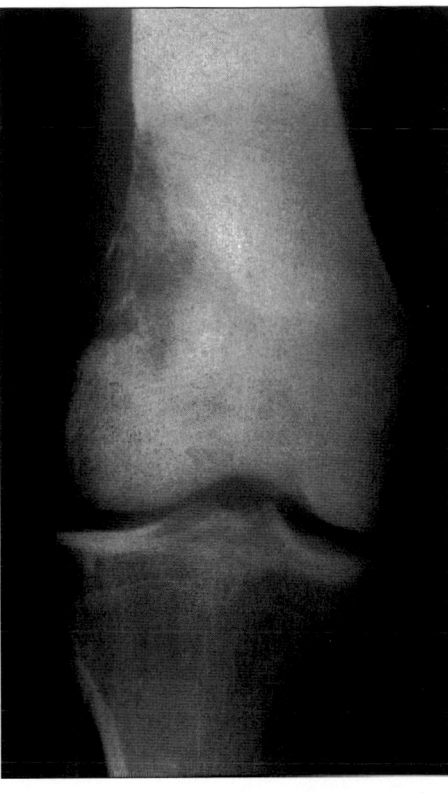

Fig. 14.82 Plain X-ray of malignant fibrous histiocytoma showing a destructive lytic mass with permeative margins extending into the soft tissues.

FNA smears obtained from desmoplastic fibromas are of low cellularity and contain a mixture of individual cells and small cell clusters. Fragments of collagenous stroma may be associated with a few, plump spindle cells in some aspirates. The individual spindle cells have fusiform nuclei showing moderate variability in size and shape. Stripped nuclei are frequent. Intact cells have elongated cytoplasmic processes. Occasional cases of desmoplastic fibroma have relatively highly cellular smears. Overall, the cytologic pattern is similar to that seen with soft tissue fibromatosis.[263–269]

Desmoplastic fibroma is locally aggressive and has a high rate of recurrence following curettage. The treatment of choice is complete local excision.[257,261] Malignant transformation is an extremely rare occurrence.[4,270]

The differential diagnosis of desmoplastic fibroma includes well differentiated fibrosarcoma and intramedullary low-grade osteosarcoma. Well differentiated fibrosarcoma grows with a permeative pattern, is more cellular than desmoplastic fibroma, and demonstrates a greater degree of nuclear atypia and more numerous mitotic figures. Low-grade intramedullary osteosarcoma, like desmoplastic fibroma, is composed of bland spindle cells. In contrast to desmoplastic fibroma, well differentiated osteosarcoma demonstrates neoplastic bone formation and extensively infiltrates the underlying cancellous bone.

BENIGN FIBROUS HISTIOCYTOMA/ XANTHOMA OF BONE

Benign fibrous histiocytoma is a tumor composed of spindled bland fibroblasts arranged in a storiform pattern with scattered foamy macrophages and osteoclast-like giant cells.[271,272] This lesion is morphologically identical to non-ossifying fibroma and the fibrohistiocytic areas that are frequently found in the periphery of giant cell tumors. These tumors should be excluded before a diagnosis of benign fibrous histiocytoma is made. When xanthomatous change predominates, the term *xanthoma* is most appropriate.[47] Benign fibrous histiocytoma arises in all ages and most frequently affects the ilium and ribs, where it presents as a radiolucent, well delineated

mass with sclerotic margins. It is controversial whether fibrous histiocytoma/xanthoma of bone is a distinct bone tumor or a secondary phenomenon seen in a pre-existing primary bone tumor that is obscured by the fibrohistiocytic proliferation. Treatment is curettage, and the rate of local recurrence is low.

MALIGNANT FIBROUS HISTIOCYTOMA/ FIBROSARCOMA

Malignant fibrous histiocytoma of bone is a non-matrix-producing fibroblastic sarcoma that was classified as fibrosarcoma in the older literature.[273] Malignant fibrous histiocytoma can arise de novo or develop in irradiated bone or against a background of Paget's disease and bone infarction. Similar to its much more common soft tissue counterpart, malignant fibrous histiocytoma of bone typically affects middle-aged and elderly adults.[273] Patients complain of pain and/or a mass.[274–277]

The tumor appears as a destructive, poorly circumscribed, nonmineralized lytic mass on imaging studies (Fig. 14.82).[273–278] Soft tissue extension is commonplace (Fig. 14.83).

Malignant fibrous histiocytoma of bone is high-grade and, like its soft tissue counterpart, is composed of fascicles of pleomorphic spindle cells arranged in a storiform pattern (Fig. 14.84).[273,274] Multinucleate tumor giant cells are frequently present. Necrosis and a high mitotic rate, including the presence of atypical mitotic figures, are common. By definition, these tumors do not produce neoplastic bone or cartilage matrix. The neoplastic cells, however, are often embedded within a collagen-rich stroma that may be hyalinized, making it very difficult to distinguish at times from bone. Myxoid change, which is a common feature of soft tissue malignant fibrous histiocytoma, is less frequently encountered among intraosseous tumors. It is also important to remember that other tumors, such as

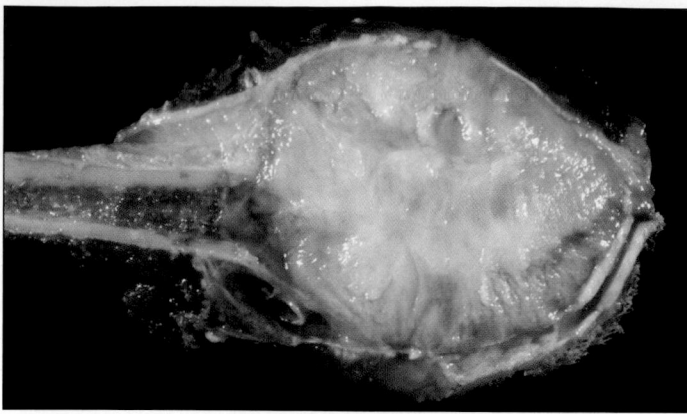

Fig. 14.83 Malignant fibrous histiocytoma. Solid tan-white mass destroying the proximal humerus and extending into adjacent soft tissue.

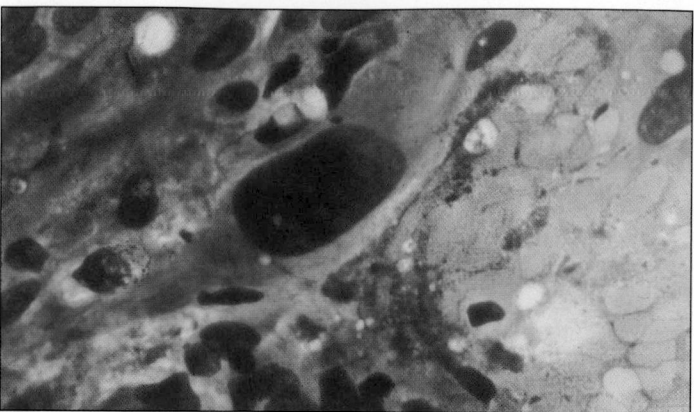

Fig. 14.85 Cellular smear showing severely pleomorphic spindle cells. (Romanowsky stain.)

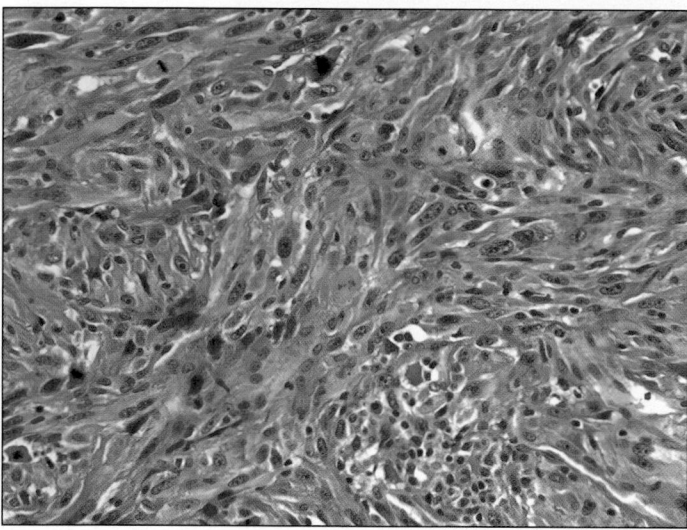

Fig. 14.84 Malignant fibrous histiocytoma. Pleomorphic spindle cells arranged in a storiform growth pattern.

osteosarcoma and dedifferentiated chondrosarcoma, may have areas indistinguishable from malignant fibrous histiocytoma.

Fine-needle aspirates from malignant fibrous histiocytoma of bone most closely resemble the storiform pleomorphic subtype found in soft tissue (Fig. 14.85). In these cases, smears contain plump, spindle-shaped cells showing marked variability in size and shape.[279] The nuclei are enlarged, irregular, and frequently contain prominent nucleoli. Nuclear pleomorphism is generally marked. Multinucleate, anaplastic tumor giant cells are characteristic and can contain from two to more than ten nuclei. The nuclei have coarse chromatin with prominent nucleoli and irregular nuclear membranes. Mitotic figures, including atypical forms, are commonly encountered. Tissue fragments with a true storiform pattern are unusual and are not specific for malignant fibrous histiocytoma. In smear preparations, examples of malignant fibrous histiocytoma are difficult to distinguish from other pleomorphic sarcomas unless multinucleate pleomorphic giant cells are prominent. The background is often rich in red blood cells and occasionally may contain necrotic debris.

In our institution, osseous malignant fibrous histiocytoma is treated like osteosarcoma of bone. The 5-year survival rate is approximately 60%.[273,278,280] The lung is the most common site for distant metastases.

FIBRO-OSSEOUS TUMORS AND ADAMANTINOMA

The hallmark of benign fibro-osseous tumors, which include fibrous dysplasia, osteofibrous dysplasia and adamantinoma, is the admixture of trabeculae of woven bone and benign fibrous tissue. The most common of these is fibrous dysplasia.

Fibrous dysplasia occurs in any bone of the body, however, osteofibrous dysplasia and adamantinoma almost always develop in the anterior tibial cortex.

Fibrous dysplasia

Fibrous dysplasia is the most common of the fibro-osseous tumors and should be viewed as a benign tumor of bone that is probably neoplastic. It has been likened to a localized developmental arrest: all the components of normal bone are present but they do not differentiate into their mature structures. Lichtenstein and Jaffe were the first to recognize it as a unique clinicopathologic entity and distinguished it from other lesions such as osteitis fibrosa cystica.[281,282] Fibrous dysplasia may involve a single bone, several bones, or many bones and may also be associated with abnormalities of the skin and endocrine glands. The skin lesions, which are café-au-lait pigmented macules, are the most common extraskeletal manifestation of fibrous dysplasia. They are present in more than half the patients with polyostotic lesions, virtually all the patients who have accompanying endocrine abnormalities, and some patients with solitary bone lesions. Infrequently, fibrous dysplasia is associated with oncogenic osteomalacia.

Monostotic solitary bone lesions are the most common clinical expression of the condition and account for 70–80% of cases. They usually arise in the rib, followed in descending order of frequency by the femur, tibia, jaw bones, calvarium, and humerus. The tumors typically develop during childhood but are only recognized in early or mid-adulthood, usually as an incidental finding. Fibrous dysplasia can cause marked enlargement and distortion of bone so that, if the craniofacial skeleton is involved, disfigurement, sometimes severe, can develop. Monostotic disease does not evolve into the polyostotic form.

Polyostotic fibrous dysplasia without endocrine dysfunction accounts for 20–30% of all cases. It manifests at a slightly earlier age than the monostotic variant, usually during childhood, and may continue to cause problems into adulthood. Polyostotic tumors may be unilateral or bilateral. The bones affected in descending order of frequency are the femur, skull, tibia, humerus, ribs, fibula, radius, ulna, mandible, and vertebrae. Craniofacial involvement is present in 50% of patients who have a moderate number of bones affected and in 100% of patients with extensive skeletal disease. All forms of polyostotic disease have a propensity to involve the shoulder and pelvic girdles, resulting in severe, sometimes crippling deformities (e.g. shepherd-crook deformity of the proximal femur) and spontaneous, often recurrent fractures. A minority of patients develop multiple soft tissue myxomas and this combination of abnormalities is known as Mazabraud syndrome.[283,284]

Polyostotic fibrous dysplasia associated with café-au-lait skin pigmentation and endocrinopathies is known as the McCune–Albright syndrome and accounts for 2–3% of all cases. The endocrinopathies include sexual precocity, hyperthyroidism, pituitary adenomas that secrete growth hormone, and primary adrenal hyperplasia.[282,284,285] The severity of manifestations in McCune–Albright syndrome depends on the number and types of cell that harbor the mutation in the G protein (see below). The most common clinical presentation is precocious sexual development and in this setting girls are affected more often than boys. The bone lesions are often unilateral and the skin pigmentation is usually limited to the same side of the body. The cutaneous macules are classically large, are dark to café-au-lait, have irregular, serpiginous borders (coastline of Maine), and are found primarily on the neck, chest, back, shoulder, and pelvic region.

In the past, fibrous dysplasia was thought to be a developmental defect in the formation of lamellar bone, such that bone formation was arrested at the stage of woven bone. Recently, however, the skeletal, skin, and endocrine lesions have been shown to result from a somatic (not hereditary) mutation, occurring during embryogenesis, that involves the gene that codes for a guanine nucleotide-binding protein (G protein).[286] The G protein normally couples receptors to the effector enzyme adenylyl cyclase and the mutation causes constitutive activation of the enzyme so that there is excess production of cyclic adenosine monophosphate (AMP), which leads to hyperfunction of cells in the involved tissues. In bone, this abnormality causes a proliferation of osteoprogenitor cells while at the same time inhibiting their differentiation. This results in an overproduction of fibrous matrix and woven bone formation.[287,288] Recent studies have also demonstrated a clonal origin for fibrous dysplasia, supporting the concept that this lesion is neoplastic in nature.[289]

Radiographically, fibrous dysplasia has a classic 'ground glass' appearance but can be radiolucent or radiodense, depending on the amount of bone present and its degree of mineralization (Fig. 14.86). In the appendicular skeleton, the margins of the lesion are usually well defined and surrounded by a rim of sclerotic bone. Fibrous dysplasia of the craniofacial skeleton seems to be less well defined and blends with the surrounding bone.[290] Extensive involvement causes bony expansion and sometimes severe deformity of the affected bone.

Grossly, fibrous dysplasia is well circumscribed and has a gritty and leather-like consistency. Occasionally, it contains cystic areas, which may occupy a small or large portion of the lesion. In a minority of instances nodules of pearly white cartilage are present. Microscopically, fibrous dysplasia is composed of cellular fibrous

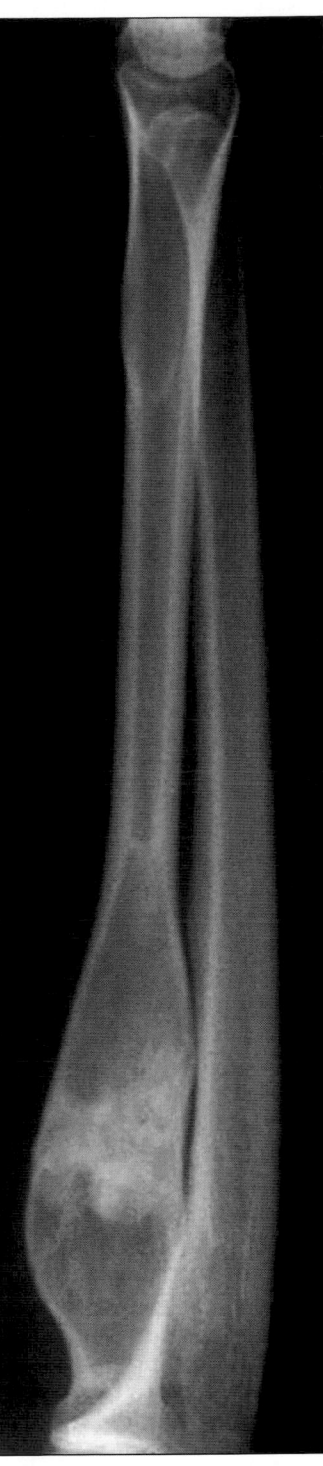

Fig. 14.86 Fibrous dysplasia. Expansile lesions involving the proximal and distal radius. Each is well circumscribed and has a ground glass appearance.

tissue surrounding irregular, curvilinear bony trabeculae (Fig. 14.87). The bony trabeculae are discontinuous and are composed of woven bone that is formed directly from the spindle cells with minimal osteoblastic rimming; however, osteoclasts may be numerous. In craniofacial tumors, the lesional bone tends to fuse with the surrounding host cancellous bone, explaining the lack of demarcation radiographically. The fibrous tissue is composed of cytologically banal, plump spindle cells without atypia or mitotic figures. The spindle cells can be arranged in a storiform pattern, especially in areas devoid of bone, and may be associated with collections of

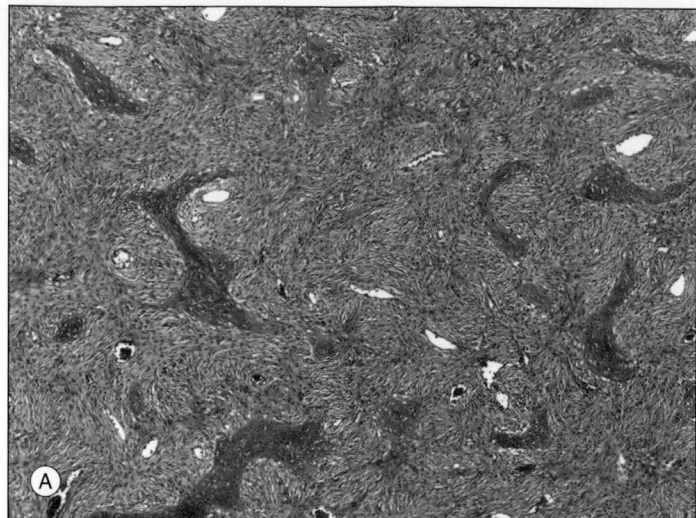

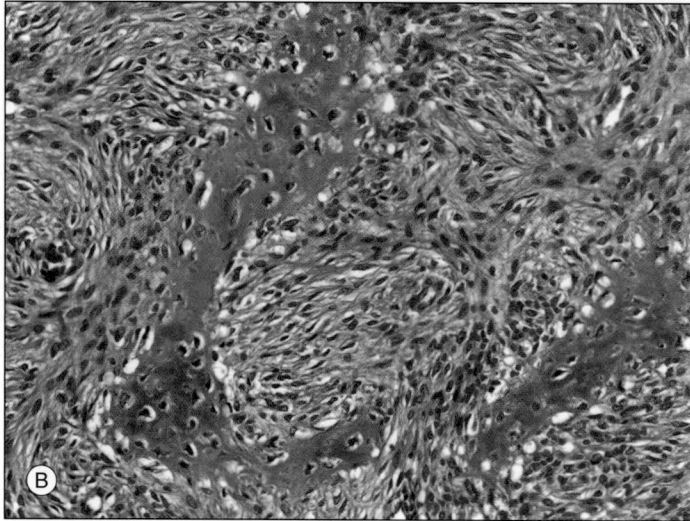

Fig. 14.87 Fibrous dysplasia. **(A)** Low power shows curvilinear trabeculae of bone surrounded by cellular fibroblastic proliferation. **(B)** High power shows that the bone is woven and lacks osteoblastic rimming. The spindle cells are cytologically bland.

foamy histiocytes, thus mimicking a xanthoma or a fibroxanthoma. Collagen fibers (Sharpey's-like fibers) are frequently seen extending from the fibrous tissue into the lesional bone. Cellular nodules of hyaline or myxoid cartilage, which can sometimes resemble cartilage in the growth plate, are present in approximately 20% of cases. Rarely, the cartilage predominates and these lesions have been designated fibrocartilaginous dysplasia.[291,292] Lesions previously designated fibrocartilaginous mesenchymoma also probably represent examples of fibrocartilaginous dysplasia.[293,294] Matrix resembling cementum may be found in lesions of the craniofacial skeleton and less frequently in the bones of the extremities. Cystic changes mimicking aneurysmal bone cyst are occasionally encountered.

Smears of aspiration specimens obtained from examples of fibrous dysplasia are of low to moderate cellularity. The individual cells are spindle-shaped and usually have short cytoplasmic processes, sometimes responsible for an overall oval appearance. The nuclei are bland and oval to spindle-shaped. Nucleoli are usually indistinct. The chromatin is finely granular and the nuclear membranes are smooth.

Mitotic activity is absent. Occasional fragments of bone or osteoid may be found and have an irregular three-dimensional shape. Rare multinucleate giant cells are present within most smears. The cytologic findings are usually insufficient for a specific diagnosis based purely on cytologic grounds but when coupled with radiographic features a diagnosis of fibrous dysplasia can generally be rendered.

Polymorphic fibro-osseous lesion of bone, also known as liposclerosing myxofibrous tumor, is a controversial entity that some investigators believe merely represents a variant of fibrous dysplasia.[295,296] A recent study identifying the mutation of the G protein characteristic of fibrous dysplasia in a case of polymorphic fibro-osseous lesion of bone probably confirms this impression.[297] Polymorphic fibro-osseous lesion of bone is almost always located in the intertrochanteric region of the proximal femur, affects adults, and has a slight male predominance. The lesions are usually asymptomatic and discovered as an incidental finding. On X-ray they appear as an irregular, oval lesion that has well circumscribed sclerotic margins. The tumors have lucent areas, as well as irregular patchy regions of marked radiodensity, and foci that have a ground glass appearance. Histologically, they frequently contain foci that closely resemble fibrous dysplasia. Additional elements include sclerotic woven bone that has a pagetoid appearance, fat, and myxoid fibrous tissue. These lesions behave in a benign fashion but rarely have been reported to undergo malignant transformation.

The treatment of fibrous dysplasia depends on the extent and severity of the disease and the problems caused by individual lesions. Therapy ranges from observation to surgical removal. Medical treatment with drugs such as bisphosphonates has yielded promising results.[298]

Malignant transformation of fibrous dysplasia is rare and is more common in patients with polyostotic disease or McCune–Albright syndrome. The sarcomas usually develop years after initial diagnosis and include osteosarcoma, fibrosarcoma, chondrosarcoma, and malignant fibrous histiocytoma.[299] Many affected patients have previously had fibrous dysplasia irradiated and some of these tumors therefore represent radiation-induced sarcomas.[299,300]

The differential diagnosis of fibrous dysplasia includes several lesions, particularly when the biopsy sample is small. Desmoplastic fibroma, a lesion composed of fascicles of spindle shaped cells, may mimic fibrous dysplasia; however, bone formation is not a component of desmoplastic fibroma. Osteofibrous dysplasia invariably arises in the anterior cortex of the tibia and fibula rather than the medullary cavity and, unlike fibrous dysplasia, shows prominent osteoblastic rimming of the lesional bone. The most important tumor to exclude is well differentiated or low-grade osteosarcoma. Well differentiated osteosarcoma shows greater cytologic atypia and has an infiltrative growth pattern, encasing pre-existing trabeculae of bone – features not present in fibrous dysplasia.

Psammomatoid (juvenile) ossifying fibroma

Psammomatoid ossifying fibroma is a fibro-osseous lesion that has a predilection for the supraorbital frontal and ethmoid bones and the ethmoid and maxillary sinuses.[301] In the literature, it is also known as ossifying fibroma, juvenile or young ossifying fibroma, juvenile active ossifying fibroma, cementifying fibroma, and cemento-ossifying fibroma.[301] This multitude of terms reflects two things: the uncertain histogenesis of the tumor and one of its defining features – numerous acellular, 'cementicle-like' structures.

Psammomatoid ossifying fibroma arises primarily in young individuals. Most patients are in their second decade of life although

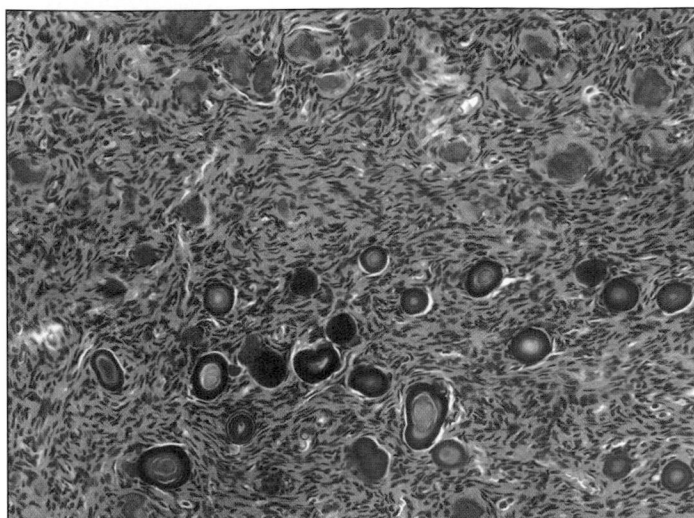

Fig. 14.88 Psammomatoid (juvenile) ossifying fibroma. Numerous psammomatoid calcifications and cementum-like matrix surrounded by spindle cells.

rare cases have been reported in patients as old as 54 years.[301,302] The male to female ratio is approximately equal. While specific localizing presenting symptoms depend on the exact site of the tumor, the most common clinical manifestation overall is proptosis. Other signs and symptoms include visual disturbances, nasal obstruction, papilledema, strabismus, headaches, ptosis, and recurrent sinusitis.[301,302]

Radiographically, psammomatoid ossifying fibroma is mixed lytic and blastic. It frequently demonstrates an aggressive growth pattern with invasion of adjacent anatomic structures; however, occasionally it is well demarcated and expansile.[301]

The tumor is usually 3–5 cm in size, well circumscribed, firm to hard, and tan-white.[301] Microscopically, it is composed of a cellular fibrous component consisting of bland, stellate or spindle cells, woven bone spicules, and small ossicular or 'cementicle-like' structures that have a concentric layering ('psammomatoid') pattern (Fig. 14.88). The ossicles contain osteocytes and some are rimmed by osteoblasts. Large specimens often reveal a zoning pattern with hypercellular areas containing 'psammomatoid' ossicles or 'cementicles' in the center, which merge peripherally with fibrous-dysplasia-like/ ossifying-fibroma-like areas that in turn merge with lamellar bone or bone that has a pagetoid pattern.[302] Cystic change and areas of hemorrhage with clustering of multinucleate osteoclast-type giant cells may be present in some cases. Ultrastructural examination reveals an admixture of fibroblasts, osteoblasts, and osteoclasts and calcium hydroxyapatite deposits either in areas occupied by collagen fibers or as amorphous dense aggregates, the latter corresponding to the 'psammoma bodies.'[303]

The clinical behavior of psammomatoid ossifying fibroma is that of repeated local recurrence.[304,305] Because of this 'aggressive' behavior, the term aggressive psammomatoid ossifying fibroma has been proposed.[301] Surgery is the treatment of choice and should be as complete as possible.

The main differential diagnosis of this tumor includes meningioma, with numerous psammoma bodies invading bone. The patient's age, anatomic location, and radiographic findings are important. Also, meningioma involving bone shows a very infiltrative growth pattern, extending in between bony trabeculae, in contrast to the relatively noninfiltrative growth pattern seen in psammomatoid ossifying

fibroma. Also, the psammoma bodies in meningiomas are not associated with osteocytes or osteoblasts.[301]

Osteofibrous dysplasia

Osteofibrous dysplasia is a benign fibro-osseous lesion of bone that characteristically occurs during childhood and arises in the anterior cortex of the tibia. It was initially considered to be a form of congenital pseudoarthrosis, fibrous dysplasia, or ossifying fibroma of the jaw bones.[306,307] It wasn't until 1976 that Campanacci recognized it as a distinct clinicopathologic entity and coined the term osteofibrous dysplasia to simultaneously signify its similarity to fibrous dysplasia and acknowledge its uniqueness.[308,309] The etiology of osteofibrous dysplasia is unknown but genetic studies have identified chromosomal abnormalities in these tumors, including trisomy 7 and 8.[310,311]

Osteofibrous dysplasia accounts for fewer than 1% of all bone tumors. It usually develops during the first two decades and only arises in the tibia and/or the fibula. In the largest reported series, the patients ranged in age from 3 weeks to 35 years; 68 lesions involved the tibia, nine involved the tibia and fibula, and three involved only the fibula.[312] Clinically, the tumors cause pain, localized swelling, bowing deformity, and, infrequently, pathologic fracture.[309,312]

Osteofibrous dysplasia produces a well delineated, intracortical lucency that is surrounded by areas of sclerosis and which may extend into the medullary cavity. (Fig. 14.89). The tumor may manifest as a single lytic lesion but more commonly consists of multiple lytic foci scattered along the anterior cortex of the tibia, which frequently results in anterior bowing.

The tumor varies in size from less than 1 cm to more than 10 cm. It is typically solid, yellow or white, gritty, and centered in the cortex, which is expanded and attenuated (Fig. 14.90). Microscopically, osteofibrous dysplasia is composed of irregular curvilinear trabeculae of woven bone, which in the periphery merge with pre-existing lamellar cancellous bone (Fig. 14.91A). The trabeculae of woven bone are rimmed by prominent osteoblasts and scattered osteoclasts. The intervening stroma is composed of bland spindle cells embedded within a collagenous matrix. Isolated single stromal cells express keratin but clusters of epithelial cells, as seen in well differentiated adamantinoma, are absent (Fig. 14.91B). The cortex may be thinned but the periosteum remains intact.

Osteofibrous dysplasia is a benign tumor that has been reported to regress with skeletal maturation.[309] Surgical treatment, either curettage or conservative en bloc excision, is indicated for: growing or extensive lesions, pathologic fracture, or significant tibial bowing.[312] The clinical, radiographic, and pathologic features of osteofibrous dysplasia overlap with those of well differentiated adamantinoma. Therefore, it may be impossible to distinguish these two tumors on needle biopsy specimens, and extensive histologic sampling may be necessary. Consequently, patients with osteofibrous dysplasia need to be clinically followed, as disease progression raises the possibility that the lesion is actually an adamantinoma.

The scattered keratin-positive cells in osteofibrous dysplasia suggest that osteofibrous dysplasia might be related to adamantinoma. The exact relation between these two tumors, however, is unclear. For example, in the study by Sweet et al.,[313] none of the 30 patients with follow-up developed adamantinoma. It is possible that the cases of osteofibrous dysplasia reported to have progressed to adamantinoma may have been adamantinomas from the onset, the initial biopsies only having sampled the osteofibrous-dysplasia-like areas. There are molecular and cytogenetic findings, however, that support the concept that these tumors are closely related to one another.

Fig. 14.89
Osteofibrous dysplasia. Plain X-ray shows multiple oval lucencies with adjacent sclerosis involving the tibial diaphysis.

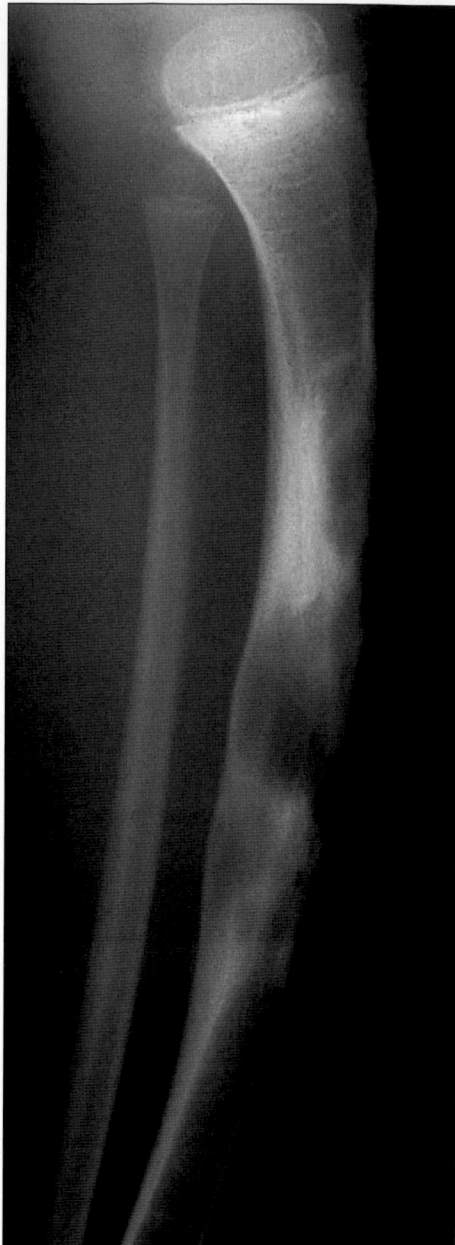

Fig. 14.90
Osteofibrous dysplasia. Gritty, tan-white tumor expands the tibia. Gray-white bone wax fills the track of the biopsy site.

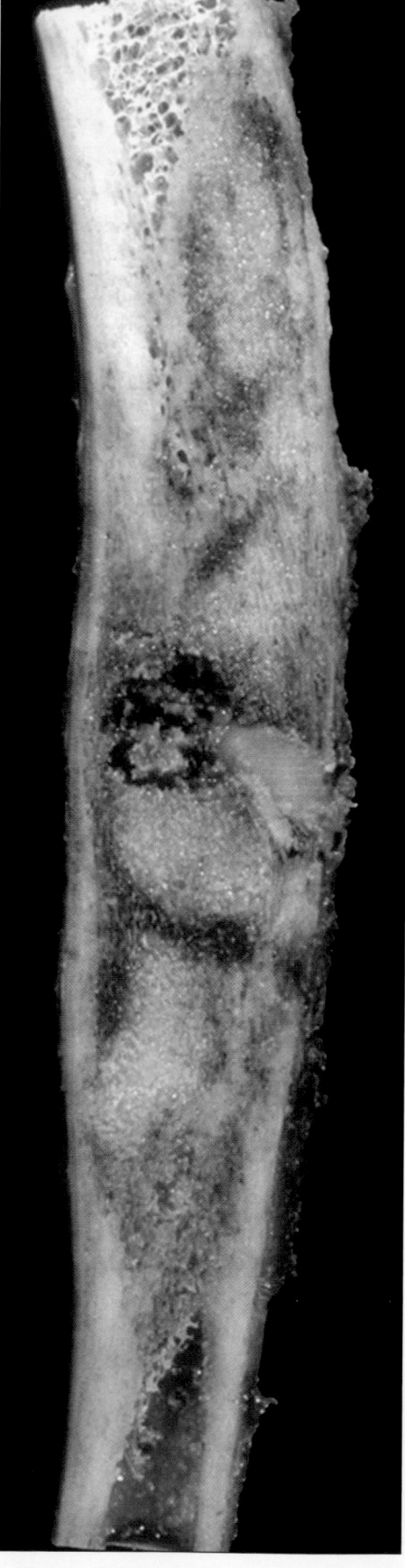

Adamantinoma

Adamantinoma is a low-grade biphasic malignant tumor of bone composed of epithelial and stromal elements. The term adamantinoma was coined to convey its similarity to ameloblastoma of the jaw bones. Adamantinoma is extremely uncommon and represents fewer than 1% of primary malignant bone tumors.[4] It occurs almost exclusively in the tibia, with or without involvement of the fibula, and rarely as a primary mass limited to the pretibial soft tissues. The diagnosis should be made with caution and only after other types of tumors have been excluded.[314] Adamantinoma is more common in males than in females.[314–316] Cytogenetic studies have shown gains of genetic material on chromosomes 7, 8, 12, and 19.[317–319] Clinically, adamantinoma causes pain, anterior bowing deformity, and a palpable mass; symptoms have often been noted for years prior to diagnosis.

Adamantinoma is divided into two main types: classic adamantinoma and well differentiated (osteofibrous-dysplasia-like)

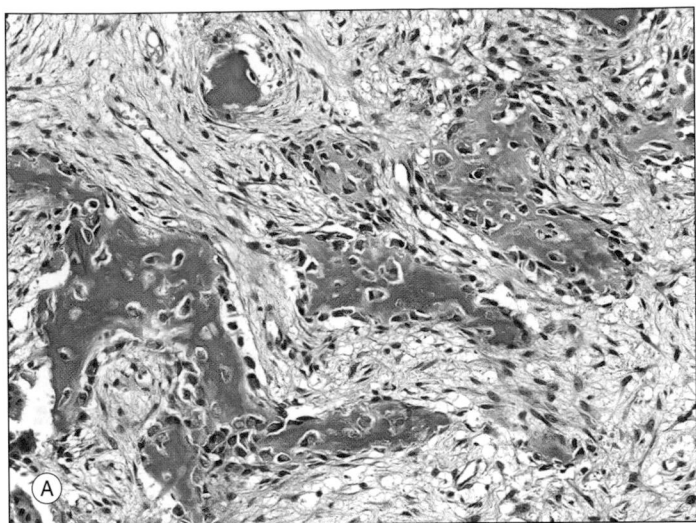

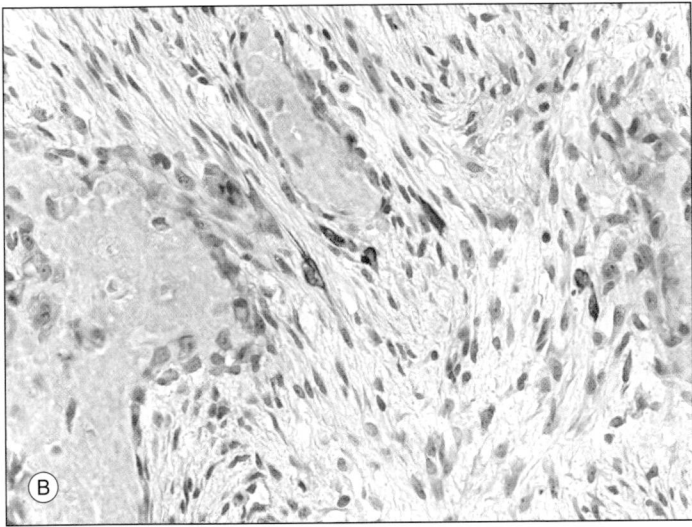

Fig. 14.91 Osteofibrous dysplasia. **(A)** Microscopically it is composed of irregular trabeculae of woven bone with prominent osteoblastic rimming. **(B)** Scattered spindle cells are keratin-positive.

adamantinoma. This distinction is important because these variants differ in their biological behaviors. Well differentiated adamantinoma was first recognized as a distinct entity in 1989[320] and characteristically occurs entirely within the anterior tibial cortex in young patients (first two decades of life). It is typically composed of a predominance of osteofibrous-dysplasia-like areas and rare clusters of epithelial cells. In contrast, classic adamantinoma affects patients older than 20 years, may have intramedullary and soft tissue components, contains prominent epithelial elements, and lacks large areas that resemble osteofibrous dysplasia.

Radiographically, both types of adamantinoma are diaphyseal and manifest as well circumscribed, cortically based, lytic foci with intervening sclerosis, which produces a characteristic 'soap-bubble' appearance and irregular thickening of the cortex (Fig. 14.92). Approximately 10% of cases lack sclerosis. Anterior bowing of the tibia is common but bowing does not usually occur in the fibula. The diagnosis can usually be made by plain X-ray. CT and MRI are of limited value in making the diagnosis but are helpful in assessing the extent of the bone and soft tissue involvement.[321]

Grossly, adamantinoma has sharp margins and is soft, gritty, red-tan, and surrounded by sclerotic bone (Fig. 14.93). The tumor varies in size from less than 1 cm to more than 10 cm and extends longitudinally along the tibial diaphysis. The involved cortex is usually thickened. Both classic and well differentiated types may be confined to the cortex but intramedullary or soft tissue extension is commonly present in the classic type.

Both subtypes have a biphasic histologic pattern composed of spindled stromal cells, groups or sheets of epithelial cells, and a variable amount of osteofibrous-dysplasia-like tissue. In classic adamantinoma the epithelial component is prominent, and osteofibrous-dysplasia-like areas are inconspicuous. The epithelial cells have four different morphologic patterns: basaloid, tubular, squamoid, and spindled (Fig. 14.94). The *basaloid* pattern is composed of nests of spindle cells surrounded by palisading basal cells, whereas the *squamoid* pattern consists of epithelial nests with obvious squamous differentiation. The *tubular* pattern is formed by groups of epithelial cells with one or more layers of cuboidal or flattened cells that delineate gland-like spaces. The *spindle* pattern is composed of spindle cells arranged in intersecting fascicles resembling fibrosarcoma. Regardless of the pattern, the epithelial cells do not demonstrate significant cytologic atypia or mitotic activity. The osteofibrous-dysplasia-like areas, if present, are limited to the periphery of the tumor. In contrast, well differentiated adamantinoma is characterized by a predominance of osteofibrous-dysplasia-like areas with only small nests of epithelial cells surrounded by fibrous tissue. The nests can be difficult to identify and may easily be confused with small vascular spaces, sometimes requiring immunohistochemistry to confirm their epithelial nature. Recently, a dedifferentiated variant of adamantinoma has been described with the dedifferentiated component having the features of a poorly differentiated matrix producing sarcoma.[322]

Ultrastructural examination confirms the epithelial nature of the nests of epithelial cells in adamantinoma. Immunohistochemical stains show that the epithelial cells are keratin-positive and have a keratin profile similar to the basal layer cells of the epidermis.[323] The keratins expressed are usually types 14 and 19 and less frequently keratins 5, 7, 13, and 17.[324] This is in contrast to other bone and soft tissue tumors with epithelial features, such as synovial sarcoma, chordoma, and epithelioid sarcoma, which usually express keratins 8 and 18.[324]

FNA smears obtained from adamantinomas are usually cellular.[18,325–327] The neoplastic cells are predominantly spindle-shaped or ovoid in morphology. The cells are dispersed singly or may be arranged in cohesive clusters and have an epithelial appearance. The neoplastic cells have absent or indistinct cytoplasmic margins and the nuclei are darkly stained with a uniformly distributed, finely granular chromatin. Chroma centers are indistinct and nucleoli are generally absent. Metachromatic stroma (Giemsa) may invest individual tumor cells. Mitotic figures are rare or absent, and nuclear pleomorphism is minimal. In rare cases, multinucleate osteoclast-like giant cells are present. Necrotic debris may be found in occasional cases.

Classic adamantinoma behaves as a low-grade malignancy with a tendency for local recurrence. Metastases usually develop after a long clinical course and occur in approximately 20% of patients. The most common site of spread is the lungs. Rarely are lymph nodes involved.[328] There does not appear to be a relationship between the clinical behavior of the tumor and the histologic pattern of the epithelial cells (basaloid, squamous, tubular, or spindle).[329] Factors associated with a more aggressive outcome include male sex, short duration of symptoms, pain, and inadequate initial treatment.[328] In the largest series from the Mayo Clinic, 31%

Fig. 14.92 Adamantinoma involving tibial diaphysis. **(A)** The tumor produces multiple oval lucencies and causing bowing of the bone. **(B)** Axial CT showing prominent cortical involvement.

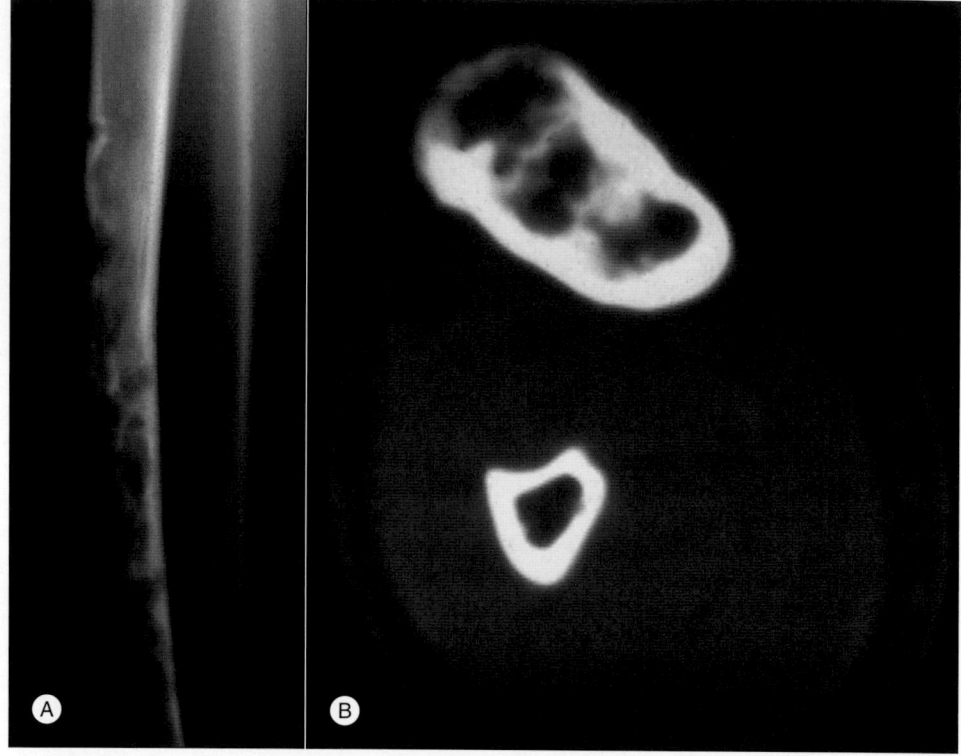

of patients experienced one or more local recurrences, 15% developed pulmonary metastases, and 13% died of disease.[328] In contrast, well differentiated adamantinoma behaves similarly to osteofibrous dysplasia and only rare cases have exhibited aggressive behavior.[330–332] The treatment of adamantinoma is wide surgical excision with reconstructive surgery. Radiation therapy and chemotherapy have not been shown to be effective in the management of this type of tumor.[321]

The differential diagnosis of adamantinoma includes metastatic carcinoma, fibrosarcoma, and osteofibrous dysplasia. Metastatic carcinoma and fibrosarcoma can be excluded on the basis of the clinicopathologic features and the radiographic appearance of the tumor. In contrast to well differentiated adamantinoma, osteofibrous dysplasia does not contain nests of epithelial cells. The presence of scattered individual keratin positive cells in osteofibrous dysplasia, however, raises questions about the relationship between these two tumors. Some investigators suggest that they may represent different ends of a spectrum of disease, only distinguishable by the quantity of epithelial elements in the tumor.[321,333]

MALIGNANT NEUROECTODERMAL TUMORS OF BONE

Malignant neuroectodermal tumors of bone frequently have the appearance of small round cell sarcomas. Their differential diagnosis is broad and includes a variety of primary and metastatic neoplasms (Table 14.9). The difficulty in diagnosing these tumors is based on a morphologic overlap that frequently requires special studies such as immunohistochemistry, electron microscopy, cytogenetics, and molecular genetics to make an accurate diagnosis. The importance of correctly identifying these neoplasms is related to the difference in their treatment and prognoses.

EWING'S SARCOMA/PRIMITIVE NEUROECTODERMAL TUMOR

Ewing's sarcoma and primitive peripheral neuroectodermal tumor are primary malignant small round cell tumors of bone and soft tissue. Current opinion is that, as both Ewing's sarcoma and primitive neuroectodermal tumor have a similar phenotype and share an identical chromosome translocation, they should be viewed as the same tumor, differing from each other only in their degree of neural differentiation. Tumors that demonstrate neural differentiation by light microscopy, immunohistochemistry, or electron microscopy have been traditionally labeled primitive neuroectodermal tumor, and those that are undifferentiated by these analyses have been diagnosed as Ewing's sarcoma.

James Ewing first described Ewing's sarcoma/primitive neuroectodermal tumor in 1921 and believed that it was a variant of diffuse endothelioma.[334] Since its recognition as a distinct clinicopathologic entity, it has been shown to account for approximately 6–10% of primary malignant bone tumors and follows osteosarcoma as the second most common bone sarcoma in children and adolescents. The annual incidence of newly diagnosed cases is 0.6 per million persons with approximately 13 cases identified per million individuals 0–24 years old.[335] Of all bone sarcomas, Ewing's sarcoma/primitive neuroectodermal tumor has the youngest average age at presentation, as most patients are 10–15 years old and approximately 80% are younger than 20 years. Boys are affected more frequently than girls at a ratio of 1.3–1.4:1, and there is a striking predilection for whites; blacks are rarely afflicted.[8]

Ewing's sarcoma/primitive neuroectodermal tumor was one of the first sarcomas found to have a specific translocation. Approximately 85% of the neoplasms harbor a t(11;22)(q24;q12) translocation, 5–10% of cases have a t(21;22)(q22;q12) translocation, and in less than 1% of tumors, a t(7;22)(p22;q12) translocation is

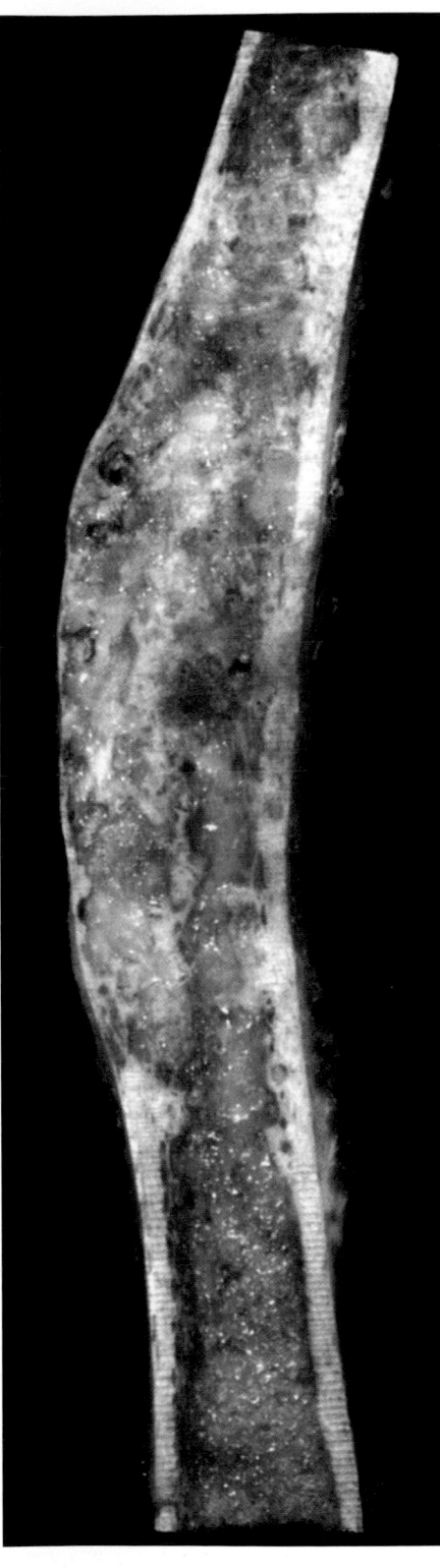

Fig. 14.93
Adamantinoma.
The tumor involves
the anterior tibial
cortex and
medullary canal.

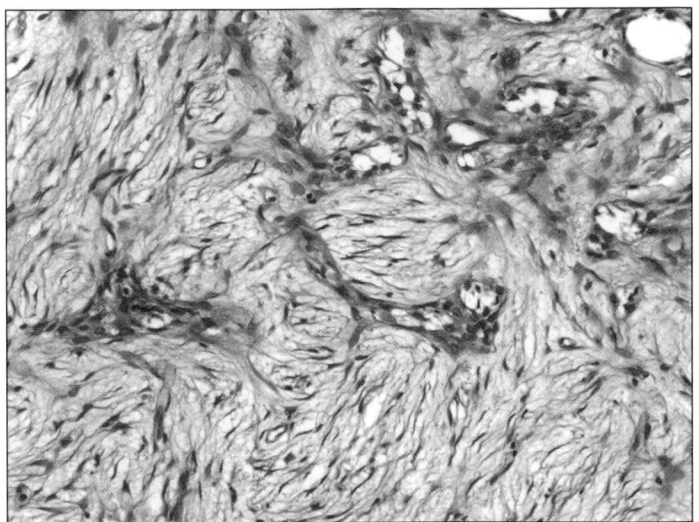

Fig. 14.94 Adamantinoma showing well defined nests of epithelial cells with early tubular formation embedded within the fibrous stroma.

Table 14.9 Malignant round cell tumors of bone

Primary	Metastatic
Ewing's sarcoma/primitive neuroectodermal tumor	Neuroblastoma
Rhabdomyosarcoma	Wilms tumor
Small cell osteosarcoma	Rhabdomyosarcoma
	Small cell carcinoma
Mesenchymal chondrosarcoma	Olfactory neuroblastoma
Lymphoma	
Leukemia	Round cell liposarcoma
Myeloma	Lymphoma
	Desmoplastic small round cell tumor

Ewing's sarcoma/primitive neuroectodermal tumor can arise in any portion of the skeleton but usually develops in the diaphysis or metadiaphysis of long tubular bones and the flat bones of the pelvis. Approximately 22% of cases originate in the femur, 12% in the ilium, 11% in the tibia, 10% in the humerus, 9% in the fibula, and 8% in the ribs. The tumor typically presents as a painful enlarging mass, and the affected site is frequently tender, warm, and swollen. Some patients have systemic findings that mimic infection: fever, elevated sedimentation rate, anemia, and leukocytosis.

Plain X-rays reveal a destructive lytic tumor that has permeative margins and extension into the surrounding soft tissues (Fig. 14.95). Extraosseous tumor erodes the outer cortex, producing 'saucerization' of the bone, and displaced periosteum deposits layers of reactive bone in an onion-skin-like fashion. CT and MRI are helpful in mapping the intra- and extraosseous extent of the tumor and the relationship of the mass to important anatomic structures. Ewing's sarcoma/primitive neuroectodermal tumor has low signal intensity in T1-weighted images and high signal intensity in T2-weighted images. These findings may be useful in assessing postchemotherapy tumor viability. Ewing's sarcoma/primitive neuroectodermal tumor has avid uptake of radionuclides and this facilitates scanning the skeleton in search of bone metastases.

present. Evidence suggests that the fusion genes (*EWS–FLI1*) generated from the translocations play a vital role in the molecular genesis of the neoplasms. These aberrant genes act as dominant oncogenes and the resultant chimeric proteins function as aberrant transcription factors that stimulate cell proliferation by regulating a network of target genes.[336]

Fig. 14.95
Ewing's
sarcoma/primitive
neuroectodermal
tumor. Plain X-ray
showing a
permeative lesion
extending into soft
tissue and
producing a
sunburst
appearance.

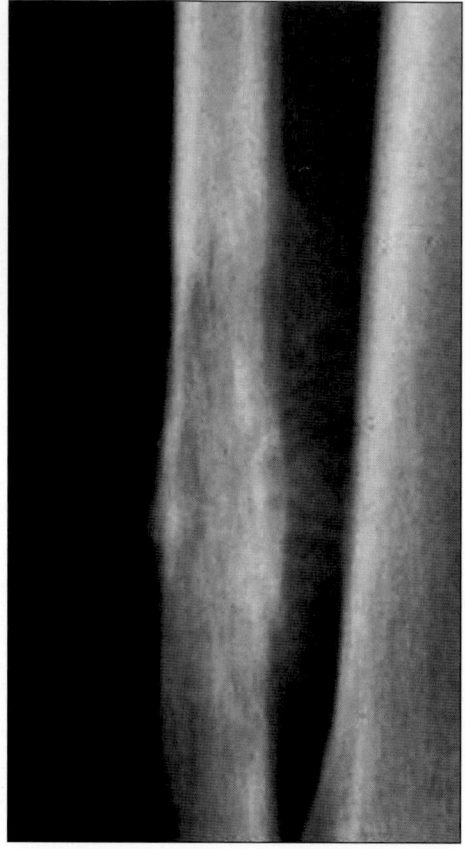

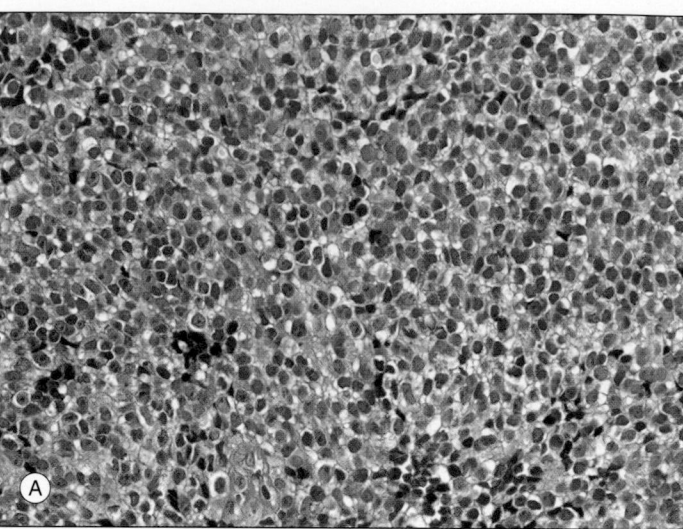

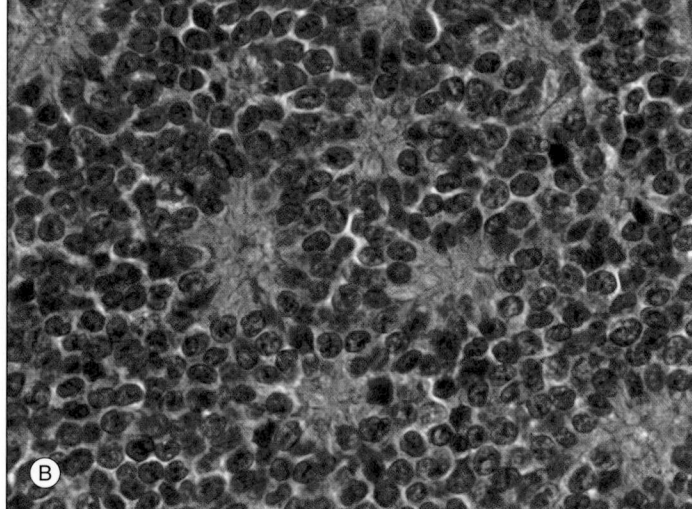

Fig. 14.97 Ewing's sarcoma/primitive neuroectodermal tumor.
(A) Ewing's sarcoma composed of sheets of small round cells.
(B) Numerous rosettes can be seen in primitive neuroectodermal tumor.

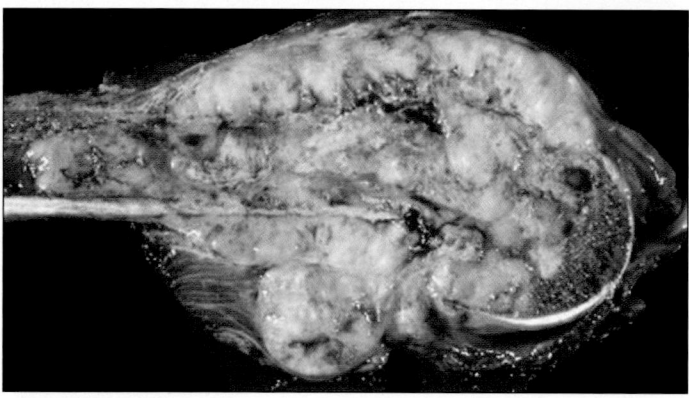

Fig. 14.96 Ewing's sarcoma/primitive neuroectodermal tumor. A
tan-white tumor destroys the proximal humerus and forms a large soft
tissue mass.

Arising in the medullary cavity, Ewing's sarcoma/primitive
neuroectodermal tumor usually transgresses the cortex and periosteum, producing a soft tissue mass. The tumor is tan-white or fish-
flesh-like in appearance and frequently contains areas of
hemorrhage and necrosis (Fig. 14.96). Thin layers of reactive bone
underpin the raised periosteum, and the underlying osseous
structure is eroded and destroyed. The intramedullary margins of the
tumor are poorly defined, whereas the soft tissue borders may be
deceptively well circumscribed by a pseudocapsule.

The classic Ewing's sarcoma/primitive neuroectodermal tumor is
composed of tumor cells that are one or two times the size of
lymphocytes. The cells grow in sheets or irregular islands delineated
by dense fibrous tissue. Architectural features suggestive of neural
differentiation traditionally included an organoid growth pattern,
within which Homer–Wright rosettes may be present (Fig. 14.97).
The tumor cell nuclei are oval and have finely distributed chromatin,
inconspicuous nucleoli, and scant eosinophilic or clear cytoplasm.
The cell nuclei in tumors with obvious neural differentiation are
frequently slightly elongated and darkly staining. Occasionally,
tumor cells are larger and have irregular nuclear contours and
prominent nucleoli. Neoplasms composed predominately of these cells
were previously designated atypical or large cell variant of Ewing's
sarcoma. In most Ewing's sarcoma/primitive neuroectodermal tumors,
mitoses are numerous and easily identified, and necrosis may be
extensive. The stroma is scant and the supportive vascular tree is
inconspicuous. Special histochemical stains demonstrate glycogen
in up to 75% of tumors.

Ultrastructurally, the tumor cells may be very primitive in
appearance, containing only abundant cytoplasmic glycogen and a
few organelles, including a small number of mitochondria, poorly

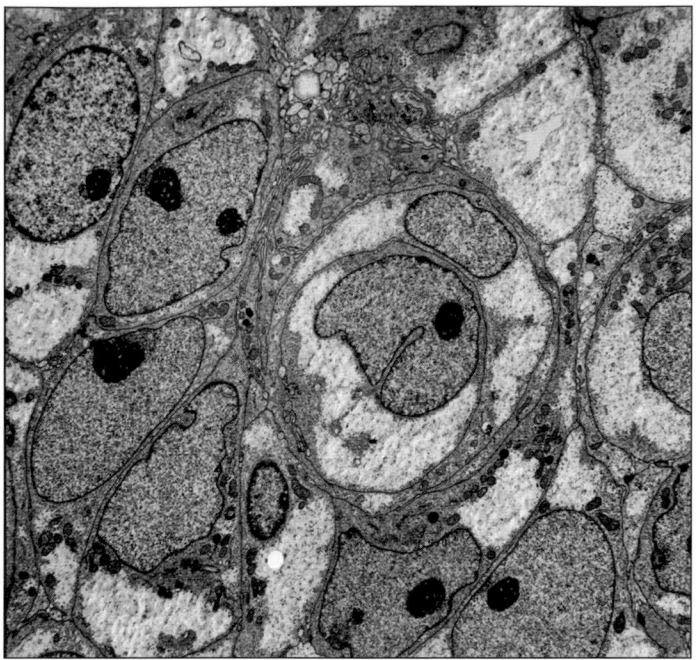

Fig. 14.98 Ewing's sarcoma. Ultrastructurally the cells are primitive in appearance and contain abundant intracytoplasmic glycogen.

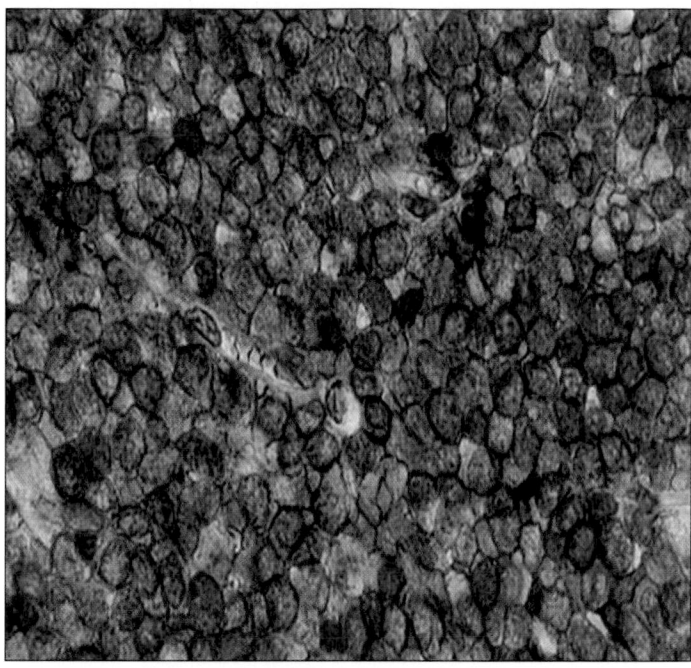

Fig. 14.99 Ewing's sarcoma/primitive neuroectodermal tumor. A Mic-2 stain shows membranous staining.

developed Golgi complexes, free ribosomes, and inconspicuous rough endoplasmic reticulum (Fig. 14.98).[337] Features indicative of neural differentiation, if present, include delicate interdigitating cytoplasmic cell processes connected by primitive junctions, scattered microtubules, intermediate filaments, and, in a minority of cases, dense core neurosecretory granules. In some keratin-positive cases we have identified definite tonofibrils and well developed basal lamina.

Ewing's sarcoma/primitive neuroectodermal tumor cells express vimentin, CD-99 (MIC-2), FLI-1, c-Kit, and one or more neural markers, including NSE, Leu-7, S-100, neurofilament, and keratin in approximately 20% of cases (Fig. 14.99).[338–341] At least 90% of Ewing's sarcoma/primitive neuroectodermal tumors stain positively for CD-99; however, many other malignant small round cell tumors, including lymphoblastic lymphoma, small cell osteosarcoma, mesenchymal chondrosarcoma, and small cell carcinoma, express this antigen as well. Therefore, a negative staining for CD-99 stain should raise the possibility that the tumor may not be Ewing's sarcoma/primitive neuroectodermal tumor.[342] It is noteworthy to remember that neuroblastoma, a tumor in the differential diagnosis, is negative for CD-99.

Smears prepared from aspirates of Ewing's sarcoma/primitive neuroectodermal tumor are highly cellular, with cells arranged both individually and in clusters (Fig. 14.100). The cell population can be separated into 'light' and 'dark' cells based on the nuclear chromatin pattern. A fine open chromatin pattern characterizes 'light' cells. The nuclei are round, with one to three small indistinct nucleoli, and are surrounded by a thin rim of scanty cytoplasm. The so-called 'dark' cells have a denser, more compact nuclear chromatin and poorly visualized nucleoli. Both cell populations have well defined cytoplasmic borders, which occasionally have large, 'punched out' clear spaces within the cytoplasm. These spaces usually lie within the perinuclear region but, in occasional cells with elongated cytoplasmic

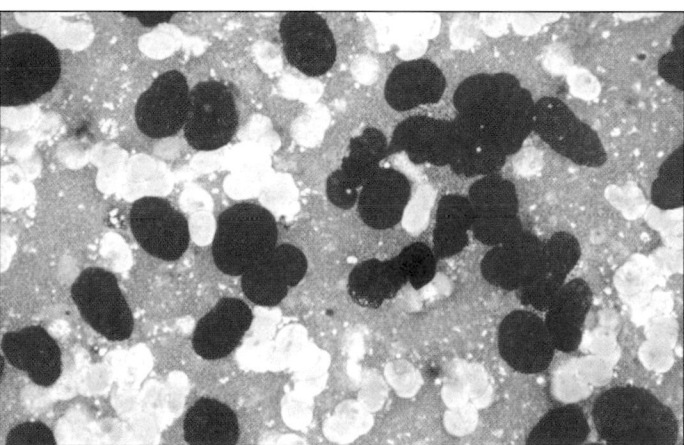

Fig. 14.100 The small round cells obtained from Ewing's sarcoma may be characterized by a bimorphic population with small, dark, pyknotic nuclei in one population and larger, paler nuclei comprising the second. The background frequently has a dirty proteinaceous appearance. (Romanowsky stain.)

processes, the vacuoles may lie more peripherally. The background often contains fine, reticular cytoplasm wisps that appear to connect the neoplastic cells, giving the background a fibrillar appearance. Nuclear molding is generally not a prominent feature. Rosette-like structures have been reported but are infrequent. The presence of glycogen is variable. In a significant number of smears, many of the neoplastic cells have a degenerative appearance. In these cells, the cytoplasm is stripped off, leaving bare, deformed nuclei. Pyknotic degeneration is common.

Ewing's sarcoma/primitive neuroectodermal tumor is usually treated with a combination of chemotherapy and surgery. Frequently the chemotherapy is given preoperatively, which allows for the pathologic assessment of the effectiveness of the drug regimen.[347] Chemotherapy-induced necrosis of 90% or greater is considered a good response.[342,343] Therapy-related cytologic changes of the tumor cells are uncommon and include ganglion cell differentiation, marked enlargement, hyperchromasia, pleomorphism, and the presence of rhabdoid-like cells. Radiotherapy is reserved for tumors that are located in inaccessible sites, surgical beds in which tumors have been excised with inadequate margins, and patient palliation.[344]

The advent of effective chemotherapy has dramatically improved the prognosis of Ewing's sarcoma/primitive neuroectodermal tumor from a dismal 5–15% 5-year survival to 75%; at least 50% are long-term cures. Important factors influencing prognosis include the patient's stage at the time of diagnosis, site and size of the tumor, type of translocation, percentage of chemotherapy-related tumor necrosis, presence of chimeric transcripts in cells from the peripheral blood or bone marrow after treatment, and the development of local recurrence.[345–348]

The main histologic differential diagnosis of Ewing's sarcoma/primitive neuroectodermal tumor includes malignant lymphoma, metastatic neuroblastoma, small cell osteosarcoma, and mesenchymal chondrosarcoma. The cells in large cell lymphoma are frequently larger than those of Ewing's sarcoma/primitive neuroectodermal tumor, have more cytoplasm, and their nuclei are irregular, cleaved, and hyperlobular. Lymphoblastic lymphoma is composed of smaller, more uniform, round cells and frequently contains benign infiltrating lymphocytes. Lymphomas express lymphoid antigens (some are MIC-2-positive) and ultrastructurally the cells have marginated chromatin, lack intercellular junctions, and do not have large amounts of glycogen. Lastly, the chromosomal translocations associated with malignant lymphoma do not include those identified in Ewing's sarcoma/primitive neuroectodermal tumor. Metastatic neuroblastoma can be very difficult to distinguish from Ewing's sarcoma/primitive neuroectodermal tumor on strict histologic grounds. Helpful findings include the presence of neuropil and evidence of ganglion cell differentiation, both of which are not usually seen in Ewing's sarcoma/primitive neuroectodermal tumor. Immunohistochemically, neuroblastoma does not stain for MIC-2 and ultrastructurally the tumor cells have numerous neurosecretory granules. Lastly, neuroblastoma expresses different oncogenes, especially N-*myc* and does not have a 11;22 or 21;22 translocation. If matrix is present, Ewing's sarcoma/primitive neuroectodermal tumor is easily distinguished from small cell osteosarcoma and mesenchymal chondrosarcoma. In the absence of matrix, both small cell osteosarcoma and mesenchymal chondrosarcoma usually contain some cells that are spindled and a vascular tree, which frequently has a hemangiopericytoma-like pattern, findings that are usually not present in Ewing's sarcoma/primitive neuroectodermal tumor.

In 1983 Lipper and Kahn coined the term 'Ewing-like adamantinoma' for a morphologically unique destructive bone tumor that arose in the radial head of a 29-year-old man.[349] The neoplasm was composed of small, round, undifferentiated cells that exhibited some light-microscopic and ultrastructural features of epithelial cells. Three histologically similar tumors were reported in the pathology and radiology literature over the subsequent 16 years under the same name of Ewing-like adamantinoma.[350–352] Subsequently, Schofield et al. described 'an unusual round cell tumor of the tibia with granular cells' in a 10-year-old boy that had many morphologic, immunohistochemical, and ultrastructural features similar to the Ewing-like

adamantinoma.[353] Most recently a new name, 'insular and trabecular round cell sarcoma', was proposed for these tumors.[354] Exactly what these neoplasms are is unclear, however. It has not been definitively proved that they are actually related to Ewing's sarcoma or adamantinoma and, although similarities exist between them, there are compelling differences as well.

MELANOTIC NEUROECTODERMAL TUMOR OF INFANCY

Melanotic tumor of infancy was first described by Krompecher in 1918 in his report of a congenital melanoma (melanocarcinoma) that arose in the maxilla of a 2-month-old infant.[355] Since that time, a variety of terms have been used for this tumor, including melanotic ameloblastoma, pigmented ameloblastoma, melanoameloblastoma, melanotic progonoma, retinal anlage tumor, congenital melanocarcinoma, ameloblastic odontoma, and retinoblastic teratoma.[153] These terms reflect the uncertain histogenesis of this neoplasm, although it is considered to be of neural crest origin.[355,356] Molecular genetic studies have not shown any specific abnormality.[357]

Most melanotic tumors of infancy arise in the head and neck region, usually in the anterior portion of the maxilla, followed in frequency by the mandible. Other locations include the brain, intracranial dura,[358–361] and testes.[362] The vast majority of tumors are diagnosed during the first year of life, with rare cases being discovered in adulthood. The distribution among genders is approximately equal. Clinically, melanotic tumor of infancy presents as a rapidly growing, painless, pigmented mass. When arising in the maxilla, it may cause anterior protrusion of the upper lip and interfere with feeding.[358,360] Some tumors secret vanillylmandelic acid, with levels returning to normal after resection of the tumor.[355,356]

Radiographically, melanotic tumor of infancy produces an osteolytic lesion that displaces teeth and tooth buds.[360,363] Macroscopically, it has a tan-gray to black cut surface and is composed of two populations of cells that are embedded in a fibrous stroma. The larger, more epithelioid-appearing cells are arranged in pseudoglandular, glandular, or tubular structures. They have abundant eosinophilic cytoplasm and many contain dark brown melanin pigment. These epithelioid cells frequently surround solid nests of smaller cells that have scant cytoplasm, are similar in appearance to lymphocytes, and occasionally also contain cytoplasmic pigment (Fig. 14.101). Some cells have tapering eosinophilic cytoplasm suggestive of neuroblastic differentiation. Mitoses are rare. Ultrastructurally, nests of cells are surrounded by an external basal lamina. The larger cells contain abundant melanosomes in different stages of development, numerous mitochondria, and free ribosomes, and are joined to one another by numerous intercellular junctions. The smaller cells are more primitive: the nuclei are slightly irregular in size and shape and have clumped chromatin. The cytoplasm is notable for mitochondria and free ribosomes.

FNA smears obtained from examples from melanotic neuroectodermal tumor of infancy are cellular, with a dual population of cell types. The predominant cell type is a small uniform neuroblastic cell possessing a round nucleus and scanty or absent cytoplasm.[364–366] The nuclei of this small cell component may be fragile with chromatin smearing in FNA preparations. The second population of cells is composed of oval to cuboidal large cells with eccentrically placed nuclei and moderate amounts of cytoplasm. The cytoplasm contains granules of melanin pigment, which stain brown on Papanicolaou or bluish with Giemsa. The background may contain a small amount of free melanin pigment.

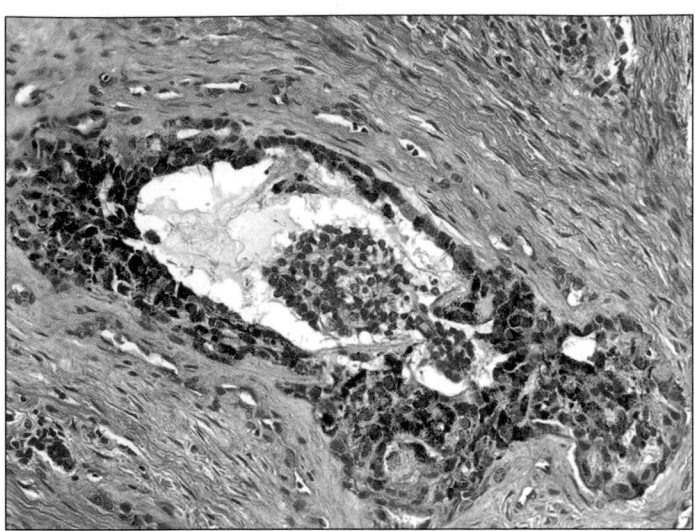

Fig. 14.101 Melanotic neuroectodermal tumor of infancy. The tumor nests are embedded in a fibrous stroma. Two populations of cells are seen– larger peripherally arranged cells with abundant intracytoplasmic melanin pigment and centrally located small round cells that lack melanin pigment.

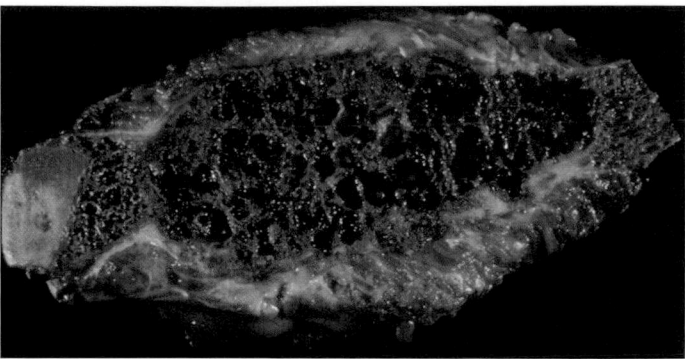

Fig. 14.102 Brown tumor of rib. The dark red tumor expands the bone and has a lobular growth pattern.

Immunohistochemically, the larger cells show epithelial and melanocytic differentiation and are positive for keratin and HMB-45. The small cells, however, have a different immunophenotype and express neuroendocrine markers.[363] Rare tumors stain for desmin, muscle actin, and glial fibrillary acidic protein, and both the small and large cells are usually negative for S-100 protein. Based on the morphology and antigen profile, melanotic tumor of infancy may represent a dysembryogenetic neoplasm that recapitulates the retina at 5 weeks gestation.[363]

The treatment of melanotic tumor of infancy is surgical removal of the tumor. The overall local recurrence rates range from 10–15%[358,359] and metastases occur in less than 5% of cases.[360] Histologically, it is not possible to predict which tumors will metastasize except for rare cases with features of neuroblastoma (malignant melanotic tumor of infancy).[355,367,368]

GIANT-CELL-RICH LESIONS

Giant-cell-rich lesions include reactive processes, such as brown tumor of hyperparathyroidism, and locally aggressive benign neoplasms including giant cell reparative granuloma and giant cell tumor. All these lesions are characterized by the presence of numerous multinucleate, osteoclast-type giant cells, but they can be distinguished from one another on the basis of their clinical findings and the morphology of the mononuclear stromal cells.

BROWN TUMOR OF HYPERPARATHYROIDISM

Brown tumors are masses of non-neoplastic reactive tissue and develop as a complication of hyperparathyroidism. The hemorrhage and hemosiderin deposits associated with the massive bone resorption and subsequent microfractures give the lesion its brown color, for which it has been named.

The association of brown tumor with parathyroid adenomas was first noted by Askanazy in 1904, and brown tumors have since been

documented in the setting of primary, secondary, and tertiary hyperparathyroidism. They usually develop in adults during the third and fourth decades of life, and females are affected more frequently than males. Brown tumors may be solitary or multiple and usually arise in the pelvis, ribs, clavicles, and extremities. Atypical locations include the sphenoid sinus,[369] vertebral column,[370] and cricoid cartilage.[371] Clinically, they may produce a mass, which can be painful.

Brown tumors manifest radiographically as expansile, lytic lesions with occasional intralesional trabeculations. The surrounding periosteum produces reactive bone and the margins of the tumor may be well defined or indistinct. Other radiographic characteristics of hyperparathyroidism are also often present, and include generalized osteoporosis, subperiosteal bone resorption of the distal phalanges, pelvis and clavicle, and diffuse granular radiolucencies in the skull. The radiographic differential diagnosis often includes metastatic disease and multiple myeloma.

Brown tumor is a well circumscribed, reddish brown, hemorrhagic mass that has a lobular architecture produced by fibrous septae that may contain reactive woven bone (Fig. 14.102). The lobules are composed of an admixture of plump fibroblasts, extravasated red blood cells, hemosiderin-laden macrophages, and scattered osteoclast-type giant cells that frequently cluster around areas of hemorrhage. This bloody mass of reactive tissue erodes the endosteum, resulting in thinning and expansion of the cortex as the periosteum deposits new bone (Fig. 14.103). In severe cases, large, blood-filled cysts develop and the resultant lesion is known as osteitis fibrosa cystica (von Recklinghausen's disease of bone). Areas of bone uninvolved by the tumor show evidence of increased osteoclastic activity in the form of dissecting osteitis (osteoclasts boring through the center of bony trabeculae), cortical cutting cones (groups of osteoclasts tunneling into and expanding haversian canals), and subperiosteal excavation.[372]

Smears prepared from needle aspirates of brown tumors associated with hyperparathyroidism have a hemorrhagic background and contain a prominent number of osteoclast-like giant cells. These cells have regular, ovoid, bland-appearing nuclei that vary in number from four to 20 per cell. A second population of mononuclear stromal cells with a spindled shape is present.[373,374] The nuclei of the stromal cells are slightly larger than those of the osteoclast-like giant cells and have a more open chromatin pattern. The background is bloody and many contain granular basophilic calcium debris.[373,374]

The prognosis of brown tumor is related to the underling cause of the lesion. With successful treatment of the hyperparathyroidism the osteoclastic activity abates, and the brown tumor eventually regresses and fills in with newly deposited bone.

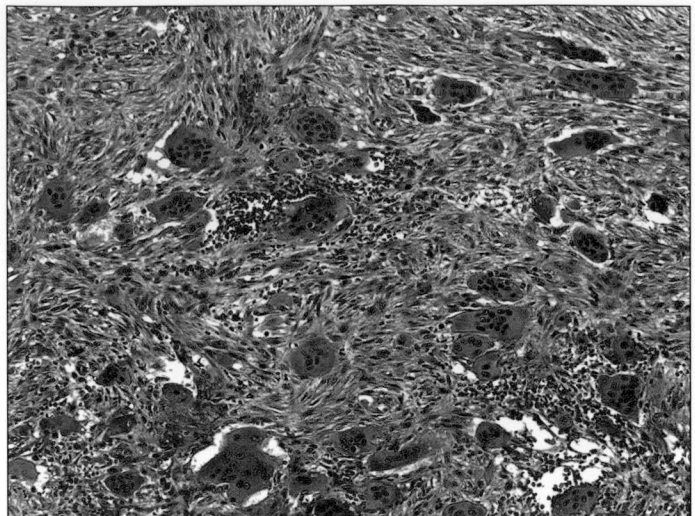

Fig. 14.103 Brown tumor. Microscopically, it is composed of mononuclear spindle shaped cells, scattered osteoclast type giant cells and stromal hemorrhage.

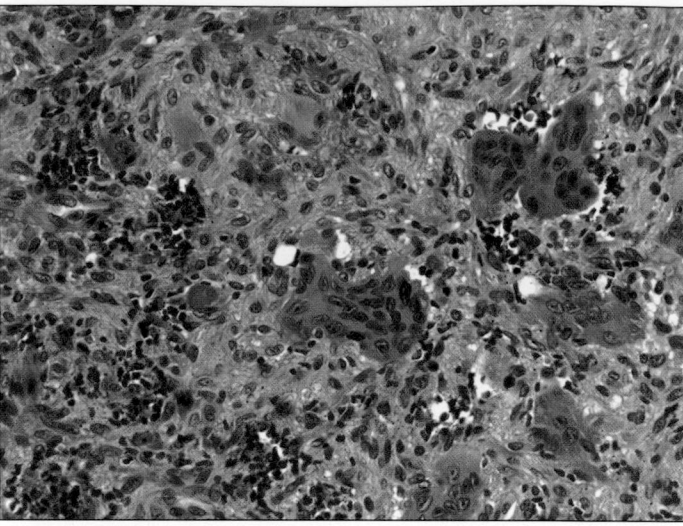

Fig. 14.104 Giant cell reparative granuloma has very similar histologic appearance to brown tumor, being composed of spindle shaped stromal cells, osteoclast type giant cells, and stromal hemorrhage.

The histologic differential diagnosis of brown tumor includes other giant-cell-rich lesions, particularly giant cell reparative granuloma and giant cell tumor of bone. Giant cell reparative granuloma can have very similar morphologic features and may be impossible to distinguish from brown tumor by light microscopy alone. One helpful feature we have noted is that brown tumors tend to have a much more lobular architectural growth pattern than giant cell reparative granuloma. In the diagnostic areas of giant cell tumor of bone, the mononuclear cells are not as spindled as the fibroblasts in brown tumor, and the nuclei of the mononuclear cells are morphologically identical to those in the osteoclasts, which is not a finding in brown tumor.

GIANT CELL REPARATIVE GRANULOMA

The term giant cell reparative granuloma was initially coined by Jaffe in 1953[375] to describe a tumor of the jaw bones that had previously been diagnosed as giant cell tumor of bone.[376] In 1962, Ackerman and Spjut described the first two cases involving the small tubular bones of the hand, for which they coined the term 'giant cell reaction.'[377] Subsequently, most reports have shown that giant cell reparative granuloma is generally limited to these two anatomic sites.

The majority of giant cell reparative granuloma that arise in the jaw bones occur in the first and second decades of life and are approximately twice as common in females as in males.[378,379] Clinically, patients complain of swelling, pain, or displacement of teeth. It is not uncommon for these lesions to be incidentally discovered on X-rays taken for other reasons. Patients with giant cell reparative granuloma involving the small tubular bones of the hand and feet are generally older, with a peak incidence in the second to third decades.[380] Signs and symptoms in this location are similar in that patients complain of pain and swelling, which is occasionally secondary to a pathologic fracture. Giant cell reparative granuloma rarely arises in other bones, and there have been isolated examples in which it has involved multiple sites.[381]

As the name implies, giant cell reparative granuloma is thought to be a non-neoplastic reparative or reactive process. The name is actually misleading, as the lesion does not contain true granulomas. Therefore, the noncommittal designation 'giant cell lesion' has been recommended by some authors.[376] The etiology of giant cell reparative granuloma is unknown and, though it has been hypothesized that the giant-cell-rich areas represent a reaction to recent hemorrhage and the fibroblastic component represents the older or the healing part of the lesion, a history of previous trauma is present in only a small percentage of cases.[379] Recently, cytogenetic abnormalities have been identified in a giant cell reparative granuloma, raising the possibility that this tumor may indeed be neoplastic.[382]

Within the head and neck region, giant cell reparative granuloma characteristically arises in the mandible and, less commonly, in the maxilla. It has a tendency to involve the anterior portions of these bones and usually does not extend posterior to the first permanent molar area. Giant cell reparative granuloma rarely affects other bones of the skull.[378,379] In the small bones of the hand and feet, giant cell reparative granuloma can involve the phalanges, metacarpals, and metatarsals as well as the carpal and tarsal bones.[380,383]

Giant cell reparative granuloma forms a well demarcated, radiolucent, often trabeculated or multiloculated ('soap bubble') lesion that may expand the bone.[375,384] The multiloculated appearance is more common in large tumors. Adjacent teeth are more frequently displaced than resorbed.[385] The cortex is usually intact, and there is no periosteal reaction.[47] In the small tubular bones of the hand and feet, giant cell reparative granuloma can involve the diaphysis, the metaphysis, the epiphysis, or the entire length of the bone, where it forms a radiolucent, expanding lesion with little or no cortical destruction.

The tumor is red-brown and hemorrhagic and consists of spindled fibroblasts and collagenous stroma with areas of hemorrhage and numerous multinucleate osteoclast-type giant cells (Fig. 14.104). The giant cells tend to be arranged in small clusters around areas of hemorrhage and usually contain 12 or fewer nuclei. Scattered lymphocytes, hemosiderin deposits, reactive woven bone rimmed by osteoblasts, and small blood-filled spaces (aneurysmal-bone-cyst-like areas) are frequently present.[379] Mitotic figures are usually few in number.

The treatment for giant cell reparative granuloma is curettage, after which the lesion usually heals and becomes ossified.[386,387] The tumor can recur locally but this is uncommon after a second curettage.[380,383,386,388] In surgically inaccessible lesions such as the skull base, partial removal of the lesion combined with radiation therapy may be indicated.[379,388]

The histologic differential diagnosis includes a variety of bone lesions that contain osteoclast-type giant cells. Morphologically, giant cell reparative granuloma is indistinguishable from brown tumor of hyperparathyroidism, and Jaffe in his original description believed that brown tumor of hyperparathyroidism 'also represents a giant-cell reparative granuloma.'[375] Accordingly, it is reasonable that a patient with giant cell reparative granuloma should have the appropriate tests performed to rule out hyperparathyroidism. The jaw lesion present in patients with Jaffe–Companacci syndrome (multiple non-ossifying fibromas, café-au-lait skin lesions, and other extra-skeletal anomalies) is also histologically similar to giant cell reparative granuloma,[389] and the possibility of Jaffe–Companacci syndrome should always be kept in mind in a patient with multiple giant cell reparative granulomas of the jaw.

Another important tumor in the differential diagnosis is conventional giant cell tumor of bone. Unlike giant cell reparative granuloma, the osteoclast-type giant cells in giant cell tumor of bone contain many more than 12 nuclei, and the nuclei in the giant cells are morphologically identical to those of the stromal cells. Another feature helpful in the distinction of these two tumors is the distribution of the giant cells. In giant cell reparative granuloma, the giant cells cluster around areas of hemorrhage, whereas they are evenly distributed in giant cell tumor of bone. The solid variant of aneurysmal bone cyst[390] is also histologically identical to giant cell reparative granuloma. It is possible that these lesions represent the same or similar entities.

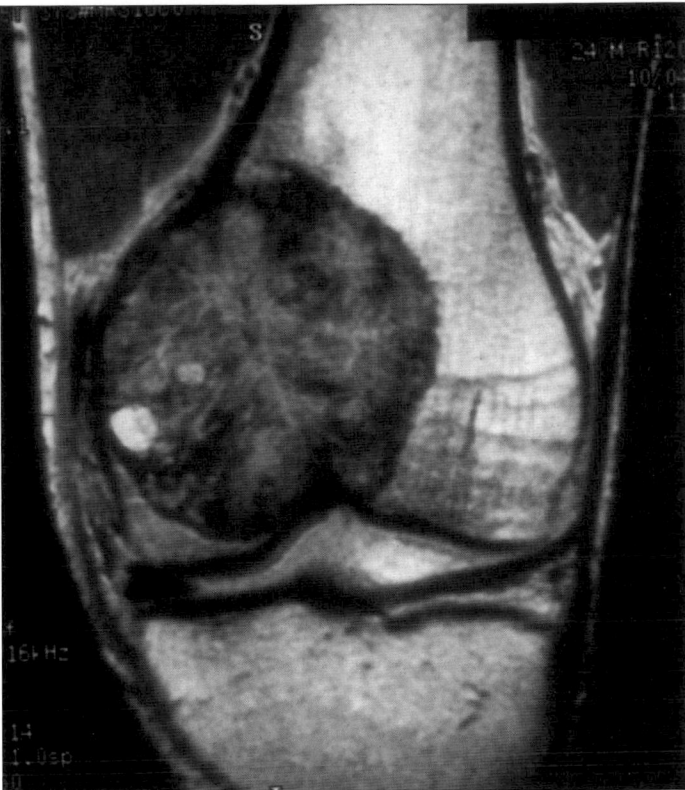

Fig. 14.105 MRI of a giant cell tumor of bone involving the distal femur. The tumor is eccentrically located, involves the distal portion of the bone, and extends to the subchondral area.

GIANT CELL TUMOR OF BONE

Giant cell tumor is the prototype of giant-cell-rich neoplasms of the skeleton. The name 'giant cell tumor' was coined by Bloodgood in 1912,[391] and in 1940 Jaffe distinguished the neoplasm from other osteoclast-rich tumors of bone.[392] Giant cell tumor accounts for approximately 4–5% of all primary bone tumors and, in the Mayo Clinic experience, represents almost 23% of benign skeletal neoplasms examined histologically.[4,393–395]

Giant cell tumor of bone is defined pathologically as a neoplasm composed of cytologically benign, oval or polyhedral mononuclear cells that are admixed with numerous, evenly distributed, osteoclast-like giant cells. The exact phenotype of the mononuclear cells is not clear and evidence suggests that they may be undifferentiated mesenchymal cells, fibroblasts, or macrophages. Cytogenetic studies have shown that telomeric associations are the most common chromosomal aberration found in these tumors.[396] The significance of this finding is unknown.

Giant cell tumor of bone usually develops during the third to fifth decades of life; it rarely occurs in children.[397] In many series, females are affected slightly more frequently than males (F:M = 1.2:1).[4] The vast majority of giant cell tumors of bone arise in the epiphyseal–metaphyseal region of long tubular bones, except in patients with open growth plates, in which the tumor is centered in the metaphysis and abuts the physeal plate.[4,393–395] Almost one half of cases develop in the vicinity of the knee, with a predilection for the distal femur followed by the proximal tibia. The third most common location is the distal end of the radius. Uncommon sites of involvement include the vertebral bodies, short tubular bones of the hands and feet, skull base, and patellae. Giant cell tumors are

usually solitary and, in the 1% of cases in which they are multifocal, they frequently affect the bones of the hands and feet.[398] Common presenting symptoms include pain and swelling; pathologic fracture occurs in a minority of cases.

Radiographically, giant cell tumor of bone manifests as an eccentric, large, lytic mass that frequently extends from the subchondral bone plate into the metaphysis; larger tumors may involve the adjacent diaphysis, focally destroy the cortex, and invade the neighboring soft tissues (Fig. 14.105).[4,393,399] The tumor often expands the bone and may elicit a periosteal reaction. Although the margins are well defined, they are usually not sclerotic and in some cases they may appear moth-eaten. Cystic degeneration is a common secondary finding.

Giant cell tumors are friable, hemorrhagic, red-brown masses that are solid or focally cystic and typically range in size from 5–15 cm (Fig. 14.106). They erode the cortex and have well delineated margins within the medullary canal and neighboring soft tissues. The histologic hallmark of giant cell tumors is the presence of innumerable multinucleate, osteoclast-like giant cells that are scattered evenly throughout the tumor (Fig. 14.107). The number of nuclei in any individual cell is variable but may be as many as 50 or more. The nuclei are ovoid and vesicular, have central nucleoli, and tend to be situated in the center of the cell where they are surrounded by abundant eosinophilic cytoplasm.

The mononuclear stromal cells are the diagnostic and neoplastic component of the tumor. These cells appear to grow in a syncytium and have ill-defined cell borders and little eosinophilic cytoplasm. The nuclei are round or ovoid and vesicular, have central nucleoli,

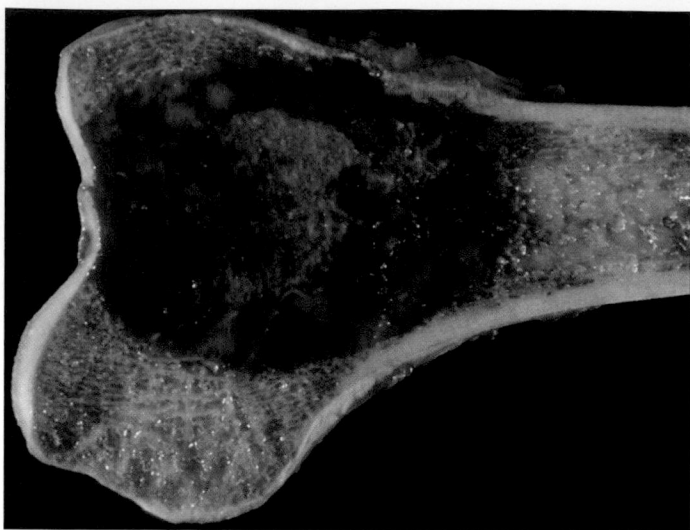

Fig. 14.106 Giant cell tumor of bone involving the distal femur. The tumor is well circumscribed. The central yellow area represents an area of necrosis.

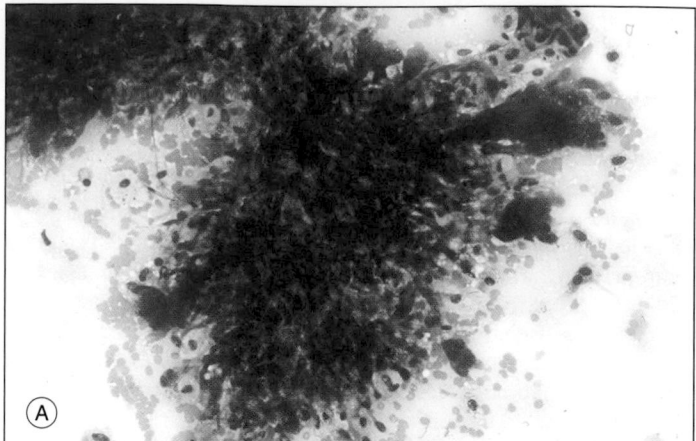

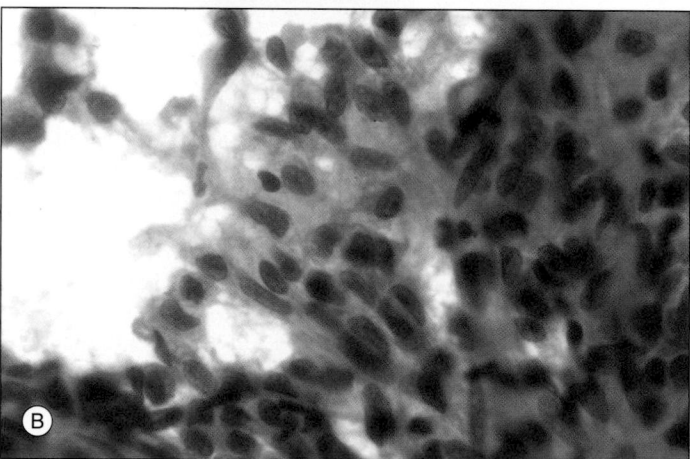

Fig. 14.108 Large tissue fragments obtained by FNA from a giant cell tumor of bone. **(A)** Note the checkerboard appearance in which multinucleate giant cells alternate with mononuclear cells **(B)**. The mononuclear cells are ovoid to spindle-shaped and possess small to moderate amounts of cytoplasm. (Romanowsky stain.) In contrast to chondroblastoma, the cells and nuclei of conventional giant cell tumors of bone demonstrate an elongated shape. (H&E stain.)

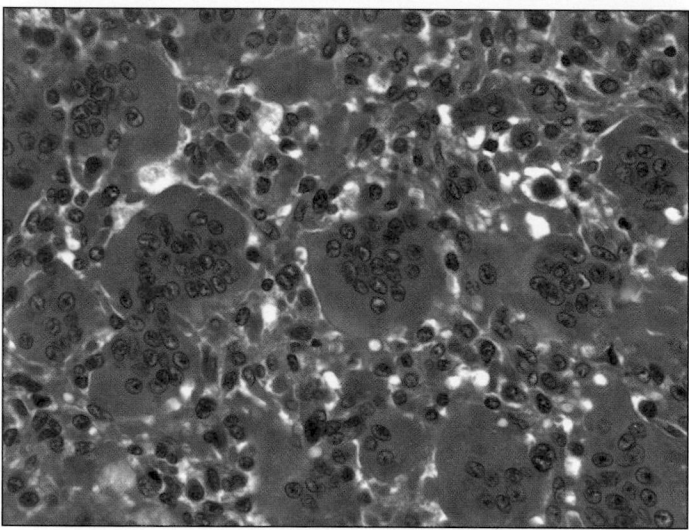

Fig. 14.107 Giant cell tumor of bone. Histologically it shows mononuclear cells and numerous osteoclast-type giant cells. The nuclei of the mononuclear cells are similar to the nuclei of the osteoclast-type giant cells.

and are morphologically identical to the nuclei of the giant cells. The mononuclear cells may be mitotically active and can show variable degrees of cytologic atypia, which may be prominent in areas admixed with previous hemorrhage and fibrin deposition. Foci of necrosis and vascular invasion are other common findings.

Most giant cell tumors also have areas that morphologically resemble benign fibrous histiocytoma or non-ossifying fibroma. These regions are characterized by cytologically banal spindle cells arranged in intersecting fascicles, forming a storiform pattern with scattered osteoclast-like giant cells. This spindle cell component is frequently located in the periphery of the tumor, and is not in itself

diagnostic of giant cell tumor. In the appropriate clinical setting, however, it is strongly suggestive of the diagnosis. Other secondary changes commonly encountered in giant cell tumor include hemosiderin deposits, aggregates of foamy macrophages, cystic change, and reactive bone formation.

Aspirate smears of conventional giant cell tumor of bone are cellular and contain a biphasic population of mononuclear ovoid to spindle stromal cells and multinucleate osteoclast-like giant cells (Fig. 14.108). These cells form clusters and small cohesive sheets often yielding a 'checkerboard' pattern.[400,401] Within the clusters, the mononuclear cells appear to attach to and surround the multinucleate giant cells, however, in the background they are often dispersed individually.

Ultrastructurally, abundant dilated rough endoplasmic reticulum, well developed Golgi apparatus, mitochondria, and occasional lipid droplets are prominent but non-specific features in the cytoplasm of the mononuclear cells.[402] The multinucleate giant cells have features similar to osteoclasts. Immunohistochemically, the mononuclear cells express vimentin and alpha-1-antitrypsin and do not stain with antibodies to S-100 protein.[403] The giant cells have an immunoprofile similar to macrophages. These findings have suggested that the mononuclear and multinucleate cells in giant cell tumor are of histiocytic derivation; however, this issue has not been resolved.

Biologically, giant cell tumors of bone are considered to be benign neoplasms. They are usually treated by curettage and less frequently by en bloc resection. Radiation is used to treat surgically inaccessible tumors or when medical problems preclude surgical intervention.[404] The local recurrence rate is approximately 25% for patients treated with curettage, and most recurrences are detected within 3 years following initial therapy.[405] Although giant cell tumors are classified as benign neoplasms, it is well recognized that 1–2% of them eventually metastasize, primarily to the lungs. The metastatic deposits, however, are frequently cured by resection. Another dreaded but uncommon complication is the development of a sarcoma within a giant cell tumor. This may occur de novo, develop in a local recurrence, or follow radiation of the tumor.

PRIMARY BONE CYSTS

Primary bone cysts are common and include several different clinicopathological entities that may be a manifestation of non-neoplastic and neoplastic processes. They should be distinguished from cysts that are a secondary phenomenon of various types of arthritis, and from bone tumors that undergo cystic degeneration. Most primary bone cysts are not true cysts, in that they lack an epithelial lining.

EPIDERMOID CYST

An epidermoid cyst forms when squamous epithelium becomes embedded in bone, proliferates, and forms a mass that expands the bone.[4,406] These lesions usually occur in the acral skeleton, the fingers and toes, followed by the skull. Many of them are thought to be traumatic and secondary to implantation of epidermis into the underlying bone. Most are solitary but infrequently they may be multiple. Radiographically, epidermoid cysts are lytic and well defined, with sclerotic margins. Grossly, they are filled with soft, cheesy material and are easily detached from the adjacent bone. The cyst wall is lined by benign squamous epithelium similarly to epithelial inclusion cysts of the skin, and similarly the lumen is filled with keratinous debris. Epidermoid cysts are benign, although squamous cell carcinomas have been reported to arise within them.[407]

INTRAOSSEOUS GANGLION

Intraosseous ganglion is a non-neoplastic, fibrous-walled cyst of uncertain etiology that develops in the subchondral regions of bone. By definition, the neighboring joint does not show significant osteoarthritis, which helps distinguish intraosseous ganglion from degenerative subchondral cysts.

Although first described by Hicks in 1956, the incidence of intraosseous ganglion is unknown because it is typically discovered as an incidental finding.[408,409] Patients are usually diagnosed during mid adulthood and males are affected more frequently than females in a ratio of approximately 1.2:1.[408,410,411] Various hypotheses that attempt to

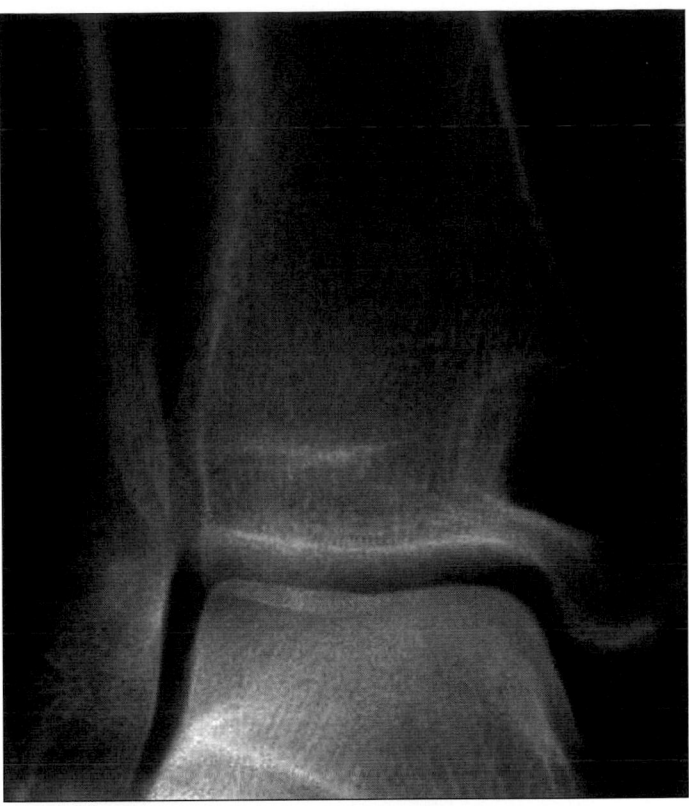

Fig. 14.109 Plain X-ray of an intraosseous ganglion shows a well defined and eccentric lytic lesion.

explain its development have been proposed, including myxomatous degeneration of adjacent inserting ligaments; however, none have been substantiated.[408,410–413] Intraosseous ganglion develops in the subchondral regions of bones of the hip, knee, ankle, wrist, and shoulder joints, but they have no connection to the joint cavity or synovial structures.[408–415] Most lesions are clinically silent but some may cause chronic pain that is exacerbated by physical activity.

X-rays of intraosseous ganglion reveal an eccentric, round, well defined radiolucency that has sclerotic margins (Fig. 14.109). Most are solitary but occasional cases may be multiple. The cysts are usually 0.5–1 cm in diameter. Lesions as large as 2–5 cm are uncommon. On MRI, the cysts have low signal intensity on T1-weighted images and high signal intensity on T2-weighted images. They are hot on bone scan.

Intact resection specimens reveal a thin-walled cyst filled with translucent gelatinous fluid sharply demarcated from the surrounding sclerotic rim of bone. Curettage specimens may consist of bloody strips of the cyst wall and globs of its mucinous contents. The cyst wall lacks a true cell lining and is composed of hypocellular fibrous tissue that contains abundant collagen. The inner portion of the cyst wall may be myxoid with scattered muciphages and the lumen is filled with amorphous basophilic remnants of the viscous fluid, which may be admixed with red blood cells and scattered inflammatory cells. The surrounding bone shows rebuttressing and remodeling of the trabecula and marrow fibrosis with myxoid change.

Asymptomatic intraosseous ganglion can be observed and does not require surgical intervention. Painful lesions are successfully treated with curettage and bone packing, which is associated with a low rate of recurrence.

Fig. 14.110
Unicameral bone
cyst of the proximal
humerus. The
lesion is well
circumscribed, has
a soap bubble
appearance, and
slightly expands
the bone.

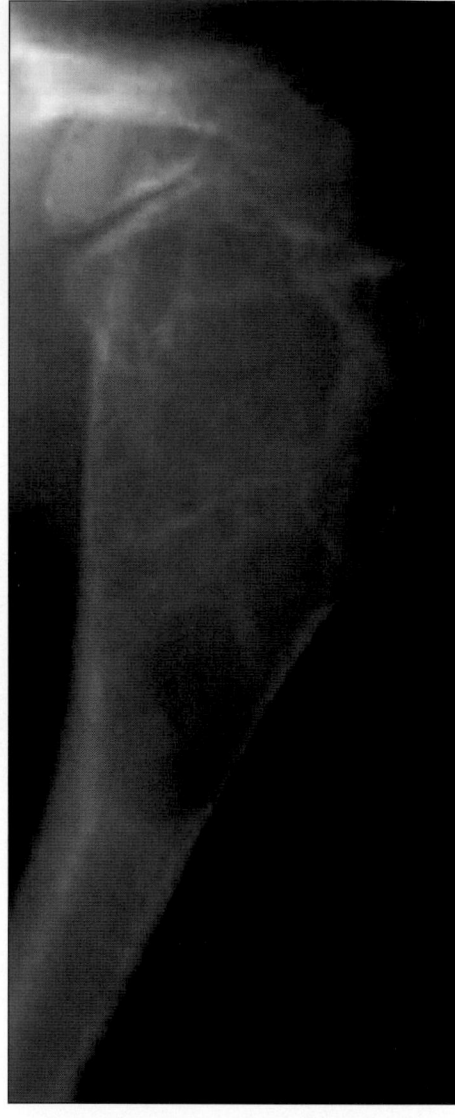

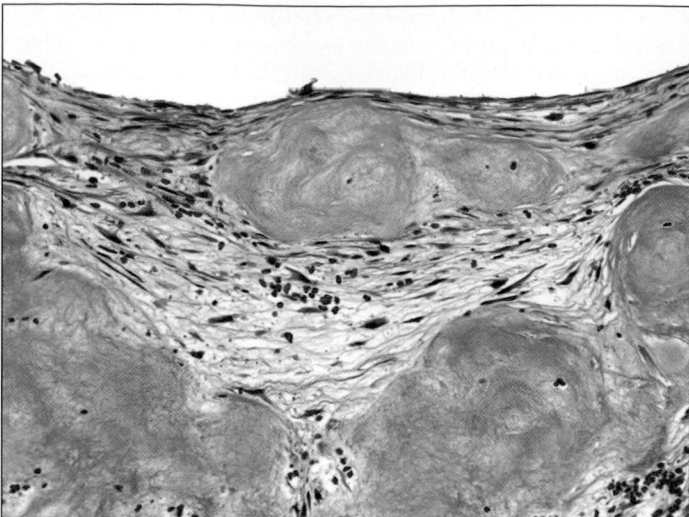

Fig. 14.111 Unicameral bone cyst. Fibrous cyst wall containing aggregates of fibrin mimicking cementum.

SIMPLE (UNICAMERAL) BONE CYST

Simple bone cyst (unicameral bone cyst) is a fluid filled cyst of unknown etiology. It usually arises in the appendicular skeleton, especially the proximal humerus, proximal femur, and proximal tibia, followed by the pelvis and calcaneus, and typically occurs in the first two decades of life. Some investigators have shown that the fluid has a biochemical composition similar to that of serum, suggesting that it forms from venous obstruction and subsequent extravasation of blood.[416,417]

Simple bone cyst is well demarcated and radiolucent, with occasional internal trabeculations (Fig. 14.110). The bone may be slightly expanded but is not greater than the width of the epiphyseal plate. The cyst usually begins in the metaphysis and extends into the diaphysis; epiphyseal involvement is rare.[418] Early lesions usually abut the growth plate; however, with skeletal growth they may become centered in the shaft. MRI is useful in confirming the fluid-filled nature of the cyst.[419] Some lesions contain a fractured piece of cortex that appears to float in the fluid, producing the fallen fragment sign.

The well delineated cyst is filled with straw-colored or bloodstained serous fluid, is lined by a thin, white wall, and minimally expands the bone. The cyst wall lacks a true cell lining and consists of a thin layer of

fibrous tissue, which is composed of scattered banal fibroblasts, collagen fibers, and in some cases deposits of fibrin, which can undergo mineralization and resemble cementum (Fig. 14.111). In the setting of a previous pathologic fracture, the cyst wall may be thickened and contain numerous reactive fibroblasts, osteoclast-type giant cells, hemosiderin deposits, and reactive woven bone.

Smears of aspirated material are markedly hypocellular and characterized by a proteinaceous granular background. In most reported cases, the aspirates have been nondiagnostic, the predominant cell type being either a lymphocyte or a histiocyte.[230,420,421]

Treatment options include resection, curettage, bone grafting, steroid injections, and percutaneous marrow grafting.[422,423] The local recurrence rate is 10–20%. The primary differential diagnosis includes aneurysmal bone cyst, which usually shows marked eccentric expansion of the affected bone and is generally hemorrhagic and multiloculated. The walls of an aneurysmal bone cyst are composed of plump fibroblasts, histiocytes, and osteoclast-type giant cells and generally appear more cellular than those of a simple bone cyst. Although 'cementum-like' material is characteristic of simple bone cyst, we have seen identical material in the wall of aneurysmal bone cysts.

ANEURYSMAL BONE CYST

Aneurysmal bone cyst is a benign tumor of bone that was first described by Jaffe and Lichtenstein in 1942.[424] It is a destructive, expansile lesion characterized by multiloculated, blood-filled cystic spaces. Despite its aggressive radiographic appearance, aneurysmal bone cyst behaves in a benign fashion. In fact, it is uncertain whether it is a true neoplasm or merely a reactive process, although the former hypothesis is supported by recent cytogenetic and molecular studies.[425–431]

Aneurysmal bone cyst affects all age groups but generally occurs during the first two decades of life and has no sex predilection.[427,428] It most frequently develops in the metaphyses of long bones and the posterior elements of vertebral bodies.[427] The most common signs and symptoms are pain and swelling or, rarely, pain secondary to a

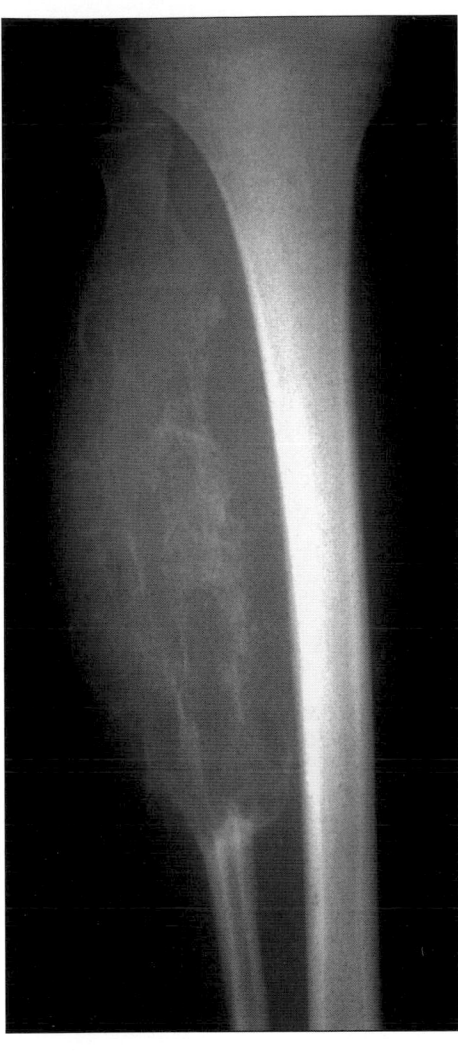

Fig. 14.112 Aneurysmal bone cyst. Plain X-ray showing an expansile lesion with internal trabeculations involving the proximal fibula.

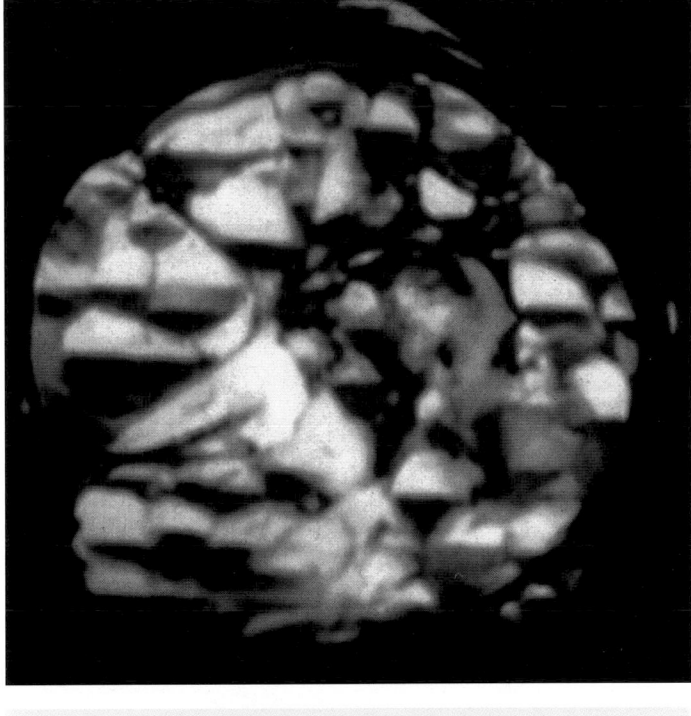

Fig. 14.113 An MRI of a large aneurysmal bone cyst of the distal femur showing prominent fluid–fluid levels.

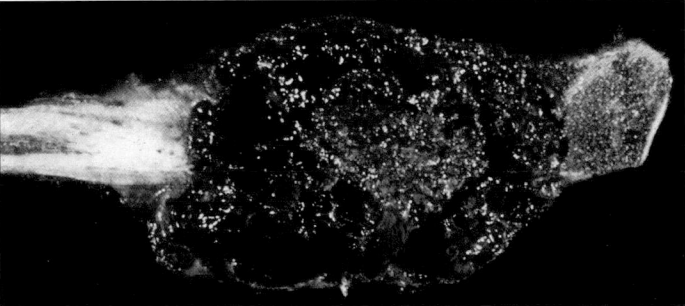

Fig. 14.114 Aneurysmal bone cyst involving the proximal fibula (same as Fig. 14.112). The tumor is hemorrhagic and cystic in appearance.

pathologic fracture. When an aneurysmal bone cyst involves the vertebrae, it can compress nerves and cause neurologic symptoms.

Aneurysmal bone cyst may arise de novo (primary aneurysmal bone cyst), or areas resembling aneurysmal bone cyst can be found in other benign and malignant bone tumors (secondary aneurysmal bone cyst) that have undergone secondary cystic change.[429] Primary aneurysmal bone cysts account for approximately 70% of cases. The majority of secondary aneurysmal bone cysts arise in association with giant cell tumor of bone, chondroblastoma, osteoblastoma, fibrous dysplasia, and osteosarcoma.[425,427,428] It is important to recognize the underlying benign or malignant condition associated with secondary aneurysmal bone cyst as it determines the behavior and treatment of the tumor.

Radiographically, aneurysmal bone cyst is usually an eccentric, expansile lesion with well defined margins (Fig. 14.112). Most lesions are completely lytic and often contain a thin shell of reactive bone at the periphery.[425,427,428] CT and MRI may demonstrate internal septa and characteristic fluid-fluid levels (Fig. 14.113).[425,427]

Grossly, aneurysmal bone cyst consists of multiple, blood-filled cystic spaces separated by thin, tan-white septa (Fig. 14.114). More solid tan-white areas can also be seen, and they may either represent a solid portion of the aneurysmal bone cyst or a primary lesion that has developed secondary aneurysmal-bone-cyst-like change. Therefore, any solid area within an aneurysmal bone cyst

should be thoroughly sampled to identify the presence of a possible underlying primary lesion.

Histologically, the walls of aneurysmal bone cyst are composed of plump uniform fibroblasts (which may be mitotically active), multinucleate osteoclast-like giant cells, and reactive woven bone (Fig. 14.115). The reactive woven bone is lined by osteoblasts and its deposition typically follows the contours of the fibrous septa (Fig. 14.116). Approximately one-third of cases contain a cartilage-like matrix called 'blue bone', which is infrequently seen in other bone lesions (Fig. 14.117).[389,427] Necrosis is uncommon unless there has been a previous pathologic fracture.

In 1983, Sanerkin and colleagues[390] described an unusual noncystic intraosseous lesion that had the morphologic features found in the more solid areas of aneurysmal bone cyst. They termed this tumor the 'solid' variant of aneurysmal bone cyst. Their four patients were 5–13 years old; three tumors arose in the spine and one

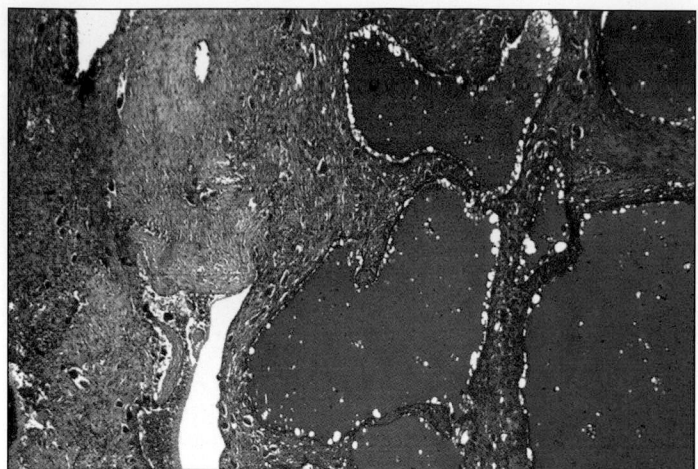

Fig. 14.115 Aneurysmal bone cyst. Low power shows blood-filled cystic spaces surrounded by cellular septae.

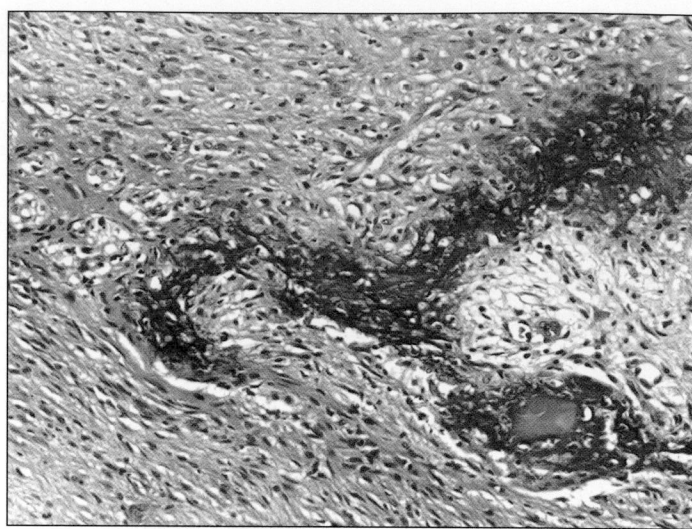

Fig. 14.117 Aneurysmal bone cyst showing the characteristic 'blue' bone.

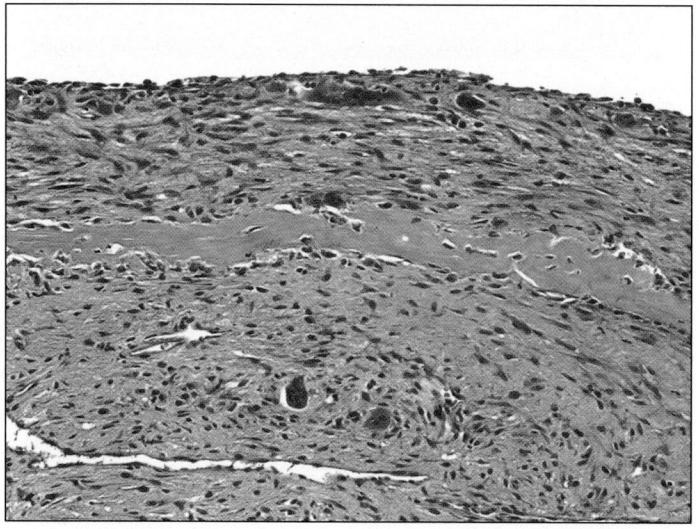

Fig. 14.116 Aneurysmal bone cyst. The wall shows spindle-shaped cells, osteoclast-type giant cells, and reactive bone formation that follows the contours of the lumen.

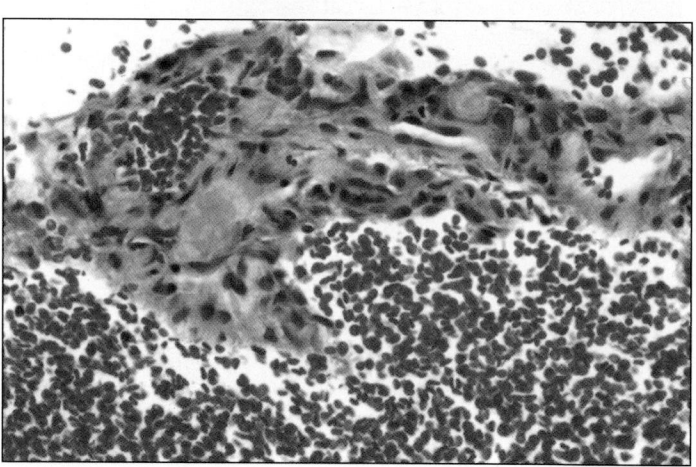

Fig. 14.118 Tissue fragment composed of spindle cells and osteoid lying within a bloody background. The tissue fragments such as the one illustrated may be obtained from aneurysmal bone cysts following vigorous aspiration. The background contains numerous red blood cells. (H&E stain.)

in the ethmoid bone. Histologically, the solid variant of aneurysmal bone cyst is very similar, if not identical, to giant cell reparative granuloma and it is unclear whether or not these two lesions represent the same entity.

FNA specimens obtained from aneurysmal bone cysts are composed predominantly of red blood cells, among which rare bipolar spindle cells with wispy cytoplasm and multinucleate, osteoclast-like giant cells are scattered (Fig. 14.118).[23,255] Rarely, small fragments of septal wall will be obtained, and they are composed of bland, spindle-shaped cells with small streamers of dense collagen or osteoid.[23]

The treatment of aneurysmal bone cyst is surgical, usually in the form of curettage or, in certain situations, en bloc resection. The recurrence rate is low and spontaneous regression may occur following incomplete removal. Rare reports of apparent malignant transformation of aneurysmal bone cyst have been described, however

it is unclear whether they represent malignant transformation or aneurysmal-bone-cyst-like change in a pre-existing sarcoma.[432]

The differential diagnosis of aneurysmal bone cyst includes giant cell reparative granuloma, telangiectatic osteosarcoma, and all entities that may contain secondary cystic changes. Although telangiectatic osteosarcoma can grossly simulate aneurysmal bone cyst, the fibrous septa in telangiectatic osteosarcoma contain overtly malignant neoplastic cells with marked pleomorphism and easily identifiable mitotic figures.

TUMORS OF THE HEMATOPOIETIC SYSTEM

Tumors of the hematopoietic system commonly present as lesions in the skeleton. The bone involvement may be the primary and only site of disease or may be a component of more widespread multi-organ dissemination. Both benign and malignant neoplasms of the hematopoietic system affect bone and each have their own unique biology and recommended forms of treatment.

SINUS HISTIOCYTOSIS WITH MASSIVE LYMPHADENOPATHY

Sinus histiocytosis with massive lymphadenopathy, also known as Rosai–Dorfman disease, was first recognized by Rosai and Dorfman in 1969 in their description of four cases involving lymph nodes that had previously been diagnosed as 'malignant reticuloendotheliosis.'[433] Subsequently, it became clear that sinus histiocytosis with massive lymphadenopathy was not limited to lymph nodes and could be seen, albeit infrequently, in virtually every organ of the body, the most common extranodal sites being the skin, upper respiratory tract, and bone.[434–436] Patients with bone involvement usually also have extraskeletal disease and the individual bone lesions usually cause localized pain and tenderness.

Radiographically, the bone lesions are lucent and have well circumscribed sclerotic margins but there may be destruction of the cortex associated with a periosteal reaction. The tumors may be solitary or multifocal and affect both the axial and appendicular skeleton. Regardless of their location, the lesions exhibit classic morphologic features and are composed of numerous large histiocytes that have abundant eosinophilic cytoplasm containing phagocytosed lymphocytes (emperipolesis). The histiocytes' nuclei have finely stippled chromatin, small nucleoli, and smooth contours that lack folds and clefts. Accompanying the histiocytes is a mixed inflammatory infiltrate that is usually rich in lymphocytes. Immunohistochemically, the histiocytes stain positively for S-100 protein and are negative for CD1a.

The natural history of the disease depends upon the extent of nodal and extranodal disease. In most cases, the clinical course is relatively benign and indolent; however, involvement of the kidneys, liver, and lungs may portend more aggressive behavior. Lesions of the skeleton have been adequately treated with curettage.

Sinus histiocytosis with massive lymphadenopathy should be considered in the histologic differential diagnosis of a mixed inflammatory process and should be distinguished from lesions such as lymphoma, Langerhans cell histiocytosis, osteomyelitis, and storage diseases. Sinus histiocytosis with massive lymphadenopathy is discussed in more detail in Chapter 11.

LANGERHANS CELL HISTIOCYTOSIS (EOSINOPHILIC GRANULOMA) OF BONE

Langerhans cell histiocytosis of bone, previously known as histiocytosis X, is defined as an intraosseous mass of proliferating Langerhans cells. Langerhans cells are dendritic cells and normally populate the skin, mucosal surfaces, lymph nodes, and other tissues where they function as specialized antigen-presenting cells. In Langerhans cell histiocytosis, the proliferating cells are monoclonal, supporting the theory that the disease is neoplastic.[437]

Langerhans cell histiocytosis is associated with a variety of clinical syndromes that vary according to the number, site, and size of the tumors. Traditionally, single or multiple lesions restricted to the skeleton have been termed 'eosinophilic granuloma.' Multifocal bone disease associated with exophthalmos and diabetes insipidus is known as Hand–Schüller–Christian disease, and Letterer–Siwe

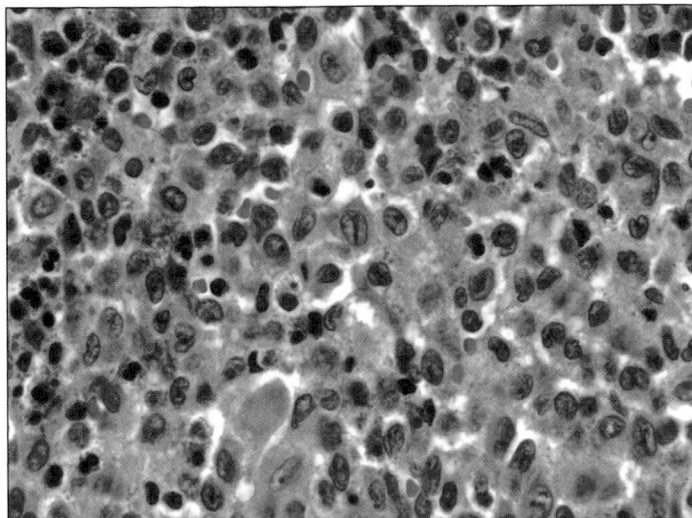

Fig. 14.119 Eosinophilic granuloma. Aggregates of Langerhans cells admixed with eosinophils. The Langerhans cells have cleaved nuclei and a moderate amount of eosinophilic cytoplasm.

disease is an aggressive disseminated form of the disorder that occurs in infants.[438–441]

Langerhans cell histiocytosis is usually diagnosed during the first three decades of life and males are affected approximately twice as frequently as females.[438–440] The disease usually manifests in the skeleton; other common sites of involvement include the skin, lung, and lymph nodes.[438–440] In general, solitary bone lesions are encountered twice as often as multiple bone lesions. The tumors can develop in any bone but most commonly originate in the skull and jaw, followed by vertebral bodies, ribs, pelvis, and long bones. Ordinarily, the lesions cause localized pain; however, in some instances they may produce a pathologic fracture.[438–440]

The lesions are well defined and lytic on radiographs; however, in a minority of cases, they have ill defined and permeative margins.[438–440] Cortical involvement may elicit a periosteal reaction.[438–440] Complete resolution of radiographic abnormalities may follow treatment or occasionally occurs spontaneously.

The lesional tissue has a non-specific, gritty, tan appearance. The proliferating Langerhans cells are ovoid or round, histiocyte-like cells 10.0–15.0 μm in diameter that are arranged in aggregates, sheets, or individually within a loose fibrous stroma. The cells have eosinophilic cytoplasm and contain central, ovoid 'coffee-bean'-shaped nuclei that have pale chromatin and inconspicuous nucleoli. The 'coffee bean' appearance is produced by deep indentations, clefts, and folds of the nuclear membranes, which form linear grooves that traverse the length of the nuclei (Fig. 14.119). Most of the Langerhans cells are mononuclear but some cells contain multiple nuclei, which tend to be centrally located. Mitotic figures are commonplace; however, atypical forms are absent. One of the morphologic hallmarks of Langerhans cell histiocytosis is an accompanying infiltrate of eosinophils, which may be so dense that the underlying Langerhans cells are obscured. The eosinophils are distributed evenly or arranged in clusters, producing eosinophilic abscesses. Other types of inflammatory cells, including lymphocytes, plasma cells, macrophages, neutrophils, and osteoclast-type giant cells, are also frequently present.[440] Necrosis may be a finding in a minority of cases and, if prominent, is usually a complication of a pathologic fracture.

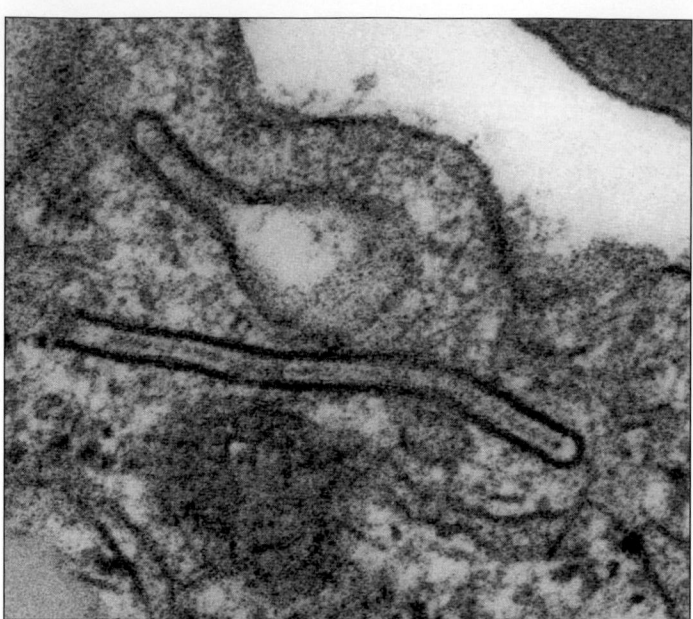

Fig. 14.120 Ultrastructurally, the Birbeck granules have a pentilaminar appearance and bulbous ends mimicking 'tennis rackets.'

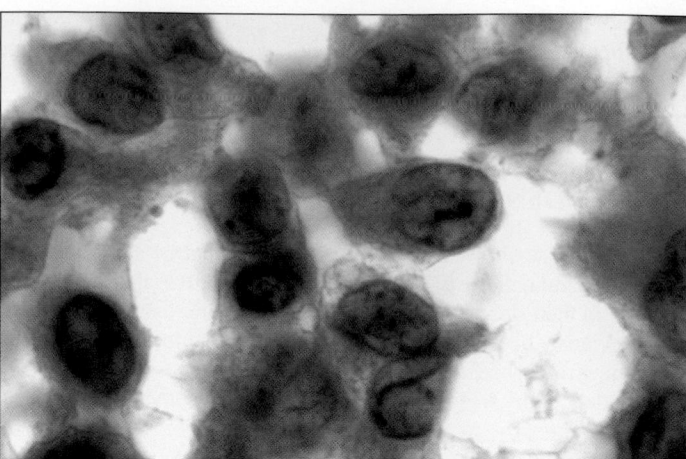

Fig. 14.121 Cytology of eosinophilic granuloma showing prominent nuclear irregularities and grooving of the neoplastic cells. (H&E stain.)

The diagnosis of Langerhans cell histiocytosis is principally based upon the light-microscopic appearance of the Langerhans cells and the appropriate mixed cellular background; however, adjuvant diagnostic techniques, including electron microscopy and immunohistochemistry, help to confirm their presence.[438,442] Langerhans cells strongly express CD1a and S-100 protein. Ultrastructurally, they contain tubular, pentilaminar, membrane-bound cytoplasmic bodies with central, electron-dense, granular material. These structures, known as Birbeck granules, frequently have terminal oval protrusions, producing an appearance that has been likened to a tennis racket or lollipop (Fig. 14.120).[438,442] They are thought to arise from an invagination and fusion of the plasma membranes and are a unique marker of Langerhans cells.[438]

Fine-needle aspirates of eosinophilic granuloma (Langerhans cell histiocytosis) are associated with smears of moderate to high cellularity. In most cases, round to ovoid histiocytes containing large pale nuclei dominate the smears. The nuclei of the histiocytes are frequently kidney-shaped and display a distinct irregular or folded nuclear outline (Fig. 14.121). The chromatin pattern is bland, and nucleoli are usually small and multiple. The cytoplasm of the histocytic cells is often vacuolated or foamy and may contain phagocytosed debris. Occasional multinucleate giant cells of similar nuclear morphology are seen in most smears. A modest number of eosinophils is commonly present but in some smears they are quite sparse.[443,444] Immunohistochemical analysis of cell block material for the expression of S-100 and CD1a can be performed to confirm the diagnosis.

The treatment and prognosis of Langerhans cell histiocytosis depends on the site and size of the lesion, the age of the patient, and the presence or absence of multifocal disease. In general, monostotic disease is usually managed by curettage but tumors located in difficult sites may be treated with low-dose radiation therapy.[438–440] Single- or multiagent chemotherapy may be administered in the setting of disseminated and fulminant disease. Patients with monostotic skeletal involvement have an excellent prognosis and usually remain disease-free after adequate therapy.[439]

The differential diagnosis of Langerhans cell histiocytosis includes osteomyelitis and malignant lymphoma. Acute osteomyelitis typically has a prominent neutrophilic and fibrinous exudate in addition to bone necrosis. Chronic osteomyelitis exhibits a mixed inflammatory infiltrate that may contain histiocytes; however, the histiocytes lack the characteristics of Langerhans cells and usually only a few scattered eosinophils are present. Primary skeletal lymphoma or secondary bone involvement by generalized disease typically occurs with non-Hodgkin's, diffuse, large B cell lymphoma. The neoplastic cells in these tumors manifest a greater degree of nuclear atypia and mitotic activity than is seen in Langerhans cell histiocytosis, and both tumors have a distinguishing immunoprofile. Other skeletal diseases that may contain numerous eosinophils include fungal and parasitic infections, foreign body giant cell reactions, and Hodgkin's disease.

PRIMARY NON-HODGKIN'S LYMPHOMA OF BONE

Primary lymphoma of bone is defined as lymphoma originating in bone with no evidence of extraskeletal disease or disseminated marrow involvement developing during a minimum of 6 months following diagnosis. It is rare, accounting for approximately 5% of primary malignant bone tumors and about 5% of all extranodal lymphomas. More commonly, lymphoma involves the skeleton as a manifestation of widespread disease, in which it may take the form of isolated destructive lesions or diffuse marrow infiltration.

Patients with primary lymphoma of bone are usually adults and approximately 50% are older than 40 years. An important minority, however, arise in older children and adolescents. There is a slight male predominance: the gender ratio ranges from 1.2–1.6:1 in larger reported series. The tumor frequently develops in the axial skeleton (pelvis 20%, vertebrae 10%) and the metadiaphyseal region of long bones (femur 20%, humerus 10%). In approximately 10–40% of cases the lymphoma is multifocal, where it manifests as several lesions either in one bone or multiple bones concurrently. Common symptoms include pain localized to the site of disease, as well as erythema, swelling, and tenderness. Tumors of the axial skeleton may cause complaints related to nerve impingement.

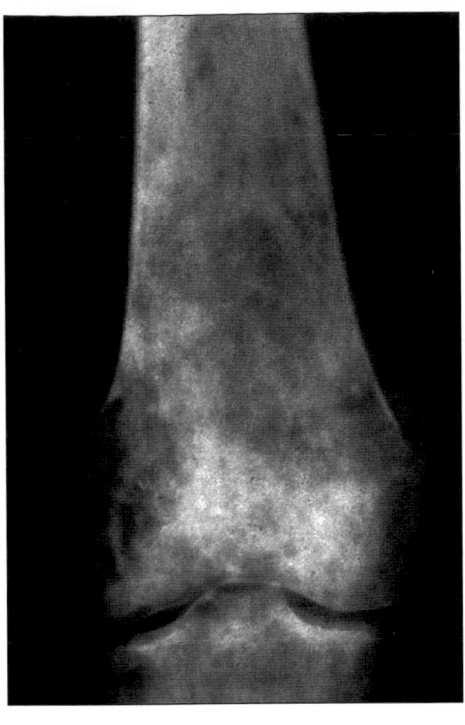

Fig. 14.122 Plain X-ray of lymphoma of bone showing a permeative mixed lytic and sclerotic tumor.

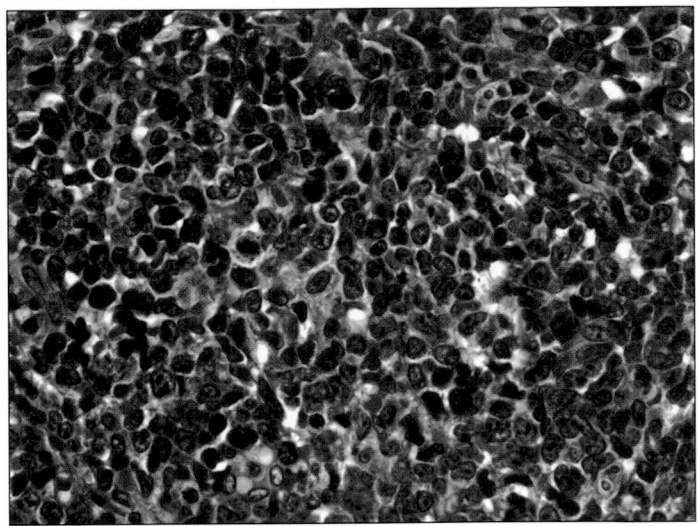

Fig. 14.123 Large cell lymphoma of bone. The neoplastic cells have large irregular cleaved nuclei, prominent nucleoli, and little eosinophilic cytoplasm. Note numerous mitotic figures.

Malignant lymphoma of bone usually produces a large, destructive, lytic mass that erodes the cortex and forms a soft tissue component (Fig. 14.122). The margins are 'moth-eaten' or permeative, and an onion skin periosteal reaction may be present. In a minority of cases, the tumor may elicit sclerosis and present as a blastic mass. CT and MRI provide important information regarding the extent of bone and soft tissue involvement. In some instances, the plain X-ray is normal, with abnormalities only recognized on bone scan, CT, or MRI.[445]

The vast majority of primary bone lymphomas are centered in the medullary cavity, and only rare cases develop beneath the periosteum.[446] The tumors destroy the cortex, extend into the neighboring soft tissue, are moderately firm, gray-white, and fleshy, and frequently have areas of necrosis. Histologically, they exhibit the same features as nodal lymphomas and are classified accordingly. Because of extensive necrosis or crush artifact that may be present, several biopsies may be required before a definitive diagnosis can be reached. The most common primary lymphoma of bone is diffuse large B-cell lymphoma (Fig. 14.123). Immunohistochemically, the tumor cells express LCA and B-cell markers. In children, lymphoblastic lymphoma may also be encountered. It is important to note that lymphoblastic lymphoma may not express LCA. Therefore, a panel of other lymphoid markers needs to be performed to confirm the diagnosis.

Aspirates of malignant lymphomas yield highly cellular smears with characteristic round cell morphology. Cytomorphologic analysis is best undertaken using Romanowsky-stained smears. The cell populations are relatively monomorphous but may be biphasic in mixed lymphomas.[447,448] The precise cytomorphology depends on the subtype of lymphoma (see Chapter 11). The presence of a significant number of lymphoglandular bodies in the background is a helpful clue to the lymphoid nature of the process.

In the past, primary large cell lymphoma of bone was treated solely with radiation. Recent studies, however, have shown a better outcome when treatment includes both radiation and chemotherapy.[449–452] Current disease-free survival rates for 10 years approach 75% and in some studies better results have been achieved. The fact that some treatment centers have not shown a statistically improved outcome for patients with primary lymphoma versus patients with systemic disease suggests that many patients with primary lymphoma of bone may have undetectable systemic disease at the time of initial diagnosis.[453] Also, there is evidence that suggests that primary bone lymphomas that have a germinal-center-like immunophenotype may have a better prognosis than those that have a different immunophenotype.[454]

The differential diagnosis of lymphoma of bone includes a spectrum of other round cell lesions such as osteomyelitis, Langerhans cell histiocytosis, Ewing's sarcoma/primitive neuroectodermal tumor, and metastatic small cell carcinoma, neuroblastoma, rhabdomyosarcoma, and other round cell malignancies. Immunohistochemistry, electron microscopy, and cytogenetic analysis may be necessary to distinguish among these possibilities.

HODGKIN'S LYMPHOMA OF BONE

Primary Hodgkin's disease of bone is extremely rare and very few cases have been reported.[455] It is much more common for the tumor to involve the skeleton as a manifestation of widespread disease.[456] The axial skeleton and proximal long bones tend to be affected, and patients present complaining of pain centered over the site of involvement. The tumor has aggressive features radiographically and may produce a blastic, lytic, or mixed lytic and blastic destructive mass. The diagnosis is based on the presence of the classic morphologic features of Hodgkin's lymphoma, including Reed–Sternberg cells that express CD15 and CD30 and are negative for other B- and T-cell antigens. In many instances, the tumor exhibits the features of the nodular sclerosing or mixed cellularity variants. The prognosis may be good with aggressive forms of treatment.

PLASMA CELL MYELOMA

Myeloma is a malignant monoclonal proliferation of plasma cells and is the most common primary malignant tumor of bone. Like lymphoma, it may present as a localized lesion (myeloma) or as a component of widespread disease (multiple myeloma). Patients are usually over 40 years of age at the time of diagnosis and males are affected more frequently than females.[4] Myeloma may involve any bone in the body but the most common sites are the vertebrae, ribs, skull, pelvis, and long bones. Patients typically present with pain, which may be associated with a pathologic fracture.

Myeloma can produce generalized osteoporosis as well as localized destructive, lytic lesions, for example in the skull, where they are well circumscribed and have a punched out appearance. The osteolysis is caused by activation of the RANK receptor–ligand system by the neoplastic plasma cells, which results in increased production and activity of osteoclasts.[457] Rarely, myeloma generates sclerotic lesions. This may occur in the setting of POEMS syndrome.[458]

Grossly, myeloma appears as a soft, friable, red mass and the underlying bone is eroded and fragile. In most cases, sheets of mature-appearing plasma cells replace the marrow, but in some cases the tumor cells are poorly differentiated and the neoplastic cells may mimic other poorly differentiated tumors such as metastatic carcinoma or high-grade lymphoma. This may sometimes be problematic on frozen sections but the diagnosis can usually be readily made on touch preps. The immunohistochemical profile and laboratory data are discussed in Chapter 12.

FNA smears obtained from the lytic lesions of solitary plasmacytoma and multiple myeloma are cytologically identical. The smears are highly cellular and are composed of round or ovoid cells with eccentric nuclei.[459] Examples of plasma cell dyscrasias reveal various degrees of differentiation. In well differentiated lesions, the plasma cells deviate little from their normal morphology and possess round nuclei with a 'spoked wheel' chromatin pattern. The nuclei are eccentric and are associated with moderate amounts of cytoplasm (Fig. 14.124). In more poorly-differentiated lesions, significant degrees of atypia are seen in which the nuclei are enlarged, hyperchromatic, and possess an irregular chromatin pattern. The plasmacytoid appearance is less well defined, and binucleate and multinucleate cells may be seen. The atypia of the plasma cell population appears to have prognostic significance.[460]

Although initially, patients can present with a single lesion and no evidence of disease elsewhere, most patients will eventually develop multiple myeloma. Localized disease is treated with resection or radiation. More disseminated disease is incurable but treatment with a combination of chemotherapy and radiation therapy may prolong survival.[461] Bone marrow transplantation is also an option for younger patients.[462]

LEUKEMIA

Leukemia diffusely affects the bone marrow and can cause a variety of skeletal manifestations, which taken together can be helpful in recognizing the disease before a tissue diagnosis is rendered (Table 14.10).[463–465] Skeletal lesions are most frequent in acute childhood leukemia but may also be a component of adult disease. In a very small number of cases, the leukemia is localized and presents as granulocytic sarcoma, which may produce a solitary, large, destructive mass.[466] Many of the bony changes seen in leukemia are associated with infiltration of the marrow, cortex, and subperiosteal space by leukemic cells, which cause secondary osteoclastic and osteoblastic reactions. Some radiographic changes, however, such as metaphyseal radiolucent and radiodense bands, are a secondary metabolic phenomenon.

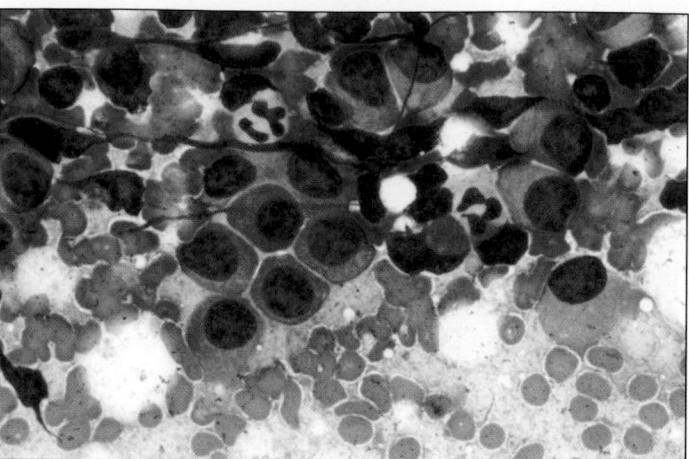

Fig. 14.124 The cells of myeloma often have a spoked or cartwheel appearance to the chromatin. The nuclei may be centrally located but are more often placed eccentrically within the cytoplasm. (Romanowsky stain.)

Table 14.10 Radiological manifestations of leukemic involvement of the skeleton

Diffuse osteopenia
Radiolucent and radiodense metaphyseal bands
Single or multiple localized lytic lesions
Periostitis
Osteosclerosis

MASTOCYTOSIS

Systemic mastocytosis is a very uncommon disorder and skeletal changes occur in approximately 80% of patients. The bone abnormalities may be the primary manifestation of the disease and may be important in making the initial diagnosis. In many instances, however, they are accompanied by characteristic skin lesions.[47] Systemic mastocytosis usually develops in adults, with both genders equally affected. The disease has a propensity for involving the bones of the trunk and proximal extremities. Patients typically present with symptoms caused by the release of chemical mediators by the proliferating mast cells. This includes edema, flushing, hypotension, tachycardia, and dyspnea. Urticaria pigmentosa is commonly seen in patients who also have cutaneous involvement.

Systemic mastocytosis may produce diffuse osteosclerosis, diffuse osteopenia, or more localized mixed sclerotic and lytic lesions.[467–469] Histamine, a substance produced in abundance by mast cells, is known to stimulate bone formation, while molecules such as prostaglandins and heparin, also secreted by mast cells, are known stimulators of osteoclastic bone resorption. The diagnostic findings of bone disease in mastocytosis are increased number of mast cells, which have a paratrabecular arrangement and are associated with fibrosis and eosinophils. The mast cells may appear normal morphologically; however, they may also be spindle-shaped and contain fewer cytoplasmic granules. The granules can be highlighted by a Giemsa stain and have characteristic features ultrastructurally; immunohistochemistry can be helpful in rendering a diagnosis in that mast cells strongly express CD117 (c-Kit).

Systemic mastocytosis usually has a long, relatively benign clinical course. Patients with the leukemic form of the disease, however, may survive for only 1–2 years. In addition, a minority of patients may die of secondary complications such as severe gastrointestinal hemorrhage. Treatment of indolent disease is based on symptom control. Chemotherapy has not been shown to be effective in any form of the disease.

CHORDOMA

Chordoma is a slow growing malignant neoplasm that has a notochordal phenotype and is thought to arise from notochordal remnants.[470–479] It accounts for 5% of primary bone tumors, and its age-adjusted incidence rate is 0.08 per 100 000.[480] Chordoma develops in the axial skeleton, most commonly the sacrum (50%), followed by the skull base (35%) and the mobile spine (15%). Rare cases have originated in bones of the extremities.[481]

The pathogenesis of chordoma is unknown. Although it is generally accepted that chordomas arise from persistent rests of notochord within rigid bony structures and not the intervertebral discs, this fact has never been proved. Chordoma has no known association with irradiation or any other environmental factor. A very small percentage of cases have a familial pattern of inheritance and in at least one case the mode of inheritance was probably autosomal dominant. Cytogenetic and genome-wide analyses have revealed loss of genetic material at chromosomes 1p21 and 36, and 3p in sporadic and familial tumors while linkage analysis found that familial chordoma linked to 7q33.[482]

Chordoma is usually diagnosed during the fourth to eighth decades of life; only 5% of tumors develop in patients less than 20 years of age.[478,479] Men are affected more frequently than women. Pain and neurologic deficits specific to the site of origin are common symptoms and some tumors, especially those arising in the sacrum or the mobile spine, may be present for years before a diagnosis is made.

Radiographically, chordoma is centered in the midline and produces a destructive lytic mass that frequently extends into the soft tissues (Fig. 14.125). In the sacrum, the soft tissue component is often anterior and may displace the rectum.

A soft, friable, tan-gray, oozing, gelatinous, hemorrhagic mass centered in bone is characteristic of chordoma (Fig. 14.126). The tumors vary in size. Those in the skull base are the smallest (2–5 cm), whereas those in the sacrum are the largest, usually greater than 10 cm in size, commonly with an anterior soft tissue component.

Pathologically, chordoma is classified into the conventional, chondroid, and dedifferentiated variants. A component of the conventional type is virtually always found in the chondroid and dedifferentiated variants. *Conventional chordoma* (Fig. 14.127) has a lobular growth pattern, infiltrates the marrow space, encases pre-existing bony trabeculae, and frequently transgresses the cortex, forming a well demarcated soft tissue mass. The tumor is composed of large epithelioid cells arranged in cohesive nests and cords in which one tumor cell may wrap around or 'hug' another. The nuclei of the neoplastic cells are of moderate size, are darkly staining, and may contain a small nucleolus or pseudoinclusion. The eosinophilic cytoplasm is abundant and sometimes contains multiple round clear vacuoles that impart a 'bubbly' appearance to the cytoplasm. Occasionally, the vacuoles coalesce into a single large structure causing the cells to mimic adipocytes. These 'bubbly' cells were termed 'physaliphorous cells' by Virchow in 1857 and since that

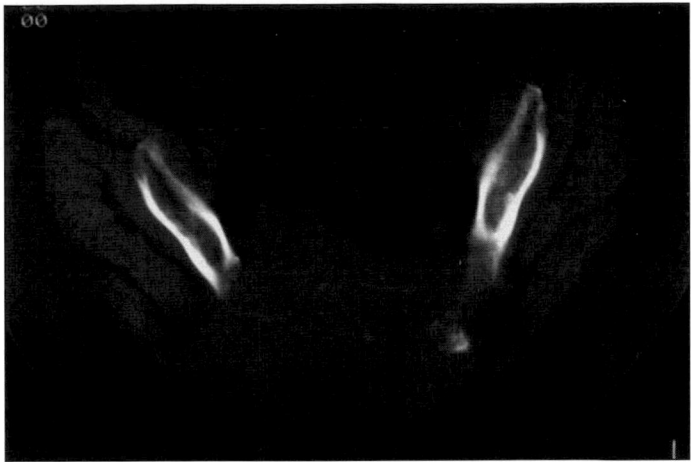

Fig. 14.125 Chordoma. A CT scan of the sacrum shows a destructive lytic mass extending into soft tissue.

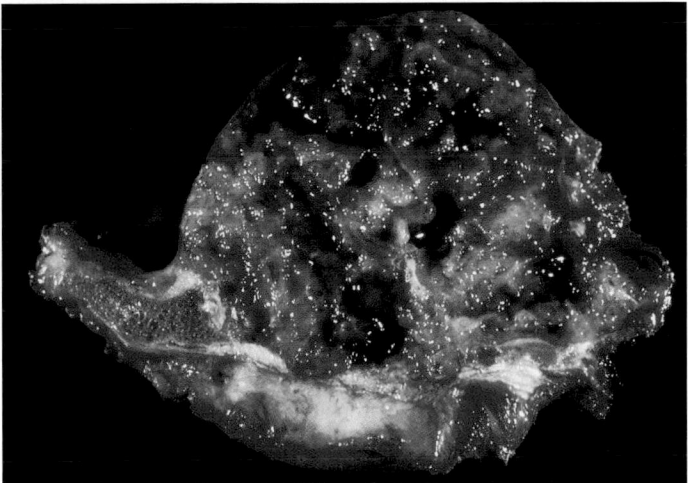

Fig. 14.126 Chordoma arising in the sacrum and forming a large anterior soft tissue mass. The tumor is red-tan and glistening.

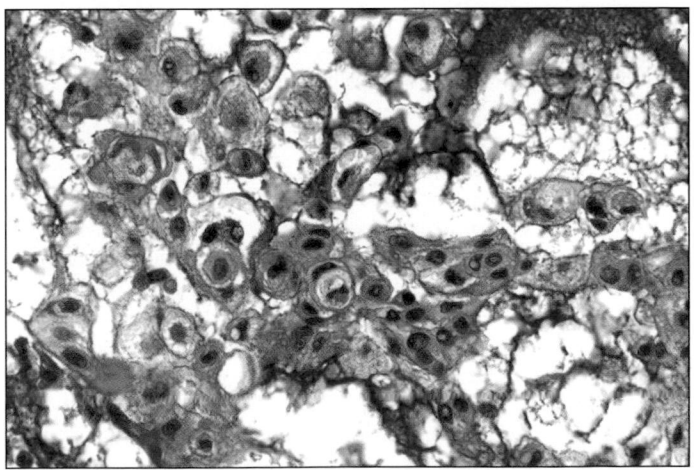

Fig. 14.127 Conventional chordoma. Cohesive nests of large cells with abundant pink cytoplasm. In some areas tumor cells wrap around one another. Cells with bubbly cytoplasm (physaliferous cells) are present.

time they have become recognized as being characteristic of chordoma. It is important to note, however, that physaliphorous cells are not always present in chordomas and that other types of tumor may have similar-appearing cells, so their diagnostic significance is limited. Additional morphologic features in otherwise conventional chordoma include pleomorphism and spindling of the tumor cells. Mitoses are usually limited in number, but foci of necrosis are common, especially in larger tumors. The stroma is myxoid, frothy, basophilic, and surrounds the cords and nests of cells. We have noted an aggressive variant of conventional chordoma in children in which the tumor cells grow in large solid sheets with little or no stroma, have vesicular nuclei, and exhibit numerous mitoses.

Ultrastructurally, the neoplastic cells in conventional chordoma have villous surface projections, abundant cytoplasmic glycogen, mitochondria–rough endoplasmic reticulum complexes, cytoplasmic processes that wrap around an adjacent cell, and epithelial features, including well developed desmosomes, intracytoplasmic lumina, and tonofilament-like bundles of intermediate filaments.[483–485] The vacuoles in the physaliphorous cells are formed by either dilated rough endoplasmic reticulum, cytoplasmic inclusions of the extracellular space, or intracellular lumina.[483–485] Immunohistochemically, conventional chordoma typically expresses the epithelial markers keratin, including keratins 8 and 19, and epithelial membrane antigen, and the vast majority also stain with antibodies to S-100 protein.[485,486] This profile can be very helpful in distinguishing chondrosarcoma from chordoma, in that chondrosarcomas are negative for epithelial markers, especially keratin. E-cadherin expression has also been found in chordoma but not in chondrosarcoma.[487]

FNA smears of conventional chordoma are characterized by myxoid matrix containing many dispersed large cells with abundant vacuolated cytoplasm. Frequently, there is a second population of smaller mononuclear cells with granular cytoplasm (Fig. 14.128A).[488–490] The physaliferous cells contain multiple cytoplasmic vacuoles and may be mono- or multinuclear, but the nuclei are of a bland morphology. With Romanowsky-stained preparations, the vacuoles contain a densely metachromatic inclusion (Fig. 14.128B). Romanowsky preparations demonstrate the background material to have a magenta color. This stroma varies in appearance from watery to thick and mucoid. The matrix surrounds and entraps both physaliferous cells and the smaller mononuclear cells. Nucleoli, when present, are small. In most cases, physaliferous cells are easily demonstrable on smear preparations but occasional cases contain only the small-cell population.[491]

Chondroid chordoma is a subtype that has generated much controversy. Historically it was originally defined as a chordoma that contained areas of conventional chordoma as well as regions that resembled low-grade hyaline type chondrosarcoma (Fig. 14.129).[492] The significance of this variant originally appeared to be that chondroid chordoma portended a better prognosis (longer survival time but similar overall survival) than conventional chordoma.[492] This original study was subsequently disputed and the very entity of chondroid chordoma was called into question, as some investigators argued that it merely represented a form of chondrosarcoma. Although the issue is not entirely resolved, several studies have convincingly shown that chondroid chordoma *is* a distinct morphologic variant of chordoma and is not a misclassified chondrosarcoma.[475,486,493–497] The survival advantage of chondroid chordoma has also been refuted, and currently the evidence supports the argument that chondroid chordoma does not behave biologically differently from conventional chordoma; therefore this subtype does not predict a better prognosis.[498] Chondroid chordoma most commonly arises in the skull base, less frequently in the mobile spine, and uncommonly in the

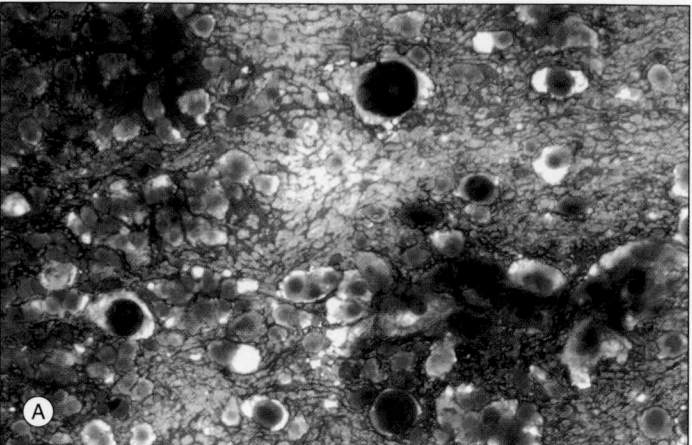

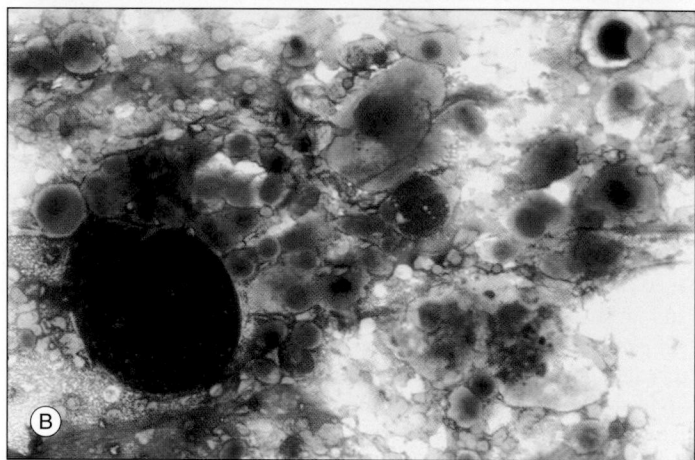

Fig. 14.128 Material aspirated from a chordoma. **(A)** The background contains a myxoid matrix that may condense into filamentous streamers or more solid aggregates. The majority of the cells are mononuclear and possess either a granular or a pale cytoplasm. Occasional large cells with abundant cytoplasm are seen. The larger cells frequently contain intracytoplasmic aggregates of dense purple matrix. (Romanowsky stain.) **(B)** Large physaliferous cells with abundant, dense, purple intracytoplasmic substance associated with smaller mononuclear cells and other large cells containing a granular purple material are common in chordomas. The larger cells represent the physaliferous cell component of the chordoma. (Romanowsky stain.)

sacrococcygeal region. Morphologically, the chondroid regions may merge with or be abruptly distinct from the conventional component. The chondroid element is characterized by neoplastic cells distributed individually in lacunar spaces that are surrounded by a solid hyalinized matrix, similar in appearance to hyaline cartilage. The amount of the chondroid component can vary in any particular tumor, and in some cases it may be abundant, causing confusion with chondrosarcoma. Ultrastructurally, the tumor cells in the chondroid areas have the same features as those of conventional chordoma. Similarly, the cells in the chondroid regions have the same immunohistochemical profile as those in the conventional areas in that they both strongly express epithelial markers as well as S-100 protein. Accordingly, the chondroid appearance in these tumors represents a morphologic change in the extracellular matrix and cell distribution and does not represent the presence of hyaline cartilage in a chordoma.

Dedifferentiated chordoma is the least common subtype of chordoma. It is composed of areas of conventional chordoma and

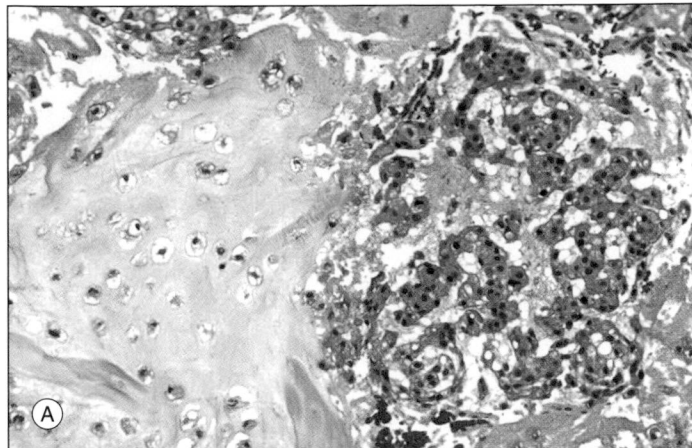

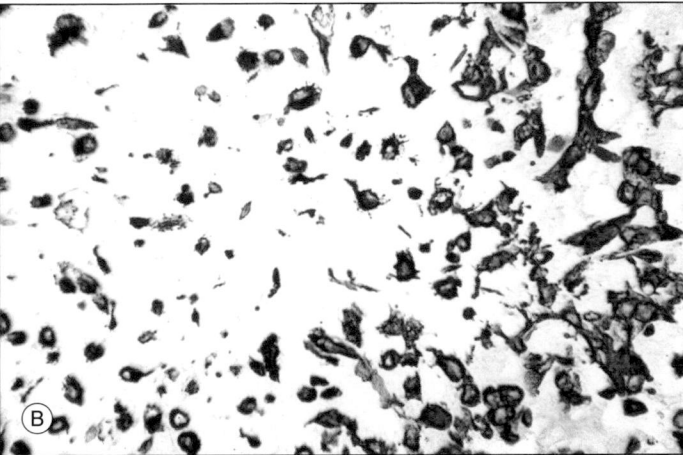

Fig. 14.129 Chondroid chordoma. **(A)** Conventional chordoma is seen adjacent to an area mimicking chondrosarcoma. **(B)** Immunohistochemical stain for keratin shows positive staining in the conventional area and in the chondroid area confirming the diagnosis of a chordoma.

regions that have the morphology of a high-grade or poorly differentiated spindle cell sarcoma. This phenomenon affects less than 5% of conventional chordomas and most frequently complicates sacrococcygeal tumors. The dedifferentiated component may arise de novo within the primary tumor, in a recurrence, or within a chordoma after it has been irradiated. Morphologically, the dedifferentiated component is usually distinct from the areas of conventional chordoma and has the light microscopic features, immunohistochemical phenotype, and ultrastructural characteristics of malignant fibrous histiocytoma; although in some tumors it has the histology of osteosarcoma. The significance of identifying the dedifferentiated component is its aggressive biological behavior. Dedifferentiated chordoma has the worst prognosis because these tumors are usually rapidly fatal and systemic spread occurs in approximately 90% of cases.

The prognosis of chordoma is affected by a variety of clinical and pathologic characteristics. Important features include tumor location, size, and resectability, as well as the age and gender of the patient. Chordomas of the sacrum have the best prognosis and the longest overall survival. The 5- and 10-year modern-era survival rates of sacrococcygeal chordoma range from 60–95% and 40–60% respectively; however, many of these patients may not have been disease- or recurrence-free.[499,500] Important prognostic findings for tumors in this location have included completeness of resection and

the level of sacral involvement; the more proximal the tumor within the sacrum, the worse the prognosis.[499] Local recurrences for sacrococcygeal chordomas are commonplace, especially after incomplete excision.

In the mobile spine, the 5-year survival rate is approximately 55% and the mean survival is about 4.7 years, only 15% of patients being alive without tumor after a mean follow-up of almost 2 years.[501] Complete excision of spinal tumors is difficult to accomplish so local recurrence rates are very high, ranging from 62–75%.[501,502]

In the skull base, important prognostic features have included the presence of necrosis, the size of the tumor, and the age and gender of the patient. Larger tumors, female gender, and age greater than 40 years have been associated with a poorer outcome.[503,504] In a large series in which the patients were treated with surgery and radiation, 46% of patients developed local progression at a median of 69 months follow-up.[503] Other investigators found that the 5-year local control rate was 59%.[504] In another analysis, the 5-year recurrence free survival was 65%[505] while the 5- and 10-year estimated overall survival rates in another study were 51% and 35% respectively.[506] Several studies have shown that skull base chordomas in young children frequently have atypical histologic features and an aggressive clinical course, particularly for children less than 5 years of age.[507,508]

The rate of metastatic spread of chordoma varies widely in the literature and ranges from less than 5% to 43%. Tumors in the sacrococcygeal region and mobile spine metastasize more frequently than those originating in the skull base. The low rate of systemic spread from skull base neoplasms, which is reported to be 0–10%, is probably related to the fact that the patients succumb to the local affects of their tumor before metastases develop. Metastases tend to occur late in the clinical course of chordoma, usually after a period of several or more years. Common sites of dissemination include the lung, skin, and bone. There are no effective chemotherapeutic agents for the treatment of this disease.

Giant vertebral notochordal rests and intraosseous benign notochordal tumors are recently described and related entities that should be distinguished from chordoma.[509–512] These intraosseous lesions are usually asymptomatic and are discovered as an incidental finding during clinical evaluation for an unrelated problem or at autopsy. They have an anatomic distribution similar to chordoma but importantly have a nonprogressive clinical course. Unlike conventional chordoma, these lesions lack lobulation, contain no extracellular myxoid matrix, and are composed of sheets of large, adipocyte-like, vacuolated cells. The tumors are well delineated but not encapsulated, and the involved bone is not destroyed, as in chordoma, but is rebuttressed and sclerotic.

VASCULAR TUMORS

Vascular tumors of bone are very common, although most involve the vertebral column and are asymptomatic. Clinically significant neoplasms are infrequent and range in their biology from those that are relatively indolent to those that are extremely aggressive and frequently fatal. An important group of vascular tumors of the skeleton are those composed of epithelioid endothelial cells, which further complicates pathologic interpretation.

HEMANGIOMA

Hemangioma is the most common vascular tumor of bone and may be found in vertebral bodies in approximately 10% of the population

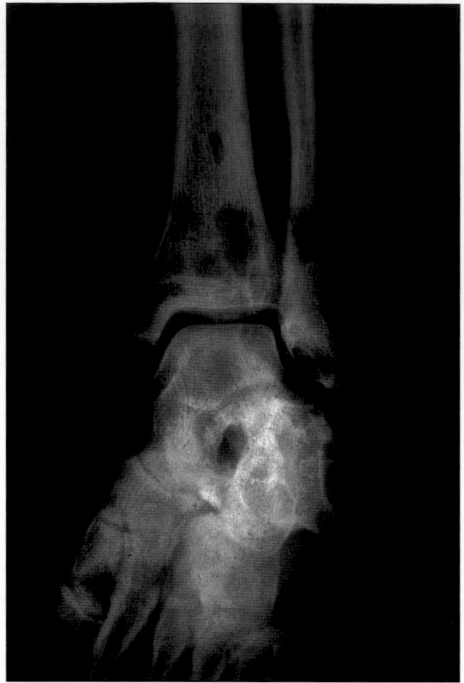

Fig. 14.130 Plain X-ray of epithelioid hemangioma of bone showing multiple lytic lesions in the bones of the ankle and foot.

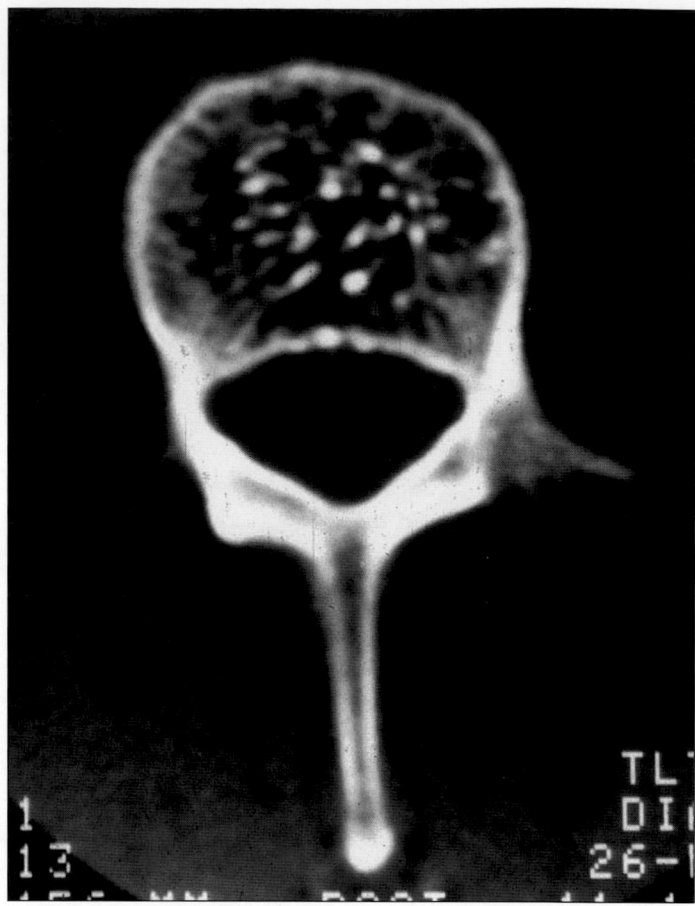

Fig. 14.131 An axial CT of a hemangioma of the vertebra. The image shows the characteristic 'polka dot' pattern.

at the time of autopsy. Clinically detectable tumors, however, are uncommon and account for less than 1% of primary bone tumors.[513] Hemangiomas may be solitary or multifocal (Fig. 14.130). Solitary lesions such as some capillary hemangiomas are usually indolent tumors and are stable or enlarge slowly. Multifocal disease has been subclassified into two distinct entities: multiple primary hemangiomas and diffuse cystic angiomatosis. *Multiple primary hemangiomas of bone* consist of collections of lesions that individually have the radiographic findings and clinical behavior of solitary hemangiomas. Aside from their multifocality they are not clinically important. In contrast, the vascular lesions in *diffuse cystic angiomatosis* are large and destructive and may appear cystic on X-rays. Visceral involvement is common and can result in fatal hemorrhage. *Gorham syndrome* ('disappearing bone disease') is a rare disorder characterized by an osseous hemangioma or lymphangioma that produces extensive osteolysis without forming a tumorous mass. The tumor can spread across joints from one bone to another and extend into adjacent soft tissues. Gorham syndrome most frequently affects the bones of the skull and extremities.[514]

Hemangiomas of bone most commonly arise in the vertebral column, followed by the craniofacial skeleton and the metaphyses of long bones.[513,515–518] The tumors are usually diagnosed in adulthood, with the peak incidence in the fifth decade of life. They are more common in women than in men.[513,515]

Radiographically, hemangiomas including epithelioid hemangioma are radiolucent and have coarse trabeculations. In the spine they produce the characteristic 'polka dot' pattern within vertebral bodies (Fig. 14.131). The craniofacial tumors are usually centered within the diploë, and have a lytic appearance, often with prominent intralesional radiating spicules of bone that create the so-called 'sunburst' appearance.[513,515] Elsewhere, the tumors are usually well circumscribed, may be expansile, and are lucent, with an internal web-like trabecular pattern.

The tumors are usually centered in the medullary cavity and are gritty and dark red with a sponge-like appearance. They resemble conventional capillary or cavernous hemangiomas of skin and soft tissue and are composed of thin-walled vascular spaces that may or may not be filled with red blood cells. The lumina are lined by a single layer of flat, uniform, cytologically bland endothelial cells (Fig. 14.132). The vessels are surrounded by loose connective tissue and typically infiltrate the pre-existing cancellous bone. Entrapped, thickened, bony trabeculae produce the radiographically detectable intralesional spicules. The endothelial cells exhibit positive immunostaining for the endothelial markers factor-VIII-related antigen, *Ulex europaeus* lectin, CD34, and CD31.[519]

Smears obtained from hemangiomas are dominated by red blood cells in which are dispersed rare individual, bland spindle cells and small tissue fragments composed of similar short, bland, spindle cells with plump, ovoid cells along the edge of the tissue fragments (Fig. 14.133).[23]

Curettage is usually the mode of therapy for symptomatic lesions and is associated with a low rate of local recurrence.

The differential diagnosis of conventional skeletal hemangioma is limited. The vascular spaces may be difficult to appreciate and, as a result, one may fail to recognize the lesion. A hemangioma should always be considered when confronting a bone biopsy that appears to be normal, as the vessels can be subtle and on biopsy may consist of a few fragments of thin-walled structures.

Epithelioid hemangioma of bone is a variant that may pose diagnostic difficulty because of the plump, 'histiocyte-like' or epithelioid appearance of the endothelial cells.[519–522] The hallmark

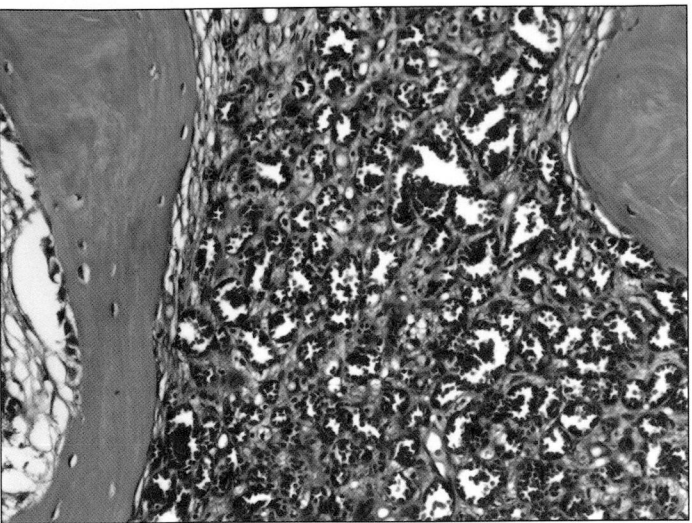

Fig. 14.132 Capillary hemangioma of bone. Numerous small capillaries filling the intertrabecular space. The vessels and lined by uniform flat endothelial cells.

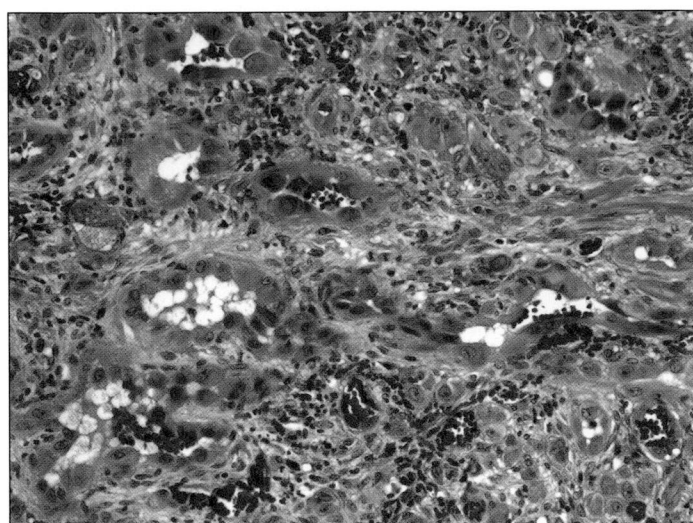

Fig. 14.134 Epithelioid hemangioma. The vascular lumens are lined by large epithelioid endothelial cells. In some areas (lower right) they grow in solid cords.

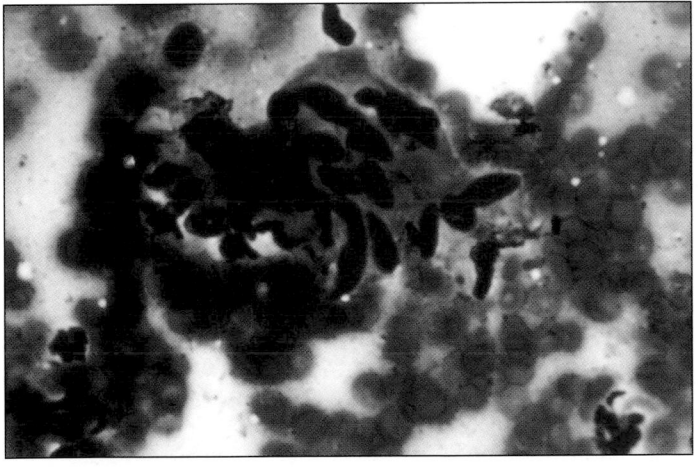

Fig. 14.133 Material aspirated from hemangiomas has a markedly hemorrhagic background in which are dispersed bland spindle cells and small aggregates of similar cells. Nuclear atypia is absent, although the nuclei are often hyperchromatic. (Romanowsky stain.)

of epithelioid endothelial cells is their polyhedral shape and their abundant densely eosinophilic cytoplasm, which frequently contains one or more large vacuoles (Fig. 14.134). The vacuoles represent the earliest stage of vessel lumen formation and may be empty or contain intact or fragmented red blood cells. As vacuoles from neighboring cells fuse they create vascular spaces of varying degrees of differentiation. Well formed vessels are numerous in epithelioid hemangioma, and the epithelioid endothelial cells bulge into their lumens in a 'tombstone ' or 'hobnail-like' fashion. In some cases, the cells are arranged in solid cords and even sheets, which can cause confusion with more aggressive lesions. Numerous inflammatory cells, including plasma cells and eosinophils present in the stroma of occasional cases, can mimic osteomyelitis. The epithelioid endothelial cells express the usual markers of endothelial cells by immunohistochemistry; however, approximately 50% also stain for keratin and epithelial membrane antigen.[519]

Local excision of epithelioid hemangioma is usually curative and recurrences are uncommon.[513,515,519]

The differential diagnosis of epithelioid hemangioma includes epithelioid hemangioendothelioma and epithelioid angiosarcoma, which are both discussed in detail below.

EPITHELIOID HEMANGIOENDOTHELIOMA

Epithelioid hemangioendothelioma is an uncommon endothelial tumor that most frequently arises in the soft tissues, liver, lung, and skeleton.[523,524] It usually behaves as a low-grade sarcoma but a minority are aggressive and life-threatening. Similarly to other skeletal vascular tumors, epithelioid hemangioendothelioma demonstrates multifocal osseous involvement in approximately one third to one half of cases.[523] Unfortunately, some of the literature analyzing skeletal epithelioid hemangioendothelioma is confusing because, in our opinion, many of the reported cases represent epithelioid hemangioma or other types of vascular neoplasms.[515,525–527]

Epithelioid hemangioendothelioma can be seen in most age groups and has its peak frequency in the second decade.[524] The tumor affects males and females equally and develops in whites disproportionately more often than in members of other races. Like other vascular tumors of bone, epithelioid hemangioendothelioma frequently involves multiple sites in a single bone or multiple bones simultaneously. The tumor tends to arise in the extremities, pelvis and spine. In the extremities, the long bones, as well as the small bones of the hands and feet, are commonly involved and typically cause localized pain, which may be associated with swelling. Some patients also have disease in the soft tissues, liver, or lung at the time of diagnosis of the skeletal disease.

The radiographic features of epithelioid hemangioendothelioma are variable. Most lesions range in size from 1–3 cm and are round or elongated and predominately lytic. The margins may be well delineated or poorly defined and the adjacent bone is usually sclerotic.[523,524,528]

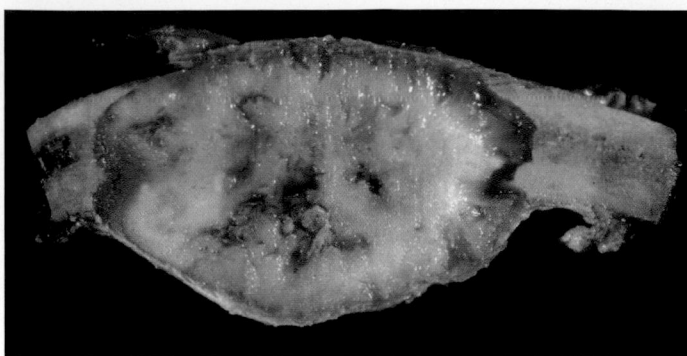

Fig. 14.135 Epithelioid hemangioendothelioma of the skull. The tumor is solid, tan and white, and expands the inner table.

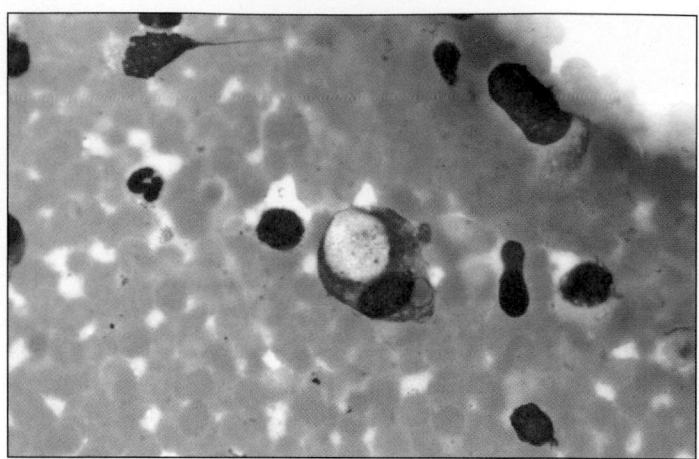

Fig. 14.137 Polygonal cells dispersed singly within a background rich in red blood cells characteristic of epithelioid hemangioendothelioma. Rare cells contain intracytoplasmic vacuoles, displacing the nucleus to one side. Nuclear hyperchromasia and irregularity is variable but is usually of moderate degree. (Romanowsky stain.)

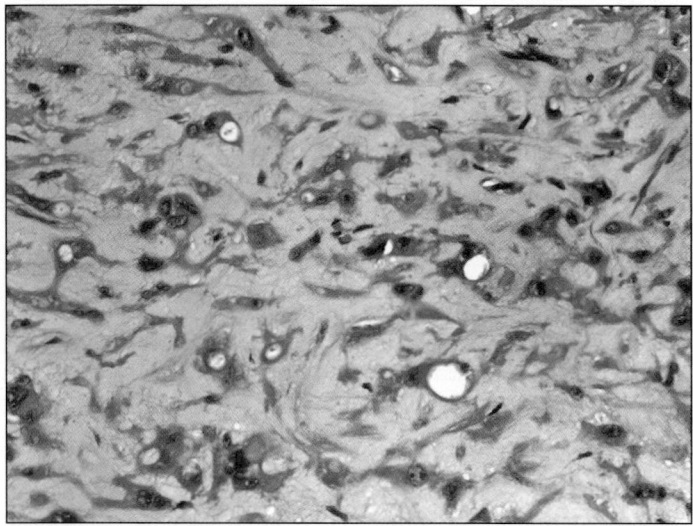

Fig. 14.136 Epithelioid hemangioendothelioma. The tumor cells are epithelioid and spindle shaped and embedded in a basophilic hyalinized stroma. Some of the tumor cells have intracytoplasmic vacuoles containing fragments of red blood cells.

Epithelioid hemangioendothelioma is pale tan in color and lacks the red, hemorrhagic appearance of conventional hemangiomas (Fig. 14.135). Microscopically, it is composed of large epithelioid and spindle endothelial cells with round or elongate nuclei, prominent nucleoli, and abundant eosinophilic cytoplasm. Intracytoplasmic lumens appear as vacuoles that may contain intact or fragmented red blood cells (Fig. 14.136). The vacuoles may coalesce to form primitive vascular channels, recapitulating embryonic angiogenesis; however, well formed blood vessels are not prominent in most cases. Instead, the tumor cells are arranged in cords and nests embedded within a myxoid to hyalinized ground substance that may resemble cartilaginous matrix.[523,524,528] The neoplastic cells generally show limited cytologic atypia and mitotic activity but, in some cases, nuclear hyperchromasia and pleomorphism are significant and mitoses numerous, making it difficult to distinguish the neoplasm from high-grade angiosarcoma.

A background rich in red blood cells, in which are dispersed a small number of single, polygonal, or even plasmacytoid-appearing cells, characterizes smears from epithelioid hemangioendotheliomas. These cells have abundant cytoplasm and eccentric nuclei. The cytoplasm frequently contains one or two vacuoles, representing an early stage in lumen formation (Fig. 14.137). Cytologic atypia is usually minimal.

The tumor cells express the full spectrum of immunohistochemical endothelial markers including factor VIII, CD34, and CD31 and, like epithelioid endothelial cells in general, may also exhibit intense and extensive positive staining for keratin and epithelial membrane antigen. The tumor cells usually do not stain with antibodies to S-100 protein and desmin. Ultrastructurally, the neoplastic cells contain abundant intermediate filaments, pinocytotic vesicles, intracytoplasmic lumens, and basal lamina material.

Epithelioid hemangioendothelioma is treated by complete surgical excision if feasible. However, multifocal lesions may be difficult to excise and may require radiation or thermal ablation. Predicting the outcome for patients with osseous epithelioid hemangioendothelioma is problematic as the clinical behavior is not always predicted by the morphologic features of the tumor. In one large series, 20% of patients succumbed to disease; of those who died most had concurrent visceral tumors.[524] In the absence of parenchymal organ involvement, epithelioid hemangioendotheliomas of bone usually behave in an indolent fashion and infrequently metastasize. They may locally recur following curettage or slowly enlarge if left untreated.

The differential diagnosis of epithelioid hemangioendothelioma includes other epithelioid vascular neoplasms, particularly epithelioid hemangioma and angiosarcoma. Epithelioid hemangioendothelioma is distinguished from epithelioid hemangioma by its characteristic hyalinized stroma and the paucity of well formed vessels. Angiosarcoma also lacks the hyalinized stroma and usually shows a greater degree of cytologic atypia and mitotic activity. The epithelioid features of the tumor cells, their cohesive nature, and intracytoplasmic vacuoles can also mimic metastatic adenocarcinoma. The staining of tumor cells of epithelioid hemangioendothelioma for epithelial markers can further complicate this distinction. Fortunately, metastatic carcinomas do not stain for endothelial markers, and the myxoid or hyalinized stroma is distinct from the desmoplastic seen in metastatic carcinoma. The cells in cartilaginous tumors do not form cohesive nests, stain immunohistochemically for S-100 protein, and are negative for endothelial markers.

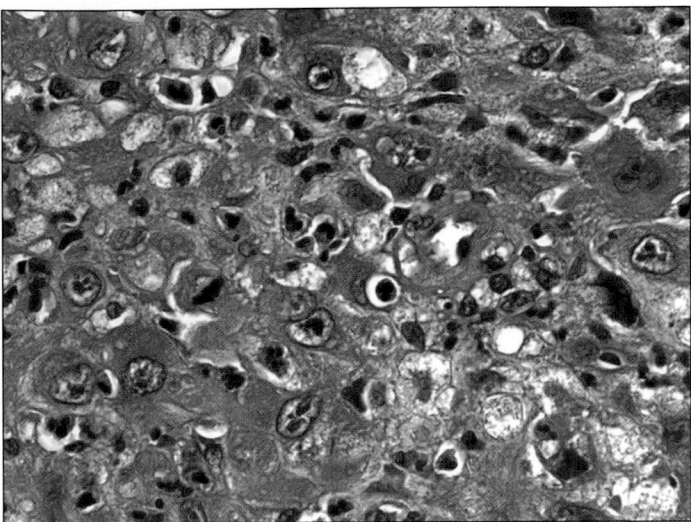

Fig. 14.138 Epithelioid angiosarcoma of bone. Sheets of cytologically malignant epithelioid cells. Note the neutrophils in the background.

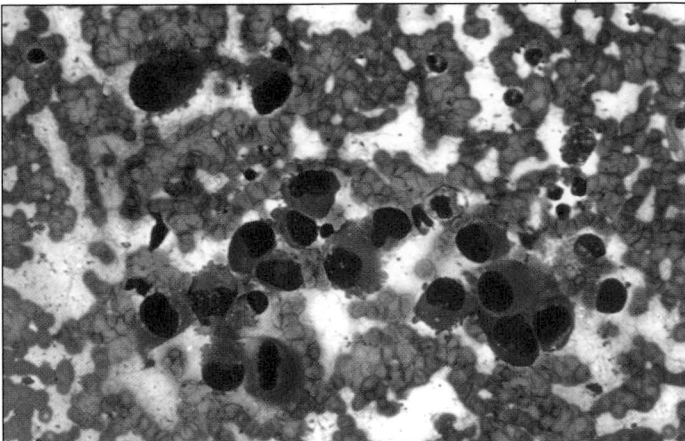

Fig. 14.139 Fine-needle aspiration material obtained from an angiosarcoma. Note the blood background in which are distributed loosely cohesive round to ovoid cells. Mitotic figures are frequent, and nuclear atypia is marked. The cytoplasm is present in moderate amounts, and the nuclei may be eccentrically located. (Romanowsky stain.)

ANGIOSARCOMA

Skeletal angiosarcoma, also known as hemangioendothelial sarcoma, is a very uncommon tumor and accounts for little more than 1% of primary bone sarcomas.[8] It is a neoplasm of adulthood and usually arises in the appendicular skeleton.[513,515,528–531] Most angiosarcomas are solitary; however, as many as a third present with involvement of multiple bones.[528] Angiosarcoma of bone is usually a high-grade, poorly differentiated neoplasm and we feel that many tumors that were previously classified as low-grade hemangioendothelial sarcoma probably represent examples of epithelioid hemangioma.[519] Angiosarcoma of bone usually presents as a painful enlarging mass, which may cause pathologic fracture. It arises rarely in association with previous radiation, Paget's disease, bone infarction, and skeletal hemangiomatosis.

The tumor manifests on X-ray as an ill-defined, lytic mass with prominent destruction of the underlying bone. The tumor may erode the cortex, elicit a periosteal reaction, and extend into the soft tissues.[513,515,528–531]

Skeletal angiosarcoma is usually 5–10 cm in size, appears dark red and hemorrhagic, has poorly defined, irregular borders, and may infiltrate the neighboring soft tissues. Frequently, the underlying bone appears ravaged and tumor necrosis may be prominent. Angiosarcoma is composed of cytologically malignant spindle and epithelioid endothelial cells that have the capacity to form rudimentary blood vessels (Fig. 14.138). In the epithelioid variant, the tumor is composed almost entirely of epithelioid cells and, as with the other epithelioid vascular tumors, some of the cells contain intracytoplasmic vacuoles.[497] A prominent neutrophilic infiltrate is occasionally noted. Mitoses are numerous and atypical mitotic figures are frequently present. The stroma is inconspicuous and consists of small amounts of fibrous tissue.

Smears from angiosarcomas are characterized by abundant background blood and contain a population of anaplastic spindle or ovoid cells (Fig. 14.139).[532] The malignant endothelial cells may form three-dimensional clusters of tightly packed cuboidal or polygonal cells forming slit-like structures.[532] The nuclear atypia is usually obvious and severe.

Immunohistochemistry shows that the neoplastic cells express one or more of the endothelial markers including factor VIII, CD31, and CD34. The neoplastic cells in epithelioid angiosarcoma may also stain prominently with antibodies to keratin and epithelial membrane antigen. Ultrastructurally, the neoplastic cells have the features of primitive endothelial cells.

Angiosarcoma of bone is best treated with complete en bloc excision. Adjuvant radiation and chemotherapy have little proven effect. The prognosis is poor, as most of the tumors are high-grade and usually metastasize.

The differential diagnosis of osseous angiosarcoma includes vascular tumors such as epithelioid hemangioma and epithelioid hemangioendothelioma, as well as metastatic carcinoma, malignant melanoma, and other high-grade sarcomas. Epithelioid angiosarcoma differs from epithelioid hemangioma because it demonstrates significantly more cytologic atypia and a paucity of well-formed blood vessels. It is distinguished from epithelioid hemangioendothelioma mainly by the lack of hyalinized or chondroid stroma. Immunohistochemistry and electron microscopy are very useful in excluding metastatic carcinoma and melanoma. In this differential diagnosis, it is important to note that most carcinomas and melanomas are negative for factor-VIII-related antigen, CD31, and CD34 and angiosarcoma does not express S-100 protein. Accordingly, immunohistochemistry employing antibodies directed against endothelial markers should be performed on unusual epithelioid tumors of bone.

HEMANGIOPERICYTOMA

The term hemangiopericytoma was coined by Stout and Murray for a unique soft tissue vascular tumor characterized by branching capillaries surrounded by what they believed to be neoplastic pericytes.[533] Although the existence of hemangiopericytoma has recently been questioned, rare examples of primary hemangiopericytoma of bone have been described.[534,535] Hemangiopericytoma accounts for significantly fewer than 0.1% of primary bone tumors, usually arises in adults and tends to involve the long bones, although any bone can be affected.

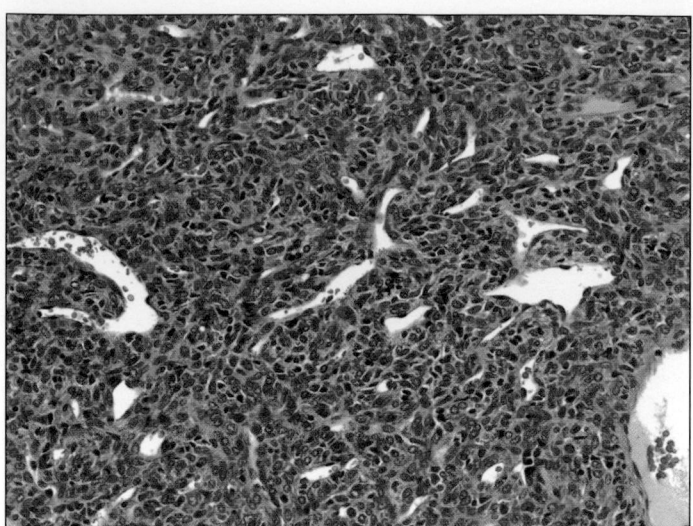

Fig. 14.140 Hemangiopericytoma of bone. Cellular neoplasm composed of oval to spindle shaped cells with a prominent branching vascular pattern.

The tumor presents as a lytic, intramedullary mass that may destroy the cortex and extend into the soft tissue. The margins are frequently permeative.

The tumor is tan-gray, with areas of hemorrhage, is centered in the medullary cavity, and may either have well defined or infiltrative margins. Histologically, it is identical to soft tissue hemangiopericytoma and is characterized by oval to spindle cells that may appear banal or cytologically atypical and are associated with a prominent vascular tree composed of small-caliber vessels or sinusoids that branch at 45° angles, causing them to have a staghorn or antler-like appearance (Fig. 14.140).

Hemangiopericytoma should be excised with negative margins. Most hemangiopericytomas of bone behave in a malignant fashion, and the 5- and 10-year survival rates are 75% and 44% respectively.[534]

Hemangiopericytoma-like areas can be seen in variety of benign and malignant primary bone tumors. Therefore, thorough sampling is necessary before the diagnosis is made. Additionally, metastatic meningeal hemangiopericytoma may present as a solitary bone tumor, and this also should be excluded clinically.

FATTY TUMORS OF BONE

Fatty tumors of bone are uncommon and the overwhelming majority are benign. In contrast to fatty tumors of the soft tissues, which exhibit a wide histologic spectrum, those developing in bone are restricted in morphology and are usually composed of neoplastic white adipocytes.

LIPOMA OF BONE (INTRAMEDULLARY AND PAROSTEAL)

Lipoma of bone is a benign neoplasm of fat that arises within the medullary cavity and cortex, or on the surface of bone (parosteal lipoma). Intraosseous tumors are uncommon, account for less than

0.1% of primary bone tumors, and occur over a wide age range (second to eighth decades), with most patients being approximately 40 years old at the time of diagnosis.[536] Males are affected more frequently than females, at a ratio of approximately 1.6:1.[536] Parosteal lipoma usually develops during adulthood (with a slight male predominance (9:7)), and most patients are in their fifth to sixth decade of life at the time of diagnosis.[537] The vast majority of intraosseous lipomas are intramedullary and arise in the metaphyseal regions of the long tubular bones, especially the femur, tibia, and fibula, and in the calcaneus. They have also been described in the pelvis, vertebrae, sacrum, skull, mandible, maxilla, and ribs. Rare cases are intracortical in origin.[538] Parosteal lipoma generally develops on the diaphyseal surface of long tubular bones, including the femur, humerus, and tibia.[537] Intramedullary lipoma may be asymptomatic or produce achy pain; patients rarely present with a pathologic fracture.[536,539,540] Parosteal lipoma is frequently asymptomatic and may be detected as a visible or palpable mass.

Intramedullary lipoma usually produces a well defined, lytic mass surrounded by a thin rim of sclerosis on plain X-ray. The lesion may also contain trabeculations or central calcifications, and bony expansion may occur in small-caliber bones.[536,539–541] CT images demonstrate the fatty component with a low attenuation value similar to that of subcutaneous fat. On MRI, the fat has high signal intensity on both T1- and T2-weighted sequences.[541] Parosteal tumors manifest as a radiolucent mass adjacent to the cortical surface that may be thickened by periosteal reactive bone. As in intraosseous lipoma, the CT and MRI findings have the same features as subcutaneous fat, with the exception that parosteal lipomas may contain calcification, cartilage, or bone.[542,543]

Intramedullary lipoma is usually 3–5 cm in size, well defined, soft, and yellow, similar grossly to a soft tissue lipoma. The surrounding bone is frequently sclerotic. Parosteal lipoma is usually 4–10 cm in greatest dimension, well defined, soft, and yellow. Some cases contain gritty spicules of bone, or firm nodules of cartilage in the base or scattered throughout the mass. Intramedullary lipoma consists of lobules of mature-appearing, white adipocytes, which may replace the marrow and encase pre-existing bony trabeculae. Each adipocyte contains a single, large, clear, cytoplasmic vacuole that displaces the crescent-shaped nucleus to the periphery. Some tumors may demonstrate fat necrosis with foamy macrophages and fibrosis. Ossifying lipomas contain delicate trabeculae of woven and lamellar bone, which may be present throughout the tumor.[544,545] Parosteal lipoma is also well defined and consists of lobules of mature-appearing, white adipocytes. Some cases contain bone and/or hyaline cartilage in the base or randomly distributed in small islands scattered throughout the mass.[537] The neoplastic fat expresses vimentin and S-100 protein, similar to extraskeletal lipomas. The translocation t(3;12)(q28;q14) and associated fusion transcript *HMGIC–LPP,* characteristic of subcutaneous lipoma, has been detected in one case of parosteal lipoma.[546,547] Lipoma of bone has an excellent prognosis and rarely recurs.

LIPOSARCOMA OF BONE

Liposarcoma of bone is an extremely rare malignant neoplasm with a phenotype that recapitulates fat. Most cases are described in the form of single case reports in the older literature, with the validity of the diagnosis questioned in some cases.[548] Liposarcoma of bone occurs in all age groups, although the majority of patients are adults. Men are affected slightly more frequently than women.[548–551] Liposarcoma of bone usually develops in the long tubular bones, notably in the tibia and femur and has been reported in the diaphysis, metaphysis, and epiphysis.[548–551] Clinically, it presents as a painful mass that may be either well delineated or poorly defined radiographically.[548–551]

Most liposarcomas are large, lobular, soft to firm, and yellow to tan-white in color. Myxoid tumors may be glistening, slimy, and mucinous. The histologic variants of liposarcoma reported in bone include well differentiated lipoma-like, myxoid, and pleomorphic types.[548–551] Well differentiated lipoma-like liposarcoma consists of sheets of mature-appearing, white adipocytes with scattered tumor cells that have enlarged hyperchromatic nuclei. Some of these atypical cells are lipoblasts and are distinguished by cytoplasmic vacuoles that are round, clear, and scallop the nucleus. Myxoid liposarcoma consists of mildly atypical stellate and spindle cells enmeshed in a myxoid stroma that contains a finely arborizing vascular tree with a plexiform pattern. Also scattered throughout the tumor are lipoblasts. Sheets of large pleomorphic cells in which the cytoplasm is either eosinophilic or filled with round clear vacuoles characterize pleomorphic liposarcoma. Mitoses are usually numerous. The cytoplasm of the neoplastic cells contains membrane-bound lipid droplets of varying size. Dilated rough endoplasmic reticulum and scattered mitochondria are also present.[552] Prognostic information regarding liposarcoma of bone is scant. Generally, the behavior of the tumor should correlate with its histologic grade.

PERIPHERAL NERVE SHEATH TUMORS OF BONE

Peripheral nerve sheath tumors of the skeleton are very uncommon. They may involve bone by secondary erosion from a neighboring soft tissue primary or by expansion of bony foramina as the nerve courses though it, or arise in the intramedullary cavity. Intraosseous peripheral nerve sheath tumors are usually benign and most are schwannomas.

Schwannoma of bone accounts for fewer than 0.2% of all primary bone tumors and only a few hundred cases have been reported in the literature. They usually affect adults and tend to develop in the mandible and sacrum but have been described in a variety of skeletal locations.[553–556] Radiographically, they produce an oval or round radiolucency with well defined margins, which may be sclerotic. At the time of excision, they are well circumscribed, soft, tan-yellow, and may have areas of hemorrhage. Histologically, they demonstrate the features characteristic of schwannoma of soft tissue, with Antoni A and Antoni B regions as well as Verocay bodies. Cellular schwannomas frequently arise in the paravertebral soft tissue and erode the vertebral column. Treatment of intraosseous schwannoma is excision by curettage or enucleation and local recurrences are uncommon.

Neurofibromas usually involve the skeleton by producing pressure erosions on the cortices of adjacent bones. Growing tumor occasionally expands neural foramina.[557]

Malignant peripheral nerve sheath tumors are one of the rarest primary sarcomas of bone.[558,559] Some patients have underlying type I neurofibromatosis. The tumors tend to develop in association with pre-existing nerves, and most have arisen in the mandible or maxilla.[558] The sarcomas are composed of malignant spindle cells arranged in fascicles that may assume a herringbone pattern. Alternating areas of relative hypo- and hypercellularity are common. Approximately 50% of malignant peripheral sheath tumors express S-100 protein. These tumors have the potential to behave in an aggressive fashion and are frequently treated with surgical excision and adjuvant radiation and chemotherapy when appropriate.

SMOOTH MUSCLE TUMORS

Smooth muscle tumors of the skeleton may be primary neoplasms or a manifestation of benign metastasizing leiomyoma or metastatic leiomyosarcoma, usually from a uterine primary.[560–563] Clinical history and examination can be very helpful in determining whether or not the lesion is primary or metastatic.

Leiomyoma of bone is extraordinarily rare. Only a few cases have been reported and they have arisen in the bones of the jaw and extremities.[561] The tumors affect adults and produce a well circumscribed and lytic mass. They are composed of intersecting fascicles of mature-appearing smooth muscle cells with fibrillar eosinophilic cytoplasm and elongated, blunt-ended nuclei. Surgical excision is usually curative.

Leiomyosarcoma of bone is also rare, fewer than 100 cases being reported.[562–568] The tumors usually affect adults in the third to fifth decade of life, with no gender predilection. A minority of cases are radiation induced. No specific cytogenetic abnormalities have been identified, although significant complex genetic alterations may be present. The sarcoma tends to develop in long tubular bones, especially the distal femur and proximal tibia, and the flat bones of the pelvis. Pain and an enlarging mass are common presenting symptoms.

Leiomyosarcoma produces a lytic destructive mass with permeative margins and soft tissue extension. Intralesional mineralization is rare.[564] The tumor is usually more than 5 cm in diameter, centered in the medullary cavity, firm, and tan-white, with areas of hemorrhage and necrosis present in high-grade neoplasms. Destruction of the cortex and an accompanying soft tissue mass are common findings. The tumor grows with infiltrative margins replacing the marrow, surrounding bony trabeculae and crawling through haversian systems. The neoplastic cells are usually spindled, with eosinophilic fibrillar cytoplasm and elongated nuclei with blunted or rounded ends. The degree of cytologic atypia, mitotic activity, and necrosis generally correlates with the grade of the tumor. Immunohistochemistry shows that the tumor cells express markers indicative of myogenic differentiation including muscle specific actin, smooth muscle actin, and desmin.[567] Thin filaments with dense bodies, subplasmalemmal attachment plaques, and pinocytotic vesicles are apparent ultrastructurally.

METASTATIC DISEASE

Metastatic tumor to bone is the most common type of skeletal malignancy. In fact, some studies have shown that as many as 85% of patients with common visceral carcinomas have bone involvement. This emphasizes the fact that a metastasis should always be considered in the differential diagnosis of a malignant bone tumor in an adult.

Carcinomas, melanomas, lymphomas, and sarcomas can all metastasize to bone. Based on sheer numbers, however, carcinomas are by far and away the most numerous and are usually diagnosed between the ages of 40 and 60 years. Of the carcinomas, most metastases originate from the prostate, breast, kidney, and lungs.[569] Skeletal metastases do occur in children and usually represent neuroblastomas originating from the adrenals or rhabdomyosarcomas arising in the soft tissues or viscera.

By the time the metastasis is diagnosed, the bone disease is usually multifocal. Renal cell carcinoma and thyroid carcinomas, however, are notorious for presenting as a solitary metastasis and causing confusion with a primary bone tumor. Metastases develop in all bones but most involve bones that have hematopoietic elements, including the axial skeleton and the proximal femur and humerus. Metastases to the short tubular bones of the hands and feet are uncommon and, when present, usually originate from the lungs. Progressive pain, swelling, and tenderness are common symptoms of metastases and in some cases an acute pathologic fracture is the presenting event.

Metastases gain access to bone by direct extension and lymphatic or hematogenous dissemination. Once in bone, the malignant cells produce substances that result in bone resorption, bone formation, or a mixture of these two processes. Based upon the activity that predominates, the metastases may appear lytic, blastic or mixed lytic and blastic on radiographs. Lytic metastases are commonly caused by tumors originating in the kidneys, lungs, and gastrointestinal tract, as well as melanomas. Prostate adenocarcinoma and carcinoid tumors typically produce sclerotic metastases. Most tumors from a variety of sites, however, elicit a mixed lytic and sclerotic reaction. Metastases are destructive and usually have poorly defined margins and elicit periosteal reactions. Bone scintigraphy is a useful and sensitive way to scan the skeleton for their presence. Abnormal uptake may be associated with obvious lesions, as well as those that have normal plain X-rays. The plain X-rays may remain unremarkable for several months before evidence of bone destruction appears and CT and MRI are helpful in this situation as they are sensitive techniques in confirming the presence of early disease. Additionally, they provide important information regarding the full extent of a mass.

The diagnosis of metastatic disease is frequently made on a biopsy or bone marrow aspirate. In most instances, the diagnosis is easy and straightforward. Sometimes, however, it may be difficult to distinguish between a keratin-positive primary sarcoma of bone and metastatic sarcomatoid carcinoma. In these instances, we have found ultrastructural examination to be very helpful. Some tumors, such as metastatic lobular carcinoma of the breast and prostatic adeno-carcinoma, may be difficult to detect in small-needle biopsies or aspirates and, in these circumstances, keratin stains may facilitate the identification of the few malignant cells present.[570] We also have experience with some metastases from the breast, in which the cancer cells are admixed with numerous osteoclast-like giant cells. This can cause confusion with giant cell tumor of bone but positive staining of the mononuclear cancer cells for keratin helps make the correct diagnosis.

The treatment of bone metastases depends on the origin of the tumor and the patients' symptoms. Combinations of chemotherapy, radiation therapy, and surgery are employed. Patients who present with bone metastases are usually incurable, although solitary metastases can sometimes be treated effectively with surgery.[571]

REACTIVE PSEUDOSARCOMATOUS LESIONS OF THE PERIOSTEUM

A group of pseudoneoplastic reactive processes that includes subungual exostosis, bizarre parosteal osteochondromatous pro-liferation, and florid reactive periostitis deserves recognition because they arise underneath the periosteum on bone surfaces and mimic neoplasms clinically, radiologically, and pathologically (Table 14.11). This group of pseudosarcomas also have in common an association with prior trauma, the propensity to affect the fingers, a limited potential for growth, morphology characterized by variable amounts of hypercellular fibrous tissue, bone and cartilage, and an excellent prognosis, in that they are usually successfully treated by simple excision. Although their nomenclature implies that they are

Table 14.11 Bone forming pseudosarcomas of periosteum and soft tissue

Florid reactive periostitis
Bizarre parosteal osteochondromatous proliferation
Subungual exostosis
Myositis ossificans
Fibro-osseous pseudotumor

distinctly different entities, the similarities in their clinicopathological features indicates that they are actually closely related processes. Unfortunately, the terminology for these lesions is confusing and many of the features used to distinguish among them are somewhat arbitrary and not based on fundamental differences in their pathobiology.

FLORID REACTIVE PERIOSTITIS

Florid reactive periostitis, also known as fibro-osseous pseudotumor, as its name implies, is a non-neoplastic reparative process that originates in the periosteum.[572,573] Historically, the term florid reactive periostitis was coined by Spjut and Dorfman in 1981[572] but lesions with the characteristics of florid reactive periostitis were described by Mallory as early as 1933.[574] Since that time, fewer than 75 examples have been described in the literature, with the three largest series accounting for more than half the cases and the remainder largely being the subject of individual case reports.[572,575,576]

Florid reactive periostitis typically presents as a mass or fusiform swelling of a finger. The lesion is usually noted for only several weeks to a couple of months prior to diagnosis and, in the larger series, a history of prior trauma has been documented in between 33% and nearly 50% of cases.[572,575,576] On physical exam, the mass is firm, immobile, and can be painful, with erythema of the adjacent skin. The majority of cases arise in the periosteum of the proximal phalanx, followed in frequency by the middle and distal phalanges. The toes are affected only in a small percentage of cases, and long bones are rarely involved.[577,578] Florid reactive periostitis has an equal gender distribution and, although all ages can be affected, most patients are in their third decade of life at the time of diagnosis.[579]

Radiographically, florid reactive periostitis is attached to the bone surface by a broad base and always demonstrates evidence of soft tissue prominence or a mass (Fig. 14.141). The soft tissue component typically has areas of calcification or ossification, and the underlying bone shows either minimal or no changes, layers of reactive periosteal bone or less commonly cortical erosion.[572,577]

Florid reactive periostitis is composed of an admixture of woven bone and hypercellular fibrous tissue (Fig. 14.142). In most cases, the bone is deposited as trabeculae rimmed by prominent osteoblasts. Frequently, the trabeculae merge with sheet-like aggregates of osseous tissue, and in these regions the rimming phenomenon of osteoblasts is less obvious or absent. The cellular fibrous component resembles nodular fasciitis and is composed of plump spindled and stellate fibroblasts. The fibroblasts are oriented randomly or arranged in short intersecting fascicles enmeshed in a loose stroma that contains extravasated red blood cells. Both the osteoblasts and fibroblasts are mitotically active, however, the mitotic figures are not atypical. Cellular hyaline cartilage is present in a small minority of cases and frequently 'caps' the periphery of the lesion.

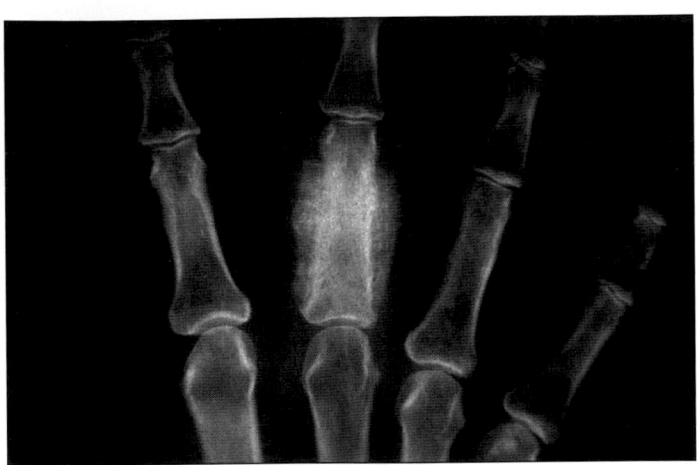

Fig. 14.141 Florid reactive periostitis. A plain X-ray showing a circumferential subperiosteal reactive new bone.

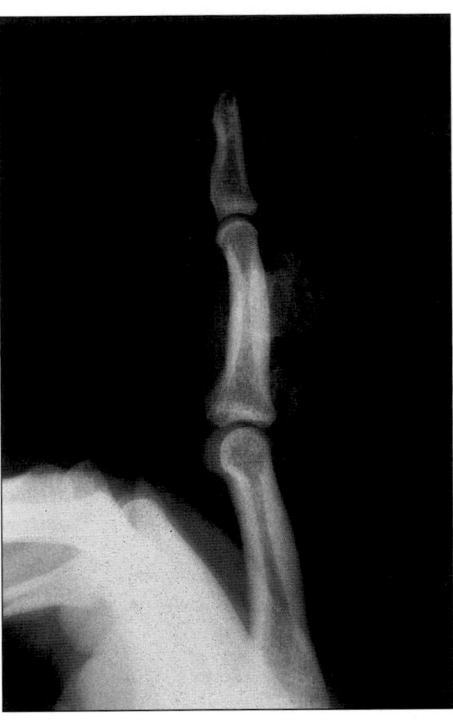

Fig. 14.143 Bizarre parosteal osteochondromatous proliferation. A plain X-ray shows a mushroom shaped mineralized mass on the surface of the phalanx.

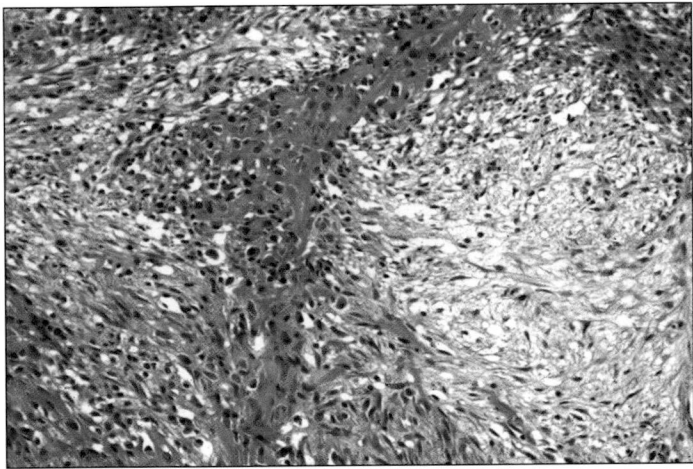

Fig. 14.142 Florid reactive periostitis. Reactive woven bone with prominent osteoblastic rimming surrounded by fibrous tissue.

The complete natural history of florid reactive periostitis is not known because most cases are excised in the early stages of evolution. Nonetheless, it is a self-limiting proliferative process, as those cases that had been known to be present for several years prior to diagnosis did not become particularly large.[572] Florid reactive periostitis behaves in a benign fashion and is usually cured by marginal excision. Recurrence is uncommon, and the few recurrences that have been reported have been successfully treated by re-excision.[575]

BIZARRE PAROSTEAL OSTEOCHONDROMATOUS PROLIFERATION AND SUBUNGUAL EXOSTOSIS

Bizarre parosteal osteochondromatous proliferation, also known as 'Nora's lesion,'[578] and subungual exostosis[580] differ from each other only in their location. Like florid reactive periostitis, they develop from the periosteum, but differ in that they have a nodular or polypoid configuration and a peripheral cap of reactive cellular hyaline cartilage.

First described by Nora in 1983, bizarre parosteal osteochondromatous proliferation typically develops on the surfaces of the short tubular bones of the hands and feet, and approximately 27% arise on long bones.[581] Subungual exostosis originates on the cortex of the distal phalanx beneath or adjacent to the nailbed. Approximately 70–80% involve the great toe, followed by the thumb and index finger.[582] Both types of lesions are diagnosed during adolescence through mid adulthood, with an equal gender distribution.[582–585] Patients with bizarre parosteal osteochondromatous proliferation present complaining of a mass, which has developed during the preceding several months and is painful in a minority of cases. Lesions arising under the nailbed produce an obvious mass that distorts the nail, is frequently painful, and can cause bleeding.[585,586] A documented history of trauma can be elicited in some cases but in most there is no obvious etiology.

Bizarre parosteal osteochondromatous proliferation and subungual exostosis produce a well delineated, pedunculated, nodular, surface-based, radiodense mass.[581–586] The cortex underlying the lesion is intact, unlike osteochondroma (Fig. 14.143). On MRI, the lesions have low signal intensity on T1 weighted and high signal on T2 weighted sequences.[584]

Intact resection specimens reveal bizarre parosteal osteochondromatous proliferation and subungual exostosis to be polypoid, well defined, firm, tan-white masses that range in size from 0.5–2 cm. Most lesions are about 1 cm in dimension and are either loosely or firmly attached to the underlying cortex. The periphery of bizarre parosteal osteochondromatous proliferation and subungual exostosis is defined by periosteum, which overlies the cap of the mass that is composed of hypercellular hyaline cartilage. The chondrocytes are enlarged with plump nuclei and are frequently binucleate. The cartilage undergoes endochondral ossification forming trabeculae of woven bone that are rimmed by prominent osteoblasts that have moderate amounts of amphophilic cytoplasm and round vesicular nuclei that sometimes contain nucleoli (Fig. 14.144). Both the periosteum and intertrabecular areas contain hypercellular fibrous

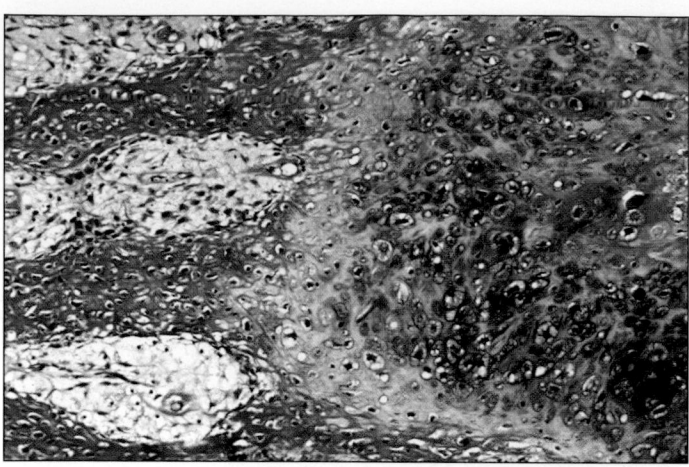

Fig. 14.144 Bizarre parosteal osteochondromatous proliferation. The lesion is composed of reactive cellular cartilage, usually located on the surface, and undergoing endochondral ossification.

tissue. The fibroblasts are arranged in short intersecting fascicles and have ill-defined eosinophilic cytoplasm and elongated nuclei with finely dispersed chromatin. Mitoses may be numerous but are not atypical.

The treatment of bizarre parosteal osteochondromatous proliferation and subungual exostosis is simple excision. Recurrences are commonplace and may develop in 50% of cases and can be adequately treated with re-excision.[578]

REFERENCES

1. Caffy J. On fibrous defects in cortical walls of growing tubular bones: their radiologic appearance, structure, prevalence, natural cause, and diagnostic significance. Ad Pediatr 1955; 7: 13.

2. Sontag LW, Pyle SI. The appearance of nature of cyst like spaces in the distal femoral metaphysis of children. American Journal of Roentgenology 1941; 46: 185.

3. Schmorl G, Junghanns H. The human spine in health and disease. New York: Grune & Stratton; 1971.

4. Unni K. Dahlin's bone tumors. General aspects of data on 11,087 cases, 5th edn. Philadelphia, PA: Lippincott-Raven; 1996.

5. Ries LAG, Kosary CL, Hankey BF, et al. SEER cancer statistics review, 1973–1996. Bethesda, MD: National Cancer Institute.

6. National Cancer Institute. Surveillance, Epidemiology, and End Results (SEER) Program, SEER*Stat database: incidence – SEER 9 regs public-use, 1973–2000. In: National Cancer Institute, DCCPS, Surveillance Research Program, Cancer Statistics Branch. Bethesda, MD: National Cancer Institute; 2003.

7. Dorfman H, Czerniak B, Kotz R, et al. WHO classification of tumours of bone: introduction. In: Fletcher CDM, Unni KK, Mertens F, eds. World Health Organization classification of tumors. Pathology and genetics of tumours of soft tissue and bone. Lyon: IARC Press; 2002.

8. Dorfman HD, Czerniak B. Bone cancers. Cancer 1995; 75(1 Suppl): 203–210.

9. Keel SB, Jaffe KA, Petur Nielsen G, Rosenberg AE. Orthopaedic implant-related sarcoma: a study of twelve cases. Mod Pathol 2001; 14: 969–977.

10. McDonald DJ, Enneking WF, Sundaram M. Metal-associated angiosarcoma of bone: report of two cases and review of the literature. Clin Orthop 2002; 396: 206–214.

11. Costa J, Wesley RA, Glatstein E, Rosenberg SA. The grading of soft tissue sarcomas. Results of a clinicohistopathologic correlation in a series of 163 cases. Cancer 1984; 53: 530–541.

12. Trojani M, Contesso G, Coindre JM, et al. Soft-tissue sarcomas of adults; study of pathological prognostic variables and definition of a histopathological grading system. Int J Cancer 1984; 33: 37–42.

13. Evans HL, Ayala AG, Romsdahl MM. Prognostic factors in chondrosarcoma of bone: a clinicopathologic analysis with emphasis on histologic grading. Cancer 1977; 40: 818–831.

14. Green FL, Page DL, Fleming ID, et al. AJCC cancer staging manual. 6th edn. New York: Springer; 2002.

15. Enneking WF, Spanier SS, Goodman MA. Current concepts review. The surgical staging of musculoskeletal sarcoma. J Bone Joint Surg 1980; 62A: 1027–1030.

16. Sanders TG, Parsons TW III. Radiographic imaging of musculoskeletal neoplasia. Cancer Control 2001; 8: 221–231.

17. Bredella MA, Caputo GR, Steinbach LS. Value of FDG positron emission tomography in conjunction with MR imaging for evaluating therapy response in patients with musculoskeletal sarcomas. AJR 2002; 179: 1145–1150.

18. Bommer KK, Ramzy I, Mody D. Fine-needle aspiration biopsy in the diagnosis and management of bone lesions: a study of 450 cases. Cancer 1997; 81: 148–156.

19. Ottolenghi CE. Diagnosis of orthopaedic lesions by aspiration biopsy. J Bone Joint Surg 1955; 37A: 443–464.

20. Jones C, Liu K, Hirschowitz S, et al. Concordance of histopathologic and cytologic grading in musculoskeletal sarcomas: can grades obtained from analysis of the fine-needle aspirates serve as the basis for therapeutic decisions? Cancer 2002; 96: 83–91.

21. Kilpatrick SE, Cappellari JO, Bos GD, et al. Is fine-needle aspiration biopsy a practical alternative to open biopsy for the primary diagnosis of sarcoma? Experience with 140 patients. Am J Clin Pathol 2001; 115: 59–68.

22. Palmer HE, Mukunyadzi P, Culbreth W, Thomas JR. Subgrouping and grading of soft-tissue sarcomas by fine-needle aspiration cytology: a histopathologic correlation study. Diagn Cytopathol 2001; 24: 307–316.

23. Layfield LJ. Cytopathology of bone and soft tissue tumors. Oxford: Oxford University Press; 2002.

24. Donahoo JS, Miller JA, Lal B, Rosario PG. Chest wall hamartoma in an adult: an unusual chest wall tumor. Thorac Cardiovasc Surg 1996; 44: 110–111.

25. Ayala AG, Ro JY, Bolio-Solis A, et al. Mesenchymal hamartoma of the chest wall in infants and children: a clinicopathological study of five patients. Skeletal Radiol 1993; 22: 569–576.

26. McDermott MB, Ponder TB, Dehner LP. Nasal chondromesenchymal hamartoma: an upper respiratory tract analogue of the chest wall mesenchymal hamartoma. Am J Surg Pathol 1998; 22: 425–433.

27. Carney JA, Boccon-Gibod L, Jarka DE, et al. Osteochondromyxoma of bone: a congenital tumor associated with lentigines and other unusual disorders. Am J Surg Pathol 2001; 25: 164–176.

28. Groom KR, Murphey MD, Howard LM, et al. Mesenchymal hamartoma of the chest wall: radiologic manifestations with emphasis on cross-sectional imaging and histopathologic comparison. Radiology 2002; 222: 205–211.

29. Serrano-Egea A, Santos-Briz A, Garcia-Munoz H, Martinez-Tello FJ. Chest wall hamartoma. Report of two cases with secondary aneurysmal bone cysts. Pathol Res Pract 2001; 197: 835–839.

30. Freeburn AM, McAloon J. Infantile chest hamartoma–case outcome aged 11. Arch Dis Child 2001; 85: 244–245.

31. Porter DE, Simpson AH. The neoplastic pathogenesis of solitary and multiple osteochondromas. J Pathol 1999; 188: 119–125.

32. Schmale GA, Conrad EU III, Raskind WH. The natural history of hereditary multiple exostoses. J Bone Joint Surg 1994; 76A: 986–992.

33. Vanhoenacker FM, Van Hul W, Wuyts W, et al. Hereditary multiple exostoses: from genetics to clinical syndrome and complications. Eur J Radiol 2001; 40: 208–217.

34. Brien EW, Mirra JM, Luck JV Jr. Benign and malignant cartilage tumors of bone and joint: their anatomic and theoretical basis with an emphasis on radiology, pathology and clinical biology. II. Juxtacortical cartilage tumors. Skeletal Radiol 1999; 28(1): 1–20.

35. Delgado E, Rodriguez JI, Rodriguez JL, et al. Osteochondroma induced by reflection of the perichondrial ring in young rat radii. Calcif Tissue Int 1987; 40(2): 85–90.

36. Feely MG, Boehm AK, Bridge RS, et al. Cytogenetic and molecular cytogenetic evidence of recurrent 8q24.1 loss in osteochondroma. Cancer Genet Cytogenet 2002; 137(2): 102–107.

37. Sandberg AA, Bridge JA. Updates on the cytogenetics and molecular genetics of bone and soft tissue tumors: osteosarcoma and related tumors. Cancer Genet Cytogenet 2003; 145(1): 1–30.

38. Taitz J, Cohn RJ, White L, et al. Osteochondroma after total body irradiation: an age-related complication. Pediatr Blood Cancer 2004; 42(3): 225–229.

39. Bottner F, Rodl R, Kordish I, et al. Surgical treatment of symptomatic osteochondroma. A three- to eight-

year follow-up study. J Bone Joint Surg 2003; 85B: 1161–1165.

40. Griffiths HJ, Thompson RC Jr, Galloway HR, et al. Bursitis in association with solitary osteochondromas presenting as mass lesions. Skeletal Radiol 1991; 20: 513–516.

41. Hudson TM, Springfield DS, Spanier SS, et al. Benign exostoses and exostotic chondrosarcomas: evaluation of cartilage thickness by CT. Radiology 1984; 152: 595–599.

42. Lange RH, Lange TA, Rao BK. Correlative radiographic, scintigraphic, and histological evaluation of exostoses. J Bone Joint Surg 1984; 66A: 1454–1459.

43. Ragsdale BD, Sweet DE, Vinh TN. Radiology as gross pathology in evaluating chondroid lesions. Hum Pathol 1989; 20: 930–951.

44. Ahmed AR, Tan TS, Unni KK, et al. Secondary chondrosarcoma in osteochondroma: report of 107 patients. Clin Orthop 2003: 193–206.

45. Park YK, Yang MH, Ryu KN, Chung DW. Dedifferentiated chondrosarcoma arising in an osteochondroma. Skeletal Radiol 1995; 24: 617–619.

46. Kilpatrick SE, Pike EJ, Geisinger KR, Ward WG. Chondroblastoma of bone: use of fine-needle aspiration biopsy and potential diagnostic pitfalls. Diagn Cytopathol 1997; 16(1): 65–71.

47. Dorfman HD, Czerniak B. Bone tumors. St Louis, MO: Mosby; 1998.

48. Jaffe HL. Solitary benign enchondroma of bone. Arch Surg. 1943; 46: 480–490.

49. Buddingh EP, Naumann S, Nelson M, et al. Cytogenetic findings in benign cartilaginous neoplasms. Cancer Genet Cytogenet 2003; 141(2): 164–168.

50. Flemming DJ, Murphey MD. Enchondroma and chondrosarcoma. Semin Musculoskelet Radiol 2000; 4(1): 59–71.

51. Crim JR, Mirra JM. Enchondroma protuberans. Report of a case and its distinction from chondrosarcoma and osteochondroma adjacent to an enchondroma. Skeletal Radiol 1990; 19: 431–434.

52. Tunc M, Ekinci C. Chondrosarcoma diagnosed by fine needle aspiration cytology. Acta Cytol 1996; 40: 283–288.

53. Walaas L, Kindblom LG. Light and electron microscopic examination of fine-needle aspirates in the preoperative diagnosis of osteogenic tumors: a study of 21 osteosarcomas and two osteoblastomas. Diagn Cytopathol 1990; 6(1): 27–38.

54. Marco RA, Gitelis S, Brebach GT, Healey JH. Cartilage tumors: evaluation and treatment. J Am Acad Orthop Surg 2000; 8: 292–304.

55. Bauer HC, Brosjo O, Kreicbergs A, Lindholm J. Low risk of recurrence of enchondroma and low-grade chondrosarcoma in extremities. 80 patients followed for 2–25 years. Acta Orthop Scand 1995; 66: 283–288.

56. Muller PE, Durr HR, Wegener B, et al. Solitary enchondromas: is radiographic follow-up sufficient in patients with asymptomatic lesions? Acta Orthop Belg 2003; 69: 112–118.

57. Ollier L. De la dyschondroplasie. Bull Soc Chir Lyon 1900; 3: 22–24.

58. Liu J, Hudkins PG, Swee RG, Unni KK. Bone sarcomas associated with Ollier's disease. Cancer 1987; 59: 1376–1385.

59. Schwartz HS, Zimmerman NB, Simon MA, et al. The malignant potential of enchondromatosis. J Bone Joint Surg 1987; 69A: 269–274.

60. Cannon SR, Sweetnam DR. Multiple chondrosarcomas in dyschondroplasia (Ollier's disease). Cancer 1985; 55: 836–840.

61. Fanburg JC, Meis-Kindblom JM, Rosenberg AE. Multiple enchondromas associated with spindle-cell hemangioendotheliomas. An overlooked variant of Maffucci's syndrome. Am J Surg Pathol 1995; 19: 1029–1038.

62. Lewis MM, Kenan S, Yabut SM, et al. Periosteal chondroma. A report of ten cases and review of the literature. Clin Orthop 1990; 256: 185–192.

63. Nojima T, Unni KK, McLeod RA, Pritchard DJ. Periosteal chondroma and periosteal chondrosarcoma. Am J Surg Pathol 1985; 9: 666–677.

64. Lichtenstein L, Hall JE. Periosteal chondroma. A distinctive benign cartilage tumor. J Bone Joint Surg 1952; 34A: 691–697.

65. Boriani S, Bacchini P, Bertoni F, Campanacci M. Periosteal chondroma. A review of twenty cases. J Bone Joint Surg 1983; 65A: 205–212.

66. Bauer TW, Dorfman HD, Latham JT Jr. Periosteal chondroma. A clinicopathologic study of 23 cases. Am J Surg Pathol 1982; 6: 631–637.

67. Ramnath RR, Rosenthal DI, Cates J, et al. Intracortical chondroma simulating osteoid osteoma treated by radiofrequency. Skeletal Radiol 2002; 31: 597–602.

68. Jaffe HL, Lichtenstein L. Benign chondroblastoma of bone: a reinterpretation of the so-called calcifying or chondromatous giant cell tumor. Am J Pathol 1942; 18: 969–991.

69. Dahlin DC, Ivins JC. Benign chondroblastoma. A study of 125 cases. Cancer 1972; 30: 401–413.

70. Turcotte RE, Kurt AM, Sim FH, et al. Chondroblastoma. Hum Pathol 1993; 24: 944–949.

71. Kurt AM, Unni KK, Sim FH, McLeod RA. Chondroblastoma of bone. Hum Pathol 1989; 20: 965–976.

72. Varvares MA, Cheney ML, Goodman ML, et al. Chondroblastoma of the temporal bone. Case report and literature review. Ann Otol Rhinol Laryngol 1992; 101: 763–769.

73. Ilaslan H, Sundaram M, Unni KK. Vertebral chondroblastoma. Skeletal Radiol 2003; 32: 66–71.

74. Ramappa AJ, Lee FY, Tang P, et al. Chondroblastoma of bone. J Bone Joint Surg 2000; 82A: 1140–1145.

75. Bridge JA, Bhatia PS, Anderson JR, Neff JR. Biologic and clinical significance of cytogenetic and molecular cytogenetic abnormalities in benign and malignant cartilaginous lesions. Cancer Genet Cytogenet 1993; 69(2): 79–90.

76. Mark J, Wedell B, Dahlenfors R, et al. Human benign chondroblastoma with a pseudodiploid stemline characterized by a complex and balanced translocation. Cancer Genet Cytogenet 1992; 58(1): 14–17.

77. Brien EW, Mirra JM, Kerr R. Benign and malignant cartilage tumors of bone and joint: their anatomic and theoretical basis with an emphasis on radiology, pathology and clinical biology. I. The intramedullary cartilage tumors. Skeletal Radiol 1997; 26: 325–353.

78. Aigner T, Loos S, Inwards C, et al. Chondroblastoma is an osteoid-forming, but not cartilage-forming neoplasm. J Pathol 1999; 189: 463–469.

79. Huang L, Cheng YY, Chow LT, et al. Receptor activator of NF-kappaB ligand (RANKL) is expressed in chondroblastoma: possible involvement in osteoclastic giant cell recruitment. Mol Pathol 2003; 56: 116–120.

80. Pohar-Marinsek Z, Us-Krasovec M, Lamovec J. Chondroblastoma in fine needle aspirates. Acta Cytol 1992; 36: 367–370.

81. Jain M, Kaur M, Kapoor S, Arora DS. Cytological features of chondroblastoma: a case report with review of the literature. Diagn Cytopathol 2000; 23: 348–350.

82. Povysil C, Tomanova R, Matejovsky Z. Muscle-specific actin expression in chondroblastomas. Hum Pathol 1997; 28: 316–320.

83. Edel G, Ueda Y, Nakanishi J, et al. Chondroblastoma of bone. A clinical, radiological, light and immunohistochemical study. Virchows Arch A Pathol Anat Histopathol 1992; 421: 355–366.

84. Erickson JK, Rosenthal DI, Zaleske DJ, et al. Primary treatment of chondroblastoma with percutaneous radio-frequency heat ablation: report of three cases. Radiology 2001; 221: 463–468.

85. Springfield DS, Capanna R, Gherlinzoni F, et al. Chondroblastoma. A review of seventy cases. J Bone Joint Surg 1985; 67A: 748–755.

86. Green P, Whittaker RP. Benign chondroblastoma. Case report with pulmonary metastasis. J Bone Joint Surg 1975; 57A: 418–420.

87. Riddell RJ, Louis CJ, Bromberger NA. Pulmonary metastases from chondroblastoma of the tibia. Report of a case. J Bone Joint Surg 1973; 55B: 848–853.

88. Wirman JA, Crissman JD, Aron BF. Metastatic chondroblastoma: report of an unusual case treated with radiotherapy. Cancer 1979; 44: 87–93.

89. Kyriakos M, Land VJ, Penning HL, Parker SG. Metastatic chondroblastoma. Report of a fatal case with a review of the literature on atypical, aggressive, and malignant chondroblastoma. Cancer 1985; 55: 1770–1789.

90. Wu CT, Inwards CY, O'Laughlin S, et al. Chondromyxoid fibroma of bone: a clinicopathologic review of 278 cases. Hum Pathol 1998; 29: 438–446.

91. Jaffe HL, Lichtenstein L. Chondromyxoid fibroma of bone. A distinctive benign tumor likely to be mistaken especially for chondrosarcoma. Arch Pathol 1948; 45: 541–551.

92. Zillmer DA, Dorfman HD. Chondromyxoid fibroma of bone: thirty-six cases with clinicopathologic correlation. Hum Pathol 1989; 20: 952–964.

93. Granter SR, Renshaw AA, Kozakewich HP, Fletcher JA. The pericentromeric inversion, inv (6)(p25q13), is a novel diagnostic marker in chondromyxoid fibroma. Mod Pathol 1998; 11: 1071–1074.

94. Dahlin DC. Chondromyxoid fibroma of bone, with emphasis on its morphological relationship to benign chondroblastoma. Cancer 1956; 9: 195–203.

95. Bahk WJ, Mirra JM, Sohn KR, Shin DS. Pseudoanaplastic chondromyxoid fibroma. Ann Diagn Pathol 1998; 2: 241–246.

96. Gupta S, Dev G, Marya S. Chondromyxoid fibroma: a fine-needle aspiration diagnosis. Diagn Cytopathol 1993; 9: 63–65.

97. Nielsen GP, Keel SB, Dickersin GR, et al. Chondromyxoid fibroma: a tumor showing myofibroblastic, myochondroblastic, and chondrocytic differentiation. Mod Pathol 1999; 12: 514–517.

98. Soder S, Inwards C, Muller S, et al. Cell biology and matrix biochemistry of chondromyxoid fibroma. Am J Clin Pathol 2001; 116: 271–277.

99. Rubin BP, Fletcher JA. Skeletal and extraskeletal myxoid chondrosarcoma: related or distinct tumors? Adv Anat Pathol 1999; 6: 204–212.

100. Lee FY, Mankin HJ, Fondren G, et al. Chondrosarcoma of bone: an assessment of outcome. J Bone Joint Surg 1999; 81A: 326–338.

101. Rizzo M, Ghert MA, Harrelson JM, Scully SP. Chondrosarcoma of bone: analysis of 108 cases and evaluation for predictors of outcome. Clin Orthop 2001: 224–233.

102. Fiorenza F, Abudu A, Grimer RJ, et al. Risk factors for survival and local control in chondrosarcoma of bone. J Bone Joint Surg 2002; 84B: 493–499.

103. Ogose A, Unni KK, Swee RG, et al. Chondrosarcoma of small bones of the hands and feet. Cancer 1997; 80: 50–59.

104. Rosenberg AE, Nielsen GP, Keel SB, et al. Chondrosarcoma of the base of the skull: a clinicopathologic study of 200 cases with emphasis on its distinction from chordoma. Am J Surg Pathol 1999; 23: 1370–1378.

105. Welkerling H, Kratz S, Ewerbeck V, Delling G. A reproducible and simple grading system for classical chondrosarcomas. Analysis of 35 chondrosarcomas and 16 enchondromas with emphasis on recurrence rate and radiological and clinical data. Virchows Arch 2003; 443: 725–733.

106. Mankin HJ, Lange TA, Spanier SS. The hazards of biopsy in patients with malignant primary bone and soft-tissue tumors. J Bone Joint Surg 1982; 64A: 1121–1127.

107. Sanerkin NG. The diagnosis and grading of chondrosarcoma of bone: a combined cytologic and histologic approach. Cancer 1980; 45: 582–594.

108. Reith JD, Horodyski MB, Scarborough MT. Grade 2 chondrosarcoma: stage I or stage II tumor? Clin Orthop 2003: 45–51.

109. Bjornsson J, McLeod RA, Unni KK, et al. Primary chondrosarcoma of long bones and limb girdles. Cancer 1998; 83: 2105–2119.

110. Lerma E, Tani E, Brosjo O, et al. Diagnosis and grading of chondrosarcomas on FNA biopsy material. Diagn Cytopathol 2003; 28(1): 13–17.

111. Olszewski W, Woyke S, Musiatowicz B. Fine needle aspiration biopsy cytology of chondrosarcoma. Acta Cytol 1983; 27: 345–349.

112. Kumar RV, Hazarika D, Mathews T, et al. Fine needle aspiration biopsy cytology of chondrosarcoma. Indian J Pathol Microbiol 1993; 36: 436–441.

113. Abdul-Karim FW, Wasman JK, Pitlik D. Needle aspiration cytology of chondrosarcomas. Acta Cytol 1993; 37: 655–660.

114. Pring ME, Weber KL, Unni KK, Sim FH. Chondrosarcoma of the pelvis. A review of sixty-four cases. J Bone Joint Surg 2001; 83A: 1630–1642.

115. Vanel D, De Paolis M, Monti C, et al. Radiological features of 24 periosteal chondrosarcomas. Skeletal Radiol 2001; 30: 208–212.

116. Papagelopoulos PJ, Galanis EC, Boscainos PJ, et al. Periosteal chondrosarcoma. Orthopedics 2002; 25: 839–842.

117. Robinson P, White LM, Sundaram M, et al. Periosteal chondroid tumors: radiologic evaluation with pathologic correlation. AJR 2001; 177: 1183–1188.

118. Inoue YZ, Frassica FJ, Sim FH, et al. Clinicopathologic features and treatment of postirradiation sarcoma of bone and soft tissue. J Surg Oncol 2000; 75(1): 42–50.

119. Megas PD, Panagopoulos AM, Tsamandas AC, Lambiris EE. Femoral chondrosarcoma complicating Paget's disease of bone. Orthopedics 2004; 27(1): 63–64.

120. Wicklund CL, Pauli RM, Johnston D, Hecht JT. Natural history study of hereditary multiple exostoses. Am J Med Genet 1995; 55(1): 43–46.

121. Pierz KA, Stieber JR, Kusumi K, Dormans JP. Hereditary multiple exostoses: one center's experience and review of etiology. Clin Orthop 2002(401): 49–59.

122. Wuisman PI, Jutte PC, Ozaki T. Secondary chondrosarcoma in osteochondromas. Medullary extension in 15 of 45 cases. Acta Orthop Scand 1997; 68: 396–400.

123. Bovee JV, Cleton-Jansen AM, Rosenberg C, et al. Molecular genetic characterization of both components of a dedifferentiated chondrosarcoma, with implications for its histogenesis. J Pathol 1999; 189: 454–462.

124. Astorino RN, Tesluk H. Dedifferentiated chondrosarcoma with a rhabdomyosarcomatous component. Hum Pathol 1985; 16: 318–320.

125. Johnson S, Tetu B, Ayala AG, Chawla SP. Chondrosarcoma with additional mesenchymal component (dedifferentiated chondrosarcoma). I. A clinicopathologic study of 26 cases. Cancer 1986; 58: 278–286.

126. Niezabitowski A, Edel G, Roessner A, et al. Rhabdomyosarcomatous component in dedifferentiated chondrosarcoma. Pathol Res Pract 1987; 182: 275–282.

127. Munk PL, Connell DG, Quenville NF. Dedifferentiated chondrosarcoma of bone with leiomyosarcomatous mesenchymal component: a case report. Can Assoc Radiol J 1988; 39: 218–220.

128. Reith JD, Bauer TW, Fischler DF, et al. Dedifferentiated chondrosarcoma with rhabdomyosarcomatous differentiation. Am J Surg Pathol 1996; 20: 293–298.

129. Estrada EG, Ayala AG, Lewis V, et al. Dedifferentiated chondrosarcoma with a noncartilaginous component

130. Dervan PA, O'Loughlin J, Hurson BJ. Dedifferentiated chondrosarcoma with muscle and cytokeratin differentiation in the anaplastic component. Histopathology 1988; 12: 517–526.

131. Lichtenstein L, Bernstein D. Unusual benign and malignant chondroid tumors of bone: A survey of some mesenchymal cartilage tumors and malignant chondroblastic tumors, including a few multicentric ones, as well as many atypical benign chondroblastomas and chondromyxoid fibromas. Cancer 1959; 12: 1142–1157.

132. Huvos AG, Rosen G, Dabska M, Marcove RC. Mesenchymal chondrosarcoma. A clinicopathologic analysis of 35 patients with emphasis on treatment. Cancer 1983; 51: 1230–1237.

133. Nakashima Y, Unni KK, Shives TC, et al. Mesenchymal chondrosarcoma of bone and soft tissue. A review of 111 cases. Cancer 1986; 57: 2444–2453.

134. Salvador AH, Beabout JW, Dahlin DC. Mesenchymal chondrosarcoma–observations on 30 new cases. Cancer 1971; 28: 605–615.

135. Wehrli BM, Huang W, De Crombrugghe B, et al. Sox9, a master regulator of chondrogenesis, distinguishes mesenchymal chondrosarcoma from other small blue round cell tumors. Hum Pathol 2003; 34: 263–269.

136. Naumann S, Krallman PA, Unni KK, et al. Translocation der(13; 21)(q10; q10) in skeletal and extraskeletal mesenchymal chondrosarcoma. Mod Pathol 2002; 15: 572–576.

137. Vencio EF, Reeve CM, Unni KK, Nascimento AG. Mesenchymal chondrosarcoma of the jaw bones: clinicopathologic study of 19 cases. Cancer 1998; 82: 2350–2355.

138. Unni KK, Dahlin DC, Beabout JW, Sim FH. Chondrosarcoma: clear-cell variant. A report of sixteen cases. J Bone Joint Surg 1976; 58A: 676–683.

139. Present D, Bacchini P, Pignatti G, et al. Clear cell chondrosarcoma of bone. A report of 8 cases. Skeletal Radiol 1991; 20: 187–191.

140. Bjornsson J, Unni KK, Dahlin DC, et al. Clear cell chondrosarcoma of bone. Observations in 47 cases. Am J Surg Pathol 1984; 8: 223–230.

141. Kalil RK, Inwards CY, Unni KK, et al. Dedifferentiated clear cell chondrosarcoma. Am J Surg Pathol 2000; 24: 1079–1086.

142. Le Charpentier Y, Forest M, Postel M, et al. Clear-cell chondrosarcoma: a report of five cases including ultrastructural study. Cancer 1979; 44: 622–629.

143. Angervall L, Kindblom LG. Clear-cell chondrosarcoma. A light- and electron-microscopic and histochemical study of two cases. Virchows Arch A Pathol Anat Histol 1980; 389(1): 27–41.

144. Onitsuka H. Roentgenologic aspects of bone islands. Radiology 1977; 123: 607–612.

145. Greenspan A. Bone island (enostosis): current concept – a review. Skeletal Radiol 1995; 24: 111–115.

146. Greenspan A, Steiner G, Knutzon R. Bone island (enostosis): clinical significance and radiologic and pathologic correlations. Skeletal Radiol 1991; 20: 85–90.

147. White LM, Kandel R. Osteoid-producing tumors of bone. Semin Musculoskelet Radiol 2000; 4: 25–43.

148. Trombetti A, Noel E. Giant bone islands: a case with 31 years of follow-up. Joint Bone Spine 2002; 69(1): 81–84.

149. Benli IT, Akalin S, Boysan E, et al. Epidemiological, clinical and radiological aspects of osteopoikilosis. J Bone Joint Surg 1992; 74B: 504–506.

150. Haddad FS, Haddad GF, Zaatari G. Cranial osteomas: their classification and management. Report on a giant osteoma and review of the literature. Surg Neurol 1997; 48: 143–147.

151. Bertoni F, Unni KK, Beabout JW, Sim FH. Parosteal osteoma of bones other than of the skull and face. Cancer 1995; 75: 2466–2473.

152. Smith ME, Calcaterra TC. Frontal sinus osteoma. Ann Otol Rhinol Laryngol 1989; 98: 896–900.

153. Fechner RE, Mills SE. Tumors of the bone and joints. Washington, DC: Armed Forces Institute of Pathology; 1993.

154. Fu YS, Perzin KH. Non-epithelial tumors of the nasal cavity, paranasal sinuses, and nasopharynx. A clinicopathologic study. II. Osseous and fibro-osseous lesions, including osteoma, fibrous dysplasia, ossifying fibroma, osteoblastoma, giant cell tumor, and osteosarcoma. Cancer 1974; 33: 1289–1305.

155. Greenspan A. Benign bone-forming lesions: osteoma, osteoid osteoma, and osteoblastoma. Clinical, imaging, pathologic, and differential considerations. Skeletal Radiol 1993; 22: 485–500.

156. Whittet HB, Quiney RE. Middle turbinate osteoma; an unusual cause of nasal obstruction. J Laryngol Otol 1988; 102: 359–361.

157. Wilkes SR, Trautmann JC, DeSanto LW, Campbell RJ. Osteoma: an unusual cause of amaurosis fugax. Mayo Clin Proc 1979; 54: 258–260.

158. Schajowicz F, Lemos C. Osteoid osteoma and osteoblastoma. Closely related entities of osteoblastic derivation. Acta Orthop Scand 1970; 41: 272–291.

159. Byers PD. Solitary benign osteoblastic lesions of bone. Osteoid osteoma and benign osteoblastoma. Cancer 1968; 22: 43–57.

160. Jackson RP, Reckling FW, Mants FA. Osteoid osteoma and osteoblastoma. Similar histologic lesions with different natural histories. Clin Orthop 1977; 128: 303–313.

161. Gitelis S, Schajowicz F. Osteoid osteoma and osteoblastoma. Orthop Clin North Am 1989; 20: 313–325.

162. Kattapuram SV, Kushner DC, Phillips WC, Rosenthal DI. Osteoid osteoma: an unusual cause of articular pain. Radiology 1983; 147: 383–387.

163. Kawaguchi Y, Sato C, Hasegawa T, et al. Intraarticular osteoid osteoma associated with synovitis: a possible role of cyclooxygenase-2 expression by osteoblasts in the nidus. Mod Pathol 2000; 13: 1086–1091.

164. Greco F, Tamburrelli F, Ciabattoni G. Prostaglandins in osteoid osteoma. Int Orthop 1991; 15(1): 35–37.

165. Mungo DV, Zhang X, O'Keefe RJ, et al. COX-1 and COX-2 expression in osteoid osteomas. J Orthop Res 2002; 20(1): 159–162.

166. Crofford LJ. COX-1 and COX-2 tissue expression: implications and predictions. J Rheumatol 1997; 24(Suppl 49): 15–19.

167. Baruffi MR, Volpon JB, Neto JB, Casartelli C. Osteoid osteomas with chromosome alterations involving 22q. Cancer Genet Cytogenet 2001; 124(2): 127–131.

168. Torriani M, Rosenthal DI. Percutaneous radiofrequency treatment of osteoid osteoma. Pediatr Radiol 2002; 32: 615–618.

169. Rosenthal DI, Alexander A, Rosenberg AE, Springfield D. Ablation of osteoid osteomas with a percutaneously placed electrode: a new procedure. Radiology 1992; 183: 29–33.

170. Rosenthal DI, Springfield DS, Gebhardt MC, et al. Osteoid osteoma: percutaneous radio-frequency ablation. Radiology 1995; 197: 451–454.

171. Rosenthal DI, Hornicek FJ, Wolfe MW, et al. Decreasing length of hospital stay in treatment of osteoid osteoma. Clin Orthop 1999; 361: 186–191.

172. Rosenthal DI, Hornicek FJ, Wolfe MW, et al. Percutaneous radiofrequency coagulation of osteoid osteoma compared with operative treatment. J Bone Joint Surg 1998; 80A: 815–821.

173. Rosenthal DI. Percutaneous radiofrequency treatment of osteoid osteomas. Semin Musculoskelet Radiol 1997; 1: 265–272.

174. Lucas DR, Unni KK, McLeod RA, et al. Osteoblastoma: clinicopathologic study of 306 cases. Hum Pathol 1994; 25: 117–134.

175. Marsh BW, Bonfiglio M, Brady LP, Enneking WF. Benign osteoblastoma: range of manifestations. J Bone Joint Surg 1975; 57A: 1–9.

176. Della Rocca C, Huvos AG. Osteoblastoma: varied histological presentations with a benign clinical course. An analysis of 55 cases. Am J Surg Pathol 1996; 20: 841–850.

177. Bertoni F, Unni KK, Lucas DR, McLeod RA. Osteoblastoma with cartilaginous matrix. An unusual morphologic presentation in 18 cases. Am J Surg Pathol 1993; 17: 69–74.

178. Dorfman HD, Weiss SW. Borderline osteoblastic tumors: problems in the differential diagnosis of aggressive osteoblastoma and low-grade osteosarcoma. Semin Diagn Pathol 1984; 1: 215–234.

179. Klein MJ, Kenan S, Lewis MM. Osteosarcoma. Clinical and pathological considerations. Orthop Clin North Am 1989; 20: 327–345.

180. Bertoni F, Bacchini P. Classification of bone tumors. Eur J Radiol 1998; 27(Suppl 1): S74–76.

181. Unni KK, Dahlin DC. Grading of bone tumors. Semin Diagn Pathol 1984; 1: 165–172.

182. Unni KK. Osteosarcoma of bone. J Orthop Sci 1998; 3: 287–294.

183. Unni KK, Dahlin DC. Osteosarcoma: pathology and classification. Semin Roentgenol 1989; 24: 143–152.

184. Ragland BD, Bell WC, Lopez RR, Siegal GP. Cytogenetics and molecular biology of osteosarcoma. Lab Invest 2002; 82: 365–373.

185. Fuchs B, Pritchard DJ. Etiology of osteosarcoma. Clin Orthop 2002; 397: 40–52.

186. Fry SA. Studies of US radium dial workers: an epidemiological classic. Radiat Res 1998; 150(5 Suppl): S21–S29.

187. Ron E. Cancer risks from medical radiation. Health Phys 2003; 85: 47–59.

188. Huvos AG, Woodard HQ. Postradiation sarcomas of bone. Health Phys 1988; 55(4): 631–636.

189. Huvos AG, Butler A, Bretsky SS. Osteogenic sarcoma associated with Paget's disease of bone. A clinicopathologic study of 65 patients. Cancer 1983; 52: 1489–1495.

190. Kitao S, Shimamoto A, Goto M, et al. Mutations in RECQL4 cause a subset of cases of Rothmund–Thomson syndrome. Nat Genet 1999; 22(1): 82–84.

191. Bridge JA, Nelson M, McComb E, et al. Cytogenetic findings in 73 osteosarcoma specimens and a review of the literature. Cancer Genet Cytogenet 1997; 95(1): 74–87.

192. Boehm AK, Neff JR, Squire JA, et al. Cytogenetic findings in 36 osteosarcoma specimens and a review of the literature. Ped Pathol Mol Med 2000; 19: 359–375.

193. Szymanska J, Mandahl N, Mertens F, et al. Ring chromosomes in parosteal osteosarcoma contain sequences from 12q13–15: a combined cytogenetic and comparative genomic hybridization study. Genes Chromosomes Cancer 1996; 16(1): 31–34.

194. Klein RM, Norman A. Diagnostic procedures for Paget's disease. Radiologic, pathologic, and laboratory testing. Endocrinol Metab Clin North Am 1995; 24: 437–450.

195. Nellissery MJ, Padalecki SS, Brkanac Z, et al. Evidence for a novel osteosarcoma tumor-suppressor gene in the chromosome 18 region genetically linked with Paget disease of bone. Am J Hum Genet 1998; 63: 817–824.

196. Bacci G, Ferrari S, Longhi A, et al. High-grade osteosarcoma of the extremity: differences between localized and metastatic tumors at presentation. J Pediatr Hematol Oncol 2002; 24: 27–30.

197. Rosenberg ZS, Lev S, Schmahmann S, et al. Osteosarcoma: subtle, rare, and misleading plain film features. AJR 1995; 165: 1209–1214.

198. Saifuddin A. The accuracy of imaging in the local staging of appendicular osteosarcoma. Skeletal Radiol 2002; 31: 191–201.

199. Seeger LL, Gold RH, Chandnani VP. Diagnostic imaging of osteosarcoma. Clin Orthop 1991; 270: 254–263.

200. Raymond AK, Simms W, Ayala AG. Osteosarcoma. Specimen management following primary chemotherapy. Hematol Oncol Clin North Am 1995; 9: 841–867.

201. Springfield DS, Schakel ME Jr, Spanier SS. Spontaneous necrosis in osteosarcoma. Clin Orthop 1991; 263: 233–237.

202. Unni KK, Dahlin DC, Beabout JW, Ivins JC. Parosteal osteogenic sarcoma. Cancer 1976; 37: 2466–2475.

203. Okada K, Frassica FJ, Sim FH, et al. Parosteal osteosarcoma. A clinicopathological study. J Bone Joint Surg 1994; 76A: 366–378.

204. Antonescu CR, Huvos AG. Low-grade osteogenic sarcoma arising in medullary and surface osseous locations. Am J Clin Pathol 2000; 114(Suppl): S90–S103.

205. Campanacci M, Giunti A. Periosteal osteosarcoma. Review of 41 cases, 22 with long-term follow-up. Ital J Orthop Traumatol 1976; 2: 23–35.

206. Hall RB, Robinson LH, Malawar MM, Dunham WK. Periosteal osteosarcoma. Cancer 1985; 55: 165–171.

207. Ritts GD, Pritchard DJ, Unni KK, et al. Periosteal osteosarcoma. Clin Orthop 1987; 219: 299–307.

208. Wold LE, Unni KK, Beabout JW, Pritchard DJ. High-grade surface osteosarcomas. Am J Surg Pathol 1984; 8: 181–186.

209. Okada K, Unni KK, Swee RG, Sim FH. High grade surface osteosarcoma: a clinicopathologic study of 46 cases. Cancer 1999; 85: 1044–1054.

210. Unni KK, Dahlin DC, McLeod RA, Pritchard DJ. Intraosseous well-differentiated osteosarcoma. Cancer 1977; 40: 1337–1347.

211. Kurt AM, Unni KK, McLeod RA, Pritchard DJ. Low-grade intraosseous osteosarcoma. Cancer 1990; 65: 1418–1428.

212. Bertoni F, Bacchini P, Fabbri N, et al. Osteosarcoma. Low-grade intraosseous-type osteosarcoma, histologically resembling parosteal osteosarcoma, fibrous dysplasia, and desmoplastic fibroma. Cancer 1993; 71: 338–345.

213. Choong PF, Pritchard DJ, Rock MG, et al. Low grade central osteogenic sarcoma. A long-term followup of 20 patients. Clin Orthop 1996; 322: 198–206.

214. Matsuno T, Unni KK, McLeod RA, Dahlin DC. Telangiectatic osteogenic sarcoma. Cancer 1976; 38: 2538–2547.

215. Huvos AG, Rosen G, Bretsky SS, Butler A. Telangiectatic osteogenic sarcoma: a clinicopathologic study of 124 patients. Cancer 1982; 49: 1679–1689.

216. Murphey MD, wan Jaovisidha S, Temple HT, et al. Telangiectatic osteosarcoma: radiologic-pathologic comparison. Radiology 2003; 229: 545–553.

217. Sim FH, Unni KK, Beabout JW, Dahlin DC. Osteosarcoma with small cells simulating Ewing's tumor. J Bone Joint Surg 1979; 61A: 207–215.

218. Ayala AG, Ro JY, Raymond AK, et al. Small cell osteosarcoma. A clinicopathologic study of 27 cases. Cancer 1989; 64: 2162–2173.

219. Dickersin GR, Rosenberg AE. The ultrastructure of small-cell osteosarcoma, with a review of the light microscopy and differential diagnosis. Hum Pathol 1991; 22: 267–275.

220. Devaney K, Vinh TN, Sweet DE. Small cell osteosarcoma of bone: an immunohistochemical study with differential diagnostic considerations. Hum Pathol 1993; 24: 1211–1225.

221. Bertoni F, Bacchini P, Staals EL. Giant cell-rich osteosarcoma. Orthopedics 2003; 26: 179–181.

222. Hasegawa T, Shibata T, Hirose T, et al. Osteosarcoma with epithelioid features. An immunohistochemical study. Arch Pathol Lab Med 1993; 117: 295–298.

223. Yoshida H, Yumoto T, Adachi H, et al. Osteosarcoma with prominent epithelioid features. Acta Pathol Jpn 1989; 39: 439–445.

224. Grimer RJ, Cannon SR, Taminiau AM, et al. Osteosarcoma over the age of forty. Eur J Cancer 2003; 39: 157–163.

225. Bertoni F, Unni KK, McLeod RA, Dahlin DC. Osteosarcoma resembling osteoblastoma. Cancer 1985; 55: 416–426.

226. Bertoni F, Bacchini P, Donati D, et al. Osteoblastoma-like osteosarcoma. The Rizzoli Institute experience. Mod Pathol 1993; 6: 707–716.

227. Wold LE, Unni KK, Beabout JW, et al. Dedifferentiated parosteal osteosarcoma. J Bone Joint Surg 1984; 66A: 53–59.

228. Pintado SO, Lane J, Huvos AG. Parosteal osteogenic sarcoma of bone with coexistent low- and high-grade sarcomatous components. Hum Pathol 1989; 20: 488–491.

229. Sheth DS, Yasko AW, Raymond AK, et al. Conventional and dedifferentiated parosteal osteosarcoma. Diagnosis, treatment, and outcome. Cancer 1996; 78: 2136–2145.

230. Peng XJ, Yan XC. Cytodiagnosis of bone tumors by fine needle aspiration. Acta Cytol 1985; 29: 570–575.

231. Wilkerson JA, Crowell WT. Intraoperative cytology of osseous lesions. Diagn Cytopathol 1986; 2(1): 5–12.

232. White VA, Fanning CV, Ayala AG, et al. Osteosarcoma and the role of fine-needle aspiration. A study of 51 cases. Cancer 1988; 62: 1238–1246.

233. Ellison DA, Silverman JF, Strausbach PS, Joshi VV. Fine-needle aspiration of chondroblastic osteosarcoma of the skull: report of a case in an 11-year-old girl. Diagn Cytopathol 1996; 14: 51–55.

234. Okada K, Hasegawa T, Yokoyama R. Rosette-forming epithelioid osteosarcoma: a histologic subtype with highly aggressive clinical behavior. Hum Pathol 2001; 32: 726–733.

235. Fanburg JC, Rosenberg AE, Weaver DL, et al. Osteocalcin and osteonectin immunoreactivity in the diagnosis of osteosarcoma. Am J Clin Pathol 1997; 108: 464–473.

236. Okada K, Hasegawa T, Yokoyama R, et al. Osteosarcoma with cytokeratin expression: a clinicopathological study of six cases with an emphasis on differential diagnosis from metastatic cancer. J Clin Pathol 2003; 56: 742–746.

237. Ferguson WS, Goorin AM. Current treatment of osteosarcoma. Cancer Invest 2001; 19: 292–315.

238. Bacci G, Bertoni F, Longhi A, et al. Neoadjuvant chemotherapy for high-grade central osteosarcoma of the extremity. Histologic response to preoperative chemotherapy correlates with histologic subtype of the tumor. Cancer 2003; 97: 3068–3075.

239. Bielack SS, Kempf-Bielack B, Delling G, et al. Prognostic factors in high-grade osteosarcoma of the extremities or trunk: an analysis of 1,702 patients treated on neoadjuvant cooperative osteosarcoma study group protocols. J Clin Oncol 2002; 20: 776–790.

240. Huvos. Bone tumors: diagnosis, treatment and prognosis. Philadelphia, PA: WB Saunders; 1991: 179–200.

241. Picci P, Bacci G, Campanacci M, et al. Histologic evaluation of necrosis in osteosarcoma induced by chemotherapy. Regional mapping of viable and nonviable tumor. Cancer 1985; 56: 1515–1521.

242. Hauben EI, Weeden S, Pringle J, et al. Does the histological subtype of high-grade central osteosarcoma influence the response to treatment with chemotherapy and does it affect overall survival? A study on 570 patients of two consecutive trials of the European Osteosarcoma Intergroup. Eur J Cancer 2002; 38: 1218–1225.

243. Frassica FJ, Sim FH, Frassica DA, Wold LE. Survival and management considerations in postirradiation osteosarcoma and Paget's osteosarcoma. Clin Orthop 1991, 270. 120–127.

244. Temple HT, Scully SP, O'Keefe RJ, et al. Clinical outcome of 38 patients with juxtacortical osteosarcoma. Clin Orthop 2000; 373: 208–217.

245. Chung EB, Enzinger FM. Infantile myofibromatosis. Cancer 1981; 48: 1807–1818.

246. Soper JR, De Silva M. Infantile myofibromatosis: a radiological review. Pediatr Radiol 1993; 23: 189–194.

247. Johnson GL, Baisden BL, Fishman EK. Infantile myofibromatosis. Skeletal Radiol 1997; 26: 611–614.

248. Foss RD, Ellis GL. Myofibromas and myofibromatosis of the oral region: A clinicopathologic analysis of 79 cases. Oral Surg Oral Med Oral Pathol Oral Radiol Endod 2000; 89(1): 57–65.

249. Inwards CY, Unni KK, Beabout JW, Shives TC. Solitary congenital fibromatosis (infantile myofibromatosis) of bone. Am J Surg Pathol 1991; 15: 935–941.

250. Chateil JF, Brun M, Lebail B, et al. Infantile myofibromatosis. Skeletal Radiol 1995; 24: 629–632.

251. Hasegawa T, Hirose T, Seki K, et al. Solitary infantile myofibromatosis of bone. An immunohistochemical and ultrastructural study. Am J Surg Pathol 1993; 17: 308–313.

252. Jaffe HL. Tumors and tumorous conditions of the bones and joints. Philadelphia, PA: Lea & Febiger; 1958.

253. Arata MA, Peterson HA, Dahlin DC. Pathological fractures through non-ossifying fibromas. Review of the Mayo Clinic experience. J Bone Joint Surg 1981; 63A: 980–988.

254. Drennan DB, Maylahn DJ, Fahey JJ. Fractures through large non-ossifying fibromas. Clin Orthop 1974; 0(103): 82–88.

255. Sanerkin NG, Jeffree GM. Cytology of bone tumors. A colour atlas with text. Philadelphia, PA: JB Lippincott; 1980.

256. Gnepp DR. Pathology of the head and neck. New York: Churchill Livingstone; 1988.

257. Hopkins KM, Huttula CS, Kahn MA, Albright JE. Desmoplastic fibroma of the mandible: review and report of two cases. J Oral Maxillofac Surg 1996; 54: 1249–1254.

258. Nussbaum GB, Terz JJ, Joy ED Jr. Desmoplastic fibroma of the mandible in a 3-year-old child. J Oral Surg 1976; 34: 1117–1121.

259. Taguchi N, Kaneda T. Desmoplastic fibroma of the mandible: report of case. J Oral Surg 1980; 38: 441–444.

260. George DI Jr, Gould AR, Miller RL, Strull NJ. Desmoplastic fibroma of the maxilla. J Oral Maxillofac Surg 1985; 43: 718–725.

261. Goldberg AN, Janecka IP, Sekhar LN. Desmoplastic fibroma of the skull: a case report. Otolaryngol Head Neck Surg 1995; 112: 589–591.

262. Inwards CY, Unni KK, Beabout JW, Sim FH. Desmoplastic fibroma of bone. Cancer 1991; 68: 1978–1983.

263. Yokoyama R, Tsuneyoshi M, Enjoji M, Hashimoto H. Extra-abdominal desmoid tumors: correlations between histologic features and biologic behavior. Surg Pathol 1989; 2: 29–42.

264. Raab SS, Silverman JF, McLeod DL, et al. Fine needle aspiration biopsy of fibromatoses. Acta Cytol 1993; 37: 323–328.

265. McLeod DL, Geisinger KR, Hopkins BM III, Silverman JF. Fine needle aspiration cytology of the fibromatoses: a clinical and cytopathologic assessment. Acta Cytol 1987; 31: 683.

266. Pettinato G, Manivel JC, Petrella G, Jassim AD. Fine needle aspiration cytology, immunocytochemistry and electron microscopy of fibromatosis of the breast: report of two cases. Acta Cytol 1991; 35: 403–408.

267. El-Naggar A, Abdul-Karim FW, Marshalleck JJ, Sorensen K. Fine-needle aspiration of fibromatosis of the breast. Diagn Cytopathol 1987; 3: 320–322.

268. Tani EM, Stanley MW, Skoog L. Fine-needle aspiration cytology presentation of bilateral mammary fibromatosis. Report of a case. Acta Cytol 1988; 32: 555–558.

269. Zaharopoulos P, Wong JY. Fine-needle aspiration cytology in fibromatoses. Diagn Cytopathol 1992; 8(1): 73–78.

270. Takazawa K, Tsuchiya H, Yamamoto N, et al. Osteosarcoma arising from desmoplastic fibroma treated 16 years earlier: a case report. J Orthop Sci 2003; 8: 864–868.

271. Bertoni F, Calderoni P, Bacchini P, et al. Benign fibrous histiocytoma of bone. J Bone Joint Surg 1986; 68A: 1225–1230.

272. Bertoni F, Unni KK, McLeod RA, Sim FH. Xanthoma of bone. Am J Clin Pathol 1988; 90: 377–384.

273. Nishida J, Sim FH, Wenger DE, Unni KK. Malignant fibrous histiocytoma of bone. A clinicopathologic study of 81 patients. Cancer 1997; 79: 482–493.

274. Sohail D, Kerr R, Simpson RH, Babajews AV. Malignant fibrous histiocytoma of the mandible: the importance of an accurate histopathological diagnosis. Br J Oral Maxillofac Surg 1995; 33: 166–168.

275. Anavi Y, Herman GE, Graybill S, MacIntosh RB. Malignant fibrous histiocytoma of the mandible. Oral Surg Oral Med Oral Pathol 1989; 68: 436–443.

276. Akai M, Ohno T, Sugano I, et al. Case report 601: Malignant fibrous histiocytoma of skull and face presenting with massive osteolysis. Skeletal Radiol 1990; 19: 154–157.

277. Narvaez JA, Muntane A, Narvaez J, et al. Malignant fibrous histiocytoma of the mandible. Skeletal Radiol 1996; 25: 96–99.

278. Link TM, Haeussler MD, Poppek S, et al. Malignant fibrous histiocytoma of bone: conventional X-ray and MR imaging features. Skeletal Radiol 1998; 27: 552–558.

279. Kannan V, von Ruden D. Malignant fibrous histiocytoma of bone: initial diagnosis by aspiration biopsy cytology. Diagn Cytopathol 1988; 4: 262–264.

280. Bielack SS, Schroeders A, Fuchs N, et al. Malignant fibrous histiocytoma of bone: a retrospective EMSOS study of 125 cases. European Musculo-Skeletal Oncology Society. Acta Orthop Scand 1999; 70: 353–360.

281. Lichtenstein L, Jaffe HL. Fibrous dysplasia of bone. Arch Pathol Lab Med 1942; 33: 777–816.

282. Albright F, Scoville B, Sulkowitch HW. Syndrome characterized by osteitis fibrosa disseminata, areas of pigmentation and gonadal dysfunction. Endocrinology 1938; 22: 411–421.

283. Cabral CE, Guedes P, Fonseca T, et al. Polyostotic fibrous dysplasia associated with intramuscular myxomas: Mazabraud's syndrome. Skeletal Radiol 1998; 27: 278–282.

284. Faivre L, Nivelon-Chevallier A, Kottler ML, et al. Mazabraud syndrome in two patients: clinical overlap with McCune–Albright syndrome. Am J Med Genet 2001; 99: 132–136.

285. Albright F, Butler AM, Hampton AO, et al. Syndrome characterized by osteitis fibrosa disseminata, areas of pigmentation and endocrine dysfunction with precocious puberty in females. N Engl J Med 1947; 216: 727–746.

286. Weinstein LS, Chen M, Liu J. Gs(alpha) mutations and imprinting defects in human disease. Ann NY Acad Sci 2002; 968: 173–197.

287. Marie PJ, de Pollak C, Chanson P, Lomri A. Increased proliferation of osteoblastic cells expressing the activating Gs alpha mutation in monostotic and polyostotic fibrous dysplasia. Am J Pathol 1997; 150: 1059–1069.

288. Weinstein LS, Shenker A, Gejman PV, et al. Activating mutations of the stimulatory G protein in the McCune-Albright syndrome. N Engl J Med 1991; 325: 1688–1695.

289. Mikami M, Koizumi H, Ishii M, Nakajima H. The identification of monoclonality in fibrous dysplasia by methylation-specific polymerase chain reaction for the human androgen receptor gene. Virchows Arch 2004; 444(1): 56–60.

290. MacDonald-Jankowski DS. Fibro-osseous lesions of the face and jaws. Clin Radiol 2004; 59(1): 11–25.

291. Kyriakos M, McDonald DJ, Sundaram M. Fibrous dysplasia with cartilaginous differentiation ('fibrocartilaginous dysplasia'): a review, with an illustrative case followed for 18 years. Skeletal Radiol 2004; 33(1): 51–62.

292. Ishida T, Dorfman HD. Massive chondroid differentiation in fibrous dysplasia of bone (fibrocartilaginous dysplasia). Am J Surg Pathol 1993; 17: 924–930.

293. Dahlin DC, Bertoni F, Beabout JW, Campanacci M. Fibrocartilaginous mesenchymoma with low-grade malignancy. Skeletal Radiol 1984; 12: 263–269.

294. Bulychova IV, Unni KK, Bertoni F, Beabout JW. Fibrocartilagenous mesenchymoma of bone. Am J Surg Pathol 1993; 17: 830–836.

295. Kransdorf MJ, Murphey MD, Sweet DE. Liposclerosing myxofibrous tumor: a radiologic-pathologic-distinct fibro-osseous lesion of bone with a marked predilection for the intertrochanteric region of the femur. Radiology 1999; 212: 693–698.

296. Ragsdale BD. Polymorphic fibro-osseous lesions of bone: an almost site-specific diagnostic problem of the proximal femur. Hum Pathol 1993; 24: 505–512.

297. Matsuba A, Ogose A, Tokunaga K, et al. Activating Gs alpha mutation at the Arg201 codon in liposclerosing myxofibrous tumor. Hum Pathol 2003; 34: 1204–1209.

298. Schoenau E, Rauch F. Fibrous dysplasia. Horm Res 2002; 57(Suppl 2): 79–82.

299. Ruggieri P, Sim FH, Bond JR, Unni KK. Malignancies in fibrous dysplasia. Cancer 1994; 73: 1411–1424.

300. Yabut SM Jr, Kenan S, Sissons HA, Lewis MM. Malignant transformation of fibrous dysplasia. A case report and review of the literature. Clin Orthop 1988(228): 281–289.

301. Wenig BM, Vinh TN, Smirniotopoulos JG, et al. Aggressive psammomatoid ossifying fibromas of the sinonasal region: a clinicopathologic study of a distinct group of fibro-osseous lesions. Cancer 1995; 76: 1155–1165.

302. Margo CE, Ragsdale BD, Perman KI, et al. Psammomatoid (juvenile) ossifying fibroma of the orbit. Ophthalmology 1985; 92: 150–159.

303. Damjanov I, Maenza RM, Snyder GG, et al. Juvenile ossifying fibroma: an ultrastructural study. Cancer 1978; 42: 2668–2674.

304. Margo CE, Weiss A, Habal MB. Psammomatoid ossifying fibroma. Arch Ophthalmol 1986; 104: 1347–1351.

305. Johnson LC, Yousefi M, Vinh TN, et al. Juvenile active ossifying fibroma. Its nature, dynamics and origin. Acta Otolaryngol Suppl 1991; 488: 1–40.

306. Campbell CJ, Hawk T. A variant of fibrous dysplasia (osteofibrous dysplasia). J Bone Joint Surg 1982; 64A: 231–236.

307. Kempson RL. Ossifying fibroma of the long bones. A light and electron microscopic study. Arch Pathol 1966; 82: 218–233.

308. Campanacci M. Osteofibrous dysplasia of long bones a new clinical entity. Ital J Orthop Traumatol 1976; 2: 221–237.

309. Campanacci M, Laus M. Osteofibrous dysplasia of the tibia and fibula. J Bone Joint Surg 1981; 63A: 367–375.

310. Bridge JA, Dembinski A, DeBoer J, et al. Clonal chromosomal abnormalities in osteofibrous dysplasia. Implications for histopathogenesis and its relationship with adamantinoma. Cancer 1994; 73: 1746–1752.

311. Bridge JA, Swarts SJ, Buresh C, et al. Trisomies 8 and 20 characterize a subgroup of benign fibrous lesions arising in both soft tissue and bone. Am J Pathol 1999; 154: 729–733.

312. Park YK, Unni KK, McLeod RA, Pritchard DJ. Osteofibrous dysplasia: clinicopathologic study of 80 cases. Hum Pathol 1993; 24: 1339–1347.

313. Sweet DE, Vinh TN, Devaney K. Cortical osteofibrous dysplasia of long bone and its relationship to adamantinoma. A clinicopathologic study of 30 cases. Am J Surg Pathol 1992; 16: 282–290.

314. Keeney GL, Unni KK, Beabout JW, Pritchard DJ. Adamantinoma of long bones. A clinicopathologic study of 85 cases. Cancer 1989; 64: 730–737.

315. Mills SE, Rosai J. Adamantinoma of the pretibial soft tissue. Clinicopathologic features, differential diagnosis, and possible relationship to intraosseous disease. Am J Clin Pathol 1985; 83: 108–114.

316. Bertoni F, Zucchi V, Mapelli S, Bacchini P. Case report 506: adamantoma of the soft tissues of leg. Skeletal Radiol 1988; 17: 522–526.

317. Hazelbag HM, Wessels JW, Mollevangers P, et al. Cytogenetic analysis of adamantinoma of long bones: further indications for a common histogenesis with osteofibrous dysplasia. Cancer Genet Cytogenet 1997; 97: 5–11.

318. Kanamori M, Antonescu CR, Scott M, et al. Extra copies of chromosomes 7, 8, 12, 19, and 21 are recurrent in adamantinoma. J Mol Diagn 2001; 3(1): 16–21.

319. Mandahl N, Heim S, Rydholm A, et al. Structural chromosome aberrations in an adamantinoma. Cancer Genet Cytogenet 1989; 42: 187–190.

320. Czerniak B, Rojas-Corona RR, Dorfman HD. Morphologic diversity of long bone adamantinoma. The concept of differentiated (regressing) adamantinoma and its relationship to osteofibrous dysplasia. Cancer 1989; 64: 2319–2334.

321. Kahn LB. Adamantinoma, osteofibrous dysplasia and differentiated adamantinoma. Skeletal Radiol 2003; 32: 245–158.

322. Hazelbag HM, Laforga JB, Roels HJ, Hogendoorn PC. Dedifferentiated adamantinoma with revertant mesenchymal phenotype. Am J Surg Pathol 2003; 27: 1530–1537.

323. Benassi MS, Campanacci L, Gamberi G, et al. Cytokeratin expression and distribution in adamantinoma of the long bones and osteofibrous dysplasia of tibia and fibula. An immunohistochemical study correlated to histogenesis. Histopathology 1994; 25: 71–76.

324. Hazelbag HM, Fleuren GJ, van der Broek LJ, et al. Adamantinoma of the long bones: keratin subclass immunoreactivity pattern with reference to its histogenesis. Am J Surg Pathol 1993; 17: 1225–1233.

325. Hales MS, Ferrell LD. Fine-needle aspiration biopsy of tibial adamantinoma: a case report. Diagn Cytopathol 1988; 4: 67–70.

326. Perez-Ordonez B, Bedard YC. Metastatic adamantinoma diagnosed by fine-needle aspiration biopsy of the lung. Diagn Cytopathol 1994; 10: 347–351.

327. Galera-Davidson H, Fernandez-Rodriguez A, Torres-Olivera FJ, et al. Cytologic diagnosis of a case of recurrent adamantinoma. Acta Cytol 1989; 33: 635–638.

328. Kenney JN, Kaugars GE, Abbey LM. Comparison between the peripheral ossifying fibroma and peripheral odontogenic fibroma. J Oral Maxillofac Surg 1989; 47: 378–382.

329. Jundt G, Remberger K, Roessner A, et al. Adamantinoma of long bones. A histopathological and immunohistochemical study of 23 cases. Pathol Res Pract 1995; 191: 112–120.

330. Hazelbag HM, Taminiau AH, Fleuren GJ, Hogendoorn PC. Adamantinoma of the long bones. A clinicopathological study of thirty-two patients with emphasis on histological subtype, precursor lesion, and biological behavior. J Bone Joint Surg 1994; 76A: 1482–1499.

331. Schneider H, Enderle A. [Differential diagnosis of a metastasizing adamantinoma of the tibia and fibula (author's transl)]. Arch Orthop Trauma Surg 1979; 94: 143–149.

332. Unni KK, Dahlin DC, Beabout JW, Ivins JC. Adamantinomas of long bones. Cancer 1974; 34: 1796–1805.

333. Maki M, Athanasou N. Osteofibrous dysplasia and adamantinoma: correlation of proto-oncogene product and matrix protein expression. Hum Pathol 2004; 35: 69–74.

334. Ewing J. Diffuse endothelioma of bone. Proc NY Pathol Soc 1921; 21: 17–24.

335. Cotterill SJ, Parker L, Malcolm AJ, et al. Incidence and survival for cancer in children and young adults in the North of England, 1968–1995: a report from the Northern Region Young Persons' Malignant Disease Registry. Br J Cancer 2000; 83: 397–403.

336. Burchill SA. Ewing's sarcoma: diagnostic, prognostic, and therapeutic implications of molecular abnormalities. J Clin Pathol 2003; 56: 96–102.

337. Peydro-Olaya A, Llombart-Bosch A, Carda-Batalla C, Lopez-Guerrero JA. Electron microscopy and other ancillary techniques in the diagnosis of small round cell tumors. Semin Diagn Pathol 2003; 20: 25–45.

338. Devoe K, Weidner N. Immunohistochemistry of small round-cell tumors. Semin Diagn Pathol 2000; 17: 216–224.

339. Gu M, Antonescu CR, Guiter G, et al. Cytokeratin immunoreactivity in Ewing's sarcoma: prevalence in 50 cases confirmed by molecular diagnostic studies. Am J Surg Pathol 2000; 24: 410–416.

340. Scotlandi K, Manara MC, Strammiello R, et al. C-kit receptor expression in Ewing's sarcoma: lack of prognostic value but therapeutic targeting opportunities in appropriate conditions. J Clin Oncol 2003; 21: 1952–1960.

341. O'Neil-Smith K, Wittenberg KH, Efird JT, et al. Ewing's sarcoma and peripheral primitive neuroectodermal tumor: a proposal for a standardized classification scheme based on morphologic, immunohistochemical and clinical features. Mod Pathol 1995; 8: 10A.

342. Bacci G, Forni C, Longhi A, et al. Long-term outcome for patients with non-metastatic Ewing's sarcoma treated with adjuvant and neoadjuvant chemotherapies. 402 patients treated at Rizzoli between 1972 and 1992. Eur J Cancer 2004; 40: 73–83.

343. Rosenberg AE, Amstalden EMJ, Nielsen GP. Ewing's sarcoma/PNET: Preoperative chemotherapy induced necrosis and outcome. Lab Invest 1996; 74: 13A.

344. Dunst J, Schuck A. Role of radiotherapy in Ewing tumors. Pediatr Blood Cancer 2004; 42: 465–470.

345. Avigad S, Cohen IJ, Zilberstein J, et al. The predictive potential of molecular detection in the nonmetastatic Ewing family of tumors. Cancer 2004; 100: 1053–1058.

346. Oberlin O, Deley MC, Bui BN, et al. Prognostic factors in localized Ewing's tumours and peripheral neuroectodermal tumours: the third study of the French Society of Paediatric Oncology (EW88 study). Br J Cancer 2001; 85: 1646–1654.

347. De Alava E, Kawai A, Healey JH, et al. EWS–FLI1 fusion transcript structure is an independent determinant of prognosis in Ewing's sarcoma. J Clin Oncol 1998; 16: 1248–1255.

348. Cotterill SJ, Ahrens S, Paulussen M, et al. Prognostic factors in Ewing's tumor of bone: analysis of 975 patients from the European Intergroup Cooperative Ewing's Sarcoma Study Group. J Clin Oncol 2000; 18: 3108–3114.

349. Lipper S, Kahn LB. Case report 235. Ewing-like adamantinoma of the left cranial head and neck. Skeletal Radiol 1983; 10: 61–66.

350. Meister P, Konrad E, Hubner G. Malignant tumor of humerus with features of 'adamantinoma' and Ewing's sarcoma. Pathol Res Pract 1979; 166: 112–122.

351. Fukunaga M, Ushigome S. Periosteal Ewing-like adamantinoma. Virchows Arch 1998; 433: 385–389.

352. Ishida T, Kikuchi F, Oka T, et al. Case report 727. Juxtacortical adamantinoma of humerus (simulating Ewing tumor). Skeletal Radiol 1992; 21: 205–209.

353. Schofield DE, Conrad EU, Liddell RM, Yunis EJ. An unusual round cell tumor of the tibia with granular cells. Am J Surg Pathol 1995; 19: 596–603.

354. O'Connell JX, Nielsen GP, Ishida T, et al. Insular and trabecular round cell sarcoma. A proposal for the recognition of a distinct bone neoplasm. Mod Pathol 2001; 14: 16A.

355. Dehner LP, Sibley RK, Sauk JJ Jr, et al. Malignant melanotic neuroectodermal tumor of infancy: a clinical, pathologic, ultrastructural and tissue culture study. Cancer 1979; 43: 1389–1410.

356. Borello ED, Gorlin RJ. Melanotic neuroectodermal tumor of infancy – a neoplasm of neural crest origin. Report of a case associated with high urinary excretion of vanilmandelic acid. Cancer 1966; 19: 196–206.

357. Khoddami M, Squire J, Zielenska M, Thorner P. Melanotic neuroectodermal tumor of infancy: a molecular genetic study. Pediatr Dev Pathol 1998; 1: 295–299.

358. Mosby EL, Lowe MW, Cobb CM, Ennis RL. Melanotic neuroectodermal tumor of infancy: review of the literature and report of a case. J Oral Maxillofac Surg 1992; 50: 886–894.

359. Cutler LS, Chaudhry AP, Topazian R. Melanotic neuroectodermal tumor of infancy: an ultrastructural study, literature review, and reevaluation. Cancer 1981; 48: 257–270.

360. Kapadia SB, Frisman DM, Hitchcock CL, et al. Melanotic neuroectodermal tumor of infancy. Clinicopathological, immunohistochemical, and flow cytometric study. Am J Surg Pathol 1993; 17: 566–573.

361. Young S, Gonzalez-Crussi F. Melanocytic neuroectodermal tumor of the foot. Report of a case with multicentric origin. Am J Clin Pathol 1985; 84: 371–378.

362. Ulbright TM, Amin MB, Young RH. Tumors of the testis, adnexa, spermatic cord and scrotum. 3rd edn. Washington, DC: Armed Forces Institute of Pathology; 1999.

363. Pettinato G, Manivel JC, d'Amore ES, et al. Melanotic neuroectodermal tumor of infancy. A reexamination of a histogenetic problem based on immunohistochemical, flow cytometric, and ultrastructural study of 10 cases. Am J Surg Pathol 1991; 15: 233–245.

364. Galera-Ruiz H, Gomez-Angel D, Vazquez-Ramirez FJ, et al. Fine needle aspiration in the pre-operative diagnosis of melanotic neuroectodermal tumour of infancy. J Laryngol Otol 1999; 113: 581–584.

365. Rao CR, Visweshwaraiah LD, Veerapaiah KS, et al. Melanotic neuroectodermal tumor of infancy initially diagnosed by fine needle aspiration cytology. Acta Cytol 1990; 34: 681–684.

366. Toda T, Sadi AM, Kiyuna M, et al. Pigmented neuroectodermal tumor of infancy in the epididymis. A case report. Acta Cytol 1998; 42: 775–780.

367. Johnson RE, Scheithauer BW, Dahlin DC. Melanotic neuroectodermal tumor of infancy. A review of seven cases. Cancer 1983; 52: 661–666.

368. Navas Palacios JJ. Malignant melanotic neuroectodermal tumor: light and electron microscopic study. Cancer 1980; 46: 529–536.

369. Kanaan I, Ahmed M, Rifai A, Alwatban J. Sphenoid sinus brown tumor of secondary hyperparathyroidism: case report. Neurosurgery 1998; 42: 1374–1377.

370. Mourelatus Z, Goldberg H, Sinson G, et al. Case of the month: March 1998 – 48 year old man with back pain and weakness. Brain Pathol 1998; 8: 589–590.

371. Blinder G, Hiller N, Gatt N, et al. Brown tumor in the cricoid cartilage: an unusual manifestation of primary hyperparathyroidism. Ann Otol Rhinol Laryngol 1997; 106: 252–253.

372. Rosenberg AE. The pathology of metabolic bone disease. Radiol Clin North Am 1991; 29: 19–36.

373. Kashkari S, Kelly TR, Bethem D, Pepe RG. Osteitis fibrosa cystica (brown tumor) of the spine with cord compression: report of a case with needle aspiration biopsy findings. Diagn Cytopathol 1990; 6: 349–353.

374. Gupta RK, Boss DM, McHutchison AGR, Hatfield PJ. Osteitis fibrosa cystica (brown tumor) in a patient with renal transplantation. Report of a case with aspiration with cyto diagnosis. Acta Cytol 1992; 36: 555–558.

375. Jaffe H. Giant cell reparative granuloma. Traumatic bone cyst and fibrous (fibro-osseous) dysplasia of the jawbones. Oral Surg Oral Med Oral Pathol 1953; 6: 159–175.

376. Whitaker SB, Waldron CA. Central giant cell lesions of the jaws. A clinical, radiologic, and histopathologic study. Oral Surg Oral Med Oral Pathol 1993; 75: 199–208.

377. Ackerman LV, Spjut HJ. Tumors of bone and cartilage. Washington, DC: Armed Forces Institute of Pathology; 1962.

378. Maruno M, Yoshimine T, Kubo T, Hayakawa T. A case of giant cell reparative granuloma of the petrous bone: demonstration of the proliferative component. Surg Neurol 1997; 48: 64–68.

379. Hirschl S, Katz A. Giant cell reparative granuloma outside the jaw bone. Diagnostic criteria and review of the literature with the first case described in the temporal bone. Hum Pathol 1974; 5: 171–181.

380. Lorenzo JC, Dorfman HD. Giant-cell reparative granuloma of short tubular bones of the hands and feet. Am J Surg Pathol 1980; 4: 551–563.

381. Caskey PM, Wolf MD, Fechner RE. Multicentric giant cell reparative granuloma of the small bones of the hand. A case report and review of the literature. Clin Orthop 1985; 193: 199–205.

382. Buresh CJ, Seemayer TA, Nelson M, et al. t(X; 4)(q22; q31.3) in giant cell reparative granuloma. Cancer Genet Cytogenet 1999; 115(1): 80–81.

383. Wold LE, Dobyns JH, Swee RG, Dahlin DC. Giant cell reaction (giant cell reparative granuloma) of the small bones of the hands and feet. Am J Surg Pathol 1986; 10: 491–496.

384. Som PM, Lawson W, Cohen BA. Giant-cell lesions of the facial bones. Radiology 1983; 147: 129–134.

385. Waldron CA, Shafer WG. The central giant cell reparative granuloma of the jaws. An analysis of 38 cases. Am J Clin Pathol 1966; 45: 437–447.

386. Quick CA, Anderson R, Stool S. Giant cell tumors of the maxilla in children. Laryngoscope 1980; 90(5 Pt 1): 784–791.

387. Abaza NA, el-Khashab MM, Fahim MS. Central giant cell reparative granuloma involving the mandible: report of case. J Oral Surg 1965; 23: 643–648.

388. Ciappetta P, Salvati M, Bernardi C, et al. Giant cell reparative granuloma of the skull base mimicking an intracranial tumor. Case report and review of the literature. Surg Neurol 1990; 33: 52–56.

389. Mirra JM, Picci P, Gold RH. Bone tumors: clinical, radiologic and pathologic correlations. Philadelphia, PA: Lea & Febiger; 1989.

390. Sanerkin NG, Mott MG, Roylance J. An unusual intraosseous lesion with fibroblastic, osteoclastic, osteoblastic, aneurysmal and fibromyxoid elements. 'Solid' variant of aneurysmal bone cyst. Cancer 1983; 51: 2278–2286.

391. Bloodgood JC. The conservative treatment of giant cell sarcomas, with the study of bone transplantation. Ann Surg 1912; 56: 210–239.

392. Jaffe HL, Lichtenstein L, Portis RB. Giant cell tumor of bone. Its pathologic appearance, grading, supposed variants and treatment. Arch Pathol 1940; 30: 993–1013.

393. Goldenberg RR, Campbell CJ, Bonfiglio M. Giant-cell tumor of bone. An analysis of two hundred and eighteen cases. J Bone Joint Surg 1970; 52A: 619–664.

394. Campanacci M, Giunti A, Olmi R. Giant-cell tumours of bone. A study of 209 cases with long-term follow-up in 130. Italian J Orthop and Traumat 1975; 1: 249–277.

395. McDonald DJ, Sim FH, McLeod RA, Dahlin DC. Giant-cell tumor of bone. J Bone Joint Surg 1986; 68A: 235–242.

396. Sciot R, Dorfman H, Brys P, et al. Cytogenetic-morphologic correlations in aneurysmal bone cyst, giant cell tumor of bone and combined lesions. A report from the CHAMP study group. Mod Pathol 2000; 13: 1206–1210.

397. Picci P, Manfrini M, Zucchi V, et al. Giant-cell tumor of bone in skeletally immature patients. J Bone Joint Surg 1983; 65A: 486–490.

398. Cummins CA, Scarborough MT, Enneking WF. Multicentric giant cell tumor of bone. Clin Orthop 1996; 322: 245–252.

399. Dahlin DC. Caldwell Lecture. Giant cell tumor of bone: highlights of 407 cases. AJR 1985; 144: 955–960.

400. Sneige N, Ayala AG, Carrasco CH, et al. Giant cell tumor of bone. A cytologic study of 24 cases. Diagn Cytopathol 1985; 1(2): 111–117.

401. Vetrani A, Fulciniti F, Boschi R, et al. Fine needle aspiration biopsy diagnosis of giant-cell tumor of bone. An experience with nine cases. Acta Cytol 1990; 34: 863–867.

402. Steiner GC, Ghosh L, Dorfman HD. Ultrastructure of giant cell tumors of bone. Hum Pathol 1972; 3: 569–586.

403. Medeiros LJ, Beckstead JH, Rosenberg AE, et al. The giant cells and mononuclear cells of giant cell tumor of bone resemble histiocytes. Applied Immunohistochemistry 1993; 1: 115–122.

404. Chakravarti A, Spiro IJ, Hug EB, et al. Megavoltage radiation therapy for axial and inoperable giant-cell tumor of bone. J Bone Joint Surg 1999; 81A: 1566–1573.

405. O'Donnell RJ, Springfield DS, Motwani HK, et al. Recurrence of giant-cell tumors of the long bones after curettage and packing with cement. J Bone Joint Surg 1994; 76A: 1827–1833.

406. Wang BY, Eisler J, Springfield D, Klein MJ. Intraosseous epidermoid inclusion cyst in a great toe. A case report and review of the literature. Arch Pathol Lab Med 2003; 127: e298–e300.

407. Bretschneider T, Dorenbeck U, Strotzer M, et al. Squamous cell carcinoma arising in an intradiploic epidermoid cyst. Neuroradiology 1999; 41: 570–572.

408. Schajowicz F, Clavel Sainz M, Slullitel JA. Juxta-articular bone cysts (intra-osseous ganglia): a clinicopathological study of eighty-eight cases. J Bone Joint Surg 1979; 61B: 107–116.

409. Hicks JD. Synovial cysts in bone. Aust NZ J Surg 1956; 26: 138–143.

410. Bauer TW, Dorfman HD. Intraosseous ganglion: a clinicopathologic study of 11 cases. Am J Surg Pathol 1982; 6: 207–213.

411. Helwig U, Lang S, Baczynski M, Windhager R. The intraosseous ganglion. A clinical-pathological report on 42 cases. Arch Orthop Trauma Surg 1994; 114(1): 14–17.

412. Schrank C, Meirer R, Stabler A, et al. Morphology and topography of intraosseous ganglion cysts in the carpus: an anatomic, histopathologic, and magnetic resonance imaging correlation study. J Hand Surg [Am] 2003; 28: 52–61.

413. Feldman F, Johnston AD. Ganglia of bone: theories, manifestations, and presentations. CRC Crit Rev Clin Radiol Nucl Med 1973; 4: 303–332.

414. Rozbruch SR, Chang V, Bohne WH, Deland JT. Ganglion cysts of the lower extremity: an analysis of 54 cases and review of the literature. Orthopedics 1998; 21: 141–148.

415. Sim FH, Dahlin DC. Ganglion cysts of bone. Mayo Clin Proc 1971; 46: 484–488.

416. Donkor P, Punnia-Moorthy A. Biochemical analysis of simple bone cyst fluid–report of a case. Int J Oral Maxillofac Surg 1994; 23: 296–297.

417. Chigira M, Maehara S, Arita S, Udagawa E. The aetiology and treatment of simple bone cysts. J Bone Joint Surg 1983; 65B: 633–637.

418. Ovadia D, Ezra E, Segev E, et al. Epiphyseal involvement of simple bone cysts. J Pediatr Orthop 2003; 23: 222–229.

419. Margau R, Babyn P, Cole W, et al. MR imaging of simple bone cysts in children: not so simple. Pediatr Radiol 2000; 30: 551–557.

420. Dollahite HA, Tatum L, Moinuddin SM, Carnesale PG. Aspiration biopsy of primary neoplasms of bone. J Bone Joint Surg 1989; 71A: 1166–1169.

421. Melkert PW. Fine needle aspiration cytology of bone lesions. Analysis of a three-year experience in rural Africa. Acta Cytol 1990; 34: 677–680.

422. Lokiec F, Wientroub S. Simple bone cyst: etiology, classification, pathology, and treatment modalities. J Pediatr Orthop B 1998; 7: 262–273.

423. Mylle J, Burssens A, Fabry G. Simple bone cysts. A review of 59 cases with special reference to their treatment. Arch Orthop Trauma Surg 1992; 111: 297–300.

424. Jaffe HL. Solitary unicameral bone cyst. Arch Surg 1942; 44: 1004–1005.

425. Kransdorf MJ, Sweet DE. Aneurysmal bone cyst: concept, controversy, clinical presentation, and imaging. AJR 1995; 164: 573–580.

426. Dal Cin P, Kozakewich HP, Goumnerova L, et al. Variant translocations involving 16q22 and 17p13 in solid variant and extraosseous forms of aneurysmal bone cyst. Genes Chromosomes Cancer 2000; 28: 233–234.

427. Vergel De Dios AM, Bond JR, Shives TC, et al. Aneurysmal bone cyst. A clinicopathologic study of 238 cases. Cancer 1992; 69: 2921–2931.

428. Martinez V, Sissons HA. Aneurysmal bone cyst. A review of 123 cases including primary lesions and those secondary to other bone pathology. Cancer 1988; 61: 2291–2304.

429. Ruiter DJ, van Rijssel TG, van der Velde EA. Aneurysmal bone cysts: a clinicopathological study of 105 cases. Cancer 1977; 39: 2231–2239.

430. Oliveira AM, Hsi BL, Weremowicz S, et al. USP6 (Tre2) fusion oncogenes in aneurysmal bone cyst. Cancer Res 2004; 64: 1920–1923.

431. Althof PA, Ohmori K, Zhou M, et al. Cytogenetic and molecular cytogenetic findings in 43 aneurysmal bone cysts: aberrations of 17p mapped to 17p13.2 by fluorescence in situ hybridization. Mod Pathol 2004; 17: 518–525.

432. Kyriakos M, Hardy D. Malignant transformation of aneurysmal bone cyst, with an analysis of the literature. Cancer 1991; 68: 1770–1780.

433. Rosai J, Dorfman RF. Sinus histiocytosis with massive lymphadenopathy. A newly recognized benign clinicopathological entity. Arch Pathol 1969; 87: 63–70.

434. Foucar E, Rosai J, Dorfman R. Sinus histiocytosis with massive lymphadenopathy (Rosai–Dorfman disease): review of the entity. Semin Diagn Pathol 1990; 7: 19–73.

435. Nielsen GP, Bjornsson J, Rosenberg AE, Unni KK. Primary Rosai–Dorfman disease of bone. A clinicopathologic study of 13 cases. Modern Pathology 2002; 15: 20A.

436. Goel MM, Agarwal PK, Agarwal S. Primary Rosai–Dorfman disease of bone without lymphadenopathy diagnosed by fine needle aspiration cytology. A case report. Acta Cytol 2003; 47: 1119–122.

437. Willman CL, Busque L, Griffith BB, et al. Langerhans'-cell histiocytosis (histiocytosis X) – a clonal proliferative disease. N Engl J Med 1994; 331: 154–160.

438. Lieberman PH, Jones CR, Steinman RM, et al. Langerhans cell (eosinophilic) granulomatosis. A clinicopathologic study encompassing 50 years. Am J Surg Pathol 1996; 20: 519–552.

439. Howarth DM, Gilchrist GS, Mullan BP, et al. Langerhans cell histiocytosis: diagnosis, natural history, management, and outcome. Cancer 1999; 85: 2278–2290.

440. Kilpatrick SE, Wenger DE, Gilchrist GS, et al. Langerhans' cell histiocytosis (histiocytosis X) of bone. A clinicopathologic analysis of 263 pediatric and adult cases. Cancer 1995; 76: 2471–2484.

441. Giona F, Caruso R, Testi AM, et al. Langerhans' cell histiocytosis in adults: a clinical and therapeutic analysis of 11 patients from a single institution. Cancer 1997; 80: 1786–1791.

442. Emile JF, Wechsler J, Brousse N, et al. Langerhans' cell histiocytosis. Definitive diagnosis with the use of monoclonal antibody O10 on routinely paraffin-embedded samples. Am J Surg Pathol 1995; 19: 636–641.

443. Van Heerde P, Maarten Egeler R. The cytology of Langerhans cell histiocytosis (histiocytosis X). Cytopathology 1991; 2: 149–158.

444. Elsheikh T, Silverman JF, Wakely PE Jr, et al. Fine-needle aspiration cytology of Langerhans' cell histiocytosis (eosinophilic granuloma) of bone in children. Diagn Cytopathol 1991; 7: 261–266.

445. Krishnan A, Shirkhoda A, Tehranzadeh J, et al. Primary bone lymphoma: radiographic–MR imaging correlation. Radiographics 2003; 23: 1371–1383; discussion 1384–7.

446. Campbell SE, Filzen TW, Bezzant SM, et al. Primary periosteal lymphoma: an unusual presentation of non-Hodgkin's lymphoma with radiographic, MR imaging, and pathologic correlation. Skeletal Radiol 2003; 32: 231–235.

447. Orucevic A, Reddy VB, Selvaggi SM, et al. Fine-needle aspiration of extranodal and extramedullary hematopoietic malignancies. Diagn Cytopathol 2000; 23: 318–321.

448. Ascoli V, Facciolo F, Nardi F. Cytodiagnosis of a primary non-Hodgkin's lymphoma of bone. Diagn Cytopathol 1994; 11: 168–173.

449. Fidias P, Spiro I, Sobczak ML, et al. Long-term results of combined modality therapy in primary bone lymphomas. Int J Radiat Oncol Biol Phys 1999; 45: 1213–1218.

450. Stein ME, Kuten A, Gez E, et al. Primary lymphoma of bone–a retrospective study. Experience at the Northern Israel Oncology Center (1979–2000). Oncology 2003; 64: 322–327.

451. Zinzani PL, Carrillo G, Ascani S, et al. Primary bone lymphoma: experience with 52 patients. Haematologica 2003; 88: 280–285.

452. Barbieri E, Cammelli S, Mauro F, et al. Primary non-Hodgkin's lymphoma of the bone: treatment and analysis of prognostic factors for Stage I and Stage II. Int J Radiat Oncol Biol Phys 2004; 59: 760–764.

453. Lewis VO, Primus G, Anastasi J, et al. Oncologic outcomes of primary lymphoma of bone in adults. Clin Orthop 2003; 415: 90–97.

454. De Leval L, Braaten KM, Ancukiewicz M, et al. Diffuse large B-cell lymphoma of bone: an analysis of differentiation-associated antigens with clinical correlation. Am J Surg Pathol 2003; 27: 1269–1277.

455. Ozdemirli M, Mankin HJ, Aisenberg AC, Harris NL. Hodgkin's disease presenting as a solitary bone tumor. A report of four cases and review of the literature. Cancer 1996; 77: 79–88.

456. Ostrowski ML, Inwards CY, Strickler JG, et al. Osseous Hodgkin disease. Cancer 1999; 85: 1166–1178.

457. Farrugia AN, Atkins GJ, To LB, et al. Receptor activator of nuclear factor-kappaB ligand expression by human myeloma cells mediates osteoclast formation in vitro and correlates with bone destruction in vivo. Cancer Res 2003; 63: 5438–5445.

458. Mulleman D, Gaxatte C, Guillerm G, et al. Multiple myeloma presenting with widespread osteosclerotic lesions. Joint Bone Spine 2004; 71(1): 79–83.

459. Cooper GL, Shaffer DW, Raval HB. Fine-needle aspiration biopsy of multiple myeloma in a patient with renal-cell carcinoma: a case report. Diagn Cytopathol 1993; 9: 551–554.

460. Greipp PR, Raymond NM, Kyle RA, O'Fallon WM. Multiple myeloma: significance of plasmablastic subtype in morphological classification. Blood 1985; 65: 305–310.

461. Sirohi B, Powles R. Multiple myeloma. Lancet 2004; 363: 875–887.

462. Attal M, Harousseau JL, Facon T, et al. Single versus double autologous stem-cell transplantation for multiple myeloma. N Engl J Med 2003; 349: 2495–2502.

463. Pear BL. Skeletal manifestations of the lymphomas and leukemias. Semin Roentgenol 1974; 9: 229–240.

464. Gallagher DJ, Phillips DJ, Heinrich SD. Orthopedic manifestations of acute pediatric leukemia. Orthop Clin North Am 1996; 27: 635–644.

465. Heinrich SD, Gallagher D, Warrior R, et al. The prognostic significance of the skeletal manifestations of acute lymphoblastic leukemia of childhood. J Pediatr Orthop 1994; 14: 105–111.

466. Hermann G, Feldman F, Abdelwahab IF, Klein MJ. Skeletal manifestations of granulocytic sarcoma (chloroma). Skeletal Radiol 1991; 20: 509–512.

467. Fallon MD, Whyte MP, Teitelbaum SL. Systemic mastocytosis associated with generalized osteopenia. Histopathological characterization of the skeletal lesion using undecalcified bone from two patients. Hum Pathol 1981; 12: 813–820.

468. Sostre S, Handler HL. Bony lesions in systemic mastocytosis: scintigraphic evaluation. Arch Dermatol 1977; 113: 1245–1247.

469. Daly JF, Stark E, Van Buskirk FW. Radiologic and pathologic bone changes associated with urticaria pigmentosa; report of a case. AMA Arch Pathol 1956; 62: 143–148.

470. Okajima K, Honda I, Kitagawa T. Immunohistochemical distribution of S-100 protein in tumors and tumor-like lesions of bone and cartilage. Cancer 1988; 61: 792–799.

471. Salisbury JR, Isaacson PG. Distinguishing chordoma from chondrosarcoma by immunohistochemical techniques [letter]. J Pathol 1986; 148: 251–252.

472. Sarasa JL, Fortes J. Ecchordosis physaliphora: an immunohistochemical study of two cases. Histopathology 1991; 18: 273–275.

473. Miettinen M, Lehto VP, Dahl D, Virtanen I. Differential diagnosis of chordoma, chondroid, and ependymal tumors as aided by anti-intermediate filament antibodies. Am J Pathol 1983; 112: 160–169.

474. Wyatt RB, Schochet SS Jr, McCormick WF. Ecchordosis physaliphora. An electron microscopic study. J Neurosurg 1971; 34: 672–677.

475. Abenoza P, Sibley RK. Chordoma: an immunohistologic study. Hum Pathol 1986; 17: 744–747.

476. Pena CE, Horvat BL, Fisher ER. The ultrastructure of chordoma. Am J Clin Pathol 1970; 53: 544–551.

477. Spjut HJ, Luse SA. Chordoma: an electron microscopic study. Cancer 1964; 17: 643–656.

478. Sibley RK, Day DL, Dehner LP, Trueworthy RC. Metastasizing chordoma in early childhood: a pathological and immunohistochemical study with review of the literature. Pediatr Pathol 1987; 7: 287–301.

479. Nielsen GP, Rosenberg AE, Liebsch NJ. Chordoma of the base of skull in children and adolescents. A clinicopathologic study of 35 cases. 1996; 9: 11A.

480. McMaster ML, Goldstein AM, Bromley CM, et al. Chordoma: incidence and survival patterns in the United States, 1973–1995. Cancer Causes Control 2001; 12(1): 1–11.

481. Nielsen GP, Mangham DC, Grimer RJ, Rosenberg AE. Chordoma periphericum: a case report. Am J Surg Pathol 2001; 25: 263–267.

482. Kelley MJ, Korczak JF, Sheridan E, et al. Familial chordoma, a tumor of notochordal remnants, is linked to chromosome 7q33. Am J Hum Genet 2001; 69: 454–460.

483. Dickersin GD. Diagnostic electron microscopy. New York: Igaku-Shoin; 1988.

484. Friedman I, Harrison DFN, Bird ES. The fine structure of chordoma with particular reference to the physaliphorous cell. J Clin Pathol 1962; 15: 116–125.

485. Persson S, Kindblom LG, Angervall L. Classical and chondroid chordoma. A light-microscopic, histochemical, ultrastructural and immunohistochemical analysis of the various cell types. Pathol Res Pract 1991; 187: 828–838.

486. Rosenberg AE, Brown GA, Bhan AK, Lee JM. Chondroid chordoma–a variant of chordoma. A morphologic and immunohistochemical study. Am J Clin Pathol 1994; 101: 36–41.

487. Mori K, Chano T, Kushima R, et al. Expression of E-cadherin in chordomas: diagnostic marker and possible role of tumor cell affinity. Virchows Arch 2002; 440: 123–127.

488. Nijhawan VS, Rajwanshi A, Das A, et al. Fine-needle aspiration cytology of sacrococcygeal chordoma. Diagn Cytopathol 1989; 5: 404–407.

489. Finley JL, Silverman JF, Dabbs DJ, et al. Chordoma: diagnosis by fine-needle aspiration biopsy with histologic, immunocytochemical, and ultrastructural confirmation. Diagn Cytopathol 1986; 2: 330–337.

490. Walaas L, Kindblom LG. Fine-needle aspiration biopsy in the preoperative diagnosis of chordoma: a study of 17 cases with application of electron microscopic, histochemical, and immunocytochemical examination. Hum Pathol 1991; 22: 22–28.

491. Thompson SK, Callery RT. Cytologic diagnosis of a chordoma without physaliforous cells. Diagn Cytopathol 1988; 4: 144–147.

492. Heffelfinger MJ, Dahlin DC, MacCarty CS, Beabout JW. Chordomas and cartilaginous tumors at the skull base. Cancer 1973; 32: 410–420.

493. Bottles K, Beckstead JH. Enzyme histochemical characterization of chordomas. Am J Surg Pathol 1984; 8: 443–447.

494. Heaton JM, Turner DR. Reflections on notochordal differentiation arising from a study of chordomas. Histopathology 1985; 9: 543–550.

495. Rutherfoord GS, Davies AG. Chordomas–ultrastructure and immunohistochemistry: a report based on the examination of six cases. Histopathology 1987; 11: 775–787.

496. Meis JM, Giraldo AA. Chordoma. An immunohistochemical study of 20 cases. Arch Pathol Lab Med 1988; 112: 553–556.

497. Ishida T, Dorfman HD. Chondroid chordoma versus low-grade chondrosarcoma of the base of the skull: can immunohistochemistry resolve the controversy? J Neurooncol 1994; 18: 199–206.

498. Mitchell A, Scheithauer BW, Unni KK, et al. Chordoma and chondroid neoplasms of the spheno-occiput. An immunohistochemical study of 41 cases with prognostic and nosologic implications. Cancer 1993; 72: 2943–2949.

499. Cheng EY, Ozerdemoglu RA, Transfeldt EE, Thompson RC Jr. Lumbosacral chordoma. Prognostic factors and treatment. Spine 1999; 24: 1639–1645.

500. Bergh P, Kindblom LG, Gunterberg B, et al. Prognostic factors in chordoma of the sacrum and mobile spine: a study of 39 patients. Cancer 2000; 88: 2122–2134.

501. Bjornsson J, Wold LE, Ebersold MJ, Laws ER. Chordoma of the mobile spine. A clinicopathologic analysis of 40 patients. Cancer 1993; 71: 735–740.

502. Boriani S, Chevalley F, Weinstein JN, et al. Chordoma of the spine above the sacrum. Treatment and outcome in 21 cases. Spine 1996; 21: 1569–1577.

503. O'Connell JX, Renard LG, Liebsch NJ, et al. Base of skull chordoma. A correlative study of histologic and clinical features of 62 cases. Cancer 1994; 74: 2261–2267.

504. Hug EB, Loredo LN, Slater JD, et al. Proton radiation therapy for chordomas and chondrosarcomas of the skull base. J Neurosurg 1999; 91: 432–439.

505. Gay E, Sekhar LN, Rubinstein E, et al. Chordomas and chondrosarcomas of the cranial base: results and follow-up of 60 patients. Neurosurgery 1995; 36: 887–896; discussion 896–897.

506. Forsyth PA, Cascino TL, Shaw EG, et al. Intracranial chordomas: a clinicopathological and prognostic study of 51 cases. J Neurosurg 1993; 78: 741–747.

507. Coffin CM, Swanson PE, Wick MR, Dehner LP. Chordoma in childhood and adolescence. A clinicopathologic analysis of 12 cases. Arch Pathol Lab Med 1993; 117: 927–933.

508. Borba LA, Al-Mefty O, Mrak RE, Suen J. Cranial chordomas in children and adolescents. J Neurosurg 1996; 84: 584–591.

509. Kyriakos M, Totty WG, Lenke LG. Giant vertebral notochordal rest: a lesion distinct from chordoma: discussion of an evolving concept. Am J Surg Pathol 2003; 27: 396–406.

510. Mirra JM, Brien EW. Giant notochordal hamartoma of intraosseous origin: a newly reported benign entity to be distinguished from chordoma. Report of two cases. Skeletal Radiol 2001; 30: 698–709.

511. Yamaguchi T, Suzuki S, Ishiiwa H, Ueda Y. Intraosseous benign notochordal cell tumours: overlooked precursors of classic chordomas? Histopathology 2004; 44: 597–602.

512. Yamaguchi T, Suzuki S, Ishiiwa H, et al. Benign notochordal cell tumors: A comparative histological study of benign notochordal cell tumors, classic chordomas, and notochordal vestiges of fetal intervertebral discs. Am J Surg Pathol 2004; 28: 756–761.

513. Wold LE, Swee RG, Sim FH. Vascular lesions of bone. Pathol Annu 1985; 20(2): 101–137.

514. Moller G, Priemel M, Amling M, et al. The Gorham–Stout syndrome (Goram's massive osteolysis). A report of six cases with histopathological findings. J Bone J Surg 1999; 91B: 501–506.

515. Dorfman HD, Steiner GC, Jaffe HL. Vascular tumors of bone. Hum Pathol 1971; 2: 349–376.

516. Pinna V, Clauser L, Marchi M, Castellan L. Haemangioma of the zygoma: case report. Neuroradiology 1997; 39: 216–218.

517. Palacios E, Valvassori G. Temporal bone hemangioma as a cause of facial paralysis. Ear Nose Throat J 1999; 78: 84.

518. Sweet C, Silbergleit R, Mehta B. Primary intraosseous hemangioma of the orbit: CT and MR appearance. Am J Neuroradiol 1997; 18: 379–381.

519. O'Connell JX, Kattapuram SV, Mankin HJ, et al. Epithelioid hemangioma of bone. A tumor often mistaken for low-grade angiosarcoma or malignant hemangioendothelioma. Am J Surg Pathol 1993; 17: 610–617.

520. Lamovec J, Bracko M. Epithelioid hemangioma of small tubular bones: a report of three cases, two of them associated with pregnancy. Mod Pathol 1996; 9: 821–827.

521. Ben Romdhane K, Khattech R, Ben Othman M. Epithelioid hemangioma of bone [letter]. Am J Surg Pathol 1994; 18: 1270–1271.

522. Cone RO, Hudkins P, Nguyen V, Merriwether WA. Histiocytoid hemangioma of bone: a benign lesion which may mimic angiosarcoma. Report of a case and review of literature. Skeletal Radiol 1983; 10: 165–169.

523. Tsuneyoshi M, Dorfman HD, Bauer TW. Epithelioid hemangioendothelioma of bone. A clinicopathologic, ultrastructural, and immunohistochemical study. Am J Surg Pathol 1986; 10: 754–764.

524. Kleer CG, Unni KK, McLeod RA. Epithelioid hemangioendothelioma of bone. Am J Surg Pathol 1996; 20: 1301–1311.

525. Boutin RD, Spaeth HJ, Mangalik A, Sell JJ. Epithelioid hemangioendothelioma of bone. Skeletal Radiol 1996; 25: 391–395.

526. Shin MS, Carpenter JT Jr, Ho KJ. Epithelioid hemangioendothelioma of bone. CT manifestations and possible linkage to vinyl chloride exposure. J Comput Assist Tomogr 1991; 15: 505–507.

527. Abrahams TG, Bula W, Jones M. Epithelioid hemangioendothelioma of bone. A report of two cases and review of the literature. Skeletal Radiol 1992; 21: 509–513.

528. Wold LE, Unni KK, Beabout JW, et al. Hemangioendothelial sarcoma of bone. Am J Surg Pathol 1982; 6: 59–70.

529. Volpe R, Mazabraud A. Hemangioendothelioma (angiosarcoma) of bone: a distinct pathologic entity with an unpredictable course? Cancer 1982; 49: 727–736.

530. Campanacci M, Boriani S, Giunti A. Hemangioendothelioma of bone: a study of 29 cases. Cancer 1980; 46: 804–814.

531. Hartmann WH, Stewart FW. Hemangioendothelioma of bone: unusual tumor characterized by indolent course. Cancer 1962; 15: 846–854.

532. Khiyami A, Green LK, Gyorkey F, Landon G. Primary angiosarcoma of the cuboidal bone: a case report. Diagn Cytopathol 1991; 7: 520–523.

533. Stout AP, Murray MR. Hemangiopericytoma. A vascular tumor featuring Zimmermann's pericytes. Ann Surg 1942; 116: 26–33.

534. Tang JS, Gold RH, Mirra JM, Eckardt J. Hemangiopericytoma of bone. Cancer 1988; 62: 848–859.

535. Wold LE, Unni KK, Cooper KL, et al. Hemangiopericytoma of bone. Am J Surg Pathol 1982; 6: 53–58.

536. Milgram JW. Intraosseous lipomas. A clinicopathologic study of 66 cases. Clin Orthop 1988; 231: 277–302.

537. Miller MD, Ragsdale BD, Sweet DE. Parosteal lipomas: a new perspective. Pathology 1992; 24: 132–139.

538. Yamamoto T, Marui T, Akisue T, et al. Intracortical lipoma of the femur. Am J Surg Pathol 2002; 26: 804–808.

539. Goto T, Kojima T, Iijima T, et al. Intraosseous lipoma: a clinical study of 12 patients. J Orthop Sci 2002; 7: 274–280.

540. Hirata M, Kusuzaki K, Hirasawa Y. Eleven cases of intraosseous lipoma of the calcaneus. Anticancer Res 2001; 21(6A): 4099–4103.

541. Propeck T, Bullard MA, Lin J, et al. Radiologic–pathologic correlation of intraosseous lipomas. AJR 2000; 175: 673–678.

542. Ramos A, Castello J, Sartoris DJ, et al. Osseous lipoma: CT appearance. Radiology 1985; 157: 615–619.

543. Kawashima A, Magid D, Fishman EK, et al. Parosteal ossifying lipoma: CT and MR findings. J Comput Assist Tomogr 1993; 17(1): 147–150.

544. Chow LT, Lee KC. Intraosseous lipoma. A clinicopathologic study of nine cases. Am J Surg Pathol 1992; 16: 401–410.

545. Barcelo M, Pathria MN, Abdul-Karim FW. Intraosseous lipoma. A clinicopathologic study of four cases. Arch Pathol Lab Med 1992; 116: 947–950.

546. Bridge JA, DeBoer J, Walker CW, Neff JR. Translocation t(3; 12)(q28; q14) in parosteal lipoma. Genes Chromosomes Cancer 1995; 12: 70–72.

547. Petit MM, Swarts S, Bridge JA, Van de Ven WJ. Expression of reciprocal fusion transcripts of the HMGIC and LPP genes in parosteal lipoma. Cancer Genet Cytogenet 1998; 106: 18–23.

548. Dawson EK. Liposarcoma of bone. J Pathol Bacteriol 1955; 70: 513–520.

549. Addison AK, Payne SR. Primary liposarcoma of bone. Case report. J Bone Joint Surg 1982; 64A: 301–304.

550. Torok G, Meller Y, Maor E. Primary liposarcoma of bone. Case report and review of the literature. Bull Hosp Jt Dis Orthop Inst 1983; 43(1): 28–37.

551. Kenan S, Lewis MM, Abdelwahab IF, et al. Case report 652: Primary intraosseous low grade myxoid sarcoma of the scapula (myxoid liposarcoma). Skeletal Radiol 1991; 20: 73–75.

552. Pardo-Mindan FJ, Ayala H, Joly M, et al. Primary liposarcoma of bone: light and electron microscopic study. Cancer 1981; 48: 274–280.

553. Mutema GK, Sorger J. Intraosseous schwannoma of the humerus. Skeletal Radiol 2002; 31: 419–421.

554. De la Monte SM, Dorfman HD, Chandra R, Malawer M. Intraosseous schwannoma: histologic features, ultrastructure, and review of the literature. Hum Pathol 1984; 15: 551–558.

555. Gordon EJ. Solitary intraosseous neurilemmoma of the tibia: review of intraosseous neurilemmoma and neurofibroma. Clin Orthop 1976; 117: 271–282.

556. Verma RR, Khan MT, Davies AM, et al. Subperiosteal schwannomas of the femur. Skeletal Radiol 2002; 31: 422–425.

557. Vitale MG, Guha A, Skaggs DL. Orthopaedic manifestations of neurofibromatosis in children: an update. Clin Orthop 2002; 401: 107–118.

558. Bullock MJ, Bedard YC, Bell RS, Kandel R. Intraosseous malignant peripheral nerve sheath tumor. Report of a case and review of the literature. Arch Pathol Lab Med 1995; 119: 367–370.

559. Terry DG, Sauser DD, Gordon MD. Intraosseous malignant peripheral nerve sheath tumor in a patient with neurofibromatosis. Skeletal Radiol 1998; 27:346–349.

560. Alessi G, Lemmerling M, Vereecken L, De Waele L. Benign metastasizing leiomyoma to skull base and spine: a report of two cases. Clin Neurol Neurosurg 2003; 105: 170–174.

561. Goldblatt LI, Edesess RB. Central leiomyoma of the mandible. Oral Surg Oral Med Oral Pathol 1977; 43: 591–597.

562. Shen SH, Steinbach LS, Wang SF, et al. Primary leiomyosarcoma of bone. Skeletal Radiol 2001; 30: 600–603.

563. Sundaram M, Akduman I, White LM, et al. Primary leiomyosarcoma of bone. AJR 1999; 172: 771–776.

564. Bush CH, Reith JD, Spanier SS. Mineralization in musculoskeletal leiomyosarcoma: radiologic-pathologic correlation. AJR 2003; 180: 109–113.

565. Berlin O, Angervall L, Kindblom LG, et al. Primary leiomyosarcoma of bone. A clinical, radiographic, pathologic-anatomic, and prognostic study of 16 cases. Skeletal Radiol 1987; 16: 364–376.

566. Jundt G, Moll C, Nidecker A, et al. Primary leiomyosarcoma of bone: report of eight cases. Hum Pathol 1994; 25: 1205–1212.

567. Antonescu CR, Erlandson RA, Huvos AG. Primary leiomyosarcoma of bone: a clinicopathologic, immunohistochemical, and ultrastructural study of 33 patients and a literature review. Am J Surg Pathol 1997; 21: 1281–1294.

568. Khoddami M, Bedard YC, Bell RS, Kandel RA. Primary leiomyosarcoma of bone: report of seven cases and review of the literature. Arch Pathol Lab Med 1996; 120: 671–675.

569. Desai S, Jambhekar N. Clinicopathological evaluation of metastatic carcinomas of bone : a retrospective analysis of 114 cases over 10 years. Indian J Pathol Microbiol 1995; 38(1): 49–54.

570. Lyda MH, Tetef M, Carter NH, et al. Keratin immunohistochemistry detects clinically significant metastases in bone marrow biopsy specimens in women with lobular breast carcinoma. Am J Surg Pathol 2000; 24: 1593–1599.

571. Althausen P, Althausen A, Jennings LC, Mankin HJ. Prognostic factors and surgical treatment of osseous metastases secondary to renal cell carcinoma. Cancer 1997; 80: 1103–1109.

572. Spjut HJ, Dorfman HD. Florid reactive periostitis of the tubular bones of the hands and feet. A benign lesion which may simulate osteosarcoma. Am J Surg Pathol 1981; 5: 423–433.

573. Craver RD, Correa-Gracian H, Heinrich S. Florid reactive periostitis. Hum Pathol 1997; 28: 745–747.

574. Mallory TB. A group of metaplastic and neoplstic bone and cartilage containing tumors of soft parts. Am J Pathol 1933; 9: 765–776.

575. Dupree WB, Enzinger FM. Fibro-osseous pseudotumor of the digits. Cancer 1986; 58: 2103–2109.

576. Ackerman LV. Extra-osseous localized non-neoplastic bone and cartilage formation (so-called myositis ossificans). J Bone Joint Surg 1958; 40A: 279–298.

577. Howard RF, Slawski DP, Gilula LA. Florid reactive periostitis of the digit with cortical erosion: a case report and review of the literature. J Hand Surg 1996; 21A: 501–505.

578. Meneses MF, Unni KK, Swee RG. Bizarre parosteal osteochondromatous proliferation of bone (Nora's lesion). Am J Surg Pathol 1993; 17: 691–697.

579. Kilpatrick SE, Koplyay PD, Pope TL, Ward WG. Clinical, radiologic, and pathologic spectrum of myositis ossificans and related lesions: a unifying concept. Adv Anat Pathol 1997; 5: 277–286.

580. Yuen M, Friedman L, Orr W, Cockshott WP. Proliferative periosteal processes of phalanges: a unitary hypothesis. Skeletal Radiol 1992; 21: 301–303.

581. Oviedo A, Simmons T, Benya E, Gonzalez-Crussi F. Bizarre parosteal osteochondromatous proliferation: case report and review of the literature. Pediatr Dev Pathol 2001; 4: 496–500.

582. Michelsen H, Abramovici L, Steiner G, Posner MA. Bizarre parosteal osteochondromatous proliferation (Nora's lesion) in the hand. J Hand Surg [Am] 2004; 29: 520–525.

583. Abramovici L, Steiner GC. Bizarre parosteal osteochondromatous proliferation (Nora's lesion): a retrospective study of 12 cases, 2 arising in long bones. Hum Pathol 2002; 33: 1205–1210.

584. Torreggiani WC, Munk PL, Al-Ismail K, et al. MR imaging features of bizarre parosteal osteochondromatous proliferation of bone (Nora's lesion). Eur J Radiol 2001; 40: 224–231.

585. Letts M, Davidson D, Nizalik E. Subungual exostosis: diagnosis and treatment in children. J Trauma 1998; 44: 346–349.

586. Landon GC, Johnson KA, Dahlin DC. Subungual exostoses. J Bone Joint Surg 1979; 61A: 256–259.

Upper respiratory system

Sinonasal and nasopharyngeal surgical pathology

Margaret Brandwein-Gensler

15

RHINITIS, SINUSITIS

The 'common cold' is the most frequent infectious upper respiratory tract malady, manifesting as profuse, watery, nasal discharge, usually persisting less than one week. Most commonly it is caused either by rhinoviruses, parainfluenza and influenza viruses, adenoviruses, or respiratory syncytial virus. The onset of mucopurulent discharge indicates bacterial superinfection, following decreased sinus aeration and changes in bacterial flora. Clinically, this is associated with pain over the affected sinus. Chronic sinusitis results from either persistent acute inflammation or repeated bouts of acute or subacute sinusitis; this may develop in up to one-third of patients. The surgical pathologist seldom evaluates specimens from acute sinusitis, but we commonly examine tissues with chronic sinusitis. We often see moderate to dense lymphoplasmacytic infiltrates. The presence of eosinophilia signifies allergic etiology. If dense eosinophilic exudates and necrotic debris are seen, then allergic fungal sinusitis should be considered.[1] All submitted tissue should then be examined by Gomori methenamine silver stain, as only sparse hyphae may be present. By contrast, a 'mycetoma' or sinus 'fungus ball' contains abundant hyphae and fruiting heads bearing conidia amidst inflammatory debris. Chronic sinusitis can also cause hypertrophic polypoid mucosa. The papillary goblet cell hyperplasia in chronic sinusitis can be so extreme as to mimic low-grade intestinal-like adenocarcinoma (ITAC). Pseudostratified respiratory epithelium lines the papillae of papillary sinusitis, and the papillae are thick and diffusely inflamed. Simple columnar epithelium with goblet cells line the papillae of low-grade ITAC; the stalks are thin and fibrous. When in doubt, correlation with the radiographic findings will resolve this dilemma, as sinus papillary hyperplasia causes diffuse sinus mucosal thickening. Though the effects of sinus obstruction may be seen, a space-occupying mass will not be present.

CYSTS, POLYPS AND MUCOCELES

Polyps and cysts are the most frequent complications of inflammatory sinusitis. Mucous retention cysts are most common, found incidentally on plain films in about 10–35% of patients. They result from the obstruction of submucosal mucinous glands. A mucocele is a mucous retention cyst that has erupted through the sinus boundaries, and expanded, causing bony remodeling in its wake. Mucus retention cysts can occur in any sinus, along any wall, but most commonly occur in the maxilla. Mucoceles most often occur in sinuses with dependent drainage: the frontal and ethmoid sinuses. Pathologically, if the mucocele is removed intact, one sees a mucous-filled cyst lined by sinonasal mucosa. Polyps result from an expansion of fluids in the lamina propria of the Schneiderian mucosa caused by allergy, vasomotor rhinitis, infectious rhinosinusitis, diabetes mellitus,

cystic fibrosis, aspirin intolerance, and nickel exposure. Occasionally, antral polyps may expand and prolapse through sinus ostia, presenting intranasally. These are referred to as antrochoanal polyps, and represent 4% to 6% of all polyps. Stalk torsion can result in singly dispersed bizarre reactive fibroblasts within the lamina propria. Between 10% and 20% of children with cystic fibrosis have nasal polyps. Generally, nasal polyps in children are uncommon, and 29% of such polyps in children are associated with cystic fibrosis. Nasal polyps may be also associated with aspirin intolerance and bronchial asthma (Sampter's triad). About 20% of patients with nasal polyps have asthma, and conversely about 30% of asthmatic patients have polyps.

SCHNEIDERIAN PAPILLOMAS

EXOPHYTIC PAPILLOMA

Clinical presentation

Exophytic papilloma (EP) (fungiform or squamous papillomas) are small gray, pink or white, sessile, warty growths representing 25–50% of all Schneiderian papillomas.[2,3] EP occur from the third decade of life onwards with a male predominance. Sinonasal EP can develop on the anterior nasal septum, vestibule, and inferior turbinate. Multiple sinonasal EP are uncommon (3.6%).[4] Paranasal sinus involvement is even less common but may be associated with multiple papillomas. EP are usually small (< 2 cm); they may be asymptomatic or cause epistaxis and nasal obstruction. There is usually no preceding history of chronic sinusitis and multiple procedures.

Pathology

EP are purely exophytic, with multiple layers of squamous epithelium lining distinct, delicate, arborizing, fibrovascular cores. The epithelium may be keratinizing or nonkeratinizing, but is more mature than that of inverted papilloma (IP) (Fig. 15.1). Goblet cells and gland formation may be seen within the epithelial ribbons. Nasal vestibule EP can resemble verruca vulgaris with a sessile, 'spiky' hyperkeratotic/parakeratotic appearance. Abundant keratinization in EP is uncommon; if present it can indicate either malignant transformation or an alternative diagnosis. Squamous cell carcinoma (SCC) can be quite papillary, and should be considered in the differential diagnosis. Papillary SCC will contain significant dysplasia, unlike benign EP. EP are usually entirely snared on biopsy. Definitive diagnosis of a squamous papillary lesion, especially one with dysplasia, should only be made after examination of the entire lesion.

Treatment and outcome

Sinonasal EP require conservative excision. The average recurrence rate cited is around 35%.[2–4] While this can be the result of incomplete excision, recurrent EP probably have a greater HPV viral

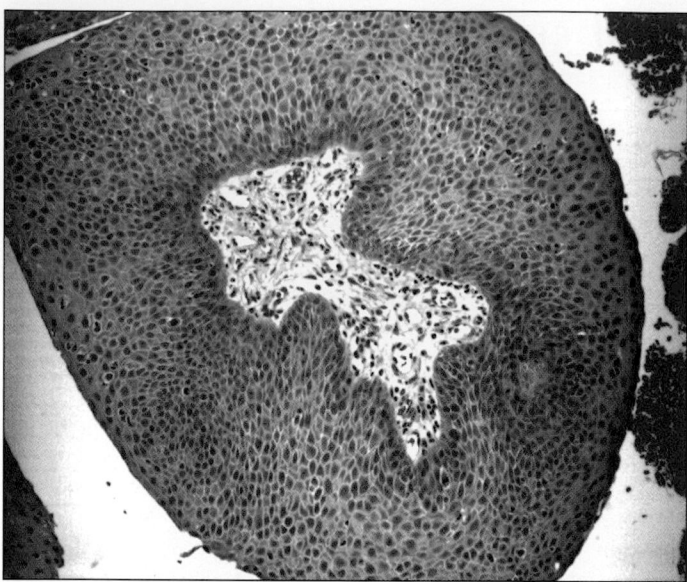

Fig. 15.1 Exophytic papilloma. These papillomas are defined by stratified squamous mucosa surrounding fibrovascular cores.

load, and might also be the result of reactivation of latent HPV infection in adjacent mucosa.[5] Malignant degeneration is uncommon, reported in 3.5% of 28 EP.[4] Buchwald reported two cases of nasal septal carcinoma ex EP.[6]

INVERTED PAPILLOMA

Clinical presentation

Inverted papilloma (IP) are white, gray 'prune-like' polypoid tumors with a pitted surface. They tend to occur from the fourth decade of life onward, with peak incidence in the sixth decade and a strong male predominance (approximately 3:1).[7] They are distinctly uncommon in children. Presenting symptoms include nasal obstruction, epistaxis, pressure, pain, rhinorrhea, and headache. A history of multiple polypectomies is commonly elicited. The most common site is the lateral nasal wall, around the middle turbinate or in the ethmoid recess. From these sites, IP may expand to fill the maxilla. Ethmoid IP can erode the lamina papyracea to involve the orbit and displace the globe. Bulky IP may extend through the posterior choanae to fill the nasopharynx.[8] Involvement of the frontal and sphenoid sinuses is uncommon, and usually results from nasal cavity extension. Likewise, isolated antral IP, without nasal cavity involvement, is uncommon (5%).[9] Bona fide nasal septal IP are also distinctly uncommon.[10] Bilateral presentation occurs in 8% of cases[7] and may be associated with malignant transformation.[11]

Pathology

IP are composed of ribbons and islands of immature, stratified squamous mucosa. The outermost layer can be composed of ciliated columnar epithelia and goblet cells or epithelial, keratinizing cells (Fig. 15.2) These ribbons invert into the loose lamina propria. Clear cell change of the squamous ribbons can be seen. Hyperkeratosis and parakeratosis are uncommon, and may portend malignant transformation. Squamous metaplasia and focal hyperplasia are common in the adjacent mucosa. Dysplasia is seen in approximately 10% of cases, ranging from focal mild to diffuse severe. A mixed exophytic/inverting pattern or mixed oncocytic/inverting pattern may be observed. However, if any inverting pattern is seen, then the mixed lesion is classified as IP. There are therapeutic implications in this, as IP are usually treated by lateral rhinotomy, whereas EP may be approached more conservatively. SCC ex IP is first recognized as an alteration in the silhouette of the inverting islands. Rather than the smooth contours of IP, the epithelial islands are larger and more confluent, with complicated shapes. Nuclear pleomorphism, increased mitotic figures, apoptosis, and necrosis are seen. IP should

Fig. 15.2 Inverted papilloma. **A**, Lateral rhinectomy specimen with typical, white, prune-like polyp with visible clefts. **B**, Thin ribbons of hyperplastic respiratory mucosa invert into the lamina propria. **C**, Hyperplastic squamous mucosa forms smooth ribbons and islands. **D**, Clear cell change due to glycogen deposition. The squamous mucosa is nonkeratinizing.

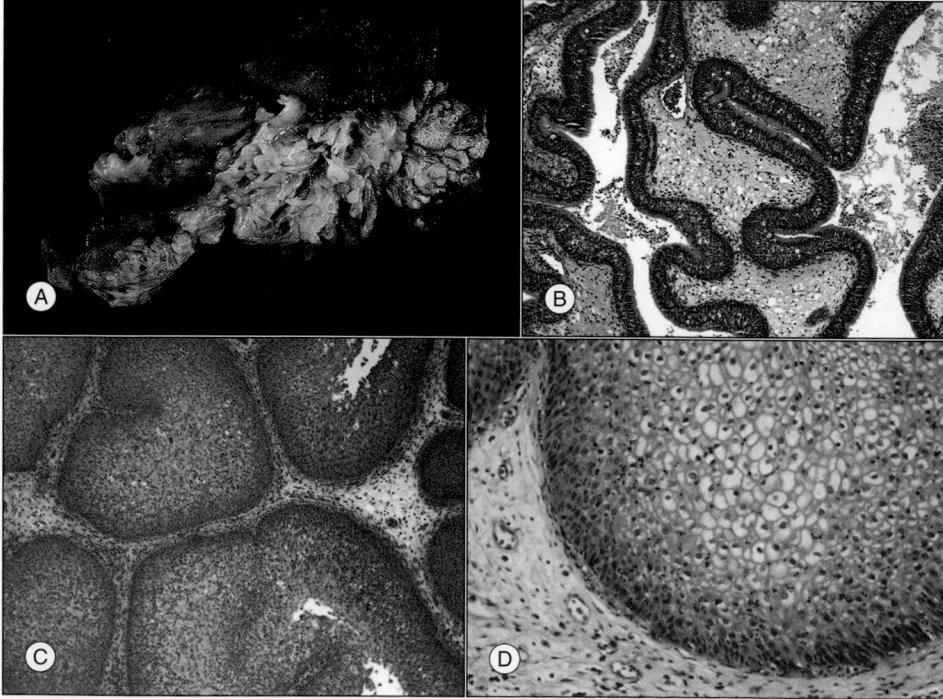

be distinguished from transitional cell carcinoma (TCC) – a variant of SCC. The islands of TCC are larger and more confluent than the discrete islands of IP. The typical hallmarks of malignancy (nuclear pleomorphism, increased mitotic figures, and necrosis) are features of TCC but not benign IP.

Treatment and outcome

IP has unlimited growth potential and can erode surrounding bone; intracranial or intraorbital erosion can cause significant morbidity. Intranasal polypectomy and Caldwell-Luc procedures have been associated with high recurrence rates,[7] as these approaches may leave IP behind in the nasofrontal duct, supraorbital ethmoid, lacrimal fossa, and infraorbital or prelacrimal recess. Lateral rhinotomy, i.e. removal of the 'party wall' between the nasal cavity and maxillary antrum, plus en bloc ethmoidectomy, is usually curative in 70–80% of cases.[12] Incomplete excision or large size predict recurrence, but disease recurrence after adequate resection is thought to be the result of multicentric disease. A compilation of 1300 cases[7] revealed that malignant degeneration develops in up to 3% of cases, and is concurrently present in 8% of all IP.

COLUMNAR CELL PAPILLOMA

Clinical presentation

Columnar cell papilloma (CCP) (1991 WHO classification), oncocytic Schneiderian papilloma, cylindrical cell papilloma, is an uncommon (3–5%) variant of Schneiderian papillomas.[2,13] The male:female predisposition (1.6:1) is less pronounced than in IP (3:1), and CCP presents over a wide age range, from the fourth decade onward.[2,13–16] CCP appear as soft, ragged, reddish tumors, grossly mimicking malignancy. They are more likely to involve the antrum alone than IP.

Pathology

CCP is comprised of pseudostratified and stratified tall oncocytes pierced with mucous microcysts containing polymorphonucleocytes (Fig. 15.3). The stratified layers of tall cells may also form a delicate lace-like pattern. Exophytic and inverted patterns are present. Inverting islands form 'star-like' glandular structures. CCP may also contain areas of typical IP; however, oncocytic epithelia predominates. On EM, CCP retains cilia and residual goblet cells amidst tall oncocytes.[13] Pleomorphism and mitoses are not routinely seen and should be considered ominous.

Treatment and outcome

CCP requires adequate surgical resection, rather than polypectomy. Although small series indicate a tendency towards recurrences,[2] en bloc resection probably is curative for most cases. Malignancy ex CCP is uncommon: while reported in 10–17% of CCP, this probably overestimates its malignant potential. The true incidence of malignancy in CCP is unknown for lack of a large reported series. Mucoepidermoid carcinoma, intestinal type adenocarcinoma, as well as SCC and undifferentiated carcinomas have been reported,[2,13–16] with disease-related mortality due to local disease or widespread metastases.[15]

SQUAMOUS CELL CARCINOMA

A review of data from the Surveillance, Epidemiology and End Results (SEER) program (1973 to 1987), demonstrates that head and neck malignancies constitute 4% of all tumors.[17] Sinonasal and

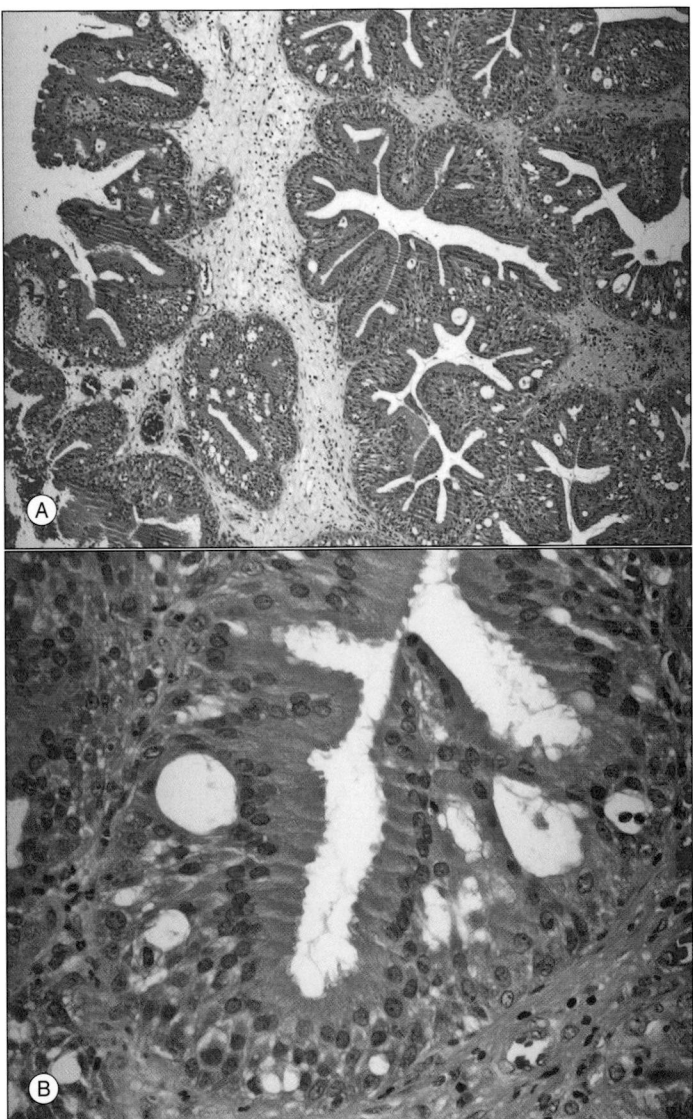

Fig. 15.3 Columnar cell papilloma. **A**, Stratified oncocytic columnar cells with ciliated and goblet cells line the surface and inverting islands of this polypoid neoplasm. **B**, 'Lace-like' glandular spaces punctuate this oncocytic, stratified mucosa.

nasopharyngeal malignancies represent a subset of 7%, (3700 cases), equally distributed between the posterior nasopharynx and anterior sinonasal tract. Most of these (approximately 64% or 2300 cases) were squamous cell carcinoma (SCC). When sinonasal cancers are stratified per site, 58% are antral (<700 cases/14 years), 30% are nasal cavity (<350 cases /14 years), 10% are ethmoidal (<115 cases/14 years) and only 1% are frontal or sphenoidal in origin (<12 cases /14 years).[18]

NASAL SEPTUM AND VESTIBULE

Clinical presentation

Nasal septal SCC is extremely rare, comprising 0.6% of almost 5000 head and neck tumors.[19] A male predominance is noted,[20,21] and there is a peak incidence in the sixth and seventh decades for

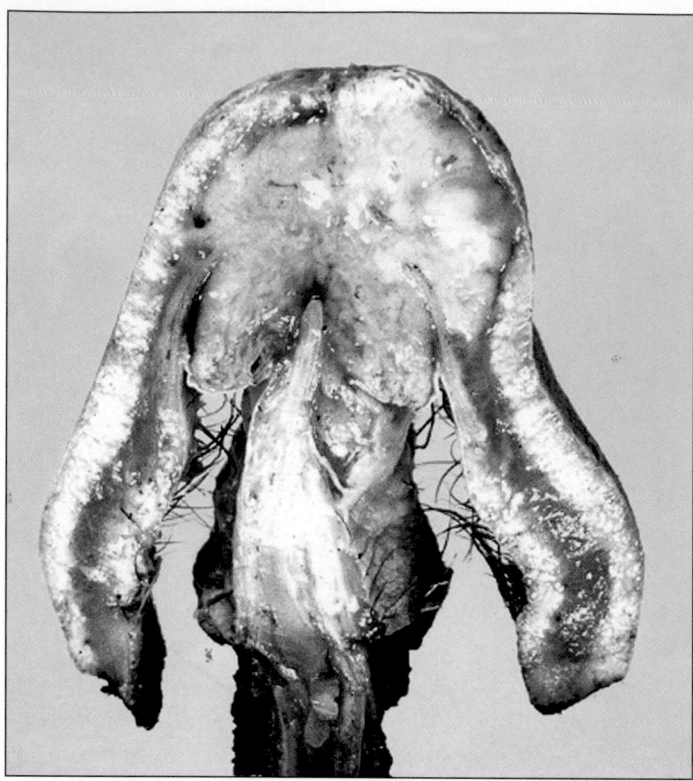

Fig. 15.4 Nasal squamous carcinoma. This septal carcinoma invades the subcutaneous tissue of the nasal dome.

septal/vestibular SCC. They present as a crusting ulcerations or 'sores' or as exophytic growths (Fig. 15.4).

Pathology

The histology of SCC applies for all sites of the sinonasal tract. SCC can vary dramatically with grade, and within various clones within a single tumor. SCC variants (basaloid-squamous, carcinosarcoma, transitional carcinoma, etc.) are discussed below. SCC is typified by keratinization and/or intercellular bridges, and lacking other features (glandular areas, goblet cells, ductal/myoepithelial component, sarcomatous areas, etc.). Keratinization is not confined to well-differentiated SCC, but may be seen in all grades. Individual cell keratinization can be seen within the cell cytoplasm as bright pink abundant 'glassy' fibrillary material. Intercellular bridges can be observed between cells as 'spider legs' or fine lines within intercellular spaces.

Treatment and outcome

Small septal/vestibule SCC can be primarily approached by either surgery or radiotherapy (RT), whereas larger tumors require surgery with adjunctive RT for inadequate margins. RT has the cosmetic advantages over surgical reconstruction.[22,23] Prophylactic, bilateral cervical RT may be indicated for N_0 patients, as this improves regional cancer control, but does not improve survival. Septal/vestibule SCC are usually deeply infiltrative and can extend into the columella, nasal dome, and lip. The rate of cervical lymph node metastasis at presentation varies from 10% to 30%.[20–22] The 5-year overall and disease-specific survival for septal/vestibule SCC is 58.5% and 87.0%,

respectively.[22] Mendenhall found the local control rates at 5 years after primary RT were: T1–T2, 94%; T4, 71%; and overall, 85%.[23] Positive lymph nodes are a poor prognosticator. Disease failure is usually locoregional; distant metastases (e.g. bone, lung) are uncommon.[20]

NASAL CAVITY, ETHMOIDS AND MAXILLARY ANTRUM

Clinical presentation

Nasal cavity/ethmoid SCC presents with nasal obstruction, anosmia, epistaxis, purulent drainage, widening of the nasal dorsum, and retro-orbital pain. Unfortunately, antral SCC is initially silent and presents late as T4 tumors with palatal ulceration, dental pain, loose teeth, facial pain, facial asymmetry or proptosis. Cranial base extension or posterior sphenoid involvement may result in facial pain (trigeminal nerve involvement) or ocular disturbances (adbucens, troclear, and oculomotor nerve palsies). Frontal sinus involvement is usually secondary to extension from the nasal cavity/ethmoids. Palpable neck nodes are initially present in 15% of cases.[24]

Pathology

See above section.

Treatment and outcome

Surgical resection is the treatment of choice, unless contraindicated by patient status. Combined otolaryngologic/neurosurgical approach is necessary for tumors eroding the cribriform plate and fovea ethmoidalis. Surgeons tend to preserve the orbital contents unless orbital apex involvement is discovered intraoperatively. Adjuvant RT is recommended for antral suprastructure SCC with orbital invasion or inadequate margins. However, the necessity for skull base RT should be balanced with the risk of radiation-induced blindness due to optic neuropathy or retinopathy. Multimodality approaches (neoadjuvant chemotherapy/RT protocol or regional chemotherapy) have been advocated and may improve survival.[25,26] Ipsilateral prophylactic cervical lymph node RT is recommended for N_0 necks.[27] The locoregional effects of antral SCC usually dominate; most patients die of tumor spread to the skull base and brain. Distant metastases (e.g. lung, brain, bone, liver) can develop in up to 25% of patients.

BASALOID SQUAMOUS CELL CARCINOMA

Clinical presentation

Basaloid squamous cell carcinoma (BSCC) is a rare, distinct variant of SCC. Only 3% of head and neck BSCC present in the sinonasal tract.[28–30] Clinically, BSCC is mostly submucosal, with little surface erosion, generally resembling salivary tumors. However, palpable cervical nodes would hint towards BSCC, as adenoid cystic carcinoma infrequently presents with enlarged lymph nodes.

Histopathology

BSCC is characterized by basaloid tumor cells with scanty cytoplasm with microcystic and reticulated growth patterns (Fig. 15.5). Invading islands exhibit prominent nuclear palisading. Stromal hyalinization (basement membrane production) is pronounced – a distinctive feature not seen in SCC. This hyalinization results in serpiginous, trabecular, and cribriform patterns of tumor infiltration imparting a salivary-type

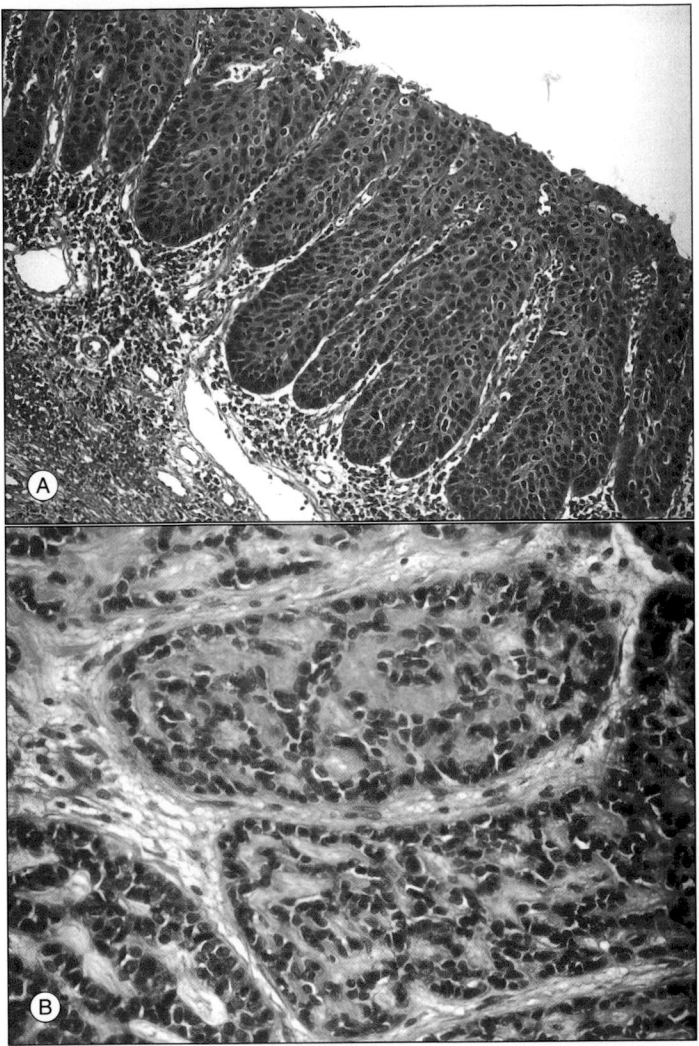

Fig. 15.5 Basaloid squamous cell carcinoma. **A,** Classical squamous carcinoma in situ bespeaks its nature as a nonsalivary tumor. **B,** Elaboration of basement membrane material within the tumor islands imparts an 'adenoid-cystic-like' appearance. However, the basement membrane material infiltrates between cells, and is not contained in a crisp, Swiss-cheese-like pattern.

appearance. The tumor infiltrates in discreet, smoothly contoured islands. Tumor cells emerge from elongated rete pegs, thus confirming its 'squamous' nature. Keratinization can be present either in the primary or metastatic tumor. The nuclei are not bland, but have coarse chromatin and prominent nucleoli. The cells may mold against one another to form a cobblestone pattern as is seen SCC. Necrosis and a high mitotic rate belie the high-grade nature of BSCC.

Treatment and outcome

The primary treatment is similar to that of SCC or adenoid cystic carcinoma – surgical resection followed by adjuvant RT. Most BSCC are diagnosed at Stage III/IV. Regional lymphatic spread is present in over 60% of patients; distant metastases develops in over 40% of cases. It is difficult to access the 5-year survival for sinonasal BSCC, as few cases have been reported. There are no convincing data to indicate that BSCC follows a distinctly more aggressive course than the SCC when matched for site, stage, and grade.

VERRUCOUS CARCINOMA

Clinical presentation

Verrucous carcinoma (VC) is an indolent, locally invasive carcinoma, which does not metastasize. In the upper aerodigestive tract it most commonly arises in the oral cavity. VC rarely originates from the nasal cavity, nasal septum, or maxillary antrum.[31–33]

Pathology

VC is characterized by a papillary, hyperkeratotic and parakeratotic surface (Fig. 15.6). The deep portion reveals pushing, broad, anastomosing rete pegs, often accompanied by a band of chronic inflammation. Adjacent mucosal hyperplasia is present with thin, elongated, anastomosing rete pegs. Nuclear pleomorphism is rare. When typical SCC develops in VC (hybrid tumor), one sees nuclear pleomorphism and irregular, infiltrating tumor islands, distinct from the typical pattern of VC.

Treatment and outcome

VC is primarily a surgical disease. Primary RT is adequate for unresectable VC, albeit associated with significant recurrence rates. The histologically benign nature of VC may contribute to delay in diagnosis; therefore, VC can become quite locally destructive before the diagnosis is established. Lymph nodes are usually palpable, but are reactive and benign. The clinical course depends on adequacy of primary resection; negative resection margins can assure cure.

SPINDLE CELL CARCINOMA

Clinical presentation

Spindle cell carcinoma (SpCC) (carcinosarcoma or pseudo-sarcomatoid carcinoma) represents 0.6% of sinonasal tumors seen at the AFIP.[34] They may arise in the nasal cavity, maxillary antrum, ethmoid, or sphenoid sinuses.[34] Presenting symptoms are nasal obstruction, discharge, epistaxis, and ocular symptoms.

Pathology

Polypoid or exophytic growth pattern is common.[34] SpCC is predominantly composed of malignant spindle cells and a variable admixture of malignant epithelial elements. If the overlying mucosa is intact, then carcinoma in situ can be seen. Keratinization may be focal, requiring extensive sectioning for demonstration (Fig. 15.7). Transition of keratinizing SCC into the spindle cell component can be appreciated. Immunohistochemical (IHC) and electron microscopic (EM) studies confirm that the spindle cells are actually transformed squamous cells, thus a 'sarcomatoid' carcinoma.[35] True mesenchymal differentiation can also be present in SpCC[36] but is not diagnostically requisite. SpCC should be distinguished from adult sinonasal teratomas (teratocarcinomas). The latter contain immature benign epithelial components, neuro-ectodermal components, variable mesenchymal components, and may also demonstrate carcinomatous and sarcomatous elements. Some adult sinonasal teratomas have abundant mesenchymal matrix (chondroid, myxoid differentiation), but for others the mesenchymal differentiation may not be obvious, manifesting only as foci of 'small blue round cells.'

Treatment and outcome

Surgical resection is indicated with combined neurosurgical approach for tumors involving the cribriform plate, anterior or

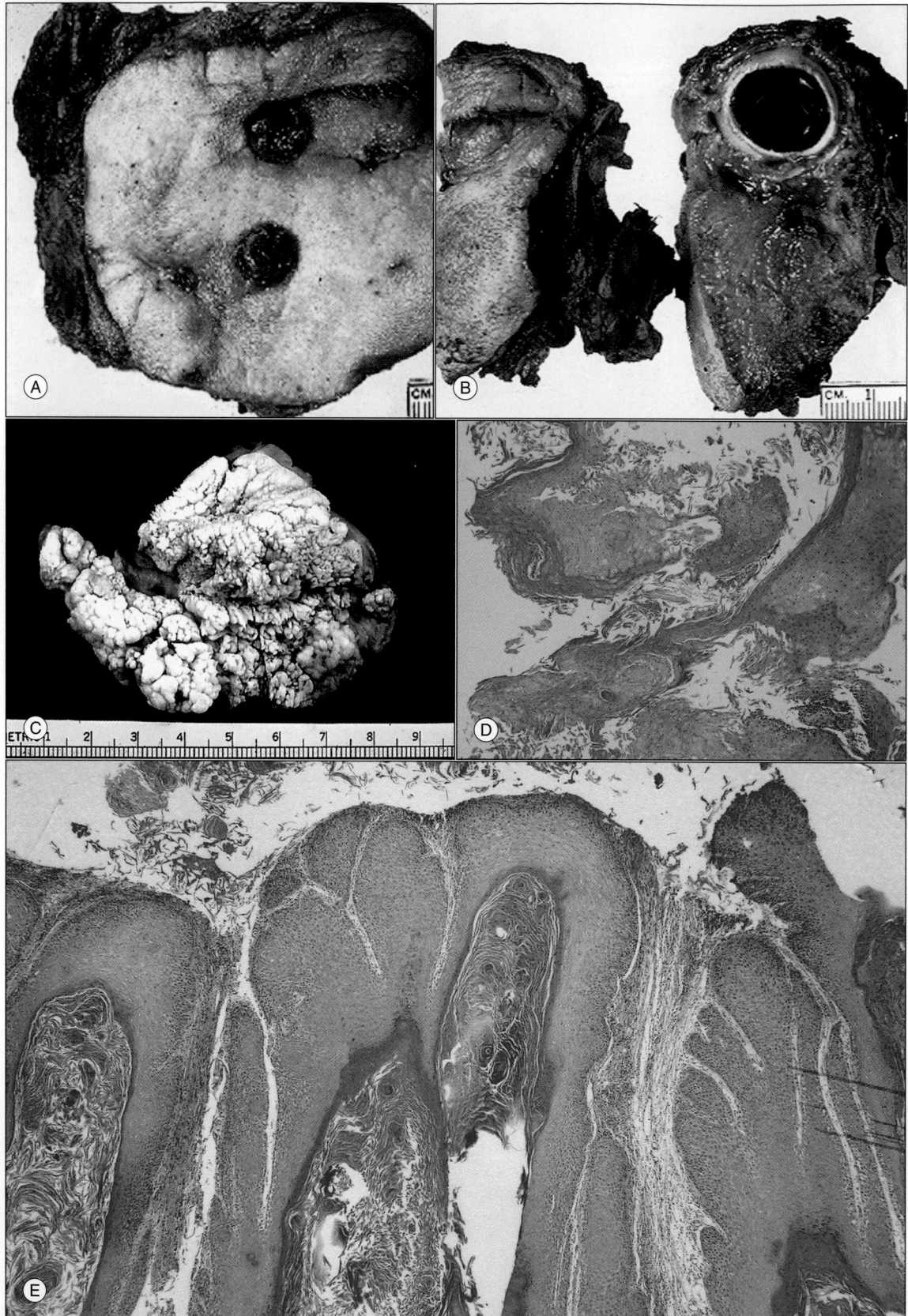

Fig. 15.6 Verrucous carcinoma (VC). **A**, This woman presented with lesions of the skin of the cheek, after multiple recurrences of a palatal tumor. **B**, En bloc maxillectomy with orbital exenteration was necessary. **C**, This buccal VC has a typical, white, gray cauliflower appearance. **D**, Superficial biopsy of an oral VC reveals only nondiagnostic, keratinized, bland tissue. **E**, Bulbous deep pushing rete pegs (pictured here) in addition to surface papillary hyperplasia with hyperparakeratosis confirm the diagnosis.

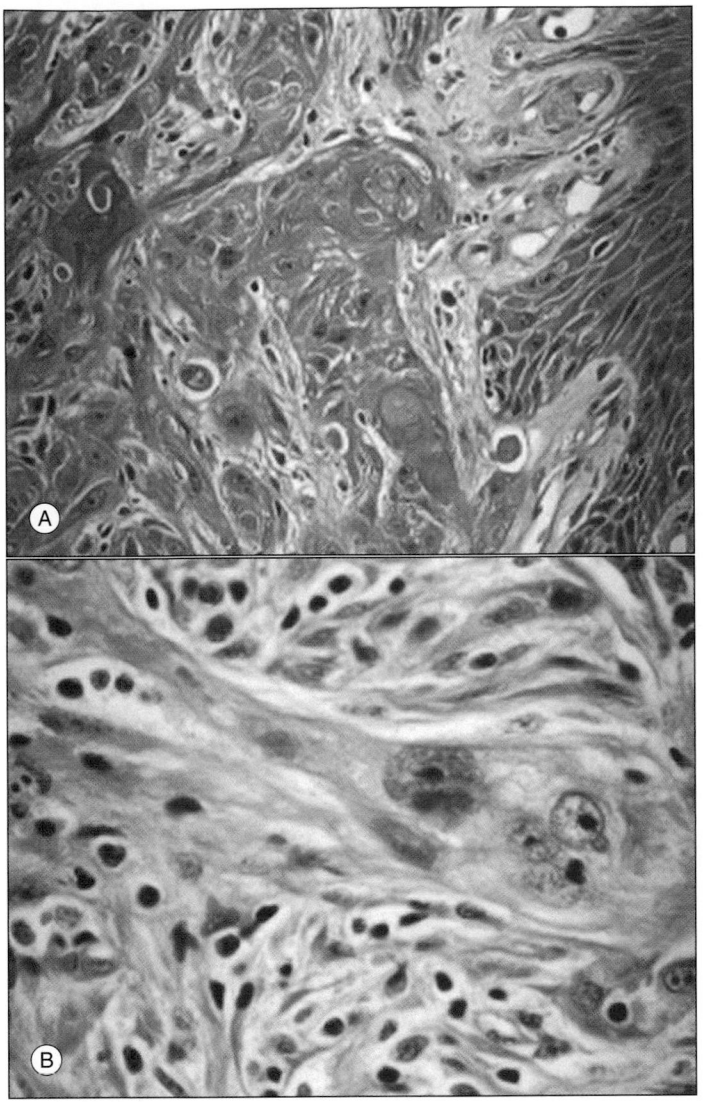

Fig. 15.7 Spindle cell carcinoma. **A**, If present, the more typical keratinizing component is seen adjacent to the surface mucosa. **B**, A significant component manifests as bizarre tumor spindle cells.

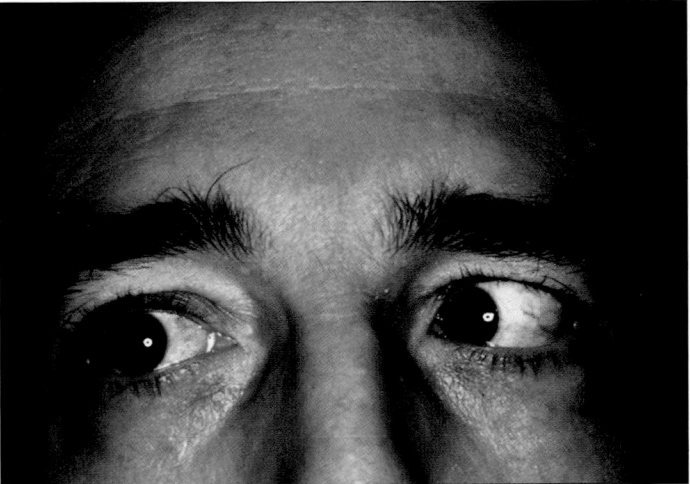

Fig. 15.8 Nasopharyngeal carcinoma. Skull base tumor extension can result in ocular disturbances (adbucens, troclear, and oculomotor nerve palsies).

NPC has a wide age range, with the peak incidence in the fourth and fifth decades, and a striking male predominance (2:1 to 3:1).[39] Familial case clustering is seen among the Chinese. Interestingly, although the US incidence is very low (1–2/100 000 men, .04/100 000 women), familial case clustering has *also* been described.[40] Early intervention for NPC is rare. More often it is diagnosed after already infiltrating the skull base or metastasizing to cervical lymph nodes. Patients complain of nasal obstruction and discharge, and present with unilateral serous otitis from Eustachian tube obstruction or oculomotor paralysis and sensorineural hearing loss from skull base infiltration (Fig. 15.8). Trotter's triad refers to the classic diagnostic triad of palatal fullness, deafness, and trigeminal neuralgia. NPC usually originates from the superior-posterior roof and superior-lateral nasopharyngeal walls. The overlying mucosa may remain intact; mucosal changes can be barely conspicuous on clinical examination. 'Blind' biopsies are often focused on the roof and fossa of Rosenmuller, directly posterior to the torus tubaris.

medial cranial fossa. The role of adjuvant therapy is uncertain. Most of the 13 patients reported by Howell[34] died within 18 months, with only one long-term survivor. Generally, superficial polypoid SpCC that lacks invasion is associated with a better prognosis than invasive SpCC.[37] Olsen reported that keratin expression adversely affected overall survival.[38] Conversely, Sonobe[36] noted that only the squamoid component was sensitive to chemotherapy/RT, while the osteosarcomatous component was unresponsive and metastasized.

NASOPHARYNGEAL CARCINOMA

Clinical presentation

Nasopharyngeal carcinoma (NPC) is endemic in Southern China: the incidence is 50/100 000 population. It is the third most common male cancer in Hong Kong. High incidences are also seen in Southeast Asia, Uganda and Kenya, Papau New Guinea, and Alaska.

Pathology

The WHO classification for NPC stratifies into 3 groups: WHO I, WHO II, and WHO III (Fig. 15.9). WHO I represents keratinizing SCC, as described above. It can be further subdivided into well, moderately, and poorly differentiated, based on the degree of nuclear pleomorphism, necrosis, and mitotic rate. WHO II represents transitional-type carcinoma or nonkeratinizing SCC. This tumor forms broad bands and anastomosing islands of tumor cells that can be tall cylindrical-shaped or cuboidal ('transitional cells'). Importantly, keratinization and intercellular bridges are not light microscopic features of WHO II. A variable lymphocytic infiltrate accompanies WHO II NPC. WHO III is an undifferentiated carcinoma ('lymphoepithelioma') with large, syncytial tumor cells having a high nuclear:cytoplasmic ratio, vesicular nuclei, large amphophilic nucleoli, and either forming nests (Rigaud tumor) or infiltrating individually (Schmincke tumor). They resemble lymphoid cells, especially immunoblasts. WHO III is typically accompanied by a dense lymphocytic infiltrate. A dendritic appearance may also be seen:

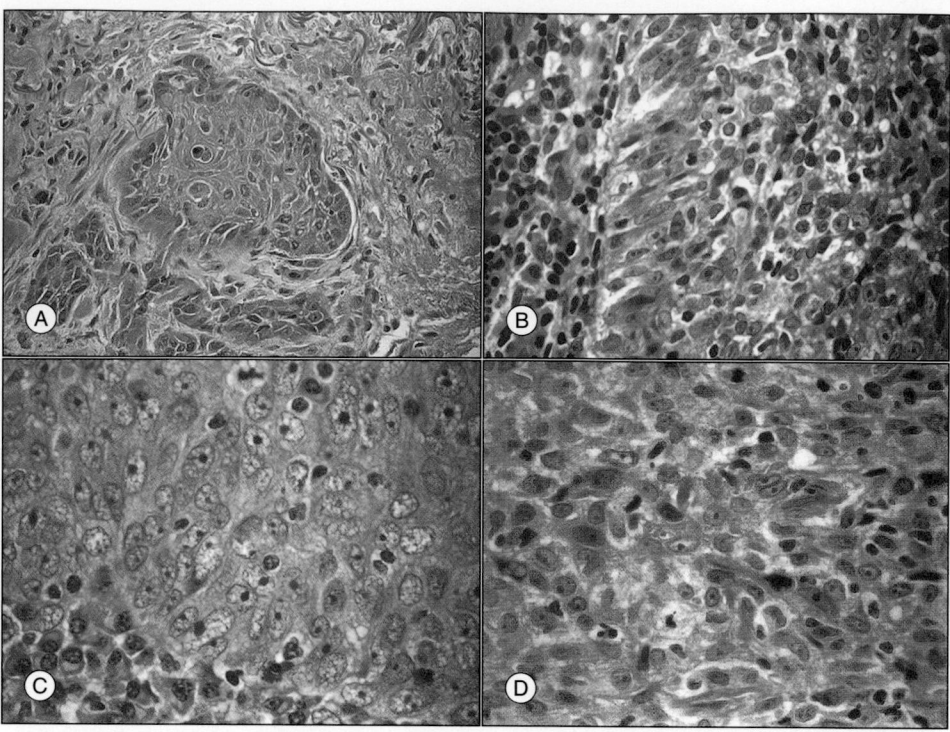

Fig. 15.9 Nasopharyngeal carcinoma. **A**, WHO I NPC is a typical keratinizing squamous carcinoma, posing no diagnostic challenge. **B**, WHO II NPC is a cohesive, nonkeratinizing squamous carcinoma with variable lymphoid components. Peripheral palisading of tumor cells can be seen. **C**, This WHO II NPC demonstrates amphophilic nucleoli and eosinophilic infiltrate, features suggestive for NPC. **D**, WHO III NPC is composed of discohesive immature tumor cells that may resemble malignant lymphoma.

interconnecting cytoplasmic processes between tumor cells are 'stretched out' and distorted by infiltrating lymphocytes. Tumors with spindled, basaloid (high nuclear:cytoplasmic ratio), syncitial cells may also be classified as WHO III. The distribution of WHO subtypes varies strongly with the populations queried. In the US, 75% of NPC are WHO I tumors, and are more likely seen in non-Asian patients, whereas the remaining 25% of patients with WHO II/WHO III are more likely to be Asian Americans.[41] By contrast, up to 98% of NPC in Asian series are WHO II/WHO III tumors.[42] Cervical metastases of WHO III NPC may mimic diffuse large cell lymphoma or Hodgkin's disease. Intermingled eosinophils can complete the mimicry.

Treatment and outcome

RT with high energy photon beams (6–10 MeV) to the nasopharynx and both necks is the mainstay therapy for NPC. Concurrent chemotherapy with cisplatin and 5-fluorouracil improves local disease control, and overall survival.[43] Patients who have failed radiochemotherapy protocols can undergo salvage resection. The prognostic value of subclassifying NPC by the WHO schema is debatable. Historically, WHO I NPC were considered less radiosensitive than WHO II/III NPC, and hence associated with a poorer prognosis than the latter.[41,44,45] Other groups have reported no significant differences in observed survival when stratified for histology.[46,47] Tumor stage is an indisputable prognosticator, and positive lymph nodes can predict propensity for distant metastasis, which typically involves the lungs, liver, and bone. Overall survival at 5 years for Stage I, II, III, and IV NPC has been reported at 89–97%, 64–70%, 53–54%, and 37–41%, respectively.[48,49] Patient demise is usually the result of local infiltration into the skull base, cranium, and middle or posterior cranial fossa.

SALIVARY TUMORS

ADENOID CYSTIC CARCINOMA

Clinical presentation

Salivary tumors comprise but a small proportion of all sinonasal malignancies, and adenoid cystic carcinoma (ACC) is most commonly encountered. The distribution is as follows: antrum, 69%; nasal cavity, 30%; nasopharynx, 2%; and ethmoids 3%.[50,51] ACC can occur over a wide age range, with a preponderance from the fourth to seventh decades and a male predominance. Typically, it is an indolent, widely infiltrative neoplasm with a propensity for perineural spread. Symptoms include long-standing pain, nasal obstruction, sinusitis, and nasal discharge (Fig. 15.10).

Pathology

ACC is composed of bland epithelial cells with oval nuclei and usually little cytoplasm, reminiscent of basal cell carcinoma. The nuclei may have coarse chromatin and prominent nucleoli. Myoepithelial cells are a variably present, and can be seen rimming infiltrating tubules and cords of tumor. ACC produces three architectural patterns: tubular (low grade), cribriform (intermediate grade) and solid (high grade) (Fig. 15.11A). The tubular pattern is characterized by slender tubules, solid cords, and glandular structures infiltrating a hyalinized background. The cribriform pattern has tumor islands with multiple 'holes' punched out in a sieve-like or Swiss cheese pattern, that are sharply demarcated from the surrounding cells. They may contain a 'rind' of dense pink basement membrane material, and central blue mucopolysaccharides or they may be entirely filled by this basement membrane material (Fig. 15.11B). The solid pattern consists of large carcinoma islands only infrequently punctuated by these 'holes.' Mitotic figures and necrosis are common in the solid pattern. Perineural spread is common to all patterns. ACC is usually composed keratinization, attachment to the rete pegs or the presence of surface carcinoma in situ. Table 15.1 includes the comparative IHC profiles between these tumors. Demonstration of myoepithelial markers (e.g. actin, calponin) will distinguish ACC from nonsalivary carcinomas.[52]

Treatment and outcome

Surgery with adjuvant RT is the standard therapy; adjuvant RT will improve local disease-free survival. Numerous reports have confirmed that the current grading system correlates with survival.[53–55] Tumor site is also an important prognosticator: minor salivary site ACC are associated with the worst prognosis.[51] Most sinonasal ACC are diagnosed at Stage III/IV, and the local recurrence rate is high (63%). While the local recurrence rate is highest within the first 5 years, many patients develop locoregional recurrence after 10–20 years. The 5, 10, and 15-year survival for sinonasal ACC is 82–70%, 55%, and 55–43%, respectively.[56,57] Distant metastasis (i.e. lung, bone) occurs in 40–50% of patients, up to two decades later, even in the absence of local recurrence.

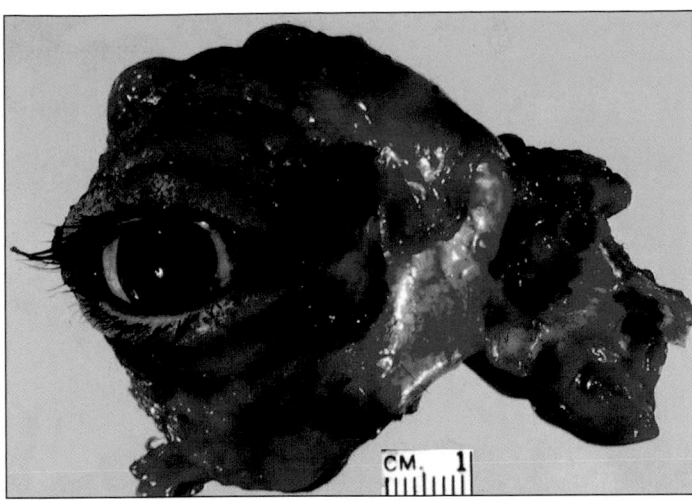

Fig. 15.10 Adenoid cystic carcinoma. En bloc resection of maxillary suprastructure with orbital exenteration.

of a mixture of two or three distinct patterns and tumors are graded (low, intermediate, or high) according to the most aggressive pattern present (30% or more). Solid ACC must be distinguished from basaloid squamous carcinoma (BSCC) and sinonasal neuroendocrine carcinoma (SNEC). Both ACC and BSCC may produce basement membrane and have cribriform and lace-like areas. Necrosis, and basaloid cells (ovoid with high nuclear:cytoplasmic ratio) with prominent nucleoli and coarse chromatin, can be seen in both. BSCC may be distinguished from solid ACC by identifying focal

PLEOMORPHIC ADENOMA

Clinical presentation

Compagno and Wong reported on 40 patients with sinonasal pleomorphic adenoma (PA),[58] demonstrating a wide age range (3 to 82 years, median 42), a slight female predominance (1.3:1), and a proclivity for the nasal septum (76%).

Pathology

Epithelial elements predominate here: bland epithelial ducts and islands can be seen rimmed and interspersed with spindled or triangular myoepithelial cells (Fig. 15.12). The mesenchymal matrix

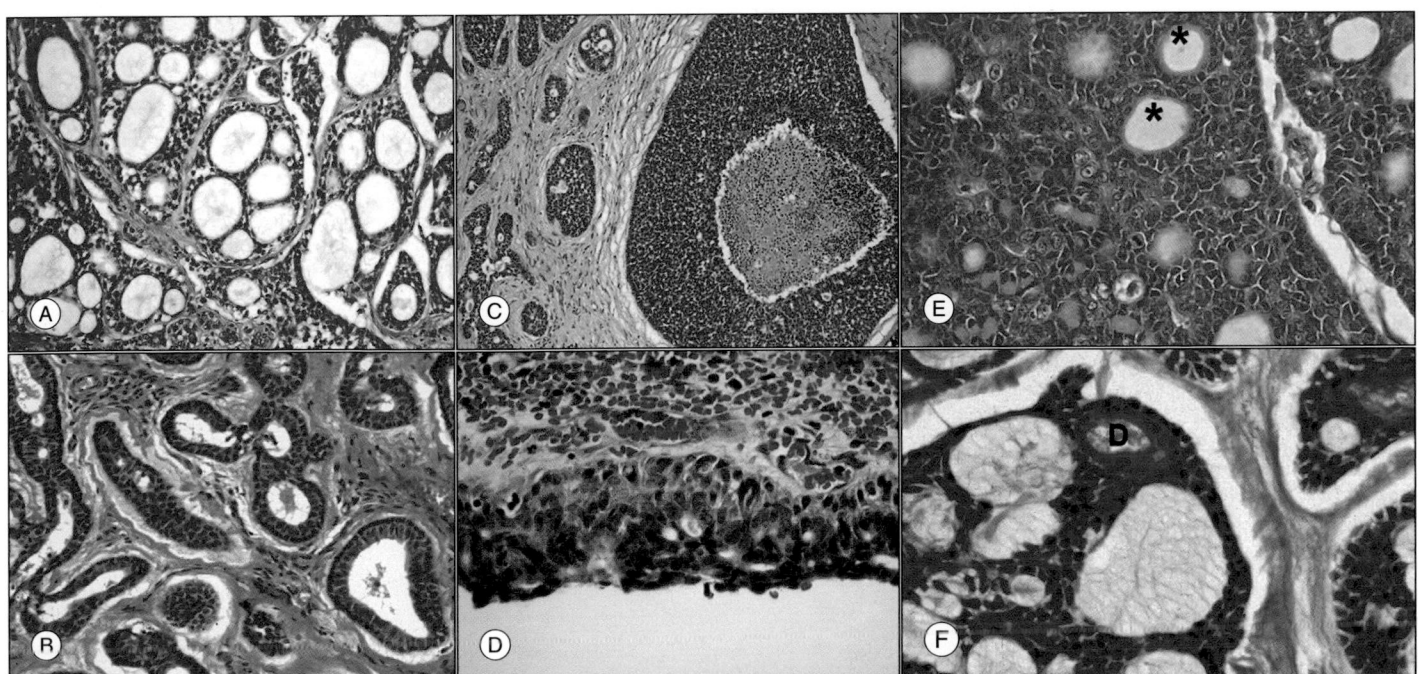

Fig. 15.11 Adenoid cystic carcinoma (ACC). **A,** Intermediate grade ACC is composed of 30% or more of the cribriform pattern. **B,** Low-grade ACC is composed of at least 70% of this infiltrating ductal architecture. **C,** High-grade ACC is composed of at least 30% solid tumor. Necrosis and numerous mitotic figures are frequently seen. **D,** In situ ACC in the maxillary sinus mucosa. **E,** The rigid cribriform spaces are pseudoglandular spaces formed by myoepithelial cells. They can be lined by a 'rind' of basement membrane material (*), or basophilic mucopolysaccharides. **F,** True ductal differentiation (D) is seen.

Table 15.1 Immunohistochemical profile for sinonasal neoplasia (modified from www.immunoquery.com)

	AE1/AE3	Cam 5.2	Keratin-Pan	EMA	CEA-P	S-100	NSE	Syn	Vim	Chrom	CD99	PGP 9.5	HMB-45	LCA	CD34	Actin-SM	FXIIIa	Calponin
Nasopharyngeal carcinoma	Yes	79	Yes	85	72	6	25	No	29	34	No	No	No	No	No	No	No	No
Spindle cell carcinoma	60	11	46	35		No			Yes		No	No	No	No	No	24		
Basaloid squamous carcinoma	88	80		83	54	40	50	2	27	No	No	No	No	No	No	No	No	No
Adenoid cystic carcinoma	Yes	78	Yes	64	30	68	No	No	Yes	No	No	No	No	No	No	60	No	Yes
Paraganglioma	No	No	11	No	No	Yes	Yes	Yes	54	Yes	No	82	No	No				
ONB	No	37	8	5	10	Yes	Yes	70	8	54	No	89	No	No	No			
SNUC	Yes	Yes	Yes	39/45	8/18	1/8	50	Neg	1/5	14/18	No	No	No					
SNEC	Yes	Yes				2/10	9/10	4/6	2/4	6/6			No	No	No	No	No	No
Melanoma	5	No	No	5	38	97	73	No	Yes	No	8	42	89	No	No		No	No
Melanocytic neuroendocrine tumor of infancy			Yes	3/9		2/8	Yes	13/17	Yes	3/17	1/8		11/17	No	No	No	No	No
Primitive neuroectodermal tumor	22		7	10		47	71	60	84	No	89		No	No	No	No	No	No
Ewing's sarcoma	16	No	9	No		32	52	39	96	No	93		No	No	No	No	No	No
ITAC	Yes	Yes		Yes	2/12		5/12	No	No	9/12								
Nerve sheath tumor	13	10	11	11		76	44	No	93	No	20	76	No	No	42	6	No	No
Pituitary adenoma	50	94	100			No	80	92		Yes	No		No	No	No	No	No	No
Chordoma	Yes	Yes	Yes	Yes	42	89	93	10	Yes	No			35	No	No	No		
Chondrosarcoma	No	7	No	6	No	Yes	65		Yes	No	13		No	No	No	No		
Hemangiopericytoma	No	No	No	9	No	10	No	No	Yes	No			No	No	No	20	Yes	20
Glomus tumor	No	No	No	No	No	No	No	6	Yes	No			No	No	30	Yes	67	80
Rhabdomyosarcoma	17	38	No	12	No	8	37	No	Yes	No	19		No	No	No	34		
Solitary fibrous tumor	5	No	No	No	No	11	38	No	Yes	No	88		No	No	94	10	85	25
Leiomyoma	16	15	13	8	No	6	No	No	92	No		No	No	No	17	89	No	82
Malignant fibrous histiocytoma	10	14	6	14	No	No	No	No	Yes	No	36	No	No	No	36	48	62	37
Inflammatory myofibroblastic tumor	27	32	33	16		No	15		Yes			No		Yes	18	78	54	
Plasmacytoma	67	0	23	65		No	No	No	Yes	No	No		No	64	No	No	No	No

Numbers represent percent cases expressing marker. Expression of <5% of tumors is designated as 'No,' marker expression in >95% of tumors is designated as 'Yes.'

can be myxoid, cartilaginous, or ossified. As with all minor salivary PA, tumors appear circumscribed but capsule formation is generally absent. Extensive oncocytic change[59] and rhabdoid differentiation[60] have been reported.

Treatment and outcome

Complete resection with negative margins is recommended. Compagno's long-term follow-up on 34 patients demonstrated that 90% were disease free after resection. This was attributed to the epithelial predominance, as myxoid-predominant PA are more likely to develop recurrence. Malignant transformation[61] or 'benign' metastasis[62] are rare events.

MYOEPITHELIOMA/MYOEPITHELIAL CARCINOMA

Clinical presentation

Myoepitheliomas are benign tumors comprised of myoepithelial cells (90% or higher). In the AFIP experience, benign and malignant myoepithelial tumors constituted only 0.025% of all salivary neoplasia. Few reports exist regarding these tumors in the sinonasal tract.[63–66]

Pathology

Myoepithelial cells can form spindled, plasmacytoid, or clear cells. They are most often seen as short, bland spindled or stellate cells. IHC and/or EM examination are necessary to confirm the salivary/

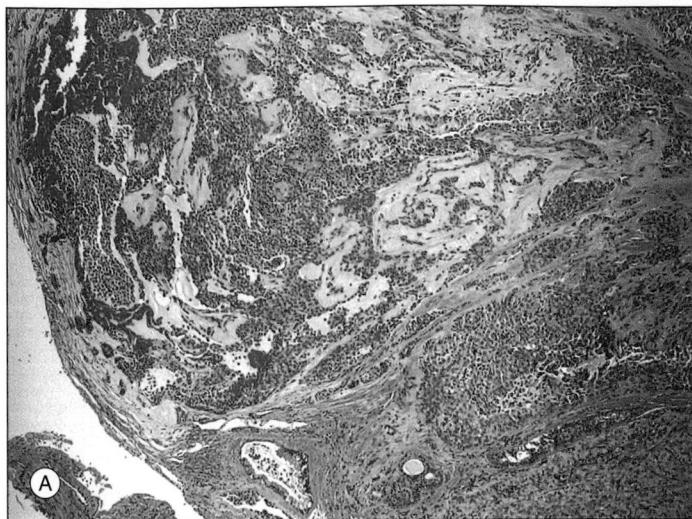

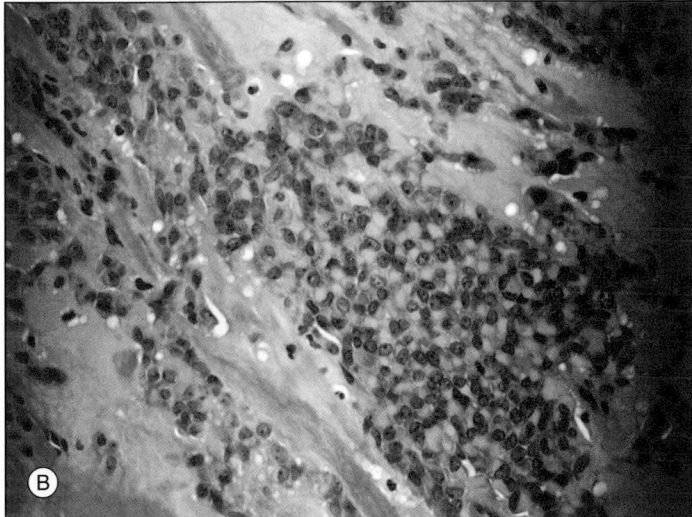

Fig. 15.12 Nasal septal pleomorphic adenoma. **A,** This tumor has a prominent myoepithelial component, with minimal chondromyxoid matrix production. **B,** The myoepithelial cells assume a plasmacytoid 'hyaline cell' appearance.

myoepithelial nature of these tumors. Myoepithelial cells express vimentin, S-100, keratin, muscle-specific actin, and calponin. This unique IHC profile is helpful in ruling out other tumors of mesenchymal origin. The malignant designation is based on evidence of aggressive growth and cellular pleomorphism.

Treatment and outcome

All salivary tumors, benign or malignant, require adequate resection. Adjuvant RT may be necessary for incomplete resection margins. Two patients reported by Begin were recurrence free 33 months and 80 months after resection.[63,64] One patient presented by Nilles was diagnosed as malignant based on a high mitotic rate. However, this patient only had limited follow-up (6 months).[65]

ACINIC CELL CARCINOMA

Clinical presentation

Most acinic cell carcinoma (AC) arise in the parotid; sinonasal AC are extremely uncommon, comprising only 0.2% of AC among almost 500 minor salivary neoplasms.[67] Three (1.3%) AC were seen among 224 sinonasal adenocarcinomas at the AFIP over 32 years.[68] Tumors are usually polypoid, and arise from the lower turbinate, nasal septum, nasal cavity, and maxilla and ethmoids.[69–75]

Pathology

Several architectural patterns may be seen: solid pattern, microfollicular with a lattice-like appearance, macrofollicular with larger follicles mimicking thyroid, and papillocystic, consisting of dominant cysts and fine papillae. The various cell types seen include the acinic cell, the vacuolated cell, the intercalated duct cell, and the glandular cell. The acinic cell has an eccentric, basally situated nucleus, and basophilic granular, bubbly cytoplasm that is strongly positive after diastase-treated periodic acid–Schiff stain. The vacuolated cell type is less basophilic and more bubbly. The 'intercalated duct' cell type has less acinar differentiation and resembles intercalated duct cells, with an occasional tendency to form ductal structures. The glandular cell type seen in the papillocystic variant tends to form hobnail cells, presumably after releasing its secretions into glandular spaces. EM examination may be the best means to establish the diagnosis.

Treatment and outcome

All salivary tumors, benign or malignant, require adequate resection. Adjuvant RT may be necessary for incomplete resection margins. The prognosis for AC is generally good. For parotid AC, the disease-free survival at 9 and 10 years is 90% and 60%, respectively, and metastatic rates of 8% and 19% have been reported.[76,77] Minor salivary AC *also* can behave as indolent tumors. No recurrences or metastases developed in 9 such cases (including two sinonasal AC).[78] Chen reported on 12 patients with minor salivary AC, wherein 3 of them developed recurrence.[79] Sparse prognostic data is available, but sinonasal AC appear also to behave in a low-grade manner. One patient developed a recurrence after 6.2 years, and was disease free after 11.3 years. The remaining 5 patients were disease free 10 months to 9.6 years after resection (mean 48 months).[69–75]

BENIGN AND MALIGNANT SINONASAL ONCOCYTIC TUMORS (OTHER THAN CYLINDRICAL CELL PAPILLOMA)

Clinical presentation

Few sinonasal oncocytomas have been reported, but they seem to have a predilection for the nasal septum, and are usually less than 1 cm.[80–83] Malignant or locally aggressive tumors have been reported in the nasal cavity, ethmoid, and maxillary sinuses.[84–90] Generally, locally aggressive sinonasal oncocytic tumors are larger than benign tumors, and usually display evidence of aggressive behavior (bony and perineural invasion) from the onset.

Pathology

Benign oncocytic tumors form follicular, papillary, and cystic structures. Tubular, cord-like, and solid areas can also be seen. General tumor circumscription is an important feature favoring benignity. Oncocytes are either cuboidal or columnar; columnar cells may have a characteristic tapered shape, a diagnostic clue for oncocytic tumors. The nuclei are round with condensed chromatin or open chromatin and prominent nucleoli. Binucleated cells may be seen. The cytoplasm is abundant and granular – this can be appreciated by flipping down the microscope condenser. Hyalinization, myoepithelial cells, or chondromyxoid matrix suggests pleomorphic adenoma-like differentiation. A tumor with these features may be classified as an oncocytic mixed tumor. Nuclear pleomorphism and increased mitotic rate can be seen in malignant oncocytomas,[88] but these features alone are insufficient criteria for malignant classification (Fig. 15.13). Alternatively, it is possible for malignant oncocytomas to be entirely bland. Malignant oncocytomas demonstrate either bony invasion and destruction, perineural invasion, or metastatic disease. Necrosis is seen in malignant but not in benign oncocytomas. If necrosis is encountered without the other hallmarks of malignancy, the tumor should be noted as atypical, and complete resection with negative margins should be recommended. The differential diagnosis includes cylindrical cell papilloma (CCP), and non-oncocytic tumors such as low-grade intestinal-type adeno-carcinoma, mucoepidermoid carcinoma, moderately differentiated neuroendocrine carcinoma, and transitional SCC. CCP may be recognized by its columnar oncocytes producing a lace-like cribriform pattern. Goblet cells are usually present in CCP but not in benign oncocytoma; CCP also frequently contains areas of inverted papilloma.

Treatment and outcome

Adequate surgical resection is indicated. Prognostic data is limited for 'locally invasive' nasal oncocytic tumors. They appear to follow the course of low-grade malignancies with multiple recurrences after a number of years.[85–87] One reported case developed locoregional metastasis.[90]

MUCOEPIDERMOID CARCINOMA

Clinical presentation

Mucoepidermoid carcinoma (MEC) comprises 39% of all minor salivary malignancies, based on the cumulative AFIP experience. The most common minor salivary site is the palate. Sinonasal MEC is rarely encountered; it is more likely for a maxillary MEC to have originated in the palate than to have arisen in the antrum. MEC comprised 15% of all sinonasal salivary tumors, 7 of them occurred in the nasal cavity, 13 in the maxillary antrum.[91] The AFIP reported on 11 patients with sinonasal MEC.[92] Healey's series of 60 patients with MEC contained 8 patients with maxillary (7) and nasal cavity (1) tumors.[93]

Pathology

MEC are composed of varying proportions of three cell types – keratinizing squamous cells with abundant eosinophilic cytoplasm, noncommited intermediate cells that are generally larger than the squamous cells and have abundant cleared-out cytoplasm, and neoplastic mucin-producing goblet cells (Fig. 15.14A). The proportion of cell types, pattern formation, and presence of features such as perineural invasion and nuclear pleomorphism determine tumor grade. Table 15.2 details the proposed weighted grading schema for MEC.[94] Low-grade MEC is predominantly cystic and composed of mucin-producing cells. Intermediate-grade MEC has a combination of cystic and solid areas, with a prominent intermediate cell component. It is more cellular than low-grade MEC, and may have some degree of nuclear pleomorphism and occasional mitotic figures. An aggressive pattern of spread at the tumor periphery may separate low-grade from intermediate-grade MEC.[94] At the other end of the spectrum, high-grade MEC is predominantly composed of solid areas and infiltrating islands of squamous cells, with a smaller

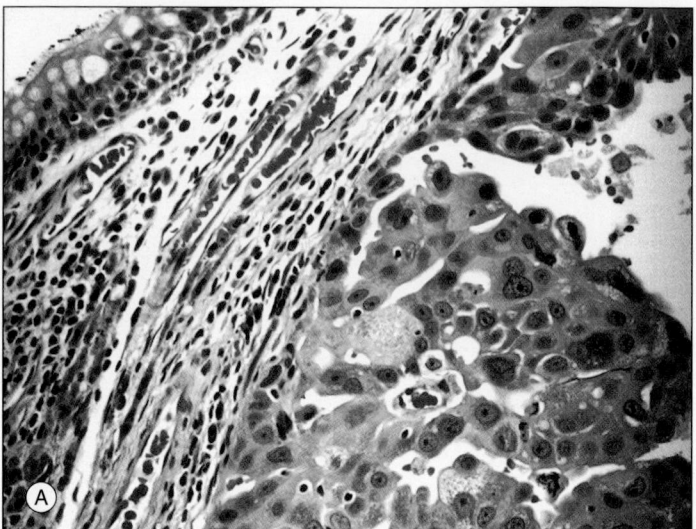

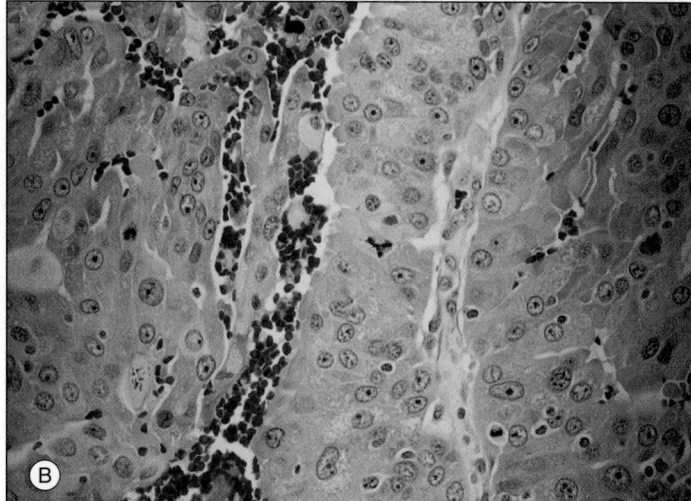

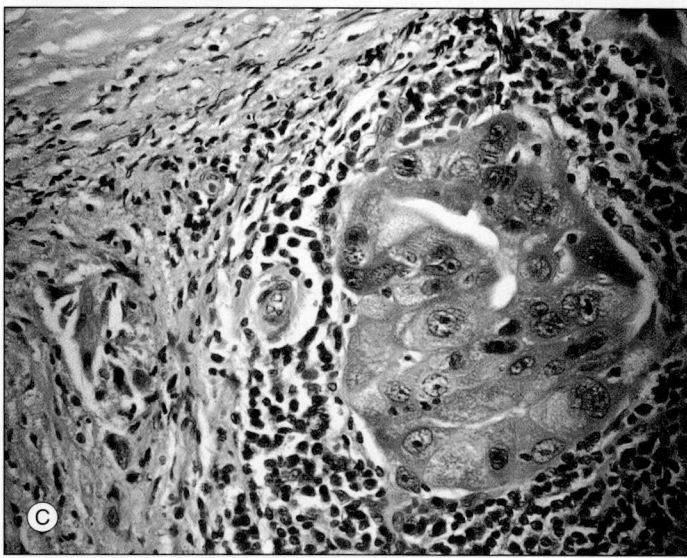

Fig. 15.13 Malignant sinonasal oncocytic carcinoma. **A,** This oncocytic maxillary tumor displayed invasion and pleomorphism. **B,** Atypical mitotic figures were abundant. **C,** Metastatic oncocytic carcinoma to cervical lymph nodes was seen at initial presentation.

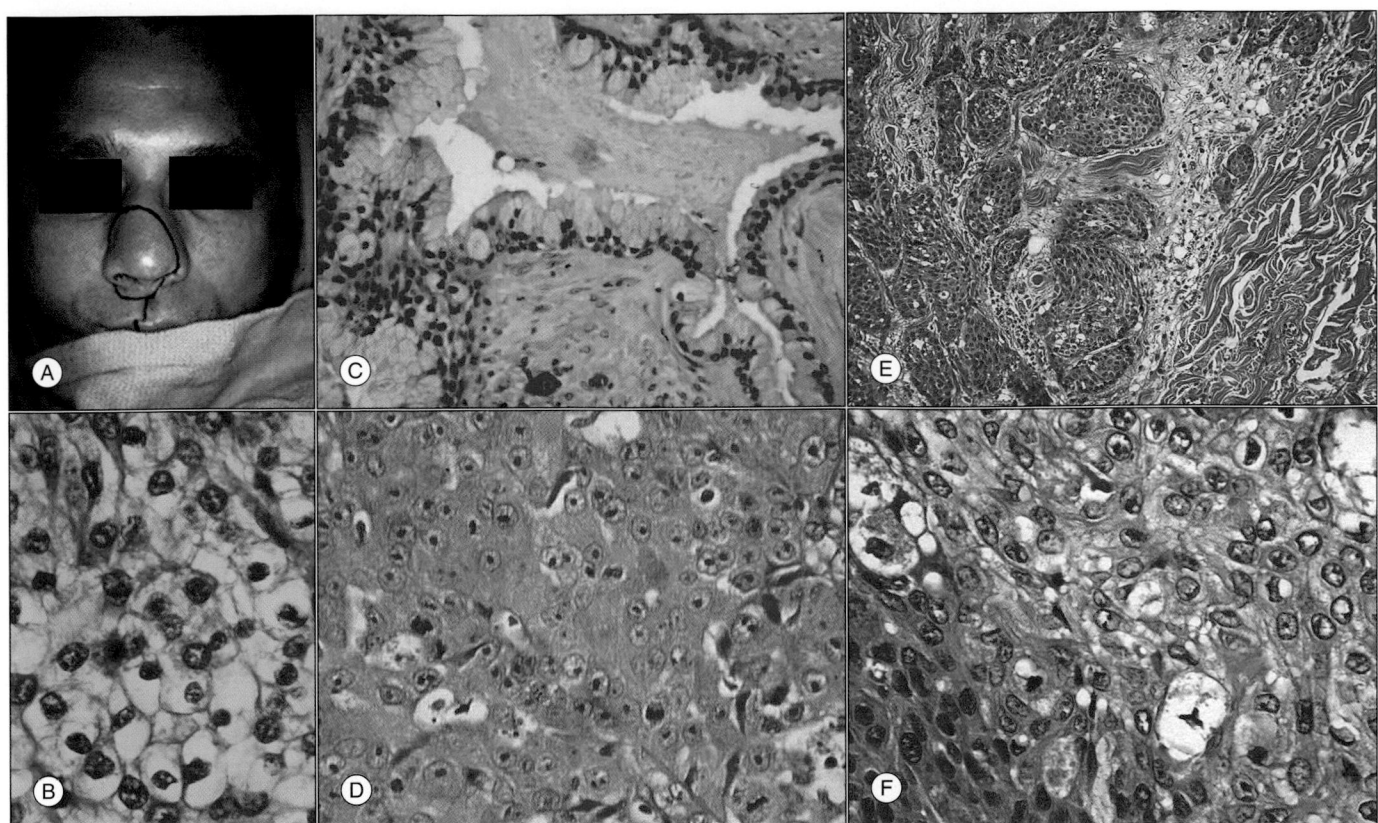

Fig. 15.14 Mucoepidermoid carcinoma (MEC). **A,** A rare example of MEC of the sinonasal tract. **B,** Clear intermediate cell component. **C,** Cystic goblet cell component. **D,** Squamoid component. **E,** Example of aggressive pattern of spread for MEC. This feature separates Grade II from Grade I MEC. **F,** Pleomorphism and atypical mitotic figures are some of the defining features of Grade III MEC.

proportion of intermediate and goblet cells. Necrosis, nuclear pleomorphism, prominent nucleoli, and abundant mitotic figures are present (Fig. 15.14B). Low-grade MEC should be distinguished from CCP and low-grade intestinal-type adenocarcinoma (LGITAC), which may also contain goblet cells. Further, the squamous component of MEC may take on an epithelial 'oncocytoid' appearance, due to the abundant pink granular cytoplasm. The predominant cells of LGITAC are also usually columnar, and papillary LGITAC, which contain goblet cells, are lined by one-cell-thick intestinal-type columnar cells. Intermediate-grade MEC may have a prominent clear cell component. The differential diagnosis here includes acinic cell carcinoma and metastatic renal cell carcinoma. The differential diagnosis of high-grade MEC includes SCC and adenosquamous carcinoma. Irradiated SCC is especially likely to produce glandular structures but does not contain goblet cells.

Treatment and outcome

Surgical resection with negative margins is the treatment of choice. Adjuvant RT is indicated for inadequately resected cases and all high-grade MEC. Elective neck dissection or cervical RT should be considered for N_0 patients with intermediate-grade MEC, and is indicated for N_0 patients with high-grade MEC. Not much data is available concerning patient survival for sinonasal MEC. Four patients from the AFIP series have follow-up; however, the details as to tumor stage and grade are unknown.[92] Two patients were disease free 4 years after surgery; 2 patients treated primarily with RT remained disease

free after 2 and 16 years. Two patients with high-grade MEC (antrum, ethmoids, one case each) were reported by Bergman;[95] both were alive with persistent disease at 3 and 5 years. In Healey's series,[93] 5 patients (1 intermediate grade, 4 high grade) died of disease within 1 to 4 years. The remaining 3 patients (1 intermediate grade, 2 high grade) were recurrence free at 1, 6, and 11 years.

POLYMORPHOUS LOW-GRADE ADENOCARCINOMA

Clinical presentation

Polymorphous low-grade adenocarcinoma (PLGA) most commonly occurs in the palate, and usually involves the maxilla secondarily. The female:male ratio is 1.6:1, with a peak incidence of diagnosis from fifth to seventh decades of life. Sinonasal PLGA comprise 2.0% of 173 reported cases of PLGA.[96]

Pathology

PLGA is composed of bland epithelial cells with fine chromatin, and myoepithelial cells, which may appear spindled, plasmacytoid, or epithelioid. A spectrum of architectural patterns is seen: solid growth, cystic, ductal/glandular, cribriform, papillary, and lobular infiltration. The background matrix can be similar to other salivary tumors, especially pleomorphic adenomas, namely hyalinized or myxoid stroma. Definite infiltration and perineural spread are features

Table 15.2 Proposed grading for mucoepidermoid carcinoma

	Characteristic features	Defining features
Grade I	Prominent goblet cell component Cyst formation Intermediate cells may be prominent Circumscribed growth pattern	Lack of grade III defining features, lack of aggressive invasion pattern
Grade II	Intermediate cells predominate over mucinous cells	Aggressive invasion pattern
	Mostly solid tumor Squamous cells may be seen	Lack of grade III defining features
Grade III	Squamous cells predominate Intermediate and mucinous cells must also be present Mostly solid	Necrosis Perineural spread Vascular invasion Bony invasion >4 mitoses/10 HPF High-grade nuclear pleomorphism

Feature	Points
Intracystic component <25%	2
†Tumor front invades in small nests and islands	2
Prounounced nuclear atypia	2
†Lymphatic and or vascular invasion	3
†Bony invasion 3 >4 mitoses/10 HPF	3
Perineural spread	3
Necrosis	3
Grade I	0
Grade II	2–3
Grade III	4 or more

† Modifications to AFIP grading criteria of mucoepidermoid carcinoma

that distinguish PLGA from benign tumors. Necrosis and abundant mitotic figures are generally not seen in PLGA. Vincent tabulated the original diagnoses submitted for 42 cases of PLGA which included monomorphic adenoma, adenoid cystic carcinoma, malignant pleomorphic adenoma, and pleomorphic adenoma.[96] Benign diagnoses may be dismissed upon finding tumor infiltration and/or perineural spread. The potential problem caused by a benign misdiagnosis would be in undertreating the patient: inadequate surgical margins might not be addressed with adjuvant RT, thus predisposing patients to recurrence. 'Overdiagnosing' PLGA as adenoid cystic or adeno-carcinoma NOS is less problematic from a therapeutic viewpoint; however, the overall patient prognosis is better for PLGA.

Treatment and outcome

Surgical resection with adjuvant RT for inadequately resection margins is indicated. PLGA may recur locally, even after many years. The overall recurrence rate is 17%, 1 to 19 years after initial surgery. A small percentage of tumors (9%) may metastasize to local cervical lymph nodes. Distant metastases have not been reported for PLGA. Too few cases of PLGA have been identified in the sinonasal tract to compare their behavior to palatal tumors, but it appears reasonable to expect at least the same propensity towards local recurrence after long periods of time.

LOW-GRADE PAPILLARY ADENOCARCINOMA

Clinical presentation

The papillary variant of PLGA (also referred to as low-grade papillary adenocarcinoma, LGPA) has received attention, as some of cases have followed a more aggressive course.[97] LGPA have a propensity to occur on the hard and soft palate.

Pathology

LGPA is more cellular than PLGA, composed of microcysts filled with papillary outgrowths. LGPA lacks the lobular breast carcinoma-like whorling and lobular arrangement typical of PLGA. The papillations of LGPA variably contain hyalinized fibrovascular cores. Local infiltration and perineural invasion are characteristic of both tumors.

Treatment and outcome

LGPA requires surgical resection. Inadequate margins require RT. Adjuvant RT for clinical N_0 necks is a consideration (see below). Slootweg compared 8 cases of LGPA to 7 cases of PLGA.[98] Three of eight patients with PLGA developed recurrence after 4 to 8 years, but no patients developed metastatic disease. By comparison, 2 of 8 patients with LGPA developed recurrence, one of whom subsequently developed locoregional and fatal distant metastasis. Likewise, Mills found that local metastatic disease developed in 3 of 5 patients up to 19 years after presentation.[99] Mostofi tabulated 22 cases in total of LGPA; 18 were from the palate, none was from the sinonasal tract.[100] The overall rate of regional metastasis was 17%. While this suggests that LGPA might have an inherently greater predisposition for metastasis, more experience and comparison with PLGA is warranted.

'SALIVARY GLAND ANLAGE TUMOR' (NASOPHARYNGEAL CONGENITAL PLEOMORPHIC ADENOMA)

Clinical presentation

Dehner originally proposed the term salivary gland anlage tumor (SGAT) for 9 babies with nasopharyngeal tumors who all presented with respiratory obstruction.[101] Feeding difficulties were also present in some babies, mimicking choanal atresia. The tumors were all pedunculated nasopharyngeal masses ranging 1.3–3 cm.

Pathology

SGAT are firm, bosselated tumors. Microscopically, they have a prominent biphasic nature. Epithelial islands, cysts, and branching duct-like structures are embedded within mesenchymal stromal-type background reminiscent of pleomorphic adenomas. Squamous metaplasia and keratinization can be seen. IHC, these tumors express salivary amylase. The stromal type cells can coexpress cytokeratin and muscle-specific actin, suggestive of myoepithelial differentiation, but definitive mature myoepithelial differentiation is not seen. The classic 'epithelial-myoepithelial' unit of mature salivary differentiation was not observed. The authors conclude that SGAT are hamartomatous or benign tumors that recapitulate developing salivary tissue. The main differential diagnosis is with a midline congenital teratoma. Histologically, SGAT lack teratomatous elements such as skin adnexal, neuronal, cartilaginous, or muscular elements.

Treatment and Outcome

Save for one baby who experienced spontaneous expulsion of the tumor during resuscitation, all were treated with localized excision.

One baby died of sepsis. None of the others experienced recurrence after follow-up (mean 3.6 years). Therefore, if the newborn survives the original insult of upper airway obstruction, these lesions, be they benign, neoplastic, or hamartomatous in nature, are associated with an excellent prognosis.

BENIGN AND MALIGNANT NEUROECTODERMAL AND NEURONAL TUMORS

PARAGANGLIOMA

Given the spectrum of neuroectodermal and neuroendocrine neoplasia that affect the sinonasal tract, one may justifiably query if true sinonasal paragangliomas actually exist. It is difficult to speculate on the nature of reported sinonasal paragangliomas prior to 1980, as they predate the evolution of the concept of sinonasal neuroendocrine carcinoma (SNEC), as well as the development of IHC. Certainly, cases of 'aggressive sinonasal paragangliomas' most likely represent SNEC. There are only a few reports of benign sinonasal paragangliomas in the literature in the past decade,[102] but few are convincingly illustrated.[103] Paragangliomas can be distinguished by IHC from SNEC by their lack of epithelial marker expression (Table 15.1). Both paragangliomas and ONB may reveal a sustentacular pattern of S-100 expression. The lack of neurofibrillary material, microscopically, corresponding ultrastructurally to the absence of neural processes, distinguishes paragangliomas from Grade I ONB. Presently, any sinonasal neuroendocrine neoplasm with paraganglioma-like areas, but with features of local invasion, are best designated as well- or moderately differentiated SNEC (see below).

OLFACTORY NEUROBLASTOMA

Clinical presentation
Olfactory neuroblastoma (ONB) are neuroectodermal tumors that arise within the superior nasal cavity. The origin for ONB has been debated. Traditionally, ONB is thought to arise from olfactory neuronal precursors, akin to neuroblastoma. However, evidence of epithelial differentiation within ONB has morphogenically distinguished it from neuroblastomas, and was the basis for nomenclature such as 'olfactory neuroepithleioma' or 'esthesioneuroblastoma.' Conflicting data also exist regarding the relationship between ONB and Ewing's sarcoma with regard to the t(11;22) or t(21;22) chromosomal translocation.[104,105] ONB occurs over a wide age range with the peak age of incidence in the sixth decade (Table 15.3).[106–118] They are usually polypoid tumors, causing nasal obstruction, epistaxis, and rhinorrhea. Larger tumors cause sinus pain, orbital symptoms, or middle ear complaints. ONB commonly extends into the ipsilateral ethmoid and antrum; large ONB can involve both sides of the nasal cavity and the paranasal sinuses.

Pathology
ONB is composed of relatively uniform cells, slightly larger than lymphocytes, with round to oval nuclei, either fine or coarse chromatin, occasional prominent nucleoli, and scanty cytoplasm (Fig. 15.15). Nuclear pleomorphism is minimal, and few mitoses are seen. The cells are embedded within a fibrillary background that corresponds to neuronal processes formed by the most differentiated of tumor cells. Homer-Wright rosettes represent tumor cells centripetally aligned around tangles of neurofibrillary processes. Flexner-Wintersteiner rosettes are gland-like structures formed by columnar or cuboidal tumor cells, and are evidence of true olfactory differentiation. Lamellated calcifications may be seen, and can occasionally be confluent. Hyams introduced a four-tiered grading system of ONB (Table 15.4).[119] It has been questioned as to whether grade IV ONB tumors are actually better classified as SNEC (see below). Generally, the less differentiated an ONB appears, the greater the need to rule out entities such as sinonasal undifferentiated carcinoma (SNUC), large cell lymphoma, melanoma, extramedullary plasmacytoma, and embryonal rhabdomyosarcoma. IHC and EM have become standard adjunctive tests to resolve these issues (see Table 15.1).[104,120] On EM, ONB contains multiple cytoplasmic processes with

Table 15.3 Clinical features and patient outcome for ONB

Author, year	Number	Age range (median)	Presentation at Kadish C (%)	Cervical lymph node metastasis (%)	Distant metastasis (%)	Actuarial survival Disease-free	Overall
Dulguerov 1992[107]	24	4–73 (41)	27	17	8	58% @ 5Y 53% @ 10Y	74% @ 5Y 60% @ 10Y
Morita 1993[109]	49	3–78 (48)	68	20	18	53% @ 5Y	69% @ 5Y
Jekunen 1996[108]	11	34–83 (59)	82		27	38% @ 5Y	51% @ 5Y
Irish 1997[110]	10	17–64 (50.5)	67				
Koka 1998[111]	40	1–67 (38)	76	18	40	38% @ 5Y	51% @ 5Y
McElroy 1998[112]	10	22–74 (45)	100				
Levine 1999[113]	35	13–77 (45.9)	62.9	25.7	11.4	80.4% @ 8Y	75% @ 8Y
Resto 2000[114]	27	17–77 (32)		33	26		
Miyamoto 2000[115]	12	17–85 (53)	58				71% @ 2Y
Eriksen 2000[116]	13	14–83 (49)	54	15			51% @ 5Y
Simon 2001[117]	13	36–81 (59)	62			56% @ 5Y 42% @ 10Y	61% @ 5Y 24% @ 10Y
Smith (in press)[118]	21	16–63 (48.9)	72	19		43% @ 11.3Y	80% @ 5

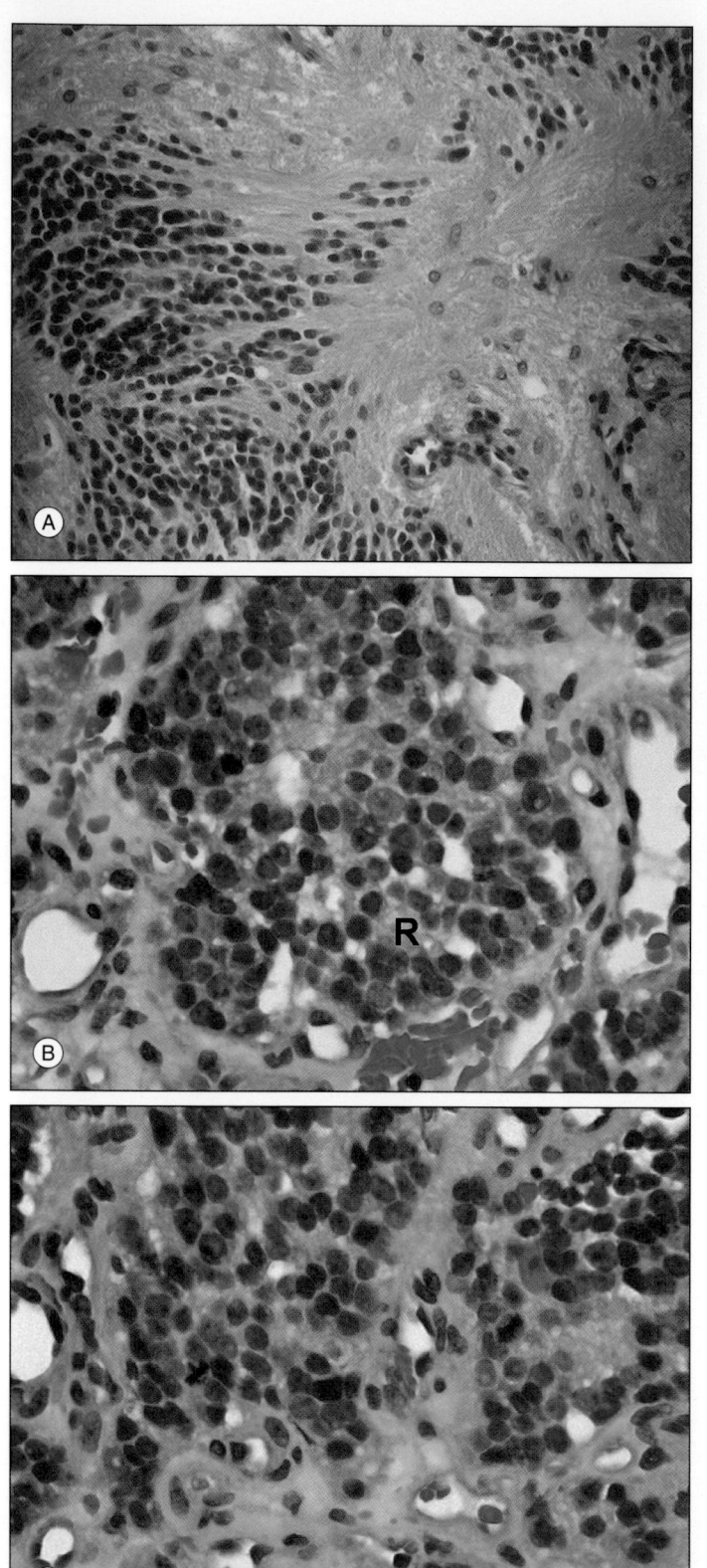

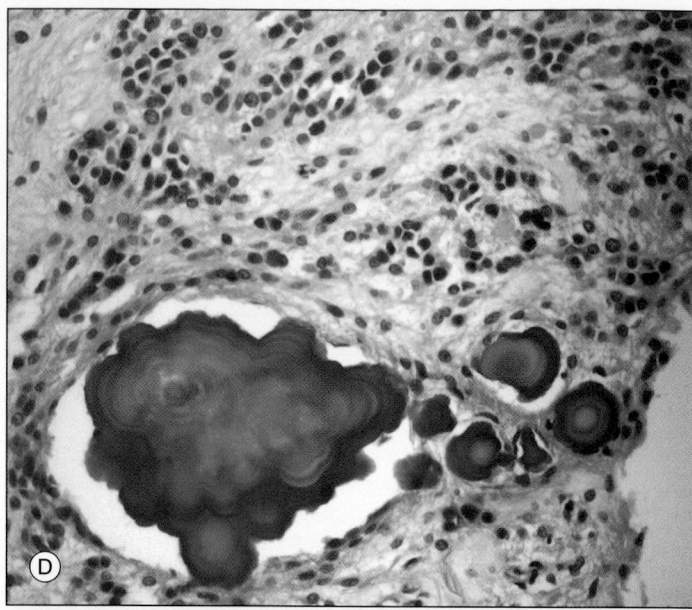

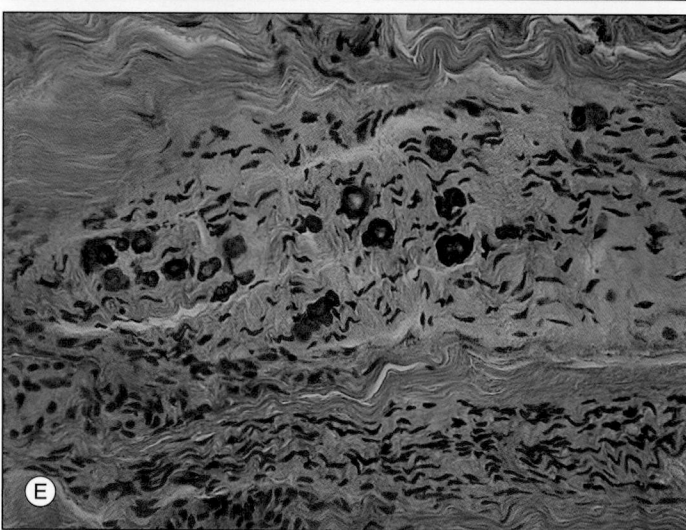

Fig. 15.15 Olfactory neuroblastoma (ONB). **A**, The fibrillary background is a significant diagnostic feature of ONB. **B**, Small, blue, bland tumor cells forming an organoid pattern with rosettes (R), representing a confluence of neural processes. **C**, Abundant mitotic figures define Grade III ONB. **D**, Psammomatoid calcifications can be seen, and sometimes are quite large and confluent. **E**, Similar psammomatoid calcifications seen in a branch of the olfactory nerve.

neurofilaments and microtubules. Neurosecretory granules about 90–240 μm in diameter are found in the cytoplasm and in neural processes. The Hyams grading system (see Table 15.4) and the Kadish staging (Table 15.5) were traditionally touted as independent predictors of outcome.[106,121] The Hyams grading has actually received relatively little attention in the literature, but its validity has been reaffirmed.[122,123] Many studies had failed to demonstrate statistically significant predictive value for both Kadish and Hyams systems. This was not due to inherent fallibility of these staging and grading systems, but rather are a result of the small number of reported patients, and skewing towards presentation at Kadish B and C. Recent meta-analysis has demonstrated a statistically significant correlation with collapsed

Table 15.4 Hyams grading for ONB

	Architecture	Rosettes	Mitoses	Necrosis	Pleomorphism
I	Lobules, abundant neurofibrillary stroma	May be abundant	None	None	None, uniform cells
II	Lobules, and more solid areas	Occasional	Can be seen	None	Moderate
III	Limited neurofibrillary stroma	Occasional	Abundant	Apoptotic cells	Yes
IV	No neurofibrillary stroma	None	Abundant	Zones of necrosis	Yes

Table 15.5 Kadish staging system for olfactory neuroblastoma

Kadish	
A	Confined to nasal cavity
B	Nasal cavity plus one or more sinus
C	Beyond nasal cavity and paranasal sinuses

Hyams grades and 5-year survival,[124] disease-free survival, and overall survival.[11] From the pathologist's viewpoint, Hyams grading should be reported to clinicians, as it may be a rationale for adjuvant therapy (see below).

Treatment and outcome

Craniofacial resection via combined neurosurgical/otolaryngologic approach can be curative, as this addresses microscopic disease at the cribriform plate and in the olfactory bulbs. By contrast, a recurrence rate of nearly 50% can be seen after an extended lateral rhinotomy for stage A and stage B patients. Patients with Kadish A ONB, negative resection margins, and Hyams I/II grade need not receive adjuvant RT. If patients have positive resection margins, and/or Kadish B or C tumors, adjuvant RT to the primary site is recommended. Palpable adenopathy requires cervical lymph node dissection. Patients without palpable adenopathy should also receive adjuvant RT to cervical lymph nodes as a preventative measure. Patients with Kadish C disease also require adjuvant chemotherapy. A Hyams grade of III/IV may also be used as a rationale for adjuvant chemotherapy. Sheehan reported *no* chemotherapy response in three patients with Hyams II ONB, but variable responses in six of seven patients with Hyams III ONB.[125] Likewise, McElroy reported tumor regression in two patients with Hyams III ONB, but tumor progression in two patients with Hyams IV ONB, and no response in all four patients with Hyams II ONB.[112] Conversely, Polin reported that patients with grade III/IV ONB tend to have less response to chemotherapy than those with Grade I/II ONB.[123] Prognosis is related to extent of disease: tumors confined to the nasal cavity have a better prognosis than those that involve adjacent sinuses. Cervical lymph node metastases are seen in about 20–25% of cases. The overall metastatic rate, including distant metastases, ranges from 38% to 62%. Local recurrence rate is around 30%, usually from incomplete excision. Table 15.3 details overall survival and disease-year survival from recent series. Recurrences or metastatic disease can occur up to two decades after initial presentation. Negative prognostic factors include female sex, age over 50 years at presentation, positive cervical lymph nodes, tumor recurrence, metastasis, high tumor grade, and Kadish stage C at presentation.

SINONASAL NEUROENDOCRINE CARCINOMA

Clinical presentation

In the 1980s, sinonasal neuroendocrine carcinoma (SNEC) became appreciated as a tumor that, histologically, did not quite seem to fit as ONB.[126,127] SNEC resides within the less-differentiated end of the spectrum of neuroendocrine tumors relative to ONB. Many cases were previously diagnosed as 'oat cell' carcinoma, atypical carcinoid, malignant paraganglioma, Merkel cell carcinoma, or anaplastic or undifferentiated carcinoma. Many SNEC occur in the same sites as ONB, (superior nasal cavity/superior turbinates/ethmoids). However, some SNEC arise from the antra or the middle turbinates – a location that would be unusual for ONB. Patients typically present with facial pain, epistaxis, nasal obstruction, and may have orbital symptoms. Smaller lesions can be polypoid and confined to one nasal fossa. Larger tumors can erode the cribriform plate and may extend into the orbit and the cranium.

Pathology

SNEC is a cellular tumor lacking the fibrillary background of ONB. Gland formation may be seen, but true Homer-Wright rosettes are not (Fig. 15.16). SNEC generally has a more compact architecture than ONB. The tumor forms either solid sheets, ribbons, or trabeculae. 'Zell-ballen' formation can be seen, ergo previous designations as 'malignant paraganglioma.' Cytologically, SNEC may differ from ONB in that cells are larger with more cytoplasm, coarser chromatin, and larger nucleoli. Necrosis and increased mitotic figures may be seen. Likewise, goblet cells or signet-ring cells may be seen.[128] However, there can be overlap between ONB and SNEC, as well as SNEC and sinonasal undifferentiated carcinoma (SNUC, see below). Table 15.1 details the IHC profile of SNEC.[129] Contrary to ONB, SNEC typically expresses markers of epithelial differentiation. Contrary to SNUC, SNEC usually expresses strong, diffuse evidence of neuroendocrine differentiation. EM is helpful, but the features of SNEC overlap, rather than distinguish it from ONB. Interdigitating neuronal processes containing dense core neurosecretory granules and occasionally microtubules, have been described in SNEC.[126,130] Membrane bound dense core neuroendocrine granules (100–250 nm) are seen. Microtubule aggregates may be present within the processes. Trull reported that a greater density of dendritic processes appeared to directly relate to prolonged survival (see below).[130] Olfactory vesicles are apical protrusions containing dense core neurosecretory granules, which protrude into rosette spaces. This feature is distinctive although not always observed in ONB. Olfactory vesicles are not observed in SNEC.

Treatment and outcome

Surgical resection with adjuvant RT is indicated. Patients with clinically N_0 necks should also receive adjuvant RT to the neck. Some

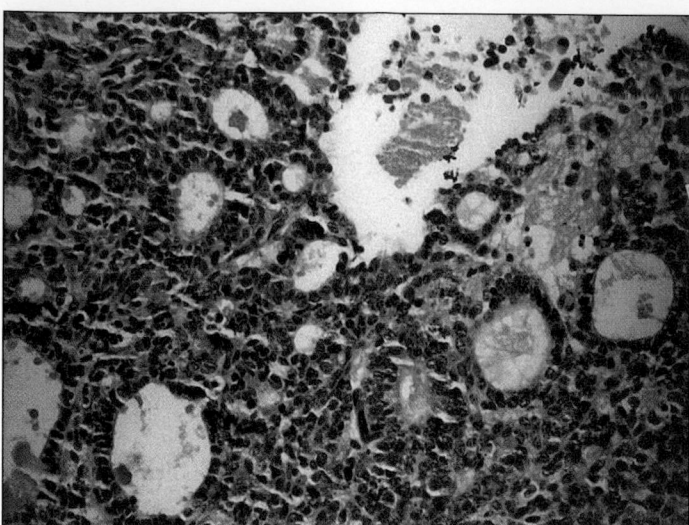

Fig. 15.16 Sinonasal neuroendocrine carcinoma (SNEC). Ultrastructurally, this glandular carcinoma revealed evidence of seromucinous glandular differentiation as well as sustentacular and neuroendocrine differentiation. It was mucin positive and expressed cytokeratin. This epithelial differentiation is beyond the realm of ONB. This patient is disease free after 5 years, which would not be expected for tumor diagnosed as sinosal undifferentiated carcinoma (SNUC).

Table 15.6 Patient outcome with sinonasal neuroendocrine carcinoma

Author	n	Overall survival	Disease-specific mortality rate (median)	Number disease-free survivors
Kameya 1980[126]	4		75% (6 years)	
Silva 1982[127]	20	100% @ 5Y 77% @ 10Y	15% (7 years)	7 (5 <3 years, but 2 at 13 and 15 years)
Perez-Ordonez 1998[129]	6			0/6
Smith 2000[138]	4		50%	2 (3 and 9 years)

patients have also received neoadjuvant or adjuvant chemotherapy. The paucity of reported cases, and the disparity in patient survival, render it difficult to formulate treatment recommendations. Kameya reported on 2 patients who developed local recurrence and locoregional metastasis, but survived 6 and 10 years, respectively.[126] Multiple local recurrences and locoregional metastasis were also seen in Silva's patient cohort.[127] Unlike SNUC, which is uniformly high grade, and usually fatal, SNEC grade is variable, as is survival rate. Some long-term disease-free survivals have been reported (Table 15.6).[127] However, greater experience with SNEC is necessary before prognosticators can be identified and confirmed. It is quite likely that, just as a classification schema has emerged for laryngeal neuroendocrine carcinomas, so too will a classification schema be developed for SNEC, which will allow for better prognostication and treatment recommendations.[131]

SINONASAL UNDIFFERENTIATED CARCINOMA

Clinical presentation

The term sinonasal undifferentiated carcinoma (SNUC) was first coined by Frierson to describe a group of tumors with no obvious differentiation, which were united by their aggressive clinical course. These tumors were previously diagnosed as anaplastic or undifferentiated.[132] They reported on 8 patients: 1 had an exposure history to heavy metals, plus coal mining, another also had been a coal miner. Gallo reported on 13 patients with SNUC; 2 worked in the chemical industry, 2 worked as shoemakers.[133] Most tumors arise in the nasal cavity, and can extend into ethmoids and antra. Presentation with orbital or intracranial tumor penetration can be common.

Pathology

SNUC is inherently high grade, and is an exclusionary diagnosis. Tumor cells have a high nuclear:cytoplasmic ratio, placing them in

the category of 'round blue cell tumors' (Fig. 15.17). SNUC may be composed of either small cells or large cells. Nucleoli are prominent and chromatin is coarse, and so the 'blandness' of ONB and PNET is not present. The tumor invariably contains numerous mitoses, necrosis, and vascular tumor emboli. Festooning ribbons, nests, and trabeculae can be present, yielding a 'neuroendocrine' appearance. Surface mucosal in situ carcinoma can be seen.[132] Features specific for other tumors (Homer-Wright rosettes, fibrillary background, keratinization, glandular formation) are absent. Osteoclast-like giant cells and spindle cells can be rarely seen.[134] Table 15.1 demonstrates the IHC profile of SNUC.[132,133,135–139] SNUC usually expresses epithelial markers, and may express some neuroendocrine markers (NSE, chromogranin); however the degree of neuroendocrine differentiation never matches that seen in SNEC or ONB. By EM, a few, sparse neurosecretory granules can be found.[132] The limited EM evidence of neuroendocrine differentiation aids in distinguishing SNUC from SNEC. The issue of EBV as a promoter of SNUC had been raised[140] and refuted by others.[139] It is unclear in many studies if the tumors at hand actually represent SNUC or nasopharyngeal carcinoma-like neoplasia (lymphoepithelial carcinomas).

Treatment and outcome

As dismal outcomes are common, the recommended treatment consists of an aggressive combination of craniofacial resection, adjuvant RT, and chemotherapy.[136,137] Some tumor response has been seen with protocols such as cyclophosphamide, doxorubicin, and vincristine,[140] and a neoadjuvant approach prior to resection has been recommended. Greater accrual of experience will hopefully determine if neoadjuvant therapy improves patient survival. Table 15.7 summarizes outcome for a number of studies, which, as mentioned, is almost uniformly poor. The possibility for distant metastasis warrants a metastatic work-up. Intracranial tumor extension has been noted as a particularly poor prognosticator. However, some long-term survivors have been reported. Helliwell compared the overall survival of 21 patients with SNUC against 24 patients with poorly differentiated SCC. They found a decreased mean survival for SNUC patients (54 weeks) as compared to poorly differentiated SCC (80 weeks).[134]

SINONASAL MELANOMAS

Clinical presentation

Sinonasal melanomas (SNM) represents less than 3.6% of sinonasal tumors; less than 2.5% of all malignant melanomas (MM) occur in the sinonasal tract. They are more common in the nasal cavity

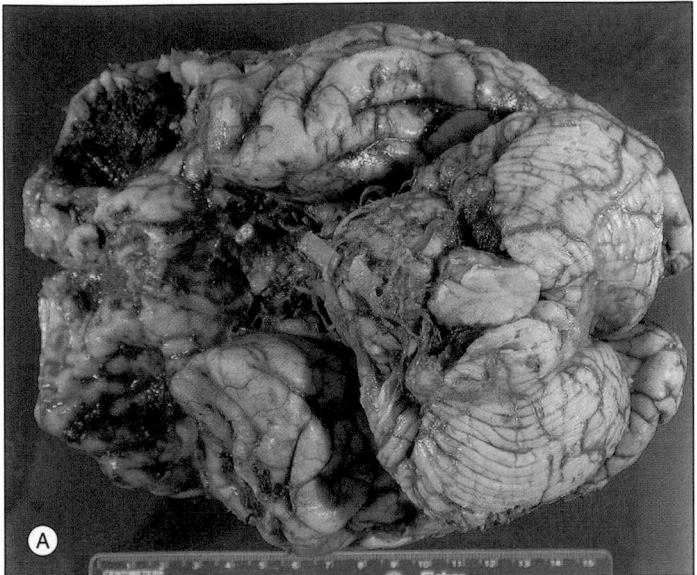

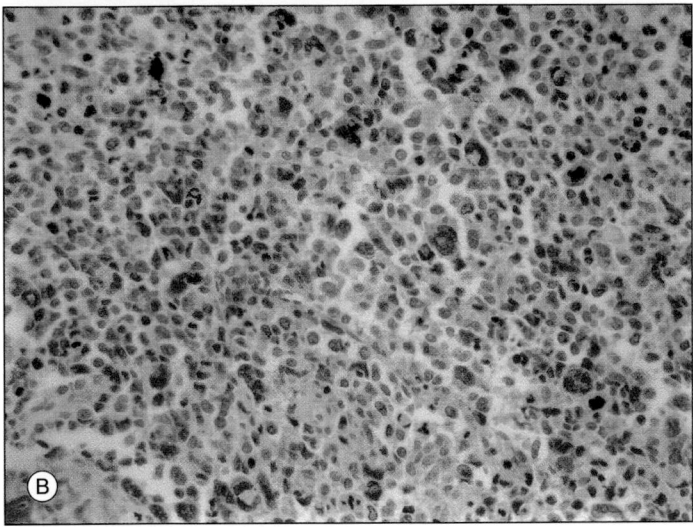

Fig. 15.17 Sinonasal undifferentiated carcinoma (SNUC). **A**, This 72-year-old man underwent craniofacial resection for SNUC with intracerebral extension. His autopsy took place two months later. **B**, This SNUC was composed of discohesive pleomorphic malignant cells, that expressed Cam 5.2, AE-1/AE-3, but not S-100, chromogranin, or synaptophysin.

Table 15.7 Patient outcome with sinonasal undifferentiated carcinoma

Author	n	Disease-specific mortality rate (median)	Number recurrence-free survivors (months)
Frierson 1986[132]	8	63% (4 months)	0/8
Helliwell 1986[134]	21		
Levine 1987	11	73% (12 months)	3 (79, 52 and 43 months)
Deutsch 1993[141]	6	33% (7.5 months)	
Gallo 1993[133]	13	77% (18 months)	2 (5 and 10 years)
Righi 1996	7	57% (11.5 months)	3 (under 18 months)
Gorelick 2000[137]	4	75% (15 months)	0/4
Smith 2000[138]	6		2 (under 18 months)
Miyamoto 2000[115]	14	50% (13 months)	4 (median 57 months)

(especially septum) than in the paranasal sinuses. The antrum is involved in 80% of sinus cases, usually together with the nasal cavity. Rare cases develop in the ethmoids; the frontal and sphenoid sinuses are virtually never primarily affected.[142] The age range is predominantly 50 to 70 years. The diagnosis of SNM need not prompt a work-up to rule out a skin primary, as this is quite unlikely. When MM metastasizes to the upper aerodigestive tract, it usually involves the larynx or pharynx, often during the disseminated phase. By contrast, dermatological screening of patients with parotid melanomas can uncover primary MM of the upper third of the face, scalp, orbit, or sinonasal tract.

Pathology

Grossly, SNM varies in color from white to gray, brown or black (Fig. 15.18). Pathologically, MM manifest a myriad of patterns composed of varying cell types: epithelioid, sarcomatoid, plasmacytoid, or clear cell. Most of these tumors grow in sheets or nests of variable size. Polygonal cells of variable size may have vesicular nuclei and prominent nucleoli. In a few cases, spindle cells predominate, mimicking sarcoma. The amount of melanin varies considerably. The differential diagnosis includes a wide range of tumors, including ONB, SNEC, SNUC, lymphoma, and sarcoma, (Table 15.1). Expression of vimentin, S-100, and HMB-45 is specific and diagnostic. Notably, 5% of MM can express epithelial markers, this should not distract the pathologist from the correct diagnosis. Of note, SCC can rarely contain melanin, mimicking melanoma.[143]

Treatment and outcome

Wide local surgical excision, possibly with adjuvant RT, is the recommended treatment. Up to 40% of patients present with positive neck nodes.[144] Radical neck dissection is indicated for palpable lymph nodes. Elective neck dissection is not indicated with clinically N_0 necks. In fact, a study from Duke University demonstrated survival benefit for patients with delayed (3 months) neck dissection and positive lymph nodes (56% 5-year survival), as compared to those patients who underwent elective neck dissection at the same time as melanoma resection, and were found to have positive lymph nodes (24% at 5 years).[145] It was postulated that microscopic tumor burden in lymph nodes over time may have a beneficial effect by conditioning the immune system, much in the same way as a vaccine. The prognosis of SNM is generally poor because of advanced local disease. In one study, only patients with MM less than 8 mm in thickness survived.[146] Five-year survival rates range from 25% to 30%.[146–149] Up to 65% of patients with SNM develop local recurrence or metastases within one year. Metastatic disease usually follows local recurrence. Distant metastases tend to involve lungs, lymph nodes, brain, adrenal glands, liver, and skin. The median survival time is 18 to 34 months.[147,149] A meta-analysis of 195 patients with SNM demonstrated a 50% survival rate at 36 months,[147] but occasional tumors may be mysteriously dormant for up to a decade before explosive recurrence. MM of the nasal cavity has a better prognosis than those of the paranasal sinuses; the average survival time of these patients is only 2 to 3 years, and the 10-year survival rate is 0.5%. Mortalities are usually preceded by local recurrence.

MELANOTIC NEUROECTODERMAL TUMOR OF INFANCY

Clinical presentation

Melanotic neuroectodermal tumor of infancy (MNTI) (progonoma, retinal anlage tumor) is a rare melanocytic neoplasm of neural crest

Fig. 15.18 Sinonasal melanomas (SNM). **A,** Typical pigmented polypoid tumor of the superior nasal cavity. **B,** Epithelioid melanoma cells with prominent eosinophilic nucleoli. **C,** Melanoma cells with prominent nuclear holes.

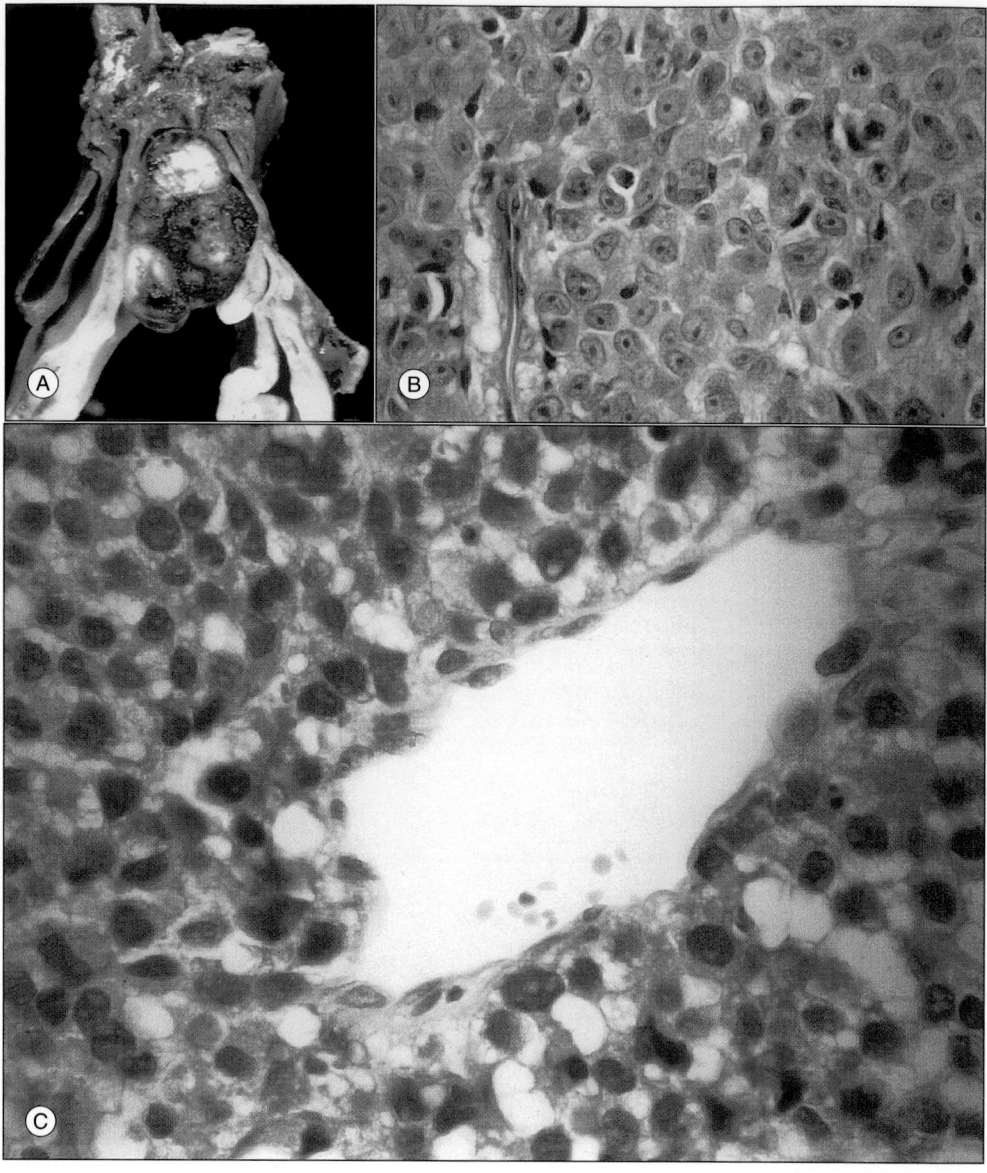

origin. The majority of MNTI arise in the maxilla, and are diagnosed within the first year of life. Less commonly, MNTI can arise from the mandible or flat bones of the skull. There is no gender predilection. They present as rapidly enlarging pigmented tumors causing bony destruction.

Pathology

MNTI is characterized by a biphasic pleomorphic tumor population consisting of epithelioid melanocytes and smaller, neuroblast-like cells which may also contain melanin. The cells may grow in an organoid nesting pattern, form pseudoglands, and may palisade. Neurofibrillary material can be seen, and MNTI may produce a hyalinized matrix. Mitotic activity can be brisk. IHC reveals that MNTI usually expresses cytokeratins and neuroendocrine markers, but S-100 and HMB-45 expression are variable (Table 15.1).[149,150] The IHC profile of cytokeratin and HMB-45 positivity, yet S-100 negativity, should bring MNTI to mind. EM analysis confirms the presence of melanosomes, premelanosomes, and neuroendocrine granules.

Treatment and outcome

MNTI require resection with negative margins. Palpable lymph nodes should be addressed as cervical lymph node metastases are possible (see below). Historically, MNTI was considered a paradox: histologically pleomorphic yet oncologically benign. However, reported recurrence rates range 10–15%. The metastatic rate ranges from 2–6%, involving either to regional lymph nodes, intracranial sites or distant sites, with resultant mortality.[150–152]

PRIMITIVE NEUROECTODERMAL TUMOR AND EWING'S SARCOMA

Clinical presentation

Primitive neuroectodermal tumor (PNET) and Ewing's sarcoma (ES) are interrelated primitive tumors, the majority of which possess rearrangements of the EWS gene 22q12, to 11q24. In the head and neck, both may rarely occur in osseous and intraosseous locations.

Sinonasal ES/PNET are rare,[153] and have been reported as second malignancies after RT for retinoblastoma.[154]

Pathology
ES/PNET are histologically similar, and composed of uniform, small, round malignant cells with little cytoplasm. Mitotic activity and necrosis can be seen, but ES/PNET tumor cells are generally bland and round, not pleomorphic and spindled. Homer-Wright rosettes are not seen in ES. Classically, ES is distinguished from PNET by the presence of glycogen, and lack of evidence of neuroectodermal differentiation. Conversely, PNET may form rosettes, and have a greater tendency towards IHC expression of neuroendocrine markers (Table 15.1). The diagnostic convention is to assign the diagnosis of PNET when at least one neuroendocrine marker is positive. However, the overlap of histology, immunophenotype, and chromosomal translocations seen in ES/PNET justify the consideration of these tumors as a related, unified entity.

Treatment and outcome
Multimodality therapy (multidrug chemotherapy, RT, surgical resection) is indicated for ES/PNET. ES/PNET are aggressive tumors with a propensity for hematogenous and lymphatic spread. ES is thought to be more chemoresponsive than PNET, and patient survival is poorer for PNET as compared to ES. Bacci recently reported the 5-year disease-free survival for patients with PNET was 54.2%, as compared to 70.6% for patients with ES treated with the identical protocol.[155]

INTESTINAL TYPE ADENOCARCINOMA

Clinical presentation
Intestinal type adenocarinoma (ITAC) resembles various gastrointestinal (GI) tumors, ranging from benign polyps to adenocarcinomas. ITAC occurs primarily in males between 55 and 60 years of age. Patients typically present with epistaxis and nasal obstruction. ITAC was first recognized among workers in the hardwood and shoe industries; individuals exposed to wood dust have increased relative risks of developing adenocarcinoma and squamous carcinoma (900 times and 20 times, respectively).[156] However, ITAC is not restricted to those with known occupational exposures. Interestingly, an association is noted between tumor site and presence of occupational exposure. Exposure-related tumors more often arise within the nasal cavity and ethmoid sinuses, whereas sporadic tumors more likely develop in the antra (Fig. 15.19). Thus, exposure-associated ITAC are more likely to become symptomatic and be diagnosed earlier than sporadic, maxillary ITAC.[157] The preoperative diagnosis of ITAC should prudently initiate clinical studies to rule out metastases from GI sources. However, such events are rare; only 6% of all metastases to the sinonasal cavities are from primary GI malignancies.

Pathology
ITAC are subclassified as either high grade, intermediate grade or low grade, designations of significant prognostic implication (Table 15.8).[158] Generally, ITAC can be papillary and noninvasive, papillary and invasive, solid and invasive, or have a mixture of components (Fig. 15.20). Kleinsasser and Schroeder advocated classifying the papillary ITAC as 'papillary tubular cylindrical cell' (PTCC), and subclassifying these as grades I, II, or III. Table 15.8 details the various histological features of ITAC, and Table 15.1 details the IHC profile.[159] ITAC may express neuroendocrine proteins such as gastrin and serotonin.[160]

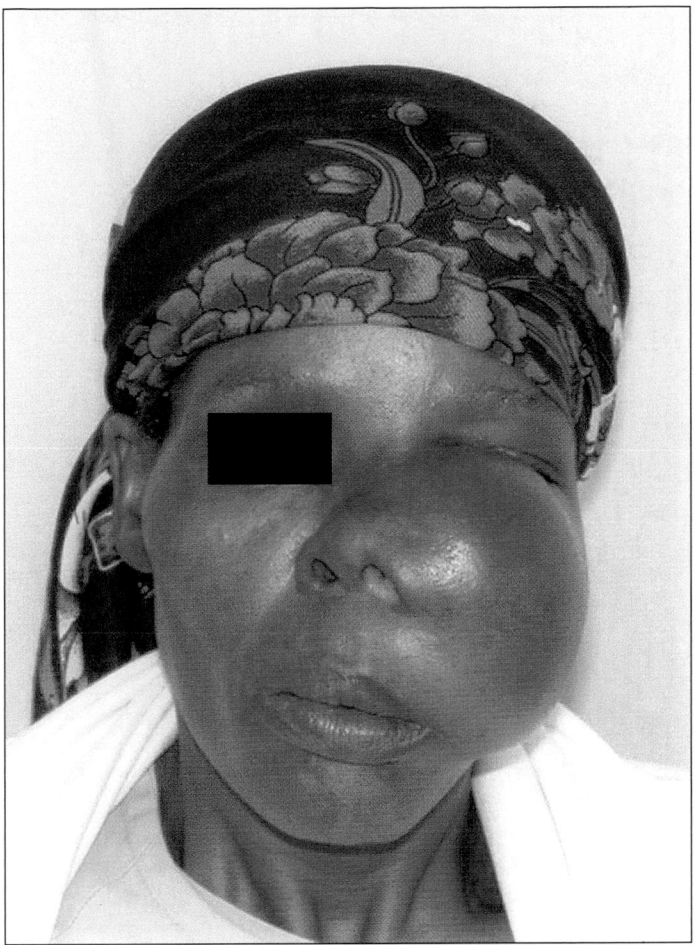

Fig. 15.19 Intestinal-type adenocarcinoma (ITAC). This woman presented with massive maxillary swelling.

McKinney compared the IHC profile of ITAC with colonic adenocarcinoma and found that ITAC was *more* likely to express neuroendocrine markers.[159] EM has demonstrated enterochromaffin-like dense-core granules.[161,162]

Treatment and outcome
Complete resection is recommended. Polypectomy is inadequate, even for low-grade ITAC. The decision for adjuvant RT should depend upon tumor grade and resection adequacy. ITAC can locally recur and invade the skull base and orbit. Metastasis to cervical lymph nodes and distant sites are rare. Barnes has noted an overall mortality rate of 60%, usually within the first 3 years. Patients with sporadic ITAC tend to have shorter survival times than those patients with occupational exposure-related tumors, which relates to delay in tumor discovery for antral tumors.

LOW-GRADE NASOPHARYNGEAL PAPILLARY ADENOCARCINOMA

Clinical presentation
Low-grade nasopharyngeal papillary adenocarcinoma (LGNPPA) are rare, exophytic, low-grade tumors of nasopharyngeal origin.

Table 15.8 Classification and outcome for ITAC (after Kleinsasser and Schroder[160])

	Type	Architecture	Cell types	Invasion & mitoses	Pleomorphism	Kleinsasser[160] et al	McKinney (n)[161] et al	Median survival (years)[158]
			Histology				3 year survival	
Low grade	PTCC - I	Thin, fibrous papillae, can be ramified, lined by single cell layer	Columnar (cylinder), goblet, cuboidal	Can be seen	Limited, most nuclei with polarity	81.8%	100% (3) (1 patient died year 4)	9 (4–18)
Intermediate	PTCC - II	Fewer papillae, more tubular glandular structures	Columnar (cylinder), goblet, cuboidal	Yes	Nuclear crowding, greater atypia	54.2%	60% (5)	3 (1–17)
	PTCC - III	Tubular glandular structures predominate	Loss of columnar cells, more cuboidal cells	Yes	Nuclear crowding, greater atypia, no polarity	36.4%		
High grade	Alveolar goblet	Solid, alveolar structures, glands, garlands of tumor cells in mucin	Goblet cells, cuboidal cells	Yes	Yes	47.6%	100% (n) (1 patient died year 4)	7 (4–14)
	Signet-ring	Solid, nests and strands, garlands, mucin	Signet-ring cells	Yes	Yes	0	100%	
	Transitional		A mixture of all types above			71.4%	(1 case)	

Wenig first drew attention to this group of papillary carcinomas akin to papillary ITAC, except for their nasopharyngeal location.[163] He reported on 5 males and 4 females, 11 to 64 years, with polypoid tumors arising from the roof, posterior, and lateral nasopharyngeal walls. Patients commonly presented with nasal obstruction, although one tumor was an incidental finding in a child at the time of adenoidectomy.

Pathology

LGNPPA forms arborizing papillary structures on fibrovascular cores, and crowded glands with a cribriform pattern. The nuclei are round to oval, vesicular and cleared, reminiscent of papillary thyroid carcinoma. Psammoma bodies can also be seen. Infiltration into surrounding tissue can be present, but no perineural or vascular invasion has been described. IHC for thyroglobulin is warranted only if there is prior thyroid carcinoma. The main differential diagnosis is with low-grade papillary adenocarcinoma (LGPA), which most commonly arises in the palate. LGPA is also cytologically bland, but architecturally heterogeneous (infiltrating lobular pattern, solid and microfollicular patterns). Perineural invasion is common to LGPA, but has not been observed for LGNPPA. LGNPPA expresses epithelial markers, but no myoepithelial antigens (S-100, calponin), thereby confirming its mucosal, not salivary, origin.

Treatment and outcome

Local surgical resection is indicated. Adjuvant RT may be unnecessary. Seven patients originally reported underwent transpalatal resection; two also received adjuvant RT.[163] All were recurrence free after 1 to 14 years (mean 7 years). One patient was initially irradiated, but had evidence of tumor persistence. She was disease-free 11 years after salvage resection. The man reported by Van Hasselt and Ng was recurrence free 2 years after transpalatal resection.[164]

SINONASAL RENAL CELL-LIKE CARCINOMA

Clinical presentation

Few sinonasal neoplasia can manifest as clear cell tumors; the one most commonly encountered is metastatic renal cell carcinoma. Primary sinonasal tumors that may contain clear cells include squamous cell carcinoma and mucoepidermoid carcinoma. Primary salivary clear cell carcinoma occurs almost exclusively in the oral cavity, and has not been previously described in the nasal cavity. We have coined the term 'sinonasal renal cell-like carcinoma' to described a new entity which was a histological 'dead ringer' for renal cell carcinoma.[165] Our patient, plus one recently reported by Hadi,[166] presented with nasal obstruction and epistaxis. Radiographically, this tumor causes bony remodeling but no destruction, features unusual for metastasis. Neither patient had evidence of any renal malignancy.

Pathology

The tumor is uniformly composed of nests of an invasive clear cell adenocarcinoma within fibrous stroma (Fig. 15.21). Tumor nests produce a follicular pattern, with dense eosinophilic secretions. Neither ductal formation nor hyaline stroma deposition is seen. The nuclei are rounded, and usually centrally located within the large polygonal cells, which have abundant clear cytoplasm and prominent cytoplasmic membranes. Nuclear pleomorphism is present. Prominent vascularity and hemorrhage was seen. EM reveals tumor myofibroblastic differentiation, and cytoplasmic glycogen, neutral lipid vacuoles, and cholesterol. Table 15.9 summarizes the findings that distinguish sinonasal renal cell-like carcinoma from renal cell carcinoma and salivary clear cell carcinoma.

Treatment and outcome

Our patient remained disease free after resection and adjuvant RT with short follow-up. The patient reported by Hadi remained disease free after 4 years.

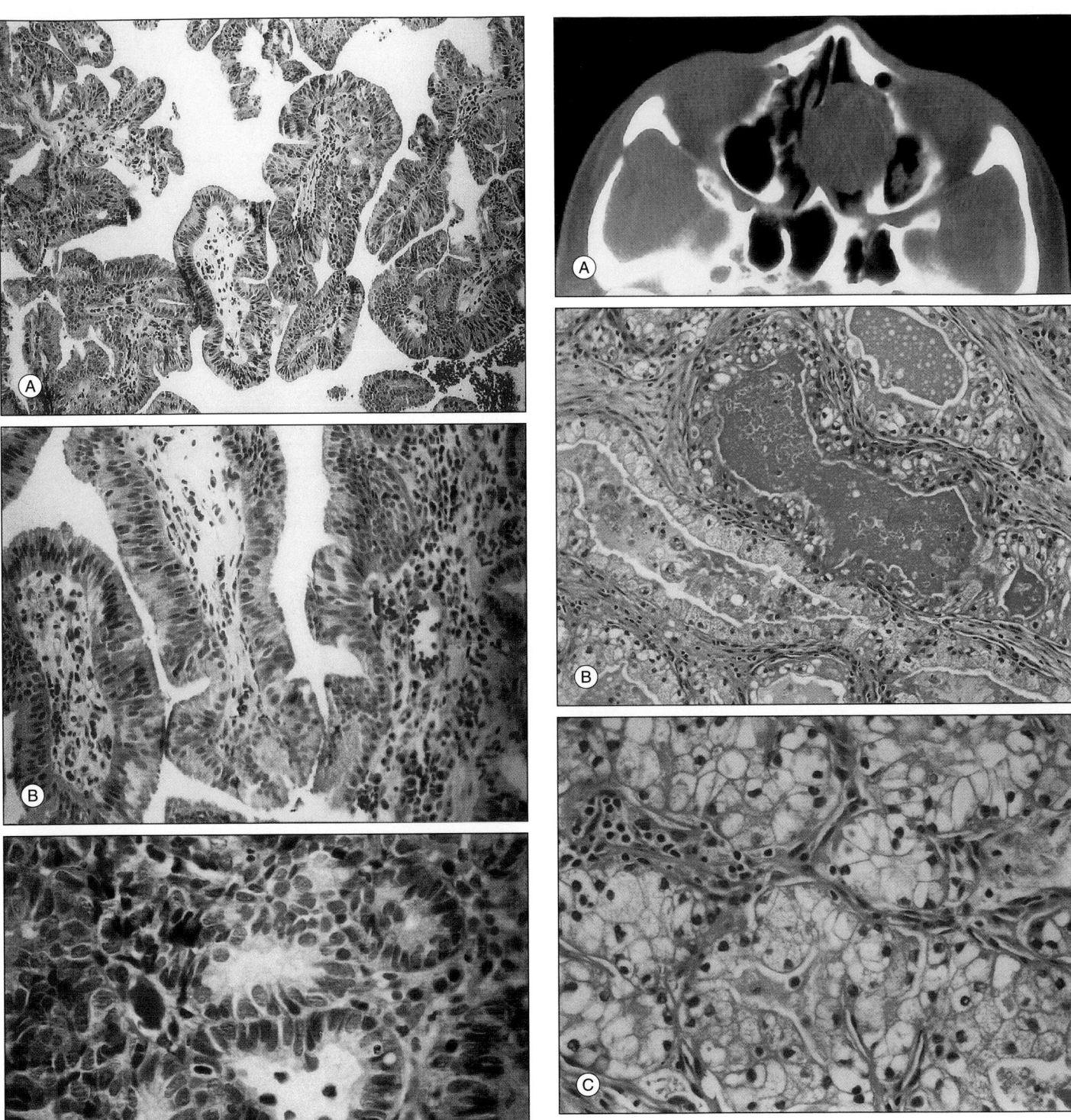

Fig. 15.20 Intestinal-type carcinoma (ITAC). **A**, Low-grade papillary ITAC consists of a single layer of columnar cells on distinct fibrovascular cores. Radiographic correlation may be necessary to distinguish this form of ITAC from hypertrophic papillary sinusitis. By contrast, Schneiderian papillomas contain stratified epithelium. **B**, The columnar epithelium here is crowded, but lacks pleomorphism. This can easily be misdiagnosed as benign. **C**, This high-grade ITAC is easily recognized as malignant. IHC aids in distinguishing it from SNEC.

Fig. 15.21 Sinonasal renal cell-like carcinoma. **A**, Radiographically, this tumor remodeled bone, rather than destroying it, an appearance inconsistent with metastatic disease. **B**, This tumor formed follicle-like glands. **C**, These clear tumor cells mimicked renal cell carcinoma.

Table 15.9 Comparison between sinonasal renal cell-like carcinoma, renal cell carcinoma and salivary clear cell carcinoma[167]

	Renal cell-like carcinoma	Renal cell carcinoma	Salivary clear cell carcinoma
Histochemistry and immunohistochemistry			
PAS	Pos	Pos	Pos
Diastase treated PAS	Neg	Neg	Neg
Mucin	Neg	Neg	Neg
Vimentin	Neg	Pos	Neg
Low mol wt keratin	Pos	Pos	Pos
High mol wt keratin	*Pos*	*Neg*	Pos
EMA	Membranous pos	Pos	Pos
CEA	Membranous pos	Pos	Pos
S-100	*Strong diffuse*	*Neg*	*Neg*
Calponin	Neg		Neg
Actin	Neg	Neg	Neg
GFAP	Neg	Neg	Neg
HMB-45	Neg	Neg	Neg
Thyroglobulin	Neg	Neg	Neg
Ultrastructure			
Lipid droplets	Pos	Pos	Neg
Glycogen	Pos	Pos	Pos
Dense bodies, cellular processes (myoepithelial differentiation)	*Pos*	*Neg*	*Neg*
Lateral interdigitating processes	Pos	Neg	Pos

PERIPHERAL NERVE SHEATH TUMORS

Peripheral nerve sheath tumors can be classified as Schwannoma or neurofibroma, (benign peripheral nerve sheath tumors, BPNST), or malignant peripheral nerve sheath tumor (MPNST). BPNST arise from Schwann cells and fibroblasts of the supporting perineurieum. As the myelinated Schwann cells are not among the olfactory nerve ensheathing cells, it is no surprise that BPNST do not arise from the olfactory nerve. Rather, sinonasal BPNST arise from the first and second branches of the trigeminal nerve, and autonomic plexi.

SCHWANNOMA

Clinical presentation

Schwannomas are benign nerve sheath tumors that present in young individuals, although any age group may be involved. Most are solitary and arise in soft tissues, including the head and neck, and sites such as the cranial or spinal nerve roots and cervical nerves (e.g. 'acoustic neuromas' of cranial nerve VIII). Sinonasal Schwannoma are extremely uncommon, representing less than 4% of all Schwannomas, and present as discrete, globular expansive, masses.[167]

Pathology

Schwannomas are composed of distinct, mixed architectural patterns: fusiform cells with wavy nuclei, moderate amounts of cytoplasm and indistinct borders, and loosely arranged fascicles having a whorled or palisading arrangement (Verocay body) with stromal hyalinization; this pattern is referred to as Antoni A. In the Antoni B pattern, the tumor cells are found in a loose matrix with microcyst formation. Mitotic activity should be rare in these tumors.

Treatment and outcome

Conservative dissection is adequate therapy.[167,168] Schwannomas are benign tumors with no propensity for malignant transformation.

NEUROFIBROMA

Clinical presentation

Neurofibromas are benign, expansile swellings contained within epineurium. Most tumors are sporadic and not associated with von Recklinghausen's disease (neurofibromatosis type 1, NF-1). Conversely, sinonasal neurofibromas are more often encountered in patients with NF-1, and are rare as isolated sporadic tumors.[169,170]

Pathology

Neurofibromas are composed of spindled cells with irregular, wavy nuclei. The overall cellularity is fairly uniform from field to field. 'Comma-shaped' cells may be seen. The cells may be arranged in fascicles in a fibrous or myxoid stroma. Plexiform neurofibromata reveal tortuous collections of diffusely hyperplastic hypercellular nerve fascicles, arising in a background of diffuse neurofibroma – spindled, wavy cells in a fibrocollagenous and myxoid background. Focal atypia or rare mitoses are not uncommon in all variants of neurofibroma. However, when seen to a marked degree, malignant transformation should be considered.

Treatment and outcome

Complete excision is the treatment of choice. Unlike Schwannomas, neurofibromas have the potential to undergo malignant change in the setting of neurofibromatosis.

MALIGNANT PERIPHERAL NERVE SHEATH TUMOR

Clinical presentation

Malignant peripheral nerve sheath tumors (MPNST) are aggressive sarcomas of neural origin. Generally, MPNST may arise de novo, from a pre-existing benign or plexiform neurofibroma, especially in patients with NF-1 or as a complication of prior RT therapy. Sinonasal MPNST are quite rare.[171,172]

Pathology

MPNST are usually high grade and cellular, composed of fascicles of spindle cells with a wavy appearance in a myxoid stroma. Nuclear atypia and mitoses can be prominent. IHC (Table 15.1) and EM (reduplicated basement membrane, abundant collagen, cell processes) may be essential to confirm their nerve sheath origin.

Treatment and outcome

Wide excision is the treatment of choice. Generally, the prognosis of MPNST is poor and is affected by tumor size, association with NF-1, and resection adequacy. Patients with MPNST and NF-1 have a poorer prognosis (21% 5-year survival), compared to those without NF-1 (56% 5-year survival). Large tumors (>5 cm) are associated with poorer prognosis.[173] For a mixed group of sinonasal fibrosarcomas and MPNST, mitotic rate >4/50 HPF, tumor cellularity, and male gender correlated with mortality.

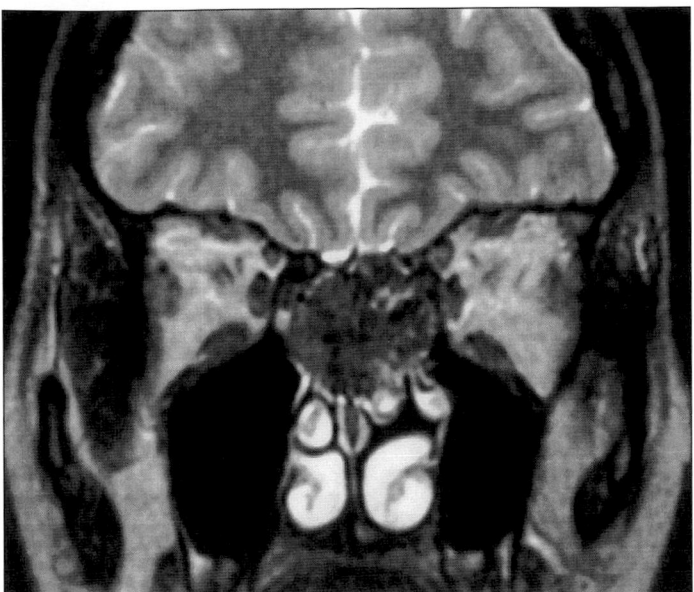

Fig. 15.22 Sinonasal meningiomas appear as expansile tumors causing bony remodeling. Most lesions are in the nasal vault. Adjacent sclerotic, reactive bone may be a dominant feature, which can, radiographically, mimic fibrous dysplasia. MR imaging (seen here): these enhancing tumors have signal intensities similar to that of the brain on all imaging sequences.

MENINGIOMA

Clinical presentation

Meningiomas are derived from meningeal arachnoid cells. Rarely, they may arise extracranially, in the sinonasal tract, temporal bone, parotid, or orbit.[174] Ectopic meningiomas probably originate from arachnoid cells trapped within or around bone as the cranial bones develop and fuse. Sinonasal meningiomas may be grouped as: Type 1, direct extension of an intracranial tumor after bony resorption; Type 2, extracranial metastasis from an intracranial tumor; Type 3, originating from arachnoid cells sequestered around suture lines, cranial nerves, or vessels exiting foramina; Type 4, no demonstrable intracranial component or association with cranial nerves or foramina. Type 4 meningiomas can be designated as ectopic. Sinonasal meningiomas produce polypoid, space-occupying masses, most often in the nasal cavity (Fig. 15.22).[175]

Pathology

Ectopic meningiomas are identical to intracranial meningiomas: meningotheliomatous, mixed, psammomatous, fibroblastic, and angioblastic. Meningotheliomatous meningiomas are most commonly seen. Psammoma bodies are variably present (Fig. 15.23). They may be confused with the psammomatous type of ossifying fibroma, especially in frozen sections. IHC expression of EMA will definitely differentiate meningiomas from fibro-osseous tumors.

Treatment and outcome

Surgical resection is indicated; meningiomas are generally not radiosensitive. The 5- and 10-year disease-free survival rates are 82.1% and 78.6%, respectively. Local recurrence developed in 14% of patients (excluding two patients with residual persistent disease).[175] Nasal meningiomas with an intracranial component have a poorer outcome, local recurrence, and disease progression is more likely.

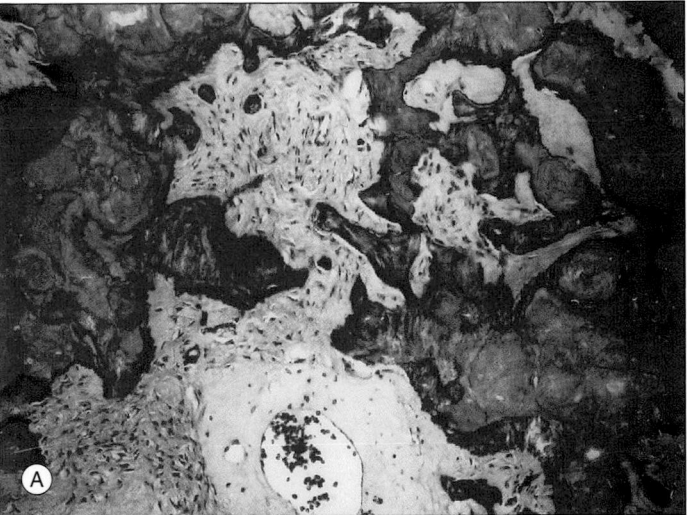

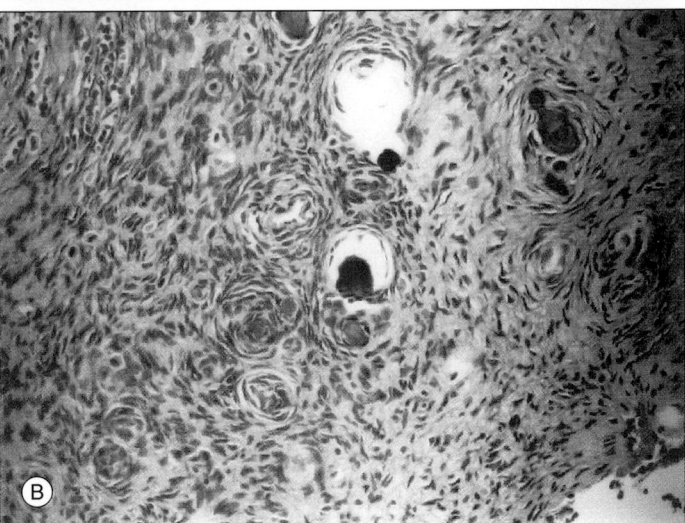

Fig. 15.23 Meningioma. **A**, This psammomatoid meningioma produced coalescent deposits of woven bone. **B**, Bland spindle cells forming meningothelial whorls and small psammoma bodies are seen. The expression of epithelial membrane antigen distinguishes meningioma from psammomatoid ossifying fibroma, solitary fibrous tumor, and hemangiopericytoma.

CHORISTOMAS

NASAL GLIAL HETEROTOPIA

Clinical presentation

Nasal glial heterotopia (NGH or nasal gliomas) are congenital malformations of displaced glial tissue in which the intracranial meningeal continuity has become obliterated. By contrast, encephaloceles represent herniation of brain tissue and leptomeninges through a bony defect of the skull, which maintain intracranial continuity. NGH usually present during infancy, but occasionally may be identified in older children and adults. Most cases present as small, firm subcutaneous nodules at or near the bridge of the nose in children or infants (Fig. 15.24). Approximately 10% have subcutaneous and intranasal components, and approximately 30% manifest as polypoid lesions within the superior

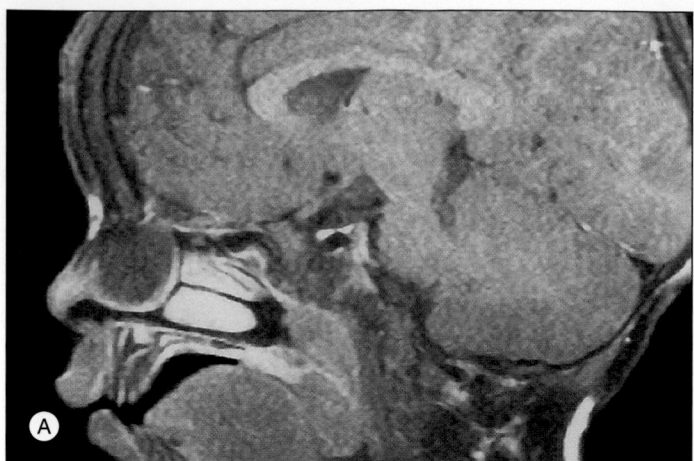

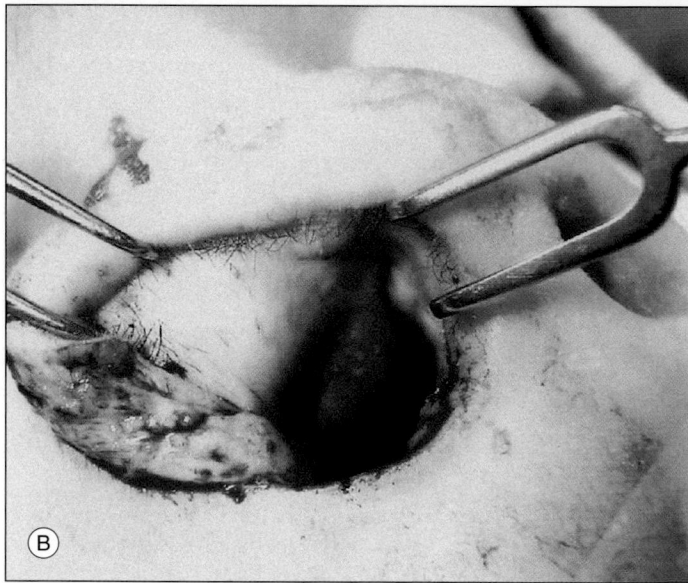

Fig. 15.24 Nasal glial heterotopia. **A**, Sagittal T1-weighted, fat-suppressed MR image of an anterior nasal fossa mass that comes up to the anterior skull base, but which has no intracranial component. There is *no* caudal distortion of the undersurface of the frontal lobe, as one would see in an encephalocele. This is a nasal glioma. **B**, Nasal glial heterotopia can present as purely intranasal polyps, without a subcutaneous mass.

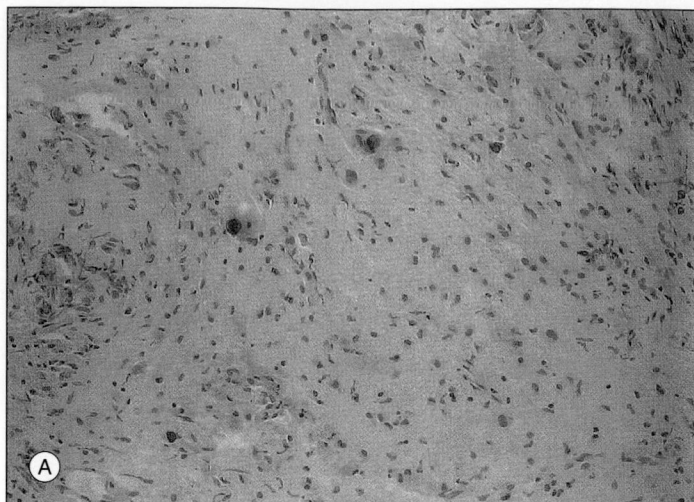

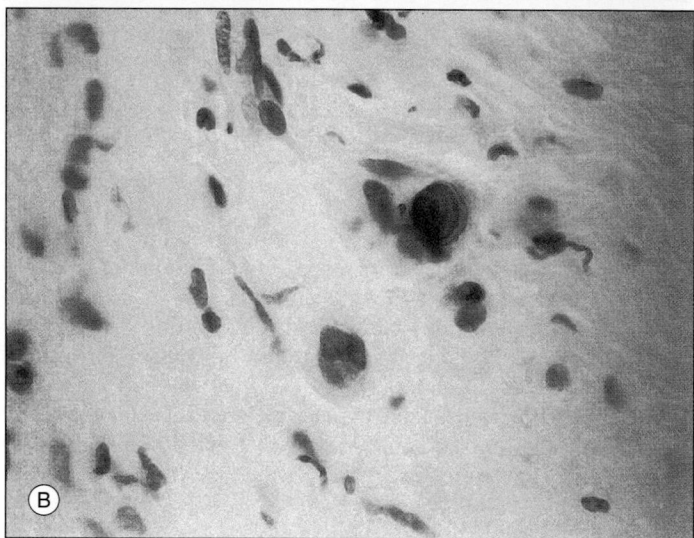

Fig. 15.25 Nasal glial heterotopia. **A**, The lesion is composed of nondescript glial cells and laminated calcifications. **B**, The clinical scenario (intranasal polyp in a child) can prompt suspicion for this diagnosis. IHC for glial fibrillary acid protein is confirmatory.

nasal cavity. A few paranasal sinus gliomas have been reported. The intranasal masses may produce symptoms of nasal obstruction.

Pathology

NGH are composed of nests and masses of fibrillary neuroglial tissue with a prominent network of glial fibers. Astrocytic cells may show gemistocytic changes (Fig. 15.25). Neuronal cells are rarely identified. Large astrocytic cells may be misinterpreted as histiocytes, but IHC expression of GFAP is diagnostic.[176,177] Choroid plexus, ependymal cells, and pigmented cells with retinal differentiation have also been reported. Encephaloceles appear identical to normal brain tissue, but degeneration may result in loss of neurons. In such cases, distinction from NGH requires radiographic correlation.

Treatment and outcome

Confirmed NGH may be resected by local excision. This should be avoided, however, if intracranial continuity is demonstrated

radiographically. NGH are slowly growing lesions. Rare postsurgical recurrences are thought to be the result of incomplete excision.

ECTOPIC PITUITARY

Clinical presentation

Pituitary tumors may occasionally infiltrate the sella turcica and extend into the sphenoid sinus, posterior nasal cavity, and/or superior nasopharynx, producing polypoid lesions or space-occupying masses leading to nasal obstruction. Alternatively, some adenomas may arise in ectopic pituitary tissue, misplaced during the migration of anterior pituitary cells from Rathke's pouch, an evagination from the nasopharyngeal roof. Both invasive and ectopic adenomas may be destructive and aggressive.

Pathology

Pituitary adenomas are composed of nests and cords of epithelioid cells that may display moderate nuclear pleomorphism and mitotic activity. The tumor cells have abundant, finely or coarsely granular cytoplasm.[178,179] IHC demonstration of pituitary hormones (usually prolactin, plus possibly growth hormone, ACTH, adrenocorticotrophic hormone, thyroid stimulating hormone, or follicular stimulating hormone) is diagnostic.

Treatment and outcome

Medical treatment (bromocriptine) may be effective in controlling prolactinomas. The majority of pituitary adenomas are benign, although some may be invasive and resistant to local control. Rare pituitary carcinomas may develop systemic metastases. A mitotic rate of >2/10 HPF, elevated proliferative indices, and p53 expression may predict those pituitary tumors which have metastatic potential.[180]

CHORDOMA

Clinical presentation

Chordomas arise mainly in the sacrococcygeal and spheno-occipital regions from notochordal remnants gone awry. In the latter site, chordomas can extend into the posterior nasal cavity, sphenoid sinus, sphenoid bone, nasopharynx, and skull base.

Pathology

Chordomas produce sheets, nests, and cords of tumor cells, often with a lobulated pattern. The characteristic physaliferous cells contain vacuolated cytoplasm, producing a bubble-like appearance. Some tumor cells have multiple, fine, cytoplasmic vacuoles, some have cleared cytoplasm, others have dense eosinophilic cytoplasm, and yet others appear as 'signet-ring' cells. Many cells contain finely granular, PAS-positive, diastase sensitive cytoplasmic glycogen. Mucicarmine stain can reveal a rim of mucin-positive material at the borders of vacuoles. In distinction, mucinous adenocarcinomas (either primary or metastatic) can demonstrate intracytoplasmic mucin positivity within the vacuolar spaces. Most chordomas demonstrate little pleomorphism, hyperchromatism, or mitotic activity. However, rare cases can demonstrate 'dedifferentiation' with sarcomatous foci. The term chondroid chordoma refers to chordomas with areas of cartilaginous differentiation. They can be distinguished from skull base chondrosarcomas by their cytokeratin expression. The significance of distinguishing chondroid chordoma from skull base chondrosarcoma lies in the improved prognosis of the latter group.

Treatment and outcome

Conventional skull base surgery rarely results in local disease control. However, the addition of adjuvant proton therapy has significantly improved local tumor control and overall survival for skull base chordomas. Chordomas are generally slow-growing and locally infiltrative, but do not metastasize. Hug reported an overall 5-year survival of 79% for skull base chordomas treated with resection and adjuvant proton therapy.[181] Smaller tumors are associated with improved outcome.

BENIGN AND MALIGNANT OSSEOUS (FIBRO-OSSEOUS) LESIONS/TUMOR

OSTEOMAS

Clinical presentation

Most sinonasal osteomas involve the frontal sinus, especially the ostium at the junction of the frontal sinus and the anterior ethmoid air cells, the floor, the roof, and the septum. The ethmoid and maxillary sinuses are less commonly affected. Most patients are asymptomatic; their osteomas are incidental radiographic findings. Larger osteomas can cause nasal obstruction, and may extend intracranially.[182]

Pathology

Osteomas consist of either dense cortical bone without Haversian canals (ivory type) or mature lamellar bone forming trabeculae (compact type) or mature lamellar bone plus fibrous tissue (fibrous type).

Treatment and outcome

Small osteomas can be conservatively removed endoscopically, whereas larger osteomas may require an external craniofacial approach. Removal is curative.

OSSIFYING FIBROMA

Clinical presentation

Ossifying fibroma (OF) (cemento-ossifying fibroma, psammomatoid OF) is a locally aggressive, invasive neoplasm. In the head and neck, the mandible is most commonly involved. Sinonasal OF is less common; most of these develop in the ethmoid sinuses and nasal cavity (one-third), frontal sinus (one-third), maxillary sinus (20%), and sphenoid sinus (rare). Psammomatoid OF has a particular predisposition for the sinonasal tract. While most OF develop in patients in their third and fourth decades of life, a subgroup of clinically aggressive OF, classified as 'juvenile aggressive OF,' is recognized and diagnosed within the first two decades of life. Radiographically, sinonasal OF presents as a well-circumscribed, mixed radiolucent, radio-opaque mass that may cause bony destruction. However, the demarcation aids in distinguishing OF from fibrous dysplasia.

Pathology

OF is composed of fibrous tissue and maturing lamellar bone with osteoblastic rimming (Fig. 15.26). The cellularity of the fibroblastic stroma varies from moderate to high, but usually with only minimal pleomorphism and mitotic activity. The osseous component can appear as cellular trabecular osteoid strands (trabecular ossifying fibroma), dark calcified globules of cementum-like material (cemento-ossifying fibroma) or psammomatoid islands with central bony tissue rimmed by pink osteoid and occasional osteoblasts.[183–185] Transition between osteoid, psammoma-like bone, and more fully developed lamellar bone may be seen.

Treatment and outcome

En bloc resection is recommended for sinonasal OF, as compared to mandibular OF which may be treated more conservatively by curettage. While OF are potentially capable of bony destruction, they do not metastasize, hence are more aggressive radiographically than oncologically. Resection is usually curative.

FIBROUS DYSPLASIA

Clinical presentation

Fibrous dyplasia (FD) represents a benign process in which osseous maturation is arrested at the woven bone stage. The craniofacial bones are normally formed via intramembranous ossification. Osteoid is first deposited in the stroma, developing into a woven

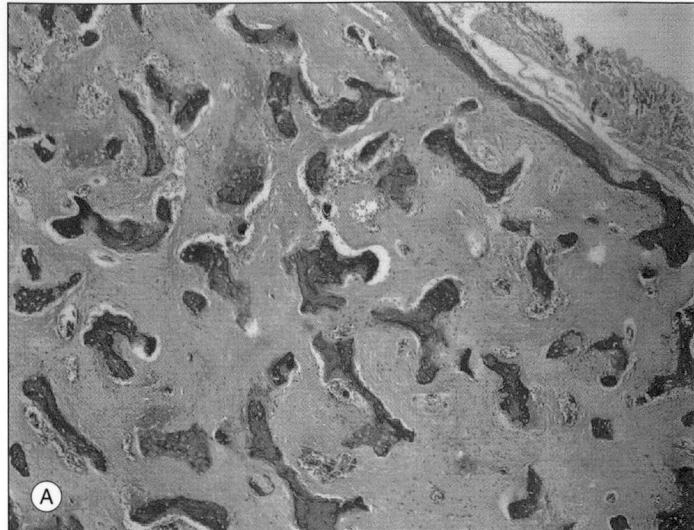

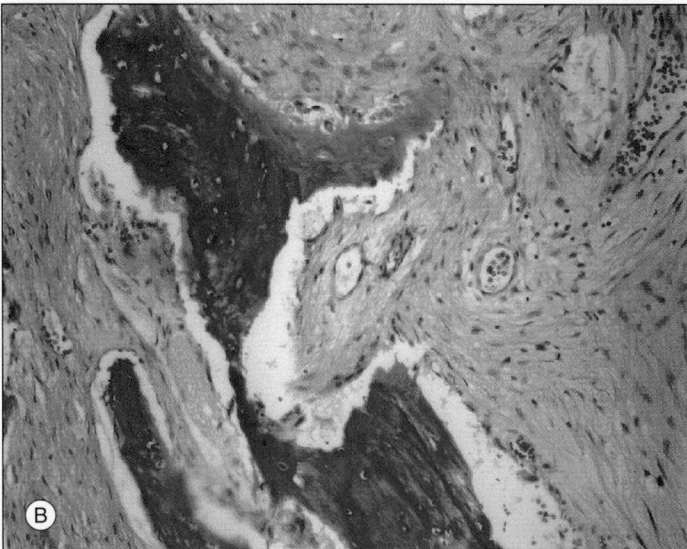

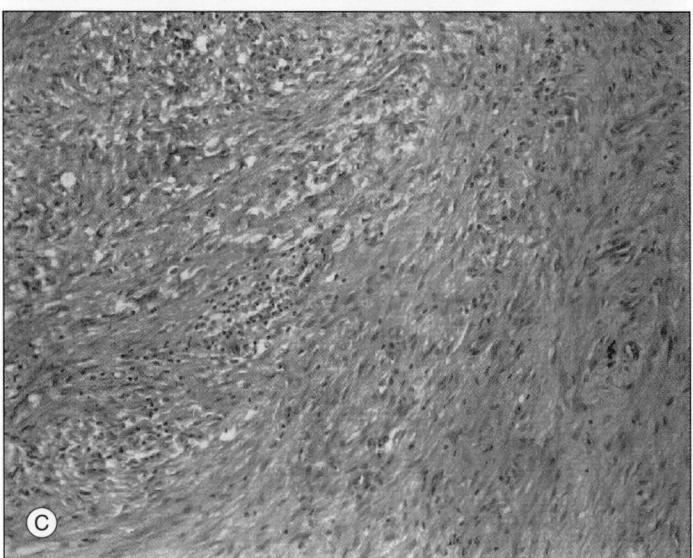

Fig. 15.26 Ossifying fibroma. **A**, Trabecular pattern of ossification is seen. **B**, Evidence of bony maturation is evident, with lamellar cement line and osteoclastic rimming of trabeculae. **C**, The 'fibromatous' element is composed of mature fibroblasts.

fibrous bone. Later, osteoblasts line the surfaces of the woven bone, remodeling it into lamellar bone with regular cement lines. In FD, lamellar bone is usually not seen, as maturation is disrupted at the woven bone stage. Monostotic FD is the most common and mildest form and is typically diagnosed in the third decade. Polyostotic FD has an earlier onset, causing more severe craniofacial involvement. The most severe form of the disorder, McCune-Albright syndrome, is rare. It has a female predilection, and is associated with short stature, endocrine abnormalities, and pigmented skin lesions. Sinonasal FD frequently involve the ethmoid sinuses.[186] Radiographically, FD appears as a radiolucent or sclerotic bony expansion which typically blends into the adjacent host bone, rather than standing out as a demarcated tumor.

Pathology

FD is composed of fibrous and osseous tissue in varying proportions. The moderately to highly cellular fibrous stroma consists of relatively mature spindle-shaped fibroblastic cells lacking hyperchromatism, pleomorphism, or mitotic activity. The osseous component contains irregular trabeculae of woven bone without osteoblasts or regular cement lines. With polarized light, woven bone with irregular birefringent fibers may be identified. The periphery of the lesion may reveal foci of reactive new bone formation with trabeculae of lamellar bone lined by osteoblasts. Similar areas may be found within recurrent lesions of FD. Thus, clinicoradiographic features may be necessary to distinguish FD from OF.

Treatment and outcome

FD can be treated with conservative local resections, usually for diagnostic or cosmetic reasons. FD may persist or 'recur' but can be managed conservatively. Sarcomatous transformation may develop in rare cases.[187,188]

GIANT CELL TUMOR

Clinical presentation

Giant cell tumour (GCT) is an uncommon, benign, yet potentially locally aggressive tumor that comprises up to 5% of all primary bone neoplasia. More than 75% develop in the long bone epiphyseae, half occur around the knee. There is a female predisposition, and most affected patients are older than 20 years. GCT of the head and neck are extraordinarily rare; most occur at the skull base, usually in the spheno-ethmoid region.[189,190] Jaw GCT has been associated with Paget's disease.

Pathology

One sees osteoclastic giant cells diffusely spread across a background of short, spindled cells, their nuclei identical to those within the giant cells. This latter point allows for distinction between GCT and the myriad of other osteoclastic giant cell-rich lesions. There may be dozens to hundreds of nuclei within the giant cells; these gargantuan cells are diagnostic. Hemorrhage and hemosiderin deposition are not prominent in GCT. Peripheral reactive bone may be seen due to remodeling. The differential diagnosis of head and neck GCT includes central giant cell reparative granuloma (CGCRG), 'brown tumor' of hyperparathyroidism or, more rarely, a giant cell-rich osteogenic sarcoma. The distinctions between these entities may be impossible without clinicoradiographic correlation. There is considerable demographic and histological overlap between GCT and CGCG, so that these two entities may represent a spectrum of a single disease process.

Treatment and outcome

Complete surgical excision for sinonasal or skull base GCT is recommended when feasible. RT should be reserved only for surgically inaccessible tumors, as generally GCT are not radiosensitive, and RT is accompanied with the threat of malignant transformation. The recurrence rate for GCT for all sites is 30–50% after curettage. Most local failures occur within 2 years. Approximately 10–15% of GCT demonstrate clinical or histological evidence of malignancy, either de novo or secondarily. Almost all secondary malignant transformations are RT induced.

CENTRAL GIANT CELL REPARATIVE GRANULOMA

Clinical presentation

Giant cell reparative granuloma is an entity of uncertain etiology that can affect either the jaws (central giant cell reparative granuloma – CGCRG) or the intraoral soft tissues (peripheral giant cell reparative granuloma – PGCRG). PGCRG is four times more common than CGCRG. CGCRG presents as an expansile, destructive intraosseous jaw mass. There is a female predisposition, and most patients present prior to fourth decade of life. There is no association with prior trauma. CGCRG can arise from either mandible or maxilla,[191,192] as compared to GCT which are more likely to arise in the skull base.

Pathology

CGCRG is characterized by a hemorrhagic fibroblastic background studded with innumerable osteoclastic giant cells. This background is helpful in distinguishing CGCRG from GCT. GCT lacks the diffuse hemorrhage, hemosiderin, and fibroblasts, and the background cells are identical to the nuclei of the osteoclastic giant cells. The giant cells of a GCT are diffusely and evenly dispersed throughout the tumor. By contrast, the brown tumor of hyperparathyroidism has uneven clumps of osteoclasts, perivascular hemorrhage, and hemosiderin deposition. It is necessary to know a patient's serum calcium and parathyroid hormone levels when evaluating any giant cell lesion.

Treatment and outcome

Complete surgical excision is recommended for maxillary CGCRG, as opposed to mandibular CGCRG, which can be treated more conservatively by curettage. Although oncologically benign, CGCRG has some potential for local recurrence, but malignant transformation has not been reported.

OSTEOBLASTOMA

Clinical presentation

Osteoblastoma (giant osteoid osteoma) is a benign tumor representing only 3% of all benign bone neoplasia. There is a peak age incidence in the second decade of life, with a male to female ratio of 2:1. The most commonly involved sites are: vertebral column (34%) and long bones (30%). However, osteoblastomas are more likely to involve the head and neck (15%) than are osteoid osteomas (0%).[193] The mandible is the most common site, followed by the cranium and maxilla. Sphenoethmoid osteoblastomas have also been reported.[194,195] Osteoblastomas may cause pain, but not with the consistent pattern encountered with osteoid osteoma, which is nocturnal and relieved with aspirin. Radiographically, osteoblastomas tend to be expansile and remodel adjacent bone. They range from 2 cm to 10 cm in diameter; in contrast, the nidus of osteoid osteomas is invariably less than 1 cm.

Pathology

Osteoblastoma is virtually identical to osteoid osteoma. One sees interconnecting trabeculae of osteoid or woven immature bone. The term aggressive osteoblastoma (juvenile aggressive osteoblastoma) is reserved for recurrent tumors or those with histological atypia. Histologically, these lesions have a denser population of epithelioid osteoblasts, with prominent mitotic activity and multifocality. At times, the distinction between aggressive osteoblastoma and a well-differentiated osteogenic sarcoma may be difficult.

Treatment and outcome

Conservative surgery, consisting of local excision or curettage, cures 80–90% of the cases. Aggressive osteoblastomas can recur locally, but do not metastasize.

OSTEOGENIC SARCOMA

Clinical presentation

Osteogenic sarcoma (OS) commonly arise after the first decade of life. Primary OS usually develops prior to growth plate closure, most often at the distal femur. In a series of over 1000 cases of OS, only 7% arose in the head and neck, usually in the jaws.[196] The age incidence peaks one to two decades later than for skeletal OS. The predilection for OS to arise within Paget's disease (PD) is well known; however, only 9% of all PD related OS arise within craniofacial bones despite the propensity for PD to affect this area. Other predisposing factors for craniofacial OS include previous RT and retinoblastoma. The association between retinoblastoma and OS is not solely due to RT, but is probably potentiated by homozygous RB gene deletion or RT-induced RB gene loss in heterozygotes.[197]

Pathology

By definition, OS is a tumor in which the malignant cells produce osteoid matrix. Histological subtypes include: (1) osteoblastic – producing abundant osteoid matrix, (2) chondroblastic – producing abundant chondroid matrix, yet the osteoid present merits the classification of OS, (3) telangiectatic – a highly vascular sarcoma with a lytic radiographic appearance, (4) fibroblastic – composed predominantly of malignant fibroblast-like cells with some osteoid production, (5) fibrohistiocytic – containing malignant multi-nuclear tumor giant cells in addition to the fibrosarcomatous component, and (6) round cell – composed predominantly of small round malignant cells with occasional osteoid production. Many OS display multiple histological patterns, thereby precluding neat categorization. Despite the wealth of clinicopathological data, there is little to indicate that histological subclassification for OS has prognostic significance over tumor staging and grading schemata.

Treatment and outcome

Surgery and adjuvant chemotherapy is indicated. The preoperative diagnosis of OS allows for neoadjuvant chemotherapy. Then chemotherapeutic effect can be accessed based on tumor viability, and the postoperative completion of chemotherapy can be tailored according to the observed response. Proton beam therapy may be considered as primary therapy for unresectable cases. Jaw OS has a 5-year disease-free survival rate between 30% and 50%. The prognosis for PD-related OS is particularly poor.[196] Fu and Perzin emphasize that sinonasal OS are less amenable to resection than OS of other sites.[198] The metastatic rate (predominantly lungs, liver, brain, bones, lymph nodes) directly correlates with tumor grade.

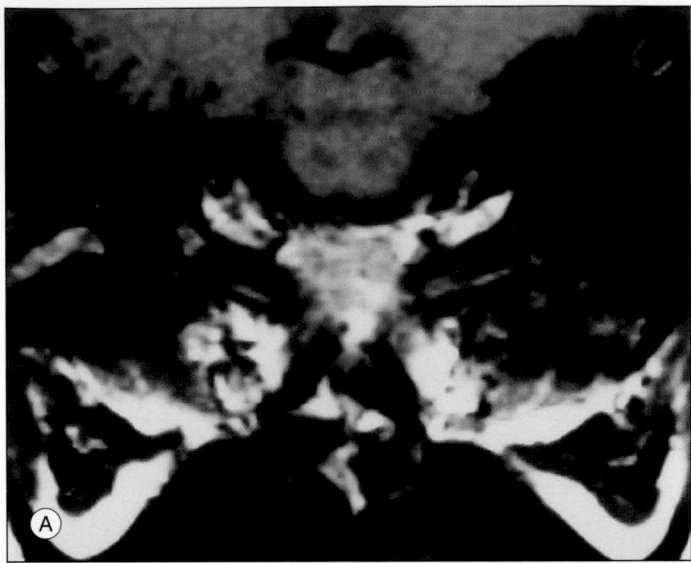

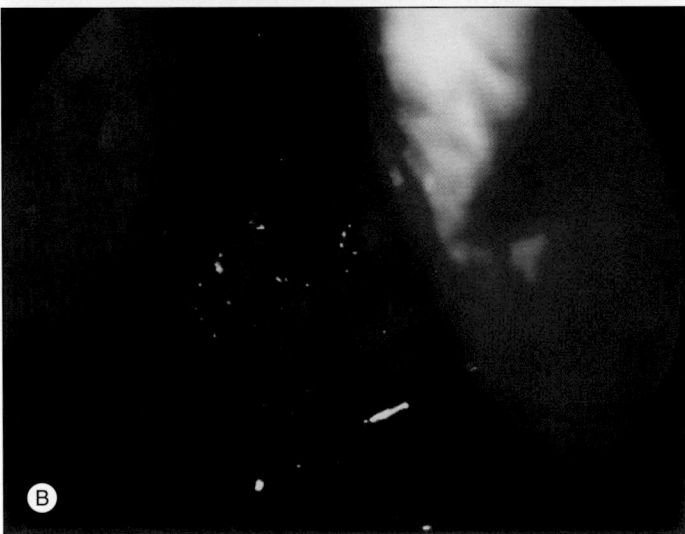

Fig. 15.27 Nasal septal chondroma. **A**, On CT, these are expansile tumors, associated with bony remodeling, and usually contain calcifications. **B**, Endoscopic view of this lobulated, glistening tumor.

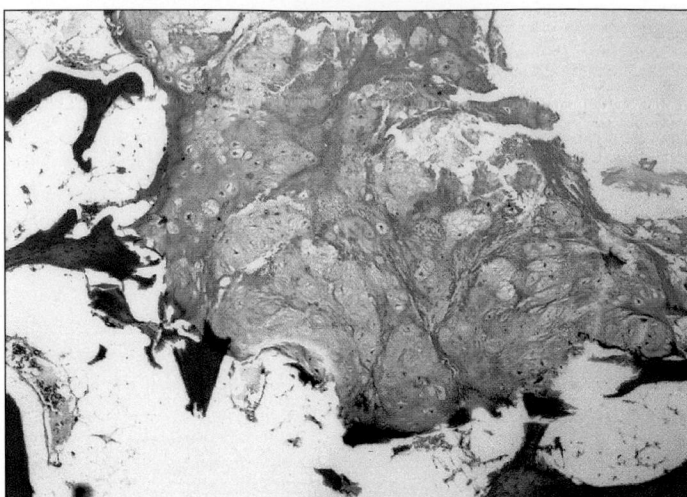

Fig. 15.28 Chondromas are composed of mature lobulated cartilaginous tissue that expands into the surrounding host tissue. On biopsy, the differential diagnosis of a sinonasal, well-differentiated cartilaginous tumor includes: chondroma, chondrosarcoma, chondroblastic osteogenic sarcoma, chondroid chordoma, and salivary mixed tumor. IHC can distinguish the latter two from the first three entities. Only analysis of the resection specimen allows for the distinction between the first three entities.

CHONDROMA

Clinical presentation

Chondromas are fully benign cartilaginous tumors. The definition of chondromas may vary with anatomic site and there may be no absolute criteria distinguishing chondromas from Grade I chondrosarcomas in some confined areas, such as the larynx. However, no diagnosis of chondroma should be associated with radiological findings of destruction or histological evidence of pleomorphism. Most head and neck chondromas (70%) arise in the nasal cavity and ethmoids. Others may occur in the maxilla, sphenoid sinuses, palate, and nasopharynx. There is no sex predilection, and about 60% occur in patients younger than 50 years.[199] Radiographically, sinonasal chondromas tend to remodel but not destroy bone (Fig. 15.27).

Pathology

Chondromas are circumscribed and not necessarily encapsulated. The bland chondrocytes grow in an expansile, lobulated fashion (Fig. 15.28). A myxoid stromal component can be seen. Cellular crowding and nuclear pleomorphism should not be present. The differential diagnosis of a bland 'cartilaginous' sinonasal tumor biopsy includes chondroma, chondrosarcoma, chondroblastic osteosarcoma, chondroid chordoma, and pleomorphic adenoma.

Treatment and outcome

Surgical resection with negative margins should be curative. A recurrent 'chondroma' was probably not a chondroma from the onset.

CHONDROSARCOMA

Clinical presentation

In a series of almost 500 chondrosarcoma (CS), only 5% occurred in the head and neck.[200] Secondary CS can be seen after RT or in association with Maffucci syndrome (multiple enchondromata and hemangiomata) or Ollier disease (dyschondroplasia without hemangiomata). In a review of 56 craniofacial CS the following sites were involved: 44.6% alveolar maxilla and maxillary sinus; 41.1% nasal septum, ethmoid, and sphenoid; 10.7% mandible; and 3.6% nasal tip.[201] Skull base CS is less common than craniofacial CS and enters into the differential diagnosis of chondroid chordomas.[202]

Pathology

Histologically, CS is more uniform as compared to OS, and abundant chondroid matrix is the rule. CS is graded according to cellularity and cytologic atypia: Grade I CS is composed of invasive lobulated tumor producing abundant matrix, with binucleate chondrocytes. Distinction from benign chondroma may be impossible on biopsy, and requires radiographic correlation. Grade II CS has greater cellularity and pleomorphism and is easily identified as both malignant and chondroid in nature. A Grade III neoplasm is very cellular and pleomorphic. Actual chondroid matrix may be limited. Spindle cell CS (so-called dediffentiated CS) is an unusual variant, in which a high-grade undifferentiated sarcoma 'springs forth' from a lower-grade CS. Mesenchymal chondrosarcoma is a rare variant, representing approximately 10% of all CS. It is a bimorphic tumor, composed of islands of well-differentiated hyaline cartilage juxtaposed with a small cell undifferentiated malignancy.

Treatment and outcome

Surgical resection with adequate margins is indicated if feasible. Patients with inadequately resected tumors will benefit from adjuvant proton beam therapy.[181] Outcome is directly influenced by tumor size, adequacy of resection, and sarcoma grade. Overall, only 7% of sinonasal CS develop metastases. Patients with mesenchymal CS, in general, have a 5-year survival rate ranging of 42–54.6% and a 10-year survival rate of 28%. Mesenchymal CS of the jaws (5- and 10-year survival rates of 82% and 56%, respectively) appears to have a more indolent course than axial skeletal or soft tissue mesenchymal CS.[203]

VASCULAR/PERIVASCULAR

HEMANGIOMA

Hemangiomas are found most often in the anterior nasal septum, followed by the turbinates and vestibule. Capillary hemangiomas are most common; cavernous and venous hemangiomas, benign hemangioendotheliomas, and angiomatoses are less common. They are usually diagnosed when small as they present with dramatic epistaxis. Rarely, intranasal hemangiomas may develop in the third trimester of pregnancy. Most of these lesions spontaneously regress within 4 to 8 weeks after delivery.[204] Hemangiomas of the paranasal sinuses are very rare; two have been described in the maxillary sinuses and two in the sphenoid sinuses. The sphenoid sinus cases showed destruction of the skull base.[204]

Pathology

These lesions have the same appearance as hemangiomas elsewhere. Vascular malformations may be easily overlooked in multiple pieces of curetted tissue. In contrast to normal vascular channels and to the vessels in hemangiomas, vascular malformations contain numerous closely packed tortuous blood vessels of variable size and configuration.

Pyogenic granuloma is generally considered a reactive process, appearing as an exophytic lesion with mucosal ulceration and lobulated vascular proliferation. When the following features are encountered, a neoplastic process should be suspected: a lobular pattern replaced by solid growth, presence of high mitotic activity, proliferation of spindle cells between blood vessels, intervascular stromal fibrosis, and epithelioid appearance of endothelial cells.

ANGIOFIBROMA

Clinical presentation

Angiofibroma is the most common nonepithelial neoplasm of the upper respiratory tract. Patients are typically male, between 10 and 18 years old, but this lesion can be diagnosed occasionally in older individuals. Symptoms include nasal obstruction, epistaxis, facial deformity, proptosis, sinusitis, nasal discharge, serous otitis media, headache, and anosmia. Almost all angiofibromas originate from the posterior choanae, near the pterygopalatine fossa and sphenopalatine foramen, and fill the nasopharynx. They grow asymmetrically, and one side is always predominantly involved. Extension into the pterygopalatine fossa is common, causing widening of the fossa with resultant anterior bowing of the posterior ipsilateral antral wall, which can be demonstrated radiographically. Although other indolent tumors may also widen the pterygopalatine fossa, the vast majority of antral bowing is caused by nasopharyngeal angiofibromas. The sphenoid sinus is involved by extension through the roof of the nasopharynx in many cases. Angiofibromas also spread into the maxillary and ethmoid sinuses, as well as intracranially (Fig. 15.29).

Pathology

Angiofibromas are composed of characteristic fibrous stromal background with numerous blood vessels of various sizes and shapes. Smaller vascular channels are surrounded only by the fibrous stroma of the tumor (Fig. 15.30). Larger vessels may have an irregular or incomplete smooth muscle walls and elastic fibers usually are not present. The stromal cells vary from mature fibroblasts with small, dense nuclei, to large reactive fibroblasts with

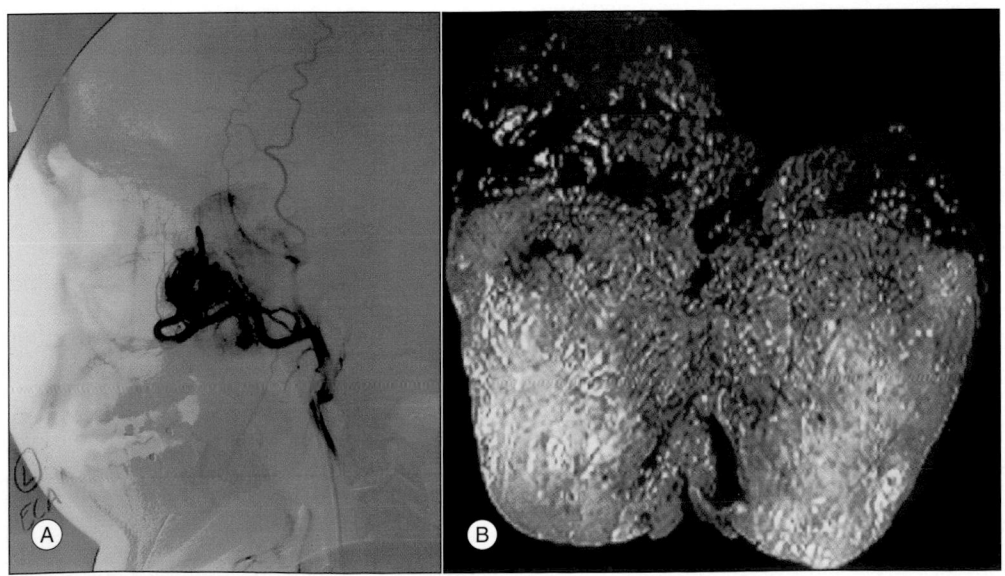

Fig. 15.29 Nasopharyngeal angiofibroma. **A**, The imaging is so characteristic it allows for preoperative embolization and progression to surgery in the absence of definitive pathologic diagnosis. This is desirable, as preoperative biopsy can be a bloody ordeal. Here we see the typical angiographic blush in the nasopharynx. **B**, These vascular tumors are firm yet spongy.

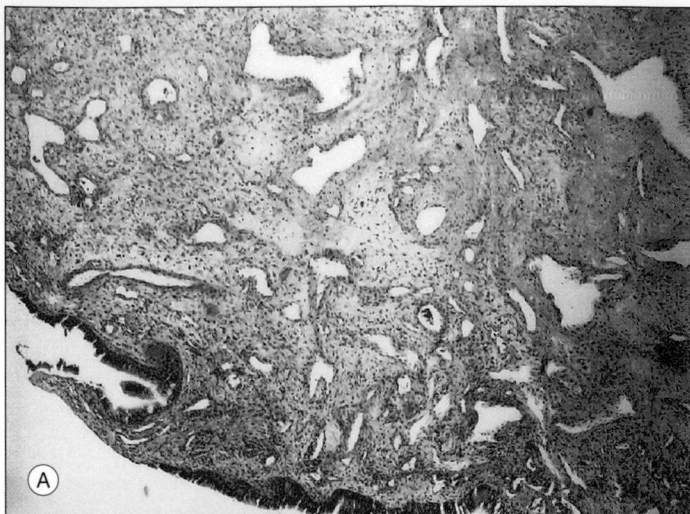

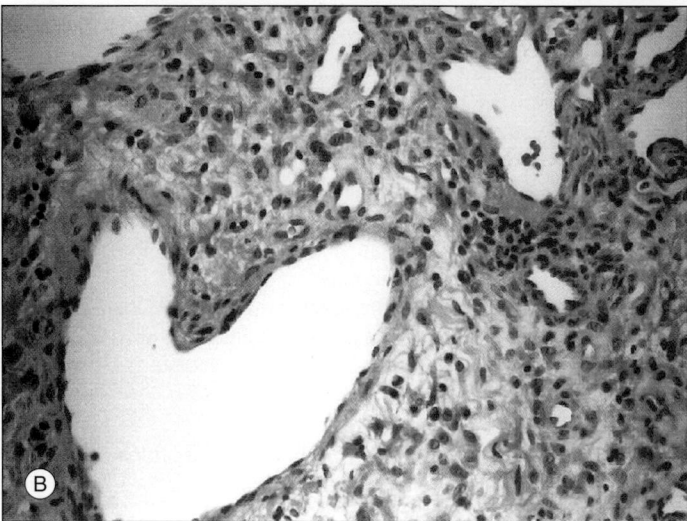

Fig. 15.30 Angiofibroma. **A**, At low power, one sees numerous irregularly shaped vessels embedded in a spindle cell background. **B**, These vessels are thin-walled, and the 'fibromatous' component is much less cellular than that of hemangiopericytoma.

regular nuclei and fine chromatin. Occasionally, the stromal cells may show focal moderate to marked hypercellularity, but are neither pleomorphic nor mitotically active. If marked stromal cellularity and numerous mitoses are seen, a sarcoma is more likely present.

Treatment and outcome

Preoperative embolization and resection, usually via a transpalatal approach, is standard therapy. Unresectable intracranial disease may be controlled with RT. Unresectable tumors respond variably to estrogen therapy. Recurrence after surgical resection ranges up to 46%.[205,206] In some cases, the lesion appears to regress after puberty. Sarcomatous transformation of angiofibroma has been associated with prior RT.[207]

ANGIOMATOUS POLYPS

Angiomatous polyps are fibrosed, vascularized nasal choanal polyps that have been traumatized. Their main significance is that they can be confused histologically with nasopharyngeal angiofibromas. Several points differentiate these two lesions. Angiomatous polyps are located primarily in the nasal fossa and not in the nasopharynx. The polyps do not extend into the pterygopalatine fossa and only rarely protrude into the sphenoid sinuses; they do not extend intracranially. On angiography, the polyps have only a few demonstrable feeding vessels compared with the rich vascular supply of the angiofibroma. Angiomatous polyps are easily 'shelled out' surgically as is a routine nasal polyp, whereas angiofibromas are difficult to remove from their primary attachment site. The pathologic distinction between an angiomatous polyp and an angiofibroma may be difficult, and hence clinicoradiographic correlation may be necessary to arrive at the correct diagnosis.

ANGIOSARCOMAS

Clinical presentation

Angiosarcomas (AS) refers to sarcomas derived from vascular tissue, this nosology includes other vascular tumors, such as hemangioendothelioma, in which endothelial differentiation is more prominent, or lymphangiosarcoma, derived from lymphatic tissue. AS account for only 2–3% of all soft tissue sarcomas. Approximately half occur in the skin and subcutaneous tissues of the head and neck, particularly scalp, legs, and trunk. Sinonasal and nasopharyngeal AS are extremely uncommon, comprising 11% of head and neck AS.[204,208,209] They present with epistaxis, nasal obstruction, headaches, and proptosis.

Pathology

Histologically, AS varies dramatically with tumor grade. Well-differentiated AS (malignant hemangioendothelioma) produces obvious blood-filled vascular spaces. There is a combination of 'closed' lumina, which are finite and delineated, as well as serpiginous 'open' lumina, which are infiltrating inter-anastomosing spaces. They produce minimal solid areas and are cytologically low grade. High-grade AS are densely cellular, infiltrative sarcomas. The amount of malignant vascular lumen formation varies, and may be focal. Cytologically, these tumors are frankly malignant with nuclear pleomorphism and atypical mitotic figures. IHC may be necessary to distinguish high-grade tumors from other sarcomas, namely the demonstration of Ulex, CD31 and CD34 expression.

Treatment and outcome

Surgical resection is indicated as the primary treatment for AS. However, the insidious infiltrating pattern of AS may render complete resection impossible; therefore, adjuvant RT may be necessary. The rate of cervical lymph node metastasis reported for cutaneous AS varies from 10% to 41%, the reported rate of distant metastasis ranges from 33% to 63%.[204] The 5-year survival is poor, ranging from 41% to 18%.[204] Inexplicably, sinonasal tumors appear to have a better prognosis than skin, soft-tissue, and osseous tumors, with a lower recurrence rate, higher salvage rate, and lower metastatic rate. Barnes reported that 6 of 10 patients with sinonasal AS were recurrence free after 0.5–5 years (median 29 months), which may be related to sarcoma grade.[204]

HEMANGIOPERICYTOMA

Clinical presentation

Hemangiopericytoma (HPC) has been recognized as a distinct neoplasm since Stout's original description, and it was thought to arise

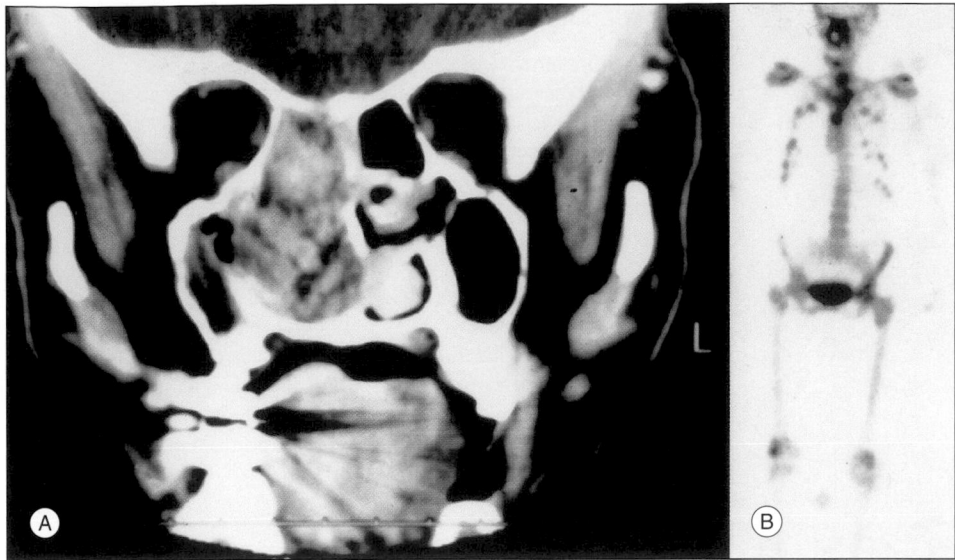

Fig. 15.31 Sinonasal hemangiopericytoma. CT scan reveals a destruction tumor of the nasal cavity **(A)**. This woman's bone scan revealed multiple 'hotspots' simulating bony metastases **(B)**. This case of hemangiopericytoma-induced osteomalacia resolved after tumor resection.

from Zimmerman's pericyte or its precursor cell.[210] Pericytes possess contractile processes. Zimmerman likened pericytes to a 'hand with slightly spread fingers gripping the other arm;' the fingers being the cellular processes.[211] The lower extremities and retroperitoneum/pelvis are the most common sites for HPC. The head and neck is the third most common site, occurring in the neck, perioral soft tissue, and lastly in the sinonasal tract, a richly vascular site. Rarer sites include the orbit, parotid gland, skull base, temporal bone, and sphenoid sinus. The reported age range is 4 to 80 years (mean 55) and an equal gender propensity.[212,213] Nasal obstruction and epistaxis are common presenting symptoms. Other presenting complaints include watery rhinorrhea, serous otitis media, proptosis, infraorbital anesthesia, and facial pain. Tumor-induced osteomalacia may also be associated with HPC (Fig. 15.31).[213] Most sinonasal HPC involve the nasal cavity only, and many arise from a turbinate. The ethmoid labyrinth, sphenoid sinus, maxillary and frontal sinuses, and nasopharynx can also be involved. Some sinonasal HPC can erode the cribriform plate and extend intracranially.

Pathology

HPC is composed of proliferating, fusiform, spindled cells that condense around large and medium-sized vessels. The tumor background has bountiful small vascular spaces (Fig. 15.32). The medium-sized vascular spaces contained elastic membrane and abundant pink hyaline-type material within their ill-defined walls, providing a border between tumor cells and vessels. The vascular spaces are round or serpiginous; the classical 'staghorn'-type vessels are rarely seen. This pattern is neither a specific nor entirely sensitive finding for HPC. Reticulin stain reveals a meshwork of reticulin fibers surrounding each tumor cell. The spindle cells generally are short to medium size, tapered, without much cytoplasm, distinguishing them from leiomyosarcomas or fibrosarcomas. Nucleoli were usually single and not prominent, chromatin was finely dispersed. The pattern of HPC is one of short fascicles, small whorls, and perpendicular orientation around vessels. The lack of long sweeping fascicles, herringbone and storiform patterns, and the lack of nuclear pleomorphism aid in distinguishing HPC from fibrosarcoma, leiomyosarcoma, monophasic synovial sarcoma, and malignant fibrous histiocytoma. The differential diagnosis includes sinonasal glomus tumor, solitary fibrous tumor, and leiomyoma. Glomus tumors are histologically most similar to HPC,

but they are composed predominantly of epithelioid cells. While HPC is uniformly composed of short, bland spindle cells, spindled elements may also be observed in glomus tumors. On IHC, glomus tumor is more likely to express smooth muscle markers (calponin, actin) than would HPC (Table 15.1).[214]

Treatment and outcome

Wide excision with adequate surgical margins is recommended to achieve local control and decrease subsequent recurrences. Combined neurosurgical/ENT craniofacial resection is required if the cribriform plate is possibly breached. Polypectomy is ill advised as it will surely lead to persistence or recurrence. Routine preoperative embolization reduces intraoperative blood loss. RT, while inadequate as primary therapy, has been recommended for unresectable HPC. Chemotherapy appears to be limited to palliation of unresectable local or metastatic disease. An overall recurrence rate of 18% has been reported for sinonasal HPC treated by either polypectomy or resection. Most of these are single recurrences within the first 5 years after resection. However, first recurrences can occur even after one decade. Multiple recurrences are rare (3%). Overall, the rate of metastatic spread is low (2.5%), usually to locoregional sites or local lymph nodes. Similarly, the mortality rate is low (3.3%), usually from a lack of local control.

GLOMUS TUMOR

Clinical presentation

Glomus tumors represent benign neoplasia that arise from perivascular glomus bodies, akin to HPC arising from hemangiopericytes. The term glomus tumors should not be confused with the misnomers 'glomus tympanicum' and 'glomus jugulare' which are paragangliomas. Glomus tumors usually present as small painful tumors of the fingers. They may rarely arise in the nasal cavity, either as polypoid vascular tumors of the nasal cavity or the soft tissues of the nasal vestibule.[215–217] Epistaxis is a common presenting complaint.

Pathology

Glomus tumors are vascularized tumors composed of tufts and sheets of epithelioid glomus cells with uniform round nuclei, clear

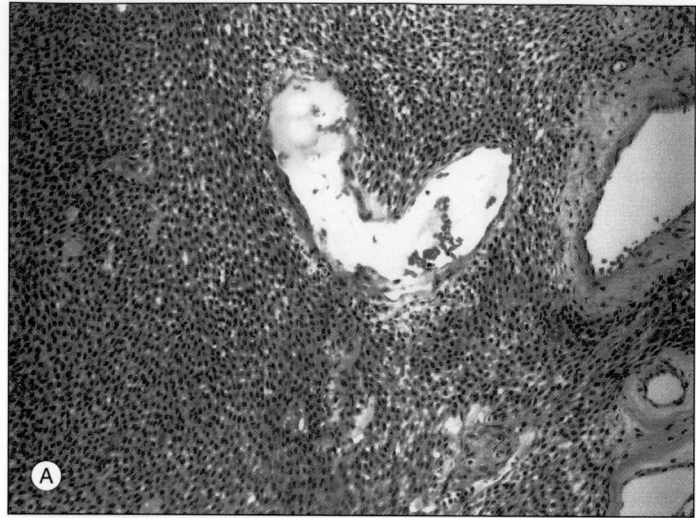

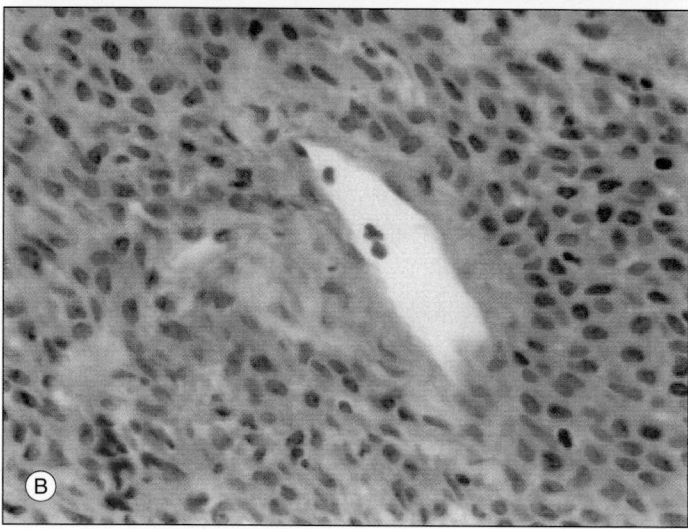

Fig. 15.32 Sinonasal hemangiopericytoma. **A**, This tumor is composed of bland, short spindle cells. 'Staghorn' vessel formation is typical, but neither specific nor sensitive for the diagnosis. **B**, More typical is the finding of perivascular hyalinization, and the perpendicular orientation of spindle cells around vessel walls.

cytoplasm, and prominent cell membranes. Tumor tufts may concentrate around larger vessels, which may be hyalinized, similar to HPC. An infiltrating pattern can be seen. Reticulin stain typically reveals a fine framework around each tumor cell, as compared to the 'zell-ballen' pattern seen with paragangliomas. EM reveals basement membrane production, contractile dense bodies, and no neuro-endocrine granules.[218] The main differential diagnosis is with HPC. While spindled elements may be observed in glomus tumors, HPC is uniformly composed of short, bland spindle cells. On IHC, glomus tumor is more likely to express smooth muscle markers (calponin, actin) than would HPC.[214]

Treatment and outcome

Glomus tumors require complete local resection. No metastatic work-up is necessary. Occasional sinonasal glomus tumors may manifest multiple local recurrences,[217] but metastatic disease has not been reported.

RHABDOMYOMA

Clinical presentation

Rhabdomyomas are rare benign tumors representing about 2% of all skeletal muscle neoplasia.[204] Clinically, rhabdomyomas can be classified as either cardiac or extracardiac. Cardiac rhabdomyomas are most commonly associated with tuberosclerosis. Extracardiac rhabdomyomas are rare, but tend to affect head and neck sites such as facial soft tissues, oral cavity, and the larynx. Rhabdomyomas are classified as either fetal type (myxoid versus cellular types), adult type, or juvenile-intermediate type, which histologically lies between fetal and adult rhabdomyomas.[219–221] Fetal rhabdomyomas occur over a wide age range, starting at birth. About half the patients with fetal rhabdomyomas are in their second decade of life or older.[205] Sinonasal rhabdomyomas have been reported in the nasopharynx, and are usually fetal type, though one adult type has also been illustrated.[220,221]

Pathology

Fetal rhabdomyomas are composed of primitive mesenchymal cells and elongated, immature rhabdomyoblasts within a myxoid stroma. They resemble fetal rhabdomyoblasts in varying stages of differentiation. Some have eosinophilic fibrillary cytoplasm, but cross-striations are rarely seen.[220] The circumscription of the mass and the lack of nuclear atypia distinguish these tumors from rhabdomyosarcoma. Fetal rhabdomyomas may be mitotically active, but atypical mitotic figures are not seen. Adult rhabdomyomas are composed of huge, polygonal skeletal muscle-like cells with vacuolated eosinophilic cytoplasm producing a characteristic spider-like appearance.

Treatment and outcome

Conservative excision should be curative for rhabdomyomas.

RHABDOMYOSARCOMA

Clinical presentation

Rhabdomyosarcoma (RMS) is a skeletal muscle sarcoma comprising 20% of all soft tissue sarcomas. It is the most common soft tissue sarcoma of childhood (75%). In the head and neck, the most common sites are the orbit (36%), nasopharynx (15.4%), middle ear and mastoid (13.8%), sinonasal cavities (8.1%), face (4.5%), neck (4.1%), larynx (4.1%), and oral cavity.[204,221] Sinonasal RMS may occur over a wide age range and commonly present with nasal obstruction.

Pathology

RMS can be classified as: embryonal, botryoid (a variant of embryonal RMS), alveolar, pleomorphic, and sclerosing. Most head and neck RMS can be classified as either embryonal type, botryoid variant, or alveolar type. Embryonal RMS (ERMS) is composed of round cells with darkly staining hyperchromatic nuclei and scant cytoplasm and short spindled cells with central elongated nuclei, tapered ends, and eosinophilic or amphophilic cytoplasm. Botryoid ERMS (5% of cases) is a noteworthy subtype which has a characteristic polypoid 'bunch of grapes' clinical appearance. It is associated with the most favorable prognosis for all RMS. Histologically, it grows as a polypoid tumor with a prominent myxoid stroma in which hypocellular and more cellular areas are seen with a subepithelial condensation of tumor cells, the 'cambium' layer. Pleomorphic RMS contains large atypical, polygonal, pleomorphic rhabdomyoblasts, which may be multinucleated. Sclerosing RMS produces a collagenous matrix that can mimic osteoid. IHC invariably plays a diagnostic role (Table 15.1). Antibodies against myogenin, fast skeletal muscle myosin (Myf4), and MyoD1 are important diagnostic adjuncts to myoglobin.[222,223]

Treatment and outcome

Resection followed by chemotherapy is the mainstay of therapy. RT therapy is not necessary after complete surgical resection with adequate margins.[224] Regional lymph node sampling is appropriate. Prophylactic lymph node dissection is not necessary. Survival depends on site (orbital better than parameningeal, nonorbital better than orbital), histological type (botryoid and embryonal better than alveolar), and stage. An overall survival rate at 5 years of 73% for parameningeal RMS has been reported.[225] Favorable prognostic factors were: age 1–9 years at diagnosis; primary tumor in the nasopharynx/nasal cavity, middle ear/mastoid or parapharyngeal areas; no meningeal involvement; and noninvasive tumors (T1).

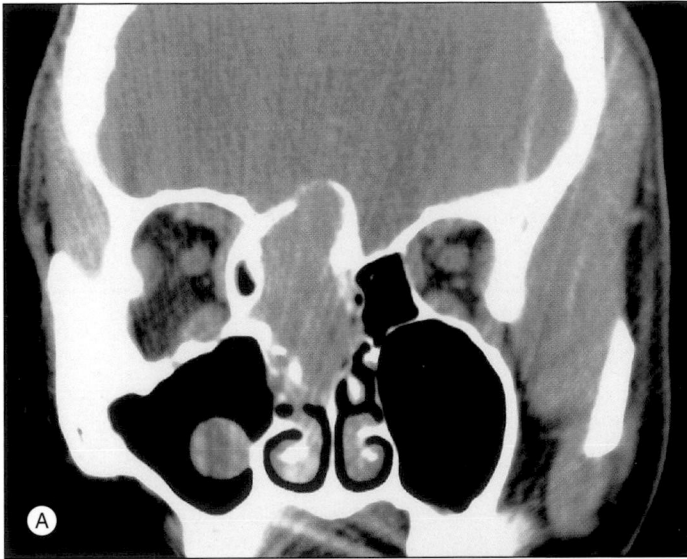

LEIOMYOMA AND LEIOMYOSARCOMAS

Clinical presentation

Sinonasal smooth muscle neoplasia are derived from the abundant perivascular smooth muscle tissue in the sinonasal tract. Both sinonasal leiomyomas and leiomyosarcomas are rare. Fu and Perzin identified only 2 leiomyomas and 6 leiomyosarcomas from 256 nonepithelial sinonasal tumors.[226] Leiomyomas have been reported to arise from the nasal septum, turbinates, vestibule, and choanae.[227–229] As the vascular component may be prominent, they can cause epistaxis. Sinonasal leiomyosarcomas are rare; fewer than 50 cases have been reported.[230–232] The AFIP reported on nine sinonasal leiomyosarcomas, which constitutes the largest such series.[232] Either the nasal cavity alone or contiguous paranasal sinuses were involved (Fig. 15.33). There is an equal sex distribution and an average age incidence of 50 years. The sinonasal symptoms are non-specific; patients complain of unilateral nasal obstruction, bleeding, and pain.

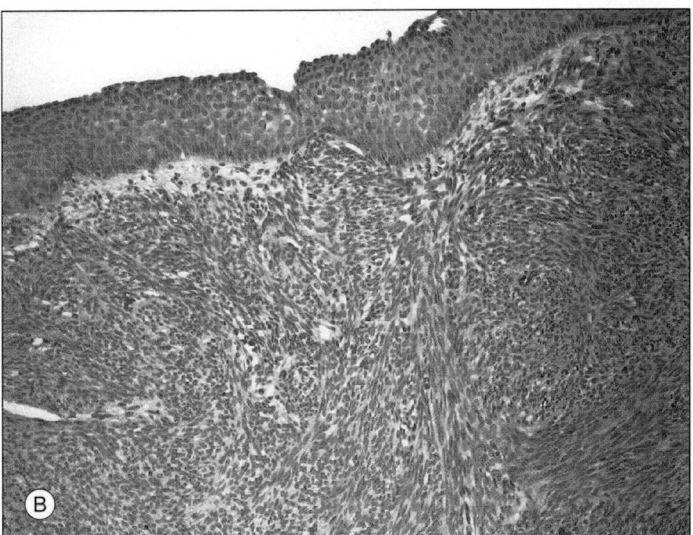

Pathology

Leiomyomas are composed of bland whorls of spindled cells with blunt cigar-shaped nuclei. Angioleiomyomas have a prominent vascular component that may be compressed or thick-walled. The absence of nuclear pleomorphism, necrosis, mitoses, and an infiltrative growth pattern separates leiomyomas from leiomyosarcomas. The malignant cells of the epithelioid variant appear less spindled and more cuboidal. This variant is more likely to arise in the stomach or the mesentery but has been found in head and neck sites.[234] IHC (Table 15.1) for CD34 and FXIIIa will aid in excluding other tumors such as solitary fibrous tumor and hemangiopericytoma.

Treatment and outcome

Both leiomyomas and leiomyosarcomas are surgical diseases. Resection can be conservative for leiomyomas, as these are curable. Leiomyosarcomas require a wide surgical approach as they are locally aggressive. About 75% of patients experience local recurrence and 35% develop metastases. At least 50% of patients die of the disease, usually within 2 years. Adjuvant RT or chemotherapy have no proven efficacy.[232] Those sinonasal leiomyosarcomas confined to the nasal cavity are associated with a better outcome as compared to those which also involve the paranasal sinuses. No leiomyosarcoma confined to the nasal cavity recurred.[232]

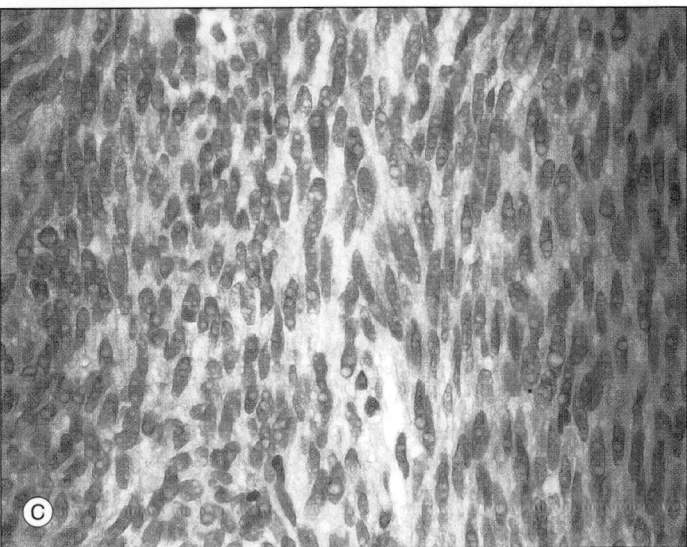

Fig. 15.33 Leiomyosarcoma. **A,** This young woman presented with a destructive, expansive tumor of the nasal cavity. **B,** Interlacing fascicles of spindled sarcoma cells are seen. The cellularity is much greater than would be seen in sinonasal hemangiopericytoma. **C,** Cigar-shaped nuclei of leiomyosarcoma. The tumor expressed muscle actin by IHC, confirming the diagnosis. A work-up was initiated after biopsy to rule out metastasis from sources.

LIPOMA

Lipomas have only rarely been reported in the sinonasal tract.[233–235] They present as pedunculated or space occupying tumors of the nasal cavity or antrum, or fat density by MRI (high signal on T1-weighted images). Neonatal nasal cavity lipomas have been reported that may be associated with other congenital abnormalities.[235] Conservative excision of lipomas should be curative.

LIPOSARCOMA

Clinical presentation

Liposarcoma is one of the most common soft tissue sarcomas of adulthood, usually occurring in the lower extremities and retroperitoneum. The head and neck is the site of origin for approximately 3–6% of all liposarcomas, most often the soft tissues of the neck and face. Hypopharyngeal and laryngeal sites were involved in 27% of cases.[204] The sinonasal tract is an extremely rare site for liposarcoma.[233]

Pathology

Liposarcomas can be polypoid, pedunculated tumors that are soft and yellow/tan/gray upon sectioning. A spectrum of histology is seen, ranging from low grade (lipoblastic liposarcoma or lipoma-like, sclerosing liposarcoma or atypical lipoma) or intermediate to high grade (myxoid liposarcoma, pleomorphic liposarcoma, round cell liposarcoma, dedifferentiated liposarcoma). Low-grade tumors are characterized by an abundance of mature, histologically benign adipose tissue, coursed by collagenous fibrous tissue. Lipoblasts may be focal, and they have characteristic 'chicken claw' shaped nuclei that are indented by cytoplasmic fat globules. Their chromatin is usually dense and pyknotic, but enlarged nucleoli may be found. Myxoid liposarcoma is another common subtype. The stromal background is loose and myxoid, perforated by a fine 'chicken-wire' meshwork of arborizing vessels. The lipoblasts appear as univacuolated signet-ring cells and multivaculolated cells.

Treatment and outcome

Generally, liposarcomas are properly treated by resection with adequate margins. Radical neck dissection is not usually warranted for low-grade tumors, but high-grade liposarcomas may develop locoregional metastases. The rarity of this tumor in the sinonasal tract precludes discussion of specific disease-free survival.

FIBROMAS (SOLITARY FIBROUS TUMORS), FIBROSARCOMA (INCLUDING DESMOID TUMOR) AND MYOFIBROSARCOMAS

Clinical presentation

Solitary fibrous tumor (SFT) is an uncommon spindle cell neoplasm derived of primitive mesenchymal or fibroblast-like cells. First recognized in the pleura (fibrous mesothelioma), SFT has gained greater recognition, and has been reported at other sites including the sinonasal tract.[238,239] Sinonasal SFT presents as a firm, polypoid well-circumscribed or encapsulated neoplasm. Fibrosarcomas (desmoid tumors, aggressive fibromatoses) are infiltrative, nonmetastasizing, unencapsulated fibroblastic tumors, which account for 12–19% of all soft tissue sarcomas. They occur most often in the lower extremities and trunk; only 2–10% occur in the head and neck, and the sinonasal tract is most commonly involved.[204] Sinonasal desmoids have a

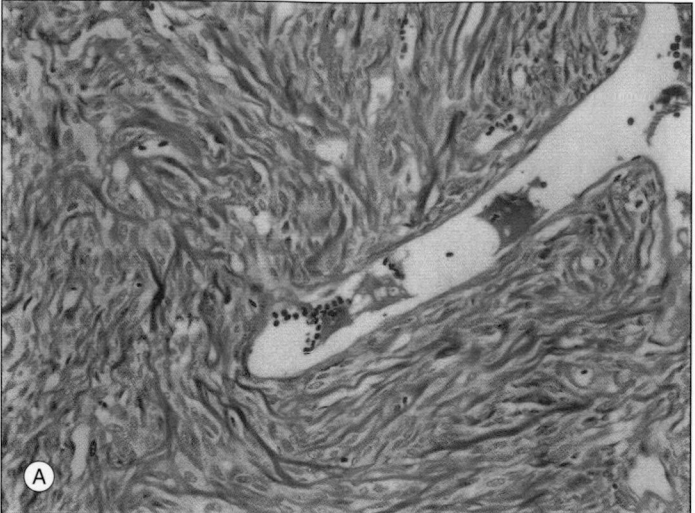

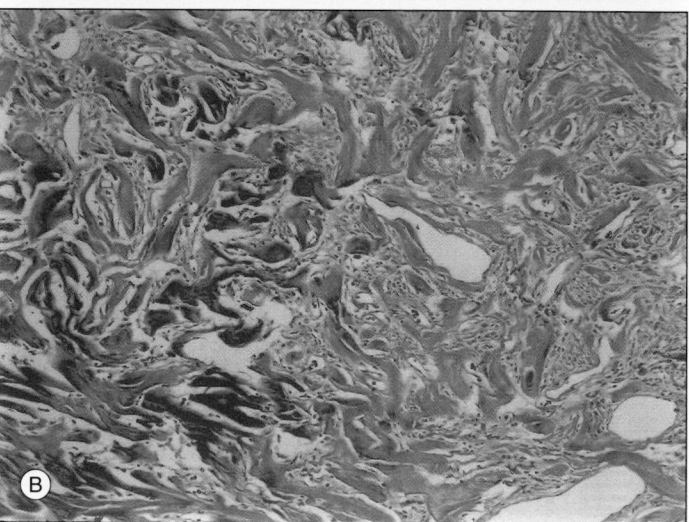

Fig. 15.34   Solitary fibrous tumor. **A,** This tumor contains abundant thin-walled vessels, and fibroblast-like spindle cells producing abundant collagen. **B,** Unlike desmoid tumors, these cells form a 'patternless' pattern rather than dense fascicles. The collagen deposition is dense, haphazard, and keloid-like.

propensity to involve the maxilla.[238] Fibromatoses (desmoid tumors, grade I fibrosarcomas) are more likely to occur in the pediatric population. Higher-grade fibrosarcomas (grade II/grade III) usually arise in patients between 20 and 60 years of age, but may also occasionally occur in the pediatric population.[204] Myofibroblastic sarcomas represent related sarcomas that demonstrate smooth muscle differentiation by IHC and EM, in addition to the fibroblastic phenotype. These may also rarely arise in the sinonasal tract.[239]

Pathology

SFT is composed of bland spindle cells arranged in a 'patternless pattern,' with a focal storiform or fascicular pattern or hemangiopericytoma-like vascular pattern. Keloid-like, collagen deposition can be seen (Fig. 15.34). Myxoid areas and rich vascularity with hyalinized vessels can be seen. The tumor boundary may be circumscribed or infiltrative. On IHC, SFT expresses vimentin, CD34 and CD99 (Table 15.1). Fibromatoses (desmoid tumors) are very bland, well differentiated, and appear as densely cellular spindle cell malignancies producing a collagenous matrix. The fascicles or bundles of tapered spindle cells grow in a variable intersecting pattern, seen on cross-section as 'herringbone' areas. The diagnosis is firmly established on biopsy when the infiltration of host tissue by bland fibroblasts is confirmed. Grades II and III fibrosarcoma are distinguished from Grade I desmoids by increased cellularity, degree of pleomorphism, mitotic rate, and necrosis. Myofibrosarcomas are composed of fusiform or tapering fibroblast-like spindle cells that can produce a collagenized matrix. IHC will confirm expression of at least one contractile marker (actin-HHF 35, muscle-specific actin, desmin, calponin, myosin) in addition to CD34 (fibroblastic).

Treatment and outcome

SFT is usually cured with resection; recurrence or progression to higher tumor grade is rare. Fibrosarcomas are best treated by complete surgical excision with ample margins. However, intraoperative examination usually reveals that this white-tan scar-like tumor sends out innumerable tentacles, making complete extirpation virtually impossible. Positive resection margins are the rule and recurrences after resection are common. Nuclear pleomorphism, a significant mitotic rate, and necrosis are generally not seen, and when present, indicate transformation to a higher grade. Grade progression may be facilitated by RT. The overall prognosis depends on the resection adequacy, sarcoma grade, size and location, male sex, and the presence of pain or cranial nerve symptoms. Of these parameters, grade and resection margin status are probably the most important. The 5-year survival rates of head and neck fibrosarcomas (all grades, all sites) ranges from 56% to 71%.[204] Of the series of sinonasal fibromatoses, 5 patients (20%) developed single or multiple recurrences from 6 to 34 months.[238]

BENIGN FIBROUS HISTIOCYTOMA

Benign fibrous histiocytoma (BFH) refers to a histologically benign lesion with fibroblastic and histiocytic component, which most commonly occurs in the dermis and subcutis. In a report of nine sinonasal fibrohistiocytic tumors (which pre-dated immuno-histochemistry), Perzin and Fu presented two tumors histologically classified as benign.[240] Basak reported an additional benign case.[241] Histologically, fibrous histiocytomas are composed of whorls of benign fibroblastic cells with a radiating, storiform pattern, admixed with multinucleated giant cells. They can be distinguished from MFH, as they are less cellular and lack nuclear pleomorphism, abnormal mitotic figures, and necrosis.

MALIGNANT FIBROUS HISTIOCYTOMAS

Clinical presentation

Malignant fibrous histiocytoma (MFH) is one of the most common soft tissue sarcomas below the clavicles. While it is recognized that MFH has become a 'waste-basket' category for some sarcomas, there remains a group of sarcomas that truly reveal both fibroblastic and histiocytic phenotype. Only about 3–10% occur in the head and neck, and most of these occur in the sinonasal tract, craniofacial bones, and soft tissues.[242]

Pathology

MFH can be classified as myxoid, angiomatoid, inflammatory, or giant cell type, and mixed patterns are common. Most MFH have a storiform/pleomorphic pattern. Whorls and fascicles of malignant fibroblastic spindle cells forming a 'rush-mat' or radiating 'star-like' (storiform) pattern characterize MFH. The putative 'histiocytic' component is composed of plump epithelioid cells and larger multinucleated giant cells that have bizarre nuclei. If a prominent myxoid background is present, these sarcomas can be classified as myxoid MFH. As with other sarcomas, focal metaplastic, mesenchymal elements (e.g. cartilaginous or osseous differentiation) may be seen. A marked inflammatory infiltrate may be present, thus warranting the designation of inflammatory MFH. Table 15.1 details the IHC profile for MFH.

Treatment and outcome

En bloc excision with adequate margins is indicated. Adjuvant RT may be indicated for close or positive resection margins. Elective neck dissection is not necessary. The 2-year survival rate for all MFH is 60%. Regarding sinonasal MFH, local recurrence, pulmonary metastases, and disease-related mortality are unfortunately common.[242–244]

FIBROMYXOMA, MYXOMA

Clinical presentation

A number of benign or low-grade neoplasms can develop from pleuripotential mesenchymal cells, producing fibromyxoid and myxoid tumors. These tumors are related to the fibro-osseous lesions; however, they lack osseous or odontogenic matrix. A myxoma is a benign mesenchymal tumor comprised of undifferentiated stellate cells producing a myxoid stroma. They are generally uncommon, and have been reported in the heart (atrial myxoma), subcutaneous tissues, bone, genitourinary tract, and skin. Head and neck myxomas are usually intraosseous jaw tumors. Mandibular myxomas have been presumed to arise from odontogenic tissue, hence are also called odontogenic myxomas. Those that arise from the maxillary bone may extend to the maxillary sinus and nasal cavity.[204,245] They grow as firm to gelatinous lobulated, erosive tumors and may reach massive proportions.

Pathology

Myxomas are composed of bland stellate fibroblastic cells producing myxoid stroma. A variable collagenizing component may be present. Bone erosion may be seen.

Treatment and outcome

Maxillary myxomas require en bloc resection, as they can be locally aggressive with a significant recurrence rate, especially if treated by curettage.[204,245,246]

INFLAMMATORY MYOFIBROBLASTIC TUMOR

Clinical presentation

Inflammatory myofibroblastic tumor (IMT) (inflammatory pseudotumor) is a tumor composed of a benign lymphoplasmacytic and myofibroblastic infiltrate. In the head and neck, IMT occurs most often in the periorbital soft tissue. A predisposition for the first two decades of life is noted.[247] Sinonasal IMT have been reported in the nasal cavity, maxilla, and nasopharynx over a wide age range from children to the elderly.[248,249] They can present as polypoid masses causing nasal obstruction, and may fill the maxilla and cause bony remodeling. Fever, weight loss, malaise, anemia, hypergammaglobulinemia, and elevated sedimentation rate may be accompanying systemic symptoms. The term 'tumefactive fibroinflammatory lesions' has also been used to describe patients with related lesions. One-third of these patients had evidence of multifocal fibro-inflammatory processes (retroperitoneal fibrosis, sclerosing cholangitis, mediastinal fibrosis, and orbital fibroinflammatory tumor).[250] Tumefactive fibroinflammatory tumors seem to fall within the histological realm of IMT.

Pathology

IMT is an exclusionary diagnosis on biopsy. Excised tumors are fleshy, whorled, firm or myxoid, and multinodular. The polymorphous appearance of IMT may reflect its shifting histology during disease course. The basic components of IMT are lymphocytes, plasma cells, histiocytes, fibroblasts, and myofibroblasts (Fig. 15.35). Four basic patterns emerge: (1) dominant lymphoplasmacytic infiltrate, (2) dominant lymphohistiocytic infiltrate, (3) predominantly 'young and active' myofibroblastic process, and (4) predominantly collagenized process with lymphoplasmacytic infiltrate. The lympho-plasmacytic IMT consists of mature lymphoid infiltrate with germinal centers, and a rich plasma cell infiltrate. Lymphohistiocytic IMT most resembles an infectious process, as foamy histiocytes are prominent. The 'young and active' IMT has a densely cellular fascicular and storiform pattern – it resembles fibrous histiocytoma save for the inflammatory infiltrate or nodular fasciitis but for the lack of necrosis. Collagenized IMT is more paucicellular and resembles a desmoid tumor, again, except for the inflammatory infiltrate. A zonation/maturation effect may be observed. Progression of patterns may also be observed in some long-standing cases necessitating multiple procedures. IHC reveals that the majority of fibroblastic spindle cells express markers of smooth muscle differentiation (muscle specific actin, smooth muscle actin, desmin) (Table 15.1). Mitotic figures and plump spindle cells are present in IMT, but nuclear pleomorphism and apoptosis are not part of IMT, and should lead one to consider inflammatory sarcomas. IMT appears to overlap with the entity described a 'low-grade inflammatory fibrosarcoma.'[251]

Treatment and outcome

In the head and neck, many IMT are initially treated and may resolve/regress with excisional biopsy and steroid therapy. However, some cases so treated may persist and worsen. Single or multiple recurrences develop in 25% of patients after excision. Sarcomatous transformation is rare. However, the recurrent or transformed cases still showed a tendency to remain localized.[247] Some patients with recurrent tumors have been treated with RT and chemotherapy.

MALIGNANT LYMPHOMA

Clinical presentation

Only 10% of head and neck lymphomas are extranodal, usually involving the tonsils, sinonasal tract, and thyroid. Sinonasal lymphoma (SNL) is more common in Asian than Western populations, where it represents the second most frequent group of extranodal lymphomas, after gastrointestinal lymphomas. It has previously been referred to as lethal midline granuloma, malignant midline reticulosis, or polymorphic reticulosis. These are clinical, inexact terms, which imply a lack of definitive pathologic diagnosis. These terms have been replaced by microscopic and phenotypic classifications. SNL can be classified as either of B-cell, T-cell natural killer cell (T/NK-cell) or T-cell natural killer precursor cell (T/null-cell) phenotypes. The revised European and American lymphoma classification (REAL) includes

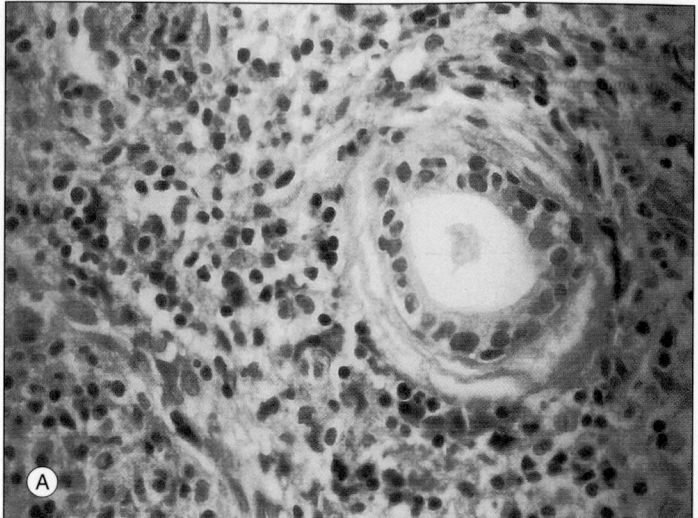

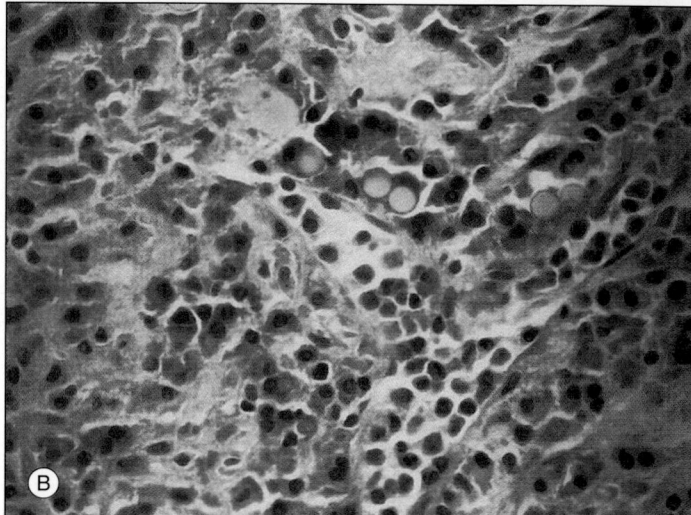

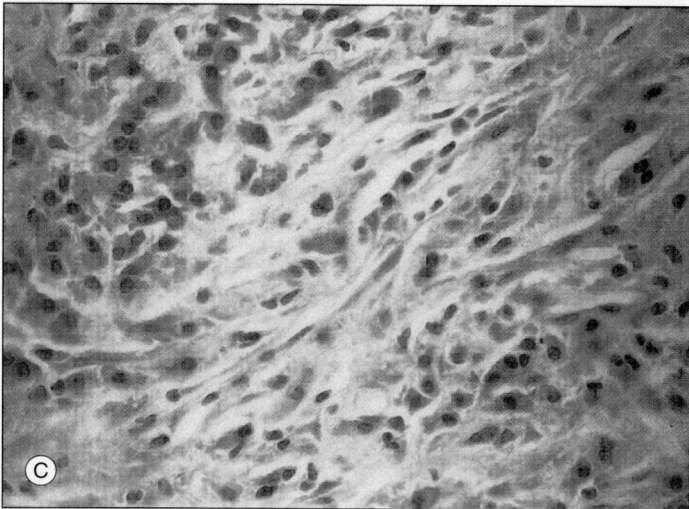

Fig. 15.35 Inflammatory myofibroblastic tumor (IMT). **A**, Sinonasal tissue involved by dense, non-specific chronic inflammation. Correlation with radiographic imaging is necessary to establish that a mass effect is seen. **B**, Plasma cells with Russell bodies. **C**, Spindled fibroblasts (myofibroblasts).

Table 15.10 Comparison of the demographics and survival of several recent series for both B-cell and T-cell SNL

Author	Year	Country	Total cases	Med age	B-cell cases	T-cell cases	Overall survival	Notes
Ko[253]	2000	Korea	48			45, plus 3 NK precursor neoplasms	1 YS 41%	Strong association with EBV Progression to extranodal disease
Quraishi[252]	2000	UK	24	72	21/24 (87%)	3/24 (13%)	5 YS 40% 10 YS 33%	
Aviles[254]	2000	Mexico	108			108 (100%)	8 year overall and disease-free survival ranged 79–90%	
Lei[255]	1999	Hong Kong	25 SNL 19 NPL		SNL: 4/16 (25%) NPL: 11/16 (69%)	SNL: 12/16 (75%) NPL: 5/16 (31%)	Overall 5 YS (33% versus 82%) and disease-free 5 YS (36% versus 76%) and worse in NSL than NPL patients, correlating with age and bulky disease.	
Yang[256]	1997	Taiwan	34	60	2/20 (10%)	18/20 (90%)	Mean survival was 84.2 months; overall 5 YS 63%	
Nakamura[257]	1997	Japan	32			32 (100%)	Overall 5 YS 49%	Strong association with EBV
Harabuchi[258]	1996	Japan	18	18		18 (100%)	Median survival 6 mo	Strong association with EBV Extranodal involvement
Davison[259]	1996	USA	30	44.5		30 (100%)	10/30 (33%) NED 12/30 (40%) DOD 6/30 (20%) DID	Strong association with EBV
Liang[260]	1995	Hong Kong	100	50	8/45 (33%)	35/45 (77%)	Improved survival correlated with age (<60), stage I disease, and absence of clinical (B) symptoms	
Abbondanzo[261]	1995	USA	120	59	101/120 (84%)	19/120 (16%)	24/66 patients, (36.4%) DOD 17/66 (25.7%) NED 13/66 (19.7%) AWD 12/66 (18.2%) DID or unknown	Extranodal involvement
Arber[262]	1993	Peru	14		2 (14%)	11 (78%)		Strong association with EBV
Kojima[263]	1992	Japan	20		9 (45%)	9 (45%)	2 YS was poorer for T-cell than B-cell lymphomas Survival correlated with stage	

SNL, sinonasal lymphoma; NPL, nasopharyngeal lymphoma; YS, year survival; EBV, Epstein-Barr virus; NED, no evidence of disease; DOD, died of disease; DID, died of intercurrent disease; AWD, alive with disease

SNL within the classification of extranodal lymphomas. Some pertinent clinicopathologic distinctions can be made between B-cell and T-cell SNL (Table 15.10).[252–263] B-cell phenotype SNL typically involves the paranasal sinuses, with a slight predominance in Western countries. Presenting symptoms relate to paranasal sinus involvement. Patients present with pain, facial or palatal mass, or ocular symptoms. These lymphomas are more likely to be associated with ocular symptoms and have orbital extension more than T/NK-cell phenotype SNL. T-cell SNL is most common in Asian and South American countries. The majority of T-cell SNL have the natural killer T-cell phenotype T/NK-cell; however, a small percentage lack this phenotype, and are classified as T/null-cell SNL. They are typically located in the nasal cavity and have an aggressive, angioinvasive growth pattern that often results in necrosis and bony erosion. The term angiocentric T-cell lymphoma refers to those T-cell lymphomas that grow around and into vessels and are associated with necrosis. In general, sinonasal T-cell lymphomas are rare in the United States and Europe, and more common in Asia and Central America. Presenting symptoms relate to nasal cavity involvement; patients present with nasal obstruction, rhinorrhea, fever, weight loss, cervical lymph adenopathy, palatal ulceration, and periorbital cellulitis. Patients with T-cell SNL are younger, with a lower male-to-female ratio than those with B-cell SNL. T-cell SNL is more commonly associated with the Epstein-Barr virus than is B-cell SNL. Typically, T-cell SNL, especially angiocentric lymphomas, may present with, or progress to involve, numerous extranodal sites such as skin, liver, larynx, kidney, breast, testis, and prostate. In addition to the development of extranodal disease, T/NK-cell SNL may be associated with hemophagocytic syndrome, a fatal complication that may be etiologically associated with EBV reactivation.[264]

Pathology
The histology of malignant lymphomas is covered in Chapter 11.

Treatment and outcome

SNL is treated with a combination of local RT and chemotherapy with an anthracycline-based regimen. B-cell SNL is usually responsive, whereas in Asian studies, T/NK-cell SNL is less responsive with a worse prognosis. Table 15.10 compares some recent series for both B-cell and T-cell SNL regarding demographics and survival. Generally, survival is dependent upon tumor stage and grade rather than phenotype.

GRANULOCYTIC SARCOMA

Clinical presentation

Granulocytic sarcoma (GS) (chloroma) represents a soft tissue infiltrate of immature myeloid elements that develops in 3% of patients with myeloid leukemia. The term 'chloroma' describes the green hue seen when these tumors are sectioned. The color, caused by the cytoplasmic enzyme myeloperoxidase, fades after exposure to air. The mean patient age is 48 years, and most (85%) present with solitary lesions. In the head and neck, osseous lesions have been reported in the skull, face, orbit, and paranasal sinuses, whereas extramedullary tumors have been reported in the nasal cavity, paranasal sinuses, nasopharynx, tonsil, mouth, lacrimal gland, salivary glands, and thyroid gland.[265]

Pathology

The histology of granulocytic sarcomas is covered in Chapter 11.

Treatment and outcome

An associated myeloproliferative disease is found in 48% of patients, and acute myeloid leukemia occurs in 22% of the cases. However, 30% of patients with chloroma have no hematological disease at initial diagnosis. Chloromas can be treated with local RT. In patients with chronic myeloid leukemia and other myeloproliferative disorders, chloroma is ominous as it is associated with the onset of acute or blastic phase of the disease. The administration of antileukemic chemotherapy at diagnosis of chloroma is associated with a significantly lower probability of developing acute myeloid leukemia and with longer survival.[266]

MULTIPLE MYELOMA

Clinical presentation

Multiple myeloma (MM) is the most common of the plasma cell dyscrasias, a group that includes Waldenström's macroglobulinemia, heavy chain disease, and primary amyloidosis. All of the above represent malignant proliferations of plasma cells or lymphocytoid plasma cells producing monoclonal immunoglobulins. MM usually affects patients over the age of 40 (median age is within sixth and seventh decades) and has a roughly equal sex distribution.[267–269] Extramedullary plasmacytoma (EMP) is the initial manifestation of MM in only 5% of patients. Eighty percent of EMP occur in the head and neck, 28% occur in the nasal cavity, and 22% occur in the paranasal sinuses. Conversely, EMP represents 3–4% of all sinonasal cavity tumors. About 20% of the head and neck EMP are initially associated with MM.[267]

Pathology

The histology of plasmacytomas is covered in Chapters 11 and 12. Poorly differentiated, anaplastic plasmacytoma can also be distinguished from anaplastic carcinomas, olfactory neuroblastomas, melanomas, and large cell lymphomas by IHC (Table 15.1).

Treatment and outcome

RT and surgery are the treatments of choice for EMP. Eventually, about 15% of patients with primary EMP develop MM;[268,269] adjuvant chemotherapy appears to have no preventive effect here. However, once multifocal or disseminated disease appears, alkylating agents and steroids can relieve the symptoms of bone pain. The 10-year disease specific and overall survival rates for EMP are excellent (87% and 61%, respectively).[270]

LANGERHANS CELL GRANULOMATOSIS

Langerhans cell granulomatosis (LCG) (histiocytosis X) is the current nomenclature for a group of childhood diseases including eosinophilic granuloma (EG), Hand-Schüller-Christian (HSC) disease, and Letterer-Siwe (L-S) disease. EG is a more localized form of LCG, often manifesting as a solitary bone lesion, whereas Hand-Schüller-Christian disease and Letterer-Siwe disease are multifocal or disseminated diseases which involve lymph nodes, skin, liver, spleen, lung, head and neck, or gastrointestinal tract. The head and neck is frequently involved in LCG, usually the flat bones of the skull or the jaws. Patients often present with otitis media and/or destructive temporal bone lesions. Sinonasal involvement is extremely rare.[269] Histology, treatment, and prognosis of LCG are covered in Chapter 11.

ROSAI-DORFMAN DISEASE

Rosai-Dorfman disease (massive lymphadenopathy with histiocytosis) is a rare, idiopathic, benign histiocytic proliferation usually seen in young patients. The massive lymphadenopathy most commonly involves the cervical lymph nodes, with a predominant infiltration of sinusoidal histiocytes. Nearly half of the patients have extranodal involvement, the majority of which (75%) occur in sites in the head and neck. Paranasal sinus involvement has been reported, usually in conjunction with cervical adenopathy and multifocal extranodal lesions.[270] Histology, treatment, and prognosis are covered in Chapter 11.

TERATOMAS AND RELATED LESIONS

Clinical presentation

The term hamartoma refers to an abnormal, oncologically benign proliferation of indigenous tissues. The sinonasal tract is the most common site for head and neck hamartomas, usually in the area of the nasal septum. Histologically, one sees benign disorganized epithelium, salivary glands, muscle, cartilaginous and vascular tissues. Respiratory epithelial adenomatoid hamartomas refers to sinonasal polypoid lesions with prominent glandular hyperplasia, but no mesenchymal component.[271] These lesions can mimic Schneiderian inverted papillomas or intestinal-type adenocarcinomas. Hairy polyps of the sinonasal tract/nasopharynx are not true tumors but represent development malformations of the first branchial arch, resulting in the presence of two germinal layers: ectoderm and mesoderm. These lesions are usually recognized at birth but can be discovered later. These lesions produce pedunculated masses attached to the lateral nasopharyngeal wall or to the nasopharyngeal portion of the soft palate. They cause difficulty in breathing, sucking, or swallowing. Histologically, hairy polyps are lined by skin, and contain accessory skin structures, fibrous and adipose tissue, smooth and skeletal muscle, and cartilage and bone. The term teratoma refers to a neoplasm that recapitulates all three germ layers (ectodermal, mesodermal, and endodermal). Teratomas may be histologically mature and oncologically benign. They may also be histologically immature but oncologically benign or they may harbor malignant components within, and have an aggressive biologic potential. As a general rule, pediatric head and neck teratomas tend to be oncologically benign, whereas adult teratomas tend to be histologically, and thus oncologically, malignant. An epignathus ('fetus-in-fetus') is an extreme example of a neonatal teratoma originating from the oropharynx, presenting as a massive protruding oral neoplasm. While neonatal teratomas are grotesquely manifest, and can cause fatal upper airway obstruction, they are usually oncologically benign. Thus, prenatal surgical intervention can convert an otherwise moribund situation. Sinonasal teratomas (teratocarcinoma, malignant teratoma, blastoma, teratocarcinosarcoma) have been reported predominantly in the adult population, with a male predominance.[273]

Pathology

Benign teratomas are cystic and solid tumors containing a mixture of immature and mature tissue trigeminal elements. The epithelial elements usually consist of mature squamous and immature intestinal or respiratory epithelia. Primitive neuroepithelium with rosettes, pseudorosettes, or neurofibrillary matrix predominate in some tumors. Pigmented retinal epithelium can be seen. The mesodermal component consists of fibroblasts and embryonal, immature spindle cells in a myxoid matrix. Islands of cartilage, smooth muscle, and skeletal muscle cells in varying degrees of maturation can be present. Malignant teratomas (teratocarcinosarcoma, teratocarcinoma) contain histologically malignant components (either carcinomatous and or sarcomatous) in addition to the immature, benign teratomatous elements.[273–277] As the malignant component of these tumors can manifest diversely, malignant teratoma should always be considered in the differential diagnosis of sinonasal 'round cell tumors' and any immature-appearing neoplasm.

Treatment and outcome

Benign dermoid tumors, hamartomas, and hairy polyps can be simply excised. Teratomas require surgical resection, and malignant teratomas require adjuvant RT. Chemotherapy has also been administered.[274–276] Heffner and Hyams reported a 60% mortality rate within 3 years, usually after aggressive local extension.[273] Regional lymph nodes and pulmonary metastases may also occur.

METASTATIC DISEASE TO THE SINONASAL TRACT

In a review of 224 sinonasal adenocarcinomas, 7 were metastatic (3%).[68] Renal cell carcinoma (RCC) is the single most common tumor, comprising 54% of sinonasal metastatic neoplasia.[277] However, only 1% of all patients with RCC develop solitary head and neck metastasis.[278] The valveless veins within the prevertebral, vertebral, and epidural venous plexuses offer little resistance to tumor emboli, and increased intra-abdominal pressure leads to retrograde blood flow to the skull base. It has been postulated that communication of these plexi with the pterygoid and pharyngeal plexi and the cavernous sinus can allow tumor emboli to reach the sinonasal tract, while bypassing the pulmonary circulation.[277] Sinonasal metastasis may represent the initial presentation of RCC or can manifest a decade after nephrectomy.[279] Usually, sinonasal metastatic RCC develops in the context of disseminated metastases, and the reported five-year survival ranges 15–30%.[280] Other carcinomas that can metastasize to the sinonasal tract originate from the breast,[281] prostate,[282] lung,[283] thyroid,[284] uterine cervix,[285] colon,[286] and testes.[287] Metastatic disease can occur in the maxillary antrum, nasal cavity/ethmoids, or nasal tip. Metastasis to the nasal tip may initially mimic an inflammatory/infectious process. As with metastatic RCC, metastases of other carcinomas to the sinonasal tract are usually associated with a very poor prognosis.

ACKNOWLEDGMENT

I would like to thank Dr. Teresa Alasio for critical review of this chapter.

REFERENCES

1. Brandwein M. The histopathology of sinonasal fungal diseases. In: Fungal diseases of the head and neck. Blitzer A, Lawson W. Otolaryngologic Clinics Vol 26 pp 1993; 26: 949–981.

2. Hyams VJ. Papillomas of the nasal cavity and paranasal sinuses. Ann Otol Rhinol Laryngol 1971; 80: 192–206.

3. Buchwald C, Franzmann MB, Tos M. Sinonasal papillomas: a report of 82 cases in Copenhagen County, including a longitudinal epidemiological and clinical study. Laryngoscope 1995; 105: 72–79.

4. Norris HJ. Papillary lesions of the nasal cavity and paranasal sinuses. Part I Exophytic (squamous) papillomas. A study of 28 cases. Laryngoscope 1962; 72: 1784–1797.

5. Ogura H, Fukushima K, Watanabe S. A high prevalence of human papillomavirus DNA in recurrent nasal papillomas. J Med Microbiol 1996; 45: 162–166.

6. Buchwald C, Franzmann MB, Jacobsen GK, et al. Carcinomas occurring in papillomas of the nasal septum associated with human papilloma virus (HPV). Rhinology 1997; 35: 74–78.

7. Bielamowicz S, Calcaterra TC, Watson D. Inverting papilloma of the head and neck: the UCLA update. Otolaryngol Head Neck Surg 1993; 109: 71–76.

8. Lawson W, Ho BT, Shaari CM, Biller HF. Inverted papilloma: a report of 112 cases. Laryngoscope 1995; 105: 282–288.

9. Peters BW, BW, O'Reilly, RC, Wilcox TO, et al. Inverted papilloma isolated to the sphenoid sinus. Otolaryngol Head Neck Surg 1995; 113: 771–777.

10. Kelly JH, Joseph M, Carroll E, et al. Inverted papilloma of the nasal septum. Arch Otolaryngol 1980; 106: 767–771.

11. Nielsen PL, Buchwald C, Nielsen LH, Tos M. Inverted papilloma of the nasal cavity: Pathological aspects in a follow-up study. Laryngoscope 1991; 101: 1094–1101.

12. Jones ME, Wackym PA, Said-Al-Naief N, et al. Clinical and molecular pathology of aggressive Schneiderian papilloma involving the temporal bone. Head Neck 1998; 20: 83–88.

13. Barnes L, Bedetti C. Oncocytic Schneiderian papilloma: A reappraisal of cylindrical cell papilloma of the sinonasal tract. Hum Pathol 1984; 15: 344–351.

14. Ward BE, Fechner RE, Mills SE. Carcinoma arising in oncocytic Schneiderian papilloma. Am J Surg Pathol 1990; 14: 364–369.

15. Kapadia SB, Barnes L, Pelzman K, et al. Carcinoma ex oncocytic Schneiderian (cylindrical cell) papilloma. Am J Otolaryngol 1993; 14: 332–338.

16. Maitra A, Baskin LB, Lee EL. Malignancies arising in oncocytic Schneiderian papillomas: a report of 2 cases and review of the literature. Arch Pathol Lab Med 2001; 125: 1365–1367.

17. Muir C, Weiland L. Upper aerodigestive tract cancers. Cancer 1995; 75: 147–153.

18. Lewis JS, Castro EB. Cancer of the nasal cavity and paranasal sinuses. J Laryngol Otol 1972; 86: 255–262.

19. Patel P, Tiwari R, Karim ABMF. Squamous cell carcinoma of the nasal vestibule. J Laryngol Otol 1992; 106: 332–336.

20. Poulsen M, Turner S. Radiation therapy for squamous cell carcinoma of the nasal vestibule. Int J Radiation Oncol Biol Phys 1993; 27: 267–272.

21. Beatty CW, Pearson BW, Kern EB. Carcinoma of the nasal septum: experience with 85 cases. Otolaryngol Head Neck Surg 1982; 90: 90–94.

22. Mazeron JJ, Chassagne D, Crook J, et al. Radiation therapy of carcinomas of the skin of nose and nasal vestibule: A report of 1676 cases by the Groupe European de Curietherapie. Radiother Oncol 1988; 13: 165–173.

23. Mendenhall WM, Stringer SP, Cassisi NJ, Mendenhall NP. Squamous cell carcinoma of the nasal vestibule. Head Neck 1999; 21: 385–393.

24. Stern SJ, Goepfert H, Clayman G, et al. Squamous cell carcinoma of the maxillary sinus. Arch Otolaryngol 1993; 119: 964–969.

25. Hayashi T, Nonaka S, Bandoh N, et al. Treatment outcome of maxillary sinus squamous cell carcinoma. Cancer 2001; 92: 1495–1503.

26. Nishino H, Miyata M, Morita M, et al. Combined therapy with conservative surgery, radiotherapy, and regional chemotherapy for maxillary sinus carcinoma. Cancer 2000; 89: 1925–1932.

27. Paulino AC, Fisher SG, Marks JE. Is prophylactic neck irradiation indicated in patients with squamous cell carcinoma of the maxillary sinus? Int J Radiat Oncol Biol Phys 1997; 39: 283–289.

28. Raslan WF, Barnes L, Krause JR, et al. Basaloid squamous cell carcinoma of the head and neck: A clinicopathologic and flow cytometric study of 10 new cases with review of the English literature. Am J Otolaryngol 1994; 15: 204–211.

29. Wan SK, Chan JKC, Tse KC. Basaloid-squamous carcinoma of the nasal cavity. J Laryngol Otol 1992; 106: 370–371.

30. Weineke JA, Thompson LD, Wenig BM. Basaloid squamous cell carcinoma of the sinonasal tract. Cancer 1999; 85: 841–854.

31. Agrawal R, Martin FW. Unusual presentation of verrucous carcinoma of maxillary antrum. J Otolaryngol 1992; 21: 371–372.

32. Vico P, Nagypal P, Rahier I, Deraemaecker R. Verrucous carcinoma of the nasal septum and columella. Acta Chir Belg 1997; 97: 50–51.

33. Pothula VB, Jones HS. Verrucous carcinoma of the nasal septum. J Laryngol Otol 1998; 112: 72–73.

34. Howell JH, Hyams VJ, Sprinkle PM. Spindle cell carcinoma of the nose and paranasal sinuses. Surgical Forum Otolaryngologic Surg Am Coll Surg 1978; 29: 565–568.

35. Zarbo RJ, Crissman JD, Venkat H, Weiss MA. Spindle-cell carcinoma of the upper aerodigestive tract mucosa. An immunohistologic and ultrastructural study of 18 biphasic tumors and comparison with seven monophasic spindle-cell tumors. Am J Surg Pathol 1986; 10: 741–753.

36. Sonobe H, Hayashi K, Takahashi K, et al. True carcinosarcoma of the maxillary sinus. Pathol Res Pract 1989; 185: 488–492.

37. Leventon GS, Evans HL. Sarcomatoid squamous cell carcinoma of the mucous membranes of the head and neck: a clinicopathologic study of 20 cases. Cancer 1981; 48: 994–1003.

38. Olsen KD, Lewis JE, Suman VJ. Spindle cell carcinoma of the larynx and hypopharynx. Otolaryngol Head Neck Surg 1997; 116: 47–52.

39. Yeh S. A histological classification of carcinomas of the nasopharynx with a critical review as to the existence of lymphoepitheliomas. Cancer 1962; 15: 895–920.

40. Levine PH, Pochinki AG, Madigan P, Bale S. Familial nasopharyngeal carcinoma in patients who are not Chinese. Cancer 1992; 70: 1024–1029.

41. Marks JE, Phillips JL, Menck HR. The national cancer data base report on the relationship of race and national origin to the histology of nasopharyngeal carcinoma. Cancer 1998; 83: 582–588.

42. Chan AT, Teo ML, Lee WY, et al. The significance of keratinizing squamous cell histology in Chinese patients with nasopharyngeal carcinoma Clin Oncol (R Coll Radiol) 1998; 10: 161–164.

43. Cheng SH, Jian JJ, Tsai SYC, et al. Prognostic features and treatment outcome in locoregionally advanced nasopharyngeal carcinoma following concurrent chemotherapy and radiotherapy. Int J Rad Oncol Biol Phys 1998; 41: 755–762.

44. Shanmugaratnam K, Chan SH, de-Thé et al.: Histopathology of nasopharyngeal carcinoma. Correlations with epidemiology, survival rates, and other biologic characteristics. Cancer 44: 1029-1044, 1979.

45. Sanguineti G, Geara FB, Garden AS et al. Carcinoma of the nasopharynx treated by radiotherapy alone.

Determinants of local and regional control. Int J Radiat Oncol Biol Phys 1997; 37: 985–996.

46. Erkal HS, Serin M, Cakmak A. Nasopharyngeal carcinomas: analysis of patient, tumor and treatment characteristics determining outcome. Radiother Oncol 2001; 61: 247–256.

47. Qin DX, Hu YH, Yan JH, et al. Analysis of 1379 patients with nasopharyngeal carcinoma treated by radiation. Cancer 1998; 61: 1117–1124.

48. Ma J, Mai H, Hong M, et al. Is the 1997 AJCC staging system for nasopharyngeal carcinoma prognostically useful for Chinese patient populations? Int J Rad Oncol Biol Phys 2001; 50: 1181–1189,

49. Chua D, Sham JST, Wei WI, et al. The predictive value of the 1997 American Joint Committee on Cancer stage classification in determining failure patterns in nasopharyngeal carcinoma. Cancer 2001; 92: 2845–2855.

50. Spiro RH, Huvos AG. Stage means more than grade in adenoid cystic carcinoma. Am J Surg 1992; 164: 623–628.

51. Conley J, Casler JD. Adenoid cystic cancer of the head and neck. New York, NY: Thieme Medical Publishers; 1991.

52. Prasad AR, Savera AT, Gown AM, Zarbo RJ. The myoepithelial immunophenotype in 135 benign and malignant salivary gland tumors other than pleomorphic adenoma. Arch Pathol Lab Med 1999; 123: 801–806.

53. Matsuba HM, Spector GJ, Thawley SE, et al. Adenoid cystic salivary gland carcinoma: a histopathologic review of treatment failure patients. Cancer 1986; 57: 519–524.

54. Nasciemento AG, Amaral ALP, Pradao LAF, et al. Adenoid cystic carcinoma of salivary glands: a study of 61 cases with clinicopathologic correlations. Cancer 1986; 57: 312–319.

55. Perzin KH, Gullane P, Clairmont AC. Adenoid cystic carcinoma arising in salivary glands: a correlation of histologic features and clinical course. Cancer 1978; 42: 265–282.

56. Goepfert H, Luna MA, Lindberg RD, et al. Malignant salivary gland tumors of the paranasal sinuses and nasal cavity. Arch Otolaryngol 1983; 109: 662–668.

57. Tran L, Sidrys J, Horton D, et al. Malignant salivary gland tumors of the paranasal sinuses and nasal cavities. Am J Clin Oncol 1989; 12: 387–392.

58. Compagno J, Wong RT. Intranasal mixed tumors (pleomorphic adenomas). A clinicopathologic study of 40 cases. Am J Clin Pathol 1977; 68: 213–218.

59. Thomas MR, Ward K, Al-Khabori M, et al. Oncocytic mixed nasal tumor. J Laryngol Otol 1993; 107: 732–734.

60. Lam PW, Chan JK, Sin VC. Nasal pleomorphic adenoma with skeletal muscle differentiation: potential misdiagnosis as rhabdomyosarcoma. Hum Pathol 1997; 28: 1299–302.

61. Cho KJ, el-Naggar AK, Mahanupab P, et al. Carcinoma ex-pleomorphic adenoma of the nasal cavity: a report of two cases. J Laryngol Otol 1995; 109: 677–679.

62. Freeman SB, Kennedy KS, Parker GS, Tatum SA. Metastasizing pleomorphic adenoma of the nasal septum. Arch Otolaryngol Head Neck Surg 1990; 116: 1331–1333.

63. Begin LR, Rochon L, Frenkiel S. Spindle cell myoepithelioma of the nasal cavity. Am J Surg Pathol 1991; 15: 184–190.

64. Begin LR, Black MJ. Salivary-type myxoid myoepithelioma of the sinonasal tract: a potential diagnostic pitfall. Histopathology 1993; 23: 283–285.

65. Nilles R, Lenarz T. Kaiserling: myoepitheliales Karzinom des Nasopharynx. Fallbreicht und Literaturübersicht HNO 1993; 41: 396–400.

66. Graadt van Roggen JF, Baatenberg-de Jong RJ, Verschuur HP, et al. Myoepithelial carcinoma (malignant myoepithelioma): first report of an occurrence in the maxillary sinus. Histopathology 1998; 32: 239–234.

67. Spiro RH, Koss LG, Hajdu SI, Strong EW. Tumors of minor salivary origin. A clinicopathologic study of 492 cases. Cancer 1973; 31: 117–129.

68. Heffner DK, Hyams VJ, Hauck KW, Lingeman C. Low grade adenocarcinoma of the nasal cavity and paranasal sinuses. Cancer 1982; 50: 312–322.

69. Manace ED, Goldman JL. Acinic cell carcinoma of the paranasal sinuses. Laryngoscope 1971; 81: 1074–1082.

70. Valerdiz-Casasola S, Sola J, Pardo-Mindan FJ. Acinic cell carcinoma of the sinonasal cavity with intracytoplasmic crystalloids. Histopathol 1993; 23: 382–384.

71. Schmitt FC, Wal R, Santos GC. Acinic cell carcinoma arising in the nasal cavity. Diagnosis by fine-needle aspiration. Diagnost Cytopathol 1994; 10: 96–97.

72. Hanada T, Moriyama I, Fukami K. Acinic cell carcinoma originating in the nasal cavity. Arch Otorhinolaryngol 1988; 245: 344–347.

73. Takimoto T, Kano M, Umeda R. Acinic cell carcinoma of the nasal cavity: A case report. Rhinology 1989; 27: 191–196.

74. Perzin KH, Cantor JO, Johannessen JV. Acinic cell carcinoma arising in nasal cavity. Report of a case with ultrastructural observations. Cancer 1981; 47: 1818–1822.

75. Ordonez NG, Batsakis JG. Acinic cell carcinoma of the nasal cavity: electron-optic and immunohistochemical observations. J Laryngol Otol 1986; 100: 345–349.

76. Ellis GL, Corio R. Acinic cell carcinoma. A clinicopathologic analysis of 294 cases. Cancer 1983; 52: 542–549.

77. Lewis JE, Olsen KD, Weiland LH. Acinic cell carcinoma. Clinicopathologic review. Cancer 1991; 67: 172–179.

78. Abrams AM, Melrose RJ. Acinic cell tumors of minor salivary gland origin. Oral Surg Oral Med Oral Pathol 1978; 46: 220–233.

79. Chen YS, Brannon RB, Miller AS, et al. Acinic cell adenocarcinoma of minor salivary glands. Cancer 1978; 42: 678–685.

80. Buchanan JA, Krolls SO, Sneed WF, et al. Oncocytoma in the nasal vestibule. Otolaryngol Head Neck Surg 1988; 99: 63–65.

81. Miracco C, Sensini I, Vessio G, et al. Oncocytic adenoma of the nasal cavity. A case report. Histol Histopath 1986; 1: 9–11.

82. Hamdan AL, Kahwagi G, Farhat F, et al. Oncocytoma of the nasal septum: a rare cause of epistaxis. Otolaryngol Head Neck Surg 2002; 126: 440–441.

83. Colreavy MP, Sigston E, Lacy PD, et al. Post-nasal space oncocytoma: a different approach to a rare tumour. J Laryngol Otol 2001; 115: 57–59.

84. Handler SD, Ward PH. Oncocytoma of the maxillary sinus. Laryngoscope 1979; 89: 372–376.

85. Mahmoud NA. Malignant oncocytoma of the nasal cavity. J Laryngol Otol 1979; 93: 729–734.

86. DiMaio SJ, DiMaio VJM, DiMaio TM, et al. Oncocytic carcinoma of the nasal cavity. Southern Medical J 1980; 73: 803–806.

87. Chui RTK, Liao SY, Bosworth H. Recurrent oncocytoma of the ethmoid sinus with orbital invasion. Otolaryngol Head Neck Surg 1985; 93: 267–270.

88. Mikhail RA, Reed DN, Bybee DB, et al. Malignant oncocytoma of the maxillary sinus – an ultrastructural study. Head and Neck Surg 1988; 10: 427–431.

89. Nayak DR, Pillai S, Balakrishnan R, et al. Malignant oncocytoma of the nasal cavity: a case report. Am J Otolaryngol. 1999; 20: 323–327.

90. Hamperl H. Benign and malignant oncocytoma. Cancer 1962;. 15: 1019–1027.

91. Tran L, Sidrys J, Horton D, et al. Malignant salivary gland tumors of the paranasal sinuses and nasal cavities. Am J Clin Oncol 1989; 12: 387–392.

92. Hyams VJ, Batsakis JG, Micheals L. Nonepidermoid epithelial neoplasms. In: Tumors of the upper

respiratory tract. Atlas of tumor pathology. 2nd Series, Fascicle 25, Washington DC: Armed Forces Institute of Pathology; 1986.

93. Healey WV, Perzin KH, Smith L. Mucoepidermoid carcinoma of salivary gland origin. Cancer 1970; 26: 368–388.

94. Brandwein MS, Ivanov K, Wallace DI, et al. Mucoepidermoid carcinoma: a clinicopathologic study of 80 patients with special reference to histological grading. Am J Surg Pathol 2001; 25: 835–845.

95. Bergman F. Tumors of the minor salivary glands. A report of 46 cases. Cancer 1969; 3: 538–543.

96. Vincent SD, Hammond HL, Finkelstein MW. Clinical and therapeutic features of polymorphous low-grade adenocarcinoma. Oral Surg Oral Med Oral Pathol 1994; 77: 41–47.

97. Slootweg PJ. Low-grade adenocarcinoma of the oral cavity: Polymorphous or papillary? J Oral Pathol Med 1993; 22: 327–330.

98. Slootweg PJ, Muller H. Low-grade adenocarcinoma of the oral cavity: A comparison between the terminal duct and the papillary type. J Cranio-Max-Fac Surg 1987; 15: 359–364.

99. Mills SE, Garland TA, Allen MS Jr. Low-grade papillary adenocarcinoma of palatal salivary gland origin. Am J Surg Pathol 1984; 8: 367–374.

100. Mostofi R, Wood RS, Christison W, Talerman A. Low-grade papillary adenocarcinoma of minor salivary glands: case report and literature review. Oral Surg Oral Med, Oral Pathol 1992; 73: 591–595.

101. Dehner LP, Valbuena L, Perez-Atayde A, et al. Salivary gland anlage tumor ('congenital pleomorphic adenoma'). A clinicopathologic, immunohistochemical and ultrastructural study of nine cases. Am J Surg Pathol 1994; 18: 25–36.

102. Welkoborsky HJ, Gosepath J, Jacob R, et al. Biologic characteristics of paragangliomas of the nasal cavity and paranasal sinuses. Am J Rhinol 2000; 14: 419–426.

103. Scott M, Brooker DS, Davis RI. Paraganglioma of the nasal cavity. Ulster Med J 2001; 70: 149–151.

104. Argani P, Perez-Ordonez B, Xiao H, et al. Olfactory neuroblastoma is not related to the Ewing family of tumors: absence of EWS/FLI1 gene fusion and MIC2 expression. Am J Surg Pathol 1998; 22: 391–398.

105. Sorensen PH, Wu JK, Berean KW, et al. Olfactory neuroblastoma is a peripheral primitive neuroectodermal tumor related to Ewing sarcoma. Proc Natl Acad Sci USA 1996; 93: 1038–1043.

106. Elkon D, Hightower SI, Lim ML, et al. Esthesioneuroblastoma. Cancer 1979; 44: 1087–1094.

107. Dulguerov P, Calcaterra T. Esthesioneuroblastoma: the UCLA experience 1970–1990. Laryngoscope 1992; 102: 843–849.

108. Jekunen AP, Kairemo KJ, Lehtonen HP, Kajanti MJ. Treatment of olfactory neuroblastoma. A report of 11 cases. Am J Clin Oncol. 1996; 19: 375–378.

109. Morita, A, Ebersold MJ, Olsen KD, et al. Esthesioneuroblastoma: prognosis and management. Neurosurgery. 1993; 32: 706–714.

110. Irish J, Dasgupta R, Freeman J, et al. Outcome and analysis of the surgical management of esthesioneuroblastoma. J Otolaryngol 1997; 26: 1–7.

111. Koka VN, Julieron M, Bourhis J, et al. Aesthesioneuroblastoma. J Laryngol Otol 1998; 112: 628–633.

112. McElroy EA Jr, Buckner JC, Lewis JE. Chemotherapy for advanced esthesioneuroblastoma: the Mayo Clinic experience. Neurosurgery. 1998; 42: 1023–1027.

113. Levine PA, Gallagher R, Cantrell RW. Esthesioneuroblastoma: reflections of a 21-year experience. Laryngoscope 1999; 109: 1539–1543.

114. Resto VA, Eisele DW, Forastiere A, et al. Esthesioneuroblastoma: the Johns Hopkins experience. Head Neck 2000; 22: 550–558.

115. Miyamoto RC, Gleich LL, Biddinger PW, Gluckman JL. Esthesioneuroblastoma and sinonasal undifferentiated carcinoma: impact of histological grading and clinical staging on survival and prognosis. Laryngoscope 2000; 110: 1262–1265.

116. Eriksen JG, Bastholt L, Krogdahl AS, et al. Esthesioneuroblastoma – what is the optimal treatment? Acta Oncol 2000; 39: 231–235.

117. Simon JH, Zhen W, McCulloch TM, et al. Esthesioneuroblastoma: the University of Iowa experience 1978–1998. Laryngoscope 2001; 111: 488–493.

118. Smith S, Iskander A, Brandwein M, et al. Treatment of esthesioneuroblastoma: the Mount Sinai experience. Laryngoscope. In press.

119. Hyams VJ, Batsakis JG, Micheals L. Tumors of the upper respiratory tract and ear. In: Atlas of tumor pathology, 2nd series, Fascicle 25. Washington DC: Armed Forces Institute of Pathology; 1988: 240–248.

120. Frierson HF Jr, Ross GW, Mills SE, Frankfurter A. Olfactory neuroblastoma. Additional immunohistochemical characterization. Am J Clin Pathol 1990; 94: 547–553.

121. Kadish S, Goodman M, Wang CC. Olfactory neuroblastoma. A clinical analysis of 17 cases. Cancer 1976; 33: 1571–1576.

122. Foote RL, Morita A, Ebersold MJ, et al. Esthesioneuroblastoma: the role of adjuvant radiation therapy. Int J Radiat Oncol Biol Phys 1993; 27: 835–842.

123. Polin RS, Sheehan JP, Chenelle AG, et al. The role of preoperative adjuvant treatment in the management of esthesioneuroblastoma: the University of Virginia experience. Neurosurgery 1998; 42: 1029–1037.

124. Dulguerov P, Allal AS, Calcaterra TC. Esthesioneuroblastoma: a meta-analysis and review. Lancet Oncol 2001; 2(11): 683–690.

125. Sheehan JM, Sheehan JP, Jane JA Sr, Polin RS. Chemotherapy for esthesioneuroblastomas. Neurosurg Clin N Am 2000; 11: 693–701.

126. Kameya T, Shimosato Y, Adachi I, et al. Neuroendocrine carcinoma of the paranasal sinuses. Morphological and endocrine study. Cancer 1980; 45: 330–339.

127. Silva EG, Butler J, MacKay B, Goepfert H. Neuroblastomas and neuroendocrine carcinomas of the nasal cavity. A proposed classification. Cancer 1982; 50: 2388–2405.

128. McCluggage WG, Napier SS, Primrose WJ, et al. Sinonasal neuroendocrine carcinoma exhibiting amphicrine differentiation. Histopathology 1995; 27: 79–82.

129. Perez-Ordonez B, Caruana SM, Huvos AG, Shah JP. Small cell neuroendocrine carcinoma of the nasal cavity and paranasal sinuses. Hum Pathol 1998; 29: 826–832.

130. Trull JL, Mckay B, Troncoso P, et al. Neuroendocrine tumors of the nasal cavity: an ultrastructural and morphometric study of 24 cases. Ultrastruct Pathol 1992; 16: 165–175.

131. Mills SE. Neuroectodermal neoplasms of the head and neck with emphasis on neuroendocrine carcinomas. Mod Pathol 2002; 15: 264–278.

132. Frierson HF, Mills SE, Fechner RE, et al. Sinonasal undifferentiated carcinoma. An aggressive neoplasm derived from Schneiderian epithelium and distinct from olfactory neuroblastoma. Am J Surg Pathol 1986; 101: 771–779.

133. Gallo O, Graziani P, Fini-Storchi O. Undifferentiated carcinoma of the nose and paranasal sinuses. An immunohistochemical and clinical study. ENT J 1993; 72: 588–595.

134. Helliwell TR, Yeoh LH, Stell P. Anaplastic carcinoma of the nose and paranasal sinuses. Light microscopy, immunohistochemistry and clinical correlation. Cancer 1986; 58: 2938–2045.

135. Zoppi J, Avagnina A, Elsner B, et al. Carcinoma indiferenciados de nariz y senos paranasales. Estudio clinicopatologico e inmunohistoquimico Medicina (Buenos Aires) 1991; 51: 222–226.

136. Righi RD, Francis F, Aron BS, et al. Detection of EBV genome in sinonasal undifferentiated carcinoma by use of in-situ hybridization. Otolaryngol Head Neck Surg 1995; 112: 659–664.

137. Gorelick J, Ross D, Marentette L, Blaivas M. Sinonasal undifferentiated carcinoma: case series and review of the literature. Neurosurgery 2000; 47: 750–754.

138. Smith SR, Som P, Fahmy A, et al. A clinicopathological study of sinonasal neuroendocrine carcinoma and sinonasal undifferentiated carcinoma. Laryngoscope 2000; 110: 1617–1622.

139. Cerilli LA, Holst VA, Brandwein MS, et al. Sinonasal undifferentiated carcinoma: immunohistochemical profile and lack of EBV association. Am J Surg Pathol 2001; 25: 156–163.

140. Shinokuma A, Hirakawa N, Tamiya S, et al. Evaluation of Epstein-Barr virus infection in sinonasal small round cell tumors. J Cancer Res Clin Oncol. 2001;1 26: 12–18.

141. Deutsch BD, Levine PA, Stewart FM, et al. Sinonasal undifferentiated carcinoma: a ray of hope. Otolaryngol Head Neck Surg 1993; 108: 697–700.

142. Javral SM, Hern JD, Mouchloulis G, Porter GC. Malignant melanoma arising in the frontal sinuses. J Laryngol Otol 1997; 111: 376–378.

143. Mathews A, Abraham EK, Amman S, Nair MK. Pigmented squamous cell carcinoma of nasal cavity. Histopathology 1998; 33: 184–185.

144. Franquemont DW, Mills SE. Sinonasal malignant melanoma. A clinicopathologic and immunohistochemical study of 14 cases. Am J Clin Pathol 1991; 96: 689–697.

145. Fisher SR. Elective, therapeutic, and delayed lymph node dissection for malignant melanoma of the head and neck: analysis of 1444 patients from 1970 to 1998. Laryngoscope 2002; 112: 99–110.

146. Trap TK, Fu YS, Calcaterra TC. Melanoma of the nasal and paranasal sinus mucosa. Arch Otolaryngol Head Neck Surg 1987; 113: 1086–1089.

147. Brandwein M, Rothstein A, Lawson W, et al. Sinonasal melanoma – a clinicopathologic study of 25 cases and literature meta-analysis. Arch Otolaryngol Head Neck Surg 1997; 123: 290–296.

148. Regauer S, Anderhuber W, Richtig E, et al. Primary mucosal melanomas of the nasal cavity and paranasal sinuses. A clinicopathological analysis of 14 cases. APMIS 1998; 106: 403–410.

149. Barrett AW, Morgan M, Ramsay AD, et al. A clinicopathologic and immunohistochemical analysis of melanotic neuroectodermal tumor of infancy. Oral Surg Oral Med Oral Pathol Oral Radiol Endod 2002; 93: 688–698.

150. Pettinato G, Manivel JC, d'Amore ES, et al. Immunohistochemical, ultrastructural, and histogenetic considerations in a patient with melanotic neuroectodermal tumor of infancy. J Oral Maxillofac Surg. 1992; 50: 186–189.

151. Cutler LS, Chaudhry AP, Topazian R. Melanotic neuroectodermal tumor of infancy: an ultrastructural study, literature review, and reevaluation. Cancer 1981; 48: 257–270.

152. Dehner LP, Sibley RK, Sauk JJ, et al. Malignant melanotic neuroectodermal tumor of infancy: a clinical, pathologic, ultrastructural and tissue culture study. Cancer 1979; 43: 1389–1410.

153. Boor A, Jurkovic I, Friedmann I, et al. Extraskeletal Ewing's sarcoma of the nose. J Laryngol Otol 2001; 115: 74–76.

154. Cope JU, Tsokos M, Miller RW. Ewing sarcoma and sinonasal neuroectodermal tumors as second malignant tumors after retinoblastoma and other neoplasms. Med Pediatr Oncol 2001; 36: 290–294

155. Bacci G, Ferrari S, Bertoni F, et al. Neoadjuvant chemotherapy for peripheral malignant neuroectodermal tumor of bone: recent experience at the Istituto Rizzoli. J Clin Oncol 2000; 18: 885–892.

156. Franquemont DW, Fechner RE, Mills SE. Histologic classification of sinonasal intestinal-type adenocarcinoma. Am J Surg Pathol 1991; 15: 368–375.

157. Barnes L. Intestinal-type adenocarcinoma of the nasal cavity and paranasal sinuses. Am J Surg Pathol 1986; 10: 192–202.

158. Kleinsasser O, Schroeder HG. Adenocarcinomas of the inner nose after exposure to wood dust. Morphological findings and relationships between histopathology and clinical behavior in 79 cases. Arch Otorhinolaryngol 1988; 245: 1–15.

159. McKinney CD, Mills SE, Franquemont DW. Sinonasal intestinal-type adenocarcinoma: immunohistochemical profile and comparison with colonic adenocarcinoma. Mod Pathol. 1995; 8: 421–426.

160. Böör A, Jurkovic I, Dudrikova K, Kavecansky V, Friedmann I. Pathology in focus: Intestinal-type sinonasal adenocarcinoma: a sporadic case. J Laryngol Otol 1996; 100: 805–810.

161. Batsakis JG, Mackay B, Ordonez NG. Enteric-type adenocarcinoma of the nasal cavity. An electron microscopic and immunocytochemical study. Cancer 1984; 54: 855–860.

162. Mills SE, Fechner RE, Cantrell RW. Aggressive sinonasal lesion resembling normal intestinal mucosa. Am J Surg Pathol 1982; 6:803–809.

163. Wenig BM, Hyams VJ, Heffner DK. Nasopharyngeal papillary adenocarcinoma. A clinicopathologic study of a low-grade carcinoma. Am J Surg Pathol 1988; 12: 946–953.

164. Van Hasselt CA, Ng HK. Papillary adenocarcinoma of the nasopharynx. J Laryngol Otol 1991; 105: 853–854.

165. Zur K, Brandwein M, Wang B, et al. A renal cell-like adenocarcinoma of the nasal cavity – a new entity? "Van Meegeren in the house of Vermeer." Arch Otolaryngol Head Neck Surg 2002; 128: 441–447.

166. Hadi UM, Kahwaji GJ, Mufarrij AA, et al. Low grade primary clear cell carcinoma of the sinonasal tract. Rhinol 2002; 40: 44–47.

167. Hasegawa SL, Mentzel T, Fletcher D. Schwannomas of the sinonasal tract and nasopharynx. Mod Pathol 1997; 10: 777–784.

168. Berlucchi M, Piazza C, Blanzuoli L, et al. Schwannoma of the nasal septum: a case report with review of the literature. Eur Arch Otorhinolaryngol 2000; 257: 402–405.

169. Moreno PM, Meseguer DH. Solitary neurofibroma of the inferior nasal turbinate. Auris Nasus, Larynx 1998; 25: 329–331.

170. Hillstrom R, Zarbo R, Jacobs JR. Nerve sheath tumors of the paranasal sinuses: electron microscopy and histopathologic diagnosis. Otolaryngol Head Neck Surg 1990; 102: 257–263.

171. Heffner DK, Gnepp DR. Sinonasal fibrosarcomas, malignant Schwannomas, and "Triton" tumors. A clinicopathologic study of 67 cases. Cancer 1992; 70: 1089–1101.

172. Hellquist H B, Lungren J. Neurogenic sarcoma of the sinonasal tract. J Laryngol Otol 1991; 105: 186–190.

173. Swanson PE, Scheithauer BW, Wick MR. Peripheral nerve sheath neoplasms. Clinicopathologic and immunochemical observations. Pathol Ann 1995; 30: 1–82.

174. Perzin KH, Pushparaj N. Nonepithelial tumors of the nasal cavity, paranasal sinuses, and nasopharynx: a clinicopathologic study. XIII. Meningiomas. Cancer 1984; 54: 1860–1869.

175. Thompson LDR, Gyure K. Extracranial sinonasal tract meningioma. Am J Surg Pathol 2000; 24: 640–650.

176. Patterson K, Kapur S, Chandra R. "Nasal gliomas" and related brain heterotopias: A pathologist's perspective. Ped Pathol 1986; 5: 353–362.

177. Cerda-Nicolas M, Fernandez de Sevilla CS, Lopez-Gines C, et al. Nasal glioma or nasal glial heterotopia? Morphological, immunohistochemical and ultrastructural study of two cases. Clin Neuropathol 2002; 21: 66–71.

178. Luk ISC, Chan JKC, Chow SM, Leung S. Pituitary adenoma presenting as sinonasal tumor: pitfalls in diagnosis. Human Pathol 1996; 27: 605–609.

179. Jingyun L, Li W, Jing G. Primary nasal ectopic pituitary adenoma: a case report. Chinese Med J 1997; 110: 731–733.

180. Pernicone PJ, Scheithauer BW, Sebo TJ, et al. Pituitary carcinoma. A clinicopathologic study of 15 cases. Cancer 1997; 79: 804–812.

181. Hug EB, Loredo LN, Slater JD, et al. Proton radiation therapy for chordomas and chondrosarcomas of the skull base. J Neurosurg 1999; 91: 432–439.

182. Koivenen P, Lopponene H, Fors A, Jokinen K. The growth rate of osteomas of the paranasal sinuses. J Otolaryngol 1997; 22: 111–114.

183. Slootweg PJ, Panders AK, Nikkels PG. Psammomatoid ossifying fibroma of the paranasal sinuses. An extragnathic variant of cemento-ossifying fibroma. Report of three cases. J Craniomaxillofac Surg 1993; 21: 294–297.

184. Wenig BM, Vinh TN, Smirniotopoulos JG, et al. Aggressive psammomatoid ossifying fibromas of the sinonasal region: a clinicopathologic study of a distinct group of fibro-osseous lesions. Cancer 1995; 76: 1155–1165.

185. El-Mofty S. Psammomatoid and trabecular juvenile ossifying fibroma of the craniofacial skeleton: Two distinct clinicopathologic entities. Oral Surg Oral Med Oral Pathol Oral Radiol Endod 2002; 93: 296–304.

186. Lustig LR, Holliday MJ, McCarthy EF, Nager GT. Fibrous dysplasia involving the skull base and temporal bone. Arch Otolaryngol Head Neck Surg 2001; 127: 1239–1247.

187. Kaushik S, Smoker WR, Frable WJ. Malignant transformation of fibrous dysplasia into chondroblastic osteosarcoma. Skeletal Radiol 2002; 31: 103–106.

188. Beuerlein ME, Schuller DE, DeYoung BR. Maxillary malignant mesenchymoma and massive fibrous dysplasia. Arch Otolaryngol Head Neck Surg 1997; 123: 106–109.

189. Rimmelin A, Roth T, George B, et al. Giant-cell tumour of the sphenoid bone: case report. Neuroradiology 1996; 38: 650–653.

190. Kujas M, Faillot T, Van Effenterre R, Poirier J. Bone giant cell tumour in neuropathological practice. A fifty year overview. Arch Anat Cytol Pathol 1999; 47: 7–12.

191. Boulaich M, Benbouzid MA, Lazrak A, et al. Central giant cell reparative granuloma of the jaw. Rev Stomatol Chir Maxillofac 1995; 96: 8–12.

192. Schlorf RA, Koop SH. Maxillary giant cell reparative granuloma. Laryngoscope 1977; 87: 1017.

193. Huvos A. Osteoblastoma. In: Huvos AG. Bone tumors: diagnosis, treatment and prognosis. 2nd edn. Philadelphia: WB Saunders; 1991: 67–83.

194. Imai K, Tsujiguchi K, Toda C, et al. Osteoblastoma of the nasal cavity invading the anterior skull base in a young child. J Neurosurg 1997; 87: 625–628.

195. Velegrakis GA, Prokopakis EP, Papadakis CE, et al. Osteoblastoma of the nasal cavity arising from the perpendicular plate of the thymoid bone. J Laryngol Otol 1997; 111: 865–868.

196. Huvos AG. Osteogenic sarcoma of the craniofacial bones. In: Huvos AG. Bone tumors. diagnosis, treatment, and prognosis. 2nd edn. Philadelphia: WB Saunders; 1991: 85–156.

197. Chauveinc L, Mosseri V, Quintana E, et al. Osteosarcoma following retinoblastoma: age of onset and latency period. Opthalmic Gen 2001; 22: 77–78.

198. Fu YS, Perzin KH. Non-epithelial tumors of the nasal cavity, paranasal sinuses and nasopharynx: a clinicopathologic study. II. Osseous and fibro-osseous lesions, including osteoma, fibrous dysplasia, ossifying fibroma, osteoblastoma, giant cell tumor and osteosarcoma. Cancer 1974; 33: 1289–1305.

199. Barnes L. Diseases of the bones and joints. In: Barnes L. Surgical pathology of the head and neck. 2nd edn. New York: Marcel Dekker; 2000: 1144.

200. Huvos A. Chondrosarcoma. In: Bone tumors: diagnosis, treatment and prognosis. Huvos AG. 2nd edn. Philadelphia: WB Saunders; 1991: 343–401.

201. Saito K, Unni KK, Wollan PC, Lund BA. Chondrosarcoma of the jaw and facial bones. Cancer 1995; 76: 1550–1558.

202. Rosenberg AE, Nielsen GP, Keel SB, et al. Chondrosarcoma of the base of skull. A clinicopathologic study of over 200 cases with emphasis on its distinction from chordoma. Am J Surg Pathol 1999; 23: 1370–1378.

203. Vencio EF, Reeve CM, Unni KK, Nascimento AG. Mesenchymal chondrosarcoma of the jaw bones. Cancer 1998; 82: 2350–2355.

204. Barnes L. Tumor and tumor-like conditions of the soft tissues. In: Barnes L. Surgical pathology of the head and neck. 2nd edn. New York: Marcel Dekker; 2000: 889–1048.

205. Lloyd G, Howard D, Phelps P, Cheesman A. Juvenile angiofibroma: the lessons of 20 years of modern imaging. J Laryngol Otol 1999; 113: 127–134.

206. Gullane PJ, Davidson J, O'Dwyer T, Forte V. Juvenile angiofibroma: a review of the literature and a case series report. Laryngoscope 1992; 102: 928–933.

207. Makek MS, Andrews JC, Fisch U. Malignant transformation of a nasopharyngeal angiofibroma. Laryngoscope 1989; 99: 1088–1092.

208. Kurien M, Nair S, Thomas S. Angiosarcoma of the nasal cavity and maxillary antrum. J Laryngol Otol 1989; 103: 874–876.

209. Wong KF, So CC, Wong N, et al. Sinonasal angiosarcoma with marrow involvement at presentation mimicking malignant lymphoma: cytogenetic analysis using multiple techniques. Cancer Genet Cytogenet 2001; 129: 64–68.

210. Stout AP, Murray MR. Hemangiopericytoma: A vascular tumor featuring Zimmermann's pericytes. Ann Surg 1942; 116: 26–33.

211. Zimmerman KW. Der feinere bau der blutcapillaren. Z Anat Entwicklungsgesch 1923; 68: 29–109.

212. Compagno J, Hyams VJ. Hemangiopericytoma-like intranasal tumors: a clinicopathologic study of 23 cases. Am J Clin Pathol 1976; 66: 672–683.

213. Catalano PJ, Brandwein M, Shah DK, et al. Sinonasal hemangiopericytomas: a clinicopathological and immunohistochemical study of seven cases. Head and Neck Surg 1996; 18: 42–53.

214. Tse LLY, Chan JKC. Sinonasal haemangiopericytoma-like tumour: a sinonasal glomus tumour or a haemangiopericytoma? Histopathology 2002; 40: 510–517.

215. Chu PG, Chang KL, Wu AY, Weiss LM. Nasal glomus tumors: Report of two cases with emphasis on immunohistochemical features and differential diagnosis. Human Pathol 1999; 30: 1259–1261.

216. Cullen RD, Hanna EY. Intranasal glomangioma. Am J Otolaryngol 2000; 21: 402–404.

217. Hayes MM, Van der Westhuizen N, Holden GP. Aggressive glomus tumor of the nasal region. Report of a case with multiple local recurrences. Arch Pathol Lab Med 1993;117: 649–652.

218. Shek TW, Hui Y. Glomangiomyoma of the nasal cavity. Am J Otolaryngol 2001; 22: 282–285.

219. Kapadia SB, Meis JM, Frisman DM, et al. Adult rhabdomyoma of the head and neck: a clinicopathologic and immunophenotypic study. Hum Pathol 1993; 24: 608–617.

220. Kapadia SB, Meis JM, Frisman DM, et al. Fetal rhabdomyoma of the head and neck: a clinicopathologic and immunophenotypic study of 24 cases. Hum Pathol 1993; 24: 754–765.

221. Fu YS, Perzin KH. Non-epithelial tumors of the nasal cavity, paranasal sinuses and nasopharynx: a clinicopathologic study. V. Skeletal muscle tumors (rhabdomyoma and rhabdomyosarcoma). Cancer 1976; 37: 364–376.

222. Cessna MH, Zhou H, Perkins SL, et al. Are myogenin and myoD1 expression specific for rhabdomyosarcoma? A study of 150 cases, with emphasis on spindle cell mimics. Am J Surg Pathol 2001; 25: 1150–1157.

223. Furlong M, Mentzel T, Fanburg-Smith JC. Pleomorphic rhabdomyosarcoma in adults: a clinicopathologic study of 38 cases with emphasis on morphologic variants and recent skeletal muscle-specific markers. Mod Pathol 2001; 14: 595–603.

224. Daya H, Chan HS, Sirkin W, Forte V. Pediatric rhabdomyosarcoma of the head and neck: is there a place for surgical management? Arch Otolaryngol Head Neck Surg 2000; 126: 468–472.

225. Raney RB, Meza J, Anderson JR, et al. Treatment of children and adolescents with localized parameningeal sarcoma: experience of the Intergroup Rhabdomyosarcoma Study Group protocols IRS-II through -IV, 1978–1997. Med Pediatr Oncol 2002; 38: 22–32.

226. Fu YS, Perzin KH. Nonepithelial tumors of the nasal cavity, paranasal sinuses, and nasopharynx: a clinicopathologic study. IV. Smooth muscle tumors (leiomyoma, leiomyosarcoma) Cancer 1975; 35: 1300–1308.

227. Huang CT, Chien CY, Su CY, Chen WJ. Leiomyoma of the inferior turbinates. J Otolaryngol 2000; 29: 55–56.

228. Nicolai P, Redaelli de Zinis LO, Facchetti F, et al. Craniofacial resection for vascular leiomyoma of the nasal cavity. Am J Otolaryngol 1996; 17: 340–344.

229. Nall AV, Stringer SP, Baughman RA. Vascular leiomyoma of the superior turbinate: first reported case. Head Neck 1997; 19: 63–67.

230. Strasser M, Gleich L, Hakim S, Biddinger P. Pathologic quiz case 2. Nasal leiomyosarcoma, low grade. Arch Otolaryngol Head Neck Surg 1998; 124: 715–717.

231. Lippert BM, Godbersen GS, Luttges J, Werner JA. Leiomyosarcoma of the nasal cavity. Case report and literature review. ORL J Otorhinolaryngol Relat Spec 1996; 58: 115–120.

232. Kuruvilla A, Wenig BM, Humphrey DM, Heffner DK. Leiomyosarcoma of the sinonasal tract. A clinicopathologic study of nine cases. Arch Otolaryngol Head Neck Surg 1990; 116: 1278–1286.

233. Fu YS, Perzin KH. Non-epithelial tumors of the nasal cavity, paranasal sinuses and nasopharynx: a clinicopathologyic study. VIII. Adipose tissue tumors (lipoma and liposarcoma). Cancer 1977; 40: 1314–1317.

234. Takasaki K, Yano H, Hayashi T, Kobayashi T. Nasal lipoma. J Laryngol Otol 2000; 114: 218–220.

235. Hollis LJ, Bailey CM, Albert DM, Hosni A. Nasal lipomas presenting as part of a syndromic diagnosis. J Laryngol Otol 1996; 110: 269–271.

236. Mentzel T, Bainbridge TC, Katenkamp D. Solitary fibrous tumour: clinicopathological, immunohistochemical, and ultrastructural analysis of 12 cases arising in soft tissues, nasal cavity and nasopharynx, urinary bladder and prostate. Virchows Arch 1997; 430: 445–453.

237. Kohmura T, Nakashima T, Hasegawa Y, Matsuura H. Solitary fibrous tumor of the paranasal sinuses. Eur Arch Otorhinolaryngol 1999; 256: 233–236.

238. Gnepp DR, Henley J, Weiss S, Heffner D. Desmoid fibromatosis of the sinonasal tract and nasopharynx. A clinicopathologic study of 25 cases. Cancer 1996; 78: 2572–2579.

239. Kondo S, Yoshizaki T, Minato H, et al. Myofibrosarcoma of the nasal cavity and paranasal sinus. Histopathology 2001; 39: 216–217.

240. Perzin KH, Fu YS. Non-epithelial tumors of the nasal cavity, paranasal sinuses and nasopharynx: a clinicopathologic study. XI. Fibrous histiocytomas. Cancer 1980; 45: 2616–2626.

241. Basak S, Mutlu C, Erkus M, et al. Benign fibrous histiocytoma of the nasal septum. Rhinol 1998; 36: 133–135.

242. Barnes L, Kanhour A. Malignant fibrous histiocytoma of the head and neck. A report of 12 cases. Arch Otolaryngol Head Neck Surg 1988; 114: 1149–1156.

243. Iguchi Y, Takahashi H, Yao K, et al. Malignant fibrous histiocytoma of the nasal cavity and paranasal sinuses: review of the last 30 years. Acta Otolaryngol Suppl 2002; 547: 75–78.

244. Rodrigo JP, Fernandez JA, Suarez C, et al. Malignant fibrous histiocytoma of the nasal cavity and paranasal sinuses. Am J Rhinol 2000; 14: 427–431.

245. Fu YS, Perzin KH. Non-epithelial tumors of the nasal cavity, paranasal sinuses and nasopharynx: a clinicopathologic study. VII. Myxomas. Cancer 1977; 39: 195–203.

246. Hunchaisri N. Myxoma of the nasal cavity and paranasal sinuses: Report of a case. J Med Assoc Thai 2002; 85: 120–124.

247. Coffin CM, Watterson J, Priest JR, Dehner LP. Extrapulmonary inflammatory myofibroblastic tumor (inflammatory pseudotumor): A clinicopathologic and immunohistochemical study of 84 cases. Am J Surg Pathol 1995; 19: 859–872.

248. Som PM, Brandwein MS, Maldjian C, et al. Inflammatory pseudotumor of the maxillary sinus: CT and MR findings in six cases. AJR 1994; 163: 689–692.

249. Ruaux C, Noret P, Godey B. Inflammatory pseudotumor of the nasal cavity and sinuses. J Laryngol Otol 2001; 115: 563–566.

250. Olsen KD, DeSanto LW, Wold LE, Weiland LH. Tumefactive fibroinflammatory lesions of the head and neck. Laryngoscope 1986; 96: 940–944.

251. Meis JM, Enzinger FM. Inflammatory fibrosarcoma of the mesentery and retroperitoneum. A tumor closely simulating inflammatory pseudotumor. Am J Surg Pathol 1991; 15: 1146–1156.

252. Quraishi MS, Bessell EM, Clark D, et al. Non-Hodgkin's lymphoma of the sinonasal tract. Laryngoscope 2000; 110: 1489–1492.

253. Ko YH, Ree HJ, Kim WS, et al. Clinicopathologic and genotypic study of extranodal nasal-type natural killer/T-cell lymphoma and natural killer precursor lymphoma among Koreans. Cancer 2000; 89: 2106–2116.

254. Aviles A, Diaz NR, Neri N, et al. Angiocentric nasal T/natural killer cell lymphoma: a single centre study of prognostic factors in 108 patients Clin Lab Haematol 2000; 22: 215–220.

255. Lei KI, Suen JJ, Hui P, et al. Primary nasal and nasopharyngeal lymphomas: a comparative study of clinical presentation and treatment outcome. Clin Oncol (R Coll Radiol) 1999; 11: 379–387.

256. Yang Y, Gau JP, Chang SM, et al. Malignant lymphomas of sinonasal region, including cases of polymorphic reticulosis: a retrospective clinicopathologic analysis of 34 cases. Chung Hua I Hsueh Tsa Chih (Taipei) 1997; 60: 236–244.

257. Nakamura S, Katoh E, Koshikawa T, et al. Clinicopathologic study of nasal T/NK-cell lymphoma among the Japanese. Pathol Int 1997; 47: 38–53.

258. Harabuchi Y, Imai S, Wakashima J, et al. Nasal T-cell lymphoma causally associated with Epstein-Barr virus: clinicopathologic, phenotypic, and genotypic studies. Cancer 1996; 77: 2137–2149.

259. Davison SP, Habermann TM, Strickler JG, et al. Nasal and nasopharyngeal angiocentric T-cell lymphomas. Laryngoscope 1996; 106: 139–143.

260. Liang R, Todd D, Chan TK, et al. Treatment outcome and prognostic factors for primary nasal lymphoma. J Clin Oncol 1995; 13: 666–670.

261. Abbondanzo SL, Wenig BM. Non-Hodgkin's lymphoma of the sinonasal tract. A clinicopathologic and immunophenotypic study of 120 cases. Cancer 1995; 75: 1281–1291.

262. Arber DA, Weiss LM, Albujar PF, et al. Nasal lymphoma in Peru. High incidence of T-cell immunophenotype and Epstein-Barr virus infection. Am J Surg Pathol 1993; 17: 392–399.

263. Kojima M, Hosomura Y, Kurabayashi Y, et al. Malignant lymphomas of the nasal cavity and paranasal sinuses. A clinicopathologic and immunohistochemical study. Acta Pathol Jpn 1992; 42: 333–338.

264. Han JY, Seo EJ, Kwon HJ, et al. Nasal angiocentric lymphoma with hemophagocytic syndrome. Kor J Intern Med 1999; 14: 41–46.

265. Prades JM, Alaani A, Mosnier J, et al. Granulocytic sarcoma of the nasal cavity. Rhinology 2002; 40: 159–161.

266. Imrie KR, Kovacs MJ, Selby D, et al. Isolated chloroma: the effect of early antileukemic therapy. Ann Intern Med 1995; 123: 351–353.

267. Fu YS, Perzin KH. Non-epithelial tumors of the nasal cavity, paranasal sinuses and nasopharynx: a clinicopathologic study. IX. Plasmacytomas. Cancer 1978; 42: 2399–2406.

268. Strojan P, Soba E, Lamovec J, Munda A. Extramedullary plasmacytoma: clinical and histopathologic study. Int J Rad Oncol Biol Phys 5. 2002; 3: 692–701.

269. Galieni P, Cavo M, Pulsoni A, et al. Clinical outcome of extramedullary plasmacytoma. Haematologica 2000; 85: 47–51.

270. Kulkani A, Lakheeram D, Haller JO, Loh JO. Histiocytosis presenting as a nasal mass. Pediatr Radiol 2000; 30: 87–89.

271. Wenig BM, Abbondanzo SL, Childers EL, et al. Extranodal sinus histiocytosis with massive lymphadenopathy (Rosai-Dorfman disease) of the head and neck. Hum Pathol 1993; 24: 483–492.

272. Wenig BM, Heffner DK. Respiratory epithelial adenomatoid hamartomas of the sinonasal tract and nasopharynx: a clinicopathologic study of 31 cases. Ann Otol Rhinol Laryngol 1995; 104: 639–645.

273. Heffner DK, Hyams VJ. Teratocarcinosarcoma (malignant teratoma?) of the nasal cavity and paranasal sinuses. A clinicopathologic study of 20 cases. Cancer 1984; 53: 2140–2154.

274. Endo H, Hirose T, Kuwamura K, Sano T. Sinonasal teratocarcinosarcoma. Pathol International 2001; 51: 107–112.

275. Deveci MS, Deveci G. Blastomatous tumor with teratoid features of nasal cavity: Report of a case and review of the literature. Pathol International 2000; 50: 71–75.

276. Pai SA, Naresh KN, Masih K, et al. Teratocarcinosarcoma of the paranasal sinuses: A clinicopathologic and immunohistochemical study. Hum Pathol 1998; 29: 718–722.

277. Bernstein JM, Montgomery WW, Balogh K. Metastatic tumors to the maxilla, nose, and paranasal sinuses. Laryngoscope 1966; 76: 621–650.

278. Boles R, Cerny J. Head and neck metastasis from renal cell carcinoma. Mich Med 1971; 70: 616.

279. Menauer F, Issing WJ. Unusual metastasis of renal cell carcinoma. A case report with review of the literature. Laryngorhinootologie 1998; 77: 525–527.

280. Montoro Martinez V, Lopez Vilas M, Gurri Freixa M, et al. [Nasal sinus metastasis of renal carcinoma. A case report] Acta Otorrinolaringol Esp 1999; 50: 653–656.

281. Wanamaker JR, Kraus DH, Eliachar I, Lavertu P. Manifestations of metastatic breast carcinoma to the head and neck. Head Neck 1993; 15: 257–262.

282. Har-El G, Avidor I, Weisbord A, Sidi J. Carcinoma of the prostate metastatic to the maxillary antrum. Head Neck Surg 1987; 10: 55–58.

283. Mota AV, Correira O, Resende C, et al. Nasal tip metastasis revealing a Pancoast tumor. Br J Dermatol 1998; 138: 559–560.

284. Yamasoba T, Kikuchi S, Sugasawa M, et al. Occult follicular carcinoma metastasizing to the sinonasal tract. ORL J Otorhinolaryngol Relat Spec 1994; 56: 239–243.

285. Itin PH, Heitzmann F, Stamm B. Metastasis to the nasal tip from a cervical carcinoma. Dermatology 1999; 199: 171–173.

286. Robiony M, Polini F, Costa F, Politi M. Disfiguring nasal metastasis from colorectal adenocarcinoma: a case report. Otolaryngol Head Neck Surg 2001; 125: 103–104.

287. Tariq M, Gluckman P, Thebe P. Metastatic testicular teratoma of the nasal cavity: a rare cause of severe intractable epistaxis. J Laryngol Otol 1998; 112: 1078–1081.

Larynx and trachea

William J. Frable

16

SPECIMEN HANDLING

Endoscopy is required in establishing a diagnosis of laryngeal and tracheal disease in the presence of a mass lesion. Biopsies are taken within a confined space and they are often small. Precise clinical information is required, including location and orientation, so that biopsies are cut perpendicular to the mucosal surface. Affixing small biopsy specimens to a support material and using a hand lens at the time of embedding will result in the correct orientation. Biopsy specimens should be fixed in 10% neutral buffered formalin, a suitable fixative for immunohistochemistry, and cut at a minimum of three initial levels with a ribbon of five or six sections on each slide. Children with recurrent respiratory tract infections may have tracheal mucosa submitted for study of ciliary dyskincsia. Improved visualization has been demonstrated by fixation in glutaraldehyde supplemented with tannic acid.[1]

Total or partial laryngectomy with or without radical or modified radical neck dissection is the most common major specimen received. Specimens for frozen section examination are submitted from these cases for the determination of tumor-free margins. Surgeons should avoid submitting margins for frozen section examination separately. It is preferable to complete the resection and then to allow the surgical pathologist to view the entire gross specimen for correct orientation and selection of critical margins.[2] Sections should be perpendicular to the nearest point of gross tumor involvement, including the deepest tumor penetration. The tumor-free margin should be marked with ink before freezing to afford the proper orientation in reviewing the subsequently prepared slides. A fast hematoxylin and eosin stain is required for a detailed assessment of the margins. A diagnosis of dysplasia or carcinoma in situ (CIS) should not be attempted, only a report of invasive carcinoma, if present. A gross margin of less than 5 mm is probably inadequate. There is no convincing evidence in the literature documenting the efficacy of frozen section review of margins in the subsequent management or outcome of the patients with carcinoma of the larynx. It is certainly not cost effective.[2] A well-planned surgical attack with a grossly adequate margin is a more practical approach.

A radical neck dissection specimen is best examined in the fresh state while the larynx is processed after fixation. Lymph nodes are easier to discriminate from fat and connective tissue within fresh tissue. Dissected nodes should be bisected in the long axis to allow penetration of fixative. Consistency is the most important part of labeling lymph nodes from radical neck dissections. One option is a numeric system referring to levels. The submaxillary salivary gland and accompanying nodes are labeled level I. Nodes from the jugular chain are divided into three equal portions from the superior to the inferior. Nodes from the upper portion are labeled level II, those from the middle part level III, and those from the lower segment level IV. (The tip of the parotid salivary gland may be included in level II.)

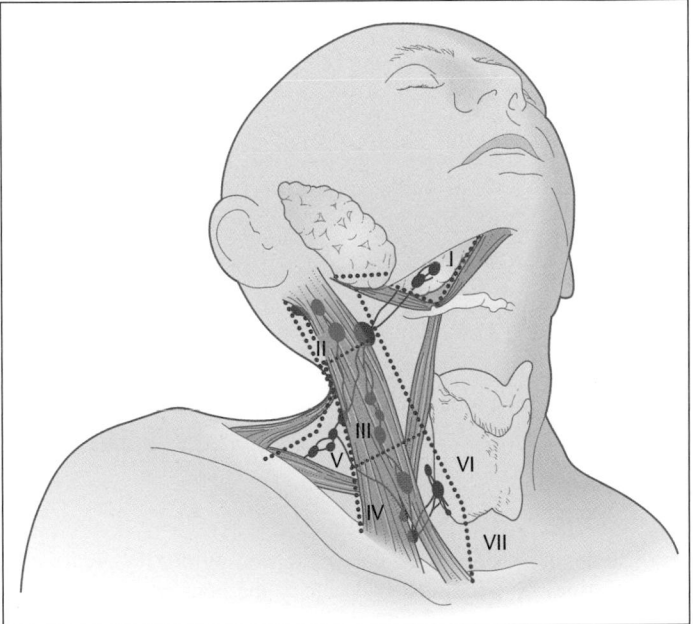

Fig. 16.1 Lymph node levels from a radical neck dissection.

Nodes from the posterior cervical chain are level V. Juxathyroid nodes, if they are part of the neck dissection, are labeled level VI, and paratracheal, paraesophageal, and superior mediastinal nodes are labeled level VII (Fig. 16.1). If lymph nodes are grossly positive within any of the levels, only two nodes from that level need to be submitted. All questionable and grossly negative nodes should be submitted from all other levels. A listing of the positive and negative nodes is incorporated into synoptic reporting formats.[3]

A laryngectomy specimen received for a diagnosis of tumor is opened posteriorly, spread with wooden applicator sticks, and then fixed in formalin. It is usually necessary to crack the thyroid cartilage to open the specimen sufficiently for good fixation. A diagram of the open larynx is useful to mark the lesion or lesions present and to indicate where sections are taken (Fig. 16.2). These diagrams can also be embedded in synoptic reporting formats.[3] Standard sections for a carcinoma of the larynx would include (1) two to four sections of the primary tumor demonstrating its depth as well as its superior and inferior margins (these sections should be taken to include some normal mucosa); (2) one section each of the right and left vocal cords (a portion not involved by tumor); (3) one section of the epiglottis; (4) one section of each thyroid lobe; (5) one section of any parathyroid discovered; and (6) sections of the tracheal margins and superior margins, particularly the area at the base of the tongue or wherever

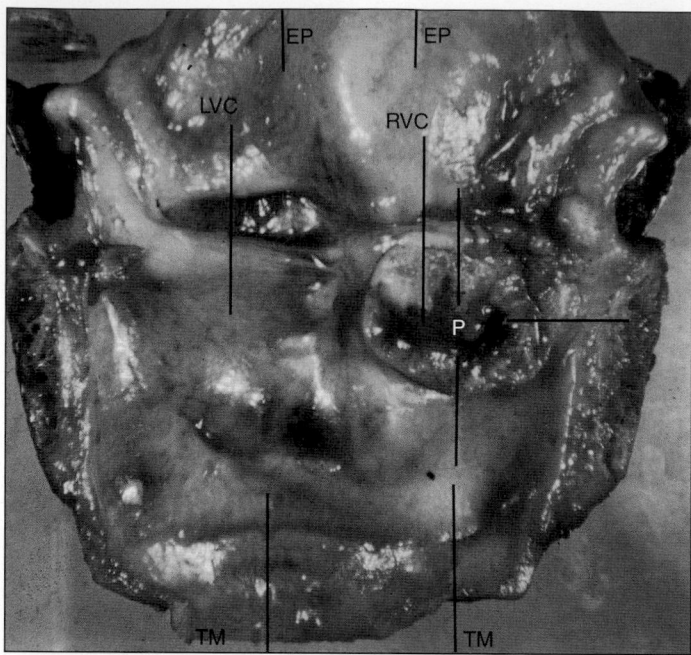

Fig. 16.2 Standard sections that should be submitted from a typical laryngectomy specimen for squamous cell carcinoma of the right true vocal cord with subglottic extension. P, primary tumor; RVC, right vocal cord; LVC, left vocal cord; EP, epiglottis; TM, tracheal margin. Sections from the thyroid and parathyroid, if present, should also be submitted.

gross tumor approximates the line of excision. With a deeply invasive lesion, it may be necessary to decalcify the bony and cartilaginous portions of the larynx to document invasion or complete penetration. A recommended synoptic format for reporting neoplasms of the larynx is found at the end of this chapter (Appendix 16.1).[3]

Vertical hemilaryngectomy specimens may be submitted as treatment of some glottic carcinomas. Supraglottic partial laryngectomy specimens may be submitted if the tumor arises in the pyriform sinus or the supraglottic region. Because tumors in these locations tend to spread to lymph nodes more quickly than tumors originating in the glottic region, they will often be submitted with a neck dissection. Hemilaryngectomy specimens should be assessed grossly before any attempt at frozen section control of margins. The relationship between the tumor and its margins is easily destroyed in this type of specimen and compromises the final interpretation as to the completeness of the resection. Only the nearest gross margin to the tumor should be taken and then only if a definite therapeutic decision for more surgery is immediately required. This margin should be carefully marked with ink before sectioning so that it may subsequently be reoriented to the total specimen. If margins are grossly tumor free, it is preferable to fix the entire specimen. Sections are then taken stepwise and perpendicular to the vocal cord to examine the entire mucosa and submucosa.

EMBRYOLOGY, ANATOMY, AND HISTOLOGY

The beginning of the respiratory tract, the laryngotracheal groove, is found in the 20 somite (3 mm) embryo. This structure runs lengthwise in the floor of the gut just distal to the pharyngeal pouches. Its epithelium is endodermal in origin, and its supporting connective tissue, striated muscle, and cartilage are derived from mesoderm. All the cartilage and both the intrinsic and extrinsic muscles of the larynx arise from the mesenchyme of the fourth and fifth branchial arches. Because of this origin, the innervation of the muscles of the larynx is primarily through branches of the vagus nerve

The trachea elongates rapidly during early fetal development, descending nearly eight body segments. The endodermally derived columnar epithelium differentiates into a pseudostratified and a ciliated columnar epithelium throughout the trachea and larynx, excluding the aryepiglottic folds laterally and ventrally, the lingual side of the epiglottis and the upper half of its laryngeal aspect, the vocal folds (true vocal cords), and the superior points of the arytenoid cartilage. These mucosal surfaces are covered by a stratified squamous epithelium. There is a transitional zone of stratified columnar epithelium between adjacent areas of pseudostratified columnar and stratified squamous mucosa.

The seromucous glands found throughout the larynx and trachea are derived by invagination of the covering columnar epithelium. They are prominently displayed along the aryepiglottic and ventricular folds and within the lamina propria of the ventricle. These glands are usually confined to the submucosa, superficial to the lamina propria, but may penetrate the cartilaginous tissue of the epiglottis. Like their counterparts found throughout the oral cavity, they are referred to as aberrant salivary glands. They may give rise to salivary gland-type tumors, hence their importance to the surgical pathologist.

NON-NEOPLASTIC CONDITIONS

INFLAMMATORY AND DEGENERATIVE DISEASE

The surgical pathologist is seldom involved in the diagnosis of acute laryngitis and epiglottitis.[4] Tracheostomy and intubation are sometimes required to treat these conditions. Biopsy specimens of granulation tissue forming either at the site of the tracheostomy or in the subglottic area after intubation may be submitted to the surgical pathologist. Typically featured is a polypoid mass of capillary blood vessels, fibrin, and acute inflammatory cells (pseudotumor). Abundant and persistent granulation tissue can lead to laryngeal and tracheal stenosis.[5,6]

Physical agents, particularly thermal burns, produce acute inflammation of the larynx and trachea as part of a generalized effect on the respiratory tract. Secretions submitted for cytologic study from these cases can show severe atypia of regeneration and repair that may be mistaken for carcinoma.[7]

Cytologic evidence of *herpes virus* may also be found. This infection in the larynx and trachea seems to be incidental in the debilitated immunosuppressed patient who develops acute tracheobronchitis.[8] The clustering of cases in time, after admission to respiratory intensive care, ventilatory assistance, or endotracheal intubation, suggests a possible patient-to-patient transmission through the use of such equipment. Unsuspected herpetic tracheitis may also be noted in biopsies from patients undergoing tracheostomy after prolonged intubation.[9] An acute bacterial or viral tracheitis may occur in children. Epiglottitis, most prevalent in children 4 to 8 years of age, results in swelling of the epiglottis and supraglottic structures. Both of these diseases can present as medical emergencies.

Chronic laryngitis, whose etiology in the past has been attributed to overuse of the voice, is more commonly associated with continuous exposure to irritating fumes and dust, alcohol abuse, cigarette smoking, and gastro-esophageal reflux.[10] Histologically, a chronic

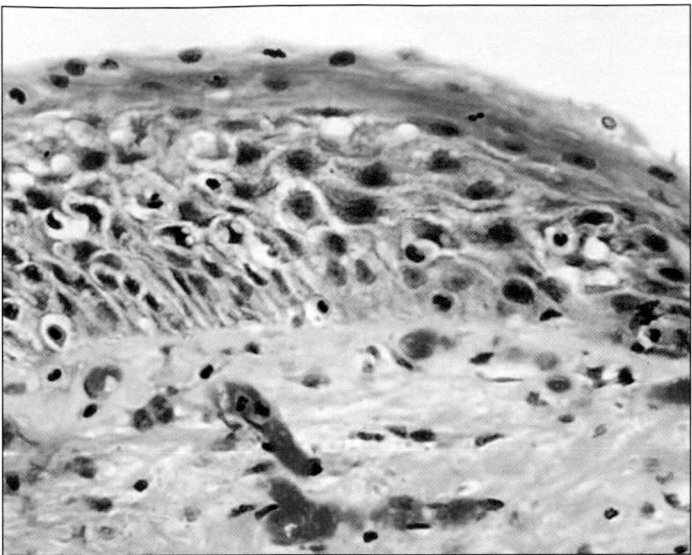

Fig. 16.3 Vocal cord biopsy specimen illustrating inflammatory atypia with active but uniform nuclei. The most prominent atypical feature of these cells is the large nucleoli. The chromatin is bland. Polarity of the cells is slightly disturbed. Compare with Figure 16.7A.

inflammatory exudate is seen. Of more importance are the epithelial alterations (hypertrophy, hyperkeratosis, and regeneration and repair atypia) that must be differentiated from carcinoma (Fig.16.3). The symptom of hoarseness and the clinical appearance of the vocal cords, with thickening and opacity of the epithelium, strongly suggest preneoplasia or early carcinoma.

Chronic laryngitis and tracheitis may also be *granulomatous*, indicating tuberculosis, sarcoidosis, leprosy, or a mycotic etiology.[11–13] Caseating granulomas strongly suggest tuberculosis, tuberculoid leprosy being quite rare in the larynx. Cases of both sarcoidosis and tuberculosis of the trachea are most often extensions from involved mediastinal lymph nodes.[11,12] The granulomas of sarcoid are very discrete, with little or no necrosis. Those of tuberculosis are less well formed, intermixed with lymphocytes, and often necrotic. Rhinoscleroma, which typically presents as a nasal granulomatous disease, may involve the larynx in at least 40% of cases. It may cause upper airway obstruction.[14,15] Blastomycosis of the larynx produces a marked pseudoepitheliomatous hyperplasia with both acute and chronic inflammation and intraepithelial abscesses. Both in the lower respiratory tract, where it is most common, and in the larynx, blastomycosis may grossly and histologically resemble carcinoma.[16] Histoplasmosis evolves as a granulomatous reaction, like tuberculosis. The latter may also present as an ulcerated lesion similar to carcinoma.[17] A vocal cord biopsy demonstrating organism of *Cryptococcus* from a patient with acquired immunodeficiency syndrome (AIDS) is illustrated in Figure 16.4. South American blastomycosis involving the larynx has been reported from Brazil.[18]

Of the saprophytic fungi, *Candida albicans (Monilia albicans)* is the most likely organism to involve mucosal surfaces of the larynx and trachea. Persistence of candidal infection may be a manifestation of immunosuppression, poorly controlled diabetes, or AIDS. If oral infection by *Candida* extends to the pharynx, trachea, and/or esophagus, investigation for human immunodeficiency virus (HIV) should be pursued.[19,20] Cases of actinomycosis and aspergillosis have been reported in an irradiated larynx.[21,22] Invasive aspergillosis

of the larynx has also been seen in AIDS and in a patient with severe aplastic anemia.[23,24]

In addition to specific granulomatous disease, other inflammatory and degenerative lesions in the larynx or trachea may form tumorous masses. Rheumatoid arthritis may result in fixation of the cricoarytenoid joint and the vocal cord by a typical rheumatoid nodule.[25] Gouty tophi of the vocal cord may produce a mass and hoarseness.[26] The larynx may also be involved in Wegener's granulomatosis. In two cases, biopsy of a subglottic mass revealed necrotizing granulomas with vasculitis and giant cells.[27] Relapsing polychondritis, a presumed autoimmune disease, affects cartilage in multiple organs including the larynx and trachea. Rarely, pathology may receive a biopsy of the larynx for diagnosis of this process.[28]

So-called amyloid tumors that result in a vocal cord nodule or polyp are not composed of true amyloid. However, the larynx and the trachea may be involved by the deposition of true amyloid.[11,29] In an unrecognized case of amyloidosis of the trachea, removal of the polypoid masses of amyloid led to a fatal tracheal hemorrhage.[30]

CYSTS

Cystic masses in the trachea and larynx may be divided into those that are true epithelium-lined structures and those that are herniations of the laryngeal ventricle, termed *laryngocele*. The latter are both internal (intrinsic to the larynx, presenting with dyspnea and hoarseness) and external (manifesting as a soft tissue mass in the neck). There are also combined forms. True cysts may be lined by either glandular, squamous epithelium or oncocytic epithelium, whereas the laryngocele is usually lined by glandular epithelium unless squamous metaplasia occurs. Those cysts arising in the adult result from duct obstruction and retention or from traumatic inclusion of epithelium. Similar cysts may arise in the newborn (congenital cysts) and cause acute airway obstruction.[31] True cysts of only the vocal cord may have a lining of mucus cells, ciliated cells, or squamous epithelium that is keratinized or nonkeratinized.[32]

PSEUDOTUMORS

The *laryngeal nodule*, or singer's node, is one of the most common lesions seen by the surgical pathologist. It is attributed to constant irritation of the vocal cord, usually by chronic misuse of the voice. Traditionally, four stages, fibrous, polypoid, varicose, and fibrinoid or amyloid-like, are described. All of them intermingle and overlap histologically. Initially, there is a fibrous thickening of the true vocal cord involving Reinke's layer. Thin-walled vessels exude increased amounts of fluid, producing a polypoid projection of the vocal cord with thinning of the overlying squamous mucosa. The vessels dilate, and there is focal hemorrhage. Organization of the hemorrhage evolves into the amyloid stage. This substance is not true amyloid, as demonstrated by either special stains or electron microscopy.[33] Several composite examples of vocal cord polyps are illustrated in Figure 16.5.

Masses composed of lymphoid tissue, *pseudolymphoma*, may arise in the upper respiratory tract.[34] These pseudotumors show lymphoid tissue with well-developed germinal centers. The presence of this exuberant lymphoid proliferation in an adult has been cause for concern, as true malignant lymphomas do occur in the larynx and upper respiratory tract. The pseudolymphoma contains a mixture of plasma cells and lymphocytes. Reaction of the overlying squamous epithelium also occurs, producing both acanthosis and hyperkeratosis. These epithelial reactions extend into the crypts,

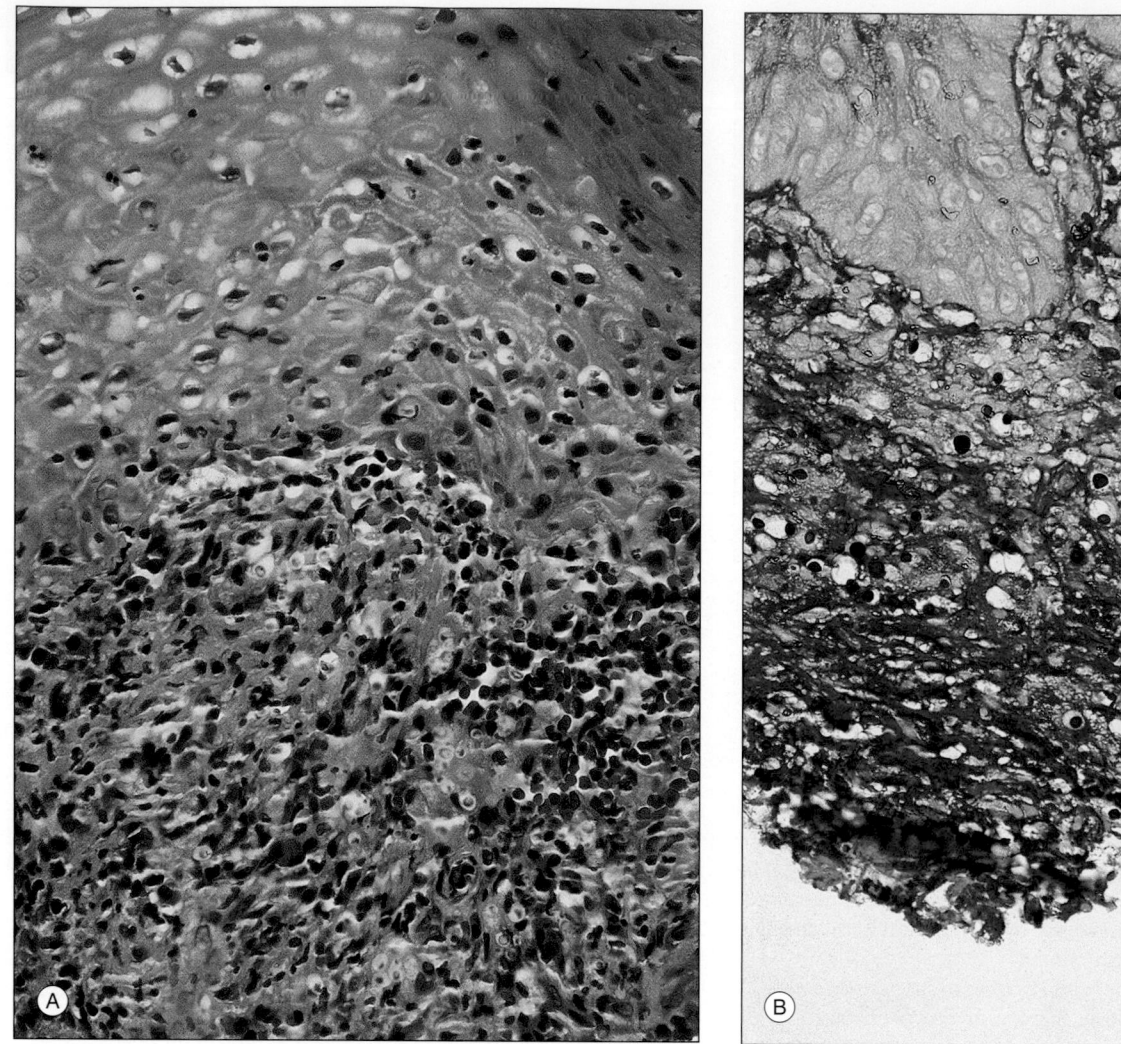

Fig. 16.4 A, Vocal cord biopsy with intense inflammation around small round organism with a thick clear capsule (H&E stain); **B,** Periodic acid–Schiff (PAS)-light green stain confirms the presence of yeast-like organisms with the morphology of *Cryptococcus*.

giving the appearance of misplaced or greatly hypertrophied tonsillar tissue. Problem cases may be resolved by immunohistochemical staining to determine monoclonality or molecular diagnostic methods to find gene rearrangements in the lymphoid infiltrate.

Granulation tissue forming a polypoid mass (pseudotumor) has been previously mentioned as a result of prolonged intubation and incorrect use of endotracheal tubes. The adjacent epithelium, usually squamous or squamous metaplastic, may be quite atypical, mimicking a true dysplasia of the vocal cords.[35]

NEOPLASMS

BENIGN EPITHELIAL NEOPLASMS: SQUAMOUS PAPILLOMA

Squamous papilloma is the most common and important entity among the benign neoplasms of the larynx and trachea. It is an easily recognized proliferation of squamous epithelium of the Malpighian layer overlying a thin, fibrovascular connective tissue stalk. Squamous papillomas comprise approximately one-sixth of

the tumors of the larynx and about one-eighth of the neoplasms of the trachea.[36] There are two clinical forms, juvenile and adult. In children, the tumors are frequently multiple, whereas in adults, they usually are single. Clinical and molecular marker observations indicate that both adult- and juvenile-onset papillomas result from exposure to the human papillomavirus.[37]

Abramson et al. tested 26 patients with laryngeal papillomas for HPV DNA by Southern blot hybridization and found it to be present in all 26. In 11 of 14 cases, latent HPV DNA was also detected in clinically uninvolved tissue. Type 6 or type 11 HPV accounted for 92% of the cases examined. The authors also reported no correlation with histopathology, age of onset, or the clinical pattern of recurrence and remission. They did not find any specific histopathology or clinical features with respect to the type of HPV infection. Transmissibility has been proven experimentally for the juvenile form. Despite a history of maternal genital infection documented in the series of Abramson and associates, it is curious that HPV type 6 is more common in genital papillomas than HPV-11, which is more common in the larynx papillomas.[38]

Malignant transformation, except for the juvenile form treated by irradiation, has been rare.[39,40] Recent studies demonstrate several

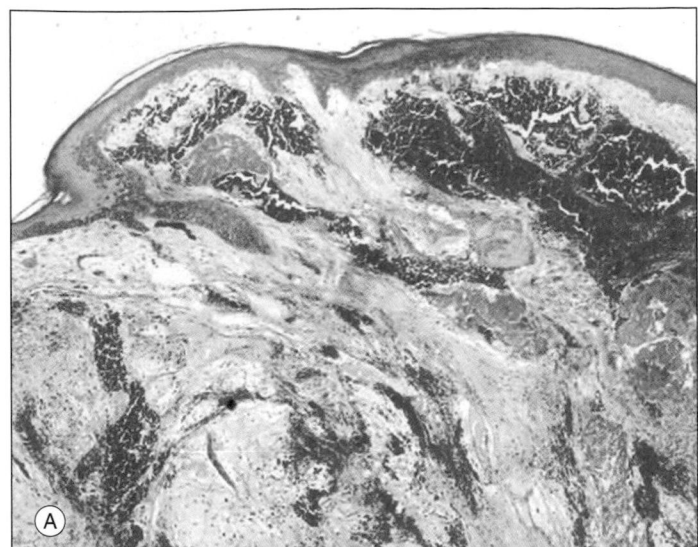

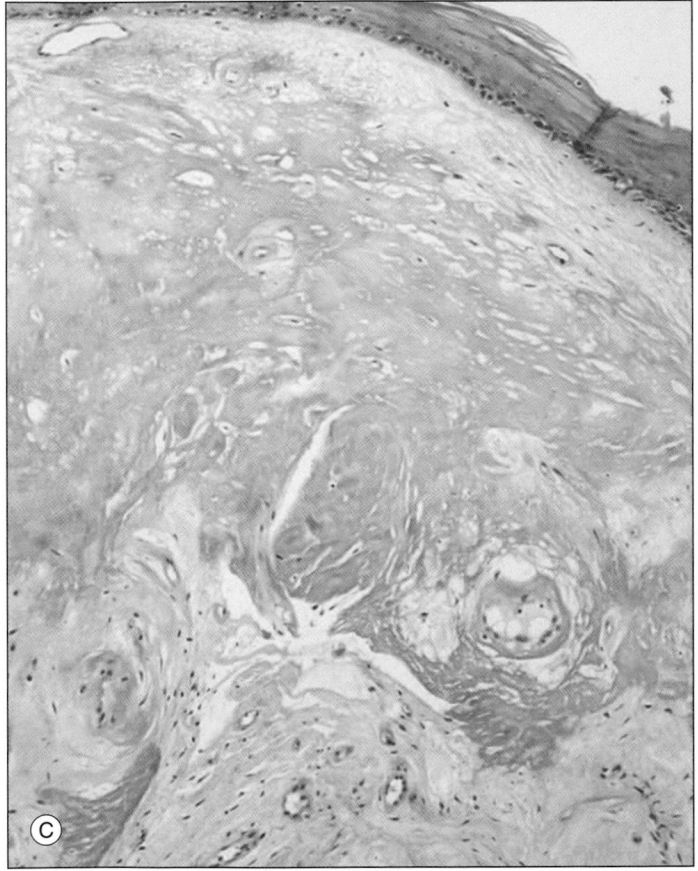

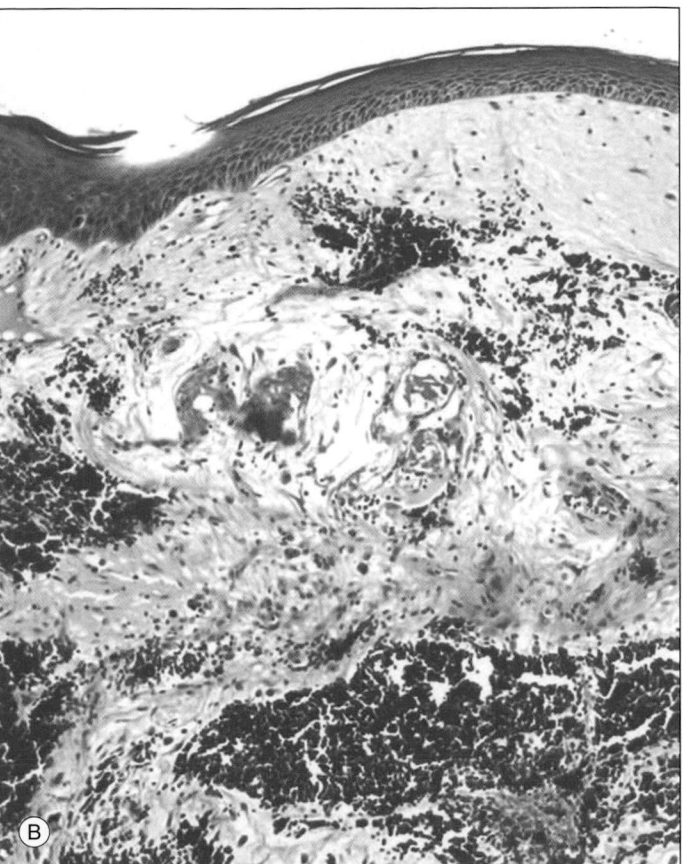

Fig. 16.5 Vocal cord polyp. **A**, Overall configuration is polypoid, with fibrous and myxoid stroma and dilated capillary vessels beneath the squamous epithelium; **B**, Detail of a polyp with many small vessels and amyloid-like stroma. There is some thickening of the squamous epithelium; **C**, Another example of a polyp with largely 'amyloid-like' stroma.

molecular transcription factors, epidermal growth factor receptor (EGFR), mitogen-activated protein kinase (MAPK), and C/EBP that are elevated in HPV-infected laryngeal papillomas.[41,42] It has been determined in one study that an overexpression of p53 occurred with increasing grades of epithelial abnormality in respiratory papillomas. Cytoplasmic staining for c-erb-2 also become more prominent with increasing epithelial dysplasia in papillomas.[43] Malignant transformation of recurrent respiratory papillomas has been documented with integration of HPV type 11 DNA and mutation of p53.[44] Coinfection

of HPV-11 and HPV-16 was found in a single case of laryngeal squamous papillomas with severe dysplasia.[45]

Recurrence of papillomas after local treatment is quite frequent and may occur rapidly in children (Fig. 16.6).[46] Adult onset of laryngeal papillomas has been linked to poor antibody response to the virus.[47] Although malignant transformation in the juvenile form has been documented in nonirradiated cases, the real threat is the spread of the process throughout the larynx and trachea, multiple recurrences, and sudden asphyxia. The localized form, if it involves the anterior segments of the vocal cords or the anterior commissure, tends to have a good prognosis, with fewer recurrences.[46]

Laryngeal papillomas are characterized by hyperplasia of the spinous epithelial layer and abnormal differentiation. The growth of the epithelial cells is regulated in part through the binding of epidermal growth factor (EGF) to the EGF receptors. If EGF is removed from in vitro cultures of papilloma cells, normal stratification and differentiation occur as determined by the synthesis of keratin.[48]

Malignant degeneration, the most serious complication of papilloma, is heralded by proliferation of dysplastic and frankly anaplastic cells. There is also hyperkeratosis and individual cell dyskaryosis with the presence of mitotic figures, some of which may be atypical. With prolonged lesions, malignant change becomes more common, being reported in up to 20% of adult cases. An example of squamous papilloma with areas of dysplasia is illustrated in

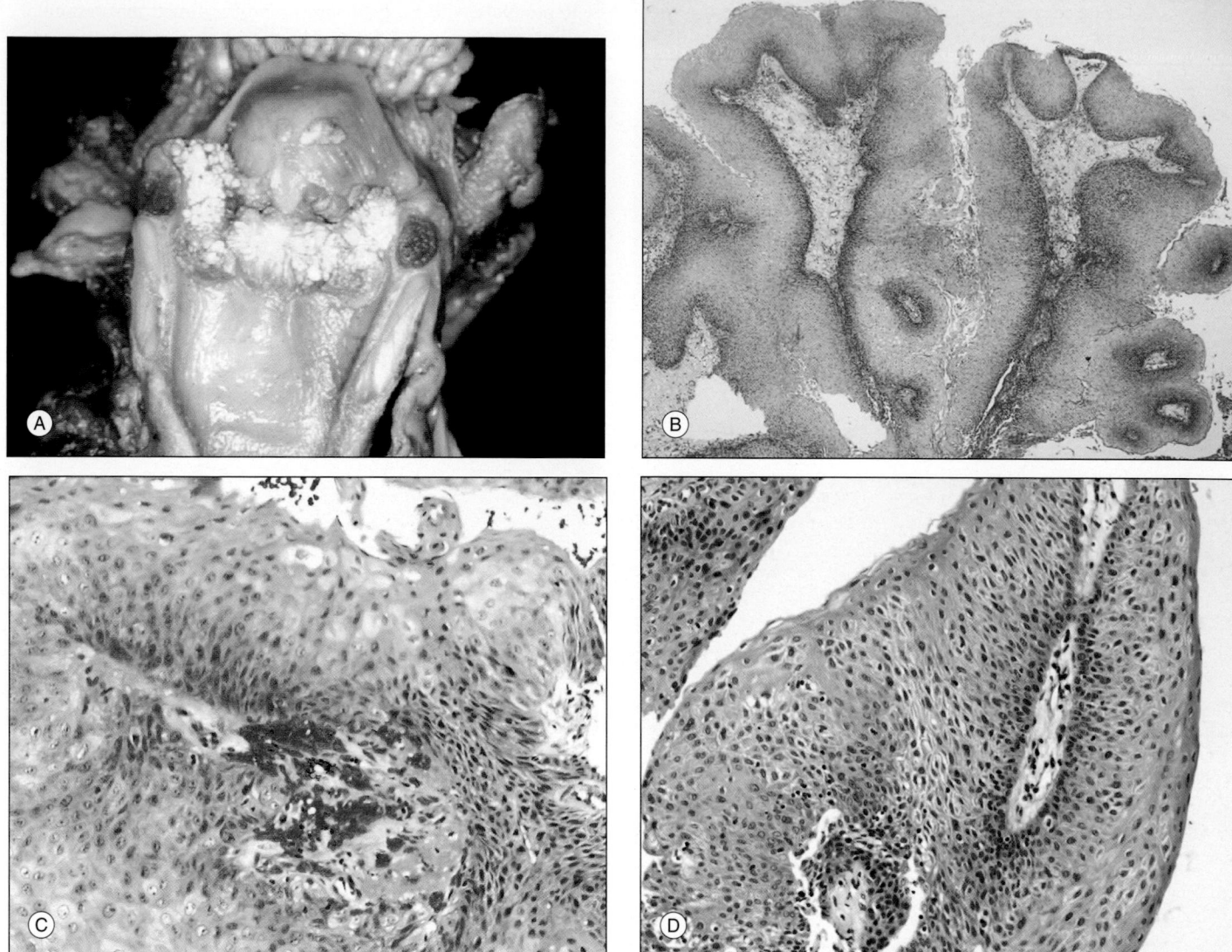

Fig. 16.6 A, Gross larynx from a child who expired from multiple papillomas throughout the respiratory tract. Multiple attempts to destroy them were eventually unsuccessful; **B**, Papillary configuration is obvious microscopically; Higher magnification (**C**) demonstrates areas of koilocytotic change within the papilloma; **D**, Fragment of papilloma with areas of mild epithelial dysplasia. Extent and degree of dysplasia when present in squamous papillomas from adults can be difficult to interpret because of orientation and the fragmented nature of the biopsies.

Figure 16.6C. As in any papillary neoplasm, invasion is difficult to evaluate unless a biopsy is performed at the base of the stalk, along with the complete removal of the tumor itself.[49]

The varieties of therapy, which include laser, electrodesiccation, cryotherapy, and continued re-excisions, confirm the difficulty of treatment. The objective is removal of tumor without destruction of the larynx and trachea. The use of radiotherapy has been condemned because of a documented increase in malignant transformation, particularly with juvenile papillomatosis.[46]

HYPERPLASIAS, PRECANCEROUS LESIONS, CARCINOMA IN SITU

The larynx is unique in that very minimal alterations of the vocal cords will produce voice changes. Therefore, the surgical pathol-ogist is likely to see biopsies with a variety of hyperplastic and preneoplastic epithelial alterations unless the patient totally ignores the symptom of hoarseness. A current classification groups laryngeal epithelial hyperplastic lesions as follows: (1) simple, (2) abnormal, (3) atypical (risky epithelium), and (4) carcinoma in situ. Both simple and abnormal are considered benign categories.[50] The risk of malignant transformation over a period of 2–12 years was 0.3% for simple and abnormal hyperplasia and 11.6% for atypical hyperplasia.[51] In the past these changes have been referred to as keratosis.

Crissman prefers the term dysplasia to indicate some precancerous potential. He divides these lesions into three grades with increasing keratin formation: acanthosis, pseudoepitheliomatous hyperplasia, and individual cellular atypia.[52] Hyperplasia combined with keratosis shows thickening of the squamous epithelium and surface keratinization, which may be orthokeratotic or parakeratotic. There is subjectivity in evaluating the degree of cellular atypia in any dysplastic (keratosis with atypia) epithelium, but these biopsies are the most important to assess. There is usually thickening of the epithelium, but not invariably. There is cellular alteration, initially confined to the base of the epithelium. Later, with increasing individual cell atypia, more layers of the epithelium are involved. Individual cells and nuclei are irregular in shape and size, and nuclei have a granular irregular chromatin distribution. Accompanying nuclear abnormalities, there is a loss of polarity of the individual cells within the epithelium. In summary, there is a variable irregularity with respect both to individual cells and to cells in relation to each other. Several comparative examples are found in Figure 16.7. These examples may be regarded as dysplastic reactions of mild, moderate, and severe degree. The term *laryngeal intraepithelial neoplasia* has also been proposed and generally accepted for this spectrum of precancerous change.[53,54] In a systematic review of a number of classification schemes for abnormal laryngeal epithelium applied to a series of biopsies with good clinical follow-up, Blackwell et al. found that there were five significantly different parameters when lesions that progressed to carcinoma were compared to those that did not: (1) abnormal mitotic figures, (2) mitotic activity, (3) stromal inflammation, (4) maturation level, and (5) nuclear pleomorphism.[55] Computer analysis of nuclear texture features has also been found to separate with reasonably accuracy benign laryngeal epithelial lesions from dysplastic and malignant lesions.[56]

Recent studies have also focused on molecular markers to reduce the subjectivity of interpretation of atypical versus truly dysplastic laryngeal epithelium and to provide information on potential progression to carcinoma. As discussed previously, these studies have also included investigation into the role of HPV infection and viral integration. Severe dysplasia overlaps with CIS of the larynx. A full-thickness involvement of intraepithelial neoplasia is seldom seen in laryngeal mucosa, unlike classic CIS of the cervix. There is almost always surface keratinization or parakeratosis. Morphological judgment must be made as to the malignant potential of the epithelium without a full-thickness epithelial alteration (Figs 16.8 and 16.9).

During the last decade the role of HPV infection in head and neck carcinoma and precancerous lesions has also been extensively studied. Sugar et al. noted in a 1996 review that HPV had been detected in carcinoma, juvenile and adult multiple and single papillomas of the larynx. Both juvenile- and adult-onset respiratory papillomatosis have HPV types 6 and 11 DNA while types 16, 18, and 33 can be found in squamous carcinoma, including the verrucous type. It was also found that p53 oncoprotein abnormalities were related to smoking-induced cancers and not HPV. The authors concluded that evidence unequivocally linking HPV infection to laryngeal squamous cell carcinoma was still lacking.[57]

However, in a follow-up study, it was found, using immuno-histochemistry, mutations, and overexpression of p53 not only in squamous cell carcinoma of the larynx but also in some keratoses and papillomas.[58] Specifically, the E7 gene of HPV-16 has been demonstrated to be immortalized in in vitro primary human laryngeal epithelial cells and that p53 gene mutations occur during this immortalization process.[59] Several additional studies have confirmed this reciprocal relationship of HPV infection and p53 overexpression.[60,61]

A sudy of 88 cases of laryngeal lesions including the spectrum of simple hyperplasia to invasive squamous cell carcinoma detected HPV infection by polymerase chain reaction (PCR) in only two cases, simple hyperplasia with HPV-6 and HPV-16 in a case of invasive squamous cell carcinoma.[62] Moore et al., studying HPV types with the E6 consensus primers, hybrid capture assays for high-

and low-risk viral types, and dot blot hybridization of generic E6 PCR products with E6 type specific probes found that respiratory papillomas may have either high- or low-risk papilloma types and that the presence of high-risk HPV types increases the long-term risk of squamous cell carcinoma.[63] Several subsequent reports detected HPV using PCR in 20% of squamous cell carcinomas of the larynx and in 14% of adjacent normal mucosa in the same group of patients;[64] by in situ hybridization (ISH) in 42% of larynx carcinoma with higher rates for HPV-16 and -18 than for HPV type 6;[65] and in 8% of 39 squamous cell carcinomas of the larynx by PCR with consensus primers (CP, My 09/11 and Gp 5+/6+) followed by both PCR and ISH of the positive cases for HPV-6, 11, 16, 18, 31, 33 or 35.[66] Using immunoperoxidase (IP) and ISH, Caruso et al. found viral related sequences to types 16 and 18 only in squamous cell carcinoma of the larynx but not in dysplastic lesions (ten cases of dysplasia examined).[60]

In 1998, McKaig et al. conducted a further review of the published literature to determine the prevalence of HPV in benign, precancerous, and neoplastic lesions of the oral cavity, pharynx, and larynx. The reported positivity for benign and precancerous lesions ranged from 18.5% to 35.9% dependent upon the detection method. Based upon the most sensitive technique, PCR, the prevalence of HPV in head and neck cancers was 34.5%. The majority of the positive cases were high-risk types, type 16 (40%) and type 18 (12%). In the larynx 33% of the cases were positive, the lowest percentage for the major head and neck sites. Important factors for the association of HPV and squamous cell carcinoma of the larynx were age <60 and male sex.[67] Cell lines from carcinoma have also been studied to detect HPV. Atula et al. used Southern blot hybridization (SBH) on 27 cell lines from 22 patients with squamous cell carcinoma of the larynx and ISH on 12 original tumor sections to detect HPV. The authors also investigated these cases by PCR using three sets of consensus primers to L1 and E1 open reading frames. All cases tested negatively except the adjacent normal epithelium in one biopsy. The study was then extended to a total of 27 carcinoma cell lines from the larynx including 18 of the original cases. A nested PCR method was used to achieve maximum sensitivity. Subsequent SBH was performed to confirm the specificity of the PCR products for both low- and high-risk HPV types with oligonucleotide probe mixtures and with HPV-16 oligorobe. Seven of 27 cell lines (26%) were positive. Seven of the 12 tumor samples (58%) were also positive for high-risk HPV types. The authors concluded that HPV copy numbers are low and that only a minority of tumors harbor HPV.[68]

Variation in detection techniques and attention to contamination of specimens may impact the results for finding HPV in larynx and head and neck carcinomas. Lindberg and Krogdahl conducted a study of cases of carcinoma of the larynx without a pre-existing laryngeal papillomas or papillomatosis. They placed particular attention on sectioning tissue blocks of the tumors and in DNA extraction methods to avoid contamination. With PCR using three consensus primers, MY9MY11, GP5+/GP6+ and CPI/CPII, they found HPV in only one of 30 cancers. The HPV type was not determinable.[69] These results conflict with others. Azzimonti et al. used PCR for capsid protein expression by ISH with a polyclonal antibody directed against the L1 protein. 56% of 50 cases of precancerous lesions of the larynx were positive. Multiple infections of two or three types were found in 17 of the 28 positive cases. Eleven cases of keratosis with no dysplasia were also positive for HPV DNA. The authors noted that fully productive HPV infection is strictly dependent on epithelial differentiation and surface keratinization. They postulated that HPV is a cofactor in the malignant progression of these lesions as three of four patients who developed carcinoma

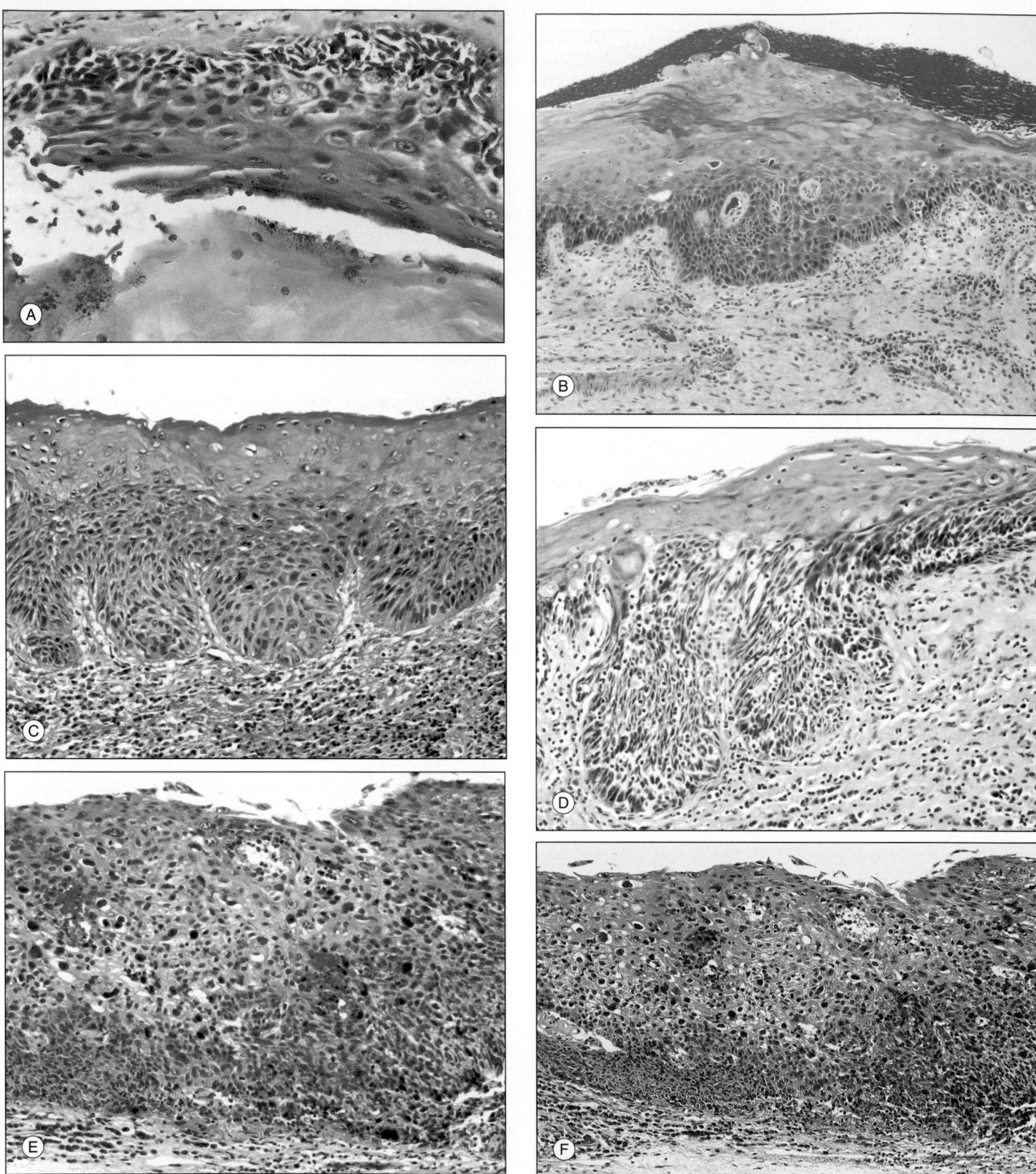

Fig. 16.7 Composite photomicrograph of vocal cord biopsy specimens demonstrating dysplasia. **A,** Mild dysplasia with thin but hyperkeratotic epithelium. Atypical cells occupy the lower one-third of the epithelium, are hyperchromatic, very in size and shape, and have some altered polarity; **B,** Mild dysplasia with thickening and hyperkeratosis of the epithelium. There is minimal nuclear atypia, some individual cell keratinization, and slight alteration of polarity; **C,** Moderate dysplasia with hyperkeratotic and parakeratotic epithelium. There is altered polarity and nuclei with hyperchromasia demonstrating some variability in size and shape. Downward growth suggests substantial biologic activity. Invasive carcinoma may occur without evolution through full-thickness neoplastic epithelium of classic carcinoma in situ; **D,** Moderate dysplasia and thickening of the epithelium with some parakeratosis. Atypical cells involve about one-half of the thickness of the epithelium. Note downgrowth of the dysplastic epithelium without full-thickness change. Biased cuts of the biopsy may isolate portions of the epithelium below the apparent mucosal surface suggesting invasive well-differentiated squamous cell carcinoma; **E,** Borderline lesion classified as severe dysplasia. Thick epithelium with marked individual cell atypia and altered polarity nearly reaching to the surface of the biopsy specimen; **F,** Severe dysplasia with thickening of the epithelium and substantial individual nuclear atypia in size, shape, and chromatin structure. Both epithelial lesions in panels E and F could be considered carcinoma in situ.

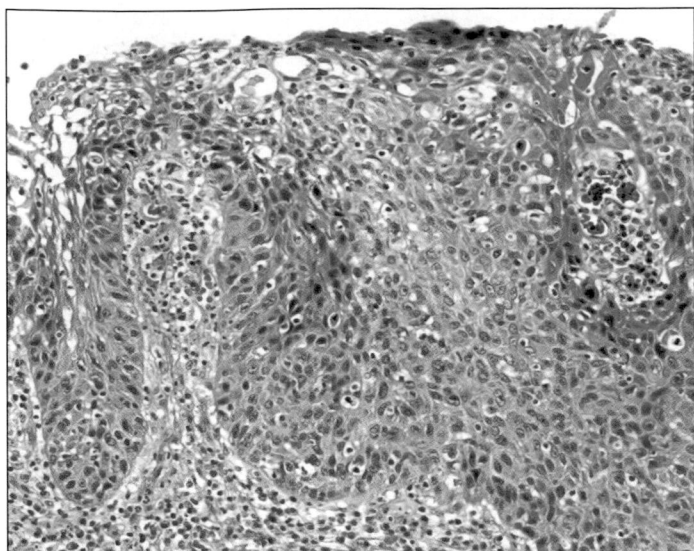

Fig. 16.8 Vocal cord biopsy specimen demonstrating carcinoma in situ (CIS) with full-thickness epithelial change. Marked individual cell atypia is present throughout the epithelium. Downgrowth of the abnormal epithelium suggests an evolution toward invasive squamous cell carcinoma.

found in HPV-16-positive tumors. The authors concluded that the pattern of expression was consistent with an active role of HPV in cellular transformation.[71] The most recent work of Jacob et al. focused on detection of p53, proliferating cell nuclear antigen (PCNA), and HPV in normal laryngeal tissues, papillomas and carcinomas. No HPV was found in normal tissue in their study but was present in 13 of 16 papillomas and 15 of 44 carcinomas. PCNA expression increased as the lesions progressed though an increasing histologic abnormality. HPV-positive tumors also showed increasing p53 accumulation. The authors concluded that changes in p53 and PCNA expression may be associated with HPV infection and could play a role in laryngeal carcinogenesis.[72]

Although excessive smoking and tobacco use have clearly been implicated as carcinogenic agents in the larynx and other head and neck sites, HPV infection seems to play a role as a cofactor in some laryngeal carcinomas and may be more obviously implicated in cases that follow upon papillomas and papillomatosis of the larynx and upper aerodigestive tract.

Regardless of the role of HPV in carcinogenesis of the larynx and head and neck, interpretative problems in high-grade dysplasias/carcinoma in situ are compounded by the projections of neoplastic epithelium, still connected to the surface, into the underlying stroma. Biased cuts will appear to isolate these neoplastic fragments, thereby leading to a false diagnosis of either microscopic or frankly invasive carcinoma. Surface keratinization may be present throughout the whole spectrum of dysplasia, CIS, and microinvasive carcinoma making a confident distinction between a well-differentiated, invasive squamous carcinoma and a severe dysplasia sometimes quite difficult. Clinical correlation with what the otolaryngologist actually visualized at laryngoscopy is very important in determining the interpretation of the biopsy for appropriate clinical management of the patient.

A large study has attempted to reduce the subjectivity of diagnosis of laryngeal squamous cell carcinoma and preneoplasia by using DNA cytophotometry. Results of DNA analysis agreed with histologic interpretation in all cases of definitively benign or

within fifty months were HPV DNA positive.[70] Venuti and colleagues focused on HPV viral integration in patients with carcinoma of the larynx. Of 25 patients, they found positive results for HPV-16, 6, and 45 in 52% of cases. There were no multiple infections in their series. Actual viral integration into the tumor cell genome was present in 43% of HPV-16-positive and 20% of HPV-6-positive cases. Viral RNA expression detected by reverse transcription PCR was only

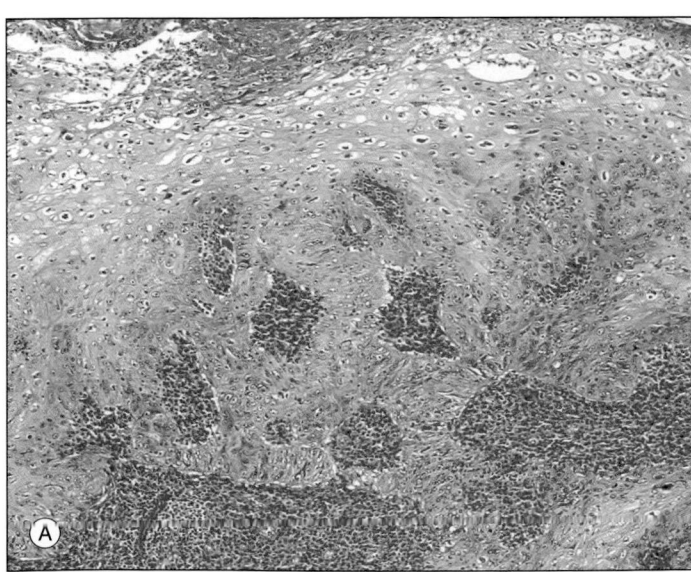
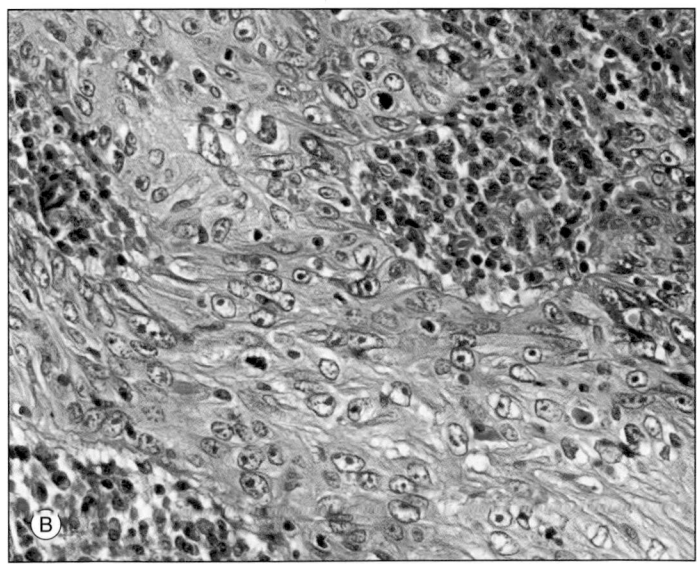

Fig. 16.9 Vocal cord biopsy illustrating carcinoma in situ without full-thickness neoplasia. **A,** Cells are spindle shaped with poorly defined cell boundaries in the lower one-third of the epithelium. There is a complex growth pattern that could represent early stromal invasion; **B,** Cells within the trabeculae at the base of the lesion have variations in size, shape, and polarity and definitively malignant nuclear features of very abnormal chromatin distribution within the nucleus and prominent nucleoli.

malignant lesions. DNA algorithms identified four cases within the group of mild-to-moderate epithelial dysplasias of the larynx that were proved to be malignant either at follow-up or from another biopsy site within the larynx. DNA measurements also divided the cases of squamous cell carcinoma into two distinct groups based on their survival.[73]

Regardless of the terminology or subjectivity of the diagnosis, the importance of CIS can be noted from studies in which the mucosa has been examined adjacent to frank invasive carcinoma. Bauer[74] in 354 cases found that 76% had CIS spreading widely from adjacent invasive carcinoma of the nonkeratinizing variety. Only 26% had CIS that was not far from the edges of a visible keratinizing carcinoma. Experience with cord stripping as reported by Miller and Fisher[75] also substantiates the importance of CIS. They reported 25 patients with CIS among whom the reappearance of carcinoma was invasive in 13 and in situ in 12. All these studies have implications for the treatment of stage I carcinomas of the larynx by hemilaryngectomy.

MALIGNANT EPITHELIAL TUMORS

Squamous cell carcinoma

Squamous cell carcinoma of the larynx is the most common malignant epithelial neoplasm of the upper respiratory tract with an estimated 8900 new cases for 2002 and with a male to female ratio of 3.4:1. The estimated deaths from larynx cancer in 2002 are 2900 males and 800 females. Primary squamous cell carcinoma of the trachea is quite rare.[76] Laryngeal squamous cancer is closely related to cigarette smoking and alcohol consumption.[54,77]

Cigarettes and alcohol together create a powerful carcinogenic effect throughout the respiratory tract, particularly on the larynx. Alcohol alone, at least in experimental studies in animals, does not appear to be a carcinogen[78] and is not linked to alcohol dehydrogenase genetic polymorphism.[79] However, the human OGG1 DNA repair enzyme showed a significantly increased risk for the hOGG1 326(Cys)/326(Cys) genotype in drinkers of alcohol, odds ratio 6:9. A similar risk was also present in cigarette smokers.[80] Experimentally, alcohol has been shown to be an important down regulator of the cell cycle inhibitor p21 leading to an increase in hyperphosphorylated pRb accelerating the cell cycle for G1 to S phase.[81]

Tobacco smoke is associated with N7-alkylguanine in the DNA of larynx tissue with levels found to be double in tumor cells of carcinoma of the larynx versus nontumor cells or in the patient's white blood cells.[82] Elevated levels of 4-aminobipheynyl-DNA adducts and p53 overexpression have also been found in larynx carcinoma in smokers versus nonsmokers or patients with laryngeal polyps.[83] Two environmental habitual pollutants, dibuylphthalate and diisobutylphthalate, also show elevated genotoxicity in cells from squamous cell carcinoma of the larynx and oropharynx,[84] but mutagen sensitivity, a risk factor for upper aerodigestive carcinoma, was found to be independent of smoking or alcohol intake.[85]

Clinical carcinoma of the larynx is *staged* by the TNM system of the American Joint Committee on Cancer (AJCC) Staging and End Results Reporting.[86] The endolarynx is divided into three regions to provide for appropriate treatment and prognosis: (1) the supraglottic compartment, which includes the arytenoids, epiglottis and its tip, aryepiglottic fold, ventricular bands (false vocal cords), and the mucosa of the ventricle; (2) the glottic compartment, which includes the true vocal cords and the anterior commissure; and (3) the subglottic compartment, which includes the area below the vocal cords to the level of the first tracheal cartilage. Squamous cell carcinomas are classified according to the region in which they arise. Changes in the latest version (6th edition) of AJCC Cancer Staging Handbook for carcinoma of the larynx divide T4 lesions into T4a (resectable) and T4b (unresectable) with the following division of Stage IV into Stage IVa, Stage IVb and Stage IVc.[86]

Studies of whole larynx sections demonstrate that laryngeal carcinomas do not respect arbitrary anatomic boundaries. Olofsson[87] determined that there are certain weak points through which carcinoma of the larynx will spread, depending on its point of origin. Glottic carcinomas tend to extend vertically but also invade intrinsic laryngeal muscles. The most common site of breakthrough is the thyroid cartilage in the anterior midline. This spread has been frequently found with extension through the cricothyroid membrane anteriorly. Supraglottic carcinomas invade both upward and laterally. Subglottic carcinomas tend to spread up into the thyroarytenoid muscle and also invade the laryngeal cartilages, particularly the cricoid and thyroid. Pre-epiglottic space invasion is quite common among the carcinomas arising on the epiglottis. This is uncommon if the supraglottic tumor begins on the ventricular bands without involvement of the epiglottic cartilage. In summary, clinical methods do not permit accurate assessment of deep invasion by larynx cancer and tend to underestimate it substantially.[77] Carcinoma of the trachea is even more lethal because it is relatively silent until clinically manifest at an advanced stage.

Squamous cell carcinoma is *graded* histologically into well-differentiated, moderately differentiated, and poorly differentiated tumors. Well-differentiated tumors contain orderly stratification and heavy keratinization and keratin pearls. Moderately differentiated tumors have prickle cells and some stratification with few or no keratin pearls. Poorly differentiated carcinomas are still recognizable as squamous but with nuclear pleomorphism, many and atypical mitoses.[88] If moderately and poorly differentiated tumors are lumped together, there are some clinical and biologic differences summarized in Table 16.1. The nonkeratinizing carcinoma has extensive intra-mucosal neoplasia and pushing margins rather than predominantly infiltrating margins as seen with keratinizing carcinoma.[87]

Prognostic pathology of squamous cell carcinoma of the larynx

Several pathologic features, in addition to site, are of prognostic importance in determining the outcome of squamous cell carcinoma of the larynx. Size and grading of squamous cell cancer of the larynx have correlated with presence of lymph node metastasis, clinical behavior, and prognosis.[77] Biopsy specimens tend to be undergraded. A sophisticated grading system, reporting on eight morphologic criteria, was developed by Jakobsson and later modified by Crissman.[89,90] Four elements represent the tumor cell population: structure, differentiation, nuclear polymorphism, and mitoses. Four elements represent tumor–host relationship: mode of invasion, stage of invasion, vascular invasion, and host cellular response. Infiltrative growth, strands, and cords versus pushing type tumor margins correlate best with the presence or absence of lymph node metastasis.[89] The status of tumor margins also influences recurrence rates, specifically a tumor-free distance of 5.0 mm versus 2.0 mm.[77] Table 16.2 indicates the major pathologic features currently of prognostic importance for carcinoma of the larynx.

DNA ploidy measurements by flow cytometry have been controversial in correlation with prognosis in laryngeal cancer. Review of studies of DNA content measured by image analysis and related to nuclear area (DNA index) have correlated with lymph node metastases, survival being best predicted by a 2c deviation index (mean square deviation from a diploid malignant tumor).[91] Results

Table 16.1 Comparison of keratinizing and nonkeratinizing carcinoma of the larynx

	Keratinizing	Nonkeratinizing
Age of patient	Same	Same
Percentage of females	4%	2%
Major site	Glottic-subglottic	Supraglottic
Gross appearance	Ulcerated, fungating, hyperkeratotic	Tumor mass with fissured mucosa, small ulcerated; may be papillary
Mucosal spread	Infrequent	Major mode of spread
Surface tumor margins	Sharply limited	Often poorly defined
Deep growth pattern	Infiltrating	About half with pushing margins
Carcinoma in situ	Less common at edge of tumor	Common and extensive

Table 16.2 Pathologic, clinical features, and prognosis of carcinoma of the larynx

Site	Glottic, supraglottic, subglottic, or transglottic
Size	Actually measured: use laryngography, CT, MRI
Extent	CT and or MRI
Tumor-free margins	Positive for tumor, 2.0 mm., 5.0 mm or greater free
Differentiation	Use of multifactorial histologic assessment
Tumor–host interface	Pushing versus infiltrating

of flow cytometry to measure proliferative activity (S-phase fraction of the cell cycle) have also been inconsistent and have not been associated with node metastases in one reported series.[91,92] Nakashima et al. reviewed cellular DNA content of human head and neck squamous tumors, finding that the DNA aneuploidy was higher among the poorly differentiated tumors. These investigators suggest that both chemosensitivity and DNA ploidy may aid in selecting effective antitumor drugs and in predicting cellular characteristics of the tumor during its course.[93] Studies of DNA in dysplastic laryngeal lesions also show mixtures of aneuploid and diploid histograms. It is believed that those biopsies demonstrating aneuploidy have undergone true malignant transformation.[94]

Over the past several years, studies of molecular and genetic markers have been reported to identify mechanisms of carcinogenesis in the larynx and relationships to prognosis. The results from a selected number of studies are summarized in Table 16.3. They support the concept of a multistep sequence in carcinogenesis but fail to identify a specific prognostic marker for any given tumor. In addition to those listed in Table 16.3, other markers that have been linked, at least by some investigators, to laryngeal carcinoma and precancerous changes include MUC2,[107] hormone related proteins ER-D5, EGFr and cathepsin D,[108,109] and downregulations of transforming growth factor beta type II.[110]

Stomal recurrence is one of the most serious complications of laryngeal carcinoma. It is associated with undetected subglottic extension after primary tumor excision and leads to uncontrolled disease, involving both local spread and a high incidence of distant metastasis.[111,112] In the patient treated by radiation the persistence of laryngeal edema beyond 3 months after completion of therapy is a poor prognostic sign. Edema makes biopsy difficult and tends to obscure persistent carcinoma.[113]

Larynx cancer is not infrequently associated with other primary carcinomas of the lung or head and neck. Approximately 11% of patients with carcinoma of the larynx will develop a second primary in these sites.[77]

Other carcinomas of surface epithelium

Other varieties of mucosal carcinoma, much less frequently seen, are verrucous squamous cell carcinoma, 'adenoid' squamous cell carcinoma, 'angiosarcoma-like' squamous cell carcinoma, basaloid squamous cell carcinoma, papillary squamous cell carcinoma, adenosquamous carcinoma, undifferentiated carcinoma (lymphoepithelioma), and neuroendocrine carcinoma. All these varieties of carcinoma are uncommon in the larynx, but can pose some problems in differential diagnosis. In the head and neck, neuroendocrine carcinoma and typical carcinoid tumors are essentially found only in the larynx.[77]

Neuroendocrine carcinoma

Terminology for this group of tumors has been controversial. Mills et al. suggest dividing them into carcinoids (typical morphology as found in other sites), moderately differentiated neuroendocrine carcinomas (replaces atypical carcinoid), and small cell neuroendocrine (undifferentiated) carcinomas. This terminology is favored, as the moderately and undifferentiated neuroendocrine carcinomas are both clinically aggressive neoplasms, are much more common in the larynx than typical carcinoids, and have a very strong association with a prominent history of cigarette smoking.[77] The neuroendocrine nature of these tumors is based on the presence of argyrophilic cytoplasmic granules and positive staining for a wide variety of neuroendocrine markers, neuron-specific enolase, chromogranin, synaptophysin, somatostatin, calcitonin, adrenocorticotropic hormone, gastrin, glucagon, and insulin, as summarized from the literature.[114] By ultrastructure, there are membrane-bound dense core neurosecretory granules in the tumor cells. Carcinoid syndrome has now been reported for one example of both a typical and an atypical carcinoid of the larynx. Other types of paraneoplastic syndromes have been documented for the small cell neuroendocrine carcinoma of the larynx.[114]

Small cell neuroendocrine carcinoma must be differentiated from malignant lymphoma, basaloid squamous cell carcinoma, and moderately differentiated neuroendocrine carcinoma of the larynx. Lymphoma is exceedingly rare. Histologically, it does not show conspicuous nuclear molding, extensive amounts of denatured DNA, or the necrosis found in typical small cell neuroendocrine carcinoma. CD45 (leukocyte common antigen) may be used to separate lymphomas from epithelial malignancies by immunohistochemistry. Basaloid squamous carcinomas have some foci of squamous differentiation and dysplasia in the overlying mucosa. This tumor lacks positive staining for chromogranin and synaptophysin but may stain for neuron-specific enolase. Moderately differentiated neuroendocrine carcinomas may have a pleomorphic pattern or spindle cell pattern that can be confusing. They have more neurosecretory granules than small cell neuroendocrine carcinoma, but stain for peptide hormones in only a fraction of the cases.[114]

Neuroendocrine carcinomas need to be differentiated from *primary paraganglioma* of the larynx, a rare tumor with a much better prognosis. Two pairs of paraganglia are located within the

Table 16.3 Molecular markers, chromosomes, and precancer and cancer of the larynx

Marker	Comment	Reference
p53	Increased in lesions preceding in situ or invasive squamous cell carcinoma.	94
	Not useful as a prognostic marker.	95
P21 ras	Not useful as a prognostic marker.	91
Proliferative cell nuclear antigen (PCNA)	Low levels expressed in dysplasia, papillomas and keratoses versus in situ and invasive carcinomas. Upregulated in early phases of carcinogenesis.	96
Retinoblastoma Rb	Progressive increase from benign lesions, keratoses and papillomas to carcinoma.	96
Ki-67 proliferation marker	Same as Rb, not predictive of clinical course, node metastases or survival.	91
Metallothionein (MT)	Same as p53 and PCNA.	97
Human telomerase catalytic subunit	Elevated twice as often in squamous cell carcinoma of larynx versus normal or hyperplastic squamous epithelium.	98
hTERT mRNA	No correlation with tumor size or node status.	
hTERT PCR TRAP assay	Levels of activity in squamous cell carcinoma of larynx correlate with stage of disease.	99
hTERT PRC TRAP assay	Levels of activity elevated in squamous cell carcinoma of the larynx, no differences in density related to tumor grade.	100
Matrix metallo-proteinase-2 (MMP-2)	Sequential increase in laryngeal epithelium beginning with atypical hyperplasia through invasive squamous cell carcinoma of the larynx. Not correlated with stage or histologic grade.	101
Stromyelysin-3 (ST-3)	Expression correlated with highly aggressive carcinomas of the larynx. Strongly expressed in squamous dysplasia that progressed rapidly to carcinoma.	102
Chromosomes 1, 7 polysomies and loss of heterozygosity	Aberrations in most cases of dysplasia and carcinoma in situ. None in normal epithelium adjacent to carcinoma or squamous epithelium from normal controls. Tetrasomy present in majority of dysplasias. Unstable chromosome content strongly predicted progression of dysplasia.	103
7, 17 polysomies	Linked to overexpression of epidermal growth factor receptor and p53 with progressive grades of hyperplastic lesions (Ljubljana classification).	104
Heterozygosity loss at 8p, 9p, 17q	Found in both benign and malignant lesions of the larynx. These chromosome arms harbor tumor suppressor genes p16 and BRCA1.	105
Loss of chromosomal material	9p21, 3p21, 17p13 (normal to dysplasia), 11q13, 13q21, 14q31 (dysplasia to carcinoma in situ), 4q26-28, 6p, 8p, 8q (in situ carcinoma to invasive carcinoma).	106

larynx, a laryngeal glomus at the upper and anterior one-third of the vestibular fold, and a second just above the division of the recurrent laryngeal nerve.[114] Twenty-four cases have been collected from the literature, only four of which were primary in the trachea.[115] These tumors are relatively benign but will bleed extensively on biopsy. Patients presented with marked spasmodic pain in the larynx, moving upward toward one ear, on swallowing. Paragangliomas were small lesions and occasionally quite difficult to see. Most of them are in the arytenoid region. They tended to recur, and cervical lymph node metastasis was a frequent feature, although taking many years to develop.[114] In a review of 78 reported cases of paraganglioma Barnes found that only 34 cases were acceptable, most of the remaining reported cases representing neuroendocrine carcinoma.[116]

Paragangliomas fail to demonstrate positive immunohistochemical staining for cytokeratin, EMA, CEA, calcitonin, and bombasin.[117] Primary small cell neuroendocrine carcinoma has been described as primary in the trachea in fewer than 20 cases.[118]

Small cell neuroendocrine carcinoma of the larynx is often rapidly fatal. In contrast to their more organoid appearance, approximately one-third of reported carcinoids of the larynx have produced distant metastasis. However, the patients have survived for long periods with distant disease.[77]

Neuroendocrine carcinomas are believed to originate from Kulchitsky cells or a common stem cell, with the ability for divergent differentiation into predominantly or exclusively a neuroendocrine type of tumor. Combination forms with differentiated squamous cell and adenocarcinoma have been reported.[114]

Verrucous carcinoma

Examples of verrucous carcinoma are illustrated in Figures 16.10 and 16.11. This specific clinical and pathologic entity can be difficult to recognize, particularly with superficial biopsies. It demonstrates an exuberant proliferation of squamous epithelium with hyperkeratosis. It is a pale, wart-like growth clinically. The absence of cell anaplasia belies the malignant nature of this lesion, which pushes and penetrates into soft tissue. Microabscesses form in response to keratin debris, while pressure of this neoplasm may actually cause necrosis of cartilage. This tumor has even invaded the thyroid. Although the amount of local neoplasm may be quite extensive, metastases from pure verrucous carcinoma are unknown. The presence of typical squamous cell carcinoma is found in 20% of cases and changes the prognosis to that of a tumor with metastatic potential.[77]

Various types of HPV have been detected in verrucous carcinoma of the larynx. Fliss et al.[119] reviewed tumor samples from 19 patients using PCR and DNA primers. They identified HPV type 16 DNA or HPV type 18 DNA, or both, in 13 patients (45%). These findings were confirmed by Southern blot hybridization. There was a trend toward HPV DNA detection in higher-stage tumors. The coexpression of p53

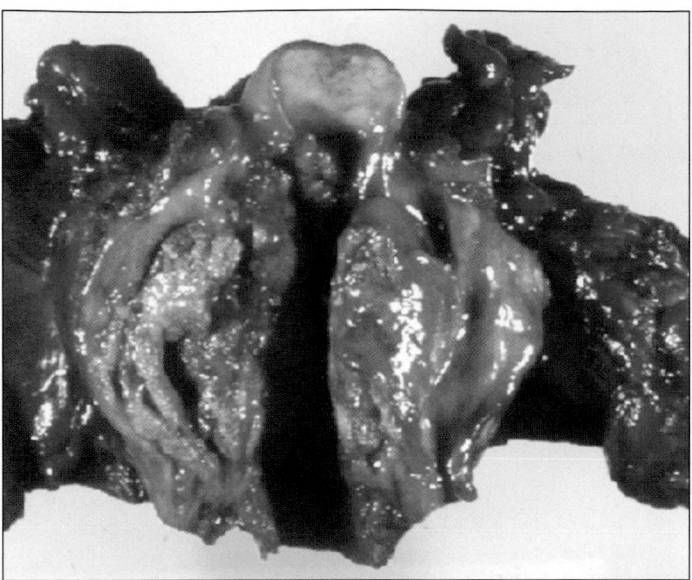

Fig. 16.10 Extensive verrucous carcinoma of the larynx. This tumor had invaded a tracheotomy site, the thyroid cartilage, which was partially ossified, the base of the epiglottis, and the pyriform sinus on the right. No clinically positive nodes were present in the cervical area.

and HPV in verrucous carcinoma of the larynx has been previously noted.[61]

In the differential diagnosis of verrucous carcinoma are a variety of verrucous lesions that appear to form a spectrum from verrucous hyperplasia, to varying degrees of dysplasia (referred to as proliferative verrucous leukoplakia), to three forms of squamous cell carcinoma: verrucous, conventional, and perhaps papillary squamous. It is believed that verrucous hyperplasia is the forerunner of verrucous carcinoma with such a consistent transition that it should be treated like verrucous carcinoma.[120] Whether other verrucous hyperplasias with features of verruca vulgaris fit into this spectrum is not clear. The most important histologic feature defining verrucous carcinomas is invasion, which cannot be evaluated by biopsies taken from the surface of the lesions.[77]

There has been some controversy over the correct treatment of verrucous carcinoma of the larynx. An extensive review of a large number of cases treated by radiotherapy initially revealed that the tumor persisted in 71% of patients.[121] Currently, the mainstay of therapy is surgical excision. There has also been the threat of radiation-induced anaplastic transformation, although this has been recently discounted.[122]

Basaloid squamous cell carcinoma

This tumor is now considered a distinct entity by the World Health Organization.[123] It was first described in 1986.[124] The tumor has

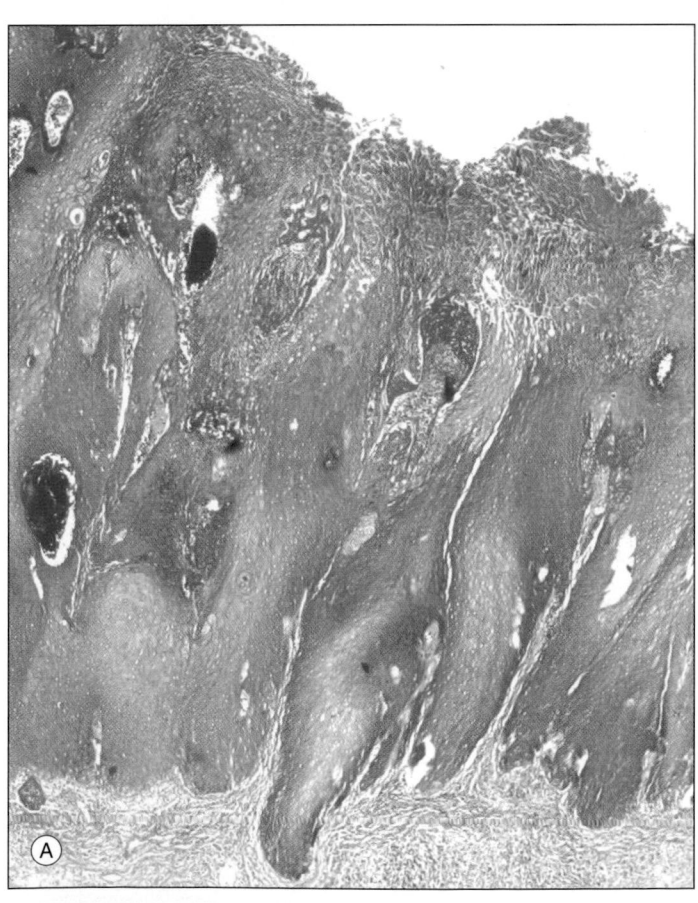

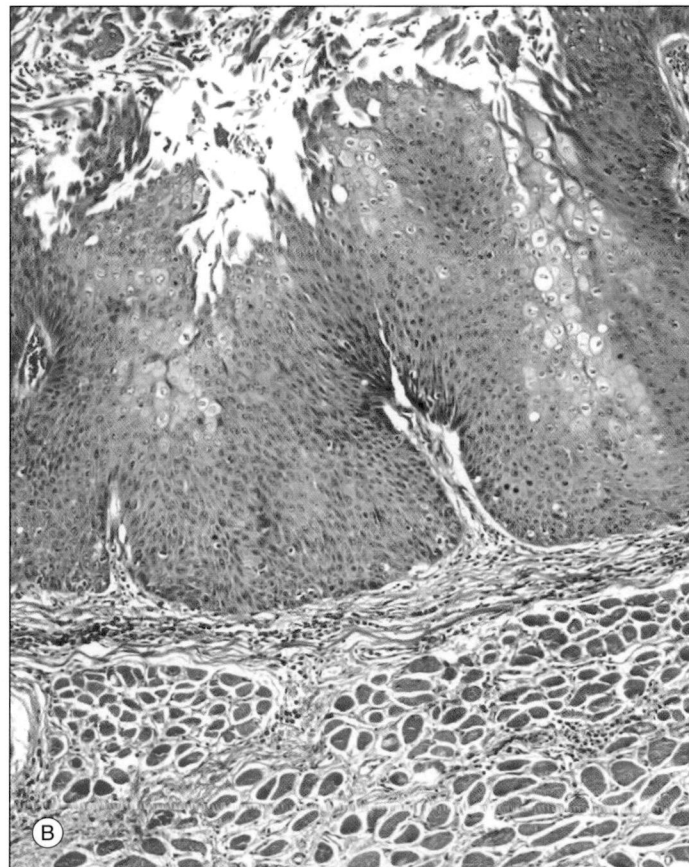

Fig. 16.11 Verrucous carcinoma. **A**, Column-like exophytic growth of squamous epithelium is seen; **B**, The base of the tumor is the only clue to true cancer as there is invasive growth into strap muscles of the neck in this case. Differentiating small tumors from squamous papillomas may be very difficult and cannot be made from superficial biopsies.

mixed basaloid and squamous components and is usually found in the supraglottic area. The basaloid cells are small, and in biopsies this tumor may be confused with adenoid cystic or neuroendocrine carcinoma of the larynx. The tumor is a high grade cancer that remains in dispute as to having a worse prognosis, stage for stage, than conventional squamous cell carcinoma.[77,125]

Papillary squamous cell carcinoma

This neoplasm is a poorly differentiated squamous carcinoma with a papillary pattern. Unlike verrucous carcinoma, the papillary fronds are covered with overtly malignant squamous cells.[77] A report of 104 cases in the larynx showed a better prognosis than for cases of conventional squamous cell carcinoma, with those tumors having a narrow base and frond-like appearance versus those having a broad base (exophytic pattern) having an even better prognosis.[126] HPV DNA was found in 5 of 14 cases using PCR in a recent series and there was a reciprocal relationship with HPV and p53 expression.[127]

Adenoid squamous cell carcinoma

This very rare variant of squamous cell carcinoma primary in the larynx demonstrates acantholysis of the tumor cells producing a pseudoglandular pattern that resemble true adenocarcinoma or, at a low-power microscopic view, an angiosarcoma. This neoplasm is also called acantholytic squamous cell carcinoma. It is found in the supraglottic portion of the larynx. It is aggressive, with a worse prognosis than conventional squamous cell carcinoma.[128]

Spindle cell carcinoma (spindle cell squamous carcinoma, sarcomatoid carcinoma, pseudosarcoma, carcinosarcoma, spindle cell carcinoma with or without pseudosarcomatous stroma)

The original report by Lane in 1957 described polypoid sarcoma-like masses in association with a squamous cell carcinoma of the mouth, fauces, and larynx.[129] After some years of study and controversy, recent electron microscopic and immunohistochemical studies indicate these tumors are spindle cell carcinomas. Their biologic behavior supports these findings.[77] These tumors are grossly exophytic or polypoid (Fig. 16.12) and are often predominantly composed of spindle cells that have malignant features including in some cases giant cells and cells with atypical mitotic figures. The identifying squamous cell carcinoma may be inconspicuously present and frequently may be only on the surface of the lesion (in situ carcinoma). The spindle cell pattern may have divergent differentiation including cartilage and bone formation as well as the storiform pattern of malignant fibrous histiocytoma.

Wick and Swanson reviewed the historical controversy and current histogenetic evidence for the concept of carcinosarcoma and carcinoma with pseudosarcomatous stroma, two among several terms applied to these tumors. They concluded that all these cases are sarcomatoid carcinomas with divergent differentiation, whether with homologous or heterologous elements.[130] A recent study supports this interpretation, including DNA analysis showing a majority of tumors have aneuploidy in both the carcinomatous and sarcomatous parts of the neoplasm.[131]

The case illustrated in Figure 16.13 demonstrates a focus of superficial squamous cell carcinoma merging with a poorly differentiated spindle cell sarcomatous neoplasm. This tumor showed reactivity for cytokeratin in some of the spindle cells.

This neoplasm may be large and bulky but with little or no invasion into the narrow stalk that is a feature of this tumor. It is important to evaluate for invasion at the base of the neoplasm as that has much more significance for determining stage and prognosis than

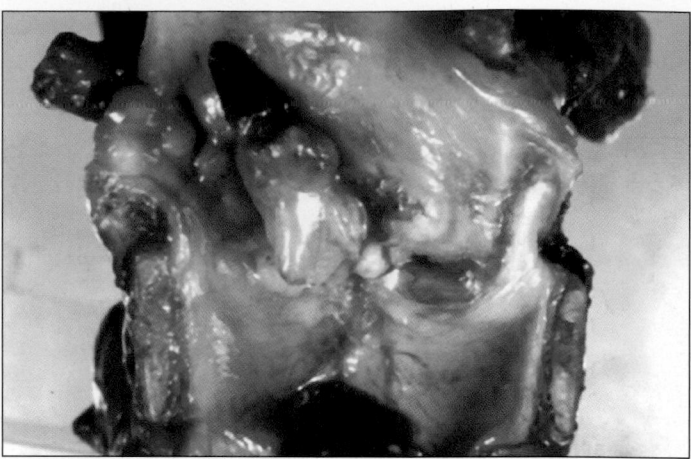

Fig. 16.12 Polypoid spindle squamous cell carcinoma. Gross polypoid configuration arising from the left vocal cord is a rather typical gross presentation.

size alone. The prognosis follows that of conventional squamous cell carcinomas of similar stage.[77]

Lymphoepithelial carcinoma

This undifferentiated carcinoma is quite rare and involves the laryngohypopharyngeal (supraglottic) area of the larynx where there is lymphoid tissue. It is discussed in detail in Chapter 15, including its association with Epstein-Barr virus.

MALIGNANT AND BENIGN GLANDULAR TUMORS

Adenocarcinoma

Throughout the larynx and trachea are collections of acini and ducts with morphologic features identical to salivary gland tissue. Tumors arising in these structures are counterparts of benign and malignant neoplasms of major salivary glands. They are quite rare (<1% of laryngeal tumors) and are most often either non-specific adenocarcinoma or adenoid cystic carcinoma.[132]

Non-specific adenocarcinomas, which have variable morphologic features and differing degrees of pleomorphism, are usually found supra- or transglottically. There is a marked male preponderance, and patients are often elderly. The location corresponds to the concentration of seromucous glands in the false cords and just inferior to the anterior commissure.[133] Although this neoplasm manifests the typical symptoms of hoarseness, most cases reported had advanced tumors when first seen. The prognosis is dismal despite radical surgery, not unlike the non-specific adenocarcinoma primary in major salivary glands.[134] Their tendency to widespread metastasis is also similar.

Adenoid cystic carcinoma

Adenoid cystic carcinoma, with its characteristic pattern of cylinders of basement membrane substance surrounded by small, uniform epithelial cells, may be grossly circumscribed but microscopically infiltrative (Fig. 16.14). It grows along tissue planes and is frequently found surrounding nerves. Olofsson and Van Nostrand[135] collected 60 cases from the literature and reported four additional examples. The tumors arose almost exclusively in the subglottic and supraglottic areas. In four cases, whole laryngeal sections demonstrated marked

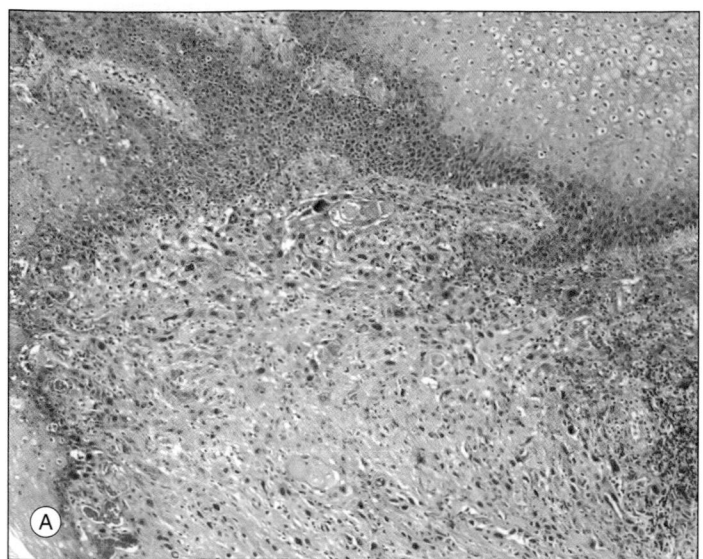
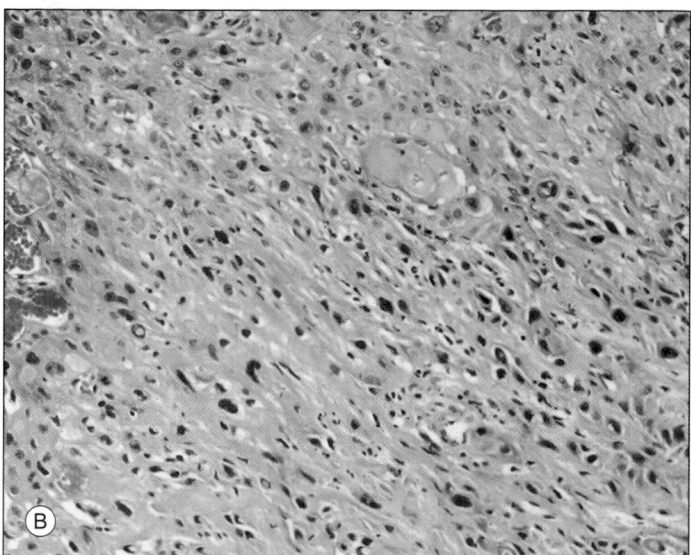

Fig. 16.13 A, Thick squamous epithelium with poorly differentiated squamous cell carcinoma seen just to the right edge of the photograph merging into a spindle cell pattern of growth beneath the intact overlying squamous epithelium. Immunohistochemical stains for cytokeratin can be helpful in determining the nature of the spindle cells though they will not be uniformly positive; **B,** Higher magnification of the undifferentiated spindle cell area with a vague keratin-like pearl at the upper center of the photograph.

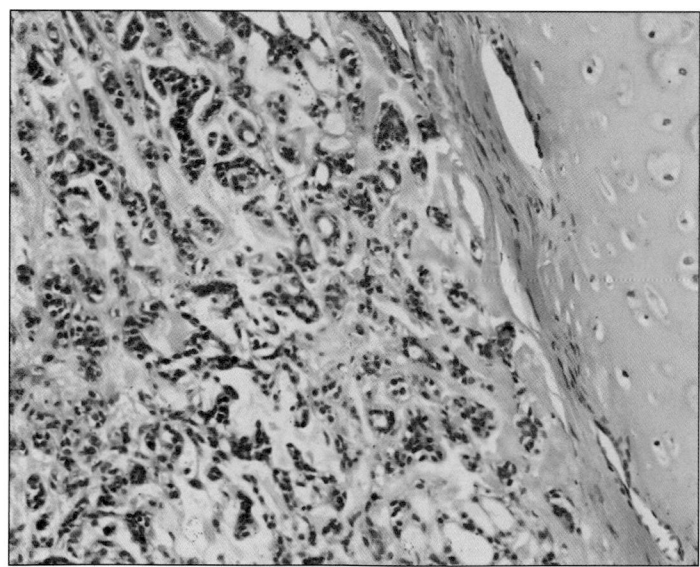

Fig. 16.14 Adenoid cystic carcinoma of the larynx. Typical pattern of the small tubular and ribbon-like nests of tumor cells surrounding eosinophilic basement membrane material. The tumor is invading into the laryngeal cartilage in this photomicrograph.

local spread of the tumor with multiple skip areas. This tumor has a protracted clinical course with multiple recurrences. Distant metastases have appeared in at least half the patients, even in reports with minimal follow-up periods.[136]

Because of the insidious nature of adenoid cystic carcinoma and its infiltrative character, patients do not usually seek medical attention until they experience dyspnea. This is particularly true of this tumor when primary in the trachea. It is the most common adenocarcinoma of the trachea. In the trachea, there is a female preponderance, but that is not true for the larynx.[137] Adenoid cystic carcinoma has an aggressive form in which the epithelial cells occur in broad sheets, there are few cylindrical structures, and marked areas of necrosis are present.[138,139]

Other salivary gland type tumors

In a comprehensive review, examples of the following benign and malignant salivary gland neoplasms occurring in the larynx are described: pleomorphic adenoma, carcinoma ex pleomorphic adenoma, pure myoepithelioma, both a benign and malignant example, mucoepidermoid carcinoma, adenosquamous carcinoma as distinct from mucoepidermoid carcinoma, acinic cell carcinoma, salivary gland duct carcinoma, epithelial-myoepithelial carcinoma, clear cell carcinoma, sebaceous carcinoma, and mucinous (mucoid) adenocarcinoma.[132]

An oncocytic carcinoma has been reported that arose in the arytenoid. Although cells had abundant eosinophilic cytoplasm, there was no indication of hyperplasia of mitochondria.[140] Benign oncocytic tumors are quite common in the larynx and pharynx, some of them forming the typical papillary cystic lesions with lymphoid tissue that are analogous to true Warthin's tumor of salivary gland type. The spectrum of oncocytic hyperplasia and metaplasia that may be seen in the larynx casts some doubt on the true neoplastic nature of these tumors.[132]

Fechner[141] is not convinced that a true malignant mixed tumor of salivary gland type has been found in the larynx. This author has not personally seen such a case, either in the larynx or the trachea, and could not find a well-documented example in the literature. A case of benign mixed tumor reported in 1986 produced ulceration and atypical squamous metaplasia of the vocal cord, resulting in an initial misdiagnosis of squamous cell carcinoma.[142]

Chan et al.[143] collected 113 acceptable and 5 probable cases of benign mixed tumor of the trachea and reported 1 additional case. The prognosis and histopathology are that of benign mixed tumors of major salivary glands. They are found predominantly in middle-aged men.

METASTATIC TUMORS

Metastatic tumors to the larynx have been reviewed by Ferlito.[144] The most common sites of primary tumor are melanoma of skin, renal cell carcinoma, and breast, lung, prostate, and colon carcinoma, in descending order of frequency. The most common sites within the larynx are the supraglottic and subglottic areas. Metastasis to the vocal cord is quite rare. Metastasis may be the initial sign of disseminate cancer when presenting with obstruction or hoarseness, or may be totally asymptomatic.[140] Although rarely metastatic, direct extension by thyroid carcinoma occasionally compromises the larynx. There were 18 cases of laryngeal invasion reported among 2000 patients treated for thyroid cancer: 7 follicular, 6 papillary, 4 anaplastic, and 1 medullary carcinomas.[145]

MISCELLANEOUS TUMORS

Malignant *melanoma*, although seen more frequently in the upper respiratory tract, is still an exceedingly rare neoplasm of both the larynx and trachea. A recent paper noted 53 reported cases of primary melanoma of the larynx in the medical literature.[146] This author has seen two similar cases primary in the larynx in 39 years of practicing surgical pathology. It is important to demonstrate junctional activity for a diagnosis of primary malignant melanoma, because the larynx is a potential site of metastatic melanoma. This tumor is seen predominantly in older men. Like cutaneous examples, the tumor cells are S-100 and HMB-45 positive in most of the cases.[146] Melanomas of the larynx may have a striking spindle cell pattern having to be differentiated from sarcomatoid carcinoma. The epithelial varieties may also have very small uniform cells, raising the differential diagnosis of neuroendocrine carcinoma. A comprehensive discussion of these diagnostic problems is presented by Mills.[147] Since the report of Mori et al.[148] of six cases of primary malignant melanoma of the trachea three additional cases have been added.[149] Like other mucous membrane melanomas, those in the upper respiratory tract and trachea are clinically aggressive.

NEUROGENIC TUMORS

Both neurofibroma and neurilemmoma have been reported in the larynx.[150–152] It is rare, however, for the larynx to be involved in neurofibromatosis (von Recklinghausen's disease).[153,154] There are over 130 reported cases in the literature with one case that presented as a primary of the trachea in a case of von Recklinghausen's disease.[155] Neurilemmoma is usually seen in females whereas neurofibroma of the larynx affects the sexes equally.[156] Most of the tumors occur in the supraglottic areas, causing hoarseness. Their histologic appearance is discussed in detail in Chapter 45. Twenty cases of solitary neurilemmoma of the trachea have been reported.[157]

The granular cell tumor has been established to be of neural origin (Fig. 16.15).[158,159] A 50-year review compiled 24 cases as primary within the trachea.[160] About 8% of all granular cell tumors are primary in the larynx. The tumor is seen predominantly in the fourth through the fifth decade and is grossly polypoid. This tumor is circumscribed but not encapsulated. Its most important pathologic feature is pseudoepitheliomatous hyperplasia of overlying squamous

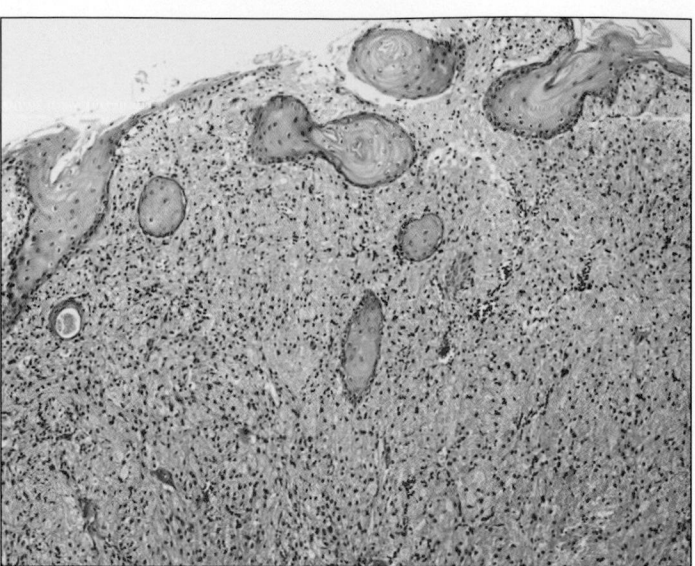

Fig. 16.15 Granular cell tumor of vocal cord. The tumor is composed of cells with small central nuclei and granular cytoplasm. Pseudoepitheliomatous hyperplasia is evident over the surface of this tumor. A superficial biopsy may lead to an erroneous interpretation of squamous cell carcinoma.

epithelium. In one review, this occurred in 64% of the cases and was severe in 22%. It is possible to mistake this hyperplasia for squamous cell carcinoma.[161] The granules are periodic acid–Schiff positive and red with Masson trichrome. Tumor cells are positive for S-100 protein, neuron-specific enolase, and nerve growth factor receptor, supporting the Schwann cell origin.[162]

A malignant example of granular cell tumor has not been described in the trachea or the larynx. This tumor does recur in a few instances.[163]

BENIGN CONNECTIVE TISSUE TUMORS

At least one case, primary in the larynx, has been reported of practically all the connective tissue tumor types. This totals about 80 cases. *Lipoma* of the larynx usually arises on the arytenoid or in the pyriform fossa. Lipomas, because their density is less than water, may be imaged by computed tomography scan.[156]

True *fibromas* are exceedingly rare and may not exist in the larynx. Cases reported as fibroma on careful examination represent other lesions: fibrous vocal cord polyps, fibromatosis, reparative granulomas, neurofibromas, or sarcomatoid squamous cell carcinoma described previously. The very rare tracheal *hamartoma* in children may be composed of a variety of soft tissues including fibrous connective tissue.[164,165]

True *benign fibrous histiocytoma* is exceedingly rare in the larynx.[156] Several cases of fibrous histiocytomas primary in the trachea have been reported. Fibrous histiocytoma has been found predominantly in children and young adults. Although reportedly benign, in several cases the tumor showed infiltration at the time of surgery.[166] This tumor may be mistaken for malignant fibrous histiocytoma.[156] A few cases of true *myxoma* of the larynx have been reported,[156] but no examples primary in the trachea; however, myxoid change is common in the laryngeal nodules (polyps). Approximately 20 cases of *leiomyoma* have been documented as primary in the larynx, and one example of epithelioid leiomyoma (leiomyoblastoma) has been reported.[156,167] Fifteen cases of leiomyoma have been reported in the trachea.[168]

There are 23 well-documented cases of extracardiac rhabdomyoma reported in the literature. Fifteen are of the adult type, four of the fetal myxoid type, and four of the fetal cellular type.[169] The tumor presents typically as a 1–2 mm submucosal polypoid or cystic nodule, most commonly involving the true vocal cord.[169] The histopathology of rhabdomyoma is discussed fully in Chapter 9. The age range of reported cases of rhabdomyoma is quite broad, 11 months to 82 years.[170] Clinical recurrence followed if the tumor was incompletely excised, but this does not indicate malignant behavior.[169]

Hemangiomas usually occur in infants as bulging masses below the vocal cords, whereas in adults they are usually proximal to the vocal cords.[33] Adults account for 90% of the cases.[156] The adult form is seen nearly exclusively in men, whereas there is a preponderance of females in the infantile form. Airway obstruction is the most common symptom in the infantile form.[33] The lesion may be compressible. In the infant, relieving airway obstruction is the most important consideration. While spontaneous regression has been noted in the infantile form after 6 months of age, tracheostomy and watchful waiting has been associated with an almost 50% mortality.[33] Histologically, this neoplasm is usually of the capillary (mostly in infants) or cavernous (mostly in adults) type, often circumscribed but occasionally infiltrating.[156] Malignant transformation in a non-irradiated case has only been reported once.[171]

Lymphangioma primary in the larynx and trachea is exceedingly rare but may cause acute airway obstruction. This tumor involving the larynx is more commonly part of large cystic hygroma involving the neck.[172] In a review of 160 cases of cystic hygroma of the neck, 10 were found to have involvement of the larynx.[173]

Chondromas, although rare, still represent the most common tumor arising in skeletal tissue within the larynx.[174] Chondromas and chondrosarcomas are discussed together as recent reviews with long-term follow-up indicate that most cartilaginous tumors of the larynx are at least low-grade malignancies.[175,176] They occur about three times as often in men versus women and are located principally in the posterior midline involving the cricoid cartilage. Radiographs reveal irregular calcification in 80% of the cases. The tumor projects as a smooth mass, which gradually enlarges and causes obstructive symptoms. This neoplasm can recur if not completely removed and one example of the mesenchymal variety disseminated widely.[177] Histologically, chondroma poses the same problem as cartilaginous tumors in other sites. Minor alterations, binucleate cells, and atypism may be considered evidence of a low-grade malignancy (Fig. 16.16). True cartilaginous tumors actually arising from laryngeal or tracheal cartilage need to be distinguished from nodules of metaplastic cartilage within soft tissue near the larynx and trachea. This latter condition is entirely benign.[33]

Most reports favor conservative therapy for true cartilaginous tumors, an attempt at local excision without laryngectomy in those chondromas that are clearly benign or at least no more than borderline malignancy.[178] Biopsy of this neoplasm is quite difficult, frequently removing only the overlying mucosa without penetration of the actual tumor.[175] This author has made the diagnosis from a fine needle aspiration biopsy in one case. Chondroma of the trachea is rare.[179] Eleven cases of primary tracheal chondrosarcoma, the majority in elderly men, have been reported.[180]

Osteoma of the larynx or trachea has not been reported. A pseudotumor, *tracheopathia osteochondroplastica*, may have to be differentiated from true chondromas or osteochondromas. In tracheopathia osteochondroplastica multiple nodules of cartilage and

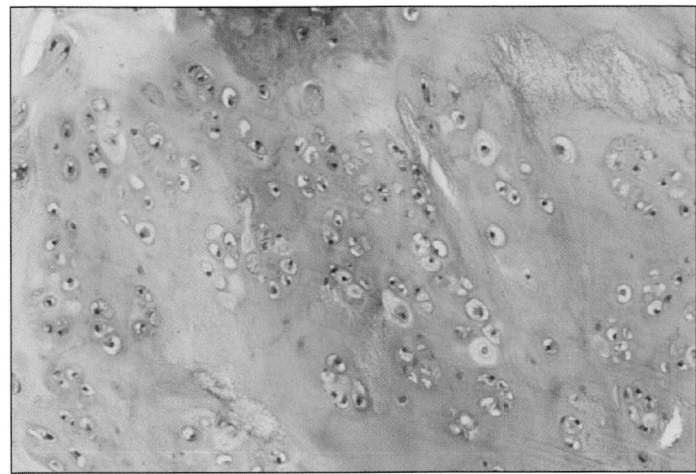

Fig. 16.16 Chondroma vs. low-grade chondrosarcoma. Well-differentiated cartilage is present with rare binucleate chrondrocyte found on multiple sections. This tumor was a smooth mass projecting from the arytenoid cartilage and measuring 1.5 cm in maximum diameter. It was removed by local excision and the follow-up, now of several years, has been negative for recurrence.

bone develop and grow between the cartilaginous rings of the trachea. These may present within the mucosa. The condition is quite rare but has been reported in conjunction with pulmonary thromboembolic disease.[33]

MALIGNANT TUMORS OF CONNECTIVE TISSUE, CARTILAGE, AND BONE

Among the malignant connective tissue tumors a majority of fibrosarcoma reported in the past have been reclassified, based on the use of immunoperoxidase stains, as sarcomatoid carcinomas.[33] Other types of sarcomas are also mistaken for fibrosarcoma, chiefly malignant fibrous histiocytoma and monophasic synovial sarcoma.[156] Many soft tissue sarcomas have now been demonstrated to have a variety of specific markers at the gene level. These are more fully discussed in Chapter 9. Prior cases of congenital or infantile fibrosarcoma should be reclassified as fibromatosis.[181] Rare cases in adults continue to be reported, indicating that fibromatosis can be locally and aggressively infiltrative without producing metastases.[182] Canalis et al.[183] reported a case of primary fibrosarcoma of the trachea, finding only three other acceptable cases in the English literature.

Thirty-five cases of *malignant fibrous histiocytoma* of the larynx have been reported, accounting for 10–15% of all examples of this neoplasm primary in the head and neck.[156] Twenty-four cases have been reported as primary in the trachea.[184] The pattern of malignant fibrous histiocytoma seems to dominate postradiation sarcomas occurring after treatment for carcinoma of the larynx.[185,186] An example is illustrated in Figure 16.17. The differential diagnosis is frequently that of sarcomatoid carcinoma.[33] Even the existence of malignant fibrous histiocytoma of soft tissue has been challenged by some contemporary pathologists.[187]

Twenty-one cases of primary *leiomyosarcoma* of the larynx and trachea have now been reported.[188] A differential diagnosis from other spindle cell sarcomas requires immunohistochemical stains and/or ultrastructural studies.[156]

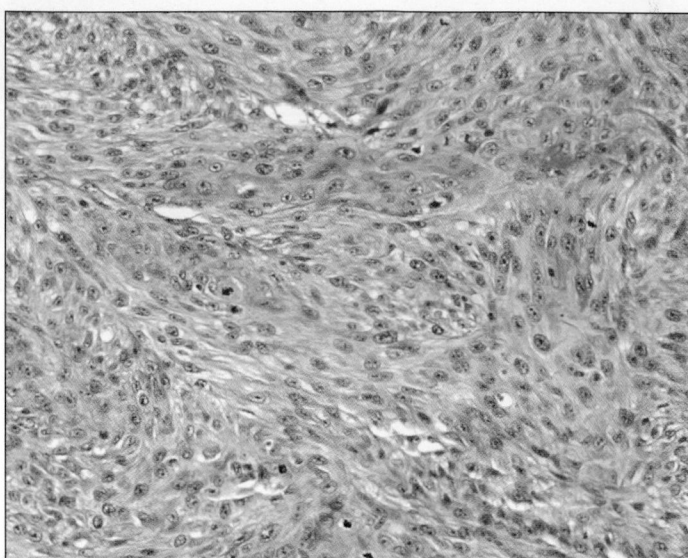

Fig. 16.17 Postradiation sarcoma. Cellular spindle cell tumor replacing the vocal cord and extending into the subglottic area. Mitotic activity is evident and there is some pleomorphism but not that usually seen with malignant fibrous histiocytoma. The patient had been treated by radiation therapy for squamous cell carcinoma of the larynx several years before. This tumor failed to stain by immunohistochemistry for any epithelial markers.

Among rare malignant neoplasms of the larynx in children and adolescents, *embryonal rhabdomyosarcoma* is the most common neoplasm.[189] Among all reported cases of this entity primary to the larynx there is a 3:1 male predominance.[156] This tumor is usually of embryonal type, and in children, like its counterpart in the orbit, seems to have a good prognosis with modern therapy protocols developed by the Intergroup Rhabdomyosarcoma Study. Pleomorphic and alveolar rhabdomyosarcomas have been reported in older patients.[190,191] Documentation of all the pleomorphic tumors is subject to close scrutiny, as only one was confirmed by ultrastructural studies.[190]

An accurate determination of the number of *hemangiosarcomas* has proved difficult, as documentation in the past has been sparse. A recent report evaluated five cases from the Armed Forces Institute of Pathology. All of these cases were confirmed by immunohistochemical stains for Factor VIII-RA and CD34.[192]

About 12 cases of *hemangiopericytoma* have been reported as primary within the larynx. Some are frankly malignant, but all of them should be considered potentially malignant, although data on biologic behavior are generally lacking.[193] Kaposi's sarcoma of the larynx has become somewhat more common, occurring in unusual sites and associated with the AIDS epidemic.[194]

Synovial sarcomas have been reported in the hypopharynx as a distinct entity, the first reported case in the larynx being that of Miller et al.[195] Only eight cases with one example in a child in the endolarynx have been authenticated in an updated review.[196] Synovial lining is not required for origin, but only mesenchymal tissue capable of divergent differentiation. The characteristic chromosome aberration t(x;18) has been detected in two examples primary in the larynx.[197] Synovial sarcoma in this location has been somewhat better differentiated, which has an impact on prognosis.[198] The monophasic pattern is rare in those cases originating in the head and neck.[156]

Thirty cases of laryngeal *liposarcoma* have been collected from the literature by Barnes and Ferlito.[156] The tumor is most commonly

supraglottic or in the pyriform sinus, only two cases having been localized to a single vocal cord.[199] The vast majority of laryngeal liposarcomas are well differentiated or of the myxoid type, with local recurrence over extended periods being the problem in management.[200]

Because of their overlapping features, primary chondromas and chondrosarcomas of the larynx have been reviewed together previously. Primary *osteosarcomas* are the rarest of the malignant mesenchymal tumors of the larynx. In a recent review twelve cases have been accepted with two additional cases, one being the first example reported in a female.[201,202] Rarely, osteosarcoma may follow radiation therapy for squamous cell carcinoma of the larynx.[201]

LYMPHOMAS AND PLASMACYTOMAS

Given the large amount of lymphoid tissue in the nasopharyngeal area, the presence of lymphoma either as a primary lesion or as part of generalized disease is not unexpected. Involvement of the larynx is extremely rare, with a total of 90 cases of non-Hodgkin's lymphoma compiled in a recent review and case report.[203] Approximately seven cases of primary non-Hodgkin's lymphoma of the trachea have now been reported. Most of the tracheal primaries have been low-grade mucosa associated lymphoid tissue (MALT) lymphomas while the majority of cases primary in the larynx have been of poorly differentiated large B-cell type.[203,204] Only three well-documented examples of T-cell lymphoma, one of gamma/delta type, have been reported as primary in the larynx.[205] When dissemination of primary laryngeal lymphoma occurs, it tends to be preferentially to other extranodal sites. Although not a lymphoma, sinus histiocytosis with massive lymphadenopathy (Rosai-Dorfman disease) has been reported to involve the larynx in seven cases.[206]

Approximately 10% of upper respiratory tract solitary plasmacytomas have occurred in the hypopharynx and larynx. Only seven cases have been reported strictly localized to one of the vocal cords,[207] and some cases have been of long clinical duration. Plasmacytomas have a male predominance with a ratio of 3:1, usually occurring in an older age group (50–70 years).[77] The differential diagnosis includes chronic inflammation with a prominent component of plasma cells. When other inflammatory cells are not present, this strongly suggests plasmacytoma. Deposits of amyloid may be striking, making the correct diagnosis of plasmacytoma difficult.[206] For typical plasmacytomas, there are broad masses of plasma cells that lie in a delicate stroma composed of thin capillary blood vessels, adjacent tissue replaced by plasma cell sheets, tumor cell nuclei with prominent red nucleoli, increase in nuclear:cytoplasmic ratio, and atypical nuclear characteristics with multinucleated cells.[77] Dissemination occurs in 35–50% of patients, sometimes after a long tumor-free interval.[77]

A report by Kuhn et al. documents a total of five cases (two of their own) of mycosis fungoides initially presenting in the larynx.[208] Dissemination of the process usually follows and transformation to large cell lymphoma may occur in up to 8% of cases.[156]

FUTURE DIRECTIONS

Although classification of some laryngeal tumors remains controversial, the most important aspect of surgical pathology is the correct interpretation of preneoplasia and intraepithelial neoplasia of the vocal cords. The limits of morphology as a predictor of biologic behavior of tumors have probably been reached, and intraobserver variability for dysplasia and in situ carcinomas will continue to be a problem.

Research into a variety of molecular and other markers has yet to uncover specific identifiers or prognosticators for individual patients for these lesions, though the general sequence of carcinogenesis of squamous mucous membranes seems better defined. Micro-laryngoscopy, precise biopsy, and therapeutic techniques using lasers make it important that progress be made in identifying individual intraepithelial lesions that have significant risk for progression to invasive cancer.

REFERENCES

1. Valletta EA, Bertini M, Sbarbati A. Tannic acid supplemented fixation improves ultrastructural evaluation of respiratory epithelium in children with recurrent respiratory tract infections. Biotech Histochem 1996; 71: 245–250.

2. Wick MR, Mills SE. Evaluation of surgical margins in anatomic pathology: Technical, conceptual, and clinical considerations. Sem in Diag Pathol 2002; 19: 207–218.

3. Gnepp DR, Barnes L, Crissman J, Zarbo R. Recommendations for the reporting of larynx specimens containing laryngeal neoplasms. Am J Clin Pathol 1998; 110: 137–139.

4. Davidson FW. Acute laryngeal obstruction in children. A fifty-year review. Ann Otol Rhinol Laryngol 1978; 87: 606–613.

5. Eschapasse H, Lacomme Y, Hassani M, et al. Laryngeal and tracheal stenosis after intubation and/or tracheotomy. A review of 32 cases including 39 lesions and 33 operations. (Authors' transl.). Acta Chir Belg 1977; 76: 381–385.

6. Smith RO, Hemenway WG, English GM. Post-intubation subglottic granulation tissue: review of the problem and evaluation of radiotherapy. Laryngoscope 1969; 79: 1227–1251.

7. Cooney W, Dzura B, Harper R. The cytology of sputum from thermally injured patients. Acta Cytol 1972; 16: 433–437.

8. Zhang S, Farmer TL, Frable MA, Powers CN. Adult herpetic laryngitis with concurrent candidal infection: a case report and literature review. Arch Otolaryngol Head Neck Surg 2000; 126: 672–674.

9. Ben-Izhak O, Ben-Arieh Y. Necrotizing squamous metaplasia in herpetic tracheitis following prolonged intubation: a lesion similar to necrotizing sialometaplasia. Histopathology 1993; 22: 265–269.

10. Contencin P, Narcy P. Gastropharyngeal reflux in infants and children. A pharyngeal pH monitoring system. Arch Otolaryngol Head Neck Surg 1992; 118: 1028–1030.

11. Mukherjee DK. Solitary tuberculoma of the larynx: a case report. Tubercle 1997; 58: 9–11.

12. Ellefsen P. Tracheal dystonia and sarcoidosis. Acta Otolaryngol (Stockh) 1970; 70: 438–442.

13. Batsakis JG. Coccidioidomycosis of the larynx. Ann Otol Rhinol Laryngol 1984; 93: 528–529.

14. Soni NK. Scleroma of the larynx. J Laryngol Otol 1997; 111: 438–440.

15. Al Jahdali H, Bamefleh H, Memish Z, et al. Upper airway obstruction due to rhinoscleroma: case report. J Chemother 2001; Suppl 1: 69–72.

16. Reder PA, Neal B III. Blastomycosis in the otolaryngology. Review of a large series. Laryngoscope 1993; 103: 53–58.

17. Rajah V, Essa A. Histoplasmosis of the oral cavity, oropharynx and larynx. J Laryngol Otol 1993; 107: 58–61.

18. Sant'Anna GD, Mauri M, Arranrte JL, Camargo H Jr. Laryngeal manifestations of paracoccidioidomycosis (South American blastomycosis). Arch Otolaryngol Head Neck Surg 1999; 125: 1375–1378

19. Tashjian LS, Peacock JE. Laryngeal candidiasis. Report of seven cases and review of the literature. Arch Otolaryngol 1984; 110: 806–809.

20. Rosenberg RA, Schneider KL, Cohen NL. Update on AIDS (editorial). Otolaryngol Head Neck Surg 1986; 95: 127-130.

21. Ogawa Y, Nishimyama N, Hagiwara A, et al. A case of laryngeal aspergillosis following radiation therapy. Auris Nasus Larynx 2002; 29: 73–76.

22. Nelson EG, Tybor AG. Actinomycosis of the larynx. Ear Nose Throat J 1992; 71: 356–358.

23. Kingdom TT, Lee KC. Invasive aspergillosis of the larynx in AIDS. Otolaryngol Head Neck Surg 1996; 115: 135–137.

24. Nagasawa M, Itoh S, Tomizawa D, et al. Invasive subglottal aspergillosis in a patient with severe aplastic anemia: a case report. J Infect 2002; 44: 198–201.

25. Tarnowska C, Amernik K, Matyja G, et al: Fixation of the crico-arythenoid joints in rheumatoid arthritis–preliminary report. Otolaryngol Pol 2004; 58: 843–849.

26. Tsikoudas A, Coatesworth AP, Martin-Hirsch DPJ. Laryngeal gout. Laryngol Otol 2002; 116: 140–142.

27. Waxman J, Bose WJ. Laryngeal manifestations of Wegener's granulomatosis: case reports and review of the literature. J Rheumatol 1986; 13: 408–411.

28. Letko E, Zafirakis P, Baltatzis S, et al. Relapsing polychondritis: a clinical review. Semin Arthritis Rheum 2002; 31: 384–395.

29. Barnes EL, Zafar T. Laryngeal amyloidosis, clinicopathologic study of seven cases. Ann Otol Rhinol Laryngol 1977; 86: 856–863.

30. Shaheen NA, Salman SD, Nassar VH. Fatal bronchopulmonary hemorrhage due to unrecognized amyloidosis. Arch Otolaryngol 1975; 101: 259–261.

31. Arens C, Glanz H, Kleinsasser O. Clinical and morphological aspects of laryngeal cysts. Eur Arch Otorhinolaryngol 1997; 254: 430–436.

32. Shvero J, Koren R, Hadar T, et al. Clinicopathologic study and classification of vocal cord cysts. Pathol Res Pract 2000; 196: 95–98.

33. Barnes L. Surgical pathology of the head and neck. 2nd edn. New York: Marcel Dekker; 2001: 128–132,204–205,151,152,612–613,1136–1144.

34. Saleem TI, Peale AR, Robbins R. Lymphocytic pseudotumor (pseudolymphoma) of the larynx. Report of a rare case and review of the literature. Laryngoscope 1970; 80: 133–136.

35. Bumber Z, Jurlina M, Manojlovic S, Jakic-Razumovic J. Inflammatory pseudotumor of the trachea. J. Pediatr Surg 2001; 36: 631–634.

36. Aaltonen LM, Rihkanen H, Vaheri A. Human papillomavirus in larynx. Laryngoscope 2002; 112: 700–707.

37. Kashima H, Shah F, Lyles A, et al. A comparison of risk factors in juvenile-onset and adult-onset recurrent respiratory papillomatosis. Laryngoscope 1992; 102: 9–13.

38. Abramson AL, Steinberg BM, Winkler B. Laryngeal papillomatosis: clinical, histopathologic and molecular studies. Laryngoscope 1987; 97: 678–685.

39. Zur Hausen H. Human papilloma viruses and their role in squamous cell carcinomas. Curr Top Microbiol Immunol 1977; 78: 1–30.

40. Shapiro RS, Marlowe FI, Butcher J. Malignant degeneration of non-irradiated juvenile laryngeal papillomatosis. Ann Otol Rhinol Laryngol 1976; 85: 101–104.

41. Johnston D, Hall H, DiLorenzo TP, Steinberg BM. Elevation of the epidermal growth factor receptor and dependent signaling in human papillomavirus-infected laryngeal papillomas. Cancer Res 1999; 59: 968–974.

42. Jin L, Yang GY, Auborn K. Differences in C/EBPs in normal tissue and papillomas of the larynx. Cell Prolif 1998; 3–4: 127–138.

43. Luzar B, Gale N, Kambic V, et al. Human papillomavirus infection and expression of p53 and c-erb-2 protein in laryngeal papillomas. Act Otolaryngol Supp 1997; 527: 120–124.

44. Rady PL, Schnadig VJ, Weiss RL, et al. Malignant transformation of recurrent respiratory papillomatosis associated with integrated human papillomavirus type 11 DNA and mutation of p53. Laryngoscope 1998; 108: 735–740.

45. Lin KY, Westra WH, Kashima HK, et al. Coinfection of HPV-11 and HPV-16 in a case of laryngeal squamous papillomas with severe dysplasia. Laryngoscope 1997; 107: 942–947.

46. Derkay CS, Darrow DH. Recurrent respiratory papillomatosis of the larynx: current diagnosis and treatment. Otolaryngol Clin North Am 2000; 33: 1127–1142.

47. Aaltonen LM, Auvinen E, Dillner J, et al. Poor antibody response against human papillomavirus in adult-onset laryngeal papillomatosis. J Med Microbiol 2001; 50: 468–471.

48. Vambutas A, DiLorenzo TP, Steinberg BM. Laryngeal papilloma cells have high levels of epidermal growth factor receptor and respond to epidermal growth factor by a decrease in epithelial differentiation. Cancer Res 1993; 53: 910–914.

49. Franceschi S, Munoz N, Bosch XF, et al. Human papillomavirus and cancers of the upper aerodigestive tract: a review of epidemiological and experimental evidence. Cancer Epidemiol Biomarkers Prev 1996; 5: 567–575.

50. Gale N, Kambie V, Michaels L, et al. The Ljubljana classification: a practical strategy for the diagnosis of laryngeal precancerous lesions. Adv Anat Pathol 2000; 7: 240–251.

51. Gale N, Zidar N, Fischinger J, Kambic V. Clinical applicability of the Ljubljana classification of epithelial hyperplastic laryngeal lesions. Clin Otolaryngol 2000; 25: 227–232.

52. Crissman JD. Laryngeal keratosis preceding laryngeal carcinoma. A report of four cases. Arch Otolaryngol 1982; 108: 445–448.

53. Friedmann I, Ferlito A. Precursors of squamous cell carcinoma. In: Ferlito A, ed. Neoplasms of the larynx. New York: Churchill Livingstone; 1993: 97–111.

54. Crissman JD, Zarbo RJ. Quantitation of DNA ploidy in squamous intraepithelial neoplasia of the laryngeal glottis. Arch Otolaryngol Head Neck Surg 1991; 117: 182–188.

55. Blackwell KE, Fu YS, Calcaterra TC. Laryngeal dysplasia. A clinicopathologic study. Cancer 1995; 75: 457–463.

56. Dreyer T, Knoblauch I, Doudkine A, et al. Nuclear texture features for classifying benign vs. dysplastic or malignant squamous epithelium of the larynx. Anal Quant Cytol Histol 2001; 23: 193–200.

57. Sugar J, Vereczkey I, Toth J. Some etio-pathogenetic factors in laryngeal carcinogenesis. J Environ Pathol Toxicol Oncol 1996; 15: 195–199.

58. Sugar J, Vereczkey I, Toth J, et al. New aspects in the pathology of the preneoplastic lesions of the larynx. Acta Otolaryngol Suppl 1997; 527: 52–56.

59. Suzuki T, Tsutsumi K, Nakajima T, et al. Spontaneous mutation of p53 gene in human papillomavirus type 16 E7-immortalized human laryngeal epithelial cells. Acta Otolaryngol Suppl 1996; 522: 94–98.

60. Caruso ML, Valentini AM. Localization of p53 protein and human papillomavirus in laryngeal squamous lesions. Anticancer Res 1997; 17: 4671–4675.

61. Lopez-Amado M, Garcia-Calballero T, Lozano-Ramirez A, Labella-Caballero T. Human papillomavirus and p53 oncoprotein in verrucous carcinoma of the larynx. J Laryngol Otol 1996; 110: 742–747.

62. Poljak M, Gale N, Kambic V. Human papillomaviruses: a study of their prevalence in the epithelial hyperplastic lesions of the larynx. Acta Otolaryngol Suppl 1997; 5 27: 66–69.

63. Moore CE, Wiatrak BJ, McClatchey KD, et al. High-risk human papillomavirus types and squamous cell carcinoma in patients with respiratory papillomas. Otolaryngol Head Neck Surg 1999; 120: 698–705.

64. Almadori G, Cadoni G, Cattani P, et al. Detection of human papillomavirus DNA in laryngeal squamous cell carcinoma by polymerase chain reaction. Eur J Cancer 1996; 32A: 783–788.

65. Cerovac Z, Sarcevic B, Kralj Z, Ban J. Detection of human papillomavirus (HPV) type 6, 16 and 18 in head and neck squamous cell carcinomas by in situ hybridization. Neoplasma 1996; 43: 185–194.

66. Lie ES, Karlsen F, Holm R. Presence of human papillomavirus in squamous cell laryngeal carcinomas. A study of thirty-nine cases using polymerase chain reaction and in situ hybridization. Acta Otolaryngol 1996; 116: 900–905.

67. McKaig RG, Baric RS, Olshan AF. Human papillomavirus and head and neck cancer: epidemiology and molecular biology. Head Neck 1998; 20: 250–265.

68. Atula S, Grenman R, Kujari H, Syrjanen S. Detection of human papillomavirus (HPV) in laryngeal carcinoma cell lines provided evidence for a heterogeneic cell population. Eur J Cancer 1999; 35: 825–832.

69. Lindeberg H, Krogdahl A. Laryngeal cancer and human papillomavirus: HPV is absent in the majority of laryngeal carcinomas. Cancer Lett 1999; 146: 9–13.

70. Azzimonti B, Hertel L, Aluffi P, et al. Demonstration of multiple HPV types in laryngeal premalignant lesions using polymerase chain reaction and immunohistochemistry. J Med Virol 1999; 59: 110–116.

71. Venuti A, Manni V, Morello R, et al. Physical state and expression of human papillomavirus in laryngeal carcinoma and surrounding normal tissue. J Med Virol 2000; 60: 396–402.

72. Jacob SE, Sreevidya S, Chacko E, Pillai MR. Cellular manifestations of human papillomavirus infection in laryngeal tissues. J Surg Oncol 2002; 79: 142–150.

73. Bocking A, Auffermann W, Vogel H, et al. Diagnosis and grading of malignancy in squamous epithelial lesions of the larynx with DNA cytophotometry. Cancer 1985; 56: 1600–1604.

74. Bauer WC. Concomitant carcinoma in situ and invasive carcinoma of the larynx. In: Alberti PW, Bryce DP (eds). Workshops from the Centennial Conference on Laryngeal Cancer. E. Norwalk, CT: Appleton & Lange; 1976: 127–134.

75. Miller AH, Fisher JR. Clues to the life history of carcinoma in situ of the larynx. Laryngoscope 1971; 81: 1475–1480.

76. Jemal A, Thomas A, Murry T, Thun M. Cancer statistics, 2002. Cancer J Clin 2002; 52: 23–47.

77. Mills SE, Gaffey MJ, Frierson Jr HF. Atlas of tumor pathology. Tumors of the upper aerodigestive tract and ear. Washington DC: Armed Forces Institute of Pathology; 1997: 62,227–230.

78. Seitz HK, Poschl G, Simanowski UA. Alcohol and cancer. Recent Dev Alcohol 1998; 14: 67–95.

79. Olshan AF, Weissler MC, Watson MA, Bell DA. Risk of head and neck cancer and the alcohol dehydrogenase 3 genotype. Carcinogenesis 2001; 22: 57-61.

80. Elahi A, Zheng Z, Park J, et al. The human OGG1 DNA repair enzyme and its association with orolaryngeal cancer risk. Carcinogenesis 2002; 23: 1229–1234.

81. Hager G, Formanek M, Gedlicka C, et al. Ethanol decreases expression of p21 and increases hyperphosphorylated pRb in cell lines of squamous cell carcinoma of the head and neck. Alcohol Clin Exp Res 2001; 25: 496–501.

82. Szyfter K, Hemminki K, Szyfter W, et al. Tobacco smoke-associated N7-alkylguanine in DNA of larynx tissue and leukocytes. Carcinogenesis 1996; 17: 501–506.

83. Flamini G, Romano G, Curigliano G, et al. 4-Aminobiphenyl-DNA adducts in laryngeal tissue and smoking habits: an immunohistochemical study. Carcinogenesis 1998; 19: 353–357.

84. Kleinsasser NH, Weissacher H, Kastenbauer ER, et al. Altered genotoxicity in mucosal cells of head and neck cancer patients due to environmental pollutants. Eur Arch Otorhinolaryngol 2000; 257: 337–342.

85. Spitz MR, McPherson RS, Jiang H, et al. Correlates of mutagen sensitivity in patients with upper aerodigestive tract cancer. Cancer Epidemiol Biomarkers Prev 1997; 6: 687–692.

86. Greene FL, Page DL, Fleming ID, et al, eds. AJCC cancer staging handbook. 6th edn. New York: Springer-Verlag; 2002: 61.

87. Olofsson J. Growth and spread of laryngeal carcinoma. In: Alberti PW, Bryce DP, eds. Workshops from the Centennial Conference on Laryngeal Cancer. E. Norwalk, CT: Appleton & Lange; 1976: 40–52.

88. Ferlito A, Friedmann L. Squamous cell carcinoma. In: Ferlito A, ed. Neoplasms of the larynx. New York: Churchill Livingstone; 1993: 113–133.

89. Jakobsson PA. Histologic grading of malignancy and prognosis in glottic carcinoma of the larynx. In: Alberti PW, Bryce DP, eds. Workshops from the Centennial Conference on Laryngeal Cancer. E. Norwalk, CT: Appleton & Lange; 1976: 847–852.

90. Crissman JF, Gluckman J, Whiteley J, Quenelle D. Squamous-cell carcinoma of the floor of the mouth. Head Neck Surg 1980; 3: 2–7.

91. Cappellari JO. Histopathology and pathologic prognostic indicators. Otolaryngol Clin North Am 1997; 30: 251–268.

92. Resnick JM, Uhlman D, Niehans GA, et al. Cervical lymph node status and survival in laryngeal carcinoma: Prognostic factors. Ann Otol Rhinol Laryngol 1995; 104: 685–694.

93. Nakashima T, Kusumoto T, Maehara Y, et al. Chemosensitivity and DNA ploidy in head and neck squamous cell carcinomas. Arch Otolaryngol Head Neck Surg 1992; 118: 1031–1036.

94. Munck-Wikland E, Kuyleustierna R, Lindholm J, Auer G. p53 immunostaining and image cytometry DNA analysis in precancerous and cancerous squamous epithelial lesions of the larynx. Head Neck 1997; 19: 107-115.

95. Assimakopoulos D, Kolettas E, Zagorianakou N, et al. Prognostic significance of p53 in the cancer of the larynx. Anticancer Res 2000; 20(5B): 3555–3564.

96. Ioachim E, Assimakopoulos D, Agnantis NJ, et al. Altered patterns of retinoblastoma gene product expression in benign, premalignant and malignant epithelium: an immunohistochemical study including correlation with p53 bcl-2 and proliferating indices. Anticancer Res 1999; 19(1A): 541–545.

97. Ioachim E, Assimakopoulos D, Peschos D, et al. Immunohistochemical expression of metallothionein in benign premalignant and malignant epithelium of the larynx: correlation with p53 and proliferative cell nuclear antigen. Pathol Res Pract 1999; 195: 809–814.

98. Luzar B, Poljak M, Marin IJ, et al. Quantitative measurement of telomerase catalytic subunit (hTERT) m RNA in laryngeal squamous cell carcinomas. Anticancer Res 2001; 21: 4011–4015.

99. Hohaus S, Cavallo S, Bellacosa A, et al. Telomerase activity in human laryngeal squamous cell carcinoma. Clin Cancer Res 1996; 2: 1895–1900.

100. Curran AJ, Gullane PJ, Irish J, et al. Telomerase activity is upregulated in laryngeal squamous cell carcinoma. Laryngoscope 2000; 110: 391–396.

101. Sarioglu S, Ozer E, Kirimca F, et al. Matrix metalloproteinase-2 expression in laryngeal preneoplastic and neoplastic lesions. Pathol Res Pract 2001; 197: 483–486.

102. Munck-Wikland E, Heselmeyer K, Lindblom J, et al. Stromelysin-3 mRNA expression in dysplastic and invasive epithelial cancer of the larynx. Int J Oncol 1998; 12: 859–864.

103. Veltman JA, Bot FJ, Huynen FC, et al. Chromosome instability as an indicator of malignant progression in laryngeal mucosa. J Clin Oncol 2000; 18: 1644-1651.

104. Gale N, Kambic V, Poljak M, et al. Chromosomes 7.17 polysomies and overexpression of epidermal growth factor and p53 protein in epithelial hyperplastic laryngeal lesions. Oncology 2000; 58: 117–125.

105. Rizos E, Sourvinos G, Spandidos DA. Loss of heterozygosity at 8p, 9p and 17q in laryngeal cytologic specimens. Oral Oncol 1998; 34: 519–523.

106. Patel V, Leethanakul C, Gutkind JS. New approaches to the understanding of the molecular basis of oral cancer. Crit Rev Oral Biol Med 2001; 12: 55–63.

107. Jeannon JP, Stafford FW, Soames JV, Wilson JA. Altered MUCI1 and MUC2 glycoprotein expression in laryngeal cancer. Otolaryngol Head Neck Surg 2000; 124: 199–202.

108. Resta L, Marsigliante S, Leo G, et al. Molecular biopathology of metaplastic, dysplastic and neoplastic laryngeal epithelium. Acta Otolaryngol Suppl 1997; 527: 39–42.

109. Maiorano E, Botticella MA, Marzullo A, Resta L. Expression of ER-D5 and EGFr in laryngeal carcinoma and pre-malignant epithelium. Acta Otolaryngol Suppl 1997; 527: 95–99.

110. Franchi A, Gallo O, Sardi I, Santucci M. Downregulation of transforming growth factor beta type II receptor in laryngeal carcinogenesis. J Clin Pathol 2001; 54: 201–204.

111. Imauchi Y, Ito K, Takasago E, et al. Stromal recurrence after total laryngectomy for squamous cell carcinoma of the larynx. Otolaryngol Head Neck Surg 2002; 126: 63–66.

112. Reddy SP, Narayana A, Melian E, et al. Stromal recurrence in patients with T1 glottic cancer after salvage laryngectomy for radiotherapy failures: role of p53 overexpression and subglottic extension. Am J Clin Oncol 2001; 24: 124–127.

113. Jordan J, Piotrowski S. Laryngeal edema after radiotherapy – radiation reaction or a property of the neoplasm (recurrence, residual neoplasm). Otolaryngol Pol 1995; 49 Suppl 20: 358–366.

114. Ferlito A, Friedman I. Neuroendocrine neoplasms. In: Ferlito A, ed. Neoplasms of the larynx. New York: Churchill Livingstone; 1993: 169–205.

115. Liew SH, Leong AS, Tang HM. Tracheal paraganglioma: a case report with review of the literature. Cancer 1981; 47: 1387–1393.

116. Barnes L. Paraganglioma of the larynx. A critical review of the literature. ORL J Otorhinolaryngol Relat Spec 1991; 53: 220–234.

117. Ferlito A, Barnes L, Rinaldo A, et al. A review of neuroendocrine neoplasms of the larynx: update on diagnosis and treatment. J Laryngol Otol 1998; 112: 827–834.

118. Kavy SD, Harrell JH. Small cell carcinoma of the trachea. Case reports and review of the literature (abst 2509). In: 1990 World Conference on Lung Health. Boston; 1990.

119. Fliss DM, Noble-Topham SE, McLachlin CM, et al. Laryngeal verrucous carcinoma: a clinicopathologic study and detection of human papillomavirus using polymerase chain reaction. Laryngoscope 1994; 104: 146–152.

120. Batsakis JG, Suarex P, el-Naggar AK. Proliferative verrucous leukoplakia and its related lesions. Oral Oncol 1999; 35: 354–359.

121. Hagan P, Lyons GD, Haindel C. Verrucous carcinoma of the larynx: role of human papilloma virus, radiation and surgery. Laryngoscope 1993; 103: 253–257.

122. McCaffrey TV, Witte M, Ferguson MT. Verrucous carcinoma of the larynx. Ann Otol Rhinol Laryngol 1998; 107: 391–395.

123. Shanmugaratnam K. Histological typing of tumours of the upper respiratory tract and ear. In: World Health

Organization, ed. International histological classification of tumours. 2nd edn. Berlin: Springer-Verlag; 1991.

124. Wain SL, Kier R, Vollmer RT, et al. Basaloid-squamous carcinoma of the tongue, hypopharynx, and larynx: report of 10 cases. Hum Pathol 1986; 17: 1158–1166.

125. Paulino AF, Singh B, Shah JP, Huvos AG. Basaloid squamous cell carcinoma of the head and neck. Laryngoscope 2000; 110: 1479–1482.

126. Thompson LD, Wenig BM, Heffner DK, Gnepp DR. Exophytic and papillary squamous cell carcinomas of the larynx: A clinicopathologic series of 104 cases. Otolaryngol Head Neck Surg 1999; 120: 718–724.

127. Suarez PA, Adler-Storthz K, Luna MA, et al. Papillary squamous cell carcinomas of the upper aerodigestive tract: a clinicopathologic and molecular study. Head Neck 2000; 22: 360–368.

128. Ferlito A. Atypical forms of squamous cell carcinoma. In: Ferlito A, ed. Neoplasms of the larynx. New York: Churchill Livingstone; 1991: 135–161.

129. Lane N. Pseudosarcoma (polypoid sarcoma-like masses) associated with squamous cell carcinoma of the mouth, fauces, and larynx. Cancer 1957; 10: 19–41.

130. Wick MR, Swanson PE. Carcinosarcoma: current perspectives and an historical review of nosological concepts. Semin Diagn Pathol 1993; 10: 118–127.

131. Lewis JE, Olsen KD, Sebo TJ. Spindle cell carcinoma of the larynx: review of 26 cases including DNA content and immunohistochemistry. Hum Pathol 1997; 28: 664–673.

132. El-Jabbour JN, Ferlito A, Friedmann I. Salivary gland neoplasms. In: Ferlito A, ed. Neoplasms of the larynx. New York: Churchill Livingstone; 1993: 231–264.

133. Cohen J, Guillamondegui OM, Batsakis JG, et al. Cancer of minor salivary glands of the larynx. Am J Surg 1985; 150: 513–518.

134. Spiro RH, Lewis JS, Jajdu SI, Strong EW. Mucus gland tumors of the larynx and laryngopharynx. Ann Otol Rhinol Laryngol 1976; 85: 498–503.

135. Olofsson J, Van Nostrand AW. Adenoid cystic carcinoma of the larynx: a report of four cases and a review of the literature. Cancer 1977; 40: 1307–1313.

136. Mahlstedt K, Ussmuller J, Donath K. Malignant sialogenic tumours of the larynx. J Laryngol Otol 2002; 6: 119–122.

137. Azar T, Abdul-Karim FW, Tucker HM. Adenoid cystic carcinoma of the trachea. Laryngoscope 1998; 108: 1297–1300.

138. Stillwagon GB, Smith RR, Highstein C. Adenoid cystic carcinoma of the supraglottic larynx: report of a case and review of the literature. Am J Otolaryngol 1985; 6: 309–314.

139. Ferlito A, Barnes L, Myers EN. Neck dissection for laryngeal adenoid cystic carcinoma: is it indicated? Ann Otol Rhinol Laryngol 1990; 99: 277–280.

140. Johns ME, Batsakis JG, Short CD. Oncocytic and oncocytoid tumors of the salivary glands. Laryngoscope 1973; 83: 1940–1952.

141. Fechner RE. Adenocarcinoma of the larynx. In: Alberti PW, Bryce DP, eds. Workshops from the Centennial Conference on Laryngeal Cancer. E. Norwalk, CT: Appleton & Lange; 1976: 466–471.

142. MacMillan RH, Fechner RE. Pleomorphic adenoma of the larynx. Arch Pathol Lab Med 1986; 110: 245–247.

143. Chan KM, Fine G, Lewis J, et al. Benign mixed tumors of the trachea. Cancer 1979; 44: 2260–2266.

144. Ferlito A. Secondary neoplasms. In Ferlito A, ed. Neoplasms of the larynx. New York: Churchill Livingstone; 1993: 349–360.

145. Djalilian M, Beahrs OH, Devine KD. Intraluminal involvement of the larynx and trachea by thyroid cancer. Am J Surg 1974; 128: 500–504.

146. Amin HH, Petruzzeli GJ, Jusain AN, Nickoloff BJ. Primary malignant melanoma of the larynx. Arch Pathol Lab Med 2001; 125: 271–273.

147. Mills SE. Neuroectodermal neoplasms of the head and neck with emphasis on neuroendocrine carcinoma. Mod Pathol 2002; 15: 264–278.

148. Mori K, Cho H, Som M. Primary "flat" melanoma of the trachea. J Pathol 1977; 121: 101–105.

149. Duarte IG, Gal AA, Mansour KA. Primary malignant melanoma of the trachea. Ann Thorac Surg 1998; 65: 559–560.

150. Schaeffer BT, Som PM, Biller HF, et al. Schwannomas of the larynx: review and computed tomographic scan analysis. Head Neck Surg 1986; 8: 469–472.

151. Mevio E, Galioto P, Scelsi M, et al. Neurofibroma of vocal cord: case report. Acta Otorhinolaryngol Belg 1990; 44: 447–450.

152. Chang-Lo M. Laryngeal involvement in von Recklinghausen's disease: a case report and review of the literature. Laryngoscope 1977; 87: 435–442.

153. Supance JS, Quenelle DJ, Crissman J. Endolaryngeal neurofibromas. Otolaryngol Head Neck Surg 1980; 88: 74–78.

154. O'Connor AFF, Freeland AP. Neonatal laryngeal neurofibromatosis. Ear Nose Throat J 1980; 59: 174–177.

155. Rosen FS, Pou AM, Quinn Jr FB. Obstructive supraglottic Schwannoma: A case report and review of the literature. Laryng 2002; 112: 997–1002.

156. Barnes L, Ferlito A. Soft tissue neoplasms. In: Ferlito A, ed. Neoplasms of the larynx. New York: Churchill Livingstone; 1993: 270–271,275–304.

157. Tiedemann R. Neurogenic tumors of the trachea, HNO 1993; 40: 41–43.

158. Fisher ER, Wechsler H. Granular cell myoblastoma, a misnomer. Electron microscopic histochemical evidence concerning its Schwann cell derivation and nature (granular cell Schwannoma). Cancer 1962; 15: 936–954.

159. Garancis JC, Komorowski RA, Kuzma JF. Granular cell myoblastoma. Cancer 1970; 25: 542-550.

160. Burton DM, Heffner DK, Patow CA. Granular cell tumors of the trachea. Laryngoscope 1992; 102: 807–813.

161. Compagno J, Hyams VJ, Ste-Marie P. Benign granular cell tumors of the larynx: a review of 36 cases with clinicopathologic data. Ann Otol Rhinol Laryngol 1975; 84: 308–314.

162. Barnes L, Ferlito A. Soft tissue neoplasms. In: Ferlito A, ed. Neoplasms of the larynx. New York: Churchill Livingstone; 1993: 270–271, 275–304.

163. Sataloff RT, Sessue JC, Portell M, et al. Granular cell tumors of the larynx. J Voice 2000; 14: 119–134.

164. Gross E, Chen MK, Hollabaugh RS, Joyner RE. Tracheal hamartoma: report of a child with a neck mass. J Pediatr Surg 1996; 11: 1584–1585.

165. Rinaldo A, Mannara GM, Fisher C, Ferlito A. Hamartoma of the larynx: a critical review of the literature. Ann Otol Rhinol Laryngol 1998; 107: 264–267.

166. Sandstrom RE, Proppe KH, Trelstad RL. Fibrous histiocytoma of the trachea. Am J Clin Pathol 1978; 70: 429–433.

167. Mori H, Kumoi T, Hashimoto M, et al. Leiomyoblastoma of the larynx: report of a case. Head Neck 1992; 14: 148–152.

168. Douzinas M, Sheppard MN, Lennox SC. Leiomyoma of the trachea – an unusual tumor. Thorac Cardiovasc Surg 1989; 37: 285–287.

169. Johansen EC, Illum P. Rhabdomyoma of the larynx: a review of the literature with a summary of previously described cases of rhabdomyoma of the larynx and a report of a new case. J Laryngol Otol 1995; 109: 147–153.

170. Granich MS, Pilch BZ, Nadol JB, et al. Fetal rhabdomyoma of the larynx. Arch Otolaryngol 1983; 109: 821–826.

171. McRae RD, Gatland DJ, McNab-Jones RF, Khan S. Malignant transformation in a laryngeal hemangioma. Ann Otol Rhinol Laryngol 1990; 99: 562–565.

172. Sobol SE, Manoukian JJ. Acute airway obstruction from a laryngeal lymphangioma in a child. Int J Pediatr Otorhinolaryngol 2001; 58: 255–257.

173. Cohen SR, Thompson JW. Lymphangiomas of the larynx in infants and children. A survey of pediatric lymphangioma. Ann Otol Rhinol Laryngol, 1986; 95: 1–20.

174. Franco Jr RA, Singh B, Har-El G. Laryngeal chondroma. J Voice 2002; 16: 92–95.

175. Devaney KO, Ferlito A, Silver CE. Cartilaginous tumors of the larynx. Ann Otol Rhinol Laryngol 1995; 104: 251–255.

176. Lewis JE, Olsen KD, Inwards CY. Cartilaginous tumors of the larynx: clinicopathologic review of 47 cases. Ann Otol Rhinol Laryngol 1997; 106: 94–100.

177. Thompson LD, Gannon FH. Chondrosarcoma of the larynx: a clinicopathologic study of 11 cases with a review of the literature. Am J Surg Pathol 2002; 26: 836–851.

178. Moran CA, Suster S, Carter D. Laryngeal chondrosarcomas. Arch Pathol Lab Med 1993; 117: 914–917.

179. Jortay AM, Bisschop P. Chondroma of the trachea. Acta Otorhinolaryngol Belg 1998; 52: 247–251.

180. Farrell ML, Gluckman JL, Biddinger P. Tracheal chondrosarcoma: a case report. Head Neck 1998; 20: 568–572.

181. Rosenberg HS, Vogler C, Close LG, et al. Laryngeal fibromatosis in the neonate. Arch Otolaryngol 1981; 107: 513–517.

182. Mirra M, Calo S, Salviato T, et al. Aggressive fibromatosis of the larynx: report of a new case in an adult patient and review of the literature. Pathol Res Pract 2001; 197: 51–55;discussion 56–58.

183. Canalis RF, Green M, Kenard HR, et al. Malignant fibrous xanthoma (xanthofibrosarcoma) of the larynx. Arch Otolaryngol 1975; 101: 135–137.

184. Vinod SK, Macleod CA, Barner DJ, Fletcher J. Malignant fibrous histiocytomas of the trachea. Respirology 1999; 4: 271–274.

185. Guney E, Yigitbasi OG, Balkanli S, Canoz OM. Postirradiation malignant fibrous histiocytoma of the larynx: A case report. Am J Otolaryngol 2002; 23: 293–296.

186. Resta L, Pennella A, Fiore MG, Botticella MA. Malignant fibrous histiocytoma of the larynx after radiotherapy for squamous cell carcinoma. Eur Arch Otorhinolaryngol 2000; 257: 260–262.

187. Hollowood K, Fletcher CDM. Malignant fibrous histiocytoma: morphologic pattern or pathologic entity? Semin Diagn Pathol 195; 12: 210–220.

188. Paczona R, Jori J, Tiszlavicz L, Czigner J. Leiomyosarcoma of the larynx. Review of the literature and report of two cases. Ann Otol Rhinol Laryngol 1999; 108: 677–682.

189. Ferlito A, Rinaldo A, Marioni G. Laryngeal malignant neoplasms in children and adolescents. Int J Pediatr Otorhinolaryngol 1999; 49: 1–14.

190. Akyol MU, Sozeri B, Kucukali T, Ogretmenoglu O. Laryngeal pleomorphic rhabdomyosarcoma. Eur Arch Otorhinolaryngol 2001; 255: 307–310.

191. Winter LK, Lorentzen M. Rhabdomyosarcoma of the larynx. Report of two cases and a review of the literature. J Laryngol Otol 1978; 92;417–424.

192. Loos BM, Wiencke JA, Thompson LD. Laryngeal angiosarcoma: a clinicopathologic study of five cases with a review of the literature. Laryngoscope 2001; 111: 1197–1202.

193. Pesavento G, Ferlito A. Hemangiopericytoma of the larynx. A clinico-pathological study with review of the literature. J Laryngol Otol 1082; 96: 1065–1073.

194. Schiff NF, Annino DJ, Woo P, Shapshay SM. Kaposi's sarcoma of the larynx. Ann Otol Rhinol Laryngol 1997; 107: 563–567.

195. Miller LH, Sanatella-Latimer L, Miller T. Synovial sarcoma of larynx. Trans Am Acad Ophthalmol Otolaryngol 1975; 80: 448–451.

196. Morland B, Cox G, Randall C, et al. Synovial sarcoma of the larynx in a child: case report and histological appearances. Med Pediatr Oncol 1994; 23: 64–68.

197. Deo Tos AP, Dal Cin P, Sciot R, et al. Synovial sarcoma of the larynx and hypopharynx. Ann Otol Rhiol Laryngol 1998; 107: 1080–1085.

198. Oda Y, Hashimoto H, Tsuneyoshi M, et al. Survival in synovial sarcoma. A multivariate study of prognostic factors with special emphasis on the comparison between early death and long-term survival. Am J Surg Pathol 1993; 17: 35–44.

199. Hurtado JF, Lopez JJ, Aranda FI, Talavera J. Primary liposarcoma of the larynx. Case report and literature review. Ann Otol Rhinol Laryngol 1994; 103: 315–318.

200. Wenig BM, Heffner DK. Liposarcomas of the larynx and hypopharynx: a clinicopathologic study of eight new cases and a review of the literature. Laryngoscope 1995; 105: 747–756.

201. Berge JK, Kapadia SB, Myers EN. Osteosarcoma of the larynx. Arch Otolaryngol Head Neck Surg 1998; 124: 207–210.

202. Myssiorek D, Patel M, Wasserman P, Rofeim O. Osteosarcoma of the larynx. Ann Otol Rhinol Laryngol 1998; 107: 70–74.

203. Cavalot AL, Preti G, Vione N, et al. Isolated primary non-Hodgkin's malignant lymphoma of the larynx. J Laryngol Otol 2001; 115: 324–326.

204. Fidias P, Wright C, Harris NL, et al. Primary tracheal non-Hodgkin's lymphoma. A case report and review of the literature. Cancer 1996; 77: 2332–2338.

205. Marianowski R, Wassef M, Amanou L, et al. Primary T-cell non-Hodgkin lymphoma of the larynx with subsequent cutaneous involvment. Arch Otolaryngol Head Neck Surg 1998; 124: 1037–1040.

206. MacLennan KA, Schofield JB. Haemopoietic neoplasms. In: Ferlito A, ed. Neoplasms of the larynx. New York: Churchill Livingstone; 1993: 327–336.

207. Rakover Y, Bennett M, David R, Rosen G. Isolated extramedullary plasmacytoma of the true vocal fold. J Laryngol Otol 2000; 114: 540–542.

208. Kuhn JJ, Wenig BM, Clark DA. Mycosis fungoides of the larynx. Report of two cases and review of the literature. Arch Otolaryngol Head Neck Surg 1992; 118: 853–858.

APPENDIX 16.1 ASSOCIATION OF DIRECTORS OF ANATOMIC AND SURGICAL PATHOLOGY RECOMMENDATIONS

To be included in the report for carcinoma of the larynx.[1]

1. Topography: type of specimen(s) received (e.g., total or partial larynx, neck contents)
2. Procedure (e.g., total or partial laryngectomy, supraglottic [horizontal] or hemilaryngectomy [vertical], radical neck dissection)
3. Exact site of tumor (supraglottic, subglottic, glottic, see No. 1)
4. Histologic type (WHO classification recommended, see No. 2) (comment on no tumor present after therapy)
5. Histologic grade as appropriate (check grading systems)
6. Tumor extent: depth of invasion with respect to landmarks (comment on neural, vascular, cartilage, pre-epiglottic space and extralaryngeal soft tissue [muscle soft tissue, cartilage] or tracheostomy involvement as well as multifocal growth)
7. Status of surgical margins
8. Lymph node metastases: number of involved nodes, size of metastatic node (comment whether extranodal spread of tumor is found; comment on keratin debris as evidence of previous tumor)
9. Preoperative treatment effects on nodes

Features optional for the final report: these are optional because they represent specific institutional preferences or are of inconclusive prognostic significance.

A. Interface with stroma; infiltrating, pushing, superficial or deep invasion
B. Extent of and location of any dysplasia (including grade)/CIS
C. Results of ancillary investigations (i.e., flow cytometry)
D. Type or density of inflammatory infiltrate
E. Distance from surgical margins

Features contained in a good gross description.

1. How the specimen was received: fresh, in formalin, opened by surgeon or pathologist, unopened, etc.
2. How the specimen was identified: labeled (with name, number) and anatomic site designation as, e.g., right partial vertical laryngectomy, modified neck dissection, etc.
3. Describe portions of larynx included with specimen including other structures that may be attached: hyoid bone, adjacent pharynx, thyroid and parathyroid glands, and tracheal rings

4. Measure the overall dimensions of all specimens received
5. Tumor description
   Size (give in three dimensions)
   Shape (ulcerating, exophytic, polypoid)
   Color
   Necrosis
   Multifocal growth
6. Location of the tumor: describe all anatomic structures involved including ventricles, which cords, right and/or left, true and/or false cord (specify clearly). Distance above and/or below false and true cords, respectively. Involvement of aryepiglottic folds: does tumor cross midline or extend more than 1 cm from below true vocal cord? If tumor crosses the midline, estimate the percentage of tumor on right and left sides. Is there submucosal spread?
7. Depth of invasion, involvement of cartilage (note specific cartilages involved)
8. Involvement of extralaryngeal structures, thyroid, soft tissue prelaryngeal (delphian) lymph node, and parathyroid glands
9. Describe tracheotomy site if present. Presence or absence of tumor
10. Lymph node dissection if included
    Type; extended radical, radical, or modified radical or selective. Inclusion of sternomastoid muscle/submandibular and/or parotid gland/jugular vein
    Palpable mass (solitary, matted)
    Size and location of gross invasion of adjacent soft tissues, muscle, and jugular vein
    Measure and describe sternomastoid muscle, major salivary glands, and internal jugular vein

Measure size of lymph nodal masses (see No. 3)

Larynx Carcinoma Check List
1. Topography
   Larynx _____
   Partial larynx _____
   Neck dissection _____
2. Procedure
   Total laryngectomy _____
   Partial laryngectomy _____
   Supraglottic (horizontal) _____
   Hemilaryngectomy (vertical) _____

Radical neck dissection _____

Partial neck dissection _____

3. Exact site of tumor

Supraglottic _____

Glottic _____

Subglottic _____

Transglottic _____

4. Histologic type

CIS/severe dysplasia only _____

Squamous cell carcinoma _____

Keratinizing _____

Nonkeratinizing _____

Undifferentiated carcinoma _____

Salivary gland carcinoma (specify) _____

Neuroendocrine carcinoma _____

Well differentiated (carcinoid) _____

Moderately differentiated (atypical carcinoid) _____

Poorly differentiated (small cell carcinoma) _____

Papillary (exophytic) squamous cell carcinoma _____

Spindle cell carcinoma _____

Verrucous carcinoma _____

Basaloid squamous carcinoma _____

Adenosquamous carcinoma _____

Adenocarcinoma, nonsalivary type _____

Other cancer (specify) _____

5. Histologic grade

Well differentiated _____

Moderately differentiated _____

Poorly differentiated _____

Undifferentiated _____

6. Tumor extent

Commissure	Anterior _____	Posterior _____
Ventricle	Right _____	Left _____
False cord	Right _____	Left _____
True cord	Right _____	Left _____
Subglottic region	Right _____	Left _____
Aryepiglottic fold	Right _____	Left _____
Vallecula _____		
Pyriform sinus	Right _____	Left _____
Epiglottis _____	Right _____	Left _____

Extralaryngeal structures

Thyroid _____

Soft tissue _____

Prelaryngeal (delphian) lymph node _____

Parathyroid glands _____

Tumor invades cartilage	Yes _____	No _____
Vascular invasion	Yes _____	No _____
Neural invasion	Yes _____	No _____
Tracheostomy invasion	Yes _____	No _____
Multicentric tumor	Yes _____	No _____
CIS/dysplasia present	Yes _____	No _____
Verrucous hyperplasia present	Yes _____	No _____

7. Status of surgical margins (specify specimen margins or margins separately submitted)

Free of tumor _____

Involved by tumor (specify) _____

8. Lymph node metastases

Number of nodes involved	Right _____	
Number of nodes involved	Left _____	
Extracapsular invasions	Present _____	
Jugular vein invasion	Present _____	
Muscle invasion	Present _____	
Keratin debris	Present _____	

9. Preoperative treatment effects on nodes Yes _____ No _____

10. Special investigations performed

Flow cytometry _____

Electron microscopy _____

Image analysis _____

Molecular diagnostics _____

Gross photograph _____

Note 1. The American Joint Committee on Cancer divides the larynx into the following three regions: supraglottis, glottis, and subglottis. The supraglottis comprises the epiglottis (both its lingual and laryngeal aspects), arytenoepiglottic folds (laryngeal aspect), arytenoids, and ventricular bands (false cords). The inferior boundary of the supraglottis is a horizontal plane passing through the apex of the ventricle. The glottis comprises the true vocal cords, including the anterior and posterior commissures. The lower boundary is the horizontal plane, 1 cm below the apex of the ventricle. The subglottis is the region extending from the lower boundary of the glottis to the lower margin of the cricoid cartilage.

Note 2. Histologic type (World Health Organization Classification, modified)

Squamous cell carcinoma, typical, keratinizing or nonkeratinizing, invasive or in situ

Spindle cell squamous (sarcomatoid) carcinoma

Verrucous carcinoma

Basaloid squamous carcinoma

Undifferentiated carcinoma (including lymphoepithelioma)

Salivary gland type tumors

Adenoid cystic carcinoma

Mucoepidermoid carcinoma

Adenosquamous carcinoma

Others

Neuroendocrine carcinoma

Well differentiated (carcinoid tumor)

Moderately differentiated (atypical carcinoid tumor)

Poorly differentiated (small cell carcinoma)

Adenocarcinoma, nonsalivary gland type

Other cancers (sarcoma, melanoma, etc.)

Note 3. It is generally recognized that most masses greater than 3 cm in diameter are not single lymph nodes but represent confluent nodes or tumor in soft tissues of the neck.

REFERENCES

1. Gnepp DR, Barnes L, Crissman J, Zarbo R. Recommendations for the reporting of larynx specimens containing laryngeal neoplasms. Am J Clin Pathol 1998; 110: 137–139.

Pulmonary and cardiovascular systems and serosal membranes

Diffuse lung diseases

17

Kevin O. Leslie   Nestor L. Müller   Thomas V. Colby

INTRODUCTION

Diffuse lung diseases comprise mainly inflammatory processes that involve the structural elements of this organ. Some of these are caused by infections, but most are a result of immune-inflammatory, environmental, or toxic mechanisms. These diseases are presented together because they all tend to produce bilateral abnormalities on chest imaging studies and are mainly non-neoplastic conditions. Historically, diffuse lung diseases have been treated empirically, typically without the need for biopsy. The advent of the AIDS epidemic and newer sampling techniques has dramatically increased the probability that the general pathologist will be confronted with a surgical lung biopsy and be called upon to help establish a specific and clinically relevant diagnosis.

It is the rare lung biopsy that arrives with a specific question such as 'Is this methotrexate toxicity?' More commonly, the clinical diagnosis is simply 'Rule out interstitial lung disease.' Using the approach outlined in the pages that follow, the general pathologist is empowered with the tools of the lung pathology specialist, and becomes capable of arriving at a narrow differential diagnosis in most cases or even a specific diagnosis in some. To use the information in this chapter most effectively, it is essential to know the clinical condition of the patient and the rapidity with which the disease has progressed. With this information in hand, Table 17.1 provides a list of the potential diseases that should be included in the differential diagnosis. The specific histopathologic abnormalities produced by each of these are presented later in the chapter to help narrow the differential diagnosis.

First, we present a brief overview of the microscopic anatomy of the lung, for without a standardized 'map' of the lung architecture, understanding distribution of disease (and thereby diagnostic patterns) is impossible. Second, we review available sampling methods used by pulmonologists and surgeons for obtaining diagnostic specimens, including guidelines for how these should be handled for optimal results. Third, we introduce basic definitions and concepts, with a special emphasis on the limited patterns of disease and how they help refine diagnostic considerations when coupled with the clinical presentation of disease. This chapter is organized into the following 10 categories:

I. Microscopic anatomy,
II. General concepts,
III. Basic lung radiology,
IV. Handling of lung tissue samples,
V. Pattern analysis approach to surgical lung biopsies,
VI. Acute, subacute and chronic diffuse parenchymal diseases,
VII. Diffuse diseases of the airways,
VIII. Diffuse pulmonary vascular diseases,
IX. Pathology of lung transplantation, and
X. Miscellaneous diffuse lung diseases.

MICROSCOPIC ANATOMY

The lung structure relevant to this chapter begins with the trachea and conducting airways and ends with the alveolar gas exchange units. This overview is intended to refresh the surgical

Table 17.1 Clinical presentation and differential diagnosis in diffuse lung disease

Acute (days to a week or two)	Subacute (weeks to many months)	Chronic (many months to years)
Diffuse alveolar damage		
Infection	Collagen vascular diseases	Idiopathic pulmonary fibrosis/UIP
Drugs/gas/fume toxicity	Some chronic infections	Collagen vascular diseases
Collagen vascular diseases	Hypersensitivity pneumonitis	Pneumoconiosis
Acute eosinophilic pneumonia	Pneumoconioses	Pulmonary Langerhans cell histiocytosis
Idiopathic (AIP)	Sarcoidosis	Non-specific interstitial pneumonia (fibrotic)
Diffuse alveolar hemorrhage	Non-specific interstitial pneumonia (cellular)	Respiratory bronchiolitis – ILD (RBILD)
	Chronic eosinophilic pneumonia	Sarcoidosis
	Diffuse alveolar hemorrhage	Small airways disease
	Pulmonary Langerhans cell histiocytosis	
	Bronchiolitis	

AIP = Acute interstitial pneumonia
UIP = Usual interstitial pneumonia
ILD = Interstitial lung disease
RBILD = Respiratory bronchiolitis associated interstitial lung disease

pathologist's existing knowledge of the normal lung. For the reader interested in greater detail, the comprehensive and authoritative review of gross and microscopic lung anatomy by Nagaishi is recommended.[1]

THE CONDUCTING AIRWAYS

Each of the major divisions of the tracheobronchial tree (trachea, bronchi, bronchioles) has a specific role in lung function.

The *trachea* is the gateway to the lung and experiences effects of exposure to environmental factors in highest concentration. This rigid tube is designed for conducting gas, with C-shaped cartilage rings that protect it from frontal injury and also prevent collapse during the changes in intrathoracic pressure that occur during respiration. The open side of the cartilage ring faces posteriorly, where the trachealis muscle completes the tracheal circumference. This arrangement allows the esophagus to abut the 'soft' side of the trachea, down to the level of the carina. Respiratory epithelium (pseudostratified, ciliated, columnar type), submucous glands, and smooth muscle combine to prepare inspired air for use in the lung by adding moisture and warmth, while trapping dust particles and chemical vapor droplets before they can reach more delicate peripheral lung. For all these reasons, when diseases affect the trachea, the potential for impact on general respiratory function is significant.

The *bronchi* are the large conducting airways with cartilage. Like the trachea, the cartilage of the mainstem bronchi is C-shaped but this configuration changes to that of puzzle piece-like cartilage plates once the bronchus enters the lung parenchyma. These cartilage plates decrease in density progressively as the bronchial diameter decreases, resulting in increasing area between individual plates. Mucous glands are positioned just beneath the surface epithelium and may be readily seen in endobronchial biopsies. When inflamed, or distorted by crush artifact, they may simulate granulomas or tumor. These glands connect to the airway lumen by a short duct. As the bronchi divide and subdivide successively, their lumens become ever smaller on their way to the air exchange units of the lung. Because each branch lumen is more than 50% of the diameter of the preceding airway, total lumenal volume actually *increases* with each successive branching, allowing for decreased resistance to airflow as one proceeds distally.

The *bronchioles* are the final air conductors and lack cartilage altogether (therefore sometimes referred to as 'membranous'). The bronchioles have no alveoli; these are acquired more distally in the pulmonary acinus. A schematic diagram of the peripheral lung is shown in Figure 17.1. The cells that line the airways down to the level of the smaller bronchioles are columnar in shape and ciliated. Each cell is polarized toward the airway lumen and touches the basement membrane, but each cell's nucleus is present at a different level relative to the basement membrane (a phenomenon referred to a *pseudostratification*). In the smallest bronchioles (the respiratory bronchioles) the lining epithelial cells become basally oriented and more cuboidal in shape. Under normal circumstances mucus-secreting cells are sparse (Fig. 17.2) and difficult to identify in the epithelium of terminal and respiratory bronchioles. Goblet cells may be prominent and distended with mucous in situations where chronic airway irritation occurs, such as seen in smokers and in asthmatic patients (Fig. 17.3).

Neuroendocrine cells are present in the conducting airway epithelium, typically as single cells with clear cytoplasm, but rarely they may be present in groups, forming so-called *neuroepithelial bodies*. Immunohistochemical stains show these cells to be reactive

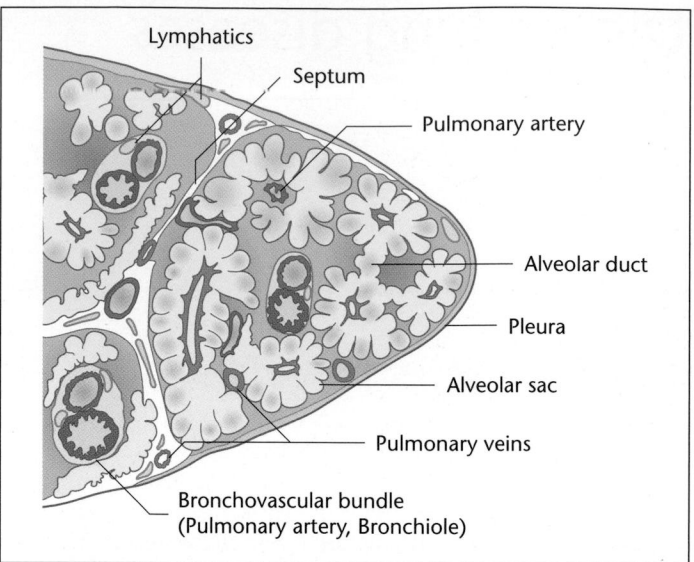

Fig. 17.1 The peripheral lung. Schematic illustration of the peripheral lung parenchyma demonstrating the general relationships that exist between elements of the secondary pulmonary lobules (not drawn to scale). (From Colby et al. Atlas of pulmonary surgical pathology. WB Saunders; 1991, with permission.)

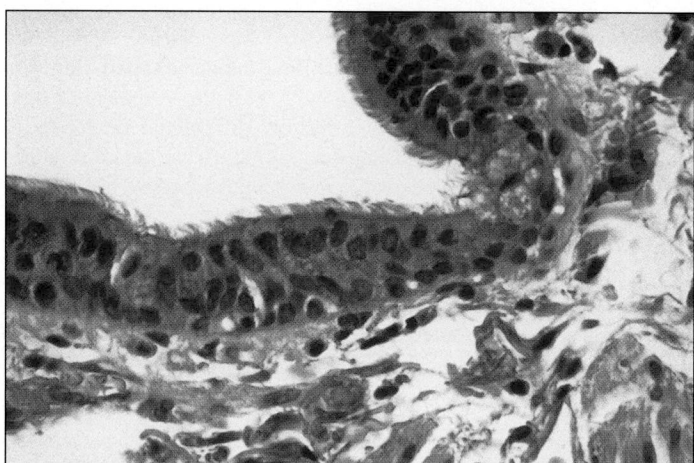

Fig. 17.2 Airway epithelium. The cells that line the airways are columnar in shape and ciliated. Their nuclei are pseudostratified down to the level of the smaller bronchioles, where they become basal with a more cuboidal cell shape. Scattered mucous cells (goblet cells) can be seen as individual pale blue globules, between columnar cells.

with antibodies directed against the common neuroendocrine markers, chromogranin A and synaptophysin, as well as more esoteric neuropeptides. The exact function of these cells is unknown. It has been hypothesized that they play a role as sensory cells in ventilation-perfusion matching and may even play a role in airway morphogenesis during gestation.[2]

Bronchus-associated lymphoid tissue (BALT) is analogous to the mucosa-associated lymphoid tissue (MALT) of the gastrointestinal tract.[3] BALT is located primarily at airway divisions where inhaled antigens and other particles are likely to impact.[4] BALT consists of specialized epithelial cells in the mucosa and closely associated

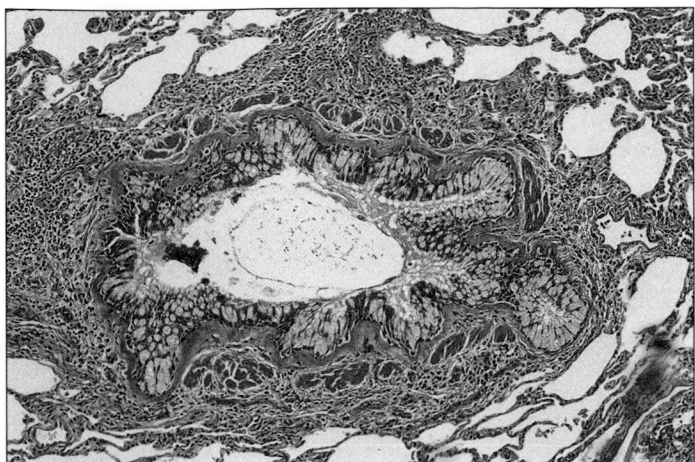

Fig. 17.3 Epithelial goblet cells. Under normal circumstances mucus-secreting cells are sparse and difficult to identify in the epithelium of small bronchioles. They may be prominent and distended with mucous in smokers or asthmatic patients, as illustrated here, where mucous cells seem to outnumber columnar cells.

aggregates of lymphocytes, with admixed macrophages, and dendritic cells. The epithelial cells of BALT likely play a role in the detection of inhaled allergens, viruses, and bacteria, the antigens of which are presented to the lymphoid tissue. BALT is a critical component of the defense mechanism of the lung. BALT may become hyperplastic, with germinal center formation, in a number of diseases. When this occurs, germinal centers may be sampled on bronchoscopic biopsies and can pose a diagnostic challenge when crushed or cut in such a way that follicular center cells appear as a nodule or sheet in the specimen. BALT may also be important in diseases of immunologic origin that produce bronchiolitis, such as Sjögren's syndrome, rheumatoid arthritis, graft-versus-host disease, and transplantation.

Lymphoid aggregates are seen commonly in lung biopsies but are uncommon (or do not exist at all) under normal conditions. They have no capsule and are composed of B cells, T cells, and dendritic cells. Lymphoid aggregates increase in the lungs of cigarette smokers,[4,5] and may be found in the interlobular septa, in the pleura, and in the subpleurally connective tissue.[6] Lymphoid aggregates may be the source of the condition known as *diffuse lymphoid hyperplasia*.

Dendritic cells throughout the body are capable of presenting antigen to T lymphocytes. Dendritic cells occur in the epithelium and subepithelial tissue of the airways. They have a reniform, eccentric nucleus, prominent cytoplasmic protrusions and they strongly express major histocompatibility antigens.[7] A subpopulation of dendritic cells carries the Langerhans cell marker[5] (and contains so-called 'Birbeck' granules ultrastructurally).[8] Langerhans cells are prominent in the lungs of smokers, and can be identified by immunohistochemical techniques using antibodies directed against S-100 protein and CD1a. These cells are involved in the smoking-related disease known as pulmonary Langerhans cell histiocytosis (formerly known as pulmonary eosinophilic granuloma or histiocytosis X.)

The *basement membrane* lies immediately beneath the airway epithelium and is visible in routine stains as a delicate eosinophilic line, mainly by association with a matrix of type III collagen. A fine layer of elastic tissue is present beneath the epithelial basement membrane. When chronic injury to the airway occurs, this elastic tissue becomes separated from the overlying basement membrane by collagen.

The *smooth muscle of the airways* is arranged in a complex spiral pattern and receives nutrition from the bronchial arteries. The *bronchovascular bundle* is composed of the airway, the accompanying pulmonary artery, a common adventitia, and a sheath of loose connective tissue. The connective tissue of the bronchovascular bundle progressively diminishes in the smallest bronchioles.

The *terminal bronchiole* is the last conducting bronchiole before alveoli begin to appear. The *acinus*, where most of the gas exchange occurs, begins distal to the terminal bronchiole. As one proceeds distally, the elements of the acinus include the *respiratory bronchioles, the alveolar ducts, and the alveolar sacs*. Respiratory bronchioles have more alveoli in their walls with each succeeding distal generation, finally culminating in the alveolar ducts, which are entirely alveolated. The *alveolar sac* is present at the end of the alveolar duct and is made up entirely of alveoli. As the airways of the acinus branch and diminish in diameter progressively, the transition from ciliated cells to flattened epithelium occurs abruptly.

THE ALVEOLI

Most of the alveolar surface is covered by extremely flat, *type I epithelial cells*, which are not easily seen with the light microscope. The thinness of the type I epithelial cell is well suited for gas exchange. *Type II epithelial cells* are cuboidal in shape and limited in number per alveolus. They are present at places where the alveolar walls form angles with each other. The surface of the type II cell facing the alveolar airspace has microvilli that may on occasion be identified by light microscopy as slight roughening. Type II cells contain large numbers of organelles and are responsible for the production of surfactant, a substance that lowers surface tension, and is essential for preventing alveolar collapse at end exhalation when intra-alveolar pressure is low. Type II cells are the progenitor cells of the alveolar type I cells and after an injury, divide and replace them. Tight junctions join adjacent type I and type II cells and represent a physical barrier between the interstitial fluid and the alveolar air.

Alveolar macrophages play an essential role as phagocytes in the lung. Under appropriate stimulation, these cells secrete soluble factors that are an essential part of the lung's defense mechanism and response to injury.

The *alveolar walls* are made up of capillaries,[9] the extracellular matrix, and sparse cellular elements, including mast cells, smooth muscle cells, pericytes, connective tissue cells, and occasional lymphocytes. The connective tissue cells of the interstitium have been the subject of considerable study. Unstimulated, they resemble fibroblasts and have few organelles. During the repair phase of an injury, actin and myosin appear allowing these *myofibroblasts* to perform a contractile role in lung repair.[10–12] *Capillary endothelial cells* within the acinus are joined by tight or semi-tight junctions. The semi-tight junctions exist to allow large molecules to traverse the capillary wall. When the type I cell is damaged, widening of these junctions allows the formation of alveolar edema. Type II cells proliferate to repopulate the alveolar lining, eventually changing shape to become flattened type I cells. A delicate capillary net is present for gas exchange.

THE VASCULAR SYSTEM

The lung has muscular arteries that carry venous blood from the right heart to the acinus. Pulmonary arteries accompany the airways, so the blood vessel next to an airway is typically an artery. In cross-

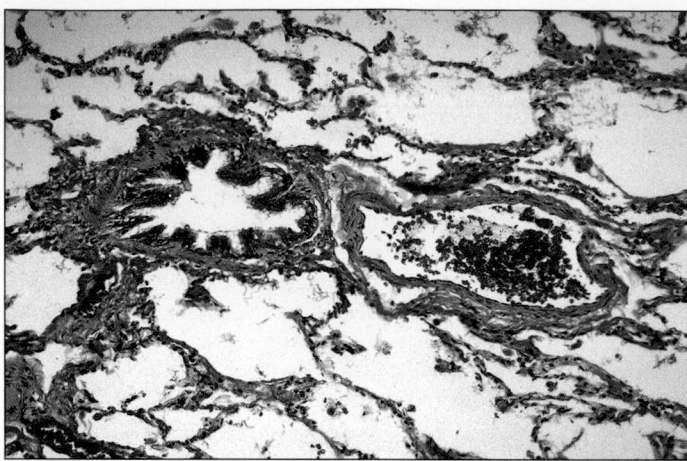

Fig. 17.4 Pulmonary arteries. In cross-sectional view, the pulmonary arterial diameter should be approximately equal to that of the accompanying airway.

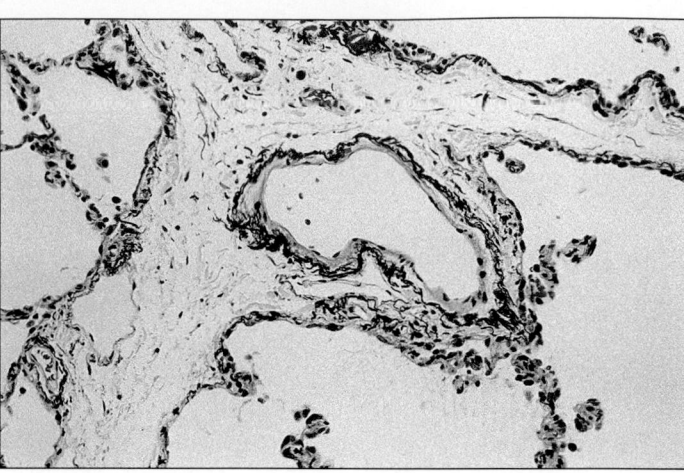

Fig. 17.5 Pulmonary veins. A pulmonary vein within an intralobular septum. The walls of veins are much thinner than those of arteries and in general have a single, poorly formed external elastic lamina and no muscle. (Elastic van Gieson's stain)

sectional view, the arterial diameter should be approximately equal to that of the accompanying airway (Fig. 17.4). The paired artery and airway are destined to arrive at the center of the acinus. In contrast, the pulmonary veins exit from the venous side of the capillary bed, beginning in the alveolar walls and travel along interlonular septa at the periphery of the secondary pulmonary lobule. To identify veins in lung tissue the simplest method is to find a pleural surface and follow an interlobular septum off this into the lung parenchyma (Fig. 17.5). In the adult, two or more elastic laminae are present in arteries larger than 1 mm in diameter. Arteries between 100 and 200 μm (0.1–0.2 mm) are muscular, and have an internal and external elastic lamina. Smaller arteries may be muscular or nonmuscular. The two elastic layers appear fused in smaller vessels owing to progressive attenuation of spiral smooth muscle fibers. Where muscle is absent, a single fragmented elastic lamina is all that separates intima from adventitia. In the adult, arterial muscle extends down to the level of the alveoli. The ratio of arterial wall thickness to external arterial diameter is often a useful marker for abnormality. Nondistended muscular arteries have a medial thickness that represents about 5% of external arterial diameter. The *pulmonary veins* begin in the alveolus, extend to the periphery of the acinus and travel along the interlobular septa carrying oxygenated blood to the hilum and finally to the left atrium. Veins coalesce on their journey to the heart, forming progressively larger structures that lie separate from arteries and airways. Pulmonary veins have very little smooth muscle, and typically have an ill-defined external elastic lamina. Elastic lamina increase in prominence and number in larger diameter veins.

THE LYMPHATIC SYSTEM

The alveoli have no defined lymphatic channels, so the interstitial space serves as the conduit for extracellular water before this encounters the opening of a lymphatic channel on the venous side of the capillary bed or centrally in the acinus in close association with small arteries. The pulmonary lymphatics typically begin at the periphery of the acinus or lobule, and where alveoli abut bronchovascular sheaths. The lymphatics are thinner than veins of equal diameter, are surrounded by a loose connective tissue matrix, and are lined by endothelial cells.

Like veins, the pulmonary lymphatics have valves that help direct the flow of lymph. As mentioned, the lymphatics proceed toward the hilum along a number of different routes, typically within the bronchovascular bundles and interlobular septa, where they are present adjacent to veins. The most peripheral regions of the lung rely on lymphatic arcades that first drain to the pleura, and then rejoin central perivenous lymphatics in the interlobular septa on their way back to the hilum.

THE INTERSTITIUM

The interstitium begins as the tissue space that exists *between* the structures of gas exchange in the alveolar wall and extends along the bronchovascular bundles, veins, and lymphatics, culminating with the connective tissue of the interlobular septa and the pleura. The interstitium can be visualized as an interconnected compartment, from the hilum to the pleura and, as might be predicted by this arrangement, pleural and septal fibrosis often accompany diseases that produce diffuse interstitial fibrosis of the alveolar parenchyma.

GENERAL CONCEPTS

THE MULTIDISCIPLINARY APPROACH

As emphasized in previous editions, the interpretation of lung biopsies for diffuse (mainly non-neoplastic) diseases is best accomplished using a multidisciplinary approach, leading to a clinico-radiologic-pathologic diagnosis. In a perfect world pathologist, radiologist, chest physician, and thoracic surgeon would discuss every patient before and after a biopsy sample was taken, with each specialist sharing their unique view of the patient's clinical problem. Unfortunately, the real world doesn't always allow such focused interaction. For neoplasms, it may be possible for the pathologist to function alone, with minimal input (e.g. knowledge as to whether a mass lesion is present or not). For the diffuse lung diseases, the pathologist must have some essential information regarding the clinical and radiologic findings in order to arrive at a clinically meaningful diagnosis. In many instances more extensive clinical and radiologic consultation may be necessary. Moreover, biopsy findings in diseases characterized by the accumulation of inflammatory cells may be interpreted as non-specific without information regarding the acuity of symptoms, the characteristics of disease onset, the distribution of radiologic abnormalities, and any critical past medical history, such as the presence of a connective tissue disease (or serologic abnormalities), types of medication used, and environmental exposures.

DIFFUSE LUNG DISEASE

There has been debate over the years regarding the best nomenclature for describing the diffuse lung diseases as a group. Our clinical colleagues have firmly entrenched the term 'interstitial lung disease' to describe diffuse parenchymal diseases. In part, this is based on the notion that disease of the lung parenchyma generally evolves from the cellular 'interstitial' compartment of the lung, even if the disease manifests primarily within the alveolar spaces (e.g. organizing pneumonia). For the pathologist rigid in the notion of strict anatomical reference, the term 'interstitial' seems too narrow, implying only disease that involves the lung interstitium. The term 'infiltrative' was proposed in a previous edition of this chapter as a more inclusive term, encompassing the acquisition of cells and matrix in any compartment of the lung, including the airspaces. A more detailed discussion of the concept of diffuse infiltrative lung disease can be found elsewhere.[13] For our purposes in this chapter, diffuse lung diseases are those that are widespread in the lung and typically result in radiologically observable increased density of lung parenchyma (opacification), typically with a multilobe and/or bilateral distribution.[14] Depending on the disease, and the timing of biopsy relative to onset of symptoms, the pathologic abnormalities seen in the diffuse lung diseases may be interstitial, airway centered, intra-alveolar, intravascular, or involve combinations of these anatomic compartments.

RESTRICTIVE LUNG DISEASE

Restrictive lung disease implies impaired maximal filling of the lung with air on inspiration, and corresponds to diminished total lung capacity by pulmonary function testing. This term is applied most often in the context of a patient with extensive bilateral pulmonary radiologic abnormalities, referred to as *infiltrative, interstitial, or diffuse* lung disease. This correlation is based in part on the notion that the lungs may be 'stiff' or noncompliant in these conditions, typically as a result of cellular infiltration with or without matrix deposition (fibrosis). Importantly, not all patients with *restrictive* lung disease have *diffuse* lung disease, or even disease of the lungs, per se. By the same token, not all patients with diffuse lung disease have a restrictive pattern on lung function testing.

BASIC LUNG RADIOLOGY

In clinical practice today, high-resolution computed tomography (HRCT) is increasingly relied upon for the evaluation of diffuse lung disease. HRCT provides a reasonable approximation of gross lung pathology as seen in sections of fixed, inflated autopsy lungs. Because of this, the nomenclature used by radiologists in the interpretation of these scans is important for the pathologist to know, in order to correlate these with traditional histopathologic findings in tissue.[15] To this end, we include here a 'glossary' of terms used by radiologists,

their implication regarding lung biopsy findings, and their relation to known diffuse lung diseases.

In general, HRCT refers to scans performed at approximately 1 mm thickness, so summation effect is minimal. Still, the pathologic abnormalities detected under the microscope for many structures (alveoli, alveolar ducts, respiratory bronchioles) are not directly discernible by this technique. Radiologists reviewing HRCT scans report two key features: composition of an observed change in density (opacity), and distribution within the anatomy of the lung.

The images obtained can be divided into categories that alone and in various combinations are strongly indicative or even diagnostic, especially when their location is taken into account. These categories are descriptive and include 5 main patterns: linear, cystic, nodular, ground glass, and consolidation.[15] Ground-glass opacity is a hazy increase in opacity through which normal vessels can still be identified.[16] It usually reflects the presence of mild interstitial thickening or partial filling of the airspaces. Consolidation is considered present when the increase in lung opacity obscures the vessels on HRCT. CT sections can be compared with surfaces of fixed, distended slices cut in the same plane as CT. This comparison has taught both pathologists and radiologists a good deal about the gross appearance of diseased lungs (Fig. 17.6). It is important to realize that, although the radiologic images are as clear as the gross specimen, the limit of resolution is about 0.3 mm. CT has the obvious advantages over the biopsy because the whole lung can be visualized, the extent and nature of the disease can be recognized, and the changes that occur over time can be appreciated.

In a study of 118 consecutive patients with chronic infiltrative lung disease, without knowledge of the clinical features or diagnosis, three radiologists were able to make a confident diagnosis in 49% of CT scans (compared with 23% in chest radiographs): in 93%, this was correct (77% in radiographs).[17] An approximately twofold improvement in diagnostic accuracy of HRCT over the chest radiograph was confirmed in a subsequent study.[18] Several studies have shown a particularly high diagnostic accuracy of HRCT in the diagnosis of idiopathic pulmonary fibrosis and cystic lung diseases such as Langerhans cell histiocytosis and lymphangioleiomyomatosis.[19,20]

TYPES OF ABNORMALITIES

Opacity/opacification: Any density visible on scan images that exceeds that expected for air and normal lung tissue.

Linear opacities: Linear opacities reflect the presence of thickening of the pulmonary interstitium by fluid, cells, or other tissue. Fluid, as seen in interstitial pulmonary edema or lymphatic obstruction by tumor, leads to smooth thickening of the interlobular septa (known on HRCT as septal lines) (Fig. 17.7). Interstitial fibrosis results in irregular linear opacities and a reticular pattern. A reticular pattern is seen in a number of fibrosing lung diseases such as UIP, NSIP, sarcoidosis, and asbestosis (Fig. 17.8). The differential diagnosis of these entities on HRCT is based on the distribution of fibrosis (e.g. typically predominately subpleural and basal in UIP) and the presence of associated findings (e.g. presence of pleural plaques in asbestosis).

Cystic opacities: Cystic opacities (also known as lung cysts) refer to circumscribed, rounded or oval lesions with well-defined walls. On HRCT, cystic opacities containing air are seen most commonly in pulmonary fibrosis (honeycomb cysts), Langerhans cell histiocytosis, and lymphangioleiomyomatosis (Fig. 17.9). Honeycomb cysts visible on HRCT range in size from approximately 3 mm to 2 cm, and are typically found in association with a reticular pattern. Cystic lung disease is distinguished from emphysema by the presence of distinct

Fig. 17.6 Radiology: CT comparison with macroscopic pathology. A comparison of the CT image of the lingula (**A**) and macroscopic lung sections taken from a biopsy of the tip of the lingula (**B**) in a patient with lymphangitic carcinoma. The scan image shows polygonal lines in the anterior lung. Nodular densities in the centers of these lines represent tumor growth along lymphatic routes of the bronchovascular sheath. Corresponding findings in the lung biopsy sections can be seen. The darker areas of septal and bronchovascular bundle thickening fibrosis (short arrows) represent tumor, while paler areas (curved arrow) represent fibrosis. (From Munk PL, Müller NL, Miller RR, Ostrow DN. Pulmonary lymphangitic carcinomatosis: CT and pathologic findings. Radiology 1988; 166:705–709.)

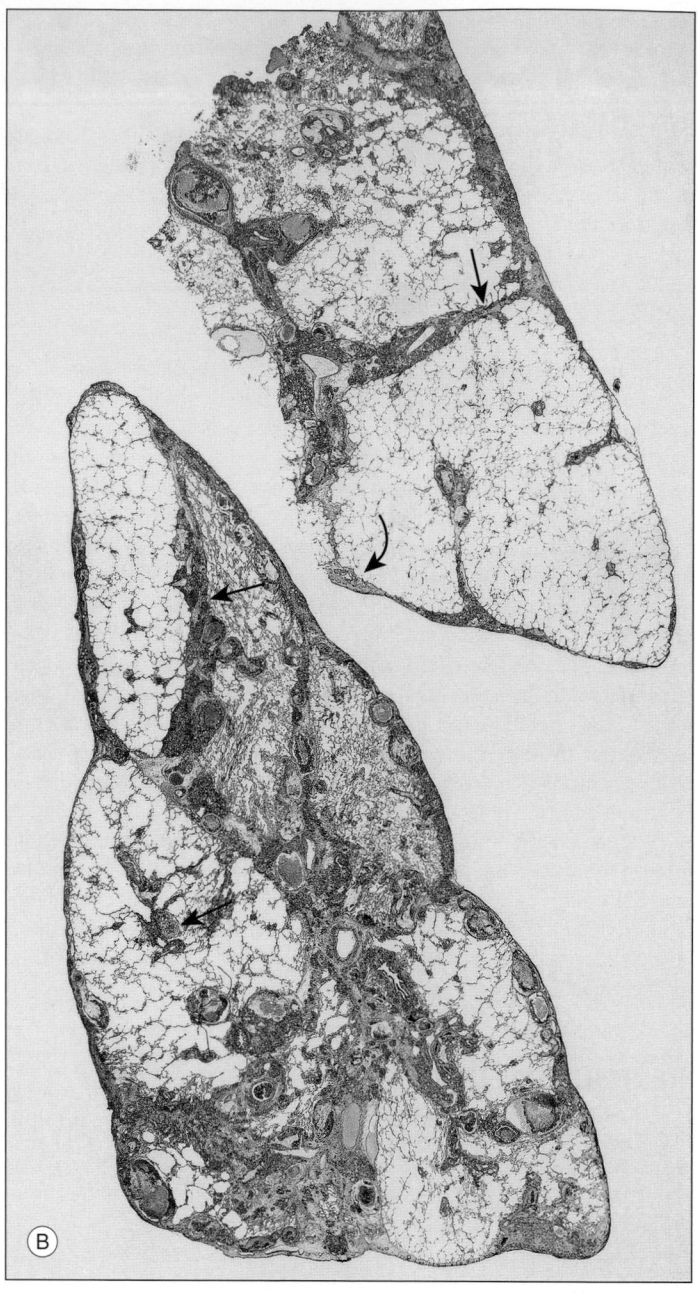

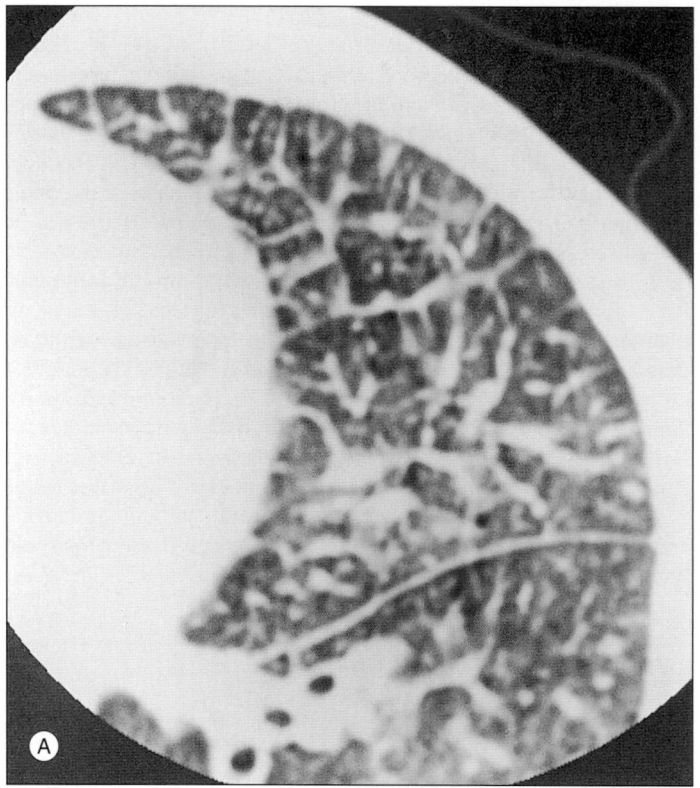

walls. Emphysema is characterized on HRCT by the presence of localized areas of low attenuation without walls.

Nodular opacities: A nodular opacity (nodule) is a rounded opacity that measures less than 3 cm in diameter. Nodular opacities measuring less than 1 cm in diameter are seen in a number of lung diseases including sarcoidosis, silicosis, Langerhans histiocytosis, pulmonary metastases, and miliary tuberculosis (Fig. 17.10). The nodules seen on HRCT in sarcoidosis reflect the presence of conglomeration of sarcoid granulomata and have a characteristic perilymphatic distribution (Fig. 17.11).

Ground-glass opacities: Ground-glass opacity refers to a hazy increase in lung density that is not sufficiently opaque so as to obscure underlying lung structure (airways, vessels). It is a relatively non-specific finding that can reflect the presence of mild interstitial thickening or mild airspace disease. Lung diseases commonly associated with ground-glass opacities are cellular non-specific

interstitial pneumonia (NSIP), hypersensitivity pneumonitis, *Pneumocystis jiroveci* pneumonia, and alveolar proteinosis (Fig. 17.12).

Consolidation: Consolidation is defined as homogenous opacification of sufficient density so as to obscure underlying lung structure normally visible on scans. Also known as *airspace filling*, this abnormality can be seen in a number of conditions, including chronic eosinophilic pneumonia, cryptogenic organizing pneumonia, diffuse alveolar damage, and diffuse pulmonary hemorrhage (Fig. 17.13).

LOCATION OF ABNORMALITIES

The radiologic differential diagnosis of diffuse lung diseases is based on pattern of abnormality, the distribution of abnormalities, and the presence of associated findings such as symmetric bilateral hilar and mediastinal lymphadenopathy in sarcoidosis and pleural

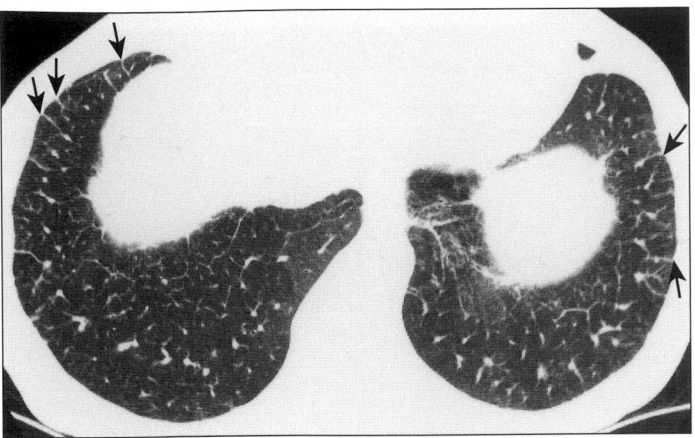

Fig. 17.7 Radiology: Septal lines. High-resolution CT image shows bilateral smooth septal lines (arrows) seen as 1–2 cm long lines extending to the pleura. These reflect the presence of thickening of the interlobular septa. The patient had interstitial edema due to fluid overload.

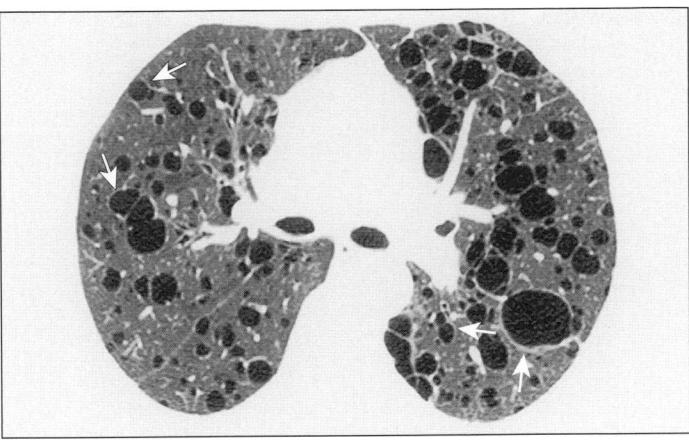

Fig. 17.9 Radiology: Cystic pattern. High-resolution CT image shows bilateral areas of air density surrounded by a thin wall (arrows). These reflect the presence of parenchymal cysts. The patient was a 51-year-old woman with lymphangioleiomyomatosis.

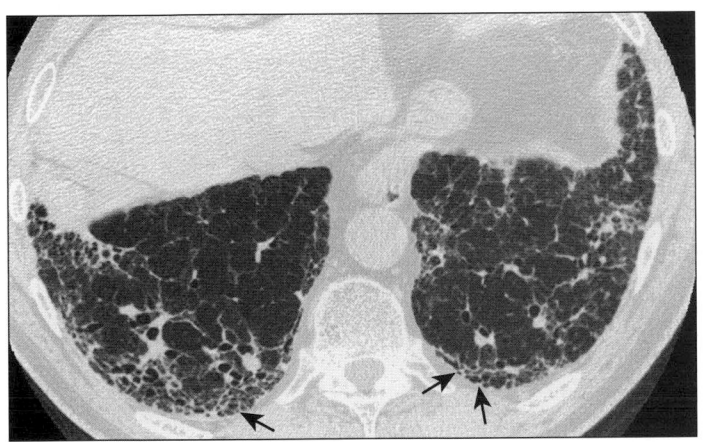

Fig. 17.8 Radiology: Reticular pattern. High-resolution CT image shows numerous small irregular lines (arrows) forming a mesh (reticular pattern). The lines are only a few millimeters long and a few millimeters apart, indicating that they are located within the secondary pulmonary lobule. A reticular pattern usually reflects the presence of fibrosis. The patient was a 79-year-old man with usual interstitial pneumonia (idiopathic pulmonary fibrosis).

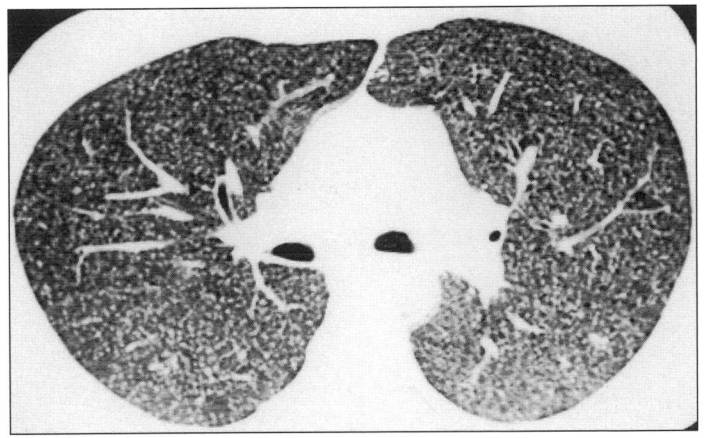

Fig. 17.10 Radiology: Nodular pattern. High-resolution CT image shows numerous nodules throughout both lungs. The nodules measure 1–2 mm in diameter and are randomly distributed. The patient was a 27-year-old woman with miliary tuberculosis.

Table 17.2 Distribution of diseases by radiologic location

Predominately upper lobe abnormalities
Sarcoidosis
Pulmonary Langerhans cell histiocytosis
Silicosis, coalworker's pneumoconiosis
Predominately mid-lung abnormalities
Hypersensitivity pneumonitis
Predominately lower lung zone abnormalities
Usual interstitial pneumonia (UIP)
Hypersensitivity pneumonitis
Asbestosis

plaques or diffuse pleural thickening in asbestosis. Although, by definition, diffuse lung diseases usually involve all lobes, some of them tend to involve mainly the upper lobes while others tend to involve mainly the lower lobes (Table 17.2).

Table 17.3 presents a list of the four major patterns of radiologic abnormality and their corresponding diseases.

HANDLING OF LUNG TISSUE SAMPLES

TECHNIQUES AND CLINICAL CONSIDERATIONS

Many patients with diffuse lung disease will ultimately require diagnostic intervention for the acquisition of cells and tissue for diagnostic evaluation. The type of procedure, site of sampling, and

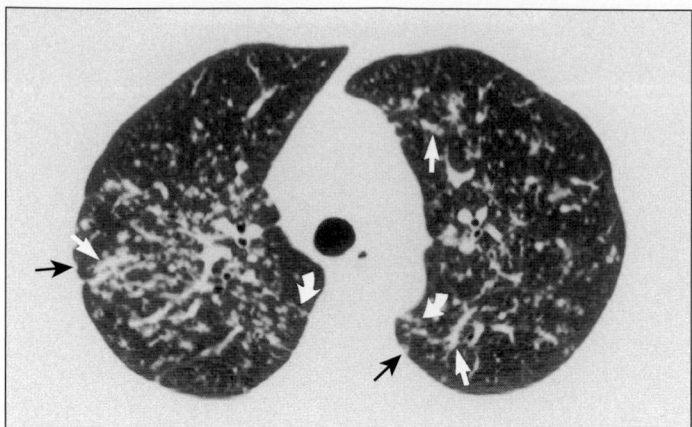

Fig. 17.11 Radiology: Nodular pattern in sarcoidosis. High-resolution CT image shows extensive nodular thickening of the pulmonary vessels (straight arrows) and minimal nodular thickening of the interlobular septa (curved arrows). Also noted are a few subpleural nodules (black arrows). The patient was a 35-year-old man with sarcoidosis.

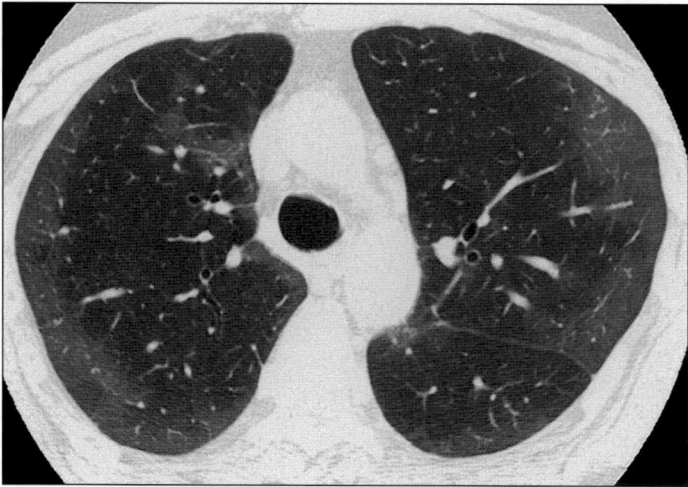

Fig. 17.12 Radiology: Ground-glass opacities. High-resolution CT image shows mild hazy increase in opacity in the peripheral lung regions. Note that the pulmonary vessels are still visible in these regions of increased opacity (ground-glass opacities). The patient was a 57-year-old woman with non-specific interstitial pneumonia (NSIP).

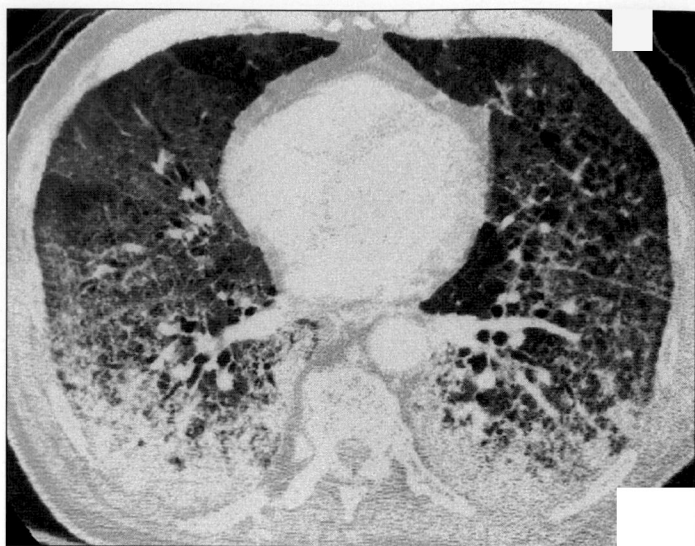

Fig. 17.13 Radiology: Airspace consolidation. High-resolution CT image shows extensive bilateral opacities. In the dorsal lung regions there is homogeneous opacification that obscures the underlying vessels. This is characteristic of airspace consolidation. In the more anterior lung regions the vessels are still visible within the areas of increased opacity (ground-glass attenuation). The patient was a 60-year-old man with diffuse alveolar damage.

Table 17.3 CT patterns of diffuse lung disease

Irregular linear pattern
Idiopathic pulmonary fibrosis
Lymphatic spread of tumor
Asbestosis
Cystic pattern
Lymphangioleiomyomatosis
Nodular pattern
Silicosis and coalworker's pneumoconiosis
Sarcoidosis
Langerhans cell histiocytosis
Hypersensitivity pneumonitis
Ground-glass pattern
Alveolar proteinosis
Chronic eosinophilic pneumonia
Cryptogenic organizing pneumonia

From Müller and Miller.[403]

laboratory techniques called upon all depend on a few basic clinical, radiologic, and pathologic questions. As a critical member of the diagnostic team, it is essential for the pathologist to understand both the advantages and limitations of the available sampling methods used for the diagnosis of lung diseases. Moreover, optimal processing for each type of sample acquired is necessary to ensure diagnostic accuracy. Fortunately, only a limited number of sampling techniques is available and the specimens they generate are few. These are presented in Table 17.4 along with optimal handling recommendations for each.

Sputum examination and bronchoalveolar lavage (BAL) have the greatest use in acute diffuse lung disease, especially in the immunocompromised host. For example, Bigby and coworkers examined saline-induced sputum in patients with the acquired immunodeficiency syndrome (AIDS) and were able to diagnose *Pneumocystis* pneumonia (PCP) in more than one-third of patients with

AIDS who had this infection, thus avoiding bronchoscopy.[21] BAL sampling in AIDS is also valuable in the diagnosis of PCP; however, it is even more useful in diagnosing other types of infection in this setting. The role of BAL in the diagnosis of chronic infiltrative disease is controversial[22] but can be effective as a diagnostic tool in a number of specific settings such as pulmonary alveolar proteinosis, eosinophilic lung disease, and sometimes in pulmonary Langerhans cell histiocytosis. Diffuse lung diseases that involve the bronchi and peribronchial tissue with a characteristic histopathologic marker (e.g. the granulomas of sarcoidosis) can be approached successfully with transbronchial biopsy (TBB). Finally, surgical lung biopsy may be required for diffuse lung diseases that involve the alveolar

Table 17.4 Diagnostic sampling techniques and their specimens

Source	Specimens and common analyses
Sputum	Cytologic smears and centrifuge preparations, cultures
Bronchoscopy with:	
Washings	Cytologic smears and centrifuge preparations, cultures
Brushings	Cytologic smears and centrifuge preparations, cultures
(Endo-) Bronchial biopsy	Forceps tissue biopsy
Transbronchial biopsy	Forceps tissue biopsy
Bronchoalveolar lavage (BAL)	Cytologic smears and centrifuge preparations, biochemical analysis, culture
Transbronchial fine needle aspiration	Cytologic smears and centrifuge preparations
Surgical 'wedge' lung biopsy (either video-assisted or open)	Tissue sample including pleura and alveolar parenchyma, material for culture
Transthoracic needle core biopsy and aspiration	Core biopsy fragment(s), and cytologic smears/centrifuge preparations
Thoracentesis	Cytologic centrifuge preparations, biochemical analysis, culture

parenchyma primarily, especially when a pattern of involvement is required for diagnosis.

The video-assisted thoracoscopic (VATS) biopsy technique is relatively new and seems to provide all of the advantages of open surgical lung biopsy (OLB), possibly with less morbidity and shorter hospitalization time.[23] Based on anecdotal observations of current pulmonary practice, it appears as though the VATS biopsy will eventually replace OLB, except in special circumstances. VATS is performed using a rigid endoscopic camera (the thoracoscope), with operator visualization accomplished using a video monitor, in contrast to the direct visualization through the thoracotomy incision used in OLB. Three short incisions are needed, one for the thoracoscope and two for the instruments (Fig. 17.14). The total amount of tissue produced by the two procedures is comparable and diagnostic accuracy is the same.[24] There are some disadvantages to the VATS technique. First, direct palpation is severely limited, so that nodular infiltrates must be visible from the pleural surface or be amenable to palpation using a single finger (once the lung is brought up to the incision.). Second, the patient must be able to withstand single lung ventilation since the lung being sampled has to be deflated by the anesthesiologist. The initial overall cost of VATS biopsy is greater than that for OLB, but shorter hospital stays after VATS biopsy may make up for this difference when comparing total costs.

A number of critical clinical questions influence the choice of a diagnostic sampling method for the patient with diffuse lung disease. Naturally, the acuity of the presentation and severity of clinical symptoms are paramount. For example, a patient seen in the clinic for slowly progressive, chronic disease with moderate symptoms might be treated empirically and handled with a 'wait and watch' attitude. By contrast, the severely ill, immunocompromised patient, on a ventilator in the intensive care unit, may require aggressive lung sampling for hour by hour management. Also, the character and distribution of infiltrates on imaging studies often provide clues that dictate the requirement for biopsy, location to be sampled, and technical approach for acquiring a sample, should this be judged necessary.

The immunocompromised host (ICH): Lung disease has become common in the current era of high-dose chemotherapy for malignant tumors, aggressive immunosuppression for autoimmune diseases and organ transplantation, and the acquired immunodeficiency of HIV infection. When immunocompromised patients present with acute respiratory symptoms, the differential diagnosis typically includes infection, drug reaction, recurrent tumor (if immunosuppression is a result of antineoplastic therapy), organ rejection (if lung transplant-

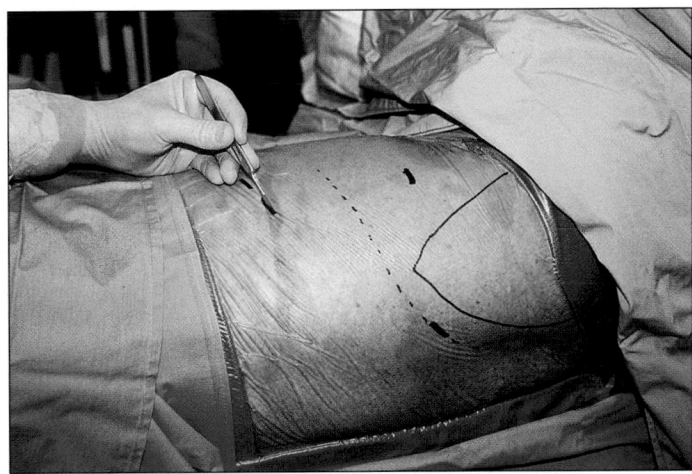

Fig. 17.14 VATS procedure. Three short incisions are needed for VATS biopsy, one for the thoracoscope and two for the instruments.

related) and new tumor (i.e. post-transplant lymphoproliferative disease) related to significant immunosuppression. The yield of different diagnostic techniques is variable. BAL is highly sensitive in detecting *Pneumocystis* pneumonia in AIDS patients[25] and may be effective in the diagnosis of cytomegalovirus (CMV) infection.[26] TBB, usually in conjunction with BAL, is a reasonably sensitive method of diagnosing infection in this setting.[27] Surgical lung biopsy is still the major means of diagnosing noninfectious infiltrates in the ICH.[28] If a wedge biopsy is required, the biopsy should be taken from the area of most prominent involvement, because this increases the probability of finding diagnostic abnormalities.[29] Preliminary microbiological results, fluorescence studies for viral antigens, and histologic examination for pattern of reaction, viral inclusions, and fungal or *Pneumocystis jiroveci* organisms should be available as soon as possible. For example, if the patient requires a biopsy after normal working hours or on a weekend, touch imprint preparations and frozen sections are typically performed by the pathologist as an intraoperative consultation. Special (e.g. silver) stains are often performed the next working day.

The patient with normal immunity: Sometimes a patient who seems to have normal immunity will present with acute diffuse lung disease, the etiology of which eludes routine diagnostic techniques.

Considerations of site of biopsy and laboratory procedure, in general, are similar to those pertaining to the ICH. Non-specific acute lung injury (diffuse alveolar damage) is often the pathologic finding, presumably due to viral or other community acquired infection, but sometimes as a lung manifestation of systemic connective tissue disease, drug toxicity, *Legionella* pneumonia, an unusual infection in an unsuspected AIDS patient, and even lymphangitic or endovascular tumor.

For chronic diffuse lung disease in the non-immunocompromised patient, the approach to type and site of biopsy, and selection of laboratory procedures, is different. For example, TBB is more likely to be diagnostic in the patient with sarcoidosis or lymphangitic carcinoma than in most other diseases. In fact, little correlation has been found between non-specific findings on TBB and definitive diagnosis established by subsequent wedge lung biopsy.[30] In the event that surgical lung biopsy should be required, the object is to sample at least one area felt to represent the 'transition zone' from normal to abnormal lung. Ideally, three biopsies should be obtained to include uninvolved, moderately involved, and more advanced disease (advanced fibrosis is an exception in the latter, given the low specificity of advanced fibrosis and significant risk for postsurgical air leak). The advent of high-resolution computed tomography (HRCT) of the lungs also allows more detailed preoperative evaluation and biopsy site selection. Moreover, HRCT is useful in distinguishing sarcoidosis and lymphangitic carcinoma from other types of chronic diffuse lung disease, assisting in the decision of whether to attempt a TBB rather than subject the patient to surgery. HRCT is also useful in assessing the distribution of disease, providing guidance to the surgeon as to the best area of accessible average involvement. Routine avoidance of the lingula and right middle lobe, once the recommended policy, no longer seems to be necessary, especially in view of the additional information provided by CT.[29] Nevertheless, selection of only middle lobe or lingula may result in less than optimal sampling. Frozen section evaluation is rarely critical in chronic diffuse lung disease, microbiologic studies may be done on a routine basis rather than urgently, and special stains for organisms may also be performed routinely on paraffin sections well after the procedure.

LUNG TISSUE PROCESSING

Once the decision has been made to acquire a lung specimen for diagnostic purposes, it is important for the pathologist to make the most of this material through appropriate handling (including microbiological cultures, if necessary), dissemination of the specimen to all required sections of the laboratory, and final processing for histopathologic examination. The suggestions provided here have been proven to be effective in our practice, but are not intended as replacements to existing functional methods the reader may already have in place. In general, bronchial washings, bronchial brushings, bronchoalveolar lavage, and needle aspirations in the diffuse lung disease setting are useful only in the diagnosis of certain infectious diseases, and rarely, metastatic cancer involving the lymphatics or vascular system of the lung. Differential cellular analysis of fluid obtained by BAL has been studied extensively, but remains primarily a research tool in current practice. In the near future, it is likely that specialized studies, such as proteomic and molecular genetic analysis, will play important diagnostic roles using these fluid samples.

Bronchial biopsy

Lesions of the trachea and proximal airways can be sampled under direct visualization using the flexible fiberoptic bronchoscope. The cupped biopsy forceps is commonly used and produces a small sample of the airway mucosa and underlying wall to variable degree. The biopsy forceps used with the flexible fiberoptic bronchoscope produce a 2–3 mm tissue sample. Careful handling is required prior to paraffin embedding, since crushing and tearing can easily occur. The biopsies are usually teased from the forceps jaws in the bronchoscopy suite, using a sterile probe or needle, and placed directly into carrying medium or fixative prior to being sent to the laboratory. A disposable styrene plastic pipette with the tip truncated by a scissors is very useful for transferring these small samples at the grossing table. All tissue received should be processed and embedded (typically in paraffin wax). Routine fixation of a sample for electron microscopy is only rarely useful. Serial sections should be obtained for routine and special stains, as required.

Transbronchial biopsy

Similar to the directed bronchoscopic biopsy, the transbronchial biopsy produces a 2–3 mm specimen. The difference between these sampling techniques resides in how these biopsies are obtained. The transbronchial biopsy commonly employs the crocodile forceps resembling the jaws of the reptile for which it is named. The goal of the transbronchial biopsy is to sample more peripheral lung tissue in an attempt to assess parenchymal lung abnormalities. The technique is performed by advancing the tip of the biopsy forceps blindly until resistance is met. The forceps is then retracted slightly, the jaws are opened, and then the forceps is forcibly advanced while closing the jaws. This results in the distal airway being turned inside out as alveolar parenchyma is gathered into the jaws as they close. The samples are delicate and can be damaged during handling. The same technical considerations for proper handling apply here as do those of bronchoscopic biopsies detailed above.

Surgical biopsy (VATS, OLBx)

The ideal surgical wedge lung biopsy measures 3–5 cm in length and 2–4 cm in thickness (as measured from pleural surface to staple line) (Fig. 17.15). Naturally, if the sample received in the laboratory is also intended for microbiological cultures, sterile precautions must be used from the outset. A number of methods have been proposed for fixing these biopsies. For some pathologists, the 'artifactual' overexpansion of the lung parenchyma produced by inflating the biopsy with fixative is to be avoided, even if some atelectasis is present on microscopic

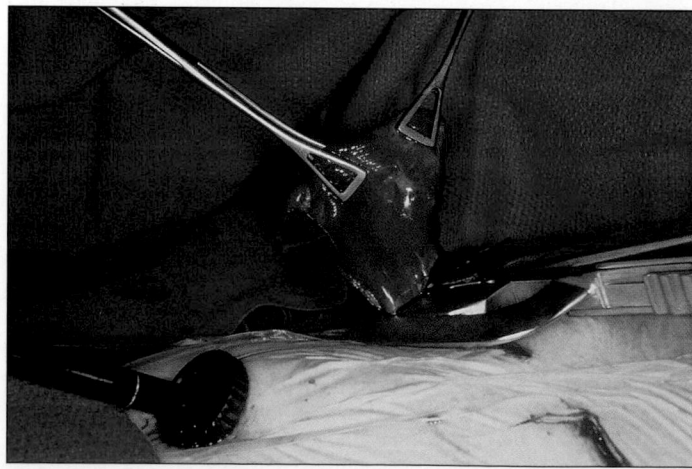

Fig. 17.15 VATS procedure. At the end of the VATS biopsy procedure, the lung biopsy is extracted through one of the incisions.

exam. For others, the atelectasis that may dominate the microscopic image in the immersion-fixed sample is intolerable and hampers accurate diagnosis. Both methods are presented here and the reader can select the method that best suits their interpretive skills and experience.

Regardless of the fixation method of choice, the surgical staples should always be removed first. If performed with sterile technique, this part of the biopsy can be used for microbiology cultures. The remainder of the wedge can be sampled as needed for frozen sections, electron microscopy, snap-freezing, or placement in special medium for immunofluorescent and other studies.

The immersion methods commonly used in practice today rely on passive transfer of fixative into the lung parenchyma. The simplest technique is to place the sample directly into a volume of fixative sufficient to completely immerse the specimen. Because some air always remains in the alveoli, these specimens tend to float. A paper towel placed over the biopsy and fixative surface ensures that the pleural surface remains covered with solution. Formalin is an excellent tissue penetrator and provides reasonable fixation even with simple immersion, while alcohol-based fixatives have a more limited capacity to fix with immersion alone. Two enhancements to immersion fixation are vigorous agitation of the specimen and fixative together (after ensuring a tight lid seal), or the addition of a small amount of carbonated water to the fixative (the gas released from solution tends to help the fixative penetrate the lung parenchyma). Fixation by immersion requires a minimum of 4 hours before sectioning for processing in the histology laboratory, although no test data are available.

Injection inflation is achieved by gentle infusion of fixative into the cut surface of the staple margin using a small-gauge needle (21–22 gauge) attached to a 5 ml syringe. Fixation after inflation should be allowed for at least 2 to 3 hours before sectioning, and similar to immersion-fixed specimens, all the tissue should be processed. If frozen sections are required, the biopsy may be 'infused' for better sectioning and structural preservation using the synthetic embedding medium used for mounting frozen sections.[31] An 18–19-gauge needle is large enough to allow the viscous material to be injected slowly in the latter scenario.

PATTERN ANALYSIS APPROACH TO SURGICAL LUNG BIOPSIES

The concept of 'losing the forest for the trees' is nowhere more evident than in the evaluation of medical pathology specimens in general, and lung wedge biopsies in particular. The age-old training method of requiring that the microscope slide be first evaluated by the naked eye may seem overly methodical, but it does force the interpreter to see the big picture before getting lost in the fine details. For non-neoplastic lung diseases, the scanning low-power objective (2× or 4×) is very useful, if not essential, because different diseases give rise to different architectural patterns, which may immediately place the case into a particular category of disease. This is the essence of pattern recognition, and for diffuse lung diseases several helpful patterns emerge.

ACUTE LUNG INJURY PATTERN (Fig. 17.16)

The prototype is diffuse alveolar damage with hyaline membranes, classically encountered in the clinical setting of the adult respiratory distress syndrome (ARDS), but also occurring as a result of infectious pneumonias, cytotoxic drug reactions, oxygen poisoning, acute manifestation of some immunologically mediated diseases

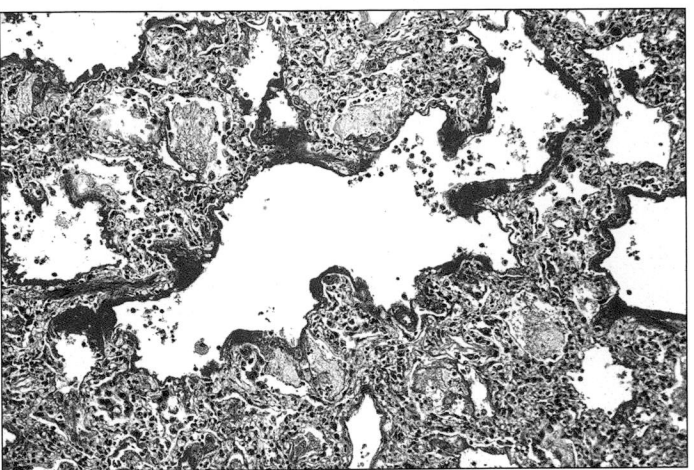

Fig. 17.16 Pattern Analysis: Acute lung injury pattern. The diagnostic components include airspace fibrin, reactive-appearing type II cells, and interstitial edema of variable degree. Hyaline membranes and variable organization may be seen. The biopsy tends to have an overall pink, or eosinophilic, appearance at scanning magnification.

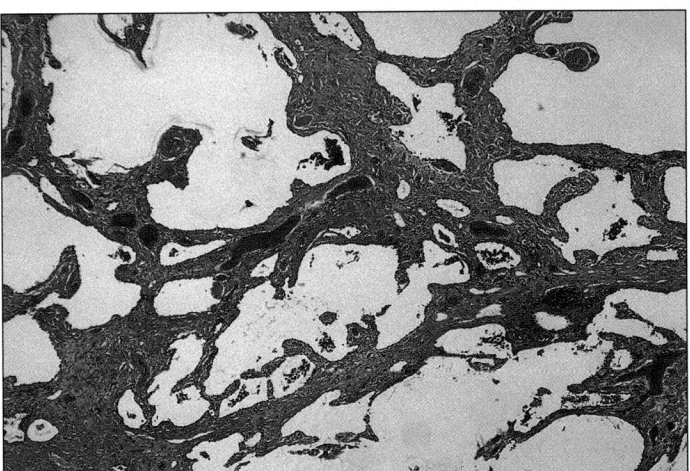

Fig. 17.17 Pattern Analysis: Fibrosis pattern. Collagen deposition in the lung can be 'interstitial' with widening of alveolar septa, lobular septa and/or pleura, or associated with structural remodeling (microscopic honeycombing). In this photomicrograph, several lobules are involved by dense fibrosis.

(such as the systemic connective tissue diseases), and as an idiopathic form (acute interstitial pneumonia).

FIBROSIS PATTERN (Fig. 17.17)

The prototype is usual interstitial pneumonia (UIP), but fibrosis can occur from a variety of causes such as systemic connective tissue diseases, chronic drug toxicity, and many others.

CELLULAR INTERSTITIAL PATTERN (Fig. 17.18)

The prototype is hypersensitivity pneumonitis (extrinsic allergic alveolitis or 'farmer's lung'). Other entities in this category include

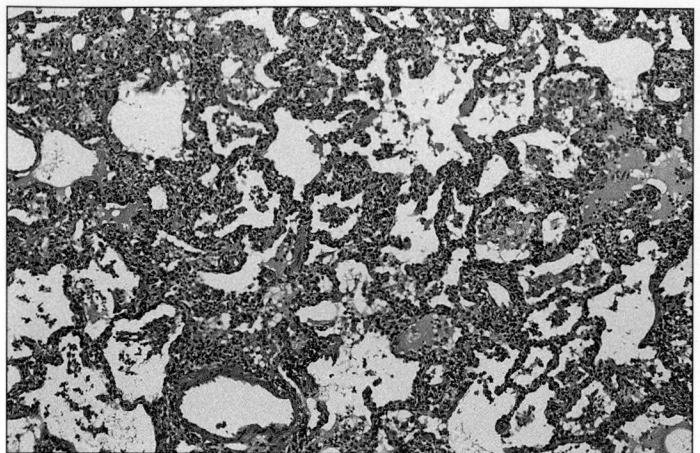

Fig. 17.18 Pattern Analysis: Cellular interstitial pattern. The alveolar walls have increased numbers of mononuclear cells. In some cases the cellular infiltrate may be dense enough to give the biopsy overall a blue, or basophilic, appearance at scanning magnification. Contrast this image with the pink overall appearance of Figure 17.16.

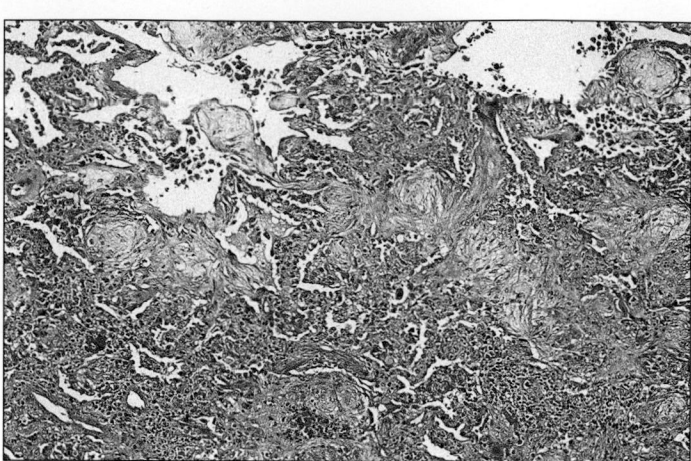

Fig. 17.20 Pattern Analysis: Airspace filling pattern. The alveoli are filled with cellular (as in organizing pneumonia) or exudative (as in alveolar proteinosis, or fibrin) material.

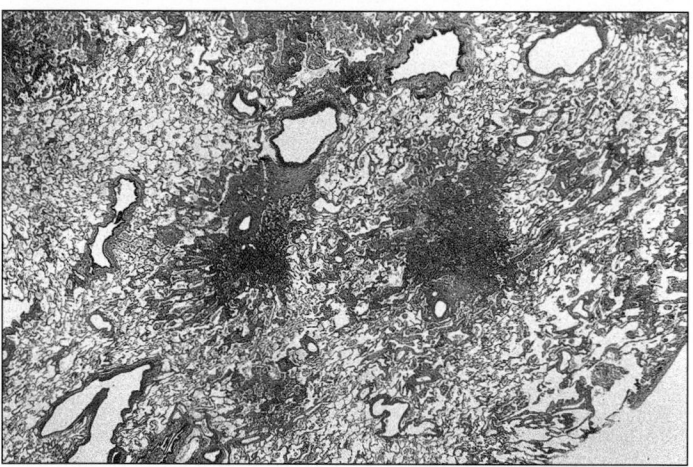

Fig. 17.19 Pattern Analysis: Nodular pattern. Nodules of abnormal tissue are seen of variable size and numbers. A defining feature is the presence of spared parenchyma around or between nodules.

viral and atypical pneumonias, cytotoxic drug reactions, low-grade lymphomas, and two idiopathic forms – nonspecific interstitial pneumonia (NSIP) of cellular type and lymphoid interstitial pneumonia (LIP).

AIRSPACE FILLING PATTERN (Fig. 17.19)

The prototype is organizing pneumonia (OP) where immature fibroblasts and matrix fill the alveoli. Depending on the alveolar content, this pattern also includes infectious bronchopneumonia (where neutrophils fill the alveoli), classic *Pneumocystis* infection in the immunocompromised host (foamy casts), pulmonary alveolar proteinosis (proteinaceous material), diffuse pulmonary hemorrhage (blood, siderophages, and OP) and desquamative interstitial pneumonia (DIP) where lightly pigmented 'smokers'-type macrophages are the dominant element, to mention a few.

NODULAR PATTERN (Fig. 17.20)

The prototype is Wegener's granulomatosis (large nodular pattern). Small (miliary) forms of disease also are included here. The differential diagnosis always includes benign and malignant neoplasms, sarcoidosis, Langerhans cell histiocytosis, lymphoma, certain infections (miliary TB, herpesvirus infection), and a variety of bronchiolocentric diseases.

NEAR NORMAL PATTERN (Fig. 17.21)

The prototype is small airways disease (SAD), where pruning, dilatation, and generalized scaring of the small airways occurs as a subtle finding difficult to appreciate at scanning magnification. Vascular diseases (pulmonary hypertension) and cystic diseases (lymphangioleiomyomatosis) can also produce subtle disease resembling 'normal' lung from scanning magnification.

HONEYCOMBING ONLY – ADVANCED LUNG REMODELING

Advanced lung remodeling with fibrosis occurs when an injury damages or destroys alveolar walls with consequent permanent changes in the lung architecture. The prototype disease of advanced lung remodeling is 'usual interstitial pneumonia' (UIP), as defined originally by Liebow.[32] UIP is diffuse, progressive lung disease of unknown etiology, attended by structural remodeling with cyst formation and fibrosis.[33] However, not all lung diseases with advanced remodeling and fibrosis are UIP. Advanced remodeling can occur in many forms of chronic inflammatory lung disease. Without the capacity to regenerate alveolar structure after irreversible injury (typically an injury that results in destruction of basement membrane), granulation tissue forms within and between alveolar walls, with subsequent collapse of the parenchyma. Proliferation of fibroblasts and secretion of collagen within the interstitium simultaneously occur, and the granulation tissue that forms eventually retracts to form dense scar. These tractional events in turn produce an effect on surrounding lung

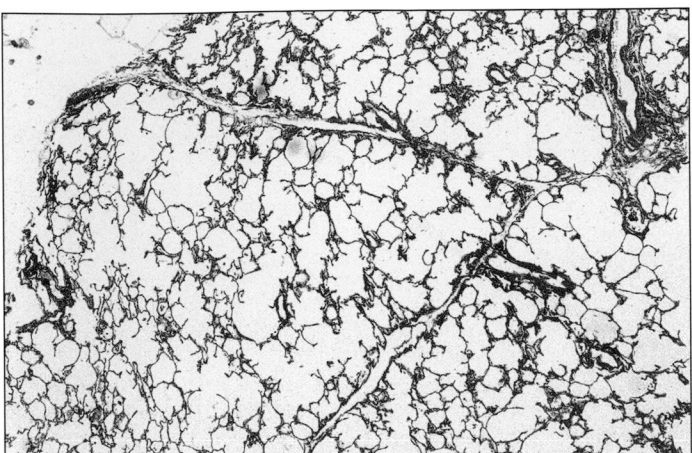

Fig. 17.21 Pattern Analysis: Near normal pattern. The general absence of findings defines this pattern. The vessels, airways, or both are usually abnormal, but the changes may be subtle at low magnification. Cysts (such as those of lymphangioleiomyomatosis) are also in the differential diagnosis for this pattern.

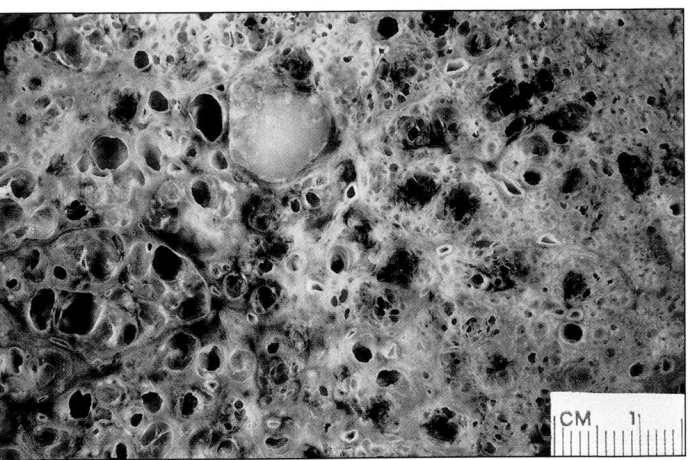

Fig. 17.22 Honeycomb lung. The term 'honeycomb lung' refers to the gross (or radiologic) manifestation of this cystic change

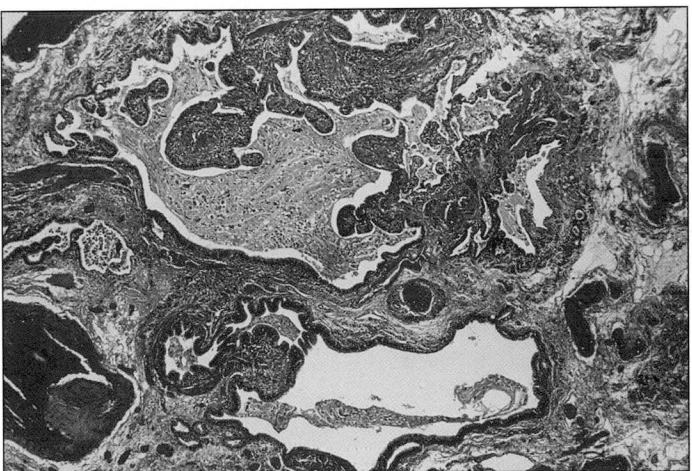

Fig. 17.23 Microscopic honeycombing. The cysts of microscopic honeycombing are about an order of magnitude smaller than those seen on high-resolution CT scans or grossly at autopsy. Microscopic honeycombing is characterized by the presence of cystic spaces lined by columnar ciliated epithelium embedded within fibrosis, typically at the periphery of the lung (subpleurally in the surgical lung biopsy).

resulting in progressive dilation of adjacent alveoli, alveolar ducts and terminal bronchioles, the latter ultimately forming small cysts with mucus in their lumen.[34] Generally, a mixture of cell types lines the cystic spaces, including goblet cells, consequently, mucous secretions accumulate. The final result of honeycomb remodeling is production of multiple cysts accompanied by residual pulmonary arteries, embedded in fibrosis occurring in subpleural lung, containing mucous secretions and variable acute and chronic inflammation. The cystic structures are separated from each other by connective tissue of varying thickness and smooth muscle (sometimes extensive).

The term 'honeycomb lung' refers to the gross (or radiologic) manifestation of this cystic change (Fig. 17.22) that occurs in irreversibly damaged lung tissue. Over the years, honeycomb remodeling has also been called 'endstage lung' by pathologists who may encounter this change as the main finding in a wedge biopsy of lung. This designation is probably best avoided since it carries a clinical implication that may not be accurate – for example, when honeycomb remodeling is localized to the middle lobe in a patient who has otherwise normal lung in other lobes. When remodeling is diffuse and bilateral, a variety of diseases may be implicated, and UIP is the diagnosis of exclusion given this disease's generally poor prognosis and lack of proven response to immunosuppressive therapy.[35] Other considerations in the presence of diffuse advanced remodeling include systemic connective tissue diseases, hypersensitivity pneumonitis, chronic drug toxicity, sarcoidosis, and even certain of the pneumoconioses. The histopathologic corollary of honeycomb remodeling is *microscopic honeycombing*, characterized by the presence of cystic spaces lined by columnar epithelium embedded within fibrosis, typically at the periphery of the lung (subpleurally in the surgical lung biopsy). The cysts of microscopic honeycombing are often an order of magnitude smaller than those seen on high-resolution CT scans or grossly (Fig. 17.23).

The general patterns of diffuse lung disease are summarized in Table 17.5. Once the dominant pattern is identified, additional specific findings visible at higher magnification are useful for narrowing the differential diagnosis. In the search for additional findings, specific attention should be given to the conducting airways, vessels, pleura, and alveoli. Polarized light microscopy should always be performed, and special stains (e.g. for organisms, elastin, fibrous tissue) should be performed as necessary. Bear in mind that the lung may be harboring pathology from more than one disease process. For example, a patient who has a fibrosing lung disease such as usual interstitial pneumonia (UIP) as their long-term problem may develop acute bronchopneumonia or acute drug toxicity, prompting urgent admission to the hospital and lung biopsy. Alternatively, a patient with a nodular lesion suspicious for lung carcinoma, may also have clinically silent background lung disease that only becomes apparent once lung tissue, removed with the tumor, is reviewed in a systematic fashion.

ACUTE, SUBACUTE, AND CHRONIC DIFFUSE PARENCHYMAL DISEASES

It is useful to divide diffuse lung diseases according to their clinical presentation. Three time periods of clinical evolution help define the

Table 17.5 Pattern approach to diffuse lung disease

Acute lung injury	Fibrosis	Cellular IP	Alveolar filling	Nodular	Minimal change
with hyaline membranes	*with variable fibrosis (normal to HC)*	*with lymphs and plasma cells*	*with macrophages*	*with lymphoid*	*with SAD*
Infection	UIP/IPF	C-NSIP, CVD	Smoking related	Follicular bronchiolitis	Constrictive bronchiolitis
CVD	Asbestosis	HSP, Drug	Local fibrosis	Wegener's	
Drug	RA	Infection		Lymphoma	
Idiopathic	Chronic HSP	Lymphoma			
with eosinophils	*with honeycombing only*	*with neutrophils*	*with neutrophils*	*with necrosis*	*with vascular pathology*
AEP	Diffuse	Infection	Infection	Infections	PHT
Drug	Late UIP	CVD	DPH	Tumor	
DAD in smoker	Focal	Hemorrhage		Wegener's	
	Many causes				
with necrosis	*with diffuse fibrosis*	*with granulomas*	*with OP*	*with atypical cells*	*with cysts*
Infections	CVD	Infection, HSP,	Infection, Drug	Infections	PLCH
Viral	Drug	Sarcoid/Berylliosis,	CVD	Carcinomas	LAM
Bacterial	Sarcoid (with granulomas)	Aspiration	*with Eosinophilic material*	Lymphomas	*with no findings*
Fungal	PLCH (with stellate scars)	*with Focal OP*	Infection, CVD,	Sarcomas	Sampling error?
	Pneumoconiosis	Infection	Drug, DPH	*with stellate scars*	
	F-NSIP	CVD	CHF, PAP	PLCH	
with siderophages	*with pleuritis*	*with pleuritis*	*with hemorrhage*	*with OP*	
DPH	CVD	CVD	CVD	Infections, CVD	
CVD			DPH	Drug, Wegener's	
				Infarct	

AEP = acute eosinophilic pneumonia	DPH = diffuse pulmonary hemorrhage	LAM = lymphangioleiomyomatosis
CHF = congestive heart failure	Drug = drug toxicity	OP = organizing pneumonia
C-NSIP = cellular nonspecific interstitial pneumonia	F-NSIP = fibrotic nonspecific interstitial pneumonia	PAP = pulmonary alveolar proteinosis
CVD = collagen vascular disease	HC = honeycomb	PLCH = pulmonary Langerhans cell
DAD = diffuse alveolar damage	HSP = hypersensitivity pneumonitis	RA = rheumatoid arthritis
		UIP = usual interstitial pneumonia/idiopathic pulmonary fibrosis

diffuse lung diseases; acute diseases (e.g. DAD) evolve over days to a few weeks and often are characterized by rapid onset. Subacute (e.g. hypersensitivity pneumonitis) and chronic diseases evolve over weeks to many months, and in some forms, many years (e.g. UIP). Unfortunately, this classification is not perfect because a number of diffuse lung diseases manifest differently in different patients, or may evolve at different rates in the same patient. For example, many collagen vascular diseases have well-recognized acute, subacute, and chronic manifestations, and this is also true of a number of drug toxicities. Nevertheless, the patient with chronic pulmonary symptoms of rheumatoid arthritis, may develop an accelerated form of the disease, and present acutely. To avoid confusion, we have grouped the subacute and chronic diseases together, and in those processes capable of more than one clinical manifestation, we have separated the acute form from those that have manifestations that evolve over many weeks, months, and sometimes years. Thus, this method of categorizing the diffuse lung diseases divides them more by acuity of onset, rather than specific duration.

ACUTE DIFFUSE LUNG DISEASE (DAYS TO WEEKS IN EVOLUTION, RAPID ONSET OF SYMPTOMS)

We begin with the acute diseases because they are dramatic clinically and engender significant anxiety on the part of patient, family members, and caregivers alike. This anxiety is transferred to the pathologist who, more than ever, is expected to arrive at a definitive, and hopefully treatable, diagnosis. The basic pattern of *acute lung injury* is characterized by variable interstitial and alveolar edema, fibrin in airspaces, and reactive type II cells (Fig. 17.24). Hyaline membranes, neutrophils, necrosis, eosinophils, and siderophages are the qualifying elements to be searched for once the pattern is identified. When hyaline membranes are present the term diffuse alveolar damage (DAD) is appropriate (see below). The differential diagnosis in the setting of DAD always includes infection at the top of the list, but a number of other causes must be considered once infection has been reasonably excluded (Table 17.6). Toxic reactions to drugs, acute lung disease produced by the systemic connective tissue diseases, acute eosinophilic pneumonia, pulmonary hemorrhage and vasculitis, and idiopathic DAD (acute interstitial pneumonia) must all be considered in the differential diagnosis.

The clinical prototype of acute lung disease is the adult respiratory distress syndrome (ARDS). The pathologic manifestation of ARDS is diffuse alveolar damage (DAD) with hyaline membranes. It is essential for the pathologist to realize that, although DAD is the prototypic manifestation of ARDS, pathologic DAD does not necessarily correspond to the clinical entity of ARDS. In current practice in the United States, most cases of DAD arise as a consequence of lung infection or immunologically mediated acute lung disease related to drug toxicity or connective tissue disease. In the immunocompromised patient, infection dominates this picture.

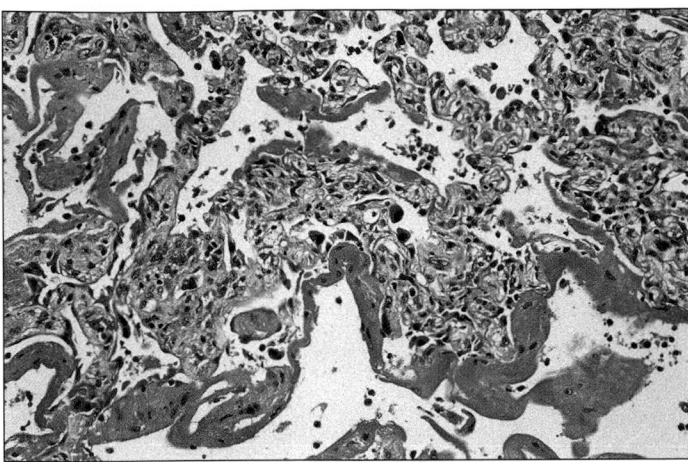

Fig. 17.24 Acute lung injury. Variable interstitial and alveolar edema, fibrin in airspaces, and reactive type II cells, with or without hyaline membranes, all combine to produce the pattern of acute lung injury.

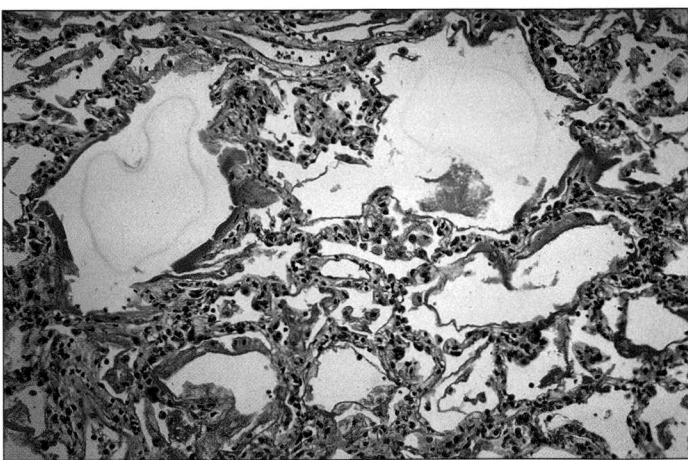

Fig. 17.25 Diffuse alveolar damage (DAD). A more specific term for generic acute lung injury is diffuse alveolar damage. In DAD, serum proteins and tissue debris accumulate in the alveolar airspaces and coalesce to form *hyaline membranes*. DAD is the pathology manifestation of ARDS, although not all patients with DAD have ARDS clinically.

Table 17.6 Causes of diffuse alveolar damage (DAD)

Infections
Pneumocystis jiroveci
Viruses (influenza, cytomegalovirus, varicella, and adenovirus)
Fungi (blastomycosis, aspergillus)
Legionella sp.

Toxins
Inhaled toxins (e.g. O_2 NO_2, household ammonia and bleach, mercury vapor)
Ingested toxins (e.g. paraquat)

Drugs
Cytotoxic (azothioprine, carmustine [BCNU], bleomycin, busulfan, lomustin [CCNU], cyclophosphamide, melphelan, methotrexate, mitomycin, procarbazine, teniposide, vinblastin, and zinostatin)
Non-cytotoxic (amiodarone, amitriptyline, colchicine, gold salts, hexamethonium, nitrofurantoin, penicillamine, streptokinase, sulphathiozole)
Illicit (heroin)

Shock
Traumatic
Septic
Cardiogenic

Radiation

Miscellaneous
Acute pancreatitis

From Dail and Hammer[404] with permission.

Diffuse alveolar damage

The lung has a limited repertoire of responses to acute injury. When severe enough, the initial specific lesion(s) become rapidly overshadowed by a final common response, and DAD results.[36] Nevertheless, the concept of diffuse alveolar damage is important for understanding inflammatory lung diseases because it provides a template for the sequential way the lung responds to a temporally limited injury, and how repair is accomplished in an organ that is mostly comprised of air.

When type I cells are damaged diffusely, the alveolar walls lose their barrier function, leading to flow of interstitial water into the airspaces.[36] Alveolar edema occurs. Serum proteins and tissue debris accumulate and coalesce to form *hyaline membranes* (Fig. 17.25). Within a few days, macrophages begin to accumulate in the airspaces and begin to clear the cellular debris. Simultaneously, interstitial fibroblast-like cells proliferate and migrate into the airspaces. These migrating fibroblasts become *myofibroblasts* capable of exerting tractional forces on surrounding cells and structures and eventually will secrete collagen matrix. This is the principal manifestation of the 'organizing' or 'proliferative' phase (Fig. 17.26) of diffuse alveolar damage.[37] In time, myofibroblasts and their associated matrix are reabsorbed into the alveolar wall by cellular contraction and eventual apoptosis. Variable collagen deposition occurs depending on the extent, severity, and duration of the initial insult. Thus, after a limited insult, such as experimental oxygen toxicity, there is only slight residual tissue alteration consistent with a return to normal, or near normal, lung function. Based on follow-up studies of patients who recover from ARDS, minimal functional deficits are reported.[38]

Adult respiratory distress syndrome

Adult respiratory distress syndrome (ARDS) is a clinically defined disease with characteristic pathologic features, usually DAD.[39] These identical features can be present in biopsies from patients who do not have clinical ARDS. There was a time when ARDS was thought to be a disease unique to oxygen therapy. Today this is not the case, and the potential causes of ARDS are numerous. The most common cause of ARDS is significant nonthoracic trauma of any type, especially when accompanied by significant hemorrhage, either spontaneous or related to surgery. This fact is a clue to the underlying mechanism of ARDS, where activation of complement in serum seems to be one of the important early events. When inhalational injury is the primary event (e.g. gases, near-drowning), presumably the type I cell is the initial target of injury. Occasional cases appear to occur spontaneously,[40] and these would now be regarded as examples of AIP, to be discussed later.[41]

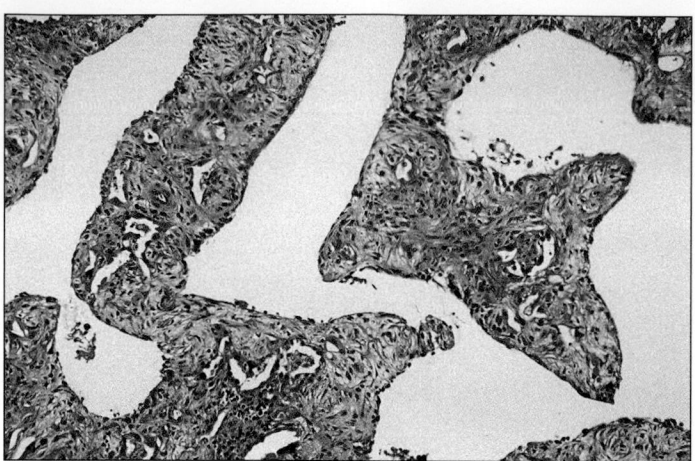

Fig. 17.26 Phases of ARDS. The proliferative phase follows the exudative phase, and is characterized by varying degrees of intra-alveolar and interstitial fibroblastic organization.

ARDS typically occurs in people without pre-existing lung disease that experience major physical trauma accompanied by shock (the rationale behind the term 'shock lung'). Once stabilized, the patient develops sudden unexplained onset of respiratory failure, with bilateral infiltrates on radiologic imaging.[42] The infiltrates progress rapidly, eventually involving all lung zones ('diffuse white out' radiologically), typically with air bronchograms evident. About half the patients who develop ARDS die in the acute phase. Unfortunately, ARDS is a common condition in the United States, where it is estimated to occur at a rate of 150 000 cases per year.

Of use in the discussion of the lung response to repair are the predictable phases that can be seen pathologically.[43] The initial damage in ARDS is thought to result from aggregation of neutrophils after activation of the complement cascade. The neutrophils damage the endothelium by release of their lysosomal enzymes and/or by generation of free radicals. Florid edema occurs in this phase. Clinically, respiratory failure has begun. The pathologic findings now follow a predictable sequence from exudation (exudative phase) to organization (proliferative phase) (see DAD above). ARDS taught us the sequence of events as they occur after a defined injury to the lung, and we have extrapolated these findings over the years to explain the appearance of DAD from any cause, even without ARDS clinically. In practice, this sequence seems to correlate well with clinical evidence of lung injury. For example, the hyaline membrane phase of DAD may be present in a patient who developed acute symptoms of pneumonia 2 or 3 days prior to biopsy. Unfortunately, we do not know the exact amount of time each phase of DAD actually lasts outside of the clinical setting of ARDS, and this may depend on the nature of the injury (i.e. continuous versus episodic, mechanism of injury, severity of injury, etc.).

ARDS may complicate infection occurring in immuno-compromised individuals, and many lung biopsies in the clinical setting of ARDS are performed under these circumstances. Naturally, biopsies are also performed in non-immunosuppressed patients who develop ARDS, if not to establish the presence of infection, then to exclude other conditions.

Infections

In the patient with normal immunity, bacterial pneumonias rarely require tissue biopsy for diagnosis. Contemporary microbiological and serologic techniques for analyzing sputum, bronchial secretions, and blood samples make the morbidity and cost of tissue biopsy unnecessary in most cases. On rare occasions a biopsy may be required for the diagnosis of an atypical pneumonia (e.g. mycoplasma pneumonia) in the normal host with diffuse lung infiltrates identified on radiologic imaging.

The immunocompromised patient is a different matter entirely. Bacterial pneumonias in these patients are often caused by Gram-negative organisms,[44] typically progress rapidly to diffuse infiltrates, and may cause extensive necrotizing pneumonia with abscess formation, if not treated expeditiously. The bacteria involved may be fastidious and/or difficult to culture from more easily accessible specimens (e.g. sputum, bronchial washings). Under these circumstances the surgical pathologist may be called upon to help provide an immediate diagnosis on lung biopsy specimens. Furthermore, mycobacterial infections, either *Mycobacterium* tuberculosis or atypical forms,[45,46] can cause disseminated disease in the host with deficient immunity, a particularly common occurrence in patients with HIV infection who develop the acquired immunodeficiency syndrome (AIDS).[47,48] To complicate matters further, the expected normal host reaction to infection, such as the production of discrete necrotizing granulomas in the case of fungal and mycobacterial infection, may not be well-developed when immunity is compromised by disease or by iatrogenic means. In these situations, the diagnosis can be easily overlooked without the use of special techniques applied to tissue sections designed to highlight the presence of organisms.

Bacterial pneumonias

Bacteria typically require extracellular substrate for reproduction. Because of this, the morphologic changes that occur in bacterial pneumonias are somewhat stereotypic. The bacteria either encounter substrate already in place, such as necrotic cellular debris resulting from some pre-existing tissue injury, or invoke tissue necrosis as part of their pathogenic mechanism, mainly through the release of toxins. The body responds to the presence of bacteria with neutrophilic migration into the airspaces, producing the morphologic pattern known as bronchopneumonia. The prototype for bronchopneumonia is streptococcal pneumonia; i.e. *typical* pneumonia (Fig. 17.27).

Bacterial infections of the respiratory tract typically begin when organisms gain access to the lung parenchyma by aerosol inhalation or aspiration of oral contents. Gram-positive organisms, predominately streptococci and staphylococci, comprise the majority of the oral flora, accompanied by certain Gram-negative organisms, such a *Hemophilus*, *Moraxella* and *Neisseria* species.[49,50] Bacterial pneumonias occur in healthy individuals when access is enhanced (e.g. aspiration, trauma), local circumstances predispose (e.g. airway obstruction, malformation), or exposure to naturally virulent organisms occurs (e.g. anthrax spore inhalation). The appearance of bacterial pneumonia typically begins as opacification in a lobular bronchiolocentric distribution. If untreated, this may spread to become confluent lobular or even completely lobar in distribution, as a consequence of progressive uncontrolled bacterial growth and concomitant cellular immune response. Bronchopneumonia generally occurs within hours of initial infection.

Legionella pneumonia (Legionnaire's disease)

Acute respiratory infection caused by the fastidious Gram-negative bacilli of the genus has been termed '*Legionnaires' disease.*' These bacteria were identified as the cause of a 1976 epidemic that occurred at an American Legion convention in Philadelphia, Pennsylvania. Several fatalities resulted from this outbreak. The same genus of

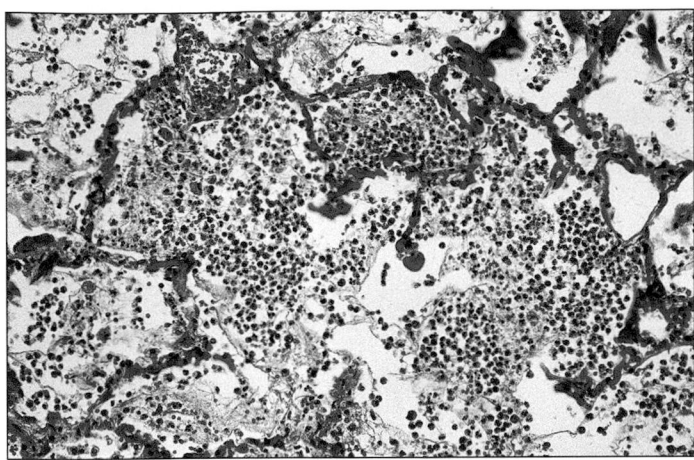

Fig. 17.27 Bacterial pneumonia. Acute bronchopneumonia of bacterial origin is characterized by neutrophils filling the alveolar spaces, and variable amounts of fibrin, edema, and necrosis.

bacteria was found to have caused earlier outbreaks of a less virulent respiratory disease known as Pontiac fever.[51]

The organism *Legionella pneumophilia* is fastidious and requires complex media for growth in culture. The organism has six antigenically different serogroups differentiated by direct fluorescence on secretions or tissue. Serotype I is by far the most common. Many patients who develop life-threatening *Legionella* pneumonia are immunocompromised. A related organism, *Legionella micdadei*, causes life-threatening pneumonia exclusively in the immuno-compromised individuals.[51]

Lobular, or confluent lobular, consolidation is evident on gross exam. Abscesses occur in approximately 25% of cases.[51] Complete lobar pneumonia is a less frequent gross pattern. Microscopically, there is alveolar filling by fibrinous exudates rich in neutrophils and macrophages (Fig. 17.28A). A morphologic clue to the diagnosis is the presence of nuclear dust in the exudates. The changes begin in the distal acinus and involve larger airways secondarily.[52] The diagnosis

must be confirmed by silver stains (e.g. Dieterle, Fig. 17.28B) or direct immunofluorescence techniques. The Gram technique used on tissue sections (Brown-Brenn, Brown-Hopps) does not stain these organisms well. Culture is definitive in most cases. Diffuse alveolar damage has been described.[53]

The atypical pneumonias

The *atypical* pneumonias are caused by a group of bacteria that are either obligate/facultative intracellular organisms, or are membrane deficient. These pneumonias are distinguishable clinically and pathologically from *typical bacterial pneumonias*, such as that caused by *Streptococcus pneumoniae*, and are difficult infections to document by growth in culture. Organisms generally included in this group include *Rickettsia*, *Mycoplasma*, and *Chlamydia*. The exact incidence of these pneumonias in the adult population is not known. Most cases are treated empirically, either on the basis of clinical and radiologic findings, or serologic studies. In biopsy specimens, the findings they produce are not specific and the changes present may resemble a chronic cellular interstitial pneumonia, unless complicated by secondary infections with more characteristic features.

Mycoplasma pneumoniae: *M. pneumoniae* may be the most common cause of pneumonia in humans, but the disease is rarely seen by the surgical pathologist. Children and adolescents are most commonly affected; for example, *M. pneumoniae* is found to be the agent responsible for as many as 74% of community acquired pneumonias in children between 9 and 15 years of age.[54] The organism is a slender motile bacterium that does not produce a Gram-staining reaction because it lacks the required cell wall constituents. *M. pneumoniae* exerts its pathogenetic effect through attachment to host cells and release of peroxide, which results in host cell membrane injury. *Mycoplasma* resists culture in the laboratory, so the diagnosis is typically confirmed by blood tests (cold agglutinins, complement fixation, DNA probe).

A productive cough, fever, diarrhea, and headache frequently accompany *Mycoplasma* pneumonia. The white blood count tends to be normal, distinguishing this pneumonia from that produced by *Streptococcus pneumoniae*.[55]

Chlamydia pneumoniae: Pneumonia produced by *C. pneumoniae* is another common pneumonia in adults, evident from serologic

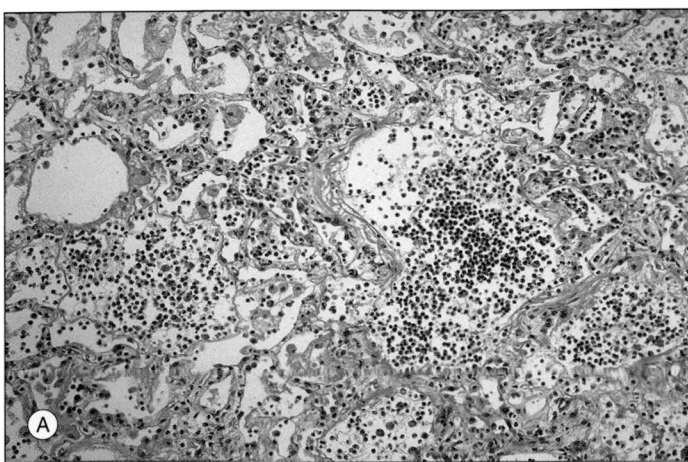
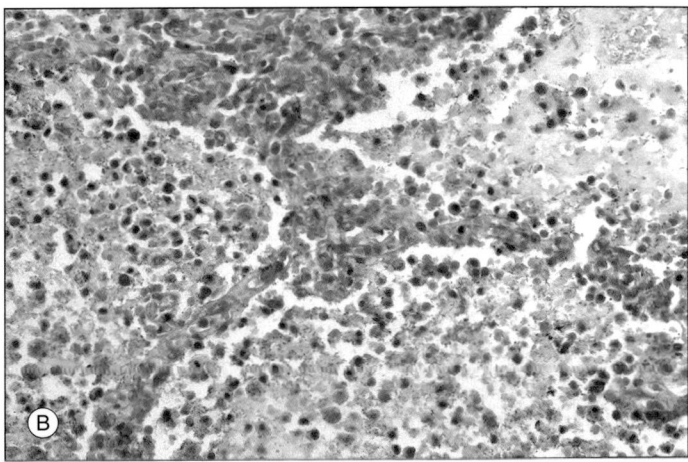

Fig. 17.28 *Legionella* pneumonia. Characteristically there is leukocytoclasis, with nuclear dust in exudates (**A**). The diagnosis must be confirmed by Dieterle stain (**B**).

Table 17.7 Viral pneumonias

Virus	Usual patient
RNA	
Influenza	NLH (adults)
Measles	ICH
Respiratory syncytial virus	NLH (infants), ICH adults (rare)
Hantavirus	NLH
DNA	
Adenovirus	NLH, NLH (children), ICH
Herpes simplex	ICH
Varicella-zoster	NLH (adults), ICH
Cytomegalovirus	ICH

NLH, normal host; ICH, immunocompromised host
From Miller et al[405] with permission.

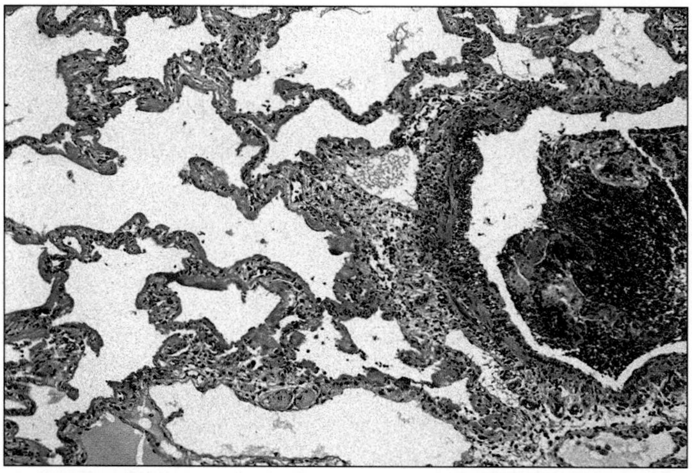

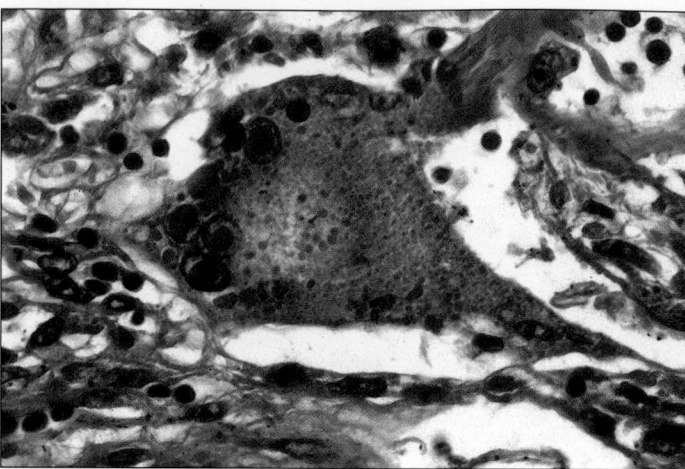

Fig. 17.30 Measles pneumonia. Distinctive viral inclusions can be seen in the cytoplasm and nuclei of submucosal glandular cells and alveolar epithelium. Inclusion-bearing cells are characteristically multinucleated.

Fig. 17.29 Influenza pneumonia. Influenza pneumonia produces diffuse alveolar damage (DAD) with necrotizing bronchitis/bronchiolitis.

studies showing a high incidence of serum antibodies to this agent in the population, presumably based on mild or minimally symptomatic infection.[54] Pharyngitis precedes cough and radiographic evidence of pneumonia. The *Chlamydiae* are obligate intracellular bacteria, so they are difficult to culture in the laboratory. Their intracellular pathogenesis resembles more a virus than bacterium, commandeering cellular resources and releasing infectious particles on cell lysis.

Viral pneumonias

The more common viruses known to produce lower respiratory tract infection[56] are presented in Table 17.7.

Influenza

In the normal adult, influenza is the most common cause of viral pneumonia.[57–59] Three patterns of disease emerge in biopsy or autopsy material: 'pure' influenza pneumonia (Fig. 17.29), influenza pneumonia followed by bacterial superinfection, and concurrent influenza and bacterial pneumonia. Influenza infection is not associated with specific viral inclusions. Moreover, concurrent or subsequent bacterial infection (bronchopneumonia) may overshadow any underlying viral effects.

Measles

Measles (rubeola) infection in the normal host is frequently associated with radiologic infiltrates, and sometimes a symptomatically mild pneumonia. Immunocompromised children are at risk for serious measles pneumonia. Absence of a rash, persistence of tissue giant cells, persistence of virus on repeated cultures, and a poor antibody response are indicators of a potentially serious clinical course. In biopsy or autopsy tissue, the lungs show a combination of bronchitis, bronchiolitis, and diffuse alveolar damage, similar to that produced by influenza virus. With measles, however, a distinctive set of viral inclusions occurs. The inclusions are present in multinucleated giant cells that arise from epithelial cells of submucous glands and of the acinus. While both intranuclear and cytoplasmic inclusions occur, the nuclear inclusions are more conspicuous and consist of an eosinophilic core surrounded by a halo. The occurrence of one inclusion in each nucleus results in a cluster of inclusions in the same multinucleated cell (Fig. 17.30), giving these a distinctive appearance.[60–63]

Respiratory syncytial virus

Although this organism is a common cause of serious lower respiratory tract infection in children, respiratory syncytial virus (RSV) rarely produces life-threatening pneumonia in normal adults. Immunocompromised adults, however, are at risk, and in these individuals the infection causes a striking acute bronchiolitis with epithelial necrosis, and chronic inflammatory peribronchiolitis (Fig. 17.31). Extension of the inflammatory process to involve alveolar walls does not typically occur. Bronchiolar epithelial cells develop a small intracytoplasmic eosinophilic inclusion that can be enhanced using immunohistochemistry (Fig. 17.32).

Adenovirus

Like RSV, adenovirus mainly causes lower respiratory tract infection in children, where pneumonia carries a high risk of long-term sequelae such as bronchiectasis. In adults, infection occurs mainly in the immunocompromised host. The histopathology is that of DAD, typically with a necrotizing bronchitis/bronchiolitis. Intranuclear and 'smudge' cell-type inclusions, can be seen in airway and alveolar epithelial cells (Fig. 17.33). Small irregular intranuclear inclusions

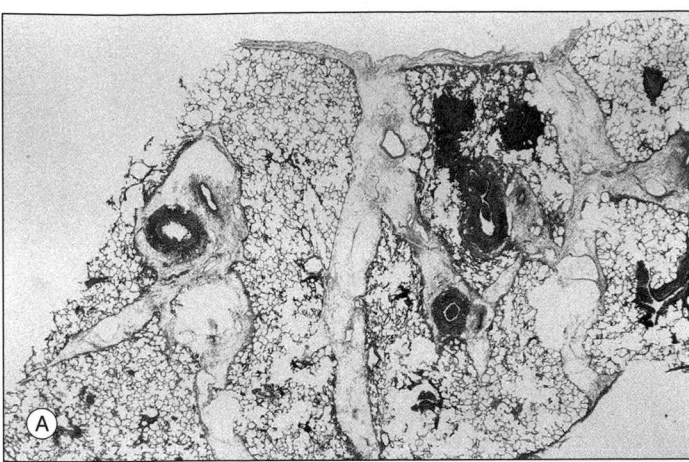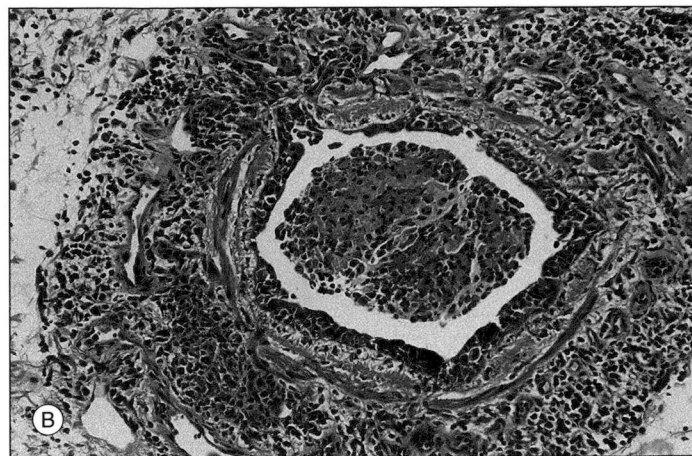

Fig. 17.31 RSV pneumonia. The histopathologic picture at scanning magnification is one of striking acute cellular bronchiolitis (**A**). At higher magnification epithelial necrosis, neutrophilic debris in bronchiolar lumens, and a mononuclear cell peribronchiolitis can be seen (**B**).

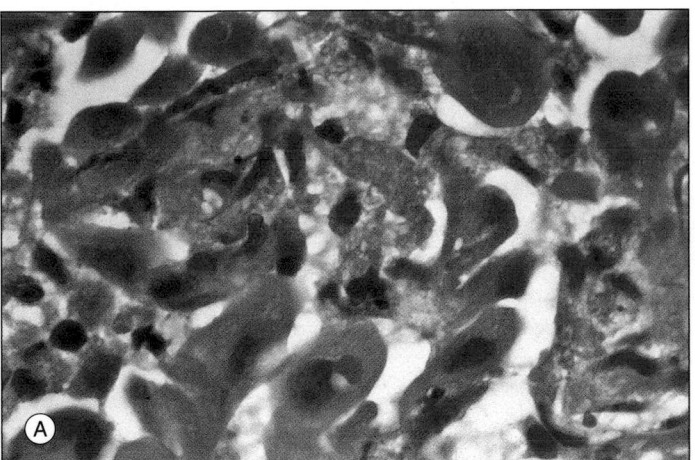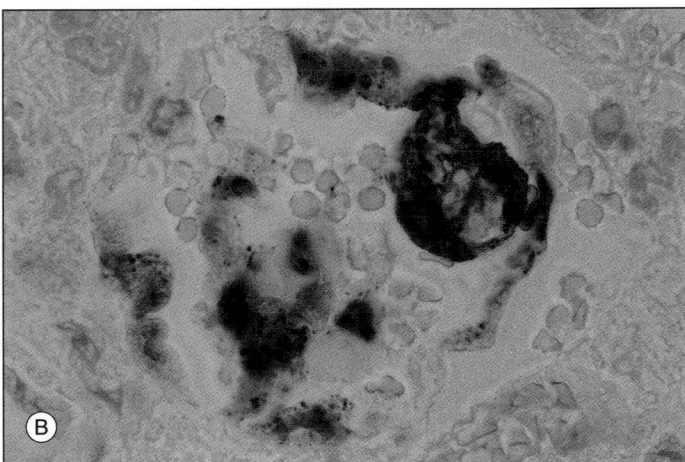

Fig. 17.32 RSV pneumonia. At very high magnification (**A**) eosinophilic globular inclusions can be seen in the cytoplasm of airway epithelial cells. Immunohistochemical stains for RSV (**B**) can be useful in confirming the morphologic impression of RSV infection. (Immuno-alkaline phosphatase immunohistochemical stain using antibodies directed against RSV, Vector red chromogen).

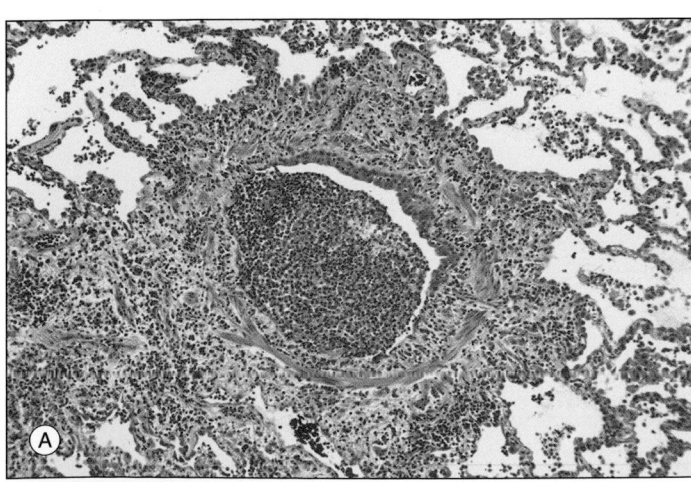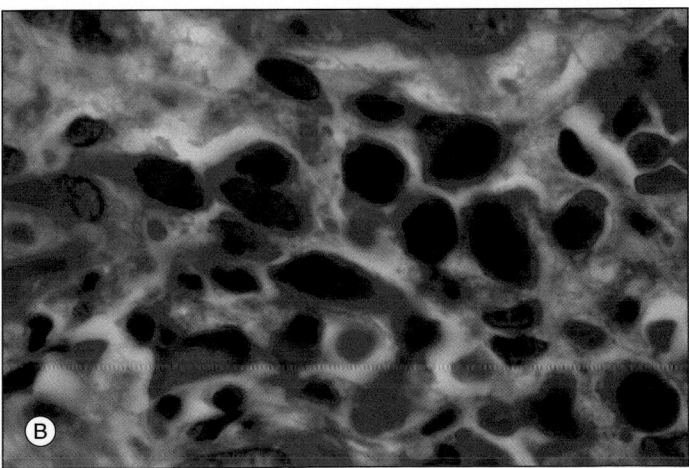

Fig. 17.33 Adenovirus pneumonia. A necrotizing bronchitis/bronchiolitis is typical (**A**). Two types of inclusions (intranuclear and 'smudge' cell types) may be found, primarily in airway and alveolar epithelial cells (**B**).

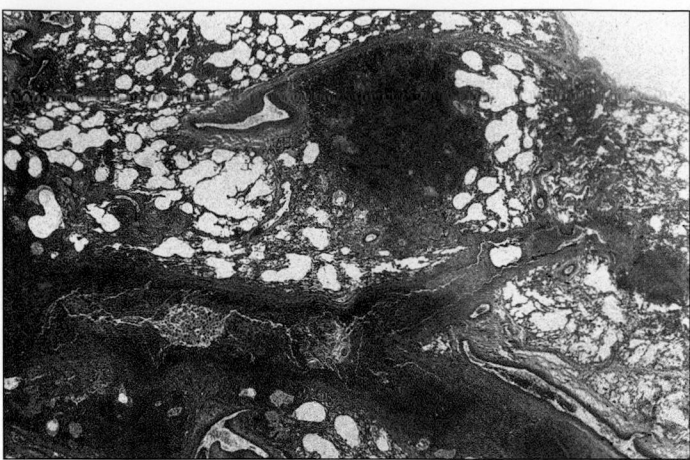

Fig. 17.34 HSV tracheobronchitis. Ulcerative lesions in the upper airways progresses distally to involve terminal bronchioles. Scanning magnification shows the linear outline of a dilated and necrotic bronchiole (below center). A nodular lesion nearby represents a separate bronchiole in cross-sectional view.

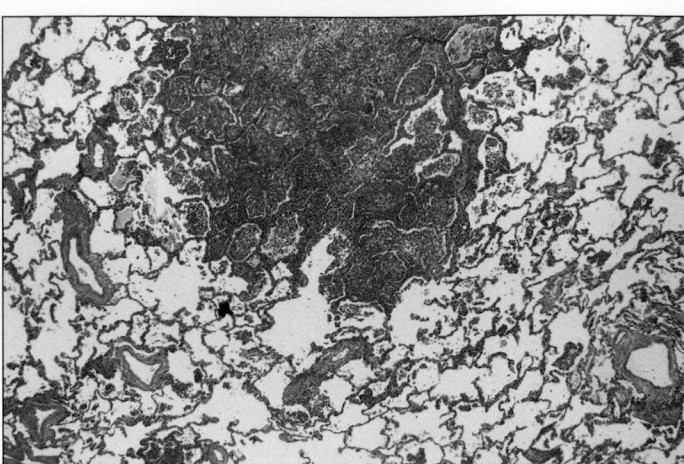

Fig. 17.35 Miliary nodular HSV. Hemorrhagic inflammatory parenchymal nodules with central necrosis are typical.

are formed early, and have a granular halo. This appearance could be mistaken for herpes simplex virus (HSV) (see below). The more numerous, 'smudge' cell inclusions, are larger and basophilic. 'Smudge' cells are produced as a result of nuclear membrane rupture. The cytoplasm of the smudge cell contains massive numbers of replicated virions. In cases where culture was either not performed or inconclusive, the morphologic impression of adenovirus (as well as several other viral infections) in tissue samples can be confirmed using immunohistochemical and molecular hybridization techniques.[64,65]

Herpes simplex virus

Herpes simplex virus (HSV) pneumonia is mainly a disease of individuals with compromised immunity. Two patterns are seen: ulcerative tracheobronchitis and miliary parenchymal nodules. HSV ulcerative tracheobronchitis begins in the upper airways (Fig. 17.34). Over time, the mucosal lesions extend distally to involve the bronchioles and eventually the peripheral lung parenchyma. This pattern of disease affects a broad spectrum of seriously ill patients. The miliary nodular type of HSV pneumonia is seen primarily in those with profound immunosuppression, and consists of hemorrhagic, variably cellular, inflammatory parenchymal nodules with central necrosis (Fig. 17.35). The airways are not directly involved.

Cells with characteristic herpetic nuclear inclusions occur in both the tracheobronchitis and the miliary nodular manifestations of HSV respiratory disease. Early inclusions arise in the nucleus and cause nuclear enlargement with a slightly basophilic, uniform ground-glass alteration of the nucleoplasm (Fig. 17.36). Later, this intranuclear material coalesces to form a single eosinophilic inclusion body surrounded by a halo. When in doubt about the presence of HSV infection, immunohistochemistry, electron microscopy, in situ hybridization, or polymerase chain reaction (PCR) may be useful in verifying the diagnosis.

Cytomegalovirus

Cytomegalovirus (CMV) pneumonia is also a disease of immunocompromised individuals. Organ transplant recipients are at high risk, particularly those who receive kidney and bone marrow transplants. Individuals with the acquired immunodeficiency

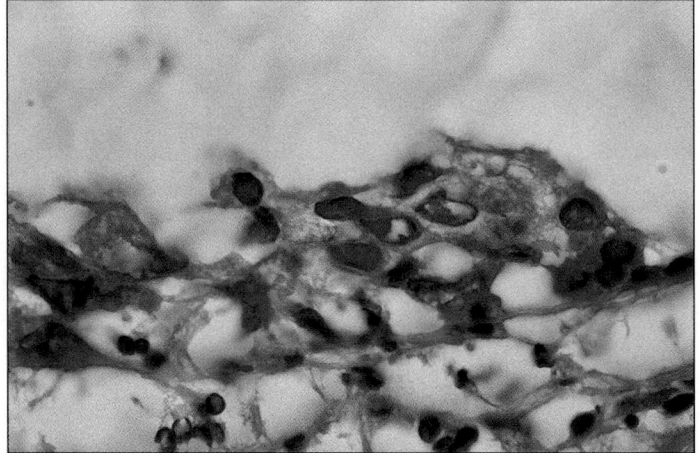

Fig. 17.36 HSV inclusions. Infected respiratory cells have characteristic nuclear herpetic inclusions. A slightly basophilic, uniform ground-glass alteration of the nucleoplasm is the first recognizable inclusion.

syndrome (AIDS) are also commonly prone to this illness. The histopathology of CMV pneumonia is similar to that caused by herpes simplex virus and herpes varicella-zoster. Hemorrhagic nodules are accompanied by diffuse alveolar damage to a variable degree (Fig. 17.37A). Bronchi and bronchioles are typically not involved. The CMV viropathic cellular change is characterized by dramatic nuclear and cellular enlargement. The nuclear inclusion is central and surrounded by a clear halo, the outer edge of which consists of marginated nuclear chromatin. Cytoplasmic inclusions occur as perinuclear basophilic dots (Fig. 17.37B).

Herpes varicella-zoster

Primary varicella infection (chickenpox) is a common infectious disease of childhood. Pulmonary complications are distinctly uncommon in children with normal immunity (less than 1% of cases),

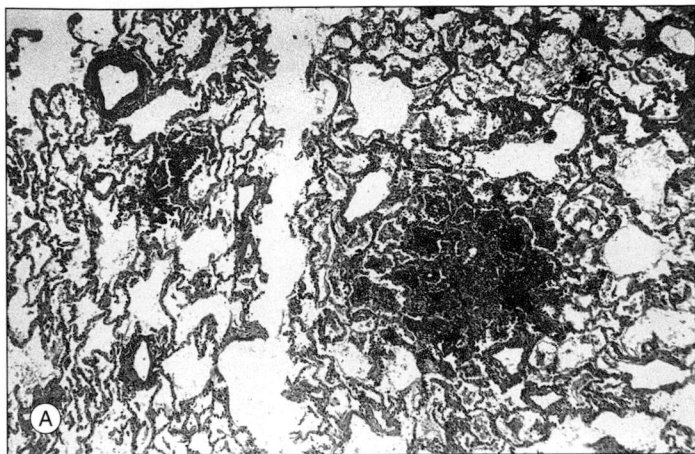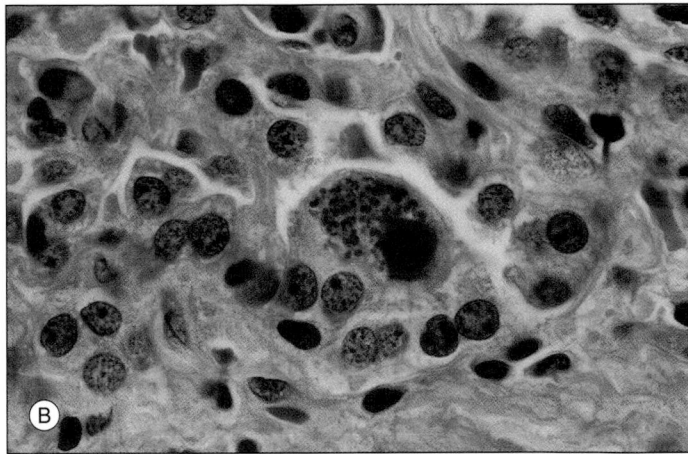

Fig. 17.37 CMV pneumonia. Hemorrhagic nodules are accompanied by variable degrees of diffuse alveolar damage (**A**). The intranuclear inclusion of CMV is distinctive (**B**).

whereas 15% of primary infections in adults are associated with radiologic evidence of pneumonia. Herpes zoster occurs as a reactivation form of varicella infection, and consists of a painful skin rash with vesicles distributed along dermatomes whose corresponding nerve ganglia harbor the latent virus. Life-threatening respiratory illness rarely occurs in otherwise healthy individuals.[66] Immunocompromised patients may develop life-threatening pneumonia following both types of infections. The pneumonia resembles the miliary hemorrhagic nodules seen in HSV infection. Ulcers of the conducting airways are uncommon in herpes varicella-zoster infection.

Hantavirus

Hantaviruses are an enveloped RNA virus of the Bunyaviridae family. Hantaviruses were known to be responsible for a group of illnesses together referred to as the 'hemorrhagic fever with renal syndrome,' but in 1993 a hantavirus with a novel nucleotide sequence was identified as the etiologic agent responsible for an epidemic of acute pulmonary edema that occurred in the southwestern United States.[67,68] The new disease was characterized by a prodrome consisting of fever, nausea, vomiting, and myalgia, followed by rapidly evolving, severe respiratory distress with pulmonary edema. The average age of affected individuals was 30 years, but there was a broad range (12–68 years). Males and females were equally affected. Viruses are spread to humans through the excrement of rodents (deer mice, field mice, voles, and rats) that are chronically infected with the virus and serve as reservoirs. During the epidemic, the mortality was high (80%), with the average interval between onset of symptoms and death being 6 days. Casual person to person spread does not occur. Since 1993, other cases have been reported in North America, including four fatal cases in British Columbia, Canada.

Initial laboratory studies are typically abnormal. Hematologic evaluation reveals a neutrophilic leukocytosis with immature forms, thrombocytopenia, an elevated hematocrit, and atypical circulating lymphoid cells (immunoblasts). At autopsy, the lungs are massively congested and edematous. Pleural effusions are universally present. The microscopic appearance differs from typical DAD by the lack of reactive type II cells, hyaline membranes or intra-alveolar debris. Instead, a delicate meshwork of intra-alveolar fibrin is seen accompanied by a distinctive infiltrate of small and large mononuclear

cells within the alveolar walls. (Fig. 17.38) Similar cells are present in other organs at autopsy. Airway epithelial injury is not an expected feature of the disease. Viral inclusions are not seen by light microscopy but spherical hantavirus-like particles, 90–110 nm in diameter, can be identified ultrastructurally within in the pulmonary capillary endothelium.

Coronaviruses

The coronaviruses are ubiquitous RNA viruses. These infectious organisms produce disease in a number of animal species. In humans, coronaviruses and rhinoviruses are responsible for the majority of common colds. In certain epidemiologic situations, they can cause pneumonia in children, in frail elderly individuals, and in immunocompromised adults.[69]

In November 2002, an atypical pneumonia outbreak was reported in China, and subsequently became known as the Severe Acute Respiratory Syndrome, or *SARS*. Over the course of a few months, the disease achieved global notoriety as a serious health problem.[70] Tissue culture isolation, electron microscopy, and molecular analysis finally identified the organism as a novel coronavirus, and the name 'Urbani strain of SARS-associated coronavirus' was proposed.[71]

Manifestations in affected individuals ranged from a non-hypoxemic febrile respiratory disease to severe respiratory compromise characterized by the adult respiratory distress syndrome clinically, and diffuse alveolar damage pathologically. Death occurred in approximately 5% of patients.[72]

Histopathologically, scant intra-alveolar fibrin deposits were sometimes present with some congestion and edema. In more severe cases, the spectrum of findings included hyaline membrane formation, interstitial lymphocytic infiltrates, desquamation of alveolar pneumocytes, and areas undergoing organization of acute lung injury. Viral cytopathic effects (multinucleated syncytial cells) were seen in some patients, similar to those of influenza, respiratory syncytial virus, and measles virus infections,[73] but viral inclusions were not identified and immunohistochemical studies failed to reveal viral antigens.

Fungal pneumonias

Fungal organisms cause significant granulomatous lung disease in both normal and immunocompromised individuals. Localized

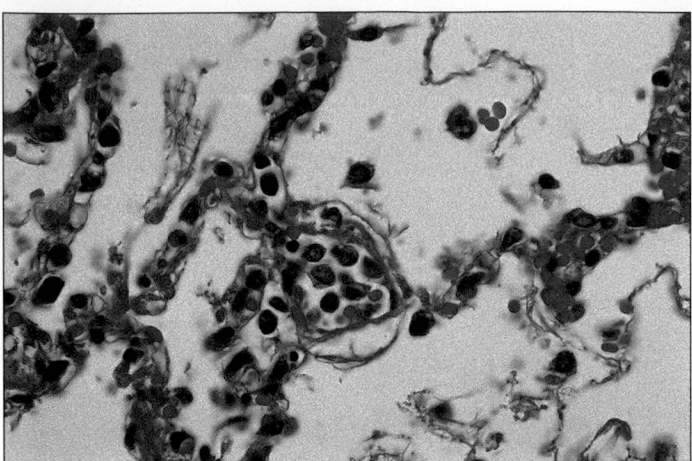

Fig. 17.38 *Hantavirus* pneumonia. A delicate meshwork of intra-alveolar fibrin is seen, accompanied by a distinctive infiltrate of small and large mononuclear cells within the alveolar walls.

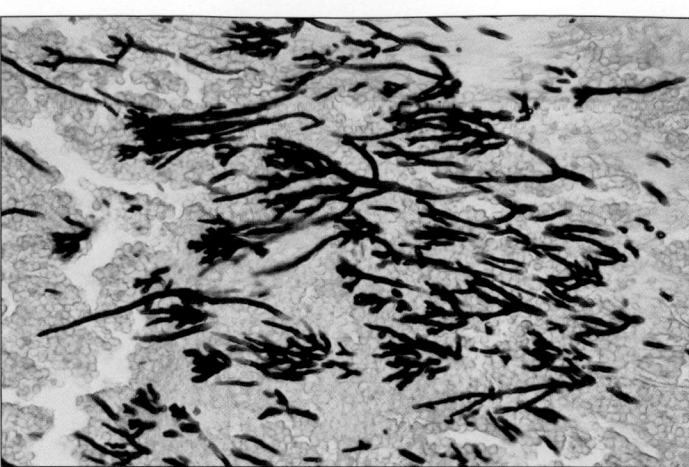

Fig. 17.40 *Aspergillus* fungal hyphae. With the Grocott methenamine silver (GMS) stain, the septate hyphae of *Aspergillus* have parallel walls and characteristic 45° angle branching.

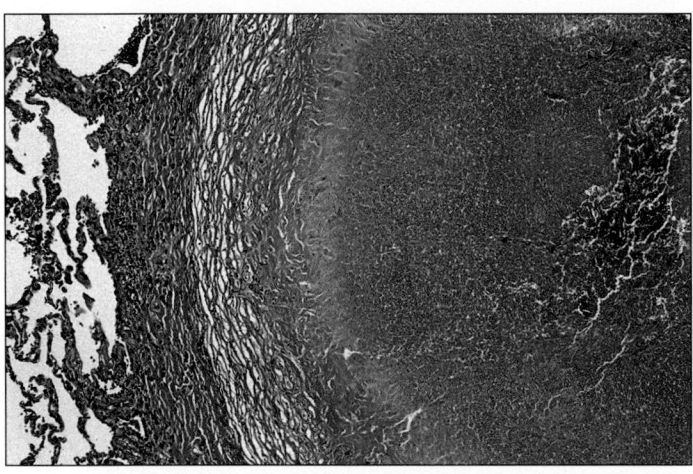

Fig. 17.39 Fungal granulomas. Fungal organisms generally produce nodular granulomatous lung lesions, characteristically with necrosis. Here, a large histoplasmoma can be seen from scanning magnification.

disease is typical in the patient with normal immunity,[74] where fungal organisms generally produce nodular granulomatous lung lesions, characteristically with necrosis. Diffuse fungal pneumonias may be life threatening for individuals with compromised immunity. Morphologic identification and/or culture of the offending organism involved are essential to accurate diagnosis. Differential diagnostic considerations in the setting of necrotizing granulomatous inflammation in the lung (Fig. 17.39) most often include infections produced by *Histoplasma capsulatum*,[75] *Cryptococcus neoformans*, *Coccidiodes immitus*, *Blastomyces dermatitidis*,[76] and *Sporothrix schenckii*.

Aspergillus, Mucormyces, and Candida

Aspergillus infection also may be seen in several forms. Allergic bronchopulmonary aspergillosis,[77] (now referred to as 'allergic bronchopulmonary *fungal* disease' because other fungi can produce identical clinical and pathologic findings) occurs when fungal hyphae colonize bronchial mucus plugs. *Aspergillus* 'fungus balls' occur when fungi colonize pre-existent pulmonary cavities resulting

from any cause (Fig. 17.40). The most serious setting in which *Aspergillus* lung infection is seen in surgical pathology material occurs in the patient with compromised immunity.[78] Typically, the organisms invade blood vessel walls, giving rise to infected infarcts, which then cavitate. *Mucormycosis*[79] is less common than aspergillosis and occurs almost exclusively in either diabetic or immunocompromised patients. Like *Aspergillus* in the immunocompromised host, septic thrombi with infarction occur. *Candidiasis* also is a common infection in immunocompromised patients.[80] The usual lung involvement occurs as either endobronchial-related fungal colonies or multiple abscesses containing yeast forms and pseudohyphae centered on the small vessels and airways. *Candida* infection can also occur as septic thrombi in large arteries, sometimes mimicking *Aspergillus*, or as granulomatous infection that mimics tuberculosis. Sometimes the pseudohyphae produced by *Candida* are difficult to distinguish from *Aspergillus* using silver stains on tissue sections. In this setting, microbiological culture is usually required for a specific diagnosis.

Pneumocystis pneumonia

Pneumocystis jiroveci (previously known as *P. carinii*) is a free-living fungal organism,[81] once thought to be a protozoan organism based on a lack of response to antifungal therapy and resistance to culture attempts in vitro. Based on molecular studies, it is now known that *P. jiroveci* is a eucaryotic fungal organism. Opportunistic pulmonary disease occurs in immunocompromised hosts.[82,83] Extrapulmonary involvement is rare.[82] Diagnosis depends on the demonstration of the organisms in sputum, bronchial biopsies, bronchial washings/lavage, and surgical wedge lung biopsies.[21,25] The presence of *P. jiroveci* can sometimes be suggested on H&E stains, but the methenamine silver stain, or other staining method, is typically required for demonstrating the cysts. The cysts of *P. jiroveci* are approximately 6 mm in diameter and frequently display a half-moon shape in tissue sections. At higher magnification, the cysts can be seen to have a pair of adjacent structures in their membranes, resembling commas (so-called 'dark bodies') (Fig. 17.41). With the Giemsa stain, six to eight individual inner bodies within each cyst (merozoites) become visible.

The classic H&E appearance of lung tissue infected with *P. jiroveci* in the immunocompromised host is one of foamy eosinophilic intra-alveolar exudates (which contain the organisms), along with a

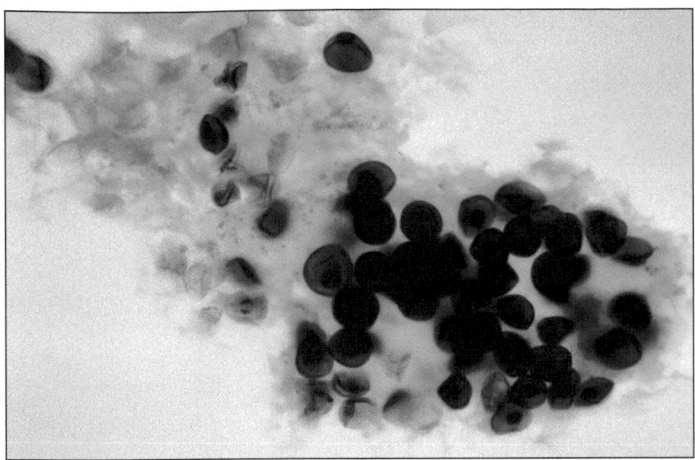

Fig. 17.41 *Pneumocystis.* While the presence of *P. jiroveci* can sometimes be suggested on H&E stains, the methenamine silver stain demonstrate the cysts, which are approximately 6 mm in diameter and often have a crescent or half-moon shape.

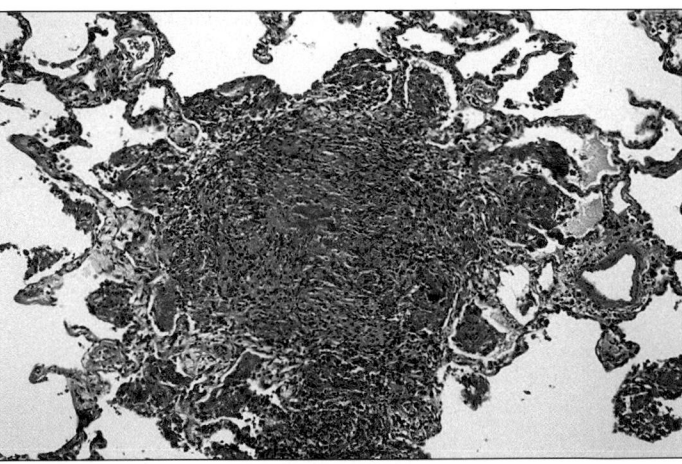

Fig. 17.42 Granulomatous *Pneumocystis. P. jiroveci* pneumonia may not be histologically classic in the minimally immunocompromised patient (by corticosteroids, for example). As illustrated here, even granulomatous inflammation may be seen.

mild mononuclear interstitial infiltrate. However, many cases of *P. jiroveci* pneumonia do not present this classic morphology, especially in patients with moderate immunocompromise (by systemic corticosteroid therapy, for example). Absence of the foamy exudate, marked interstitial inflammation, prominent intra-alveolar histiocytic reaction, and even granulomatous inflammation (Fig. 17.42) have all been described in *Pneumocystis* pneumonia[83] For these reasons, silver stains should be routinely performed in all cases of acute lung injury, especially in specimens from immunocompromised patients. Also, it is important to remember that once *Pneumocystis* pneumonia is identified, a careful search for other pathogens (such as CMV) should be undertaken. In the setting of the acquired immunodeficiency syndrome produced by HIV infection, it is worthwhile to consider the possibility of comorbid Kaposi's sarcoma (which can be a subtle finding), especially if the patient has experienced hemoptysis.

Acute eosinophilic lung disease

Acute lung injury occurring in the presence of significant numbers of tissue eosinophils is referred to as 'acute eosinophilic lung disease.' Peripheral blood and bronchoalveolar lavage eosinophils are commonly elevated in these conditions (defined in the blood as an absolute eosinophil count exceeding 450 eosinophils/μL of blood, in the presence of leukocytosis exceeding 11,000/μL). Eosinophilia may not be persistent throughout the disease and eosinophilic vasculitis is not a prerequisite for the diagnosis in lung tissue. A number of different conditions have been described (see below). Rather than regarding each as a separate disease, we prefer to consider them all to be variants of eosinophilic pneumonia, a rationale underscored by the clinical use of the term *pulmonary infiltrates with eosinophilia (PIE)*, in reference to these eosinophilic lung diseases.

Several idiopathic forms have been described over the years. The mildest form has been referred to as *Loeffler syndrome or simple eosinophilic pneumonia.* Affected individuals are asymptomatic, have blood eosinophilia, and develop transient or migratory areas of consolidation. *Ascaris* infestation was documented eventually in the initial series by Loeffler, leading to the hypothesis that simple eosinophilic pneumonia was a manifestation of hypersensitivity to *Ascaris* antigens. The second idiopathic form occurs commonly

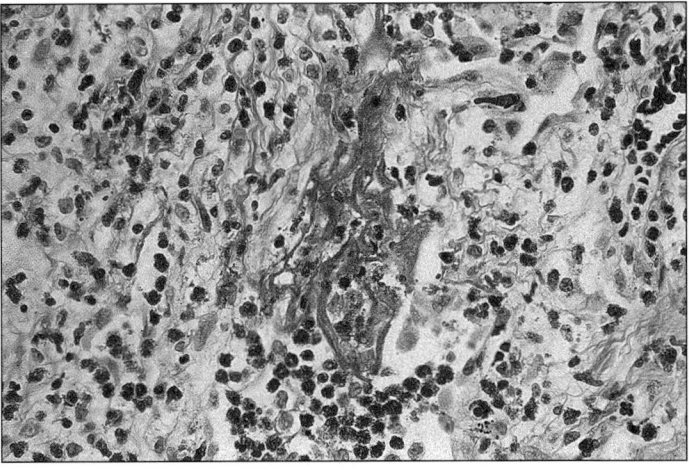

Fig. 17.43 Acute eosinophilic pneumonia. Diffuse alveolar damage may occur in acute eosinophilic pneumonia, even with the presence of hyaline membranes.

(though not exclusively) in asthmatic patients and presumably is an allergic manifestation to an unknown antigen. This manifestation is commonly associated with clinical symptoms and radiologic abnormalities, and the clinical course is more chronic, typically evolving slowly over many months. Because of this protracted course, this form of eosinophilic lung disease has been termed *chronic eosinophilic pneumonia.* Chronic eosinophilic pneumonia frequently has a characteristic radiologic appearance consisting of areas of consolidation involving mainly the subpleural regions of the upper lobes. Finally, a dramatic new manifestation of idiopathic eosinophilic lung disease has been described, characterized by rapid onset (typically over 5 days or less) of breathlessness in an otherwise healthy, nonasthmatic, young adult.[84] This form may mimic diffuse alveolar damage clinically and pathologically, even with the presence of hyaline membranes (Fig 17.43). The importance of recognizing this

Table 17.8 Drugs causing pulmonary eosinophilia and/or polyarteritis

Drug	Pulmonary eosinophilia	Polyarteritis
Allopurinol		+
Aspirin	+	
Busulfan		+
Hydantoins		+
Hydralazine		+
Imipramine	+	
Iodides		+
Gold salts		+
Nitrofurantoin	+	+
Penicillins	+	+
Sulfonamides	+	+

From Miller et al[405] with permission.

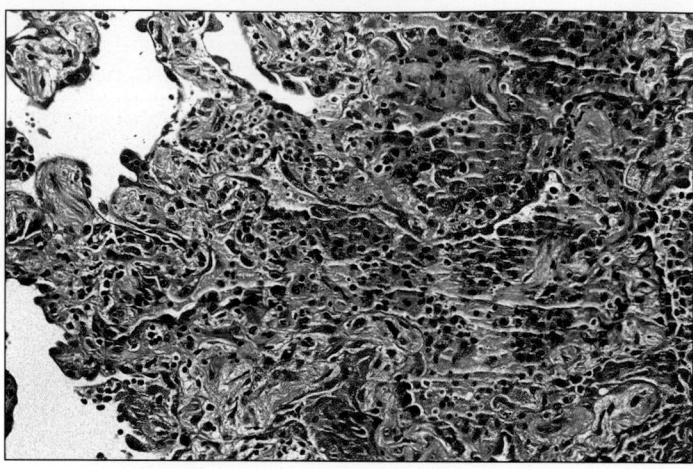

Fig. 17.44 Acute eosinophilic pneumonia. The reactive type II cells of AEP can be sufficiently prominent and atypical so as to raise concern for viropathic changes or even malignant tumor.

latter entity lies in its excellent prognosis and characteristic rapid response to corticosteroid therapy.

Some other well-recognized associations have been described with eosinophilic pneumonia. The best example is that produced by sensitivity to nitrofurantoin and other drugs. (Table 17.8). Also, pulmonary infiltrates associated with peripheral eosinophilia are common in tropical countries, presumably representing a reaction to migration of parasites through the lung, analogous to simple eosinophilic pneumonia. Finally, eosinophilic pneumonia, together with asthma, may be a manifestation of hypersensitivity to *Aspergillus* and other fungal organisms (e.g. allergic bronchopulmonary fungal disease). The chronic manifestations of eosinophilic pneumonia are discussed later in this chapter.

A distinctive and potentially life-threatening form of systemic vasculitis, accompanied by eosinophilic pneumonia, occurs in asthmatic individuals, and is worthy of mention here. Peripheral eosinophilia and eosinophilic pneumonia (typically with some degree of pulmonary eosinophilic vasculitis) are characteristic findings, but alone are not sufficient for a definitive diagnosis. Serum ANCA studies typically reveal elevated levels of P-ANCA. This condition is known as 'Churg-Strauss syndrome,'[85] and if left untreated, has particularly devastating results in the heart.

The histologic features are similar in all forms of eosinophilic pneumonia (EP), and consist of a triad of 1) variable numbers of eosinophils in the alveolar spaces, 2) plump, densely eosinophilic alveolar macrophages, and 3) reactive type II cell hyperplasia. There may be an associated mild interstitial pneumonia. In some instances, the interstitial pneumonia may be quite severe, with type II cells sufficiently prominent and atypical so as to raise concern for viropathic changes or even malignant tumor (Fig. 17.44). In these circumstances clinical and pathologic diffuse alveolar damage may be evident.

The macrophages of EP may be so densely aggregated in the airspaces as to be mistaken for desquamative interstitial pneumonia (DIP). Also, focal eosinophilic necrosis of the dense alveolar macrophage reaction can occur, and multinucleated macrophages can be present, thereby simulating a granulomatous reaction. Other expected findings in eosinophilic lung disease include eosinophilic infiltration of small vessels, and alveolar organization with loosely aggregated immature-appearing fibroblasts.

Acute fibrinous and organizing pneumonia

In 2001, Beaseley and coworkers presented clinical, radiologic, and pathologic findings from 30 patients with acute diffuse lung injury associated with a high mortality rate.[85a] These authors coined the term 'acute fibrinous and organizing pneumonia (AFOP)' for the pathologic manifestation and emphasized that the condition resembled diffuse alveolar damage to great extent, except without hyaline membranes. AFOP is rich in fibrinous alveolar exudates (Fig. 17.45), without evidence of infection or tissue eosinophils. Like DAD, AFOP can be idiopathic or associated with a number of underlying or associated conditions, such as collagen vascular disease, drug reaction, and occupational exposures. The pathologic manifestations in the 30 patients presented ranged from patchy to diffuse in surgical biopsy sections. Survival is similar to DAD in general (about 50% mortality), but was bimodal, with death being highly associated with the requirement for mechanical ventilation.

Acute manifestations of the collagen vascular diseases

The most common acute manifestation of the collagen vascular diseases is diffuse alveolar damage, but diffuse pulmonary hemorrhage also occurs. The more common collagen vascular diseases producing acute manifestations are presented here.

Rheumatoid arthritis

At least 50% of patients with rheumatoid arthritis (RA) have one or more forms of rheumatoid lung disease,[86] and patients with more severe joint involvement are more likely to develop pleuro-pulmonary manifestations. Lung disease typically follows the development of joint disease, but on occasion the lung or pleura may herald the disease. Diffuse alveolar damage is a well-recognized complication of RA.[87]

Systemic lupus erythematosus

Like RA, systemic lupus erythematosus (SLE) also commonly involves the lungs and pleura.[86] Painful pleuritis with or without effusion is the most common abnormality,[88] but acute lupus pneumonitis is a potentially disastrous complication, with a mortality of 50%.[89] Acute lupus pneumonitis is characterized morphologically by

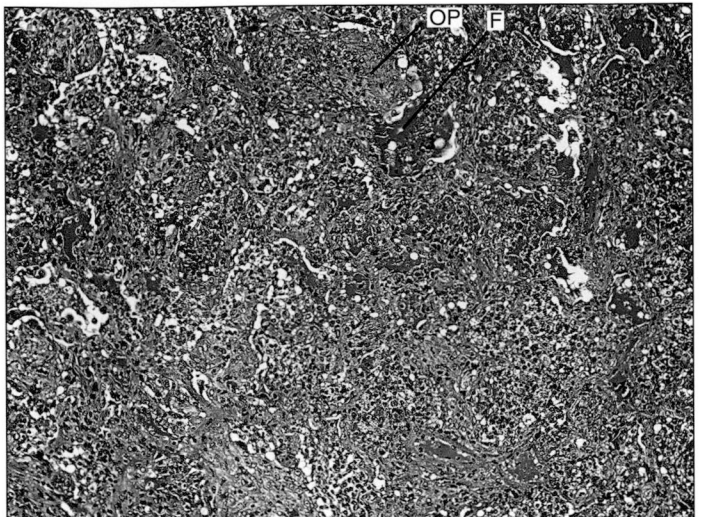

Fig. 17.45 Acute fibrinous and organizing pneumonia (AFOP). AFOP is a recently described form of acute lung injury rich in fibrinous alveolar exudates (F) with variable alveolar organization (OP), but lacking hyaline membranes, evidence of infection, or tissue eosinophils. AFOP can be idiopathic or associated with a number of underlying or associated conditions, such as collagen vascular disease, drug reaction, and occupational exposures. The pathologic manifestations can vary from patchy to diffuse in surgical biopsy sections.

diffuse alveolar damage. Diffuse pulmonary hemorrhage may also occur, usually accompanied by vasculitis and capillaritis. Immune complexes may be identified on capillary basement membranes in this setting.[90]

Dermatomyositis-polymyositis

Tazelaar and coworkers presented 14 patients with dermatomyositis-polymyositis (DM-PM) who developed lung disease.[91] Three patients developed diffuse alveolar damage, all of whom died, most frequently in the acute episode. These authors also reviewed 27 additional cases of DM-PM lung disease reported in the literature and found similar results. Interestingly, diffuse alveolar damage may be the first clinical manifestation of DM-PM, and may actually precede the clinical and serologic diagnosis of the disease by many months. The other lung manifestations of DM-PM will be discussed later under chronic lung diseases.

Acute diffuse alveolar hemorrhage

Diffuse alveolar hemorrhage (DAH) is characterized by a triad of: 1) hemoptysis, 2) anemia, and 3) bilateral ground-glass opacities (or consolidation) that rapidly wax and wane. Hemorrhage and hemosiderin-laden macrophages in alveolar spaces are essential to the pathologic diagnosis.[92–94] Because there are many etiologies of DAH, it is helpful to have a classification algorithm for the diagnostic approach to these patients (Fig. 17.46). In practice, because artifactual hemorrhage can occur commonly in lung biopsy specimens, hemosiderin-laden macrophages (with coarsely granular, golden-brown refractile pigment) should always be present in the alveolar spaces before invoking the diagnosis of DAH (Fig. 17.47).

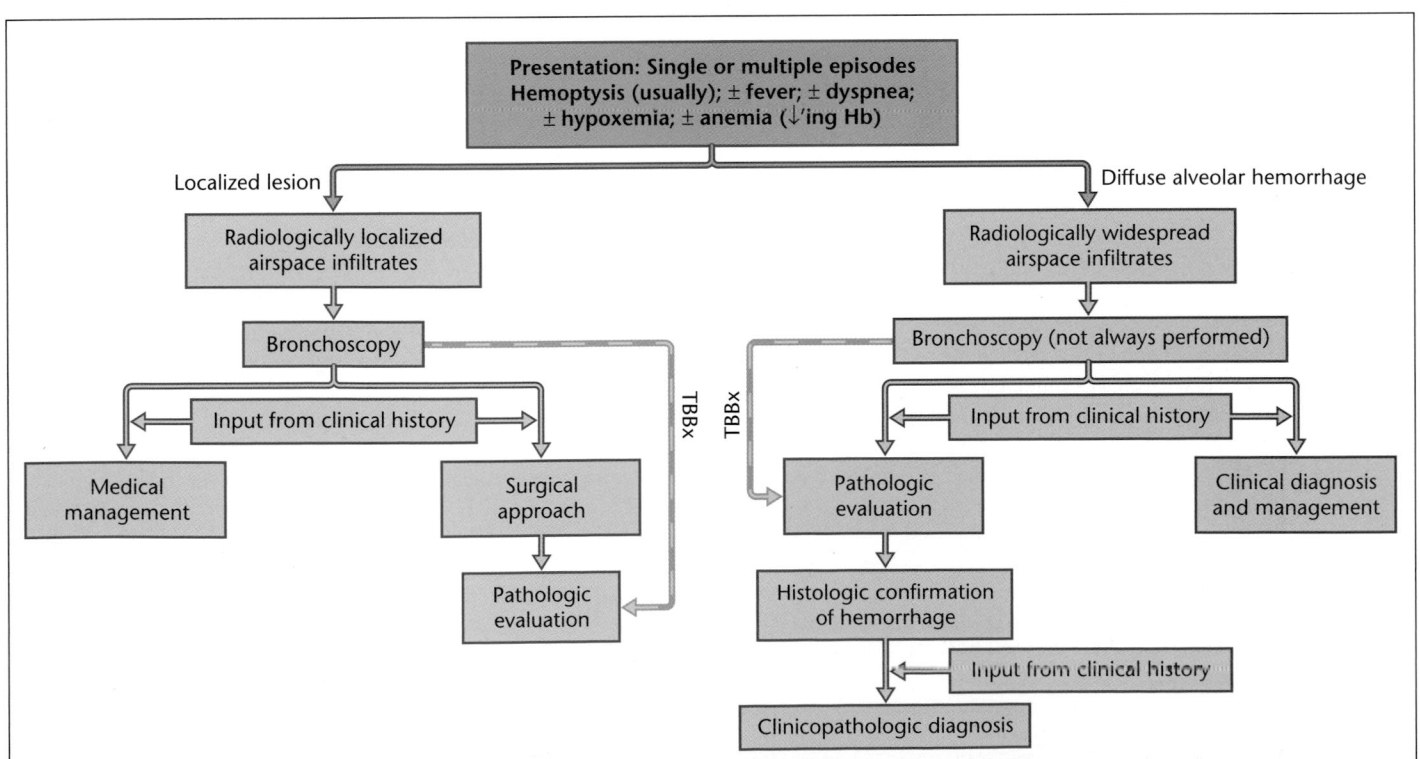

Fig. 17.46 DAH algorithm. Because there are many etiologies of DAH, it is important to have an algorithm for the diagnostic approach to these patients. (From Colby et al. Pathologic approach to pulmonary hemorrhage,[93] with permission).

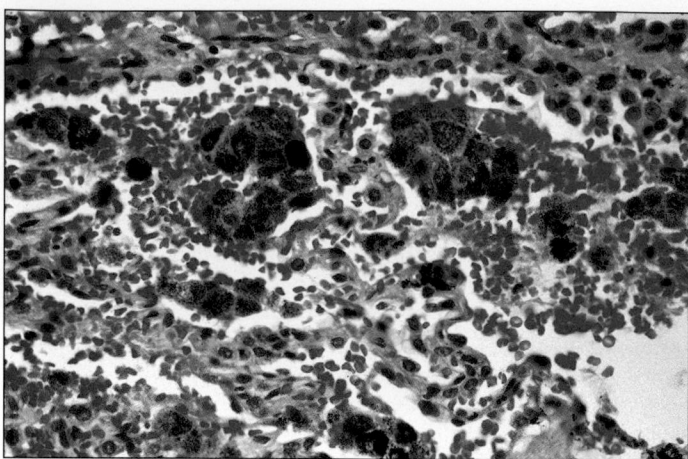

Fig. 17.47 Pulmonary hemorrhage. Blood free in the alveolar spaces may occur as a result of trauma during the biopsy procedure. Significant hemorrhage is always accompanied by siderophages – macrophages filled with 'chunky' golden-brown hemosiderin. This gross hemosiderin differs from the delicate punctate hemosiderin that may be present in smokers' macrophages.

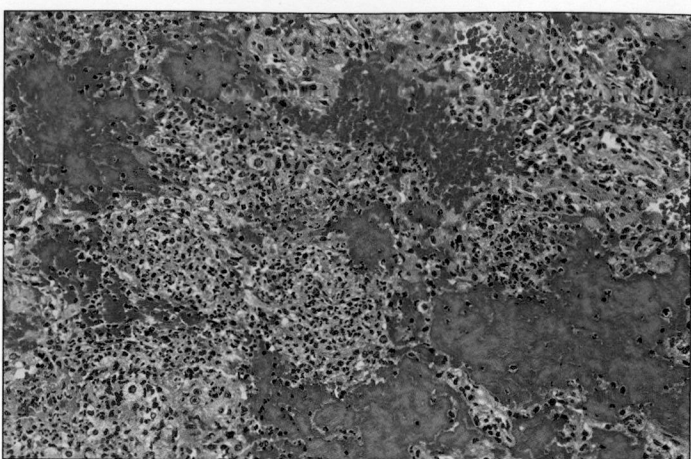

Fig. 17.48 Capillaritis. DAH may be accompanied by subtle or quite dramatic capillaritis (as seen here). The context of airspace fibrin and siderophages is often helpful in confirming the diagnosis.

DAH associated with collagen vascular disease

DAH may occur as a consequence of several immune-mediated vasculitides including those occurring in the setting of collagen vascular disease. Potential causes of DAH in this setting include microscopic polyangiitis, systemic lupus erythematosus (SLE), Wegener's granulomatosis, cryoglobulinemia, rheumatoid arthritis, crescentic glomerulonephritis, and scleroderma.[92,94–96] The common feature is acute capillaritis, with or without larger vessel lesions.

Antiglomerular basement membrane disease (Goodpasture's syndrome)

When diffuse pulmonary hemorrhage occurs with renal disease in the presence of circulating antibodies against glomerular basement membranes, the condition is referred to as 'anti-GBM disease.' (ABMD)[95–98] The disease occurs most commonly in men (frequently smokers) between the ages of 18 and 30. Hemoptysis is the presenting symptom in most affected individuals. Lung biopsy is less desirable than kidney as a diagnostic specimen in ABMD, but because renal disease is commonly occult at the time of presentation, the lung is often the first sample examined by the surgical pathologist. Unfortunately, the lung findings are relatively non-specific and consist of fresh alveolar hemorrhage, hemosiderin deposition in macrophages (siderophages), and variable interstitial inflammation and delicate fibrosis. If capillaritis (Fig. 17.48) is present, a diagnosis such as 'pulmonary hemorrhage with capillaritis' is appropriate, followed by a differential diagnosis to include anti-GBM disease, Wegener's granulomatosis, microscopic polyangiitis, certain drug reactions, and systemic connective tissue disease-related hemorrhage.[99] The presence of capillaritis in the alveolar wall is also helpful in distinguishing anti-GBM disease from idiopathic pulmonary hemosiderosis and chronic passive lung congestion. The results of immunofluorescent studies on lung tissue are not as reliable as they are on kidney tissue,[96] and for cost-effective practice, we generally recommend serologic confirmation (radioimmunoassay or enzyme-linked immunosorbent assay), even when appropriately preserved lung tissue is available. In the kidney biopsy, diagnostic linear deposits of immunoglobulin (IgG) can be demonstrated along glomerular basement membranes using immunofluorescent techniques.

Idiopathic pulmonary hemosiderosis

DAH, in the absence of renal disease or demonstrable immunologic disease, has been termed 'idiopathic pulmonary hemosiderosis (IPH).' IPH occurs most commonly in children younger than 10 years old and young adults in the second to third decades of life. Anemia is accompanied by bilateral areas of consolidation on the chest radiograph. The sexes are equally affected in the younger age group, but the disease occurs more frequently in males in the older age group. The histopathology is similar to that of anti-GBM disease, namely, alveolar hemorrhage and hemosiderin-laden macrophages, but in IPH there are lesser degrees of interstitial inflammation and more fibrosis (Fig. 17.49). By definition, tissue immunoglobulin studies and electron microscopy are nondiagnostic.

Miscellaneous causes of DAH

DAH may occur from any number of causes, especially in the immunocompromised host.[99,100] Some causes may be obvious, but in many cases a specific etiology remains elusive. Drug reactions,[94] cardiovascular disorders (e.g. mitral stenosis), pulmonary veno-occlusive disease, severe pulmonary edema,[92] and even amyloidosis can produce DAH. Disorders of coagulation and hemostasis such as those produced by blood dyscrasias, anticoagulation therapy, disseminated intravascular coagulation, and thrombocytopenia[92,101] may be complicated by DAH. A number of infections are commonly associated with DAH, including those caused by fungi (commonly *Aspergillus*), viruses (typically CMV or HSV), various bacteria (especially those causing necrotizing infection), and *P. jiroveci*.[100,102]

Other causes of acute diffuse lung disease

Drugs and radiation reactions

Medications taken orally or by injection may produce a variety of lesions within the lung including diffuse alveolar damage, pulmonary edema, asthma, eosinophilic pneumonia, and even advanced fibrosis.[103,104] For many drugs, both acute and chronic forms of toxicity

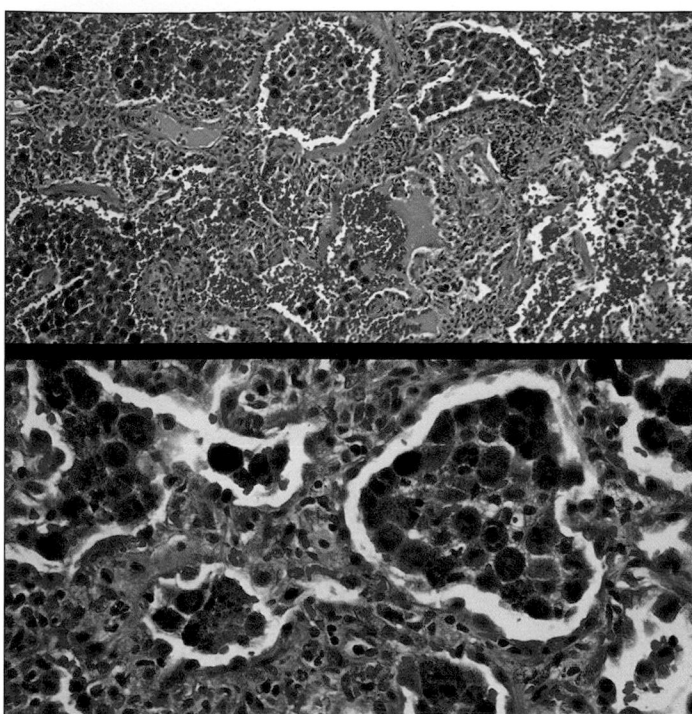

Fig. 17.49 Idiopathic pulmonary hemosiderosis. Less interstitial inflammation and more fibrosis is typical in IPH which differs from the immune-mediated causes of pulmonary hemorrhage.

have been reported. Here we will emphasize a few that classically manifest as acute lung disease and highlight those that also may produce chronic disease.

The common features of DAD induced by therapeutic agents include proliferation of alveolar type II cells, interstitial fibrosis, and relative preservation of lung structure. Advanced remodeling is not typical of the acute phase of drug injury. With antineoplastic agents, a characteristic finding may be the presence of large type II cells, with atypical hyperchromatic nuclei and prominent nucleoli. Many drugs have been associated with the occurrence of pulmonary disease. A few of the most common, and/or most distinctive drugs, from a pathologic perspective, are presented here. Because of a general lack of diagnostic clinical or pathologic features, the best method of diagnosing drug-induced disease is to combine a high index of suspicion with a thorough clinical history.

Nitrofurantoin

Nitrofurantoin is responsible for more cases of pulmonary toxicity than any other drug, with both acute and chronic reactions reported.[105,106] Nitrofurantoin is an antimicrobial agent used in the treatment of urinary tract infections. Acute reactions are accompanied by fever, dyspnea, and peripheral eosinophilia, typically appearing within two weeks of initiating therapy. Chest radiographs show a bilateral reticular pattern with a basal predominance, occasionally associated with septal lines (Kerley B lines), and small pleural effusions, findings resembling those of interstitial pulmonary edema. Gastrointestinal symptoms, headaches, or myalgia occur in approximately 20% of the patients who develop toxicity. Because acute cases rarely require a lung biopsy for diagnosis, limited information is available. From reports of cases where biopsies have been performed, the findings are descriptively similar to those of

AEP. For example, mild interstitial inflammation and vasculitis may be present (sometimes accompanied by poorly formed granulomas), and intra-alveolar eosinophils accompanied by macrophages may be present. Also similar to AEP, macrophage density in the airspaces may be sufficiently prominent to suggest a diagnosis of desquamative interstitial pneumonia.[107] Chronic reactions occur in a minority of patients taking the drug (approximately 10%) and clinical manifestations appear after 1 to 6 months of treatment. Dyspnea in these patients is mild, and systemic reactions are rare. Autoantibodies are occasionally present.[108] The chronic cases are more often subjected to biopsy and show interstitial inflammation and fibrosis accompanied by vascular sclerosis. The chest radiograph demonstrates a reticular pattern. Less commonly, nitrofurantoin may cause an organizing pneumonia[109] with patchy bilateral areas of consolidation that on CT have a predominantly peribronchial distribution.[110]

Cytotoxic chemotherapeutic drugs

The most common drugs producing acute lung injury are the antineoplastic agents. Nevertheless, from a clinical standpoint some drugs (5-fluorouracil, vinblastine, cytarabine, adriamycin, thiotepa, azathioprine) never or very rarely produce pulmonary lesions. With increasing numbers of newer antineoplastic agents being used, the number that reportedly produce pulmonary toxicity will likely increase. Excellent on-line resources provide comprehensive and up-to-date lists of these agents.[111] Two chemotherapeutic drugs are presented here for illustration purposes: bleomycin, because it is a relatively common chemotherapeutic agent and has been used as an experimental tool in the study of lung injury and fibrosis; and methotrexate, because it is also commonly used in clinical practice and produces reasonably distinctive manifestations in the lung.

Bleomycin

Bleomycin is a chemotherapeutic agent used in the treatment of a number of neoplastic diseases (e.g. epidermoid carcinoma, lymphomas, malignant testicular tumors), often in combinations with other agents. Bleomycin becomes concentrated in the skin, the lungs, and in lymphatic fluid. Pulmonary lesions appear to be dose-related,[112,113] and prior radiotherapy seems to predispose to toxicity.[114]

Toxic symptoms are characterized by dry cough accompanied by progressive dyspnea. Rales in the basal lung segments are an early physical sign and pulmonary function studies show restriction. Radiographs do not exhibit changes until symptoms are present, and then they show a diffuse reticular pattern or areas of consolidation in the lower lung zones. The initial site of injury in experimental models seems to be the venous endothelial cell[115] but it is the type I cell injury that allows fibrin and other serum proteins to leak into the alveolus. Type II hyperplasia occurs as a regenerative phenomenon, resulting in the formation of very atypical enlarged forms, and intra-alveolar fibroplasia occurs, eventually resulting in alveolar septal widening (Fig. 17.50).

Methotrexate

Methotrexate seems to manifest toxicity largely through a hyper-sensitivity reaction,[116] and there does not appear to be dose relationship to toxicity. Intravenous administration has been shown to be associated with more toxic effects. A cough occurring within the first 3 months after administration is followed by fever, malaise, and progressive breathlessness. Peripheral eosinophilia is observed in a significant number of patients who develop toxicity. In lung tissue, a mildly cellular interstitial pneumonia is

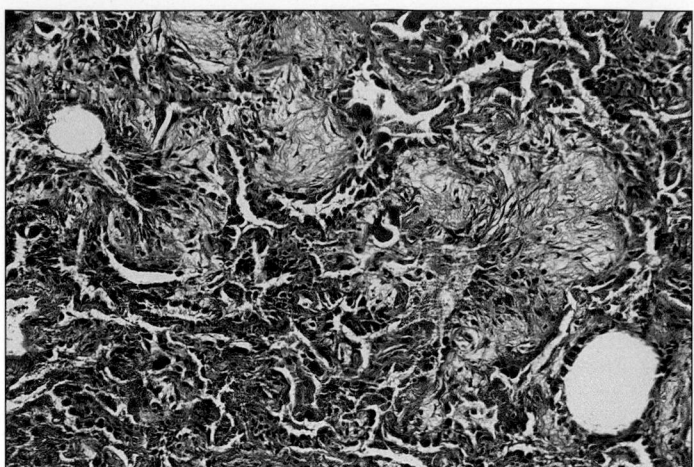

Fig. 17.50 Bleomycin toxicity. As the intra-alveolar fibrin becomes organized by fibroblasts (here seen as pale-staining plugs of loose fibroblasts and matrix) a distinctive intra-alveolar fibrosis with septal widening eventually occurs.

observed, composed of lymphocytes, plasma cells, and a few eosinophils (Fig. 17.51A). Poorly formed, non-necrotizing granulomas may be seen and scattered multinucleated giant cells are common (Fig. 17.51B). Symptoms gradually abate after the drug is withdrawn,[117] but systemic corticosteroids have also been used in some patients.

Analgesics

Heroin,[118] methadone, propoxyphene, and even aspirin, can produce similar lung reactions,[119,120] Toxicity typically results from overdose and is characterized by pulmonary edema sometimes complicated by aspiration of gastric contents. When pill binding agents such as talc or microcrystalline cellulose are injected with drug intravenously, a foreign body giant cell reaction may be seen in lung tissue in a characteristic perivascular distribution. Polarization in this setting reveals refractile intracellular particles in the perivascular macrophages (typically larger than 10 microns in size).

Radiation pneumonitis

Radiation therapy was a common cause of acute lung injury before improved technology and modifications in radiation dosing were instituted.[121] Radiation injury can be exacerbated by infection[122] and chemotherapeutic drugs.[123] Initial clinical signs and symptoms often are absent or very mild. In the acute phase, the chest radiograph and HRCT show ground-glass opacities, or airspace consolidation with some loss of lung volume. In the chronic phase of irradiation injury, fibrosis accompanied by architectural remodeling is seen, presumably a result of recurrent cycles of ischemic injury from radiation-induced vascular sclerosis. Different from many other causes of radiologically definable lung fibrosis, the fibrosis of radiation injury is relatively limited to the treatment field.

Histopathologically, irradiation causes cellular injury with the creation of atypical type II cells, often with large hyperchromatic nuclei ('radiation atypia'). Some authors have postulated that an immune mechanism is stimulated as part of a 'subacute phase' of radiation injury,[124] partially based on evidence of interstitial pneumonitis observed outside of the anticipated radiation field. There is considerable debate as to the existence of this phenomenon and its mechanism, if it does occur.[125]

Chronic radiation injury may have to be distinguished histopathologically from other causes of fibrosis, such as that produced by usual interstitial pneumonia (UIP). As mentioned earlier, the fibrosis of radiation injury is relatively limited to the treatment field, in contrast to that of UIP, where fibrosis occurs in a peripherally accentuated, bi-basilar distribution. As will become apparent later in this chapter in the discussion of UIP and other fibrosing lung diseases, the microscopic pattern of fibrosis is also very helpful in resolving the differential diagnosis.

Idiopathic diffuse alveolar damage: acute interstitial pneumonia

Clinical features: The term *acute interstitial pneumonia* (AIP) was first introduced in 1986 to describe a syndrome of rapidly evolving acute respiratory failure occurring in *immunologically normal individuals*.[126] The patients described included 3 men and 5 women (two of whom were pregnant), who developed sudden unexplained respiratory failure. Six reported a viral-like prodrome. None of the patients was reported to have underlying collagen vascular disease. By definition, AIP is of

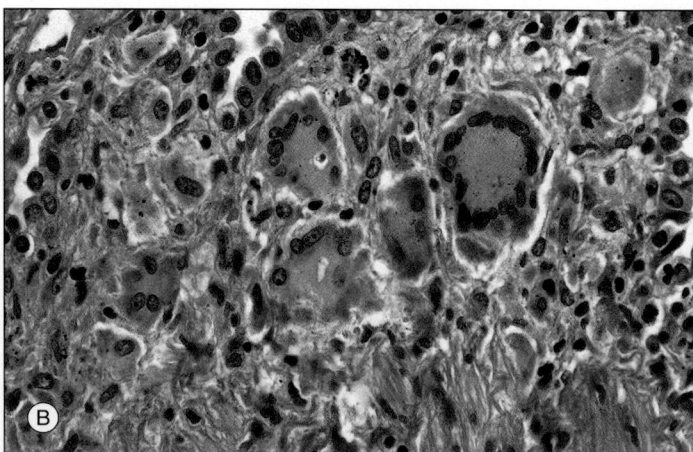

Fig. 17.51 Methotrexate toxicity. An interstitial infiltrate of lymphocytes, plasma cells, and eosinophils is present (**A**), accompanied by ill-defined granulomas with flattened multinucleated giant cells (**B**).

unknown cause and is a diagnosis of exclusion. The usual causes of ARDS, such as shock, sepsis, trauma, aspiration, or drug toxicity, can be ruled out clinically. Infection should be excluded by special stains, a search for viropathic inclusions, and microbiological cultures.

Radiologic findings: The radiologic and CT findings of AIP are similar to those of ARDS. The chest radiograph typically shows extensive, symmetric bilateral airspace consolidation. HRCT demonstrates extensive bilateral areas of ground-glass attenuation and focal areas of consolidation.[127] The areas of consolidation tend to involve mainly the dorsal lung regions.[128]

Pathologic findings: Surgical lung biopsies show diffuse alveolar damage in varying stages. The cases previously reported by Pratt et al.[129] and those reported by Hamman and Rich[130] had a similar course. Five of the cases reported by Pratt et al. had collagen vascular diseases (three of whom had rheumatoid arthritis) and four others had a history of allergic disorders. The changes observed in biopsy specimens depend on the stage at which the biopsy is taken and these tend to be relatively diffuse throughout the specimen. Like other forms of DAD, the early stages show an exudative phase with edema and hyaline membranes. Bronchioles may show squamous metaplasia extending to involve adjacent alveolar walls. Organizing arterial thrombi were seen in five of the seven patients who died in the Katzenstein series. In the last stages, fibrosis distorts the lung architecture.

Clinical course: Seven of the eight patients presented by Pratt et al. died, five within 2 months of the onset. The significant number of patients with collagen vascular disease or allergic disorders suggests that these underlying conditions may be responsible, even though they may not be clinically apparent at the time of presentation. AIP has been formally added to the classification of the idiopathic interstitial pneumonias by a recent international consensus committee.[33]

SUBACUTE AND CHRONIC DIFFUSE LUNG DISEASES (MONTHS TO YEARS IN EVOLUTION)

Table 17.1 provides a list of the more common diagnostic considerations for diffuse lung diseases that evolve slowly over weeks to months, and sometimes even years.

Subacute and chronic pulmonary manifestations of the connective tissue diseases

The collagen vascular diseases as a group involve the respiratory system frequently. Each of these diseases may involve the lung and pleura in a number of different ways. While the lung morphologic abnormalities are not specific for any one of these diseases, some features are more commonly manifested than others in each of them (Table 17.9).

Rheumatoid arthritis

As mentioned earlier in the discussion of acute lung involvement in the collagen vascular diseases, a significant proportion of patients with RA develop pleuropulmonary disease and most of these evolve over weeks to many months.[86] Sometimes these pulmonary manifestations can remain a clinical problem for years.

The most common thoracic complication of RA is pleural disease (effusion and/or pleuritis), seen in as many as 50% of patients in autopsy studies. According to a study by Walker et al., about one-third of the patients with pleural effusions also have pulmonary manifestations of RA in the form of nodules or interstitial disease.[131] In this large series, only 1.6% had radiologic evidence of fibrosis, while in other series, restrictive lung disease was present in as many as 40%.[132,133] In about one-half of these patients, the chest radiograph was normal despite interstitial fibrosis in lung biopsies,[132] attesting to the insensitivity of lung imaging relative to the presence or absence of microscopic pathology (even with 1mm high-resolution CT scans). Nodules may be seen in the lung parenchyma and occasionally in the walls of airways in RA representing lymphoid hyperplasia with germinal centers in most instances. Moreover, lymphocytic aggregates with germinal centers are often seen in biopsies of patients with RA, and while not specific for the disease, should always raise RA lung (and Sjögren syndrome) in the differential diagnosis, especially in the context of chronic inflammatory airways disease, variable interstitial inflammation, and non-specific fibrosis. The interstitial pneumonia of RA may be quite cellular with little fibrosis (cellular NSIP-like, see below), and on occasion, a macrophage-rich desquamative interstitial pneumonia (DIP) pattern may be seen.[87] Pulmonary hypertension is the rarest[86] pulmonary manifestation of

Table 17.9 Lung manifestations of the collagen vascular diseases

	RA	J-RA	SLE	PSS	DM-PM	MCTD	Sjögren	Ankylosing spondilitis
Pleural inflammation, fibrosis, effusions	X	X	X	X	X	X	X	X
Airway disease: Inflammation, obstruction, lymphoidhyperplasia, follicular bronchiolitis	X	X	X	X			X	
Interstitial disease	X	X	X	X	X	X	X	
Acute (DAD), with or without hemorrhage	X	X	X	X	X	X		
Subacute/organizing (OP pattern)	X		X	X	X		X	
Subacute cellular	X		X				X	
Chronic cellular	X	X	X	X	X	X	X	
Eosinophilic infiltrates	X							
Granulomatous interstitial pneumonia	X		X			X		
Vascular diseases; hypertension/vasculitis	X	X	X	X	X	X	X	
Parenchymal nodules	X	X						
Apical fibrobullous disease	X						X	
Lymphoid proliferation (reactive, neoplastic)			X		X	X		

Modified from Colby et al.[406] and Travis et al.[408]

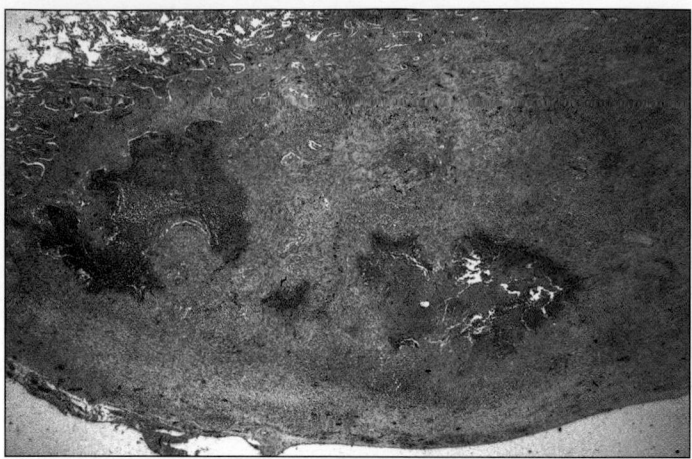

Fig. 17.52 Rheumatoid arthritis. The histologic appearance of pulmonary rheumatoid nodules is similar to that of rheumatoid nodules elsewhere in the body.

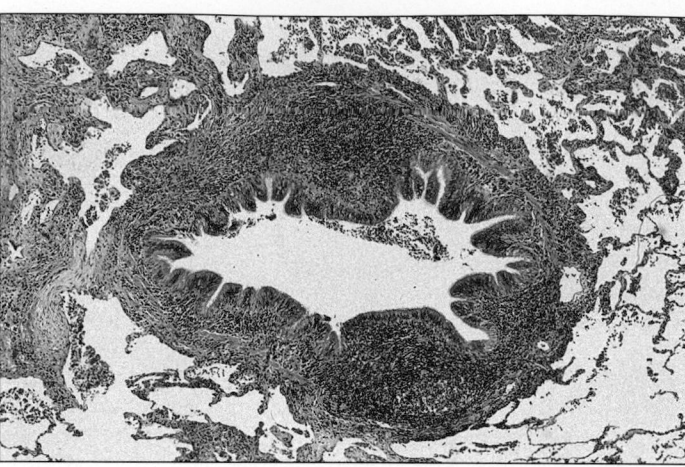

Fig. 17.53 Rheumatoid arthritis. The characteristic parenchymal abnormality is a cellular bronchiolitis with many germinal centers (follicular bronchiolitis).

RA. The clinical presentation resembles that of primary pulmonary hypertension, and the vascular lesions may be indistinguishable histologically. Some of the more typical pulmonary manifestations of RA follow:

Rheumatoid lung nodules are the most distinctive and specific histologic lung lesions seen in RA.[134] Radiologically, they may be solitary, but often appear as multiple well-defined nodules, ranging from a few millimeters to several centimeters in diameter, present throughout the lung. Rheumatoid nodules typically raise a radiologic differential diagnosis to include metastatic tumor and miliary infection. Patients with subcutaneous rheumatoid nodules are more likely to develop lung nodules, and both manifestations tend to wax and wane together.[134] Cavitation of rheumatoid nodules may occur, mimicking abscess or necrotic tumor. The histologic appearance of pulmonary rheumatoid nodules is similar to that of rheumatoid nodules elsewhere in the body (Fig. 17.52). In the RA patient being treated with systemic corticosteroids, tuberculosis and other infections must be included in the clinical and pathologic differential diagnosis. The histologic distinction may be difficult, but characteristic palisading, paucity of giant cells, and absence of identifiable organisms all favor rheumatoid nodule as the correct diagnosis.

Caplan's syndrome (rheumatoid pneumoconiosis) is the occurrence of pulmonary rheumatoid nodules in the setting of occupational pneumoconiosis. Silica and silicates are the most commonly implicated exposures. Coal miners and workers exposed to silica, aluminum, asbestos, roof tiles, and boiler scaling seem to be particularly at risk.[86] Affected individuals become seropositive for rheumatoid factor. The clinical presentation is characterized by the rapid development of one or more lung nodules, 1–5 cm in diameter. Microscopic examinations revels the nodules to have a central necrotic area surrounded by dust and fibrosis. The edge of the necrotic area has palisaded cells, and a characteristic accumulation of neutrophils can be seen at the junction of necrosis with the palisaded cellular reaction. The etiology of Caplan's syndrome is unknown, but there is speculation that genetically predisposed individuals react with the inhaled dusts and develop an abnormal immunologic reaction.[135]

Lymphoid hyperplasia with germinal centers may be found distributed along bronchovascular bundles as follicular bronchiolitis

(Fig. 17.53), and also along interlobular septa.[87] This manifestation may be helpful in creating a differential diagnosis in the setting of a 'non-specific interstitial pneumonia pattern.'

Cellular interstitial infiltrates in isolation are a relatively uncommon manifestation of RA, but when these occur, they resemble those described later in the section on non-specific interstitial pneumonia (NSIP).

Organizing pneumonia can occur as a pulmonary manifestation of RA. In a study by Yousem and coworkers, OP was seen as the primary pattern in 6 of the 40 biopsies.[87] No infectious etiology was identified in their series, and the process was attributed to RA.

Constrictive (obliterative) bronchiolitis with significant airflow obstruction is a well-recognized manifestation of RA. The exact incidence and prevalence in RA patients is unknown. Constrictive bronchiolitis is discussed later in this chapter in the section on bronchiolitis occurring in non-smokers.

Progressive systemic sclerosis

Lymphoid hyperplasia in the lung occurs in the early stages of scleroderma, but the most notable feature is the presence of extensive fibrosis without much evident inflammation.[136] A non-specific cellular interstitial pneumonia is common,[137] and some degree of diffuse lung fibrosis occurs in nearly every case.[86] Morphologically, patients with long-standing progressive systemic sclerosis-related fibrosis are at high risk of developing bronchioloalveolar carcinoma. Vascular sclerosis, usually without true vasculitis, is typical and is associated with pulmonary hypertension if sufficiently severe.[138] Onset of pulmonary hypertension at any point in the disease is associated with a significantly worse survival.[139,140] Pleural disease is considerably less common in progressive systemic sclerosis than in RA or SLE.

Mixed connective tissue disease

Mixed connective tissue disease is a relatively common collagen vascular disease associated with radiologic and functional evidence of interstitial pulmonary disease and/or pleural effusions.[86] In many cases, the abnormalities respond quite well to systemic corticosteroid

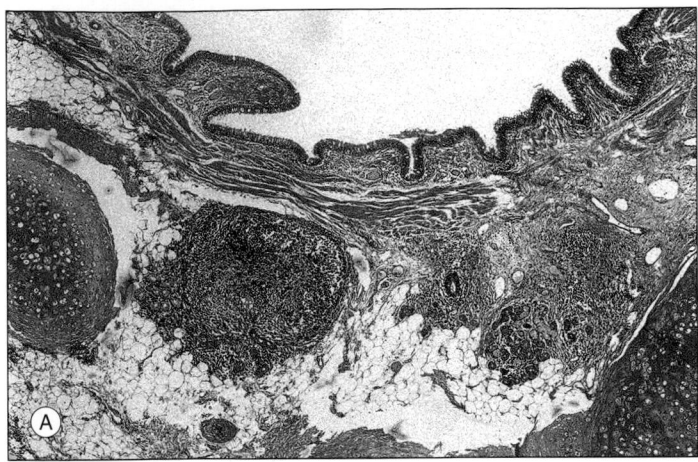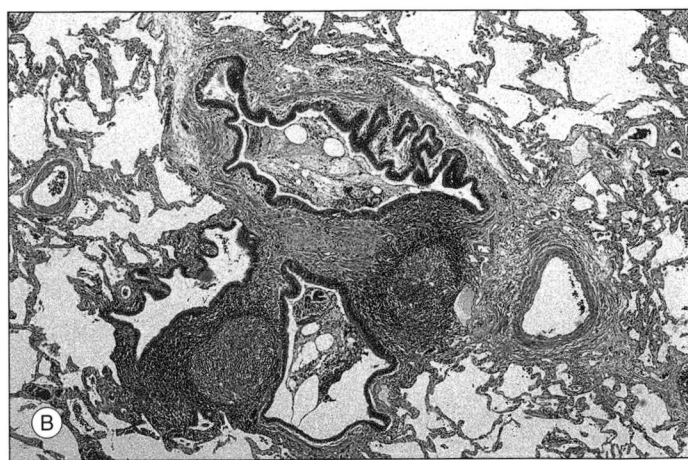

Fig. 17.54 Sjögren's syndrome. The common pulmonary lesions are analogous to the salivary gland lesions. A marked lymphoreticular infiltrate in the submucosal glands of the tracheobronchial tree (**A**). In more peripheral lung, Sjögren's syndrome is characterized by follicular bronchiolitis, similar to that seen in rheumatoid lung (**B**).

therapy, but severe and progressive pulmonary disease with fibrosis does occur. Three of the patients in one study had a pattern of fibrosis resembling that of usual interstitial pneumonia, and two had pulmonary hypertension complicated by plexiform lesions as seen in primary pulmonary hypertension.[141]

Systemic lupus erythematosus

As discussed earlier, systemic lupus erythematosus (SLE) commonly involves the respiratory system.[86] Painful pleuritis is the most common abnormality, with or without pleural effusions.[88] Organizing pneumonia[142] and cellular interstitial infiltrates have also been reported.[143,144]

Polymyositis and dermatomyositis

Systemic polymyositis/dermatomyositis is associated with four types of interstitial lung disease, and the histologic findings seen on biopsy are better predictors of prognosis than clinical or radiologic features. Tazelaar and coworkers[91] described the lung findings in 14 patients. Six developed a subacute presentation with a noninfectious organizing pneumonia pattern and this manifestation was associated with the best prognosis (67% survival). The worst prognosis was seen in five patients who had advanced lung fibrosis (40% survival).

Sjögren's syndrome

The common pulmonary lesions of Sjögren's syndrome generally evolve over weeks to months and are analogous to the salivary gland lesions, namely a marked lymphoreticular infiltrate in the submucosal glands of the tracheobronchial tree (Fig. 17.54).[86] Patients with Sjögren's syndrome also are at risk for developing pulmonary lymphoproliferative disorders, ranging from low-grade extranodal marginal zone lymphoma ('maltoma') to a high-grade lymphoma.

Certain chronic drug reactions

Many drugs are reported to produce lung fibrosis, among them bleomycin, carmustine, penicillamine, nitrofurantoin, tocainide, mexiletine, amiodarone, azathioprine, methotrexate, melphalan and mitomycin C. The list of agents grows rapidly and the reader is referred to on-line resources such as *www.pneumotox.com* for continuously updated information on reported drug reactions.

Subacute/chronic lung diseases with granulomas

Hypersensitivity pneumonitis (HSP)

Lung disease can result following inhalation of a variety of organic dusts and as a group are referred to as hypersensitivity pneumonitis. In most of these, the disease is immunologically mediated, presumably through a type III hypersensitivity reaction, although the immunologic mechanisms have not been well-documented in all conditions.[145] The prototypical example is so-called *farmer's lung*, caused by hypersensitivity to thermophilic actinomycetes (*Micromonospora vulgaris* and *Thermophylliae polyspora*) that grow in moldy hay. Farmer's lung is more common in Britain and Europe than in North America. In the United States, *Micropolyspora faeni* is the most commonly implicated organism.

Characteristically, the condition occurs when the summers are wet. Cut hay is not gathered until it is dry, and this allows sufficient time for proliferation of the organisms. Typically, exposure to the moldy hay occurs during winter feeding in a barn or other enclosed space.

Clinical features: Symptoms appear within hours of exposure and consist of fever, malaise, cough, and breathlessness. Wheezing is uncommon. The symptoms soon pass, but may reappear when the individual re-enters the offending environment. The acute symptoms may not be recognized as an environmental exposure, and following repeated episodes, the patient eventually develops progressive dyspnea. Most patients are biopsied during this stage.[146] With continued exposure, the patient enters the chronic stage and lung fibrosis occurs. Precipitating antibodies to the responsible organism are found in a high percentage of those who develop symptoms, compared with asymptomatic individuals in the same environment.[147]

Radiologic findings: The radiologic appearance depends on the stage of the disease. In the acute stage, the dominant feature is airspace consolidation. In the subacute stage, there is a fine nodular pattern or ground-glass opacification. The chronic stage is dominated by fibrosis as evidenced by irregular linear opacities resulting in a reticular pattern. CT scans add little to the chest radiograph in the acute stage. In the subacute phase, the HRCT findings are often characteristic enough to suggest the diagnosis. The HRCT manifestations consist of bilateral 3–5 mm poorly defined centrilobular nodular opacities and/or symmetric bilateral ground-glass opacities often associated

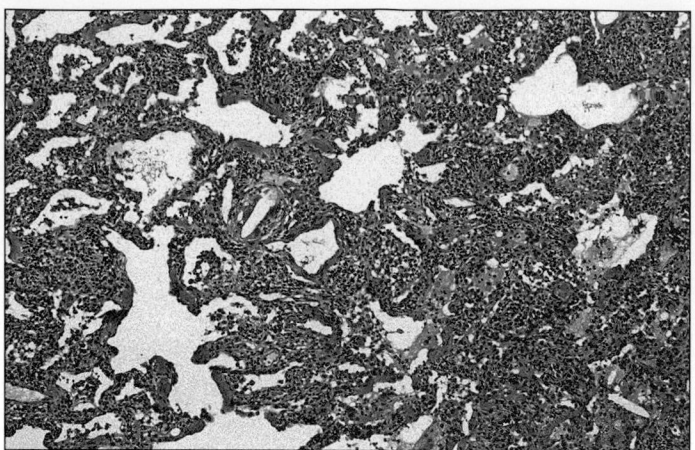

Fig. 17.55 Hypersensitivity pneumonitis. Scanning magnification shows a characteristic cellular infiltration of the alveolar interstitium associated with chronic bronchiolitis.

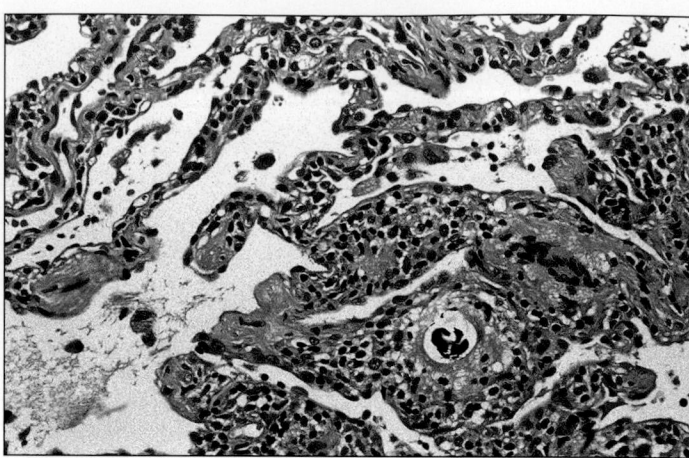

Fig. 17.56 Hypersensitivity pneumonitis. The epithelioid cells in the 'granulomas' are loosely aggregated and mixed with lymphocytes. Very characteristically, scattered giant cells of the foreign body type are seen around terminal airways and may contain cleft-like spaces or small particles that are doubly refractile.

with lobular areas of air trapping.[148] The areas of ground-glass attenuation presumably represent alveolitis, the nodules correspond to bronchiolitis, while the lobular areas of airtrapping presumably result from partial obstruction of bronchioles by bronchiolitis. The chronic phase is characterized by irregular linear opacities (reticular pattern) representing fibrosis. These may involve any lung zone but are usually most severe in the mid-lung zones.[149] Ground-glass opacities and small nodules are also still frequently seen in the chronic phase, presumably representing continued alveolitis and bronchiolitis. HRCT is superior to conventional CT, particularly in delineating areas of ground-glass attenuation.[150]

Pathologic findings: The histologic features depend on the stage in which the disease is biopsied. Because biopsy typically occurs in the subacute phase, the picture is usually one of a chronic interstitial infiltrate comprised of lymphocytes and variable numbers of plasma cells. Lung structure is preserved and alveoli can usually be distinguished. The dominant lesion is the interstitial pneumonia, with a few scattered poorly formed granulomas seen in the interstitium (Fig. 17.55). The epithelioid cells in the 'granulomas' are loosely aggregated and mixed with lymphocytes. Very characteristically, scattered giant cells of the foreign body type are seen around terminal airways and may contain cleft-like spaces or small particles that are doubly refractile (typically calcium oxalate) (Fig. 17.56). Terminal airways display chronic inflammation of their walls (bronchiolitis), often with destruction, distortion, and even occlusion. Pale, or lightly eosinophilic, vacuolated macrophages are typically found in alveolar spaces and are a common sign of bronchiolar obstruction. Similar macrophages are also seen within alveolar walls. The largest series reported[151] has been analyzed for the frequency of morphologic lesions, and these are presented in Table 17.10. It is important to recognize that the inciting allergen was not identified in 37% of patients who had unequivocal evidence of hypersensitivity pneumonitis on biopsy, even with careful retrospective search.[146] As the condition becomes more chronic, there is progressive distortion of the lung architecture by fibrosis and microscopic honeycombing, occasionally attended by extensive pleural fibrosis. At this stage, the lesions may be difficult to distinguish from other chronic lung diseases with fibrosis, because the lymphocytic infiltrate diminishes

Table 17.10 Summary of morphologic features in pulmonary biopsies of 60 farmer's lung patients (degree of involvement*)

Morphologic criteria	Present	%	±	1+	2+	3+
Interstitial infiltrate	60	100	0	14	19	27
Unresolved pneumonia	39	65				
Pleural fibrosis	29	48				
Fibrosis, interstitial	39	65	10	24	5	
Bronchiolitis obliterans	30	50	3			
Foam cells	39	65	6	24	6	3
Edema	31	52				
Granulomas	42	70				
With giant cells †	30	50				
Without giant cells	35	58				
Solitary giant cells	32	53				
Foreign bodies	36	60				
Birefringent †	28	47				
Nonbirefringent	24	40				

* Degree of involvement rated on an arbitrary but documented scale for each criterion.
† The discrepancy in the total numbers is due to the fact that in some cases granulomas with and without giant cells may be found. This discrepancy also applies with the foreign bodies. From Reyes et al.[407] with permission.

and granulomas may not be evident. The differential diagnosis of HSP is presented in Table 17.11.

Avian hypersensitivity (Bird fancier's lung) has a similar clinical presentation and pathology. The allergens are bird proteins, and precipitating serum antibodies to extracts of feathers, droppings, serum, and bird egg white may be present.[152] The condition occurs in pigeon breeders, pigeon fanciers, poultry farmers, and individuals who keep birds in their homes as pets (including parakeets, doves, parrots, and cockatiels). Hypersensitivity pneumonitis has also been

Table 17.11 Differential diagnosis of hypersensitivity pneumonitis

Histologic feature	Hypersensitivity pneumonitis	Sarcoidosis	Lymphocytic interstitial pneumonia
Granulomas			
Frequency	$^2/_3$ of open biopsies	100%	5–10% of cases
Morphology	Poorly formed	Well formed	Well formed or poorly formed
Distribution	Mostly random, some peribronchiolar	Lymphangitic, peribronchiolar, perivascular	Random
Intraluminal fibrosis	$^2/_3$ of open biopsies	Very rare	Unusual
Lymphocyte infiltrates	Mild–moderate, peribronchiolar	Absent or minimal	Extensive, diffuse
Dense fibrosis	In advanced cases	In advanced cases	Unusual
BAL lymphocytosis	CD8>CD4	CD4>CD8	Usually B cell

From Travis et al.[408] with permission.

reported to occur as a result of infestation of humidifiers and air conditioners by thermophilic actinomycetes.[153] This exposure source may be easily overlooked because no occupational or leisure activity history is present.

Occupational hypersensitivity

Hypersensitivity is likely the basic lesion in a number of reasonably well-defined occupational exposures, although the histopathology and the serum findings have not been completely worked out for all of them. Here, we present several that share clinical and histopathologic features with classical HSP.

Bagassosis is a lung disease caused by inhalation of sugar cane fiber residue. The residue, bagasse, is compressed for industrial use and the disease may result from hypersensitivity to fungal spores in stored material. Almost half of all workers exposed to large amounts of stored bagasse develop symptoms similar to those of hypersensitivity pneumonitis, although radiologically, changes are more extensive in the upper lung zones. Antibodies to thermophilic actinomycetes occur in about two-thirds of these patients.[154] The histopathology of bagassosis resembles that of HSP in early stages, with giant cells containing spindle- and rod-shaped particles. Later in the disease, extensive pulmonary fibrosis occurs, and emphysema has been described.

Byssinosis results from inhalation of cotton dust. In byssinosis, the relationship to HSP is less clear. The features differ in that bronchoconstriction is a prominent clinical feature, characteristically occurring at the beginning of the work week and diminishing over the following days. No serologic evidence for hypersensitivity to cotton dust has been identified, but extracts of the cotton pods contain a substance that causes histamine release.[155] The lung lesions are not well characterized but are said to appear different from those of HSP. Fibrous nodules occur throughout the lung, with extensive lung pigmentation and peribronchial fibrosis with bronchial distortion. Large fibers, so-called 'byssinosis bodies,' have been seen in the lung nodules, apparently representing cotton fibers.[156] When this occurs, the fiber is coated with brown, iron-containing pigment.

Metal working fluid-associated HSP is a recently defined form of diffuse lung disease occurring in metal working occupations such as those related to the automobile manufacturing industry. The proposed pathogenesis is related to bioaerosolization of bacteria, fungi, and atypical mycobacteria that colonize the recycled coolant fluid used in drilling and cutting operations. Presumably these organism produce a hypersensitivity response rather than outright infection.

Sarcoidosis

Sarcoidosis is a systemic granulomatous disease of uncertain etiology. The disease commonly affects the lungs.[157,158] The etiology, pathogenesis, and epidemiology of sarcoidosis suggest that it is a disorder of immune regulation.[159–161] The observation that sarcoid granulomas recur after lung transplantation[162–164] seems to further underscore the notion that this is an acquired systemic abnormality in immunity. It also emphasizes the fact that even profound immunosuppression (such as that used in transplantation) may be ineffective in halting disease progression for the subset of patients whose condition persists and progresses to lung fibrosis. The surgical pathologist's role is to establish the presence of non-necrotizing granulomas, most commonly with sclerosis (see below). Today it is more prudent than ever to perform tissue stains for microorganisms to exclude infection before suggesting a diagnosis of sarcoidosis.

Clinical presentation: Many patients with intrathoracic sarcoid are symptom free, with the disease being identified on routine chest X-ray. In early stages, asymptomatic intrathoracic disease may have no systemic manifestations. When systemic manifestations are present, they include granulomas in lymph nodes, eye, liver, skin, spleen, salivary glands, bone, heart, and kidneys (in decreasing frequency). Dyspnea is the most common pulmonary symptom. Sarcoidosis occurs most frequently in young adults, but has been described in all ages. There is a decreased incidence of sarcoidosis in cigarette smokers.

Radiologic findings: The plain radiograph is often characteristic with a combination of symmetric bilateral hilar and paratracheal lymph node enlargement, together with a rather varied pattern of parenchymal involvement, including linear, nodular, and ground-glass opacities.[165] In about one-quarter of the patients the radiograph is atypical, and in about 10% it is normal.[166]

Staging of the disease is based on pattern of involvement on plain chest radiographs, even though CT scans may show parenchymal involvement even when the radiograph is normal. Type I sarcoid is characterized by radiologic hilar adenopathy only, type II by hilar and parenchymal involvement, and type III by parenchymal involvement only.[158,165] Even CT images are not always able to resolve parenchymal abnormalities.[165] Type I patients are most likely to have a favorable outcome, type III patients are most likely to progress, and type II patients have an intermediate risk of progression. In a small percentage of patients, unilateral hilar adenopathy is present, and in 2–4%, nodules larger than 1.0 cm are present in the lung.

HRCT typically demonstrates small irregular nodular opacities predominately along the bronchovascular bundles, interlobular septa,

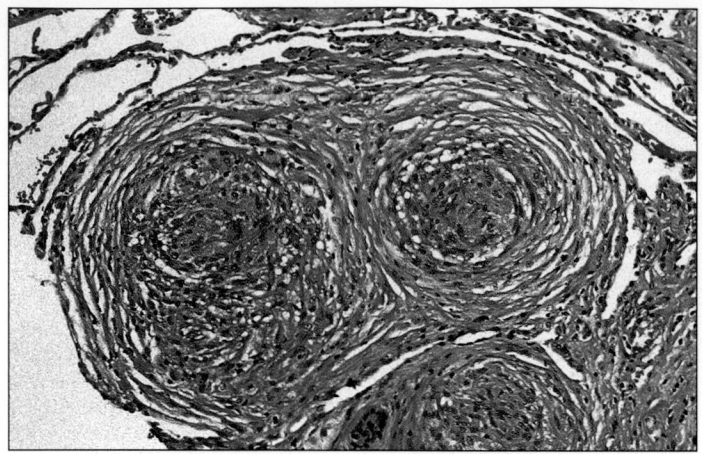

Fig. 17.57 Sarcoidosis. The hallmark of sarcoidosis is the presence of well-formed, tuberculoid granulomas without central necrosis.

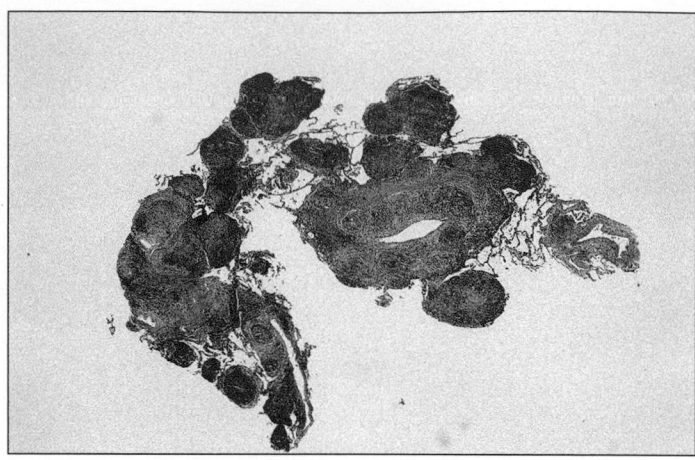

Fig. 17.59 Sarcoidosis. Because of involvement of the bronchovascular bundles and the characteristic histology, sarcoidosis is one of the few diffuse lung diseases that can be diagnosed with a high degree of success by transbronchial biopsy.

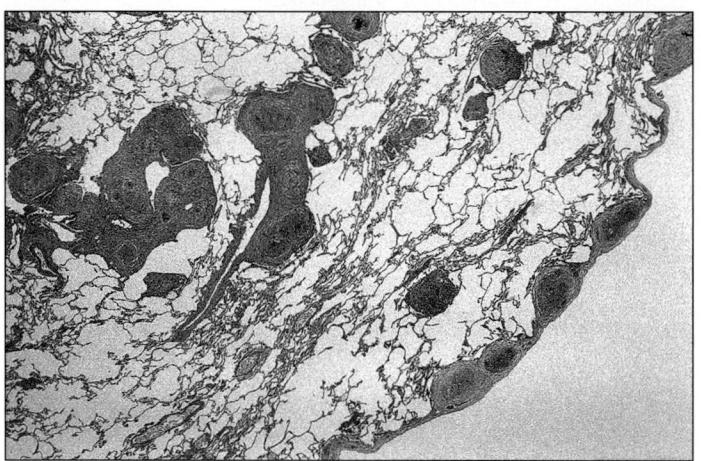

Fig. 17.58 Sarcoidosis. Granulomas are classically distributed along lymphatic channels of the bronchovascular bundles, interlobular septa, and pleura.

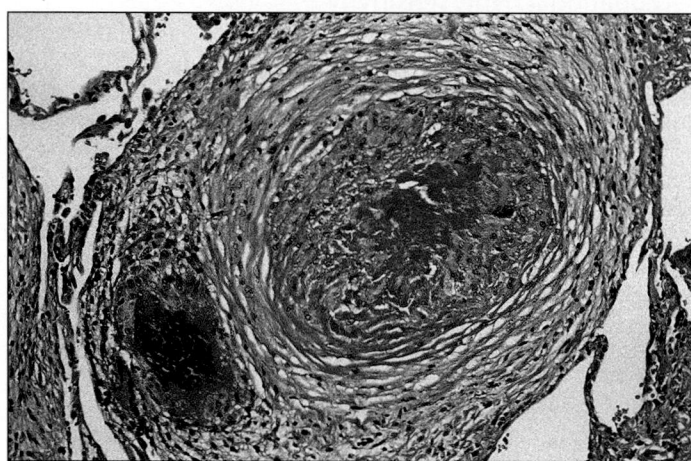

Fig. 17.60 Sarcoidosis. While necrosis is not a feature of the disease, sometimes foci of granular eosinophilic material may be seen within the granulomas.

major fissures, and subpleural regions.[167–169] These nodular opacities correspond to aggregations of microscopic sarcoid granulomas. Ground-glass opacities are seen in 16–60% of patients, depending on the stage.[168] These ground-glass opacities may represent interstitial granulomas that are seen as ground-glass opacification because of a volume averaging effect rather than alveolitis.[167] Sarcoidosis must be distinguished radiologically from lymphangitic carcinoma. Typically, thickening of the lobular septa is less marked and nodules are more irregular in sarcoidosis. In advanced disease, there may be progressive fibrosis, honeycombing, and bulla formation.

Pathologic findings: The hallmark of sarcoidosis is the presence of well-formed granulomas without central necrosis (Fig. 17.57). Granulomas are classically distributed along lymphatic channels of the bronchovascular bundles, interlobular septa, and pleura (Fig. 17.58). The area between granulomas is frequently sclerotic, producing confluence of multiple small granulomas into larger nodules with intervening normal lung. Because of involvement of the

bronchovascular bundles and the characteristic histology, sarcoidosis is one of the few diffuse lung diseases that can be diagnosed with a high degree of success by transbronchial biopsy (Fig. 17.59).[30] Although a large percentage of patients with pulmonary sarcoidosis have vascular involvement with granulomas around veins and arteries, pulmonary hypertension is rare, except in advanced fibrotic cases.[157]

While necrosis is not a feature of the disease, sometimes foci of granular eosinophilic material may be seen at the center of the granulomas (Fig. 17.60). The 'dirty' necrosis typical of mycobacterial and fungal disease is not seen. Distinctive inclusions may be present such as asteroid and Schaumann bodies (Fig. 17.61) within giant cells, but these can be seen in other granulomatous diseases. As mentioned earlier, granulomas commonly are present around arteries and veins in sarcoidosis and this features rarely if ever carries clinical implications for pulmonary hypertension (Fig. 17.62). There is a generally held belief that a mild interstitial inflammatory infiltrate

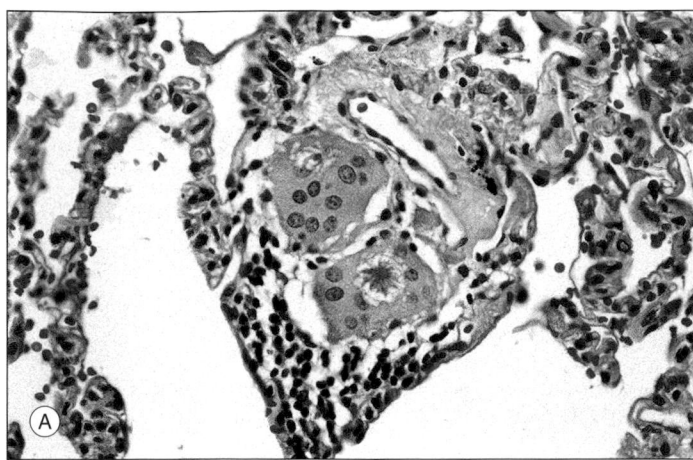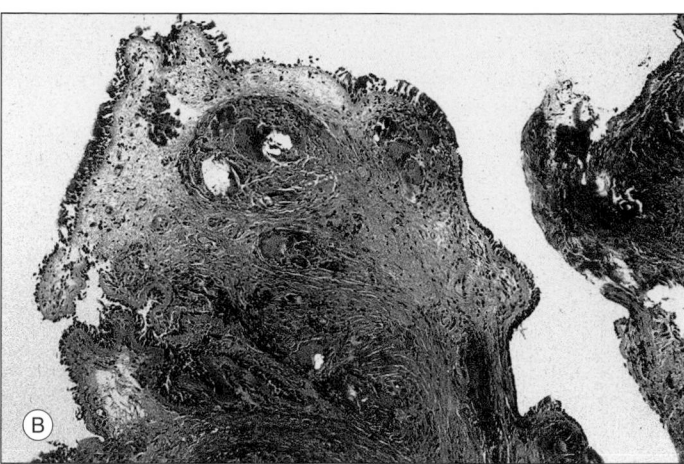

Fig. 17.61 Sarcoidosis. Distinctive inclusions may be present such as asteroid and Schaumann bodies within giant cells (**A**), but these can be seen in other granulomatous diseases. Polarizable birefringent calcification is also common in the granulomas and should not be confused with foreign material (**B**).

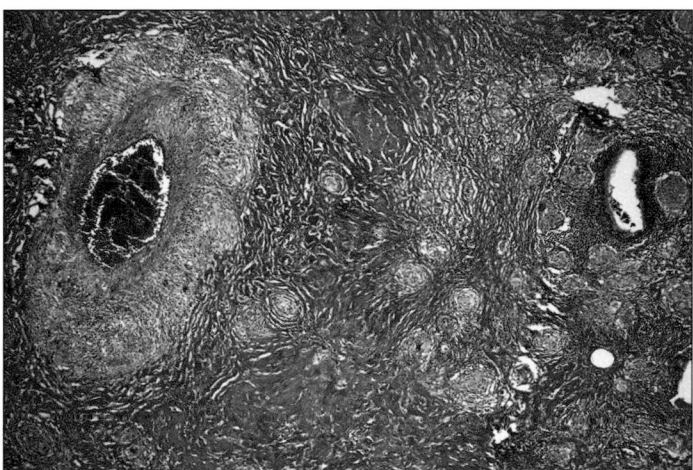

Fig. 17.62 Sarcoidosis. Because the disease follows bronchovascular bundles and interlobular veins, it is not surprising that vascular involvement by granulomas is seen in about two-thirds of cases.

frequently accompanies granulomas in sarcoidosis.[170–172] This 'interstitial pneumonia' of sarcoidosis is subtle in the best example, and consists of a few lymphocytes, mononuclear cells, and macrophages.

Differential diagnosis: When necrosis is present in granulomas, every effort must be made to exclude infection. Some forms of mycobacterial infection (e.g. *Mycobacterium avium intracellulare*) may be exceedingly difficult to identify by special stains or even culture. On occasion, even *Pneumocystis* pneumonia can produce a granulomatous infiltrate with variable amounts of necrosis. The granulomas of sarcoidosis are indistinguishable from those of chronic berylliosis, so it is prudent to always suggest this possibility. Poorly formed interstitial and alveolar granulomas can be seen in a variety of other noninfectious conditions such as hypersensitivity pneumonitis and drug reactions. In these diseases, the granulomas are less distinct than sarcoidosis and there is little to no tendency towards confluence of granulomas, or sclerosis.

In 1973, Liebow described a vasculitic form of sarcoidosis and coined the term *necrotizing sarcoid granulomatosis*.[173] The histopathologic findings included a pneumonitis with sarcoid-like granulomas having central necrosis, granulomatous or giant cell vasculitis, and variable parenchymal necrosis, sometimes with cavitation. Occlusion of vessels by extensive granulomatous inflammation was observed. Most investigators today view this disease as a rare, vasculitic manifestation of sarcoidosis, given the benign course of the disease and clinical features which more resemble sarcoidosis than a systemic vasculitis or infectious disease.

Clinical course: Steroid therapy has been used successfully in symptomatic patients. In many patients, the disease seems to run a relatively benign course and is self-limited. The prognosis for patients with sarcoidosis is excellent. The disease typically resolves or improves, with only 5–10% of patients developing significant pulmonary fibrosis. The majority of patients recover completely with minimal residual disease.

Bioaerosol-associated atypical mycobacterial infection

The classical lung manifestations of infection with *Mycobacterium tuberculosis* (MTb) are well known to pathologists and clinicians alike. Less well known are the many subacute to chronic lung manifestations of infection by nontuberculous mycobacteria (NTM) species such as *M. kansasii*, *M. avium intracellulare* complex, and *M. xenopi*; as a group they are often referred to as the *atypical* mycobacteria.[174] Being inherently less pathogenic than MTb, these organisms often flourish in the setting of immunocompromise or circumstances where there is enhanced opportunity for colonization and low-grade infection. Acute pneumonia can be produced by these organisms in patients with compromised immunity. Chronic airway disease-associated NTM infection is discussed in the section that follows on airway diseases. A distinctive and recently highlighted presentation of NTM is presented here because it may mimic hypersensitivity pneumonitis: NTM infection occurring in the normal host as a result of bioaerosol exposure ('Hot tub lung').[175]

'Chronic' eosinophilic pneumonia

As discussed earlier, several different conditions have been described in which the airspaces of the lungs contain a large number of eosinophils.[176,177] When disease manifests clinically over many weeks to months, the term 'chronic eosinophilic pneumonia' has been applied, even though the pathologic findings in biopsy specimens may not reflect this chronicity with fibrosis.

Clinical features: Patients with the 'chronic' form of eosinophilic pneumonia often manifest a typical clinical syndrome and radiographic appearance.[178] The disease frequently affects middle-aged women and presents with severe systemic effects, including fever, sweats, and loss of weight, cough and dyspnea. Asthma is present in about one-quarter of the cases, and nasal symptoms occur in about one-third. Eosinophilia of the blood can often be identified, but this may be transient or absent.

Radiologic findings: The chest radiograph shows areas of bilateral subpleural airspace consolidation with poorly defined margins, most commonly in the upper lobes. The infiltrates may disappear spontaneously and recur in the same position or elsewhere (so-called 'migratory' infiltrates). In the most extreme example, the infiltrates surround the peripheral portions of the lung and spare the central region, resulting in what has been called the 'photographic negative of pulmonary edema.'[178] The predominantly peripheral location of the infiltrates can be seen on HRCT even when is not apparent on the radiograph.[179] Once the characteristic presentation is recognized, corticosteroid administration can lead to dramatic improvement and may even be used as a diagnostic test. Lung biopsy can often be avoided, but atypical presentations occur so that surgical biopsy may be is required to establish the diagnosis.

Pathologic findings: The histologic features are remarkably similar to the acute form and it has been said that the distinction must rely on the clinical course rather than the constellation of morphologic findings. Alveolar spaces are filled with eosinophils and plump eosinophilic macrophages. There is an associated mild interstitial pneumonia. Type II hyperplasia is characteristic and fibrin is often present in the airspaces. A vaguely granulomatous accumulation of dense macrophages may be seen within the alveolar spaces, sometimes with multinucleated giant cells whose nuclei and cytoplasm closely resembles that of adjacent macrophages. Angiitis of small vessels may be seen. Patchy airspace and alveolar duct organization may be present to variable degree.

The idiopathic interstitial pneumonias

In the early years of surgical lung biopsy, a group of diffuse inflammatory diseases came to light that were not caused by infection, toxin, sarcoidosis, pneumoconiosis, or neoplasm. Liebow is credited for recognizing and classifying this group of diseases, later to become known as the 'idiopathic interstitial pneumonias.'[32]

The original classification of the interstitial pneumonias proposed by Liebow is presented for historical purposes in Table 17.12. This classification has been recently modified by an international consensus committee and is presented in Table 17.13. Much has changed in medical science over the intervening years and few of the entities proposed in Liebow's original classification are viewed today as he described them more than 30 years ago.

Usual interstitial pneumonia (cryptogenic fibrosing alveolitis)

A large number of terms have been applied over the years to describe this chronic diffuse lung disease, characterized by a clear tendency to produce fibrosis (chronic Hamman-Rich syndrome, fibrosing alveolitis, cryptogenic fibrosing alveolitis, idiopathic pulmonary fibrosis, widespread pulmonary fibrosis, idiopathic interstitial fibrosis of the lung). Usual interstitial pneumonia (UIP), as diagnosed in current practice, has been restricted to a subset of the diseases initially

Table 17.12 Liebow classification of interstitial pneumonia (1975)

Usual interstitial pneumonia (UIP)
Bronchiolitis obliterans with usual interstitial pneumonia (BIP)
Desquamative interstitial pneumonia (DIP)
Lymphoid interstitial pneumonia (LIP)
Giant cell interstitial pneumonia (GIP)
Adapted from Liebow[180]

Table 17.13 International Consensus Committee classification of idiopathic interstitial pneumonia (2002)

Usual interstitial pneumonia (UIP)
Acute interstitial pneumonia (AIP)
Desquamative interstitial pneumonia (DIP)
Respiratory bronchiolitis-associated interstitial disease (RBILD)
Cryptogenic organizing pneumonia (COP)
Non-specific interstitial pneumonia/fibrosis (NSIP)
Lymphoid interstitial pneumonia (LIP)
Adapted from Travis et al.[408]

described. Liebow considered UIP to be a form of the acute lung fibrosis syndrome described by Hamman and Rich.[130] Today that form of acute lung fibrosis more closely resembles the idiopathic form of diffuse alveolar damage, known as acute interstitial pneumonia (AIP). For Liebow, UIP was the most common, or 'usual,' form of diffuse lung fibrosis. Liebow's UIP was idiopathic in about half of the patients originally studied. In the other half, the disease was 'heterogeneous in terms of structure and causation.'[180]

Clinical features: Patients with UIP typically report an insidious onset of breathlessness. A significant percentage of affected individuals attribute the onset of their symptoms to a flu-like illness, occurring many months to years before diagnosis. UIP is a disease of older individuals, typically more than 50 years of age.[35] Men are slightly more commonly affected than women. Characteristic clinical findings include clubbing, distinctive end-inspiratory crackles ('Velcro crackles') at the lung bases, and the eventual development of lung fibrosis with cor pulmonale. The erythrocyte sedimentation rate may be elevated, but values over 100 should raise concern for a disease other than UIP. Polycythemia is rare. Many patients die of respiratory failure, often precipitated by pulmonary infection. The average duration of symptoms in one series was 3 years,[32] and mean survival after diagnosis has been reported to be 4.2 years, in a population-based study.[181] Different from other chronic inflammatory lung diseases, immunosuppressive therapy improves neither survival nor quality of life for patients with UIP.[35]

Radiologic findings: The chest radiograph in patients with UIP initially shows a fine reticular pattern involving mainly the lower lung zones. As fibrosis progresses, the reticular pattern becomes coarser and there is progressive loss of lung volume. Terminal stages show coarse reticulation, often associated with peripheral cysts, best appreciated in the lower lung zones.[182]

HRCT has added a new dimension to the diagnosis of UIP. In UIP, the abnormalities are characteristically worst in the periphery

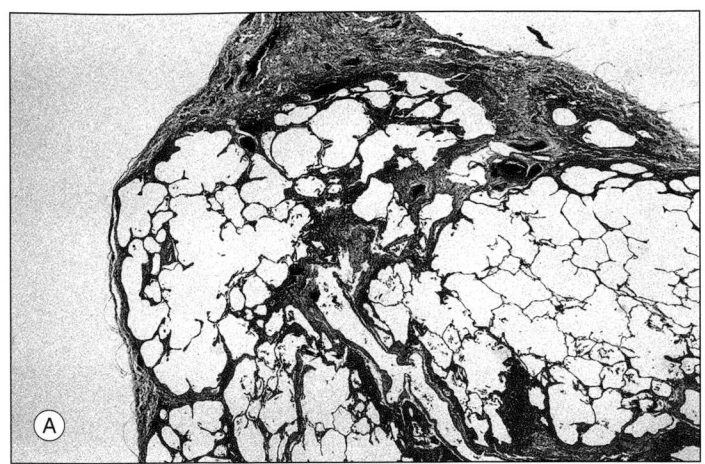
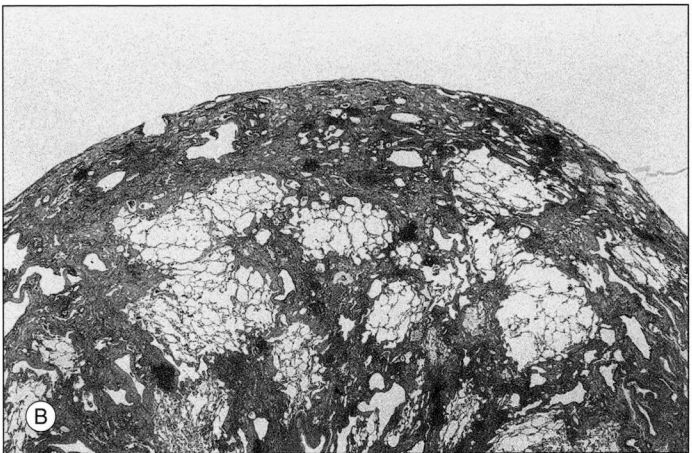

Fig. 17.63 Usual interstitial pneumonia (UIP). Fibrosis begins at the periphery of the secondary lobule (**A**) and progresses toward the center of the lobule (**B**). The individual components of the process are not specific, but this physical arrangement in the surgical biopsy is key to the diagnosis.

of the lungs and in the lung bases on CT regardless of the stage.[183] The dominant picture is of irregular linear opacities resulting in a reticular pattern. The linear opacities correspond to thin irregular scars in the lung.[183] End-stage lung (honeycombing) is much more readily identified on CT than on the plain radiograph and is seen in approximately 90% of patients at presentation on HRCT as compared with 30% on radiographs.[184] The cysts of end-stage lung are 2–20 mm in diameter. In approximately 80% of cases of UIP, but seldom extensive, ground-glass attenuation corresponds to intra-alveolar aggregates of histiocytes, interstitial alveolar wall inflammation, and young granulation tissue.[185,186] In 20% of patients with UIP, ground-glass attenuation represents fibrosis rather than inflammation.[185,186] In these cases, the fibrosis is microscopic and below the spatial resolution of CT. Other signs of fibrosis are usually seen in these patients, particularly traction bronchiectasis and bronchiolectasis.[187] Therefore, ground-glass attenuation can only be considered a marker of inflammation if it is seen away from other abnormalities. In the majority of patients, the clinical and HRCT findings are characteristic enough to allow a confident diagnosis and obviate lung biopsy.[35] In a prospective multicenter study of 91 patients with suspected IPF, the positive predictive value of a confident radiologic diagnosis on HRCT was 96%.[19]

Pathologic findings: At surgery, the lung often has a characteristic hobnailed external surface, and this appearance can also be recognized in lung biopsy tissue. Histopathologically, UIP can be described as a smoldering alveolitis of unknown cause, attended by microscopic foci of injury, repair, and lung remodeling. The disease begins at the periphery of the pulmonary lobule and has a consistent tendency to leave lung fibrosis and honeycomb cystic lung remodeling in its wake, as it progresses from the periphery to the center of the lobule (Fig. 17.63). The individual components of the process are not specific, but their physical arrangement in the surgical biopsy can be relatively compelling in the right clinical and radiological context. Accurate diagnosis requires experience with the interpretation of interstitial lung disease, appropriate terminology, and a multidisciplinary approach. As mentioned earlier, the clinical corollary of UIP is known as idiopathic pulmonary fibrosis (IPF). To our clinical colleagues, IPF is a distinct clinical lung disorder characterized by chronic progressive restriction of lung function without identifiable cause.

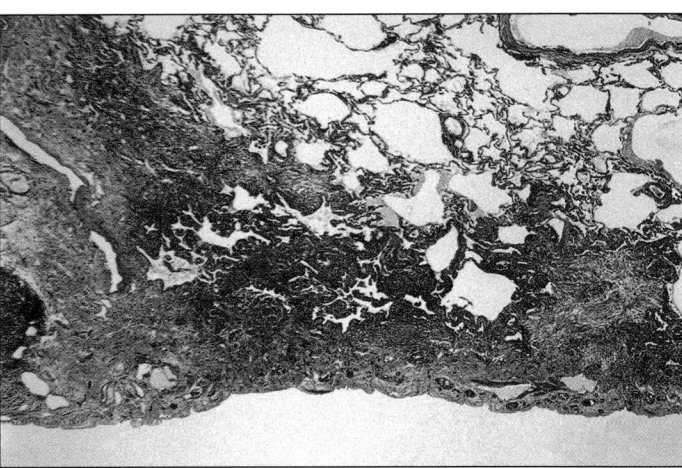

Fig. 17.64 Usual interstitial pneumonia (UIP). Fibrotic remodeling of the lung is best seen in a subpleural location.

At low magnification, the open lung biopsy mimics the radiographic findings and shows peripheral accentuation of fibrosis and fibrotic remodeling in a subpleural location (Fig. 17.64). At the interface between fibrosis and more normal lung, there are focal crescent-shaped bands of organization ('fibroblastic foci') (Fig. 17.65) accompanied by a mild alveolitis with variable numbers of lymphocytes and plasma cells in the alveolar interstitium. Although airspace organization is present to some degree, it is usually not a prominent feature unless infection or other superimposed injury is present (see acute exacerbation below). Within the biopsy, the transitions from end-stage dense fibrosis, with or without honeycombing, to near normal lung, with an intermediate stage of alveolar organization and inflammation are the histologic hallmarks of so-called 'temporal heterogeneity.' Smooth muscle within areas of fibrosis are also typical of UIP (Fig. 17.66), presumably arising as a consequence of progressive parenchymal collapse with incorporation of native airway and vascular smooth muscle into fibrosis. Less well-recognized additional features are the distortion and narrowing of

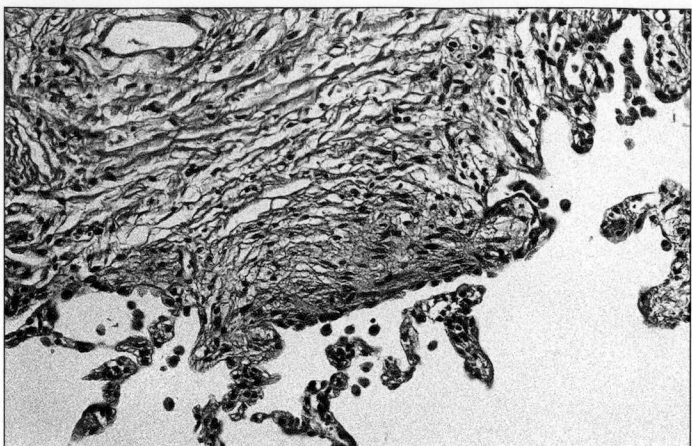

Fig. 17.65 Usual interstitial pneumonia (UIP). At the interface between fibrosis and more normal lung, there is a mild alveolitis with variable numbers of lymphocytes and plasma cells in the alveolar interstitium. A characteristic lesion of UIP is the 'fibroblastic focus,' an arc-shaped bulge of loosely aggregated immature-appearing fibroblasts, analogous to the fibroblastic proliferation seen in a healing wound. The fibroblastic foci occur at the interface between remodeled lung (top-left) and normal lung (bottom-left).

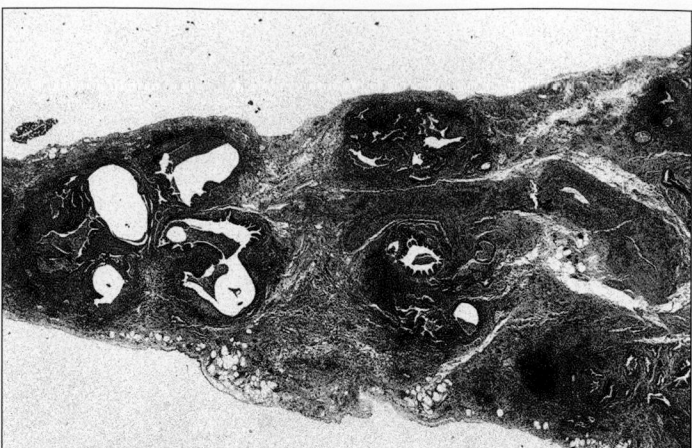

Fig. 17.67 Usual interstitial pneumonia (UIP). In late-stage UIP, all that remains is microscopic honeycombing.

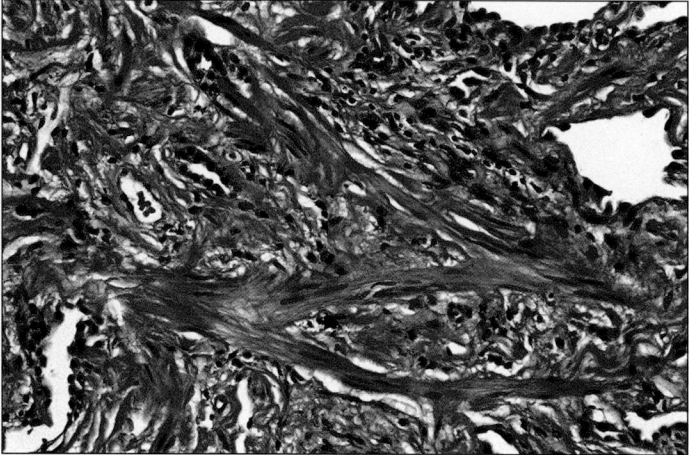

Fig. 17.66 Usual interstitial pneumonia (UIP). Smooth muscle bundles within areas of fibrosis are also typical of UIP. Presumably these arise as a consequence of progressive parenchymal collapse with incorporation of native airway and vascular smooth muscle into fibrosis.

bronchioles, together with peribronchiolar fibrosis and inflammation. This observation likely accounts for the functional evidence of small airway obstruction that is found in UIP.[188] Widespread bronchial dilation (traction bronchiectasis) may be present at postmortem examination in advanced disease and correlates with HRCT findings late in the course of IPF. In late-stage disease the surgical biopsy may consist entirely of microscopic honeycombing (Fig. 17.67).

Acute exacerbation of IPF: Episodes of clinical deterioration are expected in patients with UIP. While respiratory failure is the cause of death in about one-half of affected individuals, for a subset, death is associated with sudden acute respiratory failure and this has been termed 'acute exacerbation of IPF' when no infectious etiology is identified. The typical history is that of a patient being followed for IPF who suddenly develops acute respiratory distress, often accompanied by fever, elevation of the sedimentation rate, marked increase in dyspnea, and new infiltrates that often have an 'alveolar' character radiologically. For many years this manifestation was thought to be infectious pneumonia (possibly viral), superimposed on a fibrotic lung with marginal reserve. The fact that the cases are sufficiently common, organisms are rarely identified, and a small percentage of patients respond to pulse systemic corticosteroid therapy, have lead a number of investigators to now consider such exacerbation to be a form of fulminant progression of the disease process itself. Overall, this condition has a very poor prognosis, and death within one week is not unusual. Pathologically, acute lung injury resembling DAD and/or organizing pneumonia is superimposed on a background UIP with honeycombing and fibrosis. This latter finding can be highlighted with the Masson's trichrome stain.

Differential diagnosis: It is important to exclude other causes of pulmonary fibrosis when considering a diagnosis of UIP, especially if biopsy material consist mainly of fibrosis and microscopic honeycomb lung. A number of conditions that have a specific microscopic appearance early in their course may be non-specific in their end stage.[182] For example, chronic hypersensitivity, chronic eosinophilic pneumonia, advanced lung remodeling in collagen vascular diseases, and certain drug reactions can also produce end-stage fibrosis indistinguishable from that seen in advanced areas of fibrosis in UIP. In contrast to these latter mimics, UIP is a fatal disease in more than 90% of patients so diagnosed, and the designation should not be used as a default or 'wastebasket' diagnosis for any lung disease with inflammation and fibrosis. Today, UIP has evolved from a broad and inclusive rubric, to a more select idiopathic form.

A careful search for any specific lesions (e.g. granulomas) or clues to another etiology from the clinical history or radiographs is always in order. In particular, asbestosis may be a problem. Although asbestosis is usually easily recognized by the presence of obvious asbestos bodies and by the pattern of fibrosis, cases have been reported in which the lesions appear to be more typical of UIP, yet only an occasional asbestos body is found. Under these circumstances, the diagnosis of UIP may be considered by some to be an unreasonable one. Regardless of intellectual arguments that might suggest the possibility of coincidental UIP occurring in an individual with asbestos exposure, our practice today in a litigious society dictates that one asbestos body in a case of otherwise typical UIP is sufficient to be diagnosed as lung fibrosis resulting from asbestos exposure.

Clinical course: UIP is a fatal disease in more than 90% of patients so diagnosed.[189] We do not yet know why injury episodes occur in UIP, the underlying target of the injury, or the specific mechanisms involved. Hopefully, we have now defined the problem sufficiently well that therapeutic advances will begin to target more specific control pathways (e.g. transforming growth factor beta). Even without a defined specific etiology, such therapies may benefit IPF patients in the short run while further clarifying the required next steps in addressing the underlying cause of this disease.

Non-specific interstitial pneumonia

In the 30 years following the original Liebow classification of the idiopathic interstitial pneumonias, pulmonary pathologists realized that a number of interstitial lung diseases did not fit well into the patterns he described. A 'new' category of interstitial pneumonia thus arose and was referred to as 'unclassified or unclassifiable' by some, or simple 'cellular interstitial pneumonia' by others. In an effort to group these 'unclassifiable' patterns of interstitial pneumonia, in 1994, Katzenstein and Fiorelli published a review of 64 patients[190] whose biopsies showed diffuse interstitial inflammation and/or fibrosis that did not fit recognizable patterns. The described clinical, radiologic, and pathologic findings for these patients were grouped under the heading of 'non-specific interstitial pneumonia/fibrosis' or simply NSIP. Katzenstein and Fiorelli acknowledged that NSIP was not a specific disease entity but likely represented a number of different diseases. These diseases had in common a lack of resemblance to other recognized inflammatory lung diseases, including the subset of idiopathic interstitial pneumonias that remained from Liebow's initial classification (UIP, DIP, AIP).

Clinical features: NSIP occurs mainly in middle-aged adults with an average age at onset of 46 years (range 9–78) and, different from UIP, a slight female predominance. The average duration of symptoms prior to biopsy was 8.1 months (range 0.25–60), and the presenting symptoms included dyspnea (51%), cough (21%), and fever (14%).

Radiologic findings: The chest radiograph shows patchy parenchymal opacities involving mainly the lower lung zones. The predominant finding on HRCT consists of ground-glass attenuation involving mainly the lower and peripheral lung regions. The majority of patients have a reticular pattern superimposed on the ground-glass attenuation. Ground-glass attenuation without reticulation usually reflects active alveolitis while reticulation on HRCT correlates with the presence of fibrosis.[191]

Pathologic findings: The histologic findings in their 64 patients are presented in Table 17.14. Biopsy findings included variable amounts of interstitial chronic (lymphoplasmacellular) inflammation and fibrosis. Importantly, extensive airspace organization and/or significant areas of lung replaced by honeycomb fibrosis were generally felt to exclude patients from the spectrum of NSIP. Because the term 'non-specific interstitial pneumonia/fibrosis' implies a 'nonclassifiable' interstitial inflammatory disease, a number of patterns are evident in their series. The main emphasis was on the *temporally uniform* appearance of the disease process; that is, the pathology seemed to reflect a single injury in time.

Katzenstein and Fiorelli subdivided their cases into three groups: *Group I* had diffuse interstitial inflammation alone (Fig. 17.68), *Group II* had interstitial inflammation and early interstitial fibrosis occurring together (Fig. 17.69), and *Group III* had denser, diffuse

Table 17.14 Histopathologic findings in 64 patients with nonspecific interstitial pneumonia/fibrosis

Histopathologic Finding	Frequency
Patchy	35 (55%)
Bronchiolocentric	18 (28%)
Diffuse	29 (45%)
Granulomas	5 (8%)
Focal 'BOOP-like' areas	31 (48%)
'Marked' epithelial hyperplasia	20 (31%)
'DIP-like' reaction	19 (30%)
Germinal centers	17 (27%)
Fibroblast foci	13 (20%)
Pleuritis	20 (31%)

Data from Katzenstein & Fiorelli.[190]
BOOP = bronchiolitis obliterans organizing pneumonia

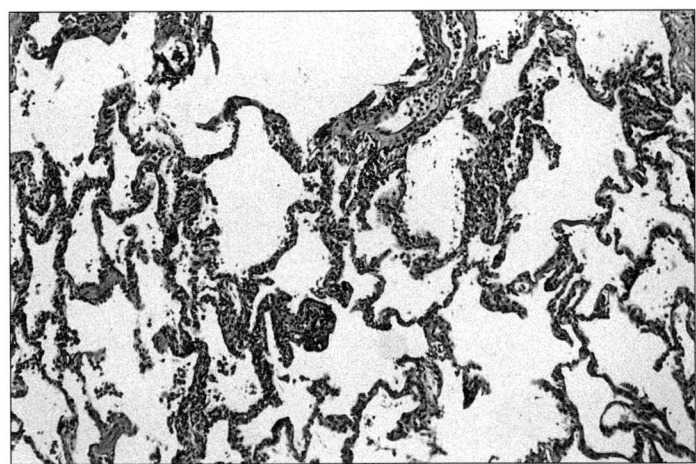

Fig. 17.68 Non-specific interstitial pneumonia. Group I was described as having diffuse interstitial inflammation alone.

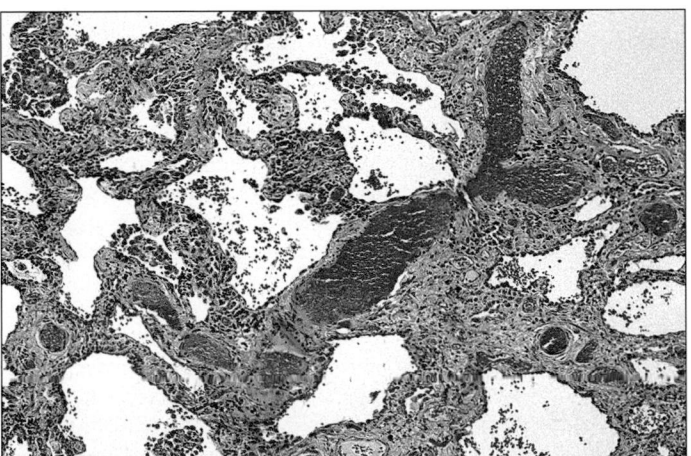

Fig. 17.69 Non-specific interstitial pneumonia. Group II biopsies had the combination of mild interstitial inflammation and early interstitial fibrosis, occurring together in a similar distribution.

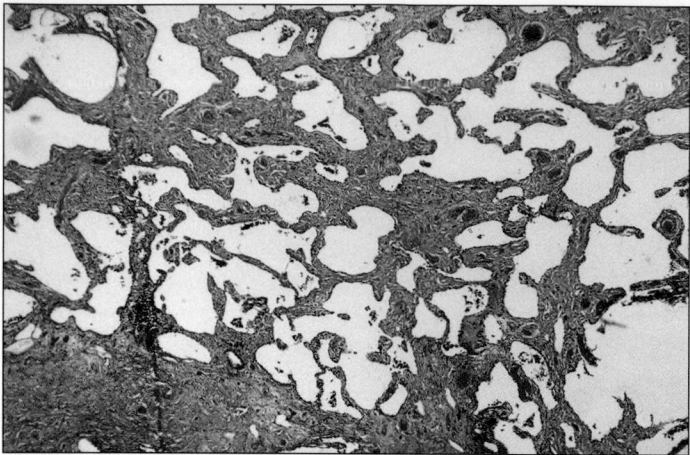

Fig. 17.70 Non-specific interstitial pneumonia. Group III was described as having denser, diffuse interstitial fibrosis, without significant active inflammation.

Table 17.15 Literature review of deaths or progression related to NSIP

Authors	# Pts	Sex	Progression	Deaths (NSIP)
Katzenstein & Fiorelli[190]	64	26/M – 38/F	13%	11%
Nagai et al.[195]	31	15/M – 16/F	16%	6%
Cottin et al.[192]	12	6/M – 6/F	33%	0%
Park, et al.[196]	7	1/M – 6/F	29%	29%
Hartman, et al[197]	39	16/M – 23/F	19%	29%
Kim, et al.[194]	23	1/M – 22/F	Not Given	Not given
Travis, et al.[198]	29	10/M – 9/F	41% (at least)	41%
Daniil, et al [193]	15	7/M – 8/F	33%	13%
Bjoraker, et al.[189]	14	8/M – 6/F	Not given	25% (5 yr) 35% (10yr)

interstitial fibrosis, without significant active inflammation (Fig. 17.70). These uniform injury patterns were judged to be separable from the temporally heterogeneous injury seen in UIP (new and old injury coexisting).

Group I disease is perhaps the least controversial pattern and easiest to identify pathologically, since it corresponds to what others have called 'cellular interstitial pneumonia.' With the addition of fibrosis to groups II and III, however, potential problems arise, since the appearance and distribution of NSIP fibrosis in lung tissue can be difficult to separate from that of UIP. The study emphasized that the distribution of fibrosis was to be uniform and primarily interstitial, with preservation of general lung architecture. When fibrous obliteration of parenchyma occurred with scarring, it was only allowed as a minor component and not in a distribution to suggest UIP.

Although many patients in this initial series had true idiopathic interstitial lung disease, several significant systemic disease associations were identified in their population. Connective tissue disease was identified in 16% of patients, including rheumatoid arthritis, systemic lupus erythematosus, polymyositis/dermatomyositis, scleroderma, and Sjögren's syndrome. Interestingly, pulmonary disease preceded the development of systemic collagen vascular disease in some of their cases; a phenomenon well documented for some collagen vascular diseases, such as polymyositis/dermatomyositis. Other autoimmune diseases occurring in their series included Hashimoto's thyroiditis, glomerulonephritis, and primary biliary cirrhosis. Beyond these systemic associations, another subset of their patients was found to have a history of chemical, organic antigen, or drug exposures, suggesting the possibility of a hypersensitivity phenomenon. Interestingly, two additional patients were status post-ARDS and two patients had suffered pneumonia months before the biopsy was performed.

Perhaps the most important finding in the Katzenstein and Fiorelli study was that their population of patients had a morbidity and mortality rate significantly different from that expected for UIP. Only 5 of 48 patients with clinical follow-up died of progressive lung disease (11%), while 39 patients either recovered or were alive with stable lung disease. For the patients with follow-up, no deaths were reported in group I patients, while 3 patients from group II and 2 patients from group III died. Unfortunately a significant number of patients were lost to follow-up and mean lengths of follow-up were quite variable. Nevertheless, this contrasts sharply with UIP, where reported mortality figures are more in the range of 90%, with median survival in the range of 3 years.

Since 1994, there have been a number of additional reported series of NSIP patients[189,192–198] with variable reported survival rates (Table 17.15). Deaths occurred in those patients with NSIP who had fibrosis (groups II and III), analogous to results reported by Katzenstein and Fiorelli. Nagai et al. restricted the scope of NSIP to those patients with idiopathic disease, primarily by excluding patients with known collagen vascular diseases and environmental exposures.[195] Two of thirty-one patients in their study (6.5%) died of progressive lung disease, both having group III disease. By contrast, the highest mortality rate was reported in the series by Travis et al., where 9 of 22 patients (41%) died with group II and III disease.[198] Importantly, these deaths occurred after 5 years, somewhat different from the course of most patients with UIP. Also, Travis et al. reported 5- and 10-year survival rates of 90% and 35%, respectively, in their patients with NSIP, compared to 5- and 10-year survival rates for UIP of 43% and 15%, respectively.[198]

Desquamative interstitial pneumonia

In 1965, Liebow et al.[199] described 18 cases of diffuse lung diseases that differed in many respects from UIP. The striking histologic feature was the presence of numerous cells filling the airspaces. Liebow et al.[199] thought that the cells were chiefly desquamated alveolar epithelial lining cells, and coined the term *desquamative interstitial pneumonia* (DIP). However, it is now known that these cells are predominately macrophages.[200] Today DIP and the cigarette smoking-related disease known as *respiratory bronchiolitis associated interstitial disease* (RBILD), are felt to be very similar if not identical diseases, possibly representing different expressions of disease severity.[201] RBILD is discussed later in this chapter in the section on smoking-related diffuse lung disease.

Clinical features: The patients originally described by Liebow and coworkers[199] were on average slightly younger than patients with UIP, and their symptoms were usually milder. Clubbing was not a characteristic feature, but in later series some clubbed patients were identified.[33] Most patients present with a subacute lung disease of weeks to months evolution.

Radiologic findings: The predominant finding on the radiograph and HRCT in patients with DIP consists of ground-glass opacities,

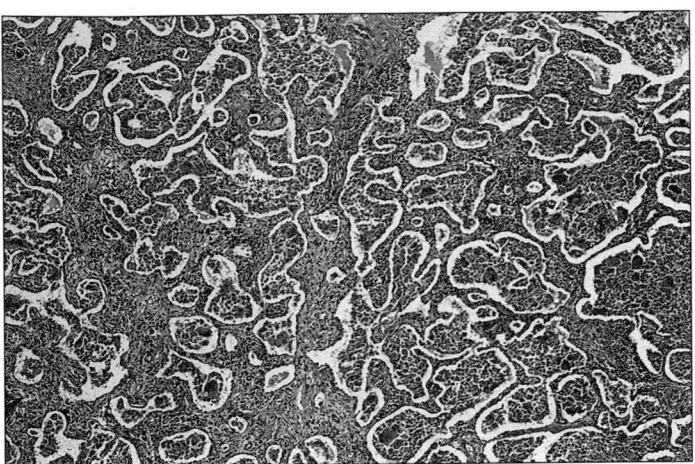

Fig. 17.71 Desquamative interstitial pneumonia (DIP). At scanning magnification, the alveolar spaces in DIP are filled uniformly with macrophages and this phenomenon is present throughout the wedge biopsy.

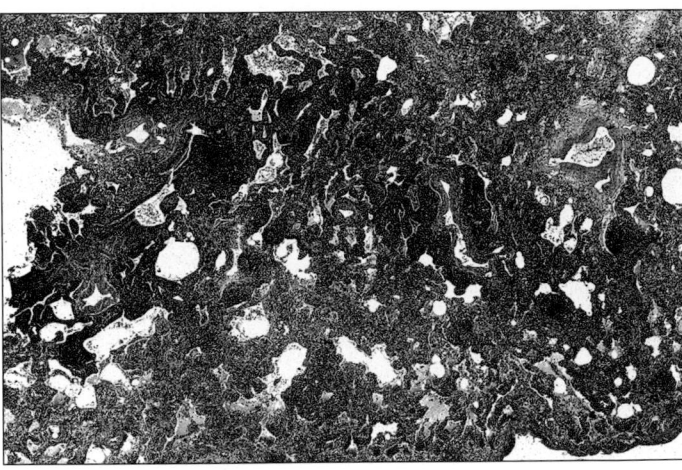

Fig. 17.72 Lymphocytic interstitial pneumonia (LIP). Described originally as an 'exquisitely interstitial infiltrate' comprised of a polymorphous population of lymphocytes, plasma cells, and large mononuclear cells, today LIP is more of a pattern of lung inflammation than a specific disease.

particularly at the bases and at the costophrenic angles.[202] Some patients have mild reticular changes superimposed on the ground-glass opacities.

Pathologic findings: In lung biopsy, the scanning magnification appearance of DIP is striking (Fig. 17.71). The alveolar spaces are filled with macrophages, and multinucleate cells are commonly present. The original description emphasized the presence of green-brown pigment in the cytoplasm of these cells, which stained strongly with periodic acid–Schiff (PAS) stain and was also diastase resistant. Occasional granules in these cells stained positively for iron. Additional important features included the relative preservation of lung architecture, with only mild thickening of alveolar walls and absence of severe fibrosis or honeycombing.[203–205] Interstitial mononuclear inflammation was seen, sometimes with scattered lymphoid follicles. Liebow and coworkers recognized intracytoplasmic 'blue bodies' in the cells in the airspaces in about 10% of the cases. These bodies are 15–25 mm in diameter, stain darkly with hematoxylin, have a central round or oval core surrounded by a clear space, and an outer rim of granular brown material.

The histologic appearance of DIP is not specific. It is commonly present in other diffuse and localized lung diseases, including UIP and asbestosis,[206] as well as other dust-related diseases.[207] DIP-like reactions occur after nitrofurantoin therapy,[107,108] and typically in airspaces adjacent to the nodules of pulmonary Langerhans cell histiocytosis (see later section on smoking-related diseases).

Cases have been reported in which classic DIP 'progressed to fibrosing alveolitis.'[204,208] It seems clear that DIP represents a non-specific reaction to injury. It is critical to distinguish between DIP and UIP, especially since these diseases are regarded as very different from one another today. It has been shown conclusively that the clinical features are different, the prognosis is much better in DIP, and DIP may respond to corticosteroid administration,[209] while UIP clearly does not.[35]

Lymphoid interstitial pneumonia

Lymphoid interstitial pneumonia (LIP) is a clinical pathologic entity that fits descriptively within the chronic interstitial pneumonias. By consensus, LIP has been included in the current classification of the idiopathic interstitial pneumonias, despite decades of controversy about what diseases are encompassed by this term. In 1969, Liebow and Carrington[32] briefly presented a group of patients and used the term *lymphoid interstitial pneumonia* (LIP) to describe their biopsy findings. The defining criteria were morphologic, and included 'an exquisitely interstitial infiltrate' that was described as generally polymorphous consisting of lymphocytes, plasma cells, and large mononuclear cells (Fig. 17.72). A number of associated clinical conditions have been described, including connective tissue diseases, bone marrow transplantation, acquired and congenital immuno-deficiency syndromes, and diffuse lymphoid hyperplasia of the intestine. This disease is considered idiopathic only when a cause or association cannot be identified.

We consider LIP to be a pattern rather than a diagnosis, since LIP, as proposed initially, has morphologic features that are difficult to accurately separate from other lymphoplasmacellular interstitial infiltrates, including low-grade lymphomas of extranodal marginal zone type (maltoma). The LIP pattern requires clinical and laboratory correlation for accurate assessment, similar to organizing pneumonia (OP), NSIP, and DIP.

Clinical presentation: The idiopathic form of LIP occurs most commonly between 50 and 70 years of age, but children may be affected. Women develop the disease more commonly than men. Respiratory symptoms include cough, dyspnea, and progressive shortness of breath, similar to other chronic interstitial pneumonias. Weight loss, fever, and adenopathy are more commonly present in LIP than in other interstitial pneumonias. LIP can affect children, although the majority of individuals affected are adults. There may be dysproteinemia with abnormalities in gammaglobulin production. Pulmonary function studies show a restrictive defect with abnormal gas exchange.

Radiologic findings: The chest X-ray shows bilateral basilar reticulonodular infiltrates, sometimes with fibrosis and honey-combing. Bilateral reticular or reticulonodular infiltrates are most common, but a coarsely nodular pattern has been described in patients who also had elevated IgG levels.[210] The predominant HRCT finding usually is ground-glass attenuation.[211] Other abnormalities commonly

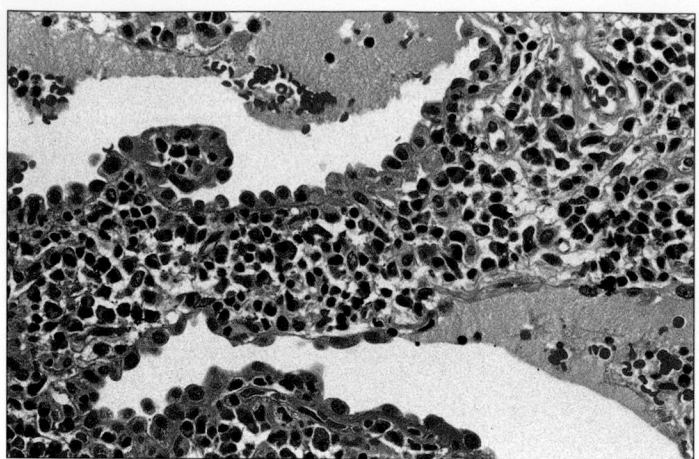

Fig. 17.73 Lymphocytic interstitial pneumonia (LIP). The characteristic appearance of LIP is that of a diffuse chronic inflammatory infiltrate, limited to the interstitium of the lung. The infiltrate is typically polymorphous and comprised of lymphocytes, plasma cells, and large mononuclear cells.

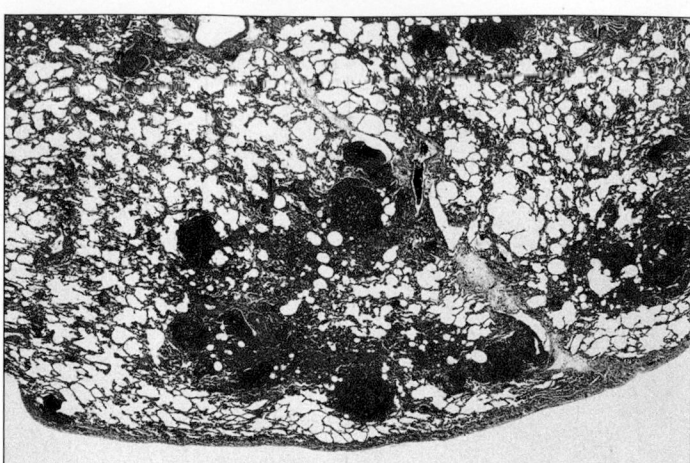

Fig. 17.74 Diffuse lymphoid hyperplasia (DLH). DLH is characterized by a proliferation of lymphoid follicles, primarily of the interstitium of the bronchovascular bundles, lobular septa, and pleura.

seen on HRCT include thickening of the bronchovascular bundles and thin-walled cysts.[211]

Pathologic findings: The hallmarks of the LIP-pattern include diffuse interstitial infiltration by a mixed chronic inflammatory cell population, comprised of lymphocytes, plasmacytoid lymphocytes, plasma cells, and histiocytes (Fig. 17.73). Giant cells and small granulomas may be present.[210] Honeycombing with interstitial fibrosis can occur. Immunophenotyping shows lack of clonality in the lymphoid infiltrate; B or T lymphocytes may predominate.

Differential diagnosis: The most challenging entity in the differential diagnosis is low-grade lymphoma. Extensive involvement of airways, with epithelial ulceration and destruction of cartilage, favors lymphoma. In lymphoma, the infiltrate is also said to follow lymphatic routes ('tracking').[212] Molecular studies are often helpful. Hypersensitivity pneumonitis can be differentiated from LIP by the extent of the lymphoid infiltrate, this being more extensive and severe in LIP. Furthermore, the characteristic bronchiolitis and the poorly formed interstitial granulomas of hypersensitivity are absent in LIP. Lymphomatoid granulomatosis (angiocentric immuno-proliferative disorder) is composed of cytologically atypical lymphoid cells, with angioinvasion and angiodestruction. Large areas of necrosis may be seen in lymphomatoid granulomatosis as a result of the angioinvasive infiltrate.

When LIP accompanies HIV infection, a wide age range occurs, and it is very commonly found in children.[213–216] These HIV-infected patients have the same non-specific respiratory symptoms, but weight loss is more common. Other features of HIV/AIDS, such as lymphadenopathy and hepatosplenomegaly, are also more common. Mean survival is worse than that of LIP alone, with adults living an average of 14 months and children, 32 months.[217] The morphology of LIP, with or without HIV, is similar.

A related condition, often included under the diagnosis of LIP, is *diffuse lymphoid hyperplasia* of the lung, characterized by a proliferation of lymphoid follicles, primarily in the interstitium of the bronchovascular bundles, lobular septa, and pleura (Fig. 17.74). Different from LIP, diffuse lymphoid hyperplasia has only slight involvement of the interstitium of the alveolar wall.[6]

Clinical course: In those patients with associated connective tissue diseases or immunodeficiency, treatment of the underlying disease may favorably affect the clinical course of LIP. With idiopathic LIP, the prognosis is variable, with some patients responding to immunosuppressive therapy. Interestingly, the prognosis of idiopathic LIP and that of low-grade lymphomas involving the lung may be similar; in fact, these forms of low-grade lung lymphoma may have a better prognosis than that reported historically for LIP.[218]

Cryptogenic organizing pneumonia

In 1983, Davison et al.[219] described a group of patients with 'cryptogenic organizing pneumonia'; and 2 years later Epler and coworkers[220] described similar cases as 'bronchiolitis obliterans organizing pneumonia' or 'BOOP.' The process described in both of these series is thought to be the same[13] as those cases described by Liebow and Carrington in 1969 as 'bronchiolitis obliterans interstitial pneumonia'.[32] Today, a reasonable consensus has emerged regarding what is now being called 'cryptogenic organizing pneumonia' (COP).[219–222] King and Mortensen[223] have recently compiled the findings from four major case series reported from North America, adding 18 of their own cases (112 cases in all). Based on these compiled data, the following description of COP emerges.

Clinical presentation: The average age for patients with COP is 58 years (range, 21 to 80 years) and there is no sex predominance. The evolution of clinical symptoms is subacute (4 months on average, and 3 months in most) and follows a flu-like illness in 40% of cases. Dyspnea and cough are present in half the patients. Fever is common and leukocytosis occurs in about one-quarter. The erythrocyte sedimentation rate is typically elevated.[224] Clubbing is rare. Restrictive lung disease is present in about half of patients with COP, and the diffusing capacity is reduced in most. Mild airflow obstruction may be present, typically in those patients who are smokers.

Radiologic findings: The chest radiographs are quite often characteristic,[225] with the appearance of patchy, bilateral (sometimes unilateral) nonsegmental airspace consolidation. These are occasionally migratory, as occurs in eosinophilic pneumonia. Linear

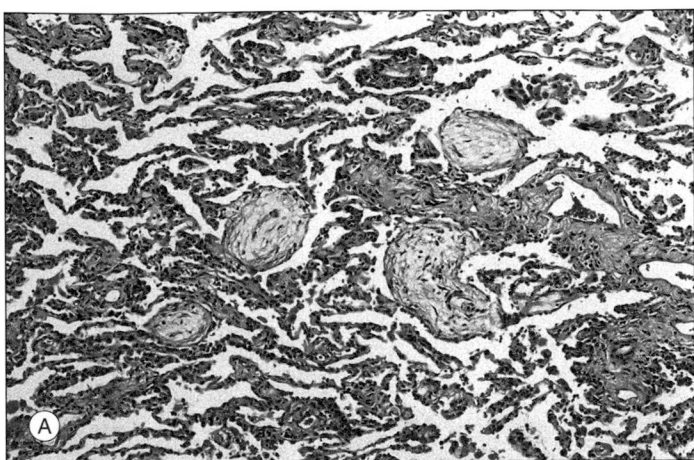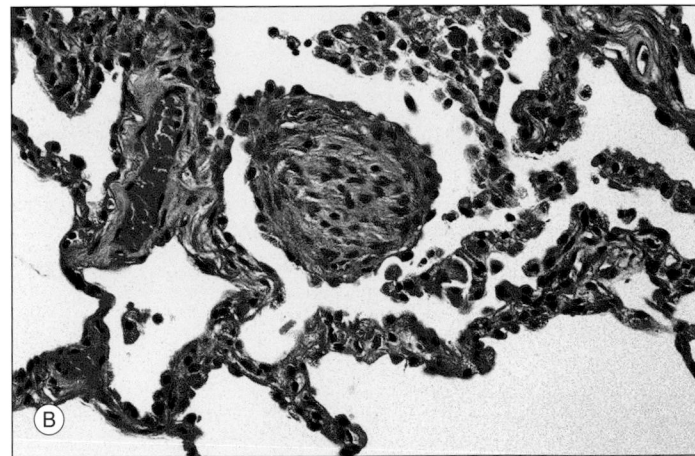

Fig. 17.75 Cryptogenic organizing pneumonia (COP). The major feature is airspace organization, mainly in alveoli (so-called *Masson bodies* or *polyps*), alveolar ducts, and respiratory bronchioles, where the lesions are characteristically of polypoid and fibromyxoid appearance. The organization is patchy and peribronchiolar, and tends to be all of similar 'age' in evolution (**A**). Masson body is present in an alveolar space (**B**).

opacities (reticulation) may be seen in 10–40% of patients but are rarely predominant.[225,226] Linear opacities are uncommon. In one series,[227] 10 of 11 cases were diagnosed correctly by radiology. The CT findings have been described by several authors.[228–231] The most characteristic HRCT features of COP are patchy unilateral or bilateral areas of consolidation, which in approximately 60% of cases have a predominantly peribronchial or subpleural distribution, or both. Small, ill-defined, nodules (3–10 mm in diameter) are seen in 30–50% of cases, and a reticular pattern is seen in 10–30% of cases. Airspace consolidation showed airspace granulation tissue histologically, whereas ground-glass opacities corresponded to alveolar wall inflammation and accumulation of alveolar macrophages with only little granulation tissue. Thus, although CT and HRCT give a better assessment of disease pattern, most of the features can be seen on the plain radiography.

Pathologic findings: The major feature is organization, mainly in alveoli (so-called Masson bodies), alveolar ducts, and respiratory bronchioles, where the exudate has a characteristic polypoid and fibromyxoid appearance (Fig. 17.75). This is patchy and peribronchiolar, and all the lesions appear to be recent, and of about the same age in evolution. Unfortunately, the term *bronchiolitis obliterans/organizing pneumonia* or '*BOOP*' has become one of the most commonly misused descriptions in lung pathology, much to the dismay of clinicians. Pathologists use the term to describe non-specific organization occurring in alveolar ducts and alveolar spaces of lung biopsies. Clinicians hear the term 'BOOP' or 'BOOP pattern' and often interpret this as a diagnosis of 'idiopathic BOOP' referred to above. Because of this, there is a growing consensus[223,232] for use of the term *cryptogenic organizing pneumonia* (COP) to describe the *clinicopathologic entity* for the following reasons: (1) while COP is primarily an organizing pneumonia, in up to 30% or more of cases, granulation tissue is not present in membranous bronchioles and at times may not even be seen in respiratory bronchioles;[219] (2) the term *bronchiolitis obliterans* has been used in so many different ways that it has become so ambiguous as to be functionally useless (this is discussed subsequently in the section on bronchiolitis); (3) bronchiolitis generally produces obstruction to air flow and COP is primarily characterized by a restrictive defect.

Differential diagnosis: The differential diagnosis of COP is long and includes many forms of lung injury in which repair occurs by intra-alveolar organization. The morphologic appearance suggests a healing infectious process, but no consistent agent has ever been found. *Nocardia asteroides* has been identified in a single case report.[233] Occult drug reaction has been raised as a possible etiology for COP.[234] Lesions resembling COP are frequently seen in a variety of conditions such as rheumatoid lung, eosinophilic pneumonia, heart-lung and lung transplants, and graft-versus-host disease (GVHD). These are not, by definition, cryptogenic. Finally, despite similarities in terminology, there is no histologic resemblance between occlusive bronchiolitis (OB, bronchiolitis obliterans) and COP.

Clinical course: The expected prognosis of COP is relatively good. In 63% of patients affected, the condition resolves, mainly as a response to steroids. Twelve percent die, typically in about 3 months. The disease persists in the remaining subset, or relapses if steroids are not tapered over a long period. Those COP patients that do poorly, frequently have comorbid disorders such as connective tissue disease or thyroiditis or have been taking nitrofurantoin.[235]

The differential diagnosis for the idiopathic diffuse lung diseases is presented in Table 17.16.

Pneumoconioses

The pneumoconioses are lung diseases that result from inhalation of inorganic dust. The reaction of the lung to inorganic dust depends on several factors, including the composition of the minerals involved, the size of the particles inhaled, and individual susceptibility. The composition of the dust determines toxicity. Some inhaled dusts are relatively inert while others are quite bioreactive. Dust particle size determines the site of deposition within the respiratory tract. Particles greater than 5 μm in diameter tend to be deposited in the nose and large airways, while particles less than 1 μm in diameter find their way to the peripheral airways and airspaces. Individual susceptibility must play a major role in pneumoconioses, since one person may be unaffected while an identically exposed individual develops significant disease.

In assessing patients with pneumoconiosis, the clinical history, pulmonary function test data, radiologic features, and pathologic

Table 17.16 Contrasting pathologic features of idiopathic interstitial pneumonias

Features	NSIP	UIP	DIP	AIP	LIP	COP
Temporal appearance	Uniform	Variegated	Uniform	Uniform	Uniform	Uniform
Interstitial inflammation	Prominent	Scant	Scant	Scant	Prominent	Scant
Interstitial fibrosis (collagen)	Variable, diffuse	Patchy	Variable, diffuse	No	Some cases	No
Interstitial fibrosis (fibroblasts)	Occas, diffuse	No	No	Yes, diffuse	No	No
OP Pattern	Occas, focal	Occas, focal	No	Occas, focal	No	Prominent
Fibroblast foci	Occas, focal	Typical	No	No	No	No
Honeycomb areas	Rare	Yes	No	No	Sometimes	No
Intra-alveolar macrophages	Occas, patchy	Occas, focal	Yes, diffuse	No	Occas, patchy	No
Hyaline membranes	No	No	No	Yes, focal	No	No
Granulomas	No	No	No	No	Focal, poorly formed	No

NSIP = non-specific interstitial pneumonia; DIP = desquamative interstitial pneumonia; UIP = usual interstitial pneumonia; AIP = acute interstitial pneumonia; Occas = occasional; LIP = lymphocytic interstitial pneumonia; COP = cryptogenic organizing pneumonia
Data from Katzenstein[190] and Travis[408]

material must all be correlated. Identification of the injurious dust may be essential to the diagnosis and this may fall within the responsibilities of the pathologist; methods of determining the specific composition of dusts within the lung, such as electron probe microanalysis, are discussed in detail in a 1987 comprehensive review of occupational lung disease.[236] Here we present only those inorganic dusts that are encountered with reasonable frequency at biopsy; for a more complete exposition, the reader is referred to several excellent published works on occupational lung disease.[236–239]

Asbestosis

The fibrous silicates occur in nature and have been utilized by humans for centuries because of their remarkable properties of heat and chemical resistance and their ability to insulate. They are comprised of varying amounts of magnesium, iron, aluminum, manganese, calcium, sodium, and potassium.[240] The distinctive properties of these minerals are related to their fibrous structure, with each particle having a length to width ratio of 3 or more. There are two main types of asbestos: serpentine and amphibole.[241] Chrysotile is the only example of the former, but the latter has many subtypes, of which crocidolite (Cape Blue asbestos) and amosite are the best known. The two types differ both in composition and lattice structure, with chrysotile fibers having a central core. Asbestos is found in many industries and in many forms, so there are abundant opportunities for exposure.[237] *Asbestosis* is the name given to the pneumoconiosis caused by inhalation of this group of mineral compounds. Asbestos fibers have an inherent tendency to split along their long axis into ever thinner and smaller forms. This property is felt to be central to the pathogenicity of the fibrous silicates.

Clinical presentation: Pneumoconiosis typically develops insidiously after exposure. Shortness of breath is often the first symptom and indication of disease. Late inspiratory crackles (rales) are found initially in the lung bases but these become widespread as the disease advances. Digital clubbing (flattening of the usually obtuse angle formed between the fingernail and cuticle) is present in about 75% of the patients, but this does not necessarily correlate with the radiologic extent of disease. Pulmonary function tests show a restrictive pattern. Early in experimental asbestosis there is fibrosis of respiratory bronchioles and/or alveolar ducts, but recent attention has been drawn to airway lesions in asbestos workers (see section on mineral dust bronchiolitis).[242]

Radiologic findings: Asbestosis predominantly affects the lower lung zones, and the earliest changes are seen in the costophrenic angles bilaterally, where there are first fine linear opacities that progress to irregular opacities. Significant morphologic and functional abnormalities may be present even when the chest radiograph is normal,[243] as may be the case in 10–20% of patients with histologically confirmed asbestosis.[244] HRCT is much more sensitive than conventional CT and the chest radiograph in recognizing pleural thickening and interstitial fibrosis.[245,246] The findings in asbestosis include subpleural lines (linear opacities of variable length within 1 cm of and parallel to the pleura); parenchymal bands (linear opacities up to 5 cm in length, usually extending to a pleural surface); thickening of lobular septal lines and small opacities within the lobules; and honeycombing.[245–247] The findings may be indistinguishable from UIP, except that pleural plaques or diffuse pleural thickening is seen in virtually all cases of asbestosis.[245]

Pathologic findings: The histopathology of asbestosis is highly variable, ranging from diffuse fine fibrosis of the alveolar walls with relative preservation of alveolar structure, to heterogeneous fibrosis of lung tissue, resembling that seen in advanced fibrotic diseases such as UIP. The inhaled fibers enter the airway wall where they impact at branch points in the terminal airways. Bronchiolocentric scarring is characteristic. Typical asbestos bodies consist of a central fiber core of asbestos encrusted with iron ('ferruginous asbestos bodies'). Asbestos bodies have knobs at each end, and a central body that appears beaded along a central thread-like fiber (Fig. 17.76). Asbestos fibers are found free in the extracellular space of the interstitium, in alveolar spaces, and surrounded by macrophages. They are not visible in polarized light. A variety of other iron-encrusted bodies of various shapes and sizes may be seen, but not all iron-coated bodies are asbestos bodies. Nevertheless, in routine sections, the classic beaded asbestos body described above is rarely encountered in other than asbestos exposure. While a significant dose-related response curve has been identified in workers occupationally exposed to asbestos, the amount of fibrosis (Fig. 17.77) present in the lung seems to have little relation to fiber burden.[248] Progressive massive fibrosis is said to occur when nodular lesions 1 cm in diameter or larger occur throughout the lungs.[249]

Pleural effusions are typically unilateral in asbestosis,[250] and there is little association between the occurrence of pleural plaques

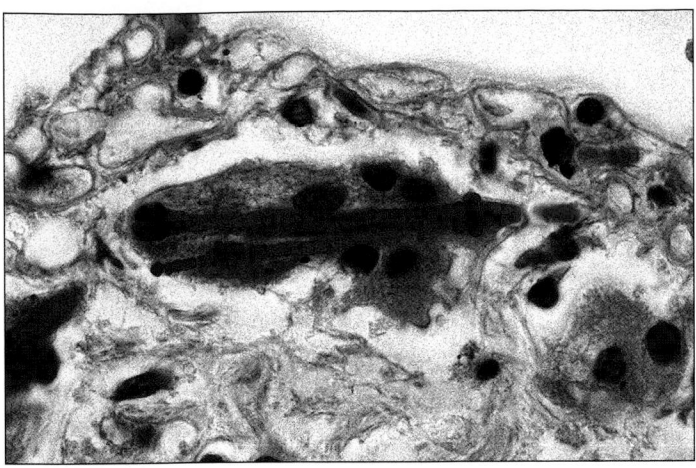

Fig. 17.76 Asbestosis. Asbestos bodies have knobs at each end, and a central body that appears beaded along a central thread-like fiber.

and pleural effusion. In fact, the cause of pleural plaques remains unknown. Plaques occur only on the parietal pleura and tend to be bilateral. Common locations involved are the area over the ribs, on surfaces abutting the lung bases, and along the aponeurotic areas of the diaphragm. On gross examination, plaques are raised, glistening, and unusually white. Microscopically, plaques are composed of acellular hyaline fibrous tissue with interlacing bands of collagen, producing a basket-weave pattern. Asbestos bodies are rarely found in plaques.

Clinical course: The pulmonary consequences of asbestos exposure include diffuse interstitial fibrosis (asbestosis), conglomerate massive fibrosis, pleural effusion, pleural plaque, mesothelioma, and lung cancer.[236–238,243]

Silicosis

Prolonged inhalation of dusts containing crystalline silicon dioxide (SiO_2) results in a chronic fibrosing pulmonary disease known as silicosis. Quartz, cristobalite, and tridymite are the three naturally occurring forms of silicon dioxide, with quartz being the most common. Minerals containing SiO_2 are ubiquitous and are found in many industries and occupations. Inhalation of particles of 0.5–5 μm in diameter are most likely to cause disease. Both the concentration and size of the particles determine the likelihood of developing silicosis.[237] Silicosis occurs in three relatively distinctive morphologic forms: acute silicosis, simple nodular silicosis, and conglomerate silicosis (progressive massive fibrosis).

Clinical presentation: Most patients develop disease over a fairly long time course (20–40 years) and symptoms often develop late in the disease. Slowly progressive shortness of breath with a productive cough is typical, but overwhelming exposure to free silica can produce the acute disease known as 'acute silicosis.' Today this is rare form of silicosis, but can occur in sandblasting if respiratory protection is not used. The inhaled particles involved are typically 1–2 μm in diameter, and are high in quartz content. The silicotic process develops rapidly in these massively exposed individuals. The exact pathogenesis of the acute lesion is not known. Simple nodular silicosis produces minor symptoms and runs a chronic course. A detailed classification of silicosis in particular, and pneumoconiosis in general, has been,[251] and continues to be, widely used in epidemiologic surveys and in establishing disability related to occupational exposure. When mycobacterial or fungal infections are superimposed, weight loss and other constitutional symptoms and signs may dominate the clinical presentation. In regards to mechanism of disease, tuberculosis is known to enhance and perpetuate cellular reactions to dust particles, thereby enhancing progression of lesions. Also, silica itself may inhibit macrophage containment of mycobacterial growth. Both *Mycobacterium tuberculosis* and atypical mycobacteria seem to be implicated in this comorbid relationship.

Radiologic findings: Nodules are readily appreciated on plain chest radiographs of patients with simple nodular silicosis. Both conventional CT and HRCT are superior to the plain chest radiograph in detecting the presence of nodules as well as coalescence of nodules.[252] CT has also shed light on the cause of pulmonary function abnormalities in simple silicosis, because emphysema can be readily recognized using CT. Abnormalities of FEV_1 and diffusing capacity correlate well to CT-determined emphysema but poorly to the profusion of nodules.[253] In another study, Kinsella et al.[254] found that the extent of emphysema as determined by CT was the strongest predictor of

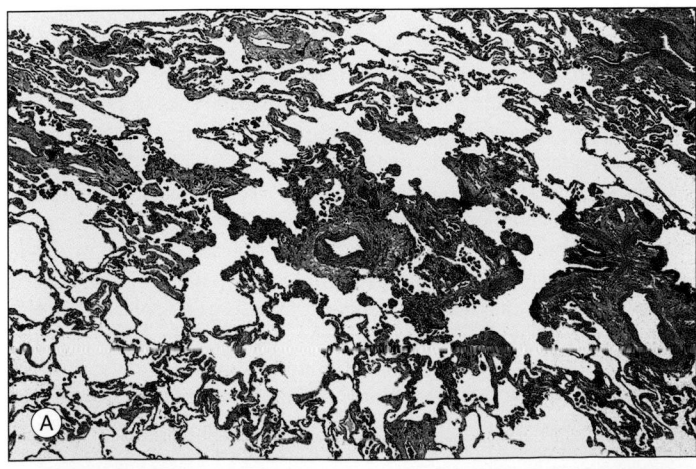

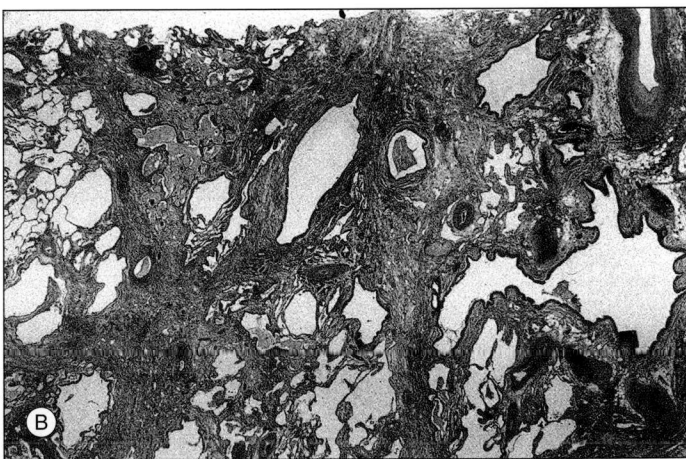

Fig. 17.77 Asbestosis. The diffuse parenchymal manifestation of asbestosis occurs as airway associated fibrosis in its early phase (**A**). Later, more confluent fibrosis occurs (**B**), and may be mistaken for UIP in late stage.

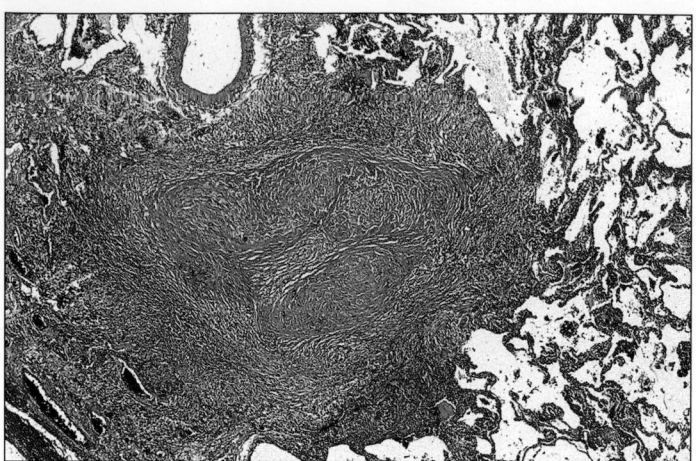

Fig. 17.78 Silicosis. The diagnostic lesion of silicosis is the silicotic nodule, which is comprised of a central whorled mass of acellular hyalinized collagen, surrounded by layers of macrophages and plasma cells.

pulmonary function impairment. They also found that the extent of silicosis was an independent predictor of impairment, but a much weaker one. Smokers had worse emphysema than nonsmokers.

Pathologic findings: In acute silicosis, the lungs have a diffuse consolidated appearance. Microscopically, the alveoli are filled by an eosinophilic foamy exudate, containing many macrophages, similar to that seen in alveolar proteinosis. In acute silicosis, there is prominent type II cell hyperplasia with interstitial fibrosis, findings not expected in alveolar proteinosis.

The gross lung specimen in *simple nodular silicosis* is remarkable for pleural fibrosis with adhesion formation. Well-circumscribed gray-black nodules, measuring 0.5–5 mm in diameter, are present consistently in the upper lung zones, posteriorly, and these areas are the earliest to show pathologic changes. The hilar lymph nodes are enlarged and may be distinctively calcified in radiographs (so called 'eggshell calcification'). Microscopically, dust particles are found within alveolar macrophages or free in the alveolar interstitium. Respiratory bronchioles often show aggregated particles in their walls.

The diagnostic lesion of silicosis is the silicotic nodule, which has a central whorled mass of acellular hyalinized collagen (Fig. 17.78) surrounded by variable numbers of macrophages and plasma cells. Small quantities of dust can usually be identified in the nodules, but if the dust is high in quartz content and the particles are small, severe fibrosis can result. Pure silica is poorly refractile in polarized light. The highly refractile, needle-like particles usually abundant in the silicotic nodule are typically composed of aluminum and magnesium *silicates*. Continued dust exposure increases the number and size of nodules. Even after exposure is ended, the nodules may continue to grow, presumably as a result of ongoing migration of macrophages to their periphery, and a continued cycle of fibrogenesis.

Conglomerate silicosis (progressive massive fibrosis) is similar to simple nodular silicosis, but by definition nodules 1 cm or more in diameter are produced. These often coalesce to form even larger masses. The time course for this occurrence in conglomerate silicosis is shorter than that for simple nodular silicosis. Superimposed tuberculosis can result in cavitation of nodules. Tuberculosis has also been implicated in the pathogenesis of conglomerate silicosis, even when cavitation is absent. To make matters more complicated, there is a

higher incidence of tuberculosis in association with the disease.[255] One of the interesting features of silicosis is that the fibrosis produced is not only confined to the regions where dust can be identified, but may also be present in the lymph nodes that drain the lung. An immunologic mechanism has been implicated in the pathogenesis of the disease.

Berylliosis

Occupational exposure to beryllium was first recognized as a health hazard in fluorescent lamp factory workers. The use of beryllium in this industry was discontinued, but because of beryllium's remarkable structural characteristics, it continues to be used in metallic, alloy, and oxide forms in numerous industries today. Berylliosis may occur as acute and chronic forms. The acute disease is usually seen in refinery workers and produces diffuse alveolar damage. Chronic berylliosis is a multiorgan disease, but the lung is most severely affected.

Radiologic findings: The findings are similar to sarcoidosis except that hilar and mediastinal adenopathy is seen in only 30–40% of cases compared with 80–90% in sarcoid.[256,257] Of 28 patients with biopsy-proven berylliosis, the chest radiograph was abnormal in 15 (54%), and the HRCT was abnormal in 25 (89%).[257]

Pathologic findings: Berylliosis is characterized by non-necrotizing lung parenchymal granulomas indistinguishable from those of sarcoidosis.[258]

Hard metal pneumoconiosis (Cobalt pneumoconiosis)

Giant cell interstitial pneumonia (GIP) was one of Liebow's original chronic interstitial pneumonias.[32] By 1972, only seven cases had been reported in detail.[259] GIP is now recognized to be a form of pneumoconiosis caused in most instances by inhalation of hard metal fumes.[260,261] *Hard metal* is an industrial term that refers to tungsten carbide, used in the manufacture of tool bits and drills. Cobalt is added to tungsten and carbon during the formation of tungsten carbide. Cobalt, alone or in combination with other metals, may produce a multitude of tissue effects.

Clinical features: An IgE-mediated asthmatic presentation (chest tightness, dyspnea, and wheezing) of hard metal disease is actually more common than the diffuse parenchymal manifestation with infiltrates.

Radiologic findings: The chest radiograph usually shows bilateral patchy, nodular infiltrates involving the middle or upper zones of the lung, with sparing of the apices and costophrenic angles. Progressive pulmonary fibrosis and respiratory insufficiency have been noted in most cases.

Pathologic findings: The histopathology of GIP is characterized by the presence of many large, rather bizarre multinucleate cells in the alveolar spaces in a airway-centered distribution. These cells characteristically engulf other cells (cannabalistic). As in DIP/RBILD (see later section on diffuse smoking-related diseases), macrophages fill the alveolar spaces, and there is an interstitial infiltrate comprised mainly of lymphocytes. Fibrosis is seen around distal bronchioles, respiratory bronchioles, and alveolar ducts, similar to that occurring in mineral dust bronchiolitis (described later). This combination of airway disease and airspace macrophages, produces a pattern of nonuniform involvement. The diagnosis is made on the basis of alveolar giant cells, coupled with the presence of distal airway fibrosis (Fig. 17.79).

Differential diagnosis: The differential diagnosis includes DIP, mineral dust-associated bronchiolitis, and even measles pneumonia (multinucleated cells mimicking measles giant cells) if a patient with GIP is biopsied during an acute episode of some other illness.

Clinical course: The distinctive relationship between hard metal exposure and GIP is illustrated by two case reports[262,263] of GIP re-occurring in a transplanted lung, despite no additional exposure to

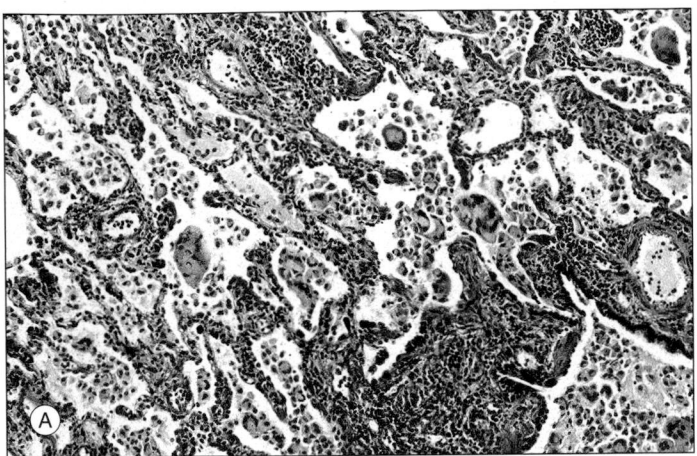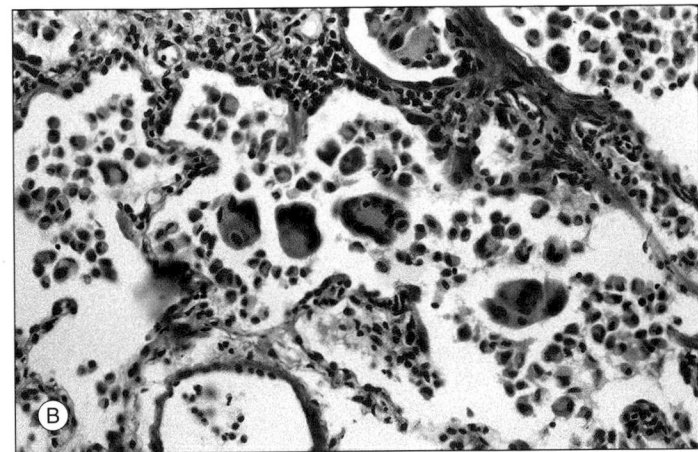

Fig. 17.79 Hard metal disease (giant cell interstitial pneumonia). The combination of airway disease and distinctive multinucleated airspace macrophages produces a variegated pattern at scanning magnification (**A**). At high magnification the giant cells have a distinctive appearance (**B**).

Table 17.17 Less common pneumoconioses

Dust	Industry	Presence of fibrosis	Characteristic features
Aluminum	Metal refining	Idiosyncratic interstitial fibrosis	Occasional granulomas, black interstitial dust
Antimony	Mining alloy	No	Dust-bearing macrophages
Coal (anthracosis)	Coal workers	No	Black dust in peribronchial aggregates
Barium (baritosis)	Miners, grinders, aspiration of dust	Minimal	Macrophages containing granules
Fiberglass	Manufacturing	No	Particle as negative space
Fuller's earth (aluminum silicate)	Toiletry manufacture	Confluent in upper lobe	No foreign body giant cells; large particle, 15–30 µm
Iron (siderosis)	Welder's oxyacetylene, silver finishers	No	Iron dusts
Magnesium silicate (talcosis)	Talc inhalation, narcotic abuse	Lower lobe fibrosis that cavitates	Doubly refractile particles, often needle shaped
Tin dioxide (stannosis)	Tin smelting, mining, refining	No	Macrophage aggregates in small nodules
Titanium dye	Dye	No	Particles within macrophages

From Previous edition. Table 28.9, p. 1151, with permission.

hard metal. In one of these reports,[262] no hard metal was found in the transplanted lung; and steroid treatment partially ameliorated the reaction in both the native and transplanted lung. These observations have suggested to some that GIP is an immunologically mediated reaction to cobalt.

Other dusts

A variety of other dusts may be encountered in the lung, some of which are fibrogenic and others of which are not. These are listed in Table 17.17.

DIFFUSE DISEASES OF THE SMALL AIRWAYS

Diseases of the conducting airways produce variable obstruction to airflow, a parameter that can be measured clinically with pulmonary function tests. Airflow obstruction is best estimated by measurements made during forced expiration. This is accomplished using the pulmonary function test known as the FEV_1 (forced expiratory volume achieved in the first second of measurement). The FEV_1 is

typically expressed as a 'percentage of predicted,' as determined by body height and age.

Lung biopsy is seldom required for patients with the common clinical forms of airflow obstruction. When unexplained airflow obstruction occurs (i.e. not clearly associated with smoking, chronic bronchitis, or emphysema) transbronchial or surgical lung biopsy may be undertaken. The term *small airways disease* (SAD) was a popular clinical term in the 1970s, originally intended as a description of disease affecting the small bronchi and bronchioles distal to the catheter used to measure peripheral airway resistance in patients with end-stage chronic airflow obstruction.[264] We have expanded the use of this term to include a wider spectrum of inflammatory and fibrotic disease of the terminal airways. From a clinical perspective, the most serious of the SAD manifestations is constrictive/occlusive bronchiolitis. Constrictive bronchiolitis may occur following respiratory infection, as a result of fume or toxin inhalation, as a manifestation of bronchiolitis in connective tissue diseases (e.g. rheumatoid arthritis), as a result of drug toxicity, in some asthmatic patients who develop bronchiolitis, in some patients with inflammatory bowel disease, in a peculiar condition of neuroendocrine

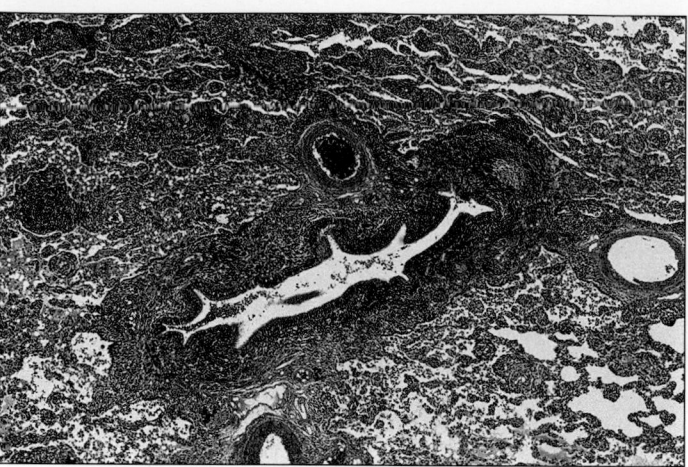

Fig. 17.80 Cellular bronchiolitis. The membranous bronchioles show an increased number of chronic inflammatory cells (lymphocytes and plasma cells), hence the term *chronic cellular bronchiolitis*.

Table 17.18 Etiologic classification of bronchiolitis

Smoking-related
Respiratory bronchiolitis
Not smoking-related
Irritants and viral infections
Rheumatoid bronchiolitis
Diffuse panbronchiolitis
Heart-lung transplantation
Bronchiolitis in IBD
Graft-versus-host disease
Mineral dust bronchiolitis
Neuroendocrine cell hyperplasia with constrictive bronchiolitis
Foreign body occlusive bronchiolitis
Cryptogenic bronchiolitis

Modified from previous edition. Table 28.10, p. 1153, with permission.

hyperplasia of the distal airways, and in lung or bone marrow transplant recipients. Naturally, when our knowledge of possible etiologies is exhausted, an idiopathic form remains.

Bronchiolitis

Bronchiolitis is defined as inflammation of the bronchioles, and generally refers to inflammation of membranous bronchioles (Fig. 17.80).[265] Bronchiolitis is an essential part of the patho-physiology of the chronic airflow obstruction that occurs in cigarette smokers. Bronchiolitis not related to cigarette smoking has become an important focus of study in the past two decades. A useful classification based on clinical associations is shown in Table 17.18. It would seem possible to classify bronchiolitis morphologically, but this is difficult because the available morphologic terms have been used in confusing ways, and the same morphologic findings may have different clinical associations. To complicate matters further, patients with the same clinical condition may have varying morphologic features. Fortunately, HRCT scanning can be very helpful in the evaluation of these patients and also may indicate physiologic

dysfunction by demonstrating air trapping in the lung in a dynamic fashion (comparison of inspiratory and expiratory scans). We begin our analysis of SAD with some definitions of morphologic terms.

ETIOLOGIC CLASSIFICATION OF SMALL AIRWAYS DISEASE

Bronchiolar lesions in smokers (tobacco bronchiolitis)

Bronchiolitis is an integral part of the lesions found in patients with typical chronic airflow obstruction. Most of these patients are smokers with chronic bronchitis and varying degrees of pulmonary dysfunction. In patients with mild airflow obstruction, bronchiolar inflammation probably plays a major role. In severe airflow obstruction, some degree of alternating constriction and dilatation (analogous to varicosity) of the bronchioles are typically the dominant lesions.[9,266] Biopsy specimens in this setting are rarely submitted to the surgical pathologist for this process alone, but these airway changes are frequently seen in biopsies taken for other reasons.

Forms of bronchiolitis in unexplained chronic air flow obstruction (nontobacco bronchiolitis)

Inhaled irritant gases and infections

Many irritant gases can produce severe bronchiolitis, sometimes with acute ulceration and inflammation. This inflammatory injury may be followed by the accumulation of loose granulation tissue and finally by complete stenosis and occlusion of the airways. The best known of these agents are nitrogen dioxide,[267] sulfur dioxide,[268] and ammonia.[269] Viral infection can also cause permanent bronchiolar injury, particularly adenovirus infection.[270] Mycoplasma pneumonia is also cited as a potential cause.[271] The course of events is similar to that for the toxic gases. Variable degrees of bronchiectasis or bronchioloectasia may result because of bronchiolar occlusion and loss. Lung biopsy is performed rarely and then usually because of clinically unusual airflow obstruction, often in a young person. Sometimes mixed obstruction and restriction may occur, presumably on the basis of peribronchiolar scarring. This latter feature may produce CT findings suggesting 'interstitial' disease. The airway lesions are not specific, but can be recognized by variable reduction in bronchiolar luminal diameter compared to the adjacent pulmonary artery branch (these should be of roughly equal diameter in complete cross-sections). The diagnosis depends on careful clinical correlation and sometimes the addition of a comparison between inspiratory and expiratory high-resolution CT scans (which show characteristic air trapping).

Rheumatoid bronchiolitis

Geddes et al.[272] described six nonsmoking females who developed rapidly progressive dyspnea and airflow obstruction. Five patients had classic RA and the sixth had a positive antinuclear antibody. The condition was progressive and death occurred 5 to 18 months after the onset of disease. Radiologically, the lungs were grossly overinflated, but without the peripheral arterial deficiency of emphysema. The diffusing capacity and volume-pressure curves were normal. Morphologically, scattered occlusion of small bronchi and bronchioles was observed, associated with the presence of loose connective tissue in their lumina. These patients were considered to have constrictive bronchiolitis as a consequence of rheumatoid

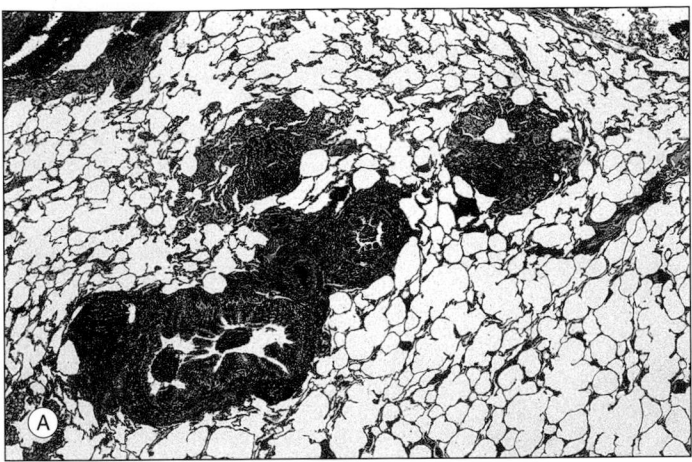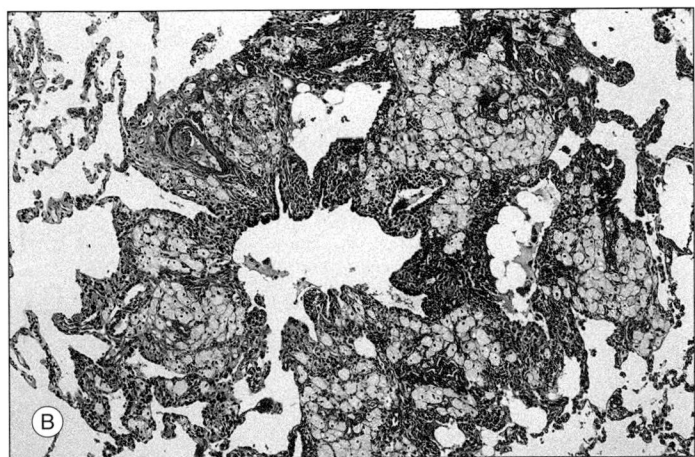

Fig. 17.81 Diffuse panbronchiolitis (DPB). Histopathologically, severe chronic inflammation is centered on respiratory bronchioles early in the disease, followed by involvement of distal membranous bronchioles and peribronchiolar alveolar spaces as the disease progresses. A characteristic low-magnification appearance is that of nodular bronchiolocentric lesions (**A**). The nearly diagnostic feature of DPB is the accumulation of many pale vacuolated macrophages in the walls and lumens of respiratory bronchioles and in adjacent airspaces (**B**).

arthritis, and this is now a well-recognized complication of RA. In some patients, necrobiotic granulomas can be seen in the walls of airways resulting in their partial or total occlusion. From a practical point of view, the lesions are focal within the airways, often in small bronchi, and therefore may not be easily visualized in the biopsy specimen. The sequence of events in constrictive bronchiolitis from an inflammatory cause is illustrated later in the section on constrictive bronchiolitis as a pathologic finding. Today, because of the widespread recognition of rheumatoid bronchiolitis, biopsy is rarely performed in these patients. Another common pulmonary manifestation of RA is follicular bronchitis/bronchiolitis (described below).

Diffuse panbronchiolitis

Diffuse panbronchiolitis (DPB) is a distinctive form of chronic bronchiolitis seen almost exclusively in people of east Asian decent (Japan, Korea, China). DPB may occur rarely in the United States.[273–275] and in patients of non-Asian descent.

Clinical presentation: DPB occurs with an age range of 20 to 60 years. Men are twice as commonly affected as women. Chronic productive cough and dyspnea are the typical presenting complaints, and most patients have sinusitis. A genetic susceptibility has been well documented over the years, and recently has been identified as a human leukocyte antigen (HLA)-associated major susceptibility gene, likely residing within the HLA-B locus on the short arm of chromosome 6 (6p21.3). HLA-B54 is the haplotype reported in Japanese patients and HLA-A11 is identified in those of Korean ancestry.[276] Repeated *Haemophilus influenzae* infections are reported to occur. *Pseudomonas aeruginosa* colonization is an ominous development and was associated with a mean survival of 2.9 years, according to one study.[274]

Radiologic findings: On CT scan there is variable hyperinflation, and multiple scattered fine opacities less than 2 mm in diameter are seen, which are more profuse in the lower zones. The radiologic findings are non-specific, but HRCT usually demonstrates characteristic findings.[277,278] These consist of 2–5 mm diameter nodules and branching linear opacities, known as tree-in-bud pattern and corresponding pathologically to dilated and inflamed bronchioles. Other common findings include bronchiectasis, and decreased vascularity and attenuation in the peripheral lung due to air trapping.

Functionally, there is chronic airflow obstruction, which is progressive, terminating in respiratory failure.

Pathologic findings: Histopathologically, severe chronic inflammation is centered on respiratory bronchioles early in the disease, followed by involvement of distal membranous bronchioles and peribronchiolar alveolar spaces as the disease progresses. A characteristic low-magnification appearance is that of nodular bronchiolocentric lesions (Fig. 17.81A). The characteristic and nearly diagnostic feature of DPB is the accumulation of many pale vacuolated macrophages in the walls and lumens of respiratory bronchioles and in adjacent airspaces (Fig. 17.81B). Japanese investigators have speculated that the condition occurs in the United States and has been unrecognized. This view has been substantiated by the finding of 7 of 81 cases (8.6%) previously diagnosed as cellular chronic bronchiolitis.[273] The reported recurrence of the disease in allografted lungs after transplantation suggests a systemic disorder, perhaps indicating persistence of a pretransplant immune cell activation.

Graft-versus-host disease

Patients who receive bone marrow transplants are by definition immunosuppressed and are at risk for lung complications related to radiation, chemotherapeutic or antirejection drugs, infection and, notably, graft-versus-host disease (GVHD).[279–281] One infection in particular, reactivation of CMV infection, is a major problem and occurs in approximately half the patients.[282] Relevant to this section, clinical chronic obstructive bronchiolitis, with its morphologic correlate of constrictive bronchiolitis, has become a well-recognized complication,[283] occurring in about 4–10% of patients.[279,284] Clinically, progressive air flow obstruction with radiologic evidence of overinflation is seen between 3 months to 2 years after transplantation. Other manifestations of GVHD are usually present,[285] and treatment directed at GVHD may be effective. A necrotizing bronchiolitis together with constrictive bronchiolitis has been described,[281,283] as well as interstitial fibrosis, mild interstitial inflammation, and peribronchiolar fibrosis.[286]

Mineral dust bronchiolitis

Mineral dust bronchiolitis is best exemplified by the so-called 'simple pneumoconiosis of coal workers.' Although typically

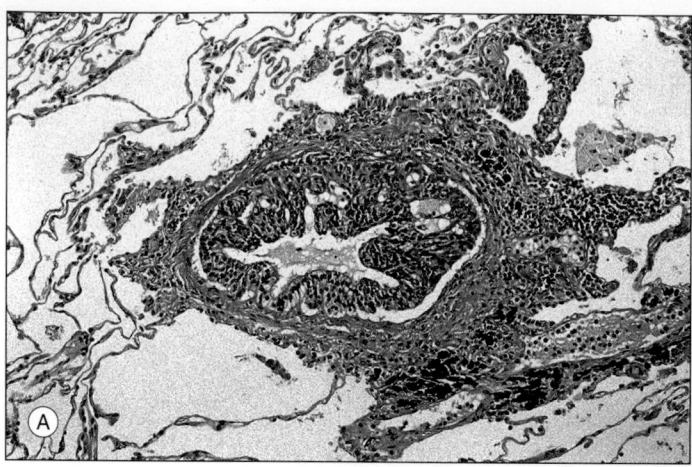
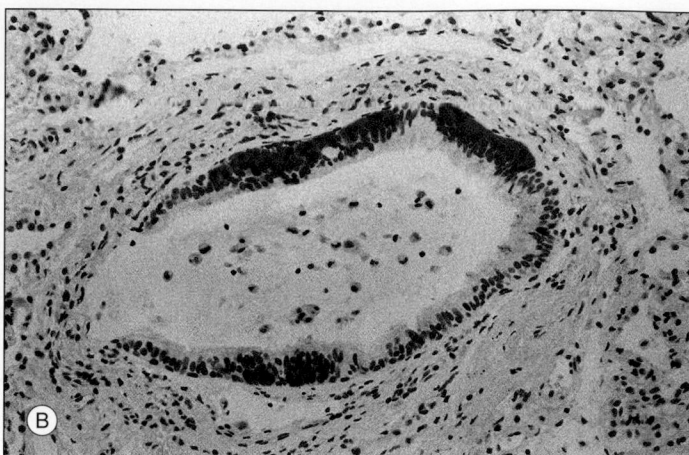

Fig. 17.82 Neuroendocrine cell hyperplasia with occlusive bronchiolar fibrosis. Diffuse neuroendocrine cell hyperplasia of the airways can produce occlusive bronchiolitis (**A**). An immunohistochemical stain for synaptophysin highlights the neuroendocrine cells, markedly increased here (**B**, antisynaptophysin, immunoalkaline phosphatase, Vector red chromogen).

recognized as the classical 'dust macule' and thought of as a form of focal emphysema, mineral dust bronchiolitis likely represents the result of bronchiolar inflammation produced by coal. Evidence of active inflammation is slight, as in emphysema. Mineral dust bronchiolitis was first clearly defined by Churg and Wright in 1983.[287] It occurs following exposure to a number of different mineral dusts and to asbestos in particular.[242] Careful clinicopathologic study[288] has implicated mineral dust bronchiolitis as a cause of chronic airflow obstruction. The basic lesion consists of fibrous thickening of the distal membranous bronchioles, respiratory bronchioles, and alveolar ducts. Fibrosis is particularly prominent in respiratory bronchioles, typically accompanied by heavy pigmentation.

Neuroendocrine cell hyperplasia with occlusive bronchiolar fibrosis

In 1992, Aguayo et al.[289] reported findings in six patients with moderate chronic airflow obstruction, all of whom were nonsmokers. Diffuse neuroendocrine cell hyperplasia of the bronchioles, associated with partial or total occlusion of airway lumens by fibrous tissue, was present in all six patients (Fig. 17.82). Three of these patients also had peripheral carcinoid tumors and three had progressive dyspnea. The association between peripheral carcinoid tumors in the lung and multiple carcinoid 'tumorlets' (by definition measuring less than 5 mm) has long been recognized, but its frequency and significance were not known. In a study of 25 peripheral carcinoid tumors occurring in both smokers and nonsmokers, 19 (76%) were found to have neuroendocrine cell hyperplasia of the airways, occurring mostly in bronchioles.[290] Eight patients (32%) were found to have occlusive bronchiolar fibrosis. Four of these patients had mild chronic airflow obstruction, and two of these were nonsmokers.

An increase in neuroendocrine cells was present in more than 20% of bronchioles examined in lung tissue adjacent to the tumor, and in tissue blocks taken well away from tumor. Less than half of these airways were partially or totally occluded. The mildest lesion consisted of linear zones of neuroendocrine cell hyperplasia with very focal subepithelial fibrosis. More obvious lesions consisted of a plaque of eccentric fibrous tissue partially occluding the airway lumen and sometimes the occlusion was caused by a proliferation of neuroendocrine cells. The most severely involved bronchioles showed total occlusion of their lumens by fibrous tissue, with few

visible neuroendocrine cells. Of interest, 17 of the 19 patients with neuroendocrine hyperplasia (8 of whom had associated bronchiolar fibrosis) reported by Miller and Müller were women,[290] as were all three of Aguayo's patients with bronchiolar fibrosis and carcinoid tumors.[289] Presumably fibrosis in this setting of neuroendocrine hyperplasia is related to one or more peptides secreted by neuroendocrine cells and these cells are more effective in stimulating fibrosis in women.

Foreign body bronchiolitis

Aspiration of exogenous material into the lungs can produce dramatic bronchiolitis with variable amounts of fibrosis.[291,292] Aspiration of gastric contents containing activated charcoal was accompanied by pneumatoceles and death from respiratory failure 14 weeks after aspiration.[293] Severe centrilobular pigmentation was noted grossly, and massive black pigmentation, doubly refractile material, and a foreign body giant cell reaction were seen in most of the bronchioles that demonstrated obliterative bronchiolitis. Foreign body bronchiolitis can occur other than from gastric aspiration. Obeid et al.[294] described such a case in a cocaine sniffer.

Inflammatory bowel disease-associated bronchiolitis

The lungs may be affected by inflammatory reactions in the setting of inflammatory bowel disease.[295] They include acute and chronic bronchitis with associated bronchiectasis (Fig. 17.83),[296,297] occlusive or constrictive bronchiolitis,[297,298] and COP.[299] The process can be likened to the occurrence of sclerosing cholangitis in patients with ulcerative colitis. In the lung, inflammation of the central airways may progress to fibrosis with narrowing and destruction of the tracheobronchial tree.[298]

Cryptogenic bronchiolitis

The frequency of unexplained (idiopathic) chronic airflow obstruction is probably quite low, at least as inferred from a study by Turton et al.[300] who identified 10 patients (9 women) with chronic airflow obstruction unexplained by any known cause in a review of 2094 patients with an FEV_1 of less than 60% of predicted. Asthma, chronic bronchitis, emphysema, smoking, and other specific lung diseases were excluded. The ages ranged from 27 to 60 years. Five of the 10 were found to have RA and presumably rheumatoid

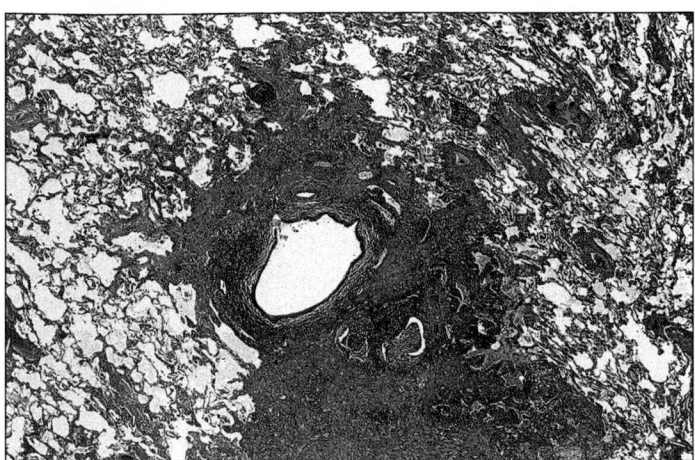

Fig. 17.83 Bronchiolitis in inflammatory bowel disease. Some patients with inflammatory bowel disease develop bronchiolitis. The changes identified include acute and chronic bronchiolitis, and bronchiectasis.

Table 17.19 Pathologic classification of bronchiolitis

Cellular bronchiolitis
Follicular bronchiolitis
Constrictive/occlusive bronchiolitis
Bronchiolar loss
Foreign body bronchiolitis
From previous edition. Table 28.11, p. 1153, with permission.

bronchiolitis, and the others had airflow obstruction of unknown cause, but thought to be due to bronchiolitis. Other studies have also identified a cryptogenic form of bronchiolar disease that produces airflow obstruction,[301,302] When biopsies have been performed, constrictive bronchiolitis seems to be the common pathologic manifestation. We may conclude that there exists a fairly distinct clinical syndrome consisting of mild airflow obstruction usually affecting middle-aged women who manifest non-specific respiratory symptoms such as cough and dyspnea. These cryptogenic cases of constrictive bronchiolitis may represent as yet undeclared systemic connective tissue disease or the sequelae of prior undetected infections (e.g. viral, mycoplasma, chlamydia).

RADIOLOGIC CLASSIFICATION OF SMALL AIRWAYS DISEASE

The following description of radiologic findings in the setting of airway disease has been proposed,[303] and each is presented here with corresponding pathologic considerations.

1. Nodules and branching lines: The CT changes are due to severe bronchiolar and peribronchiolar disease. Infectious bronchiolitis, diffuse panbronchiolitis, and bronchial diseases with distal bronchiolitis can produce these patterns.

2. Ground-glass attenuation (i.e. hazy increase in opacity without obscuring normal vessels) and consolidation (i.e. more marked density obscuring vessels): The CT changes are mainly due to alveolar filling. Organizing infections, COP, and respiratory bronchiolitis interstitial lung disease enter the differential diagnosis.

3. Low attenuation and mosaic perfusion: Partial airway obstruction typically leads to air trapping, best seen in expiratory scans. Mosaic perfusion is due to decreased vascular perfusion with bronchiolar obstruction and flow redistribution to normal areas. OB and constrictive bronchiolitis can produce this pattern.

4. Mixed: linear, nodular, ground-glass: These are due to combined alveolar and bronchiolar disease or fine nodules in the peribronchiolar interstitial space and parenchyma. Histopathologic causes include extrinsic allergic alveolitis, sarcoidosis, follicular bronchiolitis, pneumoconiosis, and giant cell interstitial pneumonia.

MORPHOLOGIC CLASSIFICATION OF DIFFUSE SMALL AIRWAYS DISEASE

The morphologic classification of bronchiolitis is presented in Table 17.19.

1. Cellular bronchiolitis (see Fig. 17.80) is a morphologic abnormality in which the bronchioles show an increased number of associated inflammatory cells only. These cells are usually chronic inflammatory cells (lymphocytes and plasma cells, hence the term *chronic cellular bronchiolitis*). Cellular bronchiolitis is seen commonly in smoking-induced bronchiolitis, bronchiolitis associated with immune disorders, certain collagen vascular diseases manifesting in the lung, viral bronchiolitis (notably that produced by respiratory syncytial virus), the specific condition known as diffuse panbronchiolitis, and the bronchiolitis of lung transplantation rejection.

2. Follicular bronchitis/bronchiolitis (Fig. 17.84): In a review of a large series of surgical lung biopsies, Yousem and coworkers identified a group of 19 that showed prominent lymphoid follicles, with coalescent germinal centers, adjacent to small bronchi and/or bronchioles, occurring in the absence of bronchiectasis or clinical airflow obstruction.[304] These authors identified three groups of patients: (1) seven with autoimmune disorders (six with RA and one with unclassifiable collagen-vascular disease); (2) four with immunodeficiency; and (3) eight with hypersensitivity reactions (seven of whom had peripheral eosinophilia). Thirteen patients were female and ages ranged from 1.5 to 77 years. The most common symptom was progressive breathlessness, occurring in 15 patients. Radiographically, bilateral reticular or nodular interstitial infiltrates were seen. In general, progressive disease was more common in younger patients and corticosteroid response was variable.

Kinane et al. identified follicular bronchiolitis in surgical lung biopsies from five young children.[305] Different from those reported by Yousem and coworkers, two of these patients had mild acute inflammation and occasional mucus plugs. All five patients had symptoms by 6 weeks of age, and these worsened until age 2. All improved by 4 years of age without significant effect of treatment. At present, this group should be regarded as a subset of follicular bronchitis/bronchiolitis arising in infancy and having a favorable outcome.

3. Constrictive (occlusive/obliterative) bronchiolitis (Fig. 17.85): This poorly defined morphologic entity has airway inflammation accompanied by bronchiolar luminal narrowing, typically as a result of subepithelial fibrosis. In some instances, cellular infiltration may be minimal, such as when the condition is related to mineral dust exposure. Myers and Colby[232] have used the term *constrictive bronchiolitis* synonymously with what has been referred to as

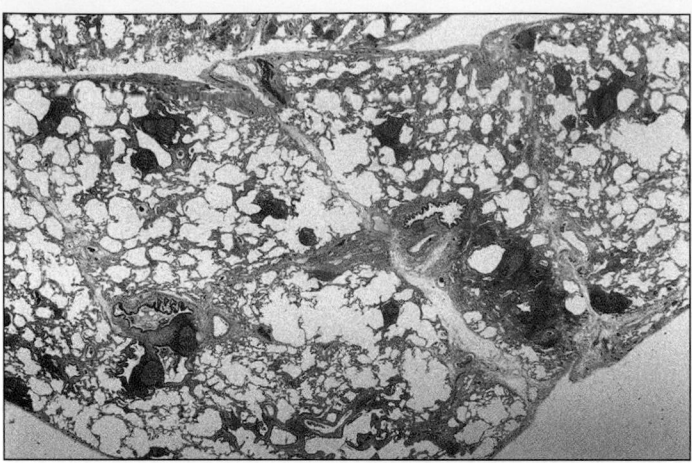

Fig. 17.84 Follicular bronchiolitis. Prominent lymphoid follicles with germinal centers occur adjacent to small bronchi and/or bronchioles.

occlusive bronchiolitis (OB). Constrictive bronchiolitis is most commonly found in smokers, where it tends to be mild. It also occurs in mineral dust bronchiolitis, lung transplant rejection, ulcerative colitis, neuroendocrine hyperplasia of the bronchioles (where fibrosis is associated with neuroendocrine hyperplasia of the small airways in non-smokers), and as an idiopathic form.

4. Bronchiolar loss (Fig. 17.86): Occlusion and destruction of bronchioles may occur, resulting in a reduction in the number of bronchioles visible in two-dimensional sections of peripheral lung. The loss is usually inferred or established by quantitative methods. The process is best documented in chronic bronchiectasis, in which bronchiolar loss is well described[306] and leads to air flow obstruction, parenchymal collapse, and bronchial dilation. Bronchiolar loss is also suspected to occur as an end result of constrictive bronchiolitis.

5. Foreign body bronchiolitis is the one form of bronchiolitis that is specific in appearance, given the presence of giant cells and recognizable foreign material within and around them. Foreign body bronchiolitis is discussed as an entity later in this chapter.

6. Small airways-associated fibrosis (Fig. 17.87) occurs relatively commonly in certain pneumoconioses and as a common relatively

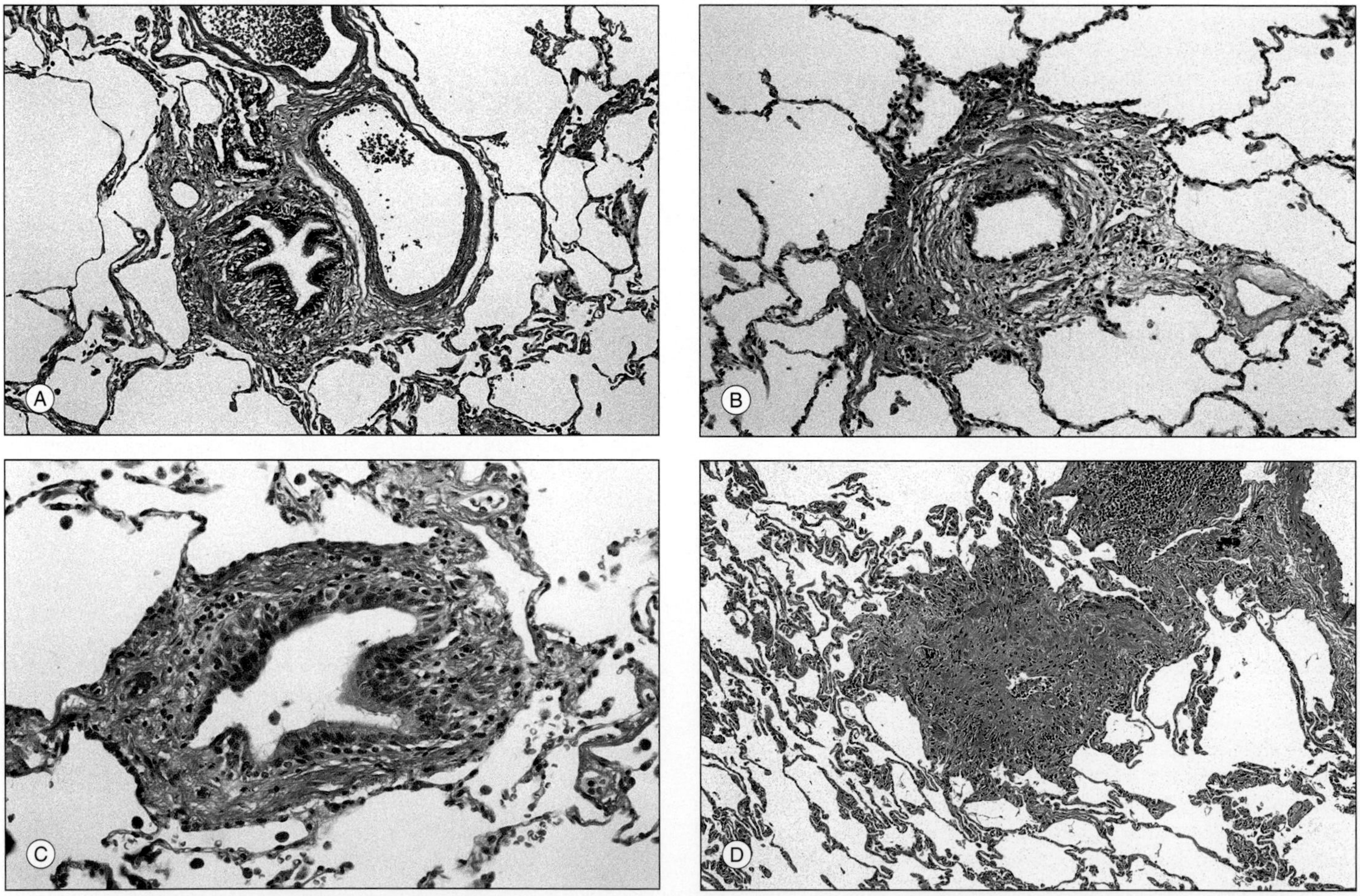

Fig. 17.85 Constrictive bronchiolitis and occlusive (obliterative) bronchiolitis. The morphologic entity in which airway inflammation (**A**) is accompanied by bronchiolar narrowing (**B**), typically due to subepithelial fibrosis (**C**), Collagen stained green, Gomori's one-step trichrome). In late stages there may be complete obliteration by concentric narrowing and fibrosis (**D**).

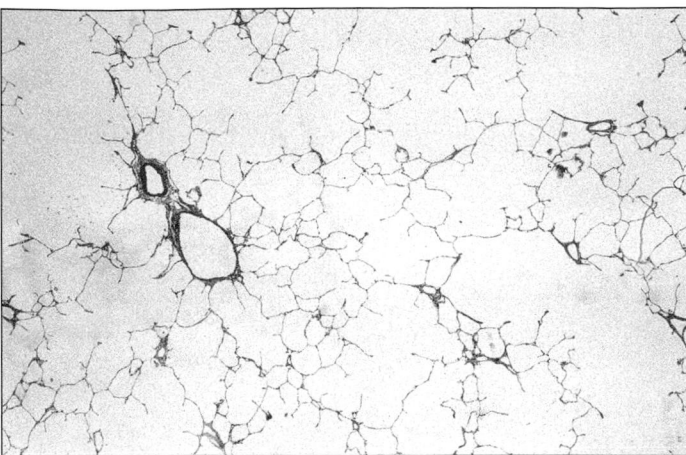

Fig. 17.86 Bronchiolar loss. The occlusion and destruction of bronchioles results in a dramatic decrease in the number of bronchioles visible at scanning magnification.

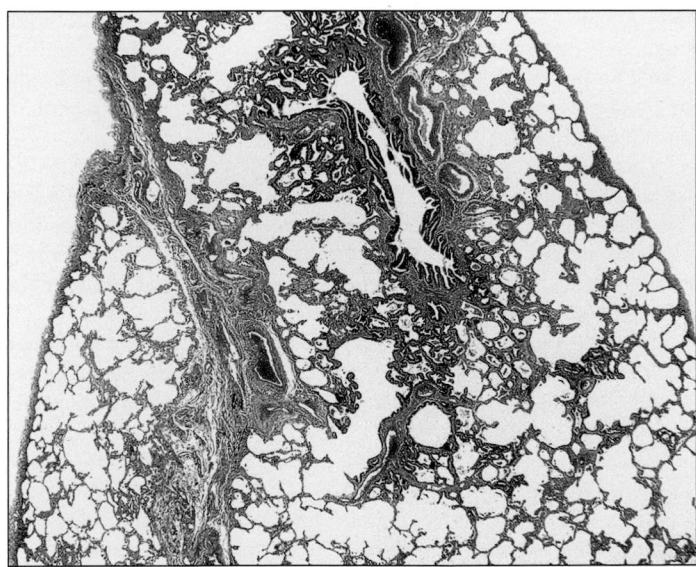

Fig. 17.87 Small airways-associated fibrosis. A recently described idiopathic form of fibrotic lung disease is distinguished by the presence of peribronchiolar fibrosis, and associated with an unusually poor prognosis. The disease seems to affect middle-aged women, similar to 'cryptogenic bronchiolitis.' Morphologically, fibrosis radiates from the centrilobular airways, accompanied by variable chronic inflammation.

asymptomatic pathologic manifestation observed in heavy smokers. An idiopathic form associated with an unusually poor outcome was first described by Yousem and Dacic in 2002[307] in 10 patients who presented with unexplained hypoxia, restrictive lung function studies, and increased interstitial markings radiologically. The disease affected middle aged women, similar to 'cryptogenic bronchiolitis' described earlier. Morphologically, fibrosis was seen to radiate from the centrilobular airways, accompanied by variable chronic inflammation. A similar airway-centered fibrosis was later described by Churg and coworkers.[308] The importance of these studies, regardless of the lack of defined causation, is that they underscore the potential for airway-associated fibrosis to credibly imitate fibrosing interstitial lung disease clinically and radiologically.

Table 17.20 Non-neoplastic disorders of the large airways

Asthma
Bronchitis
Infectious
Irritant (e.g. cigarettes, dust, aspiration)
Collagen vascular diseases (especially Sjögren's syndrome)
Miscellaneous (e.g. inflammatory bowel disease-related bronchitis, Wegener's granulomatosis)
Bronchiectasis
Bronchocentric granulomatosis
Mucoid impaction of bronchi
Allergic bronchopulmonary fungal disease
Plastic bronchitis
Tracheobronchomegaly
Congenital bronchial cartilage deficiency
Relapsing polychondritis
Broncholithiasis, bronchostenosis
Miscellaneous (e.g. tracheobronchial amyloid, tracheopathia osteochondroplastica)

Modified from Travis[408] with permission.

Diffuse large airway lesions

A list of the diseases that involve the large central airways is presented in Table 17.20. Chronic bronchitis and asthma are important common lung diseases that are diagnosed based on clinical parameters. These diseases may produce characteristic lesions on bronchial biopsy, and a subset of patients with asthma may develop peripheral airway disease with bronchiolitis. While the diagnosis of chronic bronchitis and/or asthma may be suggested by dense chronic inflammation beneath airway epithelium, bronchial gland hyperplasia and basement membrane thickening (Fig. 17.88), these diagnoses should not be made based on biopsy findings alone. It is beyond the scope of this chapter to discuss these clinical entities in detail and the interested reader is referred elsewhere.[309]

Similarly, the *ciliary dyskinesia syndrome* and *Kartagener's syndrome* are two central airway processes that may be diagnosed at biopsy, but the techniques involved and expertise required are highly specialized. Suffice it to say that inherited disorders of ciliary ultrastructure can result in chronic lung disease from chronic airway inflammation and or bronchiectasis.[310] When the general surgical pathologist is confronted with a mucosal biopsy for the evaluation of ciliary ultrastructure, it is advisable to refer the specimen to specialists familiar with the potential artifacts and normal variations that may be seen.[311]

DIFFUSE PULMONARY VASCULAR DISEASE

Few lung biopsy specimens create as much anxiety on the part of surgical pathologists then those performed for the evaluation of pulmonary hypertension (PHT). Historically, pulmonary hypertension has been conceptualized according to the anatomy of the pulmonary vascular system, with the alveolar capillary bed at the center. Thus

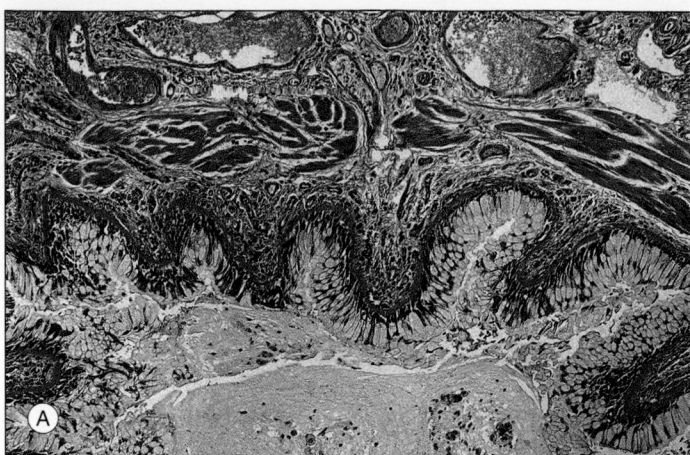
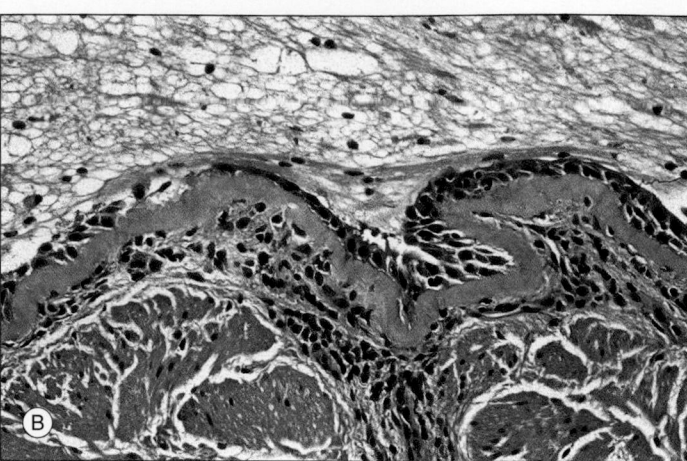

Fig. 17.88 Bronchitis/bronchiolitis in asthma. Asthma may be suggested by dense chronic inflammation beneath central airway epithelium, epithelial mucous cell hyperplasia, and bronchial gland hyperplasia (**A**). Basement membrane thickening is often striking (**B**).

precapillary hypertension is related to increased flow or increased resistance to flow, with a normal or nearly normal capillary bed; *capillary hypertension* is produced by destruction of alveoli or distortion of the alveolar capillary bed, such as occurs in emphysema or pulmonary fibrosis; and *postcapillary hypertension* resulting from veno-occlusive disease or venous outflow obstruction. The most recent WHO classification[312] proposes five categories of disease based on a combination of clinical, epidemiologic, and pathologic data (Table 17.21). Grading of PHT using historical schemes (see below) has not proven to be of prognostic value outside of the setting of congenital heart disease. Descriptive terms are recommended for observed arterial lesions in other settings of PHT (e.g. concentric intimal fibrosis).

PULMONARY ARTERIAL HYPERTENSION

Primary pulmonary hypertension (sporadic type)

Although the cause of primary pulmonary hypertension (plexogenic pulmonary arteriopathy) is by definition unknown, the disease has well-documented clinical features[313–315] and risk factors (Table 17.22). In individuals over the age of 12, there is a striking female predominance, whereas in those patients younger than 12, the sex incidence is roughly equal. Primary pulmonary hypertension is typically a disease of young adults, with a median age at death of 34 years.[316] Increased pulmonary arterial pressure with a normal wedge pressure is definitional.

Clinical findings: Clinical symptoms are inconsistent, but shortness of breath is characteristic. Hypoxia may be associated with anginal pain and signs of congestive heart failure. More dramatic, but less frequent, manifestations include hemoptysis, syncope, and palpitations. The electrocardiogram shows evidence of right ventricular hypertrophy.

Radiologic findings: Enlargement of the main pulmonary artery branches and decreased vascularity of the peripheral lung are typical findings.

Secondary pulmonary hypertension

Congenital heart disease

With the advent of cardiovascular surgery, much attention has been paid to the morphologic changes that occur in the pulmonary arterial tree of patients with congenital heart disease and sporadic adult pulmonary hypertension. Surgical wedge biopsy has been used to search for pathogenesis, for prognostic purposes,[317] and as a indicator of disease severity for determining the safety of surgical correction of anomalous flow.[318]

The Heath-Edwards[319] classification described six grades of disease based on structural changes in the pulmonary arteries. Over the years, the proposed grading *sequence* has come into question. Here we present the grading system as described by Wagenvoort[318] as a more accurate reflection of disease severity, at least in the setting of congenital heart disease.

Grade I: Muscular hypertrophy: Muscular arteries have thickened walls. The smooth muscle may appear hypereosinophilic, standing out at scanning magnification. Luminal narrowing is typically present and may be prominent. (Fig. 17.89).

Grade II: Intimal proliferation: subintimal proliferation and thickened media. (Fig. 17.90).

Grade III: Concentric intimal fibrosis: Concentric bands of collagen and spindle-shaped cells form in the subintimal space. Dramatic luminal narrowing is characteristically present (Fig. 17.91).

Grade IV: Necrotizing vasculitis: Increased pressure results in fibrinoid necrosis of the arterial wall (Fig. 17.92). Destruction of elastic laminae can be highlighted with special stains.

Grade V: Plexiform lesions: are identified at branch points of the small muscular arteries and may be sparse. Plexiform lesions resemble cellular granulation tissue or recanalizing thrombus (Fig. 17.93). Destruction of elastic lamina helps distinguish primary plexogenic lesions from similar appearing post-thrombotic lesions, where the elastica is typically preserved.

Grade VI: Dilatation and angiomatoid lesions: Thin-walled, dilated arterial lesions appear. When tortuous, these are referred to as *angiomatoid lesions* (Fig. 17.94). A single elastic lamina is present.

In the evaluation of pulmonary hypertension in the setting of congenital heart disease, reversible findings include medial hypertrophy, cellular intimal proliferation, and the early stages of concentric laminar intimal fibrosis. Severe intimal fibrosis does not reverse, and the presence of dilation lesions and/or fibrinoid necrosis are ominous findings.[320,321]

Table 17.21 WHO nomenclature and classification of pulmonary hypertension

Pulmonary arterial hypertension
Primary pulmonary hypertension
  Sporadic
  Familial
Related to:
  Collagen vascular disease
  Congenital systemic to pulmonary shunts
  Portal hypertension
  Human immunodeficiency virus (HIV) infection
  Drugs/toxins
    Anorexigens
    Other
  Persistent pulmonary hypertension of the newborn
  Other

Pulmonary venous hypertension
Left-sided atrial or ventricular heart disease
Left-sided valvular heart disease
Extrinsic compression of central pulmonary veins
  Fibrosing mediastinitis
  Adenopathy/tumors
Pulmonary veno-occlusive disease
Other

Pulmonary hypertension associated with disorders of the respiratory system and/or hypoxemia
Chronic obstructive pulmonary disease
Interstitial lung disease
Sleep disordered breathing
Alveolar hypoventilation disorders
Chronic exposure to high altitude
Neonatal lung disease
Alveolar-capillary dysplasia
Other

Pulmonary hypertension due to chronic thrombotic and/or embolic disease
Thromboembolic obstruction of proximal pulmonary arteries
Obstruction of distal pulmonary arteries
  Pulmonary embolism (thrombus, tumor, ova and/or parasites, foreign material)
  In situ thrombosis
  Sickle cell disease

Pulmonary hypertension due to disorders directly affecting the pulmonary vasculature
Inflammatory
  Schistosomiasis
  Sarcoidosis
  Other
Pulmonary capillary hemangiomatosis

From Travis[408] with permission.

Table 17.22 Risk factors for primary pulmonary hypertension

Drugs and toxins
Definite: aminorex, fenfluramine, dexfenfluramine, toxic rape seed oil
Very likely: amphetamines, L-tryptophan
Possible: meta-amphetamines, cocaine, chemotherapeutic agents
Unlikely: antidepressants, oral contraceptives, estrogen therapy, cigarette smoking

Demographics and medical conditions
Definite: gender
Possible: pregnancy, systemic hypertension
Unlikely: obesity

Diseases
Definite: HIV infection
Very likely: portal hypertension/liver disease, collagen vascular diseases, congenital systemic pulmonary cardiac shunts
Possible: thyroid disorders

From Travis[408] with permission.

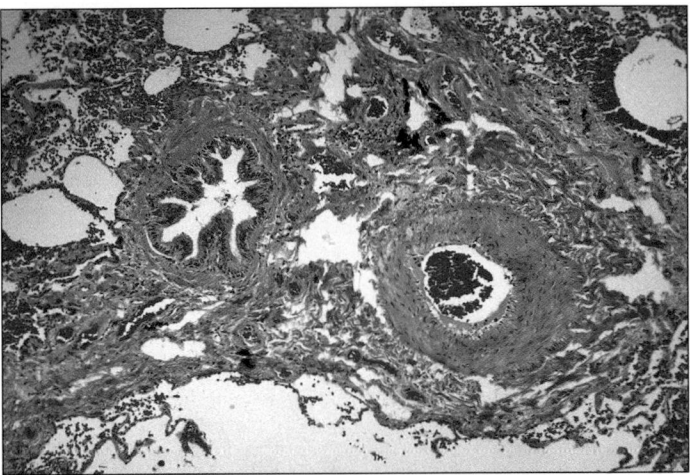

Fig. 17.89 Pulmonary hypertension, Grade I. Muscular hypertrophy: muscular arteries have thickened walls. Luminal narrowing is typically present and may be prominent.

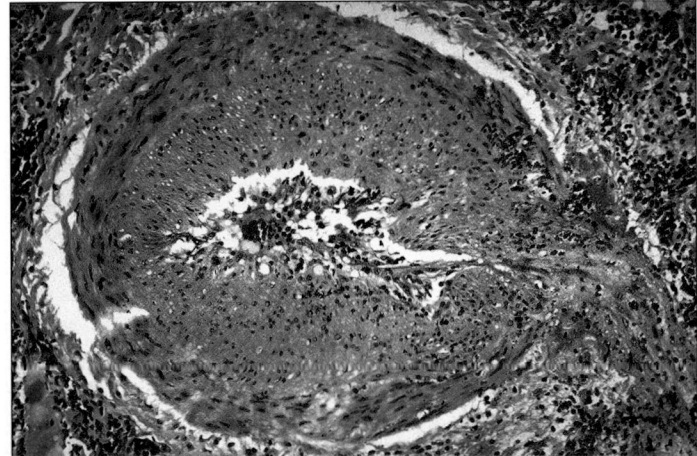

Fig. 17.90 Pulmonary hypertension, Grade II. Intimal proliferation: subintimal proliferation is combined with a thickened arterial media.

Other causes

In a study of 156 patients with the diagnosis of primary pulmonary hypertension, Wagenvoort and Wagenvoort[321] were able to exclude 46 cases on the basis of other histologically recognizable diseases. For example, a number of drugs, including Aminorex,[322] Crotalaria,[323] and fenfluramine/phentermine,[324] have been identified as causing pulmonary hypertension, either epidemiologically or by experi-

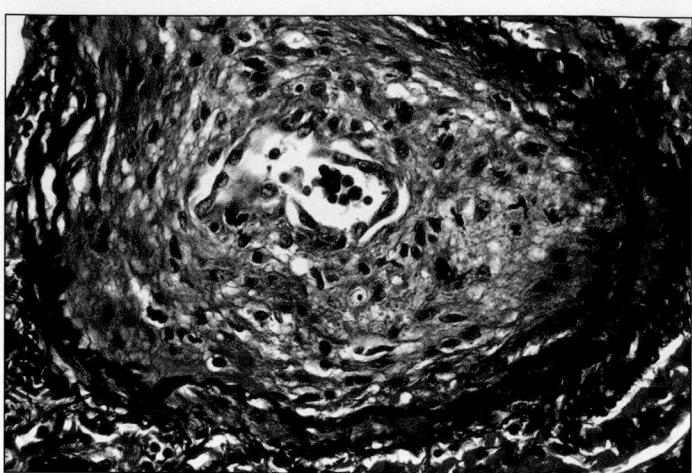

Fig. 17.91 Pulmonary hypertension, Grade III. Concentric intimal fibrosis: concentric bands of collagen and spindle-shaped cells form in the subintimal space. Dramatic luminal narrowing is characteristically present.

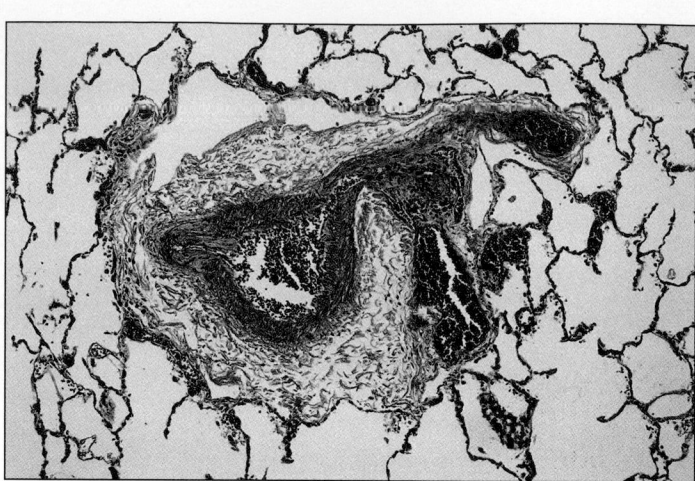

Fig. 17.93 Pulmonary hypertension, Grade V. Plexiform lesions: are identified at branch points of the small muscular arteries and may be sparse. Plexiform lesions resemble cellular granulation tissue or recanalizing thrombus.

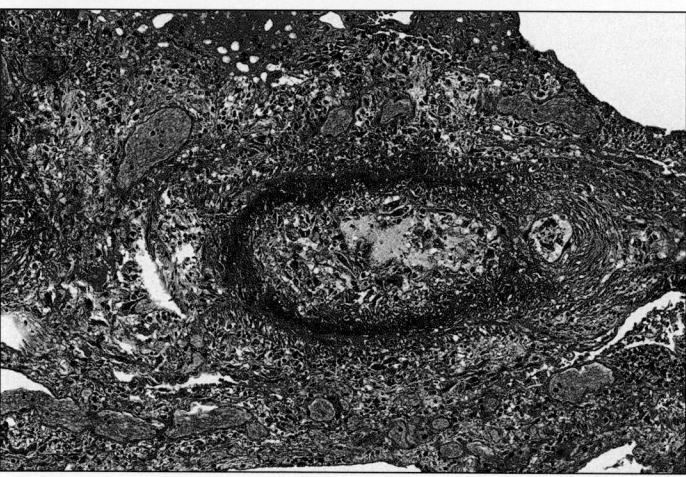

Fig. 17.92 Pulmonary hypertension, Grade IV. Necrotizing vasculitis: increased pressure results in fibrinoid necrosis of the arterial wall.

mental studies. HIV infection has been recently implicated in secondary plexogenic arteriopathy.[325,326] The disease may manifest as long as 3 years after infection and tends to be fatal. A pathogentic role for human herpesvirus type 8 (HHV-8) has also been suggested.[327,328]

PULMONARY VENOUS HYPERTENSION

Left sided heart disease or extrinsic compression

Venous hypertension typically is a result of chronic cardiac disease, especially left ventricular failure and mitral valve disease. Nevertheless, any chronic cause of restriction to venous outflow from the lung can potentially result in so-called 'congestive vasculopathy' seen in lung specimens.[318,320,329,330]

Clinical features: A number of clinical scenarios must be considered in the context of venous hypertension. Beyond cardiac

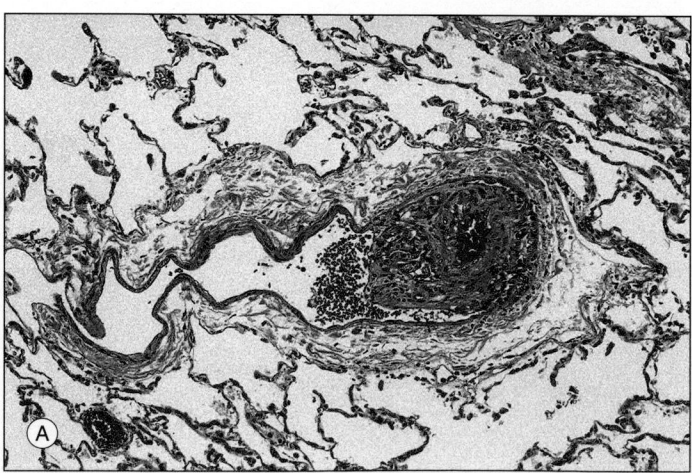

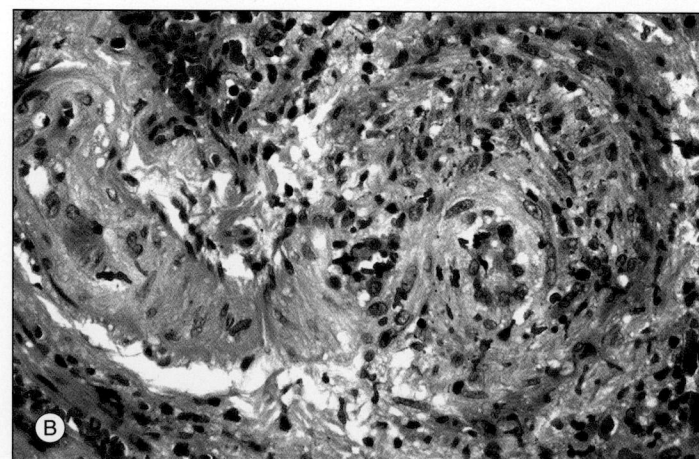

Fig. 17.94 Pulmonary hypertension, Grade VI. Dilatation and angiomatoid lesions: thin-walled, dilated arterial lesions appear (**A**). When tortuous these are referred to as *angiomatoid lesions* (**B**). A single elastic lamina is present.

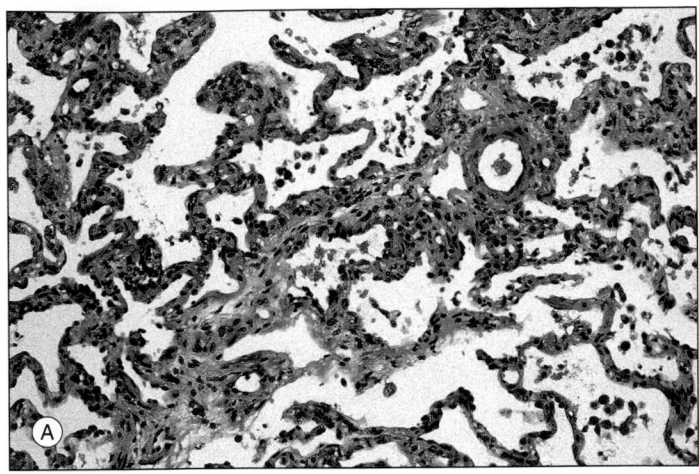
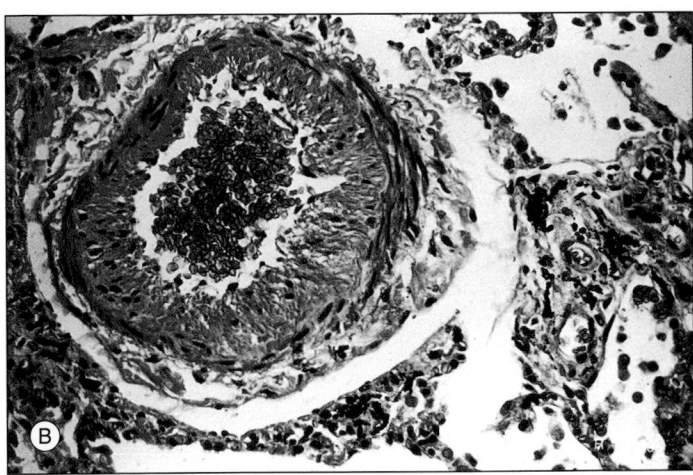

Fig. 17.95 Chronic passive congestion (CPC). At scanning magnification, diffuse alveolar congestion, variable hemosiderosis (sometimes striking) and fibrosis (**A**). Metaplastic bone and venous infarcts may be present in CPC. Arterial and venous abnormalities are a constant finding, more prominently evident in veins that become muscularized (**B**).

etiologies, congestive pulmonary vasculopathy can be a result of extrinsic compression of the mediastinal or perihilar pulmonary veins (e.g. sclerosing mediastinitis, adenopathy). Pulmonary veno-occlusive disease (see below) is also an etiology for the observed vascular changes.

Radiologic findings: Blood flow redistribution to the upper lobes results in enlargement of these, making them appear of similar diameter to the lower lobe vessels (these are typically larger than their upper lobe counterparts). Pulmonary edema and cardiomegaly may be evident.

Pathologic findings: The lung biopsy in this setting can be confusing, with fibrosis, hemosiderosis, and capillary congestion (Fig. 17.95). This latter feature causes the interstitium of the alveolar walls to appear cellular, sometimes simulating interstitial inflammation or veno-occlusive disease (see below). The pulmonary arteries show intimal fibrosis that is often eccentric, and this can be especially prominent in the elastic arteries. Veins become muscularized and also show eccentric intimal fibrosis. The concentric intimal fibrosis of primary pulmonary hypertension is not seen. When the disease is bilateral in the lung the clinical diagnosis is usually made without biopsy. On occasion a lung lobe may suffer extrinsic venous outflow obstruction related to a hilar or mediastinal mass (such as sclerosing mediastinitis or lymphoma). In this setting the radiologic images may suggest an 'interstitial' lung disease, chronic infection, or even a parenchymal tumor. These lung manifestations may require a surgical biopsy for resolution.

Pulmonary veno-occlusive disease

Pulmonary veno-occlusive disease (PVOD) accounts for 10–15% of unexplained pulmonary hypertension cases according to retrospective[313] and prospective studies.[314] The disease typically affects young individuals with an average age of 30 years, but the reported age spectrum ranges from birth to old age. Males are more commonly affected than females, and symptoms often begin with an influenza-like illness.[331]

Clinical features: The clinical presentation is very similar to that of primary pulmonary hypertension, with progressive shortness of breath with evidence of pulmonary hypertension and, finally, cor pulmonale.

Radiologic findings: The lung parenchyma is abnormal, with evidence of chronic passive congestion, typified by the presence of edematous interlobular septa (Kerley B lines). The venous pressure as measured by pulmonary wedge pressure is typically normal.

Pathologic findings: Microscopic examination reveals alveolar walls thickened by increased cellularity with associated pulmonary hemosiderosis. Sometimes the disease is attended by considerable interstitial fibrosis (Fig. 17.96A). Closer inspection reveals the alveolar walls to be thickened by congested alveolar capillaries (Fig. 17.96B). PVOD is often strikingly focal in the surgical lung biopsy (Fig. 17.97), likely corresponding to a lobular distribution. Distinctive granulomas may be present, the giant cells of which contain fragmented elastic fibers encrusted with iron (Fig. 17.98) and calcium (so-called 'endogenous pneumoconiosis'). The small pulmonary veins show varying degrees of intimal proliferation, partial recanalization, eccentric proliferation, and sometimes complete occlusion (Fig. 17.99). The lesions appear inactive in most cases. As indicated, venous changes may not be very obvious, especially in H&E-stained sections. Fibrous occlusion of pulmonary arteries may be seen in about half the cases,[332] because the patients typically have severe secondary pulmonary arterial hypertension.[333] The condition should always be suspected when a biopsy specimen shows hemosiderosis in addition to pulmonary fibrosis and/or evidence of pulmonary arterial hypertension. In order to examine the pulmonary veins specifically, the easiest way to identify them is to scan the pleura of the biopsy until an interlobular septum is identified. The veins can be most easily seen within these structures.

It is more than likely that there are multiple causes of veno-occlusive disease;[334] however, most cases are idiopathic. The disease may occur as a complication of other conditions such as bone marrow transplantation,[335] where it likely results as a toxic complication of myeloablative drugs such as carmustine, etoposide and others.

DISORDERS OF THE RESPIRATORY SYSTEM AND/OR HYPOXEMIA (COPD, INTERSTITIAL DISEASES, SLEEP DISORDERED BREATHING, OTHERS)

Disorders of the respiratory system are the most frequent cause of pulmonary hypertension but disease is typically unrecognized until

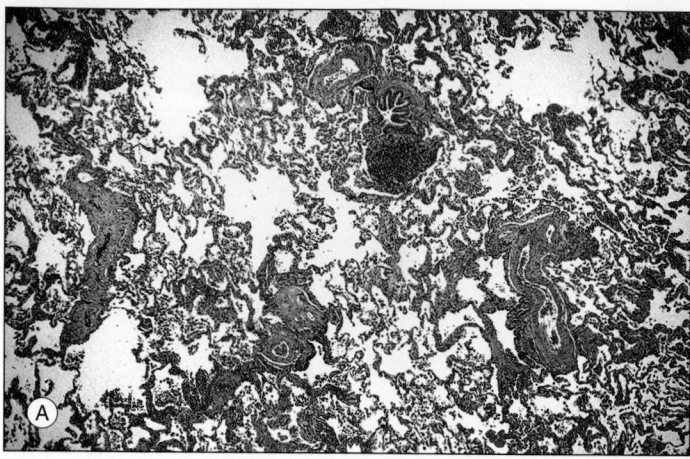
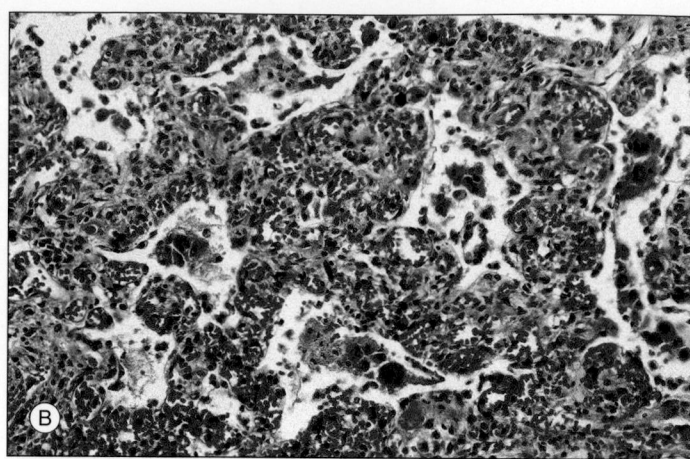

Fig. 17.96 Pulmonary veno-occlusive disease (PVOD). Scanning magnification suggests interstitial fibrosis with alveolar septal widening (**A**) and interlobular thickening. Closer inspection reveals markedly dilated (and seemingly redundant) capillaries in the alveolar walls and hemosiderin-laden macrophages in airspaces (**B**).

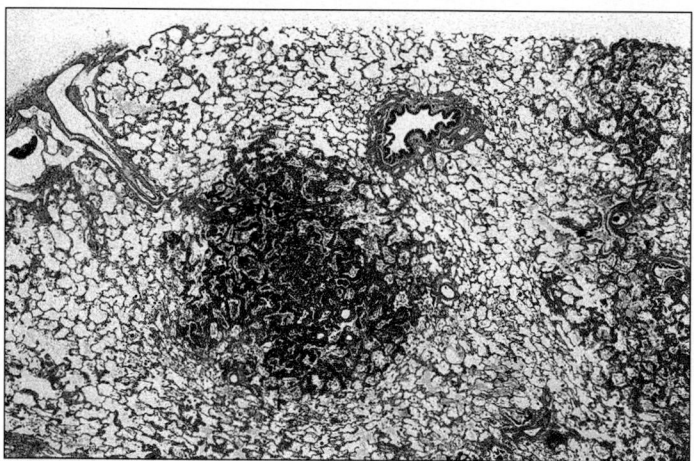
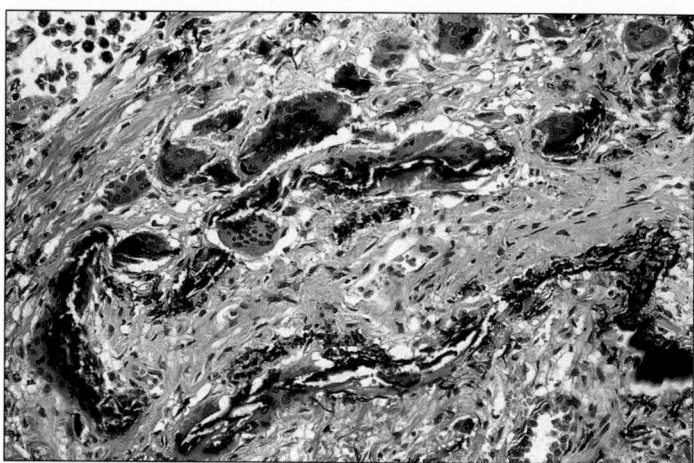

Fig. 17.97 Pulmonary veno-occlusive disease (PVOD). PVOD can be very focal in the surgical lung biopsy, possibly reflecting selective lobular venous injury.

Fig. 17.98 Pulmonary veno-occlusive disease (PVOD). Iron incrustation of the elastica of pulmonary veins may be prominent (Prussian blue iron stain, red counterstain).

late in the particular disease in question (e.g. COPD). Arterial hypertension is generally mild in most instances and mainly small arteries are affected (and easily overlooked).

CHRONIC THROMBOTIC OR EMBOLIC DISEASE

Blockage of pulmonary blood flow at the precapillary level results in increased pulmonary artery pressure. This phenomenon can be the result of any form of embolization, but most often is the result of multiple recurrent pulmonary thrombotic emboli. The clinical presentation depends on a number of factors including the size, number, and location of the emboli; the time interval between embolic episodes; whether vascular occlusion is complete or partial; and whether cardiopulmonary disease is present or absent. The possibility of unrecognized pulmonary emboli producing the hypertension has been a consistent problem, especially so because

thrombi are often seen in the vessels in both primary and secondary forms of plexogenic arteriopathy. Recent evidence suggests that the differentiation can be made at lung biopsy.[320] In primary pulmonary hypertension, there seems to be a decrease in the number of arteries that measure less than 40 μm in diameter, whereas this does not occur in the setting of recurrent pulmonary thromboemboli. In both primary and secondary forms, there is thickening of the media of the pulmonary arteries, but in primary pulmonary hypertension there is no neomuscularization of nonmuscular arteries. Some authors believe that the occurrence of *concentric* laminar intimal fibrosis is specific for primary pulmonary hypertension.[334] *Eccentric* intimal fibrosis is not specific for multiple recurrent pulmonary emboli; however, the presence of organizing thromboemboli (in the context of an intact vascular elastica) are highly suggestive (Fig. 17.100A), and intravascular fibrous septal 'webs' are diagnostic (Fig. 17.100B).

Clinical features: Symptoms range from absent to severe and include cardiac arrhythmias, hypotension, and sudden death. Pul-

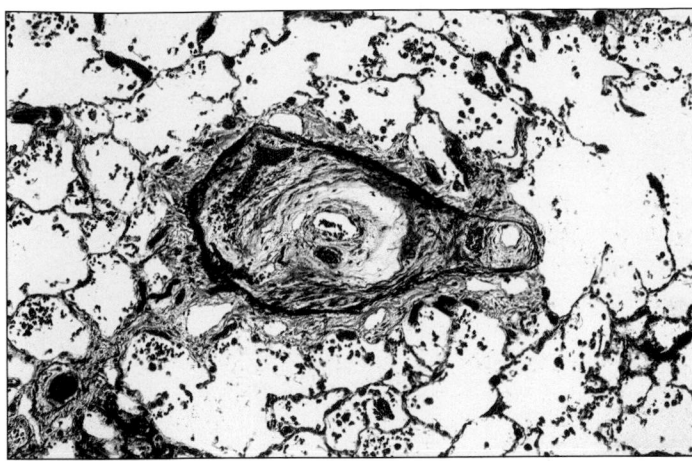

Fig. 17.99 Pulmonary veno-occlusive disease (PVOD). The diagnostic feature is sclerosis and variable occlusion of pulmonary veins (elastic van Gieson's stain, green counterstain).

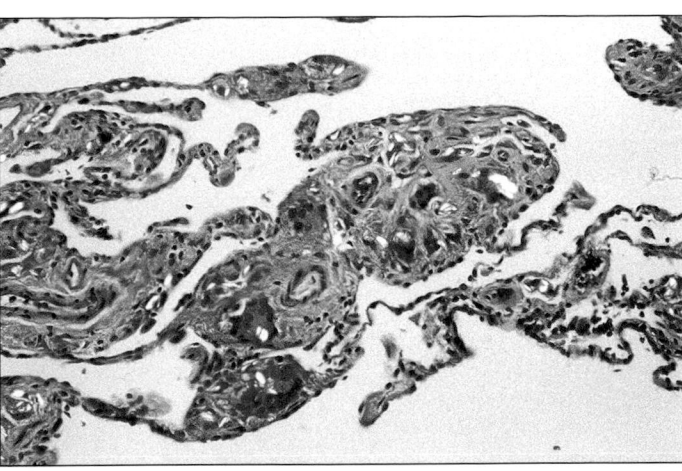

Fig. 17.101 Embolic vascular disease from i.v. drug abuse. Intravenous talcosis produces distinctive arterial lesions with birefringent particles in vessel-associated giant cells (H&E stain, polarized light microscopy).

monary hypertension is not sustained until 50–70% of the pulmonary vascular bed is damaged.

Radiologic findings: Patients have mid-zonal, well-defined, small (2–3 mm) nodules that coalesce to form larger nodules. The radiologic appearance may mimic sarcoidosis or the progressive massive fibrosis of silicosis. HRCT demonstrates a fine granular pattern or multiple small nodules. When the nodules coalesce, high attenuation material can be seen that is consistent with talc.[336]

Pathologic findings: Muscular arteries are more commonly obstructed than elastic ones. Although present throughout the lung, the lesions are focal and typically vary in age.[337] It is not unusual to find coexistent early thrombi, organized and recanalized vessels, and fibrous bands and intimal plaques, marking the sites of embolic episodes.

A variety of other materials may lodge by embolism in the pulmonary arteries, including fat, brain tissue, and amniotic fluid.

In most instances, such findings are of less importance to the surgical pathologist then is talc embolization. Talc embolization has been discussed earlier in relation to foreign body bronchiolitis. The talc is centered on vessels in intravenous drug abusers and on bronchioles in inhalational exposure. Talc penetrates through the walls of vessels in the case of intravenous injection and penetrates the walls of bronchioles in the case of inhalational exposure (Fig. 17.101). Regardless of exposure route however, talc particles eventually reach the interstitium. As pointed out in the section on foreign body bronchiolitis, the talc particles are of different size in the two conditions – in intravenous drug users the particles are longer than the typically 2.5–5 μm particles seen in cocaine sniffers. The eventual consequences of talc embolization include pulmonary fibrosis, emphysema, and pulmonary hypertension.

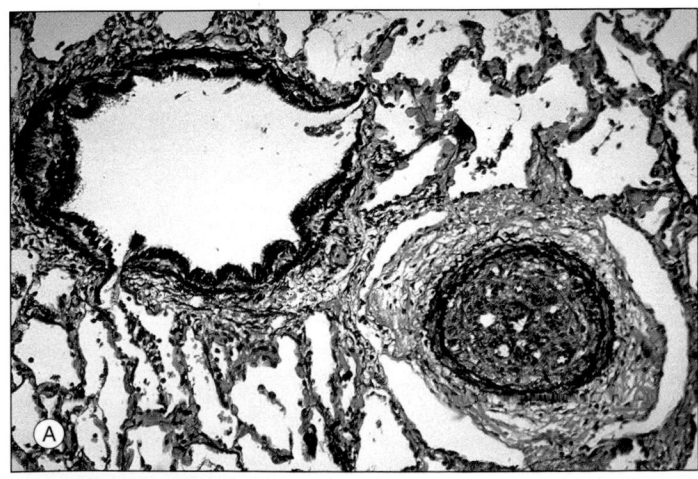

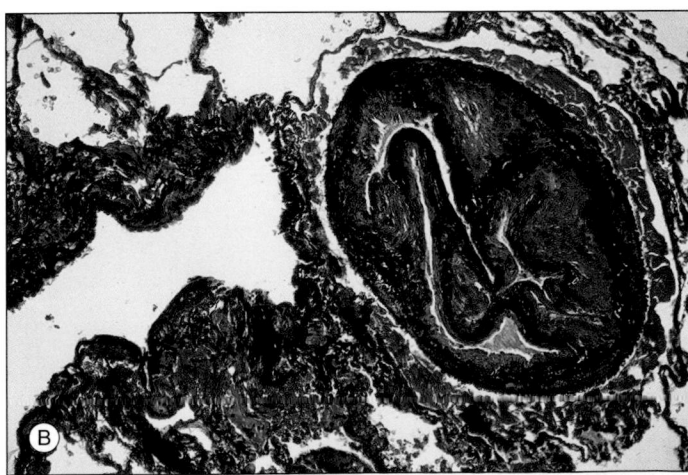

Fig. 17.100 Chronic thromboembolic pulmonary hypertension. When thromboemboli lodge in small arteries, they are eventually recanalized (**A**, note the intact elastic lamina. Elastic van Gieson's stain, red counterstain) and later may become web-like septations crossing the vessel lumen (**B**, Elastic van Gieson's stain, red counterstain). These latter findings are virtually diagnostic of thromboembolic-type pulmonary hypertension.

DISORDERS DIRECTLY AFFECTING THE PULMONARY VASCULATURE

Pulmonary capillary hemangiomatosis

Pulmonary capillary hemangiomatosis (PCH) is a rare and perhaps related condition to PVOD. The disease can be suspected clinically, may be diagnosed pathologically, and is amenable to treatment. Wagenvoort et al. reported the first case of capillary hemangiomatosis in 1978,[338] and a significant number of cases have been described since that time.[339,340]

Clinical features: The average age at presentation is 28 years, with a range of 12 to 71 years.[339] Patients present with unexplained pulmonary hypertension, typically with evidence of intrapulmonary bleeding and hemoptysis.

Radiologic findings: Evidence of intra-alveolar bleeding is suggested by scattered airspace opacities. Diffusely distended lymphatics are seen, indicating severe pulmonary venous hypertension. Pulmonary veno-occlusive disease is typically in the clinical differential diagnosis.

Pathologic findings: Gross examination reveals punctate miliary nodules throughout the lung.[340] Surgical lung biopsy specimens may show subpleural hemorrhagic nodules.[339] Microscopically, there is histologic evidence of pulmonary arterial hypertension, although the advanced hypertensive lesions are not typically seen. Signs of recent and/or old intra-alveolar hemorrhage (siderophages) typically raise concern pathologically for congestive arteriopathy of cardiac origin or a pulmonary hemorrhage syndrome with vasculitis/capillaritis. Prominent venous changes may be seen with intimal fibrosis and 'arterialization.' The most recognizable lesion of PCH is an intense proliferation of capillary-like structures (Fig. 17.102) involving all parts of the lung interstitium. Involvement of veins is thought to produce the most serious consequence with venous obstruction and intrapulmonary bleeding. The abnormal new vessels are thin-walled and seem to infiltrate the structures they involve, sometimes raising concern for a vasoproliferative neoplasm. The histologic differential diagnosis, when alveolar wall capillaries are prominent, includes pulmonary veno-occlusive disease, Kaposi's sarcoma, and pulmonary hemangiomatosis or lymphangiomatosis of children.

Table 17.23 Complications of lung transplantation

Cellular rejection	Occlusive bronchiolitis
Infection	Foreign body bronchiolitis
Cellular (rejection) bronchiolitis	Chronic graft rejection
Acute bronchitis/bronchiolitis	Lymphoproliferative disorders
Eosinophilic bronchiolitis	Recurrence of original disease
Lymphocytic bronchitis/bronchiolitis	New tumors
Organizing pneumonia	

The nature of PCH is unknown. Death occurs within 1 to 4 years of the onset of symptoms in most cases. It is possible that venous hypertension is the true cause of PCH, and therefore this could qualify PCH as a condition related to PVOD. The treatment of PCH is lung or heart-lung transplantation. Administration of interferon-alpha-2a has been effective in some cases.[341]

PATHOLOGY OF LUNG TRANSPLANTATION

Lung transplantation became a viable therapeutic option for patients with end-stage lung disease in the last decade of the twentieth century. A wide variety of lung diseases have been treated using heart-lung, single lung, and bilateral lung transplantation, with reasonable overall success. US survival data for 1999 show a 1-year survival rate for heart-lung transplantation of 59% and single/double lung transplants of 77%.[342] Furthermore, the 5-year reported survival rates for transplantation that occurred during 1995 were 56% for heart lung and 44% for single/double lung transplants. Complications associated with lung transplantation (Table 17.23) pose significant diagnostic challenges for the surgical pathologist, and these include infection, rejection, chronic airway diseases, post-transplant lymphoproliferative disorders, and recurrence of pretransplant disease.

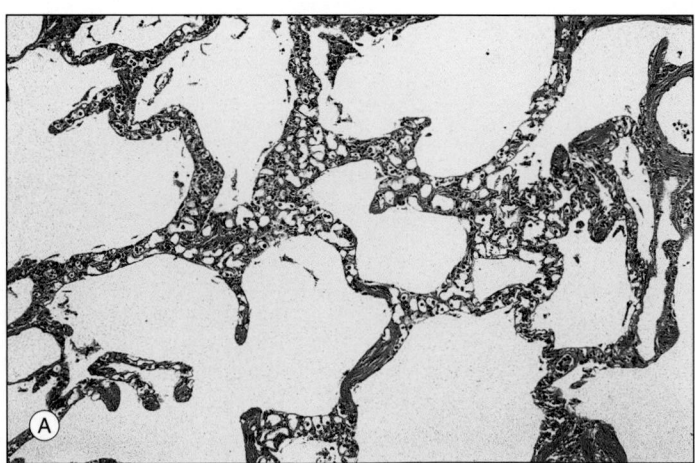
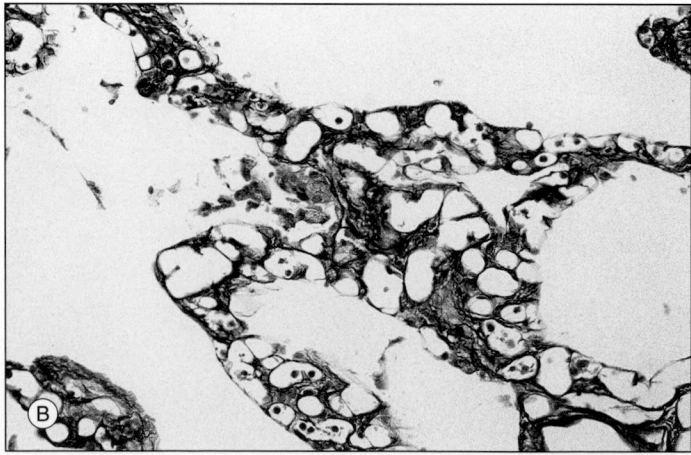

Fig. 17.102 Pulmonary capillary hemangiomatosis. An intense proliferation of capillary-like structures involves all parts of the lung interstitium (**A**), including the interlobular septa, the walls of arteries, veins, and lymphatics, and even nerves. A reticulin silver stain (**B**) helps outline the redundant capillary channels (reticulin silver stain, red counterstain).

COMPLICATIONS OF TRANSPLANTATION

Reperfusion injury (reimplantation response): occurs immediately after surgical implantation and results from ischemic capillary injury. When severe, reperfusion injury resembles diffuse alveolar damage (DAD).

Allograft rejection

Acute cellular rejection occurs in nearly every lung transplant recipient, typically within the first month postoperatively.[343] The radiographic findings are non-specific and may be mimicked by infection, especially by CMV, and after the first month the chest radiograph may be normal in the face of biopsy-proven rejection.[344] The use of newer immunosuppressive strategies has reduced the frequency of acute rejection and substantially lowered the histologic rejection grade during the first 30 days post-transplant.[345]

In transbronchial lung biopsy specimens, acute cellular rejection is characterized by the presence of perivascular lymphocytes, plasma cells, and activated mononuclear cells (Fig. 17.103). Venules are typically involved, but arterioles may also be affected. With increasing severity, these cells increase in number and extend beyond the peribronchiolar adventitia to involve adjacent alveolar walls.[346] A formal grading system (Table 17.24) was originally proposed by the Working Formulation for Lung Rejection Study Group in 1990.[347] Lesions are assessed by the severity and nature of the perivascular infiltrates from 0 (normal) to 4 (severe). At each numerical level, a suffix (a to d) is assigned to indicate the nature of involvement of airways that may or may not accompany the perivascular infiltrates in all stages of rejection.

Grading rejection

Grade 1 (minimal acute rejection): There are infrequent, and minimally cellular, perivascular infiltrates not obvious at scanning magnification. Venules are surrounded by a cuff of small round lymphocytes, plasmacytoid lymphocytes, and transformed lymphocytes, typically two to three cells in thickness.

Grade 2 (mild acute rejection): There are larger perivascular infiltrates readily visible at scanning magnification. The cellular composition resembles that of grade 1, but occasional eosinophils are typically present. Subendothelial accumulation of lymphoid cells attended by endothelial reactive changes ('endothelialitis') is seen in this grade.

Grade 3 (moderate acute rejection): Perivascular infiltrates of mononuclear cells, eosinophils, and neutrophils are common and densely cellular. Infiltrates extend to involve adjacent alveolar walls or spaces. Larger activated lymphoid cells are typically present.

Grade 4 (severe acute rejection): Beyond those findings listed for grade 3, there is also evidence of alveolar epithelial degeneration, often associated with cellular necrosis, macrophages, hyaline membranes, and neutrophils. More severe cytotoxic injury may be evident as parenchymal necrosis, infarction, or a necrotizing vasculitis.

Bronchi and bronchioles are also involved in rejection and show a progression from perivascular lymphocyte cuffing to extensive lymphoid infiltrates, referred to as lymphocytic bronchitis/bronchiolitis (LBB).[348] These mural changes are followed by epithelial injury, with ulceration, neutrophilic infiltration, and finally ulceration.

Chronic injury to the small airways with consequent life-threatening obstructive ventilatory defect is the most significant long-term complication of both heart-lung and lung transplantation.[349] Pathologic findings of constrictive and obliterative bronchiolitis (OB), referred to clinically as *bronchiolitis obliterans syndrome (BOS),* are the hallmarks of this chronic ventilatory defect and

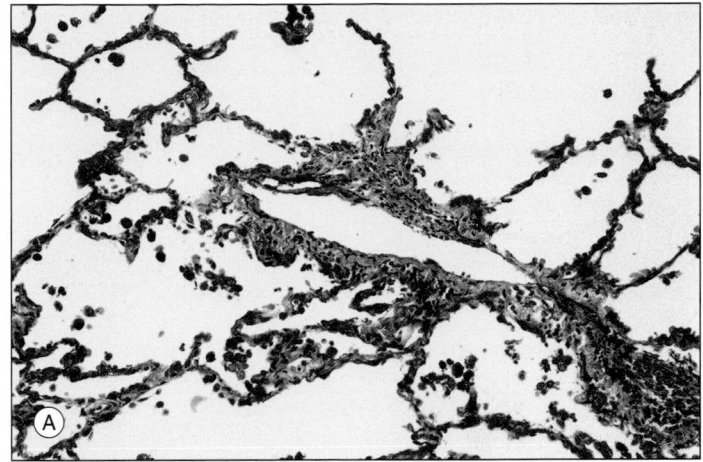

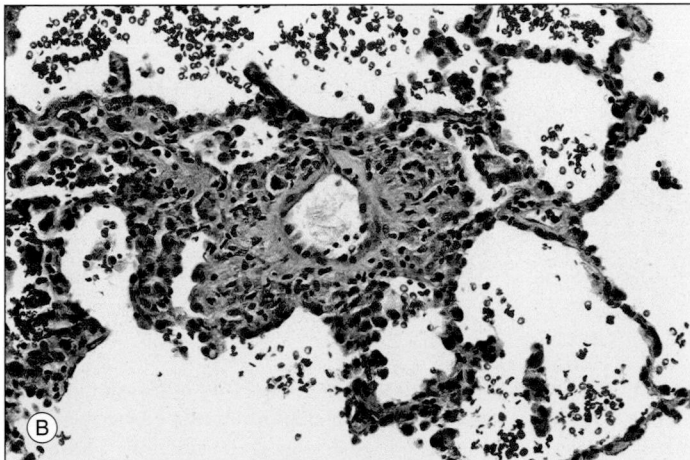

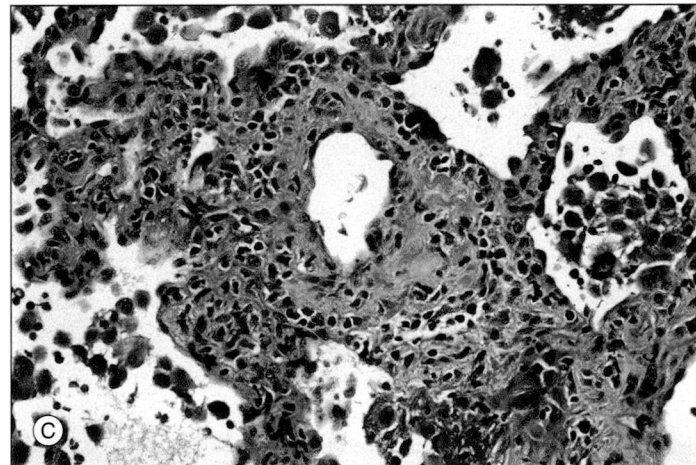

Fig. 17.103 Lung transplant rejection. Acute cellular rejection is characterized by the presence of perivascular lymphocytes, plasma cells, and activated mononuclear cells. The infiltrates begin eccentrically (**A**, mild rejection) and progress with the severity of the grade (**B**, moderate rejection). Severe rejection is characterized by the development of endothelialitis and vascular necrosis (**C**, severe rejection), coupled with extension of the mononuclear infiltrate to involve adjacent alveolar walls.

Table 17.24 Grading scheme for lung allograft rejection[409]

Acute cellular rejection
Grade A-0 – No evidence for rejection
Grade A-1 – Minimal rejection
Grade A-2 – Mild rejection
Grade A-3 – Moderate rejection
Grade A-4 – Severe rejection
Associated airway inflammation
Grade B-0 – No airway inflammation
Grade B-1 – Rare lymphocytes in subepithelial region
Grade B-2 – Circumferential band of subepithelial lymphocytes – no epithelial inflammation or necrosis
Grade B-3 – Circumferential band of subepithelial lymphocytes – with epithelial inflammation or necrosis
Grade B-4 – Circumferential band of subepithelial lymphocytes – with epithelial inflammation *and* ulceration *and* necrosis
Grade B-X – Not gradable
Chronic airway rejection
Grade C-a (active) – Fibrosis with mononuclear cell infiltrates
Grade C-b (inactive) – Fibrosis with minimal inflammation
Chronic vascular rejection (graft vasculopathy)
Grade D

Adapted from Travis[408] with permission.

appear to be related to organ rejection.[349] Other inflammatory airway conditions arise in lung transplantation as a consequence of infection or as comorbid of rejection and infection. These are presented below in the context of their current terminology and potential etiology.

Sampling by transbronchial biopsy

As in all sampling techniques, the likelihood of achieving a successful result in the biopsy assessment of rejection depends on a number of variables, such as the known general distribution of the disease process in the lung, the probability of acquiring a diagnostic finding via the airway, and the quality of the sample. For example, Scott and coworkers calculated that 18 biopsy specimens were required to provide a high confidence of diagnosing rejection (95%).[350] While there is no specific requirement regarding the number of specimens that must be obtained, the Lung Rejection Study Group[347] recommended a minimum of five, with a minimum of three section levels on each slide. Trichrome, elastic tissue, and silver stains for organisms are best performed as a routine (similar to the proscribed approach to renal or liver biopsy specimens obtained for assessment of non-neoplastic disorders). If these and other special stains are to be ordered on an as-needed basis, unstained sections should be made during the first sectioning of the biopsy block(s) to avoid losing tissue during repeated block refacing each time a new 'staining round' is initiated.

Infection

Lung infections are a common problem in lung transplant recipients and are similar to those of other immunocompromised hosts (see earlier section on infections of the lung). The transplant recipient is most vulnerable to infection during the first 6 months postoperatively, given mucociliary dysfunction and decreased cough reflex related to transplantation. Commonly identified infections include those

produced by CMV (37%) and *Aspergillus* (26%), and when these occur they are frequently serious with a high mortality.[350] Rejection and infection may facilitate one another to some degree, such that the separation of one from the other may be difficult on occasion. To further complicate the interpretation, perivascular infiltrates in the transplant setting have been reported to occur as a result of conditions other than rejection.[351–354] Infections may also produce acute bronchitis/bronchiolitis, bronchiolitis with inflammatory polyps, organizing pneumonia-like lesions, or more rarely even obliterative bronchiolitis.

Airway diseases

Acute bronchitis/bronchiolitis (ABB): ABB is characterized by neutrophilic infiltration of the airways, with variable necrosis of the airway epithelium, dilation of airways, mucus plugging, and early granulation tissue.[355] In one series, infection was the etiology of the ABB in about one-third of cases, rejection in one-third, and the remaining third had either histology suggesting rejection (but with BAL cultures confirming infection), or histology suggesting infection, with a negative BAL.[355]

Cellular bronchiolitis in rejection and infection: Cellular bronchiolitis is most commonly due to lung rejection but may also be due to infection. When cellular bronchiolitis is a manifestation of rejection, it is usually accompanied by vasculitis.

Eosinophilic bronchiolitis (graft eosinophilia): Yousem reviewed 145 biopsy specimens from lung allograft recipients, 112 of which had evidence of acute cellular rejection, and found prominent tissue eosinophils in nine of the biopsies that also showed evidence of acute rejection.[356] Five of these individuals had moderate to severe acute rejection and responded well to steroid treatment. The intensity of tissue eosinophilia correlated with severity of rejection.

Lymphocytic bronchitis/bronchiolitis: Diffuse or patchy infiltrates of lymphocytes, histiocytes, and plasma cells in the submucosa of bronchi and/or bronchioles in lung transplant recipients has been termed lymphocytic bronchitis/bronchiolitis (LBB). LBB was preceded by acute rejection in 20 of the 26 cases reported by Yousem,[348] and the condition appeared on average 1 year after transplantation. The infiltrate extended into the airway epithelium and smooth muscle in about half of the cases. Loose subepithelial granulation tissue was present in about one-third. Patients with LBB frequently developed subsequent OB, especially when the LBB was more severe. LBB bears some resemblance to follicular bronchitis and also to the lymphocytic airway infiltrate seen in graft-versus-host disease (GVHD) manifesting in the lungs of patients who have received non-lung transplants.

Bronchiolitis with organizing pneumonia: In a review of post-transplant biopsies, Yousem et al.[357] identified 23 patients whose biopsied showed patchy plugs of fibromyxoid granulation tissue in airways and airspaces resembling organizing pneumonia. Eleven of these patients were felt to have acute rejection on the basis of associated histologic and clinical features. Nine of these patients responded to bolus steroid therapy, and the organizing granulation tissue resolved within 3 to 4 weeks. In the remaining two, persistent rejection occurred, accompanied by OB. Organizing pneumonia is clearly a recognizable entity and may occur as a result of a variety of injuries. It may resolve or progress to OB, especially if accompanied by rejection.[358]

Constrictive and occlusive bronchiolitis (OB): OB is recognized as the major limiting factor to long-term survival in heart-lung and lung transplantation, so much so that this occurrence has been codified as "bronchiolitis obliterans syndrome" (BOS or BO).[349] The reported incidence of OB has been quite variable in the literature and depends on a number of factors such as the duration of follow-

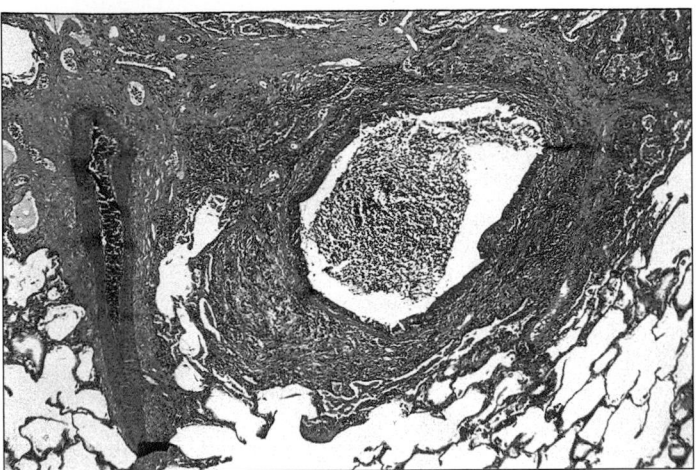

Fig. 17.104 Lung transplant rejection, bronchiolitis obliterans (BO). The histopathology of BO is distinctive. The earliest stage is characterized by eccentric subepithelial fibrosis with scattered mononuclear cells.

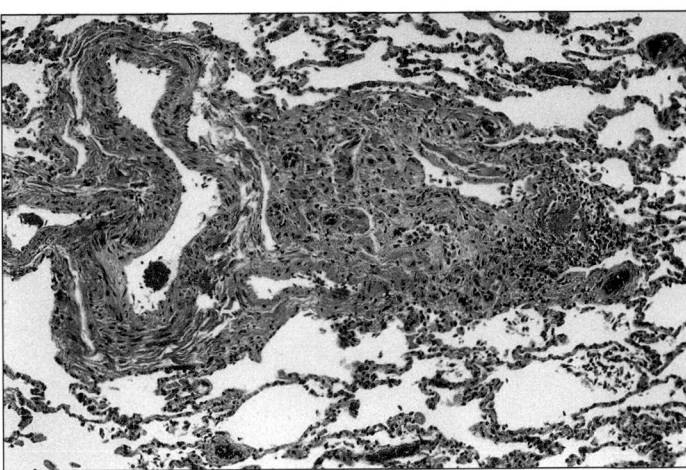

Fig. 17.105 Lung transplant rejection, bronchiolitis obliterans (BO). BO progresses over time until the lumen becomes markedly narrowed or completely occluded.

up, the exact nature of the cases studied, when they were reported (the incidence may be decreasing), and whether it was considered as a separate lesion from 'chronic rejection.' It has been estimated that OB will be present in 30–50% of patients surviving more than 6 months post-transplantation.[349] The frequency of OB may be as high as 80% in pediatric lung transplantation.[359]

The incidence of OB increases with the duration of the transplant, but cases can occur as soon as 2 months post-transplant. The peak incidence of occurrence is between 7 and 12 months.[349] The clinical onset is usually insidious, with non-specific symptoms such as cough and dyspnea. An acute respiratory episode may herald the onset of OB. Within several months of onset, dyspnea becomes rapidly progressive, with deterioration from normal lung function to severe air flow obstruction.[360] Plain chest radiographs may be normal or show small nodular or linear opacities or, less commonly, areas of airspace consolidation. Bronchial dilation is frequently seen on chest radiography or CT.[361,362]

The histopathology of OB is distinctive.[363] Bronchioles throughout the lung are variably involved, and affected bronchioles show lesions of different ages. Cagle proposed a sequence of events in the pathogenesis of OB[363] in which the earliest stage is characterized by eccentric subepithelial fibrosis with scattered mononuclear cells (Fig. 17.104). This concentric fibrosis progresses over time until the lumen becomes markedly narrowed (Fig. 17.105). In other instances, the lumen may be occluded by loose fibrous tissue. Some have distinguished these latter lesions as more typical of bronchiolitis obliterans, where the outer dimension of the bronchiole is relatively normal (i.e. not necessarily constricted). Given the limited repertoire of airway repair after injury, it seems likely that constrictive forms of bronchiolitis in the setting of lung transplantation simple represent a later evolution of the repair process. On transbronchial biopsies, small airways included in the sample may show dramatic luminal scarring and obliteration (Fig. 17.106). In addition to OB, extensive bronchiectasis (Fig. 17.107) was present in two of the five cases presented by Burke et al., and in their series, mucus plugging was also seen.[364] They also found pleural scars, patchy interstitial fibrosis, and accelerated arterial and venous arteriosclerosis in association with OB.

The risk of developing OB increases with the incidence of more frequent and severe rejection episodes,[360] and aggressive

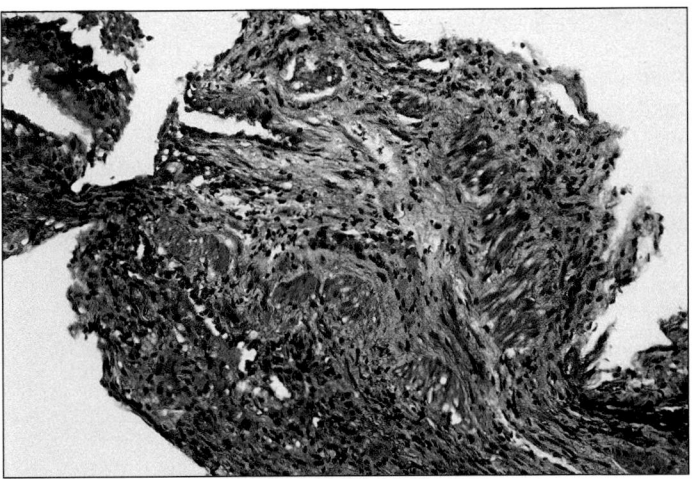

Fig. 17.106 Lung transplant rejection, bronchiolitis obliterans (BO). In transbronchial biopsies, a trichrome stain for collagen accentuates the luminal fibrosis of otherwise constricted airways.

treatment of rejection significantly reduces the frequency OB.[365] There is a statistically significant relationship between the occurrence of OB and nonviral infection,[357] leading some to suspect that infection may in fact act in a synergistic way with rejection.

OTHER COMPLICATIONS OF LUNG TRANSPLANTATION

Lymphoproliferative disorders

Post-transplant lymphoproliferative disorders (PTLD) may complicate the course of lung transplant patients as they do other organ transplantation. Yousem et al.[366] found 5 cases in 54 patients (9.4%) who had received heart-lung transplants. These lesions occurred relatively early in the post-transplant period (0.9–2.2 months), and

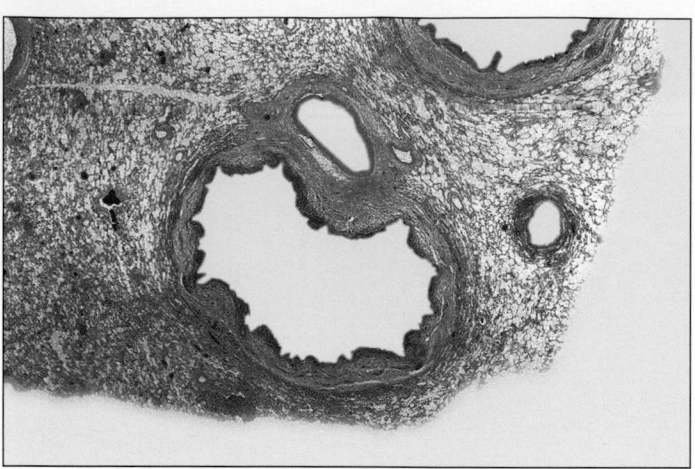

Fig. 17.107 Lung transplant rejection, bronchiolitis obliterans (BO). The late BO of chronic rejection may show bronchiolectasis.

consisted of a mixture of large lymphoid cells, plasma cells, and immunoblasts. Epstein-Barr virus was present in all of the cases. Reduction of immunosuppression and addition of acyclovir led to rapid clinical resolution in two patients.

It is now clear that a wide spectrum of immunoproliferative diseases occur in the transplant setting. These disease manifestations may be polyclonal or monoclonal and can have plasmacytic, B-cell, and T-cell immunophenotypes. Some of these processes are indistinguishable by any means from large cell lymphomas occurring in the absence of transplantation or severe immunosuppression. A recent Cleveland Clinic review of all PTLD cases in their organ transplant history showed earlier occurrence of PTLD in lung transplant patients, more frequent involvement of the transplanted organ in the case of lung transplants, and large B-cell lesions to be the most common manifestation.[367]

Re-occurrence of original disease

A number of diseases have been reported to re-occur in the transplanted lung. Most prominent among these are hard metal disease/giant cell interstitial pneumonia (GIP), lymphangiomyomatosis (LAM), and sarcoidosis.

MISCELLANEOUS DIFFUSE LUNG DISEASES

DISEASES RELATED TO CIGARETTE SMOKING

Respiratory bronchiolitis-associated interstitial lung disease

Respiratory bronchiolitis (RB) is a common finding in the lungs of cigarette smokers and some authorities considered this lesion to be a precursor of centri-acinar (smoker's) emphysema. RB lesions are centered on the terminal airways and are characterized by delicate fibrous bands, which radiate from the peribronchiolar connective tissue into the surrounding lung. Accompanying this are tan-brown pigmented alveolar macrophages, present in the adjacent airspaces, and a mild amount of interstitial chronic inflammation including lymphocytes and plasma cells. Bronchiolization (extension of terminal airway epithelium to alveolar ducts) is usually present to

some degree. In the bronchioles, variable amounts of submucosal fibrosis may be present, but constrictive changes are not a characteristic finding. When RB becomes much more extensive, involves appreciable amounts of lung tissue, and the patients have signs and symptoms of interstitial lung disease, the term respiratory bronchiolitis-associated interstitial lung disease (RBILD) has been suggested.[368,369] The relationship between RBILD and desquamative interstitial pneumonia (DIP) is unclear, and in smokers these two conditions are probably part of a continuous spectrum of disease.

Clinical presentation: By definition, all patients with RBILD are cigarette smokers. Symptoms include dyspnea, excess sputum production, and cough.[370] Rare patients may be asymptomatic with functional or radiographic abnormalities. In small series, men are slightly more commonly affected than women, and the mean age of onset is approximately 36 years (range 22–53). The average pack-year smoking history is 32 (range 7–75).

Radiologic findings: The majority of patients with respiratory bronchiolitis have normal radiologic findings. In one investigation of 41 heavy smokers, ground-glass opacities were evident on HRCT in 27% patients and micronodules in 10%.[371] The commonest radiographic and HRCT findings in RBILD are thickening of the bronchial walls, ground-glass opacities, and poorly defined centrilobular nodular opacities.[371] Because the patients are heavy smokers, centrilobular emphysema is commonly seen on HRCT.

Pathologic findings: In RB, a mild inflammatory process is centered on the membranous and respiratory bronchioles, typically associated with delicate scarring and pigmented macrophages (Fig. 17.108). In RBILD, sequelae of COPD, including mucostasis and mucinous metaplasia of bronchial epithelium, can be seen. The finding of lightly pigmented macrophages filling airspaces around the terminal airways with variable bronchiolization is characteristic (Fig. 17.109). Iron stains may show finely delicate positivity within these pigmented cells. The relatively patchy nature of the disease is extremely important in differentiating it from DIP (Fig. 17.110). A spectrum of pathologic severity emerges with the isolated lesions of RB on one end and the diffuse macrophage accumulation in DIP on the other, with RBILD somewhere between. The diagnosis of RBILD should be reserved for those situations where RB is prominent, with associated clinical and pathologic interstitial lung disease (ILD).[372] No other cause for ILD should be apparent.

Differential diagnosis: The differential diagnosis includes incidental RB, pulmonary Langerhans cell histiocytosis (PLCH), and desquamative interstitial pneumonia (DIP). In PLCH (see below) the characteristic large stellate scars and microcyst formation should stand out as distinguishing features. Also, in PLCH the presence of aggregated eosinophils and Langerhans cells is important in making the diagnosis. Distinguishing RBILD from DIP is more difficult in small biopsies, but comparison between these two diseases radiologically shows ground-glass alveolar infiltrates on X-ray more commonly in DIP than in RBILD, and alveolar macrophages are more diffuse in DIP on histologic exam. On physical examination, patients with DIP have clubbing much more frequently than patients who have RBILD.

Clinical course: The prognosis is excellent and there does not appear to be evidence for progression to end-stage fibrosis, in the absence of other lung disease.

PULMONARY LANGERHANS CELL HISTIOCYTOSIS

Pulmonary Langerhans cell histiocytosis (PLCH, formerly known as pulmonary eosinophilic granuloma or histiocytosis X) is now

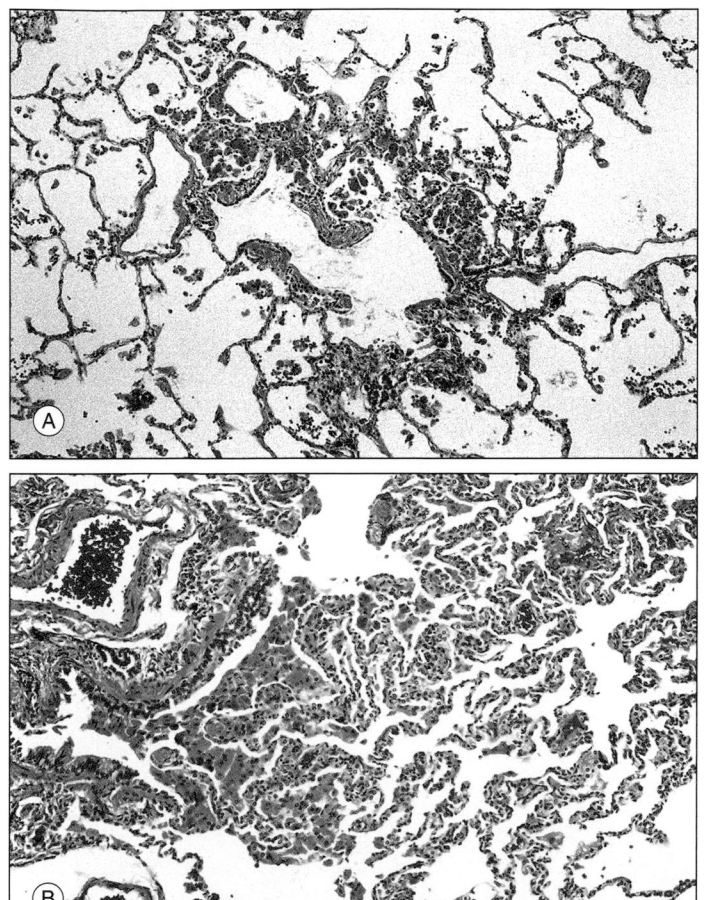

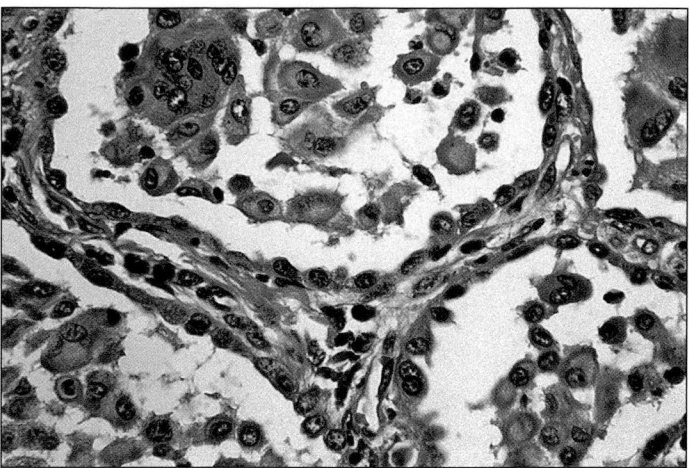

Fig. 17.110 Desquamative interstitial pneumonia (DIP). In DIP, not only is the macrophage accumulation more diffuse, but at high magnification there is mild interstitial widening with inactive-appearing fibrous tissue.

Fig. 17.108 Respiratory bronchiolitis (RB) is a smoking-related lesion that is centered on the terminal airways. (**A**) RB is characterized by delicate fibrous bands which radiate from the peribronchiolar connective tissue into the surrounding lung. Pigmented macrophages are present to variable degree in peribronchiolar airspaces. (**B**)

recognized to be a lung disease strongly associated with cigarette smoking. PLCH arises as a proliferation of Langerhans cells, which results in the formation of stellate lung scars and cystic change in affected individuals. The incidence of the disease is unknown but it is generally considered to be a rare complication of cigarette smoking.[373]

Clinical presentation: PLCH is a disease that most commonly affects smokers between the ages of 20 and 40. Some patients are asymptomatic despite chest X-ray abnormalities. The most common presenting symptom is cough with dyspnea. Chest pain, fever, weight loss, and even hemoptysis can occur. Pneumothorax has been reported in some series as a common presentation, but in others it is relatively uncommon. A relatively frequent clinical scenario for the discovery of PLCH is the patient with treated carcinoma (breast carcinoma, for example) being seen in follow-up surveillance for metastatic disease. In these patients, the nodules of PLCH typically

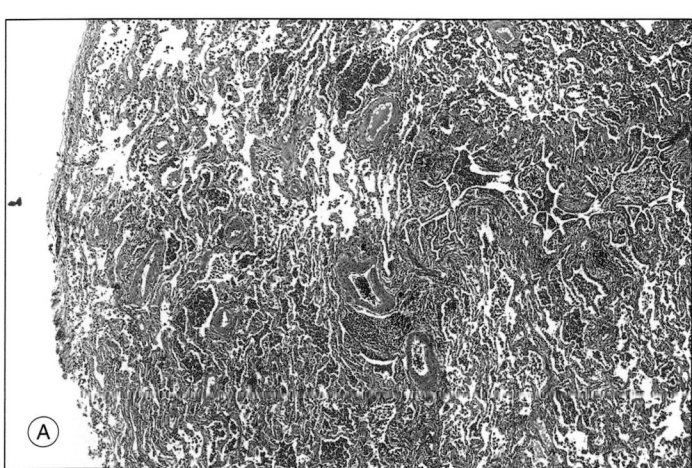

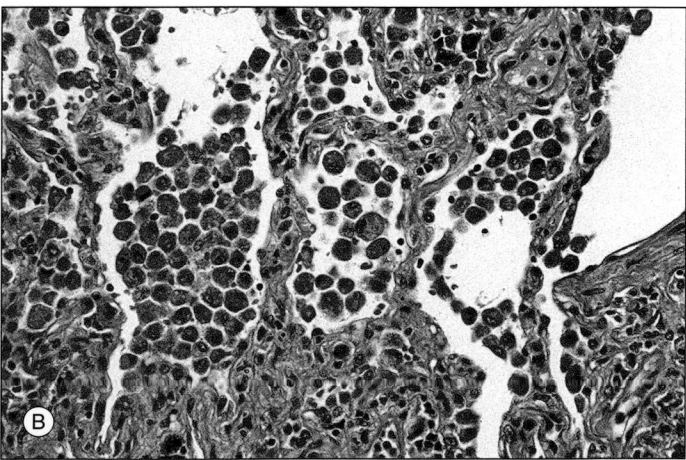

Fig. 17.109 Respiratory bronchiolitis-associated interstitial lung disease (RBILD). In RBILD the airspace accumulation of macrophages expands to involve adjacent alveoli over more of the lobule (**A**), but spared interlobular zones are still apparent. At high magnification, more pigmented macrophages are present than are seen in RB (**B**).

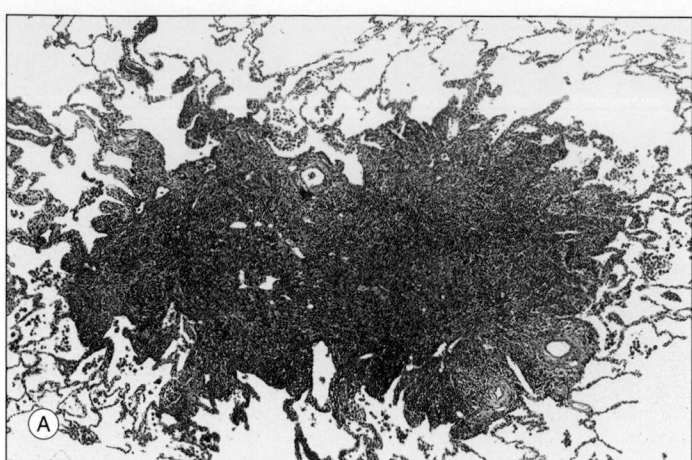
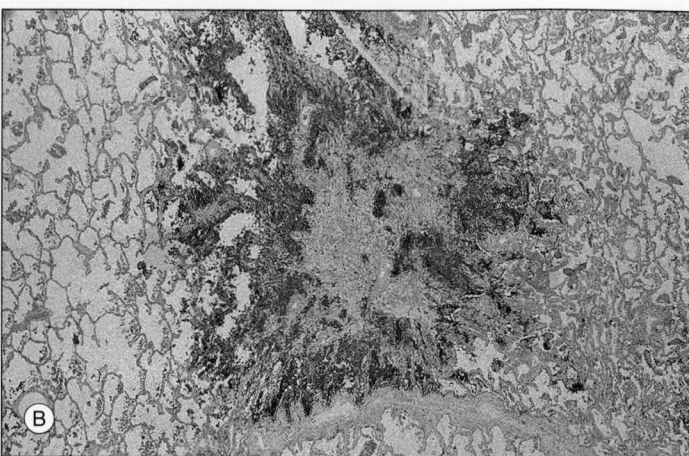

Fig. 17.111 Pulmonary Langerhans cell histiocytosis (PLCH). The diagnostic lesion of PLCH is a nodular scar with stellate fibrous ramifications into surrounding lung (**A**). Immunohistochemical stains for S-100 protein and CD1a are strongly positive in Langerhans cells, typically densest at the periphery of early cellular lesions (**B**, brown-stain immunohistochemistry using S-100 protein antibody and streptavidin-biotin labeling with diaminobenzidene chromogen).

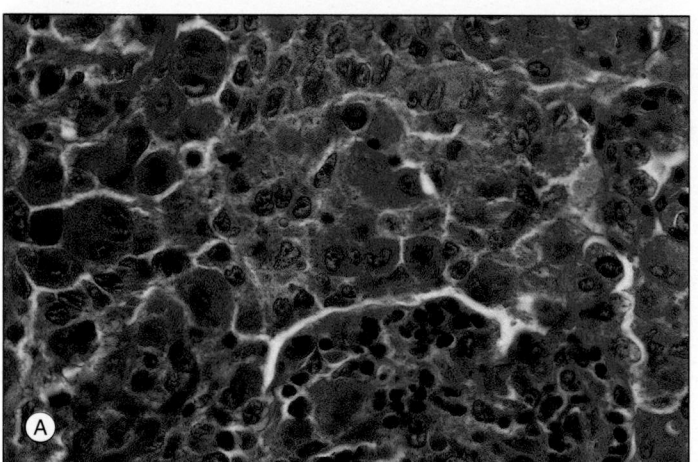
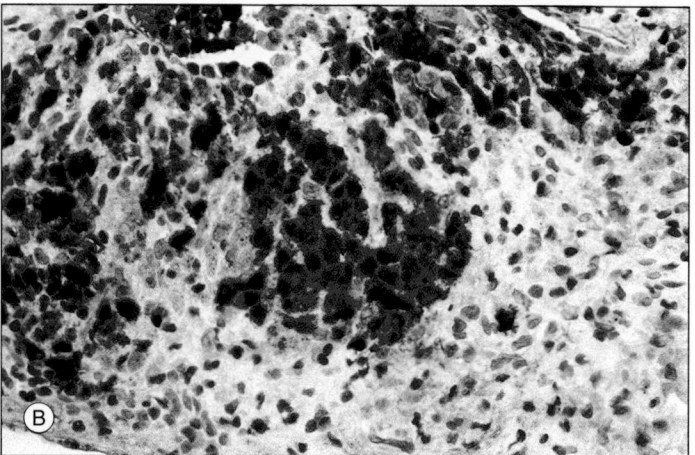

Fig. 17.112 Pulmonary Langerhans cell histiocytosis (PLCH). The Langerhans cell has a slightly pale basophilic nucleus with characteristic sharp nuclear folds (**A**). The nuclear folds have been likened to the appearance of crumpled tissue paper. Immunohistochemical stains for S-100 protein and CD1a highlight the Langerhans cells (**B**, immunohistochemistry using S-100 protein antibody and streptavidin-biotin labeling with Vector red chromogen).

suggest the occurrence of pulmonary metastasis, thereby engendering a lung biopsy.

Radiologic findings: The infiltrates of PLCH are bilateral and are worst in the upper lung zones, characteristically sparing the costophrenic angles. Reticular, nodular, and cystic opacities are seen, often together. HRCT is superior to plain radiography in showing the lesions. In particular, linear opacities on radiographs were the walls of cysts on CT.[374] In approximately 80% of cases, widely scattered, small (<5 mm) nodules with indistinct margins are distributed irregularly through the lungs. These are usually solid but may have a central small lucency, corresponding to cavities seen histologically in the center of the nodules and may represent a stage in the development of the cysts.[375] The cysts seen on CT range from a few millimeters to 3 cm in diameter, and involve mainly the upper and mid-lung zones, with relative sparing of the lung bases.[374] High-resolution CT scan shows nearly pathognomonic changes

including predominately upper and middle lung zone nodules and cysts.[373,376]

Pathologic findings: The diagnostic lesion of PLCH is illustrated in Figure 17.111A. These nodular scars with stellate fibrous ramifications into surrounding lung have been likened to a starfish or 'medusa' head. Pigmented alveolar macrophages and variable numbers of eosinophils surround and permeate the lesions. Immunohistochemistry using antibodies directed against S-100 protein/CD1a highlight numerous positive Langerhans cells at the periphery of the 'early' cellular lesions (Fig. 17.111B). The Langerhans cell has a slightly pale, basophilic nucleus with characteristic sharp nuclear folds resembling crumpled tissue paper (Fig. 17.112). One or two small nucleoli are usually present. The cytoplasm is abundant and finely vacuolated or faintly eosinophilic. In the cellular lesions of PLCH, Langerhans cells may be sufficiently numerous as to be confused with neoplasm. Late lesions (so-called 'burned out' or

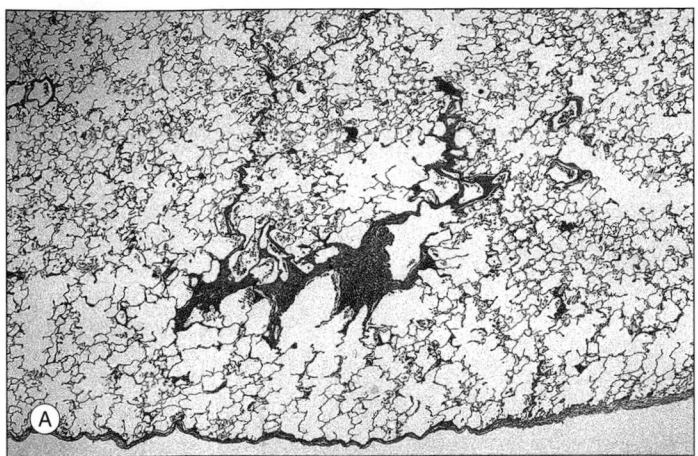
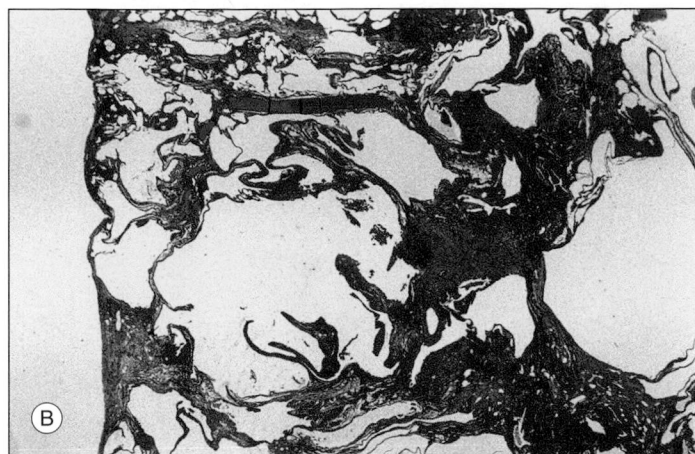

Fig. 17.113 Pulmonary Langerhans cell histiocytosis (PLCH). Late lesions (so-called 'burned out' or resolved PLCH) consist only of fibrotic centrilobular scars with a stellate configuration (**A**). If progressive fibrosis occurs, cysts and large stellate scars may be the only evidence of PLCH (**B**).

resolved PLCH) consist only of fibrotic centrilobular scars[377] with a stellate configuration (Fig. 17.113). Microcysts and honeycombing may be present. Immunohistochemistry for S-100 protein and CD1a may be used to confirm the diagnosis, but this is usually unnecessary and even may be confounding in late lesions where Langerhans cells may be sparse and the stellate scar is the diagnostic lesion.

Up to 20% of transbronchial biopsies in patients with PLCH may have diagnostic changes. Greater than 5% Langerhans cells in bronchoalveolar lavage is considered diagnostic of PLCH in the appropriate clinical setting. Unfortunately, cigarette smokers without PLCH have increased numbers of Langerhans cells in their BAL.

Differential diagnosis: Respiratory bronchiolitis-associated interstitial lung disease (RBILD) is in the differential diagnosis since both RBILD and PLCH are diseases of smokers, and respiratory bronchiolitis may be prominent in both conditions. Active cellular lesions may mimic lymphoma or other tumors. When eosinophils are numerous, eosinophilic pneumonia is a consideration, but the latter is an airspace disease, without nodules. Pleural reaction to pneumothorax from any cause may mimic PLCH with proliferation of mesothelial cells and eosinophils ('eosinophilic pleuritis'). Late-stage lesions simulate fibrosing interstitial pneumonias. When alveolar macrophages are prominent, desquamative interstitial pneumonia (DIP) enters into the differential diagnosis. In DIP the disease is more diffuse, with ground-glass radiographic infiltrates. When pigmentation of macrophages is striking, pulmonary hemorrhage may be suspected. Iron stains may be weakly positive in the 'smokers' macrophages' of PLCH, contrasting with the strong granular positivity of hemorrhage-associated macrophages. PLCH may be associated with pulmonary neoplasms, especially lung cancer, since smoking is a cause of both.

Clinical course: Smoking cessation is the primary 'therapy.' The prognosis is excellent, with less than 20% of patients progressing to end-stage fibrosis. Corticosteroid therapy has been used for symptomatic patients.

PULMONARY ALVEOLAR PROTEINOSIS

Pulmonary alveolar proteinosis (PAP, alveolar lipoproteinosis), is a rare diffuse lung disease characterized by an intra-alveolar accumulation of lipid-rich eosinophilic material.[378] PAP presumably occurs as a result of overproduction of surfactant by type II cells, impaired clearance of surfactant by alveolar macrophages, or a combination of these mechanisms.

Clinical presentation: The disease can occur as an idiopathic form, and also in the settings of occupational disease (especially dust-related), drug-induced injury, hematologic diseases, and in many settings of immunodeficiency.[378–381] The disease is commonly associated with exposure to crystalline material and silica, although other substances have also been implicated.[379] The idiopathic form is the most common presentation, where there is a male predominance and an age range of 30 to 50 years. The usual presenting symptom is insidious dyspnea, sometimes with cough.[382]

Radiologic findings: Chest radiographs show extensive bilateral airspace consolidation, involving mainly the perihilar regions, and often the symptoms belie the severe radiographic abnormalities. CT demonstrates what appears to be smooth thickening of lobular septa that is not seen on the chest radiograph. The thickening of lobular septa within areas of ground-glass attenuation is characteristic of alveolar proteinosis on CT and is referred to as the 'crazy paving pattern.'[383] The areas of ground-glass attenuation and consolidation are often sharply demarcated from the surrounding normal lung without an apparent anatomic reason.[383–385]

Pathologic findings: The gross lung shows firm yellow-white nodules, some as large as 2 cm in diameter. Microscopically, the scanning magnification appearance is distinctive, if not diagnostic. Pink granular material fills the airspaces, sometimes with a rim of retraction that separates the alveolar wall slightly from the exudate (Fig. 17.114A). Closer inspection of this material shows embedded clumps of dense globular material and cholesterol clefts (Fig. 17.114B). The PAS stain may be useful in demonstrating a diastase resistant, positive reaction in the proteinaceous material of PAP. Immunohistochemistry can be used to demonstrate staining using antibodies directed against surfactant. There may be few other associated changes in the lung biopsy, although patients with long-standing disease may develop some interstitial fibrosis and chronic inflammation. More dramatic inflammatory changes should suggest comorbid infection. For example, *Nocardia* infection is known to be associated with PAP. PAP can be patchy in

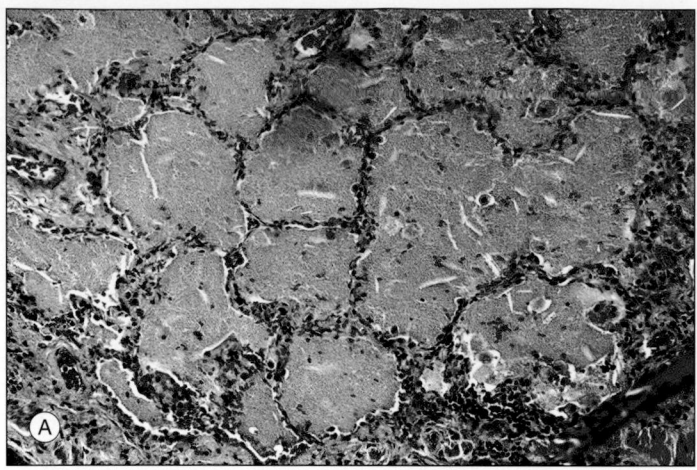
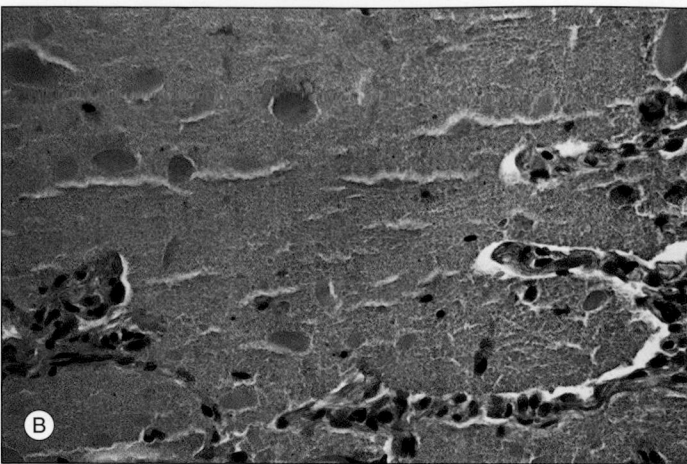

Fig. 17.114 Pulmonary alveolar proteinosis (PAP). Pink granular material fills the airspaces, sometimes with a rim of retraction that separates the alveolar wall slightly from the exudate (**A**). Closer inspection of this material shows embedded clumps of dense globular material and cholesterol clefts (**B**).

the lungs and in biopsy specimens, so a high index of suspicion, coupled with good clinical and radiologic data, are often necessary.

Differential diagnosis: Pulmonary edema lacks the globular material and cellular debris seen in PAP. *Pneumocystis* pneumonia can be distinguished from PAP by exudates that appear finely vacuolated or foamy, and background lung with significantly more inflammatory changes.

Clinical course: Despite significant radiologic abnormalities, the disease may be unusually silent, producing little if any clinical manifestations in the absence of superinfection. In the patient with severe dyspnea and hypoxemia, treatment can be accomplished with one or more sessions of whole-lung lavage, which usually induces remission and excellent long-term survival.[386]

LYMPHANGIOLEIOMYOMATOSIS

Pulmonary lymphangioleiomyomatosis (LAM) is a rare disease in the lung, characterized by an abnormal proliferation of smooth muscle cells in the pulmonary interstitium associated with the formation of cysts.[387–390] The disease is centered on lymphatic channels, blood vessels, and airways.

Clinical presentation: LAM is a disease of women of childbearing age, although the disease does occur in older women and there has been one case report of LAM in a man.[391] Some patients with LAM also have tuberous sclerosis complex (TSC), an inherited autosomal dominant condition. TSC is characterized by mental retardation, epilepsy, and adenoma sebaceum of the skin. About one-fourth of patients with TSC have LAM by chest HRCT,[392] but most LAM patients do not have TSC. The most common presenting symptoms are spontaneous pneumothorax and exertional dyspnea. Others symptoms include chyloptosis, hemoptysis, and chest pain. Pulmonary function reveals airflow obstruction and decreased DLC_O.

Radiologic findings: The radiographic appearance is that of fine linear and nodular densities, mainly at the lung bases, which progress to bullous and cystic changes throughout the lungs. As opposed to most other causes of infiltrative lung disease, lung volumes progressively increase radiologically. The characteristic findings on

CT are presence of numerous cysts separated from one another by normal-appearing lung parenchyma. The cysts are seen much better with HRCT and usually measure 2–10 mm in diameter, have well-defined margins, and thin walls.[388,393]

Pathologic findings: The appearance of the abnormal smooth muscle in LAM is sufficiently characteristic that, once recognized, is rarely forgotten. Cystic spaces are present at low magnification (Fig. 17.115A). The walls of these spaces have variable amounts of bundled spindled cells (Fig. 17.115B). The nuclei of these spindled cells (Fig. 17.116A) are larger than those of normal smooth muscle bundles seen around alveolar ducts or in the walls of airways or vessels. In larger proliferations of this muscle, irregular slit-like channels lined by endothelium can be seen, consistent with lymphatic vessels. Immunohistochemical staining using the melanoma marker antibodies HMB-45 and Mart-1 are positive in the abnormal smooth muscle of LAM (Fig. 17.116B). These findings may be useful in the evaluation of transbronchial biopsy where only a few spindled cells may be present. Actin, desmin, estrogen, and progesterone receptors can also be demonstrated in the spindled cells of LAM.[394] In a subset of patients with LAM, other lung parenchymal abnormalities may be present, including peculiar nodules of hyperplastic pneumocytes (Fig. 17.117) that do not show immunoreactivity for HMB-45 or Mart-1, but instead show immunoreactivity for cytokeratins and surfactant apoprotein.[395] These epithelial lesions have been referred to as 'micronodular pneumocyte hyperplasia.'

Differential diagnosis: There is some resemblance of the CT appearance of LAM to both UIP and pulmonary Langerhans cell histiocytosis (PLCH). However, in UIP the cysts are seen mostly in the peripheral part of the lower lobes, whereas in LAM the cysts are more diffuse. In addition, the remaining lung shows linear opacities in UIP. In PLCH, the cysts are most prominent in the upper two-thirds of the lung, sparing the costophrenic angles, and the intervening lung shows irregular nodules. The presence of stellate scars, eosinophils, and characteristic Langerhans cells is useful in separating this disease from LAM.

Clinical course: The disease is progressive with average survival of more than 10 years. All of the patients who died in one large series did so within five years of disease onset,[396] suggesting the rate of progression can vary widely among patients.

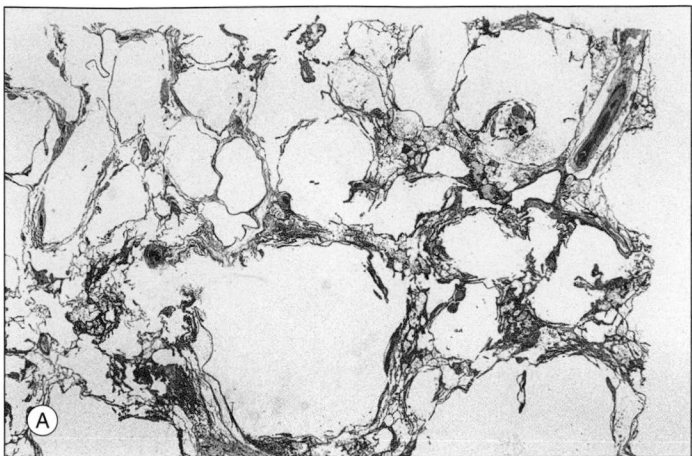
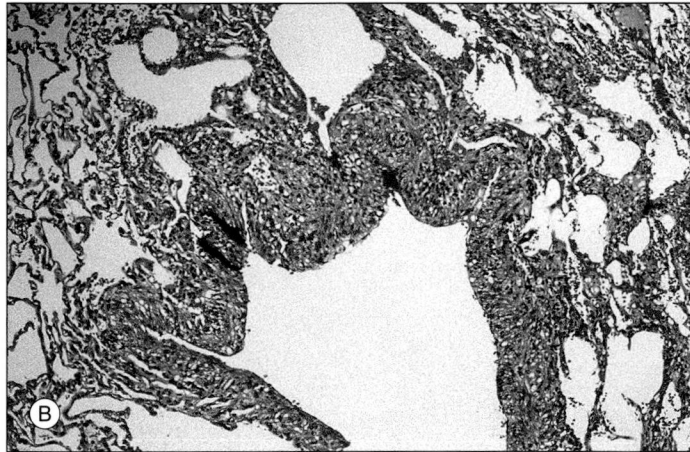

Fig. 17.115 Lymphangioleiomyomatosis (LAM). Cystic spaces are present at low magnification (**A**). The walls of these spaces have variable amounts of bundled spindled cells (**B**).

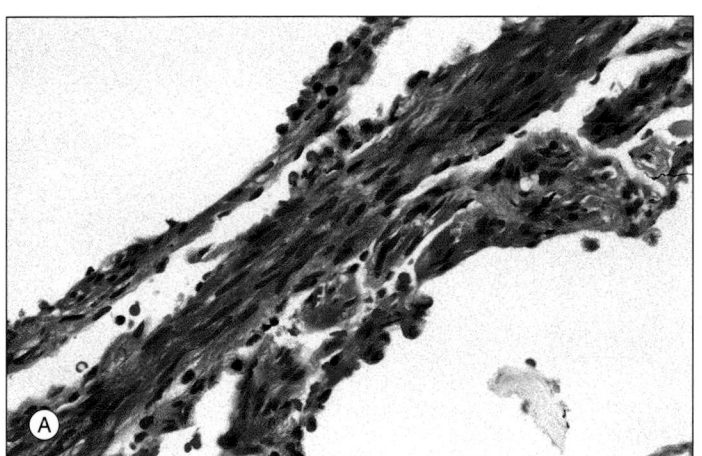
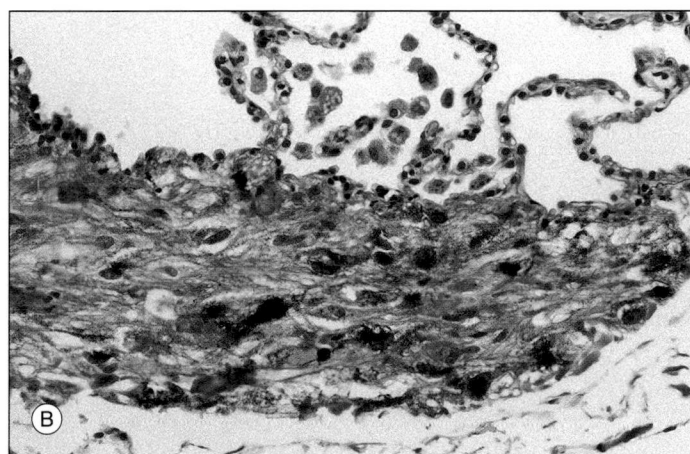

Fig. 17.116 Lymphangioleiomyomatosis (LAM). The nuclei of these spindled cells are larger nuclei than those of normal smooth muscle bundles of the alveolar ducts (**A**). Immunohistochemical stains for melanoma markers HMB-45 and Mart-1 highlight the LAM cells (**B**, immunohistochemistry using HMB-45 and streptavidin-biotin labeling with Vector red chromogen).

LYMPHANGITIC CARCINOMATOSIS

Pulmonary lymphangitic carcinomatosis (lymphangitis carcinomatosa) is a form of metastatic carcinoma involving the lung, primarily within lymphatics. Lymphangitic carcinoma is typically adenocarcinoma and this phenomenon accounts for as many as 8% of all metastatic disease to the lung. The most common sites of origin are breast, lung, and stomach, although primary disease in pancreas, ovary, kidney, and uterine cervix can also give rise to this manifestation of metastatic spread.[397,398] The published reports on the subject are found predominately in the radiology literature.[397–400]

Clinical presentation: Patients often present with insidious onset of dyspnea, frequently accompanied by an irritating cough.

Radiologic findings: The plain chest radiograph appearances are often subtle and non-specific, and a correct diagnosis was only made in 20 of 87 of cases (23%); 50% were normal.[401] The radiographic abnormalities include linear opacities, Kerley B lines (horizontal linear lines abutting on the pleura, mostly in the lower lobes), subpleural edema, and commonly hilar and mediastinal lymph node enlargement.[399] By contrast, the HRCT findings are highly characteristic and accurately reflect the macroscopic abnormalities in this disease. Because the major lymphatic vessels in the lung are located in the pleura, interlobular septa, and bronchovascular bundles, the obvious abnormalities are found primarily in this distribution and consist of thickening and accentuation of these structures. HRCT scanning shows uneven thickening of the bronchovascular bundles and lobular septa, giving them a beaded appearance.[398,400] Intersecting thickened lobular septa produce polygonal lines,[402] often with a central dot representing the lobular artery and thickened bronchovascular bundle (see Fig. 17.6). Increased linear opacities are seen in all cases, and polygonal densities in half.[400]

Pathologic findings: Tumor cells are typically present in small aggregates within lymphatic channels of the bronchovascular sheath

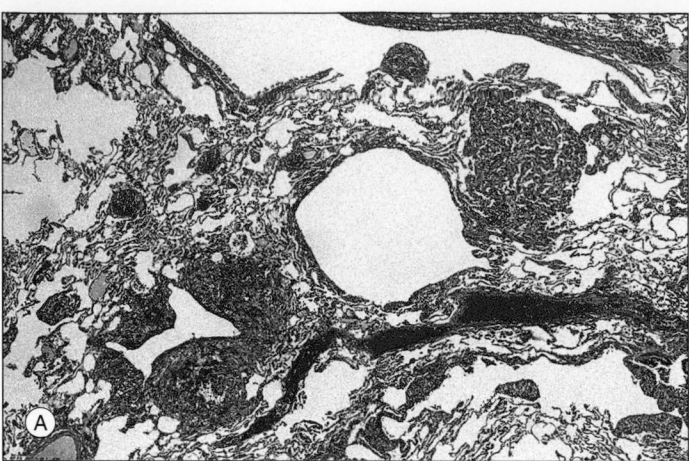
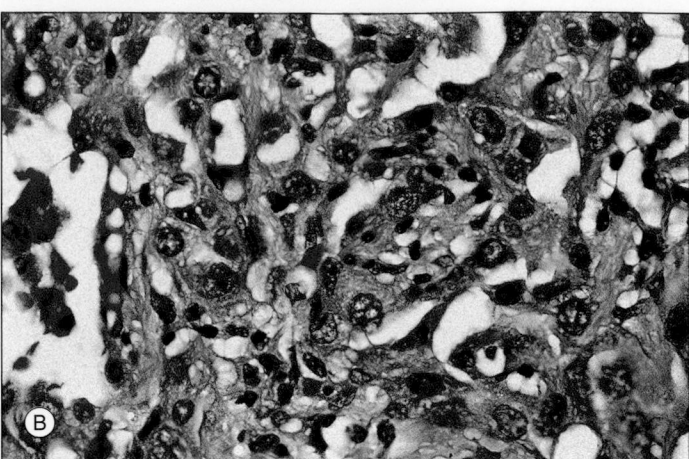

Fig. 17.117 Lymphangioleiomyomatosis (LAM) and multinodular pneumocyte hyperplasia (MNPH). In a subset of patients with LAM, other lung parenchymal abnormalities may be present, including peculiar nodules of hyperplastic pneumocytes (**A**, upper right) referred to as MNPH. These lesions have cells with a cuboidal appearance (**B**). The cells of MNPH do not react with antibodies directed against HMB-45 or Mart-1, but instead show immunoreactivity for cytokeratins and surfactant apoprotein.

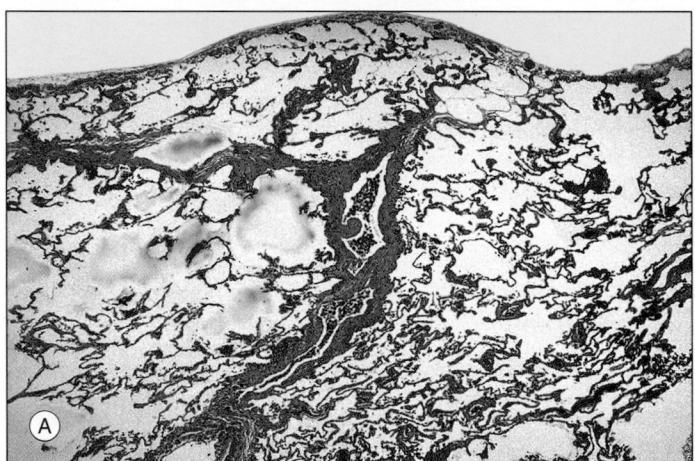
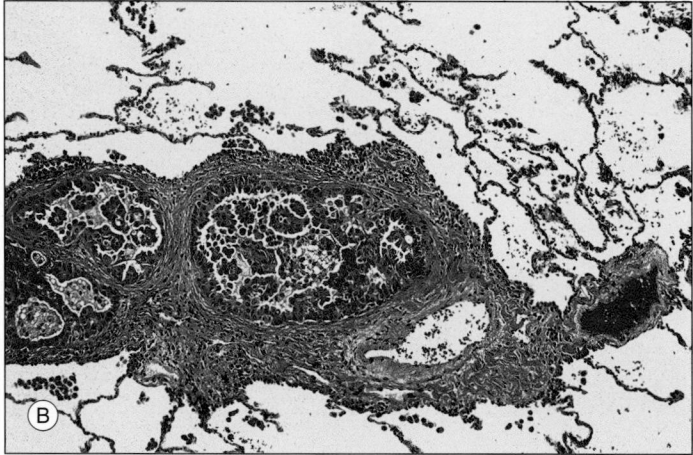

Fig. 17.118 Lymphangitic carcinomatosis: Tumor cells resemble thromboembolus at scanning magnification (**A**). At higher magnification, the cellular composition of these endovascular and endolymphatic emboli becomes clear, in this case, metastatic adenocarcinoma with mucinous and micropapillary features (**B**).

and pleura (Fig. 17.118). Tumor cells are present in the lymphatics of the bronchi in this process, making lymphangitic carcinoma one of the few diffuse lung diseases that can be diagnosed by bronchial or transbronchial biopsy.[30]

Variable amounts of tumor may be present throughout the lung in the interstitium of the alveolar walls, in the air spaces, and in small muscular pulmonary arteries. This latter finding (microangiopathic obliterative endarteritis) may be the origin of the edema, inflammation, and interstitial fibrosis that frequently accompanies the disease, and likely accounts for the clinical and radiologic impression of non-neoplastic diffuse lung disease.[397,399] The pathogenesis of this peculiar manifestation of metastatic carcinoma is unknown. Seeding of the lung lymphatics from retrograde spread of microvascular tumor emboli is the likely pathogenesis, supported by observations of hematogenous tumor found in the lungs and other organs of patients with pulmonary lymphangitic carcinoma.[397,399]

Differential diagnosis: Intravascular lymphoma, thromboembolic disease, and foreign material from intravenous injection.

Clinical course: The prognosis is grim, with most patients dying before 6 months. Rarely, long-term survivors are reported.[397]

REFERENCES

1. Nagaishi C. Functional anatomy and histology of the lung. 1st edn. Baltimore: University Park Press; 1972.

2. Aguayo S, Schuyler W, Murtagh J, et al. Regulation of branching morphogenesis by bombesin-like peptides and neutral endopeptidase. Am J Respir Cell Mol Biol 1994; 10: 635–642.

3. Bienenstock J, Johnston N, Perey D. Bronchial lymphoid tissue I. Morphological characteristics. Lab Invest 1973; 28: 686–692.

4. Richmond I, Pritchard G, Ashcroft T, et al. Bronchus associated lymphoid tissue (BALT) in human lung. Its distribution in smokers and non-smokers. Thorax 1993; 48: 1130–1134.

5. van Haarst J, de Wit H, Drexhage H, et al. Distribution and immunophenotype of mononuclear phagocytes and dendritic cells in the human lung. Am J Respir Cell Mol Biol 1994; 10: 487–492.

6. Kradin R, Mark E. Benign lymphoid disorders of the lung, with a theory regarding their development. Hum Pathol 1983; 14: 857–867.

7. Van Voorhis W, Hair L, Steinman R, et al. Human dendritic cells, enrichment and purification from peripheral blood. J Exp Med 1982; 155: 1172–1187.

8. Soler P, Moreau A, Basset F, et al. Cigarette smoking-induced changes in the number and differentiated state of pulmonary dendritic/Langerhans cells. Am Rev Respir Dis 1989; 139: 1112–1117.

9. Thurlbeck W. Chronic airflow obstruction. In: Churg A, ed. Pathology of the lung. 2nd edn. New York: Thieme Medical Publishers; 1995: 739–825.

10. Fukuda Y, Ishizaki M, Masuda Y, et al. The role of intraalveolar fibrosis in the process of pulmonary structural remodeling in patients with diffuse alveolar damage. Am J Pathol 1987; 126(1): 171–182.

11. Leslie K, King TE Jr, Low R. Smooth muscle actin is expressed by air space fibroblast-like cells in idiopathic pulmonary fibrosis and hypersensitivity pneumonitis. Chest 1991; 99(3 Suppl): 47S–48S.

12. Leslie KO, Mitchell J, Low R. Lung myofibroblasts. Cell Motil Cytoskeleton 1992; 22(2): 92–98.

13. Colby TV, Carrington CB. Interstitial lung disease. In: Churg A, ed. Pathology of the lung. 2nd edn. New York: Thieme Medical Publishers; 1995: 589–737.

14. Carrington CB, Gaensler EA. Clinical-pathologic approach to diffuse infiltrative lung disease. In: Abell M, ed. The lung structure, function and disease. Baltimore: Williams & Wilkins; 1978: 58–67.

15. Müller N. Differential diagnosis of chronic diffuse infiltrative lung disease on high-resolution computed tomography. Semin Roentgenol 1991; 26: 132–142.

16. Webb W, Müller N, Naidich D. Standardized terms for high resolution computed tomography of the lung: a proposed glossary. J Thorac Imaging 1993; 8: 167–175.

17. Mathieson JR, Mayo JR, Staples CA, et al. Chronic diffuse infiltrative lung disease: comparison of diagnostic accuracy of CT and chest radiography. Radiology 1989; 171(1): 111–116.

18. Grenier P, Valeyre D, Cluzel P, et al. Chronic diffuse interstitial lung disease: diagnostic value of chest radiography and high-resolution CT. Radiology 1991; 179: 123–132.

19. Hunninghake G, Zimmerman M, Schwartz D, et al. Utility of a lung biopsy for the diagnosis of idiopathic pulmonary fibrosis. Am J Respir Crit Care Med 2001; 164: 193 196.

20. Bonelli F, Hartman T, Swensen S, et al. Accuracy of high-resolution CT in diagnosing lung diseases. Am J Roentgenol 1998; 170: 1507–1512.

21. Bigby TD, Margoleskee D, Curtis JL, et al. The usefulness of induced sputum in the diagnosis of Pneumocystis carinii pneumonia in patients with AIDS. Am Rev Respir Dis 1986; 133: 515–518.

22. Raghu G. Interstitial lung disease: A diagnostic approach. Are CT scan and lung biopsy indicated in every patient? Am J Respir Crit Care Med 1995; 151: 909–914.

23. Dijkman J, van der Meer W, Bakker W, et al. Transpleural lung biopsy by the thoracoscopic route in patients with diffuse lung interstitial pulmonary disease. Chest 1982; 82: 76–83.

24. Bensard DD, McIntyre RCJ, Waring BJ, et al. Comparison of video thoracoscopic lung biopsy to open lung biopsy. Chest 1993; (103): 765–770.

25. Ognibene F, Shelhamer J, Gill V, et al. The diagnosis of Pneumocystis carinii pneumonia in patients with the acquired immunodeficiency syndrome using subsegmental bronchoalveolar lavage. Am Rev Respir Dis 1984; 129: 929–932.

26. Clark JG, Crawford SW. Diagnostic approaches to pulmonary complications of marrow transplantation. Chest 1987; 91: 477–479.

27. Canham EM, Kennedy TC, Merrick TA. Unexplained pulmonary infiltrates in the compromised patient. Cancer 1983; 52: 325–329.

28. Wetstein L. Sensitivity and specificity of lingular segmental biopsies of the lung. Chest 1986; 90: 383–386.

29. Miller R, Nelems B, Müller N, et al. Lingular and right middle lobe biopsy in the assessment of diffuse lung disease. Ann Thorac Surg 1987; 44: 269–273.

30. Wall C, Gaensler E, Carrington C, et al. Comparison of transbronchial and open biopsies in chronic infiltrative lung disease. Am Rev Respir Dis 1981; 123: 280–285.

31. Gianoulis M, Chan N, Wright J. Inflation of lung biopsies for frozen sections. Mod Pathol 1988; 1: 357–358.

32. Liebow A, Carrington C. The interstitial pneumonias. In: Potchen E, LeMay M, eds. Frontiers of pulmonary radiology pathophysiologic, roentgenographic and radioisotopic considerations. Orlando, FL: Grune & Stratton; 1969: 109–142.

33. Travis W, King T, Bateman E, et al. ATS/ERS international multidisciplinary consensus classification of the idiopathic interstitial pneumonias. Am J Respir Crit Care Med 2002; 165(2): 277 304.

34. Pimentel J. Tridimensional photographic reconstruction in a study of the pathogenesis of honeycomb lung. Thorax 1967; 22: 444–452.

35. American Thoracic Society. Idiopathic pulmonary fibrosis: diagnosis and treatment. International consensus statement. American Thoracic Society (ATS), and the European Respiratory Society (ERS). Am J Respir Crit Care Med 2000; 161(2 Pt 1): 646–664.

36. Katzenstein A, Bloor C, Liebow A. Diffuse alveolar damage. The role of oxygen, shock and related factors. Am J Pathol 1976; 85: 210–222.

37. Pache JC, Christakos PG, Gannon DE, et al. Myofibroblasts in diffuse alveolar damage of the lung. Mod Pathol 1998; 11(11): 1064–1070.

38. Lakshminarayan S, Stanford R, Petty T. Prognosis after recovery from adult respiratory distress syndrome. Am Rev Respir Dis 1976; 113: 7–16.

39. Ashbaugh DG, Bigelow DB, Petty TL, et al. Acute respiratory distress in adults. Lancet 1967; 2: 319–321.

40. Petty T, Ashbaugh D. The adult respiratory distress syndrome clinical features, factors influencing prognosis and principles of management. Chest 1971; 60: 233–239.

41. Bouros D, Nicholson AC, Polychronopoulos V, et al. Acute interstitial pneumonia. Eur Respir J 2000; 15(2): 412–418.

42. Kobayashi H, Itoh T, Sasaki Y, et al. Diagnostic imaging of idiopathic adult respiratory distress syndrome (ARDS)/diffuse alveolar damage (DAD) histopathological correlation with radiological imaging. Clin Imaging 1996; 20(1): 1–7.

43. Tomashefski JF Jr. Pulmonary pathology of acute respiratory distress syndrome. Clin Chest Med 2000; 21(3): 435–466.

44. Rosenow E, Wilson W, Cockerill F. Pulmonary disease in the immunocompromised host (Part 1). Mayo Clin Proc 1985; 60: 473–487.

45. Kaplan M, Armstrong D, Rosen P. Tuberculosis complicating neoplastic disease. A review of 201 cases. Cancer 1974; 33: 850–858.

46. Wolinsky E. State of the art nontuberculous mycobacteria and associated diseases. Am Rev Respir Dis 1979; 119: 107–159.

47. Murray J, Garay S, Hopewell P, et al. Pulmonary complications of the acquired immunodeficiency syndrome: an update. Am Rev Respir Dis 1987; 135: 504–509.

48. Handwerger S, Mildvan D, Senie R, et al. Tuberculosis and the acquired immunodeficiency syndrome at a New York City hospital 1978–1985. Chest 1987; 91: 176–180.

49. Winther F, Horthe K, Lystad A, et al. Pathogenic bacterial flora in the upper respiratory tract of healthy students. Prevalence and relationship to nasopharyngeal inflammatory symptoms. J Laryngol Otol 1974; 88: 407–412.

50. Mackowiac P. The normal microbial flora. N Engl J Med 1982; 307: 83–93.

51. Winn WJ, Myerowitz R. The pathology of the Legionella pneumonias A review of 74 cases and the literature. Hum Pathol 1981; 12: 401–422.

52. Hicklin M, Thomason B, Chandler F, et al. Pathogenesis of acute Legionnaires' disease pneumonia. Am J Clin Pathol 7 1980; 3: 480–487.

53. Hernandez F, Kirby B, Stanley T, et al. Legionnaires' disease: Postmortem pathologic findings of 20 cases. Am J Clin Pathol 1980; 7: 488–495.

54. Leigh M, Clyde W Jr. Chlamydial and mycoplasmal pneumonias. Semin Resp Infect 1987; 2: 152–158.

55. Woodhead MA, Macfarlane JT. Comparative clinical and laboratory features of Legionella with pneumococcal and mycoplasma pneumonias. Br J Dis Chest 1987; 81: 133–139.

56. Miller R. Viral infections of the respiratory tract. In: Churg A, ed. Pathology of the lung. 2nd edn. New York: Thieme Medical Publishers; 1995: 195–222.

57. Dowdle WR, Coleman MT, Gregg MB. Natural history of influenza type A in the United States, 1957–1972. Prog Med Virol 1974; 17: 91–135.

58. Fry J. Influenza 1959: The story of an epidemic. Br Med J 1959; 2: 135–138.

59. Yeldandi AV, Colby TV. Pathologic features of lung biopsy specimens from influenza pneumonia cases. Hum Pathol 1994; 25(1): 47–53.

60. Haram K, Jacobsen J. Measles and its relationship to giant cell pneumonia (Hecht pneumonia). Acta Pathol Microbiol Immunol Scand [A] 1973; 81: 761–769.

61. Enders JF, McCarthy K, Mitus A, et al. Isolation of measles virus at autopsy in cases of giant-cell pneumonia without rash. N Engl J Med 1959; 261: 875–881.

62. Sobonya RE, Hiller FC, Pingleton W, et al. Fatal measles (rubeola) pneumonia in adults. Arch Pathol Lab Med 1978; 102: 366–371.

63. Mitus A, Enders JF, Craig JM, et al. Persistence of measles virus and depression of antibody formation in patients with giant-cell pneumonia after measles. N Engl J Med 1959; 261: 882–889.

64. Kenny D, Shen L, Kolberg J. Detection of viral infection and gene expression in clinical tissue specimens using DNA (bDNA) in situ hybridization. J Histochem Cytochem 2002; 50(9): 1219–1227.

65. Natarajan K, Shepard L, Chodosh J. The use of DNA array technology in studies of ocular viral pathogenesis. DNA Cell Biol 2002; 21(5-6): 483–490.

66. Pugh RN, Omar RI, Hossain MM. Varicella infection and pneumonia among adults. Int J Infect Dis 1998; 2(4): 205–210.

67. Duchin J, Koster F, Peters C, et al. Hantavirus pulmonary syndrome. A clinical description of 17 patients with a newly recognized disease. N Engl J Med 1994; 330: 949–955.

68. Nolte K, Feddersen R, Foucar K, et al. Hantavirus pulmonary syndrome in the United States. A new pathological description of a disease caused by a new agent. Hum Pathol 1995; 26: 110–120.

69. Falsey A, Walch E, Hayden F. Rhinovirus and coronavirus infection-associated hospitalization among older adults. J Infect Dis 2002; 185: 1338–1341.

70. Wenzel R, Edmund M. Managing SARS amidst uncertainty. N Engl J Med 2003; 348: 1947–1950.

71. Ksiazek T, Erdman M, Goldsmith C. A novel coronavirus associated with severe acute respiratory syndrome. N Engl J Med 2003; 348: 1953–1966.

72. Booth C, Marukas L, Tomlinson G. Clinical features and short-term outcomes of 144 patients with SARS in the greater Toronto area. JAMA 2003; 289: 2801–2809.

73. Lee N, Hui D, Wu A, et al. A major outbreak of severe acute respiratory syndrome in Hong Kong. N Engl J Med 2003; 348(20): 1986–1994.

74. England DM, Hochholzer L. Primary pulmonary sporotrichosis. Am J Surg Pathol 1985; 9: 193–204.

75. Goodwin R, Des Prez R. State of the art histoplasmosis. Am Rev Respir Dis 1978; 117: 929–956.

76. Atkinson JB, McCurley TL. Pulmonary blastomycosis: filamentous forms in an immunocompromised patient with fulminating respiratory failure. Human Pathol 1983; 14: 186–188.

77. Greenberger P, Patterson R. Allergic bronchopulmonary aspergillosis. Chest 1987; 91: 165S–171S.

78. Orr D, Myerowitz R, Dubois P. Pathoradiologic correlation of invasive pulmonary *Aspergillosis* in the compromised host. Cancer 1978; 41: 2028–2039.

79. Bigby TD, Serota ML, Tierney LMJ, et al. Clinical spectrum of pulmonary mucormycosis. Chest 1986; 89: 435–439.

80. Dubois P, Myerowitz R, Allen C. Pathoradiologic correlation of pulmonary candidiasis in immunosuppressed patients. Cancer 1977; 40: 1026–1036.

81. Stringer J, Beard C, Miller R, et al. A new name (*Pneumocytis jiroveci*) for pneumocytis from humans. Emerg Infect Dis 2002; 8(9): 891–896.

82. Grimes M, LaPook J, Bar MH, et al. Disseminated *Pneumocystis carinii* infection in a patient with acquired immunodeficiency syndrome. Hum Pathol 1987; 18: 307–308.

83. Weber W, Askin F, Dehner L. Lung biopsy in *Pneumocystis carinii* pneumonia. A histopathologic study of typical and atypical features. Am J Clin Pathol 1977; 67: 11–19.

84. Buchheit J, Eid N, Rodgers GJ, et al. Acute eosinophilic pneumonia with respiratory failure. A new syndrome? Am Rev Respir Dis 1992; 145: 716–718.

85. Lanham J, Elkon K, Pusey C, et al. Systemic vasculitis with asthma and eosinophilia: a clinical approach to the Churg-Strauss syndrome. Medicine 1983; 62: 142–158.

85a. Beasley MB, Franks TJ, Galvin JR, et al. Acute fibrinous and organizing pneumonia: a histological pattern of lung injury and possible variant of diffuse alveolar damage. Arch Pathol Lab Med 2002: 126(9): 1064–70.

86. Hunninghake G, Fauci A. Pulmonary involvement in the collagen vascular diseases. Am Rev Respir Dis 1979; 119: 471–503.

87. Yousem S, Colby T, Carrington C. Lung biopsy in rheumatoid arthritis. Am Rev Respir Dis 1985; 131: 770–777.

88. Sahn S. The pleura. Am Rev Respir Dis 1988; 138: 184–234.

89. Matthay R, Schwarz M, Petty T, et al. Pulmonary manifestations of systemic lupus erythematosus: review of twelve cases with acute lupus pneumonitis. Medicine 1974; 54: 397–409.

90. Myers JL, Katzenstein AA. Microangiitis in lupus-induced pulmonary hemorrhage. Am J Clin Pathol 1986; 85(5): 552–556.

91. Tazelaar HD, Viggiano RW, Pickersgill J, et al. Interstitial lung disease in polymyositis and dermatomyositis. Clinical features and prognosis as correlated with histologic findings. Am Rev Respir Dis 1990; 141(3): 727–733.

92. Albelda SM, Gefter WB, Epstein DM, et al. Diffuse pulmonary hemorrhage: a review and classification. Radiology 1984; 154: 289–297.

93. Colby TV, Fukuoka J, Ewaskow SP, et al. Pathologic approach to pulmonary hemorrhage. Ann Diagn Pathol 2001; 5(5): 309–319.

94. Miller R. Diffuse pulmonary hemorrhage. In: Pathology of the lung. 2nd edn. Churg A, ed. New York: Thieme Medical Publishers; 1995: 365–373.

95. Leatherman J, Davies S, Hoida J. Alveolar hemorrhage syndromes: diffuse microvascular lung hemorrhage in immune and idiopathic disorders. Medicine (Baltimore) 1984; 63: 343–361.

96. Leatherman J. Immune alveolar hemorrhage. Chest 1987; 91: 891–897.

97. Wilson CB. Recent advances in the immunological aspects of renal disease. Fed Proc 1977; 36(8): 2171–2175.

98. Young KJ. Pulmonary-renal syndromes. Clin Chest Med 1989; 10: 655–672.

99. Travis WD, Colby TV, Lombard C, et al. A clinicopathologic study of 34 cases of diffuse pulmonary hemorrhage with lung biopsy confirmation. Am J Surg Pathol 1990; 14(12): 1112–1125.

100. Kahn F, Jones J, England D, et al. Diagnosis of pulmonary hemorrhage in the immunocompromised host. Am Rev Respir Dis 1987; 136: 155–160.

101. Martinez A, Maltby J, Hurst D. Thrombotic thrombocytopenic purpura seen as pulmonary hemorrhage. Arch Intern Med 1983; 143: 1818–1822.

102. Cordonnier C, Bernaudin JF, Bierling P, et al. Pulmonary complications occurring after allogeneic bone marrow transplantation: a study of 130 consecutive transplanted patients. Cancer 1986; 58: 1047–1054.

103. Gillett D, Ford G. Drug-induced lung disease. In: Abell M, ed. The lung structure, function and disease. Baltimore: Williams & Wilkins; 1978: 21–42.

104. Myers JL. Diagnosis of drug reactions in the lung. Monogr Pathol 1993; 36: 32–53.

105. Sovijarvi A, Lemola M, Stenius B. Nitrofurantoin-induced acute, subacute and chronic pulmonary reactions. Scand J Respir Dis, 1977; 58: 41–50

106. Cooper J, White D, Mathay R. Drug-induced pulmonary disease (Parts 1 and 2). Am Rev Respir Dis 1986; 133: 321–338; 488–502.

107. Bone RC, Wolfe J, Sobonya RE, et al. Desquamative interstitial pneumonia following chronic nitrofurantoin therapy. Chest 1976; 69(suppl 2): 296–297.

108. Lundgren R, Back O, Wiman L. Pulmonary lesions and autoimmune reactions after long-term nitrofurantoin treatment. Scand J Respir Dis 1975; 56: 208–216.

109. Yousem SA, Lohr RH, Colby TV. Idiopathic bronchiolitis obliterans organizing pneumonia/cryptogenic organizing pneumonia with unfavorable outcome: pathologic predictors. Mod Pathol 1997; 10(9): 864–871.

110. Padley S, Adler B, Hansell D, et al. High resolution computed tomography of drug induced lung disease. Clin Radiol 1992; 46: 232–236.

111. Camus PH, Foucher P, Bonniaud PH, et al. Drug-induced infiltrative lung disease. Eur Respir J Suppl 2001; 32: 93s–100s.

112. Holoye P, Luna M, MacKay B, et al. Bleomycin hypersensitivity pneumonitis. Ann Intern Med 1978; 8: 47–49.

113. Borzone G, Moreno R, Urrea R, et al. Bleomycin-induced chronic lung damage does not resemble human idiopathic pulmonary fibrosis. Am J Respir Crit Care Med 2001; 163(7): 1648–1653.

114. Samuels M, Johnson D, Holoye P, et al. Large-dose bleomycin therapy and pulmonary toxicity. A possible role of prior radiotherapy. JAMA 1976; 235: 1117–1120.

115. Adamson I, Bowden D. The pathogenesis of bleomycin-induced pulmonary fibrosis in mice. Am J Pathol 1974; 77: 185–198.

116. Clarysse AM, Cathey WJ, Cartwright GE, et al. Pulmonary disease complicating intermittent therapy with methotrexate. JAMA 1969; 209: 1861–1864.

117. Imokawa S, Colby TV, Leslie KO, et al. Methotrexate pneumonitis: review of the literature and histopathological findings in nine patients. Eur Respir J 2000; 15(2): 373–381.

118. Siegel H. Human pulmonary pathology associated with narcotic and other addictive drugs. Hum Pathol 1972; 3: 55–70.

119. Rosenow E. Drug-induced pulmonary disease. Clin Notes Respir Dis 1977; 16: 3–12.

120. Davis P, Burch R. Pulmonary edema and salicylate intoxication (letter). Ann Intern Med 1974; 80: 553–554.

121. Abid SH, Malhotra V, Perry M. Radiation-induced and chemotherapy-induced pulmonary injury. Curr Opin Oncol 2001; 13(4): 242–248.

122. Bennett DE, Million PR, Ackerman LV. Bilateral radiation pneumonitis a complication of the radiotherapy of bronchogenic carcinoma (A report and analysis of seven cases with autopsy). Cancer 1969; 23: 1001–1018.

123. Phillips T, Wharham M, Margolis L. Modification of radiation injury to normal tissues by chemotherapeutic agents. Cancer 1975; 35: 1678–1684.

124. Roswit B, White D. Severe radiation injuries of the lung. AJR 1977; 129: 127–136.

125. Fujita J, Bandoh S, Ohtsuki Y, et al. The role of anti-epithelial cell antibodies in the pathogenesis of bilateral radiation pneumonitis caused by unilateral thoracic irradiation. Respir Med 2000; 94(9): 875–880.

126. Katzenstein A, Myers J, Mazur M. Acute interstitial pneumonia: a clinicopathologic, ultrastructural, and cell kinetic study. Am J Surg Pathol 1986; 10: 256–267.

127. Johkoh T, Muller NL, Cartier Y, et al. Idiopathic interstitial pneumonias: diagnostic accuracy of thin-section CT in 129 patients. Radiology 1999; 211(2): 555–560.

128. Primack S, Hartman T, Ikezoe J, et al. Acute interstitial pneumonia: radiographic and CT findings in nine patients. Radiology 1993; 188: 817–820.

129. Pratt D, Schwartz M, May J, et al. Rapidly fatal pulmonary fibrosis: the accelerated variant of interstitial pneumonitis. Thorax 1979; 34: 587–593.

130. Hamman L, Rich A. Acute diffuse interstitial fibrosis of the lungs. Bull Johns Hopkins Hosp 1944; 74: 177–214.

131. Walker W, Wright V. Rheumatoid pleuritis. Ann Rheum Dis 1967; 26: 467–473.

132. Frank S, Weg J, Harkleroad L, et al. Pulmonary dysfunction in rheumatoid disease. Chest 1973; 63: 27–34.

133. Laitinen O, Nissila M, Salorinne Y, et al. Pulmonary involvement in patients with rheumatoid arthritis. Scand J Respir Dis 1975; 56: 297–304.

134. Portner M, Gracie W. Rheumatoid lung disease with cavitary nodules, pneumothorax, and eosinophilia. N Engl J Med 1966; 275: 697–700.

135. Ondrasik M. Caplan's syndrome. Baillieres Clin Rheumatol 1989; 3(1): 205–210.

136. Harrison N, Myers A, Corrin B, et al. Structural features of interstitial lung disease in systemic sclerosis. Am Rev Respir Dis 1991; 144: 706–713.

137. Kim DS, Yoo B, Lee JS, et al. The major histopathologic pattern of pulmonary fibrosis in scleroderma is nonspecific interstitial pneumonia. Sarcoidosis Vasc Diffuse Lung Dis 2002; 19(2): 121–127.

138. Yousem SA. The pulmonary pathologic manifestations of the CREST syndrome. Hum Pathol 1990; 21(5): 467–474.

139. MacGregor AJ, Canavan R, Knight C, et al. Pulmonary hypertension in systemic sclerosis: risk factors for progression and consequences for survival. Rheumatology (Oxford) 2001; 40(4): 453–459.

140. Kawut SM, Taichman DB, Archer-Chicko CL, et al. Hemodynamics and survival in patients with pulmonary arterial hypertension related to systemic sclerosis. Chest 2003; 123(2): 344–350.

141. Wiener-Kronish J, Solinger A, Warnock M, et al. Severe pulmonary involvement in mixed connective tissue disease. Am Rev Respir Dis 1981; 124: 499–503.

142. Gammon R, Bridges T, Al-Nezir H, et al. Bronchiolitis obliterans organizing pneumonia associated with systemic lupus erythematosus. Chest 1992; 102: 1171–1174.

143. Kim JS, Lee KS, Koh EM, et al. Thoracic involvement of systemic lupus erythematosus: clinical, pathologic, and radiologic findings. J Comput Assist Tomogr 2000; 24(1): 9–18.

144. Lamblin C, Bergoin C, Saelens T, et al. Interstitial lung diseases in collagen vascular diseases. Eur Respir J Suppl 2001; 32: 69s–80s.

145. Bourke SJ, Dalphin JC, Boyd G, et al. Hypersensitivity pneumonitis: current concepts. Eur Respir J Suppl 2001; 32: 81s–92s.

146. Coleman A, Colby TV. Histologic diagnosis of extrinsic allergic alveolitis. Am J Surg Pathol 1988; 12(7): 514–518.

147. Pepys J, Jenkins P. Precipitin (FLH) test in farmer's lung. Thorax 1965; 20: 21–35.

148. Hansell D, Wells A, Padley S, et al. Hypersensitivity pneumonitis: correlation of individual CT patterns with functional abnormalities. Radiology 1996; 199: 123–128.

149. Adler BD, Padley SPG, Müller NL, et al. Chronic hypersensitivity pneumonitis: high resolution CT and radiographic features in 16 patients. Radiology 1992; 185: 91–95.

150. Silver S, Müller N, Miller R, et al. Computed tomography in hypersensitivity pneumonitis. Radiology 1989; 173: 441–445.

151. Reyes C, Wenzel F, Lawton B, et al. Pulmonary pathology in farmers' lung. Chest 1982; 81: 142–146.

152. Moore V, Fink J, Barboriak J, et al. Immunologic events in pigeon breeders' disease. J Allergy Clin Immunol 1974; 53: 319–327.

153. Fink JN, Banaszak EF, Thiede WH, et al. Interstitial pneumonitis due to hypersensitivity to an organism contaminating a heating system. Ann Intern Med 1971; 74: 80–85.

154. Salvaggio J, Arquembourg G, Seabury J, et al. Bagassosis IV precipitins against extracts of thermophilic actinomycetes in patients with bagassosis. JAMA 1969; 46: 538–543.

155. Nicholls P, Nicholls G, Bouhuys A. Histamine release by compound 48/80 and textile dust from lung tissue in vitro. In: Davies C, ed. Inhaled particles and vapors 2nd edn. Oxford: Pergamon Press; 1967: 69–74.

156. Ruttner J, Spycher M, Engeler M. Pulmonary fibrosis induced by cotton fibre inhalation. Pathol Microbiol 1968; 32: 1–9.

157. Carrington CB, Gaensler EA, Mikus JP, et al. Structure and function in sarcoidosis. Ann NY Acad Sci 1977; 278: 265–283.

158. Hunninghake G. Staging of pulmonary sarcoidosis. Chest 1986; 89: 178S–180S.

159. Daniele R, Rossman M, Kern J, et al. Pathogenesis of sarcoidosis. Chest 1986; 89: 174S–177S.

160. Sharma OP, Alam S. Diagnosis, pathogenesis, and treatment of sarcoidosis. Curr Opin Pulm Med 1995; 1(5): 392–400.

161. Moller DR. Cells and cytokines involved in the pathogenesis of sarcoidosis. Sarcoidosis Vasc Diffuse Lung Dis 1999; 16(1): 24–31.

162. Johnson B, Duncan S, Ohori N, et al. Recurrence of sarcoidosis in pulmonary allograft recipients. Am Rev Respir Dis 1993; 148: 1373–1377.

163. Martinez FJ, Orens JB, Deeb M, et al. Recurrence of sarcoidosis following bilateral allogeneic lung transplantation. Chest 1994; 106(5): 1597–1599.

164. Judson MA. Lung transplantation for pulmonary sarcoidosis. Eur Respir J 1998; 11(3): 738–744.

165. Müller NL, Kullnig P, Miller RR. The CT findings of pulmonary sarcoidosis: analysis of 25 patients. AJR Am J Roentgenol 1989; 152(6): 1179–1182.

166. McLoud T, Epler G, Gaensler E, et al. A radiographic classification of sarcoidosis: physiologic correlation. Invest Radiol 1982; 17: 129–138.

167. Müller N, Kullnig P, Miller R. The CT findings of sarcoidosis: analysis of 25 patients. AJR 1989; 152: 1179–1182.

168. Lynch D, Webb W, Gamsu G, et al. Computed tomography in pulmonary sarcoidosis. J Comput Assist Tomogr 1989; 13: 405–410.

169. Brauner MW, Grenier P, Mompoint D, et al. Pulmonary sarcoidosis: evaluation with high resolution CT. Radiology 1989; 172: 467–471.

170. Judd PA, Finnegan P, Curran RC. Pulmonary sarcoidosis: a clinicopathological study. J Pathol 1975; 115: 191–198.

171. Rosen Y, Athanassiades T, Moon S, et al. Non-granulomatous interstitial inflammation in sarcoidosis: Relationship to development of epithelioid granulomas. Chest 1978; 74: 122–125.

172. Takemura T, Hiraga Y, Oomechi M, et al. Ultrastructural features of alveolitis in sarcoidosis. Am J Respir Crit Care Med 1995; 152: 367–373.

173. Liebow A. The J Burns Amberson lecture. Pulmonary angiitis and granulomatosis. Am Rev Respir Dis 1973; 108: 1–18.

174. Marchevsky A, Damsker B, Gribetz A, et al. The spectrum of pathology of nontuberculous mycobacterial infections in open lung biopsy specimens. Am J Clin Pathol 1982; 78: 695–700.

175. Khoor A, Leslie KO, Tazelaar HD, et al. Diffuse pulmonary disease caused by nontuberculous mycobacteria in immunocompetent people (hot tub lung). Am J Clin Pathol 2001; 115(5): 755–762.

176. Carrington CB, Addington WW, Goff AM, et al. Chronic eosinophilic pneumonia. Engl J Med 1969; 280: 787–798.

177. Liebow A, Carrington C. The eosinophilic pneumonias. Medicine (Baltimore) 1969; 48: 251–285.

178. Gaensler E, Carrington C. Peripheral opacities in chronic eosinophilic pneumonia. The photographic negative of pulmonary edema. AJR 1977; 128: 1–13.

179. Mayo J, Müller N, Road J, et al. Chronic eosinophilic pneumonia: CT findings in six cases. AJR 1989; 153: 727–730.

180. Liebow AA. Definition and classification of interstitial pneumonias in human pathology. Prog Respir Res 1975; 8: 1–31.

181. Mapel DW, Hunt WC, Utton R, et al. Idiopathic pulmonary fibrosis: survival in population based and hospital based cohorts. Thorax 1998; 53(6): 469–476.

182. Genereux G. The end-stage lung: pathogenesis, pathology, and radiology. Radiology 1975; 116: 279–289.

183. Müller N, Miller R, Webb W, et al. Fibrosing alveolitis: CT-pathologic correlation. Radiology 1986; 160: 585–588.

184. Staples C, Müller N, Vedal S, et al. Usual interstitial pneumonia: correlations of CT with clinical, functional and radiologic findings. Radiology 1987; 162: 377–381.

185. Müller NL, Staples CA, Miller RR, et al. Disease activity in idiopathic pulmonary fibrosis: CT and pathologic correlation. Radiology 1987; 165(3): 731–734.

186. Leung A, Miller R, Müller N. Parenchymal opacification in chronic infiltrative lung diseases: CT-pathologic correlation. Radiology 1993; 188: 209–214.

187. Remy-Jardin M, Giraud F, Remy J, et al. Importance of ground glass attenuation in chronic diffuse infiltrative lung disease: pathologic-CT correlation. Radiology 1993; 189: 693–698.

188. Ostrow D, Cherniack R. Resistance to airflow in patients with diffuse interstitial lung disease. Am Rev Respir Dis 1973; 108: 205–210.

189. Bjoraker JA, Ryu JH, Edwin MK, et al. Prognostic significance of histopathologic subsets in idiopathic pulmonary fibrosis. Am J Respir Crit Care Med 1998; 157(1): 199–203.

190. Katzenstein A, Fiorelli R. Nonspecific interstitial pneumonia/fibrosis: histologic features and clinical significance. Am J Surg Pathol 1994; 18: 136–147.

191. Johkoh T, Müller N, Ichikado K, et al. Nonspecific interstitial pneumonia: correlation between thin-section CT findings and pathologic subgroups in 55 patients. Radiology 2002; 225: 199–204.

192. Cottin V, Donsbeck AV, Revel D, et al. Nonspecific interstitial pneumonia. Individualization of a clinicopathologic entity in a series of 12 patients. Am J Respir Crit Care Med 1998; 158(4): 1286–1293.

193. Daniil ZD, Gilchrist FC, Nicholson AG, et al. A histologic pattern of nonspecific interstitial pneumonia is associated with a better prognosis than usual interstitial pneumonia in patients with cryptogenic fibrosing alveolitis. Am J Respir Crit Care Med 1999; 160(3): 899–905.

194. Kim T, Lee K, Chung M, et al. Nonspecific interstitial pneumonia with fibrosis: high resolution CT and pathologic findings. Roentgenol 1998; 171: 949–953.

195. Nagai S, Kitaichi M, Itoh H, et al. Idiopathic nonspecific interstitial pneumonia/fibrosis: comparison with idiopathic pulmonary fibrosis and BOOP. Eur Respir J 1998; 12(5): 1010–1019.

196. Park J, Lee K, Kim J, et al. Nonspecific interstitial pneumonia with fibrosis: radiographic and CT findings in 7 patients. Radiology 1995; 195: 645–648.

197. Hartman TE, Swensen SJ, Hansell DM, et al. Nonspecific interstitial pneumonia: variable appearance at high-resolution chest CT. Radiology 2000; 217(3): 701–705.

198. Travis WD, Matsui K, Moss J, et al. Idiopathic nonspecific interstitial pneumonia: prognostic significance of cellular and fibrosing patterns: survival comparison with usual interstitial pneumonia and desquamative interstitial pneumonia. Am J Surg Pathol 2000; 24(1): 19–33.

199. Liebow A, Steer A, Billingsley J. Desquamative interstitial pneumonia. Am J Med 1965; 39: 369–404.

200. Farr G, Harley R, Henningar G. Desquamative interstitial pneumonia. An electron microscopic study. Am J Pathol 1970; 60: 347–354.

201. Katzenstein AL, Myers JL. Idiopathic pulmonary fibrosis: clinical relevance of pathologic classification. Am J Respir Crit Care Med 1998; 157(4 Pt 1): 1301–1315.

202. Hartman TE, Primack SL, Swensen SJ, et al. Desquamative interstitial pneumonia: thin-section CT findings in 22 patients. Radiology 1993; 187(3): 787–790.

203. Yousem S, Colby T, Gaensler E. Respiratory bronchiolitis and its relationship to desquamative interstitial pneumonia. Mayo Clin Proc 1989; 64: 1373–1380.

204. Patchefsky A, Israel H, Hock W, et al. Desquamative interstitial pneumonia: relationship to interstitial fibrosis. Thorax 1973; 28: 680–693.

205. Carrington C, Gaensler EA, Coutu RE, et al. Natural history and treated course of usual and desquamative interstitial pneumonia. N Engl J Med 1978; 298: 801–809.

206. Corrin B, Price AB. Electron microscopic studies in desquamative interstitial pneumonia associated with asbestos. Thorax 1972; 27: 324–331.

207. Coates EO, Watson JHL. Diffuse interstitial lung disease in tungsten carbide workers. Ann Intern Med 1971; 75: 709–716.

208. McCann B, Brewer D. A case of desquamative interstitial pneumonia progressing to "honeycomb lung." J Pathol 1974; 112: 199–202.

209. Carrington CB, Gaensler EA, Coutu RE, et al. Natural history and treated course of usual and desquamative interstitial pneumonia. N Engl J Med 1978; 298(15): 801–809.

210. Liebow AA, Carrington CB. Diffuse pulmonary lymphoreticular infiltrations associated with dysproteinemia. Med Clin North Am 1973; 57: 809–843.

211. Johkoh T, Müller N, Pickford H, et al. Lymphocytic interstitial pneumonia: thin-section CT findings in 22 patients. Radiology 1999; 212: 567–572.

212. Colby TV, Carrington CB. Lymphoreticular tumors and infiltrates of the lung. Pathol Annu 1983; 18 Pt 1: 27–70.

213. Joshi V, Oleske J. Pulmonary lesions in children with the acquired immunodeficiency syndrome: a reappraisal based on data in additional cases and follow-up study of previously reported cases. Hum Pathol 1986; 17: 641–642.

214. Joshi V, Oleske J, Minnefor A, et al. Pathologic pulmonary findings in children with the acquired immunodeficiency syndrome. Hum Pathol 1985; 16: 241–246.

215. Solal-Celigny P, Coudere L, Herman D, et al. Lymphoid interstitial pneumonitis in acquired immunodeficiency syndrome-related complex. Am Rev Respir Dis 1985; 131: 956–960.

216. Grieco M, Chinoy-Acharya P. Lymphoid interstitial pneumonia associated with the acquired immune deficiency syndrome. Am Rev Respir Dis 1985; 131: 952–955.

217. Saldana M, Mones J. Lymphoid interstitial pneumonia in HIV infected individuals. Prog Surg Pathol 1991; 12: 181–215.

218. Julsrud P, Brown L, Li C-Y, et al. Pulmonary processes of mature-appearing lymphocytes: pseudolymphoma, well-differentiated lymphocytic lymphoma, and lymphocytic interstitial pneumonitis. Radiology 1978; 127: 289–296.

219. Davison A, Heard B, McAllister W, et al. Cryptogenic organizing pneumonitis. Q J Med 1983; 52: 382–394.

220. Epler GR, Colby TV, McLoud TC, et al. Bronchiolitis obliterans organizing pneumonia. N Engl J Med 1985; 312(3): 152–158.

221. Guerry-Force M, Müller N, Wright J, et al. A comparison of bronchiolitis obliterans with organizing pneumonia, usual interstitial pneumonia and small airways disease. Am Rev Respir Dis 1987; 135: 705–712.

222. Katzenstein A, Myers J, Prophet W, et al. Bronchiolitis obliterans and usual interstitial pneumonia. A comparative clinicopathologic study. Am J Surg Pathol 1986; 10: 373–376.

223. King TJ, Mortensen R. Cryptogenic organizing pneumonitis. Chest 1992; 102: 8S–13S.

224. Yoshinouchi T, Ohtsuki Y, Kubo K, et al. Clinicopathological study on two types of cryptogenic organizing pneumonia. Respir Med 1995; 89: 271–278.

225. Müller NL, Guerry-Force ML, Staples CA, et al. Differential diagnosis of bronchiolitis obliterans with organizing pneumonia and usual interstitial pneumonia: clinical, functional, and radiologic findings. Radiology 1987; 162(1 Pt 1): 151–156.

226. Chandler PW, Shin MS, Friedman SE, et al. Radiographic manifestations of bronchiolitis obliterans with organizing pneumonia vs usual interstitial pneumonia. AJR 1986; 147(5): 899–906.

227. Möller N, Guerry-Force M, Staples C, et al. Differential diagnosis of bronchiolitis obliterans with organizing pneumonia and usual interstitial pneumonia. Clinical, functional and radiologic findings. Radiology 1987; 162: 151–156.

228. Müller N, Staples C, Miller R. Bronchiolitis organizing pneumonia. CT features in 14 patients. AJR 1990; 154: 983–987.

229. Nishimura K, Itoh H. High-resolution computed tomographic features of bronchiolitis obliterans organizing pneumonia. Chest 1992; 102: 26S–31S.

230. Bouchardy LM, Kuhlman JE, Ball WC, et al. CT findings in bronchiolitis obliterans organizing pneumonia (BOOP) with radiographic, clinical, and histologic correlation. J Comput Assist Tomogr 1993; 17: 352–357.

231. Lee K, Kullnig P, Hartman T, et al. Cryptogenic organizing pneumonia. CT findings in 43 patients. AJR 1994; 62: 543–546.

232. Myers JL, Colby TV. Pathologic manifestations of bronchiolitis, constrictive bronchiolitis, cryptogenic organizing pneumonia, and diffuse panbronchiolitis. Clin Chest Med 1993; 14(4): 611–622.

233. Camp M, Mehta JB, Whitson M. Bronchiolitis obliterans and *Nocardia asteroides* infection of the lung. Chest 1987; 92: 1107–1108.

234. Camus P, Lombard JN, Perichon M, et al. Bronchiolitis obliterans organizing pneumonia in patients taking acebutol or amiodarone. Thorax 1989; 44: 711–715.

235. Cohen AJ, King TEJ, Downey GP. Rapidly progressive bronchiolitis obliterans with organizing pneumonia. Am J Respir Crit Care Med 1994; 149: 1670–1675.

236. Churg A, Green FHY. Pathology of occupational lung disease. In: Green F, ed. New York: Igaku-Shoin; 1987.

237. Parkes W. Occupational lung disorders. London: Butterworths-Heineman; 1994.

238. Morgan WKC, Seaton A (eds). Occupational lung diseases, 2nd edition. Philadelphia: WB Saunders; 1984.

239. Churg A, Green FHY. Occupational lung disease. In: Churg AM, ed. Pathology of the lung. New York: Thieme Medical; 1995: 851–929.

240. Hendry N. The geology, occurrences and major uses of asbestos. Ann NY Acad Sci 1965; 132: 12–22.

241. Gaze R. The physical and molecular structure of asbestos. Ann NY Acad Sci 1965; 132: 23–30.

242. Wright J, Churg A. Morphology of small-airway lesions in patients with asbestos exposure. Hum Pathol 1984; 14: 68–74.

243. Gaensler E. Pathological, physiological and radiological correlations in the pneumoconioses. Ann NY Acad Sci 1972; 200: 574–607.

244. Kipen H, Lilis R, Suzuki Y, et al. Pulmonary fibrosis in asbestos insulation workers with lung cancer: a radiological and histopathological evaluation. Br J Ind Med 1987; 44: 96–100.

245. Aberle DR, Gamsu G, Ray CS, et al. Asbestos-related pleural and parenchymal fibrosis: detection with high-resolution CT. Radiology 1988; 166: 729–734.

246. Friedman A, Fiel S, Fisher M, et al. Asbestos-related pleural disease and asbestos: a comparison of CT and chest radiography. AJR 1988; 150: 269–275.

247. Staples C, Gamsu G, Ray C, et al. High resolution computed tomography and lung function in asbestos-exposed workers with normal chest radiographs. Am Rev Respir Dis 1989; 139: 1502–1508.

248. Ashcroft T, Heppleston AG. The optical and electron microscopic determination of pulmonary asbestos fiber concentration and its relations to the human pathological reaction. J Clin Pathol 1973; 26: 224–234.

249. Gough J. Differential diagnosis in the pathology of asbestosis. Ann NY Acad Sci 1965; 132: 368–372.

250. Gaensler E, Kaplin A. Asbestos pleural effusion. Ann Intern Med 1971; 74: 178–191.

251. UICC Committee. Cincinnati classification of the radiographic appearance of the pneumoconioses. A cooperative study of the UICC committee. Chest 1970; 58: 57–65.

252. Begin R, Ostiguy G, Fillon R, et al. Computed tomography scan in the early detection of silicosis. Am Rev Respir Dis 1991; 144: 697–705.

253. Bergin CJ, Müller NL, Vedal S, et al. CT in silicosis: correlation with plain films and pulmonary function tests. AJR 1986; 146: 477–483.

254. Kinsella M, Müller N, Vedal S, et al. Emphysema in silicosis: a comparison of smokers and nonsmokers using pulmonary function testing and computed tomography. Am Rev Respir Dis 1990; 141: 1497–1500.

255. Snider D. The relationship between tuberculosis and silicosis. Am Rev Respir Dis 1978; 118: 455–460.

256. Aronchik JM, Rossman MD, Miller WT. Chronic beryllium disease: diagnosis, radiographic findings, and correlation with pulmonary function tests. Radiology 1987; 163: 677–678.

257. Newman L, Buschman D, Newell J, et al. Beryllium disease: assessment with CT. Radiology 1994; 190: 835–840.

258. Matilla A, Galera H, Pascual E, et al. Chronic berylliosis. Br J Dis. Chest 1973; 67: 308–314.

259. Sokolowski J, Cordray D, Cantow E, et al. Giant cell interstitial pneumonia. A report of a case. Am Rev Respir Dis 1972; 105: 417–420.

260. Ohori N, Sciurba F, Owens G, et al. Giant-cell interstitial pneumonia and hard-metal pneumoconiosis. A clinicopathologic study of four cases and review of the literature. Am J Surg Pathol 1989; 13(7): 581–587.

261. Abraham JL, Hertzburg MA. Exposure to hard metal (letter). Chest 1985; 87: 554.

262. Frost A, Keller C, Brown R, et al. Giant cell interstitial pneumonitis: disease recurrence in the transplanted lung. Am Rev Respir Dis 1993; 148: 1401–1404.

263. Barberii M, Harari S, Tironi A, et al. Recurrence of primary disease in a single lung recipient. Transplant Proc 1992; 24: 2660–2662.

264. Hogg J, Macklem P, Thurlbeck W. Site and nature of airway obstruction in chronic obstructive lung disease. N Engl J Med 1968; 278: 1355–1360.

265. Epler G. Diseases of the bronchioles. New York: Raven Press; 1994.

266. Thurlbeck W. Chronic airflow obstruction. In: Petty TL, ed. Correlation of structure and function in chronic obstructive pulmonary disease. 2nd edn. New York: Marcel Dekker; 1985: 129–203.

267. Horvath E, DoPico G, Barbee R, et al. Nitrogen dioxide-induced pulmonary disease. J Occup Med 1978; 20: 103–110.

268. Woodford DM, Coutu RE, Gaensler E. Obstructive lung disease from acute sulphur-dioxide exposure. Respiration 1979; 38: 238–245.

269. Close LG, Catlin FI, Gohn AM. Acute and chronic effects of ammonia burns of the respiratory tract. Arch Otolaryngol 1980; 106: 151–158.

270. Becroft DMO. Bronchiolitis obliterans, bronchiectasis and other sequelae of adenovirus type 21 infection in young children. J Clin Pathol 1971; 24: 72-79.

271. Edwards C, Penny M, Newman J. Mycoplasma pneumonia, Stevens-Johnson syndrome and chronic obliterative bronchiolitis. Thorax 1983; 38: 867–869.

272. Geddes D, Corrin B, Brewerton D, et al. Progressive airway obliteration in adults and its association with rheumatoid disease. Q J Med 1977; 46: 427–444.

273. Iwata M, Colby TV, Kitaichi M. Diffuse panbronchiolitis: diagnosis and distinction from various pulmonary diseases with centrilobular interstitial foam cell accumulations. Hum Pathol 1994; 25(4): 357–363.

274. Randhawa P, Hoagland M, Yousem S. Diffuse panbronchiolitis in North America. Am J Surg Pathol 1991; 15: 43–47.

275. Baz MA, Kussin PS, Davis RD, et al. Recurrence of diffuse panbronchiolitis after lung transplantation. Am J Respir Crit Care Med 1995; 151: 895–898.

276. Keicho N, Ohashi J, Tamiya G, et al. Fine localization of a major disease-susceptibility locus for diffuse panbronchiolitis. Am J Hum Genet 2000; 66(2): 501–507.

277. Akira M, Kitani F, Yong-Sik L, et al. Diffuse panbronchiolitis: evaluation with high-resolution CT. Radiology 1988; 168: 433–438.

278. Nishimura K, Kitaichi M, Izumi T, et al. Usual interstitial pneumonia: histologic correlation with high-resolution CT. Radiology 1992; 182(2): 337–342.

279. Krowka M, Rosenow EI, Hoagland H. Reviews of pulmonary complications of bone marrow transplantation. Chest 1986; 87: 237–246.

280. Ettinger N, Trulock E. Pulmonary considerations of organ transplantation Part 2. Am Rev Respir Dis 1991; 144: 213–223.

281. Yousem S. The histologic spectrum of pulmonary graft-versus-host disease in bone marrow transplant recipients. Hum Pathol 1995; 26: 668–675.

282. Winston D, Ho W, Champlin R. Cytomegalovirus after allogenic bone marrow transplantation. Rev Infect Dis 1992; 12(suppl): S776–S792.

283. Roca J, Granana A, Rodriguez-Roisin R, et al. Fatal airway disease in an adult with chronic graft-versus-host disease. Thorax 1982; 37: 77–78.

284. Ralph D, Springmeyer S, Sullivan K, et al. Rapidly progressive air-flow obstruction in marrow transplant recipients. Possible association between obliterative bronchiolitis and chronic graft-versus-host disease. Am Rev Respir Dis 1984; 129: 641–644.

285. Kurzrock R, Zander A, Kanojia M, et al. Obstructive lung disease after allogenic bone marrow transplantation. Transplantation 1984; 37: 156–160.

286. Johnson F, Stokes D. Chronic obstructive airways disease after bone marrow transplantation. J Pediatr 1984; 105: 370–376.

287. Churg A, Wright JL. Small airways disease and mineral dust exposure. Part 2. Pathol Annu 1983; 18: 233–251.

288. Churg A, Wright JL, Wiggs B, et al. Small airways disease and mineral dust exposure. Am Rev Respir Dis 1985; 131: 139–143.

289. Aguayo SM, Miller YE, Waldron JAJ, et al. Brief report: idiopathic diffuse hyperplasia of pulmonary neuroendocrine cells and airways disease. N Engl J Med 1992; 327: 1285–1288.

290. Miller R, Müller N. Neuroendocrine cell hyperplasia and obliterative bronchiolitis in patients with peripheral carcinoid tumors. Am J Surg Pathol 1995; 19: 653–658.

291. Wynne J, Modell J. Respiratory aspiration of stomach contents. Ann Intern Med 1977; 87: 466–474.

292. Schwartz D, Wynne J, Gibbs C, et al. The pulmonary consequences of aspiration of gastric contents of pH greater than 2.5. Am Rev Respir Dis 1980; 121: 119–126.

293. Eliot C, Colby T, Kelly T, et al. Charcoal lung bronchiolitis obliterans after aspiration of activated charcoal. Chest 1989; 96: 672–674.

294. Obeid M, Bickel J, Ingram E, et al. Pulmonary talc granulomatosis in a cocaine sniffer. Chest 1990; 98: 237–239.

295. Camus P, Colby TV. The lung in inflammatory bowel disease. Eur Respir J 2000; 15(1): 5–10.

296. Kraft S, Earle E, Roesler M, et al. Unexplained bronchopulmonary disease with inflammatory bowel disease. Arch Int Med 1976; 136: 454–459.

297. Higgenbottam T, Cochrane G, Clarke T, et al. Bronchial disease in ulcerative colitis. Thorax 1980; 35: 581–585.

298. Wilcox P, Miller R, Nelems B, et al. Airway involvement in ulcerative colitis. Chest 1987; 92: 18–22.

299. Williams T, Eidus L, Thomas P. Fibrosing alveolitis, bronchiolitis obliterans and sulfalazine therapy. Chest 1982; 81: 766–768.

300. Turton C, Williams G, Green M. Cryptogenic obliterative bronchiolitis in adults. Thorax 1981; 36: 805–810.

301. Kraft M, Mortensen R, Colby T, et al. Cryptogenic constrictive bronchiolitis. A clinicopathologic study. Am Rev Respir Dis 1992; 148: 1093–1101.

302. Edwards C, Cayton R, Bryan R. Chronic transmural bronchiolitis: a nonspecific lesion of small airways. J Clin Pathol 1992; 45: 993–998.

303. Müller N, Miller R. Diseases of the bronchioles: CT and histopathologic findings. Radiology 1995; 196: 3–12.

304. Yousem SA, Colby TV, Carrington CB. Follicular bronchitis/bronchiolitis. Hum Pathol 1985; 16(7): 700–706.

305. Kinane B, Mansell A, Zwerdling R, et al. Follicular bronchitis in the pediatric population. Chest 1993; 104: 1183–1186.

306. Reid L. Reduction in bronchial subdivisions in bronchiectasis. Thorax 1950; 5: 233–247.

307. Yousem SA, Dacic S. Idiopathic bronchio;ocentric interstitial pneumonia. Mod Pathol 2002; 15(11): 1148–1153.

308. Churg A, Myers J, Suarez T, et al; Airway-centered interstitial fibrosis: a distinct form of aggressive diffuse lung disease. Am J Surg Pathol 2004; 28(1): 62–68.

309. Thurlbeck W. Chronic airflow obstruction in lung disease. Philadelphia: WB Saunders; 1976.

310. McDowell E, Barrett L, Harris C, et al. Abnormal cilia in human bronchial epithelium. Arch Pathol Lab Med 1976; 100: 429–436.

311. Verra H, Escudier L, Lebargy F, et al. Ciliary abnormalities in bronchial epithelium of smokers, ex-smokers and nonsmokers. Am J Respir Crit Care Med 1995; 151: 630–634.

312. Primary pulmonary hypertension. In: Executive summary from the world symposium – primary pulmonary hypertension 1998. Evian, France: World Heath Organization; 1998.

313. Burke AP, Farb A, Virmani R. The pathology of primary pulmonary hypertension. Mod Pathol 1991; 4: 269–282.

314. Rich S, Dantzker D, Ayres S, et al. Primary pulmonary hypertension. A national prospective study. Ann Intern Med 1987; 107: 216–223.

315. Pietra G, Edwards W, Kay J, et al. Histopathology of primary pulmonary hypertension. A qualitative and quantitative study of pulmonary blood vessels from 58 patients in the National Heart, Lung, and Blood Institute primary pulmonary hypertension registry. Circulation 1989; 80: 1198–1206.

316. Walcott G, Burchell H, Brown AL. Primary pulmonary hypertension. Am J Med 1970; 49: 70–82.

317. Reid L. The pulmonary circulation: remodeling in growth and disease. The 1978 J. Burns Amberson lecture. Am Rev Respir Dis 1979; 119: 531–534.

318. Wagenvoort C. Lung biopsy specimens in the evaluation of pulmonary vascular disease. Chest 1980; 77: 614–625.

319. Heath D, Edwards J. The pathology of hyperactive pulmonary vascular disease. A description of six grades of structural changes in the pulmonary arteries with special reference to congenital cardiac septal defects. Circulation 1958; 18: 533–547.

320. Wagenvoort C. The pathology of human pulmonary hypertension pattern recognition and specificity. In: Buckner C, ed. The pulmonary circulation in health and disease. San Diego: Academic Press; 1987: 15–25.

321. Wagenvoort C, Wagenvoort N. Primary pulmonary hypertension A pathologic study of the lung vessels in 156 clinically diagnosed cases. Circulation 1970; 42: 1163–1184.

322. Kay J, Smith P, Heath D. Aminorex and the pulmonary circulation. Thorax 1971; 26: 262–270.

323. Kay J, Heath D, Smith P, et al. Fulvine and the pulmonary circulation. Thorax 1971; 26: 249–261.

324. Fishman A. Aminorex to Fen/Phen: an epidemic foretold. Circulation 1999; 99: 156–161.

325. Mehta N, Khan L, Mehta R, et al. HIV-related pulmonary hypertension: analytic review of 131 cases. Chest 2000; 118: 1133–1141.

326. Pellicelli A, Barbaro G, Palmieri F, et al. Primary pulmonary hypertension in HIV patients: a systematic review. Angiology 2001; 51: 31–41.

327. Cool CD, Rai PR, Yeager ME, et al. Expression of human herpesvirus 8 in primary pulmonary hypertension. N Engl J Med 2003; 349(12): 1113–1122.

328. Bull TM, Cool CD, Serls AE, et al. Primary pulmonary hypertension, Castleman's disease and human herpesvirus-8. Eur Respir J 2003; 22(3): 403–407.

329. Wagenvoort C, Wagenvoort N. Pathology of pulmonary hypertension. New York: John Wiley & Sons; 1977.

330. Wagenvoort C, Wagenvoort N. Pulmonary vascular bed: normal anatomy and responses to disease. In: Moser K, ed. Pulmonary vascular diseases: lung biology in health and disease. New York: Marcel Dekker; 1979: 1–110.

331. Carrington CB, Liebow AA. Pulmonary veno-occlusive disease. Hum Pathol 1970; 1: 322–324.

332. Wagenvoort C, Wagenvoort N, Takahashi T. Pulmonary veno-occlusive disease: involvement of pulmonary arteries and review of the literature. Hum Pathol 1985; 16: 1033–1041.

333. Heath D, Scott O, Lynch J. Pulmonary veno-occlusive disease. Thorax 1971; 26: 663–674.

334. Kay J. Vascular disease. In: Churg A, ed. Pathology of the lung. 2nd edn. New York: Thieme Medical Publishers; 1995: 931–1066.

335. Hackman R, Madtes D, Petersen F, et al. Pulmonary veno-occlusive disease following bone marrow transplantation. Transplantation 1989; 47: 989–992.

336. Padley S, Adler B, Staples C, et al. Pulmonary talcosis: CT findings in three cases. Radiology 1993; 186: 125–127.

337. Edwards W, Edwards J. Recent advances in the pathology of the pulmonary vasculature. In: Abell M, ed. The lung, structure, function and disease. Baltimore: Williams & Wilkins; 1978: 235–261.

338. Wagenvoort C, Beetstra A, Spijker J. Capillary haemangiomatosis of the lungs. Histopathology 1978; 2: 401–406.

339. AI-Fawaz IM, AI Mobaireek KF, AI-Suhahaibani M, et al. Pulmonary capillary hemangiomatosis: a case report and review of the literature. Pediatr Pulmonol 1995; 19: 243–248.

340. Masur Y, Remberger K, Hoefer M. Pulmonary capillary hemangiomatosis as a rare cause of pulmonary hypertension. Pathol Res Pract 1996; 192: 290–295.

341. White C, Sondheimer H, Crouch E, et al. Treatment of pulmonary hemangiomatosis with interferon alpha-2a. N Engl J Med 1989; 320: 1197–1200.

342. Bennett L, Keck B, Hertz M, et al. Worldwide thoracic organ transplantation: a report from the UNOS/ISHLT international registry for thoracic organ transplantation. Clin Transpl 2001; 1: 25–40.

343. Griffith B, Paradis H, Zeevi A, et al. Immunologically-mediated disease of the airways after pulmonary transplantation. Ann Surg 1988; 208: 371–378.

344. Ettinger N, Trulock E. State of the art pulmonary considerations of organ transplantation Part 3. Am Rev Respir Dis 1991; 144: 433–451.

345. Griffith B, Hardesty R, Armitage J, et al. Acute rejection of lung allografts with various immunosuppressive protocols. Ann Thorac Surg 1992; 54: 846–851.

346. Chaparro C, Maurer JR, Chamberlain DW, et al. Role of open lung biopsy in lung transplant recipients: ten-year experience. Ann Thorac Surg 1995; 59: 928–932.

347. Yousem S, Berry G, Brunt E, et al. A working formulation for the standardization of nomenclature in the diagnosis of heart and lung rejection. Lung Rejection Study Group. J Heart Transplant 1990; 9: 593–601.

348. Yousem S. Lymphocytic bronchitis/bronchiolitis in lung allograft recipients. Am J Surg Pathol 1993; 17: 491–496.

349. Kramer M. Topical review of bronchiolitis obliterans following heart-lung and lung transplantation. Respir Med 1994; 88: 9–15.

350. Scott J, Fradet G, Smyth R, et al. Prospective study of transbronchial biopsies in the management of heart-lung and single lung transplant patients. J Heart Lung Transplant 1991; 10: 626–637.

351. Cagle PT, Truong LD, Holland VA, et al. Factors contributing to mortality in lung transplant recipients: an autopsy study. Mod Pathol 1989; 2: 85–89.

352. Starnes V, Theodore J, Oyer P, et al. Evaluation of heart-lung transplant recipients with prospective, serial transbronchial biopsies and pulmonary function studies. J Thorac Cardiovasc Surg 1989; 98: 689–690.

353. Starnes V, Theodore Y, Oyer P, et al. Pulmonary infiltrates after heart-lung transplants: evaluation by serial biopsies. J Thorac Cardiovasc Surg 1989; 1998: 945–950.

354. Sibley R, Berry G, Tazelaar H, et al. The role of transbronchial biopsies in the management of lung transplant recipients. J Heart Lung Transplant 1993; 12: 308–324.

355. Ohori N, Iacono A, Grgurich W, et al. The significance of acute bronchitis/bronchiolitis in the lung transplant recipient. Am J Surg Pathol 1994; 18: 1192–1204.

356. Yousem S. Graft eosinophilia in lung transplantation. Hum Pathol 1992; 23: 1172–1177.

357. Yousem S, Duncan S, Griffith B. Interstitial and airspace consolidation tissue reactions in lung transplant recipients. Am J Surg Pathol 1992; 16: 877–884.

358. Milne D, Gascoine A, Ashcroft T, et al. Organizing pneumonia following pulmonary transplantation and the development of obliterative bronchiolitis. Transplantation 1994; 57: 1752–1762.

359. Starnes V, Marshall S, Lewiston N, et al. Heart-lung transplantation in infants, children and adolescents. J Pediatr Surg 1991; 26: 4–11.

360. Scott J, Higgenbottam T, Hutter J, et al. Natural history of chronic rejection in heart-lung transplants. J Heart Transplant 1990; 9: 510–515.

361. Skeens J, Fuhrman C, Yousem S. Bronchiolitis obliterans in heart-lung transplantation patients. AJR 1989; 153: 253–256.

362. Lentz D, Bergin C, Berry G, et al. Diagnosis of bronchiolitis obliterans in heart-lung transplantation: importance of bronchial dilatation on CT. AJR 1992; 159: 463–467.

363. Cagle PT. Lung transplant pathology. In: Churg A, ed. Pathology of the lung. 2nd edn. New York: Thieme Medical Publishers; 1995: 827–849.

364. Burke CM, Theodore J, Dawkins SD, et al. Post-transplant obliterative bronchiolitis and other late sequelae in human heart-lung transplantation. Chest 1984; 86: 824–839.

365. Hutter J, Stewart S, Higgenbottam T, et al. Histologic changes in heart-lung transplants during rejection episodes and at routine biopsy. J Heart Transplant 1988; 7: 440–444.

366. Yousem S, Randhawa P, Locker J, et al. Post-transplant lymphoproliferative disorders in heart-lung transplant recipients. Hum Pathol 1989; 20: 361–369.

367. Ramalingam P, Rybicki L, Smith M, et al. Posttransplant lymphoproliferative disorders in lung transplant patients: The Cleveland Clinic experience. Modern Pathol 2002; 15(6): 647–656.

368. Myers J, Katzenstein A. Wegener's granulomatosis presenting with massive pulmonary hemorrhage and capillaritis. Am J Surg Pathol 1987; 11: 895–898.

369. Yousem S, Colby T, Gaensler E. Respiratory bronchiolitis-associated interstitial lung disease and its relationship to desquamative interstitial pneumonia. Mayo Clin Proc 1989; 64: 1373–1380.

370. Myers J, Veal C, Shin M, et al. Respiratory bronchiolitis causing interstitial lung disease. A clinicopathologic study of six cases. Am Rev Respir Dis 1987; 135: 880–884.

371. Heyneman L, Ward S, Lynch D, et al. Respiratory bronchiolitis, respiratory-bronchiolitis-associated interstitial lung disease, and desquamative interstitial pneumonia: different entities or part of the spectrum of the same disease process? Am J Roentgenol 1999; 173: 1617–1622.

372. Moon J, du Bois RM, Colby TV, et al. Clinical significance of respiratory bronchiolitis on open lung biopsy and its relationship to smoking related interstitial lung disease. Thorax 1999; 54(11): 1009–1014.

373. Vassallo R, Ryu JH, Colby TV, et al. Pulmonary Langerhans'-cell histiocytosis. N Engl J Med 2000; 342(26): 1969–1978.

374. Moore A, Godwin J, Müller N, et al. Pulmonary histiocytosis X: comparison of radiographic and CT findings. Radiology 1989; 172: 249–254.

375. Brody AR, Kanich RE, Graham WG, et al. Cyst wall formation in pulmonary eosinophilic granuloma. Chest 1974; 66: 576–578.

376. Brauner M, Grenier P, Tijani K, et al. Pulmonary Langerhans cell histiocytosis: evolution of lesions on CT scans. Radiology 1997; 204: 497–502.

377. Basset F, Soler P, Wyllie L, et al. Langerhans' cells and lung interstitium. Ann NY Acad Sci 1976; 278: 599–611.

378. Singh G, Katyal S, Bedrossian C, et al. Pulmonary alveolar proteinosis; staining for surfactant apoprotein in alveolar proteinosis and in conditions simulating it. Chest 1983; 83: 82–86.

379. Miller R, Churg A, Hutcheon M, et al. Pulmonary alveolar proteinosis and aluminum dust exposure. Am Rev Respir Dis 1984; 130: 312–315.

380. Bedrossian CWM, Luna MA, Conklin RH, et al. Alveolar proteinosis as a consequence of immunosuppression. A hypothesis based on clinical and pathologic observations. Hum Pathol 1980; 11(5 Suppl): 527–535.

381. Wang B, Stern E, Schmidt R, et al. Diagnosing pulmonary alveolar proteinosis. Chest 1997; 111: 460–466.

382. Davidson J, MacLeod W. Pulmonary alveolar proteinosis. Br J Dis. Chest 1969; 63: 13–16.

383. Murch C, Carr D. Computed tomography appearances of pulmonary alveolar proteinosis. Clin Radiol 1989; 40: 240–243.

384. Godwin J, Müller N, Tagasuki J. Pulmonary alveolar proteinosis: CT findings. Radiology 1989; 169: 609–614.

385. Lee K, Levin D, Webb W, et al. Pulmonary alveolar proteinosis: high resolution CT, chest radiographic, and functional correlations. Chest 1997; 111: 989–995.

386. Claypool W, Roger R, Matuschak G. Update on the clinical diagnosis, management, and pathogenesis of pulmonary alveolar proteinosis (phospholipidosis). Chest 1984; 85: 550–558.

387. Carrington CB, Cugell DW, Gaensler EA, et al. Lymphangioleiomyomatosis: physiologic-pathologic-radiologic correlations. Am Rev Respir Dis 1977; 116: 977–995.

388. Templeton P, McLoud T, Müller N, et al. Pulmonary lymphangioleiomyomatosis: CT and pathologic findings. J Comput Assist Tomogr 1989; 13: 54–57.

389. Kitaichi MNK, Itch H, Izumi T. Pulmonary lymphangioleiomyomatosis: a report of 46 patients including a clinicopathologic study of prognostic factors. Am J Resp Crit Care Med 1995; 151: 527–533.

390. Chu S, Horiba K, Usuki J, et al. Comprehensive evaluation of 35 patients with lymphangioleiomyomatosis. Chest 1999; 115: 1041–1052.

391. Aubry MC, Myers JL, Ryu JH, et al. Pulmonary lymphangioleiomyomatosis in a man. Am J Respir Crit Care Med 2000; 162(2 Pt 1): 749–752.

392. Costello L, Hartman T, Ryu J. High frequency of pulmonary lymphangioleiomyomatosis in women with tuberous sclerosis complex. Mayo Clin Proc 2000; 75: 591–594.

393. Lenoir S, Grenier P, Brauner M, et al. Pulmonary lymphangiomyomatosis and tuberous sclerosis: comparison of radiographic and thin section CT. Radiology 1989; 175: 329–334.

394. Ohori N, Yousem S, Sonmez-Alpan E, et al. Estrogen and progesterone receptors in lymphangioleiomyomatosis, epithelioid hemangioendothelioma, and sclerosing hemangioma of the lung. Am J Clin Pathol 1991; 96(4): 529–535.

395. Muir TE, Leslie KO, Popper H, et al. Micronodular pneumocyte hyperplasia. Am J Surg Pathol 1998; 22(4): 465–472.

396. Taylor JR, Ryu J, Colby TV, et al. Lymphangioleiomyomatosis. Clinical course in 32 patients. N Engl J Med 1990; 323(18): 1254–1260.

397. Heitzman E. The lung: radiologic-pathologic correlations. 2nd vol. St. Louis: CV Mosby; 1984.

398. Munk P, Müller N, Miller R, et al. Pulmonary lymphangitic carcinomatosis: CT and pathologic findings. Radiology 1988; 166: 705–709.

399. Janower M, Blennerhassett J. Lymphangitic spread of metastatic cancer to the lung. A radiologic-pathologic classification. Radiology 1971; 101: 267–273.

400. Stein M, Mayo J, Müller N, et al. Pulmonary lymphangitic spread of carcinoma: appearance on CT scans. Radiology 1987; 162: 371–375.

401. Goldsmith S, Bailey H, Callahan E, et al. Pulmonary metastases from breast carcinoma. Surgery 1967; 94: 483–488.

402. Zerhouni E, Naidich D, Stitik F, et al. Computed tomography of the pulmonary parenchyma. II Interstitial disease. J Thorac Imaging 1985; 1: 54–64.

403. Müller NL, Miller RR. Computed tomography of chronic diffuse infiltrative lung disease (Part 1). Am Rev Respir Dis 1990; 142(5): 1206–1215.

404. Dail D, Hammer S. Pulmonary pathology. 2nd edn. New York: Springer-Verlag; 1994.

405. Miller R, Müller N, Thurlbeck W. Diffuse diseases of the lungs. In: Silverberg S, ed. Silverberg's principles and practice of surgical pathology and cytopathology. Philadelphia: WB Saunders; 1995: 1099–1186.

406. Colby T, Lombard C, Yousem S, et al. Atlas of pulmonary surgical pathology. In: Bordin G, ed. Atlases in diagnostic surgical pathology, vol. 2, Philadelphia: WB Saunders; 1991: 380.

407. Reyes C, Wenzel F, Lawton D, et al. The pulmonary pathology of farmer's lung disease. Chest 1982; 81: 142–151.

408. Travis W, Colby T, Koss M, et al. Non-neoplastic disorders of the lower respiratory tract. In: King D, ed. Atlas of nontumor pathology. Vol. 2. Washington, DC: American Registry of Pathology and the Armed Forces Institute of Pathology: 2002: 939.

409. Yousem S, Berry G, Cagle P, et al. Revision of the 1990 working formulation for the classification of pulmonary allograft rejection: Lung Rejection Study Group. J Heart Lung Transplant 1996; 15(1): 1–15.

Localized diseases of the bronchi and lung

Arthur S. Patchefsky   Hormoz Ehya   Hong Wu

18

This chapter deals primarily with the cytology and histopathology of tumors and tumor-like conditions of the bronchi and lung. The scope of coverage includes only those non-neoplastic conditions that may enter into the differential diagnosis of tumors, but is not encyclopedic and therefore such entities as granulomatous disease, or those infections that may cause localized lung masses are not discussed. Such topics as tuberculosis, fungal infections, parasitic infestations and autoimmune diseases are well reviewed in other resources or elsewhere in this text.

EPIDEMIOLOGY OF LUNG CANCER

Lung cancer was a rare disease until the early 1900s, but is now the most common cancer in the United States and worldwide. In the US, in the year 2002, an estimated 169 400 people (90 200 males and 79 200 females) were diagnosed with lung cancer, and 154 900 people died.[1] The incidence and mortality rates are nearly equivalent because of the high case-fatality rate. Lung cancer is, by far, the leading fatal cancer in both men (31%) and women (25%), compared to prostate (10%), colon and rectum (10% in men and 11% in women) and breast (15%).[2] It began a sharp rise around 1930 in men and in the 1960s in women. Since the early 1950s the disease has become the most common cause of cancer death, rising steadily until 1991 when the mortality rate in men began to decline. In women, the mortality rate has continued to increase. Interestingly, over the years, the incidence by histologic type has significantly changed with adenocarcinoma increased in all race-sex groups.[3]

ETIOLOGY OF LUNG CANCER

The causes of lung cancer can be divided into genetic and environmental. The increased incidence in the 20th century followed the explosive growth of cigarette smoking. In comparison with cigar and pipe smoking, the milder tobacco leaf used for cigarettes and the more acidic smoke lends itself to deeper inhalation. This results in increased deposition and absorption of particles and gases in the lung. Cigarette smoke contains irritants, oxidants, free radicals, and a variety of other toxins and carcinogens. Greater than 400 compounds in cigarette smoke have been identified to be tumorigenic agents.[4] In 1964, the US Surgeon General's report concluded that cigarette smoking caused lung cancer.[5] In the US and other countries where cigarette smoking is common, it is estimated that this accounts for approximately 90% of lung cancer cases.[3] Compared to nonsmokers, the risk of developing lung cancer is increased 10-fold for average smokers and at least 15–25-fold for heavy smokers. The risk increases with both average number of cigarettes smoked and number of years of smoking. The duration of smoking is estimated to increase the lung cancer risk exponentially, which has special implication on assessing the likelihood of having lung cancer in young patients who started smoking early in life.[3,6] The risk also increases with depth of inhalation, the tar content of the cigarette, and early age of smoking initiation.[7] Lung cancer risk begins to fall after smoking cessation, and decreases with increasing years of abstinence. Ten years after quitting, the risk decreases by approximately 50%, but it never returns to that of 'never-smokers.'[8] In many studies, the risk of lung cancer in pipe and cigar smokers is less than cigarette smokers, probably because of less inhalation, related to the harsher and more alkaline smoke. In 1986, the Surgeon General announced passive smoking to be a cause of lung cancer. The Environmental Protection Agency (EPA) estimates that approximately 3000 lung cancer deaths per year in the US can be attributed to passive smoking. Close to one-fourth of lung cancer cases among never-smokers are estimated to be attributable to exposure to passive smoking.[3]

Although cigarette smoking accounts for the majority of lung cancers, a proportion (9–15% in various studies) has been attributed to occupational exposures. The International Agency for Research on Cancer (IARC) has identified over 20 occupational substances as established or suspected lung carcinogens. One of the most common, asbestos, is a group of naturally occurring fibrous materials that in the past was commonly used for insulation, fireproofing, shipbuilding, construction materials, water pipes, brake linings, floors, and textiles. Since the 1950s, numerous epidemiologic studies have established that asbestos exposure independently increases the risk of lung cancer. A study on a cohort of asbestos insulation workers shows that the peak incidence occurs 30 to 35 years after the initial exposure. The risk is dose-dependent in workers with occupational exposure. There is a synergistic and multiplicative effect between tobacco smoking and asbestos. In smokers with asbestos exposure, the lung cancer rate is approximately 50 times that of nonexposed individuals.[3,7,9] Current evidence suggests that the causal relationship is a function of the finding of pulmonary asbestosis and not simply environmental exposure. All histologic tumor types are seen.[10]

Radon is an inert radioactive gas produced by the natural decay of radium. It is present in most soils and rocks in various concentrations and can be found in both indoor and outdoor air. Two of the decay products of radon emit high-energy alpha particles that can enter the lung and cause DNA damage. Epidemiologic studies on underground miners have established a causal relationship to lung cancer. Recent meta-analysis has supported a statistically significant association between indoor radon exposure and lung cancer in the general population, which is estimated to account for up to 10–15% of lung cancers in non-smokers.[3,7,8] Efforts to educate the public on the dangers of radon and the efficacy of indoor radon testing have been earnestly undertaken.[11] Other occupational exposures with an associated increased risk for lung cancer include: arsenic (used in copper smelting, pesticides, veterinary medications, electronic and semiconductor devices), bischloromethyl ether and chloromethyl ether (used in textile and paint industries), cadmium (encountered in electroplating, welding, and smelting), chromium (in chromate pigment production, welding, and chrome plating), nickel sulfides and oxides (in nickel refineries), soot (in chimney sweeps), and vinyl chloride. Limited evidence also exists for carcinogenic effect of acrylonitirile, diesel exhaust, and crystalline silica.[3,7,8] Four large prospective cohort studies suggest that air pollution increases the incidence of lung cancer.[7]

Since only 10–15% of smokers develop lung cancer, host factors other than environmental exposures must influence the development of lung cancer. Studies have shown that female in comparison with male never-smokers have between two and seven times the risk for lung cancer. Also, female smokers have an increased likelihood for developing lung cancer and a sharper increase in risk with increasing cigarette consumption compared to male smokers.[7] Some epidemiologic studies have shown that a family history of lung cancer also predicts increased risk. Genetic polymorphisms may affect many factors such as smoking behavior, carcinogen metabolism and detoxification, DNA repair, cell cycle control, other aspects of cellular function, as well as immune response to transformed cells.[12]

The relative prevalence of lung cancer by histologic subtypes has changed over the years. Squamous cell carcinoma was the most common type in the earlier decades of the 20th century, but now adenocarcinoma is the most common type. This occurred during the five-year period between 1992 and 1998, which saw a decline in the incidence of squamous cell carcinoma, accompanied by an increase in that of adenocarcinoma. Adenocarcinoma is now the most frequent tumor type seen in women; data from 1973 to 1996 indicate that the rate for adenocarcinoma is still rising, while that of other types has reached a plateau. Associated with the change in histologic types, there is also a relative decrease in the percentage of central tumors. Studies have postulated that the changes in histologic types and location are related to the changes in cigarette design and in smoking behavior. Many people who smoke 'low tar and nicotine' cigarettes compensate for lower nicotine delivery by smoking more cigarettes per day and deeper inhalation.[12] Deep inhalation has been found to be associated with increased risk of peripheral tumors and a decreased risk of central tumors.[3]

CLINICAL FEATURES OF LUNG CANCER

Symptoms and signs related to the presence of the primary tumor include cough that is often chronic, hemoptysis that can be due to ulceration of tumor into the bronchial mucosa or massive bleeding due to direct invasion of blood vessels (a rare event), and dyspnea. Tumors with regional extrapulmonary extension may cause chest pain, pleural effusion, superior vena cava syndrome, lymphadenopathy, hoarseness, dysphagia, pericardial effusion or tamponade, and Pancoast syndrome. A wide range of systemic symptoms can be caused by distant metastases. Small cell carcinoma is the most common tumor type associated with paraneoplastic syndromes including digital clubbing and hypertrophic osteoarthropathy, fatigue and cachexia, cerebellar degeneration, cancer-related retinopathy, sensory neuropathy and encephalomyelitis, Eaton-Lambert syndrome, syndrome of inappropriate antidiuretic hormone, and Cushing's syndrome. Hypercalcemia is most common in squamous cell carcinoma.[13]

RADIOLOGIC FEATURES OF LUNG CANCER

Twenty to thirty percent of cancer patients present with a solitary lung lesion on chest X-ray, routine non-enhanced and contrast-enhanced computerized tomography (CT) and magnetic resonance (MR) imaging. Lesions that are suspicious, but indeterminate for malignancy can be further evaluated with positron emission tomography (PET). PET is significantly more accurate than CT and MR in local and regional staging, particularly in detecting metastasis in normal-sized lymph nodes. However, false-positive PET can be seen in inflammatory diseases. False-negative PET can be seen in lesions less than 1 cm, or slow-growing tumors such as carcinoid or bronchioloalveolar carcinoma.[14,15]

Rapid, relatively low-dose spiral CT can detect peripheral nodules in the 2–3 mm range. The radiation exposure is similar to that of mammography. The Early Lung Cancer Action Project used spiral CT to screen 1000 high-risk individuals for lung cancer, and has shown that CT can be used to detected small lung cancers.[16] Similar studies in Japan and Germany have also documented that low-dose spiral CT can detect lung cancers that cannot be seen on a chest X-ray. Screening of asymptomatic individuals with low-dose CT results in an approximately 3-fold higher detection rate than with chest X-ray. Not surprisingly, CT detected more stage I cancers. The cancers detected in the CT screening trials are predominantly peripherally located adenocarcinomas (79.6%). The detection rate of benign noncalcified pulmonary nodules is, however, also high. Randomized, controlled trials are currently underway to evaluate the effect of screening on disease-specific mortality, which despite enhanced tumor detection has not been clearly shown by current studies.[17]

MOLECULAR PATHOGENESIS OF LUNG CANCER

Lung cancer develops as a result of largely unknown complex interactions between environmental carcinogens and inherited predisposition. There is typically a latent period between exposure to carcinogens and the clinical appearance of a tumor, which is felt to be a reflection of the multistage process of tumorigenesis. Statistical analysis based on the age-specific mortality for different types of human cancers indicates that usually 3–12 critical alterations accumulate before the appearance of clinically diagnosable tumors.[18] Multiple clinical and experimental data support the theory of 'field cancerization' and multistep tumorigenesis. This is the result of accumulation of various genetic and epigenetic alterations that lead to outgrowth of clonal populations within the lung that may eventually produce a clinically evident cancer. Molecular studies have shown that there are multiple genetic lesions in the respiratory epithelium of current and former smokers. Benzopyrene, a polycyclic aromatic hydrocarbon, is the most well-known carcinogen in cigarette smoke and induces guanine (G) to thymine (T) nucleotide transversions in genes. There is a dose–response relationship between tobacco smoking and G to T nucleotide transversions in *p53* mutations. Recent studies have also shown an association of smoking with hypermethylation of promoter regions of tumor suppressor genes.[12] Hanahan and Weinberg suggest that at least six major functional pathways must be affected for successful tumorigenesis. These consist of regulation-independent growth (through overexpression of growth factor receptors), insensitivity to antigrowth signals (defects in Rb pathway), evasion from apoptosis (alterations in p53 or bcl-2), limitless replicative potential (continued telomerase expression), sustained angiogenesis (upregulation of vascular growth factors), and tissue invasion and metastasis (alterations in cell adhesion molecules, cell matrix proteases, etc.).[19] Molecular studies on lung cancer cell lines and primary human lung cancer tissues have shown that common genetic and epigenetic changes

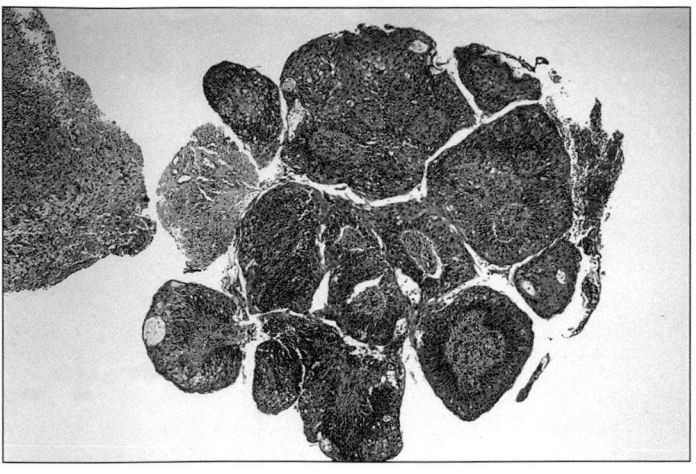

Fig. 18.1 Squamous papilloma. Endobronchial papillary tumor with well-developed fibrovascular stroma. The squamous epithelium shows dysplasia, a common feature.

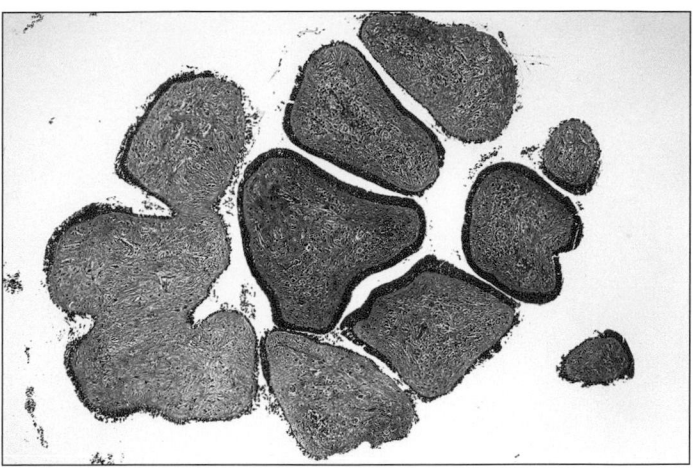

Fig. 18.3 Fibroepithelial polyp. Endobronchial papillary lesion composed predominantly of fibrous stroma covered by a thin layer of benign respiratory or squamous epithelium.

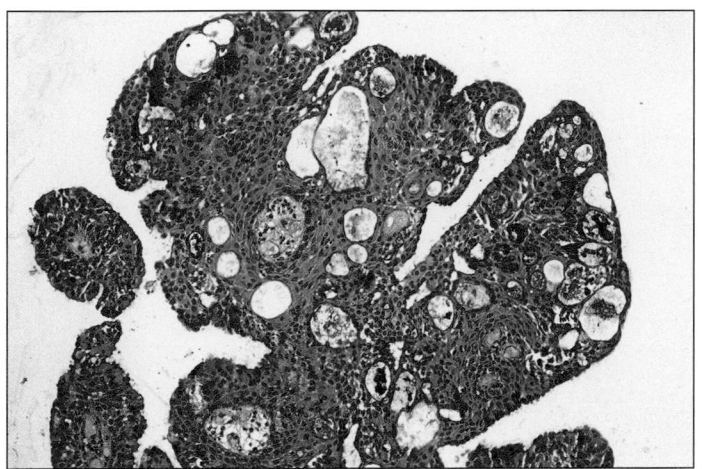

Fig. 18.2 Mixed squamous cell and glandular papilloma. Endobronchial tumor removed because of hemoptysis. Note combination of squamous and glandular epithelium.

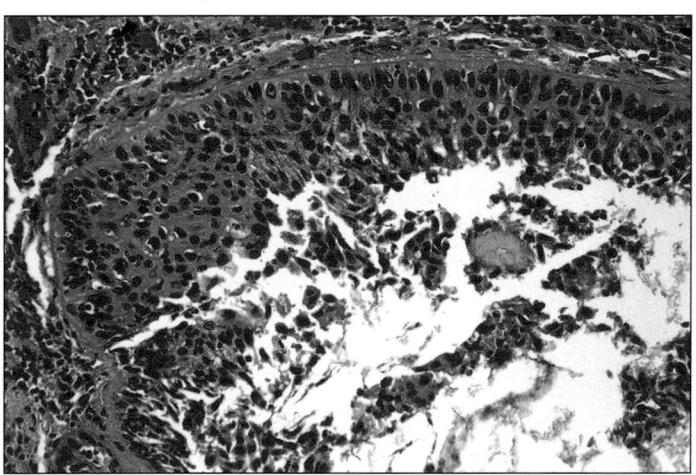

Fig. 18.4 In situ squamous cell carcinoma. Respiratory mucosa is replaced by highly abnormal squamous cells showing disorganized growth and nuclear atypia throughout the full thickness of the epithelium. Malignant surface cells shed into the bronchial lumen enabling cytologic detection.

Squamous cell carcinoma

Squamous cell carcinoma most often involves the central portion of the lung, arising from the larger bronchi. Approximately a third, however, are peripheral tumors. There is a strong relationship with cigarette smoking and other carcinogens. Squamous cell carcinoma accounts for approximately 30% of lung cancer in the United States. HPV DNA has been observed in approximately 18–30% of cases using in situ hybridization techniques.[118] Squamous cell carcinoma has a long natural history and evolves from gradually accumulating epithelial changes throughout the bronchial tree over many years. This enables the identification of precursor cellular abnormalities by cytology in a higher proportion of cases than for other tumor types. Squamous metaplasia and dysplasia precede carcinoma by up to a decade, but it is important to recognize that even severe degrees of dysplasia may regress over time.[119] Squamous cell carcinoma in situ is differentiated from dysplasia by severe full-thickness cellular atypia in the epithelium accompanied by significant disorganization

and dyskeratosis (Fig. 18.4). In situ squamous cell carcinoma may not be recognized grossly or endoscopically. Examples have been described as opacification of the usually glistening translucent bronchial mucosa by white or hyperemic discoloration associated with loss of the longitudinal mucosal folds or rarely as a polypoid excrescence or micronodular abnormality. It progresses to early invasion of the subepithelial connective tissue and further to invasion of bronchial cartilage and into the pulmonary parenchyma. The incidence of lymph node metastases is directly proportional to tumor size even in occult or early invasive tumors. In radiographically occult endobronchial lesions over 20 mm in length, over one-fourth had lymph node metastases, while none under this size metastasized.[120,121] The preclinical or occult phase of the tumor is often multicentric in the tracheobronchial tree and second primary tumors have been observed in 20–36% of early squamous cell carcinomas.[122–124]

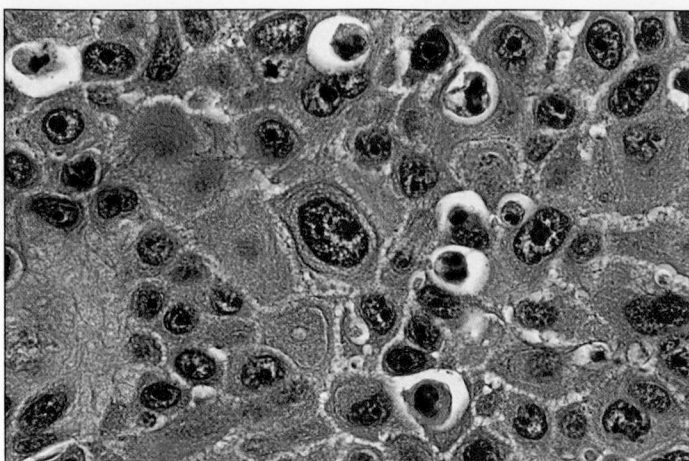

Fig. 18.5 Invasive well-differentiated squamous cell carcinoma. Abnormal squamous cells with prominent intercellular bridges.

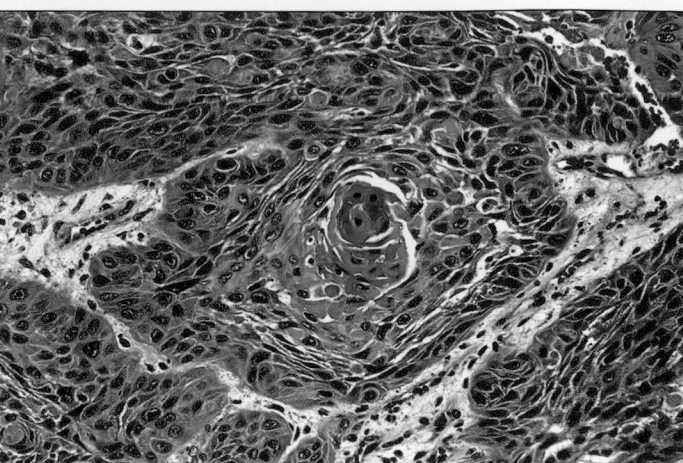

Fig. 18.6 Invasive well-differentiated squamous cell carcinoma. Infiltrating tumor nest shows well-developed keratin pearl.

As the tumor progresses, it forms an endobronchial mass causing bronchial obstruction with clinical manifestations of cough, hemoptysis, atelectasis, and obstructive pneumonia. Grossly, the tumors are characteristically firm, solid, and gray-white with flecks of hemorrhage and necrosis. Squamous cell carcinomas occurring in the periphery of the lung are often cavitary due to extensive necrosis.[125] The prognosis of squamous cell carcinoma of the lung is related to both cellular grade and clinical stage. Recurrences following therapy are more likely to be localized within the thorax than with adenocarcinoma.[126–128] The prognosis is better for squamous cell carcinoma in stage I and stage II as compared with adenocarcinoma and other cell types. The five-year survival rate for squamous cell carcinoma versus aden20carcinoma in stage I is 83% versus 69% and for stage II 75% versus 52%, respectively.[28] Unlike adenocarcinoma, regional (N1) lymph node metastases do not seem to effect prognosis.[129]

Histologically, squamous cell carcinoma shows varying degrees of keratinization, as exemplified by intracytoplasmic keratin rings, and intercellular bridges (Fig. 18.5). Discrete squamous pearls are more common in well-differentiated tumors (Fig. 18.6). Lesions that show large areas of sheet-like growth but without pearls or intercellular bridges are best regarded as large cell undifferentiated carcinoma.

Variants of squamous cell carcinoma have been described that have prognostic significance. The papillary variant of squamous cell carcinoma is characterized grossly by an exophytic growth pattern within the bronchial lumen, similar to squamous papilloma (Fig. 18.7). This tumor tends to be well differentiated and sometimes difficult to differentiate from dysplastic papilloma. Papillary squamous cell carcinoma is most often diagnosed in stage I and has an excellent prognosis. Over 60% of the patients survive five years.[130]

The small cell variant reveals areas that contain small tumor cells with little cytoplasm and without intercellular bridges that call to mind the diagnosis of small cell anaplastic carcinoma (Fig. 18.8). However, such areas gradually blend with more clear-cut evidence of squamous differentiation. Tumors tend to show better-developed fibrous stroma and discrete cell nests and nuclei show coarser chromatin and more frequent nucleoli than do small cell carcinomas. Ultrastructurally, there is squamous differentiation without neurosecretory granules.[131]

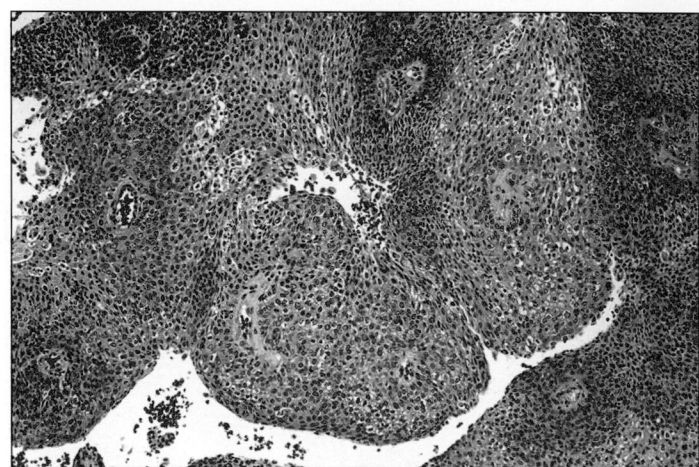

Fig. 18.7 Papillary squamous cell carcinoma. Highly atypical endobronchial squamous tumor with papillary configuration and fibrovascular stroma, showing epithelial thickening and full-thickness cellular abnormality diagnostic of carcinoma.

The basaloid variant of squamous cell carcinoma resembles its counterpart in the upper aerodigestive tract and is distinguished by nodular or trabecular growth with palisading of the basal layer of malignant squamous epithelium along the basement membrane, reminiscent of basal cell carcinoma (Fig. 18.9).[132,133] Both the basaloid and small cell variants of squamous cell carcinoma are poorly differentiated and have a poor prognosis. Other variants such as clear cell, giant cell, and spindle cell squamous carcinomas have been observed (Fig. 18.10).[134]

Cytology of squamous cell carcinoma

Squamous cell carcinomas have variable morphology in cytologic samples, depending on the degree of tumor differentiation, collection method, and preparation technique. In general, tumor cells appear singly or in small groups in exfoliative cytology (i.e. sputum, bronchial washing), whereas in bronchial brushings and needle aspirates larger

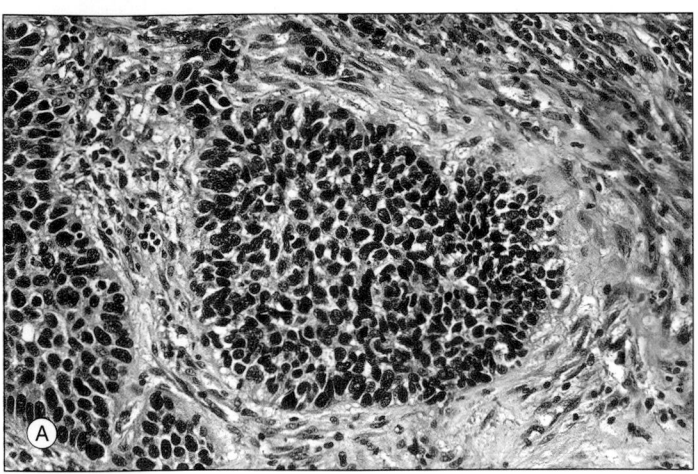

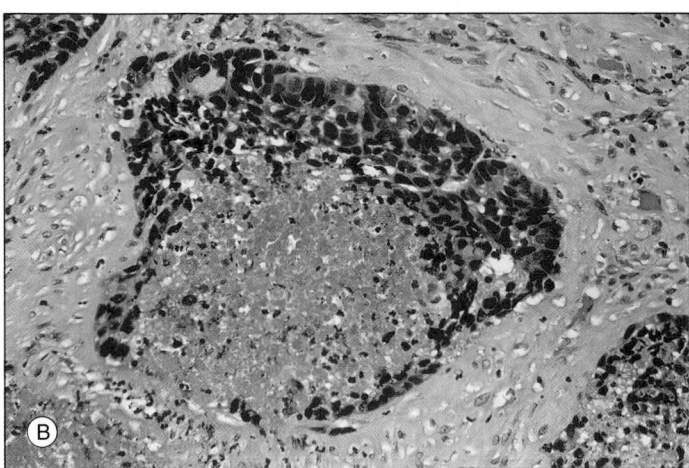

Fig. 18.8 A, Squamous cell carcinoma, small cell variant. Cells show enlarged, hyperchromatic nuclei with small to moderate amount of pink cytoplasm. Areas like this blend imperceptibly with easily recognizable squamous cell carcinoma; **B,** Abundant necrosis in nest of poorly differentiated squamous cell carcinoma, small cell variant.

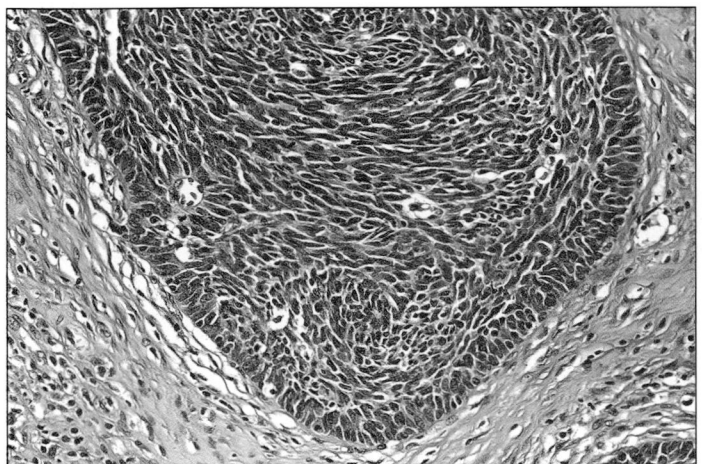

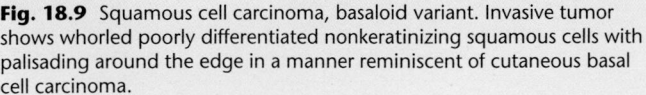

Fig. 18.9 Squamous cell carcinoma, basaloid variant. Invasive tumor shows whorled poorly differentiated nonkeratinizing squamous cells with palisading around the edge in a manner reminiscent of cutaneous basal cell carcinoma.

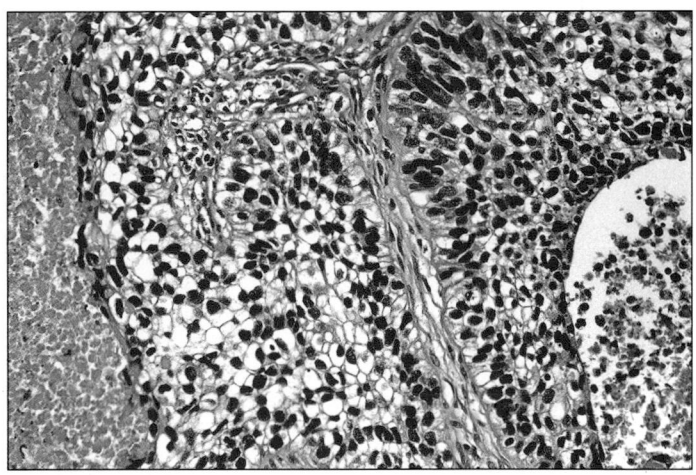

Fig. 18.10 Squamous cell carcinoma, clear cell variant. Tumor cells show distinct cell borders and optically clear cytoplasm, which bears some similarity to other types of clear cell tumors such as metastatic renal cell adenocarcinoma.

tissue fragments are present in addition to single cells. Loss of cohesiveness is more pronounced in well-differentiated than in poorly differentiated tumors; thus the former presents with single tumor cells, while the latter sheds large cell clusters. Tumor cells are readily identifiable in sputum and bronchoscopic samples.

Well-differentiated, keratinizing squamous cell carcinoma is characterized by the presence of large pink and orangiophilic cells that exhibit marked variation in shape and size. The cytoplasm is dense and devoid of mucin vacuoles (Fig. 18.11A,B). Some cells may show small cytoplasmic vacuoles, but these are generally different from mucin vacuoles seen in adenocarcinoma, in that they do not have the bluish hue of mucin and usually do not cause indentation of the nucleus. Long, slender, tadpole-shaped, angulated and irregular 'fiber' cells are frequently seen (Fig. 18.11C). Significant anisonucleosis and pleomorphism are common. Nuclei are hyperchromatic and exhibit

uneven distribution of chromatin and irregularity of the nuclear membrane. Nucleoli are present, but not usually prominent. Squamous pearls composed of concentric clusters of elongated eosinophilic cells with hyperchromatic nuclei are characteristic of this tumor (Fig. 18.11D). Degenerated tumor cells, and acellular orangiophilic keratin debris is present in the background. Because of the tendency of these tumors to form large necrotic centers, FNA samples sometimes show only necrotic material. It is extremely important not to render a diagnosis of malignancy when a sample contains only necrotic debris and degenerated or 'ghost' cells, since degenerated non-neoplastic cells may exhibit eosinophilic cytoplasm and pyknotic nuclei that can mimic malignancy. During on-site evaluation of FNA, if the sample is largely necrotic, the radiologist should be instructed to avoid the center and instead obtain a sample from the periphery of the tumor.

Fig. 18.11 Fine needle aspirate of moderately well-differentiated keratinizing squamous cell carcinoma. **A**, Sheet of pleomorphic epithelial cells exhibiting marked variation in nuclear size and shape, hyperchromasia, and nuclear membrane irregularity. Prominent nucleoli are not seen (Papanicolaou stain); **B**, The cytoplasm is dense, eosinophilic, or amphophilic with scattered orangiophilic cells indicating keratinization (Papanicolaou stain); **C**, Pleomorphic malignant squamous cells with markedly elongated and hyperchromatic nuclei. Necrotic cells are seen in the background (Papanicolaou stain); **D**, Cell-block section depicting malignant cells forming a 'squamous pearl' in a background of necrotic debris (H&E stain).

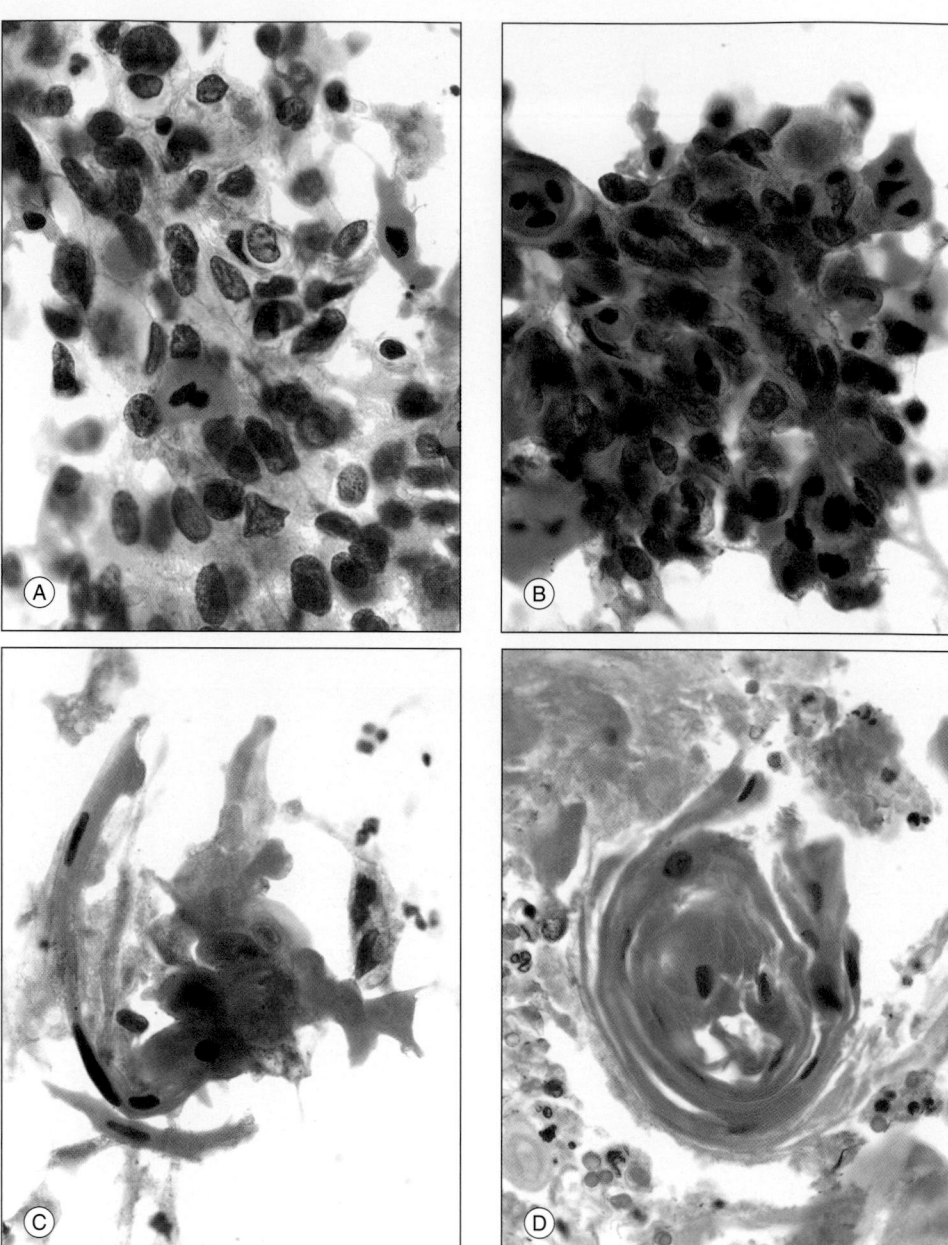

Poorly differentiated squamous cell carcinoma is characterized by malignant cells that are generally smaller than the well differentiated variant and exhibit more basophilic cytoplasm (Fig. 18.12A, B). The nuclei have coarse chromatin and prominent nucleoli and the nuclear:cytoplasmic (N/C) ratio is high. Cell borders are distinct and cells lack secretory vacuoles, which are helpful in classification of this tumor, but significant overlap of morphologic features with poorly differentiated adenocarcinoma or large cell carcinoma (Fig. 18.12C, D) often precludes distinction of these tumor types in cytologic samples.

Differential diagnosis: The differential diagnosis of squamous cell carcinoma includes atypical squamous metaplasia secondary to irradiation, chronic inflammatory conditions, reparative processes resulting from necrotizing tracheobronchitis, and chronic irritation of tracheal epithelium in patients with tracheostomy tube.[135] In necrotizing infections, degenerated cells with dark pyknotic nuclei and eosinophilic cytoplasm in a background of necrotic debris may mimic keratinizing squamous cell carcinoma. In viral infections clusters of degenerated upper respiratory tract epithelial cells, referred to as 'Pap cells,' shed into the sputum and can mimic cancer.[136] The respiratory epithelium in irradiated lung undergoes squamous metaplasia with marked cytoplasmic enlargement, cellular pleomorphism, and sometimes orangiophilia, that can also be mistaken for squamous carcinoma. Finally, chronic bronchitis, bronchiectasis, and mycetoma are usually associated with pronounced squamous metaplasia, at times with marked nuclear atypia. Unfortunately, no single cytologic criterion can distinguish such reactive conditions from lung cancer, and a constellation of findings must be used to avoid a false-positive diagnosis. Most importantly, a definitive diagnosis of cancer should not be rendered in the absence of well-preserved cells with nuclear features of malignancy. When nuclei are pyknotic or smudged, inflammation is present in the background,

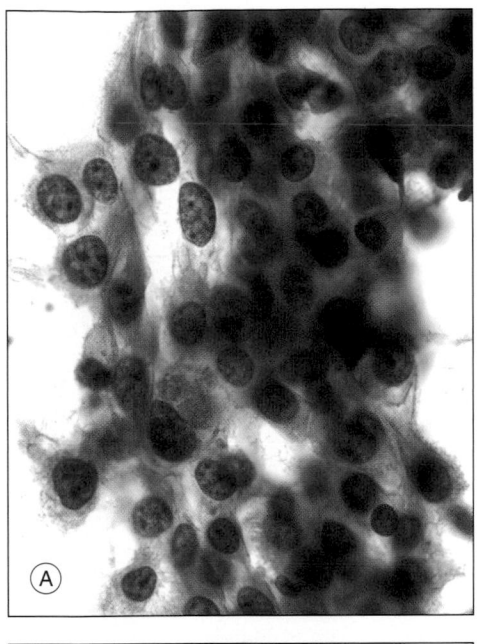

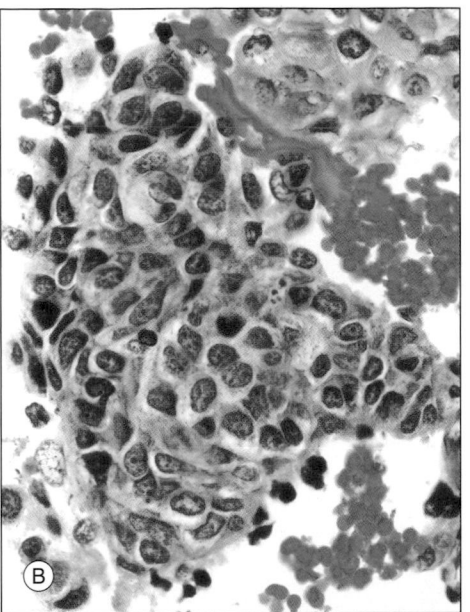

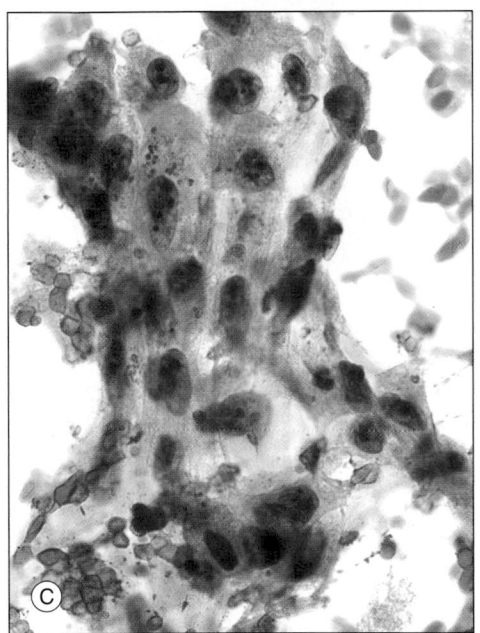

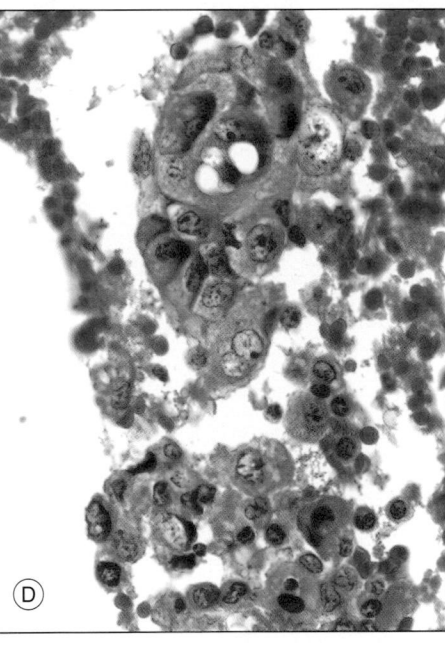

Fig. 18.12 Cytopathology of poorly differentiated non-small cell carcinoma. **A**, FNA smear of a poorly differentiated squamous cell carcinoma. Malignant epithelial cells vary in arrangement from monolayer sheet to three-dimensional cluster. Prominent nucleoli are seen in some cells. No obvious squamous differentiation is appreciated, although there is some suggestion of intercellular bridges (Papanicolaou stain); **B**, Cell block section of the same sample showing relatively small malignant epithelial cells without evidence of keratinization. The tumor cells in the right upper corner have more abundant cytoplasm with squamoid features (H&E stain); **C**, FNA smear of a poorly differentiated adenocarcinoma showing a sheet of large cells with obviously malignant-appearing nuclei and prominent nucleoli. There are no secretory vacuoles or gland formations and it is difficult to distinguish the tumor from a poorly differentiated squamous carcinoma (Papanicolaou stain); **D**, Cell-block section of the same specimen exhibiting occasional vacuoles (H&E stain).

and there is no loss of cohesion, the possibility of reactive conditions should be raised.

Aside from reactive conditions, squamous dysplasia and carcinoma in situ (CIS) must be differentiated from invasive squamous cell carcinoma in sputum or bronchoscopic samples. High-grade dysplasia and CIS shed relatively small to medium-sized, round cells singly or in small groups. In bronchial brushing samples sheets of atypical squamous cells are seen. The nucleus is enlarged, the chromatin is coarse, there is slight irregularity of the nuclear membrane, and small nucleoli and cytoplasmic keratinization can be seen (Fig 18.13). While overlapping cellular features preclude definitive distinction of these lesions from invasive squamous cell carcinoma, there are some criteria that can be helpful in the differential diagnosis. Significant pleomorphism of the cells, prominent nucleoli, and a necrotic background are generally absent in dysplasia and CIS and favor invasive carcinoma.[137] It is also important to correlate the cytology

with radiographic findings, as noninvasive squamous lesions do not form a mass. One exception, however, is when dysplasia or CIS is associated with a benign, mass-producing condition such as a granuloma.

GLAND FORMING-LESIONS (Table 18.3)

Benign gland-forming lesions of the bronchi and lung are rare and include the bronchial gland adenoma and mixed tumor (pleomorphic adenoma) of the bronchi, as well as the alveolar adenoma and so-called sclerosing hemangioma of peripheral lung tissue.

Bronchial gland adenoma

The bronchial gland adenoma arises from the seromucous bronchial glands in the main lobar and segmental bronchi. Only about 30 cases

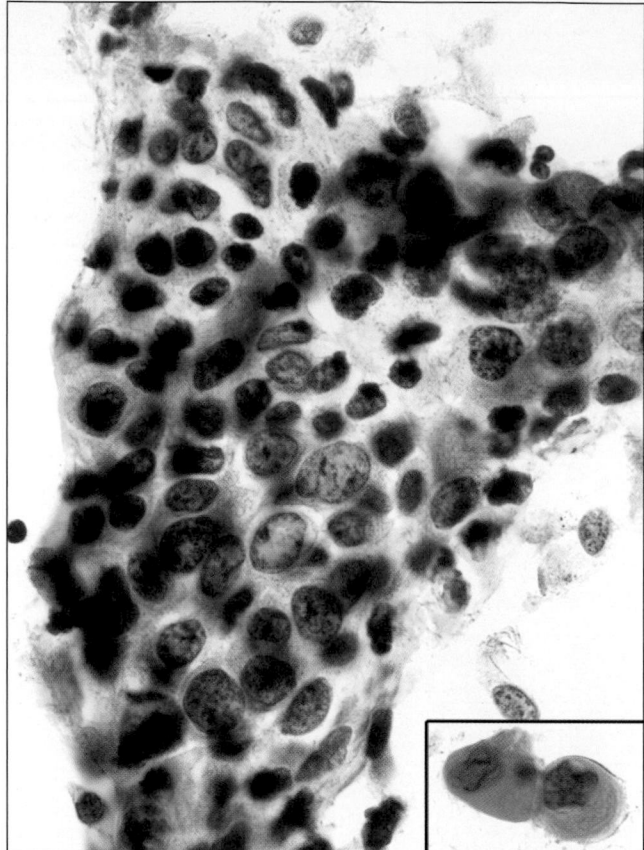

Fig. 18.13 Cytopathology of squamous cell carcinoma in situ in a bronchial brushing sample. A sheet of medium-sized cells with enlarged, hyperchromatic nuclei exhibiting coarse chromatin and irregular nuclear membrane. The inset depicts single dysplastic squamous cells with dark, irregular nuclei (H&E stain).

Table 18.3 Gland-forming lesions of bronchi and lung

Benign	Malignant
Bronchial gland adenoma	Mucoepidermoid carcinoma
Mixed tumor (pleomorphic adenoma)	Adenoid cystic carcinoma
Alveolar adenoma	Endobronchial polypoid adenocarcinoma
Sclerosing hemangioma	Peripheral adenocarcinoma
Papillary adenoma	Bronchioloalveolar carcinoma
Cystic mucinous tumor	Papillary, acinar, solid, clear cell
	Other

have been reported.[138,139] They commonly appear in adults as soft mucoid endobronchial tumors. Clinically, wheezing is common. This tumor may present as a radiographic coin lesion. Histologically, they are composed of flat, cuboidal, or columnar epithelial cells that form papillae and small cysts and glands containing mucus (Fig. 18.14A,B). Squamous metaplasia is an uncommon finding. Nuclei are small with small indistinct nucleoli and mitotic figures are rare. Resection is curative. Bronchial gland adenoma must be differentiated from low-grade mucoepidermoid carcinoma with which it shares many histologic features. The most critical point in the differential diagnosis is the presence of nonglandular, nonsquamous intermediate cells in mucoepidermoid carcinoma and their absence in bronchial gland adenoma (see below).

Benign mixed tumor (pleomorphic adenoma)

Benign mixed tumor or pleomorphic adenomas are seen in the trachea and major bronchi, but also rarely can form peripheral lung nodules.[140–143] They are tumors of middle-aged adults with an equal sex distribution. The size varies widely, up to 4.5 cm. Histologically, tumors resemble their counterparts in major salivary glands, but often show areas of more epithelial, glandular differentiation compared with stromal, cartilaginous matrix. Mitoses may be seen. Tumors tend to be

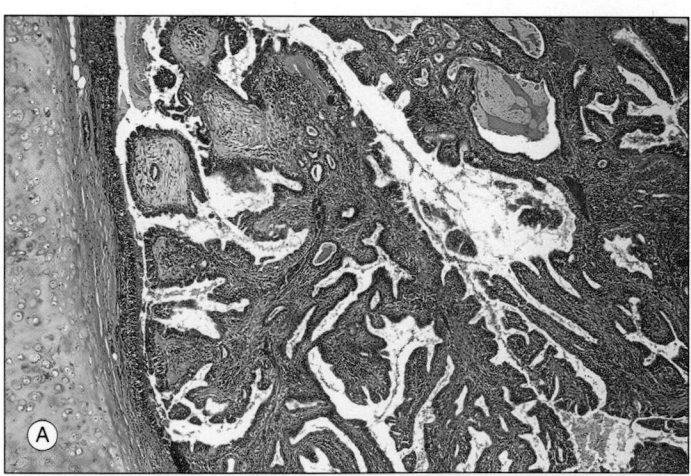

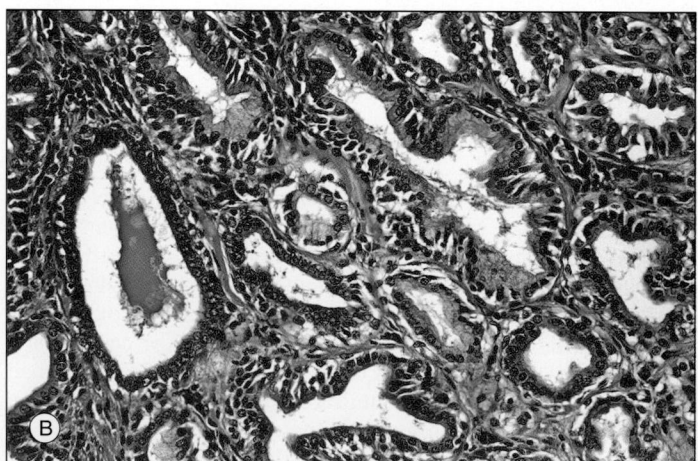

Fig. 18.14 A, Bronchial gland adenoma. Endobronchial papillary-glandular tumor; **B**, Bronchial gland adenoma. Glands composed of benign mucinous and cuboidal cells containing intraluminal secretions. They are interspersed in fibrous stroma without stromal reaction. Intermediate cells are absent, which helps differentiate this tumor from low-grade mucoepidermoid carcinoma. (Courtesy of Dr. Douglas Flieder, NYC).

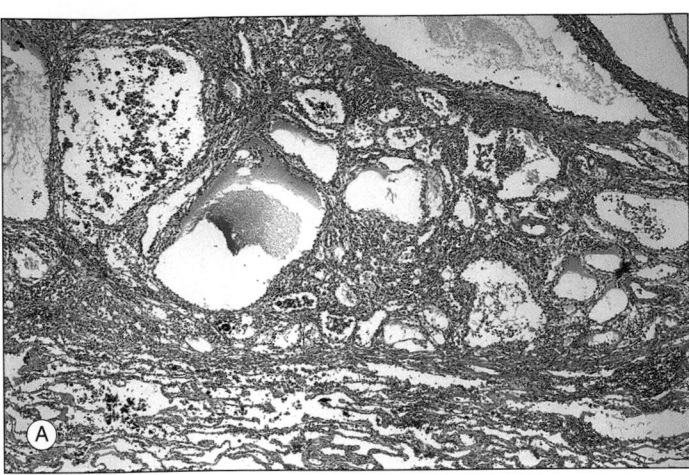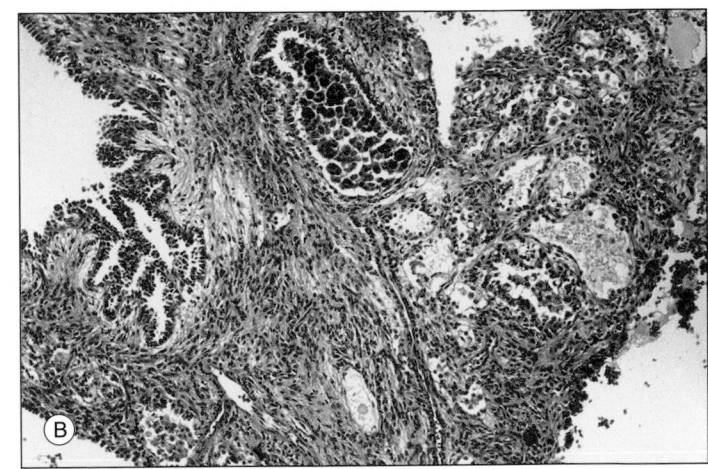

Fig. 18.15 A, Alveolar adenoma. Tumor appears microcystic and well demarcated from surrounding lung tissue. It is composed of small dilated spaces lined by a single layer of benign pink hob-nailed epithelium. Focal areas show cellular spindle cell stroma; **B**, Alveolar adenoma. Focus of hypercellular spindled stroma seen focally in the tumor. Sometimes this can be extensive, giving rise to a biphasic appearance. (Courtesy of Dr. Douglas Flieder, NYC)

well circumscribed, grossly. Mixed tumors of the lung are rare and the proportion of histologically malignant lesions appears to be greater than in major salivary glands. Complete resection is recommended. The differential diagnosis includes metastases from a previous or concomitant salivary gland tumor and such malignancies as metastatic malignant mixed mesodermal tumor, teratoma, and metaplastic lung cancer.

Alveolar adenoma

The alveolar adenoma is a well-circumscribed but unencapsulated solitary peripheral tumor that contains a combination of proliferating nonmucinous epithelium, often having a bland interstitial spindle cell component, which gives some tumors a biphasic appearance (Fig. 18.15A,B).[144] It characteristically has a microcystic appearance histologically. The epithelium is composed of a single layer of simple, TTF-1-positive alveolar-type II cells, while the spindled stroma has ultrastructural characteristics of fibroblasts.[145] A combined alveolar adenoma-sclerosing hemangioma has been reported.[146] Lesions may be shelled out from the surrounding lung tissue, surgically. The tumor is cured by wedge resection or lobectomy.

Sclerosing hemangioma

The most common peripheral benign glandular tumor is sclerosing hemangioma. This was first reported by Liebow and Hubbell as a well-circumscribed tumor having a prominent vascular pattern containing blood lakes, which they considered as having a vascular origin.[147] Subsequent studies, however, have shown that the tumor cells are actually type II pneumocytes, as evidenced by electron microscopy and immunohistochemistry.[148–151] Sclerosing hemangiomas are mostly solid solitary tumors that have a confusing variety of histologic patterns that occur either in pure form or mixed, described as papillary, solid, vascular, and sclerotic. The age range is wide, from adolescence to old age. Female predominance has been noted. Histologically, the characteristic cells are relatively large with clear or pink cytoplasm, centrally placed nuclei, and inconspicuous nucleoli. Mitoses are rare. Blood-filled spaces are common, lined by epithelial cells that are positive with vimentin, cytokeratin, EMA, TTF-1, and surfactant apoprotein (Fig. 18.16A,B).[146] Tumor cells are negative for endothelial markers CD31 and factor VIII, which

stain tumor blood vessels, but not the cells lining the spaces. Blood lakes, although characteristic, are not essential for the diagnosis and tumors may entirely lack this feature. Rare tumors with mediastinal or hilar lymph node metastases have been reported.[146,152,153] Combined carcinoid-sclerosing hemangioma has been described.[146]

Cytology of sclerosing hemangioma

There are only a few case reports describing the microscopic features of sclerosing hemangioma in FNA material.[154–160] FNA samples are usually cellular and exhibit a characteristic biphasic pattern (Fig. 18.17). The first pattern is the presence of loosely cohesive sheets of round or polygonal epithelioid cells with moderate amount of cytoplasm and bland nuclei. Chromatin is evenly distributed and nucleoli are indistinct. Intranuclear cytoplasmic inclusions are occasionally seen.[154–156] The second pattern has papillary structures covered by round, cuboidal, columnar, or polygonal cells with clear or granular cytoplasm and uniform nuclei, which may contain distinct nucleoli (Fig. 18.17B).[154,155,160] The core of the papillae may contain a hyalinized sclerotic stroma, which is best seen in cell block preparations (Fig. 18.17D).[156] Blood and hemosiderin-laden macrophages are commonly seen in the background (Fig. 18.17C, inset).[154–156] Some authors have reported the presence of 'blood spaces' filled by red blood cells and surrounded by aggregates of tumor cells.[160] Mitoses are virtually absent. Focal nuclear pleomorphism or hyperchromasia may be seen.[154] Positive immunocytochemical staining for cytokeratin establishes the epithelial nature of tumor cells (Fig. 18.17D, inset).

Differential diagnosis: In cytologic specimens sclerosing hemangioma may be mistaken for bronchioloalveolar carcinoma,[154,155] carcinoid tumor,[158,161] or metastatic papillary thyroid carcinoma.[155] In bronchioloalveolar carcinoma, although the tumor cells can be remarkably uniform, the nuclei still exhibit malignant criteria. In sclerosing hemangioma nuclear atypia is usually absent and, when present, is only focal. In carcinoid tumor the cells are monotonous and nuclei exhibit the characteristic salt and pepper appearance. The presence of angiomatous and sclerotic patterns support the diagnosis of sclerosing hemangioma and is unusual in bronchioloalveolar carcinoma, carcinoid, and metastatic papillary carcinoma. Iyoda and

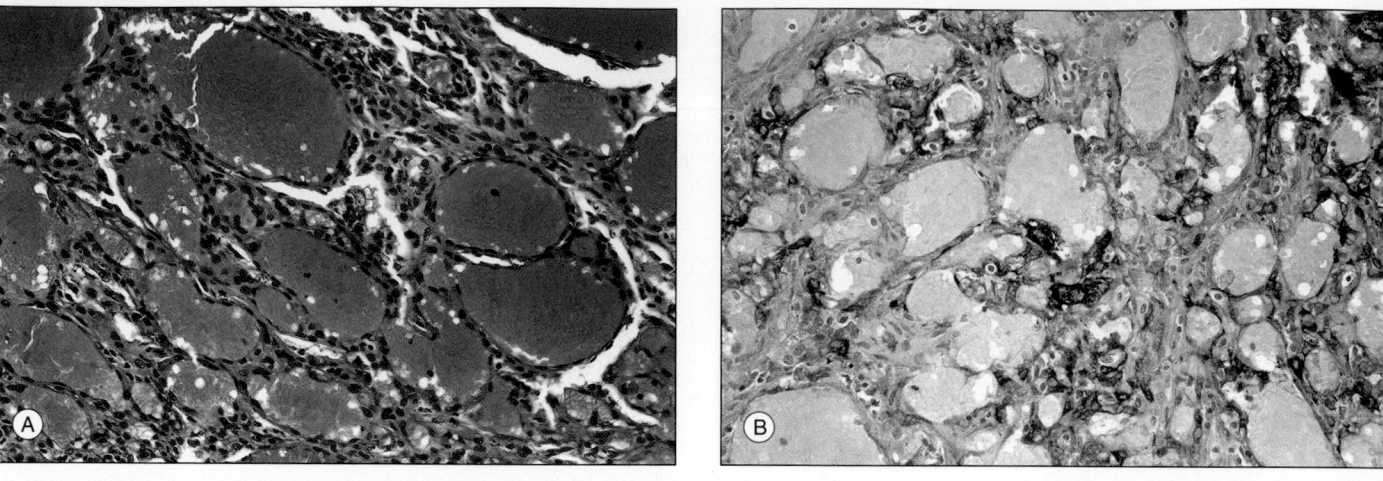

Fig. 18.16 A, Sclerosing hemangioma. Blood-filled spaces lined by single flattened or cuboidal epithelial cells; **B**, Sclerosing hemangioma. Cytokeratin stains showing positivity in the epithelial lining cells.

Fig. 18.17 FNA cytology of sclerosing hemangioma. **A**, Arborizing papillary structures covered by epithelioid cells; **B**, Higher magnification showing the endothelial cells of capillaries in the core of papillary structures and medium-sized round to polygonal epithelial cells with bland nuclei and small nucleoli; **C**, A loosely cohesive sheet of epithelial cells with round nuclei, relatively low N:C ratio, finely granular chromatin, and indistinct nucleoli. The inset depicts a hemosiderin-laden macrophage from another field (A–C: Papanicolaou stain); **D**, Cell block section demonstrating papillary structures with hyalinized, sclerotic cores, covered by epithelioid cells (H&E stain). Inset depicts immunostaining for cytokeratin.

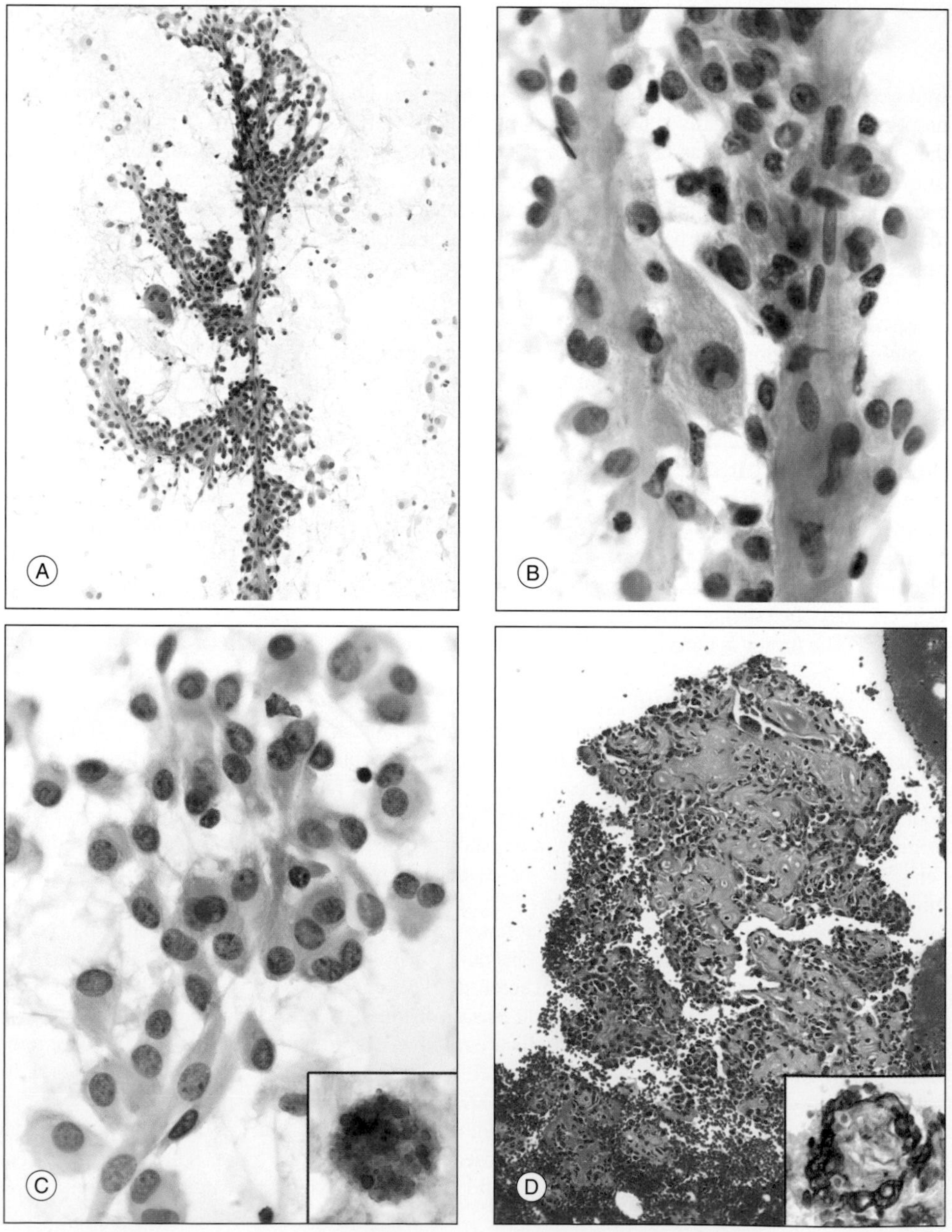

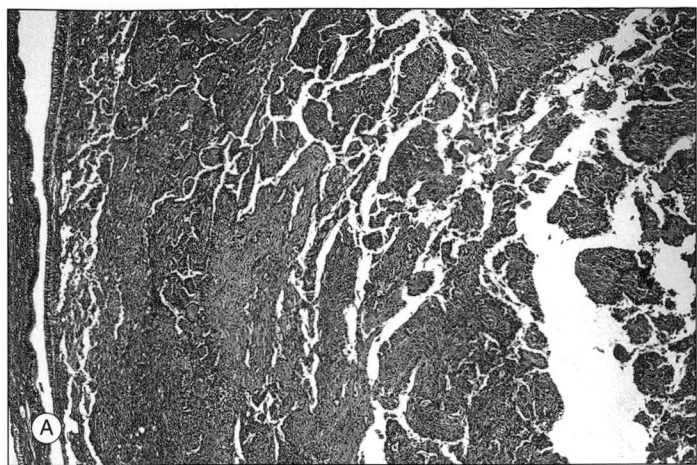
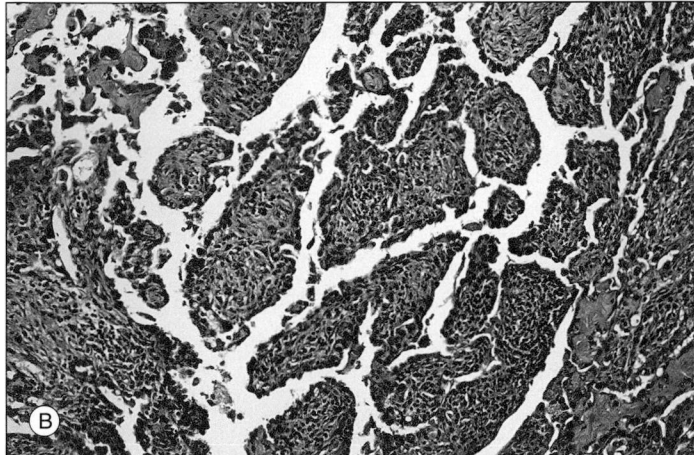

Fig. 18.18 A, Papillary adenoma. Well-demarcated tumor with circumscribed pushing borders that compress surrounding lung. Fat club-shaped papillae that project toward the center of the lesion are seen; **B**, Papillary adenoma. Papillae are lined by a single layer of type II pneumocytes. Fibrous stroma contains lymphocytes.

coworkers[162] compared imprint smears of resected sclerosing hemangiomas and well-differentiated papillary adenocarcinomas of the lung and found that the presence of blood and round cells was more commonly associated with sclerosing hemangioma, whereas the presence of nucleoli, irregularity of nuclear membrane, nuclear indentation, anisokaryosis, necrosis, and high N:C ratio were more common in adenocarcinoma than sclerosing hemangioma.[162] Immunocytochemical stains for neuroendocrine markers and thyroglobulin are helpful in differentiating this tumor from carcinoid or papillary thyroid carcinoma. Immunoreactivity to TTF-1 is seen in sclerosing hemangioma and, therefore, is not helpful in the differential diagnosis.[154]

Papillary adenoma

Lesions designated as papillary adenoma have been described in the periphery of the lung and characterized by well-circumscribed papillary proliferations of nonmucinous epithelium derived from type II pneumocytes that compresses surrounding lung tissue (Fig. 18.18A,B).[163] They have been reported rarely and their clear separation from nonhemorrhagic sclerosing hemangioma is sometimes difficult. Histologically, the tumor shows filiform and club-shaped papillae, with ample stroma, covered by a single layer of flat or raised simple epithelium. Ultrastructure shows lamellar bodies, consistent with type II pneumocytes. Examples of alveolar adenoma, sclerosing hemangioma, and papillary adenoma may have histologic features in common and would appear to represent a closely related group of tumors.

Malignant gland forming tumors

From a clinicopathologic standpoint, it is convenient to separate the malignant gland-forming tumors into those that most commonly arise endobronchially and those that present in the lung periphery. The endobronchial malignancies are most commonly recognized as variants of salivary gland-type tumors that originate in the analogous seromucous glands of the bronchus. These include mucoepidermoid carcinoma, adenoid cystic carcinoma, and acinic cell carcinoma. Acinic cell carcinoma can also be seen in the lung parenchyma as well as endobronchially, while peripheral presentation of adenoid cystic carcinoma is less frequent.

Mucoepidermoid carcinoma

Mucoepidermoid carcinoma of the bronchus is rare, accounting for 1% or less of all lung tumors.[164] Somewhat less than half are associated with cigarette smoking. They are divided into low- and high-grade types, which has a direct bearing on prognosis.[165] Mucoepidermoid carcinoma is characterized by the presence of mucus and squamous cells, as well as transitional or intermediate-type cells consisting of solid, nonmucinous, but nonkeratinizing epithelium without intercellular bridges. The recognition of this cell type is important in differentiating the low-grade mucoepidermoid carcinoma from bronchial gland adenoma, which does not contain intermediate cells. High- and low-grade neoplasms are separated by the degree of cellular atypia, mitotic activity, necrosis, and other histologic features that otherwise distinguish low-grade from high-grade carcinoma. In the largest series thus far reported by Yousem and Hochholzer,[165] the majority of tumors were low grade. For low-grade tumor, the age ranges from childhood to old age with almost half of patients under 30 years. Women predominate slightly over men. Patients most commonly present with cough and hemoptysis. Grossly, low-grade tumors are endobronchial polypoid masses. They may contain cystic mucus-filled spaces. Microscopically, they are predominantly glandular and microcystic, lined by columnar and mucin-filled goblet cells that alternate with bland pink intermediate-type cells. There is no significant cellular atypia, necrosis, or mitotic activity (Fig. 18.19A,B). Tumors tend to remain localized to the bronchus and show limited invasion. In almost all cases regional lymph nodes are uninvolved. Complete surgical removal is curative. Aggressive behavior, however, has been rarely reported.[166]

High-grade mucoepidermoid carcinomas, on the other hand, are more often associated with cigarette smoking than low-grade tumors and are characterized histologically by significant nuclear pleomorphism, mitotic activity, and necrosis and are more likely to invade the lung (Fig. 18.20A,B). Patients with high-grade mucoepidermoid carcinoma have a greater incidence of hilar and mediastinal lymph node involvement, dissemination, and death. In one series of twelve patients, all died in less than one year.[167] Rare examples of intrapulmonary mucoepidermoid tumors have been reported.[168] High-grade mucoepidermoid carcinoma is distinguished from adenosquamous carcinoma of the lung by their endobronchial location compared with

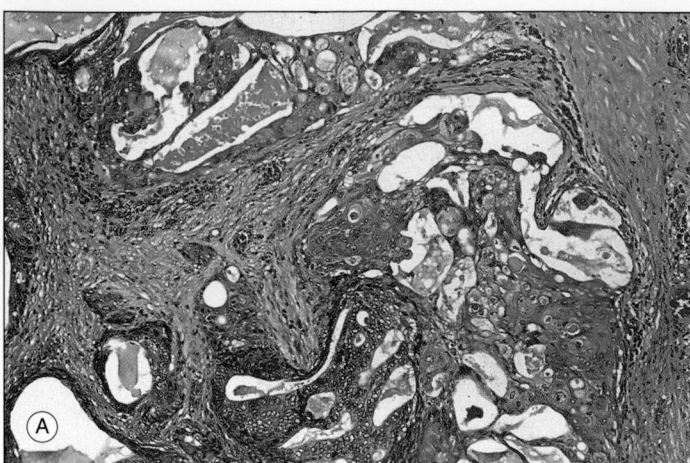
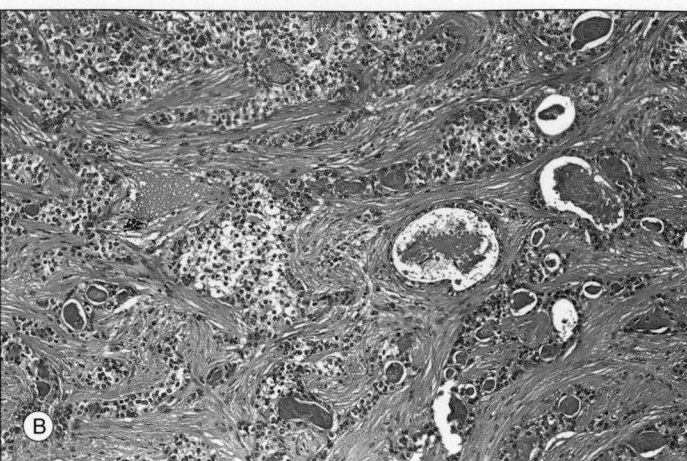

Fig. 18.19 A, Low-grade mucoepidermoid carcinoma. Tumor shows pushing architecture with an abundant mucinous-glandular component. Small areas of keratinizing squamous and intermediate cells are seen; **B**, Low-grade mucoepidermoid carcinoma. Bland intermediate cells and glands are in approximately equal distribution. No mitoses, necrosis, or nuclear pleomorphism.

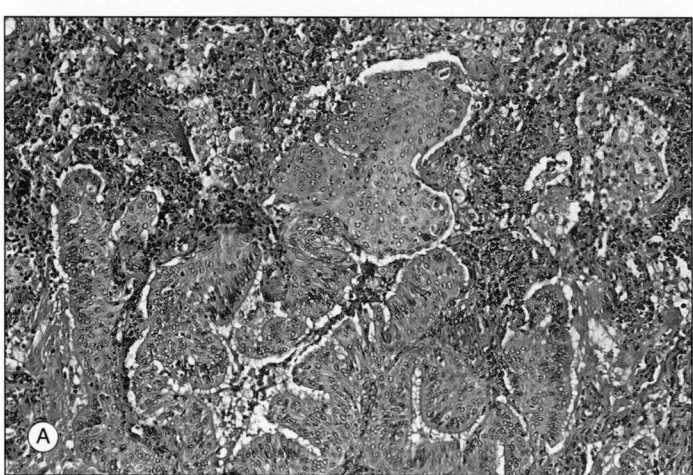
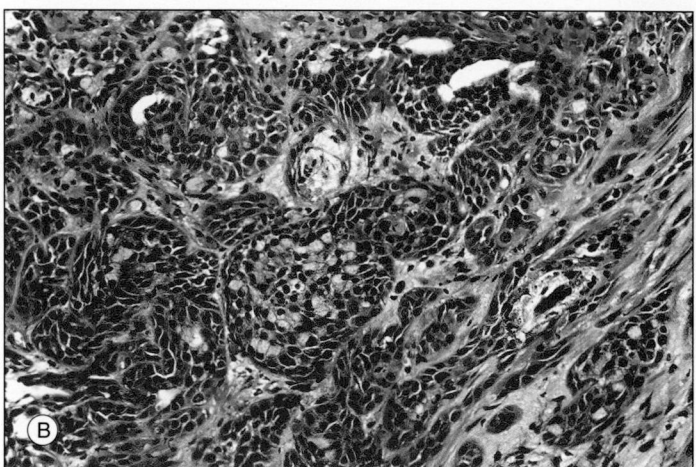

Fig. 18.20 A, High-grade mucoepidermoid carcinoma invading lung parenchyma. Intermediate cells are dominant. Nuclei show enlargement and discernible nucleoli; **B**, High-grade mucoepidermoid carcinoma. Invasive tumor penetrates the bronchial wall. Tumor has only a minor mucinous component. Nuclei show hyperchromasia and more atypia than low-grade tumors.

the more common peripheral localization and presence of keratinizing cells with intercellular bridges in adenosquamous carcinoma.

Cytology of mucoepidermoid carcinoma

Sputum and bronchial washings are not useful in the diagnosis of mucoepidermoid carcinoma, because the tumors are frequently covered by intact bronchial epithelium and therefore do not shed cells.[169] In FNA and bronchial brushing specimens the tumors occur as an intimate mixture of three cell types: nonkeratinizing squamous cells, intermediate cells, and mucus-secreting cells (Fig. 18.21).[170–172] In FNA samples, tissue fragments composed of spindle cells in the center and squamous or intermediate cells at the periphery can be seen.[172] The squamous cells are large and polygonal, occur in cohesive sheets, and have dense cytoplasm, distinct cell borders, and round to ovoid nuclei with a low N:C ratio (Fig. 18.21A,B). The intermediate cells appear in cohesive sheets of small to medium-sized, round to polygonal cells with distinct cell borders, and solitary, round, central

nuclei. The chromatin is finely granular, N:C ratio is high, and small nucleoli may be present (Fig. 18.21C). Mucus-secreting cells occur singly or in clusters. They have moderate amount of cytoplasm containing large solitary mucin vacuoles and eccentric, indented nuclei, and may be seen intermingled with squamous or intermediate cells (Fig. 18.21B). In low-grade mucoepidermoid carcinoma, mucinous cells are abundant and mucin may be present in the background. Mitoses, nuclear pleomorphism, and necrosis are absent. In high-grade tumors mucinous cells are scant, the transitional and squamous cells show a higher degree of pleomorphism and mitotic activity, and necrosis may be seen.

Differential diagnosis: Low-grade mucoepidermoid carcinoma is difficult to diagnose in cytologic samples because of the lack of obvious malignant criteria. Different cellular components of the tumor may be mistaken for reactive changes, particularly in bronchial brushings. The mucus cells may mimic benign goblet cells or clusters of reactive bronchial cells.[172] The squamous cells do not

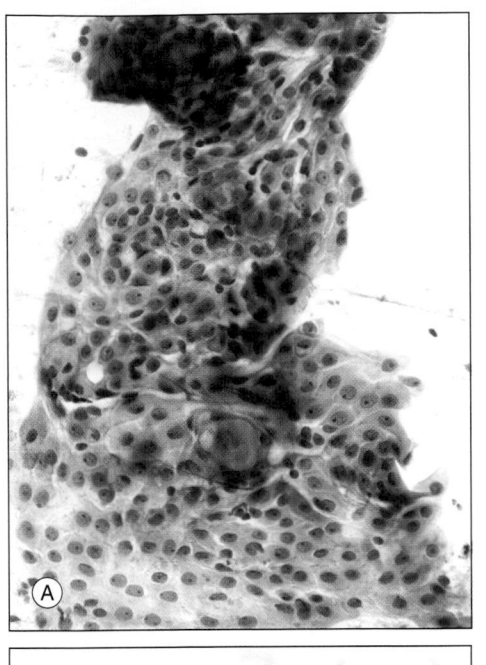

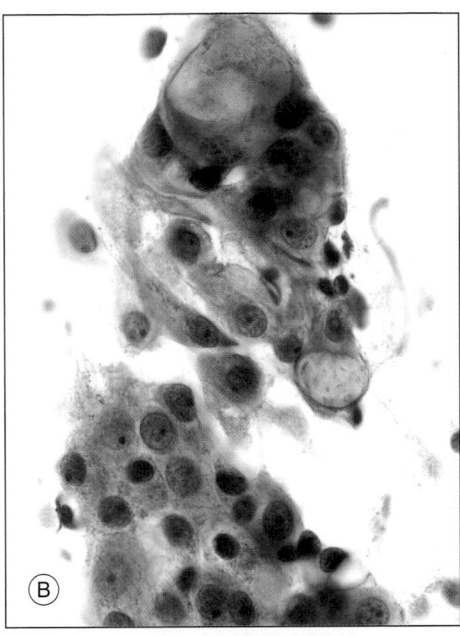

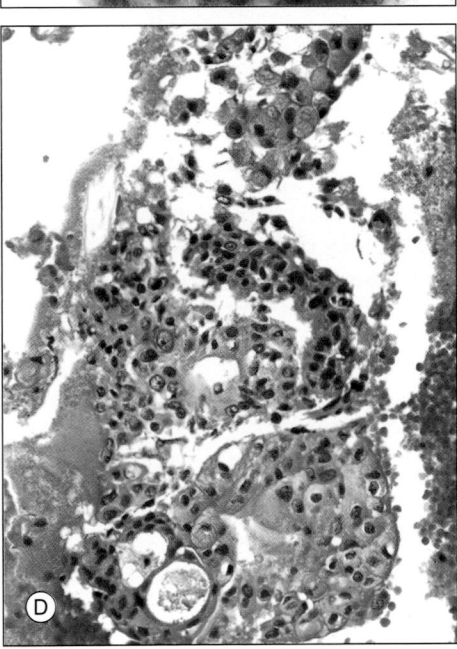

Fig. 18.21 FNA cytology of mucoepidermoid carcinoma. **A**, A large sheet of squamoid cells interspersed with a few mucus cells; **B**, Higher magnification showing cohesive, large, polygonal squamoid cells with low N:C ratio and bland nuclei. The mucus cells possess single large vacuoles that displace the nuclei; **C**, Intermediate cells with moderate amount of cytoplasm, well-defined cell borders, high N:C ratio and small nucleoli (A–C: Papanicolaou stain); **D**, Cell-block section showing a mixture of squamous, mucus, and intermediate cells (H&E stain).

exhibit significant nuclear pleomorphism, hyperchromasia, or mitoses, and therefore may be mistaken for squamous metaplasia of bronchial epithelium. The intermediate cells may look like immature squamous metaplasia. Low-grade mucoepidermoid carcinoma is easier to diagnose in FNA samples than by bronchoscopy because of the classic admixture of different cell types and of the unlikelihood of having large numbers of reactive bronchial cells in aspirated material. High-grade mucoepidermoid carcinoma, on the other hand, is composed of cells that are cytologically malignant, but are difficult to differentiate from adenosquamous carcinoma.[169]

Adenoid cystic carcinoma

Adenoid cystic carcinoma of the bronchus shares morphologic features with its more common counterpart in the salivary glands. It is the most common of the salivary gland-type tumors of the bronchus and is not associated with cigarette smoking.[173] Grossly, these tumors tend to be infiltrative, which thickens and constricts the bronchial wall or forms a nodular mass. Like salivary gland tumors, insidious microscopic spread and perineural invasion within the bronchus makes any form of local endobronchial resection difficult. Patients present with symptoms as the result of bronchial obstruction with cough, hemoptysis and shortness of breath. Peripheral tumors have been described, but these should be viewed cautiously as they may actually represent metastases from an occult or previously treated head and neck primary.[174]

Histologically, the tumors include glandular-cribriform, trabecular, and solid types (Fig. 18.22). Commonly, combinations occur. Tumor cells are typically small with scant cytoplasm. Mitoses are variable. Recently, attempts to stratify adenoid cystic carcinoma by histologic grade have shown that the cribriform type (grade I), the solid subtype (grade III), and the intermediate type showing combinations of grades

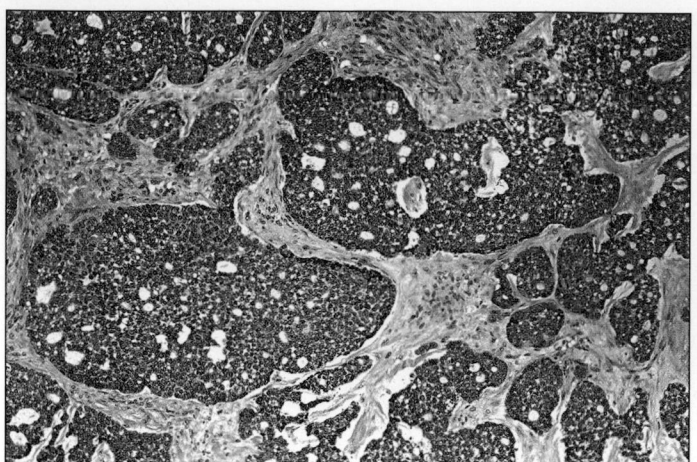

Fig. 18.22 Adenoid cystic carcinoma. Irregularly shaped nests of basaloid cells with cylindromatous and glandular features invade the bronchus.

I and III (grade II) may accurately predict outcome. Grade III carcinomas characteristically grow in solid sheets or trabeculae with necrosis and abundant mitotic activity. Distant metastases are more likely to be encountered with high-grade lesions.[175,176] Others have suggested that stage rather than histologic pattern is more predictive of outcome.[141,173]

The age range of adenoid cystic carcinoma is wide, and isolated pediatric cases have been reported.[177] Tumor size ranges from under 1 cm to up to 4 cm, and lesions may significantly infiltrate the pulmonary parenchyma. By immunohistochemistry, tumor cells are positive with low molecular weight cytokeratin, vimentin, and actin. S-100 protein may also be positive in varying proportions of the cells. Collagen type IV antibody outlines the prominent basement membrane seen most commonly in the glandular or cylindromatous areas. GFAP has been reported as negative.[178]

The prognosis of adenoid cystic carcinoma is not good. In one series of sixteen cases, three patients had disseminated tumor at the time of diagnosis, three patients had recurrence in the ipsilateral or contralateral thorax, and only three patients were alive and well without evidence of disease during the follow-up interval.[173] As in the salivary gland, recurrences may appear more than a decade after first treatment.[179]

Cytology of adenoid cystic carcinoma

Adenoid cystic carcinoma has characteristic cytologic features that are best seen in bronchial washing and brushing or FNA specimens.[169,172,180–185] Sputum samples are either devoid of tumor cells or, when present, they are difficult to classify.[40,184] Bronchoscopic and needle aspirate samples are usually cellular and contain tightly cohesive clusters of small, uniform tumor cells (Fig. 18.23). Several patterns have been described that correspond to architectural variations seen histologically, including solid groups, cribriform clusters, branching cylinders, and acellular hyalin spheres surrounded by tumor cells. Usually, more than one of these patterns are seen.[182] Tumor cells have scant cytoplasm resulting in a very high N:C ratio. Nuclei are ovoid and uniform with finely granular, evenly distributed chromatin (Fig. 18.23B). Nuclear molding and prominent nucleoli are not seen. The hyalin spheres stain bright magenta with Giemsa and pale bluish-green with the Papanicolaou

method. 'Naked' hyalin spheres without the surrounding tumor cells are occasionally seen, particularly in bronchial washings.[182]

Differential diagnosis: In bronchoscopic samples adenoid cystic carcinoma cells can be mistaken for reserve cell hyperplasia and vice versa. Reserve cells are generally smaller, may show an intimate association with ciliated bronchial cells, and do not exhibit complex architectural patterns or hyalin spheres.[172] In scant samples adenoid cystic carcinoma cells can mimic small cell carcinoma. However, the characteristic cytologic features of small cell carcinoma that include lack of cell uniformity and cohesiveness, coarse chromatin, high mitotic activity, nuclear molding, apoptosis, necrotic background, as well as the absence of hyalin spheres, are helpful in distinguishing this tumor from adenoid cystic carcinoma.

Acinic cell carcinoma

Acinic cell carcinoma of the bronchus, first reported by Fechner in 1972, is an extremely rare tumor.[186] Circumscribed tumor nodules ranging from slightly over 1 cm to over 4 cm have been described within the trachea and bronchi, but can also be seen peripherally within the pulmonary parenchyma. Histologically, there is a range of morphologic expression similar to its salivary gland counterpart (Fig. 18.24). Tumor cells show bland cytologic features and often show prominent PAS-positive intracytoplasmic secretory granules. They are reported to be immunohistochemically positive for amylase and alpha-1-chymotrypsin, but this is inconsistent.[187] The prognosis is excellent, with only one reported case having evidence of local lymph node metastasis.[141,188]

The differential diagnosis of acinic cell carcinoma includes other tumors that have eosinophilic granular cytoplasm, such as granular cell tumor and carcinoid.[189,190] This can be troublesome because each of these tumor types occur primarily in the larger bronchi, and therefore biopsy material is usually small. Granular cell tumor tends to be unencapsulated but benign. Histologically, tumor cells are round or polygonal with pink granular cytoplasm and eccentric small dark nuclei (Fig. 18.25). Immunohistochemistry may be helpful, since granular cell tumors characteristically are strongly positive with S-100 protein and negative with cytokeratin, while acinic cell tumors show the opposite. Both carcinoid and acinic cell tumors, however, are positive with cytokeratin and chromogranin.[187,191,192] Electron microscopy also shows that the cytoplasmic granularity of acinic cell tumor is due to large secretory granules as compared with smaller membrane-bound granules of carcinoid or abundant intracytoplasmic mitochondria of granular cell tumor.[141] Unusual, rare examples of combined acinic cell-carcinoid tumors of the lung have been reported that show immunohistochemical and ultrastructural features of both tumors.[187]

Endobronchial polypoid adenocarcinoma

Endobronchial polypoid adenocarcinoma is rare, accounting for approximately 3% of adenocarcinomas in the lung.[193] This tumor does not seem to be associated with cigarette smoking. It is characterized by endobronchial polypoid growth of tall columnar epithelial cells showing mild atypia and mitotic activity overlying fine fibrovascular papillary stalks (Fig. 18.26A,B). These tumors penetrate the bronchus and metastasize to mediastinal lymph nodes and cause death in 40% of cases. Electron microscopy shows that the cells contain numerous mitochondria and secretory mucus granules consistent with bronchial surface cell and goblet cell differentiation.

Bronchioloalveolar carcinoma

Central to the evolution of more common types of pulmonary adenocarcinoma is the role of atypical alveolar cell hyperplasia and

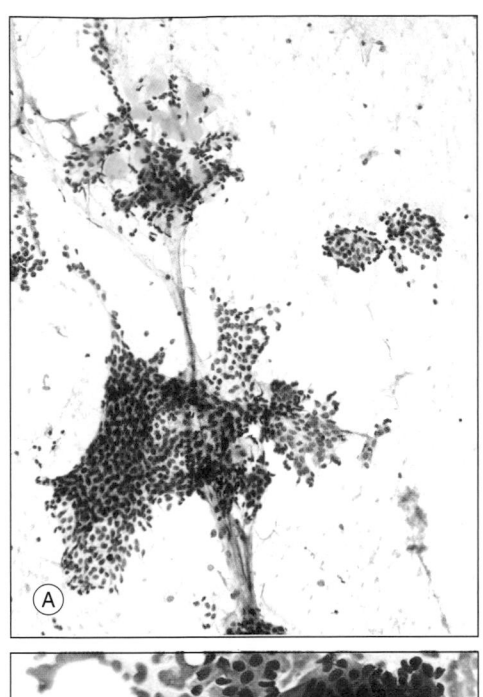
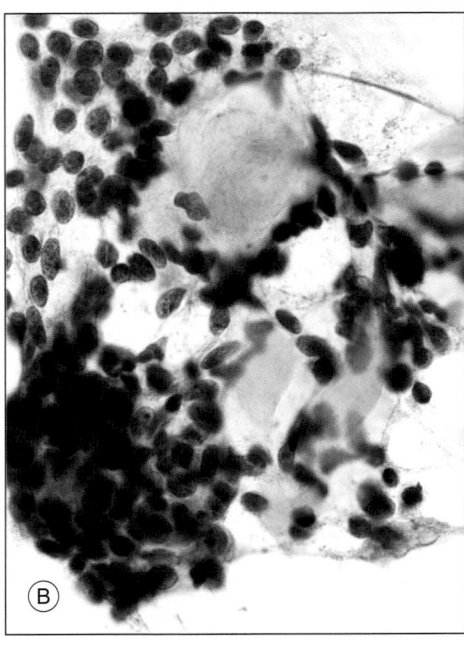
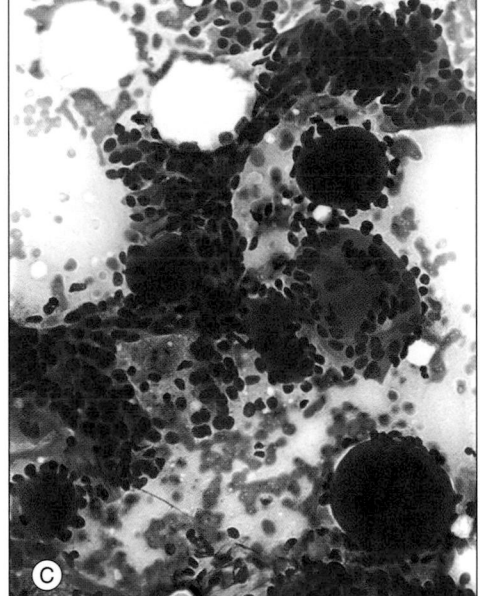
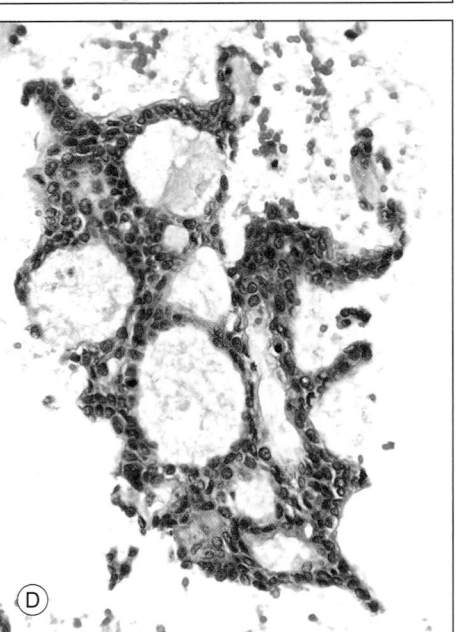

Fig. 18.23 FNA cytology of adenoid cystic carcinoma. **A**, Low magnification showing sheets and clusters of small tumor cells and a few acellular hyalin spheres in the left upper part of the field (Papanicolaou stain); **B**, Higher magnification depicting small cells surrounding blue-green hyalin material. Tumor cells have scant, indistinct cytoplasm and uniform, hyperchromatic, oval nuclei. Chromatin is evenly dispersed and nucleoli are inconspicuous (Papanicolaou stain); **C**, Hyalin material shows a brilliant magenta color with Romanowsky stains (Diff-Quik stain); **D**, Cell-block section exhibiting characteristic cribriform configuration of the tumor (H&E stain).

bronchioloalveolar carcinoma (BAC). Evidence suggests that these are indeed precursor lesions to invasive adenocarcinoma and represent the dysplastic and in situ phase of glandular lung neoplasia analogous to dysplasia and in situ squamous carcinoma in the bronchial mucosa.[194]

Noguchi and colleagues laid the groundwork for this concept in their 1995 paper, in which they studied 236 surgically resected small peripheral adenocarcinomas measuring 2 cm or less and separated them into six separate types that represent a progressive tumor model, ranging from localized bronchioloalveolar carcinomas that grew in lepidic fashion along normal preserved alveolar septa (Type A) (Fig. 18.27A), cases with lepidic growth but also with areas of structural alveolar collapse, thereby forming thickened interstitial stroma (Type B) (Fig. 18.27B), cases with foci of stromal alteration and fibroblastic proliferation resulting in architectural disarray of the underlying lung structure (Type C), and poorly differentiated adenocarcinoma, including tubular and papillary adenocarcinomas that showed more advanced disruption of the alveolar architecture, stromal disorganization, and little if any bronchoalveolar pattern at the periphery (Types D, E, and F) (Fig. 18.27C).[195] Types A and B showed 100% five-year survival rates while survival was shown to progressively decline for Types C, D, E, and F. It has been postulated that Types A and B represent the equivalent of in situ carcinoma, whereas the other subtypes show invasive adenocarcinoma with concomitant stromal disruption and alteration. The term bronchioloalveolar carcinoma should be reserved for only those tumors showing lepidic growth without nodular scar formation or an irregular pattern of glandular distribution and stromal proliferation that indicates invasion. The others are regarded as full-fledged adenocarcinoma with or without bronchoalveolar features depending on the presence of lepidic growth at the periphery of the tumor mass. Cases studied for loss of heterozygosity (LOH) have demonstrated

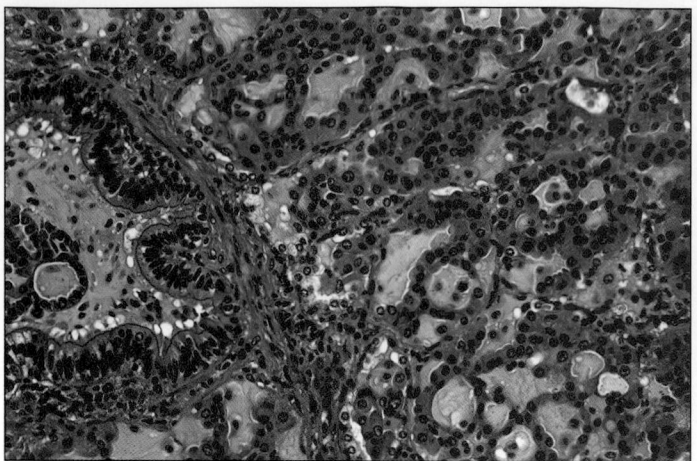

Fig. 18.24 Acinic cell carcinoma. Peripheral lung nodule showing glandular pattern of granular eosinophilic cells containing intraluminal mucinous material that stains faintly with mucicarmine. There is little cellular pleomorphism and only rare mitoses.

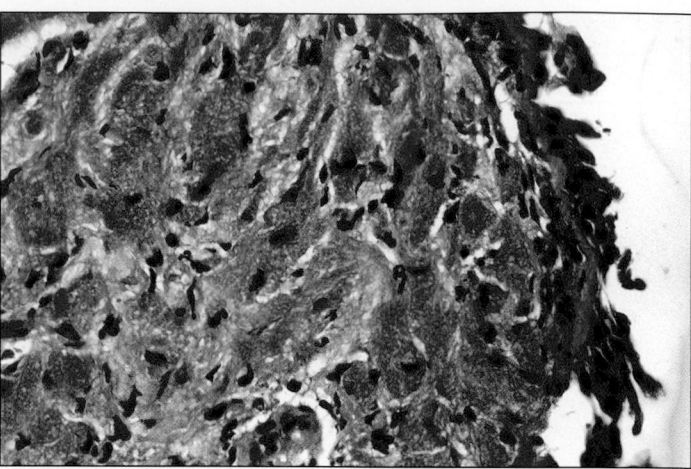

Fig. 18.25 Granular cell tumor. Bronchoscopic biopsy showing typical picture of large pink cells with granular cytoplasm and eccentric, small, dark nuclei. Tumors are strongly S-100 positive.

increasing allelic loss in eight chromosomal loci in types A, B, and C tumors. Tumor cells in the fibrotic areas of type C lesions showed the greatest number of chromosomal changes. These findings are consistent with a progression of genetic alterations as tumors invade the stroma.[196,197]

Immunohistochemical studies have also shown destruction and loss of basement membrane in type C tumors compared with types A and B using antibodies to collagen type IV, S collagen, and laminin, as well as progressive disruption of the elastic framework.[198,199] In addition, increasing nuclear accumulation of p53 has been shown. These observations support the in situ carcinoma concept of early BAC.

Bronchioloalveolar adenocarcinoma is composed of several cell types that are usually pure, but which may show a mixed phenotype. These are mucus-producing BACs that contain mucin-filled cells and intra-alveolar mucin secretion, and nonmucinous tumors composed of either Type II pneumocytes, Clara cells, or a combination of the two (Fig. 18.28A–C).[200] There is a wide range of cellular differentiation but usually tumors are composed of cells having relatively small low-grade nuclei, cellular uniformity, and little mitotic activity.

Grossly, bronchioloalveolar carcinomas are gray-white, poorly circumscribed lesions having a diffuse consolidating appearance that resembles organizing bronchopneumonia. Mucinous tumors often have a slimy, mucoid cut surface. Tumors are either single or multinodular, presumably as a result of intra-alveolar tumor spread.[201]

Recent studies have correlated the high-resolution CT scan appearance of small tumors with the histologic amount of bronchoalveolar pattern compared to invasive tumor growth. There is strong correlation between the proportion of bronchoalveolar growth pattern seen histologically and the presence of radiographic ground-glass opacity. Patients with tumors having radiographic ground-glass opacity were predominantly bronchoalveolar and had no relapses at

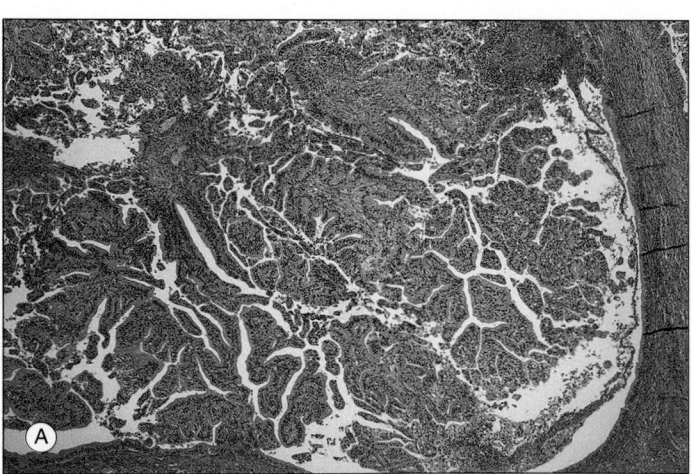

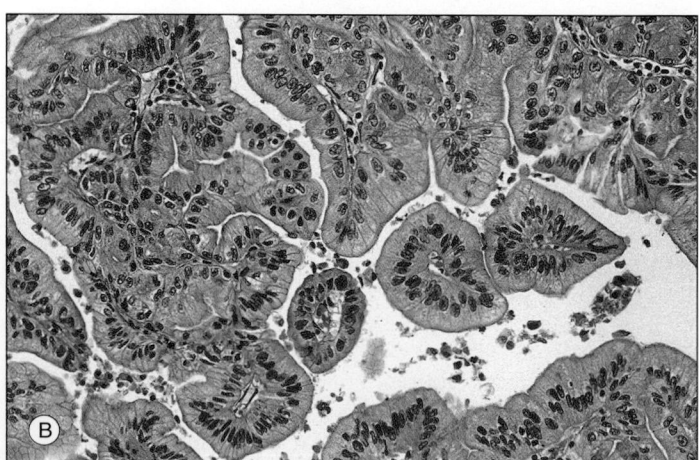

Fig. 18.26 **A,** Endobronchial polypoid adenocarcinoma. Intricately arborizing endobronchial growth; **B,** Higher magnification showing mildly atypical columnar tumor cells with basally oriented nuclei and fine fibrovascular stroma.

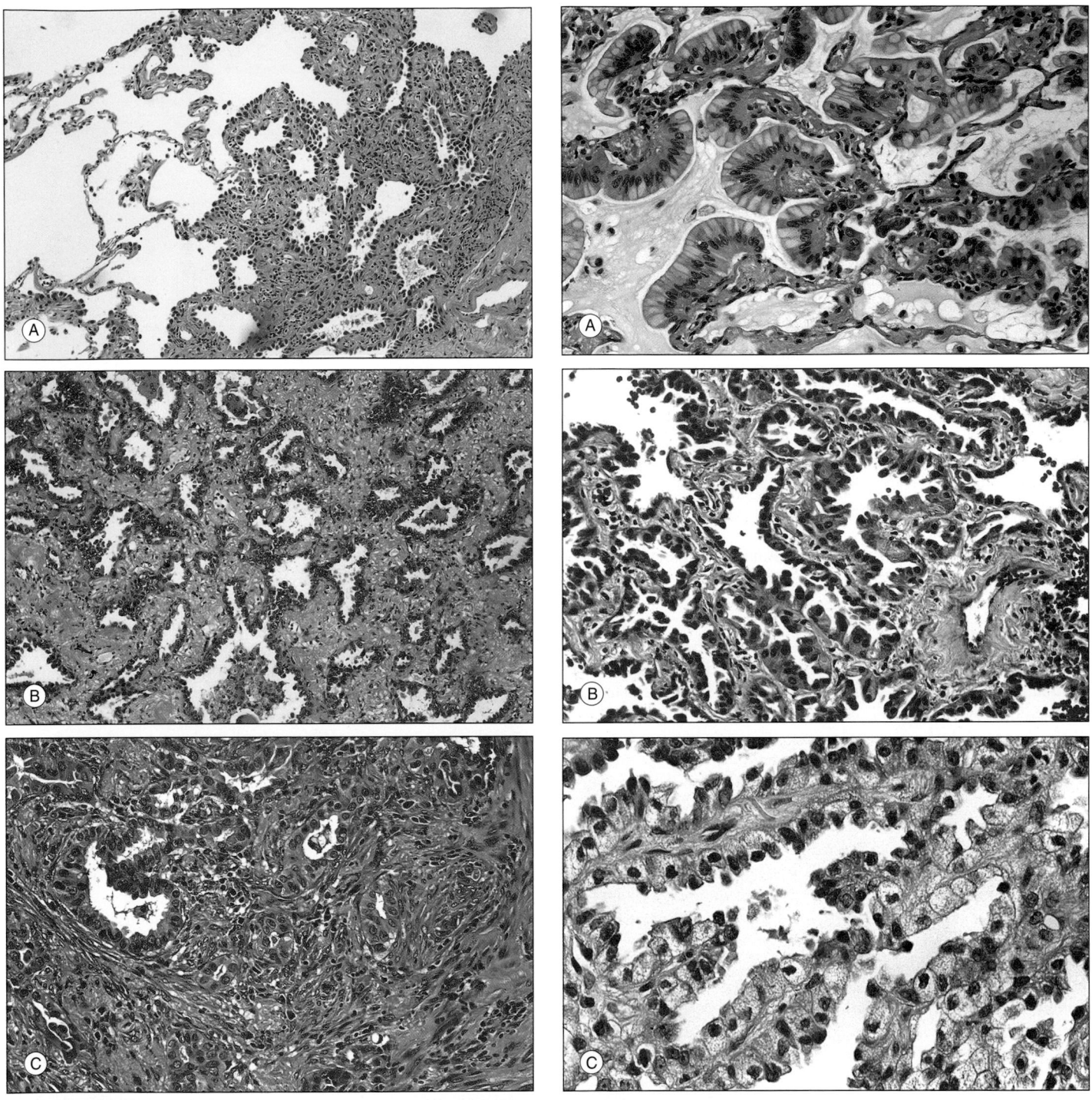

Fig. 18.27 A, Bronchioloalveolar adenocarcinoma. Nonmucinous tumor demonstrating growth along intact alveolar septae (lepidic growth) and increased interstitial fibrous tissue, but with intact alveolar architecture and no invasion; **B**, Bronchioloalveolar adenocarcinoma. Interstitial fibrosis is increased, but tumor cells maintain alveolar arrangement with lung architecture intact. Stromal fibrosis traps epithelium causing distortion of alveolar outlines, but without stromal invasion; **C**, Invasive adenocarcinoma in bronchioloalveolar adenocarcinoma. Glands show invasive growth with disruption of stroma.

Fig. 18.28 A, Mucinous bronchioloalveolar adenocarcinoma. Well-differentiated columnar mucinous epithelium growing along intact alveolar septae; **B**, Nonmucinous bronchioloalveolar adenocarcinoma. Pink cuboidal cells without vacuoles showing lepidic growth with mild fibrous thickening of alveolar septae; **C**, Clara cell differentiation in bronchioloalveolar adenocarcinoma. Tumor is made up predominantly of clear cuboidal cells showing little atypia.

two-year follow-up compared with tumors with more nodular-appearing CT scans, which tended to be solid adenocarcinomas and showed recurrence rates of almost 30% at two years.[202] Such radiographic findings seem to correlate with recent histopathologic observations that compare the degree of invasion and fibrosis in small adenocarcinoma with survival.[203] Tumors under 2.0 cm that microscopically show only minimal invasion, either in the lepidic portion of BAC or at the peripheral interface of bronchoalveolar and fibrotic areas, showed 100% 5-year disease-free survival. Nodular tumors with more ample invasion in the center of a fibrous nodule have a significantly worse outcome.

The prognosis of BAC is predominantly related to tumor size and multicentricity. Multinodular tumors have markedly decreased survival when compared with single tumors (4% versus 61% at five years).[204] Mucinous tumors have a greater tendency to multicentricity and a worse prognosis than nonmucinous tumors. Histologic features that influence survival include the presence of stromal sclerosis and invasion, nodal involvement, degree of lymphocytic infiltrate, as well as the completeness of resection. Nuclear grade and mitoses do not correlate with survival.[201] Completely resected stage I bronchioloalveolar carcinomas have demonstrated 100% survival.[195,203] Recent investigations, mostly in Japan, have studied the efficacy of limited wedge resection for small tumors, under 2 cm, and have shown no recurrences after short (less than three years) follow-up.[205,206] The need to clearly limit the definition of this tumor type by thorough histologic examination of small tumors is of obvious importance.

The differential diagnosis of BAC includes metastatic carcinoma from distant sites and atypical alveolar cell hyperplasia (atypical adenomatous hyperplasia). Many different types of adenocarcinomas, particularly from the gastrointestinal tract, may metastasize to the lung and demonstrate mucinous cells with lepidic growth similar to that of BAC. Some colonic metastases may be indistinguishable from mucinous BAC, even at the ultrastructural level.[207] Immunohistochemistry may aid in this differentiation since the majority of mucinous BAC stain positively with CK7 and CK20 while CK7 is usually negative in metastatic colonic adenocarcinoma. Also, TTF-1 (thyroid transcription factor) is positive in up to 90% of nonmucinous pulmonary adenocarcinomas and is usually negative in nonpulmonary tumors.[208-210] It is less useful in defining primary and metastatic mucinous tumors where the positivity rate is much less.[209]

The criteria for the differentiation of well-differentiated nonmucinous BAC from atypical alveolar cell hyperplasia (atypical adenomatous hyperplasia) is the subject of debate. Strict morphologic definitions have not been developed and are prone to observer bias. Nevertheless, one tentative criterion has been set at 5 mm size by several observers.[200,211-213] Some authors have included lesions up to several centimeters, however. Atypical adenomatous hyperplasia should have only mild nuclear atypia, no nuclear crowding, few mitoses, and does not demonstrate discohesive papillary tufts of epithelial cells in the alveolar space, which are features usually associated with carcinoma (Fig. 18.29).

The relationship of atypical adenomatous hyperplasia to BAC has been studied by molecular and other techniques and it has been shown to be a putative precursor. The majority of lesions studied from both groups of cases show progressive increase in nuclear size, CEA staining, aneuploidy, abnormalities in RAS oncogene, chromosomal deletions, and p53 expression.[214-218] There is significant overlap among the groups, which is indicative of a close association.

Atypical adenomatous hyperplasia is seen in approximately 10–60% of resected lung cancers specimens, depending on the definition and methods employed in detection.[219,220] The prognosis

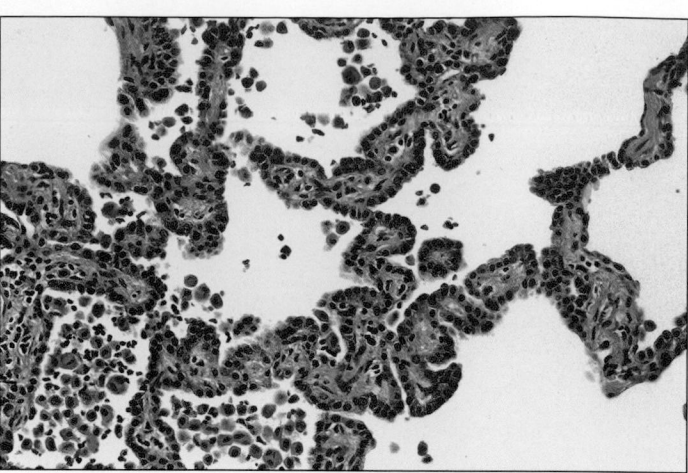

Fig. 18.29 Atypical adenomatous hyperplasia. Slightly enlarged, pink cuboidal nonmucinous epithelium lining slightly thickened alveolar septae. Nuclei are bland appearing. This lesion measures less than 5.0 mm in greatest diameter and was found incidentally in a lobectomy specimen for adenocarcinoma. Intra-alveolar macrophages are noted.

of patients with this finding was not significantly impacted when compared with lung cancer cases without atypical adenomatous hyperplasia, however.

Cytology of bronchioloalveolar carcinoma

Despite their peripheral location, BACs readily shed cells into the alveolar spaces, which can be detected in sputum cytology. Bronchoalveolar lavage also has a high tendency to yield tumor cells, but bronchial washing and brushing are less effective in the diagnosis. The sensitivity of bronchoscopic samples for BAC is 50–60% as compared to 70–75% for sputum cytology.[40,221,222] Because of the subtle cytologic abnormalities associated with well-differentiated BAC, a definitive diagnosis of malignancy can be difficult in exfoliative cytology, but these tumors are diagnosed with a high degree of accuracy by FNA.[104,221,223-226]

Mucinous BAC presents in cytologic specimens as sheets and cohesive papillary clusters of epithelial cells in a background of abundant mucin (Fig. 18.30). Tumor cells are uniform with abundant clear or foamy cytoplasm and round to ovoid nuclei. Large vacuoles are less common. Nuclear crowding is seen in the center of the cell clusters while at the periphery of such groups the columnar shape of the cells and basal nuclei can be appreciated. Nuclei are moderately enlarged, but the N:C ratio is low. Nuclear abnormalities may be quite subtle and appreciated only under high magnification (Fig. 18.30B). Nuclear membrane irregularity and grooves are present, chromatin is finely granular, and prominent nucleoli may be observed. Necrosis is generally absent.

Nonmucinous BAC appears as monolayer sheets and loose clusters of relatively small, round, or polyhedral cells (Fig. 18.31A). Tumor cells are generally uniform and possess round or ovoid nuclei with a high N:C ratio. The chromatin is finely granular and intranuclear cytoplasmic invagination is present (Fig. 18.31B). Prominent nucleoli are seen at least in some cells. Cytoplasmic vacuoles and extracellular mucin are absent. Sometimes large numbers of benign macrophages are present, which may provide a clue to this type of neoplasm.

Unlike well-differentiated bronchioloalveolar carcinomas, poorly differentiated BACs exhibit hyperchromasia, pleomorphism, and

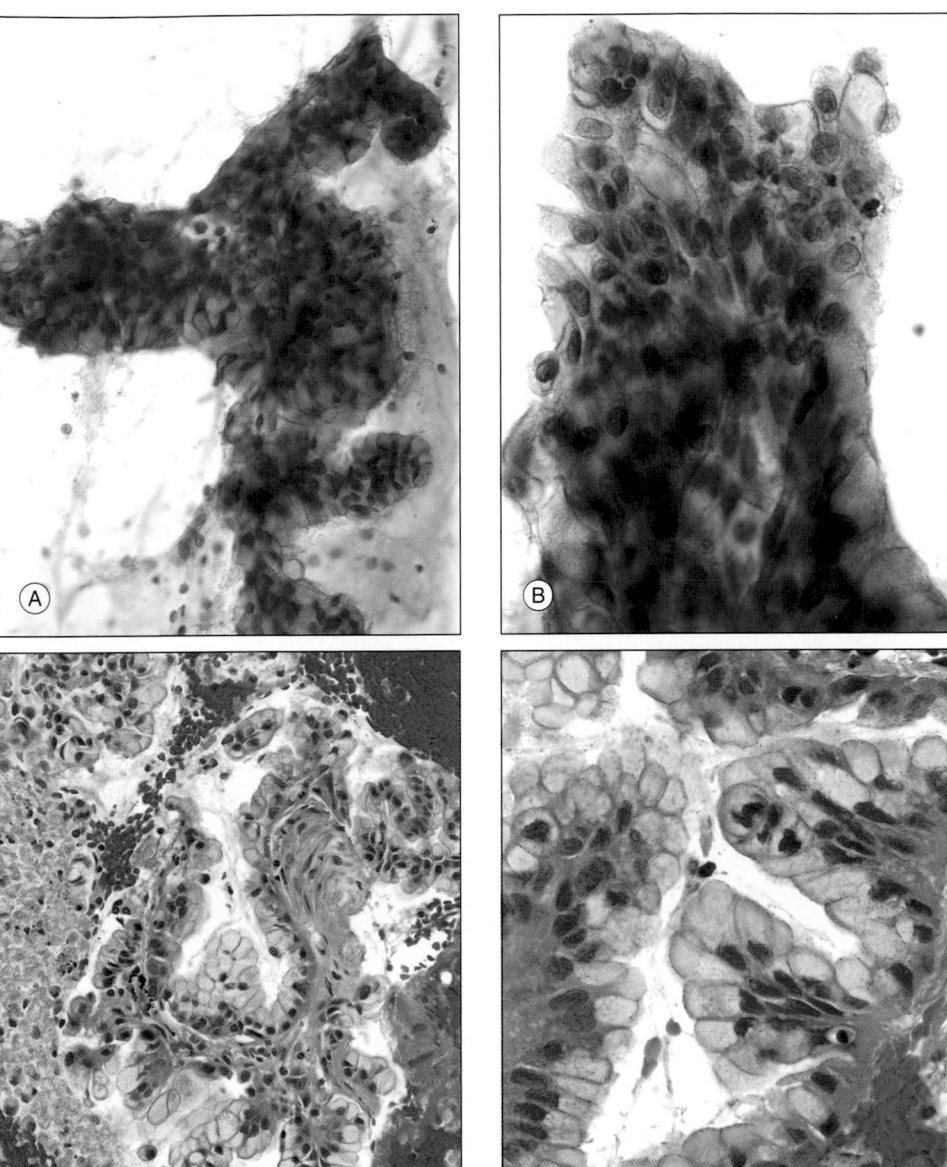

Fig. 18.30 FNA cytology of mucinous bronchioloalveolar carcinoma. **A**, Papillary clusters of cohesive glandular cells in a mucinous background; **B**, Higher magnification showing a three-dimensional cluster of cells with foamy cytoplasm and round to oval nuclei. The cells on the edge of the group are columnar with basically located nuclei. Within the cluster, the nuclei appear crowded and disorganized. Nuclear membrane irregularity is evident (A & B: Papanicolaou stain); **C**, Cell-block section of the same case showing the alveolar architecture of the tissue fragment; **D**, A single layer of atypical mucinous cells lining the alveolar spaces (C & D: H&E stain).

loss of cohesiveness, making their distinction from ordinary adenocarcinoma or metastatic tumors impossible.

Differential diagnosis: BAC is to be distinguished from other types of cancer on the one hand and from benign reactive conditions on the other. While the criteria described above are generally helpful in distinguishing BAC from adenocarcinoma, overlap of cytologic criteria precludes such a distinction in all cases. Auger et al. found that prominence of monolayer sheets, fine chromatin pattern and mild cellular pleomorphism correlated significantly with nonmucinous BAC, whereas the prominence of nuclear grooves and the abundance of extracellular mucin correlated significantly with mucinous BAC when compared to adenocarcinoma.[104] Cell blocks are often helpful in the diagnosis of BAC, as minute tissue fragments may enable visualization of small portions of alveolar walls lined by malignant cells (Figs. 18.30C,D and 18.31C,D). Primary and metastatic adenocarcinomas usually exhibit a higher degree of pleomorphism and loss of cohesiveness than BAC. Distinguishing BAC from metastatic papillary carcinoma of the thyroid is difficult as these tumors share many cytologic features including papillary or monolayer arrangement, uniformity of the cells, nuclear grooves, and occasionally psammoma bodies.[227] However, this differential diagnosis rarely comes into play in practice and when it does, clinical correlation and immunocytochemical staining for thyroglobulin can solve the problem.

In exfoliative cytology (sputum, bronchial washing, bronchial brushing) reactive and hyperplastic bronchial epithelium may mimic BAC. In bronchoscopic samples of reactive conditions, usually a spectrum of cellular abnormalities are seen that range from minimally atypical cells easily recognizable as benign to more severely atypical cells. This is not the case in malignant tumors, in which two distinct populations of cells, separate from each other and

Fig. 18.31 FNA cytology of nonmucinous bronchioloalveolar carcinoma. **A,** Sheets of highly uniform, round to polygonal epithelial cells (Papanicolaou stain); **B,** Higher magnification demonstrating round nuclei with bland chromatin and minimal nuclear membrane irregularity. Nucleoli are prominent and occasional mitoses are present. Inset depicts intranuclear cytoplasmic invagination; **C, D,** Cell block section of the same case. Minute tissue fragments have an alveolar pattern with thin septa, lined by a single layer of cuboidal or columnar tumor cells. Intracytoplasmic mucin is not observed (H&E stain).

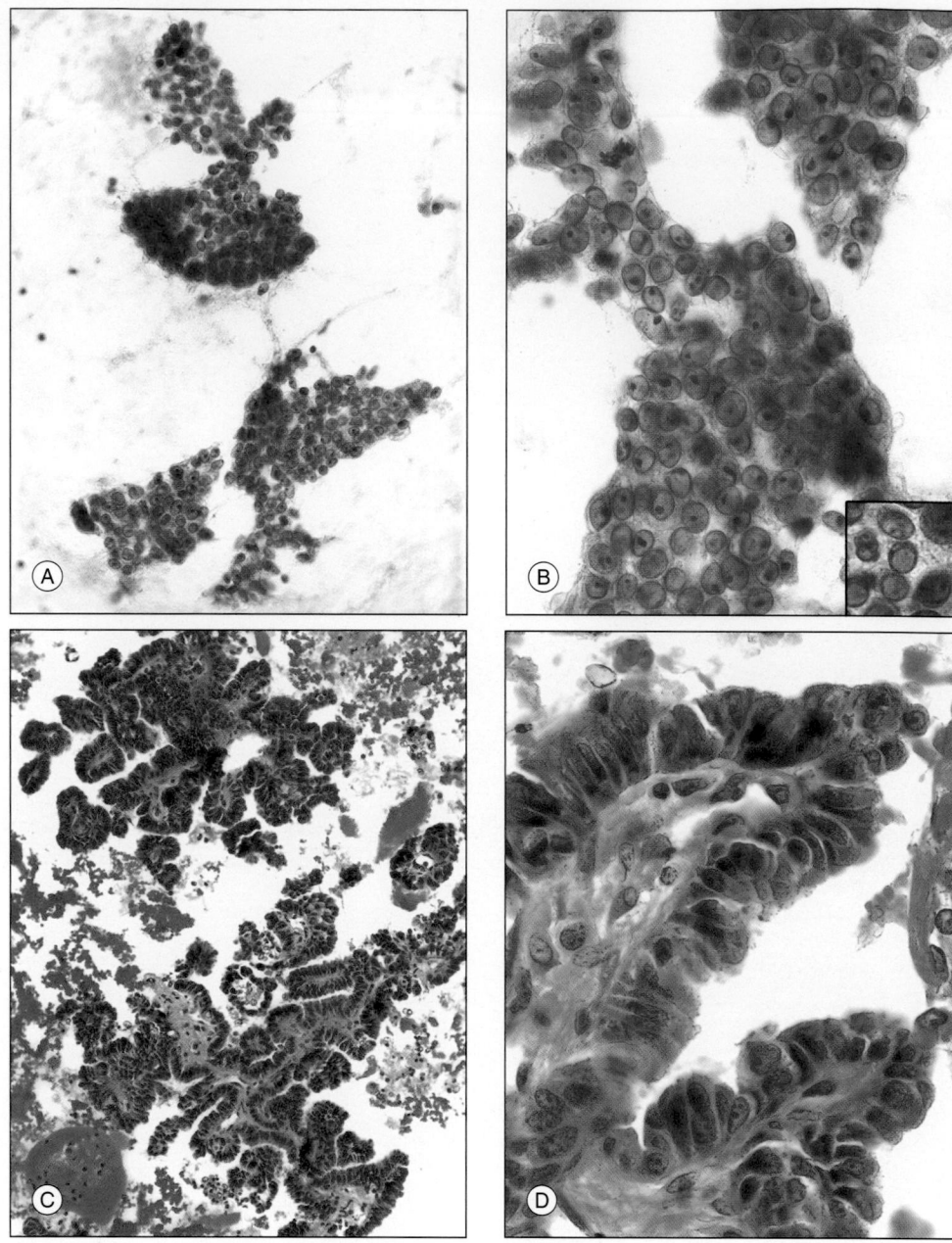

without a transition between them are often found. When doubt exists in interpretation of bronchoscopic samples, fine needle aspiration should be performed, which has a higher sensitivity and is easier to evaluate because a pure population of tumor cells can be collected.

In FNA specimens, reactive and hyperplastic pneumocytes caused by inflammatory processes, chemotherapy, radiation, acute alveolar damage, infarct, and other benign conditions may mimic BAC. Reactive cells, however, are generally fewer in number, less commonly form three-dimensional clusters, exhibit little or no hyperchromasia, have lower N:C ratio, and rarely possess prominent nucleoli compared to malignant cells. A morphometric study reported by Zaman et al. showed statistically significant differences between the mean nuclear area of reactive cells and that of BAC,[228] but another study by Fiorella et al. did not support this finding.[229]

Cystic mucinous tumors

There is a group of cystic mucinous tumors in the lung that bear close similarity to mucinous tumors of the ovary and appendix and present similar problems in classification. All are extremely rare. The benign mucinous cystadenoma is a unilocular, well-circumscribed, cystic, mucus-filled lesion lined by a simple layer of bland goblet cell epithelium.[230] At the other end of the spectrum is the mucinous cystadenocarcinoma, which is grossly similar to mucinous cystadenoma, but with malignant-appearing epithelium or free-floating tumor cells in the mucinous pools, and evidence of capsular or parenchymal invasion (Fig. 18.32A,B).[231,232]

The place of mucinous cystic tumor of borderline malignancy in the spectrum of these lesions is somewhat controversial. First reported by Graeme-Cook and Mark, they described a well-differentiated, grossly mucinous and colloid-appearing lung tumor microscopically composed of large areas of acellular mucus similar to a mucocele or

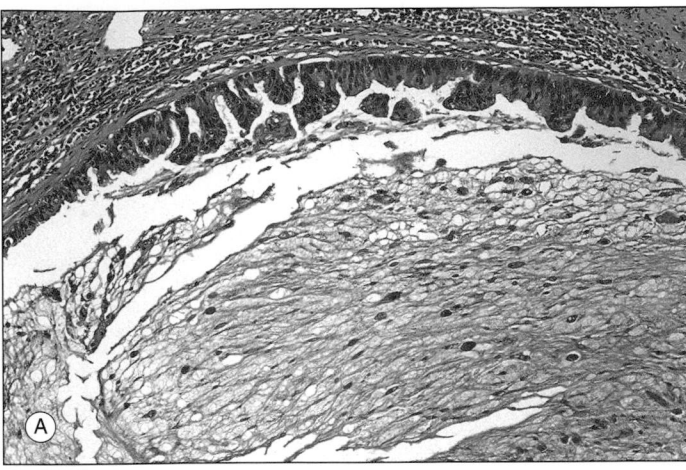

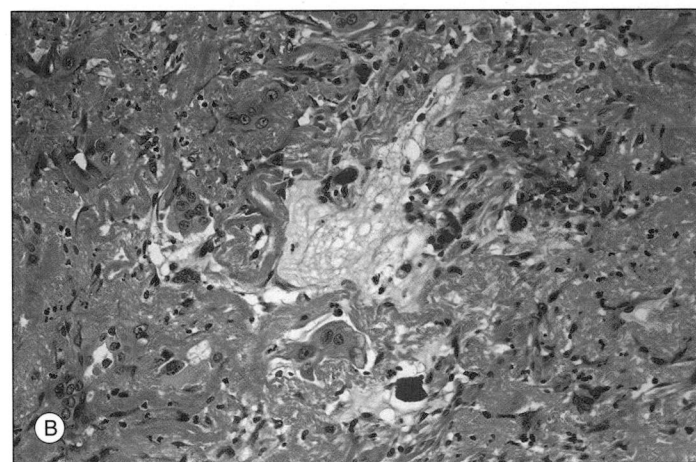

Fig. 18.32 **A**, Mucinous cystadenocarcinoma. Predominantly cystic tumor lined by hyperchromatic tumor cells arranged in noninvasive papillary configuration; **B**, Mucinous cystadenocarcinoma. Portions of fibrous capsule containing invasive adenocarcinoma.

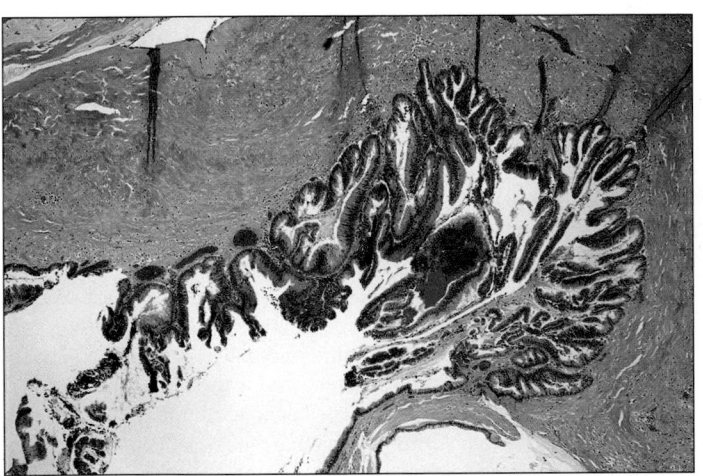

Fig. 18.33 Mucinous cystic tumor of borderline malignancy. Noninvasive cystic mucinous tumor lined by complex glandular-papillary arrangement of mucinous epithelium. No cellular atypia or mitoses.

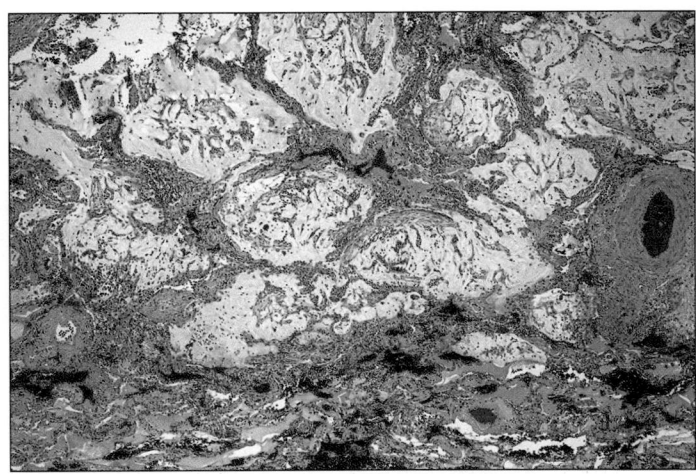

Fig. 18.34 Mucinous cystic tumor of borderline malignancy. Alveolar spaces are distended by acellular mucinous material at edge of tumor. Regions like this can be seen in borderline and malignant mucinous tumors, as well as in mucinous bronchioloalveolar adenocarcinoma. Distinct separation of these tumors is sometimes difficult and arbitrary.

cystadenoma (Fig. 18.33).[233] The majority of cases show at least focal mucin-producing vacuolated tumor cells lining up along the alveolar septae with varying degrees of atypia similar to borderline mucinous tumors of the ovary. Tumors are usually well circumscribed, but not encapsulated, and acellular mucus is seen within intact alveoli at the margin (Fig. 18.34). The prognosis of mucinous cystadenoma, borderline tumor, and cystadenocarcinoma has been uniformly good, but rare local recurrences have been observed.[234]

Pulmonary colloid carcinomas have been defined as showing clusters of malignant tumor cells floating free in the mucinous pools, when compared with the mucinous cystic borderline and mucinous cystadenocarcinoma, but this definition seems arbitrary.[231] Recent studies have suggested that those colloid carcinomas that contain signet-ring cells and show GI immunophenotype have a poor prognosis. Tumors showing intestinal-type goblet cells with combined lung and GI immunophenotype have a good prognosis similar to other

mucinous cystic tumors. Of thirteen such cases recently studied, two patients with signet-ring carcinoma cells died of disease, while all patients with goblet cell tumors survived.[235] Clear separation of cystic mucinous tumors from solitary, well-differentiated mucinous BAC and colloid carcinoma may be difficult.

Pulmonary adenocarcinoma

Pulmonary adenocarcinomas are invasive tumors and show varying morphology as reflected in the nomenclature adopted by the WHO.[200] Papillary, acinar, and solid patterns are common (Fig. 18.35A,B). Mixed forms are frequent, particularly in larger tumors. In addition, rare variants such as well-differentiated fetal adenocarcinoma and clear cell adenocarcinoma have been described (Fig. 18.36). The previously discussed cystic mucinous carcinomas are also included in this group.[200] Adenocarcinomas generally share similar clinical and radiographic features, being more common in women than men,

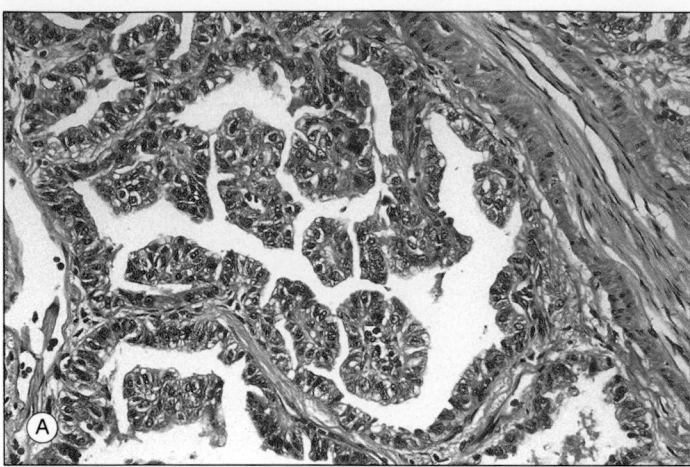 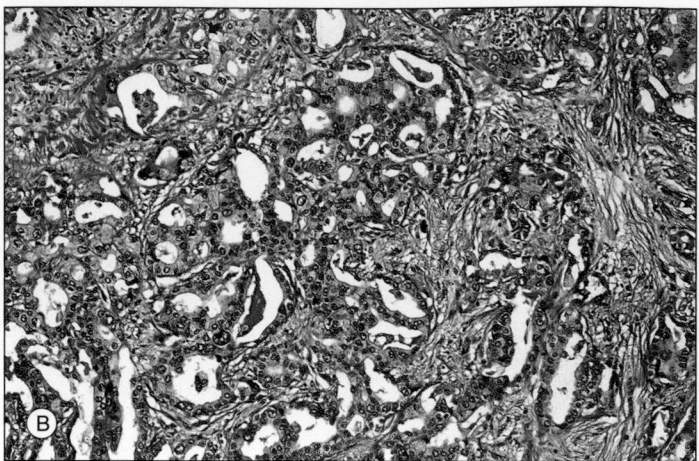

Fig. 18.35 A, Adenocarcinoma, papillary pattern; **B**, Adenocarcinoma, acinar pattern.

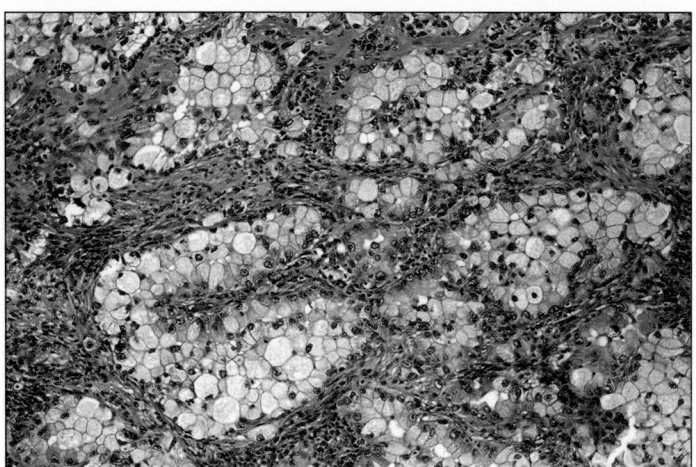

Fig. 18.36 Adenocarcinoma, clear cell pattern.

and associated with cigarette smoking. They tend to be more often peripheral in location than squamous cell carcinoma or small cell carcinoma. Tumors may vary in size from under a centimeter to lesions that opacify the lung, radiographically. Even small tumors under 1.0 cm may metastasize, however.[236] The degree of differentiation from tumor to tumor and within a single lesion may vary greatly from areas of well-developed gland formation to solid undifferentiated tumor recognizable as adenocarcinoma only by associated company or histochemical demonstration of mucin by mucicarmine or PAS stains. Nuclei are enlarged with peripheral clumping of chromatin and commonly have prominent nucleoli, in contrast to squamous cell carcinoma where the nuclear chromatin is denser, more diffuse, and nucleoli are less conspicuous. The coexistence of invasive adenocarcinoma and BAC, (noninvasive lepidic growth) is common, particularly in tumors less than 2.0 cm.[195,237] The DNA labeling index correlates with degree of cellular atypia, mitotic count, and clinical stage.[238] It may be low in many cases, however, and therefore is not useful in distinguishing well-differentiated adenocarcinoma from reactive epithelial changes.[238] Tumor cells characteristically stain with antibodies to polyclonal

CEA, LeuM1 (CD15), BerEP4, and B72.3 in over 90% of cases.[239–241] This immunoprofile, however, is not specific for lung cancer. Antibody to thyroid transcription factor 1 (TTF-1), on the other hand, is highly specific for adenocarcinoma of the lung, with a sensitivity of over 70%. The majority of lung tumors show the keratin profile CK7 positive, CK20 negative.[239–241] Some adenocarcinomas may show focal areas of signet ring, spindle cell, giant cell, and hepatoid differentiation or may be composed entirely of these elements (Fig. 18.37A,B).[242–244] Abundant lymphoid stroma is seen in some cases (Fig. 18.38).

Multicentricity may be seen in approximately 20% of cases with separate tumor nodules present in other areas of the lung tissue.[245]

The differential diagnosis of pulmonary adenocarcinoma is wide. Nonmucinous tumors must be differentiated from malignant mesothelioma. Instances of small peripheral adenocarcinomas that thicken the pleural surface, thereby mimicking malignant mesothelioma (pseudomesoepitheliomatous adenocarcinoma), have been described (Fig. 18.39).[246] Here again, immunohistochemistry can play an important role since mesotheliomas most often are positive for calretinin and negative with markers commonly associated with pulmonary adenocarcinoma, such as polyclonal CEA, CD15, and TTF-1.[210] Metastatic carcinoma to the lung from many different sites must always be considered. In general, the clinical history is extremely important in evaluating whether a tumor is primary or metastatic. In patients with a prior history of breast or colon cancer who have new solitary lung masses, approximately half have been shown to have new independent lung tumors.[247] Immunohistochemistry may greatly aid in localizing the site of a solitary pulmonary metastasis (Table 18.4).

The prognosis of adenocarcinoma of the lung is poor and is related to clinical stage at presentation.[248] Most patients present with advanced-stage disease. Small resectable tumors, under 2 cm, may be expected to have between 65% and 80% five-year survival.[248,249]

Cytology of adenocarcinoma

Because of their peripheral location in the lung, adenocarcinomas are less commonly diagnosed in sputum and bronchoscopic specimens and more often in FNAs compared to squamous cell carcinoma. In cytologic specimens, adenocarcinomas generally appear as three-dimensional clusters of cells (Fig. 18.40A–C). Tumor cells are medium-sized and round, cuboidal, or columnar in shape. Nuclei are enlarged as compared to normal epithelial cells, resulting in an

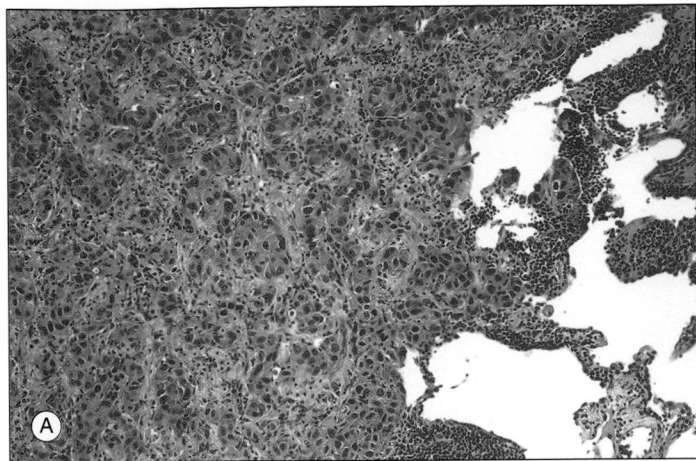

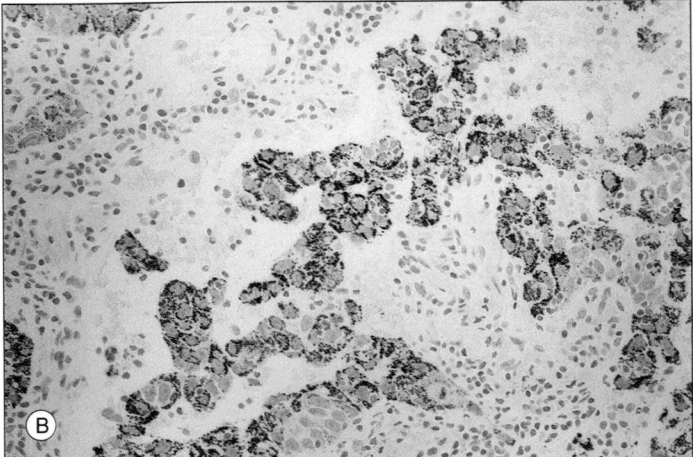

Fig. 18.37 **A**, Adenocarcinoma, hepatoid variant. Cords of large, eosinophilic tumor cells with liver-like appearance; **B**, Hepatocyte antigen is positive in cytoplasm of tumor. AFP may also be positive in tumors with hepatoid differentiation.

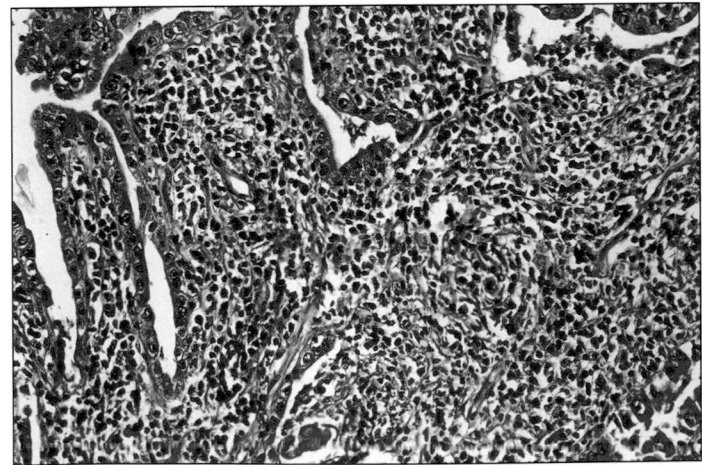

Fig. 18.38 Adenocarcinoma with lymphoid stroma.

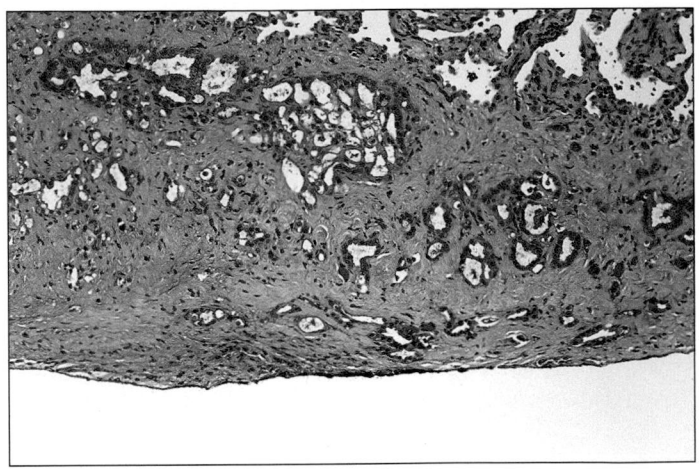

Fig. 18.39 Adenocarcinoma with extensive pleural invasion. Such tumors may radiographically and grossly mimic malignant mesothelioma, (pseudomesotheliomatous carcinoma).

increase in N:C ratio. The nucleus may not exhibit significant hyperchromasia or chromatin clumping, but irregularity of the nuclear membrane is evident under high magnification. Single or multiple prominent nucleoli are usually present. The cytoplasm is pale and basophilic and frequently contains small and, less often, single large vacuoles. Well-differentiated adenocarcinomas are usually characterized by the presence of relatively uniform and cohesive cells, whereas poorly differentiated tumors exhibit a higher degree of anisocytosis and loss of cohesiveness. Unlike squamous carcinoma, the presence of necrosis in the background is not a common feature.

The differential diagnosis of adenocarcinoma includes reactive changes secondary to chronic inflammatory conditions, infections, asthma, treatment effect, and drug reactions (i.e. chemotherapy, radiation, amiodarone). In chronic bronchitis and asthma, papillary hyperplasia of bronchial epithelium sheds three-dimensional clusters of epithelial cells known as Creola bodies, which can be mistaken for adenocarcinoma in sputum cytology.[250] Creola bodies are characterized by cellular cohesiveness, mild nuclear enlargement and the presence of small nucleoli, but generally do not exhibit significant pleomorphism, nuclear membrane irregularity, and chromatin abnormalities as seen in malignant tumors (Fig. 18.40D). Correlation with clinical and radiologic data, as well as well-prepared specimens, are of utmost importance in this differential diagnosis. Bronchoscopic sampling and FNA should be employed to confirm the diagnosis in unclear circumstances. In chemotherapy or irradiation related atypias there is usually a range of abnormalities from cells that appear to be reactive to those with marked enlargement and nuclear abnormalities; however, N:C ratio is low and nuclei often exhibit degenerative changes. In amiodarone toxicity the abundance of large cells with numerous small vacuoles and slightly enlarged nuclei may raise the suspicion of adenocarcinoma, but they exhibit features of pulmonary macrophages, do not form cohesive clusters, and lack mucin. In lipid pneumonia, single and small groups of cells with variable-sized vacuoles and abnormal nuclei can mimic adenocarcinoma. In the organizing stage of adult respiratory distress syndrome reactive and hyperplastic type II pneumocytes show marked atypical features that may be mistaken for adenocarcinoma in bronchoalveolar lavages.[251] The cells may appear singly or in small clusters, and have high N:C ratio and prominent nucleoli. Many macrophages and other

Table 18.4 Differential immunohistochemistry profile of primary and metastatic adenocarcinoma

Primary site	Antibody profile					
	TTF-1	CK7	CK20	p-CEA	CD15	Other
Lung adenocarcinoma	+^	+	–*	+	+	villin –/+
Colon	–	–	+	+	+	villin +
Breast	–	+	–	+	+	ER +, PR +, Brst-2 +
Kidney	–	–**	–	–	+	CD10 +, vimentin +, EMA +
Mesothelioma	–	+	–	–	–	calretinin +, vimentin +, CK5/6+
Pancreas	–	+	+	+	+	CA19-9 +
Anaplastic large cell lymphoma	–	–	–	–	–	LCA+, CD30+, ALK-1+, EMA+
Germ cell tumors	Seminoma: CAM 5.2 –, EMA–, PLAP +					
	Non-seminomatous GCTs: CAM5.2 +, EMA – (except choriocarcinoma),					
	AFP +, HCG +, CD30+, PLAP +					

^ TTF-1 nuclear positivity is generally seen in up to 75% of pulmonary adenocarcinomas.

* 70–80% of mucinous BACs are negative for TTF-1 and positive for CK20 in contrast to nonmucinous BAC. A CK7–/CK20+/villin+ /TTF-1– pattern is most commonly seen with colonic carcinoma.[564,565]

** Conventional (clear cell) renal cell carcinoma is negative for CK7. However, papillary, chromophobe and collecting duct variants may be positive for CK7.[566]

inflammatory cells are present in the background. Familiarity with this pitfall and careful correlation with clinical and radiologic findings are essential in preventing a false-positive diagnosis. Repeat sampling also can be helpful as the number of atypical cells and degree of atypia decreases after a few weeks. In a series reported by Stanley et al. hyperplastic pneumocytes were not seen in BAL specimens collected a month after the onset of injury.[251] The cytologic features that distinguish adenocarcinoma from malignant mesothelioma are discussed elsewhere in this book.

CLEAR CELL AND LARGE CELL TUMORS (Table 18.5)

A variety of lung lesions, both benign and malignant, either primary or metastatic, are characterized by large cells with or without optically clear cytoplasm.

Benign clear cell tumor

The benign clear cell tumor was first reported in 1963 by Liebow and Castleman and named 'sugar' tumor of the lung.[252,253] Patients are characteristically asymptomatic and present with a solitary peripheral radiographic abnormality. Grossly, tumors are well circumscribed, variably colored, and without necrosis. Microscopically, they are composed of nests or fascicles of optically clear epithelioid and spindle cells, often having sharp cell borders, and sometimes showing a perivascular arrangement (Fig. 18.41). Nuclei are small without prominent nucleoli or significant mitotic activity. The cells characteristically contain large amounts of glycogen, easily demonstrated by the PAS stain with diastase digestion and by electron microscopy, which demonstrates complex membrane-bound glycogen granules.[254]

The origin of the tumor has long been the subject of speculation, but current evidence points to a close relationship of benign clear cell tumor to angiomyolipoma of the kidney and to tuberous sclerosis.[255] Clear cell tumors have been described in patients with tuberous sclerosis in association with pulmonary lymphangioleiomyomatosis and micronodular pneumocyte hyperplasia.[256,257] Some suggest they are part of the spectrum of so-called perivascular epithelioid cell tumors (PEComas).[258]

Immunohistochemistry shows most clear cell tumors to be strongly positive with melanoma antigen, HMB-45, and some cases are positive with NSE, synaptophysin, and CD57, similar to angiomyolipoma of the kidney and lymphangioleiomyomatosis of the lung. In addition, clear cell tumors can also be focally positive for S-100.[259,260] Almost all tumors have been cured by local resection. One report describes metastases to the liver.[261]

Benign clear cell tumor must be differentiated from large cell carcinoma of the lung with clear cell changes and metastatic renal cell carcinoma. Katzenstein analyzed a large group of squamous cell adenocarcinomas and large cell undifferentiated carcinomas, and found foci of clear cells in approximately 30% of the cases.[134] In the majority of cases, clear cell change was only focal, however. Clear cell morphology is usually a reflection of glycogen content of the cytoplasm.

Metastatic clear cell adenocarcinoma of the kidney is perhaps the most common epithelial malignancy to present clinically as pulmonary metastases from an occult primary tumor. The most characteristic appearance is that of nests of clear epithelial cells surrounded by fine fibrovascular stroma, sometimes combined with spindled and granular cell components (Fig. 18.42).[262] Immunohistochemistry is helpful in identifying this tumor, which shows positivity for vimentin and CD10 and most often negative staining with CEA, CD15, B72.3, and BerEP4, in contrast to lung cancer.

Large cell carcinoma

Large cell carcinoma of the lung is characterized by sheets of large cuboidal epithelial cells without evidence of cytoplasmic differentiation on routine stains. Not surprisingly, this tumor category shows the greatest degree of interobserver variability among pathologists. It is a diagnosis of exclusion after ruling out tumors with recognizable squamous, glandular, or neuroendocrine appearance, which to a certain extent is dependent on the volume of tissue available for microscopic study.[263] At the ultrastructural level, evidence for squamous or glandular differentiation is common, however.

The tumors are usually large and peripherally located, and often show necrosis and hemorrhage. Involvement of the major bronchi is not usually seen. Microscopically, the tumor cells are large and have

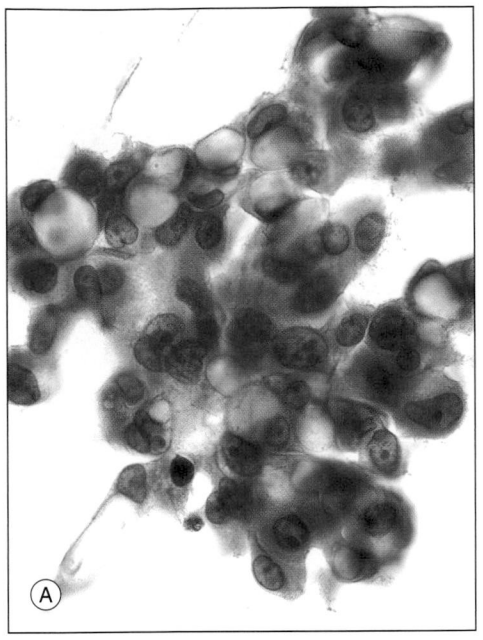

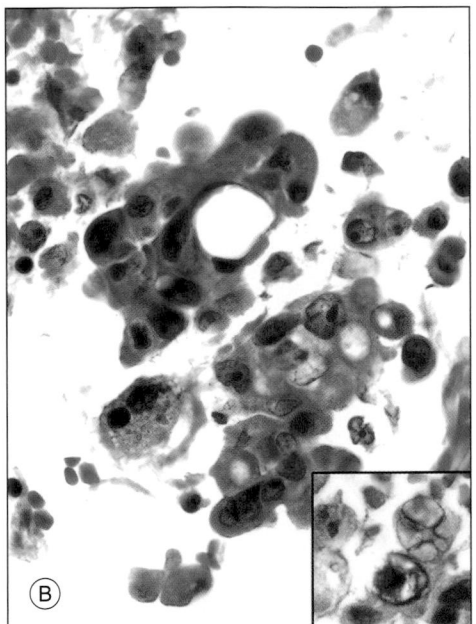

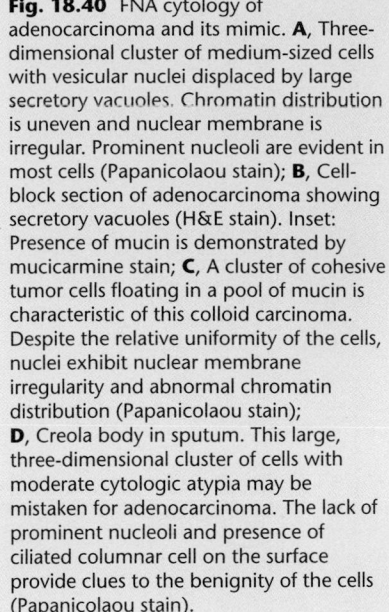

Fig. 18.40 FNA cytology of adenocarcinoma and its mimic. **A**, Three-dimensional cluster of medium-sized cells with vesicular nuclei displaced by large secretory vacuoles. Chromatin distribution is uneven and nuclear membrane is irregular. Prominent nucleoli are evident in most cells (Papanicolaou stain); **B**, Cell-block section of adenocarcinoma showing secretory vacuoles (H&E stain). Inset: Presence of mucin is demonstrated by mucicarmine stain; **C**, A cluster of cohesive tumor cells floating in a pool of mucin is characteristic of this colloid carcinoma. Despite the relative uniformity of the cells, nuclei exhibit nuclear membrane irregularity and abnormal chromatin distribution (Papanicolaou stain); **D**, Creola body in sputum. This large, three-dimensional cluster of cells with moderate cytologic atypia may be mistaken for adenocarcinoma. The lack of prominent nucleoli and presence of ciliated columnar cell on the surface provide clues to the benignity of the cells (Papanicolaou stain).

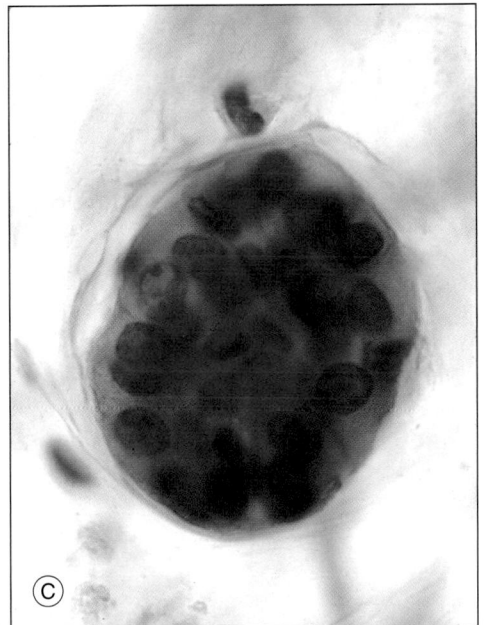

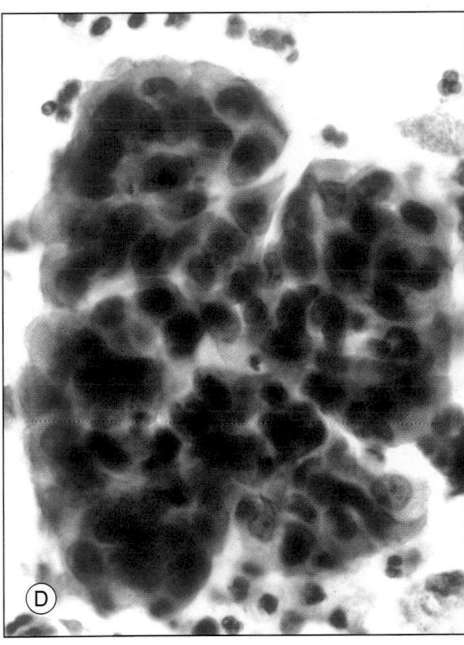

Table 18.5 Clear cell and large cell tumors

Benign clear cell tumor

Metastatic renal cell carcinoma

Large cell carcinoma
  Large cell carcinoma with neuroendocrine features
  Giant cell carcinoma
  Lymphoepithelioma-like carcinoma

round or cuboidal shapes with abundant clear or pink cytoplasm and large nuclei containing prominent nucleoli. Small amounts of intracellular mucin, as evidenced with mucicarmine stains, can be seen, but there is no evidence of glandular differentiation and no intercellular bridges (Fig. 18.43).

The outcome of large cell carcinoma is poor. The majority of patients present in advanced stages and the prognosis is worse than that of squamous cell carcinoma or adenocarcinoma. Approximately 40% of resectable cases survive five years; the survival for all patients is closer to 10%.[264–266] Giant cell carcinoma of the lung is felt by most to be a variant of large cell carcinoma and is characterized by large multinucleated giant tumor cells with huge nucleoli. Demographics and anatomic location are similar to ordinary large cell carcinoma. In order for a tumor to qualify as giant cell carcinoma, this feature should predominate over all others, histologically (Fig. 18.44). One peculiar, yet characteristic, histologic feature is the finding of

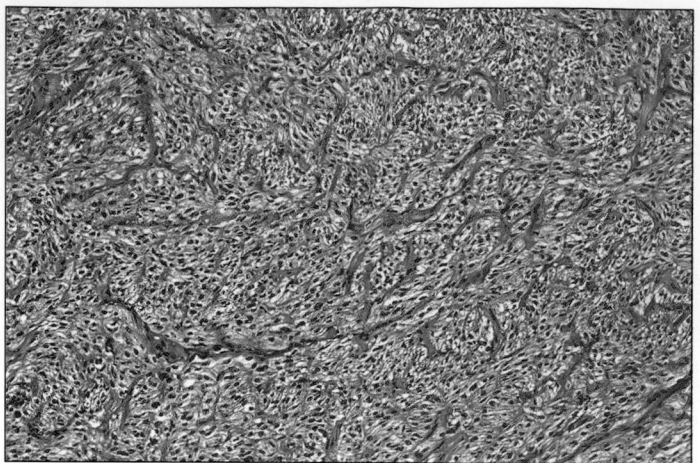

Fig. 18.41 Benign clear cell tumor. Nests of spindled clear cells with fine fibrovascular stroma. Nuclei are dark staining, small, and uniform without mitoses.

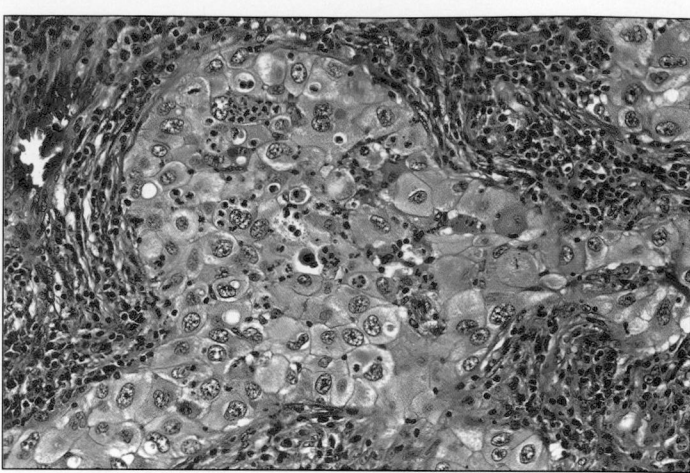

Fig. 18.43 Large cell carcinoma. Tumor cells have large nuclei with prominent nucleoli. Cell borders are distinct but lack intercellular bridges.

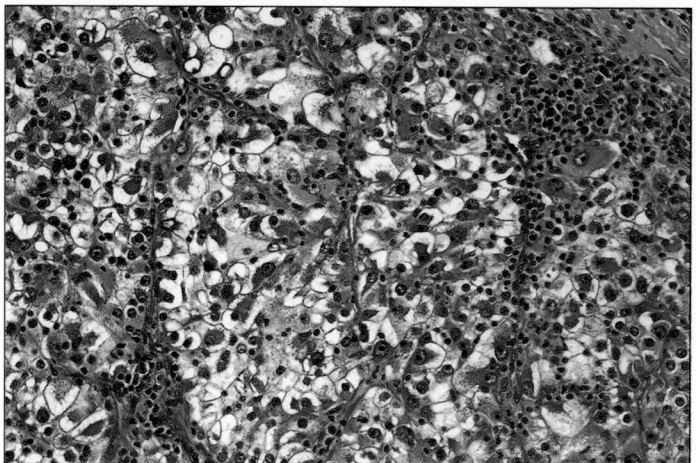

Fig. 18.42 Metastatic clear cell adenocarcinoma from the kidney. Tumor is composed of solid nests of pleomorphic clear cells surrounded by finely vascularized stroma. The patient had a prior renal tumor.

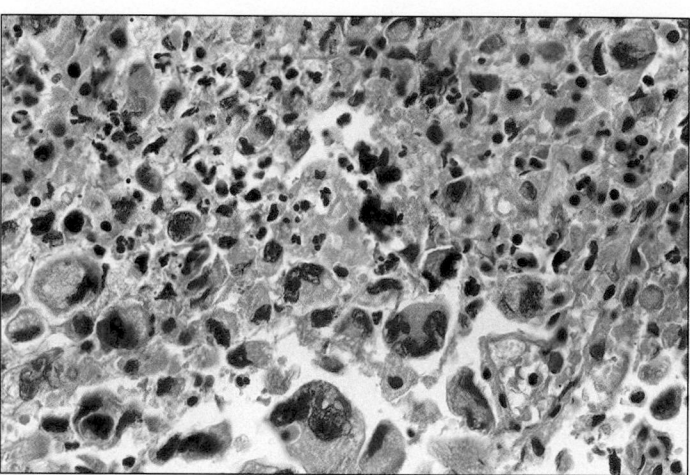

Fig. 18.44 Giant cell carcinoma. Large multinucleated tumor cells are seen in association with polymorphonuclear cell infiltration, a common feature.

inflammatory infiltrates composed of polymorphonuclear cells, eosinophils, and to a lesser extent lymphocytes within the cytoplasm of the tumor giant cells. This is felt to be due to chemotactic effect of colony stimulating factor produced by the giant cells.[267] Giant cell carcinomas of lung can show features that mimic choriocarcinoma and produce human chorionic gonadotrophin (Fig. 18.45). Patients have been reported to have experienced uterine bleeding secondary to ectopic hormone production.[268,269] These tumors have a propensity to metastasize to the GI tract, causing obstruction and severe bleeding.[270]

Large cell carcinoma with neuroendocrine features and large cell neuroendocrine carcinoma offer confusing terminology, but are entirely different tumors. Large cell carcinoma with neuroendocrine features has similar appearance to ordinary large cell carcinoma with the additional findings that neuroendocrine markers (chromogranin, synaptophysin, NSE) are positive by immunohistochemistry or neurosecretory granules are observed by electron microscopy.[200] The prognosis is worse than for large cell carcinoma without neuroendocrine features and is similar to that of small cell carcinoma.[271–273]

Lymphoepithelioma-like carcinoma

Lymphoepithelioma-like carcinomas of the lung were first reported in 1987 by Begin et al. and are rare.[274] They are usually subpleural peripheral nodules that present as asymptomatic coin lesions. A few cases have shown more widespread lung disease.

Histologically, the tumors look identical to lymphoepithelial carcinomas of the nasopharynx and elsewhere in the upper aerodigestive tract. There are cohesive nests or cords of large epithelial cells growing in a syncytial pattern or isolated cells separated by a richly cellular infiltrate of plasma cells and lymphocytes (Fig. 18.46A,B). Nuclei are usually round or oval with prominent nucleoli. Ultrastructurally, the epithelial cells show tonofilaments and desmosomes indicative of poorly differentiated squamous carcinoma. The tumors vary in size from 1cm to 6 cms. Forty percent of

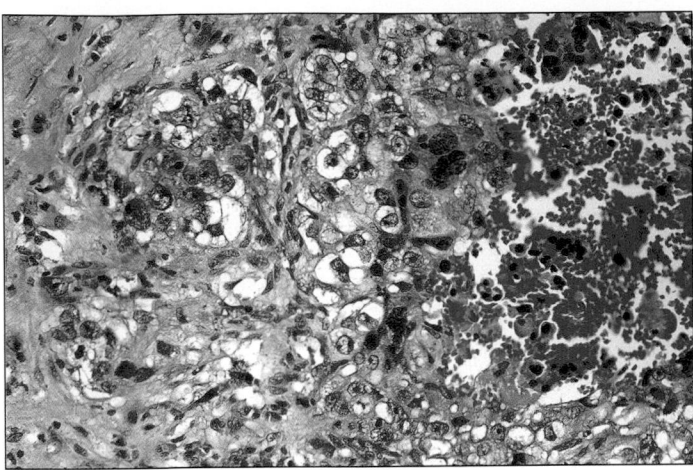

Fig. 18.45 Large cell carcinoma of lung with choriocarcinoma-like features. There is a two-cell population composed of multinucleated giant cells and clear cells associated with hemorrhage reminiscent of syncytial and cytotrophoblast.

patients are current or ex-cigarette smokers. Lymphoepithelioma-like carcinoma has a predilection for Asian patients; it has been described in only four Caucasians. In Asian cases there is a strong association with Epstein-Barr virus (EBV) analogous to similar tumors of the nasopharynx. In contrast, Caucasian patients have tested negative for EBV-related DNA using in situ hybridization techniques.

The majority of patients present with early-stage disease; 70% were in stage I. The prognosis seems to be better than for the more usual large cell carcinoma.[258,275–277]

Cytology of large cell carcinoma

The cells of large cell carcinoma are easily recognized as malignant in bronchoscopic and needle aspirate specimens. A large number of single and poorly cohesive groups of tumor cells are present in a background of necrosis. Tumor cells have abundant cytoplasm and contain one or more large, pleomorphic nucleus with marked irregularities of chromatin distribution and nuclear membrane. Single or multiple prominent nucleoli are usually seen.[137] Secretory vacuoles, acinar or papillary formations, keratinization, and intercellular bridges that would indicate glandular or squamous differentiation are not present. The giant cell variant of large cell carcinoma is characterized by huge, pleomorphic tumor cells containing multiple malignant-looking nuclei (Fig. 18.47).[278–281] Neutrophils are frequently present in the background and within the cytoplasm.[278,280,281] Lymphoepithelioma-like carcinoma appears as cohesive sheets of moderately pleomorphic spindle cells with vesicular nuclei and prominent nucleoli in a background of numerous small lymphocytes.[282]

Differential diagnosis: The cells of large cell carcinoma exhibit obvious malignant criteria and are not mistaken for benign conditions. However, there is a significant degree of overlap between the cytologic features of this tumor and those of poorly differentiated adenocarcinoma and squamous carcinoma, which together with sampling error is responsible for only a 42% correlation between cytologic and histologic typing in a large series.[283] Therefore, it is best to use the more noncommittal term 'poorly differentiated non-small cell carcinoma' and defer final classification until histologic examination of the excised tumor in such cases. Malignant melanoma and sarcomas should also be considered in the differential diagnosis. Lymphoepithelioma-like carcinoma should be differentiated from granulomatous inflammation, malignant lymphoma, Hodgkin's disease, melanoma, and germ cell tumors. The mixture of epithelioid cell aggregates and lymphocytes in this neoplasm may mimic a granulomatous process, but prominent nucleoli seen in the tumor cells provide a clue in distinguishing them from histiocytes. The cohesive nature of tumor cells is against the diagnosis of Hodgkin's or non-Hodgkin's lymphoma. In difficult cases immunohistochemical stains assist in correct diagnosis of this neoplasm, as tumor cells react positively for cytokeratin and epithelial membrane antigen.[282]

SPINDLE CELL LESIONS (Table 18.6)

Many different pulmonary lesions of diverse origin may show spindle cell morphology. These range from epithelial tumors such as

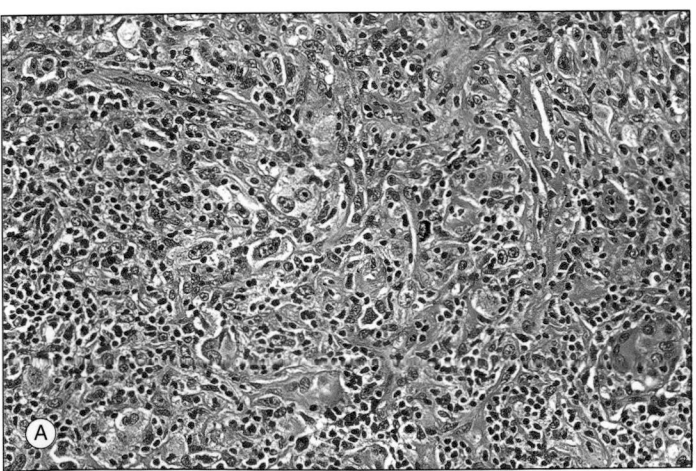

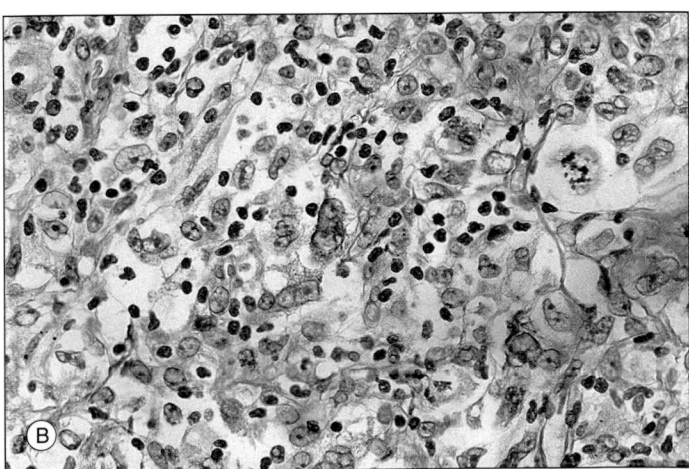

Fig. 18.46 **A**, Lymphoepithelial carcinoma. Scattered large atypical tumor cells are obscured by an extensive lymphoplasmacytic infiltrate; **B**, Lymphoepithelial carcinoma. Cytokeratin stains tumor cells.

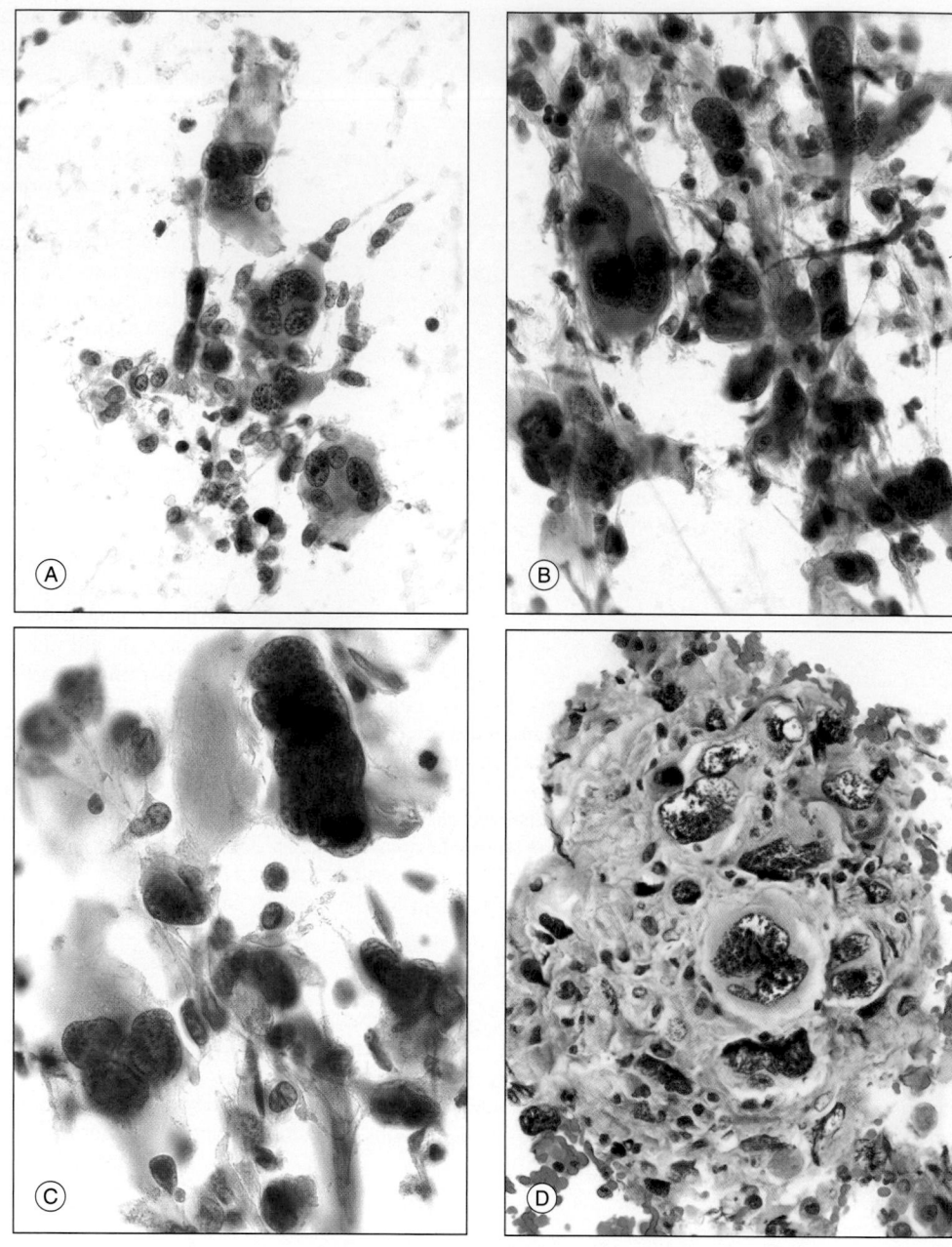

Fig. 18.47 FNA cytology of giant cell carcinoma. **A**, Mixed population of spindle and multinucleated giant cells with marked variation in size and shape (Papanicolaou stain); **B,C**, Higher magnification showing highly pleomorphic nuclei with marked hyperchromasia, clumped chromatin and irregular nuclear membrane; **D**, Cell-block section of the same sample. Small lymphocytes are admixed with giant tumor cells (H&E stain).

Table 18.6 Spindle cell tumors and tumor-like conditions

Benign	Malignant
Inflammatory pseudotumor	Benign metastasizing leiomyoma
Pulmonary hyalinizing granuloma	Spindle cell carcinoma
Nodular amyloid	Spindle cell sarcoma
Eosinophilic granuloma	Malignant fibrous histiocytoma
Malakoplakia	Monophasic synovial sarcoma
Mycobacterial pseudotumor	
Solitary fibrous tumor	
Meningothelial-like nodules (chemodectoma)	
Lymphangioleiomyomatosis	

spindle cell carcinoma to various mesenchymal tumors and tumor-like proliferations.

Inflammatory pseudotumor

Inflammatory pseudotumors are rare. The classic 1973 paper of Bahadori and Liebow described forty cases and set the standard for the subsequent literature.[284–288] They occur at any age but tend to be seen in younger people, including children, and have a peak incidence in the third decade. Most cases are solitary, well-circumscribed tumor-like masses radiographically. Occasional patients may show more than a single lesion. Invasion of surrounding structures such as the esophagus and vertebrae has been rarely described.[284,289] Microscopically, the characteristic findings are a cellular spindle cell proliferation arranged in interlacing fascicles, sometimes with a storiform pattern, intimately mixed with varying proportions of mature plasma cells, often with Russell bodies, foam cells, and other

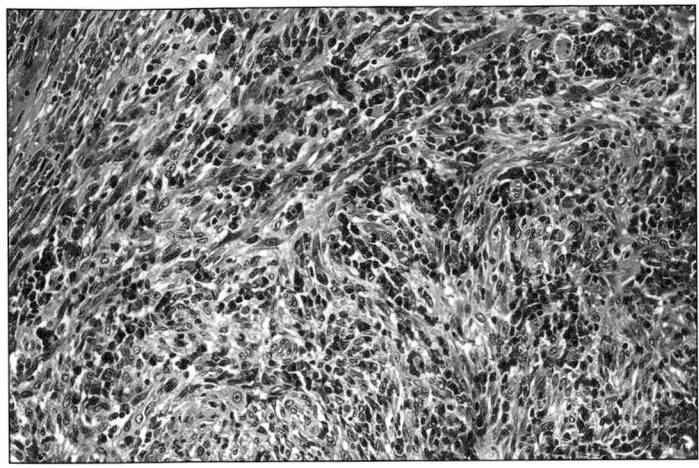

Fig. 18.48 Inflammatory pseudotumor. Fascicles of benign-appearing spindle cells are intimately admixed with lymphocytes and plasma cells.

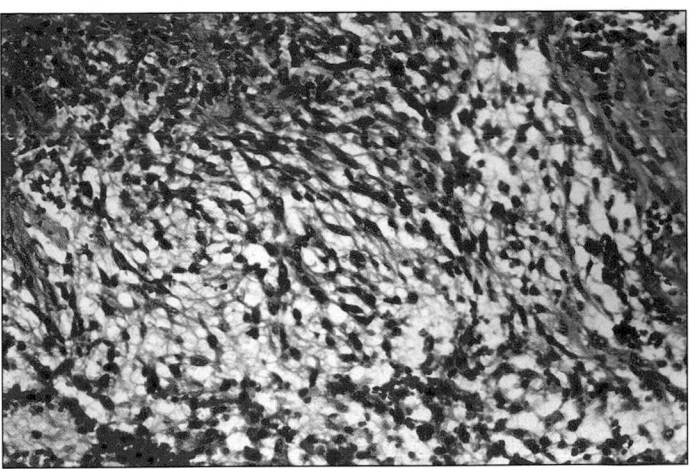

Fig. 18.49 Inflammatory pseudotumor. Myxoid stroma may be a prominent feature of some cases.

inflammatory elements including lymphocytes, mast cells, and eosinophils. The spindle cells show no significant atypia and mitoses are rare or absent (Fig. 18.48). The periphery is well circumscribed, but not encapsulated. Inflammatory elements, including germinal centers, are mostly concentrated at the edge of the lesion, while the central portion usually shows more spindle cells and fibrosis. Calcification, hemorrhage and necrosis may be seen on occasion. Some lesions may show myxoid change in the spindle cell component (Fig. 18.49). Depending on the relative proportion of spindle cells to inflammatory cells, some examples look decidedly inflammatory while others suggest a spindle cell tumor. This idea is further strengthened by gross and microscopic invasion of pulmonary blood vessels in some cases.[284,290] Some lesions are predominantly endobronchial and invade the lung (Fig. 18.50). The spindle cell component has been shown to be a mixture of fibroblasts and myofibroblasts by electron microscopy and by immunohistochemistry, and hence the lesion is now regarded as an inflammatory myofibroblastic process by many authorities.[291–294] Characteristically, the cells stain positively with only vimentin or with vimentin and actin and occasionally with desmin.[285,295] Occasional cases may show abnormal laboratory findings such as anemia, elevated erythrocyte sedimentation rate, serum immunoglobulin elevation, leukocytosis, and thrombocytosis, which may be reversed by complete removal of the lesion.[284] This suggests that these effects are caused by cytokines produced by the inflammatory portion of the tumor.[296] Most patients have been treated by resection. The clinical course is most often benign. The debate about whether inflammatory pseudotumor is a postinflammatory reaction or actually a neoplasm has been ongoing. Recent evidence derived from both pulmonary and extrapulmonary lesions has shown clonal abnormalities and acquired Epstein-Barr virus genomic material on the 2p23 locus of the alk gene as well as more complex genetic clonal abnormalities that point to myofibroblastic tumor.[291–294]

Pulmonary hyalinizing granuloma

Another unusual entity that should be differentiated from inflammatory pseudotumor is pulmonary hyalinizing granuloma, first described in 1977 by Engleman et al.[297] This is a putative inflammatory fibrotic process composed predominantly of laminated hyalinized collagen, sparse fibroblasts, and chronic inflammatory

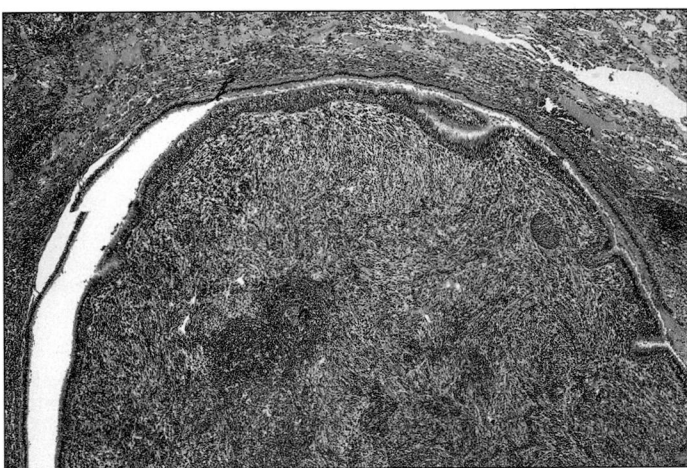

Fig. 18.50 Inflammatory pseudotumor. Polypoid endobronchial growth.

cells (Fig. 18.51). The histologic pattern is very similar to that seen in sclerosing mediastinitis, and indeed coexisting sclerosing mediastinitis has been diagnosed in a minority of patients.[297,298] Radiographically, most cases show multiple pulmonary nodules suggestive of metastatic disease, but solitary masses have also been observed. Patients usually have mild symptoms and a few are asymptomatic. The clinical course is marked by a stable chest X-ray or slowly progressive enlargement of the pulmonary lesions. No deaths have been reported from this disease. Pathologically, the features are fairly constant. The lesions are discrete, but not encapsulated firm white to gray nodules. Histologically, the most characteristic feature is the presence of dense hyalinized lamellar collagen bundles arranged in parallel arrays, sometimes with a storiform pattern. The interface between the lesion and the uninvolved lung tissue shows active fibrosis and chronic inflammation that matures into dense collagen towards the center. Trapped bronchiolar epithelium may be seen in the fibrotic process. The collagen may have the tinctorial quality of amyloid, but amyloid stains are usually negative.[297,298] The etiology of pulmonary hyalinizing granuloma

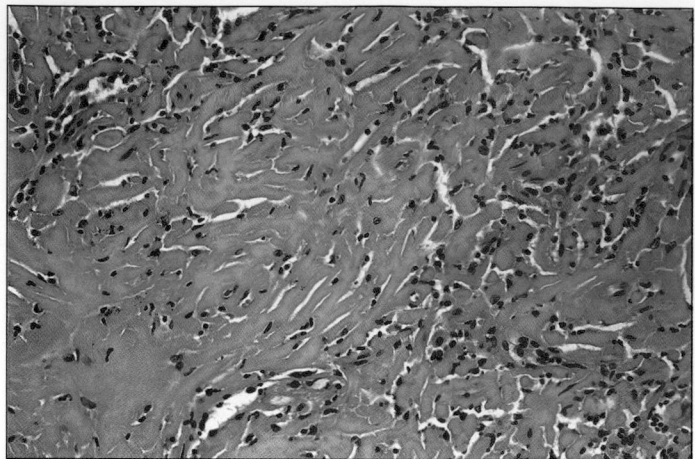

Fig. 18.51 Pulmonary hyalinizing granuloma. Lesion is predominantly composed of thick collagen with interspersed spindled fibroblasts and chronic inflammatory cells.

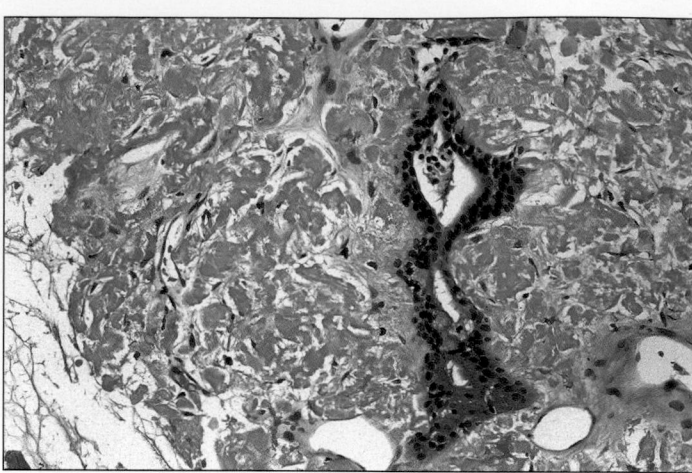

Fig. 18.52 Nodular amyloid tumor. Amorphous waxy pink material surrounding terminal bronchiole. Multinucleated giant cells that appear to ingest the amyloid are commonly seen.

has long been discussed, but no cohesive theory has been forthcoming. An association with amyloidosis, Castleman's disease, lymphoma, and autoimmunity with circulating immune complexes has been described.[299–301] There have also been reports of association with retroperitoneal fibrosis and Reidel's trauma, lesions with similar microscopic pathology.[302,303]

Nodular amyloid tumor

The differential diagnosis of pulmonary hyalinizing granuloma includes nodular pulmonary amyloidosis.[304] Unfortunately, the Congo red stain may not be an absolute means to separate these two lesions since some cases of pulmonary hyalinizing granuloma may be positive, while some cases of bona fide amyloidosis may be negative. Amyloid usually is amorphous and does not show the characteristically laminated fibrillary collagen seen in pulmonary hyalinizing granuloma (Fig. 18.52). Also, multinucleated giant cells are commonly associated with nodular pulmonary amyloid. Radiographically, amyloid tumor is most often a single lesion, while a majority of pulmonary hyalinizing granulomas are multiple. Nodular amyloid tumor is localized and self-limiting and is not part of systemic amyloidosis.

Eosinophilic granuloma, malakoplakia and mycobacterial pseudotumor

Several other tumor-like conditions composed of spindled and epithelioid histiocytes may present as spindle cell masses. Pulmonary eosinophilic granuloma most often occurs in the form of diffuse interstitial lung disease, but rare instances of it manifesting as a solitary coin lesion have been observed (Fig. 18.53A,B).[305,306] Pulmonary malakoplakia is caused by the organism *Rhodococcus Equi* in 70% of cases, usually in patients with acquired immunodeficiency syndrome, but also with organ transplantation, alcoholism, and malignant lymphoma. The hallmark of malakoplakia is the presence of Michaelis-Gutmann bodies, laminated calcified concretions seen microscopically. These are positive with PAS, iron, and calcium stains and represent the results of altered degradation of bacteria and cell products. The lesion is composed of epithelioid and spindled histiocytes with scattered inflammatory cells and is the result of an abnormal response to infection (Fig. 18.54A,B).[307,308]

Radiographically, there may be single or multiple masses, or infiltrative lesions.

Mycobacterial pseudotumor, also seen in immunocompromised patients, is composed of spindled, whorled histiocytes with scattered plasma cells and lymphocytes that appear very similar to some cases of inflammatory pseudotumor. The clinical setting of immunodeficiency, however, should alert the pathologist to do acid-fast stains, which clearly show large numbers of stainable acid-fast organisms (Fig. 18.55A,B).[309,310]

Solitary fibrous tumor

The solitary fibrous tumor most often involves the pleura, but can invade into the lung parenchyma. Occasionally, it may be entirely intrapulmonary (Fig. 18.56).[311,312] The majority of tumors located in the pleura are benign. England et al. describe a higher percentage of malignant solitary fibrous tumors in 'atypical locations' such as when inverted into the lung tissue.[312] These lesions are discussed more fully in Chapter 19.

Primary pulmonary hemangiopericytoma has been reported; the largest series has been 18 cases reported from the AFIP.[313] The majority of cases were recorded before the widespread recognition of solitary fibrous tumor as a distinct entity and the place of pulmonary hemangiopericytoma as separate from solitary fibrous tumor must now be called into question. The 2004 World Health Organization International Histologic classification of tumors no longer lists hemangiopericytoma as a separate entity.[200]

Meningothelial-like nodules (chemodectoma)

Meningothelial-like nodules are small, incidental findings measuring usually 1–3 mm found at autopsy or in surgically removed lung specimens. They have been found in 3% of lung reduction surgical specimens and in a similar percentage of autopsies.[314] They were first described in 1960 as multiple minute pulmonary chemodectomas and for many years had been felt to be derived from intrapulmonary chemoreceptors.[315] Subsequent studies, however, have recognized that these lesions actually bear close similarity to meningioma by ultrastructure and by immunohistochemistry and, therefore, meningothelial-like nodule is now the preferred nomenclature.[316,317]

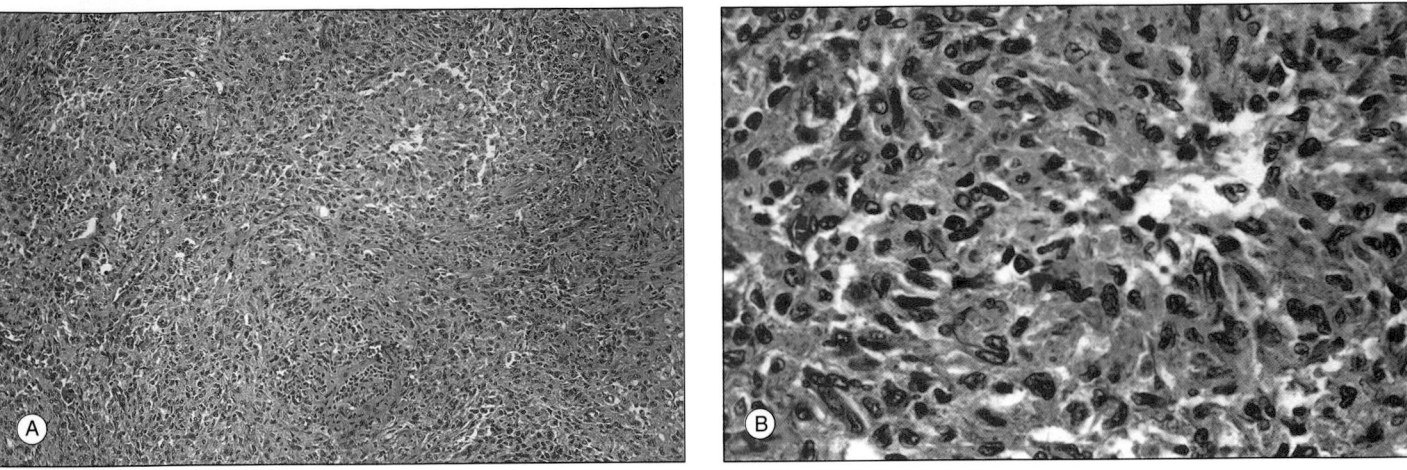

Fig. 18.53 A, Eosinophilic granuloma. Solid mass of pink epithelioid and spindled Langerhans histiocytes with scattered eosinophils; **B**, Eosinophilic granuloma. Langerhans histiocytes showing indistinct cell borders and wrinkled or grooved nuclei associated with scattered eosinophils. Langerhans cells are strongly S-100 positive.

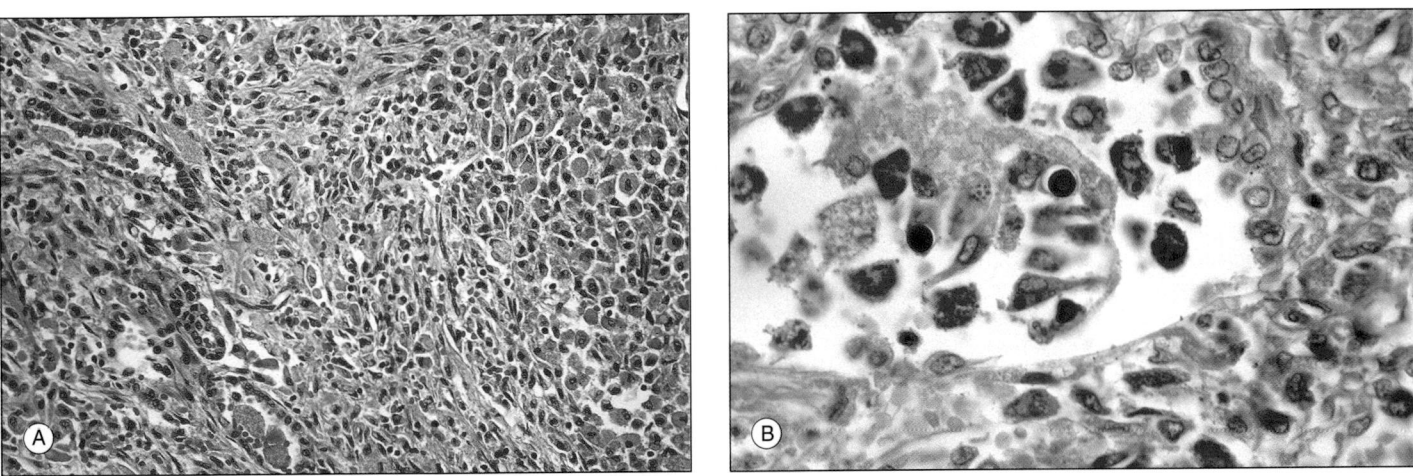

Fig. 18.54 A, Pulmonary malakoplakia. Discohesive sheets of spindled and epithelioid histiocytes that form a solid mass or infiltrate. Patient was HIV positive; **B**, Pulmonary malakoplakia. PAS stain highlights the concentrically laminated extracellular Michaelis-Gutman bodies.

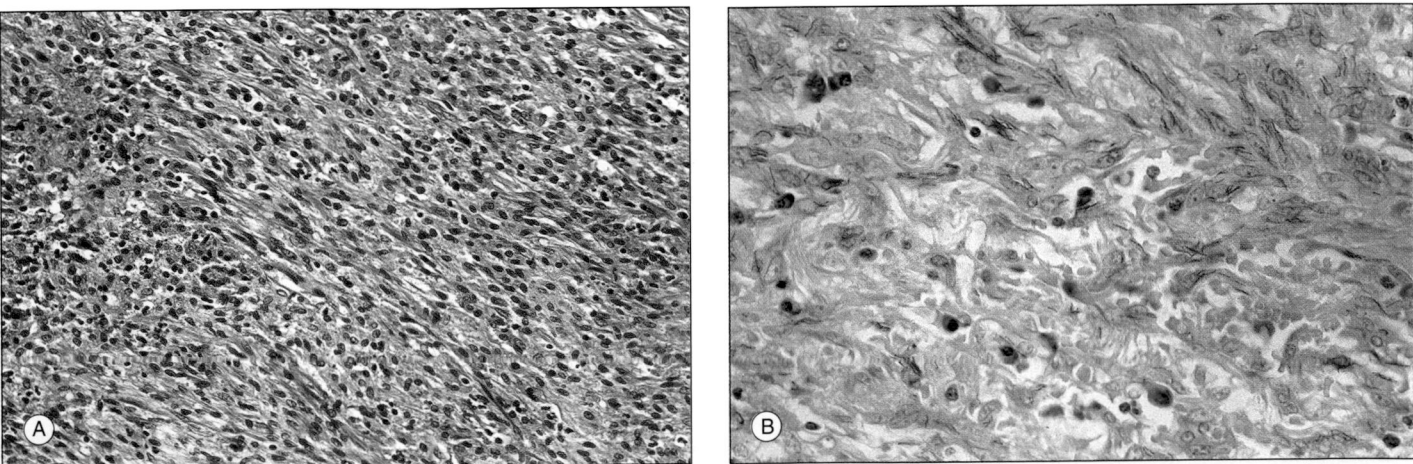

Fig. 18.55 A, Mycobacterial pseudotumor. Solid spindle cell nodule containing scattered chronic inflammatory cells. There is close similarity to the histology of inflammatory pseudotumor (see Figure 18.48); **B**, Acid-fast stain showing many positive mycobacteria.

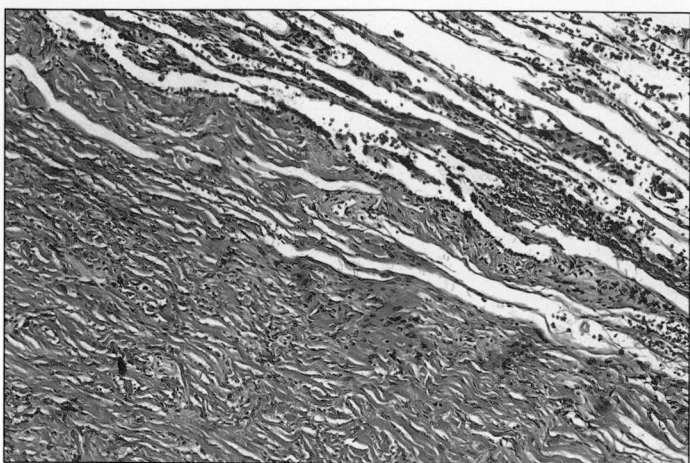

Fig. 18.56 Solitary fibrous tumor. This tumor was almost entirely within the lung parenchyma, but abutted on the visceral pleura. Tumor is well circumscribed but not encapsulated. The spindle cells within the lesion reveal the characteristic 'patternless pattern.'

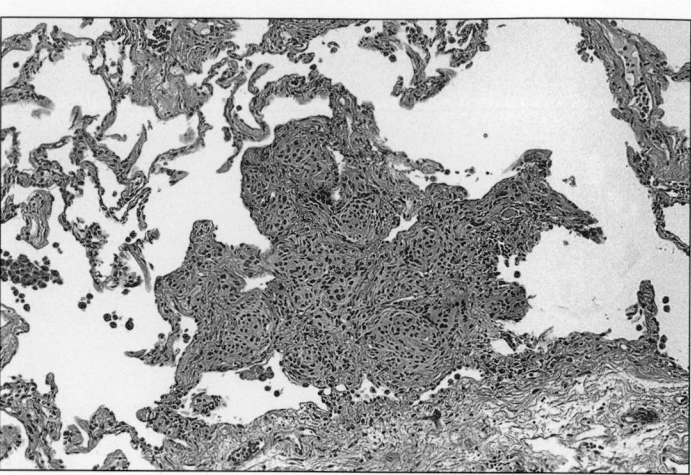

Fig. 18.57 Meningothelial-like nodule. Small interstitial proliferation of nested round to spindle cells having a 'zellballen' pattern. Similarity to chemodectoma is apparent.

They are seen in association with many different intrapulmonary conditions including granulomas and carcinoma. An etiologic relationship has been postulated with thromboembolic disease.[318] Grossly, most lesions are so small that they are not visible on gross examination. Lesions that measure more than a few millimeters may reveal indistinct, gray-white indurated nodules scattered in the pulmonary parenchyma. Microscopically, meningothelioma-like nodules appear as discrete rounded, swirled nests of pink spindle cells within the interstitium, often around small blood vessels (Fig. 18.57). They have a distinctive 'zellballen' appearance reminiscent of nonchromophobe paraganglioma, but which also resemble the meningothelial whorls seen typically in intracranial tumors. The immunophenotype and ultrastructure are also similar to meningioma. Cells characteristically decorate with EMA and vimentin and are negative with cytokeratin, S-100 protein, and neuroendocrine markers, such as NSE, chromogranin, and synaptophysin.[316,319,320] Ultrastructurally, numerous interdigitating cytoplasmic processes attached by desmosomes are seen and intracytoplasmic organelles are sparse, without evidence of neuroendocrine-type secretory granules.

Recent clonal analysis utilizing the HUMARA assay or microsatellite polymorphic markers for loss of heterozygosity have shown that some lesions are monoclonal, consistent with a tumor-like proliferation, while others are polyclonal, consistent with a reactive process.[319,320]

Meningothelial-like nodules have no clinical significance, as far as can be determined, but might be mistaken for carcinoid tumorlets or lymphangioleiomyomatosis histologically. Importantly, the lesions of lymphangioleiomyomatosis are interstitial, larger, and more extensive and can easily be differentiated by immunohistochemistry (see below).

Rare examples of primary pulmonary meningioma and ependymoma that cause single radiographically visible space-occupying masses in the lung have been reported.[321,322]

Lymphangioleiomyomatosis

Lymphangioleiomyomatosis (LAM) is seen exclusively in women, usually of reproductive age. It rarely presents as tumor-like nodules, but rather as diffuse infiltrative interstitial and microcystic lesions. The majority of patients present with shortness of breath,

hemoptysis, chylous pleural effusion, chest pain, or pneumothorax. It is felt to be a forme fruste of tuberous sclerosis. From 10% to almost 50% of patients have associated renal angiomyolipomas, whereas only 1% or 2% of patients with clinical tuberous sclerosus have full-blown pulmonary LAM. Sensitive pulmonary CT scans, however, have shown a much higher incidence of occult pulmonary disease in patients with tuberous sclerosis.[323–325] The lesion is composed of short fascicles with whorled plump spindled smooth muscle cells that arise from blood vessels, lymphatics, and distal airways that can sometimes form nodules (Fig. 18.58). LAM stains positively with antibodies to smooth muscle as well as HMB-45, the melanoma-associated antigen.[326,327] Mutations in the TSC-1 and TSC-2 genes (tuberous sclerosis complex) have been reported in both pulmonary LAM and angiomyolipomas of the kidney.[328–330]

Benign metastasizing leiomyoma

Rarely, patients present with multiple, circumscribed, bland appearing smooth muscle nodules that may contain entrapped indigenous epithelial cells for which the term benign metastasizing leiomyoma or fibroleiomyomatous hamartoma has been used.[331,332] The nature of this lesion has been controversial, with some believing that it represents an indigenous smooth muscle tumor of the lung, while currently the majority favors the concept that they are metastatic smooth muscle tumors, most often from the uterus.[331,332] The lesion almost always occurs in females, usually in the reproductive years, and in this regard is similar to LAM. The great majority of patients have had a prior history of hysterectomy for benign leiomyomas. Microscopically, the lung tumors are usually round or nodular, with only minimal mitotic activity (Fig. 18.59). Significant pleomorphism, necrosis or overt signs of malignancy are absent. Most often when the uterine tumors are examined they also lack malignant criteria. Sometimes, however, there is discordance between the uterine and pulmonary lesions with apparently bland uterine smooth muscle tumors giving rise to mitotically active pulmonary lesions.[333]

Grossly, the size ranges from a few millimeters up to 10 cm. About two-thirds of the cases are multiple and bilateral. The average

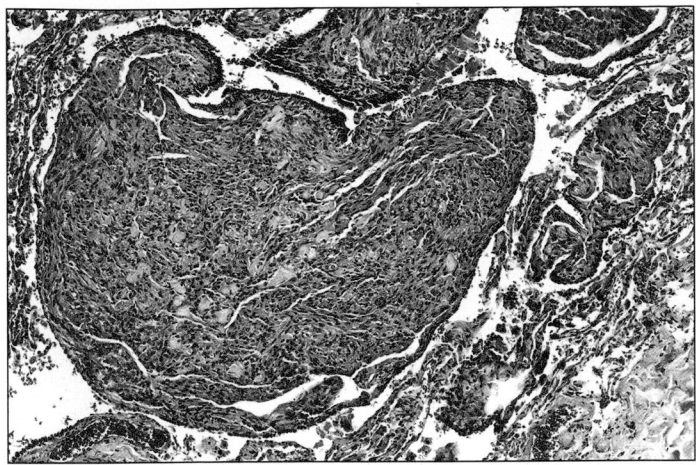

Fig. 18.58 Lymphangioleiomyomatosis. Nodular proliferation of smooth muscle cells involving terminal bronchiole. Smaller interstitial nodules are seen adjacent to the larger lesion.

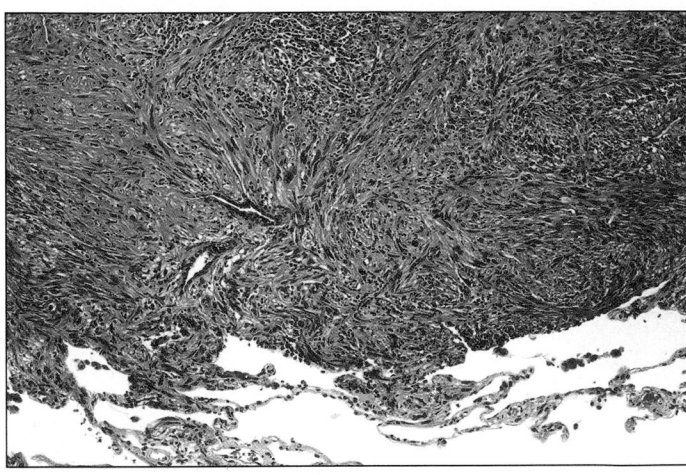

Fig. 18.59 Benign metastasizing leiomyoma. One of several pulmonary nodules that appeared years after hysterectomy for leiomyoma. Lung tumor is composed of smooth muscle cells showing slight nuclear pleomorphism, but no mitoses.

age of patients is 47 years. The majority of patients have been asymptomatic.

Lung tumors are characterized by low proliferative activity as measured with Ki-67 immunohistochemistry, while over 80% of cases stain positively with estrogen and progesterone specific receptors. The median survival of patients is over 8 years.[334] The presence of identical X-chromosome inactivation patterns in the uterus and in the lung lesions of a reported case supports the metastatic nature of the pulmonary nodules.[335] The prognosis is worse for younger women, with approximately a third of patients under age 50 showing progressive pulmonary insufficiency or death.[331] The disease is usually more stationary in older women. Some patients have experienced regression after hormonal manipulation with antiestrogen substances, but the response may not be permanent.[336] We believe the majority of these lesions are low-grade malignancies and cases with mitotically active uterine tumors and pulmonary lesions are simply metastatic leiomyosarcomas.

The differential diagnosis must include metastasis from low-grade endometrial stromal sarcoma, some of which may demonstrate smooth muscle differentiation. Such tumors characteristically show a solid peritheliomatous appearance of short bland spindle cells grouped around prominent blood vessels with collagen formation between individual cells and cell groups (Fig. 18.60). Both endometrial stromal sarcoma metastatic to the lung and smooth muscle tumors may be positive for muscle specific actin and desmin, but CD10 positivity can usually identify a metastatic lesion as endometrial stromal sarcoma, while h-Caldesmon positivity is very sensitive for identifying smooth muscle tumors.[337]

Spindle cell carcinoma

Spindle cell carcinomas of the lung are most often located in the lung periphery rather than the bronchi and by definition are composed entirely of elongated spindled or sarcomatoid cells. These may grow as a solid tumor mass or infiltrate the interstitium between the alveoli. The histologic pattern is most often fascicular and/or storiform (Fig. 18.61A,B). By definition, immunohistochemistry for epithelial elements such as cytokeratin and EMA are positive. When spindle cell carcinoma is combined with another recognizable epithelial type such as giant cell carcinoma or adenocarcinoma, the

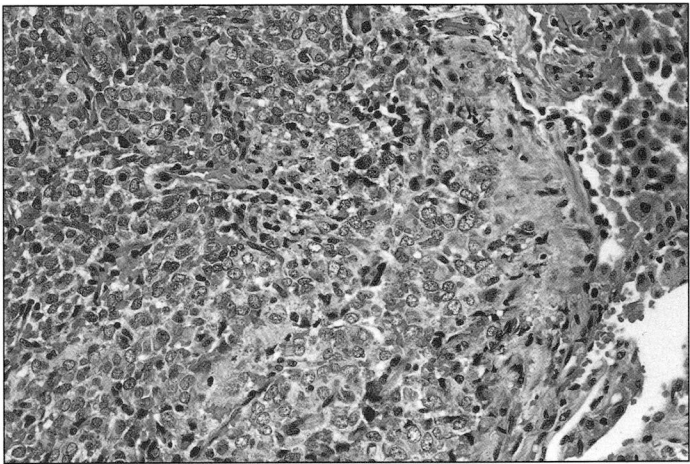

Fig. 18.60 Metastatic endometrial stromal sarcoma. Patient had prior history of low-grade uterine tumor. Lesion shows short spindle and round cells with sparse intercellular collagenous stroma.

term pleomorphic carcinoma is appropriate. Rare cases of spindle cell carcinoma accompanied by a significant inflammatory component that resembles inflammatory pseudotumor have been reported.[338] The prognosis is poor.[338,339]

Spindle cell sarcomas

A wide variety of malignant mesenchymal tumors have been reported in the lung, many, however, before the widespread use of immunohistochemistry which makes the true nature of the tumors in older reports open to question. Such entities as liposarcoma, chondrosarcoma, osteosarcoma, angiosarcoma, leiomyosarcoma and rhabdomyosarcoma as well as malignant fibrous histiocytoma and fibrosarcoma have all been described.[340–345] The majority of intraparenchymal pulmonary sarcomas are actually metastatic deposits from a visceral or somatic primary and it is important that this be kept in mind when faced with the possibility of a lung sarcoma.

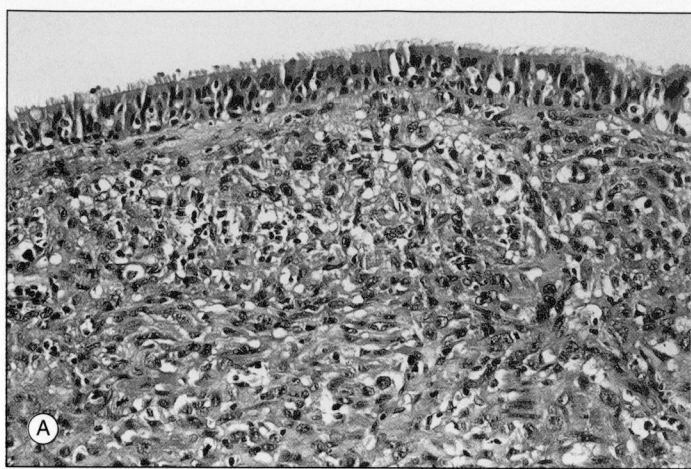

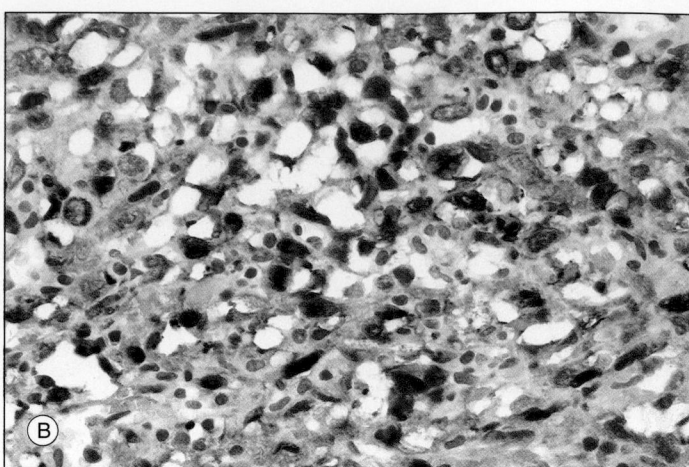

Fig. 18.61 A, Spindle cell carcinoma of lung. Large spindle cell carcinoma that infiltrates the bronchus; **B**, Cytokeratin stain shows focal positive reaction in tumor cells. Many spindle cell carcinomas demonstrate focal, rather than diffuse cytokeratin staining.

Indeed, some authors believe that all intrapulmonary angiosarcomas represent metastases from an occult primary tumor.[346] Primary pulmonary sarcomas are very rare and account for less than 0.2% of lung tumors.[347] There is nothing microscopically that differentiates metastatic from primary lung sarcomas. The clinical history and knowledge of the radiographs is critical, since the large majority of primary sarcomas are solitary lesions whereas most metastases consist of multiple pulmonary nodules.

Malignant fibrous histiocytoma

Malignant fibrous histiocytoma (MFH) has been reported as primary in the lung.[340,348] This diagnosis must be approached with some wariness by the pathologist, however, since other more common lesions such as primary spindle cell or metastatic carcinoma and sarcoma may show similar histologic patterns. The age range of patients has been wide, from children to octogenarians. The mean age is approximately 55 years. Males and females are about equally affected and up to a third of patients may be asymptomatic. Radiographically, most tumors are solitary and located in the lung periphery. Size varies from 2.0 cm to 12.0 cm. Grossly, the lesions are solid, well-circumscribed, soft, fleshy masses with myxoid areas, hemorrhage, and necrosis. Histologically, classic cases differ little from their soft tissue counterparts and are characterized by storiform architecture composed of pleomorphic spindle cells showing numerous mitoses, atypical mitotic figures, and sometimes giant cells. Some authors have included tumors showing similarity to inflammatory pseudotumor, but with more significant nuclear pleomorphism and mitotic activity within the MFH category (Fig. 18.62).[286,288] We feel that such lesions are part of the biologic spectrum of inflammatory pseudotumors, however. Immunohistochemistry is rarely contributory. The most commonly positive antibody is vimentin and sometimes actin. S-100, epithelial markers, and CD34 are usually negative. Isolated cases may show positive keratin staining.[349] Surgical resection is the treatment of choice. Approximately half of reported patients have died of their tumor.[340,348]

Monophasic synovial sarcoma

Monophasic synovial sarcoma has been reported in both the lung and pleura.[350,351] Cases are equally divided between the sexes. The

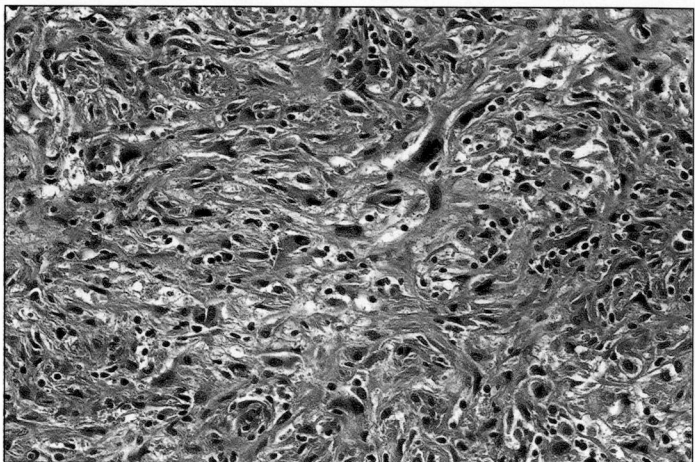

Fig. 18.62 Malignant fibrous histiocytoma. Tumor is composed of fascicles and whorls of spindle cells showing nuclear enlargement, hyperchromasia, and atypia mixed with scattered inflammatory cells. There is marked similarity to inflammatory pseudotumor. Such tumors might be considered as examples of malignant myofibroblastic tumor (inflammatory pseudotumor), but have been reported as malignant fibrous histiocytoma.

size varies from quite small, under 1 cm, up to 20 cm in diameter. A few tumors involve major bronchi, but most are peripheral. Histologically, tumors are identical to monophasic synovial sarcoma seen in soft tissue and display interlacing fascicles of atypical mitotically active, hyperchromatic spindle cells with a myxoid, neuroid, and hemangiopericytic growth pattern (Fig. 18.63). Most cases stain positively with epithelial membrane antigen, pancytokeratin and vimentin. Tumors have the same chromosomal translocation t(X18) and SYT/SSX fusion transcripts detected by RT-PCR as somatic synovial sarcoma.[352–355] They are highly aggressive, with the majority of patients ultimately succumbing to widespread metastases. Rarely, biphasic synovial sarcoma has been observed, usually involving the pleura and adjacent lung tissue.[356]

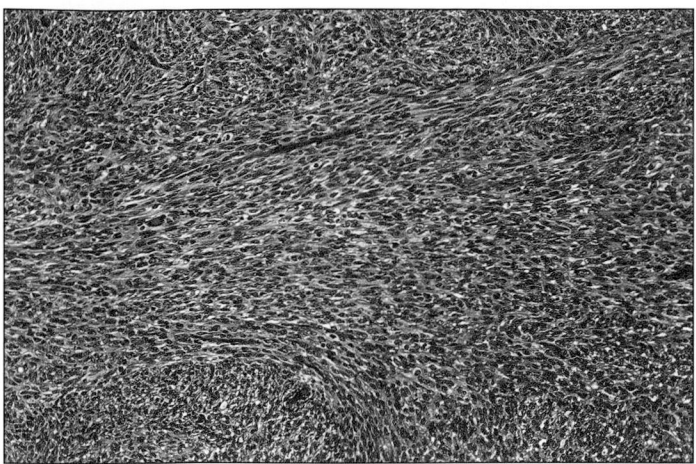

Fig. 18.63 Monophasic synovial sarcoma of lung. Cellular tumor with little or no stroma composed of fascicles of dark staining, short spindle cells. Tumors are identical to lesions in soft tissue.

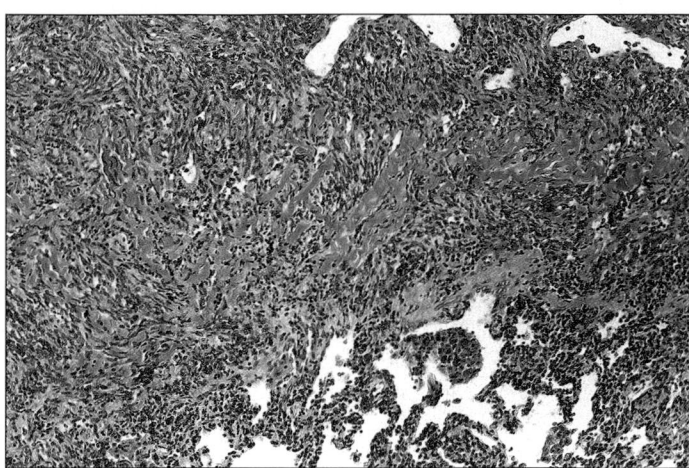

Fig. 18.64 Kaposi's sarcoma. Nodular interstitial tumor composed of spindled endothelial cells with slit-like spaces containing red blood cells.

Table 18.7 Tumors with vascular pattern

Kaposi's sarcoma
Angiosarcoma
Epithelioid hemangioendothelioma

TUMORS WITH VASCULAR PATTERN (Table 18.7)

Kaposi's sarcoma

Kaposi's sarcoma is almost invariably found in patients with AIDS or organ transplantation, particularly kidney transplant recipients. In Western countries it is estimated to involve 4% of renal transplant patients.[357] In AIDS patients, approximately 3–5% of patients will have clinical lung involvement, while the incidence approaches 50% post-mortem. It may effect the lung alone in between 10% and 15% of AIDS patients.[358–361] Pulmonary involvement is usually a late development in the course of the disease and is usually associated with coexisting *Pneumocystis carinii* or cytomegalovirus pneumonia.[360,361] There is a strong association with male homosexuals.[362] The diagnosis is often made by thoracoscopic biopsy, but between 35% and 70% of patients may be diagnosed by fiber optic bronchoscopy.[358] Patients have fever, cough, shortness of breath, pleural effusion, and hemoptysis. Chest radiographs are variable and may show linear densities, reticular nodular infiltrates, or discrete masses.

At bronchoscopy, flat, violet-red discoloration or nodules may be seen in the tracheobronchial tree.[360] The microscopic features of nodular or interstitial Kaposi's sarcoma often show lymphangitic distribution in the lung and are comprised of interlacing fascicles of short spindle cells with bland hyperchromatic nuclei associated with slit-like vascular spaces lined by flattened endothelium and inflammatory cells (Fig. 18.64). The morphology is identical to that of tumor-stage cutaneous Kaposi's sarcoma.[363] Immuno-histochemistry shows that the endothelial cells of Kaposi's sarcoma are usually positive only with endothelial markers CD31 and CD34 and are negative for factor VIII and Ulex europaeus agglutinin 1 (UEA-1).[364]

In male homosexual AIDS patients, evidence of herpes virus type 8 has consistently been found in the endothelial cells of Kaposi's sarcoma as demonstrated by polymerase chain reaction, in situ hybridization, and Southern blot analysis.[362,365] The virus results in endothelial cell proliferation through complex interaction with a G protein coupled receptor homologous to the interleukin-8 receptor. The prognosis of Kaposi's sarcoma with pulmonary involvement is poor; most patient die within 1 year.[366]

Angiosarcoma

The differential diagnosis of pulmonary Kaposi's sarcoma includes high-grade angiosarcoma. Primary pulmonary angiosarcoma is exceedingly rare, if it exists at all. Most authors feel that the overwhelming majority or perhaps all examples of this entity actually represent disease of the pleura or metastases from skin, breast, liver, or elsewhere.[346,367,368] High-grade angiosarcomas in the lung show prominent rounded or anastomosing sieve-like vascular channels lined by atypical mitotically active endothelial cells with enlarged hyperchromatic and irregular nuclei (Fig. 18.65). Tumor cells have a predilection to infiltrate the media of muscular pulmonary blood vessels and form discrete tumor nodules as well as more diffuse interstitial infiltrative lesions. All cases of suspected pulmonary angiosarcoma should be investigated for a primary tumor somewhere else. Histologically, these tumors lack the characteristic flattened, bland spindle cells with slit-like vascular spaces that characterize Kaposi's sarcoma.

Epithelioid hemangioendothelioma (intravascular bronchoalveolar tumor)

Epithelioid hemangioendothelioma was first described in 1983 by Dail and colleagues as intravascular bronchoalveolar tumor in recognition of the intra-alveolar growth pattern and endothelial nature of the lesion.[369] These tumors are rare and occur predominantly in women in the reproductive years, but children and older people have been reported, as have men. Most patients are symptomatic and present with cough or shortness of breath. Radiographically, there are multiple, well-circumscribed bilateral pulmonary nodules. The

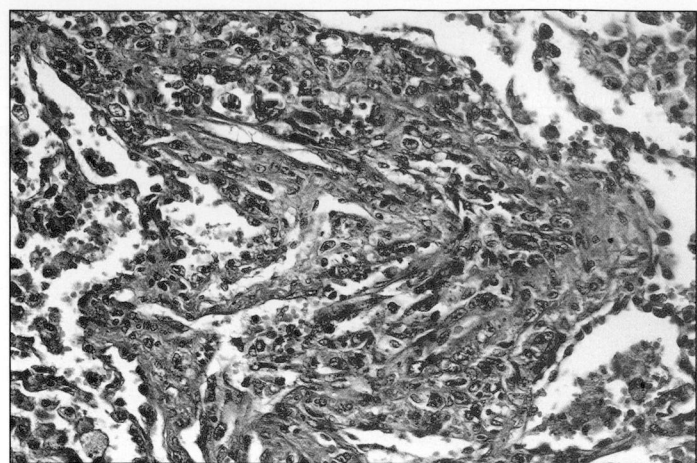

Fig. 18.65 High-grade angiosarcoma. Anaplastic endothelial tumor cells infiltrate the lumen of a small pulmonary blood vessel. These tumors tend to involve the lung vasculature. A primary angiosarcoma elsewhere should be excluded in all such cases.

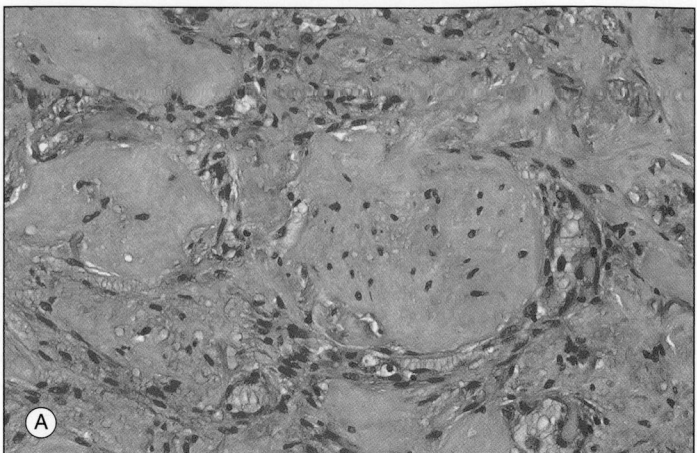

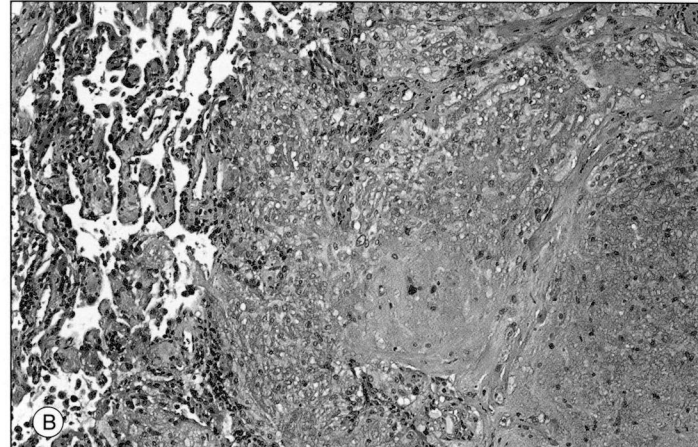

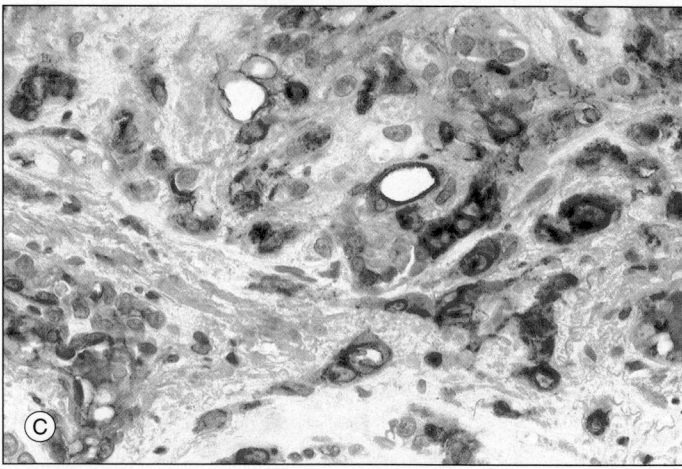

Fig. 18.66 A, Epithelioid hemangioendothelioma. Nodules of tumor replace contiguous alveoli. Collagen tumor matrix is abundant and tends to compress and obscure tumor cells; **B**, Epithelioid hemangioendothelioma. Some tumors have predominantly myxoid or mucinous matrix; **C**, Epithelioid hemangioendothelioma. CD31 immunohistochemistry that decorates neoplastic endothelial cells. Intracytoplasmic vacuoles can be appreciated.

microscopic appearance reveals round or polygonal tumor cells with ample pink cytoplasm and central or eccentric nuclei. Intracytoplasmic vacuoles indicative of incipient vascular lumen formation are sometimes seen. The tumor cells are embedded within a slightly basophilic or myxoid matrix and grow within alveolar spaces in an intraluminal polypoid configuration (Fig. 18.66A–C). They have a distinct epithelioid appearance but have been shown by electron microscopy and immunohistochemistry to be endothelial in nature with Wiebel-Palade bodies and the presence of factor VIII related antigen, CD31, and other endothelial markers (Fig. 18.66C). Recently, evidence of glucocorticoid receptors and 11 beta hydroxysteroid dehydrogenase has been demonstrated in the tumor cells by immunohistochemistry, which holds some promise for hormonal therapy.[370] The clinical course is characteristically one of slow progression with approximately 40% of the patients dying at five years' follow-up. Some patients, however, have very indolent disease.[369–372]

TUMORS WITH A BIPHASIC PATTERN (Table 18.8)

Biphasic tumors comprise combinations of spindled and epithelioid cells showing a clearly distinctive separation of these elements microscopically. Such tumors are rare with the exception of benign hamartoma. Malignancies such as pulmonary carcinosarcoma, pulmonary blastoma, biphasic malignant mesothelioma (discussed elsewhere), and metastatic synovial sarcoma comprise most of the entities seen in clinical practice.

Hamartoma

Pulmonary hamartomas are almost always found as incidental findings. The age range is broad and the lesion has occasionally been reported in children. The majority of patients are adults in the forth to sixth decades of life.[373] Most examples are in the lung periphery, but approximately 10% of hamartomas are endobronchial and therefore may be associated with symptoms of cough, hemoptysis, or bronchial obstruction.[374] Grossly, tumors are well circumscribed and measure from as little as a few millimeters to several centimeters in

size, averaging approximately 3 cm in diameter. They may be easily shelled out from the surrounding lung parenchyma. Microscopically, they are composed of lobules of sparsely cellular, spindled, fibro-myxoid or fibrous stroma, often with a cartilage and adipose tissue component, associated with bland entrapped glandular epithelium

Table 18.8 Tumors with a biphasic pattern

Hamartoma

Carcinosarcoma

Pulmonary blastoma

Malignant mesothelioma

Metastatic biphasic synovial sarcoma

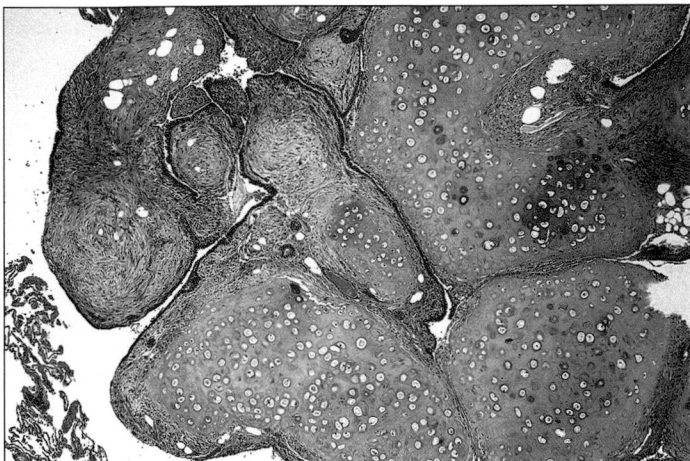

Fig. 18.67 Hamartoma. Lobulated nodules of cartilage associated with invaginated respiratory-type epithelium. There is no perichondrium around the cartilage, which is consistent with cartilaginous metaplasia from fibrous stroma, a finding characteristic of pulmonary hamartoma.

that appears to invaginate into the stromal component of the lesion (Fig. 18.67). The cartilage characteristically lacks a layer of perichondrium. The epithelial component is composed of either ciliated bronchial cells or simple, flattened epithelial cells. Calcification is often present.

Hamartomas are the most common incidentally found tumors in the lung. They are characterized by very slow growth and are treated by simple enucleation. Local recurrence is extremely rare. Endobronchial tumors may be locally resected.

Pulmonary hamartoma can be part of Carney's triad of gastric epithelioid leiomyosarcoma, functioning extra-adrenal paraganglioma, and pulmonary 'chondroma.'[375]

Cytology of hamartoma

Pulmonary hamartomas can be accurately diagnosed by FNA.[376–381] The most commonly seen elements are fibromyxoid tissue, cartilage, and clusters of benign epithelial cells (Fig. 18.68). The fibromyxoid material consists of spindle-shaped and stellate cells with slender bland nuclei and long cytoplasmic processes, loosely dispersed in a fibrillary, myxoid matrix in a haphazard pattern (Fig. 18.68B). The chondroid material varies from myxocartilage to mature cartilage. The epithelial component consists of cohesive sheets of small cuboidal or short columnar, ciliated or nonciliated cells with round, uniform nuclei and finely dispersed chromatin (Fig. 18.68C). Wiatrowska et al.[381] found positive immunostaining of the fibromyxoid material for S-100 protein a useful tool in diagnosis of pulmonary hamartoma by FNA.

Carcinosarcoma

This tumor is classified under the heading of sarcomatoid carcinomas with pleomorphic, or sarcomatous elements in the latest WHO classification of lung and pleural tumors and actually represents metaplastic carcinoma analogous to similar lesions of the breast or elsewhere.[200] Tumors show histologic features of carcinoma in combination with spindle cell elements that grow in broad fascicles resembling noncommitted spindle cell sarcoma (Fig. 18.69A,B). Rare examples, however, may show heterologous elements such as bone, skeletal muscle, and cartilage.[382,383] Morphologically, biphasic carcinosarcomas most often show squamous cell carcinoma with spindle cell sarcomatoid elements, but adenocarcinoma, undifferentiated carcinoma, and small cell carcinoma have been described. These tumors can be endobronchial polypoid growths or present as large peripheral pulmonary tumors. Carcinosarcomas are rare, accounting for less than 1% of lung cancers.[384] They are often large and clinically aggressive with high mortality.

Immunohistochemically, the epithelioid tumor cells as well as focal areas of the spindle cell component are usually positive for cytokeratin or epithelial membrane antigen. CEA is generally positive in the epithelial component, but negative in the spindle cells.[385]

Pulmonary blastoma

Biphasic carcinosarcoma should be differentiated from pulmonary blastoma.[386] This tumor is characterized by distinctly separate glandular and spindle cell components, but in contrast to carcinosarcoma that features adult-appearing tissue components, those seen in pulmonary blastoma resemble fetal lung. Similarity to fetal lung tissue is also seen ultrastructurally.[387] Characteristically, the tumor presents as a single large peripheral lung mass often over 5 cm in diameter. A minority of cases show multiple nodules.[388] The mean age of cases is 39 years with a third occurring in children under 10 years. The majority are in stage I. Of 24 cases reported from the AFIP, only 9 patients were alive with no evidence of disease after an average of four-year follow-up.[388] Others have also shown a poor prognosis similar to carcinosarcoma.[390] Microscopically, they characteristically show a primitive undifferentiated malignant mesenchymal component composed predominantly of small spindle cells with abrupt juxtaposition of fetal-appearing glandular structures resembling embryonal bronchial epithelium (Fig. 18.70A,B). These glandular elements show intracytoplasmic vacuolization, in many respects similar to that of secretory endometrium. The vacuoles contain glycogen as evidenced by strong PAS positivity that is abolished by diastase digestion. Rarely, cartilage, bone, and smooth muscle may be identified in the mesenchymal component. Isolated areas of yolk sac carcinoma have also been seen in pulmonary blastoma.[389]

The proportion of glands to stroma varies widely but both components are seen in all cases. Necrosis and mitotic activity are common. Immunohistochemically, the epithelial component is strongly reactive for keratin, CEA, and human milk fat globulin. Chromogranin and NSE is seen in slightly over 70% of cases.[388] The mesenchymal component usually is positive for vimentin and actin, while desmin is positive in a third of cases.

The differential diagnosis of pulmonary blastoma includes the fetal adenocarcinoma and metastatic Wilms' tumor, hepatoblastoma, pancreaticoblastoma, and other biphasic embryonal tumors of childhood as well as pleuropulmonary blastoma. By definition, fetal adenocarcinomas contain only a glandular component, which is identical to that of biphasic pulmonary

Fig. 18.68 FNA cytology of pulmonary hamartoma. **A,** Low magnification showing an intimate association of a fibromyxoid tissue, cartilage, and benign epithelial cells (Diff-Quik stain); **B,** High magnification of fibromyxoid tissue showing a fibrillary matrix and spindle cells with indistinct cytoplasm and elongated nuclei with finely granular chromatin (Papanicolaou stain); **C,** A cohesive sheet of small, uniform epithelial cells with round nuclei, high N:C ratio, bland chromatin, and indistinct nucleoli (Papanicolaou stain); **D,E,** Cell-block sections exhibiting benign-appearing fibromyxoid tissue and cartilage, respectively (H&E stain).

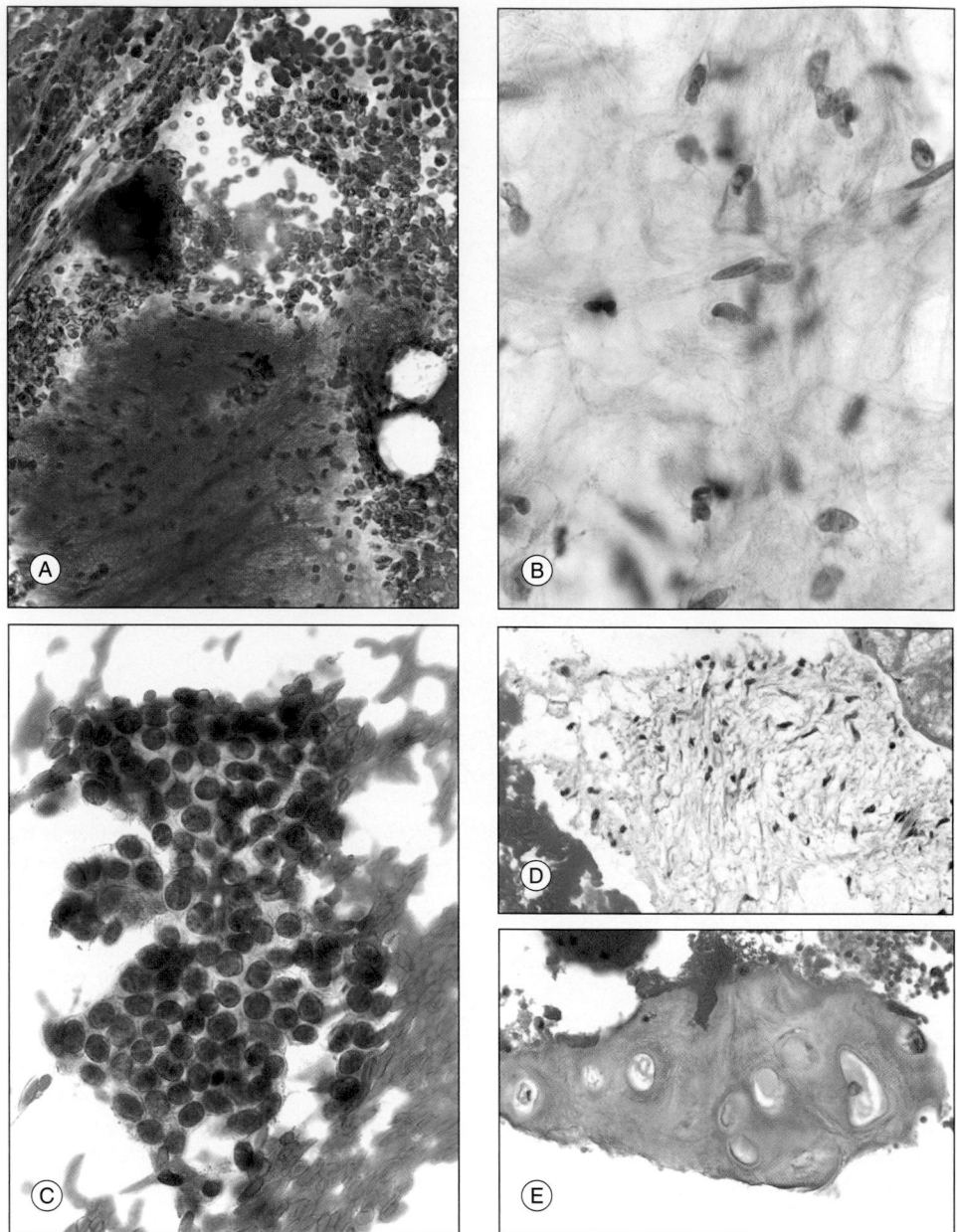

blastoma, complete with glycogen-rich clear cytoplasmic vacuoles (Fig. 18.71). Grossly, both tumors usually present as large peripheral lung masses limited to the lung in young adults. In contrast to pulmonary blastoma, however, fetal adeno-carcinoma is unusual in children under 10 years. Seventeen of 21 patients with fetal adenocarcinoma were free of disease after a follow-up period that averaged 8 years.[388] The prognosis therefore seems to be much better.

Both pulmonary blastoma and fetal adenocarcinoma have beta-catenin gene mutations demonstrated by immunohistochemistry implying histogenetic similarity between these tumors, despite differences in survival.[391]

Rare examples of pleuropulmonary blastoma of children have been reported.[392] These tumors are composed of blastomatous stroma similar to that seen in biphasic pulmonary blastoma, but without an epithelial component. Tumors involve lung and pleura and rarely the

mediastinum. The prognosis is poor; seven of the eleven patients originally reported died within two years of diagnosis. We have not seen a case.

Metastatic Wilms' tumor and other blastomas can usually be differentiated on clinical grounds by their high incidence in childhood, history of a tumor elsewhere, and the presence of multiple pulmonary nodules.

Biphasic malignant mesothelioma can sometimes present as a localized tumor mass in the pleura in contrast to the vast majority, which involve it diffusely.[393] These tumors show none of the fetal appearance of pulmonary blastoma and can usually be separated from carcinoma by virtue of both histologic and immunohistochemical evidence. Clinical history of a soft tissue sarcoma easily distinguishes metastatic synovial sarcoma from the other entities. We have seen examples of biphasic epithelioid and spindled endometrial stromal sarcoma that have metastasized to the lung.

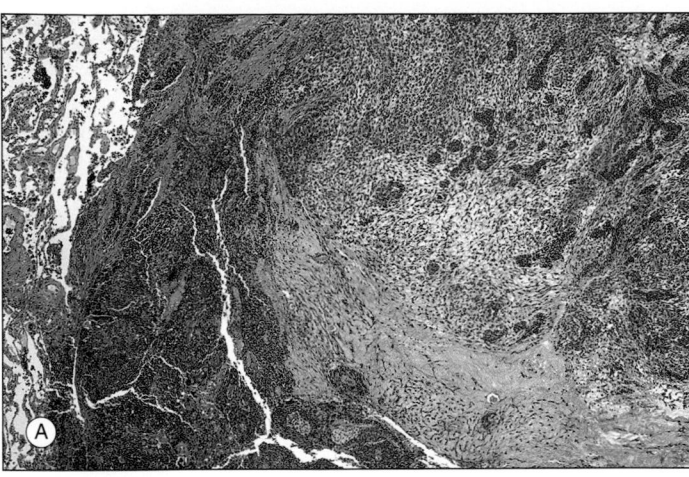
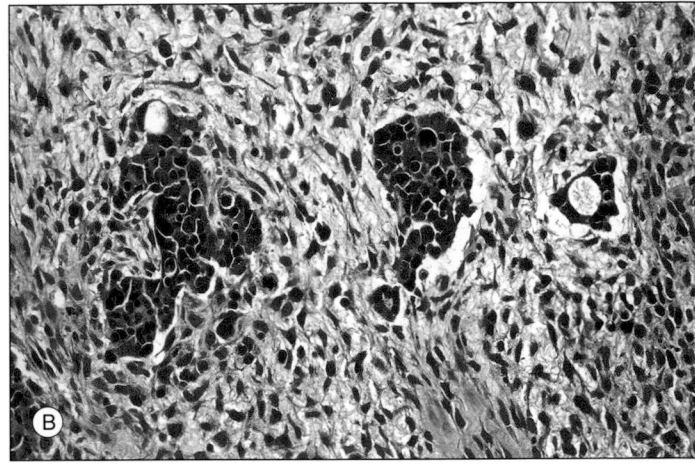

Fig. 18.69 A, Carcinosarcoma. Solid undifferentiated carcinoma in juxtaposition with spindle cell sarcoma; **B**, Higher magnification showing transition of epithelioid to spindle cells.

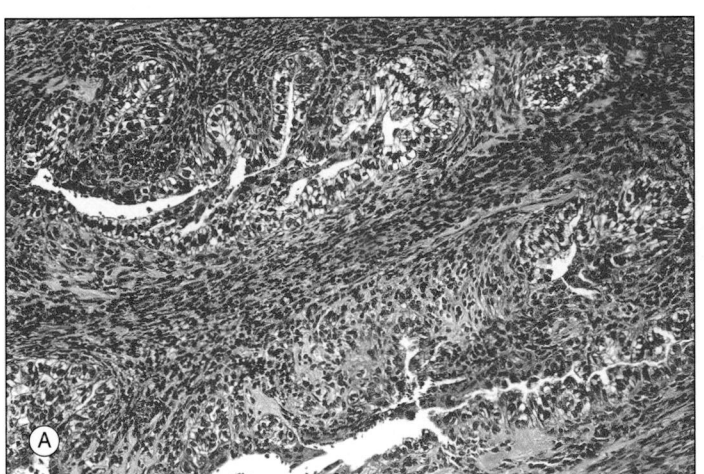
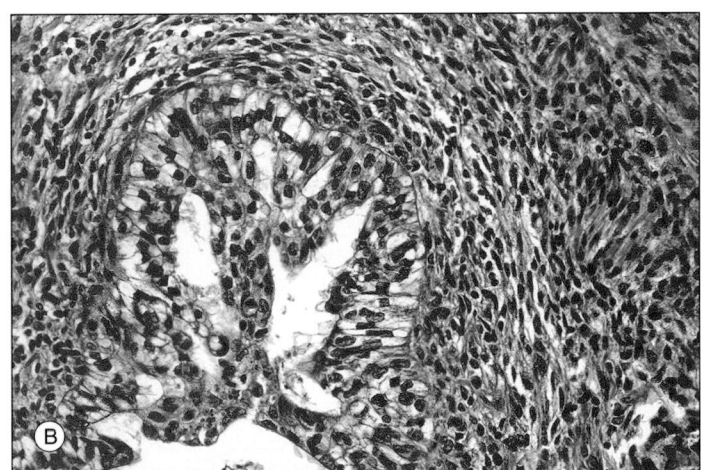

Fig. 18.70 A, Pulmonary blastoma. Biphasic tumor showing separate spindle and epithelial components with similarity to embryonal lung tissue; **B**, Pulmonary blastoma. Higher magnification of glandular component demonstrating characteristic intracytoplasmic clear vacuoles similar to fetal respiratory epithelium. (Courtesy of Dr. Douglas Flieder, NYC)

LYMPHOID LESIONS (Table 18.9)

Because benign lymphoid lesions are rare and must be differentiated from the vast majority, which are low-grade lymphoma, discussion of lymphoma of bronchial-associated lymphoid tissue (BALT) is undertaken first in this section.

Low-grade BALT lymphoma

Primary pulmonary lymphoma accounts for only 1% of all malignant lymphomas.[394] Seventy to eighty percent of these are BALT lymphomas.[395,396] Benign lymphocytic proliferations, such as lymphocytic interstitial pneumonia (LIP) and nodular lymphoid hyperplasia (pseudolymphoma) are relatively rare compared to the incidence of low-grade BALT lymphoma. These account for 70–80% of small lymphocytic proliferations in the lung.[396–398] Clinically, the disease equally affects men and women of middle to older age.

Approximately half of patients are asymptomatic, being discovered after a routine chest X-ray. Others complain of shortness of breath, cough, hemoptysis, or chest pain. Weight loss and fever are unusual. Collagen vascular disease or Sjögren's syndrome occur in about 10% of cases.[399,400] Radiographically, approximately 70% of patients show solitary nodules or infiltrates. Up to one-fifth of cases show bilateral pulmonary involvement. Tumor size varies from only a few centimeters to huge tumors that may opacify a lung.[396,401] Pleural effusion has been reported in up to 28% of cases.[396] Approximately 30% of patients have monoclonal gammopathy. [96,402]

The disease is slowly progressive and tends to remain localized in the lung for years, although a few patients may have simultaneous tumors in other extranodal sites.[396,397,400] The majority of tumor relapses or progression occur in the lung, pleura, or mediastinum, but spread to other areas such as the GI tract, skin, orbit, and salivary gland can occur.[396,398] Recurrent tumors may also involve the peripheral

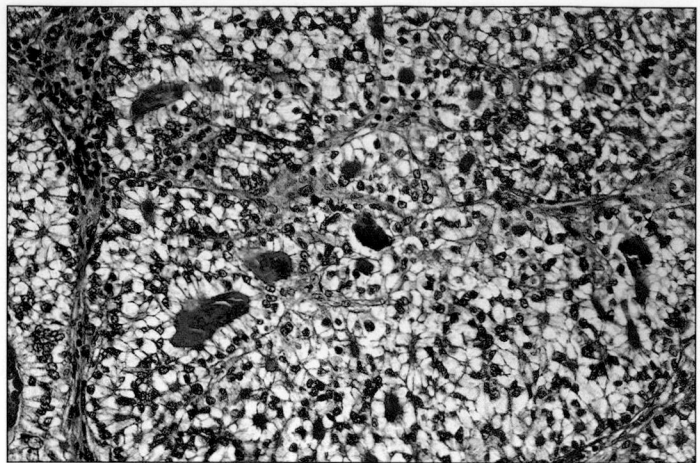

Fig. 18.71 Fetal adenocarcinoma. Solid peripheral lung tumor composed entirely of glands containing clear intracytoplasmic vacuoles identical to the epithelial cells of pulmonary blastoma.

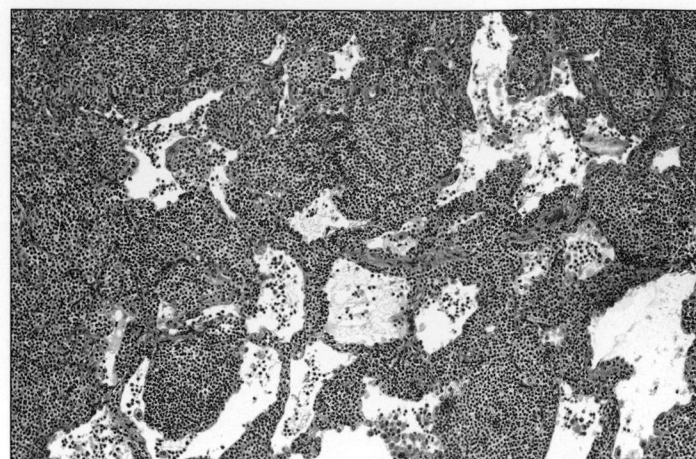

Fig. 18.72 Low-grade BALT lymphoma. Nodular-interstitial infiltration of monotonous small lymphocytes is the characteristic architecture of this tumor in the lung.

Table 18.9 Pulmonary lymphoid lesions

Benign	Malignant
Follicular bronchitis-bronchiolitis	Low-grade BALT lymphoma
Lymphocytic interstitial pneumonia	Large cell lymphoma
Nodular lymphoid hyperplasia	Intravascular large cell lymphoma
Castleman's disease	Lymphomatoid granulomatosis
	Hodgkin's disease

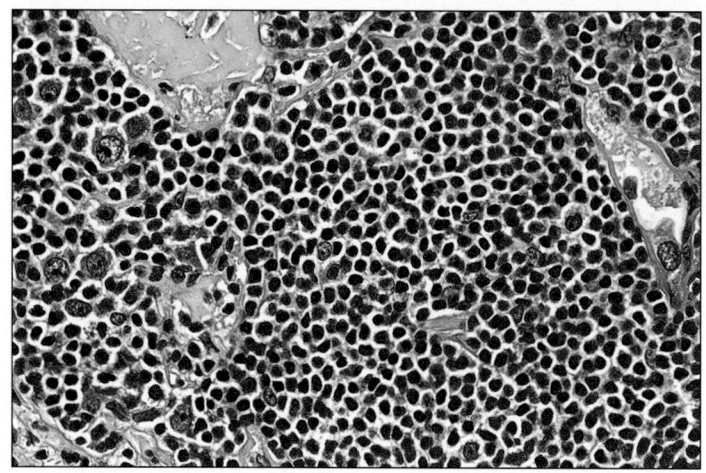

Fig. 18.73 Low-grade BALT lymphoma. Monotonous small lymphocytes, slightly larger than normal, that widen the interstitium and coalesce into solid sheets of cells.

lymph nodes and bone marrow in approximately 25% of patients who relapse.[396] The prognosis of low-grade BALT lymphoma is excellent, ranging from over 95% at five years to between 75% and 85% at ten years.[396,398,401,403] Treatment options vary widely from observation alone for cases with indolent disease, to resection, radiation therapy, and chemotherapy in various combinations for symptomatic cases with progressive disease.

Microscopically, the hallmark of low-grade BALT lymphoma is the recognition of nodular nests of infiltrating monotonous small lymphoid cells that show only slight nuclear abnormality (Fig. 18.72). Some cases bear resemblance to small cleaved cell lymphoma (centrocytic lymphoma).[404] Other tumors may be composed of small lymphocytes with round nuclei similar to small lymphocytic lymphoma or monocytoid cells with abundant pale-staining cytoplasm, plasmacytoid cells with or without Dutcher bodies, or mixtures of these cell types (Fig. 18.73).[400,404] Mature plasma cells may be prominent. Lymphoepithelial lesions consisting of foci of proliferative respiratory epithelium infused with lymphocytes are a common feature of lymphoma but are also seen in benign conditions (Fig. 18.74).

On low-power magnification, tumors often have a multinodular interstitial growth pattern that coalesces into more solid masses. In lung tissue away from mass lesions, lymphatic tracking characterized by perivascular cuffs of tumor lymphocytes may be prominent in more than 75% of cases (Fig. 18.75).[399,405] Germinal centers are commonly seen in well-documented pulmonary lymphomas as are epithelioid granulomas, isolated multinucleated giant cells, and granulomatous vasculitis (Fig. 18.76).[396,398,399,403,406] Dense penetration of the visceral pleura has been reported in 20–85% of cases.[396,398,400,406] Hilar lymph nodes may be histologically positive in 30% of cases, but are rarely sampled.[398]

The immunohistochemistry of low-grade BALT lymphoma reveals that the tumor is composed of CD20-positive lymphocytes with liberal admixtures of CD3-positive T cells. BALT lymphomas characteristically do not express CD5, CD10, or bcl-1 (cyclin D-1).[407–409] Several studies have shown that 20–70% of BALT lymphomas demonstrate light chain restriction by kappa and lambda staining of paraffin sections.[396,400,406] There is often an admixture of polyclonal plasma cells. A majority of cases show immunoglobulin heavy chain (JH) gene rearrangement by molecular diagnostic techniques.[400,409,410] Immunohistochemistry for light chain restriction and the polymerase chain reaction (PCR) for gene rearrangements have been found to be complimentary,

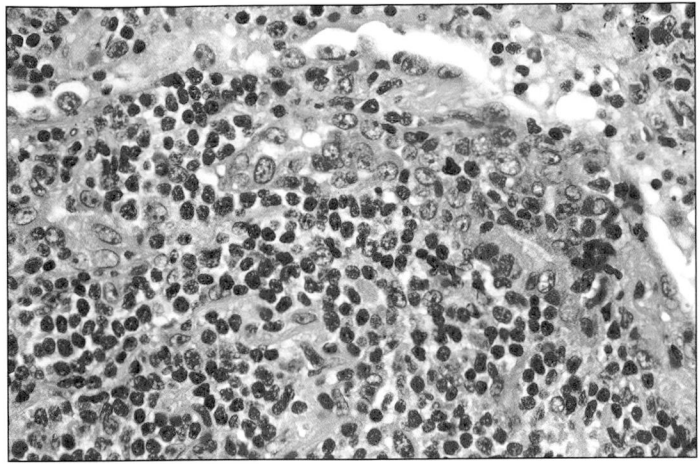

Fig. 18.74 Low-grade BALT lymphoma. Lymphoepithelial lesion showing lymphocytic infiltration of terminal airway associated with swelling and prominence of epithelial cells.

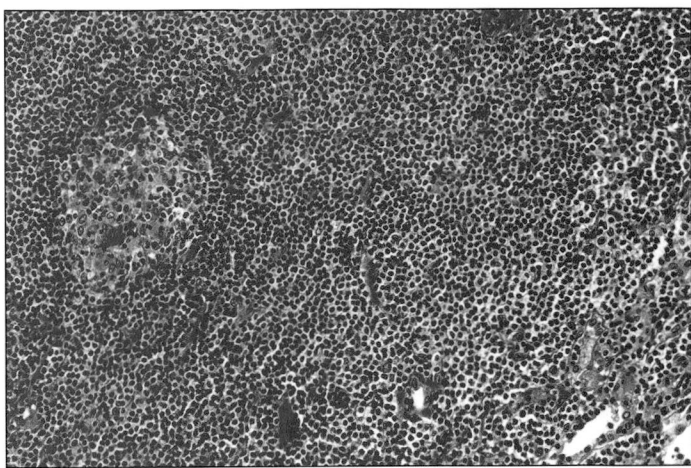

Fig. 18.76 Low-grade BALT lymphoma. Germinal centers are commonly seen within the tumor. Normal marginal and mantle zones are obscured by malignant infiltrate.

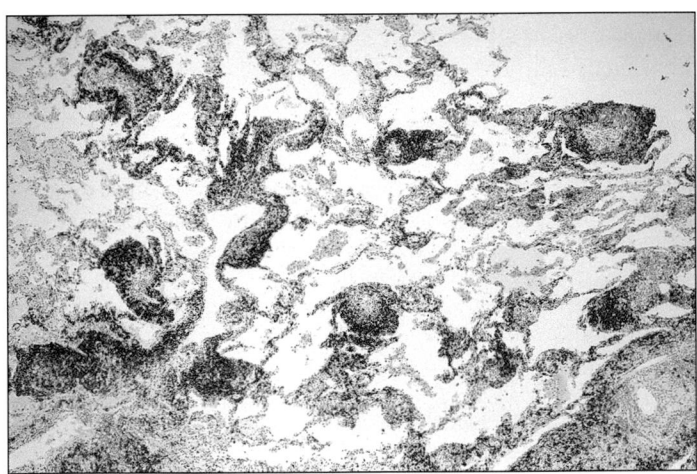

Fig. 18.75 Low-grade BALT lymphoma. Lymphatic tracking showing CD20-positive tumor cells infiltrating perivascular tissue.

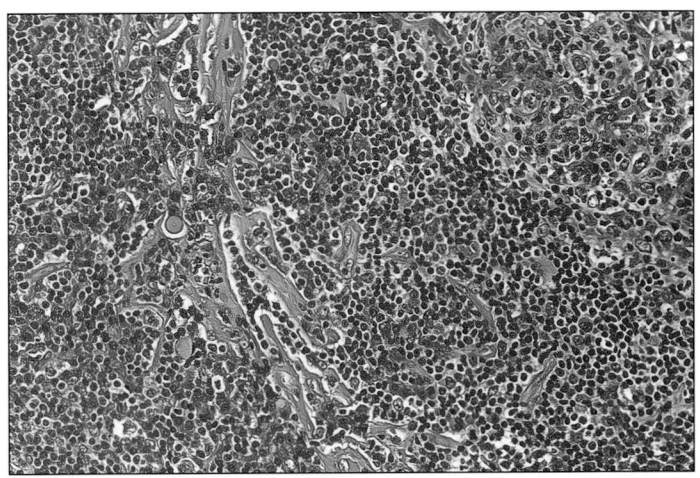

Fig. 18.77 Nodular lymphoid hyperplasia. Germinal centers in upper corner surrounded by mantle of small lymphocytes that mature into polytypic plasma cells.

some cases being positive by only one modality.[400,410] Flow cytometry is useful in characterizing these tumors and can successfully be used in either solid biopsy material or needle aspiration cytology.[411]

Nodular lymphoid hyperplasia

The differential diagnosis of low-grade BALT lymphoma includes benign lymphocytic lesions such as lymphocytic interstitial pneumonia (LIP), follicular bronchitis-bronchiolitis, nodular lymphoid hyperplasia (pseudolymphoma) and Castleman's disease.[412] Both LIP and follicular bronchiolitis are diffuse interstitial and small airway diseases that are discussed elsewhere. A recent study, however, using immunohistochemical and molecular diagnostic techniques, has identified patients with tumor-like nodular lymphoid masses consistent with reactive nodular lymphoid hyperplasia of lung.[413] Ages range from the second to the eighth decade, with most patients being approximately 60 years of age.

Seventy percent of cases are detected as incidental radiographic findings. Most lesions are solitary pulmonary nodules or an area of consolidation ranging 2–5 cm.

Grossly, they are described as firm to fleshy nodules. Characteristically, the lesion is located in the periphery under the pleura, but it fails to invade the visceral pleura in contrast to low-grade BALT lymphoma. Numerous reactive germinal centers are seen throughout that have normal-appearing mantle and marginal zones. The interfollicular tissue is filled with sheets of mature plasma cells, often with numerous Russell bodies (Fig. 18.77). Some cases show significant interfollicular laminated fibrosis that surrounds lymphoid nodules, separating the lesion into smaller lymphoid aggregates (Fig. 18.78). A minor degree of lymphatic tracking can be seen, but it is never as exuberant as in BALT lymphoma. Immunohistochemical studies show a normal reactive pattern with polytypic plasma cells and CD20-positive lymphoid follicles. Interfollicular T cells have a normal immunophenotype showing CD3, CD43, and CD5 positivity,

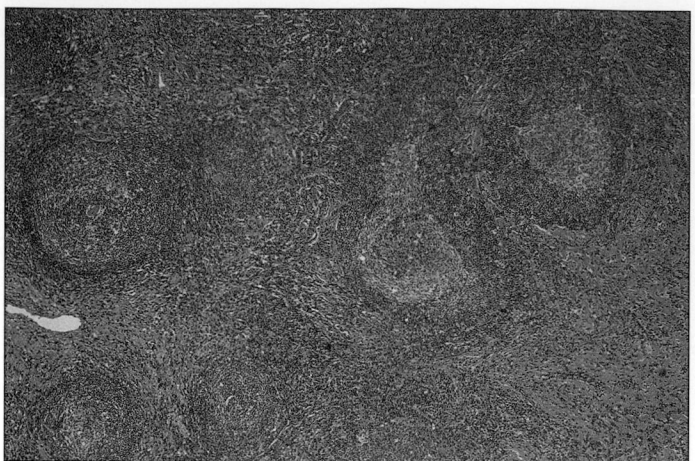

Fig. 18.78 Nodular lymphoid hyperplasia. Numerous reactive germinal centers showing normal perifollicular lymphocyte maturation including mature plasma cells. Increased collagen surrounds these foci, which is a characteristic finding.

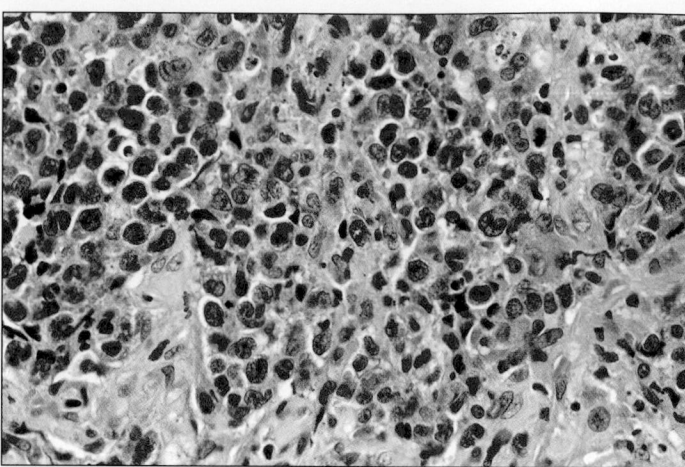

Fig. 18.79 Large cell lymphoma. Solid mass of large atypical lymphoid cells with necrosis and mitotic activity is similar in lung and extrapulmonary sites.

while molecular genetics reveals no evidence of immunoglobulin heavy chain gene rearrangement. Follow-up has shown no recurrence after surgical resection.

Castleman's disease

Castleman's disease may affect the lung as a solitary mass usually located near the hilum due to involvement of lymph nodes.[414,415] The hyaline vascular type of Castleman's disease is most commonly seen and is characterized by a well-circumscribed soft lymphoid nodule that may have a thick fibrous capsule. Microscopically, hyperplastic germinal centers show prominent onion-skin layering of lymphocytes and collagen similar to extrapulmonary lesions.[416] The plasma cell variant of Castleman's disease may be seen in the lung as part of multisystemic involvement.[417]

Other malignant lymphomas

Malignant lymphomas other than BALT tumors such as follicular center cell lymphoma have been described, but most reports have lacked immunologic studies. Waldenström's macroglobulinemia has been reported in the lung.[418] Mantle cell lymphoma has not yet been reported as a primary lung neoplasm.

Large cell lymphoma

Primary large cell lymphomas in the lung are uncommon and are histologically similar to their counterparts in systemic lymph nodes. Pulmonary spread from generalized lymphoma is much more common than primary large cell lymphoma and is indistinguishable microscopically.[394] In primary large cell lymphoma of the lung, evidence of pre-existing low-grade BALT lymphoma is seen in a significant number of patients.[406] Tumors most often show a single mass on chest radiography. Histologically, there are sheets of mitotically active atypical large cells often with necrosis (Fig. 18.79). Lymphatic tracking is inconspicuous compared with low-grade BALT lymphoma.[419] Both B- and T-cell subtypes have been recognized as has anaplastic large cell lymphoma (Ki-1 positive) in the lung.[420] Evidence for EBV in large cell pulmonary lymphoma has been shown to be largely restricted to B-cell lymphomas in nonimmuno-compromised patients while in patients with significant immuno-suppression, including those with AIDS, both T- and B-cell lineages

may reveal evidence of EBV-related DNA by in situ hybridization or immunohistochemistry.[421]

Intravascular large B-cell lymphoma

Intravascular large B-cell lymphoma may rarely affect the lung primarily, but is usually part of widespread systemic disease. In the lung, the chest radiograph usually shows diffuse bilateral involvement, but occasionally localized nodular densities may be seen. The diagnosis can be made with lung biopsy.[39,422–424] Tumor cells are for the most part confined to intrapulmonary capillaries and small blood vessels and are composed of large atypical B cells positive for CD20, negative for CD5 and CD10 (Fig. 18.80). Vascular involvement may be so pronounced as to cause pulmonary hypertension.[425] A minority of intravascular large cell lymphomas appear to be T-cell lesions.[426] The disease is a high-grade malignant lymphoma with poor prognosis.

Lymphomatoid granulomatosis

Lymphomatoid granulomatosis (LYG) is by far the most common large cell lymphoma that affects the lung. The disease is now recognized as a clonal EBV virus-associated large B-cell lymphoma with a heavy reactive T-cell response similar to that seen in post-transplant immunoproliferative lesions.[427–431] By convention, however, the original term lymphomatoid granulomatosis first coined by Liebow and colleagues is maintained in the current WHO tumor classification.[432] A minority of cases appear to be variants of peripheral T-cell lymphoma without evidence of EBV-associated material.[429,430]

Clinically, LYG affects a wide age range, but it is rare in children and adolescents. The mean age at diagnosis is between 50 and 60 years without sex predilection. The vast majority of patients are symptomatic, most commonly demonstrating fever, cough, shortness of breath, weight loss, hemoptysis, or chest pain. Extrapulmonary manifestations in the central nervous system, skin, and peripheral neuropathy are common. Involvement of lymph nodes is unusual. Rare cases can be asymptomatic.[433] Radiographically, the most common pattern is of multiple pulmonary nodules usually mistaken for metastatic tumor. Solitary masses, diffuse pneumonia-like infiltrates, and unilateral lesions are less common.

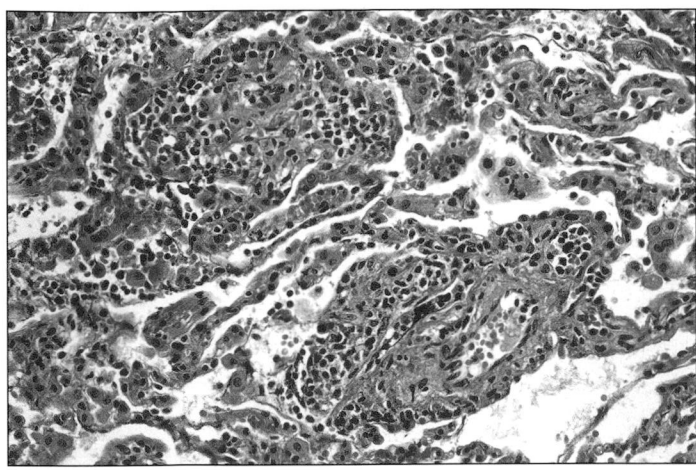

Fig. 18.80 Intravascular large B-cell lymphoma. Tumor cells are seen to selectively infiltrate pulmonary capillaries and perivascular lymphatics.

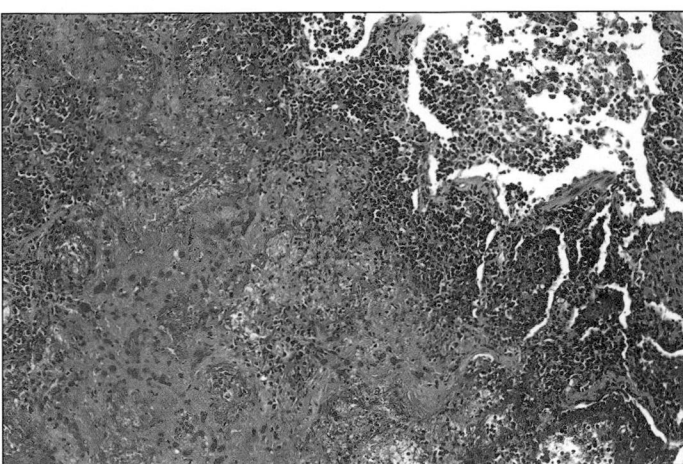

Fig. 18.82 Lymphomatoid granulomatosis. Largely necrotic tumor nodule.

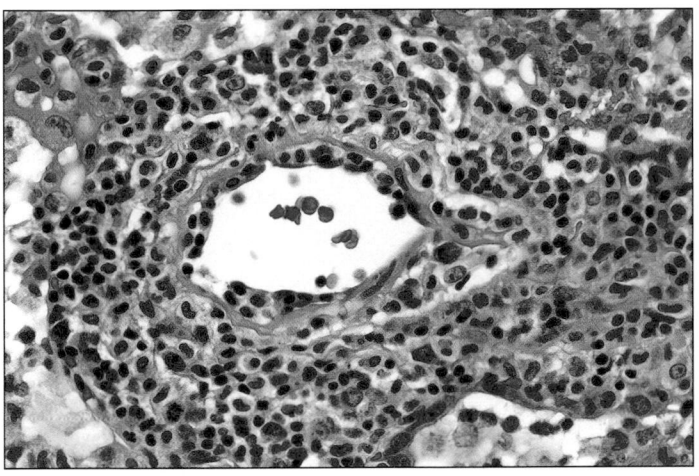

Fig. 18.81 Lymphomatoid granulomatosis. Polymorphous lymphoid infiltrate has predilection for blood vessels, causing vascular occlusion with subsequent tumor necrosis.

The microscopy of LYG is characterized by a polymorphic cell infiltrate composed of large malignant lymphoid cells showing prominent nucleoli and mixed with varying numbers of small lymphocytes, plasma cells, epithelioid histiocytes, and other inflammatory cells (Fig. 18.81). Blood vessel invasion is the hallmark of LYG, with transmural invasion of large and medium-sized arteries and veins that may cause occlusion and necrosis of the infiltrate (Fig. 18.82). Fibrinoid necrosis in the blood vessels is not seen in LYG in contrast to Wegener's granulomatosis. There is a morphologic spectrum of lymphocyte populations from case to case and sometimes within a single biopsy, which has lead to a three-tiered histologic grading system. Increased numbers of large malignant lymphoid cells have been found to correspond to a poor response to therapy.[429,434,435]

In the past the treatment of LYG has been difficult, with most patients succumbing to their disease. More current multiagent chemotherapy has resulted in some long-term control.[436] Autologous hematopoietic stem cell transplantation has resulted in some complete remissions as has cyclosporine and interferon.[427,437–439]

A case of T-cell-rich B-cell lymphoma of the lung has been reported which seems to bear a close kinship to LYG, particularly since Epstein-Barr virus DNA has been demonstrated in the neoplastic B cells in both tumors.[429,431,440]

Hodgkin's disease

Large cell lymphomas and LYG should be differentiated from pulmonary Hodgkin's disease. Primary pulmonary Hodgkin's disease is very rare, accounting for only about 1% of all Hodgkin's disease cases. Most often, Hodgkin's involvement of the lung results from direct extension from disease in the mediastinum or pulmonary spread after treatment failure.[441,442] Nodular sclerosis is the most common histologic type. The Reed-Sternberg cells characteristically are negative for CD45 (LCA) and positive for CD15 and CD30, similar to the pattern seen in lymph nodes. Immunohistochemistry for EBV-latent membrane protein is often positive in the Reed-Sternberg cells. In contrast, the large cells of LYG are usually positive for CD45 and CD20 and negative for CD15. CD30 positivity is variable.[427,443]

Cytology of pulmonary lymphoma

Traditionally, the diagnosis of pulmonary lymphoma has been made on the basis of histologic examination. Particularly, the diagnosis and subclassification of small cell lymphomas was extremely difficult. In recent years, however, the availability of lymphocyte marker studies by immunocytochemical stains and flow cytometry has led to the increased use of FNA for the diagnosis of lymphoma.[411,444–453]

In FNA samples BALT lymphomas appear as a monotonous population of small to medium-sized lymphocytes with mild nuclear membrane irregularity and slight chromatin condensation (Fig. 18.83A,B).[411] Some lymphocytes may exhibit small nucleoli and scattered plasmacytoid cells, and larger lymphoid cells can be seen. Additionally, there are sheets of reactive epithelial cells characterized by uniform nuclei, bland chromatin, and indistinct or small nucleoli (Fig. 18.83A,B). A definitive diagnosis of BALT lymphoma should not be made on the basis of cytology alone, however. Establishing the monoclonal nature of the lymphocytes by demonstrating immunoglobulin light chain restriction by flow cytometry or immunohistochemistry is essential for diagnosis

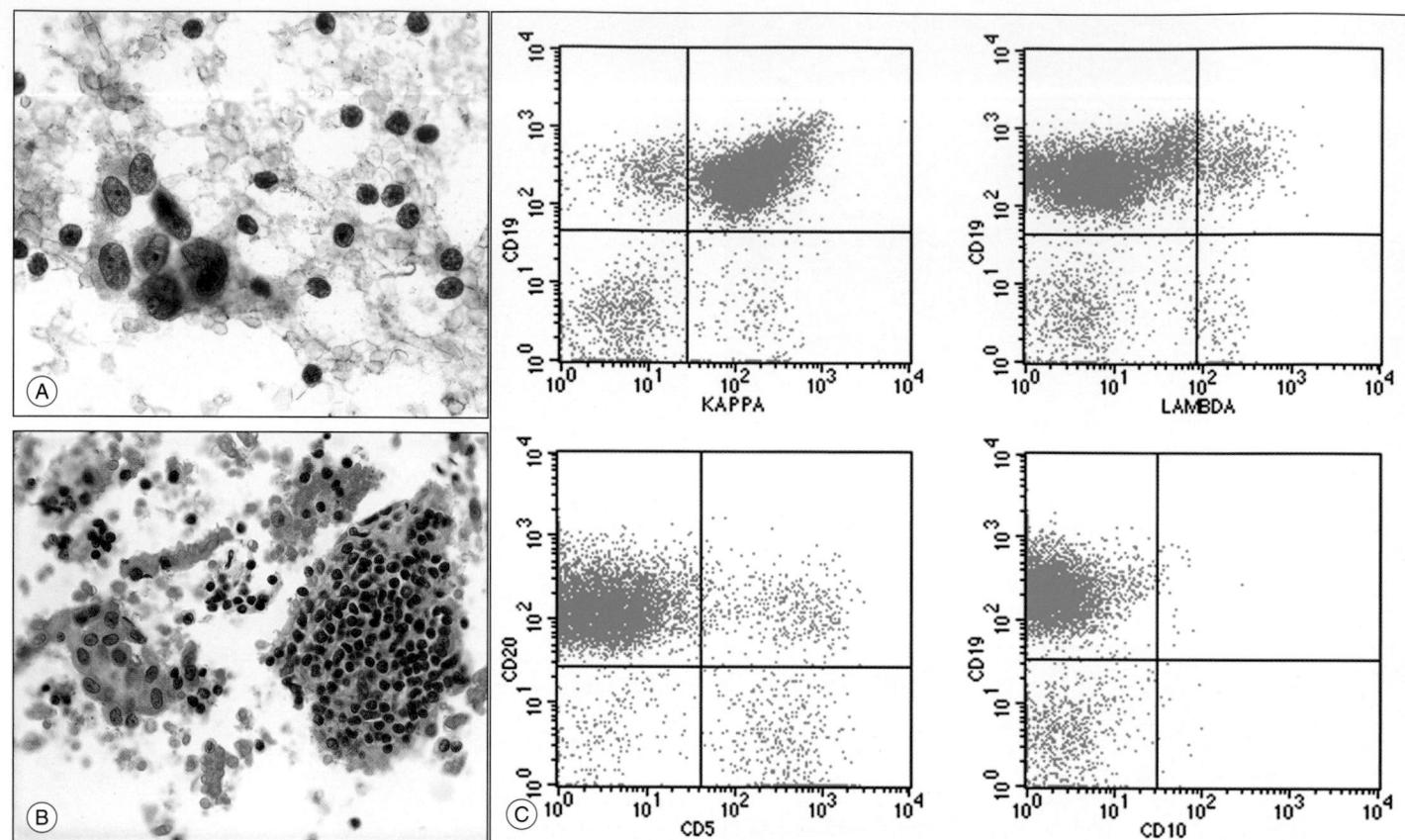

Fig. 18.83 FNA cytology of BALT lymphoma. **A,** Monotonous population of small lymphocytes exhibiting slight nuclear membrane irregularity and chromatin condensation. A group of reactive epithelial cells with bland chromatin and small nucleoli is also present (Papanicolaou stain); **B,** Cell block section showing an aggregate of small lymphocytes in a nodular pattern and a group of benign epithelial cells (H&E stain); **C,** Flow cytometry shows a population of CD5-negative, CD10-negative, kappa light chain restricted B lymphocytes.

(Fig. 18.83C). Negative staining for CD5 and CD10 distinguishes BALT from other low-grade lymphomas.[446]

In contrast to small cell lymphomas, large cell lymphomas can be readily diagnosed by FNA because of their characteristic morphologic features. These tumors occur as a monotonous population of single, round, malignant-looking cells (Fig. 18.84A,B). Nuclear morphology varies depending on the type of lymphoma.[446] Poorly differentiated carcinoma and malignant melanoma are considered in the differential diagnosis, but some tendency for cohesive cell grouping is almost always present in these tumors, while lymphoma cells always appear singly in cytologic specimens. An exception is anaplastic large cell lymphoma, which may mimic carcinoma because of the abundance of cytoplasm, marked pleomorphism, multinucleation, and occasional clustering of cells (Fig. 18.84C,D).[448,454] Immunohistochemical stains on cell-block preparations are highly useful in distinguishing this tumor from carcinoma and melanoma.

NEUROENDOCRINE NEOPLASMS (Table 18.10)

The histologic classification of neuroendocrine tumors of the lung is one of the most vexing problems for the diagnostic pathologist. As a group, they are generally defined by their microscopic appearance, having a 'neuroendocrine look,' consisting of nests, ribbons, festoons, trabeculae, rosettes, and spindle cells as well as by the presence of dense core granules ultrastructurally and the neuroendocrine immuno-

phenotype. Diagnostic problems are not infrequent and arise as a result of small biopsy samples, frequent artifacts, overlap of histologic patterns, and mixed tumor types, and the difficulty in applying imprecise morphologic definitions to put small round cell tumors into small square boxes.

Carcinoid tumor

The carcinoid tumor represents the least aggressive, best-differentiated tumor of the neuroendocrine spectrum. These tumors appear in younger patients than do more ordinary lung carcinomas; the average age at diagnosis is approximately 50 years.[455] There is about an equal sex distribution. There is no known association with cigarette smoking. Pulmonary carcinoids have been rarely observed with multiple endocrine neoplasia syndrome type I, an autosomal dominant syndrome often associated with pituitary, parathyroid, and pancreatic islet cell adenomas.[456,457] In addition, evidence of neuro-peptide and hormone production in the form of ACTH, VIP, ADH, and neurotensin have been described.[458] Cushing's syndrome has also been reported with pulmonary carcinoid tumor.[459]

Grossly, approximately 75% of typical carcinoid tumors arise in the lobar bronchi, while 10% originate in the mainstem bronchi and 15% in the lung periphery.[460] They have also been reported in the trachea.[461] Patients commonly present with hemoptysis or with fever and chills due to obstructive pneumonia distal to an occluded bronchus. Tumors are characteristically polypoid endobronchial lesions that may also penetrate into the adjacent lung parenchyma.

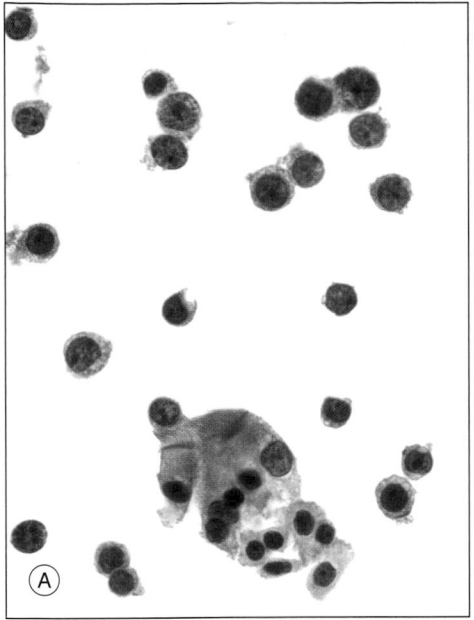

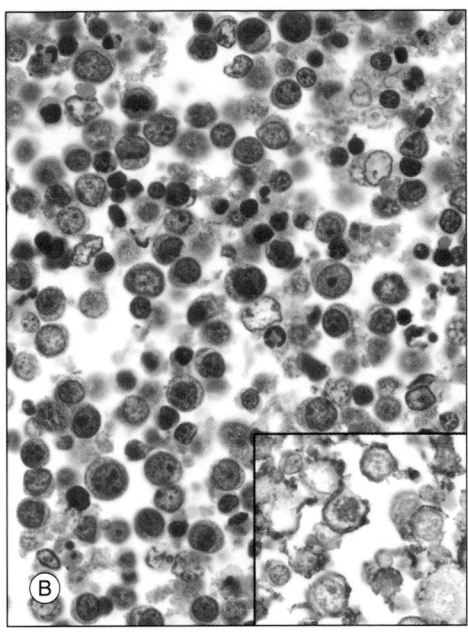

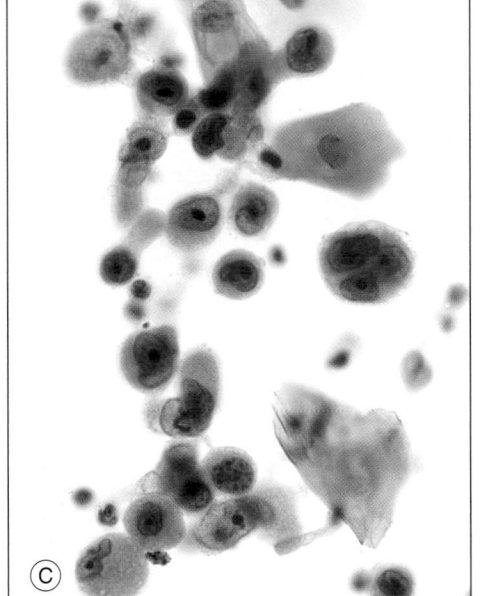

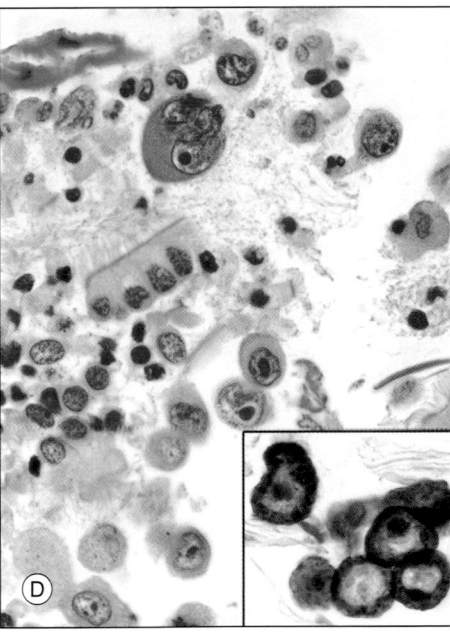

Fig. 18.84 Cytopathology of large cell lymphoma. **A**, Bronchial washing on a case of large B-cell lymphoma of the lung. Single, round, large lymphoid cells showing high nuclear:cytoplasmic ratio and coarse chromatin. A few normal bronchial epithelial cells are present in the lower part of the field (Papanicolaou stain); **B**, Cell block section of transbronchial needle aspirate of the same case showing large lymphoid cells, some of which possess prominent nucleoli. Many apoptotic cells are seen in this field (H&E stain); Inset: Positive immunostaining for CD20; **C**, Bronchoalveolar lavage in a case of large cell anaplastic lymphoma of the lung. Tumor cells appear as large, round cells, about the size of pulmonary macrophages (left lower corner). The nuclei exhibit irregular membrane, coarse chromatin, and large nucleoli. An occasional multinucleated tumor cell is present (Papanicolaou stain); **D**, Cell-block section of the same case showing single, large tumor cells admixed with pulmonary macrophages and ciliated bronchial epithelial cells (H&E stain); Inset: Positive staining for CD30.

Table 18.10 Neuroendocrine carcinoma

Carcinoid tumorlet

Carcinoid tumor

Atypical carcinoid

Large cell neuroendocrine carcinoma

Small cell carcinoma

Mixed small /large cell neuroendocrine carcinoma

Combined small cell carcinoma and squamous cell carcinoma, adenocarcinoma, or other types

Askin's tumor

Histologically, carcinoids show the signature pattern of neuroendocrine differentiation by light microscopy. It has been described as organoid, insular, rosetting or festooned, composed of uniform groups of cells with small centrally placed nuclei and cuboidal eosinophilic or amphophilic granular cytoplasm. These cells are surrounded by a single, often inapparent, layer of spindled, sustentacular cells and sustained by fine fibrovascular stroma. Patterns may be mixed and associated with spindled carcinoid cells. Mitoses are absent or rare, as is evidence of cell necrosis (Fig. 18.85). Occasional cases may show cells with pronounced nuclear pleomorphism, but without mitotic activity, prominent nucleoli, or any other nuclear features of malignancy (Fig. 18.86). Lymphatic space invasion is unusual in otherwise ordinary carcinoid tumors, but can be seen.

Histologic variants of carcinoid tumors occur that may sometimes cause confusion with other tumor types. Rarely, carcinoid tumors

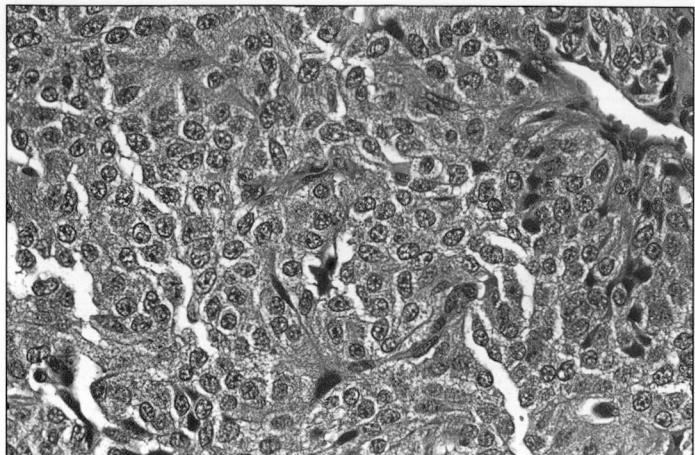

Fig. 18.85 Carcinoid tumor. Lesion is composed of nests of uniform epithelial cells. Sparse spindle cells surround several of these nests in a sustentacular cell pattern.

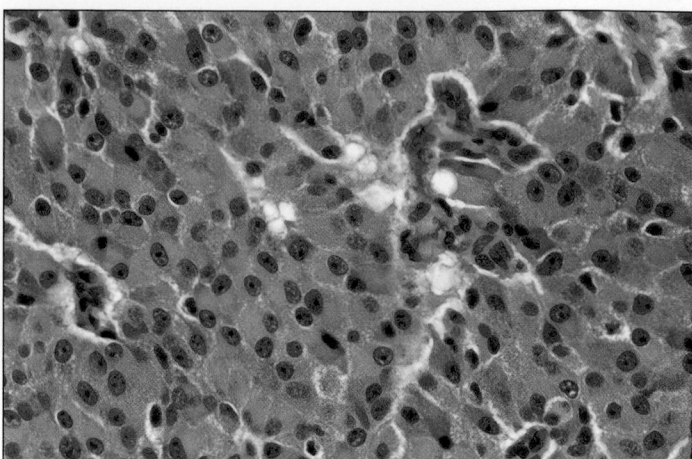

Fig. 18.87 Carcinoid tumor. Oncocytic differentiation.

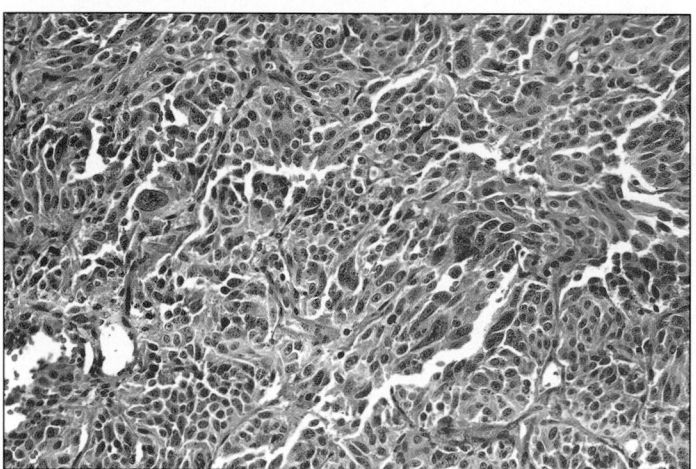

Fig. 18.86 Carcinoid tumor. Nuclei show enlargement and pleomorphism, but the majority of the tumor otherwise has characteristics of typical carcinoid without mitoses or necrosis, and with a solid nested pattern.

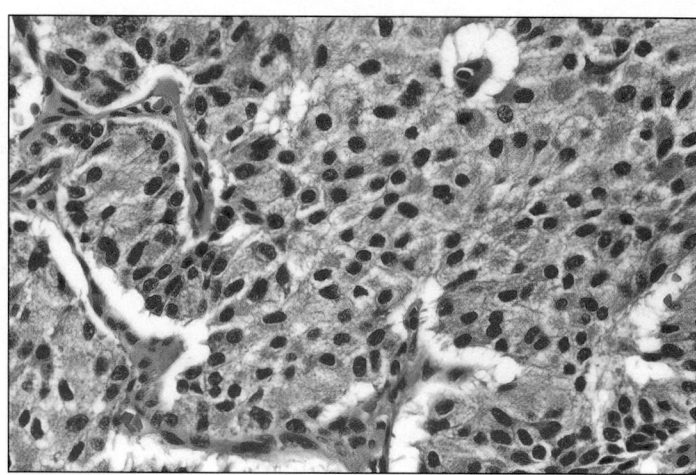

Fig. 18.88 Carcinoid tumor. Clear cell differentiation.

may show oncocytic properties composed of cells with ample eosinophilic cytoplasm (Fig. 18.87).[191,192] This tumor has been shown to have both dense core neurosecretory granules characteristic of carcinoid tumor and numerous swollen mitochondria typical of oncocytoma, ultrastructurally.[192,462] Rarely, carcinoids show clear cytoplasm (Fig. 18.88).

Occasional tumors have a papillary pattern,[463] or are glandular with mucin production similar to mucinous or goblet cell carcinoids of the appendix (Fig. 18.89A,B).[464,465] Other rare variations are pneumocyte-like carcinoid,[466] melanin producing showing cells that ultrastructurally contain both neurosecretory type granules and melanosomes,[467,468] and paraganglioma-like carcinoids.[469]

The immunohistochemical reaction seen in carcinoids defines the neuroendocrine phenotype. The majority of tumors stain positively for chromogranin A, synaptophysin, and neuron-specific enolase.[470–472] Carcinoids contain various classes of intermediate filaments that stain positively with neurofilaments and keratin.[473] Other antibodies have been studied in carcinoid tumors including monoclonal CEA. In a

study of 31 patients, positive staining with anti-CEA antibodies was predictive of treatment failure.[474]

Ultrastructurally, carcinoid cells are uniform in appearance and have centrally placed nuclei, course clumped chromatin, and abundant cytoplasm that contains numerous dense core granules ranging in diameters from 90 nanometers to 380 nanometers.[475] These granules are bounded by a double-layered membrane usually separated from the central dense core by a clear circumferential space. The cells show basal lamina formation and intermediate filaments, and many tumors show spindle-shaped cells containing smooth muscle filaments adjacent to the basal lamina that appear to be sustentacular cells. Dense core granules are usually numerous and are the most reliable criterion for neuroendocrine differentiation in carcinoid tumors.

In contrast to central endobronchial carcinoids, carcinoid tumors that arise in the periphery of the lung show more spindle cells that sometimes infiltrate the lung tissue in an interstitial pattern (Fig. 18.90). Nuclei tend to be round or spindled with few or no mitoses. There is no necrosis or significant cellular pleomorphism.

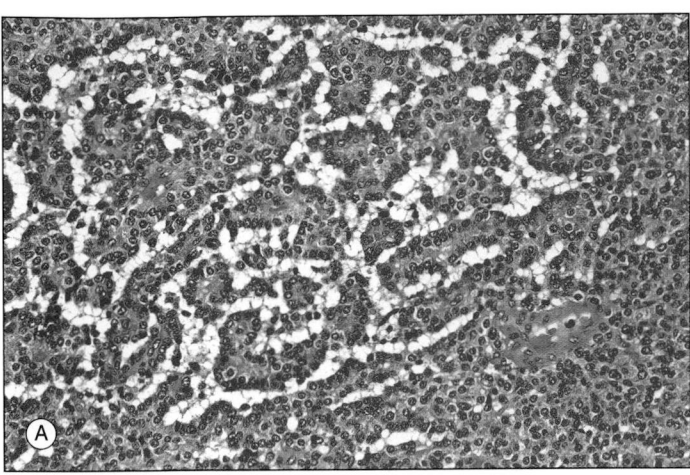 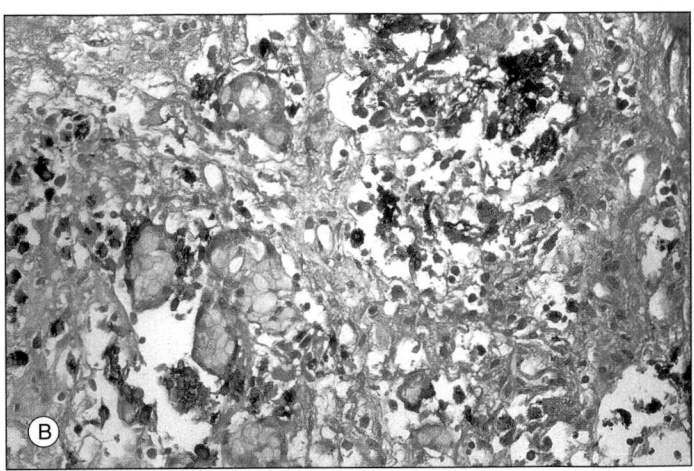

Fig. 18.89 A, Carcinoid tumor. Papillary pattern; **B**, Carcinoid tumor. Mucinous carcinoid. Typical carcinoid cells stain positively with chromogranin, while goblet cells are negative.

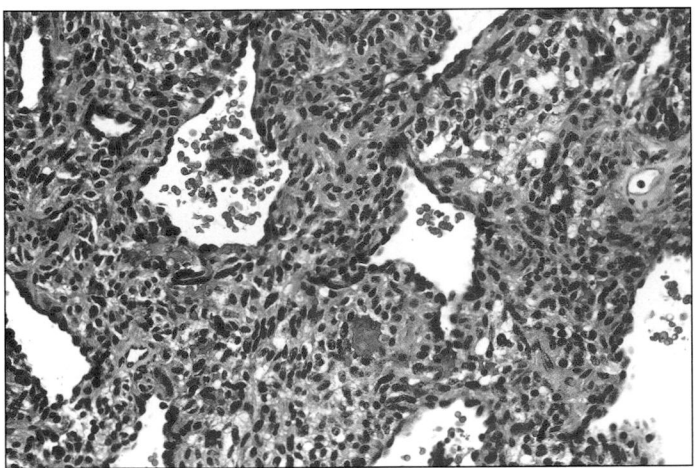 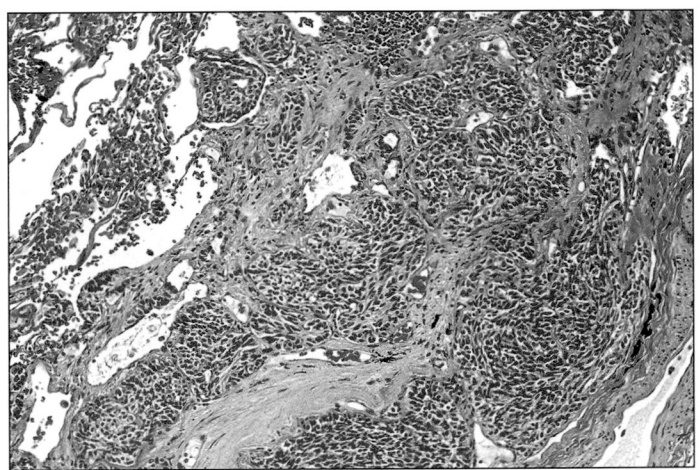

Fig. 18.90 Peripheral spindle cell carcinoid. Tumor cells show an interstitial pattern of lung involvement.

Fig. 18.91 Carcinoid tumorlet. Lesion shows all of the features of a peripheral spindle cell carcinoid except that it measures less than 5.0 mm.

Unlike endobronchial carcinoid, the majority of peripheral carcinoid tumors are incidental findings in asymptomatic patients.[476] Patients with both central and peripheral carcinoid tumors may show more than one tumor and may also have multiple foci of carcinoid tumorlets or neuroendocrine hyperplasia in the lung tissue.[477,478] Carcinoid tumorlets are small and arbitrarily defined by their size. Lesions larger than 5 mm in diameter are designated as small carcinoid tumors (Fig. 18.91). Some tumorlets may cause diffuse lung disease with multiple bilateral lesions. Rarely, they can metastasize to regional lymph nodes.[479]

Cytology of carcinoid tumor

Central carcinoid tumors are accessible by bronchoscopy because of their intrabronchial location. Tumor cells are rarely found in sputum because of an intact bronchial epithelium. Bronchial brushing is a useful method and complementary to biopsy for the diagnosis of carcinoids.[137] Peripheral lesions are best diagnosed by FNA. Tumor cells appear as loose aggregates of uniform, medium-sized, round or spindle-shaped cells (Fig. 18.92).[480,481] Cytoplasm is pale and granular

with poorly outlined boundaries. The cells possess single, central or mildly eccentric, round to ovoid nuclei. Chromatin is slightly coarse, but evenly dispersed, producing a 'salt and pepper' look. Small nucleoli may be seen. Occasionally, a cell with a considerably larger nucleus may be observed, but the chromatin detail is similar to the other cells (Fig. 18.92B,C). Acinus-like structures or rosette formations are evident in some tumors (Fig. 18.92C).[481] Prominent nucleoli, mitoses, and necrosis are not features of this tumor. In the spindle cell variant the nuclei are elongated, but exhibit the same chromatin pattern as the more common round cell type.[161]

Differential diagnosis: Because they lack pleomorphism, hyperchromasia, nuclear membrane irregularity, abnormality of chromatin distribution, and prominent nucleoli, carcinoid tumor cells may be missed in bronchoscopic cytology samples as the cells may be mistaken for normal or reactive bronchial cells, particularly in poorly prepared smears. Bronchial epithelial cells show a higher degree of cohesiveness, columnar appearance, and cilia or at least brush borders. The eccentric nuclei and the chromatin appearance of carcinoid may mimic plasmacytoma. However, benign and neoplastic plasma cells

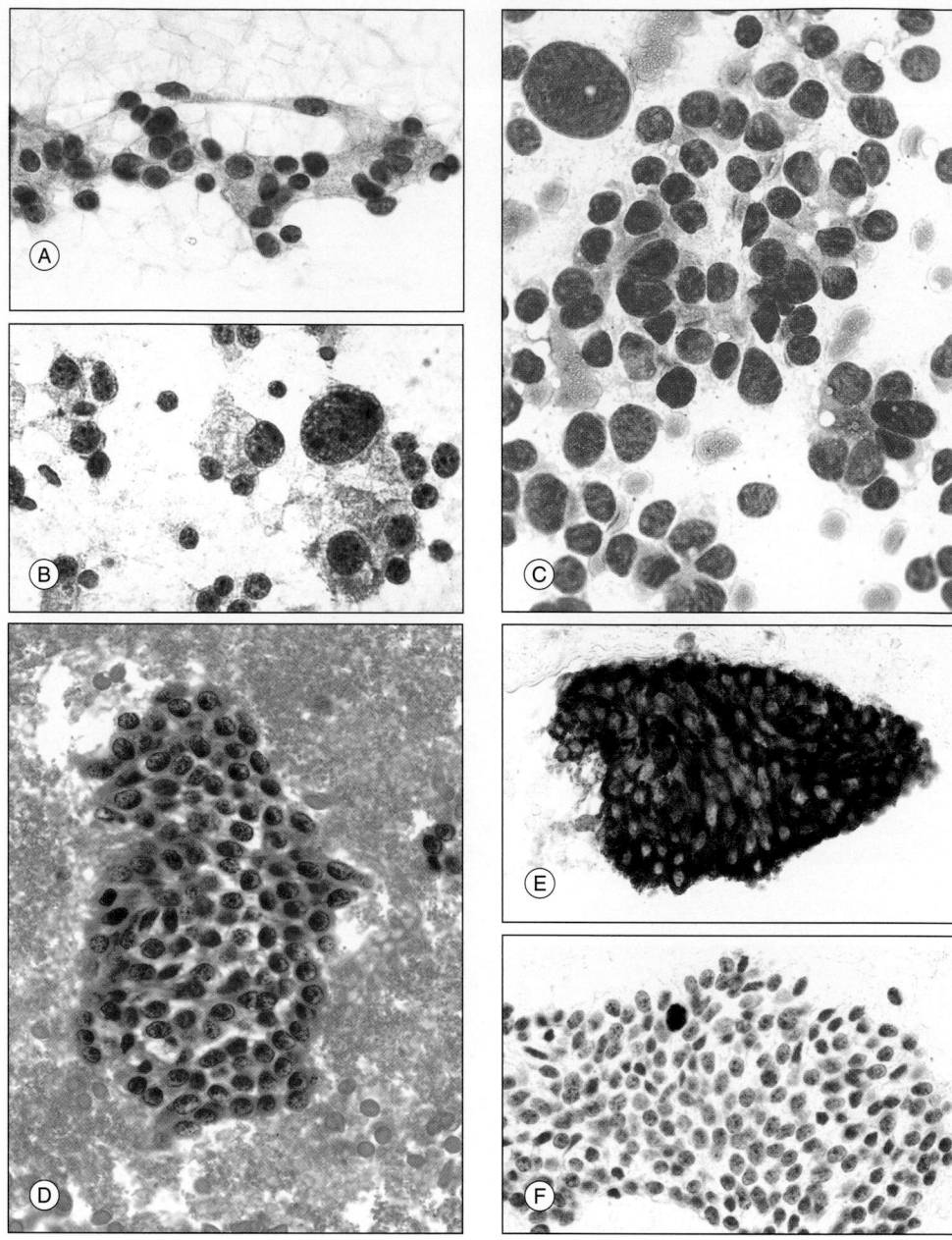

Fig. 18.92 FNA cytology of carcinoid tumor. **A**, A sheet of medium-sized, uniform epithelial cells with granular cytoplasm and round to oval nuclei. Chromatin is evenly dispersed and nucleoli are not seen (Papanicolaou stain); **B**, Loosely cohesive cells with granular cytoplasm and 'salt and pepper' chromatin. An occasional large nucleus is seen with the same chromatin appearance as the smaller nuclei (Papanicolaou stain); **C**, Loosely cohesive cells with characteristic nuclear features of carcinoid tumor. A pseudorosette formation is present in right lower and a large nucleus in the left upper portion of this field (Diff-Quik stain); **D**, Cell-block section showing remarkable uniformity of the cells (H&E stain); **E**, Tumor cells demonstrate strong immunostaining for chromogranin; **F**, Very low proliferative activity is demonstrated by MIB-1 immunostaining.

always occur singly in cytologic preparations, whereas in carcinoid tumor some degree of cohesiveness is usually present. On rare occasions, particularly in scant samples, smearing or crush artifacts combined with overstaining may lead to the erroneous diagnosis of small cell carcinoma.[481–483] Careful correlation with clinical, radiologic, and endoscopic findings is essential in avoiding such a misdiagnosis.

The clinical behavior of carcinoid tumors is indolent. The older literature suggested that they were benign, hence the designation of 'bronchial adenoma.' Indeed, most reports have demonstrated that the majority of bronchopulmonary carcinoid tumors do not metastasize. One study of 93 resected typical carcinoid tumors followed for 25 years showed 100% survival at 5, 10, and 15 years. One patient died as a result of metastatic carcinoid tumor at 17 years, however, while another was alive at 9 years with evidence of distant metastases. Almost 10% of patients had positive regional lymph nodes. These clinical findings have been reflected in other series. Recurrence and metastases tend to occur late so that limited follow-up does not accurately reflect their potential for malignant behavior.[484,485] Small tumor size and the absence of lymph node metastasis are predictive of survival without recurrence.[485]

Atypical carcinoid

The concept of atypical carcinoid was introduced by Arrigoni and colleagues from the Mayo Clinic in 1972.[486] They reported a series of 215 carcinoid tumors of the lung among which approximately 10% were regarded as atypical carcinoid. These tumors looked histologically like carcinoids showing the nested and ribboned architectural appearance typical of carcinoids but differed in several respects by one or more of the following features: (a) increased numbers of mitotic figures, (b) pleomorphism of the nuclei with prominent nucleoli, (c) hyperchromasia and increased N:C ratio,

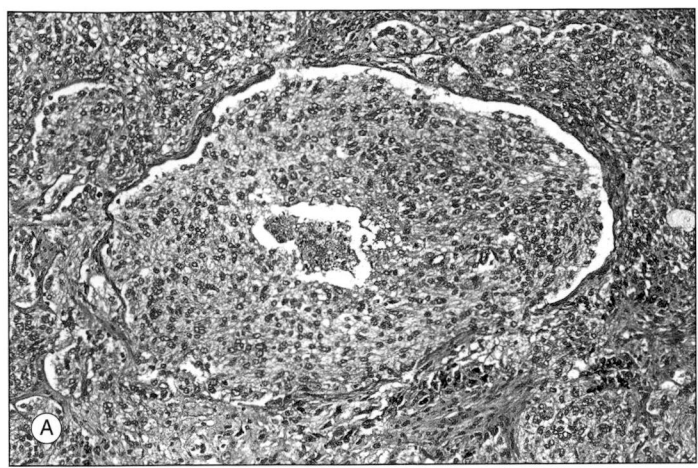
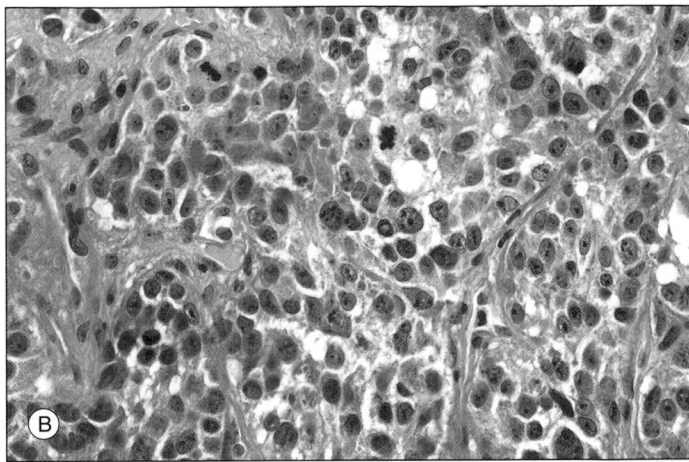

Fig. 18.93 A, Atypical carcinoid. Nest of tumor cells show punctate central necrosis, a common finding; **B**, Atypical carcinoid. Tumor cells have the basic architecture of carcinoid tumor, but show several mitoses and individual cell necrosis.

(d) areas of increased cellularity with disorganized architecture, and (e) areas of tumor necrosis (Fig. 18.93A,B). They commented on the focal nature of these findings and the need for thorough sampling of carcinoid tumors to detect their presence. Comparison of atypical with typical carcinoid tumors showed that 70% of patients with atypical carcinoids had metastases compared with 3% of the typical carcinoids. The mortality rate was 30% for the atypical carcinoids whereas no patient with typical carcinoid died of tumor. Other series have substantiated the more aggressive nature of atypical carcinoid.[487–490] Generally speaking, patients with atypical carcinoids are a decade older than those with typical carcinoids and demonstrate a more positive correlation with cigarette smoking.[455] Tumors tend to be larger, and are more likely to be in stage II or III than their typical carcinoid counterparts. More recently, histologic criteria that separate typical carcinoid from atypical carcinoid have been further refined. The presence of cellular pleomorphism no longer is considered a major differentiating feature, but the presence of necrosis in atypical carcinoid, and, most importantly, the mitotic rate (fewer than two mitoses per 10 high-power fields for typical carcinoid and ten mitoses for atypical carcinoid), have been found to be predictive and reproducible criteria.[491] Nuclear characteristics such as DNA content as measured by image analysis and MIB-1 (Ki-67) immunohistochemistry staining show strong correlation with this classification.[483,489,492]

Several series have reported unusual tumors with combined features of atypical carcinoid and small cell carcinoma.[493,494] Survival rates range from approximately 45% to 50% and appear to be stage dependent.

Cytology of atypical carcinoid

Cytologic features of atypical carcinoid fall between those of classic carcinoid and high-grade neuroendocrine carcinomas.[495,496] Tumor cells appear in small clusters of medium-sized, polygonal or fusiform cells that occasionally form acinus-like or palisading structures (Fig. 18.94).[496] Single cells are also present in most cases. Cytoplasm is pale and granular. The nuclei have a chromatin structure reminiscent of carcinoid tumor, but show a greater variation in size and shape and contain small or prominent nucleoli.[161,481,495,496] Most importantly, mitoses and necrosis are present in atypical carcinoid in contrast to ordinary carcinoid tumor.

Differential diagnosis: The distinction of atypical carcinoids from high-grade neuroendocrine neoplasms (small cell carcinoma and large cell neuroendocrine carcinoma) is not always possible in small samples.[481,483,495] In histologic sections, mitotic count is used to distinguish these tumors, but the number of mitoses per high-power field is not a reliable criterion in cytologic samples because cell concentration is variable from one case to another case and from one field to another field. Proliferation rate assessed by immunocytochemical stain for Ki-67 has proven feasible and may be useful in cytologic specimens.[483] In a cytology series reported by Lin et al., proliferation activity by Ki-67 immunostaining was less than 25% in all low-grade neuroendocrine neoplasms (classic and atypical carcinoids) and higher than 50% in all high-grade tumors.[483] Unlike small cell carcinomas, nuclear molding is not present in atypical carcinoid. When distinction from small cell carcinoma is uncertain, the report should include the differential diagnosis. Either additional biopsies or resection can then be done.

Large cell neuroendocrine carcinoma

The spectrum of neuroendocrine carcinomas ranging from typical carcinoid to small cell anaplastic carcinoma has been largely defined by light microscopy appearance combined with mitotic rate.[497] Large cell neuroendocrine carcinoma (LCNEC) represents the most recent subdivision of this group of neuroendocrine lung cancer, having been described in 1985 and in subsequent reports.[273,498] They are high-grade tumors that behave aggressively even when initially confined to the lung. In one series, only one of nine stage I cases was alive and free of disease at the time of last follow-up.[273]

LCNEC is described as showing microscopic similarity to carcinoid, but is composed of large cells having course nuclear chromatin and frequent prominent nucleoli along with a high mitotic rate and areas of necrosis (Fig. 18.95A–C). There is no squamous or glandular differentiation. Immunohistochemistry or electron microscopy documents neuroendocrine differentiation. It is distinguished from atypical carcinoid predominantly by mitotic counts. LCNEC shows greater than ten mitoses per 10 high-power fields compared with atypical carcinoid that shows between two and ten mitoses. This lends some degree of objectivity and reproducibility to the histologic separation of atypical carcinoid from LCNEC, but divergent differentiation does occur and problems in classifying some tumors

Fig. 18.94 FNA cytology of atypical carcinoid. **A**, A cluster of medium-sized cells with granular cytoplasm, round to oval nuclei and occasional nucleoli (Papanicolaou stain); **B**, Chromatin exhibits 'salt & pepper' appearance. Some cells have eccentric nuclei reminiscent of plasma cells (Papanicolaou stain); **C**, In this cell-block section tumor cells show an overall resemblance to carcinoid tumor, but there is a moderate degree of variation in size and shape of the nuclei, some having prominent nucleoli. Necrosis is seen in the lower portion of the field. The inset shows higher magnification (H&E stain); **D**, Strong immunostaining of tumor cells for chromogranin; **E**, MIB-1 immunostaining demonstrating a higher proliferative activity than classic carcinoid and much lower activity that high-grade neuroendocrine carcinomas.

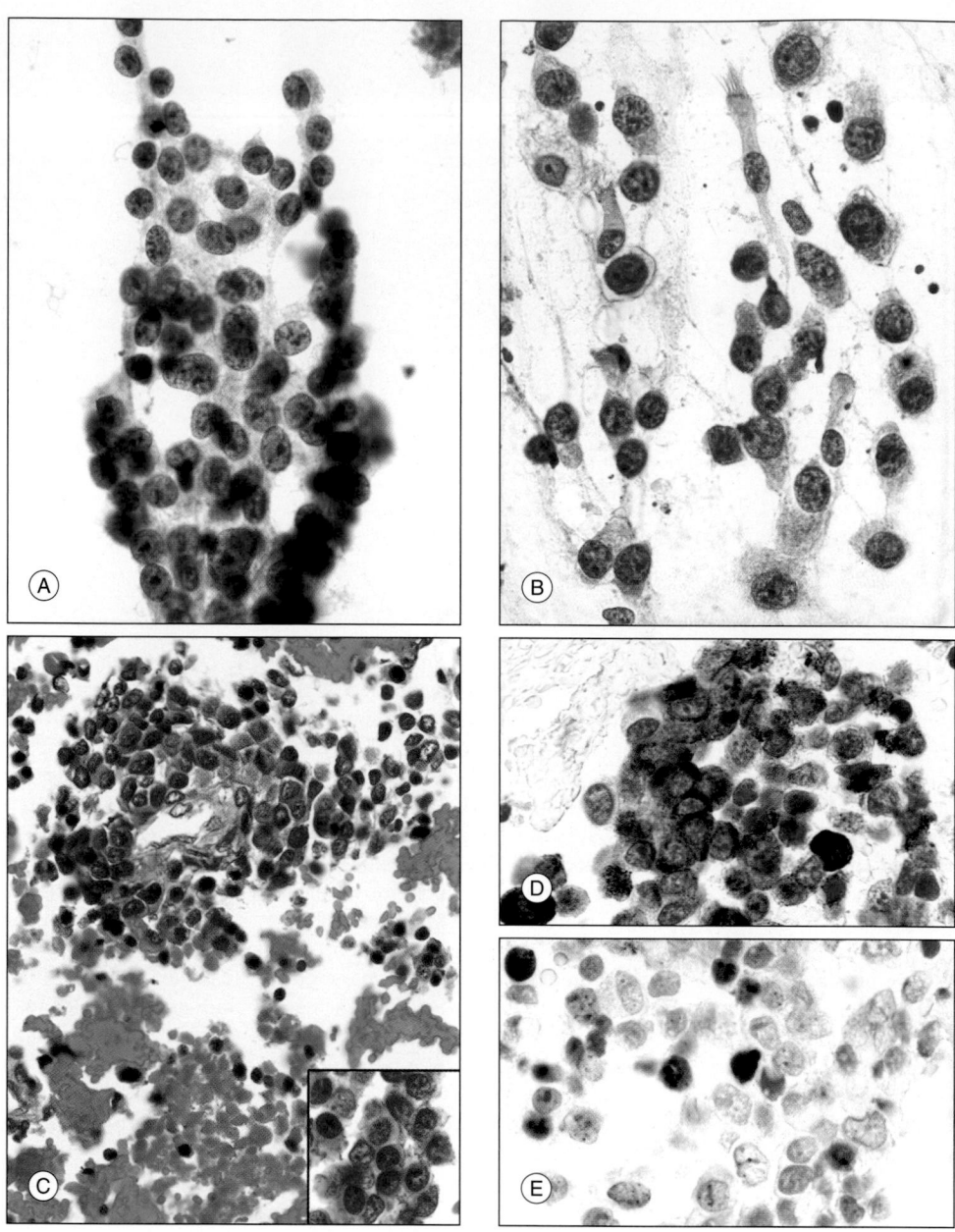

remain.[499] Studies of DNA index and DNA ploidy have shown progressive differences from typical carcinoid, atypical carcinoid, and LCNEC and found excellent correlation with morphology and survival.[500–502]

Cytology of large cell neuroendocrine carcinoma

In cytologic specimens LCNEC appears as single- and three-dimensional clusters of medium-sized epithelial cells in a background of necrosis and/or inflammation. Cell clusters show peripheral palisading.[503] Nuclei are oval or polygonal and N:C ratio is moderate to high. Chromatin varies from finely to coarsely granular and nuclear molding is uncommon. Nucleoli are commonly seen and are occasionally prominent, an important feature in differentiating LCNEC from small cell carcinoma (Fig. 18.96).[503] Immunostaining with Ki-67 is helpful in distinguishing this tumor from atypical carcinoid (Fig. 18.96E).[483]

Small cell carcinoma

Small cell lung carcinoma (SCLC) was first described by Barnard in 1926 in a report of 19 cases.[386] Azzopardi in 1959 further refined the morphologic criteria. He noted the histologic features of ribbons, rosettes, tubules, and spindle cells as well as the peculiar deposition of basophilic material in and around stromal blood vessels that has subsequently been called 'Azzopardi effect' and has been shown to represent foci of DNA deposition from tumor necrosis.[504] The importance of distinguishing small cell carcinoma was shown in the 1973 report of Fox and Scadding that demonstrated the ineffectiveness of surgery in this disease by comparing patients treated by surgery alone with surgery plus radiation therapy.[505] No patients treated with surgery survived while there were a few survivors in the radiation therapy group. This study lead to the recognition that SCLC is not curable by surgery and represents a systemic disease at the outset, requiring systemic chemotherapy.

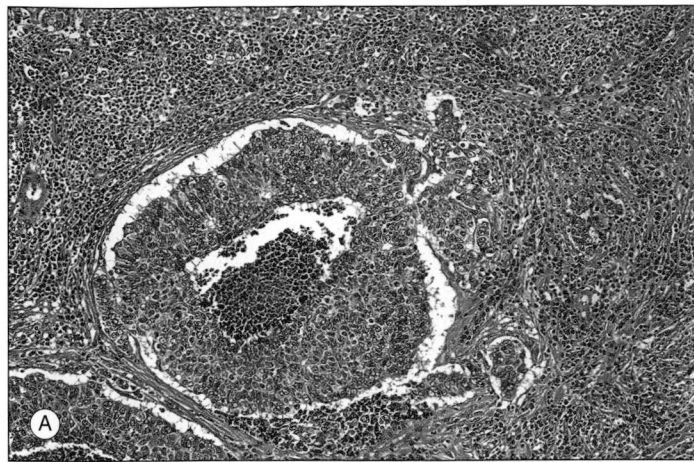

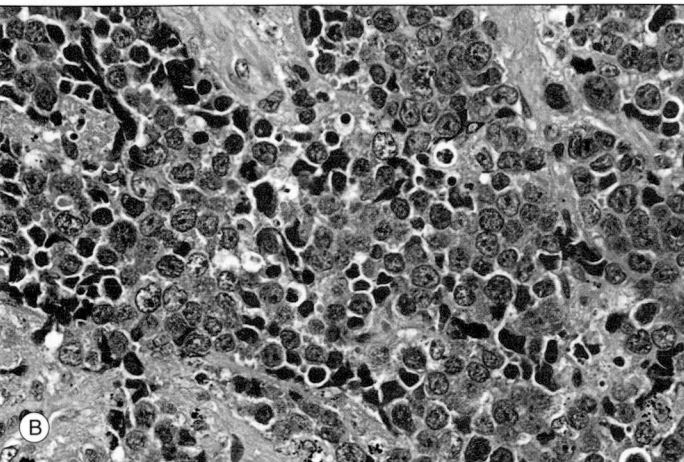

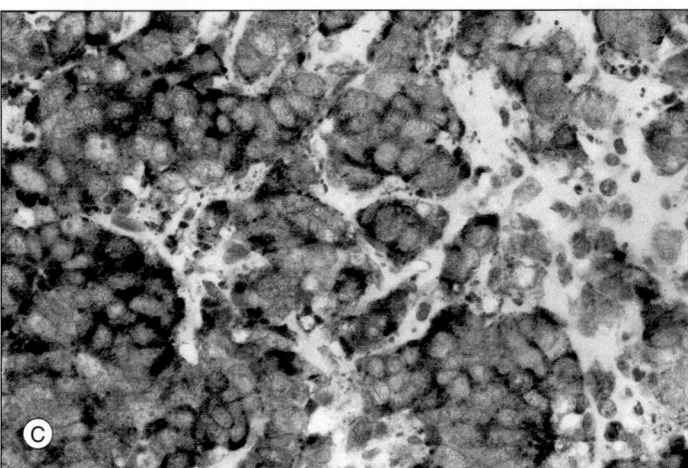

Fig. 18.95 A, Large cell neuroendocrine carcinoma. Tumor architecture is similar to that of atypical carcinoid with solid nests of cells showing central necrosis; **B**, Tumor nuclei reveal easily observed nucleoli and cells are uniformly large; **C**, Chromogranin stain that demonstrates neuroendocrine nature of the tumor.

SCLC accounts for approximately 25% of lung cancers. The median age is approximately sixty years with male predominance. There is a strong association with cigarette smoking; so much so that if a patient is a non-smoker, the diagnosis of small cell carcinoma should be regarded skeptically. The incidence of small cell carcinoma

increases with the amount of cigarettes smoked, and the early onset of cigarette smoking.[263,506–508] Ionizing radiation also has a strong association with SCLC in patients exposed to atomic radiation, radon gas, and in uranium miners.[509,510] Cigarette smoking and radiation exposure appear to be synergistic in tumorigenesis.[510] Exposure to bischloromethyl ether has also been found to be associated with relative increase in the incidence of small cell carcinoma.[511] Most patients are symptomatic due to cough, dyspnea, hemoptysis, or chest pain. Superior vena caval syndrome may be seen due to mediastinal involvement. Most patients have regional or systemic spread at the time of diagnosis with only approximately 5% of cases presenting as a solitary pulmonary nodule or in stage I.[512]

Most SCLC of the lung arise in proximal bronchi and show circumferential narrowing of the bronchus, thickening or roughening of the bronchial mucosa, or extraneous compression. Enlarged mediastinal lymph nodes are common.

Histologically, small cell carcinoma consists of small tumor cells with scant cytoplasm and round, spindled, or elongated nuclei exhibiting finely granular nuclear chromatin and inconspicuous nucleoli (Fig. 18.97). Nuclear molding is a characteristic feature as is a high mitotic rate and focal individual cell necrosis or apoptosis. Mitotic counts are in the 70–80 mitoses per 10 high-power fields range. Very often biopsies show the Azzopardi effect of blue powdery disassociated DNA in scant tumor stroma (Fig. 18.98). Overall, tumors are very cellular and tend to show characteristic crush artifact in small biopsy material. The architecture of the cells demonstrates the neuroendocrine phenotype with discrete nests, ribbons, rosettes and pseudorosettes, and spindled areas that are discernible to varying degrees depending on the type of biopsy sample examined. Tumors diagnosed by lymph node biopsy where the tissue is generally ample may show a variety of separate or combined patterns, while a small bronchoscopic biopsy may not. Nuclear size tends to be smaller and crush artifact more apparent in cases diagnosed by bronchoscopic biopsy or core needle biopsy compared with larger excision specimens where the cells are better preserved and tend to be larger with more cytoplasm and sometimes even contain nucleoli.[513]

Cell and nuclear size alone does not define SCLC as some examples may show focal areas where measurements approach those of non-small cell carcinoma or even large cell carcinoma.[462] However, these larger cells still have the characteristic finely granular nuclear chromatin, absent or inconspicuous nucleoli, high mitotic rate, and individual cell necrosis that is characteristic of and defines SCLC.

The diagnostic criteria of small cell carcinoma have undergone several revisions over the years. The classification of Kreyberg in 1961 considered oat cell carcinoma and a large cell type termed polygonal.[514] The 1967 WHO classification subclassified small cell carcinoma into oat cell carcinoma (lymphocytic-like), fusiform, polygonal, and other. This last category included small cell carcinomas combined with elements of squamous cell carcinoma, giant cells, or tubules.[515] In 1982, the World Health Organization further revised the classification, combining the polygonal, fusiform, and other groups into what was termed intermediate carcinoma, while retaining the lymphocytic-like or oat cell designation for the classic morphology.[516]

Currently, the WHO incorporates all these subtypes under the designation of small cell carcinoma.

It is not surprising that given the shifting criteria for classification of these tumors that problems concerning their definition and distinction from other tumor types may be expected. The report of an expert panel of pathologists classifying the same tumors showed a high level of overall consensus in the diagnosis of small cell carcinoma, but a poor level of agreement in differentiating it from large

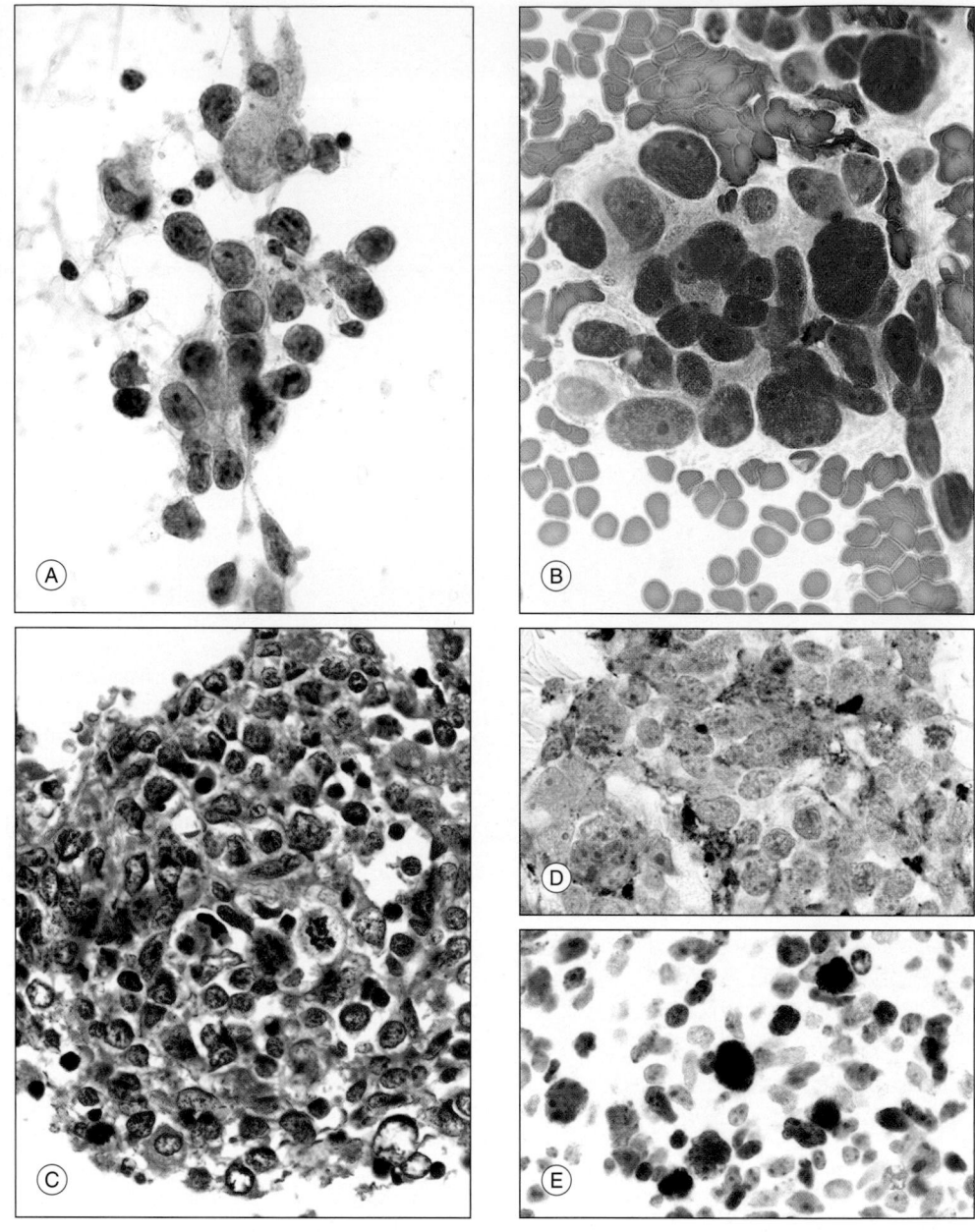

Fig. 18.96 FNA cytology of large cell neuroendocrine carcinoma. **A**, A cluster of cells with ill-defined, granular cytoplasm and high N:C ratio. Chromatin varies from finely to coarsely granular. Nucleoli are evident in many of the cells (Papanicolaou stain); **B**, Nuclear pleomorphism and prominent nucleoli are more pronounced in this air-dried smear (Diff-Quik stain); **C**, Cell-block section showing nuclear pleomorphism, nucleoli, and high mitotic activity (H&E stain); **D**, Positive immunostaining for synaptophysin; **E**, MIB-1 immunostaining shows a very high proliferative activity.

cell neuroendocrine carcinoma.[491] Such observations have lead to the proposal of a three-tiered classification scheme for neuroendocrine carcinoma consisting of grade I (carcinoid), grade II (atypical carcinoid), and grade III (large and small cell neuroendocrine carcinoma) that lumps together the more aggressive tumor types into a single high-grade category.[273,458,462,491,513,517,518] This concept may have clinical practicality since the survival and treatment of high-grade lesions is about the same and there are many similar genetic and other biological changes that are distinct from carcinoids.[499,519–522]

Nevertheless, we believe that adherence to traditional nomenclature has the advantage of being understood by treating physicians.[200]

Some have recognized a separate subtype of mixed small/large cell neuroendocrine carcinoma, which shows features of typical small cell carcinoma mixed with foci of LCNEC.[523] As might be expected, there has been controversy about whether this represents a separate tumor type worth distinguishing from SCLC. Follow-up

studies have shown that there is little difference in survival between the mixed small cell-large cell category and typical small cell carcinoma.[524] Cell culture studies have also shown the kinship of the small and large cells.[525–527] A category of combined small cell carcinoma, tumors with biphasic populations of small cell carcinoma and either adenocarcinoma or squamous cell carcinoma, has been recognized and incorporated into the current WHO classification (Fig. 18.99A,B). Combined tumors tend to be more often peripherally located in the lung than classic small cell carcinoma and, therefore, are more likely to be thoroughly examined after resection compared to proximal SCLC that are most often diagnosed by biopsy. This could partly account for the heterogeneity of these cases.[528]

The morphologic plasticity of this neoplasm has also been demonstrated in autopsy study of biopsy-proven SCLC, where approximately 28% of cases had either an entirely different morphology (squamous carcinoma, adenocarcinoma, or giant cell carcinoma) or

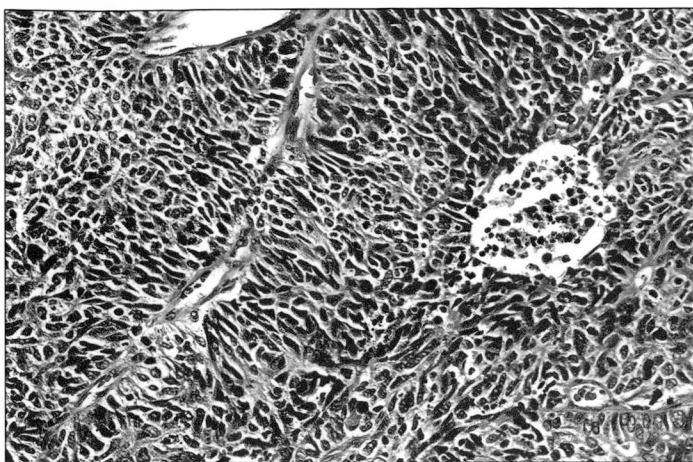

Fig. 18.97 Small cell carcinoma. Tumor cell nests with fusiform nuclei and central necrosis, similar to large cell neuroendocrine carcinoma and atypical carcinoid. Nuclear chromatin is finely granular and evenly dispersed and there are no nucleoli. These nuclear features define the tumor as small cell carcinoma.

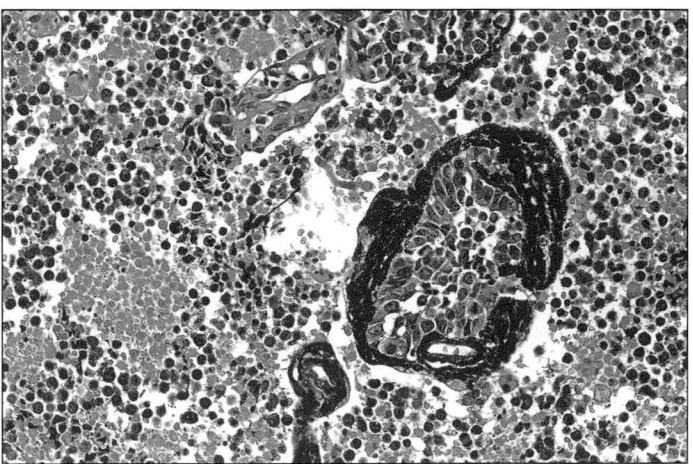

Fig. 18.98 Small cell carcinoma. Loosely cohesive small tumor cells with little cytoplasm and necrosis. Purple-staining DNA material is seen impregnating blood vessels and stroma (Azzopardi effect).

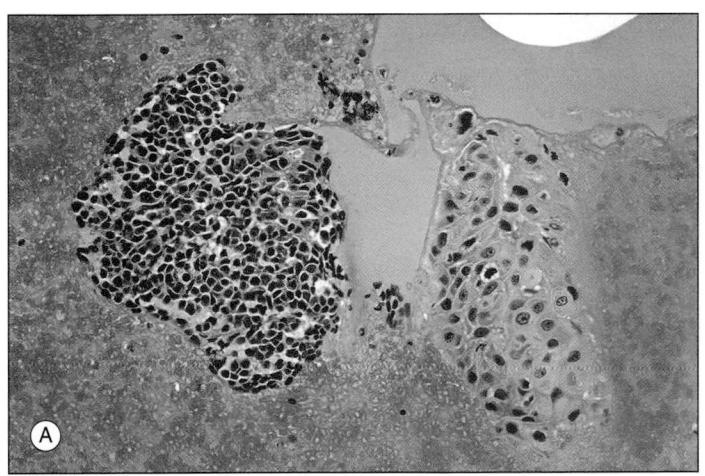

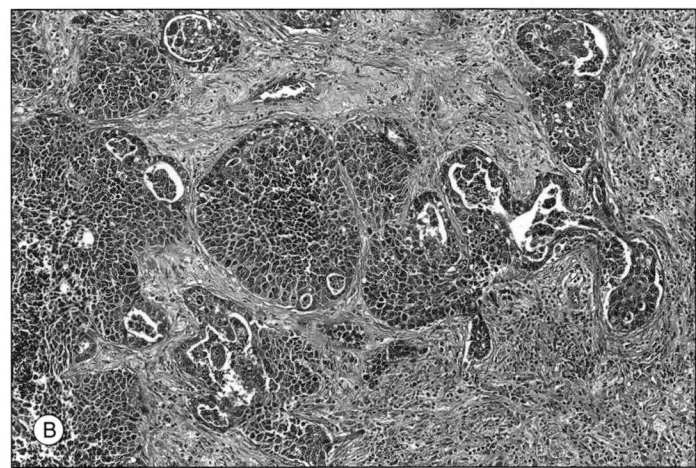

Fig. 18.99 **A**, Combined small cell-squamous cell carcinoma. Needle aspiration biopsy cell block; **B**, Combined small cell-adenocarcinoma. Cuboidal cell glands intimately associated with small cell carcinoma.

one of these elements combined with small cell carcinoma. It was suggested that cellular differentiation in small cell carcinoma may be affected by chemotherapy.[529] Others have noticed a similar shift in morphology after therapy.[530] Recent study of nontreated cases, however, has also found a similar incidence of mixed morphology.[531]

The ultrastructural findings in SCLC have been well characterized. Nuclei have dispersed uniform chromatin with small or absent nucleoli. Dense core granules are present in the cytoplasm but are far fewer than the number seen in carcinoid tumors. They range in size from 100 nanometers to 130 nanometers. In up to 35% of cases, these granules may be absent. Interdigitating cell processes characterize the cells borders which are attached by desmosomes.[532,533]

Most, but not all, examples of SCLC show immuno-histochemistry evidence of neuroendocrine markers.[534] NSE stains the majority of cases but is the least specific neuroendocrine marker since it stains many examples of non-small cell lung cancer.[497]

Chromogranin A, synaptophysin, and Leu7 stain from 5% to 60% of cases.[531] Bombesin is positive in 80% of cases and neurofilaments in 69%.[533] NCAM (CD56) has been shown to stain up to 100% of SCLC.[535] A more recently used antibody, TTF-1, has been shown to stain almost 90% of pulmonary small cell carcinomas, while showing no staining of poorly differentiated squamous cell carcinoma.[536] Combined with p63, which stained no cases of small cell carcinoma but all cases of poorly differentiated squamous cell carcinoma, it has been suggested that the two antibodies are useful in distinguishing between these two tumor types.[536] TTF-1 antibody also appears useful in separating high-grade neuroendocrine tumors from lower-grade lesions as well. In one study, positive TTF-1 staining was detected in over 85% of pure small cell carcinomas, in 49% of large cell neuroendocrine carcinomas, and in 95% of mixed small/large cell neuroendocrine carcinomas, but there was no staining of carcinoids or neuroendocrine hyperplasias.[537] Earlier studies, however, have

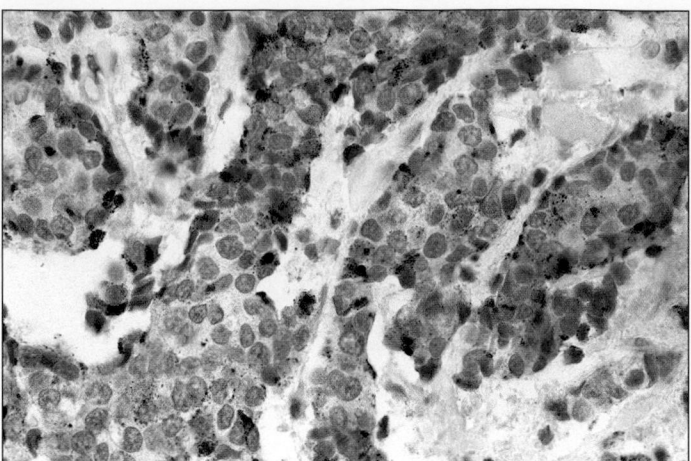

Fig. 18.100 Small cell carcinoma. Dot-like cytoplasm staining with CAM 5.2 (low MW cytokeratin).

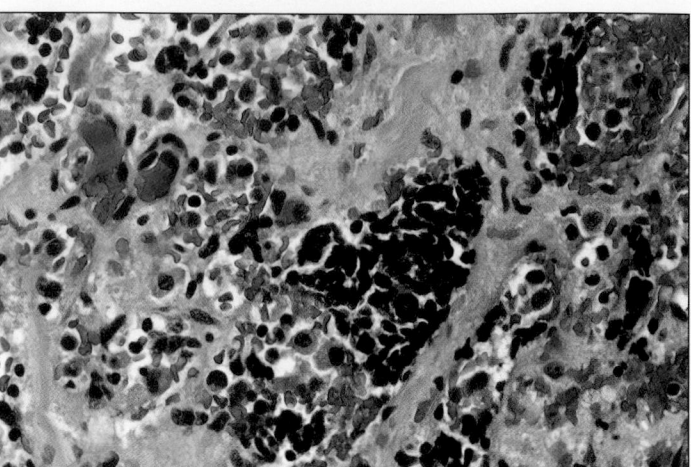

Fig. 18.101 Carcinoid tumor showing focus of crushed, dark cells that can be easily mistaken for small cell carcinoma. We have seen instances of entire bronchoscopic biopsies composed of such cells.

shown that TTF-1 does not discriminate between pulmonary neuroendocrine tumors, and resulted in 35% of typical carcinoids, 100% of atypical carcinoids, and 75–95% of the large cell neuroendocrine and small cell carcinomas staining positively with this antibody.[538] TTF-1 is of little help in distinguishing pulmonary small cell carcinoma from those arising in extrapulmonary sites.[539,540] Class III Beta-Tubulin, an antibody associated with fetal neuronal differentiation, has been found to be a potentially useful marker for small cell carcinoma compared with carcinoid tumor.[541] Practically all small cell carcinomas stain positively with either pan cytokeratin (AE1/AE3), low molecular weight cytokeratin (CAM 5.2), or EMA, often with a 'dot like' staining pattern (Fig. 18.100).[534] CEA is rarely positive.[542]

As mentioned earlier, the prognosis of SCLC is extremely poor and the treatment is both local and systemic at the time of initial diagnosis. A recent study of limited-stage SCLC patients entered into a Southwest Oncology Group protocol treated with concomitant chemotherapy and radiation therapy showed a 40% one-year progression-free survival and a two-year progression-free survival of 21%. The overall response rate to the treatment was 86% with a third of cases showing a complete response.[543] Patients with extensive disease rarely survive two years.[544] Rare isolated cases of SCLC presenting as peripheral lung nodules may benefit from surgical resection, with pathological stage I patients having an actuarial survival rate of approximately 25% at three years.[545–547]

The molecular and genetic relationship between the neuroendocrine tumors and those without neuroendocrine differentiation has been the subject of recent intense study. The frequencies of molecular alterations of many genes vary between SCLC and non-small cell lung cancer (NSCLC), as well as within the neuroendocrine group.[548] Studies have shown that the carcinoids (classic and atypical) can be segregated from high-grade neuroendocrine carcinomas (SCLC and LCNEC). Inactivation of *MEN1* gene, located on chromosome 11q13, is commonly seen in carcinoids, particularly in atypical type. However, this genetic alteration is uncommon in SCLC and LCNEC, supporting the hypothesis that SCLC and carcinoids develop via distinct molecular pathways. SCLC and LCNEC have significantly more genetic alterations, and are characterized by a different pattern of DNA losses and gains.[520,521,549] Ullmann et al.,

using a statistical meta-analysis of published chromosomal studies, have also shown that carcinoids are segregated from other lung carcinomas, including SCLC and LCNEC.[550] *p53* mutations and aberrant p53 IHC positivity are seen in practically all SCLC and LCNEC. In contrast, *p53* mutations have not been detected in classic or atypical carcinoids. RB or p16 expression is absent in high-grade neuroendocrine tumors, but is present in classic and atypical carcinoids.[551–553] Gene profiling study also shows that SCLC differs from carcinoids and is related more to cultured bronchial epithelial cells, whereas the carcinoids are more related to neural crest-derived brain tumors suggesting different progenitor cells for these tumors.[554]

Among the carcinoid tumors, atypical carcinoid has more genetic alterations. Several studies have shown that the changes in chromosome 11q are more frequent and extensive in atypical carcinoid than in classic carcinoid. Atypical carcinoid cases also show a higher frequency and more extensive genetic losses in regions of chromosome 3p.[549,555]

The high-grade neuroendocrine tumors, while apparently related, may nevertheless show some genetic differences. Comparative genomic hybridization (CGH) and LOH analyses have in general shown similar complex abnormal chromosomal patterns in LCNEC and SCLC.[520,549] Investigations of several oncogenes, including *p53*, *RB*, and *p16*, have also indicated similar genetic abnormalities.[552] However, one study using CGH showed divergent chromosomal aberration between the two tumor types among many other shared chromosomal changes. The most significant differences were gains at chromosomal arm 3q and loss of 10q and 17p, which were more frequent in SCLC.[556] SCLC also showed more frequent (86%) LOH at chromosomal 5p21 region than LCNEC (46%).[549]

The diagnosis of SCLC may not be straightforward in small biopsies where cells may be distorted or necrotic. We have seen examples of tumors mistakenly diagnosed as SCLC in bronchoscopic biopsies, but the resected specimen showed typical carcinoids or even lymphoid lesions (Fig. 18.101). It cannot be emphasized enough that clinical history, which indicates tumor location, history of cigarette smoking, extent of disease and, importantly, coincident site correlation with any cytology material by the pathologist, may help in solving some otherwise difficult cases. Some differential diagnostic points are illustrated in Table 18.11.

Fig. 18.102 FNA cytology of small cell carcinoma. **A**, Clusters of cohesive small cells with very scant cytoplasm and nuclear molding. Chromatin is evenly dispersed. Mitoses and apoptotic nuclei are evident (Papanicolaou stain); **B**, Pronounced nuclear molding, evenly dispersed chromatin, and lack of prominent nucleoli are well demonstrated in this air-dried smear (Diff-Quik stain); **C**, Cell-block section showing nests of small cells with nuclear molding, and lack of prominent nucleoli (H&E stain); **D**, Positive immunostaining for CD56; **E**, MIB-1 immunostaining shows a very high proliferative activity.

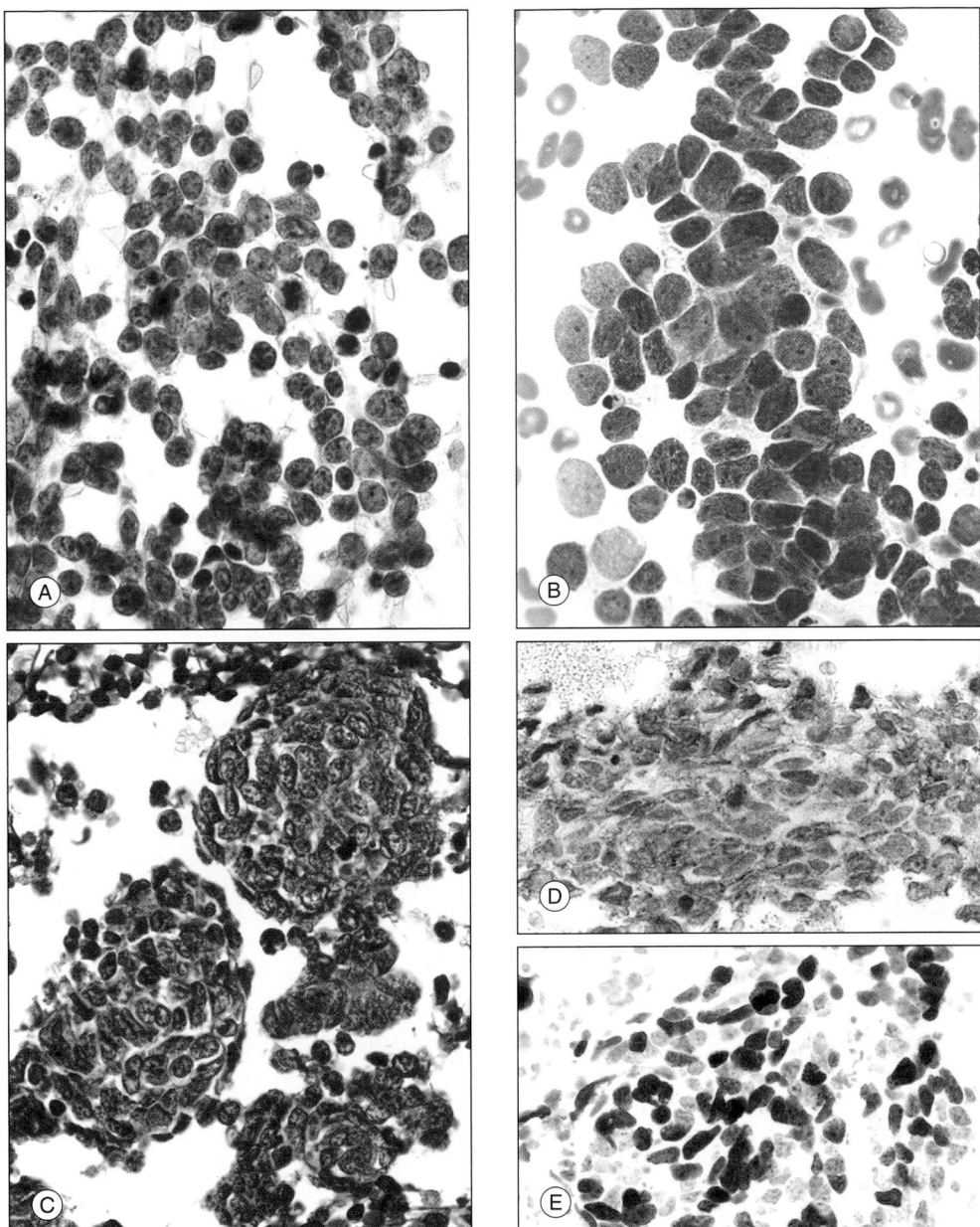

Cytology of small cell lung carcinoma

The cytologic diagnosis of SCLC is highly accurate and reliable in most instances. Tumors readily shed cells into the sputum and are easily accessible by the bronchoscope as most involve large bronchi. For this reason sputum and bronchoscopic specimens are very sensitive for the diagnosis of SCLC.[40,222,283] The less common peripheral tumors are best diagnosed by FNA, which also is very accurate. Among all lung cancers SCLC has the highest degree of agreement between cytologic and histologic diagnoses, over 95% in a series reported by Johnston et al.[283] Cytologic samples often are complementary, and in some cases superior to small biopsies, as crush artifact commonly seen in histologic samples are uncommon in cytologic preparations.

In sputum, SCLC appears as single and small groups of tumor cells that are slightly larger than lymphocytes and vary in size.[137] The cells have little or no visible cytoplasm. Nuclei are hyperchromatic and frequently mold against each other. Some of the nuclei are pyknotic and have a smudged appearance as the result of degeneration. Nucleoli are uncommon. Necrotic debris is commonly seen in the background. In bronchoscopic and FNA samples, tumor cells are better preserved and appear larger, approximately 2–4 times the size of lymphocytes (Fig. 18.102). Larger cell clusters are seen in addition to single and small groups of tumor cells. Nuclear features are largely the same as in the sputum specimens, but sometimes in areas where tumor cells are more spread out, the chromatin appears more open and small nucleoli may be seen.

Differential diagnosis: Reserve cell (basal cell) hyperplasia, a reactive process commonly associated with cigarette smoking and chronic inflammatory conditions, may mimic SCLC in bronchial washings and brushings. Hyperplastic basal cells are covered by bronchial columnar cells and do not exfoliate spontaneously. Therefore, such cells do not create a problem in sputum cytology except in postbronchoscopic samples. They appear as cohesive clusters of small cells with high N:C ratio. Unlike SCLC, reserve cells are seen only in

Table 18.11 Microscopic features of neuroendocrine neoplasms

	Cell size	Nucleoli	Necrosis	Mitoses (per 10 HPF)	Positive neuroendocrine stains
Carcinoid	Intermediate	Uncommon	No	0– less than 2	Yes
Atypical carcinoid	Intermediate	Yes	Yes	2–10	Yes
Large cell neuroendocrine carcinoma	Large	Yes	Yes	11 or more	Yes
Small cell carcinoma	Small to intermediate*	No	Yes	Many	15% of cases may be negative [531]

* Some large cells may be present, but usually lack nucleoli.

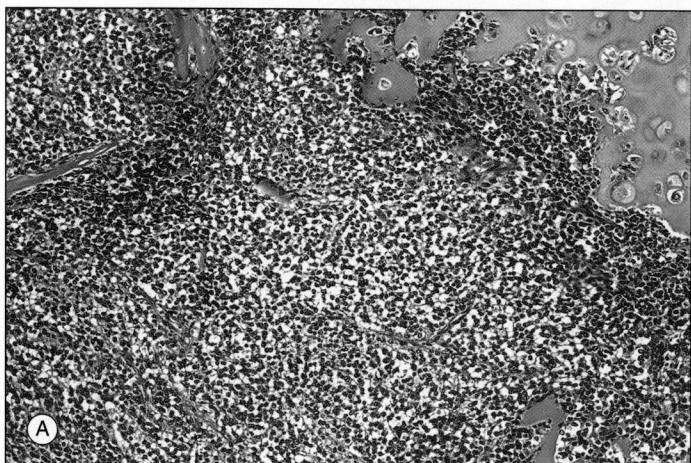
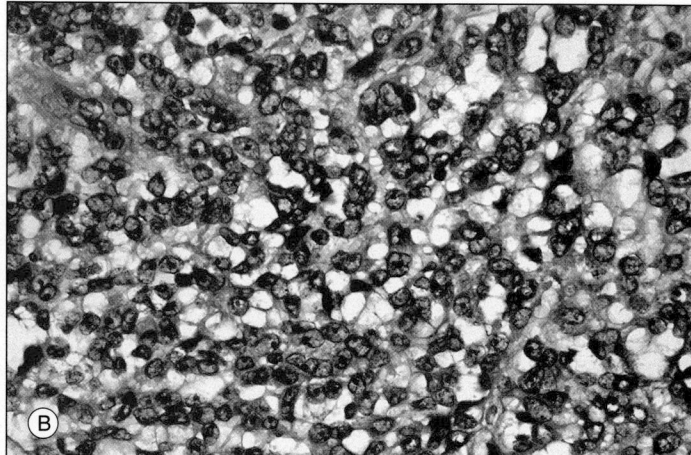

Fig. 18.103 A, Askin's tumor. Uniform small tumor cells infiltrate bronchial cartilage; **B**, Tumor cells show scant cytoplasmic processes, a vague pseudorosette pattern, and open nuclei with easily observed nucleoli.

very compact clusters with uniform nuclei. Loss of cohesiveness, abnormalities of chromatin texture and distribution, irregularity of nuclear membrane, necrosis, and mitotic activity that are important features of SCLC are not seen in reserve cell hyperplasia. This distinction may be very difficult in poorly prepared specimens, however. Reserve cell hyperplasia does not present a problem in FNA specimens, because only rare clusters of cells may be seen in this type specimen.

Unlike small biopsies, the distinction between SCLC and lymphocytic lesions is relatively easy in well-fixed cytologic specimens. Lymphocytes are noncohesive, round cells that do not show abnormal chromatin pattern, necrosis, or nuclear molding, unlike SCLS.

SCLC also should be distinguished from other neuroendocrine and non-neuroendocrine neoplasms. Carcinoid tumor has characteristic morphologic features that allow accurate classification in cytologic specimens, but sometimes, particularly in scanty cellular specimens, crushed and smudged tumor cells can mimic SCLC.[483] Atypical carcinoids may resemble the so-called 'intermediate variant' of SCLC.[481,483,495] As discussed previously, immunocytochemical staining for proliferation marker Ki-67 can be helpful in distinguishing low-grade neuroendocrine neoplasms (carcinoid and atypical carcinoid) from SCLC.[483] Immunocytochemical stains for neuroendocrine differentiation are very helpful in distinguishing SCLC from non-neuroendocrine neoplasms (Fig. 18.102D). The most common reason for diagnostic difficulties is the technical quality of the sample, such as scant cellularity, suboptimal fixation, and poor staining. Diagnostic mistakes can be minimized by

employing good laboratory techniques, using multiple preparation techniques (i.e. direct smears, concentration methods, cell block), and combination of multiple sampling methods (i.e. washing, brushing, biopsy). When samples are too scant for reliable classification of the tumor, the pathologist should not hesitate to request more material.

Askin tumor

In 1979, Askin and colleagues reported a series of malignant small cell tumors of the thoracopulmonary region in children.[557] They described 20 cases, all of which were within the thorax and involved the chest wall and pleura. Only one case showed involvement limited to the lung. These highly malignant tumors are primitive small cell malignancies that histologically resemble neuroblastomas and Ewing's tumors (Fig. 18.103). Electron microscopy shows neurosecretory-type granules and microtubules.

Further reports revealed similar lesions in young patients, confined to the ribs and soft tissues of the thorax that conform to the Askin report. Rare lung tumors have been reported in adults.[557–563] Evidence that Askin tumor is identical to Ewing's sarcoma-PNET was the finding of the characteristic t(11;22) (q24;q12) translocation characteristic of Askin tumor, and also shared with Ewing's-PNET lesions. Reverse transcriptase-polymerase chain reaction (RT-PCR) demonstrates Ewing's-PNET fusion transcripts, EWS/FLI-1.[562,563] Immunohistochemistry shows positivity with NSE and MIC-2 gene product (O13) and is usually negative for chromogranin and synaptophysin.[561,562]

REFERENCES

1. Society AC. Cancer facts and figures 2002. Atlanta, GA: American Cancer Society; 2002.

2. Jemel A, Thomas A, Murray T, et al. Cancer Statistics, 2002. CA Cancer J Clin 2002; 512: 22.

3. Alberg AJ, Samet JM. Epidemiology of lung cancer. Chest 2003; 123(1 Suppl): 21S.

4. Burns DM. Tobacco Smoking. In: Samet JM, ed. Epidemiology of lung cancer. New York: Marcel Dekker; 1994: 15.

5. Services DDoHaH. The health consequences of smoking: Cancer. A report of the Surgeon General. Report No.: DHHS Publication number 82-50179 ed.

6. Doll R, Peto R. Cigarette smoking and bronchial carcinoma: dose and time relationships among regular smokers and lifelong non-smokers. J Epidemiol Community Health 1978; 32: 303.

7. Josen K, Siegal R, Kamp D. Incidence and etiology. In: Weitberg AB, ed. Cancer of the lung: from molecular biology to treatment guidelines. New Jersey: Humana Press; 2002: 3.

8. Bach PB, Ginsberg RB. Epidemiology of lung cancer. In: Ginsberg RB, ed. Lung cancer, American Cancer Society atlas of clinical oncology. London: BC Decker; 2002: 1.

9. Hughes JM, Weill H. Asbestos and man-made fibers. In: Samet JM, ed. Epidemiology of lung cancer. New York: Marcel Dekker; 1984.

10. Churg A. Chapter 10. Neoplastic asbestos induced disease. In: Green FHY, ed. Pathology of occupational lung disease. 2nd edn. Baltimore: Williams & Wilkins; 1998: 339.

11. Indoor air pollution. If you think your home is a bastion of clean air in a polluted world – think again. Consumer Reports 1985; 50: 600–603.

12. Shields PG. Molecular epidemiology of smoking and lung cancer. Oncogene 2002; 21(45): 6870.

13. Feinstein MB, Stover D. Clinical features of lung cancer. In: Ginsberg RB, ed. Lung cancer, American cancer society atlas of clinical oncology. London: BC Decker; 2002: 43.

14. Akhurst T, Heelan RT. Imaging work-up of lung cancer: Utility and comparison of computed tomography and FDG positron emission tomography. In: Ginsberg RB, ed. Lung cancer, American cancer society atlas of clinical oncology. London: BC Decker; 2002: 71.

15. Munden RF, Erasmus JJ. Thoracic imaging techniques for non-small cell and small cell lung cancer. In: Putnam JJB, ed. Lung cancer, M. D. Anderson Cancer Care Series. New York: Springer; 2002: 35.

16. Henschke CI, McCauley DI, Yankelevitz DF, et al. Early Lung Cancer Action Project: overall design and findings from baseline screening. Lancet 1999; 354(9173): 99.

17. Bepler G, Goodridge Carney D, Djulbegovic B, et al. A systematic review and lessons learned from early lung cancer detection trials using low-dose computed tomography of the chest. Cancer Control 2003; 10(4): 306.

18. Renan MJ. How many mutations are required for tumorigenesis? Implications from human cancer data. Mol Carcinog 1993; 7: 139.

19. Hanahan D, Weinberg RA. The hallmarks of cancer. Cell 2000; 100: 57.

20. Hittelman WN, Kurie JM, Swisher SG. Molecular events in lung cancer and implications for prevention and therapy. In: Putnam JJB, ed. Lung cancer, M. D. Anderson Cancer Care Series. New York: Springer-Verlag; 2003.

21. Mao L. Molecular abnormalities in lung carcinogenesis and their potential clinical implications. Lung Cancer 2001; 34: S27.

22. Forgacs E, Zochbauer-Muller S, Olah E, et al. Molecular genetic abnormalities in the pathogenesis of human lung cancer. Pathol Oncol Res 2001; 7(1): 6.

23. Kaye FJ. Molecular biology of lung cancer. Lung Cancer 2001; 34 Suppl 2: S35.

24. Rom WN, Tchou-Wong KM. Molecular and genetic aspects of lung cancer. Methods Mol Med 2003; 75: 3.

25. Brennan J, O'Connor T, Makuch RW, et al. *myc* family DNA amplification in 107 tumors and tumor cell lines from patients with small cell lung cancer treated with different combination chemotherapy regimens. Cancer Res 1991; 51(6): 1708.

26. Gandara DR, Lara Jr PN, Lau DH, et al. Molecular-clinical correlative studies in non-small cell lung cancer: application of a three-tiered approach. Lung Cancer 2001; 34: S75.

27. AJCC. Thorax. In: Greene F, et al., eds. Cancer staging manual. 6th edn. New York: Springer-Verlag; 2002: 167.

28. Mountain C. Histologic and anatomic classification of lung cancer and regional lymph nodes. In: Calten D, Patchefsky AS, eds. Tumors and tumor-like lesions of the lung. Philadelphia: WB Saunders; 1998: 5.

29. Gledhill A, Bates C, Henderson D, et al. Sputum cytology: a limited role. J Clin Pathol 1997; 50(7): 566.

30. Sing A, Freudenberg N, Kortsik C, et al. Comparison of the sensitivity of sputum and brush cytology in the diagnosis of lung carcinomas. Acta Cytol 1997; 41(2): 399.

31. Steffee CH, Segletes LA, Geisinger KR. Changing cytologic and histologic utilization patterns in the diagnosis of 515 primary lung malignancies. Cancer 1997; 81(2): 105.

32. Raab SS, Hornberger J, Raffin T. The importance of sputum cytology in the diagnosis of lung cancer: a cost-effectiveness analysis. Chest 1997; 112(4): 937.

33. Goldberg-Kahn B, Healy JC, Bishop JW. The cost of diagnosis: a comparison of four different strategies in the workup of solitary radiographic lung lesions. Chest 1997; 111(4): 870.

34. Bechtel JJ, Kelley WR, Petty TL, et al. Outcome of 51 patients with roentgenographically occult lung cancer detected by sputum cytologic testing: a community hospital program. Arch Intern Med 1994; 154(9): 975.

35. Bocking A, Biesterfeld S, Chatelain R, et al. Diagnosis of bronchial carcinoma on sections of paraffin-embedded sputum. Sensitivity and specificity of an alternative to routine cytology. Acta Cytol 1992; 36(1): 37.

36. Erozan YS, Frost JK. Cytopathologic diagnosis of cancer in pulmonary material: a critical histopathologic correlation. Acta Cytol 1970; 14(9): 560.

37. Gagneten CB, Geller CE, Del Carmen Saenz M. Diagnosis of bronchogenic carcinoma through the cytologic examination of sputum, with special reference to tumor typing. Acta Cytol 1976; 20(6): 530.

38. Koss LG, Melamed MR, Goodner JT. Pulmonary cytology – A brief survey of diagnostic results from July 1st, 1952 until December 31st, 1960. Acta Cytol 1964; 8(2): 104.

39. Liang XM. Accuracy of cytologic diagnosis and cytotyping of sputum in primary lung cancer: analysis of 161 cases. J Surg Oncol 1989; 40(2): 107.

40. Ng AB, Horak GC. Factors significant in the diagnostic accuracy of lung cytology in bronchial washing and sputum samples. II. Sputum samples. Acta Cytol 1983; 27(4): 397.

41. Pilotti S, Rilke F, Gribaudi G, et al. Sputum cytology for the diagnosis of carcinoma of the lung. Acta Cytol 1982; 26(5): 649.

42. Rosa UW, Prolla JC, Gastal Eda S. Cytology in diagnosis of cancer affecting the lung. Results in 1,000 consecutive patients. Chest 1973; 63(2): 203.

43. Truong LD, Underwood RD, Greenberg SD, et al. Diagnosis and typing of lung carcinomas by cytopathologic methods. A review of 108 cases. Acta Cytol 1985; 29(3): 379.

44. Delarue NC, Anderson W, Sanders D, et al. Bronchiolo-alveolar carcinoma. A reappraisal after 24 years. Cancer 1972; 29(1): 90.

45. Roger V, Nasiell M, Linden M, et al. Cytologic differential diagnosis of bronchiolo-alveolar carcinoma and bronchogenic adenocarcinoma. Acta Cytol 1976; 20(4): 303.

46. Kern WH, Schweizer CW. Sputum cytology of metastatic carcinoma of the lung. Acta Cytol 1976; 20(6): 514.

47. Bedrossian CW, Rybka DL. Bronchial brushing during fiberoptic bronchoscopy for the cytodiagnosis of lung cancer: comparison with sputum and bronchial washings. Acta Cytol 1976; 20(5): 446.

48. Steinmann G, Greul W. Effect of methods of sample taking on the cytologic diagnosis of lung tumors. Acta Cytol 1978; 22(5): 425.

49. Oswald NC, Hinson KF, Canti G, et al. The diagnosis of primary lung cancer with special reference to sputum cytology. Thorax 1971; 26(6): 623.

50. Hayata Y, Oo K, Ichiba M, et al. Percutaneous pulmonary puncture for cytologic diagnosis – its diagnostic value for small peripheral pulmonary carcinoma. Acta Cytol 1973; 17(6): 469.

51. Arroliga AC, Matthay RA. The role of bronchoscopy in lung cancer. Clin Chest Med 1993; 14(1): 87.

52. Naryshkin S, Daniels J, Young NA. Diagnostic correlation of fiberoptic bronchoscopic biopsy and bronchoscopic cytology performed simultaneously. Diagn Cytopathol 1992; 8(2): 119.

53. Savage C, Morrison RJ, Zwischenberger JB. Bronchoscopic diagnosis and staging of lung cancer. Chest Surg Clin N Am 2001; 11(4): 701.

54. Govert JA, Kopita JM, Matchar D, et al. Cost effectiveness of collecting routine cytologic specimens during fiberoptic bronchoscopy for endoscopically visible lung tumor. Chest 1996; 109(2): 451.

55. Kvale PA, Bode FR, Kini S. Diagnostic accuracy in lung cancer; comparison of techniques used in association with flexible fiberoptic bronchoscopy. Chest 1976; 69(6): 752.

56. Shure D. Fiberoptic bronchoscopy – diagnostic applications. Clin Chest Med 1987; 8(1): 1.

57. Levy H, Horak DA, Lewis MI. The value of bronchial washings and bronchoalveolar lavage in the diagnosis of lymphangitic carcinomatosis. Chest 1988; 94(5): 1028.

58. Linder J, Radio SJ, Robbins RA, et al. Bronchoalveolar lavage in the cytologic diagnosis of carcinoma of the lung. Acta Cytol 1987; 31(6): 796.

59. Pirozynski M. Bronchoalveolar lavage in the diagnosis of peripheral, primary lung cancer. Chest 1992; 102(2): 372.

60. Baaklini WA, Reinoso MA, Gorin AB, et al. Diagnostic yield of fiberoptic bronchoscopy in evaluating solitary pulmonary nodules. Chest 2000; 117(4): 1049.

61. Chechani V. Bronchoscopic diagnosis of solitary pulmonary nodules and lung masses in the absence of endobronchial abnormality. Chest 1996; 109(3): 620.

62. Chin R Jr, Cappellari JO, McCain TW, et al. Increasing use of bronchoscopic needle aspiration to diagnose small cell lung cancer. Mayo Clinic Proceedings 2000; 75(8): 796.

63. de Gracia J, Bravo C, Miravitlles M, et al. Diagnostic value of bronchoalveolar lavage in peripheral lung cancer. American Review of Respiratory Disease 1993; 147(3): 649.

64. Jones AM, Hanson IM, Armstrong GR, et al. Value and accuracy of cytology in addition to histology in the diagnosis of lung cancer at flexible bronchoscopy. Respiratory Medicine 2001; 95(5): 374.

65. Pilotti S, Rilke F, Gribaudi G, et al. Cytologic diagnosis of pulmonary carcinoma on bronchoscopic brushing material. Acta Cytol 1982; 26(5): 655.

66. Karahalli E, Yilmaz A, Turker H, et al. Usefulness of various diagnostic techniques during fiberoptic bronchoscopy for endoscopically visible lung cancer:

should cytologic examinations be performed routinely? Respiration 2001; 68(6): 611.

67. Bhat N, Bhagat P, Pearlman ES, et al. Transbronchial needle aspiration biopsy in the diagnosis of pulmonary neoplasms. Diagn Cytopathol 1990; 6(1): 14.

68. Salathe M, Soler M, Bolliger CT, et al. Transbronchial needle aspiration in routine fiberoptic bronchoscopy. Respiration 1992; 59(1): 5.

69. Schenk DA, Bryan CL, Bower JH, et al. Transbronchial needle aspiration in the diagnosis of bronchogenic carcinoma. Chest 1987; 92(1): 83.

70. Govert JA, Dodd LG, Kussin PS, et al. A prospective comparison of fiberoptic transbronchial needle aspiration and bronchial biopsy for bronchoscopically visible lung carcinoma. Cancer 1999; 87(3): 129.

71. Katis K, Inglesos E, Zachariadis E, et al. The role of transbronchial needle aspiration in the diagnosis of peripheral lung masses or nodules. Eur Respir J 1995; 8(6): 963.

72. Dasgupta A, Jain P, Minai OA, et al. Utility of transbronchial needle aspiration in the diagnosis of endobronchial lesions. Chest 1999; 115(5): 1237.

73. Reichenberger F, Weber J, Tamm M, et al. The value of transbronchial needle aspiration in the diagnosis of peripheral pulmonary lesions. Chest 1999; 116(3): 704.

74. Caya JG, Wollenberg NJ, Clowry LJ, et al. The diagnosis of pulmonary small-cell anaplastic carcinoma by cytologic means: a 13-year experience. Diagn Cytopathol 1988; 4(3): 202.

75. Popp W, Rauscher H, Ritschka L, et al. Diagnostic sensitivity of different techniques in the diagnosis of lung tumors with the flexible fiberoptic bronchoscope. Comparison of brush biopsy, imprint cytology of forceps biopsy, and histology of forceps biopsy. Cancer 1991; 67(1): 72.

76. Johnston WW, Bossen EH. Ten years of respiratory cytopathology at Duke University Medical Center. I. The cytopathologic diagnosis of lung cancer during the years 1970 to 1974, noting the significance of specimen number and type. Acta Cytol 1981; 25(2): 103.

77. Jones DF, Chin R Jr, Cappellari JO, et al. Endobronchial needle aspiration in the diagnosis of small-cell carcinoma. Chest 1994; 105(4): 1151.

78. Lam B, Wong MP, Ooi C, et al. Diagnostic yield of bronchoscopic sampling methods in bronchial carcinoma. Respirology 2000; 5(3): 265.

79. Shure D, Fedullo PF. Transbronchial needle aspiration in the diagnosis of submucosal and peribronchial bronchogenic carcinoma. Chest 1985; 88(1): 49.

80. Wang KP. Transbronchial needle aspiration and percutaneous needle aspiration for staging and diagnosis of lung cancer. Clin Chest Med 1995; 16(3): 535.

81. Bilaceroglu S, Cagiotariotaciota U, Gunel O, et al. Comparison of rigid and flexible transbronchial needle aspiration in the staging of bronchogenic carcinoma. Respiration 1998; 65(6): 441.

82. Schenk DA, Bower JH, Bryan CL, et al. Transbronchial needle aspiration staging of bronchogenic carcinoma. Am Rev Respir Dis 1986; 134(1): 146.

83. Wang KP, Brower R, Haponik EF, et al. Flexible transbronchial needle aspiration for staging of bronchogenic carcinoma. Chest 1983; 84(5): 571.

84. Castella J, Buj J, Puzo C, et al. Diagnosis and staging of bronchogenic carcinoma by transtracheal and transbronchial needle aspiration. Ann Oncol 1995; 6(Suppl 3): S21.

85. Blumenfeld W, Singer M, Glanz S, et al. Fine-needle aspiration as the initial diagnostic modality in malignant lung disease. Diagn Cytopathol 1996; 14(3): 268.

86. Denley H, Singh N, Clelland CA. Transthoracic fine needle aspiration cytology of lung for suspected malignancy: an audit of cytological findings with histopathological correlation. Cytopathology 1997; 8(4): 223.

87. Hayes MM, Zhang DY, Brown W. Transthoracic fine-needle aspiration biopsy cytology of pulmonary neoplasms. Diagn Cytopathol 1994; 10(4): 315.

88. Hsu WH, Chiang CD, Hsu JY, et al. Ultrasound-guided fine-needle aspiration biopsy of lung cancers. J Clin Ultrasound 1996; 24(5): 225.

89. Johnston WW. Percutaneous fine needle aspiration biopsy of the lung. A study of 1,015 patients. Acta Cytol 1984; 28(3): 218.

90. Mitchell ML, King DE, Bonfiglio TA, et al. Pulmonary fine needle aspiration cytopathology. A five-year correlation study. Acta Cytologica 1984; 28(1): 72.

91. Pilotti S, Rilke F, Gribaudi G, et al. Transthoracic fine needle aspiration biopsy in pulmonary lesions. Updated results. Acta Cytol 1984; 28(3): 225.

92. Simpson RW, Johnson DA, Wold LE, et al. Transthoracic needle aspiration biopsy. Review of 233 cases. Acta Cytol 1988; 32(1): 101.

93. Stanley JH, Fish GD, Andriole JG, et al. Lung lesions: cytologic diagnosis by fine-needle biopsy. Radiology 1987; 162(2): 389.

94. Swischuk JL, Castaneda F, Patel JC, et al. Percutaneous transthoracic needle biopsy of the lung: review of 612 lesions. J Vascul Intervent Radiol 1998; 9(2): 347.

95. Tao LC, Pearson FG, Delarue NC, et al. Percutaneous fine-needle aspiration biopsy. I. Its value to clinical practice. Cancer 1980; 45(6): 1480.

96. Westcott JL. Direct percutaneous needle aspiration of localized pulmonary lesions: result in 422 patients. Radiology 1980; 137(1 Pt 1): 31.

97. Zarbo RJ, Fenoglio-Preiser CM. Interinstitutional database for comparison of performance in lung fine-needle aspiration cytology. A College of American Pathologists Q-Probe Study of 5264 cases with histologic correlation. Arch Pathol Lab Med 1992; 116(5): 463.

98. Afify A, Davila RM. Pulmonary fine needle aspiration biopsy. Assessing the negative diagnosis. Acta Cytol 1999; 43(4): 601.

99. Delgado PI, Jorda M, Ganjei-Azar P. Small cell carcinoma versus other lung malignancies: diagnosis by fine-needle aspiration cytology. Cancer 2000; 90(5): 279.

100. Zakowski MF, Gatscha RM, Zaman MB. Negative predictive value of pulmonary fine needle aspiration cytology. Acta Cytologica 1992; 36(3): 283.

101. Layfield LJ, Coogan A, Johnston WW, et al. Transthoracic fine needle aspiration biopsy. Sensitivity in relation to guidance technique and lesion size and location. Acta Cytologica 1996; 40(4): 687.

102. Austin JH, Cohen MB. Value of having a cytopathologist present during percutaneous fine-needle aspiration biopsy of lung: report of 55 cancer patients and metaanalysis of the literature. AJR Am J Roentgenol 1993; 160(1): 175.

103. Santambrogio L, Nosotti M, Bellaviti N, et al. CT-guided fine-needle aspiration cytology of solitary pulmonary nodules: a prospective, randomized study of immediate cytologic evaluation. Chest 1997; 112(2): 423.

104. Auger M, Katz RL, Johnston DA. Differentiating cytological features of bronchioloalveolar carcinoma from adenocarcinoma of the lung in fine-needle aspirations: a statistical analysis of 27 cases. Diagn Cytopathol 1997; 16(3): 253.

105. Padhani AR, Scott WW, Cheema M, et al. The value of immediate cytologic evaluation for needle aspiration lung biopsy. Investigative Radiology 1997; 32(8): 453.

106. Chhieng DC, Cangiarella JF, Zakowski MF, et al. Use of thyroid transcription factor 1, PE-10, and cytokeratins 7 and 20 in discriminating between primary lung carcinomas and metastatic lesions in fine-needle aspiration biopsy specimens. Cancer 2001; 93(5): 330.

107. Bocking A, Klose KC, Kyll HJ, et al. Cytologic versus histologic evaluation of needle biopsy of the lung, hilum and mediastinum. Sensitivity, specificity and typing accuracy. Acta Cytologica 1995; 39(3): 463.

108. Greif J, Marmur S, Schwarz Y, et al. Percutaneous core cutting needle biopsy compared with fine-needle aspiration in the diagnosis of peripheral lung malignant lesions: results in 156 patients. Cancer 1998; 84(3): 144.

109. Greif J, Marmur S, Schwarz Y, et al. Percutaneous core needle biopsy vs. fine needle aspiration in diagnosing benign lung lesions. Acta Cytol 1999; 43(5): 756.

110. Klein JS, Salomon G, Stewart EA. Transthoracic needle biopsy with a coaxially placed 20-gauge automated cutting needle: results in 122 patients. Radiology 1996; 198(3): 715.

111. Magid MS, Chen YT, Soslow RA, et al. Juvenile-onset recurrent respiratory papillomatosis involving the lung: A case report and review of the literature. Pediatr Dev Pathol 1998; 1(2): 157.

112. Flieder DB, Koss MN, Nicholson A, et al. Solitary pulmonary papillomas in adults: a clinicopathologic and in situ hybridization study of 14 cases combined with 27 cases in the literature. Am J Surg Pathol 1998; 22(11): 1328.

113. Shah H, Garbe L, Nussbaum E, et al. Benign tumors of the tracheobronchial tree. Endoscopic characteristics and role of laser resection. Chest 1995; 107(6): 1744.

114. Popper HH, el-Shabrawi Y, Wockel W, et al. Prognostic importance of human papilloma virus typing in squamous cell papilloma of the bronchus: comparison of in situ hybridization and the polymerase chain reaction. Hum Pathol 1994; 25(11): 1191.

115. Popper HH, Wirnsberger G, Juttner-Smolle FM, et al. The predictive value of human papilloma virus (HPV) typing in the prognosis of bronchial squamous cell papillomas. Histopathology 1992; 21(4): 323.

116. Cook JR, Hill DA, Humphrey PA, et al. Squamous cell carcinoma arising in recurrent respiratory papillomatosis with pulmonary involvement: emerging common pattern of clinical features and human papillomavirus serotype association. Mod Pathol 2000; 13(8): 914.

117. Colby TV, Koss MN, Travis WD. Tumors of the lower respiratory tract. In: Rosai J, ed. Atlas of tumor pathology, 3rd Series. Washington, DC: Armed Forces Institute of Pathology; 1995.

118. Yousem SA, Ohori NP, Sonmez-Alpan E. Occurrence of human papillomavirus DNA in primary lung neoplasms. Cancer 1992; 69(3): 693.

119. Saccomanno G, Archer VE, Auerbach O, et al. Development of carcinoma of the lung as reflected in exfoliated cells. Cancer 1974; 33(1): 256.

120. Nagamoto N, Saito Y, Ohta S, et al. Relationship of lymph node metastasis to primary tumor size and microscopic appearance of roentgenographically occult lung cancer. Am J Surg Pathol 1989; 13(12): 1009.

121. Nagamoto N, Saito Y, Suda H, et al. Relationship between length of longitudinal extension and maximal depth of transmural invasion in roentgenographically occult squamous cell carcinoma of the bronchus (nonpolypoid type). Am J Surg Pathol 1989; 13(1): 11.

122. Martini N, Melamed MR. Occult carcinomas of the lung. Ann Thorac Surg 1980; 30(3): 215.

123. Carter D, Marsh BR, Baker R, et al. Relationships of morphology to clinical presentation in ten cases of early squamous cell carcinoma of the lung. Cancer 1976; 37(3): 1389.

124. Woolner LB, David E, Fontana RS, et al. In situ and early invasive bronchogenic carcinoma. Report of 28 cases with postoperative survival data. J Thorac Cardiovasc Surg 1970; 60(2): 275.

125. Chaudhuri MR. Primary pulmonary cavitating carcinomas. Thorax 1973; 28(3): 354.

126. Stanley KE, Matthews MJ. Analysis of a pathology review of patients with lung tumors. J Natl Cancer Inst 1981; 66(6): 989.

127. Stanley K, Cox JD, Petrovich Z, et al. Patterns of failure in patients with inoperable carcinoma of the lung. Cancer 1981; 47(11): 2725.

128. Kirsh MM, Kahn DR, Gago O, et al. Treatment of bronchogenic carcinoma with mediastinal metastases. Ann Thorac Surg 1971; 12(1). 11.

129. Gail MH, Eagan RT, Feld R, et al. Prognostic factors in patients with resected stage I non-small cell lung cancer. A report from the Lung Cancer Study Group. Cancer 1984; 54(9): 1802.

130. Dulmet-Brender E, Jaubert F, Huchon G. Exophytic endobronchial epidermoid carcinoma. Cancer 1986; 57(7): 1358.

131. Hammar S. The use of electron microscopy and immunohistochemistry in the diagnosis and understanding of lung neoplasms. Clin Lab Med 1987; 7(1): 1.

132. Brambilla E, Moro D, Veale D, et al. Basal cell (basaloid) carcinoma of the lung: a new morphologic and phenotypic entity with separate prognostic significance. Hum Pathol 1992; 23(9): 993.

133. Moro D, Brichon PY, Brambilla E, et al. Basaloid bronchial carcinoma. A histologic group with a poor prognosis. Cancer 1994; 73(11): 2734.

134. Katzenstein AL, Prioleau PG, Askin FB. The histologic spectrum and significance of clear-cell change in lung carcinoma. Cancer 1980; 45(5): 943.

135. Nunez V, Melamed MR, Cahan W. Tracheo-bronchial cytology after laryngectomy for carcinoma of larynx. II. Benign atypias. Acta Cytol 1966; 10(1): 38.

136. Koss LG, Richardson HL. Some pitfalls of cytological diagnosis of lung cancer. Cancer 1955; 8(5). 937.

137. Erozan YS. Cytopathologic diagnosis of pulmonary neoplasms in sputum and bronchoscopic specimens. Semin Diagn Pathol 1986; 3(3): 188.

138. England DM, Hochholzer L. Truly benign "bronchial adenoma." Report of 10 cases of mucous gland adenoma with immunohistochemical and ultrastructural findings. Am J Surg Pathol 1995; 19(8): 887.

139. Heard BE, Corrin B, Dewar A. Pathology of seven mucous cell adenomas of the bronchial glands with particular reference to ultrastructure. Histopathology 1985; 9(7): 687.

140. Moran CA, Suster S, Askin FB, et al. Benign and malignant salivary gland-type mixed tumors of the lung. Clinicopathologic and immunohistochemical study of eight cases. Cancer 1994; 73(10): 2481.

141. Moran CA. Primary salivary gland-type tumors of the lung. Semin Diagn Pathol 1995; 12(2): 106.

142. Davis PW, Briggs JC, Seal RM, et al. Benign and malignant mixed tumours of the lung. Thorax 1972; 27(6): 657.

143. Hayes MM, van der Westhuizen NG, Forgie R. Malignant mixed tumor of bronchus: a biphasic neoplasm of epithelial and myoepithelial cells. Mod Pathol 1993; 6(1): 85.

144. Yousem SA, Hochholzer L. Alveolar adenoma. Hum Pathol 1986; 17(10): 1066.

145. Burke LM, Rush WI, Khoor A, et al. Alveolar adenoma: a histochemical, immunohistochemical, and ultrastructural analysis of 17 cases. Hum Pathol 1999; 30(2): 158.

146. Nicholson AG, Magkou C, Snead D, et al. Unusual sclerosing haemangiomas and sclerosing haemangioma-like lesions, and the value of TTF-1 in making the diagnosis. Histopathology 2002; 41(5): 404.

147. Liebow AA, Hubbell DS. Sclerosing hemangioma (histiocytoma, xanthoma) of the lung. Cancer 1956; 9(1): 53.

148. Hill GS, Eggleston JC. Electron microscopic study of so-called "pulmonary sclerosing hemangioma." Report of a case suggesting epithelial origin. Cancer 1972; 30(4): 1092.

149. Satoh Y, Tsuchiya E, Weng SY, et al. Pulmonary sclerosing hemangioma of the lung. A type II pneumocytoma by immunohistochemical and immunoelectron microscopic studies. Cancer 1989; 64(6): 1310.

150. Yousem SA, Wick MR, Singh G, et al. So-called sclerosing hemangiomas of lung. An immunohistochemical study supporting a respiratory epithelial origin. Am J Surg Pathol 1988; 12(8): 582.

151. Nagata N, Dairaku M, Sueishi K, et al. Sclerosing hemangioma of the lung. An epithelial tumor composed of immunohistochemically heterogenous cells. Am J Clin Pathol 1987; 88(5): 552.

152. Spencer H, Nambu S. Sclerosing haemangiomas of the lung. Histopathology 1986; 10(5): 477.

153. Lee ST, Lee YC, Hsu CY, et al. Bilateral multiple sclerosing hemangiomas of the lung. Chest 1992; 101(2): 572.

154. Ng WK, Fu KH, Wang E, et al. Sclerosing hemangioma of lung: A close cytologic mimicker of pulmonary adenocarcinoma. Diagn Cytopathol 2001; 25(5): 316.

155. Wang SE, Nieberg RK. Fine needle aspiration cytology of sclerosing hemangioma of the lung, a mimicker of bronchioloalveolar carcinoma. Acta Cytol 1986; 30(1): 51.

156. Wojcik EM, Sneige N, Lawrence DD, et al. Fine-needle aspiration cytology of sclerosing hemangioma of the lung: case report with immunohistochemical study. Diagn Cytopathol 1993; 9(3): 304.

157. Gal AA, Nassar VH, Miller JI. Cytopathologic diagnosis of pulmonary sclerosing hemangioma. Diagn Cytopathol 2002; 26(3): 163.

158. Krishnamurthy SC, Naresh KN, Soni M, et al. Sclerosing hemangioma of the lung: a potential source of error in fine needle aspiration cytology. Acta Cytol 1994; 38(1): 111.

159. Kaw YT, Nayak RN. Fine needle aspiration biopsy cytology of sclerosing hemangioma of the lung. A case report. Acta Cytol 1993; 37(6): 933.

160. Chow LT, Chan SK, Chow WH, et al. Pulmonary sclerosing hemangioma. Report of a case with diagnosis by fine needle aspiration. Acta Cytol 1992; 36(3): 287.

161. Anderson C, Ludwig ME, O'Donnell M, et al. Fine needle aspiration cytology of pulmonary carcinoid tumors. Acta Cytol 1990; 34(4): 505.

162. Iyoda A, Baba M, Saitoh H, et al. Imprint cytologic features of pulmonary sclerosing hemangioma: comparison with well-differentiated papillary adenocarcinoma. Cancer 2002; 96(3): 146.

163. Noguchi M, Kodama T, Shimosato Y, et al. Papillary adenoma of type 2 pneumocytes. Am J Surg Pathol 1986; 10(2): 134.

164. Miller DL, Allen MS. Rare pulmonary neoplasms. Mayo Clin Proc 1993; 68(5): 492.

165. Yousem SA, Hochholzer L. Mucoepidermoid tumors of the lung. Cancer 1987; 60(6): 1346.

166. Barsky SH, Martin SE, Matthews M, et al. "Low grade" mucoepidermoid carcinoma of the bronchus with "high grade" biological behavior. Cancer 1983; 51(8): 1505.

167. Turnbull AD, Huvos AG, Goodner JT, et al. Mucoepidermoid tumors of bronchial glands. Cancer 1971; 28(3): 539.

168. Green LK, Gallion TL, Gyorkey F. Peripheral mucoepidermoid tumour of the lung. Thorax 1991; 46(1): 65.

169. Nguyen GK. Cytology of bronchial gland carcinoma. Acta Cytol 1988; 32(2): 235.

170. Brooks B, Baandrup U. Peripheral low-grade mucoepidermoid carcinoma of the lung – needle aspiration cytodiagnosis and histology. Cytopathology 1992; 3(4): 259.

171. Tao LC, Robertson DI. Cytologic diagnosis of bronchial mucoepidermoid carcinoma by fine needle aspiration biopsy. Acta Cytol 1978; 22(4): 221.

172. Segletes LA, Steffee CH, Geisinger KR. Cytology of primary pulmonary mucoepidermoid and adenoid cystic carcinoma. A report of four cases. Acta Cytol 1999; 43(6): 1091.

173. Moran CA, Suster S, Koss MN. Primary adenoid cystic carcinoma of the lung. A clinicopathologic and immunohistochemical study of 16 cases. Cancer 1994; 73(5): 1390.

174. Inoue H, Iwashita A, Kanegae H, et al. Peripheral pulmonary adenoid cystic carcinoma with substantial submucosal extension to the proximal bronchus. Thorax 1991; 46(2): 147.

175. Nomori H, Kaseda S, Kobayashi K, et al. Adenoid cystic carcinoma of the trachea and main-stem bronchus. A clinical, histopathologic, and immunohistochemical study. J Thorac Cardiovasc Surg 1988; 96(2): 271.

176. Ishida T, Nishino T, Oka T, et al. Adenoid cystic carcinoma of the tracheobronchial tree: clinicopathology and immunohistochemistry. J Surg Oncol 1989; 41(1): 52.

177. Ahel V, Zubovic I, Rozmanic V. Bronchial adenoid cystic carcinoma with saccular bronchiectasis as a cause of recurrent pneumonia in children. Pediatr Pulmonol 1992; 12(4): 260.

178. Moran CA, Suster S, Koss MN. Acinic cell carcinoma of the lung ("Fechner tumor"). A clinicopathologic, immunohistochemical, and ultrastructural study of five cases. Am J Surg Pathol 1992; 16(11): 1039.

179. Conlan AA, Payne WS, Woolner LB, et al. Adenoid cystic carcinoma (cylindroma) and mucoepidermoid carcinoma of the bronchus. Factors affecting survival. J Thorac Cardiovasc Surg 1978; 76(3): 369.

180. Radhika S, Dey P, Rajwanshi A, et al. Adenoid cystic carcinoma in a bronchial washing. A case report. Acta Cytol 1993; 37(1): 97.

181. Buchanan AJ, Fauck R, Gupta RK. Cytologic diagnosis of adenoid cystic carcinoma in tracheal wash specimens. Diagn Cytopathol 1988; 4(2): 130.

182. Chen KT. Exfoliative cytology of tracheobronchial adenoid cystic carcinoma. Diagn Cytopathol 1996; 15(2): 132.

183. Gupta RK, McHutchison AG. Cytologic findings of adenoid cystic carcinoma in a tracheal wash specimen. Diagn Cytopathol 1992; 8(2): 196.

184. Hajdu SI, Koss LG. Cytology of carcinoma of the trachea. Acta Cytol 1969; 13(5): 255.

185. Lozowski MS, Mishriki Y, Solitare GB. Cytopathologic features of adenoid cystic carcinoma. Case report and literature review. Acta Cytol 1983; 27(3): 317.

186. Fechner RE, Bentinck BR, Askew JB Jr. Acinic cell tumor of the lung. A histologic and ultrastructural study. Cancer 1972; 29(2): 501.

187. Rodriguez J, Diment J, Lombardi L, et al. Combined typical carcinoid and acinic cell tumor of the lung: a heretofore unreported occurrence. Hum Pathol 2003; 34(10): 1061.

188. Ukoha OO, Quartararo P, Carter D, et al. Acinic cell carcinoma of the lung with metastasis to lymph nodes. Chest 1999; 115(2): 591.

189. Deavers M, Guinee D, Koss MN, et al. Granular cell tumors of the lung. Clinicopathologic study of 20 cases. Am J Surg Pathol 1995; 19(6): 627.

190. Thomas de Montpreville V, Dulmet EM. Granular cell tumours of the lower respiratory tract. Histopathology 1995; 27(3): 257.

191. Sklar JL, Churg A, Bensch KG. Oncocytic carcinoid tumor of the lung. Am J Surg Pathol 1980; 4(3): 287.

192. Scharifker D, Marchevsky A. Oncocytic carcinoid of lung: an ultrastructural analysis. Cancer 1981; 47(3): 530.

193. Kodama T, Shimosato Y, Koide T, et al. Endobronchial polypoid adenocarcinoma of the lung. Histological and ultrastructural studies of five cases. Am J Surg Pathol 1984; 8(11): 845.

194. Goto K, Yokose T, Kodama T, et al. Detection of early invasion on the basis of basement membrane destruction in small adenocarcinomas of the lung and its clinical implications. Mod Pathol 2001; 14(12): 1237.

195. Noguchi M, Morikawa A, Kawasaki M, et al. Small adenocarcinoma of the lung. Histologic characteristics and prognosis. Cancer 1995; 75(12): 2844.

196. Aoyagi Y, Yokose T, Minami Y, et al. Accumulation of losses of heterozygosity and multistep carcinogenesis in pulmonary adenocarcinoma. Cancer Res 2001; 61(21): 7950.

197. Yoshioka H, Takeuchi T, Matsuno Y, et al. Analysis of loss of heterozygosity in small adenocarcinomas of the lung. Jpn J Clin Oncol 1998; 28(4): 240.

198. Kawasaki M, Noguchi M, Morikawa A, et al. Nuclear p53 accumulation by small-sized adenocarcinomas of the lung. Pathol Int 1996; 46(7): 486.

199. Eto T, Suzuki H, Honda A, et al. The changes of the stromal elastotic framework in the growth of peripheral lung adenocarcinomas. Cancer 1996; 77(4): 646.

200. Travis WD et al., eds. Pathology and genetics of tumors of the lung, pleura, thymus and heart. World Health Organisation classification of tumors. Lyon: IARC Publications; 2004.

201. Okubo K, Mark EJ, Flieder D, et al. Bronchoalveolar carcinoma: clinical, radiologic, and pathologic factors and survival. J Thorac Cardiovasc Surg 1999; 118(4): 702.

202. Kodama K, Higashiyama M, Yokouchi H, et al. Prognostic value of ground-glass opacity found in small lung adenocarcinoma on high-resolution CT scanning. Lung Cancer 2001; 33(1): 17.

203. Sakurai H, Maeshima A, Watanabe S, et al. Grade of stromal invasion in small adenocarcinoma of the lung: histopathological minimal invasion and prognosis. Am J Surg Pathol 2004; 28(2): 198.

204. Clayton F. Bronchioloalveolar carcinomas. Cell types, patterns of growth, and prognostic correlates. Cancer 1986; 57(8): 1555.

205. Yamato Y, Tsuchida M, Watanabe T, et al. Early results of a prospective study of limited resection for bronchioloalveolar adenocarcinoma of the lung. Ann Thorac Surg 2001; 71(3): 971.

206. Watanabe S, Watanabe T, Arai K, et al. Results of wedge resection for focal bronchioloalveolar carcinoma showing pure ground-glass attenuation on computed tomography. Ann Thorac Surg 2002; 73(4): 1071.

207. Engstrand DA, England DM, Oberley TD. Limitations of the usefulness of microvillous ultrastructure in distinguishing between carcinoma primary in and metastatic to the lung. Ultrastruct Pathol 1987; 11(1): 53.

208. Hecht JL, Pinkus JL, Weinstein LJ, et al. The value of thyroid transcription factor-1 in cytologic preparations as a marker for metastatic adenocarcinoma of lung origin. Am J Clin Pathol 2001; 116(4): 483.

209. Kaufmann O, Dietel M. Thyroid transcription factor-1 is the superior immunohistochemical marker for pulmonary adenocarcinomas and large cell carcinomas compared to surfactant proteins A and B. Histopathology 2000; 36(1): 8.

210. Ordonez NG. Value of thyroid transcription factor-1, E-cadherin, BG8, WT1, and CD44S immunostaining in distinguishing epithelial pleural mesothelioma from pulmonary and nonpulmonary adenocarcinoma. Am J Surg Pathol 2000; 24(4): 598.

211. Vazquez MF, Flieder DB. Small peripheral glandular lesions detected by screening CT for lung cancer. A diagnostic dilemma for the pathologist. Radiol Clin North Am 2000; 38(3): 579.

212. Miller RR. Bronchioloalveolar cell adenomas. Am J Surg Pathol 1990; 14(10): 904.

213. Kitamura H, Kameda Y, Nakamura N, et al. Proliferative potential and p53 overexpression in precursor and early stage lesions of bronchioloalveolar lung carcinoma. Am J Pathol 1995; 146(4): 876.

214. Kitamura H, Kameda Y, Ito T, et al. Atypical adenomatous hyperplasia of the lung. Implications for the pathogenesis of peripheral lung adenocarcinoma. Am J Clin Pathol 1999; 111(5): 610.

215. Kitamura H, Kameda Y, Nakamura N, et al. Atypical adenomatous hyperplasia and bronchoalveolar lung carcinoma. Analysis by morphometry and the expressions of p53 and carcinoembryonic antigen. Am J Surg Pathol 1996; 20(5): 553.

216. Anami Y, Matsuno Y, Yamada T, et al. A case of double primary adenocarcinoma of the lung with multiple atypical adenomatous hyperplasia. Pathol Int 1998; 48(8): 634.

217. Ritter JH. Pulmonary atypical adenomatous hyperplasia. A histologic lesion in search of usable criteria and clinical significance. Am J Clin Pathol 1999; 111(5): 587.

218. Mori M, Rao SK, Popper HH, et al. Atypical adenomatous hyperplasia of the lung: a probable forerunner in the development of adenocarcinoma of the lung. Mod Pathol 2001; 14(2): 72.

219. Suzuki K, Nagai K, Yoshida J, et al. The prognosis of resected lung carcinoma associated with atypical adenomatous hyperplasia: a comparison of the prognosis of well-differentiated adenocarcinoma associated with atypical adenomatous hyperplasia and intrapulmonary metastasis. Cancer 1997; 79(8): 1521.

220. Koga T, Hashimoto S, Sugio K, et al. Lung adenocarcinoma with bronchioloalveolar carcinoma component is frequently associated with foci of high-grade atypical adenomatous hyperplasia. Am J Clin Pathol 2002; 117(3): 464.

221. Lozowski W, Hajdu SI. Cytology and immunocytochemistry of bronchioloalveolar carcinoma. Acta Cytol 1987; 31(6): 717.

222. Ng AB, Horak GC. Factors significant in the diagnostic accuracy of lung cytology in bronchial washing and sputum samples. I. Bronchial washings. Acta Cytol 1983; 27(4): 391.

223. MacDonald LL, Yazdi HM. Fine-needle aspiration biopsy of bronchioloalveolar carcinoma. Cancer 2001; 93(1): 29.

224. Silverman JF, Finley JL, Park HK, et al. Fine needle aspiration cytology of bronchioloalveolar-cell carcinoma of the lung. Acta Cytol 1985; 29(5): 887.

225. Tao LC, Weisbrod GL, Pearson FG, et al. Cytologic diagnosis of bronchioloalveolar carcinoma by fine-needle aspiration biopsy. Cancer 1986; 57(8): 1565.

226. Elson CE, Moore SP, Johnston WW. Morphologic and immunocytochemical studies of bronchioloalveolar carcinoma at Duke University Medical Center, 1968–1986. Anal Quant Cytol Histol 1989; 11(4): 261.

227. Chen C, Hoda RS, Hoda SA. Intranuclear cytoplasmic inclusions in the differential diagnosis of papillary thyroid carcinoma and bronchioloalveolar carcinoma. Diagn Cytopathol 1998; 18(5): 384.

228. Zaman SS, van Hoeven KH, Slott S, et al. Distinction between bronchioloalveolar carcinoma and hyperplastic pulmonary proliferations: a cytologic and morphometric analysis. Diagn Cytopathol 1997; 16(5): 396.

229. Fiorella RM, Gurley SD, Dubey S. Cytologic distinction between bronchioalveolar carcinoma and reactive/reparative respiratory epithelium: a cytomorphometric analysis. Diagn Cytopathol 1998; 19(4): 270.

230. Kragel PJ, Devaney KO, Meth BM, et al. Mucinous cystadenoma of the lung. A report of two cases with immunohistochemical and ultrastructural analysis. Arch Pathol Lab Med 1990; 114(10): 1053.

231. Moran CA, Hochholzer L, Fishback N, et al. Mucinous (so-called colloid) carcinomas of lung. Mod Pathol 1992; 5(6): 634.

232. Ishibashi H, Moriya T, Matsuda Y, et al. Pulmonary mucinous cystadenocarcinoma: report of a case and review of the literature. Ann Thorac Surg 2003; 76(5): 1738.

233. Graeme-Cook F, Mark EJ. Pulmonary mucinous cystic tumors of borderline malignancy. Hum Pathol 1991; 22(2): 185.

234. Mann GN, Wilczynski SP, Sager K, et al. Recurrence of pulmonary mucinous cystic tumor of borderline malignancy. Ann Thorac Surg 2001; 71(2): 696.

235. Rossi G, Murer B, Cavazza A, et al. Primary mucinous (so-called colloid) carcinomas of lung. A clinicopathologic and immunohistochemical study with special reference to CDX2 homiobox gene and muck II expression. Am J Surg Pathol 2004; 28: 442.

236. Yoshida J, Nagai K, Yokose T, et al. Primary peripheral lung carcinoma smaller than 1 cm in diameter. Chest 1998; 114(3): 710.

237. Higashiyama M, Kodama K, Yokouchi H, et al. Prognostic value of bronchiolo-alveolar carcinoma component of small lung adenocarcinoma. Ann Thorac Surg 1999; 68(6): 2069.

238. Yoshida K, Morinaga S, Shimosato Y, et al. A cell kinetic study of pulmonary adenocarcinoma by an immunoperoxidase procedure after bromodeoxyuridine labeling. Cancer 1989; 64(11): 2284.

239. Sheibani K, Battifora H, Burke JS, et al. Leu-M1 antigen in human neoplasms. An immunohistologic study of 400 cases. Am J Surg Pathol 1986; 10(4): 227.

240. Sheibani K, Shin SS, Kezirian J, et al. Ber-EP4 antibody as a discriminant in the differential diagnosis of malignant mesothelioma versus adenocarcinoma. Am J Surg Pathol 1991; 15(8): 779.

241. Loy TS, Nashelsky MB. Reactivity of B72.3 with adenocarcinomas. An immunohistochemical study of 476 cases. Cancer 1993; 72(8): 2495.

242. Ishikura H, Kanda M, Ito M, et al. Hepatoid adenocarcinoma: a distinctive histological subtype of alpha-fetoprotein-producing lung carcinoma. Virchows Arch A Pathol Anat Histopathol 1990; 417(1): 73.

243. Hayashi Y, Takanashi Y, Ohsawa H, et al. Hepatoid adenocarcinoma in the lung. Lung Cancer 2002; 38(2): 211.

244. Fan Z, van de Rijn M, Montgomery K, et al. Hep par 1 antibody stain for the differential diagnosis of hepatocellular carcinoma: 676 tumors tested using tissue microarrays and conventional tissue sections. Mod Pathol 2003; 16(2): 137.

245. McElvaney G, Miller RR, Muller NL, et al. Multicentricity of adenocarcinoma of the lung. Chest 1989; 95(1): 151.

246. Koss M, Travis W, Moran C, et al. Pseudomesotheliomatous adenocarcinoma: a reappraisal. Semin Diagn Pathol 1992; 9(2): 117.

247. Cahan WG, Castro EB, Hajdu SI. Proceedings: The significance of a solitary lung shadow in patients with colon carcinoma. Cancer 1974; 33(2): 414.

248. Cibas ES, Melamed MR, Zaman MB, et al. The effect of tumor size and tumor cell DNA content on the survival of patients with stage I adenocarcinoma of the lung. Cancer 1989; 63(8): 1552.

249. Takise A, Kodama T, Shimosato Y, et al. Histopathologic prognostic factors in adenocarcinomas of the peripheral lung less than 2 cm in diameter. Cancer 1988; 61(10): 2083.

250. Naylor B, Railey C. A pitfall in the cytodiagnosis of sputum of asthmatics. J Clin Pathol 1964; 17: 84.

251. Stanley MW, Henry-Stanley MJ, Gajl-Peczalska KJ, et al. Hyperplasia of type II pneumocytes in acute lung injury. Cytologic findings of sequential bronchoalveolar lavage. Am J Clin Pathol 1992; 97(5): 669.

252. Liebow AA, Castleman B. Benign "clear cell tumors" of the lung. Am J Pathol 1963; 43: 13a.

253. Liebow AA, Castleman B. Benign clear cell ("sugar") tumors of the lung. Yale J Biol Med 1971; 43(4): 213.

254. Hoch WS, Patchefsky AS, Takeda M, et al. Benign clear cell tumor of the lung. An ultrastructural study. Cancer 1974; 33(5): 1328.

255. Bonetti F, Pea M, Martignoni G, et al. Clear cell ("sugar") tumor of the lung is a lesion strictly related to angiomyolipoma – the concept of a family of lesions characterized by the presence of the perivascular epithelioid cells (PEC). Pathology 1994; 26(3): 230.

256. Flieder DB, Travis WD. Clear cell "sugar" tumor of the lung: association with lymphangioleiomyomatosis and multifocal micronodular pneumocyte hyperplasia in a patient with tuberous sclerosis. Am J Surg Pathol 1997; 21(10): 1242.

257. Chuah KL, Tan PH. Multifocal micronodular pneumocyte hyperplasia, lymphangiomyomatosis and clear cell micronodules of the lung in a Chinese female patient with tuberous sclerosis. Pathology 1998; 30(3): 242.

258. Vang R, Kempson RL. Perivascular epithelioid cell tumor ('PEComa') of the uterus: a subset of HMB-45-positive epithelioid mesenchymal neoplasms with an uncertain relationship to pure smooth muscle tumors. Am J Surg Pathol 2002; 26(1): 1.

259. Gaffey MJ, Mills SE, Askin FB, et al. Clear cell tumor of the lung. A clinicopathologic, immunohistochemical, and ultrastructural study of eight cases. Am J Surg Pathol 1990; 14(3): 248.

260. Gaffey MJ, Mills SE, Zarbo RJ, et al. Clear cell tumor of the lung. Immunohistochemical and ultrastructural evidence of melanogenesis. Am J Surg Pathol 1991; 15(7): 644.

261. Sale GE, Kulander BG. 'Benign' clear-cell tumor (sugar tumor) of the lung with hepatic metastases ten years after resection of pulmonary primary tumor. Arch Pathol Lab Med 1988; 112(12): 1177.

262. Katzenstein AL, Purvis R Jr, Gmelich J, et al. Pulmonary resection for metastatic renal adenocarcinoma: pathologic findings and therapeutic value. Cancer 1978; 41(2): 712.

263. Yesner R, Gelfman NA, Feinstein AR. A reappraisal of histopathology in lung cancer and correlation of cell types with antecedent cigarette smoking. Am Rev Respir Dis 1973; 107(5): 790.

264. Downey RJ, Deschamps C, Asakura S, et al. Large cell carcinoma of the lung: results of surgical treatment. Lung Cancer 1994; 11: 153.

265. Ishida T, Kaneko S, Tateishi M, et al. Large cell carcinoma of the lung. Prognostic implications of histopathologic and immunohistochemical subtyping. Am J Clin Pathol 1990; 93(2): 176.

266. Travis WD, Travis LB, Devesa SS. Lung cancer. Cancer 1995; 75(1 Suppl): 191.

267. Suzuki H, Miyasaka H, Ota H, et al. Purification and partial primary sequence of a chemotactic protein for polymorphonuclear leukocytes derived from human lung giant cell carcinoma LU65C cells. J Exp Med 1989; 169: 1895.

268. Rabson AS, Rosen SW, Tashijan AH Jr, et al. Production of human chorionic gonadotropin in vitro by a cell line derived from a carcinoma of the lung. J Natl Cancer Inst 1973; 50(3): 669.

269. Smith LG, Lyubsky SL, Carlson HE. Postmenopausal uterine bleeding due to estrogen production by gonadotropin-secreting lung tumors. Am J Med 1992; 92(3): 327.

270. Ginsberg SS, Buzaid AC, Stern H, et al. Giant cell carcinoma of the lung. Cancer 1992; 70(3): 606.

271. Iyoda A, Hiroshima K, Baba M, et al. Pulmonary large cell carcinomas with neuroendocrine features are high-grade neuroendocrine tumors. Ann Thorac Surg 2002; 73(4): 1049.

272. Iyoda A, Hiroshima K, Toyozaki T, et al. Clinical characterization of pulmonary large cell neuroendocrine carcinoma and large cell carcinoma with neuroendocrine morphology. Cancer 2001; 91(11): 1992.

273. Wick MR, Berg LC, Hertz MI. Large cell carcinoma of the lung with neuroendocrine differentiation. A comparison with large cell "undifferentiated" pulmonary tumors. Am J Clin Pathol 1992; 97(6): 796.

274. Begin LR, Eskandari J, Joncas J, et al. Epstein-Barr virus related lymphoepithelioma-like carcinoma of lung. J Surg Oncol 1987; 36(4): 280.

275. Chan JK, Hui PK, Yip TT, et al. Detection of Epstein-Barr virus only in lymphoepithelial carcinomas among primary carcinomas of the lung. Histopathology 1995; 26(6): 576.

276. Gal AA, Unger ER, Koss MN, et al. Detection of Epstein-Barr virus in lymphoepithelioma-like carcinoma of the lung. Mod Pathol 1991; 4(2): 264.

277. Pittaluga S, Wong MP, Chung LP, et al. Clonal Epstein-Barr virus in lymphoepithelioma-like carcinoma of the lung. Am J Surg Pathol 1993; 17(7): 678.

278. Broderick PA, Corvese NL, LaChance T, et al. Giant cell carcinoma of lung: a cytologic evaluation. Acta Cytol 1975; 19(3): 225.

279. Craig ID, Desrosiers P, Lefcoe MS. Giant-cell carcinoma of the lung. A cytologic study. Acta Cytol 1983; 27(3): 293.

280. Laforga JB. Giant cell carcinoma of the lung. Report of a case with cytohistologic and clinical correlation. Acta Cytol 1999; 43(2): 263.

281. Nonomura A, Mizukami Y, Shimizu J, et al. Small giant cell carcinoma of the lung diagnosed preoperatively by transthoracic aspiration cytology. A case report. Acta Cytol 1995; 39(1): 129.

282. Chow LT, Chow WH, Tsui WM, et al. Fine-needle aspiration cytologic diagnosis of lymphoepithelioma-like carcinoma of the lung. Report of two cases with immunohistochemical study. Am J Clin Pathol 1995; 103(1): 35.

283. Johnston WW, Bossen EH. Ten years of respiratory cytopathology at Duke University Medical Center. II. The cytopathologic diagnosis of lung cancer during the years 1970 to 1974, with a comparison between cytopathology and histopathology in the typing of lung cancer. Acta Cytol 1981; 25(5): 499.

284. Bahadori M, Liebow AA. Plasma cell granulomas of the lung. Cancer 1973; 31(1): 191.

285. Pettinato G, Manivel JC, De Rosa N, et al. Inflammatory myofibroblastic tumor (plasma cell granuloma). Clinicopathologic study of 20 cases with immunohistochemical and ultrastructural observations. Am J Clin Pathol 1990; 94(5): 538.

286. Gal AA, Koss MN, McCarthy WF, et al. Prognostic factors in pulmonary fibrohistiocytic lesions. Cancer 1994; 73(7): 1817.

287. Matsubara O, Tan-Liu NS, Kenney RM, et al. Inflammatory pseudotumors of the lung: progression from organizing pneumonia to fibrous histiocytoma or to plasma cell granuloma in 32 cases. Hum Pathol 1988; 19(7): 807.

288. Spencer H. The pulmonary plasma cell/histiocytoma complex. Histopathology 1984; 8(6): 903.

289. Hong HY, Castelli MJ, Walloch JL. Pulmonary plasma cell granuloma (inflammatory pseudotumor) with invasion of thoracic vertebra. Mt Sinai J Med 1990; 57(2): 117.

290. Warter A, Satge D, Roeslin N. Angioinvasive plasma cell granulomas of the lung. Cancer 1987; 59(3): 435.

291. Snyder CS, Dell'Aquila M, Haghighi P, et al. Clonal changes in inflammatory pseudotumor of the lung: a case report. Cancer 1995; 76(9): 1545.

292. Su LD, Atayde-Perez A, Sheldon S, et al. Inflammatory myofibroblastic tumor: cytogenetic evidence supporting clonal origin. Mod Pathol 1998; 11(4): 364.

293. Yousem SA, Shaw H, Cieply K. Involvement of 2p23 in pulmonary inflammatory pseudotumors. Hum Pathol 2001; 32(4): 428.

294. Coffin CM, Patel A, Perkins S, et al. ALK1 and p80 expression and chromosomal rearrangements involving 2p23 in inflammatory myofibroblastic tumor. Mod Pathol 2001; 14(6): 569.

295. Barbareschi M, Ferrero S, Aldovini D, et al. Inflammatory pseudotumour of the lung. Immunohistochemical analysis on four new cases. Histol Histopathol 1990; 5(2): 205.

296. Rohrlich P, Peuchmaur M, Cocci SN, et al. Interleukin-6 and interleukin-1 beta production in a pediatric plasma cell granuloma of the lung. Am J Surg Pathol 1995; 19(5): 590.

297. Engleman P, Liebow AA, Gmelich J, et al. Pulmonary hyalinizing granuloma. Am Rev Respir Dis 1977; 115(6): 997.

298. Yousem SA, Hochholzer L. Pulmonary hyalinizing granuloma. Am J Clin Pathol 1987; 87(1): 1.

299. Atagi S, Sakatani M, Akira M, et al. Pulmonary hyalinizing granuloma with Castleman's disease. Intern Med 1994; 33(11): 689.

300. Drasin H, Blume MR, Rosenbaum EH, et al. Pulmonary hyalinizing granulomas in a patient with malignant lymphoma, with development nine years later of multiple myeloma and systemic amyloidosis. Cancer 1979; 44(1): 215.

301. Guccion JG, Rohatgi PK, Saini N. Pulmonary hyalinizing granuloma. Electron microscopic and immunologic studies. Chest 1984; 85(4): 571.

302. Dent RG, Godden DJ, Stovin PG, et al. Pulmonary hyalinising granuloma in association with retroperitoneal fibrosis. Thorax 1983; 38(12): 955.

303. Gans SJ, van der Elst AM, Straks W. Pulmonary hyalinizing granuloma. Eur Respir J 1988; 1(4): 389.

304. Laden SA, Cohen ML, Harley RA. Nodular pulmonary amyloidosis with extrapulmonary involvement. Hum Pathol 1984; 15(6): 594.

305. Fichtenbaum CJ, Kleinman GM, Haddad RG. Eosinophilic granuloma of the lung presenting as a solitary pulmonary nodule. Thorax 1990; 45(11): 905.

306. ten Velde GP, Thunnissen FB, van Engelshoven JM, et al. A solitary pulmonary nodule due to eosinophilic granuloma. Eur Respir J 1994; 7(8): 1539.

307. Colby TV, Hunt S, Pelzmann K, et al. Malakoplakia of the lung: a report of two cases. Respiration 1980; 39(5): 295.

308. Kwon KY, Colby TV. *Rhodococcus equi* pneumonia and pulmonary malakoplakia in acquired immunodeficiency syndrome. Pathologic features. Arch Pathol Lab Med 1994; 118(7): 744.

309. Loo KT, Seneviratne S, Chan JK. Mycobacterial infection mimicking inflammatory 'pseudotumour' of the lung. Histopathology 1989; 14(2): 217.

310. Sekosan M, Cleto M, Senseng C, et al. Spindle cell pseudotumors in the lungs due to *Mycobacterium tuberculosis* in a transplant patient. Am J Surg Pathol 1994; 18(10): 1065.

311. Yousem SA, Flynn SD. Intrapulmonary localized fibrous tumor. Intraparenchymal so-called localized fibrous mesothelioma. Am J Clin Pathol 1988; 89(3): 365.

312. England DM, Hochholzer L, McCarthy MJ. Localized benign and malignant fibrous tumors of the pleura. A clinicopathologic review of 223 cases. Am J Surg Pathol 1989; 13(8): 640.

313. Yousem SA, Hochholzer L. Primary pulmonary hemangiopericytoma. Cancer 1987; 59(3): 549.

314. Duarte IG, Gal AA, Mansour KA, et al. Pathologic findings in lung volume reduction surgery. Chest 1998; 113(3): 660.

315. Korn D, Bensch K, Liebow AA. Multiple minute pulmonary tumors resembling chemodectomas. Am J Pathol 1960; 37: 641.

316. Gaffey MJ, Mills SE, Askin FB. Minute pulmonary meningothelial-like nodules. A clinicopathologic study of so-called minute pulmonary chemodectoma. Am J Surg Pathol 1988; 12(3): 167.

317. Kuhn C 3rd, Askin FB. The fine structure of so-called minute pulmonary chemodectomas. Hum Pathol 1975; 6(6): 681.

318. Ichinose H, Hewitt RL, Drapanas T. Minute pulmonary chemodectoma. Cancer 1971; 28: 692.

319. Ionescu DN, Sasatomi E, Aldeeb D, et al. Pulmonary meningotholial-like nodules: a genotypic comparison with meningiomas. Am J Surg Pathol 2004; 28(2): 207.

320. Niho S, Yokose T, Nishiwaki Y, et al. Immunohistochemical and clonal analysis of minute pulmonary meningothelial-like nodules. Hum Pathol 1999; 30(4): 425.

321. Robinson PG. Pulmonary meningioma. Report of a case with electron microscopic and immunohistochemical findings. Am J Clin Pathol 1992; 97(6): 814.

322. Crotty TB, Hooker RP, Swensen SJ, et al. Primary malignant ependymoma of the lung. Mayo Clin Proc 1992; 67(4): 373.

323. Kitaichi M, Nishimura K, Itoh H, et al. Pulmonary lymphangioleiomyomatosis: a report of 46 patients including a clinicopathologic study of prognostic factors. Am J Respir Crit Care Med 1995; 151(2 Pt 1): 527.

324. Bernstein SM, Newell JD Jr, Adamczyk D, et al. How common are renal angiomyolipomas in patients with

pulmonary lymphangiomyomatosis? Am J Respir Crit Care Med 1995; 152(6 Pt 1): 2138.

325. Castro M, Shepherd CW, Gomez MR, et al. Pulmonary tuberous sclerosis. Chest 1995; 107(1): 189.

326. Chan JK, Tsang WY, Pau MY, et al. Lymphangiomyomatosis and angiomyolipoma: closely related entities characterized by hamartomatous proliferation of HMB-45-positive smooth muscle. Histopathology 1993; 22(5): 445.

327. Guinee DG Jr, Feuerstein I, Koss MN, et al. Pulmonary lymphangioleiomyomatosis. Diagnosis based on results of transbronchial biopsy and immunohistochemical studies and correlation with high-resolution computed tomography findings. Arch Pathol Lab Med 1994; 118(8): 846.

328. Johnson SR, Clelland CA, Ronan J, et al. The TSC-2 product tuberin is expressed in lymphangioleiomyomatosis and angiomyolipoma. Histopathology 2002; 40(5): 458.

329. Sato T, Seyama K, Fujii H, et al. Mutation analysis of the TSC1 and TSC2 genes in Japanese patients with pulmonary lymphangioleiomyomatosis. J Hum Genet 2002; 47(1): 20.

330. Strizheva GD, Carsillo T, Kruger WD, et al. The spectrum of mutations in TSC1 and TSC2 in women with tuberous sclerosis and lymphangiomyomatosis. Am J Respir Crit Care Med 2001; 163(1): 253.

331. Horstmann JP, Pietra GG, Harman JA, et al. Spontaneous regression of pulmonary leiomyomas during pregnancy. Cancer 1977; 39(1): 314.

332. Wolff M, Silva F, Kaye G. Pulmonary metastases (with admixed epithelial elements) from smooth muscle neoplasms. Report of nine cases, including three males. Am J Surg Pathol 1979; 3(4): 325.

333. Gal AA, Brooks JS, Pietra GG. Leiomyomatous neoplasms of the lung: a clinical, histologic, and immunohistochemical study. Mod Pathol 1989; 2(3): 209.

334. Kayser K, Zink S, Schneider T, et al. Benign metastasizing leiomyoma of the uterus: documentation of clinical, immunohistochemical and lectin-histochemical data of ten cases. Virchows Arch 2000; 437(3): 284.

335. Tietze L, Gunther K, Horbe A, et al. Benign metastasizing leiomyoma: a cytogenetically balanced but clonal disease. Hum Pathol 2000; 31(1): 126.

336. Horstmann JP, Hague WM, Abdulwahid NA, et al. Use of LHRH analog to obtain reverse castration in a patient with benign metastasizing leiomyoma. Br J Obstet Gynecol 1986; 93: 455.

337. Yilmaz A, Rush DS, Soslow RA. Endometrial stromal sarcomas with unusual histologic features: a report of 24 primary and metastatic tumors emphasizing fibroblastic and smooth muscle differentiation. Am J Surg Pathol 2002; 26(9): 1142.

338. Wick MR, Ritter JH, Nappi O. Inflammatory sarcomatoid carcinoma of the lung: report of three cases and clinicopathologic comparison with inflammatory pseudotumors in adult patients. Hum Pathol 1995; 26(9): 1014.

339. Ro JY, Chen JL, Lee JS, et al. Sarcomatoid carcinoma of the lung. Immunohistochemical and ultrastructural studies of 14 cases. Cancer 1992; 69(2): 376.

340. Yousem SA, Hochholzer L. Malignant fibrous histiocytoma of the lung. Cancer 1987; 60(10): 2532.

341. Nascimento AG, Unni KK, Bernatz PE. Sarcomas of the lung. Mayo Clin Proc 1982; 57(6): 355.

342. Lee SH, Rengachary SS, Paramesh J. Primary pulmonary rhabdomyosarcoma: a case report and review of the literature. Hum Pathol 1981; 12(1): 92.

343. Gal AA, Marchevsky AM, Koss MN. Unusual tumors of the lung. In: Marchevsky AM, ed. Surgical pathology of lung neoplasms. New York: Marcel Dekker; 1990: 325.

344. Sun CC, Kroll M, Miller JE. Primary chondrosarcoma of the lung. Cancer 1982; 50(9): 1864.

345. Colby TV, Bilbao JE, Battifora H, et al. Primary osteosarcoma of the lung. A reappraisal following

immunohistologic study. Arch Pathol Lab Med 1989; 113(10): 1147.

346. Patel AM, Ryu JH. Angiosarcoma in the lung. Chest 1993; 103(5): 1531.

347. Attanoos RL, Appleton MA, Gibbs AR. Primary sarcomas of the lung: a clinicopathological and immunohistochemical study of 14 cases. Histopathology 1996; 29(1): 29.

348. Halyard MY, Camoriano JK, Culligan JA, et al. Malignant fibrous histiocytoma of the lung. Report of four cases and review of the literature. Cancer 1996; 78(12): 2492.

349. Litzky LA, Brooks JJ. Cytokeratin immunoreactivity in malignant fibrous histiocytoma and spindle cell tumors: comparison between frozen and paraffin-embedded tissues. Mod Pathol 1992; 5(1): 30.

350. Zeren H, Moran CA, Suster S, et al. Primary pulmonary sarcomas with features of monophasic synovial sarcoma: a clinicopathological, immunohistochemical, and ultrastructural study of 25 cases. Hum Pathol 1995; 26(5): 474.

351. Aubry MC, Bridge JA, Wickert R, et al. Primary monophasic synovial sarcoma of the pleura: five cases confirmed by the presence of SYT-SSX fusion transcript. Am J Surg Pathol 2001; 25(6): 776.

352. Kaplan MA, Goodman MD, Satish J, et al. Primary pulmonary sarcoma with morphologic features of monophasic synovial sarcoma and chromosome translocation t(X;18). Am J Clin Pathol 1996; 105(2): 195.

353. Roberts CA, Seemayer TA, Neff JR, et al. Translocation (X;18) in primary synovial sarcoma of the lung. Cancer Genet Cytogenet 1996; 88(1): 49.

354. Mikami Y, Nakajima M, Hashimoto H, et al. Primary poorly differentiated monophasic synovial sarcoma of the lung. A case report with immunohistochemical and genetic studies. Pathol Res Pract 2003; 199(12): 827.

355. Hisaoka M, Hashimoto H, Iwamasa T, et al. Primary synovial sarcoma of the lung: report of two cases confirmed by molecular detection of SYT-SSX fusion gene transcripts. Histopathology 1999; 34(3): 205.

356. Gaertner E, Zeren EH, Fleming MV, et al. Biphasic synovial sarcomas arising in the pleural cavity. A clinicopathologic study of five cases. Am J Surg Pathol 1996; 20(1): 36.

357. Harwood AR, Osoba D, Hofstader SL, et al. Kaposi's sarcoma in recipients of renal transplants. Am J Med 1979; 67(5): 759.

358. Huang L, Schnapp LM, Gruden JF, et al. Presentation of AIDS-related pulmonary Kaposi's sarcoma diagnosed by bronchoscopy. Am J Respir Crit Care Med 1996; 153(4 Pt 1): 1385.

359. White DA, Matthay RA. Noninfectious pulmonary complications of infection with the human immunodeficiency virus. Am Rev Respir Dis 1989; 140(6): 1763.

360. O'Brien RF, Cohn DL. Serosanguineous pleural effusions in AIDS-associated Kaposi's sarcoma. Chest 1989; 96(3): 460.

361. Murray JF, Felton CP, Garay SM, et al. Pulmonary complications of the acquired immunodeficiency syndrome. Report of a National Heart, Lung, and Blood Institute workshop. N Engl J Med 1984; 310(25): 1682.

362. Aboulafia DM. The epidemiologic, pathologic, and clinical features of AIDS-associated pulmonary Kaposi's sarcoma. Chest 2000; 117(4): 1128.

363. Purdy LJ, Colby TV, Yousem SA, et al. Pulmonary Kaposi's sarcoma. Premortem histologic diagnosis. Am J Surg Pathol 1986; 10(5): 301.

364. Russell Jones R, Orchard G, Zelger B, et al. Immunostaining for CD31 and CD34 in Kaposi sarcoma. J Clin Pathol 1995; 48(11): 1011.

365. Chan JK. Vascular tumors with prominent spindle cell component. Curr Diagn Pathol 1997; 4: 76.

366. Cadranel J, Mayaud C. AIDS and the lung: update 1995. 3. Intrathoracic Kaposi's sarcoma in patients with AIDS. Thorax 1995; 50(4): 407.

367. Falconieri G, Bussani R, Mirra M, et al. Pseudomesotheliomatous angiosarcoma: a

pleuropulmonary lesion simulating malignant pleural mesothelioma. Histopathology 1997; 30(5): 419.

368. Sheppard MN, Hansell DM, Du Bois RM, et al. Primary epithelioid angiosarcoma of the lung presenting as pulmonary hemorrhage. Hum Pathol 1997; 28(3): 383.

369. Dail DH, Liebow AA, Gmelich JT, et al. Intravascular, bronchiolar, and alveolar tumor of the lung (IVBAT). An analysis of twenty cases of a peculiar sclerosing endothelial tumor. Cancer 1983; 51(3): 452.

370. Kumazawa Y, Maeda K, Ito M, et al. Expression of glucocorticoid receptor and 11beta hydroxysteroid dehydrogenase in a case of pulmonary epithelioid haemangioendothelioma. Mol Pathol 2002; 55(1): 61.

371. Corrin B, Manners B, Millard M, et al. Histogenesis of the so-called "intravascular bronchioloalveolar tumour." J Pathol 1979; 128(3): 163.

372. Ledson MJ, Convery R, Carty A, et al. Epithelioid haemangioendothelioma. Thorax 1999; 54(6): 560.

373. Murray J, Kielkowski D, Leiman G. The prevalence and age distribution of peripheral pulmonary hamartomas in adult males. An autopsy-based study. S Afr Med J 1991; 79(5): 247.

374. Ribet M, Jaillard-Thery S, Nuttens MC. Pulmonary hamartoma and malignancy. J Thorac Cardiovasc Surg 1994; 107(2): 611.

375. Carney JA. The triad of gastric epithelioid leiomyosarcoma, functioning extra-adrenal paraganglioma, and pulmonary chondroma. Cancer 1979; 43(1): 374.

376. Azua Blanco J, Azua Romeo J, Ortego J, et al. Cytologic features of pulmonary hamartoma. Report of a case diagnosed by fine needle aspiration cytology. Acta Cytol 2001; 45(2): 267.

377. Hamper UM, Khouri NF, Stitik FP, et al. Pulmonary hamartoma: diagnosis by transthoracic needle-aspiration biopsy. Radiology 1985; 155(1): 15.

378. Ludwig ME, Otis RD, Cole SR, et al. Fine needle aspiration cytology of pulmonary hamartomas. Acta Cytol 1982; 26(5): 671.

379. Ramzy I. Pulmonary hamartomas: cytologic appearances of fine needle aspiration biopsy. Acta Cytol 1976; 20(1): 15.

380. Sinner WN. Fine-needle biopsy of hamartomas of the lung. AJR Am J Roentgenol 1982; 138(1): 65.

381. Wiatrowska BA, Yazdi HM, Matzinger FR, et al. Fine needle aspiration biopsy of pulmonary hamartomas. Radiologic, cytologic and immunocytochemical study of 15 cases. Acta Cytol 1995; 39(6): 1167.

382. Zimmerman KG, Sobonya RE, Payne CM. Histochemical and ultrastructural features of an unusual pulmonary carcinosarcoma. Hum Pathol 1981; 12(11): 1046.

383. Nappi O, Glasner SD, Swanson PE, et al. Biphasic and monophasic sarcomatoid carcinomas of the lung. A reappraisal of 'carcinosarcomas' and 'spindle-cell carcinomas'. Am J Clin Pathol 1994; 102(3): 331.

384. Bergmann M, Ackerman L, Kemier R. Carcinosarcoma of the lung. Review of the literature and report of two cases treated by pneumonectomy. Cancer 1951; 4: 919.

385. Matsui K, Kitagawa M, Miwa A. Lung carcinoma with spindle cell components: sixteen cases examined by immunohistochemistry. Hum Pathol 1992; 23(11): 1289.

386. Barnard W. Embryoma of the lung. Thorax 1952; 7: 229.

387. Fung CH, Lo JW, Yonan TN, et al. Pulmonary blastoma: an ultrastructural study with a brief review of literature and a discussion of pathogenesis. Cancer 1977; 39(1): 153.

388. Koss MN, Hochholzer L, O'Leary T. Pulmonary blastomas. Cancer 1991; 67(9): 2368.

389. Siegel RJ, Bueso-Ramos C, Cohen C, et al. Pulmonary blastoma with germ cell (yolk sac) differentiation: report of two cases. Mod Pathol 1991; 4(5): 566.

390. Rossi G, Cavazza A, Sturm N, et al. Pulmonary carcinomas with pleomorphic, sarcomatoid, or sarcomatous elements: a clinicopathologic and

immunohistochemical study of 75 cases. Am J Surg Pathol 2003; 27(3): 311.

391. Sekine S, Shibata T, Matsuno Y, et al. Beta-catenin mutations in pulmonary blastomas: association with morule formation. J Pathol 2003; 200(2): 214.

392. Manivel JC, Priest JR, Watterson J, et al. Pleuropulmonary blastoma. The so-called pulmonary blastoma of childhood. Cancer 1988; 62(8): 1516.

393. Crotty TB, Myers JL, Katzenstein AL, et al. Localized malignant mesothelioma. A clinicopathologic and flow cytometric study. Am J Surg Pathol 1994; 18(4): 357.

394. L'Hoste RJ Jr, Filippa DA, Lieberman PH, et al. Primary pulmonary lymphomas. A clinicopathologic analysis of 36 cases. Cancer 1984; 54(7): 1397.

395. Isaacson P, Wright DH. Extranodal malignant lymphoma arising from mucosa-associated lymphoid tissue. Cancer 1984; 53(11): 2515.

396. Li G, Hansmann ML, Zwingers, T et al. Primary lymphomas of the lung: morphological, immunohistochemical and clinical features. Histopathology 1990; 16(6): 519.

397. Addis BJ, Hyjek E, Isaacson PG. Primary pulmonary lymphoma: a re-appraisal of its histogenesis and its relationship to pseudolymphoma and lymphoid interstitial pneumonia. Histopathology 1988; 13(1): 1.

398. Koss MN, Hochholzer L, Nichols PW, et al. Primary non-Hodgkin's lymphoma and pseudolymphoma of lung: a study of 161 patients. Hum Pathol 1983; 14(12): 1024.

399. Turner RR, Colby TV, Doggett RS. Well-differentiated lymphocytic lymphoma. A study of 47 patients with primary manifestation in the lung. Cancer 1984; 54(10): 2088.

400. Nicholson AG, Wotherspoon AC, Diss TC, et al. Pulmonary B-cell non-Hodgkin's lymphomas. The value of immunohistochemistry and gene analysis in diagnosis. Histopathology 1995; 26(5): 395.

401. Cordier JF, Chailleux E, Lauque D, et al. Primary pulmonary lymphomas. A clinical study of 70 cases in nonimmunocompromised patients. Chest 1993; 103(1): 201.

402. Kennedy JL, Nathwani BN, Burke JS, et al. Pulmonary lymphomas and other pulmonary lymphoid lesions. A clinicopathologic and immunologic study of 64 patients. Cancer 1985; 56(3): 539.

403. Herbert A, Wright DH, Isaacson PG, et al. Primary malignant lymphoma of the lung: histopathologic and immunologic evaluation of nine cases. Hum Pathol 1984; 15(5): 415.

404. Isaacson PG, Spencer J. Malignant lymphoma of mucosa-associated lymphoid tissue. Histopathology 1987; 11(5): 445.

405. Colby TV, Carrington CB. Pulmonary lymphomas: current concepts. Hum Pathol 1983; 14(10): 884.

406. Fiche M, Caprons F, Berger F, et al. Primary pulmonary non-Hodgkin's lymphomas. Histopathology 1995; 26(6): 529.

407. Wotherspoon AC, Soosay GN, Diss TC, et al. Low-grade primary B-cell lymphoma of the lung. An immunohistochemical, molecular, and cytogenetic study of a single case. Am J Clin Pathol 1990; 94(5): 655.

408. Isaacson PG, Wotherspoon AC, Diss T, et al. Follicular colonization in B-cell lymphoma of mucosa-associated lymphoid tissue. Am J Surg Pathol 1991; 15(9): 819.

409. Wotherspoon AC, Pan LX, Diss TC. et al. A genotypic study of low grade B-cell lymphomas, including lymphomas of mucosa associated lymphoid tissue (MALT). J Pathol 1990; 162(2): 135.

410. Subramanian D, Albrecht S, Gonzalez JM, et al. Primary pulmonary lymphoma. Diagnosis by immunoglobulin gene rearrangement study using a novel polymerase chain reaction technique. Am Rev Respir Dis 1993; 148(1): 222.

411. Ehya H, Patchefsky AS. Bronchus-associated lymphoid tissue (BALT) lymphoma: Diagnosis by fine

412. Kradin RL, Mark EJ. Benign lymphoid disorders of the lung, with a theory regarding their development. Hum Pathol 1983; 14(10): 857.

413. Abbondanzo SL, Rush W, Bijwaard KE, et al. Nodular lymphoid hyperplasia of the lung: a clinicopathologic study of 14 cases. Am J Surg Pathol 2000; 24(4): 587.

414. Pejaver RK, Watson AH. Castleman's disease. Respir Med 1994; 88(4): 309.

415. Bragg DG, Chor PJ, Murray KA, et al. Lymphoproliferative disorders of the lung: histopathology, clinical manifestations, and imaging features. AJR Am J Roentgenol 1994; 163(2): 273.

416. Barrie JR, English JC, Muller N. Castleman's disease of the lung: radiographic, high-resolution CT, and pathologic findings. AJR Am J Roentgenol 1996; 166(5): 1055.

417. Johkoh T, Muller NL, Ichikado K, et al. Intrathoracic multicentric Castleman disease: CT findings in 12 patients. Radiology 1998; 209(2): 477.

418. Lin P, Bueso-Ramos C, Wilson CS, et al. Waldenstrom macroglobulinemia involving extramedullary sites: morphologic and immunophenotypic findings in 44 patients. Am J Surg Pathol 2003; 27(8): 1104.

419. Koss MN. Pulmonary lymphoid disorders. Semin Diagn Pathol 1995; 12(2): 158.

420. Rush WL, Andriko JA, Taubenberger JK, et al. Primary anaplastic large cell lymphoma of the lung: a clinicopathologic study of five patients. Mod Pathol 2000; 13(12): 1285.

421. Sabourin JC, Kanavaros P, Briere J, et al. Epstein-Barr virus (EBV) genomes and EBV-encoded latent membrane protein (LMP) in pulmonary lymphomas occurring in nonimmunocompromised patients. Am J Surg Pathol 1993; 17(10): 995.

422. Yamagata T, Okamoto Y, Ota K, et al. A case of pulmonary intravascular lymphomatosis diagnosed by thoracoscopic lung biopsy. Respiration 2003; 70(4): 414.

423. Goh SG, Chuah KL, Tan PH. Intravascular lymphomatosis of the lung and liver following eyelid lymphoma in a Chinese man and review of primary pulmonary intravascular lymphomatosis. Pathology 2002; 34(1): 82.

424. Chim CS, Choy C, Ooi GC, et al. Two unusual lymphomas. Case 2: pulmonary intravascular lymphomatosis. J Clin Oncol 2000; 18(21): 3733.

425. Evert M, Lehringer-Polzin M, Mobius W, et al. Angiotropic large-cell lymphoma presenting as pulmonary small vessel occlusive disease. Hum Pathol 2000; 31(7): 879.

426. Ko YH, Han JH, Go JH, et al. Intravascular lymphomatosis: a clinicopathological study of two cases presenting as an interstitial lung disease. Histopathology 1997; 31(6): 555.

427. Wilson WH, Kingma DW, Raffeld M, et al. Association of lymphomatoid granulomatosis with Epstein-Barr viral infection of B lymphocytes and response to interferon-alpha 2b. Blood 1996; 87(11): 4531.

428. Nicholson AG, Wotherspoon AC, Diss TC, et al. Lymphomatoid granulomatosis: evidence that some cases represent Epstein-Barr virus-associated B-cell lymphoma. Histopathology 1996; 29(4): 317.

429. Myers JL, Kurtin PJ, Katzenstein AL, et al. Lymphomatoid granulomatosis. Evidence of immunophenotypic diversity and relationship to Epstein-Barr virus infection. Am J Surg Pathol 1995; 19(11): 1300.

430. Guinee D Jr, Jaffe E, Kingma D, et al. Pulmonary lymphomatoid granulomatosis. Evidence for a proliferation of Epstein-Barr virus infected B-lymphocytes with a prominent T-cell component and vasculitis. Am J Surg Pathol 1994; 18(8): 753.

431. Brousset P, Chittal SM, Schlaifer D, et al. T-cell rich B-cell lymphoma in the lung. Histopathology 1995; 26(4): 371.

432. Liebow AA, Carrington CR, Friedman PJ.

433. Saldana MJ, Patchefsky AS, Israel HI, et al. Pulmonary angiitis and granulomatosis. The relationship between histological features, organ involvement, and response to treatment. Hum Pathol 1977; 8(4): 391.

434. Donner LR, Dobin S, Harrington D, et al. Angiocentric immunoproliferative lesion (lymphomatoid granulomatosis). A cytogenetic, immunophenotypic, and genotypic study. Cancer 1990; 65(2): 249.

435. Jaffe ES. Pulmonary lymphocytic angiitis: a nosologic quandary. Mayo Clin Proc 1988; 63(4): 411.

436. Katzenstein AL, Peiper SC. Detection of Epstein-Barr virus genomes in lymphomatoid granulomatosis: analysis of 29 cases by the polymerase chain reaction technique. Mod Pathol 1990; 3(4): 435.

437. Lemieux J, Bernier V, Martel N, et al. Autologous hematopoietic stem cell transplantation for refractory lymphomatoid granulomatosis. Hematology 2002; 7(6): 355.

438. Baldi A, Groeger AM, Esposito V, et al. Lymphomatoid granulomatosis of the lung: a clinico-pathological study. Anticancer Res 1998; 18(6B): 4621.

439. Raez LE, Temple JD, Saldana M. Successful treatment of lymphomatoid granulomatosis using cyclosporin-A after failure of intensive chemotherapy. Am J Hematol 1996; 53(3): 192.

440. Loke SL, Ho F, Srivastava G, et al. Clonal Epstein-Barr virus genome in T-cell-rich lymphomas of B or probable B lineage. Am J Pathol 1992; 140(4): 981.

441. Radin AI. Primary pulmonary Hodgkin's disease. Cancer 1990; 65(3): 550.

442. Yousem SA, Weiss LM, Colby TV. Primary pulmonary Hodgkin's disease. A clinicopathologic study of 15 cases. Cancer 1986; 57(6): 1217.

443. Guinee DG Jr, Perkins SL, Travis WD, et al. Proliferation and cellular phenotype in lymphomatoid granulomatosis: implications of a higher proliferation index in B cells. Am J Surg Pathol 1998; 22(9): 1093.

444. Dong HY, Harris NL, Preffer FI, et al. Fine-needle aspiration biopsy in the diagnosis and classification of primary and recurrent lymphoma: a retrospective analysis of the utility of cytomorphology and flow cytometry. Mod Pathol 2001; 14(5): 472.

445. Young NA, Al-Saleem TI, Ehya H, et al. Utilization of fine-needle aspiration cytology and flow cytometry in the diagnosis and subclassification of primary and recurrent lymphoma. Cancer 1998; 84(4): 252.

446. Young NA, Al-Saleem T. Diagnosis of lymphoma by fine-needle aspiration cytology using the revised European-American classification of lymphoid neoplasms. Cancer 1999; 87(6): 325.

447. Zaer FS, Braylan RC, Zander DS, et al. Multiparametric flow cytometry in the diagnosis and characterization of low-grade pulmonary mucosa-associated lymphoid tissue lymphomas. Mod Pathol 1998; 11(6): 525.

448. Sgrignoli A, Abati A. Cytologic diagnosis of anaplastic large cell lymphoma. Acta Cytol 1997; 41(4): 1048.

449. Reyes CV, Jensen JA, Chinoy M. Pulmonary lymphoma in cardiac transplant patients treated with OKT3 for rejection: diagnosis by fine-needle aspiration. Diagn Cytopathol 1995; 12(1): 32.

450. Kuruvilla S, Gomathy DV, Shanthi DV, et al. Primary pulmonary lymphoma. Report of a case diagnosed by fine needle aspiration cytology. Acta Cytol 1994; 38(4): 601.

451. Collins BT. Cavitary lung mass representing primary pulmonary malignant lymphoma with initial diagnosis by fine needle aspiration biopsy. Acta Cytol 2001; 45(5): 901.

452. Gattuso P, Castelli MJ, Peng Y, et al. Posttransplant lymphoproliferative disorders: a fine-needle aspiration biopsy study. Diagn Cytopathol 1997; 16(5): 392.

453. Sprague RI, deBlois GG. Small lymphocytic

pulmonary lymphoma. Diagnosis by transthoracic fine needle aspiration. Chest 1989; 96(4): 929.

454. Zakowski MF, Feiner H, Finfer M, et al. Cytology of extranodal Ki-1 anaplastic large cell lymphoma. Diagn Cytopathol 1996; 14(2): 155.

455. Godwin JD 2nd, Brown CC. Comparative epidemiology of carcinoid and oat-cell tumors of the lung. Cancer 1977; 40(4): 1671.

456. Farhangi M, Taylor J, Havey A, et al. Neuroendocrine (carcinoid) tumor of the lung and type I multiple endocrine neoplasia. South Med J 1987; 80(11): 1459.

457. Snyder N 3rd, Scurry MT, Deiss WP. Five families with multiple endocrine adenomatosis. Ann Intern Med 1972; 76(1): 53.

458. Gould VE, Linnoila RI, Memoli VA, et al. Neuroendocrine components of the bronchopulmonary tract: hyperplasias, dysplasias, and neoplasms. Lab Invest 1983; 49(5): 519.

459. Limper AH, Carpenter PC, Scheithauer B, et al. The Cushing syndrome induced by bronchial carcinoid tumors. Ann Intern Med 1992; 117(3): 209.

460. Davila DG, Dunn WF, Tazelaar HD, et al. Bronchial carcinoid tumors. Mayo Clin Proc 1993; 68(8): 795.

461. Briselli M, Mark GJ, Grillo HC. Tracheal carcinoids. Cancer 1978; 42(6): 2870.

462. Marchevsky AM, Gal AA, Shah S, et al. Morphometry confirms the presence of considerable nuclear size overlap between "small cells" and "large cells" in high-grade pulmonary neuroendocrine neoplasms. Am J Clin Pathol 2001; 116(4): 466.

463. Mark EJ, Quay SC, Dickersin GR. Papillary carcinoid tumor of the lung. Cancer 1981; 48(2): 316.

464. Pilotti S, Rilke F, Lombardi L. Pulmonary carcinoid with glandular features. Report of two cases with positive fine needle aspiration biopsy cytology. Acta Cytol 1983; 27(5): 511.

465. Isaacson P. Crypt cell carcinoma of the appendix (so-called adenocarcinoid tumor). Am J Surg Pathol 1981; 5(3): 213.

466. Geller SA, Gordon RE. Peripheral spindle-cell carcinoid tumor of the lung with type II pneumocyte features. An ultrastructural study with comments on possible histogenesis. Am J Surg Pathol 1984; 8(2): 145.

467. Gal AA, Koss MN, Hochholzer L, et al. Pigmented pulmonary carcinoid tumor. An immunohistochemical and ultrastructural study. Arch Pathol Lab Med 1993; 117(8): 832.

468. Grazer R, Cohen SM, Jacobs JB, et al. Melanin-containing peripheral carcinoid of the lung. Am J Surg Pathol 1982; 6(1): 73.

469. Barbareschi M, Frigo B, Mosca L, et al. Bronchial carcinoids with S-100 positive sustentacular cells. A comparative study with gastrointestinal carcinoids, pheochromocytomas and paragangliomas. Pathol Res Pract 1990; 186(2): 212.

470. Linnoila RI, Mulshine JL, Steinberg SM, et al. Neuroendocrine differentiation in endocrine and nonendocrine lung carcinomas. Am J Clin Pathol 1988; 90(6): 641.

471. Said JW, Vimadalal S, Nash G, et al. Immunoreactive neuron-specific enolase, bombesin, and chromogranin as markers for neuroendocrine lung tumors. Hum Pathol 1985; 16(3): 236.

472. Gould VE. Synaptophysin. A new and promising pan-neuroendocrine marker. Arch Pathol Lab Med 1987; 111(9): 791.

473. Blobel GA, Gould VE, Moll R, et al. Coexpression of neuroendocrine markers and epithelial cytoskeletal proteins in bronchopulmonary neuroendocrine neoplasms. Lab Invest 1985; 52(1): 39.

474. Bishopric GA Jr, Ordonez NG. Carcinoembryonic antigen in primary carcinoid tumors of the lung. Cancer 1986; 58(6): 1316.

475. Mackay B, Osborne B, Wilson R. Ultrastructure of lung neoplasms. In: Strauss M, ed. Lung cancer. New York: Grune and Stratton; 1997: 71.

476. Ranchod M, Levine GD. Spindle-cell carcinoid tumors of the lung: a clinicopathologic study of 35 cases. Am J Surg Pathol 1980; 4(4): 315.

477. Miller MA, Mark GJ, Kanarek D. Multiple peripheral pulmonary carcinoids and tumorlets of carcinoid type, with restrictive and obstructive lung disease. Am J Med 1978; 65(2): 373.

478. Skinner C, Ewen SW. Carcinoid lung: diffuse pulmonary infiltration by a multifocal bronchial carcinoid. Thorax 1976; 31(2): 212.

479. D'Agati VD, Perzin KH. Carcinoid tumorlets of the lung with metastasis to a peribronchial lymph node. Report of a case and review of the literature. Cancer 1985; 55(10): 2472.

480. Lozowski W, Hajdu SI, Melamed MR. Cytomorphology of carcinoid tumors. Acta Cytol 1979; 23(5): 360.

481. Szyfelbein WM, Ross JS. Carcinoids, atypical carcinoids, and small-cell carcinomas of the lung: differential diagnosis of fine-needle aspiration biopsy specimens. Diagn Cytopathol 1988; 4(1): 1.

482. Kyriakos M, Rockoff SD. Brush biopsy of bronchial carcinoid – a source of cytologic error. Acta Cytol 1972; 16(3): 261.

483. Lin O, Olgac S, Green I, et al. Immunohistochemical staining of cytologic smears with MIB-1 helps distinguish low-grade from high-grade neuroendocrine neoplasms. Am J Clin Pathol 2003; 120(2): 209.

484. Schreurs AJ, Westermann CJ, van den Bosch JM, et al. A twenty-five-year follow-up of ninety-three resected typical carcinoid tumors of the lung. J Thorac Cardiovasc Surg 1992; 104(5): 1470.

485. McCaughan BC, Martini N, Bains MS. Bronchial carcinoids. Review of 124 cases. J Thorac Cardiovasc Surg 1985; 89(1): 8.

486. Arrigoni MG, Woolner LB, Bernatz PE. Atypical carcinoid tumors of the lung. J Thorac Cardiovasc Surg 1972; 64(3): 413.

487. Carter D, Yesner R. Carcinomas of the lung with neuroendocrine differentiation. Semin Diagn Pathol 1985; 2(4): 235.

488. DeCaro LF, Paladugu R, Benfield JR, et al. Typical and atypical carcinoids within the pulmonary APUD tumor spectrum. J Thorac Cardiovasc Surg 1983; 86(4): 528.

489. Paladugu RR, Benfield JR, Pak HY, et al. Bronchopulmonary Kulchitzky cell carcinomas. A new classification scheme for typical and atypical carcinoids. Cancer 1985; 55(6): 1303.

490. Grote TH, Macon WR, Davis B, et al. Atypical carcinoid of the lung. A distinct clinicopathologic entity. Chest 1988; 93(2): 370.

491. Travis WD, Rush W, Flieder DB, et al. Survival analysis of 200 pulmonary neuroendocrine tumors with clarification of criteria for atypical carcinoid and its separation from typical carcinoid. Am J Surg Pathol 1998; 22(8): 934.

492. Costes V, Marty-Ane C, Picot MC, et al. Typical and atypical bronchopulmonary carcinoid tumors: a clinicopathologic and KI-67-labeling study. Hum Pathol 1995; 26(7): 740.

493. Mills SE, Cooper PH, Walker AN, et al. Atypical carcinoid tumor of the lung. A clinicopathologic study of 17 cases. Am J Surg Pathol 1982; 6(7): 643.

494. Valli M, Fabris GA, Dewar A, et al. Atypical carcinoid tumour of the lung: a study of 33 cases with prognostic features. Histopathology 1994; 24(4): 363.

495. Frierson HF Jr, Covell JL, Mills SE. Fine needle aspiration cytology of atypical carcinoid of the lung. Acta Cytol 1987; 31(4): 471.

496. Jordan AG, Predmore L, Sullivan MM, et al. The cytodiagnosis of well-differentiated neuroendocrine carcinoma. A distinct clinicopathologic entity. Acta Cytol 1987; 31(4): 464.

497. Travis WD, Linnoila RI, Tsokos MG, et al. Neuroendocrine tumors of the lung with proposed criteria for large-cell neuroendocrine carcinoma. An ultrastructural, immunohistochemical, and flow cytometric study of 35 cases. Am J Surg Pathol 1991; 15(6): 529.

498. Hammond ME, Sause WT. Large cell neuroendocrine tumors of the lung. Clinical significance and histopathologic definition. Cancer 1985; 56(7): 1624.

499. Brambilla E, Negoescu A, Gazzeri S, et al. Apoptosis-related factors p53, Bcl2, and Bax in neuroendocrine lung tumors. Am J Pathol 1996; 149(6): 1941.

500. Yousem SA, Taylor SR. Typical and atypical carcinoid tumors of lung: a clinicopathologic and DNA analysis of 20 tumors. Mod Pathol 1990; 3(4): 502.

501. Larsimont D, Kiss R, de Launoit Y, et al. Characterization of the morphonuclear features and DNA ploidy of typical and atypical carcinoids and small cell carcinomas of the lung. Am J Clin Pathol 1990; 94(4): 378.

502. el-Naggar AK, Ballance W, Karim FW, et al. Typical and atypical bronchopulmonary carcinoids. A clinicopathologic and flow cytometric study. Am J Clin Pathol 1991; 95(6): 828.

503. Wiatrowska BA, Krol J, Zakowski MF. Large-cell neuroendocrine carcinoma of the lung: proposed criteria for cytologic diagnosis. Diagn Cytopathol 2001; 24(1): 58.

504. Azzopardi JG. Oat-cell carcinoma of the bronchus. J Pathol Bacteriol 1959; 78: 513.

505. Fox W, Scadding JG. Medical Research Council comparative trial of surgery and radiotherapy for primary treatment of small-celled or oat-celled carcinoma of bronchus. Ten-year follow-up. Lancet 1973; 2(7820): 63.

506. Auerbach O, Garfinkel L, Parks VR. Histologic type of lung cancer in relation to smoking habits, year of diagnosis and sites of metastases. Chest 1975; 67(4): 382.

507. Huhti E, Sutinen S, Reinila A, et al. Lung cancer in a defined geographical area: history and histological types. Thorax 1980; 35(9): 660.

508. Morabia A, Wynder EL. Cigarette smoking and lung cancer cell types. Cancer 1991; 68(9): 2074.

509. Land CE, Shimosato Y, Saccomanno G, et al. Radiation-associated lung cancer: a comparison of the histology of lung cancers in uranium miners and survivors of the atomic bombings of Hiroshima and Nagasaki. Radiat Res 1993; 134(2): 234.

510. Saccomanno G, Auerbach O, Kuschner M, et al. A comparison between the localization of lung tumors in uranium miners and in nonminers from 1947 to 1991. Cancer 1996; 77(7): 1278.

511. Weiss W, Moser RL, Auerbach O. Lung cancer in chloromethyl ether workers. Am Rev Respir Dis 1979; 120(5): 1031.

512. Kreisman H, Wolkove N, Quoix E. Small cell lung cancer presenting as a solitary pulmonary nodule. Chest 1992; 101(1): 225.

513. Cerilli LA, Ritter JH, Mills SE, et al. Neuroendocrine neoplasms of the lung. Am J Clin Pathol 2001; 116 Suppl: S65.

514. Kreyberg L. Main histological types of primary epithelial lung tumours. Br J Cancer 1961; 15: 206.

515. Kreyberg L. Histological typing of lung tumours. Geneva: WHO (World Health Organization); 1967.

516. The World Health Organization histological typing of lung tumours. 2nd edn. Am J Clin Pathol 1982; 77(2): 123.

517. Warren WH, Memoli VA, Jordan AG, et al. Reevaluation of pulmonary neoplasms resected as small cell carcinomas. Significance of distinguishing between well-differentiated and small cell neuroendocrine carcinomas. Cancer 1990; 65(4): 1003.

518. Wick MR. Neuroendocrine neoplasia. Current concepts. Am J Clin Pathol 2000; 113(3): 331.

519. Haruki N, Yatabe Y, Travis WD, et al. Characterization of high-grade neuroendocrine tumors of the lung in relation to menin mutations. Jpn J Cancer Res 2000; 91(3): 317.

520. Walch AK, Zitzelsberger HF, Aubele MM, et al. Typical and atypical carcinoid tumors of the lung are characterized by 11q deletions as detected by comparative genomic hybridization. Am J Pathol 1998; 153(4): 1089.

521. Debelenko LV, Swalwell JI, Kelley MJ, et al. MEN1 gene mutation analysis of high-grade neuroendocrine lung carcinoma. Genes Chromosomes Cancer 2000; 28(1): 58.

522. Helpap B, Kollermann J. Immunohistochemical analysis of the proliferative activity of neuroendocrine tumors from various organs. Are there indications for a neuroendocrine tumor-carcinoma sequence? Virchows Arch 2001; 438(1): 86.

523. Hirsch FR, Matthews MJ, Aisner S, et al. Histopathologic classification of small cell lung cancer. Changing concepts and terminology. Cancer 1988; 62(5): 973.

524. Fraire AE, Johnson EH, Yesner R, et al. Prognostic significance of histopathologic subtype and stage in small cell lung cancer. Hum Pathol 1992; 23(5): 520.

525. Gazdar A, Carney D, Baylin SB. Small cell carcinoma of the lung. Altered morphological, biological and biochemical characteristics in long term cultures and heterotransplanted tumors. Proc Am Assoc Cancer Res 1980; 21: 51.

526. Gazdar A. Endocrine tumors of the lung: biology. In: Becker K, Gasdar A, eds. The endocrine lung in health and disease. Philadelphia: WB Saunders; 1984: 546.

527. de Leij L, Postmus PE, Buys CH, et al. Characterization of three new variant type cell lines derived from small cell carcinoma of the lung. Cancer Res 1985; 45: 6024.

528. Mangum MD, Greco FA, Hainsworth JD, et al. Combined small-cell and non-small-cell lung cancer. J Clin Oncol 1989; 7(5): 607.

529. Abeloff MD, Eggleston JC, Mendelsohn G, et al. Changes in morphologic and biochemical characteristics of small cell carcinoma of the lung. A clinicopathologic study. Am J Med 1979; 66(5): 757.

530. Matthews MJ. Effects of therapy on the behavior and morphology of small cell carcinoma of the lung. Prog Cancer Res Ther 1979; 11: 155.

531. Nicholson SA, Beasley MB, Brambilla E, et al. Small cell lung carcinoma (SCLC): a clinicopathologic study of 100 cases with surgical specimens. Am J Surg Pathol 2002; 26(9): 1184.

532. Mackay B, Ordonez NG, Bennington JL, et al. Ultrastructural and morphometric features of poorly differentiated and undifferentiated lung tumors. Ultrastruct Pathol 1989; 13(5-6): 561.

533. Shy SW, Lee WH, Chou MC, et al. Small cell lung carcinoma: clinicopathological, immunohistochemical, and ultrastructural study. J Surg Oncol 1990; 45(3): 146.

534. Guinee DG Jr, Fishback NF, Koss MN, et al. The spectrum of immunohistochemical staining of small-cell lung carcinoma in specimens from transbronchial and open-lung biopsies. Am J Clin Pathol 1994; 102(4): 406.

535. Komminoth P, Roth J, Lackie PM, et al. Polysialic acid of the neural cell adhesion molecule distinguishes small cell lung carcinoma from carcinoids. Am J Pathol 1991; 139(2): 297.

536. Wu M, Wang B, Gil J, et al. p63 and TTF-1 immunostaining. A useful marker panel for distinguishing small cell carcinoma of lung from poorly differentiated squamous cell carcinoma of lung. Am J Clin Pathol 2003; 119(5): 696.

537. Sturm N, Rossi G, Lantuejoul S, et al. Expression of thyroid transcription factor-1 in the spectrum of neuroendocrine cell lung proliferations with special interest in carcinoids. Hum Pathol 2002; 33(2): 175.

538. Folpe AL, Gown AM, Lamps LW, et al. Thyroid transcription factor-1: immunohistochemical evaluation in pulmonary neuroendocrine tumors. Mod Pathol 1999; 12(1): 5.

539. Cheuk W, Chan JK. Thyroid transcription factor-1 is of limited value in practical distinction between pulmonary and extrapulmonary small cell carcinomas. Am J Surg Pathol 2001; 25(4): 545.

540. Cheuk W, Kwan MY, Suster S, et al. Immunostaining for thyroid transcription factor 1 and cytokeratin 20 aids the distinction of small cell carcinoma from Merkel cell carcinoma, but not pulmonary from extrapulmonary small cell carcinomas. Arch Pathol Lab Med 2001; 125(2): 228.

541. Katsetos CD, Kontogeorgos G, Geddes JF, et al. Differential distribution of the neuron-associated class III beta-tubulin in neuroendocrine lung tumors. Arch Pathol Lab Med 2000; 124(4): 535.

542. Tabatowski K, Vollmer RT, Tello JW, et al. The use of a panel of monoclonal antibodies in ultrastructurally characterized small cell carcinomas of the lung. Acta Cytol 1988; 32(5): 667.

543. Edelman MJ, Chansky K, Gaspar LE, et al. Phase II trial of cisplatin/etoposide and concurrent radiotherapy followed by paclitaxel/carboplatin consolidation for limited small-cell lung cancer: Southwest Oncology Group 9713. J Clin Oncol 2004; 22(1): 127.

544. Chak LY, Daniels JR, Sikic BI, et al. Patterns of failure in small cell carcinoma of the lung. Cancer 1982; 50(9): 1857.

545. Quoix E, Fraser R, Wolkove N, et al. Small cell lung cancer presenting as a solitary pulmonary nodule. Cancer 1990; 66(3): 577.

546. Spira A, Ettinger DS. Extensive-stage small-cell lung cancer. Semin Surg Oncol 2003; 21(3): 164.

547. Zimmermann FB, Bamberg M, Molls M, et al. Limited-disease small-cell lung cancer. Semin Surg Oncol 2003; 21(3): 156.

548. Virtanen C, Ishikawa Y, Honjoh D, et al. Integrated classification of lung tumors and cell lines by expression profiling. Proc Natl Acad Sci USA 2002; 99(19): 12357.

549. Onuki N, Wistuba, II, Travis WD, et al. Genetic changes in the spectrum of neuroendocrine lung tumors. Cancer 1999; 85(3): 600.

550. Ullmann R, Petzmann S, Klemen H, et al. The position of pulmonary carcinoids within the spectrum of neuroendocrine tumors of the lung and other tissues. Genes Chromosomes Cancer 2002; 34(1): 78.

551. Sampietro G, Tomasic G, Collini P, et al. Gene product immunophenotyping of neuroendocrine lung tumors. No linking evidence between carcinoids and small-cell lung carcinomas suggested by multivariate statistical analysis. Appl Immunohistochem Mol Morphol 2000; 8(1): 49.

552. Przygodzki RM, Finkelstein SD, Langer JC, et al. Analysis of p53, K-ras-2, and C-raf-1 in pulmonary neuroendocrine tumors. Correlation with histological subtype and clinical outcome. Am J Pathol 1996; 148(5): 1531.

553. Cagle PT, el-Naggar AK, Xu HJ, et al. Differential retinoblastoma protein expression in neuroendocrine tumors of the lung. Potential diagnostic implications. Am J Pathol 1997; 150(2): 393.

554. Anbazhagan R, Tihan T, Bornman DM, et al. Classification of small cell lung cancer and pulmonary carcinoid by gene expression profiles. Cancer Res 1999; 59(20): 5119.

555. Kovatich A, Friedland DM, Druck T, et al. Molecular alterations to human chromosome 3p loci in neuroendocrine lung tumors. Cancer 1998; 83(6): 1109.

556. Ullmann R, Petzmann S, Sharma A, et al. Chromosomal aberrations in a series of large-cell neuroendocrine carcinomas: unexpected divergence from small-cell carcinoma of the lung. Hum Pathol 2001; 32(10): 1059.

557. Askin FB, Rosai J, Sibley RK, et al. Malignant small cell tumor of the thoracopulmonary region in childhood: a distinctive clinicopathologic entity of uncertain histogenesis. Cancer 1979; 43(6): 2438.

558. Contesso G, Llombart-Bosch A, Terrier P, et al. Does malignant small round cell tumor of the thoracopulmonary region (Askin tumor) constitute a clinicopathologic entity? An analysis of 30 cases with immunohistochemical and electron-microscopic support treated at the Institute Gustave Roussy. Cancer 1992; 69(4): 1012.

559. Fuzesi L, Heller R, Schreiber H, et al. Cytogenetics of Askin's tumour. Case report and review of the literature. Pathol Res Pract 1993; 189(2): 235.

560. Baumgartner FJ, Omari BO, French SW. Primitive neuroectodermal tumor of the pulmonary hilum in an adult. Ann Thorac Surg 2001; 72(1): 285.

561. Imamura F, Funakoshi T, Nakamura S, et al. Primary primitive neuroectodermal tumor of the lung: report of two cases. Lung Cancer 2000; 27(1): 55.

562. Mikami Y, Nakajima M, Hashimoto H, et al. Primary pulmonary primitive neuroectodermal tumor (PNET). A case report. Pathol Res Pract 2001; 197(2): 113.

563. Tsuji S, Hisaoka M, Morimitsu Y, et al. Peripheral primitive neuroectodermal tumour of the lung: report of two cases. Histopathology 1998; 33(4): 369.

564. Goldstein NS, Thomas M. Mucinous and nonmucinous bronchioloalveolar adenocarcinomas have distinct staining patterns with thyroid transcription factor and cytokeratin 20 antibodies. Am J Clin Pathol 2001; 116: 319–325.

565. Nambu Y, Iannettoni MD, Orringer MB, et al. Unique expression patterns and alterations in the intestinal protein villin in primary and metastatic pulmonary adenocarcinomas. Mol Carcinog 1998; 23(4): 234.

566. Cameron RI, Ashe P, O'Rourke DM, et al. A panel of immunohistochemical stains assists in the distinction between ovarian and renal clear cell carcinoma. Int J Gynecol Pathol. 2003; 22: 272.

19

Pleura, pericardium, and peritoneum

Victor L. Roggli   Philip Cagle

THE PLEURA

ANATOMY, DEVELOPMENT AND NORMAL FUNCTION

The pleura is a continuous membrane that covers the pleural cavities. The parietal pleura covers the chest wall, diaphragm, and mediastinal structures. The visceral pleura covers the entire pulmonary surface.[1] The visceral and parietal pleura are connected at the pulmonary hilum. Histologically, a single layer of low cuboidal to flattened mesothelial cells lines the pleura. These cells have abundant eosinophilic cytoplasm, well-defined cell borders, and small, centrally located nuclei with a homogeneous chromatin pattern. Ultrastructurally, mesothelial cells are characterized by the presence of long surface microvilli measuring up to 3 μm in length and 0.1 μm in diameter.[1] The cells are connected by tight junctions and abundant desmosomes, and the cytoplasm contains ribosomes, rough endoplasmic reticulum, mitochondria, and intermediate filaments. The latter are usually arranged in a perinuclear distribution.[1]

The submesothelial layer of the pleura consists of collagen, elastin, and subserosal cells that have morphologic and ultrastructural features of fibroblasts.[1] Mesothelial cells produce glycosaminoglycans, primarily hyaluronic acid, thought to be important in the normal lubricating function of the pleura. Mesothelial cells contain abundant cytokeratins and may express the intermediate filament vimentin, which may be detected immunohistochemically. Nonproliferating submesothelial cells contain vimentin but lack cytokeratins. However, in reactive processes, these cells may also express low molecular weight cytokeratins, suggesting their potential for mesothelial cell differentiation.[2]

The parietal pleura receives its blood supply from the systemic circulation, and the visceral pleura is supplied by the pulmonary and bronchial arterial systems.[1] Pleural membranes are a selective barrier for cellular elements and fluids. Stomata in the parietal pleura result in direct continuity between the mesothelium and underlying lymphatic vessels. A variety of pathologic processes may alter the permeability of the pleural surface, which may in turn result in pleural effusion (i.e. accumulation of fluid within the pleural space).[1]

DIAGNOSTIC SPECIMENS

Cope needle biopsy

The Cope needle biopsy or closed pleural biopsy is the usual method used by pulmonologists to obtain biopsy specimens of the parietal pleura. This procedure produces a core biopsy specimen that can then be examined histologically, histochemically, immunohistochemically, or ultrastructurally. Importantly, such specimens also allow assessment of invasion when one is trying to determine the presence of malignancy. Because this is a blind procedure, diagnostic material may or may not be obtained. If diagnostic material is obtained, an accurate diagnosis is possible in a large percentage of cases. Nonetheless, it is the authors' experience that needle biopsy of the pleura is only occasionally sufficient to make an unequivocal premortem diagnosis of malignant mesothelioma.[3]

Thoracoscopic biopsy

Thoracoscopic biopsies are obtained by direct inspection of the pleura through the pleuroscope or thoracoscope. Consequently, such biopsies provide in most instances a sufficient diagnostic sample.[4] The procedure is less invasive than an open biopsy and the hospital stay is on average less than that of patients who have had a thoracotomy. The accuracy of diagnosis is reported to be very high among patients with malignant mesothelioma.[4]

Open biopsy

An open pleural biopsy is obtained by direct inspection of the pleural space by the surgeon during a thoracotomy. The superior visualization allows for a more thorough sampling of the pleura and, at least theoretically, a more accurate diagnosis. The amount of material available provides the opportunity for a wide range of ancillary diagnostic tests, including immunohistochemical and ultrastructural studies. In practice, however, it is the authors' experience that both thoracoscopic and open biopsies provide adequate material for diagnosis in the vast majority of cases. When thoracoscopic visualization is inadequate, the surgeon typically converts to a thoracotomy so that adequate material is obtained. In those rare cases where inadequate material is obtained by thoracoscopy, additional samples may be obtained by thoracotomy.

Valuable information may also be obtained from cytologic preparations such as smears, cytospins, cell blocks, or fine needle aspirations (FNA).[4–7] In addition to routine cytologic evaluation, immunocytochemical, flow cytometric, and molecular biologic studies can be performed on cytologic specimens. The reported accuracy of FNA in the diagnosis of malignant pleural mesothelioma varies from 39% to 73%.[6,7] The diagnostic accuracy is greater when a core sample is obtained. It should be noted that assessment of invasion is crucial to the accurate diagnosis of mesothelioma.[8] Therefore, the authors do not recommend the use of cytologic specimens for the diagnosis of mesothelioma.[9]

NON-NEOPLASTIC PLEURAL DISEASES

Inflammation

Inflammation of the pleura is usually a consequence of inflammation of the subjacent lung. The morphologic features range from acute inflammation to chronic non-specific inflammation to granulomatous inflammation. Granulomatous inflammation may be seen in patients with mycobacterial or fungal infections of the pleura.[10] These are particularly common in immunocompromised patients, especially among patients with the acquired immunodeficiency syndrome.[11] A granulomatous foreign body reaction occurs following talc pleurodesis. Granulomatous inflammation of the pleura is rarely caused by sarcoidosis.[12] Collagen vascular diseases such as lupus erythematosus and rheumatoid arthritis may also result in pleural effusion and reactive changes in the pleura.[13,14] Reactive eosinophilic pleuritis is an unusual variant of pleural inflammation that is associated with pneumothorax. It is characterized by infiltrates of histiocytes and eosinophils in the pleura and must be distinguished from pulmonary Langerhans cell histiocytosis (eosinophilic granuloma).[15]

Reactive mesothelial hyperplasia

Mesothelial hyperplasia occurs as a response to injury to the serosal membranes. In some cases, the response can be quite pronounced and must be distinguished from a malignant process. Reactive mesothelium can show marked cytologic atypia and pleomorphism (Fig. 19.1). Mitotic figures may be present. On the other hand, the tumor cells within a mesothelioma may be quite bland. The single most useful feature for distinguishing reactive mesothelium from mesothelioma or a well-differentiated adenocarcinoma involving the pleura is the presence of invasion.[8] This may be difficult to identify on a needle biopsy and is especially problematic in cytologic preparations, in which features such as the pattern of infiltration and stromal invasion cannot be determined.

Histochemical and immunohistochemical studies are of little help in distinguishing reactive atypical mesothelial proliferations from neoplastic processes, since the basic immunophenotype of reactive mesothelial cells is essentially identical to that of epithelial mesothelioma.[8,16] Several studies have reported on markers that might be useful in this regard, such as nucleolar organizer regions (AgNORs),[17] p53 protein,[18,19] platelet-derived growth factor (PDGF),[20] p-170 glycoprotein, bcl-2,[21] and epithelial membrane antigen.[22] None of these has been accepted as a reliable marker of malignancy, and considerably more work is needed in this diagnostically difficult area. In some cases, keratin immunostaining may demonstrate subtle invasion of adipose tissue by tumor cells, an indicator that the process is malignant.[8]

Parietal pleural plaque

Pleural plaques are localized scars, typically located on the parietal pleura, often on the surface of the diaphragm or posterolaterally, running along the direction of the ribs.[23] They are firm, sharply circumscribed, raised, and ivory colored. Their surface may be either smooth or knobby, resembling 'candle wax' drippings (Fig. 19.2). They are often calcified and are associated with asbestos exposure in the vast majority of cases. Histologically, plaques consist of layers of acellular hyalinized collagen arranged in a 'basket-weave' pattern (Fig. 19.3). Plaques are relatively acellular, although a focal collection of lymphocytes is often seen at the interface between the plaque and adipose tissue of the chest wall. Plaques should be distinguished from localized fibrous tumors and the desmoplastic variant of malignant mesothelioma.

Diffuse visceral pleural fibrosis

Diffuse pleural fibrosis typically involves the visceral pleura and may occur as a consequence of a variety of clinical conditions, including infections, collagen vascular disorders, drug-induced reactions, and exposure to asbestos.[23] The antecedent process is

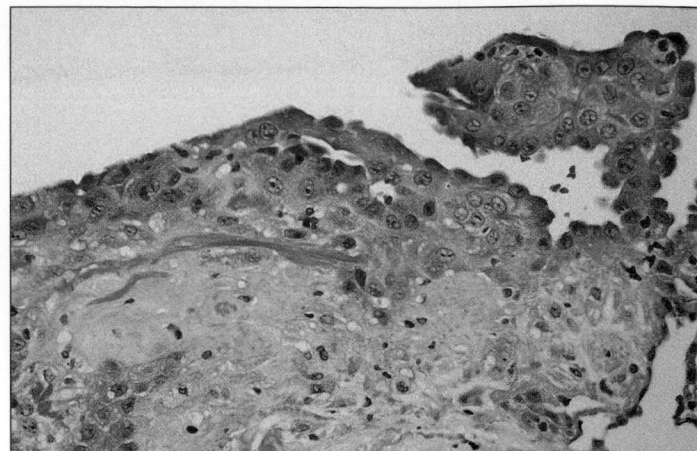

Fig. 19.1 Atypical mesothelial hyperplasia with focal papillary formation. Note prominent nucleoli. (H&E)

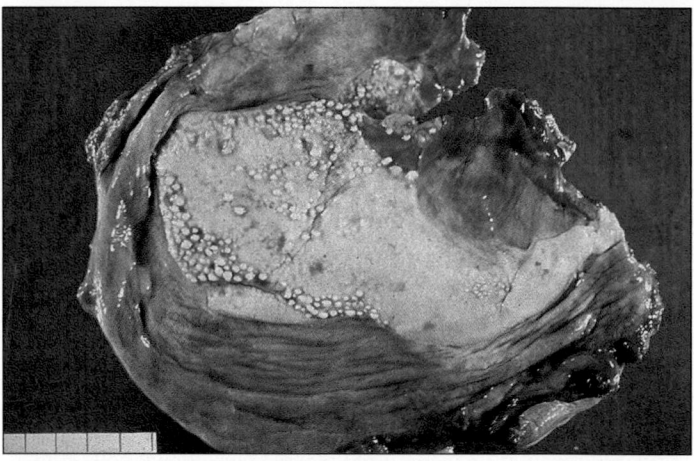

Fig. 19.2 Parietal pleural plaque on surface of diaphragm. Plaque is sharply circumscribed, tan, and focally nodular, giving a 'candle-wax dripping' appearance.

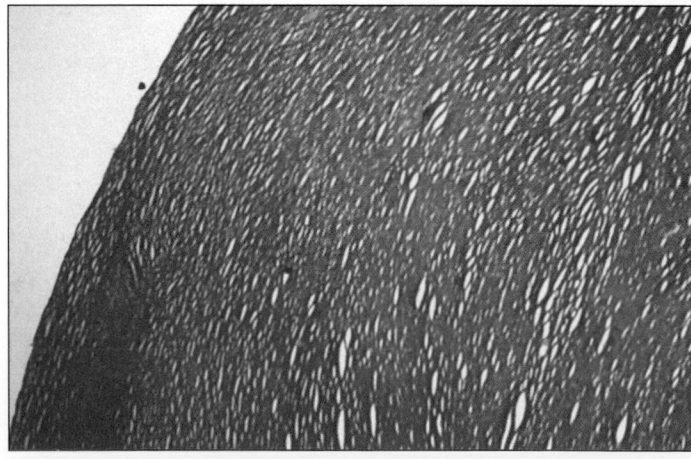

Fig. 19.3 Histology of parietal pleural plaque, which is composed of layers of acellular hyalinized collagen arranged in a 'basket-weave' pattern.

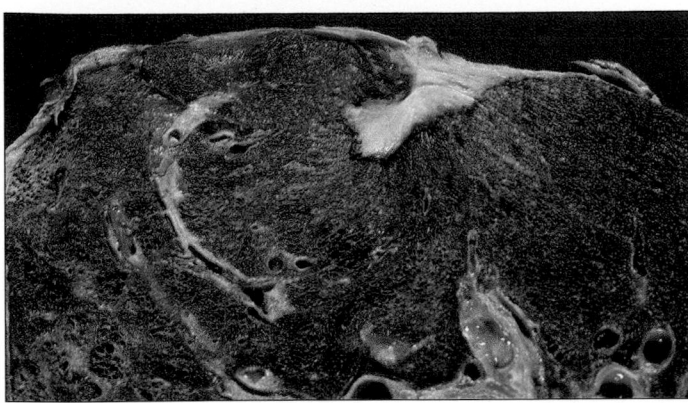

Fig. 19.4 Rounded atelectasis in a patient who received radiation for Hodgkin's disease. There is pleural thickening with buckling into the lung parenchyma. The adjacent lung is atelectatic.

believed to be a chronic exudative pleural effusion that has undergone organization. The histologic pattern is non-specific regardless of the etiology. Early lesions show reactive mesothelial cell proliferation and inflammation. Later lesions show diffuse uniform fibrotic thickening of the visceral pleura. In advanced cases, a fibrothorax may develop resulting in a 'trapped lung' and restrictive pulmonary physiology.[24] Tuberculosis formerly was a common cause of fibrothorax. Chronic empyema, asbestos-induced diffuse pleural fibrosis, and organized hemothorax may all result in fibrothorax.[24]

Rounded atelectasis

Rounded atelectasis, also known as folded lung or Blesovsky's syndrome, is a localized area of atelectatic lung parenchyma that has been entrapped by an overlying focus of fibrotic visceral pleura (Fig. 19.4).[23] These lesions typically occur posteriorly and may be bilateral. Most cases are caused by exposure to asbestos, but rare cases may be related to hemothorax, pleural infection, uremia, or radiation.[25] Rounded atelectasis has a distinctive radiographic appearance, and can occasionally be mistaken clinically for a neoplasm.[26]

Amyloidosis

Pleural involvement is rarely seen in amyloidosis, and may be associated with the development of a pleural effusion.[27] Involvement of the underlying lung parenchyma with diffuse interstitial amyloidosis usually coexists. The diagnosis may be made by Cope needle biopsy with appropriate ancillary studies (e.g. Congo red stain, electron microscopy).

NEOPLASTIC PLEURAL DISEASES

Primary pleural neoplasms

The most common primary pleural neoplasm is diffuse malignant mesothelioma. This tumor must be distinguished from several other less common diffuse primary pleural malignancies as well as malignancies that involve the pleura secondarily. In addition, mesothelioma must be distinguished from a number of localized pleural tumors with which it may be confused, especially in small biopsy specimens.

Malignant mesothelioma

Malignant pleural mesothelioma is a relatively rare neoplasm that has received a great deal of attention because of its relationship to occupational and environmental exposure to asbestos. Because of these medicolegal implications, much effort has been expended to improve the diagnostic accuracy of this disease. Distinguishing mesothelioma from other histologically similar tumors involving the pleura may be extremely difficult based on traditional morphologic features. Consequently, numerous studies have reported on histochemical, immunohistochemical, and ultrastructural features that permit an accurate premortem diagnosis of malignant mesothelioma.

Epidemiology and pathogenesis

The relationship between asbestos exposure and the subsequent development of malignant pleural mesothelioma has been established in epidemiologic, pathologic, and experimental animal studies.[28] The risk of disease appears to be a function of both total cumulative fiber dose and fiber type. For example, the risk of mesothelioma among insulators is about 8–10%, among shipyard workers 2–3%, and among chrysotile miners and millers about 0.5%.[29] Asbestos appears to be the cause of mesothelioma in the United States in about 80–90% of cases.[30] There is a long latency period between exposure to asbestos and the appearance of disease, ranging from about 15 to more than 70 years, with an average of 30–40 years.[28] The disease has been reported in children.[31,32]

The precise mechanisms by which asbestos induces mesothelioma of the pleura are unknown. It is generally believed that direct contact between asbestos fibers and mesothelial cells is an important part of the process, and long thin asbestos fibers have in fact been identified within pleural tissues.[33–35] A clastogenic process is likely, whereby asbestos fibers interfere with normal chromosomal segregation during cell division. Mutations caused by reactive oxygen species generated by asbestos fibers or inflammatory cells may also play a role.[36] A few cases have been reported as a consequence of prior thoracic radiation or long-standing smoldering pleural inflammation.[28,37] More recent studies have identified simian virus 40 (SV40)-like DNA sequences within human pleural mesothelioma, and experimental studies have shown a high incidence of mesothelioma in animals infected with SV40.[38,39] The possible role of SV40 in the pathogenesis is intriguing, but its precise role (if any) is currently unknown.

Clinical and radiographic features

Malignant pleural mesothelioma typically presents in elderly males with complaints of chest pain, dyspnea, weight loss, or cough. Pleural effusion is frequently detected on physical examination. Distant metastases are unusual at the time of initial presentation, but are frequently identified at autopsy.[40] Thrombocytosis is present in the majority of cases. The prognosis is poor, with most patients dying within a year or two of the diagnosis. Patients with limited disease may be treated with radical extrapleural pneumonectomy, with prolonged disease-free interval in some cases. Radiation and chemotherapy are generally ineffective.[28]

Radiographic findings provide important information to the pathologist regarding the gross distribution of tumor. Chest roentgenograms typically show a large unilateral pleural effusion, and may also show diffuse pleural thickening or a localized pleural-based mass. Computed tomography (CT) of the thorax and magnetic resonance imaging provide significantly more detailed information, including invasion of adjacent structures such as ribs or pericardium, metastases to mediastinal lymph nodes, or extension of tumor into the peritoneal cavity (Fig. 19.5).[41,42] CT may also demonstrate the

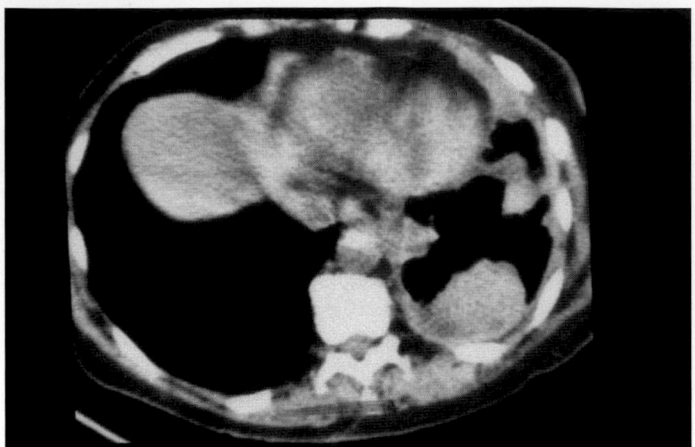

Fig. 19.5 Computed tomographic scan of the thorax in a patient with malignant mesothelioma. There are multiple pleural-based masses in the left hemithorax.

presence of pleural plaques or calcification as evidence of prior asbestos exposure.

Macroscopic features

The gross distribution of tumor is a critical feature in the accurate diagnosis of pleural mesothelioma. These tumors tend to grow over the surface of the pleura, predominantly on the parietal pleura. The tumor forms sheets of irregular pleural thickening or confluent nodules, and eventually encases the lung in a rind of tumor (Fig. 19.6). In advanced stages, the tumor spreads throughout the visceral and parietal pleura with obliteration of the pleural cavity. A localized pleural-based mass is seen less commonly. The tumor extends into the major fissures and may involve the contralateral pleural or peritoneal cavities. Involvement of bony structures of the thorax, mediastinal structures, pericardium, and subcutaneous tissues of the chest wall may be observed. Lymph node metastases are common, and there may be lymphangitic spread involving the subjacent lung parenchyma. Hematogenous spread of tumor to distant sites is commonly observed at autopsy, although metastases to the brain are unusual.[28,43]

Histology

The histologic spectrum of malignant mesothelioma is broad, and diagnostic traps abound for the unwary. The histologic classification is presented in Table 19.1. Mesothelioma has classically been divided into three large categories: epithelial, sarcomatoid, and mixed or biphasic. Approximately 50% of tumors are epithelial, 20% sarcomatoid, and 30% mixed or biphasic.[44] A variety of patterns may be observed in each of these major categories.

Epithelial mesothelioma A highly characteristic pattern for mesothelioma is the tubulopapillary pattern, consisting of relatively uniform cuboidal cells with oval nuclei, single nucleoli, and moderately abundant cytoplasm (Fig. 19.7). Both tubules and papillary structures are observed, and either pattern may predominate. The tubules often contain wispy basophilic secretions consisting of hyaluronic acid. The material is water-soluble and may be removed by prolonged fixation in formalin prior to sectioning. In some cases, the formation of tubules may closely mimic an adenoid cystic pattern (Fig. 19.8). Epithelial mesotheliomas often grow as solid

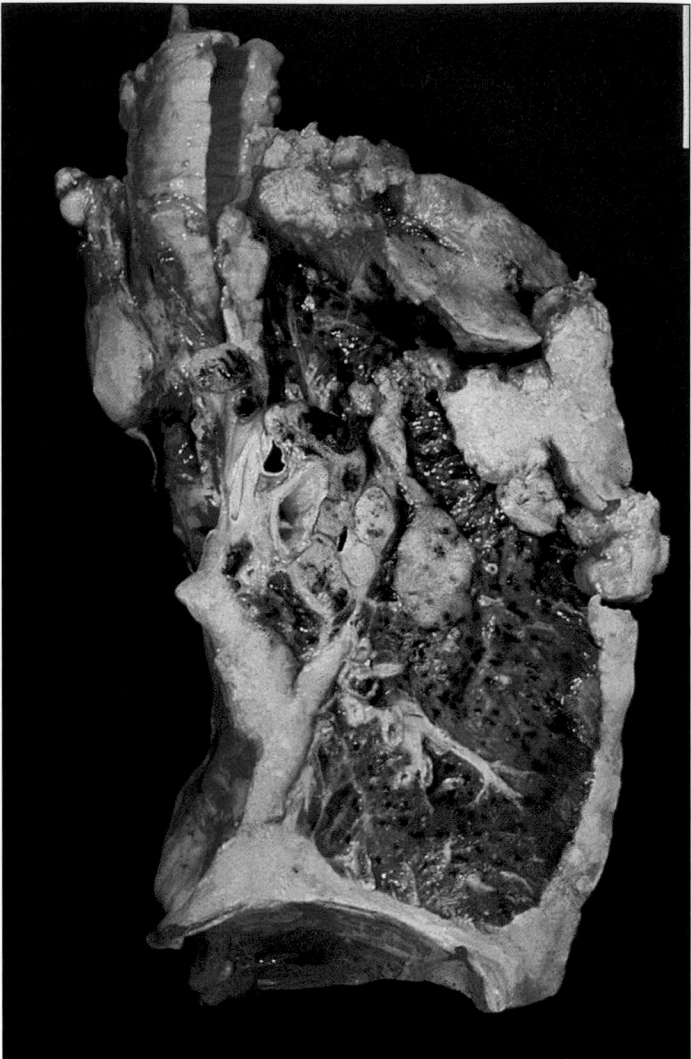

Fig. 19.6 Gross appearance of malignant mesothelioma at autopsy. The tumor has encased the lung in a rind of tumor. (From Roggli VL, Kolbeck J, Sanfilippo F, Shelbourne JD. Pathology of human mesothelioma: etiologic and diagnostic considerations. Pathol Annu 1987; Part 2, 22: 91–131.)

Table 19.1 Histologic classification of malignant mesothelioma

Epithelial
  Tubulopapillary
  Adenoid cystic
  Solid variant
  Deciduoid
  Small cell
  Pleomorphic
  Well-differentiated papillary*
Sarcomatoid
  Fibrosarcomatoid
  Heterologous elements (chondrosarcomatoid, osteosarcomatoid)
  Desmoplastic
  Lymphohistiocytoid
Biphasic (mixed)

*This variant is considered to be a tumor of low-grade malignant potential.

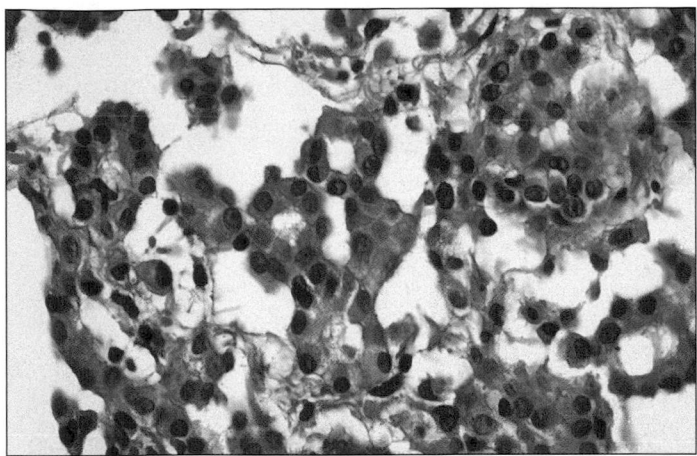

Fig. 19.7 Tubulopapillary variant of malignant mesothelioma. Tumor cells are cuboidal with uniform nuclei. (H&E)

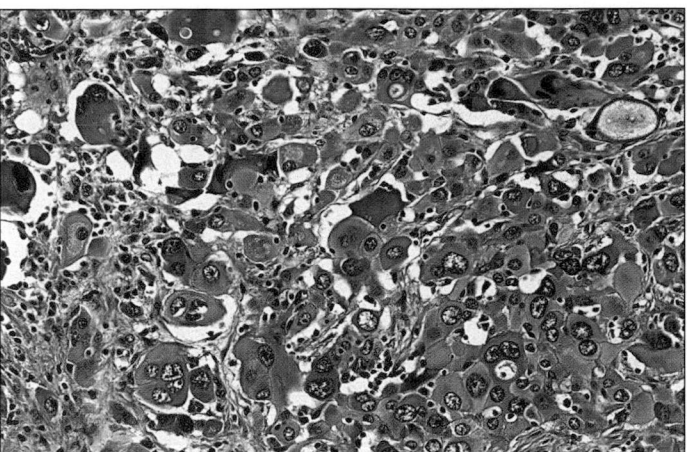

Fig. 19.9 Pleomorphic variant of malignant mesothelioma. The tumor cells are large with anaplastic, often multiple nuclei and prominent nucleoli. Compare tumor size with background inflammatory cells. (H&E)

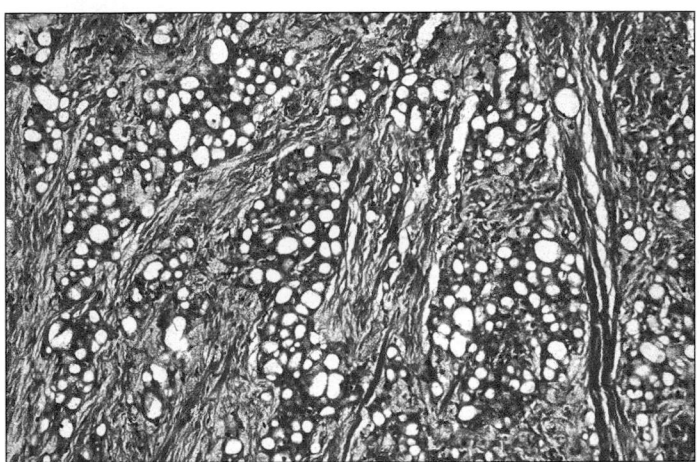

Fig. 19.8 Microcystic variant of malignant mesothelioma, resembling adenoid cystic carcinoma. Figure courtesy Dr. Sam Hammar, Bremerton, WA. (H&E)

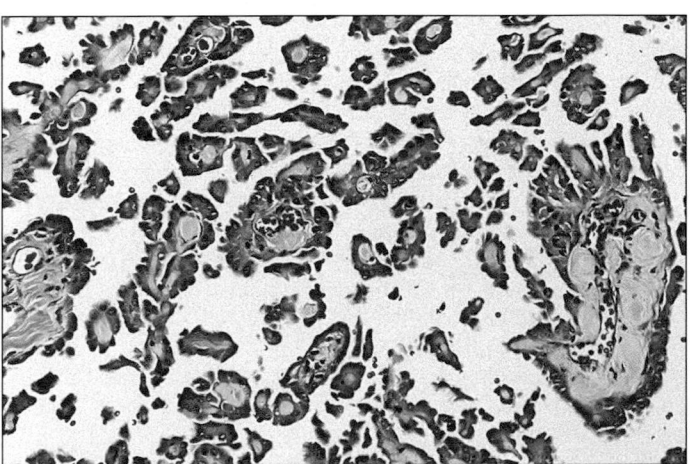

Fig. 19.10 Well-differentiated papillary mesothelioma of the pleura. A single layer of cuboidal uniform tumor cells lines the surface of fibrovascular cores. (H&E)

sheets or as nests of tumor cells in a desmoplastic stroma. In some cases, these sheets of tumor cells have abundant glassy eosinophilic cytoplasm with distinct cell borders, a pattern that has been referred to as deciduoid mesothelioma.[45] In others, the tumor cells may be quite small, a pattern that has been described as the small cell variant.[43] These latter tumors look quite different from small cell carcinoma of the lung, with which they should not be confused. In some cases, the tumor cells may be rather pleomorphic with anaplastic tumor giant cells highly suggestive of carcinoma of the lung (Fig. 19.9).

A histologic variant that should be distinguished from other forms of epithelial mesothelioma is well-differentiated papillary mesothelioma. This tumor consists of a single layer of cuboidal mesothelial cells lining a fibrovascualr papillary core (Fig. 19.10). Tumors in which this is the only pattern present are rather uncommon and are noninvasive. Consequently, the prognosis is good and patients with this pattern may survive for decades after the diagnosis, although recurrent disease is often noted.[46] However, we

have on a number of occasions observed this pattern in association with otherwise invasive tubulopapillary mesothelioma. In some cases, an initial biopsy shows only a well-differentiated papillary pattern, while subsequent biopsies show an invasive component. Whether this is due to inadequate sampling initially or progression of the tumor is unknown. When an invasive component is detected, the clinical course is less predictable and the prognosis guarded.

Some authors have noted the presence of an in-situ (noninvasive) component in some cases of mesothelioma, and have proposed the term mesothelioma in situ.[47] This finding is of considerable interest, since it suggests that mesothelioma begins as an in-situ process prior to the development of invasive disease. However, the distinction of this pattern from atypical reactive mesothelial hyperplasia in biopsy specimens is difficult if not impossible.[8]

Sarcomatoid mesothelioma The sarcomatoid variant typically consists of anaplastic spindle cells arranged in a haphazard distribution in a pattern reminiscent of fibrosarcoma (Fig. 19.11). Heterologous elements such as osteosarcomatoid or chondrosarcomatoid

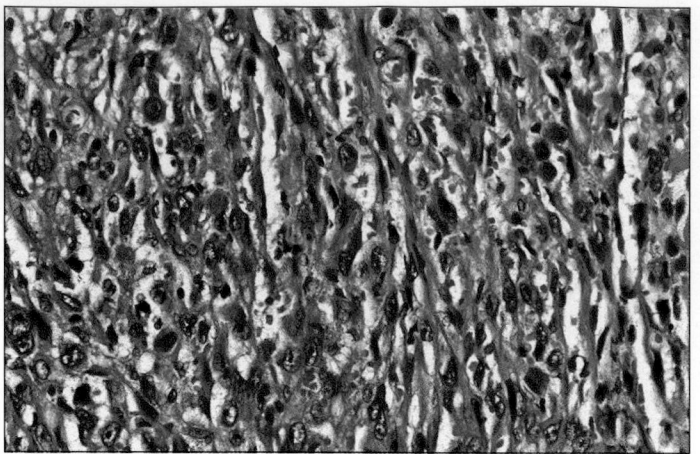

Fig. 19.11 Sarcomatoid variant of malignant mesothelioma. The tumor cells are spindle-shaped with anaplastic, hyperchromatic nuclei, resembling fibrosarcoma. (H&E)

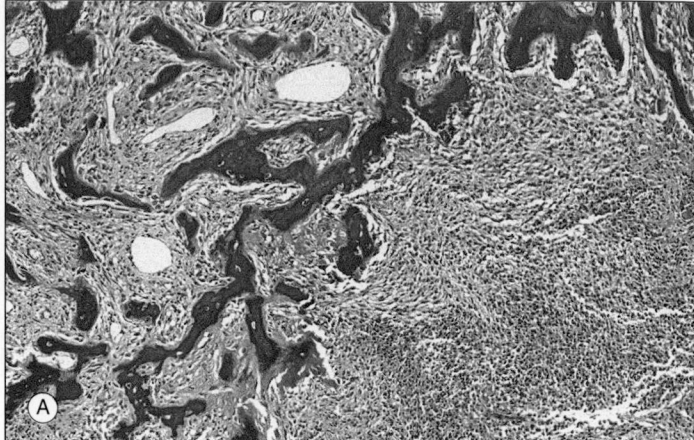

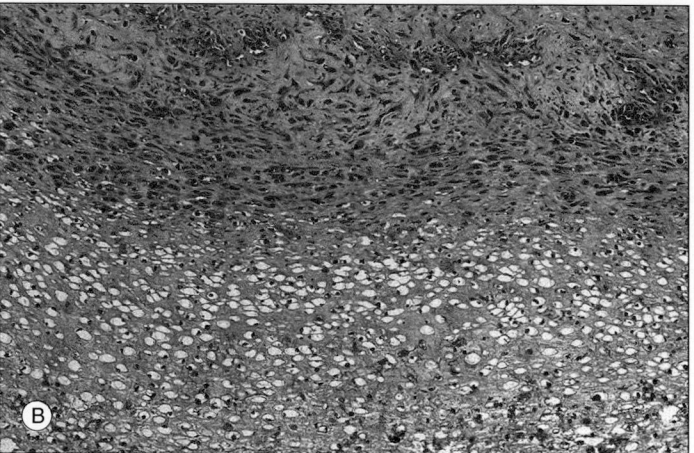

Fig. 19.12 Sarcomatoid mesothelioma with heterologous elements. **A**, Ostesarcomatoid differentiation, with spicules of bone lined by anaplastic spindle cells; **B**, Malignant spindle cells (above) with abrupt transition to chondrosarcomatoid area (below). (H&E)

differentiation may occasionally be observed (Fig. 19.12). Less often, the pattern may resemble malignant fibrous histiocytoma, leiomyosarcoma, neurogenic sarcoma, liposarcoma, or rhabdomyosarcoma. A particularly deceptive variant is that of desmoplastic mesothelioma, consisting of atypical spindle cells separated by abundant collagen fibers arranged in a storiform pattern or in the 'patternless pattern' of Stout (Fig. 19.13). This pattern may be difficult to distinguish from fibrous pleurisy, especially in small biopsy specimens. The distinction is based on the findings of frankly sarcomatoid foci, areas of bland necrosis, or invasion of chest wall or underlying lung parenchyma.[48] This may require extensive sampling in order to identify diagnostic areas. Furthermore, the distinction may be complicated by the presence of an organizing fibrinous exudate overlying desmoplastic mesothelioma.

A rare variant of sarcomatoid mesothelioma known as lymphohistiocytoid mesothelioma was first described by Henderson et al.[49] This morphologic subtype is important because it may be confused with a malignant lymphoma secondarily involving the pleura. It is composed of large cells that exhibit cytologic features resembling histiocytes. These large cells are typically obscured by a dense lymphocytic infiltrate admixed with eosinophils and plasma cells. Immunohistochemical stains are useful for making the distinction, in that the large neoplastic cells of lymphohistiocytoid mesothelioma stain strongly positive for cytokeratins.

Mixed (biphasic) epithelial and sarcomatoid mesothelioma This is a highly characteristic pattern of mesothelioma in which both epithelial and sarcomatous elements are present and often intimately admixed (Fig. 19.14). Any combination of subtypes noted in Table 19.1 is theoretically possible, although these tumors are usually poorly differentiated so that well-differentiated elements are typically lacking. The more a mesothelioma is sampled, the greater is the likelihood that a biphasic nature will be revealed. However, caution should be taken so that benign epithelium entrapped by a sarcomatoid mesothelioma or reactive fibroblastic stroma in an epithelial mesothelioma is not confused with a true biphasic malignant mesothelioma.

Histochemistry

The histochemical basis for the diagnosis of mesothelioma lies in the identification of neutral mucin, often produced by adenocarcinomas, and hyaluronic acid, produced by a subset of epithelial mesotheliomas.

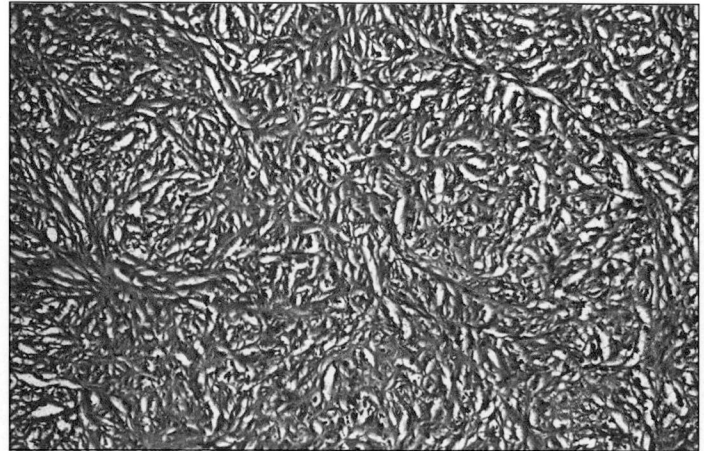

Fig. 19.13 Desmoplastic variant of malignant mesothelioma. Collagen bundles are arranged in a storiform pattern and separated by sparse hyperchromatic spindle cells. (H&E)

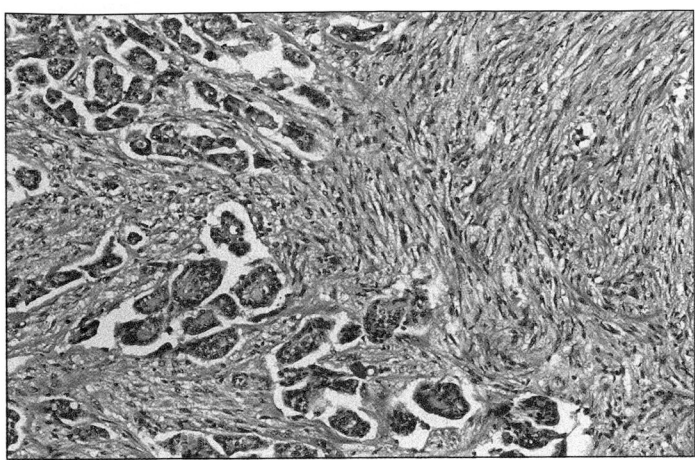

Fig. 19.14 Biphasic variant of malignant mesothelioma. Epithelial islands with papillary features are surrounded by neoplastic spindle cells. (H&E)

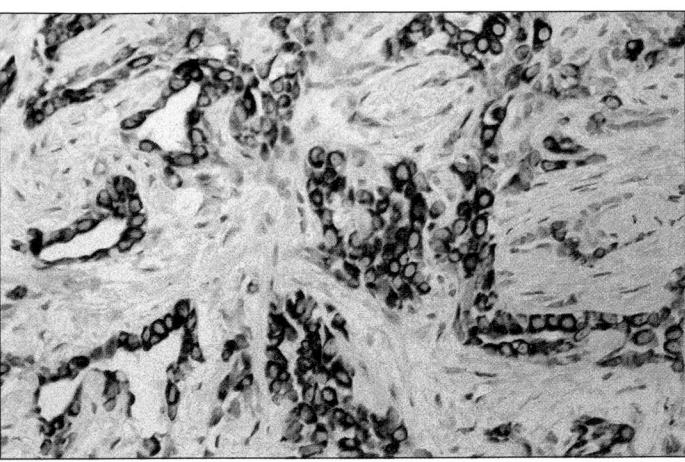

Fig. 19.15 Epithelial mesothelioma shows strong cytoplasmic staining for cytokeratins 5/6. (IHC)

The preferred stain for the detection of neutral mucin is periodic acid–Schiff (PAS) following predigestion with diastase (DPAS). Mucicarmine should be avoided, since it will occasionally stain hyaluronic acid produced by mesotheliomas. Alcian blue stains acid mucopolysaccharides, and the stain is made specific for hyaluronic acid by treating a serial section with hyaluronidase. Adenocarcinomas often produce acid or neutral mucins within intracellular or glandular lumens, and this material stains positive with DPAS and Alcian blue, but is resistant to hyaluronidase pretreatment. In contrast, the wispy basophilic intraluminal secretions of mesotheliomas stain negative with DPAS but positive for Alcian blue. The latter staining is sensitive to hyaluronidase.[28]

It should be noted that rare cases have been reported of epithelial mesothelioma that stain positive with DPAS and show Alcian blue positivity that is resistant to hyaluronidase.[50,51] This is apparently due to the formation of crystalline structures of hyaluronic acid and/or peptidoglycans within the tumor cells. Because such cases are so uncommon, a diagnosis of mucin-positive mesothelioma should only be made when the gross distribution of tumor is typical for mesothelioma and all other immunohistochemical and ultrastructural findings favor mesothelioma (see below).

Some caution needs to be employed in the interpretation of DPAS stains. Some mesotheliomas produce a thick circumferential basal lamina that will stain with DPAS. In addition, granular staining due to incomplete removal of glycogen should not be confused with neutral mucin. Occasional tumors will have eosinophilic intracytoplasmic globules that stain positive with DPAS but do not have the spidery intraluminal appearance of mucin.[52] Most epithelial mesotheliomas do not produce significant amounts of hyaluronic acid. Therefore, we reserve histochemical staining for those tumors that have identifiable luminal secretions on hematoxylin and eosin-stained sections. In these cases, the results of histochemical studies are usually supportive of the diagnosis of mesothelioma.

Immunohistochemistry

Because of the broad spectrum of histologic patterns of mesothelioma, difficulty of distinction from other neoplasms involving the pleura, and medicolegal implications of the diagnosis, a variety of immunostains have been developed to assist in distinguishing mesothelioma from other pleural tumors. Several review articles

have dealt with the application of these antibodies to the differential diagnosis of mesothelioma.[53–59] The following is a brief review of the most commonly used antibodies that have been shown to have diagnostic utility in the distinction between mesothelioma and morphologically similar malignant neoplasms.

Cytokeratin Virtually all malignant epithelial mesotheliomas stain diffusely and strongly positive for cytokeratins when a broad-spectrum cocktail of antikeratin antibodies is used. Our laboratory uses a cocktail that includes AE1/AE3, Cam 5.2, and MNF.116. Such staining is not useful to distinguish mesothelioma from adenocarcinoma, since the latter will also stain for cytokeratins. However, absence of staining for cytokeratins will prevent one from mistaking the occasional large cell lymphoma, melanoma, or epithelioid hemangioendothelioma secondarily involving the pleura for an epithelial mesothelioma.

Some authors have reported that antibodies to certain subsets of cytokeratins preferentially stain mesotheliomas. Antibodies to cytokeratins 5/6 react moderately to strongly with most epithelial mesotheliomas.[60–62] In our experience, the staining is usually diffuse but may be focal (Fig. 19.15). In contrast, most adenocarcinomas, including those originating from the lung, are negative for CK 5/6. On the other hand, squamous cell and large cell lung carcinomas usually do stain for CK 5/6, as do most transitional cell carcinomas of the urinary bladder.[61] The sarcomatoid component of mesotheliomas usually stains negative for CK 5/6. Epithelial mesotheliomas tend to stain strongly positive for cytokeratin 7 and are either weakly positive or negative for cytokeratin 20.[63] This staining pattern is similar to that for adenocarcinomas of pulmonary origin, and therefore is not useful for distinguishing mesothelioma from adenocarcinoma of the lung. However, the staining pattern of mesotheliomas differs from that of most carcinomas of gastrointestinal origin.[63]

Keratin stains are also useful for distinguishing sarcomatoid mesotheliomas from other sarcomas that may secondarily involve the pleura. Sarcomatoid mesotheliomas typically stain moderately to strongly positive for broad-spectrum cytokeratins (Fig. 19.16). Most sarcomas are cytokeratin negative, although focal positivity has occasionally been reported in leiomyosarcomas and malignant fibrous histiocytomas.[64,65] Exceptions to this include epithelioid sarcoma and synovial sarcoma, both of which stain positive for cytokeratins. Cytokeratins staining does not distinguish sarcomatoid

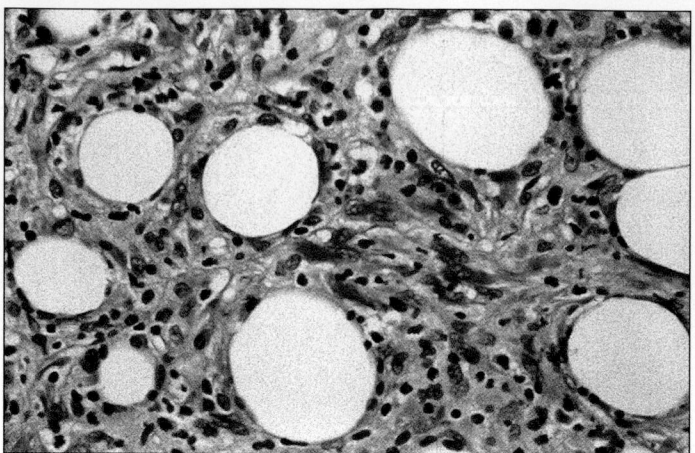

Fig. 19.16 Malignant spindle cells of sarcomatoid mesothelioma invading adipose tissue of chest wall. The tumor cells stain strongly positive for cytokeratins using a monoclonal cocktail. (IHC)

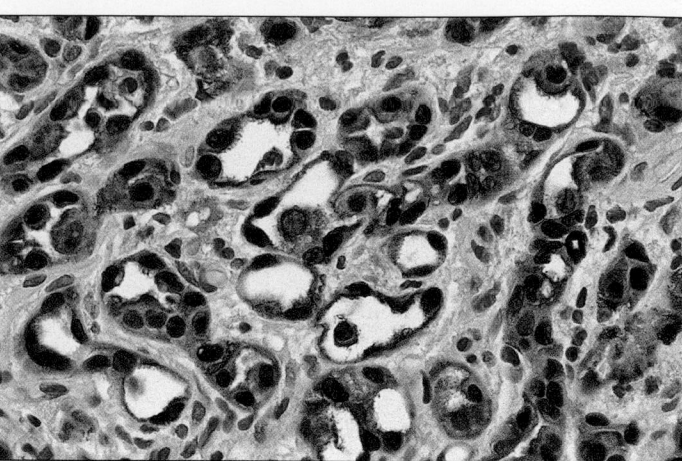

Fig. 19.17 Epithelial mesothelioma shows strong nuclear staining for calretinin. Cytoplasmic staining is also apparent. (IHC)

mesothelioma from sarcomatoid carcinomas of pulmonary origin.[66] In this circumstance, the gross distribution of the tumor as determined by radiographic studies is a helpful differential diagnostic feature. Cytokeratin staining may be useful for distinguishing desmoplastic mesothelioma from fibrous pleurisy by demonstrating the presence of keratin-positive spindle cells invading into adipose tissue of the chest wall or subjacent lung.[8] Rarely, a sarcomatoid malignancy diffusely involving the pleural space with no known primary site will be keratin negative. Such tumors probably represent a dedifferentiated sarcomatoid mesothelioma that has lost the capacity to make cytokeratins. Similarly, areas of osteosarcomatoid or chondrosarcomatoid differentiation in mesotheliomas may stain negative for cytokeratins.[67]

Calretinin Several studies have demonstrated the usefulness of antibodies to calretinin for distinguishing mesothelioma from adenocarcinoma.[62,68,69] Epithelial mesotheliomas typically stain moderately to strongly positive for calretinin. Both nuclear and cytoplasmic staining is highly sensitive for epithelial mesothelioma (>90%), but nuclear staining is more specific (Fig. 19.17).[62] The vast majority of adenocarcinomas stain negative for this antibody, although cytoplasmic staining is occasionally seen.[68] Sarcomatoid mesotheliomas are often negative for calretinin, but focal nuclear staining is observed in some cases.

Thrombomodulin A high percentage of epithelial mesotheliomas stain positive for antibodies to thrombomodulin.[62,70] The staining is typically in a surface membrane distribution. In contrast, most adenocarcinomas do not stain positive with this antibody. Ordonez reported that only three of 27 (11%) lung adenocarcinomas were positive for thrombomodulin, whereas 16 of 20 (80%) epithelial mesotheliomas reacted.[70] Blood vessels also stain positive for thrombomodulin, which can make interpretation of surface membrane staining of tumor cells difficult in some cases.[62]

Wilms' tumor antigen (WT1) Epithelial mesotheliomas stain positive for antibodies directed at the product of the Wilms' tumor susceptibility gene 1 (WT1). Amin et al. reported that 20 of 21 mesotheliomas stained positive, whereas all 20 non-small cell lung cancers tested stained negative.[71] The staining in mesotheliomas is characteristically in a nuclear distribution. This observation is of particular interest since several cases have been reported of mesothelioma developing many years following treatment for Wilms' tumor.[37]

Antimesothelioma antibodies A number of monoclonal antibodies have been developed and raised against mesothelioma-associated antigens that show partial specificity for mesothelial cells.[72-78] The pattern of immunoreactivity of these antibodies typically shows peripheral accentuation. Many of these antibodies require frozen sections, and none is entirely specific for malignant mesothelioma. HBME-1 does work on paraffin sections and has been reported to be useful for distinguishing mesothelioma from adenocarcinoma by some authors[56,78] but not by others.[70] The specificity for mesothelioma is best when this antibody is used at dilutions from 1:5000 to 1:15 000 (personal communication, Drs. Hector Battifora, Sam Hammar, and Doug Henderson).

Glycoprotein markers A wide variety of glycoprotein markers have been used to help distinguish mesothelioma from metastatic adenocarcinoma. These markers typically stain adenocarcinomas but fail to stain the vast majority of mesotheliomas (Fig. 19.18). Included among the markers that have been found to be useful are carcinoembryonic antigen (CEA),[79-82] BerEP4,[83-88] Leu M1,[16,89-91] B72.3,[90,92-94] Bg8,[95,96] and MOC-31.[59] These markers stain adenocarcinomas from different primary sites to varying degrees, and may also stain a small percentage of mesotheliomas.[28,43] Therefore, these markers are typically incorporated into a panel of antibodies used for diagnosing mesothelioma. Some caution is necessary in the interpretation of these stains, since infiltrating inflammatory cells and foci of necrosis often stain positive with some of these markers (i.e. CEA and Leu M1). In addition, invasion of mesothelioma into subjacent lung tissue may entrap alveolar or bronchiolar epithelium that may stain positive with these markers. Finally, the focal nature of the immunoreaction may give false-negative results on small biopsy samples.

Glycoproteins isolated from human milk fat globule membranes have been detected immunohistochemically in a variety of epithelial neoplasms.[81,97-99] The most commonly used antibodies are to epithelial membrane antigen (EMA) and HMFG-2 and give quite similar results. Both antibodies will react with mesotheliomas and adenocarcinomas in a high percentage of cases. Therefore, the detection of positive staining is of no benefit in distinguishing between adenocarcinoma and mesothelioma. However, the pattern of staining is reportedly different, with mesothelioma demonstrating a membrane pattern of staining, often referred to as a 'thick membrane

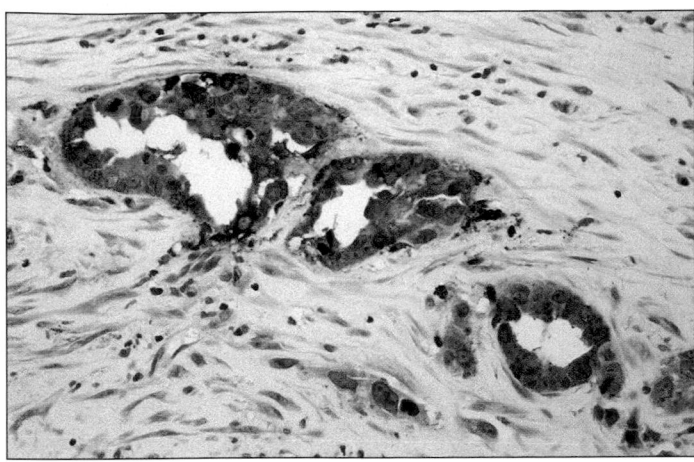

Fig. 19.18 Pseudomesotheliomatous adenocarcinoma of the lung showing strong cytoplasmic staining for carcinoembryonic antigen. Mesotheliomas typically stain negative for this marker. (IHC)

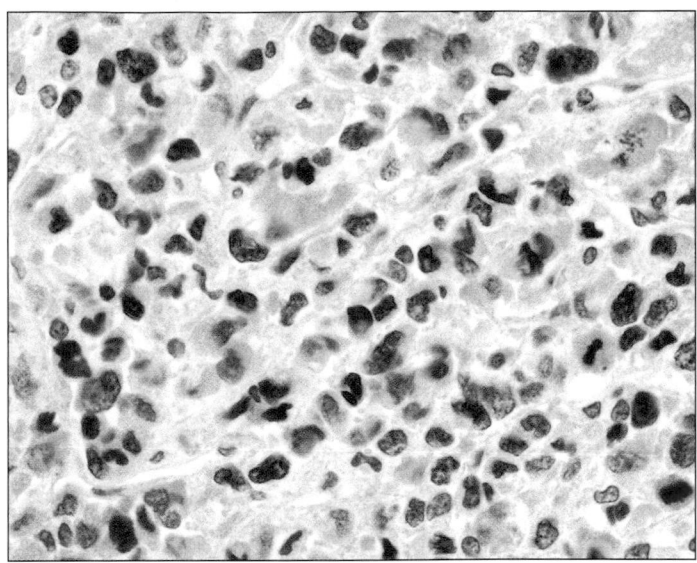

Fig. 19.19 Nuclear staining for p53 in a mesothelioma. Reactive mesothelium typically stains negative for this marker. ((IHC)

pattern.' In contrast, most adenocarcinomas demonstrate diffuse cytoplasmic staining with these markers.

Blood group antigens Blood group-related antigens also can be found in cells of nonhematopoietic tissues. Monoclonal antibodies with specific reactivity for blood group antigens are reported to be useful for discriminating between adenocarcinoma and mesothelioma.[95,96,100,101] Antibodies reactive with Lewis blood group antigens are more useful than other blood group antigens in this regard.[101]

Vimentin Some investigators have reported that immunostaining for vimentin is useful for distinguishing between mesothelioma and adenocarcinoma, with mesotheliomas expressing both cytokeratins and vimentin.[102,103] However, others have found that a number of adenocarcinomas will also stain for vimentin, giving this marker limited differential diagnostic utility.[43] On the other hand, vimentin is a good marker for antigen preservation in tissue sections. We especially use it in the evaluation of sarcomatoid tumors, the vast majority of which are vimentin positive. Thus in a case in which vimentin staining is negative, one must be wary regarding the interpretation of negative results for other markers, which may be the result of false-negative staining secondary to poor antigen preservation.

Muscle actins, desmin, and S-100 Sarcomatoid mesotheliomas frequently stain positive for muscle-specific actin (MSA) and smooth muscle actin (SMA).[104] This is an important point to remember when trying to distinguish sarcomatoid mesotheliomas from other sarcomas that secondarily involve the pleura. Sarcomatoid mesotheliomas may also stain focally positive for desmin and may stain for S-100 protein. Such markers are of limited utility when trying to distinguish sarcomatoid mesotheliomas from leiomyosarcomas or Schwannomas. In addition, S-100 is not useful for distinguishing epithelioid mesothelioma from melanoma involving the pleura. In this differential diagnostic setting, markers for cytokeratins and HMB-45 would be the more appropriate choice.

p53 protein p53 is a human nuclear protein with oncogene-suppressing activity. It has been identified immunohistochemically in some mesotheliomas but is present much less frequently in reactive mesothelial cells or subpleural fibroblasts.[19,48,105–107] The immunostaining pattern typically has a distinct nuclear distribution

(Fig. 19.19). However, most mesotheliomas are negative for this oncoprotein, thus significantly limiting its diagnostic potential. Immunostaining for p53 protein is not useful to differentiate carcinoma from mesothelioma.

Miscellaneous antibodies Numerous other antibodies have been reported to be useful in the differential diagnosis of malignant mesothelioma. These include 44-3A6,[108,109] neuron-specific enolase, and Leu-7,[110] parathyroid hormone-related protein,[111] secretory component,[112] human placental glycogen and CA-19-9 antigen,[113] lectins,[114] epidermal growth factor,[115] vascular cell adhesion molecule,[116] K1,[117] β chain of platelet derived growth factor receptor,[118] P-170 glycoprotein,[119] E-cadherin and N-cadherin,[120] CA-125,[1,93] and telomerase reverse transcriptase (TERT).[121] These antibodies offer no obvious advantages to the more established markers discussed in previous sections, and more work needs to be done before they can be incorporated into commonly used antibody panels.

A systematic approach to immunodiagnosis of malignant mesothelioma No single antibody has sufficient sensitivity and specificity to be diagnostic for mesothelioma. Consequently, investigators have proposed the use of various panels of antibodies to aid in the distinction between mesothelioma and other diseases with which it may be confused.[80,96,122] The panel used by one of the authors (VLR) is shown in Table 19.2. The cornerstone of the panel is a cocktail of anticytokeratin antibodies to insure that the rare lymphoma, melanoma, or epithelioid hemangioendothelioma involving the pleura is not missed. Epithelial and most sarcomatoid mesotheliomas stain strongly and diffusely positive with this antibody cocktail. For epithelial pleural tumors, two antibodies that stain most epithelial mesotheliomas positive (calretinin and CK 5/6) are used, along with two antibodies that stain most mesotheliomas negative but most lung adenocarcinomas positive (CEA and TTF-1 [Fig. 19.20]). We hold BerEP4, B72.3, and Leu M1 in reserve for the occasional case with discordant immunohistochemical staining with the original panel.

For epithelial peritoneal tumors, a slightly different panel is used. Many intra-abdominal carcinomas are CEA negative, and TTF-1

Table 19.2 Immunohistochemical diagnostic panel for mesothelioma

Malignant pleural mesothelioma, epithelial, or biphasic

First Line: Cocktail of anticytokeratin antibodies
Calretinin
Cytokeratin 5/6
Polyclonal carcinoembryonic antigen (CEA)
Thyroid transcription factor (TTF-1)

Second Line: BerEP4
B72.3
Leu M1

Malignant peritoneal mesothelioma, epithelial, or biphasic

First Line: Cocktail of anticytokeratin antibodies
Calretinin
Cytokeratin 5/6
BerEP4
B72.3

Second Line: Leu M1
HBME-1
Thrombomodulin

Sarcomatoid mesothelioma

Cocktail of anticytokeratin antibodies
Vimentin

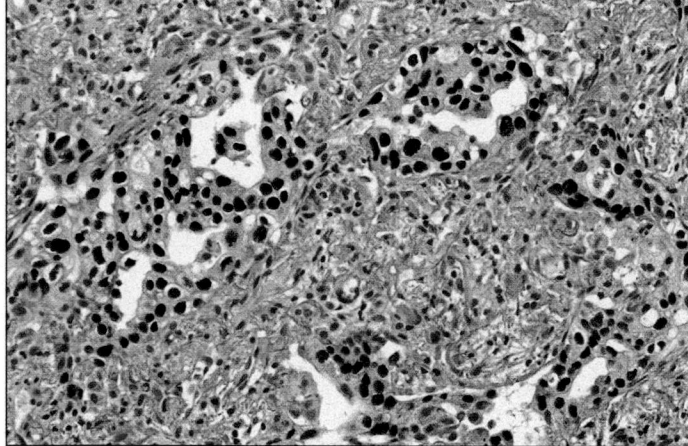

Fig. 19.20 Nuclear staining for thyroid transcription factor (TTF-1) in an adenocarcinoma of the lung. Mesotheliomas typically stain negative for this marker. (IHC)

Table 19.3 Most commonly expected immunohistochemical staining results for mesothelioma and adenocarcinoma

Antibody	Mesothelioma	Adenocarcinoma
Keratin cocktail	Pos	Pos
Cytokeratins 5/6	Pos	Neg[a]
Cytokeratin 7	Pos	Pos/Neg[b]
Cytokeratin 20	Neg	Pos/Neg[b]
Calretinin	Pos (N)	Neg
Thrombomodulin	Pos	Neg
WT1	Pos (N)	Neg
HBME-1	Pos	Neg
CEA	Neg	Pos
BerEP4	Neg	Pos
Leu M1	Neg	Pos
B72.3	Neg	Pos
Bg8	Neg	Pos
MOC-31	Neg	Pos
EMA	Pos	Pos[c]
HMFG-2	Pos	Pos[c]
Lewis^x/Lewis^y	Neg	Pos
Vimentin	Pos/Neg	Pos/Neg
Muscle actins	Pos[d]	Neg
Desmin	Pos[d]	Neg
S-100	Pos[d]	Neg
p53	Pos	Pos
44-3A6	Neg	Pos
NSE	Pos	Neg
Leu 7	Pos	Neg
PTH-related protein	Pos	Neg
Secretory component	Neg	Pos
Human placental lactogen	Neg	Pos
CA-19-9	Neg	Pos
CA-125	Neg	Pos
Lectins	Neg[e]	Pos
Vascular cell adhesion molecule	Pos	Neg
K1	Pos	Neg
E-cadherin	Neg	Pos
N-cadherin	Pos	Neg

a. Many adenocarcinomas of extrapulmonary origin may stain positive. See Ref. 124.
b. Varying combinations of CK 7 and CK 20 positivity are seen in adenocarcinomas, depending upon primary site. See Ref. 63.
c. Distribution of staining is primarily membranous in mesothelioma, cytoplasmic in adenocarcinoma.
d. Positive staining primarily seen in sarcomatoid mesotheliomas
e. Most mesotheliomas stain positive for wheat germ and peanut agglutinins. See Ref. 114.
Pos, positive staining; Neg, negative staining; N, nuclear staining

primarily stains lung and thyroid adenocarcinomas, less likely differential diagnostic considerations for an intra-abdominal malignancy. Therefore, B72.3 and BerEP4 are substituted for CEA and TTF-1 in the peritoneal panel. Many intra-abdominal malignancies other than mesothelioma will stain positive for CK 5/6,[123] so one must use care interpreting cases that are CK 5/6 positive but calretinin negative in the abdomen. For pure sarcomatoid tumors, we use only an anticytokeratin cocktail and vimentin.

The most common differential diagnostic consideration is between mesothelioma and metastatic adenocarcinoma. Most commonly expected staining results with the various antibodies discussed above are summarized in Table 19.3. It must be emphasized that one should not fall into the trap of over-reliance on immunohisto-chemical results! Although the diagnosis of mesothelioma may be difficult at times, the most important information for the practicing pathologist is the gross distribution or appearance of the tumor in combination with the histologic findings. Histochemistry, immuno-histochemistry, and ultrastructural studies (see below) are primarily designed to avoid misdiagnosis of the occasional mimic of the gross and histologic features of mesothelioma.

Ultrastructure

The ultrastructural hallmark of mesothelioma is the presence of long thin surface microvilli with a length to diameter ratio greater than 10.[124–130] These microvilli may be branching and lack a fuzzy glycocalyx. In contrast, the microvilli of adenocarcinomas tend to be blunt, sparse, and possess a fuzzy glycocalyx, often in association with glycocalyceal bodies. Rootlets at the base of the microvilli similarly favor adenocarcinoma. Scanning electron microscopy may also be useful for identifying the microvillous structure of epithelial mesotheliomas.[131] Other ultrastructural features commonly seen in epithelial mesotheliomas are cytoplasmic tonofilaments, often in a perinuclear distribution, and long desmosomes. Mesotheliomas lack lamellar bodies and mucous, Clara cell, or dense core neuroendocrine-type granules, and these findings are evidence against a diagnosis of mesothelioma. Electron microscopy is less helpful in more poorly differentiated mesotheliomas, which may have shorter microvilli or lack microvilli entirely.[129] Sarcomatoid mesotheliomas ultrastructurally most commonly resemble fibrosarcomas. In some cases, epithelial differentiation (i.e. occasional microvilli, incomplete basal lamina, intercellular junctions, or tonofilaments) may suggest the diagnosis of mesothelioma. Ultrastructural features may also help differentiate sarcomatoid mesotheliomas from angiosarcoma, schwannoma, leiomyosarcoma, rhabdomyosarcomas, or spindle cell melanomas that secondarily involve the pleura.[130] Although cellular preservation is often poor in tissues retrieved from paraffin blocks, many of the important ultrastructural features of mesothelioma (e.g. tonofilaments and long surface microvilli) are still preserved in such specimens.[132]

Molecular Biology

The molecular pathogenesis of diffuse malignant mesothelioma has some unique features compared to most cancers.[133] The role of asbestos in the pathogenesis of most mesotheliomas is discussed above. Diffuse malignant mesothelioma is characterized by chromosomal defects that can be found on karyotypes, DNA cytometry, and comparative genomic hybridization studies.[134] Interestingly, of the many chromosomal abnormalities found in each tumor, no single cytogenetic defect is specific to mesothelioma, although the resultant pattern of genomic defects is fairly typical. Mutations of p16, p14ARF, and NF2 have been described in diffuse malignant mesothelioma. A recent series found p16 alterations in 31% of diffuse malignant mesotheliomas.[135] Although the WT1 protein is used as a diagnostic antibody for diffuse malignant mesothelioma, mutations of the Wilms' tumor gene (WT1) occur only in a small minority of mesotheliomas.[136] Mutations of basic tumor suppressor genes like p53 and RB characteristic of so many cancers are rarely found in diffuse malignant mesothelioma. This has led to theories that the T-antigen of the SV40 virus identified in many human mesotheliomas may bind the p53 and/or RB products and inhibit them without causing mutation. This would produce the same effect as mutations seen in these tumor suppressor genes in other cancers. The SV40 virus has also been reported to induce telomerase activity in human mesothelial cells.[137] Additional investigations of the unique molecular steps in the development and progression of mesothelioma are underway at this time.

Adenomatoid tumor

Adenomatoid tumors are benign tumors of mesothelial origin occurring primarily in the male and female genital tract. These tumors

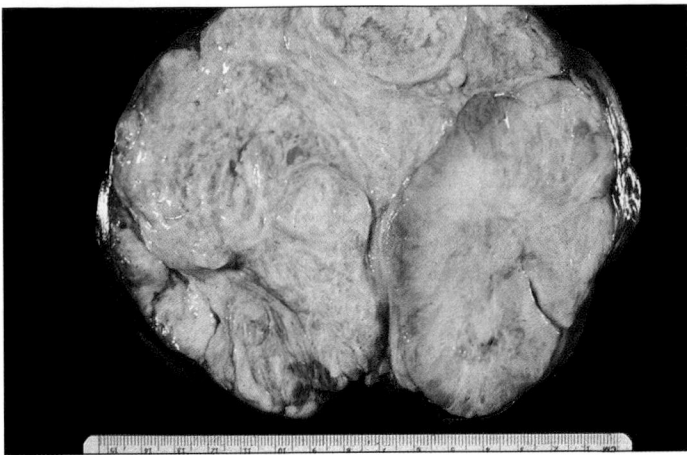

Fig. 19.21 Typical gross appearance of localized fibrous tumor. The lesion is sharply circumscribed with a tan, homogeneous cut surface. (From Roggli VL, Kolbeck J, Sanfilippo F, Shelbourne JD. Pathology of human mesothelioma: etiologic and diagnostic considerations. Pathol Annu 1987; Part 2, 22: 91–131.)

have rarely been described as primary pleural neoplasms.[138,139] They present as a solitary nodule on the visceral or parietal pleura, discovered incidentally during surgery for other causes. Histologically, these tumors are composed of epithelioid cells forming vacuoles and tubular spaces in a desmoplastic stroma. Immunohistochemical and ultrastructural features are those of mesothelial cells. These tumors must be distinguished from diffuse epithelial mesotheliomas. The presence of clinical symptoms, a pleural effusion, or multiple nodules would favor the latter diagnosis.

Localized fibrous tumor

Localized fibrous tumor of the pleura (LFT), also known as submesothelial fibroma, localized fibrous mesothelioma, or solitary fibrous tumor, is a relatively rare neoplasm first described in 1931.[140] Patients present with cough, dyspnea, or fever. Hypoglycemia due to the production of insulin-like growth factor may also be a presenting finding.[141] The tumor is sometimes discovered incidentally on routine examination.[142–154] Pleural effusion is uncommon.[145,146] Localized fibrous tumors typically arise from the visceral pleura and average 6.0 cm in diameter.[142] They are usually pedunculated, rounded, and well circumscribed (Fig. 19.21). The tumor may project into the adjacent pulmonary parenchyma, and rarely the entirety of the tumor may be intrapulmonary.[147,148]

Histologically, LFT consists of spindle cells resembling fibroblasts in a collagenous or myxoid stroma (Fig. 19.22). Bundles of hyalinized ropey collagen arranged in a storiform or haphazard pattern are characteristic, and the cellularity often varies from site to site within the tumor. Areas of cystic degeneration may be observed. Most of these tumors are benign, but malignant variants have been reported. Malignant LFT has a broad base of attachment to the pleura and is less often pedunculated. Histologic features favoring malignancy include large size, invasion of adjacent structures, increased mitotic activity, foci of necrosis, and nuclear pleomorphism.[142–145]

LFT is a mesenchymal neoplasm believed to originate from submesothelial fibroblasts.[66,149] The tumor cells express vimentin and CD34, but lack cytokeratins (Fig. 19.23).[66,149–154] These immunohistochemical features are useful for distinguishing LFT from sarcomatoid mesothelioma, especially in small biopsy specimens.

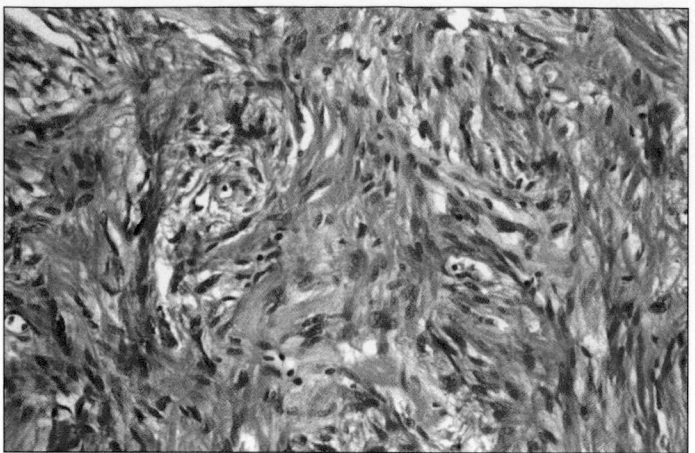

Fig. 19.22 Localized fibrous tumor of the pleura. The tumor consists of spindle cells arranged in a haphazard distribution with variable amounts of extracellular collagen. (H&E)

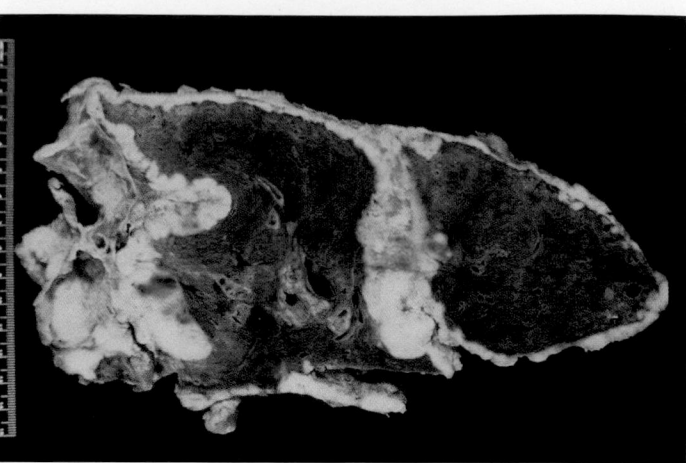

Fig. 19.24 Gross appearance of epithelioid hemangioendothelioma of the pleura at autopsy. The tumor encases the lung in a manner quite similar to that of malignant mesothelioma.

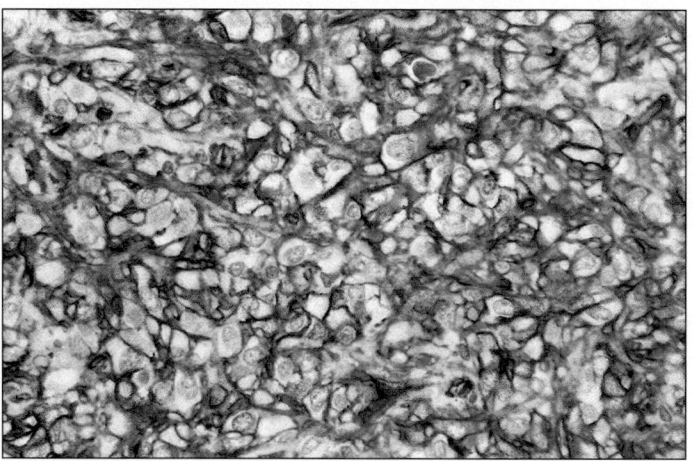

Fig. 19.23 Malignant localized fibrous tumor with strong cytoplasmic staining for CD34. Figure courtesy Dr. William Travis. AFIP, Washington, DC. (IHC)

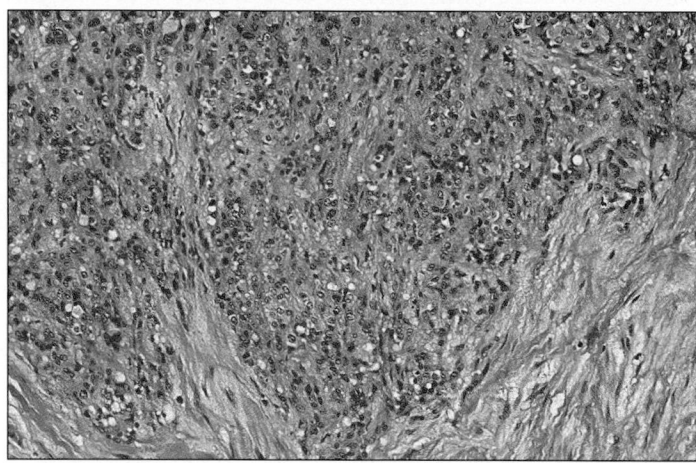

Fig. 19.25 Epithelioid hemangioendothelioma of the pleura, showing nests of tumor cells surrounded by a desmoplastic stroma. Note red blood cells associated with the tumor cells. (H&E)

Sarcomatoid mesotheliomas typically stain positive for cytokeratins but negative for CD34. The localized nature of LFT also distinguishes it from mesothelioma, which is typically diffuse. No conclusive relationship has been identified between LFT and exposure to asbestos. Surgical resection is the treatment of choice. Local recurrences are uncommon after wide resection.[150]

Epithelioid hemangioendothelioma

Epithelioid hemangioendothelioma is a malignant tumor of vascular origin that has been described in a variety of sites, including skin, bone, liver, lung, and soft tissue. Several cases have been described that appeared to arise in the serosal membranes, mimicking mesothelioma (Fig. 19.24).[155–158] Histologically, the tumor cells form sheets or nests in a desmoplastic stroma (Fig. 19.25). There may be a spindle cell component. Closer examination often demonstrates the presence of cytoplasmic luminal spaces, some of which may contain red blood cells. The first clue to the diagnosis is often failure of the tumor cells to stain for cytokeratins (Fig. 19.26),

although focal positivity is seen in some cases. Immunostaining for vascular markers (CD31, CD34, and Factor VIII) will then confirm the diagnosis (Fig. 19.27).[155–158] Mesotheliomas and adenocarcinomas are typically negative for these markers.[159] Ultrastructural studies show pinocytotic vesicles, intermediate filaments, Weibel-Palade bodies, and an absence of surface microvilli.[130] Although this tumor in other sites often has an indolent clinical course, those arising in the pleura have a poor prognosis similar to that of mesothelioma. A causal relationship to asbestos exposure has not been established.[157]

Pleuropulmonary blastoma

Pleuropulmonary blastoma is a malignant tumor that involves the peripheral lung, parietal pleura, and/or the mediastinum.[160–165] They occur in children with the exception of one case reported in a 36-year-old patient.[164] Patients typically present with respiratory distress, fever, or pneumonia. Grossly, the tumors may be entirely cystic (Type I), entirely solid (Type III), or a mixture of solid and

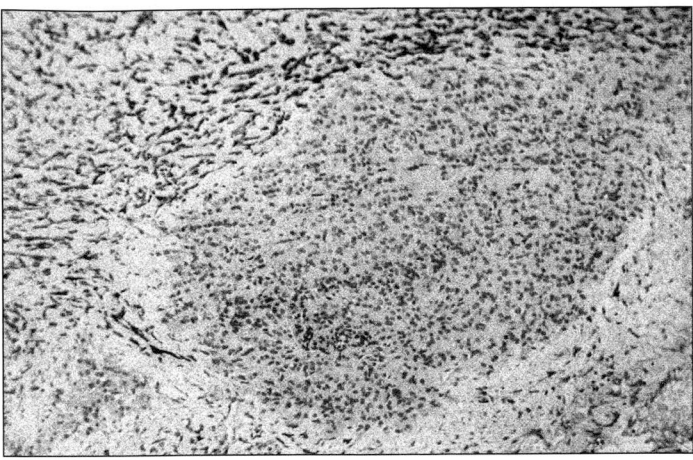

Fig. 19.26 The tumor cells of this epithelioid hemangioendothelioma stain negative for cytokeratins using a monoclonal cocktail. Note the positive staining of the spindle cells in the surrounding desmoplastic stroma. (IHC)

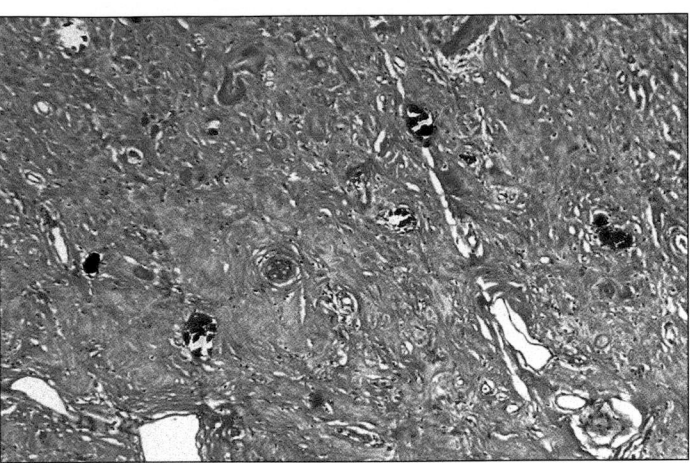

Fig. 19.28 Calcifying fibrous pseudotumor of the pleura consists of dense hyalinized collagen with scattered punctate calcifications. (H&E)

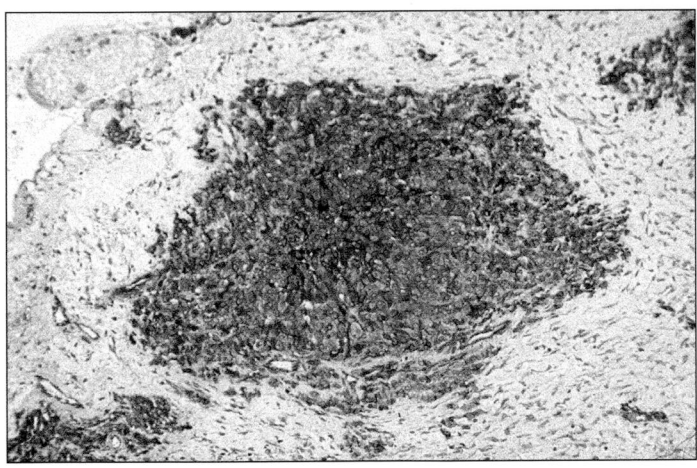

Fig. 19.27 The tumor cells of epithelioid hemangioendothelioma stain strongly positive for CD31, an endothelial marker. (IHC)

cystic elements (Type II). Histologically, the tumors are entirely mesenchymal and lack a malignant epithelial component. Diverse differentiation may be present, including blastema cells, rhabdomyoblasts, fibrosarcoma-like cells, immature cartilage, lipoblasts, and histiocytoid cells with bizarre giant cells. Benign entrapped airway epithelium may line cystic structures. Depending upon the differentiation, the mesenchymal cells may stain immunohistochemically for vimentin, desmin, actin, S-100 protein, alpha-1-antitrypsin or antichymotrypsin, lysozyme, or CD68. Benign entrapped epithelium stains for cytokeratins and epithelial membrane antigen. Cytogenetic studies show an association with trisomy 2 or 8.[165] Treatment is resection with chemotherapy and/or radiotherapy. The overall 5-year survival is 45%, with cystic tumors having a better prognosis than tumors with a solid component.

Calcifying fibrous pseudotumor

Calcifying fibrous pseudotumor is a tumor originally described in soft tissue. A few cases have been reported in the pleura or mediastinum.[166–168] Patients have ranged in age from 23 to 54 years. Radiographic studies show single or multiple pleural-based masses with central calcifications. The lesions are sharply circumscribed and range up to 12 cm in diameter.[169] Histologically, these tumors consist of bundles of densely hyalinized collagen interspersed with a lymphoplasmacytic infiltrate and punctate calcifications (Fig. 19.28). Immunohistochemical stains are positive for vimentin but negative for cytokeratins and CD34.[167] Ultrastructural studies show fibroblasts and collagen. Calcifying fibrous pseudotumors must be distinguished from localized fibrous tumors, pleural plaques, desmoplastic mesothelioma, fibrous pleurisy, pulmonary hyalinizing granuloma, inflammatory pseudotumors, and nodular amyloidosis. Local excision is the treatment of choice.

Desmoplastic small round cell tumor

Desmoplastic small round cell tumor is an aggressive malignancy of young adults with distinctive histologic and immunohistochemical features. The tumor typically involves the abdominal cavity, but a few cases have been described in the pleura.[170–172] These tumors are characterized by angulated nests of small cells in a desmoplastic stroma. Focal areas of central necrosis may be present. Immunohistochemical studies show evidence of epithelial, mesenchymal, and neural differentiation. Dot-like perinuclear positivity for vimentin and desmin is characteristic for this neoplasm. The tumor cells also stain positive for cytokeratins, epithelial membrane antigen, and neuron-specific enolase. Focal positivity for S-100 and rare cells staining for GFAP are also observed. Ultrastructurally, aggregates of intermediate filaments are present in a perinuclear distribution. Desmosomes are also present. Cytogenetic studies have identified the EWS-WT1 fusion product.[171] Desmoplastic small round cell tumors must be distinguished from small cell carcinoma secondarily involving the pleura and from the small cell variant of mesothelioma. The prognosis is poor.

Synovial sarcoma

Gaertner et al. reported five cases of primary synovial sarcomas involving the pleura.[173] The patients had an average age of 25 years and presented with a pleural-based intrathoracic mass. The tumors were 5–21 cm in size and had areas of hemorrhage and/or necrosis on the cut surface. Two tumors were attached to the pleura by a pedicle. Histologically, both biphasic and monophasic variants have been recognized.[173,174] These tumors share a number of immuno-histochemical features with malignant mesothelioma. Both tumors stain positive for broad-spectrum cytokeratins, calretinin, and cytokeratins 5/6. Distinguishing features include strong positivity of synovial sarcomas for BerEP4 and cytokeratin 14, but rarity or lack of staining for WT1 and CD141.[175] Presentation as a localized mass and presence of the SYT-SSX fusion transcripts also help distinguish synovial sarcoma from mesothelioma.[174] These tumors may behave aggressively, with nearly half of the reported patients dying of disease.

Secondary pleural neoplasms

Metastatic carcinoma is the most common malignancy that occurs within the pleura. Most of these metastases originate within the lung or the breast. Adenocarcinoma is the most common lung primary to involve the pleura because of its frequent peripheral location. Metastatic carcinoma usually consists of multiple small nodules or granulations on the visceral pleura, often accompanied by malignant pleural effusion. Rarely, a primary adenocarcinoma of the lung may diffusely infiltrate the pleural cavity exhibiting clinical, radiologic, and pathologic features closely mimicking mesothelioma (Fig. 19.29). These tumors are designated pseudomesotheliomatous adenocarcinomas.[176]

The morphologic distinction of pseudomesotheliomatous adenocarcinoma from mesothelioma is based on histologic, histochemical, immunohistochemical, and ultrastructural studies (see section on mesothelioma above).[177,178] In brief, adenocarcinomas often stain positive for neutral mucins and acid mucopolysaccharides other than hyaluronic acid (Fig. 19.30). In addition, they stain positive for glycoprotein markers such as CEA, BerEP4, Leu M1, and B72.3. Nuclear staining for TTF-1 is particularly helpful, being present in approximately 90% of pulmonary adenocarcinomas but absent in mesotheliomas.[179] Ultrastructurally, adenocarcinomas tend to have short, stubby microvilli coated with a glycocalyx and often associated with glycocalyceal bodies. Mucin or Clara cell granules may be present as well. The clinical course of these tumors is aggressive, with a prognosis similar to that of mesothelioma. An association with asbestos exposure has been suggested in some cases.[178]

Renal cell carcinoma may on occasion result in a differential diagnostic problem. We have seen examples of renal cell carcinoma that metastasized to the ipsilateral or contralateral pleura and mimicked mesothelioma.[180] The usual markers listed in Tables 19.2 and 19.3 may be of limited use in making this distinction. Therefore, extreme caution should be used in making a diagnosis of mesothelioma in a patient with a known renal mass (other than cysts). In this circumstance, the most reliable way to make an accurate diagnosis is to compare the histology of the pleural and renal tumors to determine whether they are similar or distinct. Other malignancies that may involve the pleura and result in pleural effusion include leukemia, lymphoma, melanoma, and sarcomas.[181]

THE PERICARDIUM

The anatomic features of the pericardium are essentially similar to those of the pleura. The parietal pericardium forms a sac that surrounds the heart, and the visceral pericardium forms the epicardium. As in the pleura, the pericardium is lined by a continuous layer of flattened mesothelial cells that rest on a basal lamina and submesothelial connective tissue layer.[1]

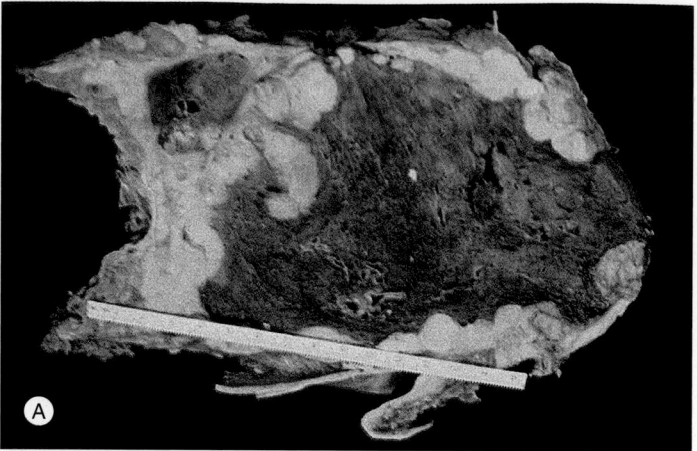

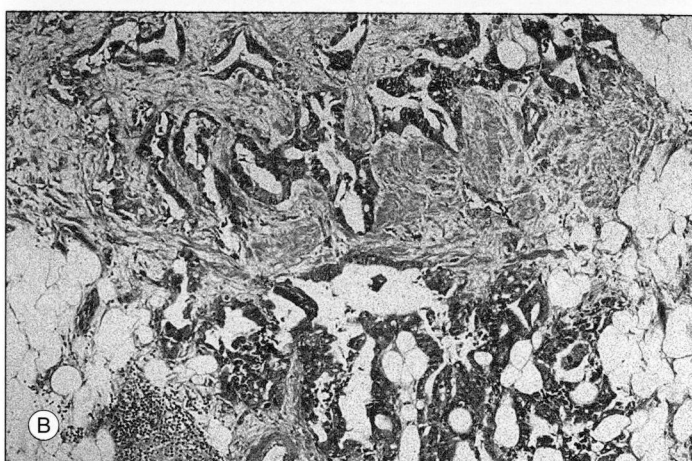

Fig. 19.29 A, Gross appearance of pseudomesotheliomatous adenocarcinoma of the lung after radical extrapleural pneumonectomy. The appearance closely mimics that of malignant mesothelioma; **B**, The tumor consists of irregularly shaped glands in a desmoplastic stroma with invasion of adipose tissue. Case provided by Dr. Sam Hammar, Bremerton, WA.

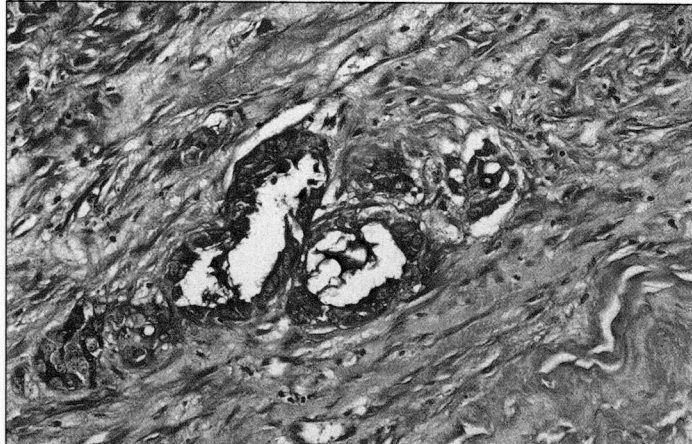

Fig. 19.30 The glandular lumens of this pseudomesotheliomatous adenocarcinoma contain neutral mucin, as demonstrated by periodic acid–Schiff (PAS) stain following diastase. Same case as Figure 19.29. (PASD)

NON-NEOPLASTIC PERICARDIAL DISEASES

Congenital cysts and defects

Pericardial cysts are the most common cystic lesions of the pericardium. They are typically unilocular, and may be of mesothelial or bronchogenic origin. Radiographically, they produce costophrenic mass lesions that may cause clinical confusion. Occasionally, multiple cysts are present. Certain congenital abnormalities such as partial or complete absence of the pericardium have been reported.[182] In rare cases, the pericardial sac may have a diverticulum that clinically and radiographically resembles a mass lesion.[183] Ectopic tissues may rarely be found in pericardium.[182]

Inflammation

Inflammatory diseases of the pericardium are similar to those of the pleura.[183] Suppurative pericarditis usually develops as a result of bacterial infection, caused mainly by complication of surgical procedures or trauma. The most common organisms are staphylococci, pneumococci, and streptococci. Fibrinous pericarditis may be caused by myocardial infarction, renal failure, collagen vascular diseases, rheumatic fever, radiation, or chemotherapy. Granulomatous pericarditis may be due to mycobacterial or fungal infections or sarcoidosis. It must be kept in mind that pericardial inflammation may also be due to malignant neoplasms secondarily involving the pericardium.

Fibrosis and calcification

Any of the causes of pericardial inflammation noted above may eventuate in pericardial fibrosis. In the past, severe fibrosis and calcification of the pericardium was related to infection by *Mycobacterium tuberculosis*, a process referred to as concretio cordis. Severe pericardial fibrosis with or without calcification may lead to cardiac tamponade by interfering with cardiac filling during diastole. Pericardial plaque formation with calcification has also been associated with exposure to asbestos.[184,185]

NEOPLASTIC PERICARDIAL DISEASES

Primary pericardial neoplasms

Malignant mesothelioma

Malignant mesothelioma of the pericardium is a very rare disease, with approximately 150 cases reported in the literature.[44,186–188] The ratio of reported cases of pleural mesothelioma to reported cases of pericardial mesothelioma is greater than 100:1.[44] The epidemiology, pathogenesis, and pathologic features of pericardial mesothelioma are similar to those of pleural mesothelioma. Most patients present with pericardial effusion or compromised cardiac function. A history of asbestos exposure has been documented in some cases.[189–191] These tumors typically encase the heart in a rind of tumor (Fig. 19.31) and occasionally invade the myocardium. Invasion of adjacent structures, extension into the peritoneal cavity, and involvement of mediastinal lymph nodes can occur. The spectrum of histologic types is similar to that seen in pleural mesotheliomas (Fig. 19.32), although biphasic patterns seem to predominate.[44] The prognosis for these patients is poor, with a mean survival time of 3.5 months.[186]

Pericardial mesothelioma must be distinguished from metastatic malignancies to the heart, which are far more common than primary pericardial tumors.[187] They should also be distinguished from rare cases of angiosarcoma, fibrosarcoma, rhabdomyosarcoma, Kaposi's sarcoma,[192] lymphoma,[193] synovial sarcoma, malignant Schwannoma,[187] well-differentiated papillary mesothelioma,[194] and malignant germ cell tumors[195] that have been reported in the pericardium. In addition, primary pericardial mesothelioma must not be confused with the much more common pleural mesothelioma that secondarily extends to involve and even encase the heart.[1,28] Finally, pericardial mesothelioma should be distinguished from benign mesothelial hyperplasia of the pericardium. The criteria for making these distinctions, including histochemical, immunohistochemical, and ultrastructural studies, are outlined in the section on pleural diseases.

Benign tumors

Benign primary tumors of the pericardium are extremely rare.[196] Lipomas,[196] germ cell tumors,[197] lymphangioma,[187] thymomas,[187] giant lymph node hyperplasia,[198] and giant intraparacardial localized fibrous tumors[199] have been reported. A distinctive cardiovascular lesion that resembles histiocytoid (epithelioid) hemangioma involving the endocardium and pericardial cavity has also been described.[200,201] Based on its immunologic and morphologic features, a possible mesothelial origin for this lesion has been suggested.

Secondary pericardial neoplasms

Most neoplasms involving the pericardium are metastatic carcinomas, usually from lung, breast, stomach, or esophageal primaries.[187] In addition, direct extension from adjacent organs may occur.[187] Leukemia, lymphoma, and melanoma occasionally involve the pericardium. The gross appearance of metastatic tumors may resemble mesothelioma in these cases, and a distinction should be made histochemically, immunohistochemically, and/or ultrastructurally. In addition, malignant pleural mesothelioma may invade the adjacent pericardium and even encase the heart in a pattern that mimics pericardial mesothelioma.

THE PERITONEUM

The peritoneum is a continuous membrane that lines the abdominal wall and intra-abdominal organs.[1] The visceral peritoneum covers the intra-abdominal viscera and mesenteries. The parietal peritoneum covers the abdominal wall, the anterior aspects of the retroperitoneal viscera, the inferior diaphragm, and the pelvis.[1] Inguinal and umbilical hernias and the tunica vaginalis testis are out-pouchings of the peritoneum.[1] The morphologic, histochemical, immunohistochemical, and ultrastructural features of peritoneal mesothelial cells are similar to those of mesothelial cells of the pleura and pericardium.

NON-NEOPLASTIC PERITONEAL DISEASES

Inflammation

Acute and chronic inflammation of the peritoneum can be caused by a variety of infectious and noninfectious agents. Primary bacterial peritonitis is usually seen in children with streptococcal infection or in alcoholics with cirrhosis and ascites. Secondary bacterial peritonitis is caused by intestinal perforation. Rarely, infectious agents such as *Actinomyces*, *Candida*, and amebae may cause acute peritonitis. The cause of tuberculous peritonitis may be either systemic infection or direct extension within the abdominal cavity.[202] Granulomatous peritonitis may on rare occasions be caused by fungi.

Foreign or other irritant material can lead to granulomatous peritonitis of noninfectious origin. Examples include talc introduced into the peritoneum surgically, ruptured bowel contents, ruptured ovarian dermoid cyst,[203] meconium, pancreatic and intestinal secretions, and bile. Rare cases of granulomatous peritonitis have

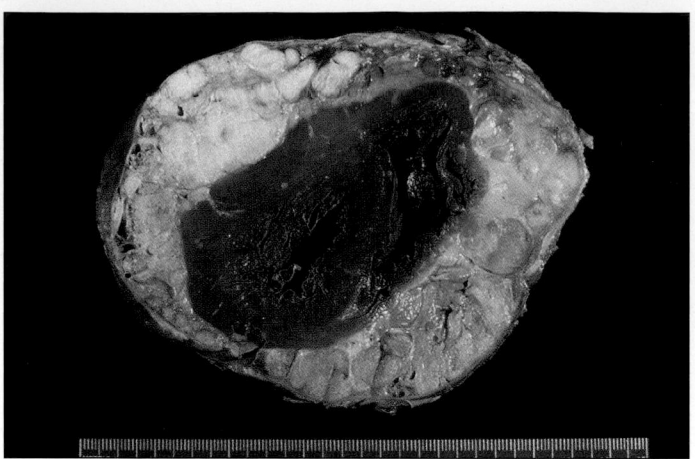

Fig. 19.31 Gross appearance of pericardial mesothelioma at autopsy. The heart has been encased in a rind of tumor. This patient had no history of asbestos exposure.

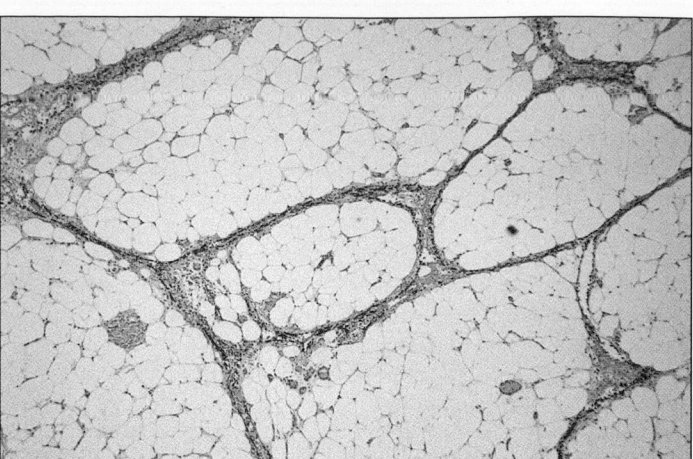

Fig. 19.33 Reactive mesothelium in the peritoneal cavity. The reactive cells surround lobules of fat in the omentum. This pattern should not be confused with invasion. Courtesy Dr. Andrew Churg, Vancouver, BC. (Keratin IHC)

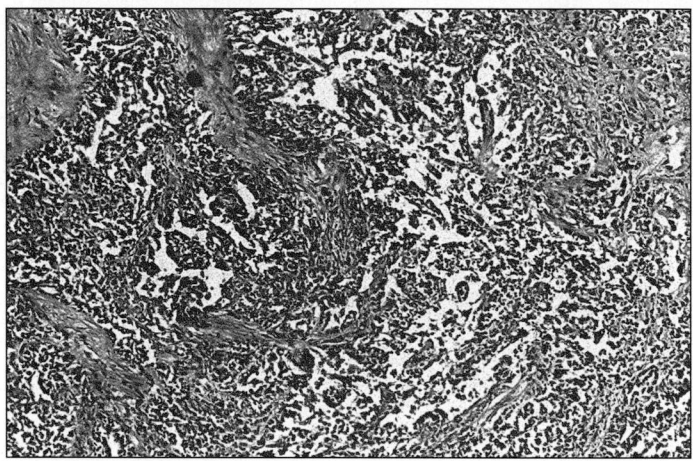

Fig. 19.32 Papillary epithelial variant of malignant pericardial mesothelioma. Same case as Figure 19.31. (H&E)

been reported secondary to sarcoidosis[204] and Crohn's disease.[205] Other rare forms of peritonitis include eosinophilic peritonitis,[206] peritonitis in patients with collagen vascular disease,[207] and recurrent acute peritonitis in periodic disease (familial Mediterranean fever).[208]

Reactive mesothelial hyperplasia

Reactive mesothelial cells may show marked cytologic atypia that can be confused with malignant mesothelioma, especially in small biopsy specimens. Striking proliferation and atypia may be observed in individuals with cirrhosis and ascites. Localized atypical proliferation of mesothelial cells (nodular mesothelial hyperplasia) may simulate mesothelioma in hernia sacs.[209] The presence of grossly visible nodules and invasion of adjacent tissues favors mesothelioma over reactive processes.[8] However, hyperplastic mesothelial cells surrounding lobules of fat in the omentum may result in a pattern that can be confused with invasion by the unwary (Fig. 19.33).[8] Occasionally, psammoma bodies are observed in conditions associated with reactive mesothelial hyperplasia.

Marked focal mesothelial hyperplasia may be seen in association with various ovarian neoplasms.[210] The presence of mesothelial hyperplasia overlying a borderline papillary serous tumor may be misinterpreted as invasion by an ovarian neoplasm.[211] Similarly, papillary mesothelial cell hyperplasia with vascular stroma may resemble an ovarian serous tumor involving the omentum.[211]

Adhesions and peritoneal fibrosis

Adhesions and reactive fibrosis occur as complications of inflammation and intra-abdominal surgery and may cause intestinal obstruction. Localized peritoneal fibrosis histologically similar to parietal pleural plaques may occur on the surface of the liver or spleen in patients with hepatic cirrhosis, pulmonary tuberculosis, or asbestos exposure.[212] In sclerosing or fibrosing peritonitis, diffuse and extensive fibrosis is present throughout the peritoneal cavity. Most cases are idiopathic, but occasional cases have been reported in patients with asbestos exposure,[213] carcinoid syndrome, chronic peritoneal dialysis,[214] and in patients who have been treated with beta-adrenergic blocking agents.[215] Marked reactive peritoneal fibrosis must be distinguished from desmoplastic peritoneal mesothelioma. Criteria for the differential diagnosis are similar to those described for distinguishing pleural fibrosis from desmoplastic mesothelioma of the pleura.[8,48]

Metaplastic conditions

Metaplastic changes may occasionally occur in mesothelial cells, including those of the peritoneum.[216] Proliferative epithelial peritoneal lesions associated with some low-grade ovarian serous neoplasms are considered by some investigators to represent examples of mesothelial cell metaplasia. Other examples include endometriosis, endosalpingiosis, and Walthard rests. Metaplastic changes may also occur in submesothelial cells. Decidual reaction of pregnancy, chondroid metaplasia, and a rare condition called leiomyomatosis peritonealis disseminata are considered to be examples of metaplasia of submesothelial cells.

Endometriosis and endosalpingiosis

Endometriosis involving the peritoneum usually appears as hemorrhagic, fibrotic, blue or brown lesions that often form nodules or cysts.[217] These lesions are characterized by a benign endometrial type of epithelium with associated endometrial-type stroma. Foci of endometriosis may exhibit changes similar to those of the cycling endometrium and undergo atrophy in postmenopausal women. Hyperplastic and metaplastic changes may occur, and glandular elements may develop variable degrees of nuclear atypia. The lesions may become necrotic, with pseudoxanthoma cells and fibrosis. Abundant smooth muscle may be present, thought to be of Müllerian stromal origin. When muscle is prominent, the lesion is referred to as endomyometriosis. Malignant neoplasms may arise from endometriosis, with endometrioid and clear cell carcinoma being the most common types.[218] Endometrial stromal sarcoma, carcinosarcoma (malignant mesodermal mixed tumor), pelvic adenosarcoma, yolk sac tumor, and sex cord tumor with annular tubules have also been reported.[219–223]

Endosalpingiosis has a characteristic microscopic appearance. The lesion is found mainly in the pelvic peritoneum, omentum, and on ovarian surfaces.[224] However, it may involve any area of the peritoneum as well as intra-abdominal lymph nodes. The lesions are typically small and may become cystic. The glands are lined by a single layer of bland-appearing ciliated epithelial cells associated with a fibrotic stroma that lacks the characteristics of endometrial-type stroma. In addition, benign glands of endocervical type may be encountered in the pelvic peritoneum.[224]

Deciduosis

Ectopic decidual reaction may be seen in pelvic submesothelial stroma and, more rarely, in abdominal sites remote from the pelvis in women.[225] Peritoneal decidual reaction is similar morphologically to that seen in the uterine cervix and oviduct. The finding of necrosis and nuclear atypia may cause confusion with deciduoid malignant mesothelioma. However, the nuclear atypia observed in ectopic decidua is usually less severe than that seen in deciduoid mesothelioma.

Leiomyomatosis peritonealis disseminata

Leiomyomatosis peritonealis disseminata is another example of metaplasia of submesothelial cells.[226] Grossly, the lesion appears as well-demarcated white firm nodules. Microscopically, it is composed of smooth muscle cells with bland, uniform nuclei. The lesion has a benign clinical course, but rarely shows progression to leiomyosarcomas. Rare foci of endometriosis may be present in the nodules, and these may be associated with clinical symptoms.[226]

Chondroid and osseous metaplasia

Foci of osseous or cartilaginous (chondroid) metaplasia have rarely been described in the peritoneal cavity.[227,228] These consist of single or multiple nodules of well-circumscribed mature bone or cartilage, ranging from 2 mm to 2 cm in size. Histologically, there is no evidence of cytologic atypia, and the lesions are covered by intact mesothelium. Most patients have had a history of prior surgery. These lesions presumably represent metaplasia of submesothelial mesenchyme. Interestingly, reported cases of heterotopic mesenteric ossification have occurred primarily in men whereas cartilaginous metaplasia has been reported in women.[227,228]

Walthard rests

Walthard rests arising in the serosa of the fallopian tubes and adnexal structures probably derive from foci of transitional epithelium of Müllerian origin. Rarely, Brenner tumors may arise from this transitional epithelium.[229]

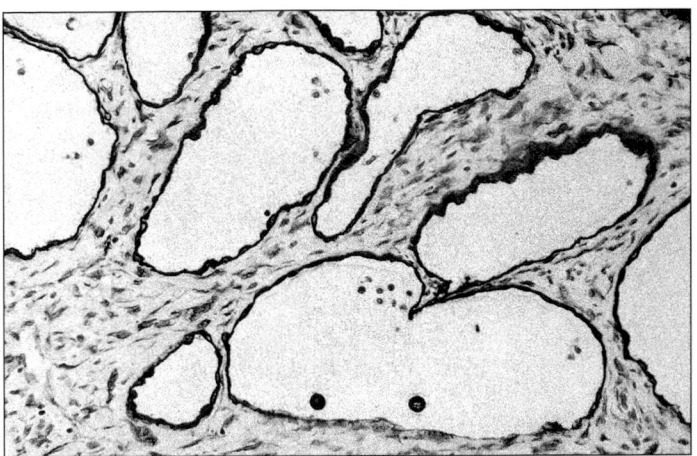

Fig. 19.34 Multilocular peritoneal inclusion cyst is lined by a single layer of flattened to cuboidal mesothelium. (Keratin IHC)

Unilocular and multilocular peritoneal cysts

Peritoneal inclusion cysts usually are an incidental finding in the peritoneal cavity of women. They are generally small and unilocular, have a translucent wall, and contain a watery, clear fluid. They may be either single or multiple and range from 1.5 cm to 6.0 cm in diameter. The cysts have a thin connective tissue wall lined by a single layer of flattened, uniform mesothelial cells.[230]

Multilocular peritoneal inclusion cyst (MPIC) is a controversial entity that has gone by many names, including cystic mesothelioma, multicystic peritoneal mesothelioma, postoperative peritoneal cysts, multicystic peritoneal inclusion cysts, and inflammatory cysts of the peritoneum.[231–244] It most commonly involves the pelvic peritoneum[211] but may also involve the surface of the intra-abdominal organs and, rarely, the retroperitoneum. Involvement of the liver, spleen, or pancreas has also been reported.[240] Similar lesions have been described in the pleural cavity.[245]

The lesion occurs predominantly in young women, but may also occur in men[243] and even in children.[240] Patients may present with abdominal or pelvic pain, and most patients have a tender, palpable mass simulating an ovarian tumor.[211] A history of pelvic surgery, inflammatory pelvic disease, or endometriosis can be elicited in the majority of cases.[240,241] The lesions occasionally are discovered incidentally at laparotomy.[240] In most patients, the clinical course is benign.[241] Recurrences, however, have been noted in approximately half of cases, and some patients have been reported to die of the disease.[231,240] There was no correlation between the extent of disease and survival in the series studied by Weiss and Tavassoli.[240] Some authors consider the lesion to be neoplastic,[235] while others believe that it is reactive.[236,238]

Grossly, MPIC consists of a confluent mass of multiple translucent, membranous cysts, arranged in grape-like clusters, located on the surface of the peritoneum. The cysts vary in size from a few millimeters up to 20 cm.[211] They usually contain clear fluid, although blood-tinged and, rarely, gelatinous or mucinous intracystic fluid may be present.[211] Histologically, the cysts are separated by fibrous septa and lined by a single or several layers of cuboidal to flattened mesothelial cells (Fig. 19.34).[241] Cells with a hobnail appearance are occasionally observed. Focal mesothelial cell hyperplasia, adenomatoid change, or squamous metaplasia can occur.[211,240] Rarely, the mesothelial lining shows atypical proliferation with cytologic atypia, which may be confused with malignant mesothelioma or serous carcinoma.

The differential diagnosis includes malignant mesothelioma, lymphangioma, and adenomatoid tumors. Mesotheliomas occasionally are associated with marked microcystic changes, but usually exhibit papillary or tubulopapillary patterns with pronounced cellular proliferation and cytologic atypia.[211] Cystic lymphangioma may grossly resemble MPIC but can be distinguished microscopically by the presence of smooth muscle and lymphoid cells in the cyst wall. The lining cells of lymphangioma typically express endothelial cell-associated antigens and lack cytokeratins.[211] Moreover, ultrastructural studies of MPIC show typical features of mesothelial cells.[233,238,242] Rarely, adenomatoid tumors show cystic changes and may be confused with MPIC.[211]

There is no documented evidence that MPIC is related to asbestos exposure. In one of the authors' (VLR) series of more than 1800 mesotheliomas consisting mostly of medicolegal cases of individuals allegedly exposed to asbestos, not a single case of so-called 'multicystic mesothelioma' was observed. We believe that this represents further evidence of the reactive rather than neoplastic nature of this entity.

Splenosis

Splenosis typically occurs as a result of implantation of splenic tissue after traumatic rupture of the spleen.[246] The clinical picture and gross appearance in women may resemble endometriosis or peritoneal carcinomatosis, with nodules ranging from microscopic size to several centimeters in diameter.[246] Thoracic splenosis has also been described.[247]

Melanosis

Benign peritoneal melanosis is a rarely reported entity consisting of focal or diffuse brown peritoneal pigmentation or dark tumor-like nodules within the pelvis and omentum. All documented cases have been associated with ovarian mature cystic teratomas.[248]

Trophoblastic implants

Trophoblastic implants occur as a postoperative complication of treatment for tubal pregnancy.[249] Implants of villi and trophoblastic tissue occur in the pelvic peritoneum or omentum. These implants are more likely to occur in cases managed by laparoscopy than in those managed by laparotomy.

Gliomatosis peritonei

Benign mature glial implants have been reported to occur on the peritoneal surfaces.[250] The condition is known as gliomatosis peritonei and is a complication of ovarian immature teratoma. The lesion may persist or eventually disappear. Rare malignant transformation has been reported.[250]

Inflammatory myofibroblastic tumor (plasma cell granuloma)

Inflammatory myofibroblastic tumors have been identified in multiple sites of the body, including the abdomen.[251,252] The lesion, also known as inflammatory pseudotumor and plasma cell granuloma, consists of myofibroblastic spindle cells with interspersed plasma cells and small lymphocytes. Patients are usually young and present with a mesenteric mass, fever, weight loss, anemia, thrombocytosis, and polyclonal hypergammaglobulinemia. The disease has a benign clinical course, with symptoms typically disappearing after surgical resection.[251,252]

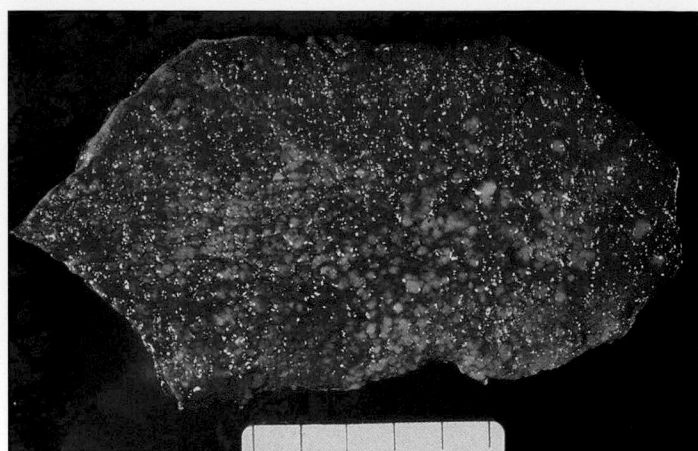

Fig. 19.35 Gross appearance of the undersurface of the diaphragm in a patient with malignant peritoneal mesothelioma, showing a myriad of confluent nodules of tumor.

Omental-mesenteric myxoid hamartoma

Omental-mesenteric myxoid hamartoma is a novel entity first described by Gonzalez-Crussi et al.[253] The lesion is characterized by multiple omental and mesenteric nodules, which may be confused with malignant neoplasm. Microscopically, these lesions consist of a richly vascularized, myxoid stroma with plump mesenchymal cells. Follow-up has demonstrated a benign clinical course without recurrence.[253] It may represent a variant of inflammatory myofibroblastic tumor.[251]

NEOPLASTIC PERITONEAL DISEASES

Primary peritoneal neoplasms

Malignant mesothelioma

Malignant mesotheliomas of the peritoneum are far less common than pleural mesotheliomas, accounting for 10–20% of all mesotheliomas.[44,254] Most patients have a history of asbestos exposure, and on average, a greater cumulative exposure is seen with peritoneal as compared to pleural tumors.[255,256] Rare cases have been reported after recurrent peritonitis[257] or after radiation to the abdominal and pelvic areas.[258–260] The tumor occurs primarily in middle-aged or elderly adults, but may occur in young adults and even children.[31,261–263] Patients typically present with non-specific clinical symptoms, including weight loss, abdominal discomfort, and ascites.

In its early stages, malignant peritoneal mesothelioma consists of numerous small plaques and nodules of various sizes, indistinguishable from those of carcinomatosis peritonealis (Fig. 19.35).[264,265] In advanced stages, mesothelioma encases the abdominal viscera in a thick cake of tumor. Invasion of underlying structures such as the outer aspect of the intestine is not unusual. Invasion of the pancreas rarely occurs. Occasionally, there is involvement of both the peritoneal and pleural cavities, making determination of the primary site difficult or impossible. Metastases to abdominal lymph nodes and, rarely, to axillary lymph nodes, liver, and lung occur as late complications of the disease. Although most peritoneal mesotheliomas are diffuse, occasional patients may present with a localized mass.[266] Rarely, patients may present with ovarian masses.[267] The tunica vaginalis testis is an extension of the peritoneal cavity, and in exceptional cases mesotheliomas may occur at this site. These lesions typically present as a hydrocele or paratesticular mass. The tumor may spread to the peritoneal surface, and metastases to inguinal and retroperitoneal lymph nodes have been reported.[268–270]

Malignant peritoneal mesothelioma has similar histologic features to those of pleural mesothelioma. However, the sarcomatoid variant is quite uncommon in the peritoneum, accounting for only 4% of 185 peritoneal mesotheliomas from one of the authors' series (VLR). One histologic variant of peritoneal mesothelioma that merits further discussion is the deciduoid variant. This pattern consists of sheets of large epithelioid cells with sharply delimited cell borders and abundant glassy cytoplasm, resembling peritoneal deciduosis (see above). Originally described in the peritoneum of young women,[271,272] this variant is now recognized to occur in the pleura or peritoneum of both sexes.[273–275] Rare morphologic variants of peritoneal mesothelioma with dense lymphocytic and granulomatous stroma or mesothelioma associated with large numbers of foamy lipid-rich histiocytes have been reported.[262,276] The ultrastructural, histochemical, and immunohistochemical features of peritoneal mesothelioma are similar to those of the pleural and pericardial mesothelioma as noted previously.

The most frequently encountered differential diagnoses of peritoneal mesothelioma are metastatic adenocarcinoma with diffuse involvement of the peritoneum and primary serous carcinoma of the peritoneum in women. The morphologic distinction can be quite difficult, and appropriate ancillary studies should be performed. The presence of psammoma bodies and diastase-resistant periodic acid–Schiff-positive intracellular mucin supports the diagnosis of papillary serous carcinoma. As is the case for pleural mesothelioma, immunohistochemical studies are helpful for supporting or excluding the diagnosis of peritoneal mesothelioma. We use a slightly different panel for peritoneal mesotheliomas (see Table 19.2), since many of the malignancies in the differential diagnosis are also negative for CEA, and TTF-1 is less useful since metastatic lung cancer is less likely a differential diagnostic consideration. One must also be cautious not to rely too heavily on CK 5/6, since many of the tumors that involve the abdomen or peritoneum will stain positive for this antibody.[123] Adenocarcinoma of the rete testis, when it involves the tunica vaginalis, may also be confused with mesothelioma.[277]

The prognosis for peritoneal mesothelioma is poor, and most patients die of the disease within a year of the diagnosis.[278] However, a recent study has shown that the prognosis of peritoneal mesothelioma in women is highly variable, and morphologic features cannot reliably identify tumors with a favorable prognosis.[279]

Serous carcinoma

The clinical presentation and pattern of peritoneal involvement of primary serous carcinoma of the peritoneum are similar to those of serous carcinoma of the ovary with secondary involvement of the peritoneum. The tumor extensively involves the peritoneal surfaces, particularly in the pelvis and omentum, mimicking a malignant peritoneal mesothelioma. In most patients, the ovaries are grossly unremarkable or may have small granules on their surfaces.

Histologically, primary serous carcinoma of the peritoneum is identical to ovarian serous carcinoma.[280] The tumors typically exhibit complex papillary formations with 'tufting' (Fig. 19.36), and psammoma bodies are often present. In some cases, these may be so numerous that the term psammocarcinoma has been suggested.[281,282] Mucin positivity is also a helpful feature, with the identification of intracytoplasmic PAS-positive, diastase-resistant vacuoles supporting a diagnosis of serous papillary carcinoma (Fig. 19.37). Nuclear anaplasia may be moderate to marked. However, there is sufficient

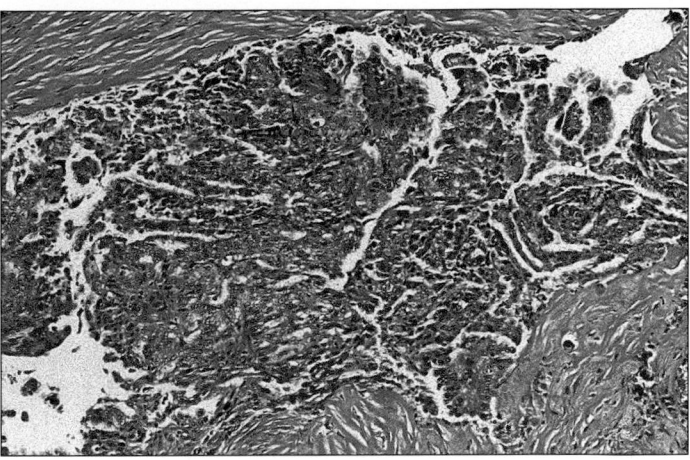

Fig. 19.36 Serous papillary carcinoma of the peritoneum in a woman shows complex papillary structures with tufting. The tumor cells are surrounded by a desmoplastic stroma. (H&E)

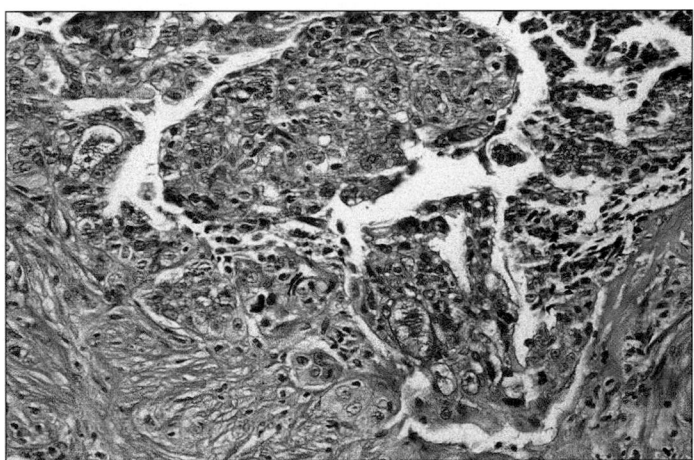

Fig. 19.37 Neutral mucin is present within this serous carcinoma of the peritoneum, as demonstrated by periodic acid–Schiff (PAS) stain following diastase. Same case as Figure 19.36. (PASD)

overlap in the histologic features of mesothelioma and serous carcinoma that immunohistochemical studies are often required to make the distinction (Fig. 19.38).[283–286] In a recent study, Ordonez found that calretinin, thrombomodulin, CK 5/6, MOC-31, B72.3, BerEP4, CA-19-9, and Leu M1 are the best antibodies for distinguishing serous papillary carcinoma of the peritoneum from malignant peritoneal mesothelioma (see also Table 19.3).[286]

The prognosis is poor and probably is the same as that of advanced ovarian serous carcinoma with a similar degree of peritoneal involvement.

Well-differentiated papillary mesothelioma

Well-differentiated papillary mesothelioma is a rare and clinically indolent neoplasm that occurs mainly in the peritoneum of young women.[287] A few cases have been reported in the pleura, epicardium, and tunica vaginalis.[46,269,287] Most patients have multiple pelvic and omental nodules, ranging in size from 0.5 cm to several centimeters. Histologically, tumors consist of papillary structures with a

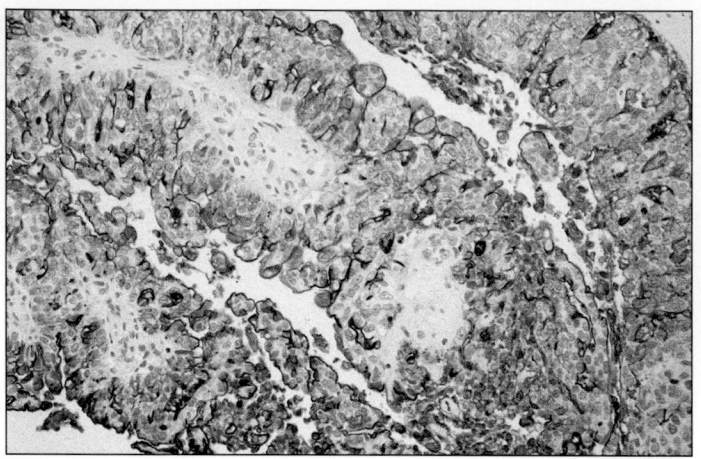

Fig. 19.38 Serous papillary carcinoma of the peritoneum showing positive staining for CA-125. Same case as Figures 19.36 and 19.37. (IHC)

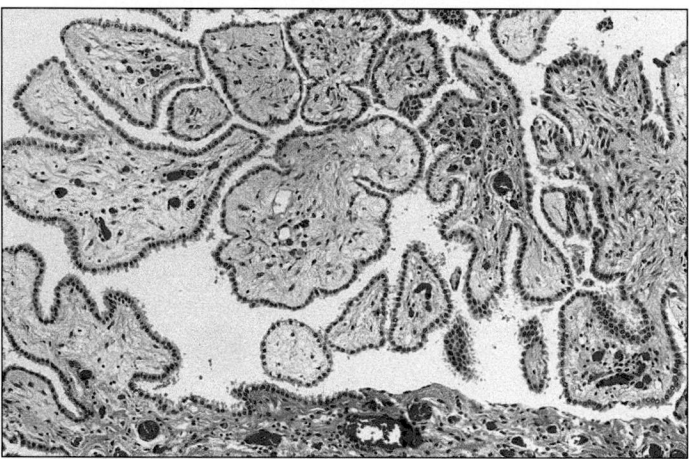

Fig. 19.39 Well-differentiated papillary mesothelioma of the peritoneum. A single layer of cuboidal uniform tumor cells lines the surface of fibrovascular cores. (See also Figure 19.10) (H&E)

fibrovascular core and lined by a single layer of uniform flattened to cuboidal mesothelial cells (Fig. 19.39). The histochemical, immuno-histochemical, and ultrastructural features of the tumor support a mesothelial origin.

The distinction of well-differentiated papillary mesothelioma from malignant mesothelioma is critical, since the prognosis is vastly different for these two tumor types. The distinction is not as straightforward as it may seem, since we have observed the well-differentiated papillary pattern in tumors that were otherwise typical tubulopapillary mesotheliomas. Furthermore, some well-differentiated papillary mesotheliomas have behaved aggressively, causing the death of the patient, whereas some epithelial peritoneal mesotheliomas in women pursue a more indolent clinical course.[46,279,287] Consequently, we suggest that the term well-differentiated papillary mesothelioma be reserved exclusively for those cases lacking an invasive component. Tumors that contain an invasive component are more likely to behave aggressively and would have a more guarded prognosis. Such tumors should be designated as epithelial mesotheliomas with a focal well-differentiated papillary component.

Adenomatoid tumor

Adenomatoid tumor is a distinctive benign tumor, commonly found around the genital tract.[288] They are typically discrete, tan-yellow nodules ranging from a few millimeters to several centimeters in size. In women, most are found adjacent to the fallopian tubes, serosal surfaces of the uterus, or broad ligaments. Occasionally, they are found in the ovarian hilus or ovary.[289] In men, most are found in relation to the epididymis, but some occur in the spermatic cord or on the surface of the testis. Rare tumors have been reported in the omentum.[290] A number of histologic variants have been described, including solid, adenoid, angiomatoid, and cystic patterns. Multicentric adenomatoid tumors and rare malignant adenomatoid tumors have been reported.[291] The mesothelial nature of this tumor is supported by immunohistochemical and ultrastructural studies.[292,293]

Localized fibrous tumor

Localized fibrous tumors of the peritoneum are extremely rare, only a few cases having been reported.[294] The gross appearance and microscopic features of peritoneal localized fibrous tumors are identical to those of localized fibrous tumors of the pleura. Young et al.[295] reported three cases and reviewed an additional seven previously reported cases. The patients' ages ranged from 27 to 68 years. Seven tumors occurred in men and three in women. Most were large (>9 cm), solid, and encapsulated masses with a whorled, homogeneous cut surface. There was no recurrence in any of the cases for which follow-up information was available. The immunohistochemical features in the cases studied were similar to the established immunophenotype of solitary fibrous tumors of the pleura.[146,147] These tumors are immunoreactive with vimentin, CD34, and bcl-2 but fail to stain for cytokeratins, actin, or desmin. Localized fibrous tumors should be distinguished from gastrointestinal stromal tumors and gastrointestinal autonomic nerve tumors, with which they may be confused.[296] There is no evidence for an asbestos etiology of peritoneal localized fibrous tumors.[295]

Desmoplastic small round cell tumor

Desmoplastic small round cell tumor (DSRCT) is an extremely rare and distinctive peritoneal tumor that has an uncertain histogenesis, although a possible mesothelial origin has been suggested.[297] This tumor is typically found in young males in the first or second decade.[297,298] At laparotomy, DSRCT appears as an enlarged mass associated with smaller peritoneal nodules. Histologically, the tumor is composed of sharply demarcated masses of basophilic cells embedded in a desmoplastic stroma (Fig. 19.40). Neoplastic cells are uniform and round with scanty cytoplasm, ill-defined cell borders, and round to oval hyperchromatic nuclei. Nucleoli are inconspicuous. The tumors have a high mitotic activity and there are foci of necrosis. Clear cell change or rhabdoid features may be seen focally in some cases.

Immunohistochemically, the tumor cells stain positive for cytokeratins, neuron-specific enolase, vimentin, and desmin.[297,299] Ultrastructurally, tumor cells contain intermediate cytoplasmic filaments packed in perinuclear bundles. The Ewing's sarcoma and Wilms' tumor-1 genes are activated in neoplastic cells of DSRCT.[300] The tumor is highly aggressive, with extra-abdominal metastases reported in some cases. The tumor has also been reported to originate in the pleura (see above). The treatment usually consists of debulking, followed by postoperative radiation and chemotherapy.

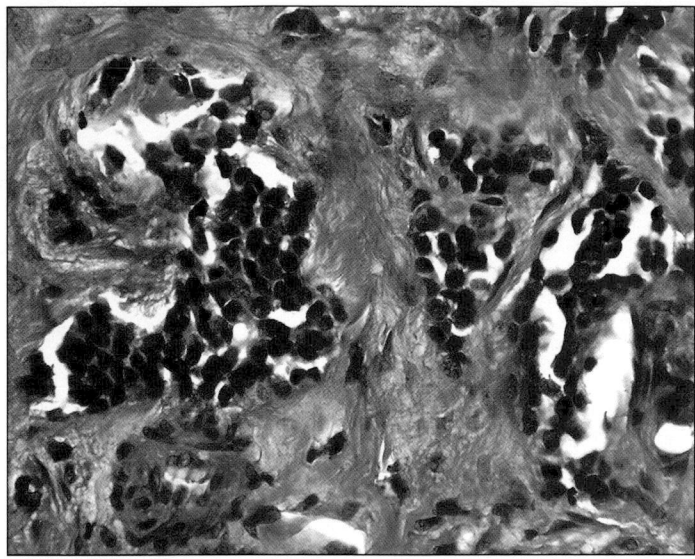

Fig. 19.40 Desmoplastic small round cell tumor of the peritoneum consists of nests of small blue tumor cells surrounded by a desmoplastic stroma. (H&E)

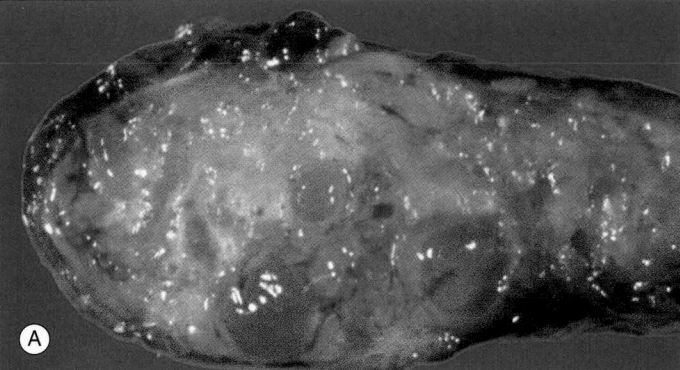

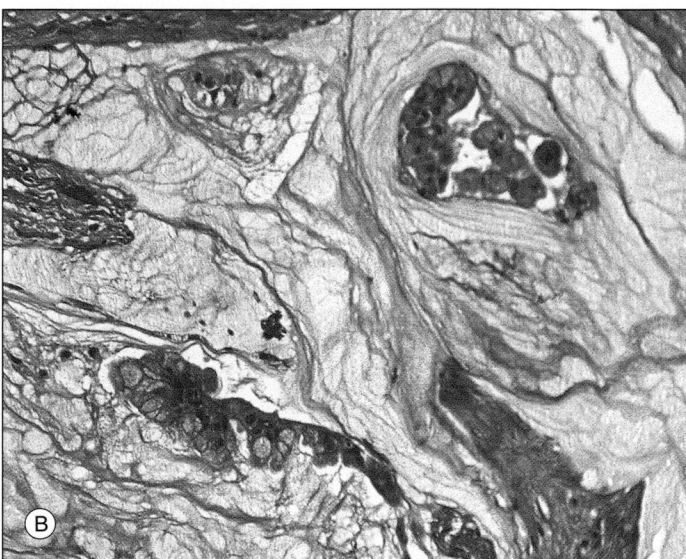

Fig. 19.41 **A**, Gross appearance of pseudomyxoma peritonei. Multiple deposits throughout the abdomen give this lesion the name 'jelly belly;' **B**, Microscopic appearance, showing abundant mucin in association with scattered clusters of tumor cells. (H&E)

Secondary peritoneal neoplasms

The peritoneum is a common site of metastatic implantation of tumors.[301–303] The most common primary sites include ovaries, stomach, colon, and breast.[1] The omentum is often involved at an early stage and may be converted to an indurated mass, sometimes referred to as an omental cake. The appearance may closely mimic that of a mesothelioma. Histochemical and immunohistochemical stains (see Table 19.3) usually permit the distinction to be made. Ultrastructural studies may also be helpful in difficult cases.

Pseudomyxoma peritonei

Diffuse involvement of the peritoneal cavity by mucinous implants is called pseudomyxoma peritonei (Fig. 19.41). These lesions typically arise from a primary mucinous cystadenoma or cystadeno-carcinoma of the ovary or appendix, or, in some cases, both. The implants grossly have a gelatinous appearance, giving rise to the term 'jelly belly'. Ronnett et al. separated pseudomyxoma peritonei into two diagnostic categories.[304] Those cases in which peritoneal lesions were composed primarily of extracellular mucin were designated *disseminated peritoneal adenomucinosis*. Lesions that were characterized by the presence of abundant atypical mucinous epithelium were classified as *peritoneal mucinous carcinomatosis*. A statistically significant difference in survival was noted between these two categories.[304]

CYTOPATHOLOGY OF EFFUSIONS

GENERAL CONSIDERATIONS OF SPECIMEN PREPARATION AND REPORTING

Excess fluid accumulations within the serous cavities are referred to as effusions. Effusions in the pleural cavity are the most common clinically, followed by peritoneal effusions or ascites, and finally pericardial effusions. Effusions are divided into transudates and exudates, with exudates distinguished from transudates by a ratio of effusion protein to serum protein that is greater than 0.5.[305–307] Differentiation between transudates and exudates is a clinical laboratory procedure, but provides insight into the etiology of effusions.

Transudates result from changes in hydrostatic or oncotic pressures that cause physiologic imbalances in the formation and reabsorption of fluid resulting in fluid accumulation generally as a result of systemic factors. On cytology, transudates generally have scanty cellularity. The most frequent cause of transudative pleural effusion is congestive heart failure, that accounts for approximately 500 000 of the roughly 1 340 000 pleural effusions in the United States each year (about 37%). Other etiologies of transudates include cirrhosis, nephrotic syndrome, glomerulonephritis, hypoalbuminemia and pulmonary emboli.[305–307]

Exudates result from factors localized to the serosal membranes and adjacent tissues that produce leakage of proteins and cells from damaged capillaries. The most frequent cause of exudative pleural effusion is infection. About 300 000 bacterial pneumonias, 100 000 viral infections and 2500 cases of tuberculosis result in exudative pleural effusions in the United States each year. The next most common etiology of exudative pleural effusion is malignancy with approximately 200 000 caused by pleural metastases and 1500 caused by diffuse malignant mesothelioma per year in the US.[305]

Pulmonary embolization can cause transudative or exudative pleural effusions and accounts for 150 000 cases annually. Interestingly, malignancies can indirectly cause benign transudates or benign exudates by blocking pleural lymphatics or from peritumoral reactions in overlying pleural tissues.[305]

There are numerous other causes of nonmalignant pleural exudates, including collagen vascular diseases, drug reactions, trauma, and asbestos exposure. Cirrhosis and gastrointestinal diseases may cause ascites and also pleural effusion with fluid entering the pleural cavity through defects in the diaphragm. For the same reason, patients undergoing peritoneal dialysis may also develop pleural effusions.

When an effusion fluid is received in the laboratory, the amount of the fluid and the gross features should be recorded. For example, fluids may be bloody, serous, serosanguinous or cloudy, and these gross features may be suggestive of the differential diagnosis. Bloody pleural effusions are characteristic of malignancy, pulmonary embolus, and chest trauma. Cloudy pleural effusion is seen with chylothorax and pseudochylothorax. Knowledge of the clinical setting, clinical suspicions, and any previous or concurrent histopathologic or cytologic diagnoses help put the specimen into proper perspective prior to interpretation.[305–307]

Fluid specimens prepared as cytospins are typically stained with Papanicolaou and Wright's (Diff-Quik) stains. Depending on the volumes received, cell blocks may be prepared for paraffin embedding, sectioning, and staining with H&E or special stains, including immunostains. Fluid specimens can also be submitted for flow cytometry, molecular studies or other specialized tests. Diagnosis of specimens that are poorly preserved or poorly prepared should be avoided since these are subject to misinterpretation.

The primary role of cytopathology is to exclude or diagnose malignancy in effusion fluids. About 30–40% of pleural diffuse malignant mesotheliomas are diagnosed by pleural fluid cytology and about 60–70% of cancers metastatic to the pleura can be diagnosed on fluid cytology.[308] The list of possible etiologies of transudates and exudates means that many fluid samples examined by the cytopathologist will be negative for malignancy. In some situations, the diagnosis of malignancy may be equivocal due to the paucity of the neoplastic cells, obscuring by blood or other cells and/or overlap of cytologic features with reactive atypia. In these situations, depending on the level of concern, diagnoses of 'suspicious for malignancy' or even 'malignancy cannot be ruled out' may be used. Correlation with the clinical setting or with other cytologic or histologic samples may help put findings into their proper context, and communication with the clinician is encouraged in any difficult or unusual case. It should be noted that sometimes cytology specimens may be positive for malignancy when the biopsy is negative and vice versa. It is generally best to err on the conservative side in a questionable case, and if a diagnosis of malignancy cannot be made but is suspected cytologically or clinically, then additional cytology samples or biopsies will typically clarify the diagnosis.[305–307,309]

If a fluid is positive for malignancy, the primary site of the malignancy may be apparent on the basis of the cytologic features. The cytopathologist may wish to do additional studies such as immunohistochemistry to identify or confirm a primary site. A differential of likely primary sites can also be suggested in a report if the specific primary site is not identifiable. If available, correlation of the cytopathology with a previous or concurrent tumor biopsy or resection specimen may be helpful in determining a primary site.

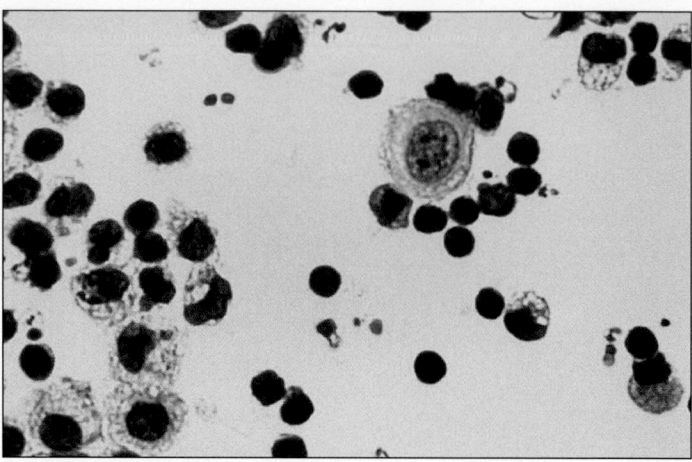

Fig. 19.42 Benign effusion showing a mesothelial cell with fluffy cytoplasmic rim surrounded by lymphocytes and a nearby group of histiocytes with eccentric nuclei and foamy cytoplasm. (Papanicolaou)

When a fluid is negative for malignancy, the cytopathologist may sometimes assist in the diagnosis of effusions by reporting findings such as eosinophilia that have specific differential diagnoses. Specific infectious organisms may be recognized in a fluid, for example viral inclusions or organisms detected with special stains.[309]

BENIGN EFFUSIONS

Cell components

Mesothelial cells

Mesothelial cells are shed into serosal fluids in both transudates and exudates (Fig. 19.42). Particularly in exudates, mesothelial cells may display reactive atypia that is worrisome for malignancy as discussed below. Exfoliated mesothelial cells are usually seen as individual cells or in small aggregates with adjacent cells separated by spaces traditionally referred to as 'windows.' They are round to oval with abundant dense darkly staining cytoplasm and the peripheral cytoplasm may stain darker than the central. Microvilli around the periphery of the cell may cause a characteristic fuzzy rim or border. Cytoplasmic vacuoles may be present and should not cause confusion with mucin-producing adenocarcinoma cells (Fig. 19.43). Nuclei are round to oval with thin distinct nuclear membranes and vesicular to finely granular chromatin. Binucleation or mutinucleation is not uncommon and nuclei within the same cell appear essentially identical. Round uniform nucleoli are apparent and may also be multiple within a single nucleus.[309]

Red blood cells

Blood elements including red blood cells are seen in many effusions when examined microscopically. Red blood cells may merely be a procedural artifact. As noted above, grossly bloody effusions are associated with malignancy, pulmonary embolization, and chest trauma. A pleural effusion hematocrit of more than 50% of the patient's peripheral blood indicates hemothorax.[305,306] On occasion, hemosiderin particles may form aggregates and are referred to as Heinz bodies.[309]

Leukocytes

As noted, the pleural fluid may contain blood elements and small numbers of neutrophils and lymphocytes. Abundant neutrophils

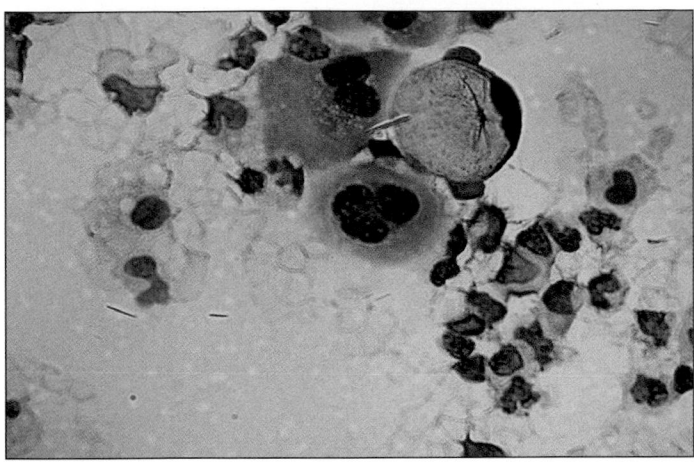

Fig. 19.43 Group of mesothelial cells in benign effusion. Two of the mesothelial cells are binucleated and trinucleated, respectively. One mesothelial cell has a large intracytoplasmic vacuole that compresses the nucleus against the cell membrane mimicking adenocarcinoma. (Papanicolaou)

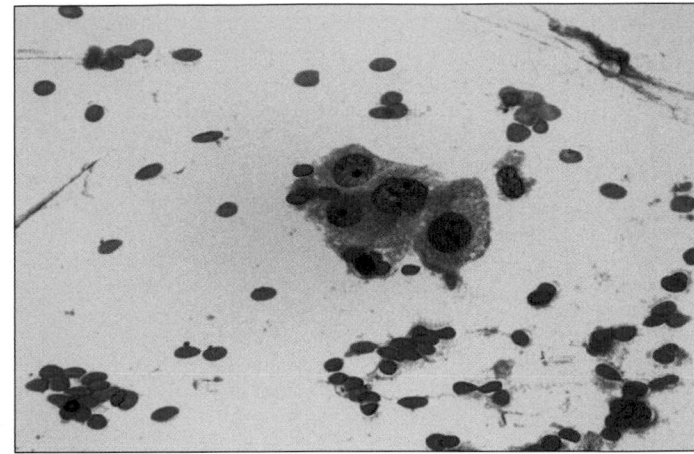

Fig. 19.44 Mesothelial cell hyperplasia in pleural effusion consisting of small cluster of mesothelial cells with simple reactive changes. (H&E)

generally indicate infection, especially bacterial infection. Intra-abdominal abscesses can not only cause ascites, but can also cause exudative pleural effusion with neutrophils.[305]

A finding of abundant pleural fluid lymphocytes is a classic finding in tuberculous pleural effusion and is believed to be a secondary immunologic response to the rupture of bacillary tubercles in most cases. Tuberculous pleural effusions occur in about 30% of patients with tuberculosis, and 65% of patients with tuberculous pleural effusions develop active tuberculosis within 5 years even if their effusion resolves.[310,311] Few bacilli are found in most tuberculous pleural effusions,[312] and a recent study reported sensitivities of 6% for acid-fast staining, 17% for cultures, and 50% for polymerase chain reaction amplification-assay for detection of *Mycobacteria* in tuberculous pleural effusions.[313]

Other causes of lymphocyte-rich exudates include fungal infections, sarcoidosis, and collagen vascular disease.[305,314,315] Lymphocyte-rich pleural effusions can also be seen in lung transplant patients with graft rejection. Pleural malignancy other than lymphoma can cause a lymphocyte-rich pleural effusion even when malignant cells are not detected in the fluid cytology.[305]

Eosinophilia of the pleural fluid occurs when more than 10% of the cells are eosinophils.[305] Eosinophilic pleuritis is a relatively common reaction to pneumothorax, and the most common causes of eosinophilia of the pleural fluid are air or blood in the pleural space. Eosinophils in the pleural fluid may also indicate drug reaction. Less often, pleural eosinophils are seen with infections (parasites, tuberculosis, fungus), Churg-Strauss syndrome, or malignancy.[309]

Lupus erythematosus also may cause effusions containing characteristic cells (lupus cells) formed by a leukocyte with its nucleus displaced by a phagocytized neutrophil.[309,314]

Histiocytes

Histiocytes can be seen in many effusions and may be numerous in the exudates caused by malignancy or chronic inflammation (see Fig. 19.42). Histiocytes have some superficial resemblance to mesothelial cells, but histiocyte nuclei tend to be reniform rather than round and have irregular rather than smooth nuclear borders. The cytoplasm of histiocytes may be foamy in contrast to the dense cytoplasm of mesothelial cells. Whereas mesothelial cells may contain a single large cytoplasmic vacuole, histiocytes are more likely to contain multiple tiny cytoplasmic vacuoles. Similar to mesothelial cells, histiocytes can be binucleated. Histiocytes are characteristic of effusions caused by rheumatoid arthritis in which they are seen with neutrophils and necrotic debris.[307,309,315] When nodular histiocytic hyperplasia of a serosal surface is a histologic mimic of malignancy, present effusions may show vaguely nodular aggregates of bland mononuclear cells with entrapped mesothelial cells.[316]

Reactive mesothelial hyperplasia

Benign mesothelial cells may proliferate and display a spectrum of reactive changes. These range from minimal simple reactive changes to highly atypical reactive changes that enter into the differential diagnosis for malignancy. With simple mesothelial hyperplasia, the mesothelial cells may shed in clusters or sheets and maintain the morphologic features of normal mesothelial cells. With simple reactive mesothelial hyperplasia, the mesothelial cells tend to maintain round to oval nuclei with smooth nuclear contours and fine chromatin (Fig. 19.44).[307,309]

Atypical mesothelial hyperplasia

With increasing cytologic atypia, differentiation of reactive mesothelial cells from malignancies including malignant mesothelioma and metastatic carcinomas can become more difficult (Fig. 19.45).[317–319] Cytologic changes may include enlarged nuclei, coarse chromatin, prominent nucleoli, and frequent mitoses. Nuclear contours may show some variation, but are still generally round to oval with smooth nuclear membranes. Vacuoles in the cytoplasm, already mentioned as a cytologic feature of mesothelial cells, may compress the nucleus and, in the setting of cytologic atypia, mimic signet-ring cells of an adenocarcinoma (see Fig. 19.43).[320] Atypical mesothelial cells may shed as papillary excrescences from the pleural surface or form rosettes or three-dimensional clusters within the fluid, architecturally mimicking adenocarcinoma.[321] Acinar structures have been reported in 6% of benign effusions with atypical reactive mesothelial cells.[317]

Differentiating atypical mesothelial hyperplasia from malignancy may be very difficult. Reactive mesothelial cells stain for the same markers of mesothelial differentiation as do diffuse malignant

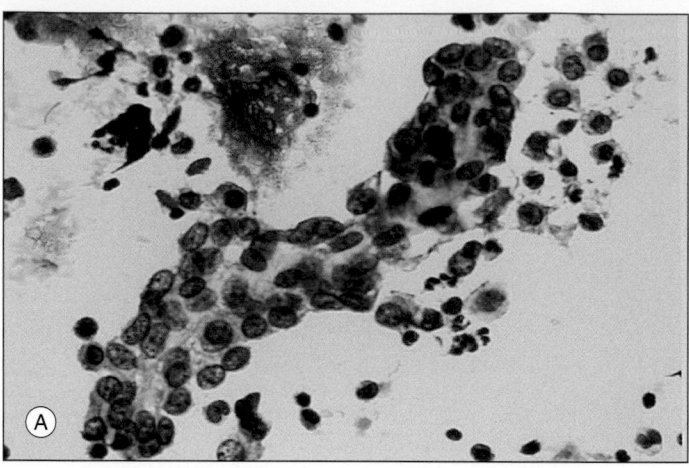
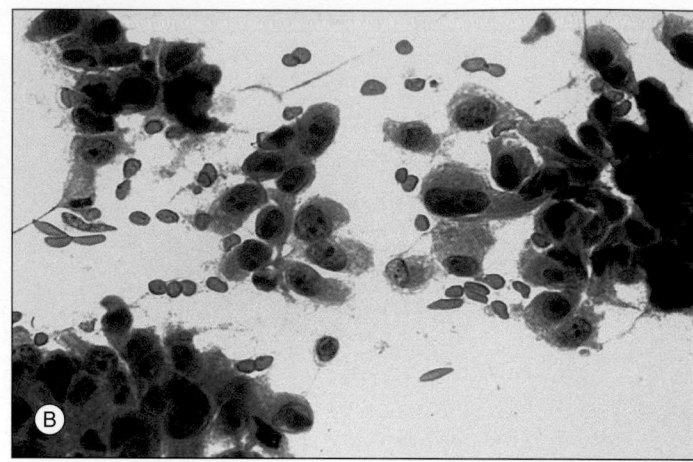

Fig. 19.45 Atypical mesothelial hyperplasia within pleural effusion consisting of (**A**) papillary frond composed of mesothelial cells with reactive atypia (Papanicolaou) and (**B**) large clusters of mesothelial cells with worrisome cytologic atypia mimicking malignancy. (H&E)

mesotheliomas (keratin, CK 7, CK 5/6, calretinin, HBME-1, etc.) and, therefore, merely proving that the cells are mesothelial in origin does not determine if the cells are benign or malignant. It is also imprudent to make a diagnosis of malignancy purely on the basis of apparently positive immunostains for carcinoma markers. One should first determine if the cells are truly malignant before secondarily determining the type of cancer. Regular round to oval nuclei with smooth nuclear membranes favor benign mesothelial cells. Generally, atypical reactive mesothelial cells blend with cells of lesser degrees of reactive atypia within a benign effusion. On the other hand, when a cancer is present, there are two separate and distinct populations of cells – reactive mesothelial cells and frankly malignant cells.

Since there are early mesotheliomas and we believe that mesothelial cell dysplasias and mesothelioma in situ likely exist, some atypical mesothelial proliferations in effusions may represent these entities even when a tumor mass is not present. On the other hand, obstruction of lymphatics by cancer or reactive serosal changes overlying a cancer can produce benign effusions with benign reactive mesothelial hyperplasias even though the patient has a tumor mass. The inability to assess invasion of underlying tissues makes diagnosis of mesothelioma difficult in many effusions. Not only can atypical mesothelial hyperplasias mimic cancer cytologically, but many epithelial mesotheliomas can be very bland cytologically.[1,307,309]

MALIGNANT EFFUSIONS

Malignant effusions are effusions that contain malignant cells.[322–324] As already noted, cancers can obstruct lymphatics or cause peritumoral reactions and inflammation in overlying serosal tissues and thereby produce benign effusions.

The differential diagnosis for an effusion is first between benign and malignant effusion. If a diagnosis of malignancy is made, then the differential diagnosis potentially becomes between one type of cancer and another.[325]

As with other tissues, cancers of the serosal membranes and their malignant effusions can be primary or metastatic. Metastatic cancers are overwhelmingly the most common cancers in malignant effusions. As discussed earlier in this chapter, diffuse malignant mesothelioma is the most common primary cancer of the serosal membranes, but, even so, it is a relatively uncommon cancer. In the United States, diffuse malignant mesothelioma causes about 1500 pleural effusions annually. In contrast, metastatic cancers cause about 200 000 pleural effusions each year for a ratio of about 133 malignant pleural effusions from metastatic cancers for every malignant pleural effusion caused by diffuse malignant mesothelioma.[305,306] A diagnosis of mesothelioma may be suggested when malignant cells consistent with mesothelioma are identified on cytologic smears and cell blocks, with confirmation of mesothelial origin of the malignant cells with immunocytochemistry (Fig. 19.46).[326–332] Cytologic preparations may be used for immunocytochemistry employing cell blocks or smears and cytospins, although the latter have some technical nuances depending on fixatives, preparations, etc.[333,334] The antibodies used for phenotypic evaluation of malignant cells in effusions are the same as those used for histologic sections discussed earlier, and numerous studies have evaluated the efficacy of these antibodies in malignant effusions.[335–359]

In addition to diffuse malignant mesothelioma, there are a few other rare primary cancers of the serosal membranes discussed earlier in this chapter. These rare cancers include serous carcinoma of the peritoneum, occasional sarcomas such as synovial sarcoma and angiosarcoma, and exotic tumors such as desmoplastic small round cell tumor. These cancers can cause malignant effusions and, therefore, although rare, the cytopathologist should be aware of them.

Of the 200 000 malignant pleural effusions caused by metastatic cancers each year, about 60 000 are lung carcinomas, 50 000 are breast carcinomas, 40 000 are lymphoma, and 50 000 are from other primary sites, particularly gastrointestinal and genitourinary carcinomas. In the abdomen, gastrointestinal and genitourinary carcinomas are likely causes of malignant effusions.[305–307,309]

Cancer cells in malignant effusions are most often seen as separate individual cancer cells, in sheets, and in spherical three-dimensional highly cellular clusters called morulae (Fig. 19.47). By focusing up and down, the three-dimensional structure of the morulae is apparent and confirms the compact cellularity. Depending on the morphology of the tumor, cancer cells may be arranged in papillary or acinar structures. Psammoma bodies may be present with papillary cancers including papillary adenocarcinomas from

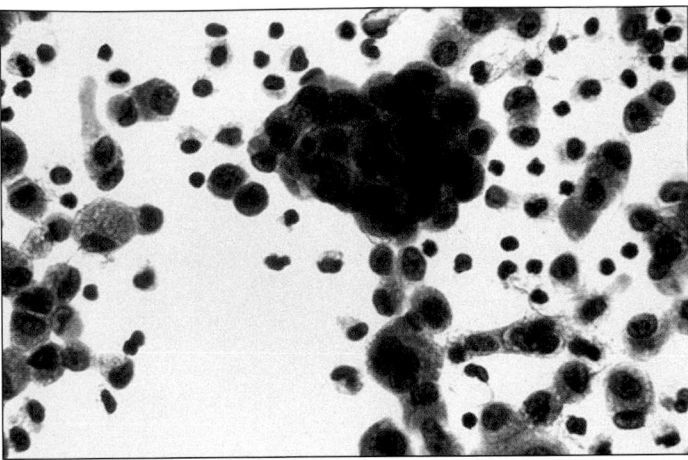

Fig. 19.46 Morulae and individual cells of diffuse malignant mesothelioma in a malignant pleural effusion. (Papanicolaou)

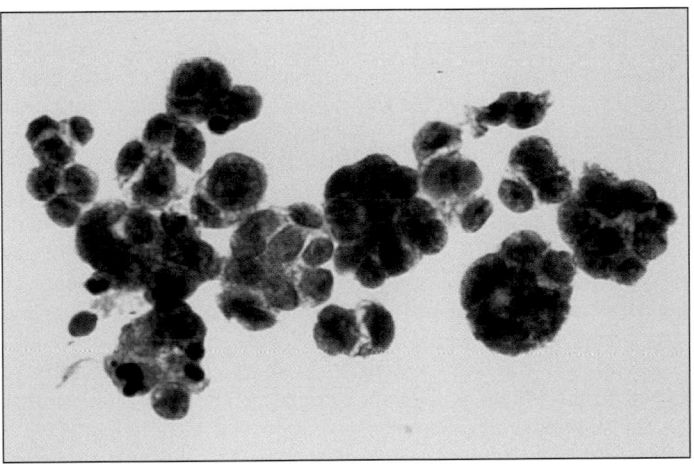

Fig. 19.47 Morulae or three-dimensional clusters of adenocarcinoma cells in a malignant effusion. (Papanicolaou)

various organs and papillary diffuse malignant mesotheliomas. Classic cytologic features of individual cancer cells in malignant effusions include enlarged cells with high N:C ratios, coarse chromatin, enlarged and multiple nucleoli, and irregular or indented nuclear contours. Mitoses and/or atypical mitoses may be present. Cancers of particular types or from particular primary sites often show features consistent with their specific phenotype. For example, adenocarcinomas may have intracytoplasmic mucin vacuoles. The diagnosis of malignancy is based on a combination of these individual cell cytologic features and the architectural arrangements of the cells. As previously noted, atypical mesothelial hyperplasia can mimic many of these cytologic and architectural features.[1,307,309]

Malignant effusions with special cytologic features

In addition to the general cytologic and architectural features of malignancy, some cancers have cytologic or architectural features that suggest their primary site. Immunostains may be useful in identifying primary sites of cancers in malignant effusions, although for many cancers there are still no specific markers.[335–359]

Mesothelioma

As noted previously, diffuse malignant mesotheliomas cause about 1% of malignant pleural effusions. There is recent interest in diagnosing diffuse malignant mesothelioma at an early stage in the hope that aggressive and investigational therapies may improve survival. It is not unusual for a diffuse malignant mesothelioma to present as a recurrent pleural effusion diagnosed on cytology repeatedly as negative for malignancy, perhaps for months, before a diagnosis of mesothelioma is finally made on pleural biopsy.

Mesothelioma cells in malignant effusions are virtually always of epithelial type (see Fig. 19.46).[326–332] Sarcomatous mesotheliomas may cause pleural effusions, but these are typically not malignant effusions since the malignant sarcomatous cells seldom shed into the effusion fluid. Presumably these effusions are caused by local effect of the sarcomatous mesothelioma on serosal membranes and obstructed lymphatics.[305]

Epithelial malignant mesothelioma cells may have a recognizably mesothelial appearance, sharing cytologic features of nonmalignant mesothelial cells as described above combined with varying degrees of cytologic features of malignancy.[320–326] Epithelial malignant mesothelioma cells may be in sheets, clusters, morulae, or papillary structures. Papillary malignant mesotheliomas, like other papillary cancers, can form psammoma bodies.[321–327] Confirmation that malignant cells are of mesothelial origin can be done with immunostains.

Since the malignant mesothelioma cells are virtually always of epithelial type, they share characteristic 'mesothelial' features with benign mesothelial cells. In addition, these malignant mesothelioma cells generally lack the significant degree of pleomorphism seen with carcinoma cells and in some cases they are frankly bland. Therefore, it is not surprising that the primary differential diagnosis for diffuse malignant mesothelioma is often reactive atypical mesothelial hyperplasia.[1,307,309]

Breast cancer

Breast carcinoma accounts for about 25% of malignant pleural effusions.[305,306] The hallmark of breast cancer cells in malignant pleural effusions is the three-dimensional morulae or spherical clusters of cells that make up a population distinct from the mesothelial cells (Fig. 19.48).[1,309,360] In most, but not all, breast cancer effusions, these morulae are abundant. The cells in these morulae have irregularly shaped nuclei and multiple nucleoli, but are generally not as cytologically bizarre as adenocarcinomas from other organs. Breast cancer cells can also be arranged in papillary structures or appear as individual cells with malignant cytologic features.[360]

Lobular carcinomas may appear as chains of small uniform hyperchromatic cells. Lobular carcinoma cells may sometimes form signet-ring cells with the nucleus compressed to the side by a large intracytoplasmic vacuole. These cells are generally smaller than the signet-ring cells of gastrointestinal adenocarcinoma.[307,309]

Ovarian cancer

Ovarian carcinoma is the most common cause of malignant peritoneal effusions. In effusions, ovarian serous carcinomas usually consist of papillary structures made up of large cells with often strikingly enlarged and irregular nuclei and prominent intracytoplasmic vacuoles. Psammoma bodies are often present with ovarian serous carcinomas in effusions and, although psammoma bodies can be seen with other papillary cancers, they are most frequent with ovarian serous carcinomas (Fig. 19.49).[309,360]

Ovarian mucinous carcinomas in effusions consist of individual mucin-containing cells and small clusters of such cells floating in a

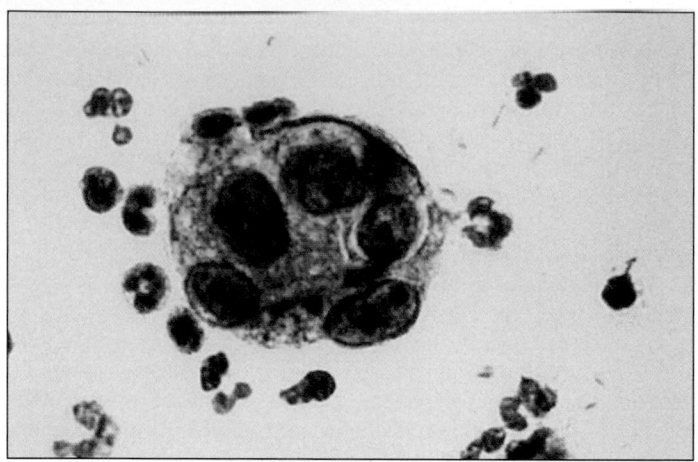

Fig. 19.48 Classic morula of metastatic breast carcinoma cells in an effusion. (Papanicolaou)

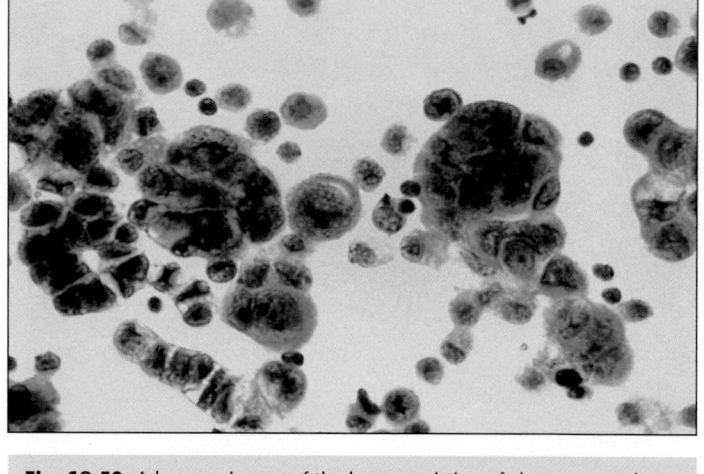

Fig. 19.50 Adenocarcinoma of the lung consisting of clusters, morulae, and individual tumor cells in a malignant pleural effusion. (Papanicolaou)

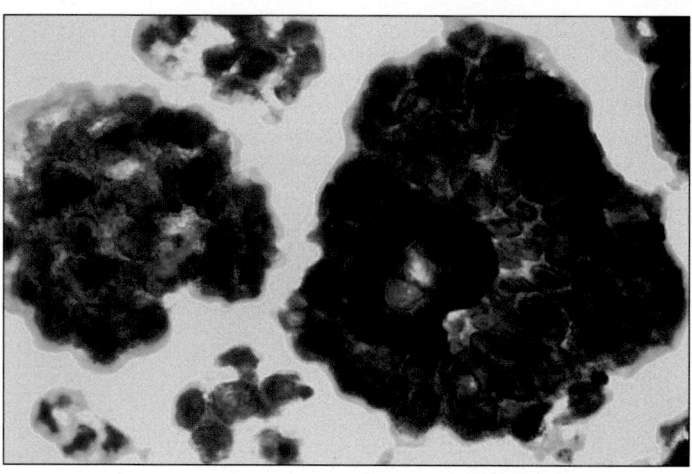

Fig. 19.49 Papillary clusters of metastatic serous papillary ovarian carcinoma in a malignant effusion. A psammoma body is present within one cluster. (Papanicolaou)

mucoid basophilic background. These cells often lack significant cytologic features of malignancy, unless they are poorly differentiated, in which case they may resemble poorly differentiated mucinous adenocarcinomas of other organs. The mucinous carcinoma cells may be columnar or may appear rounded in the effusion fluid.[307,309]

Lung cancer

Carcinomas of the lung are the most frequent cause of malignant pleural effusions and account for about 30% of these.[305,306] Adenocarcinomas make up the largest group of lung cancers in malignant pleural effusions. Adenocarcinomas of the lung often form papillary or acinar structures composed of large cells with pale chromatin, thickened nuclear membrane and an enlarged nucleolus (Fig. 19.50). Mucin vacuoles are often present in the cytoplasm. Cancers that invade the pleura can no longer be classified as bronchioloalveolar, but well-differentiated peripheral adenocarcinomas may be composed of relatively uniform columnar cells with enlarged, but relatively uniform, nuclei and prominent nucleoli.[309]

Large cell carcinoma consists of large pleomorphic cells with obvious cytologic features of malignancy. These cells often have large very prominent nucleoli in an enlarged nucleus with coarse chromatin. The cells may be seen as individual malignant cells or in clusters.[309]

Squamous cell carcinomas of the lung are found in malignant pleural effusions less often than adenocarcinomas. The better-differentiated squamous cell carcinomas will consist of cells with thick cytoplasm, and keratinization is diagnostic. It may be difficult to distinguish poorly differentiated squamous cell carcinomas from adenocarcinomas, and poorly differentiated squamous cell carcinomas may even have cytoplasmic vacuoles.[309]

Small cell carcinomas consist of short chains or clusters of hyperchromatic cells with scant cytoplasm. The chromatin tends to be finely stippled in appearance, so-called 'salt and pepper.' There is often nuclear molding of cells with adjacent cells fitting together somewhat like pieces of a puzzle. Although most cells of small cell carcinoma are relatively small compared to the cells of many other carcinomas, and when individual might somewhat resemble lymphocytes, the cells are larger than lymphocytes and have irregular shapes (Fig. 19.51).[309]

Gastrointestinal cancer

Gastrointestinal carcinomas in malignant effusions are usually mucin-containing adenocarcinomas and may be made up of columnar cells or so-called signet-ring cells. Signet-ring cells have large intracytoplasmic vacuoles containing mucin that compress the nucleus to one side, creating an appearance that resembles a signet ring. The cells usually have frankly malignant cytologic features discussed previously (Fig. 19.52). Signet-ring cells are most often associated with gastric cancers, but can occur in metastatic adenocarcinomas from other primary sites. Mucinous adenocarcinomas may consist of only a few clusters of relatively bland mucin-containing cells with a basophilic mucoid background. When a primary site is sought from the effusion specimen, immunostains may be of limited help.[309]

Melanoma

Malignant effusions due to metastatic melanoma are relatively common. Melanoma cells in effusions are typically very pleomorphic with enlarged eccentric nuclei often containing large prominent

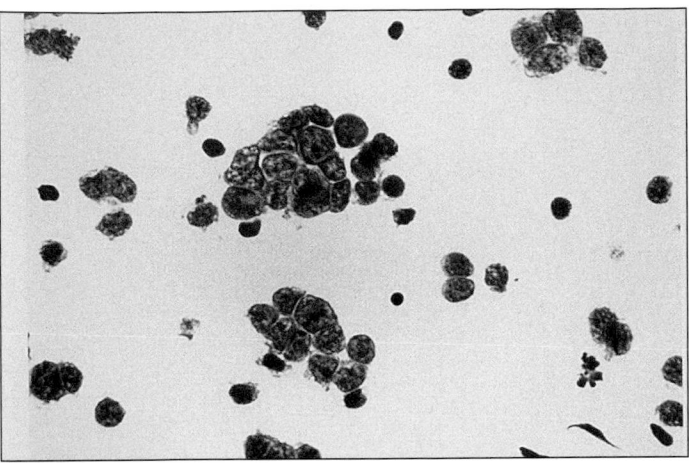

Fig. 19.51 Metastatic small cell carcinoma of the lung in a malignant effusion consisting of cells with stippled chromatin, scant cytoplasm, and nuclear molding. (Papanicolaou)

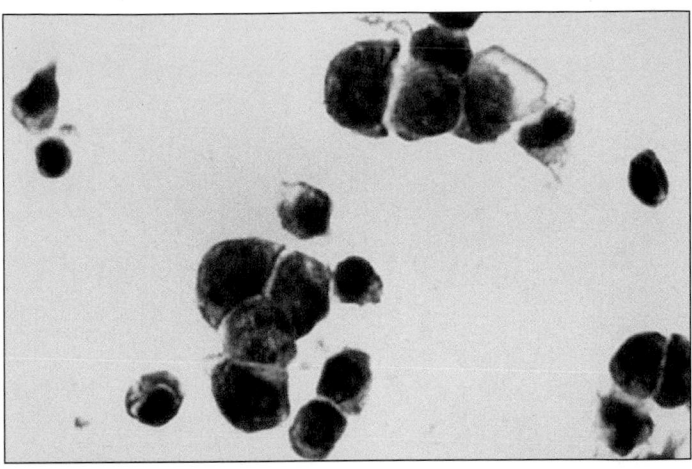

Fig. 19.53 Metastatic melanoma in pleural effusion showing enlarged malignant cells in small groups. (Papanicolaou)

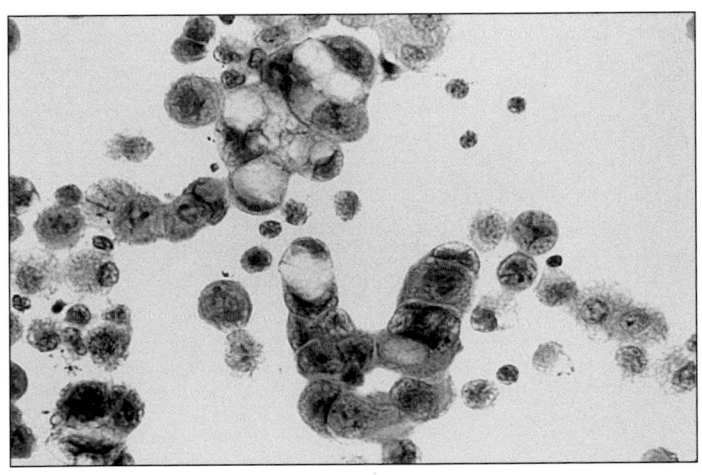

Fig. 19.52 Metastatic gastric adenocarcinoma in malignant effusion showing multiple signet-ring cells with nuclei compressed by intracytoplasmic mucin vacuoles. (Papanicolaou)

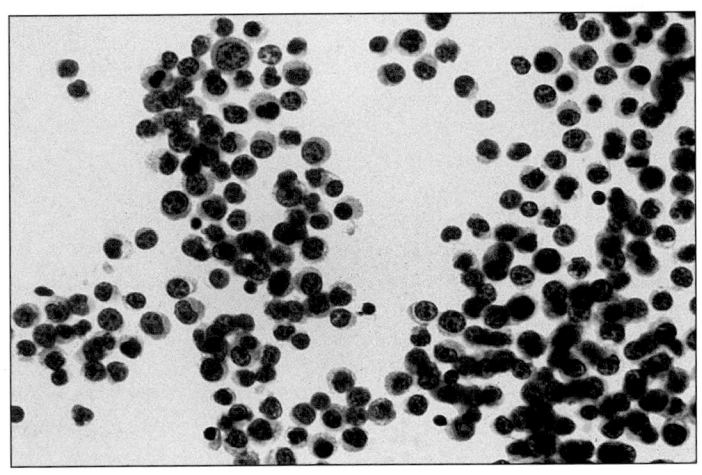

Fig. 19.54 Abundant lymphoid cells of a non-Hodgkin's lymphoma in a pleural effusion. (Papanicolaou)

nucleoli. Binucleate cells are common and intranuclear cytoplasmic inclusions are characteristic. The melanoma cells are often in small clusters, but may be single and cell 'cannibalism' may be observed (Fig. 19.53). Melanin pigment may be seen in the cytoplasm of occasional cells but is often absent. Immunostains are helpful in confirming a diagnosis of melanoma.[361]

Hematologic neoplasms

Lymphomas cause about 20% of malignant pleural effusions.[305] Today, most lymphomas and other hematologic malignancies are characterized by leukocyte antigens using flow cytometry, by cytogenetics, or by molecular genetics. In situ hybridization for Epstein-Barr virus may be important for some types of lymphoma. Lymphomas in malignant effusions are characterized by their lack of cellular cohesion and are composed of many single cells without forming morulae, glands, or other tissue structures. Several morphologic variants can be seen on cytology. Well-differentiated small cell lymphomas are composed of uniform populations of cells with features of small, mature-appearing lymphocytes (Fig. 19.54). The differential diagnosis includes benign effusions characterized by numerous lymphocytes, such as effusions caused by tuberculosis, viruses, and post-transplant rejection. Phenotypic and genetic studies, including flow cytometric studies and gene rearrangement studies by PCR or Southern blot, help differentiate well-differentiated lymphomas from benign reactive lymphocytic effusions.[307,309]

High-grade lymphomas have variation in lymphocyte size, including larger cells and enlarged nuclei, irregular nuclear shapes, presence of one or more nucleoli, and mitoses. Large cell lymphomas have large vesicular nuclei that are irregularly shaped and may have nuclear protrusions. Cytoplasm is scant but recognizable and occasionally vacuolated. Nucleoli are prominent, often multiple and irregularly shaped. The cells are typically variable in size.[309]

Hodgkin's lymphoma usually has a polymorphous background of lymphocytes, plasma cells, and eosinophils. The presence of Reed-Sternberg cells or mononuclear variants is required for cytologic diagnosis.

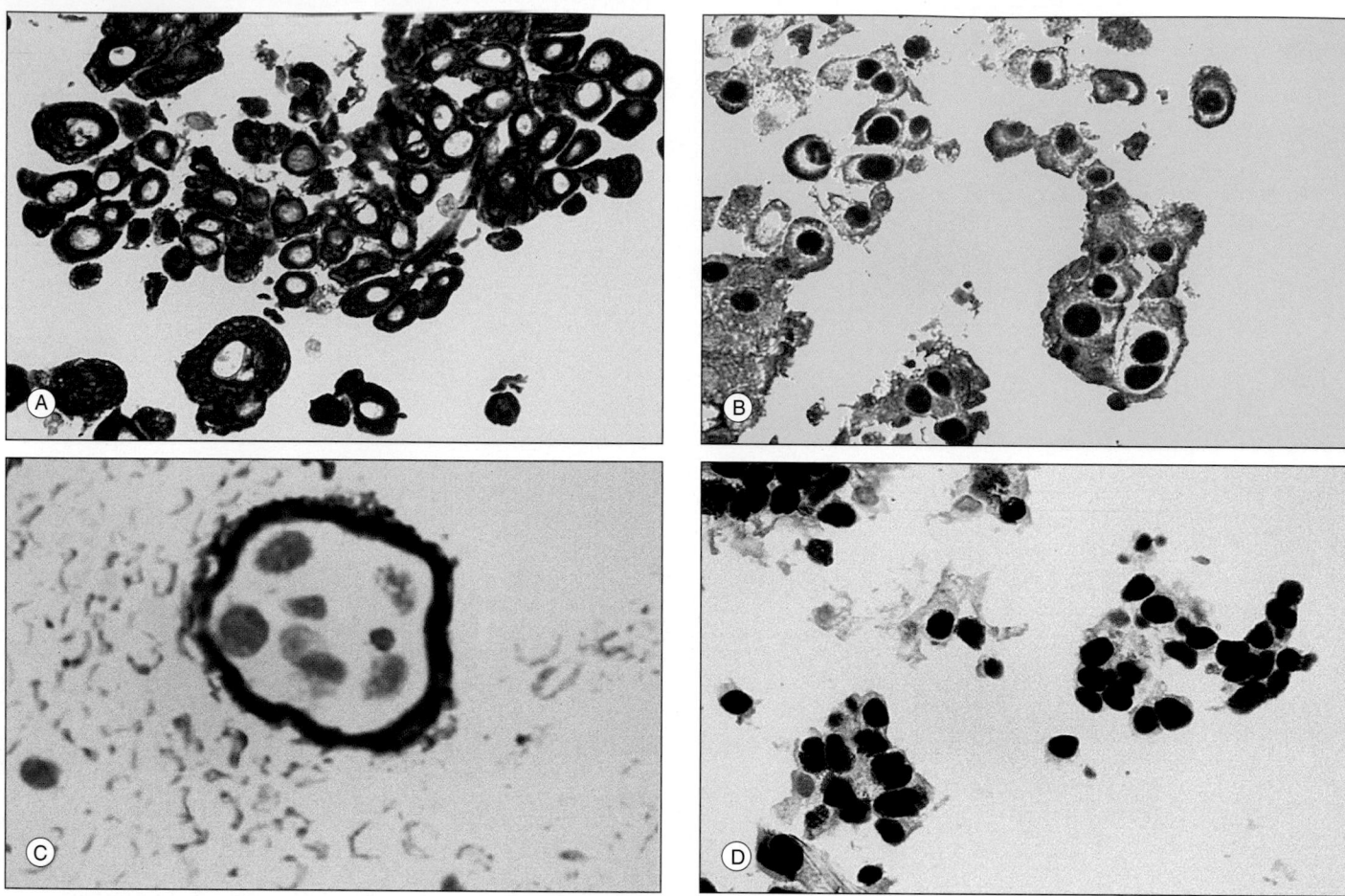

Fig. 19.55 A, Cytoplasmic expression of keratin in diffuse malignant mesothelioma cells in a pleural effusion (antipankeratin); **B,** Nuclear and cytoplasmic expression of calretinin in diffuse malignant mesothelioma cells in a pleural effusion (anticalretinin); **C,** Membranous expression of HBME-1 in diffuse malignant mesothelioma cells in a pleural effusion (anti-HBME-1); **D,** Nuclear expression of TTF-1 in metastatic adenocarcinoma of the lung in a pleural effusion (anti-TTF-1).

Leukemic effusions contain cells representative of the specific type of leukemia and, therefore, may contain primitive blast cells and mitoses. As with lymphomas, phenotypic studies with flow cytometry, cytogenetics, and molecular genetics are usually used to further characterize the leukemia.[307,309]

Multiple myeloma rarely causes malignant effusion. The effusions contain a uniform population of atypical plasma cells.[309]

Rare neoplasms

Sarcomas cause malignant effusions only rarely. Sarcoma cells are typically frankly malignant by cytologic criteria and may be bizarre. Diagnosis of a malignancy is usually not difficult with sarcoma and further classification can be done with immunostains (See below).[309]

Immunocytochemistry

Uses of immunohistochemistry in tissue sections have been discussed above and numerous studies have shown that the same antibodies are generally useful in the immunocytochemistry of effusions (Figure 19.55).[335-359] Cell blocks are preferred for immunocyto-chemistry and more closely resemble paraffin-embedded tissue sections so that protocols and conditions do not need alterations. Immunocytochemistry can be performed on smears and cytospins,

but one must be aware that proteins in the fluid may coat cells and create false staining.[333,334]

The primary reasons that immunocytochemistry is performed on malignant effusion specimens is to differentiate epithelial mesothe-lioma from metastatic cancers, primarily carcinomas, and to determine the primary site of metastatic cancers. Problems of sarcomatous mesotheliomas versus other types of sarcomatous cancers are much less likely to be encountered in malignant effusions since these types of tumors are much less likely to shed cells into the serosal cavity fluid.[305,309]

Immunostains can be very helpful in making a diagnosis of a type of cancer, but should always be interpreted with appropriate caution since there are exceptions to the specificity and sensitivity of antibodies and potentially technical issues with any given immuno-stain. Some antibodies can be used to limit the differential diagnosis of a malignant effusion. For example, expression of cytokeratin may help limit the differential diagnosis to primarily one of metastatic carcinoma versus mesothelioma. However, there can be even occasional exceptions to this broader use of antibodies.

An increasing number of antibodies have proven useful for specific primary sites, but these are still limited and, as noted, exceptions to specificity and sensitivity occur. For example, TTF-1 expression is seen predominantly with thyroid cancers and lung cancers. However, many lung cancers are not positive for TTF-1 and, therefore, a negative TTF-1 does not rule out a lung primary. Rare cases of other types of carcinomas have been reported to express TTF-1, and so the rare TTF-1-positive carcinoma will not be from either a lung or thyroid primary. Therefore, TTF-1 is useful in diagnosing metastatic lung carcinomas in effusions provided that one is aware of these caveats.[359,362] Due to these limitations of specificity and sensitivity, and the observation that many antigens are expressed by more than one type of tumor, it is best to perform a panel of several antibodies in many situations. The panel of antibodies helps address variations in expression of expected markers by a tumor. A panel may also occasionally point to a diagnosis not previously considered when the combination of antigens that are expressed and not expressed fail to match with the original differential diagnosis.

The immunostains useful for diagnosis of mesothelioma have already been discussed. Use of calretinin and other antibodies (HBME-1, mesothelin, thrombomodulin, CK 5/6) that are relatively specific for mesothelioma in a panel that includes antibodies typically positive in the differential diagnosis is the usual approach. Many panels include markers for adenocarcinoma of the lung, a frequent differential diagnosis for epithelial malignant mesothelioma and, prior to markers for mesothelial cells, mesothelioma was favored if the panel failed to disclose any positive markers for adenocarcinoma of the lung. Obviously, the cancers that might enter into the differential diagnosis of epithelial malignant mesothelioma include more than lung cancer, and so the use of markers for mesothelial cells has proven advantageous. A panel of antibodies is still needed, however, since markers of mesothelial cells may be positive in other types of cancers, particularly thrombomodulin and CK 5/6.

Common pitfalls in the cytologic diagnosis of malignant effusions

As already emphasized, the most common difficulty in diagnosing malignant effusions is making an accurate diagnosis of malignancy in the first place. Reactive mesothelial cells may mimic malignant cells in effusions from many etiologies. Reactive mesothelial cells are known to be particularly worrisome in effusions caused by pulmonary infarcts, cirrhosis, radiation, and chemotherapy. Pleural effusions from pulmonary infarcts have the finding of a unilateral bloody effusion, a feature also found with many malignant effusions, in addition to florid atypical mesothelial hyperplasia.[363] Reactive mesothelial cells with radiation changes may be particularly bizarre,

often consisting of enlarged or giant cells with normal N:C ratios and vacuolated cytoplasm.[364,365] Giving consideration to the clinical context of an effusion specimen is generally recommended especially for equivocal cases, but ultimately the cytology must be diagnosed on its own merits. Cytologic characteristics of malignant cells in effusions have already been described above. As previously noted, the presence of two populations of cells with distinct cytologic features, one of which is malignant, is a very useful observation. Situations in which the malignant cells mimic benign cells are less frequent problems than reactive mesothelial cells mimicking cancer. However, some cancers, for example, lobular carcinoma of the breast and some epithelial diffuse malignant mesotheliomas, can be cytologically bland.[309]

The use of immunocytochemistry to identify malignant cells has risks and should not be the only basis for making a malignant diagnosis on cytology. False-positive and false-negative stains for carcinoma markers such as CEA or B72.3 can lead the cytopathologist astray. Immunostains for genetic molecular markers such as p53[366–368] or telomerase activity[369] have been proposed as adjuncts in the cytologic diagnosis of malignant effusions, but should not be considered the only basis for making a cytologic diagnosis of cancer. At present, no immunocytochemical stain is recognized as a completely reliable marker for cancer independent of the morphologic and other features. Other ancillary studies such as AgNOR have been evaluated as a basis for differentiating benign and malignant cells in effusion cytology. While they may have some value as an adjunct study, like immunostains, they also cannot be used alone as a basis for diagnosis of malignancy, but only add additional information.[370–371]

On occasion, malignant cells are present but are too few to permit a reliable diagnosis.[309] As with other equivocal situations, it is considered best to err on the side of caution, and diagnoses such as 'cannot rule out,' 'suspicious for' or 'suggestive of' can be used.

Abundant lymphocytes lacking frankly malignant features may represent an inflammatory process such as tuberculosis or collagen vascular disease or may be a well-differentiated lymphoma. Flow cytometry or other studies to determine clonality can assist in differentiating lymphoma from inflammatory lymphocytic effusions.[309]

Epithelial cells from endometriosis and endosalpingiosis rarely shed into the peritoneal fluid and even more rarely into the pleural fluid. These consist of relatively small cuboidal cells arranged in tight clusters, occasionally with stromal cells as well. Although these cells lack cytologic features of malignancy, their detail may be obscured by the compactness of the clusters.[309]

REFERENCES

1. Battifora H, McCaughey WTE. Tumors of the serosal membranes, Fascicle 15, Third Series, Washington, DC: AFIP; 1995.

2. Bolen JW, Hammar SP, McNutt MA. Reactive and neoplastic serosal tissue. A light-microscopic, ultrastructural, and immunohistochemical study. Am J Surg Pathol 1986; 10: 34–38.

3. Roggli VL. Role of closed needle biopsy in the diagnosis of malignant mesothelioma of the pleura. Chest 1994; 105: 321–322.

4. Boutin C, Rey F. Thoracoscopy in pleural malignant mesothelioma: a prospective study of 188 consecutive patients. Cancer 1993; 72: 389–393.

5. Parakash UBS, Reiman HM. Comparison of needle biopsy with cytologic analysis for evaluation of pleural

effusion. Analysis of 414 cases. Mayo Clin Proc 1985; 60: 158–164.

6. Nance KV, Shermer RW, Askin FB. The diagnostic efficacy of pleural biopsy as compared to that of pleural fluid examination. Mod Pathol 1991; 4: 320–324.

7. Beauchamp HD, Kundra NK, Aranson R, et al. The role of closed pleural needle biopsy in the diagnosis of malignant mesothelioma of pleura. Chest 1992; 102: 1110–1112.

8. Churg A, Colby TV, Cagle PT, et al. The separation of benign and malignant mesothelial proliferations. Am J Surg Pathol 2000; 24: 1183–1200.

9. Johnston WW. Cytologic correlations, Ch 31. In: Dail DH, Hammar SP, eds. Pulmonary pathology. New York: Springer-Verlag; 1988: 1029–1094.

10. Sahn SA. The pleura. Am Rev Respir Dis 1988; 138: 184–234.

11. Soriano E, Mallolas J, Gatell JM, et al. Characteristics of tuberculosis in HIV-infected patients. AIDS 1988; 2: 420–432.

12. Wilen SB, Rabinowitz JG, Ulrich S, Lyons HA. Pleural involvement in sarcoidosis. Am J Med 1974; 57: 200–209.

13. Petty TL, Wilkins M. The five manifestations of rheumatoid lung. Dis Chest 1966; 49: 75–82.

14. Aru A, Engel U, Francis D. Characteristic and specific histological findings in rheumatoid pleurisy. Acta Pathol Microbiol Immunol Scand [A] 1986; 94: 57–62.

15. Askin FB, McCann BG, Kuhn C. Reactive eosinophilic pleuritis. A lesion to be distinguished

from pulmonary eosinophilic granuloma. Arch Pathol Lab Med 1977; 101: 187–192.

16. Sheibani K, Battifora H, Burke J. Antigenic phenotype of malignant mesotheliomas and pulmonary adenocarcinomas: an immunohistologic analysis demonstrating the value of Leu-M1 antigen. Am J Pathol 1986; 123: 212–219.

17. Ayers JG, Crocker JG, Skilbek NQ. Differentiation of malignant from normal and reactive mesothelial cells by the argyrophil technique for nucleolar organizer region associated proteins. Thorax 1988; 43: 366–370.

18. Mayall FG, Goddard DH, Gibbs AR. p53 in the distinction between benign and malignant mesothelial proliferations using formalin-fixed paraffin sections. J Pathol 1992; 168: 377–381.

19. Cagle PT, Brown R, Lebovitz R. p53 immunostaining in the differentiation of reactive processes from malignancy in pleural biopsy specimens. Hum Pathol 1994; 25: 443–448.

20. Ramael M, Buysse C, Van Den Bossche J, et al. Immunoreactivity for the beta chain of the platelet-derived growth factor receptor in malignant mesothelioma and non-neoplastic mesothelium. J Pathol 1992; 167: 1–4.

21. Segers K, Ramael M, Singh SK, et al. Immunoreactivity for bcl-2 protein in malignant mesothelioma and non-neoplastic mesothelium. Virchows Arch [A] 1994; 424: 631–634.

22. Hammar SP, Bolen JW, Bockus D, et al. Ultrastructural and immunohistochemical features of common lung tumors: An overview. Ultrastruct Pathol 1985; 9: 283–318.

23. Oury TD. Benign asbestos-related pleural diseases. In: Roggli VL, Oury TD, Sporn TA, eds. Pathology of Asbestos-Associated Diseases, 2nd Ed. New York: Springer; 2004; 169–192.

24. Siebens AA, Storey CF, Newman MM, et al. The physiologic effects of fibrothorax and the functional results of surgical treatment. J Thorac Surg 1956; 32: 53–62.

25. Hillerdal G. Rounded atelectasis: clinical experience with 74 patients. Chest 1989; 95: 836–841.

26. Lynch DA, Gamsu G, Ray CS, Aberle DR. Asbestos related focal lung masses: manifestations on conventional and high resolution CT scans. Radiology 1988; 169: 603–607.

27. Knapp MJ, Roggli VL, Kim J, et al. Pleural amyloidosis. Arch Pathol Lab Med 1988; 112: 57–60.

28. Sporn TA, Roggli VL. Mesothelioma. In: Roggli VL, Oury TD, Sporn TA, eds. Pathology of Asbestos-Associated Diseases, 2nd Ed. New York: Springer; 2004; 104–168.

29. Churg A, Green FHY. Pathology of occupational lung disease, 2nd ed. Baltimore: Williams & Wilkins; 1998.

30. Srebro SH, Roggli VL, Samsa GP. Malignant mesothelioma associated with low pulmonary tissue asbestos burdens: A light and scanning electron microscopic analysis of 18 cases. Mod Pathol 1995; 8: 614–621.

31. Fraire AE, Cooper S, Greenberg SD, et al. Mesothelioma of childhood. Cancer 1988; 62: 838–847.

32. Nishioka H, Furusho K, Yasunaga T, et al. Congenital malignant mesothelioma: A case report and electron microscopic study. Eur J Pediatr 1988; 147: 428–430.

33. Dodson RF, Williams MG, Corn CI, et al. Asbestos content of lung tissue, lymph nodes, and pleural plaques from former shipyard workers. Am Rev Respir Dis 1990; 142: 843-847.

34. Gibbs AR, Stephens M, Griffiths DM, et al. Fibre distribution in the lungs and pleura of subjects with asbestos related diffuse pleural fibrosis. Br J Ind Med 1991; 48: 762–770.

35. Boutin C, Dumortier P, Rey F, et al. Black spots concentrate oncogenic asbestos fibers in the parietal pleura: Thoracoscopic and mineralogic study. Am J Respir Crit Care Med 1996; 153: 444–449.

36. Jaurand MC, Bignon J, eds. The mesothelial cell and mesothelioma. New York: Marcell Dekker, 1994.

37. Austin MB, Fechner RE, Roggli VL. Pleural malignant mesothelioma following Wilms' tumor. Am J Clin Pathol 1986; 86: 227–230.

38. Cicala C, Pompetti F, Carbone M. SV 40 induces mesotheliomas in hamsters. Am J Pathol 1993; 142: 1524–1533.

39. Carbone M, Pass HI, Rizzo P, et al. Simian virus 40-like DNA sequences in human pleural mesotheliomas. Oncogene 1994; 9: 1781–1790.

40. Roggli VL, McGavran MH, Subach J, et al. Pulmonary asbestos body counts and electron probe analysis of asbestos body cores in patients with mesothelioma: A study of 25 cases. Cancer 1982; 50: 2423–2432.

41. Mirvis S, Dutcher JP, Haney PJ, et al. CT of malignant pleural mesothelioma. Am J Roentgenol 1983; 140: 665–670.

42. Lorigan JG, Libshitz HI. MR imaging of malignant pleural mesothelioma. J Comput Asst Tomogr 1989; 13: 617–620.

43. Hammar SP. Pleural diseases, Ch 34. In: Dail DH, Hammar SP, eds. Pulmonary pathology, 2nd edn. New York: Springer-Verlag; 1994: 1463–1579.

44. Hillerdal G. Malignant mesothelioma 1982: Review of 4710 published cases. Br J Dis Chest 1983; 77: 321–343.

45. Ordonez NG. Epithelial mesothelioma with deciduoid features: Report of four cases. Am J Surg Pathol 2000; 24: 816–823.

46. Butnor KJ, Sporn TA, Hammar SP, Roggli VL. Well differentiated papillary mesothelioma. Am J Surg Pathol 2001; 25: 1304–1309.

47. Whitaker D, Henderson DW, Shilkin KB. The concept of mesothelioma in situ: implications for diagnosis and histogenesis. Semin Diagn Pathol 9: 1992; 151–161.

48. Mangano WE, Cagle PT, Churg A, et al. The diagnosis of desmoplastic mesothelioma and its distinction from fibrous pleurisy: A histologic and immunohistochemical analysis of 31 cases including p53 immunostaining. Am J Clin Pathol 1998; 110: 191–199.

49. Henderson DW, Attwood DH, Constance TJ, et al. Lymphohistiocytoid mesothelioma: a rare lymphomatoid variant of predominantly sarcomatoid mesothelioma. Ultrastruct Pathol 1988; 12: 367–384.

50. MacDougall DB, Wang SE, Zidar BL. Mucin-positive epithelial mesothelioma. Arch Pathol Lab Med 1992; 116: 874–880.

51. Hammar SP, Bockus DE, Remington FL, Rohrbach KA. Mucin-positive epithelial mesotheliomas: A histochemical, immunohistochemical, and ultrastructural comparison with mucin-producing pulmonary adenocarcinomas. Ultrastruct Pathol 1996; 20: 293–325.

52. Scroggs MW, Roggli VL, Fraire AE, Sanfilippo F. Eosinophilic intracytoplasmic globules in pulmonary adenocarcinomas: A histochemical, immunohistochemical, and ultrastructural study of six cases. Hum Pathol 1989; 20: 845–849.

53. Wick MR, Loy T, Mills SE, et al. Malignant epithelioid pleural mesothelioma versus peripheral pulmonary adenocarcinoma: a histochemical, ultrastructural, and immunohistologic study of 103 cases. Hum Pathol 21: 1990; 759–766.

54. Wirth PR, Legier J, Wright GL. Immunohistochemical evaluation of seven monoclonal antibodies for differentiation of pleural mesothelioma from lung adenocarcinoma. Cancer 1991; 67: 655–662.

55. Bedrossian CWM, Bonsib S, Moran C. Differential diagnosis between mesothelioma and adenocarcinoma: a multimodal approach based on ultrastructure and immunocytochemistry. Semin Diagn Pathol 1992. 9: 124–140.

56. Sheibani K, Esteban JM, Bailey A, et al. Immunopathologic and molecular studies as an aid to the diagnosis of malignant mesothelioma. Hum Pathol 1992; 23: 107–116.

57. Leong ASY, Vernon-Roberts E. The immunohistochemistry of malignant mesothelioma. Pathol Annu 1994; 29: 157–179.

58. Ordonez NG, Mackay B. The roles of immunohistochemistry and electron microscopy in distinguishing epithelial mesothelioma of the pleura from adenocarcinoma. Adv Anat Pathol 1996; 3: 273–293.

59. Carella R, Deleonardi G, D'Errico A, et al. Immunohistochemical panels for differentiating epithelial malignant mesothelioma from lung adenocarcinoma: A study with logistic regression analysis. Am J Surg Pathol 2001; 25: 43–50.

60. Moll R, Dhouailly D, Sun T-T. Expression of keratin 5 as a distinctive feature of epithelial and biphasic mesotheliomas: An immunohistochemical study using monoclonal antibody AE14. Virch Arch B Cell Pathol 1989; 58: 129–145.

61. Ordonez NG. Value of cytokeratin 5/6 immunostaining in distinguishing epithelial mesothelioma of the pleura from lung adenocarcinoma. Am J Surg Pathol 1998; 22: 1215–1221.

62. Cury PM, Butcher DN, Fisher C, et al. Value of the mesothelium-associated antibodies thrombomodulin, cytokeratin 5/6, calretinin, and CD44H in distinguishing epithelioid pleural mesothelioma from adenocarcinoma metastatic to the pleura. Mod Pathol 2000; 13: 107-112.

63. Chu P, Wu E, Weiss LM. Cytokeratin 7 and cytokeratin 20 expression in epithelial neoplasms: A survey of 435 cases. Mod Pathol 2000; 13: 962–972.

64. Gown AM, Boyd HC, Chang Y, et al. Smooth muscle cells can express cytokeratins of "simple" epithelium: Immunocytochemical and histochemical studies in vitro and in vivo. Am J Pathol 1988; 132: 223–232.

65. Weiss SW, Bratthauer GL, Morris PA. Postirradiation malignant fibrous histiocytoma expressing cytokeratin. Am J Surg Pathol 1988; 12: 554–558.

66. Cagle PT, Truong L, Roggli VL, Greenberg SD. Immunohistochemical differentiation of sarcomatoid mesotheliomas from other spindle cell neoplasms. Am J Clin Pathol 1989; 92: 566–571.

67. Yousem SA, Hochholzer L. Malignant mesotheliomas with osseous and cartilaginous differentiation. Arch Pathol Lab Med 1987; 111: 62–66.

68. Doglioni C, Dei Tos AP, Laurino L, et al. Calretinin: A novel immunocytochemical marker for mesothelioma. Am J Surg Pathol 1996; 20: 1037–1046.

69. Ordonez NG. Value of calretinin immunostaining in differentiating epithelial mesothelioma from lung adenocarcinoma. Mod Pathol 1998; 11: 929–933.

70. Ordonez NG. The value of antibodies 44-3A6, SM3, HBME-1, and thrombomodulin in differentiating epithelial pleural mesothelioma from lung adenocarcinoma: A comparative study with other commonly used antibodies. Am J Surg Pathol 1997; 21: 1399–1408.

71. Amin KM, Litzky KA, Smythe WR, et al. Wilms' tumor 1 susceptibility (WT1) gene products are selectively expressed in malignant mesothelioma. Am J Pathol 1995; 146: 344–356.

72. Donna A, Bettar PG, Bellingeri O, Marchesiai A. New marker for mesothelioma; an immunoperoxidase study. J Clin Pathol 1986; 39: 961–968.

73. Anderson TM, Holmes AC, Kosaka CG, et al. Monoclonal antibodies to human malignant mesothelioma. J Clin Immunol 1987; 7: 254–261.

74. Stahel RA, O'Hara CJ, Waibel R, Martin A. Monoclonal antibodies against mesothelial membrane antigen discriminate between malignant mesothelioma and lung adenocarcinoma. Int J Cancer 1988; 41: 218–223.

75. Hsu SM, Hsu PL, Zhau X, et al. Establishment of human mesothelioma cell lines (MS-1, -2) and production of a monoclonal antibody (anti-MS) with diagnostic and therapeutic potential. Cancer Res 1988; 48: 5228–5236.

76. Donna A, Bettar PG, Jones JS. Verification of the histologic diagnosis of malignant mesothelioma in relation to the binding of an antimesothelial cell antibody. 1989; Cancer 63: 1331–1336.

77. O'Hara CJ, Corson JM, Pinkus GS, et al. ME1: A monoclonal antibody that distinguishes epithelial-type malignant mesothelioma from early adenocarcinoma and extrapulmonary malignancies. Am J Pathol 1990; 136: 421–428.

78. Miettinen M, Kobatich AJ. HBME-1: a monoclonal antibody useful in the differential diagnosis of mesothelioma, adenocarcinoma, and soft-tissue and bone tumors. Appl Immunohistochem 1995; 3: 115–122.

79. Corson JM, Pinkus GS. Mesothelioma: profile of keratin and carcinoembryonic antigen: An immunoperoxidase study of 20 cases and comparison with pulmonary adenocarcinoma. Am J Pathol 1982; 108: 80–87.

80. Battifora H, Kopinski N. Distinction of mesothelioma from adenocarcinoma: An immunohistochemical approach. Cancer 1985; 55: 1679–1685.

81. Tron V, Wright JL, Churg A. Carcinoembryonic antigen and milk fat globule protein staining of malignant mesothelioma and adenocarcinoma of the lung. Arch Pathol Lab Med 1987; 111: 291–293.

82. Otis CN, Carter D, Cote S, et al. Immunohistochemical evaluation of pleural mesothelioma and pulmonary adenocarcinoma: a bi-institutional study of 47 cases. Am J Surg Pathol 1987; 11: 445–456.

83. Latza U, Niedobitek G, Schwarting R, et al. Ber-Ep4: new monoclonal antibody which distinguishes epithelia from mesothelia. J Clin Pathol 1990; 43: 213–219.

84. Sheibani K, Shin S, Kazarian J, Weiss LM. Ber-Ep4 antibody as a discriminant in the differential diagnosis of malignant mesothelioma versus adenocarcinomas. Am J Surg Pathol 1991; 15: 779–784.

85. Kuhlmann L, Berhäuser KH, Schäfer R. Distinction of mesothelioma from carcinoma in pleural effusions. An immunohistochemical study on routinely processed preparations. Path Res Pract 1991; 187: 467–471.

86. Gaffy MJ, Neals SE, Swenson PE, et al. Immunoreactivity for Ber-Ep4 in adenocarcinomas, adenomatoid tumors, and malignant mesotheliomas. Am J Surg Pathol 1992; 16: 593–599.

87. Baily MD, Brown RW, Moley DR, et al. Ber-Ep4 differentiates adenocarcinoma from reactive and neoplastic mesothelial cells in serous effusion: a comparison with CEA, B72.3 and Leu-M1 (abstract). Am J Clin Pathol 1994; 101: 387.

88. Ordonez NG. Value of the BerEP4 antibody in differentiating epithelial pleural mesothelioma from adenocarcinoma. Am J Clin Pathol 1998; 109: 85–89.

89. Strickler JG, Herndier BG, Rous RV. Immunohistochemical staining of malignant mesotheliomas. Am J Clin Pathol 1987; 88: 610-614.

90. Warnock ML, Stoloff A, Thor A. Differentiation of adenocarcinoma of the lung from mesothelioma: Periodic acid-Schiff, monoclonal antibodies B72.3, and Leu M1. Am J Pathol 1988; 133: 30–38.

91. Arber DA, Weiss LM. CD15: a review. Appl Immunohistochem 1993; 1: 17–30.

92. Szpak CA, Johnston WW, Roggli V, et al. The diagnostic distinction between malignant mesothelioma of the pleura and adenocarcinoma of the lung as defined by a monoclonal antibody, B72.3. Am J Pathol 1986; 122: 252–260.

93. Khoury N, Raju U, Crissman JD, et al. A comparative immunohistochemical study of peritoneal and ovarian serous tumors, and mesothelioma. Hum Pathol 1990; 21: 811–819,

94. Wirth PR, Legler J, Wright GL Jr. Immunohistochemical evaluations of 7 monoclonal antibodies for differentiation of pleural mesothelioma from lung adenocarcinoma. Cancer 1991; 67: 655–662.

95. Jordon D, Jagirdar J, Kaneko M. Blood group antigens, Lewis^x and Lewis^y in the diagnostic discrimination of malignant mesothelioma versus adenocarcinoma. Am J Pathol 1989; 135: 931–937.

96. Riera JR, Astengo-Osuna C, Longmate JA, Battifora H. The immunohistochemical diagnostic panel for epithelial mesothelioma: A reevaluation after heat-induced epitope retrieval. Am J Surg Pathol 1997; 21: 1409–1419.

97. Marshall RJ, Herbert A, Braye SG, Jones DB. Use of antibodies through carcinoembryonic antigen and human milk fat globule to distinguish carcinoma, mesothelioma and reactive mesothelium. J Clin Pathol 1984; 37: 1215–1221.

98. Pinkus GS, Kurtin PJ. Epithelial membrane antigen – A diagnostic discriminant in surgical pathology: Immunohistochemical profile in epithelial, mesenchymal, and hematopoietic neoplasms using paraffin sections and monoclonal antibodies. 1985; Hum Pathol 16: 929–940,

99. Cibas ES, Corson JM, Pinkus GS. The distinction of adenocarcinoma from mesothelioma in cell blocks of effusions: the role of routine mucin histochemistry and immunohistochemical assessment of carcinoembryonic antigen, keratin proteins, epithelial membrane antigen and milk fat globule derived antigen. Hum Pathol 1987; 18: 67–74.

100. Kawai T, Suzuki M, Torikata C, Suzuki Y. Expression of blood group-related antigens and Helix pomatia agglutinin in malignant pleural mesothelioma and pulmonary adenocarcinoma. Hum Pathol 1991; 22: 118–124.

101. Noguchi M, Nakajima J, Hirohashi S, et al. Immunohistochemical distinction of malignant mesothelioma from pulmonary adenocarcinoma with anti-surfactant apoprotein, anti-Lewis$_a$ and anti-Tn antibodies. 1989; Hum Pathol 20: 52–57.

102. Churg A. Immunohistochemical staining for vimentin and keratin in malignant mesothelioma. Am J Surg Pathol 1985; 9: 360–365.

103. Mullink H, Henzen-Longmans SC, Alons-van Kordelaar JJM, et al. Simultaneous immunoenzyme staining of vimentin and cytokeratins with monoclonal antibodies as an aid in differential diagnosis of malignant mesothelioma from pulmonary adenocarcinoma. Virchows Arch [B] 1986; 52: 55–65.

104. Kung ITM, Thallas V, Spencer EJ, Wilson SM. Expression of muscle actins in diffuse mesothelioma. Hum Pathol 1995; 26: 565–570.

105. Kafiri G, Thomas DM, Shepherd NA, et al. p53 expression is common in malignant mesothelioma. Histopathology 1992; 21: 331–334.

106. Ramael M, Lemons G, Aerdekens C, et al. Immunoreactivity for p53 protein in malignant mesothelioma and non-neoplastic mesothelium. J Pathol 1992; 168: 371–375.

107. Hall PA, Lane DP. p53 in tumor pathology. Can we trust immunohistochemistry?-revisited. J Pathol 1994; 172: 1–4.

108. Lee I, Radosevich JA, Chejfec G, et al. Malignant mesotheliomas: Improved differential diagnosis from lung adenocarcinoma using monoclonal antibodies 44-3A6 and 624A12. Am J Pathol 1986; 123: 497–507.

109. Spagnolo DV, Whitaker D, Carrello S, et al. The use of monoclonal antibody 44-3A6 in cell blocks in the diagnosis of lung carcinoma, carcinomas metastatic to lung and pleura, and pleural malignant mesothelioma. Am J Clin Pathol 1991; 95: 322–329.

110. Mayall FG, Jassani B, Gibbs AR. Immunohistochemical positivity for neuron-specific enolase and Leu-7 in malignant mesotheliomas. J Pathol 1991; 165: 325–328.

111. Clark SP, Chout ST, Martin TJ, Danks JA. Parathyroid hormone-related protein antigen localization distinguishes between mesothelioma and adenocarcinoma of lung. J Pathol 1995; 176: 161–165.

112. Ernest CS, Brooks JJ. Immunoperoxidase localization of secretory component in reactive mesothelium and mesotheliomas. J Histochem Cytochem 1981; 29: 1102–1104.

113. Ordonez NG. The immunohistochemical diagnosis of mesothelioma: differentiation of mesothelioma and lung adenocarcinoma. Am J Surg Pathol 1989; 13: 276–291.

114. Kawai T, Greenberg SD, Truong LD, et al. Differences in lectin-binding of malignant pleural mesothelioma and adenocarcinoma of the lung. Am J Pathol 1988; 130: 401–410.

115. Ramael M, Segers K, Buysse C, et al. Immunohistochemical distribution patterns of epidermal growth factor receptor in malignant mesothelioma and non-neoplastic mesothelium. Virchows Arch [A] 1991; 419: 171–175.

116. Yamada T, Jiping J, Endo R, et al. Molecular cloning of a cell-surface glycoprotein that can potentially discriminate mesothelium from epithelium: its identification as vascular cell adhesion molecule 1. Br J Cancer 1995; 71: 562–570.

117. Chang K, Pai LH, Pass H, et al. Monoclonal antibody K1 reacts with epithelial mesothelioma but not with lung adenocarcinoma. Am J Surg Pathol 1992; 16: 259–266.

118. Ramael M, Buysse C, van den Bosche J, et al. the β chain of the platelet-derived growth factor receptor in malignant mesothelioma and non-neoplastic mesothelium. J Pathol 1992; 167: 1–4.

119. Ramael M, van den Bosche J, Buysse C, et al. Immunoreactivity for p-170 glycoprotein in malignant mesothelioma and in non-neoplastic mesothelium of the pleura using the murine monoclonal antibody JSB-1. J Pathol 1992; 167: 5–8.

120. Soler AP, Knudsen KA, Jaurand M-C, et al. The differential expression of N-Cadherin and E-Cadherin distinguishes pleural mesotheliomas from lung adenocarcinomas. Hum Pathol 1995; 26: 1363–1369.

121. Kumaki F, Kawai T, Churg A, et al. Expression of telomerase reverse transcriptase (TERT) in malignant mesotheliomas. Am J Surg Pathol 2002; 26: 365–370.

122. Ghosh AK, Gatter KC, Dunnill MS, Mason DY. Immunohistological staining of reactive mesothelium, mesothelioma, and lung carcinoma with a panel of monoclonal antibodies. J Clin Pathol 1987; 40: 19–25.

123. Chu PG, Weiss LM. Expression of cytokeratin 5/6 in epithelial neoplasms: An immunohistochemical study of 509 cases. Mod Pathol 2002; 15: 6–10.

124. Wang NS. Electron microscopy in the diagnosis of pleural mesotheliomas. Cancer 1973; 31: 1046–1054.

125. Warhol MJ, Hickey WF, Corson JM. Malignant mesothelioma: Ultrastructural distinction from adenocarcinoma. Am J Surg Pathol 1982; 6: 307–314.

126. Dardick I, El-Jabbi M, McCaughey WT, et al. Ultrastructure of poorly differentiated diffuse epithelial mesotheliomas. Ultrastruct Pathol 1984; 7: 151–160.

127. Warhol MJ, Corson JM. An ultrastructural comparison of mesotheliomas with adenocarcinomas of the lung and breast. Hum Pathol 1985; 16: 50–55.

128. Burns TR, Greenberg D, Mace ML, Johnson EH. Ultrastructural diagnosis of epithelial malignant mesothelioma. Cancer 1985; 56: 2036–2040.

129. Dardick I, El-Jabbi M, McCaughey WT, et al. Diffuse epithelial mesothelioma: a review of the ultrastructural spectrum. Ultrastruct Pathol 1987; 11: 503–533.

130. Oury TD, Hammar SP, Roggli VL. Ultrastructural features of diffuse malignant mesotheliomas. Hum Pathol 1998; 29: 1382–1392.

131. Jandik WR, Landas SK, Bray CK, Lager DJ. Scanning electron microscopic distinction of pleural mesotheliomas from adenocarcinomas. Mod Pathol 6; 1993: 761–764.

132. Roggli VL, Kolbeck J, Sanfilippo F, Shelburne JD. Pathology of human mesothelioma: Etiologic and diagnostic considerations. Pathol Annu Part 2, 1987; 22: 91–131.

133. Carbone M, Kratzke RA, Testa JR. The pathogenesis of mesothelioma. Semin Oncol 2002; 29: 2–17.

134. Krismann M, Muller KM, Jaworska M, Johnen G. Molecular cytogenetic differences between histological subtypes of malignant mesotheliomas: DNA cytometry and comparative genomic hybridization of 90 cases. J Pathol 2002; 197: 363–371.

135. Hirao T, Bueno R, Chen C-J, et al. Alterations of the p16^{INK4} locus in human malignant mesothelial tumors. Carcinogenesis 2002; 23: 1127–1130.

136. Scharnhorst V, van der Eb AJ, Jochemsen AG. WT1 proteins: functions in growth and differentiation. Gene 2001; 273: 141–161.

137. Foddis R, De Rienzo A, Broccoli D, et al. SV40 infection induces telomerase activity in human mesothelial cells. Oncogene 2002; 221: 1434–1442.

138. Ikuta N, Tano M, Iwata M, et al. A case of adenomatoid mesothelioma of the pleura. Nippon Kyobu Shikkan Gakkai Zasshi (Japanese Journal of Thoracic Diseases) 1989; 27: 1540–1544.

139. Kaplan MA, Tazelaar HD, Tomayoshi H, et al. Adenomatoid tumors of the pleura. Am J Surg Pathol 1996; 20: 1219–1223.

140. Klemperer P, Rabin CB. Primary neoplasms of the pleura. Arch Pathol 1931; 11: 385–401.

141. Strom EH, Skjorten F, Aarseth LB, et al. Solitary fibrous tumor of the pleura: An immunohistochemical, electron microscopic, and tissue culture study of a tumor producing insulin-like growth factor-1 in a patient with hypoglycemia. Path Res Pract 1991; 187: 109–113.

142. England DM, Hochholzer L, McCarthy MJ. Localized benign and malignant fibrous tumors of the pleura: A clinical pathologic review of 223 cases. Am J Surg Pathol 1989; 13: 640–658.

143. Okike N, Bernatz PE, Woolner LB. Localized mesothelioma of the pleura: Benign and malignant variants. J Thorac Cardiovasc Surg 1978; 75: 363–372.

144. Briselli M, Mark AJ, Dickerson GR. Solitary fibrous tumors of the pleura: 8 new cases and review of 360 cases in the literature. Cancer 1981; 47: 2678–2689.

145. Dalton WT, Zolliker AS, McCaughey WTE, et al. Localized primary tumors of the pleura: An analysis of 40 cases. Cancer 1979; 44: 1465–1475.

146. Foster EA, Ackerman LV. Localized mesotheliomas of the pleura: The pathologic evaluation of 18 cases. Am J Clin Pathol 1960; 34: 349–364.

147. Yousem SA, Flynn SD. Intrapulmonary localized fibrous tumor: Intraparenchymal so called localized fibrous mesothelioma. Am J Clin Pathol 1988; 89: 365–369.

148. Aufiero TX, McGary SA, Campbell DB, Phillips PP. Intrapulmonary benign fibrous tumor of the pleura. J Thorac Cardiovas Surg 1995; 110: 549–551.

149. El-Naggar AK, Ro JY, Ayala AG, et al. Localized fibrous tumor of the serosal cavities: Immunohistochemical, electron microscopic and flow cytometric DNA study. Am J Clin Pathol 1989; 92: 561–565.

150. Moran CA, Suster, S, Koss MA. The spectrum of histologic growth patterns in benign and malignant fibrous tumors of the pleura. Semin Diagn Pathol 1992; 9: 169–180.

151. van de Rijn M, Lombard CM, Rouse RV. Expression of CD34 by solitary fibrous tumors of pleura, mediastinum and lung. Am J Surg Pathol 1994; 18: 814–820.

152. Hanau CA, Miettinen M. Solitary fibrous tumor: Histological and immunohistochemical spectrum of benign and malignant variants presenting at different sites. Hum Pathol 1995; 26: 440–449.

153. Vallat-Decouvelaere A-V, Dry SM, Fletcher CDM. Atypical and malignant solitary fibrous tumors in extrathoracic locations: Evidence of their comparability to intra-thoracic tumors. Am J Surg Pathol 1998; 22: 1501–1511.

154. Chang Y-L, Lee Y-C, Wu C-T. Thoracic solitary fibrous tumor: Clinical and pathological diversity. Lung Cancer 1999; 23: 53–60.

155. Lin BT-Y, Colby T, Gown AM, et al. Malignant vascular tumors of the serous membranes mimicking mesothelioma: A report of 14 cases. Am J Surg Pathol 1996; 20: 1431–1439.

156. Zhang PJ, LiVolsi VA, Brooks JJ. Malignant epithelioid vascular tumors of the pleura: Report of a series and literature review. Hum Pathol 2000; 31: 29–34.

157. Attanoos RL, Suvarna SK, Rhead E, et al. Malignant vascular tumors of the pleura in "asbestos workers" and endothelial differentiation in mesothelioma. Thorax 2000; 55: 860–863.

158. Sporn TA, Butnor KJ, Roggli VL. Epithelioid hemangioendothelioma of the pleura: An aggressive vascular malignancy and clinical mimic of mesothelioma. Histopathology 2002; 41 (Suppl 2): 173–177.

159. De Young BR, Frierso HF, Ly MN, et al. CD31 immunoreactivity in carcinoma and mesothelioma. Am J Clin Pathol 1998; 110: 374–377.

160. Dehner LP, Watterson J, Priest J. Pleuropulmonary blastoma: A unique intrathoracic-pulmonary neoplasm of childhood. Perspect Pediatr Pathol 1995; 18: 214–226.

161. Priest JR, McDermott MB, Bhatia S, et al. Pleuropulmonary blastoma: A clinicopathologic study of 50 cases. Cancer 1997; 80: 147–161.

162. Romeo C, Impellizzeri P, Grosso M, et al. Pleuropulmonary blastoma: Long term survival and literature review. Med Pediatr Oncol 1999; 33: 372–376.

163. Baraniya J, Desai S, Kane S, et al. Pleuropulmonary blastoma. Med Pediatr Oncol 1999; 32: 52–56.

164. Hill DA, Sadeghi S, Schultz MZ, et al. Pleuropulmonary blastoma in an adult: An initial case report. Cancer 1999; 85: 2368–2374.

165. Yang P, Hasegawa T, Hirose T, et al. Pleuropulmonary blastoma: Fluorescence in situ hybridization analysis indicating trisomy 2. Am J Surg Pathol 1997; 21: 854–859.

166. Pinkard NB, Wilson RW, Lawless N, et al. Calcifying fibrous pseudotumor of the pleura: A report of three cases of a newly described entity involving the pleura. Am J Clin Pathol 1996; 105: 189–194.

167. Jeong HS, Lee GK, Sung R, et al. Calcifying fibrous pseudotumor of mediastinum – A case report. J Korean Med Sci 1997; 12: 58–62.

168. Hainaut P, Lesage V, Weynaud B, et al. Calcifying fibrous pseudotumor: A patient presenting with multiple pleural lesions. Acta Clin Belg 1999; 54: 162–164.

169. Erasmus JJ, McAdams HP, Patz EF, et al. Calcifying fibrous pseudotumor of pleura: Radiologic features in three cases. J Comput Asst Tomogr 1996; 20: 763–765.

170. Parkash V, Gerald WL, Parma A, et al. Desmoplastic small round cell tumor of the pleura. Am J Surg Pathol 1995; 19: 659–665.

171. Sapi Z, Szentirmay Z, Orosz Z. Desmoplastic small round cell tumor of the pleura: A case report with further cytogenetic and ultrastructural evidence of 'mesothelioblastemic' origin. Eur J Surg Oncol 1999; 25: 633–634.

172. Cagle PT, Hicks MJ, Haque A. Desmoplastic small round cell tumor of the pleura: Report of two cases and review of the literature. Histopathology 2002; 41 (Suppl 2): 164–170.

173. Gaertner E, Zeren EH, Fleming MV, et al. Biphasic synovial sarcomas arising in the pleural cavity: A clinicopathologic study of five cases. Am J Surg Pathol 1996; 20: 36–45.

174. Aubry M-C, Bridge JA, Wickert R, Tazelaar HD. Primary monophasic synovial sarcoma of the pleura: Five cases confirmed by the presence of SYT-SSX fusion transcript. Am J Surg Pathol 2001; 25: 776–781.

175. Miettinen M, Limon J, Niezabitowski A, Lasota J. Calretinin and other mesothelioma markers in synovial sarcoma: Analysis of antigenic similarities and differences with malignant mesothelioma. Am J Surg Pathol 2001; 25: 610–617.

176. Harwood TR, Gracey DR, Yokoo H. Pseudomesotheliomatous carcinoma of the lung. A variant of peripheral lung cancer. Am J Clin Pathol 1986; 65: 159–167.

177. Koss M, Travis W, Moran C, Hochholzer L. Pseudomesotheliomatous adenocarcinoma. A reappraisal. Semin Diagn Pathol 1992; 9: 117–123.

178. Hammar SP. Pseudomesotheliomatous carcinoma of the lung: A report of three unusual cases and review of the literature. Histopathology 2002; 41(Suppl 2): 159–164.

179. Yatabe Y, Mitsudomi T, Takahashi T. TTF 1 expression in pulmonary adenocarcinomas. Am J Surg Pathol 2002; 26: 767–773.

180. McCaughey WTE, Colby TV, Battifora H, et al. Diagnosis of diffuse malignant mesothelioma: Experience of a US/Canadian mesothelioma panel. Mod Pathol 1991; 4: 342–353.

181. Leuallen EC, Carr DT. Pleural effusion: A statistical study of 436 patients. N Engl J Med 1955; 252: 79–83.

182. McAllister HA Jr, Fenoglio JJ. Tumors of the cardiovascular system. In: Atlas of tumor pathology. Series 2, Fasc 15. Washington, DC: Armed Forces Institute of Pathology; 1978.

183. Waller BF, Taliercio CP, Howard J, et al. Morphologic aspects of pericardial heart disease. Clin Cardiol 1992; 15: 203–209.

184. Fischbein L, Namade M, Sachs RN, et al. Chronic constrictive pericarditis associated with asbestosis. Chest 1988; 94: 646–647.

185. Davies D, Andrews MI, Jones JS. Asbestos induced pericardial effusion and constrictive pericarditis. Thorax 1991; 46: 429–432.

186. Thompson R, Schlegel W, Lucca M, et al. Primary malignant mesothelioma of the pericardium. Case report and literature review. Texas Heart Inst J 1994; 21: 170–174.

187. Burke A, Virmani R. Tumors of the heart and great vessels. In: Atlas of tumor pathology. Series 3, Fasc 16. Washington, DC: Armed Forces Institute of Pathology; 1996.

188. Vigneswaran WT, Stefanacci PR. Pericardial mesothelioma. Curr Treat Options Oncol 2000; 1: 299–302.

189. Beck B, Konetzke G, Ludwig V, et al. Malignant pericardial mesotheliomas and asbestos exposure: A case report. Am J Ind Med 1982; 3: 149–159.

190. Kahn EI, Rohl A, Barnett EW, Suzuki Y. Primary pericardial mesothelioma following exposure to asbestos. Environ Res 1980; 23: 270–281.

191. Churg A, Warnock ML, Bersch KG. Malignant mesothelioma arising after direct application of asbestos and fiberglass to the pericardium. Am Rev Respir Dis 1978; 118: 419–424.

192. Cammarasano C, Lewis W. Cardiac lesions in acquired immunodeficiency syndrome (AIDS). J Am Coll Cardiol 1985; 5: 703–706.

193. Case records of the Massachusetts General Hospital. Case 22-1987. N Engl J Med 1987; 316: 1394–1404.

194. Sane AC, Roggli VL. Curative resection of a well-differentiated papillary mesothelioma of the pericardium. Arch Pathol Lab Med 1995; 119: 226–267.

195. Nelson E, Stenzel P. Intrapericardial yolk sac tumor in an infant girl. Cancer 1987; 60: 1567–1569.

196. Chan HSL, Sonley MJ, et al. Primary and secondary tumors of childhood involving the heart, pericardium and great vessels: a report of 75 cases and review of the literature. Cancer 1985; 56a: 825–836.

197. Cox JN, Friedle B, Mechmeche R, et al. Teratoma of the heart: a case report and review of the literature. Virchows Arch [A] 1983; 402: 163–174.

198. Virmani R, Bewtra C, McAllister HA, Schulte RD. Intrapericardial giant lymph node hyperplasia. Am J Surg Pathol 1982; 6: 475–481.

199. Bortolotti U, Calabro F, Loy M, et al. Giant intrapericardial solitary fibrous tumors. Ann Thorac Surg 1992; 54: 1219–1220.

200. Luthringer DJ, Virmani R, Weiss SW, Rosai J. A distinctive cardiovascular lesion resembling histiocytoid (epithelioid) hemangioma. Evidence suggesting mesothelial participation. Am J Surg Pathol 1990; 14: 993–1000.

201. Veinot JP, Tazelaar HD, Edwards WD, Colby TV. Mesothelial/monocytic incidental cardiac excrescences: cardiac MICE. Mod Pathol 1994; 7: 9–15.

202. Haded FS, Ghossain A, Sawaya E, et al. Abdominal tuberculosis. Dis Colon Rectum 1987; 30: 724–725.

203. Waxman M, Boyce JG. Intraperitoneal rupture of benign cystic ovarian teratoma. Obstet Gynecol 1976; (suppl. 1)48: 9S–13S.

204. Trimble EN, Siago PE, Freeberg GW, et al. Peritoneal sarcoidosis and elevated CA-125. Obstet Gynecol 1991; 78: 976–977.

205. Daum F, Boney SG, Cohen MI. Crohn's disease. Gastroenterology 1974; 67: 527–530.

206. Adams HW, Kaing EL. Eosinophilic ascites: Case report and review of literature. Dig Dis 1977; 22: 40–42.

207. Metzger AL, Coyme N, Lee S, et al. LE cell formation in peritonitis due to systemic lupus erythematosus. J Rheumatol 1974; 1: 130–133.

208. Sohar E, Gafni J, Pras M, et al. Familial Mediterranean fever: a survey of 470 cases and review of the literature. Am J Med 1967; 43: 227–253.

209. Rosai J, Dehner LP. Nodular mesothelial hyperplasia in hernia sacs: A benign reactive condition simulating a neoplastic process. Cancer 1975; 35: 165–175.

210. Clement PB, Young RH. Florid mesothelial hyperplasia associated with ovarian tumors: A potential source of error in tumor diagnosis and staging. Int J Gynecol Pathol 1993; 12: 51–58.

211. Daya D, McCaughey WT. Pathology of peritoneum: A review of selected topics. Semin Diagn Pathol 1991; 8: 277–289.

212. Mollo F, Bellis D, Magnani C, et al. Hyaline splenic and hepatic plaques: Correlation with cirrhosis, pulmonary tuberculosis, and asbestos exposure. Arch Pathol Lab Med 1993; 117: 1017–1021.

213. Castelli MG, Armin AR, Husain A, Orfei E. Fibrosing peritonitis in a drug abuser. Arch Pathol Lab Med 1985; 109: 767–769.

214. Bradley JA, McWhinnie DL, Hamilton DNH. Sclerosing obstructive peritonitis after continuous ambulatory peritoneal dialysis. Lancet 1983; 2: 113–114.

215. Brown P, Baddeley H, Read AE, et al. Sclerosing peritonitis: An unusual reaction to a beta-adrenergic blocking drug (Practolol). Lancet 1974; 2: 1477–1481.

216. Lauchlan SC. The secondary mullerian system revisited. Int J Gynecol Pathol 1994; 13: 73–79.

217. Clement PB. Pathology of endometriosis. Pathol Annu 1990; 25(1): 245–295.

218. Heaps JM, Nieberg RK, Berek JS. Malignant neoplasms arising in endometriosis. Obstet Gynecol 1990; 75: 1023–1028.

219. Toki T, Fujii S, Silverberg SG. A clinicopathologic study on the association of endometriosis and carcinoma of the ovary using a scoring system. Int J Gynecol Cancer 1996; 6: 68–75.

220. Mahoney AD, Waisman J, Zeldis LJ. Adenomyoma: A precursor of extrauterine mullerian adenocarcinoma? Arch Pathol Lab Med 1977; 101: 579–584.

221. Lankerani MR, Aubrey RW, Reid JD. Endometriosis of the colon with mixed "germ cell" tumor. Am J Clin Pathol 1982; 78: 555–559.

222. Rutgers JL, Young RH, Scully RE. Ovarian yolk sac tumor arising from an endometrioid carcinoma. Hum Pathol 1987; 18: 1296–1299.

223. Griffith LM, Carcangiu M. Sex cord tumor with annular tubules associated with endometriosis of fallopian tube. Am J Clin Pathol 1991. 96: 259–262.

224. Burmeister RE, Fechner RE, Franklin RR. Endosalpingiosis of the peritoneum. Obstet Gynecol 1969; 34: 310–318.

225. Zaytsev P, Taxy JB. Pregnancy-associated ectopic decidua. Am J Surg Pathol 1987; 11: 526–530.

226. Kuo T, London Sn, Dinh TV. Endometriosis occurring in leiomyomatosis peritonealis disseminate: Ultrastructural study and histogenetic consideration. Am J Surg Pathol 1980; 4: 197–204.

227. Fadare O, Bifulco C, Carter D, Parkash V. Cartilaginous differentiation in peritoneal tissues:

Report of two cases and a review of the literature. Mod Pathol 2002; 15: 777–780.

228. Wilson JD, Montague CJ, Salcuni P, et al. Heterotopic mesenteric ossification ("intraabdominal myositis ossificans"): Report of five cases. Am J Surg Pathol 1999; 23: 1464–1470.

229. Roth LM. The Brenner tumor and the Walthard cell nest: An electron-microscopic study. Lab Invest 1974; 31: 15–23.

230. Lascano EF, Villamayor RD, Llauer T. Loose cysts of peritoneal cavity. Ann Surg 1960; 152: 836–844.

231. Manjo W, Goldfarb W. Postoperative peritoneal cyst. Surgery 1963; 53: 470–473.

232. Lees RF. Inflammatory cysts of the pelvic peritoneum. Aust Radiol 1978; 22: 319–324.

233. Mennemeyer R, Smith M. Multicystic, peritoneal mesothelioma: A report with electron microscopy of a case mimicking intra-abdominal cystic hygroma (lymphangioma). Cancer 1979; 44: 692–698.

234. Moore JH, Crum CP, Chandler JG, Feldman PS. Benign cystic mesothelioma. Cancer 1980; 45: 2395–2399.

235. Katsube Y, Mukai K, Silverberg SG. Cystic mesothelioma of peritoneum: A report of five cases and review of literature. Cancer 1982; 50: 1615–1622.

236. Gussman D, Thickman D, Wheeler JE. Postoperative peritoneal cysts. Obstet Gynecol 1986; 68: 535–555.

237. McFadden DE, Clement PE. Peritoneal inclusion cysts with mural mesothelial proliferation: A clinical pathologic analysis of 6 cases. Am J Surg Pathol 1986; 10: 844–854.

238. Sienkowski IK, Russel AJ, Dilby SA, et al. Peritoneal cystic mesothelioma: An electron microscopic and immunohistochemical study of 2 male patients. J Clin Pathol 1986; 39: 440–445.

239. Kjellevold K, Nesland JM, Holm R, et al. Multicystic peritoneal mesothelioma. Pathol Res Proc 1986; 181: 767–771.

240. Weiss SW, Tavassoli FA. Multicystic mesothelioma: An analysis of pathologic findings and biologic behavior in 37 cases. Am J Surg Pathol 1988; 12: 737–746.

241. Ross MJ, Welsh WR, Skully RE. Multilocular peritoneal inclusion cysts (so called cystic mesothelioma). Cancer 1989; 64: 1326–1346.

242. Santucci M, Biancalani M, Dini S. Multicystic peritoneal mesothelioma: A fine structure study with special reference to the spectrum of phenotypic differentiation exhibited by mesothelial cells. J Submicrosc Cytol Pathol 1989; 21: 749–764.

243. Kanty MD, Williams J, Volpe RJ, et al. Benign cystic mesothelioma in males. Am J Gastrenterol 1990; 85: 311–315.

244. Clement PB. Reactive tumor-like lesions of the peritoneum. J Clin Pathol 1995; 103: 673–675.

245. Ball NJ, Urbanski S, Green F, Kieser T. Pleural multicystic mesothelial proliferation: The so-called multicystic mesothelioma. Am J Surg Pathol 1990; 14: 375–378.

246. Fleming CR, Dickson FR, Harrison EG Jr. Splenosis: Autotransplantation of splenic tissue. Am J Med 1976; 61 414–419.

247. O'Connor JV, Brown CC, Thomas JK, et al. Thoracic splenosis. Ann Thorac Surg 1998; 66: 552–553.

248. Fukushima M, Sharpe L, Okagaki T. Peritoneal melanosis secondary to benign dermoid cyst of the ovary: A case report with ultrastructural study. Int J Gynecol Pathol 1984; 2: 403–409.

249. Thatcher SS, Granger DA, True ID, DeCherney AH. Pelvic trophoblastic implants after laparoscopic treatment of tubal ectopic pregnancy. Fertil Steril 1989; 52: 337–339.

250. Truong LD, Jurco S, McGavran MH. Gliomatosis peritonei. Am J Surg Pathol 1982; 6: 443–449.

251. Coffin CM, Watterson J, Priest JR, Dehner LP. Extrapulmonary inflammatory myofibroblastic tumor (inflammatory pseudotumor): A clinicopathologic and immunohistochemical study of 84 cases. Am J Surg Pathol 1995; 19: 859–872.

252. Pettinato G, Manivel JC, De Rosa N, Dehner LP. Inflammatory myofibroblastic tumor (plasma cell granuloma): Clinicopathologic study of 20 cases with immunohistochemical and ultrastructural observations. Am J Clin Pathol 1990; 94: 537–546.

253. Gonzalez-Crussi F, deMello DE, Sotelo-Avila C. Omental mesenteric myxoid hamartomas. Am J Surg Pathol 1983; 7: 567–578.

254. Kannerstein M, Churg J. Peritoneal mesothelioma. Hum Pathol 1977; 8: 83–93.

255. Browne K, Smither WJ. Asbestos related mesothelioma: Factors discriminating between pleural and peritoneal sites. Br J Indust Med 1983; 40: 145–152.

256. Roggli VL, Sharma A, Butnor KJ, et al. Malignant mesothelioma and occupational exposure to asbestos: A clinicopathological correlation of 1445 cases. Ultrastruct Pathol 2002; 26: 55–65.

257. Riddell RH, Goodman MJ, Moosa AR. Peritoneal malignant mesothelioma in a patient with recurrent peritonitis. Cancer 1981; 48: 134–139.

258. Maurer R, Egloff B. Malignant peritoneal mesothelioma after cholangiography with Thorotrast. Cancer 1975; 36: 1381–1385.

259. Stark RJ, Fu YS, Carter JR. Malignant peritoneal mesothelioma following radiotherapy for seminoma of the testis. Cancer 1979; 44: 914–919.

260. Horie A, Hiraoka K, Yamamoto O, et al. An autopsy case of peritoneal malignant mesothelioma in a radiation technologist. Acta Pathol Jpn 1990; 40: 57–62.

261. Niggli FK, Gray TJ, Faafat F, Stevens MCG. Spectrum of peritoneal mesothelioma in childhood: Clinical and histopathologic features including DNA cytometry. Pediatr Hematol Oncol 1994; 11: 399–408.

262. Berry PT, Favara BE, Odom LF. Malignant peritoneal mesothelioma in a child. Pediatr Pathol 1986; 5: 397–409.

263. Armstrong GR, Raafat F, Ingram L, Mann JR. Malignant peritoneal mesothelioma in childhood. Arch Pathol Lab Med 1988; 112: 1159–1162.

264. Asensio JA, Goldblatt P, Thomford NR. Primary malignant peritoneal mesothelioma: A report of 7 cases and a review of the literature. Arch Surg 1990; 125: 1477–1481.

265. McCaughey WT. Criteria for a diagnosis of diffuse mesothelial tumors. Ann NY Acad Sci 1965; 132: 603–613.

266. Goldblum J, Hart W. Localized and diffuse mesotheliomas of the genital tract and peritoneum in women: A clinicopathologic study of 19 true mesothelial neoplasms, other than adenomatoid tumors, multicystic mesotheliomas and localized fibrous tumors. Am J Surg Pathol 1995; 19: 1124–1137.

267. Clement PB, Young RH, Scully RE. Malignant mesotheliomas presenting as ovarian masses: A report of nine cases, including two primary ovarian mesotheliomas. Am J Surg Pathol 20: 1067–1080. 1996;

268. Walker AM, Mills SE. Surgical pathology of tunica vaginalis testis and embryologically related mesotheliomas. Pathol Annu 1988; 23: 125–152.

269. Grow A, Jenson ML, Dona A. Mesotheliomas of the tunica vaginalis, testis and hernia sacs. Virchows Arch [A] 1989; 415: 283–292.

270. Japko L, Horta AA, Schreiber K, et al. Malignant mesothelioma of the tunica vaginalis testis: Report of first case with preoperative diagnosis. Cancer 1982; 49: 119–127.

271. Nascimento AG, Keeny GL, Fletcher CDM. Deciduoid peritoneal mesothelioma: An unusual phenotype affecting young females. Am J Surg Pathol 1994; 18: 439–445.

272. Talerman A, Montero JR, Chilcotte RR, Okagaki T. Diffuse malignant peritoneal mesothelioma in a 13 year old girl: Report of a case and review of the literature. Am J Surg Pathol 1985; 9: 73–80.

273. Shanks JH, Harris M, Banerjee SS, et al. Mesotheliomas with deciduoid morphology: A

morphologic spectrum and a variant not confined to young females. Am J Surg Pathol 2000; 24: 285–294.

274. Ordonez NG. Epithelial mesothelioma with deciduoid features: Report of four cases. Am J Surg Pathol 2000; 24: 816–823.

275. Diaz-Cascajo C, Hoos A. Deciduoid epithelial mesothelioma of the pleura with focal rhabdoid change (letter). Am J Surg Pathol 2000; 24: 1440–1444.

276. Kitazawa M, Kaneko H, Toshima M, et al. Malignant peritoneal mesothelioma with massive foamy cells. Acta Pathol Jpn 1984; 34: 687–692.

277. Nochomowitz LE, Orenstein JM. Adenocarcinoma of the rete testis: Case report, ultrastructural observations and clinicopathologic correlates. Am J Surg Pathol 1984; 8: 625–634.

278. Fox H. Primary neoplasia of the female peritoneum. Histopathology 1993; 23: 103–110.

279. Kerrigan SAJ, Turnnir RT, Clement PB, et al. Diffuse malignant epithelial mesotheliomas of the peritoneum in women: A clinicopathologic study of 25 patients. Cancer 2002; 94: 378–385.

280. Wick MR, Mills SE, Swanson PE. Expression of myelomonocytic antigens in mesotheliomas and adenocarcinomas involving the serosal surfaces. Am J Clin Pathol 1990; 94: 18–26.

281. McCaughey WTE, Schryer MJ, Lin X, Al-Jabi M. Extraovarian pelvic serous tumor with marked calcification. Arch Pathol Lab Med 1986; 110: 78–80.

282. Gilks CB, Bell DA, Scully RE. Serous psammocarcinoma of the ovary and peritoneum. Int J Gyn Pathol 1990; 9: 110–121.

283. Khoury N, Raju U, Crissman JD, et al. A comparative immunohistochemical study of peritoneal and ovarian serous tumors and mesotheliomas. Hum Pathol 1990; 21: 811–819.

284. Zhou J, Iwasa Y, Konishi I, et al. Papillary serous carcinoma of the peritoneum in women. A clinicopathologic and immunohistochemical study. Cancer 1995; 76: 429–436.

285. Bollinger DJ, Wick MR, Dehner LP, et al. Peritoneal malignant mesothelioma versus serous papillary adenocarcinoma: A histochemical and immunohistochemical comparison. Am J Surg Pathol 1989; 13: 659–670.

286. Ordonez NG. Role of immunohistochemistry in distinguishing epithelial peritoneal mesotheliomas from peritoneal and ovarian serous carcinomas. Am J Surg Pathol 1998; 22: 1203–1214.

287. Daya D, McCaughey WT. Well differentiated papillary mesothelioma of the peritoneum: A clinicopathologic study of 22 cases. Cancer 1990; 65: 292–296.

288. Golden A, Ash J. Adenomatoid tumors of genital tract. Am J Pathol 1945; 21: 63–80.

289. Young RH, Silva EG, Scully RE. Ovarian and juxtaovarian adenomatoid tumors: A report of 6 cases. Int J Gynecol Pathol 1991; 10: 364–371.

290. Craig JR, Hart WR. Extragenital adenomatoid tumor: Evidence for the mesothelial theory of origin. Cancer 1979; 43: 1678–1681.

291. Souderstrom J, Liederberg CF. Malignant adenomatoid tumor of the epididymis. Acta Pathol Microbiol Immunol Scand 1966; 67: 165–168.

292. Mackay B, Benton JL, Skoglund RW. The adenomatoid tumor: Fine structural evidence for a mesothelial origin. Cancer 1971; 27: 109–115.

293. Stevenson TJ, Mills PM. Adenomatoid tumors: An immunohistochemical and ultrastructural appraisal of the histogenesis. J Pathol 1986; 148: 327–335.

294. Ibrahim NBN, Briggs JC, Corrin B. Double primary localized fibrous tumors of the pleura and peritoneum. Histopathology 1993; 22: 282–284.

295. Young RH, Clement PB, McCaughey WT. Solitary fibrous tumor ("fibrous mesothelioma") of peritoneum: A report of 3 cases and a review of literature. Arch Pathol Lab Med 1990; 114: 493–495.

296. Berman J, O'Leary TJ. Gastrointestinal stromal tumor workshop. Hum Pathol 2001; 32: 578–582.

297. Gerald WL, Miller HK, Battifora H, et al. Intraabdominal desmoplastic small round-cell tumor: Report of 19 cases of a distinctive type of high grade polyphenotypic malignancy affecting young individuals. Am J Surg Pathol 1991; 15: 499–513.

298. Layfield LJ, Lenarsky C. Desmoplastic small cell tumor of peritoneum coexpressing mesenchymal and epithelial markers. Am J Clin Pathol 1991; 96: 536–543.

299. Young RH, Eichhorn JH, Dickersin GR, Scully RE. Ovarian involvement by the intraabdominal desmoplastic small round cell tumor with divergent differentiation: A report of three cases. Hum Pathol 1992; 23: 454–464.

300. Brodie S, Stocker SJ, Wardow JC, et al. EWS and WT-1 gene fusion in desmoplastic small round cell tumor of the abdomen. Hum Pathol 1995; 26: 1370–1374.

301. Young RH, Gilks CB, Scully RE. Mucinous tumors of the appendix associated with mucinous tumors of the ovary and pseudomyxoma peritonei: A clinicopathological analysis of 22 cases supporting an origin in the appendix. Am J Surg Pathol 1991; 15: 415–429.

302. Campbell JS, Lou P, Ferguson JP, et al. Pseudomyxoma peritonei et ovarii with occult neoplasms of appendix. Obstet Gynecol 1973; 42: 897–902.

303. Qizilbash AH. Mucoceles of the appendix: Their relationship to hyperplastic polyps, mucinous cystadenomas, and cystadenocarcinomas. Arch Pathol 1975; 99: 548–555.

304. Ronnett BM, Zahn CM, Kurman RJ, et al. Disseminated peritoneal adenomucinosis and peritoneal mucinous carcinomatosis: a clinicopathologic analysis of 109 cases with emphasis on distinguishing pathologic features, site of origin, prognosis and relationship to "pseudomyxoma peritonei." Am J Surg Pathol 1995; 19: 1390–1408.

305. Light RW. Clinical diagnosis of pleural disease. In: Cagle PT, ed. Diagnostic pulmonary pathology. New York: Marcel Dekker; 2000: 571–581.

306. Light RW, MacGregor MI, Luchsinger PC, Ball WC. Pleural effusions: the diagnostic separation of transudates and exudates. Ann Intern Med 1972; 77: 507–513.

307. Battifora H. The pleura. In: Sternberg S, ed. Diagnostic surgical pathology. New York; Raven Press; 1994: 1095–1123.

308. Wick MR, Moran CA, Mills SE, Suster S. Immunohistochemical differential diagnosis of pleural effusions, with emphasis on malignant mesothelioma. Curr Opin Pulm Med 2001; 7: 187–192.

309. Ramzy I, ed. Clinical cytopathology and aspiration biopsy. 2nd edn. New York: McGraw Hill; 2001.

310. Light RW. Tuberculous pleural effusions. In: Light RW, ed. Pleural diseases. 3rd edn. Baltimore: Williams & Wilkins; 1995: 154–156.

311. Ferrer-Sancho J. Pleural tuberculosis. Eur Respir J 1997; 10: 942–947.

312. Light RW. Establishing the diagnosis of tuberculous pleuritis. Arch Intern Med 1998; 158: 1967–1968.

313. Reechaipichitkul W, Lulitanond V, Sungkeeree S, Patjanasoontorn B. Rapid diagnosis of tuberculous pleural effusion using polymerase chain reaction. Southeast Asian J Trop Med Public Health 2000; 31: 509–514.

314. Metzger AL, Coyme N, Lee S, et al. LE cell formation in peritonitis due to systemic lupus erythematosus. J Rheumatol 1974; 1: 130–133.

315. Petty TL, Wilkins M. The five manifestations of rheumatoid lung. Dis Chest 1966; 49: 75–82.

316. Choi Y-L, Song S-Y. Cytologic clue of so-called nodular histiocytic hyperplasia of the pleura. Diagn Cytopathol 2001; 24: 256–259.

317. Luse SA, Reagan J. A histocytological study of effusions. Effusions not associated with malignant tumors. Cancer 1958; 7: 1155–1166.

318. Kho-Duffin J, Tao L-C, Cramer H, et al. Cytologic diagnosis of malignant mesothelioma with particular emphasis on the epithelial noncohesive cell type. Diagn Cytopathol 1999; 20: 57–62.

319. Lee A, Baloch ZW, Yu G, Gupta PK. Mesothelial hyperplasia with reactive atypia: Diagnostic pitfalls and role of immunohistochemical studies – a case report. Diagn Cytopathol 2000; 22: 113–116.

320. Boon M, Veldhuizen RW, Ruinaard C, et al. Qualitative distinctive differences between the vacuoles of mesothelioma cells and of cells from metastatic carcinoma exfoliated in pleural fluid. Acta Cytol 1984; 28: 443–449.

321. Stevens M, Leong A, Fazzalari N, Dowling KD. Cytopathology of malignant mesothelioma: a stepwise logistic regression analysis. Diagn Cytopathol 1992; 8: 333–341.

322. Monte S, Ehya H, Lang W. Positive effusion cytology as the initial presentation of malignancy. Acta Cytol 1987; 31: 448–452.

323. DiBonito L, Falconieri G, Colautti I, et al. The positive pleural effusion. Acta Cytol 1992; 36: 329–332.

324. Sears D, Hajdu S. The cytologic diagnosis of malignant neoplasms in pleural and peritoneal effusions. Acta Cytol 1995; 31: 85–97.

325. Murphy W, Ng A. Determination of primary site by examination of cancer cells in body fluids. Am J Clin Pathol 1972; 58: 479–488.

326. Klempman S. The exfoliative cytology of diffuse pleural mesothelioma. Cancer 1962; 15: 691–704.

327. Berge T, Grontoft O. Cytologic diagnosis of malignant pleural mesothelioma. Acta Cytol 1965; 9: 207–212.

328. Tao LC. The cytopathology of mesothelioma. Acta Cytol 1979; 23: 209–213.

329. Whitaker D, Shilkin KB. Diagnosis of pleural malignant mesothelioma in life – a practical approach. J Pathol 1984; 143: 147–175.

330. Triol JH, Conston AS, Chandler SV. Malignant mesothelioma. Cytopathology of 75 cases seen in a New Jersey community hospital. Acta Cytol 1984; 28: 37–45.

331. Pedio G, Landolt-Weber U. Cytologic presentation of malignant mesothelioma in pleural effusion. Exp Cell Biol 1988; 56: 211–216.

332. Sherman M, Mark E. Effusion cytology in the diagnosis of malignant epithelioid and biphasic pleural mesothelioma. Arch Pathol Lab Med 1990; 114: 845–851.

333. Cheepsumon S, Leong AS-Y, Vinyuvat S. Immunostaining of cell preparations: a comparative evaluation of common fixatives and protocols. Diagn Cytopathol 1996; 15: 167–174.

334. Leong AS-Y. Immunostaining of cytologic specimens. Am J Clin Pathol 1996; 105: 139–140.

335. Ghosh AK, Spriggs AI, Taylor-Papadimitriou J, et al. Immunocytochemical staining of cells in pleural and peritoneal effusions with a panel of monoclonal antibodies. J Clin Pathol 1983; 36: 1154–1164.

336. Bramwell ME, Ghosh AK, Smith WD, et al. New monoclonal antibodies evaluated as tumor markers in serous effusions. Cancer 1985; 56: 105–110.

337. Banner BF, Warren WH, Gould VE. Cytomorphology and marker expression of malignant neuroendocrine cells in pleural effusions. Acta Cytol 1986; 30: 99–104.

338. Hilborne LH, Cheng L, Nieberg RK, et al. Evaluation of an antibody of human fat globule antigen in the detection of metastatic carcinoma in pleural, pericardial and peritoneal fluids. Acta Cytol 1986; 30: 245–250.

339. Martin SE, Moshiri S, Thor A, et al. Identification of adenocarcinoma in cytospin preparations of effusions using monoclonal antibody B72.3. Am J Clin Pathol 1986; 86: 10–18.

340. Pinto MM. An immunoperoxidase study of S-100 protein in neoplastic cells in serous effusions. Use as a marker for melanoma. Acta Cytol 1986; 30: 240–244.

341. Ching-Yang L, Lazcano-Villareal O, Pierre RV, et al. Immunocytochemical identification of cells in serous effusions. Am J Clin Pathol 1987; 88: 696–706.

342. Mason MR, Bedrossian CWM, Fahey CA. Value of immunocytochemistry in the study of malignant effusions. Diagn Cytopathol 1987; 3: 215–221.

343. Silverman JF, Nance K, Phillips B, et al. The use of immunoperoxidase panels for cytologic diagnosis of malignancy in serous effusions. Diagn Cytopathol 1987; 3: 134–140.

344. Walts AE, Said JW, Shintaku IP. Epithelial membrane antigen in the cytodiagnosis of effusions and aspirates: immunocytochemical and ultrastructural localization in benign and malignant cells. Diagn Cytopathol 1987; 3: 41–49.

345. Van Niekerk CC, Jap PHK, Thomas CMG, et al. Marker profile of mesothelial cells *versus* ovarian carcinoma cells. Int J Cancer 1989; 43: 1065–1071.

346. Esteban JM, Yokota S, Husain S, et al. Immunocytochemical profile of benign and carcinomatous effusions: a practical approach to difficult diagnosis. Am J Clin Pathol 1990; 94: 698–705.

347. Gioanni J, Caldani C, Zanghellini E, et al. A new epithelial membrane antigen (Calam 27) as a marker of carcinoma in serous effusions. Acta Cytol 1991; 35: 315–319.

348. Cuijpers V, Boerman O, Salet M, et al. Immunocytochemical detection of ovarian carcinoma cells in serous effusions. Acta Cutol 1993; 37: 272–279.

349. Ascoli V, Carnovale Scalzo C, Taccogna S, Nardi F. The diagnostic value of thrombomodulin immunolocalization in serous effusions. Arch Pathol Lab Med 1995; 119: 1136–1140.

350. Fetsch PA, Abati A, Hijazi Y. Utility of the antibodies CA 19-9, HBME-1 and thrombomodulin in the diagnosis of malignant mesothelioma and adenocarcinoma in cytology. Cancer (Cancer Cytopathol) 1998; 84: 101–108.

351. Nagel H, Hemmerlein B, Ruschenburg I, et al. The value of anti-calretinin antibody in the differential diagnosis of normal and reactive mesothelia versus metastatic tumors in effusion cytology. Pathol Res Pract 1998; 194: 759–764.

352. Miedouge M, Rouzaud P, Salama G, et al. Evaluation of seven tumour markers in pleural fluid for the diagnosis of malignant effusions. Br J Cancer 1999; 81: 1059–1065.

353. Simsir A, Fetsch PA, Mehta D, et al. E-cadherin, N-cadherin and calretinin in pleural effusions: the good, the bad, the worthless. Diagn Cytopathol 1999; 20: 125–130.

354. Chhiend DC, Yee H, Schaefer D, et al. Calretinin staining pattern aids in the differentiation of mesothelioma from adenocarcinoma in serous effusions. Cancer 2000; 90: 194–200.

355. Wieczorek TJ, Krane JF. Diagnostic utility of calretinin immunohistochemistry in cytologic cell block preparations. Cancer 2000; 90: 312–319.

356. Fetsch PA, Simsir A, Abati A. Comparison of antibodies to HBME-1 and calretinin for the detection of mesothelial cells in effusion cytology. Diagn Cytolpathol 2001; 25: 158–161.

357. Fetsch PA, Abati A. Immunocytochemistry in effusion cytology: a contemporary review. Cancer 2001; 93: 293–308.

358. Lozano MD, Panizo A, Toledo GR, et al. Immunocytochemistry in the differential diagnosis of serous effusions: a comparative evaluation of eight monoclonal antibodies in Papanicolaou stained smears. Cancer 2001; 93: 68–72.

359. Ng WK, Chow JC, Ng PK. Thyroid transcription factor-1 is highly sensitive and specific in differentiating metastatic pulmonary from extrapulmonary adenocarcinoma in effusion fluid cytology specimens. Cancer 2002; 96: 43–48.

360. Mallonee M, Lin F, Hassanein R. A morphologic analysis of the cells of ductal carcinoma of the breast and of adenocarcinoma of the ovary in pleural and abdominal effusions. Acta Cytol 1987; 31: 441–447.

361. Beaty M, Fetsch PA, Wilder AM, et al. Effusion cytology of malignant melanoma. Cancer (Cancer Cytopathol) 1997; 81: 57–63.

362. Khoor A, Whitsett JA, Stahlman MT, et al. Utility of surfactant protein B precursor and thyroid transcription factor 1 in differentiating adenocarcinoma of the lung from malignant mesothelioma. Hum Pathol 1999; 30: 695–700.

363. Romero Candeira S, Hernandez Blasco L, Soler MJ, et al. Biochemical and cytologic characteristics of pleural effusions secondary to pulmonary embolism. Chest 2002; 121: 465–469.

364. Casarett G. Radiation histopathology. Boca Raton, FL: CRC Press; 1980.

365. Wojno K, Olson J, Sherman M. Cytopathology of pleural effusions after radiotherapy. Acta Cytol 1994; 38: 1–8.

366. Tiniakos D, Healicon R, Hair T, et al. p53 immunostaining as a marker of malignancy in cytologic preparations of body fluids. Acta Cytol 1995; 39: 171–176.

367. Zoppi J, Pellicer E, Sundblad A. Diagnostic value of p53 protein in the study of serous effusions. Acta Cytol 1995; 39: 721–724.

368. Mullick SS, Green LK, Ramzy I, et al. p53 gene product in pleural effusions. Practical use in distinguishing benign from malignant cells. Acta Cytol 1996; 40: 855–860.

369. Mu XC, Brien TP, Ross JS, et al. Telomerase activity in benign and malignant cytologic fluids. Cancer 1999; 87: 93–99.

370. Carrillo R, Sneige N, El-Naggar A. Interphase nucleolar organizer regions in the evaluation of serosal cavity effusions. Acta Cytol 1994; 38: 367–372.

371. Huang M, Tsai M, Hwang J, et al. Comparison of nucleolar organizer regions and DNA flow cytometry in the evaluation of pleural effusion. Thorax 1994; 49: 1152–1156.

The cardiovascular system

Allen Burke   Renu Virmani

20

ENDOMYOCARDIAL BIOPSY

GENERAL COMMENTS

Indications for biopsy and specimen processing

The most common indications for endomyocardial biopsy are to evaluate unexplained congestive heart failure, to diagnose transplant rejection, and to evaluate drug (especially anthracycline) toxicity.[1–3] Occasionally, biopsy is used to evaluate restrictive cardiomyopathy, especially in confirming the diagnosis of amyloid. Typical diagnoses rendered by biopsies for the evaluation of unexplained cardiomyopathy include idiopathic cardiomyopathy (i.e. non-specific changes consistent with dilated cardiomyopathy), myocarditis, amyloid, ischemic cardiomyopathy, anthracycline toxicity, and (in tertiary centers) hemochromatosis.[3] Less common indications include the investigation of idiopathic arrhythmias[4] and biopsies of neoplasms.[5]

The indications for biopsy affect tissue processing (Table 20.1). For the evaluation of cardiomyopathy, four to five biopsy fragments should be processed routinely, and one fragment processed for ultrastructure. Ultrastructure is unnecessary in the evaluation of transplant biopsies; all fragments should be processed routinely, unless vascular rejection is suspected, in which case one fragment may be frozen for immunofluorescence. For the evaluation of anthracycline toxicity, all fragments should be processed for electron microscopy; similarly, the diagnosis of chloroquine and amiodarone toxicity requires ultrastructural analysis.

Tissue evaluation

One of the major limitations of endomyocardial biopsy is that of sampling. The bioptome is generally guided towards the septum of the right ventricle, yielding tissue from the ventricular septum. Many inflammatory and infiltrative processes, such as myocarditis, hemochromatosis, sarcoidosis, and amyloidosis, are focal and may easily be missed by biopsy. For this reason, serial cuts of multiple sections are sometimes recommended for adequate evaluation.

To evaluate endomyocardial biopsies for acute rejection, it is essential that multiple sections representing all levels of the tissue in the paraffin block be examined. Three to five 'step' levels should therefore be cut and stained with hematoxylin and eosin (H&E).

Special stains for amyloid and iron are sometimes recommended as a routine adjunct for the evaluation of heart biopsies. Because Congo red stains require thick sections, one 7–10 μm thick section should be cut before the block is exhausted. In cases of myocarditis, cardiomyopathy, and transplant rejection, a Masson trichrome stain is helpful in identifying areas of cellular necrosis and in assessing the degree of interstitial fibrosis. Ultrastructural examination is considered routine in the evaluation of endomyocardial biopsies other than those performed for transplant rejection. Myocyte hypertrophy is diagnosed if the myocyte is larger than a 3,000 × field, if there is irregularity of the nuclear membrane, if there are multiple nuclei, and if there are two or more nucleoli. Significant myofibrillar loss is indicative of myocyte atrophy and is a non-specific finding present in failing hearts. Specific note should be made of mitochondrial morphology, which is abnormal in some forms of congenital cardiomyopathies, and lysosomes, which may degenerate into lamellar bodies characteristic of Fabry's disease and chloroquine toxicity. The interstitium, especially in areas around capillaries, should routinely be evaluated for the presence of amyloid. Sarcotubular dilatation characteristic of anthracycline toxicity is best appreciated on ultrastructural examination.

Artifacts and non-specific findings

Myofiber disarray is normally present in the right ventricle, which is heavily trabeculated. Right ventricular myofiber disarray should not be confused with the myofiber disarray of hypertrophic cardiomyopathy, which usually affects the mid-portion of the ventricular septum. The myofiber disarray of hypertrophic cardiomyopathy is associated with marked hypertrophy, fibrosis, and intramural coronary thickening and is not amenable to the bioptome.

Acute fibrin platelet thrombi may occur on the endocardial surface; these are usually secondary to the procedure and not indicative of

Table 20.1 Specimen handling, endomyocardial biopsy

Indication for biopsy	Formalin fixation	Frozen	EM fixative
Heart failure (dilated)	All fragments, except (optional) 1 frozen and 1 EM fragment	1 (optional), to evaluate HLA upregulation	1 (optional); for amyloid, mitochondrial disease
Heart failure (restrictive)	All fragments except 1	0	1 (corroborate amyloid, desmin cardiomyopathy)
Transplant rejection	All fragments, except 1 (optional)	1 (optional), in cases of suspected acute vascular (humoral) rejection	
Anthracycline toxicity	0	0	All fragments, to evaluate 10 thick sections

mural thrombus. Rarely, thrombus rich in eosinophils may be helpful in diagnosis of hypereosinophilic syndrome. In patients undergoing repeat biopsies, particularly patients with orthotopic transplants, sampling of previous biopsy site is not uncommon. Previous biopsy sites are histologically characterized by surface inflammation granulation tissue, which progresses to scarring. Typically, disorganized myofibers underlie the lesion.

Mesothelial cells may be present and do not generally result in hemopericardium. Contraction bands are extremely common, and are especially marked when cold fixative has been used. Contraction bands often result in artifactual loss of contractile elements in adjacent areas of the myocyte; this change should not be misdiagnosed as myocytolysis or myofibrillar loss. Tangential orientation of the endocardium may mimic endocardial thickening; the presence of multiple, layered endocardial elastic lamellae is required for the diagnosis of endocardial fibroelastosis.

ROLE OF ENDOMYOCARDIAL BIOPSY IN UNEXPLAINED HEART FAILURE AND POSSIBLE MYOCARDITIS

In the nontransplant setting, the primary reason for endomyocardial biopsy is for the evaluation of unexplained heart failure. In a large series of such biopsies, just over 50% of patients were ultimately given a diagnosis of idiopathic dilated cardiomyopathy (Table 20.2). In nontertiary centers, this percentage is likely higher. In this series, only 16% of biopsies demonstrated a specific diagnosis; most of these were myocarditis or infiltrative diseases (notably amyloid).[6] The remainder of the biopsies showed non-specific diagnoses, and the ultimate clinical diagnosis rested on history, such as the presence of AIDS, hypertension, or drug abuse.

Because of the very high proportion of non-specific findings in endomyocardial biopsies for unexplained heart failure, the utility of biopsy has been questioned.[7] The specificity and sensitivity of making the diagnosis of myocarditis in patients with endomyocardial biopsy has been estimated at 95% and 63%, respectively.[7] In addition, there is a very wide variation in the reported incidence of myocarditis in endomyocardial biopsies;[8] in one careful study, only 4% of patients biopsied with idiopathic congestive heart failure showed myocarditis.[9] Therefore, a negative biopsy is not particularly helpful in determining if a patient should receive anti-inflammatory treatment for suspected myocarditis. Furthermore, there has been little difference shown in clinical outcome between patients with the endomyocardial biopsy diagnosis of lymphocytic myocarditis and patients with non-specific biopsy findings (dilated cardiomyopathy), despite treatment with prednisone.[10,11] These findings have led to a steady decline in the numbers of nontransplant heart biopsies. However, a recent study demonstrated that 31% of clinical diagnoses are altered by endomyocardial biopsy, many of which are unsuspected myocarditis; typical diagnoses confirmed by endomyocardial biopsy are myocarditis, idiopathic cardiomyopathy (non-specific findings), ischemic cardiomyopathy, amyloidosis and hemochromatosis.[3]

Recently, the clinical subclassification of biopsy-proven myocarditis into fulminant and nonfulminant forms has bolstered the rationale for endomyocardial biopsy to establish a diagnosis of myocarditis.[6] Somewhat paradoxically, fulminant myocarditis has been demonstrated to respond well to steroids and have a good prognosis.[6] Another potential benefit of biopsy is to establish the rare diagnosis of giant cell myocarditis, which is especially fulminant and requires early transplantation. In order to reconcile the awareness of several clinical categories of myocarditis, the Mayo clinic has established an algorithm for indications for biopsy in cases of unexplained (angiogram-negative) heart failure and possible myocarditis. In this algorithm,[8] patients with rapidly progressive symptoms, recent ventricular tachycardia or conduction system disturbances, or extracardiac symptoms including autoimmune manifestations are selected for biopsy, while other patients with unexplained heart failure are treated without biopsy. Those patients with positive biopsy and clinical indicators of fulminant myocarditis (severe hemodynamic compromise, rapid onset of symptoms, and fever) have been shown to respond to anti-inflammatory regimens.[12]

In addition to purely histologic determination of an inflammatory component of dilated cardiomyopathy (i.e. myocarditis), identification of immunoglobulin[11] or HLA expression[13] on frozen endomyocardial biopsies has been utilized to diagnose forms of dilated cardiomyopathy that may respond to anti-inflammatory agents. In the former study[11] there was no apparent diagnostic use, but in the latter study[13] patients with biopsies lacking overt inflammation but expressing HLA antigen responded to steroid and azathioprine treatment. Expression of HLA class I and class II molecules occurs 3–4 times as frequently as overt myocarditis in biopsies from patients with idiopathic heart failure, and is uniformly present if overt myocarditis is seen. Other investigators have demonstrated that the detection of viral genome by polymerase chain reaction (PCR) correlates with poor survival in biopsy positive myocarditis.[14]

MYOCARDITIS: HISTOLOGIC FEATURES

Lymphocytic myocarditis

The term 'myocarditis' denotes lymphocytic myocarditis, characterized by lymphocytic infiltration and myocyte necrosis. Lymphocytic myocarditis is believed in most patients to be a sequela of enteroviral (often Coxsackievirus B) or adenoviral infection.

Table 20.2 Clinicopathologic diagnoses in 1230 patients with unexplained cardiomyopathy evaluated by endomyocardial biopsy and clinical studies

Diagnosis	Number of patients	%
Idiopathic dilated cardiomyopathy	616	50
Myocarditis*	111	9
Ischemic cardiomyopathy	91	7
Infiltrative diseases	59	5
Amyloid*	36	
Sarcoid*	14	
Hemochromatosis*	9	
Peripartum cardiomyopathy	51	4
Hypertension	49	4
Human immunodeficiency virus infection	45	4
Substance abuse	37	3
Doxorubicin related	15	1
Other causes†	117	10

* Conditions in which biopsy was helpful in establishing a specific diagnosis
† These included a number of conditions not resulting in dilated cardiomyopathy, such as restrictive cardiomyopathy and tumors, and cases that ultimately were non-myocardial
Adapted from Felker GM, Thompson RE, Hare JM et al. Underlying causes and long-term survival in patients with initially unexplained cardiomyopathy. N Engl J Med 2000; 342: 1077–1084.

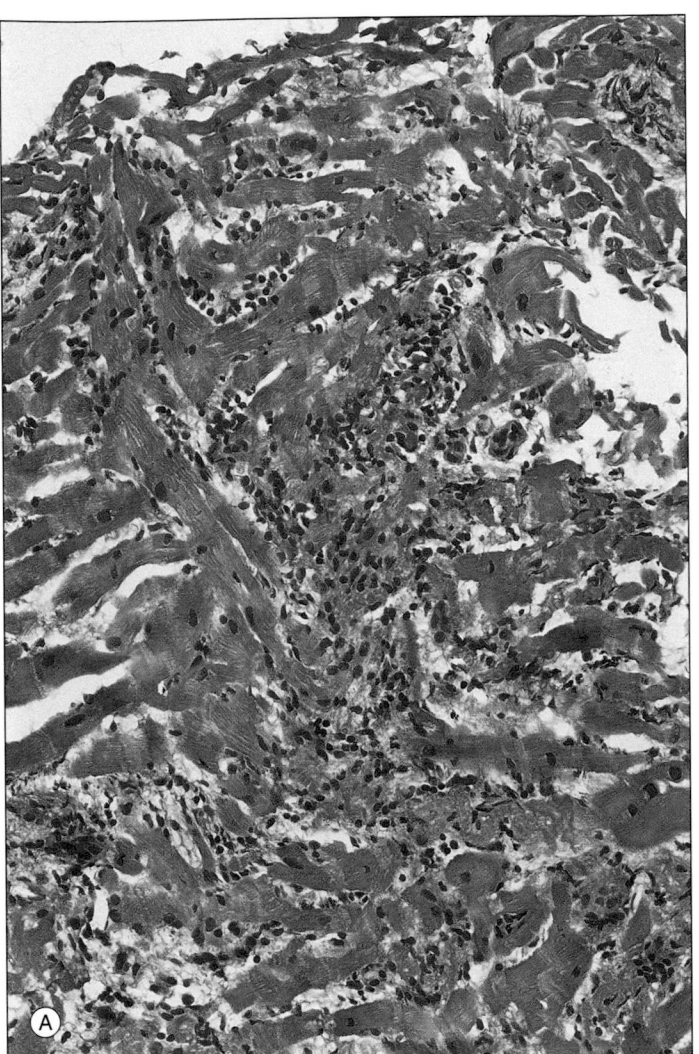
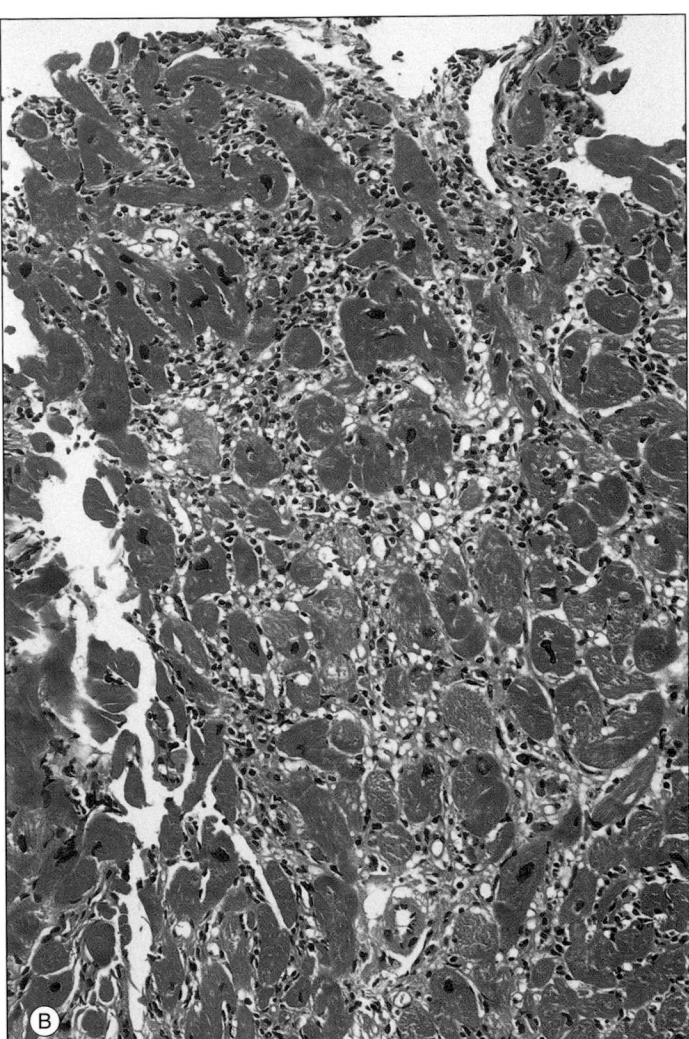

Figure 20.1 Lymphocytic myocarditis. **(A)** There is an extensive infiltrate composed predominantly of lymphocytes. **(B)** Ongoing lymphocytic myocarditis denotes the presence of replacement fibrosis with a lymphocytic infiltrate.

However, a similar histologic form of myocarditis may occasionally be seen in patients with systemic lupus erythematosus, polymyositis, Kawasaki disease, Lyme disease, the acquired immune deficiency syndrome, and as a drug-related response. Drugs that have been associated with a lymphocytic type of myocarditis include cocaine, anthracyclines, 5-fluorouracil and antiretroviral agents.

The identification of specific viruses in myocardial biopsies demonstrating lymphocytic myocarditis is problematic and difficult. Enteroviruses and possibly adenoviruses are transient invaders of the myocardium, and are presumably absent at the time of biopsy in many patients. Their small size makes them difficult to identify even by ultrastructure, RNA in situ hybridization techniques are not diagnostically helpful, and reverse transcriptase PCR (RT-PCR) for the identification of enteroviral RNA sequences currently lacks sensitivity and specificity. Recent reports of a high rate of virus positivity by PCR are to be viewed skeptically.[14]

The most common clinical presentation of lymphocytic myocarditis is heart failure, but arrhythmias and chest pain may be prominent manifestations of the disease. As mentioned above, the clinical distinction between fulminant and acute forms may have prognostic and therapeutic implications. A further clinical separation into acute, fulminant, chronic active, and chronic persistent, has not been universally accepted.[6]

In endomyocardial biopsies, lymphocytic myocarditis has been separated into two histologic forms: myocarditis and borderline myocarditis. In overt myocarditis, there are focal infiltrates of lymphocytes and macrophages with accompanying myocyte necrosis (Fig. 20.1). Necrosis is characterized by cytoplasmic degeneration with floccular changes. Necrotic myocytes are bluish-gray with Masson trichrome stains, facilitating their identification; trichrome stains are also helpful in identifying interstitial fibrosis. Serial sectioning of the block increases the yield of detection of myocarditic foci. If there is inflammation with no convincing necrosis, borderline myocarditis is diagnosed, with a suggestion for rebiopsy.[15] Healing myocarditis denotes the presence of inflammation and fibrosis without active necrosis.

Immunohistochemical studies of endomyocardial biopsies with myocarditis reveal T-lymphocytes with occasional macrophages and few B cells. B-lymphocytes, macrophages, activated T-lymphocytes, and endothelial cells of capillaries and arterioles express MHC class

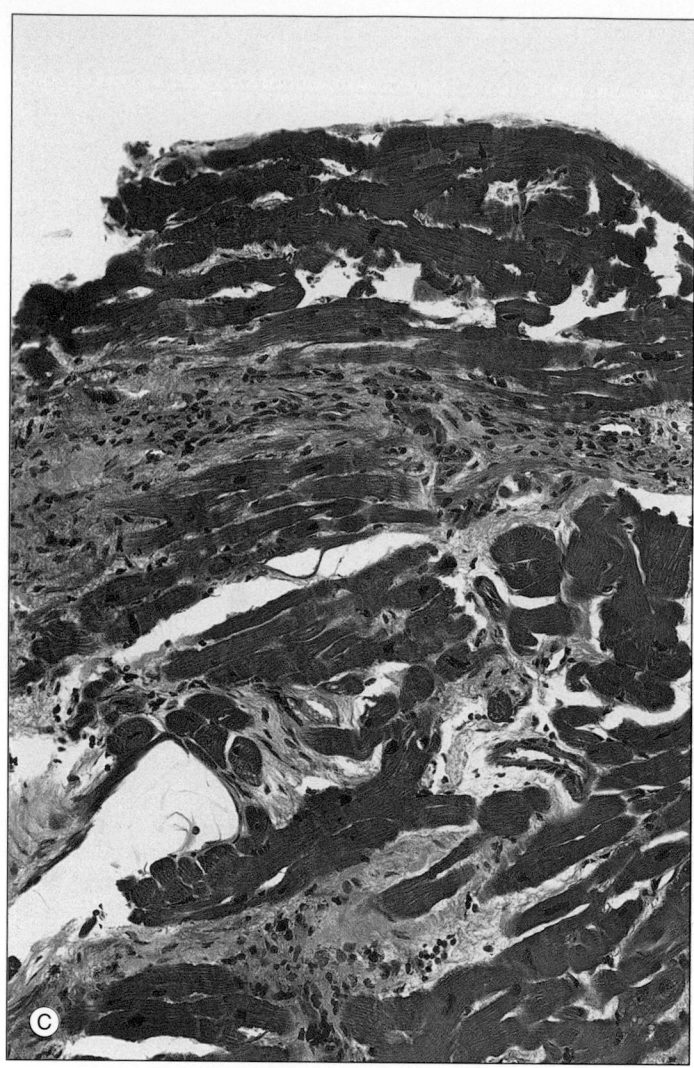

Figure 20.1 *(cont'd)* **(C)** In healing myocarditis, the predominant feature is fibrosis, with a sparse lymphohistiocytic infiltrate.

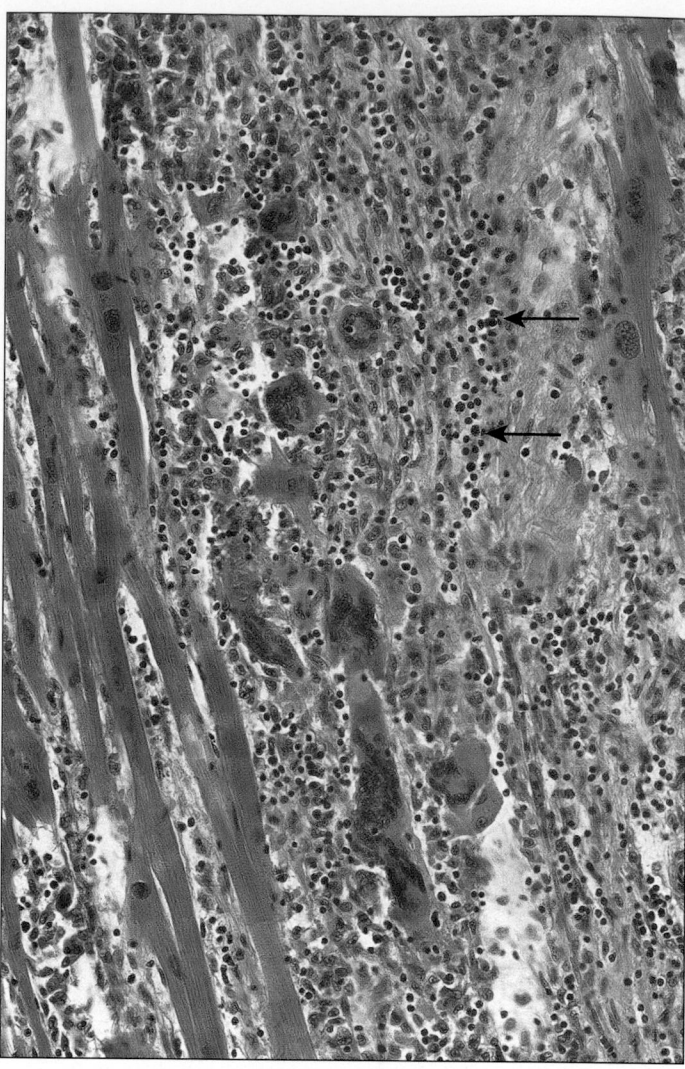

Figure 20.2 Giant cell myocarditis. There is extensive myocyte necrosis, fibrosis and giant cells with a sparse eosinophilic infiltrate (arrows).

II HLA DR molecules. HLA DR expression has been utilized as a diagnostic adjunct in the diagnosis of myocarditis in biopsies.[9]

Giant cell myocarditis

Giant cell myocarditis is an idiopathic inflammatory process resulting in myocyte necrosis associated with an inflammatory infiltrate composed of histiocytic giant cells, lymphocytes and scattered eosinophils. In biopsy series, giant cell myocarditis comprises less than 5% of cases of myocarditis. Clinically, most patients are young and middle-aged adults, and the disease is usually rapidly fatal and treated with intensive immunosuppression and transplantation.[16–18] Unlike sarcoidosis, giant cell myocarditis is localized to the heart, although there is a rare association with skeletal muscle inflammation, thymoma, systemic lupus erythematosus and thyrotoxicosis. Rare recurrences in allografts have been reported.[19]

Histologically, there is myocardial necrosis, a mixed infiltrate of lymphocytes, plasma cells, macrophages, eosinophils, and numerous multinucleated giant cells, most of which are histiocytic in origin (Fig. 20.2). In contrast to sarcoidosis, well-formed granulomas are absent, eosinophils are frequently seen, and there is abundant necrosis. Similar to sarcoidosis, there may be healing with fibrosis.

Hypersensitivity myocarditis

Allergic reactions may manifest as an eosinophilic myocarditis characterized by interstitial infiltrates of histiocytes, lymphocytes, and eosinophils. Patients are often elderly with known allergies, and are on multiple medications, making identification of the specific allergic agent difficult. More than 20 drugs have been implicated in hypersensitivity myocarditis; classically, methyldopa, sulfonamide, and penicillin have been cited as causes of hypersensitivity myocarditis. Symptoms include arrhythmias, sudden death, and rarely congestive heart failure. Because it is only rarely clinically suspected, hypersensitivity myocarditis is only rarely diagnosed by biopsy. In biopsy series, hypersensitivity myocarditis comprises less than 5% of myocarditis.[9]

In contrast to lymphocytic myocarditis, there is little ongoing necrosis and fibrosis in hypersensitivity myocarditis. In general, the degree of necrosis reflects the degree of inflammation; if there is abundant inflammation, the degree of necrosis may be moderate, although, in typical cases, necrosis is absent. The single most important diagnostic criterion is the distribution of the infiltrates, which, in hypersensitivity reactions, is exclusively within the interstitium, in perivascular regions, and in the subendocardium. The infiltrates are typically polymorphic and are composed of variable numbers of macrophages, eosinophils, lymphocytes, and Anitschkow cells. There may be collections of histiocytes suggesting poorly formed granulomas.

Other forms of myocarditis that may demonstrate variable numbers of eosinophils include hypereosinophilic syndrome, sarcoidosis, giant cell myocarditis, parasitic myocarditis, and idiopathic myocarditis.

Sarcoidosis

Cardiac involvement occurs in 20–30% of patients with sarcoidosis, as determined by autopsy. Less than 5% of patients with sarcoidosis have cardiac manifestations, which include heart block, congestive heart failure, ventricular arrhythmias, and sudden death; both restrictive and congestive cardiomyopathy may occur. The granulomas of sarcoid primarily affect the ventricular septum and left ventricular free wall, although any area may be involved.

Endomyocardial biopsy is positive in only a small proportion of patients with suspected sarcoid cardiomyopathy and is most probably positive (up to one-third) in patients with sarcoid-induced dilated cardiomyopathy.[20] In patients with known sarcoid and new-onset congestive heart failure, a negative biopsy does not exclude sarcoid as the cause of heart failure, although a positive biopsy essentially confirms sarcoid as the cause of dilated cardiomyopathy. The granulomas of sarcoid typically heal as large scars, and areas of lymphocytic infiltrates may occur adjacent to granulomas, simulating lymphocytic myocarditis. The differential diagnosis includes giant cell myocarditis, which demonstrates myocyte necrosis without well formed granulomas; mycobacterial infections, which are rare in the USA; and hypersensitivity myocarditis, which generally does not demonstrate distinct granulomas or scars.

Toxic myocarditis

Most toxic insults to the heart result in non-inflammatory cardiomyopathy. In the acute phase of damage from dose-related drug injury, there may be acute and chronic inflammation, interstitial edema and single cell necrosis. So-called toxic myocarditis, which demonstrates these histologic features, is classically seen in catecholamine toxicity, and there are anecdotal reports of toxic myocarditis associated with amphetamines, arsenic, lithium, emetine, paraquat, acetaminophen (paracetamol), solvents, anthracyclines, and 5-fluorouracil.

CARDIOMYOPATHY

Dilated cardiomyopathy

Clinically, dilated cardiomyopathy occurs when there is increased left ventricular end diastolic volume, decreased ejection fraction, and diffuse hypokinesis of the ventricles. End-stage hypertensive heart disease, coronary artery disease, and valvular heart disease are generally excluded by history, echocardiography and angiography before endomyocardial biopsy is performed to determine the etiology of dilated cardiomyopathy. Diseases that may clinically resemble dilated cardiomyopathy and that may be diagnosed by biopsy include myocarditis, storage diseases, amyloidosis, hemochromatosis, and toxic cardiomyopathy.

In cases of idiopathic dilated cardiomyopathy, a family history is elicited in up to 30% of cases.[21] The genetics of familial cardiomyopathy is complex; the few described mutations often involve sarcolemmal proteins.[22] In cases of X-linked cardiomyopathy associated with dystrophin disorders, skeletal muscle biopsy may be helpful in demonstrating absence of sarcolemmal dystrophin. Up to 5% of men with dilated cardiomyopathy may have latent skeletal muscular dystrophy[23] and dystrophin mutations. When dilated cardiomyopathy occurs during the last 3 months of pregnancy or within 6 months post-partum, the term peripartum cardiomyopathy is used, but the clinical and histologic features are identical to those of dilated cardiomyopathy in men. There is an association between dilated cardiomyopathy and long-term alcohol abuse, diabetes mellitus, chronic substance use, and HIV infection; the histologic features of dilated cardiomyopathy associated with these entities are not specific and biopsy does not help in establishing these diagnoses.

The histologic features of idiopathic dilated cardiomyopathy include myocyte hypertrophy, myocyte atrophy with myofibrillar loss, and interstitial fibrosis (Fig. 20.3). The degree of morphologic changes is quite variable and, in some documented cases of dilated cardiomyopathy, the endomyocardial biopsy is normal. The pathologic diagnosis by biopsy is one of exclusion: the absence of intracellular iron deposition, interstitial amyloid, and forms of myocarditis should be mentioned in the surgical pathologic description. About one-third of patients with idiopathic dilated cardiomyopathy and negative biopsies for myocarditis will demonstrate class I and II HLA activation of endothelial cells and/or myocytes by immunohistochemical studies of biopsy samples. Whether these patients have an inflammatory form of dilated cardiomyopathy – myocarditis with false-negative biopsy – and respond better to antiinflammatory treatment remains to be determined.[13]

Ultrastructural findings in cases of idiopathic dilated cardiomyopathy are non-specific and include increased mitochondria, sarcotubular dilatation, enlarged nuclei with irregular nuclear membranes, Z-band streaming, and cytoplasmic fat. Myofibrillar loss is more accurately identified by ultrastructure than by light microscopy and is characterized by large areas of cytoplasm devoid of contractile elements. Electron microscopy may be especially useful in excluding drug toxicity, storage disorders, and amyloid deposition. Morphometric analysis of ultrastructurally determined parameters (interstitial structured tissue, myofibril volume fraction, and myocytic fiber diameters) has not been shown to be correlated with prognosis in idiopathic dilated cardiomyopathy, even in left ventricular biopsies.[24]

Hemochromatosis

Hemochromatosis is a congenital disorder of iron metabolism that causes a dilated, or less commonly restrictive cardiomyopathy. Secondary forms of hemosiderosis may occur from excessive blood transfusion, thalassemia major, hemolytic anemia or increased iron intake. Histologically, there are iron deposits in the perinuclear region of the myocyte. The diagnosis is straightforward, because the normal myocyte does not contain iron. Care must be taken in the distinction between lipofuscin, the wear and tear pigment, and iron, as both are typically perinuclear in location. A Prussian blue stain for iron should also be performed if the diagnosis of hemochromatosis is considered. The cardiomyopathy of hemochromatosis may be missed by biopsy in early stages of disease, because iron deposition tends to begin in the epicardium and later progress to the endocardium. In cases of iron overload due to thalassemia, endomyocardial biopsy has been shown to correlate with serum ferritin and may help guide therapy.[25]

Restrictive cardiomyopathy

Restrictive cardiomyopathy results from any of a number of processes that are hemodynamically characterized by decreased ventricular compliance, decreased cardiac output, and normal systolic function. Pathologically, the term 'restrictive cardiomyopathy' is sometimes

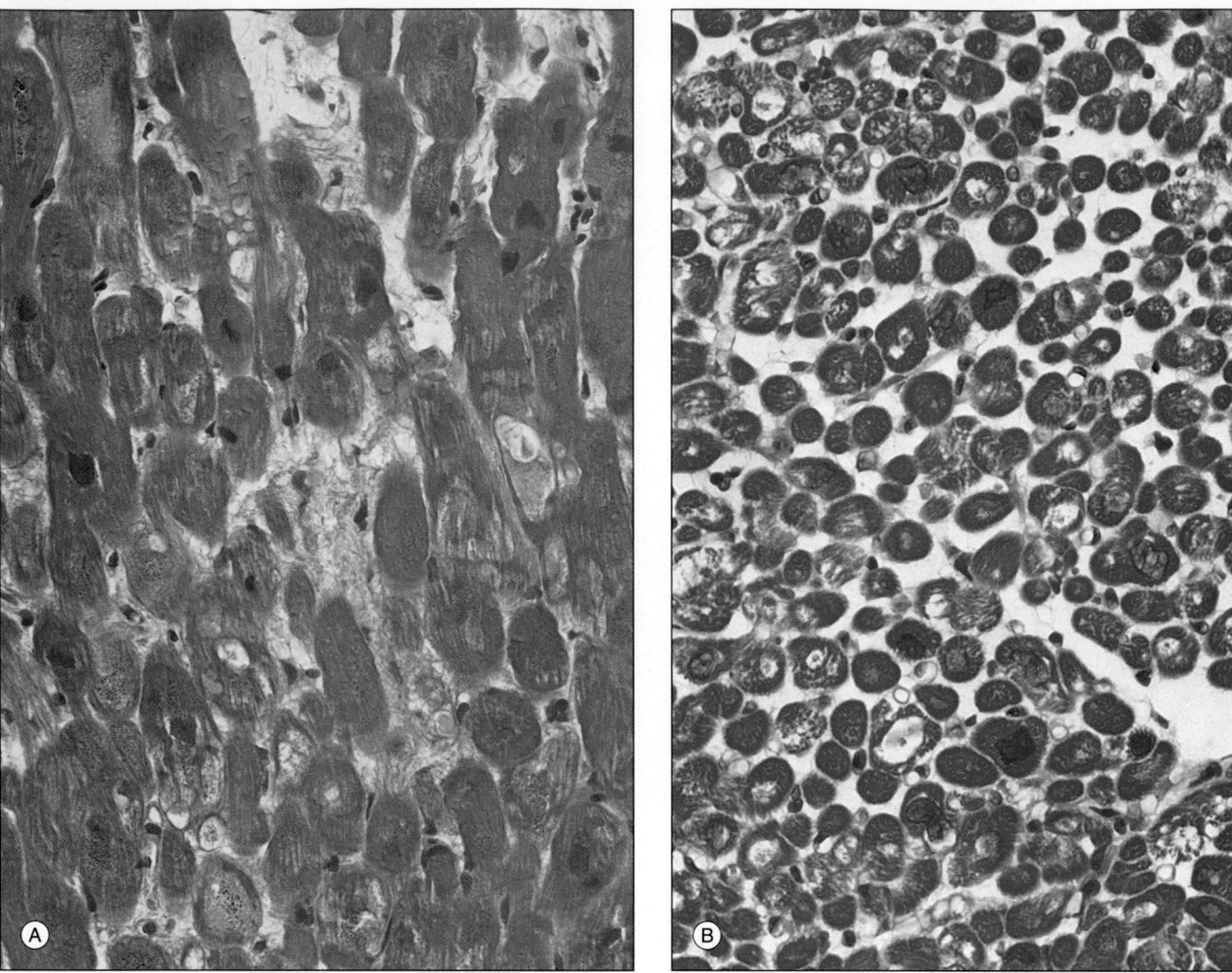

Figure 20.3 Dilated cardiomyopathy. **(A)** A longitudinal section demonstrates myocyte hypertrophy, areas of cytoplasmic clearing indicative of myofibrillar loss; interstitial fibrosis may be prominent or absent. **(B)** A cross-section highlights varying diameters of myofibers with vacuolar change and myofibrillar loss. The histologic features of dilated cardiomyopathy are non-specific; the diagnosis is essentially one of exclusion.

reserved for idiopathic restrictive cardiomyopathy. Infiltrative processes that result in restrictive hemodynamic parameters may be difficult to distinguish clinically from chronic pericardial disease, but magnetic resonance imaging and computed tomography scans of mediastinum are quite sensitive in diagnosing constrictive pericarditis. Most restrictive cardiomyopathy is secondary, caused by amyloidosis, endocardial fibrosis, and hypereosinophilic syndrome. Less commonly, hemochromatosis, sarcoidosis, storage diseases, hypertrophic cardiomyopathy, carcinoid heart disease, radiation induced myocardial fibrosis, and methylsergide-induced endocardial fibrosis may result in restrictive cardiomyopathy.

Idiopathic restrictive cardiomyopathy demonstrates non-specific histologic features and is the most common form in children. Histologic features are non-specific, and include myocyte hypertrophy and interstitial fibrosis.[26] Some cases of familial idiopathic restrictive cardiomyopathy are associated with heart block, and demonstrate characteristic desmin inclusion on endomyocardial biopsy.[27] Electron microscopic evaluation is necessary to establish the diagnosis of desmin cardiomyopathy. There is some evidence that a subset of

patients with idiopathic restrictive cardiomyopathy may actually suffer from hypertrophic cardiomyopathy with restrictive hemodynamic patterns.[28] Secondary causes of restrictive cardiomyopathy that can be diagnosed by biopsy include hypereosinophilic syndrome and idiopathic endocardial fibrosis (Davies disease). The latter is seen almost exclusive in developing regions, such as India and Africa, and is histologically characterized by a thick collagen layer under the endocardium, with relative sparing of the myocardium. In cases of isolated left ventricular involvement, right ventricular biopsy may be negative in cases of endocardial fibrosis. In the differential diagnosis of endocardial fibrosis is radiation-induced heart disease, methysergide cardiomyopathy, and carcinoid heart disease, although these conditions prominently involve the valve surfaces.

Hypereosinophilic syndrome is a systemic illness characterized by persistent peripheral eosinophilia ($>1500/mm^2$) and multiorgan infiltration by eosinophils. There is a male predominance, with a peak incidence in the fourth decade of life. Some 75% of patients have cardiac involvement (Löffler's endocarditis) characterized by congestive heart failure and arrhythmias. Mural thrombi, which

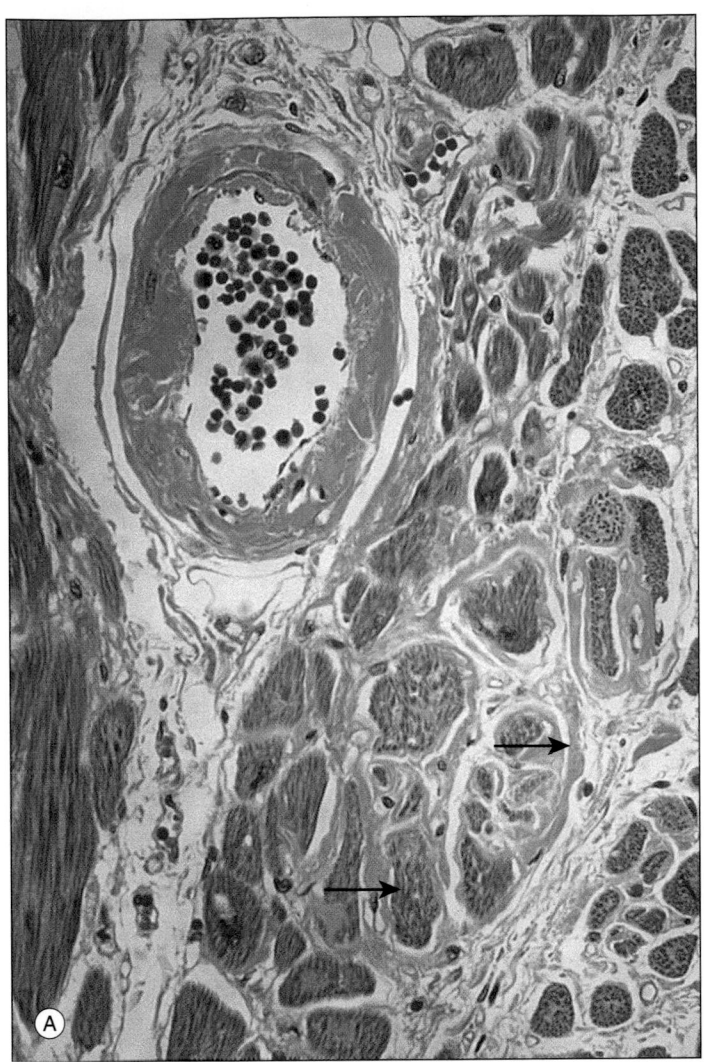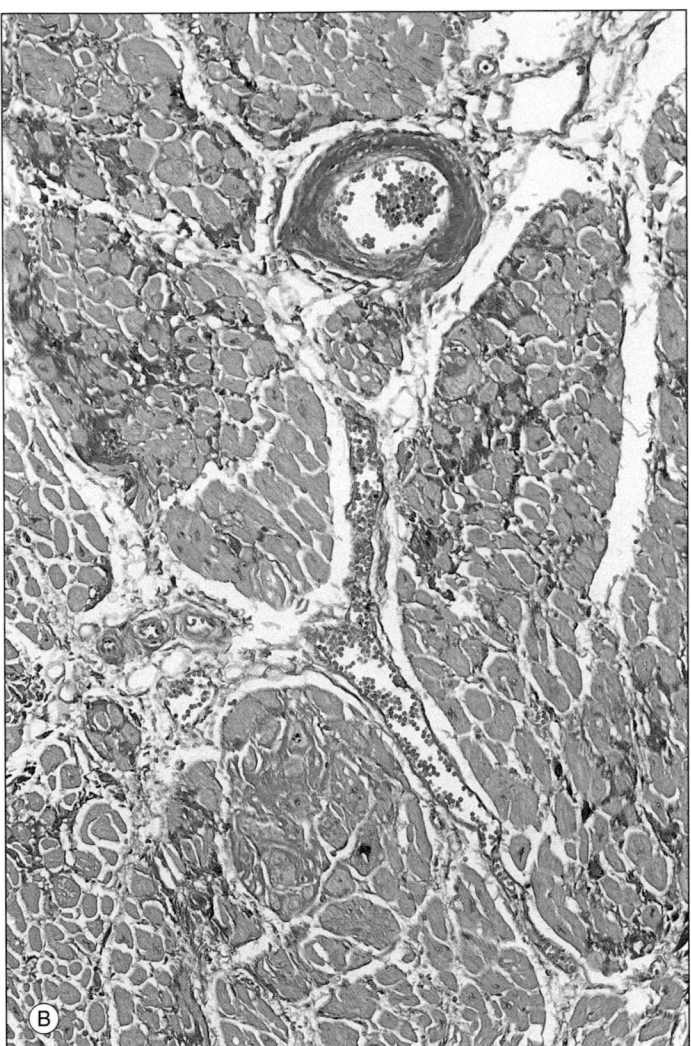

Figure 20.4 Cardiac amyloidosis. **(A)** There is diffuse amyloid in the media of the small artery, as well as focal interstitial amyloid surrounding myocytes (arrows). **(B)** A sulfated Alcian blue stain highlights vascular and nodular amyloid (blue-green).

occur in early stages of disease, may encroach upon the base of the mitral valve, resulting in mitral insufficiency.

Histologically, there are endocardial and myocardial infiltrates of eosinophils, initially present in organizing mural thrombi or within thrombi in intramural coronary vessels. Typically, there are eosinophilic microabscesses with granulomas forming around extracellular deposits of eosinophil granules (Charcot–Leyden crystals). In contrast to hypersensitivity myocarditis, endomyocardial fibrosis, eosinophilic microabscesses, and granulomas are characteristic of hypereosinophilic syndrome.

Amyloidosis

Cardiac involvement by amyloidosis accounts for up to 10% of all noncoronary cardiomyopathies. One-third to one-half of patients with amyloidosis of the AL (immunoglobulin light chains) type will develop cardiac symptoms, in contrast to less than 10% of patients with secondary amyloidosis (non-immunoglobulin amyloid AA).[29] The most common cause of cardiac amyloidosis in the elderly is senile amyloidosis, which is formed by the deposition of transthyretin (prealbumin). Although most patients with senile amyloidosis are

older that 70 years of age, rare familial forms of cardiac amyloidosis occur in patients as young as 35 years and are characterized by amyloid AS deposits in the heart and visceral arteries.

The clinical cardiac manifestations and the histologic features of the three biochemical types of amyloidosis are similar. Although classically considered to cause a restrictive type of cardiomyopathy, some patients present with congestive heart failure and dilated cardiomyopathy. The mean survival of patients with primary amyloidosis (AL) is less than 6 months, compared to a mean survival of over 2 years with senile amyloidosis.[29] Histologically, there are four patterns of amyloid deposition in the heart: interstitial, nodular, subendocardial, and vascular; there is often an overlap of patterns (Fig. 20.4).

The diagnosis of amyloid is confirmed by Congo red staining with apple green birefringence with polarized light on 7–10-μm thick sections. Other special stains that may be used include methyl violet, thioflavin T (viewed with ultraviolet fluorescence) and the sulfated Alcian blue stain. It is important for patient management to type the amyloid present within the heart. In most cases of primary amyloidosis, light chains are detected in the serum or urine. However, 10–15% of patients are non-secretors, and typing can be performed by

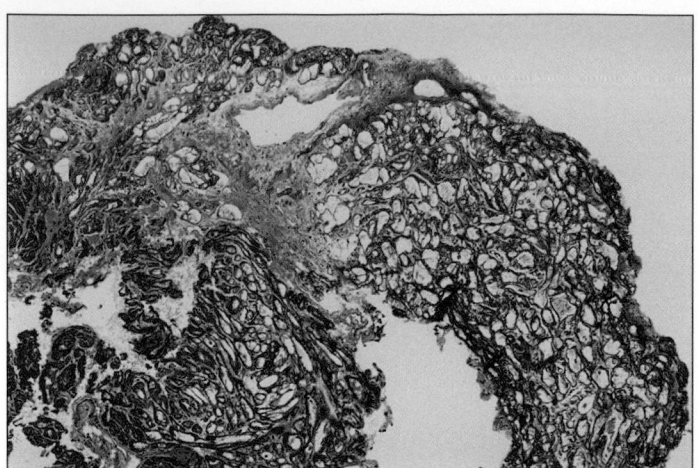

Figure 20.5 Glycogen storage disease. Diffuse vacuolization of myocytes suggests a storage disorder. Glycogen storage disease, especially Pompe's disease, often causes cardiac symptoms in children, and Fabry's disease, or angiokeratoma corporis diffusum universale, seen only in adults, may cause cardiac symptoms. This biopsy was taken from a 10-year-old girl with a glycogen storage disease.

immunohistochemical methods. AL and AS may be distinguished by immunohistochemical stains for kappa and lambda free light chains (the antibodies used differ from those detecting cytoplasmic kappa and lambda light chain restriction in lymphoid cells) and transthyretin.[29]

Occasionally, cardiomyopathy that mimics amyloidosis (restrictive parameters, conduction disturbances) may result from light chain deposition without amyloid formation (light chain deposition disease). The histologic findings including perivascular thickening, which on ultrastructural examination shows characteristic flocculent perivascular deposits.[30] Immunohistochemical stains on frozen of paraffin-embedded specimens confirm the type of light chain (kappa, lambda).

Fabry's disease

Also known as angiokeratoma corporis diffusum universale, Fabry's disease is an X-linked disorder that manifests as symptomatic cardiovascular disease by middle age. Cardiac symptoms may mimic amyloidosis, mitral valve prolapse, hypertrophic cardiomyopathy, or restrictive cardiomyopathy. Endomyocardial biopsy will demonstrate a vacuolar myopathy.[31] Hypertrophied myocytes demonstrate large periodic acid–Schiff and Sudan black positive perinuclear vacuoles, shown at electron microscopy to consist of lamellated cytoplasmic figures. The disease is confirmed by diagnostic low activity of alpha-galactosidase A in the peripheral lymphocytes.

The differential diagnosis of vacuolar cardiomyopathy includes glycogen storage disease (Fig. 20.5) and drug-induced cardiomyopathy. The most common glycogen storage disease involving the myocardium is Pompe's disease, which is easily distinguished from Fabry's disease because patients are infants or children, and there is abundant glycogen by histochemical stains and ultrastructural analysis. Chloroquine may result in a vacuolar cardiomyopathy which ultrastructurally may mimic Fabry's disease.

Histiocytoid cardiomyopathy

Also known as oncocytic cardiomyopathy and Purkinje cell hamartoma, histiocytoid cardiomyopathy is a congenital hamartoma of multiple microscopic clusters of modified myocytes with an appearance similar to histiocytes.[32] Patients present in infancy and

early childhood, with a mean age of 12 months; there is a 4:1 female predominance. Symptoms include tachyarrhythmias, sudden death, and congestive heart failure. All portions of the heart may be involved, including valves, conduction system, subendocardium, and subepicardium. Microscopically, cells are large, pale, vacuolated, rounded or oval, and are faintly PAS-positive. They are clearly of cardiac myocyte origin, and express muscle antigens, possess numerous mitochondria, and few contractile elements.

Hypertrophic cardiomyopathy

Hypertrophic cardiomyopathy is characterized by cardiomegaly, a small left ventricular cavity, and asymmetric septal hypertrophy manifest histologically by myofiber hypertrophy and disarray. Approximately 50% of patients will suffer from subaortic stenosis (idiopathic hypertrophic subaortic stenosis). The diagnosis is generally made by echocardiography. Endomyocardial biopsy is useful in excluding rare causes of septal asymmetry, such as Fabry's disease, amyloidosis, and cardiac tumors; histologic features of hypertrophic cardiomyopathy are usually out of reach of the bioptome.

Hypertrophic cardiomyopathy may be treated surgically by myectomy and by percutaneous intra-arterial injection of 100% ethanol if there is significant subaortic stenosis. The surgical specimen will demonstrate marked endocardial fibrosis, and myofiber disarray in the underlying myocardium is generally identified histologically. The finding of thickened intramural coronary arteries corroborates the diagnosis. The role of pathologist in evaluating these myectomy samples is to exclude uncommon causes of subaortic obstruction, including Fabry's disease and amyloid.

DRUG-INDUCED CARDIOMYOPATHY

Anthracycline toxicity

The incidence of doxorubicin (Adriamycin®) cardiotoxicity is 1.7%, compared to 4.4% for daunorubicin (Cerubidine®). The upper limit of toxic dose is 550 mg/m² for doxorubicin; some patients develop toxicity at lower doses, especially if there is a history of heart disease, radiation therapy, advanced age, or systemic hypertension.[33] Endomyocardial biopsy is the gold standard for assessing cardiac damage, but nuclear scans with indium-111-antimyosin scintigraphy represent an alternative non-invasive method.[34]

In biopsies performed for the evaluation of doxorubicin toxicity, the entire specimen should be submitted for ultrastructural examination, and ten plastic embedded blocks should be reviewed. The toxic myocardial damage is dose-dependent and progressive, and pathologic changes in the myocardium may persist for months or years after initial damage. Continued drug may be given if the biopsy shows grade 2 damage or less. There are two hallmarks of anthracycline toxicity (Fig. 20.6). Sarcotubular dilatation is reflected by cytoplasmic vacuolization on thick toluidine-blue-stained sections, and myofibrillar loss is characterized by pale, granular cytoplasm. On thin sections, dilated T-tubules appear as membrane-bound vacuoles, and myofibrillar loss as large areas within the myocyte that are almost devoid of contractile elements.

In grade 1 damage, there are isolated myocytes affected by distended sarcotubular system or early myofibrillar loss, with damage to fewer than 5% of all cells. Grade 1.5 denotes changes similar to those in grade 1 but with damage to 6–15% of all cells. In grade 2 damage, there are clusters of myocytes affected by myofibrillar loss or vacuolization, with damage to 16–25% of all cells in ten plastic embedded blocks of tissue. Grade 2.5 indicates that 26–35% of all cells are affected by vacuolization or myofibrillar loss. At this

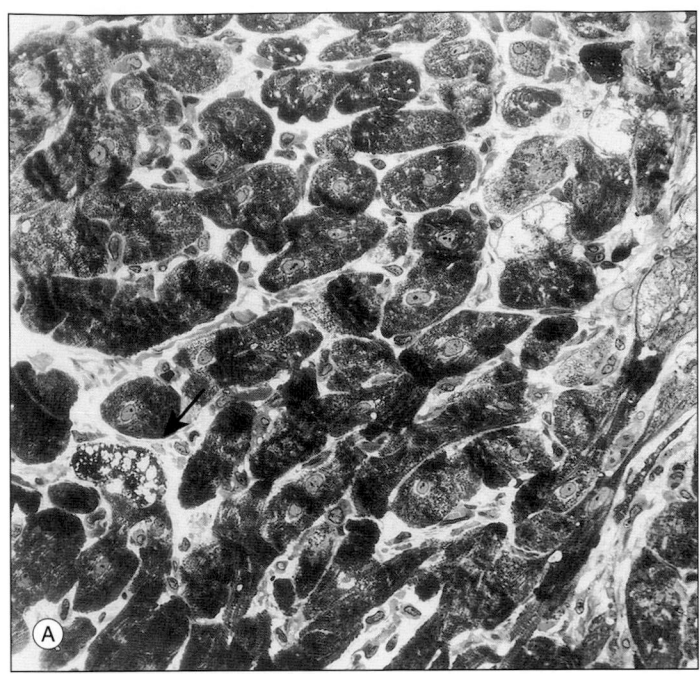

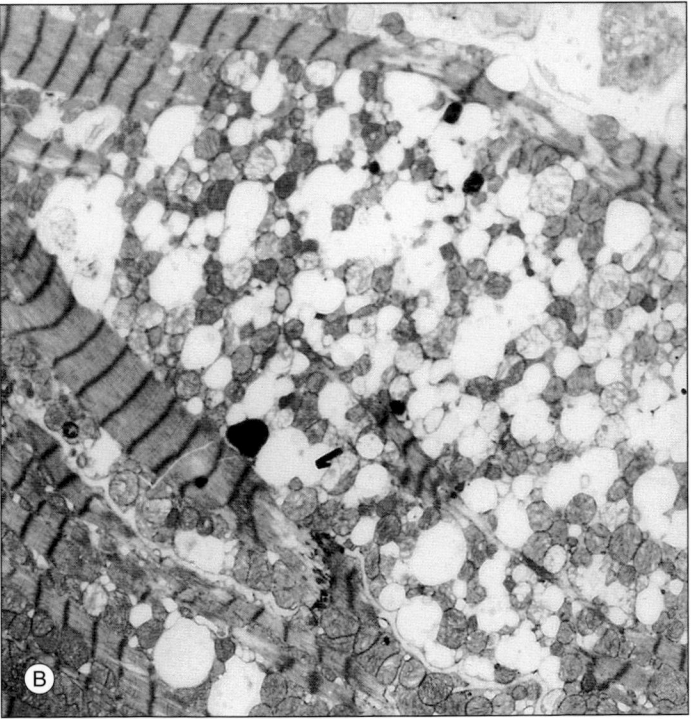

Figure 20.6 Anthracycline toxicity. **(A)** A toluidine-blue-stained section demonstrated scattered vacuolated cells indicating grade 2 toxicity (arrow). **(B)** Ultrastructural examination demonstrates membrane-bound vacuoles characteristic of dilated sarcolemma.

stage, only one more dose of anthracycline should be given without further evaluation.[1] Maximum anthracycline toxicity (grade 3) is characterized by severe and diffuse myocyte damage affecting more than 35% of all cells; no more anthracyclines are to be given.[34]

Other forms of drug-induced cardiomyopathy

Long-term administration of chloroquine and hydroxychloroquine may produce cardiotoxicity with a dilated or restrictive cardio-myopathy. The diagnosis of hydroxychloroquine or chloroquine cardiotoxicity may be made by ultrastructural examination of endomyocardial biopsies, which reveal curvilinear bodies, myelin figures, and large secondary lysosomes, similar to findings in skeletal muscle. Curvilinear bodies are closely associated with lysosomes, are membrane-bound, and consist of numerous regular, curved profiles, suggesting the presence of partially digested lipids in secondary lysosomes. Myelin figures are lamellated electron-dense bodies that demonstrate alternating light and dark bands, similar to those seen in Fabry's disease and paclitaxel-induced cardiomyopathy.[35]

ACUTE TRANSPLANT REJECTION

General features of acute rejection

The clinical signs and symptoms of rejection do not reliably correlate with the presence or severity of rejection, particularly in cyclosporine-treated patients.[36] Endomyocardial biopsy is the gold standard for diagnosis of acute rejection; at least four pieces of myocardium from a standard bioptome are required, and at least 50% of the samples should consist of myocardium and not previous biopsy site or scar tissue.

The histopathologic features of acute cardiac rejection consist of inflammation with or without myocyte necrosis. The severity of rejection is classified according to the extent, pattern, and type of inflammation, and the presence or absence of myocyte necrosis. Large, 'activated' lymphocytes (predominantly T cells) comprise the inflammatory cell infiltrate.

Grading of acute rejection

In an effort to standardize the grading of acute rejection, a working formulation was devised by pathologists at a study group sponsored by the International Society for Heart and Lung Transplantation in 1990.[37] The diagnostic feature of each grade of rejection is outlined in Table 20.3 and illustrated in Figure 20.7A–I. The infiltrate is predominantly a mixture of CD4 and CD8 lymphocytes. Because the proportion of CD4 to CD8 cells is not useful in management, routine lymphocytic subtyping is not warranted in diagnostic evaluation.

Difficulties in grading of acute rejection involve determination of myocyte necrosis, which may be difficult to identify in milder forms of rejection, and the precise definition of grade 2 rejection, which requires the presence of necrosis or myocyte damage.[38] Progression of grade 2 rejection is unusual, especially in biopsies obtained more than 2 years after transplant.

Additional diagnostic categories may be required for biopsies that are obtained after episodes of acute rejection. 'Ongoing' rejection implies no improvement from the previous biopsy, while 'resolved' rejection indicates complete resolution. 'Resolving' acute rejection implies that the degree of inflammation is less than that seen in the previous biopsy. As rejection episodes 'resolve,' the lymphocytes evolve from large, immunoblastic-like cells to small lymphocytes. In some instances, methyl green pyronin stains may be useful to determine the relative number of 'activated' cells versus small lymphocytes, although this differentiation can usually be made with H&E-stained sections.

The therapeutic implications of rejection grades vary from institution to institution. In general, low grades of rejection do not warrant a change in immunosuppression, although repeat biopsy may be earlier than scheduled. Moderate rejection (with the possible exception of grade 2) is often treated with increased steroids, and severe rejection with monoclonal antibodies, such as OKT3.[39]

Table 20.3 International Society for Heart and Lung Transplantation grading for acute cardiac rejection

Grade 0	**No rejection**
	Normal myocardium with no evidence of inflammation or myocyte damage
Grade 1	**Mild rejection**
1A	*Focal* (interstitial or perivascular) lymphocytic infiltrate involving one or more pieces and no myocyte damage
1B	*Diffuse*, sparse lymphocytic infiltrate involving one or more pieces with no myocyte damage.
Grade 2	**Focal moderate rejection**
	One focus with an aggressive, sharply circumscribed infiltrate, usually associated with myocyte damage or architectural distortion of the myocardium. The infiltrate is comprised of lymphocytes and immunoblasts, with occasional eosinophils.
Grade 3	**Moderate rejection**
3A	Multifocal lymphocytic inflammatory infiltrates with myocyte damage; eosinophils may be present, and there are areas of normal myocardium between foci of inflammation. These changes can be seen in one or more pieces of myocardium. The distinction of grade 3A from grade 1A (where one or more pieces are involved by inflammation) is made by finding multifocal infiltrates within single pieces in grade 3A rejection, as well as the presence of myocyte damage.
3B	In addition to changes seen in 3A, there may be eosinophils and rare neutrophils. There are fewer areas of normal myocardium separating areas of inflammation than in grade 3A.
Grade 4	**Severe rejection**
	Diffuse, aggressive inflammation consisting of lymphocytes, eosinophils and neutrophils; myocyte necrosis is always present; edema, hemorrhage, and vasculitis are also seen.
Nonrejection biopsy findings:	
Quilty effect A or B	
Ischemic injury	
Early (≤3 mo)	
Late (>3 mo)	
Infection	
Post-transplant lymphoproliferative disorder.	

Effect of treatment on transplant rejection

Immunosuppressive therapy other than standard cyclosporine and corticosteroids may influence interpretation of endomyocardial biopsies performed for the evaluation of acute transplant rejection. Monoclonal antibody OKT3 effect is characterized by reduced cellularity of the infiltrates, edema, increased vascular rejection, and increased incidence of Quilty effect. Flow cytometric evaluation of sera from such patients demonstrates anti-OKT3 antibody that blocks adherence of LKT3 to CD3 cells.

Photopheresis, or administration of autologous lymphocytes treated with 8-methoxypsoralen activated by extracorporeally-administered ultraviolet-A irradiation, may result in extensive, persistent inflammatory infiltrates in the face of clinical resolution of acute rejection.

Acute vascular rejection

While the vast majority of rejection episodes in cardiac allografts are 'cellular,' Hammond and her colleagues at Utah have demonstrated a 'vascular' or 'humoral' form of rejection in some patients.[39] Vascular rejection should be considered if the allograft is not functioning optimally, particularly in the immediate postoperative period (first 6 weeks after transplantation), the classic signs of cellular rejection are absent in the endomyocardial biopsy, and other causes of graft dysfunction (postoperative ischemia, infection) have been excluded.

The diagnosis of vascular rejection is suggested when endothelial cells are prominent; inflammation is sparse and interstitial, or absent; and there is neutrophil margination. Confirmation of the diagnosis is made when capillary deposits of IgM and C3 and prominent HLA-DR expression are demonstrated by immunofluorescence on fresh-frozen, unfixed biopsies. In renal biopsies, immunohistochemical localization of complement component CD4d is strongly associated with humoral rejection[40]; whether this marker will aid in the diagnosis of cardiac humoral rejection remains unclear.[41]

The significance of the diagnosis of vascular rejection involves treatment, which may differ from that for cellular rejection. Plasmapheresis and alternative forms of immunosuppression has shown beneficial results.

Previous biopsy site

One of the most common pitfalls in diagnosing acute cardiac rejection is misinterpretation of previous biopsy sites (Fig. 20.8), which are histologically characterized by the presence of fibrin, necrosis and granulation tissue at or near the endocardial surface. Healed biopsy sites demonstrate fibrosis with underlying myocyte disarray.

Ischemic injury

Ischemic changes are classified as early (≤3 months) and late (>3 months).[37] Early changes are generally related to operative ischemia, whereas later ischemic lesions are associated with allograft coronary disease. The major findings in acute ischemia are focal myocyte necrosis, with a sparse, predominantly neutrophilic, inflammatory infiltrate. In contrast to acute rejection, myocyte damage precedes an acute inflammatory response and the extent of myocyte damage exceeds the degree of inflammation seen in acute rejection. Late changes are manifest by subendomyocardial myocyte vacuolization, and subendocardial microinfarcts. Both of these lesions are specific for allograft coronary disease, but lack sensitivity.[42]

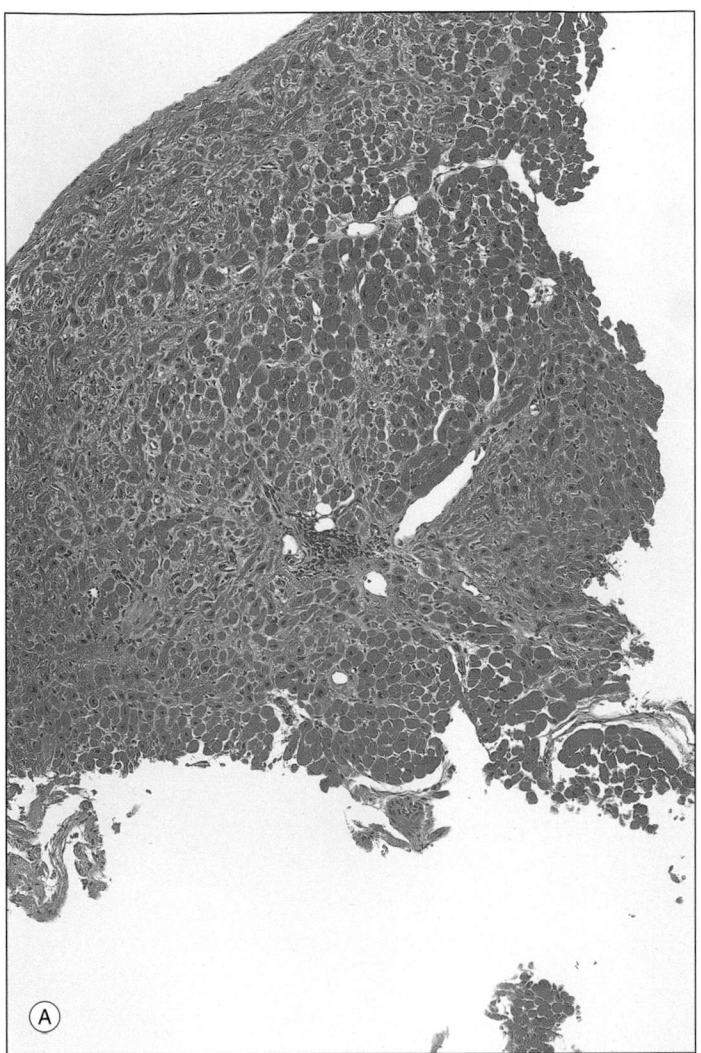
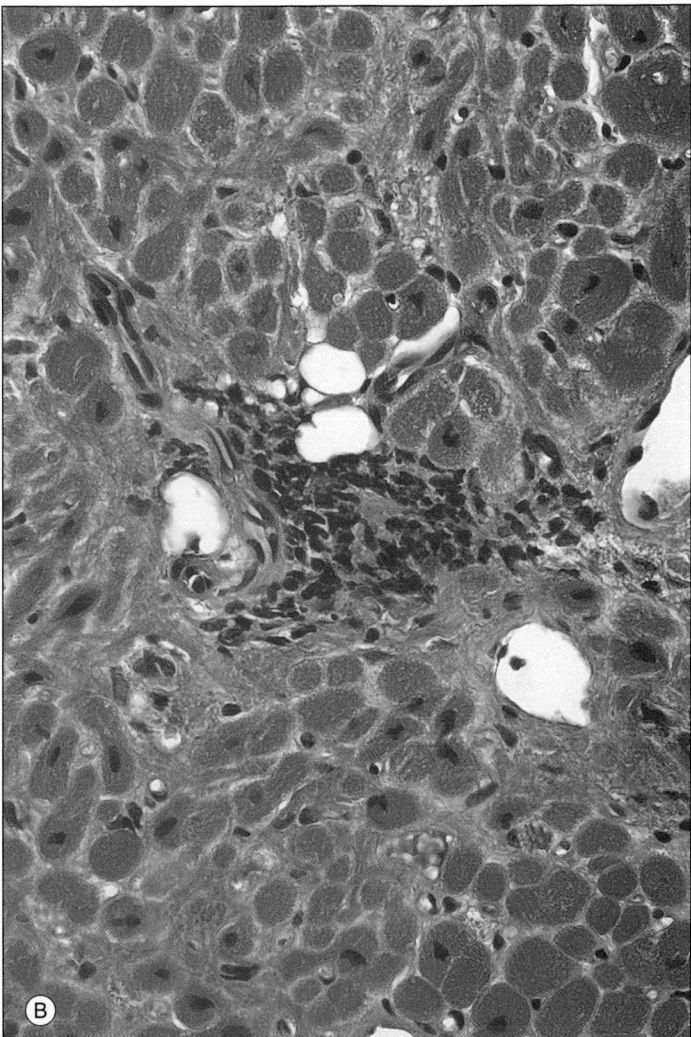

Figure 20.7 Acute transplant rejection. **(A)** A single focus of interstitial lymphoid aggregates without myocyte damage in one or more pieces indicates a grade 1A rejection. **(B)** A higher magnification of Figure 20.7A demonstrating grade 1A focus of rejection. In contrast to grade 2 rejection (not shown), which is also characterized by a single focus, it is a small focus and there is no destruction of surrounding myocytes.

Quilty effect

In 10–20% of patients receiving cyclosporine, the biopsy may have a dense endocardial collection of lymphocytes ('Quilty' effect, named after the first patient at Stanford noted to have these changes) (Fig. 20.9). Histologically, Quilty lesions are flat or nodular, densely cellular endocardial nodules consisting predominantly of T lymphocytes, with scattered clusters of B cells, macrophages, plasma cells, and small blood vessels. Two subtypes have been defined: Quilty A, with the infiltrate confined to the endocardium; and, Quilty B, when the infiltrate encroaches into the myocardium. When the inflammatory infiltrate extends into the subendocardium, the distinction from acute rejection or transplant-associated lymphoproliferative disorder may be difficult.

Possible mechanisms of the Quilty effect include a drug-specific effect, and drug-specific alteration in the immune response to the allograft, or a secondary response to cyclosporine-induced endothelial cell injury. The association between Quilty effect and acute and chronic rejection is controversial, but there is yet no convincing data to suggest a cause and effect relationship between endocardial infiltrates and either form of rejection.

Opportunistic infections

Infections may occur in the cardiac allograft and can be recognized in endomyocardial biopsy samples, especially when the inflammatory infiltrate in a cardiac biopsy is mixed and not characteristic of acute rejection.

Toxoplasma infections in immunocompromised patients can produce myocarditis as well as necrotizing encephalitis and pneumonia. The endomyocardial biopsy will show a mixed inflammatory infiltrate and tachyzoites or bradyzoites encysted in myocytes.

Although infection with cytomegalovirus is an important problem in cardiac transplant recipients, it is rare that typical inclusions are found in the myocardium, and serologic diagnosis may be unreliable. The diagnosis of cytomegalovirus infection is often made by demonstrating inclusions in biopsies of other organs. In small biopsy samples, cytopathic changes suggestive of cytomegalovirus can be confirmed by immunoperoxidase techniques or by in situ hybridization. The role of PCR in detecting DNA sequences specific for cytomegalovirus remains to be established.

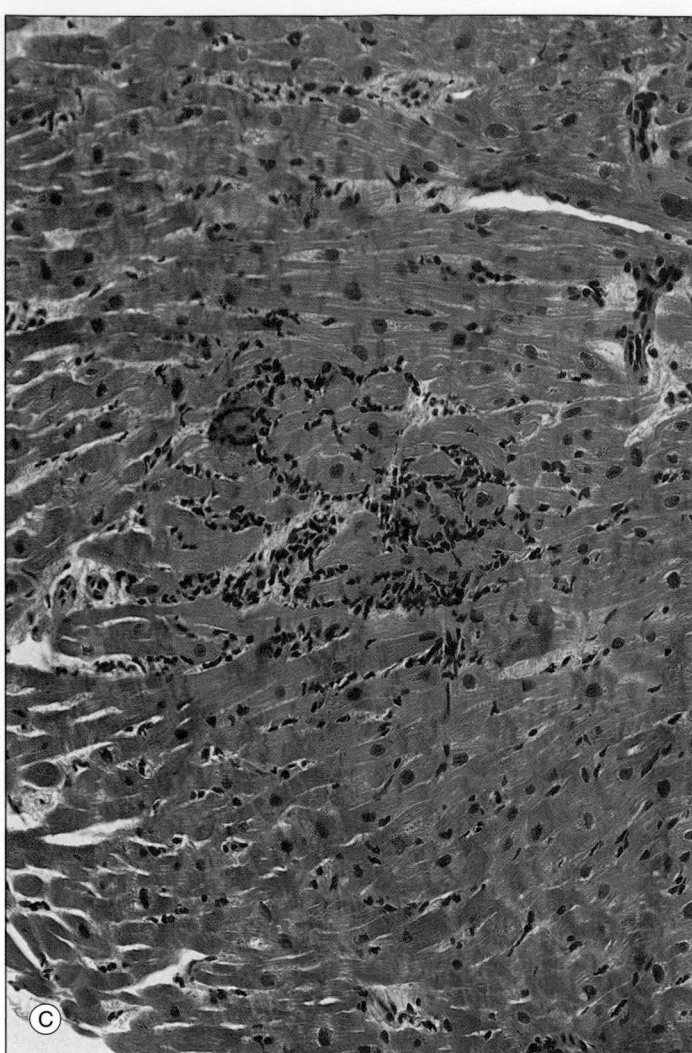

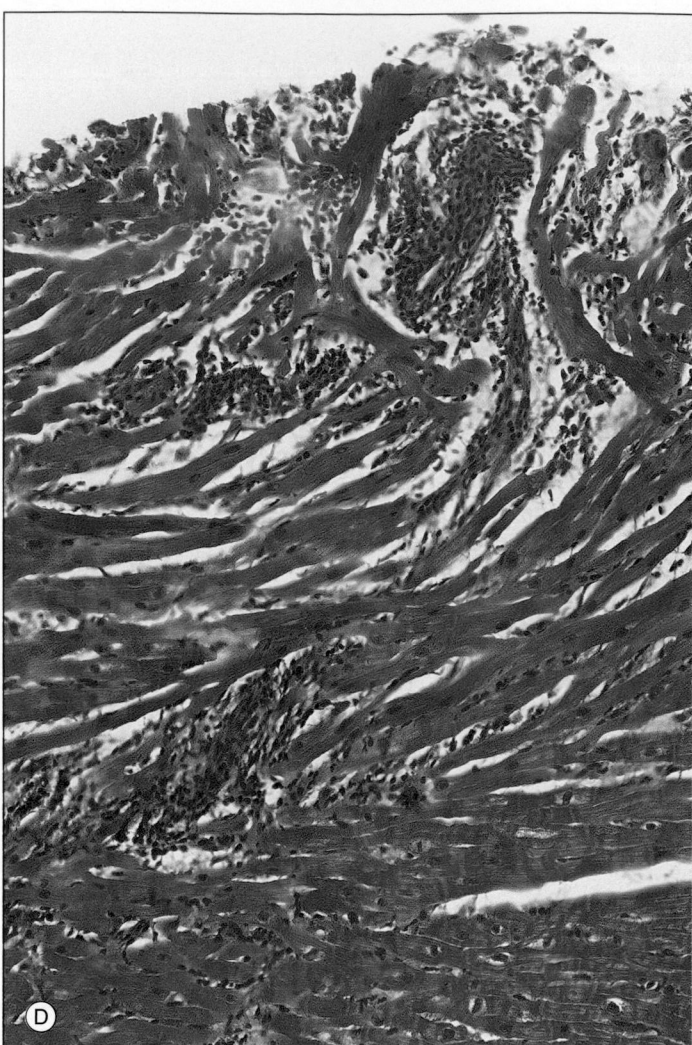

Figure 20.7 *(cont'd)* **(C)** Grade 1B rejection is characterized by scattered sparse interstitial infiltrates, no myocyte necrosis, and large areas of normal cardiac muscle. **(D)** Grade 3A rejection demonstrates multifocal infiltrates with myocyte damage and intervening normal areas; in contrast to grade 1A, there are several infiltrates in a single piece of myocardium.

EXAMINATION OF CARDIAC VALVES

GENERAL APPROACH TO CARDIAC VALVES

Clinical history

For optimal evaluation of all surgically excised cardiac valves, the pathologist should know the patient's age, sex, if there is a history of rheumatic fever or endocarditis, and the degree of insufficiency and/or stenosis. For atrioventricular valves, a history of ischemic heart disease, mitral prolapse, and chordal rupture are important. For semilunar valves, the pathologist should know if there is aortic root dilatation.

Gross examination

The gross examination is the most important aspect of the pathologic examination of valves. The intact valve structure should be recreated, if possible, in its probable functional condition, in order to estimate the annular circumference. If only a portion of the valve has been submitted, this should be noted. Heavily calcified aortic valves are often submitted in pieces, making a definitive morphologic diagnosis impossible.

A surgical pathologic report should specify the number of excised pieces; approximate annular circumference, if possible, by apposing leaflets; number of commissures and presence of raphes (aortic valve); presence of commissural fusion or calcification; the presence of leaflet or cuspal fibrosis, calcification, destruction, or perforation; and the presence, size, location, and shape of vegetations, with or without underlying valve destruction. The chordae tendineae of atrioventricular valves should be described as normal, thickened, or fused, thinned or elongated, and the presence of rupture noted.

Microscopic examination

Microscopic evaluation is essential for valves with vegetations, carcinoid heart disease, valvular amyloidosis, connective tissue diseases (especially in unexplained aortic insufficiency) and ochronosis. If there is any clinical suspicion of endocarditis, the valve should be sectioned even in the absence of gross vegetations.

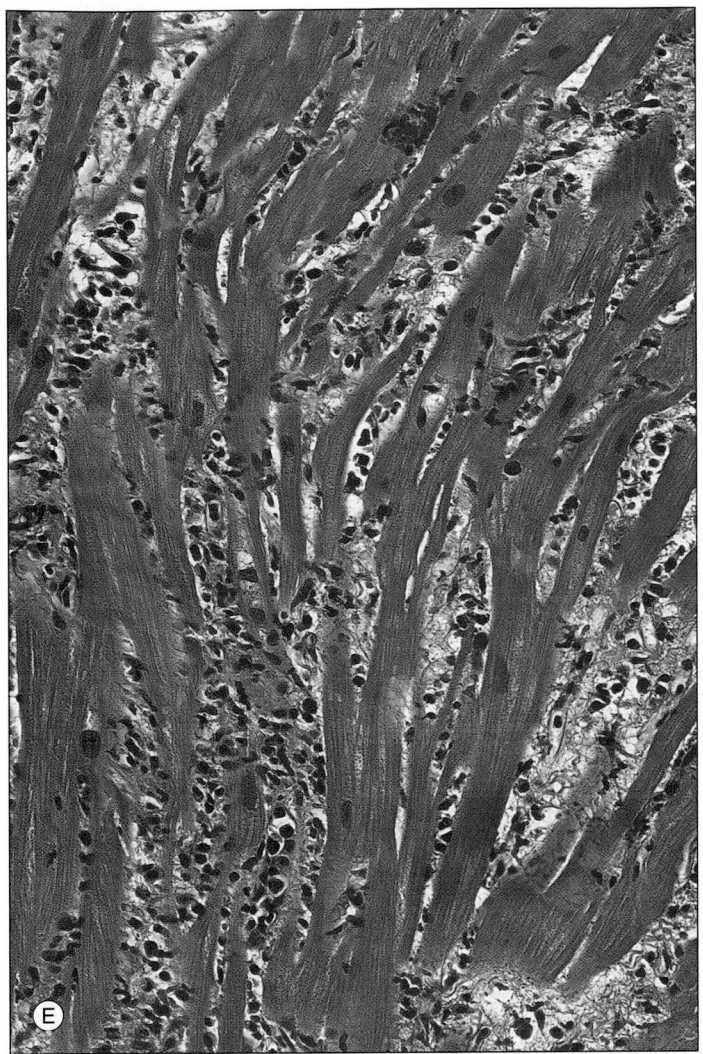
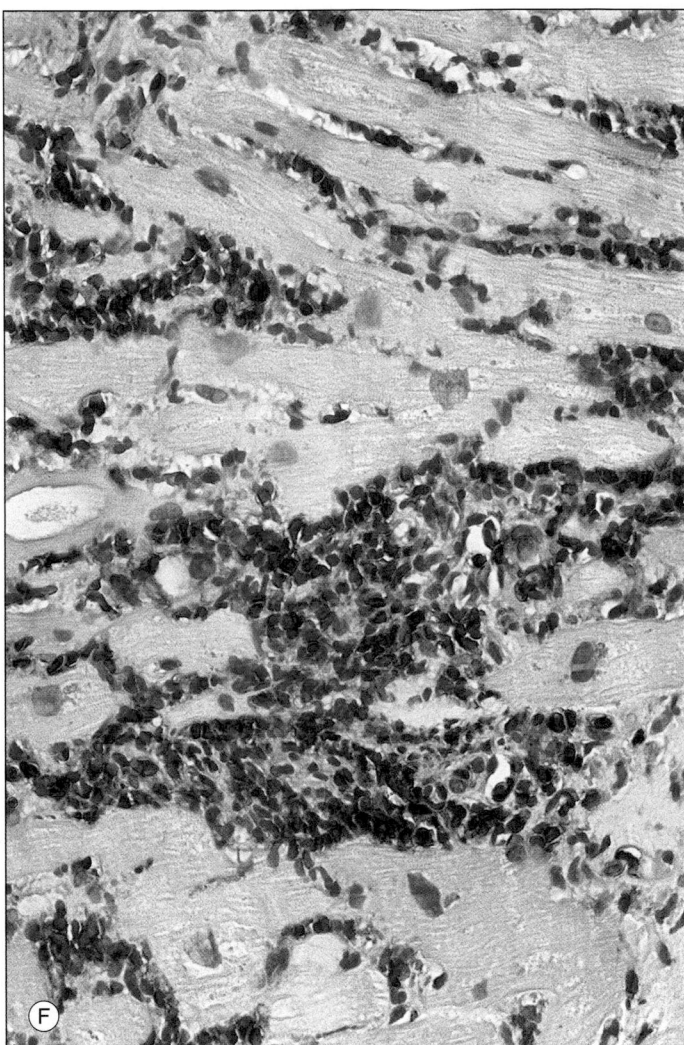

Figure 20.7 *(cont'd)* **(E)** If there are few areas of normal intervening myocardium, grade 3B rejection is diagnosed (borderline severe). **(F)** The lymphocytic infiltrate of acute rejection is primarily that of T-cells (avidin-biotin, anti-CD3). Grade 3B rejection.

Histologic evaluation of any aortic tissue submitted with the valve, especially aortic valve, is mandatory to exclude healed dissection, cystic medial change, and inflammatory lesions.

Other studies

Gross valve photography is an important tool to document the valve disease for the patient record, especially indicated in cases that will be sectioned for microscopy. Cultures of vegetations should be sent to the laboratory for organism identification and antibiotic sensitivity testing; this should preferably be done in the operating suite to avoid contamination.

MITRAL VALVE

Approach to specimen

A clinical history is essential in the proper evaluation of excised mitral valves. Virtually all cases of mitral stenosis in adults are secondary to post-inflammatory or postrheumatic mitral disease (Table 20.4). The causes of mitral insufficiency are more varied. In previous years, post-rheumatic valve disease was considered the most common cause of mitral insufficiency as well as stenosis. Currently, mitral valve prolapse has become the most frequent indication for surgical manipulation of incompetent mitral valve, both because of increased awareness of the condition and because of the decreased prevalence of rheumatic disease in the population.[43] Other causes of mitral insufficiency include ischemic damage to the posteromedial papillary muscle (in which case the valve may appear entirely normal) and infectious endocarditis.

There are several surgical options in the treatment of mitral valve disease. A complete valve replacement is generally performed if the valve cannot be repaired. Valve repair is especially difficult in cases of post-rheumatic disease and diffuse scarring and fibrosis of valve leaflets. In many cases of mitral valve replacement, a portion of the posterior leaflet is allowed to remain in situ and the pathologist receives only the anterior leaflet with or without a portion of the posterior leaflet. Valve repair, or valvuloplasty, involves removal only of a part of the posterior leaflet of the mitral valve and is often performed in patients with mitral valve prolapse or incompetence, or, less commonly, endocarditis.

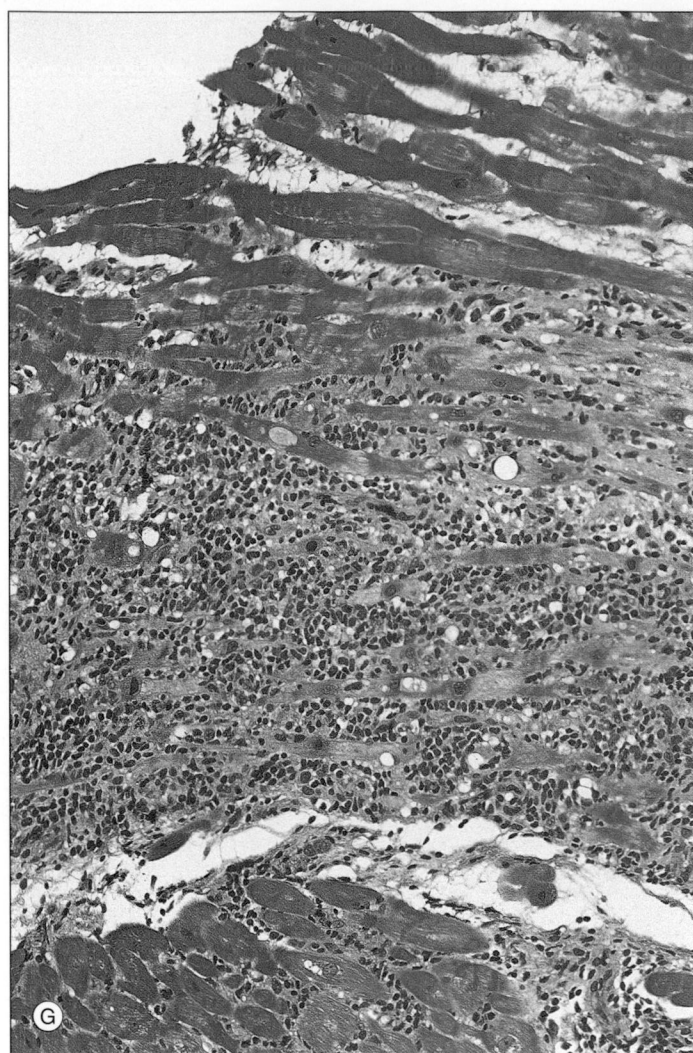

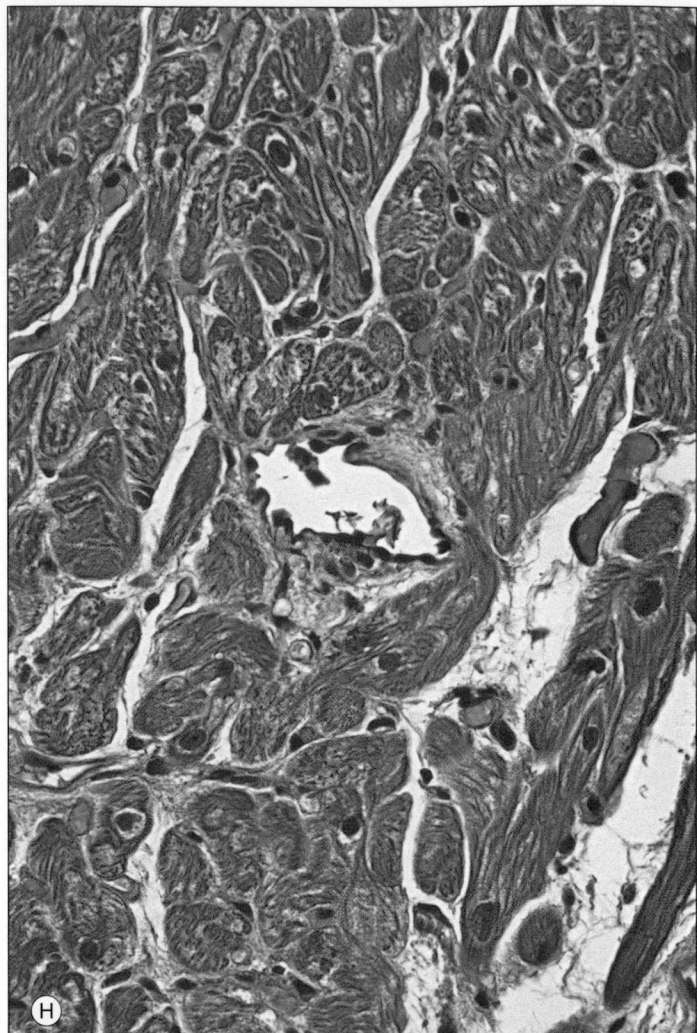

Figure 20.7 *(cont'd)* **(G)** Grade 4 (severe rejection) is characterized by diffuse inflammation with neutrophils, and edema. **(H)** Vascular rejection may occur in the absence of inflammation, and is characterized by endothelial swelling. **(I)** The diagnosis of vascular rejection is confirmed by immunofluorescent staining of endothelial cells by immunoglobulins and complement. (Courtesy of Dr James B. Atkinson.)

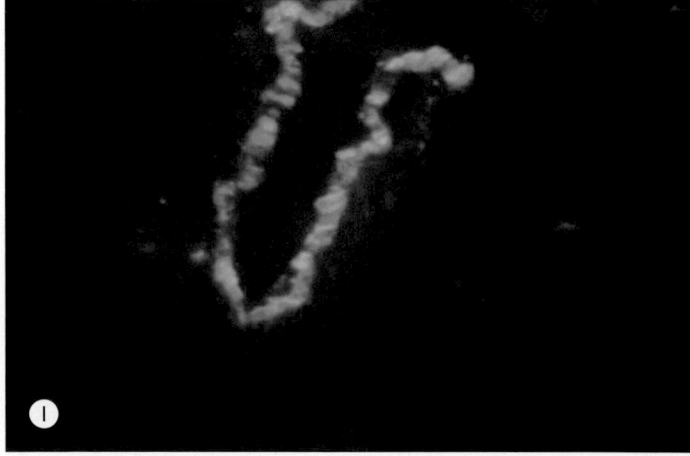

Mitral valve prolapse

The most common valvular abnormality in the United States, mitral valve prolapse affects 0.5–3% of the population. Most patients are asymptomatic but progressive mitral regurgitation occurs in 10–15% of patients, necessitating valve replacement. Symptomatic patients have myxomatous degeneration of the valve, which may be associated with myxoid deposits in other cardiac sites, including the conduction tissues. Although usually an isolated cardiac lesion, mitral valve prolapse is associated with Marfan syndrome, hypertrophic cardiomyopathy, ostium secundum atrial septal defect, Ehlers–Danlos syndrome, and Ebstein's tricuspid anomaly.[44]

If technically feasible, valve repair with segmental valve resection (mitral valvuloplasty) and/or placement of a prosthetic ring (annuloplasty) is recommended, rather than total valve replacement. The surgical specimen may consist of the entire valve, the entire or a large portion of the anterior or posterior leaflet and attached chordae, or a wedge resection of valve tissue. Features characteristic of mitral valve prolapse are myxomatous thickening of the valve leaflets, interchordal hooding, increase in leaflet length, abnormal chordal insertion, elongation of chordae, and chordal rupture (Fig. 20.10). The valve is typically glistening white, or whitish-blue. The middle scallop of the posterior leaflet is most frequently involved.[44]

Histologic examination is not required unless endocarditis is suspected. Excessive accumulation of proteoglycans in the spongiosa

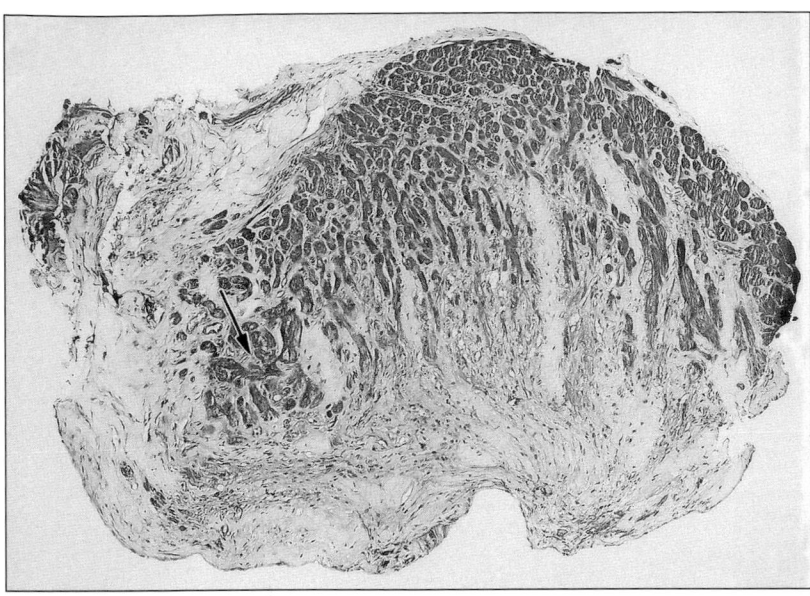

Figure 20.8 Biopsy site. Previous biopsy sites are commonly encountered in transplant biopsies. There is granulation tissue along the endocardial surface and there is often underlying disorganization of myocytes (arrow).

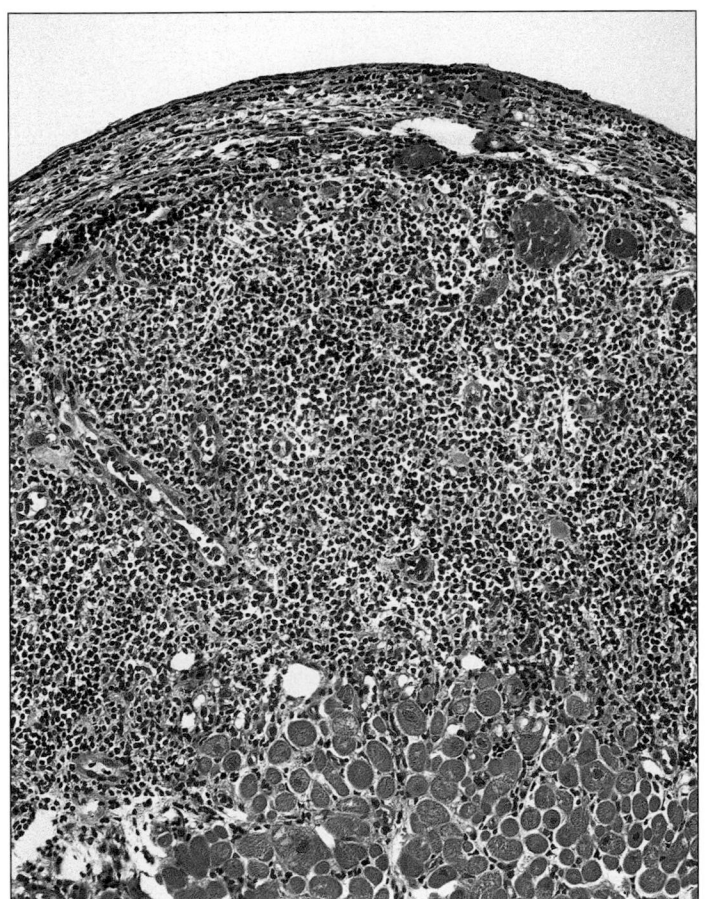

Figure 20.9 Quilty effect. There is a subendocardial collection of lymphocytes. In contrast to rejection, the infiltrate is relatively contained and there is prominent vascularity. (Courtesy of Dr James B. Atkinson.)

Table 20.4 Indications for mitral valve replacement

Condition	Usual functional disturbance	Approximate frequency (% of valve replacements)	Typical age range (years)
Mitral valve prolapse	Insufficiency	40	50–70
Postinflammatory	Stenosis	40	40–60
	Insufficiency	10	40–60
Ischemic	Insufficiency	5	60–80
Endocarditis	Insufficiency	5	Variable, 25–60

'Stenosis' includes valves with or without a degree of insufficiency

results in disruption of the fibrosa and expansion and elongation of valve leaflets. The atrial surface shows elastic fiber duplication and fibrosis.

The differential diagnosis includes post-rheumatic disease, which will demonstrate commissural fusion, disorganized valve architecture, leaflet retraction, and chordal thickening and fusion. A precise diagnosis is not always possible, especially if only a portion of valve is resected.

Chronic rheumatic mitral valve disease

A documented history of previous rheumatic fever is present in less than half of patients with mitral stenosis presumed to be post-rheumatic. After acute rheumatic valvulitis, chronic rheumatic valve disease becomes manifest after a latent period of 10–25 years, with symptoms most typically appearing in the third to fourth decade. The risk of developing chronic rheumatic valvulitis after an episode of acute rheumatic fever varies widely and is highest in patients with rheumatic carditis that results in congestive heart failure.[45]

Rheumatic mitral stenosis is the most important clinical manifestation of chronic rheumatic heart disease; mixed stenosis and regurgitation is common and pure regurgitation is rare. Concurrent involvement of the aortic valve is common, often resulting in concomitant excision of the aortic valve. The surgical specimen may

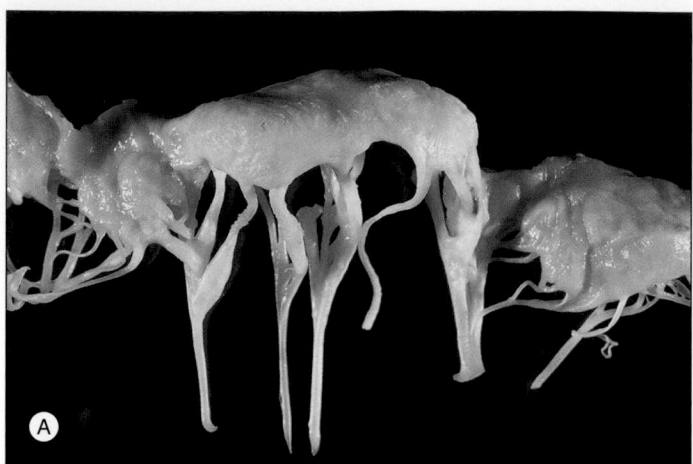

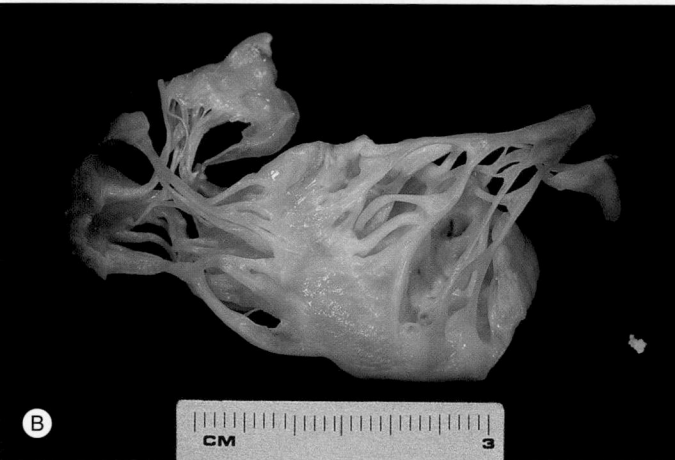

Figure 20.10 Mitral valve prolapse. **(A)** The posterior leaflet is primarily involved in mitral valve prolapse, and demonstrates hooding and redundancy. **(B)** The undersurface of the valve demonstrates chordal disarray. The valve is typically glistening white. Only the anterior leaflet of the valve may be resected if there is valve replacement, and may appear relatively normal.

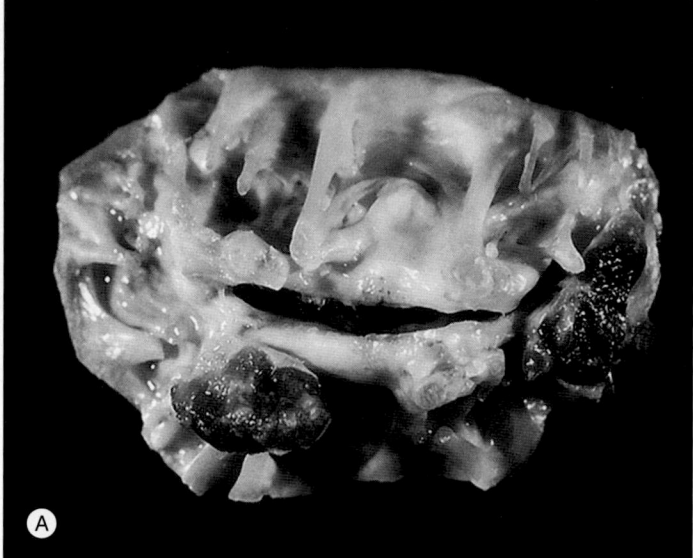

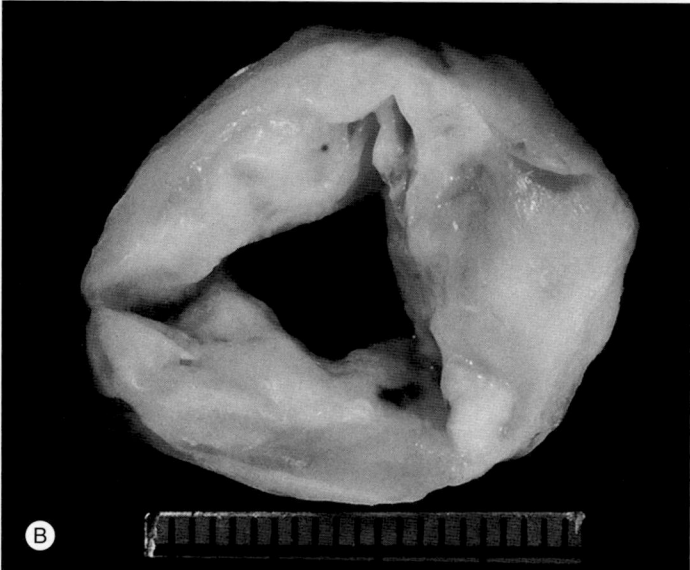

Figure 20.11 Chronic rheumatic valve disease. The mitral valve **(A)** demonstrates thickened, shortened chordae, fusion of the commissures, and a stenotic valve opening often likened to a fishmouth. The aortic valve **(B)** demonstrates fibrous thickening and fusion of the commissures resulting in a valve that is both stenotic and incompetent.

consist of only the anterior leaflet, because retention of the posterior leaflet and its chordal attachments to the papillary muscles is associated with improved cardiac function and reduced risk of postoperative left ventricular rupture.

Characteristic pathologic findings are commissural fusion; retracted, fibrotic leaflets; and thickened, fibrotic, matted, and shortened chordae tendineae (Fig. 20.11). Leaflets are markedly fibrotic, and calcification may be severe, mild, or absent, and is most prominent in the commissures.

Mitral regurgitation secondary to ischemic heart disease

Coronary artery bypass is usually performed at the time of valve replacement for ischemic mitral regurgitation. The posteromedial papillary muscle becomes infarcted more frequently than the anterolateral papillary muscle because of its relatively limited blood supply. It receives blood only from the right, in contrast to the anterolateral muscle, which is supplied by both the anterior descending and left circumflex.

The surgical specimen may consist of the entire valve or just the anterior leaflet, or sometimes only chordae tendineae. There are often no pathologic abnormalities in the resected valve. Occasionally, fragments of infarcted papillary muscle are present in the resection specimen. In chronic ischemic mitral regurgitation, the papillary muscle is thin and atrophic, and on histologic examination there is replacement of the papillary muscle by scar; in papillary muscle rupture, coagulation necrosis of the papillary muscle is present associated with a layer of fibrin and platelets along the ruptured muscular surface.

Miscellaneous lesions

Mitral annular calcification is a degenerative condition primarily seen in women older that 70 years; most surgically resected valves with annular calcification have been removed because of mitral valve prolapse or ischemic heart disease.

Table 20.5 Indications for aortic valve replacement

Condition	Usual functional disturbance	Approximate frequency (% of valve replacements)	Typical age range (years)
Degenerative valve disease	Stenosis	38	70–80
Bicuspid valve	Stenosis	25	50–70
	Insufficiency	3	40–60
Aortic root disease	Insufficiency	12	20–70
Postinflammatory valve disease	Stenosis	8%	40–70
	Insufficiency	3%	30–60
Endocarditis	Insufficiency	5	Variable, 5–60
Unicuspid valve	Stenosis	1–3	10–50

'Stenosis' includes valves with or without a degree of insufficiency

The heart is commonly involved in rheumatoid arthritis but rarely does it produce clinical cardiac dysfunction. Valvular regurgitation is produced when large nodules in the leaflets interfere with closure.

Case reports have been published that document the repair or replacement of mitral valves for amyloidosis, Whipple's disease, methylsergide-induced fibrosis, mucopolysaccharidoses, Fabry's disease, pseudoxanthoma elasticum, congenital mitral stenosis, hypertrophic cardiomyopathy, hypereosinophilic syndrome, trauma, postradiation therapy, and Kawasaki disease.[43]

AORTIC VALVE

Calcific valves

The presence of calcification is indicative of aortic stenosis or combined stenosis and insufficiency; there are three major diagnostic considerations: degenerative, congenital bicuspid, and post-inflammatory (post-rheumatic) valve disease[46] (Table 20.5). Heavily calcified valves may be removed in numerous small pieces; in this case, the diagnosis of fragments of calcified valve cusps, consistent with degenerative aortic stenosis, is made. For relatively intact valves with only two cusps present, it is helpful to search for evidence of a median raphe in congenitally bicuspid aortic valves.

Commissural fusion and fibrosis are indicative of post-inflammatory aortic stenosis; in these valves, calcification begins at the commissures and extends on to the cuspal surface and less often forms bulky nodules at the base of the cusps as seen in degenerative valve disease. Because rheumatic disease affects the mitral valve before the aortic valve, there may be concomitant mitral valve replacement for postrheumatic valve disease.

Septal myomectomy is performed for hemodynamically significant hypertrophy of the ventricular septum in fewer than 10% of patients with aortic stenosis and aortic valve replacement. Myomectomy may be surgical, or by injection of 100% ethanol via the septal perforator arterial branch, to induce ischemic necrosis of the septum. In most cases, the septal hypertrophy is a secondary change; occasionally, there may be coexistent hypertrophic cardiomyopathy.

Congenital aortic valve disease

Congenitally unicuspid aortic valves generally present with aortic stenosis early in childhood or adolescence and represent 6% of aortic

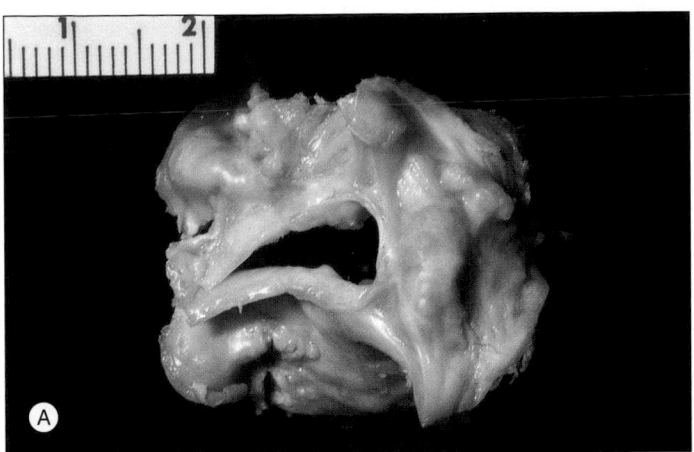

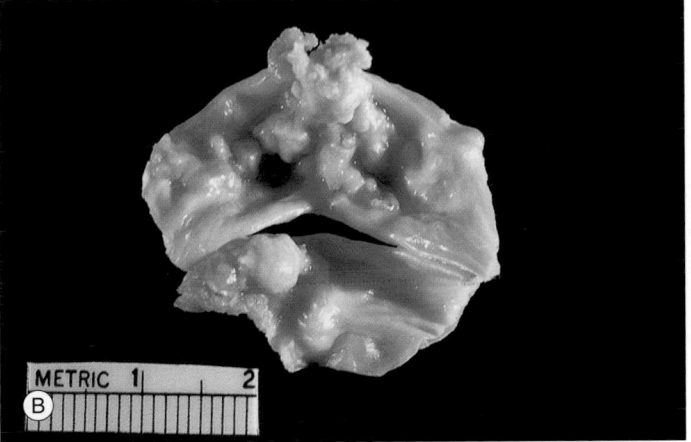

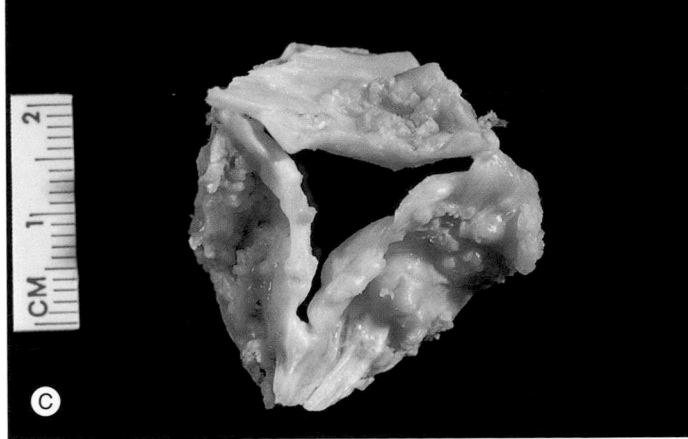

Figure 20.12 Congenital and acquired aortic stenosis. **(A)** Unicuspid aortic stenosis results in a 'teardrop'-shaped valve, usually with two raphes present and one commissure. **(B)** Bicuspid aortic stenosis will result in excision of two leaflets and nodular calcification (aortic surface). Note presence of raphe in the upper leaflet. **(C)** Senile calcific aortic stenosis is characterized by nodules of calcium, which form on the aortic surface of the valve cusps in the sinuses. The underlying valve has a normal structure; commissural fusion is not prominent.

stenosis in adults. The excised valve demonstrates either a dome shape or a slit-like opening with a tear drop shape ('exclamation point') and often possesses two aborted commissures (raphes) (Fig. 20.12A). The leaflet may be dysplastic with or without calcification, and histologic evaluation is not necessary unless endocarditis is suspected.

Occasionally the valve will be both incompetent and stenotic, or, rarely, entirely incompetent.

Congenitally bicuspid aortic valves are present in 1–2% of general population and approximately 50% of patients will develop complications of stenosis or insufficiency. Patients with congenitally bicuspid aortic valves generally become symptomatic in the fifth to eighth decades. The most common complication is aortic stenosis; bicuspid valves are the most frequent cause of aortic stenosis in age 50–70 years. Similar to unicuspid valves, patients with congenitally bicuspid valves are at increased risk for aortic dissection and endocarditis.

Pathologically, a stenotic bicuspid aortic valve will be composed of two separate cusps in intact valve resections; a diagnostic feature is the identification of a *median raphe* (aborted third commissure) in the conjoint cusp, present in approximately 60% of cases. Characteristics of the raphe are lack of extension to free edge of valve, lack of separation into two cusp margins, and a relatively straight free edge of conjoint cusp (Fig. 20.12B).

Bicuspid aortic valve accounts for 16–24% of cases of aortic incompetence.[47,48] The pathologic features of incompetent valves are similar to those of stenotic valve. However, calcification is mild or absent and the valve cusps show varying degrees of fibrous thickening, retraction, and rolled edges. Because of an increased incidence of structural abnormalities of the aortic root (cystic medial change), valvular regurgitation may be primarily caused by aortic root dilatation rather than by lesions in the valve cusps themselves.

Acquired degenerative aortic valve disease (excluding congenitally malformed valves)

Degenerative aortic valve disease is generally a disease of senescence, currently accounting for over one-half of surgical valve replacements in patients older than 70 years.[49] Degenerative aortic valve disease rarely affects patients under the age of 50 years, and is the most frequent indication for isolated aortic valve replacement. There is a male predominance of approximately 1.6:1. Most patients suffer from aortic stenosis, although often the valve is mildly insufficient as well.

Pathologically, the valve may be fragmented during surgical removal due to heavy calcification, which forms nodules on the aortic surfaces most prominently in the base of the cusps extending up towards the mid-portion, ending proximal to the free edge (Fig. 20.12C). Commissural fusion is rare and a median raphe is absent. Histologic examination is not necessary unless endocarditis suspected

Postinflammatory aortic valve disease

Inflammatory scarring of the aortic valve, similar to that of the mitral valve, is presumed to be post-rheumatic in origin, although less than 50% of patients have a history of rheumatic fever. Some cases of inflammatory scarring of the aortic valve, especially if there is single commissural fusion, may be the result of healed endocarditis. The proportion of aortic valves removed for postrheumatic disease is declining, because of a higher rate of operations on elderly patients with degenerative aortic disease and a decrease in the incidence of rheumatic disease.[49] Of aortic valves removed because of post-inflammatory changes, 35% are purely stenotic; 25% are regurgitant, and 40% are stenotic and regurgitant.

In aortic valves removed for postinflammatory stenosis, commissural fusion is the most important diagnostic feature. There may be fusion of one, two or all three commissures. The cusps are thickened, fibrotic, and cusp calcification may occur beginning in the fused commissures and extending into the cusp body. Rarely, fibrosis may

involve the valve cusps exclusively, without involvement of the commissures.

It may be difficult to distinguish acquired bicuspid aortic valves resulting from postinflammatory fusion of a single commissure from congenital bicuspid aortic valve. In general, the free edge of the conjoint cusp is smooth in cases of congenital bicuspid valves and indented in cases of acquired bicuspid valve. Additional features of postinflammatory conjoint cusps not present in congenitally bicuspid valves include extension of the commissure to the free edge of the valve, large size of the conjoint cusp – nearly twice that of the uninvolved leaflet, and the destruction of elastic layers of valve as seen histologically.

Miscellaneous causes of aortic stenosis

Ochronosis is a rare cause of aortic stenosis resulting in aortic valve replacement. Other rare causes of aortic stenosis resulting in aortic valve replacement include irradiation, familial hypercholesterolemia, Fabry's disease, and systemic lupus erythematosus.[49]

Aortic insufficiency secondary to diseases of the ascending aorta

The most common cause of pure aortic insufficiency resulting in valve replacement is not related to intrinsic valve disease but to dilatation of the aortic root. The cause of valvular insufficiency is often not apparent on examination of valve; histologic examination of the aortic wall, if submitted, may reveal a specific diagnosis. The valve itself may appear normal or show non-specific myxoid changes histologically.

Causes of aortic root dilatation are numerous but the major histologic differential is between non-inflammatory disease, specifically medial degeneration, and aortitis. If there is healed or ongoing dissection in cases of hypertension- or medial-degeneration-induced aortic rupture, secondary inflammatory changes with the presence of lymphocytes, plasma cells, and eosinophils should not be misinterpreted as aortitis.

In cases of non-inflammatory aortic root dilatation in patients with Marfan syndrome, idiopathic annuloaortic ectasia, hypertension, and bicuspid aortic valve, there is a variable degree of medial degeneration ('cystic medial necrosis'), characterized by loss of medial elastic lamella and accumulations of proteoglycans. In occasional cases of Marfan syndrome the aortic wall will appear histologically normal. There may be superimposed changes of acute or chronic dissection, with splitting of the outer media and accumulation of acute hemorrhage or granulation tissue. In cases of aortitis, there will be inflammatory changes within the media, suggesting features of either syphilis, giant cell arteritis, Takayasu's disease, or non-specific aortitis.

Miscellaneous causes of aortic insufficiency

Rarely, idiopathic aortic incompetence occurs in the absence of obvious valvar or aortic disease. In patients with membranous or subpulmonic ventricular septal defects, aortic incompetence may lead to surgical resection of the aortic valve. In patients with hypertrophic cardiomyopathy and prior myomectomy, aortic insufficiency may result.

The seronegative spondyloarthropathies (ankylosing spondylitis, Reiter syndrome, and psoriatic arthritis) are associated with HLA-B27 histocompatibility antigen and may result in inflammation of the aortic root and aortic valve cusps to produce aortic regurgitation. The valve cusps are scarred and fibrotically thickened, particularly in their basal portion, which results in cusp retraction. Foci of chronic inflammation may be seen in histologic sections, sometimes with interspersed neutrophils.

Case reports of valve repair or replacements have been published for rheumatoid arthritis, Behçet syndrome, hypereosinophilic syndrome, mucopolysaccharidoses (Hunter–Hurler phenotype), amyloidosis, radiation therapy, and postmethylsergide therapy.

TRICUSPID VALVE

Postinflammatory (rheumatic) valve disease

Post-rheumatic disease is the most common indication for surgical removal of the tricuspid valve, most often resulting in valvular regurgitation (56%), followed by combined stenosis and regurgitation (41%), and isolated tricuspid stenosis (3%).[50] Postrheumatic scarring of the tricuspid valve never occurs as an isolated valve lesion, and there is frequently removal of the mitral and/or aortic valves as well. Currently, valvotomy for stenosis or annuloplasty for regurgitation is preferred to valve replacement, if technically feasible.

Pathologically, the changes of postinflammatory tricuspid valve disease are analogous to those occurring on the mitral valve and include commissural fusion, especially of the anteroseptal commissure, leaflet fibrosis, and chordal fusion, thickening, and shortening. Leaflet fibrosis is generally diffuse in stenotic valves but may be limited to lines of valve closure in incompetent valves. Histologic evaluation is not necessary unless endocarditis is suspected.

Pulmonary venous hypertension resulting in tricuspid insufficiency

Pulmonary venous hypertension commonly results in tricuspid incompetence, although surgical replacement is rarely required. Tricuspid annuloplasty is a more common procedure. The causes of pulmonary venous hypertension are numerous; most cases result from mitral stenosis and/or regurgitation. Therefore, there may be concomitant resection of the mitral valve (for whatever cause) in addition to tricuspid valve resection or tricuspid annuloplasty.

Pathologically, tricuspid regurgitation is generally a result of annular dilatation, generally greater than 12 cm, with minimal gross changes in the valve. There may be focal leaflet thickening but the appearance of the tricuspid valve is essentially normal.

Carcinoid tricuspid valve disease and anorexigen-induced valve disease

Carcinoid heart disease occurs in 20–50% of patients with carcinoid syndrome and is an important cause of morbidity and mortality in these patients.[51] Accumulation of carcinoid plaques deposited on the valve surface results in tricuspid regurgitation with or without stenosis, and rarely pure stenosis, occasionally necessitating valve replacement. Tricuspid valve plaques occur with equal frequency to pulmonic valve plaques; the mitral valve is only rarely involved.

The pathogenesis of carcinoid plaques is unknown but may be related to endothelial injury from vasoactive agents produced by the carcinoid tumor or mitogenic effects of serotonin on subendocardial cells.[52] Grossly, white plaques first accumulate on the ventricular endocardial surface, spreading to the atrial and chordal surfaces in severe cases. Histologically, carcinoid plaques consist of smooth muscle cells within a proteoglycan matrix, which are deposited upon the underlying normal valve tissue, with intact valve layers.

Similar endocardial plaques (often referred to as 'onlay' lesions) have been described in patients receiving fenfluramine–phentermine.[53] Although non-specific, these lesions have been described as extensive in fenfluramine–phentermine-related mitral and tricuspid

stenosis.[54] Whether these lesions are related to the mild increase in cardiac valve insufficiency, especially aortic insufficiency, has not been established.[55,56] However, it is essential that valve tissue be evaluated histopathologically to attempt to differentiate chronic rheumatic valve disease, floppy mitral valve, infective endocarditis, carcinoid heart disease and valve disease associated with ergotamine and methylsergide therapy.

Miscellaneous tricuspid valve diseases

Myxomatous degeneration (floppy tricuspid valve) accounts for 2–5% of tricuspid insufficiency that results in valve replacement.[50] Floppy tricuspid valve is usually accompanied by mitral valve prolapse. A number of other congenital heart diseases unrelated to Ebstein's anomaly that may result in tricuspid incompetence and valve replacement, include complete transposition, tetralogy of Fallot, pulmonary stenosis and atresia, dysplastic tricuspid valve and other congenital heart diseases.

PULMONARY VALVE

Congenital pulmonic stenosis

Congenital pulmonary stenosis accounts for more than 90% of excised pulmonary valves.[57] The acommissural dome-shaped stenotic valve is amenable to balloon dilatation, is usually an isolated lesion, and is rarely seen by the surgical pathologist. Pathologically, excised dysplastic bicuspid and tricuspid valves show variable degrees of leaflet thickening and dysplasia, and valvular calcification in older patients.

VALVULAR VEGETATIONS

Infectious endocarditis

The majority of cases of infectious endocarditis occur in the setting of an anatomically abnormal valve or abnormal flow dynamics across valve or congenital shunts. High-risk disease includes cyanotic congenital heart lesions, previous bacterial endocarditis, aortic valve disease (including bicuspid aortic valve), mitral regurgitation and uncorrected left-to-right shunt, but not atrial septal defect; moderate risk includes mitral valve prolapse with valvar regurgitation or leaflet thickening, isolated mitral stenosis, tricuspid valve disease, pulmonary stenosis, and hypertrophic cardiomyopathy.[58] Approximately one-fourth of infectious endocarditis cases occur on normal valves; many of these cases arise in patients with predisposing noncardiac conditions, such as intravenous drug abuse, alcoholism, immuno-suppression, and colon cancer. There has been a recent increase in the frequency of *Staphylococcus aureus* endocarditis; other common isolates include streptococci, Gram-negative rods, and fungi.[59]

Grossly, there are typically friable vegetations that may be present anywhere on the valve surface, often attached to the line of closure (Fig. 20.13). In cases of chronic endocarditis, there may be valve leaflet ulceration, perforation, or rupture. The appearance of active vegetations varies from soft gray-pink to firm yellow-brown. In healed lesions, there may be focal leaflet fibrotic thickening, calcification, and/or perforation without residual vegetations.

Histologically, the vegetation typically consists of platelets, fibrin, and acute and chronic inflammatory cells. The organisms are generally present in areas of inflammation, and are often intracellular within neutrophils or macrophages. Organizing vegetations contain chronic inflammatory cells (lymphocytes, macrophages, giant cells) and fewer neutrophils. There is typically destruction of the

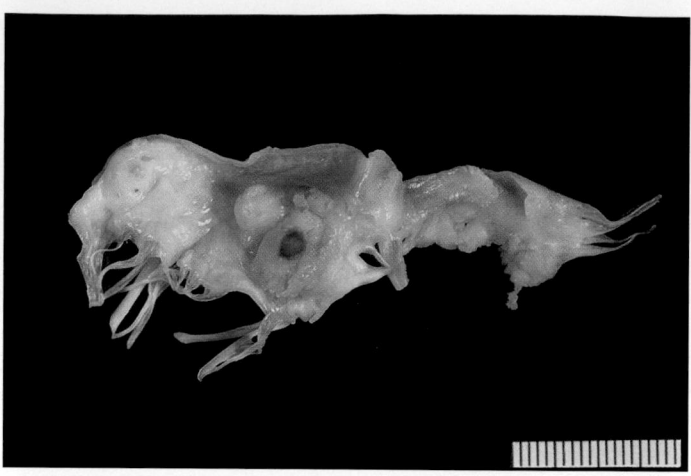

Figure 20.13 Bacterial endocarditis. The anterior leaflet and a portion of the posterior leaflet of the mitral valve demonstrating destruction of the free edge of valve as well as a bulky vegetation on the anterior valve surface (kissing lesion).

underlying valve structure, both in acute and healed lesions. It is not unusual that organisms are not identified, either because of unusual bacteria that are difficult to stain or because of antibiotic treatment.

Tissue Gram, Gomori methenamine silver, and periodic acid–Schiff stains of histologic sections should be performed to identify microorganisms. It is often helpful to perform both Brown and Brenn and Brown and Hopps Gram stains. The Brown and Brenn stain is superior for Gram-positive organisms, which, upon death, may stain reddish with the Brown and Hopps, which is more sensitive for Gram-negatives.

Culture-negative endocarditis occurs in approximately 10–25% of clinically diagnosed endocarditis[60] and comprises a group of infections that include partly treated streptococcal[61] or staphylococcal infections, fastidious organisms such as abiotrophia, HACEK group bacteria (*Haemophilus parainfluenzae, aphrophilus,* and *paraphrophilus, Actinobacillus actinomycetemcomitans,*[62] *Cardiobacterium hominis, Eikenella corodens,* and *Kingella kingae*), *Clostridium, Brucella, Legionella, Mycobacterium,* and intracellular organisms (*Bartonella,*[63] Whipple's,[64] *Chlamydiae pneumoniae,*[65] and Q fever).[66] Those that may be diagnosed by pathologic evaluation include Whipple's disease and *Bartonella*; silver impregnation stains and periodic acid–Schiff stains are imperative in the diagnoses of these entities. Immunohistochemical stains and PCR technique for the identification of culture-resistant organisms may also be helpful.[61,67]

The differential diagnosis of infectious endocarditis includes marantic or nonbacterial thrombotic endocarditis, and autoimmune endocarditis. The latter entity comprises lupus-related endocarditis (Libman–Sacks endocarditis), Wegener's granulomatosis,[68] and rheumatoid endocarditis; autoimmune and nonbacterial thrombotic endocarditis are sometimes considered to be the same entity.[69] The absence of apparent valve perforation, the distribution of the neutrophils within the core of the leaflet (and not within the fibrin vegetation), favor an autoimmune process over an infection. Serologic studies such as antineutrophil cytoplasmic antibodies and antinuclear antibodies are helpful in establishing a diagnosis of autoimmune disease, although antinuclear autoantibodies may occur in patients with infectious endocarditis. In fact, some cases of partly treated

infectious endocarditis, or endocarditis caused by unusual, low-virulence organisms (such as *Actinobacillus*) cannot histologically be distinguished reliably from marantic vegetations.

Libman–Sacks lesions are seen exclusively in patients with systemic lupus erythematosus and may occur on the mitral and tricuspid and, less commonly, aortic valve. They are rarely present in excised valve specimens, because functional valve abnormalities are uncommon. Many patients have coexisting antiphospholipid syndrome. Microscopically, vegetations consist of fibrin, cellular debris, degenerating valve tissue, and inflammatory cells; hematoxylin bodies may be present in the acute phase.

Nonbacterial thrombotic endocarditis

Also referred to as marantic endocarditis, nonbacterial thrombotic endocarditis occurs most often in the setting of an underlying malignancy, chronic inflammatory disease, or coagulopathy. Tricuspid or pulmonic vegetations may occur secondary to central-venous-catheter-induced trauma. Embolization is not uncommon and is the usual indication for surgery.

Pathologically, the aortic and mitral valves are most commonly affected along the lines of closure. Vegetations may be large or small, and friable or firm. In contrast to infectious vegetations, they appear 'tacked on' without destruction of the underlying valve. Histologically, marantic vegetations consist predominantly of fibrin with a few trapped erythrocytes and rare acute and chronic inflammatory cells, and the underlying valve is usually normal.

Papillary fibroelastoma

Also referred to as fibroelastic papillomas, these are usually incidental nodules, found at echocardiography or at autopsy, that are grossly and histologically related to giant Lambl's excrescences.[70,71] Papillary fibroelastomas occurring on the left-sided valves may result in embolic symptoms of stroke and cardiac ischemia.[72–74] The mitral valve is most commonly involved, although any valve or area of the endocardium may be affected and multiple tumors are not uncommon. An association with iatrogenic disturbances in hemodynamics has been proposed.[75,76] The papillary nature of the excrescence is best appreciated when the valve is submerged in water. Histologically, the papillae are avascular (unlike myxoma excrescences), containing occasional fibroblasts and smooth muscle cells, and lined by endothelial cells (Fig. 20.14). Most tumors show proteoglycan deposition and elastic fibers within the papillary cores. The differential diagnosis includes cardiac myxoma, which is also rich in proteoglycan matrix. However, the lack of vascularity and inflammation and the usual location on the valve allow for ready distinction from myxoma in most cases.

PROSTHETIC HEART VALVES

Bioprosthetic valves

The most common tissue valves implanted in humans are porcine aortic valves mounted on a circular mechanical stent, and pericardial valves constructed from strips of bovine pericardium mounted on a similar circular stent. Bioprosthetic valves are prone to gradual tissue degeneration, or primary tissue failure related to cusp mineralization, which occurs at a rate of about 50% at 15 years in adults and at a much faster rate in children. The surgical pathologist should X-ray the specimen to determine the extent of calcification, and describe any tissue tears, which may originate from the free edge of the valve or occur as a perforation within a valve leaflet. The latter type of tear is often a result of endocarditis and a histologic examination of such

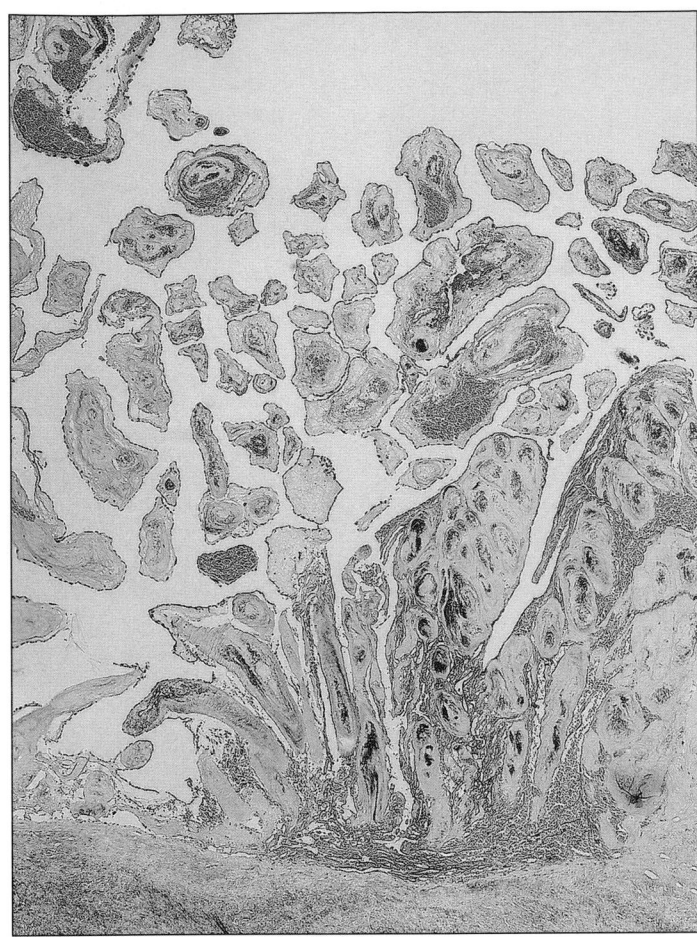

Figure 20.14 Papillary fibroelastoma. There are avascular papillary fronds lined by a single layer of endothelium. The papillary cores are composed of proteoglycans, smooth muscle cells, collagen, and elastic tissue is frequently present, especially towards the base of the tumor (Movat pentachrome).

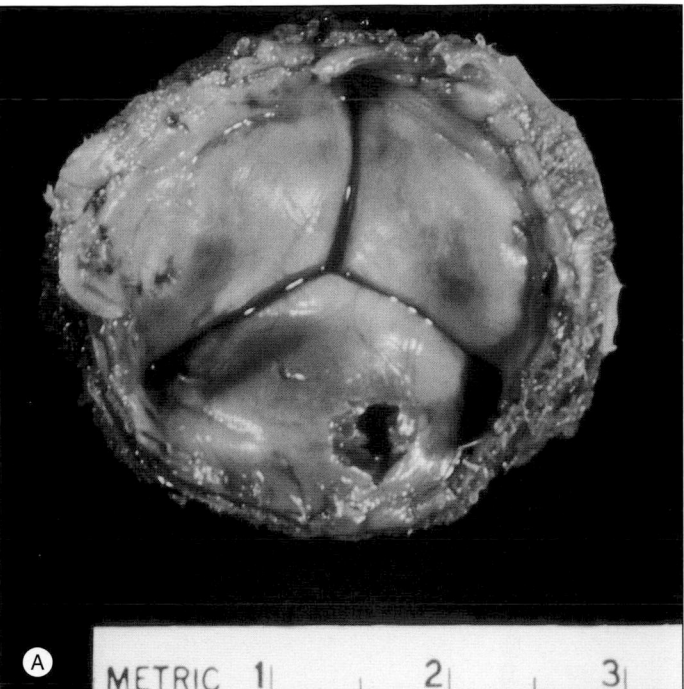

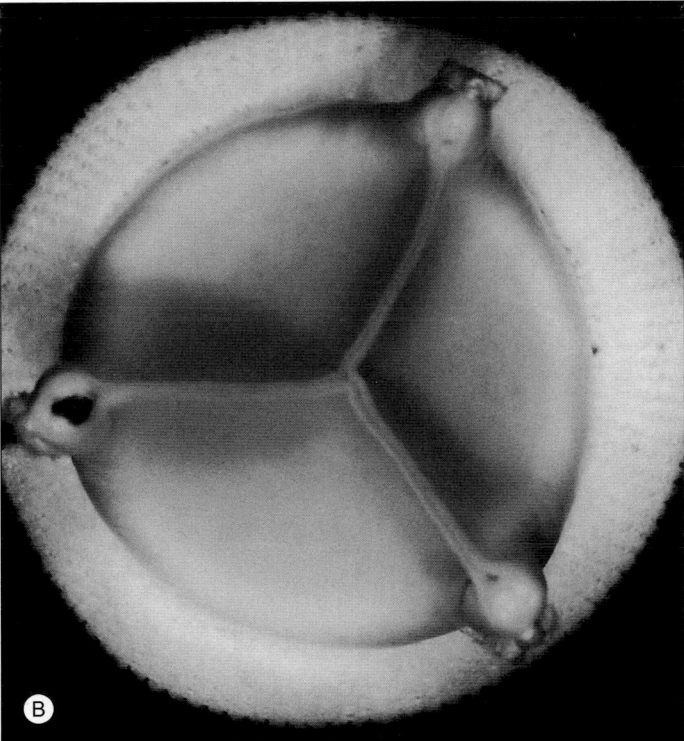

Figure 20.15 Prosthetic heart valves. **(A)** Porcine bioprosthetic valve explanted for insufficiency. Note perforation in one cusp, possibly secondary to healed endocarditis. **(B)** Bioprosthetic pericardial valve, preimplantation. In contrast to porcine valves, which are biologic aortic valves, the cusps of pericardial valves are made of xenograft tissue (usually bovine) and attached to struts.

tears is indicated. Thrombosis is an uncommon complication of bioprosthetic valves; however, it may be the sole indication for surgical removal.

Mechanical valves

Mechanical valves in current use are of three basic types: caged ball prostheses (Starr–Edwards valve), tilting disc valves (Bjork–Shiley, Medtronic-Hall, and Omniscience valves), and bileaflet valves (St Jude, CarboMedics, Sorin Allcarbon, and ATS Medical Open Pivot valve) (Fig. 20.15). The major advantage of mechanical valves is their superior durability compared with bioprosthetic valves. However, there is significantly increased risk of thromboembolic events, especially in the mitral position. The most common indication for removal of a mechanical valve is thrombosis; rarely, there may be mechanical failure resulting in disc escape and embolization. Swelling of ball poppets and unraveling of protective cloth coverings resulting in occlusion were complications seen in older models of prosthetic valves. A relatively common complication of both bioprosthetic and mechanical valves is the ring abscess, which may progress to a chronic paravalvular leak. In prosthetic valves removed for paravalvular leak, the excised valve may appear normal, and the pathologist must rely on clinical history for an explanation of surgical removal. In such cases, histologic examination of soft tissue removed with the valve may demonstrate ongoing inflammation or organisms.

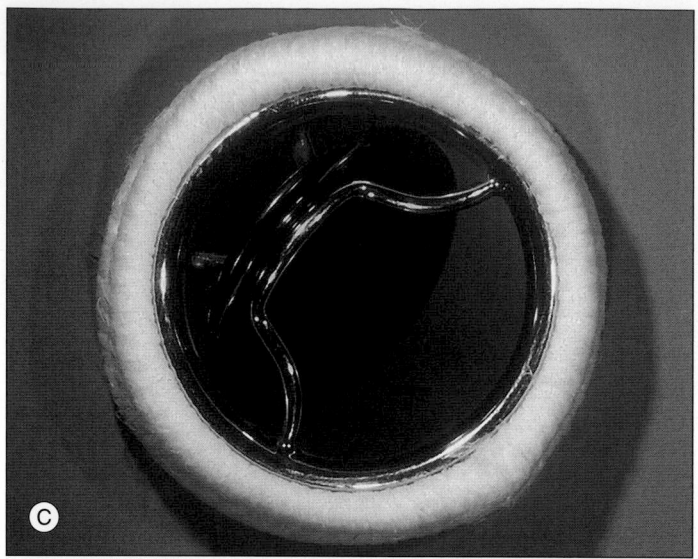

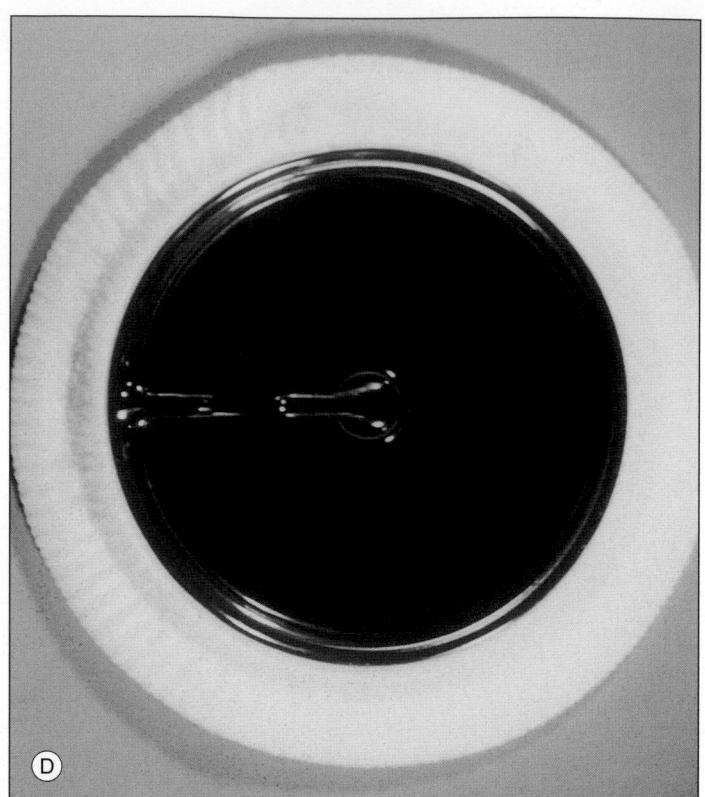

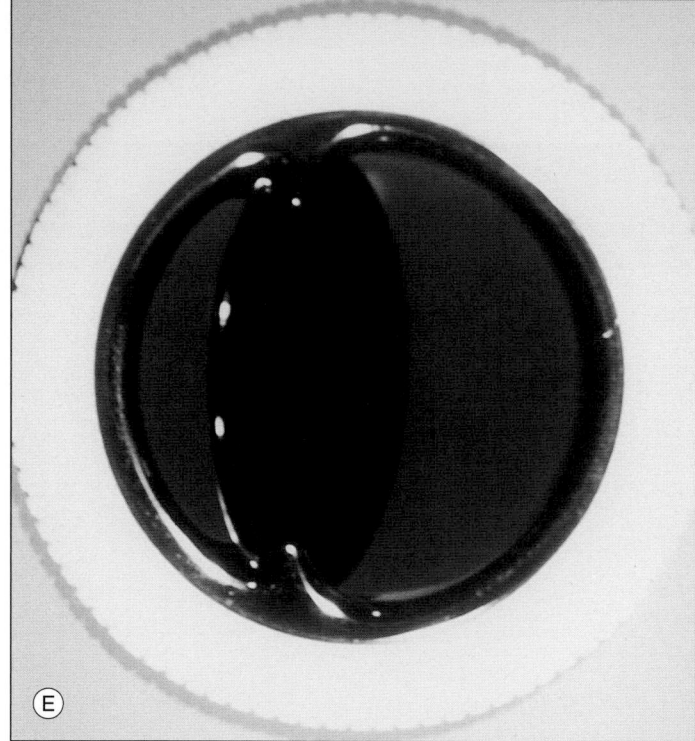

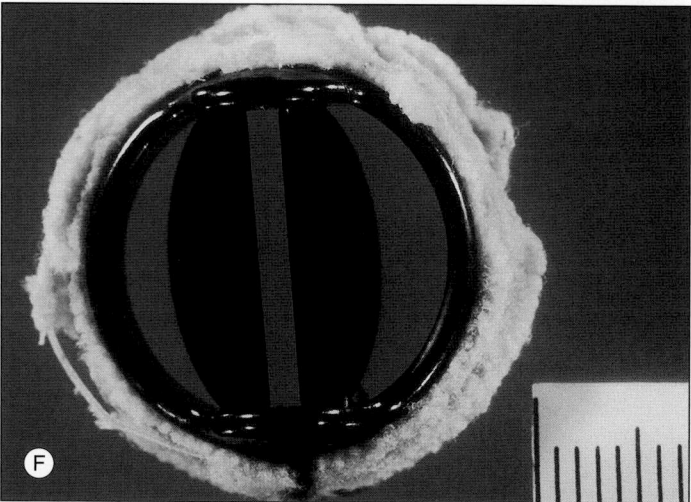

Figure 20.15 *(cont'd)* **(C)** Tilting disk valve, Bjork–Shiley. There are two struts (major and minor) which hold the occluder in place. **(D)** Medtronic-Hall tilting disk valve. The occluder passes through a hole in the pyrolytic carbon disk. **(E)** OmniScience tilting disk valve. The titanium orifice ring holds a pyrolytic carbon disc controlled by short struts. **(F)** Bileaflet mechanical valve. The St Jude's valve, which currently enjoys widespread use, is a bileaflet valve composed of pyrolytic carbon coated graphite; the leaflets open to 85°.

PATHOLOGY OF CARDIAC MASSES

INTRODUCTION

Primary cardiac tumors are rare and occur in 0.001–0.03% of autopsies. Metastatic cardiac tumors are between 40 and 500 times more common than primary tumors in autopsy series; however, in surgical series of cardiac tumors, primary benign and malignant cardiac tumors outnumber metastatic neoplasms.[77]

Some 80% of surgically resected cardiac tumors are myxomas (Table 20.6). In adults, most of the remaining tumors are either sarcomas, metastatic tumors, or organizing mural thrombi. Most tumors excised from children are rhabdomyomas, fibromas, or teratomas.

In general, open heart surgery is required for excision of cardiac tumors. Occasionally, large inoperable tumors will be biopsied using a needle, for tissue diagnosis only. Right-sided tumors may be diagnosed by endomyocardial biopsy, but inadequate tissue sampling may cause problems in establishing a definitive diagnosis.

Table 20.6 Cardiac tumors: surgical series

Tumor type	n*	%*	Mean age at presentation
Myxoma	995	77	50–55 years
Sarcoma	139	11	40–50 years
Fibroma	41	3	10–20 years
Angioma	30	2	40–45 years
Lipoma/lipomatous hypertrophy, interatrial septum	27	2	60–65 years
Rhabdomyoma†	24	1	<6 months
Histiocytoid cardiomyopathy (Purkinje cell hamartoma)	14	1	<6 months
Papillary fibroelastoma	11	<1	50–55 years
Lymphoma	7	<1	60 years
Hamartoma	5	<1	‡
Ectopic thyroid	2	<1	‡
Malignant mesothelioma	1	<1	‡
Pheochromocytoma (paraganglioma)	1	<1	40 years
Cystic tumor, atrioventricular node	1	<1	‡
Totals	1298	100	

*Data from references 97, 224–235.

‡ Few data for surgically excised tumors

† Most common surgically excised tumor in children;[98] in addition, teratomas represent approximately 5% of surgically excised pediatric cardiac tumors

For all tumors, especially myxomas and other polypoid tumors, it is best to ink surgical margins at the endocardial attachment site, to determine completeness of excision. A variety of cardiac masses, especially myxomas, may be calcified, necessitating decalcification. Sterile dissection of cardiac sarcomas and preservation of a portion of tumor in culture medium will allow cytogenetic studies that are occasionally helpful in the differential diagnosis of sarcomas. In addition, saving an unfixed portion of a malignancy for DNA ploidy studies and flow cytometry may be of research or potential clinical relevance.

CARDIAC MYXOMA

Introduction and clinical findings

Cardiac myxomas are benign intracavitary neoplasms that are found uniquely in the heart, usually attached to the atrial septum.[78] They account for 80% of surgically excised heart tumors. The origin of the myxoma cell remains controversial; possibilities include primitive endocardial cushion cells and endothelial cells.[79] The majority of cardiac myxomas are found in the left atrium, typically causing symptoms of mitral stenosis.[80] Other modes of presentation include tumor embolization resulting in strokes or cerebral ischemia, and pulmonary embolism from right-sided tumors. A variety of constitutional symptoms, including fever, weight loss, and anorexia, may occur, possibly related to the elaboration of growth factors by the neoplasm. In sporadic myxomas, the recurrence rate is less than 2%. Rarely, cardiac myxomas are part of a syndrome characterized by familial, multiple, recurrent myxomas in young individuals with spotty skin pigmentation and endocrine abnormalities.[81] The Carney complex disease gene

identifying patients at risk for familial myxoma has been localized to chromosome region 17q2.[82,83]

Gross findings

Some 75% of cardiac myxomas occur in the left atrium at the level of the fossa ovalis, 20% in the right atrium, and 5% at other endocardial sites.[84] Sporadic myxomas arising on the surface of a cardiac valve are exceedingly rare. Grossly, cardiac myxomas are attached to the endocardium by a broad stalk, often necessitating atrial patching during resection, or by a narrow pedicle (Fig. 20.16A). Cardiac myxomas may be classified as smooth-surfaced or friable; the latter are more likely to embolize. Tumors occurring in patients with myxoma syndrome are always of the friable, gelatinous type and are more likely to occur in areas remote from the atrial septum, including valves and ventricular surfaces.

Microscopic diagnosis

The microscopic diagnosis of cardiac myxoma rests on the identification of 'myxoma' cells, which are stellate or ovoid, with eosinophilic cytoplasm, and indistinct cell borders. The nuclei of myxoma cells contain open chromatin, and nucleoli are indistinct or prominent. Characteristically, myxoma cells form rings, cords, and nests that seem to emanate from and merge imperceptibly with capillaries, often infiltrated by lymphocytes and histiocytes (Fig. 20.16B). The ring-like structures are often surrounded by an acellular halo, where the proteoglycans are less dense than surrounding tissue. The myxoid background is infiltrated by a sparse or focally dense collection of histiocytes, plasma cells, mast cells, and lymphocytes; hemosiderin is invariably present within macrophages. Mitotic figures are rare.

Smooth surfaced myxomas are histologically characterized by fibrosis, relatively little myxoid matrix, and degenerative changes of calcification, ossification, and Gamna–Gandy body formation (calcific elastic fiber degeneration with hemosiderosis). Calcification is present more commonly in right-sided, as compared to left-sided tumors. Extramedullary hematopoiesis is present in approximately 7% of cardiac myxomas.[84]

Immunohistochemical studies of cardiac myxomas are not particularly helpful in the differential diagnosis. Myxoma cells may express a variety of antigens, but are generally cytokeratin-negative and variably S-100-, thrombomodulin-, and smooth muscle actin-positive.[85] When forming ring structures, the inside is often CD34-positive, with apparent differentiation to CD31-positive endothelial cells at the periphery; this change is best appreciated near the attachment at the oval fossa. The inflammatory infiltrate is rich in factor XIIIa dendritic cells,[86] but such cells are often present in cardiac sarcomas as well. One helpful diagnostic feature is the expression of calretinin in most, if not all cardiac myxomas.[87,88] Calretinin positivity is generally restricted to the myxoma cells, whether they are single, in cords, or in rings. In cases of organized thrombi, in which there are reactive, plump endothelial cells that may be mistaken for myxoma cells, negativity for calretinin is evidence that the lesion is not a myxoma. Furthermore, cardiac sarcomas are generally calretinin-negative, further adding to the utility of calretinin staining in myxomas.

About 1% of myxomas have intestinal-like glands that express cytokeratin and carcinoembryonic antigen, often present at the base of the tumor.[89] The origin of these inclusions is unclear, as is the histogenesis of myxoma itself. Immunohistochemical studies of this component of cardiac myxoma are consistent with gastrointestinal type mucosa, often with interspersed endocrine cells.[90,91] The differential diagnosis of cardiac myxoma includes both benign and

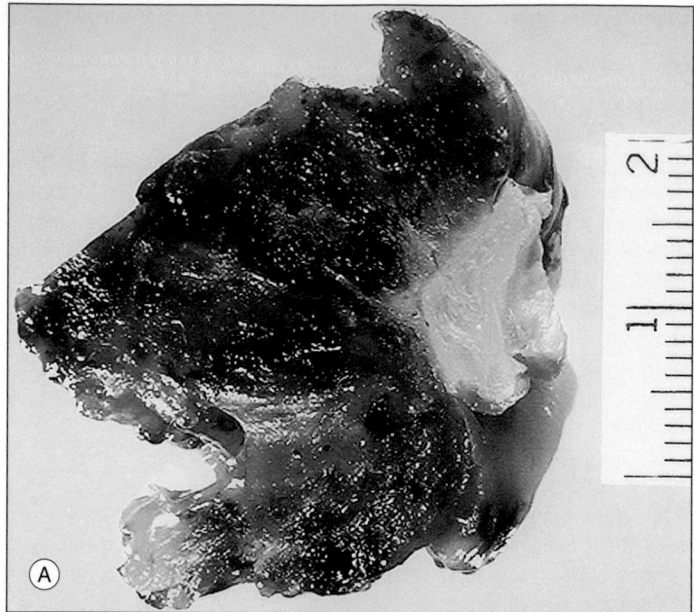

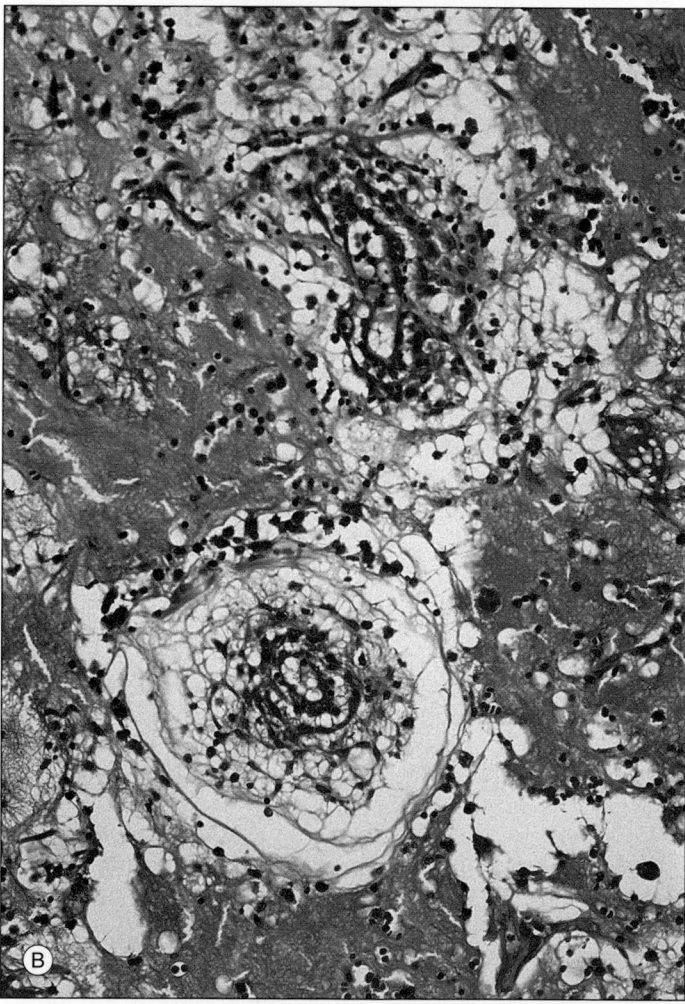

Figure 20.16 Cardiac myxoma. **(A)** A gross section demonstrates an exophytic, focally hemorrhagic mass that does not infiltrate the atrial wall. The yellow tint is a result of fixation in Bouin's solution. **(B)** Myxomas of the heart are histologically distinct from those of soft tissue. Myxoma cells form rings emanating from vascular channels and are generally infiltrated with lymphocytes and hemosiderin-laden macrophages.

malignant lesions. Cardiac sarcomas frequently possess a myxoid matrix but lack characteristic myxoma cells and myxoma structures, contain cellular areas with pleomorphism and atypical mitotic figures, and lack abundant inflammation and hemosiderin-laden macrophages. Papillary fibroelastomas are distinguished by their frequent location on cardiac valves and are avascular, unlike myxomas, which contain abundant capillaries. Metastatic adenocarcinoma may be confused with the rare case of a myxoma with glandular structures; however, the glands of myxoma lack atypia and mitotic figures, and areas of typical myxoma should be identified.

CARDIAC FIBROMA

Introduction and clinical findings

Cardiac fibroma is a congenital, solitary, mural hamartoma of fibrous tissue that generally occurs in the ventricle or ventricular septum.[92] It comprises about one-third of childhood heart tumors, the most common being rhabdomyoma.[93] Fibromas may be diagnosed from birth to adulthood, usually in infancy or childhood; mean age at presentation is approximately 13 years. Symptoms include arrhythmias, sudden death, congestive heart failure; some cardiac fibromas are incidental findings during evaluation of a cardiac murmur. There is an association between cardiac fibroma and Gorlin syndrome (nevoid basal cell carcinoma syndrome); manifestations include enlarged occipital circumference, odontogenic keratocysts of the jaws, epidermal cysts, rib anomalies, and multiple basal cell carcinomas of the skin.

Surgical therapy is the preferred treatment, which can cause normalization of cardiac rhythm in patients with ventricular tachy-arrhythmias. In some patients, tumors are not resectable, and partial excision is performed with good long-term prognosis.[93] There appears to be little if any propensity for increased growth of cardiac fibroma after infancy, but spontaneous regression is not the rule as with rhabdomyoma,. Unresectable tumors have been treated by cardiac transplantation, occasionally with preoperative ventricular bridges to afford time before a suitable organ donor is located.[94]

Gross pathology

Cardiac fibromas are bulging masses of rubbery white tissue resembling uterine 'fibroids'. Although they are often grossly circumscribed, the microscopic borders are invariably infiltrating. Sites of involvement, in order of decreasing frequency, are left ventricular free wall, right ventricle, and atria. Occasionally, fibromas may bulge into the ventricular outflow, resulting in subaortic stenosis.

Microscopic findings

In infants, cardiac fibromas are cellular with relatively little collagen; mitotic figures may be present but are generally not numerous. In children and adults, there is extensive collagen deposition; some tumors histologically resemble scars. Elastic fibers are often prominent in 50% of tumors, and calcification is present in one-third of cases.[92] Inflammation is sparse, generally limited to perivascular regions and at the margin of the tumor, usually mononuclear.

There are few entities in the microscopic differential diagnosis. In adults, the histologic appearance is similar to scar; however, unlike scars, fibromas are tumors that bulge on section and infiltrate into surrounding tissues. In infants, it may be difficult to distinguish cardiac fibroma from fibrosarcoma, because of the high cellularity of cardiac fibromas in the newborn period. In general, most fibrous infantile cardiac tumors do not recur or metastasize and are probably best classified as fibromas.

RHABDOMYOMA

Introduction and clinical findings

Cardiac rhabdomyoma is a hamartoma that occurs exclusively in the heart, often as multiple nodules, composed of altered cardiac myocytes with large vacuoles and abundant glycogen. It is the most common pediatric heart tumor, comprising over two-thirds of cases.[93] Up to 90% of cardiac tumors diagnosed in utero are rhabdomyomas, which are extremely rare in patients older than 10 years. There is a strong association with tuberous sclerosis (intracranial hamartomas, facial angiofibromas, subungual fibromas, linear epidermal nevi, renal angiomyolipomas, and other hamartomas). Virtually 100% of infants with tuberous sclerosis have echocardiographic evidence of cardiac rhabdomyoma; this number decreases to 60% in children and less than 25% in adults, because of spontaneous regression of cardiac lesions. Presenting symptoms include congestive heart failure, arrhythmias, fetal hydrops, or sudden death. In cases of intrauterine diagnosis, there is rarely a family history of tuberous sclerosis, although infants generally develop the complex, and multiple tumors are the rule, with frequent regression.[95]

Gross pathology

Virtually all rhabdomyomas occurring in patients with tuberous sclerosis are multiple, in contrast to sporadic rhabdomyomas, 60% of which are multiple.[96] They are pale, circumscribed nodules ranging from 1 mm to several centimeters in size. Rhabdomyomas in patients with tuberous sclerosis are usually intramural lesions that do not obstruct blood flow and are not surgically resected; solitary tumors are more frequent in sporadic cases, which account for most surgical resections.

Microscopic findings

Cardiac rhabdomyomas are well-demarcated nodules of vacuolated myocytes that have cross-striations and abundant glycogen. The typical cell of rhabdomyoma is the 'spider cell,' with strands of cytoplasm extending from the periphery of the cell to the nucleus (Fig. 20.17). Ultrastructurally, cells are similar to myoblasts, with intercalated disk-like structures around the cell periphery, and plentiful glycogen particles.

The differential diagnosis of cardiac rhabdomyoma includes histiocytoid cardiomyopathy and glycogen storage diseases. Pompe's disease results in diffuse vacuolization of myocytes with central vacuoles and peripheral location of myofibrils; discrete tumors and spider cells are absent. The cells of histiocytoid cardiomyopathy are finely vacuolated with abundant mitochondria and little glycogen or myofilaments.

MISCELLANEOUS BENIGN CARDIAC TUMORS

Hemangioma

Hemangiomas are rare tumors of the heart and represent about 2% of resected tumors.[97,98] Presenting symptoms include arrhythmias, syncope, sudden death, pericardial effusion, and shortness of breath.[99] Surgical excision is curative. Pathologically, they are one of two types. Endocardial-based hemangiomas resemble capillary or cavernous hemangiomas. These lesions often have a myxoid background leading to the erroneous diagnosis of atrial myxoma. In contrast to myxoma, immunohistochemical stains will demonstrate a diffuse actin-positive pericyte population of cells supporting the endothelial proliferation. Intramural hemangiomas are similar to extracardiac intramuscular hemangiomas, with the presence of fat and occasionally fibrous tissue;

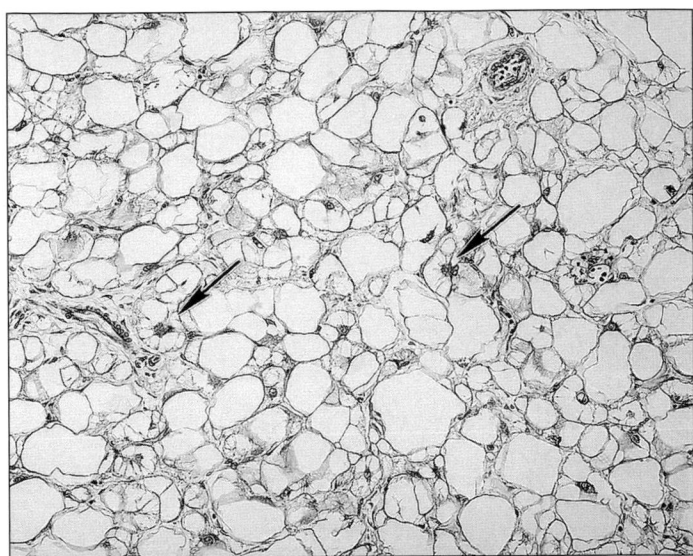

Figure 20.17 Cardiac rhabdomyoma. Cells are diffusely vacuolated and strands of myofiber cytoplasm are seen in occasional 'spider' cells (arrows).

these are poorly circumscribed infiltrative tumors. In either case the lesions are benign, but complete excision may be difficult because of their cardiac location.

Lipomatous hypertrophy of the atrial septum

Lipomatous hypertrophy of the interatrial septum is a non-encapsulated hamartomatous lesions composed of vacuolated 'brown' fat cells, mature fat, and hypertrophied myocytes. Patients are usually middle-aged or elderly, and may present with supraventricular arrhythmias, sudden death, and congestive heart failure, sometimes necessitating surgical removal.[100] Imaging studies will demonstrate a right atrial mass. Microscopically, there is a triad of vacuolated 'brown' fat cells, bizarre hypertrophic myocytes, and normal fat cells (Fig. 20.18). The major differential diagnosis is liposarcoma, which can be excluded by the absence of lipoblasts.

Monocyte/macrophage incidental cardiac excrescence

This curious entity, dubbed cardiac 'MICE', is a collection of detached mesothelial cells, histiocytes, and other blood cells that are most often artifacts from bypass surgery extracorporeal circulation.[101] They are incidental findings within atria or ventricles, usually during open heart surgery for other conditions. Microscopically, there is an absence of stroma or vascular supply in detached clusters of mesothelial cells, monocytes and lymphocytes (Fig. 20.19). The mesothelial cells are strongly cytokeratin-positive, and the monocytes/macrophages express macrophage markers such as KP-1.

Non-neoplastic cardiac lesions rarely requiring surgical removal

Some 50% of patients with hypertrophic cardiomyopathy will have significant left ventricular outflow tract obstruction with a significant hemodynamic gradient that may be relieved by septal myotomy/myectomy.

Organizing mural thrombi commonly occur in hypokinetic ventricles (after myocardial infarcts, in patients with cardiomyopathy,

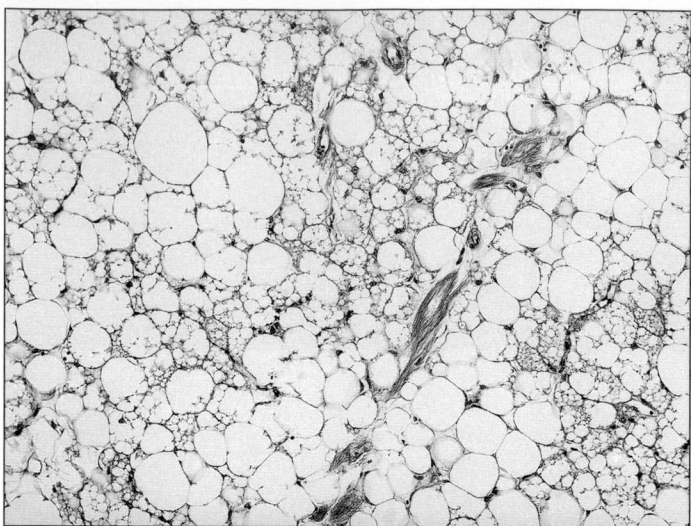

Figure 20.18 Lipomatous hypertrophy, atrial septum. These tumors may be occasionally excised surgically and are composed of brown fat cells, myocytes, and occasional inflammatory cells (not present in this example).

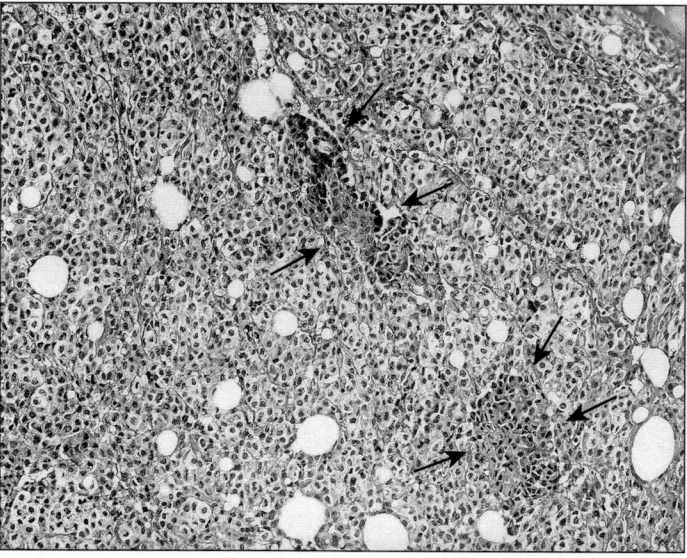

Figure 20.19 Mesothelial/monocytic incidental cardiac excrescence. These are avascular collections of macrophages, fat globules, and mesothelial cells (arrows) that are usually artifacts of cardiac bypass surgery.

etc.), and in the atria, especially in patients with atrial fibrillation. These thrombi are generally not excised surgically, and patients are placed on anticoagulants without a tissue diagnosis. Rarely, organizing thrombi may occur in the right or left ventricle in patients without obvious cardiac disease, and surgical removal is performed to exclude a neoplastic process. Some of these patients may have occult clotting disorders but occasionally no reason for thrombosis is identified.

Calcifying intracardiac pseudoneoplasm, or *cardiac calcifying amorphous tumor*, is a term used for mural calcific nodules, which probably represent organized mural thrombi, that may form in any cardiac chamber and result in embolic phenomena. Patients often have underlying diseases predisposing to thrombosis or calcification.[102] Histologically, there is nodular calcium, surface fibrin thrombi in a paucicellular fibrous matrix. This lesion should not be confused with calcifying fibrous (pseudo)tumor, which may occur on the pleural surfaces and, rarely, the pericardium.[103]

Infectious cysts, such as hydatid or echinococcal cysts, must be considered in the differential diagnosis of cardiac cystic masses, and are relatively common in endemic areas of developing countries. Blood cysts of the tricuspid and mitral valve are common incidental findings at infant autopsy. Rarely, they may persist and achieve a size of several centimeters, resulting in tricuspid stenosis. They are dark red, thin-walled unicavitary cysts that on microscopic examination are simple endothelial lined cysts filled with blood and may represent varicosities of veins around the fossa ovalis.

Amyloid tumors are rare masses that may occur in the heart, generally the atria. They presumably have a similar relationship to plasmacytoma and risk for development of multiple myeloma as amyloidomas in other soft tissue sites.[104,105] We have encountered amyloid tumors that are composed of transthyretin-derived amyloid. Although their rarity precludes generalization, cardiac amyloid tumors are not associated with cardiac amyloidosis, partly by definition. In order to be considered an amyloid tumor, the lesion should come to attention because of a mass lesion in the absence of hemodynamic changes of cardiomyopathy.

Miscellaneous soft tissue neoplasms/endocrine tumors

A variety of benign neoplasms of soft tissue may occur in the heart, with pathologic features identical to their more common soft tissue counterparts. Cardiac paragangliomas usually present in the atria or on the epicardial surfaces; 50% are functional, causing hypertension, resulting in the designation 'cardiac pheochromocytoma'.[106–108] They occasionally have a malignant course.[109] Neurofibromas and schwannomas may occur within the myocardium, causing ventricular outflow obstruction. Encapsulated cardiac lipomas are usually epicardial tumors and asymptomatic; rare examples are large and multiple, necessitating surgical removal. Inflammatory pseudotumors (inflammatory myofibroblastic tumors) are low-grade lesions, which may represent neoplasms of myofibroblastic derivation, that occur rarely in the heart, often as endocardial-based masses.[110–112] They may be associated with hypergammaglobulinemia and fever, and usually occur in children and young adults. We have seen examples extend into the coronary ostia, resulting in ischemic symptoms and sudden cardiac death. The utility of ALK-1 immunohistochemical staining in corroborating the diagnosis of inflammatory myofibroblastic tumor of the heart has yet to be demonstrated.

MALIGNANT CARDIAC TUMORS

Cardiac sarcomas

Virtually all types of sarcoma have been shown to arise within the heart. Cardiac sarcomas represent 10% of surgically resected cardiac tumors, second to cardiac myxomas (Table 20.7). Because more than half of cardiac sarcomas are located in the left atrium, the most common presenting symptom is dyspnea secondary to left ventricular inflow obstruction. Other modes of presentation for cardiac sarcoma include pericardial tamponade, especially if there is extensive pericardial involvement, embolic phenomena, chest pain, syncope, fever of unknown origin, and peripheral edema. Distant metastases commonly develop in patients with primary cardiac sarcoma and are sometimes the presenting symptom. Metastatic sites are most

Table 20.7 Surgically resected cardiac sarcomas: incidence and location of histologic subtypes

Histologic type	n	Mean age, years	Age range, years	Male: Female	Left atrium, %	Right atrium, %
Angiosarcoma	68	43	15–80	46:22	5	85
Unclassified	56	42	0–77	29:27	58	14
Malignant fibrous histiocytoma	34	44	12–86	13:21	84	8
Leiomyosarcoma	24	35	1–69	13:11	75	8
Rhabdomyosarcoma	11	22	0–63	5:6	41	21
Myxoid fibrosarcoma	15	40	2–66	3:12	80	5
Fibrosarcoma	11	44	2–68	5:6	40	0
Osteosarcoma	15	33	16–67	7:8	100	0
Synovial sarcoma	6	39	30–48	5:1	33	17
Liposarcoma	2	67	64–70	1:1	0	100
Malignant peripheral nerve sheath tumor	2	52	48–55	2:0	0	0
Totals	244	42	0–80	129:115	50	30

Data from references 77, 114, 226, 230–233, 236, 237.

commonly lungs, followed by vertebrae, liver, brain, bowel, long bones, spleen, adrenal, and skull.[113]

The intracardiac location of sarcomas has some effect on the histologic subtype. In general, angiosarcomas are right-sided tumors that often infiltrate the pericardium and metastasize to the lungs early in the course of disease. The most common location of cardiac sarcomas other than angiosarcoma is the left atrium. The gross and imaging characteristics of left atrial sarcomas often mimic those of cardiac myxoma, and the clinical diagnosis is frequently that of a benign tumor. The vast majority of left atrial sarcomas demonstrate predominantly myofibroblastic differentiation, and there is frequently a myxoid background that may lead to the erroneous pathologic diagnosis of myxoma. These sarcomas are often varieties of malignant fibrous histiocytoma, myxoid fibrosarcoma, or unclassifiable sarcomas with areas of fibrous differentiation; rarely, the histologic and immunohistochemical profile is that of leiomyosarcoma. Malignant osteoid and areas of chondrosarcoma are not rare in left atrial sarcomas and may therefore be classified as osteo- or chondrosarcoma. Rhabdomyosarcomas of the heart are rare, and have no predilection for a particular site.

The prognosis of cardiac sarcomas is poor and generally measured in months. Pathologic grading of cardiac sarcomas is similar to soft tissue sarcomas[114] and histologic features such as necrosis and mitotic rate have shown some correlation with survival.[113] Both chemotherapy and radiation therapy[115] have been used for the treatment of cardiac sarcoma, in conjunction with surgical removal. Heart transplantation is an option if metastatic disease is not present at the time of diagnosis.[116,117]

The classification of cardiac sarcoma follows that of soft tissue sarcoma, with one exception. The term 'myxosarcoma' has occasionally been used to described a subset of cardiac sarcomas that typically occur in the left atrium and are initially diagnosed clinically and even pathologically as myxoma.[118] It is best to avoid the term 'myxosarcoma' and use terms established for sarcomas of the soft tissue, such as myxoid fibrosarcoma and myxoid malignant fibrous histiocytoma. The existence of a malignant form of cardiac myxoma is controversial; most, if not all cases of malignant transformation of cardiac myxoma represent myxoid sarcomas, especially myxoid chondrosarcomas, that were initially misdiagnosed as myxoma.

Cardiac lymphomas

Cardiac lymphomas are distinctly rare but may be encountered by the surgical pathologist as resected lesions apparently localized to the heart.[119–121] Approximately one-third of newly reported cardiac lymphomas occur in immunosuppressed patients.[122] Virtually all lymphomas that have been reported in the heart are B-cell in origin, and are most frequently large cell lymphomas, although a wide variety of lesions, including Burkitt's lymphoma, have been reported.[121,123] Those lymphomas occurring in immunosuppressed patients may evolve through a polyclonal proliferation of B-cells (post-transplant lymphoproliferative disorder); these precursor lesions may be difficult to distinguish from severe transplant rejection, and are related to Epstein–Barr virus infection.

Metastatic cardiac tumors

Approximately 35% of excised cardiac masses are metastatic tumors removed for palliation, often because of obstruction of atrial inflow or ventricular outflow. The most common cardiac sites are the right ventricle and right atrium, followed by the left atrium and ventricular septum. Virtually all types of malignancy have been surgically excised from the myocardium, including carcinomas of a variety of primary sites. There is an increased frequency of unusual or slow-growing metastases resected from the heart, including soft tissue sarcomas, skeletal sarcomas, endocrine tumors, and malignant melanoma. In the case of right atrial masses, the surgical pathologist should consider metastatic hepatocellular carcinomas and renal cell carcinomas that have extended from the inferior vena cava.

SURGICAL PATHOLOGY OF THE PERICARDIUM

INDICATIONS FOR TISSUE SAMPLING

Pericardial effusions

The majority of isolated pericardial effusions result from acute pericarditis. In hospitalized patients, the most common cause of pericardial effusions resulting in tamponade is malignancy, followed by radiation pericarditis, viral pericarditis, collagen vascular disease, uremia, and idiopathic pericarditis.

The indications for pericardiocentesis are generally for diagnostic purposes and for therapeutic relief of pericardial tamponade. *Subxiphoid pericardiotomy* is usually performed under local anesthesia, an incision is made in the apical pericardium excising a small amount of tissue, and a catheter is placed for gravity drainage. To increase the diagnostic yield when pericardiocentesis is performed for malignancy and granulomatous disease, percutaneous pericardial biopsy has been advocated, using bioptomes for bronchoscopic and endomyocardial biopsy under fluoroscopic guidance, with the use of flexible fiberoptic endoscopes. *Partial or limited pericardiectomy* is removal at thoracotomy of a portion of anterior pericardium/left parietal pleura, resulting in drainage to the left hemithorax. The term *pericardial* or *pleuropericardial window* is usually applied to partial pericardiectomy but has also been used for subxiphoid pericardiotomy (*subxiphoid pericardial window*). In general, therapeutic options for draining pericardial fluid include pericardiocentesis, pleuropericardial window, subxiphoid pericardial drainage, and pericardioscopy.[124]

Pericardial constriction

Constrictive pericarditis is defined by fibrotic thickening of the pericardium that results in obliteration of the pericardial space and restriction of diastolic filling. The most common cause of constrictive pericarditis is idiopathic pericarditis, which may be characterized by a protracted clinical course lasting decades. Other causes of pericardial constriction include radiation pericarditis, postsurgical pericarditis, chronic renal failure treated with hemodialysis, connective tissue diseases, neoplasms, purulent and other forms of infectious pericarditis, and myocardial infarction.

Constrictive pericarditis is generally treated by *complete pericardiectomy*, which involves removal of pericardium under general anesthesia from the right phrenic nerve to the left pulmonary veins, and from the great vessels to the mid-diaphragm.

NON-NEOPLASTIC PERICARDIAL DISEASE

Non-specific pericarditis

In most cases of pericarditis resulting in effusions or pericardial constriction, there are no specific histologic findings pointing to an etiologic diagnosis. An etiology for most cases of non-specific pericarditis is never found, leading to an ultimate diagnosis of idiopathic pericarditis. The histopathologic findings of idiopathic pericarditis include fibrin deposition and a mixed inflammatory infiltrate in early stages (Fig. 20.20), progressing to scarring. Hemosiderin deposits and cholesterol crystals may also be prominent histologic features. Most diagnostic biopsies are taken for the relief of pericardial constriction after chronic changes, including mesothelial proliferation and fibrosis, have occurred.

Pericarditis caused by uremia and autoimmune diseases generally result in non-specific histologic changes similar to those of idiopathic pericarditis. Hematoxylin bodies, lupus cells (LE cells) may occasionally be seen in lupus pericarditis, rheumatoid granulomas are only occasionally found in pericarditis of rheumatoid arthritis, and perivascular deposits of complement and immunoglobulins may be demonstrated by immunofluorescence in cases of pericarditis associated with lupus, rheumatoid arthritis, scleroderma, and mixed connective tissue diseases.

The major diagnostic problem confronting the surgical pathologist is the distinction between reactive mesothelial hyperplasia in cases of idiopathic pericarditis and metastatic carcinoma. Stains for mucin are helpful to exclude the presence of intracytoplasmic lumina diagnostic of adenocarcinoma. Immunohistochemical panels for carcinoembryonic antigen, calretinin, B72.3 antigen and leu-M1 are markers employed as in the distinction between mesothelial hyperplasia and carcinoma in the pleura. In our experience, BerEP4 and related antigens are not helpful, as they are often expressed in reactive mesothelial cells in the pericardium.

Cholesterol pericarditis

Cholesterol pericarditis is classically associated with the pericardial effusions in patients with myxedema, and patients with hypercholesterolemia may be at increased risk for the development of cholesterol pericarditis. Cholesterol crystals surrounding chronic infiltrates have been described in various types of pericarditis, including tuberculosis, postinfarction, and rheumatoid pericarditis. The majority of patients with cholesterol pericarditis, however, have no known predisposing cause and suffer from a form of idiopathic pericarditis. Grossly, the pericardial fluid in patients with cholesterol pericarditis has glittering gold appearance.

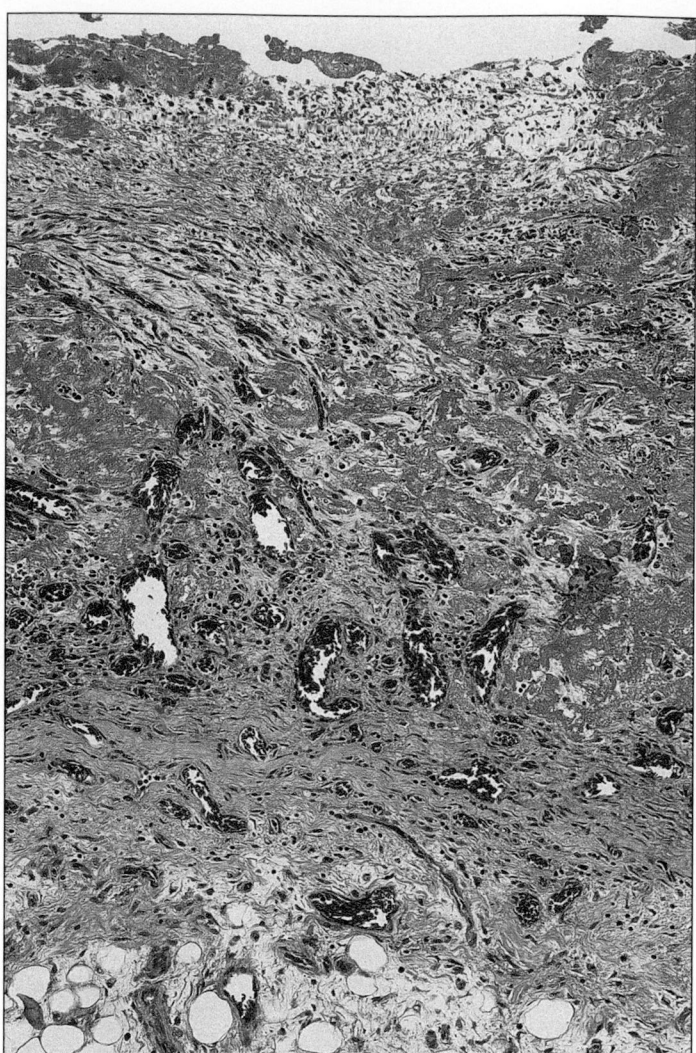

Figure 20.20   Fibrinous pericarditis. Note the granulation tissue, prominent vascularity, chronic inflammation and surface fibrin. The etiology of many cases of fibrinous pericarditis is unknown.

Calcific pericarditis

In surgical series of pericardial resections for constriction, approximately 40% of patients will demonstrate pericardial calcification.[125] Most cases of calcific pericarditis are idiopathic and are associated with a protracted clinical course. Calcification rarely complicates pericarditis of specific etiology, including rheumatoid pericarditis, postoperative pericarditis, uremic pericarditis in patients on dialysis, and rheumatic pericarditis. Pathologically, the pericardium is markedly thickened as a result of dense fibrosis involving both the pericardial and visceral layers. Histologically, there are diffuse layers or nodules of calcification of the parietal pericardium, generally with involvement of the epicardium (Fig. 20.21).

Mycobacterial pericarditis

Tuberculous pericarditis occurs in 1% of patients with active tuberculosis; approximately 4% of cases of acute pericarditis are due to tuberculosis. Virtually all patients with pericardial tuberculosis develop constrictive pericarditis without treatment. Because of the high risk of constrictive pericarditis, early pericardiectomy has been

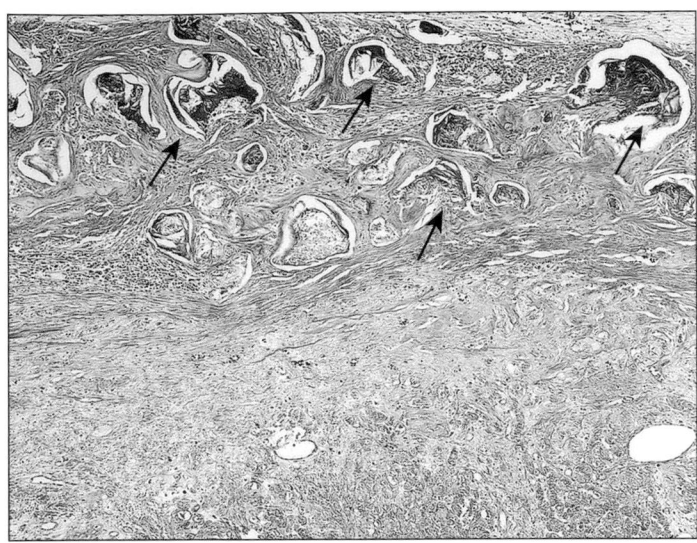

Figure 20.21 Calcific pericarditis. Fibrinous pericarditis of virtually any etiology may progress to fibrosing constrictive pericarditis which may calcify. Note masses of calcium (arrows) with intervening collagen overlying surface of the myocardium.

recommended in all patients with tuberculous pericarditis, although medical management is effective in many cases.[126] Between 30% and 75% of cultures of pericardial fluid will demonstrate positive growth; the positive culture rate is greater if cultures are taken early in the course of disease and if a portion of pericardial tissue is submitted for culture. Acid-fast stains of pericardial fluid are notoriously unrewarding. The demonstration of necrotizing granulomas on pericardial biopsy is virtually diagnostic in the appropriate clinical setting, even in the absence of demonstrable acid-fast bacilli. The characteristics of the granuloma range from large, necrotic areas of liquefactive necrosis with few or no granulomas to compact aggregates of macrophages with little necrosis.

Purulent pericarditis

Bacterial pericarditis (excluding mycobacteria) represents less than 5% of acute pericarditis. The most frequent pathogens causing purulent pericarditis are streptococci, and less commonly Gram-negative rods. A wide variety of rare pathogens have been isolated from pericardial fluid in immunosuppressed and postoperative patients with pericarditis. Risk factors for the development of bacterial pericarditis are chronic illness and immunocompromised states, postoperative infection, chronic renal failure, malignancy, diabetes mellitus, and myeloproliferative diseases. In over 95% of patients, a primary infective site is found, including pneumonia, bacterial endocarditis, pleuritis, otitis media, meningitis, and skin infections. Pathologically, there are usually sheets of neutrophils with abundant fibrin deposition. The degree of neutrophilic infiltration is generally greater than that seen in acute autoimmune or viral pericarditis; a tissue Gram stain may demonstrate intracytoplasmic organisms. In chronic organizing purulent pericarditis, the histologic findings are non-specific and consist of organizing fibrin, fibrosis, and granulation tissue.

Sarcoidal pericarditis

Pericardial involvement occurs in 3% of patients with sarcoidosis at autopsy. Occasionally, sarcoidosis may result in pericardial tamponade or pericardial constriction. Grossly, there is studding of the pericardial surfaces with pericardial adhesions in symptomatic pericardial sarcoidosis. Histologically, noncaseating granulomas are present In small biopsies, the distinction between sarcoid and tuberculosis may be impossible and definitive diagnosis depends on results on culture and clinical findings.

Radiation pericarditis

Pericardial effusions occur in approximately 20% of patients following radiation therapy, and are usually transient. Constrictive pericarditis occurs less commonly, at a time interval ranging from several months to 45 years (mean 7 years). The most common antecedent tumor is Hodgkin's disease, followed by non-Hodgkin's lymphoma and carcinoma of the lung.

Features of acute radiation pericarditis include atypical fibroblasts, endothelial cell proliferation, and fibrinous pericarditis. In later stages of radiation pericarditis, there is vascular thickening, which consists primarily of medial hypertrophy and intimal proliferation, and diffuse fibrosis. The parietal pericardium is generally affected to a greater degree than the visceral pericardium.

Radiation-induced changes may be superimposed on the findings of recurrent tumor. If pericardial symptoms occur years after radiation in patients with a history of lymphoma or in patients with breast cancer in remission, radiation-induced pericarditis is the likely diagnosis. Recurrent tumor generally causes large effusions, in contrast to fibrosis and constrictive pericarditis, and is usually not isolated to the pericardium.[127,128]

Miscellaneous pericardial lesions

Occasionally, reactive fibroinflammatory masses may be encountered in the pericardium. In these cases, in infectious process (e.g. *Actinomycetes*, tuberculosis) or non-specific processes (e.g. sclerosing mediastinitis) should be considered and excluded by appropriate special stains and clinical evaluation. Rarely, histiocytic proliferations, such as Chester–Erdheim disease, may present as pericardial masses that are clinically suspicious for metastasis.[129] In such cases, immunohistochemical staining for CD1a, factor XIIIa, S100 protein, and macrophage markers are useful in the differential diagnosis, as well as skeletal survey to document the characteristic bony lesions. Other hematologic processes that may occur in the pericardium and should be included in the differential diagnosis of inflammatory pericardial lesions are Castleman's disease, and, very rarely, Hodgkin's lymphoma.

NEOPLASTIC PERICARDIAL DISEASE

Metastatic carcinoma

Pericardial tamponade is a frequent complication of pericardial metastases and has been reported for a large number of tumor types. Pericardial fluid in patients with malignant tamponade is usually hemorrhagic; accumulations are typically 500–1000 ml. Effusions in cancer patients may be idiopathic or secondary to radiation or chemotherapy. In patients with breast cancer, small, asymptomatic effusions are probably benign and, of those that are clinically apparent, only one-half are malignant

Of tumors that metastasize to the pericardium, the most common site of origin is the lung; of lung tumors, large cell or adenocarcinomas are the most common histologic types. A surprisingly high percentage of malignant pericardial biopsies occur in patients in whom the diagnosis of malignancy has not yet been made clinically. Most adenocarcinomas presenting as pericardial metastases originate either in the lung or an undetermined primary site. Breast carcinoma, unlike lung carcinoma, usually manifests as pericardial disease only after the primary site is known.[130]

The sensitivity of cytologic examination in the diagnosis of malignant pericardial effusions ranges from 50–95%, and averages 87%.[131] High rates of false-negative cytology are associated with pericardial lymphoma and mesothelioma. The additional diagnostic sensitivity achieved by biopsy in addition to cytologic examination is small. Routine immunohistochemical staining to differentiate adenocarcinomas from reactive mesothelial proliferations is useful in cell block specimens. Pericardial biopsy may be negative in the face of positive cytology, presumably because of tissue sampling error; the converse is distinctly less common.

Malignant mesothelioma

Pericardial mesotheliomas represent approximately 0.7% of malignant mesotheliomas.[77] Cardiac tamponade is unusual at the time of presentation but often develops during the course of disease. The pericardial cavity may be obliterated by tumor, explaining the lack of fluid at pericardiocentesis in some cases. Repeated pericardiocentesis may be necessary before the diagnosis of malignancy is made, because of non-specific cytologic findings. With adequate tissue sampling, most pericardial mesotheliomas are biphasic. The epithelial component of tubules, papillary structures, and cords of infiltrating cells with a desmoplastic response typically predominates.

Primary pericardial sarcomas

The most common sarcoma that arises within the pericardium is angiosarcoma. Grossly, angiosarcomas may diffusely infiltrate the pericardium but, unlike mesothelioma, typically form variegated hemorrhagic masses. The diagnosis may be missed on repeated pericardial biopsy because there is often marked reactive mesothelial hyperplasia. In practice, it may be difficult to determine the precise primary site of angiosarcomas of the heart and pericardium because of diffuse infiltration of both structures.

Other mesenchymal neoplasms arising within the pericardial space include localized (solitary) fibrous tumors (hemangiopericytomas) and synovial sarcomas. The latter diagnosis is confirmed by the chromosomal translocation (x;18), which can be determined on RNA extracted from paraffin-embedded tissue. Localized fibrous tumors and synovial sarcomas may also involve the myocardium.

PERICARDIAL CYSTS

Mesothelial cysts

Mesothelial cysts are considered to represent pericardial diverticula, in which the site of communication with the pericardium is no longer intact. Surgical management has been recommended for patients with symptoms of chest pain, dyspnea, or airway obstruction, or if the mass is increasing in size. Mesothelial cysts of the pericardium are usually unilocular, thin-walled, and translucent, ranging in diameter from 2–16 cm. The cysts contain clear fluid and are lined by a flattened, single layer of mesothelial cells and, occasionally, hyperplastic mesothelial cells. The cyst wall is made up of connective tissue rich in collagen with scattered elastic fibers.

Bronchogenic cyst

Bronchogenic or enteric cysts located within the pericardium are rare. At the time of diagnosis, approximately one-third of patients are infants and one half are over the age of 15. Bronchogenic cysts in infants are often symptomatic, whereas those in adults are generally incidental findings. Intrapericardial bronchogenic cysts are located on the epicardial surface over the right side of the heart, and are 1–3 cm in diameter. Microscopically, the cyst lining is ciliated columnar or cuboidal epithelium, often resembling ciliated respiratory epithelium. Both goblet cells and squamous epithelium may be present. The wall of the cyst generally contains a wall of smooth muscle and cartilage; lymphoid nodules, seromucinous glands, gastric mucosa, and pancreatic tissue are variably present. Unlike teratomas, which rarely occur in the pericardium, bronchogenic cysts lack ectodermal elements, such as hair, teeth, or neural tissue.

DISEASES OF BLOOD VESSELS

SURGICAL PATHOLOGY OF ATHEROSCLEROSIS

Atherosclerotic aneurysm

The majority of atherosclerotic aneurysms occur in the abdominal aorta distal to the renal arteries; most of the remainder occur in the iliac, femoral, and popliteal arteries and ascending aorta. A large number of splenic artery aneurysms demonstrate calcification and atherosclerosis, although these changes may be secondary. The major risk factors for the development of atherosclerotic aneurysms are hypertension and cigarette smoking, although many atherosclerotic aneurysms occur in patients with neither risk factor. The etiology of atherosclerotic aneurysms is multifactorial, and there are associations with hereditary factors, increased collagenase and elastase activity, and alpha-1-antitrypsin deficiency. Atherosclerotic aneurysms are most common in Caucasian males. Unfortunately, patients are usually asymptomatic until there is rupture, which results in back and abdominal pain, hypovolemic shock, or sudden death. In patients with aneurysms measuring larger than 5 cm, rupture occurs at a rate of 25% at 5 years.[132]

Grossly, atherosclerotic aneurysms are partly filled with laminated yellow-brown thrombus. Generally, the surgeon will leave the aneurysm in place while performing a bypass, and the pathologist will receive luminal thrombus in one or multiple pieces. Histologic examination will demonstrate severe atherosclerosis of adjacent aorta, destruction of elastic lamellae, and smooth muscle cell atrophy. Calcification is common, and there is luminal thrombus with little organization.

Penetrating atherosclerotic ulcer

In contrast to atherosclerotic aneurysms, atherosclerotic ulcers generally occur in the descending thoracic aorta, penetrate the elastic lamellae and result in hematoma formation within the aortic wall. Most patients are elderly, hypertensive, and suffer from severe atherosclerosis and frequently abdominal aneurysms. Clinically, the sudden onset of severe chest or back pain mimics classic aortic dissection, but contrast-enhanced computed tomography shows intramural hematoma, focal ulcer, displaced intimal calcification, and a thick or enhancing aortic wall in the absence of a double lumen as seen in dissection. Histologically, there is a discrete ulcer crater with atherosclerotic plaque and mural hemorrhage. There may be focal dissection of blood within the media but it is limited to 1–2 cm or less. Because of the risk of rupture and hemothorax, which has been said to be even higher than with typical aortic dissections,[133] surgical repair or endoluminal graft stenting is usually undertaken.

Coronary atherectomy and endarterectomy

Atherectomy, or the percutaneous removal of plaque at the time of catheterization and ballooning procedures, is now only rarely performed in the coronary arteries, because stenting is the current preferred method of enlarging the lumen of diseased vessels. In contrast, endarterectomy is the intraoperative removal of athero-sclerotic plaque, and is occasionally performed at the time of bypass graft surgery enabling diffusely diseased, inoperable arteries to be grafted. The histologic features of coronary endarterectomy that should be described in the surgical pathologic report are similar to those of carotid endarterectomy (see next section). Removal of media is generally avoided in surgical endarterectomy, and the presence of media should be carefully evaluated by the pathologist.

Carotid endarterectomy

Symptomatic carotid artery disease is usually located at the carotid sinus and at the origin of the internal carotid artery. Primary carotid endarterectomy is performed in patients with a history of transient ischemic attacks and in asymptomatic patients with severe stenosis. Most surgeons remove the carotid plaques from the common carotid artery bifurcation along with 10–15 mm of the internal and, if necessary, the external carotid artery. Some specimens are excised as a single large piece through a single incision along the lateral aspect of the carotid artery, but the pathologist often receives multiple or two/three pieces of plaque. Specimen X-rays allow the identification of calcification and may help determine the degree of luminal narrowing. Following decalcification, which is often necessary, the specimen is cut transversely at 3–4 mm intervals, identifying on the cassettes if possible the bifurcation, internal, external, and common carotid arteries. These efforts may identify the source of the embolus or the plaque characteristics that gave rise to the symptoms.[134] The pathologist should report the presence of calcification, necrotic atheroma, hemorrhage into plaque, plaque rupture, ulceration, and thrombosis. Asymptomatic patients with more than 75% stenosis and morphologically soft plaques are at risk of transient ischemic attack or stroke. The presence of plaque hemorrhage and thrombosis is more frequent in symptomatic patients than asymptomatic patients.

Plaque morphology of recurrent carotid disease is dependent on the time interval between primary and reoperative endarterectomy. Lesions that recur within 36 months are characterized by smooth muscle cells in a proteoglycan matrix (Fig. 20.22), and intralesional and surface thrombi are extremely common. Late recurrent lesions have features of disorganized atherosclerosis (foam cells, cholesterol clefts, dense collagen, and calcification) with pultaceous debris without a fibrous cap; thrombi tend to show organization with neovascularization.

There are several pathologic features of carotid endarterectomy that correlate with clinical presentation (Table 20.8). Severely calcified carotid plaques are less likely to be symptomatic than those with mild or moderate calcification.[135] Characteristics associated with plaque instability and thrombosis include ulceration, inflammation, large necrotic core, thin fibrous cap, and hemorrhage, similar to coronary arteries.[136] Rupture of the fibrous cap in carotid artery lesions is associated with increased numbers of macrophages and activated T lymphocytes.[137] Pathologic findings that should be mentioned in histologic evaluation of carotid endarterectomies have been recently reviewed, and include plaque hemorrhage, calcification, the presence of foam cells within a fibrous cap, intraplaque fibrin, luminal thrombus, and the presence of smooth muscle cell-rich areas.[134]

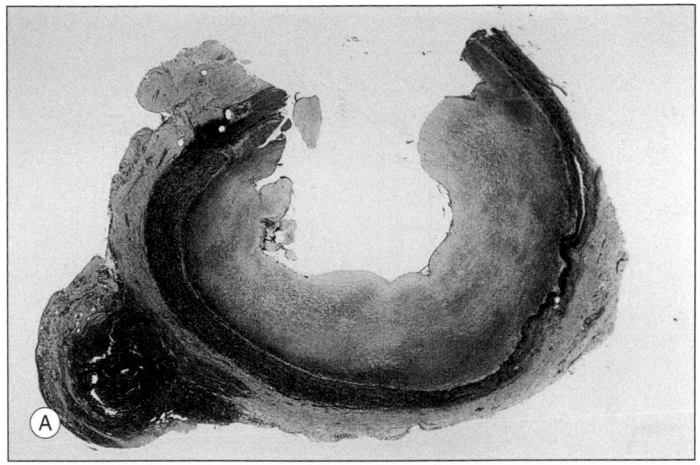

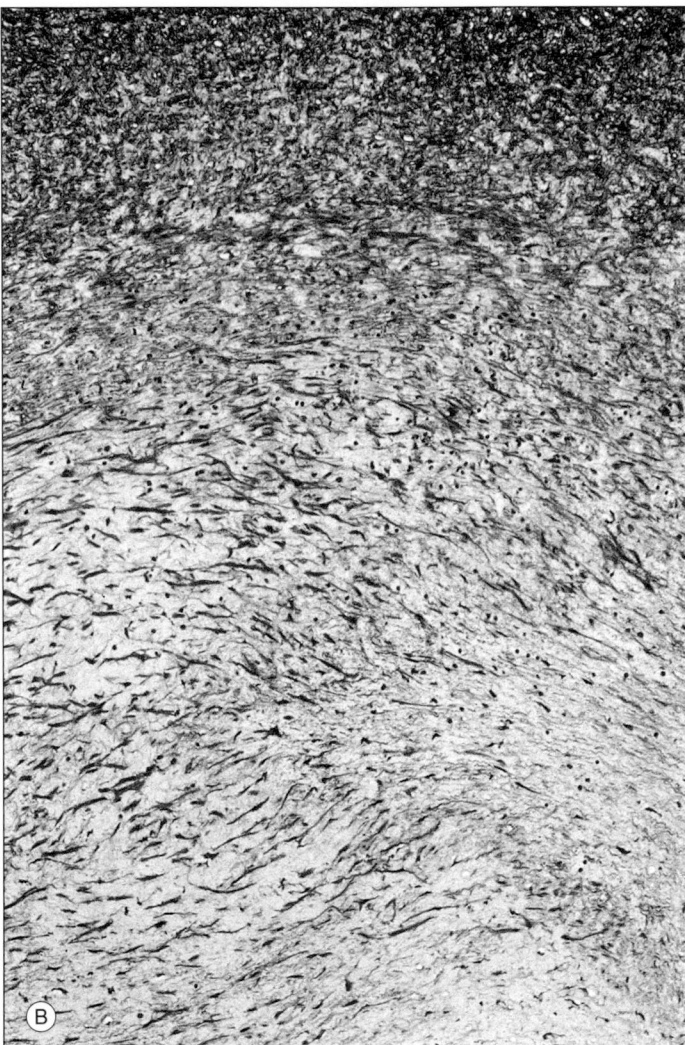

Figure 20.22 Restenosis lesion, carotid artery. **(A)** Low magnification of artery resected 6 months after carotid endarterectomy. **(B)** Restenosis is characterized by a proliferation of smooth muscle cells in a proteoglycan matrix.

Table 20.8 Gross and microscopic plaque characteristics in symptomatic and asymptomatic patients undergoing carotid endarterectomy

Gross morphology	Symptomatic, % (n = 25)	Asymptomatic, % (n = 17)	P value
% stenosis (duplex)	74 ± 17	77 ± 15	ns
Ulceration	94	64	0.02
Plaque hemorrhage	47	52	ns
Microscopic characteristics			
Plaque rupture	74	32	0.004
Thin fibrous cap	95	48	0.003
Cap foam cells	84	44	0.006
Intraplaque fibrin	100	68	0.008
Intraplaque hemorrhage.	84	56	0.06
Necrotic core	84	72	ns
Ulceration	11	8	ns
Calcified nodule	7	7	ns
Thrombus	63	80	ns
SMC-rich area	5	0	ns
Eccentric shape	68	64	ns

With permission from Virmani R, Kolodgie F, Farb A, Burke AP. Pathologic evaluation of carotid endarterectomy. Pathol Case Rev 2001; 6: 241.

Saphenous vein bypass grafts

Approximately 8–12% of saphenous vein grafts will occlude prior to hospital discharge. By 1 year, 12–20% of vein grafts will become occluded from fibrointimal proliferation and superimposed thrombosis or from thrombosis alone. Beyond 1 year, the histologic appearance is that of atherosclerotic disease, which is seen in over 70% of vein grafts examined histologically. The vein graft atherosclerosis is characterized by a large number of foam cells, necrotic core, cholesterol clefts, and a thin, delicate fibrous cap, which may or may not be ruptured with or without superimposed thrombosis.[138] By 10 years, at least 50% of vein grafts that were patent at 5 years will have become occluded. The attrition rate for vein grafts between 6 and 11 years after operation increases to 4% per year. Because of high occlusion rates from atherosclerotic disease in vein grafts, as well as progression of native coronary disease and incomplete revascular-

ization, approximately 6–10% of coronary artery surgery procedures are reoperations.

The surgeon often elects to remove the occluded vein graft during the reoperation and vein graft is sent for pathologic examination. It is recommended that the diameter and length of the graft be measured and the graft be cut at 3–4 mm intervals transversely after decalcification, if necessary. The pathologist should report the extent of severest narrowing (% cross-sectional area narrowing) and the nature of the intimal plaque (foam-cell-rich, necrotic core with cholesterol clefts, extent and type of inflammation, hemorrhage, and superimposed thrombus). Prominent development of the internal elastic lamina has been described as the arterialization of the vein graft. Because of the large amount of lipid typically present in vein graft atherosclerosis, stenting is accompanied by a high rate of embolization. Occasionally, the surgeon with remove the stented vein graft and send it for pathologic examination. In such cases, the specimen should be evaluated in a reference laboratory where plastic embedding is available to section metallic prostheses, or where stents can be carefully removed prior to paraffin embedding

VASCULITIS INVOLVING ELASTIC ARTERIES

A classification of vasculitis which involves elastic and muscular arteries is given in Table 20.9.

Giant cell arteritis

Giant cell arteritis is the most common vasculitic syndrome and affects muscular and elastic arteries. A granulomatous inflammation of muscular and elastic arteries, giant cell arteritis usually affects cranial vessels in older individuals. There is overlap with the clinical syndrome polymyalgia rheumatica (shoulder and pelvic pain and stiffness, fever, and elevated erythrocyte sedimentation rate).[139,140] The etiology of giant cell arteritis is unknown, and may involve a cell-mediated T-cell-regulated granulomatous reaction. There is a female predominance, and most patients are over 50 years of age. New onset of localized headache, tenderness of temporal artery or decreased temporal artery pulse, and elevated Westergren erythrocyte sedimentation rate above 50 mm/h are typical clinical features. Polymyalgia rheumatica occurs in 50% of patients late in the disease course, but only a small fraction of patients with polymyalgia rheumatica develop temporal arteritis.[141]

Table 20.9 Classification of large vessel vasculitic syndromes

Type of vasculitis	Vessel type involved	Typical distribution	Inflammation	Necrosis	Features
Vasculitis involving elastic arteries					
Giant cell arteritis	Muscular, elastic	Cranial, aorta, visceral, iliofemoral	Chronic, usually with giant cells	Nonfibrinoid	Elastic lamellar destruction
Takayasu's disease	Elastic, occasionally muscular extension	Aorta, proximal branches	Chronic, usually with giant cells	Nonfibrinoid	Medial destruction, prominent inflammation of vasa vasorum, intimal and adventitial scarring
Vasculitis involving muscular arteries					
Kawasaki disease	Muscular	Coronary, visceral, others	Acute in initial phases, chronic	Only in initial stages	Aneurysm formation, luminal thrombus, concentric inflammation
Polyarteritis nodosa	Muscular	Visceral, renal	Acute, chronic	Fibrinoid	Segmental, with areas of healing

changes in the temporal artery itself did aid in the diagnosis[145]; other studies differ, indicating that small vessel inflammation is suggestive of a giant cell arteritis syndrome.[144,146] In general, necrotizing inflammation of branch vessels suggests a vasculitic syndrome other than giant cell arteritis, whereas significant lymphocytic infiltrates may be associated with a higher likelihood of giant cell arteritis.

The role of biopsy in the diagnosis of giant cell arteritis of the temporal artery has been debated, because many patients are treated empirically with steroids and because 25–50% of patients with presumed temporal arteritis will have negative biopsy results. Patients with positive biopsy are more likely to have headaches, jaw claudication, and prior polymyalgia rheumatica than patients with negative biopsies, and a negative biopsy may prompt the clinician to consider alternate diagnoses before instituting steroid therapy.[147] It has been recently concluded that biopsy is helpful in the appropriate clinical setting.[148]

Age-related changes of the temporal artery include mild fibrointimal proliferation and duplication of the internal elastic lamina, with or without medial calcification (Mönckeberg's medial calcification). Intimal proliferation resulting in more than 75% reduction of the luminal area or significant loss of the internal elastic lamina should raise the possibility of healed arteritis. In such cases, step sections of the artery are especially important to detect diagnostic areas. If not found, the surgical pathologist's diagnosis should be descriptive and mention that healed arteritis is in the differential diagnosis. Significant atherosclerosis is uncommon in the temporal artery and is characterized by eccentric fibrointimal proliferation, foam cells, cholesterol clefts, calcification, and a fibrous cap overlying pultaceous debris.

Rare forms of vasculitis that may involve the temporal artery include Buerger's disease, polyarteritis nodosa, Wegener's granulomatosis and rheumatoid vasculitis. Nonvasculitic processes that may present in temporal artery biopsies include amyloidosis, vascular calcinosis (typically present in patients with chronic renal failure and diabetes), and traumatic pseudoaneurysms.

Giant cell arteritis involves the aorta in 10–15% of patients, resulting in aortic arch syndrome, aortic aneurysms, aortic dissection, or aortic valve insufficiency. Microscopically, the inflammatory infiltrate consists of lymphocytes, plasma cells, histiocytes, and giant cells in areas of elastic lamellar disruption and fragmentation, most pronounced in the inner half of the aorta. Intimal and/or adventitial fibrosis is present but usually not to the degree seen in Takayasu's aortitis.

Upper extremity involvement with giant cell arteritis is the third most common site of presentation after the cranial arteries and aorta. Such cases of 'large vessel giant cell arteritis' have a relatively low rate of polymyalgia rheumatica and temporal involvement and an overrepresentation of the HLA-DRB1*0404 allele,[149] suggesting that giant cell arteritis may be a heterogeneous disorder. Other organs that may be affected by giant cell arteritis include the uterus and breast; in such cases, the diagnosis of systemic giant cell arteritis should be considered. Isolated giant cell/granulomatous arteritis has also been reported in the central nervous system, skin, lungs, and kidney. Visceral giant cell arteritis is an extremely rare condition involving small arteries and arterioles of the internal organs.

Takayasu's arteritis

Also known as aortic arch syndrome, pulseless disease, occlusive thromboaortopathy, and young female arteritis, Takayasu's disease affects the aortic arch in young women. The acute phase of illness is characterized by malaise, weakness, fever, night sweats, arthralgias, arthritis, myalgias, weight loss, pleuritic pain, and anorexia. The late

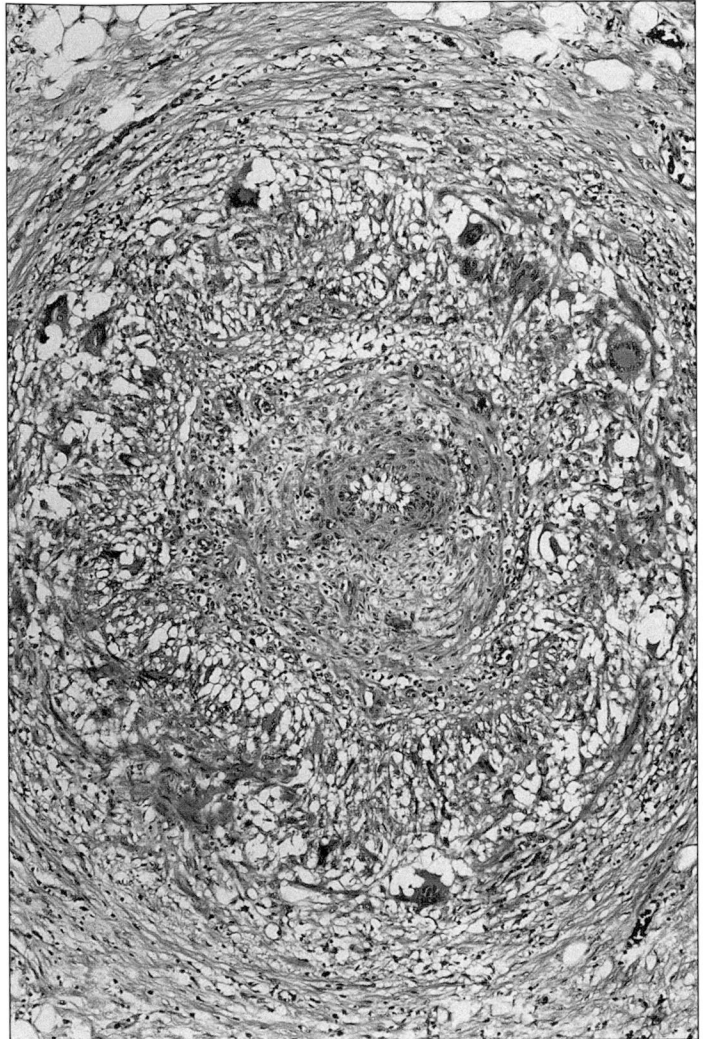

Figure 20.23 Giant cell arteritis. There is destruction of the media by a granulomatous infiltrate. Giant cells, as seen here, are present in 50% of cases.

The characteristic lesion is the destruction of the internal elastic lamina by a granulomatous infiltrate (Fig. 20.23). Despite the name, giant cells are present in only 50% of cases.[142] Lymphocytes and histiocytes are usually plentiful; eosinophils are sparse. Fibrointimal proliferation is common in healed stages. The diagnostic criteria of healed giant cell arteritis are debated, but any healed vasculitic syndrome is characterized by destruction of the elastica and medial fibrosis. In the case of giant cell arteritis, healed lesions generally have diffuse marked intimal thickening, often eccentric; intimal and medial fibrosis; loss of internal elastic lamina; adventitial scarring; and neovascularization of the scarred areas.[141] In the majority of such cases, macrophages will be identified in areas of elastic destruction. Histologic changes often decrease after treatment, but there is little correlation between histologic stage and history of steroid therapy. It is generally accepted that steroid treatment for up to 2 weeks does not increase the false negativity rate of biopsy.[143]

Not infrequently, lymphocytic infiltrates of branch vessels will be seen in temporal artery biopsies. The significance and incidence of such infiltrates is debated.[144–146] A large retrospective study concluded that perivascular infiltrates in the absence of diagnostic phase follows in weeks to months and is characterized by arterial occlusions resulting in absent pulses, bruits, hypertension, heart failure, and retinopathy. Aneurysms occur in 30% of patients and may result in pulsatile masses, embolism from mural thrombus, and rupture of aneurysm leading to hemothorax. Type I Takayasu's disease is characterized by involvement of the aortic arch and arch vessels, type II by disease of the descending thoracic and abdominal aorta, type III by involvement of all portions of the aorta, and type IV by concomitant disease of the pulmonary arteries.

The most common specimen the surgical pathologist will encounter is a fragment of aorta excised during aortic valve replacement in the case of ascending aortic aneurysms (see below, 'Approach to the surgical pathology of the ascending aorta'). Pathologically, there is marked fibrointimal proliferation and adventitial thickening, accompanied by intimal proliferation of smooth muscle cells in a myxoid, proteoglycan-rich background leading to stenoses[150] (Fig. 20.24). The elastica of the media is focally destroyed and replaced by fibrous tissue. The inflammatory infiltrate is mixed and may be accompanied by giant cells. There are no reliable histologic criteria separating Takayasu's disease from giant cell aortitis; however, patient age less than 50 years and presence of marked adventitial and intimal fibrosis, with prominent thickening of vasa vasorum, are more typical of Takayasu's disease than of giant cell arteritis.[151] Occasionally, inflammatory adventitial reactions to hemorrhage and dissections may be difficult to distinguish from aortitis. However, in these cases, inflammatory destruction of the media is absent.

VASCULITIS OF MUSCULAR ARTERIES

Polyarteritis nodosa

Polyarteritis nodosa is a systemic syndrome characterized by idiopathic inflammation of large and medium-sized muscular arteries. Clinical manifestations include weight loss, livedo reticularis, testicular pain or tenderness, myalgias and weakness, mononeuropathy or polyneuropathy, hypertension, and elevated creatinine. Hepatitis B surface antigenemia is present in less than 10% of patients. Patients with acute hepatitis B as an inciting event undergo remission only with antiviral treatment.[152,153] Arteriograms showing multiple visceral aneurysms are characteristic of polyarteritis nodosa. There is a rare association with antiphospholipid syndrome [154] and familial Mediterranean fever.[155]

Pathologically, lesions are limited to muscular arteries and arterioles; smaller vessels are not involved.[156,157] Affected vessels include testicular arteries, visceral arteries, and arteries of the lower extremities, other skeletal muscles, skin, kidneys, and liver. Lungs are involved in approximately 30% of patients at autopsy but clinical pulmonary involvement is rare.

Fibrinoid necrosis of muscular arteries (Fig. 20.25), which is often segmental, is the characteristic histologic feature of polyarteritis nodosa. Typically, other arteries in the same biopsy show healing lesions. Secondary changes include thrombosis and occlusive fibrointimal proliferation with infarction of the involved organ, and arterial aneurysms with or without rupture.

In biopsies of peripheral nerve and muscle, the only manifestations are inflammation of smaller arteries and arterioles. In nerve biopsies, a positive diagnosis confirms vasculitis as a cause of mononeuritis multiplex, peripheral motor and sensory nerve deficits that occur in a multifocal and random fashion, which is seen primarily in vasculitis or diabetic neuropathy.[158] The differential diagnosis of a positive biopsy in the setting of mononeuritis multiplex includes, in addition to polyarteritis nodosa, lupus, rheumatoid vasculitis, Wegener's

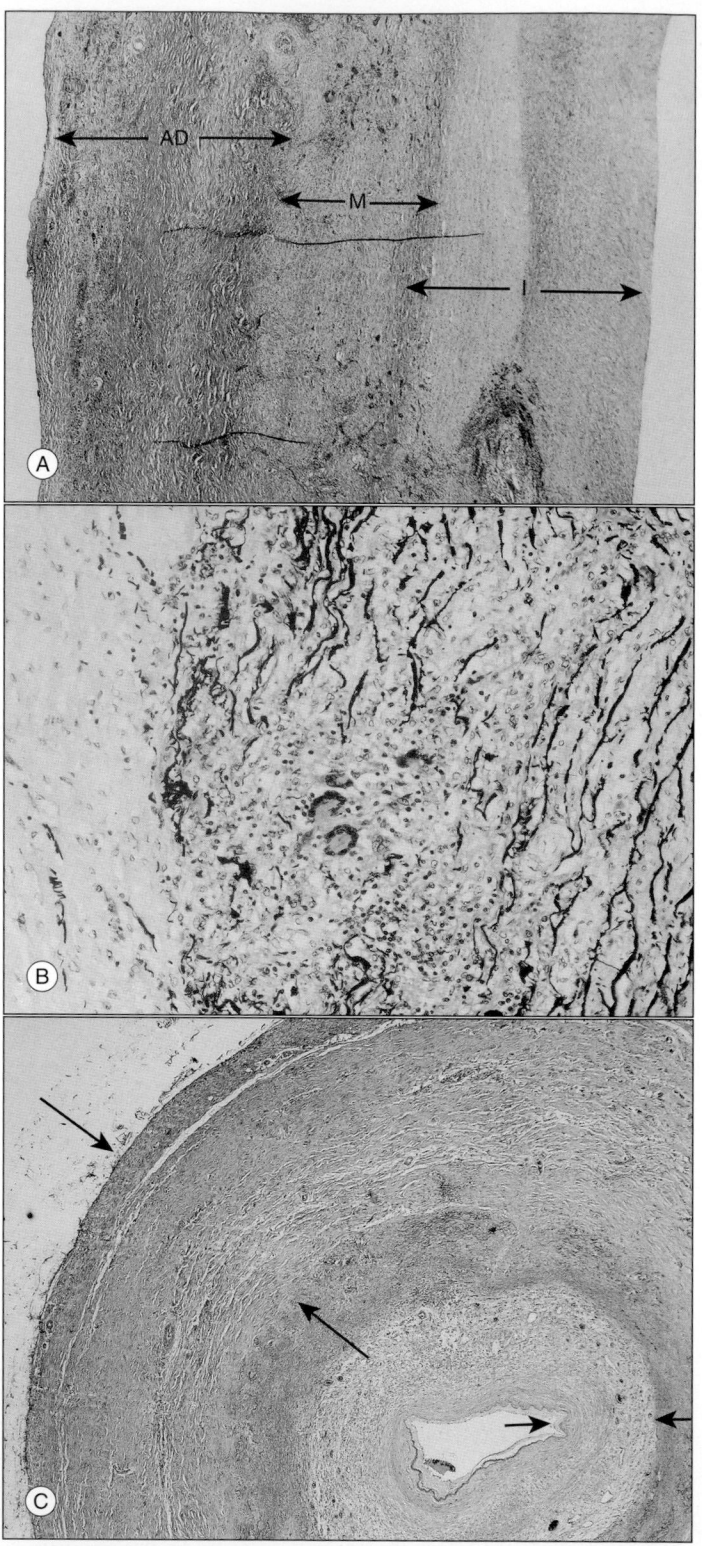

Figure 20.24 Takayasu's arteritis. **(A)** The healing phase demonstrates scarring with focal inflammation of the aorta. I = intima, M = media, and AD = adventitia. **(B)** In the acute stages, there is lymphoplasmacytic infiltrate with granulomatous destruction of aortic elastic laminae and giant cells may be present. **(C)** In healed stages, there is little inflammation and pronounced fibrosis of the intima (small arrows) and adventitia (large arrows) (subclavian artery).

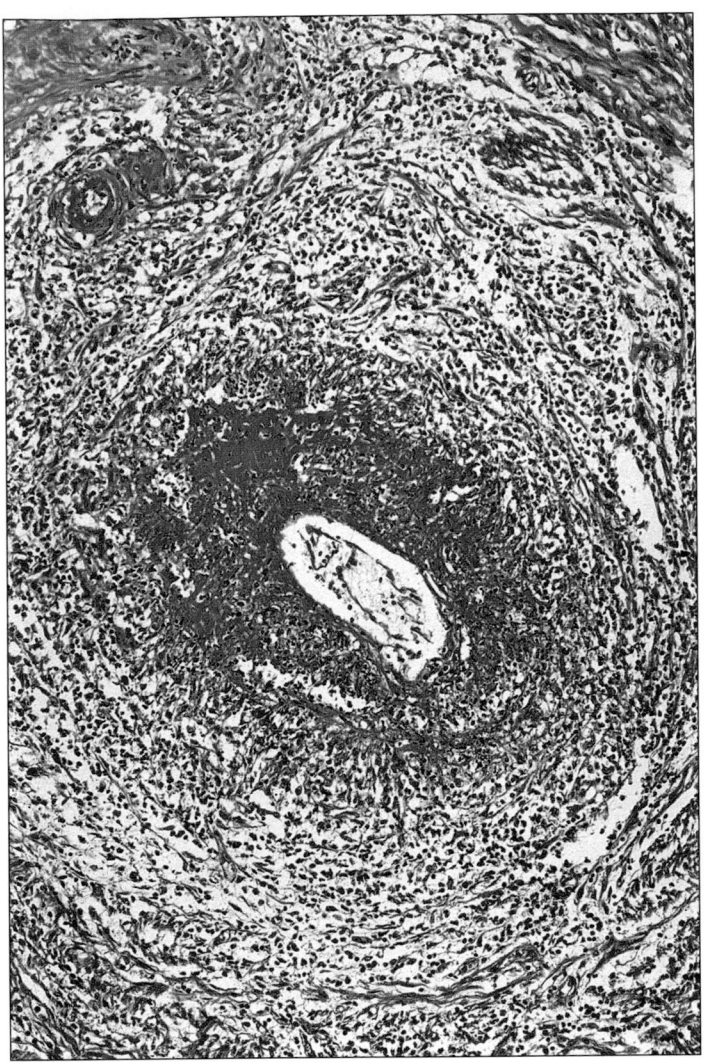

Figure 20.25 Polyarteritis nodosa. There is fibrinoid necrosis with surrounding inflammation destroying a vessel, which on step sections was demonstrated to be an artery.

granulomatosis, and microscopic polyangiitis. In muscle biopsies, inflammation of small arteries and arterioles is characteristic of polyarteritis nodosa, whereas arteriolar and capillary inflammation are more characteristic of mixed connective tissue disease vasculitis. Wegener's, rheumatoid, and lupus vasculitis may involve arteries and arterioles of all sizes.

The differential diagnosis of polyarteritis includes Wegener's granulomatosis, which is characterized by a higher incidence of antineutrophil cytoplasmic antibodies, more severe kidney involvement, prominent lung involvement, and the presence of extravascular necrotizing granulomas. In fact, necrotizing arteritis of muscular arteries may be a minor component of Wegener's granulomatosis. Churg–Strauss angiitis differs from polyarteritis nodosa in that there is generally a history of allergic symptoms and peripheral eosinophilia, veins may be involved, and extravascular granulomas with eosinophil breakdown products are present.

Localized forms of polyarteritis nodosa have been described in the bowel, gallbladder, pancreas, skeletal muscle, skin, testis, breast, uterus, and cervix.[159] Unlike classic polyarteritis nodosa, patients do not suffer from systemic illness, present with symptoms referable to a single organ, and are generally cured by removal of involved tissue. From a surgical pathologist's standpoint, localized necrotizing arteritis is more likely to be encountered than systemic polyarteritis nodosa, which is a rare disease diagnosed largely by clinical criteria. The estimated incidence is 2.5/100 000 adults in a Caucasian population.[160]

Kawasaki disease

Also known as mucocutaneous lymph node syndrome and infantile polyarteritis nodosa, Kawasaki disease is an idiopathic inflammatory disease that exclusively affects infants and children. Most cases are sporadic, although several American outbreaks have been described. The acute phase of illness is characterized by fever, rash, palmar and plantar erythema, conjunctivitis, fissuring of lips, oropharyngitis, and cervical lymphadenopathy. The latent phase is characterized by inflammatory and necrotizing lesions of muscular arteries, especially coronary arteries. Coronary artery aneurysms are present in 15–30% of patients after the acute phase of illness, and virtually all muscular arteries may be involved, including testicular, pulmonary, splenic, iliac, intercostal, mesenteric, renal, cerebral, axillary, pancreatic, and hepatic arteries.[161]

Histologically, affected arteries show in the acute phase thrombosis, medial destruction, fibrointimal proliferation, and aneurysmal dilatation. The inflammation may be at different stages or there may a healed arteritis manifest by fibrointimal proliferation, destruction of elastic laminae, and scarring of the media and adventitia. The differential diagnosis includes congenital and traumatic aneurysms; in general, any arteritis in a child involving muscular arteries should raise the possibility of Kawasaki disease. A stenotic form of Kawasaki disease has been described, in which the vasculitis results in cord-like, thickened arteries, without discrete aneurysm formation.[162]

VASCULITIS THAT INVOLVES CAPILLARIES AND VENULES

Small vessel vasculitis: definitions and concepts

Terms such as hypersensitivity vasculitis and microscopic polyarteritis have been used in the past to describe vasculitis syndromes involving capillaries and venules. Certain terms for small vessel vasculitis are fairly specific to the target organ (capillaritis for the lung, leukocytoclastic vasculitis for the skin, and crescentic glomerulonephritis to encompass entities including glomerular capillaritis). Currently, the small vessel vasculitic syndromes are grouped into pauci-immune types and those with immune complex deposits.[157,163,164] The former include entities with extravascular necrotizing lesions (Wegener's granulomatosis and Churg–Strauss angiitis) and microscopic polyangiitis (formerly called microscopic polyarteritis). The term polyangiitis is preferred because the target vessels include capillaries and venules. Polyarteritis nodosa does not generally involve small vessels, so is not in the differential diagnosis of these lesions. The immune-complex-mediated small vessel vasculitis groups are heterogeneous. The most common are serum-sickness-type reactions to drugs, often confined to the skin; Henoch–Schonlein purpura, cryoglobulinemic purpura, lupus vasculitis (which may also involve larger vessels), and mixed connective tissue vasculitis (Table 20.10).

The histologic findings of these lesions are similar and include leukocytoclastic inflammation of arterioles, capillaries, and veins. There are no histologic features that reliably distinguish the vasculitis syndromes involving capillaries and venules. However, in

Table 20.10 Classification of vasculitis involving capillaries and venules

Type of vasculitis	Vessel type involved	Typical distribution	Features
Immune-mediated vasculitis			**Usually immune-complex-mediated**
Henoch–Schonlein purpura	Arterioles Capillaries Venules	Skin, bowel, glomeruli	LCV, venular thrombosis DH-like lesions IgA-specific
Cryoglobulinemia	Arterioles Capillaries Venules	Skin (pandermal) Glomeruli Lung	LCV, venular thrombosis Globular endovascular deposits
Mixed connective tissue disease	Arterioles Capillaries Venules	Muscles	Arterioles of ? μm in size in muscle biopsies
Lupus vasculitis	Panvasculitis	Skin (pandermal) Glomeruli Nervous system	May mimic PAN, LCV
Rheumatoid vasculitis	Panvasculitis, as lupus	Skin (pandermal) Viscera Nervous system	Occasionally, rheumatoid nodules in elastic arteries, otherwise like lupus
Pauci-immune vasculitis			**Frequently ANCA-positive**
Wegener's granulomatosis	Panvasculitis	Upper airways, lungs, glomeruli, various others	Extravascular necroinflammatory lesions typical, especially in lung
Churg–Strauss angiitis	Panvasculitis	Lungs, various viscera	Extravascular eosinophilic microabscesses in association with necrotizing arteritis
Microscopic polyangiitis/polyarteritis	Arterioles Capillaries	Glomeruli, lungs, kidney, others	Typically limited to renal capillaries (crescentic GN), lungs (capillaritis), skin

the skin, pandermal involvement, venular thromboses, and arteriolar fibrinoid necrosis are associated with chronic systemic vasculitic syndromes that need long-term immunosuppressive treatment.[165] Purely chronic inflammation confined more distally in venules and larger veins, without thrombi or venous necrosis, is more typical of short-term drug reactions.

Wegener's granulomatosis

Wegener's granulomatosis is a clinicopathologic syndrome of necrotizing granulomatous vasculitis of the upper and lower respiratory tract and glomerulonephritis.[166] There is a strong association with antineutrophil cytoplasmic antibodies (ANCA), which are measured for diagnostic purposes and for monitoring disease.[163] Cytoplasmic staining generally reflects the presence of autoantibodies to anti-proteinase 3 and is present in over 75% of patients with Wegener's granulomatosis. Perinuclear staining reflects the presence of antimyeloperoxidase, which is less frequently seen in patients with Wegener's granulomatosis. Antineutrophilic cytoplasmic antibodies are fairly specific for Wegener's granulomatosis and microscopic polyarteritis, and have also been described in association with classic polyarteritis nodosa, relapsing polychondritis, Kawasaki disease, and Churg–Strauss angiitis.

Clinically, patients with Wegener's granulomatosis have fever, weight loss, anorexia, malaise, arthralgias, and myalgias. Upper respiratory tract symptoms include sinusitis, epistaxis, rhinitis, nasal perforation, and subglottic stenosis, and lung manifestations include cough, hemoptysis, pleuritis, and infiltrates.

Histologically, lung parenchyma shows necrotizing inflammation surrounded by palisading histiocytes; there are scattered giant cells but well-formed sarcoid-like granulomas are absent. The vasculitic component may be inconspicuous and is characterized by granulomatous infiltrates of arterial media (Fig. 20.26) or fibrinoid necrosis

similar to that seen in polyarteritis nodosa. The small vessel involvement of Wegener's granulomatosis includes pulmonary capillaritis, glomerular capillary involvement (crescentic glomerulonephritis), and palpable purpura (cutaneous leukocytoclastic vasculitis). Pulmonary capillaritis, characterized by infiltrates of neutrophils in capillary walls with intra-alveolar hemorrhage, may occur. Patients often suffer from severe renal damage, manifested by segmental necrotizing glomerulonephritis and glomerular thrombosis. Peripheral arteries may occasionally show changes indistinguishable from polyarteritis.

Microscopic polyangiitis (polyarteritis)

Microscopic polyangiitis is an ANCA-positive, pauci-immune vasculitis similar to Wegener's granulomatosis, but necrotizing lung lesions are absent and the dominant lesion is a small vessel vasculitis. Upper airway involvement occurs in only one-third of patients.[167] Peripheral neuropathy and gastrointestinal involvement is far less common than in polyarteritis nodosa.[168] Perinuclear ANCA by indirect immunofluorescence, corresponding to autoantibodies to myeloperoxidase by ELISA, is more frequent than cytoplasmic ANCA in patients with microscopic polyangiitis.[167] The estimated incidence is similar to that of polyarteritis and Wegener's granulomatosis, approximately 2.4/100 000 population.[160] It is characterized by pulmonary capillaritis without necrotizing lung lesions,[169] glomerulonephritis (rapidly progressive glomerulonephritis with crescents or segmental glomerular fibrinoid necrosis), and leukocytoclastic vasculitis. The skin is involved in 20–70% of patients. Gross skin lesions include purpura and petechiae, livedo, and erythema, especially erythema on the hands and fingers.[170] Microscopic polyangiitis without renal involvement is unusual.[171] Panbronchiolitis has been rarely reported.[172] In contrast to classic polyarteritis nodosa, patients are not typically hypertensive, lung involvement often

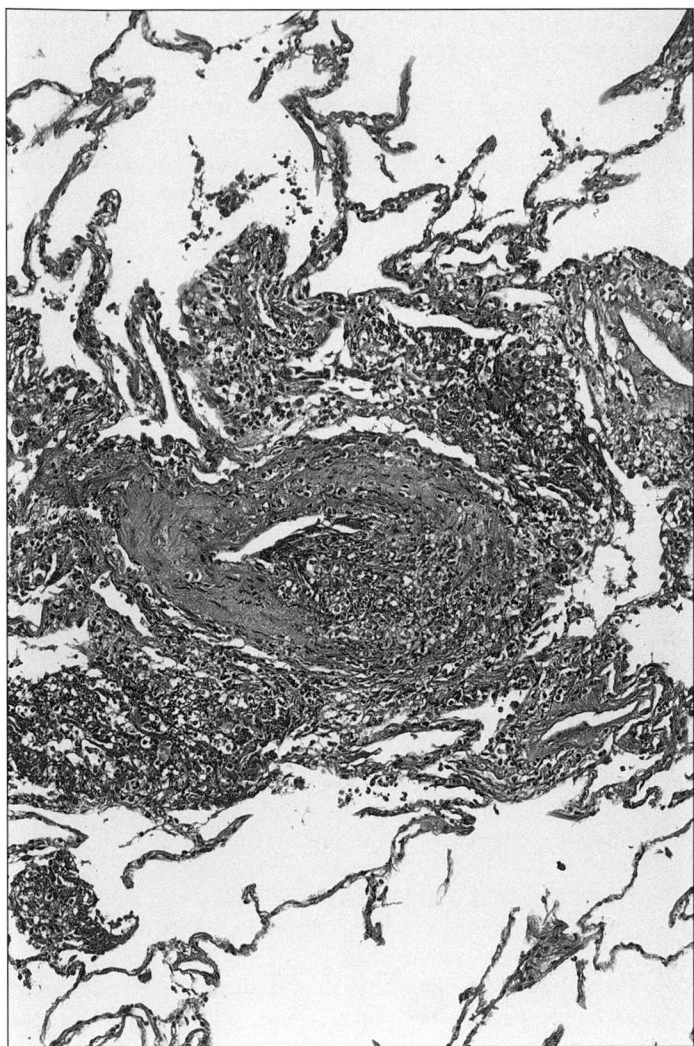

Figure 20.26 Wegener's granulomatosis. The vascular lesions of Wegener's granulomatosis are non-specific; the major lesions are extravascular necrotizing granulomas (not shown). This photomicrograph shows focal destruction of a pulmonary arterial wall by a mixed infiltrate.

causes clinical symptoms, and involvement of muscular arteries is unusual. Those cases with renal muscular arterial involvement have a lesser incidence of crescentic glomerulonephritis and a higher rate of complete remission with immunosuppressive treatment.[173] The diagnosis is typically made in patients with immune-complex-negative glomerulonephritis and pulmonary hemorrhage (capillaritis) who have serologic evidence of antineutrophil cytoplasmic auto-antibodies. There has been an association with bone marrow transplantation [171] and primary biliary cirrhosis.[174]

Histologically, the diagnosis is based on finding necrotizing glomerular lesions in kidney biopsies, capillaritis in open lung biopsy, or small vessel vasculitis in skin biopsy. There is a wide range of findings in skin biopsy, ranging from leukocytoclastic vasculitis to more non-specific inflammation of arterioles and venules.[170] Treatment consists of combined therapy of granulocytapheresis or leukocytapheresis for rapidly progressive glomerulonephritis and lung hemorrhage.[175] Cyclophosphamide is used in patients refractory to treatment to these agents.[176]

Churg–Strauss angiitis

Also known as allergic angiitis and granulomatosis, Churg–Strauss angiitis is a systemic necrotizing vasculitis associated with severe asthma that was originally considered to be a subset of polyarteritis nodosa.[177,178] Most patients are young adults. Typically, there is a prodromal phase of allergic rhinitis, sinusitis, asthma, and blood eosinophilia, followed by an infiltrative phase of fleeting, patchy, irregular lung densities and eosinophilic gastroenteritis. The end-stage manifestation is that of vasculitis, manifest by fever, malaise, weight loss, fixed pulmonary infiltrates, neuropathy, and various signs and symptoms attributable to systemic vascular lesions.[157]

The etiology of Churg–Strauss angiitis is unknown. Both eosinophils and neutrophils probably participate in skin lesion development.[179] Prolonged survival of eosinophils due to inhibition of CD95-mediated apoptosis by soluble CD95 seems to contribute to eosinophilia in Churg–Strauss syndrome, and there may be a possible role of T lymphocytes secreting eosinophil-activating cytokines.[180] Churg–Strauss syndrome has been described in association with the treatment of asthmatic patients with leukotriene receptor antagonist. Whether leukotriene receptor antagonist treatment has allowed unmasking of the disease by corticosteroid tapering or if there is a direct adverse effect of the antileukotriene is unknown.[181,182]

Histologically, there are inflammatory infiltrates of arteries, often with fibrinoid necrosis and an infiltrate of eosinophils, macrophages, and lymphocytes. In contrast to polyarteritis, veins may be involved and there are extravascular eosinophilic microabscesses. Similar to Wegener's granulomatosis, Churg–Strauss angiitis may present as soft tissue masses.[183] The differential diagnosis includes drug reactions and visceral larva migrans. In the absence of confirming clinical criteria, a histologic diagnosis of Churg–Strauss angiitis can be made only on the basis of necrotizing arteritis with prominent eosinophils, in addition to eosinophilic microabscesses. The latter are characterized by masses of apoptotic, degranulated eosinophils surrounded by a granulation tissue or granulomatous reaction. Eosinophilia may be prominent in polyarteritis nodosa and is, in itself, not diagnostic. Churg–Strauss angiitis in surgical specimens obtained from patients who do not have clinical supportive criteria has been termed localized or isolated Churg–Strauss angiitis.[159] There may be an overlap with eosinophilic endomyocardial fibrosis (Löffler's endocardial fibrosis).[184]

The accepted definition of Churg–Strauss syndrome requires the finding of necrotizing vasculitis accompanied by granulomas with eosinophilic necrosis in the setting of asthma and eosinophilia. However, Churg himself accepts an early, prevasculitic phase that is characterized by tissue infiltration by eosinophils without overt vasculitis.[185]

The general treatment of Churg–Strauss disease includes methylprednisolone and cyclophosphamide.[186] Severe cases are treated with anti-TNF blocking agents such as infliximab or etanercept, or interferon-alpha.[187] Relapses occur in more than 25% of all patients.[188]

Immune-related necrotizing polyangiitis

In contrast to pauci-immune small vessel necrotizing vasculitic syndromes of Wegener's, Churg–Strauss, and microscopic polyangiitis, there are a variety of diseases that result from immune complex deposition in the microcirculation. In general, they involve not only capillaries but venules as well, and serum ANCA is negative. Leukocytoclasia is prominent but fibrinoid necrosis of arterioles is unusual. Necrotizing inflammation of capillaries and venules, with venular thrombosis, is more frequent

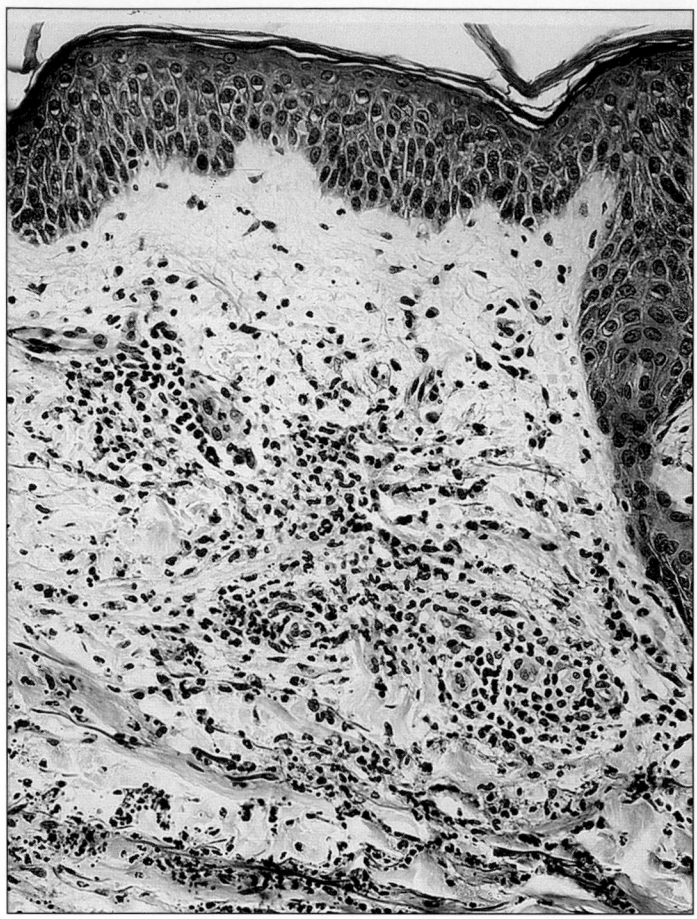

Figure 20.27 Small vessel vasculitis. Most frequently involving the skin, small vessel vasculitis is characterized by a perivascular infiltrate with neutrophils and nuclear dust.

in systemic disease than a self-limited drug reaction, as well as full dermal involvement in this skin, as opposed to involvement of the superficial plexuses typical of serum sickness.[165] However, there are no reliable distinguishing features from pauci-immune vasculitis, and capillaritis, leukocytoclastic vasculitis, and glomerulonephritis are similar. For this reason, immunofluorescence and serologic tests for ANCA are important in the differential diagnosis.

Immune vasculitis of small vessels includes drug reactions, lupus vasculitis, mixed connective tissue disease vasculitis, rheumatoid vasculitis, Henoch–Schonlein purpura, and cryoglobulinemic vasculitis, as well as others. The typical organ distributions of these syndromes is outlined in Table 20.7. The skin is the most common site of involvement, usually manifest as palpable purpura or a maculopapular rash.[165]

Histologically, there is involvement exclusively of arterioles, venules, and capillaries (Fig. 20.27). There are two histologic forms of hypersensitivity vasculitis: a leukocytoclastic type, presumably the early lesion, characterized by karyorrhectic debris and fibrinoid necrosis; and a later non-necrotizing form characterized by cuffing of vessels with neutrophils and lymphocytes and prominent endothelial swelling. Scattered eosinophils are common in both types. Immunofluorescence will demonstrate the deposition of immunoglobulins and complement.

MISCELLANEOUS INFLAMMATORY DISEASES OF BLOOD VESSELS

Vasculitis of collagen vascular disease

Rheumatoid vasculitis is more prevalent than either polyarteritis nodosa or Wegener's granulomatosis and usually occurs in patients with long-standing disease and high levels of rheumatoid factor.[189] Clinical manifestations of vasculitis in patients with rheumatoid arthritis include fever, peripheral neuropathy (particularly mononeuritis multiplex), gangrene and leg ulcers, coronary vasculitis, mesenteric ischemia, and cerebral infarcts. Unlike polyarteritis nodosa, renal involvement is rare. Digital vasculitis may occur and be relatively benign and localized, and does not in itself indicate the presence of disseminated vasculitis. Histologically, there is a range of vasculitis from a small vessel vasculitis to necrotizing arteritis similar to polyarteritis nodosa.

The incidence of vasculitis in patients with systemic lupus erythematosus is lower than in rheumatoid arthritis. The most common manifestation is cutaneous small vessel vasculitis. Gastrointestinal vasculitis mimicking polyarteritis nodosa may affect the gastrointestinal tract, resulting in ischemia or bowel perforation. Other manifestations of lupus vasculitis are coronary arteritis and pulmonary capillaritis.

In scleroderma, the predominant vascular changes are obliterative with little inflammation. There may be an acute phase of acellular fibrinoid necrosis. In dermatomyositis, vasculitis is particularly common in the childhood variant. Vascular involvement in mixed connective tissue diseases may be similar to that seen in lupus erythematosus, scleroderma, or dermatomyositis.

Thromboangiitis obliterans

Also known as Buerger's disease, thromboangiitis obliterans is a form of peripheral vascular disease seen virtually exclusively in cigarette smokers.[190] Compared to the peripheral vascular disease of atherosclerosis, patients are young adults, and distal, rather than proximal arteries of the extremities are primarily involved angiographically. Histologically, both arteries and veins are involved in an inflammatory process that rapidly progresses to occlusive organized thrombi. The thrombi are often infiltrated by chronic inflammatory cells, and the internal elastic lamina remains intact. Giant cells within organized thrombi in medium-sized arteries and veins are virtually diagnostic of Buerger's disease (Fig. 20.28) but are often not identified.

Inflammatory abdominal aortic aneurysm

First described by Walker et al in 1972 as a variant of abdominal atherosclerotic aneurysm, inflammatory aneurysms account for approximately 5% of operated abdominal aortic aneurysms.[191] Similar to atherosclerotic aneurysms, there is a male predominance. Patients typically complain of chronic abdominal and back pain and weight loss, and medial deviation of the ureters may be demonstrated by radiographic techniques. The erythrocyte sedimentation rate is typically elevated.

Histologically, there is atherosclerotic plaque lining the luminal surface, medial attenuation with replacement by scar tissue, and adventitial and periadventitial fibrosis and inflammation with entrapped lymphoid aggregates, nerves, fat, and lymph nodes. The histologic appearance is reminiscent of idiopathic retroperitoneal fibrosis, and there may be a pathogenetic relationship between the two entities. Although regression of the inflammatory layer surrounding the aneurysm, as detected by imaging, is the rule after surgery, progression with retroperitoneal

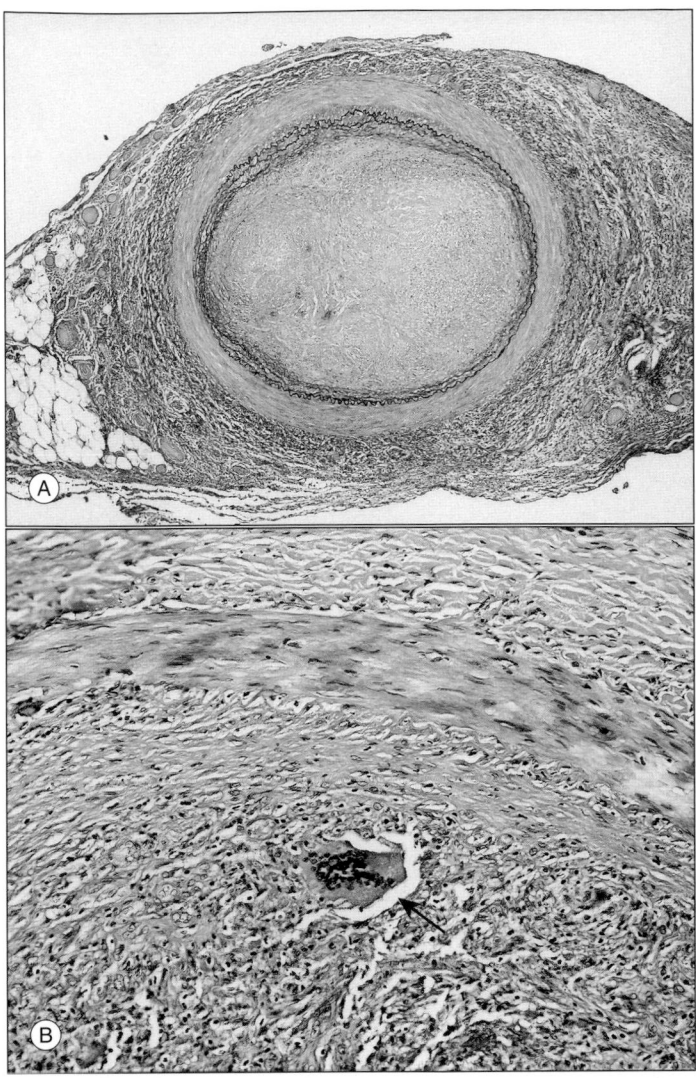

Figure 20.28 Buerger's disease. **(A)** A low magnification of an artery involved with Buerger's disease demonstrates a cellular thrombus without destruction of the elastic lamina. **(B)** The pathognomonic lesion is the presence of giant cells (arrow) within an organized thrombus. Giant cells are otherwise present within arterial lumina only as a foreign body reaction to injected substances or cholesterol clefts of atherosclerotic plaques.

fibrosis and ureteral obstruction occurs postoperatively in about one-third of patients.[191]

Mimickers of vasculitis

There are several conditions that may result in vascular inflammation that is not caused by a vasculitis process. Vessels adjacent to abscesses or acutely ulcerated mucosa may become infiltrated by acute inflammatory cells and even show fibrinoid necrosis. Infarction may result in acute inflammation of veins, and later arteries, with subsequent chronic inflammatory infiltrate in vessel walls. Acute margination of neutrophils occurs quite rapidly with surgical trauma and may simulate a vasculitis. T-cell lymphomas and other lymphoproliferative processes may invade blood vessels, mimicking vasculitis.

Infectious vasculitis

Syphilitic aortitis may result in aortic insufficiency and aortic aneurysms, which may rupture and rarely dissect.[192] Other manifestations of syphilitic aortitis include coronary ostial stenosis and aortic insufficiency. The latency period between infection and aneurysm formation is between 15 and 20 years. Only 10–30% of patients have a history of syphilis or other manifestations of tertiary syphilis, emphasizing the need for serologic diagnosis. Treponemal tests are reactive in more than 90% of cases. Because of the lack of specificity of histologic findings, the diagnosis of syphilitic aortitis should not be made in the absence of serologic confirmation.

Syphilitic aneurysms are saccular or fusiform, and 90% occur in the thoracic aorta, with a predilection for the ascending aorta. Microscopically, there are perivascular lymphocytes and plasma cells around vasa vasorum with endarteritis, and rarely areas of acute necrosis of aortic wall with neutrophilic infiltrates (microgummas). Occasionally, the abscesses may contain treponemes, demonstrated by Warthin–Starry stain.

Nonsyphilitic infectious aneurysms, or so-called mycotic aneurysms, may occur in the aorta, especially thoracic aorta, and muscular arteries, especially those in the splanchnic bed. There is a predilection for areas of structural anomalies, such as aortic coarctation and graft anastomoses. Mycotic aneurysms are most commonly related to bacterial endocarditis, and may be diagnosed years after endocarditis treatment; they affect, in descending order of frequency: aorta, superior mesenteric, splenic,[193] coronary, posterior tibial, common iliac, popliteal, radial, ulnar, and renal arteries. The most frequent organisms are salmonella, staphylococci, and enterococci. Histologically, there is medial destruction with microabscess formation; often organisms are not identified because of antibiotic therapy.

Phlebitis

Deep venous thrombosis is characterized by pain, swelling, and tenderness, and may result in pulmonary embolism. Although the term 'thrombophlebitis' is commonly used for venous thrombosis syndromes, inflammation is generally secondary to the thrombosis and may not be histologically prominent, unless there is bacterial infection (septic phlebitis). Histologically, there are acute and organizing thrombi in veins of affected vessels, and there may be associated acute and chronic inflammation of the venous wall.

Superficial thrombophlebitis may be classified as migratory, nonmigratory (often associated with varicosities), Mondor's disease (limited to chest wall), and traumatic (associated with intravenous lines). Risk factors for superficial thrombophlebitis include hypercoagulable states, Behçet's disease, inflammatory bowel disease, secondary syphilis, and Buerger's disease; many cases, however, are idiopathic.

Giant cell phlebitis is an uncommon disease of the bowel that most commonly affects the right colon and omentum.[194] Giant cell phlebitis typically presents as a mass lesion, perforation or hemorrhage; histologically, there is a pronounced mixed inflammatory infiltrate of lymphocytes, eosinophils, and macrophages involving large muscular veins, and there is a giant cell component. It is essential to differentiate this lesion from giant cell arteritis, as steroid treatment is not indicated. Lymphocytic phlebitis of the colon may be a related entity, and is associated with hypersensitivity to medications; in contrast to the giant cell variant, smaller veins are involved and giant cells are not present. Intestinal phlebitis appears to have a relatively benign course, without development of a systemic illness. It is probably a variant of immune-related small vessel vasculitis, in which capillary and venular involvement is minimal but more distal veins are targeted.

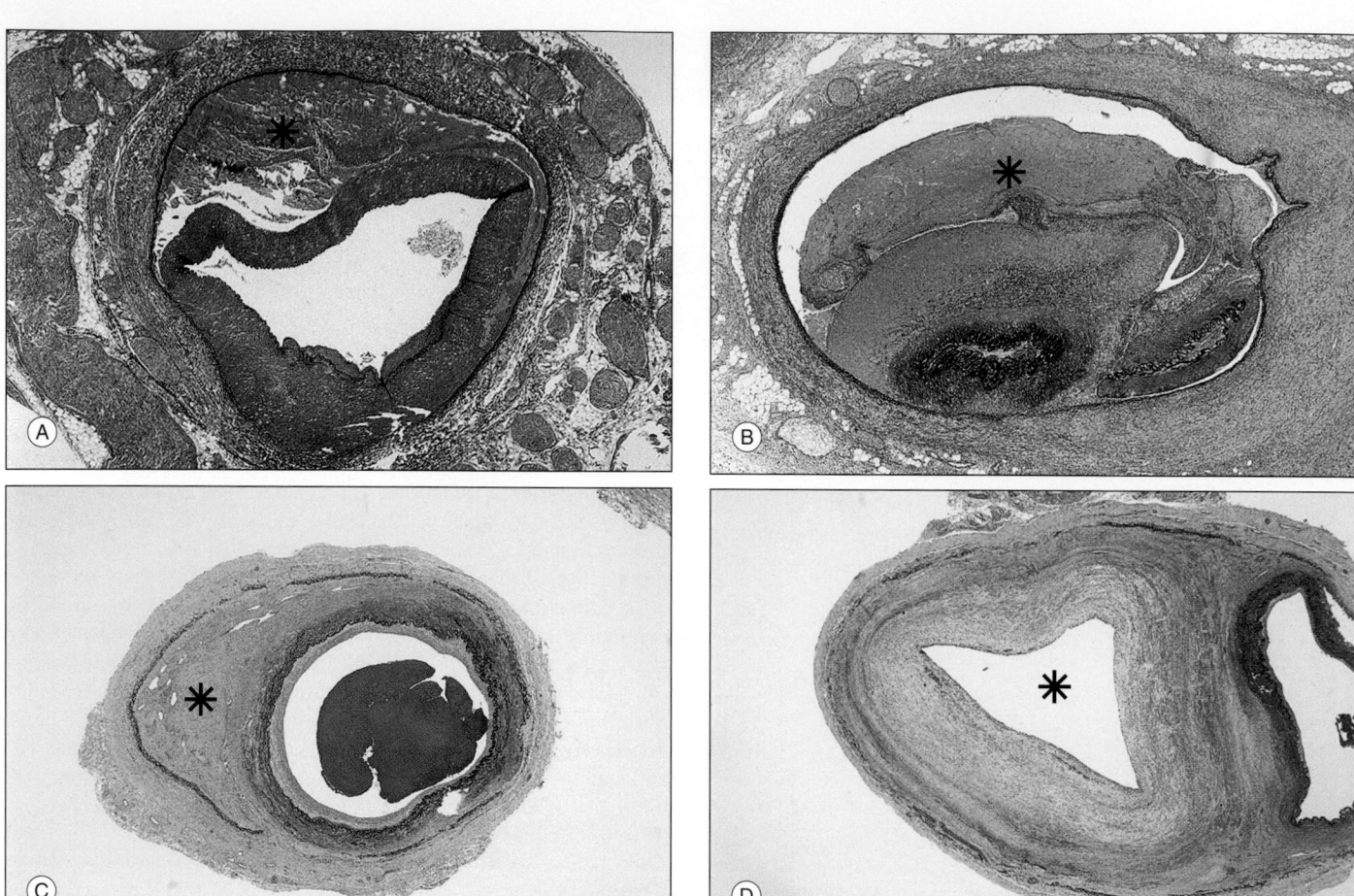

Figure 20.29 Arterial dissections. **(A)** Note acute hematoma (asterisk) in the outer media of a patient with renal artery dysplasia and dissection. **(B)** There is acute and organizing dissection (asterisk) in the mesenteric artery of a patient who developed retroperitoneal hemorrhage after iatrogenic dissection following catheterization. **(C)** Healed dissection, carotid artery. Note granulation tissue indicative of organized thrombus (asterisk) filling dissected space. The underlying disease was fibromuscular dysplasia. **(D)** Healed dissection with false lumen, fibromuscular dysplasia of carotid artery. Note false lumen (asterisk) lined by organized thrombus.

NON-INFLAMMATORY DISEASES OF BLOOD VESSELS

FIBROMUSCULAR DYSPLASIA

Fibromuscular dysplasia is a heterogeneous group of non-inflammatory disorders characterized by disorganization of muscular arterial walls resulting in arterial luminal narrowing and arterial aneurysms. Most patients are young Caucasian females, and there is an association with estrogen exposure, pregnancy, hereditary factors, and neurofibromatosis. The etiology and genetic basis are currently unknown.

Renal arterial dysplasia accounts for 75% of cases of symptomatic fibromuscular dysplasia, and 75% of cases of renal artery dysplasia are isolated to the kidneys.[195] It is an important cause of renovascular hypertension, especially in children and young adults. The right renal artery is more often involved than the left; when bilateral, there is strong association with extrarenal arterial dysplasia. The distal two-thirds of the renal artery is typically involved by areas of narrowing and aneurysms. Complications include renovascular hypertension, renal infarction, arterial dissection (Fig. 20.29), embolization, and thrombosis.

Dysplasia involving the brachiocephalic arteries (carotid, subclavian, and vertebral arteries) accounts for the majority of the remaining patients, many of whom are asymptomatic. Occasionally, there may be symptoms of cerebral or upper extremity ischemia arising from thrombosis of aneurysms, embolization, and arterial dissections. The internal carotid artery is typically involved at the level of C1 and C2, distal to the most frequent site of atherosclerosis.

Uncommon sites of arterial dysplasia include the visceral arteries (celiac, mesenteric, hepatic, and splenic), iliofemoral arteries, coronary arteries, brachial arteries, and aorta.[196]

Pathologically, there is segmental interrupted arterial narrowing resulting in an angiographic 'string of beads'. Histologically, there are two dominant patterns: medial dysplasia (accounting for 90% of cases), characterized by focal medial absence and disorganization without destruction of elastic laminae (Fig. 20.30), and intimal dysplasia, characterized by concentric fibrointimal proliferation (often segmental alternating with normal areas).[197,198] Rarely, the media and intima are normal and there is adventitial fibrosis. In practice, the histopathologic diagnosis is quite difficult, because of

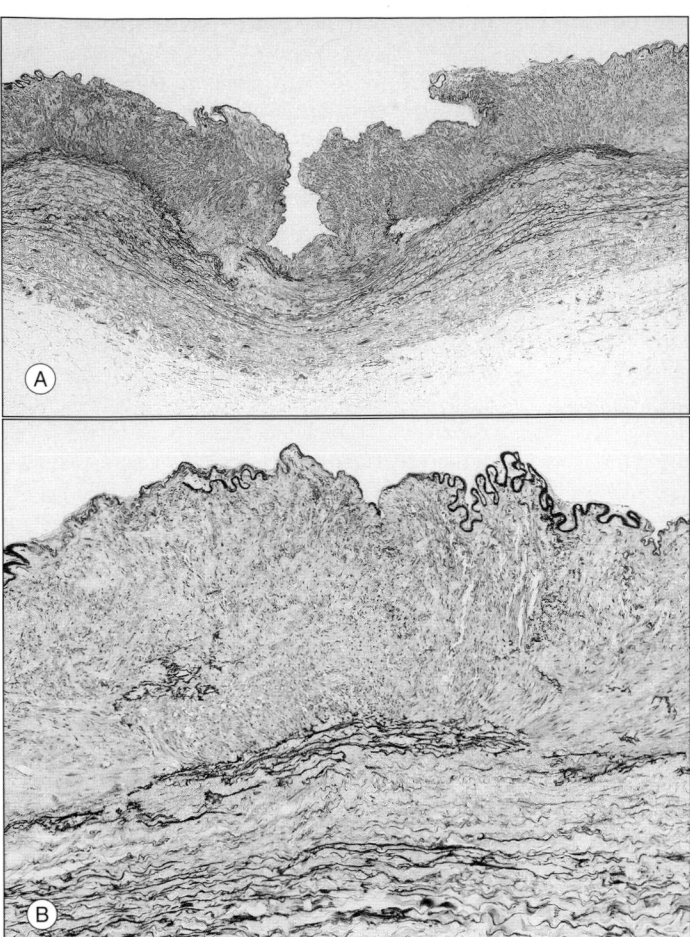

Figure 20.30 Arterial dysplasia. **(A)** A low magnification of a longitudinally oriented section demonstrates a focal defect in the media, which may account for aneurysms or a string-of-beads appearance on angiography. **(B)** There is disorganization of the smooth muscle cells and uneven thickness of the media. In contrast to postinflammatory or post-traumatic disruptions, there is no granulation tissue or fibrosis.

frequent superimposed changes of aneurysm, luminal thrombosis, and healed dissection. Optimally oriented sections with elastic stains are essential in arriving at a presumptive diagnosis of fibromuscular dysplasia. In the majority of cases, the diagnosis is made angiographically and the lesions are treated with percutaneous stents without tissue sampling. The differential diagnosis includes atherosclerosis, which, unlike medial dysplasia, results in lipid deposition and an inflammatory cell infiltrate, with destruction of the elastic laminae; and healed arteritis, which results in focal medial destruction with scarring and obliteration of the elastic laminae.

Segmental arterial mediolysis

Currently believed to be a form of medial dysplasia,[199] segmental arterial mediolysis (or segmental mediolytic arteritis) is a degenerative process of mesenteric arteries characterized by replacement of segments of the media by hemorrhage and fibrin, without inflammatory changes of fibrinoid necrosis.[200–203] The primary differential diagnosis is polyarteritis nodosa, but lesions at various stages of healing, and true fibrinoid necrosis, is absent. Patients are typically elderly, with symptoms of acute abdomen or hemoperitoneum.

INHERENT NON-INFLAMMATORY MEDIAL DISEASE (MEDIAL DEGENERATION)

Marfan syndrome

Marfan syndrome is an autosomal dominant disease resulting from a deficiency of the microfibril component of elastic fibers, specifically fibrillin-1, related to mutations of the fibrillin gene located on chromosome 15. The histologic manifestation of the defect is multifocal, patchy areas of elastin loss within the media, accompanied by an increase in proteoglycans and eventual smooth muscle cell loss. This change has many names, including medial degeneration, cystic medial necrosis, and cystic medial degeneration; the term 'necrosis' is currently not favored. Cardiovascular manifestations of Marfan syndrome are fusiform ascending aortic aneurysms (39%), aortic dissections (36%), mitral regurgitation without other cardiovascular involvement (21%), and peripheral arterial aneurysms and dissections (4%).[204] Marfan syndrome accounts for approximately 10% of all proximal aortic aneurysms and dissections, and 25–50% of those occurring in patients under the age of 30.

The histologic hallmark of Marfan aneurysms is medial degeneration (cystic medial change) (Fig. 20.31). Cystic medial change was the term initially used by Erdheim in patients with annuloaortic ectasia and aortic rupture without dissection, and denotes large pools or lakes of proteoglycans with loss of elastic fibers. Medionecrosis, or laminar medial necrosis, refers to loss of smooth muscle cells with resultant close apposition of intervening elastic laminae, and is present in 10% of aortic dissections. A grading system of medial degeneration, ranging from 1+ (mild patchy elastin loss) to 4+ (transmural involvement) has been employed.[205] Sampling issues render the comparison of the degree of cystic medial change among different risk groups (Marfan, hypertensive, and bicuspid aortic valve disease) problematic.[206] A Movat pentachrome stain, which demonstrates elastic fibers and proteoglycans, is the optimal method for the demonstration of degenerative medial changes. In addition to medial change, there may also be histologic evidence of acute dissection in aortic specimens removed from patients with Marfan syndrome and aortic root aneurysms.

Idiopathic aortic root dilatation

Idiopathic aortic root dilatation, or annuloaortic ectasia, is the most common cause of proximal aortic aneurysms that may rupture or dissect. The molecular basis for idiopathic aortic root dilatation has yet to be determined. A small proportion of non-Marfan aortic root disease appears to be related to mutations in the fibrillin gene. The term 'fibrillinopathy' has been employed for non-Marfan diseases, with similar cardiovascular manifestations, without the full-blown syndrome.[207] The genetic basis for these diseases, however, and related familial dissections in families without Marfan syndrome, has yet to be fully elucidated.[208,209] The distinction from Marfan syndrome is made on the patient's age (generally two to three decades older at presentation than the patient with Marfan syndrome) and the absence of extracardiac manifestations of Marfan syndrome. Although there is a weaker hereditary predisposition in idiopathic aortic root dilatation, as compared to Marfan syndrome, familial aortic root dissections in patients without Marfan syndrome have been reported.[210]

Hypertension-induced medial degeneration

In older adults with medial degeneration and aortic dissection, hypertension plays a major role, and any contribution by fibrillin abnormalities in pathogenesis are speculative at best. Hypertension is present in 70% of all cases of aortic dissection, and is present in more than 80% of dissections of the descending thoracic aorta and

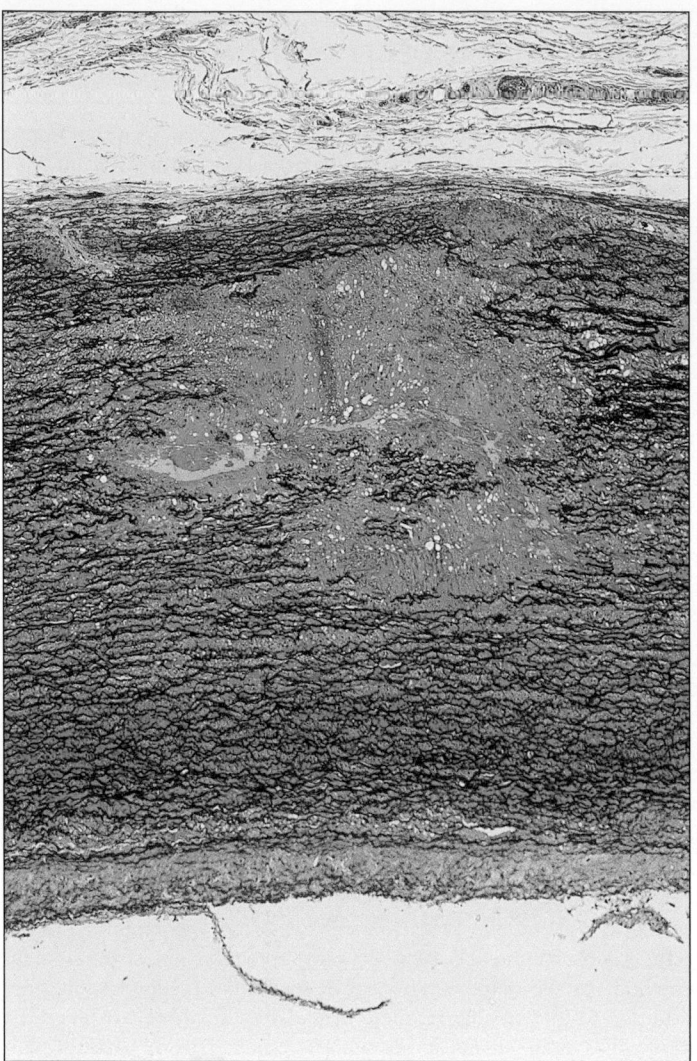

Figure 20.31 Medial degeneration, aorta. Often designated as cystic medial necrosis, medial degeneration is characterized by multifocal absence of elastic laminae and deposition of proteoglycan ground substance. Medial degeneration predisposes to aneurysms and dissections and is often seen in Marfan syndrome, idiopathic aortic root dilatation, and hypertension.

Miscellaneous causes of medial degeneration

There are several factors in addition to Marfan syndrome and hypertension that predispose to non-inflammatory ascending aortic aneurysms. The risk of ascending aortic dissection in patients with bicuspid aortic valves is nine times that of patients with normal aortic valves and, for unicuspid aortic valves, 18 times greater. Because the aortic valve in Marfan syndrome is tri-leaflet, the genetic basis for familial bicuspid aortic valve[211] and aortic dissections in patients with bicuspid aortic valve is presumably not related to fibrillin defects. 40% of aortic valves in ascending aortic dissections are bicuspid or unicuspid, and are usually, but not always stenotic. 25% of dissections in women occur during pregnancy but a firm association has not been established. Coarctation of the aorta is associated with aortic dissections but may not be independent of the association with bicuspid aortic valve and hypertension. Turner syndrome is associated with dissection, bicuspid aortic valve, and coarctation of the aorta. Familial dissections of the descending thoracic aorta have been reported but are rare. Aortic dissections in weightlifters have been described, suggesting that strenuous isometric exercise may precipitate aortic intimal damage.

The histologic findings in aortic dissections and aneurysms associated with bicuspid aortic valve are non-specific; most reports suggest that the degree of cystic medial necrosis is less than that seen in full-blown Marfan syndrome or hypertension-related dissections in older patients.[206]

Aneurysms of muscular arteries may occasionally show medial degeneration on histologic examination. In such cases, hypertension and connective tissue disorders should be clinically ruled out, although often no predisposing cause is identified.

Approach to surgical pathology of the ascending aorta

Aneurysms of the ascending aorta are surgically repaired, often with aortic valve replacement. The surgeon will typically submit a portion of aortic wall with the valve specimen, if there is one. There may be a history of acute aortic dissection, which has caused emergent surgery for aortic root dilatation, impending aortic rupture, and aortic valve insufficiency.

The role of the surgical pathologist in this setting is to describe the histologic findings of the aortic wall, which is often aided by elastic stains, with or without concomitant stains for proteoglycans (e.g. Movat pentachrome). The histologic evaluation of the valve itself is generally not as rewarding. There are two classes of findings: non-inflammatory aortic disease (embracing cystic medial necrosis, or medial degeneration) and inflammatory aneurysms. In both scenarios, but especially the former, superimposed changes of prior healed dissections, or those of atherosclerosis, may be present.

Inflammatory aneurysms of the ascending aorta (see above, vasculitis) fall into three categories: syphilitic aortitis, non-specific aortitis/Takayasu's disease, and giant cell aortitis. The first can be for the most part dismissed in developed countries, because tertiary syphilis is rare. However, a statement in the surgical pathology report to the effect that syphilis should be excluded by serologic testing is appropriate. Non-specific aortitis is histologically characterized by zonal necrosis with surrounding giant cells, often imparting a disordered smooth muscle cell reaction in the media of healed lesions, essentially indistinguishable from syphilis. Whether this entity represents an aneurysmal form of Takayasu's disease is a current controversy, but most patients have isolated surgical disease, do not have systemic vasculitis, and range in age from young adults to elderly without gender predilection. Giant cell aortitis lacks zonal necrosis of non-specific aortitis and adventitial endarteritis obliterans, and occurs exclusively in elderly adults, usually women.

transverse aortic arch.[205] The dissection results in a false lumen, lined by a thin outer wall and the inner media. The histologic assessment of the media surrounding dissections caused by systemic hypertension is generally not rewarding; changes of medial degeneration are often less marked than aneurysms present in patients with Marfan syndrome or annuloaortic ectasia, but are present in over 50% of cases.[206] Relative to ascending aortic dissections, distal dissections have a high frequency of healed tears (approximately 40%), and aneurysms of the false channel occur in 20% of cases. The histologic appearance of healed dissection is that of a double-lumen (double-barreled) aorta. The false channel is lined by granulation tissue with diffuse elastic deposition, in contrast to the regular elastic laminae of the true media.

Hypertension-related medial degeneration is also considered to be a predisposing cause for aneurysms of muscular arteries, including the splanchnic circulation.

Non-inflammatory aneurysms of the ascending aorta represent an overlapping spectrum of genetic disease (full-blown Marfan syndrome in young adults, presumed incomplete forms of Marfan syndrome, including non-Marfan familial aortic dissections, and isolated aortic dissection, in the absence of known connective tissue disorder, in older adults (usually hypertensives)). The role of fibrillin-1 mutations have been firmly established in the first group (Marfan syndrome), but are currently under investigation in the second and third groups.[207,209] The role of the surgical pathologist is primarily to ascertain the non-inflammatory nature of the dissection, as histologic extent of cystic medial necrosis does not predict the presence or absence of a genetic syndrome in an individual case. It is important to try to establish, by contacting the surgeon or reading the operative report, whether the valve is bicuspid. The genetics of bicuspid aortic valve,[211–213] which is associated with an increased risk of aortic dissection and which has a hereditary basis, is distinct from that of Marfan syndrome and related fibrillinopathies.

TRAUMATIC DISEASES OF BLOOD VESSELS

Aortic pseudoaneurysms

Pseudoaneurysms are localized arterial dilatations lined by granulation tissue or scar tissue overlying a rupture in the media. Most cases of pseudoaneurysms are caused by trauma, although any healed rupture of a vessel secondary to vasculitis, medial degeneration, or pancreatitis, may result in a pseudoaneurysm. The trauma may result from external injury or iatrogenic causes such as arterial cannulation, aortotomy, aortic cross-clamping, and vascular anastomoses.

Although most traumatic lacerations of the aorta result in sudden death, a minority heal and may not be diagnosed for years. Most patients have a history of some trauma, although 60% do not have a history of apparent thoracic trauma. Approximately 50% of chronic dissections are asymptomatic; symptoms in the remaining half of patients include chest and back pain and hypotension related to leakage or rupture. Most are located at the aortic isthmus near the ligamentum arteriosum. Grossly, an intimal tear is found, which is generally transverse, and circumferential in 50% of cases. The lining of the aneurysm is organized hematoma and fibrous tissue, with a sharp demarcation between normal media and fibrous lining of the pseudoaneurysm.

Pseudoaneurysms of the peripheral arteries

Traumatic (pseudo) aneurysms of peripheral arteries are typically superficial and are found most frequently on the face, followed by lower and upper extremities. In the consultation files at the Armed Forces Institute of Pathology, pseudoaneurysms comprise the largest groups of surgically resected aneurysms.[214] The mean age at presentation is 26 years and there is a male predominance. A history of trauma is not always elicited. Histologically, there is typically an abrupt interruption in the vessel wall, with granulation tissue or scar replacing a portion of the vessel (Fig. 20.32). The pseudoaneurysm is often several diameters larger than the parent artery, which may be difficult to identify without elastic stains and proper orientation of the specimen.

MISCELLANEOUS VASCULAR DISEASES

Idiopathic non-inflammatory aneurysms

The histologic examination of a large number of surgically resected aneurysms will not reveal a specific cause for the arterial dilatation.

The differential diagnosis is generally hypertension-induced medial degeneration, congenital syndromes such as Marfan and Ehlers–Danlos syndrome, medial or fibromuscular dysplasia, infectious, and vasculitis aneurysms. It is often difficult to histologically subclassify aneurysms in surgical arterial resections, because of inadequate sampling, improper orientation of the specimen, or extensive secondary changes, such as atherosclerosis, calcification, or healed rupture. If there are no identifiable abnormalities of uninvolved media, the aneurysm is considered congenital or idiopathic and a hereditary or connective tissue disorder should be excluded clinically.

Occasionally, spontaneous idiopathic dissections of visceral arteries may occur, resulting in hemoperitoneum and emergency laparotomy. In the absence of catheter-induced trauma and radiographic or histopathologic features of fibromuscular dysplasia, the differential diagnosis includes rare cases of cystic medial necrosis involving muscular arteries, and so-called segmental mediolytic arteriopathy. Also known as segmental mediolytic arteritis, segmental arteriopathy is a form of idiopathic arterial dissection that is often mistaken histologically for polyarteritis nodosa,[200] because of fibrin deposition in the dissected portion. The etiology is unknown but vacuolar degeneration of medial smooth muscle cells is a histologic feature of the disease.

Berry aneurysms in the circle of Willis are generally considered congenital in origin, although this is a matter of debate. Splenic artery aneurysms are found most often in women in the distal artery; there is usually superimposed calcification and one-third are multiple. Pregnancy and estrogen exposure are considered predisposing factors to the development of non-inflammatory aneurysms, but the mechanism underlying this association is unknown.

Medial calcification: Mönckeberg's and vascular calcinosis

Age-related, modest calcification of the media of small and medium sized muscular arteries (Mönckeberg's medial calcification) is a common finding in the elderly. Many arterial beds may be involved. The surgical pathologist may frequently see medial calcification in arteries of the thyroid gland, lower leg amputations, in breast biopsies, in the genitourinary tract, and in temporal artery biopsies. Calcification involves the media and elastic laminae, and there is little if any inflammatory reaction or intimal thickening. Significant luminal narrowing or obliteration does not occur.

More severe forms of calcification of the media, which result in a marked giant cell reaction and elevation of acute phase reactants, are termed vascular calcinosis or calciphylaxis.[215] Obstruction of the vessel occurs because of an intimal fibrotic reaction, causing ischemia symptoms or progressive ischemic gangrene.[216] Most patients have end-stage renal disease and diabetes; antiphospholipid syndrome has been reported in some patients.[217] Radiographs demonstrate diffuse vascular calcifications of vessels of the extremities. The pathologist may encounter calcinosis in amputation specimens, or biopsies of necrotic skin, breast, or even temporal artery biopsies. The histologic features are those of marked calcification of the media, a giant cell reaction with lymphocytes, and intimal thickening. In smaller arteries and arterioles, concentric calcifications may be the only finding. Because aggressive treatment is indicated to prevent complications of gangrene, the submitting physician should be notified immediately if the diagnosis is considered.

Cystic adventitial disease, popliteal artery

Cystic adventitial disease is an idiopathic accumulation of mucinous ground substance in the adventitia of the popliteal arterial wall, accounting for approximately 1 in 1200 cases of claudication.[218]

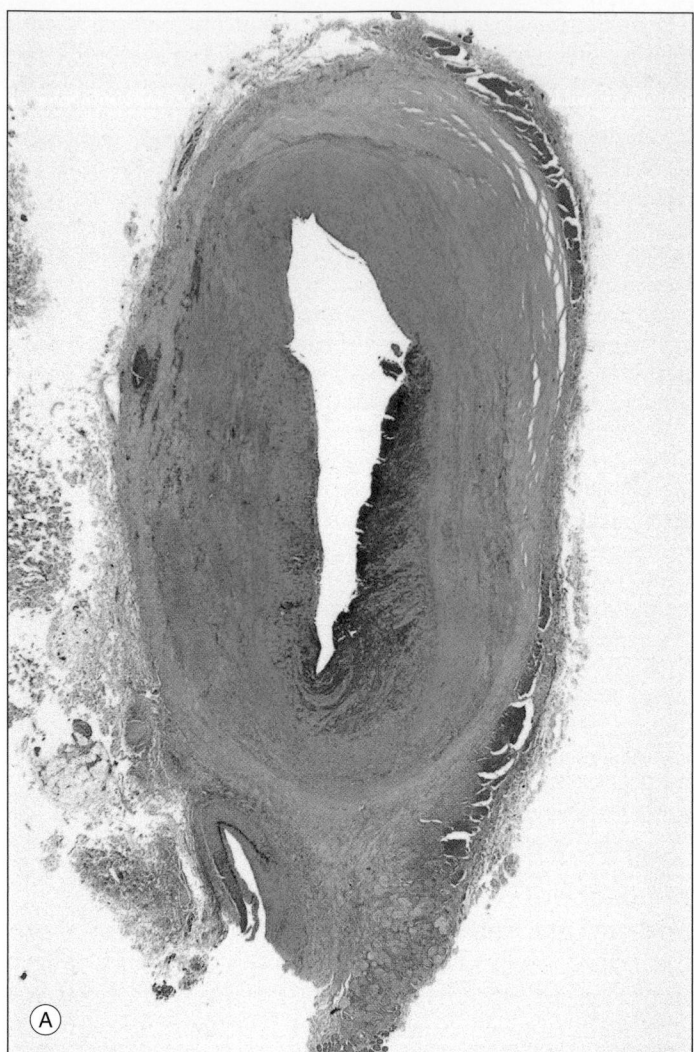
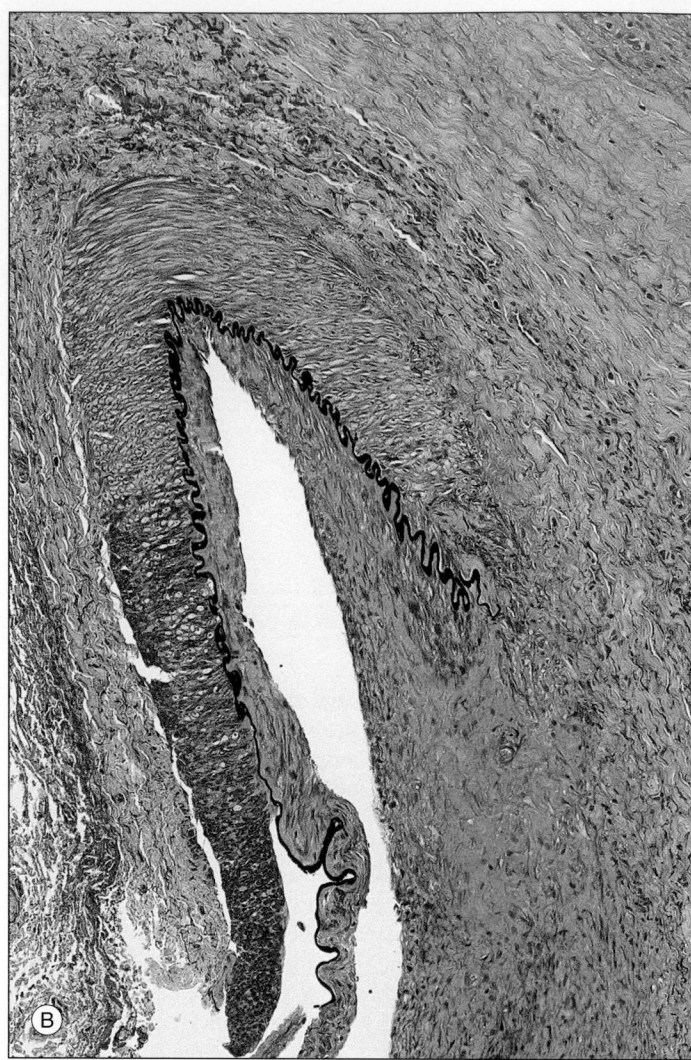

Figure 20.32 Arterial pseudoaneurysm. **(A)** Low magnification demonstrates a large channel lined by fibrous tissue and granulation tissue. **(B)** Higher magnification of the native artery shows an abrupt interruption of the internal elastic lamina and surrounding scar.

There is a male:female preponderance of 5–8:1. Arteriography demonstrates a smooth-walled narrowing or a non-specific complete occlusion. Pathologically, there are mucus filled cysts of the adventitial layer of the popliteal artery and surrounding popliteal fossa (Fig. 20.33), resulting from mucin-secreting synovial cells originating from the neighboring joint capsule or tendon sheath. The media may be involved with the mucinous degeneration, and rare involvement of other arteries and veins in the extremities has been reported.[218]

Arterial thrombosis

Occasionally, the pathologist will encounter thrombosed arterial resections and be asked to comment on possible etiologies for the thrombus. Intrinsic arterial diseases that predispose to thrombus formation include atherosclerosis and vasculitis syndromes, such as Takayasu's disease and Behçet's disease in elastic arteries, and Kawasaki disease in smaller vessels. Thrombus formation without underlying vascular disease is less common in arteries than in veins. Idiopathic arterial thrombosis may occur in virtually any artery, including the aorta. Risk factors in otherwise normal arteries include hypercoagulable states and estrogen use. Hypercoagulable states

include antiphospholipid syndrome, protein C deficiency, protein S deficiency, decreased factor XII, antithrombin III deficiency, heparin-induced thrombopathy, myeloproliferative syndromes, and other malignancies. In some cases, especially when the biopsy is small, inflammatory infiltrates reactive to the thrombus may be difficult to distinguish from inherent vasculitis; in such cases, fibroinflammatory medial destruction with interruption of elastic layers may be helpful in establishing a diagnosis of vasculitis.

The histopathologic alterations in antiphospholipid syndrome, an acquired autoimmune disorder in which patients present with thrombosis together with antibodies that recognize anionic phospholipid–protein complexes,[219] are somewhat distinctive.[220] The large vessel changes include calcified mural thrombi in the atria,[102] Libman–Sacks vegetations on heart valves, and venous and arterial thrombosis with embolism. A small number of patients develop disseminated arterial thrombosis with intimal proliferation of smaller arterioles similar to hypertensive vascular disease.[220]

Atheroembolism

The atheroembolic syndrome in the lower extremities is characterized by bluish discoloration of toes and painful bilateral foot ulcers.

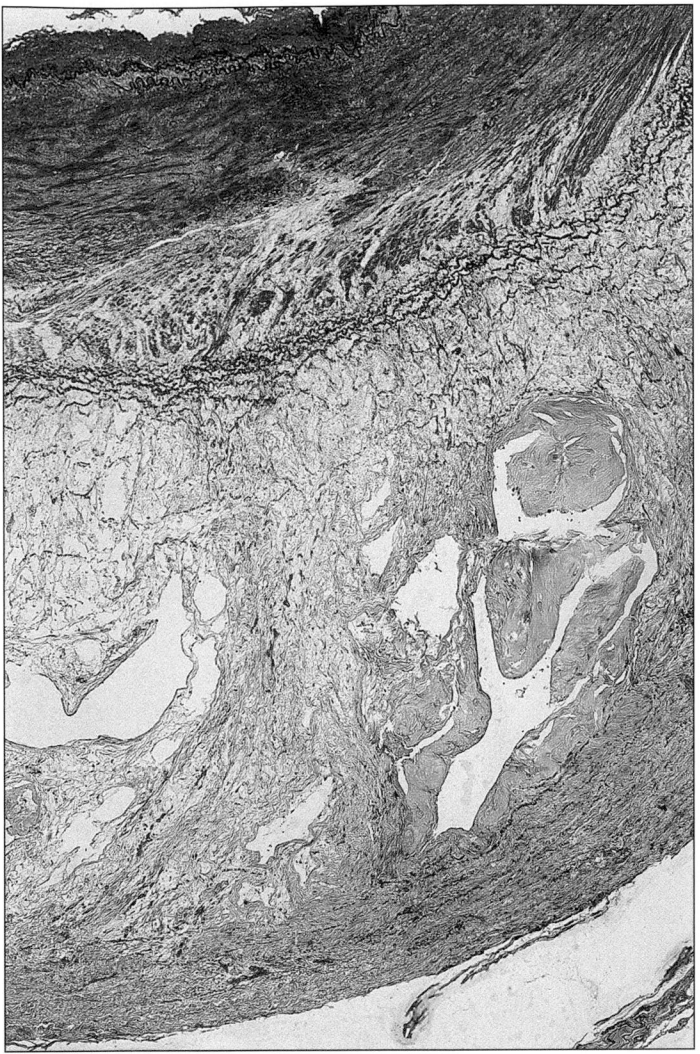

Figure 20.33 Cystic adventitial disease, popliteal artery. There is loose edematous tissue in the arterial adventitia with cystic spaces lined by flattened cells reminiscent of synovium. Cystic adventitial disease is a rare cause of claudication of the lower extremities.

Systemic atheroembolism occurs spontaneously in patients with ulcerative aortic atherosclerosis but is often precipitated by catheterization, surgery, or other manipulation of the aorta. Renal failure and visceral infarction may occur and the diagnosis may be clinically suspected if there is elevated erythrocyte sedimentation rate and transient amaurosis secondary to cholesterol emboli in the ocular fundi. The histopathologic diagnosis may be made by the examination of surgically excised intestine, mucosal biopsy,[221] skin biopsies, or renal biopsies. The histologic findings are characterized by the presence of cholesterol clefts, with or without giant cells and thrombus in small arteries, at different stages of organization. Acute atheroemboli are surrounded by fibrin and blood cells; in later stages, the thrombi surrounding the cholesterol crystals show organization.

Varicose veins

Venous varicosities are most common in the superficial veins of the leg and are characterized by dilatation and loss of valvular function. Most patients are female and there is an association with obesity and multiple pregnancies. A family history is present in almost 50% of cases. Saphenous veins express the progesterone receptor, which may be related to the hormonal predisposition to venous varicosities.[222] Children with the Klippel–Trenaunay syndrome typically suffer from venous varicosities, in addition to cutaneous hemangiomas and soft tissue and/or skeletal hypertrophy.

Histologically, there is fibrointimal proliferation with elastosis, with or without calcification.[223] Treatment of varicose veins consists of surgical removal by stripping or excision and is recommended for the prevention of thrombosis with propagation into the deep venous system and pulmonary embolism

REFERENCES

1. Veinot JP. Diagnostic endomyocardial biopsy pathology: secondary myocardial diseases and other clinical indications – a review. Can J Cardiol 2002; 18: 287–296.

2. Veinot JP. Diagnostic endomyocardial biopsy pathology – general biopsy considerations, and its use for myocarditis and cardiomyopathy: a review. Can J Cardiol 2002; 18: 55–65.

3. Ardehali H, Qasim A, Cappola T, et al. Endomyocardial biopsy plays a role in diagnosing patients with unexplained cardiomyopathy. Am Heart J 2004; 147: 919–923.

4. Nishikawa T, Ishiyama S, Sakomura Y, et al. Histopathologic aspects of endomyocardial biopsy in pediatric patients with idiopathic ventricular tachycardia. Pediatr Int 1999; 41: 534–537.

5. Alter P, Grimm W, Tontsch D, Maisch B. Diagnosis of primary cardiac lymphoma by endomyocardial biopsy. Am J Med 2001; 110: 593–594.

6. Felker GM, Hu W, Hare JM, et al. The spectrum of dilated cardiomyopathy. The Johns Hopkins experience with 1278 patients. Medicine (Baltimore) 1999; 78: 270–283.

7. Hrobon P, Kuntz KM, Hare JM. Should endomyocardial biopsy be performed for detection of myocarditis? A decision analytic approach. J Heart Lung Transplant 1998; 17: 479–486.

8. Wu LA, Lapeyre AC III, Cooper LT. Current role of endomyocardial biopsy in the management of dilated cardiomyopathy and myocarditis. Mayo Clin Proc 2001; 76: 1030–1038.

9. Arbustini E, Gavazzi A, Dal Bello B, et al. Ten-year experience with endomyocardial biopsy in myocarditis presenting with congestive heart failure: frequency, pathologic characteristics, treatment and follow-up. G Ital Cardiol 1997; 27: 209–223.

10. Grogan M, Redfield MM, Bailey KR, et al. Long-term outcome of patients with biopsy-proved myocarditis: comparison with idiopathic dilated cardiomyopathy. J Am Coll Cardiol 1995; 26: 80–84.

11. Parrillo JE, Cunnion RE, Epstein SE, et al. A prospective, randomized, controlled trial of prednisone for dilated cardiomyopathy. N Engl J Med 1989; 321: 1061–1068.

12. McCarthy RE III, Boehmer JP, Hruban RH, et al. Long-term outcome of fulminant myocarditis as compared with acute (nonfulminant) myocarditis. N Engl J Med 2000; 342: 690–695.

13. Wojnicz R, Nowalany-Kozielska E, Wojciechowska C, et al. Randomized, placebo-controlled study for immunosuppressive treatment of inflammatory dilated cardiomyopathy: two-year follow-up results. Circulation 2001; 104: 39–45.

14. Angelini A, Crosato M, Boffa GM, et al. Active versus borderline myocarditis: clinicopathological correlates and prognostic implications. Heart 2002; 87: 210–215.

15. Aretz H, Billingham ME, Edwards WD, et al. Myocarditis: a histologic definition and classification. Am J Cardiovasc Pathol 1987; 1: 3–14.

16. Cooper LT Jr. Giant cell myocarditis: diagnosis and treatment. Herz 2000; 25: 291–298.

17. Cooper LT Jr., Berry GJ, Shabetai R. Idiopathic giant cell myocarditis–natural history and treatment.

Multicenter Giant Cell Myocarditis Study Group Investigators. N Engl J Med 1997; 336: 1860–1866.

18. Davies RA, Veinot JP, Smith S, et al. Giant cell myocarditis: clinical presentation, bridge to transplantation with mechanical circulatory support, and long-term outcome. J Heart Lung Transplant 2002; 21: 674–679.

19. Scott RL, Ratliff NB, Starling RC, Young JB. Recurrence of giant cell myocarditis in cardiac allograft. J Heart Lung Transplant 2001; 20: 375–380.

20. Uemura A, Morimoto S, Hiramitsu S, et al. Histologic diagnostic rate of cardiac sarcoidosis: evaluation of endomyocardial biopsies. Am Heart J 1999; 138: 299–302.

21. Arbustini E, Morbini P, Pilotto A, et al. Genetics of idiopathic dilated cardiomyopathy. Herz 2000; 25: 156–160.

22. Towbin JA, Bowles NE. Molecular genetics of left ventricular dysfunction. Curr Mol Med 2001; 1: 81–90.

23. Arbustini E, Diegoli M, Morbini P, et al. Prevalence and characteristics of dystrophin defects in adult male patients with dilated cardiomyopathy. J Am Coll Cardiol 2000; 35: 1760–1768.

24. Grimm W, Rudolph S, Christ M, et al. Prognostic significance of morphometric endomyocardial biopsy analysis in patients with idiopathic dilated cardiomyopathy. Am Heart J 2003; 146: 372–376.

25. Lombardo T, Tamburino C, Bartoloni G, et al. Cardiac iron overload in thalassemic patients: an endomyocardial biopsy study. Ann Hematol 1995; 71: 135–141.

26. Katritsis D, Wilmshurst PT, Wendon JA, et al. Primary restrictive cardiomyopathy: clinical and pathologic characteristics. J Am Coll Cardiol 1991; 18: 1230–1235.

27. Arbustini E, Morbini P, Grasso M, et al. Restrictive cardiomyopathy, atrioventricular block and mild to subclinical myopathy in patients with desmin-immunoreactive material deposits. J Am Coll Cardiol 1998; 31: 645–653.

28. Angelini A, Calzolari V, Thiene G, et al. Morphologic spectrum of primary restrictive cardiomyopathy. Am J Cardiol 1997; 80: 1046–1050.

29. Crotty TB, Li C-Y, Edwards WD, Suman VJ. Amyloidosis and endomyocardial biopsy: correlation of extent and pattern of deposition with amyloid immunophenotype in 100 cases. Cardiovasc Pathol 1995; 4: 39–42.

30. Buxbaum JN, Genega EM, Lazowski P, et al. Infiltrative nonamyloidotic monoclonal immunoglobulin light chain cardiomyopathy: an underappreciated manifestation of plasma cell dyscrasias. Cardiology 2000; 93: 220–228.

31. Chimenti C, Ricci R, Pieroni M, et al. Cardiac variant of Fabry's disease mimicking hypertrophic cardiomyopathy. Cardiologia 1999; 44: 469–473.

32. Shehata BM, Patterson K, Thomas JE, et al. Histiocytoid cardiomyopathy: three new cases and a review of the literature. Pediatr Dev Pathol 1998; 1: 56–69.

33. Meinardi MT, van der Graaf WT, van Veldhuisen DJ, et al. Detection of anthracycline-induced cardiotoxicity. Cancer Treat Rev 1999; 25: 237–247.

34. Ganz WI, Sridhar KS, Ganz SS, et al. Review of tests for monitoring doxorubicin-induced cardiomyopathy. Oncology 1996; 53: 461–470.

35. Shek TW, Luk IS, Ma L, Cheung KL. Paclitaxel-induced cardiotoxicity. An ultrastructural study. Arch Pathol Lab Med 1996; 120: 89–91.

36. Rosenthal DN, Chin C, Nishimura K, et al. Identifying cardiac transplant rejection in children: diagnostic utility of echocardiography, right heart catheterization and endomyocardial biopsy data. J Heart Lung Transplant 2004; 23: 323–329.

37. Winters GL. The challenge of endomyocardial biopsy interpretation in assessing cardiac allograft rejection. Curr Opin Cardiol 1997; 12: 146–152.

38. Winters GL. Grade 2 cardiac rejection: pathologic clinical controversies. Pathol Case Rev 1998; 3: 66–72.

39. Hammond EH, Yowell RL. Pathologic evaluation of early cardiac allograft dysfunction. Pathol Case Rev 1998; 3: 73–79.

40. Crespo M, Pascual M, Tolkoff-Rubin N, et al. Acute humoral rejection in renal allograft recipients: I. Incidence, serology and clinical characteristics. Transplantation 2001; 71: 652–658.

41. Duong Van Huyen JP, Fornes P, Guillemain R, et al. Acute vascular humoral rejection in a sensitized cardiac graft recipient: diagnostic value of C4d immunofluorescence. Hum Pathol 2004; 35: 385–388.

42. Winters GL. Allograft coronary disease: a major limitation to long-term heart transplant recipient survival. Pathol Case Rev 2001; 6: 274–280.

43. Dare AJ, Harrity PJ, Tazelaar HD, et al. Evaluation of surgically excised mitral valves: revised recommendations based on changing operative procedures in the 1990s. Hum Pathol 1993; 24: 1286–1293.

44. Virmani R, Atkinson JB, Forman MB, Robinowitz M. Mitral valve prolapse. Hum Pathol 1987; 18: 596–602.

45. Marcus RH, Sareli P, Pocock WA, Barlow JB. The spectrum of severe rheumatic mitral valve disease in a developing country. Correlations among clinical presentation, surgical pathologic findings, and hemodynamic sequelae. Ann Intern Med 1994; 120: 177–183.

46. Passik CS, Ackermann DM, Pluth JR, Edwards WD. Temporal changes in the causes of aortic stenosis: a surgical pathologic study of 646 cases. Mayo Clin Proc 1987; 62: 119–123.

47. Olson LJ, Subramanian R, Edwards WD. Surgical pathology of pure aortic insufficiency: a study of 225 cases. Mayo Clin Proc 1984; 59: 8935–8941.

48. Sabet HY, Edwards WD, Tazelaar HD, Daly RC. Congenitally bicuspid aortic valves: a surgical pathology study of 542 cases (1991 through 1996) and a literature review of 2,715 additional cases. Mayo Clin Proc 1999; 74: 14–26.

49. Dare A, Veinot JP, Edwards WD, et al. New observations on the etiology of aortic valve disease: a surgical pathologic study of 236 cases from 1990. Hum Pathol 1993; 24: 1330–1338.

50. Hauck AJ, Freeman DP, Ackermann DM, et al. Surgical pathology of the tricuspid valve: a study of 363 cases spanning 25 years. Mayo Clin Proc 1988; 63: 851–863.

51. Simula DV, Edwards WD, Tazelaar HD, et al. Surgical pathology of carcinoid heart disease: a study of 139 valves from 75 patients spanning 20 years. Mayo Clin Proc 2002; 77: 139–147.

52. Rajamannan NM, Caplice N, Anthikad F, et al. Cell proliferation in carcinoid valve disease: a mechanism for serotonin effects. J Heart Valve Dis 2001; 10: 827–831.

53. Connolly HM, Crary JL, McGoon MD, et al. Valvular heart disease associated with fenfluramine-phentermine. N Engl J Med 1997; 337: 581–588.

54. Steffee CH, Singh HK, Chitwood WR. Histologic changes in three explanted native cardiac valves following use of fenfluramines. Cardiovasc Pathol 1999; 8: 245–253.

55. Silvestry FE, St John Sutton M. Anorectic therapy and valvular heart disease: a reappraisal. Eur Heart J 1999; 20: 917–920.

56. McDonald PC, Wilson JE, McManus BM. Fen-Phen valve disease: a real entity? Pathol Case Rev 2001; 6: 281–286.

57. Altrichter PM, Olson LJ, Edwards WD, et al. Surgical pathology of the pulmonary valve: a study of 116 cases spanning 15 years. Mayo Clin Proc 1989; 64: 1352–1360.

58. Michel PL, Acar J. Native cardiac disease predisposing to infective endocarditis. Eur Heart J 1995; 16: 2–6.

59. Bouza E, Menasalvas A, Munoz P, et al. Infective endocarditis – a prospective study at the end of the twentieth century: new predisposing conditions, new etiologic agents, and still a high mortality. Medicine (Baltimore) 2001; 80: 298–307.

60. Werner M, Andersson R, Olaison L, Hogevik H. A clinical study of culture-negative endocarditis. Medicine (Baltimore) 2003; 82: 263–273.

61. Voldstedlund M, Pedersen LN, Fuursted K, Nielsen LP. Different polymerase chain reaction-based analyses for culture-negative endocarditis caused by *Streptococcus pneumoniae*. Scand J Infect Dis 2003; 35: 757–759.

62. Paturel L, Casalta JP, Habib G, et al. *Actinobacillus actinomycetemcomitans* endocarditis. Clin Microbiol Infect 2004; 10: 98–118.

63. Avidor B, Graidy M, Efrat G, et al. *Bartonella koehlerae*, a new cat-associated agent of culture-negative human endocarditis. J Clin Microbiol 2004; 42: 3462–3468.

64. Richardson DC, Burrows LL, Korithoski B, et al. *Tropheryma whippelii* as a cause of afebrile culture-negative endocarditis: the evolving spectrum of Whipple's disease. J Infect 2003; 47: 170–173.

65. Gdoura R, Pereyre S, Frikha I, et al. Culture-negative endocarditis due to *Chlamydia pneumoniae*. J Clin Microbiol 2002; 40: 718–720.

66. Lamas CC, Eykyn SJ. Blood culture negative endocarditis: analysis of 63 cases presenting over 25 years. Heart 2003; 89: 258–262.

67. Khulordava I, Miller G, Haas D, et al. Identification of the bacterial etiology of culture-negative endocarditis by amplification and sequencing of a small ribosomal RNA gene. Diagn Microbiol Infect Dis 2003; 46: 9–11.

68. Choi HK, Lamprecht P, Niles JL, et al. Subacute bacterial endocarditis with positive cytoplasmic antineutrophil cytoplasmic antibodies and anti-proteinase 3 antibodies. Arthritis Rheum 2000; 43: 226–231.

69. Eiken PW, Edwards WD, Tazelaar HD, et al. Surgical pathology of nonbacterial thrombotic endocarditis in 30 patients, 1985–2000. Mayo Clin Proc 2001; 76: 1204–1212.

70. Boone S, Campagna M, Walley V. Lambl's excrescences and papillary fibroelastomas: are they different? Can J Cardiol 1992; 8: 372–376.

71. Boone S, Higginson L, Walley V. Endothelial papillary fibroelastomas arising in and around the aortic sinus, filling the ostium of the right coronary artery. Arch Pathol Lab Med 1992; 116: 135–137.

72. Sun JP, Asher CR, Yang XS, et al. Clinical and echocardiographic characteristics of papillary fibroelastomas: a retrospective and prospective study in 162 patients. Circulation 2001; 103: 2687–2693.

73. Mann J, Parker D. Papillary fibroelastoma of the mitral valve: a rare cause of transient neurological defects. Br Heart J 1994; 71: 6.

74. Valente M, Basso C, Thiene G, et al. Fibroelastic papilloma: a not-so-benign cardiac tumor. Cardiovasc Pathol 1992; 1: 161–166.

75. Kurup AN, Tazelaar HD, Edwards WD, et al. Iatrogenic cardiac papillary fibroelastoma: a study of 12 cases (1990 to 2000). Hum Pathol 2002; 33: 1165–1169.

76. Gowda RM, Khan IA, Nair CK, et al. Cardiac papillary fibroelastoma: a comprehensive analysis of 725 cases. Am Heart J 2003; 146: 404–410.

77. Burke AP, Virmani R. Tumors of the cardiovascular system. Washington, DC: Armed Forces Institute of Pathology; 1996.

78. Amano J, Kono T, Wada Y, et al. Cardiac myxoma: its origin and tumor characteristics. Ann Thorac Cardiovasc Surg 2003; 9: 215–221.

79. Acebo E, Val-Bernal JF, Gomez-Roman JJ. Prichard's structures of the fossa ovalis are not histogenetically related to cardiac myxoma. Histopathology 2001; 39: 529–535.

80. Grebenc ML, Rosado-de-Christenson ML, Green CE, et al. Cardiac myxoma: imaging features in 83 patients. Radiographics 2002; 22: 673–689.

81. Edwards A, Bermudez C, Piwonka G, et al. Carney's syndrome: complex myxomas. Report of four cases and review of the literature. Cardiovasc Surg 2002; 10: 264–275.

82. Goldstein MM, Casey M, Carney JA, Basson CT. Molecular genetic diagnosis of the familial myxoma syndrome (Carney complex). Am J Med Genet 1999; 86: 62–65.

83. Mahilmaran A, Seshadri M, Nayar PG, et al. Familial cardiac myxoma: Carney's complex. Texas Heart Inst J 2003; 30: 80–82.

84. Burke AP, Virmani R. Cardiac myxomas: a clinicopathologic study. Am J Clin Pathol 1994; 100: 671–680.

85. Pucci A, Gagliardotto P, Zanini C, et al. Histopathologic and clinical characterization of cardiac myxoma: review of 53 cases from a single institution. Am Heart J 2000; 140: 134–138.

86. Berrutti L, Silverman JS. Cardiac myxoma is rich in factor XIIIa positive dendrophages: immunohistochemical study of four cases. Histopathology 1996; 28: 529–535.

87. Acebo E, Val-Bernal JF, Gomez-Roman JJ. Thrombomodulin, calretinin and c-kit (CD117) expression in cardiac myxoma. Histol Histopathol 2001; 16: 1031–1036.

88. Terracciano LM, Mhawech P, Suess K, et al. Calretinin as a marker for cardiac myxoma. Diagnostic and histogenetic considerations. Am J Clin Pathol 2000; 114: 754–759.

89. Lindner V, Edah-Tally S, Chakfe N, et al. Cardiac myxoma with glandular component: case report and review of the literature. Pathol Res Pract 1999; 195: 267–272.

90. Pucci A, Bartoloni G, Tessitore E, et al. Cytokeratin profile and neuroendocrine cells in the glandular component of cardiac myxoma. Virchows Arch 2003; 443: 618–624.

91. Chopra P, Ray R, Singh MK, Venugopal P. Cardiac myxoma with glandular elements: a histologic, histochemical, and immunohistochemical evaluation. Indian Heart J 2003; 55: 182–184.

92. Burke AP, Rosado-de-Christenson M, Templeton PA, Virmani R. Cardiac fibroma. Clinicopathologic correlates and surgical treatment. J Thorac Cardiovasc Surg 1994; 108: 862–870.

93. Stiller B, Hetzer R, Meyer R, et al. Primary cardiac tumours: when is surgery necessary? Eur J Cardiothorac Surg 2001; 20: 1002–1006.

94. Waller BR, Bradley SM, Crumbley AJ III, et al. Cardiac fibroma in an infant: single ventricle palliation as a bridge to heart transplantation. Ann Thorac Surg 2003; 75: 1306–1308.

95. Pipitone S, Mongiovi M, Grillo R, et al. Cardiac rhabdomyoma in intrauterine life: clinical features and natural history. A case series and review of published reports. Ital Heart J 2002; 3: 48–52.

96. Burke AP, Virmani R. Cardiac rhabdomyoma, a clinicopathologic study. Mod Pathol 1991; 4: 70–74.

97. Fernandes F, Soufen HN, Ianni BM, et al. Primary neoplasms of the heart. Clinical and histological presentation of 50 cases. Arq Bras Cardiol 2001; 76: 231–237.

98. Sallee D, Spector ML, van Heeckeren DW, Patel CR. Primary pediatric cardiac tumors: a 17 year experience. Cardiol Young 1999; 9: 155–162.

99. Burke AP, Johns J, Virmani R. Hemangiomas of the heart: a clinicopathologic study of 10 cases. Am J Cardiovasc Pathol 1991; 13: 283–290.

100. Burke AP, Litovsky S, Virmani R. Lipomatous hypertrophy of the atrial septum presenting as a right atrial mass. Am J Surg Pathol 1996; 20: 678–685.

101. Veinot JP, Tazelaar HD, Edwards WD, et al. Mesothelial/monocytic incidental cardiac excrescences (cardiac MICE). Mod Pathol 1994; 7: 9–16.

102. Reynolds C, Tazelaar HD, Edwards WD. Calcified amorphous tumor of the heart (cardiac CAT). Hum Pathol 1997; 28: 601–606.

103. Pinkard NB, Wilson RW, Lawless N, et al. Calcifying fibrous pseudotumor of pleura. A report of three cases of a newly described entity involving the pleura. Am J Clin Pathol 1996; 105: 189–194.

104. Torstveit J, Bennett W, Hinchcliffe SW, Cornell W. Primary plasmacytoma of the atrium: report of a case

with successful surgical management. J Thorac Cardiovasc Surg 1977; 74: 563–566.

105. Warner KJ, Blackwell GG, Herrera GA, et al. Cardiac amyloidoma with IgM-kappa gammopathy. Arch Pathol Lab Med 1994; 118: 1148–1150.

106. Cruz P, Mahidhara S, Ticzon A, Tobon H. Malignant cardiac paraganglioma: follow-up of a case. J Thorac Cardiovasc Surg 1984; 87: 942–944.

107. Aravot D, Banner N, Cantor A, et al. Location, localization and surgical treatment of cardiac pheochromocytoma. Am J Cardiol 1992; 69: 283–285.

108. Johnson T, Shapiro B, Beierwalters W, et al. Cardiac paragangliomas. A clinicopathologic and immunohistochemical study of four cases. Am J Surg Pathol 1985; 11: 827.

109. Yamaguchi S, Hida K, Nakamura N, et al. Multiple vertebral metastases from malignant cardiac pheochromocytoma–case report. Neurol Med Chir (Tokyo) 2003; 43: 352–355.

110. Jenkins PC, Dickison AE, Flanagan MF. Cardiac inflammatory pseudotumor: rapid appearance in an infant with congenital heart disease. Pediatr Cardiol 1996; 17: 399–401.

111. Hartyanszky IL, Kadar K, Hubay M. Rapid recurrence of an inflammatory myofibroblastic tumor in the right ventricular outflow tract. Cardiol Young 2000; 10: 271–274.

112. Rose AG, McCormick S, Cooper K, Titus JL. Inflammatory pseudotumor (plasma cell granuloma) of the heart. Report of two cases and literature review. Arch Pathol Lab Med 1996; 120: 549–554.

113. Burke AP, Cowan D, Virmani R. Cardiac sarcomas. Cancer Treat Rev 1992; 9: 387–395.

114. Donsbeck AV, Ranchere D, Coindre JM, et al. Primary cardiac sarcomas: an immunohistochemical and grading study with long-term follow-up of 24 cases. Histopathology 1999; 34: 295–304.

115. Movsas B, Teruya-Feldstein J, Smith J, et al. Primary cardiac sarcoma: a novel treatment approach. Chest 1998; 114: 648–652.

116. Grandmougin D, Fayad G, Decoene C, et al. Total orthotopic heart transplantation for primary cardiac rhabdomyosarcoma: factors influencing long-term survival. Ann Thorac Surg 2001; 71: 1438–1441.

117. Reardon MJ, DeFelice CA, Sheinbaum R, Baldwin JC. Cardiac autotransplant for surgical treatment of a malignant neoplasm. Ann Thorac Surg 1999; 67: 1793–1795.

118. Liu S, Wang Z, Chen AQ, et al. Cardiac myxoma and myxosarcoma: clinical experience and immunohistochemistry. Asian Cardiovasc Thorac Ann 2002; 10: 8–11.

119. Rolla G, Bertero MT, Pastena G, et al. Primary lymphoma of the heart. A case report and review of the literature. Leuk Res 2002; 26: 117–120.

120. Nakakuki T, Masuoka H, Ishikura K, et al. A case of primary cardiac lymphoma located in the pericardial effusion. Heart Vessels 2004; 19: 199–202.

121. Cohen Y, Daas N, Libster D, et al. Large B-cell lymphoma manifesting as an invasive cardiac mass: sustained local remission after combination of methotrexate and rituximab. Leuk Lymphoma 2002; 43: 1485–1487.

122. Chalabreysse L, Berger F, Loire R, et al. Primary cardiac lymphoma in immunocompetent patients: a report of three cases and review of the literature. Virchows Arch 2002; 441: 456–461.

123. Meshref M, Sassolas F, Schell M, et al. Primary cardiac Burkitt lymphoma in a child. Pediatr Blood Cancer 2004; 42: 380–383.

124. Campione A, Cacchiarelli M, Ghiribelli C, et al. Which treatment in pericardial effusion? J Cardiovasc Surg 2002; 43: 735–739.

125. Anyanwu CH, Umeh BU. Pericarditis: a persisting surgical problem. Cardiovasc Surg 1994; 2: 711–715.

126. Clifford CP, Davies GJ, Scott J, et al. Tuberculous pericarditis with rapid progression to constriction. Prompt diagnosis and treatment are needed. Br Med J 1993; 307: 1052–1054.

127. Cameron J, Oesterle SN, Baldwin JC, Hancock EW. The etiologic spectrum of constrictive pericarditis. Am Heart J 1987; 113: 354–360.

128. Veinot JP, Edwards WD. Pathology of radiation-induced heart disease: a surgical and autopsy study of 27 cases. Hum Pathol 1996; 27: 766–773.

129. Gupta A, Kelly B, McGuigan JE. Erdheim–Chester disease with prominent pericardial involvement: clinical, radiologic, and histologic findings. Am J Med Sci 2002; 324: 96–100.

130. Loire R, Hellal H. Neoplastic pericarditis. Study by thoracotomy and biopsy in 80 cases. Presse Med 1993; 22: 244–248.

131. Meyers DG, Bouska DJ. Diagnostic usefulness of pericardial fluid cytology. Chest 1989; 95: 1142–1143.

132. Bengtsson H, Nilsson P, Bergqvist D. Natural history of abdominal aortic aneurysm detected by screening. Br J Surg 1993; 80: 718–720.

133. Troxler M, Mavor AI, Homer-Vanniasinkam S. Penetrating atherosclerotic ulcers of the aorta. Br J Surg 2001; 88: 1169–1177.

134. Virmani R, Kolodgie F, Farb A, Burke AP. Pathologic evaluation of carotid endarterectomy. Pathol Case Rev 2001; 6: 236–243.

135. Hunt JL, Fairman R, Mitchell ME, et al. Bone formation in carotid plaques: a clinicopathological study. Stroke 2002; 33: 1214–1219.

136. Lammie GA, Wardlaw J, Allan P, et al. What pathological components indicate carotid atheroma activity and can these be identified reliably using ultrasound? Eur J Ultrasound 2000; 11: 77–86.

137. Carr SC, Farb A, Pearce WH, et al. Activated inflammatory cells are associated with plaque rupture in carotid artery stenosis. Surgery 1997; 122: 757–763; discussion 763–764.

138. Virmani R, Atkinson JB, Forman MB. Aortocoronary bypass grafts and extracardiac conduits. In: Silver MD, ed. Cardiovascular pathology, 2nd ed. New York: Churchill Livingstone; 1991: 1607–1647.

139. Gonzalez-Gay MA. Giant cell arteritis and polymyalgia rheumatica: two different but often overlapping conditions. Semin Arthritis Rheum 2004; 33: 289–293.

140. Cantini F, Niccoli L, Storri L, et al. Are polymyalgia rheumatica and giant cell arteritis the same disease? Semin Arthritis Rheum 2004; 33: 294–301.

141. McDonnell PJ, Moore GW, Miller NR, et al. Temporal arteritis. A clinicopathologic study. Ophthalmology 1986; 93: 518–530.

142. Burke AP, Virmani R. Temporal artery biopsy of giant cell arteritis. Pathol Case Rev 2001; 6: 265–273.

143. Achkar AA, Lie JT, Hunder GGO, et al. How does previous corticosteroid treatment affect the biopsy findings in giant cell (temporal) arteritis? Ann Intern Med 1994; 120: 987–992.

144. Disdier P, Pellissier JF, Harle JR, et al. Significance of isolated vasculitis of the vasa vasorum on temporal artery biopsy. J Rheumatol 1994; 21: 258–260.

145. Corcoran GM, Prayson RA, Herzog KM. The significance of perivascular inflammation in the absence of arteritis in temporal artery biopsy specimens. Am J Clin Pathol 2001; 115: 342–347.

146. Kowalewski RM, Maddox JC, Kowalewska J, et al. Isolated temporal small vessel inflammation: an important clue to the diagnosis of giant cell arteritis. Arthr Rheum 2002; 46: S192.

147. Gonzalez-Gay MA, Garcia-Porrua C, Llorca J, et al. Biopsy-negative giant cell arteritis: clinical spectrum and predictive factors for positive temporal artery biopsy. Semin Arthritis Rheum 2001; 30: 249–256.

148. Varma D, O'Neill D. Quantification of the role of temporal artery biopsy in diagnosing clinically suspected giant cell arteritis. Eye 2004; 18: 384–388.

149. Brack A, Martinez-Taboada V, Stanson A, et al. Disease pattern in cranial and large-vessel giant cell arteritis. Arthritis Rheum 1999; 42: 311–317.

150. Hall S, Barr W, Lie JT, et al. Takayasu's arteritis. A study of 32 North American patients. Medicine 1985; 64: 89–99.

151. Virmani R, Lande A, McAllister HA. Pathologic aspects of Takayasu's arteritis. In: Lande A, Berkman YM, McAllister HA, eds. Aortitis: clinical, pathologic and radiographic aspects. New York: Raven Press; 1986: 55–79.

152. Janssen HL, Van Zonneveld M, Van Nunen AB, et al. Polyarteritis nodosa associated with hepatitis B virus infection. The role of antiviral treatment and mutations in the hepatitis B virus genome. Eur J Gastroenterol Hepatol 2004; 16: 801–807.

153. Deeren DH, De Backer AI, Malbrain ML, et al. Treatment of hepatitis B virus-related polyarteritis nodosa: two case reports and a review of the literature. Clin Rheumatol 2004; 23: 172–176.

154. Valeyrie L, Bachot N, Roujeau JC, et al. Neurological manifestations of polyarteritis nodosa associated with the antiphospholipid syndrome. Ann Med Interne (Paris) 2003; 154: 479–482.

155. Akar S, Goktay Y, Akinci B, et al. A case of familial Mediterranean fever and polyarteritis nodosa complicated by spontaneous perirenal and subcapsular hepatic hemorrhage requiring multiple arterial embolizations. Rheumatol Int 2004; 8: 8.

156. Bonsib SM. Polyarteritis nodosa. Semin Diag Pathol 2001; 18: 14–23.

157. Jennette JC, Falk RJ, Andrassy K, et al. Nomenclature of systemic vasculitides. Proposal of an international consensus conference. Arthritis Rheum 1994; 37: 187–192.

158. Gescuk BD, Davis JC. Diagnosis and management of vasculitis. J Musculoskel Med 2002; 19: 407–418.

159. Burke AP, Virmani R. Localized vasculitis. Semin Diag Pathol 2001; 18: 59–66.

160. Mahr A, Guillevin L, Poissonnet M, Ayme S. Prevalences of polyarteritis nodosa, microscopic polyangiitis, Wegener's granulomatosis, and Churg–Strauss syndrome in a French urban multiethnic population in 2000: a capture–recapture estimate. Arthritis Rheum 2004; 51: 92–99.

161. Taubert KA, Shulman ST. Kawasaki disease. Am Fam Physician 1999; 59: 3093–3102, 3107–3108.

162. Burke AP, Virmani R, Perry LW, et al. Fatal Kawasaki disease with coronary arteritis and no coronary aneurysms. Pediatrics 1998; 101: 108–112.

163. Jennette JC, Falk RJ. Anti-neutrophil cytoplasmic autoantibodies: discovery, specificity, disease associations and pathogenic potential. Adv Pathol Lab Med 1995; 8: 363–377.

164. Jennette JC, Thomas DB, Falk RJ. Microscopic polyangiitis (microscopic polyarteritis). Semin Diag Pathol 2001; 18: 3–13.

165. Magro CM, Crowson AN. The cutaneous neutrophilic vascular injury syndromes: a review. Semin Diag Pathol 2001; 18: 47–58.

166. Yi ES, Colby TV. Wegener's granulomatosis. Semin Diag Pathol 2001; 18: 34–46.

167. Pradhan VD, Badakere SS, Pawar AR, Almeida AF. Anti-myeloperoxidase antibodies in patients with microscopic polyangiitis. Indian J Med Sci 2003; 57: 479–486.

168. Agard C, Mouthon L, Mahr A, Guillevin L. Microscopic polyangiitis and polyarteritis nodosa: how and when do they start? Arthritis Rheum 2003; 49: 709–715.

169. Franks T, Koss MN. Pulmonary capillaritis. Curr Opin Pulm Med 2000; 6: 430–435.

170. Seishima M, Oyama Z, Oda M. Skin eruptions associated with microscopic polyangiitis. Eur J Dermatol 2004; 14: 255–258.

171. Almoallim H, Patterson AC. Microscopic polyangiitis sparing the kidneys in a long-term survivor after allogeneic bone marrow transplantation and graft-versus-host disease. Clin Rheumatol 2004; 19: 19.

172. Park J, Banno S, Sugiura Y, et al. Microscopic polyangiitis associated with diffuse panbronchiolitis. Intern Med 2004; 43: 331–335.

173. Zhao MH, Sun QZ, Wang HY. Clinical and pathological characterization of patients with microscopic polyangiitis with medium artery involvement. Ren Fail 2003; 25: 989–995.

174. Iannone F, Falappone P, Pannarale G, et al. Microscopic polyangiitis associated with primary biliary cirrhosis. J Rheumatol 2003; 30: 2710–2712.

175. Hasegawa M, Kawamura N, Murase M, et al. Efficacy of granulocytapheresis and leukocytapheresis for the treatment of microscopic polyangiitis. Therap Apher Dial 2004; 8: 212–216.

176. Guillevin L, Cohen P, Mahr A, et al. Treatment of polyarteritis nodosa and microscopic polyangiitis with poor prognosis factors: a prospective trial comparing glucocorticoids and six or twelve cyclophosphamide pulses in sixty-five patients. Arthritis Rheum 2003; 49: 93–100.

177. Abril A, Calamia KT, Cohen MD. The Churg Strauss syndrome (allergic granulomatous angiitis): review and update. Semin Arthritis Rheum 2003; 33: 106–114.

178. Noth I, Strek ME, Leff AR. Churg–Strauss syndrome. Lancet 2003; 361: 587–594.

179. Drage LA, Davis MD, De Castro F, et al. Evidence for pathogenic involvement of eosinophils and neutrophils in Churg–Strauss syndrome. J Am Acad Dermatol 2002; 47: 209–216.

180. Hellmich B, Ehlers S, Csernok E, Gross WL. Update on the pathogenesis of Churg–Strauss syndrome. Clin Exp Rheumatol 2003; 21: S69–S77.

181. Guilpain P, Viallard JF, Lagarde P, et al. Churg–Strauss syndrome in two patients receiving montelukast. Rheumatology (Oxford) 2002; 41: 535–539.

182. Kobayashi S, Ishizuka S, Tamura N, et al. Churg–Strauss syndrome (CSS) in a patient receiving pranlukast. Clin Rheumatol 2003; 22: 491–492.

183. Moor JW, U-King Im J, MacDonald AW, Whitehead E. Limited form of Churg–Strauss syndrome presenting as a mass in the neck. J Laryngol Otol 2002; 116: 966–968.

184. McGavin CR, Marshall AJ, Lewis CT. Churg–Strauss syndrome with critical endomyocardial fibrosis: 10 year survival after combined surgical and medical management. Heart 2002; 87: E5.

185. Churg A. Recent advances in the diagnosis of Churg–Strauss syndrome. Mod Pathol 2001; 14: 1284–1293.

186. Della Rossa A, Baldini C, Tavoni A, et al. Churg–Strauss syndrome: clinical and serological features of 19 patients from a single Italian centre. Rheumatology (Oxford) 2002; 41: 1286–1294.

187. Gross WL. Churg–Strauss syndrome: update on recent developments. Curr Opin Rheumatol 2002; 14: 11–14.

188. Hellmich B, Gross WL. Recent progress in the pharmacotherapy of Churg–Strauss syndrome. Expert Opin Pharmacother 2004; 5: 25–35.

189. Watts RA, Carruthers DM, Symmons DPM, Scott DGI. The incidence of rheumatoid vasculitis in the Norwich Health Authority. Br J Rheumatol 1994; 33: 832–833.

190. Szuba A, Cooke JP. Thromboangiitis obliterans. An update on Buerger's disease. West J Med 1998; 168: 255–260.

191. Von Fritschen U, Malzfeld E, Clasen A, Kortmann H. Inflammatory abdominal aortic aneurysm: a postoperative course of retroperitoneal fibrosis. J Vasc Surg 1999; 30: 1090–1098.

192. Heggtveit HA. Syphilic aortitis: a clinicopathologic autopsy study of 100 cases. Circulation 1965; 29: 346–359.

193. Corbi P, Manic H, Donal E, et al. Mycotic aneurysm of the splenic artery. A rare complication of surgically treated infective endocarditis and its causative cardiac lesion. Arch Mal Coeur Vaiss 1999; 92: 1221–1224.

194. Burke AP, Sobin LH, Virmani R. Localized vasculitis of the gastrointestinal tract. Am J Surg Pathol 1995; 19: 338–349.

195. Fenves AZ, Ram CV. Fibromuscular dysplasia of the renal arteries. Curr Hypertens Rep 1999; 1: 546–549.

196. Suzuki H, Daida H, Sakurai H, Yamaguchi H. Familial fibromuscular dysplasia of bilateral brachial arteries. Heart 1999; 82: 251–252.

197. Alimi Y, Mercier C, Pellissier JF, et al. Fibromuscular disease of the renal artery: a new histopathologic classification. Ann Vasc Surg 1992; 6: 220–224.

198. Luschner TF, Lie JT, Stanson AW, et al. Arterial fibromuscular dysplasia. Mayo Clin Proc 1987; 62: 931–952.

199. Lie JT. Segmental mediolytic arteritis. Not an arteritis but a variant of arterial fibromuscular dysplasia. Arch Pathol Lab Med 1992; 116: 238–241.

200. Chan RJ, Goodman TA, Aretz TH, Lie JT. Segmental mediolytic arteriopathy of the splenic and hepatic arteries mimicking systemic necrotizing vasculitis. Arthritis Rheum 1998; 41: 935–938.

201. Slavin RE, Saeki K, Bhagavan B, Maas AE. Segmental arterial mediolysis: a precursor to fibromuscular dysplasia? Mod Pathol 1995; 8: 287–294.

202. Kato T, Yamada K, Akiyama Y, et al. Ruptured inferior mesenteric artery aneurysm due to segmental mediolytic arteritis. Cardiovasc Surg 1996; 4: 644–646.

203. Juvonen T, Niemela O, Reinila A, et al. Spontaneous intraabdominal haemorrhage caused by segmental mediolytic arteritis in a patient with systemic lupus erythematosus – an underestimated entity of autoimmune origin? Eur J Vasc Surg 1994; 8: 96–100.

204. Roberts WC, Honig HS. The spectrum of cardiovascular disease in the Marfan syndrome: a clinico-morphologic study of 18 necropsy patients and comparison to 151 previously reported necropsy patients. Am Heart J 1982; 104: 115–135.

205. Larson EW, Edwards WD. Risk factors for aortic dissection: a necropsy study of 161 cases. Am J Cardiol 1984; 53: 849–855.

206. Homme JL, Aubry M-C, Kral CA, et al. Surgical pathology of the ascending aorta: A clinicopathologic study of 514 autopsy cases (1985–1999). Mod Pathol 2001; 14: 45A.

207. Katzke S, Booms P, Tiecke F, et al. TGGE screening of the entire FBN1 coding sequence in 126 individuals with Marfan syndrome and related fibrillinopathies. Hum Mutat 2002; 20: 197–208.

208. Robinson PN, Booms P. The molecular pathogenesis of the Marfan syndrome. Cell Mol Life Sci 2001; 58: 1698–1707.

209. Robinson PN, Booms P, Katzke S, et al. Mutations of FBN1 and genotype-phenotype correlations in Marfan syndrome and related fibrillinopathies. Hum Mutat 2002; 20: 153–161.

210. Nicod P, Bloor C, Godfrey M, et al. Familial aortic dissecting aneurysm. J Am Coll Cardiol 1989; 13: 811–819.

211. Clementi M, Notari L, Borghi A, Tenconi R. Familial congenital bicuspid aortic valve: a disorder of uncertain inheritance. Am J Med Genet 1996; 62: 336–338.

212. McDonald K, Maurer BJ. Familial aortic valve disease: evidence for a genetic influence? Eur Heart J 1989; 10: 676–677.

213. Huntington K, Hunter AG, Chan KL. A prospective study to assess the frequency of familial clustering of congenital bicuspid aortic valve. J Am Coll Cardiol 1997; 30: 1809–1812.

214. Virmani R, Burke AP, Farb A. Arterial dysplasia, aneurysms and dissections. In: Atlas of cardiovascular pathology. Philadelphia: WB Saunders; 1996:184.

215. Tomson C. Vascular calcification in chronic renal failure. Nephron Clin Pract 2003; 93: c124–c130.

216. El-Reshaid K, Madda JP, al-Duwairi Q, Sugathan T. Progressive ischemic gangrene in dialysis patients: a clinicopathological correlation. Ren Fail 1995; 17: 437–447.

217. Rubinger D, Friedlaender MM, Silver J, et al. Progressive vascular calcification with necrosis of

extremities in hemodialysis patients: a possible role of iron overload. Am J Kidney Dis 1986; 7: 125–129.

218. Lie JT, Jensen PL, Smith RE. Adventitial cystic disease of the lesser saphenous vein. Arch Pathol Lab Med 1991; 115: 946–948.

219. Rand JH. Molecular pathogenesis of the antiphospholipid syndrome. Circ Res 2002; 90: 29–37.

220. Hughson MD, McCarty GA, Brumback RA. Spectrum of vascular pathology affecting patients with the antiphospholipid syndrome. Hum Pathol 1995; 26: 716–724.

221. O'Briain DS, Jeffers M, Kay EW, Hourihane DO. Bleeding due to colorectal atheroembolism. Diagnosis by biopsy of adenomatous polyps or of ischemic ulcer. Am J Surg Pathol 1991; 15: 1078–1082,.

222. Perrot-Applanat M, Cohen-Solal K, et al. Progesterone receptor expression in human saphenous veins. Circulation 1995; 92: 2975–2983.

223. Charles AK, Gresham GA. Histopathological changes in venous grafts and in varicose and non-varicose veins. J Clin Pathol 1993; 46: 603–606.

224. Blondeau P. Primary cardiac tumors – French studies of 533 cases. Thorac Cardiovasc Surg 1990; 38: 192–195.

225. Centofanti P, Di Rosa E, Deorsola L, et al. Primary cardiac tumors: early and late results of surgical treatment in 91 patients. Ann Thorac Surg 1999; 68: 1236–1241.

226. Dein JR, Frist WH, Stinson EB, et al. Primary cardiac neoplasms. Early and late results of surgical treatment in 42 patients. J Thorac Cardiovasc Surg 1987; 93: 502–511.

227. Kamiya H, Yasuda T, Nagamine H, et al. Surgical treatment of primary cardiac tumors: 28 years' experience in Kanazawa University Hospital. Jpn Circ J 2001; 65: 315–319.

228. Mathur A, Airan B, Bhan A, et al. Non-myxomatous cardiac tumours: twenty-year experience. Indian Heart J 2000; 52: 319–323.

229. Melo J, Ahmad A, Chapman R, et al. Primary tumors of the heart: a rewarding challenge. Am Surg 1979; 45: 681–683.

230. Miralles A, Bracamonte L, Soncul H, et al. Cardiac tumors: clinical experience and surgical results in 74 patients. Ann Thorac Surg 1991; 52: 886–895.

231. Murphy MC, Sweeney MS, Putnam JB, et al. Surgical treatment of cardiac tumors: a 25-year experience. Ann Thorac Surg 1990; 49: 612–617.

232. Reece IJ, Cooley DA, Frazier OH, et al. Cardiac tumors. J Thorac Cardiovasc Surg 1984; 88: 439–446.

233. Tazelaar HD, Locke TJ, McGregor CG. Pathology of surgically excised primary cardiac tumors. Mayo Clin Proc 1992; 67: 957–965.

234. Veinot JP, Burns BF, Commons AS, Thomas J. Cardiac neoplasms at the Canadian Reference Centre for Cancer Pathology. Can J Cardiol 1999; 15: 311–319.

235. Verkkala K, Kupari M, Maamies T, et al. Primary cardiac tumours – operative treatment of 20 patients. Thorac Cardiovasc Surg 1989; 37: 361–364.

236. Bear PA, Moodie DS. Malignant primary cardiac tumors. The Cleveland Clinic experience, 1956 to 1986. Chest 1987; 92: 860–862.

237. Putnam JBJ, Sweeney MS, Colon R, et al. Primary cardiac sarcomas. Ann Thorac Surg 1991; 51: 906–910.

The thymus and mediastinum

21

Mark R. Wick   Celeste N. Powers

Over the past 30 years, the definition, diagnosis, and treatment of thymic epithelial tumors has been refined. That group of neoplasms formerly designated generally as 'thymomas' has now been divided into several clinicopathological entities.[1] The true gamut of the histological appearances and behavior of thymomas (defined herein as cytologically bland tumors of the thymic epithelium) has been better defined in this process.

The pathologic features of both microscopically bland and cytologically malignant thymic epithelial tumors are considered in the following discussion, along with those of other neoplasms and pseudoneoplastic conditions that may arise in the anterior mediastinum. Microscopic differential diagnostic possibilities will also be described, together with appropriate methods for separating them from one another. Neoplasms that show a preference for the posterior mediastinum typically belong to the spectrum of mesenchymal or neuroectodermal proliferations, which are discussed elsewhere in this monograph.

PART I: CYSTIC LESIONS OF THE THYMIC REGION AND MEDIASTINUM

Even if potentially cystic mediastinal neoplasms (e.g. Hodgkin's lymphoma, thyroid tumors, thymoma, teratoma, and seminoma) are included, cystic lesions of the mediastinum are uncommon; they account for 10–15% of roentgenographically found intrathoracic masses.[2,3] Several tissue types can be represented in such cysts, including pericardial, thymic, enteric, and bronchogenic elements; in fact, some mediastinal cysts may harbor more than one of these components. Many cysts in the chest cavity are developmental rather than acquired, and their multipotential tissue constituency reflects the proximity of the embryologic foregut, pleuropericardial membranes, and branchial pouches in early morphogenesis.[4]

THYMIC CYSTS

Thymic cysts are encountered clinically mainly in patients between 20 and 50 years of age, most of whom are asymptomatic. It is now known that congenital unilocular cysts and acquired multilocular cysts of the thymus both exist as distinct entities.[5] In imaging studies, they are rounded and circumscribed masses in the anterior mediastinum (Fig. 21.1). Unilocular cysts have a water-like density on computed tomograms, but multilocular cysts demonstrate a higher attenuation. Both types may demonstrate calcification of the lesional periphery, and their maximum size extends up to 18 cm.

Gross examination demonstrates a thin fibrous wall enclosing unilocular thymic cysts and a thick wall in multilocular lesions

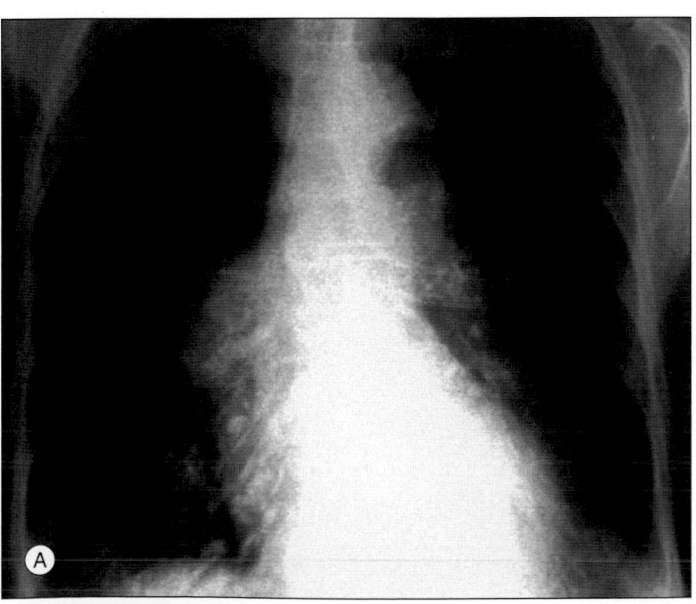
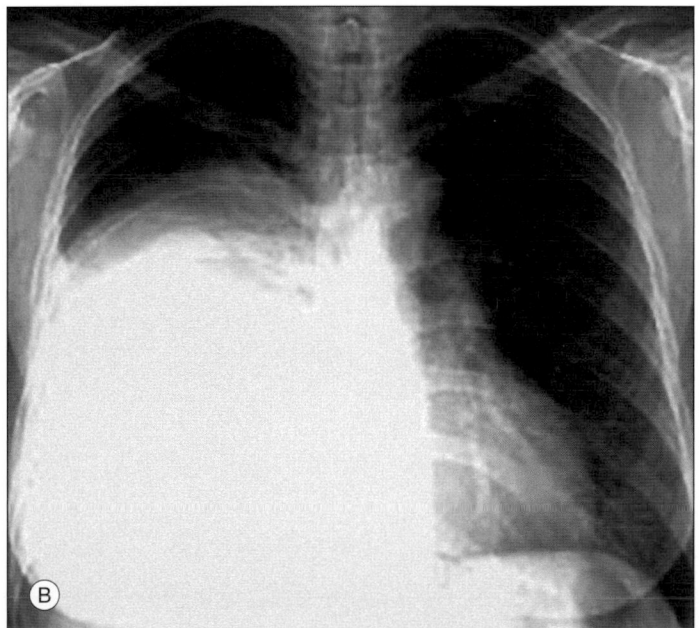

Fig. 21.1 Chest radiographs of thymic cysts **(A & B)**, showing mediastinal lesions that project into the right hemithorax.

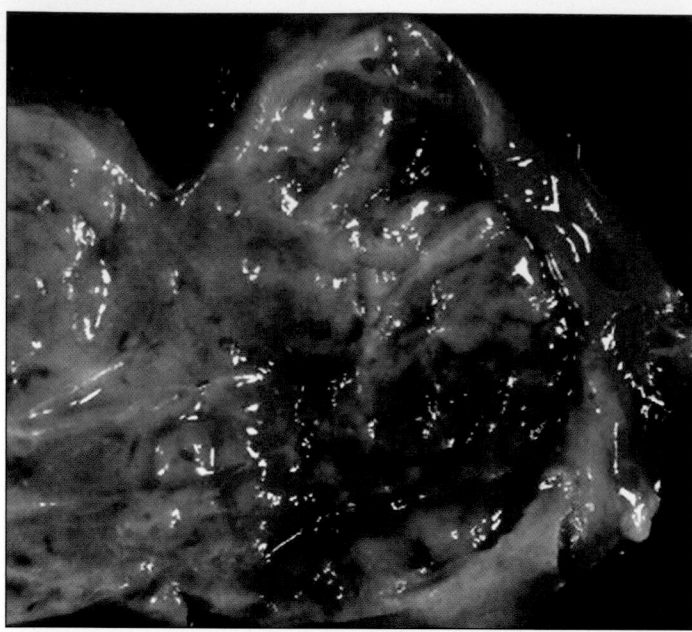

Fig. 21.2 Gross photograph of thymic cyst, demonstrating septated internal cavity and mural tissue with a variegated appearance.

(Fig. 21.2). The latter commonly show pericystic fibrous adhesions as well. Both types of thymic cyst may be centered on the thymus or connected to that gland by a pedicle. Contents of thymic cysts are variably dense; unilocular lesions typically contain serous fluid, and multilocular cysts enclose keratinous, turbid, or hemorrhagic material.

These appearances also correspond to the integrity of the lining as seen microscopically. In unilocular thymic cysts, the epithelial surface of the cyst cavity is only a few layers in thickness – consisting of bland squamoid cells – and the fibrous wall lacks inflammation, hemorrhage, and cholesterol granulomas. The epithelial component of multilocular thymic cysts is commonly proliferative in nature, with multiple layers of squamous cells, or squamous elements admixed with cuboidal, columnar, or micropapillary glandular epithelium

(Fig. 21.3). Small foci of parathyroid or salivary glandular epithelium can be observed rarely. In that eventuality, one may wish to employ the diagnostic terms 'third pharyngeal pouch cyst' or 'mixed multilocular thymic cyst.' Mature lymphocytes, granulation tissue, hemorrhage, and cholesterol granulomas are consistently present in the walls and cavities of multilocular thymic cysts. The cause of the inflammatory process that is felt to be the etiology of these lesions is currently undetermined. Hassall's corpuscles and residual thymic tissue are apparent in up to 50% cases, but cartilage and smooth muscle are absent.[5]

A distinctive subtype of multilocular thymic cyst is the 'proliferating' variant.[6,7] It is similar morphologically to cysts that are seen in the skin and called 'proliferating epidermoid cyst' and 'proliferating trichilemmal cyst' (see Chapter 8). Narrow, interconnecting tongues of squamoid epithelium extend outward from the cyst lining into the surrounding connective tissue. This change reflects the presence of pseudoepitheliomatous hyperplasia in thymic cysts. The cytologic features of the proliferating epithelium are bland rather than dysplastic, and there is no true invasion of the intervening stroma. Mitoses are often observed but they are physiological in nature. The significance of proliferating thymic cysts is, obviously, the danger that they may be overinterpreted as carcinomas. True malignant alteration in thymic cysts is rare,[8,9] and the tumors in those cases have been patently invasive at a clinical level.

Another morphological variation in multilocular thymic cysts is that of lymphoid hyperplasia, with the formation of germinal centers in a prominent stromal lymphocytic infiltrate. This eventuality should bring the possibility of acquired immunodeficiency syndrome to mind, inasmuch as it is associated with systemic infection by the human immunodeficiency virus.[10]

Thymus glands that are involved by Hodgkin's disease (HD) also may undergo cystic transformation, as may others that have been traumatized by surgery or other physical injuries. The coexistence of thymic cysts with mediastinal HD was originally felt to represent the effects of therapeutic irradiation or systemic chemotherapy.[11] However, this concurrence has also been observed in untreated Hodgkin's lymphoma cases.[12] Hence, the preferred interpretation is now that the tumor alters the integrity of the thymic epithelium, producing acquired cystic changes in the gland. The added effects of cytotoxic therapy may well facilitate this phenomenon by producing a loss of

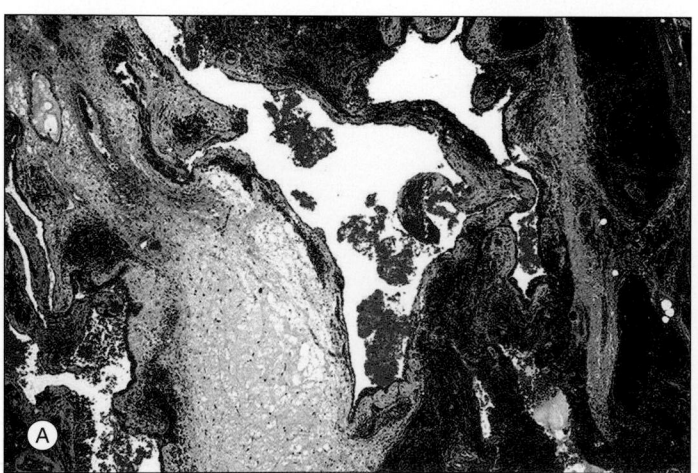

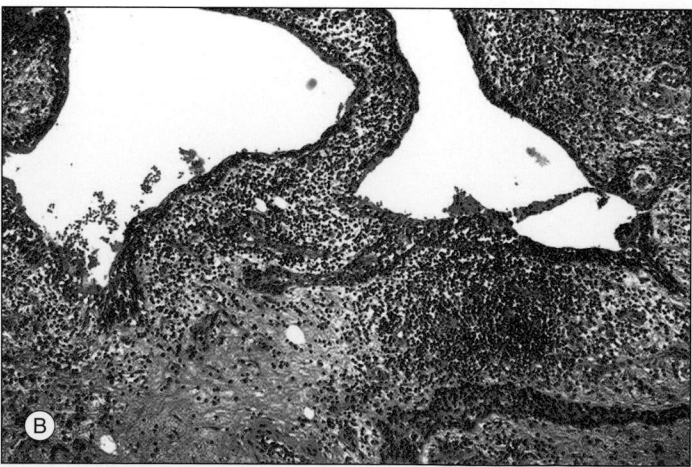

Fig. 21.3 (A) Multilocular thymic cyst, showing stromal lymphocytosis and squamoid epithelial lining. **(B)** The bland nature of the cyst lining is better seen in this photograph.

volume in the neoplastic mass. Nevertheless, the curious fact that thymic cysts have not been described in connection with mediastinal *non*-Hodgkin's lymphomas would argue against that mechanism. Another type of acquired thymic cyst is seen after thoracotomies that are done for a variety of reasons. A postulated reason for this occurrence is that surgical trauma to the thymus causes cystic epithelial alteration, perhaps by means of microscopic vascular damage.[13]

BRONCHOGENIC CYSTS

Bronchogenic cysts can arise in the anterior, superior, middle, or posterior mediastinum, or even within the pericardium, and they may be discovered potentially at any age.[2,3,14–16] Although cysts of this type in the lung parenchyma are often connected to large airways, intramediastinal bronchogenic cysts are typically self-contained. Radiographically, one sees a rounded mass that molds itself to adjacent organs; the internal portion of the cyst is hypodense and the wall may be calcified. Angiograms may demonstrate a separate vascular supply to bronchogenic cysts, differing from that of other mediastinal cysts.

Grossly, bronchogenic cysts can be uniloculated or multiloculated with internal fibrous septa. The contents are turbid or viscous.

Histologically, these lesions show the presence of respiratory-type columnar epithelium, often ciliated, juxtaposed to small aggregates of hyaline cartilage (Fig. 21.4). Smooth muscle also is potentially seen in admixture with the chondroid elements, but cholesterol granulomas are not apparent in bronchogenic cysts.[2,3,16] Their overall organization, resembling that of the normal bronchi, is sufficient to eliminate the possibility of cystic teratoma (see below) from diagnostic consideration.

PERICARDIAL CYSTS

Mediastinal pericardial cysts are found most often in the cardiophrenic angle. They are seen throughout life as generally asymptomatic masses that are discovered radiographically.[17,18] Rare cases produce dyspnea or substernal chest pain. On chest films, pericardial cysts abut the contours of the heart and are irregularly shaped with a water-like density. They can be observed in any of the mediastinal subcompartments.

Excised pericardial cysts exhibit thin fibrous walls, and they collapse when opened. The internal surfaces are smooth, with serous fluid contents. Microscopically, one sees laminated fibrous tissue that is usually covered by a single layer of bland mesothelium (Fig. 21.5).[2,3] On occasion, it may undergo focal papillary hyperplasia. Specialized mesenchymal tissues and cholesterol granulomas are absent.

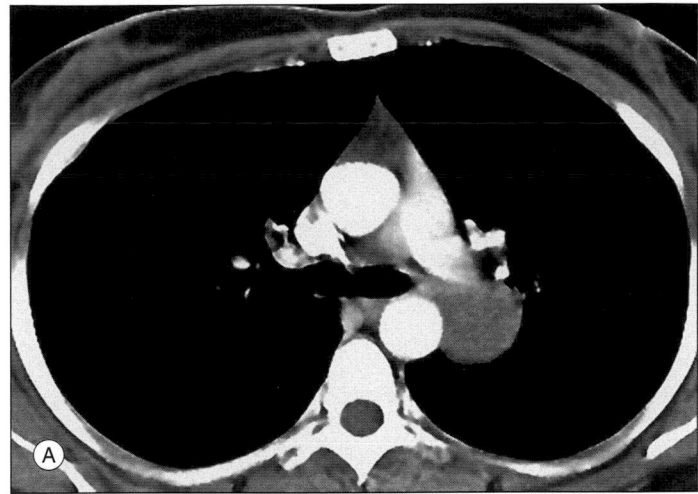

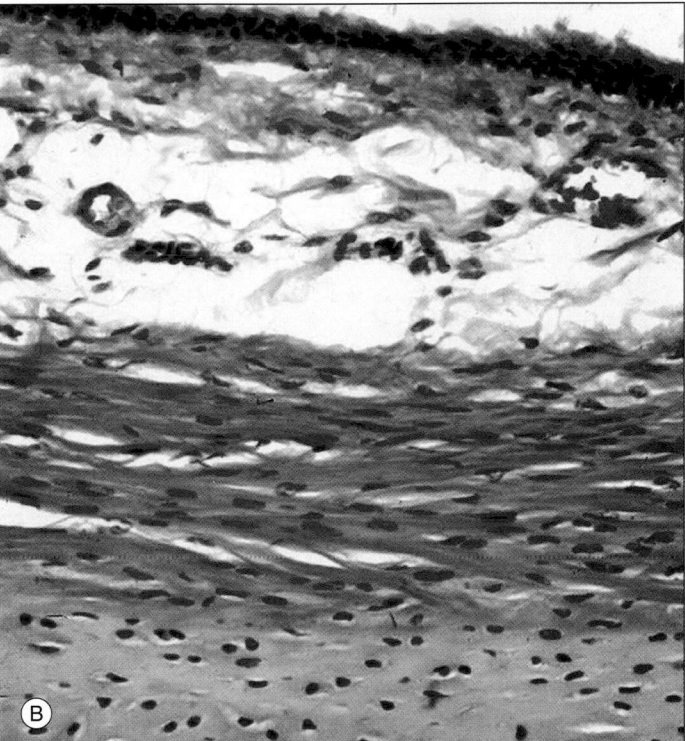

Fig. 21.4 Computed tomogram **(A)** and microscopic image **(B)** of bronchogenic cyst, with respiratory epithelial lining and mature smooth muscle and cartilage in cyst wall.

ENTERIC CYSTS

Enteric cysts are almost always localized to the posterior mediastinum, and they typically affect children or adolescents.[2,3,19,20] Patients with paraesophageal cysts may complain of dysphagia or subnormal weight gain; gastroesophageal enteric cysts can produce cough, vomiting, fever, and pneumonia or empyema. Enterogenous mediastinal cysts also may be associated with vertebral anomalies such as hemivertebrae and spina bifida.[21]

Radiographically, enteric cysts measure up to 10 cm in greatest dimension. They are usually rounded and may show internal loculation on computed tomography. If leakage of cyst contents has occurred,

pleural effusions or pulmonary consolidation can be present in the posterior lung fields.

Grossly, enteric cysts have a thick fibromuscular wall and a smooth lining, with or without multiloculation. The cyst contents are variably viscous, and they have an acidic pH in some examples where functional fundic-type gastric mucosa is well represented. Spontaneous cystic rupture may be apparent.[2,3,20]

Microscopically, enteric cysts show a double layer of mural smooth muscle, as seen in normal gut. Cartilage and cholesterol granulomas are absent. The mucosal epithelium may be squamous, columnar, or mixed, but gastroesophageal lesions usually contain at least some specialized gastric glandular mucosa.

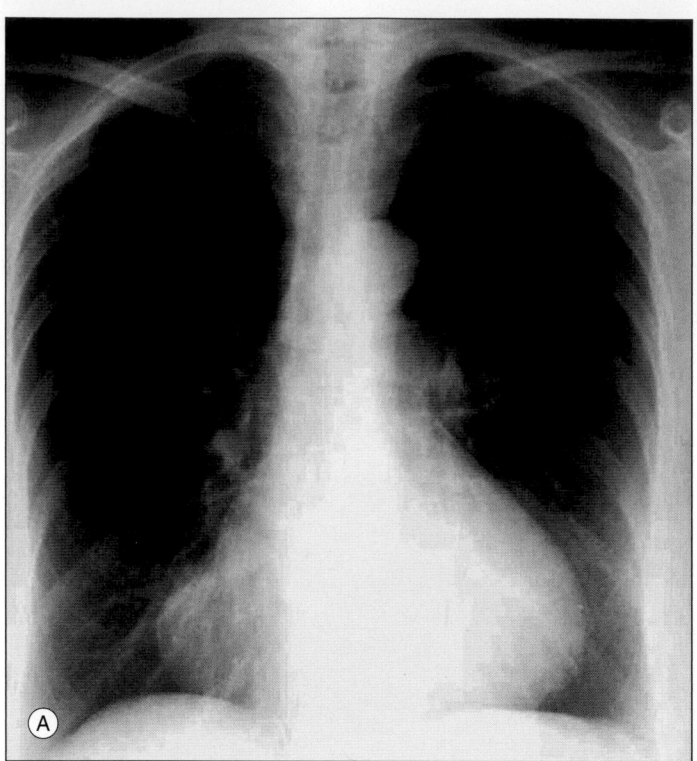

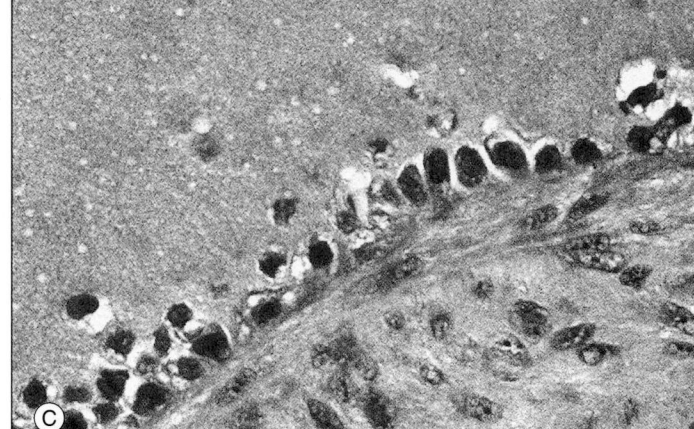

Fig. 21.5 Chest radiograph **(A)** and computed tomogram **(B)** of pericardial cyst, showing a rounded supradiaphragmatic mass at the right heart border. The cyst is lined by a plump mesothelial cell layer **(C)**.

CYTOPATHOLOGY OF MEDIASTINAL CYSTS

Aspiration of mediastinal cysts is seldom diagnostic. Regardless of which type of cyst is sampled, one typically sees only mature lymphocytes, with or without isolated epithelial cells.[10,16,17,22,23] The latter may be squamoid, cuboidal, or columnar in nature. On the other hand, cystic *neoplasms* such as thymoma, seminoma, Hodgkin's lymphoma, etc., may indeed yield characteristic aspirates, as described below and elsewhere in this book (see Chapter 11).

PART II: THYMIC HYPERPLASIAS

Thymic hyperplasia has been a controversial diagnosis for over 100 years, as a consequence of the suggestion made in the 1890s that enlargement of the thymus was a potential cause of death in childhood (so-called '*status thymicolymphaticus*'). Hofmann et al. subscribe to the premise that there are four forms of true thymic hyperplasia (TH): 'massive' hyperplasia; 'rebound' thymic hyperplasia of childhood and adolescence; hyperplasia associated with endocrinopathies; and lymphoid hyperplasia of the thymus.[24]

'Massive' TH is rare, and it is seen exclusively in children. Chest radiographs demonstrate a lobulated anterosuperior mediastinal mass. Clinically, these patients are often asymptomatic, but some of them develop dyspnea, cough, lymphadenopathy, or hepatosplenomegaly. Peripheral lymphocytosis also may be seen.[25] Pathologic examination of resected thymuses in such cases shows no abnormality in the

compartmentalization of the glands into cortex and medulla, nor are the constituent lymphoid cells and thymic epithelium aberrant. The process seems to represent a simple augmentation of all normal thymic components, with a resulting increase in glandular mass. The cause is unknown.[24]

'Rebound' TH is seen in children after burn injuries, administration of exogenous steroids or cytoreductive therapy for malignancies, cardiac surgery, or recovery from systemic infections such as tuberculosis.[26–28] The radiographic and pathologic findings in this form of glandular hyperplasia are identical to those described in connection with 'massive' TH. Similar comments apply to hyperplasia of the thymus seen in patients with Graves' disease, Addison's disease, acromegaly, and congenital panhypopituitarism.[24]

Lymphoid hyperplasia of the thymus is, by far, the most common form of TH. It is associated potentially with myasthenia gravis,

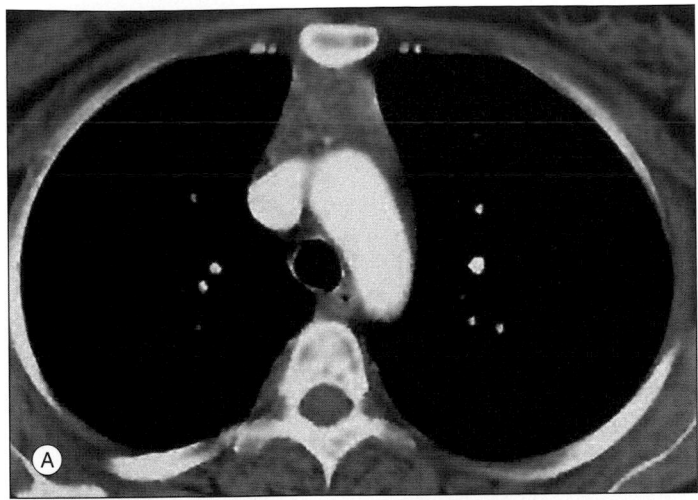

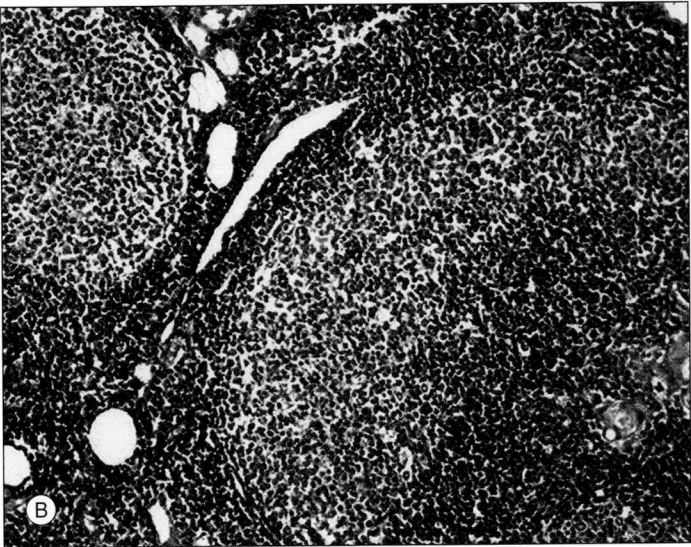

Fig. 21.6 Computed tomogram **(A)** and photomicrograph **(B)** of thymic hyperplasia. Germinal centers are present in the lymphocytic population of the thymus.

multiple sclerosis, inflammatory bowel disease, hepatopathies, thyrotoxicosis, hypoadrenalism, acromegaly, diabetes mellitus, and toxoplasmosis.[24,29,30] Importantly, it may also be seen in non-neoplastic portions of thymuses that contain thymomas. Microscopically, the sine qua non of lymphoid hyperplasia is the presence of germinal centers among the lymphoid population (Fig. 21.6). These contain immunoblasts and 'tingible-body' histiocytes, as well as accentuated mantles of small lymphocytes. Differential diagnosis centers on 'micronodular' thymoma, as described in the next section. However, unlike the latter lesion, no form of TH features the presence of thymic *epithelial* proliferation.

CYTOPATHOLOGY OF THYMIC HYPERPLASIA

Fine needle aspiration of thymic hyperplasia yields either lymphoid cells alone, or in admixture with rare thymic epithelial elements.[31,32] The former components are potentially represented by a spectrum of lymphocytic elements ranging from immunoblasts to mature thymo-cytes, and are therefore not distinguishable morphologically from lymphoid hyperplasias of mediastinal lymph nodes. Thymic epithelial cells are typified by a tendency to cohesion, pale dispersed chromatin, oval nuclei, and the presence of small chromocenters[33,34] They may be difficult to separate from histiocytes on cytological grounds, but immunoreactivity for keratin is helpful in that regard. A definitive distinction between 'true' TH and thymoma cannot be made by fine needle aspiration because the microscopic images associated with those conditions are closely similar.

PART III: THYMIC EPITHELIAL NEOPLASMS

THYMOMAS

Thymomas usually are anterosuperior mediastinal masses that may be discovered incidentally by chest radiography during routine medical examinations. Alternately, they can produce symptoms such as cough, dyspnea, palpitations, and substernal or interscapular pain. A number of paraneoplastic syndromes (myasthenia gravis, pure erythroid aplasia, acquired hypogammaglobulinemia, etc.) may herald the presence of a thymoma.[34–36] Rarely, thymomas may occur in ectopic locations, such as the posterior mediastinum,[37] the pulmonary parenchyma[38] the pleura,[39] and the base of the neck.[40] Indeed, because of that peculiarity, a simulation of such other tumors as mesothelioma or carcinoma of the lung may be produced.[41] These phenomena relate to flaws in thymic embryologic development.

Classically, thymomas are encapsulated, circumscribed, lobulated neoplasms. Their cut surfaces are firm, tan-pink, and homogeneous, and subdivision into macroscopic lobules by thick fibrous internal bands is common (Fig. 21.7). The capsule is also characteristically thick and collagenized. Up to 50% of thymomas may contain gross internal cysts, often filled with fluid or grumous cellular debris, and these may be so prominent as to simulate true cysts of the mediastinum (see below). Limited foci of necrosis may be present, but extensive necrotic changes, with or without hemorrhage, are unusual and suggest the possibility of another diagnosis. Occasional thymomas exhibit macroscopic foci of calcification or an incomplete peripheral rim of calcification or ossification. Other tumors (particularly lymphocyte-predominant thymomas) sometimes lack obvious capsules and internal septations, and assume a tan-gray, homogeneous appearance like that of 'fish flesh.' Rarely, small, nodular thymomas may be seen within a single lobe of an otherwise normal thymus; this is commonest in glands which have been excised in the treatment of myasthenia gravis. Thymomatous nodules have likewise been observed in the walls of thymic cysts.[42]

An important feature of the gross assessment of thymomas is the surgeon's detailed description of the tumor in situ. Thymomas that are totally encapsulated and therefore easily resectable differ behaviorally from those that show invasion of contiguous mediastinal structures.[43] The prognostic significance of these findings will be discussed subsequently. Tumor size is extremely variable, and it corresponds to the presence or absence of clinical symptoms. Rosai and Levine[42] described one thymoma that was merely 1 mm in diameter; conversely, Smith et al. observed one that weighed 5700 g and measured 34 cm in diameter.[44]

Thymomas are comprised by varying proportions of epithelial cells and lymphocytes. However, the epithelial cells are the only *neoplastic* elements in such tumors. These are at least three times the size of mature lymphocytes, and contain a moderate amount of amphophilic cytoplasm. Their nuclear membranes are slightly indented, and chromatin is evenly dispersed, with inconspicuous

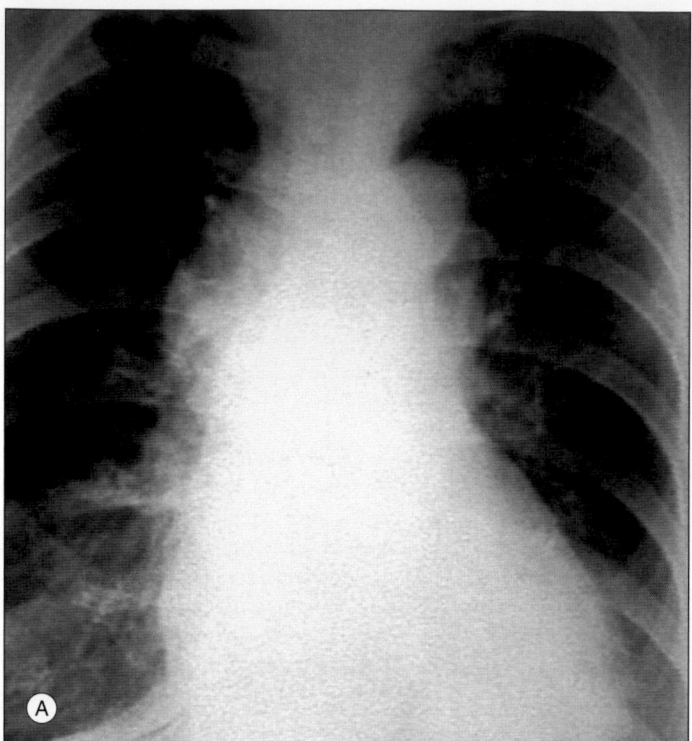

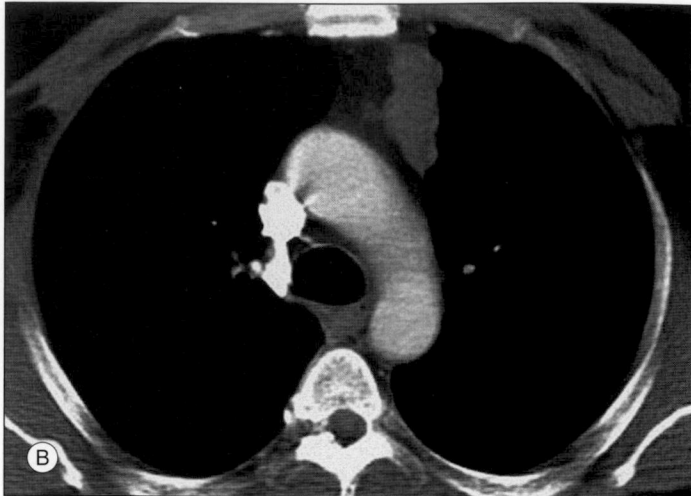

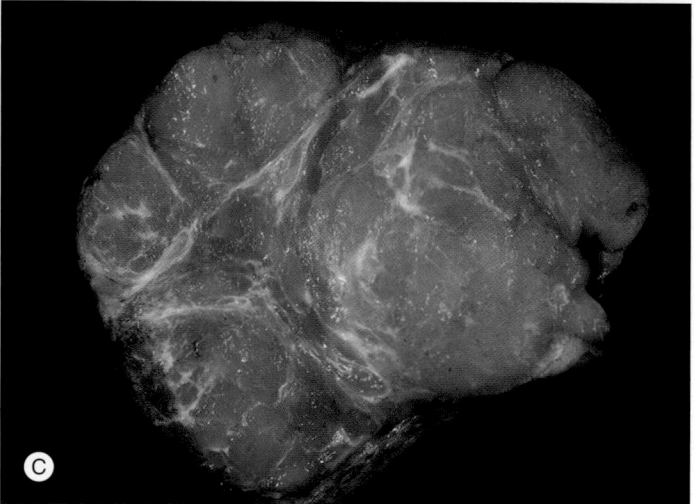

Fig. 21.7 **(A)** Chest radiograph of thymoma, demonstrating a lobulated anterosuperior mediastinal mass. **(B)** Computed tomogram showing involvement of the anterior chest wall by an invasive thymoma. **(C)** Gross photograph of an encapsulated thymoma, showing internal fibrous septa.

nucleoli. Mitoses are usually scanty in the epithelial cells of thymomas, with no atypical division figures.

Because they relate usefully to histological differential diagnosis, we prefer the terms 'predominantly lymphocytic,' 'mixed lympho-epithelial,' and 'predominantly epithelial' to describe types of thymoma, following the system introduced by Bernatz et al. (Fig. 21.8).[45] These subtypes are arbitrarily defined as neoplasms in which lymphocytes comprise respectively two-thirds or more, one-third to two-thirds, and less than one-third of the intratumoral cell population. Spindle-cell thymomas are regarded as a special variant of the last of these three groups.

As an aside, the authors believe that the Bernatz system generally does not represent – and was not intended to be – a prognostic classification. Indeed, there is currently no way of sorting thymomas microscopically which correlates perfectly with their biologic attributes.[46] That comment includes a scheme introduced by Marino, Muller-Hermelink, and coworkers.[47,48] It is usually abbreviated as the MMH classification and is predicated on the alleged resemblance of epithelial elements in thymomas to those of the normal thymic cortex ('cortical" thymomas – usually synonymous with Bernatz lymphocyte-predominant, mixed lymphoepithelial, and most epithelial-predominant lesions) or the normal thymic medulla ('medullary" thymomas, equivalent in most cases to spindle-cell lesions in the Bernatz system). It has been suggested that 'medullary' thymomas are associated with a good prognosis, whereas 'cortical' tumors (including those with modest cytologic atypia, also called 'well-differentiated thymic carcinoma'[49]) have a more adverse evolution. 'Mixed cortical-medullary' thymomas are said to demonstrate intermediary behavioral features. As synopsized by Shimosato and

Mukai,[1] it would appear that the MMH system is actually a simple redesignation of entities contained in the Bernatz classification scheme, using different terms.[50] One could therefore question whether the MMH strategy is actually progressive, as portrayed in the recent literature. Spindle-cell ('medullary') thymomas have long been known to demonstrate generally innocuous behavior; accordingly, it would seem advisable to reassess the contentions of MMH system advocates after pure spindle-cell tumors have been *excluded* from statistical evaluations.

Problems with interobserver reproducibility in the classification of thymomas are also considerable. Moran and Suster have considered the effects of sampling bias in the microscopic interpretation of such neoplasms,[51] and suggested that histological variants thereof are best defined after examination of several tissue blocks from several areas of the lesion.

In 1999, Rosai published the second edition of *Histological Typing of Tumors of the Thymus*,[52] sponsored by the World Health Organization (WHO) International Histological Classification of Tumors project. An attempt to reconcile the Bernatz and MMH schemes was introduced, producing yet another 'hybrid' system. It describes thymomas as '*type A*' (spindle-cell or medullary), 'composed of a population of neoplastic thymic epithelial cells having spindle/oval shape, lacking nuclear atypia, and accompanied by few or no non-neoplastic lymphocytes;' '*type AB*,' 'in which foci having

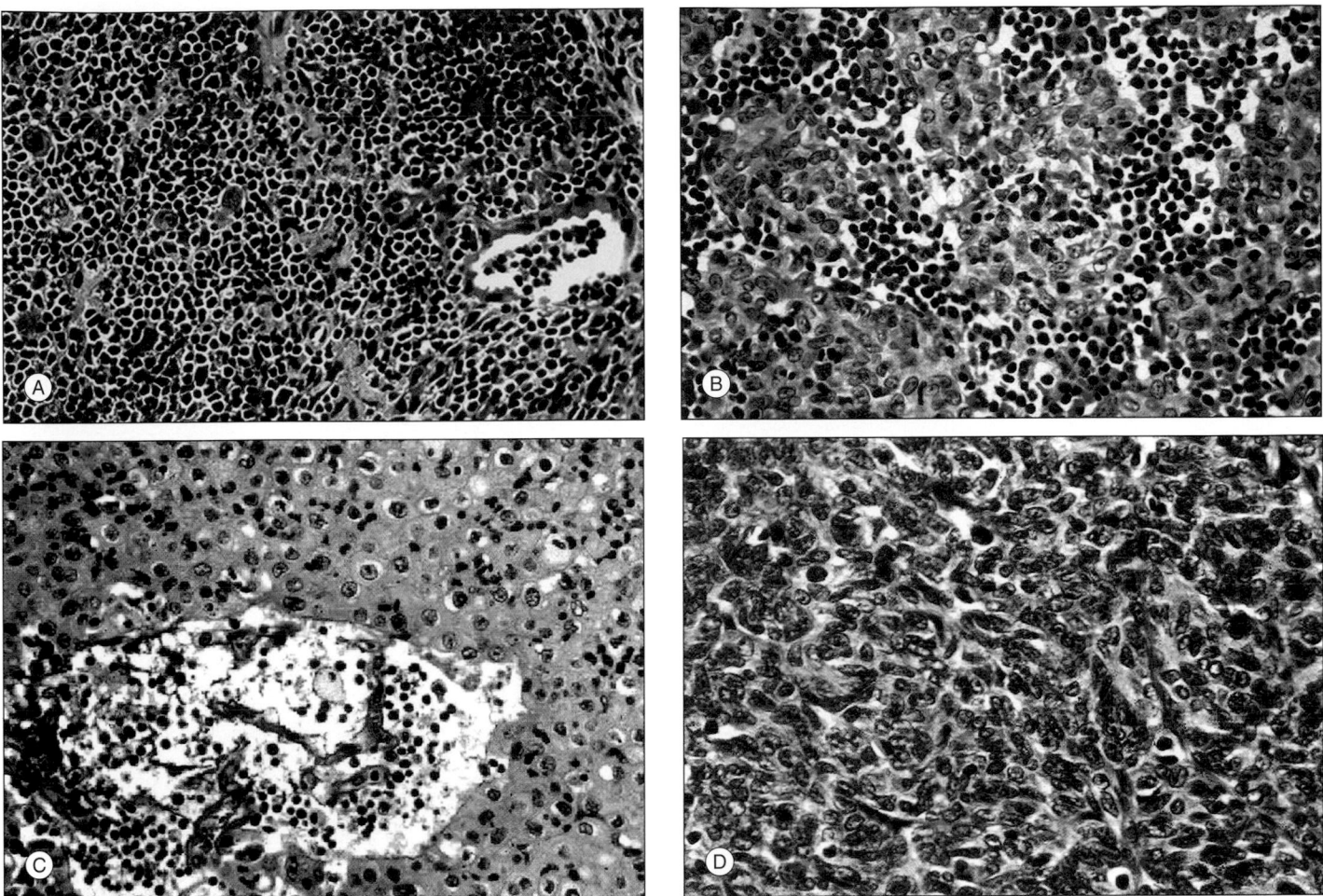

Fig. 21.8 Representative photomicrographs of **(A)** predominantly lymphocytic thymoma; **(B)** mixed lymphoepithelial thymoma; **(C)** predominantly epithelial thymoma with perivascular serum 'lake' and **(D)** spindle cell epithelial thymoma [Bernatz classification].

the features of type A thymoma are admixed with foci rich in lymphocytes;' 'type B1,' 'which resembles the normal functional thymus in that it combines large expanses having an appearance practically indistinguishable from normal thymic cortex with areas resembling thymic medulla;' 'type B2,' 'in which the neoplastic epithelial component appears as scattered plump cells with vesicular nuclei and distinct nucleoli among a heavy population of lymphocytes. Perivascular spaces are common and sometimes very prominent. A perivascular arrangement of tumor cells resulting in a palisading effect may be seen;' and 'type B3,' 'predominantly composed of epithelial cells having a round or polygonal shape and exhibiting no or mild atypia. They are admixed with a minor component of lymphocytes, resulting in a sheet like growth of the neoplastic cells.' The last of these histotypes is synonymous with 'well-differentiated thymic carcinoma,' as cited above. 'Type C' 'thymomas' are outright thymic carcinomas, with obvious cytological anaplasia.

Selected publications have since implied that the WHO paradigm is a prognostically oriented system,[53,54] but it was not intended to have that function.[55] Its primary purpose was to improve consistency in histological diagnosis. Still another scheme for the classification of thymic tumors – which has substantial practical merit, in our opinion – appeared contemporaneously with the WHO publication

and was advanced by Suster and Moran. It presented the view that thymic epithelial neoplasms could simply be divided into 'thymomas' (corresponding to WHO 'types A, AB, B1, and B2' tumors); 'atypical thymomas' (WHO 'type B3' lesions); and 'thymic carcinomas' (WHO 'type C' tumors).[56]

A salient microscopic feature of most thymomas is their internal fibrous septations, which are composed of paucicellular tissue that subdivides them into lobules. The septa characteristically form acute angles at points of intersection (Fig. 21.9). Peripherally, a fibrous capsule is typically apparent as well. Remnants of non-neoplastic thymus may be included in operative specimens of thymoma. These are distinguishable from tumor tissue by their normal cortico-medullary relationship, which is not seen in the thymoma. Intra-tumoral lymphocytes are generally small and mature, but may sometimes manifest an 'activated' appearance. In those instances, their nuclei are enlarged with folded membranes and mitotic activity. However, they never attain the convoluted nuclear appearance of lymphoblasts, nor do they exhibit increased nucleocytoplasmic ratios. Thymomas of the predominantly lymphocytic variety may also contain numerous scattered 'tingible-body' macrophages. As a result, a 'starry-sky' pattern is seen on scanning microscopic examination. However, the intervening lymphoid cells are cytologically mature,

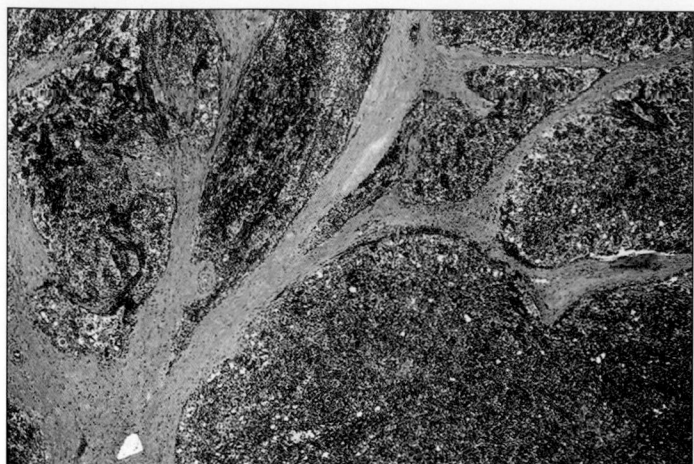

Fig. 21.9 Internal fibrous septa intersect one another at acute angles in thymoma.

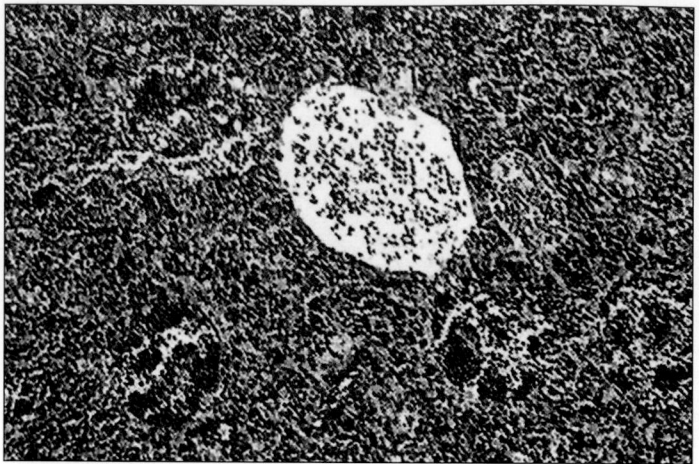

Fig. 21.11 A perivascular serum lake, containing suspended erythrocytes and leukocytes, is present in this predominantly lymphocytic thymoma. That feature is not expected in lymphoproliferative lesions of the mediastinum.

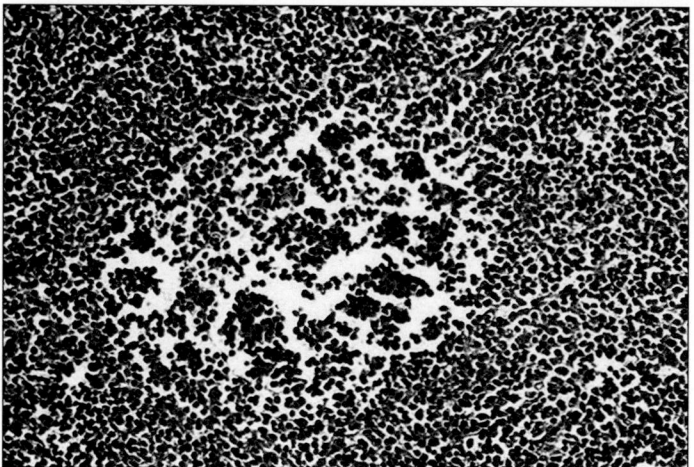

Fig. 21.10 A focus of loosely aggregated stromal lymphocytes is seen in this thymoma with 'medullary differentiation.

differing from those of small-noncleaved cell (Burkitt's) lymphoma, which is associated with a similar morphological image.[57] Moreover, epithelial cells are usually obvious in those variants of thymoma with a 'starry-sky' pattern.

Other focal or subtle microscopic features of predominantly lymphocytic thymomas are helpful in recognizing them. One has been called 'medullary differentiation' (MD)[42] because it recalls the image of the normal thymic medulla. Thymomas with MD exhibit rounded, low-density areas in the lymphocytic population on scanning microscopy (Fig. 21.10). These foci vaguely resemble germinal centers or neoplastic follicles of follicular lymphomas. Nevertheless, immunoblasts and tingible-body macrophages are not present in them, and, in contrast to the follicles seen in lymphoma, which contain small, closely apposed 'cleaved' follicular center cells, areas of MD show loosely aggregated, small, mature lymphocytes. In addition, Hassall's corpuscle-like structures may also be seen in foci of MD.

Another important diagnostic attributes that separates predominantly lymphocytic thymomas from thymic small cell lymphomas is

the presence of perivascular 'serum lakes' and microcystic changes in thymomas. The perivascular spaces are seen around capillary or venule-sized intratumoral vessels. The area between the vessels and the basement membrane of contiguous epithelial cells is filled with proteinaceous, lightly eosinophilic transudate. Lymphocytes, erythrocytes, and foamy macrophages may be suspended in the contents of the 'lakes' (Fig. 21.11). Sometimes, perivascular spaces may contain hyaline-like material as well. Microcysts are usually admixed with lymphocytes in the substance of the neoplasm. These structures are small, clustered, lucent areas which may contain degenerative epithelial cells or lymphocytes. True germinal centers are seen in roughly 10% of all thymomas, again usually of the predominantly lymphocytic type. Rarely, they may be part of lesions showing micronodular proliferations of thymic epithelium suspended in sheets of lymphoid cells, termed 'micronodular thymoma' by Suster and Moran.[58] The germinal center content of thymomas has also been reported to have some relationship to clinical myasthenia gravis.[42]

The primary differential diagnosis in such cases is that of angiofollicular lymph node hyperplasia (Castleman's disease)[59] (see Chapter 11). In both that condition and in micronodular thymoma, one may observe an 'onion-skin' configuration of plasma cells and lymphocytes around germinal center-like structures (Fig. 21.12). However, micronodular thymoma is keratin positive, in contrast to Castleman's disease, and thymoma also lacks intercellular eosinophilic material in follicular lymphoid zones, as seen in the hyaline-vascular subtype of angiofollicular hyperplasia.

At the other end of the histological spectrum of thymoma, predominantly epithelial tumors may cause diagnostic confusion with an entirely different group of neoplasms. Neuroendocrine thymic tumors (thymic 'carcinoids;' neuroendocrine carcinomas) may contain cellular rosettes or pseudorosettes.[60] Because epithelial thymomas likewise may assume a vaguely organoid growth pattern with formation of rosettes or pseudorosettes, it may be difficult to distinguish these lesions from one another. We have seen several tumors with such attributes in which electron microscopy, histochemistry, and immunohistochemistry were needed to achieve a definitive diagnosis of thymoma. Squamous metaplasia is also relatively common in thymomas; in those lesions, the tumor cells acquire acidophilic,

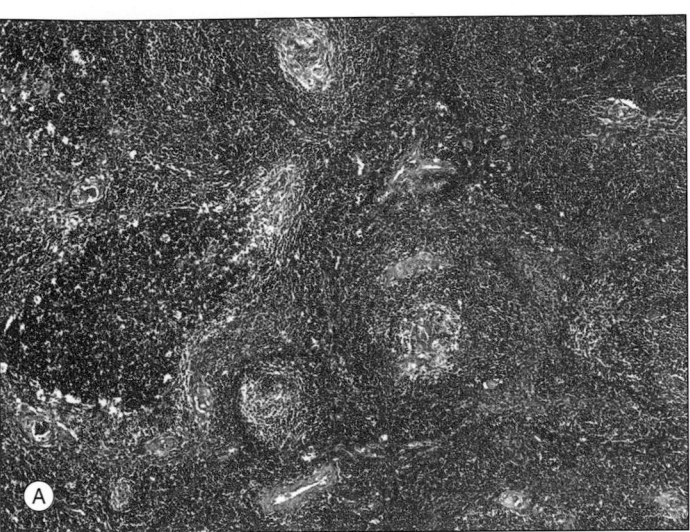
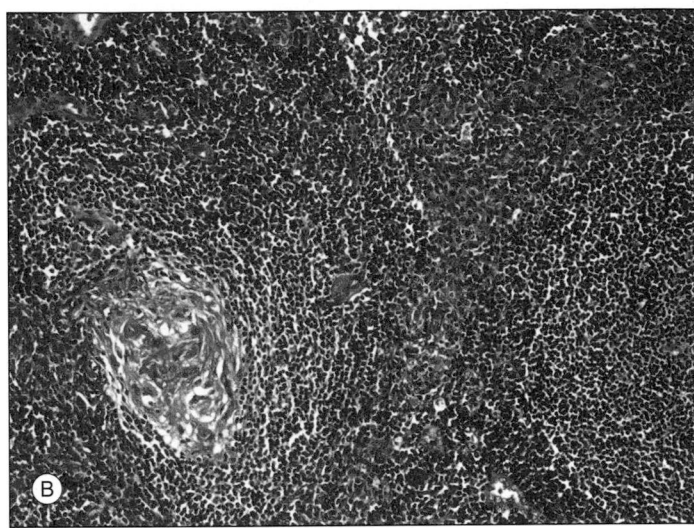

Fig. 21.12 Micronodular, or 'Castlemanoid' thymoma, showing concentric arrays of lymphocytes surrounding germinal center-like structures **(A)**. Between those structures, there are also small groups of epithelioid cells with eosinophilic cytoplasm **(B)**, representing the neoplastic thymic epithelium.

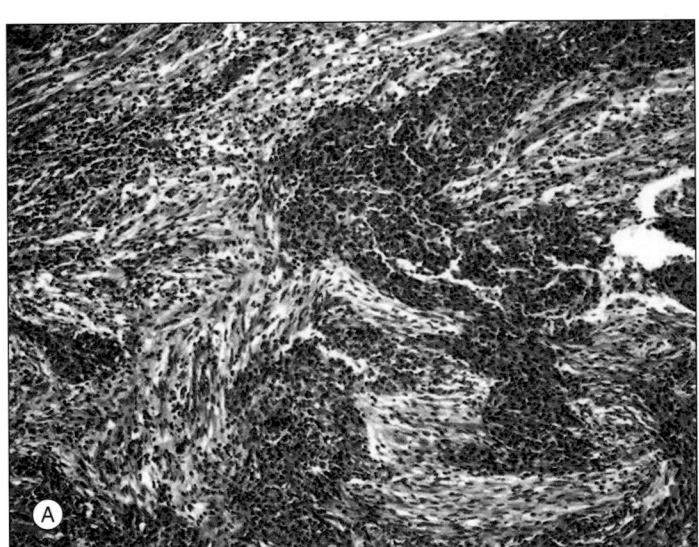
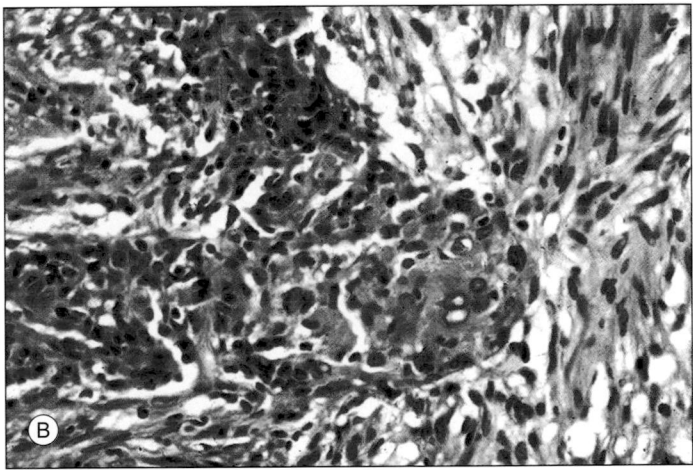

Fig. 21.13 (A) Thymoma with 'pseudosarcomatous' spindle-cell stroma. **(B)** The bland nature of the stromal cells is apparent here.

glassy cytoplasm and show a tendency to be arranged in incipient keratin 'pearls.' When that property is combined with a cellular fibroblastic stroma, a peculiar image is obtained which superficially simulates that of an invasive carcinoma; tumors with this image have been termed 'thymoma with pseudosarcomatous stroma (Fig. 21.13).[61]

Gland-like foci are observed in up to 20% of epithelial thymomas.[1,42] They are lined by low columnar or cuboidal epithelial cells, and may resemble thyroid follicles lacking colloid. Papillary epithelial structures may sometimes be present as well. The pseudoglandular spaces represent secondary change in true thymic epithelium, but may cause confusion with primary or metastatic adenocarcinoma.[62] That possibility can be eliminated by attention to the overall appearance of the tumor when a sufficient volume of it has been sampled; however, the diagnosis of small biopsy samples may require additional studies, as considered below.

A distinctive variant of spindle-cell epithelial thymoma is one in which the tumor cells assume a decidedly fusiform appearance, imparting a resemblance to mesenchymal tumors.[1,42] If prominent vascular stroma or a storiform growth pattern is also part of such lesions, the diagnoses of hemangiopericytoma (Fig. 21.14) or fibrous histiocytoma may be entertained. Nonetheless, experience indicates that most spindle-cell tumors of the anterosuperior mediastinum demonstrate thymic epithelial differentiation.[42,63] Nuclei of the tumor cells in spindle-cell thymomas may also be arranged in parallel with one another, producing a palisaded appearance. Hence, the image of neural neoplasms may also be recapitulated.

As alluded to earlier in reference to 'well-differentiated thymic carcinoma,' a range of cytologic atypia is seen in the epithelial cells of thymomas (Fig. 21.15).[52,56] In other words, nuclear pleomorphism, hyperchromasia, and limited nucleolar prominence are a part of the spectrum. These changes may be focal or diffuse. In some instances,

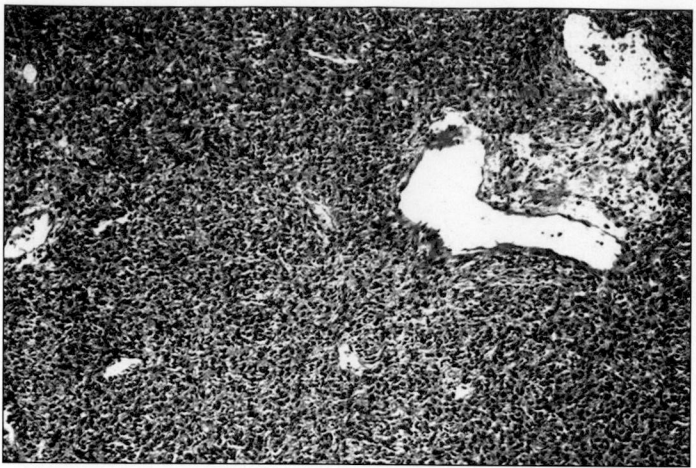

Fig. 21.14 Thymoma with hemangiopericytoma-like growth pattern.

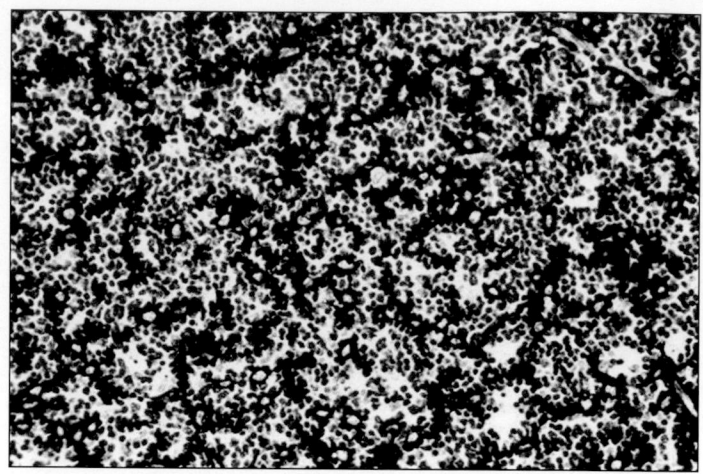

Fig. 21.16 Immunoreactivity for keratin in thymoma, showing characteristic interlocking pattern of cellular positivity.

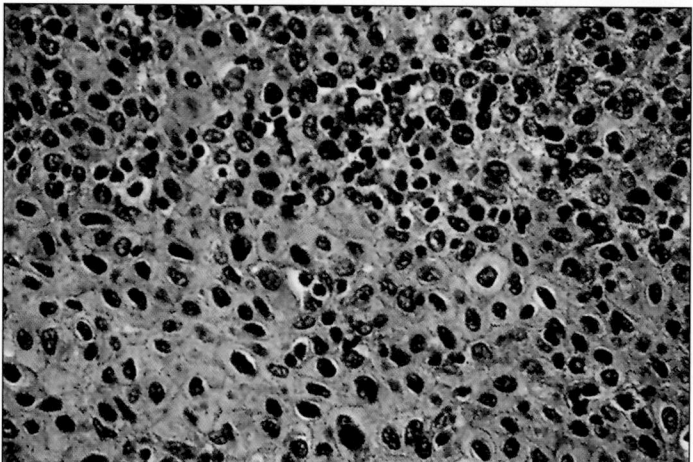

Fig. 21.15 'Atypical' thymoma with nuclear irregularity, hyperchromasia, and nucleoli. The overall image of the lesion is not aberrant enough to qualify for a diagnosis of thymic carcinoma.

it can be challenging to decide whether an atypical thymic epithelial neoplasm is a thymoma or a thymic carcinoma. However, thymic carcinomas usually manifest striking nucleolar prominence, brisk mitotic activity, high nuclear:cytoplasmic ratios, and multifocal spontaneous necrosis. The distinction between thymoma and thymic carcinoma is an important one because of the marked difference in their clinical behaviors, but, in selected cases, a final interpretation of 'atypical thymoma' may be the most appropriate.[56]

The ultrastructural attributes of thymoma are very similar to those of the normal thymus.[64,65] The proliferating elements in these tumors are thymic epithelial cells, and the electron microscopic diagnosis of thymoma is based on their identification. Thymic epithelial cells contain oval or slightly irregular nuclei, with dispersed heterochromatin and compact nucleoli. There are the usual metabolic organelles, as well as broad, electron-dense bundles of keratin-containing intermediate filaments (tonofibrils). Long, interdigitating cytoplasmic extensions, which may traverse relatively large spaces before joining to each other, are typical. Junctions between the epithelial cells are well defined and desmosomal in type. Tono-

filaments may insert into them. Basal lamina is present along the plasma membranes of cytoplasmic extensions. In predominantly lymphocytic or lymphoepithelial thymomas, the reactive lymphoid population is composed of cells with smooth borders, compact nuclei, and few organelles. Careful study may be necessary to find epithelial cells or their extensions in order to make a definite diagnosis of predominantly lymphocytic thymoma.

Immunocytochemical studies may be of great value in selected cases in confirming the thymomatous nature of a mediastinal mass. The epithelial cells of thymomas express keratin proteins[66] and epithelial membrane antigen (EMA)[67] in contrast to the large lymphoid cells and histiocytes with which they may be confused in predominantly lymphocytic lesions. In particular, keratin reactivity is distinctive in thymomas, with a delicately interlocking pattern of labeling that reflects the presence of cytoplasmic extensions of the tumor cells (Fig. 21.16). Conversely, leukocyte common antigen (LCA; CD45) is lacking in thymic epithelial cells, but this determinant is expressed by virtually all hematopoietic elements.[68,69] Hence, a panel of anticytokeratin, anti-EMA, and CD45 antibodies will usually suffice to distinguish between predominantly lymphocytic or mixed lymphoepithelial thymoma and lymphoma. This differential diagnosis is one that is typically problematic in needle biopsy or aspiration cytology specimens. Anticytokeratins are also quite useful in differentiating pure spindle cell thymomas – which are keratin reactive – from mesenchymal tumors, which usually are not. Furthermore, antivimentin will bind to the latter of these groups of neoplasms,[70] whereas, in our experience, thymomas are typically vimentin negative.[71,72] These profiles are useful in recognizing variants of spindle-cell thymoma that resemble mesenchymal neoplasms.

The lymphocytic population in thymomas has been evaluated in detail. It contains a preponderance of CD1a-positive, CD99-positive, and terminal deoxynucleotidyl transferase (TdT)-positive cells, with a paucity of CD3-reactive lymphocytes (mature T lymphocytes).[72,73] A variable number of cells with the CD8+ ('suppressor') phenotype have been observed, and this subpopulation is particularly small in thymomas that are associated with myasthenia gravis. Both the reactive lymphocytes and epithelial cells of predominantly lymphocytic thymomas have been shown to express the CD57 and HLA-DR antigens. The former of those markers is usually detected focally on epithelial cells bordering perivascular serum lakes.[73]

Another issue concerns the use of immunohistology to separate 'atypical thymomas' (see above) from outright thymic carcinomas, as considered in the next section of this chapter. Although it is most typical of thymic carcinoma,[74,75] CD5 is also potentially seen in the epithelial cells of atypical thymomas and therefore is not an absolute discriminant. However, if the intratumoral lymphocytes in such a lesion are also CD99 negative, a diagnosis of carcinoma would be favored because 'ordinary' thymomas contain CD99-positive lymphoid elements consistently (Fig. 21.17).[76]

In particular reference to the last of these points, data on leukocyte antigen immunoreactivity could well cause diagnostic misadventures if they are overemphasized in the evaluation of mediastinal tumors. Lymphoblastic lymphoma is also characterized by reactivity for CD1a, CD99, and TdT.[77] This fact underscores the indispensable need for the inclusion of keratin immunostains in the assessment of lymphoid-rich masses of the anterior mediastinum in small biopsy specimens. Immunoreactivity for such thymic 'hormones' as thymosin and serum thymic factor in normal thymic epithelium has been reported.[78] However, no convincing reports are available on the presence of these hormones in thymomas. Information on the differential diagnostic aspects of thymoma are summarized in Tables 21.1–21.3.

Reports also have been made on the use of immunostains for various gene products and proliferation markers in thymomas, with the goal of predicting the behavior of such tumors.[79,80] It is our

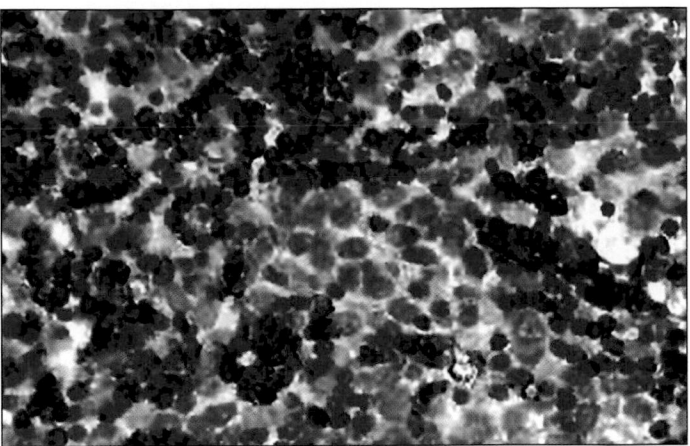

Fig. 21.17 CD99 reactivity in the intratumoral lymphocytes of thymoma.

Table 21.1 Light microscopic findings in thymoma and its differential diagnostic alternatives

Tumor	Lobulation	MD	PSL	Microcysts	Lymphoid cells	Rosettes/ pseudo-rosettes	Organoid growth	Stromal hemorrhage/ cholesterol
Predominantly lymphocytic thymoma	+ + to + + +	+ +	+	±	+ + +	0	0	0
Epithelial thymoma	+ + to + + +	0	+ +	±	± to +	± to +	0 to ±	0 to + +
Angiofollicular lymphoid hyperplasia	0	0	0	0	+ + +	0	0	0
Small or mixed small and large cell lymphomas	0	0	0	0	+ + +	0	0	0
Hemangiopericytoma	0	0	0	0	0	0	0	0
Fibrous histiocytoma	0	0	0	0	0	0	0	0
Carcinoid of thymus	0	0	0	0	±	+ + to + + +	+ + to + + +	0

MD, medullary differentiation; PSL, perivascular serum lakes; 0 absent; + focally present or observed in less than all cases; ± variably present; + + uniformly present; + + + uniformly present and prominent.

Table 21.2 Electron microscopic features of thymoma and its differential diagnostic alternatives

Tumor	ECP	PBM	Tonofil	CIF	ICJ	PCL	Pinocytosis	CDB	NSG
Thymoma (all variants)	+ +	+ +	+ +	±	+ + (D)	0	0	0	0
Malignant lymphoma	0	0	0	±	0	±	0	0	0
Thymic carcinoid	0	+	±	+ [a]	+ (MA)	0	0	0	+ + to + + +
Hemangiopericytoma	±	+	0	+	+ (AP)	0	+ to + +	+ +	0
Fibrous histiocytoma	±	0	0	±	± (AP)	+ to + +	0	0	0

ECP, elongated cellular processes; PBM pericellular basement membrane; Tonofil, cytoplasmic tonofilaments; CIF, cytoplasmic intermediate filaments; ICJ, intercellular junctions; D, desmosomes; MA, maculae adherents; AP, appositional plaques; PCL, prominent cytoplasmic lysosomes; CDB, cytoplasmic dense bodies; NSG, neurosecretory granules; 0 absent; ± variably present; + present focally; + + uniformly present; + + + uniformly present and prominent.
[a] Intermediate filaments in thymic carcinoid are often localized to perinuclear cytoplasm, and whorled.

Table 21.3 Immunohistologic differential diagnosis of thymoma & histologic alternatives

Tumor	EMA	CKER	SYN	VIM	CD45	Chromogranin
Thymoma (all variants)	+	+	0	0	+	0
Malignant lymphoma	0	0	0	±	+	0
Thymic carcinoid	±	±	+	0	0	+
Hemangiopericytoma	0	0	0	+	0	0
Fibrous histiocytoma	0	0	0	+	0	0
Angiofollicular lymphoid hyperplasia	0	0	0	±	+	0

opinion that these do not contribute to clinical practice in a meaningful way. We continue to believe that the most valuable predictive factor in thymoma cases is whether the tumor invades its capsule at a macroscopic or microscopic level.[81–83] A codification of that behavior has been published by Masaoka et al.,[84] producing a formal staging scheme. Masaoka stage I lesions are encapsulated, whereas stage II tumors invade microscopically through their capsules, stage III tumors show macroscopic and/or microscopic infiltration of lung, great vessels, or pericardium, and stage IV thymomas have seeded the pleura or pericardium extensively by 'drop' metastasis or have spread outside of the chest. In our experience, <10% of thymomas manifest the last of those behaviors. The Masaoka system has subsequently been restructured[85] with the aim of paralleling standard 'TMN' protocols, and the clinical value of staging thymic tumors is now clear.[86] For those who wish to use all-encompassing reporting formats in thymoma cases, *both* the Masaoka and AJCC-type stages can be provided, along with *both* the Bernatz and MMH classifications.[87] As mentioned above, we feel that additional studies such as cytometric measurement of DNA content, immunohisto-chemical determination of proliferation indices, and analysis of various genes and gene products add little to the prognostication of thymomas after staging has been taken into consideration.

THYMIC CARCINOMAS

'Thymic carcinoma' is the best designation for tumors derived from thymic epithelium that are cytologically malignant.[1,88–90] Thus, an adequate distinction is made from the invasive (and thus biologically malignant) but cytologically bland neoplasms (i.e. thymomas). These two groups of tumors differ significantly in their clinical behavior, making such a separation both justifiable and desirable.

Many pathologists are still unconfident regarding their knowledge of primary thymic carcinomas. There are three reasons for this:

1. Many tumors in early reports on 'carcinomas of the thymus' were later recognized to have been in reality malignant lymphomas, germ cell tumors, or carcinomas metastatic to the thymus. This discredited the concept of primary thymic carcinoma for many years;
2. Thymic carcinomas are rare. Even large thoracic surgical practices encounter fewer than one case per year;
3. There are relatively few specific pathologic findings that can be used to distinguish primary thymic carcinomas from metastatic neoplasms to which they are histologically similar.

The clinical presentation of thymic carcinomas is similar to that of thymomas, with the exception that symptoms of mediastinal structural displacement are more frequent and may evolve more rapidly;[90] radiographic or clinical evidence of extrathoracic metastasis is also more likely to be present at diagnosis. Myasthenia gravis, acquired erythroid hypoplasia, or hypogammaglobulinemia are generally not seen in association with thymic carcinoma.

In general, thymic carcinomas lack the well-defined fibrous encapsulation and internal septation of thymomas, although occasional specimens may appear to be totally encapsulated at initial presentation. The cut surfaces of thymic carcinomas are typically rubbery or gritty and gray-white; areas of necrosis and hemorrhage are common (Fig. 21.18). Mucoepidermoid carcinoma of the thymus may have a gelatinous or 'slimy' cut surface, and basaloid thymic carcinoma may be grossly cystic as well.[89–91] Leong and Brown[8] and Yamashita et al.[9] documented carcinomas of the thymus that apparently arose in pre-existing thymic cysts.

Although thymic carcinomas are extremely rare, several distinctive microscopic variants are currently recognized.[89–91] These will be discussed in order of their relative frequency.

Lymphoepithelioma-like squamous carcinoma is composed of sheets or nests of oval or round cells, with large, vesicular nuclei and prominent eosinophilic nucleoli. Nucleocytoplasmic ratios are high, the cytoplasm is amphophilic with indistinct cell borders, and mitoses are numerous (Fig. 21.19). Areas of spontaneous intratumoral necrosis are commonly seen. As this description is virtually identical to that of 'lymphoepithelioma' of the nasopharynx (poorly differentiated squamous carcinoma) (see Chapter 15), the term 'lymphoepithelioma-like thymic carcinoma' is appropriate for diagnostic use.

Keratinizing and non-keratinizing squamous carcinoma shows tumor cells with large, hyperchromatic nuclei and a moderate amount of acidophilic, occasionally 'glassy' cytoplasm. Nucleocytoplasmic ratios are again high, and mitoses are easily found (Fig. 21.20). These neoplasms variably manifest the formation of keratin pearls, which are concentric arrangements of tumor cells in association with extracellular keratin. Either a sheet-like or an organoid growth pattern may be seen; occasionally there is a predominantly spindle-cell, yet obviously clustered, epithelial appearance.

Basaloid squamous carcinoma is composed of small, uniform, polygonal cells with scanty amphophilic cytoplasm. Nuclei are oval, with equally distributed chromatin, indistinct nucleoli, and high nucleocytoplasmic ratios. Mitoses are abundant, and small foci of metaplastic-type keratinizing squamous cells may be interspersed throughout these neoplasms. Tumor cells are arranged in nests or trabeculae, with a palisaded nuclear configuration at their periphery (Fig. 21.21). Gland-like spaces may also be observed, the contents of which contain weakly periodic acid–Schiff (PAS)- and muci-carmine-positive material. Basaloid thymic carcinomas may be intimately related to thymic cyst-like structures lined by squamoid, focally dysplastic cells, and associated with contiguous cholesterol clefts and hemorrhage.

Clear cell thymic carcinomas have been documented infrequently. These lesions may exhibit a striking morphological similarity to renal cell carcinoma; they consist of sheets of polygonal cells with an abundant, optically clear cytoplasm which are occasionally subdivided by fibrovascular septa (Fig. 21.22). The nuclei in most lesions are oval with evenly dispersed chromatin, whereas in others they are more vesicular and contain prominent eosinophilic nucleoli. Mitoses are relatively rare. The cytoplasm of the tumor cells shows inconsistent PAS reactivity and stains for mucin are negative.

Sarcomatoid carcinoma of the thymus is also extremely un-common. In this subtype, variably prominent foci of cytologically

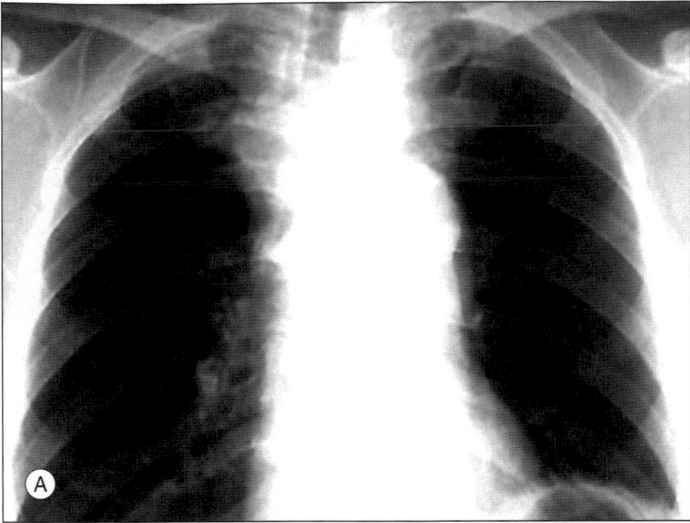

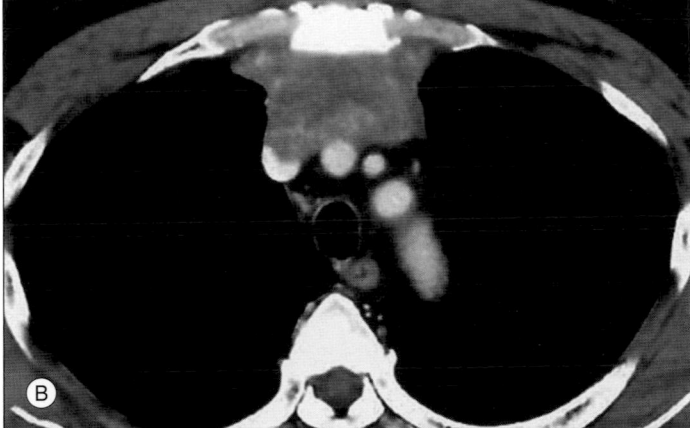

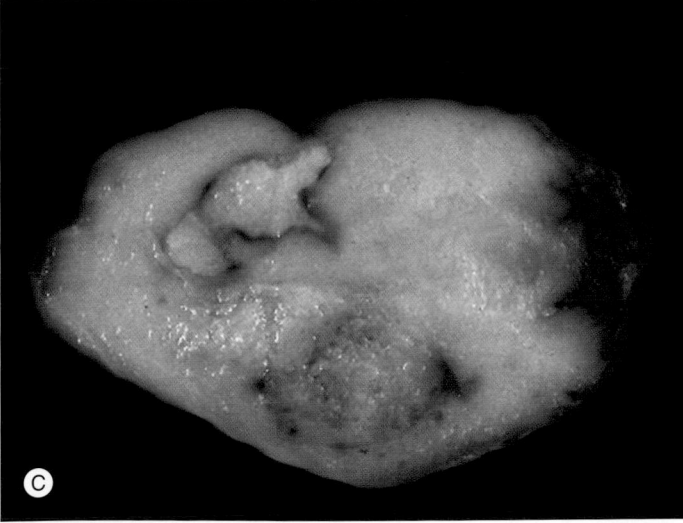

Fig. 21.18 Chest radiograph **(A)**, computed tomogram **(B)**, and gross photograph **(C)** of thymic carcinoma, demonstrating uniform gray-white tumor tissue with no lobulation or internal septation.

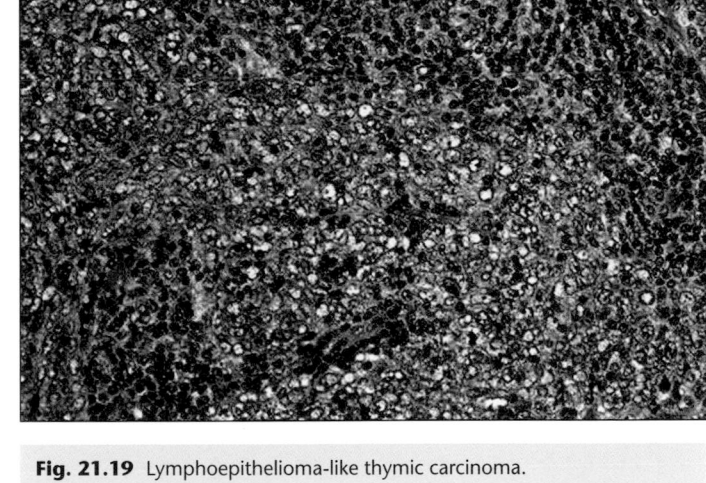

Fig. 21.19 Lymphoepithelioma-like thymic carcinoma.

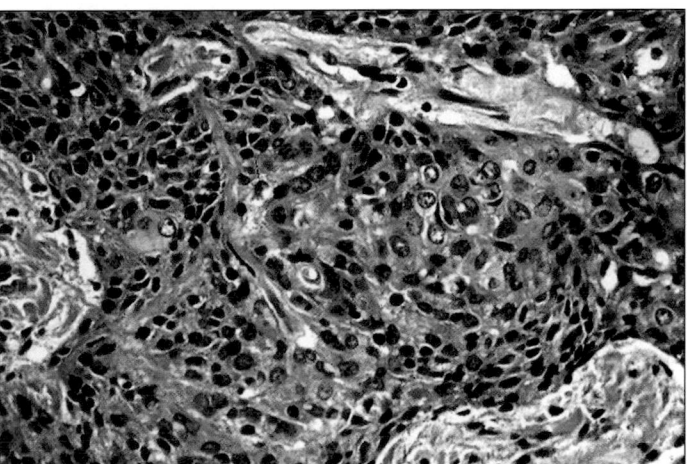

Fig. 21.20 Non-keratinizing squamous cell carcinoma of the thymus.

malignant squamous epithelium are admixed with fascicles of nondescript spindle cells (Fig. 21.23). One may see a storiform pattern or focal cytoplasmic cross-striations and acidophilia.[89] In one documented case, skeins of spindle cells regularly punctuated a background population of epithelial elements, yielding a distinctly biphasic image.[92] The nuclei of the fusiform elements are hyperchromatic, with occasionally prominent nucleoli and high nucleocytoplasmic ratios.

Mucoepidermoid and adenosquamous carcinomas of the thymus demonstrate an image essentially microscopically identical to mucoepidermoid or adenosquamous carcinomas of salivary gland origin. Mucoepidermoid tumors are composed of three cell types. One is polygonal with moderate eosinophilic cytoplasm; another contains slightly basophilic, PAS-positive (diastase-resistant) cytoplasmic vacuoles which compress the nuclei; and the third is squamoid, with intercellular 'bridges,' nuclear hyperchromasia and enlargement, and mitotic activity (Fig. 21.24). Occasional dyskeratotic cells are scattered throughout these masses. The tumor cells are arranged in partially cystic, partially necrotic nests that are separated by fibrous bands; the microcysts contain mucinous material that labels with the PAS method. Adenosquamous carcinomas are similar, except that the level of cytologic anaplasia in such lesions is much higher. Accordingly, mucin production is more limited and may only be demonstrable with special stains.

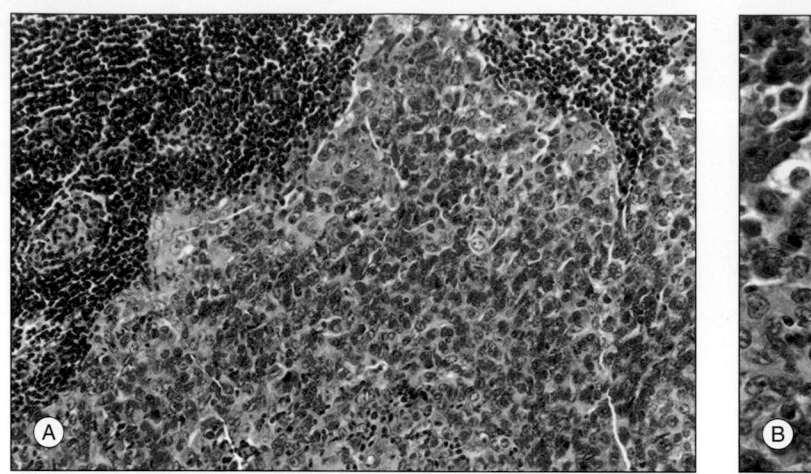

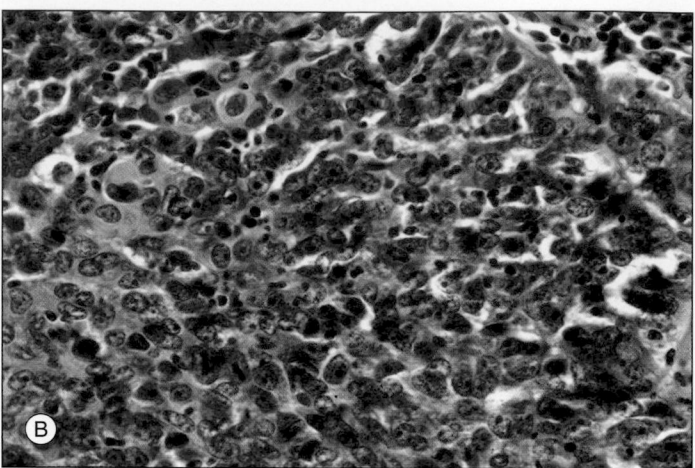

Fig. 21.21 **(A)** Basaloid squamous cell carcinoma of the thymus, demonstrating an abrupt transition between tumor tissue (lower right) and adjacent thymus gland (upper left). **(B)** The tumor cells have scant cytoplasm and high nucleocytoplasmic ratios, and show brisk apoptosis and mitotic activity.

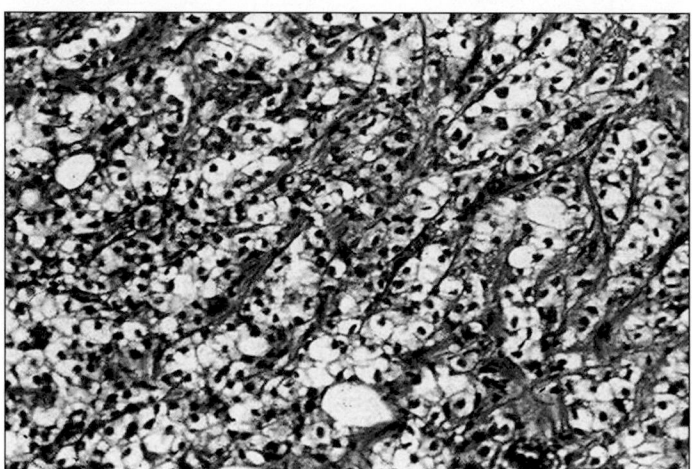

Fig. 21.22 Clear cell carcinoma of the thymus.

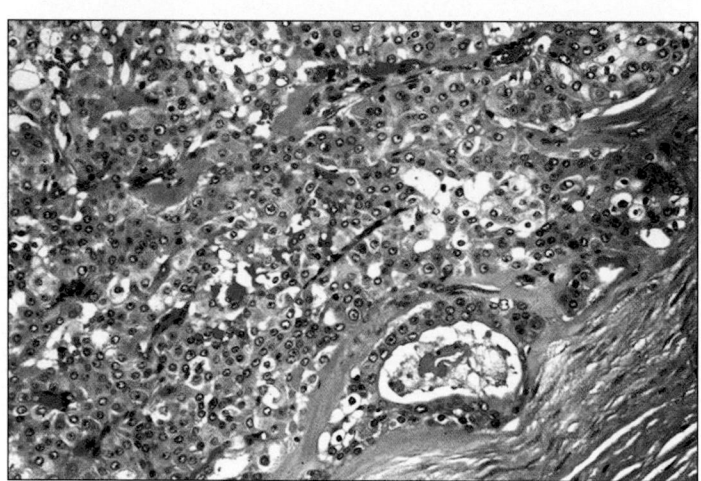

Fig. 21.24 Mucoepidermoid carcinoma of the thymus.

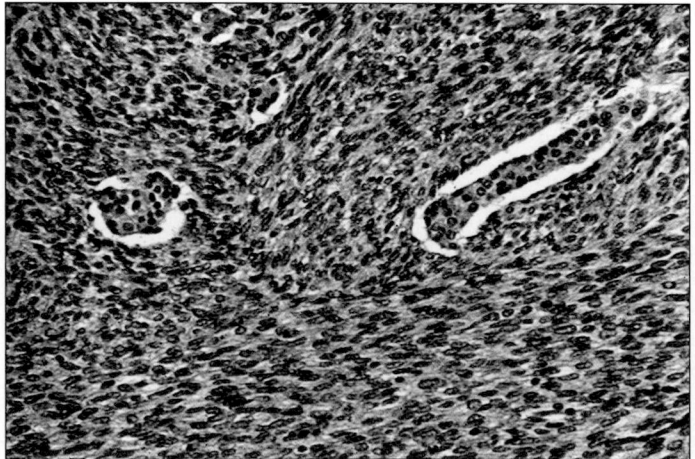

Fig. 21.23 Sarcomatoid (spindle-cell) thymic carcinoma, with only small foci of obviously epithelioid tumor cells.

Primary Adenocarcinoma of the Thymus (Not Further Specified): We have seen only one case of thymic carcinoma in which a purely adenocarcinomatous image was evident, like the two neoplasms documented by Shimosato and Mukai.[1] One of the lesions in that report arose in apparent transition from an epithelial-predominant thymoma, and demonstrated micropapillary growth and focal psammomatous calcification. The overtly malignant portion of that lesion was immunoreactive for carcinoembryonic antigen, as seen potentially in other forms of thymic carcinoma.[71] The other lesion described by Shimosato and Mukai,[1] and the one in our files, were somewhat more uniform histologically with admixed foci of micropapillary and solid growth (Fig. 21.25).

Lymphoepithelioma-like, keratinizing squamous, basaloid, and clear cell thymic carcinomas have similar ultrastructural features. They all display high nucleocytoplasmic ratios, coarsely distributed heterochromatin, and complex nucleoli. The cytoplasm of the tumor cells contains the usual metabolic organelles and some glycogen, as well as variable numbers of tonofilaments which insert into numerous well-formed desmosomes, as in thymomas. Indeed, reliance must be

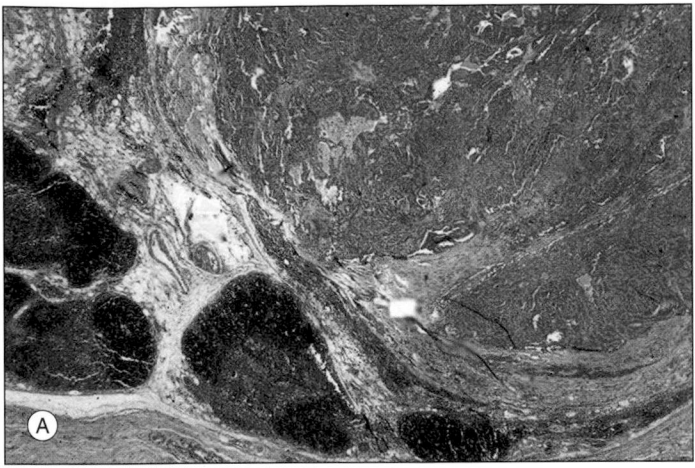
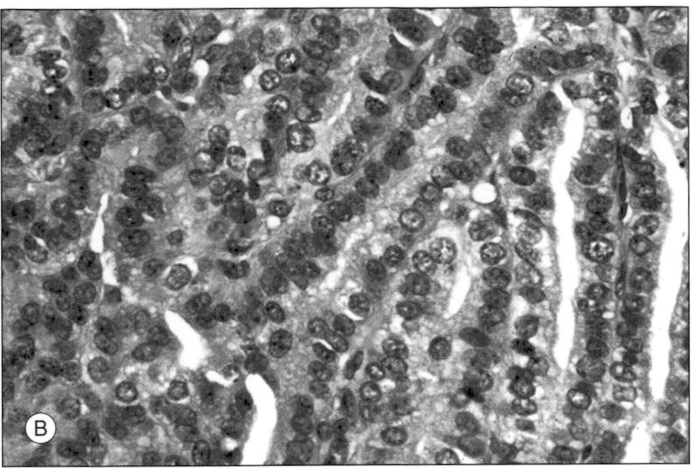

Fig. 21.25 **(A)** Adenocarcinoma of the thymus, showing interface between the tumor (right upper) and non-neoplastic glandular tissue (lower left). **(B)** The tumor has a micropapillary appearance which superficially resembles that of papillary thyroid carcinoma; however, immunostains in this case were negative for thyroglobulin and thyroid transcription factor-1, and positive for carcinoembryonic antigen.

placed solely on nuclear characteristics and the relative cell volume which they occupy in distinguishing between thymomas and thymic carcinoma.

Occasionally, one encounters carcinomas of the thymus that have the light microscopic appearance of lymphoepithelioma-like thymic carcinoma but which contain a moderate number of cytoplasmic neurosecretory granules ultrastructurally.[92] Current opinion favors the classification of such lesions as 'large cell carcinoma with neuroendocrine features,' in analogy to certain tumors of the lung.[93] This duality of cellular differentiation is also manifested immuno-histologically.

Snover et al.[89] demonstrated fine structural cytoplasmic sarcomeric development in a case of sarcomatoid thymic carcinoma, correlating with cross-striations that had been observed by light microscopy. No epithelial features such as intercellular junctional complexes were observed, but this was attributed to sampling limitations. To date, mucoepidermoid, adenosquamous, and adenocarcinomatous thymic carcinomas have not been studied ultrastructurally.

Immunohistochemistry provides a useful method for characterizing thymic carcinomas. All forms of these tumors are immunoreactive for epithelial membrane antigen and keratin;[72] reactivity for myogenous determinants such as desmin, actin, and myoglobin may also be seen in sarcomatoid thymic carcinomas with divergent differentiation.[89] Lymphoepithelioma-like tumors may be associated with positive serologic studies for Epstein-Barr virus (EBV) infection, and that agent may also be detectable in the tumor cells by in situ hybridization. These findings are similar to those seen in 'lymphoepitheliomas' of the nasopharynx and other anatomic locations.[94] However, at an immunohistochemical level, studies for EBV-latent membrane protein are uniformly nonreactive in thymic carcinomas, in our experience.

It has been shown that the lymphoid cells in thymic carcinoma are CD99 negative, contrasting with those seen in thymomas.[76] Moreover, the epithelial cells of thymic carcinomas demonstrate a tendency to express CD5 and CD70, for currently unknown reasons (Fig. 21.26). This property again differs from the attributes of thymoma, but, more importantly, CD5 and CD70 reactivity are absent in other epithelial tumors that enter differential diagnosis with carcinomas of the thymus.[75,95] These lesions principally are represented by metastatic somatic carcinomas and germ cell tumors.

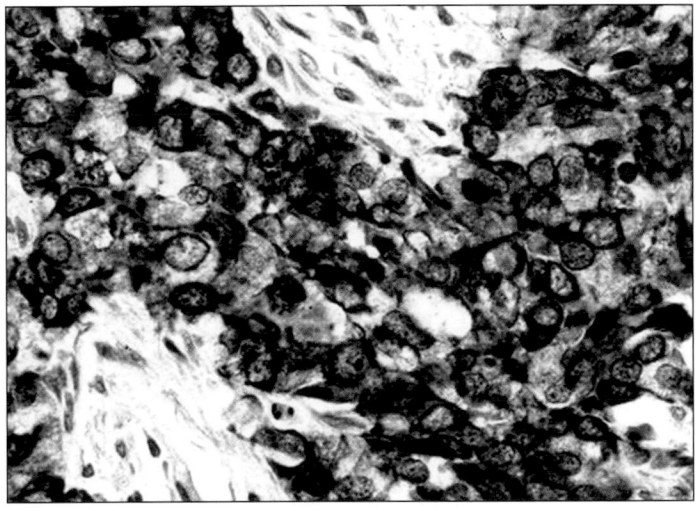

Fig. 21.26 CD5 immunoreactivity in primary thymic carcinoma.

The differential diagnostic considerations in cases of thymic carcinoma are summarized in Tables 21.4–21.6. The most important diagnostic alternative, because of the close similarity of variants of thymic carcinoma to nasopharyngeal, pulmonary, renal, salivary glandular, genital, and anorectal neoplasms, is a *mediastinal metastasis from an occult carcinoma* located in one of these sites. Electron microscopy is of limited value in distinguishing primary from secondary tumors. The only form of thymic carcinoma which is dissimilar ultrastructurally to its extrathymic counterpart is clear cell carcinoma of the thymus; unlike clear cell carcinomas of the kidney and female urogenital tract, it contains abundant cytoplasmic tonofilaments and well-formed desmosomes, and generally lacks microvillous development and copious amounts of glycogen.[96,97] As cited above, immunostains for CD5, CD70, and selected other markers are useful in addressing the possibility of a carcinomatous metastasis to the thymic region.[98] In addition, thyroid transcription factor-1 (TTF-1) is a selective marker of pulmonary carcinomas (Fig. 21.27), which are the most common sources of mediastinal metastases; in contrast, primary

Table 21.4 Points of histologic distinction between thymic carcinoma and other primary mediastinal neoplasms

Tumor	Nesting growth	Round/ oval nuclei	Complex nucleoli	Rudimentary glands	Lymphoid infiltrate	Prominent angioinvasion	PAS positivity
Thymic carcinoma (polygonal cell)	+ to + +	+ +	0	0	±	0	±
Thymic carcinoma (sarcomatoid)	± (focal)	±	0	0	±	0	±[a]
Large cell lymphoma	0[b]	0	0	0	+ +	+ +	0
Seminoma	+	+	+ +	0	+	0	+ to + +
Embryonal carcinoma	+ to + +	+	±	+ to + +	±	0	+
True sarcomas	0	0	0	0	0	0	0

0 absent; ± variably present; + present; ++ present and prominent.
[a] Isolated cells with densely eosinophilic cytoplasm may be strongly PAS-positive and show cross-striations.
[b] Some examples of large cell lymphoma with sclerotic stroma may have a clustered growth pattern.

Table 21.5 Ultrastructural features of thymic carcinoma and differential diagnostic alternatives[a]

Tumor	ICJ	Tonofil	CIF	PBM	Complex nucleolonemas	Cytopl glycogen	Cytopl AFP glob
Thymic carcinoma	+ + (D)	+ to + +	±	±	0	±	0
Large cell lymphoma	0	0	±	0	0	0	0
Seminoma	± to + (AP)	0	0	0	+ to + +	+ to + +	0
Embryonal carcinoma	+ (MA)	0	+	±	±	+	+ to + +
True sarcomas	0	0	±	±	0	0	0

ICJ, intercellular junctions; Tonofil, tonofilaments; CIF, cytoplasmic intermediate filaments; PBM, pericellular basement membrane; Cytopl, cytoplasmic; AFP glob, α-fetoprotein globules; 0 absent; ± variably present; + present; + + present and prominent.
[a] There are no electron microscopic findings which reliably distinguish primary thymic carcinomas from metastases to the thymus

Table 21.6 Immunocytochemical features of thymic carcinoma and differential diagnostic alternatives[a]

Tumor	EMA	CKER	CD45	PLAP	CD117/CD30	VIM
Thymic carcinoma	+ to + +	+ to + +	0	0	0/0	0[b]
Large cell lymphoma	0	0	+ to + +	0	0/±	±
Seminoma	0	0[c]	0	+ to + +	++to 0	0
Embryonal carcinoma	0	+ to + +	0	+ to + +	0 to+/++	0
True sarcomas	0	0	0	0	0 to +	+ to + +

EMA, epithelial membrane antigen; CKER, cytokeratin; CLA, common leukocyte antigen; PLAP, placenta alkaline prosphatase; AFP, α-fetoprotein; VIM, vimentin; 0 absent; ± variably present or weakly reactive; + present; + + present and prominent.
[a] There are no reliable immunocytochemical markers to distinguish primary thymic carcinomas from metastases to the thymus.
[b] Sarcomatoid thymic carcinomas may be focally vimentin-positive in areas of mesenchymal differentiation, and may also show myoglobin-reactivity in such foci.
[c] Approximately 10% of seminomas show focal keratin-positivity

thymic carcinomas are TTF-1-negative.[99] Despite the availability of these markers, any patient thought to have a thymic carcinoma should also undergo extensive clinical investigation to rule out a primary extrathymic neoplasm before definitive therapy is undertaken.

Another major problem in the differential diagnosis of thymic carcinoma lies in the similarity between lymphoepithelioma-like squamous carcinoma and *large cell lymphoma* of the thymic region.[100] This is one of the most common problems referred for evaluation in our consultation practices. Fortunately, the availability of antibodies directed at cytokeratin, EMA, CD20, and CD45 provides a simple yet satisfactory solution to this dilemma in most cases.[71,72] Thymic carcinoma is immunoreactive for keratin and EMA, but not CD20 and CD45; the converse of these findings typifies large cell lymphoma of the thymic region.

Extragonadal germ cell tumors of the mediastinum such as seminoma and embryonal carcinoma may also be confused with thymic carcinoma.[101] Detailed histopathologic examination will usually resolve this uncertainty (Table 21.4), but occasional cases require the use of electron microscopy (Table 21.5) and immunocytochemistry (Table 21.6). Seminomas do not contain cytoplasmic tonofilaments or fully formed desmosomes,[102] as do thymic carcinomas; on the other hand, seminomatous lesions demonstrate

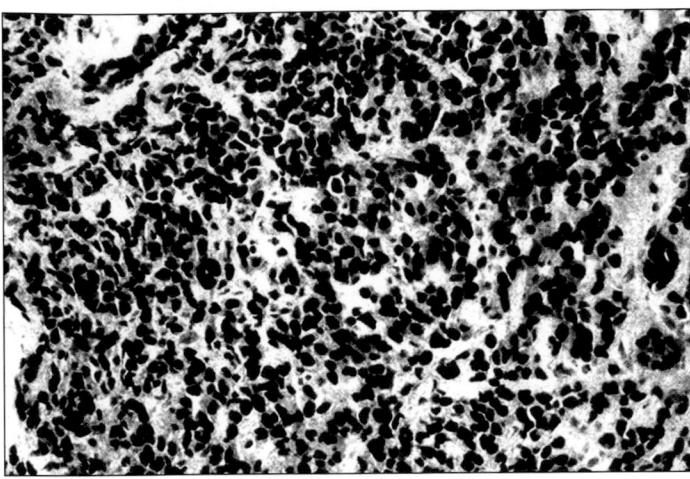

Fig. 21.27 Immunolabeling of poorly differentiated pulmonary adenocarcinoma for thyroid transcription factor-1; this marker is not seen in primary thymic carcinomas.

abundant cytoplasmic glycogen and complex nucleolar forms. Embryonal carcinoma commonly shows microvillous differentiation ultrastructurally, and lacks true tonofilaments.[103] Immunohistochemically, seminoma is positive for CD117 and placental alkaline phosphatase (PLAP),[72,104] but is nonreactive for CD5 and EMA,[72,75] and usually for keratin as well.[72] Embryonal carcinoma lacks EMA and CD5,[72,75] but is keratin positive[105] and contains PLAP as well.[72] Neither of these profiles of immunoreactivity is similar to that of thymic carcinoma.[72,75,98]

Cases of sarcomatoid thymic carcinoma could easily be confused with true sarcomas of the mediastinum. The latter tumors are generally vimentin positive but nonreactive for keratin;[72] the opposite of these findings characterizes sarcomatoid thymic carcinoma.[72,89,106] One notable exception to this characterization is represented by *monophasic synovial sarcoma* (MSS), a tumor whose immunoprofile is largely similar to that of sarcomatoid carcinomas.[107] Thus, cytogenetic analysis or fluorescent in situ hybridization studies may be necessary to detect the characteristic t(X;18) chromosomal translocation of MSS,[108] which is not expected in carcinomas.

Primary adenocarcinomas of the thymus may additionally resemble metastases of thyroid, or ovarian neoplasms. There have been no systematic comparisons of these tumors in the published literature, but it may be inferred that immunostains for thyroglobulin and CA-125 (a Müllerian epithelial marker) could contribute favorably to their differential diagnosis.[109]

An earlier section in this chapter has considered the difficulty that may be encountered in separating 'atypical thymoma' from thymic carcinoma morphologically. This problem is further exemplified by rare cases in which carcinomas of the thymus appear to arise *from* thymomas.[110] As one might expect, immunostains for CD5, CD70, and CD99 contribute to the recognition of these separate lesional elements.[111]

In aggregate, thymic carcinomas often demonstrate metastasis to lungs, liver, bones, adrenal glands, and extrathoracic lymph nodes.[1,91,112] Some have also caused death through uncontrollable mediastinal recurrence. Radiotherapy and chemotherapy have offered variable therapeutic benefit.

As already stated, the paraneoplastic syndromes which may be associated with thymoma have generally not been reported in conjunction with thymic carcinoma. However, we have seen one case in which acute myelomonocytic leukemia appeared 1 year after the diagnosis of a squamous carcinoma of the thymus which had metastasized widely.[92] Whether or not this observation was coincidental is a matter of speculation at present. As an aside, however, it would be more common to see acute leukemia in association with a mediastinal *germ cell tumor* than with primary thymic carcinoma (see below).[101,113] In any event, the potentially adverse behavior of thymic carcinoma is a compelling justification for its diagnostic separation from thymoma.

PROGNOSIS OF THYMIC CARCINOMAS

Until recently, prevailing opinion held that *all* primary thymic carcinomas (PTCs) had a dismal prognosis, regardless of their histotype.[92,112] However, current studies have examined that contention in detail and concluded that there are, in fact, some tumor variants that may be cured surgically.[114,115] Well-differentiated squamous cell carcinoma, mucoepidermoid carcinoma, and basaloid carcinoma principally represent that group.[91,114] It has been suggested that aggressive surgical excision and current adjuvant therapy may be curative in low-stage cases of *other* types of PTC as well.[114,115]

CYTOPATHOLOGY OF THYMIC EPITHELIAL NEOPLASMS

The cytologic attributes of thymic epithelial neoplasms have been adeptly summarized by Wakely[33] and others,[34,116–123] as seen in fine needle aspiration (FNA) specimens. Thymomas are morphologically heterogeneous in that context, paralleling their histological appearances. Mature lymphocytes are admixed with thymic epithelial cells, the latter of which show a tendency to cohesion (Fig. 21.28). However, scattered single epithelial cells also may be evident. As in tissue sections, epithelial cell nuclei are generally monomorphic, with dispersed chromatin and small chromocenters. Cytoplasm is amphophilic, with indistinct cell borders. A fusiform cellular shape may be encountered in spindle-cell tumors, but the grouping of such cells into small clusters helps to distinguish them from mesenchymal proliferations (Fig. 21.29). The lymphoid elements in thymoma are a potential diagnostic pitfall, in that nuclear 'activation' may be seen with increases in the nuclear:cytoplasmic ratios. Convolution of the nuclear borders also can be present, as may mitotic figures. The overall image of 'activated' intratumoral lymphocytes is quite similar to that of lymphoblastic lymphoma,[124] and a misdiagnosis may ensue unless immunostains for keratin are performed to detect the epithelial elements of thymoma. Predictably, invasive thymomas cannot be distinguished from encapsulated tumors using FNA technique.[33]

The cytopathologic characteristics of thymic carcinomas have been only rudimentarily described in the pertinent literature, especially in reference to the histologic subtypes outlined above.[33,120] Broadly speaking, the tumor cells in such lesions differ from those of thymoma in showing coarser chromatin, prominent nucleoli, and higher nuclear:cytoplasmic ratios (Fig. 21.30). Orangeophilic keratinization may be observed in the cytoplasm in overtly squamous neoplasms. In extrapolation of surgical pathologic findings, occasional cases of thymoma demonstrate relative nucleolar prominence and nuclear enlargement in cytological samples, but their overall images are not fully diagnostic of thymic carcinoma. Even after application

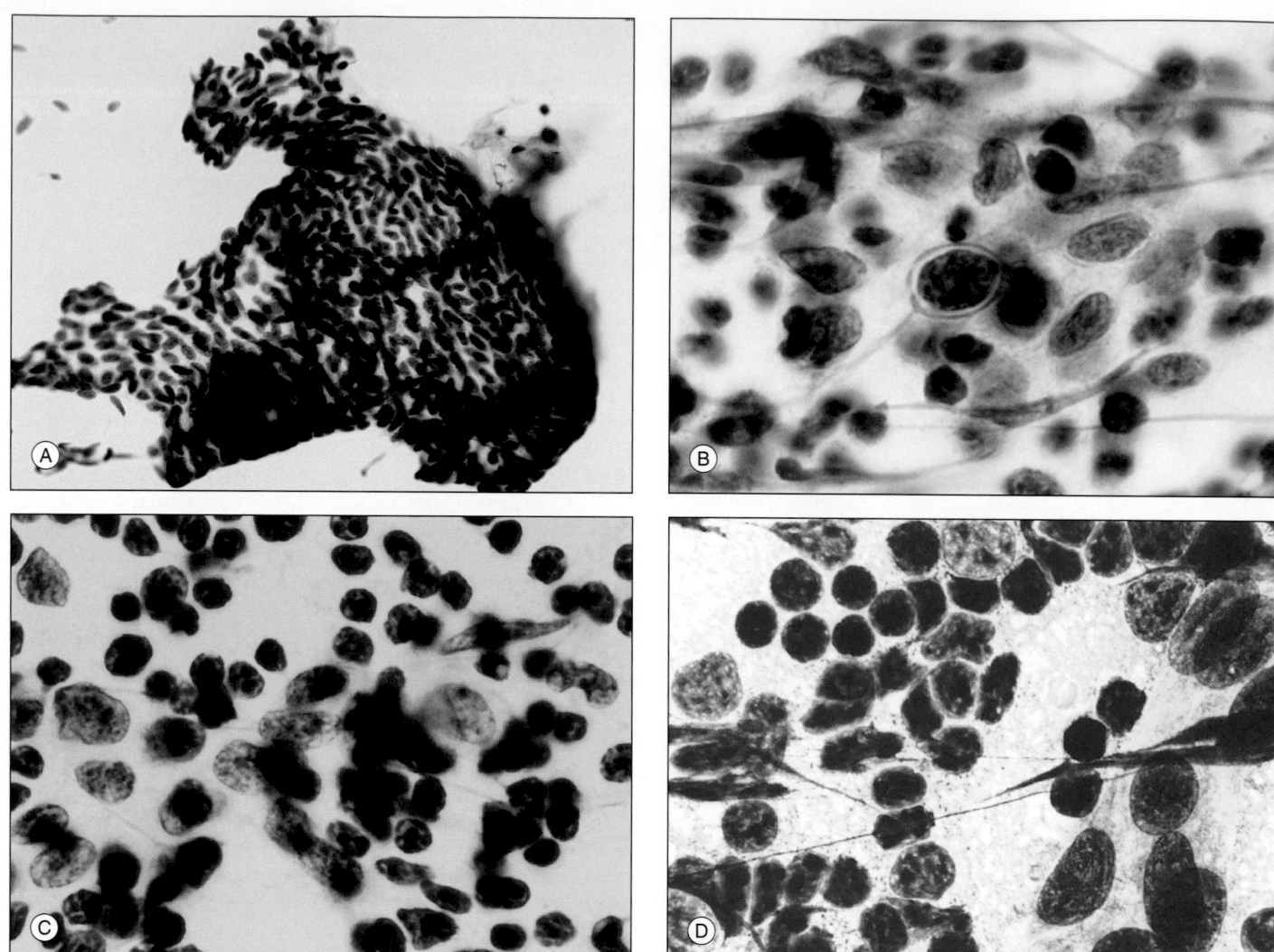

Fig. 21.28 Fine needle aspiration biopsies of thymoma: **(A)** A cohesive epithelial cell group is present; **(B)** Other tumor cells have a vaguely squamoid character; **(C)** Nuclei of epithelial cells in 'ordinary' thymoma show dispersed chromatin and inconspicuous nucleoli; **(D)** 'Atypical' thymomas show nuclear enlargement and irregularity, with discernible nucleoli (right of figure).

of immunohistologic studies in such cases, a diagnosis of 'atypical thymoma' may be necessary.[56]

Electron microscopy or immunohistology are also required to distinguish between carcinoma of the thymus and other malignant epithelioid lesions in FNA specimens. This process has been described earlier in this discussion in reference to surgical tissue samples.

PART IV: NEUROENDOCRINE, GERM-CELL, AND NONEPITHELIAL LESIONS

NEUROENDOCRINE THYMIC TUMORS ('CARCINOIDS' AND SMALL CELL NEUROENDOCRINE CARCINOMAS)

Although it had been known for many years that some thymic neoplasms were associated with clinical endocrinopathies such as

Cushing's syndrome,[125,126] these tumors were not distinguished from thymomas until 1972. At that time, Rosai and Higa remarked on their morphological similarity to neuroendocrine tumors of other sites, and suggested that they be called 'thymic carcinoids.'[127] We will retain that traditional terminology in the following discussion, although it is now felt that a more apt designation for such tumors is that of 'neuroendocrine carcinoma.'[128]

Duguid and Kennedy reported the existence of primary mediastinal 'oat cell' carcinoma (high-grade neuroendocrine carcinoma, small-cell type; small cell neuroendocrine carcinoma [SCNC]) in 1930.[129] However, this rare lesion went unstudied for nearly 50 years, because of skepticism owing to the well-known phenomenon of metastasis to the mediastinum from occult SCNCs of the bronchi.

Roughly 30% of carcinoid tumors of the thymus are associated clinically with Cushing's syndrome.[130,131] In addition, inappropriate ectopic production of antidiuretic hormone,[132] hypertrophic osteoarthropathy,[133] and the Eaton-Lambert syndrome[134] have been occasionally seen in patients with these neoplasms. Extremely high serum levels of adrenocorticotropic hormone (ACTH)

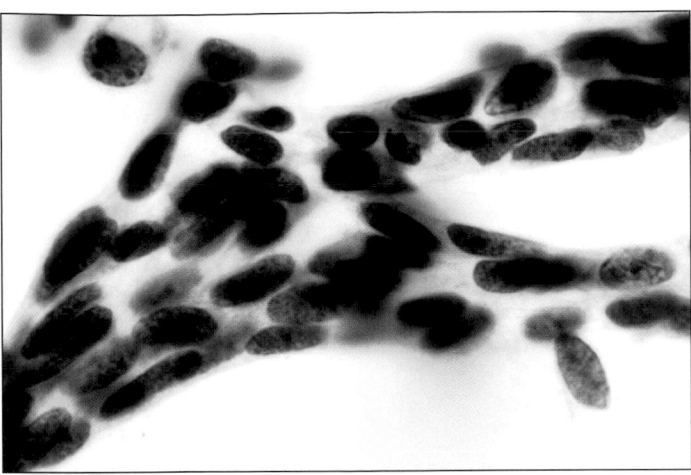

Fig. 21.29 Fine needle aspiration biopsy of spindle cell thymoma, demonstrating fascicles of epithelial cells with fusiform nuclear contours and dispersed chromatin.

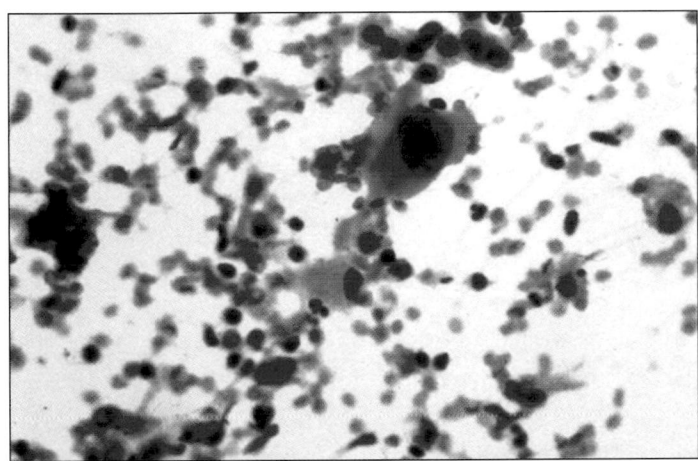

Fig. 21.30 Fine needle aspiration biopsy of sarcomatoid carcinoma, demonstrating scant cellularity with dispersed pleomorphic tumor cells. Nuclei are hyperchromatic and irregular in shape. Differential diagnosis with true sarcoma or other nonepithelial lesions would be virtually impossible without special studies.

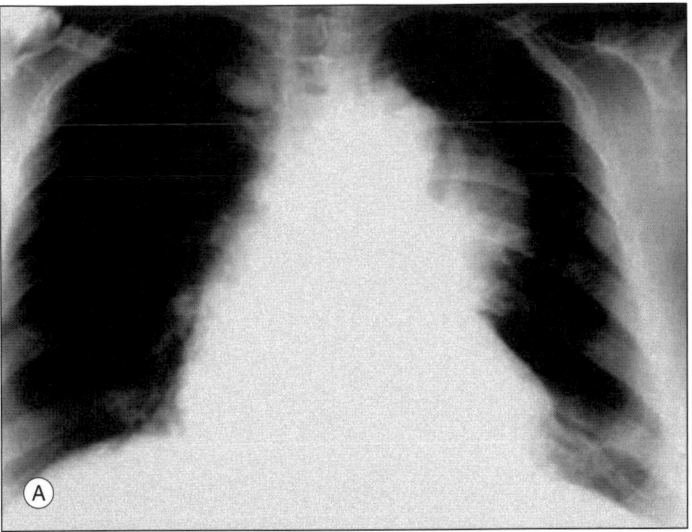

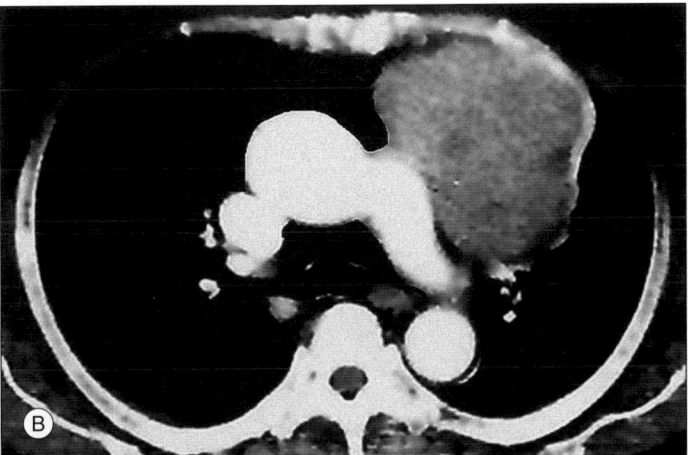

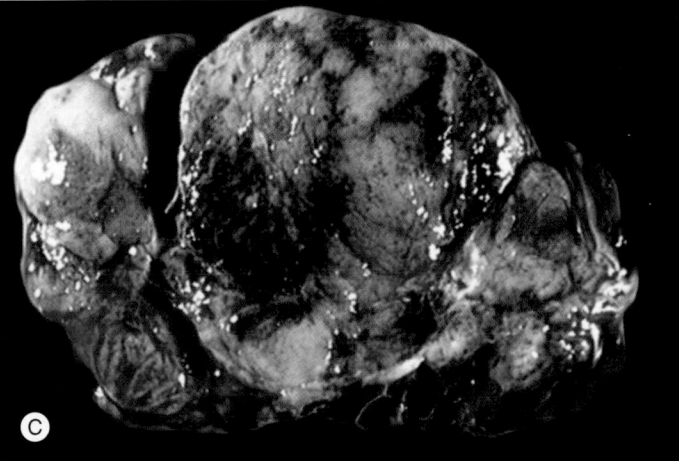

Fig. 21.31 Chest radiograph (**A**), computed tomogram (**B**), and gross photograph (**C**) of grade II neuroendocrine carcinoma of the thymus ('thymic carcinoid'), showing foci of necrosis and a lack of internal lobulation or septation as expected in thymomas.

(greater than 1000 pg/ml) are often recorded in patients with Cushing's syndrome along with cutaneous hyperpigmentation.[135] The latter conditions are enhanced after misdirected adrenalectomy, and that clinical constellation may be designated as 'pseudo-Nelson's syndrome.' The vast majority of thymic carcinoids and all reported SCNCs have presented with symptoms and signs of thoracic structural displacement, such as dyspnea, cough, chest pain, the superior vena cava syndrome, or are found incidentally on chest roentgenograms.[136] Rarely, metastasis to the cervical lymph nodes, bones, or skin may be the first manifestation of thymic carcinoids.[137]

Thymic carcinoids and SCNCs are virtually identical macroscopically, and they differ in appearance from thymomas. The majority are unencapsulated and average 8–10 cm in their greatest dimension.[138] They are gray-white and firm on cut section, often have a gritty consistency, and lack internal fibrous septation

(Fig. 21.31). Foci of hemorrhage and necrosis are apparent in approximately 70% of cases. When associated with Cushing's syndrome, carcinoid tumors of the thymus tend to be smaller at diagnosis (3–5 cm in diameter), and may be totally confined within the capsule of one thymic lobe.[135]

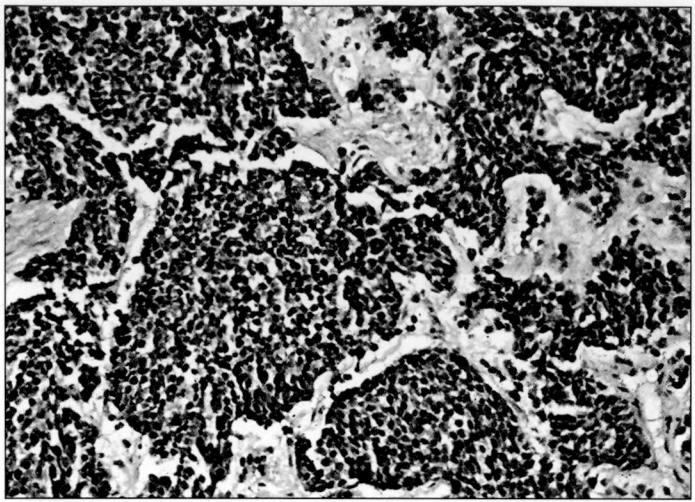

Fig. 21.32 Organoid growth in thymic carcinoid.

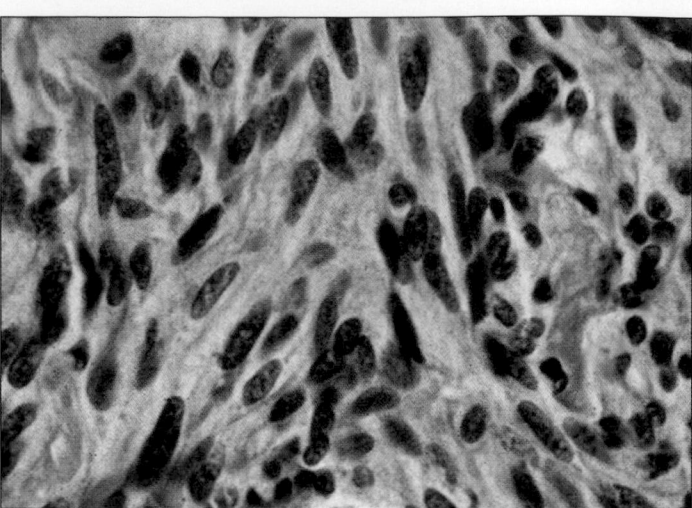

Fig. 21.34 Spindle-cell thymic carcinoid, with dispersed 'salt and pepper' chromatin pattern.

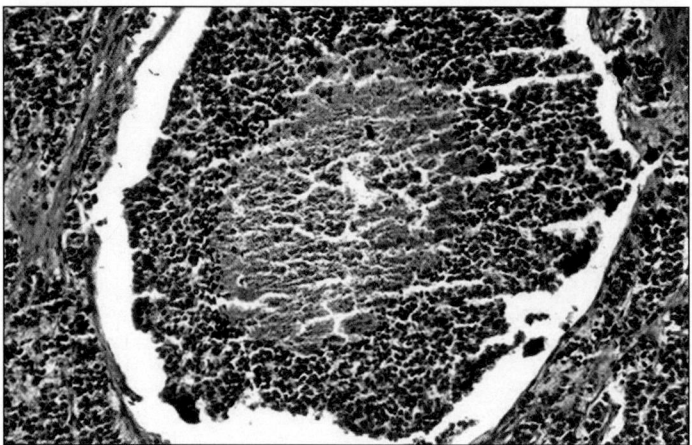

Fig. 21.33 Central necrosis is present in this cell group in thymic carcinoid (grade II neuroendocrine carcinoma), with artifactual retraction from the surrounding stroma. These are common findings in such tumors.

Thymic 'carcinoids'

Most thymic carcinoids display an 'organoid' growth pattern, characterized by nests of relatively uniform tumor cells separated by a fine fibrovascular stroma (Fig. 21.32). Individual cell borders are indistinct, cytoplasm is slightly eosinophilic and granular, and nuclei are round to oval with evenly distributed chromatin and indistinct nucleoli. Mitotic activity is variable, but is usually readily apparent; abnormally shaped division figures may be seen uncommonly.

Over 50% of thymic carcinoids show areas of trabecular growth and the formation of true rosettes.[131,136–138] The lumina of rosettes may contain material that is stainable with the Alcian blue or colloidal iron methods.[138] Another typical feature is the presence of central necrosis within tumor cell nests which manifest dystrophic calcification (Fig. 21.33);[127,137] this is the histological basis for the gritty consistency that may be observed in gross examination of carcinoid tumors of the thymus. In analogy to pulmonary neuroendocrine carcinomas, the regular presence of necrosis and mitotic activity in thymic 'carcinoids' makes most of them at least intermediate-grade lesions (so-called 'atypical' carcinoids).[139,140]

Application of argyrophilic techniques such as the Churukian-Schenk or Sevier-Munger stains yields positive results in virtually all cases,[137,138] whereas argentaffin methods such as the Fontana-Masson stain give negative results. These findings are consistent with those obtained in other neuroendocrine neoplasms of foregut derivation.[141]

Ancillary microscopic features typical of thymomas, such as significant lymphoid infiltrates, microcyst formation, perivascular serum lakes, medullary differentiation, and a hemangiopericytoma-like vascular pattern, are not seen in thymic carcinoids.[131,136,138,142] However, the latter lesions do share with thymoma a capacity for spindle cell growth (Fig. 21.34),[132,143] and occasional cases of either tumor type may require extensive special study to make a definitive diagnosis. Nonetheless, attention to the nuclear chromatin pattern in spindle cell carcinoid of the thymus usually allows this distinction to be made with conventional microscopy, since it is like that of 'classic' carcinoid cells. The use of touch preparations made from resected tumor tissue facilitates this facet of pathologic evaluation.

Stromal amyloid, demonstrated by the Congo red or crystal violet stains, has been reported in rare examples of thymic carcinoid with a spindle-cell growth pattern.[138] The similarity of these neoplasms to medullary carcinoma of the thyroid has been striking. However, the thyroid glands in the affected patients were entirely normal in both location and structure.

Other microscopic variants of thymic carcinoid have been described: some have intracytoplasmic lipofuscin-like or melanin pigment;[144,145] others have an extensively fibrous 'scirrhous' stroma, abundant intercellular mucin, diffuse oncocytoid change, prominent intracellular lipidization, a strikingly angiectoid vascular stroma, or focally cribriform or diffuse growth patterns.[131,136,142,146–149] The significance of these histologic subtypes lies in their potential confusion with a variety of tumors having dissimilar lineages.

Small cell neuroendocrine (oat cell) carcinoma

There are relatively few examples of primary thymic neoplasms with the histologic appearance of bronchogenic small cell carcinoma.[129,138,139,150–154] These differ from carcinoid tumors in that

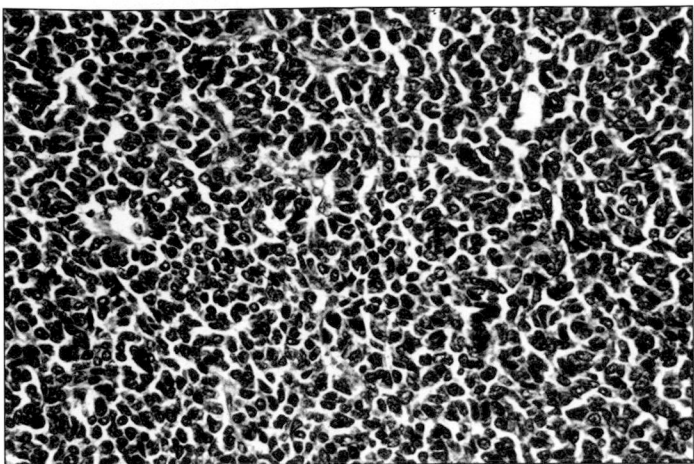

Fig. 21.35 Medullary growth of anaplastic tumor cells, with extremely high nucleocytoplasmic ratios, in primary small cell neuroendocrine carcinoma of the thymus.

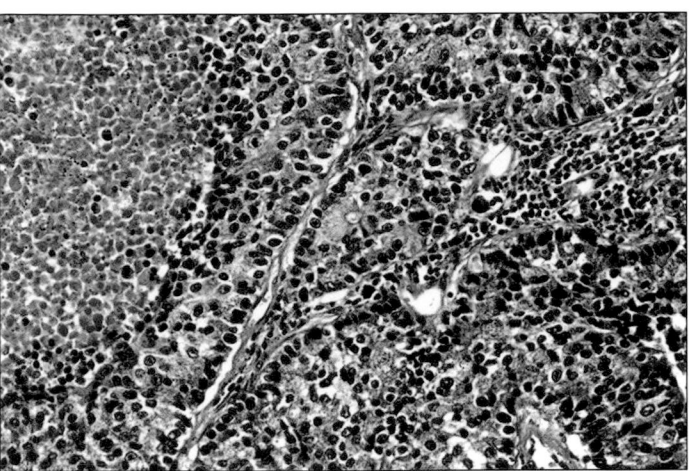

Fig. 21.37 Large cell neuroendocrine carcinoma of the thymus (grade III neuroendocrine carcinoma, large-cell type), showing typical zones of 'infarct-like' necrosis.

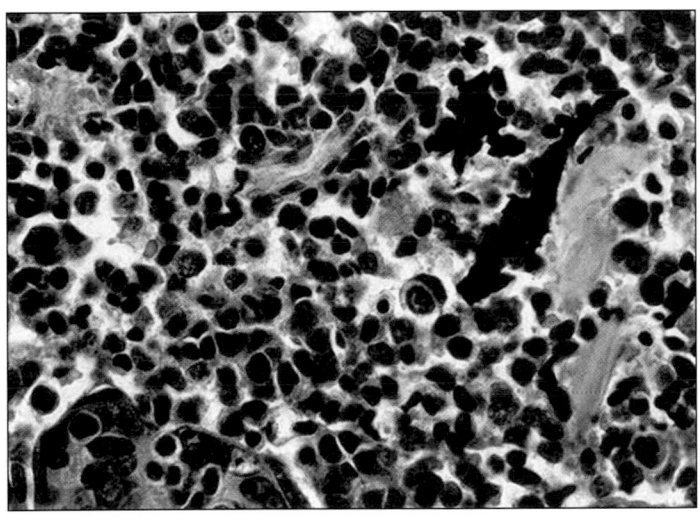

Fig. 21.36 Nuclear molding, crush artifact, and apoptosis are evident in this primary small cell neuroendocrine thymic carcinoma.

their cytoplasm is extremely scanty, mitoses are more numerous, and organoid growth is less apparent (Figs 21.35, 21.36). Tumors with an intermediate form of cytologic morphology may also be encountered, making it difficult to decide whether they should be classified as 'carcinoids' or 'small cell carcinomas.'[155] In such cases, the terms 'atypical carcinoid' or '"neuroendocrine carcinoma, not further specified' have been employed. These neoplasms have not been discussed above, under the heading of 'thymic carcinoma,' because they do not show differentiation toward thymic epithelium. Nevertheless, they are felt to be ultrastructurally and immunohistochemically similar to Kulchitzky-type neuroendocrine cells.[138] However, this is a fine point, and, in practical terms, SCNC is indeed a form of primary thymic carcinoma in the sense that it arises within the thymus.

We cannot stress the fact too strongly that most apparent SCNCs of the thymic region are actually metastases from occult bronchial neoplasms. There are few reliable pathologic points of distinction

between primary thymic and primary pulmonary SCNC, making exhaustive clinical exclusion of the latter mandatory before accepting a definitive diagnosis of the former. TTF-1 is regularly observed in small-cell lung cancers, but it has not yet been seen in SCNC of the thymus.[156,157] This marker may ultimately prove to be helpful in the cited distinction between those tumors.

Snover et al.[89] and others[158] have described cases of primary, combined SCNC-squamous carcinoma of the thymus. Squamous elements in these tumors were confined to small, randomly distributed cell nests amid the small-cell population; the boundary between the two was sharp microscopically. Again, because similar mixed differentiation has been observed in primary pulmonary neoplasms, the exclusion of metastasis to the mediastinum is necessary in such cases.

A few cases of primary thymic 'large cell neuroendocrine carcinoma' (high-grade neuroendocrine carcinoma, large-cell type) have been documented, in analogy to neoplasms arising in the lungs.[159] This tumor type is characterized by an individual cell size which is at least three times that seen in SCNCs. It also shows brisk mitotic activity, moderate nuclear pleomorphism, and peculiar infarct-like foci of spontaneous necrosis (Fig. 21.37).

Special studies of thymic neuroendocrine carcinomas

Ultrastructurally, thymic carcinoids are composed of closely apposed polygonal cells. Adjacent cells may display blunt, interdigitating cytoplasmic processes, and are incompletely invested by basement membrane material.[160] The interstitium consists of a mixture of collagen and flocculogranular matrix. Rarely, pseudoacini, formed by individual cell necrosis within cellular nests, may be evident. Intercellular junctions are invariably present, but are not abundant, and are of the *maculae adherentes* type. Nuclei are ovoid, or only slightly irregular in shape, with evenly distributed chromatin. Cytoplasmic invaginations within the nuclear contours may produce 'pseudoinclusions.' Nucleoli are characteristically inconspicuous. Typical membrane-bound dense-core neurosecretory granules are usually abundant in the cytoplasm of tumor cells (Fig. 21.38). These measure between 140 nm and 500 nm in diameter, although the size of such inclusions is usually rather uniform in any given

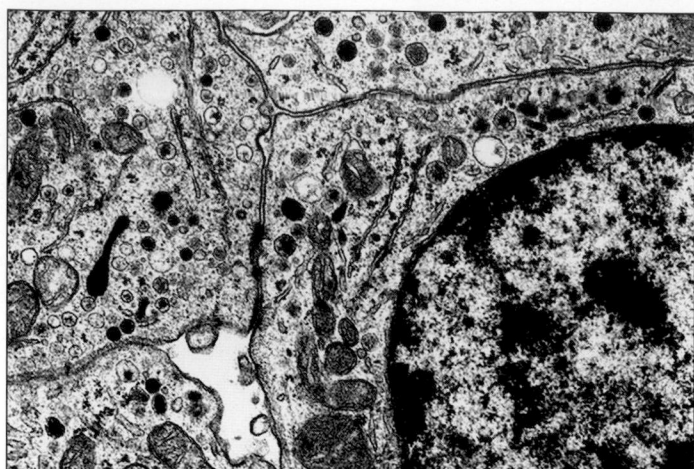

Fig. 21.38 Electron photomicrograph of thymic carcinoid, demonstrating numerous cytoplasmic dense-core (neurosecretory) granules and intercellular maculae adherens.

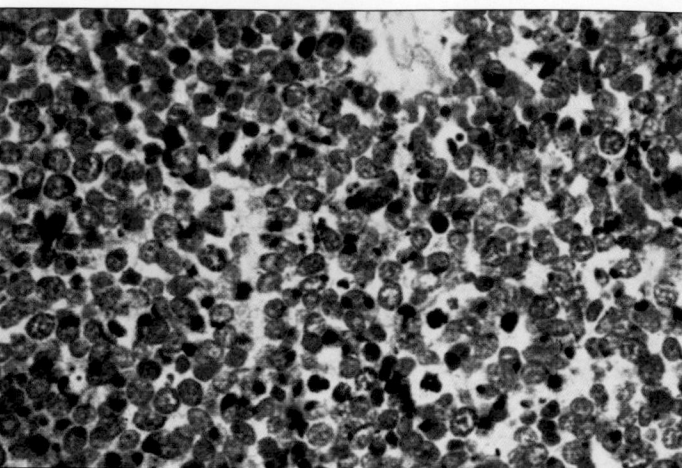

Fig. 21.39 Immunoreactivity for keratin in primary thymic small cell neuroendocrine carcinoma. Distinct perinuclear 'globules' of keratin are apparent, constituting evidence sufficient unto itself of neuroendocrine differentiation.

neoplasm. 'Misplaced' exocytosis, similar to that seen in pituitary prolactinomas, may be observed occasionally.[160] Other cytoplasmic organelles are rather nondescript, with three exceptions. Rough endoplasmic reticulum may be abundant and arranged in parallel arrays or concentric formations, particularly in hormonally active tumors. In these neoplasms, Golgi bodies are also numerous and prominent. Thymic carcinoids that synthesize ACTH also appear to show an abundance of smooth endoplasmic reticulum. Cytoplasmic filaments of the intermediate type are often present in thymic carcinoids, and not uncommonly assume a whorled, perinuclear configuration, in which dense-core granules may be enmeshed. Short, scanty tonofilaments may also be evident in thymic carcinoids, although they never assume the prominence seen in thymomas.

The electron microscopic features of thymic SCNC are generally similar to those of carcinoid tumors, except that their cytoplasm is more scanty, and neurosecretory granules are much less numerous;[92] detection of those inclusions may require diligent searching. Somewhat unexpectedly, intercellular junctional complexes may be more prominent in thymic SCNC than in carcinoid tumors. Tumors showing focal squamous differentiation by light microscopy manifest an abundance of cytoplasmic tonofilaments in such areas ultrastructurally.[89] It should be noted that dense-core granules may also be seen within the squamoid cells.

Immunohistochemically, there are similarities and important differences between thymic neuroendocrine carcinomas and true thymomas. Both tumor types display reactivity for keratin.[71,72] Some SCNCs, like thymomas, express epithelial membrane antigen (EMA), and this determinant is seen in 50% of thymic carcinoids as well.[71] A particular *pattern* of immunoreactivity for keratin is important in recognizing SCNC diagnostically; namely, the presence of globular perinuclear positivity for that intermediate filament group (Fig. 21.39). This finding is unique to neuroendocrine epithelial tumors among small-cell neoplasms. Two other markers are valuable in separating epithelial thymoma from thymic carcinoid or SCNC – synaptophysin and chromogranin-A.[72] The first of these substances is a synaptic vesicle protein that is found in neurons and the diffuse neuroendocrine cellular system. Chromogranin-A is an integral part of the membranes of neurosecretory granules. In our experience, both have been consistently present in thymic neuro-

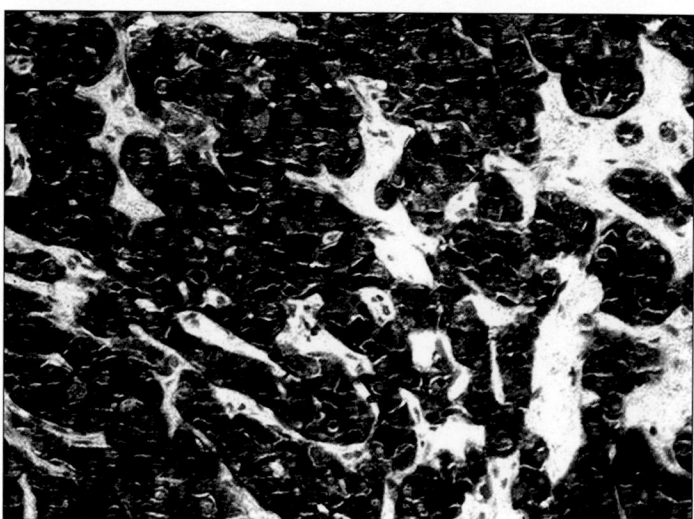

Fig. 21.40 Diffuse immunolabeling for chromogranin-A in thymic carcinoid.

endocrine neoplasms (Fig. 21.40). Other determinants that may be seen in such lesions but not in thymomas include CD56 (neural cell adhesion molecule) and neurofilament protein. Importantly, it should be noted that 'occult' neuroendocrine differentiation is relatively common in *other* forms of thymic carcinoma as well, such that scattered chromogranin-reactive cells may be observed in morphologically typical examples of lymphoepithelioma-like, nonkeratinizing squamous, or other forms of thymic carcinoma.[161-163] Hence, not only the presence but the *scope* of immunoreactivity for neuroendocrine markers is pertinent diagnostically.

In keeping with their line of differentiation, thymic carcinoids and SCNCs may exhibit immunoreactivity for any of the neuropeptide hormones or for serotonin;[131,160] ACTH, somatostatin, and calcitonin have been the neuropeptides most frequently observed.[160,164]

Thymomas do not manifest synthesis of any of these peptides, and we believe that all previous reports of 'thymomas' showing ACTH production were, in fact, examples of thymic carcinoid. Positive immunostaining results for neuropeptides are clinically valuable to confirm the origin of endocrinopathies, but also to provide useful data on hormonally 'silent' tumors. In both circumstances, patient serum may be assayed for the hormone(s) concerned (e.g. somatostatin) as a potential marker of tumor progression or recurrence.

Diagnostic confusion with malignant lymphoma may be encountered in rare cases of carcinoid tumor of the thymus showing a diffuse growth pattern.[136] However, thymic carcinoid and primary thymic SCNC fail to show immunoreactivity for CD20, CD45 or CD99, as seen in lymphomas of the thymic region, and instead are keratin positive.

Behavior of thymic neuroendocrine tumors

The primary reason for emphasizing the distinction between thymic carcinoid and SCNC on the one hand, and true thymoma on the other, is the disparity in their respective biologic behaviors. Whereas at least 30–40% of thymic neuroendocrine neoplasms demonstrate extrathoracic metastases to bones, skin, lymph nodes, and liver[131,139,142] (which are usually refractory to adjuvant chemotherapy or radiotherapy), thymomas show such behavior in <10% of all cases.[43] On the other hand, localized primary SCNC of the thymus has at least hypothetical curability with surgery and adjuvant therapy. In contrast, *metastatic pulmonary SCNC* in the thymic region is almost always fatal.

The mortality rate for carcinoid tumor of the thymus is higher in patients with the multiple endocrine neoplasia (MEN) syndrome, type I (pituitary adenoma, parathyroid adenoma or hyperplasia, and pancreatic islet cell tumor).[165–168] Individuals with ectopic Cushing's syndrome due to tumoral synthesis of ACTH also have a poorer outlook than those without clinical endocrinopathy.[130,137] Thymic carcinoid has the potential to act aggressively even if it is encapsulated at initial diagnosis; this statement also applies to SCNC of the thymus.[131,136] Thus, encapsulation does not have the same prognostic significance that it does in cases of true thymoma. Since metastasis of thymic carcinoid may occur as late as 10 years after initial presentation,[136] long-term clinical follow-up is necessary. The few cases of SCNC of the thymus that have been reported have not shown the rapidly fatal behavior of histologically identical pulmonary tumors, and average survival in one series was 36 months.[92]

Carcinoid tumors (low-grade neuroendocrine carcinomas) of the thymus are unpredictable, but all of them are felt to have the potential for distant metastasis.[136,139,142,168] An association with the multiple endocrine neoplasia syndromes or ectopic ACTH production is linked to a worsened prognosis in such cases, when compared with stage- and grade-matched nonsyndromic tumors.[137] Yamakawa et al.[180] and Gal and colleagues[139] have suggested that tumor size, mitotic activity, capsular invasion, and the presence of regional lymph node metastasis at diagnosis are likewise adverse prognostically.

Differential diagnosis

Several other pathologic entities enter into the differential diagnosis with thymic carcinoid and SCNC. *Predominantly epithelial and organoid thymoma* has been extensively discussed in the preceding sections. To recapitulate, that tumor type does not display the uniformity of nuclear chromatin seen in thymic carcinoids, and commonly shows lobulation by internal fibrous bands. Thymic carcinoids are immunoreactive for chromogranin-A, in contrast to thymomas.

Intrathymic parathyroid adenoma and carcinoma usually have a clinical association with hypercalcemia, betraying the nature of these endocrine lesions.[169–173] However, occasional cases may be hormonally silent, thereby causing possible confusion with thymic carcinoid. Several points of distinction between these lesions are evident microscopically. Most notably, parathyroid adenomas do not contain the focal necrosis, organoid growth pattern, or rosette formation, and they are usually strongly PAS-positive, in contrast to carcinoids.[173] Electron microscopy shows far fewer neurosecretory granules in parathyroid adenoma than in thymic carcinoid. Parathyroid hormone may be demonstrated immunohistochemically in the former, but usually not the latter of these lesions.[174]

Paraganglioma of the mediastinum is also morphologically similar to thymic carcinoid; however, it does not characteristically occur in the thymic bed, but rather is seen in association with large blood vessels because of its presumed origin from the aortico-pulmonary bodies or intravascular paraganglia.[131,175–177] A more tightly clustered cellular growth pattern (formation of *Zellballen*) typifies paragangliomas, as compared with the larger organoid cell nests of thymic carcinoids. Furthermore, whereas paragangliomas are usually devoid of mitotic activity, division figures are readily visible in thymic carcinoids. Argentaffin reactions are likely to yield positive results in paragangliomas, but not in thymic carcinoids. Finally, both neoplasms are immunoreactive for chromogranin-A, but paraganglioma lacks the keratin positivity of neuroendocrine carcinomas.[176]

Metastases to the thymus have been mentioned previously; they pose a difficult diagnostic problem in some cases because of their potential mimicry of thymic carcinoid tumors. Conversely, the variants of thymic carcinoid which display a cribriform growth pattern or mucinous stroma may suggest the presence of a secondary tumor rather than a primary thymic lesion. It is extremely unusual for carcinoids of the lung or intestine to metastasize selectively to the mediastinum, in the absence of overt disease at the primary site. Nevertheless, bronchoscopy and radiologic evaluation of the alimentary tract should be considered before making a definitive diagnosis of thymic carcinoid. Immunostains for TTF-1 and selected other markers of nonthymic carcinomas are also potentially helpful.[178] The problems in separating primary and secondary SCNCs in the thymus, as well as the necessity to do so, have already been discussed.

To restate, some examples of *malignant lymphoma* or *mediastinal germ cell tumor* may be confused with thymic neuroendocrine tumors. In these circumstances, immunohistologic evaluation *is* helpful diagnostically. Lymphomas display the presence of CD20, CD45, or CD99 and germinomas contain CD117 and placental alkaline phosphatase,[179] all of which are absent in neuroendocrine carcinomas.

Cytopathology of thymic neuroendocrine tumors

Thymic carcinoids exhibit a monomorphic neoplastic population of round to ovoid cells in FNA specimens,[181] sometimes with nuclear eccentricity that yields a plasmacytoid appearance on scanning microscopy (Fig. 21.41). There is a tendency to cohesion, but large groups of tumor cells are typically absent. Nuclei are round to oval with dispersed euchromatin and heterochromatin, yielding a characteristic 'salt and pepper' image (Fig. 21.42). Nucleoli are inconspicuous, and mitoses may be seen; the number of division figures, as well as the presence of background necrosis in the

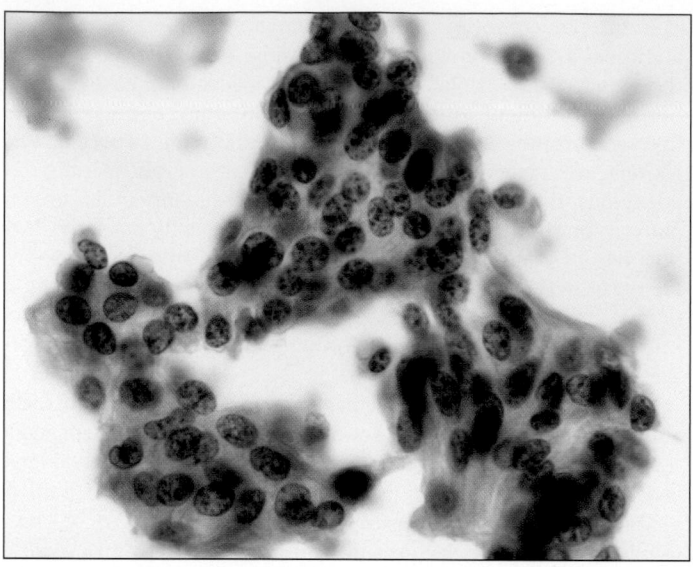

Fig. 21.41 Fine needle aspiration biopsy of thymic carcinoid, showing organoid cell groups with dispersed chromatin and inconspicuous nucleoli.

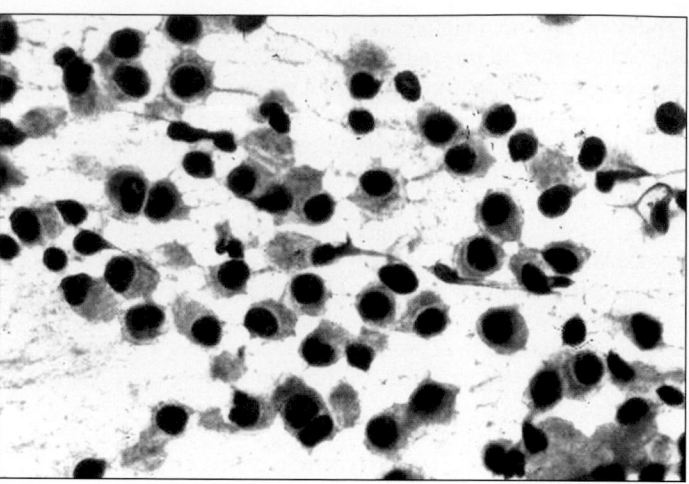

Fig. 21.42 Fine needle aspiration of thymic carcinoid, demonstrating a more dyscohesive pattern and a plasmacytoid character to the tumor cells.

specimen, parallel the grade of the tumor and are more typical of intermediate-grade neoplasms ('atypical carcinoids'). Cytoplasm is generally finely granular and amphophilic, but some tumor oncocytoid variants may exhibit abundant acidophilic granular cytoplasm. Cytoplasmic lipid droplets, intracellular pigment, and stromal amyloid are additional potential cytological findings in thymic carcinoids.[146,181]

Primary SCNCs of the thymus are identical in virtually every respect to those seen in the lungs in FNA specimens (Fig. 21.43), and the reader is referred to Chapter 18 for a discussion of their cytological features.

GERM CELL TUMORS OF THE THYMUS

It is not surprising that neoplasms showing germ cell differentiation should arise in the thymus, in view of the embryologic development of the gonads. In early fetal life, the germinal ridges are paired midline structures, which extend virtually throughout the axial dimension of the developing human.[182] With time, the cells in these ridges migrate caudally, to reach an eventual destination in the gonadal anlage. However, if they are arrested in this process, the surviving germinal cells may serve as a focus for subsequent neoplasia; this most typically evolves in the cranial sellar region,[183] thymic bed,[101,184,185] and retroperitoneum.[186,187]

The terminology of germ cell neoplasia is potentially confusing, as it has gone through several permutations and changes over the

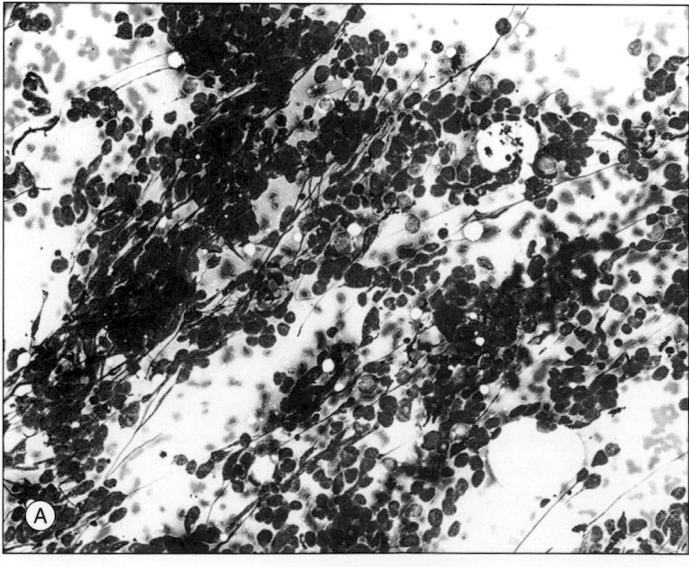

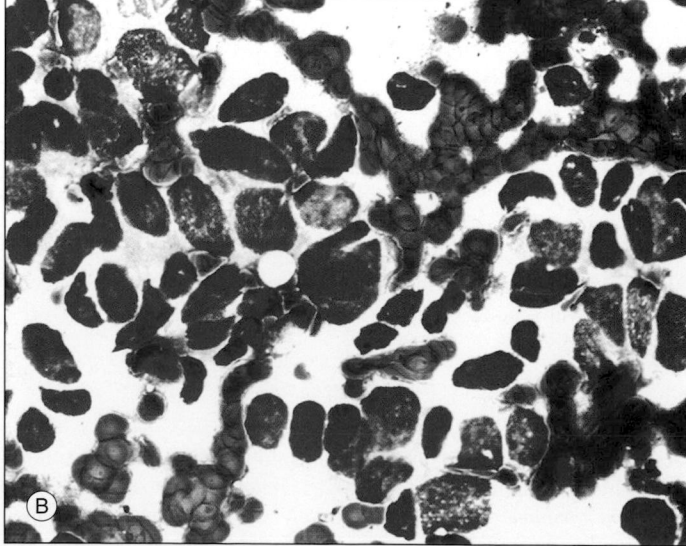

Fig. 21.43 Fine needle aspiration biopsies of primary thymic small cell neuroendocrine carcinoma, showing **(A)** characteristic 'smear' artifact, and **(B)** nuclear molding, bare nuclei, and high nucleocytoplasmic ratios.

years. We shall use the following nosologic system, which has been chosen because of its simplicity and general acceptance:

1. Mature teratomas: tumors composed of mature tissues showing differentiation representative of at least two of the three embryonal germinal layers.
2. Immature teratomas: tumors containing primitive, embryonic neuroepithelial tissues as well as mature elements, as just described, but without undifferentiated components.
3. Seminomas: tumors composed of cells showing monodifferentiation into spermatogonia-like elements.
4. Embryonal carcinomas: tumors comprised of undifferentiated cellular elements, showing a tendency to form primitive glands or ducts. The germinal origin of such neoplasms must be substantiated by the use of special techniques, and may not be obvious on conventional microscopy.
5. Yolk sac tumors (endodermal sinus tumors): neoplasms in which morphogenesis recapitulates such extraembryonic structures as the yolk sac endoderm and extraembryonic mesoblasts, in the absence of other lines of differentiation.
6. Choriocarcinomas: tumors showing sole differentiation into placental tissues, including the cytotrophoblast and syncitiotrophoblast.
7. Mixed malignant germ cell tumors (MMGCTs): combinations of any two or more of the following – mature or immature teratomas, embryonal carcinoma, yolk sac tumor, seminoma, or choriocarcinoma.

A well-known feature of germ cell neoplasms is their tendency to display more than one of these patterns. In a review of 56 cases of mediastinal germ cell tumors seen at the Mayo Clinic, Knapp et al.[188] found mixed tumors in 34% of their cases. Hence, use of the term MMGCT is preferable to attempts to force tumors into other nosologic categories, and it is also helpful to clinicians in planning therapeutic interventions and determining accurate prognoses. With this caveat in mind, we shall nonetheless provide more detailed descriptions of each form of germ cell neoplasia, in the following sections. The premise that they represent tumors of the thymus, in a topographic sense, is substantiated by the observations that they may be totally confined within the capsule of this gland,[42] or that thymic elements are intermingled within the tumors.[189]

Mature teratomas

Mature teratomas are the commonest germ cell tumors of the mediastinum, accounting for 9–20% of all tumors in this location.[190-192] They occur with equal frequency in men and women, with a peak during the third decade of life.[191] An increased incidence has been reported in men with Klinefelter's syndrome.[193] Roughly one-third are asymptomatic, and are found during routine chest radiography. The remainder present with chest, back, or shoulder pain, dyspnea, the superior vena cava syndrome, or cough. Rupture of such neoplasms into the bronchi may produce the dramatic symptom of trichoptysis, if hair is contained within the mass, and lipid pneumonia may also ensue. Foci of calcification are evident on roentgenograms of mediastinal teratomas in roughly 25% of all cases.[191]

Grossly, mature teratomas are encapsulated, internally cystic masses averaging 10–11 cm in their greatest dimension. The cyst cavities often contain keratinous debris, with or without hair; cartilage or bone may also be macroscopically obvious (Fig. 21.44).[192] Histologically, the predominant elements are usually integumentary, including keratinizing squamous epithelium with pilosebaceous and

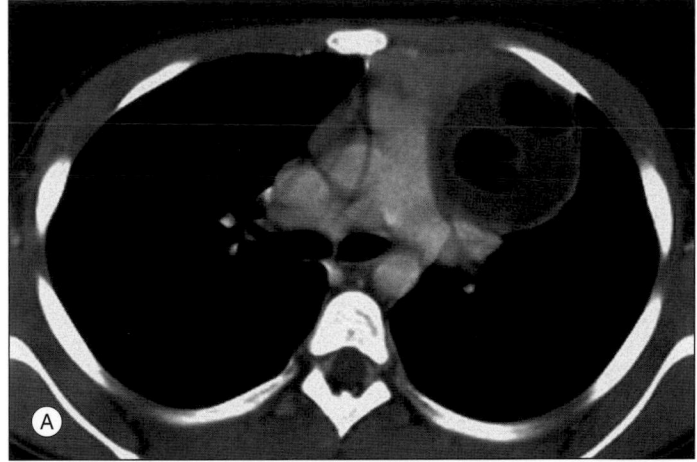

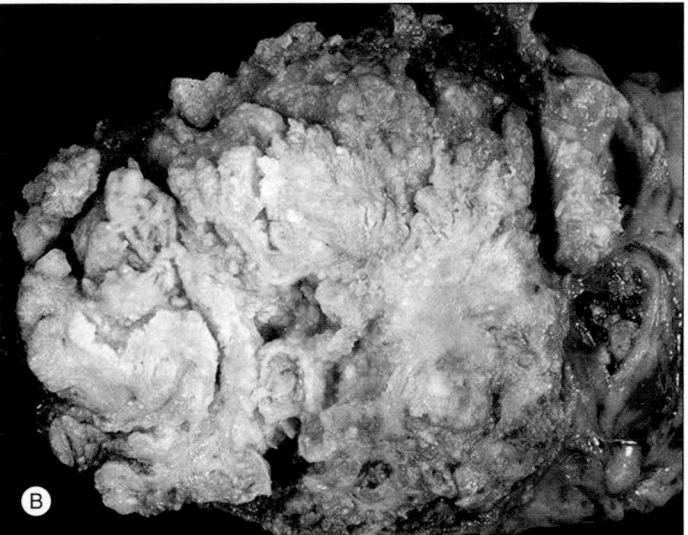

Fig. 21.44 **(A)** Computed tomogram of the thorax demonstrating a partially cystic, anterior mediastinal mature teratoma that projects into the left hemithorax. **(B)** Gross photograph of mature anterior mediastinal teratoma, showing abundant keratinous content.

sudoriferous adnexa. Respiratory and gut epithelium and pancreatic tissue are also frequently observed, along with fibroblastic or smooth muscular mesenchymal tissue, or cartilage and bone, as mentioned already. Less than 10% of mature teratomas contain teeth, choroid plexus, nervous tissue, bone marrow, striated muscle, renal tissue, or retinal tissue (Fig. 21.45).[191]

Care must be taken to sample these tumors thoroughly for microscopic examination, since the finding of foci of seminoma or other tumor types changes not only their classification but their prognosis. In addition, rare examples of mature mediastinal teratomas harboring squamous cell carcinoma, adenocarcinoma, or sarcoma have been reported.[194] In the absence of these complicating elements, surgery is curative and the prognosis is excellent.

Immature teratomas

Immature teratomas, defined as showing embryonic neuroepithelial, mesenchymal, and epithelial elements in varying combinations, account for only 1% of mediastinal teratomas.[195] In other locations, particularly in the gonads and the sacrococcygeal region, the quantity

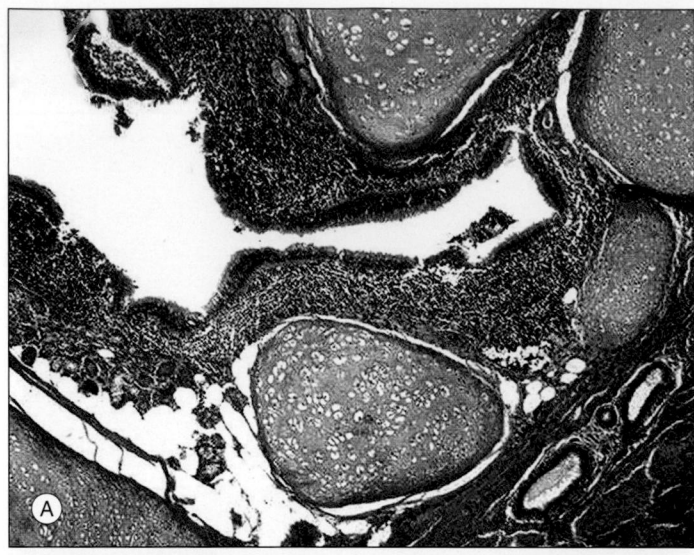

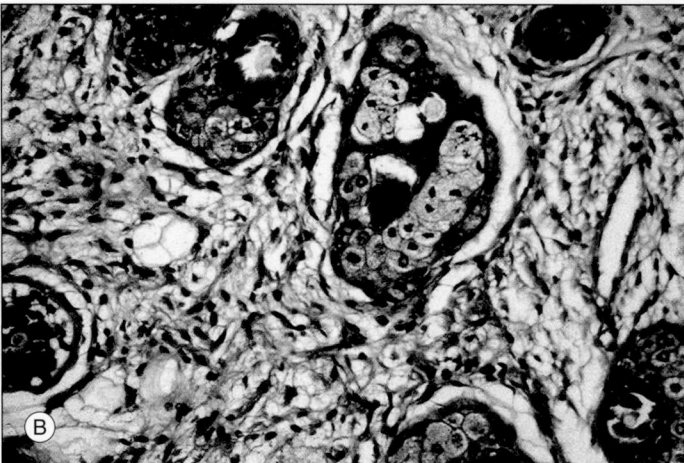

Fig. 21.45 **(A)** Mature thymic teratoma, containing respiratory epithelium, hyaline cartilage, and enteric-type epithelial profiles. **(B)** Another mature teratoma of the anterior mediastinum shows nondescript mesenchyme punctuated by cutaneous adnexal (sebaceous) tissues.

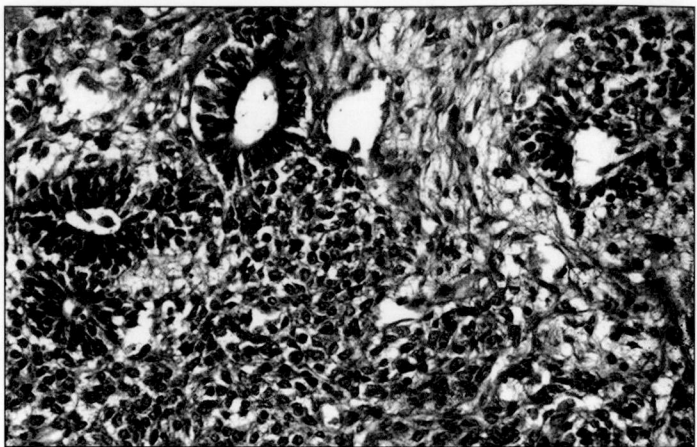

Fig. 21.46 Immature thymic teratoma, containing primitive neuroepithelial profiles resembling neural tube (upper left & right of figure).

of primitive neuroectodermal tissue in immature teratomas is thought to be an important prognostic feature.[196] The microscopic appearance of this element will be described later. In the mediastinum, however, it would appear that the patient's age is the most meaningful factor in predicting the clinical evolution.[195] The immature teratomas occurring after age 15 have tended to behave aggressively,[190,197] whereas those in younger individuals have pursued an innocuous course after surgery alone.[195,198–200] This point is an interesting one because it correlates with the behavior of gonadal germ cell tumors such as yolk sac tumors, which are generically less aggressive in infants and children than in adults.

Grossly, there are no significant differences between mature and immature teratomas. Microscopically, the latter contain foci of fetal-appearing cartilage or primitive neuroectodermal tissue,[195] which is represented by clusters of basaloid cells with high nucleocytoplasmic ratios and mitotic activity (Fig. 21.46). Neuroectodermal tissue may show a tendency to form rudimentary neural tube-like structures, and may be embedded in a fibrillar, neuroglial-like stroma. The presence of overt embryonal carcinoma, choriocarcinoma, yolk sac tumor, seminoma, or somatic carcinoma/sarcoma in an otherwise typical teratoma mandates its exclusion from this group.

Seminomas

Seminoma of the thymus is the commonest pure germ cell tumor of the mediastinum, and has been confused in the past with true thymoma (seminomatous thymoma).[101,102,184,201] However, compelling evidence has accrued which dispels any notion that this neoplasm is of thymic epithelial origin and establishes its pathologic identity with seminoma of the testis and dysgerminoma of the ovary.

This neoplasm occurs almost exclusively in males, mostly in the third and fourth decades of life. Like other space-occupying lesions of the mediastinum, it commonly presents with chest or back pain, dyspnea, cough, superior vena cava obstruction, fever, weight loss, or bone pain, although 15–40% of cases are asymptomatic.[188,197,202,203] Cervical and supraclavicular lymph nodes may be involved by metastases at diagnosis in a minority of cases.[188] It is felt that palpably normal gonads and a radiographically unremarkable retroperitoneum constitute sufficient evidence for the primary nature of thymic seminoma in any given case,[204] because of the statistical unlikelihood of selective metastasis to the thymic region from an occult gonadal tumor of this type.

Grossly, thymic seminoma is usually unencapsulated, and freely invades mediastinal great vessels, pleura, or pericardium.[1,42,201] On cut section, it is solid, rubbery, and gray-white, without the internal lobulation which characterizes true thymoma (Fig. 21.47). Foci of necrosis and hemorrhage are common, and cysts can occasionally be seen.[205]

Histologically, sheets of uniform tumor cells are subdivided by fine fibrovascular septa, which are typically invested by reactive lymphocytes. The cells of seminoma contain abundant, clear or slightly eosinophilic cytoplasm (Fig. 21.48), which is PAS-positive and labile to diastase digestion. Nuclei are round or oval, with thick membranes, coarse chromatin, and complex nucleoli. Mitotic activity is variable. A peculiar feature, which, like the lymphoid infiltrates of such neoplasms, is thought to reflect a host immune response, concerns the admixture of noncaseating epithelioid granulomas throughout some thymic seminomas. These may be prominent enough to obscure the tumor proper, and may result in erroneous diagnoses of granulomatous inflammatory processes such as sarcoidosis.[189]

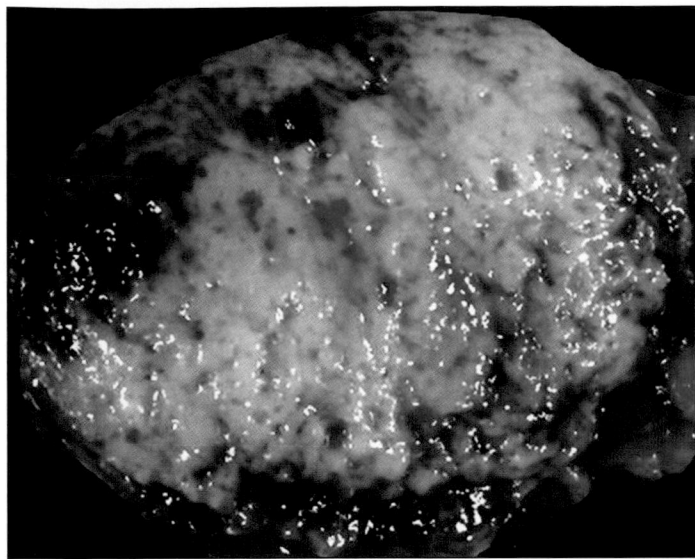

Fig. 21.47 Gross photograph of thymic seminoma, showing 'fleshy' gray-tan tumor tissue lacking internal septation or lobulation and with foci of stromal hemorrhage.

Occasional cases contain syncytiotrophoblastic cells, scattered randomly among the typical seminomatous cells. If unassociated with cytotrophoblastic elements, this finding does not alter diagnosis or prognosis. However, it should be noted in pathologic reports, since production of beta-human chorionic gonadotropin (HCG) by the syncytiotrophoblastic cells may account for elevated serum levels of this hormone.[206]

On ultrastructural examination, seminoma does not display the overt features of epithelial differentiation (tonofilaments and desmosomes) as seen in true thymomas.[102] Only primitive appositional plaques serve to join adjacent tumor cells, and basal lamina is absent. The cytoplasm contains few metabolic organelles, and lacks neurosecretory granules, but 'lakes' of glycogen particles may be abundant. The most distinctive feature of seminomas on electron microscopy is the aspect of the nucleoli in this tumor – they are complex, with dispersed nucleolonemas, and are present in nearly all neoplastic cells.

Immunohistochemically, seminoma is typified by a relative lack of positive findings. It does not express EMA[207] and cytokeratin is absent in most cases;[105] similarly, this tumor lacks alpha-fetoprotein (AFP), alpha-1-antitrypsin (A1AT), chromogranin, CD30, and CD45.[105,208] Indeed, aside from the aforementioned presence of HCG immunoreactivity in rare cases, the only determinants that are consistently exhibited by seminoma are CD117 (Fig. 21.49) and

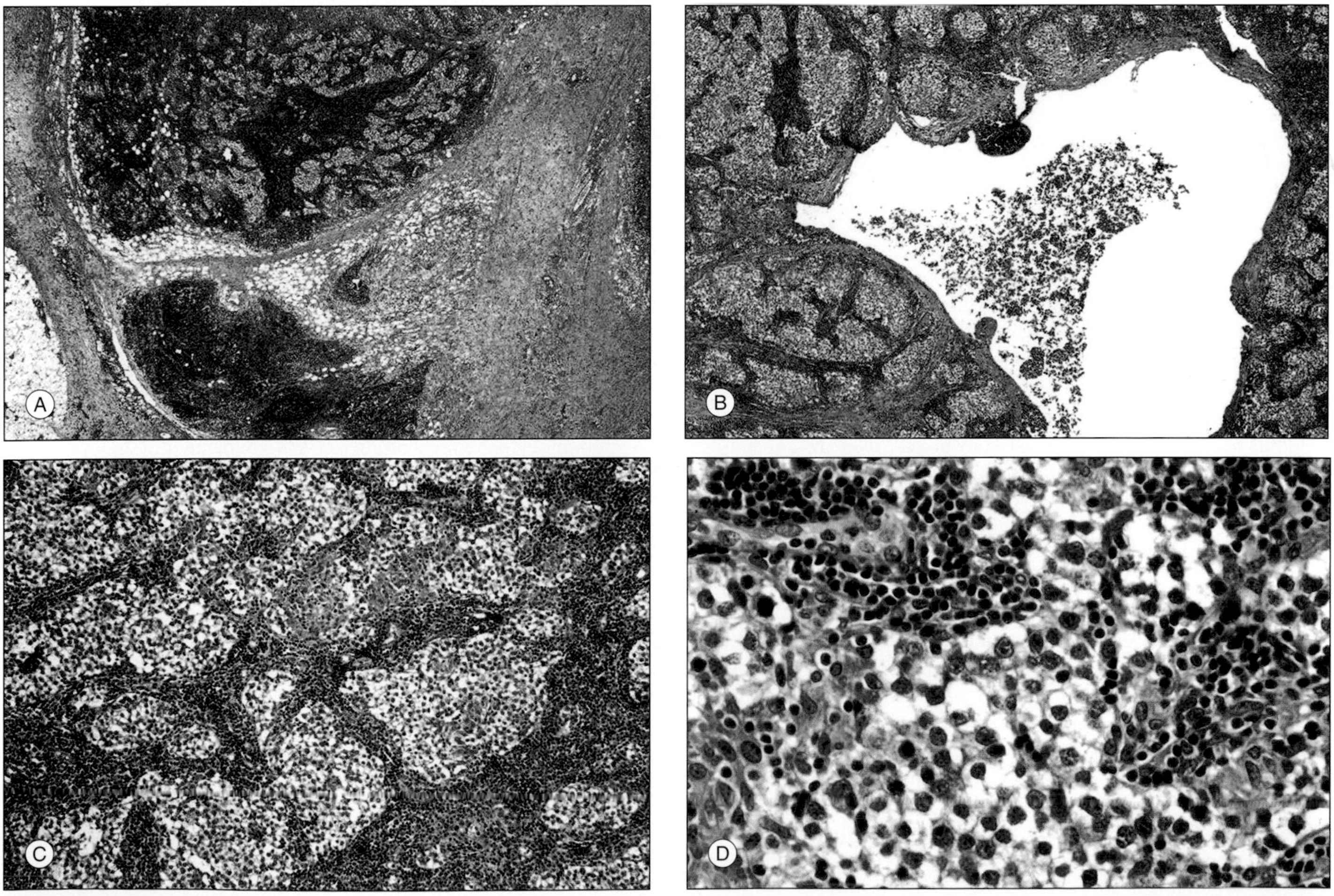

Fig. 21.48 Photomicrographs of thymic seminoma, showing **(A)** partial replacement of thymic glandular lobules by tumor; **(B)** cystic change in the tumor; **(C)** compartmentalization by lymphocytic-rich stroma; and **(D)** tumor cells with abundant clear cytoplasm and prominent nucleoli ('nucleolonemas').

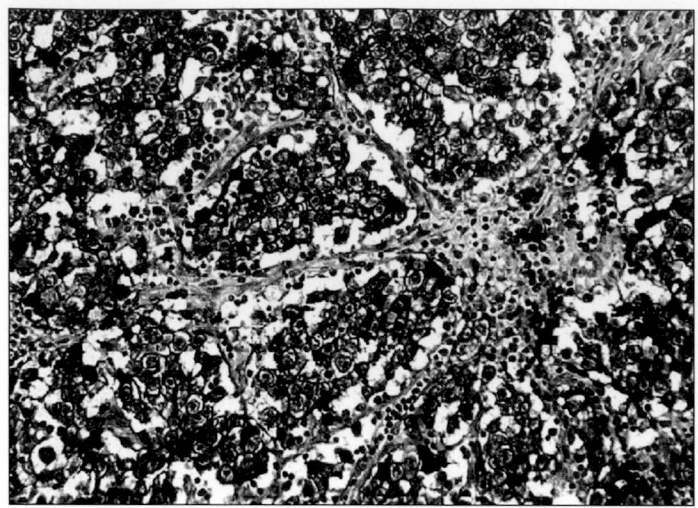

Fig. 21.49 CD117 (c-*kit* protein) immunoreactivity in primary thymic seminoma.

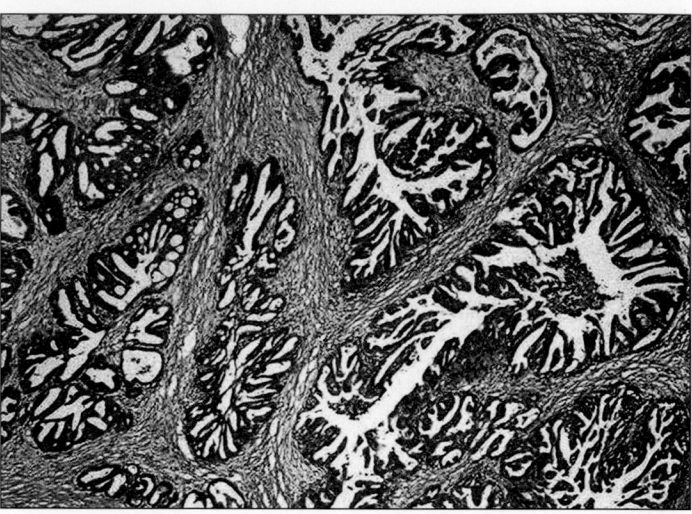

Fig. 21.50 Papillary differentiation in primary thymic embryonal carcinoma.

PLAP.[104,105,206] These two markers are present together in the great majority of such tumors, a finding that is invaluable in defining their germinal nature and which aids in excluding the differential diagnostic alternatives of *malignant lymphoma, atypical thymoma,* and *thymic carcinoma.* Keratin-specific antibodies may highlight nests of thymic epithelial cells that may be intermingled with the seminoma cells, representing a potential diagnostic trap.[189]

Another potentially useful adjuvant diagnostic technique in the recognition of germinomas is in situ hybridization for isochromosome 12p i[12p], a characteristic karyotypic marker of germ cell tumors.[209,210] This evaluation can be done on either fresh tissue or paraffin sections.[211] It should be recognized, however, that i[12p] is present in only 60–70% of these neoplasms.

Aygun et al. reviewed the clinical features of mediastinal seminoma, with particular attention to prognosis and response to treatment.[204] As with gonadal tumors of this type, radiation therapy is recommended as the primary modality. Although seminoma is thought to be equally sensitive to treatment regardless of its site of origin, a small proportion of primary mediastinal tumors fail to respond to therapy and metastasize to bones, liver, brain, and soft tissue. The 5-year survival for patients with thymic seminoma is approximately 90%.[212]

Mediastinal embryonal carcinomas (MECs)

Pure embryonal carcinoma arising in the thymus is relatively rare, and this neoplasm is most commonly encountered in combination with seminoma, yolk sac tumor, choriocarcinoma, or teratomatous elements.[188] Like seminoma, mediastinal embryonal carcinoma (MEC) is commoner in male patients, and has a peak incidence in early adulthood. Males with Klinefelter's syndrome may have a higher risk of developing this neoplasm.[213] Symptoms and signs of MEC are similar to those of thymic seminoma, but may evolve more rapidly.

Grossly, MEC presents a similar appearance to that of seminoma, except that intratumoral necrosis and hemorrhage are somewhat commoner findings. Invasion of other mediastinal structures is frequently observed at surgery. Microscopically, this neoplasm is composed of nests, sheets, or cords of undifferentiated cells with large vesicular nuclei, scanty amphophilic cytoplasm, and abundant

mitotic activity.[188,214] Papillary and duct-like structures may also be apparent (Fig. 21.50). This description is generally quite similar to that of *thymic carcinoma,* and, therefore, the two tumors may be easily confused. Nevertheless, careful sampling of MEC will almost always reveal foci of primitive glandular differentiation, a feature that is not present in most thymic epithelial tumors.

Ultrastructural findings in cases of embryonal carcinoma are generally nondescript, and may lead to an erroneous diagnosis of 'undifferentiated carcinoma, not otherwise specified.'[215] Desmosomal intercellular junctions are more prominent than in cases of thymic seminoma, but cytoplasmic tonofilaments and pericellular basal lamina are again lacking. Occasional nuclei may display focally complex nucleoli. The most distinct feature of MEC on electron microscopy is probably the presence of cytoplasmic AFP globules. These are moderately electron dense, and relatively large, and often found in close association with rough endoplasmic reticulum.[216] Rare cases of MEC may demonstrate microvillous plasmalemmal differentiation, but intracytoplasmic lumina are not evident.

Immunocytochemical studies reveal a typical antigenic profile in cases of MEC, and these pathologic investigations are the most likely to yield an accurate diagnosis. Embryonal carcinoma is EMA negative but positive for cytokeratin and CD30 (Fig. 21.51),[72] and it usually shows immunoreactivity for PLAP as seen in seminoma.[217] These results are unlike those obtained in *primary thymic carcinoma* or *metastatic carcinomas* from other sites, which represent the major differential diagnostic alternatives to MEC. CD30 is not expected in seminoma, and can therefore be used to help separate that tumor type from MEC in selected instances. The i[12p] karyotype is also seen in the majority of embryonal carcinomas and may be helpful in excluding other differential diagnoses.

The clinical course of thymic embryonal carcinoma is aggressive.[188,201] It is often refractory to surgical resection, radiotherapy, and aggressive combination chemotherapy, and proves fatal through massive intrathoracic growth and/or metastasis to the lungs, bones, liver, and brain. Median survival for patients with MEC is less than 24 months.[218] This pattern of behavior is worse than that of histologically identical gonadal tumors.

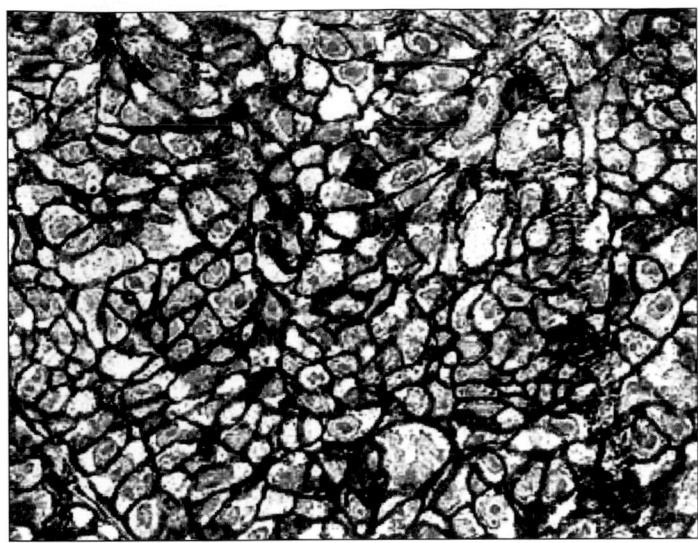

Fig. 21.51 CD30 (Ki-1) immunoreactivity in primary thymic embryonal carcinoma.

Yolk sac tumors (endodermal sinus tumors)

The clinical and gross pathologic features of yolk sac tumor (YST) of the mediastinum are virtually identical to those of embryonal carcinoma; indeed, the two tumor types are commonly admixed with one another within the same mass.[188,218–220] Pure thymic YST is rare and relatively few cases have been documented, only two of which were in females.[188,221] Interestingly, an association has been noted between acute leukemia and mediastinal germ cell neoplasms containing yolk sac tumor elements.[222] The leukemic cells are felt to derive *directly* from the neoplastic germinal elements, inasmuch as both are known to exhibit i[12p] karyotypically.[223]

Microscopically, yolk sac tumor is characterized by thin anastomosing cords composed of cuboidal cells with oval, hyperchromatic nuclei. Reticular or microcystic patterns may be evident. A distinctive structure in YST is the Schiller-Duval body, which resembles the embryonic yolk sac (Fig. 21.52). It is composed of one or two layers

of tumor cells mantling a central fibrovascular core, with an overall papillary configuration.[224] Another salient feature is the formation of embryoid bodies,[225] composed of small groups of flattened tumor cells within microcystic spaces, and reminiscent of the embryonic growth plate. Extracellular, eosinophilic basement membrane material is sometimes abundant in YST, and is PAS-positive.[220] In addition, PAS-positive, diastase-resistant globules are commonly evident within the cytoplasm of the tumor cells.

Ultrastructurally, YST is nearly identical to MEC, except that extracellular basement membrane material is much more prominent.[220,226] Cytoplasmic globules of AFP are also more numerous than in the latter neoplasm.[227] Immunocytochemical features parallel those of MEC qualitatively, but AFP and A1AT positivity is stronger and more uniform in YST.[105,216,220,226] The A1AT reactivity corresponds to PAS-positive intracytoplasmic material seen on conventional microscopy.[220]

The prognosis of thymic YST is generally poor. It is commonly unresectable at diagnosis, and the majority of documented cases have shown metastases to the lungs, liver, brain, lymph nodes, and bones.[218] Response to radiotherapy and chemotherapy is uncommon, and patients with residual mediastinal or metastatic disease have a median survival of <12 months. However, after reviewing the literature, Mukai and Adams[220] proposed clinicopathologic criteria that may correlate with a better prognosis in YST. These include an asymptomatic status at diagnosis, surgical resectability of the neoplasm, and the absence of metastatic spread at presentation. Serum levels of AFP are useful monitors of therapeutic efficacy in cases of YST of the mediastinum.[228]

Choriocarcinomas

Choriocarcinoma as a pure thymic germ cell neoplasm is vanishingly rare, and this tumor type is almost invariably admixed with MEC, YST, or both.[185,188,218] Nevertheless, any focus of choriocarcinoma in a thymic germ cell neoplasm, no matter how small, assumes major prognostic importance. Patients with such lesions are nearly all males, in their 30s or 40s, who may present with rapidly enlarging mediastinal masses and superior vena cava obstruction if the choriocarcinoma component of their tumors is sizable.[229] Erosion into bronchi by the mass may produce hemoptysis, and the synthesis of HCG by choriocarcinomas produces gynecomastia, decreased

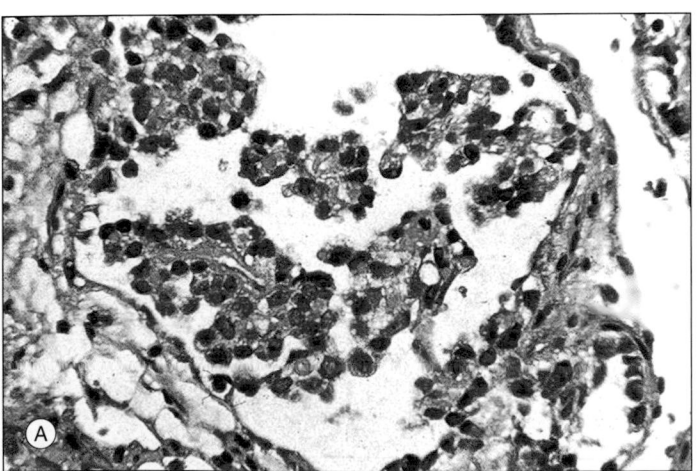
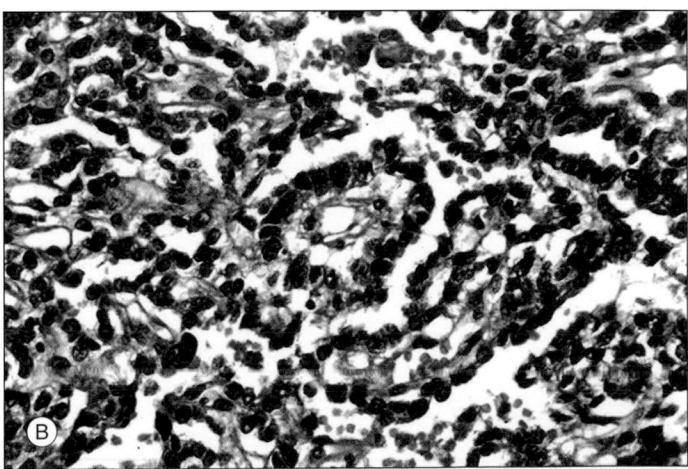

Fig. 21.52 Yolk sac tumor of the thymus, showing **(A)** micropapillary differentiation and **(B)** characteristic perivascular disposition of tumor cells, forming a Schiller-Duvall body.

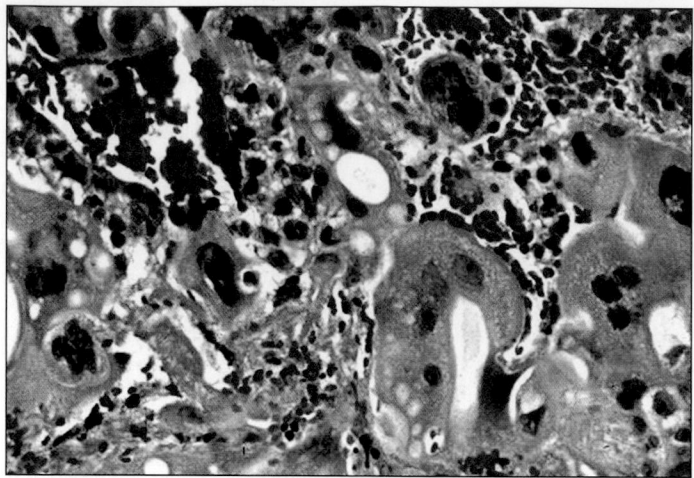

Fig. 21.53 Primary choriocarcinoma of the thymus, containing cytotrophoblastic and syncytiotrophoblastic elements.

libido, and testicular atrophy.[230] The rare tumors that occur in females cause menstrual irregularities.

Grossly, choriocarcinoma is a friable, reddish-gray, largely necrotic invasive neoplasm. Hence, any areas resembling this description in mediastinal germ cell tumors should be sampled thoroughly. Microscopically, choriocarcinoma is defined by the presence of cytotrophoblast, represented by sheets and nests of polygonal cells with single, large, vesicular nuclei and a moderate amount of amphophilic cytoplasm, and by syncytiotrophoblast, which is composed of multinucleated cellular elements occurring in apposition to the cytotrophoblastic elements (Fig. 21.53).[188,218] Spontaneous necrosis and hemorrhage are common, and cytotrophoblastic mitotic activity is typically brisk. As mentioned previously, occasional seminomas of the thymus may contain syncytiotrophoblastic cells; however, unless unequivocal cytotrophoblast is also present, such neoplasms should not be labeled as choriocarcinomas.

In distinct contrast to thymic seminoma, MEC, and YST, the absence of a palpable gonadal mass does not confirm the primary nature of a mediastinal choriocarcinoma,[231] because choriocarcinomas have a well-known tendency to form early distant metastases while only a miniscule primary tumor is present in the ovary or testis. This issue currently has little prognostic importance, but it may influence the decision of the thoracic surgeon as to whether or not a therapeutic thoracotomy is warranted.

Ultrastructural study is of little benefit in the pathologic identification of thymic choriocarcinoma. However, immunocytochemistry may be invaluable in confirming the presence of syncytiotrophoblastic elements. As one would expect, antibodies to beta-HCG are employed for this purpose.[105,188,218]

Other immunohistologic markers may be useful in excluding selected differential diagnostic alternatives. *Metastases* of anaplastic, pleomorphic carcinomas to the thymic region, which may mimic choriocarcinoma, are EMA positive, but usually PLAP negative. Choriocarcinomas usually exhibit the converse of these findings, but exceptions do occur.[71,72,105,218] Rare examples of *pleomorphic sarcomas* of the mediastinum, which may contain syncytiotrophoblast-like giant cells, are expected to show vimentin reactivity and lack keratin,[72,179] whereas choriocarcinoma has the opposite profile.[71,72,105,]

As stated previously, the diagnosis of choriocarcinoma of the mediastinum has grave prognostic implications, even if the size of

this neoplastic element is small. Thymic choriocarcinoma is invariably refractory to even the most heroic treatment regimens, and rapidly metastasizes to the lungs, liver, bones, and brain. Indeed, pulmonary metastases are commonly present at initial diagnosis. The median survival in reported cases of this entity is <1 year after presentation.[118,218]

Mixed malignant germ cell tumors

As might be anticipated, the clinical and macroscopic features of mediastinal MMGCTs resemble those of either mature or immature teratoma, embryonal carcinoma, yolk sac tumor, or seminoma, depending on the relative proportions of these elements in any given case.[188,218,232] Similarly, the histologic aspects of MMGCT represent an amalgam of the aforementioned tumor types.

As mentioned earlier, one may see the development of non-germ cell malignancies (NGCM) in mediastinal germ cell tumors containing teratoid elements. Ulbright et al.[194] described four cases in which rhabdomyosarcoma, liposarcoma, fibrosarcoma, angiosarcoma, or glioblastoma multiforme occurred in this setting. We have seen several other examples, all of which featured rhabdomyosarcoma or angiosarcoma in conjunction with malignant germ cell elements (Fig. 21.54).[233] Whether or not these tumor tissues reflect differentiation induced by therapy or are present de novo (we strongly favor the latter paradigm because the sarcomatous tissue shows the i[12p] marker of germ cell tumors[223]), they do not respond to standard germ cell tumor treatment protocols and are associated with a high rate of therapeutic failure and mortality. Similar comments apply to the equally rare circumstance of squamous cell carcinoma or adenocarcinoma arising in a teratoid tumor of the mediastinum.[194]

Until two decades ago, the outlook for uncomplicated thymic MMGCT was said to be dismal. However, a report by Parker et al. in 1983 documented the efficacy of aggressive surgical intervention for that tumor type after cyclic chemotherapy had been given.[234] Surgery is performed after serum AFP levels have fallen, indicating the cytolysis of MEC or YST components in such tumors.[235] Most patients treated with this regimen are apparently cured; patients who have chemotherapy alone do significantly less well.[236]

Cytopathology of mediastinal germ cell tumors

FNA specimens of mediastinal germinoma are hypercellular, demonstrating the presence of numerous large polygonal cells. These are principally disposed singly, but occasional small nests may be observed as well. The tumor cells contain rounded nuclei with coarse chromatin and prominent complex nucleoli (so-called nucleolonemas) (Fig. 21.55).[226,237–241] Cytoplasm is granulated, because of its content of abundant PAS-positive material. Vacuoles may be observed that project outward from the tumor cells (so-called 'blisters'), and bare nuclei are not infrequent.[33] A peculiar feature of germinoma in cytologic preparations is its 'tigroid' pattern, wherein detached cytoplasm is disposed in a linear or networked fashion (Fig. 21.56). Lymphoglandular bodies also may be appreciated if numerous lymphocytes are present in the tumor.[242] Other 'variant' features of germinoma in FNA samples include the presence of granulomas, and extreme hypo cellularity in cases where the lesion is extensively fibrotic.

As stated by Wakely,[33] the characteristic constellation of cytological features in germinoma is usually sufficient to make a definite diagnosis. However, cases departing from the classic image can be confused with large cell lymphoma, melanoma, or anaplastic carcinoma, and adjunctive studies will be required to obtain a final interpretation.[243] Those evaluations have been described above and will not be recounted here.

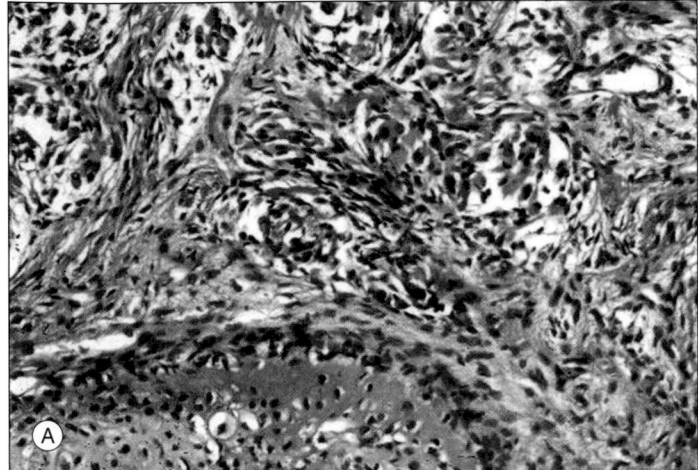

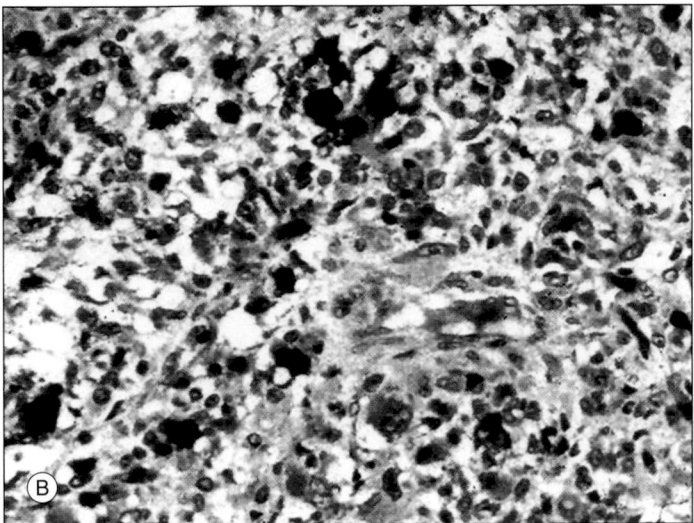

Fig. 21.54 Mature teratoma of the thymus with sarcomatous 'transformation.' **(A)** Compact, anaplastic polygonal cells and spindle cells are juxtaposed to mature cartilage. **(B)** Immunostaining for desmin shows that the anaplastic elements are myogenous in nature, representing rhabdomyosarcoma.

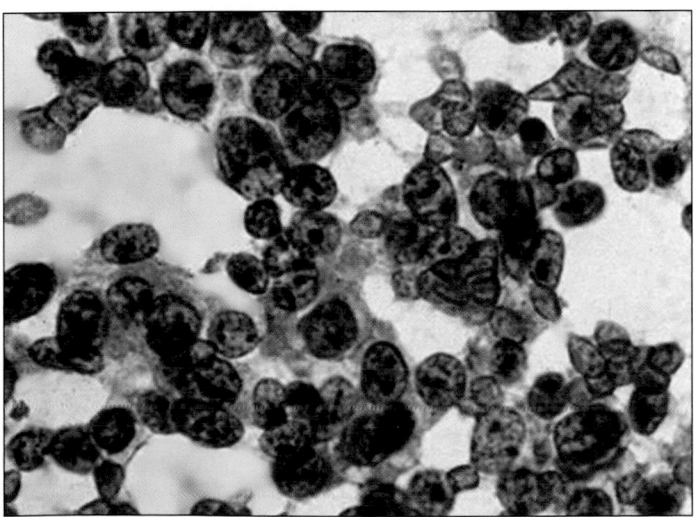

Fig. 21.55 Fine needle aspiration biopsy of thymic seminoma, showing cohesive cell groups having prominent nucleoli and pale cytoplasm.

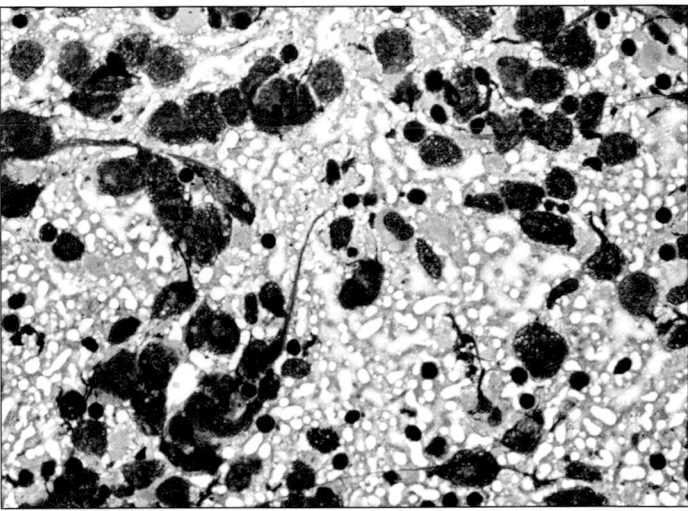

Fig. 21.56 A characteristic striated ('tigroid') mucoid background is seen in this fine needle aspiration biopsy of seminoma.

Nonseminomatous germ cell tumors are more heterogeneous cytologically, but they generally show macronucleoli, vacuolated cytoplasm, and a background tumor diathesis with necrosis.[237–241] The neoplastic cells have more tendency to cohesion than do those of seminomas, and micropapillary structures or gland-like formations may be observed in cases of MEC or YST (Fig. 21.57).[241] Metachromatic background material also can be seen in some instances, probably representing basal lamina. Interestingly, the eosinophilic globules that are often appreciated in tissue sections of YST are not seen in most FNA specimens of that lesion.[33,241]

The overall cytological image of nonseminomatous germ cell tumors is closely similar to that of poorly differentiated somatic carcinomas. Thus, a high level of diagnostic suspicion – based on patient age, location, and other clinical findings – is required along with special pathologic studies to make a definite cytopathological interpretation.

MALIGNANT LYMPHOMAS OF THE THYMIC REGION

Most types of malignant lymphoma may potentially involve the anterior mediastinum, and can present various problems in differential diagnosis with other neoplasms. The majority of mediastinal hematolymphoid proliferations are no different than those seen in lymph nodes or nonthymic extranodal tissues; accordingly, the reader is referred to the corresponding chapters for a discussion of those entities. Such lesions include, but are not limited to, Hodgkin's lymphoma,[244] small-lymphocytic- and mucosal-type lymphomas,[245] follicular non-Hodgkin's lymphoma (NHL),[246] Castleman's disease,[59,247] mixed small and large-cell NHL,[246] anaplastic large cell lymphoma,[248] lymphoblastic lymphoma,[249] Burkitt's lymphoma,[250] large cell lymphoma (not further specified),[100] plasmacytoma,[251] granulocytic sarcoma,[252] Langerhans cell histiocytosis,[253,254] and tumefactive extramedullary hematopoiesis.[255] However, large-cell NHL and lymphoblastic lymphoma may demonstrate unusual features when seen in the thymic region, and these two neoplasms are therefore particularly considered in the following sections.

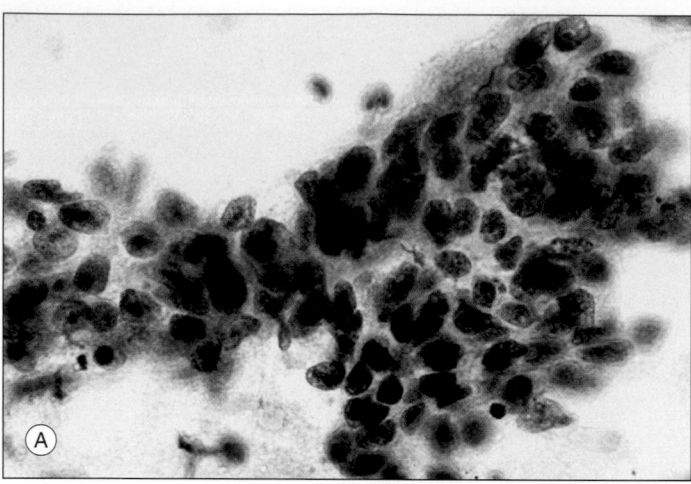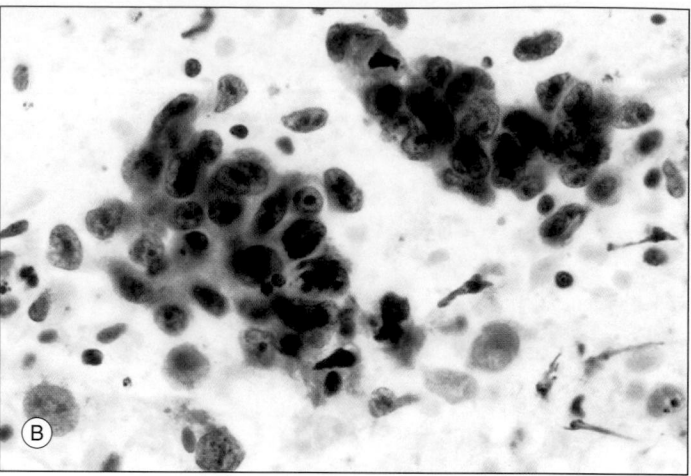

Fig. 21.57 Fine needle aspiration biopsies of primary thymic embryonal carcinoma **(A)** and yolk sac tumor **(B)**, showing cohesive groups of anaplastic epithelial cells, with metachromatic extracellular globules also seen in (B). Distinction from other epithelial malignancies would require adjunctive studies in both instances.

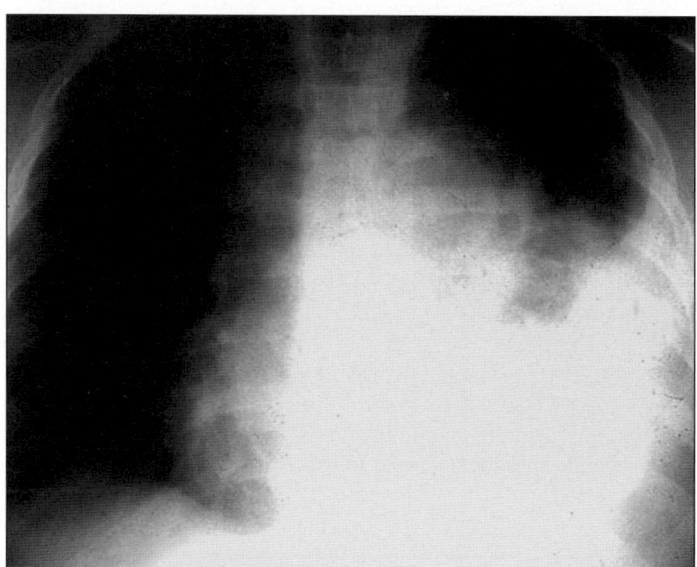

Fig. 21.58 Chest radiograph of lymphoblastic lymphoma, showing a massive anterosuperior mediastinal mass that also occupies a significant portion of the left hemithorax.

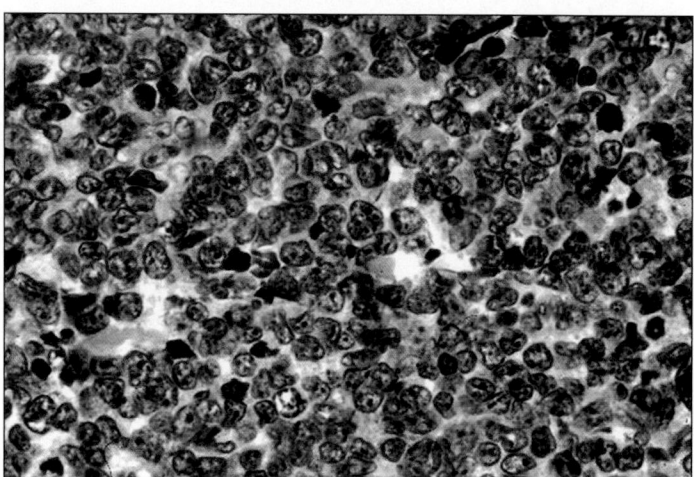

Fig. 21.59 Photomicrograph of lymphoblastic lymphoma, showing irregularity of nuclear membranes, numerous mitoses, and brisk apoptosis.

Lymphoblastic lymphomas (LBLs)

LBL is commonest in children and adolescents, and often presents with respiratory embarrassment due to a quickly growing and bulky intrathoracic mass (Fig. 21.58).[256] Typically, the disease is confined within the mediastinum, and is centered in the thymus ('Sternberg's sarcoma').[257]

LBL is characterized by a monomorphic infiltrate of small lymphoid cells, with 'convoluted' or round nuclei and a high mitotic rate (Fig. 21.59).[249,256,258] A major pitfall associated with this lesion is its potential confusion with *predominantly lymphocytic thymoma*.[124] However, several points of pathologic distinction separate the two classes of tumors. NHL does not show the encapsulation or internal fibrous septation of thymoma, either grossly or microscopically, and

it lacks perivascular serum lakes. Ultrastructurally, there are no epithelial cells in NHL, which are recognized by desmosomal attachments, pericellular basal lamina, and cytoplasmic tonofilaments. Immunohistochemical stains reveal a delicately interlocking pattern of cytokeratin-reactive tumor cells in thymoma but not in LBL.[71,72] In the latter tumor type, residual thymic epithelial cells may be entrapped by the lymphomatous infiltrate, but they tend to be distributed in small, widely-separated clusters.[259] The reactive cells of predominantly lymphocytic thymoma are thymocytes, with reactivity for CD1a, TdT, and CD99.[77,260,261] That profile may lead to confusion with LBL in small biopsy specimens unless keratin stains are performed and the pattern of resulting reactivity is closely noted.

LBL is a rapidly evolving, potentially lethal neoplasm that disseminates widely to lymph nodes, viscera, and bone marrow, commonly with the appearance of acute leukemia.[249,256] Aggressive, multiagent chemotherapy must be instituted promptly after diagnosis to offer any chance of cure.

Large cell lymphomas (not further specified)

Large cell lymphoma (LCL) is the type of NHL which, except for LBL, is most likely to present clinically with localized disease in the thymic region and anterior mediastinum.[262–269] Females are affected 1.2–2.5 times more frequently than males; the mean age at diagnosis is 27 years, although this tumor may occur in children and elderly individuals.[262] Unlike other types of NHL, aside from LBL, mediastinal LCL most commonly produces symptoms and signs that are directly related to tumor growth, including superior vena cava obstruction, chest pain, dyspnea, and cough.[263] These are generally of brief duration (1–8 weeks) before the patient comes to medical attention.[268] Evidence of extrathoracic disease is present at diagnosis in approximately 25% of cases.[263]

Grossly, mediastinal LCLs are typically large, lobulated, firm, gray-white masses that may show internal necrosis. They are usually unencapsulated, and invade contiguous lung, great vessels, or pericardium. The internal fibrous bands of thymoma or nodular sclerosing Hodgkin's lymphoma are absent. Histologically, this variant of NHL is virtually always diffuse in its pattern of growth,[264] rather than nodular, as seen in some cases of follicular lymphoma. The tumor cells have indistinct borders, scanty amphophilic or slightly basophilic cytoplasm, and irregular nuclear outlines (Fig. 21.60). Nuclear chromatin may be vesicular or coarsely clumped with occasionally prominent nucleoli, and easily found mitoses. Multi-lobulated nuclear forms are also common. If nucleoli are uniformly evident, large, and eosinophilic, the diagnosis of the immunoblastic subtype of LCL should be considered.

Secondary features which are characteristic of thymic LCL are represented by the persistence of foci of thymic epithelium – with or without cyst formation – expanded thymic lobules, and the presence of compartmentalizing fibrous stroma, which gives the neoplasm a pseudoepithelial, clustered appearance (Fig. 21.61).[263] Based on these findings, the unwary microscopist may render a diagnosis of *primary or metastatic carcinoma*; however, attention to other observations such as nuclear detail, and prominent invasion of blood vessels walls or permeation of mediastinal fat, neither of which is common in carcinomas, usually allows an avoidance of that error. Occasional cases in which the distinction between LCL and anaplastic carcinoma is problematic with conventional microscopy can often be correctly diagnosed by electron microscopy and immunohistochemistry.[71,72,103,179]

Ultrastructurally, thymic LCL does not show intercellular junctions in the vast majority of cases. Rarely, appositional plaques may be observed between cells;[263] however, the well-formed cytoplasmic tonofilaments of thymic carcinoma are uniformly absent, as is the pericellular basal lamina. Furthermore, LCL exhibits a paucity of specialized intracellular organelles except for free polyribosomes, and a limited amount of rough endoplasmic reticulum.[270]

Immunohistology is the most useful tool in the differential diagnosis of carcinoma versus LCL. *Epithelial malignancies* display reactivity for keratin, whereas thymic large cell lymphoma expresses CD45;[263,264,266,267] those results are mutually exclusive. *Thymic seminoma*, which can enter the differential diagnosis in some cases, shows immunoreactivity for CD117 and PLAP,[72] which are lacking in lymphomas and thymic carcinomas. LCL of the mediastinum, as in other sites, is usually a CD20-positive B-cell neoplasm.[266,267] A potential pitfall in the diagnosis of this tumor is represented by its additional tendency to show CD30 immunoreactivity.[271] That observation could result in the misinterpretation of thymic LCL as

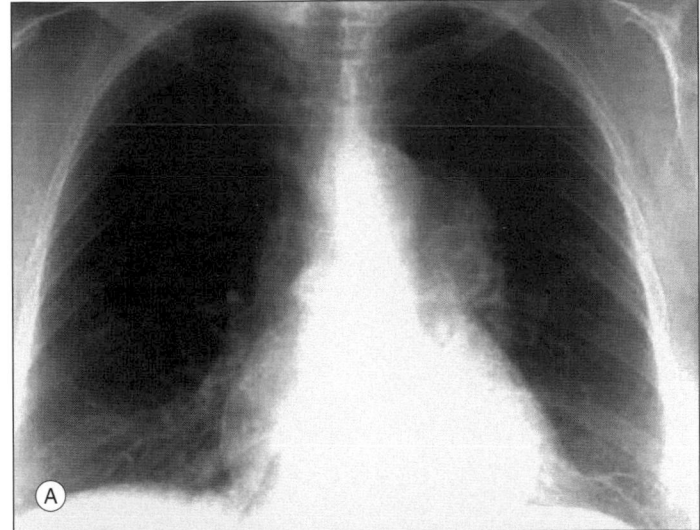

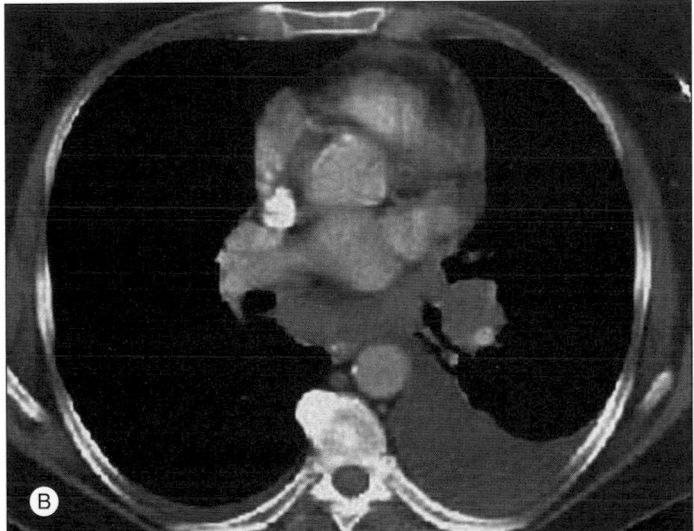

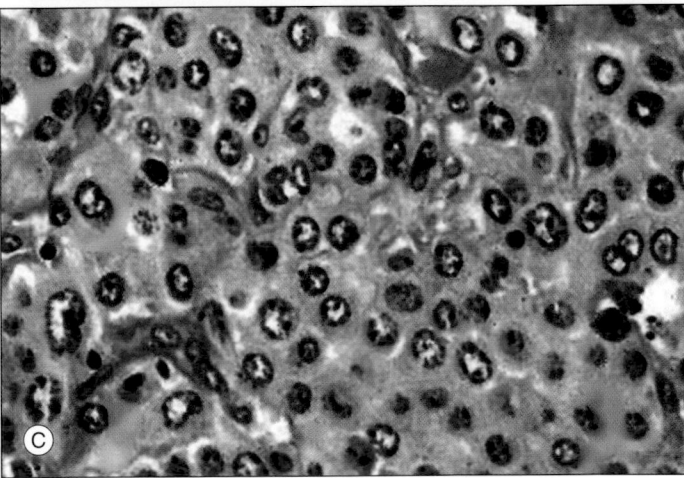

Fig. 21.60 **(A)** Chest radiograph of thymic large cell lymphoma (LCL), showing an anterosuperior mediastinal mass. **(B)** Another tumor of the same type involves other nodal groups in the thorax as seen in this computed tomogram, and a left pleural effusion is apparent. **(C)** This photomicrograph of thymic LCL demonstrates vague clustering of the tumor cells, with open nuclear chromatin and slight irregularity of the nuclear membrane. Differential diagnosis with epithelial tumors may be difficult without special studies.

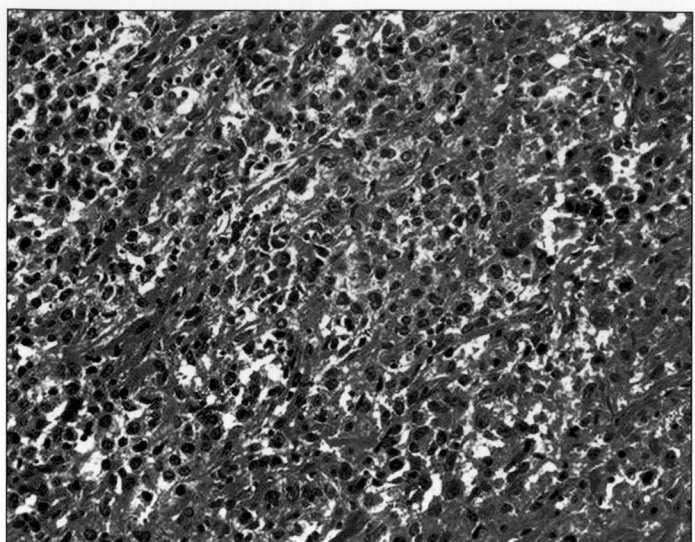

Fig. 21.61 Compartmentalizing stromal sclerosis in thymic large cell lymphoma, heightening the potential resemblance of this tumor to carcinoma.

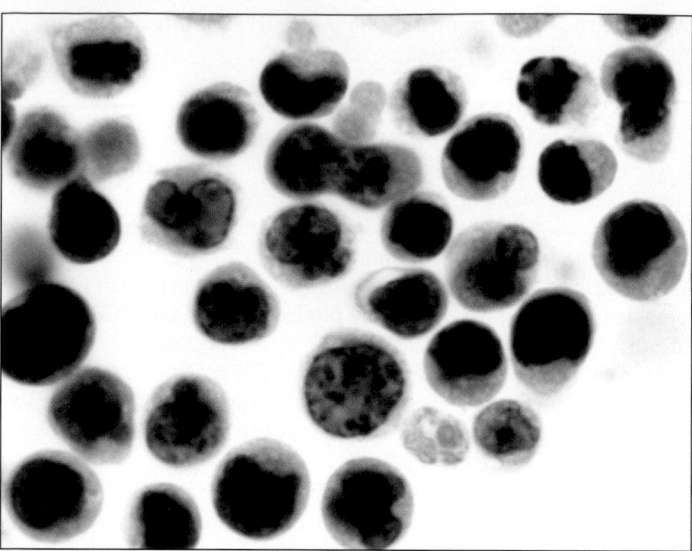

Fig. 21.62 Fine needle aspiration biopsy of lymphoblastic lymphoma, showing dyscohesive, highly atypical lymphoid cells with high nucleo-cytoplasmic ratios, folding of nuclear membranes, and dispersed chromatin.

syncytial HD.[272] Incidentally, we believe that CD30 labeling does not constitute sufficient evidence unto itself for the classification of such tumors as 'anaplastic large cell lymphoma' (Ki-1 lymphoma).[273]

Mediastinal LCL must be treated with aggressive multiagent chemotherapy protocols and adjuvant radiotherapy has also been recommended.[274] Even with appropriate therapy, 20%–30% of patients will have subsequent mediastinal tumor recurrence or extrathoracic involvement of lymph nodes, kidney, liver, pancreas, gastrointestinal tract, and gonads.[263,274] A study by Perrone et al.[263] showed that the presence of extrathoracic disease at diagnosis, incomplete response to initial therapy, and immunoblastic histologic features were poor prognostic indicators in thymic LCL, whereas the degree of intratumoral sclerosis correlated directly with a favorable response to treatment. The overall disease-free survival in cases of mediastinal LCL is approximately 70% at 5 years after diagnosis and institution of chemotherapy, but intrathoracic recurrence is an adverse event which reduces that statistic.

Cytopathology of lymphomas of the thymic region

LBL presents a characteristic cytologic configuration in FNA specimens, being typified by a uniform population of blastic lymphocytes with high nuclear:cytoplasmic ratios. The tumor cells are 1.5 to 2 times the size of mature lymphocytes (Fig. 21.62). Nuclear chromatin is evenly distributed, and nucleoli are inconspicuous.[33,275–277] Mitotic figures may be observed in the malignant lymphoid cells, but that finding is inconsistent. Tumors with an 'L1' or 'L2' morphologic image (according to the French-American-British classification system) lack cytoplasmic vacuolization, and the cytoplasm is instead uniformly amphophilic. Convolution of nuclear membranes and the presence of lymphoglandular bodies are additional findings that may be appreciated in aspirates of LBL (Fig. 21.63); however, those findings are only variably present.

The principal differential diagnostic alternative to LBL is that of predominantly lymphocytic thymoma (see above), in which

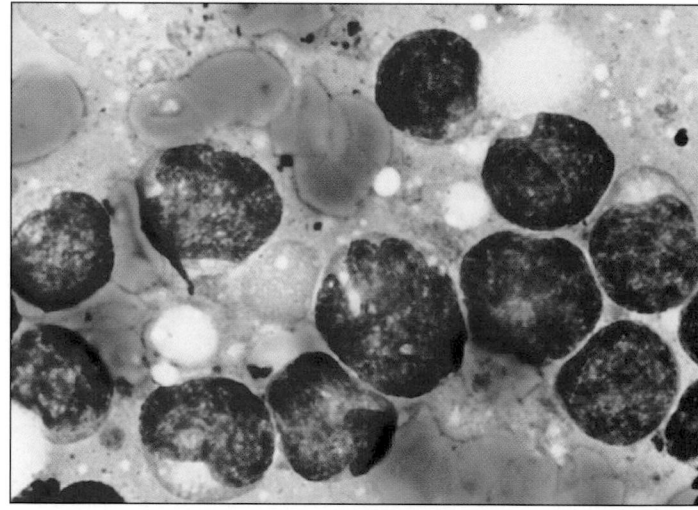

Fig. 21.63 Fine needle aspiration biopsy of lymphoblastic lymphoma, emphasizing the blastic nature of the tumor cells in this Romanowsky-stained preparation.

morphologically similar lymphoid cells may be seen.[124] At the risk of an annoying level of redundancy, we again would stress that keratin immunostains should always be obtained before rendering a final diagnosis of LBL, to avoid confusion of those two entities.

FNA specimens of mediastinal LCL show a predominant cell population that is comprised of atypical large lymphoid elements with folded nuclear contours or multilobated nuclei.[33,278,279] Nucleoli are typically prominent, and cytoplasm is nondescript, other than showing intense basophilia with Romanowsky methods (Fig. 21.64). A minor spectrum of smaller lymphocytes is typically apparent as well, which may or not exhibit atypical nuclear features. Lympho-glandular bodies are variably evident. FNA of those examples

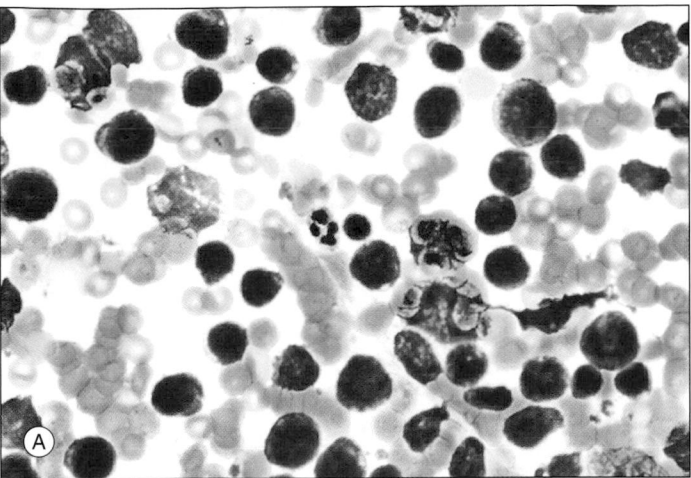
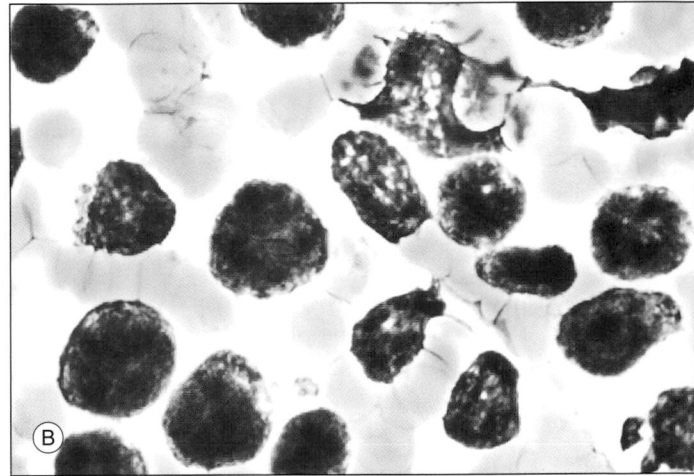

Fig. 21.64 Fine needle aspiration biopsy of large cell lymphoma of the thymus, showing **(A)** dispersed tumor cells with irregular nuclear membranes, each measuring 2–3 times the size of background mature lymphocytes. **(B)** Some of the tumor cells have a vaguely plasmacytoid appearance, owing to their B-cell lineage.

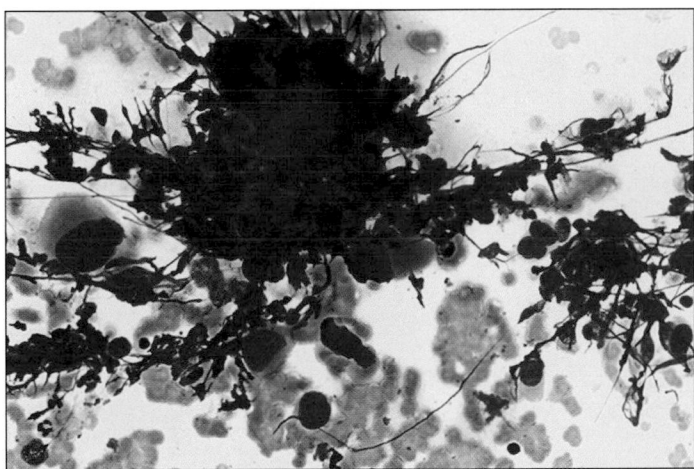

Fig. 21.65 Fine needle aspiration biopsy of large cell lymphoma of the mediastinum with sclerosis, yielding a distorted tissue fragment with only scant numbers of intact lymphoid tumor cells.

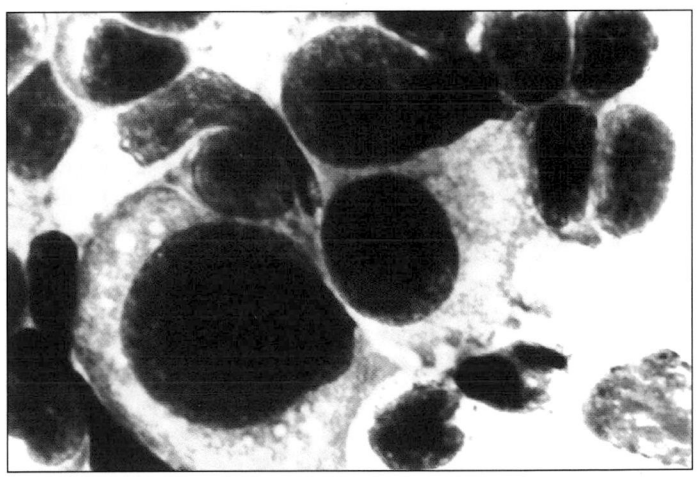

Fig. 21.66 Fine needle aspiration biopsy of 'syncytial' Hodgkin's disease of the thymic region, demonstrating apposed mononuclear Reed cell variants that are very similar morphologically to the tumor cells seen in Figures 21.63 and 21.64. Immunostains or flow cytometric studies would be necessary to identify this tumor type.

of thymic LCL with intense lesional sclerosis can yield scantily cellular specimens that are not particularly diagnostic or which may cause confusion with mesenchymal proliferations (Fig. 21.65).[279] Another pitfall in the cytopathologic interpretation of such lesions is that non-neoplastic thymic epithelium may again be admixed with the tumor cells. This finding can lead to an erroneous diagnosis of a thymic epithelial lesion unless a panel of immunostains is performed. The lymphoid elements in LCL are CD20-positive B cells, unlike those in most thymomas; moreover, thymic epithelium in LCL is arranged in small clusters, rather than the extensively interlocking network that is typical of thymoma.[263]

'Syncytial' Hodgkin's lymphoma[280] enters into differential diagnosis with mediastinal LCL, as cited previously, because the cytopathologic appearance of those tumor types is virtually identical (Fig. 21.66). Unlike syncytial HD, LCL demonstrates uniform immunoreactivity for CD45 and CD20.[72]

MESENCHYMAL PROLIFERATIONS

In analogy to the above-cited situation concerning hematopoietic lesions of the mediastinum, there is nothing unique about most mesenchymal neoplasms that can be encountered in that topographic location; however, most of them have a predilection to arise in the posterior compartment rather than in the thymic region. These include such tumors as desmoid-type fibromatosis,[281,282] lipoma,[283,284] hemangiomas,[285] lymphangioma,[286,287] myelolipoma,[288] inflammatory myofibroblastic tumor ('inflammatory pseudotumor'),[289] lipoblastoma,[290] neurofibroma,[291] neurilemmoma,[291] solitary fibrous tumor,[292] hemangioendothelioma variants[293] ganglioneuroma,[291,294] chordoma,[295] leiomyosarcoma,[296] rhabdomyosarcoma,[297] malignant fibrous histiocytoma,[298] malignant peripheral nerve sheath tumors,[291] extraosseous osteosarcoma and chondroid neoplasms,[299,300] primitive neuroectodermal tumor,[301] synovial sarcoma,[302] angiosarcoma,[303] liposarcoma,[304,305] and malignant rhabdoid tumor.[306,307] All of these neoplasms are discussed in Chapter 9, and will not be covered here. Nevertheless, two mediastinal mesenchymal tumors are singular, in that they intimately involve the thymus and contain incorporated thymic tissue, namely *thymolipoma* and *thymoliposarcoma*. Another lesion – fibrosing mediastinitis – is a non-neoplastic pseudotumor that can be confused with other diagnostic entities.

Thymolipoma and thymoliposarcoma

Thymolipoma, a tumor distinct from simple lipoma of the mediastinum, was first described by Lange in 1916.[308] It is composed of both histologically normal thymic tissue and mature fat and is contained within the thymic capsule.[1,42,309–311] However, the contention that the lesion is simply lipomatous is contradicted by the fact that the absolute mass of thymic tissue is increased in cases of thymolipoma.[42] In addition, cases of aplastic anemia,[312] pure red cell aplasia,[313,314] hypogammaglobulinemia,[314] and myasthenia gravis[309,314,315] have been reported in association with thymolipoma, but not with lipomas of the mediastinum. Nevertheless, thymolipoma is not a form of thymoma, since its nonlipomatous, epithelial element has the configuration of non-neoplastic, nonhyperplastic thymic tissue. Hence, its histogenetic nature is still the subject of controversy.

Thymolipoma may occur at any age, but the mean age for its appearance is 33 years.[309] There is no sex predilection. In the majority of cases, the lesion is found incidentally on routine chest roentgenograms, but approximately 10% are associated with paraneoplastic syndromes or present with dyspnea and cough.[309,314] Thoracic computerized tomography demonstrates the fatty density that characterizes thymolipoma (Fig. 21.67).[316]

Grossly, thymolipomas are lobated, yellowish, soft, and encapsulated. They may be adherent to contiguous mediastinal structures, but are not invasive.[1,42] Roughly 70% of thymolipomas weigh over 500 g, and 23% are in excess of 2000 g.[314] Microscopically, 75–90% of a given thymolipoma is made up of mature adipose tissue, whereas the remainder consists of unremarkable thymic tissue (Fig. 21.68) containing Hassall's corpuscles. Germinal centers are never evident. The Hassall's corpuscles in this lesion may demonstrate secondary cystification or calcification. In another tumor variant, the constituent thymic epithelium forms elongated cords or nests, yielding the designation of 'proliferating' thymolipoma.[317] Still other thymolipomas may exhibit prominent intralesional sclerosis or vascular proliferation, and have been termed 'thymofibrolipomas' and 'thymohemangiolipomas,' respectively.[318,319] Argani et al. have described the singular and simultaneous coincidence of a thymolipoma and a thymoma.[320]

Because of its distinctive histologic appearance, differential diagnostic considerations for thymolipoma are very limited. The principal alternative is that of simple lipoma of the anterior mediastinum, which does not contain internal thymic tissue.

Thymolipoma is curable with simple excision.[309–311] Even patients with tumor-related paraneoplastic syndromes have done well clinically after surgery.[314]

Two examples of a related tumor entity were described by Havlicek and Rosai[321] in adult patients. Both of those neoplasms had the overall gross appearance of thymolipoma but showed a malignant mesenchymal aspect histologically. The tumors contained areas resembling codified forms of liposarcoma, which differed from the adipose tissue of thymolipoma in that obvious nuclear atypia and hypercellularity were evident (Fig. 21.69). In addition, areas of unclassified spindle cell or pleomorphic sarcoma were observed in

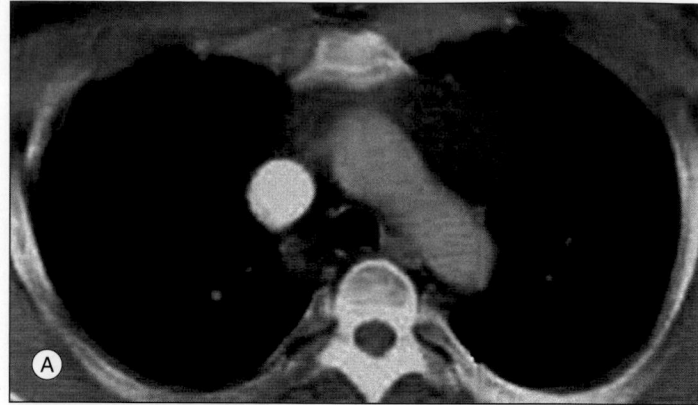

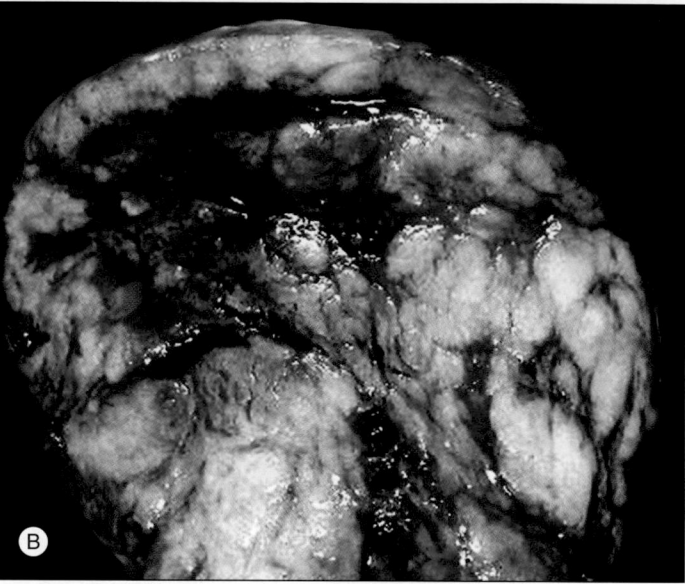

Fig. 21.67 Computed tomograph of the thorax in a case of thymolipoma **(A)** showing an anterior mediastinal mass with an internal density like that of adipose tissue. **(B)** A gross photograph of the lesion shows internal mottling of otherwise mature adipose tissue.

both cases, and one contained rosettes composed of spindle cells, which suggested neuroepithelial differentiation. Bland thymic tissue was also present in these tumors. After a recurrence (and possibly an osseous metastasis), one of the patients was well following administration of radiotherapy, 32 years after initial diagnosis and 4 years after re-excision of a thymic tumor with postoperative radiotherapy. Follow-up on the other patient was incomplete.

Another tumor reported by Okumori et al.[322] may have represented a thymoliposarcoma, although it was described as a mixed 'spindle cell thymoma' and liposarcoma. This lesion was grossly invasive, and had metastasized to supraclavicular lymph nodes, leading to death several months after diagnosis. Its exact nature is unclear, however, owing to suboptimal illustration and a lack of specialized pathologic studies.

Differential diagnosis in cases of suspected thymoliposarcoma should include *sarcomatoid thymic carcinoma*,[90] and *liposarcoma*.[323] Sarcomatoid thymic carcinoma does not contain normal thymic tissue, or liposarcoma-like differentiation; in contrast to true sarcomas, it is cytokeratin positive immunohistochemically. Mediastinal liposarcomas also lack a thymic tissue component.

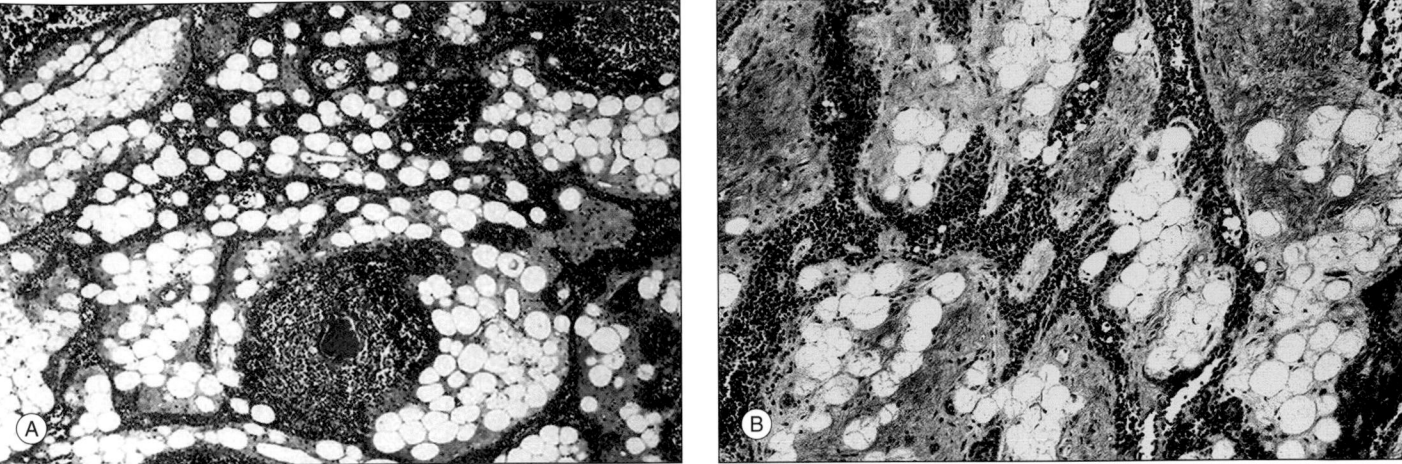

Fig. 21.68 **(A)** Photomicrograph of thymolipoma, with features of the 'proliferating' variant. **(B)** The tumor is comprised by mature fat and islands of mature thymic cortex, which in this particular case also includes cords of interconnecting thymic epithelium.

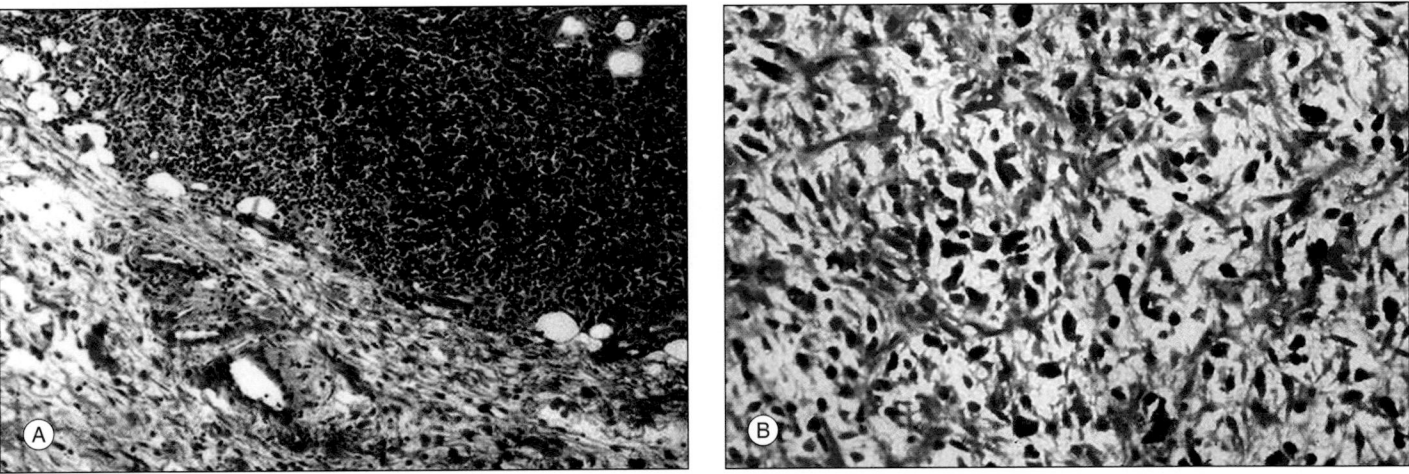

Fig. 21.69 Photomicrographs of thymoliposarcoma, showing **(A)** juxtaposition of mature thymic tissue (upper right) to an atypical adipocytic proliferation (lower left). **(B)** The lipocytic neoplasm features obvious nuclear atypia and cellular immaturity.

Cytopathology of thymolipoma and thymoliposarcoma

The literature on FNA specimens of thymolipomatous tumors is extremely scanty.[33,324] It would appear that if a characteristic mixture of mature adipose cells with bland thymic epithelial elements is present, the diagnosis could be made by such means. However, radiographic information would be essential to that process, inasmuch as simple atrophic thymus gland would have very much the same cytological image. There have been no reports on the cytological features of thymoliposarcoma.

Sclerosing (fibrosing) mediastinitis

Sclerosing mediastinitis (SM) may present itself clinically with symptoms and signs of the superior vena cava syndrome, pulmonary infarction, pulmonary hypertension, or cardiorespiratory insufficiency, and it may be observed at any time of life.[325–334] This disorder is typically reflected by the presence of asymmetric mediastinal widening on chest radiographs, usually with projection of a mass into an upper lung field.[325,328,334] and it belongs to the family of conditions known as

'tumefactive fibrobinflammatory lesions' along with such lesions as Riedel's thyroiditis and sclerosing retroperitonitis.[335]

The macroscopic findings in sclerosing mediastinitis are like those of dense but ordinary fibrosis seen in other settings. Firm, white tissue is present on sectioning, with no evidence of fascicular growth; in addition, the interface between this disease process and adjacent soft tissue is sharp.

The histologic image of SM depends on its stage of evolution. Early lesions demonstrate edematous and fibromyxoid tissue with numerous capillary-sized blood vessels and a mixed inflammatory infiltrate. Intermediate proliferations show a heterogeneous fibro-inflammatory cell population with random collagen deposition, and mature SM manifests the presence of dense, fibrohyaline, avascular, poorly cellular tissue (Fig. 21.70). In the last stage, aggregates of mature lymphocytes are trapped within the zones of fibrosis and probably play a role in their formation through the elaboration of collagenogenic cytokines.[336] Granulomas (either caseating or non-caseating) are also sometimes seen; this is not unexpected because

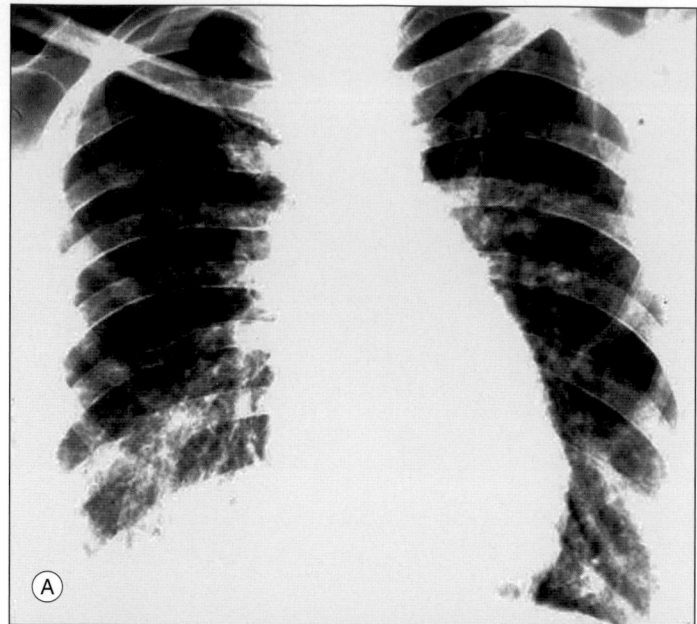

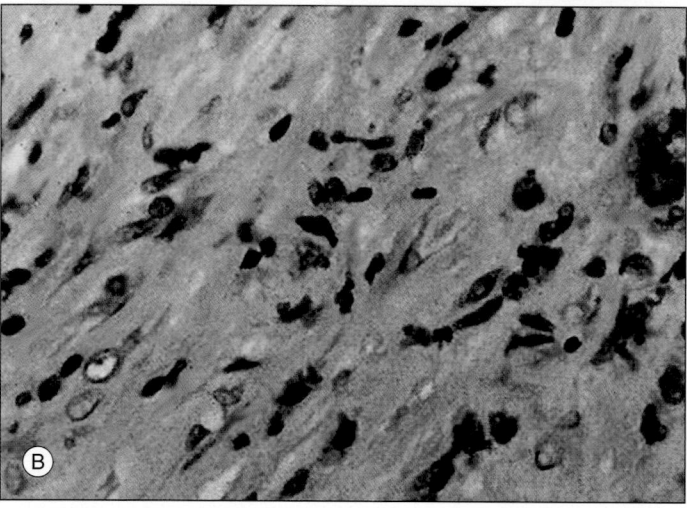

Fig. 21.70 Chest radiograph **(A)** and photomicrograph **(B)** of sclerosing (fibrosing) mediastinitis, showing proliferating fibroblasts, dense stromal collagen, and interspersed mature lymphocytes.

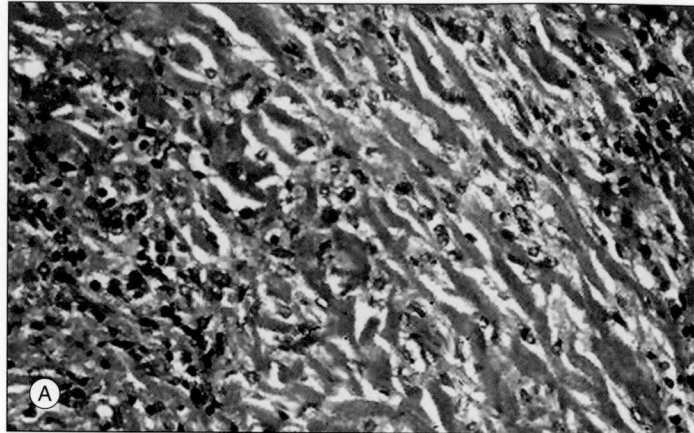

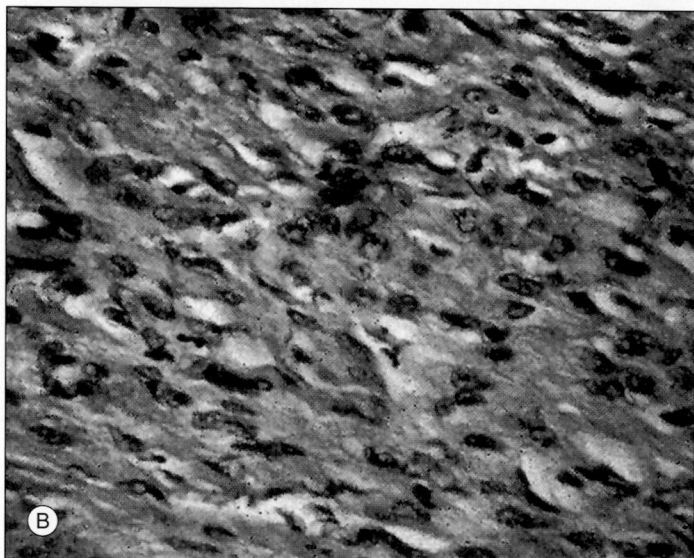

Fig. 21.71 Photomicrographs of mediastinal desmoplastic mesothelioma simulating sclerosing mediastinitis. This neoplasm is comprised by only modest-atypical spindle cells, dense collagen, and stromal lymphocytes **(A)**; Nuclear atypia in the spindle cell component is seen to better advantage in this field **(B)**.

sclerosing mediastinitis is, in a proportion of cases, a response to lymph nodal or pulmonary infection.[337]

The most common etiological microorganism is *Histoplasma capsulatum*,[338,339] which can be detected with silver or periodic acid–Schiff stains. Fungal infection is associated with <50% of mediastinitis cases overall; other implicated organisms include those in the genuses *Aspergillus*, *Cryptococcus*, and *Zygomyces*.[340,341] SM has also been described in patients with tuberculosis, sarcoidosis, nocardiosis, actinomycosis, and syphilis, or others who have had therapy with methysergide (an antimigraine agent), or chest trauma.[325,328,337] The remaining examples of this disorder are idiopathic. The postulated pathogenesis in all instances concerns a variant form of delayed cell-mediated hypersensitivity reaction. A condition with similarities to SM can sometimes involve the substance of the thymus gland itself, and may be called 'inflammatory thymic pseudotumor.'[342] Other mediastinal 'pseudotumors'

have been described by Brachet et al.[343] and by Dehner and Coffin,[344] but these proliferations had the attributes of 'inflammatory myofibroblastic tumor' (currently regarded as a clonal neoplastic lesion) (see Chapter 9) rather than those of SM.

One more important diagnostic pitfall must be remembered in connection with SM; namely, the capacity for tumor cells in some malignant lymphomas (e.g. 'obliterative total sclerosis' Hodgkin's disease), seminomas, metastatic carcinomas, or malignant desmoplastic mesotheliomas to cause obfuscating fibrosis in the mediastinum and thereby closely simulate the clinicopathological image of SM (Fig. 21.71).[345] Neoplastic elements in those conditions are sparse and may be surprisingly bland morphologically; hence, they are easily overlooked. Immunostains for keratin, CD15, CD20, CD30, and CD45 are, therefore, a wise inclusion in the evaluation of lesions thought to represent SM.

Cytopathology of sclerosing mediastinitis

No systematic studies on FNA specimens from sclerosing mediastinitis have been published. However, based on our personal experience, aspirates of this condition are nondiagnostic. They are paucicellular, showing only rare fibroblasts and mature lymphocytes.

in this book. Such proliferations include mixed tumors (pleomorphic adenomas),[346] malignant mesotheliomas,[347] neuroblastic tumors,[348] paragangliomas,[349,350] ectopic thyroid masses,[3,351] anterior mediastinal parathyroid lesions.[60,173,352] malignant melanoma,[353,354] and meningoceles.[355]

PART V: OTHER NEOPLASMS POTENTIALLY SEEN IN THE MEDIASTINUM

Lesions with several additional cellular lineages also may be seen in the mediastinum, but they are again considered in detail elsewhere

REFERENCES

1. Shimosato Y, Mukai K. Tumors of the mediastinum. In: Rosai J, ed. Atlas of tumor pathology, series 3, fascicle 21. Washington, DC: Armed Forces Institute of Pathology; 1997: 333–273.

2. Salyer DC, Salyer WR, Eggleston JC. Benign developmental cysts of the mediastinum. Arch Pathol Lab Med 1977; 101: 136–139.

3. Wick MR. Mediastinal cysts and intrathoracic thyroid tumors. Semin Diagn Pathol 1990; 7: 285–294.

4. Gilmour JR. The embryology of the parathyroid glands, the thymus, and certain associated rudiments. J Pathol Bacteriol 1937; 45: 507–522.

5. Suster S, Rosai J. Multilocular thymic cyst: an acquired reactive process. Study of 18 cases. Am J Surg Pathol 1991; 15: 388–398.

6. Suster S, Barbuto D, Carlson G, Rosai J. Multilocular thymic cysts with pseudoepitheliomatous hyperplasia. Hum Pathol 1991; 22: 455–460.

7. Michal M, Havlicek F. Pseudoepitheliomatous hyperplasia in thymic cysts. Histopathology 1991; 19: 281–282.

8. Leong ASY, Brown JH. Malignant transformation in a thymic cyst. Am J Surg Pathol 1984; 8: 471–475.

9. Yamashita S, Yamazaki H, Kato T, et al. Thymic carcinoma which developed in a thymic cyst. Intern Med 1996; 35: 215–218.

10. Chhieng DC, DeMaria S, Yee HT, Yang GC. Multilocular thymic cyst with follicular lymphoid hyperplasia in a male infected with human immunodeficiency virus: a case report with fine needle aspiration cytology. Acta Cytol 1999; 43: 1119–1123.

11. Baron RL, Sagel SS, Baglan RJ. Thymic cysts following radiation therapy for Hodgkin's disease. Radiology 1981; 41: 593–597.

12. Kaesburg PR, Foley DB, Pellett J, et al. Concurrent development of a thymic cyst and mediastinal Hodgkin's disease. Med Pediatr Oncol 1988; 16: 293–294.

13. Jaramillo P, Perez-Atayde A, Griscom NT. Apparent association between thymic cysts and prior thoracotomy. Radiology 1989; 172: 207–209.

14. Rice TW. Benign neoplasms and cysts of the mediastinum. Semin Thorac Cardiovasc Surg 1992; 4: 25–33.

15. Davis RD Jr, Oldham HN Jr, Sabiston DC Jr. Primary cysts and neoplasms of the mediastinum: recent changes in clinical presentation, methods of diagnosis, management, and results. Ann Thorac Surg 1987; 44: 229–237.

16. Kumar PV, Ashraf MJ, Safaei A, et al. Fine needle aspiration diagnosis of bronchogenic cysts. Acta Cytol 2001; 45: 656–658.

17. Cangemi V, Volpino P, Gualdi G, et al. Pericardial cysts of the mediastinum. J Cardiovasc Surg 1999; 40: 909–913.

18. Lillie WI, McDonald JR, Clagett OT. Pericardial celomic cysts and pericardial diverticula: a concept of etiology and report of cases. J Thorac Surg 1950; 20: 494–504.

19. Ladd WE, Scott HW Jr. Esophageal duplications or mediastinal cysts of enteric origin. Surgery 1944; 16: 815–835.

20. Black RA, Benjamin EL. Enterogenous abnormalities: cysts and diverticula. Am J Dis Childh 1936; 51: 1126–1137.

21. Fallon M, Gordon ARG, Lendrum AC. Mediastinal cysts of foregut origin associated with vertebral abnormalities. Br J Surg 1954; 41: 520–533.

22. Nath PH, Sanders C, Holley HC, McElvein RB. Percutaneous fine needle aspiration in the diagnosis and management of mediastinal cysts in adults. South Med J 1988; 81: 1225–1228.

23. Weisbrod GL. Percutaneous fine needle aspiration biopsy of the mediastinum. Clin Chest Med 1987; 8: 27–41.

24. Hofmann WJ, Moller P, Otto HF. Hyperplasia. In: Givel JC, ed. Surgery of the thymus. Berlin: Springer-Verlag; 1990: 59–70.

25. Arliss J, Scholes J, Dickson PR, Messina JJ. Massive thymic hyperplasia in an adolescent. Ann Thorac Surg 1988; 45: 220–222.

26. Gelfand DW, Goldman AS, Law EJ, et al. Thymic hyperplasia in children recovering from thermal burns. J Trauma 1972; 12: 813–817.

27. Rizk G, Cueto L, Amplatz K. Rebound enlargement of the thymus after successful corrective surgery for transposition of the great vessels. Am J Roentgenol 1972; 116: 528–530.

28. Bertoye A, Beraud C, Depierre A, et al. Hypertrophie thymique et primo-infection du nourisson. Pediatrie 1956; 11: 545–549.

29. Tridente G. Immunopathology of the human thymus. Semin Hematol 1985; 22: 56–57.

30. Grody WW, Jobst S, Keesey J, et al. Pathologic evaluation of thymic hyperplasia in myasthenia gravis and Lambert-Eaton syndrome. Arch Pathol Lab Med 1986; 110: 843–846.

31. Hoerl HD, Wojtowycz M, Gallagher AA, Kurtycz DF. Cytologic diagnosis of true thymic hyperplasia by combined radiologic imaging and aspiration cytology: a case report including flow cytometric analysis. Diagn Cytopathol 2000; 23: 417–421.

32. Bangerter M, Behnisch W, Griesshammer M. Mediastinal masses diagnosed as thymus hyperplasia by fine needle aspiration cytology. Acta Cytol 2000; 44: 743–747.

33. Wakely PE. Cytopathology-histopathology of the mediastinum: epithelial, lymphoproliferative, and germ cell neoplasms. Ann Diagn Pathol 2002; 6: 30–43.

34. Powers CN, Silverman JF, Geisinger KR, Frable WJ. Fine needle aspiration biopsy of the mediastinum: a multiinstitutional analysis. Am J Clin Pathol 1996; 105: 168–173.

35. Souadjian JV, Enriquez P, Silverstein MN, Pepin JM. The spectrum of diseases associated with thymoma: coincidence or syndrome? Arch Intern Med 1974; 134: 374–379.

36. Slater G, Papatestas AE, Genkins G, et al. Thymomas in patients with myasthenia gravis. Ann Surg 1978; 188: 171–174.

37. Cooper GN Jr, Narodick BG. Posterior mediastinal thymoma: case report. J Thorac Cardiovasc Surg 1972; 63: 561–563.

38. Green WR, Pressoir R, Gumbs RV, et al. Intrapulmonary thymoma. Arch Pathol Lab Med 1987; 111: 1074–1076.

39. Moran CA, Travis WD, Rosado-de-Christenson M, et al. Thymomas presenting as pleural tumors: report of eight cases. Am J Surg Pathol 1992; 16: 138–144.

40. Rosai J, Limas C, Husband EM. Ectopic hamartomatous thymoma: a distinctive benign lesion of lower neck. Am J Surg Pathol 1984; 8: 501–513.

41. Attanoos RL, Galateau-Salle F, Gibbs AR, et al. Primary thymic epithelial tumors of the pleura mimicking malignant mesothelioma. Histopathology 2002; 41: 42–49.

42. Rosai J, Levine GD. Tumors of the thymus. In: Atlas of tumor pathology, series 2, fascicle 13. Washington, DC: Armed Forces Institute of Pathology; 1976: 5–205.

43. Lewis JE, Wick MR, Scheithauer BW, et al. Thymoma: a clinicopathologic review. Cancer 1987; 60: 2727–2743.

44. Smith WF, DeWall RA, Krumholz RA. Giant thymoma. Chest 1970; 58: 383–385.

45. Bernatz PE, Harrison EG Jr, Clagett OT. Thymoma: a clinicopathologic study. J Thorac Cardiovasc Surg 1961; 42: 424–444.

46. Kornstein MJ. Controversies regarding the pathology of thymomas. Pathol Annu 1992; 27(Part II): 1–15.

47. Marino M, Muller-Hermelink HK. Thymoma and thymic carcinoma: relation of thymoma epithelial cells to the cortical and medullary differentiation of thymus. Virchows Arch Pathol Anat 1985; 407: 119–149.

48. Muller-Hermelink HK, Marino M, Palestro G. Pathology of thymic epithelial tumors. Curr Topics Pathol 1986; 75: 207–268.

49. Kirchner T, Schalke B, Buchwald J, et al. Well-differentiated thymic carcinoma: an organotypical low-grade carcinoma with relationship to cortical thymoma. Am J Surg Pathol 1992; 16: 1153–1169.

50. Koga K, Matsuno Y, Noguchi M, et al. A review of 79 thymomas: modification of staging system and reappraisal of conventional division into invasive and noninvasive thymoma. Pathol Int 1994; 44: 359–367.

51. Moran CA, Suster S. On the histologic heterogeneity of thymic epithelial neoplasms: impact of sampling in subtyping and classification of thymomas. Am J Clin Pathol 2000; 114: 760–766.

52. Rosai J. Histological typing of tumors of the thymus. World Health Organization. 2nd edn. Berlin: Springer; 1999: 9–15.

53. Chen G, Marx A, Wen-Hu C, et al. New WHO classification predicts prognosis of thymic epithelial tumors: a clinicopathologic study of 200 thymoma cases from China. Cancer 2002; 95: 420–429.

54. Okumura M, Ohta M, Tateyama H, et al. The World Health Organization histologic classification on human thymic epithelial neoplasms: a study of 146 consecutive tumors. Am J Surg Pathol 2001; 25: 103–110.

55. Dadmanesh F, Sekihara T, Rosai J. Histologic typing of thymoma according to the new World Health Organization classification. Chest Surg N Am 2001; 11: 407–420.

56. Suster S, Moran CA. Thymoma, atypical thymoma, and thymic carcinoma: a novel conceptual approach to the classification of thymic epithelial neoplasms. Am J Clin Pathol 1999; 111: 826–833.

57. Banks PM, Arseneau JC, Gralnick HR, et al. American Burkitt's lymphoma: a clinicopathologic study of 30 cases. II. Pathologic correlations. Am J Med 1975; 58: 322–329.

58. Suster S, Moran CA. Micronodular thymoma with lymphoid B-cell hyperplasia: clinicopathologic and immunohistochemical study of eighteen cases of a distinctive morphologic variant of thymic epithelial neoplasm. Am J Surg Pathol 1999; 23: 955–962.

59. Frizzera G. Castleman's disease and related disorders. Semin Diagn Pathol 1988; 5: 346–364.

60. Wick MR, Rosai J. Neuroendocrine neoplasms of the mediastinum. Semin Diagn Pathol 1991; 8: 35–51.

61. Suster S, Moran CA, Chan JKC. Thymoma with pseudosarcomatous stroma: report of an unusual histologic variant of thymic epithelial neoplasm that may simulate carcinosarcoma. Am J Surg Pathol 1997; 21: 1316–1323.

62. Oertel YC. Thymoma mimicking thyroid papillary carcinoma: another pitfall in fine needle aspiration. Diagn Cytopathol 1997; 17: 61–63.

63. Lowenhaupt E. Tumors of the thymus in relation to the thymic epithelial anlage. Cancer 1948; 1: 547–563.

64. Hammond EH, Flinner RL. The diagnosis of thymoma: a review. Ultrastruct Pathol 1991; 15: 419–438.

65. Shier KJ. The thymus according to Schambacher: medullary ducts and reticular epithelium of thymus and thymomas. Cancer 1981; 48: 1183–1199.

66. Lee D, Wright DH. Immunohistochemical study of 22 cases of thymoma. J Clin Pathol 1988; 41: 1297–1304.

67. Fukai I, Masaoka A, Hashimoto T, et al. The distribution of epithelial membrane antigen in thymic epithelial neoplasms. Cancer 1992; 70: 2077–2081.

68. Kodama T, Watanabe S, Sato Y, et al. An immunohistochemical study of thymic epithelial tumors. I. Epithelial component. Am J Surg Pathol 1986; 10: 26–33.

69. Kurtin PJ, Pinkus GS. Leukocyte common antigen – a diagnostic discriminant between hematopoietic and non-hematopoietic neoplasms in paraffin sections using monoclonal antibodies: correlation with immunologic studies and ultrastructural localization. Hum Pathol 1985; 16: 353–365.

70. Osborn M, Weber K. Tumor diagnosis by intermediate filament typing: a novel tool for surgical pathology. Lab Invest 1983; 48: 372–394.

71. Wick MR, Simpson RW, Niehans GA, Scheithauer BW. Anterior mediastinal tumors: a clinicopathologic study of 100 cases, with emphasis on immunohistochemical analysis. Prog Surg Pathol 1990; 11: 79–119.

72. Wick MR. Immunohistology of the mediastinum. In: Dabbs DJ, ed. Diagnostic immunohistochemistry. New York: Churchill Livingstone; 2002: 241–265.

73. Chan WC, Zaatari GS, Tabei S, et al. Thymoma: an immunohistochemical study. Am J Clin Pathol 1984; 82: 160–166.

74. Hishima T, Fukuyama M, Fujisawa M, et al. CD5 expression in thymic carcinomas. Am J Pathol 1994; 145: 268–275.

75. Kornstein MJ, Rosai J. CD5 labeling of thymic carcinomas and other nonlymphoid neoplasms. Am J Clin Pathol 1998; 109: 722–726.

76. Chan JKC, Tsang WY, Seneviratne S, et al. The MIC2 antibody O13: practical application for the study of thymic epithelial tumors. Am J Surg Pathol 1995; 19: 1115–1123.

77. Soslow RA, Bhargava V, Warnke RA. MIC2, TdT, bcl-2, and CD34 expression in paraffin-embedded high grade lymphoma/acute lymphoblastic lymphoma distinguishes between distinct clinicopathologic entities. Hum Pathol 1997; 28: 1158–1165.

78. Wara DW. Thymic hormones and the immune system. Adv Pediatr 1981; 28: 229–270.

79. Yang WI, Efind JT, Quintanilla-Martinez L, et al. Cell kinetic study of thymic epithelial tumors using PCNA (PC10) and Ki-67 (MIB-1) antibodies. Hum Pathol 1996; 27: 70–76.

80. Tateyama H, Eimoto T, Tada T, et al. Apoptosis, bcl-2 protein, and fas antigen in thymic epithelial tumors. Mod Pathol 1997; 10: 983–991.

81. Wick MR. Assessing the prognosis of thymomas. Ann Thorac Surg 1990; 50: 521–522.

82. Lam PN Jr. Malignant thymoma: current status and future directions. Cancer Treat Rev 2000; 26: 127–131.

83. Mehran R, Ghosh R, Maziak D, et al. Surgical treatment of thymomas. Can J Surg 2002; 45: 25–30.

84. Masaoka A, Monden Y, Nakahara K, et al. Followup study of thymomas with special reference to their clinical stages. Cancer 1981; 48: 2485–2492.

85. Masaoka A, Yamakawa Y. TNM classification of thymic epithelial tumors. Gan To Kataku Ryoho 1997; 24: 749–754.

86. Cowen D, Richaud P, Mornex F, et al. Thymoma: results of a multicentric retrospective series of 149 non-metastatic irradiated patients and review of the literature. Radiother Oncol 1995; 34: 9–16.

87. DeMontpreville VT, Dulmet E. Thymomas and carcinomas of the thymus: which classification should be used? Ann Pathol 1996; 16: 159–166.

88. Suster S, Moran CA. Primary thymic epithelial neoplasms: spectrum of differentiation and histological features. Semin Diagn Pathol 1999; 16: 2–17.

89. Snover DC, Levine GD, Rosai J. Thymic carcinomas: five distinctive histological variants. Am J Surg Pathol 1982; 6: 451–470.

90. Ritter JH, Wick MR. Primary carcinomas of the thymus gland. Semin Diagn Pathol 1999; 16: 18–31.

91. Suster S, Rosai J. Thymic carcinoma: a clinicopathologic study of 60 cases. Cancer 1991; 15: 1025–1032.

92. Wick MR, Weiland LH, Scheithauer BW, Bernatz PE. Primary thymic carcinomas. Am J Surg Pathol 1982; 6: 613–630.

93. Wick MR, Berg LC, Hertz MI. Large-cell carcinoma of the lung with neuroendocrine differentiation: a comparison with large-cell 'undifferentiated' pulmonary tumors. Am J Clin Pathol 1992; 97: 796–805.

94. Iezzoni JC, Gaffey MJ, Weiss LM. The role of Epstein-Barr virus in lymphoepithelioma-like carcinomas. Am J Clin Pathol 1995; 103: 308–315.

95. Hishima T, Fukuyama M, Hayashi Y, et al. CD70 expression in thymic carcinoma. Am J Surg Pathol 2000; 24: 742–746.

96. Wolfe JT III, Wick MR, Banks PM, Scheithauer BW. Clear cell carcinoma of the thymus. Mayo Clin Proc 1983; 58: 365–370.

97. Hasserjian RP, Klimstra DS, Rosai J. Carcinoma of the thymus with clear cell features: report of eight cases and review of the literature. Am J Surg Pathol 1995; 19: 835–841.

98. Dorfman DM, Shahsafaei A, Chan JKC. Thymic carcinomas, but not thymomas and carcinomas of other sites, show CD5 immunoreactivity. Am J Surg Pathol 1997; 21: 936–940.

99. Pomplun S, Wotherspoon AC, Shah G, et al. Immunohistochemical markers in the differentiation of thymic and pulmonary neoplasms. Histopathology 2002; 40: 152–158.

100. Barth TF, Leithauser F, Joos S, et al. Mediastinal (thymic) large B-cell lymphoma: where do we stand? Lancet Oncol 2002; 3: 229–234.

101. Weidner N. Germ cell tumors of the mediastinum. Semin Diagn Pathol 1999; 16: 42–50.

102. Levine GD. Primary thymic seminoma: a neoplasm ultrastructurally similar to testicular seminoma and distinct from epithelial thymoma. Cancer 1973; 31: 729–741.

103. Ordonez NG, Mackay B. Electron microscopy in tumor diagnosis: indications for its use in the immunohistochemical era. Hum Pathol 1998; 29: 1403–1411.

104. Leroy X, Augusto D, Leteurte E, Gosselin B. CD30 and CD117 (c-kit) used in combination are useful for distinguishing embryonal carcinoma from seminoma. J Histochem Cytochem 2002; 50: 283–285.

105. Niehans GA, Manivel JC, Copland GT, et al. Immunohistochemistry of germ cell and trophoblastic neoplasms. Cancer 1988; 62: 1113–1123.

106. Suster S, Moran CA. Spindle cell thymic carcinoma: clinicopathologic and immunohistochemical study of a distinctive variant of primary thymic epithelial neoplasm. Am J Surg Pathol 1999; 23: 691–700.

107. Trupiano JK, Rice TW, Herzog K, et al. Mediastinal synovial sarcoma: report of two cases with molecular genetic analysis. Ann Thorac Surg 2002; 73: 628–630.

108. DeLeeuw B, Suijkerbuijk RF, Olde-Weghuis D, et al. Distinct Xp11.2 breakpoint regions in synovial sarcoma revealed by metaphase and interphase FISH: relationship to histologic subtypes. Cancer Genet Cytogenet 1994; 73: 89–94.

109. DeYoung BR, Wick MR. Immunohistologic evaluation of metastatic carcinomas of unknown origin: an algorithmic approach. Semin Diagn Pathol 2000; 17: 184–193.

110. Suster S, Moran CA. Primary thymic epithelial neoplasms showing combined features of thymoma and thymic carcinoma: a clinicopathologic study of 22 cases. Am J Surg Pathol 1996; 20: 1469–1480.

111. Kuo TT, Chan JKC. Thymic carcinoma arising in thymoma is associated with alterations in immunohistochemical profile. Am J Surg Pathol 1998; 22: 1474–1481.

112. Liu HC, Hsu WH, Chen YJ, et al. Primary thymic carcinoma. Ann Thorac Surg 2002; 73: 1076–1081.

113. Berruti A, Paze E, Fara E, et al. Acute myeloblastic leukemia associated with mediastinal nonseminomatous germ cell tumors: report on two cases. Tumori 1995; 81: 299–301.

114. Chung DA. Thymic carcinoma – analysis of nineteen clinicopathologic studies. Thorac Cardiovasc Surg 2000; 48: 114–119.

115. Ogawa K, Toita T, Uno T, et al. Treatment and prognosis of thymic carcinoma: a retrospective analysis of 40 cases. Cancer 2002; 94: 3115–3119.

116. Chhieng DC, Rose D, Ludwig ME, Zakowski MF. Cytology of thymomas: emphasis on morphology and correlation with histologic subtypes. Cancer 2000; 90: 24–32.

117. Shin HJ, Katz RL. Thymic neoplasia as represented by fine needle aspiration biopsy of anterior mediastinal masses: a practical approach to the differential diagnosis. Acta Cytol 1998; 42: 855–864.

118. Ali SZ, Erozan YS. Thymoma: cytopathologic features and differential diagnosis on fine needle aspiration. Acta Cytol 1998; 42: 845–854.

119. Slagel DD, Powers CN, Melaragno MJ, et al. Spindle cell lesions of the mediastinum: diagnosis by fine needle aspiration biopsy. Diagn Cytopathol 1997; 17: 167–176.

120. Kaw YT, Esparza AR. Fine needle aspiration cytology of primary squamous cell carcinoma of the thymus: a case report. Acta Cytol 1993; 37: 735–739.

121. Shabb NS, Fahl M, Shabb B, et al. Fine needle aspiration of the mediastinum: a clinical, radiologic, cytologic, and histologic study of 42 cases. Diagn Cytopathol 1998; 19: 428–436.

122. Geisinger KR. Differential diagnostic considerations and potential pitfalls in fine needle aspiration biopsies of the mediastinum. Diagn Cytopathol 1995; 13: 436–442.

123. Finley JL, Silverman JF, Strausbauch PH, et al. Malignant thymic neoplasms: diagnosis by fine needle aspiration biopsy with histologic, immunocytochemical, and ultrastructural confirmation. Diagn Cytopathol 1986; 2: 118–125.

124. Friedman HD, Hutchison RE, Kohman LJ, Powers CN. Thymoma mimicking lymphoblastic lymphoma: a pitfall in fine needle aspiration biopsy interpretation. Diagn Cytopathol 1996; 14: 165–171.

125. Leyton O, Turnbull HM, Bratton AB. Primary cancer of the thymus with pluriglandular disturbance. J Pathol Bacteriol 1931; 34: 635–660.

126. Scholz DA, Bahn RC. Thymic tumors associated with Cushing's syndrome: review of three cases. Mayo Clin Proc 1959; 34: 433–441.

127. Rosai J, Higa E. Mediastinal endocrine neoplasm, of probable thymic origin, related to carcinoid tumor: clinicopathologic study of 8 cases. Cancer 1972; 29: 1061–1074.

128. Wick MR. Neuroendocrine neoplasia: current concepts. Am J Clin Pathol 2000; 113: 331–335.

129. Duguid JB, Kennedy AM. Oat-cell tumors of mediastinal glands. J Pathol Bacteriol 1930; 33: 93–99.

130. DePerrot M, Spiliopoulos A, Fischer S, et al. Neuroendocrine carcinoma (carcinoid) of the thymus associated with Cushing's syndrome. Ann Thorac Surg 2002; 73: 675–681.

131. Suster S, Moran CA. Neuroendocrine neoplasms of the mediastinum. Am J Clin Pathol 2001; 115(Suppl): S17–S27.

132. Levine GD, Rosai J. A spindle cell variant of thymic carcinoid tumor: a clinical, histologic, and fine structural study with emphasis on its distinction from spindle cell thymoma. Arch Pathol Lab Med 1976; 100: 293–300.

133. Lowenthal RM, Gumpel JM, Kreel L, et al. Carcinoid tumor of the thymus with systemic manifestations: a radiological and pathological study. Thorax 1974; 29: 553–558.

134. Zenone T, Bady B, Souquet PJ, Bernard JP. The Lambert-Eaton syndrome. Rev Mal Respir 1992; 9: 483–490.

135. Brown LR, Aughenbaugh GL, Wick MR, et al. Roentgenologic diagnosis of primary corticotropin-producing carcinoid tumors of the mediastinum. Radiology 1982; 142: 143–148.

136. Wick MR, Carney JA, Bernatz PE, Brown LR. Primary mediastinal carcinoid tumors. Am J Surg Pathol 1982; 6: 195–205.

137. Wick MR, Scott RE, Li CY, Carney JA. Carcinoid tumor of the thymus: a clinicopathologic report of seven cases with a review of the literature. Mayo Clin Proc 1980; 55: 246–254.

138. Rosai J, Levine GD, Weber WR, Higa E. Carcinoid tumors and oat-cell carcinomas of the thymus. Pathol Annu 1976; 11: 201–226.

139. Gal AA, Kornstein MJ, Cohen C, et al. Neuroendocrine tumors of the thymus: a clinicopathological and prognostic study. Ann Thorac Surg 2001; 72: 1179–1182.

140. Fujiwara K, Segawa Y, Takigawa N, et al. Two cases of atypical carcinoid of the thymus. Intern Med 2000; 39: 834–838.

141. Williams ED, Sandler M. The classification of carcinoid tumors. Lancet 1963; 1: 238–239.

142. Moran CA, Suster S. Neuroendocrine carcinomas (carcinoid tumors) of the thymus: a clinicopathologic analysis of 80 cases. Am J Clin Pathol 2000; 114: 100–110.

143. Moran CA, Suster S. Spindle-cell neuroendocrine carcinomas of the thymus (spindle-cell thymic carcinoids): a clinicopathologic and immunohistochemical study of seven cases. Mod Pathol 1999; 12: 587–591.

144. Klemm KM, Moran CA, Suster S. Pigmented thymic carcinoids: a clinicopathological and immunohistochemical study of two cases. Mod Pathol 1999; 12: 946–948.

145. Ho FC, Ho JC. Pigmented carcinoid tumor of the thymus. Histopathology 1977; 1: 363–369.

146. Smith NL, Finley JL. Lipid-rich carcinoid tumor of the thymus gland: diagnosis by fine needle aspiration biopsy. Diagn Cytopathol 2001; 25: 130–133.

147. Moran CA, Suster S. Primary neuroendocrine carcinoma (thymic carcinoid) of the thymus with prominent oncocytic features: a clinicopathologic study of 22 cases. Mod Pathol 2000; 13: 489–494.

148. Moran CA, Suster S. Angiomatoid neuroendocrine carcinoma of the thymus: report of a distinctive morphological variant of neuroendocrine tumor of the thymus resembling a vascular neoplasm. Hum Pathol 1999; 30: 635–639.

149. Suster S, Moran CA. Thymic carcinoid with prominent mucinous stroma: report of a distinctive morphologic variant of thymic neuroendocrine neoplasm. Am J Surg Pathol 1995; 19: 1277–1285.

150. Hekimgil M, Hamulu F, Cagirici U, et al. Small cell neuroendocrine carcinoma of the thymus complicated by Cushing's syndrome. Pathol Res Pract 2001; 197: 129–133.

151. Galanis E, Frytak S, Lloyd RV. Extrapulmonary small cell carcinoma. Cancer 1997; 79: 1729–1736.

152. Shimizu J, Hayashi Y, Morita K, et al. Primary thymic carcinoma: a clinicopathological and immunohistochemical study. J Surg Oncol 1994; 56: 159–164.

153. Truong LD, Mody DR, Cagle PT, et al. Thymic carcinoma: a clinicopathologic study of 13 cases. Am J Surg Pathol 1990; 14: 151–166.

154. Wick MR, Scheithauer BW. Oat cell carcinoma of the thymus. Cancer 1982; 49: 1652–1657.

155. Moran CA, Suster S. Thymic neuroendocrine carcinomas with combined features ranging from well-differentiated (carcinoid) to small cell carcinoma: a clinicopathologic and immunohistochemical study of 11 cases. Am J Clin Pathol 2000; 113: 345–350.

156. Lau SK, Luthringer DJ, Eisen RN. Thyroid transcription factor-1: a review. Appl Immunohistochem Molec Morphol 2002; 10: 97–102.

157. Cheuk W, Kwan MY, Suster S, Chan JKC. Immunostaining for thyroid transcription factor-1 and cytokeratin 20 aids in the distinction of small cell carcinoma from Merkel cell carcinoma, but not pulmonary from extrapulmonary small cell carcinomas. Arch Pathol Lab Med 2001; 125: 228–231.

158. Kuo TT, Chang JP, Lin FJ, et al. Thymic carcinomas: histopathological varieties and immunohistochemical study. Am J Surg Pathol 1990; 14: 24–34.

159. Chetty R, Batitang S, Govender D. Large cell neuroendocrine carcinoma of the thymus. Histopathology 1997; 31: 274–276.

160. Wick MR, Scheithauer BW. Thymic carcinoid: a histologic, immunohistochemical, and ultrastructural study of 12 cases. Cancer 1984; 53: 475–484.

161. Kuo TT. Frequent presence of neuroendocrine small cells in thymic carcinoma: a light microscopic and immunohistochemical study. Histopathology 2000; 37: 19–26.

162. Lauriola L, Erlandson RA, Rosai J. Neuroendocrine differentiation is a common feature of thymic carcinoma. Am J Surg Pathol 1998; 22: 1059–1066.

163. Hishima T, Fukayama M, Hayashi Y, et al. Neuroendocrine differentiation in thymic epithelial tumors with special reference to thymic carcinoma and atypical thymoma. Hum Pathol 1998; 29: 330–338.

164. DeLellis RA, Wolfe HJ. Calcitonin in spindle cell thymic carcinoid tumors. Arch Pathol Lab Med 1976; 100: 340.

165. Hirai S, Hamanaka Y, Mitsui N, et al. Thymic carcinoids in multiple endocrine neoplasia, type I. Jpn J Thorac Cardiovasc Surg 2001; 49: 525–527.

166. Teh BT. Thymic carcinoids in multiple endocrine neoplasia, type I. J Intern Med 1998; 243: 01–504.

167. Teh BT, McArdle J, Chan SP, et al. Clinicopathologic studies of thymic carcinoids in multiple endocrine neoplasia, type I. Medicine 1997; 76: 21–29.

168. deMontpreville VT, Macchiarini P, Dulmet E. Thymic neuroendocrine carcinoma (carcinoid): a clinicopathologic study of fourteen cases. J Thorac Cardiovasc Surg 1996; 111: 134–141.

169. Nudelman IL, Dentsch AA, Reiss R. Primary hyperparathyroidism due to mediastinal parathyroid adenoma. Int Surg 1987; 72: 104–108.

170. Massac E Jr, Righini M, Seremetis M. Mediastinal hyperfunctioning parathyroid adenoma. J Natl Med Assoc 1982; 74: 385–387.

171. Hofbauer LC, Spitzweg C, Aruholdt H, et al. Mediastinal parathyroid tumor: giant adenoma or carcinoma? Endocr Pathol 1997; 8: 161–166.

172. Kelly MD, Sheridan BF, Farnsworth AE, Palfreeman S. Parathyroid carcinoma in a mediastinal sixth parathyroid gland. Aust NZ J Surg 1994; 64: 446–449.

173. Murphy MN, Glennon PG, Diocee MS, et al. Nonsecretory parathyroid carcinoma of the mediastinum. Cancer 1986; 58: 2468–2476.

174. Wick MR, Ritter JH, Humphrey PA, Nappi O. Clear cell neoplasms of the endocrine system and thymus. Semin Diagn Pathol 1997; 14: 183–202.

175. Olson JL, Salyer WR. Mediastinal paragangliomas (aortic body tumors): a report of four cases and a review of the literature. Cancer 1978; 41: 2405–2412.

176. Moran CA, Suster S, Fishback N, Koss MN. Mediastinal paragangliomas: a clinicopathologic and immunohistochemical study of 16 cases. Cancer 1993; 72: 2358–2364.

177. Hartmann CA, Minck C, Dienemann D, et al. Thymic carcinoid and mediastinal paraganglioma: differential diagnosis and immunohistologic study. Pathologe 1989; 10: 323–331.

178. Oliveira AM, Tazelaar HD, Myers JL, et al. Thyroid transcription factor-1 distinguishes pulmonary from well-differentiated neuroendocrine tumors of other sites. Am J Surg Pathol 2001; 25: 815–819.

179. Wick MR, Cerilli LA. Applications of immunohistochemistry in the diagnosis of undifferentiated tumors. In: Lloyd RV, ed. Morphology methods. Totawa, NJ: Humana Press; 2001: 323–360.

180. Yamakawa Y, Masaoka A, Hashimoto T, et al. A tentative tumor-node-metastasis classification of thymoma. Cancer 1991; 68: 1984–1987.

181. Gherardi G, Marveggio C, Placidi A. Neuroendocrine carcinoma of the thymus: aspiration biopsy, immunocytochemistry, and clinicopathologic correlates. Diagn Cytopathol 1995; 12: 158–164.

182. Gillman J. The development of the gonads in man, with a consideration of the role of fetal endocrines and histogenesis of ovarian tumors. Contrib Embryol 1948; 32: 81–131.

183. Jaing TH, Wang HS, Hung IJ, et al. Intracranial germ cell tumors: a retrospective study of 44 children. Pediatr Neurol 2002; 26: 369–373.

184. Dehner LP. Germ cell tumors of the mediastinum. Semin Diagn Pathol 1990; 7: 266–284.

185. Billmire D, Vinocur C, Roscorla F, et al. Malignant mediastinal germ cell tumors: an intergroup study. J Pediatr Surg 2001; 36: 18–24.

186. Bokemeyer C, Nichols CR, Droz JP, et al. Extragonadal germ cell tumors of the mediastinum and retroperitoneum: results from an international analysis. J Clin Oncol 2002; 20: 1864–1873.

187. Berkman F, Peker AF, Ayyildiz A, et al. Extragonadal germ cell tumors: clinicopathologic findings, staging, and treatment experience in 14 patients. J Exp Clin Cancer Res 2000; 19: 281–285.

188. Knapp RH, Hurt RD, Payne WS, et al. Malignant germ cell tumors of the mediastinum. J Thorac Cardiovasc Surg 1985; 89: 82–89.

189. Burns BF, McCaughey WT. Unusual thymic seminomas. Arch Pathol Lab Med 1986; 110: 539–541.

190. Ringertz N, Lidholm SO. Mediastinal tumors and cysts. J Thorac Cardiovasc Surg 1956; 31: 458–487.

191. Lewis BD, Hurt RD, Payne WS, et al. Benign teratoma of the mediastinum. J Thorac Cardiovasc Surg 1983; 86: 727–731.

192. Adebonojo SA, Nicola ML. Teratoid tumors of the mediastinum. Am Surg 1976; 42: 361–365.

193. Lachman MF, Kim K, Koo BC. Mediastinal teratoma associated with Klinefelter's syndrome. Arch Pathol Lab Med 1986; 110: 1067–1071.

194. Ulbright TM, Loehrer PJ Jr, Roth LM, et al. The development of non-germ cell malignancies within germ cell tumors: a clinicopathologic study of 11 cases. Cancer 1984; 54: 1824–1833.

195. Carter D, Bibro MC, Touloukian RJ. Benign clinical behavior of immature mediastinal teratoma in infancy and childhood: report of two cases and review of the literature. Cancer 1982; 49: 398–402.

196. Gonzalez-Crussi F, Winkle RF, Mirkin DL. Sacrococcygeal teratomas in infants and children: relationship of histology and prognosis in 40 cases. Arch Pathol Lab Med 1978; 102: 420–425.

197. Oberman HA, Libcke JH. Malignant germinal neoplasms of the mediastinum. Cancer 1964; 17: 498–507.

198. Berry CL, Keeling J, Hilton C. Teratoma in infancy and childhood: a review of 91 cases. J Pathol 1969; 98: 241–252.

199. Carney JA, Thompson DP, Johnson CL, Lynn HB. Teratomas in children: clinical and pathologic aspects. J Pediatr Surg 1972; 7: 271–282.

200. Gobel U, Calaminus G, Engert J, et al. Teratomas in infancy and childhood. Med Pediatr Oncol 1998; 31: 8–15.

201. Moran CA, Suster S. Primary germ cell tumors of the mediastinum. I. Analysis of 322 cases with special emphasis on teratomatous lesions and a proposal for histopathologic classification and clinical staging. Cancer 1997; 80: 681–690.

202. Schantz A, Sewall W, Castleman B. Mediastinal germinoma: a study of 21 cases with an excellent prognosis. Cancer 1972; 30;1189–1194.

203. Hainsworth JD, Greco FA. Germ cell neoplasms and other malignancies of the mediastinum. Cancer Treat Res 2001; 105: 303–325.

204. Aygun C, Slawson RG, Bajaj K, Salazar OM. Primary mediastinal seminoma. Urology 1984; 23: 109–117.

205. Moran CA, Suster S. Mediastinal seminomas with prominent cystic changes: a clinicopathologic study of 10 cases. Am J Surg Pathol 1995; 19: 1047–1053.

206. Moran CA, Suster S, Przygodzki RM, Koss MN. Primary germ cell tumors of the mediastinum. II. Mediastinal seminomas – a clinicopathologic and immunohistochemical study of 120 cases. Cancer 1997; 80: 691–698.

207. Sloane JP, Ormerod MG. Distribution of epithelial membrane antigen in normal and neoplastic tissues and its value in diagnostic tumor pathology. Cancer 1981; 47: 1786–1795.

208. Nazeer T, Ro JY, Amato RJ, et al. Histologically pure seminoma with elevated alpha-fetoprotein: a clinicopathologic study of 10 cases. Oncol Rep 1998; 5: 1425–1429.

209. Looijenga LH, Oosterhuis JW. Pathogenesis of testicular germ cell tumors. Rev Reprod 1999; 4: 90–100.

210. Bussey KJ, Lawce HJ, Olson SB, et al. Chromosome abnormalities of eighty-one pediatric germ cell tumors: sex-, age-, site-, and histopathology- related differences: a Children's Cancer Group study. Genes Chromosomes Cancer 1999; 25: 134–146.

211. Summersgill B, Goker H, Osin P, et al. Establishing germ cell origin of undifferentiated tumors by identifying gain of 12p material using comparative genomic hybridization analysis of paraffin embedded samples. Diagn Molec Pathol 1998; 7: 260–266.

212. Bokemeyer C, Droz JP, Horwich A, et al. Extragonadal seminoma: an international multicenter analysis of prognostic factors and long-term treatment outcome. Cancer 2001; 91: 1394–1401.

213. McNeil MM, Leong ASY, Sage RE. Primary mediastinal embryonal carcinoma in association with Klinefelter's syndrome. Cancer 1981; 47: 343–345.

214. Wick MR, Siegal GP. Primary mediastinal embryonal carcinoma. Minn Med 1980; 63: 723–726.

215. Hainsworth JD, Greco FA. Poorly differentiated carcinoma and germ cell tumors. Hematol Oncol Clin North Am 1991; 5: 1223–1231.

216. Sass M, Jao W, Horn T, Keh PC. Mediastinal yolk sac tumor: ultrastructural and immunofluorescent studies. Ultrastruct Pathol 1983; 4: 67–73.

217. Suster S, Moran CA, Dominguez-Malagon H, Quevado-Blanco P. Germ cell tumors of the mediastinum and testis: a comparative immunohistochemical study of 120 cases. Hum Pathol 1998; 29: 737–742.

218. Moran CA, Suster S, Koss MN. Primary germ cell tumors of the mediastinum. III. Yolk sac tumor, embryonal carcinoma, choriocarcinoma, and combined nonteratomatous germ cell tumors of the mediastinum: a clinicopathologic and immunohistochemical study of 64 cases. Cancer 1997; 80: 699–707.

219. DeSmet AA, Silver TM, Hart WR. Endodermal sinus tumor of the anterior mediastinum. South Med J 1977; 70: 757–758.

220. Mukai K, Adams WR. Yolk sac tumor of the anterior mediastinum. Am J Surg Pathol 1979; 3: 77–83.

221. Gooneratne S, Keh PC, Sreekanth S, et al. Anterior mediastinal endodermal sinus (yolk sac) tumor in a female infant. Cancer 1985; 56: 1430–1433.

222. Orazi A, Neiman RS, Ulbright TM, et al. Hematopoietic precursor cells within the yolk sac tumor component are the source of secondary hematopoietic malignancies in patients with mediastinal germ cell tumors. Cancer 1993; 71: 3873–3881.

223. Motzer RJ, Amsterdam A, Prieto V, et al. Teratoma with malignant transformation: diverse malignant histologies arising in men with germ cell tumors. J Urol 1998; 159: 133–138.

224. Teilum G. Endodermal sinus tumors of the ovary and testis: comparative morphogenesis of the so-called mesonephroma ovarii (Schiller) and extraembryonic (yolk sac-allantoic) structures of the rat's placenta. Cancer 1959; 12: 1092–1105.

225. Jondle DM, Shahin MS, Sorosky J, Benda JA. Ovarian mixed germ cell tumor with predominance of polyembryoma: a case report with literature review. Int J Gynecol Pathol 2002; 21: 78–81.

226. Collins KA, Geisinger KR, Wakely PE Jr, et al. Extragonadal germ cell tumors: a fine needle aspiration biopsy study. Diagn Cytopathol 1995; 12: 223–229.

227. Javadpour N. Serum and cellular biologic tumor markers in patients with urologic cancer. Hum Pathol 1979; 10: 557–568.

228. Garzotto M, Nichols CR. Current concepts in risk factor assessment for advanced germ cell cancer. Semin Urol Oncol 2001; 19: 165–169.

229. Wenger ME, Dines DE, Ahmann DL, Good CA. Primary mediastinal choriocarcinoma. Mayo Clin Proc 1968; 43: 570–575.

230. Greenwood SM, Goodman JR, Schneider G, et al. Choriocarcinoma in a man: the relationship of gynecomastia to chorionic somatomammotropin and estrogens. Am J Med 1971; 51: 416–422.

231. Knapp RH, Fritz SR, Reiman HM. Primary embryonal carcinoma and choriocarcinoma of the mediastinum: a case report. Arch Pathol Lab Med 1982; 106: 507–509.

232. Bergh NP, Gatzinsky P, Larsson S, et al. Tumors of the thymus and thymic region. III. Clinicopathological studies on teratomas and tumors of germ cell type. Ann Thorac Surg 1978; 25: 107–111.

233. Manivel JC, Wick MR, Abenoza P, Rosai J. The occurrence of sarcomatous components in primary mediastinal germ cell tumors. Am J Surg Pathol 1986; 10: 711–717.

234. Parker D, Holford CP, Begent RHJ, et al. Effective treatment for malignant mediastinal teratoma. Thorax 1983; 38: 897–902.

235. Murakawa Y, Satake N, Kato S, et al. Alpha-fetoprotein normalization as a prognostic factor for mediastinal origin embryonal carcinoma: report of five cases. Intern Med 2002; 41: 883–888.

236. Vuky J, Bains M, Bacik J, et al. Role of postchemotherapy adjunctive surgery in the management of patients with nonseminoma arising from the mediastinum. J Clin Oncol 2001; 19: 682–688.

237. Chao TY, Nieh S, Huang SH, Lee WH. Cytology of fine needle aspirations of primary extragonadal germ cell tumors. Acta Cytol 1997; 41: 497–503.

238. Chhieng DC, Lin O, Moran CA, et al. Fine needle aspiration biopsy of nonteratomatous germ cell tumors of the mediastinum. Am J Clin Pathol 2002; 118: 418–424.

239. Motoyama T, Yamamoto O, Iwamoto H, Watanabe H. Fine needle aspiration cytology of primary mediastinal germ cell tumors. Acta Cytol 1995; 39: 725–732.

240. Stanley MW, Powers CN, Pitman MB, et al. Cytology of germ cell tumors: extragonadal, extracranial masses and intraoperative problems. Cancer 1997; 81: 220–227.

241. Mizrak B, Ekinci C. Cytologic diagnosis of yolk sac tumor: a report of seven cases. Acta Cytol 1995; 39: 936–940.

242. Caraway NP, Fanning CV, Amato RJ, Sniege N. Fine needle aspiration cytology of seminoma: a review of 16 cases. Diagn Cytopathol 1995; 12: 327–333.

243. Saleh H, Masood S. Value of ancillary studies in fine needle aspiration biopsy. Diagn Cytopathol 1995; 13: 310–315.

244. Krugmann J, Feichtinger H, Greil R, Fend F. Thymic Hodgkin's disease: a histological and immunohistochemical study of three cases. Pathol Res Pract 1999; 195: 681–687.

245. Parrens M, Dubus P, Danjoux M, et al. Mucosa-associated lymphoid tissue of the thymus – hyperplasia versus lymphoma. Am J Clin Pathol 2002; 117: 51–56.

246. Peckham MJ, Guay JP, Hamlin IM, Lukes RJ. Survival in localized nodal and extranodal non-Hodgkin's lymphoma. Br J Cancer 1975; 31(Suppl 2): 413–424.

247. Palestro G, Turrini F, Pagano M, Chiusa L. Castleman's disease. Adv Clin Pathol 1999; 3: 11–22.

248. Massimino M, Gasparini M, Giardini R. Ki-1 (CD30) anaplastic large cell lymphoma in children. Ann Oncol 1995; 6: 915–920.

249. Thomas DA, Kartarjian HM. Lymphoblastic lymphoma. Hematol Oncol Clin North Am 2001; 15: 51–95.

250. Murphy SB, Frizzera G, Evans AE. A study of childhood non-Hodgkin's lymphoma. Cancer 1975; 36: 2121–2131.

251. Niwa K, Tanaka T, Mori H, Takahashi M. Extramedullary plasmacytoma of the mediastinum. Jpn J Clin Oncol 1987; 17: 95–100.

252. Tagasugi JE, Godwin JD, Marglin SI, Petersdorf SH. Intrathoracic granulocytic sarcomas. J Thorac Imaging 1996; 11: 223–230.

253. Gilcrease MZ, Rajan B, Ostrowski ML, et al. Localized thymic Langerhans' cell histiocytosis and its relationship with myasthenia gravis: immunohistochemical, ultrastructural, and cytometric studies. Arch Pathol Lab Med 1997; 121: 134–138.

254. Siegal GP, Dehner LP, Rosai J. Histiocytosis X (Langerhans' cell granulomatosis) of the thymus. A clinicopathologic study of four childhood cases. Am J Surg Pathol 1985; 9: 117–124.

255. Catinella FP, Boyd AD, Spencer FC. Intrathoracic extramedullary hematopoiesis simulating anterior mediastinal tumor. J Thorac Cardiovasc Surg 1985; 89: 580–584.

256. Nathwani BN, Kim H, Rappaport H. Malignant lymphoma, lymphoblastic. Cancer 1976; 38: 964–983.

257. Smith JL, Barker CR, Clein GP, Collins RD. Characterization of malignant mediastinal lymphoid neoplasm (Sternberg's sarcoma) as thymic in origin. Lancet 1973; 1: 74–77.

258. Mazza P, Bertini M, Macchi S, et al. Lymphoblastic lymphoma in adolescents and adults: clinical, pathological, and prognostic evaluation. Eur J Cancer Clin Oncol 1986; 22: 1503–1510.

259. Yu GH, Salhany KE, Gokaslan ST, et al. Thymic epithelial cells as a diagnostic pitfall in the fine needle aspiration diagnosis of primary mediastinal lymphoma. Diagn Cytopathol 1997; 16: 460–465.

260. Freedman AS, Nadler LM. Immunologic markers in non-Hodgkin's lymphoma. Hematol Oncol Clin North Am 1991; 5: 871–879.

261. Robertson PB, Neiman RS, Worapongpaiboon S, et al. O13 (CD99) positivity in hematologic proliferations correlates with TdT positivity. Mod Pathol 1997; 10: 277–282.

262. Levitt LJ, Aisenberg AC, Harris NL, et al. Primary non-Hodgkin's lymphoma of the mediastinum. Cancer 1982; 50: 2486–2492.

263. Perrone T, Frizzera G, Rosai J. Mediastinal diffuse large cell lymphoma with sclerosis: a clinicopathologic study of 60 cases. Am J Surg Pathol 1986; 10: 176–191.

264. Addis BJ, Isaacson PG. Large cell lymphoma of the mediastinum: a B-cell tumor of probable thymic origin. Histopathology 1986; 10: 379–390.

265. Lamarre L, Jacobson JO, Aisenberg AC, Harris NL. Primary large cell lymphoma of the mediastinum: a histologic and immunophenotypic study of 29 cases. Am J Surg Pathol 1989; 13: 730–739.

266. Strickler JG, Kurtin PJ. Mediastinal lymphoma. Semin Diagn Pathol 1991; 8: 2–13.

267. Suster S. Primary large cell lymphomas of the mediastinum. Semin Diagn Pathol 1999; 16: 51–64.

268. Aisenberg AC. Primary large cell lymphoma of the mediastinum. Semin Oncol 1999; 26: 251–258.

269. Petersdorf SH, Wood DE. Lymphoproliferative disorders presenting as mediastinal neoplasms. Semin Thorac Cardiovasc Surg 2000; 12: 290–300.

270. Peiper SC, Kahn LB. Ultrastructural comparison of Hodgkin's and non-Hodgkin's lymphoma. Histopathology 1982; 6: 93–109.

271. Higgins JP, Warnke RA. CD30 expression is common in mediastinal large B-cell lymphoma. Am J Clin Pathol 1999; 112: 241–247.

272. Pai NB, Kim S, Pathak R, et al. Syncytial variant of nodular sclerosing Hodgkin's lymphoma. Lymphology 1999; 32: 75–79.

273. Hirano H, Ichimura T, Hanibuchi M, et al. Anaplastic large cell lymphoma (Ki-1 lymphoma): ultrastructural and immunohistochemical studies. Med Electron Microsc 2002; 35: 153–159.

274. Nguyen LN, Ha CS, Hess M, et al. The outcome of combined-modality treatments for stage I and II primary large B-cell lymphoma of the mediastinum. Int J Radiat Oncol Biol Phys 2000; 47: 1281–1285.

275. Kardos TF, Sprague RI, Wakely PE Jr, et al. Fine needle aspiration biopsy of lymphoblastic lymphoma and leukemia: a clinical, cytologic, and immunologic study. Cancer 1987; 60: 2448–2453.

276. Jacobs JC, Katz RL, Shabb N, et al. Fine needle aspiration of lymphoblastic lymphoma: a multiparameter diagnostic approach. Acta Cytol 1992; 36: 887–894.

277. Wakely PE Jr, Kornstein MJ. Aspiration cytopathology of lymphoblastic lymphoma and leukemia: the MVC experience. Pediatr Pathol Lab Med 1996; 16: 243–252.

278. Hughes JH, Katz RL, Fonseca GA, et al. Fine needle aspiration cytology of mediastinal non-Hodgkin's nonlymphoblastic lymphoma. Cancer 1998; 84: 26–35.

279. Silverman JF, Raab SS, Park HK. Fine needle aspiration cytology of primary large cell lymphoma of the mediastinum: cytomorphologic findings with potential pitfalls in diagnosis. Diagn Cytopathol 1993; 9: 209–215.

280. Stanley MW, Powers CN. Syncytial variant of nodular sclerosing Hodgkin's disease: fine needle aspiration findings in two cases. Diagn Cytopathol 1997; 17: 477–479.

281. Tam CG, Broome DR, Shannon RL. Desmoid tumor of the anterior mediastinum: CT and radiologic features. J Comput Assist Tomogr 1994; 18: 499–501.

282. Dosios TJ, Angouras DC, Floros DG. Primary desmoid tumor of the posterior mediastinum. Ann Thorac Surg 1998; 66: 2098–2099.

283. Handorf CR. Intrathoracic lipomas in children. South Med J 1982; 75: 1403–1405.

284. Coulomb M, Terraube P, Vincent J, Lebas JF. Fatty masses in the mediastinum: a report on 21 cases including 16 after computer tomography investigations. J Radiol 1980; 61: 13–26.

285. Mineo TC, Biancari F, Cristino B, D'Andrea V. Benign vascular tumors of the mediastinum: presentation of three cases and review of the literature. Thorac Cardiovasc Surg 1995; 43: 361–364.

286. Oshikiri T, Morikawa T, Jinushi E, et al. Five cases of lymphangioma of the mediastinum in adults. Ann Thorac Cardiovasc Surg 2001; 7: 103–105.

287. Fishman SJ. Vascular anomalies of the mediastinum. Semin Pediatr Surg 1999; 8: 92–98.

288. Krag D, Reich SB. Heterotopic bone marrow (myelolipoma) of the mediastinum. Chest 1972; 61: 514–515.

289. Corneli G, Alifano M, FortiParri S, et al. Invasive inflammatory pseudotumor involving the lung and the mediastinum. Thorac Cardiovasc Surg 2001; 49: 124–126.

290. Whyte AM, Powell N. Mediastinal lipoblastoma of infancy. Clin Radiol 1990; 42: 205–206.

291. Marchevsky AM. Mediastinal tumors of peripheral nervous system origin. Semin Diagn Pathol 1999; 16: 65–78.

292. Witkin GB, Rosai J. Solitary fibrous tumor of the mediastinum: a report of 14 cases. Am J Surg Pathol 1989; 13: 547–557.

293. Suster S, Moran CA, Koss MN. Epithelioid hemangioendothelioma of the anterior mediastinum: clinicopathologic, immunohistochemical, and ultrastructural analysis of 12 cases. Am J Surg Pathol 1994; 18: 871–881.

294. Mondal A. Cytopathology of neuroblastoma, ganglioneuroblastoma, and ganglioneuroma. J Indian Med Assoc 1995; 93: 340–343.

295. Suster S, Moran CA. Chordomas of the mediastinum: clinicopathologic, immunohistochemical, and ultrastructural study of six cases presenting as posterior mediastinal masses. Hum Pathol 1995; 26: 1354–1362.

296. Moran CA, Suster S, Perino G, et al. Malignant smooth muscle tumors presenting as mediastinal soft tissue masses: a clinicopathologic study of 10 cases. Cancer 1994; 74: 2251–2260.

297. Suster S, Moran CA, Koss MN. Rhabdomyosarcomas of the anterior mediastinum: report of four cases unassociated with germ cell, teratomatous, or thymic carcinomatous components. Hum Pathol 1994; 25: 349–356.

298. Murakawa T, Nakajima J, Fukami T, et al. Malignant fibrous histiocytoma in the anterior mediastinum. Jpn J Thorac Cardiovasc Surg 2001; 49: 722–727.

299. Venuta F, Pesacarmona EO, Rendina EA, et al. Primary osteogenic sarcoma of the posterior mediastinum: case report. Scand J Thorac Cardiovasc Surg 1993; 27: 169–173.

300. Suster S, Moran CA. Malignant cartilaginous tumors of the mediastinum: clinicopathological study of six cases presenting as extraskeletal soft tissue masses. Hum Pathol 1997; 28: 588–594.

301. Matsuyama W, Wakimoto J, Nakagawa M, et al. An autopsy case of peripheral neuroepithelioma in the posterior mediastinum with p53 point mutation. Intern Med 1998; 37: 324–329.

302. Witkin GB, Miettinen M, Rosai J. A biphasic tumor of the mediastinum with features of synovial sarcoma: a report of four cases. Am J Surg Pathol 1989; 13: 490–499.

303. Meis-Kindblom JM, Kindblom LG. Angiosarcoma of soft tissue: a study of 80 cases. Am J Surg Pathol 1998; 22: 683–697.

304. Mase T, Kawawaki N, Narumiya C, et al. Primary liposarcoma of the mediastinum. Jpn J Thorac Cardiovasc Surg 2002; 50: 252–255.

305. Swanson PE. Soft tissue neoplasms of the mediastinum. Semin Diagn Pathol 1991; 8: 14–34.

306. Maschek H, Werner M, Busche G, Weinel P. Congenital rhabdoid tumor in the mediastinum and liver: case report and review of the literature. Pathologe 1992; 13: 172–178.

307. Lemos LB, Hamoudi AB. Malignant thymic tumor in an infant (malignant histiocytoma). Arch Pathol Lab Med 1978; 102: 84–89.

308. Lange I. Uber ein Lipom des Thymus. Zentralbl Allg Pathol 1916; 27: 97–101.

309. Moran CA, Rosado-de-Christenson ML, Suster S. Thymolipoma: a clinicopathologic review of 33 cases. Mod Pathol 1995; 8: 741–744.

310. Nishimura O, Naito Y, Noguchi Y, et al. Thymolipoma: a report of three cases. Jpn J Surg 1990; 20: 234–237.

311. Ringe B, Dragojevic D, Frank G, Borst HG. Thymolipoma – a rare benign tumor of the thymus gland: two case reports and review of the literature. Thorac Cardiovasc Surg 1979; 27: 369–374.

312. Barnes RDS, O'Gorman P. Two cases of aplastic anemia associated with tumors of the thymus. J Clin Pathol 1962; 15: 264–268.

313. Lebrun E, Ajchenbaum F, Troussard X, et al. Chronic lymphocytic leukemia, erythroblastopenia, and thymolipoma. Nouv Rev Fr Hematol 1985; 27: 29–37.

314. Otto HF, Loning T, Lachenmayer L, et al. Thymolipoma in association with myasthenia gravis. Cancer 1982; 50: 1623–1628.

315. Takamori S, Hayashi A, Tayama K, et al. Thymolipoma associated with myasthenia gravis. Scand Cardiovasc J 1997; 31: 241–242.

316. Rosado-de-Christenson ML, Pugatch RD, Moran CA, Galobardes J. Thymolipoma: analysis of 27 cases. Radiology 1994; 193: 121–126.

317. Hull MT, Warfel KA, Kotylo P, et al. Proliferating thymolipoma: ultrastructural, immunohistochemical, and flow cytometric study. Ultrastruct Pathol 1995; 19: 75–81.

318. Moran CA, Zeren H, Koss MN. Thymofibrolipoma: a histologic variant of thymolipoma. Arch Pathol Lab Med 1994; 118: 281–282.

319. Ogino S, Franks TJ, Deubner H, Koss MN. Thymohemangiolipoma, a rare histologic variant of thymolipoma: a case report and review of the literature. Ann Diagn Pathol 2000; 4: 236–239.

320. Argani P, deChiocca IC, Rosai J. Thymoma arising with a thymolipoma. Histopathology 1998; 32: 573–574.

321. Havlicek F, Rosai J. A sarcoma of thymic stroma with features of liposarcoma. Am J Clin Pathol 1984; 82: 217–224.

322. Okumori M, Mabuchi M, Nakagawa M. Malignant thymoma associated with liposarcoma of the mediastinum: a case report. Jpn J Surg 1983; 13: 512–518.

323. Klimstra DS, Moran CA, Perino G, et al. Liposarcoma of the anterior mediastinum and thymus: a clinicopathologic study of 28 cases. Am J Surg Pathol 1995; 19: 782–791.

324. Heimann A, Sneige N, Shirkhoda A, DeCaro LF. Fine needle aspiration cytology of thymolipoma: a case report. Acta Cytol 1987; 31: 335–339.

325. Rossi SE, McAdams HP, Rosado-de-Christenson ML, et al. Fibrosing mediastinitis. Radiographics 2001; 21: 737–757.

326. Baslaim G, DeVarennes B. Localized idiopathic fibrosing mediastinitis as a cause of superior vena cava syndrome: a case report. Can J Surg 1998; 41: 68–71.

327. Kalweit G, Huwer H, Straub U, Gams E. Mediastinal compression syndromes due to idiopathic fibrosing mediastinitis – report of three cases and review of the literature. Thorac Cardiovasc Surg 1996; 44: 105–109.

328. Sherrick AD, Brown LR, Harms GF, Myers JL. The radiographic findings of fibrosing mediastinitis. Chest 1994; 106: 484–489.

329. Williamson WA, Tronic BS, Levitan N, et al. Pulmonary venous infarction. Chest 1992; 102: 937–940.

330. Ahmad S. Pulmonary hypertension secondary to fibrosing mediastinitis. Cleve Clin J Med 1991; 58:475.

331. Farmer DW, Moore E, Amparo E, et al. Calcific fibrosing mediastinitis: demonstration of pulmonary

vascular obstruction by magnetic resonance imaging. Am J Roentgenol 1984; 143: 1189–1191.

332. Katzenstein AL, Mazur MT. Pulmonary infarct: an unusual manifestation of fibrosing mediastinitis. Chest 1980; 77: 521–524.

333. Connell JV, Muhm JR. Radiographic manifestations of pulmonary histoplasmosis: a 10-year review. Radiology 1976; 121: 281–285.

334. Hewlett TH, Steer A, Thomas DE. Progressive fibrosing mediastinitis. Ann Thorac Surg 1966; 2: 345–357.

335. Cartier Y, Nogueira HA, Muller NL. Fibrosing mediastinitis associated with Riedel's thyroiditis – computed tomographic findings: case report. Can Assoc Radiol J 1998; 49: 408–410.

336. Flieder DB, Suster S, Moran CA. Idiopathic fibroinflammatory (fibrosing/sclerosing) lesions of the mediastinum: a study of 30 cases with emphasis on morphologic heterogeneity. Mod Pathol 1999; 12: 257–264.

337. Dines DE, Payne WS, Bernatz PE, Pairolero PC. Mediastinal granuloma and fibrosing mediastinitis. Chest 1979; 75: 320–324.

338. Wieder S, Rabinowitz JG. Fibrous mediastinitis: a late manifestation of mediastinal histoplasmosis. Radiology 1977; 125: 312–315.

339. Strauss SE, Jacobson ES. The spectrum of histoplasmosis in a general hospital: a review of 55 cases diagnosed at Barnes Hospital between 1966 and 1977. Am J Med Sci 1980; 279: 147–158.

340. Robertson BD, Bautista MA, Russell TS, et al. Fibrosing mediastinitis secondary to zygomycosis in a twenty-two-month-old child. Pediatr Infect Dis J 2002; 21: 441–442.

341. Lagerstrom CF, Mitchell HG, Graham BS, Hammon JW Jr. Chronic fibrosing mediastinitis and superior vena caval obstruction from blastomycosis. Ann Thorac Surg 1992; 54: 764–765.

342. Harpaz N, Gribetz AR, Krellenstein DJ, Marchevsky AM. Inflammatory pseudotumor of the thymus. Ann Thorac Surg 1986; 42: 331–333.

343. Brachet A, Thevenet F, Gilly FN, et al. Inflammatory pseudotumor of the superior vena cava: rare etiology of mediastinal tumor. Ann Chir 1993; 47: 170–173.

344. Dehner LP, Coffin CM. Idiopathic fibrosclerotic disorders and other inflammatory pseudotumors. Semin Diagn Pathol 1998; 15: 161–173.

345. Ritter JH, Humphrey PA, Wick MR. Malignant neoplasms capable of simulating inflammatory (myofibroblastic) pseudotumors and tumefactive fibroinflammatory lesions: pseudopseudotumors. Semin Diagn Pathol 1998; 15: 111–132.

346. Feigin GA, Robinson B, Marchevsky A. Mixed tumor of the mediastinum. Arch Pathol Lab Med 1986; 110: 80–81.

347. Crotty TB, Colby TV, Gay PC, Pisani RJ. Desmoplastic malignant mesothelioma masquerading as sclerosing mediastinitis: a diagnostic dilemma. Hum Pathol 1992; 23: 79–82.

348. Argani P, Erlandson RA, Rosai J. Thymic neuroblastoma in adults: report of three cases with special emphasis on its association with the syndrome of inappropriate secretion of antidiuretic hormone. Am J Clin Pathol 1997; 108: 537–543.

349. Reeder LB. Neurogenic tumors of the mediastinum. Semin Thorac Cardiovasc Surg 2000; 12: 261–267.

350. Odze R, Begin LR. Malignant paraganglioma of the posterior mediastinum. A case report and review of the literature. Cancer 1990; 65 564–569.

351. Bacha EA, Chapelier AR, Macchiarini P, et al. Surgery for invasive primary mediastinal tumors. Ann Thorac Surg 1998; 66: 234–239.

352. Cupisti K, Dotzenrath C, Simon D, et al. Therapy of suspected intrathoracic parathyroid adenomas: experiences using open transthoracic approach and video-assisted thoracoscopic surgery. Langenbecks Arch Surg 2002; 386: 488–493.

353. Alli PM, Crain BJ, Heitmiller R, Argani P. Malignant melanoma presenting as an intrathymic tumor: a primary thymic melanoma? Arch Pathol Lab Med 2000; 124: 130–134.

354. Vlodavsky E, Ben-Izhak O, Best LA, Kerner H. Primary malignant melanoma of the anterior mediastinum in a child. Am J Surg Pathol 2000; 24: 747–749.

355. Dolynchuk KN, Teskey J, West M. Intrathoracic meningocele associated with neurofibromatosis: case report. Neurosurgery 1990; 27: 485–487.

Oral cavity and salivary glands

The oral cavity

Robert O. Greer, Jr.   Sherif Said

22

NATURE AND HANDLING OF SURGICAL SPECIMENS FROM THE ORAL CAVITY

The vast majority of tissue samples received from the oral cavity will represent one of the following: (1) excisional biopsy, (2) incisional biopsy, (3) bone biopsy, (4) aspiration biopsy, (5) punch biopsy, (6) exfoliative cytology, (7) curettage biopsy, and (8) brush biopsy.

The punch biopsy specimen is rarely encountered because of the nearly unlimited access that the clinician has to oral sites using a scalpel. The aspiration or needle biopsy is typically used in the oral cavity to obtain fluid from a cavity of soft tissue or bone for chemical analysis.

Bone biopsy specimens are commonly encountered material from the oral cavity. The hard tissue, of course, requires decalcification before processing. The tissue sample sizes that the surgical pathologist must deal with are frequently rather small (<1 cm in diameter). Commercial rapid decalcification solutions can be used; however, they tend to compromise cellular detail. Five percent nitric acid in neutral buffered formalin can be a reasonable alternative; decalcification, of course, takes longer, but cytologic detail is maintained. The tissue is considered properly decalcified when the decalcification solution that has been in contact with the hard tissue is mixed with 5 ml of ammonium hydroxide and 5% ammonium oxalate and a clear solution results. A cloudy or milky solution indicates that further decalcification is necessary. Tissue submitted as curettings from a tooth socket often contain bone fragments. It is wise to decalcify this material to avoid sectioning difficulty.

Most soft tissue biopsy specimens from the oral cavity are small elliptical or wedge-shaped samples. If the tissue is received unfixed, it may be necessary to place thin, flat biopsy specimens (e.g. floor of the mouth lesions) on a thin sheet of cardboard to prevent folding.

The scalpel biopsy remains the gold standard when it comes to diagnostic surgical pathology.

The more recently introduced brush biopsy is similar to exfoliative cytology. If it is done properly, it can be an effective screening technique that enables the clinician to capture transepithelial cells. Typically, the brush biopsy involves rotational manipulation of a wheel-like brush that results in slight tissue bleeding until cells from the parabasalar and basalar basement membrane zone are captured. The cellular accumulation is then transferred to a glass slide where it is fixed and ultimately analyzed by computer analysis with the assistance of pathologists skilled in brush biopsy evaluation. It is important for pathologists and surgeons to recognize that the brush biopsy remains a screening tool only. It does not replace the scalpel biopsy and even when atypical cells are identified via a brush biopsy, a follow-up scalpel biopsy is mandatory.

In suspected vesiculobullous lesions, overaggressive handling of the delicate tissue can cause separation of epithelium from the underlying connective tissue, which, of course, impairs histopathologic interpretation.

Teeth are frequently only examined grossly. Often when teeth are submitted, the surgeon is interested in the microscopic findings in soft tissue attachments to the root or crown of the tooth (e.g. dentigerous cyst, periapical cyst, odontogenic keratocyst). It is of paramount importance to submit the attached soft tissue when the submitting physician entertains such differential diagnoses.

Fine needle aspiration can be performed on oral mass lesions, which are defined either through palpation or radiological means. Using this procedure, described elsewhere in this book, a sample of the cells forming the mass can be obtained using a fine needle for the purpose of diagnosis and analysis. Although some people advocate use of FNA in the head and neck only to confirm recurrence or metastasis of an already diagnosed cancer, many others, including the authors, advocate this method as a quick and effective method for first-time diagnosis to aid the clinician in planning further diagnostic and surgical steps and prepare the patients for the treatment modalities to ensue.

Frozen section specimens are handled in much the same manner as tissue from elsewhere throughout the body. Anatomically, considerable fatty tissue can be encountered in oral soft tissue specimens. These can be difficult samples on which to prepare frozen sections. The smaller the quantity of adipose tissue included, the simpler the sectioning process.

Although hard tissues from the mandible or maxilla require decalcification prior to processing, frozen sections can be obtained from a margin of bone. Since most tumors advance, invade, and metastasize through bone within the marrow cavity, the preferred area to sample when sampling for a hard tissue frozen section diagnosis is marrow rather than cortex. Marrow can be curetted from the marrow cavity quite easily at a resection margin and examined.

Very often, artifact occurs as a result of the handling of oral tissues. Several types of artifact can be encountered, including crush artifact, which occurs most commonly in the manipulation of the tissue when it is removed by using forceps or dull scalpel blades. This type of artifact is very dangerous in that it alters tissue morphology and squeezes the chromatin out of the cell nuclei.[1] Inflammatory and tumor cells are the most susceptible to crush damage, and therefore this artifact can render an otherwise adequate specimen nondiagnostic. To prevent crush artifact, tissue has to be handled very delicately, both at removal and at the surgical bench.

A second very common artifact seen in oral tissue specimens is electrosurgery artifact. Electrosurgery provides adequate and prompt tissue hemostasis when a tissue sample is removed; however, the effect of electrosurgery on the tissue cytologically is to cauterize it, thereby precipitating protein and causing the resultant cauterization artifact, which microscopically appears as coagulated or shredded tissue. A third type of artifact seen in oral tissue samples is the artifact produced by the application of dyes or colored medicaments to the tissues at the time of surgery. Such medicaments can be introduced by the injection of a local anesthetic in or around the biopsy site. A fourth kind of artifact is dehydration artifact, caused by improper fixatives or air drying of the specimen. Ten percent neutral buffered formalin remains the fixative of choice for routine biopsy specimens. The last type of frequent artifact that can inadvertently occur in oral tissue samples is freezing artifact. This frequently occurs in the winter when outpatient biopsy specimens are sent in for evaluation by mail. Ten percent formalin will freeze at −11°C, producing a clefting artifact that appears in the epithelium. Freezing artifact can be avoided by using Lillie's acetic alcohol formalin; this fixative contains 10 parts 40% formaldehyde, 5 parts glacial acetic acid, and 5 parts absolute ethyl alcohol. The solution will not freeze until it reaches −30°C.[1]

Many of the vesiculobullous diseases of skin and mucous membranes are mediated by immunologic injury. Immunofluorescence has thus become increasingly valuable in the study of the mucous membrane diseases. Immunomicroscopic techniques that are commonly used for detecting tissue-bound immunoreactants include (1) direct immunofluorescence, (2) direct immunoperoxidase, and (3) the peroxidase/antiperoxidase technique.[2]

Direct immunofluorescence is the most commonly accepted technique for evaluating mucous membrane tissue samples for vesiculobullous disease. Specimens must be received in a fresh state, unfixed. Tissue may be submitted in Michel's solution or snap frozen in liquid nitrogen as soon as possible after excision. The preferred biopsy technique involves submission of perilesional tissue. Direct lesional biopsies are not recommended for immunofluorescence evaluation, except for disseminated lupus erythematosus and vasculitis. Lesions from blistering diseases usually contain so much cellular damage that it is frequently impossible to determine if there is a deposit of immunoreactants. A biopsy extending into perilesional mucosa can be bisected to provide satisfactory biopsies for routine hematoxylin and eosin evaluation and immunofluorescent evaluation. Indirect immunofluorescence relies on identifying a concentration of circulating antibodies within serum. Indirect immunofluorescence is not widely used in association with oral lesions. Direct immunofluorescence is much more sensitive.

THE ROLE OF ONCOGENES, TUMOR SUPPRESSORS, VIRUSES, AND OTHER INFECTIOUS AGENTS IN ORAL DISEASE

It has become increasingly important to establish the role of viruses, cellular oncogenes and their products, and tumor suppressors in the growth and control mechanisms of oral disease, especially oral cancer. It has not, however, been possible to collate the role of all of these factors into a central theory of neoplastic development. To do so, it will be necessary to develop more significant studies that evaluate cell differentiation, clonality, oncogene effects, and cell cycle markers. Hundreds of antibody markers are available from commercial biotechnology laboratories that can be used to identify preneoplastic differentiation and neoplastic changes in cells. Clonality studies are but one. If one postulates that malignant cells are derived from a single mutated cell, then markers that can be developed to identify clonality early in the disease process may even prove effective in the early diagnosis or prevention of disease.[3] Because studies have demonstrated that epidermal growth factor receptors (EGFR) can be overexpressed in tumor cell lines, sometimes in conjunction with gene amplification, would it not be important then to determine if there is overexpression of EGFR in oral precancer and cancer? It is well documented that both transforming growth factor-alpha (TGF-alpha) and EGF bind to EGFR and that ultimately the receptor is internalized and degraded. Recent studies have shown that oral squamous cell carcinomas that produce high levels of TGF-alpha express only low levels of EGFR,[4] which implies that the autocrine or paracrine growth control loop involving TGF-alpha and EGFR may contribute to the growth of a significant proportion of neoplasms. Scientists are currently investigating a correlation between TGF-alpha production, EGFR expression, and the clinical behavior of oral neoplasms in an attempt to determine if there is a correlation that might be of significant prognostic value.[4]

Although it is well known that tobacco, alcohol, and genetic aberrations play a role in oral disease and particularly cancer, it is clear that human oral cancer does not result from a single exposure or even several brief exposures of the oral mucous membranes to exogenous insults, largely because the affected DNA can easily be repaired by DNA polymerase enzymes. However, extended exposures to certain carcinogens can cause enough longitudinal DNA damage to result in gene mutations. Typically DNA-damaged cells die, but in those instances when the cells do not die, malignant neoplasia can be an outcome. Most investigators suggest that six genetic mutations are mandated before a cancer cell can be activated.[5] These mutations are eventually passed on to daughter cells, which over time and multiple additional carcinogenic insults become neoplastic. Tumor-suppressor genes play a significant role in human cancer surveillance. The p53 tumor-suppressor gene, the most common gene associated with tumor abeyance, and telomerase, an enzyme responsible for cell longevity, play important roles in oral neoplasia.[6] Whereas oncogenes accumulate to eventually initiate cancer, tumor-suppressor genes such as p53 and the enzyme telomerase ultimately promote cancer because either genetic loss or inactivation makes them incapable of carrying out their essential role in cellular protection.

Keratinocytes in head and neck squamous cell cancer (HNSCC) produce molecules that induce angiogenesis including interleukin-I (IL-8). Other cytokines, including vascular endothelial growth factor (VEGF) and colony stimulating factor (CDF-1), granulocyte macrophage colony stimulating factor (GM-CSF) and transforming growth factor beta (TGFβ-1), recruit peripheral blood monocytes (PBM) to the tumor microenvironment to modulate tumor growth.[7] Macrophages also secrete basic fibroblast growth factor (bFGF) and tumor necrosis factor-alpha (TNF-α). Recently Greer, Weed, Hoernig, et al.[8] have demonstrated that cortactin, a tyrosine kinase inhibitor, may play a role in tumor cell motility and may play a potential role in the metastatic spread of head and neck cancer.

In addition to these gene product investigations, studies have been instituted to identify the role of viral latency in oral cancer. Human papillomavirus (HPV), types 16 and 18, have been implicated in the etiology of oral neoplasia for over a decade.[9,10]

HISTOLOGIC AND TAXONOMIC CONSIDERATIONS

The mucous membrane that lines the oral cavity and contiguous structures is composed of a layer of stratified squamous epithelium, which overlies a fibrous connective tissue lamina propria and fibrofatty submucosa. Nerves, capillaries, and minor salivary glands are abundant throughout the supporting connective tissue. Subjacent to the mucous membrane, one may encounter muscle, as in the tongue or buccal mucosa, or bone or cartilage, as in the mandibular or maxillary alveolar processes that support the teeth.

TOOTH GERM APPARATUS

In order to understand the pathology of tumors arising from the tooth germ apparatus, it is necessary to understand the development of the tooth. The developing tooth germ originates as an invagination of a tubular epithelial extension of basal cells from the stomadeal ectoderm overlying the developing alveolar ridges. This tubular extension is composed of cuboidal epithelial cells enveloped by a basal lamina.

The dynamic relationships observed between tissues of the developing odontogenic apparatus are markedly influenced by epitheliomesenchymal interactions. As the dental lamina progressively invades the underlying connective tissue, differentiation at the terminal end ensues. The lamina degenerates to form the inner enamel epithelium, outer enamel epithelium, and a central zone encased by these two epithelial layers. The central region is composed of an aggregate of stellate cells termed the stellate reticulum. The inner enamel epithelium differentiates further to become a layer of tall columnar cells with oval nuclei polarized away from the basal lamina. This characteristic cell, an ameloblast, is a hallmark of enamel epithelium. In juxtaposition to this ameloblastic layer and interposed between the ameloblasts and stellate reticulum is an intermediate layer of cuboidal cells termed the stratum intermedium.

As the epithelial element differentiates in this fashion, the underlying connective tissue assumes a unique quality. Subjacent to the epithelial cap of the tooth germ is a condensation of mesenchyme, which will become the vital tooth pulp. The cells are spindle shaped, and the fibrous element is delicate. At this stage, a layer of connective tissue cells begins to differentiate in juxtaposition to the ameloblastic layer. These cells are derivatives of the neural crest and are referred to as ectomesoderm. At the interface, the ectomesodermal cells (odontoblasts) become elongated and begin to elaborate an eosinophilic matrix, which will become dentin, the principal calcified substance of the tooth. Subsequent to the elaboration of a predentin layer by odontoblasts, the ameloblasts begin to synthesize a keratin matrix, which will eventually calcify as enamel, the surface structure of the tooth. The integrated efforts of the odontoblastic and ameloblastic layers eventually generate the crown of the tooth.

The radicular (root) region is formed in a similar fashion, whereby tubular extensions from the enamel epithelium progressively grow deeper into the developing alveolar bone, accompanied by continued differentiation of odontoblasts. After dentin is synthesized along this lattice, the epithelial component degenerates. The connective tissue adjacent to the developing root region buttresses the dentin layer, which was previously shielded by an epithelial layer; these mesenchymal cells differentiate into cementoblasts and generate a layer of cementum, which coats the radicular dentin. Sharpey's fibers become inserted into the cemental tissues and pass through the adjacent fibrous tissue, interlacing with fibers inserted into the developing alveolar osseous tissue to create the periodontal ligament of the tooth. As root development proceeds, an eruptive force is created, pushing the tooth toward the surface epithelium until it erupts into the oral cavity.

As tooth development proceeds, remnants of progenitor cells remain entrapped within the jaws. Three primary sources for oncogenic change remain:

1. Remnants of the dental lamina residing in the mature adult gingiva (rests of Serres);

2. Remnants of the radicular epithelial projections of the tooth germ residing throughout the periodontal ligament (rests of Malassez); and
3. Remnants of the ameloblastic layer overlying the crown of a tooth that failed to erupt (reduced enamel epithelium surrounding the crown of impacted teeth).

Thus cysts of odontogenic origin are ultimately derived from epithelial rests, dental laminal remnants, degenerated epithelium surrounding a tooth that is impacted or unerupted, or from the tooth germ itself.

All these odontogenic epithelial sources can undergo neoplastic transformation. It is theorized that during odontogenic oncogenesis, the epithelial component alone may proliferate; the epithelial component may influence surrounding connective tissue to differentiate and to proliferate in the absence of the epithelium itself; or the neoplasm may recapitulate tooth formation by neoplastic proliferation of both epithelial and mesenchymal tissues. These three possibilities account for classifying tumors as epithelial, mesenchymal, or mixed neoplasms, respectively. Figures 22.1 through 22.3 delineate the proposed histogenesis of odontogenic neoplasms.

CYSTS OF ODONTOGENIC ORIGIN

The bulk of the cysts that develop within the jaws arise from odontogenic epithelium and are classified as odontogenic cysts. Odontogenic cysts can broadly be categorized as developmental or inflammatory. In the strictest sense, a cyst that occurs at the root apex in association with a nonvital tooth is also odontogenic in origin, but custom continues to dictate that such cysts are classified as inflammatory cysts. Odontogenic cysts can develop during any stage of odontogenesis, including development within the enamel organ, in reduced enamel epithelium or in epithelial odontogenic remnants. The etiology of cyst formation is unknown. Figure 22.4 shows a schematic representation of the various odontogenic cysts. Table 22.1 delineates the classification of the most common odontogenic cysts. The periapical cyst and dentigerous cyst are far and away the most frequently occurring lesions. Nonodontogenic cysts are discussed later in this chapter.

Table 22.1 Odontogenic cysts

Classification schema
Developmental
Dentigerous cyst
Eruption cyst
Odontogenic keratocyst
Gingival cyst
Lateral periodontal cyst
Calcifying odontogenic cyst[a]
Botryoid odontogenic cyst
Inflammatory
Radicular (periapical) cyst
Residual cyst
Paradental cyst

[a] Classified as a neoplasm by the World Health Organization.[18]
From Kramer IRH, Pindborg JJ, Shear J. Histological typing of odontogenic tumors, 2nd edn. Berlin: Springer-Verlag; 1992.

Fig. 22.1 Histogenesis of epithelial odontogenic tumors.

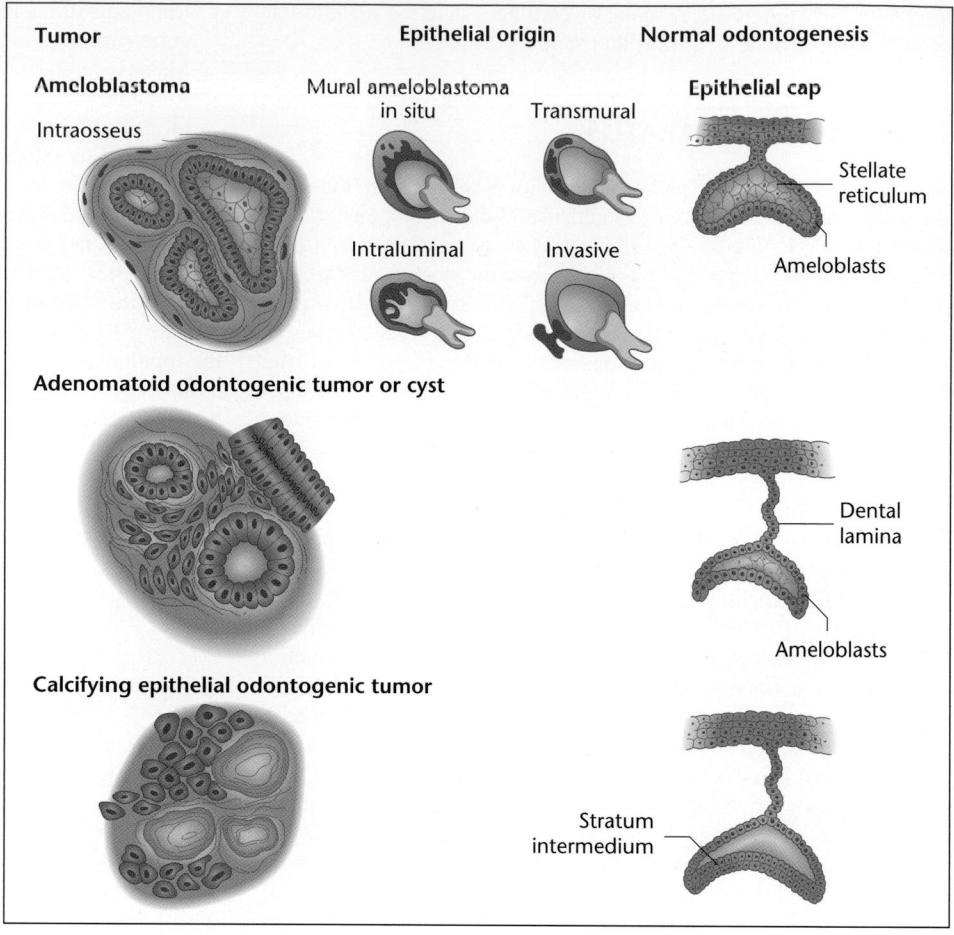

DENTIGEROUS CYST

The dentigerous cyst (follicular cyst) is a common odontogenic cyst that occurs in association with the crown of an unerupted tooth. This cyst develops when the enamel-forming apparatus (enamel organ) has been reduced to a few layers of epithelial cells surrounding the tooth crown. Fluid accumulates within the potential follicular space of the organ, and a cyst eventuates. Typically, the crown of the tooth protrudes into the cystic cavity.

Clinical and radiologic features

The dentigerous cyst is most commonly found in association with impacted or partially impacted mandibular third molars, maxillary canine teeth (cuspid teeth), and maxillary third molars. Radiologically, the dentigerous cyst will present as a well-defined radiolucent area surrounding the crown of a tooth. The lesion may be displaced to one side of the tooth crown and need not always arise superficial to it.

The radiolucency may be unilocular or multilocular. The lesion has the potential to expand bone, and the cyst may cause extensive destruction of bone, with almost complete replacement of the medullary portion of the ramus and body of the mandible by the cyst. It is not always possible to definitively diagnose a dentigerous cyst radiologically, because odontogenic keratocysts and certain odontogenic tumors such as ameloblastoma and odontogenic myxoma may have similar appearances.

Stanley[11] reviewed a 20 year series of 11 598 radiographs from patients with dentigerous cysts and found little evidence of internal resorption, bone loss adjacent to the distal surface of the approximating second molar teeth, or resorption of adjacent second molars. These data seem to dispute the current practice of early extraction of totally embedded third molars when adverse signs and symptoms are absent. Nonetheless, from a diagnostic point of view a unicystic lesion with clinical and radiologic characteristics of a dentigerous cyst may, in fact, prove to be an ominous lesion. Ameloblastoma has been shown to be a real consequence of dentigerous cyst formation in South African blacks.

Pathologic features

Grossly, the lesion will appear as a sac enveloping the tooth. The distinction between a dentigerous cyst and a hyperplastic dental follicle with cystic degeneration is often an arbitrary one because of the histologic similarity between the two. The diagnosis of dentigerous cyst is often based on the size of the gross specimen and the degree of radiologic involvement.

It is extremely important to examine the cyst wall for thickenings and outgrowths because there are well-documented instances of ameloblastoma or even squamous cell carcinoma arising in the walls of dentigerous cysts.

Histologically, the dentigerous cyst consists of lining epithelium supported by a fibrous connective tissue wall. The epithelium is generally of the stratified squamous variety and only a few cell layers thick. Occasionally, columnar or mucus-secreting cells may line the cyst.

The cyst wall may be diffusely inflamed or totally free of an inflammatory infiltrate. Frequently, the cyst wall contains extensive

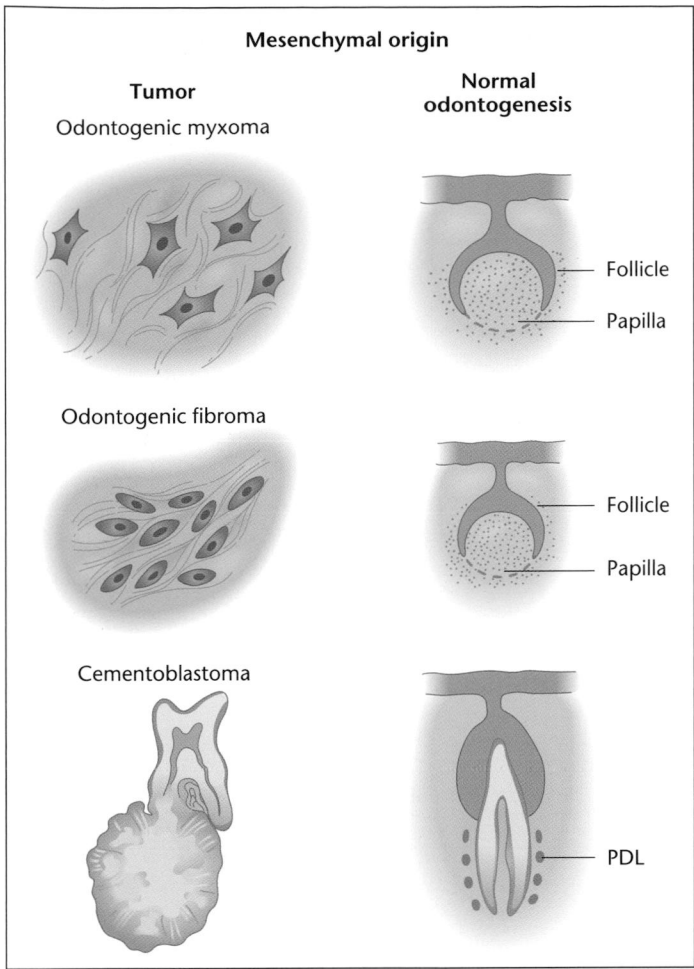

Fig. 22.2 Histogenesis of odontogenic tumors of mesenchymal origin.

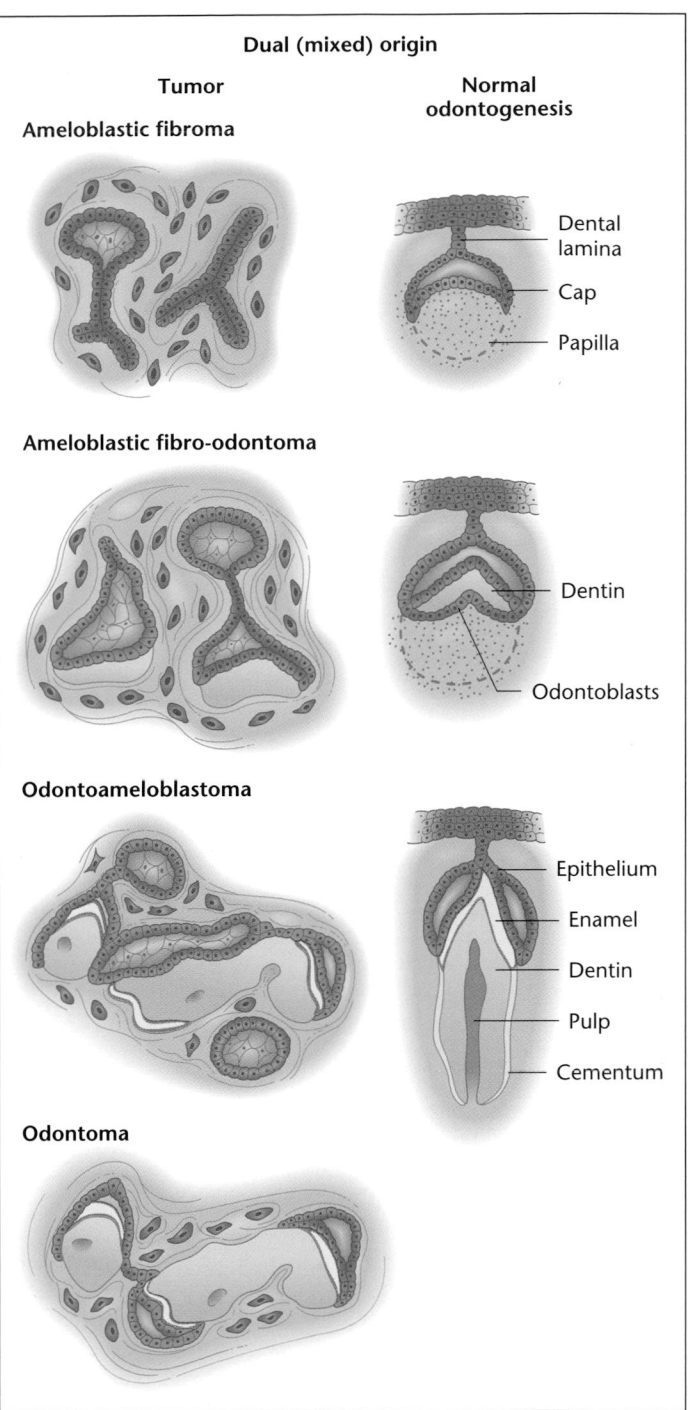

Fig. 22.3 Histogenesis of odontogenic tumors of mixed epithelial and mesenchymal origin.

cholesterol clefting so as to resemble a radicular or periapical cyst; when such clefting is noted microscopically, only the anatomic location allows one to differentiate between a dentigerous and a periapical cyst.

It is quite common to observe odontogenic epithelial rests in the walls of dentigerous cysts. There is considerable debate as to whether these rests have the potential to develop along neoplastic lines; nonetheless, it is very important to relay to the clinician the presence of rest activity in the walls of all odontogenic cysts. All dentigerous cysts should be examined with multiple histologic sections for ameloblastoma.

Behavior and management

The dentigerous cyst is most often adequately managed by complete removal of the lesion from its bony cavity via enucleation, and bony curettage. Occasionally, lesions that show extensive bony involvement are managed by multiple surgical enucleation procedures. Recurrence is a possibility in all cysts that have odontogenic epithelial remnants within bone at surgery.

Eruption cyst

The eruption cyst is simply a variant of the dentigerous cyst that is found in association with an erupting tooth. The lesion is most often seen in childhood, presenting as a bluish nodular excrescence above the erupting tooth. Eruption cysts most often rupture spontaneously. When they do not, excision of the roof of the cyst usually results in eruption of the tooth.

GINGIVAL CYSTS

Gingival cysts occur as two distinct entities, those of the newborn and those of the adult.[12] Gingival cysts of the newborn present as

Fig. 22.4 Schematic representation of the anatomic locations of the various cysts of odontogenic origin.

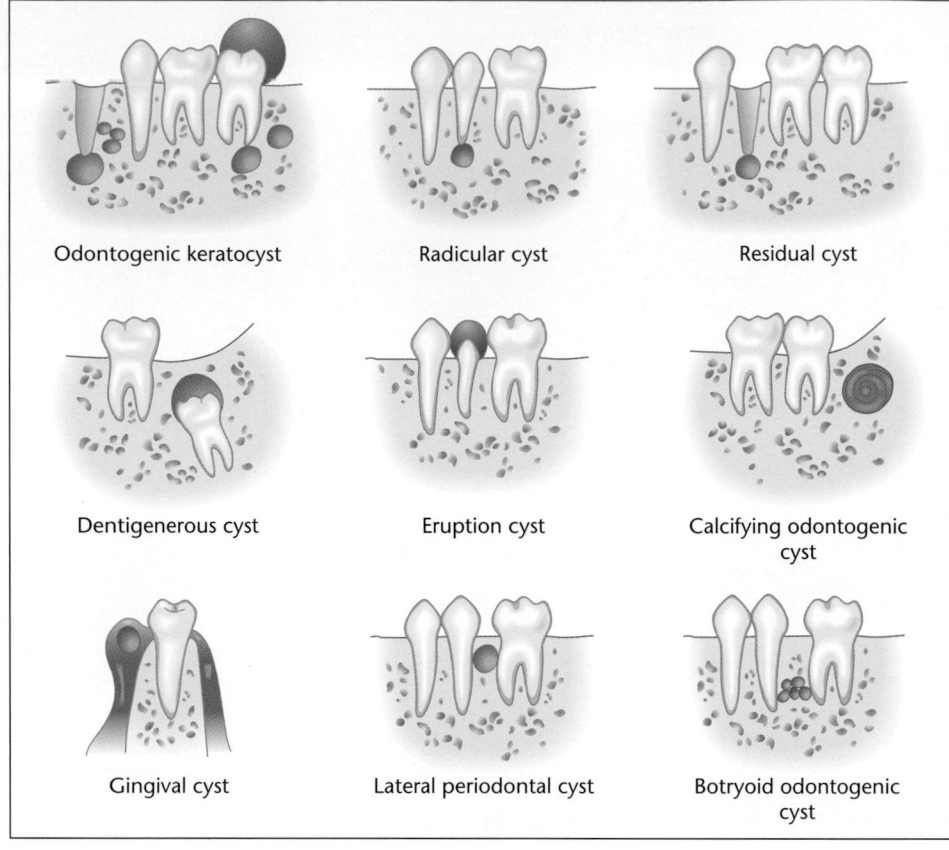

Odontogenic keratocyst   Radicular cyst   Residual cyst

Dentigenerous cyst   Eruption cyst   Calcifying odontogenic cyst

Gingival cyst   Lateral periodontal cyst   Botryoid odontogenic cyst

single or multiple small white nodules along the crest of the alveolar ridge. These excrescences have been variously reported in the literature as microcysts of the gingiva, Bohn's nodules, and Epstein's pearls.[13] These outgrowths, in fact, represent cystic degeneration of remnants of the dental lamina. They are usually asymptomatic and exfoliated without consequence. Histologically, they appear as keratin-filled cysts lined by stratified squamous epithelium. The lesions most often involute on their own.

Gingival cysts of the adult are quite common. They also are thought to originate from dental lamina remnants and represent the soft tissue counterpart of the lateral periodontal cyst. Gardner and Sapp[14] point out that these lesions may also arise from traumatic implantation of surface epithelium from the oral cavity into the underlying connective tissue. The most frequent site for the gingival cyst of the adult is in the mandibular cuspid and premolar area; interestingly, this is a frequent site for supernumerary teeth as well. Gingival cysts usually present clinically as painless swellings. Histologically, the gingival cyst of the adult mimics that of the newborn. Gingival cysts have little, if any, potential for recurrence, and simple enucleation is curative.

BOTRYOID ODONTOGENIC CYST AND LATERAL PERIODONTAL CYST

The botryoid odontogenic cyst was first described by Weathers and Waldron in 1973.[15] They defined this cyst as an unusual multilocular cyst of the anterior jaw. Since that time, additional cases have been reported in the literature. Many authorities consider the lesion to be simply a variant of a lateral periodontal cyst,[16] a rare unilocular cyst

of odontogenic origin that develops most often in the mandibular cuspid/bicuspid region adjacent and lateral to the teeth.[17] Kaugers[17] reviewed the limited number of discussions of botryoid odontogenic cysts available in the literature and found a marked predilection for occurrence in the mandibular canine-premolar region in patients older than 50 years of age. The most common symptoms were clinical expansion and tenderness, but occasionally the lesions were asymptomatic.

The botryoid odontogenic cyst is thought to arise from proliferating rests of the dental lamina or displaced rests of Serres. Kaugers[17] maintains that to render a diagnosis of botryoid odontogenic cyst, the following criteria are necessary: (1) histologic features similar to those of the lateral periodontal cyst; (2) a multilocular radiographic pattern, which is most often noted but need not absolutely be present (Fig. 22.5); and (3) no evidence of inflammatory origin from either pulpal or periodontal elements.

The histologic appearance of the botryoid odontogenic cyst is characterized by multiple cystic areas within a lesion showing no evidence of atypia and overlying epithelial keratinization. The polycystic areas are lined by two to three layers of cells with abundant cytoplasm and a lack of keratinization. The cells often pile up in a lobular or plaque-like pattern, extending into the lumen of the cyst (Fig. 22.6) and showing linkage and positivity with periodic acid–Schiff staining. The lateral periodontal cyst demonstrates similar histologic findings but remains unilocular.

Treatment and prognosis

The treatment of choice is surgical enucleation for either of the two lesions. Because the botryoid odontogenic cyst is often radiographically multilocular, there may be an increased risk of recurrence

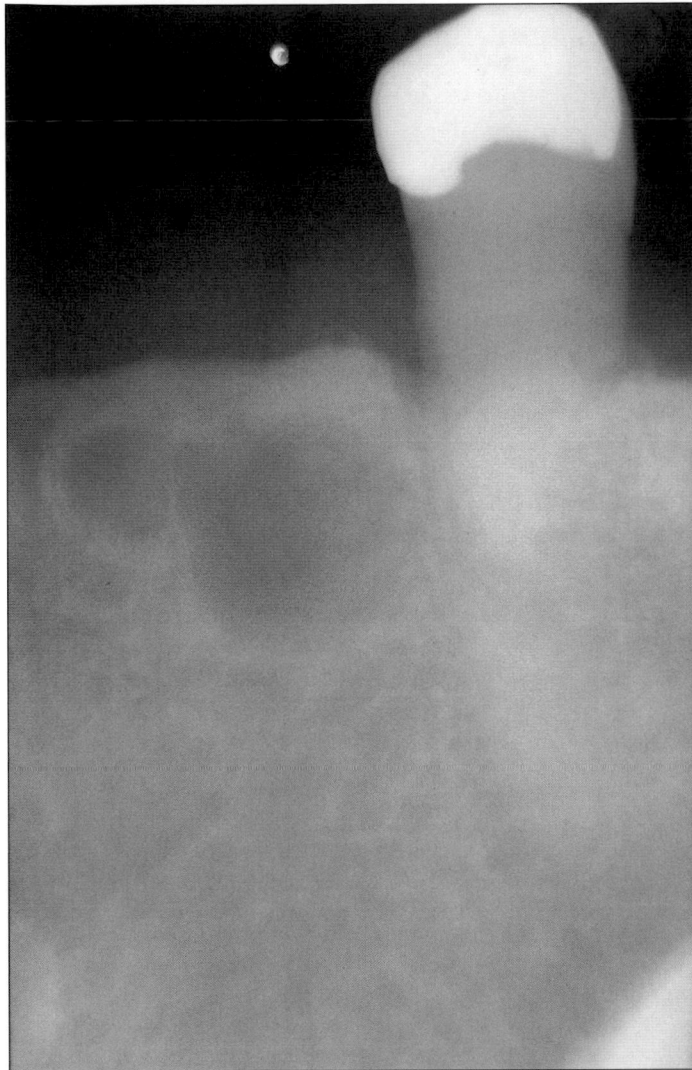

Fig. 22.5 Loculated botryoid odontogenic cyst of the mandible.

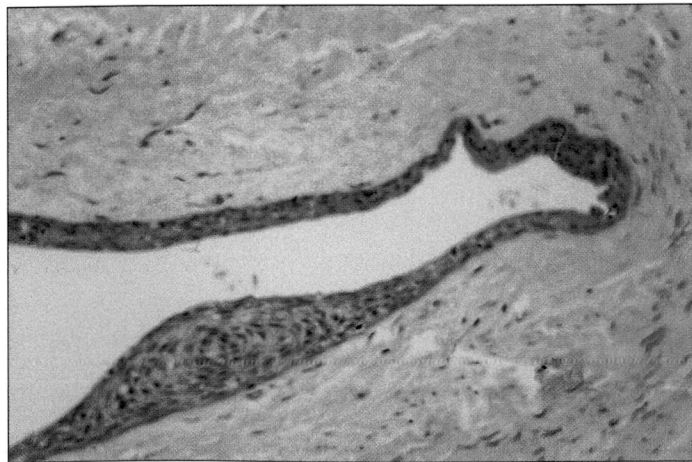

Fig. 22.6 Characteristic plaque-like extension of epithelial cells into the lumen of a botryoid odontogenic cyst.

or of persistence, and it is recommended that patients who have this diagnosis be given periodic clinical and radiographic examinations. The lateral periodontal cyst has a lower recurrence rate.

ODONTOGENIC KERATOCYST

The odontogenic keratocyst is a unique developmental odontogenic cyst with a defining histopathology and distinctive clinical behavior. The term odontogenic keratocyst was once used interchangeably with *primordial* cyst, but the current World Health Organization (WHO) taxonomy no longer uses the two terms synonymously.[18]

The etiology and pathogenesis of the odontogenic keratocyst remain undetermined, although most investigators suggest that the lesion arises from remnants of the dental lamina, from basal cells of oral epithelium (60%), or reduced enamel epithelium of the dental follicle (40%).[19] Eversole and associates[20] have suggested that the odontogenic keratocyst and other odontogenic cysts can arise from reduced enamel epithelium as well as from other follicular odontogenic remnants derived from lining epithelial cells. Stoelinga and Peters[21] conclude, however, that some of these cysts arise from other sources, perhaps oral epithelium, especially in areas of the mandible, such as the ascending ramus, where it is difficult to identify residual dental laminal tissues.

This terminology presupposes that only a cyst arising without association to a tooth can be a keratocyst. Although this may, in fact, be the general rule, exceptions certainly do occur, and numerous well-documented reports in the literature support the fact that dentigerous cysts (those cysts associated with the crown of a tooth[22]) and even residual cysts (those remaining after previous extraction of a tooth or enucleation of a cyst[23]) may have the histologic features and a behavioral pattern identical to that of the insidious odontogenic keratocyst.

A critical fact for the surgical pathologist to remember is that the odontogenic keratocyst may be in direct association with a tooth, or it may occur after tooth extraction. It need not always occur when there is a history of failure of a tooth to develop, as with the primordial variety.

Clinical and radiologic features

Philipsen[24] first used the term odontogenic keratocyst in 1956 to describe any odontogenic cyst displaying microscopic keratinization of the epithelial lining. The lesion has since been reported to account for anywhere from 8% to 10% of all jaw cysts.[25,26] These cystic lesions show a marked predilection for the posterior body of the mandible and occur most frequently in the second and third decades of life. The lesion shows a variable radiologic pattern. Browne[27] described three distinct radiologic appearances in a series of 83 cases. He documented 56% as having a unilocular pattern, 20% as a solitary cavity with a locular periphery, and 23% as multilocular. Figure 22.7 demonstrates a largely unilocular lesion of the mandible. The peak incidence is in the teenage years and twenties although the odontogenic keratocyst can occur in all ages.

The odontogenic keratocyst can have a peripheral radiographic border that is smooth or scalloped. Aggressive lesions may result in displacement of impacted teeth or resorption of the roots of teeth. Extrusion of erupted teeth has also been reported.

The odontogenic keratocyst tends to grow slowly. The patient is frequently symptomless. When a complaint is encountered, it is usually the notation of swelling by the patient, pain, or tooth mobility. Large cysts can provoke a marked inflammatory response because of keratin leakage.

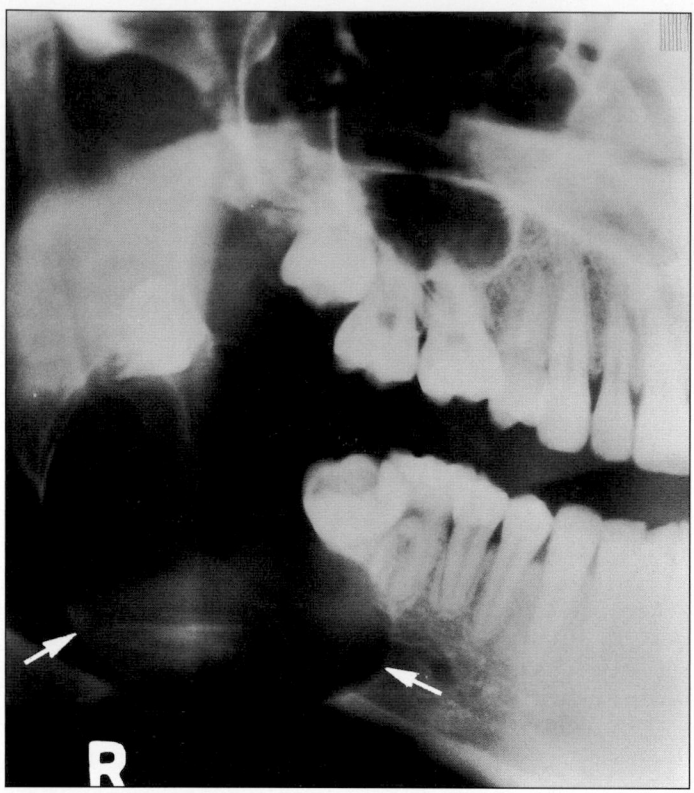

Fig. 22.7 Odontogenic keratocyst of the mandible.

Pathologic features

The salient histologic features of odontogenic keratocyst have been discussed by many authorities but probably were most succinctly described by Gardner and Sapp,[14] who indicate that the following microscopic features are necessary to arrive at a diagnosis: (1) a thin stratified squamous epithelial lining six to eight cells thick, without rete ridge formation; (2) prominent columnar or cuboidal, often budding, basal cells with dense nuclear staining; (3) a corrugated surface layer of parakeratin; and (4) a thin connective tissue wall. Figure 22.8 shows the classic histopathology of an odontogenic keratocyst. So-called 'satellite' or 'daughter' cysts may occur within the connective tissue wall.

Not all cysts displaying keratinization are odontogenic keratocysts. One cannot therefore render a diagnosis of odontogenic keratocyst simply because the cyst lumen is filled with keratin. If the salient features described above are not present, the lesion should not be designated an odontogenic keratocyst. It is probably some other form of odontogenic, fissural, or inflammatory jaw cyst. Keratinizing odontogenic cysts mimic the true odontogenic keratocyst, but they have a flat basal layer and they are orthokeratinized.

Nonetheless, two specific histologic variants of the odontogenic keratocyst are often recognized: the parakeratotic and the orthokeratotic subtypes. The predominant form is parakeratotic.[28] Wright[29] reviewed a series of odontogenic keratocysts and demonstrated a peak incidence in the third decade of life, with a male predominance. The vast majority of the lesions he identified (72%) were unilocular. The keratotic variant was found to be somewhat less aggressive than the parakeratotic type and recurred in only 1 of 24 patients, who were followed for periods ranging from 6 months to 8 years. Some investigators report that orthokeratinizing lesions are a separate lesional subtype,[28] but Crowley and Kaugars[30] suggest that separate subclassification is probably unwarranted.

The high rate of recurrence of this lesion may be related to the frequency of proliferation of daughter cysts in the wall, the penetration or budding of exceedingly thin epithelium into the connective tissue (often resulting in incomplete removal), or the reinitiated proliferation of cyst lining from remnants of the dental lamina.

A frequently noted histologic feature associated with the odontogenic keratocyst has been the separation of the epithelial cyst lining from the supporting connective tissue capsule. Wilson and Ross[31] examined this feature ultrastructurally because it had been hypothesized that the separation very likely accounted for the difficulty in surgical removal and resultant elevated recurrence rate. These investigators found the basal lamina complex in odontogenic keratocyst to be ultrastructurally normal and could not fully explain the separation phenomenon except to hypothesize that there is somehow increased enzymatic collagen degradation.

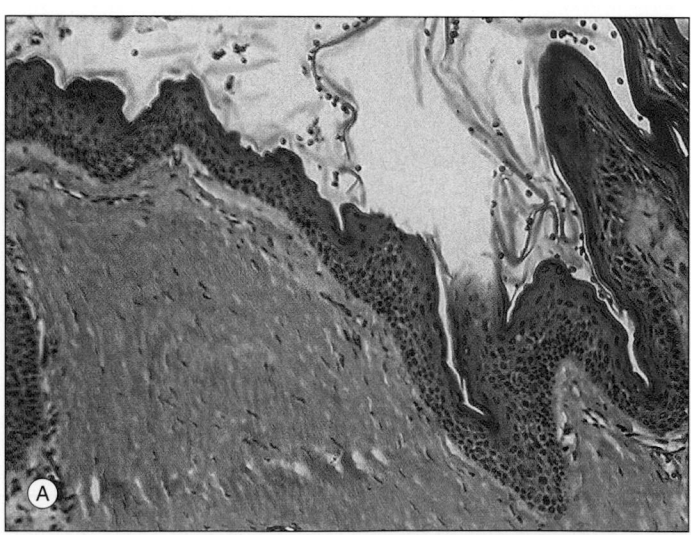
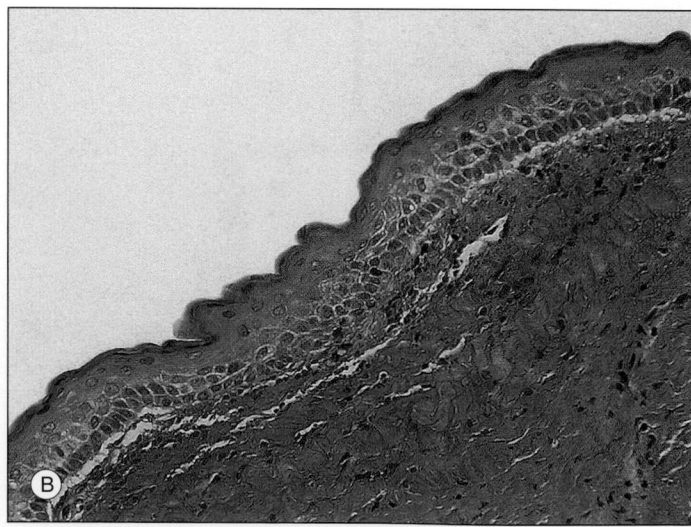

Fig. 22.8 A,B, Characteristic parakeratinized corrugated lining of the odontogenic keratocyst.

Behavior and management

The most striking clinical feature of the odontogenic keratocyst is its propensity for recurrence. The consistent recurrence rate documented in large reported series is about 25%, although reports in the literature range from 6% to 60%.[28]

Treatment has ranged from enucleation of unilocular lesions to marsupialization and shrinkage cystectomy, or resection of a considerable portion of the affected jaw in large multilocular, expanding, or erosive lesions.[25]

Marx[19] maintains that the two most common reasons for recurrence of odontogenic keratocytes are failure to remove the original cyst lining in toto and new primary cyst formations from pluripotential odontogenic rests of oral basal layer epithelium.

It has been well documented that odontogenic keratocysts can be a component of the nevoid basal cell carcinoma syndrome, with its concomitant multiple cutaneous nevoid basal cell carcinomas and skeletal abnormalities, dyskeratotic pitting of the hands and feet, and ectopic soft tissue calcifications. It is exceedingly important that the clinician and pathologist consider the possibility of this syndrome in any patient with an established diagnosis of odontogenic keratocyst. It is essential to have a high index of syndrome suspicion in patients with multiple odontogenic keratocysts or with a family history of multiple cysts of the jaws.

CALCIFYING ODONTOGENIC CYST

Clinical and radiologic features

The calcifying odontogenic cyst is a curious lesion that was first thoroughly described by Gorlin and associates[26] in 1962, although they document that it was reported by Rywland much earlier. The calcifying odontogenic cyst typically presents as a slow-growing asymptomatic central osseous jaw lesion that is thought to arise from rests of Serres. Extraosseous examples have been documented in the literature, but they represent fewer than 25% of reported lesions.[32-36] The lesions have a marked predilection of the maxilla and they occur more frequently in females. The lesions can occur at any age but are most common in teenagers. Regardless of a maxillary or mandibular occurrence, over 75% of the lesions reported in the series of Freedman and associates[28] occurred anterior to the first molar.

Radiologically, the intraosseous lesion appears as a unilocular or multilocular cystic radiolucent area. The margins may be well defined or poorly demarcated, and small irregular calcified bodies of varying sizes have been reported in 29–37% of all reported cases (Fig. 22.9).[35,36]

These calcifications may fill the cyst cavity entirely or may be totally absent; therefore, the presence or absence of such calcifications is of questionable value in unequivocally establishing a radiologic diagnosis. Numerous odontogenic tumors can have radiologic features that are quite similar to the calcifying and keratinizing odontogenic cyst. Such lesions should be included in the radiologic differential diagnosis. They include the calcifying epithelial odontogenic tumor, adenomatoid odontogenic tumor, ameloblastic odontoma, and the so-called cystic odontoma.

Keszler and Gugliemotti[35] reported two calcifying odontogenic cysts associated with odontomas. The WHO International Classification of Odontogenic Tumors and Allied Lesions defines the calcifying odontogenic cyst as a neoplastic lesion that can occur in association with other odontogenic lesions, including odontomas.[18]

There has been extended debate in the literature as to whether the calcifying odontogenic cyst represents a cyst or a tumor, because the lesion can present grossly as a cyst or a solid mass. The calcified

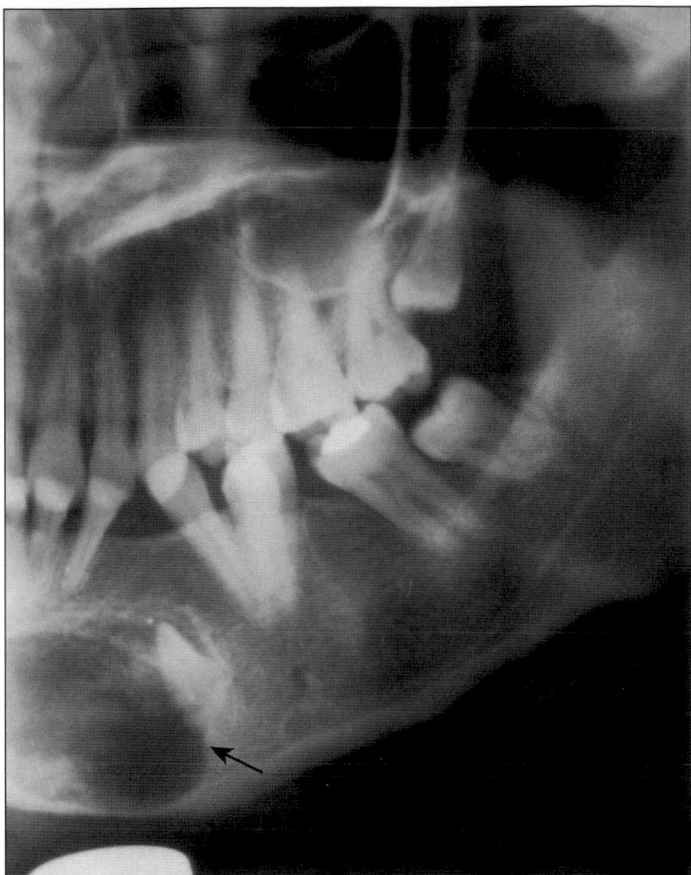

Fig. 22.9 Calcifying odontogenic cyst with rudimentary tooth structure at periphery.

structures identified radiologically can have the gross appearance of irregular hard tissue fragments or even small teeth or denticle-like structures.

Gorlin and colleagues[26] have reported the lesion originating from the dental epithelium of a developing unerupted tooth. Lesions that develop in an extraosseous site likely develop from remnants of odontogenic epithelium in the gingiva or alveolar mucosa.

Pathologic features

The calcifying odontogenic cyst can present grossly as a sac-like soft tissue structure or as a solid mass with calcified foci. Histologically, tissue sections reveal a cavity or potential cavity lined by a prominent and well-defined basal layer of cuboidal or columnar cells that have some resemblance to ameloblasts. These cells stain deeply basophilic. Overlying the basal epithelial layer, loosely arranged epithelial cells that resemble the central stellate reticulum of the tooth germ can be identified. Interspersed among these cells are large eosinophilic cells, which have been termed ghost cells (Fig. 22.10). These cells are thought to have undergone aberrant keratinization, and occasionally they flatten out in a manner similar to normal keratin. The entire lumen of the cyst may be filled with aberrant keratin, and on occasion foreign body giant cell activity is prominent in the cyst lumen and in the supporting capsular connective tissue wall.

Sauk[36] and Freedman et al.[28] have documented that the basal epithelial layer can show prominent budding and that odontogenic

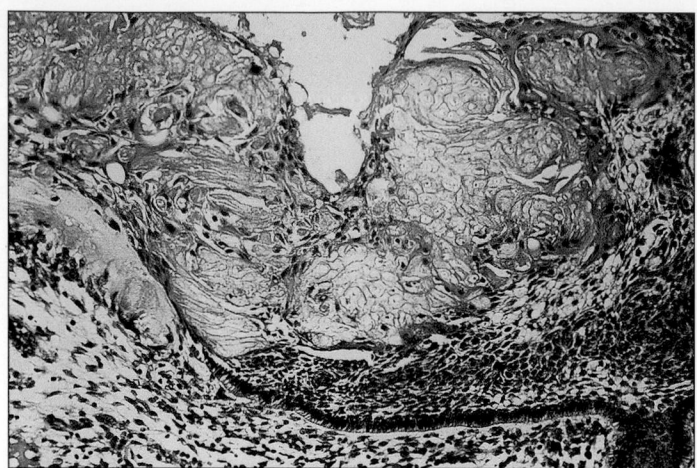

Fig. 22.10 Calcifying odontogenic cyst displaying ghost-like cells, aberrant keratin, and calcifications. Note prominence of basal layer.

epithelium frequently penetrates deeply into the supporting collagenous wall. Dentin, enamel, and even melanin have been reported proliferating within the wall of calcifying odontogenic cysts.

Behavior and management

Recurrence of the calcifying odontogenic cyst is exceedingly rare. Even the most conservative form of enucleation appears to be curative. There appears to be little potential for the lesion to develop into an odontogenic tumor, and although there are cases reported in the literature of the cyst occurring in association with an ameloblastic fibro-odontoma, there is concern that the reported cases may not represent a true calcifying odontogenic cyst.[36] The more likely sequence is that the lesion represented cystic change in a true odontogenic tumor.

CARCINOMA ARISING IN ASSOCIATION WITH ODONTOGENIC CYSTS

Malignant neoplasia arising in concert with an odontogenic cyst is rare. Neville et al.[37] have suggested that fewer than 100 adequately documented cases appear in the world literature but caution that epithelial atypia in the epithelial lining of odontogenic cysts may be appreciated more frequently than it is reported.

The most commonly documented form of neoplasia reported to occur in and with the walls of an odontogenic cyst is squamous cell carcinoma. Treatment has ranged from marginal resection to radical resection in association with radiation or chemotherapy. Five-year survival rates are no greater than 50%.[38]

GLANDULAR ODONTOGENIC CYST (SIALO-ODONTOGENIC CYST)

The glandular odontogenic cyst remains an enigma in the literature. Most authorities suggest that the lesion, which was first described in 1990, is in fact actually a low-grade mucoepidermoid carcinoma. Nonetheless, some investigators continue to suggest that the lesion is a true cyst of glandular origin.[39] It has been our experience, based on seeing multiple recurrences of these lesions,

that the glandular odontogenic cyst is not a cyst at all but a low-grade mucoepidermoid carcinoma. Too few of these cases have been reported in the literature to definitely establish a prognosis for the lesion. Until more lesions are accessioned, discussion of whether or not the lesion is a truly unusual odontogenic cyst with a glandular component or a low-grade mucoepidermoid carcinoma will remain.

INFLAMMATORY, FISSURAL, AND NONODONTOGENIC CYSTS

RADICULAR CYST

Radicular cysts account for approximately 10% of all inflammatory cysts.[40] The radicular cyst is far and away the most common cyst of the jaws. It is also known as periapical cyst, apical periodontal cyst, and dental cyst. Classically, the lesion is the end result of extensive dental caries and pulpal death.

When a carious lesion extends uncontrolled beyond the hard tissue of the tooth, the pulp subsequently becomes inflamed. Ultimately, the process can extend along the root canal of the tooth, beyond the apical foramen, and into the periapical ligamental tissues and bone. The localized inflammatory process that results from the extension of noxious stimuli beyond the apex of the tooth is typically called an apical granuloma. It is, of course, not a true granuloma but an accumulation of chronic inflammatory granulation tissue. Epithelial rests (rests of Malassez) are commonly found around the root apices, and as the inflammatory process continues, these rests frequently proliferate as strands of epithelium into the granulation tissue, with subsequent central degeneration and ultimate cyst formation.

Clinical and radiologic features

By the time a periapical cyst has formed, the patient is usually symptom free. Typically, the pulp is dead and the tooth is nonvital. Radicular cysts expand slowly, and there is usually little if any expansion of the jaw associated with them.

Radiologically, the lesion will present as a fairly well-circumscribed area of radiolucency generally measuring 0.5–2.0 cm at the root apex. It is impossible to determine from radiologic findings alone whether the lesion represents a periapical cyst, periapical granuloma, or some other form of pathologic alteration.

Pathologic features

The surgical specimen usually consists of fragments of glistening or granular soft tissue. Rarely is the tooth removed with the cyst intact. If surgical root canal therapy has been performed, the periapical remnants may be submitted as fragments from the surgical site. The cyst lining is only rarely appreciated as a shiny surface, and a lumen containing fluid or cheesy material is seen only when the specimen is submitted intact.

Microscopically, one usually finds fragments of lining and penetrating squamous epithelium supported by a diffusely and chronically inflamed connective tissue wall. Cholesterol clefts are frequently present in the cyst lumen or wall. Foam cells, plasma cells, lymphocytes, and foreign body-type giant cells are also commonly identified. Hyalinized Rushton bodies, thought to be unique to odontogenic cysts, can be identified in about 10% of the lesions.[41] This unique finding is often helpful in attempting to separate odontogenic from fissural cysts.

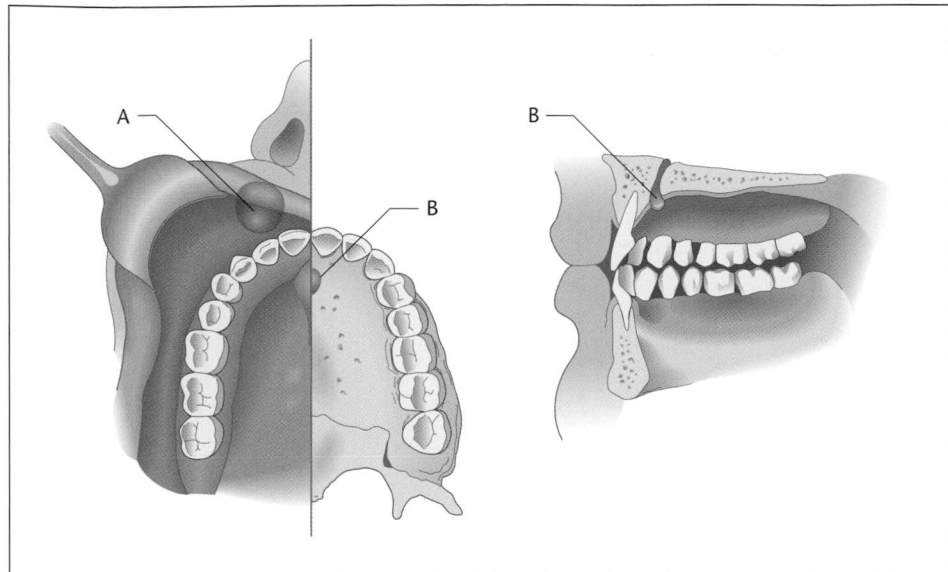

Fig. 22.11 Diagram illustrating the typical location of the nasolabial cyst (**A**) and the nasopalatine duct cyst (**B**).

The *residual radicular cyst* is thought to represent a cystic remnant that remains in the jaw after the associated tooth or teeth have been extracted or after failure of root canal therapy. Most often this term is used to indicate that the lesion is a residual radicular cyst; however, a residual cyst could certainly occur after incomplete removal of any cystic lesion. Most residual radicular cysts remain asymptomatic within the jaws and are only identified via a routine radiologic examination of the area.

Radicular cysts are not considered to have the potential to differentiate along odontogenic tumor lines, as do the odontogenic keratocyst and dentigerous cyst. Exceedingly rare cases of squamous cell carcinoma have been reported, apparently arising in association with the wall of radicular cysts.[11]

PARADENTAL CYST

The paradental cyst is a unique inflammatory odontogenic cyst that arises in association with mandibular third molar teeth that are partially erupted and thus it is a clinical variant of the dentigerous cyst. The cyst is almost exclusive to males, rarely exceeds 2 cm in diameter, and is generally adherent to the upper one-third of the affected tooth root.[42] This cyst rarely expands or destroys bony tissue and is treated adequately by enucleation.

FISSURAL AND DEVELOPMENTAL NON-ODONTOGENIC CYSTS

For decades, it has been postulated that fissural cysts are those cysts that arise from remnants of epithelium that were trapped within fusion lines during formation of the face or from remnants of embryologic ductal elements.[43–45] A schematic representation of the anatomic sites of each of these cysts is presented in Figure 22.11.

Today, most authorities recognize that fissural cysts arise not from bony entrapment but simply from embryonic epithelial remnants.[19] It has been documented that epithelial entrapment along suture lines occurs only along the medial palatal raphe, leading to the conclusion that the classification of fissural cysts is more in deference to convenience than to developmental biology. Notwithstanding the controversy concerning their origin, so-called fissural cysts have the potential to expand and destroy bone, thus they remain of considerable biologic significance.

NASOPALATINE DUCT CYST

The nasopalatine duct cyst, also known as the *incisive canal cyst*, is the most commonly encountered of the fissural cysts, and the most common nonodontogenic oral cavity cyst as well. It is thought to be derived from residua of the nasopalatine duct, an embryonic structure that actually is housed within the incisive canals of the maxilla.

Clinical and radiologic features

Linear radiologic surveys of large groups of patients indicate that the nasopalatine duct cyst occurs in approximately 1% of those persons examined.[37] The lesions commonly present as well-circumscribed, oval, heart-shaped, or occasionally elliptical radiolucencies behind the central incisors in the mid-maxilla.

Clinically, an obvious intraoral swelling can be identified, but rarely is the lesion symptomatic unless it is secondarily infected. The lesion occurs most often between the fourth to sixth decades of life and affects men twice as often as women.

At times, it is rather difficult to separate a true nasopalatine duct cyst from the normal radiologic shadow of the incisive canal. Gardner and Sapp[14] suggest that any lesion with a diameter greater than 6 mm should certainly be suggestive of a cyst. Cysts occurring in this same area that are wholly within soft tissue and present no radiologic picture are known as *cysts of palatine papilla*. Exceedingly large nasopalatine duct cysts with extensive posterior limits have been variously referred to as *median palatal cysts or mid-palatine cysts*.

Pathologic features

Microscopically, the nasopalatine duct cyst is an epithelially lined cavity rimmed by stratified squamous or respiratory epithelium. Occasionally, mucus glands, cartilage, bone, and nerve bundles are identified within or adjacent to the supporting connective tissue wall.

Nasopalatine duct cysts are treated by surgical enucleation and seldom recur.

NASOLABIAL CYST

The nasolabial cyst is a lesion of soft tissue rather than bone. It is thought to arise from embryonic residual epithelium derived from the nasolacrimal duct.

Clinical and radiologic features

The nasolabial cyst will usually present as a painless swelling in the nasolabial fold or as a swelling within the nostril itself. Most patients with the lesion are adults in the second, third, or fourth decades of life. The patient may complain of fullness in the area of the upper lip; pain is seldom a presenting symptom. The lesion may become so large that it totally fills the intraoral labial sulcus. Radiologically, there are usually no findings, unless the lesion has become so large that pressure resorption of the underlying alveolar bone has occurred. Although most nasolabial cysts are unilateral, bilateral occurrences have been documented.

Nearly three-quarters of all documented cases of nasolabial cyst have occurred in females, and there is a documented predilection for blacks.

Pathologic features

The nasolabial cyst may be lined by stratified squamous, cuboidal, or respiratory-type epithelium. Goblet secretory cells are also frequently encountered within the more prominent squamous epithelial lining. The supporting wall is generally one of avascular, often hyaline-appearing collagen.

For nasolabial cysts, the management modality of choice is surgical excision and enucleation; recurrence is uncommon.

LYMPHOEPITHELIAL CYST OF THE ORAL CAVITY

The lymphoepithelial cyst, similar histologically to the cervical lymphoepithelial cyst except for its smaller size, is thought to arise as a result of a developmental entrapment phenomenon. A popular developmental theory is that the cyst arises from crypts of lymphoid tissue that become occluded, resulting in ultimate cystic proliferation of the epithelium.[46–49] A second theory is that during embryogenesis, epithelium of glandular or ductal origin becomes included with lymphoid tissue, and subsequently this glandular epithelium undergoes cystic proliferation.[50] The oral lymphoepithelial cyst is histologically similar to the *branchial cyst* or *cervical lymphoepithelial cyst* but much smaller.

Clinical features

The cyst, which is usually yellow or white, is most often encountered in the floor of the mouth; in addition, it has been reported in nearly all other oral sites and in the parotid gland. Lymphoepithelial cysts are usually described clinically as freely movable nodular masses that are totally asymptomatic and rarely attain a size greater than 1 cm in diameter. Pain is seldom a feature, and the lesion is most often identified in young adults.

Pathologic features

Most lymphoepithelial cysts are relatively small. Guinta and Cataldo[48] reviewed a series of 21 lesions and found the average lesion to measure only 6 mm in diameter. The mucosal surface usually

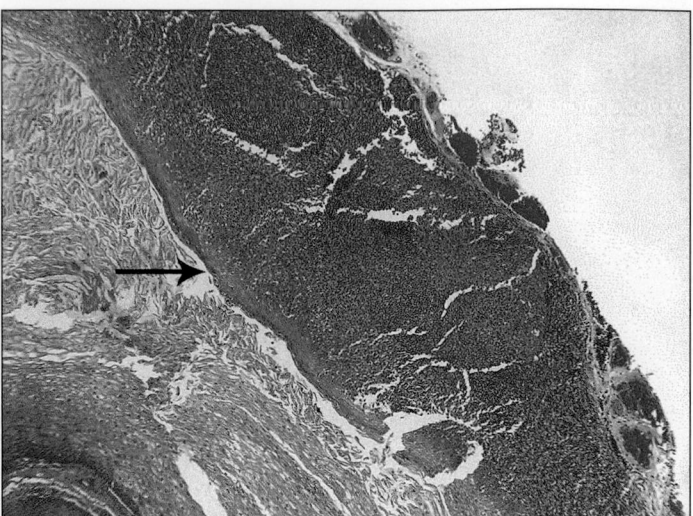

Fig. 22.12 Benign lymphoepithelial cyst demonstrating an epithelial lining (arrow) and a peripheral lymphoid rim.

appears normal. On sectioning, one may encounter yellow, cheesy material.

The histopathologic findings are rather consistent. Underlying normal oral epithelium is a cyst that is usually lined by a thin flattened layer of stratified squamous epithelium. The lumen is usually filled with amorphous eosinophilic coagulum, proteinaceous debris, and varying degrees of inflammatory cells. Subjacent to the epithelium one finds well-organized lymphoid tissue, usually encircling the entire cyst (Fig. 22.12). The lymphoid tissue, which often has a typical follicular pattern, is distributed throughout a supporting wall of loose areolar connective tissue.

Total surgical excision is the treatment of choice for oral lymphoepithelial cysts. In most large reported series, long-term follow-up has documented little tendency for recurrence.[48] *Branchial cysts*, which are usually filled with thin brown fluid, may be lined by respiratory-type epithelium. They require excision with ligation of their residual tract.

The lymphoepithelial cyst may also occur in the preauricular region in the parotid gland. Very rarely, branchial carcinomas have been reported in lymphoepithelial cysts.[51]

THYROGLOSSAL TRACT CYST

The thyroglossal tract cyst is a rather uncommon cyst that is thought to arise from residual epithelium after formation of the thyroid gland and is the most common cyst of the neck. Entrapment of this epithelium occurs during a period when the thyroglossal duct extends as a hollow tract from the foramen cecum at the base of the tongue to the thyroid gland. The cyst is commonly identified in close approximation and subjacent to the hyoid bone and usually arises after an upper respiratory tract infection, with most occurring over the thyroid membrane.

Thyroglossal tract cysts tend to be midline structures, typically arising as subcutaneous soft tissue swellings. They can develop at any age but are most frequent in the first two decades of life. Rarely do the lesions attain a size in excess of 5 cm, but there are cases reported in excess of 10 cm.[52]

Pathologic features

The typical thyroglossal tract cyst is lined by ciliated respiratory epithelium, pseudostratified columnar epithelium, or squamous epithelium. The supporting wall of the cyst will frequently contain accumulations of chronic inflammatory cells, and occasionally thyroid acini can be found in the cyst wall. Occasionally, mucus glands can be found in the wall. A few instances of carcinoma arising in thyroglossal remnants have been documented; therefore, evaluation of the specimen for excrescences or grossly thickened areas is mandatory. The most common carcinomas have been papillary adenocarcinomas.[53] As a differential diagnosis, the rare thymic cyst also has to be considered in the face of a midline neck swelling and a biopsy specimen that shows a cystic cavity. Usually, recognizable thymic tissue allows the separation of these two entities.

Surgical excision is the treatment of choice for thyroglossal duct cysts.

MUCOCELE AND ANTRAL CYSTS

Clinical and radiologic features

Although in the strictest sense the mucocele is a form of non-neoplastic salivary gland disease, not a developmental cyst, the lesion is presented here because it is one of the most frequently encountered cyst-like lesions of the oral cavity and it can occur in bone. The mucocele (mucus extravasation phenomenon, mucous retention cyst) is a common lesion that typically presents as an asymptomatic swelling with a central collection of mucus. Frequently, mucoceles have a so-called blue dome appearance. The etiology of the mucocele has been the subject of considerable scrutiny. One theory postulates that the mucocele occurs as a result of a salivary ductal stenosis or obstruction, which ultimately results in the accumulation of mucin and ductal dilation that presents clinically as a swelling. This theory assumes that all mucoceles would therefore be epithelially lined; in fact, when they are examined closely, most are not. A second theory suggests that some mucoceles result as a consequence of true rupture of the salivary gland duct system, allowing extravasation or precipitation of mucus into the surrounding connective tissue and submucosa. This theory suggests that most mucoceles are not, therefore, true mucous cysts because they have no epithelial lining.

The most frequent site for the mucocele is the labial mucosa of the lower lip. The upper lip is seldom, if ever, affected, probably because it is not subjected to the amount or degree of trauma that the lower lip and its minor salivary glands receive.[54]

Cysts similar to mucoceles have been reported in the maxillary sinus, including the *mucous retention cyst of the maxillary sinus* and the *surgical ciliated cyst of the maxilla*. The former lesion is best visualized on panoramic radiographs as a smooth, uniform, ovoid dome-shaped radiopacity of the sinus. The surgical ciliated cyst generally occurs as a unilocular or multilocular cystic lesion arising after surgical entry into the maxillary sinus. The maxillary sinus mucous retention cyst fails to have an epithelial lining and is instead lined by flattened fibroblasts and occasionally histiocytes. The surgical ciliated cyst is typically lined by respiratory-type epithelium.

Pathologic features

Histologically, the typical microscopic picture is that of benign squamous epithelium overlying a connective tissue lamina propria that contains either a dilated duct-like structure that is rimmed by flattened fibroblasts or, very rarely, epithelium. The channel-like structure will contain extravasated mucin, proteinaceous debris, and acute and chronic inflammatory cells. Mucoceles may present in a manner such that all that is identified histologically is extravasated mucin and inflammatory cells in a connective tissue stroma. Minor salivary gland acinar and ductal structures may be identified deep or lateral to the extravasated mucin.

Another common histologic feature is granulation tissue; in fact, granulation tissue frequently fills central areas of mucoceles, so that 80–90% of the tissue sample may represent granulation tissue, with very little evidence of extravasated mucin. A differential diagnosis that must be entertained in such instances is pyogenic granuloma, and frequently it is difficult to differentiate pyogenic granuloma from mucocele on the basis of histologic characteristics alone.

At times, it is difficult to distinguish a mucocele from a low-grade mucoepidermoid tumor histologically. In such instances, it is important to remember that grossly the mucoepidermoid tumor will nearly always have the appearance of a solid mass even when a large portion of the tumor is quite mucinous. The mucocele almost always manifests as a cyst. Mucoceles that occur in the floor of the mouth are termed *ranulas*.

Treatment and prognosis

Treatment is often problematic with mucoceles because it necessitates total removal of the damaged gland in addition to the associated cystic lining. If the gland is not removed as well as the cyst, mucus may continue to be extravasated into the tissues, and the mucocele will frequently recur. Two management modalities have been used. Most often, total surgical excision of the mucocele and the gland will remove the cause and the pathologic condition. A second surgical procedure that is often used is a marsupialization procedure, whereby the cyst is collapsed and its contents aspirated. Alginate is injected into the lesion so it becomes firm and the anatomic outline can be adequately visualized. Finally, excision at the borders of the alginate is used. The technique of marsupialization is one that is reserved for large lesions, typically in the floor of the mouth. The ranula typically develops in either of the two manners that a mucocele does, and surgical excision or marsupialization is the treatment modality of choice.

RARE NONONDONTOGENIC CYSTS

A host of rare, nonodontogenic cysts can occur in the oral cavity, including the *epidermal cyst (sebaceous cyst)*, thought to arise from hair follicle epithelium. Epidermal cysts are typically lined by stratified squamous epithelium and induced by trauma or embryonic inclusion. The *dermoid cyst*, which is a rare developmental cyst, is most often identified as a swelling in the floor of the mouth, and the *heterotopic oral gastrointestinal cyst* is a rare inclusion cyst which can be found throughout the length of the gastrointestinal tract, including the mouth. These lesions are all treated by complete surgical excision.

ODONTOGENIC TUMORS

Odontogenic tumors are a unique aggregate of lesions that range from true neoplasms to growths that are more accurately described as hamartomatous. The vast majority of these lesions are benign, but there are a few malignant variants. In the past, this diverse and interesting group of lesions has been classified according to tissue origin and inductive interaction between ectodermal and mesodermal components of the tooth germ appropriates. In 1992, the WHO

Table 22.2 Odontogenic tumors

A simplified classification for the surgical pathologist
A. Benign
I. Epithelial
a. Ameloblastoma and its variants
b. Calcifying epithelial odontogenic tumor
c. Odontogenic adenomatoid tumor (cyst)
d. Squamous odontogenic tumor
II. Mesenchymal
a. Odontogenic myxoma
b. Odontogenic fibroma and its variants
c. Cementoblastoma
III. Mixed
a. Ameloblastic fibroma
b. Ameloblastic fibro-odontoma
c. Odontoameloblastoma
d. Odontoma and its variants
B. Malignant
I. Odontogenic carcinoma
II. Malignant ameloblastoma
III. Ameloblastic carcinoma
IV. Ameloblastic fibrosarcoma

established a classification that defined this group of lesions according to ectomesenchymal interactions.[18] For the purposes of the practicing surgical pathologists, that classification, with the lesional headings simplified for more practical diagnostic purposes, can be found in Table 22.2. For a detailed discussion of odontogenesis please refer to the discussion of histologic and taxonomic considerations at the beginning of this chapter.

EPITHELIAL ODONTOGENIC TUMORS

Ameloblastoma

Ameloblastoma is an odontogenic neoplasm, the etiology of which is unknown. Some authorities believe that the lesion arises in association with the difficult eruption of a third molar or in association with a previous infection or cyst. Hertz[55] and Forsberg[56] suggest that trauma or inflammations are common etiologic agents. Tumors that appear to be histologically compatible with ameloblastoma in humans have been produced in mice by the injection of polyoma virus extracts.[57–59]

Although the root *amelo* is derived from the old French word for enamel, there is little consensus about the histogenesis of the ameloblastoma. Most investigators agree that the tumor is derived from odontogenic epithelium or certain derivatives or residua thereof. The histomorphologic structure is reminiscent of the dental lamina, as it penetrates the ectomesenchyme of the forming fetal jaw and differentiates into the epithelial enamel organ. The dental lamina thus remains the most likely parent tissue. The most convincing support for a dental lamina origin centers around the fact that the biologic and physiologic characteristics of the tumor remarkably parallel those of the dental lamina, a structure that continued to grow from surface oral epithelium, pushing out columns of epithelial cells in an orderly fashion into the supporting connective tissue until the site of ultimate tooth germ formation is reached within bone.

Other sources have been suggested as potential tissues of origin for the ameloblastoma. They include surface oral epithelium, odontogenic cyst epithelium, epithelial rests of Malassez, and the enamel organ.[60] All these, except the enamel organ origin, remain reasonable and likely tissues of origin.[61] Perhaps the most convincing factor against direct enamel organ origin is that enamel deposition is conspicuously absent from the histopathologic features of the ameloblastoma.

Less than 2% of all odontogenic tumors and cysts are estimated to be ameloblastoma, yet the lesion continues to fascinate pathologists because of its diversity of microscopic features and surgeons because of its defiance of complete eradication.

Clinical and radiologic features

In 1974, Sehdev and associates[62] compiled a comprehensive review of the clinicopathologic statistics on ameloblastoma. They reviewed 92 lesions, the vast majority of which occurred in the mandible. Maxillary ameloblastomas accounted for slightly less than 20% of their reported cases, consistent with other large reported series in the literature.[63] Men and women appear to be affected in nearly equal numbers, and the vast majority of all tumors show a peak incidence in the third and fourth decades.

These reviews document that painless swelling is the most common early symptom of ameloblastoma in either jaw. Sehdev et al.[62] found that in 14 of 20 patients with maxillary ameloblastoma, the duration of symptoms was less than 1 year. Nasal obstruction and epistaxis occurred late in the course of the disease. In mandibular ameloblastomas, the typical lesion presents as a slowly expanding swelling that usually causes thin-walled bulging cortical plates. The lesion appears to be a locally invasive tumor that has a tendency to recur if surgical removal is inadequate. It is estimated that 30–35% of all ameloblastomas arise within the wall of or in association with a follicular cyst.[64] There appears to be no racial predilection for ameloblastoma, although some single case reports document a greater frequency in blacks.

Radiologically, most ameloblastomas present as intraosseous multilocular or soap bubble-type radiolucencies, which may communicate with the oral cavity via destruction of the cortical plates (Fig. 22.13). Thus, the lesion is often subclassified as the conventional multicystic solid central osseous form. Occasionally, the lesions can have a unilocular cystic presentation, or the crown of a tooth may be found in association with the tumor. In the latter instance, the lesion may appear to have a radiopaque quality, but if calcifications are found radiologically, the lesion is probably not an ameloblastoma. When establishing a differential diagnosis for ameloblastoma on the basis of radiologic information, it is important to remember that lesions such as central giant cell granuloma, aneurysmal bone cyst, odontogenic myxoma, and odontogenic keratocyst may all have similar radiologic appearance.

Marx[65] has recently done much to help clarify the confusing terminology associated with ameloblastomas arising within cysts. He has defined ameloblastoma in situ as limited to the epithelial lining of a cyst. This entity once referred to as mural ameloblastoma represents an ameloblastoma arising from the epithelial lining of a cyst and projecting into the lumen. In situ ameloblastomas can be *microinvasive*, in which case the tumor proliferates into the connective tissue lining of the cyst, or *transmural and microinvasive* in which case tumor arises from the epithelial lining and proliferates through the complete thickness of the supporting connective tissue wall of the cyst. When the neoplasm proliferates throughout the total thickness of the supporting connective tissue wall to invade adjacent bone, it has been termed *invasive* by Marx.

These three subclassifications are important for the pathologist because they help to better define the behavior of the neoplasm and

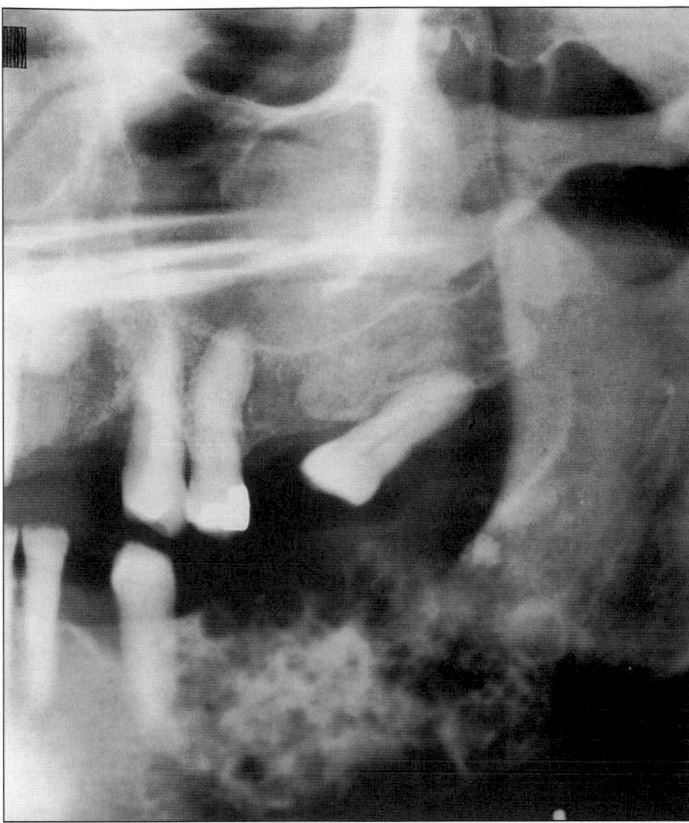

Fig. 22.13 Note the classic multilocular appearance of ameloblastoma. (Courtesy of Richard Nelson, DDS, Denver, Colorado.)

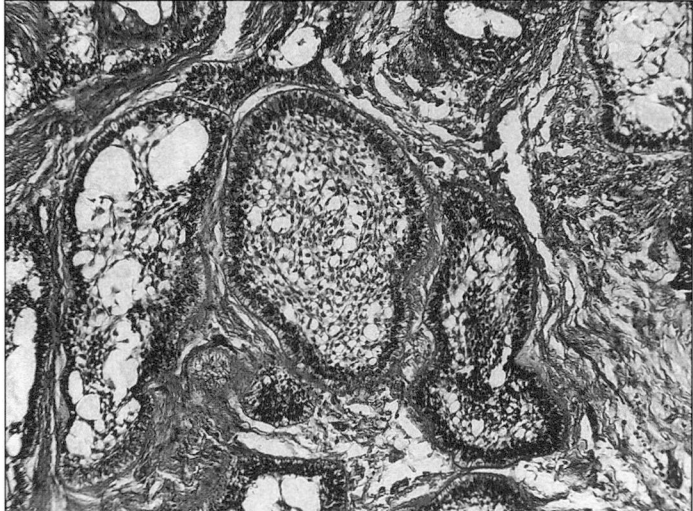

Fig. 22.14 Follicular ameloblastoma demonstrating discrete islands and nests of tumor cells set in a loose collagenous stroma.

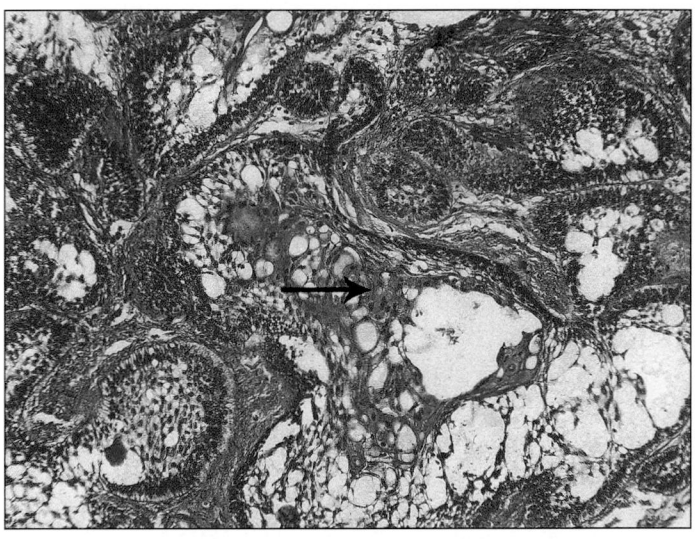

Fig. 22.15 Acanthomatous ameloblastoma. Note central tumor island keratinization (arrow).

guide the clinical management. It is important to note that when Marx defines these various subclassifications of ameloblastoma he is discussing ameloblastomas that arise from cyst lining epithelium only. The vast majority of the ameloblastomas arise within bone, as central osseous neoplasms. Ameloblastomas, regardless of subtype, generally occur in patients between twenty and thirty-five years of age. They favor the mandible, and they invade bone as insidious, poorly marginated tumors.

Pathologic features

Ameloblastomas that arise in association with the lining of a cyst generally present as plaques, excrescences, or nodular growths within the cyst wall or lumen. Central osseous ameloblastomas on the other hand typically present as solid tumor masses within a margin of maxillary or mandibular bone. They are expansible lesions within bone, and may perforate the cortical plate. When this occurs, there may be extraosseous tumor extending beyond the bony margins and proliferating into soft tissue structures.

On sectioning, the ameloblastoma is usually gray-white to gray-brown, depending on the amount of central hemorrhage within the tumor itself. It cuts readily, although there may be a gritty consistency to the tissue. Ameloblastomas do not produce a calcified odontogenic product, and therefore odontogenically derived hard tissue structures such as dentin and enamel will not be identified histologically. Occasionally, the tissue sample submitted may be a cyst. In such instances, one frequently finds a sac-like lining with elevated white nodular areas within. The white nodular areas represent mural ameloblastoma proliferation. It is important for the pathologist to examine the entire tissue sample so as not to overlook neoplastic proliferation in the wall of a cyst.

Six common histologic patterns have been described for ameloblastoma. The most common pattern, the *follicular* variant, is composed of tumor epithelium arranged in islands or sheets with a central area of cells that resemble primitive stellate reticulum (Fig. 22.14). The *plexiform pattern* consists of irregular strands of epithelium bordered by columnar cells that surround an admixture of cells resembling stellate reticulum. The *basal cell*, *granular cell*, and *acanthomatous* variants contain central tumor island cells that are basaloid, granular, or squamous or keratinaceous in character (Figs 22.15 and 22.16).

Waldron and El Mofty[66] reviewed a series of 116 ameloblastomas and identified 14 examples of a *desmoplastic* variant of ameloblastoma. The histologic features described for the lesion were

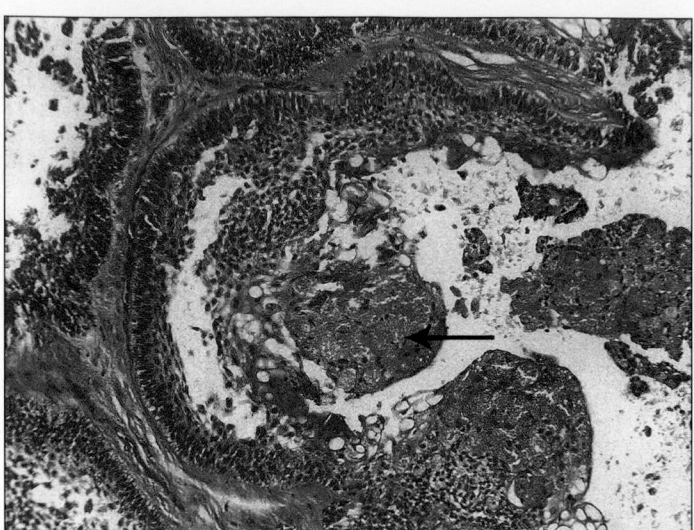

Fig. 22.16 Granular cell ameloblastoma. Note granular cells in tumor cell nests (arrow).

unique, and characterized by a rather extensive collagenized stroma containing small islands of true epithelium with a rare tendency to form cystic structures. The lesion is most often identified in the anterior portions of the jaws (uncharacteristic for ameloblastoma), and one-half of all reported examples have occurred in the maxilla. The desmoplastic ameloblastoma may have the radiographic presentation of a fibro-osseous lesion rather than an ameloblastoma, demonstrating a mixed radiolucent and radiopaque pattern that may resemble ossifying fibroma or fibrous dysplasia.[67]

Cystic degeneration is not uncommon within the central portion of the epithelial component of ameloblastomas, and quite frequently the tumor may show one or more of the six histologic patterns as it proliferates. Cells that rim individual tumor islands are usually columnar or cuboidal cells resembling preameloblasts. Individual tumor cells usually have oval to vesicular nuclei that are polarized toward the central portion of the follicular tumor nests. The cytoplasm ranges from granular to homogeneous; it is usually eosinophilic. Mitotic activity is minimal in most tissue sections.

Treatment and prognosis

The management modality of choice for the conventional central osseous ameloblastoma, be it solid or cystic, is bony marginal resection. Curettage of this type of ameloblastoma is ineffective. When such therapy is used, recurrence rates often exceed 50%. Because of this potential for recurrence, surgical margins are frequently established 1 cm beyond the tumor's apparent radiographic extension.

Variants of ameloblastoma

Gardner and Corio[68] coined the term *plexiform unicystic ameloblastoma* in 1984 to describe a variant of ameloblastoma with a low recurrence rate that usually arises in the posterior mandible. This form of ameloblastoma is thought to account for as many as 15% of all central osseous forms of the neoplasm. Clinically, most of these lesions had previously been thought to be dentigerous cysts. Eversole et al.[69] further characterized the lesion as cystogenic ameloblastoma, with findings similar to those of Gardner and Corio except that their cases demonstrated that the lesion did not have to

be radiographically unilocular and could, in fact, be multilocular. Although the unicystic ameloblastoma is most often associated with unerupted teeth, it can arise in relationship to an erupted tooth. Continued use of the term unicystic ameloblastoma is deemed appropriate, considering the more accurate terminology proposed by Marx[65] for cystic ameloblastomas.

Cystic variants of ameloblastoma have been reported to manifest a less aggressive behavior and more favorable prognosis than the classic intraosseous ameloblastoma, but recurrence rates of 10–20% have been reported, and local resection as opposed to enucleation has been proposed by some surgeons.

Gardner and Corio[68] recommend that the surgical site of a so-called cystic ameloblastoma be radiographed annually for 10 years after surgery. Should the lesion recur, the appropriate treatment should involve an en bloc resection with a 1 cm margin of normal bone at that time.

This *extraosseous or peripheral ameloblastoma*, a variant of the central osseous ameloblastoma, is a rare entity that accounts for no more than 1% of all ameloblastomas.[61,70] The most common presentation of the extraosseous tumor is as a nodular or papillary growth of the gingiva or alveolar mucosa. The posterior mandibular gingiva is favored. The histopathologic features of this lesion are similar to the central osseous form of the tumor.

Malignant variants of ameloblastoma[71,72] are discussed later in this chapter.

Differential histopathologic diagnosis for ameloblastoma

Ameloblastoma is frequently confused histologically with *ameloblastic fibroma*. Considerable care should be taken to separate the two entities because the ameloblastic fibroma behaves in a much less aggressive manner than ameloblastoma, and management is correspondingly more conservative. The ameloblastic fibroma is composed of both epithelial and mesenchymal tooth germ components. Like the ameloblastoma, it produces no calcified dental structure. Histologically, ameloblastic fibroma consists of islands and cords of odontogenic epithelium that resemble the dental lamina of early tooth development. The stroma is generally composed of fibromyxoid embryonic connective tissue, which closely resembles the dental papilla of a developing tooth germ. Both the epithelial and mesenchymal components of the lesion are considered neoplastic. One useful histologic feature that separates ameloblastic fibroma from ameloblastoma is the fact that the supporting tumor stroma of the former remains primitive and exceedingly cellular, whereas the connective tissue stroma of the ameloblastoma more closely resembles mature collagen. Ameloblastic fibroma also occurs in a much younger age group than ameloblastoma, with an average age of 15.5 years. The mean age of patients with ameloblastoma is about two decades older. Conservative surgical excision remains the treatment of choice for ameloblastic fibroma.

The *craniopharyngioma* is a rare benign lesion found in the bone beneath the sella turcica. It is histologically similar to ameloblastoma and is often referred to as a pituitary ameloblastoma. The origins of the two tumors are somewhat similar because Rathke's pouch does originate embryologically by invagination of oral epithelium, and craniopharyngioma is composed of a follicular or plexiform accumulation of epithelial cells mimicking ameloblastoma. However, one microscopic feature of the craniopharyngioma not generally found in ameloblastoma is the almost universal occurrence of irregular calcified masses of bone and/or cartilage in the former. The craniopharyngioma also tends to occur before the age of 25, much earlier than ameloblastoma.

Adamantinoma of long bones

The so-called adamantinoma of long bones bears a superficial microscopic resemblance to ameloblastoma. It is doubtful whether any valid relationship between the two can be established. Adamantinomas are low-grade malignancies that occur most often in the tibia. They resemble ameloblastomas in that they are multilocular and their histology consists of basal epithelial cells arranged in nests and cords. The tumor, however, most likely arises from skin ectoderm.[73] These tumors are treated by en bloc resection.

Malignant ameloblastoma

Ameloblastomas displaying malignant transformation are rare, and the terminology describing such lesions has been awkward at best. Two methods of defining this form of odontogenic malignancy are common. The term *malignant ameloblastoma* is best reserved for tumors that show histologic features of classic ameloblastoma in both the primary neoplastic disease at the site of origin and in any metastasis. Cellular cytologic atypia need not be present.[74]

Ameloblastic carcinoma, on the other hand, is a term reserved for ameloblastomas that demonstrate the classic histopathologic features of cancer including cytologic atypia, recurrence, and metastasis.[75] Malignant ameloblastomas and ameloblastic carcinomas have been reported over a wide age range. In most instances, metastasis is to lungs, with the cervical lymph node metastasis being the second most common metastatic site. Both lesions are treated by a wide marginal resection, but there are so few cases reported that it is not possible to determine long-term prognosis. In those cases that have been reported, half of the patients died of their disease during the course of long-term follow-up.

Slootweg and Muller[74] reviewed a series of 26 cases of malignant ameloblastoma and found that the patients had metastatic involvement in 20 instances. The vast majority of the metastases were to the lungs. The second most common site involved was lymph nodes. Patients had a mean age of 31.3 years, and follow-up showed that 11 of 16 patients died during a period of up to 9 years.

Ameloblastic carcinoma, as defined by Elzay,[75] showed a slightly older mean age of 33.2 years; 80% of the tumors were located in the mandible; the most common site of metastasis was to the lungs, just as in malignant ameloblastoma as defined by Slootweg and Muller; and patients died between 1 and 45 years after initial diagnosis of the tumor.

Ikemura et al.[72] have also described a malignant potential for ameloblastoma. They reviewed 14 cases of metastatic ameloblastoma and reported a case of their own in a 54-year-old woman with lung and lymph node metastases.

Histologically, ameloblastomas that may metastasize cannot always be differentiated from the more classic benign ameloblastoma. It appears that inadequate surgical resection and a long duration of the tumor have a significant relationship to ultimate metastatic disease occurrence.

Sound judgment is needed to distinguish between malignant ameloblastoma and central osseous jaw tumors of salivary gland origin. Occasionally, squamous cell carcinoma can occur in association with a benign ameloblastoma. When this occurs, it may be extremely difficult to determine whether the carcinoma arose within the ameloblastoma or whether, in fact, two tumors exist.

Finally, in the ill-defined realm of malignant ameloblastoma, it is worth noting that a so-called *clear cell odontogenic carcinoma* has been reported.[76] This rare jaw tumor resembles ameloblastoma and it is composed of tumor islands with clear cells inside a central acanthomatous zone that is rimmed by a peripheral margin of columnar cells resembling ameloblasts. There are so few of these cases reported,

however, that clinical classification and management modalities have not been clearly defined. Most patients have been managed by a radical surgery and succumb to pulmonary lymphoid metastasis.

Calcifying epithelial odontogenic tumor

The calcifying epithelial odontogenic tumor (CEOT) was first described in 1958 by Pindborg[77] and is now recognized as a distinct entity by WHO.[18] Until recently, the growth potential and biologic behavior of this neoplasm was authoritatively stated to be similar to that of ameloblastoma,[78] indicating the probability of invasiveness and a prediction of local recurrence if conservatively removed in an advanced developmental stage. However, new reports suggest that this tumor, which has a peak incidence in the 40s, is less aggressive than previously suggested and clearly less biologically aggressive than ameloblastoma or myxoma. Histogenesis of the calcifying epithelial odontogenic tumor is open to debate. The tumor shows a propensity for development in association with a tooth, usually in patients 30 to 50 years of age. Pindborg[77] suggests that the lesion develops from reduced enamel epithelium or from stratum intermedium.

Clinical and radiologic features

Clinically, the lesion typically appears as a locally invasive central osseous neoplasm, but extraosseous lesions have been reported,[79] usually on the anterior gingiva, and like their extraosseous ameloblastoma counterpart, they have a low biologic aggressiveness.

The mandible appears to be affected more often than the maxilla, and the most frequent site of occurrence is the premolar/molar region. Typically, the lesion appears as a radiolucent expansile lesion that is fairly well delineated peripherally. A calcified central area is frequently identified (Fig. 22.17). One-half of the lesions that have been reported in the world literature have been in association with an unerupted tooth.[80] Typically, a differential diagnosis of ameloblastoma, calcifying odontogenic cyst, odontoma, and odonto-ameloblastoma is entertained.

Pathologic features

The CEOT is typically composed of a white homogeneous tumor mass, which may contain calcified material. A tumor capsule is not always appreciated, and frequently the invasive properties of the tumor beyond the periphery into bone are not identified on gross inspection.

The basic histologic pattern of the calcifying epithelial odontogenic tumor is characteristic and unique. Histopathologically, the tumor is composed of sheets and masses of polyhedral epithelial cells with deeply eosinophilic cytoplasm supported by a well-vascularized connective tissue stroma. Intracellular bridging is an often noted characteristic, and there may be a moderate degree of cellular pleomorphism, as well as considerable variance in chromaticity of individual cell nuclei (Fig. 22.18). Foci of amorphous, faintly eosinophilic cell product and small round or irregular calcified aggregates (Liesegang ring calcifications), which may also be massively coalescent, are an invariable feature of the classic tumor histology.

The eosinophilic homogeneous material has been variously described as amyloid, keratin, basal lamina, and enamel matrix.[81,82] The substance stains positively with amyloid stains (thioflavin T and Congo red), and most investigators consider it an amyloid-like product very likely resulting from destruction of lamina densa material of epithelial cell origin.[83,84]

A survey of 23 cases from the files of the Armed Forces Institute of Pathology with a discussion of histologic variation was reported

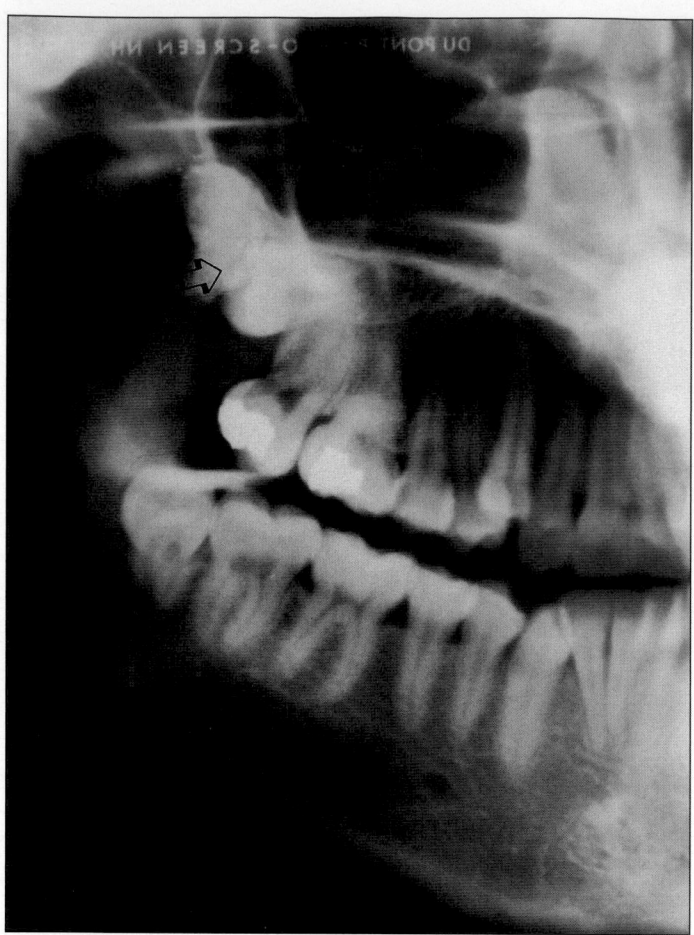

Fig. 22.17 Calcifying epithelial odontogenic tumor. Multilocular radiolucent maxillary lesion associated with impacted molar tooth with prominent calcification around the crown (arrow).

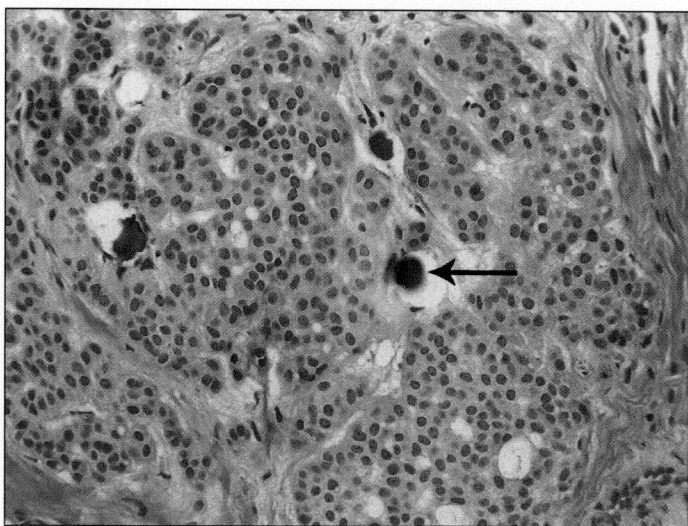

Fig. 22.18 Calcifying epithelial odontogenic tumor. Note the sheets of polygonal cells with prominent focal calcifications (arrow).

by Krolls and Pindborg.[80] They commented on the diagnostic challenge of a 'clear cell' variant and found two such tumors in their series. It is significant to note that in both cases there were transition areas to unequivocal classic tumor histology. Abrams and Howell[83] reported a single instance of clear cell calcifying epithelial odontogenic tumor in a 1967 review of four tumors. In their case, a bimorphic cytoplasmic appearance was observed. The pathologist confronted with a clear cell calcifying odontogenic tumor must consider clear cell types of salivary gland neoplasms, metastatic hypernephroma, and glycogen-rich adenocarcinoma in a differential microscopic diagnosis.

Treatment and prognosis

Krolls and Pindborg[80] maintain that the treatment of choice for the calcifying epithelial odontogenic tumor is conservative surgical resection, with an adequate margin of normal bone, but one must remember that calcifying epithelial odontogenic tumors with a classic histology have a potential for an aggressive infiltrative course. Recurrence rates vary but are generally reported to be in the 15% range.

Adenomatoid odontogenic tumor (adenomatoid odontogenic cyst)

Clinical and radiologic features

The adenomatoid odontogenic tumor (AOT) or cyst, is much more common than ameloblastoma or the calcifying epithelial odontogenic tumor, and accounts for 3–7% of all odontogenic tumors.[85] Once known by the misleading term *adenoameloblastoma*, the adenomatoid odontogenic tumor is a neoplasm of young people, with a propensity to occur between the ages of 10 and 20. Occasionally, cases have been reported in older individuals, but this represents the exception rather than the rule. Marx[86] favors the term adenomatoid odontogenic cyst for this lesion because of its typical encapsulation and the presence of a lumen. Females are affected much more commonly than males (2:1), and the most common clinical finding is that of a painless, slowly expansile lesion of bone.[86,87] The tumor is usually identified in the maxillary canine, premolar, or incisor area, although a few cases have been reported along the angle of the mandible. Seventy-five percent of the reported cases have been associated with an unerupted or impacted tooth, the most common tooth being the maxillary cuspid.[88,89] Instances of an extraosseous AOT variant have been documented.[87]

Radiologically, the lesion usually presents as a solitary cyst-like growth (Fig. 22.19). As a differential diagnosis, one should include dentigerous cyst, odontogenic keratocyst, and inflammatory cyst of dental origin (radicular cyst). Frequently, calcifications are seen in association with the tumor, producing a faintly detectable radiopacity. The lesion rarely grows to a size that results in penetration of the cortical plates, and if such is the appearance, then the differential diagnosis should include a more aggressive odontogenic neoplasm.

Current theory suggests that the adenomatoid odontogenic tumor is derived from the enamel organ or remnants of Hertwigs epithelial root sheath. There also seems to be a very distinct morphologic correspondence between the cells that line the duct-like structures of the tumor and the cells of the interenamel epithelium in the tooth germ. The duct-like structures in the tumor may, in fact, represent nothing more than an abortive attempt at the formation of the enamel organ. The WHO classifies this tumor as an epithelial tumor with an inductive effect on odontogenic ectomesenchyme,[18] and most diagnostic surgical pathologists prefer to classify the lesion with other tumors of epithelial odontogenic origin.

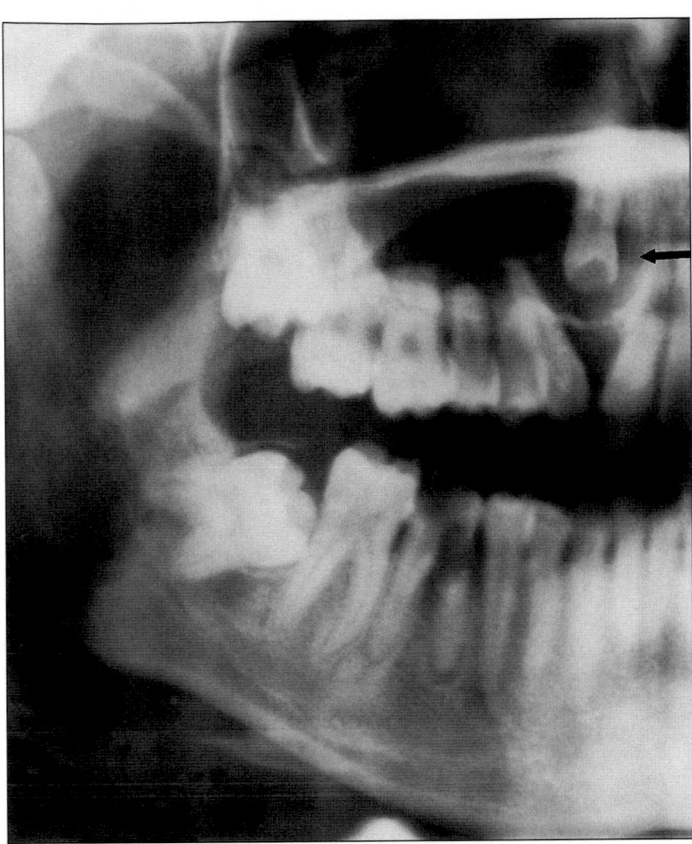

Fig. 22.19 Adenomatoid odontogenic tumor demonstrating a radiolucent lesion of the maxilla involving an unerupted tooth (arrow). Unlike the typical dentigerous cyst, the radiolucency extends nearly to the root apex.

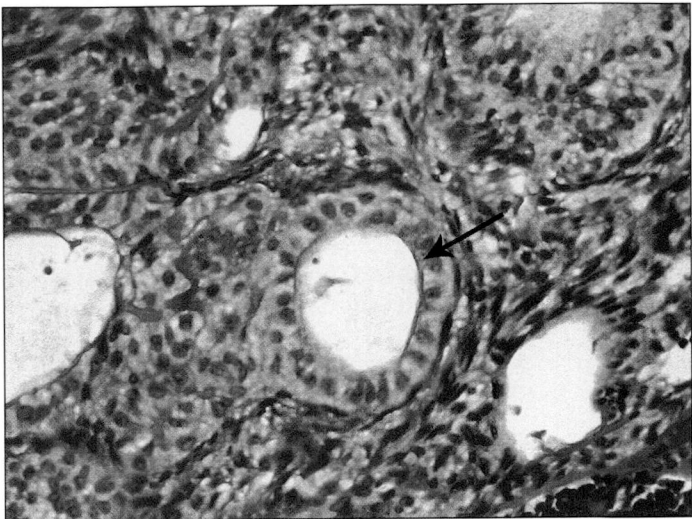

Fig. 22.20 Prominent duct-like structures of the adenomatoid odontogenic tumor (arrow).

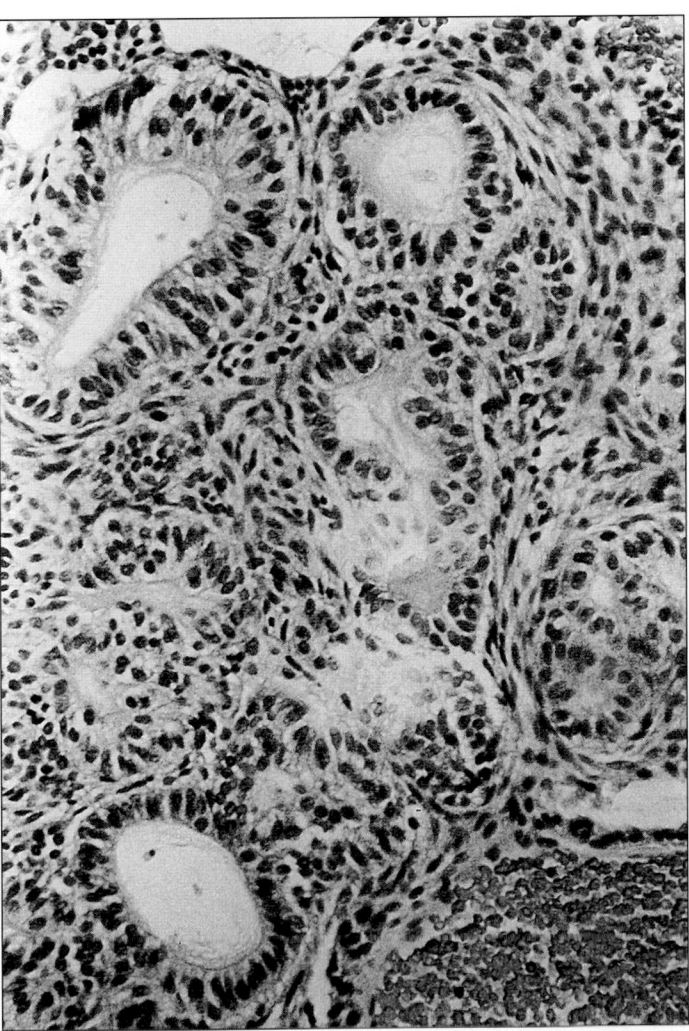

Fig. 22.21 Note prominent spindle cells surrounding duct-like spaces in the AOT.

Pathologic features

Most adenomatoid odontogenic tumors are small, measuring 1–3 cm in diameter. The tumor may or may not be encapsulated by a peripheral rim of mature collagen. On cut section, one usually identifies a white to yellow firm surface, which may have cystic areas that contain central gelatinous material. The calcified material that is often identified on radiographs may represent poorly formed tooth structure or an aberrant dystrophic type of calcification grossly, so the cut section on occasion may be quite gritty or granular, resembling the cut surface of a mature central giant cell granuloma.

The dominant histologic feature of the tumor is proliferation of sheets, nests, and cords of neoplastic epithelial cells that differentiate along columnar lines in numerous places to resemble ameloblasts. Frequently, these columnar cells form ducts or tubules, with the central lumen ultimately encased by columnar cells (Fig. 22.20). The peripheral cells stain deeply, and their nuclei are polarized away from the central portion of the neoplasm in a manner similar to that found in ameloblastoma. In addition to the tubular and ductal structures, bands, sheets, and clusters of cells arranged in a spindle-like pattern may be identified (Fig. 22.21). These areas can take on a cartwheel or cribriform pattern reminiscent of salivary gland tumors, especially the mixed tumor. Tumor nests are supported by a scant connective tissue stroma. On occasion, tumor cells are arranged in a rosette pattern lined by cuboidal or columnar epithelium. Calcified material is common throughout the tumor. These calcifications develop primarily at junctions between aggregates of epithelial cells that form the tumor and the adjacent vascularized stromal tissues. The calcific foci have been shown to resemble enamel, pre-enamel, or dentin morphologically and have similar staining and tinctorial qualities.

Poulson and Greer[89] reviewed the electron microscopic findings of two adenomatoid odontogenic tumors and identified two distinctly different cell types. One cell was polygonal to columnar and tended to surround the tumor's duct-like structures to form small nodules. These cells seemed to share common features with preameloblasts in that ultrastructurally an abundance of free ribosomes and a paucity of endoplasmic reticulum was identified. A second cell type was identified that appeared similar to cells of the stratum intermedium and stellate reticulum of the tooth germ. These cells were spindle shaped with ovoid nuclei and appeared to be perpendicular to luminal cells. Their ultrastructure showed dense cytoplasm and numerous filaments and ribosomes.

Histochemical attempts to identify the nature and source of the eosinophilic material that is often observed in the adenomatoid odontogenic tumor suggest that the material is amyloid-like.[87]

Treatment and prognosis

The adenomatoid odontogenic tumor grows slowly and generally enucleates readily from the surrounding bone. It shows little tendency toward recurrence, and conservative surgical enucleation remains the treatment of choice. It must be pointed out that some investigators including Marx[86] believe that this lesion represents a hamartoma and not a true odontogenic tumor. It is exceedingly important to separate this lesion from the ameloblastoma because the behavior patterns are diametrically opposed. Although there is a close morphologic correlation between the cells of the adenomatoid odontogenic tumor and the ameloblastoma, the lesions are unique entities, and the management of each is surgically distinctive.

Squamous odontogenic tumor

The squamous odontogenic tumor is an exceedingly rare odontogenic tumor of epithelial origin. First reported in 1975, the lesion is thought to arise from residual rests of Malassez.[90]

Clinical and radiographic features

The tumor can present as a solitary or multifocal growth. Fully 30% of patients have no symptoms, and when symptoms do occur, they fall into the category of a focal swelling that may or may not be associated with pain.

Radiographically, the tumor often results in a focal radiolucent area of destruction lateral to the roots of adjacent teeth. These defects are usually triangular in shape and rarely exceed a diameter of more than 3 cm.

Pathologic features

The squamous odontogenic tumor has a unique histopathologic appearance that consists of interconnected islands of well-differentiated acanthotic-appearing squamous epithelium lacking peripheral columnar cells. Tumor cell nests are set in a mature collagenous matrix. Individual tumor islands may contain nodules of dystrophic calcification or globular bodies of keratin. Rare extraosseous variants have been reported.[90]

Differential diagnosis and treatment

The most significant microscopic feature of this neoplasm relates to the fact that the tumor islands can mimic the islands of ameloblastoma. The key to the diagnostic separation of the two entities is

that the peripheral cells of the epithelial islands in the squamous odontogenic tumor do not demonstrate the classic polarization seen with ameloblastoma. Treatment includes curettage or conservative surgical excision, but it should be noted that new lesions arise in a different location as frequently as 20% of the time.

BENIGN MESENCHYMAL TUMORS

Odontogenic myxoma

Myxomas (odontogenic myxoma, myxofibroma) of bone are uncommon neoplasms, and the controversy as to whether myxomas of the jaws are odontogenic in origin or of central osseous mesenchymal origin continues. The distinction appears to be primarily of academic interest because the behavior pattern of myxoma of bone tends to remain the same whether or not an odontogenic origin can be demonstrated and whether or not odontogenic epithelial rests are present within the tumor. If one concurs that true myxomas do occur, one would conversely have to consider that a distinctive and unique cell gives rise to the tumor. In fact, most authorities who have evaluated the ultrastructure of myxomas support the theory that the lesion arises from fibroblasts and that the myxomatous appearance occurs because of the abundant amount of intercellular mucin within the tumor.[91,92] Thus, the preferred taxonomy for the neoplasm is probably best simple 'myxoma.' The abundant primitive mesenchymal tissue that is the source for the primary and eventually the permanent teeth is largely the reason that myxoma favors the jaws over long bones.

Clinical and radiologic features

Myxomas of the jaw favor the posterior mandible although they are more evenly distributed throughout the jaws than the ameloblastoma. Maxillary myxomas are less common. The tumors present as slow-growing, expansile, nonpainful lesions, most often in the second or third decade of life. Most myxomas appear as sessile swelling of the jaws, with a thin eggshell covering of the cortical bone. Women appear to be affected slightly more often than men.[93] Clinically, the most common finding is that of a multilocular radiolucency or a compartmentalized soap bubble radiolucency; however, there are reported cases in which myxomas have presented as solitary unilocular cyst-like lesions (Fig. 22.22). The tumor borders may be well defined or poorly delineated radiologically. It is not uncommon for the lesion to show scalloping and interdigitation between the teeth. Myxomas have been reported in association with unerupted teeth and congenitally missing teeth; however, the lesion may very well arise in association with fully developed dental structures. Tooth displacement, nerve displacement, and root resorption can recur with the myxoma.

Pathologic features

The lesion may appear grossly as a gray-white to yellow fibrous mass without a peripheral capsule. The cut surface in such instances will be firm and glistening and will fail to bulge beyond surrounding tissues on sectioning. Myxomas may also present as rather mucoid, slimy specimens with a gelatinous appearance when fixed. In such instances, a capsule is not identified. Areas of bone are often present within the cut surface.

Microscopically, myxomas consist of accumulations of triangular to stellate fibroblasts with rather lengthy anastomosing processes and loose mucoid intracellular material (Fig. 22.23). The cytoplasm ranges from slightly basophilic to deeply eosinophilic, depending on the degree of collagenization that has taken place. The supporting

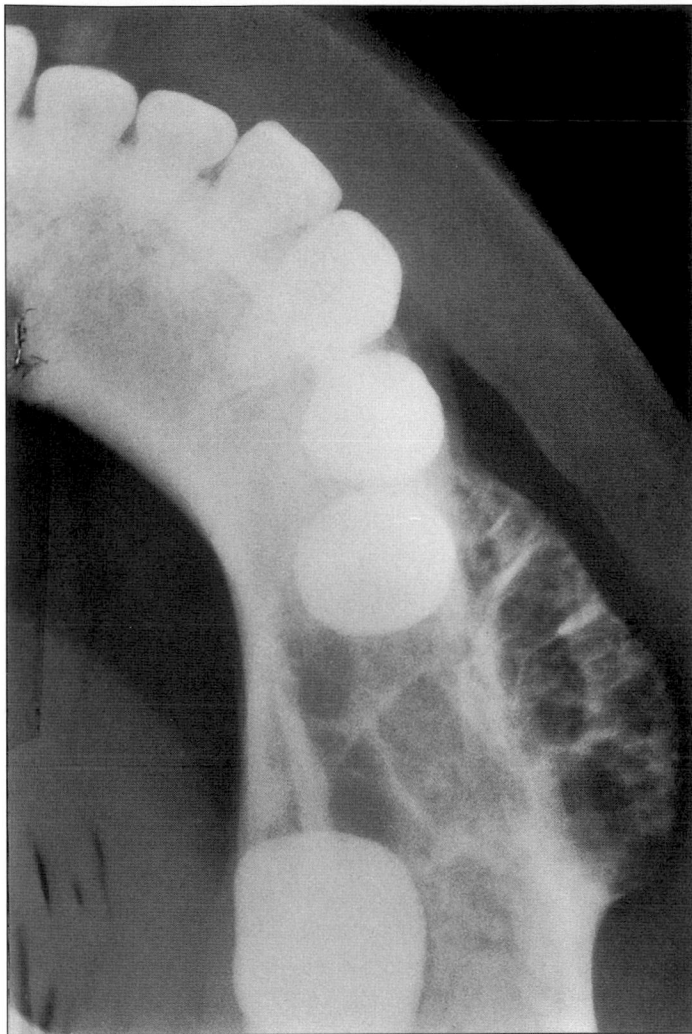

Fig. 22.22 Odontogenic myxoma. Multilocular lesion of the mandible expanding the labial cortex. (Courtesy of Michael Roher, DDS, and Stephen Young, DDS, Oklahoma City, Oklahoma.)

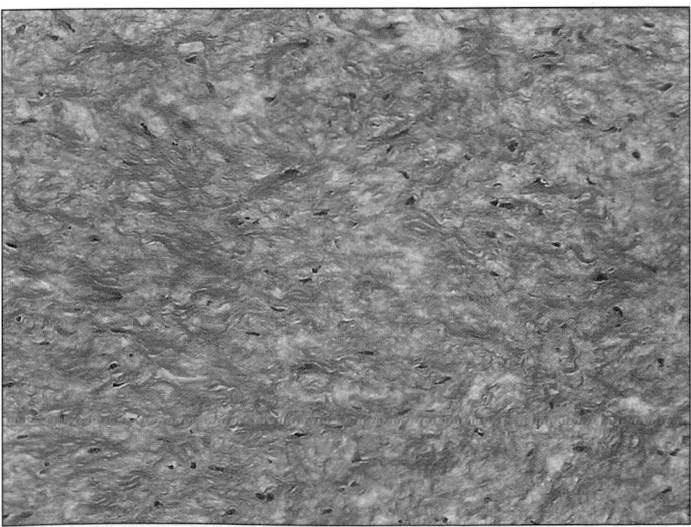

Fig. 22.23 Odontogenic myxoma. Note the delicate fibrillar stroma, stellate cells, and myxoid matrix.

stroma is typically that of a mucopolysaccharide complex that may contain odontogenic epithelium. Hasleton and colleagues[92] reported islands of odontogenic epithelium at all intervals throughout cases they reported. Although odontogenic epithelium can be found in a high percentage of cases of central myxoma of bone involving the jaws, it may represent nothing more than a fetal remnant and is not necessarily important in the genesis of the tumor or requisite for diagnosis. It is nearly impossible to distinguish between jaw myxomas that will behave aggressively and those that will have a totally benign biologic behavior. Farman et al.[93] reviewed 213 cases of jaw myxofibromas and found no mortality related to the tumor. We are aware of several cases resulting in eventual orbital exenteration and maxillectomy. Lesions of the maxilla spread rapidly throughout the surrounding cancellous bone and tend to have a more aggressive behavior than their mandibular counterparts.

The ultrastructural features of the odontogenic myxoma have shed light on the cell of origin. The tumor cell of origin closely resembles a fibroblast, a cell known to have an active secretory function. Goldblatt[94] has described two types of cells in odontogenic myxomas: a nonsecretory (type I) and a secretory (type II) cell. Both of these cells appear to be of connective tissue origin. Redman et al.[95] have ultrastructurally identified cells resembling myofibroblasts in odontogenic myxomas. Their findings support the theory that the cell of origin for the tumor may be periodontal ligament fibroblasts, which have also been shown to have such microfilament systems. The exact function of the myofibroblasts in the tumor is not known, although it has been postulated that their contractile mechanism may be the device for allowing cell motility in the granulation tissue that is often associated with this tumor. Zimmerman and Dahlin[96] have attempted to define benign and 'malignant' varieties of central jaw myxomas on the basis of the cytologic appearance of nuclei and anisocytosis. They have met with only limited success and have been unable to distinguish benign and malignant variants. There is some suggestion that the greater the fibrous component of the tumor, the less aggressive the tumor's biologic behavior.

A few examples of myxomas of the oral soft tissue have been reported. Elzay and Duntz[97] believe that soft tissue myxomas are derived from early embryonic mesenchymal tissues. These investigators maintain that the neoplasms remain quiescent for long periods of time and have the ability to suddenly enlarge. The recommended therapy is surgical excision with adequate margins. The lesion is thought not to have the aggressive potential of its central osseous counterpart.

The complex of soft tissue myxomas, spotty skin pigmentation, and endocrine overactivity has recently been recognized as a syndrome, transmitted as an autosomal dominant trait.[98] A serious component of this syndrome is the so-called cardiac myxoma. Many of the patients with this myxoma syndrome complex have clearly visible markers, including mucocutaneous pigmentation. Finally, the myxoma must not be confused with a developing tooth follicle or the chondromyxoid fibroma. Clinicopathologic correlation with radiographs or computed tomographic scans should prevent this diagnostic confusion.

Treatment and prognosis

Marx[86] suggests that the treatment of choice for most myxomas is marginal resection with a 1.0–1.5 cm bony margin and one non-involved anatomic barrier margin. Although some authorities favor curettage for small lesions, most surgeons consider such therapy inadequate. Recurrence for this neoplasm is in the 20% range, largely due to treatment with enucleation or curettage.

Central odontogenic fibroma

Clinical and radiologic features

There are to be two distinct histologic variants of the central osseous odontogenic fibroma: (1) the simple central odontogenic fibroma, and (2) the WHO central odontogenic fibroma (WHO type). The simple type, as described by Gardner,[99] is a very rare neoplasm composed of a uniform proliferation of mature, relatively dense connective tissue, which may or may not have an admixture of small entrapped epithelial odontogenic rests. The WHO variant consists of mature collagenous fibrous connective tissue with prominent islands, strands, and nests of odontogenic epithelium and occasional aggregates of dysplastic dentin, cementum, and calcifications.[18]

Dunlap and Barker[100] reviewed a series of 11 odontogenic fibromas and found the age distribution to range from 11 to 80 years. The mean age of their patients was 34 years. Five cases were identified in females and six in males. Wesley et al.[101] have documented an age range of 11 to 67 years in their clinical and morphologic studies. The lesion showed the mean age of all patients was 22 years. Handlers et al.,[102] however, report a female and maxillary predilection for the tumor. The lesion thus remains perhaps the most ill defined and least understood of all odontogenic neoplasms. Wesley and colleagues gleaned only seven cases from the world literature; all tumors were found in close association with the crown of an impacted tooth and presented clinically as slowly enlarging swellings. The tumors usually presented as multilocular radiolucencies (Fig. 22.24), although unilocular lesions were identified. Larger lesions are usually associated with expansion of the bone and movement or loosening of the teeth.

The central osseous odontogenic fibroma can contain calcified material that is visible radiologically,[103] and Allen et al.[104] have reported a giant cell granuloma type of response in association with central odontogenic fibromas.

Pathologic features

The odontogenic fibroma most often presents as an encapsulated neoplastic mass with a homogeneous white cut surface that usually glistens. Typically, it is identified in association with an impacted tooth. Microscopically, one usually finds a moderately dense and relatively cellular proliferation of interlacing collagen bundles with a uniform distribution of bland fibroblasts (Fig. 22.25). Occasionally, amorphous calcifications can be identified in the tissue sample. Odontogenic epithelium may also be identified. The presence of odontogenic epithelium should not negate a diagnosis of odontogenic fibroma. One significant difference between the WHO odontogenic fibroma and the lesion that closely resembles it microscopically, odontogenic myxoma, is that in the latter the stroma exhibits only scant amounts of collagen and abundant ground substance, whereas in the odontogenic fibroma, the stroma is more frequently collagenous and less cellular. The simple odontogenic fibroma can more closely resemble a myxoma, and distinction can be difficult. A whorled pattern of fibroblastic activity favors simple odontogenic fibroma.

Vincent and associates[105] have described a variant of odontogenic fibroma using the term *central granular cell odontogenic fibroma*. All of their cases occurred in women as well-circumscribed radiolucencies. The age range was 53 to 65 years. Seven tumors occurred in the posterior body of the mandible and one in the premolar region of the maxilla. The lesions were treated by surgical excision, and no recurrences were identified during a follow-up period ranging from 6 to 144 months. Microscopically, the lesions consisted of an abundance of polygonal cells with eosinophilic granular cytoplasm and eccentric ovoid nuclei and an occasional

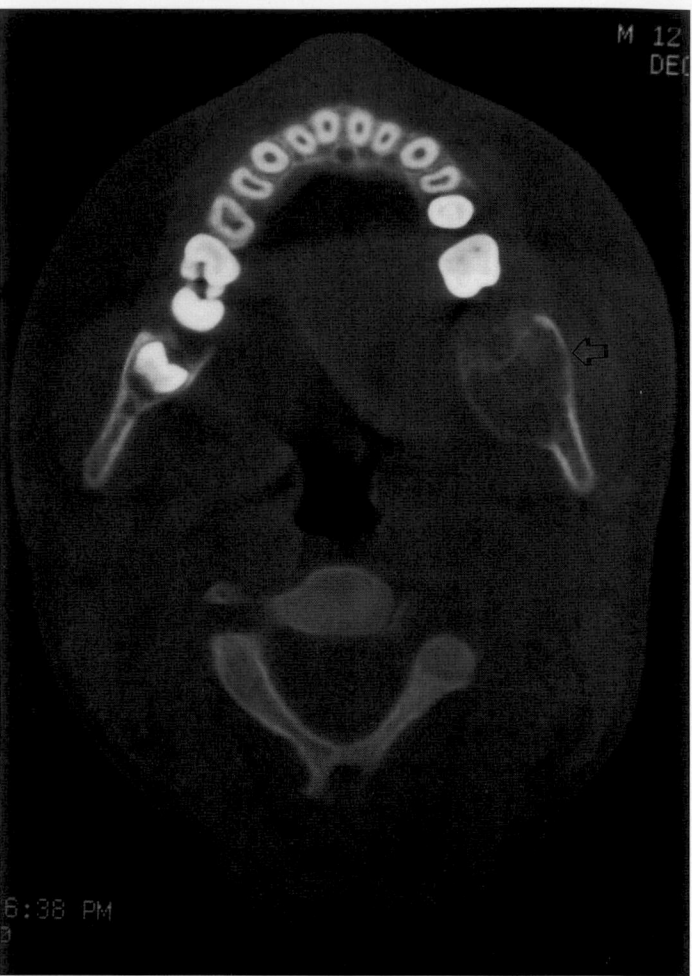

Fig. 22.24 Odontogenic fibroma. CT scan demonstrating expansile multilocular destruction of the posterior mandible.

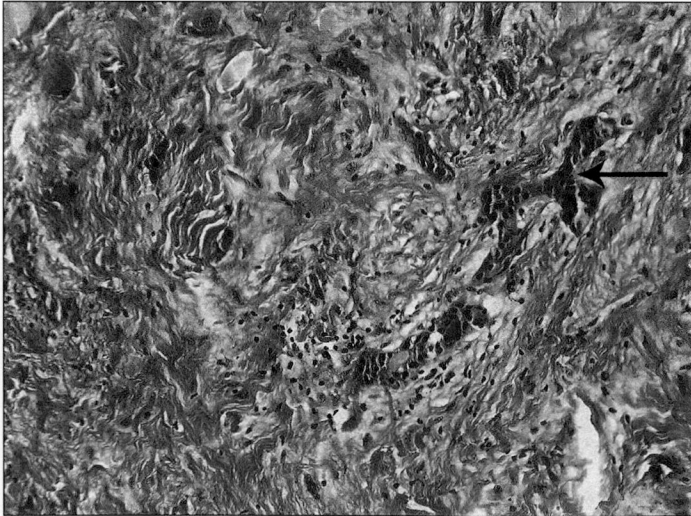

Fig. 22.25 Odontogenic fibroma. WHO type showing odontogenic rests (arrow) within a cellular fibroblastic lesion.

entrapped epithelial odontogenic rest. Rarely, ovoid calcifications could be identified.

Ultrastructurally, the morphologic characteristics of odontogenic fibroma are quite similar to those of odontogenic myxoma in that cells in both neoplasms exhibit large amounts of endoplasmic reticulum. Two cell types have not been identified in odontogenic fibroma, in contrast to odontogenic myxoma.

Peripheral odontogenic fibroma is an extraosseous variant of the central odontogenic fibroma. It most often presents as a gingival nodule, and the mandibular arch is favored over the maxilla. There is no apparent sex or age predilection, and lesion histology is similar to that of the WHO type of central odontogenic fibroma. The lesion must be distinguished histopathologically from the far more common peripheral ossifying fibroma, which is often dominated histologically by the presence of reactive bone. The treatment of choice for peripheral odontogenic fibroma is local excision with an adequate margin of normal tissue, and recurrence is rare.

Treatment and prognosis

The central odontogenic fibroma is benign and responds well to surgical enucleation and curettage, although recurrences have been reported that have required more aggressive surgery. Malignant transformation has not been reported.

Cementoblastoma

The cementoblastoma has long been classified as an odontogenic neoplasm but it is more likely a hamartoma resulting from cementoblasts amassing cementum at the apex of a tooth root.

Clinical and radiologic features

The cementoblastoma, initially described in 1930 by Norberg,[106] typically presents as a slow-growing mass tenaciously attached to the cementum of molar or premolar teeth (Fig. 22.26). Corio et al.[107] recently reviewed a series of 24 cases of cementoblastoma presented in the world literature and added a case of their own and found that the lesion was not as uncommon as might be thought given its infrequent documentation in the world literature. Their investigations found an age range of 10 to 63 years, the mean age being 23 years.

Some authorities consider the cementoblastoma and osteoblastoma to be no more than variations of the same neoplasm, but the clinical presentation of the cementoblastoma is so unique as to warrant a distinct odontogenic tumor classification.

In most instances, pain is a significant feature of cementoblastoma. More than one-half of the documented case reports indicate that pain was a primary presenting symptom.[108,109] The cementoblastoma has a distinctive radiologic appearance, that of a large radiopaque mass attached to the root of a molar or premolar tooth. A thin radiolucent line usually surrounds the opaque mass.

Pathologic features

Grossly, cementoblastoma specimens usually consist of a sectioned tooth with an attached globular mass resembling hypercementosis. The microscopic appearance of cementoblastoma is fairly consistent, characterized histologically by a peripheral rim of radiating columns of cementum lined by large pleomorphic (cemento) blastic cells. At the peripheral border, islands of cementum and cementum-like substance can be seen set in a fibrous capsular stroma. Frequently, the peripheral cementoblasts have hyperchromatic nuclei and marked pleomorphism and appear to be stacked in a layer or lattice-like pattern. A portion of the tumor may show reactive cementum with marked reversal line activity. Giansanti[110] documented a fine birefringence compatible with that of cementum in large case studies.

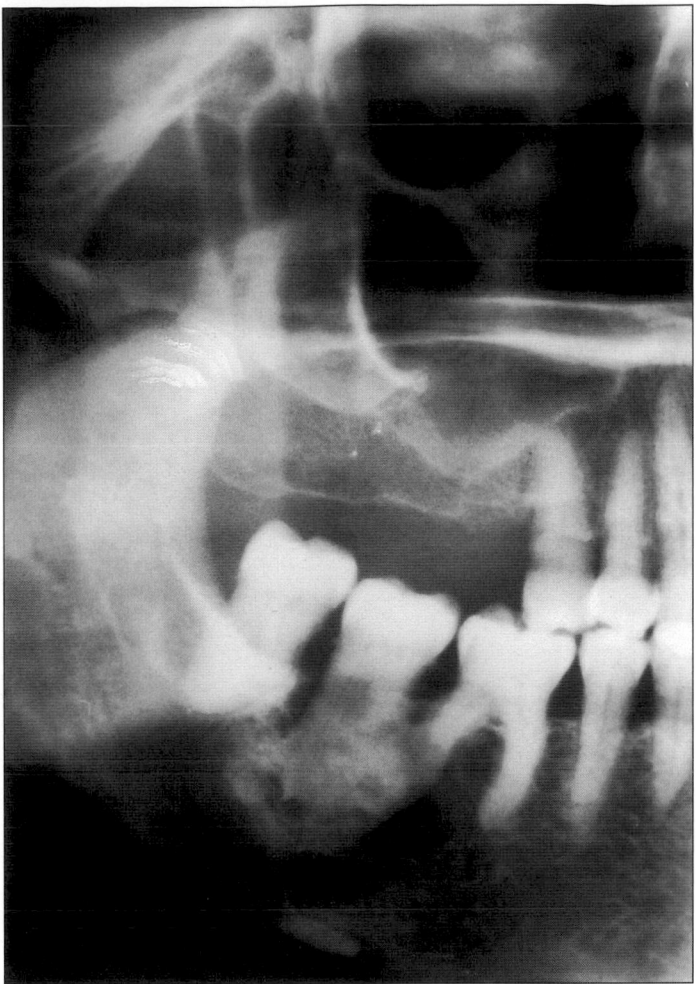

Fig. 22.26 Expansile radiopaque mass characteristic of cementoblastoma. Note adherence to the mandibular second molar roots.

Treatment and prognosis

Cementoblastoma is thought to have a relatively unlimited growth potential, with a tendency for expansion of the jaw, root resorption, and bone erosion. Even with this potential for growth, a conservative surgical approach is the treatment of choice. Extraction of the associated tooth with the intact tumor mass is indicated regardless of whether one encounters a vital or nonvital pulp. The tumor can easily be enucleated from adjacent bone, which reinforces the concept that a conservative surgical approach is the treatment of choice.

DUAL (MIXED) EPITHELIAL AND MESENCHYMAL ODONTOGENIC TUMORS

Ameloblastic fibroma

Clinical and radiologic features

The ameloblastic fibroma is an odontogenic neoplasm derived from both epithelial (ameloblastic) and connective tissue (fibroma) elements of the odontogenic apparatus. Most authorities consider that as the two cell types proliferate, they tend to undergo patterns of

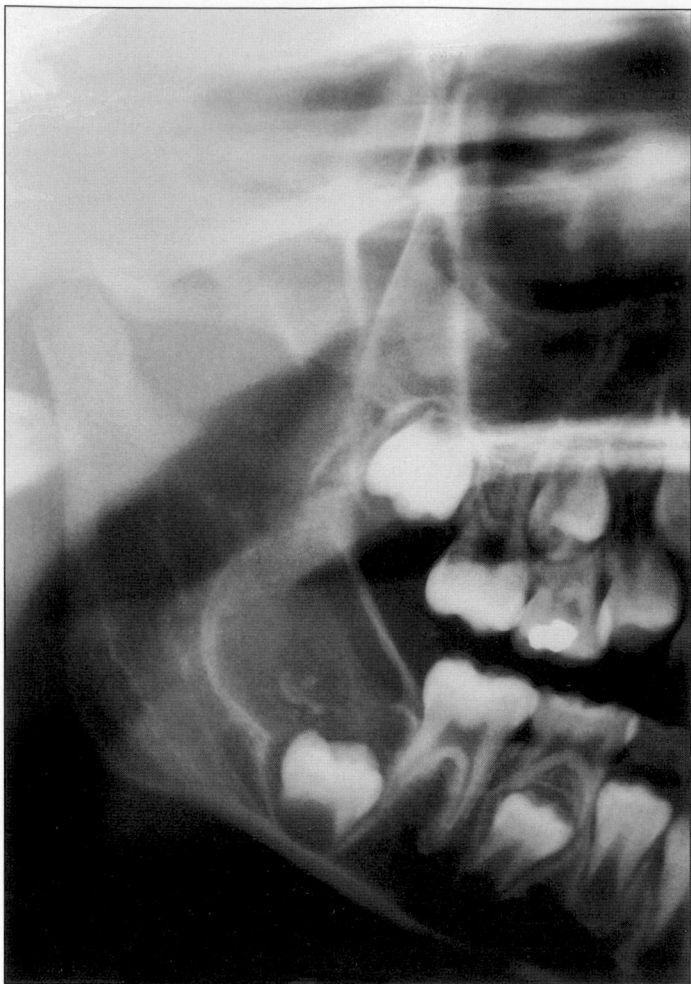

Fig. 22.27 Ameloblastic fibroma. Note radiolucent defect with focal calcification surrounding an unerupted second molar.

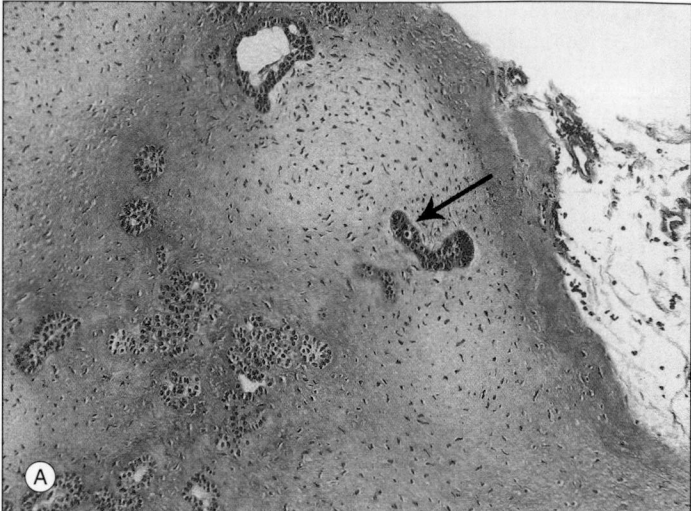

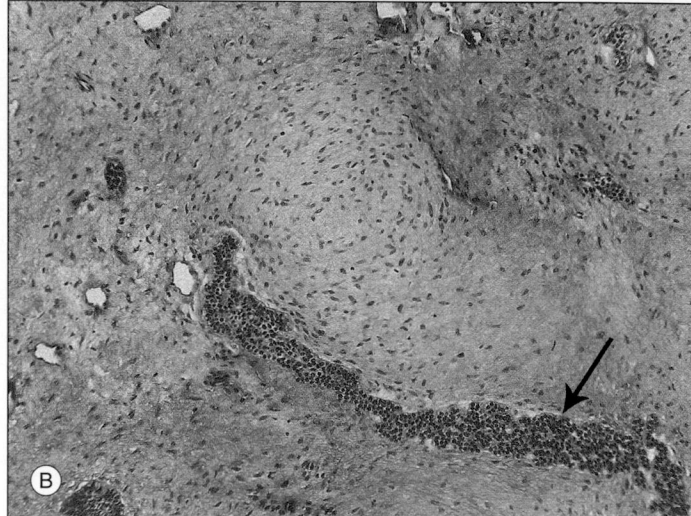

Fig. 22.28 A,B, Ameloblastic fibroma showing cell-rich embryonic stroma with odontogenic epithelial islands (arrows).

normal odontogenesis. Chaudry and associates[111] and Trodahl[112] found that odontogenic fibromas occur primarily in patients younger than the age of 20 and that the average age was 15. Marx[86] reports a mean age range of 6 to 12. Males are slightly favored.

The classic manifestation of the tumor is that of a painless swelling. The tumor usually manifests radiologically as either a unilocular or multilocular radiolucency (Fig. 22.27). There may be considerable cortical expansion in the case of larger lesions. Trodahl[112] found that 75% of the lesions that he identified were associated with the crown of an impacted tooth and that most lesions displayed a multilocular radiologic pattern.

Pathologic features

Grossly, the ameloblastic fibroma has the consistency of a solid fibrous tumor. The lesion may or may not be rimmed by a definitive collagenous capsule. Microscopically, one is able to identify sheets, nests, strands, and cords of epithelial cells set in a cellular embryonal-appearing connective tissue stroma (Fig. 22.28). The epithelial cells usually are surrounded by a prominent basement membrane and are composed predominantly of cuboidal or low columnar cells arranged back to back. The epithelial cells are quite similar to the peripheral layer of cells seen around the follicles in the

developing tooth germ. Frequently, the epithelial cells are arranged in a branching or linking chain-like pattern. At times, the epithelial cells are composed only of double rows of cells without a central stellate layer, although it is possible for the epithelial component to proliferate to such an extent that a central stellate reticulum akin to that seen in ameloblastoma can be found. Stellate cells, however, are never so prominent as in ameloblastoma. On occasion, the central stellate areas may undergo cystic degeneration.

Van Wyk and Uyver[113] reported finding an amorphous, eosinophilic, hyaline-like material in ameloblastic fibroma. The material typically surrounds epithelial islands. Edwards and Coubran[114] reported a cystic ameloblastic fibroma with melanin pigment entrapment. The pigment appeared similar to what Richardson et al.[115] described in their pigmented calcifying epithelial odontogenic tumor.

Differential diagnosis

One of the most important distinguishing histologic features that separate ameloblastic fibroma from ameloblastoma is the fact that the supporting connective tissue stroma in an ameloblastic fibroma is composed of a loose stellate proliferation of connective tissue cells that resemble that of the normal dental papilla. There is rarely any evidence of the dense collagen formation seen in the supporting stroma of the ameloblastoma.

Ameloblastic fibroma can also be confused histologically with calcifying epithelial odontogenic tumor, adenomatoid odontogenic tumor, and odontoma. The calcifying epithelial odontogenic tumor is also composed of sheets and cords of neoplastic epithelial cells; however, these cells can be differentiated from the epithelial cells in ameloblastoma because of their strikingly eosinophilic cytoplasm. Columnar ameloblasts with nuclear polarization are also absent in the calcifying epithelial odontogenic tumor. The calcifying epithelial odontogenic tumor also features a mature collagenous stroma, not the immature mesenchymal stroma of ameloblastic fibroma.

Adenomatoid odontogenic tumor occurs in the same age groups as the ameloblastic fibroma. It may also contain elongated and anastomosing cords of epithelium similar to that found in ameloblastic fibroma. The adenomatoid odontogenic tumor usually has a thick, cyst-like fibrous capsule, however. Such a capsule is usually not encountered in ameloblastic fibroma. The adenomatoid odontogenic tumor also often resembles a cyst with luminal epithelial proliferations, a feature that is not seen in ameloblastic fibroma. The stroma of the adenomatoid odontogenic tumor is extremely sparse and does not constitute a major portion of the neoplasm, whereas a loose stellate connective tissue stroma is exceedingly prominent in the ameloblastic fibroma. Finally, the ameloblastic fibroma has no organoid rosettes or ductal structures, prominent features of the adenomatoid odontogenic tumor.

Treatment and prognosis

The ameloblastic fibroma is generally considered to be a non-aggressive benign odontogenic tumor, which can easily be enucleated. Transition of ameloblastic fibroma to ameloblastic fibrosarcoma has been reported, but such transformation is exceedingly rare.[112] All such malignant transitions have been reported in adults.

Ameloblastic fibro-odontoma

Clinical and radiologic features

The ameloblastic fibro-odontoma is a rare neoplasm that most often manifests radiologically as a unilocular or multilocular cystic-appearing lesion with radiopaque central zones. WHO recognizes this tumor as a distinct odontogenic tumor, which affects both sexes equally and occurs at an early age, usually within the second decade of life.[18] There remains, nonetheless, considerable debate as to whether the lesion should be classified as a separate odontogenic tumor. Some investigators believe the tumor to be no more than a hamartomatous transitional phase in the development of an odontoma.

Ameloblastic fibro-odontoma was first described in 1967 by Hooker,[116] who differentiated it from ameloblastic odontoma. Because of the tumor's histologic resemblance to ameloblastic fibroma and/or a developing odontoma, an appreciation of its clinical presentation is paramount if a proper diagnosis is to be rendered. A small lesion abutting the occlusal surface of an erupting tooth is in all likelihood no more than a developing odontoma and not an ameloblastic fibroma or ameloblastic fibro-odontoma. Tsataras[117] reviewed a series of ameloblastic fibro-odontomas and found the median age to be 13 years, with 73.3% of the cases occurring in individuals younger than 20 years.

Pathologic features

Histologically, the ameloblastic fibro-odontoma is composed of three principal elements: (1) a stroma rich in an immature cellular

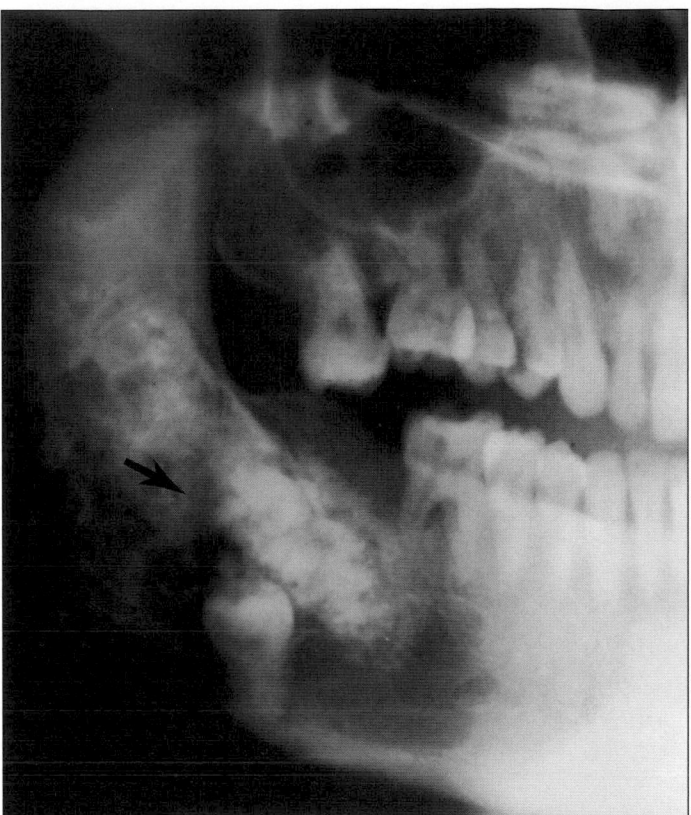

Fig. 22.29 Odontoameloblastoma showing impacted tooth, dense calcifications, and multilocular osseous destruction.

connective tissue resembling developing dental pulp or dental papilla; (2) an ectodermal component characterized by islands of epithelium composed of palisading columnar or cuboidal cells at the periphery and loosely arranged cells in the central stroma; and (3) a mineralized component made up of dental structures that include either dentin, enamel, or cementum.

Treatment and prognosis

Because ameloblastic fibro-odontomas are usually well circumscribed, management centers on enucleation with curettage and/or curettage with eburnation of the surrounding bone. A few cases of transitional ameloblastic fibrosarcoma have been documented that require more aggressive therapy.

Odontoameloblastoma

Clinical and radiographic features

This rare tumor of mixed epithelial and mesenchymal origin is thought to have the same destructive potential as the ameloblastoma. There are only a few large series reports of this lesion in the literature. The neoplasm presents most commonly in children and young adults, and it is frequently associated with bony expansion, pain, and eruption delays of the teeth. The most frequent radiographic presentation of the tumor is as a unilocular or multilocular destructive process that contains calcified masses that may resemble teeth (Fig. 22.29). Some investigators suggest that the odontoameloblastoma is a collision tumor between a simultaneously occurring ameloblastoma and odontoma.[86]

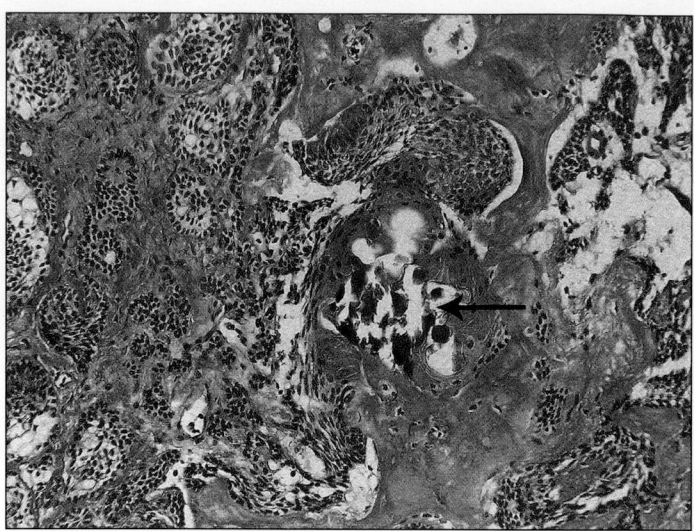

Fig. 22.30 Odontoameloblastoma. Note ameloblastic islands surrounding a central calcified odontogenic product (arrow).

Pathologic features

The tumor is composed of a mixture of dental tissues ranging from primitive mesenchymal product to dentin, pulp, periodontal ligament, and enamel. The odontoma portion of the neoplasm may predominate so that rudimentary tooth-like foci are observed, or the tumor may be largely composed of classic ameloblastoma islands within only minimal inductive calcified product (Fig. 22.30).

Treatment and prognosis

Because the odontoameloblastoma is considered to have a biologic behavior similar to that of ameloblastoma, marginal resection is the treatment of choice. Recurrence is high when curettage or enucleation are employed.

Odontoma

Clinical and radiologic features

The odontoma is the most common of all odontogenic tumors or hamartomatous growth of the jaws. The odontoma represents an aborted attempt at tooth formation and in the past the lesion has been subclassified into *compound* and *complex* subtypes. Clinically, most odontomas are identified in adolescents. Budnick[118] reviewed a series of 149 odontomas and found that 76 were of the complex type and composed of a mass of haphazardly arranged dentin, enamel, cementum, and connective tissue with little resemblance to normal tooth morphology. The remainder of his cases were of the compound variety and composed of tooth-like structures arranged in an organized pattern.

Regezi and associates[119] found that 30% of 706 odontogenic tumors they reviewed were odontomas. Complex odontomas are more common in the mandible, usually posterior to the mental foramen, whereas compound odontomas show a predilection for the anterior maxilla. The most common age for diagnosis and treatment is the second decade of life.

Clinically, the lesions are usually asymptomatic, and the most common complaint, if there is one, is intraoral swelling. Most lesions are identified on the basis of routine radiographs and appear as radiopaque masses, sometimes surrounded by lytic areas. Small denticles or tooth-like structures may also be surrounded by a radiolucent area.

Pathologic features

Odontomas are composed of enamel, enamel matrix, dentin, cementum, and pulpal tissue arranged in either or haphazard pattern or resembling normal tooth formation.

Grossly, one usually receives a hard tissue structure, often with attached firm soft tissue or, on occasion, granulation tissue. The presence of a calcified dental product in the tissue samples negates a diagnosis of ameloblastoma. It is often exceedingly difficult to distinguish between ameloblastic fibro-odontoma and an early developing complex odontoma, and the distinction may be of academic interest only. Epithelial odontogenic remnants may be prominent within odontomas.

Treatment and prognosis

All odontomas have a limited growth potential, and even though they may enlarge dramatically, for the most part they behave in a quiescent and totally benign biologic fashion. Enucleation and curettage are the treatment of choice for the odontoma and both are curative.

RARE MALIGNANT ODONTOGENIC TUMORS OF NONEPITHELIAL ORIGIN

The only odontogenic cancer of mesenchymal origin to occur with any frequency is the *ameloblastic fibrosarcoma*, the most common of all malignant odontogenic tumors.

Leider and colleagues[120] regard the lesion to be a transitional malignant counterpart of the ameloblastic fibroma. In a review of seventeen such lesions, they found the tumor occurring most frequently in young individuals, with an average age of 30 years. The tumor shows no sex predilection, and occurs more often in the mandible rather than in the maxilla. The ameloblastic fibrosarcoma can arise de novo as well.

Kramer and associates[18] define the ameloblastic fibrosarcoma as a neoplasm that appears similar to ameloblastic fibroma, with the distinction that the mesodermal component shows sarcomatous features. Some investigators[121,122] note that a calcified component may be present within the neoplasm.

Most patients with an ameloblastic fibrosarcoma present with a chief complaint of pain or swelling. Occasionally, paresthesia may also be reported. The lesions have been described most often as multilocular, occasionally showing zones of root resorption. The tumor is composed histologically of an odontogenic epithelial component that may show atypical features and a cellular stroma composed of malignant palisading spindle cells. Dysplastic dentin may occasionally be observed. Ameloblastic fibrosarcoma is a low-grade malignant neoplasm, and there are few reports of tumors metastasizing. The tumor is most often treated by marginal resection.

LESIONS OF ORAL SOFT TISSUES

DEVELOPMENTAL CONDITIONS

Median rhomboid glossitis

Clinical features

Median rhomboid glossitis is a relatively common disorder that appears clinically as a red, angular, diamond-shaped or ovoid area on the dorsal surface of the tongue. It is usually identified at the junction of the anterior two-thirds and posterior one-third of the tongue. The etiology of the condition is unknown, although most authorities postulate that it arises from a failure of the tuberculum impar to retract at the time of formation of the two lateral halves of the tongue, resulting in a central depapillated overgrowth. It has been proposed that the lesion arises from salivary gland inclusions, odontogenic epithelial rests, and even candidal infection.[123]

The condition is usually symptomless, unless the patient eats hot spicy foods or drinks exceedingly hot fluids, and it is brought to the patient's attention by the clinician. A differential diagnosis often includes squamous cell carcinoma; however, squamous cell carcinoma is exceedingly rare on the central portion of the dorsal surface of the tongue.

Pathologic features

Histologically, findings include acanthotic epithelium devoid of papillae. There may be marked branching and elongation of rete ridges as they penetrate into the supporting connective tissue. The connective tissue is usually mildly inflamed, with increased vascularity.

Treatment usually involves management of symptoms when they occur.

Lingual thyroid nodule (persistent lingual thyroid gland)

Clinical features

Functioning ectopic lingual thyroid tissue can be found in the oral cavity in the form of a tumor-like mass. It frequently presents a differential diagnostic challenge. Such nodules have been reported on the posterolateral and dorsal surfaces of the tongue and on the floor of the mouth.[124] Lingual thyroid nodules may remain dormant until puberty and then begin to proliferate as nodular masses that can be quite alarming. It is important that the clinician evaluate these nodules thoroughly because, on occasion, they have been described as the only functioning thyroid tissue in the body.[125]

Pathologic features

Lingual nodules resemble normal thyroid tissue, but when enlargement occurs there may be changes that resemble those seen in a colloid goiter. Sauk[126] implemented a study to determine the frequency of ectopic oral thyroid tissue. In a series of 200 consecutively accessioned autopsies, Sauk was able to identify thyroid tissue in 10% of the cases, a rather high frequency.

LESIONS OF EPITHELIAL ORIGIN

Squamous papilloma

Clinical features

Papillomatous proliferation of squamous epithelium is a common morphologic feature of squamous papilloma, verruca vulgaris, condyloma acuminatum, inflammatory papillary hyperplasia, papillary squamous cell carcinoma and verrucous carcinoma. It is well documented that one or more of more than 100 types of human papillomavirus (HPV), a double-stranded DNA virus, serve as the causative infectious agent in verruca vulgaris of the skin and in anogenital condylomata acuminata.[127] Eversole and associates[128] have been able to demonstrate type 2 DNA in oral and labial verruca vulgaris, and HPV DNA has been found in host oral papillary lesions, including the oral squamous papilloma.[129] HPV type 6 and 11 are found in most cases. A number of studies have also alluded to

the presence of *ras* p21[130] *c-myc* [131] oncogene products in these lesions, in addition to the wild type *p53* suppressor gene and proliferating cell nuclear antigen (*PCNA*).[132]

The oral squamous papilloma is a surface epithelial neoplasm and represents one of the most frequently encountered benign lesions in the oral cavity.[133,134] The prevalence rate is documented between 1–4.6/100 000 with equal frequency among men and women.[134–136] Bhaskar[137] and Jones[138] report that papillomas represent 80% of all the tumors of the oral cavity in children, and Kohn and associates[139] indicate that they are the most frequent benign neoplasm of the soft palate and uvula. Waldron, in a review of 125 papillomas (unpublished data), noted that more than 50% occurred in the second to fifth decades of life, with the lip being the most common site. They can present clinically as broad-based, raised, oval swellings, or they may be pedunculated. The surface is typically corrugated or villous. Most tumors in the oral cavity take on a marked degree of keratinization and appear as white lesions, although red lesions may occur in nonkeratinized regions, especially in the posterior pharynx.

Although most lesions present as single lesions, multiple coalescent oral papillomas can occur in association with verruca vulgaris or condyloma acuminatum of the skin,[140,141] focal dermal hyperplasia syndrome (Goltz-Gorlin syndrome), and Heck's disease. Florid oral papillomatosis (FOP) can be seen in association with other lesions such as traumatic lesions or lichen planus and in occasions may be associated with conditions such as nevus unius lateris, acanthosis nigricans and Cowden syndrome. Eversole and Sorenson[142] have reported florid oral papillomatosis in Down syndrome patients. The exact etiology in these florid lesions is unclear and may be related to reasons other than HPV (irritation, trauma, diabetes, etc.).

In an evaluation of 110 oral papillomas, Greer and Goldman[143] found the age range to be 6 to 85, with 38 as the median age. They documented one exceedingly rare inverted oral papilloma, histologically similar to the inverted papilloma of the paranasal sinuses and bladder.

The most frequent location for oral squamous papilloma documented by Greer and Goldman was the tongue. Together the palate and buccal mucosa accounted for nearly as many lesions. The three sites combined accounted for two-thirds of the lesions.

Pathologic features

The papilloma is classically an exophytic lesion demonstrating a complex pattern of multiple finger-like projections of stratified squamous epithelium surrounding a central vascular connective tissue core. The epithelium may be hyperkeratotic or acanthotic, and the supporting collagen usually contain chronic inflammatory cells, especially if there has been superficial ulceration of the lesion due to trauma. Occasionally, lesions that are much more biologically aggressive than papillomas may take on a papillomatous appearance clinically. Wertheimer and Stroud[144] have reported a case of peripheral ameloblastoma occurring in a papilloma, but the relationship of this lesion to the more benign papilloma is purely morphologic. Greer and Goldman were unable to detect evidence of dysplasia in a large series, thus contradicting some reports that indicated that some oral papillomas might display a malignant change.

Other benign papillomatous lesions

Verruca vulgaris, or the common skin wart, is HPV induced, with HPV-2, HPV-4, or HPV-40 most often implicated.[145] It only rarely occurs in the oral cavity. *Condyloma acuminatum* or the venereal wart is most frequently initiated by HPV-6, HPV-11, HPV-16, or HPV-18, although other viruses have been identified in tissue samples evaluated

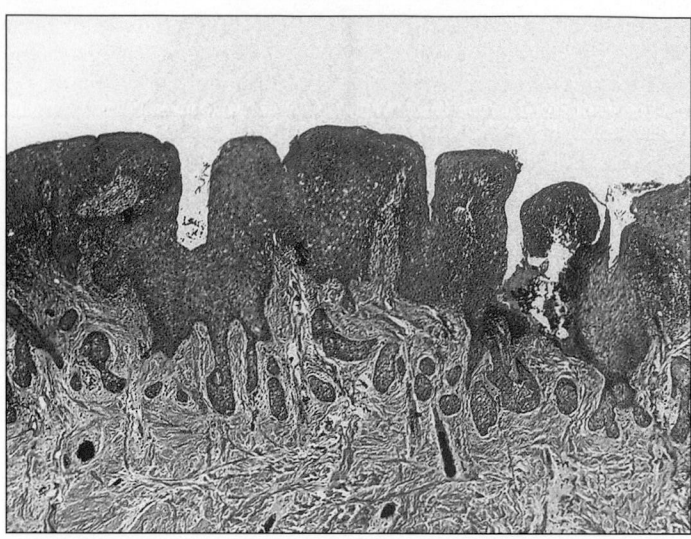

Fig. 22.31 Inflammatory papillary hyperplasia. Note the nodular projections of thickened squamous epithelium and the underlying interface chronic inflammatory infiltrate.

by PCR assay. The disorder is sexually transmitted, and although it is most common in the anogenital region, the oral cavity can be affected. Oral lesions, like their anogenital counterparts, tend to be larger than squamous papillomas. They are clustered as opposed to solitary, and histologically their epithelial fronds tend to be broad and blunt with keratin plugging in between. Surgical excision is the treatment of choice for verrucae and condyloma. Although genital condyloma have been reported to undergo malignant transformation, oral condyloma show little propensity to undergo malignant change.[146]

Treatment and prognosis

Excision of the oral squamous papilloma at its base is mandatory to prevent recurrence. Although this is the most prevalent form of treatment, cryosurgery has been used as well.

Inflammatory papillary hyperplasia

Clinical features

Inflammatory papillary hyperplasia most often occurs in the oral cavity in association with an ill-fitting maxillary denture or in association with poor oral hygiene. The typical site is the palate, although cases have been reported in the cheeks.[147] It is rather uncommon to find inflammatory papillary hyperplasia in patients who do not wear dentures, but it does occur, with the same clinical appearance as the lesion in a denture-bearing area. Greer and associates[148] identified HPV DNA in smokeless tobacco-associated keratoses from juveniles, adults, and older patients, using papillary hyperplasia cases as control tissue samples. In none of 35 instances of papillary hyperplasia were they able to identify HPV DNA.

Typically, the lesions appear as diffuse papillary or warty exophytic lesions affecting denture-bearing areas (Fig. 22.31). They may be so extensive as to take on the appearance of verrucous carcinoma; thus, verrucous carcinoma is often included in a differential diagnosis of such lesions. Frequently, the epithelium is ulcerated owing to the trauma from ill-fitting dentures. The chief complaint may be pain when ulceration occurs. Rarely, the disorder has been documented in the palate of nondenture wearers who are mouth breathers.

There has been debate in the literature as to whether papillary hyperplasia is a premalignant lesion. Although there are reported cases of the development of squamous cell carcinoma arising in lesions that were thought to be papillary hyperplasia,[147] there is little evidence to support the theory that this lesion actually leads to the development of squamous cell carcinoma. Differential diagnoses that should be considered on the basis of clinical examination include florid oral papillomatosis, multifocal condyloma acuminatum, and verrucous carcinoma.

Pathologic features

Papillary hyperplasia presents as a proliferation of multiple exophytic papillary projections, supported by a connective tissue core that is nearly always chronically inflamed. Very often, the chronic inflammatory infiltrate is limited to the superficial connective tissue layer and is composed predominantly of plasma cells and lymphocytes. The epithelium may show marked hyperkeratosis, parakeratosis, or acanthosis. Atypical epithelial changes are rarely, if ever, identified.

Treatment and prognosis

The treatment of choice is surgical excision unless the lesion is very small, in which case it may respond to denture relief, relining of the denture, or reconstruction of the denture.

Keratoacanthoma

Clinical features

Keratoacanthoma, also known as self-healing carcinoma, is a lesion that typically occurs on sun-exposed skin surfaces. The most common perioral site is the lip. It can occur in the oral cavity, but it is an exceedingly rare intraoral phenomenon. Svirsky et al.[149] have reported a solitary keratoacanthoma on the maxillary gingiva in a 12-year-old boy, and few additional cases of solitary intraoral keratoacanthoma have been reported in the English literature. Periorally, keratoacanthoma usually occurs along the vermilion border of the lip, where it presents as a painless, usually rapidly growing, 1–2 cm, firm, raised nodule with a central keratin-filled crater. It tends to occur most frequently in middle-aged and older patients, but there are reports in infants and children.[150] Males appear to be affected twice as frequently as females. Actinic damage to the skin and HPV, subtypes 26 and 27, have been suggested as etiologic agents for sun-exposed surfaces in which keratoacanthomas arise.[151] Two variants of keratoacanthoma are recognized: solitary and multiple.[150,152] In the multiple keratoacanthomatous state, the oral mucous membranes are rarely involved; when they are, the histologic appearance of the multifocal keratoacanthomas is similar to that of solitary cutaneous or mucosal keratoacanthoma.[153] Muir-Torre syndrome is a symptom complex of multiple keratoacanthomas, sebaceous tumors, and carcinomas of the gastrointestinal tract. Oral lesions in association with the syndrome are rare.

Most investigators concur that keratoacanthomas of the skin arise from a portion of the adnexal hair follicle. There is some debate as to origin of the lesion when it presents entirely on the mucosal surface of the oral cavity. Svirsky and coworkers[149] postulate that an adnexal structure other than a hair follicle may be responsible for the development of intraoral keratoacanthoma, and it is their contention that perhaps sebaceous glands, which are common to the mucous membranes as well as to the skin, may be responsible for the development of keratoacanthoma. In the small number of well-documented intraoral cases, it has been rather difficult to demonstrate sebaceous glands in tissue sections; therefore, the hypothesis that the lesion

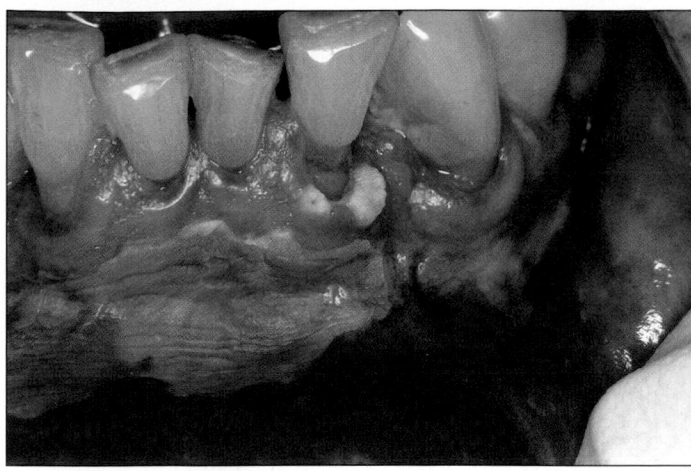

Fig. 22.32 Oral leukoplakia. Note the white patch covering part of the gingiva. (Courtesy of John McDowell, DDS, Denver, Colorado.)

Table 22.3 Leukoplakia of the oral cavity – clinical types

Authors	Leukoplakia subtype
Pindborg et al.[156]	Homogeneous; white patch with a variable appearance, smooth or wrinkled; smooth areas may have small cracks or fissures Speckled or nodular: erythematous base with white patches or nodular excrescences
Sugar and Banocyz[157]	Leukoplakia simplex: white, homogeneous keratinized lesion, slightly elevated Leukoplakia verrucosa: white, verrucous lesion, with wrinkled surface Leukoplakia erosiva: white lesion with erythematous areas, erosions, fissures

arises from sebaceous adnexal structures remains unsupported histologically. The distinctive features of keratoacanthoma are described elsewhere.

LEUKOPLAKIA AND ERYTHROPLAKIA

The term *leukoplakia* is used to classify a white patch or plaque on the oral mucous membrane (Fig. 22.32) that cannot be removed by scraping and cannot be classified clinically or microscopically as another disease entity.[154,155]

Leukoplakia has further been defined to have multiple subtypes by Pindborg and associates[156] and Sugar and Banocyz.[157] Table 22.3 depicts the various types of leukoplakia described by these investigators. Leukoplakia appears to occur most often before age 40 and shows a predilection for males. In Sugar and Banocyz's study of 670 leukoplakic patients who were followed for more than 3 years, 31% of the lesions disappeared, 30% improved, and 25% remained unchanged. Their study and those of Pindborg and others revealed that approximately 6% of oral leukoplakias became malignant. Leukoplakia has been reported in all oral sites but appears to be most common in the tongue, lips, and floor of the mouth.

Burkhardt[158] has separated leukoplakia into three microscopic forms, corresponding to the verrucous and erosive clinical forms that have been described: (1) plain, (2) papillary endophytic, and (3) papillomatous exophytic. However, most authorities consider leukoplakia to be exclusively a clinical term and suggest that there is no histologic picture that is uniquely characteristic of this process.

Erythroplakia is defined as a red patch that is characteristically velvety and cannot be clinically or pathologically ascribed to any other disease entity. It is considered by many investigators to be the earliest sign of asymptomatic oral cancer.[159] It is important to consider both leukoplakia and erythroplakia together, as both in the past have been considered premalignant lesions. Figure 22.33 is a schematic representation of a clinical leukoplakia/erythroplakia continuum that also depicts the microscopic findings that can be seen in association with these oral changes, from benign keratosis through carcinoma in situ.

Although various systemic diseases may appear as white plaques (lichen planus, syphilitic mucous patches, moniliasis, lupus erythematosus), such entities do not, in fact, represent leukoplakia as defined by WHO, because they have a distinctive histologic appearance.[155]

The prevalence of oral leukoplakia in the general population is unknown, although there are studies that indicate it affects from 0.2–0.5% of the population.[155,160,161] Typically, patients with leukoplakia are totally asymptomatic, and the lesions are most commonly discovered on routine examination of the oral cavity or because the patient may be aware of a roughness or color change within the mouth. It is mandatory in nearly all instances to do a biopsy of such white lesions to determine their exact nature. The agents that are most commonly implicated as causal are cigarette smoking, tobacco chewing, snuff dipping, and the concomitant use of alcohol in excess.

Greer and associates[148] have identified a special form of leukoplakia (smokeless tobacco leukoplakia) associated with the use of smokeless tobacco products. These investigators have identified HPV DNA in 15% of smokeless tobacco keratoses and suggest that the HPV may play a synergistic role with tobacco to produce such clinically discernible leukoplakic lesions. Dysplasia was only rarely identified in their series. The possible premalignant nature of leukoplakia has been debated for many years. Silverman and Galante[154] contend that between 2.5% and 6% of lesions properly ascribed the name *leukoplakia* transform into carcinoma. Mashberg and Meyers[159] suggest that erythroplakia is even more likely to develop into cancer than leukoplakia. Intermediate forms (speckled leukoplakia or erythroplakia) have also been reported.[162]

Hansen et al.[163] in 1985 described a lesion they defined as *proliferative verrucous leukoplakia*, a series of irregular white patches or plaques that progress slowly across the oral mucosa membranes with nearly a 100% risk of malignant transformation and a high risk of recurrence after removal. In 1980, Shear and Pindborg[164] described a series of 68 precancerous lesions described clinically as indistinguishable from verrucous carcinomas, which they termed *verrucous leukoplakia*. Histologic findings in these so-called leukoplakic lesions range from simple benign hyperkeratosis through carcinoma in situ.

Although oral leukoplakia is defined quite simply as a white patch; most investigators consider it to have precancerous potential. Factors that potentiate that risk include tobacco, alcohol, microorganisms including viruses, nutrition, and actinic radiation. These etiologic factors are discussed more fully under the heading Squamous cell carcinoma.

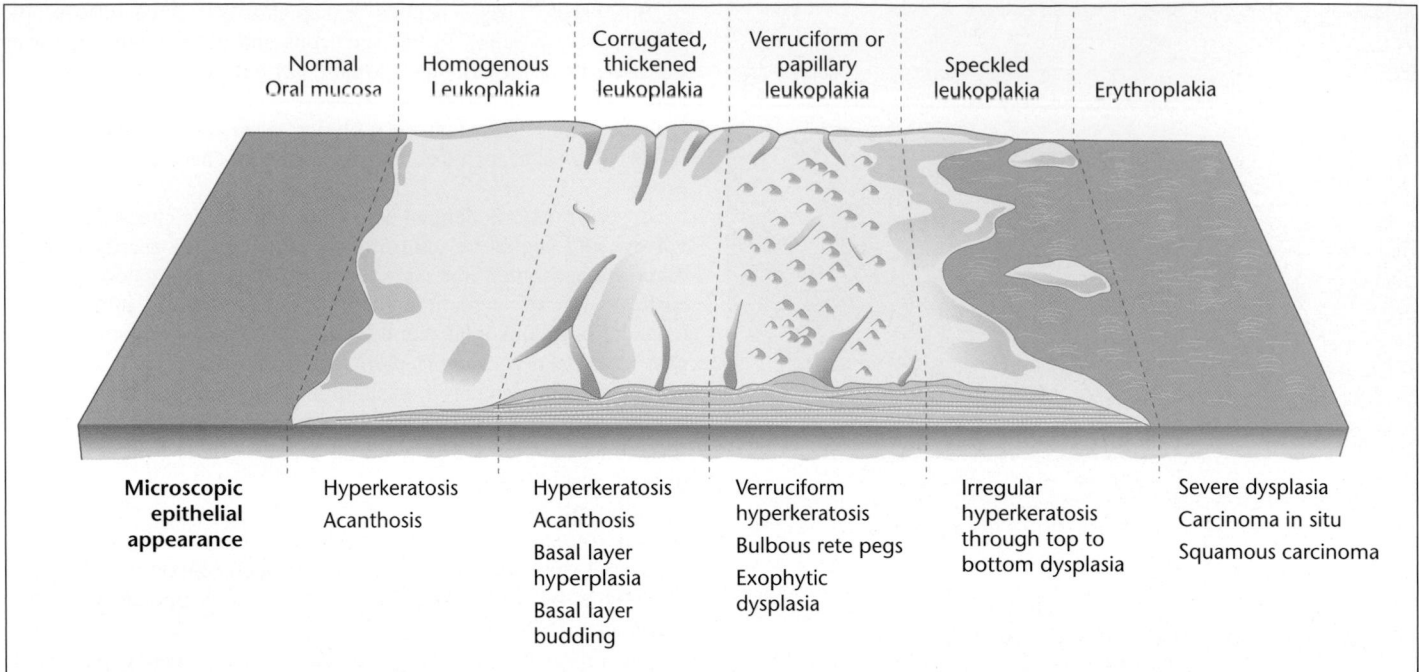

Fig. 22.33 Leukoplakia/erythroplakia continuum showing various clinical and histopathologic alterations ranging from hyperkeratosis through carcinoma in situ.

Nicotine stomatitis (stomatitis nicotina)

Clinical features

Smoking, particularly cigar and pipe smoking, is the etiologic agent responsible for nicotine stomatitis, and it occurs almost exclusively in men. This lesion has been linked to the heat and other combustion products [165–167] resulting from tobacco smoking. Interestingly, it is also reported in patients who are not smokers but drink hot liquids.[168] Nicotine stomatitis is characterized by palatal hyperkeratosis with central red areas representing inflamed or obstructed minor salivary gland ducts. The surrounding and intervening mucosa is frequently also white and may show desquamation.

Pathologic features

Histologically, the pathologist can appreciate hyperkeratinized epithelium and marked squamous metaplasia with deep rete ridge penetration into the connective tissue lamina propria, with diffuse inflammation that frequently surrounds small ducts and associated minor salivary glands. It is often difficult to identify a section showing salivary gland to surface epithelial communication, the classic histologic marker of the disorder.

The lesion is benign and shows no progression toward dysplasia. Although nicotine stomatitis is thought to be a reversible benign transformation, the continued use of the tobacco irritant may in fact potentiate a de novo palatal carcinoma, unassociated with the previous nicotine stomatitis.

The treatment of choice is cessation of smoking and/or drinking hot liquids, as most of these lesions regress after employing these measures.

Lichen planus

Lichen planus is a mucocutaneous disease, characterized by the development of white or lacy striae in the oral cavity. Although in the strictest sense its origin is immunologically mediated, the disorder is discussed here because its clinical features so closely mimic those of leukoplakia. Lichen planus can mimic traumatic hyperkeratosis, leukoedema, geographic tongue of the ectopic variety, or white sponge nevus. Lesions may also occur on the skin or oral cavity as bullae or ulcers, or as plaque-like abrasions. Skin lesions may not precede oral lesions (15–35% of patients).

The pathologic process in lichen planus is unknown. However, it is likely that antigen-specific and non-specific mechanisms are involved. Antigen specific mechanisms include a cell-mediated response localized to the basement membrane zone and characterized by degeneration of the epithelial cells in the basal layer and disruption of the basement membrane. An atypical, possibly premalignant form of lichen planus termed *lichenoid dysplasia* has been investigated by Eisenberg and colleagues.[168B] These investigators suggest that, although superficial similarities exist at the clinical and microscopic levels between lichen planus and lichenoid dysplasia, lichenoid dysplasia is characterized by classic cytologic alterations of dysplasia and the features of lichen planus may only be coincident. They further suggest that immunostaining may allow distinction between the two disorders. Greer et al.[168C] have reported a 2% transformation rate of oral lichen planus to oral squamous cell carcinoma. The principal treatment has been local and systemic corticosteroids; however, recent research suggests that erosive lichen planus can be treated with systemic isotretinoin and topical retinoic acid.[169] Others find the relationship coincidental.[170] The pathologic features of lichen planus are discussed at length in Chapter 7.

Oral epithelial dysplasia

Features characteristic of oral epithelial dysplasia are the classic cytologic abnormalities associated with most epithelial atypias: basal layer hyperchromatism, atypical mitoses, altered nuclear: cytoplasmic ratios, loss of cellular polarity, nuclear pleomorphism,

Table 22.4 Oral epithelial dysplasia

Microscopic features
An increased nuclear:cytoplasmic ratio
Sharp angled rete processes
Loss of cellular polarity
Cellular pleomorphism
Nuclear pleomorphism
Enlarged nucleoli
Reduction of cellular cohesion
Individual spinous layer cell keratinization
Increased number of mitotic figures
Presence of mitotic figures in the superficial half of the epithelium
Basal cell layer hyperplasia
Loss of polarity of the basal cells

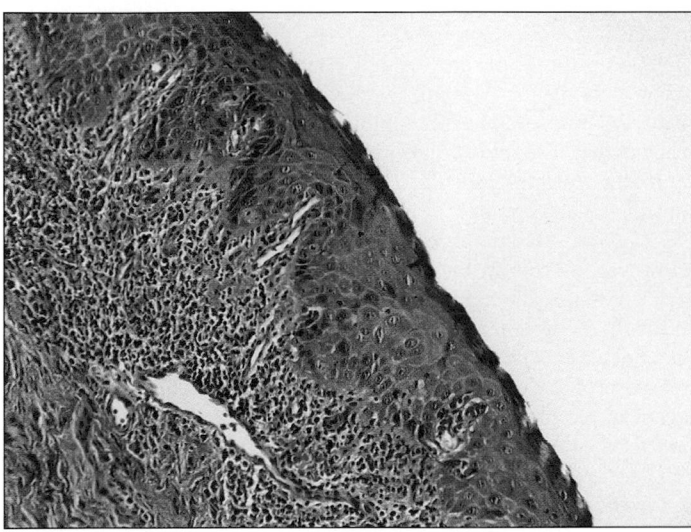

Fig. 22.34 Moderate epithelial dysplasia.

hyperchromatic nucleoli, and basal layer hyperplasia to name a few (Table 22.4). The WHO Collaborating Center for Oral Precancerous Lesions has defined a battery of such histologic features that are characteristic of squamous oral dysplasia.

Epithelial dysplasia of the oral cavity has not undergone the close scrutiny and extensive categorization that dysplasia of the uterine cervix has. Oral epithelial dysplasia is usually classified as mild, moderate, or severe. In mild dysplasia, the severity of atypical change is minimal; the most prominent features may include only basal layer hyperplasia, loss of cellular polarity, and atypical mitoses. The surface layer is usually hyperkeratinized, so the lesion appears white clinically. As the atypical cytologic changes increase to include a greater frequency of altered nuclear:cytoplasmic ratios, dyskeratoses, basal layer hyperchromatism, and mitoses, the degree of severity of the dysplasia increases proportionately (Fig. 22.34). It has been suggested that the term oral intraepithelial neoplasia (OIN), synonymous with the cervix (CIN system) and the vulva (VIN system), should be used to characterize the dysplastic changes in the oral mucosa.

There is considerable debate as to whether lesions that affect the mucosa in continuity with the skin surface should be categorized as actinic keratosis or as a mild, moderate, or severe dysplastic change. It is our position that lesions involving the mucosal surface, regardless of contiguous skin surface findings, must be classified according to dysplastic criteria and not simply as an actinic change. The biologic behavior of a dysplastic lesion of the oral mucosa is inherently more aggressive than a corresponding atypical change in skin.

Once dysplasia is diagnosed, the risk of transformation increases. In one large study, there was a 23.4% malignant transformation rate in lesions with an erythroplakic component as compared with a 6.5% rate in lesions that were homogeneous leukoplakia.[158] Additionally, malignant transformation was highest (36.4%) in lesions that showed histopathologic dysplastic changes. The anatomic location of a dysplasia is another important factor in accessing the risk for malignant transformation. Lesions of the tongue (28.9%), gingiva (24.4%), and floor of mouth (15.6%) are at a greater risk of transformation than lesions located in the palate (11.1%), buccal mucosa (11.1%), and lip (8.9%).[171]

Carcinoma in situ (intraepithelial carcinoma)

The diagnosis of carcinoma in situ of the oral mucosa should be based on rigid histologic criteria; however, the distinction between carcinoma in situ and severe epithelial dysplasia is often arbitrary. Classically, a carcinoma in situ tissue sample should show all the atypical cytologic criteria necessary for a malignant diagnosis, but these atypical changes must be confined to the epithelial layer. With carcinoma in situ, one must identify an intact basement membrane and top to bottom or through and through epithelial dysplasia. Lesions that are diagnosed as carcinoma in situ may appear red, white, blue, or black clinically, and on occasion they may present as a tumor mass. Mashberg and Meyers[159] indicate that a large percentage of early epithelial changes that present as red lesions clinically show at least some degree of dysplasia, and a large percentage of the lesions represents carcinoma in situ.

Squamous cell carcinoma

Cancer statistics compiled by the National Cancer Institute and more recently by the American Cancer Society estimates that 28 900 to 30 000 new cases of oral cancer will occur in the United States in the year 2002 and predicts approximately 7 400 deaths from this disease. These statistics are based on annual surveys of oral cancers that include cancer of the lips, tongue, floor of mouth, salivary glands, oropharynx, and other unspecified sites within the mouth. Over 90% of these tumors are squamous cell carcinomas.[172] Nearly 2–3 % of all new cancer cases seen in both men and women are of the squamous cell type,[154] making it the tenth most common malignancy in the United States. Although primarily a disease of the middle and older age groups, a younger patient population presenting with oral cancers has increased alarmingly in recent years. In this younger group, the etiologic factors associated with oral cancer development remain poorly defined with proposed familial, occupational, immune deficiency, and viral-linked factors most often favored.

The male to female ratio for oral cancer is approximately 2:1,[172–174] with higher incidence seen among the African-American population (12.4 cases/100 000 population) than Caucasians (9.7 cases/100 000 population). The highest incidence is seen in the African-American males (20.5 cases/100 000 population).[174,175]

Oral cancers are estimated to account for 6.2% of all carcinomas in men and 1.9% of all carcinomas in women in the United States.[176,177] Worldwide, over 500 000 cases occur annually with a higher percentages in certain world locations, particularly Asian countries,[178] where there are reports that oral cancer represents 50% of all recorded cancers.[175,179]

Despite marked advances in treatment modalities of oral cancers in recent years, the overall five-year survival rate remains a disappointing 50–55%. Early detection and treatment remains the most important positive prognostic factor. This discussion centers on squamous epithelial lesions. Rare sarcomas of the oral cavity occur. They are discussed in Chapter 9, Soft Tissue Tumors.

Etiologic factors

Tobacco: The voluminous data establishing the link between oral cancers and the use of tobacco/cigarettes, pipes, cigars, and smokeless tobacco, including chewing tobacco and snuff,[179] reflects the continuous national and international interest in the effect of tobacco, smoking, and other related products on health and cancer development.

Studies have shown that aromatic hydrocarbons, potent carcinogens in tobacco products, contribute to tobacco's neoplastic potential, along with more than 20 other carcinogens.[180]

Investigators are continuously evaluating the molecular effects of these carcinogens and their various proposed or established mechanisms in the development of cancers. Cigarette smoking is considered to be the major cause of oral cancer in the United States.[180] The risk of developing oral cancer is three times greater for smokers than the general population of nonsmokers. Mortality rates from oral cancer increase with the number of cigarettes smoked daily and diminishes with the cessation of smoking.[177] A 1986 comprehensive evaluation of tobacco smoking completed by the International Agency for Research on Cancer demonstrated that pipe and/or cigar use increases the cancer risk to the patient at approximately the same rate as cigarette smoking.[184]

The use of tobacco in the United States has gone through many phases, and although reports from the US Surgeon General and others[176,177] have concluded that cigarette smoking is a principal cause of cancer mortality in the United States, new data suggest that smokeless tobacco consumption also puts patients at risk.[181] There has been a 40% increase in the consumption of moist snuff from 1972 to 1991.[182] The significant carcinogenic agents in smokeless tobacco include carbon monoxide, nicotine, hydrogen cyanide, ammonia, benzyl, phenol, pyridine *N*-nitrosonorinicotine, *N*-nitrosoanabasine, benzanthrene, benzanthracene, and benzopyrene.[183]

The mixed habit of using chewing tobacco and smoking is relatively rare in the United States, but it has been studied in India and Pakistan,[185] where there appears to be a synergistic reaction between chewing and smoking that increases cancer development risk.[186] Molecular studies recently conducted in Japan linked the genotoxic effect of this mixed habit on the development of mutations on oncogenes and tumor suppressor genes.[187]

A 1986 report of the US Surgeon General, *The Health Consequences of Using Smokeless Tobacco*,[188] concluded that the use of smokeless tobacco increases the risk of oral cancer. Other cancers that may be associated with smokeless tobacco use include esophageal, laryngeal, and stomach cancers.[189] Smokeless tobacco users, in addition to their cancer risk, also may become addicted to nicotine.[188]

Longitudinal studies have demonstrated an increased risk for oral cancer among smokers, including the American Cancer Society cancer prevention studies I and II, each of which followed about one million adults.[190] Numerous case control studies have also demonstrated an increased risk for oral cancer with increased use of tobacco products.[191]

Although there is a significant database suggesting a cause and effect relationship between the use of tobacco products and oral cancer,[191–195] there are certain gaps in our knowledge that need to be pursued. Additional prospective studies among tobacco users followed for extended periods, especially in the area of smokeless tobacco, need to be undertaken; and dose response-related studies are needed to determine whether there are links between the extent of exposure to tobacco and the risk of oral cancer. One such study demonstrating the relative risks for oral cancer, completed by Hirayama,[196] showed that the risk for developing oral cancer after using betel quid, a practice particularly prevalent in large populations of Southeast Asia and India, more than doubled when the frequency of use rose to six or more times per day as opposed to twice per day. Similarly, Ho[197] has linked the rising trend in oral cancer in Taiwan to rising consumption of betel quid in that country.

Experimental evidence in animals using the hamster cheek pouch model to evaluate the role of tobacco in the production of cancer in the oral cavity has long demonstrated such a link.[198,199] The model of multistage skin carcinogenesis has proven to be useful in understanding the evolution of squamous cell carcinoma and its surrogate model in the interpretation of etiologic factors responsible for the development of oral carcinoma as well.

A number of studies have also discussed the effect of environmental tobacco smoking (ETS) on the development of cancer including those of the United States environmental protection agency in 1992.[200] Zhang[201] found a dose-response relationship between exposure to ETS and elevated cancer risk in the head and neck region. The role of marijuana smoking has also been emphasized in recent years, in particular as it relates to the development of cancer in younger age groups.[202]

Alcohol: Alcohol has long been linked to a host of diseases. However, its role in the development of oral cancer as a singular agent remains the subject of continuous investigation. It has been difficult to design research that can determine how tobacco and alcohol act independently or in synergy to produce oral cancer. One of the problems associated with identifying alcohol as a singular agent in the production of oral cancer is that many heavy drinkers are also heavy users of tobacco products in one of its forms. In 1957, Wynder et al.[203] reported that excessive alcohol consumption may be a significant factor in the development of cancer of the oral cavity. Since that time, there has been a host of studies, including case–control studies that support the premise that alcohol consumption elevates oral cancer risk.[203–212] Although most scientific data suggest that alcohol consumption seems to have a potentiating effect with smoking, the mechanisms by which alcohol produces cancer in the oral cavity are poorly understood. Interestingly, Hindle has suggested that alcohol might be more important in the development of oral cancer than the use of tobacco.

Blot[213] has proposed that there are nine mechanistic pathways by which alcohol consumption causes cancer: (1) certain oncogenes and other contaminants are present in alcohol that may be carcinogenic; (2) alcohol may generate metabolites that are carcinogenic to humans, particularly as it enhances liver metabolizing activity; (3) alcohol may act as a solvent, increasing penetration of other carcinogens into target tissues; (4) alcohol may reduce intake and bioavailability of nutrients that may inhibit cancer and enhance nutritional deficiencies that increase the risk of cancer; (5) alcohol may inhibit the detoxification of carcinogenic compounds; (6) alcohol may catalyze the metabolic activation of some compounds into carcinogens as acetaldehyde; (7) alcohol may affect the hormonal status of the host; (8) alcohol may increase cellular exposure to oxidants; and (9) alcohol may suppress host immune function. Recent evidence suggests that there may be a genetic link[214–217] between alcohol dehydrogenase-2 and aldehyde dehydrogenasegenes-2 genotypes and alcohol consumption in the development of oral cancers.

Alcohol's role in the development of cancer in younger age groups is much debated. While certain studies[218] show a high percentage of their young cancer patients to be abusers of alcohol and tobacco, others[219,220] report that inherent genetic determinants play more of a role in oral cancer development in young patients.

Gaps still remain in our knowledge concerning the association between alcohol consumption and cancer of the oral cavity. Winn et al.[221] has reported that alcohol appears to increase oral cancer risk in humans regardless of the form it takes (i.e. hard liquor, beer, wine, dark or light color liquor, or mouthwash). However, alcoholic mouth rinses, which often contain as high as 25% alcohol, have not been shown definitively to increase the oral cancer risk for regular users of those products. These incongruent findings suggest a need for further clarifying how alcohol acts as a carcinogen. Perhaps, as Blot[213] suggests, contaminants or metabolites in alcohol itself may be responsible for promoting oral mucous membrane cancer. To determine how significant a factor alcohol is in the development of cancer of the oral cavity, a comprehensive study needs to be completed that evaluates its effect on the mucous membrane alone, as well as in synergy with tobacco, at the same time controlling for growth factors and growth factor receptors, expression of cancer-related genes, and genetic alterations. Studies that can identify a dose-response relationship also need to be completed prospectively, taking into account that one of the problems with designing such studies would be the enormous number of subjects who would need to be recruited and the long-term period of follow-up needed to investigate a disease of such low incidence.

Actinic radiation: The role of actinic radiation in the development of cancer in the oral cavity relates most directly to the role sunlight plays in producing cancer along the vermilion border of the lip. Johnson has demonstrated that in some countries, including the United States, Canada, Romania, Hungary, and Yugoslavia, cancer of the vermilion border of the lip is common.[222] The incidence of these 'sunlight'-induced cancers is much higher in fair-skinned individuals who are constantly exposed to the outdoor life. These cancers are much less frequent in individuals who have a darker skin pigment, and it is believed that darker pigment acts as a protective agent against actinic radiation damage.[222] The actual wavelengths of the light responsible for the actinic damage are usually considered to be those in the 2900–3200 Å range. However, experimental attempts to produce similar lesions with infrared levels of radiation have been unsuccessful.[223] The mechanism of cancer development in this area is not fully understood. It has been suggested that subepithelial collagen becomes degraded by long-term exposure to ultraviolet light, but the actual epithelial neoplastic transformation is less well understood. There are significant gaps in knowledge in this area, especially related to whether cigarette smoking and actinic radiation act in synergy. There is also little information concerning whether actinic damage to the collagen in some way potentiates epithelial neoplasia. Certain agents have been used to protect tissue from the damaging effects of ultraviolet light, including sunscreens and sun blocks.

Nutrition: Although certain nutritional deficiencies or excesses have been associated with mucous membrane cancers elsewhere in the body, particularly the colon, there are few studies directly linking food or dietary factors to oral cancer. One nutritional abnormality that predisposes to oral cancer is the sideropenia dysphasia of patients with Plummer-Vinson syndrome. This disorder is rare in the United States but common in Europe. This special form of iron deficiency anemia can be seen in oral cancer patients who are neither alcohol abusers nor tobacco users.[224] The mechanism by which iron deficiency potentiates mucous membrane cancer is not fully understood, although there are some investigators who suggest that increased mitotic activity tends to diminish the repair mechanism of epithelium, promoting mucosal atrophy and enhancing neoplastic potential.[225]

Recent epidemiologic and case–control studies confirm the protective role played by certain micronutrients (e.g vitamins, beta-carotene, iron, zinc, magnesium), vegetables, fruits, cereals and certain oils such as olive oil in preventing the development of oral cancers.[226–235] McLaughlin et al.[233] have suggested that carotenes and other vitamins may reduce one's risk for oral and pharyngeal cancer. Gupta et al.[234] in two epidemiologic studies in India found that lack of certain nutritional factors are probably contributory to the development of oral mucous membrane cancer rather than the primary functional etiologic agent, and that certain food groups have a protective role.

Also Gridley and colleagues[235] found that vitamins E, A, B, and C seemed to be related to a reduced incidence of oral and pharyngeal cancer in a large population-based study that was controlled for other oral cancer risk factors.

Orodental and occupational factors: Investigators have long debated whether poor oral hygiene, improperly fitting dental prostheses, defective dental restorations, and malaligned or sharp teeth are agents that might promote oral and pharyngeal cancer. Occasionally, oral cancer can be identified directly in the area of these proposed mitigating factors, but there is little evidence to suggest that they predispose to oral cancer.[236] Gorsky and Silverman[237] evaluated 400 patients with oral cancer at the University of California Oral Medicine Clinic to determine if denture wearing might be a risk factor in their disease. These investigators could find no correlation between the wearing of dentures and the patient's oral cancer. Numerous other studies have shown similar results.[238,239] However, reports in the literature demonstrate that hamster cheek pouch mucosa that is subjected to trauma in concert with a known carcinogen develops cancer more readily than mucosa that is not subjected to such trauma.[240] There are no clear-cut studies in humans to suggest that these findings might be transferable.

Finally, occupational exposure to certain chemicals including formaldehyde, nickel, chromium, and leather-tanning products to name a few has been implicated as factors in the development of oral cancer.[241–243]

Oncogenes, tumor suppressors, viruses, and other infectious agents: Although malignant neoplasms are thought by many investigators to be derived from a single monoclonal mutated cell,[244] squamous cancers have been shown to consist of either monoclonal or polyclonal phenotypes. Thus, neoplasia may progress without clonal dominance, resulting in composite tumors composed of a balanced growth of several cell populations. Yet cell growth simulations of preneoplastic lesions suggest that with time, polyclonal populations tend toward monoclonality when there are variations in the growth properties of cells in the original population.[244] Because oral cancer involves damage to genetic material at the cellular level, a thorough understanding of how cells maintain stability in the face of carcinogenic insults is imperative.

The role of genetic changes in neoplastic disease has been a source of scientific inquiry for a century. Alterations of cellular oncogenes, leading to altered expression of their products, have been implicated in the pathology of human cancers.[245] Cellular oncogenes, also known as proto-oncogenes, acquire their transforming properties or become activated by various mechanisms, such as gene amplification, point mutations, and gene rearrangements. Subsequently, activated alleles or oncogenes, which differ from the normal proto-oncogene counterparts by single nucleotides substitutions, ensue. Only within the past three decades have these oncogenes been a source of investigation. Oncogenes can encode growth factors and growth factor receptors, act on internal signaling molecules, and regulate DNA transcription factors. Altered oncogenes are expressed in cancer cells and may eventually become important markers of tumor progression. Antioncogenes are proteins that can also be mutated in certain tumors. Once mutated, these gene products may not monitor mitoses as they should, resulting in neoplastic transformation. Science now has the technology to identify such mutations in gene products. Scores of oncogenes have now been described, but the ones most often considered to be of significance in oral cancer are the H-*ras*, c-*myc*, and c-*erbB-1* oncogenes. There is also a family of transforming growth factors that can modulate cell growth: EGF, TGF-alpha, and TGF-beta, all of which have been implicated in oral cancer.[246]

The role of altered cell proliferation and its effect on genetic change during premalignant progression are related to local expression of growth factors. Neoplastic cells have been shown to become unresponsive to growth regulation by TGF-beta. This may then result in clonal overgrowth of selected cell populations and further accumulation of genetic changes. Inactivation of tumor suppressor genes may lead to a similar effect on neoplastic progression. Thus, a common pathway, characterized by altered control of proliferation, appears to lie central to the etiology of squamous cell carcinoma.[246]

The *myc* family of oncogenes has also been noted to show increased copy numbers in head and neck and oral cancers, as has the H-*ras* oncogene situated on chromosome 11.[247] There remains a significant debate as to whether overexpression of these oncogenes is an important step in oral cancer and whether they are activated or their function suppressed by exogenous carcinogens such as tobacco or alcohol.

It is highly possible that multiple oncogenes may be involved in oral cancer initiation including H-*ras*, c-*myc*, and c-*erbB-1*. Recent studies suggest that as many as one-half of the oral cancers studied demonstrate amplification of one or more gene products.[248,249] These data suggest that multiple mutations of certain oncogenes and tumor suppressor genes are a necessary step in the oral cancer process.

The most widely evaluated tumor suppressor gene postulated to be linked to oral cancer is the p53 oncosuppressor gene.[250] Mutations in this oncosuppressor appear to be one of the most common changes in all of human cancer. The p53 oncogene plays its role in oral cancer carcinogenesis by undergoing mutation in association with exogenous carcinogens, such as tobacco and alcohol, or viruses.[251]

If it is assumed that cancer of the oral cavity is a multiple-step process that can involve tumor suppressor genes, oncogenes, and exogenous agents, clearly the role of viruses as one group of exogenous promoters must be studied. The viruses most commonly implicated in oral cancer transformation have been human papillomavirus (HPV),[252,253] herpes simplex virus (HSV),[254] and the adenoviruses.[255] Of these, HPV and HSV have been the most thoroughly studied and are now considered to be the most likely 'synergistic viruses' involved in human oral cancer. The herpes viruses that have been most often linked to oral cancer are the Epstein-Barr virus (EBV) and the cytomegalovirus (CMV).[254] Both EBV DNA and CMV DNA have been demonstrated in oral squamous cell carcinoma tissue.[254] Debate continues as to whether the presence of HSV in such tissue mirrors a cause and effect association between virus and cancer.

The role of HPV in oral cancer has been studied exhaustively in the past two decades, using a host of science's most sophisticated molecular biologic techniques. In excess of 100 different HPV types have been isolated from benign and malignant neoplasms. HPV antigens and gene products have been detected in biopsies of oral cancer and precancer by a host of workers.[256,257] HPV has also been identified in nodal metastases from oral and head and neck cancers.[257] However, HPV can also be found in normal oral mucosa, and a cause and effect relationship to oral cancer has yet to be proved. Whether HPV plays an active role in the initiation of oral cancer, whether it is simply a passenger virus, or whether the virus acts in synergy with exogenous agents such as tobacco or alcohol to promote neoplasia needs to be studied more fully.

Recent evidence suggest that the HPV-16 E-5 gene can induce malignant transformation in epithelial cells, possibly acting by enhancing growth factor-mediated intercellular signal transduction.[258] Given this large milieu of oncogenes, viruses, oncosuppressors, and exogenous promoters, Scully[246] has postulated a hypothesis for oral carcinogenesis, suggesting that oncosuppressor genes can act in cyclic association with growth factors and viruses, chemical carcinogens, and oncogenes to result in a process that can initiate cancer through the dependence of each.

Immune competence: Compromised immunity related to HIV infection, organ transplantation, or chemotherapy or radiation therapy may act as contributory factors in the development of oral cancer.[259–263] Studies also suggest HIV-16 transfectants play a significant role in oral cancer development by altering intercellular immune surveillance mechanisms.[264]

Genetic and familial influences: Genetic defects associated with a number of inherited cancer syndromes have been linked to the development of oral cancer. Syndromes associated with defective DNA repair including xeroderma pigmentosa, ataxia telangiectasia, Bloom syndrome and Fanconi's anemia all have an increased rate of second primary malignancies including oral cancer.[265] Li-Fraumeni syndrome with its significant p53 mutations has a known association with head and neck cancers[265] and p53 germ line mutations have been reported in patients with multiple head and neck primary cancers and their first-degree relatives.[266–270]

Clinical and radiologic presentation of oral squamous cell carcinoma

Although the clinical presentation of oral squamous cell carcinoma can be quite varied, the vast majority of oral cavity lesions present as red patches, white patches, ulcers, tumor masses, or some other color variation in the tissue. Some investigators have divided the lesions into three specific subtypes: leukoplakic and erythroplakic plaques, endophytic nodules, and exophytic tumor masses. The lesions that are plaque-like tend to have a leathery feel to them on clinical examination. The endophytic and exophytic lesions can be firm, rock hard, or granulomatous. Occasionally, the two lesions can simulate non-specific chronic ulcers or mimic the ulcers seen in tuberculosis or granulomas seen in Crohn's disease. When lesions extend to involve subjacent bone, the most common presentation is that of an ill-defined moth-eaten radiolucency.

In general, the most frequent sites for cancer of the oral cavity are ventral and lateral aspects of the tongue. More than 75% of all oral cancer cases are unfortunately discovered in an advanced stage of development (stage III–IV; see discussion on staging).

Staging and general prognostic parameters

The most consistent manner of determining patient prognosis for squamous cell carcinoma of the oral cavity is by evaluating the initial tumor size and the extent of metastasis to either regional or distant lymph nodes. This TNM system for the clinical staging of squamous cell carcinoma is the most commonly used method of defining prognosis (Table 22.5).

Table 22.5 Staging system for oral squamous carcinoma, TNM classification*

Primary tumor size (T)

TX	Primary tumor not assessed
T0	No evidence of primary tumor
T1S	Carcinoma in situ
T1	Tumor is less than 2 cm in greatest diameter
T2	Tumor is 2 to 4 cm in greatest dimension
T3	Tumor is more than 4 cm in greatest dimension
T4	Tumor (lip) invades through the cortical bone, inferior alveolar nerve, floor of mouth, or skin of face
T4a	Tumor (oral cavity) invades into adjacent structures (e.g. through cortical bone, deep tongue muscles, maxillary sinus, skin of face)
T4b	Tumor invades into masticator space, pterygoid plates, or skull base and/or encases internal carotid artery

Regional lymph node involvement (N)

NX	Nodes not evaluated
N0	No clinically positive nodes
N1	Single clinically positive ipsilateral node less than 3 cm in greatest dimension
N2	Single clinically positive ipsilateral node 3 to 6 cm in greatest dimension or multiple clinically positive ipsilateral nodes, none more than 6 cm in greatest dimension
N2a	Single clinically positive ipsilateral node 3 to 6 cm in greatest dimension
N2b	Multiple clinically positive ipsilateral nodes, none more than 6 cm in greatest dimension
N2c	Metastasis in bilateral or contralateral nodes, none more than 6 cm in greatest dimension
N3	Metastasis in a lymph node more than 6 cm in greatest dimension

Involvement by distant metastases (M)

MX	Distant metastasis was not assessed
M0	Distant metastasis not evident
M1	Distant metastasis is evident

* From AJCC Cancer Staging Manual, 6th edition, Springer, 2002

There is not a common correlated histopathologic method that allows the pathologist to relate tumor staging directly to microscopic appearance, and most staging protocols for oral and head and neck cancer do not definitively use histologic findings. The overall 5-year survival rate for oral cancer remains 50–55%. However, there is a very significant difference in the 5-year survival rate for oral cancers that are clinically staged: stage I, 85%; stage II, 66%; stage III, 41% and stage IV; 9%.[271] The incidence of distant metastasis from patients with oral squamous cell carcinoma, who initially had no evidence of lymph node involvement at the time of their surgery, ranges between 30% and 60%. This rate of distant metastasis is probably largely related to current treatment modalities that allow such patients to survive much longer than they have in the past.

Early detection, together with the development of organized screening programs similar to those employed effectively in detecting prostate and breast cancer are equally as important in oral cancer.

Histologic features of prognostic significance

Two significant histologic features of oral squamous cell carcinoma are predictive of patient outcome: (1) the pattern of tumor invasion within the supporting collagenous stroma, and (2) the depth of tumor invasion into that collagenous stroma. An infiltrative pattern that is associated with regular noncohesive nests of tumor cells and individual tumor cell spread have been associated with a greater frequency of lymph node metastasis according to Yamamoto et al.[272] and Crissman and associates.[273]

A second feature, depth of invasion, has also been determined to be of prognostic significance. Shingaki et al.[274] reviewed squamous cell carcinomas from mixed oral cavity and oral pharyngeal sites and demonstrated that tumors with depths of invasion less than 4 mm had a rate of metastasis that was 8.3%, whereas tumors that showed a 4–8 mm depth of invasion demonstrated metastatic rates of 35%. Those tumors that showed invasion greater than 8 mm in depth had metastatic rates of 83%. It is apparent that the depth of invasion is an exceedingly important marker in defining whether metastasis will be problematic in any patient's therapy.

There are certain site-specific considerations that may account for variations in the behavior pattern of squamous cell carcinomas of the oral cavity. Shear et al.[275] reviewed a series of 898 squamous cell carcinomas of the oral cavity and oral pharynx and demonstrated that tumors that were of the same size and that affected the lip, floor of the mouth, buccal mucosa, hard palate, and gingiva had a risk of metastatic spread to regional lymph nodes that was quite similar. However, some site-specific differences with squamous cell carcinoma of the oral cavity are discussed as individual anatomic locations in the section that follows.

Pathologists must be aware that cervical lymph node metastasis, extracapsular lymph node extension, angiolymphatic invasion, and perineural invasion are associated with worse prognosis.

Finally, it has been reported by Byers and others[276] that in cases of invasive squamous cell carcinoma and carcinoma in situ, where there are positive margins with frozen section control, recurrence can be demonstrated for oral cavity and oral pharyngeal tumors that approaches 80%. Conversely, cases that have margins free of tumor have recurrence rates that are 12% and 18%, respectively.

Methods are evolving that attempt to evaluate positive margins for oral and squamous cell carcinomas of the oral cavity using sophisticated genetic and molecular biologic markers, including attempts to identify the presence of certain oncogene products and viruses at tumor margins to predict prognosis. Recent attempts have used a telomerase assay as a molecular biologic marker for identifying positive resection margins in oral squamous cell carcinomas in which microscopic evidence of disease is not present. Chromosomal microsatellite markers (e.g. at chromosomes 3, 8, 9, 17, and 18) and evidence of p53 mutations in histologically normal-appearing tissue are being used to demonstrate the genetically altered tissue that may proceed to recurrent squamous cell carcinoma.

General pathologic features

Grossly, squamous cell carcinoma of the oral cavity can present as an ulcer, an alteration of mucosal color, or a tumor mass (Fig. 22.35). Ulcerative lesions usually have a crateriform appearance with rolled elevated borders that are firm because of the infiltration of tumor along the margins. The cut section usually has a gray-white glistening appearance with little tendency to bulge beyond the cut margins. Lesions that appear red clinically often have a granular or gritty appearance, and the cut section frequently has the consistency of granulation tissue as opposed to the firm cut section of a tumor ulcer.

A proliferation of sheets, nests, cords, and neoplastic islands of epithelium that penetrate into the supporting connective tissue lamina propria and submucosa characterize squamous cell carcinoma (Fig. 22.36). The neoplasm is usually identified histologically as being well differentiated, moderately differentiated, poorly differentiated, or undifferentiated (nonkeratinizing). Tumors are generally graded

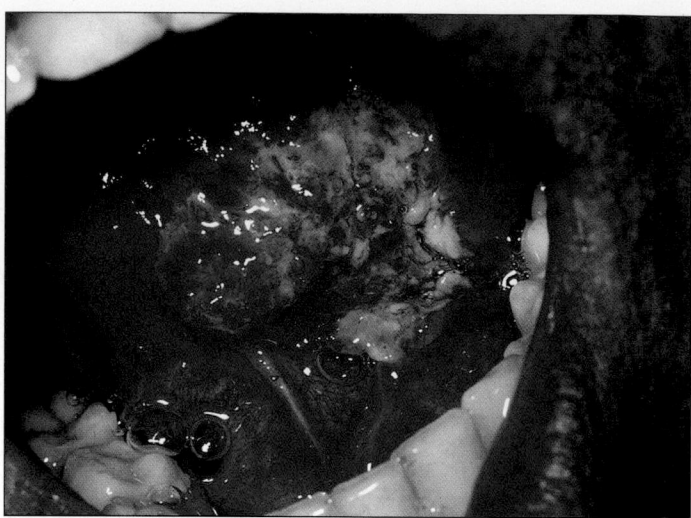

Fig. 22.35 Exophytic ulcerated squamous cell carcinoma of the ventral tongue.

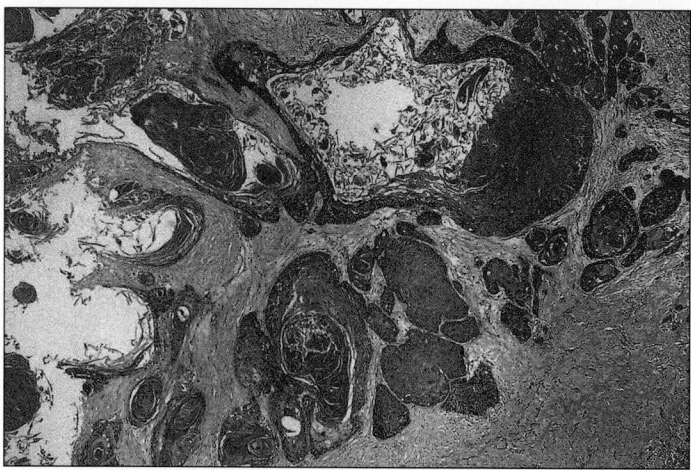

Fig. 22.36 Well-differentiated squamous cell carcinoma with keratin formation infiltrating throughout a stroma with desmoplastic reaction.

as grades I to IV,[277] in which grade I tumors closely resemble the tissue of origin and grade IV tumors demonstrate very few features that resemble tissue of squamous epithelial origin.

The neoplastic cells of well-differentiated squamous carcinomas bear a striking similarity to the cells of normal squamous epithelium. The cells are generally large with vesicular to oval nuclei and eosinophilic cytoplasm, intracellular bridging is usually easily discernible, and the degree of nuclear hyperchromatism and bizarre mitotic activity is minimal. Keratin pearl formation is usually quite prominent in well-differentiated squamous cell carcinoma, and individual cell keratinization tends to be a hallmark of this form of the disease. The connective tissue lamina propria and supporting fibromuscular submucosa into which neoplastic islands penetrate often show a marked degree of chronic inflammation, predominantly plasma cells and lymphocytes. Squamous cell carcinomas that show a moderate degree of differentiation display a much more varied histologic pattern, and although the tumor cells resemble normal

squamous epithelial cells, hyperchromatism, pleomorphism, anisocytosis, and loss of attachment of cells are more prominent. As a rule, the frequency of atypical mitoses is increased, and the frequency of individual cell keratinization and keratin pearl formation is decreased. In poorly differentiated squamous cell carcinomas, there is very little evidence that the tumor is of squamous origin. Individual cell keratinization is lacking; nuclear:cytoplasmic ratios are markedly altered; and there is significant pleomorphism and atypical mitoses. Tumor giant cells may also be prominent in poorly differentiated tumors.

Undifferentiated squamous cell carcinomas have also been referred to as nonkeratinizing squamous cell carcinoma. They have little if any resemblance to a neoplasm of squamous epithelium with the cells resembling histiocytes, atypical lymphocytes, or spindled fibroblasts. The characteristic histologic features that identify the tumor cells as epithelial may be totally lacking. Electron microscopic evaluation and immunohistochemical staining for keratin may be the only method of documenting that the tumor is of squamous epithelial origin. Stromal changes may include desmoplastic fibrosis, vascular hyperplasia, and a diffuse infiltrate of chronic inflammatory cells. Histologic grading of squamous cell carcinoma is somewhat subjective, and clinical staging has proved to correlate more favorably with prognosis than microscopic grading.

Anatomic sites

Squamous cell carcinoma of the tongue: Squamous cell carcinoma of the tongue usually manifests as an ulcerative mass or papillary-like lesion in the mid-third of the lateral tongue border and accounts for greater than 25–50% percent of all intraoral squamous cell carcinomas.[278] More than 70% of tongue cancers occur in the anterior two-thirds of the tongue while the posterior third accounts for 25–30%. These tumors are two to five times more common in men then women, with an average age of 60 years.[278,279] In the anterior tongue, the lateral border contributes the most common site of occurrence (approximately 75%), followed by the ventral aspect, dorsum, and the tip, respectively. Lymph node metastasis in tongue cancer is frequent. In the anterior two-thirds of tongue, patients with T2 or T3 lesions have a metastatic risk of 40% and 75%, respectively. The risk is higher with T4 lesions. In the posterior tongue 50–80% of patients have metastasis at the time of diagnosis.[278,280] Seventy percent of patients with squamous cell carcinoma of the tongue have unilateral or bilateral metastasis at the time of first examination. In the anterior tongue, the 3-year survival rate for tumors less than 4 cm is 80%, and in tumors more than 4 cm survival drops to 50%.[278,281] In the posterior tongue the overall 5-year survival rate is 20–40%.[278,282–284] If lymph node metastases are identified at initial surgery, the recurrence rate ranges as high as 40–50%.

Squamous cell carcinoma of the lip: Approximately 25–30% of all squamous cell carcinomas of the oral cavity affect the lip. Squamous cell carcinoma affects the lower lip (85%) much more commonly than the upper lip (2–7%). There is a male predominance with an average age of 60–70 years.[285,286] The lesion typically presents as an ulcer or warty growth along the vermilion border. The first lymph nodes to be involved are the submandibular and submental nodes, with extension into the deeper cervical lymph nodes if the lesion is not managed early. Histologically, most squamous cell carcinomas of the lip are well differentiated. Poorly differentiated and highly anaplastic lesions are rare. This form of cancer carries with it a very high 5-year survival rate. Cross and colleagues[287] reported an 80–85% 5-year survival rate when such lesions were identified without nodal involvement. When squamous cell carcinomas of the lip are identified in concert with lymph node metastases, the survival rate drops to less than 50% and tumors greater than 6 mm in thickness tend to behave more aggressively, with subsequent regional lymph node metastasis and perineural invasion.[288]

Knapel et al.[289] report that carcinomas of the upper lip and commissures are usually less differentiated than those of the lower lip and are thought to grow more insidiously and rapidly. Lymph node metastases of upper lip carcinomas are also thought to be more diffuse.

Squamous cell carcinoma of the buccal mucosa: The most common buccal mucosal site for squamous cell carcinoma is the retromolar area posterior or adjacent to the third molar teeth. The tumor favors males and accounts for approximately 2% of all intraoral squamous cell carcinomas.[290] Most tumors occur in patients between 60 and 70 years of age.[291,292] Very frequently, these lesions present as long-standing white or red lesions, which eventually develop into warty, papillary, or ulcerative growths. Long-standing lesions may invade alveolar mucosa and bone, so it is often difficult to determine where the lesion first began. Microscopically, buccal mucosal lesions usually present as well-differentiated tumors, with early spread to the submandibular and upper cervical nodes.

Vanderwall[290] has reported that squamous cell carcinomas of the buccal mucosa, left untreated, are extensively destructive lesions and can show rapid invasion into the pterygomaxillary fossa. Metastasis to regional lymph nodes will occur in about 50% of such cases. Five-year cure rates for these lesions are generally in the range of 20–30%, but lesions in the posterior third of the buccal mucosa have cure rates of only 10%.[293] Tumor thickness of greater than 6 mm favors a poor prognosis.[294]

Squamous cell carcinoma of the gingiva: Squamous cell carcinoma of the gingiva usually presents in the molar and premolar areas. Krolls and Hoffman[285] report that gingival squamous cell carcinoma represents approximately 6% of intraoral squamous cancers. The vast majority of cases afflict male patients who are 50 years or older,[295] although recent trends show an increase among females.[296] Ulcerations and papillary growths are the most common findings. This lesion can be exceedingly vexing because of its close proximity to bone, and its ability to rapidly spread into bone. Five-year survival rates are poor and are only in the range of 20–40%.[297] Cady and Catlin[295] reviewed 600 patients with carcinoma of the gingiva and found that those with lesions less than 3 cm without invasion of the underlying bone or lymph node metastasis lived longer than 5 years. Most gingival squamous cell carcinomas are well differentiated, and some have been linked to the habit of snuff dipping or tobacco chewing.[298]

Squamous cell carcinoma of the floor of the mouth: Carcinoma of the floor of the mouth is usually identified in the anterior portion of the mouth beneath the ventral surface of the tongue. Excluding lip cancer, it is the second most common oral cancer after tongue carcinoma, constituting approximately 15% of oral cancers.[299,300] It may present as a red velvety, wart-like, or ulcerative lesion. It is the third most common site for intraoral squamous cell carcinoma, exceeded only by the lip and tongue. Some reports show the floor of mouth cancer show an ethnic predisposition, with black Americans favored,[301] although some other reports dispute this claim.[299] Men are affected two to three times more than women.[299,300] Squamous cell carcinoma of the floor of the mouth tends to more frequently involve the mucous membrane anterior to the openings of the submandibular ducts, and erythroplakic lesions are common clinically. Spiro et al.[302] reviewed a series of squamous cell carcinomas in which they evaluated prognosis as it related to tumor thickness. Tumors less than 2 mm in thickness had the highest rates of survival. In a similar study, Mohit-Tabatabai et al.[303] determined that tumors greater than 3.6 mm in thickness had metastatic rates of 60%, whereas those that measured less than 1.5 mm on histologic examination showed a metastatic rate of only 2%. There is, therefore, a marked difference in the five-year survival rate depending on the depth of invasion and tumor extension. In this regard, superficial tumors have a five-year survival rate of 92%, whereas extension to the tongue or mandible decreased the survival rate to 52%.[297]

Squamous cell carcinoma of the palate: Squamous cell carcinoma is more frequently identified in the soft palate than in the hard palate. It generally presents as an ulcer or papillary growth and accounts for 5.5% of intraoral squamous cell cancers according to Krolls and Hoffman.[299] Because more than 50% of palatal squamous cell carcinomas involve bone at the time of detection, adequate sampling and decalcification of an osseous specimen are mandatory. Evans and Shah[304] report that one-third of the patients with this form of oral squamous cancer have cervical lymph node metastasis at the time of diagnosis. The overall 5-year survival rate ranges 50–77%.[304–306]

Squamous cell carcinoma of the tonsil and oropharynx: Tonsillar squamous cell carcinoma tends to affect the same population of patients as squamous cell carcinoma involving other oral cavity sites. Tumors in these areas, however, seem to demonstrate a higher rate of lymph node metastasis than other oral sites, and tumors in this area are more often undifferentiated on nonkeratinizing carcinomas resembling those of the nasopharyngeal type.[307–309] The five-year survival rate ranges from 21% to 54%.[309–311] Carcinoma of the oropharynx include oropharyngeal and palatine arch carcinomas. Squamous cell carcinomas of the palatine arch are not as aggressive as their true oropharyngeal counterparts. Tumors in this region metastasize to distant sites twice as frequently as palatine arch lesions. Squamous cell carcinomas in this entire region tend to be less well differentiated than tumors in other oral sites, and because of the abundant lymphatic drainage of the region, lymph node metastasis is early in the course of the disease and survival is poor.[285,312]

Squamous cell carcinoma arising in odontogenic cysts and the maxillary sinuses: Malignant transformation of the lining of odontogenic cysts is rare, although there are reports in the literature that document such occurrences.[313] It may be difficult to differentiate squamous cell carcinoma in the wall of the cyst from exuberant odontogenic epithelial rest activity. Characteristically, classic odontogenic epithelial rest activity tends to proliferate as a thin ribbon or small nest-like cluster of cells without the multiphasic finger-like expansions of squamous cell carcinoma.

Toller[314] postulates that the cystic lesion is most likely to undergo malignant transformation than is the odontogenic keratocyst.

Carcinoma of the maxillary antrum arises from an unknown source, although HPV, nasal polyps, and tobacco use have been suggested as possible etiologic sources. Tumors usually result in irregular poorly circumscribed destructive lesions of the sinus. The histopathologic features of this neoplasm are similar to squamous cell carcinomas elsewhere in the oral cavity. The treatment of choice is most often partial maxillectomy, and 5-year survival rates are less than 30%.

Nasopharyngeal carcinoma arises from epithelium lining the nasopharynx. This neoplasm is discussed in detail in Chapter 15.

Variants of oral squamous cell carcinoma

Verrucous carcinoma

Clinical features: Verrucous carcinoma was first reported by Friedell and Rosenthal[315] and popularized by Ackerman[316] as a variant of squamous cell carcinoma. It is chiefly identified after the sixth decade of life and is most common in the mandibular buccal sulcus and along the alveolar mucosa of the mandibular ridge. Verrucous

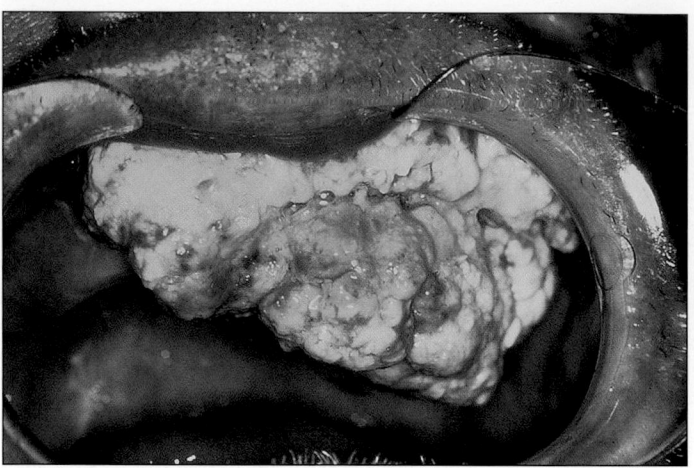

Fig. 22.37 Verrucous carcinoma demonstrating exophytic papillary mass of the anterior maxilla.

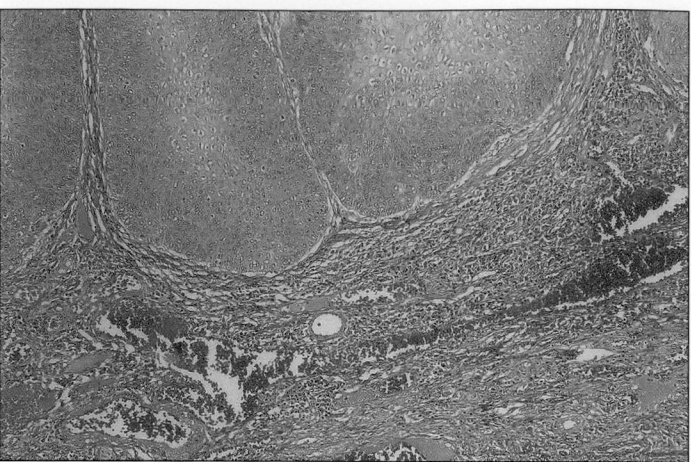

Fig. 22.38 Verrucous carcinoma. Note the interface showing the broad pushing borders, which characterize the lesion base, and the surrounding stroma, which exhibits a chronic inflammatory response.

carcinoma accounts for 2–8% of all oral squamous cell carcinomas.[317,318] A few cases of verrucous carcinoma of the maxillary alveolar mucosa have been documented.[319] Material from our laboratory, largely from white western ranchers, indicates a male predominance; other investigators document a female predominance.

Verrucous carcinoma is best defined as a clinicopathologic entity. Frequently, it goes unrecognized in its earliest stages because of its simple localized papillary or verruciform appearance, often thought to be consistent with a papilloma or verruca vulgaris (Fig. 22.37). Verrucous carcinoma is most likely part of a histologic spectrum in which the definitive lesion arises from a papillary verrucoid leukoplakia over a course of some years.[320] Shear and Pindborg[321] have suggested that the term *verrucous hyperplasia* be considered part of this continuum and propose verrucous hyperplasia as a separate and distinct clinicopathologic entity. Batsakis[320] has suggested, however, that verrucous hyperplasia is simply an early form of verrucous carcinoma. I (ROG) have had the opportunity to see several cases of verrucous hyperplasia develop into classic verrucous carcinoma.

Verrucous carcinoma can undergo multiple phases of clinical development, so that it can appear either as a soft circumscribed lesion, as a fibrotic, rather red granular lesion, as a rough stippled lesion, or as a papillomatous corrugated growth.

Frankly invasive squamous cell carcinoma can be identified in verrucous carcinoma in approximately 38% of cases as hybrid lesions. It is exceedingly important, therefore, that verrucous carcinomas be multiply sectioned to ensure diagnostic certainty.

Much information in the literature suggests that smokeless tobacco use predisposes to the development of verrucous carcinoma of the oral cavity. Shroyer and Greer[322] reviewed a series of 30 smokeless tobacco leukoplakias and were unable to demonstrate even mild dysplasia. Smokeless tobacco use alone did not appear to initiate verrucous carcinoma development in short-term users. However, papillomavirus capsid antigens were present in many of the specimens tested, and in situ DNA hybridization showed HPV types 2 and 6 in 5 of the 30 cases.

Verrucous carcinoma has been identified in chronic users of smokeless tobacco products as well as in cigarette smokers, pipe smokers, and cigar smokers; however, up to 20% of verrucous carcinomas of the oral cavity are documented in nontobacco users. Shroyer and Greer[323] demonstrated that 29% of 14 cases of verrucous hyperplasia that they evaluated for HPV DNA using in situ hybridization and PCR analysis were positive for HPV-16. They followed up this study with a review of 17 verrucous carcinomas and found, using PCR techniques, that 49% harbored HPV-16 or -11 DNA. These studies add support to the concept that HPV may often be overlooked as a cofactor in the development of verrucous carcinoma.

Pathologic features: Grossly, verrucous carcinoma presents as a papillary or corrugated mass composed of folds of tissue with finger-like clefts between tissue extensions that are all too often histopathologically benign in appearance. These papillary folds on cut section are usually gray-white and homogeneous. Microscopically, verrucous carcinoma is characterized by a proliferation of elevated layers of squamous epithelium, which typically penetrate superficially and broadly into the supporting collagen as elongated rete pegs (Fig. 22.38). The cytologic characteristics of the penetrating epithelium are often far from malignant appearing. More often than not, the pathologist is not able to appreciate the classic cytologic hallmarks of cancer in the tissue sample. The basement membrane is usually intact, which makes a diagnosis of infiltrating carcinoma difficult, and the epithelium will often extend as a blunt proliferation into the supporting connective tissue along a characteristic broad, pushing front as described by Ackerman.[316] Jacobson and Shear[324] indicate that a second characteristic feature of verrucous carcinoma is the manner in which the normal epithelium at the edge of the lesion is bent on itself by the continued proliferation of the neoplastic epithelium. If verrucous carcinoma is part of a suspected diagnosis, appropriate sampling is mandatory for diagnostic purposes, because as great as 20% of verrucous carcinomas have a routine squamous cell carcinoma developing concurrently. The supporting collagen typically shows a dense chronic inflammatory infiltrate. Shafer[325] points out that another characteristic feature of verrucous carcinoma is the distinct wedge-like parakeratin plugging between individual finger-like processes of the neoplasm. Keratohyaline granules, which are seen in verruca vulgaris or occasionally in hyperplastic epithelium, are also rarely seen, if not at all in verrucous carcinomas. It is exceedingly important for the pathologist to review an adequate sample of the lesion to render an accurate diagnosis.

Differential diagnosis: When a diagnosis of verrucous carcinoma is entertained, the most common differential diagnoses considered are pseudoepitheliomatous hyperplasia, oral florid papillomatosis as described by Eversole and Sorenson,[326] papillary hyperplasia, papillary squamous cell carcinoma (see below), and keratoacanthoma. Keratoacanthoma is an exceedingly rare entity within the oral cavity. The characteristic lipping at the periphery of keratoacanthoma and the glassy hyalinized appearance of keratoacanthoma nearly always serve to separate it from verrucous carcinoma. The distinct parakeratin plugging that is commonly seen in verrucous carcinoma is not identified in keratoacanthoma. A feature characteristic of both lesions is the broad, pushing front at the connective tissue margin of growth. Oral florid papillomatosis is characterized histologically by multiple papillary growths supported by a richly vascularized supporting connective tissue stroma. Such vascularity is an unusual finding in verrucous carcinoma. Some authorities believe that cases reported as *oral florid papillomatosis* were, in fact, verrucous carcinoma. In differentiating pseudoepitheliomatous hyperplasia from verrucous carcinoma, Kraus and Perez-Mesa[327] point out that the bulbous rete ridge pattern of verrucous carcinoma serves to differentiate it from pseudoepitheliomatous hyperplasia, in which the rete ridges tend to proliferate as sharp, pointed, elongated, or knife-like structures as they infiltrate the supporting connective tissue. Papillary hyperplasia is usually associated with an ill-fitting denture, is usually palatal, and shows no epithelial atypia.

Verrucous carcinoma must be distinguished from well-differentiated squamous carcinoma. A lesion that shows cytologic atypia, penetration of the growth beyond the basement membrane, lack of a broad, pushing front of neoplastic growth, and no evidence of parakeratin plugging is a well-differentiated squamous carcinoma. Development of a second oral cancer is not uncommon in patients with a diagnosis of verrucous carcinoma.

Treatment and prognosis: There is considerable debate in the literature as to whether verrucous carcinoma should be treated by surgery or radiotherapy. Most data indicate that the treatment of choice is wide surgical excision. This management modality is supported by Fonts et al.[328] After proper surgical excision, more than 85% of patients are disease free after 5 years. Greer[329] has reported management of a case of long-standing multifocal verrucous carcinoma in a 75-year-old woman using a chemotherapeutic regimen that included methotrexate therapy with citrovorum rescue. Although not the primary management modality of choice, this protocol may prove beneficial in problematic late-stage cases, in which usually there may be involvement of bone.

Papillary (exophytic) squamous cell carcinoma   Papillary SCC is a distinctly uncommon form of squamous cell carcinoma that usually presents as a single lesion. Although the larynx seems to be the preferred site, origin in the oro/hypopharynx has also been documented.[330–332] These lesions usually arise de novo, although on rare occasions they may arise in the background of existing benign papilloma.[331] Microscopically, the lesion is composed of exophytic, thin, short or long finger-like projections with identifiable fibrovascular cores (Fig. 22.39). The squamous epithelium shows malignant features suggestive of an in situ carcinoma and basaloid features and many of the tumors remain as in situ carcinomas. Surface keratinization is not prominent and is usually absent. The identification of invasion at times can be difficult. However, some consider these lesions as invasive even without the identification of definitive invasion. Prognostically, they are comparable to the conventional squamous cell carcinoma, although some reports suggest an overall better prognosis when matched stage for stage.[333]

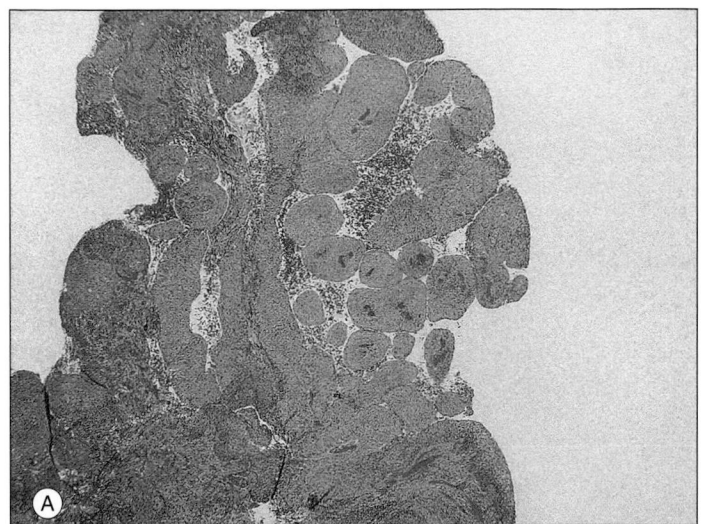

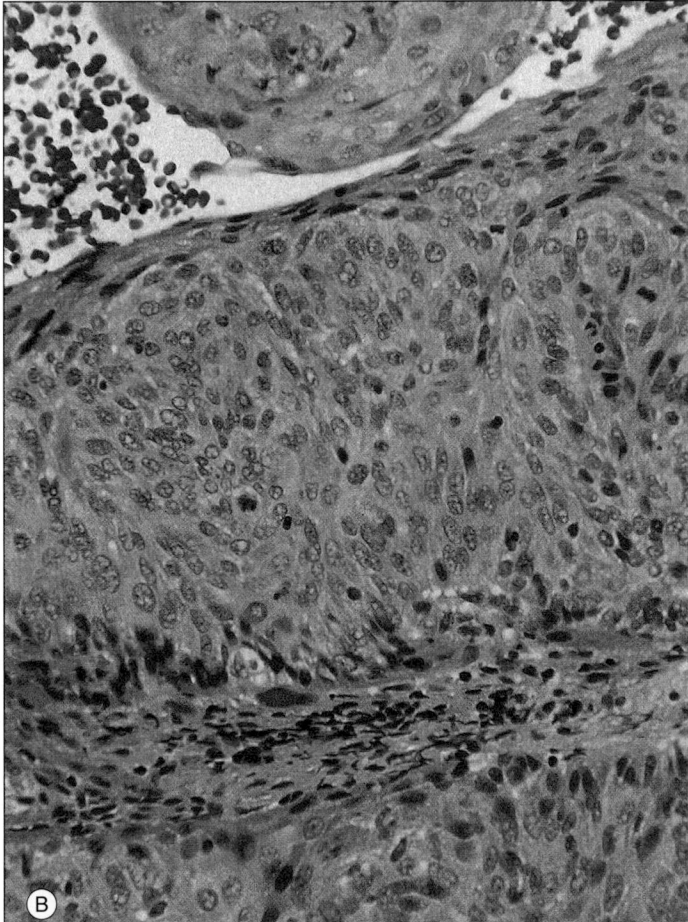

Fig. 22.39 Papillary SCC. **A**, Note papillary formations, which constitute the bulk of this exophytic tumor; **B**, The abnormal squamous epithelium lining the papillary formations shows both dysplasia and mitotic activity.

Adenoid (acantholytic) squamous cell carcinoma   This morphologic variant of squamous cell carcinoma has been initially documented by Jacoway et al.[334] and Tomich and Hutton.[335] The lesions that have been reported in relation to oral cancer were identified mainly on the lip.[323,324,336] Rare cases involving tongue, floor of mouth, and gingiva have also been reported.[337,338] These

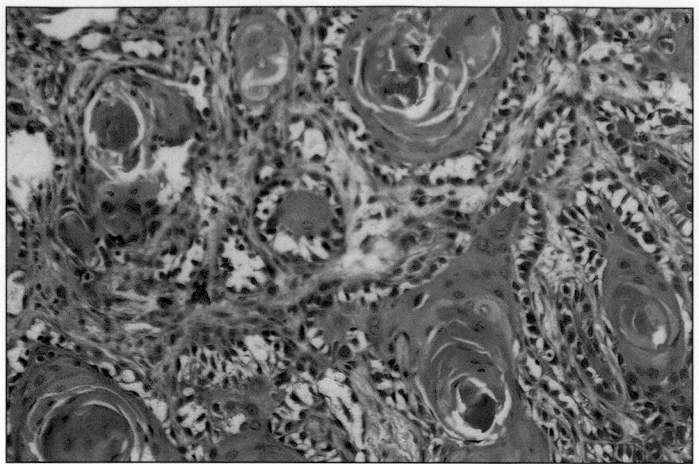

Fig. 22.40 Adenoid SCC. Note the dehiscence between the tumor cells which give the impression of cystic space that could be mistakenly interpreted as a gland lumen.

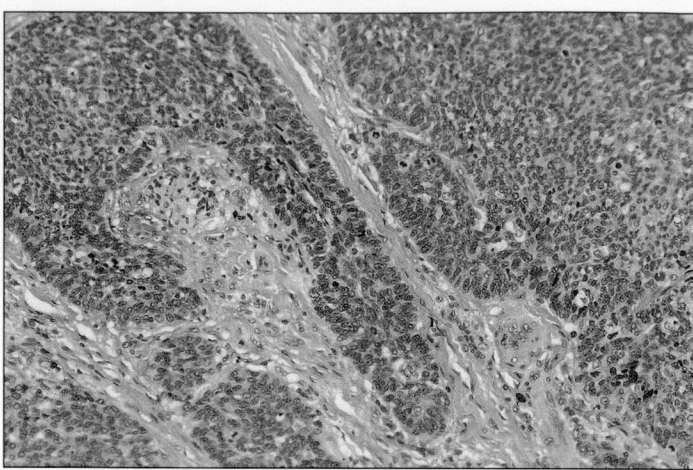

Fig. 22.41 Basaloid SCC. Note the peripheral palisading, brisk mitotic activity, and the smooth lobule contour.

lesions usually present as ulcerations or elevated slightly crusted nodules. Most cases have been reported in men older than 50 years of age.[339,340] A number of investigators have proposed its development in association with actinic keratosis.[339,340]

Microscopically, the lesions are characterized by a proliferation of squamous cell carcinoma with central acantholysis and the development of cystic spaces filled with desquamated cells, particularly in the deeper aspects of the tumor. Many cystic spaces have a pseudoglandular arrangement and are rimmed by cuboidal epithelium, hence the name *adenoid squamous carcinoma* (Fig. 22.40). Typically, the stroma shows a chronic inflammatory infiltrate and degeneration of the collagen typical of the basaloid solar degeneration found in actinic keratosis.

Many of the oral lesions documented in the lips were accompanied by excellent prognosis. However, reported cases in the floor of mouth, gingiva, and tongue have a worse clinical course. This may be due to earlier and easier recognition of the lip lesions. It is probably advisable to use the term acantholytic squamous cell carcinoma over adenoid squamous cell carcinoma, if only to resolve the confusion encountered by many, particularly nonpathologists, with this nomenclature (see below).

Adenosquamous carcinoma   It is appropriate to mention this variant here, if only to highlight the major differences between it and adenoid squamous cell carcinoma mentioned above. The two share similar sounding names, which is often confusing. This is compounded by the knowledge that both variants are rare, a fact that lends more credence to identifying the difference between both. Adenosquamous carcinoma is a rare, high-grade, aggressive, dimorphic variant that shows both squamous carcinoma and adenocarcinoma components. It is thought that the squamous component arises from the surface epithelium in the form of dysplasia, in situ carcinoma, or invasive squamous carcinoma, while the adenocarcinoma arises from the minor salivary gland ducts in the form of malignant gland formations in various grades of differentiation. Gerughty et al. first recognized this tumor in 1968.[341] According to Scully et al. approximately 15 cases have been reported in the oral cavity. Sixty percent of the patients have died from their disease.[342] The overall five-year survival rate of adenosquamous

carcinoma from all head and neck sites is only 25%. Most cases occurred in the tongue and floor of mouth.[342] Napier et al.[343] suggested that adenosquamous carcinoma may not be as rare as generally thought, and suggested that the volume of the adenocarcinoma component is usually significantly smaller than the squamous counterpart, which renders its dual recognition in many cases difficult.

Basaloid squamous cell carcinoma   This lesion, first described by Wain and coworkers in 1986,[344] is a rare, aggressive neoplasm that generally arises in the larynx (75% of cases). Approximately 40 cases have been described in the oral cavity.[345] Intraoral sites include tongue base, hypophyarnx, floor of mouth, buccal mucosa, and palate. The mean age has been reported to be 62 years, and most patients with this disease have been smokers.[346] Histopathologically, the tumor has two distinct components: (1) a component of well- or moderately differentiated squamous cell carcinoma, and (2) infiltrating tumor cell nests with basaloid features. The basaloid component is infiltrative with smoothly contoured lobules that may show peripheral palisading and often shows central necrosis (comedo pattern) and high mitotic rate (Fig. 22.41). A spindle cell component is sometimes seen. The stroma between the cell nests can be myxoid or show hyalinosis. The cells have scant cytoplasm with round to oval hyperchromatic or vesicular nuclei. Seidman[347] and Raslan[346] documented a high incidence of second primary tumors arising, particularly in the upper aerodigestive tracts.

The major differential diagnoses for basaloid carcinoma can be quite challenging. They include adenoid cystic carcinoma, small cell carcinoma, adenosquamous and mucoepidermoid carcinoma. The treatment of choice for this neoplasm is generally a combination of radical surgical excision and adjunctive chemo- or radiotherapy. The tumor is biologically aggressive with early regional and distant metastasis. The lesion has a poor prognosis and the median survival times after diagnosis rarely approach 2 years.

Spindle cell squamous cell carcinoma   Spindle cell carcinoma has also been referred to as pleomorphic carcinoma, metaplastic carcinoma, sarcomatoid squamous cell carcinoma, and polypoid squamous cell carcinoma.

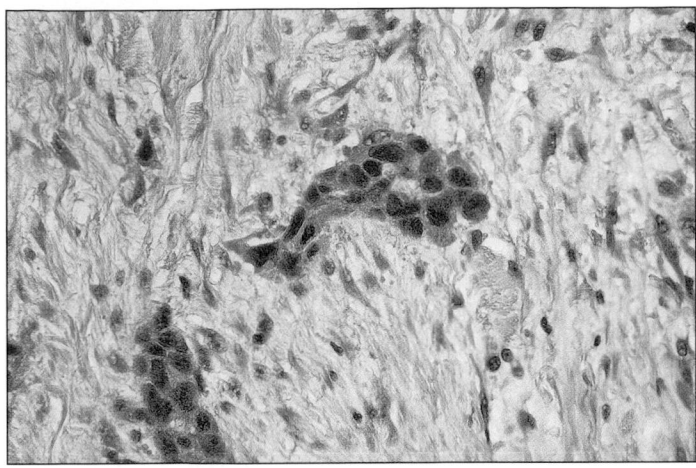

Fig. 22.42 Squamous cell carcinoma with benign reactive desmoplastic stromal reaction. Note the malignant islands infiltrating a fibroblast (spindle cells) rich reactive stroma.

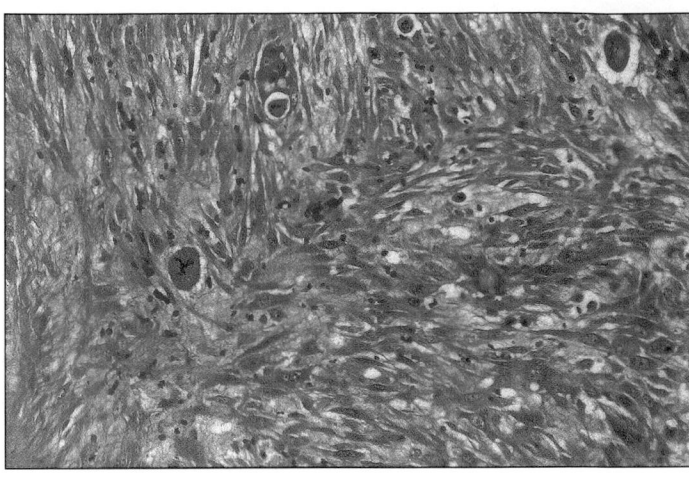

Fig. 22.43 Spindle cell SCC. Note the malignant highly abnormal spindle cells and the atypical mitotic activity. The cells in this case stained positive for pancytokeratin.

Most patients with spindle cell carcinoma are men in the sixth or seventh decade of life[348–350,353] and occurrence in younger age groups is unusual.[351] This form of squamous cell carcinoma has been documented consistently in the world literature only recently in the past thirty years, although similar lesions have long been identified in the breast and skin. Etiologically, spindle cell carcinoma is related to smoking, alcohol abuse, and prior irradiation.[352–354] No relation to HPV has so far been found.

Spindle cell carcinomas are most frequently identified on the lips. The lower lip is the most commonly involved oral site. Clinically, they present as polypoid nodular or fleshy lesions.[352]

Grossly, the lesions have a smooth, glistening, often whorled pattern on cut surface. Leifer and Miller[355] have reviewed a series of spindle cell carcinomas of the oral mucosa using both light and electron microscopy. They conclude that the lesions are of squamous epithelial derivation. Histologically, the lesion presents as an undifferentiated or anaplastic proliferation of spindle and stellate cells often arranged in interlacing fascicles, thus resembling a tumor of connective tissue origin. Usually a component of conventional squamous cell carcinoma is seen, on occasions multiple sections may be required to demonstrate it and indeed many authorities indicate that this spindle cell proliferation can always be traced to continuity with surface epithelium.[356]

Barnes[357] in his review of spindle cell carcinoma believes that the term spindle cell carcinoma is a generic term that encompasses four different categories of tumors that can potentially be separated by immunocytochemistry and/or electron microscopy. This includes (1) squamous cell carcinoma with benign reactive desmoplastic stromal reaction (Fig. 22.42); (2) spindle cell squamous cell carcinoma, in which the spindle cell component would show immunoreactivity for cytokeratin immunocytochemical stain indicating its epithelial derivation (Fig 22.43); (3) carcinosarcoma, in which a component of conventional squamous cell carcinoma is seen along a true sarcomatous spindle cell component with occasional sarcomatous foci (e.g. osteosarcoma, chondrosarcoma, rhabdomyosarcoma). The tumor in this instance arises from the same clone of cells, one epithelial and the other mesenchymal (4) collision tumors, which are rare neoplasms that arise from two different clones of malignant cells, coincidentally in adjacent areas.

Postradiation squamous cell carcinomas can often take on a spindled appearance, and it may be difficult to tell a recurrent neoplasm from a proliferation of mature fibrogranulation tissue. In the pseudotumor, giant cells seem to be found with a greater degree of frequency than in recurrent squamous cell carcinoma, and is most helpful in the differential diagnosis. Another lesion that can be confused with spindle cell carcinoma is nodular fasciitis. A striking histologic feature of nodular fasciitis that differentiates it from spindle cell carcinoma is the random arrangement of bundles of fibroblasts in a mucoid matrix; such a mucoid matrix is not a feature of spindle cell carcinoma. Another important feature that separates the two is stromal vascularity. The marked vascularity of nodular fasciitis with its fine capillary network is rarely seen in spindle cell carcinoma.

Spindle cell carcinomas can prove exceedingly aggressive. Ellis and Corio[358] found mean survival rates of patients with this disease to be less than 2 years. Batsakis et al.[359,360] found that 27% of 166 sarcomatoid carcinomas they studied metastasized. Five-year disease free survival is around 30%.

ORAL MELANOCYTIC AND OTHER PIGMENTED LESIONS

A host of pigmented lesions affect the oral mucosa. The amalgam tattoo is by far the most commonly encountered exogenous form of oral pigmentation. It is associated with the entrapment of dental amalgam granules in the oral mucosa and presents as a flat pigmented spot.

Melanoma

Malignant melanoma of the oral cavity is rare, accounting for about 1–8% of all melanomas. The annual incidence of melanoma is 1.2/10 million people. Rapini et al.[361A] reviewed a series of 171 cases reported in the oral literature and reported six new cases in 1985. Three of their six patients showed a well-developed radial growth phase. Hicks and Flaitz[361B] reported a male predilection with a mean age of 56 years. Eighty percent of oral melanomas occur on the hard palate, alveolar mucosa, or gingiva. The prognosis for oral melanoma

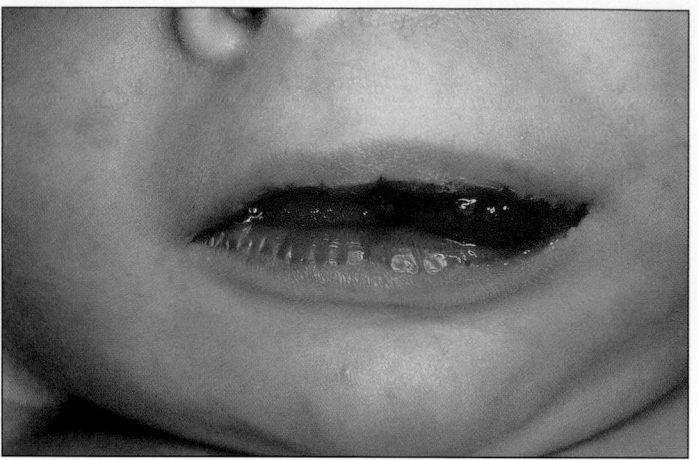

Fig. 22.44 Melanotic neuroectodermal tumor of infancy. (Courtesy of Michael Roher, DDS; Stephen Young, DDS; and Richard Glass, DDS, Oklahoma City, Oklahoma.)

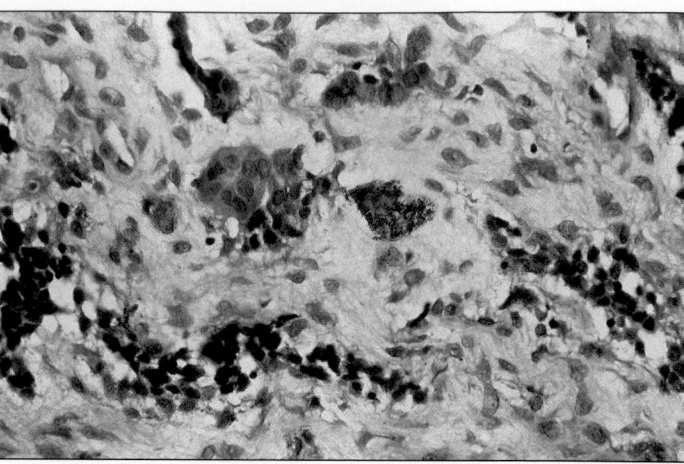

Fig. 22.45 Melanotic neuroectodermal tumor showing large epithelial tumor cells with scattered melanin and smaller lymphocyte-like cells without melanin.

is quite poor, with the average survival after diagnosis often no longer than 2 years. Melanoma and other melanocytic tumors and dysplasias are discussed in further detail in Chapter 8.

Melanotic neuroectodermal tumor of infancy

Krompecher first described melanotic neuroectodermal tumor of infancy in 1918.[362] Since that time, more than 200 cases have been documented in the world literature. There has been considerable confusion as to the origin of the tumor. The most common of the proposed origins have been the odontogenic tissues and the neural crest. It is generally considered by most authorities today that the lesion is a tumor of neural crest origin. The neoplasm has also been referred to as melanotic ameloblastoma, retinal anlage tumor, and melanotic progonoma.

The neoplasm is benign, with recurrence rates in the range of approximately 15%. However, Dehner et al.[363] reported a malignant melanotic neuroectodermal tumor in a 4-month-old boy. The tumor eventually metastasized, and the patient died 3 months later. There is some debate concerning whether the tumor was originally a neuroblastoma. Nagase and associates[364] reviewed a series of 17 recurrent melanotic neuroectodermal tumors, 12 of which they interpreted as being rapidly growing tumors, but none of which metastasized.

Clinical and radiologic features

The tumor occurs most often in infants younger than one year old. Kapadia et al. reported a female predominance.[365] Other studies reported the opposite.[366] Clinically, the lesion usually presents as a tumor mass with a subjacent radiographic lucency in the premaxilla (Fig. 22.44). More than 80% of all tumors have been identified in this area, although reports in the literature indicate that the lesion can be found in long bones or the bones of the skull. Often, the teeth in association with the tumor appear to be floating in space, and a differential diagnosis of idiopathic histiocytosis is therefore entertained. Most of the tumors occur in the first decade of life.[365–368] They may be locally destructive of bone but are benign and do not metastasize.[369,370] Elevated vanillylmandelic acid levels are frequently seen in patients. Alpha-fetoprotein serum elevation has also been reported in rare instances.[371]

Pathologic features

The tumor generally separates quite easily from the bone and is usually only partially encapsulated. On cut section, one will usually find a firm glistening cut surface that is gray-white with numerous speckles or streaks of black and brown material distributed throughout. Occasionally, there may be multiple tumor nodules instead of a single tumor mass.

Microscopically, the tumor is composed of two cell types, pigmented and nonpigmented (Fig. 22.45), both of which are set in a loose connective tissue stroma. The pigmented cells tend to be cuboidal or flattened and are much larger than the smaller nonpigmented cells. The larger cells often contain melanotic granules, whereas the nonpigmented cells tend to be arranged in solid groups and often form the lining of cleft-like spaces. The nonpigmented cells are typically round and contain a nucleus that stains deeply basophilic and usually fills up most of the cell. Pigmented spindle-shaped cells may also be identified within the tumor mass. Misugi et al.[372] have documented ultrastructurally that the pigment-containing cells are quite consistent with melanocytes and that the nonpigmented cells resemble neuroblasts.

Molecular studies on this lesion have been rare. A study in 1998 by Khodammi et al.[373] detected amplification of *MYCN* gene and 1p deletion and the presence of t (11:22)(q24:q12) and t (11:22)(13p:q12) translocations.

Treatment and prognosis

The tumor is usually treated by conservative surgical excision with a 5 mm margin of normal tissue. Recurrence is in the 15% range, and rare malignant variants have been reported.

BENIGN EPITHELIAL LESIONS RESEMBLING MALIGNANT TUMORS

Pseudoepitheliomatous hyperplasia

Occasionally, hyperplastic odontogenic epithelial cells may resemble squamous cell carcinoma, as can the organ of Chievitz, typically seen in the buccal-temporal space.[374] More common, however, is pseudoepitheliomatous hyperplasia, which may accompany oral mucosal ulceration or be seen alone. It also occurs frequently in association with granular cell tumor as a reactive proliferation. Elzay and O'Keefe[375] have reported an instance of primary pseudoepitheliomatous hyperplasia involving the gingiva. Preliminary pathologic diagnoses of inverted papilloma, verrucous carcinoma, squamous odontogenic tumor, verruca vulgaris, and keratoacanthoma need to be entertained when confronted with a possible pseudoepitheliomatous hyperplasia.

Histologic features that separate this entity from verrucous carcinoma and keratoacanthoma have been discussed previously. Rete ridge penetration into the connective tissue is typically a knife-like pseudoepitheliomatous hyperplasia; this is an unusual feature in verrucous carcinoma or keratoacanthoma, in which penetration is broad.

Inverted oral papilloma may be a reasonable differential diagnosis, although only a few cases have been reported in the world literature.[376] Inverted papilloma in the oral cavity typically shows proliferation of acantholytic squamous epithelium without cystic activity, whereas with oral pseudoepitheliomatous hyperplasia, especially the type identified in young individuals, there are often cystic areas filled with keratin. Finally, paracoccidioidomycosis (South American blastomycosis) may demonstrate pseudoepitheliomatous hyperplasia.

Usually, when pseudoepitheliomatous hyperplasia is removed, there is no recurrence. Nonetheless, my colleagues and I have had the opportunity to review a case, similar to that reported by Elzay and O'Keefe,[375] that has required three surgical procedures.

Necrotizing sialometaplasia

Clinical features

Necrotizing sialometaplasia is a benign, self-healing, inflammatory process of the salivary glands, which typically presents clinically as a deeply excavated, sharply demarcated ulcer. The disorder was first described in 1973 by Abrams and colleagues.[377] Most reported cases have been in the hard palate, but cases have been documented involving the mucosa of the mandible,[378] major salivary glands, and respiratory tract.

Necrotizing sialometaplasia usually is identified in adults and could be bilateral. Most patients indicate that the lesion is painful, but there are reported cases in which the lesions were seen without pain as a chief complaint. Occasionally, cases are reported in which there is little or no evidence of ulceration.[379] The cause of necrotizing sialometaplasia is unknown, but trauma has been implicated as an initiating factor. It is postulated that trauma causes intermittent ischemia, followed by infarction and a subsequent mucosal ulcer. Philipsen et al.[380] consider necrotizing sialometaplasia to be the ulcerative or terminal stage of leukokeratosis nicotini palati. Occasionally, patients have prodromal symptoms that include fever, malaise, and swelling. The disease is a benign one, which heals spontaneously in 6 to 10 weeks, usually without treatment.

Poulson et al.[381] reported a case of necrotizing sialometaplasia obscuring an underlying embryonal rhabdomyosarcoma in which they postulated that the extremely rapid growth of the malignant tumor in the peripharyngeal space probably resulted in physical obstruction or impingement of blood vessels supplying tissues of the oral pharynx, with consequent tissue infarction and a superimposed necrotizing sialometaplasia.

Pathologic features

Microscopically, necrotizing sialometaplasia is characterized by a central ulcer with a proliferation of reactive pseudoepitheliomatous hyperplasia at the edge. The supporting lamina propria may be filled

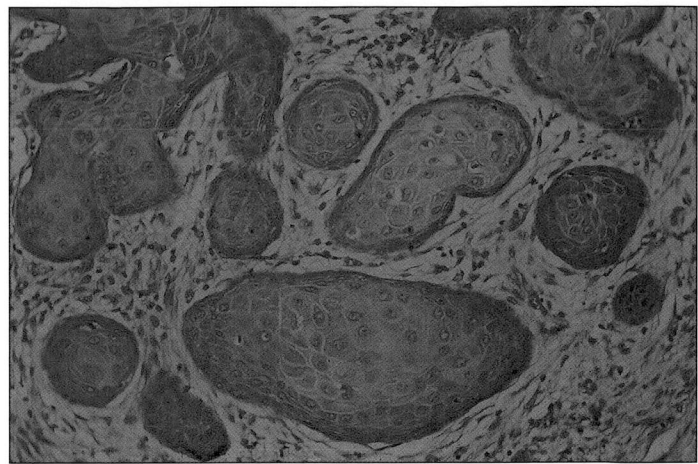

Fig. 22.46 Necrotizing sialometaplasia. Note the smooth rounded contour of lobular squamous metaplasia, which conforms to the salivary gland acinar outline in the tissue.

with acute and chronic inflammatory cells. Neutrophils and foamy histiocytes are usually prominent.[377] Within the connective tissue stroma, salivary acinar and ductal elements show marked lobular squamous metaplasia (Fig. 22.46). Lobular ischemic necrosis may be identified and is thought to be a histologic hallmark of the disease. Salivary gland mucin is frequently distributed in microcysts throughout the supporting lamina propria.

Necrotizing sialometaplasia must be differentiated from squamous cell carcinoma and mucoepidermoid carcinoma because mixtures of islands of squamous epithelium with residual mucous cells may lead to a mistaken diagnosis of mucoepidermoid carcinoma. One of the principal histologic differences between necrotizing sialometaplasia and both mucoepidermoid carcinoma and squamous cell carcinoma is the regular nuclear morphology of squamous cells in necrotizing sialometaplasia, without cytologic atypia.

Abrams et al.[377] document the following chief histologic features that help differentiate necrotizing sialometaplasia from squamous and mucoepidermoid carcinoma: (1) lobular infarction and necrosis, (2) benign-appearing squamous cells, (3) metaplasia of ducts and mucinous acini, (4) a prominent granulation tissue reaction with extensive inflammatory components, and (5) maintenance of lobular architecture. Although necrotizing sialometaplasia is thought to involve on its own, in most cases it is surgically excised because of the difficulty in differentiating it from squamous cell carcinoma or a carcinoma of salivary gland origin on clinical grounds.

METASTASIS TO THE ORAL CAVITY

Cancer that is metastatic from a primary site to the oral tissues is an infrequent finding. Such metastases account for no more than 1% of the neoplasms found in the oral cavity. Meyer and Shklar,[382] in a review of the literature, found only 25 instances out of a series of more than 2400 malignant oral tumors. Castigliano and Rominger[383] reviewed the literature from 1902 through 1953 and found only 175 reported examples of metastases to the jaws from other primary sites.

Meyer and Shklar found the most common site of the primary lesion to be breast, followed by lung, kidney, thyroid, colon and rectum, prostate, and stomach. Few metastases from primary sites in the liver, testis, bladder, or female urogenital organs were encountered.

McDaniel et al.[384] found lung carcinoma to be the most common metastatic tumor to the jaws, followed by carcinoma of the thyroid and prostate, malignant melanoma, and osteogenic sarcoma.

Oral soft tissue metastases are much rarer than bony metastases. Hatziotis and colleagues[385A] in a 1973 review of the literature found only 48 cases of soft tissue metastases between the years 1945 and 1970. Hirshberg[385B] reviewed 157 cases and found that the most common site of metastasis was the gingiva. The tongue was the next most common site. Males are more often affected, and the lung is responsible for more than one-third of all lesions. Metastatic tumors to the oral cavity occur late in the course of malignant disease and, except for those that are known to grow slowly, they generally receive only palliative treatment. Radiotherapy and chemotherapy are often used to decrease the size of the bony expansion if the deformity is interfering with vital function.

LESIONS OF MESENCHYMAL SOFT TISSUE ORIGIN

Fibroma

Many of the lesions outlined here are inflammatory hyperplastic responses that show a marked inductive connective tissue or mesenchymal change. Thus, many of these lesions can also be considered inflammatory in origin.

Clinical features

Fibromas of the oral soft tissues are not true neoplasms because they only have limited growth potential. Fibromas are more appropriately classified as inflammatory hyperplasias, generally due to trauma or irritation from cheek biting or ill-fitting dentures. They are the most common tumors of the oral cavity. When a fibrous overgrowth occurs clinically as a solitary nodular lesion, it is generally termed an 'irritation fibroma.' The irritation fibroma usually presents as a solitary nodular lesion that is typically pink and takes on the color of the associated mucosa. On occasion, the lesion may be traumatized and thus become markedly hyperparakeratotic and white. Fibromas can occur at any site within the oral cavity, and there seems to be no age or sex predilection. The irritation fibroma probably represents the most common benign fibrous overgrowth that is identified in the oral cavity. The lesions are typically asymptomatic. Occasionally, multiple lesions can be identified. Fibromas have often been called fibroid epulis in the literature. Unfortunately, this non-specific term has also been used for such lesions as peripheral giant cell granuloma and the congenital fibroid epulis of the newborn.

Pathologic features

The gross surgical specimen is usually that of a soft tissue nodule with a firm, glistening, white cut surface. Histologically, the fibroma is composed of benign keratinizing squamous epithelium overlying a lamina propria composed of interlacing fascicles of collagen. The mass often has a well-defined pseudocapsule at the periphery. Stellate giant cells may be present in some nontraumatic induced fibromas, in which case the growths are classified as *giant cell fibroma*. Although these histologic characteristics mimic those of a true neoplasm, the proliferation represents nothing more than a form of hyperplasia. On occasion, the hyperplastic connective tissue is exceedingly well vascularized, and it may be difficult to separate the fibroma from a pyogenic granuloma. Some authors indicate that lesions of this type tend to become more fibrous as they mature, and in fact, the irritation fibroma in many instances represents only the terminal stage of a pyogenic granuloma.

Treatment and prognosis

The accepted treatment for the irritation fibroma or the giant cell fibroma is local surgical excision, and recurrence is rare.

Inflammatory fibrous hyperplasia

Clinical features

Inflammatory fibrous hyperplasia, also known as *epulis fissuratum* or *denture hyperplasia*, is a very common reactive hyperplastic lesion of the oral mucosa. It is most often caused by overextension of a denture into the supporting oral soft tissue structures so that the surrounding connective tissue becomes hyperplastic. The most common sites are the maxillary and mandibular buccal vestibular mucosa adjacent to the overextended denture border. The lesions appear clinically as polypoid exophytic redundant masses of tissue along the denture border. They can become so prominent that the lateral border of the denture may be totally covered, and quite frequently the lesions become ulcerated.

Most lesions are asymptomatic, the patient may be unaware of their presence, and they do not have the firm consistency of a neoplasm. Nondenture-associated inflammatory fibrous hyperplasias may affect the gingiva as inflammatory developmental enlargements known as *fibromatosis gingivae* or as a drug-induced enlargements such as *Dilantin hyperplasia*.

Pathologic features

The gross appearances of these inflammatory hyperplasias are all quite similar. The lesions present as a polypoid piece of soft tissue, which may or may not be ulcerated. The cut section is often glistening, white, and occasionally calcified.

The lesions consists of a polypoid mucosal ellipse covered by keratinizing squamous epithelium and supported by a connective tissue lamina propria composed of interlacing fascicles of collagen. Osseous metaplasia may be seen, and a chronic inflammatory infiltrate is usually identified throughout the connective tissue stroma. Very rarely, a giant cell component may be described.

On occasion, inflammatory fibrous hyperplasia may regress on its own if it is a very small lesion. Most lesions, however, are greater than 2 cm in length and will not resolve without surgical excision. The lesions do not have malignant potential; however, there are reports of carcinoma arising in adjacent tissue unrelated to the fibrous hyperplasia. These hyperplasias, whether developmental or drug induced, are usually managed by a combination of surgery and elimination of the offending drug.

Pyogenic granuloma

Clinical features

The pyogenic granuloma is a common intraoral reactive proliferation, which classically arises from long-standing chronic irritation and abortive repair. It can be found on any surface of the oral cavity. Chronic irritants may include calculus along the gingival tissues surrounding teeth, ill-fitting prosthetic appliances, fractured teeth with jagged surfaces due to long-standing caries, or a chronic habit such as cheek biting. The lesion is not a true granuloma of the epithelioid type and production of pus in association with it is rare.

Most of the lesions appear as polypoid, nodular, hemorrhagic growths. The most frequent site is the gingiva, accounting for more than three-quarters of all cases. Frequently, interdental papillae are affected, and the patient may complain of spontaneous bleeding from that area or of blood in the mouth on awakening in the morning. Palpation or probing of the lesion will usually elicit the bleeding quite readily. On occasion, the lesions can undergo a rapid growth rate that is alarming, mimicking the growth characteristics of a true neoplasm. Children are more frequently affected than adults.

Pathologic features

Typically, the specimen consists of a nodular, granular, or gritty lesion, which may show surface erosion. The supporting connective tissue usually contains a very marked proliferation of exuberant granulation tissue composed predominantly of vascular channels, proliferating fibroblasts, acute and chronic inflammatory cells, and hemorrhage. The periphery of the specimen may show maturing collagen and osseous metaplasia. The reactive process is not a true granuloma but simply a proliferation of granulation tissue.

On occasion, a few giant cell aggregates can be found, but the dominant giant cell proliferation characteristic of giant cell granuloma is not identified. In addition, the supporting stroma does not have the fibroblastic background that is typical of a giant cell granuloma. Frequently, the endothelial cell proliferation may be so prominent as to mimic a hemangioma. Pyogenic granuloma can undergo partial fibrosis or sclerosis. Such lesions have been termed sclerosing pyogenic granulomas for the sake of convenience.

Occasionally, oral pyogenic granulomas are identified in association with pregnancy; the common terminology for such lesions is *pregnancy tumor*. The distinction is of academic interest only. Pyogenic granulomas are best treated by simple surgical excision. Pregnancy tumors usually regress postpartum, but on occasion they have to be surgically excised. Non-pregnancy associated pyogenic granulomas require surgical excision.

Differential diagnosis

The increased incidence of acquired immunodeficiency syndrome (AIDS) makes it mandatory for pathologists reviewing a suspected pyogenic granuloma of the oral cavity to obtain a thorough patient history. Kaposi's sarcoma can present as a solitary soft tissue nodule in the oral cavity, mimicking pyogenic granuloma. Histologically, Kaposi's sarcoma demonstrates vascular channels lined by endothelial cells and spindle cells, but unlike pyogenic granuloma, the spindle cell element typically has an anaplastic sarcomatous appearance. A chronic inflammatory infiltrate may make it more difficult to distinguish Kaposi's sarcoma from a non-specific reactive inflammatory granulomatous inflammation such as pyogenic granuloma. The peripheral giant cell lesion or tumor and the peripheral ossifying fibroma also mimic pyogenic granuloma clinically.

Papillary endothelial hyperplasia may also be mistaken for a pyogenic granuloma or angiosarcoma.[386] This condition, also referred to as intravascular angiomatosis, has been reported in the head and neck with some frequency.[387]

Peripheral ossifying fibroma (peripheral fibroma with calcification)

The peripheral ossifying fibroma and peripheral giant cell granuloma can closely mimic pyogenic granuloma. Clinical and microscopic distinctions are outlined in the discussion that follows.

Clinical features

The peripheral ossifying fibroma is a soft tissue tumor that characteristically presents as a focal gingival overgrowth. Like the pyogenic granuloma, it is classified as a reactive fibrocollagenous process and not a true neoplasm. Cundiff,[388] in a review of 365 lesions, noted that 8% occurred anterior to the molar area, and he documented a 16% recurrence rate. Greer and Zarlengo[389] suggest

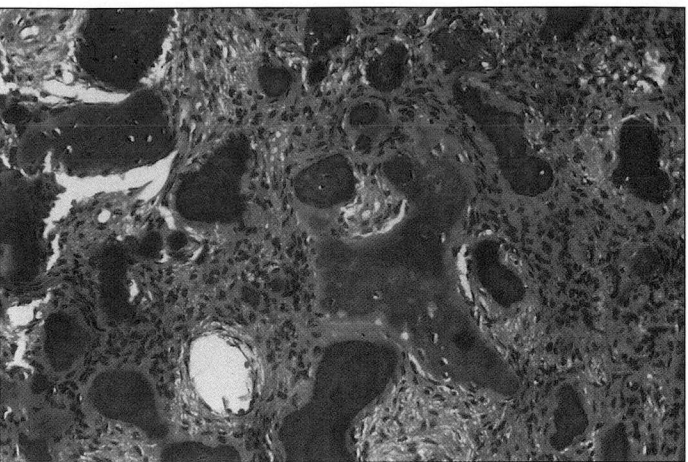

Fig. 22.47 Ossifying fibroma. Reactive fibrous proliferation with focal calcification and bone formation.

that the peripheral fibroma with calcification is simply an irritation fibroma arising from connective tissues of the periodontium with the added odontogenic potential of that tissue. This pluripotential feature is seen in the formation of bone, cementum, and other calcified tissues.

In a review of 22 cases of peripheral fibroma with ossification, Greer and Zarlengo[389] identified the lesions most often in young adults. Women were affected more often then men. A median age of 27 and an age range of 11 to 28 were documented. Twenty lesions occurred in whites, and only 2 lesions were reported in blacks. The lesions appeared as exophytic, sessile, or pedunculated soft tissue growths of the gingiva, occurring most often anterior to the molars with no predilection for either arch. These investigators documented a 27% recurrence rate.

Pathologic features

These polypoid lesions are usually covered by benign keratinizing squamous epithelium and are supported by an active fibrous proliferation with focal calcified areas. In the series of Greer and Zarlengo,[389] 18 of the 22 lesions contained calcified material that was either bone, dystrophic calcification, or cementum (Fig. 22.47). Stellate fibroblasts as well as plump endothelial cells often dominate the stromal histology. Epithelial odontogenic rests were observed in 9 of the 22 lesions reviewed.

There is considerable debate in the literature as to whether the lesion is a true neoplasm of periodontal ligament origin or a reactive lesion due to injury. Most authorities favor the second theory and maintain that the odontogenic rests identified histologically are only fortuitous findings.

Treatment and prognosis

Complete surgical excision to the base and lateral margins of the lesion is the treatment of choice if recurrence is to be avoided. A recurrence rate of 15–20% has been reported.

Peripheral giant cell granuloma (peripheral giant cell tumor)

This soft tissue tumor has often been referred to as giant cell epulis, a non-specific term that should be avoided. Although the lesion is histologically identical to the central giant cell granuloma of bone, it is more than likely a reactive soft tissue lesion and not related to the central osseous lesion it mimics histologically.

Clinical and radiologic features

The peripheral giant cell granuloma most often occurs as a soft tissue overgrowth in the tooth-bearing areas of the jaws. The lesions classically have a hemorrhagic, polypoid appearance and bleed readily on probing. Frequently, the surface is ulcerated. The tumor only rarely exceeds 2 cm in diameter, although 5–7 cm lesions have been reported and it can be clinically identical in appearance to the pyogenic granuloma and peripheral ossifying fibroma.

The peripheral giant cell granuloma may cause a radiologically evident cup or saucerization defect in the underlying bone; therefore, a periapical radiograph may aid in establishing a clinical diagnosis.

Peripheral giant cell granulomas are much more common in women than in men, and they tend to involve the anterior portion of the jaws, frequently presenting in the mandibular symphyseal region. Giansanti and Waldron[390] reviewed 720 cases of peripheral giant cell granuloma and found the average age to be 30. Edentulous areas of the jaw are most often affected.

Pathologic features

The gross appearance of peripheral giant cell granuloma is typically that of a polypoid mass, which on cut section has a firm or gritty and often hemorrhagic appearance. The texture of the cut surface, although firm, is not solid, and pressure can frequently elicit hemorrhage. Microscopically, the lesion usually consists of a nonencapsulated proliferation of stellate and reticular fibrous connective tissue with a dominance of ovoid or spindle cells and plump endothelial cells. The stroma contains an abundant proliferation of multinucleate giant cells. The supporting stromal cells may show considerable mitotic activity, and capillary proliferation throughout the mass is usually quite prominent. Hemorrhage, chronic inflammatory cells, and hemosiderin are dominant features, and quite frequently metaplastic bone and calcified structures arranged in globular and trabecular patterns can be identified.

There has been considerable debate in the literature concerning the origin of the giant cells in this lesion. Some authors believe that the giant cells arise from endothelial cells, whereas others debate an osteoclastic origin. Sapp[391] has shown ultrastructurally that the giant cells have features resembling those of osteoclasts.

The histologic differential diagnoses that most often have to be entertained when reviewing a giant cell granuloma microscopically are pyogenic granuloma and hemangioma. These lesions, however, do not contain the characteristic giant cell proliferation seen in giant cell granuloma.

Treatment and prognosis

The treatment of peripheral giant cell granuloma is local and complete surgical excision with a margin of normal tissue and inclusion of periosteum or periodontal ligament associated with the lesion. Recurrences have been reported, fueling the debate as to whether teeth adjacent to the lesion should be removed in association with the soft tissue mass. Most authorities consider this contraindicated. A decrease in the reported recurrence rate has been documented since practitioners managing this lesion have gained better understanding of its biologic behavior and realized that scaling of teeth adjacent to the lesion to remove calculus or associated debris can reduce the risk of recurrence.

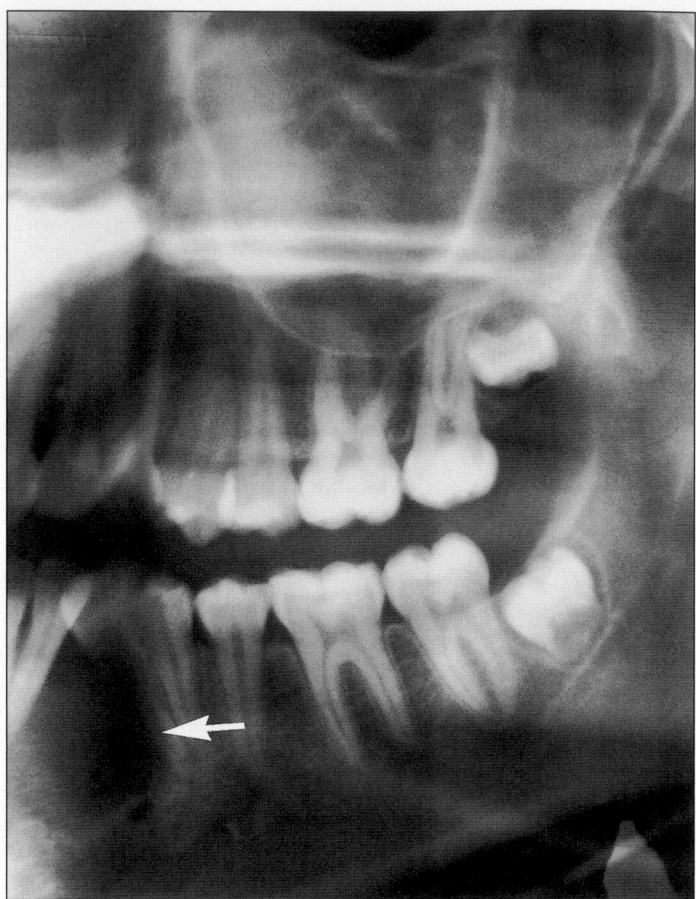

Fig. 22.48 Central giant cell granuloma. Pear-shaped radiolucency of the mandible, spreading cuspid and incisor teeth apart (arrow).

Central giant cell tumor

Although the central giant cell tumor is not a soft tissue lesion, it is discussed here because of its close relationship to the peripheral giant cell granuloma.[392] This central bony growth once known as central giant cell granuloma is an aggressive bony lesion that occurs in children and young adults, principally between the ages of 7 and 20, although Waldron and Shafer[393] have documented age extremes of 7 and 67.

Austin et al.[394] reviewed a series of 968 benign tumors of the jaws and found that central giant cell tumors accounted for only 3.5% of the lesions. Greer and others[395] documented a 3.6% incidence in a review of 109 tumors of the oral mucosa and jaws in children.

The tumor, which is not a true granuloma, usually presents as a swelling or expansile lesion within bone and is commonly associated with a sensation of increased pressure or pain. The classic radiologic appearance is that of a soap bubble, honeycomb, or locular central osseous radiolucency (Fig. 22.48). The cortical bone may be eggshell thin, and the lesion appears to affect the jaw anterior to the molars much more frequently than the posterior jaw. The mandible is much more frequently affected than the maxilla. On occasion, the lesion can perforate the cortical plates, mimicking an aggressive malignant neoplasm. The soap bubble or honeycomb appearance of the lesion is not pathognomonic, because a host of lesions, including ameloblastoma, odontogenic myxoma, aneurysmal bone cyst, and hemangioma can have the same radiologic features.

Perhaps the most heated of the long-standing debates about central giant cell tumor of bone is whether or not a percentage of these tumors represent true giant cell tumors of bone similar to those described by Austin et al.[394] Even after classifying all giant cell lesions of bone, including the brown tumor of hyperparathyroidism, variants of fibrous dysplasia, cherubism, and central giant cell tumor, there remain a small group of true neoplasms that are exceedingly aggressive and, in fact, have shown metastasis. Dahlin[396] refers to these lesions as 'true' giant cell tumors of bone, causing some investigators to classify the lesion as either nonaggressive or aggressive. Some investigators speculate that perhaps a few 'true' giant cell tumors represent exceedingly reactive osteogenic sarcomas with nearly undetectable malignant osteoid.

Batsakis[397] concludes that the following features separate the giant cell granuloma from a 'true' giant cell tumor: (1) osteoid formation or the presence of osteogenic activity is not a characteristic of the 'true' giant cell tumor except where a peripheral fracture has occurred; (2) true giant cell tumors are typically devoid of hemosiderin, histiocytes that are laden with lipid, or an inflammatory cellular component; and (3) giant cell granulomas are predominantly lesions of the first two decades of life, whereas the 'true' giant cell tumor of bone occurs most often in the third or fourth decade.

Giant cell tumors or granulomas of the jaws are considered benign tumors of osteoclastic origin. The 'true' giant cell tumor of bone is more often a neoplasm of long bones, usually identified at the lower end of the femur, upper end of the tibia, and lower end of the radius. Giant cell tumors or granulomas of the jaws may, on occasion, behave aggressively, but unequivocal metastases from such lesions have been documented in only one instance.[392]

Pathologic features

Grossly, the central giant cell tumor or granuloma is identified as loose, gritty, hemorrhagic tissue that may contain spicules of bone. Histologically, it is composed of a loose fibrillar connective tissue stroma with a prominent proliferation of endothelial cells and vascular channels. The collagen fibers are loosely arranged and only occasionally are they collected in bundles. Distributed throughout this fibrillar network are numerous giant cells that contain nuclei abundantly distributed around the periphery of the cell (Fig. 22.49). The cytoplasm of the giant cell is usually granular, and vacuoles can sometimes be identified. Bone and osteoid are frequently identified distributed randomly throughout the tumor. Hemosiderin pigment and extravasated blood are prominent findings in the lesion, particularly at the periphery. Lesions that have perforated the bone may show necrosis or extensive hemorrhage and fibrosis at their periphery.

From a differential diagnostic standpoint, several lesions have to be considered when entertaining a diagnosis of central giant cell tumor. A diagnosis of cherubism should be entertained whenever evaluating a central giant cell lesion of the jaws; however, the classic multifocal radiologic presentation of cherubism in the jaws allows distinction between the two, although histologic findings very often are identical. The brown tumor of hyperparathyroidism should also be considered as a diagnosis; its radiologic and microscopic characteristics and those of giant cell tumor are nearly identical. The brown tumor of hyperparathyroidism tends to occur a decade or two later than the central giant cell tumor of the jaws. The establishment of a definitive diagnosis of brown tumor is dependent on demonstrating parathyroid disease, kidney abnormalities, or associated systemic disease. Serum calcium level determinations are mandatory when such a diagnosis is entertained. The central giant cell tumor rarely, if ever, results in elevated serum calcium levels. The term *aneurysmal*

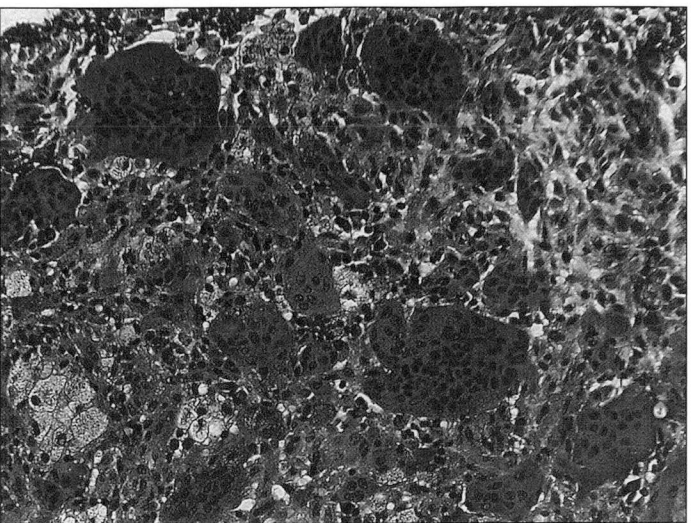

Fig. 22.49 Central giant cell granuloma displaying an abundance of multinucleated giant cells, and capillaries in a background of richly nucleated stoma. Note the similar appearing nuclei of the giant cells and the stromal cells.

bone cyst is an outdated term for a giant cell tumor with large sinusoidal spaces and should be avoided.

Treatment and prognosis

The management of the central giant cell tumor is generally considered to be thorough curettage or surgical excision to the margins of the lesion. Andersen and coworkers[398] document a recurrence rate of 13%. Most reports state a range of recurrence of 10–20%.[392] Those lesions that do recur may require marginal resection.

Nodular fasciitis

Nodular fasciitis, also known as pseudosarcomatous fasciitis, is a rather uncommon fibroblastic proliferation that histologically resembles a well-differentiated fibrosarcoma.[399] The lesion was first described by Konwaler et al;[400] since their original description, it has been documented that approximately 10% of all cases of nodular fasciitis occur in the head and neck area.[401] The lesion arises from submucosa or subcutaneous fascia and is rapidly growing.

Werning[402] reported a series of 41 cases from the Armed Forces Institute of Pathology and stated that most occurred in the subcutaneous tissues overlying the zygoma and mandible. A few were reported in the parotid sheath. The lesions are characterized microscopically by an abundant proliferation of fibroblasts set in a richly vascular myxoid matrix containing an abundance of mucopolysaccharide ground substance. The proliferation of fibroblasts is relatively haphazard, with a considerable variation in size and shape. Multinucleated giant cell forms are frequently present. The lesion may be confused with fibrosarcoma or angiosarcoma. The distinction from fibrosarcoma is probably most important. Nodular fasciitis displays a typical haphazard, random feathered arrangement of the fibroblasts; with fibrosarcoma, a more classic herringbone pattern predominates. The prominent clinical presentation in nodular fasciitis in the oral cavity is that of a rather discrete nodule.[403] The lesions range from slightly tender to asymptomatic and range in size from less than 1 cm to more than 10.5 cm.[404] There appears to be no sex predilection, and the lesion can occur at any age. The salient pathologic features are discussed in Chapter 9.

Fibromatoses of the oral and maxillofacial region

The fibromatoses are a group of fibroproliferative lesions that behave in a fashion intermediate to that of fibrosarcoma and the host of fibrous lesions of the oral cavity with limited growth potential.

Juvenile or congenital fibromatosis is most often a soft tissue lesion,[405] whereas *desmoplastic fibroma* is a central osseous lesion of the jaws. Freedman and associates[406] reviewed 25 reported cases of desmoplastic fibroma reported in the world literature and documented an additional case of their own. The lesion is predominantly seen in young persons, with a peak incidence in the second decade; there is no apparent sex predilection. More than 75% of the desmoplastic fibromas reviewed by Freedman et al. had eroded the buccal or lingual cortical plates, and approximately one-third of the cases recurred.

The etiology of this lesion is unknown, although abdominal desmoid-type fibromatosis is very likely related to trauma and to the endocrine influences of pregnancy. Of the lesions reviewed by Freedman and associates,[406] 34% showed some evidence of root resorption, and the radiographic findings were most often a unilocular, well-defined radiolucency of bone. The lesion is characteristically composed of whorls of fibroblasts and myofibroblasts, with oval or fusiform nuclei distributed between collagen bundles. The lesion is poorly circumscribed, scattered multinucleated giant cells may be present, and cytologic atypia is rare. Treatment usually includes wide local excision, and recurrences range from 25% to 65%. The characteristic histologic features are discussed in greater detail in Chapter 9.

Fibrosarcoma

Fibrosarcoma is a rare lesion of the oral and maxillofacial region. The peak incidence is in the 20s and 30s and the lesions most often are painful fleshy masses. Fibrosarcoma of the jaw is histologically graded as elsewhere in the body (grades I, II, and III). See Chapter 9 for details.

Lipoma

Lipoma, a benign neoplasm of fat cells, is the most common mesenchymal tumor of the human body, but it is not a common oral lesion.[407–409] In a 10-year study of benign tumors of the oral cavity, Dockerty and coworkers[407] found that lipomas constituted 4.4% of the total. MacGregor and Dyson[410] and Greer and Richardson[411] report similar percentages.

Lipomas are generally described as soft, freely movable, or spongy asymptomatic masses. The most frequent location of the tumor appears to be the buccal mucosa. There is no age or sex predilection. The histologic features of lipoma are delineated in Chapter 9.

Granular cell tumor

Clinical features

Granular cell 'myoblastoma' (granular cell tumor) is an uncommon oral soft tissue tumor, most often identified in the body of the tongue,[412] although it has been described in the lip, palate, gingiva, and in extraoral locations including the breast, skin, and gastrointestinal tract. The lesion is found in all ages, although adults are most often affected, and the lesion usually presents as a solitary nodule that is not painful and grows very slowly. The tumor favors females 2:1.

Pathologic features

Granular cell tumors are usually less than 2 cm in diameter and 10–15% of patients have more than one lesion. Histologically, the

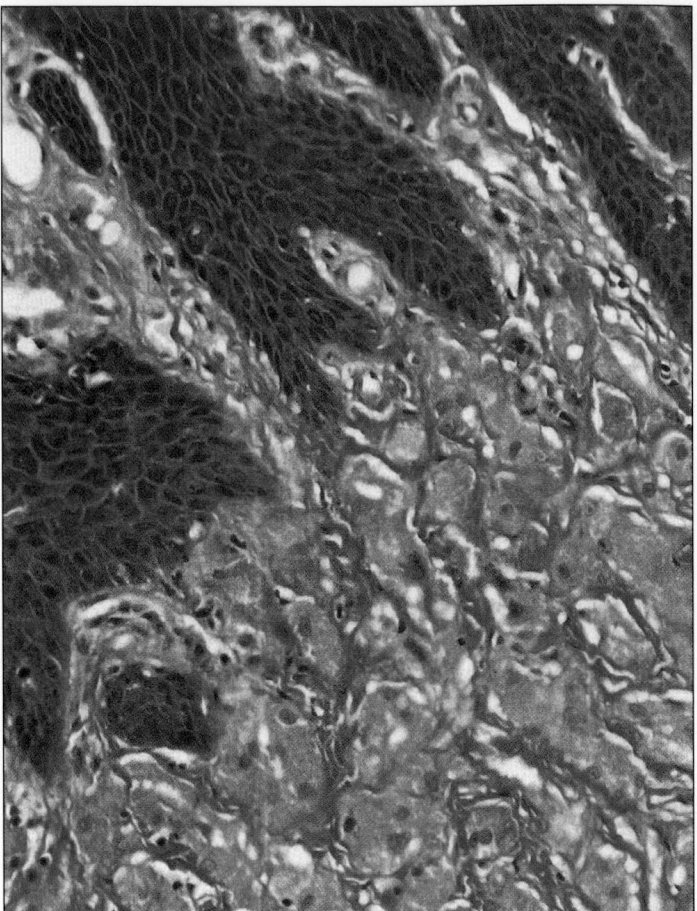

Fig. 22.50 Granular cell tumor. Large cells with eosinophilic granular cytoplasm and small nuclei are arranged in nests below surface epithelium.

granular cell tumor presents as a soft tissue nodule that is usually covered by benign keratinizing squamous epithelium. The epithelium may be quite hyperplastic and may show a marked degree of pseudoepitheliomatous hyperplasia, rendering a differentiation from squamous cell carcinoma a problem. The supporting connective tissue contains a distinct proliferation of large granular lysosomal-appearing cells, which may be arranged in sheets, cords, strands, or nests. The cytoplasm is typically filled with eosinophilic granules, and the nucleus is usually small, round to oval, and vesicular (Fig. 22.50). Mitotic activity is infrequently seen and the lesion has poorly marginated borders.

Histochemically, the granules in the granular tumor myoblastoma are nonlipid and appear to be composed of a glycoprotein substance.[413,414]

There is some controversy about the histogenesis of the granular cell tumor. Some theories suggest a muscle origin for the lesion;[415] others suggest that the condition is a degenerative process affecting muscle fibers. Histologically, cross-striations have not been conclusively demonstrated in any of the papers indicating a muscle origin. Azzopardi[416] favors a histiocytic origin. Histochemical studies have not supported this theory. The most prevalent theory in the literature suggests that the granular cell tumor is of Schwann cell origin;[417] however, even electron microscopic evaluation has not absolutely confirmed the origin of this tumor.[418]

The most important feature for the surgical pathologist to keep in mind is not to characterize the associated pseudoepitheliomatous hyperplasia seen in this lesion as a squamous epithelial neoplasm. A second important point to remember is that a superficial biopsy of the lesion is unacceptable. When the lesion is described clinically as a nodule and only a superficial fragment is submitted, a second biopsy is mandatory.

Treatment and prognosis
Recurrence of this neoplasm is rare, and surgical excision with 5 mm margins is the treatment of choice.

Congenital granular cell tumor

Clinical features
The congenital granular cell tumor is a lesion typically found in the anterior maxilla on the alveolar ridges as a pedunculated or sessile soft tissue swelling. Rarely, the lesion may occur on the mandibular mucosal surface. There is a marked female predominance. The etiology is unknown, although an origin from vascular pericytes or smooth muscle has been speculated. The tumor, which arises from primitive mesenchymal cells, is also known as gingiva granular cell tumor. Rarely does the congenital epulis, which usually presents as a nodular or polypoid mass, exceed 3 cm in diameter, although multiple tumors and lesions greater than 4 cm in diameter have been reported.

Pathologic features
The pathologic features of the congenital epulis of the newborn are quite similar to those of the granular cell tumor, but the typical pseudoepitheliomatous hyperplasia that is seen with granular cell tumor is not identified and the lesion tends to be more richly vascular. On occasion, odontogenic epithelium has been identified interspersed among the granular cells, and of osseous metaplasia reported.

The congenital granular cell tumor must be distinguished from the rare, well-differentiated rhabdomyoma.[419] Histochemically, the lesions can be differentiated in that the intracellular granules seen in congenital epulis of the newborn are not composed of glycogen and glycoproteins as they are in rhabdomyoma. The intracellular granules of congenital epulis appear to be glycolipid and stain periodic acid–Schiff positive. Campbell[420] suggests that there might be a relationship between ameloblastoma and congenital epulis of the newborn in that the granular cells that are present in the granular cell type of ameloblastoma have identical histochemical reactions to those of congenital epulis. This hypothesis has not been proved, and certainly there is no parallel in terms of biologic behavior. Schwann cells and axon fibers have not been identified in cases of congenital granular cell tumor that have undergone ultrastructural scrutiny, which negates a neurogenic origin.[421] Immunohistochemical studies show that granular cells of the granular cell tumor of the newborn, unlike those of the adult granular cell tumor, do not react with antisera against S-100 protein.[422,423]

Treatment and prognosis
The congenital granular cell tumor is a benign lesion that is amenable to conservative surgical excision with 5 mm margins. It does not appear to recur with any frequency. Progression after birth is slow, and occasional regression without treatment has been documented.

Myogenic tumors
Rhabdomyoma of the adult fetal type occurs in the oral cavity. These lesions are generally considered to be hamartomas that present as well-defined lobulated masses. The cells in these lesions are usually large, granular, and eosinophilic, but can occasionally be clear. The treatment of choice is surgical excision, and recurrence is rare.

The *leiomyoma* is a benign tumor of smooth muscle origin that rarely occurs in the oral cavity. Variations of this lesion, such as the *vascular leiomyoma* and the leiomyoma of deep soft tissue are most common in the tongue. Leiomyomas are true neoplasias composed of interlacing bands of Masson trichrome-positive spindle cells. Surgical excision with a 5 mm margin of the normal tissue is the treatment of choice.

Neurogenic tumors
Tumors arising from neural tissue, specifically tumors of nerve sheath origin, are quite common in the head and neck region.[424] These tumors can occur as both soft tissue and bony lesions. Typically, they remain asymptomatic unless they attain appreciable size. When they arise as bony lesions, they generally cause a sensation of pressure, often the patient's chief complaint. Soft tissue tumors typically begin as nodular convex swellings, the tongue being the most common site of involvement.[425]

The three types of tumors documented most frequently are Schwannoma, neurofibroma, and the c-fiber neuroma or traumatic neuroma. Schwannoma can occur at any age, typically as a solitary tumor. Generally, the lesion presents in subcutaneous tissues, and it may on occasion be multifocal. Spindle interlacing fascicles of Antoni A-type tissue and hyalinized Antoni B-type tissue are the histologic hallmarks of this neoplasm. Rarely is Schwannoma associated with von Recklinghausen's neurofibromatosis, although cases have been reported.

The *neurofibroma* occurs only rarely as a solitary tumor. It is the most common peripheral nerve tumor. It presents principally as a multifocal tumor, usually in association with multiple neurofibromatosis of the skin and internal organs. Both tumors are neoplastic proliferations of neuroectodermal Schwann cells and perineural fibroblasts with a collagenous fibrillar matrix. Detailed histology and natural history of these tumors can be found in Chapter 45.

The traumatic neuroma, or c-fiber neuroma is a rarely encountered oral lesion, which does not represent a true neoplasm but rather an exuberant overgrowth of nerve fibers occurring after nerve severance. Considering the amount of trauma that the oral cavity is exposed to through extractions of teeth, prosthetic appliances, and extensive manipulative dental procedures, it is surprising that the lesions are not more common than the literature documents.

The chief symptom of *traumatic or c-fiber neuroma* is usually isolated pain associated with a pre-existing surgical procedure. The most common sites tend to be the posterior mandibular areas adjacent to the mandibular canal and the tongue.

Harkin and Reed[426] have described a neoplasm termed *myxoma of nerve sheath* (neurothecoma). These tumors are most often lobulated tumors of the skin composed of spindled cells and an abundant mucoid matrix.[427] The nerve sheath myxoma is only rarely identified in the oral cavity. In this location, it is usually described clinically as a gradually enlarging painless growth arising on the lower lip. To date, seven cases have been reported involving the oral cavity.[428]

The *palisaded encapsulated* neuroma has a predilection for the palate and perioral facial skin. This lesion, which is lobular in appearance, is never associated with neurofibromatosis or multiple endocrine neoplasia syndrome type III (MEN III), however it can be seen with MEN II. It usually does not demonstrate the classic Anatoni A tissue or Verocay bodies of the Schwannoma. It usually presents as a non-painful submucosal mass in patients in the fourth through sixth decades of life. Local surgical excision is the treatment of choice.

Vascular and lymphatic lesions

Benign tumor-like proliferations of vascular tissues are exceedingly common in the oral cavity. These tumors probably do not represent true neoplasms but more properly represent developmental anomalies or hamartomas. The hemangioma is the most common of all these lesions. The arteriovenous hemangioma is the most problematic of these lesions and it can be life threatening.

An important fact that must be remembered by the surgical pathologist is that many oral angiomatous proliferations are found in association with syndromes that have a systemic vascular counterpart. These syndromes include hereditary hemorrhagic telangiectasia, Kasabach-Merritt syndrome, Sturge-Weber syndrome, and Maffucci's syndrome, blue rubber bleb nevus syndrome, and Cherry hemangiomas. Juvenile capillary hemangioma and cavernous hemangioma are the common subtypes. *Lymphangiomas*, hamartomas of malformed lymphatics, are rare in the oral cavity. Three subtypes exist: the congenital cystic hygroma of the neck, the deep cavernous type, and the multicystic lymphangioma.

It is also important for the surgical pathologist to recognize that AIDS may be associated with atypical vascular proliferations in the oral cavity. Close scrutiny of vascular-appearing oral soft tissue lesions for atypical cytologic features suggestive of Kaposi's sarcoma, including back to back proliferation of vascular channels and proliferation of apparent sarcomatous cells along the walls of thin slit-like spaces, is important.

Other malignant vascular tumors, including malignant hemangiopericytoma and angiosarcoma, have rarely been reported in the oral cavity.[429] The nasopharyngeal angiofibroma is an important fibrovascular lesion of teenagers and young adults, as discussed in Chapter 15.

TUMORS OF SALIVARY GLANDS

Salivary gland tumors account for approximately 1–4% of all tumors in the head and neck region. Frazell[430] has further documented that salivary gland tumors account for 5% of all the benign and malignant tumors in the human body, excluding those of the skin. Minor salivary gland tumors are much less common than major salivary gland tumors, accounting for approximately 20% of all salivary gland tumors. Documentation of the behavior and pathology of the various histologic types of salivary gland neoplasms and their histopathology can be found in Chapter 23;

however, certain characteristics of minor salivary gland tumors are unique to an intraoral presentation.

When salivary gland tumors are identified intraorally, the most common site will be the palate, followed by the lip. Pleomorphic adenomas account for more than 60% of all salivary gland tumors in major or minor salivary glands. Adenoid cystic carcinoma and mucoepidermoid carcinoma account for a much larger percentage of minor salivary gland malignancies than major salivary gland malignancies.

It is important to recognize that salivary gland tumors arise centrally within the mandible, a feature of note when the pathologist is confronted with a clear cell or apparent mucus-producing intraosseous tumor of the jaw.

Most salivary gland tumors are thought to arise from either acinar or reserve stem cells in the salivary gland duct system (Fig. 22.51). These neoplasms can be difficult to evaluate and diagnose because more than one cell type can be involved. Most salivary gland tumors arise in the parotid and most are benign. In the submandibular gland approximately half the tumors are benign while in the sublingual gland, most tumors are malignant.

A working classification schema for salivary gland tumors is included here and can also be found in Chapter 23. This classification includes both benign and malignant salivary gland tumors. Certain tumors, however, such as Warthins' tumor, basal cell adenoma, oncocytoma, acinic cell carcinoma, and sebaceous adenoma dramatically favor major salivary glands. Polymorphous low-grade adenocarcinoma shows a preference for development in intraoral minor salivary glands of the palate, while canalicular adenoma is most often identified in the upper lip. The discussion will be limited to those neoplasms that show a propensity for intraoral minor salivary gland development. Although the vast majority of salivary gland tumors are epithelial in origin, connective tissue tumors such as hemangioma, lipoma, neurogenic tumors, and lymphomas can occur in salivary glands. Here we selectively discuss some of the salivary gland tumors more frequently encountered in the oral cavity.

BENIGN TUMORS

Pleomorphic adenoma (mixed tumor)

The mixed tumor is the most common of all salivary gland neoplasms. The AFIP reports that mixed tumors of minor salivary

Fig. 22.51 Salivary gland duct system.

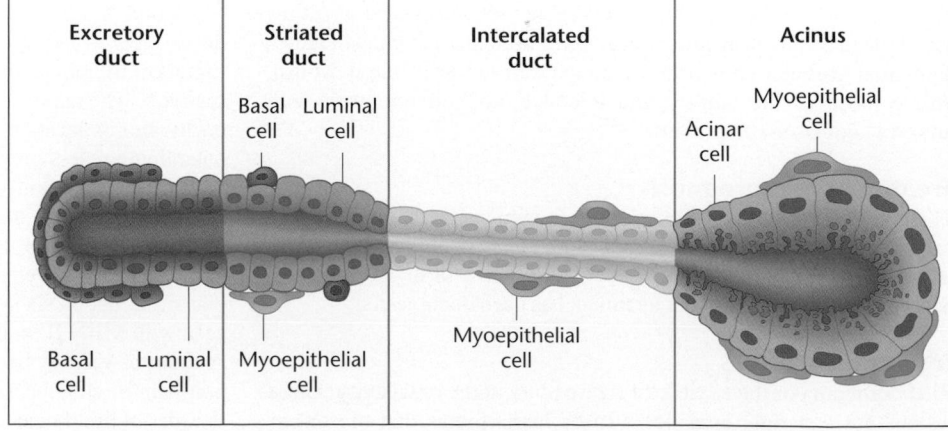

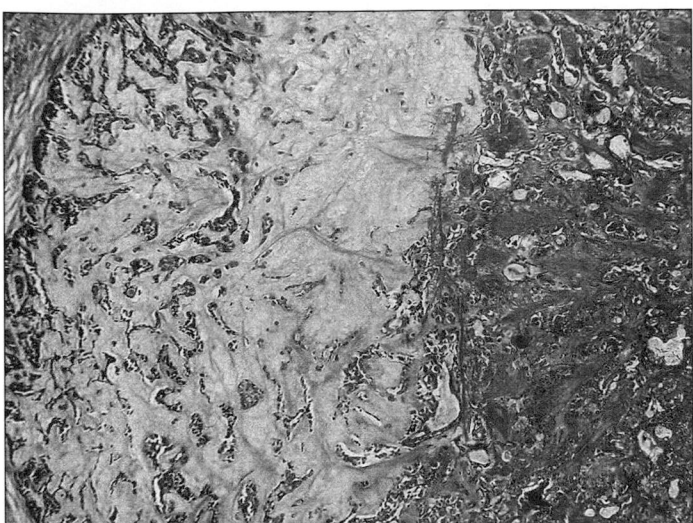

Fig. 22.52 Pleomorphic adenoma. The epithelial component is seen in the form of cords, nests, and tubules in the background of a myxochondroid stroma. Note the hyalinization of the stroma in the right half of the picture.

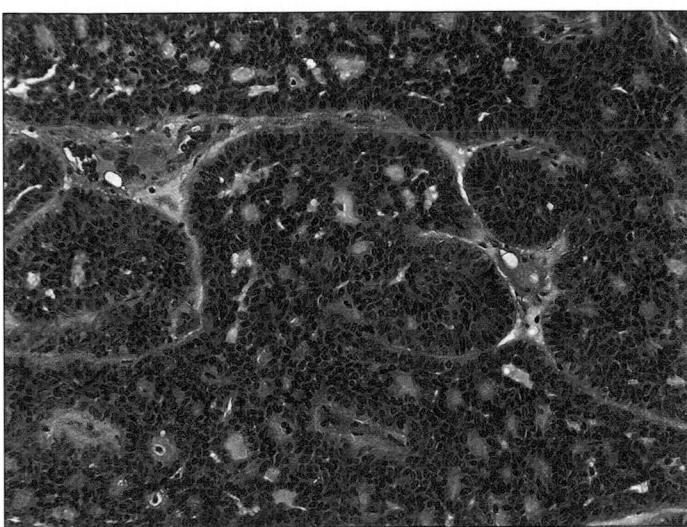

Fig. 22.53 Membranous basal cell adenoma. Note the basophilic islands displaying cells with peripheral palisading and the prominent basement membrane at the periphery of the interdigitating islands.

glands account for 72% of all minor salivary gland tumors.[431] The mixed tumor is rare in the submandibular and sublingual glands, accounting for less than 5% of tumors in these sites.

Clinical and radiographic features

Most intraoral pleomorphic adenomas occur in the mucosa overlying the posterior palate and present as painless masses. These tumors do not invade bone and are typically encapsulated. Mixed tumors can also be found in the submandibular gland, the lips, cheek, and tongue, where they most often present as freely movable nodules.

Pathologic features

Grossly, pleomorphic adenomas appear encapsulated. The cut surface of the tumor is usually glistening, white, and mimics the surface of a cut potato. Pleomorphic adenomas can contain focal zones of calcified product, gelatinous material, or mucin.

Histologically, mixed tumors are typically composed of sheets, nests, cords, and islands of epithelial cells set in a supporting matrix that tends to be either myxoid, mucoid, chondroid, myxochondroid, osseous, or hyalinized (Fig. 22.52). Spindle cells or myoepithelial cells frequently ramify throughout the tumor's epithelial component and it is common to find basophilic mucoid material or eosinophilic hyalinized material as part of the peripheral substrate of these cells. This diverse histopathology helps to account for the name mixed tumor. Benign mixed tumors occasionally undergo malignant transformation in approximately 2% of cases. The malignancy may involve only the epithelial component or may involve both the epithelial and stromal component. Features indicating malignant change include accumulation of atypical hyalinized material, cellular atypia within tumor cell nests, necrosis, calcification, and neural invasion.

Treatment and prognosis

Pleomorphic adenomas are best treated by excision with controlled frozen sections. A rare benign variant of the mixed tumor,

myoepithelioma, is composed wholly of (1) spindle-shaped or (2) plasmacytoid cells. The plasmacytoid histologic variant favors the palate. Up to 25% of the pleomorphic adenomas within the oral cavity recur, probably as a result of enucleation of the tumor instead of marginal excision of the mass.

Basal cell adenoma

Clinical features

The basal cell adenoma occurs most frequently in the parotid gland, with 30% of these tumors being reported in the oral cavity.[432] Most patients who develop basal cell adenoma are men and the average age is 60. Basal cell adenomas are usually well circumscribed and have a marked predilection for the upper lip. The tumor usually presents as a soft tissue nodule that is rubbery and compressible. The cut section is most often homogeneous, but there can be focal areas of cystic degeneration.

Pathologic features

Basal cell monomorphic adenomas are composed of an accumulation of islands of tumor cells with peripheral columnar palisading cells that marginate a stellate central zone (Fig. 22.53). The central stellate areas can contain keratin. The tumor can be divided into trabecular, tubular, and membranous subtypes in which case tumor cell nests resemble basal cell carcinoma or take on trabecular or tubular patterns. Regardless of histologic subtype, the tumor islands are generally quite bulky and there is very sparse connective tissue stroma. The stroma that is evident is generally well vascularized. A few basal cell adenomas have been reported to undergo transformation to basal cell adenocarcinoma.

Treatment and prognosis

Basal cell adenomas are best treated by marginal surgical excision and they rarely recur. The highest recurrence rates have been reported with the membranous subtype.

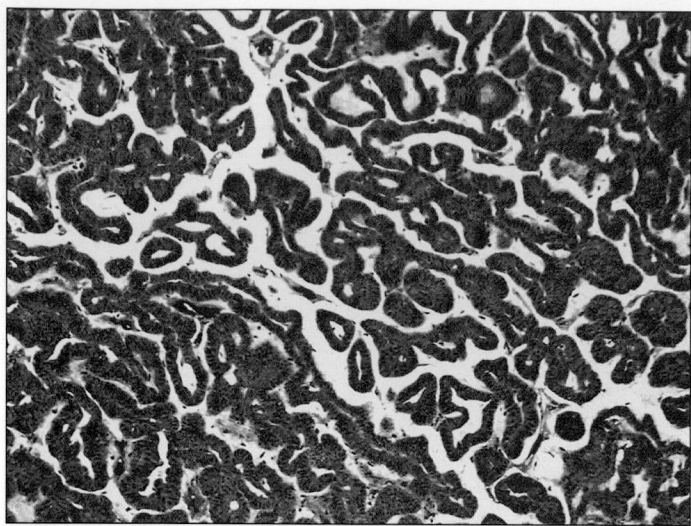

Fig. 22.54 Canalicular adenoma. Note the complex branching and interconnecting cords, which line narrow canalicular lumens marginated by columnar cells. The lumena are focally dilated, giving a beaded appearance.

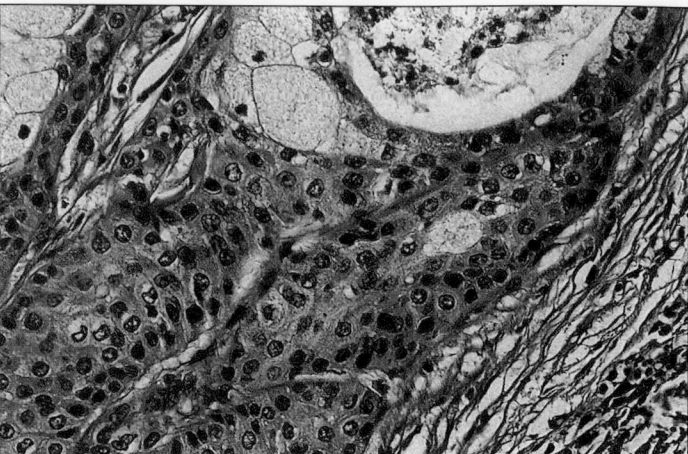

Fig. 22.55 Intermediate-grade mucoepidermoid carcinoma. Note cyst formation, intermediate cells (smaller nuclei), mucous cells, and the epidermoid cells (with prominent nucleoli).

Canalicular adenoma

Clinical and radiographic features

The canalicular adenoma is a neoplasm that occurs exclusively in the minor salivary glands of the oral cavity. The vast majority of these tumors have been reported in the upper lip. The tumor shows a marked predilection for women in the fifth or sixth decades of life. Most tumors present as painless freely movable swellings in the lip submucosa. These tumors rarely attain a size greater than 3 cm in diameter and rarely do the tumors cause erosion or ulceration of the overlying epithelium.

Pathologic features

The canalicular adenoma is most often a discrete well-marginated nodule. The cut surface can be white, gelatinous, firm, or occasionally cystic. The cells forming the tumor usually form tumor islands with a double row of marginating columnar epithelial cells. The tumor islands often take on a ductal pattern as they ramify throughout a sparse collagenous stroma (Fig. 22.54). Occasionally, tumor cells are arranged in a singular chain fence-like pattern. Individual tumor cells tend to be eosinophilic and quite uniform with elliptical nuclei. Basaloid cells may be seen between rows of the more prominent columnar cells of the tumor. The canalicular adenoma demonstrates S-100 protein and cytokeratin reactivity.[431]

Treatment and prognosis

The treatment for the canalicular adenoma is conservative surgical excision with a margin of normal tissue. Recurrences are rare.

MALIGNANT SALIVARY GLAND TUMORS

Mucoepidermoid carcinoma

Clinical and radiographic features

Mucoepidermoid carcinoma, the most common malignant salivary gland tumor, favors the parotid; however, 30% of mucoepidermoid carcinomas occur as minor salivary gland tumors of the oral cavity or the submandibular gland.[432] Mucoepidermoid carcinoma is the most common malignant salivary gland tumor of children and the tumor shows a distinct predilection for females (3:1) regardless of age.[432]

Mucoepidermoid carcinomas are thought to arise from reserve cells within the salivary gland duct system and because of that they have the potential to differentiate along both mucous-producing epidermoid cell lines, resulting in a tumor with an epidermoid, and mucous-secreting cells. Very few neoplasms lend themselves to a histopathologic grading system that is predictive of behavior. Mucoepidermoid carcinoma is one of only a few tumors where such a grading system is effective.

Tumors of the oral cavity can present as soft tissue nodules, ulcerative exophytic masses, papillary growths, or tumors that invade bone. Higher-grade tumors tend to show greater tissue destruction, ulceration, and bony invasion.

Pathologic features

Mucoepidermoid carcinoma can be divided into three distinct histologic grades: high grade, intermediate grade, and low grade. The tumors are composed of four classic components: (1) mucous-secreting cells with abundant foamy cytoplasm, (2) epidermoid cells that are arranged in sheets, nests, and cords, (3) intermediate cells which tend to be basaloid in appearance and have darker staining than epidermoid cells, and (4) clear cells which can occur as individual cell clusters within epidermoid nests. The grading of this neoplasm is based upon assessing the admixture of these various cell types. Low-grade tumors tend to be slow growing. They tend to have a bluish tint and appear to be cystic largely because they contain an abundance of mucin within dilated cystic spaces. Intermediate and high-grade tumors tend to be firmer masses, less often bluish, and relatively rapidly growing. The low-grade tumors are typically encapsulated and well circumscribed where as high-grade tumors are usually ulcerative and infiltrative.

Low-grade mucoepidermoid carcinomas tend to be cystic and are composed predominantly of mucous-filled cysts with a minimal accumulation of epidermoid and intermediate cell types. Intermediate-grade tumors are composed of fewer cysts and contain a greater abundance of intermediate cell types, and epidermoid type cells (Fig. 22.55). The mucous component in intermediate-grade tumors is much less than with the low-grade tumors. High-grade mucoepidermoid carcinomas show an abundant accumulation of epidermoid cell types (Fig. 22.56). They contain very little mucin

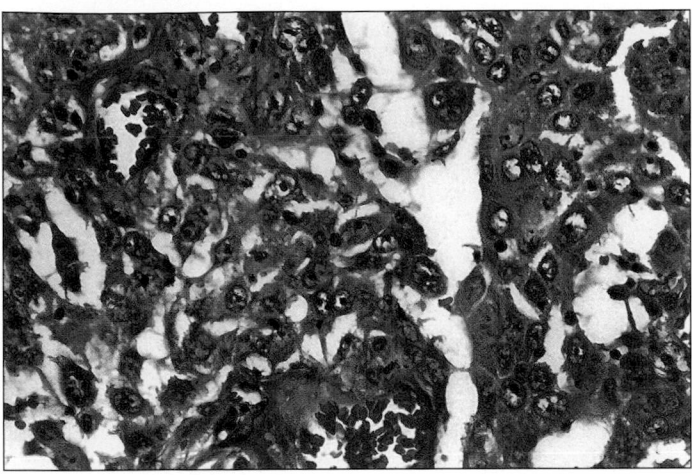

Fig. 22.56 High-grade mucoepidermoid carcinoma. Note the degree of nuclear pleomorphism, and absence of cyst formation and mucous cells.

and they tend to show the most dramatic cytologic atypia of any tumor grade. High-grade tumors may require mucicarmine staining in order to differentiate them from squamous cell carcinoma.

Treatment and prognosis

Low-grade tumors are usually treated by excision with a 1 cm margin of normal tissue, whereas intermediate and high-grade tumors are most often treated with wide surgical excision or a marginal resection of tumor and bone followed by radiation therapy doses between 5000 and 7000 cGy. Five-year survival rates for high-grade tumors rarely exceed 35%, whereas, five-year survival rate for low-grade tumors are generally above 90%.

Central osseous mucoepidermoid carcinoma is a rare variant of mucoepidermoid carcinoma that occurs exclusively within the mandible. These lesions usually occur in the tooth-bearing areas of the mandible, generally within the molar and premolar region, and they are thought to arise from either entrapment of salivary gland rests within the mandible during jaw development, or neoplastic transformation of mucous cells within the walls of the odontogenic cysts. The vast majority of central mucoepidermoid carcinomas are low-grade tumors and they are best managed by marginal resection of bone to clear margins.

Adenoid cystic carcinoma

Clinical and radiographic features

In the oral cavity, adenoid cystic carcinoma occurs most frequently as a palatal nodule or ulcer. Patients may complain of an array of symptoms that range from localized swelling to a burning sensation to a feeling of nasal stuffiness. The tumor can mask its insidious malignant potential by proliferating as a small, slow-growing neoplasm for several years. In spite of its tendency to grow slowly, adenoid cystic carcinoma is a very aggressive neoplasm with a marked propensity for perineural and intraneural spread (Fig. 22.57A). Males outnumber females with this tumor approximately 3 to 2 and the vast majority of patients present with tumors in the fourth through sixth decades of life. Although the palate is the most common oral site, the lesion can occur on any oral mucosal surface as well as within the submandibular and sublingual glands. Lesions have also been reported within the body of the tongue, a very rare presentation for a salivary gland neoplasm.

Pathologic features

Adenoid cystic carcinoma is usually an unencapsulated growth that presents as an infiltrative tumor mass. Histologically, the tumor is composed of cuboidal-appearing cells with round, very strikingly hyperchromatic nuclei and minimal cytoplasm. The tumor manifests three specific histologic patterns: cribriform, tubular, and solid. The cribriform pattern, the most common histologic pattern, grows as multiple Swiss-cheese-like cystic spaces whose lumina contain inspissated mucin, glycosaminoglycan, and basal lamina material. The stroma is generally hyalinized and eosinophilic. The tubular pattern consists of aggregates of tumor cells that lack multiple large cystic spaces. Single ductal structures set in a hyalinized matrix dominate the histopathology. Solid sheets and islands of tumor cells characterize the solid histologic subtype, and it is the most biologically aggressive of the three subtypes (Fig. 22.57B).

Treatment and prognosis

The tumor cells of adenoid cystic carcinoma frequently extend beyond the radiographic and clinical margins of the tumor, thus the

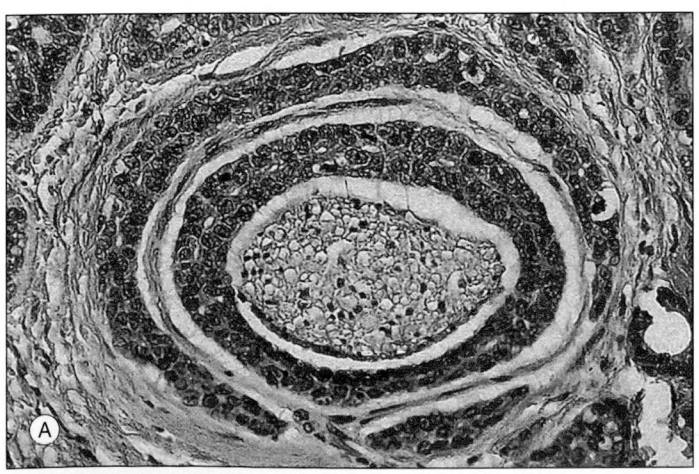
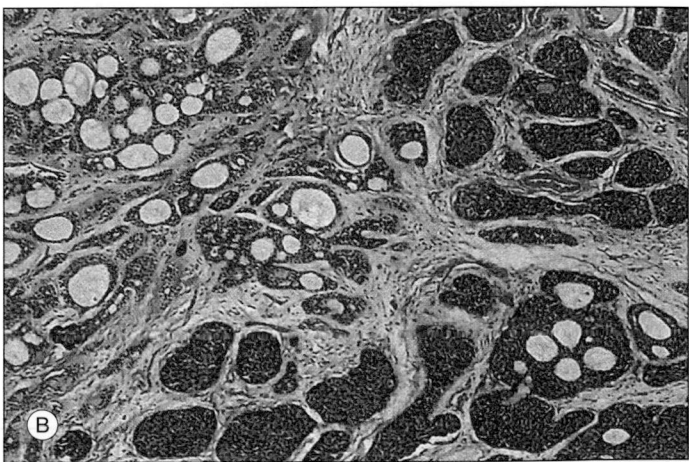

Fig. 22.57 Adenoid cystic carcinoma. **A,** Perineural invasion; **B,** The cribriform and solid pattern.

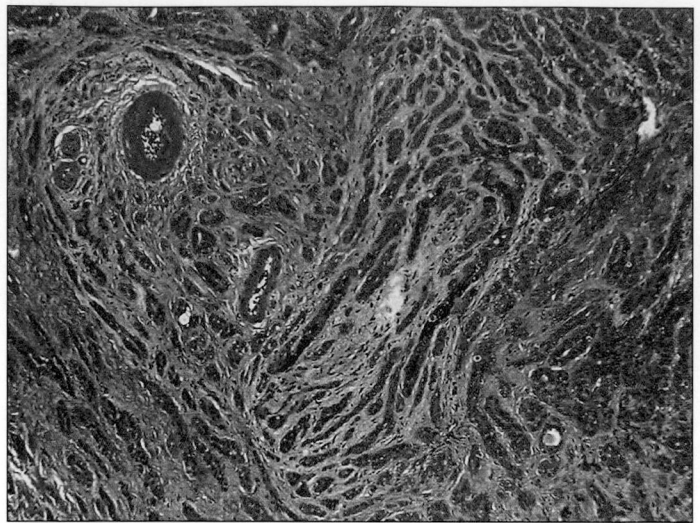

Fig. 22.58 Polymorphous low-grade adenocarcinoma, tubular pattern. Note the whorled targetoid appearance of the tumor.

management modality of choice includes wide surgical excision, generally with margins that are 3 cm around the tumor mass, followed by radiation therapy. Combined treatments that now include surgery and radiotherapy have resulted in the five-year survival rates for adenoid cystic carcinoma rising to 40%. Metastases associated with adenoid cystic carcinoma generally occur as metastatic foci within the lungs.

Polymorphous low-grade adenocarcinoma

Clinical and radiographic features

Freedman and Lumerman first described polymorphous low-grade adenocarcinoma in 1983 using the term lobular carcinoma.[433] Polymorphous low-grade adenocarcinoma is largely a tumor of minor salivary glands and it occurs only rarely in major salivary glands. The neoplasm is twice as common as adenoid cystic carcinoma in minor salivary glands and shares its perineural predilection but, unlike adenoid cystic carcinoma, it has limited metastatic potential.

Polymorphous low-grade adenocarcinoma usually presents as a firm painless oral mucosal mass that only rarely ulcerates. The palatal mucosa is the most common oral site followed by the buccal mucosa. The tumor has a marked female predilection and the vast majority of the patients who develop polymorphous low-grade adenocarcinoma are fifty years or older.

Pathologic features

Polymorphous low-grade adenocarcinomas are slow growing. They are usually encapsulated, and rarely do they show marginal infiltration of surrounding tissues but if the tumor occurs in an area adjacent to bone, it can cause bony invasion. The tumor is composed of tumor cells that are bland in appearance with a uniform nuclear pattern and few atypical cytologic features. These cells are most often arranged in solid, ductal, trabecular, and tubular patterns (Fig. 22.58). Individual tumor cell nests are generally composed of small duct-like structures with central lumina that are lined by cuboidal-appearing cells. Occasionally tumor cells are arranged in a whorled, so-called targetoid, pattern. In some instances the tumor cells can be arranged in a single-file pattern in a dense collagenous

stroma that mimics the pattern seen in breast carcinomas. Tumor cells can be round, oval, or fusiform and the chromatin pattern is often stippled. The tumor cells are generally set in a collagenous hyalinized stroma or mucocollagenous stroma.

Polymorphous low-grade adenocarcinoma can easily be confused histologically with adenoid cystic carcinoma and the tumor can infiltrate small nerves in a pattern similar to adenoid cystic carcinoma. However, necrosis is not seen in polymorphous low-grade adenocarcinoma and the nuclei in polymorphous low-grade adenocarcinoma are generally larger and more uniform and round than the tumor cells of adenoid cystic carcinoma. In addition, the cytoplasm of the cells of polymorphous low-grade adenocarcinoma is typically eosinophilic, whereas the cytoplasm of cells in adenoid cystic carcinoma is most often clear. The classic cribriform pattern of adenoid cystic carcinoma dominates the overall histology of that tumor, whereas the cribriform pattern seen in polymorphous low-grade adenocarcinoma is more random and segmented.

Treatment and prognosis

Polymorphous low-grade adenoid carcinoma is best treated by a soft tissue excision with adequate margins. If the tumor involves underlying palatal or alveolar bone, excision of that bone may be necessary. This tumor is not amenable to radiation therapy. Long-term survival rates for polymorphous low-grade adenocarcinoma are greater than 80%.[432]

FIBRO-OSSEOUS DYSPLASIAS AND RELATED CONDITIONS OF BONE

Fibro-osseous lesions are reactive bony lesions that show replacement of normal bone architecture with benign cellular fibrous tissue containing varying amounts of mineralized material. There is considerable variation among pathologists in the terminology and classification of these lesions. At present, the concepts about the lesions are not totally uniform. Three specific lesions will be considered here because of their frequent appearance in the jaws: fibrous dysplasia, ossifying fibroma, and cherubism. Central giant cell granuloma has been included under this heading by some investigators. That lesion is discussed elsewhere in this chapter along with the peripheral giant cell granuloma.

FIBROUS DYSPLASIA

Clinical and radiologic features

Fibrous dysplasia is a developmental condition of bone first described by von Recklinghausen in 1891 using the term *osteitis fibrosa disseminata*.[434] The terms fibrous dysplasia and polyostotic fibrous dysplasia, however, were proposed by Lichtenstein in 1938.[435] The disease affects the craniofacial skeleton, commonly the jaw, as a *monostotic* lesion, although *polyostotic* forms have been reported. Presentations in the context of McCune-Albright syndrome have also been seen.[436,437] In Waldron and Giansanti's review of 22 lesions,[434] the most classic findings were painless enlargement of involved bones. Ages ranged from 5 to 65, with a mean of 27 years, but the lesion is usually identified in the second and third decades of life, with males and females affected equally. A more recent review by Lustig et all.[438] of 22 patients with fibrous dysplasia involving the skull base and temporal bone, showed a similar mean age of 22 years with a male to female ratio of 2:1. In their cases, the most classic presentation was of unexplained facial pain (57%), while the

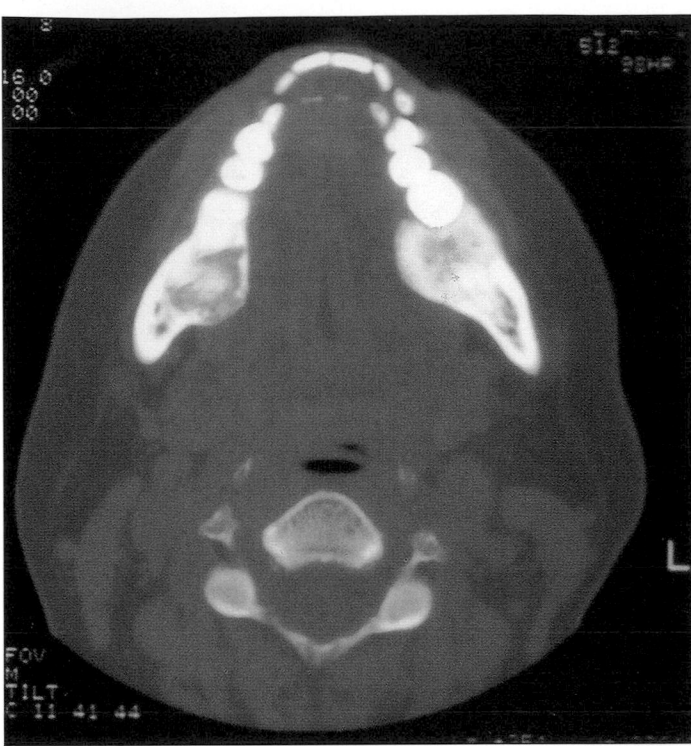

Fig. 22.59 Fibrous dysplasia. CT scan of fibrous dysplasia showing cortical expansion and mixed radiolucent/radiopaque presentation.

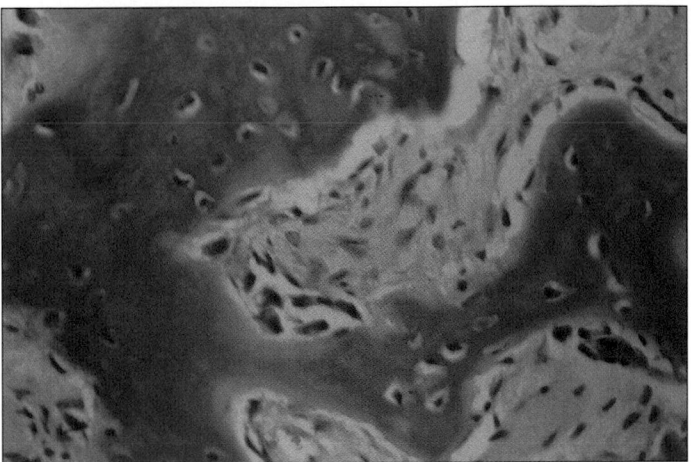

Fig. 22.60 Fibrous dysplasia with proliferating fibrous tissue and irregular osseous trabeculae that in this field shows focal rimming by plump osteoblasts.

presence of an expanding mass was present in 24% of the patients.

The characteristic radiological appearance (Fig. 22.59) is that of a ground-glass or 'orange peel' radiopacity. The borders of lesions are often difficult to define, and frequently there appears to be a transitional zone between normal and abnormal bone. Multilocular radiolucencies are occasionally seen.

With disseminated polyostotic disease, 75% of the skeleton can be affected. The monostotic form in which a solitary bone is involved is more commonly seen. Three to five percent of patients with polyostotic disease have skin pigmentation and endocrine gland hyperactivity and are classified as having McCune-Albright syndrome.

Considerable recent emphasis has been on attempts to separate head and neck fibrous dysplasia from other fibro-osseous lesions; consequently, the term *craniofacial fibrous dysplasia* has been popularized. Craniofacial fibrous dysplasia represents fibrous dysplasia of the maxilla, mandible, and bones of the skull. Eversole et al.,[439] in a review of 512 fibro-osseous lesions, found a predilection of craniofacial fibrous dysplasia for the mandible; however, the cases that were adequately documented as polyostotic fibrous dysplasia showed a predilection for the maxilla. Eversole and colleagues point out that the criteria that distinguish between monostotic fibrous dysplasia and ossifying fibroma of the jaws are varied. Their review of the literature indicates that, based on radiologic findings alone, it is often impossible to separate monostotic fibrous dysplasia radiologically from the supposedly better delineated ossifying fibroma.

The diagnosis of fibrous dysplasia is a clinicopathologic one. It is often less than productive for the surgical pathologist to attempt to diagnose fibrous dysplasia (or most fibro-osseous lesions, for that matter) by simple histologic examination of tissue samples. Accurate diagnosis is based on a very thorough evaluation of clinical, radiographic, and histologic parameters. There are no clinical laboratory tests that are absolute in diagnosing fibrous dysplasia, and bone chemistries, including calcium, phosphorus, and alkaline phosphatase, may be normal or increased. Radiographically, fibrous dysplasia of the jaws usually has a so-called ground-glass appearance, but mottled opaque and multilocular radiolucent lesions have been reported.

Pathologic findings

Grossly, the tissue received for pathologic evaluation usually is yellow, gray, or brown, with a gritty cut surface. Normal bone may be replaced by yellow to white homogeneous areas, and occasionally there may be central areas that appear cystic.

Classically, fibrous dysplasia is composed of a stroma that is fibrous in nature. The stroma may be highly cellular or have the appearance of maturing collagen. Distributed randomly throughout the supporting collagenous stroma are unconnected bone trabeculae, which usually have large osteocytes within lacunae. The margins of the bone trabeculae often show a streaming of collagen bundles and fibers from the trabeculae into the surrounding stroma (Fig. 22.60). Most of the lesions examined will show areas of woven bone. Many authorities consider the presence of woven bone mandatory for a diagnosis of fibrous dysplasia.[440] However, most reports on craniofacial fibrous dysplasia document that it is not necessary to identify woven bone to render this diagnosis.[434,439] In a series of 150 cases of craniofacial dysplasia, Eversole et al.[439] were able to identify 19 cases in which there were multiple spheroid calcifications in a connective tissue setting, 85 had woven osteoid, 27 had lamellar bone, and 19 showed osteoblastic rimming. These authors also reviewed 75 cases of monostotic fibrous dysplasia and found that once again there was a variance of pattern of bone in the lesions, ranging from spheroid calcifications to woven osteoid to lamellar bone, with areas of osteoblastic rimming. Thus, the old adage that osteoblastic rimming often negates a diagnosis of fibrous dysplasia is best discarded or considered in context.

Waldron and Giansanti[434] paid particular attention to the relative amounts of woven and lamellar bone in each section of the 65 lesions that they reviewed. They also paid considerable attention to the evidence of osteoblastic rimming in bone. Although they found that most of the bone they identified was of the woven type, lamellar bone was constantly seen among the tissue samples. It is important to realize that fibrous dysplasia represents a dynamic series of events in the maturation of bone, as opposed to permanent maturation arrest in the woven bone stage. Spjut et al.[441] have noted that occasional lamellar transformation can be identified in fibrous dysplasia and that this finding should not detract from a diagnosis of fibrous dysplasia if other criteria, especially radiologic and clinical criteria, are fulfilled.

Recently, this entity has received increasing attempts to define its molecular[442,443] and genetic abnormalities. These include the identification of mutation in the (GNASI) gene[444,445] affecting the intrinsic GTPase activity or the Gs protein signal transduction pathway and abnormal cellular regulation of cyclic AMP and protein kinase A.

Treatment and prognosis

Most lesions diagnosed as fibrous dysplasia tend to stabilize after the completion of normal skeletal development, although continuous growth has been documented in some cases. Small isolated lesions are often completely surgically resected, but most patients have a slow-growing deformity that may require multiple recontouring/cosmetic surgical interventions until the disease stabilizes. Nearly one-third of all patients demonstrate regrowth after surgical recontouring. The lesions are not radiosensitive, and radiotherapy has been shown, in fact, to predispose to postradiation sarcoma.

OSSIFYING FIBROMA

Clinical and radiologic features

Ossifying fibroma is a distinct pathologic entity that can be separated quite easily from fibrous dysplasia in cases in which Albright's syndrome or polyostotic disease are identified. However, the distinction is much more difficult when these two features are not appreciated. Ossifying fibroma occurs most commonly in the third or fourth decades of life, with females being favored dramatically and the mandible more often affected than the maxilla. The tumor usually causes a painless swelling when it is small, but facial asymmetry may result in large lesions. Waldron and Giansanti[434] found a distinct paucity of lesions reported in the anterior maxilla in their review. A large proportion of ossifying fibromas are found in intimate relationship to the roots of teeth or in the periapical regions of the jaws. There can be quite a variation in the radiologic features of ossifying fibroma, ranging from totally lytic lesions with varying amounts of radiopaque calcific foci to lesions that are totally radiopaque (Fig. 22.61). Most often, ossifying fibroma is well circumscribed radiologically, but occasionally, the lesion can have a 'punched out' appearance. On rare occasions, the lesions tend to blend into normal bone, causing some difficulty in distinguishing them from fibrous dysplasia. Waldron and Giansanti[434] and Hammer and coworkers[446] consider ossifying fibroma to be a lesion of periodontal ligament origin in the jaws.

Pathologic features

Grossly, ossifying fibroma usually consists of multiple gritty or partially calcified gray-white pieces of tissue. Histologically, one is able to identify a component of fibrous and osseous tissue. The supporting stroma may be composed of interlacing fascicles of collagen or loose proliferating fibroblasts that can have a stellate character. A varying amount of vascularity can be appreciated, ranging from areas in which there is total lack of endothelial-lined channels to areas of multiple capillary proliferations.

Lamellar trabeculae may be appreciated either as a distinct osseous component separate from the fibrocellular stroma or as an anastomosing retiform osseous component that tends to blend into the

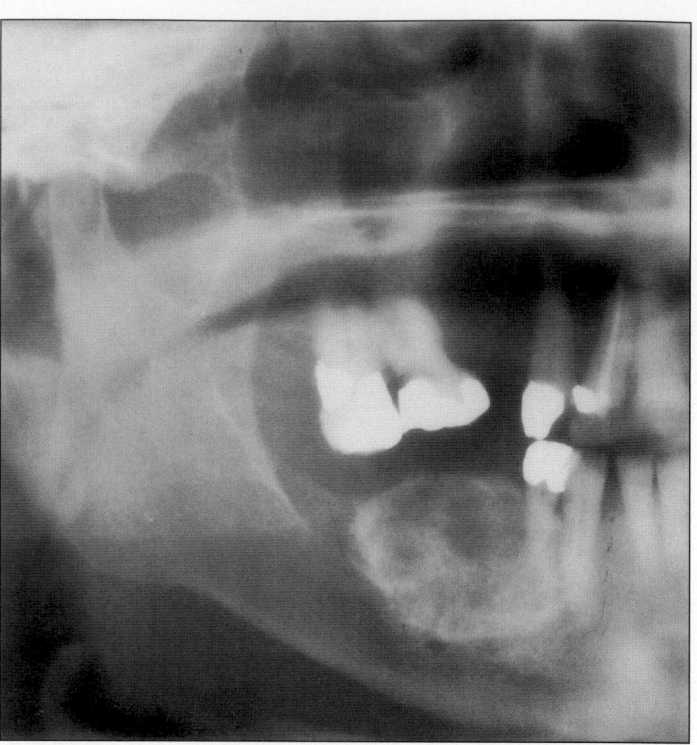

Fig. 22.61 Well-circumscribed ossifying fibroma abutting and encroaching on a mandibular bicuspid tooth.

surrounding stroma. Woven bone may also be identified. Globular calcifications frequently described as cementoid may also be seen in the tissue sample. When such globules are seen, the term *cemento-ossifying fibroma* or *cementifying fibroma* has been used. In fact, this terminology probably serves only to further confuse the spectrum of fibro-osseous lesions. The differentiation between cementoid and osteoid material is only of academic interest and does not alter the biologic behavior of the tumor. Surgical excision and occasionally en bloc resection in instances of a recurrent lesion are the accepted therapy.

Differential diagnosis

A lesion referred to as juvenile active ossifying fibroma and characterized by the accumulation of psammoma body-like aggregates histologically, has been reported at various times in the literature.[434] The lesion, most often encountered in patients in their teens or younger, is considered to be an aggressive one that has the potential to be lethal. Many pathologists, however, consider the lesion to be a low-grade osteosarcoma.

Most pathologists involved in subclassifying fibro-osseous lesions indicate that the distinction between fibrous dysplasia and ossifying fibroma is essentially a clinical and not a histopathologic one. It is important to evaluate the symptomatology and behavior of the lesion and to evaluate thoroughly the radiologic findings. Lesions that are classically identified as ossifying fibroma usually have a thin bony peripheral shell and a distinct boundary on the radiograph, whereas fibrous dysplasia tends to be much more diffuse.

The most significant feature separating ossifying fibroma from fibrous dysplasia is the classic circumscribed nature of the former. However, clinical and radiographic appearances of the two conditions can occasionally be identical. Waldron and Giansanti[434] report that the stroma of fibrous dysplasia is somewhat more fibrous than that of ossifying fibroma.

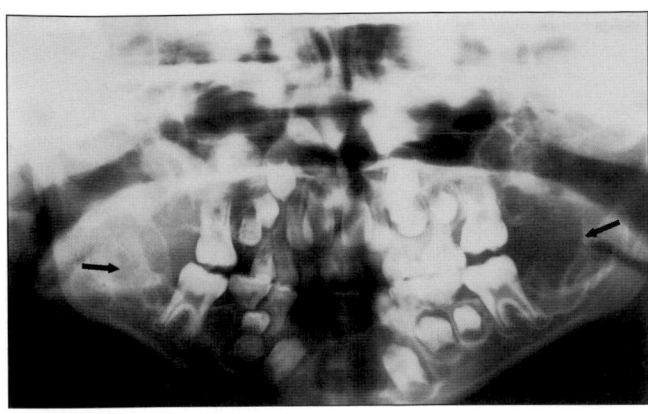

Fig. 22.62 Cherubism. Destructive multilocular lesions are seen involving all four quadrants of the jaws in this panoramic radiograph (arrows).

Cementoblastoma can also mimic ossifying fibroma, from which it is best differentiated by the observations that cementoblastoma is attached to root surfaces and that globules of cementum and layered zones of cementogenesis are typical histologically. Periapical cemental dysplasia (see odontogenic tumors) and florid cemento-osseous dysplasia can be confused with ossifying fibroma based on histology. Therefore, proper clinical input from the managing physician or dentist is mandatory to establish a correct diagnosis. *Osteomas* are exceedingly rare in the jaws and most likely are hamartomatous in nature.

Treatment and prognosis
Complete enucleation with eburnation of surrounding bone is the recommended surgical treatment. Recurrence is uncommon.

CHERUBISM

Clinical and radiologic features
Cherubism is a rare genetic disorder that is typically inherited as an autosomal dominant trait with variable expressivity.[447] Recent genetic investigations by Mangion et al.[448] and Tiziani et al.[449] have mapped the cherubism gene to chromosome 4p16. More recently, Ueki et al.[450] described seven mutations on chromosome 4p16 thought to cause cherubism. Most patients with cherubism are identified in early childhood, with the mean age of detection being 7. Boys appear to be affected more often than girls. When the lesion was first described, it was documented as a solitary lesion in one quadrant of the jaw. Since that time, it has been found that lesions frequently progress to involve all four quadrants of the jaws, additional portions of the craniofacial complex, and the long bones. Radiologically, the lesions have a typical soap bubble, multilocular, or compartmentalized appearance (Fig. 22.62). The mandible or the maxillary alveolar processes may be expanded, causing occasional perforation of the cortex. Teeth may be irregularly spaced, totally absent, or unerupted. The fact that the lesions are expansile is of special importance in the maxilla because the orbit may be impinged on, causing upward displacement of the eyeball. This classic clinical appearance, with the eyes of the child turned toward the sky and expanded cheeks, is often likened to an angelic or cherubic appearance.

Pathologic features
Typically, the specimen consists of friable mottled red-brown, sometimes gritty tissue. The cut surface may show a whorled or lobulated pattern. Microscopically, the typical appearance is that of an admixture of loosely arranged fibrous connective tissue, multinucleate giant cells, and occasional fragments of poorly mineralized bone. Giant cells of the type seen in giant cell granulomas are a predominant feature of the neoplasm. Thin-walled vessels are often prominent throughout the supporting stroma, and in many cases, giant cells tend to aggregate around small vascular spaces. Hemosiderin may also be prominent. When the lesions are mature, the histologic features are often those of mature interlacing collagen fascicles, with only a few scattered giant cells.

Several lesions can appear histologically identical to cherubism, including central giant cell granuloma, and the brown tumor of hyperparathyroidism. Thorough histories and adequate clinical work-up are absolutely mandatory in differentiating these lesions. When a familial history is demonstrable along with the classic histologic picture, a diagnosis of cherubism can usually be established.

Treatment and prognosis
The lesions of cherubism tend to show marked growth immediately after their appearance, especially in the first decade of life. After puberty, growth tends to slow, but total regression is not always appreciated and the disease may persist into adulthood. Treatment is not standardized. Curettage has proved beneficial in some instances, whereas some lesions have progressed rapidly at surgical intervention. Cosmetic osseous recontouring may be instituted when the active growth phase has terminated.[451]

CEMENTO-OSSEOUS DYSPLASIA

Cemento-osseous dysplasia is a broad, encompassing term that defines a sclerotic abnormality of bone that has in the past been variously referred to as periapical cemental dysplasia and florid osseous dysplasia. The term cemento-osseous dysplasia is considered more appropriate because it takes into account the fact that the associated dysmorphic abnormalities occur in two mineralized products, cementum and bone. These two products are often very difficult to distinguish histologically, and thus the cemento-osseous descriptor is considered very appropriate.

These so-called dysplasias of bone are clearly not true preneoplastic dysplasias but are in fact forms of bony dysmorphogenesis. Cemento-osseous dysplasias tend to be bony abnormalities that are generally identified in women of African-American descent who are most often in the third or fourth decades of their life. Men are less frequently affected by the conditions and the lesions rarely, if ever, cause expansion of the bone, tooth resorption, or tooth mobility.

Clinical and radiographic features
Periapical cemento-osseous dysplasia can present in one of three radiographic phases: radiolucent, radiopaque, or mixed. The diagnosis of this disorder is largely a clinico-radiographic one that requires close interaction between the radiologist, pathologist, and the clinician. Periapical cemento-osseous dysplasia is unique in that it tends to affect only the bone subjacent to the anterior mandibular teeth. Radiographically, one finds lucent, mixed, or opaque lesions at the apices of the anterior mandibular teeth

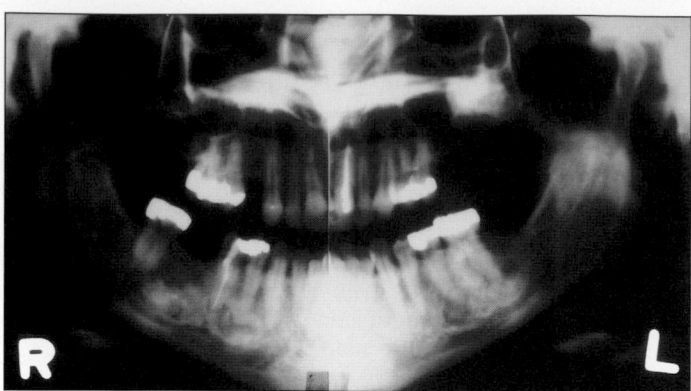

Fig. 22.63 Cemento-osseous dysplasia. Panoramic radiograph demonstrating multiple mixed radiopaque and radiolucent intraosseous lesions. (Courtesy of John McDowell, DDS, Denver, Colorado.)

(Fig. 22.63). These areas of lucency or sclerosis can extend from cuspid to cuspid.

Pathologic features

Histologically, the lesions of periapical cemento-osseous dysplasia are composed of a demineralized product set in a densely collagenous well-vascularized matrix. Osseous trabecular or cementum-like lobules can be seen set in the collagenous matrix. The calcified product can range from normal trabecular bone to immature woven bone to cemental globules, mature cementum, or solid, sclerotic avascular bone.

Treatment and prognosis

Periapical cemento-osseous dysplasia can usually be diagnosed on the basis of radiographs and a good clinical history. In most instances a biopsy is unnecessary. If the radiologist, pathologist, and the clinician work together in establishing a diagnosis then unwarranted extraction of teeth or mandibular bone can be avoided.

FLORID CEMENTO-OSSEOUS DYSPLASIA

Florid cemento-osseous dysplasia is a unique form of bone dysmorphogenesis. As with periapical cemento-osseous dysplasia, the diagnosis is more often than not rendered on the basis of clinico-radiographic findings. The disease process represents as a more diffuse extension of periapical cemento-osseous dysplasia in which radiolucent, radiopaque, and mixed bony lesions occur throughout the basalar bone. Unlike periapical cemento-osseous dysplasia, these lesions show two significant variations. The lesions of florid cemento-osseous dysplasia do not limit themselves to the periapical alveolar bone or the anterior mandible and in fact they can easily extend into the intraradicular bone to the height of the crowns of teeth. Secondarily, the lesions of florid cemento-osseous dysplasia become symptomatic in 10–20% of cases as a result of infection from microorganisms within the periodontal ligament space or in association with tooth extraction. Patients with this disorder tend to be black or of African heritage, and women are affected more often than men. The age range is essentially the same as with periapical cemento-osseous dysplasia and the histologic features are identical to periapical cemento-osseous dysplasia.

Treatment and prognosis

Asymptomatic florid cemento-osseous dysplasia is best left untreated. If the disease process does becomes symptomatic due to secondary infection, then antibiotic therapy is warranted. It is not necessary to surgically excise asymptomatic areas based upon radiographic findings in any instance. Solitary isolated forms of cemento-osseous dysplasia have been referred to as *condensing osteitis* or *bone scarification* and also require no treatment.

TUMORS OF BONE AND CARTILAGE

The principal neoplasms of bone that affect the jaws have essentially the same clinical and microscopic features that are discussed in Chapter 14. Salient clinical and histologic features exclusive to jaw lesions are discussed below.

Osteosarcoma of the jaw tends to present a different biological behavior from those seen in other bones. In the jaw, it tends to occur a decade later than in the long bones, generally shows more favorable histological types, has late metastasis, and a much higher survival rate. Previous radiation exposure,[452] Paget's disease,[453] fibrous dysplasia,[454] and giant cell tumors[455] are some of the conditions thought to predispose to osteosarcoma in this region. Theories related to the etiology of osteosarcoma include viral causes as well.[456,457] Analysis of the chromosome 12 region q13-15 containing SAS, CDK4, and MDM2 genes suggest that these genes may be implicated in the tumorigenesis and progression of low-grade osteosarcoma.[458] Homozygosity of the RB gene on chromosome 13 has also been related to the development of osteosarcoma.

An exclusive early clinical feature of osteosarcoma reported by Garrington et al.[459] is the relatively reproducible symmetric widening of the periodontal ligament around one or more teeth. Garrington contends that this radiologic feature of osteosarcoma appears before any other radiologic change.

Osteosarcoma in the maxilla or the mandible has a mean age of presentation of 34.1 years, with 44% of the tumors affecting the maxilla and 55% the mandible according to Forteza and associates.[460] Most lesions grow exceedingly rapidly and are painless or minimally painful. Histologically, the osteoblastic and chondroblastic subtypes of the tumor are the most common. The overall survival rate for all therapeutic categories is 75%, with a mean disease-free interval of 8 years, according to these investigators. The rare *parosteal osteosarcoma* of the jaws behaves in a less aggressive fashion than the central osseous variety.

Osteoid *osteoma* and *osteoblastoma* can be identified in the jaws. They have essentially the same histopathologic and clinical features as those found in long bones and other parts of the skeleton. Pain is a characteristic feature of both osteoid osteoma and osteoblastoma. Greer and Berman[461] reviewed all the existing literature on osteoblastoma of the jaws in 1975; information on age and sex was available in 10 of 12 published cases. Ages ranged from 6 to 22, with a mean of 14.7 years. An interesting finding in their review of jaw lesions was that pain was a characteristic feature in 75% of the cases. There is a growing body of evidence that suggests that there is no definitive histologic difference between osteoid osteoma and osteoblastoma except for size. This appears to be an even more acceptable proposition in view of the fact that in our review, pain, a feature that is always associated with osteoid osteoma, was a significant finding in 9 of 13 cases of osteoblastoma. Farman and coworkers[462] also deemed the distinction between osteoblastoma and osteoid osteoma so difficult that they consider the two lesions a single entity.

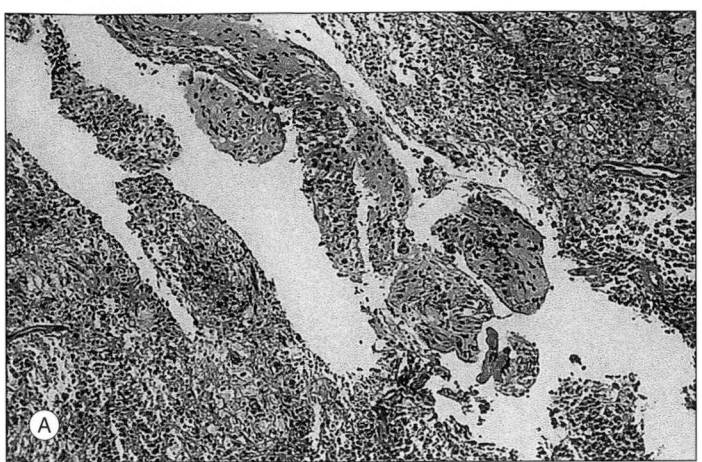
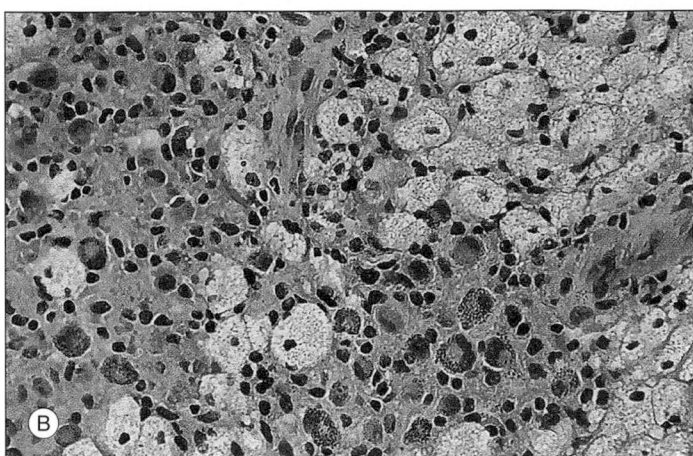

Fig. 22.64 Pigmented villonodular synovitis (PVNS). **A**, Note the papillary formations; **B**, Note the abundance of macrophages, some of which contain hemosiderin (brown pigment) and a foamy mononuclear inflammatory infiltrate.

Chondrosarcoma and *mesenchymal chondrosarcoma* are occasionally found in the jaws; they are also discussed in Chapter 14.

Pigmented Villonodular Synovitis (PVNS) of the Temporomandibular Joint: It is important to mention this entity in our discussion here, in spite of its rarity, because it can be misinterpreted as a neoplastic jaw lesion when encountered in the temporomandibular joint region. Originally described by Jaffe et al. in 1941,[463] PVNS is an idiopathic, benign, yet locally aggressive disorder of the synovium. Trauma, reactive change, inflammation, and neoplasia have been proposed as etiologic factors for PVNS. Two forms exist: the diffuse type, which constitutes the majority of reported cases; and a rarer, localized form. Both forms are exceedingly rare in the temporomandibular joint with approximately 20 cases reported in the literature worldwide.[464,465] Macroscopically, the lesion is usually a yellow-brown sessile or shaggy, villiform outgrowth of the synovium, which microscopically shows papillary formations lined by hyperplastic synovial cells. The tumor stroma is well vascularized with accumulations of histiocytes including foamy histiocytes, multinucleated giant cells, neutrophils, and mononuclear inflammatory cells. Hemosiderin is another feature and may be seen either in the cytoplasm of the synovial cells, in histiocytes, or deposited free in the interstitium (Fig. 22.64). Awareness of this entity is important in the differential diagnosis of neoplastic lesions in this region. Complete removal of the lesion and curettage of the adjacent bone is sufficient to cure the lesion; however, extensive joint destruction may require joint replacement.

REFERENCES

1. Bernstein ML. Biopsy technique: the pathological considerations. J Am Dent Assoc 1978; 96: 438–443.

2. Valenzuela R, Bergfeld WF, Deodhar SD. Interpretation of immunofluorescent patterns in skin diseases. Chicago: American Society of Clinical Pathology Press; 1984.

3. Shroyer KR, Gundlangsson E. Determination of clonality in endometrial adenocarcinoma by PCR amplification of PGK-1. Hum Pathol 1994; 25: 287–292.

4. Vambutas A, Lorenzo TP, Steinberg B. Laryngeal papilloma cells have high levels of epidermal growth factor receptor and respond to epidermal growth factor by a decrease in epithelial differentiation. Cancer Res 1993; 53: 910–914.

5. Marx RE, Stern D. Oral and maxillofacial pathology. a rationale for diagnosis and treatment. Chicago: Quintessence Publishing Co; 2002.

6. Greer RO, Hoernig G, Heinz, D, Shroyer KR. Telomerase expression in oral squamous cell carcinoma. 56th Annual Meeting AAOP, New Orleans, April 22, 2002.

7. Hasing R, Lingen MW. Angiogenesis in oral cancer. J Dent Education 2001; 65: 1282–1290.

8. Greer RO, Weed S, Hoernig G, et al. Cortactin over expression and p53 gene abnormalities in adenoid cystic carcinoma. 56th Annual Meeting, AAOP, New Orleans, April 22, 2002.

9. Greer RO, Shroyer KR, Hoernig G. EGFR in HPV infected oral smokeless tobacco keratoses, dysplasia and cancer. AAOP #19, 48th Annual Meeting, May 13, 1994.

10. Greer RO, Shroyer KR, Frankhouser CA, et al. Detection of human papillomavirus in oral verrucous carcinoma by polymerase chain reaction. Abstract #23, AAOP 49th Annual Meeting, May, 1993.

11. Stanley HR. Consequence of neglected 'impacted third molars,' abstract 25. American Academy of Oral Pathology, 41st Annual Meeting. Scottsdale, AZ, 1987.

12. Ritchey B, Orban B. Cysts of the gingiva. Oral Surg 1953; 6: 765–768.

13. Fromm A. Epstein's pearls, Bohn's nodules and inclusion cysts of the oral cavity. J Dent Child 1967; 34: 275–289.

14. Gardner DG, Sapp JP. Odontogenic and fissural cysts of the jaws. Part 1. Pathol Annu 1978; 13: 177–200.

15. Weathers DR, Waldron CA. Unusual multilocular cysts of the jaws (botryoid odontogenic cysts). Oral Surg 1973; 36: 235–241.

16. Standish SM, Shafer WG. The lateral periodontal cyst. J Periodontal 1958; 29: 27–33.

17. Kaugers SGE. Botryoid odontogenic cysts. Oral Surg 1986; 62: 555–559.

18. Kramer IRH, Pindborg JJ, Shear M. Histological typing of odontogenic tumors. 2nd edn. Berlin: Springer-Verlag; 1992.

19. Marx RE, Stern D. Oral and maxillofacial pathology. a rational for diagnosis and treatment. Chicago IL: Quintessence Publishing; 2002: 590.

20. Eversole LR, Saves WR, Rovin S. Aggressive growth and neoplastic potential of odontogenic cysts with special reference to central epidermoid and mucoepidermoid carcinomas. Cancer 1975; 35: 270–282.

21. Stoelinga PJW, Peters JH. A note on the origin of keratocysts of the jaws. Int J Oral Surg 1973; 2: 37–44.

22. Pindborg JJ, Hansen J. Studies on odontogenic cyst epithelium. 2. Clinical and roentgenological aspects of odontogenic keratocysts. Acta Pathol Microbiol Scand 1963; 58: 283–294.

23. Mosby EL, Sugg WE Jr. Residual odontogenic keratinizing cyst: report of a case. US Navy Med 1976; 67: 22–23.

24. Philipsen HP. Om keratocyster (kolesteatomer) i kaeberne. Tandlaegebladet 1956; 60: 963.

25. Bramley PA. Treatment of cysts of the jaws. Proc R Soc Med 1971; 64: 547–550.

26. Gorlin RJ, Pindborg JJ, Clausen FP, et al. Calcifying odontogenic cyst – a possible analogue of the cutaneous calcifying epithelioma of Malherbe (an analysis of fifteen cases). Oral Surg 1962; 15: 1235–1240.

27. Browne RM. The odontogenic keratocyst: clinical aspects. Br Dent J 1970; 128: 225–231.

28. Freedman PD, Lumerman H, Gee JK. Calcifying odontogenic cyst. A review and analysis of seventy cases. Oral Surg 1975; 40: 93–106.

29. Wright JM. The odontogenic keratocyst: orthokeratinized variant. Oral Surg 1981; 51: 609–618.

30. Crowley TE, Kaugars GE, Gunsolley JC. Odontogenic keratocysts: a clinical and histologic comparison of the parakeratin and orthokeratin variants. J Oral Maxillofac Surg 1992; 50: 22–26.

31. Wilson DF, Ross AS. Ultrastructure of odontogenic keratocysts. Oral Surg 1978; 45: 887–893.

32. Herd JR. The calcifying odontogenic cyst. Aust Dent J 1972; 17: 421–428.

33. Fejerskov O, Krogh J. The calcifying ghost cell odontogenic tumor – or the calcifying odontogenic cyst. J Oral Pathol 1972; 1: 273–287.

34. Altini M, Farmon AG. The calcifying odontogenic cyst. Eight new cases and a review of the literature. Oral Surg 1975; 40: 751–759.

35. Keszler A, Gugliemotti NB. Calcifying odontogenic cyst associated with odontoma: report of two cases. J Oral Surg 1987; 45: 457–459.

36. Sauk JJ. Calcifying and keratinizing odontogenic cyst. J Oral Surg 1972; 30: 893–897.

37. Neville BW, Damm DD, Allen CM, Bouquot JE. Oral and maxillofacial pathology. Philadelphia: WB Saunders; 1995.

38. Muller S, Waldron CA. Primary intraosseous carcinoma: report of two cases. Int J Oral Maxillofac Surg 1991; 20: 362–365.

39. Hussain K, Edmonson HV, Rowne RM. Glandular odontogenic cysts: diagnosis and treatment. Oral Surg Oral Med Oral Pathol 1995; 79: 592–602.

40. High AS, Hirschman PN. Age changes in residual radicular cysts. J Oral Pathol 1986; 15: 524–528.

41. Rushton MA. Hyalin bodies in the epithelium of dental cysts. Proc R Soc Med 1955; 48: 407–409.

42. Ackerman G, Cohen MA, Altini M. The paradental cyst: a clinicopathologic study of 50 cases. Oral Surg 1987; 64: 308–312.

43. Little JW, Jakoben J. Origin of the globulomaxillary cyst. J Oral Surg 1973; 31: 188–195.

44. Christ TF. The globulomaxillary cyst: an embryologic misconception. Oral Surg 1970; 30: 515–526.

45. Stafne EC, Austin LT, Gardner BS. Median anterior maxillary cysts. J Am Dent Assoc 1936; 23: 801–809.

46. Knapp MJ. Pathology of oral tonsils. Oral Surg 1970; 29: 295–304.

47. Bhaskar SN. Lymphoepithelial cysts of the oral cavity: report of 24 cases. Oral Surg 1966; 21: 120–128.

48. Guinta J, Cataldo E. Lymphoepithelial cysts of the oral mucosa. Oral Surg 1973; 35: 77–78.

49. Weitzner S. Lymphoepithelial (branchial) cyst of parotid gland. Oral Surg 1973; 35: 85–88.

50. Stewart S, Levy R, Karpel J, Stoopack J. Lymphoepithelial (branchial) cyst of the parotid gland. J Oral Surg 1974; 32: 100–106.

51. Burnstein A, Scardinio PT, Tomaszewski MM, Cohen MH. Carcinoma arising in a branchial cleft cyst. Cancer 1976; 37: 2417–2420.

52. Issa MM, deVries P. Familial occurrence of thyroglossal duct cysts. J Pediatr Surg 1991; 26: 30–31.

53. Fernandez JR. Thyroglossal duct carcinoma. Surgery 1991; 110: 928–935.

54. Jensen JL. Superficial mucoceles of the oral mucosa. Am J Dermatopathol 1990; 12: 88–92.

55. Hertz J. Adamantinoma. Histopathologic and prognostic studies. Acta Chir Scand 1951; 102: 405–432.

56. Forsberg A. A contribution to the knowledge of the histology, histogenesis and etiology of adamantinomas. Acta Odontol Scand 1954; 12: 39–64.

57. Stanley HR, Bear PN, Kilham L. Oral tissue alterations in mice inoculated with the Rose stain of polyoma virus. Periodontics 1965; 3: 178–183.

58. Main JHP, Dawe CJ. Tumor induction in transplanted tooth buds infected with polyoma virus. JNCI 1966; 36: 1121–1136.

59. Lucas RB. Odontogenic tumors in polyoma virus-infected mice. Fourth Annual Proceedings of the International Academy Oral Pathology. Scientific Program, New York, 1969.

60. Spouge JD. Oral pathology. St. Louis: CV Mosby; 1973.

61. Greer RO, Richardson JF. Ameloblastoma of mucosal origin. A pathobiologic re-evaluation. Arch Otolaryngol 1974; 100: 174–175.

62. Sehdev MK, Huvos AG, Strong EW, et al. Ameloblastoma of maxilla and mandible. Cancer 1974; 33: 324–333.

63. Rockoff WM. A statistical analysis of ameloblastoma. Oral Surg 1963; 16: 1100–1101.

64. Kane JP. Odontogenic tumors. A statistical and morphological study of 88 cases. Thesis. Georgetown University, Washington, DC, 1951.

65. Marx RE, Stern D. Oral and maxillofacial pathology. a rationale for diagnosis and treatment. Chicago: Quintessence Publishing Co; 2002: 642.

66. Waldron CA, El Mofty SK. A histopathologic study of 116 ameloblastomas with special reference to the desmoplastic variant. Oral Surg 1987; 63: 441–451.

67. Philipsen HP, Ormiston IW, Reicharg PA. The desmo and osteoblastic ameloblastoma: histologic variant or clinicopathologic entity. Int J Oral Maxillofac Surg 1992; 21: 352–357.

68. Gardner DG, Corio RL. Plexiform unicystic ameloblastoma: a variant of ameloblastoma with a low recurrence rate after enucleation. Cancer 1984; 53: 1730–1735.

69. Eversole LR, Leider AS, Straub D. Radiographic characteristics of cystogenic ameloblastoma. Oral Surg 1984; 57: 572–577.

70. Woo S-B, Smith-Williams JE, Schiubba JJ, Lipper S. Peripheral ameloblastoma of the buccal mucosa: report and review of the English literature. Oral Surg 1987; 63: 78–84.

71. Yamamoto H, Inui M., Mori A, et al. Clear cell odontogenic carcinoma. a case report and literature review of odontogenic tumors with clear cells. Oral Surg Oral Med Oral Pathol 1998; 86: 86–89.

72. Ikemura K, Tashiro H, Fugino H, et al. Ameloblastoma of the mandible with metastasis to the lungs and lymph nodes. Cancer 1972; 29: 930–940.

73. Neville BW, Damn DE, Allen CM. Bouquot JE. Oral and maxillofacial pathology. Philadelphia: WB Saunders; 2002: 619.

74. Slootweg PJ, Muller H. Malignant ameloblastoma or ameloblastic carcinoma. Oral Surg 1984; 57: 168–176.

75. Elzay RP. Primary interosseous carcinoma of the jaws: review and update of odontogenic carcinomas. Oral Surg 1982; 54: 299–303.

76. Thomas G, Panday M, Mathew A, et al. Primary intraosseous carcinoma of the jaws: pooled analysis of the world literature and report of two cases. Int J Oral Maxillo & Facial Surg 2001; 30: 349–355.

77. Pindborg JJ. A calcifying epithelial odontogenic tumor. Cancer 1958; 11: 838–839.

78. Greer RO, Richardson JF. Clear-cell calcifying odontogenic tumor viewed relative to the Pindborg tumor. Oral Surg 1976; 42: 775–779.

79. Patterson JT, Martin TH, DeJean EK, et al. Extraosseous calcifying epithelial odontogenic tumor. Report of a case. Oral Surg 1969; 27: 363–367.

80. Krolls JO, Pindborg JJ. Calcifying epithelial odontogenic tumor. A survey of 23 cases and discussions of histomorphologic variations. Arch Pathol 1974; 98: 206–211.

81. Liu AR, Liu Z, Shao J. Calcifying epithelial odontogenic tumors: a clinico-pathologic study of nine cases. J Oral Pathol 1982; 11: 399–406.

82. El-Labban NG, Lee KW, Kramer IRH, Harris M. The nature of the amyloid-like material in a calcifying epithelial odontogenic tumor: an ultrastructural study. J Oral Pathol 1983; 12: 366–374.

83. Abrams AM, Howell FV. Calcifying epithelial odontogenic tumor: report of four cases. J Am Dent Assoc 1967; 74: 1231–1240.

84. Anderson HC, Kim B, Minkowitz S. Calcifying epithelial odontogenic tumor of Pindborg: an electron microscopic study. Cancer 1969; 24: 585–596.

85. Philipsen HP. Adenomatoid odontogenic tumor: biologic profile on 499 cases. J Oral Pathol Med 1991; 20: 149–158.

86. Marx RE, Stern D. Oral and maxillofacial pathology: A rationale for diagnosis and treatment. Chicago: Quintessence Publishing; 2002.

87. Courtney RM, Kerr DA. The odontogenic adenomatoid tumor. A comprehensive study of twenty new cases. Oral Surg 1975; 39: 424–435.

88. Giansanti JS, Someren A, Waldron CA. Odontogenic adenomatoid tumor (adenoameloblastoma). Survey of 111 cases. Oral Surg 1970; 30: 69–88.

89. Poulson TC, Greer RO. Adenomatoid odontogenic tumor: clinicopathologic and ultrastructural concepts. J Oral Surg 1983; 41: 818–824.

90. Pullon PA. Squamous odontogenic tumor. Report of six cases of a previously undescribed lesion. Oral Surg Oral Med Oral Pathol 1975; 40: 616–630.

91. White DK, Chess SY, Mohnac AM, et al. Odontogenic myxoma. A clinical and ultrastructural study. Oral Surg 1975; 39: 901–917.

92. Hasleton PS, Simpson W, Craig RDP. Myxoma of the mandible – a fibroblastic tumor. Oral Surg 1978; 46: 396–406.

93. Farman AG, Nortje CJ, Groteposs FW, et al. Myxofibroma of the jaws. Br J Oral Surg 1977; 15: 3–18.

94. Goldblatt LI. Ultrastructural study of an odontogenic myxoma. Oral Surg 1976; 42: 206–220.

95. Redman RS, Greer RO, Rutherford RB. Myofibroblasts in odontogenic myxoma, abstracted. Scientific Program, American Academy of Oral Pathology Annual Meeting, Fort Lauderdale, FL, 1978

96. Zimmerman DC, Dahlin DC. Myxomatous tumors of the jaws. Oral Surg 1958; 11: 1069–1075.

97. Elzay RP, Duntz W. Myxomas of the perioral soft tissues. Oral Surg 1978; 45: 246–254.

98. Cook CA, Lund BA, Carney JA. Mucocutaneous pigmented spots and oral myxomas: the oral manifestations of the complex myxomas, spotty pigmentation, and endocrine over-activity. Oral Surg 1987; 63: 175–183.

99. Gardner DG. The central odontogenic fibroma, an attempt at clarification. Oral Surg 1980; 50: 425–432.

100. Dunlap CL, Barker BF. Central odontogenic fibroma of the WHO-type. Oral Surg 1984; 57: 390–394.

101. Wesley RD, Wysachi GP, Mintz SM. The central odontogenic fibroma. Clinical and morphologic studies. Oral Surg 1975; 40: 235–245.

102. Handlers JP, Abrams A, Melrose RJ. Central odontogenic fibroma: clinicopathologic features of 19 cases and a review of the literature. J Oral Maxillofac Surg 1991; 47: 46–54.

103. Mallow RD, Spatz JJ, Zubrow HJ, et al. Odontogenic fibroma with calcification. Oral Surg 1964; 22: 564–568.

104. Allen CM, Hammond H, Stimson PG. Antral odontogenic fibroma WHO type. A report of 3 cases with an unusual associated giant cell reaction. Oral Surg Oral Med Oral Pathol 1992; 73: 62–66.

105. Vincent SD, Hammond HL, Ellis GL, Juhlin JP. Central granular cell odontogenic fibroma. Oral Surg 1987; 63: 715–721.

106. Norberg O. Zur Kenntis der dysontogenetischen Geschwulste der Zieferknochen. Vierteljahrsschrift Zahnh 1930; 46: 321.

107. Corio RL, Crawford BE, Schaberg SJ. Benign cementoblastoma. Oral Surg 1976; 41: 524–530.

108. Cherrick HM, King OH Jr, Lucatorto FM, et al. Benign cementoblastoma. Oral Surg 1974; 37: 54–63.

109. Abrams AM, Kirby JW, Melrose RJ. Cementoblastoma. Oral Surg 1974; 38: 394–403.

110. Giansanti JS. The pattern and width of collagen bundles in bone and cementum. Oral Surg 1970; 30: 508–514.

111. Chaudry AP, Stickel FR, Gorlin RJ, et al. An unusual odontogenic tumor. Report of a case. Oral Surg 1962; 15: 86–88.

112. Trodahl JN. Ameloblastic fibroma. A survey of cases from the Armed Forces Institute of Pathology. Oral Surg 1972; 33: 547–558.

113. Van Wyk CW, Uyver PC. Ameloblastic fibroma with dentinoid formation/immature dentinoma: a microscopic and ultrastructural study of the epithelial connective tissue interface. J Oral Pathol 1983; 12: 37–46.

114. Edwards MB, Coubran CF. Cystic, melanotic ameloblastic fibroma with granulomatous inflammation. Oral Surg 1980; 49: 333,336.

115. Richardson JF, Balogh K, Merk F, et al. Pigmented odontogenic tumors of jawbone. A previously undescribed expression of neoplastic potential. Cancer 34: 1974; 1244–1251.

116. Hooker SP. Ameloblastic odontoma: an analysis of 26 cases (abstract). Oral Surg 1967; 24: 375.

117. Tsataras GT. A review of ameloblastic fibro-odontoma. Thesis. George Washington University, Washington, DC, 1972.

118. Budnick SD. Compound and complex odontomas. Oral Surg 1976; 42: 501–506.

119. Regezi JA, Kerr DA, Courtney RM. Odontogenic tumor: analysis of 706 cases. J Oral Surg 1978; 36: 771–778.

120. Leider AS, Nelson JF, Trodahl JN. Ameloblastic fibrosarcoma of the jaws. Oral Surg 1972; 33: 559–569.

121. Adekey EO, Edwards NB, Goubran GF. Ameloblastic fibrosarcoma. Oral Surg 1978; 46: 254–259.

122. Chomette G, Auriol M, Guilbert F. Ameloblastic fibrosarcoma: a clinical and anatomopathological study of three cases. Histoenzymological and ultrastructural data. Arch Anat Cytol Pathol 1982; 30: 172–178.

123. Cooke BED. Median rhomboid glossitis—candidiasis and not a developmental anomaly. Br J Dermatol 1975; 93: 399–405.

124. Knoblich R. Accessory thyroid in the lateral floor of the mouth. Report of a case with embryologic considerations. Oral Surg 1965; 19: 234–241.

125. Marx RE, Stern D. Oral and maxillofacial pathology: A rationale for diagnosis and treatment. Chicago: Quintessence Publishing; 2002.

126. Sauk JJ Jr. Ectopic lingual thyroid. J Pathol 1970; 102: 239–243.

127. Melnick JL, Bunting H, Banfield WS, et al. Electron microscopy of viruses of human papilloma, molluscum contagiosum, and vaccinia, including observations on the formation of virus within cell. Ann NY Acad Sci 1952; 54: 1214–1225.

128. Eversole LR, Laipis PJ, Green TJ. Human papillomavirus, type II DNA in oral and labial verruca vulgaris. J Cutan Pathol 1987; 14: 319–325.

129. Jing YT, Toto PD. Detection of human papovavirus antigen in papillary lesions. Oral Surg 1984; 58: 702–705.

130. Satoh M, Hatakeyama S, Sashima M, et al. Immunohistochemical detection of ras p21 in oral papilloma. J Oral Pathol Med 1990; 19: 490–491.

131. Satoh M, Sashima M, Hatakeyna S, et al. Immunohistochemical localization of c-myc oncogene product. J Oral Pathol Med 1992; 21: 97–99.

132. Sulkowska M, Famulski W, Stasiak A, et al. PCNA and P53 expression in relation to clinicopathological features of oral papilloma. Folia Histochem Cytobiol 2001; 39 (suppl 2): 193–194.

133. Greer R, Goldman H. Oral papillomas: clinicopathologic examination and retrospective examination for dyskeratosis in 110 lesions. Oral Surg Oral Med Oral Pathol 1974; 38: 435–440.

134. Knapp M. Oral disease in 181,338 consecutive oral examinations. J Am Dent Assoc 1971; 83: 1288–1293.

135. Ross N, Gross E. Oral findings based on an automated multiphasic health screen program. J Med 1971; 26: 21–26.

136. Bouquot J, Gundlach K. Oral exophytic lesions in 23,616 white Americans over 35 years of age. Oral surg Oral Med Oral Pathol 1986; 62: 284–291.

137. Bhaskar SN. Oral tumors of infancy and childhood. J Pediatr 1963; 64: 195–205.

138. Jones JH. Non-odontogenic tumors in children. Br Dent J 1965; 119: 439–447.

139. Kohn EM, Dahlin DC, Erich JB. Primary neoplasms of the hard and soft palates and uvula. Mayo Clin Proc 1963; 38: 233.

140. Orlean SL, DaDow CS. Superficial keratoses: verruca vulgaris and pachyderma oris. J Dent Med 1960; 15: 108–112.

141. Orfuss AJ. Profuse warts of the skin and mucous membranes. Arch Dermatol 1966; 93: 776–777.

142. Eversole LR, Sorenson HW. Oral florid papillomatosis in Down's syndrome. Oral Surg 1974; 37: 202–207.

143. Greer RO, Goldman HM. Oral papillomas: clinicopathologic evaluation and retrospective examination for dyskeratosis in 110 lesions. Oral Surg 1974; 38: 435–440.

144. Wertheimer FW, Stroud DE. Peripheral ameloblastoma in a papilloma with recurrence. Report of a case. J Oral Surg 1972; 30: 47–49.

145. Zunt SL, Tomich CE. Oral condyloma acuminatum. J Dermatol Surg Oncol 1989; 15: 591–594.

146. Premoli-de-Percoco G, et al. Detection of human papillomavirus type 2 DNA in oral labial verruca vulgaris among Venezuelans. J Oral Pathol Med 1993; 22: 113–116.

147. Waite DE. Inflammatory papillary hyperplasia. J Oral Surg 1961; 19: 210–214.

148. Greer RO, Eversole LR, Poulson TC, et al. Identification of human papillomavirus DNA in smokeless tobacco-associated keratoses from juveniles, adults, and other adults using immunocytochemical and in situ DNA hybridization techniques. Gerodontics 1987; 3: 87–98.

149. Svirsky JA, Freedman PD, Lumerman H. Solitary intraoral keratoacanthoma. Oral Surg 1977; 43: 116–122.

150. Scofield HH, Werning JT, Shukes RC. Solitary intraoral keratoacanthoma. Oral Surg 1974; 37: 889–898.

151. Schwartz RA. Keratoacanthoma. J Am Acad Dermatol 1994; 30: 1–19.

152. Smith JF. A case of multiple primary squamous cell carcinomata in the skin in a young man with spontaneous healing. Br J Dermatol 1934; 46: 267–271.

153. Young SK, Larsen PE, Markowitz NR. Generalized eruptive keratoacanthoma. Oral Surg 1986; 62: 422–426.

154. Silverman S Jr, Galante M. Oral cancer. 6th edn. University of California at San Francisco: San Francisco Press; 1977.

155. Pindborg JJ. World Health Organization Collaborating Center for Oral Precancerous Lesions: definition of leukoplakia and related lesions: an aid to studies on oral precancer. Oral Surg 1978; 46: 518–539.

156. Pindborg JJ, Renstrup G, Poulsen HE, Silverman S Jr. Studies in oral leukoplakias: five clinical and histologic signs of malignancy. Acta Odontol Scand 1963; 21: 407–414.

157. Sugar L, Banocyz J. Untersuchungen bei Prakanzerose der Mundschleimhaut. Dtsch Zahn Mund Kieferheilk 1959, 30.132–137.

158. Burkhardt A. Der Mundhohlenkrebs und seine Vorstadien. New York: G. Fisher; 1980.

159. Mashberg A, Meyers H. Anatomical site and size of 222 early asymptomatic oral squamous cell carcinomas: a continuing prospective study of oral cancer. II. Cancer 1976; 37: 2149–2157.

160. Gerry RG, Smith ST, Calton ML. The oral characteristics of Guamians including the effect of betel chewing on oral tissue. Oral Surg Oral Med Oral Pathol 1952; 5: 762–781.

161. Silverman S, Bhargava K, Mani N, et al. Malignant transformation and natural history of oral leukoplakia in 57,518 industrial workers of Gujarat, India. Cancer 38: 1976; 1790–1795.

162. Greer RO. Lesions of the oral cavity. In: Wood RP, Northern JL, eds. Manual of otolaryngology. a symptom oriented text. Baltimore: Williams & Wilkins; 1979: 127.

163. Hansen JL, Olsen JA, Silverman S. Proliferative verrucous leukoplakia: a long-term study. Oral Surg 1985; 60: 285–290.

164. Shear M, Pindborg JJ. Verrucous hyperplasia of the oral mucosa. Cancer 1980; 46: 1855–1862.

165. Cummer CL. Leukoplakia (lekokeratosis) of the palate. JAMA 1946; 132: 493–498.

166. Thoma KH. Stomatitis nicotina and its effects on the palate. Am J Orthodont Oral Surg. 1941; 27: 38–47.

167. Forsey RR, Sullivan TH. Stomatitis nicotina. Arch Dermatol 1961; 83: 99–104.

168a. Rossie KM, Guggenheimer J. Thermally induced 'nicotine' stomatitis. Oral Surg Oral Med Oral Pathol 70: 1990; 597–599.

168b. Eisenberg E, Murphy GE, Krutchkoff DJ. Involucrin as a diagnostic marker on oral lichenoid lesions (abstract). American Academy of Oral Pathology 41st Annual Meeting, Scottsdale, AZ, 1987.

168c. Greer R, McDowell J, Hoerig G. Oral lichen planus, a premalignant disease? Pathology case reviews 1999; 4: 28–43.

169. Camisa C, Allen CM. Treatment of oral erosive lichen planus with systemic isotretinoin. Oral Surg 1986; 62: 393–396.

170. Silverman S, Gorsky M, Lozado-Nur F. A prospective followup study of 570 patients with oral lichen planus: persistence, remission, and malignant association. Oral Surg Oral Med Oral Pathol 1985; 60: 30–34.

171. Malaowalla AM, Silverman S, Mani NJ, et al. Oral cancer in 57,518 industrial workers in Gujarat India. A prevalence and follow-up study. Cancer 1976; 37: 1882–1886.

172. Neville BW, Allen CM, et al. Oral and maxillofacial patholol. 2nd edn. Philadelphia, PA: Saunders; 2002: 337–369.

173. Swango PA. Cancers of the oral cavity and pharynx in the United States: an epidemiologic overview. J Public Health Dent 1996; 56: 309–318.

174. Ries LAG, Hankey BF, Miller BA, et al. Cancer statistics review 1973–1988. National Cancer Institute, NIH Publication No. 91-2789, 1991.

175. Silverman S Jr. Demographics and occurrence of oral and pharyngeal cancers. The outcome of trends, the challenge. J Am Dent Assoc 2001; 132: 7s–11s.

176. US Surgeon General. The health consequences of smoking. Cancer. A report of the Surgeon General. US Department of Health and Human Services, 1982.

177. US Surgeon General. Reducing the health consequences of smoking: twenty-five years of progress. A report of the Surgeon General DHHS Publication 898411. US Department of Health and Human Services, Public Health Service, Centers for Disease Control and Prevention, Rockville, MD, 1989.

178. Parkin DM, Laara E, Muir CS. Estimates of worldwide frequency of sixteen major cancers in 1980. Int J Cancer 1988; 41: 184–197.

179. Pindborg JJ. Oral cancer from an international point of view. Can Dent Assoc J 1965; 31: 219–222.

180. International Agency for Research on Cancer. Tobacco smoking. IARC monographs on the evaluation of carcinogenic risk of chemicals to humans. Vol. 38. Lyon: IARC; 1986.

181. Winn DM, Blot WJ, Shy CWM, et al. Snuff dipping and oral cancer among women in the southern United States. N Eng J Med 1981; 304: 745–749.

182. Glover E, Glover P. The smokeless tobacco problem: risk groups in North America. In: Monograph II, Smokeless Tobacco or Health. NIH Publication

92–3461. US Department of Health and Human Services. Rockville, MD: Public Health Service; 1992: 3–9.

183. Brunneman K, Hoffmann D. Chemical composition of smokeless tobacco products. In: Monograph II, Smokeless Tobacco or Health. NIH Publication 92–3461. US Department of Health and Human Services. Rockville, MD: Public Health Service; 1992: 96–105.

184. Tobacco smoking. IARC monographs on the evaluation of carcinogenic risk of chemicals to humans. Vol. 38. International Agency for Research on Cancer, 1986.

185. Jussawalla DJ, Deshpane VA. Evaluation of cancer risk in tobacco chewers and smokers: an epidemiologic assessment. Cancer 1971; 28: 244–252.

186. Baralam P, Sridhar H, Rajkumar T, et al. Oral cancer in southern India: influence of smoking, drinking, paan chewing and oral hygiene. Int J Cancer 2002; 98(3): 440–445.

187. Shwe M, Chiguchi G, Yuamada S, et al. P53 and MDM2 coexpression in tobacco and betel chewing-associated oral squamous cell carcinoma. J Med Dent Sci 2001; 48(4): 113–119.

188. US Department of Health and Human Services. The health consequences of using smokeless tobacco: a report of the advisory committee to the Surgeon General. DHHS Publication (NIH) 86-2874, US Department of Health and Human Services, Public Health Service, National Institutes of Health, National Cancer Institute, 1986.

189. Mattson ME, Winn D. Smokeless tobacco: association with increased cancer risks (NCI monograph). NIH Publication 89-3055. Vol. 8. US Department of Health and Human Services, 1989.

190. US Department of Health and Human Services. Reducing the health consequences of smoking: twenty-five years of progress. A report of the Surgeon General, 1989. DHHS Publication (CDC) 89-8411. US Department of Health and Human Services, Public Health Service, Center for Disease Control, Center for Chronic Disease Prevention and Health Promotion, Office of Smoking and Health, 1989.

191. Elwood JM, Pearson JG, Skippen DH. Alcohol, smoking, social and occupational factors in the etiology of cancer of the oral cavity, pharynx and larynx. Int J Cancer 1984; 34: 603–612.

192. Blot WJ, Fraumenti JF. Geographic patterns of oral cancer in the United States: etiologic implications. J Chronic Dis 1977; 30: 745–757.

193. Blot WJ, McLaughlin JK, Winn DM, et al. Smoking and drinking in relation to oral and pharyngeal cancer. Cancer Res 1988; 48: 3282–3287.

194. Mashberg A, Boffetta P, Winkelman R, et al. Tobacco smoking, alcohol drinking, and cancer of the oral cavity and oropharynx among US veterans. Cancer 1993; 72: 1370–1375.

195. Blot WJ, McLaughlin JK, Winn DM, et al. Smoking and drinking in relation to oral and pharyngeal cancer. Cancer Res 1988; 48: 3282–3287.

196. Hirayama T. An epidemiologic study of oral and pharyngeal cancer in Central and South-East Asia. Bull WHO 1966; 34: 41–69.

197. Ho PS, Yang YH, et al. The incidence of oropharyngeal cancer in Taiwan: an endemic betel liquid chewing area. J Oral Pathol Med 2000; 31(4): 213–219.

198. Salga TJ, Gimenez-Conti IB. An animal model for oral cancer (review). Monogr Natl Cancer Inst 1993; 13: 55–60.

199. Shklar G. Experimental oral pathology in the Syrian hamster. Prog Exp Tumor Res 1972; 16: 518–538.

200. United States Environmental Protection Agency. Respiratory health effects of passive smoking: Lung cancer and other disorders. Washington, DC. 1992.

201. Zhang Z, Morgenstern H, Spitz M, et al. Environmental tobacco smoking, mutagen sensitivity, and head and neck squamous cell carcinoma. Cancer Epidemiol Biomark & Prevent 2000; 9: 1043–1049.

202. Carriot F, Sasco AJ. Cannabis and cancer. Rev Epidemiol Sante Publique 2000; 48(5): 473–83.

203. Wynder EL, Bross IJ, Feldman RM. A study of etiologic factors in cancer of the mouth. Cancer 1957; 10: 1300–1322.

204. Slaga TJ, Gimenez-Conti IB. An animal model for oral cancer. NIH Monogr 1992; 13: 55–60.

205. Gimenez-Conti IB, Slaga TJ. The hamster cheek pouch carcinogesis model. J Cell Biochem Suppl 1993; 17F: 83–90.

206. Elwood JM, Pearson JG, Skippen DH. Alcohol, smoking, social and occupational factors in the etiology of cancer of the oral cavity, pharynx and larynx. Int J Cancer 1984; 34: 603–612.

207. Mashberg A, Boffetta P, Winkelman R, et al. Tobacco smoking, alcohol drinking, and cancer of the oral cavity and oropharynx among US veterans. Cancer 1993; 72: 1370–1375.

208. Brugere J, Guenel P, LeClerc A. Differential effects of tobacco and alcohol in cancer of the larynx, pharynx and mouth. Cancer 1986; 57: 391–395.

209. Miyazaki M, Ohno S, Futatsugi M, et al. The relation of alcohol consumption and cigarette smoking to the multiple occurrence of esophageal dysplasia and squamous cell carcinoma. Surgery 2002; 131(1 suppl): s7–s13.

210. Johnson NW. Aetiology and risk factors for oral cancer, with special reference to tobacco and alcohol use. Magy Onkol 2001; 45(2): 115–122.

211. Tuyns AJ. Alcohol and cancer. Pathol Biol (Paris) 2001; 49(9): 759–763.

212. McCoy GD, Wydner EL. Etiology and preventative implications in alcoholic carcinogenesis. Cancer Res 1979; 39: 2844–2850.

213. Blot WJ. Alcohol and cancer. Cancer Res 1992; 52: 2119s–2123s.

214. Hindle I, Downer M, et al. Is alcohol responsible for more intraoral cancer? Oral Oncol 2000; 36(4): 328–333.

215. Schwartz S, Doody D, Fitzgibbons E, et al. Oral squamous cell cancer risk in relation to alcohol consumption and alcohol dehydrogenase-3 genotype. Cancer Epidemiol Biomarkers Prev 2001; 10(11): 1137–1144.

216. Seitz H, Matsuzaki S, Yokoyama A, et al. Alcohol and cancer. Alcohol Clin Exp Res 2001; 25(5 suppl ISBRA): 137s–143s.

217. Zavras A, Laskaris G, Wang Y, et al. Interaction between a single nucleotide polymorphism in the alcohol dehydrogenase 3 gene, alcohol consumption and oral cancer risk. Int J Cancer 2002; 97(4): 526–530.

218. Slotman G, Swaminathan B, Rush B. Head and neck cancer in young age group: high incidence in black patients. 1983; 5(4): 293–298.

219. Schantz S, Hsu T, Ainslie N, Moser R. Young adults with head and neck cancer express increased susceptibility to mutagen-induced chromosome damage. JAMA 1989; 262: 3313–3315.

220. Schantz P, Liu F. An immunologic profile of young adults. Cancer 64: 1232–1237. 1989;

221. Winn DM, Blot WJ, McLaughlin JK. Mouthwash use and oral conditions in the risk of oral and pharyngeal cancer. Cancer Res 1991; 51: 3044–3047.

222. Johnson NW. Detection of patients and lesions at risk. Oral Cancer 1991; 2: 47.

223. Regezi J, Sciubba JJ. Oral pathology: clinical pathologic correlations. Philadelphia: WB Saunders; 1989.

224. Rich AM, Radden BG. Squamous cell carcinoma of the oral mucosa, a review of 244 cases in Australia. J Oral Pathol 1984; 13: 459–471.

225. Rennie JS, MacDonald DG, Dagg JH. Iron and oral epithelium: a review. J R Soc Med 1984; 77: 602–607.

226. Tavani A, Gallus S, Vecchia C, et al. Diet and risk of oral and pharyngeal cancer. An Italian case-control study. Eur J Cancer 2001; 10(2): 191–195.

227. Petridou E, Zavras A, Lefatzis D, et al. The role of diet and specific micronutrients in the etiology of oral carcinoma. Cancer 2002; 94(11): 2981–2988.

228. Negri E, Franceschi S, Bosetti C, et al. Selected micronutrients and oral and pharyngeal cancer. Int J Cancer 2000; 86(1): 122–127.

229. Morse D, Pendrys D, Katz R, et al. Food group intake and risk of oral epithelial dysplasia in the United States population. Cancer Causes Control 2000; 11(8): 713–720.

230. Wynder EL, Bross RM, Feldman RM. A study of etiological factors in cancer of the mouth. Cancer 1957; 10: 1300–1323.

231. Grahm S, Mettlin C, Marshall JR. Dietary factors in the epidemiology of cancer of the larynx. Am J Epidemiol 1981; 113: 675–680.

232. Marshall JR, Grahm S, Haughery BP, et al. Smoking, alcohol, dentition, and diet in the epidemiology of oral cancer. Eur J Cancer Oral Oncol 1992; 28b: 9–15.

233. McLaughlin JK, Gridley G, Block G, et al. Dietary factors in oral and pharyngeal cancer. J Natl Cancer Inst 1988; 80: 1237–1243.

234. Gupta PC. Incidence of oral cancer and natural history of oral precancerous lesions in a ten-year follow-up of Indian villagers. Community Dent Oral Epidemiol 1980; 8: 287–333.

235. Gridley G, McLaughlin JK, Block G, et al. Vitamin supplementation and the reduced risk of oral and pharyngeal cancer. Am J Epidemiol 1992; 135: 1083–1092.

236. Silverman S. Oral cancer. 3rd edn. Atlanta, GA: American Cancer Society; 1990.

237. Gorsky M, Silverman S. Denture wearing and oral cancer. J Prosthet Dent 1984; 52: 164–170.

238. Wynder EL, Bross IJ, Feldman RM. A study of etiological factors in cancer of the mouth. Cancer 1957; 10: 1300–1319.

239. Browne RN, Cansey MC, Waterhouse JAH. Etiological factors in oral squamous cell carcinoma. Community Dent Oral Epidemiol 1977; 5: 301–306.

240. Odukoya O, Shklar G. Initiation and promotion in experimental oral carcinogenesis. Oral Surg Oral Med Oral Pathol 1984; 58: 315–320.

241. Huebner W, Schoenberg J, Kelsey J, et al. Oral and pharyngeal cancer and occupation: a case-control study. Epidemiology 1992; 3(4): 300–309.

242. Tisch M, Enderle G, Zoller J, et al. Cancer and oral cavity in machine workers. Laryngootologie 1996; 75(12): 759–763.

243. Scildt E, Eriksson M, Hardell L, et al. Occupational exposure as risk factors for oral cancer evaluated in a Swedish case control study. Oncol Rep 1999; 6(2): 317–320.

244. Shroyer KR, Gundlaugsson E. Determination of clonality in endometrial adenocarcinoma by PCR amplification of PGK-1. 1994; Hum Pathol 25: 287–292.

245. Milasin JT, Dedovic N, Nickloic Z. High incidence of H-ras oncogene mutations in squamous cell carcinoma of lip vermilion. J Oral Pathol Med 1994; 23: 298–301.

246. Scully C. Oncogenes, tumor suppressors and viruses in oral squamous cell carcinoma. J Oral Pathol Med 1993; 22: 337–347.

247. Spandidos DA, Anderson ML. Oncogenes and onco-suppressor genes: their involvement in cancer. J Oral Pathol 1989; 197: 1–10.

248. Saranath D. Oncogene amplification in squamous cell carcinoma of the oral cavity. Jpn J Cancer Res 1989; 80: 430–437.

249. Somers KD, Glickman S, Cartwright S. Oncogenes in head and neck cancer. Smokeless tobacco and health. Monograph II, NIH Publication 92-3461. Department of Health and Human Services, Public Health Service, 1992.

250. Hollstein T, Sidransky D, Vogelstein B, et al. p53 mutations in human cancers. Science 1991; 253: 49–53.

251. Field JK, Spandidos A, Malliri A, et al. Elevated p53 expression correlates with history of heavy smoking in squamous cell carcinoma of the head and neck. Br J Cancer 1991; 64: 573–577.

252. Greer RO, Douglas JM, Breese P, et al. Evaluation of oral and laryngeal specimens for human papillomavirus (HPV) DNA by dot blot hybridization. J Oral Pathol Med 1990; 19: 35–38.

253. Greer RO, Shroyer K, Crosby L. Identification of human papillomavirus DNA in smokeless tobacco keratoses and premalignant and malignant oral lesions by PCR amplification with consensus sequence primers. Smokeless tobacco and health. Monograph II. NIH Publication 92-3461. National Institutes of Health, National Cancer Institute, 1992.

254. Park NH, Byung MM, Sheng LL, et al. Role of viruses in oral carcinogenesis. Smokeless tobacco and health. Monograph II. NIH Publication 92-3461. Bethesda, MD: National Institutes of Health, National Cancer Institute; 1992.

255. Johnson NW. Risk Markers for oral disease, oral cancer detection of patients and lesions at risk. Cambridge, England: Cambridge University Press; 1991.

256. Greer RO, Eversole S, Crosby LK. Detection of papillomavirus genomic DNA in oral epithelial dysplasias, oral smokeless tobacco associated leukoplakias and epithelial malignancy. J Oral Maxillofac Surg 1990; 48: 1201–1205.

257. Shroyer KR, Greer RO. Detection of human papillomavirus DNA by in situ DNA hybridization and polymerase chain reaction in premalignant and malignant oral lesions. Oral Surg Oral Med Oral Pathol 1991; 71: 708–713.

258. Vambutas A, Lorenzo TP, Steinberg B. Laryngeal papilloma cells have high levels of epidermal growth factor receptor and respond to epidermal growth factor by a decrease in epithelial differentiation. Cancer 1993; 53: 910–914.

259. Malone J, Snyderman C. Arachidonic metabolites in saliva of patients with squamous cell carcinoma of the head and neck. Oral Surg Oral Med Oral Path 1994; 77: 636–640.

260. Lee YW, Gisser S. Squamous cell carcinoma of the tongue in a nine-year renal transplant survivor. Cancer 1978; 41: 1–6.

261. Wallner K, Liebel S, Wara W. Squamous cell carcinoma of the head and neck after radiation therapy for Hodgkin's disease. Cancer 1985; 56: 1052–1056.

262. Curtis R, Rowlings P, Deeg H, et al. Solid cancers after bone marrow transplantation. N Engl J Med 1997; 336: 897–904.

263. King G, Healy C, Glover M, et al. Increased prevalence of dysplastic and malignant lip lesions in renal-transplant recipients. N Engl J Med 1995; 332: 1052–1057.

264. Woods KV, Shillitoe EJ, Spitz MR. Analysis of human papillomavirus DNA in oral squamous cell carcinomas. J Oral Pathol Med 1993; 22: 101–108.

265. Prime S, Thakker N, Pring M, et al. A review of inherited cancer syndromes and their relevance to oral squamous cell carcinoma. Oral Oncol 2001; 37(1): 1–16.

266. Tashiro H, Abe K, Tanioka H. Familial occurrence of cancer of the mouth. J Oral Maxillofacial Surg 1986; 44: 332–323.

267. Hara H, Ozeki S, Shiratsuchi H, et al. Familial occurrence of oral cancer, report of cases. J Oral Maxillofacial Surg 1988; 46: 1098–1102.

268. Ankathil R, Mathew A, Joseph F, et al. Is oral cancer susceptibility inherited? Report of five oral cancer families. Oral Oncol Europ J Cancer 1996; 32B: 63–67.

269. Ide F, Shimoyama T, Horie N. Carcinoma of the tongue in two siblings. J Oral Maxilofacial Surg 1999; 57: 66–68.

270. Gallo O, Sardi I, Pepe G, et al. Multiple primary tumors of the upper aerodigestive tract: is there a role for constitutional mutations in the P53 gene? Int J Cancer 1999; 82: 180–186.

271. Beahrs GH, Henderson DE, Hutter RVP, Myers A. Manual for staging cancer. 4th edn. Philadelphia; Lippencott-Raven; 1992.

272. Yamamoto E, Miyakawa A, Kohama GI. Mode of invasion and lymph node metastasis in squamous cell carcinoma of the oral cavity. Head Neck Surg 1984; 6: 938–947.

273. Crissman JD, Liu WY, Gluckman JL, et al. Prognostic value of histopathologic parameters in squamous cell carcinoma of the oropharynx. Cancer 1984; 54: 2995–3001.

274. Shingaki S, Syzuki I, Nakajiima T, et al. Evaluation of histologic parameters in predicting cervical lymph node metastasis of oral and oropharyngeal carcinoma. Oral Surg 1988; 66: 683–688.

275. Shear M, Hawkins DM, Farr HW. The prediction of lymph node metastasis from oral squamous cell carcinoma. Cancer 1976; 37: 1901–1907.

276. Byers RM, Bland KI, Borlase B, et al. The prognostic and therapeutic value of frozen section determinations in the surgical treatment of squamous cell carcinomas of the head and neck. Am J Surg 1978; 136: 525–528.

277. Broders AC. Carcinomas of the mouth: type and degrees of malignancy. AJR 1927; 17: 90–93.

278. Frazell EL, Lucas JC. Cancer of the tongue. Report of management of 1,554 patients. Cancer 1962; 15: 1085–1095.

279. Parker S, Tong T, Bolden S, Wingo P. Cancer statistics. CA Cancer J Clin 1997; 47: 5–27.

280. Decroix Y, Ghossein N. Experience of the Curie Institute in treatment of cancer of the mobile tongue. II. Management of neck nodes. 1981; 47(3): 503–508.

281. Alvi A, Myers E, Johnson J. Cancer of the oral cavity. Cancer of the head and neck. 3rd edn. Philadelphia: Saunders; 1996: 321–360.

282. Strong E. Carcinoma of the tongue. Otolaryngology Clin North Am 1979; 12: 107–114.

283. Harrold C. Surgical treatment of cancer of the base of tongue. Am J Surg 1976; 114: 493–497.

284. Ildstad ST, Bigelow M, Remensnyder J. Squamous cell carcinoma of the tongue: a comparison of the anterior two-thirds of the tongue with its base. Am J Surg 1983; 146: 456–461.

285. Krolls SO, Hoffman S. Squamous cell carcinoma of the oral soft tissues: a statistical analysis of 14,253 cases by age, sex and race of patients. J Am Dent Assoc 1976; 92: 571–574.

286. Cruse C, Radocha R. Squamous cell carcinoma of the lip. Plast Reconstr Surg 1987; 80: 787–791.

287. Cross JE, Guralnick E, Daland EM. Carcinoma of the lip. A review of 563 case records of carcinoma of the lip at the Pondville Hospital. Surg Gynecol Obstet 1948; 87: 153–162.

288. Frierson HF, Cooper PH. Prognostic factors in squamous cell carcinoma of the lower lip. Hum Pathol 1986; 17: 346–354.

289. Knapel MR, Koranda FC, Panje WR, Grand DJ. Squamous cell carcinoma of the upper lip. J Dermatol Surg Oncol 1982; 8: 487–491.

290. Vanderwall I. Squamous cell carcinoma: clinical and histopathological aspects. In: Vanderwall I, Snow GB, eds. Oral oncology. Boston: Martinus Nijhoff; 1984: 33–52.

291. Conly J, Sadoyama J. Squamous cell carcinoma of the buccal mucosa. A review of 90 cases. Arch Otolaryngol 1973; 97: 330–333.

292. O'Brien P, Catlin D. Cancer of the cheek. Cancer 1965; 18: 1392–1398.

293. Cernea, P, Billet J. Epitheliomas of the buccal mucosa; study of 60 cases. Rev Stomatol (Paris) 1962; 63: 222–228.

294. Urist M, O'Brien CJ, Soung SJ, et al. Squamous cell carcinoma of the buccal mucosa, analysis of prognostic factors. Am J Surg 1987; 154: 411–414.

295. Cady B, Catlin D. Epidermoid carcinoma of the gum. A 20-year survey. Cancer 1969; 23: 551–569.

296. Barasch A, Morse D, Krutchkoff D, Eisenberg E. Smoking, gender, and age risk factors for site-specific intraoral squamous cell carcinoma. Cancer 1994; 73: 509–513.

297. Silverman S. Oral Cancer. Semin Dermatol 1994; 13: 132–137.

298. Greer RO, Shroyer KR. Detection of human papillomavirus DNA in oral verrucous carcinoma by polymerase chain reaction. Mod Pathol 1993; 6: 669–672.

299. Krolls SO, Hoffman S. Squamous cell carcinoma of the oral soft tissues: a statistical analysis of 14,253 cases by age, sex and race of patients. J Am Dent Assoc 1976; 92: 571–574.

300. Appelbaum E, Callins W, Bytell D. Carcinoma of the floor of the mouth. Arch Otolaryngol 1980; 106: 419–421.

301. Lefall L, White J. Cancer of the oral cavity in African Americans. Surg Gynaecol Obstet 1965; 120: 70–72.

302. Spiro RH, Huvos AG, Wong GY, et al. Predictive value of tumor thickness in squamous cell carcinoma confined to the tongue and floor of the mouth. Am J Surg 1986; 152: 345–350.

303. Mohit-Tabatabai MA, Sobel HJ, Rush BF. Relation of thickness of floor of the mouth stage I and II cancers to regional metastasis. Am J Surg 1986; 152: 351–353.

304. Evans JF, Shah JP. Epidermoid carcinoma of the palate. Am J Surg 1981; 142: 451–455.

305. Chung C, Constable W. Squamous cell carcinoma of the soft palate and uvula. Int J Radiol Oncol Biol Phys 1979; 5: 845–850.

306. Weber R, Peters L, Wolf P, Guillamondegui O. Squamous cell carcinoma of the soft palate, uvula, and anterior faucial pillar. Otolaryngol Head and Neck Surg 1988; 99: 16–23.

307. Vanka V, Sibl O, Suchankova A, et al. Epstein-Barr Virus antibodies in tonsillar carcinoma patients. Laryngoscope 1974; 84: 90–97.

308. Whicker J, DeStefano L, Devine D. Surgical treatment of squamous cell carcinoma of the tonsil. Laryngoscope 1974; 84: 90–97.

309. Givens C, Johns M, Cantrell R. Carcinoma of the tonsil. Analysis of 162 cases. Arch Otolaryngol 1981; 107: 730–734.

310. Fleming P, Matz G, Powell W, Chen J. Carcinoma of the tonsil. Surg Clin North Am 1976; 56: 125–136.

311. Mak-Kreger S, Hilger F, Baris G, et al. Carcinoma of the tonsillar region. Laryngoscope 1990; 100: 634–638.

312. Barnes L, Verbin R, Guggenheimer J. Cancer of the oral cavity and oropharynx. In: Barnes L, Verbin R, Guggenheimer J, eds. Surgical pathology of the head and neck. 2nd edn. New York: Marcel Dekker; 2001: 406.

313. Baker R, D'Onofrio ED, Corio RL, et al. Squamous cell carcinoma arising in a lateral periodontal cyst. Oral Surg 1979; 47: 495–499.

314. Toller PA. Origin and growth of cysts of the jaws. Ann R Coll Surg Engl 1967; 40: 306–311.

315. Friedell HL, Rosenthal LM. The etiologic role of chewing tobacco in cancer of the mouth. Report of eight cases treated with radiation. JAMA 1941; 116: 2130–2135.

316. Ackerman LV. Verrucous carcinoma of the oral cavity. Surgery 1948; 23: 670–678.

317. Batsakis J, Hybels R, Crissman J, Rice D. The pathology of head and neck tumors. Verrucous carcinoma. Part 15. Head Neck Surg 1982; 5: 29–38.

318. Goethals P, Harrison E, Devine D. Verrucous carcinoma of the oral cavity. Am J Surg 1963; 106: 845–851.

319. Biller HF, Ogura JH, Bauer WC. Verrucous carcinoma of the larynx. Laryngoscope 1971; 81: 1323–1329.

320. Batsakis JG, Hybels R, Crissman JD, Rice PH. The pathology of head and neck tumors: verrucous carcinoma. Part 15. Head Neck Surg 1982; 5: 29–38.

321. Shear M, Pindborg JJ. Verrucous hyperplasias of the oral mucosa Cancer 1980, 46: 1855–1862.

322. Shroyer KR, Greer RO. Detection of human papillomavirus DNA by in situ DNA hybridization and polymerase chain reaction in premalignant and malignant oral lesions. Oral Surg Oral Med Oral Pathol 1991; 71: 708–713.

323. Shroyer KR, Greer RO. Detection of human papillomavirus DNA in oral verrucous carcinoma by polymerase chain reaction. Mod Pathol 1993; 6: 669–672.

324. Jacobson S, Shear M. Verrucous carcinoma of the mouth. J Oral Pathol 1972; 1: 66–75.

325. Shafer WG. Verrucous carcinoma. Int Dent J 1972; 22: 451–459.

326. Eversole LR, Sorenson JW. Oral florid papillomatosis in Down's syndrome. Oral Surg 1974; 37: 202–207.

327. Kraus FT, Perez-Mesa C. Verrucous carcinoma. Clinical and pathologic study of 105 cases involving oral cavity, larynx, and genitalia. Cancer 1966; 19: 26–38.

328. Fonts EA, Greenlaw RH, Rush BF, et al. Verrucous squamous cell carcinoma of the oral cavity. Cancer 1969; 23: 152–160.

329. Greer RO. Oral cancer: an overview. Colo Oral Cancer Bull 1978; 1: 5–9.

330. Ishiyama A, Eversole L, Ross D, et al. Papillary squamous neoplasms of the head and neck. Laryngoscope 1994; 104(12): 1446–1452.

331. Suarez P, Adler-Storthz K, Luna M, et al. Papillary squamous cell carcinoma of the upper aerodigestive tract: a clinicopathologic and molecular study. Head Neck 2000; 22(4): 360–368.

332. Takeda Y, Satoh M, Nakamura S, Yamamato H. Papillary squamous cell carcinoma of the oral mucosa. J Oral Sci 2001; 43(3): 165–169.

333. Thompson L, Wenig B, Heffner D, Gnepp D. Exophytic and papillary squamous cell carcinoma of the larynx: a clinicopathologic series of 104 cases. Otolaryngol Head Neck Surg 1999; 120: 718–24.

334. Jacoway JR, Nelson JF, Boyers RC. Adenoid squamous cell carcinoma (adenoacanthoma) of the oral labial mucosa. A clinicopathologic study of fifteen cases. Oral Surg 1971; 32: 444–449.

335. Tomich CE, Hutton CE. Adenoid squamous cell carcinoma of the lip. Report of cases. J Oral Surg 1972; 30: 592–598.

336. Weitzner S. Adenoid squamous cell carcinoma of vermilion mucosa of lower lip. Oral Surg Oral Med Oral Pathol 1974; 37: 589–593.

337. Jones A, Freedman P, Kerpel S. Oral adenoid squamous cell carcinoma: a report of three cases and a review of the literature. J Oral Maxillofac Surg 1993; 51: 676–681.

338. Goldman R, Klein H, Sung M. Adenoid squamous cell carcinoma of the oral cavity. Report of first case arising in the tongue. Arch Otolaryngol 1977; 103: 496–498.

339. Muller S, Wilhelmj C, Harrison E, Winkelmann R. Adenoid squamous cell carcinoma. Report of seven cases and review. Arch Dermatol 1964; 89: 589–597.

340. Johnson W, Helwig E. Adenoid squamous cell carcinoma. A clinicopathologic study of 155 patients. Cancer 1966; 19: 1639–1650.

341. Gerughty R, Henninger Brown F. Adenosquamous carcinoma of the oral, nasal, and laryngeal cavities. A clinicopathologic survey of ten cases. Cancer 1968; 22: 1140–1154.

342. Scully C, Porter S, Speight P, et al. Adenosquamous carcinoma of the mouth: a rare variant of squamous cell carcinoma. J Maxillofac Surg 1999; 28(2): 125–128, review.

343. Napier S, Gormely J, Newlands C, Ramsey P. Adenosquamous carcinoma. A rare neoplasm with an aggressive course. Oral Surg Oral Med Oral Pathol Oral Radiol Endod 1995; 79(5): 607–611.

344. Wain SL, Kier R, Vollmer KT, et al. Basaloid squamous carcinoma of the tongue, hypopharynx, and larynx: report of 10 cases. Hum Pathol 1986; 17: 1155–1166.

345. Coletta R, Cotrim P, Almeida O, et al. Basaloid squamous carcinoma of the oral cavity: a histologic and immunohistochemical study. Oral Oncol 2002; 38(7): 723.

346. Raslan W, Barnes L, Krause J, et al. Basaloid squamous cell carcinoma of the head and neck: a clinicopathologic and flow cytometric study of 10 cases with a review of the literature. Am J Otolaryngol 1994; 15: 204–211.

347. Seidman J, Breman J, Yost B, Isri O. Basaloid squamous cell carcinoma of the hypopharynx and larynx associated with second primary tumors. Cancer 1991; 68: 1545–1549.

348. Zarbo R, Crissman J, Venkat H, Weiss M. Spindle cell carcinoma of the upper aerodigestive tract mucosa. An immunohistologic and ultrastructural study of 18 biphasic tumors. Am J Surg Pathol 1986; 10: 741–753.

349. Ellis G, Langloss J, Heffner D, Hyams V. Spindle cell carcinoma of the aerodigestive tract. An immunohistochemical study of 21 cases. Am J Surg Pathol 1987; 11: 335–342.

350. Goellner J, Devine D, Weiland L. Pseudosarcoma of the larynx. Am J Clin Pathol 1973; 59: 312–326.

351. Kessler S, Bartley M. Spindle cell squamous cell carcinoma of the tongue in the first decade of life. Oral Surg Oral Med Oral Pathol 1988; 66: 470–474.

352. Larsen E, Duggan M, Inque M. Absence of human papilloma virus DNA in oropharyngeal spindle cell squamous carcinoma. Am J Clin Pathol 1994; 101: 514–518.

353. Ellis G, Corio RL. Spindle cell carcinoma of the oral cavity. A clinicopathologic study of 59 cases. Oral Surg Oral Med Oral Pathol 1980; 50: 522–534.

354. Wharton J, Boguniewicz A, Jennings T. Sarcomatoid tumors of the upper respiratory tract after irradiation: a comparative study (abstract). Am J Clin Pathol 1994; 102: 525.

355. Leifer C, Miller AS. Spindle cell carcinomas of the oral mucosa. A light and electron microscopic study of apparent sarcomatous metastasis to cervical lymph nodes. Cancer 1974; 34: 597–605.

356. Greene GW, Bernier JL. Spindle cell squamous carcinoma of the lip. Report of four cases. Oral Surg 1959; 12: 1008–1010.

357. Barnes L, Verbin R, Guggenheimer J, eds. Surgical pathology of the head and neck. 2nd edn. New York: Marcel Dekker; 2001: 174–182.

358. Ellis GL, Corio RL. Spindle cell carcinoma of the oral cavity: a clinicopathologic assessment of 59 cases. Oral Surg 1980; 50: 523–533.

359. Batsakis JG. Pathology of tumors of the oral cavity. In: Thawley SE, Panje WR, eds. Comprehensive management of head and neck tumors. Philadelphia: WB Saunders; 1987: 480–515.

360. Batsakis JG, Rice DH, Howard DR. The pathology of head and neck tumors: spindle cell lesions (sarcomatoid carcinomas, nodular fasciitis, and fibrosarcoma) of the aerodigestive tracts. Part 14. Head Neck Surg 1982; 4: 499–513.

361a. Rapini RP, Golitz LE, Greer RO Jr, et al. Primary malignant melanoma of the oral cavity. A review of 177 cases. Cancer 1985; 55: 1543–1551.

361b. Hicks M, Flaitz C. Oral mucosal melanoma. Epidemiology and pathobiology. Oral oncology 2000, 36(2): 152–169.

362. Krompecher E. Zur Histologenese und morphologie der admantinoma und sowstiger kiefergeschwulste. Beitre Pathol Anat 1918; 64: 165–167.

363. Dehner LP, Sibley RK, Sauk JJ Jr, et al. Melanotic neuroectodermal tumor of infancy: a clinicopathologic, ultrastructural and tissue culture study. Cancer 1979; 43: 1389–1410.

364. Nagase M, Ueda K, Fukushima M, Nakajima T. Recurrent melanotic neuroectodermal tumor of infancy: case reported survey of 16 cases. J Maxillofac Surg 1983; 11: 131–136.

365. Kapadia S, Frisman D, Hichcock C, Popek E. Melanotic neuroectodermal tumor of infancy. Clinicopathological, immunohistochemical and flow cytometric study. Am J Surg Pathol 1993; 17: 566–573.

366. Pttinato G, Manivel C, D'Amore E, et al. Melanotic neuroectodermal tumor of infancy. Am J Surg Pathol 1991; 15: 233–245.

367. Bastakis J. Melanotic neuroectodermal tumor of infancy (retinal anlage tumor). Ann Otol Rhinol Laryngol 1987; 96: 128–129.

368. Johnson R, Scheithauer B, Dahlin D. Melanotic neuroectodermal tumor of infancy: A review of seven cases. Cancer 1983; 52: 661–667.

369. Borello ED, Gorlin R. Melanotic neuroectodermal tumor of infancy: a neoplasm of neural crest origin. Report of a case associated with high urinary excretion of Vallinyl mandelic acid. Cancer 1966; 19: 196–206.

370. Hoshino S, Takashi H, Shimura T, et al. Melanotic neuroectodermal tumor of infancy in the skull associated with high serum levels of catecholamines. Case report. J Neurosurg 1994; 80(5): 919–924.

371. Dourov N, Mayer R, De Martelare F, et al. Melanotic neuroectodermal tumor of infancy with high serum levels of alphfetoproteins. An ultrastructural and immunological evidence of glial fibrillary protein and alpha-fetoprotein. J Oral Pathol 1987; 16: 251–255.

372. Misugi K, Okajima H, Newton WA, et al. Mediastinal origin of a melanotic progonoma or retinal anlage tumor. Ultrastructural evidence for neural crest origin. Cancer 1965; 18: 477–507.

373. Khoddami M, Squire J, Zeilenska M, Thorner P. Melanotic neuroectodermal tumor of infancy: a molecular genetic study. Pediatr Dev Pathol 1998; 1(4): 295–299.

374. Tschen JA, Fechner RE. The juxtaoral organ of Chievitz. Am J Surg Pathol 1979; 3: 147–150.

375. Elzay RP, O'Keefe EM. Unusual gingival proliferation: primary pseudoepitheliomatous hyperplasia. Oral Surg 1979; 47: 436–440.

376. Greer RO. Inverted oral papilloma. Oral Surg 1973; 36: 400–403.

377. Abrams AM, Melrose RJ, Howell FV. Necrotizing sialometaplasia. A disease simulating malignancy. Cancer 1973; 32: 130–135.

378. Forney SK, Foley JM, Sugg WE, et al. Necrotizing sialometaplasia of the mandible. Oral Surg 1977; 43: 720–726.

379. Bronstein SL, Greer RO, Steffen K. Necrotizing sialometaplasia. A benign disease simulating malignancy. Colo Oral Cancer Bull 1978; 1: 12–16.

380. Philipsen HP, Peterson JK, Simonsen BH. Necrotizing sialometaplasia of the palate. Int J Oral Surg 1976; 5: 292–299.

381. Poulson TC, Greer RO, Ryser RW. Necrotizing sialometaplasia obscuring an underlying malignancy: report of a case. J Oral Maxillofac Surg 1984; 44: 570–574.

382. Meyer I, Shklar G. Malignant tumors metastatic to the mouth and jaws. Oral Surg 1969; 20: 350–358.

383. Castigliano SG, Rominger CJ. Metastatic malignancy of the jaws. Am J Surg 1954; 87: 496–507.

384. McDaniel RK, Luna MA, Stimson PG. Metastatic tumors of the jaws. Oral Surg 1971; 31: 380–386.

385a. Hatziotis J, Constantinidou H, Papanayotou PH. Metastatic tumors of the oral soft tissue. Review of the literature and report of a case. Oral Surg 1973; 36: 544–550.

385b. Hirshberg A, Buchner A. Metastatic tumors to the oral region, an overview. Eur J Cancer B Oral Oncol 1995; 31b(6): 355–360.

386. McClatchey KD, Batsakis JG, Young SK. Intravascular angiomatosis. Oral Surg 1978; 46: 70–73.

387. Heyden G, Dahl I, Angervall L. Intravascular papillary endothelial hyperplasia in the oral mucosa. Oral Surg 1978; 45: 83–87.

388. Cundiff EJ. Peripheral ossifying fibroma. A review of 365 cases. Thesis. Indiana University, Bloomington, 1972.

389. Greer RO, Zarlengo WD. Peripheral odontogenic fibroma. A reappraisal of biologic behavior. J Colo Dent Assoc 1979; 57: 11–14.

390. Giansanti JS, Waldron CA. Peripheral giant cell granuloma: review of 720 cases. J Oral Surg 1969; 27: 787–791.

391. Sapp JP; Ultrastructure and histogenesis of peripheral giant cell reparative granuloma of the jaws. Cancer 1972; 30: 1119–1129.

392. Whitaker SB, Waldron CA. Giant cell lesions of the jaws: a clinical, radiologic and histopathologic study. Oral Surg Oral Med Oral Pathol 1993; 75: 199–208.

393. Waldron CA, Shafer WG. The central giant cell reparative granuloma of the jaws. An analysis of 38 cases. Am J Clin Pathol 1966; 45: 437–447.

394. Austin LT, Dahlin DC, Royer RQ. Giant cell reparative granuloma and related conditions affecting the jawbones. Oral Surg 1959; 12: 1285–1291.

395. Greer RO, Mierau GW, Favara B. Tumors of the head and neck in children. New York: Praeger; 1983.

396. Dahlin DC. Bone tumors. 2nd edn. Springfield, IL: Charles C Thomas; 1967.

397. Batsakis JG. Tumors of the head and neck. clinical and pathologic considerations. 2nd edn. Baltimore: Williams & Wilkins; 1979.

398. Andersen L, Fejerskov O, Philipsen HP. Oral giant cell granulomas. A clinical and histologic study of 129 new cases. Acta Pathol Microbiol Scand 1973; 81A: 606–616.

399. Vickers RA. Mesenchymal (soft) tissue tumors of the oral region. In: Gorlin RJ, Goldman HM, eds. Thoma's oral pathology. Vol. 1. 6th edn. St. Louis: CV Mosby; 1970.

400. Konwaler WE, Keasler L, Kaplan L. Subcutaneous pseudosarcomatous fibromatosis (fasciitis). Am J Pathol 1955; 24: 241–247.

401. Stout AP, Lattes R. Tumors of the soft tissue. In: Atlas of tumor pathology. Series 2, Fasc. 1. Washington, DC: Armed Forces Institute of Pathology; 1967.

402. Werning JT. Nodular fasciitis of the orofacial region. Oral Surg 1979; 48: 441–446.

403. Miller R, Cheris L, Stratigos GT. Nodular fascitis. Oral Surg 1975; 40: 399–403.

404. Shuman R. Mesenchymal tumors of soft tissue. In: Anderson WAD, ed. Pathology. 6th edn. St. Louis: CV Mosby; 1971: 565.

405. Takagi M, Ishikawa G. Fibrous tumor of infancy – report of a case originating in the oral cavity. J Oral Pathol 1973; 2: 293–300.

406. Freedman PD, Cardo V, Kerpel SM, et al. Desmoplastic fibroma (fibromatosis) of the jawbones. Oral Surg 1978; 46: 386–395.

407. Dockerty MB, Parkhill EM, Dahlin DC, et al. Tumors of the oral cavity and pharynx. In: Atlas of tumor pathology. Fasc. 106. Washington, DC: Armed Forces Institute of Pathology; 1968: 155.

408. Osment LS. Cutaneous lipomas and lipomatosis. Surg Gynecol Obstet 1962; 127: 129–131.

409. Gellhorn A, Marks PA. The composition and biosynthesis of lipids in human adipose tissue. J Clin Invest 1961; 40: 925–932.

410. MacGregor AJ, Dyson DP. Oral lipomas. A review of the literature and a report of twelve new cases. Oral Surg 1966; 21: 770–776.

411. Greer RO, Richardson JF. The nature of lipomas and their significance in the oral cavity. Oral Surg 1973; 36: 551–557.

412. Herschfus L, Wolter JG. Granular cell myoblastoma of the oral cavity. Oral Surg 1970; 29: 341–352.

413. Matthews JB, Mason GI. Oral granular cell myoblastoma: an immunohistochemical study. J Oral Pathol 1982; 11: 343–352.

414. Stefansson K, Wollman RL. S-100 protein in granular cell tumors (granular cell myoblastomas). Cancer 1982; 49: 1634–1639.

415. Willis RA. Pathology of tumors. 4th edn. London: Butterworths; 1967.

416. Azzopardi JG. Histogenesis of the granular cell myoblastoma. J Pathol Bacteriol 1956; 71: 85–93.

417. Fisher ER, Wechsler H. Granular cell myoblastoma – a misnomer. Electron microscopic and histochemical evidence concerning its Schwann cell derivation and nature. Cancer 1962; 15: 936–942.

418. Garancis JC, Komorowski RA, Kuzma JF. Granular cell myoblastoma. Cancer 1970; 25: 542–550.

419. Misch KA. Rhabdomyoma purum: a benign rhabdomyoma of tongue. J Pathol Bacteriol 1958; 75: 105–108.

420. Campbell JAH. Congenital epulis. J Pathol Bacteriol 1955; 70: 233–238.

421. Kay S, Elzay RP, Willson MA. Ultrastructural observations on a gingival granular cell tumor (congenital epulis). Cancer 1971; 27: 674–680.

422. Armin A, Connelly E, Rowden G. An immunoperoxidase investigation of S-100 protein in granular cell myoblastomas: evidence for Schwann cell derivation. Am J Clin Pathol 1983; 79: 37–44.

423. Monteil RA, Loubiere R, Charbit Y, Gillette JY. Gingival granular cell tumor of the newborn: immunoperoxidase investigation with anti-S-100 antiserum. Oral Surg 1987; 64: 78–81.

424. Ellis GL, Abrams AM, Melrose RJ. Intraosseous benign neural sheath neoplasms. Report of seven cases and review of the literature. Oral Surg 1977; 44: 731–743.

425. Cherrick HM, Eversole LR. Benign neurosheath neoplasms of the oral cavity: report of 37 cases. Oral Surg 1971; 32: 900–909.

426. Harkin JC, Reed JJ. Tumors of the peripheral nervous system. In: Atlas of tumor pathology. Series 2. Fasc. 3. Washington, DC: Armed Forces Institute of Pathology; 1969.

427. Gallager RL, Helwig EB. Neurothekoma – a benign cutaneous tumor of nerve origin. Am J Clin Pathol 1980; 74: 759–764.

428. Mason MR, Knepp DR, Herbold DR. Nerve sheath myxoma (neurothekoma): a case involving the lip. Oral Surg 1986; 62: 185–186.

429. Wesley RK, Mintz SM, Wertheimer FW. Primary malignant hemangioendothelioma of the gingiva. Oral Surg 1975; 39: 103–112.

430. Frazell E. Clinical aspects of tumors of the major salivary glands. Cancer 1954; 7: 637–643.

431. Ellis GL, Auclair PL, Gnepp DR, et al. Salivary gland neoplasms: general considerations. In: Ellis GL, Auclair PL, Gnepp DR, eds. Surgical pathology of salivary glands. Philadelphia: WB Saunders; 1991: 135–164.

432. Marx R, Stern D. Oral and maxillofacial pathology. A rationale for diagnosis and treatment. Chicago: Quintessence Publishing; 2003: 527–572.

433. Freedman PD, Lumerman H. Lobular carcinoma of intraoral minor salivary gland origin. Report of twelve cases. Oral Surg Oral Med Oral Pathol 1983; 56: 157–165.

434. Waldron CA, Giansanti JS. Benign fibro-osseous lesions of the jaws. A clinical and radiologic-histologic review of sixty-five cases. Part I. Oral Surg 1973; 35: 190–201.

435. Lichtenstein L. Polystotic fibrous dysplasia. Arch Surg 1938; 36: 874–898.

436. Albright F, Butler A, Hampton A, Smith P. Syndrome characterized by osteis fibrosa dissiminata, areas of pigmentation and endocrine dysfunction with precocious puberty in females. N Eng J Med 1937; 216: 727–746.

437. McCune D, Bruch H. Osteodystrophia fibrosa: report of a case in which the condition was accompanied with precocious puberty, pathologic pigmentation of the skin and hyperthyroidism, with a review of the literature. Am J Dis Child 1937; 54: 806–848.

438. Lustig L, Holliday M, McCarthy E, Nager G. Fibrous dysplasia involving the skull base and temporal bone. Arch Otolaryngol Head Neck Surg 2001; 127(10): 1239–1247.

439. Eversole LR, Sabes WR, Rovin S. Fibrous dysplasia: a nosologic problem in the diagnosis of fibro-osseous lesions of the jaws. J Oral Pathol 1972; 1: 189–220.

440. Reed RJ. Fibrous dysplasias of bone. Arch Pathol 1963; 75: 480–495.

441. Spjut JJ, Dorfman HD, Fechner RE, et al. Tumors of bone and cartilage. In: Atlas of tumor pathology. Series 2. Fasc. 5. Washington, DC: Armed Forces Institute of Pathology; 1970.

442. Rao V, Schnittger S, Hansmann I. G protein Gs alpha (GNAS1), the palpable candidate gene for Albright hereditary osteodystrophy, is assigned to human chromosome 20q 12-q13.2. Genomics 1991; 10(1): 257–261.

443. Yu D, Yu S, Schuster V, et al. Identification of two novel deletion mutations within the Gs alpha gene (GNAS1) in Albright hereditary osteodystrophy. J Clin End Metab 1999; 84(9): 3254–3259.

444. Rimminucci M, Fisher L, Majolagbe A, et al. A novel GNAS1 mutation, R201G, In McCune-Albright syndrome. J Bone Miner Res 1999; 14(11): 1987–1989.

445. Bianco P, Rimminucci M, Majolabe A, et al. Mutations of the GNAS1 gene, stromal cell dysfunction, and osteomalacic changes in non-McCune-Albright fibrous dysplasia of bone. J Bone Miner Res 2000; 15(1): 120–128.

446. Hammer JE, Scofield HH, Cornyn J. Benign fibro-osseous jaw lesions of periodontal membrane origin. Cancer 1968; 22: 861–878.

447. Jones W. Familial multilocular cystic disease of the jaws. Am J Cancer 1933; 17: 946–950.

448. Mangion J, Rahman N, Edkins S, et al. The gene for cherubism maps to chromosome 4p16.3. Am J Hum Genet 1999; 65(1): 151–157.

449. Tiziani V, Reichenberger E, Buzzo C, et al. The gene for cherubism maps to chromosome 4.p16. Am J Hum Genet 1999; 65(1): 158–166.

450. Ueki Y, Tiziani V, Santanna C, et al. Mutations in the gene encoding c-Abl-binding protein SH3BP2 cause cherubism. Nature Genetics 2001; 28(2): 125–126.

451. Eversole LR. Clinical outline of oral pathology: diagnosis and treatment. Philadelphia: Lea & Febiger; 1978.

452. Arlen M, Higinbotham N, Huvos A, et al. Radiation-induced sarcoma of bone. Cancer 1971; 28: 1087–1099.

453. Wick M, McLoed R, Seigal G, et al. Sarcoma of the bone complicating osteitis deformans (Paget's disease). Fifty-year experience. Am J Surg Pathol 1981; 5: 47–59.

454. Schwartz D, Alpert M. The malignant transformation of fibrous dysplasia. Am J Med Sci 1964; 247: 35–54.

455. Unni K. Osteosarcoma. In: Unni KK, ed. Dahlin's bone tumors. General aspects and data on 11,087 cases. 5th edn. Philadelphia: Lippincott Williams & Wilkins; 1996: 143–183.

456. Finkel M, Biskis B, Farrell C. Pathogenic effects of extracts of human osteosarcomas. Arch Pathol 1967; 84: 425–428.

457. Reilly C, Pritchard D, Biskis B, et al. Immunohistologic evidence suggesting a viral etiology of human osteosarcoma. Cancer 1972; 30: 603–609.

458. Regazzini P, Gamberi G, Benassi M, et al. Analysis of SAS gene and CDK4 and MDM2 proteins in low-grade osteosarcoma. Cancer Dtect Prev 1999; 23(2):129–136.

459. Garrington GE, Scofield HH, Cornyn J, et al. Osteosarcoma of the jaws. Analysis of 56 cases. Cancer 1967; 20: 377–391.

460. Forteza G, Colmenero B, Lopez-Barea F. Osteosarcoma of the maxilla and mandible. Oral Surg 1987; 62: 179–184.

461. Greer RO, Berman DN. Osteoblastoma of the jaws: current concepts and differential diagnosis. J Oral Surg 1978; 36: 304–307.

462. Farman AG, Nortje CJ, Grotepass F. Periosteal benign osteoblastoma of the mandible: report of a case and review of the literature pertaining to benign osteoblastic neoplasms of the jaws. Br J Oral Surg 1976; 14: 12–22.

463. Jaffe H, Lichtenstein L, Sutro C. Pigmented villonodular synovitis, bursitis, and tenosynovitis: a discussion of the synovial and bursal equivalents of tenosynovial lesion commonly denoted as xanthoma, xanthogranuloma, giant cell tumor or myeloplaxoma of the tendon sheath. Arch Pathol 1941; 31: 731–765.

464. Youssef R, Roszkowski M, Richter K. Pigmented villonodular synovitis of the temporomandibular joint. J Oral Maxillofac Surg 1996; 54: 224–227.

465. Makek M, Drommer R. Localized villonodular synovitis of the temporomandibular joint. A case report. J maxillofacia Surg 1987; 6: 302–305.

Major and minor salivary glands

23

Paul L. Auclair   Gary L. Ellis   Michael W. Stanley

SALIVARY GLAND TUMORS

Salivary gland tumors account for 2–6.5% of all neoplasms of the head and neck,[1–5] and have an annual incidence throughout the world of 0.4–6.5 cases per 100 000 people.[6–8] Despite their rarity, they perhaps exhibit a greater degree of histomorphologic diversity than tumors from any other site. This diversity is manifest among the many different tumor types and even within individual tumors and complicates their diagnostic interpretation.

Between 64% to 80% of all primary epithelial tumors occur in the parotid glands, while 7–11% occur in the submandibular glands, less than 1% occur in the sublingual glands, and 9–23% occur in the minor glands.[2,8–11] Among several large series, the proportion of salivary gland tumors that are benign varies from 63% to 78%.[2,8,12] In the files of the Armed Forces Institute of Pathology (AFIP), about one-third of major gland and one-half of minor gland tumors are malignant. The ratio of malignant to benign tumors is greatest (>2.3:1) in the sublingual gland, tongue, floor of the mouth, and retromolar area.

SPECIMENS

Frozen sections can be useful to confirm fine needle aspiration interpretation, that a mass represents primary rather than secondary disease prior to resection, and to evaluate surgical margins. However, accurate classification, especially of malignant tumors, can be difficult and is usually best after review of the entire specimen.[13,14] Typical gross specimens for the parotid and submandibular glands are superficial parotidectomy and submandibulectomy with contents of the submandibular triangle, respectively. Gross examination should include assessment of tumor size, presence or absence of cysts, necrosis, multifocal disease, and possible extension to tissue margins (marked with ink to help in microscopic evaluation). Tissue sections should include as much of the interface of tumor with surrounding tissue as possible and any area that appears different from the rest of the tumor. Lymph nodes in or around the parotid and submandibular glands should be included for microscopic sections because of the possibility of secondary involvement.

STAINS

Routine hematoxylin and eosin-stained slides of adequate specimens are usually sufficient for accurate interpretation. Histochemical analysis has limited value in diagnosis and classification of salivary gland tumors. Mucicarmine or Alcian blue, at pH 2.5, are useful for identification of intracytoplasmic mucin that can help distinguish mucoepidermoid carcinoma from squamous cell carcinoma. Phos-

photungstic acid-hematoxylin (PTAH) helps identify oncocytes, and periodic acid–Schiff (PAS) after diastase digestion highlights secretory granules in acinic cell adenocarcinoma. Immunohistochemical studies are most useful in the identification of metastatic tumors, such as malignant melanomas, confirmation of epithelial differentiation in undifferentiated carcinomas or the lack thereof in sarcomas, and classification of malignant lymphomas. They have not been particularly useful in the classification of primary epithelial salivary gland tumors or in separating benign from malignant disease, but their usefulness will be mentioned where appropriate under the discussion of specific tumors.

GRADING

Tumor grade is an independent predictor of behavior for salivary gland carcinomas and often has an important role in optimizing treatment.[15–17] In general, grading of salivary gland tumors includes four different methods. (1) For most carcinomas, there is only a single grade, and classification alone identifies the grade. Included in this group are acinic cell adenocarcinoma, basal cell adenocarcinoma, and polymorphous low-grade adenocarcinoma (PLGA), which have low-grade biologic behavior. Diagnoses of salivary duct carcinoma, primary squamous cell carcinoma, and undifferentiated carcinoma denote high-grade tumors. The next three methods are uniquely applied to specific types of tumors. (2) Adenocarcinoma, not otherwise specified, is graded on the basis of cytomorphologic features. (3) Intermediate-grade and high-grade adenoid cystic carcinomas are determined, respectively, on the recognition of the predominant growth as either cribriform-tubular or solid. (4) Mucoepidermoid carcinomas are graded on the basis of specific criteria that include the presence or absence of growth characteristics and cytomorphologic features.[18,19] The malignant component in carcinoma ex mixed tumor is graded according to the carcinoma type present.

STAGING

Clinical staging of major salivary gland carcinoma is a valuable predictor of patient outcome.[20–23] The clinical parameters include tumor size, local extension of tumor, metastasis to regional nodes, and distant metastases, as shown in Table 23.1. T4 lesions are now divided into those that are resectable with grossly clear margins (4a) and those that are not (4b).[23] Although there are no comparable staging guidelines for tumors of the intraoral minor glands, Spiro and coworkers[17,24] have successfully applied the criteria used for epidermoid carcinoma of the oral cavity, pharynx, larynx, and sinus to mucoepidermoid carcinoma.

Table 23.1 Staging system for major salivary glands

Primary tumor (T)

TX	Primary tumor cannot be assessed
T0	No evidence of primary tumor
T1	Tumor 2 cm or less in greatest dimension without extraparenchymal extension*
T2	Tumor more than 2 cm but not more than 4 cm in greatest dimension without extraparenchymal extension*
T3	Tumor more than 4 cm and/or tumor having extraparenchymal extension*
T4a	Tumor invades skin, mandible, ear canal, and/or facial nerve
T4b	Tumor invades skull base and/or pterygoid plates and/or encases carotid artery

Regional lymph nodes (N)

NX	Regional lymph nodes cannot be assessed
N0	No regional lymph node metastasis
N1	Metastasis in a single ipsilateral lymph node, more than 3 cm or less in greatest dimension
N2	Metastasis in a single ipsilateral lymph node, more than 3 cm but not more than 6 cm in greatest dimension, or in multiple ipsilateral lymph nodes, none more than 6 cm in greatest dimension, or in bilateral or contralateral lymph nodes, none more than 6 cm in greatest dimension
N2a	Metastasis in a single ipsilateral lymph node more than 3 cm but not more than 6 cm in greatest dimension
N2b	Metastasis in multiple ipsilateral lymph nodes, none more than 6 cm in greatest dimension
N2c	Metastasis in bilateral or contralateral lymph nodes, none more than 6 cm in greatest dimension
N3	Metastasis in a lymph node, more than 6 cm in greatest dimension

Distant metastasis (M)

MX	Distant metastasis cannot be assessed
M0	No distant metastasis
M1	Distant metastasis

Stage grouping

I	T1 N0 M0
II	T2 N0 M0
III	T3 N0 M0
	T1 N1 M0
	T2 N1 M0
	T3 N1 M0
IVA	T4a N0 M0
	T4a N1 M0
	T1 N2 M0
	T2 N2 M0
	T3 N2 M0
	T4a N2 M0
IVB	T4b Any N M0
	Any T N3 M0
IVC	Any T Any N M1

* Extraparenchymal extension is clinical or macroscopic evidence of invasion of soft tissues. Microscopic evidence alone does not constitute extraparenchymal extension for classification purposes.

(Used with the permission of the American Joint Committee on Cancer (AJCC), Chicago, Illinois. The original source for this material is the AJCC Cancer Staging Manual, Sixth Edition (2002) published by Springer-Verlag New York, www.springer-ny.com.[23]

CLASSIFICATION

Salivary gland tumor classification is a dynamic process that has undergone several modifications since the classification of salivary gland neoplasms that was formulated by Foote and Frazell[25] in the early 1950s. The revised World Health Organization's (WHO's) classification in 1991[26] showed significant modification and expansion from the first WHO classification[27] in 1972. The classification of Ellis and Auclair[28] (Table 23.2) varied only slightly from the revised WHO classification, and recent published classifications closely conform to that of Ellis and Auclair.[29–31]

FINE NEEDLE ASPIRATION

Approach: Technical aspects of performing fine needle aspiration (FNA), as well as detailed information regarding specific potential

complications, have recently been discussed and illustrated in detail.[32] These subjects will not be covered in depth, but a few points deserve emphasis in the context of salivary gland FNA. The small-gauge needles that are employed are usually 25 or 23 gauge (0.5 or 0.6 mm diameter, respectively), and the smaller size is preferred. Patients readily accept the procedure when thin needles are used. Extensive sampling with abundant tissue can be obtained without significant hemorrhage, nerve damage, or infection.[33–37] Occasionally, small hematomas and local tenderness may be noted.[35] Metastases attributable to tumor cell dissemination by FNA do not occur, and local implantation and recurrence are almost always associated with larger-gauge instruments.[34] Nonetheless, some continue to express concern about these issues.[38]

High-quality preparations are essential if meaningful diagnoses are to be based on FNA material.[32] Attention to the details of smearing, cell-block embedding, and allocation of material for ancillary testing (flow cytometry, immunocytochemistry, electron microscopy, etc.)

Table 23.2 Classification of salivary gland neoplasms (alternative terminology used in WHO classification of 1991, where applicable)

Benign epithelial neoplasms
　Mixed tumor (pleomorphic adenoma)
　Myoepithelioma
　Warthin's tumor
　Basal cell adenoma
　Canalicular adenoma
　Oncocytoma
　Cystadenoma (papillary and mucinous cystadenomas)
　Sialadenoma papilliferum
　Inverted ductal papilloma
　Intraductal papilloma
　Lymphadenomas[†] and sebaceous adenomas
　Sialoblastoma[†]

Malignant epithelial neoplasms
　Mucoepidermoid carcinoma
　Adenocarcinoma NOS
　Acinic cell adenocarcinoma
　Adenoid cystic carcinoma
　Polymorphous low-grade adenocarcinoma
　Carcinoma ex mixed tumor
　Carcinosarcoma
　Metastasizing mixed tumor
　Squamous cell carcinoma
　Basal cell adenocarcinoma
　Epithelial-myoepithelial carcinoma
　Clear cell adenocarcinoma[†]
　Cystadenocarcinoma (papillary cystadenocarcinoma)
　Small cell undifferentiated carcinoma (small cell carcinoma)
　Large cell undifferentiated carcinoma (undifferentiated carcinoma)
　Lymphoepithelial carcinoma (undifferentiated carcinoma with lymphoid stroma)
　Oncocytic carcinoma
　Salivary duct carcinoma
　Sebaceous adenocarcinoma and lymphadenocarcinoma
　Myoepithelial carcinoma (malignant myoepithelioma)
　Adenosquamous carcinoma
　Mucinous adenocarcinoma[†]

Mesenchymal neoplasms
　Benign
　Sarcomas

Malignant lymphomas

Metastatic tumors (secondary tumors)

† not included in WHO classification

is important. Time-consuming processing of material rinsed from needles after smears and cell blocks have been prepared does little to improve diagnostic yield.[39]

Anatomic factors in salivary gland aspiration: The complexity of head and neck anatomy complicates interpretation of masses detected at physical examination. Those not adept at head and neck examinations occasionally mistake normal anatomic structures for pathologic masses. The pathologist who is asked to perform aspirations in these cases must bring skill and caution to the procedure.

The complexity of head and neck anatomy sometimes makes it difficult to determine the site of some lesions. For example, a mass inferior to the angle of the mandible could be a parotid lesion, an intraparotid or high cervical lymph node lesion, a lateral neck cyst,

or a soft tissue mass. Cytologic confirmation of the mass's location may help focus clinical decision-making, even if a specific diagnosis is not obtained by FNA.[40]

Cervical ribs occur in approximately 1.5% of individuals[41] and may be mistaken for supraclavicular lymphadenopathy.[42] Bones of the cervical spine are sometimes mistaken for lymph nodes or cysts.[42] Radiographic studies can add confidence to this evaluation, and careful consultation among the pathologist, the clinician, and the radiologist may prevent unnecessary surgery.

After the anatomy has been altered by combinations of surgery and radiation therapy, physical assessment of the neck becomes difficult. Following radical dissections, lesions may lie close to an unexpectedly prominent carotid artery. Fibrous tissue, damaged skeletal muscle, suture granulomas, and postoperative neuromas may need to be distinguished from recurrent malignancy.

Microbiologic evaluation of aspirated material: Cultures should be initiated when grossly purulent material is aspirated.[43] Infection must also be considered when there is redness, tenderness, ill-defined swelling, immunosuppression, or other factors that raise the possibility of infection.[44] The need for cultures may not be apparent until after initial aspiration, and repeat aspiration may be necessary for microbiology. Techniques and specimen requirements have been discussed in detail.[45] It is helpful to consult with the microbiologist prior to obtaining material for culture regarding special handling requirements. At the microscope, potentially infectious aspirates must be examined carefully so that organisms are not missed.[46]

FNA-associated tissue damage: Problems with histologic interpretation of head and neck tissues excised after FNA are uncommon. Rarely, a mass will undergo near total infarction shortly after FNA, often leaving a thin peripheral rim of viable tissue.[32–55]

It has been suggested that vascular compromise, perhaps mediated by thrombosis, is responsible for such occurrences, and that squamous metaplasia in pleomorphic adenomas may in part be due to ischemia.[56] Sudden onset of pain is often a feature.[56] There is no way to predict which masses may be at risk for this rare complication of FNA. It is noteworthy that spontaneous infarction unattended by FNA or other procedures has been described in pleomorphic adenomas, monomorphic adenomas, and lymph nodes replaced by malignant lymphoma.[56] Both spontaneous and FNA-associated infarctions are rare.[57] It has been suggested that in the latter event, aspiration should be regarded as the cause of infarction.[58]

While small areas of hemorrhage or granulation tissue are readily recognized in section material, cytologic atypia and increases in mitotic activity are more problematic. A thin peripheral rim of viable tissue is usually available for study, but in cases of total infarction, only the FNA results are available for diagnosis. In a few cases, a florid, fasciitis-like proliferation of reparative connective tissue may be accompanied by varying amounts of identifiable but necrotic tumor tissue.

Approaches to application of FNA to salivary gland masses: The literature outlines three approaches to using FNA for salivary gland masses. The optimistic information just presented suggest that FNA should be used early and often, perhaps playing a role in most masses in this area. However, others cite significant false-negative and false-positive rates, and believe that this method should be applied almost exclusively for triage of new masses that arise in patients with a known history of head and neck malignancy.[39] Others are even more restrictive[60] and cite limited diagnostic accuracy and post-FNA infarction and repair that limit ultimate histologic interpretation. Thus, while agreeing that FNA has a place in evaluation of lymph node and thyroid disease, confirmation of suspected infectious or inflammatory masses, and demonstration of recurrent malignancy, these investigators argue that FNA does not merit inclusion as routine evaluation of salivary gland masses.

Accuracy of diagnosis by FNA; comparison with frozen section studies: Several studies illustrate the improvement in diagnostic accuracy for FNA of salivary gland masses that comes with increased experience, in both collecting and interpreting samples.[32,40,61–68] Understanding of accuracy figures is difficult because some series are small. Furthermore, some workers exclude unsatisfactory or nondiagnostic cases from summary calculations while others do not. In some papers, numerous aspirations of normal tissues are listed. Lacking more detailed information, many reviewers would consider these unsatisfactory. Definitions of false-negative aspiration also differ. Some, for example, would consider that a Warthin's tumor interpreted as chronic inflammation as a false-negative diagnosis; others would not. True false-negative aspirations, however, remain a problem.[60] Most involve malignancies that yield few diagnostic cells or are low cytologic grade.[56,62,69,70] Others result from sampling error,[71] particularly when small metastatic deposits are evaluated.

Published accuracy figures for salivary gland FNA should be cautiously interpreted. With detection of malignancy as the goal, sensitivity figures range from 64% to 100%, while those for specificity are usually higher in most series (94–100%).[38,62] Rates for unsatisfactory aspirations are also subject to interpretation, and reflect the procedural and interpretive skills and experience of the individuals involved. Overall, nondiagnostic rates for salivary gland or general head and neck FNA are approximately 10% in most series,[33,36,59,71,72] but some report up to 21%.[71]

It is useful to compare FNA with the only other means for rapid tissue diagnosis, the frozen section.[73] Aspiration actually allows more time for reflection, consultation, and special studies than do frozen sections that are performed during an operative procedure.[61] The rates for correct diagnosis of malignancy by these two procedures are similar in many studies and can be as low as 60%.[13,61,62,69,71,74–77] Some series show FNA to be slightly more accurate, while others indicate that frozen section leads to fewer interpretive errors. Each method is associated with false-positive[76] and false-negative diagnoses,[73] and both have been blamed for unnecessarily radical surgery due to false-positive interpretations.[73]

Higher-grade malignancies are more easily interpreted on both FNA and frozen section, so that accuracy figures for both tests depend in part on the case mix of the material under review.[13] Malignancies that are uncommon, low grade, cystic or partially cystic, or complex may be very difficult to interpret in either rapid diagnostic medium. Masses with substantial inflammatory or fibrotic components are also likely to be difficult. That is, diagnostic problems at the time of FNA may not be ameliorated by frozen section, even though recommending cryostat 'confirmation' for difficult cytologic diagnosis is a common practice.[78]

Some have found that using both FNA and frozen section improves the overall accuracy of these two imperfect tests.[71,73] Heller and coworkers suggest that both tests should be applied to 'virtually all patients in whom surgery for salivary gland tumors is performed.'[13] Since the complication rate of aspiration is negligible, repeated aspiration of clinically worrisome masses can be safely employed when necessary.

Many workers now feel that FNA is a useful test for preoperative evaluation of salivary gland masses. However, FNA has areas of interpretational difficulty with occasional false-positive and false-negative results. Reasons for this difficulty include the extraordinary diversity of salivary gland neoplasms, many of which are rare. The low-grade cytology of some malignancies and frequent problems of inflammation or cystic change in masses of many types exacerbate this problem. The former is in contrast with the fact that the most common cause of false-positive diagnoses is 'atypia' in benign mixed tumors.[79,80]

The diagnostic categories and their major entrants are summarized in Table 23.3. This table also include a few lesions that are not salivary gland tumors, but that arise for consideration in certain clinical or cytologic situations. Pleomorphic adenoma and Warthin's tumor are sufficiently common and distinctive to be listed as primary considerations that organize much of our thinking. The other categories result from our initial impressions of an aspirate, and may lead one to consider a variety of final diagnoses. Several entities are listed under more than one category, reflecting the complexity of certain differential diagnoses.

Clinical expectations: Most salivary gland masses are located in the parotid, with a smaller number in the submandibular gland and minor glands and occasional lesions in the sublingual gland.[40,43,62,72] Many individuals harbor accessory parotid tissue along Stenson's duct, and heterotopic salivary gland tissue occurs in several head and neck sites.[32] Thus, salivary gland masses are found in unusual locations.

Cytologic commonalities: Table 23.3 indicates that several cytologic findings overlap a number of diagnoses; this information is expanded in Table 23.4. Lymphoid stroma,[81] sebaceous differentiation,[82–85] cystic change,[37,40,43,61,74,86–88] squamous metaplasia,[87,89–94] clear cell change[43,95–101] and oncocytic features[102] are cytologic findings shared by diverse groups of lesions. This overlap contributes to the difficulty of salivary gland cytology and serves to emphasize both the need for excellent specimen collection and the diagnostic limitations of the method.

Aspiration of normal salivary gland tissue or adipose tissue: In some series, up to 20% of salivary gland aspirates yield only normal tissue.[40,72,103] Cytologically, acinar cells have characteristic round, basket-like arrangements. These round to wedge-shaped cells feature small, uniform, eccentrically-placed nuclei set in abundant granular or vacuolated cytoplasm. Groups of duct cells, with a typical honeycomb cell arrangement, may be associated with acinar tissue or may lie singly, often with large branching duct fragments. Variable numbers of adipocytes accompany the epithelial elements. Some acinar cells are damaged in the smearing process so that their naked nuclei and granulovacuolar cytoplasmic debris litter the smear. These naked nuclei should not be mistaken for lymphocytes.[104] Both lymphocytes and the cytoplasmic residua of damaged acinar cells are more prominent in air-dried than in fixed material.

Sialosis: This noninflammatory, non-neoplastic salivary gland enlargement is painless and slowly progressive, often present for months or years prior to diagnosis. The parotid glands, and occasionally the submandibular glands, are enlarged and doughy without distinct borders.[104,43,105–107] These enlargements are associated with nutritional deficiencies, diabetes mellitus, alcoholism, cirrhosis, endocrine deficiencies, and drugs, including phenylbutazone, iodine-containing compounds, some antibiotics, and adrenergic drugs.[43,106–108]

In the early stages, the acinar cells are hypertrophic,[106,107] and the mean acinar diameter is greater than that of normal parotid tissue.

CLINICAL SIGNIFICANCE OF ASPIRATES WITH NORMAL TISSUE

Whether or not a small lesion has been missed may be difficult to ascertain. In a series reviewing normal tissue aspirated from 18 unilateral and 2 bilateral parotid or submandibular gland enlargements, the only missed neoplasm was a single pleomorphic adenoma measuring 0.5 cm in diameter,[104] which was correctly diagnosed by repeat FNA.

If physical examination, FNA, and follow-up are expertly performed and carefully coordinated, the chance of missing a

Table 23.3 Classification of salivary gland aspirates[a]

Initial smear pattern	Major differential diagnoses
Normal tissue	Sialosis
	Lipoma or lipomatosis
	Technical miss
Inflammation	
Acute	Non-specific
	Infection
	Necrotic tumor
Chronic	Reactive, NOS
	Lymphoepithelial lesion
	Tumor associated
	Low-grade malignant lymphoma
Granulomatous	Infection
	Sarcoidosis
	Foreign body reaction
	Malignancy associated
Special type	With crystalloid formation
Pleomorphic adenoma	
Myoepithelial predominant	Plasmacytoma
	Myoepithelioma
	Other low-grade spindle cell neoplasm
Epithelial predominant	Low-grade carcinoma of several types (see text)
Atypical or aggressive	Benign atypia
	Benign metastasizing pleomorphic adenoma
	Carcinoma ex pleomorphic adenoma
	True malignant mixed tumor (carcinosarcoma)
	Malignant myoepithelioma
Warthin's tumor	
Epithelium deficient aspirate	Cysts of several types
Metaplastic alterations	Squamous cell carcinoma
Cyst	
Squamous, non-neoplastic	Lymphoepithelial cysts
	non-HIV associated
	HIV associated
	Congenital[+]
Obstructive	Stones or other obstructions
Neoplastic	
Mucoid	Low-grade MEC
Primary, benign	Pleomorphic adenoma
	Monomorphic adenoma
	Warthin's tumor
Primary, malignant	Acinic cell carcinoma
Metastatic	Squamous cell carcinoma
	Papillary thyroid CA
	Others
Epithelial neoplasm, small cell	Monomorphic adenoma
	Pleomorphic adenoma with little chondromyxoid matrix
	Carcinoma ex monomorphic adenoma
	Adenoid cystic Ca.
	Dermal eccrine cylindroma
	Pilomatrixoma
	Basal cell adenocarcinoma
	Primary small cell carcinoma
	Primary lymphoepithelioma-like carcinoma

Table 23.3 Classification of salivary gland aspirates[a] *(cont'd)*

Initial smear pattern	Major differential diagnoses
	Metastatic carcinoma
	Small cell carcinoma
	Cutaneous basal cell carcinoma
	Nasopharyngeal carcinoma
	Merkle cell carcinoma
	Malignant lymphoma
Epithelial neoplasm, large cell	
Low grade	Acinic cell carcinoma*
	Oncocytic lesions
	Polymorphous low grade carcinoma
	Epithelial-myoepithelial carcinoma
	Predominantly sebaceous neoplasms
	Squamous cell carcinoma
	Clear cell carcinoma*
	Metastases
High grade	High grade mucoepidermoid carcinoma
	High grade carcinoma, NOS
	Squamous cell carcinoma
	Primary
	Metastatic
	Direct extension from adjacent sites
	Ductal carcinoma
	Metastatic carcinoma
	Metastatic malignant melanoma
Spindle cell process	
Low grade	Reactive, NOS
	Nodular fasciitis
	Hemangioma
	Myoepithelioma
	Kaposi's sarcoma
Spindle cell neoplasm	
High grade	Primary sarcoma
	Sarcoma invasion from adjacent tissues
	Malignant myoepithelioma
	Squamous cell carcinoma
	Metastatic carcinoma
	Metastatic malignant melanoma

[+] Includes branchial cleft, thyroglossal, and thymic cysts.
[a] Some of these entities are not salivary gland lesions in the strict sense. However, they are included in the table for the sake of generating differential diagnoses for lesions that occur in this area. Clinically, for example, it may be difficult to distinguish a cervical lymph node from a salivary gland lesion. Furthermore, some 'parotid masses' are actually located in lymph nodes adjacent to or within the gland.

significant neoplasm is low. Normal tissue on a salivary gland aspirate should be considered evidence that the lesion has probably not been targeted successfully.

BENIGN TUMORS

MIXED TUMOR (PLEOMORPHIC ADENOMA)

Mixed tumors greatly outnumber all other forms of salivary gland neoplasms. Several large series have shown that they represent

Table 23.4 Cytologic features of salivary gland lesions

Cytologic feature	Lesions that may show feature
Lymphoid stroma	Sialadenitis
	Cystic lesions due to duct obstruction
	Warthin's tumor
	Sebaceous lymphadenoma
	Lymphoepithelial cyst
	Lymphoepithelial lesion
	Oncocytic lesions
	Acinic cell carcinoma
	Mucoepidermoid carcinoma
	Primary lymphoepithelioma-like carcinoma
	Metastatic lymphoepithelioma
	Other metastatic malignancies
Sebaceous differentiation	Normal salivary tissue (all sites)
	Sebaceous adenoma
	Sebaceous lymphadenoma
	Monomorphic adenoma
	Pleomorphic adenoma
	Warthin's tumor
	Mucoepidermoid carcinoma
Cystic change	Congenital
	HIV associated
	Stones or other obstructive lesions
	Pleomorphic adenoma
	Monomorphic adenoma
	Warthin's tumor
	Mucoepidermoid carcinoma
	Acinic cell carcinoma
	Metastatic carcinoma
Clear cell change	Mucoepidermoid carcinoma
	Acinic cell carcinoma
	Oncocytic lesions
	Epithelial-myoepithelial carcinoma
	Adenocarcinoma
	Clear cell carcinoma
Oncocytic cells	Warthin's tumor
	Pleomorphic adenoma
	Mucoepidermoid carcinoma (rarely)
	Acinic cell carcinoma
	Oncocytic lesions
	Oncocytoid adenocarcinoma (see text)

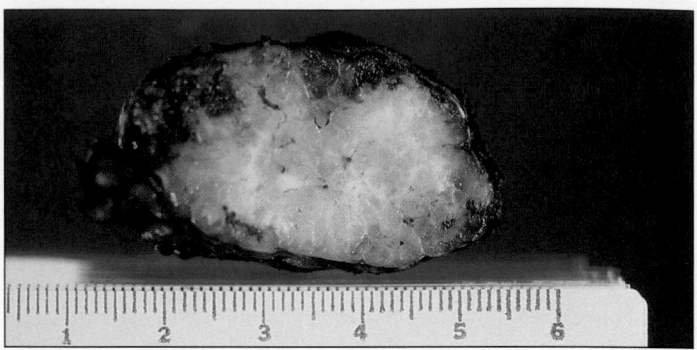

Fig. 23.1 This mixed tumor grossly shows a circumscribed but irregular mass surrounded by salivary gland tissue. The white and blue-gray cut surface varies from opaque to translucent. (Courtesy of Dr. Robert Foss, Naval Dental School, Bethesda, MD)

the tumors in the AFIP files occurred in individuals younger than 30 years of age. Mixed tumor is the most common salivary gland tumor in children and adolescents,[117] and women are more likely to be affected than men.[11,118] Rarely, a familial association has been reported.[119]

Mixed tumors usually grow slowly, are asymptomatic, and are discrete masses that may reach a large size if left untreated (Fig. 23.1). Large tumors are often irregularly nodular masses that stretch the overlying skin or mucosa. Recurrent lesions are less mobile than the original tumors and are often multiple discrete nodules within connective tissue, fat, and salivary gland. Except for predominantly myxoid lesions, mixed tumors are firm and only slightly compressible. In the parotid gland, they occur most often in the lower pole of the superficial (lateral) lobe of the gland. Some that arise in the deep lobe of the gland expand into the parapharyngeal space and produce swelling in the region of the tonsillar fossa, soft palate, or lateral pharynx.[120,121] Rarely, facial paralysis occurs, apparently as a result of extrinsic compression of the facial nerve.[122,123]

In the palate, they are typically located lateral to the midline, only rarely appear as midline masses, and exhibit very limited mobility with palpation. In other minor gland sites, such as the upper lip or buccal mucosa, mixed tumors are mobile and covered by normal mucosa unless traumatized.

Microscopic features: Mixed tumors in both the major and minor glands are usually well defined, but in contrast to most major gland tumors, the capsule is incomplete or absent in minor gland mixed tumors. The cut surface is homogeneously tan to white but may have shiny, partly translucent zones that represent myxochondroid or cartilaginous areas. Hemorrhage and infarction may result from prior surgical manipulation, such as biopsy or fine needle aspiration.

The cytomorphologic and architectural diversity of mixed tumors is extreme. Nevertheless, each case contains both epithelial and mesenchymal-like elements (Fig. 23.2). The epithelial elements manifest as well-formed ductal structures that have closely associated nonductal cells (Fig. 23.3), including spindle, round, stellate, plasmacytoid, polygonal, and clear forms. The nonductal element demonstrates varying degrees of myxoid, hyalin, cartilaginous, or osseous differentiation. The proportion of these two elements varies among different tumors and in different locations within a single tumor. Some investigators[124] designate mixed tumors as 'cellular' if the epithelial element predominates or 'myxoid' if largely composed of myxomatous or myxochrondromatous mesenchymal-like elements. There is no therapeutic significance in this distinction. Most mixed tumors have a myxoid component that comprises 30% or more of

45–74% of all salivary gland tumors.[2,9–11,109] Among AFIP cases, mixed tumors comprise slightly less than one-half of all benign and malignant salivary gland tumors, represent 50% of all parotid neoplasms, and account for 78% of the benign tumors from all salivary gland sites – 79% of major gland tumors and 72% of minor gland tumors. This is similar to the findings from other large series from several different countries.[2,11,110–114]

Clinical features: The hard and soft palates are the most common intraoral sites. Other common minor gland locations are the upper and lower lips and the buccal mucosa. Rare mixed tumors have been reported that were presumed to have arisen from ectopic salivary gland tissue present in lymph nodes, the mandible, or the maxilla.[115,116]

Patients average about 43 years of age, which is young compared with patients with most other salivary gland tumors.[11] Nearly 30% of

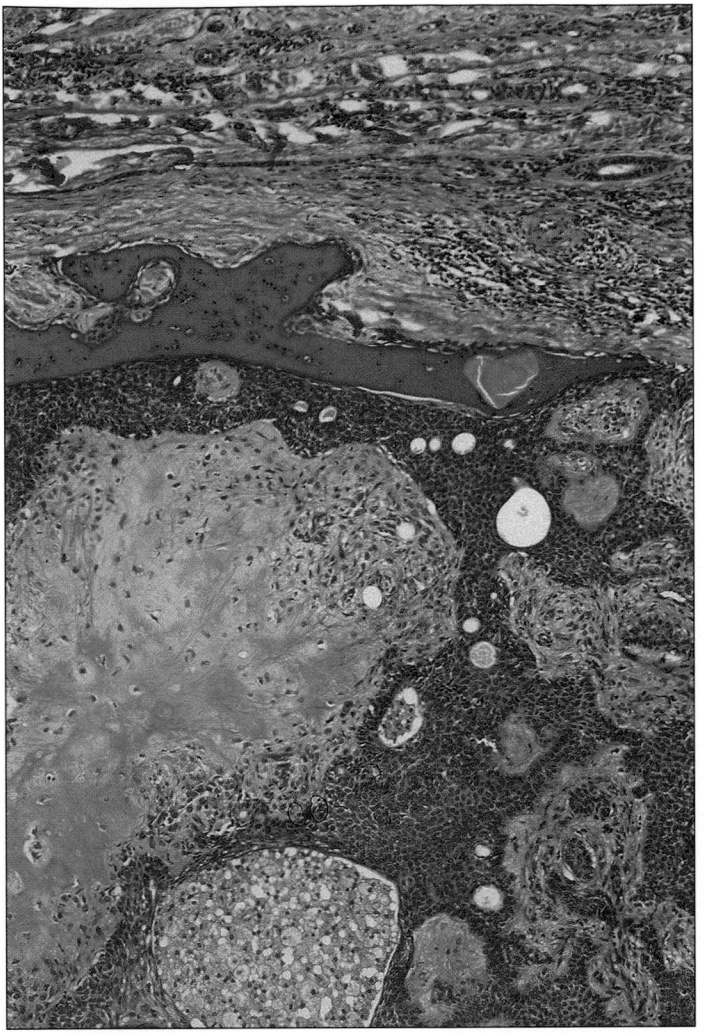

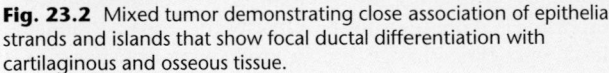

Fig. 23.2 Mixed tumor demonstrating close association of epithelial strands and islands that show focal ductal differentiation with cartilaginous and osseous tissue.

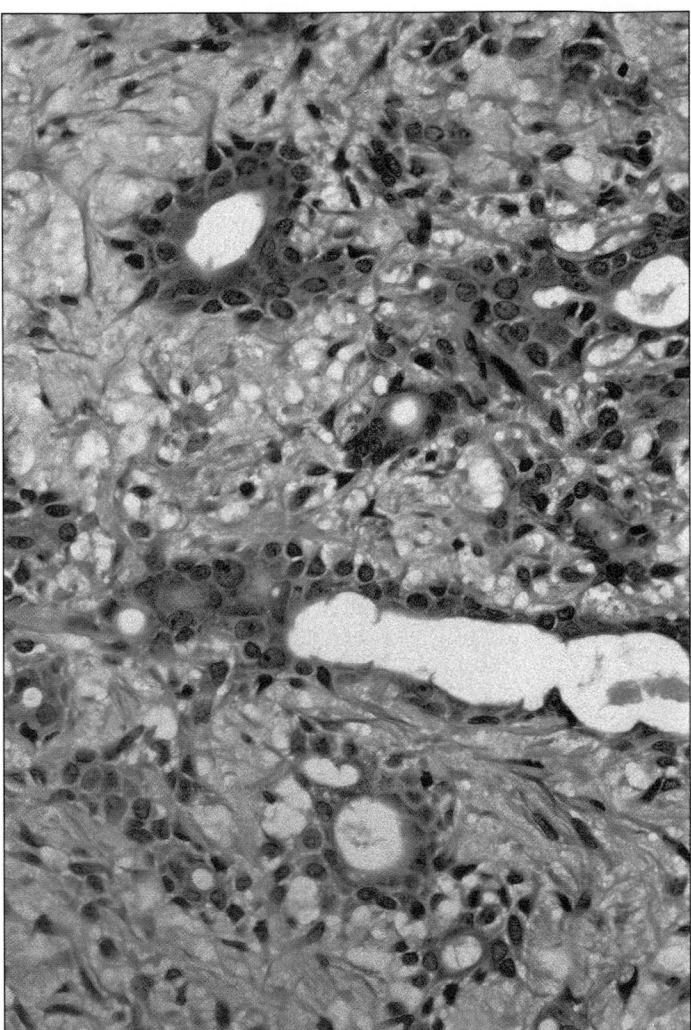

Fig. 23.3 Mixed tumor with well-formed ductal elements surrounded by stellate cells that extend into myxoid areas.

the neoplasm, whereas only 12–15% have an epithelial element that constitutes more than 80% of the tumor.[125] Epithelial cell forms include spindle, clear, squamous, basaloid, cuboidal, plasmacytoid, oncocytoid, mucous, and sebaceous. In all cell types, the nuclear features are typically bland, nucleoli are small or absent, and mitoses are rare. Exceptions occur in some tumors that have been previously manipulated by biopsy or fine needle aspiration and in which infarction may be evident. Although spontaneous necrosis in mixed tumor has been reported,[51,56] necrosis in the absence of previous surgical manipulation suggests malignant transformation and warrants thorough review of additional sections. In rare cases, tumor cells are within capsular vascular spaces, presumably due to surgical manipulation, but this feature has not been correlated with a greater likelihood of metastasis.[125,126]

Architectural configurations include anastomosing trabeculae of epithelial cells with occasional well-formed ductal structures and a closely associated, interposed stromal component. The epithelium may form broad solid sheets with mesenchymal-like stromal component between and around the epithelial elements, which are often isolated as individual ovoid or trabecular epithelial islands as well as individual

epithelial cells. Spindle cells form fibrous-like interlacing fascicles and, rarely, demonstrate Schwannoma-like palisading of nuclei.

The mesenchymal-like element includes myxoid, hyaline, chondroid, and rarely, osseous areas. The myxoid or myxochondroid areas are rich in heparan sulfate.[127] Amorphous to slightly fibrillar eosinophilic hyaline stroma may be sparsely distributed between epithelial cells or dominates large epithelium-poor areas. Cartilaginous zones result from the accumulation of myxohyaline material around individual cells and only rarely resemble mature hyaline cartilage.

Immunohistochemical and ultrastructural studies suggest that mixed tumors are entirely of epithelial origin, and the mesenchymal-like areas represent neoplastic modified myoepithelial cells.[128–130] Evidence supporting this concept includes tonofilaments and microfilaments within the cytoplasm of 'mesenchymal' cells, linear densities of the plasma membrane, pinocytotic vesicles, and remnants of basement membrane.[131,132] Morphologic diversity occurs because the epithelial element expresses ductal and myoepithelial differentiation, produces variable quantities of mucopolysaccharide matrix, and undergoes chondroid and osseous metaplasia.[133,134]

Normal myoepithelial cells are typically immunoreactive with antibodies to smooth muscle actin and calponin[135] and variably immunoreactive for cytokeratin, glial fibrillary acidic protein (GFAP), vimentin, and S-100 protein. GFAP reactivity is usually prominent in the myxoid areas of mixed tumors and limited or absent in cellular tumors. Immunoreactivity of S-100 protein is seen in all cell types in epithelial and stromal regions and is not specific for myoepithelial differentiation.[136] Mixed tumor is one of the few salivary gland tumors that have been cytogenetically well characterized. Some have an apparently normal diploid stemline, but others have reciprocal translocations, with breakpoints at 8q12, 3p21, and 12q13-15.[137–139] In those with 8q12 translocations, the pleomorphic adenoma gene 1 (PLAG1), a zinc finger transcription factor gene, is consistently rearranged and overexpressed.[140,141] Overexpression is seen in about one-half of mixed tumors and much less often in malignant salivary tumors.[141] Overexpression of p53 oncoprotein has been found in only about 13% of mixed tumors but in 75% of carcinoma ex mixed tumors. Interestingly, the benign and malignant elements of each tumor often demonstrate an identical loss of heterozygosity, suggesting that the p53 mutation is an early event in the malignant transformation.[142,143] Similarly, overexpression of the HMGIC and MDM2 genes has also been described as important.[144] There is some flow cytometric evidence that high S-phase fractions (>5%) correlate with larger tumor size and a greater likelihood for recurrence.[145]

Differential diagnosis: Epithelial and mesenchymal-like elements together allow distinction of mixed tumors from other salivary gland adenomas. Mixed tumors that contain foci of squamous and mucous cells are distinguished from mucoepidermoid carcinoma by absence of infiltration, limited cystic component, and presence of myxochondroid elements. In the minor salivary glands, it may be difficult to distinguish mixed tumor from polymorphous low-grade adenocarcinoma (PLGA). Both may be circumscribed, have uniform bland cytomorphology, and contain myxoid areas. However, PLGA frequently has perineural growth, infiltrates adjacent fibrous connective tissue, fat, and salivary parenchyma, and forms small tubular structures or single-file cords of tumor cells at the periphery. Most mixed tumors are diffusely immunoreactive for glial fibrillary acidic protein whereas PLGA typically shows limited, patchy reactivity.[146]

Malignant transformation in mixed tumor is distinguished from atypical but benign features. Capsular involvement, by itself, is not indicative of cancer, but penetration of parenchyma by individual tumor cells or by clusters of tumor cells is. Morphologic atypia, such as enlarged, pleomorphic or hyperchromatic nuclei and frequent or abnormal mitoses, is indicative of carcinomatous transformation. Tumors with mild or focally limited cytologic atypia may be designated as atypical mixed tumor, indicating a suspicion of an increased likelihood of malignant transformation. Hypercellularity without abnormal cytomorphologic features is acceptable for benignity. In one study of 65 cases of benign mixed tumors with atypical features, those with prominent zones of hyalinization or at least moderate mitotic activity were more likely to develop carcinoma than those that lacked either of those features.[147] The rare finding of morphologically normal intravascular tumor has not correlated with metastatic potential.[148] When prominent abnormal cytologic features are confined within the capsule, the terms *intracapsular carcinoma, carcinoma in situ*, or *noninvasive carcinoma ex mixed tumor* are appropriate.[118,149] Recurrent mixed tumors often are multinodular, but these foci are usually discrete, circumscribed, and without cytologic atypia.

Although some claim usefulness, immunohistochemical studies in general have not proved particularly helpful in separating mixed tumors from other types of salivary gland tumors because of similar immunoreactivity of neoplastic cells among many types of benign

and malignant salivary gland tumors.[150,151] Although coexpression of cytokeratin and smooth muscle actin supports myoepithelial differentiation, other tumor types have a myoepithelial element that immunostains similarly.

Prognosis and treatment: Studies have shown that enucleated mixed tumors of the parotid have a high recurrence rate.[152–155] There is controversy, however, over whether superficial (lateral) parotidectomy or extracapsular dissection (lumpectomy) with a margin of normal tissue is most successful in controlling the tumor and minimizing surgical complications. Both show similar recurrence rates in the range of 0 to 8%.[156–165] With either procedure, great care is needed to prevent surgical compromise of the tumor margin. Recurrence increases the risk of facial nerve injury from additional surgery. Further, recurrent mixed tumors typically are associated with scar tissue that may be adhesive to the facial nerve, complicating dissection. Total parotidectomy and excision of the scar tissue with preservation of the facial nerve are recommended for recurrent tumor.[166–171] In a large series of recurrent mixed tumors, Phillips and Olsen[172] reported recurrence rates of 32.5%, 7.1%, and 1.6% after one, two and three operations, respectively, and total or partial facial paralysis in 13.5% and 5.5%.

Submandibular gland mixed tumors are treated by complete resection of the gland.[166] In the minor glands, mixed tumors seem to have little propensity for recurrence. Chau and Radden[173] found no recurrences among 27 cases despite many of the tumors having been treated by excisional biopsy. Complete excision with a rim of normal tissue is recommended.

Cytopathology of mixed tumor (pleomorphic adenoma)

As noted previously, a substantial majority of aspirates will represent this entity. The diagnosis is usually straightforward.

Smears contain quantitatively variable combinations of three components (Figs 23.4 and 23.5). Small cuboidal duct cells form flat sheets, glandular associations, trabeculae or branching tissue fragments. In most cases, they are cytologically uniform, but moderate pleomorphism is common in a minority of cells.[174] Squamous metaplasia, oncocytic change, mucin production, or sebaceous differentiation occur.

The epithelial elements of mixed tumor are complex and diverse and not very specific. The chondromyxoid matrix is a more specific and helpful feature (Figs 23.6 and 23.7). On fixed smears, it is pale cyanophilic and closely resembles the chondroid material as it appears in histologic sections. In air-dried preparations, it is metachromatic and fibrillary. The latter feature often manifests as frayed edges. Myoepithelial cells sequestered within the matrix are well visualized on Papanicolaou-stained slides, where they appear spindled or stellate, with small dense nuclei. They are often widely dispersed through abundant matrix, which imparts a distinctly chondro-osseous appearance to tissue particles. In air-dried preparations, cells have pale smudgy blue outlines, being largely obscured by the densely staining matrix. Despite the difficulty in visualizing these cells on air-dried smears, the appearance of these tissue particles is characteristic and diagnostic. When the matrix is scanty, the risk of an incorrect diagnosis increases considerably. Identification of small amounts of this material is facilitated by review of air-dried, Romanowsky-stained slides, where its presence is trumpeted by bright metachromasia rather than the muted translucent quality in fixed preparations.[175]

Free-lying myoepithelial cells are associated with the duct cells or situated independently. They may be either spindled or plasma-

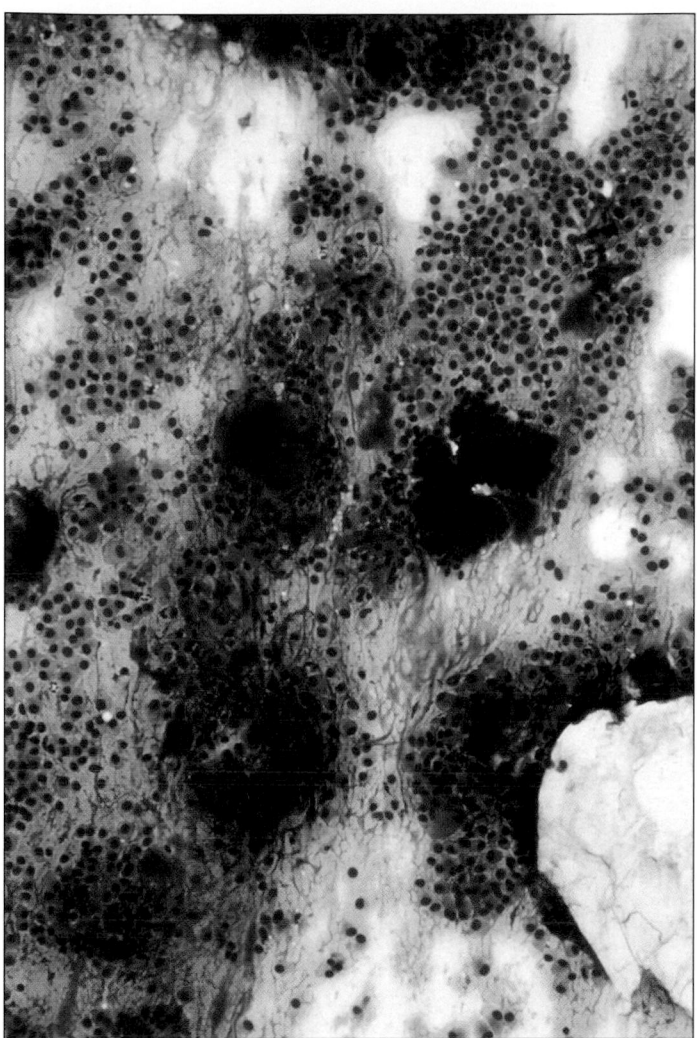

Fig. 23.4 This very low-magnification view of a pleomorphic adenoma aspirate shows all three components of this tumor's cytology. Fragments of deep purple metachromatic stromal material are set in the background showing large numbers of discohesive myoepithelial cells. The dark cellular clusters represent large fragments of ductal epithelium. Very little cytologic detail is apparent at this low magnification. However, this pattern is diagnostic of pleomorphic adenoma (40×).

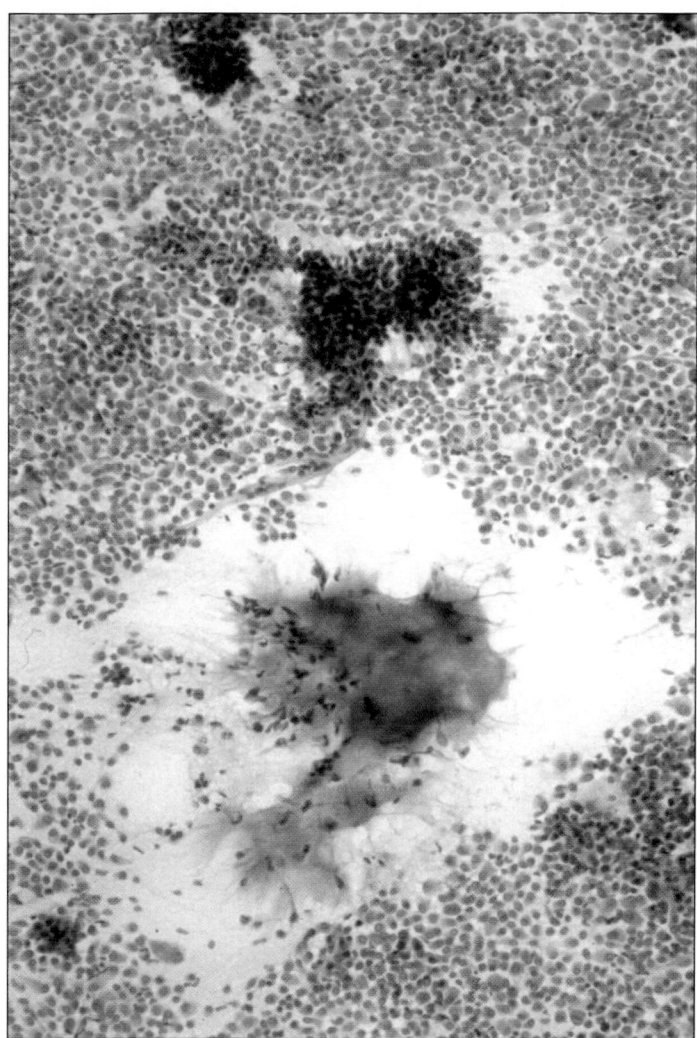

Fig. 23.5 This Papanicolaou-stained preparation shows a field similar to that seen in Figure 23.4. Fragments of chondroid matrix are readily apparent, as are darkly staining three-dimensional clusters of duct cells in a background of disassociated myoepithelial cells (40×).

cytoid (Figs 23.8–23.11). The latter are considerably dissociated and are sometimes mistaken for hematopoietic cells (see below). Myoepithelial cells can appear stellate when entrapped in the chondromyxoid matrix of the mixed tumor.

Other findings occasionally embellish the cytology of pleomorphic adenoma. Intranuclear cytoplasmic inclusions are similar to those in meningioma, paraganglioma, and papillary thyroid carcinoma.[176] Tyrosine is concentrated by the normal parotid gland, and its crystals are common in pleomorphic adenomas. These thin, needle-like or rosette-forming crystals are rare in FNA samples, however. They are not, as previously suggested, diagnostic of this tumor, having been identified in carcinoma ex pleomorphic adenoma, cysts, and polymorphous low-grade adenocarcinoma.[88,177,178]

Pleomorphic adenomas are less often affected by post-FNA infarction than Warthin's tumors.[51] Post-FNA infection is very rare, so other etiologies should be considered for these clinical findings.

Spontaneous infarction of a pleomorphic adenoma followed by FNA is an even less commonly described event. In the case described by Layfield and coworkers,[51] pain, tongue paresthesia, cystic change on CT scan, and necrosis with atypia on cytology all pointed toward malignancy. FNA diagnoses of squamous cell carcinoma or mucoepidermoid carcinoma were considered prior to excision.

Differential diagnostic considerations for pleomorphic adenoma: Any of pleomorphic adenoma's three cytologic components can suggest other diagnoses. The matrix can be mistaken for mucus, suggesting mucoepidermoid carcinoma, especially if squamous metaplasia is present. Cystic change with foam cells and a predominance of epithelium over matrix may heighten this concern. However, mucus lacks the fibrillary quality and staining density of true matrix material. The opposite occurs when the non-specific collagenous stoma of many lesions is thought to represent mixed tumor matrix. Thus, sialadenitis and sialolithiasis with fibrosis, metastases of basal cell carcinoma and squamous cell carcinoma, and

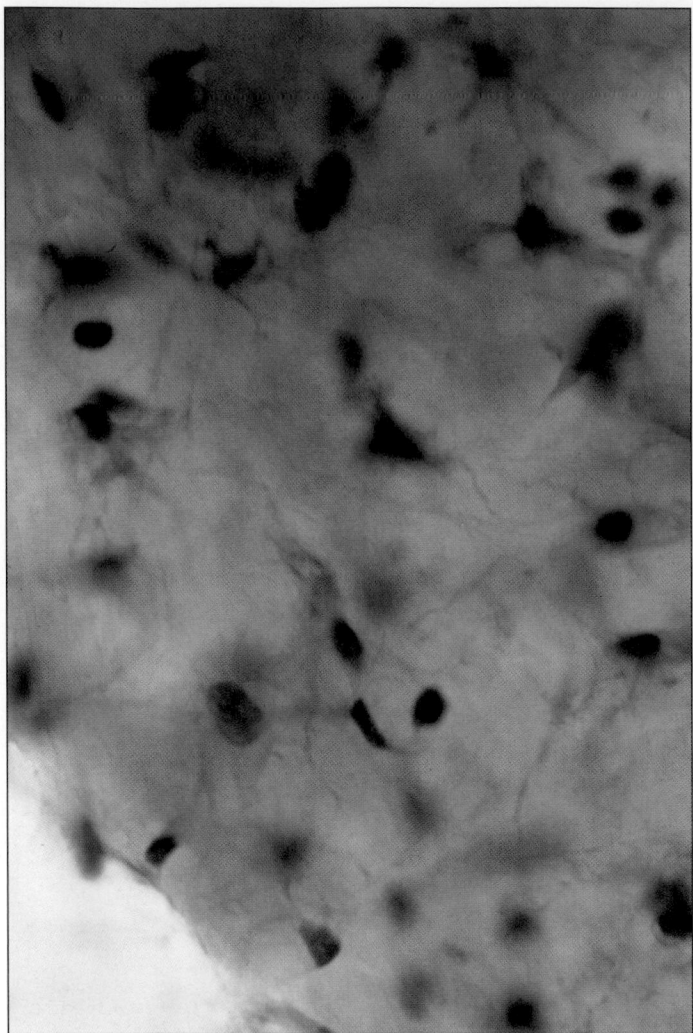

Fig. 23.6 This high-magnification illustration of Papanicolaou-stained chondroid matrix material from a pleomorphic adenoma shows dense matrix with scattered myoepithelial cells. The latter are stellate or spindle shaped and show extremely bland nuclear features (400×).

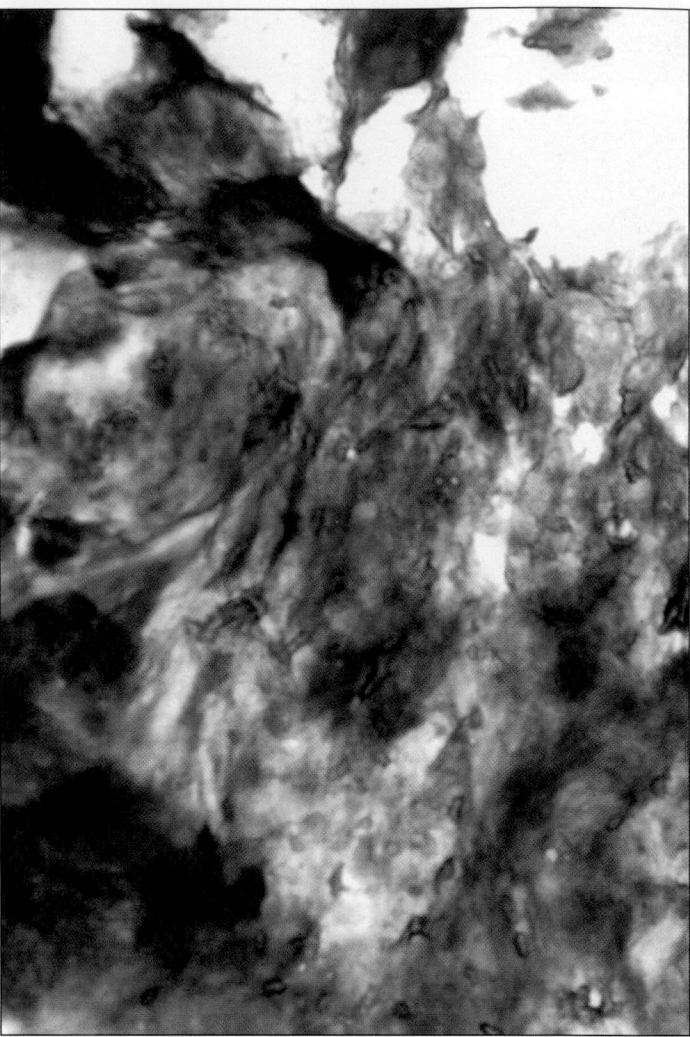

Fig. 23.7 This air-dried Diff–Quik-stained smear from a pleomorphic adenoma shows metachromatic fibrillary matrix material. Myoepithelial cells are embedded within this but their cytologic details are largely obscured by the dense matrix material (400×).

a single case of malignant peripheral nerve sheath tumor have all been interpreted as pleomorphic adenoma at the time of FNA.[76,150,179] In another instance, the necrosis of metastatic carcinoma was mistaken for this matrix material.[180] A chordoma that invades the parotid may also be mistaken for mixed tumor.[181]

Diagnostic problems related to the epithelial or myoepithelial cells are more common than those stemming from difficulties in assessment of stromal components and represent one of the most common problems leading to false-positive diagnoses in salivary gland FNA. Cells suggestive of malignancy or carcinoma ex pleomorphic adenoma feature enlarged irregular nuclei, clumped chromatin, and macronucleoli. These cells originate in either the ductal or the myoepithelial compartment. Also, highly vacuolated cells with sebaceous features suggest alternative interpretations. Whenever features (usually matrix material) suggest pleomorphic adenoma, these should override concern over focal atypia; in most instances, mixed tumor will be the correct interpretation. In our experience, mixed tumors with striking but prognostically meaningless atypia are relatively common, while carcinoma ex pleomorphic adenoma is

rarely encountered in FNA samples. Paradoxically, as discussed below, many examples of the latter give falsely negative cytology due to sampling error.

Pleomorphic adenomas are sometimes mistaken for adenoid cystic carcinoma. This usually occurs with hypercellular examples when the matrix is scanty or absent, when ductal lumen formation mimics cylinders, or when frankly cylindromatous foci are present[48,51,175,182] (Figs 23.12 and 23.13). These cellular mixed tumors approach the histology of basal cell adenomas in that they have scant foci of diagnostic chondromyxoid matrix. The term 'minimally pleomorphic adenoma' illustratively describes this histologic circumstance. Distinction of these cases from adenoid cystic carcinoma, particularly its sqlid variant, is very difficult at the time of FNA and will be discussed subsequently.

Polymorphous low-grade adenocarcinomas sometimes closely resemble pleomorphic adenoma.[183] The mass's location can be very helpful, as the former almost exclusively occurs in the minor salivary glands while the latter is often found in the major glands. When this malignancy does arise in the parotid, it is usually an element

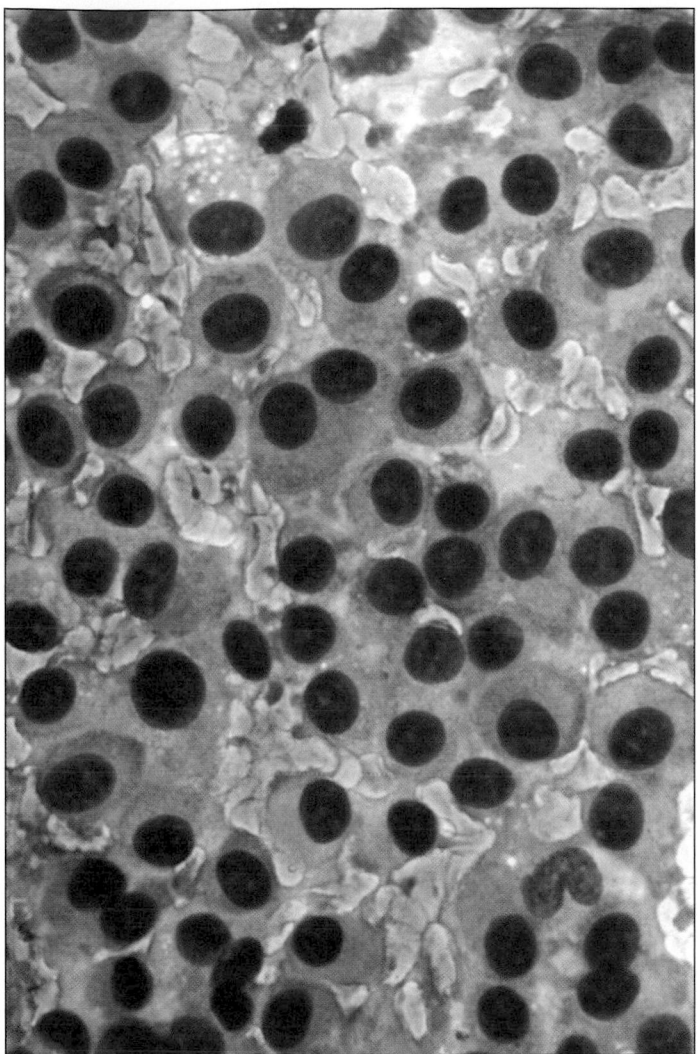

Fig. 23.8 These plasmacytoid myoepithelial cells lie singly, feature eccentric nuclei with bland chromatin, and show a moderate amount of cytoplasm (400×).

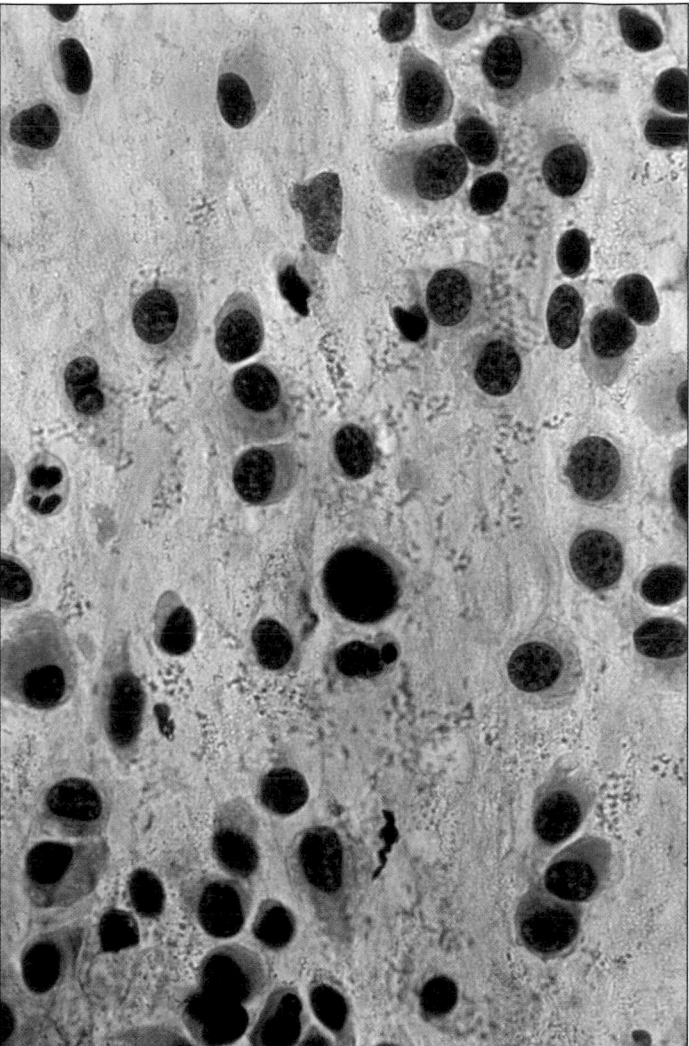

Fig. 23.9 In this Papanicolaou-stained preparation, plasmacytoid myoepithelial cells vary somewhat in size and shape and feature dense nuclei and a higher apparent nucleocytoplasmic ratio than appreciated in air dried material from the same case (400×).

of carcinoma ex pleomorphic adenoma. Epithelial-myoepithelial carcinoma may have mixed tumor-like foci, necessitating several FNA samples.[101]

Spindled myoepithelial cells cytologically resemble smooth muscle cells and may suggest a differential diagnosis that includes myoepithelioma and malignant myoepithelioma. Some myoepithelial cells are plasmacytoid, and this appearance can be very striking in air-dried smear preparations, where they have been mistaken for plasmacytoma or plasmacytoid malignant lymphoma. In some cases, individual cells are large and multinucleated and very suggestive of malignancy were it not for their occurrence in what is by other criteria a pleomorphic adenoma.

These descriptions of difficulties that occasionally attend the cytologic diagnosis of pleomorphic adenoma emphasize not only the complexity and variability of this neoplasm but also the need to base definitive cytologic diagnoses on as many criteria as possible. It has been suggested that the frequent positivity of cells within the chondromyxoid matrix of mixed tumors with immunostains for GFAP

may form the basis for resolution of some diagnostic difficulties related to myoepithelial cells.[150,184] Furthermore, positivity of pleomorphic adenoma epithelia for the breast antigen GCDFP-15 (gross cystic disease fluid protein) might be exploited to exclude diagnoses of polymorphous low-grade adenocarcinoma and adenoid cystic carcinoma, both of which are expected to be negative for this marker.[185]

MYOEPITHELIOMA

Myoepithelioma is a benign tumor composed of sheets and islands of various proportions of spindle, plasmacytoid, epithelioid, and clear cells that exhibit myoepithelial but not ductal differentiation.[186–189] It represents one end of the spectrum of mixed tumor and has a similar biologic behavior. Distinction between mixed tumor and myoepithelioma is primarily academic, but awareness of this entity can prevent misdiagnosis as malignant epithelial and mesenchymal neoplasms.

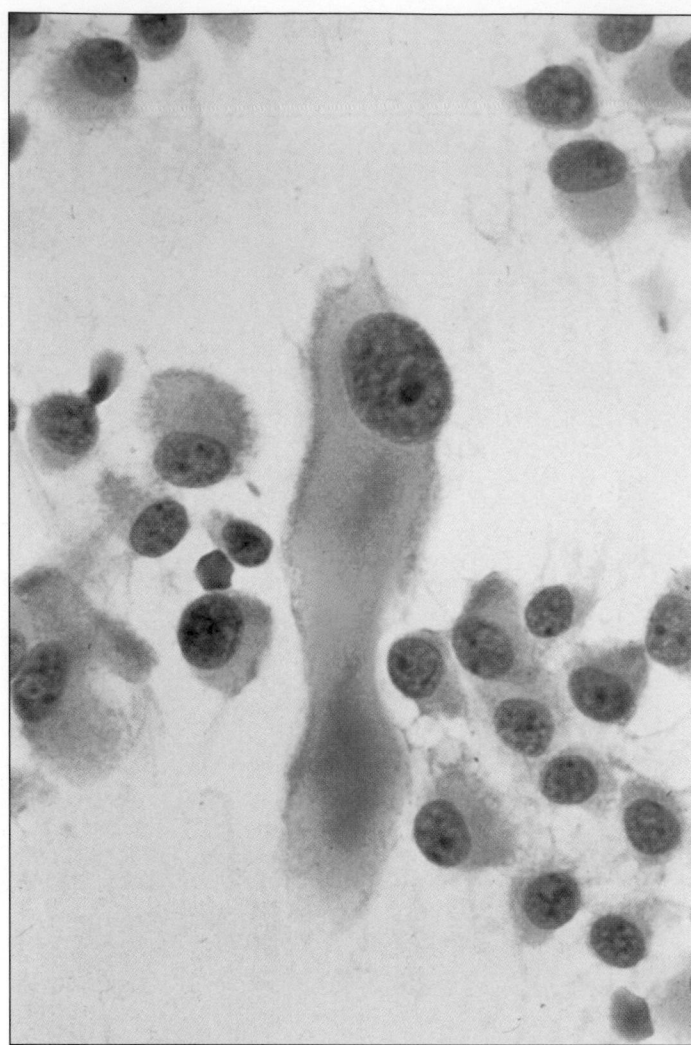

Fig. 23.10 The background of this smear shows large numbers of discohesive plasmacytoid myoepithelial cells. A single very large cell with abundant cytoplasm and a prominent nucleolus is also present. This degree of myoepithelial cell atypia is of no concern in a pleomorphic adenoma aspirate (400×).

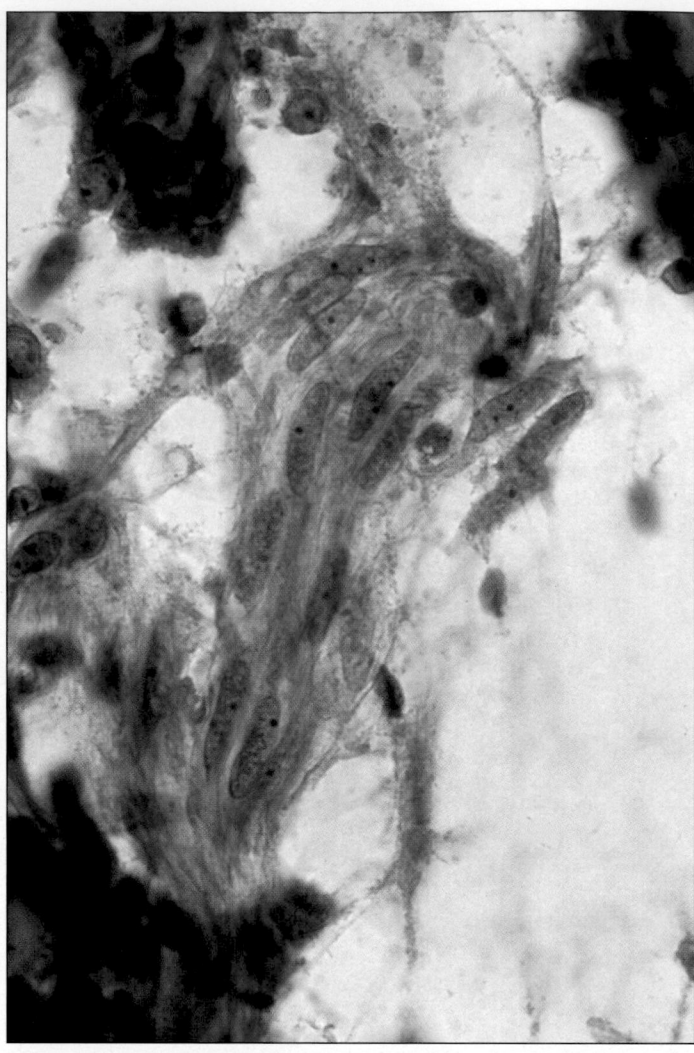

Fig. 23.11 This Papanicolaou-stained preparation shows spindled myoepithelial cells. This can lead to consideration of a pure myoepithelioma or other low-grade spindle cell proliferations. However, also present about the periphery of this illustration are cohesive three-dimensional clusters of benign ductal epithelial cells. The presence of both components indicates a pleomorphic adenoma (400×).

Spindle and epithelioid cell predominant myoepitheliomas are often hypercellular and have limited myxoid or mucoid stroma. Plasmacytoid cells are loosely cohesive and often surrounded by abundant hematoxyphilic mucoid stroma (Fig. 23.14). The plasmacytoid cells are round to ovoid and have abundant eosinophilic, so-called hyaline cytoplasm, and eccentrically placed nuclei, which are slightly pyknotic with small nucleoli.

Cytopathology of myoepithelioma

In needle aspiration material, the cells of myoepithelioma may be spindled or, less commonly, hyaline (plasmacytoid).[190,191] The cytology of these cells is identical to that illustrated for mixed tumor. These cells often lack ultrastructural or immunocytochemical evidence of myoepithelial differentiation.[192] Cytologic distinction between myoepithelioma and pleomorphic adenoma is without clinical significance, but inclusion in the differential diagnosis may prevent serious diagnostic errors, especially in the setting of atypical plasmacytoid cells. Even though myoepithelioma is rare, it is more common than other spindle cell neoplasms in the parotid. One other primary lesion that may be encountered is cellular hemangioma.[193]

WARTHIN'S TUMOR (PAPILLARY CYSTADENOMA LYMPHOMATOSUM)

Warthin's tumor, or papillary cystadenoma lymphomatosum, is the second most common benign parotid salivary gland tumor and accounts for 4–11.2% of all salivary gland tumors.[2,10,11] Although rare examples of Warthin's tumor have been reported in sites other than the parotid gland,[194–197] nearly all Warthin's tumors occur in the parotid gland. Most involve the tail of the gland, but about 10% occur in the deep lobe.[194] In the United States, they account for about 13.6% of benign parotid tumors,[2] lower than that of several other

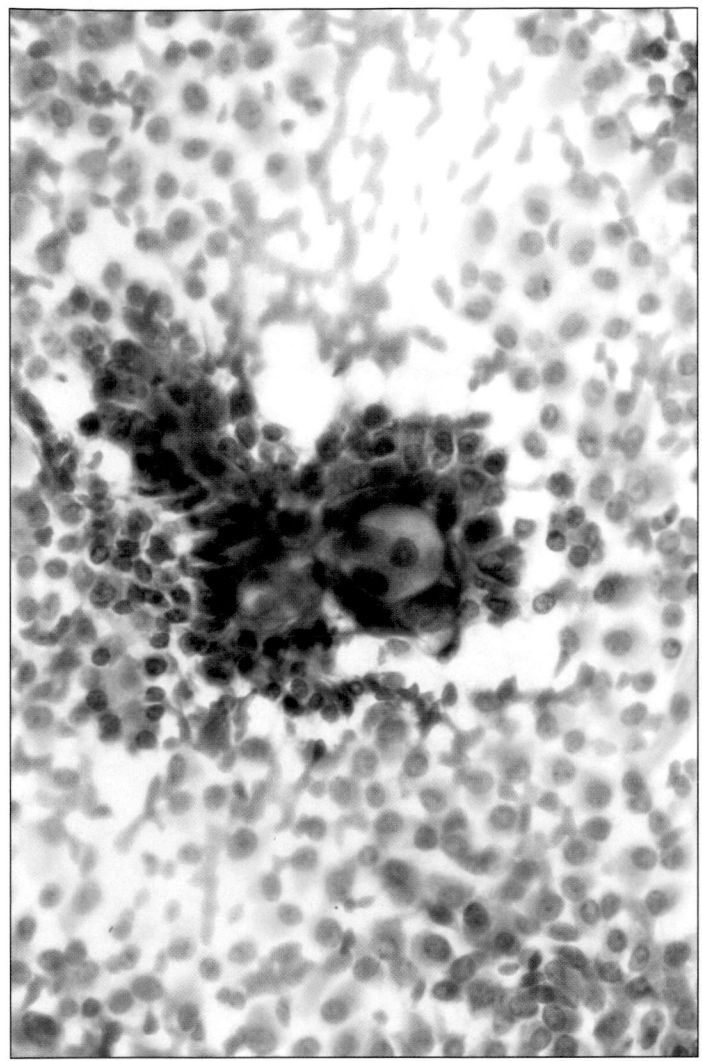

Fig. 23.12 This aspirate from a pleomorphic adenoma shows prominent ductal differentiation. The finding of small hyperchromatic uniform cells surrounding nonstaining or translucent spheres of extracellular material can be strongly evocative of adenoid cystic carcinoma. The background myoepithelial cells in this aspirate should lead to a correct interpretation (100×).

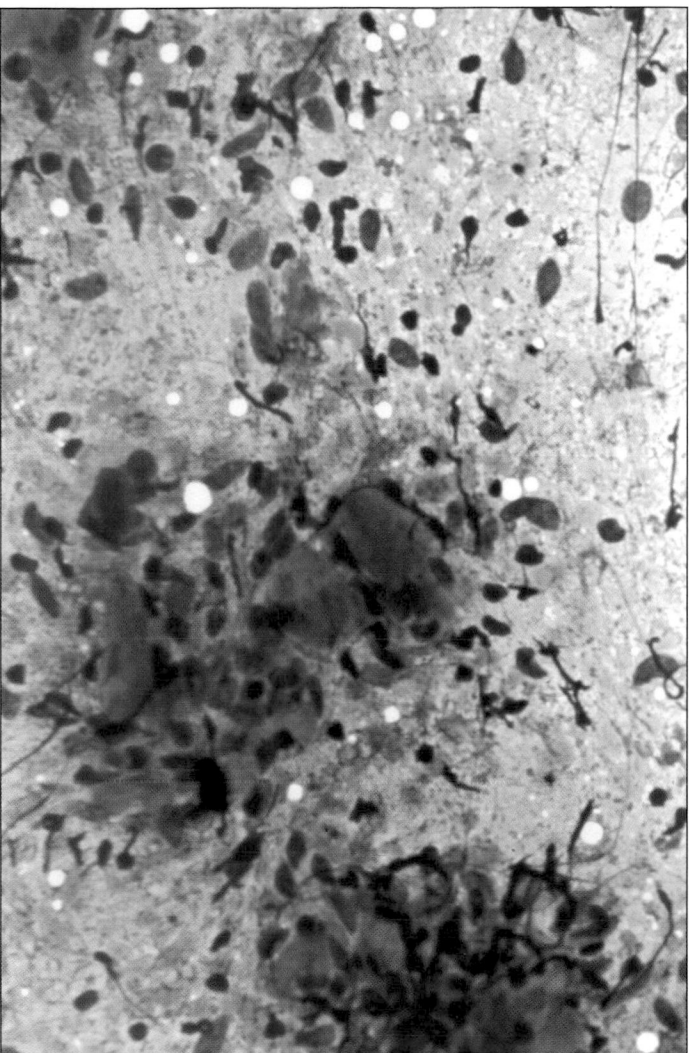

Fig. 23.13 This air-dried preparation shows small cells with uniform nuclei and scanty cytoplasm. These surround rounded fragments of metachromatic extracellular material in a pattern suggestive of possible adenoid cystic carcinoma. Examination of other portions of the aspirate for features diagnostic of pleomorphic adenoma is required to prevent an erroneous diagnosis (100×).

countries.[11,112,198–200] They have a relatively low incidence in blacks.[198]

The most popular pathogenetic concept is that Warthin's tumor develops from heterotopic salivary ducts within pre-existing intraparotid or paraparotid lymphoid tissue.[201] According to some, as many as 8% occur in paraparotid lymph nodes.[202,203] An alternative view is that the epithelium or epithelial product in Warthin's tumor incites a lymphocytic response.[204,205] In support of this proposal are several other types of salivary gland tumors that often have a prominent tumor-associated lymphoid proliferation.[81] This suggests a dependent relationship between the two elements, and an antigen-induced response is plausible.[206,207] The B- and T-cell populations are polyclonal but in some lesions both show oligoclonal expansion.[208]

Clinical features: Warthin's tumors are multicentric, synchronous or metachronous, and bilateral more often than any other salivary gland tumor.[209] About 12% of the patients develop more than one Warthin's tumor.[194,203] As many as six separate tumor foci have been

reported in a single patient, and in about one-quarter of the patients with multicentric tumors, the tumors were synchronous and bilateral.[194] Overall, Warthin's tumors are bilateral in 5–7.5% of patients.[198,210–212]

Male/female ratios of 26:1,[199] 10:1,[213] and 5:1[214] have been reported. However, recent studies claim a markedly reduced male predilection of between 1.1:1 and 1.6:1.[194,198,210,214–216] Recent evidence strongly suggests that the increasing relative incidence of Warthin's tumor in women parallels their increased smoking[216–218] and incidence of pulmonary carcinoma.[194] Compared with nonsmokers, smokers have eight times the risk of developing Warthin's tumor.[219]

In Armed Forces Institute of Pathology (AFIP) material, the average age of patients is about 62 years (range, 29 to 88 years) and is nearly identical for men and women. Warthin's tumors usually present as painless, sometimes fluctuant, swellings in the lower portion of the parotid gland, but pain is experienced by about 9% of patients.[198] These tumors are normally 2–4 cm in diameter but may achieve

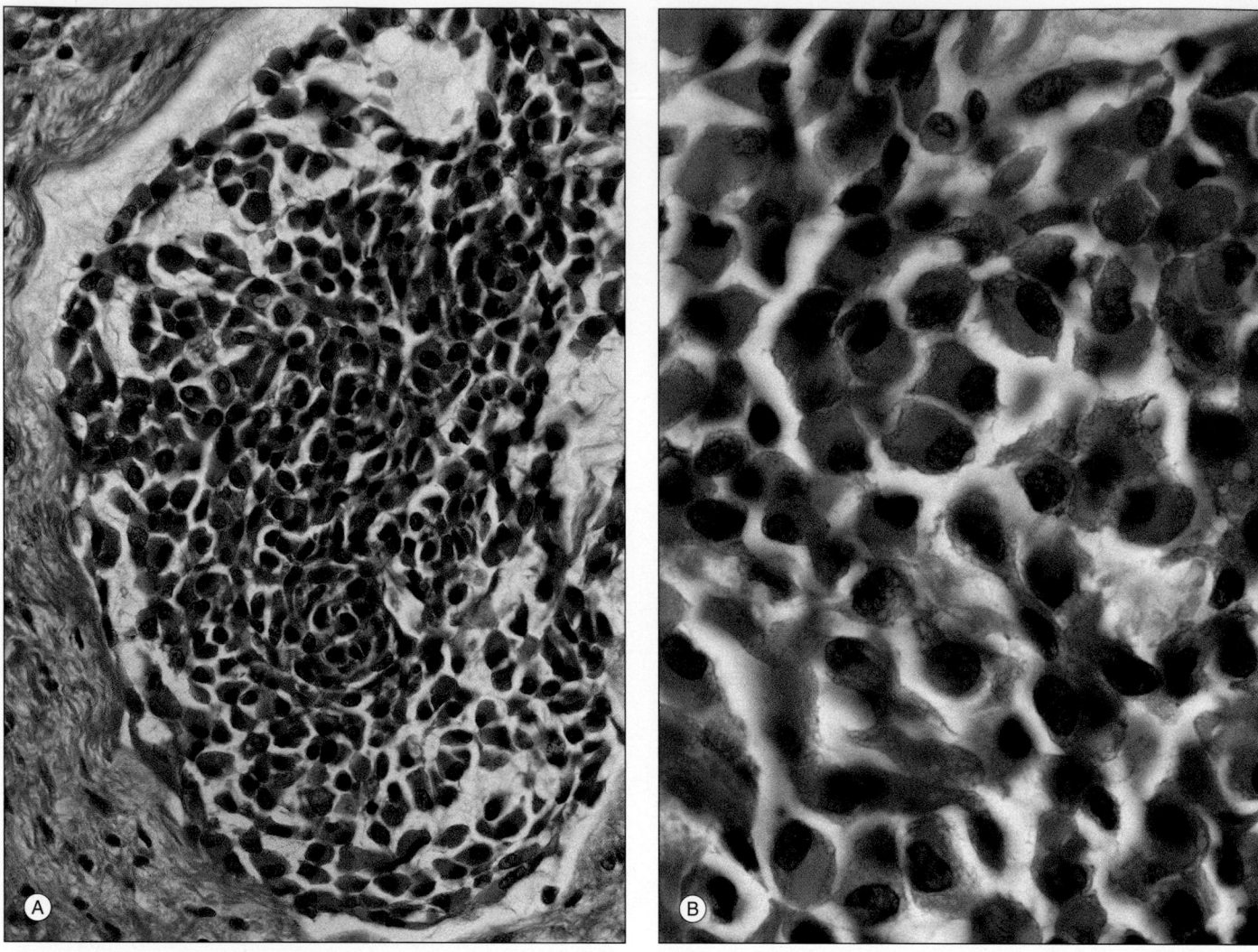

Fig. 23.14 Plasmacytoid myoepithelioma (**A**) of the hard palate reveals (**B**) aggregates of loosely cohesive cells that have eccentrically located nuclei and abundant cytoplasm.

considerable size.[220] Fluctuation sometimes suggests abscess or other inflammatory disorders. The average duration of the tumor is 21 months, but more than 40% are present less than 6 months.[198]

Warthin's tumor concentrates sodium pertechnetate and is amenable to scintigraphic examination.[221–225] However, oncocytomas also concentrate sodium pertechnetate.

Microscopic features: Grossly, parotidectomy specimens should be examined thoroughly for separate tumor foci.[194] The cut surface of Warthin's tumor reveals a variable number of cysts that exude clear, mucoid, or brown fluid or caseous semisolid debris.[226] Microscopically, Warthin's tumor is characterized by cystic spaces lined by a papillary proliferation of bilayered oncocytic epithelium whose supporting stroma is largely lymphoid tissue (Fig. 23.15). Luminal epithelium is tall columnar cells that have palisaded, ovoid nuclei, which are in the centers or apical ends of the cells. Cytoplasmic granularity is due to abundant mitochondria, which may be verified with PTAH stain or electron microscopy. Smaller basaloid cells are evident beneath and between the columnar cells. They are ovoid or triangular and often have fusiform nuclei arranged perpendicular to the long axis of the tall columnar cells. In more than one-half of the

tumors, the lymphoid element has well-formed germinal centers and distinct mantles. Some variation in the proportions of the epithelial and lymphoid components can be noted.[211] Occasionally, squamous, mucous, or sebaceous cells are found among the luminal columnar cells. Squamous metaplasia, necrosis, and fibrosis related to previous fine needle aspiration are sometimes present.[227]

In rare cases, squamous cell carcinoma[60,228–231] or other carcinomas[232–236] may arise from the epithelial component of Warthin's tumor. Similarly, lymphoma may arise or involve the lymphoid component.[237–240]

Differential diagnosis: Diagnostic difficulties occur when (1) other salivary gland lesions have a papillary oncocytic epithelial component; (2) Warthin's tumors have severe secondary reactive changes; and (3) other epithelial lesions have abundant lymphoid tissue associated with them. Papillary oncocytic cystadenoma resembles Warthin's tumor but usually arises from minor glands and lacks a well-organized lymphoid element. Fibrosis and squamous and mucinous metaplasia in infarcted Warthin's tumors resemble squamous cell and mucoepidermoid carcinoma. Outlines of necrotic, intracystic papillae of tall columnar and basal cells and absence of infiltrative growth are

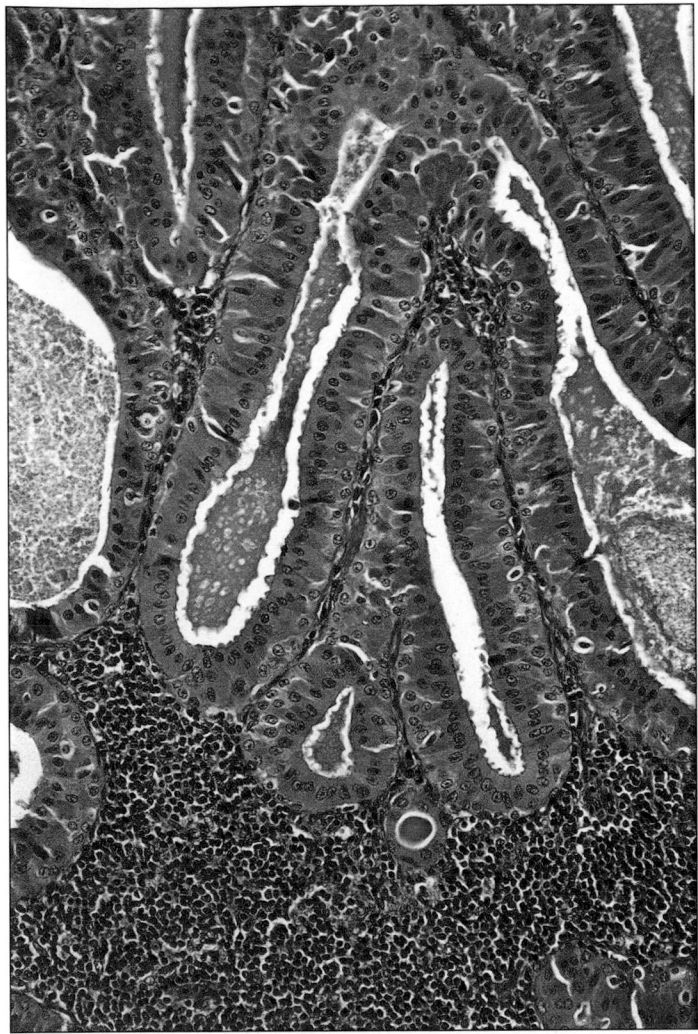

Fig. 23.15 Warthin's tumor with characteristic bilayered papillary oncocytic epithelium with prominent lymphoid element.

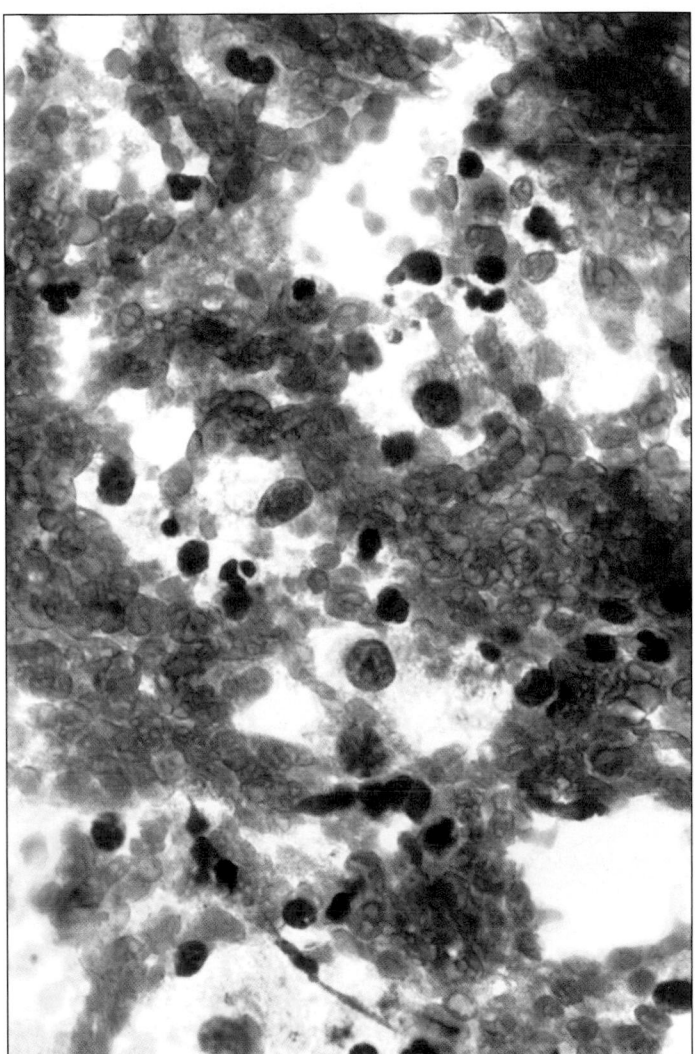

Fig. 23.16 This non-specific cyst-fluid background is usually the most prominent component in aspirates of Warthin's tumor. In addition to red blood cells, there are a few acute inflammatory cells and macrophages. Without lymphoid tissue and oncocytes, this represents a non-specific cyst fluid that could be aspirated from a wide variety of lesions (400×).

diagnostic. In addition to Warthin's tumor, parotid lesions that have a prominent lymphoid element and cystic configuration include lymphoepithelial cyst, human immunodeficiency virus (HIV)-related sialadenopathy, lymphadenoma, metastatic carcinoma, and tumor-associated lymphoid proliferation.[81] The epithelium of these lesions does not have the characteristic bilayered epithelium of Warthin's tumor.

Prognosis and treatment: Most recent studies indicate a recurrence rate of 2% or less.[198,210,211,241] Because of the propensity of Warthin's tumor to develop multifocal lesions, wide surgical exposure and careful inspection and palpation of parotid gland and paraparotid tissues have been recommended.[194] Concern for multifocal tumor has led some investigators to recommend total parotidectomy.[242] However, because of the risk of facial nerve paralysis and Frey's syndrome associated with parotidectomy, others recommend enucleation in cases in which the diagnosis is known preoperatively and if the location is amenable to such a procedure.[210,241]

Cytopathology of Warthin's tumor

At physical examination, these tumors resemble lipomas, or are boggy because of the fluid-filled cystic spaces. Most aspirates yield a small amount of very dark fluid that should be concentrated by centrifugation (Fig. 23.16). In some cases, several smears of a centrifuge pellet had only rare diagnostic oncocyte clusters. Diagnostic aspirates of Warthin's tumor have both oncocytic epithelium and lymphocytes (Figs 23.17 and 23.18). These elements are scattered through a cyst-fluid background of histiocytes and a few inflammatory cells. Rarely, the epithelium of papillary tissue fragments overlies lymphoid tissue in a manner similar to histologic preparations (Fig. 23.19). Nondiagnostic aspirates have non-specific cyst fluid, with or without lymphoid tissue, without oncocytes.

Oncocytes usually lie in flat cohesive sheets. Their nuclei are relatively large and variable, in a manner analogous to similar cells in other lesions, such as chronic lymphocytic thyroiditis. Nucleoli are sometimes prominent, but these changes do not indicate malignancy.[43,227,243] The abundant cytoplasm of these cells is usually sufficient to give them a low nuclear:cytoplasmic ratio. The cytoplasm appears dense in air-dried smears. On fixed smears it is

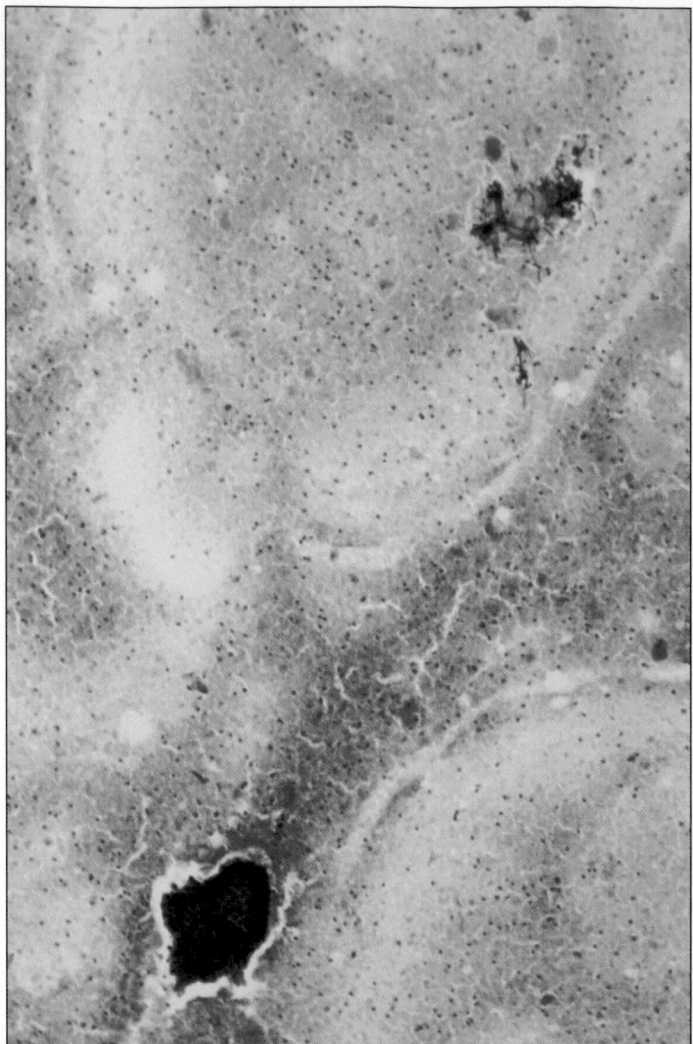

Fig. 23.17 This very low-magnification image shows a background of cyst fluid with a slightly mucoid appearance. At one edge a darkly staining cluster of oncocytes contrasts with a smaller fragment of lymphoid tissue at the opposite end of the illustration (40×).

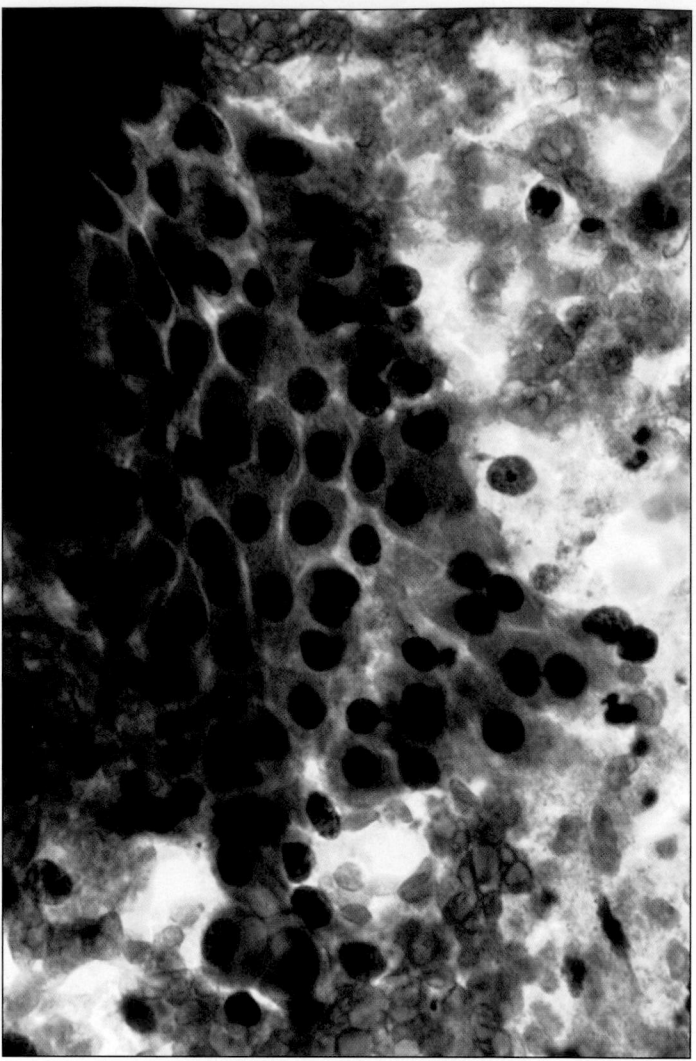

Fig. 23.18 In a background of cyst fluid similar to that illustrated previously, this image shows a cohesive flat sheet of oncocytes with abundant granular cytoplasm and relatively uniform nuclei (400×).

finely granular. The eosinophilia of oncocytes in hematoxylin and eosin-stained sections may not be recapitulated in Papanicolaou-stained FNA samples. Instead, they are often cyanophilic, so that eosinophilia is not a requirement for designating cells as oncocytic. Epithelial cells in Warthin's tumor sometimes also have sebaceous, squamous, mucinous, or pleomorphic adenoma-like foci.[82] Overall diagnostic accuracy in one recent series was 70.4%, with a 10% rate of nondiagnostic aspirates; no false-positive or false-suspicious interpretations occurred.[243]

The lymphoid tissue has mostly single small cells with densely hyperchromatic nuclei and a thin rim of basophilic to cyanophilic cytoplasm. Other manifestations, such as crushed cell aggregates ('lymphoid tangles') and detached cytoplasmic droplets ('lympho-glandular bodies'), are as described in lymph node cytology. The lymphocytic tissue of Warthin's tumors has less polymorphism and fewer germinal center fragments than expected in smears from benign lymphoepithelial lesions.[244] In some instances, however, it is polymorphous and resembles more conventional examples of

reactive lymphoid tissue. Rarely, a relatively monotonous field of small cells leads to consideration of malignant lymphoma.

The diagnosis is straightforward when each of these elements is in place. If oncocytes are prominent, an oncocytic neoplasm is a consideration,[73] especially since the latter sometimes contains various amounts of lymphoid stroma.[245] Conversely, cyst fluid with debris and lymphocytes is suggestive of Warthin's tumor, but diagnosis is not possible without positive identification of oncocytic epithelium since the entire diagnostic spectrum of cystic salivary gland lesions is raised (see Tables 23.3 and 23.4). Repeat aspiration often helps since most Warthin's tumors are only partially cystic. It is an error to interpret non-specific fluids as benign cysts without other compelling evidence. Furthermore, neutrophils in the fluid do not automatically connote an infection or other inflammatory process.

Warthin's tumors sometimes have foam cells and mucinous metaplasia, as well as precipitated material that can resemble extracellular mucus. Thus, oncocyte-deficient examples are confused

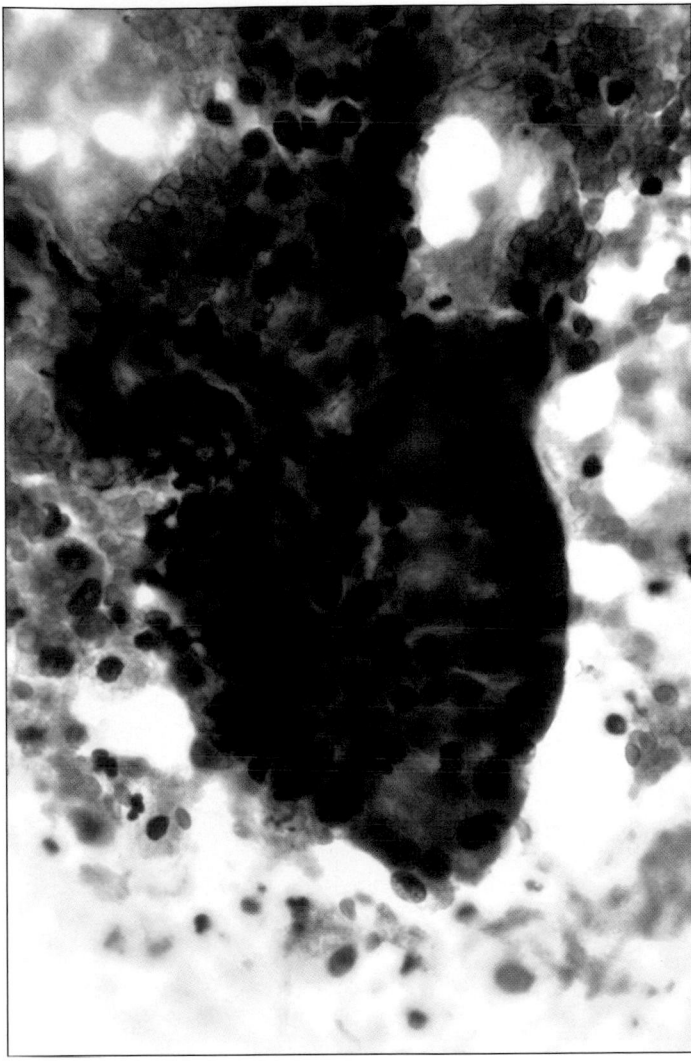

Fig. 23.19 This Warthin's tumor aspirate shows a background of cyst fluid. There is a large tissue fragment with layers of oncocytes overlying darkly staining lymphoid tissue. The latter is somewhat crushed and has the appearance of a lymphoid tangle. This tissue particle recapitulates the histologic appearance of Warthin's tumor (400×).

The cells of acinic cell carcinoma closely resemble oncocytes. Furthermore, lymphocytes and cystic change occur in this carcinoma, furthering its similarity to Warthin's tumor in aspirate smears.[43,248] This is an uncommon but very difficult problem, as is the distinction between other oncocytic lesions and acinic cell carcinoma.

Oncocytic lesions, including rare malignant examples, and oncocytic carcinoma are discussed below, where they are placed in the context of other large cell epithelial neoplasms of low nuclear grade, as summarized in Table 23.3.

BASAL CELL ADENOMA

Basal cell adenoma is a benign neoplasm dominated by basaloid epithelial cells and a uniform, monomorphous architecture. It lacks the myxochondroid tissue and cellular characteristics of mixed tumor. One study suggests a histogenesis from basal cells of the striated ducts.[249]

Clinical features: The reported incidence is uniformly low but has varied from less than 1% to 4% of all primary salivary gland tumors.[12,250–252] Over 75% occur in the parotid gland while another 5% arise in the submandibular gland. About 6 % develop in the upper lip, and they are quite rare in other intraoral locations.[250,253] The mean age of patients is 58 years with a peak incidence in the seventh decade of life. They are extremely rare in children.[250,254,255] Female patients predominate over male patients except among patients with the membranous type of basal cell adenoma.[253,256,257] Swelling is the most constant clinical sign or symptom.

A diathesis of skin eccrine tumors and basal cell adenomas of the parotid gland has been observed in several patients.[257–260] Most of the basal cell adenomas associated with the diathesis have been the membranous type, and most of the skin tumors have been dermal cylindromas.

Most tumors are less than 3.0 cm in diameter at the time of excision and sharply circumscribed. Except for some membranous types, which may be multinodular, most basal cell adenomas are single, circumscribed masses. In the parotid gland, they usually have a well-defined capsule, but encapsulation is less often grossly apparent in intraoral tumors. The cut surface is usually homogeneous and gray-white, tan-white, pink-red, or brown. A few tumors are cystic.

Microscopic features: The 'monomorphous' character of these tumors is a result of uniform, monotonous growth patterns. Electron microscopic and immunohistochemical studies have found that basal, ductal, and myoepithelial cell differentiation occurs to variable degrees in basal cell adenomas, just as in other types of salivary gland tumors,[258,261–267] but by light microscopy, a basaloid appearance predominates. The cells are uniform and small with pale eosinophilic to amphophilic cytoplasm, indistinct cell borders, and round to oval nuclei. There are frequently both dark and light basaloid cells. The dark cells have less cytoplasm and more basophilic nuclei. While the light cells usually predominate, the dark cells give the tissue a more basophilic appearance and are often clustered near the peripheral, stromal interface, where there is often palisading of the nuclei of the epithelial cells (Fig. 23.20). Although generally few in number, cuboidal ductal cells that surround small lumens are evident in most basal cell adenomas.

Based on a predominating pattern, basal cell adenomas can be subtyped into solid, trabecular, tubular, and membranous categories. Except for the membranous type, the specific subtype does not imply any predicable variation in biologic behavior. In the solid pattern, the tumor cells are arranged as large, nodular sheets, broad bands, or small nodules, which may be juxtaposed or separated by

with low-grade mucoepidermoid carcinoma.[244,246,247] When lymphocytes are prominent, these cases can suggest chronic inflammation, follicular hyperplasia, or low-grade malignant lymphoma.[62,73] Conversely, it is easy to mistake small cell lymphoma for the much more common Warthin's tumor. Except for cell marker studies, very little can be done to resolve these diagnostic problems prior to surgical excision.

Squamous metaplasia is common in Warthin's tumor. In some cases, this is thought to be related to papillary tip infarcts and is associated with considerable cytologic atypia that mimics squamous cell carcinoma or mucoepidermoid carcinoma.[43,93,94,227] DiPalma and coworkers[227] suggest that this alteration occurs not only de novo but as a sequela of needle aspiration. High standards in cyst aspiration and cytopreparation and a search for even a few oncocytic cells is required. When there are only a few isolated atypical cells, caution about the diagnosis of carcinoma in a cyst fluid is indicated. Repeat aspirations should be used liberally in doubtful cases.

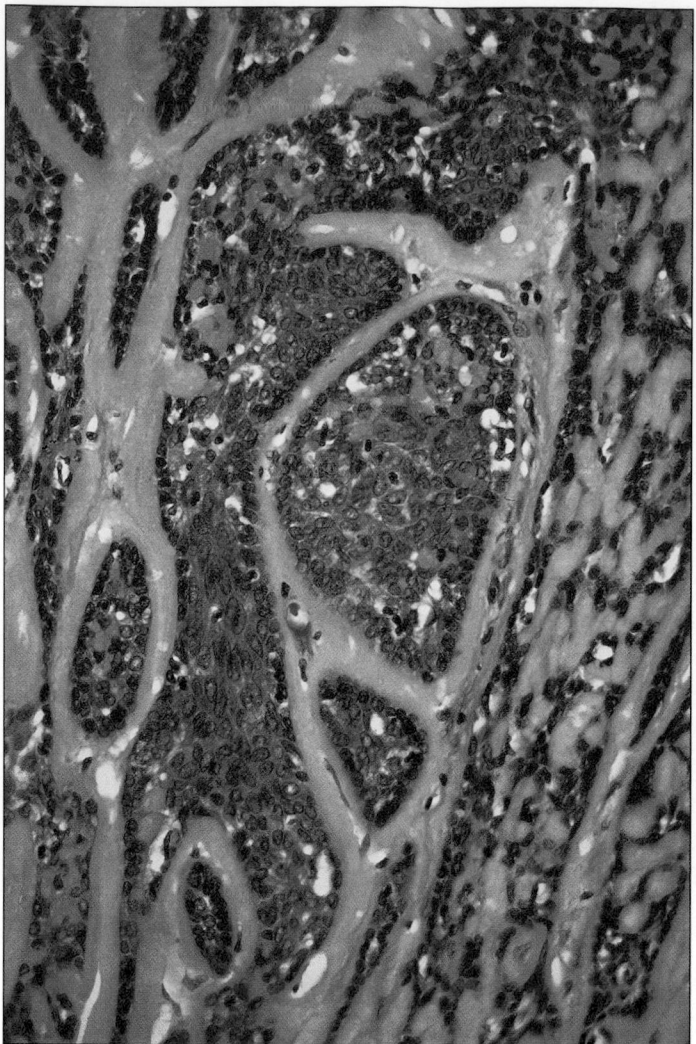

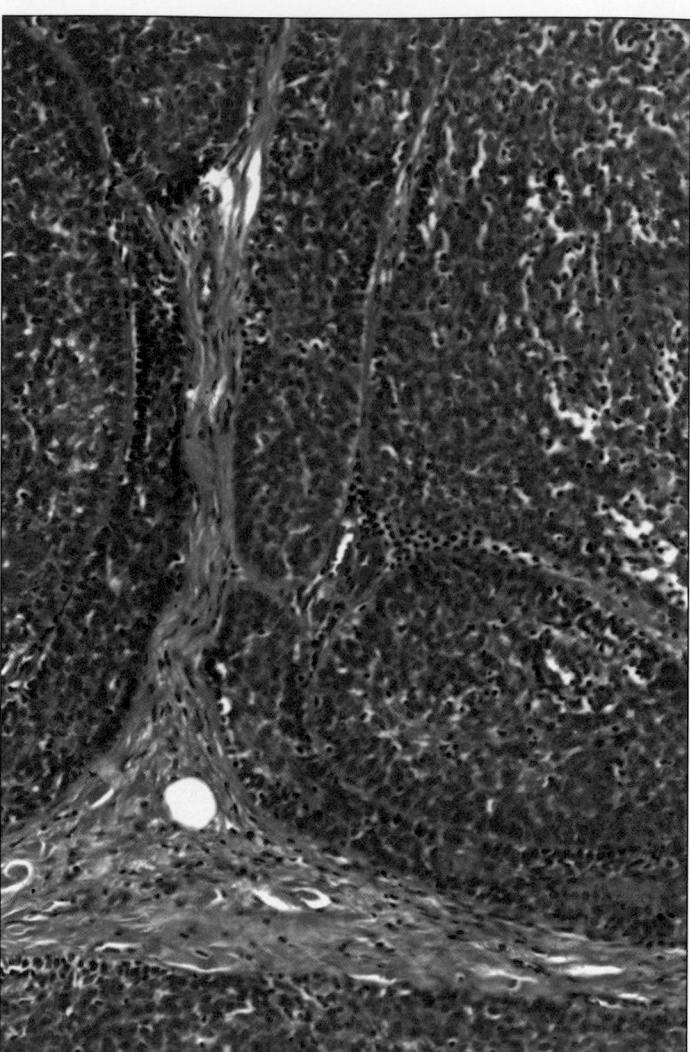

Fig. 23.20 In this membranous type of basal cell adenoma, some cells, which are mostly located toward the periphery of the epithelial islands, have small, very basophilic nuclei and scant cytoplasm. There is some palisading of the nuclei of epithelial cells along the stromal interface. More numerous are larger cells with large, pale staining nuclei, some of which have one or two small, basophilic nucleoli. Conspicuous hyaline membranes of basal lamina surround and separate irregularly shaped nests of basaloid cells, and multiple, small, round, intercellular hyaline droplets are present within the epithelial islands.

Fig. 23.21 In this solid type of basal cell adenoma, the basaloid epithelial cells form irregular nodules that are closely apposed but focally slightly separated by a fibrous stroma.

fibrous tissue (Fig. 23.21). Rounded foci of epidermoid cells, sometimes keratinized, occasionally are found among the basaloid cells. The stroma is usually moderately to markedly collagenous. In the trabecular type, basaloid cells form an interlacing network of narrow bands. Palisaded nuclei are frequently less conspicuous, and small, dark cells are typically fewer than in the solid type. In the tubular type, which is the least common, duct cell differentiation is most prominent. Since the trabecular pattern often has small cysts or ductal lumens, some investigators group the trabecular and tubular types into one *tubulotrabecular type* (Fig. 23.22).[253] The stroma in the trabecular and tubular types is often less collagenous than in the solid type and in some tumors is very loose. Cystic degeneration within basal cell adenomas varies from none to, rarely, marked.

The membranous type of basal cell adenoma is characterized by prominent intercellular droplets and thick bands at the periphery of the basaloid cell islands of eosinophilic, PAS-positive, hyalinized basal lamina (Fig. 23.20). The membranous type is frequently multinodular, and the stroma is usually densely collagenous.

Very little cytogenetic data are available for this group of tumors. Choi et al.[260] found loss of heterozygosity at chromosome 16q12-13 (CYLD), which has been associated with dermal cylindromas, in 80% of membranous-type basal cell adenomas studied, including two familial cases. Germline CYLD mutation may account for the diathesis of eccrine cylindromas and salivary basal cell adenomas. El-Naggar et al. identified loss of heterozygosity on chromosomes 8p22 and 19q13.4 in one of four monomorphic adenomas studied.[268] Basal cell adenomas do not overexpress p53.[269]

Differential diagnosis: Mixed tumor, adenoid cystic carcinoma, and basal cell adenocarcinoma are the principal entities to be differentiated from basal cell adenoma of salivary gland. Basal cell adenomas are often markedly similar to dermal eccrine tumors, but the site of a tumor should resolve the dermal versus salivary origin

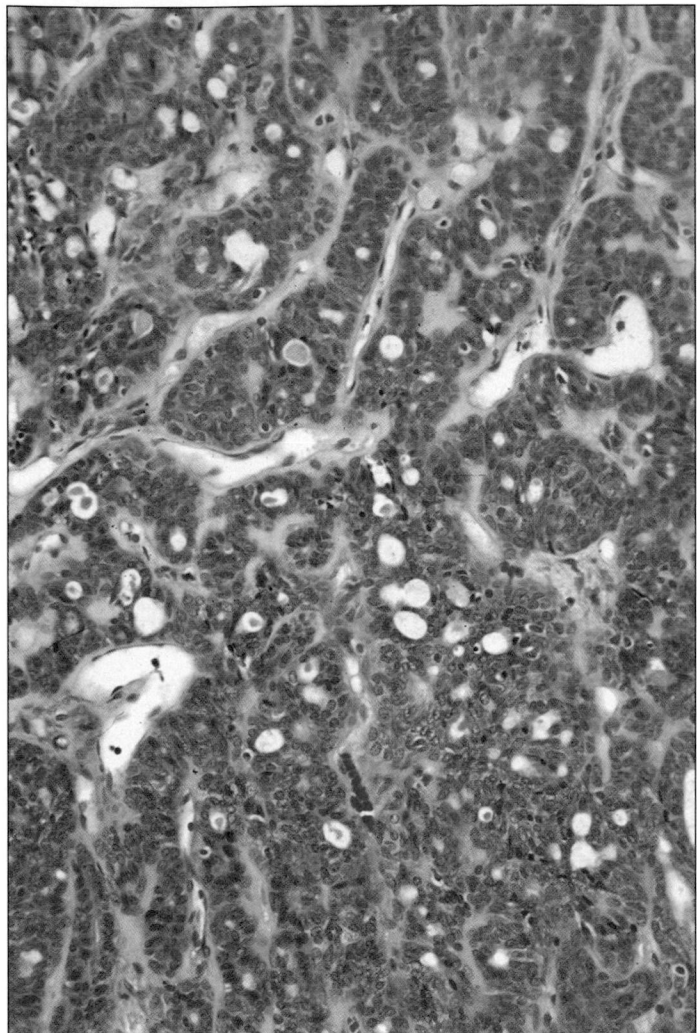

Fig. 23.22 Many small lumens are evident within the trabecular cords of basaloid cells in this tubulotrabecular-type tumor. In contrast to the solid and membranous patterns, the stroma associated with the trabecular and tubular patterns is often loose, scantily collagenous tissue.

question in most cases. Chondromyxoid tissue readily distinguishes mixed tumors and is absent from basal cell adenomas. In addition, the plasmacytoid and spindled myoepithelial cells characteristic of cellular mixed tumors and myoepitheliomas are absent from basal cell adenomas. Unlike mixed tumors, the boundaries between the epithelial tumor cells and the stroma are usually quite distinct in basal cell adenomas. The characteristic cribriform pattern of adenoid cystic carcinoma is rare and only a minor component in basal cell adenoma. Basal cell adenomas lack cells with pale to clear cytoplasm and irregular, angular-shaped nuclei that are common and characteristic in adenoid cystic carcinomas. Infiltration and perineural invasion definitely distinguish adenoid cystic carcinoma from basal cell adenoma. Basal cell adenocarcinoma is the malignant counterpart to basal cell adenoma, and its distinction from basal cell adenoma is primarily based upon infiltration of parotid parenchyma and adjacent tissues such as fat, muscle, skin, bone, nerves, and vessels. Basal cell adenocarcinomas often, but not always, have an increased mitotic count.

Prognosis and treatment: The prognosis is good. Except for the membranous type, the recurrence rate is near zero when conser-vatively but adequately excised. In contrast, the recurrence rate for the membranous subtype has been reported to be 25–37%.[253,260] Its tendency to be multifocal and unencapsulated may make complete excision more difficult.

Malignant transformation of benign basal cell adenomas has been reported,[253,270] but due to the bland cytologic features of most basal cell adenocarcinomas, it is very difficult to determine whether a malignant basal cell tumor arose within a pre-existing benign basal cell tumor or de novo.

Cytopathology of basal cell adenoma

As noted previously, basal cell adenomas (BCA) are histologically subclassified based on architectural features, but each is composed of similar small uniform cells that lack striking atypia. Some examples of pleomorphic adenoma have only small foci of chondromyxoid matrix and otherwise resemble basal cell adenomas. Such cases have been illustratively designated as 'minimally pleomorphic adenomas' to explain the cytologic diagnosis of basal cell adenoma to their ultimate histopathologic classification as mixed tumors.

FNA of BCA has uniform small blue cells associated with variable amounts of collagenous stroma (Figs 23.23–23.25).[271–274] The solid variant may lack the stromal component.[180] Sometimes, single cells and naked nuclei are numerous. Occasional features include basosquamous whorls and sebaceous differentiation.[82] Spontaneous infarction has been described.[69]

The interface between the tumor cells and the collagenous stroma is irregular, with frayed stromal filaments interdigitating among the peripheral cells in a tissue particle (Fig. 23.26). Furthermore, the stroma often contains spindle cell nuclei or small capillaries. These features are important for distinguishing basal cell adenoma from the cribriform architecture of adenoid cystic carcinoma (ACC). The latter is also characterized by uniform small blue cells associated with stroma. In both neoplasms, the stroma is brightly metachromatic in air-dried smears, and basal cell adenomas often lead to incorrect diagnoses of ACC in FNA material.[78,271] The extracellular basement membrane material in ACC has a very sharp, linear interface with the surrounding cells and is always acellular and avascular. Thus, it has been suggested that features of the cell–stroma interface are useful in distinguishing between basal cell adenoma and ACC. Unfortunately, this criterion has very limited utility since many ACC aspirates have little of the typical matrix. Furthermore, the desmoplastic stroma that is associated with invasion mimics the cell–stroma interface of BCA. These observations are especially true when the solid or anaplastic variant of ACC is considered. Some authors suggest that ACC can be recognized if sufficient attention is given to subtle nuclear features, but both BCA and ACC are composed of uniform cells that completely lack the traditional cytomorphologic features of malignancy.[78]

The small blue cell pattern of basal cell adenomas resembles other tumors, as listed in Table 23.3. Those that have clinical, radiographic, or historical features suggestive of primary or metastatic malignancy or have cytologic necrosis or other features of high-grade carcinoma are usually distinguishable from basal cell adenoma.

The membranous form of basal cell adenoma closely resembles that of dermal cylindroma. Aspiration yields aggregates of small blue cells with surrounding sheaths of hyaline material that are difficult to distinguish from adenoid cystic carcinoma.[272,274] The differential diagnosis between BCA and ACC is one of the most difficult and potentially disastrous in all of cytology. We will return to this issue during our discussion of ACC.

FNA samples of basal cell adenocarcinoma have essentially the same picture as basal cell adenoma and solid adenoid cystic

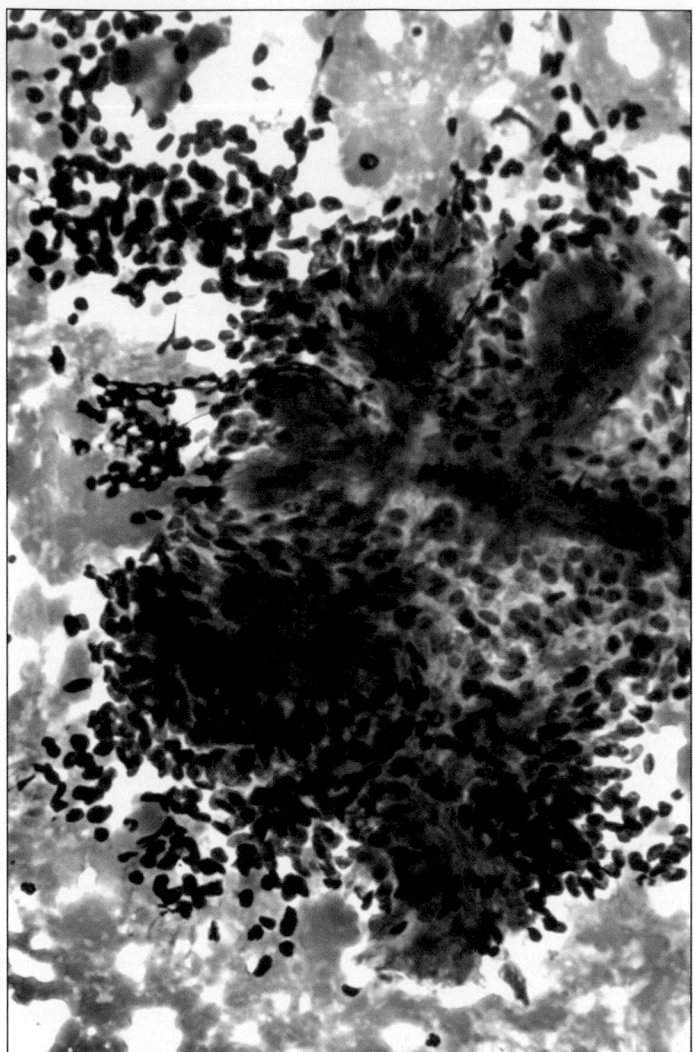

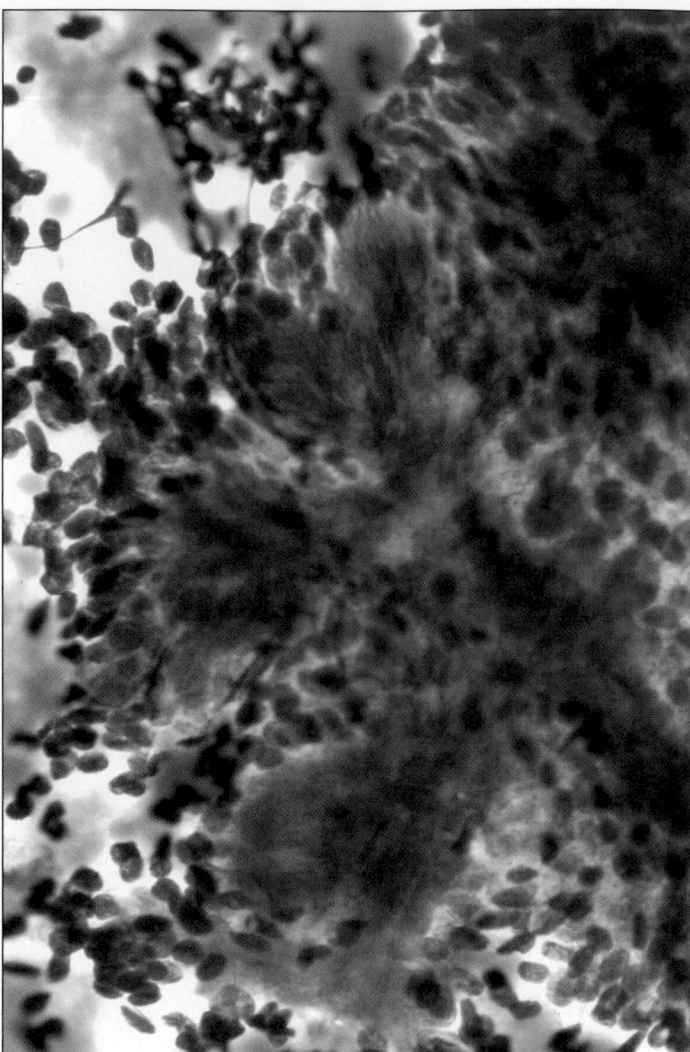

Fig. 23.23 This intermediate magnification image shows smear material from a basal cell adenoma in an air-dried preparation. It features a large number of small darkly staining cells with scanty cytoplasm and arborizing stromal material. The latter is metachromatic and appears to form spheres and cylinders in a manner that superficially resembles adenoid cystic carcinoma (100×).

Fig. 23.24 The higher magnification of the tissue particles shown in Figure 23.23 emphasizes the bland cytology and uniformity of the tumor cells (400×).

carcinoma.[275–277] Cytologic features include papillary and filiform tissue particles with peripheral palisading. Individual cells have a high nuclear:cytoplasmic ratio, fine chromatin, prominent nucleoli, and mitoses. The cells are set in a myxoid background that sometimes includes necrosis, suggesting solid adenoid cystic carcinoma. A relationship with carcinoma ex monomorphic adenoma has been suggested.[270]

CANALICULAR ADENOMA

Although canalicular adenoma has been included within the histologic spectrum of basal cell adenoma,[278,279] it has unique clinical and histological features and is best considered a distinct type of adenoma.[280,281]

Clinical features: In AFIP's and others' data, canalicular adenoma represents about 4–6% of all tumors in minor salivary glands, where

nearly all canalicular adenomas occur.[110,281] About 85% of canalicular adenomas occur in the upper lip or buccal mucosa adjacent to the lip. The male to female ratio is about 1:1.8.[280] The peak incidence is in the seventh decade of life, and they are uncommon in patients under 50 years old. They are asymptomatic, slowly enlarging, movable, compressible nodules, which are sometimes multinodular.[282] They typically range from 0.5 cm to 2.0 cm in diameter, and tumors larger than 3 cm are rare.

Microscopic features: Although most tumors are well circumscribed and encapsulated, some are only partially encapsulated, especially multinodular tumors. The tumors are composed of double rows of short to tall columnar epithelial cells that form a meshwork of branching and interconnecting cords in a very loose stroma (Fig. 23.27). Along the course of the cords of epithelium, the proximity of the two rows of cells to one another varies, so for short distances they can be tightly abutted, slightly separated to produce narrow channels, or more widely separated to produce small cysts. Cross-sectioned cords appear as unconnected small ducts or cysts without connection to adjacent epithelium. The cells are amphophilic

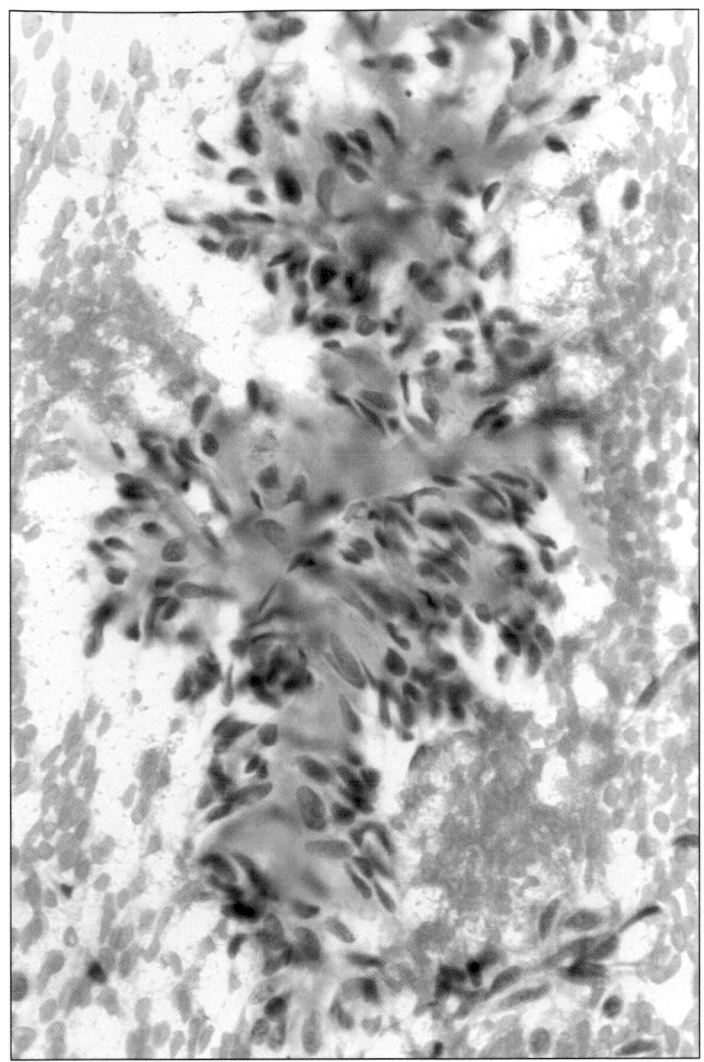

Fig. 23.25 This Papanicolaou-stained preparation shows small uniform cells with arborizing collagenous stroma (100×).

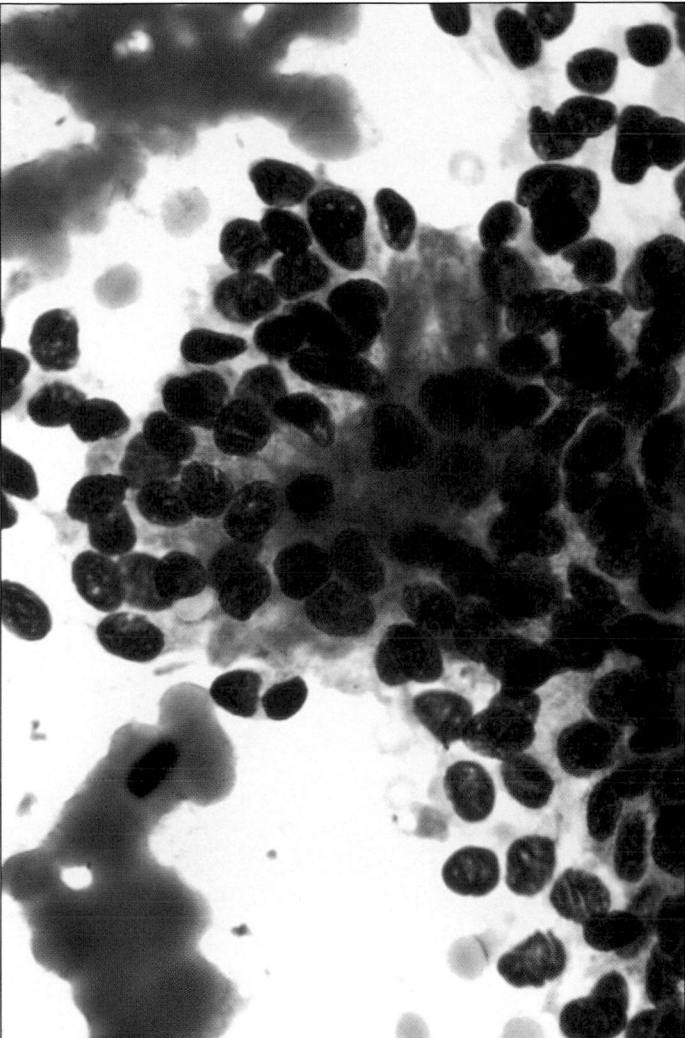

Fig. 23.26 The metachromatic stroma in this basal cell adenoma interdigitates intimately with these small tumor cells. At this magnification, it is possible to see the uniformity, small size, and bland nuclear features of the tumor cells (400×).

to eosinophilic with uniform, round to elliptical nuclei. Foci of basaloid cells can be found between rows of columnar cells in some tumors. The stroma is a very loose, lightly fibrillar collagenous tissue with few fibroblasts and many scattered small capillaries.

The few immunohistochemical studies of canalicular adenomas have demonstrated consistent immunoreactivity for S-100 protein and cytokeratin and only very limited reactivity for GFAP.[283–285] Both immunohistochemical and electron microscopic data confirm the light-microscopic impression that there is little or no myoepithelial differentiation.[267,280,286]

Differential diagnosis: Basal cell adenoma and adenoid cystic carcinoma are the principal considerations in the differential diagnosis. Distinguishing canalicular adenoma from basal cell adenoma has little therapeutic significance, but distinction from adenoid cystic carcinoma has important prognostic and therapeutic implications.

Foci of basaloid cells, occasionally many, are present in some canalicular adenomas, but columnar cells and canaliculi that characterize canalicular adenoma are absent from basal cell adenomas.

The cribriform-tubular pattern of adenoid cystic carcinoma has some resemblance to canalicular adenoma; however, adenoid cystic carcinoma lacks rows of columnar cells, has pale to clear cells with indistinct cell boundaries and irregular-shaped nuclei, has stroma pseudocysts that contain basophilic glycosaminoglycans or eosinophilic basal lamina but no capillaries, and has infiltrative, destructive growth.

Prognosis and treatment: Recurrence is uncommon and probably more related to multifocal lesions than aggressive growth. Local excision is appropriate therapy.[280,282,287]

ONCOCYTOMA

Oncocytomas are benign neoplasms of large, granular, eosinophilic epithelial cells, called oncocytes or oxyphil cells, that contain numerous, atypical mitochondria. Paradoxically, some oncocytomas may be predominantly composed of clear cells.

Oncocytic metaplasia in the parotid gland is an aging-related process. The percentage of the population with focal oncocytosis

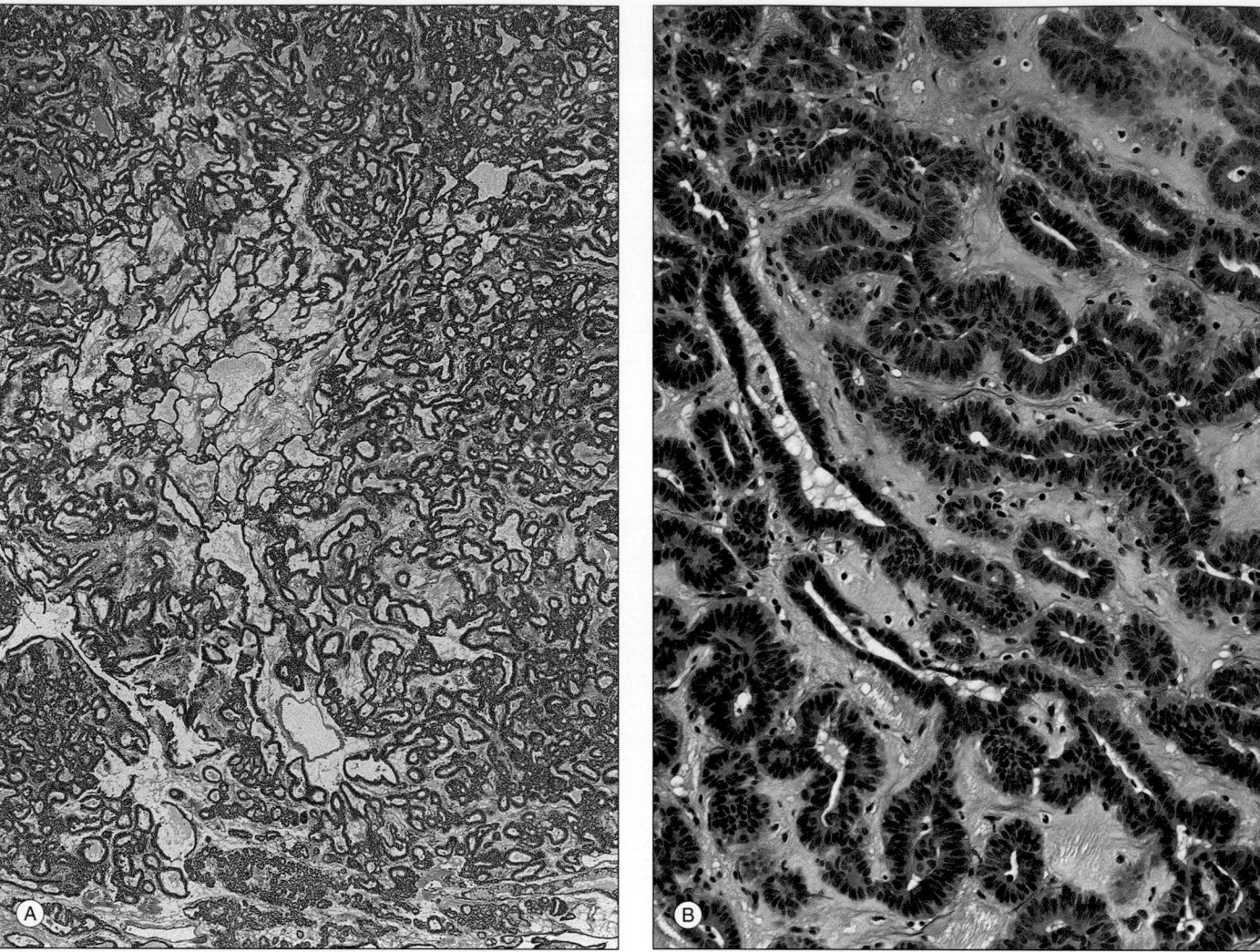

Fig. 23.27 Low magnification of canalicular adenoma (**A**) shows branched and interconnected cords of cells that have formed variably sized channels and cysts within a pale, loose stroma. Higher magnification (**B**) shows double rows of columnar cells with variable luminal space between the rows. Some of the cords are cut in cross-section and appear as isolated tubules.

increases with age until nearly universal in the population over the age of 70 years.[288] In rare cases, nearly the entire parotid gland can be affected.[289] Oncocytic cells in salivary glands can be categorized as *oncocytic metaplasia* (*oncocytosis*), *nodular oncocytic hyperplasia*, and *oncocytoma*.[290,291] Brandwein and Huvos[292] defined oncocytoma as a single nodule, and nodular oncocytic hyperplasia as two or more distinct tumor nodules. Hartwick and Batsakis[290] stated that hyperplastic nodules are less organized and circumscribed than oncocytoma, are lobular rather than lobar, and do not present a single dominant nodule. Because of the distinctive papillary cystic architecture and lymphoid stroma, Warthin's tumor is classified separately from oncocytoma.

Clinical features: Oncocytomas constitute about 1% of salivary gland neoplasms.[2,252,293–295] About 85–90% occur in the parotid gland,[291,292,294,296] and they are rare in the minor salivary glands.[110,294,297] The peak incidence is in the seventh to ninth decades of life, and oncocytomas are rare in patients younger than 50 years.[288,290,291] There is a slight female predominance.[288,294] Among patients with clear cell dominant oncocytomas, there is a marked female

predilection.[298,299] Swelling is usually the only sign. The tumors range in size from 1 cm to 7 cm, but 3–4 cm is typical. The duration has been from a few weeks to 20 years but less than 2 years is typical.[291] Bilateral parotid gland or submandibular gland disease has been estimated to be at least 7%.[292] Ionizing radiation has been cited as an etiologic factor.[292]

Microscopic features: Oncocytoma is typically a single mass but may be a dominant mass in a setting of multinodular oncocytic hyperplasia. The cells are usually arranged in an organoid pattern in which clusters of cells are separated by thin fibrovascular strands and often surround small lumens (Fig. 23.28), but some tumors are arranged in short serpentine cords. Occasional tumors contain small cysts. The cells are one to two times the size of normal acinar cells and usually have distinct cell boundaries. They are conspicuously eosinophilic, but the intensity of the eosinophilia varies. Paradoxically, clear cells dominate some lesions due to the accumulation of cytoplasmic glycogen (Fig. 23.29).[298,299] Because of its affinity for mitochondria, phosphotungstic acid-hematoxylin (PTAH) stain is often useful for identifying oncocytes,[288,292,296] although anti-

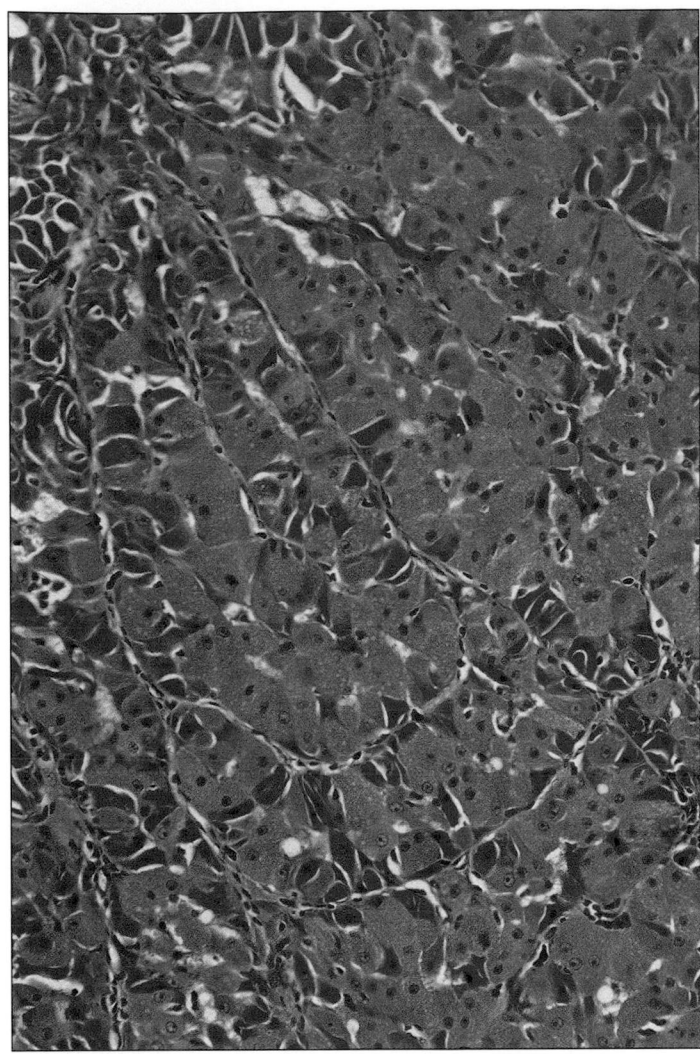

Fig. 23.28 Very thin capillaries separate organoid clusters of oncocytes, which are large polygonal cells with granular eosinophilic cytoplasm and centrally placed nuclei, in oncocytoma. The intensity of cytoplasmic staining is variable, and darker and lighter cells can be identified.

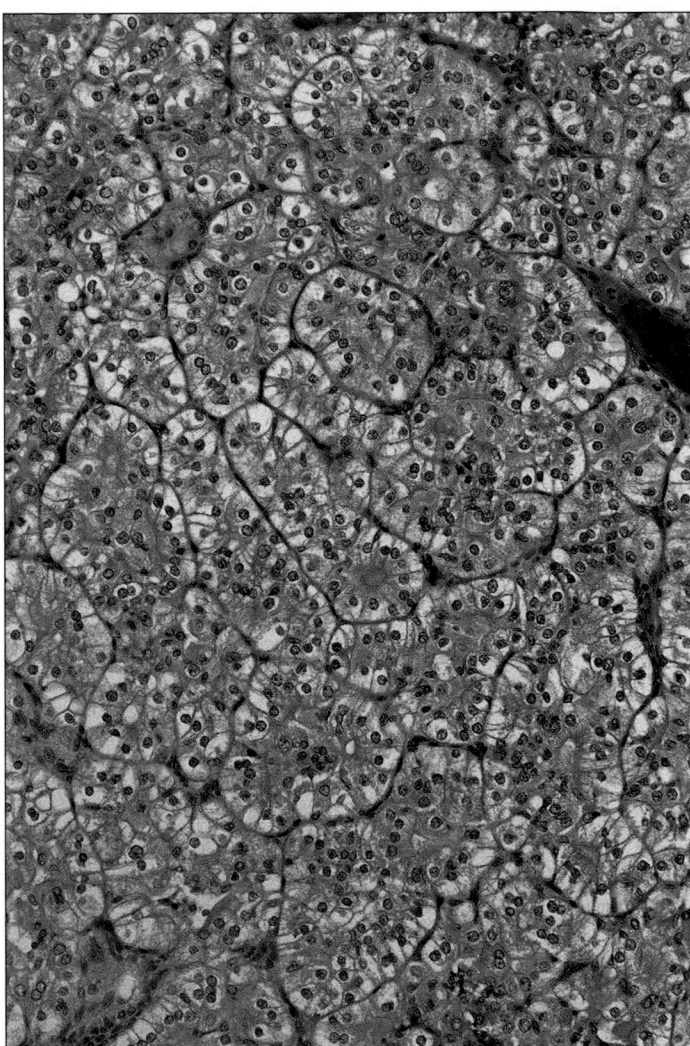

Fig. 23.29 A typical organoid architecture and cellular morphology is evident in this clear cell variant of oncocytoma. Some eosinophilic cytoplasm is evident. Small lumens are evident within some of the clusters.

mitochondrial immunohistochemistry is more sensitive and specific.[300] Although mitotic figures are rare, some cellular and nuclear pleomorphism is acceptable and has no prognostic significance.

Ultrastructurally, abundant cytoplasmic mitochondria are conspicuous and occupy 60% or more of the cytoplasmic compartment.[301] The mitochondria are frequently abnormally sized and shaped. Desmosomal cell attachments are usually evident. Tight junctions and microvilli are present on cells that border glandular lumens.

Differential diagnosis: Oncocytic metaplasia occasionally occurs in tumor cells of salivary gland neoplasms other than oncocytoma, especially mixed tumor and mucoepidermoid carcinoma.[302] Oncocytomas lack the pleomorphic architectural patterns, myxochondroid tissue, and proliferation of noncohesive myoepithelial type cells that typify mixed tumors. Mucous cell and squamous differentiation that are characteristic of mucoepidermoid carcinoma are rare in oncocytomas while the organoid architectural pattern of oncocytomas is uncharacteristic of mucoepidermoid carcinoma.

Other neoplasms that contain clear cells, such as mucoepidermoid carcinoma, clear cell adenocarcinoma, epithelial-myoepithelial carcinoma, acinic cell adenocarcinoma, and metastatic renal cell carcinoma, that need to be distinguished from clear cell oncocytoma are malignant and usually infiltrative. Most of these tumors have characteristic histomorphology and are unreactive with PTAH stain. Since metastatic renal cell carcinoma contains both abundant glycogen and mitochondria, it may be difficult to differentiate from clear cell oncocytoma. Infiltrative growth, prominent vascularity, and more extensive cellular and nuclear pleomorphism help distinguish metastatic renal cell carcinoma. Recently, immunostaining with CD10 and RCC antibodies has shown a high level of reactivity in clear cell renal cell carcinomas, but there are few data on the reaction of these antibodies in salivary gland tumors.[303] Evaluation of the patient for a primary kidney tumor is prudent in cases with any doubt about the origin of the tumor.

Prognosis and treatment: Recurrence rates have ranged from 0 to 30% of patients up to 13 years after excision.[288,291,292,304] Multifocal tumor growth and incomplete excision are factors in the incidence of recurrence.[292] Excision is the principal modality of therapy for primary and recurrent tumors. Kosuda et al.[305] recommended radioiodine therapy after finding reduction in tumor volume of an oncocytoma in a patient treated with therapeutic doses of [131]Iodide.

CYSTADENOMA

Cystadenoma is a rare benign epithelial tumor showing unicystic or multicystic growth and focal intraluminal papillary proliferation of the lining epithelium. Sometimes interpreted as intraductal hyperplasia rather than neoplasia,[306–308] the neoplastic nature of cystadenomas is supported by their occasional large size and capacity to displace and compress normal tissues.

In the AFIP files, cystadenoma represents about 4% of all benign epithelial tumors and is relatively more frequent among such tumors in the minor than major glands (7% vs. 3%, respectively). Waldron and colleagues[110] found that cystadenoma represented 8.1% of the 245 benign minor gland tumors in their series. More than one-half of all minor gland cystadenomas in AFIP's material occurred in the lips and buccal mucosa, a distribution similar to that reported by Waldron and coworkers.[110] This distribution in minor glands is unusual when compared with other salivary gland tumors, which are much more common in the palatal area. Patients average about 57 years of age at the time of diagnosis, with a range of 12 and 89 years.

Clinical features: In the major glands, cystadenomas are typically slowly enlarging, asymptomatic masses that may be slightly compressible.[309] In oral mucosa, these tumors sometimes produce smooth-surfaced nodules that resemble mucoceles. In the minor glands, cystadenomas are nearly always less than 1 cm in greatest dimension.[309]

Microscopic features: Cystadenomas are well circumscribed, and about 25% have a distinct fibrous capsule.[110] About 20% are unilocular, and the rest are multilocular. The luminal epithelium is typically cuboidal or columnar (Fig. 23.30), but sometimes there are focal mucous and oncocytic cells, which even predominate occasionally.[310] About 15% of the tumors in the AFIP files have some oncocytic change, but in one series, nearly three-quarters did so.[110] Squamous epithelium is sometimes focal but rarely predominates. The nuclei of all cell types are uniformly bland, and mitotic figures are extremely rare. About two-thirds of tumors demonstrate intraluminal papillary growth, but extraluminal sheet-like growth is not characteristic of cystadenoma.

Differential diagnosis: In contrast to Warthin's tumors, cystadenomas with oncocytic epithelium (so-called papillary oncocytic cystadenomas) usually do not have bilayered epithelium, sometimes have other types of epithelium admixed with the oncocytic cells, and lack a diffuse and dense lymphoid stroma with germinal centers, although there are patchy inflammatory infiltrates in some tumors.[311] Unlike cystadenomas, intraductal papillomas are always unicystic because they occur in a dilated salivary gland duct, and their papillary fronds are more numerous and complex than those in cystadenomas.[310,312,313] Distinction from cystadenocarcinoma depends on the lack of frank invasion of salivary gland parenchyma or connective tissue.

Some low-grade mucoepidermoid carcinomas are prominently cystic, papillary, partly circumscribed, and composed of several cell types also seen in cystadenomas. The most important distinguishing criterion is noncystic epithelium that forms extraluminal solid islands of tumor in mucoepidermoid carcinomas. In addition, in mucoepidermoid carcinoma, the epithelium lining the cystic structures is more often markedly thickened, and the cellular proliferation

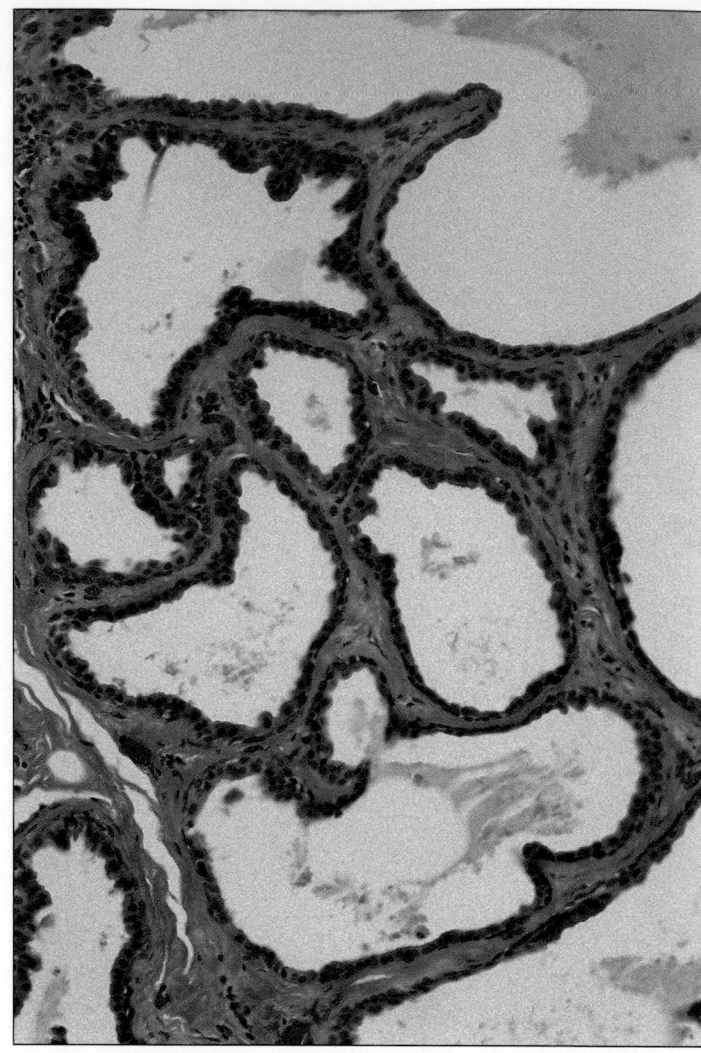

Fig. 23.30 Cystic structures in cystadenoma are lined by uniform, cuboidal to low columnar epithelium that forms simple papillary projections.

is more varied with combinations of epidermoid, mucous, and smaller intermediate or basaloid cells.

Prognosis and treatment: Data from case reports and small series of cystadenomas over the past two decades and AFIP's cases indicate that this tumor is unlikely to recur.[312–314] Conservative but complete surgical removal is recommended.

SEBACEOUS ADENOMA

Sebaceous glands are found in about 10% of normal parotid glands and 6% of submandibular glands,[315] and are described in major glands that are involved by inflammatory, cystic, and neoplastic disease.[309,315,316] Despite their frequency in normal glands, tumors with sebaceous differentiation are exceptionally rare and comprise less than 0.2% of all benign and malignant salivary gland tumors.[317] Most sebaceous adenomas occur in the parotid gland, but the submandibular and minor glands are also affected.[309] Microscopically, they are composed of epithelial cells that form solid, variably shaped islands and cysts that have focal sebaceous differentiation. A predominance of squamous cells with limited focal sebaceous differentiation is typical. Sebaceous lymphadenoma is microscopically similar to sebaceous adenoma except that the neoplastic epithelial elements are surrounded by abundant lymphoid stroma. Most occur in the parotid gland. In both tumors, foreign body reaction is occasionally present.[318] Conservative excision is appropriate.[309]

SIALOBLASTOMA

Reported under a variety of other names such as *embryoma* and *congenital carcinoma*, sialoblastoma is a rare, congenital or perinatal, aggressive, and potentially low-grade malignant basaloid salivary gland neoplasm that occurs in the major salivary glands.[319–329] Variation in cytomorphologic atypia, mitotic rate, necrosis, and infiltration among these tumors indicates they are not all identical.[319,330,331] It has been suggested that they be separated into benign and malignant, based on the absence or presence of invasion of nerves or vascular spaces, necrosis, and cytologic atypia beyond that expected for embryonic epithelium.[322,327] Alternatively, others suggest they are neither benign nor malignant but are tumors with local infiltrative potential.[332]

Typically, sialoblastoma presents at birth, or shortly thereafter, as a firm asymptomatic mass of the parotid (75%) or submandibular (25%) gland. Microscopically, sialoblastoma is composed of numerous small hypercellular islands or solid sheets of primitive basaloid cells separated by fibrous or fibromyxomatous stroma (Fig. 23.31). Small ducts lined by cuboidal or low columnar cells form distinct lumens within some of the epithelial islands.

In contrast to basal cell adenoma, sialoblastoma is congenital, is composed of more primitive cells, demonstrates cytomorphologic atypia, has much greater mitotic activity, and often infiltrates surrounding tissues. One study reported a case that demonstrated a marked increased in the MiB1 (Ki-67) proliferative index in the recurrent tumor.[326] The same tumor had moderate cytoplasmic immunostaining for Her-2/neu protein but only occasional labeling of nuclei for p53. Other basaloid neoplasms that share some features with sialoblastoma, such as adenoid cystic carcinoma and basal cell adenocarcinoma, are extremely rare in the first decade of life. Conservative excision with tumor-free margins has been recommended.[332]

MALIGNANT TUMORS

MUCOEPIDERMOID CARCINOMA

Mucoepidermoid carcinoma is the most common malignant salivary gland tumor. It represents about 22% and 41% of the malignant tumors in the major and minor glands, respectively. Because even the low-grade neoplasms may metastasize, the term *mucoepidermoid tumor* is considered inappropriate.[2,24,333,334]

Clinical features: More than one-half of mucoepidermoid carcinomas occur in the major glands, and most of those are found in the parotid gland. Of minor gland sites, the palate, buccal mucosa, upper and lower lips, and retromolar region are most commonly involved.[333,335] Patients average about 47 years of age, but there is a relatively uniform frequency between the third and seventh decades of life.[8] Women outnumber men in most large published studies.[24,336–340]

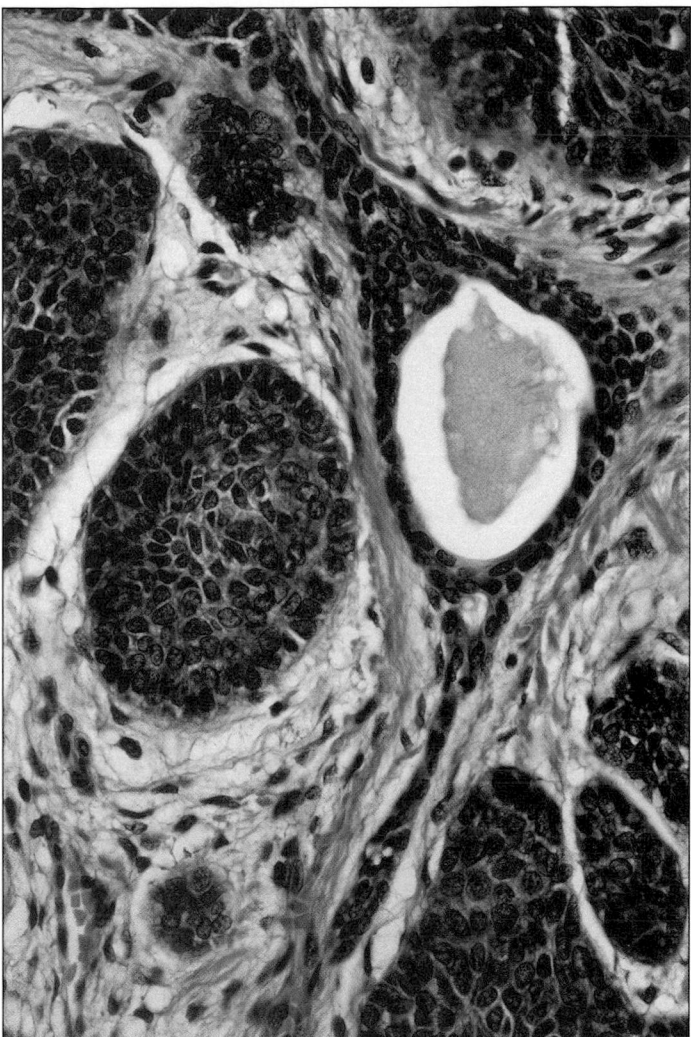

Fig. 23.31 Sialoblastoma is typically composed of individual nests of basaloid epithelium that focally may exhibit ductal differentiation.

In the parotid and submandibular glands, mucoepidermoid carcinomas typically are solitary painless masses. About one-third of patients, however, experience tenderness, pain, drainage from the ipsilateral ear, dysphagia, trismus, or facial paralysis. Minor gland tumors have many different clinical appearances. Those of the palate are often fluctuant, blue, smooth-surfaced swellings that resemble mucoceles. Others have a magenta color, which suggests a vascular or melanin-containing lesion. Some tumors discharge fluid through a small mucosal opening, resembling draining dental abscesses. Symptoms include dysphagia, pain, paresthesia, numbness of teeth, ulceration, and hemorrhage. In both major and minor glands, high-grade tumors are more likely to be symptomatic.[18,19]

Microscopic features: Grossly, the cut surface of mucoepidermoid carcinoma is usually firm, gray, tan-yellow, or pink, lobulated, and cystic. Microscopically, the tumor consists of mucous, epidermoid, intermediate, columnar, and clear cells in both solid and cystic configurations (Fig. 23.32). In most tumors, intermediate cells, which include basal cells and cells between basal cells and the larger polygonal epidermoid cells in size and appearance (Fig. 23.33), outnumber the other cell types. Mucous cells comprise less than

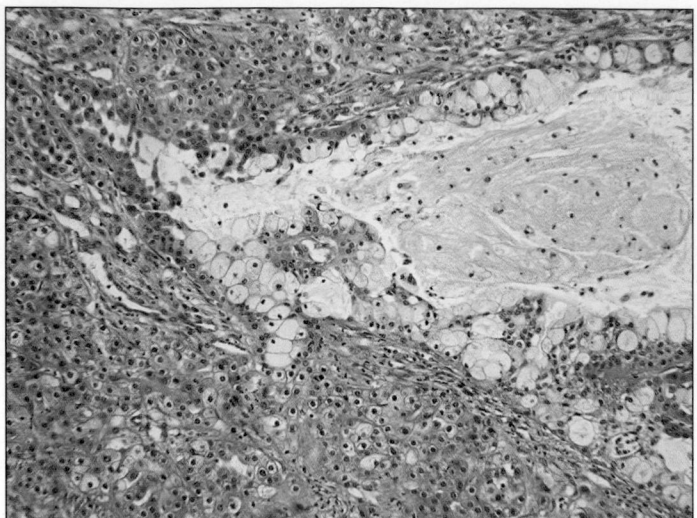

Fig. 23.32 This low-grade mucoepidermoid carcinoma had numerous mucin-filled cysts similar to the one shown lined mostly by mucous cells and surrounded by a variety of other cell types.

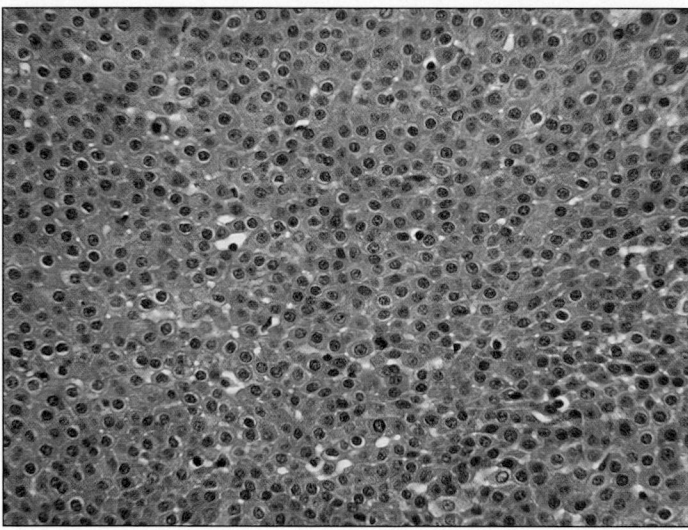

Fig. 23.33 In this low-grade mucoepidermoid carcinoma many areas were composed of solid sheets of intermediate cells. They are slightly smaller and round in contrast to the distinctly polygonal, larger squamous cells.

10% of most tumors. Typically, they are numerous in the lining of mucus-filled cystic spaces, which sometimes have an intraluminal papillary proliferation.[18] The contents of these spaces often spill into adjacent tissues. Epidermoid differentiation is typically limited to small focal areas. Examples of mucoepidermoid carcinomas exhibiting prominent oncocytic differentiation have been reported.[341–344] A dense fibrous stroma usually surrounds the neoplastic epithelium and, rarely, is prominently sclerotic.[345] The various cell types vary in cytokeratin expression.[346]

Mucoepidermoid carcinomas are divided into low, intermediate, and high-grade types on the basis of morphologic and cytologic features. The histologic features that are most useful in predicting high-grade, aggressive behavior are the presence of an intracystic component of less than 20%, four or more mitotic figures per 10 high-power fields, neural invasion, necrosis, and cellular anaplasia. The simultaneous assessment of these features improves prognostic correlation over individual parameters.[18] Some investigators have proposed also including the presence or absence of vascular invasion and the pattern of tumor infiltration to the criteria.[347] The proportion of cell types does not correlate well with behavior.

Most low-grade tumors have numerous cystic spaces and a variety of cell types but are usually solid when they are predominated by intermediate cells. Mitoses are rare and nuclei bland. Intermediate-grade tumors often have cellular anaplasia and either cystic space that comprises less than 20% of the entire tumor or neural invasion. Necrosis and solid growth occur more often in tumors of major than minor glands. Most high-grade mucoepidermoid carcinomas are relatively solid and anaplastic and have four or more mitoses per 10 high-power fields (Fig. 23.34). Necrosis and neural invasion are frequent features. Grading of mucoepidermoid carcinomas in the submandibular gland does not correlate as well with biologic behavior as it does for tumors in parotid or minor gland sites. In a study of 23 low-grade tumors in the submandibular gland, it was found that 6 either metastasized or caused the death of the patient.[19] Spiro and colleagues[22,24] and others[348] have also found that submandibular gland tumors were the least predictable with respect to grade and stage.

Compared to normal salivary tissue and benign tumors, mucoepidermoid carcinomas demonstrate increased cellular proliferation as defined by Ki-67 and proliferating cell nuclear antigen (PCNA).[349] One study has shown that patients whose tumors overexpressed HER-2/neu had a lower five-year survival rate (25%) than patients whose tumors had weaker immunoreactivity (89%).[350] Similarly, aneuploid tumors exhibited higher recurrence rates than diploid tumors.[351] Cytogenetic studies have shown deletions, translocations, and numerical chromosomal abnormalities.[352–356] Only one of eight mucoepidermoid carcinomas, however, showed a homozygous deletion of the p16 tumor suppressor gene.[352]

Differential diagnosis: Compared with mucoepidermoid carcinoma, necrotizing sialometaplasia has metaplastic squamous epithelial nests that vary in size, have smooth regular edges, are often within a necrotic salivary gland lobule, and are admixed with ductal remnants. Neither cystic growth nor other cell types, notably intermediate cells, are usually seen. Epidermoid cells are a much greater proportion of inverted papilloma than mucoepidermoid carcinoma. Furthermore, papillomas do not infiltrate surrounding tissues. Mucoepidermoid carcinomas have a more variable cell population and infiltrative, noncystic epithelial proliferation than cystadenomas. Cystadenocarcinomas usually lack epidermoid differentiation and do not have the variety of cell types typically present in mucoepidermoid carcinoma. Primary or metastatic squamous cell carcinoma lacks histochemically demonstrable mucus cells. Squamous cell carcinomas are also much more likely to have keratinization.

Prognosis and Treatment: Prognosis of mucoepidermoid carcinoma is largely dependent on the clinical stage, tumor grade, and adequacy of treatment. In AFIP data on mucoepidermoid carcinomas of the major and minor salivary glands, 5% and 2.5%, respectively, of the low-grade tumors either metastasized to regional lymph nodes or resulted in the death of the patient, whereas 55% and 80%, respectively, of the high-grade tumors did so.[18] Many patients with low-grade tumors that developed recurrences or metastases had advanced-stage tumors. However, submandibular tumors were the exception. Thirteen percent of patients with low-grade tumors in that site died of disease.

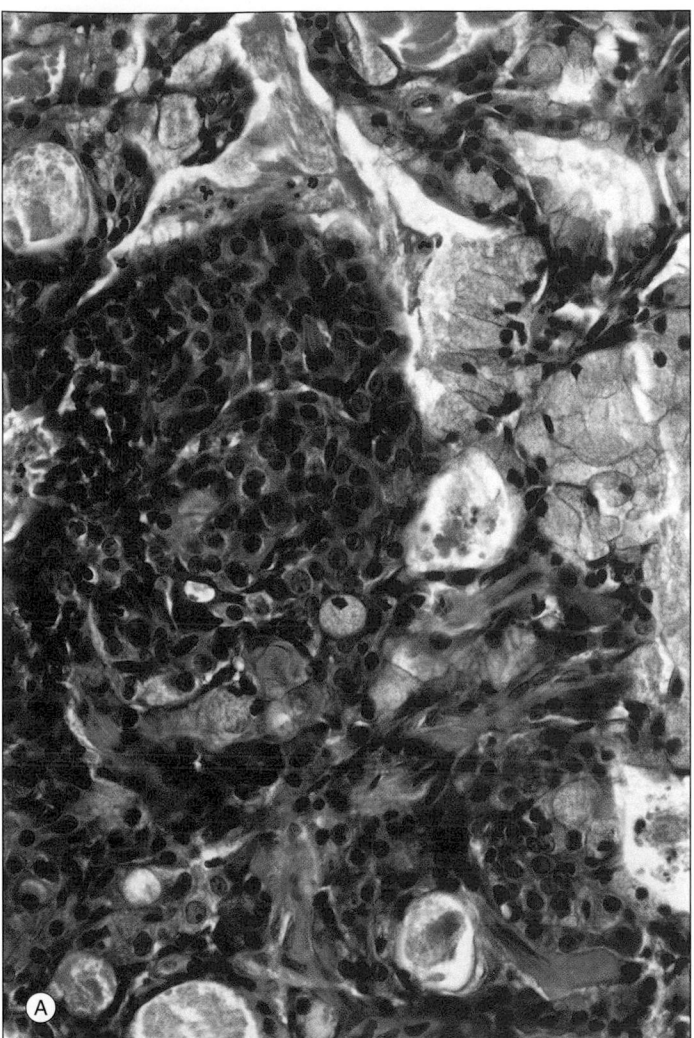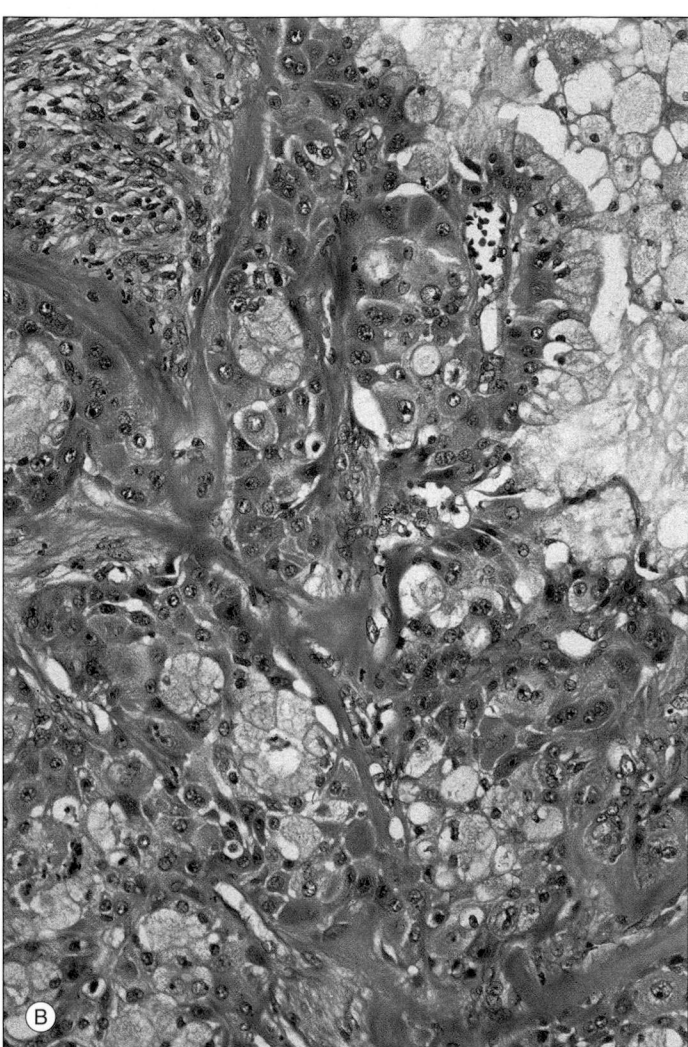

Fig. 23.34 A, Low-grade mucoepidermoid carcinoma is shown. Although this tumor lacked a large cystic component, other features indicating more aggressive behavior were not found; **B**, Intermediate-grade mucoepidermoid carcinoma is anaplastic with enlarged variably sized and variably shaped nuclei with prominent nucleoli. The tumor was predominantly solid. Clusters of mucous cells are evident.

Recurrences are much more likely if the margins of surgical resection contain tumor.[357] Regional metastasis of low-grade, minor gland tumors is extremely rare and does not necessarily imply a poor prognosis, even if multiple nodes are involved.[18] Patients who die of disease survive, on average, 2.3 and 2.6 years with minor and major gland tumors, respectively;[18] however, the survival of patients with high-grade tumors continues to decline for at least 8 years after primary treatment.[161,334,336–338,358,359]

Conservative excision with preservation of the facial nerve is recommended for stage I and II mucoepidermoid carcinomas of the parotid gland.[24] Postoperative radiotherapy using high-energy electrons with photons may improve local and regional control rates in high-risk patients.[360] An affected submandibular gland should be entirely extirpated, but radiotherapy may also be indicated for tumors in this site because of its worse prognosis.[361] Radical neck dissection is suggested for patients with T3 disease and indicated for patients with clinical evidence of cervical node metastases. Spiro and colleagues[24] performed elective neck dissection for selected patients with high-grade tumors of both major and minor glands and found that two-thirds had occult metastases. Wide surgical excision that ensures tumor-free margins is appropriate for minor gland tumors. If tumor erodes or infiltrates underlying bone, removal of a portion of the maxilla or mandible is required to ensure complete removal. Melrose and colleagues[340] suggest local excision with block excision of underlying bone only if there is evidence of bone destruction. Others agree with this approach for small, low-grade tumors[362–365] and suggest that wide excision down to periosteum with at least 1 cm tumor-free lateral margins is appropriate therapy. High-grade and advanced-stage tumors must be treated aggressively.

Cytopathology of mucoepidermoid carcinoma

The grade of mucoepidermoid carcinoma (MEC) greatly affects the cytology. Intermediate and high-grade tumors are often readily recognized as non-small cell carcinomas, even if specific classification as mucoepidermoid is not achieved. Low-grade MEC is a very difficult diagnosis.[247,366,367] The older literature is often unclear about grading, and various histologic appearances are frequently combined so as to render the accuracy of antecedent FNA uninterpretable.

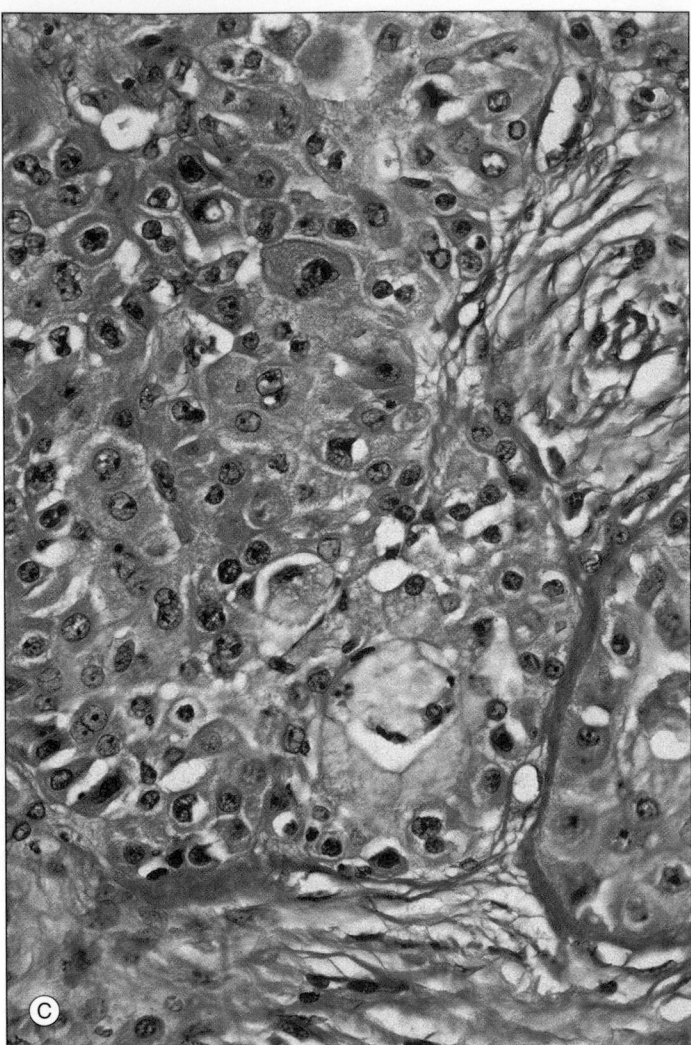

Fig. 23.34 *(cont'd)* **C**, High-grade mucoepidermoid carcinoma is anaplastic and has a mitotic rate of more than 4 per 10 high-power fields. Additionally, necrosis, neural invasion, and solid growth were found.

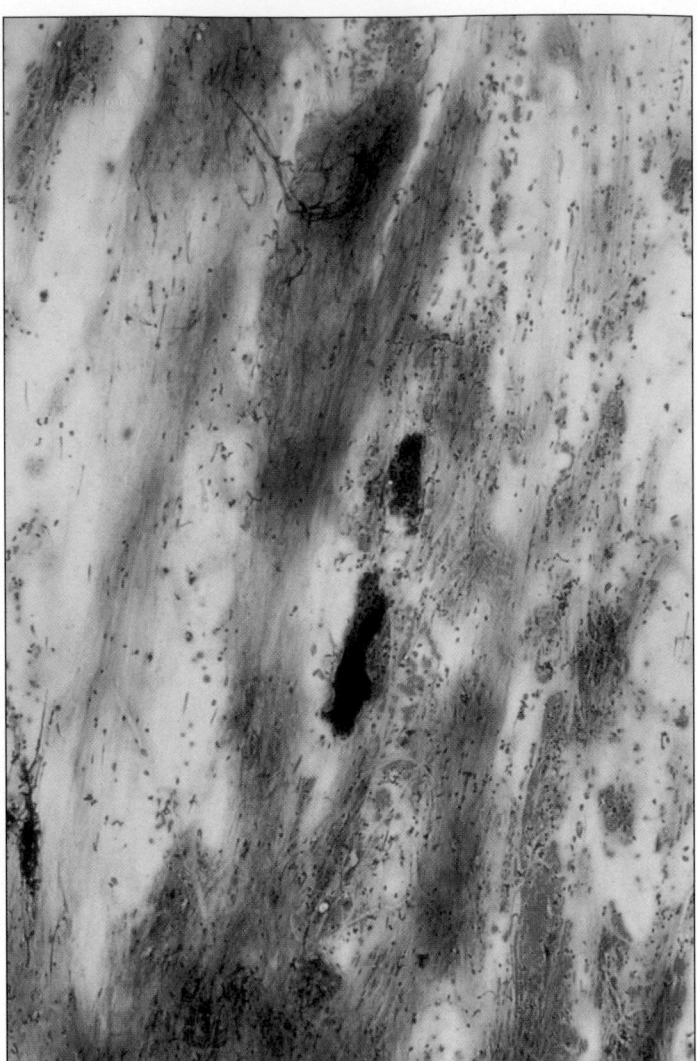

Fig. 23.35 This very low-magnification image shows abundant wispy mucinous material. Near the center are two darkly staining cell clusters. This is a typical, sparsely cellular aspirate of low-grade mucoepidermoid carcinoma (Diff-Quik, 40×).

Aspiration of low-grade MEC usually yields clear to turbid mucoid fluid. Smears have a few cells or cell clusters set in a background of abundant mucus (Fig. 23.35). The cells often have degenerative nuclear smudging and cytoplasmic vacuolization (Fig. 23.36). They are often indistinguishable from macrophages that inhabit most cyst fluid and occur as single cells or cell clusters. Intermediate and squamous cells have a relatively high nuclear: cytoplasmic ratio and closely resemble immature squamous meta- plastic cells in gynecologic cytology specimens.

Inflammation in this neoplasm further confuses the cytologic picture. Oncocytic variants are rare, but important, since most other oncocytic masses are benign. Clear cell change may be present. Cytologic recognition of these altered forms of low-grade mucoepidermoid carcinoma is difficult, and identification of characteristic features of this tumor is usually needed. Aspiration of low-grade mucoepidermoid carcinoma ex pleomorphic adenoma has been described rarely.

Aspirates of sparsely cellular mucoid material should be diagnosed as mucinous cyst with a differential diagnosis that includes low-grade MEC and various non-neoplastic duct obstructing lesions.

ACINIC CELL ADENOCARCINOMA

Acinic cell adenocarcinoma is a malignant epithelial neoplasm in which at least some of the neoplastic cells demonstrate serous acinar cell differentiation.

Clinical features: In the AFIP's experience, acinic cell adeno- carcinoma is the third most common epithelial malignancy of salivary glands and comprises about 10% of primary malignant salivary gland tumors, although the reported incidence is quite variable.[2,11,293,368–370] Over 80% of acinic cell adenocarcinomas occur in the parotid gland. Only about 4% arise in the submandibular gland, and most of the remainder develops in the intraoral minor salivary glands.[251,369,371–373] Several bilateral acinic cell adenocarcinomas have been reported.[209,374]

It is one of the few malignant salivary gland tumors to affect children.[255,369] The mean age of patients is 44 years, but the age distribution of patients is fairly even from the second to the seventh decades of life.[369,375] The female to male ratio is 3:2.

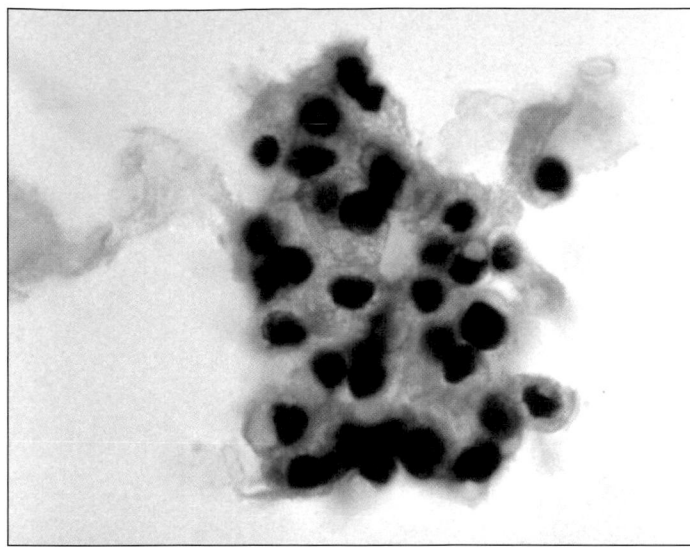

Fig. 23.36 The cells of mucoepidermoid carcinoma often show degenerative nuclear smudging and cell cluster collapse (Papanicolaou, 400×).

Tumors have ranged in size from 0.5 cm to 13.0 cm in largest dimension, but the majority of tumors are 1–3 cm. They typically enlarge slowly, but pain or tenderness is a symptom for over a third of patients.[376–379] Facial muscle weakness occurs in 5–10% of patients.[376,377,379]

Microscopic features: While serous acinar cell differentiation characterizes this group of tumors, they have a broad spectrum of architectural and cytologic features.[26,369,377,380–382] *Solid, microcystic, papillary-cystic*, and *follicular* growth patterns (Fig. 23.37) may contain *acinar, intercalated ductal, vacuolated, clear*, and *nonspecific glandular* cells (Fig. 23.38).[369] While each tumor has a predominance of one pattern and cell type, most tumors have a mixture of features.

Cytoplasmic zymogen secretory granules identify acinar differentiation. Neoplastic acinar cells typically have abundant, pale basophilic cytoplasm with purplish cytoplasmic granules and eccentrically located nuclei. They are usually polygonal with nuclei that vary from darkly basophilic to slightly vesicular. Some cells have a finely reticular or foamy cytoplasm. Periodic acid–Schiff (PAS) stain highlights the cytoplasmic secretory granules, which are resistant to diastase digestion. The zymogen-type granules are unstained by

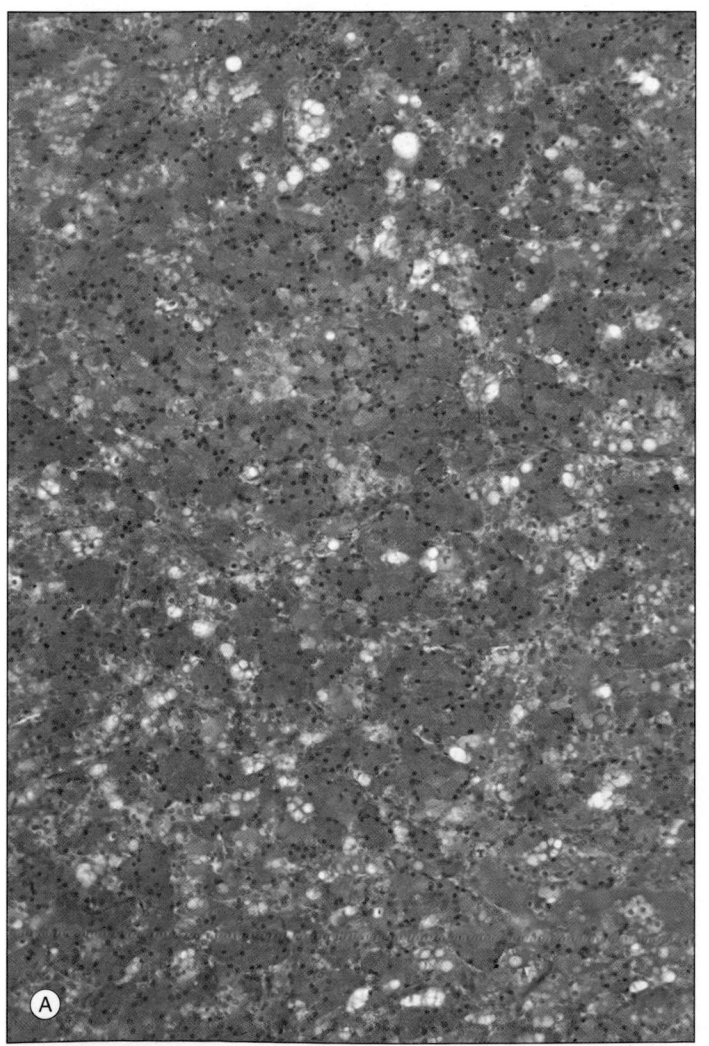

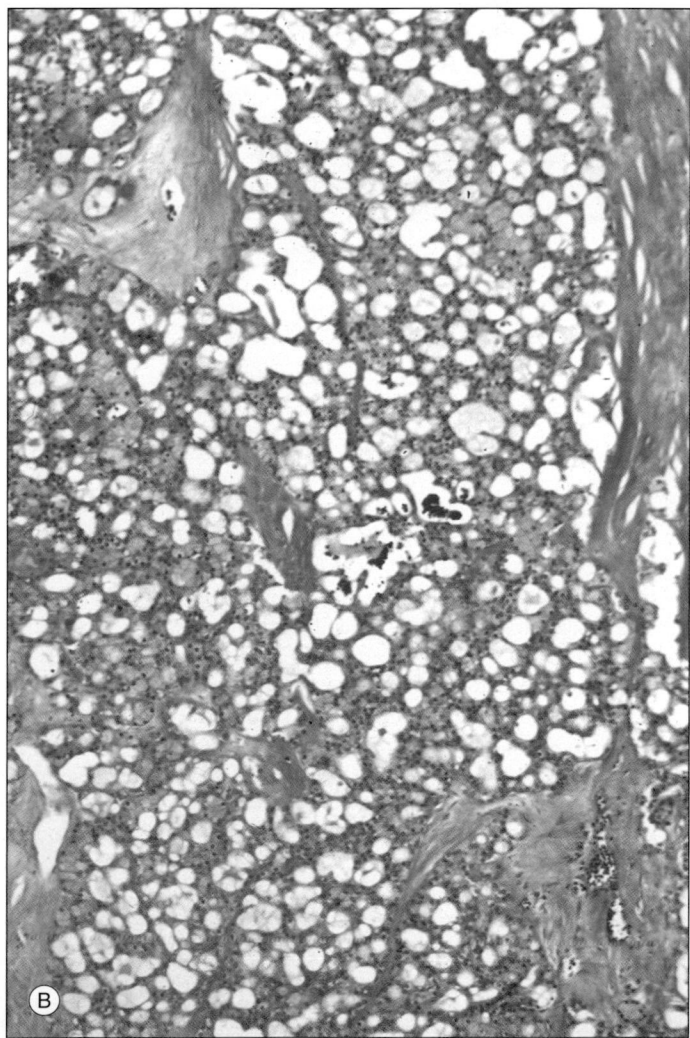

Fig. 23.37 The growth pattern of acinic cell adenocarcinoma is commonly solid sheets or nests of tumor cells (**A**), but a microcystic pattern (**B**) occurs more frequently.

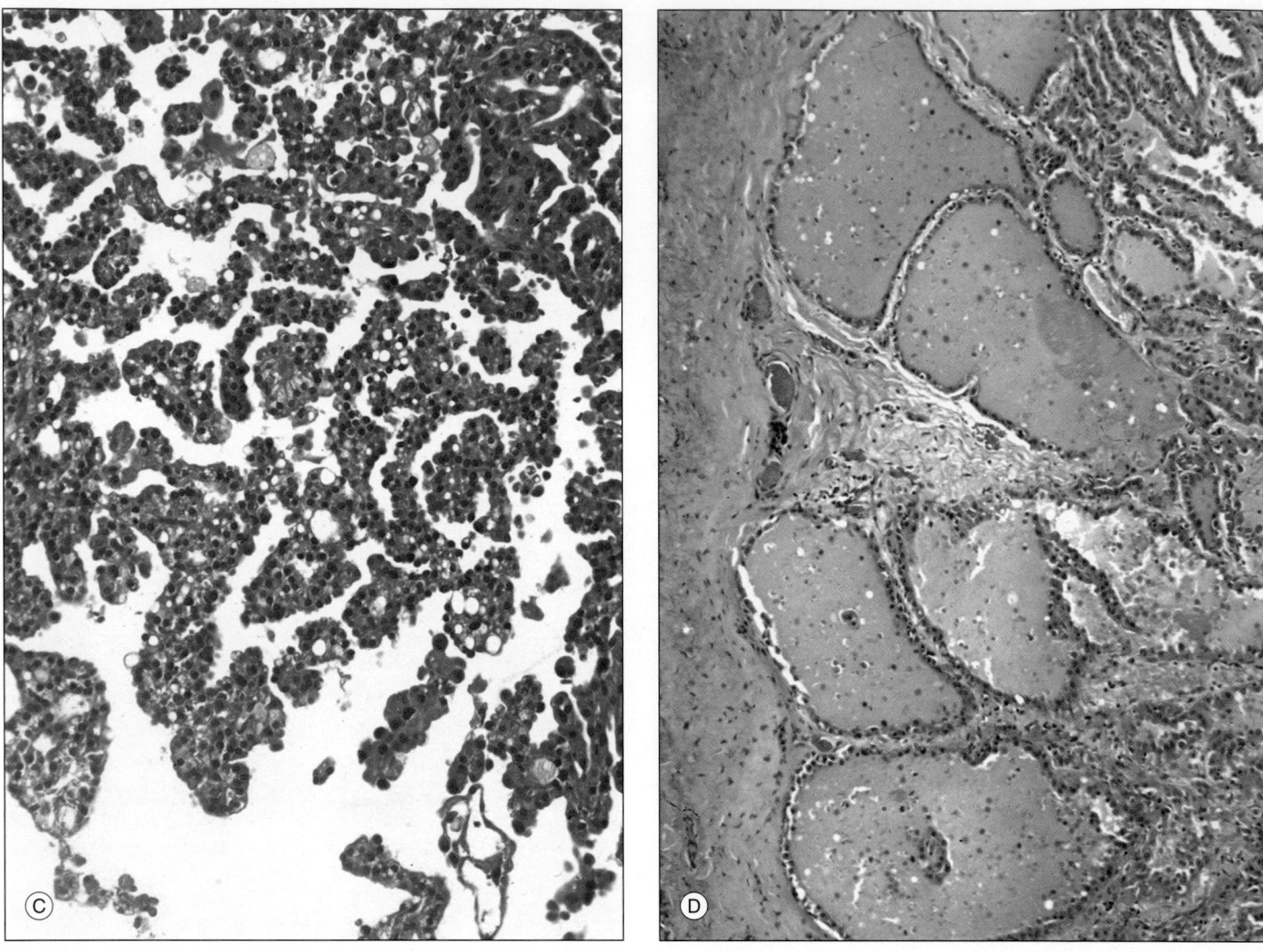

Fig. 23.37 *(cont'd)* A papillary-cystic architecture (**C**) is a less frequent pattern, and the follicular pattern (**D**) is uncommon.

mucicarmine, which helps distinguish them from the mucin in mucous cells. Acinar cells predominate in over 40% of acinic cell adenocarcinomas but are only a small minority in many tumors.

Cuboidal intercalated duct-like cells are smaller and their nuclear:cytoplasmic ratio is greater than the acinar type cells. The cytoplasm is eosinophilic to amphophilic with central, deeply basophilic to vesicular nuclei, and they surround varying sized luminal spaces. They are the predominant cell type in about a third of tumors but are in most acinic cell adenocarcinomas.

As the term implies, vacuolated cells have cytoplasmic vacuoles, and the membranes of some cells appear expanded by the vacuoles. They are the predominant cell type in less than 10% of acinic cell adenocarcinomas. The nuclear features are similar to the intercalated duct-like cells.

Clear cells are a component of only 6% of acinic cell adeno-carcinomas and are prominent in only about 1% of these tumors.[369,376,383] They do not contain glycogen, and the clear cytoplasm is due to dilatation of endoplasmic reticulum and fixation and tissue processing artifact.[384]

Non-specific glandular cells are rounded to polygonal cells with amphophilic to eosinophilic cytoplasm and round, basophilic to vesicular nuclei. They lack cytoplasmic granules and are unreactive with PAS stain. They typically occur in syncytial sheets with poorly demarcated cell borders. Nuclear pleomorphism and mitotic activity are more prominent in this cell population than the other cell types. Acinar cells are often scattered among the non-specific glandular cells. Non-specific glandular cells occur in most acinic cell adeno-carcinomas, but they are predominant in only about 15% of tumors.

A solid histomorphologic growth pattern predominates in over one-third of acinic cell adenocarcinomas. The tumor cells are closely apposed to form sheets, nodules, or aggregates. The acinar-type cell is often the predominant cell type in the solid pattern.

A microcystic pattern is slightly more frequent than the solid pattern. Numerous small spaces within sheets or nodules of tumor cells vary from several microns to a millimeter or more in size. The microcystic spaces are usually empty but sometimes contain amorphous, eosinophilic, or pale basophilic material that stains with PAS stain and, sometimes, mucicarmine stain.

The papillary-cystic pattern has large cystic lumens that are partially filled with sparse to extensive papillary epithelial growths. Some of the epithelial cells bulge into the lumen and produce an undulating, 'tombstone row' luminal surface. Many tumors contain intraluminal mucinous material, but cytoplasmic mucicarminophilia of a few cells is only occasionally observed.

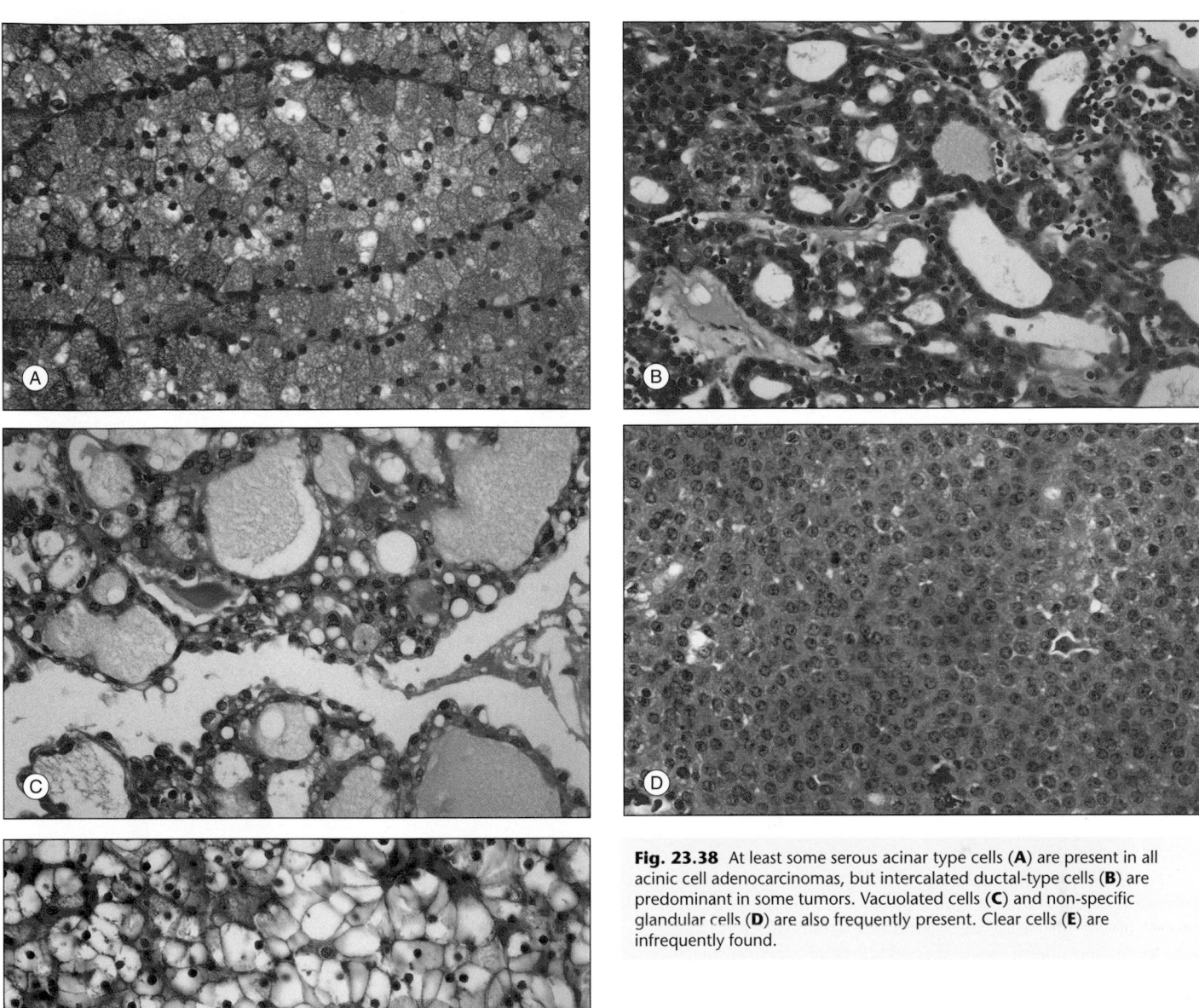

Fig. 23.38 At least some serous acinar type cells (**A**) are present in all acinic cell adenocarcinomas, but intercalated ductal-type cells (**B**) are predominant in some tumors. Vacuolated cells (**C**) and non-specific glandular cells (**D**) are also frequently present. Clear cells (**E**) are infrequently found.

A thyroid-like appearance of multiple cystic lumens filled with eosinophilic proteinaceous material characterizes the follicular pattern. It is the least frequent pattern and is prominent in only about 5% of the tumors. The cystic spaces are larger than those of the microcystic pattern and generally lack luminal papillary epithelial proliferation.

Areas of 'dedifferentiated' or undifferentiated carcinoma have rarely been described as a component of acinic cell adenocarcinomas.[374,381,385,386] Some acinic cell adenocarcinomas are associated with prominent lymphoid infiltrates of their stroma, even including lymphoid follicle formation that appears to have proliferated along with the neoplastic epithelium as it infiltrates adjacent tissues.[81] This should not be misinterpreted as lymph node metastasis.

Some small acinic cell adenocarcinomas are well circumscribed and some even have an apparent fibrous capsule, but most infiltrate adjacent normal tissues. The stroma varies from delicate fibrovascular tissue to very collagenous tissue. Hemorrhage is most often noted in association with the papillary-cystic tumors, and hemosiderin is sometimes evident not only in the connective tissue but in many of the epithelial tumor cells. There are spherical calcifications in a few tumors.

Ultrastructurally, the characteristic feature of acinar differentiated cells is multiple, round, electron dense cytoplasmic secretory granules.

Ductal cells often border lumens and have apical junctional complexes and microvilli.[380,384]

Immunohistochemical studies have found acinic cell adeno-carcinomas to be reactive for cytokeratin, transferrin, lactoferrin, alpha-1-antitrypsin, alpha-1-antichymotrypsin, IgA, carcinoembryonic antigen, Leu M1 antigen, and amylase.[387,388] Some investigators have advocated the use of antiamylase for acinic cell adeno-carcinomas,[389,390] but with formalin-fixed and paraffin-embedded tissue in others' laboratories, antiamylase has not been very useful.[391,392] Among various types of salivary gland tumors, vasoactive intestinal polypeptide and bone morphogenetic protein have been reported to be specifically reactive in acinic cell adenocarcinoma.[387,393]

Several molecular and cytogenetic studies have evaluated acinic cell adenocarcinomas in attempts to determine prognostic factors, but most studies have evaluated only a few cases.[394–402] el-Naggar et al.[403] found that 84% of tumors had cytogenetic alterations that most commonly involved chromosomes 4p, 5q, 6p, and 17p, and loss of heterozygosity suggested involvement of tumor suppressor genes. p53 expression has been variably reported at low and high levels while c-erbB-2 has been reported at a high level of expression when evaluated for mRNA and at a low level when immunohistochemically evaluated for the protein.[269,404–406] In most studies, neither the mean number of argyrophilic nucleolar organizer regions nor ploidy has been useful for predicting biologic behavior.[394,407,408] Reports on S-phase fraction have been contradictory.[407,408] Among all the cellular studies, the cell proliferation marker Ki-67 has shown the most promise as a predictor of biologic behavior.[409,410]

Differential diagnosis: In tumors where acinar type cells are not obvious, attention must be given to a differential diagnosis. A differential diagnosis for the papillary cystic and follicular patterns includes cystadenocarcinoma, mucoepidermoid carcinoma, and metastatic thyroid carcinoma. In minor salivary glands, polymorphous low-grade adenocarcinoma is also considered. Although abundant clear cells are infrequent, acinic cell adenocarcinoma is included in a differential diagnosis of clear cell neoplasms. In all cases, recognition of acinar differentiated cells, sometimes with the help of special stains or electron microscopy, is a key to diagnosis.

Prognosis and treatment: Some investigators have attempted a grading system,[377,378,381,411–414] but the biologic behavior of acinic cell adenocarcinomas cannot be reliably predicted on the basis of histomorphologic features.[376,382,415–419] In general, features that have often been associated with tumors that recurred or metastasized include frequent mitoses, focal necrosis, neural invasion, pleomorphism, infiltration (not circumscribed), stromal hyalinization, incomplete resection, large size, solid growth pattern, and involvement of the deep lobe of parotid gland.[376,378,381,383,385,411,420] Staging is a better predictor of outcome than histologic grading. As noted above, assessment of the proliferation index with Ki-67 immunostaining may be useful as a prognostic indicator.

Reported incidences vary, but on average among several studies, these tumors have a recurrence rate of about 35% and a metastatic rate and death incidence of about 16%.[161,376,377,379,382,408–410,414–416,420] Multiple recurrences, metastasis, and short duration of symptoms are associated with a poor prognosis.[376,411] Studies have noted tumor metastases and deaths of patients many years after initial treatment, and five-year survival is not a reliable indicator of cure.[382,421] Acinic cell adenocarcinomas arising in minor salivary glands are less aggressive than those that occur in the major glands.[371–373] Complete surgical excision of the primary tumor offers the best opportunity for cure.[378,411,415,422]

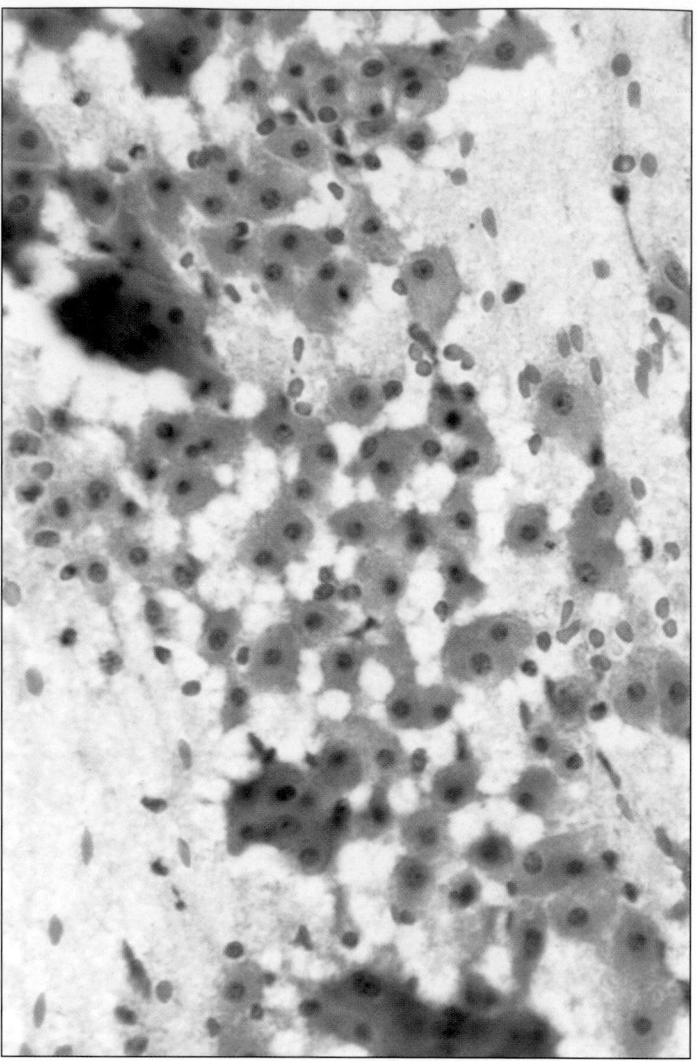

Fig. 23.39 This intermediate-magnification image shows a highly cellular smear typical of acinic cell carcinoma. The cells are loosely cohesive and feature uniform nuclei with abundant granular cytoplasm (Papanicolaou stain, 100×).

Cytopathology of acinic cell adenocarcinoma

Aspirates of acinic cell adenocarcinoma are usually quite cellular (Fig. 23.39). Large cells with abundant, finely granular cytoplasm lie singly and in groups.[423] Acinar arrangements are evident in some cases. Larger tissue particles often have a wide, thin-walled, venule-sized central vessel that ramifies through tissue fragments of considerable size (Fig. 23.40). These fragments have frayed edges, as tumor cells fall away to lie singly in the background. Numerous naked nuclei litter the smear. Nucleoli range from inconspicuous to prominent, but striking cytologic features of malignancy are not usually noted, and some cases will be falsely interpreted as negative. The coarse granules described in histopathology are more easily identified in paraffin-embedded cell-block sections than in smear material (Fig. 23.41). In two recent series, the correct cytologic diagnosis was given in under 70% of cases.[423,424]

The cytologic appearance of normal salivary gland cells, including acinar elements, was reviewed previously. Acinic cell adenocarcinoma differs in part from this picture by the absence of

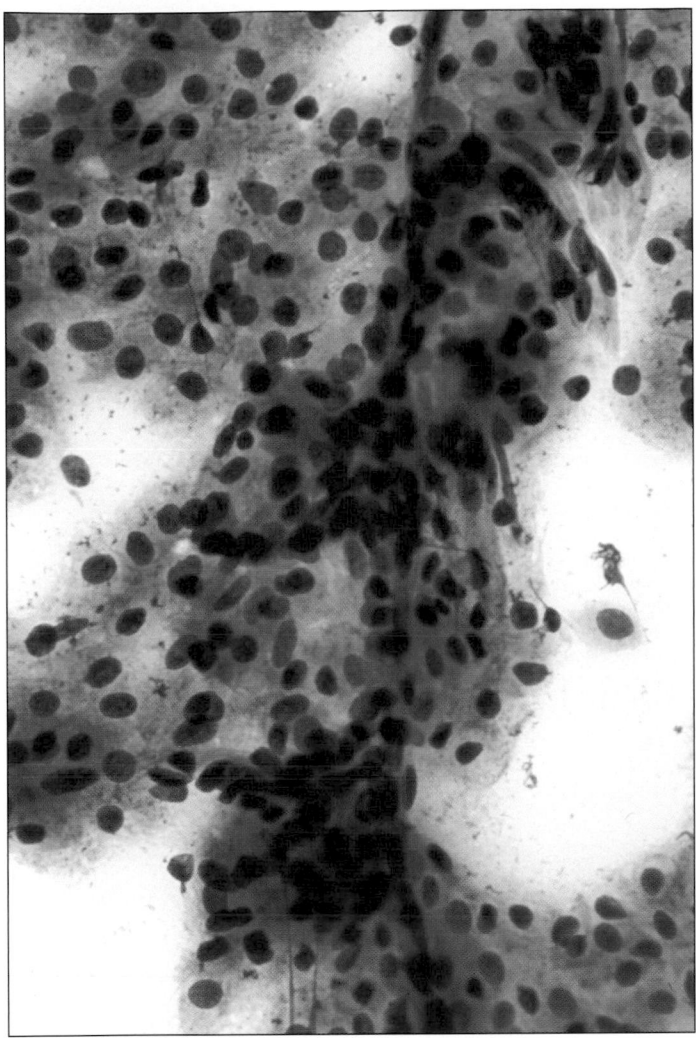

Fig. 23.40 Large tissue fragments are sometimes traversed by thin-walled dilated blood vessels. This finding is characteristic of acinic cell carcinoma but not diagnostic (Diff-Quik, 100×).

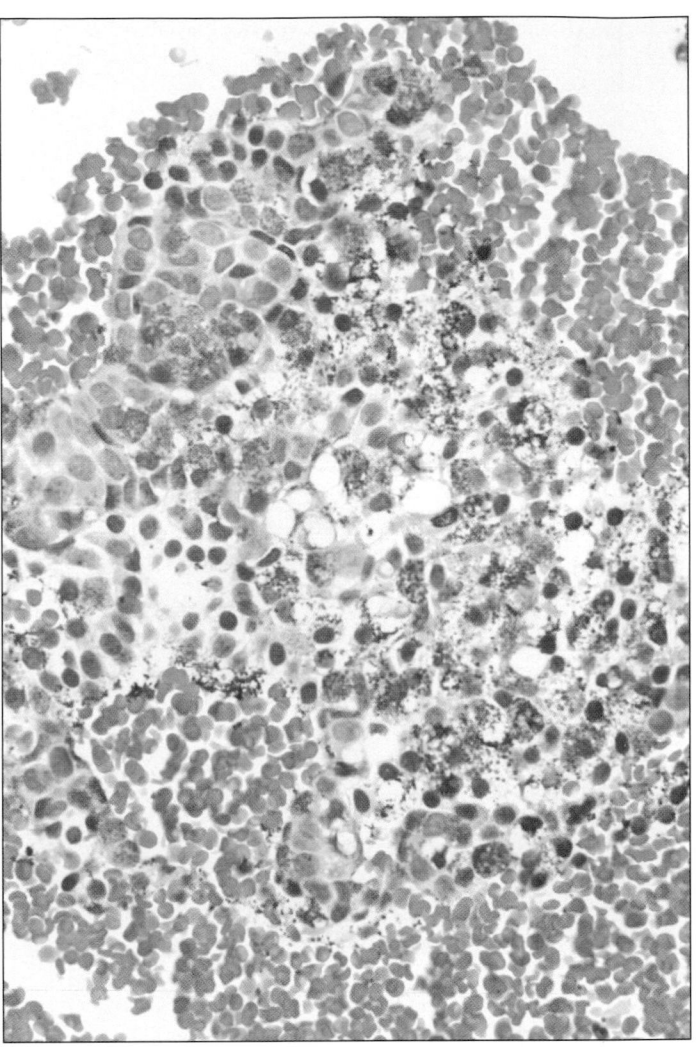

Fig. 23.41 This paraffin-embedded cell-block section shows the characteristic coarse zymogen granules very clearly (H&E, 100×).

normal duct cells and adipocytes. However, a mixture of neoplastic cells and cells from the surrounding normal gland complicates the smear pattern considerably. Occasionally, acinic cell adenocarcinomas are interpreted as normal tissue. Sometimes, numerous naked nuclei are mistaken for lymphocytes from sialadenitis, Warthin's tumor, or a lymph node. The background debris of Warthin's tumor is absent. The distinction between naked epithelial cell nuclei and lymphocytes was discussed earlier. These difficulties are compounded when lymphocytic infiltrates accompany an acinic cell adenocarcinoma.[424]

The histopathology of acinic cell adenocarcinoma is highly varied, and several alterations have been describe in FNA material. Clear cell change may be sufficiently extensive to suggest metastatic renal cell carcinoma but will usually be associated with cells more typical of acinic cell adenocarcinoma. The papillary cystic variant is difficult to recognize in a cytologic sample.[425] Smears with flat sheets of large granular cells and evidence of cyst fluid suggest Warthin's tumor, and vacuolated cells resemble low-grade mucoepidermoid carcinoma. Some aspirates have psammoma bodies, but other features that might suggest metastatic papillary thyroid carcinoma are absent.

The large granular cells of acinic cell adenocarcinoma resemble oncocytes. Distinction from oncocytic lesions is quite difficult. In most cases, however, the therapeutic approach to acinic cell adenocarcinoma and oncocytoma will not differ, and the impact of this difficulty is minimal. Acinic cell adenocarcinoma often recurs several years after initial diagnosis, and patient's history is very important for the cytopathologist.

ADENOCARCINOMA NOT OTHERWISE SPECIFIED

The salivary gland adenocarcinoma termed not otherwise specified (NOS) fails to exhibit prominence of any of the histomorphologic features that characterize the other, more specific carcinoma types. The diagnosis is one of exclusion, and the possibility of metastatic disease often has to be considered. It is difficult to establish the frequency of occurrence for this group of tumors because of reporting variability. In the literature, they represent between 8.8% and 44.7% of malignant tumors.[426]

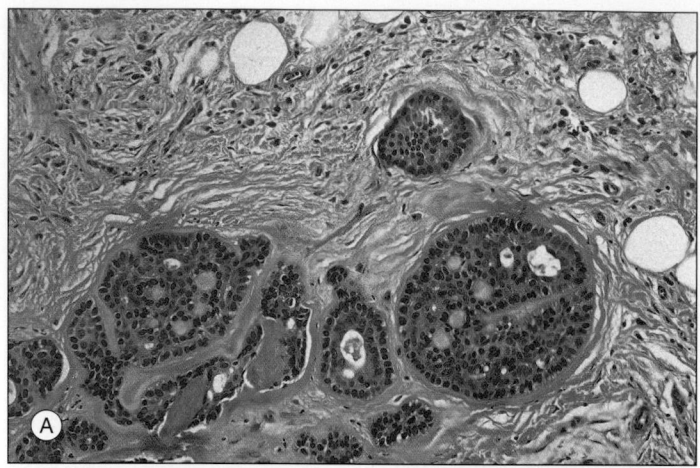

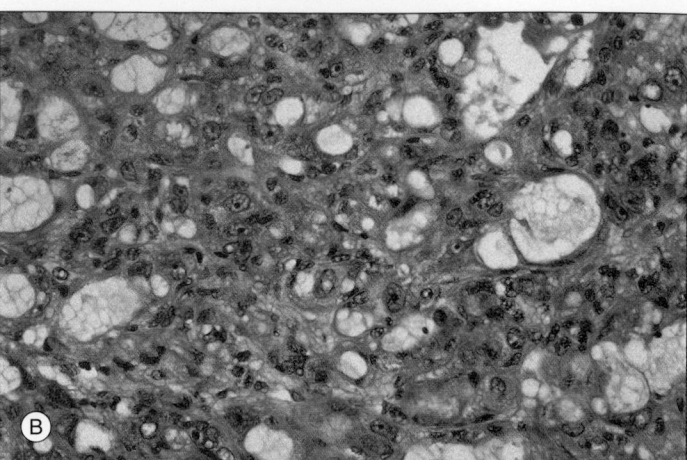

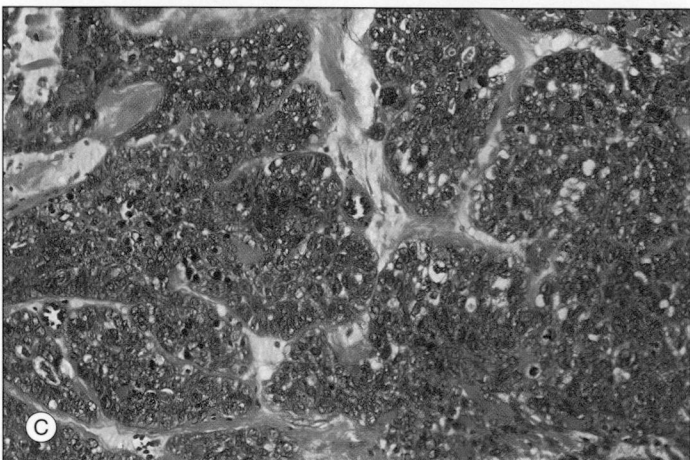

Fig. 23.42 Comparison of low, intermediate, and high-grade adenocarcinoma, not otherwise specified. **A**, A low-grade tumor demonstrates obvious infiltration of surrounding tissues but has well-formed ductal structures and relatively uniform nuclear features; **B**, The intermediate-grade tumor has enlarged, somewhat pleomorphic nuclei with prominent nucleoli. **C**, The high-grade tumor is composed of solid sheets of anaplastic cells that have a high mitotic rate. Focal ductal differentiation was evident in some areas of the tumor.

Clinical features: Of the AFIP's cases reviewed since 1985, NOSs account for about 9% of all salivary gland tumors and 17% of all carcinomas. In these cases, patients averaged 58 years of age, and about 40% and 60% occurred in the minor and major glands, respectively. Nearly 90% of the major gland tumors occurred in the parotid, and the palate, buccal mucosa, and lips were the most common minor gland sites.

Tumors in the major glands usually are solitary asymptomatic masses, but about 20% cause pain or facial weakness. Pain occurs more frequently with submandibular tumors, and ulceration often occurs with those of minor glands.[427]

Microscopic features: Although this is a heterogeneous group of tumors, glandular or duct-like structures, infiltrative growth, and absence of features diagnostic of other types of carcinoma are required features. The neoplastic epithelium forms small nests, islands, ramifying cords, tubules, or densely cellular, solid sheets. Small to medium-sized cysts may be evident in some areas of the tumor, and their lining is sometimes papillary.

A study by Spiro and coworkers[427] of 204 patients with 'adenocarcinoma' included 108 patients with adenocarcinoma NOS that arose in the major or intraoral minor salivary glands. Their study showed a correlation of histologic grade with biologic behavior and indicated that grading on the basis of cytomorphology is worthwhile.

Well-formed ductal and tubular structures, minimal variation in size, shape, and staining of nuclei, and few mitoses characterize low-grade adenocarcinomas. Intermediate-grade tumors have moderate nuclear morphologic variability and more frequent mitoses. In high-grade tumors, cells are large and pleomorphic, nuclei are hyperchromatic, mitoses are frequent and often atypical, and necrosis and hemorrhage are frequent (Fig. 23.42). Ductal and glandular differentiation is usually limited but distinguishes high-grade adenocarcinoma NOS from undifferentiated carcinoma.

Prognosis and treatment: Although limited follow-up data are available on these tumors, there is some evidence that tumors of the oral cavity have a more favorable prognoses than those of the parotid or submandibular glands.[428] Recurrence and distant metastasis, primarily to the lungs, are most frequent in patients with high-grade tumors but other metastatic sites have been reported.[429] Spiro and coworkers[427] found that the 15-year survival for low, intermediate, and high-grade tumors was 54%, 31%, and 3%, respectively. Interestingly, the cure rate for low-grade adenocarcinoma NOS was similar to acinic cell adenocarcinoma, emphasizing the importance of separating this group from high-grade adenocarcinoma NOS, a group that is one of the most aggressive of salivary gland carcinomas. Although surgery remains the primary treatment modality, adjuvant postoperative radiotherapy is indicated in intermediate and high-grade tumors that have advanced clinical stage.[428]

ADENOID CYSTIC CARCINOMA

Adenoid cystic carcinoma is a malignant neoplasm of salivary ductal and myoepithelial cells. *Cylindroma* is an undesirable synonym because of possible confusion with the benign dermal eccrine tumor of the same name.

Clinical features: Since the addition of polymorphous low-grade adenocarcinoma (PLGA) to the classification of salivary gland carcinomas, the relative incidence of adenoid cystic carcinoma has declined.[110,430,431] Although the reported incidence varies considerably, at the AFIP, it constitutes about 7.5% of all epithelial malignancies and 4% of all benign and malignant epithelial salivary gland tumors.[251,430,432,433]

The ratio of female to male patients has been just slightly higher than 3:2.[252,295,430] All ages of patients have been affected, but the peak incidence is in the fourth through sixth decades of life.[430,434] The parotid gland, submandibular gland, and palate, in descending order, are the sites of most frequent occurrence. Nearly half of the intraoral tumors occur in the palate. Tenderness, pain, and even facial nerve paralysis frequently develop during the course of the disease. Ulceration of the mucosa overlying intraoral tumors is common, especially palatal tumors.

Grossly, small tumors occasionally appear well circumscribed and even encapsulated. Circumscription is deceptive because tumor tissue has often infiltrated beyond the tumor margin that is evident by unaided visual examination. Because of the propensity for adenoid cystic carcinoma to extend insidiously along nerve tracts, surgeons often request multiple frozen section examinations of peripheral nerve segments removed from regions beyond the visual extent of the tumor.

Histologic features: The morphologic growth patterns observed in adenoid cystic carcinomas can be categorized as cribriform, tubular, and solid. The cribriform pattern is the most common whereas the solid pattern is the least common; however, a mixture of patterns within a single neoplasm is typical.

The cribriform pattern imparts a sieve-like appearance to the tumor. Islands of neoplastic cells contain several small, round, pseudocystic structures. The size of the cystic structures varies slightly, but they are rarely very large. These cyst-like spaces are contiguous with the connective tissue stroma of the tumor (Fig. 23.43). They usually contain an accumulation of basophilic glycosaminoglycans (chondroitin sulfate and heparan sulfate) or eosinophilic, hyalinized basal lamina material (laminin, fibronectin, and type IV collagen), or both.[435–440] The pseudocysts are typically Alcian blue positive. The tubular pattern lacks the complex cribriform structures, and cells are arranged in small nests that may surround individual cyst-like spaces (Fig. 23.44). The stroma is frequently hyalinized. The solid pattern is characterized by aggregates of tumor cells in which cyst-like spaces are absent or very few (Fig. 23.45), and cellular necrosis and mitotic figures are typically more frequent.

The majority of the neoplastic cells are myoepithelial differentiated.[441] They vary from amphophilic to clear, and cell borders are indistinct. Although the nuclei are fairly uniform in size, they vary from darkly to lightly basophilic and from smoothly round to angular and irregular. This angular nuclear pattern is a characteristic of adenoid cystic carcinoma (Fig. 23.46). Among the basaloid myoepithelial cells are scattered foci of ductal cells that surround tiny lumens (Fig. 23.46). True duct-type lumens are most conspicuous in the tubular pattern.

Adenoid cystic carcinomas are usually quite infiltrative, but small adenoid cystic carcinomas occasionally appear well circumscribed. Peripheral nerve invasion is characteristic but not pathognomonic. While nerve invasion is usually within the nerve sheath, some tumors invade within the nerve itself.

Ultrastructural studies have agreed with the light microscopic and immunohistochemical findings of luminal (ductal) and abluminal (myoepithelial and basal) cell differentiation.[442,443]

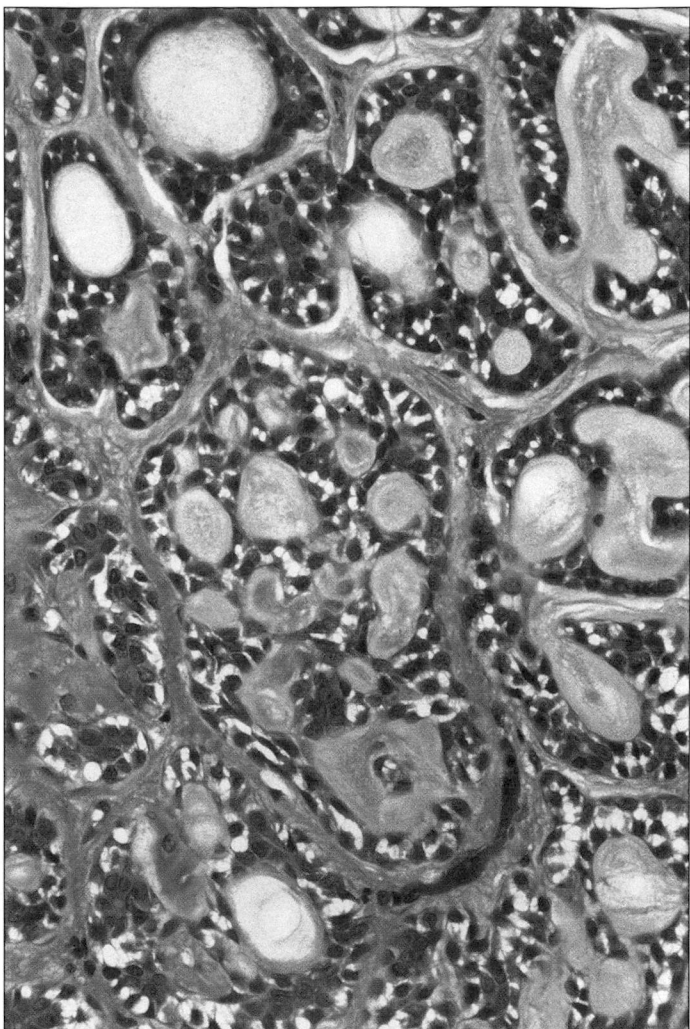

Fig. 23.43 In the cribriform pattern of adenoid cystic carcinoma interconnecting cords and nests of tumor cells surround multiple, variably sized, small cyst-like structures. Although the cyst-like spaces resemble duct lumens, they are actually pseudolumens and are in continuity with the stroma of the tumor. The basophilic and hyalinized eosinophilic material within the pseudocysts is glycosaminoglycans and basal lamina produced by the epithelial cells.

Although disparate immunohistochemical results have been reported, S-100 protein, glial fibrillary acidic protein, keratin, vimentin, muscle actin, calponin, and myosin have been identified in adenoid cystic carcinomas and are indicative of myoepithelial differentiation.[441,444,445] The ductal differentiated cells that line true lumens are reactive for carcinoembryonic antigen, epithelial membrane antigen, and lactoferrin and unreactive for muscle actin, vimentin, and alpha-1-antichymotrypsin.[439,441,446–449] Estrogen, progesterone, and progesterone receptor have been immunohistochemically localized in adenoid cystic carcinomas,[450,451] but other investigators were unable to demonstrate estrogen receptors in formalin-fixed adenoid cystic carcinomas.[451–453] Some investigators have found that over half of these tumors are immunoreactive for c-erbB-2 protein while others have found few, if any, positive tumors.[454–458] The c-Kit protein has been identified in a high percentage of adenoid cystic carcinomas in one study.[459]

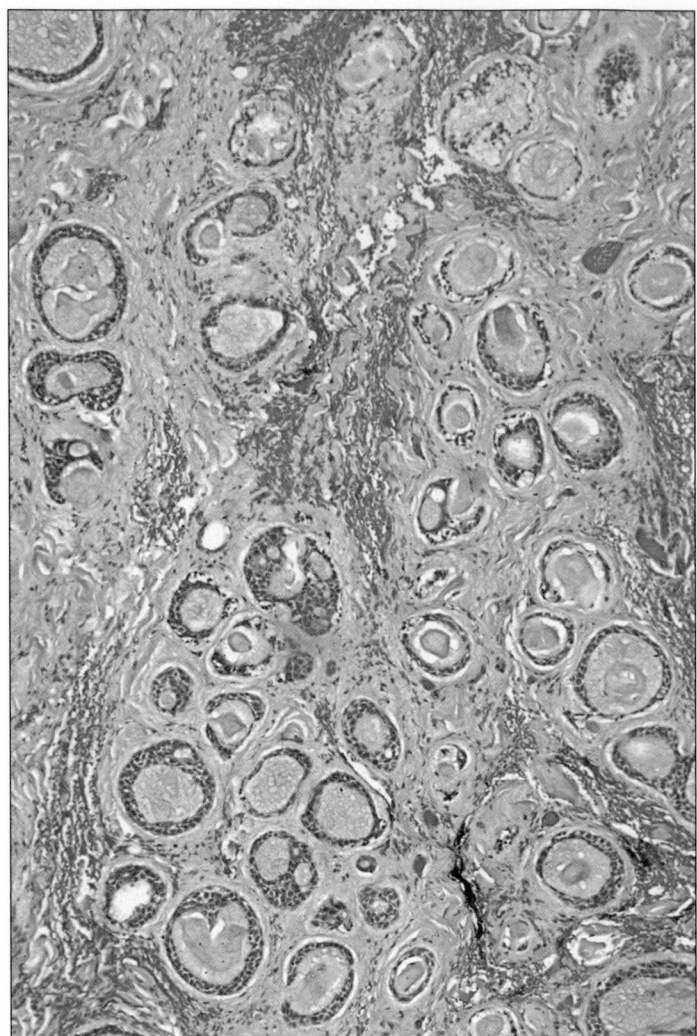

Fig. 23.44 In the tubular pattern of adenoid cystic carcinoma individual nests of tumor cells are surrounded by stroma, often hyalinized, and form circular (tubular) structures around eosinophilic, hyalinized, or basophilic material.

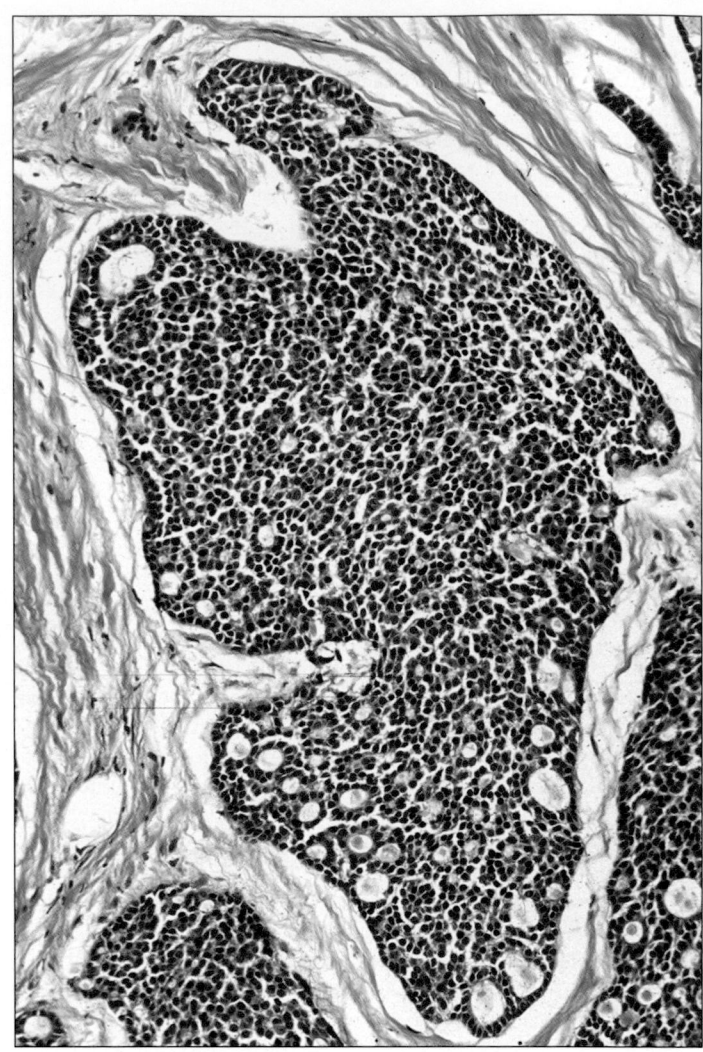

Fig. 23.45 Irregularly shaped, cellular islands of tumor contain only a few small pseudocysts in the solid pattern of adenoid cystic carcinoma.

Anomalies of chromosomes 1p, 2p, 3, 5p, 6q, 8q, 9p, 12q, 13q, 17p, 19q, and 20p have been reported for adenoid cystic carcinomas with alterations of 6q most frequently described.[268,400,460–467] The argyrophil staining technique for nucleolar organizer regions (AgNORs) has shown a significantly increased number of AgNORs in adenoid cystic carcinomas over the number in normal salivary gland tissue and benign salivary gland tumors and may have prognostic value.[394,468–473]

Differential diagnosis: Polymorphous low-grade adenocarcinoma (terminal duct carcinoma) (PLGA) is one of the principal considerations in the differential diagnosis of adenoid cystic carcinoma, and distinguishing between these two tumors is important because of their significantly different biologic behaviors. Both tumors are composed of ductal and abluminal cells and have a marked propensity to infiltrate around peripheral nerves. PLGA has a very uniform population of epithelial cells with round, vesicular to euchromatic nuclei and eosinophilic cytoplasm. Mitotic figures and cellular pleomorphism are distinctly rare in PLGA. PLGA lacks the characteristic pale to clear cells with hyperchromatic, angular nuclei

of adenoid cystic carcinoma. In PLGA, the cells are arranged in variable patterns, which include cribriform, hyalinized, cystic, sheet-like, glandular, tubular, canalicular, and single-file cords. At low magnification PLGA often has a swirled appearance. Pseudocystic, cribriform, and tubular patterns that characterize most adenoid cystic carcinomas are limited when present in PLGA. The Ki-67 labeling index is lower in PLGA than adenoid cystic carcinoma. The myoepithelial markers, smooth muscle actin, calponin, and myosin, and the c-Kit protein that characterize adenoid cystic carcinoma are weak or absent in PLGA.[441,459,474,475]

Like adenoid cystic carcinoma, epithelial-myoepithelial carcinoma (EMC) has a biphasic cell pattern of ductal cells surrounded by abluminal (myoepithelial) cells. The periductal cells in EMC are large, polygonal clear cells with rounded nuclei rather than the smaller, angular cells of adenoid cystic carcinoma. These large clear cells often dominate EMC, often grow in sheets, and contain notable amounts of glycogen. EMC does not grow in a cribriform pattern.

Foci within mixed tumors may resemble adenoid cystic, but the characteristic myxochondroid areas and the plasmacytoid and

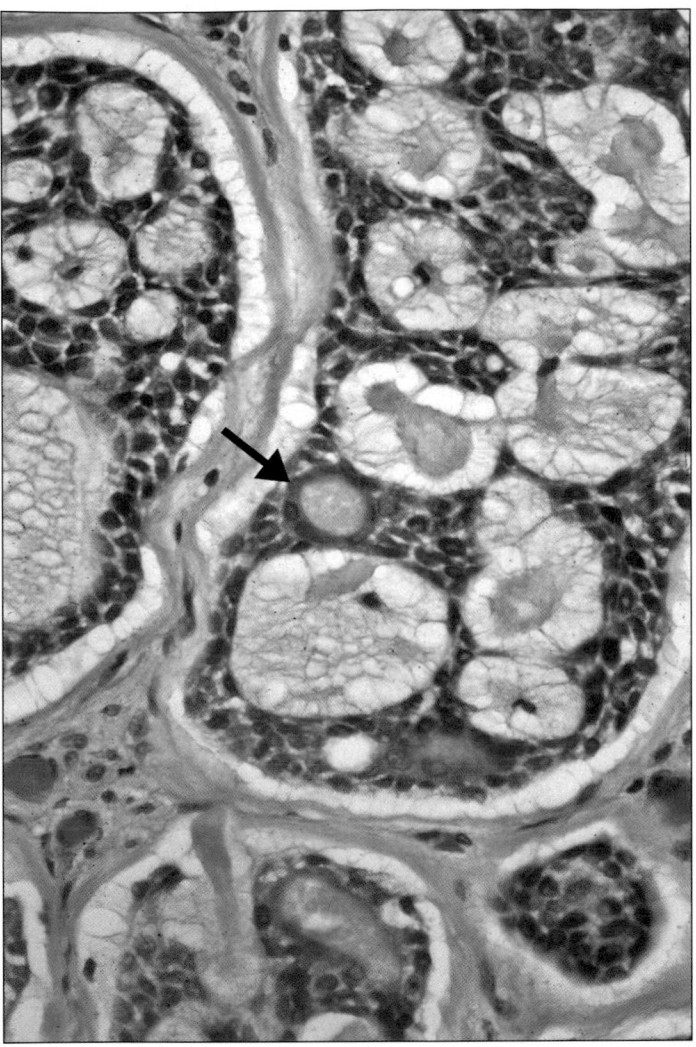

Fig. 23.46 Characteristic of adenoid cystic carcinoma, many epithelial cells have clear cytoplasm with poorly defined borders and irregular shaped nuclei. These cells surround extraepithelial cyst-like spaces. Foci of ductal-type cells (arrow) with true lumens can be found within these groups of myoepithelial differentiated cells.

Prognosis and treatment: Adenoid cystic carcinoma is often slow to metastasize but persistent and relentless in growth. In general, it has a good five-year survival rate but a poor ten-to-twenty-year survival rate. Nevertheless, different biologic courses can be predicted for adenoid cystic carcinoma by morphologic growth patterns. Tubular and cribriform growth patterns are associated with longer survival than the solid growth pattern.[484–489] Carcinomas with a solid growth pattern have the most fulminant course, which is characterized by early metastases and poor five-year survival statistics. Tumors with more than 30% solid areas have the worst prognosis,[484,487] and 15-year cumulative survival rates for patients with tumors that had none, less than 30%, and more than 30% solid areas has been reported to be 39%, 26%, and 5%, respectively.[484] Contradictory results have been reported on the relationship between perineural tumor invasion and development of metastases and survival.[490–492] Clinical stage has a major influence on prognosis.[486,489] Cumulative 10-year survivals of 75%, 43%, and 15% for stage I, stage II, and stage III and IV patients, respectively, has been reported.[489] Parotid gland tumors have a better prognosis than submandibular gland tumors. Distant metastases are more frequent than regional lymph node metastases. About 40–60% of patients develop distant metastases, most commonly to the lung, bone, and soft tissues, and distant metastases often develop despite local control of the tumors.[485,493–496]

Cytophotometry to evaluate nuclear DNA content has had mixed results as a predictor of clinical outcome.[486,487,492,497–499] Tumors with higher AgNOR counts, in general, have had a worse outcome than tumors with lower AgNOR counts.[470–473] A proliferation index assessed with immunostaining for Ki-67, proliferating cell nuclear antigen (PCNA), or topoisomerase type II alpha has been higher in tumors from patients with poorer outcome than in those with better survival while reduced expression of p27 (Kip1) has indicated a poorer prognosis.[457,477,478,480,500]

Wide to radical surgical excision and postoperative radiation therapy offer the best chance for long-term survival.[501,502] As an adjunct to surgery, radiation therapy, including fast neutron therapy, has been shown to improve local control of tumor, especially when there is microscopic residual tumor.[503–513] However, gross residual tumor portends a poor outcome. Chemotherapeutic treatment of adenoid cystic carcinoma has received only limited attention, but some tumors have responded. At present, chemotherapy must still be regarded as experimental.[514–517]

Cytopathology of adenoid cystic carcinoma

Adenoid cystic carcinoma is the most common small blue cell tumor encountered in salivary gland cytology. When the cribriform component is prominent, smears have a characteristic appearance, with spheres and cylinders of extracellular matrix material surrounded by uniform small cells (Fig. 23.47).[271,518–520] Single cells lie in the background, mostly in the form of naked nuclei. As noted in the discussion of basal cell adenomas, the interface between these spheres and the associated cells is very sharp and lacks the interdigitations of basal cell adenoma tissue particles.

Some have held that the cylindromatous appearance is pathognomonic of adenoid cystic carcinoma, and some previous writings on the subject indicate that this diagnosis should be straightforward. However, as more tumors have been studied in FNA samples, it has become clear that several other neoplasms can mimic adenoid cystic carcinoma. These usually have numerous small cells and often have frankly cylindromatous areas. Such lesions include pleomorphic adenomas, basal cell adenomas, basal cell adenocarcinoma, epithelial-myoepithelial carcinoma, and polymorphous low-grade

spindled myoepithelial cells that are common in mixed tumor are not evident in adenoid cystic carcinoma. Mixed tumors are not infiltrative and have lower Ki-67, PCNA, and AgNOR indexes and higher p27 (Kip1) index.[474,476–480]

Basaloid squamous carcinoma is a variant of squamous cell carcinoma of the upper aerodigestive tract that resembles adenoid cystic carcinoma.[481,482] It has a predilection for the hypopharynx, base of tongue, and supraglottic larynx where adenoid cystic carcinoma occurs infrequently. Basaloid squamous carcinoma has a squamous component that distinguishes it from the solid type of adenoid cystic carcinoma. The squamous component usually involves the mucosal epithelium in the form of epithelial dysplasia, carcinoma in situ, or invasive squamous cell carcinoma, but foci of squamoid cells also occur in the basaloid lobules. Immunohistochemically, basaloid squamous cell carcinoma is reported to be unreactive for muscle actin and cytokeratin (CK) 8, reactive for CK19, and reactive for CEA in the squamoid cells rather than the ductal cells in contrast to adenoid cystic carcinoma.[482,483]

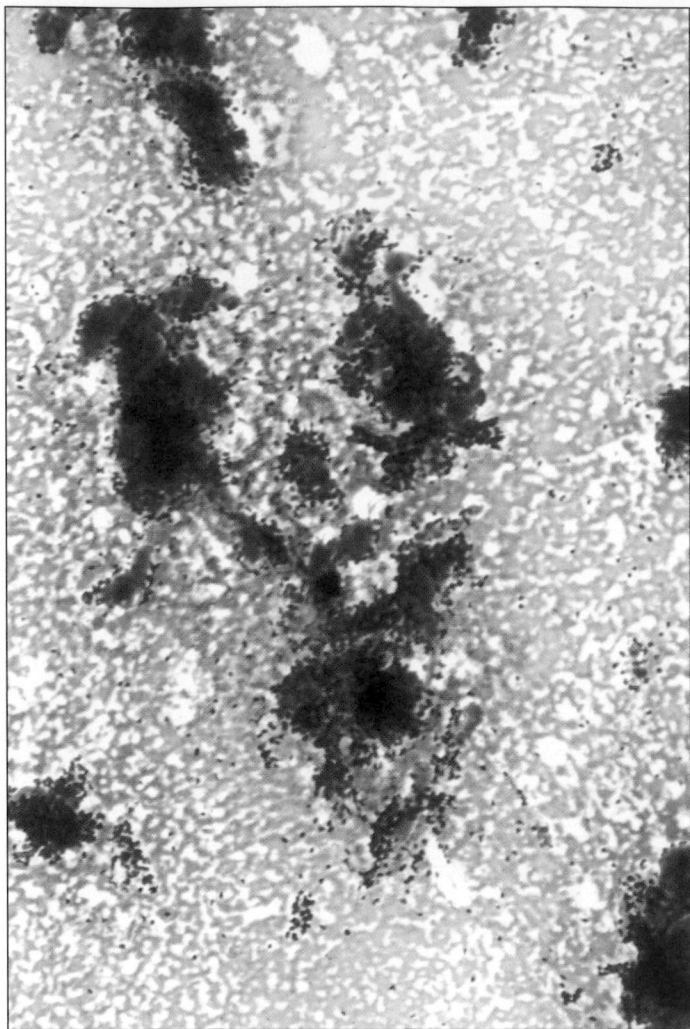

Fig. 23.47 This low-magnification image shows cribriform adenoid cystic carcinoma. Numerous uniform small cells surround spheres and cylinders of brightly metachromatic extracellular material (Diff Quik, 40×).

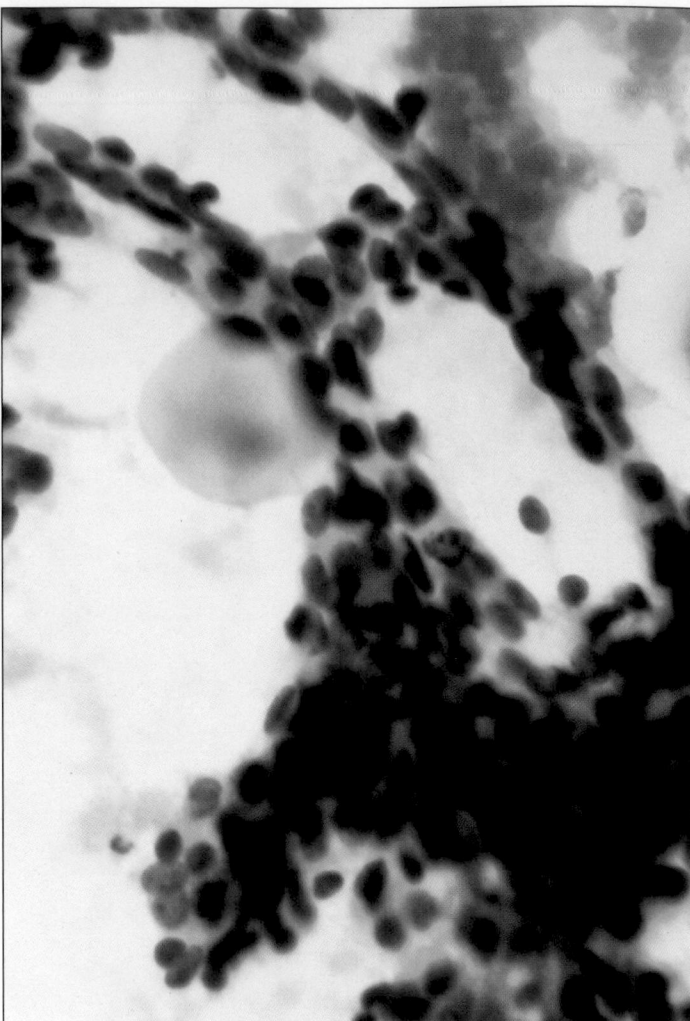

Fig. 23.48 This example of solid (anaplastic) adenoid cystic carcinoma shows uniform small cells that lack the traditional nuclear cytomorphologic features of malignancy. Spheres of extracellular matrix material are very rare (Papanicolaou, 400×).

adenocarcinoma. Similar difficulties occur with interpretation of frozen sections. The low nuclear grade of adenoid cystic carcinoma is easily misinterpreted as benign, especially if the sample is sparsely cellular and the matrix component is not well represented. The small cell pattern can also be mistaken for small cell undifferentiated carcinoma. Lee and coworkers emphasize identification of plasmacytoid cells as a key feature in distinguishing pleomorphic adenoma from adenoid cystic carcinoma.[518]

Cribriform adenoid cystic carcinoma of salivary gland origin is cytologically identical to dermal eccrine cylindroma. Both occur in the external auditory canal, which is the most common location for primary cutaneous adenoid cystic carcinoma. FNA has a limited role in their distinction.

As noted previously, the uncommon solid type of adenoid cystic carcinoma resembles basal cell adenoma. It is less often described in FNA reports than the cribriform type. The smears are usually very cellular with small uniform blue cells singly and in groups. Cylinders and spheres of extracellular matrix are absent (Fig. 23.48). Fragments of desmoplastic tumor stroma are collagenous, fibrillary, and metachromatic. They have been mistaken for the matrix of

pleomorphic adenoma and for the extracellular connective tissue of basal cell adenoma (Fig. 23.49). The stromal interface that is useful in distinguishing basal cell adenoma from cribriform adenoid cystic carcinoma is not useful with the solid variant. Some suggest that these tumors can be distinguished by careful attention to subtle nuclear features indicative of malignancy; others have not found this to be the case.[68, 271, 519, 521, 522] Necrosis strongly suggests adenoid cystic carcinoma rather than basal cell adenoma, but other small cell lesions (see Table 23.1) must also be considered. In our experience, only about half of aspirates of solid adenoid cystic carcinoma have necrosis.

Based on this information, Löwhagen et al[523] indicate considerable reluctance to render an unequivocal diagnosis of adenoid cystic carcinoma on cytologic evidence alone. They write that 'in our institution, we refuse to take the full diagnostic responsibility for a radical surgical procedure in which sacrifice of the facial nerve may be necessary in cases where there may be classic cytologic findings of adenoid cystic carcinoma but the patient is symptom free.' If this stance is justified for the cribriform pattern, it is much more appropriate for the solid variant.

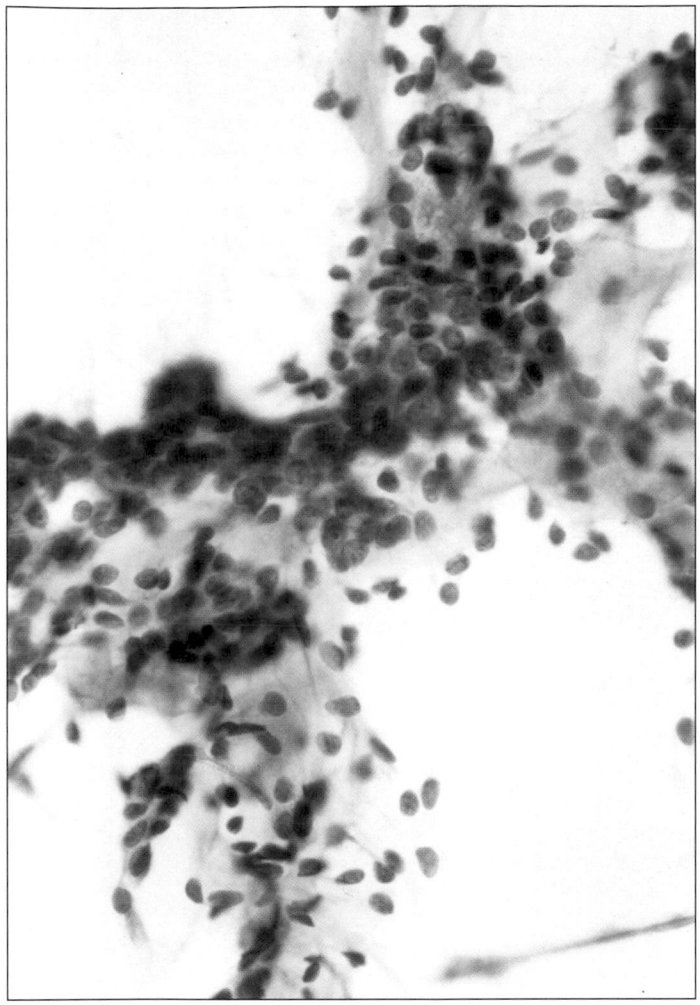

Fig. 23.49 This solid adenoid cystic carcinoma features intimate interdigitation of tumor cells and stroma in a manner that mimics basal cell adenoma (Papanicolaou, 100×).

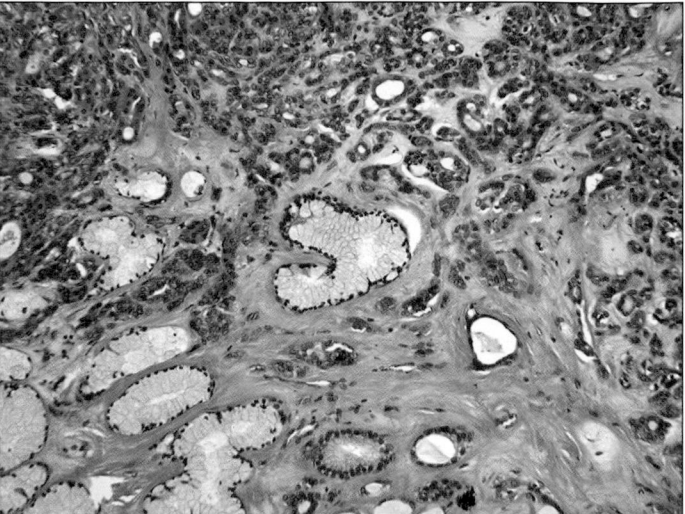

Fig. 23.50 Polymorphous low-grade adenocarcinoma with numerous small tubular duct-like structures infiltrating and replacing minor salivary gland parenchyma.

POLYMORPHOUS LOW GRADE ADENOCARCINOMA

PLGA was first reported in 1983 by Freedman and Lumerman[524] as *lobular carcinoma* and the following month by Batsakis et al.[525] as *terminal duct carcinoma*. The following year the term *polymorphous low-grade adenocarcinoma* was suggested as a clinically and morphologically descriptive term[526] and is currently preferred.[527]

Although some examples of PLGA have been reported in the major glands,[183,528–534] this tumor is mostly limited to occurrence in minor salivary gland sites, where their frequency is substantial. PLGA represents 20–25% of all malignant minor gland tumors.[110,535,536] Among AFIP cases accessioned since 1985, PLGA is twice as frequent as adenoid cystic carcinoma in minor glands. Of all benign and malignant minor salivary gland tumors, only mixed tumor and mucoepidermoid carcinoma are more common in this material.

Clinical features: The female/male ratio is about 2:1.[537] More than 70% of patients are between the ages of 50 and 79 years, and the mean age is 59 years.[537] Some evidence indicates a predilection for this tumor to occur in blacks. Whereas less than 11% of all malignant salivary gland tumors in AFIP's files occurred in blacks,

27% of these tumors did so. At least one other study of Americans has reported a similar observation,[526] and a preponderance of PLGA in an African population has been noted.[536] Multiple, synchronous tumors occasionally occur.[538] Clinically, PLGA typically is an asymptomatic firm nontender swelling of otherwise normal mucosa of the hard and soft palates, cheek, or upper lip. Mild pain or ulceration occurs in some cases. Radiographs of those overlying bone sometimes show bone erosion or infiltration.

Microscopic features: Grossly, PLGA is a circumscribed but unencapsulated mass that often approximates the mucosal epithelium. Microscopically, it is often deceptively well circumscribed at low magnification, but on closer evaluation, the tumor is at least focally infiltrative. In addition to infiltrative growth, PLGA is characterized by bland, uniform nuclear features, diverse but characteristic architecture, and prominent neurotropism. It has solid, trabecular, ductular, and tubular architectural growth. Small tubular structures with distinct central lumens lined by a single layer of cuboidal cells are more numerous peripheral to the central area of the tumor, where they infiltrate muscle, connective tissues, and salivary glands (Fig. 23.50). They are often closely associated and aligned with streaming columns and trabeculae of cells that display concentric whirling, sometimes creating a target-like appearance. This concentric arrangement is present in about one-third of the tumors.[524] Collagenous, hyaline, or mucohyaline stroma often are prominent around widely spaced epithelial structures (Fig. 23.51). Tumor cells have isomorphic, round, ovoid, or fusiform nuclei, finely stippled chromatin, and either inconspicuous or slightly enlarged nucleoli (Fig. 23.52). Mitoses are rare, and atypical mitoses are absent.[539] Transformation to high-grade adenocarcinoma has been reported following radiotherapy and multiple locoregional recurrences.[540]

PLGA has had considerable variability in the percentage of cells positive for proliferative cell nuclear antigen (0.5–70%), p53 reactivity, and ploidy status.[541] Cell proliferation indicators, including mitotic index and PCNA reactivity, of adenoid cystic carcinoma, epithelial myoepithelial carcinoma, and PLGA, were similar overall, but were largely dependent on the growth pattern.[542] Solid areas of growth exhibited the highest indices.

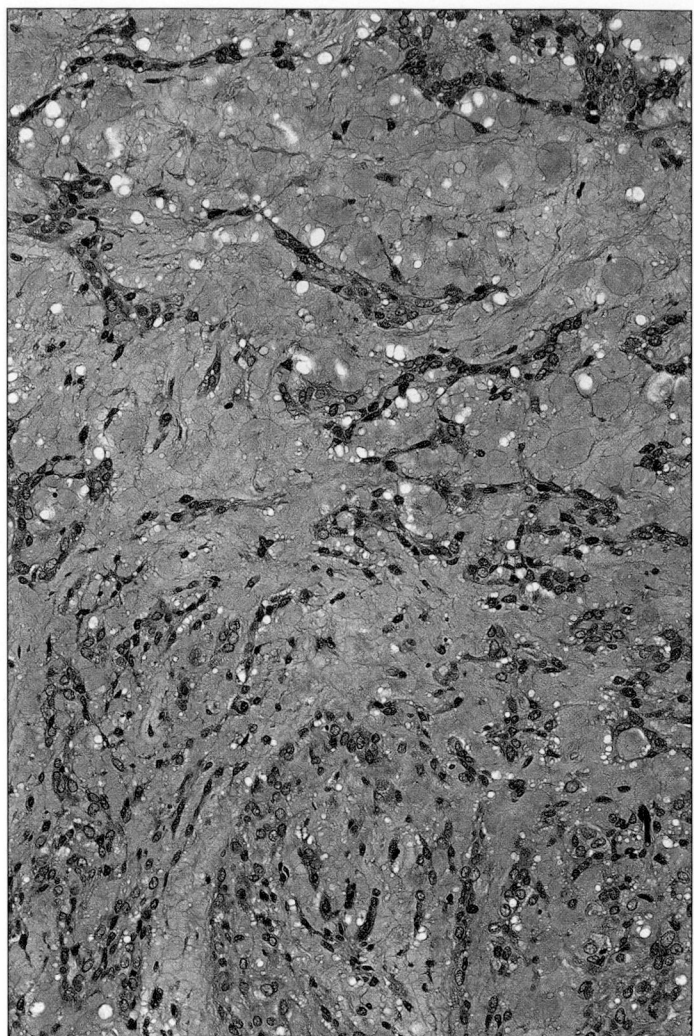

Fig. 23.51 Abundant mucohyaline stroma is present in this polymorphous low-grade adenocarcinoma, which resembles mixed tumor.

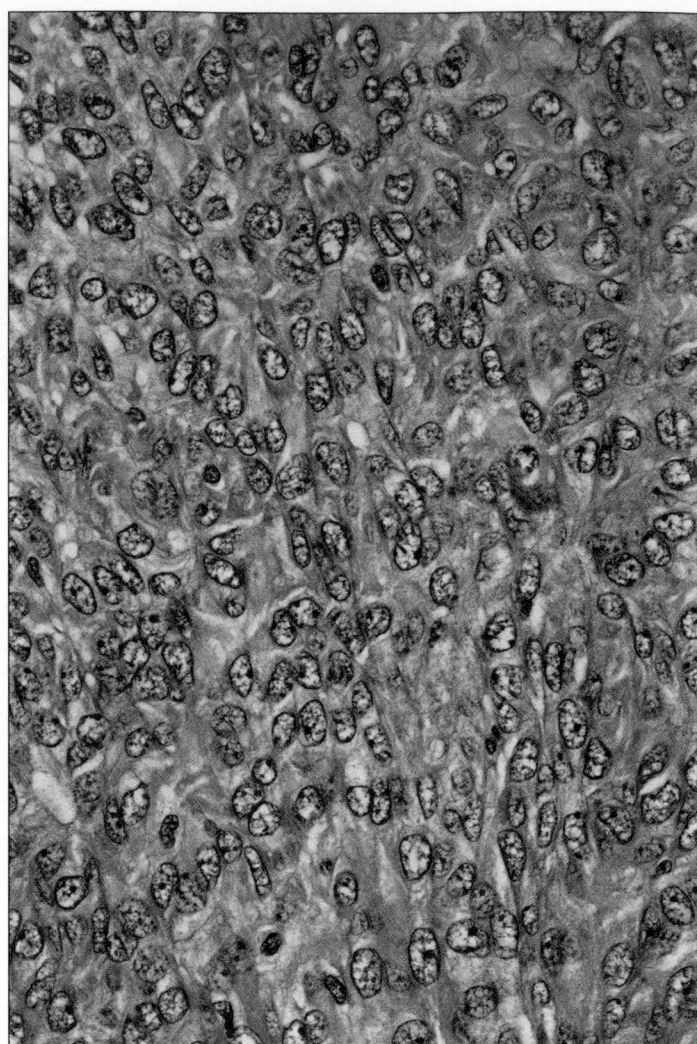

Fig. 23.52 The nuclei in this example of polymorphous low-grade adenocarcinoma show very limited variation. They are round to ovoid and have only slightly irregular contours, finely dispersed chromatin, and either inconspicuous or small single nucleoli.

Differential diagnosis: PLGA can be difficult to distinguish from mixed tumors and adenoid cystic carcinomas. Both mixed tumors and PLGAs have hyaline or mucohyaline stroma, sheets of neoplastic epithelial cells with morphologically bland nuclei, and well-formed ductal or tubular structures. Further complicating distinction, mixed tumors of the minor glands are typically not encapsulated. However, mixed tumors do not infiltrate surrounding connective tissue, fat, parenchyma, nerves, or blood vessels like PLGA. This emphasizes the need to include the interface of tumor with surrounding tissue in the biopsy specimen. Additionally, unlike mixed tumor, the tubular or ductular structures in PLGA often are entirely isolated from the more solid tumor areas. Greater GFAP immunoreactivity in mixed tumors, including of the stromal-like cells, has been reported.[543]

Like PLGA, most adenoid cystic carcinomas have isomorphic nuclei, little mitotic activity, focal mucohyaline stroma, infiltration of adjacent tissues, prominent neurotropism, and cribriform, tubular, and solid growth. However, the nuclei in PLGA are slightly larger and more round and uniform than the angular hyperchromatic nuclei in adenoid cystic carcinoma. The cytoplasm of the cells usually stain eosinophilic in PLGA and clear in adenoid cystic carcinomas. PLGA has only focal cribriform growth and lacks the large cribriform pseudocystic spaces that contain pools of hematoxyphilic glycosaminoglycans. It has been suggested that calponin is the most sensitive marker of modified, neoplastic myoepithelial cells.[135] In one related study calponin was useful in distinguishing between adenoid cystic carcinomas, tumors whose rich modified myoepithelial component stained consistently, and polymorphous low-grade adenocarcinomas, all of which were nonreactive.[441] Similarly, it has been suggested that c-kit expression may help in this distinction.[544] One group of investigators have shown that the MIB-1 index is significantly higher in adenoid cystic carcinoma than in PLGA (mean of 21.4% verses 2.4%, respectively).[475]

Prognosis and treatment: A review of 204 published cases revealed a 17% recurrence rate and a regional metastasis rate of 9%.[537] Recurrences develop from months to many years after initial treatment, indicating a need for long-term follow-up. Metastasis to distant sites is extremely unusual.[539,545,546] Treatment consists of wide but conservative surgical excision, depending on the size of the tumor and whether it demonstrates bone involvement. Soft tissue and bony surgical margins should be free of tumor. Neck dissection is not warranted unless clinical evidence of lymph node involvement is present.[547] There has been no benefit derived from postoperative radiation or adjuvant chemotherapy, although both modalities have been used.[524–526,548]

Cytopathology of polymorphous low grade adenocarcinoma

Uniform cells have fine chromatin, tiny nucleoli, and scant to moderate cytoplasm.[549,550] Cytologically, polymorphous low-grade adenocarcinoma can be very difficult to distinguish from adenoid cystic carcinoma, since it features small uniform cells that can be arranged around central hyaline cores. Hyaline stroma can be mistaken for the matrix material of pleomorphic adenoma, and small uniform cells mimic basal cell adenoma. This is a very difficult cytologic diagnosis because the infiltrative growth that typifies histologic sections cannot be appreciated in aspirate material. Great care must be exercised in making an unequivocally benign diagnosis based on aspiration of a minor salivary gland mass.

MALIGNANT MIXED TUMORS

The broad heading *malignant mixed tumor* includes three different tumors, discussed separately below.

Carcinoma ex mixed tumor (carcinoma ex pleomorphic adenoma)

Among the group of tumors referred to as malignant mixed tumors, carcinoma ex mixed tumor accounts for the vast majority. Diagnosis of carcinoma ex mixed tumor requires that (1) at least a focus of benign mixed tumor be identified; or (2) a previously operated benign mixed tumor had been excised from the site in which recurrent tumor is carcinomatous.

The frequency of carcinoma ex mixed tumor approximates 6–9% of all mixed tumors.[551,552] Mixed tumors of long duration and those that recur have the greatest risk for malignant transformation. The incidence of cancer in mixed tumors is 1.6% in those with durations of 5 years or less but 9.6% in those present for more than 15 years.[553,554] Microspectrophotometric analysis indicates that mixed tumors of long duration develop a tetraploid fraction similar to that found in the carcinomas.[553,555] Carcinomas ex mixed tumor occur, on average, about 13 years later than the adenomas (46.9 vs. 60.1 years) and are extremely unusual in patients younger 30 years of age.[551] Compared to the benign element, the carcinoma exhibits a reduced level of the CD44 cell adhesion molecules.[556]

Most patients with carcinoma ex mixed tumor present with a previously untreated painless mass of many years' duration.[557,558] About one-third of patients note recent rapid growth or ulceration, and some patients experience facial paralysis.[9]

Microscopically, foci of benign mixed tumor are associated with a characteristic carcinomatous element that is usually undifferentiated carcinoma or adenocarcinoma, not otherwise specified (Fig. 23.53). Occasionally, other carcinoma types, including mucoepidermoid carcinoma, adenoid cystic carcinoma, polymorphous low-grade, epidermoid, clear cell, and acinic cell, occur,[9,550,557–564] and in one series salivary duct carcinoma was the second most common type.[565] Extensive hyalinization in benign mixed tumors is one feature that correlates with an increased risk for malignant transformation.[147,565] It has been suggested that a series of genetic events that lead to amplification and overexpression of the HMGIC and MDM2 genes may contribute to malignant transformation.[144]

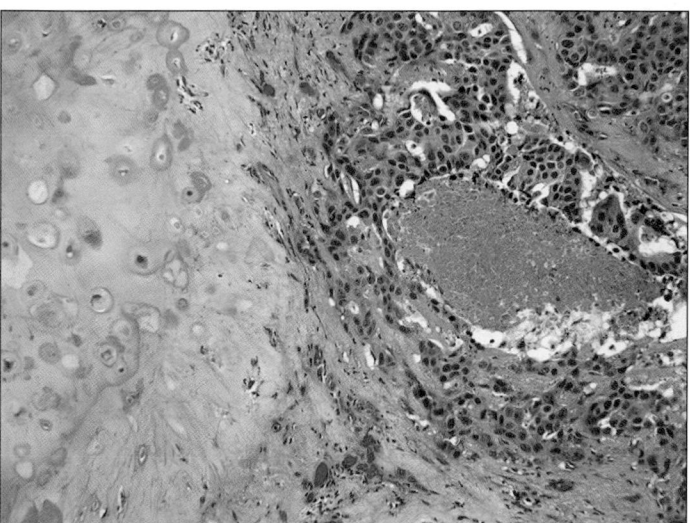

Fig. 23.53 Carcinoma ex mixed tumor in which the cartilaginous component of residual benign mixed tumor is seen at the left and high-grade adenocarcinoma, not otherwise specified, on the right. A large focus of necrosis is seen in the adenocarcinoma that destroyed both the normal gland and benign tumor.

Subclassification requires that features of a specific carcinoma predominate within the malignant component.[558] In rare instances in which the carcinoma is confined by the capsule, it is designated as *in situ* or *non invasive*,[149] but one such case was associated with metastasis.[566] These cases should be extensively sampled for extracapsular involvement. Grading of the carcinoma appears to have prognostic importance.[563] Furthermore, Tortoledo et al.[563] have shown that the distance of invasion of the carcinoma has prognostic importance. They demonstrated that patients in whom the carcinoma extended for more than 8 mm beyond residual capsule or benign tumor died of their disease, whereas none of those with less invasive tumor died.

Carcinosarcoma

Carcinosarcoma is a rare neoplasm that manifests both carcinomatous and sarcomatous components and is sometimes referred to as *true malignant mixed tumor*.[567–571] Some develop de novo while others arise in association with benign mixed tumors.[567,571–576]

Clinical features: Most reports identify only one or two cases, and these rare neoplasms represent less than 0.1% of salivary gland neoplasms.[570] About 65% have occurred in the parotid gland, and another 22% have developed in the submandibular gland. The remainder, of course, have been minor salivary gland tumors. There is no sex predilection, and patients have ranged from 14 to 87 years in age with a mean age of 57 years. Swelling, pain, nerve palsy, and ulceration have been signs and symptoms. The mean size has been about 4 cm, but primary neoplasms have been up to 13 cm in largest dimension.[567–569,572–574,577–582]

Microscopic features: The sarcomatous constituent most often has been chondrosarcoma, but osteosarcoma, fibrosarcoma, myxosarcoma, malignant fibrous histiocytoma, liposarcoma, and rhabdomyosarcoma have been identified.[567,571,575,579,583–586] The sarcomatous component usually dominates over the carcinomatous component. Ductal carcinoma is the most frequent carcinomatous element, but squamous cell carcinoma and undifferentiated carcinoma have also been identified (Fig. 23.54). Most of the carcinomatous

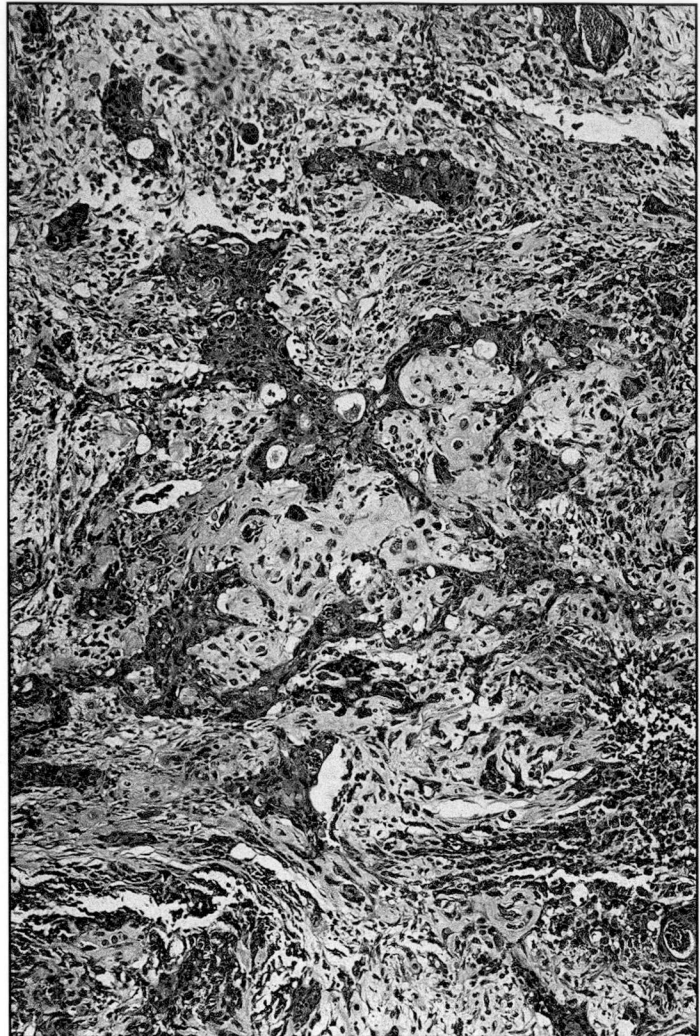

Fig. 23.54 Chondrosarcoma in carcinosarcoma. Cords of high-grade adenocarcinoma are intermingled with spindle cell and chondroid sarcomatous tissue in a carcinosarcoma of the parotid gland.

elements are high grade on the basis of cytomorphologic pleomorphism and mitoses. Metastatic and recurrent tumors usually manifest both carcinomatous and sarcomatous elements.

Ultrastructural studies have described chondrocytic and epithelial differentiation.[573,578,579] In addition, myoepithelial features have been identified in the chondrocytic areas. These latter features suggest that the sarcomatous component is derived from modulation of myoepithelial cells.

Immunohistochemical studies have generally demonstrated reactivity for cytokeratin, epithelial membrane antigen, and S-100 protein in the carcinomatous cells and reactivity for vimentin and S-100 protein in the sarcomatous tissue.[569,572,579,580] Toynton et al.[569] reported reactivity for glial fibrillary acidic protein in both sarcomatous and carcinomatous elements of a carcinosarcoma from the upper lip, but other investigators have not identified markers of neoplastic myoepithelium.[584] Only one tumor has been studied for expression of p53, and it was variably positive.[587]

Differential diagnosis: Marked cytologic atypia, including cellular and nuclear pleomorphism, hyperchromatism, and mitotic figures, and invasive growth distinguish carcinosarcoma from

benign mixed tumor. In some tumors both benign mixed tumor and carcinosarcoma are evident. The presence of both carcinomatous and sarcomatous tissues differentiates these neoplasms from carcinoma ex mixed tumors in which only carcinomatous elements are present.

Sarcomas of the major salivary glands are uncommon but not as rare as carcinosarcomas.[588,589] Anticytokeratin immunohistochemistry can be helpful for identification of carcinomatous elements in sarcomatoid salivary gland tumors. Synovial sarcoma would be an exception.

Spindled cell carcinomas of the oral mucosa need to be differentiated from carcinosarcoma. Malignant dysplasia or overt epidermoid carcinoma of the mucosal epithelium, continuity with atypical basaloid cells of the surface epithelium, and absence of adenocarcinomatous features characterizes spindle cell carcinoma.

Prognosis and treatment: Carcinosarcoma is an aggressive, high-grade malignancy. Among the limited number of patients with follow-up data reported, 58% died of disease, and 17% were living with disease.[567–569,572,573,577,578,582] Survival is usually less than five years.[586] Two-thirds of patients develop recurrences, and 50% develop metastases. Lung, rather than regional lymph nodes, has been the most common site of metastases. Radical surgery with and without adjunctive radiation therapy and chemotherapy has been utilized. Since hematogenous metastases are more common than lymphatic metastases, radical neck dissection is reserved for patients with clinical lymphadenopathy.

Metastasizing mixed tumor

Metastasizing mixed tumor is a very rare salivary gland neoplasm that histologically appears benign but inexplicably metastasizes. The diagnosis is established retrospectively after metastasis. Wenig et al.[126] reported the largest series (11 cases), and occasional case reports continue to appear in the literature. About 50 cases have been reported.

Clinical features: There is usually a long interval, on average 20 years, between diagnosis of the primary mixed tumor and its metastases.[126,590] Recurrences in the primary site precede or coincide with metastases in 90% of cases.[126,591–595] The parotid gland has been the primary site of 80% of the tumors while the submandibular gland was the primary site in 12%. Bone, lung, and lymph nodes have been the most common sites of metastatic disease.[126,590,596] There is no sex predilection. The mean age of patients at diagnosis of their primary tumors has been about 28 years, but patients have ranged from young to old. Clinical signs and symptoms of malignancy are absent in the primary tumors, which have ranged from 0.5 cm to 15 cm in largest dimension.

Radiation therapy and vascular infiltration, either natural or iatrogenic during surgery have been suggested as possible factors that may contribute to subsequent metastases,[593,597–599] but no etiologic factors have been definitely identified.[126]

Microscopic features: The histologic features of the primary neoplasms are characteristic of benign mixed tumors with mesenchymal-like myxoid and myxochondroid tissue intermixed with epithelial areas. There is both ductal and myoepithelial differentiation. In most cases, no specific histologic features distinguish the primary tumors from conventional mixed tumors, and the appearance and immunohistochemical reactions of the metastatic foci are similar to the primary salivary gland neoplasms.[126,594,595] One report has described carcinomatous transformation within a portion of a metastatic focus.[590]

The Ki-67 proliferation index was described in one report as greater in the metastatic tumor focus than the primary submandibular gland tumor.[590] Cytogenetic analysis of the skeletal metastases of a metastasizing mixed tumor identified two hypodiploid clones with abnormalities of chromosomes 1, 3, 9, 13, 21, and 22.[600] Flow cytometric analysis has not proven useful for identifying potentially metastasizing mixed tumors.[126,597,601]

Differential diagnosis: A long interval between diagnosis of the primary tumor and discovery of metastatic tumor sometimes makes it difficult to link them to one another, and skeletal and extraskeletal chondrosarcoma, chordoma, or chondroid hamartoma of the lung can be diagnostic considerations. A ductal epithelial component distinguishes metastatic mixed tumor from chondrosarcoma; characteristic physaliphorous cells of chordoma are absent in mixed tumors; and the merging of epithelial elements with adjacent alveoli or bronchioles characterizes hamartomas of the lung. Still, a complete and accurate medical history is most helpful in the differential diagnosis.

Prognosis and treatment: Twenty-two percent of patients have died of their metastatic tumors at an interval of 2 to 8 years after diagnosis of metastases.[126,594,596,602] Most metastasizing mixed tumors recur in the primary tumor site prior to metastasis, and recurrence of primary mixed tumors correlates with conservative enucleation.[595] Therefore, wide surgical excision is probably the best preventive measure. Surgery has been the principal treatment modality for metastatic foci.

Cytopathology of malignant mixed tumor

As mentioned previously, benign mixed tumors with prognostically meaningless cytologic atypia are much more common than any form of malignant mixed tumor.[603] In those aspirates that are recognized as malignant, the benign elements of pleomorphic adenoma are often either not sampled or not recognized.[604–606] False-negative interpretations after failure to sample what can be focal malignancy are reported more often than are unqualified diagnoses of carcinoma in which the mixed tumor component is not sampled. When aspirated, most, but not all, carcinosarcomas are recognized as malignant, but simultaneous cytologic identification of both carcinomatous and sarcomatous components is unusual.

EPITHELIAL-MYOEPITHELIAL CARCINOMA

This is a biphasic neoplasm of ductal and myoepithelial cells in which large, clear, myoepithelial-type cells predominate. At one time these tumors were thought to be benign,[607–609] but they are now recognized as low-grade adenocarcinomas.[26,609–612]

Clinical features: Evaluations indicate an average incidence of about 1% of salivary gland neoplasms.[370,432,610,613–617] Three-quarters of these tumors occur in the parotid gland, and the remainder develop about equally in the submandibular gland and minor salivary glands.[610,612,615,617,618] The peak incidence is in the seventh decade of life, and the mean age of patients is about 60 years. A majority of patients are women. Although tumors have been up to 12 cm in largest dimension, 2–3 cm is typical. Occasionally, patients have experienced pain or facial weakness.[619,620]

Microscopic features: A few epithelial-myoepithelial carcinomas are well circumscribed or even partially encapsulated, but nests of tumor typically infiltrate adjacent tissues. Many are multilobular. The characteristic histomorphology is a biphasic cellular pattern of ductal elements, composed of cuboidal, intercalated duct-like cells that usually border small lumens, surrounded by large, clear-staining myoepithelial cells (Fig. 23.55). A variable amount of pale eosinophilic or amphophilic cytoplasm is present in some cells. The clear cells contain glycogen that can be demonstrated with PAS

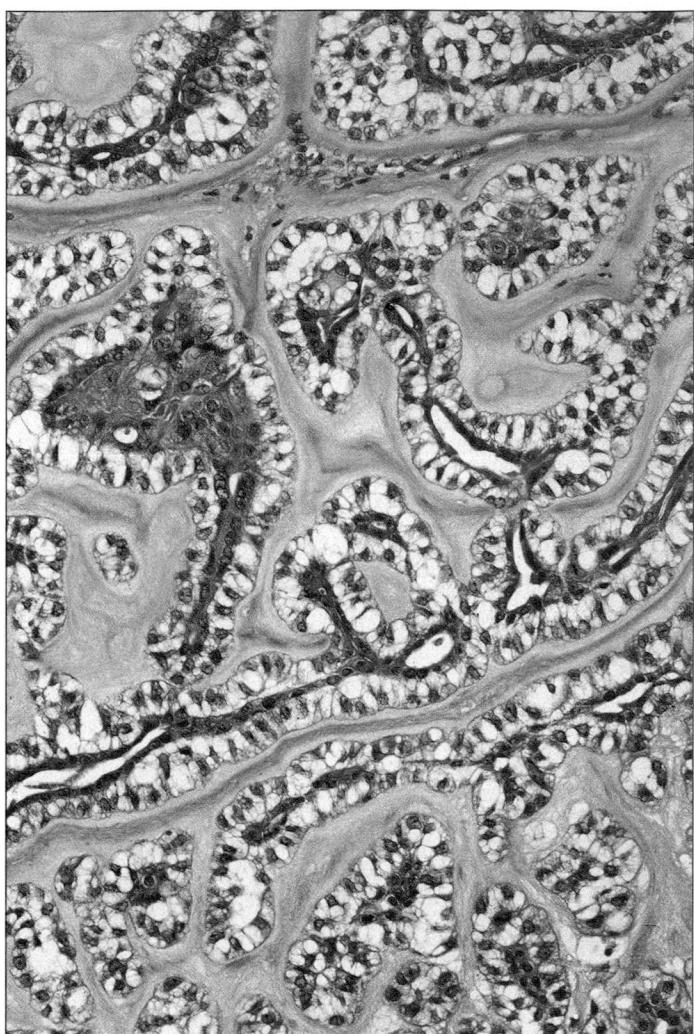

Fig. 23.55 In this epithelial-myoepithelial carcinoma relatively numerous and conspicuous, eosinophilic, cuboidal intercalated duct-like cells border lumens and are themselves surrounded by larger, polygonal cells with clear cytoplasm. The periepithelial stromal tissue is hyalinized.

staining. The ductal structures are usually conspicuous among the more numerous clear cells but are sparse in some tumors. The architecture of the tumors varies from sheets to organoid nodules to discrete tumor nests, and they may be solid or cystic. The stroma varies from loose fibrous tissue to hyalinized.

Immunohistochemical studies usually report the ductal cells as immunoreactive for cytokeratin and the clear cells as immunoreactive for S-100 protein, but these reactions are variable.[612,613,616,618,620] The clear, myoepithelial-differentiated cells are typically reactive for smooth muscle actin, which is frequently intense, and calponin while reactivity for myosin and vimentin is more variable.[441,619,621,622] Most studies have found these tumors do not express immunoreactivity for c-erbB-2 and rarely over express p53 protein, but one report described a mutation in the p53 gene.[456,623,624] The immunohistochemical Ki-67 proliferation index is generally low.[623,625]

The bicellular features are also evident with electron microscopy. Electron dense cells border small lumens and have features of duct luminal cells and are surrounded by more electron lucent cells with features of myoepithelium.[611,620,621]

Most studied tumors have been diploid or near diploid.[400,616,623,625] Cytogenetic analyses have been very limited. One tumor had a normal karyotype, and another exhibited numerical chromosome alterations without structural anomalies.[400]

Differential diagnosis: Many types of salivary gland neoplasms contain ductal and myoepithelial cells, most notably mixed tumor and adenoid cystic carcinoma. Epithelial-myoepithelial carcinomas lack the characteristic myxochondroid tissue of mixed tumors, and the myoepithelial cells of mixed tumors are usually smaller and not optically clear. The cells in adenoid cystic carcinomas are usually smaller with more irregular, angular, hyperchromatic nuclei, and the characteristic cribriform pattern of adenoid cystic carcinomas is not a feature of epithelial-myoepithelial carcinomas. Some clear cells can be found in polymorphous low-grade adenocarcinomas, but they are not a predominant component and are not arranged in a bicellular pattern with ductal cells.

Clear cells are sometimes a prominent component of mucoepidermoid carcinomas, acinic cell adenocarcinomas, sebaceous carcinomas, and oncocytomas, but these tumors lack the characteristic biphasic cellular pattern of epithelial-myoepithelial carcinomas. The characteristic epidermoid and mucous cells of mucoepidermoid carcinomas and acinar differentiated cells of acinic cell adenocarcinomas are absent in epithelial-myoepithelial carcinomas. Unlike epithelial-myoepithelial carcinoma, the clear cells are negative for glycogen in acinic cell adenocarcinomas and sebaceous carcinomas, in which frozen sections stain for lipids. Clear cell oncocytomas usually have eosinophilic oncocytes associated with the clear cells. Clear cell adenocarcinomas lack the unique bicellular differentiation of epithelial-myoepithelial carcinomas. Rare in the salivary glands, metastatic renal cell carcinoma lacks the biphasic cell pattern, contains intracellular lipid, and has a more prominent vascularity.[299]

Prognosis and treatment: In general, epithelial-myoepithelial carcinoma is a low-grade malignancy with recurrences in over 3%, lymph node metastases in about 20% of patients, and occasional distant metastasis and deaths.[610,611,613–619,623,626] Most investigators have been unable to correlate a poor prognosis with specific histologic features, but nuclear atypia, DNA aneuploidy, and high proliferative activity indicated by Ki-67 immunostaining have been associated with more aggressive behavior.[612,616,623,625]

Little data for treatment recommendations are available, but most tumors have been treated by surgical excision. Adjunctive radiation therapy is sometimes used, especially when the completeness of excision is in doubt.[621]

Cytopathology of epithelial-myoepithelial carcinoma

Smears of this neoplasm reflect its histology and have a combination of large myoepithelial cells and tubules formed by uniform small dark duct cells.[627–629] Specimens in which either component predominates cause diagnostic difficulties. A cellular hyaline material is sometimes associated with the cell clusters, and sometimes there are numerous naked nuclei. A predominance of small cells and hyaline suggests adenoid cystic carcinoma, while the clear myoepithelial cells suggest clear cell carcinoma. Other tumors in the differential diagnosis are acinic cell adenocarcinoma with clear cell change and sebaceous carcinoma, but neither has a component of small duct cells. Klijanienko and Vielh reported that all five of their cases were recognized as malignant at the time of FNA, but none was classified correctly; the cytologic interpretations were either adenoid cystic carcinoma or adenocarcinoma.[629]

PRIMARY SQUAMOUS CELL CARCINOMA

Diagnosis of primary salivary gland squamous cell carcinoma requires exclusion of primary disease in some other site, particularly the head and neck. The diagnosis is not made in the minor salivary glands because distinction from mucosal squamous cell carcinoma is not possible.

Past exposure to radiotherapy appears to increase the risk of developing this tumor, and the median time between irradiation and diagnosis of the salivary carcinoma is 15.5 years.[334,630–634] The reported frequency of primary squamous cell carcinoma among all major gland tumors in large series has varied from 0.9% to 4.7%.[11,634]

The average age of patients is about 64 years.[630,635–637] In nearly 90%, the parotid gland is affected, and there is a strong male predilection.[630,637,638] Just over one-half of patients with parotid gland disease are asymptomatic, but pain or preoperative facial nerve paralysis occurs frequently.[9,630]

Microscopically, these tumors are typical keratinizing squamous cell carcinomas that are usually well to moderately differentiated. Special stains disclose no intracytoplasmic mucin, which helps distinguish them from mucoepidermoid carcinoma.

Metastatic squamous cell carcinomas in the parotid gland from the skin or upper airway and digestive tracts outnumber primary squamous cell carcinomas.[504,631,635,639–642] In a study of 2802 patients with squamous cell carcinoma of the skin of the head and neck, the parotid gland was involved in 1.5% of the cases.[643] The skin regions of the preauricular area, ear (including the external auditory canal), cheek, neck, nose, temple, and forehead were frequent primary sites.[631,643] Most patients with metastatic carcinomas had primary skin lesions greater than 2 cm in diameter of long duration, implying that it is unusual for small or occult skin cancers to manifest first in the parotid gland.[643] Radical surgery for patients with metastatic disease remains controversial.[644,645]

Cytopathology of primary squamous cell carcinoma

Primary squamous cell carcinoma is suspected when a cytologic preparation is obtained from a patient with no evidence of a tumor at another site.[646] Occasional specimens are difficult to classify as pure squamous cell carcinoma, and a few aspirates are suspicious, but nondiagnostic, when only necrotic material is identified.

(HYALINIZING) CLEAR CELL ADENOCARCINOMA

While clear cells are a feature of a wide variety of salivary gland neoplasms, such as mucoepidermoid carcinoma, acinic cell adenocarcinoma, and epithelial-myoepithelial carcinoma, some uncommon monomorphous clear cell neoplasms lack features that are characteristic of other types of carcinomas and are classified separately.[647–654] Many of these monomorphic clear cell adenocarcinomas have densely collagenous and hyalinized stroma and the term *hyalinizing clear cell carcinoma* has been used to describe them.[652]

Clinical features: Classification of clear cell adenocarcinomas has been inconsistent and often absent from large series of salivary gland neoplasms, and incidence rates are difficult to derive. It is clear, however, that these are very uncommon salivary gland neoplasms.[12,110,251,295,427,433,653] Most reported cases have involved the minor salivary glands, but they also occur in the major salivary glands.[299,647,649,652,653,655] The palate, buccal mucosa, tongue, floor of the mouth, lip, and retromolar and tonsillar areas have been involved.

The peak incidence is in the fifth to seventh decades of life, and only one case has been reported in a child.[656] There is no sex predilection. Mucosal ulceration and pain occur with some tumors, but swelling is the only sign in most cases. Duration of the tumors has ranged from 1 month to 15 years.[649] The size of the primary tumor is usually 3.0 cm or less.

Microscopic features: Clear cell adenocarcinomas are composed of a monomorphous population of polygonal to round cells with clear cytoplasm (Fig. 23.56), although some cells have pale eosinophilic cytoplasm. The cells are generally larger than normal acinar cells with round, eccentric nuclei that frequently contain small nucleoli. Some tumors have a moderate degree of nuclear pleomorphism, but mitotic figures are uncommon. Cytoplasmic glycogen varies from marked to not demonstrable with PAS staining. Only rarely will a tumor have a rare cell with intracytoplasmic mucins.[652] The tumor cells are arranged in sheets, nests, or cords. Although microcysts occasionally occur, ductal structures are generally absent. The stroma varies from interconnecting, thin fibrous septa to thick bands that may be cellular, hyalinized, or loosely collagenous. The tumors are poorly circumscribed and usually infiltrate adjacent tissues, including the mucosal surface, bone, and nerves.

Immunohistochemical studies have given variable results.[647,649,651,652,654,656] Most tumors are at least focally immunoreactive for cytokeratin, but both positive and negative immunoreactivity for S-100 protein, glial fibrillary acidic protein, actin, and vimentin have been reported. Those tumors that are positive for S-100 protein, GFAP, and smooth muscle actin are probably more appropriately classified as clear cell myoepitheliomas or myoepithelial carcinomas.[657] Ultrastructural investigations report features of duct cell differentiation but not myoepithelial differentiation.[647,6497,651,652,658–660] Cytogenetic and molecular pathologic studies are lacking for this group of tumors.

Differential diagnosis: Clear cell adenocarcinoma is distinguished by its monomorphous population of clear cells. Mucocytes, demonstrable with mucicarmine and Alcian blue, and epidermoid cells identify mucoepidermoid carcinomas. The clear cells in acinic cell adenocarcinomas are glycogen negative, acinar cell differentiation is evinced by diastase-resistant, PAS-positive, intracytoplasmic granules, and microcystic, papillary-cystic, and follicular patterns are often present. Epithelial-myoepithelial carcinoma has a biphasic cell population of luminal duct cells surrounded by larger clear-staining myoepithelial cells, and it generally lacks the small nests, cords, and isolated clear cells that are common in clear cell adenocarcinoma. Immunohistochemical markers for neoplastic myoepithelial cells, such as smooth muscle actin, calponin, S-100 protein, and GFAP, are usually positive. Oncocytomas with clear cells lack infiltration, usually contain some intensely eosinophilic cells, are reactive with phosphotungstic acid-hematoxylin stain, and demonstrate excessive mitochondria with ultrastructural examination. The rare sebaceous adenomas and adenocarcinomas are glycogen negative, and they generally have foamy rather than water-clear cytoplasm that contains cytoplasmic lipids. The uncommon clear cell myoepithelial carcinoma is immunohistochemically reactive for markers of neoplastic myoepithelium.

Metastatic renal cell carcinoma may be difficult to distinguish from clear cell adenocarcinoma. Cytologic atypia is usually more prominent in renal cell carcinoma, but another subtle difference is the often conspicuous, dilated, and even sinusoidal vascular channels in metastatic renal cell carcinoma. Renal cell carcinomas are often immunoreactive for CD10 and RCC antigen, but information on these immunostains applied to salivary clear cell adenocarcinomas is

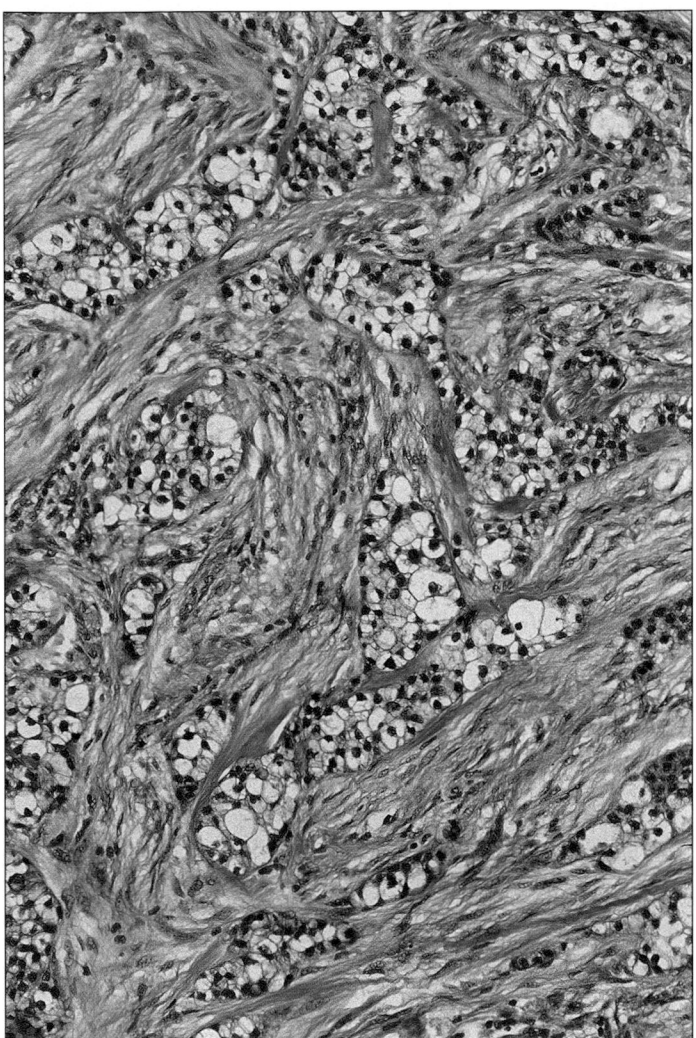

Fig. 23.56 A clear cell adenocarcinoma is characterized by nests and cords of polygonal cells with optically clear cytoplasm that have well-defined cell boundaries and eccentrically located nuclei with a mild degree of variability in nuclear size. The clear cells are separated by moderately cellular and collagenous bands of fibrous connective tissue.

lacking. Clinical evaluation for a renal primary tumor may need to be performed.

In mucosa near the maxillary or mandibular alveolar ridges, distinction from clear cell odontogenic carcinoma requires clinical, radiologic, and histopathologic correlation.[661,662] Although intra-osseous salivary-type hyalinizing clear cell carcinoma has been reported,[663] its occurrence remains in doubt, and radiographic evidence of a centralized, destructive osseous lesion indicates odontogenic rather than salivary gland origin.

Prognosis and treatment: Clear cell adenocarcinomas are low-grade neoplasms. Only a few tumors have metastasized to cervical lymph nodes. While no deaths attributable to clear cell adeno-carcinoma are known, a patient with pulmonary metastases was reported by Grenevicki et al.[664] Excision is the primary therapy.

Cytopathology of clear cell carcinoma

As noted previously, many salivary gland neoplasms, as well as metastatic renal cell carcinoma, have extensive clear cell features.

Milchgrub and colleagues described the FNA findings in four cases of the hyalinizing type of primary clear cell adenocarcinoma.[665] Although somewhat variable in size, the cells showed low-grade nuclear features and distinct cell borders. These investigators concluded that this remains a difficult diagnosis, even when paraffin-embedded cell-block sections are available.

BASAL CELL ADENOCARCINOMA

Histopathologically, basal cell adenocarcinomas are similar to basal cell adenomas except they are infiltrative and have a potential for metastasis. The largest series reported was that of Ellis and Wiscovitch,[666] but smaller series and several individual cases have been reported under various terms.[270,667–672] Tumors in infants that have been described as basal cell adenoma/carcinoma or hybrids with adenoid cystic carcinoma are best classified as *sialoblastomas*.

Most basal cell adenocarcinomas probably arise de novo, but some arise in basal cell adenomas.[270,672]

Clinical features: Few large series of salivary gland neoplasms have included basal cell adenocarcinomas, so data on the incidence are limited.[12,252,370,433,673] It has comprised about 1.5% of all salivary neoplasms and 3% of malignant salivary neoplasms in the files at the AFIP since its inclusion in the classification of salivary neoplasia. Nearly 90% occur in the parotid gland, usually the superficial lobe. They are rare in the minor salivary glands.[666,673,674] There is no sex predilection, and the average age of patients is 60 years.

Rarely, patients have complained of pain or tenderness, but most have asymptomatic swellings. Durations of tumors before excisions have been weeks to many years. Similar to some patients with basal cell adenomas, several patients have expressed a diathesis of multiple dermal adenomas and parotid basal cell adenocarcinomas.[270,666,668,673,674]

Microscopic features: Basal cell adenocarcinomas manifest histomorphologic patterns, described as solid, membranous, trabecular and tubular, similar to basal cell adenomas. Most have a solid pattern. Infiltration of nodules, nests, or cords of tumor cells from the main tumor mass into adjacent lobules of parotid parenchyma, dermis, skeletal muscle, or periglandular fat (Fig. 23.57) distinguishes basal cell adenocarcinoma from basal cell adenoma. Peripheral palisading of nuclei is less frequent and less prominent than in basal cell adenomas but is most evident in the solid and membranous patterns. Cytologic atypia and the number of mitotic figures are usually minimal but in some tumors are moderate. Vessel or peripheral nerve invasion is evident in about a fourth of the tumors. Foci of squamous differentiation are present in some tumors. A fibrous stroma usually accompanies the infiltrating adenocarcinoma and frequently contains lymphocytic and plasmacytic inflammatory cells.

Tumors are immunohistochemically reactive for cytokeratins and often at least focally reactive for S-100 protein, epithelial membrane antigen, and carcinoembryonic antigen. Immunohistochemical staining for smooth muscle actin and vimentin is variable but, when present, is usually at the periphery of islands of tumor cells and supports myoepithelial differentiation of some of the basaloid cells.[263,675,676] Immunohistochemistry is not useful for distinguishing basal cell adenocarcinomas from basal cell adenomas. Basal cell adenocarcinomas are negative for c-erbB-2, and only occasionally express accumulation of p53 protein.[406,456,676]

The limited analyses for DNA ploidy have found these tumors generally to be diploid,[276,677,678] and there has been very little cytogenetic analysis.[400,679]

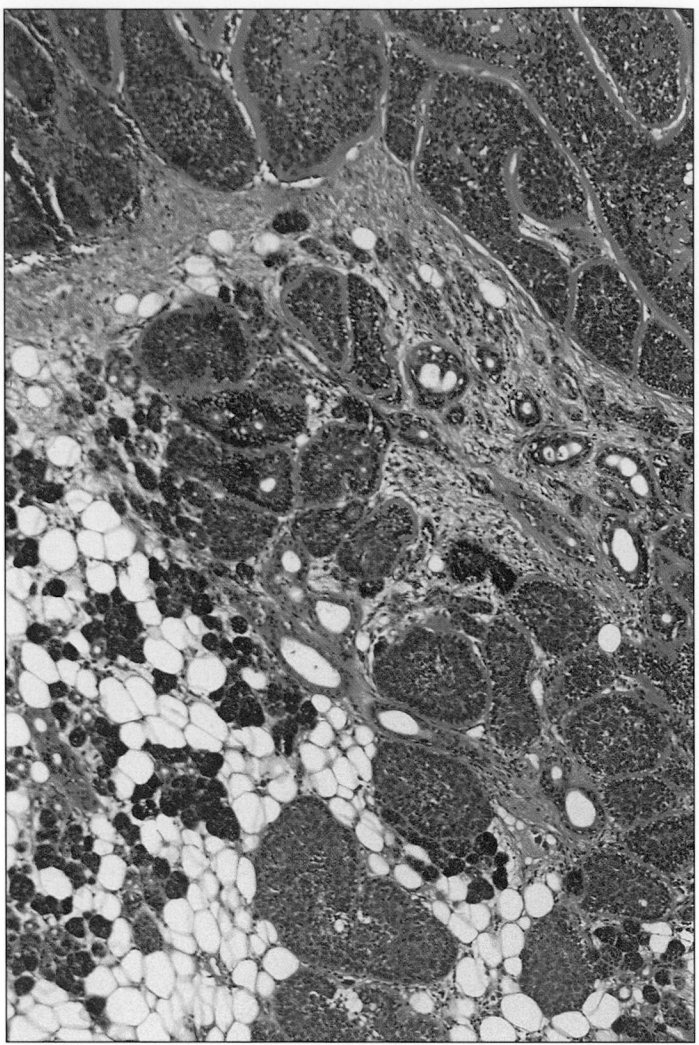

Fig. 23.57 In this basal cell adenocarcinoma numerous nests of basaloid epithelial cells, some in a fibrous stroma, infiltrate into the parotid parenchyma and adipose tissue without any evidence of a capsule.

Differential diagnosis: Basal cell adenoma is the principal entity in the differential diagnosis and, as stated, is ruled out by infiltrative growth of the tumor, although cellular atypia and mitotic figures, in general, are greater in basal cell adenocarcinomas than basal cell adenomas.

Basal cell adenocarcinoma lacks the cribriform pattern, pseudocysts that contain amorphous, basophilic glycosaminoglycans, and pale to clear cells with irregular, angular nuclei that are characteristic of adenoid cystic carcinoma.

Like basal cell adenocarcinoma, basaloid squamous carcinoma has basaloid cell features but has a predilection for sites where basal cell adenocarcinoma is absent, such as hypopharynx, base of tongue, and supraglottic larynx.[481,482,680] In contrast to basal cell adenocarcinoma, basaloid squamous carcinoma has a malignant squamous component that involves the mucosal epithelium in the form of epithelial dysplasia, carcinoma in situ, and/or invasive squamous cell carcinoma. Immunohistochemically, basaloid squamous cell carcinoma is reported to be unreactive for muscle actin, and anti-CEA reactivity occurs in the epidermoid cells rather than the ductal and basaloid cells as in basal cell adenocarcinoma.[482]

Prognosis and treatment: These are low-grade carcinomas that are locally destructive and tend to recur but only occasionally metastasize.[270,666,668–670,672,681,682] The few tumors that have been studied for proliferating cell nuclear antigen and Ki-67 had low proliferation indices.[542,676] Surgical excision is appropriate treatment.

Cytopathology of basal cell adenocarcinoma

FNA samples have essentially the same features as basal cell adenoma and solid adenoid cystic carcinoma.[276,277] Cytologic features include papillary and filiform tissue particles with peripheral palisading. Individual cells have a high nuclear:cytoplasmic ratio, fine chromatin, prominent nucleoli, and mitoses. The cells are in a myxoid background that may include necrosis, further suggesting a diagnosis of solid adenoid cystic carcinoma. Basal cell adenocarcinoma is very difficult to distinguish from metastatic basal cell carcinoma of cutaneous origin.[179]

UNDIFFERENTIATED CARCINOMAS

Undifferentiated carcinomas of salivary glands have neither glandular nor epidermoid features although electron microscopy may demonstrate some features associated with ductal, epidermoid, or neuroendocrine differentiation in some tumors. They are segregated into *small cell* and *large cell* types. In addition, some large cell undifferentiated carcinomas are characterized by an extensive, dense lymphoid stroma and are separately classified as *lymphoepithelial carcinoma*. These latter tumors have a racial predilection and an association with Epstein-Barr virus (EBV) infection that has not been identified in other salivary gland carcinomas.

Large cell undifferentiated carcinoma

Clinical features: Possibly due to varying criteria, the reported incidence of undifferentiated carcinoma has varied, but a composite of several investigations indicates that undifferentiated carcinoma accounts for about 1% of epithelial salivary gland neoplasms.[2,293,368,370,433,683–687] The majority of undifferentiated carcinomas occur in the parotid gland, but about 25% arise in the submandibular gland.[5,683,684,686] The peak incidence is in the seventh and eighth decades of life. Men and women are probably equally affected although different sex predilections have been reported.[5,684,686] Unlike the lymphoepithelial type of undifferentiated carcinoma, no ethnic predilection or association with Epstein-Barr virus infection has been identified.[688–690] Short duration and rapid growth is a common clinical presentation, and many patients have cervical lymphadenopathy at the time of diagnosis. The tumors have ranged 2–10 cm in diameter.

Microscopic features: Histopathologically, these tumors are characterized by the absence of distinct features of specific differentiation, such as acinar, ductal, epidermoid, or myoepithelial, although ultrastructural examinations have described adenomatous, epidermoid, and neuroendocrine features among undifferentiated tumor cells.[5,691,692] Tumor cells are arranged in sheets, nests, and trabecular cords separated by fibrous connective tissue stroma. No keratinization is evident.

These tumors are infiltrative and frequently extend into adjacent lobules of salivary gland, fat, skeletal muscle, dermis, and even facial and cranial bones. Vascular and neural invasion are frequent. The stroma often contains inflammatory cells but not the diffuse, dense lymphocytic infiltrates characteristic of lymphoepithelial carcinoma.

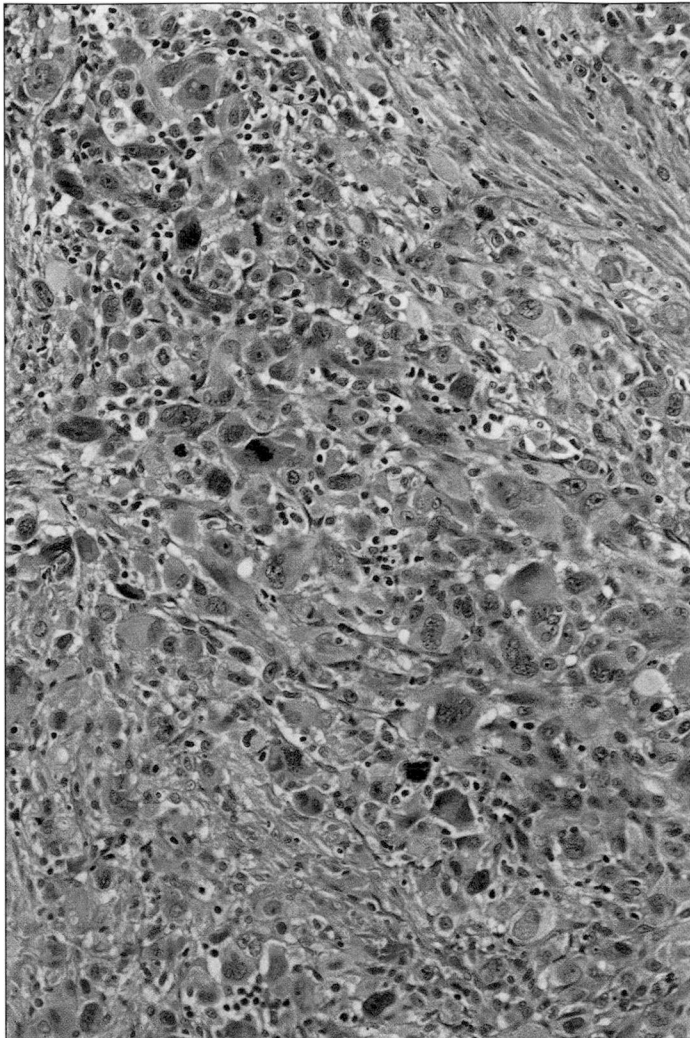

Fig. 23.58 A sheet of closely apposed but loosely arranged, pleomorphic tumor cells have a large amount of amphophilic to eosinophilic cytoplasm with vesicular nuclei that contain prominent nucleoli in this large cell undifferentiated carcinoma. The cell boundaries are relatively distinct, and some cells are multinucleated. Three mitotic figures are evident at the upper left.

Although some spindled forms occur, the tumor cells are mostly polygonal with abundant amphophilic to eosinophilic cytoplasm, which is sometimes vacuolated (Fig. 23.58). Nuclei are large and vesicular and frequently contain one or more nucleoli. Osteoclast-like, bizarre giant cells have been described.[692,693] Most cells are two or more times the size of those of small cell carcinoma. Mitoses are usually common, but the degree of anaplasia is variable. Cellular density varies from tightly packed to loosely arranged.

c-erbB-2 expression has been identified in a majority of undifferentiated carcinomas studied but has not had prognostic significance.[454] Expression of p53 protein and p53 gene mutations have been detected in about 40% of the small number of tumors studied.[269] These tumors have a high proliferation index with proliferation markers such as proliferating cell nuclear antigen.[479] Insufficient cytogenetic information is available.[694]

Differential diagnosis: Poorly differentiated squamous cell carcinoma, adenocarcinoma, large cell and anaplastic types of malignant lymphoma, and metastatic melanoma are considerations in the differential diagnosis.

Focal ductal, organoid, papillary, or cystic architectural features distinguish adenocarcinomas. Metastatic poorly differentiated squamous cell carcinoma and undifferentiated carcinoma can sometimes only be differentiated from primary undifferentiated carcinoma by identification of another primary tumor site. Face and scalp are common sites of carcinomas and melanomas that metastasize to the parotid gland.

Large cell and anaplastic lymphomas are immunohistochemically reactive to one or more lymphoid markers, such as CD45, CD20, CD45RO, CD3, and CD30 (Ki-1), while undifferentiated carcinomas are typically reactive for cytokeratins but little else. In the absence of melanin pigment, metastatic melanoma can frequently be identified by immunostains for S-100 protein, HMB-45 antigen, Melan-A, and tyrosinase.

Prognosis and treatment: Undifferentiated carcinomas are aggressive, frequently metastasize, and have a poor prognosis.[695] Ten-year survival has varied from 0 to 35% of patients.[696,697] Hui et al.[5] and Batsakis and Luna[683] reported that tumor size was the single most important prognostic factor, and neoplasms 4 cm or larger had a very poor outcome. Combined radical surgery and postoperative radiation therapy seem to offer the best chance of survival, although chemotherapy with agents such as vinorelbine and cisplatin has shown some effect.[515,517,696–699]

Small cell carcinoma

Small cell carcinoma is a rare primary malignant tumor composed of undifferentiated cells with conventional light microscopy, but ultrastructural or immunohistochemical analysis reveals neuroendocrine differentiation. Small cell carcinoma represents about 2% of primary malignant epithelial parotid tumors, submandibular cancers, and all major gland cancers in the AFIP's files accessioned since 1985.[700] More than 80% of recent cases occurred in the parotid gland. The mean age of patients is about 56 years, and men outnumber women.[700–702]

The tumor cells are about twice as large as lymphocytes and uniform in size and shape. They have limited cytoplasm and dense round to oval nuclei with diffuse chromatin and small inconspicuous nucleoli. Nuclear molding, duct-like structures, pseudoglandular spaces, and rarely, pseudorosettes can be evident (Fig. 23.59). Hui and colleagues[5] have designated tumors composed of cells smaller than 30 μm as small cell carcinoma and those with larger cells as large cell carcinoma. Focal squamous differentiation has been reported.[703] In addition to perinuclear staining with anticytokeratin, neuroendocrine differentiation is also indicated by immunoreactivity of tumor cells with anti-Leu-7, synaptophysin, chromogranin, and neuron-specific enolase.[704–708] Gnepp and Wick[709] found that 11 of 11 salivary gland small cell carcinomas reacted with at least one of these five markers despite finding that only four tumors had secretory granules by electron microscopy. Similar to Merkel cell carcinoma, but unlike small cell carcinomas from most other sites, including the lung, many salivary gland small cell carcinomas are immunoreactive with cytokeratin 20.[710] This may help confirm or rule out the rare examples of primary pulmonary disease metastatic to the major salivary glands.[711–713]

Salivary gland small cell carcinoma behaves aggressively. Among 189 published cases, 121 patients died of tumor.[5] Gnepp and colleagues[702] found that the 2-year and 5-year survival for major gland tumors was 70% and 46%, respectively. Unlike one previous report,[714] Hui and coworkers[5] found that neither the presence nor absence of neuroendocrine differentiation nor cell size (small vs. large) influenced prognosis.

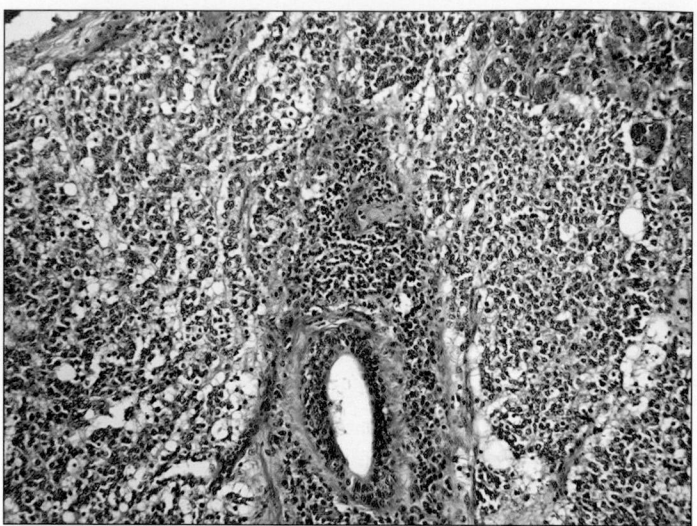

Fig. 23.59 Small cell carcinoma of the parotid gland surrounds a centrally located excretory duct and infiltrates and replaces serous acini seen in the upper right corner. The neoplastic cells are considerably larger than lymphocytes, a collection of which is evident just above the duct.

Cytopathology of undifferentiated carcinomas

Small cell[715] and large cell,[716] as well as the lymphoepithelial type[717] of undifferentiated carcinomas have been described in salivary gland aspiration samples.

Small cell carcinomas are identical to their counterparts that occur more frequently in other sites. The most important differential diagnostic considerations involve neoplasms with small uniform cells and necrosis. These include solid adenoid cystic carcinoma, metastatic small cell carcinoma, metastatic Merkel cell carcinoma, and metastatic basal cell carcinoma of cutaneous origin.[179] Clinical history is the most important guide to metastatic malignancy, while a search for rare extracellular spheres or cylinders helps identify solid adenoid cystic carcinoma. Air-dried, Romanowsky-stained smears are very helpful in this effort. It should be noted that cutaneous basal cell carcinoma sometimes have metastases many years after excision of the primary lesion, leading to considerable clinical confusion.

It is doubtful that an unequivocal diagnosis of large cell undifferentiated carcinoma will occur at the time of initial FNA. The differential diagnosis is lengthy, requiring consideration of numerous primary and metastatic lesions. It can be therapeutically important to exclude malignant melanoma, and this is best accomplished with immunohistochemistry. The need for additional material for special tests is a valid reason for repeat FNA.

Lymphoid stroma is characteristic of lymphoepithelial carcinoma but occurs in other tumors. A metastasis from an occult lesion located elsewhere must be clinically evaluated. In some cases, what was clinically believed to be a parotid mass was actually a high cervical lymph node or an intraparotid lymph node.

Lymphoepithelial carcinoma

Lymphoepithelial carcinomas are undifferentiated carcinomas associated with a dense lymphoid stroma. The term *malignant lymphoepithelial lesion* has been used for these tumors, but this term is ambiguous about whether the epithelial or lymphoid component is malignant. Others have identified these tumors as *undifferentiated carcinoma with lymphoid stroma*,[26,718] *carcinoma ex lymphoepithelial lesion*,[719] and undifferentiated carcinoma not further subclassified.[720,721] Some of these carcinomas arise in lympho-epithelial sialadenitis (benign lymphoepithelial lesions),[722–726] but most develop de novo. It is the only salivary gland carcinoma in which a definite association with Epstein-Barr virus infection has been established.[688,721,727–732]

Clinical features: Over 170 cases have been identified in the literature,[720,722,723,733] but lymphoepithelial carcinoma comprises only about 0.4% of the salivary gland neoplasms.[730,733] Unlike other salivary gland neoplasms, lymphoepithelial carcinoma has a marked ethnic predilection. Three-quarters of affected patients have been of Mongoliod ancestry, about 75% Eskimos/Inuits and 25% Asians, and familial clustering has been reported.[734–736] There is a modest female predilection, and patients ages have ranged from 10 to 86 years.[722,733] Over 80% of tumors occur in the parotid gland with most of the remainder in the submandibular gland. A tumor in the minor salivary gland has been reported.[737] They have varied from 1 cm to 10 cm in largest dimension. Pain is a frequent symptom, and facial nerve palsy occurs in up to 20% of patients.[722] Forty percent of patients have had cervical lymphadenopathy at presentation.[722,738]

Microscopic features: The malignant epithelial cells are similar to those described for large cell undifferentiated carcinoma. Irregularly shaped islands of eosinophilic, epithelioid cells are within and permeated by a lymphocyte-rich stroma (Fig. 23.60), and the epithelial islands are frequently widely separated by the lymphoid stroma. The architectural patterns of these carcinoma cells can be small islands, syncytial masses, cords, trabeculae, or isolated cells. Lymphoid follicles are often recognized. A variable amount of collagenous tissue is usually present within the lymphoid component. The histochemical, immunohistochemical, and electron microscopic features of the carcinomatous cells are similar to those of large cell undifferentiated carcinomas. In situ hybridization detects EBV-encoded RNAs in the carcinoma cells of most, but not all, cases.[670,689,727–729]

Differential diagnosis: Because of marked histologic similarity, metastatic undifferentiated nasopharyngeal carcinoma of the so-called lymphoepithelioma type is the principal consideration in the differential diagnosis.[718,720,722,734,738–741] The association with EBV infection and the predilection for people of Mongoloid ancestry suggests a common pathogenesis. Since histologic, histochemical, immunohistochemical, and ultrastructural studies cannot reliably distinguish between these two carcinomas, careful evaluation of the nasopharynx and Waldeyer's ring region are necessary. Fortunately, the parotid gland is an infrequent site of metastasis for nasopharyngeal carcinoma.

Metastatic amelanotic melanoma of the face or scalp can be distinguished from lymphoepithelial carcinoma with immunostains for cytokeratin, S-100 protein, HMB-45, Melan-A, and tyrosinase. Lymphocytic and histiocytic immunohistochemical markers, such as antibodies to CD20, CD45RO, CD68, Leu M1, and Ki-1, along with epithelial markers help differentiate large cell lymphocytic and histiocytic neoplasms from lymphoepithelial carcinoma.

Lymphoepithelial sialadenitis (benign lymphoepithelial lesion) has a similar histopathologic architecture to lymphoepithelial carcinoma. Cytologic features, as well as an absence of invasion of adjacent tissues and detectable EBV-infected cells, distinguish lymphoepithelial sialadenitis.

Prognosis and treatment: Reported survival rates have varied, but lymphoepithelial carcinoma seems to have a better prognosis than large cell undifferentiated carcinoma without lymphoid stroma. Twenty percent of patients experience distant metastases, usually to lung but also to liver, bone, and brain, within 3 years following therapy.[718,722,738,742] Survival statistics have ranged from 17% to 86%.[738] Indicators of poor prognosis include high mitotic rate,

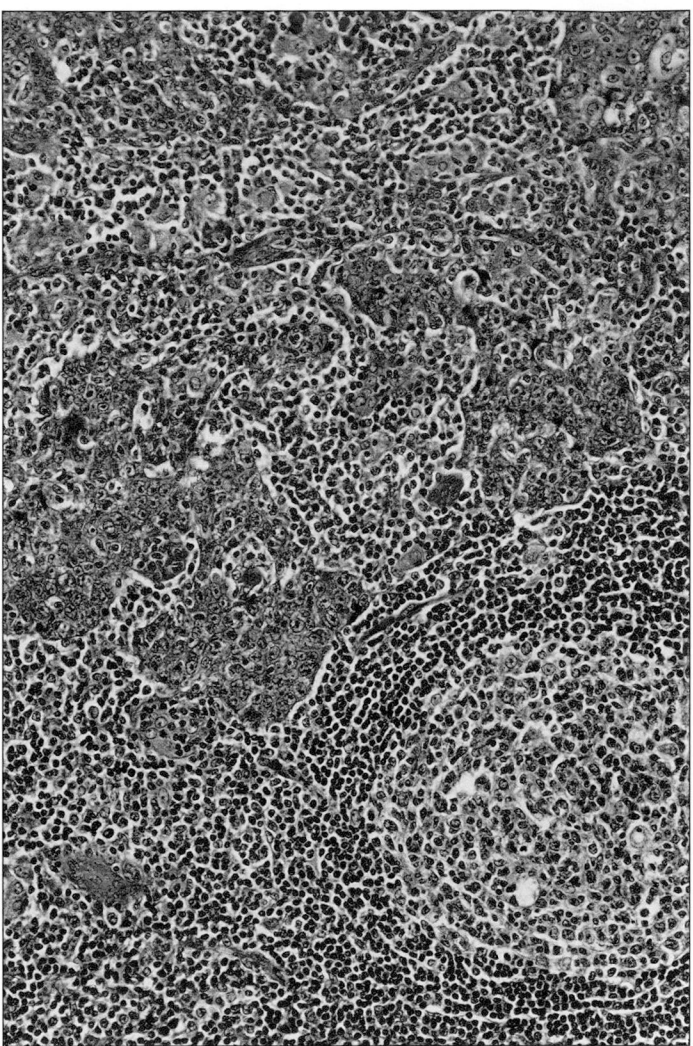

Fig. 23.60 This lymphoepithelial carcinoma is characterized by irregularly shaped nests of undifferentiated epithelial cells that are permeated and separated from one another by a dense lymphocytic stroma in which a lymphoid follicle is evident (lower right).

anaplasia, and necrosis,[718] while features of benign lymphoepithelial lesion have been found to correlate with a better prognosis.[723] Large size and lymph node metastasis have corresponded to poor survival.[718] Better survival has been reported when combined surgery, which often includes neck dissection, and radiation therapy has been employed.[722,742]

CYSTADENOCARCINOMA

Cystadenocarcinoma is a rare malignant tumor that until recently[527,743,744] had not been included in salivary gland classification schemes.[27,308,745] Conceptually, cystadenocarcinoma is the malignant counterpart of benign cystadenoma. A review of 57 cases showed that men and women are affected equally, the average age of patients is about 59 years, and nearly 65% occur in the major salivary glands.[746] In descending order of frequency, the minor gland sites include the lips, buccal mucosa, palate, tongue, retromolar area, and floor of the mouth.

Microscopically, cystadenocarcinomas are composed of numerous cystic spaces and duct-like structures separated by connective tissue. The cyst lining in about 75% of cases has a conspicuous papillary component.[746] Small cuboidal cells predominate in more than 60% of the tumors, but large cuboidal and tall columnar cells are common. Mucous, clear, oncocytic, and rarely, even epidermoid cells sometimes occur focally.

Cystadenocarcinoma is a low-grade tumor.[746–749] In one series, all 39 patients with follow-up information were either alive or had died of other causes and were free of tumor.[746] Three patients (7.7%) had recurrence, and four patients suffered metastases to regional lymph nodes (10%), three at the time of diagnosis and one 55 months later. Therapy includes superficial parotidectomy, glandectomy for submandibular or sublingual disease, and wide excision of minor gland tumors with bone resection only when involved by tumor.

SALIVARY DUCT CARCINOMA

Histologically, salivary duct carcinoma has a striking resemblance to intraductal carcinoma of the breast, and the term *intraductal carcinoma* has been used synonymously for salivary duct carcinoma.[750–752] However, the term intraductal carcinoma indicates a noninvasive tumor without potential to metastasize, similar to breast tumors of the same name. To the contrary, salivary duct carcinomas are aggressive neoplasms with a poor prognosis.

Clinical features: Salivary duct carcinoma is uncommon and constitutes 0.5–3.9% of salivary gland carcinomas.[370,750,753–757] About 90% have developed in the parotid gland, and facial nerve dysfunction has occurred in over one-fourth of patients. Rapid growth is common among these tumors, and over a third of patients have had cervical lymphadenopathy. Three-quarters of patients have been men. The peak incidence is in the sixth and seventh decades of life.[757–760]

Microscopic features: Variably sized, circular nodules of tumor that resemble intraductal carcinoma of the breast are characteristic (Fig. 23.61). Most tumor nodules are cystic, but some small nodules may be solid. Central comedonecrosis is a frequent finding within the cystic nodules. The cuboidal and polygonal epithelial tumor cells have moderately abundant eosinophilic cytoplasm and form band-like, papillary, and cribriform patterns. In the cribriform pattern, thin bands of neoplastic epithelium often appear arched over small luminal spaces along the periphery of the cysts. Small nests of epithelium, which resemble infiltrating ductal carcinoma of the breast, are often found adjacent to the cystic tumor nodules. Cytologic pleomorphism and mitotic activity vary from slight to marked. Perineural infiltration and intralymphatic infiltration are frequent findings. The stroma is typically a dense collagenous tissue.

Immunohistochemically, the tumor cells are reactive for epithelial antigens such as cytokeratin, epithelial membrane antigen, and carcinoembryonic antigen, and most investigators have reported little or no staining for S-100 protein, myosin, and smooth muscle actin.[441,626,750,754,755,760–762] Brandwein et al.,[761] however, reported reactivity for S-100 protein. Only a few tumors have been positive for estrogen receptor or progesterone receptor, but most studied tumors have been positive for androgen receptor and gross cystic disease fluid protein.[760,763–768] Some of the few tumors studied were immunoreactive for prostate specific antigen and prostatic alkaline phosphatase.[767,769] Results of immunostaining for c-erbB-2 protein and p53 have varied, but the majority of salivary duct carcinomas have been immunoreactive.[406,759,763,764,766,770,771]

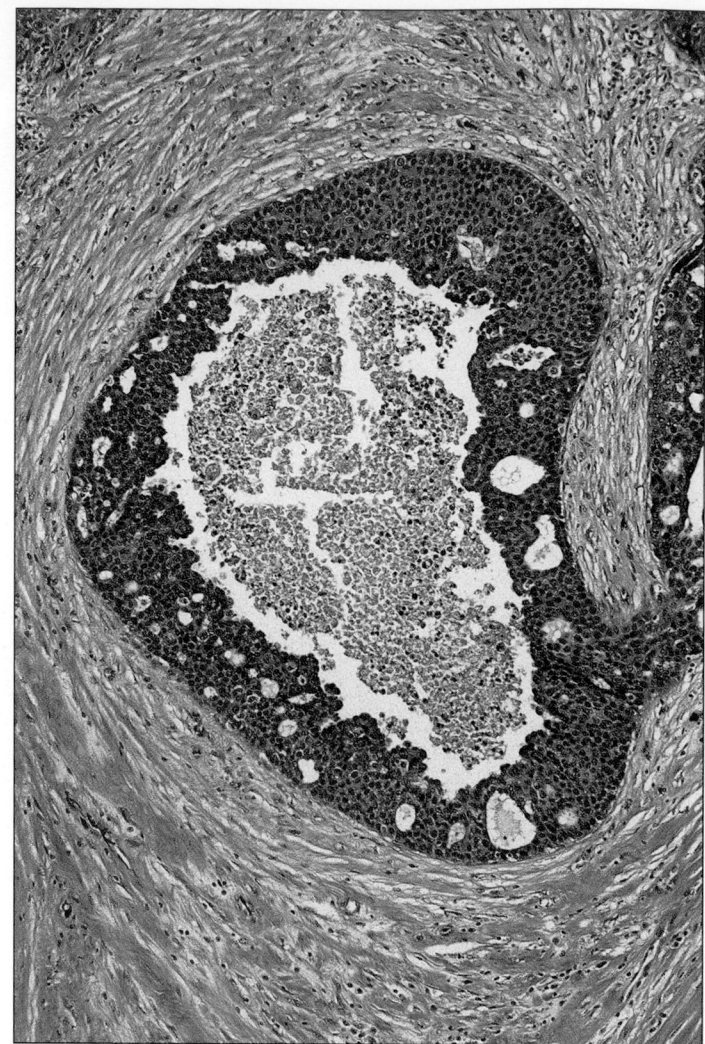

Fig. 23.61 Comedonecrosis is present in a salivary duct carcinoma within a round, circumscribed nodule of ductal epithelium that has both a cribriform and solid band-like architecture. The fibrous stroma has a mild lymphoplasmacytic infiltrate.

Salivary duct carcinomas, generally, have a high proliferative index with immunostaining for Ki-67 or PCNA, and a majority have an aneuploid DNA content.[406,758–760,764,770–772]

Ultrastructurally, salivary duct carcinomas have features of ductal cells with basal lamina, luminal cells with microvilli, desmosomes, tight junctions, rough endoplasmic reticulum, a moderate number of mitochondria, and some glycogen.[751,754,762,773]

Differential diagnosis: Tumors with eosinophilic cells and cystic, papillary, or cribriform morphologic growth patterns are considered in the differential diagnosis. Ultrastructurally, oncocytic carcinoma is distinguished by mitochondria-rich cells, and phosphotungstic acid-hematoxylin stain can help identify oncocytic differentiation. Oncocytic carcinoma typically lacks comedonecrosis and papillary, cystic, and cribriform growth patterns. High-grade mucoepidermoid carcinoma has demonstrable mucocytes and epidermoid cells and an absence of papillary-cystic and cribriform growth patterns. Acinic cell adenocarcinomas contain acinar differentiated cells and often have multiple cell types and growth patterns that are not components of the essentially isocellular salivary duct carcinomas. Cystadenocarcinomas lack comedonecrosis and cytologic pleomorphism, rarely have a cribriform growth pattern, and often have a population of columnar cells. The cribriform type of adenoid cystic carcinoma lacks comedonecrosis and forms stromal pseudolumens that contain glycosaminoglycans and basal lamina material. The cells of adenoid cystic carcinoma are less eosinophilic and have more irregular, angular nuclei.

Prognosis and treatment: About 60% of patients succumb to this neoplasm,[626,750,752–755,758–760,774–776] and most patients die within 5 years. Regional lymph node and more distant metastases develop in over 60% and 40% of patients, respectively, which are higher than the local recurrence rate.[758–760,772,776] The large majority of salivary duct carcinomas are aneuploid and have a high proliferative index with Ki-67 or PCNA.[758–760,764,770–772] Tumor size, distant metastasis, and c-erbB-2 amplification have been identified as prognostic factors.[758,759] Aggressive combination therapy of wide surgical excision, radical neck dissection, and radiation is indicated.[756,764,776]

Cytopathology of salivary duct carcinoma

The resemblance of this tumor to breast carcinoma is reflected in smears by obviously malignant cells with hyperchromatic nuclei, prominent nucleoli, and moderate pleomorphism. Necrosis resembling that in aspirates of comedo breast carcinoma is very common. The cells are in solid, cribriform or micropapillary patterns and often lie in flat sheets.[777–780] Most cases are readily interpreted as non-small cell carcinomas, but specific classification is very difficult.[781,782] The differential diagnosis includes other high-grade salivary gland malignancies, as well as metastases of several types. Rarely, abundant hyalinized stoma is very prominent and easily mistaken for the matrix of pleomorphic adenoma.[782] Positive staining of salivary duct carcinoma aspirate material for androgen receptor may be diagnostically useful, but will probably not alter the clinical team's initial approach to management of a clearly high-grade salivary gland carcinoma.[768]

ONCOCYTIC CARCINOMA

Oncocytic carcinoma represents less than 1% of salivary gland tumors.[783] They occur predominantly in the parotid gland, but any salivary gland site may be involved.[292,784–788] Patients average 63 years of age.

Microscopically, large round or polyhedral cells are arranged in solid sheets, islands, and cords. The cells have abundant, finely granular eosinophilic cytoplasm and moderately pleomorphic, medium-sized or large nuclei that are often located centrally within the cytoplasm (Fig. 23.62). Nucleoli are often large and irregular. Histochemical (PTAH) or ultrastructural confirmation of the cytoplasmic mitochondrial excess is needed because accumulation of smooth endoplasmic reticulum, lysosomes, or secretory granules may cause a similar cytoplasmic appearance.[342,789] Tumors usually demonstrate unequivocal evidence of infiltrative growth, and this is helpful in the distinction of oncocytic carcinomas that lack obvious cellular pleomorphism from oncocytomas. Oncocytic carcinoma is a high-grade neoplasm that warrants aggressive surgical intervention.[245,784,790,791]

SEBACEOUS CARCINOMAS

Because of the proximity of skin overlying the parotid gland, direct extension or metastasis of a sebaceous carcinoma of cutaneous

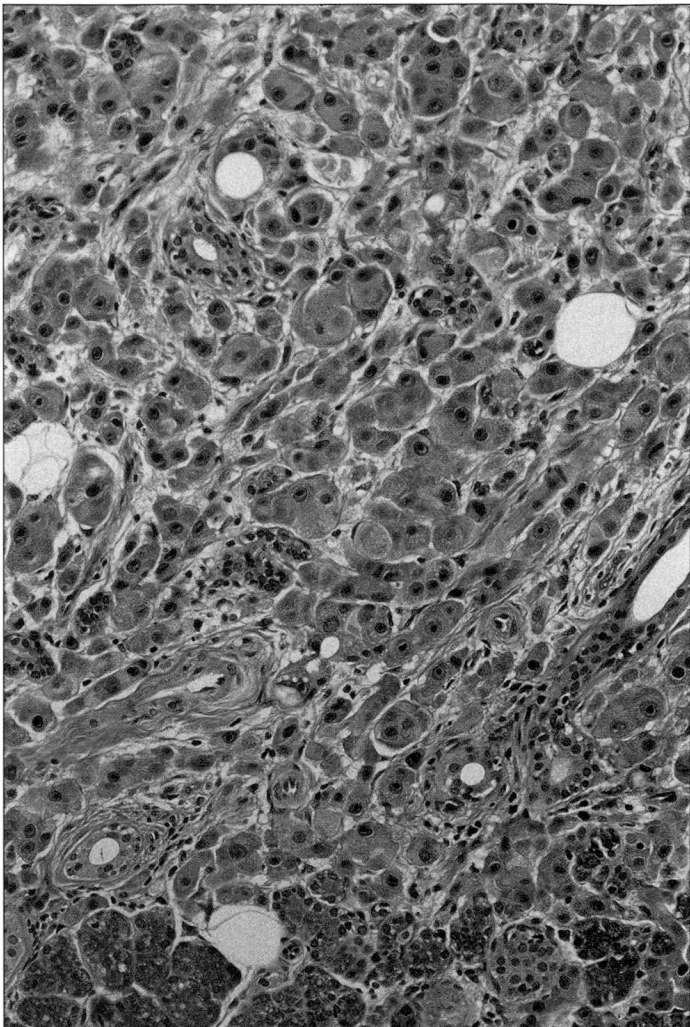

Fig. 23.62 Oncocytic carcinoma reveals small groups of cells with abundant, finely granular cytoplasm that infiltrate and destroy the parotid parenchyma.

origin must be considered any time such a tumor is found in the parotid region. Sebaceous adenocarcinoma of salivary gland origin is extremely rare.[744] It is characterized by cords and small islands that infiltrate adjacent connective tissue and salivary gland parenchyma. The degree of sebaceous differentiation is variable and may be limited to scattered cells. Usually, sebaceous nests or individual cells are among the islands of cytomorphologically atypical basaloid and squamous cells. Of the 19 reported patients with parotid tumors with available follow-up information treated with various but generally aggressive modalities, 5 died as a result of their tumor, all within 5 years of diagnosis.[318,744,792] The submandibular gland is rarely involved.[793]

The extremely rare sebaceous lymphadenocarcinoma represents carcinomatous transformation of a sebaceous lymphadenoma.[315,318] The carcinomatous element may be sebaceous carcinoma or some other specific or non-specific form of salivary gland carcinoma. A lymphadenocarcinoma without sebaceous differentiation has been reported.[794]

MYOEPITHELIAL CARCINOMA

Representing the malignant counterpart of benign myoepitheliomas, the tumor cells almost exclusively manifest myoepithelial differentiation. Cytologic abnormalities and infiltrative growth are the histopathologic features that distinguish these carcinomas from myoepitheliomas.

Clinical features: These rare neoplasms of salivary glands constitute less than 0.4% of all epithelial neoplasms of salivary glands.[795–797] In about two-thirds of the cases the parotid gland is the primary site of occurrence while the minor salivary glands and submandibular gland are involved in about 25% and 10% of cases, respectively. The palate is the most common intraoral site. Patients have ranged in age from 14 to 86 years, and no significant sex predilection is evident. Tumor size has ranged from 2 cm to 20 cm.

Microscopic features: Most investigators have used a combination of morphologic, ultrastructural, and immunohistochemical criteria to ascribe myoepithelial differentiation to these tumors.[657,795,797–800] The cellular morphologies are the same as those in benign myoepitheliomas and include spindle, plasmacytoid, clear, and epithelioid types (Fig. 23.63). The spindle cell type is most common, but many myoepithelial carcinomas manifest more than one cell morphology. Purely clear cell myoepithelial carcinomas have been reported.[657] Immunoreactivity to cytokeratin, S-100 protein, smooth muscle actin, muscle specific actin, calponin, vimentin, and glial fibrillary acidic protein is useful for identifying myoepithelial differentiation.[795,797,799–805] Longitudinally oriented 6–8 nm fine filaments with focal dense bodies, pinocytotic vesicles, desmosomes, and basal lamina are features of myoepithelial differentiated cells.[128,797,799,800,802,804–808] Since neoplastic myoepithelial cells can manifest squamous features, foci of epidermoid cells are acceptable in myoepithelial carcinomas. A rare ductal structure is also permissible.

A significant number of myoepithelial carcinomas arise from pre-existing pleomorphic adenomas and myoepitheliomas, as well as de novo.[795,797,799] Cellular and nuclear pleomorphism, as well as mitotic figures, are indicative of malignancy in myoepithelial neoplasms but vary from slight to severe. Infiltrative, destructive growth is denotative of malignancy in most cases. The cell density varies from moderate to high, and less cellular tumors frequently have mucoid or myxoid stroma.

In contrast to benign myoepitheliomas, a majority of myoepithelial carcinomas are aneuploid.[798,799] Interestingly, myoepithelial carcinoma was one of only three types of salivary gland tumor to express c-kit protein in one study.[459]

Differential diagnosis: Loosely cohesive, spindled tumor cells and absence of glandular features suggest sarcoma, and leiomyosarcoma, fibrosarcoma, malignant Schwannoma, synovial sarcoma, and malignant fibrous histiocytoma are often considered in a differential diagnosis. The immunohistochemical profile of neoplastic myoepithelial cells given above can be helpful for distinguishing myoepithelial from mesenchymal differentiation.

Likewise, metastatic amelanotic malignant melanomas are unreactive for cytokeratin, smooth muscle actin, calponin, and GFAP while myoepithelial carcinomas are unreactive for the melanocytic markers such as HMB-45, Melan-A, and tyrosinase. Both tumor types are reactive for S-100 protein. Characteristic ultrastructural melanosomes are absent in myoepithelial carcinoma.

Prognosis and treatment: In about 30% of cases patients died as a result of their disease while another 33% were living with disease at last follow-up.[795,797,801,802,805–810] The interval to death ranged from 3 months to 35 years. Two-thirds of the patients experienced recurrence and one-third developed distant metastases, which were

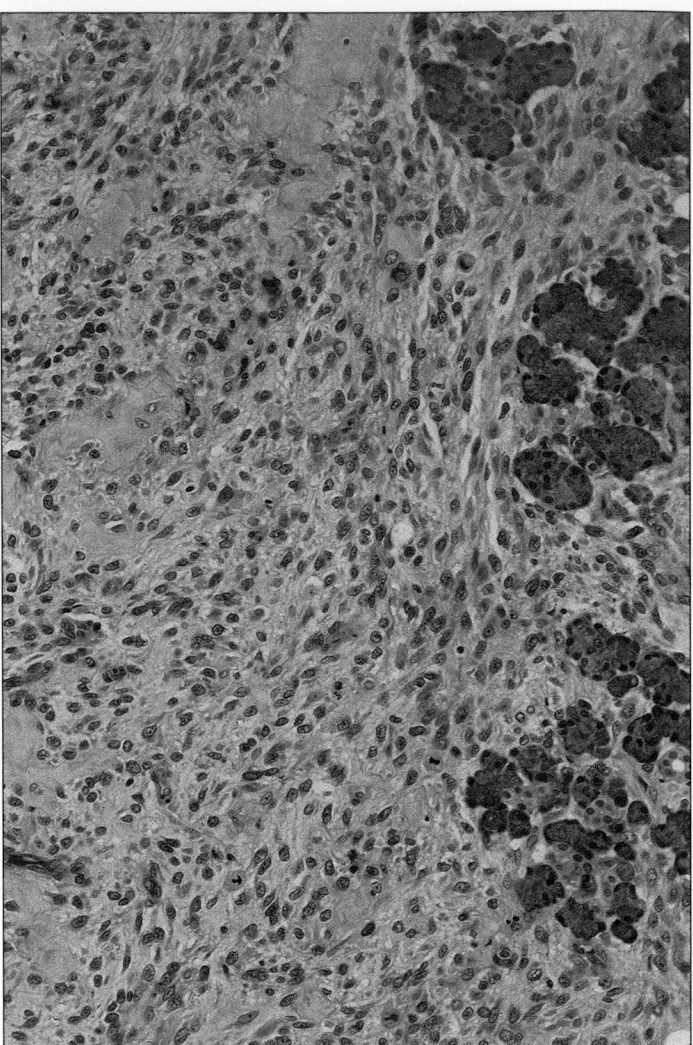

Fig. 23.63 Myoepithelial carcinoma of the parotid gland is unencapsulated and has infiltrated adjacent parotid gland parenchyma (right). Elongated, spindled, and round cells demonstrate mild to moderate atypia and a lack of cohesion. A few mitotic figures are present.

most often to lung. Carrillo et al.[809] found no correlation between the average number of silver-stained nucleolar organizing regions (AgNORs) per cell and the clinical outcome. el-Naggar et al.[811] found that a flow cytometric high S-phase fraction was a better indicator of aggressiveness than DNA content (aneuploidy). Marked cellular pleomorphism, p53 expression, and high proliferative index with Ki-67 correlated with poor outcome in the study by Nagao et al.[797]

Wide excision is recommended.[795,809] Chemotherapy was unsuccessful in controlling extensive disease in two cases but may have been helpful in another.[801,810,811] Radiation therapy has had mixed results.[801,807,808,810]

ADENOSQUAMOUS CARCINOMA

Oral adenosquamous carcinoma is a rare neoplasm that simultaneously demonstrates carcinoma of the mucosal surface squamous epithelium and salivary gland-type adenocarcinoma. While several types of benign and malignant salivary gland neoplasms can

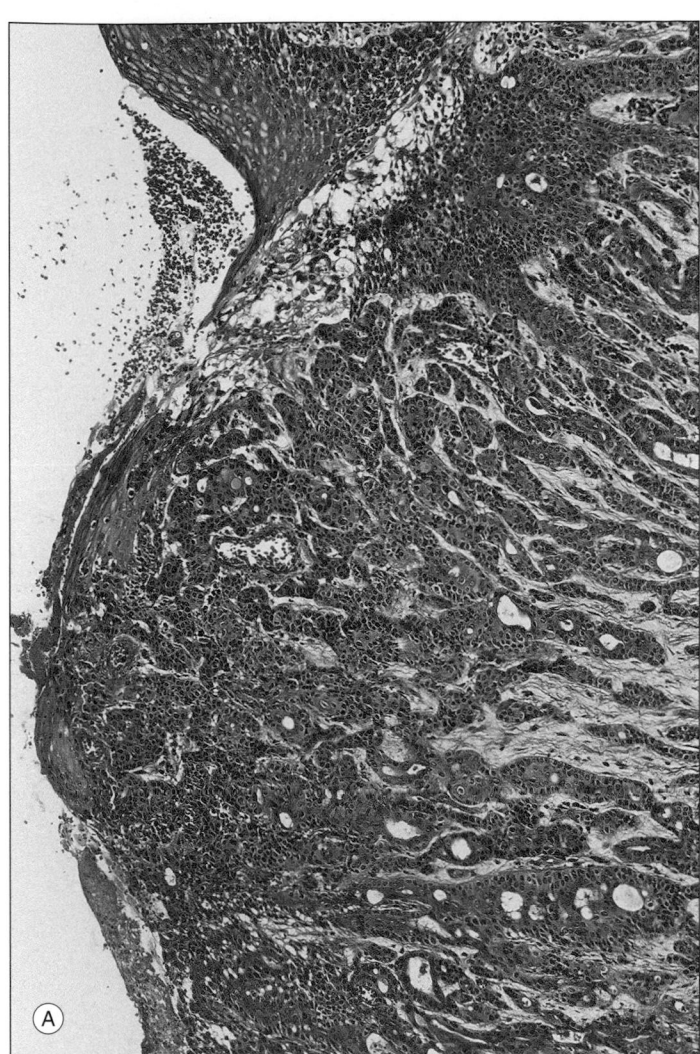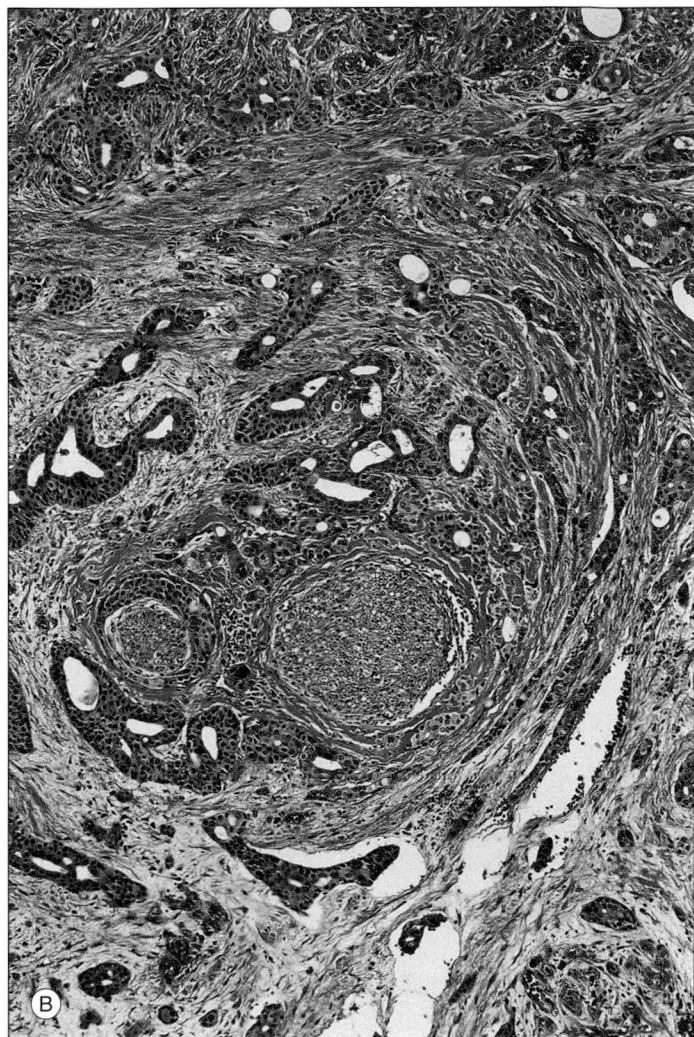

Fig. 23.64 Adenosquamous carcinoma. **A**, Epidermoid carcinoma of the mucosal surface of the floor of the mouth (upper portion) shows some areas of transition to adenocarcinoma (bottom portion); **B**, In deeper parts of the tumor there is perineural invasion by adenocarcinoma.

manifest both ductal and squamous differentiation, most notably mucoepidermoid carcinomas, oral adenosquamous carcinoma is distinguished by carcinomatous changes in the mucosal surface epithelium that are combined with adenocarcinoma in the lamina propria. Adenocarcinomas with foci of squamous differentiation should not be classified as adenosquamous carcinomas.

Clinical features: Only a handful of reports have discussed this oral neoplasm.[742,812–818] The posterior tongue, tonsillar pillars, and floor of mouth have been the sites most often involved. The ratio of male to female patients is three to one. The peak incidence is in the sixth decade of life, and all of the patients have been over 45 years old. Unlike most other salivary gland neoplasms, adenosquamous carcinomas produce changes in the mucosa that vary from erythema to ulceration and induration. Pain often accompanies ulceration.

Pathologic features: Epidermoid carcinoma and ductal adenocarcinoma are intermixed, but most of the superficial portion of the tumor is squamous cell carcinoma while adenocarcinoma occupies the deeper portion of the tumor (Fig. 23.64). The squamous carcinoma component is usually moderately well to poorly differentiated.

Carcinomatous changes in the mucosal surface epithelium manifest as severe epithelial dysplasia, carcinoma in situ, or invasive squamous cell carcinoma, and similar changes are often evident in the superficial portion of salivary gland excretory ducts. The adenocarcinoma is composed of ductal and tubular structures formed by one to several layers of moderately pleomorphic cuboidal or basaloid cells around varying sized lumens. Intraluminal and intracellular mucin is present in some tumors. Zones of transition from squamous carcinoma to adenocarcinoma are usually evident. These tumors infiltrate and invade adjacent tissues. A fibrous stroma frequently has a lymphocytic inflammatory infiltrate.

Martinez-Madrigal et al.[814] found the epidermoid component of adenosquamous carcinomas to be immunoreactive for high molecular weight cytokeratin and unreactive or only focally reactive for low molecular weight cytokeratin and carcinoembryonic antigen, while the adenocarcinoma portions were reactive for high and low molecular weight cytokeratin and carcinoembryonic antigen.

Differential diagnosis: Mucoepidermoid carcinoma, adenoid (acantholytic) squamous carcinoma, and basaloid squamous carcinoma are considered in the differential diagnosis.

In mucoepidermoid carcinoma, the glandular and epidermoid components are inseparable and present in the same nests of tumor, keratinization is an uncommon feature, and carcinomatous changes along the mucosal surface epithelium are absent. In adenosquamous carcinoma, ductal elements proliferate as independent elements, keratinization within the epidermoid component is common, and cytologic features of malignancy are present in the mucosal epithelium.

Adenoid squamous carcinoma of the oral mucosal epithelium arises primarily on the vermilion of the lips.[819] Acantholysis of epidermoid cells produces pseudoglandular structures within the carcinoma, and no mucin is produced. The pseudoglandular spaces often contain acantholytic, dyskeratotic epithelial cells. The tumor cells are immunoreactive for cytokeratin but are unreactive for carcinoembryonic antigen.

Basaloid squamous carcinoma has a predilection for the hypopharynx, base of tongue, and supraglottic larynx and is composed of small, hyperchromatic, basaloid cells that form solid lobules, adenomatoid arrangements, and cords that resemble solid adenoid cystic carcinoma.[481,482,680] It involves the mucosal epithelium in the form of epithelial dysplasia, carcinoma in situ, and invasive squamous cell carcinoma, and foci of epidermoid cells also occur in the basaloid lobules. Eosinophilic hyaline material and comedonecrosis are common. Unlike adenosquamous carcinoma, the cells are predominantly basaloid, and the duct-like structures are within the basaloid and epidermoid proliferation and not a separate component. Reportedly, in basaloid squamous carcinoma, immunoreactivity for CEA occurs in the epidermoid cells rather than the ductal cells.[482]

Prognosis and treatment: Regional lymph node metastases are often present at the time of diagnosis of the primary tumors and develop in 80% of patients. Limited follow-up information indicates that adenosquamous carcinoma is a highly aggressive neoplasm with a poor prognosis.[812–814] Little data are available, but multimodality therapy may be appropriate for such an aggressive tumor.

NON-HODGKIN LYMPHOMAS OF THE MAJOR SALIVARY GLANDS

Nodal and extranodal lymphomas represent a significant proportion of malignant tumors encountered in the major salivary glands. They account for 1.7–16% of all malignant tumors in this site.[820–823] The AFIP and others have noted an increasing proportion of salivary gland lymphomas recently relative to other tumor types.[824,825] The overall incidence of 4% in the series of Schusterman and colleagues[824] increased from 1.5% initially to 6% in the most recent period.

The most frequent types of lymphoma of the major glands include follicular and diffuse large B-cell lymphomas.[8208,821,826–829] Microscopically, the normal lobular salivary gland architecture is altered. The infiltrate replaces acini and ducts, surrounds nerves, and spills into fat and interlobular and periglandular connective tissues. Periductal fibrosis is often evident, and the lymphoid cells frequently demonstrate significant crush artifact. Primary T-cell lymphomas are extremely rare.[830]

A type of lymphoma that also often occurs in the major glands is derived from mucosa-associated lymphoid tissue (MALT). It normally is a localized, clinically indolent lymphoma. The Revised European-American Classification of Lymphoid Neoplasms proposed the term *extranodal marginal zone B-cell lymphoma of MALT type*, with or without monocytoid B cells.[831,832] It has been suggested that both MALT lymphomas and monocytoid B-cell lymphomas are derived from postgerminal center memory B cells that can differentiate into

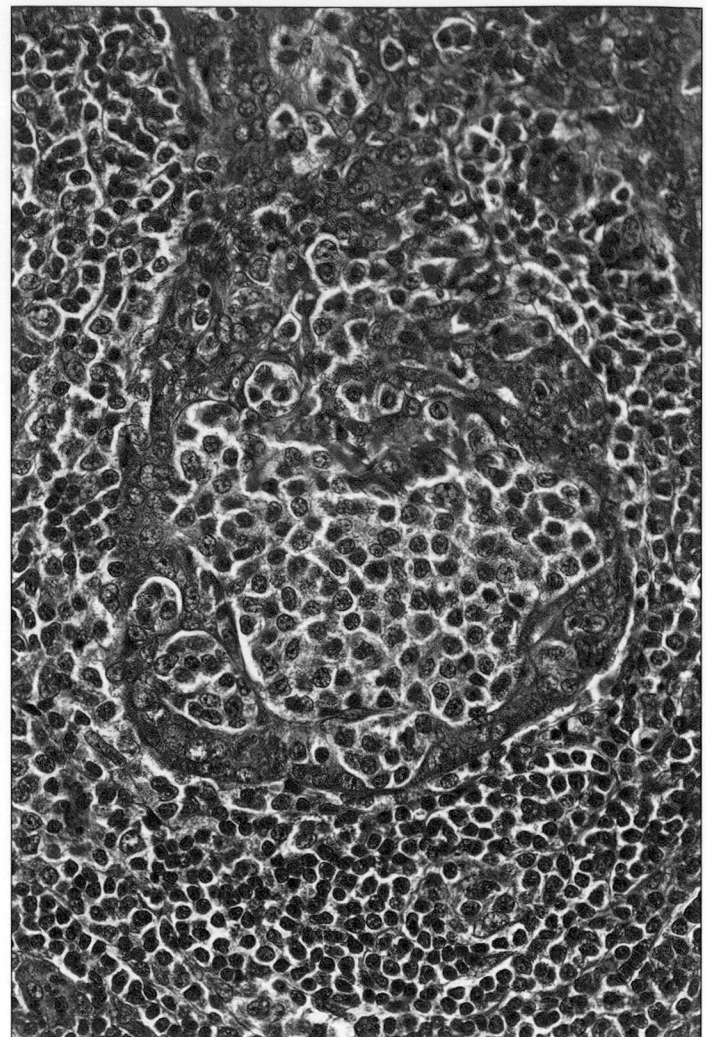

Fig. 23.65 A lymphoepithelial lesion reveals ductal epithelium with central and peripheral clusters of neoplastic cells compatible with marginal zone B-cell lymphoma of MALT origin.

plasma cells.[829,833–841] Although both cell types may be present, the neoplastic marginal zone B cells usually predominate over monocytoid B cells. They are small to medium sized, usually slightly larger than small lymphocytes, and have dense nuclei with irregular outlines and abundant pale-staining cytoplasm with distinct cell membranes.[842–845] It is usually these cells that invade the randomly scattered epithelial islands forming 'lymphoepithelial lesions' (LEL). They eventually surround the epithelial islands and extend into the surrounding parenchyma, a characteristic feature of this lymphoma (Fig. 23.65).[846] Probably because of antigen dependence, benign lymphoid follicles are often present.[847] Sheets of plasma cells, with or without Dutcher bodies, is a second important feature in some cases.[829] The epithelial complexes are eventually replaced by tumor, and the residual epithelial elements are often obscured by the infiltrate. They are occasionally cystic.[848] Transformation of low-grade MALT lymphomas to higher grade, large cell lymphomas occurs in some cases.[826,842,849,850]

Immunohistochemically, as with nodal disease, CD45RA (MT-2) and bcl-2 can help distinguish follicular lymphoid hyperplasia from follicular lymphoma.[851,852] Unlike other low-grade B-cell lymphomas, those that arise from marginal zone cells are CD5, CD10, and cyclin D1 negative.[829,835,853] This facilitates distinction of MALT-derived lymphomas from small lymphocytic lymphoma (SLL), chronic lymphocytic leukemia, and mantle zone lymphoma.[854,855] Because of the diagnostic complexity, Harris and Isaacson have suggested that for treatment purposes, exclusion of one of the other types of small B-cell lymphomas (SLL, follicular, and mantle cell) may be sufficient.[856]

Differential diagnosis: MALT-derived lymphoma should be considered whenever a lymphoid infiltrate of the major salivary glands contains sheets of monomorphic medium-sized cells with abundant pale cytoplasm and bland uniform nuclei. Unlike the benign lymphoid element of lymphoepithelial sialadenitis, lymphomas infiltrate and replace lymphoepithelial lesions and extend into paraglandular fibroadipose tissue or perineural spaces. In patients with lympho-epithelial sialadenitis, immunoglobulin gene clonality alone does not appear to correlate strongly with the morphologic or clinical diagnosis of lymphoma.[857–861] Kurtin has suggested that important features of extranodal low-grade B-cell lymphomas in such a setting include a clinical mass, tissue architectural effacement, cellular monomorphism, cytologic atypia, proliferation centers, plasma cells with Dutcher bodies, and immunoglobulin light chain restriction or aberrant B-cell phenotype.[861] Hsi and colleagues concluded that in patients with lymphoepithelial sialadenitis broad, interconnecting strands of monocytoid B cells are a predictor for the development of extrasalivary lymphoma.[846]

NON-NEOPLASTIC CONDITIONS

LYMPHOEPITHELIAL SIALADENITIS

Historically, lymphoepithelial sialadenitis (LESA) has been known as *benign lymphoepithelial lesion* and, more recently, as *myoepithelial sialadenitis*. The term *sialadenitis* more accurately identifies an inflammatory process than the term *lesion*, but myoepithelial sialadenitis is a misnomer.[829,862,863] It is a disease process that occurs most often, but not exclusively, in patients with Sjögren's syndrome. Sjögren's syndrome is an autoimmune disease complex that involves lacrimal and salivary glands and is often associated with other autoimmune diseases, such as rheumatoid arthritis. Detailed discussions of the syndrome have been published.[864,865]

Women are affected 3:1 over men. The peak incidence is in the fourth to seventh decades of life. LESA involves the parotid glands in about 85% of cases and the submandibular glands in 15%.[866] Patients have recurring and persistent, firm swelling of the affected glands, which is sometimes associated with discomfort or pain. Sjögren's syndrome patients typically manifest keratoconjunctivitis sicca and xerostomia.

Histologically, LESA is characterized by lymphoid infiltrates, acinar atrophy, and foci of ductal hyperplasia, which have been inappropriately referred to as epimyoepithelial islands,[829,862,863,867] permeated by lymphocytes (thus, the term *lymphoepithelial*). The disease may progress to total replacement of acinar tissue by lymphoid tissue, but the lobular architecture of the gland is usually retained (Fig. 23.66). Lymphoid follicles vary from prominent to absent. The lymphoid infiltrate has a predominance of T cells, but the lymphocytes within the lymphoepithelial complexes are B cells.[868,869] The irregular shaped epithelial islands frequently have deposits of intercellular eosinophilic, hyalin, basement membrane

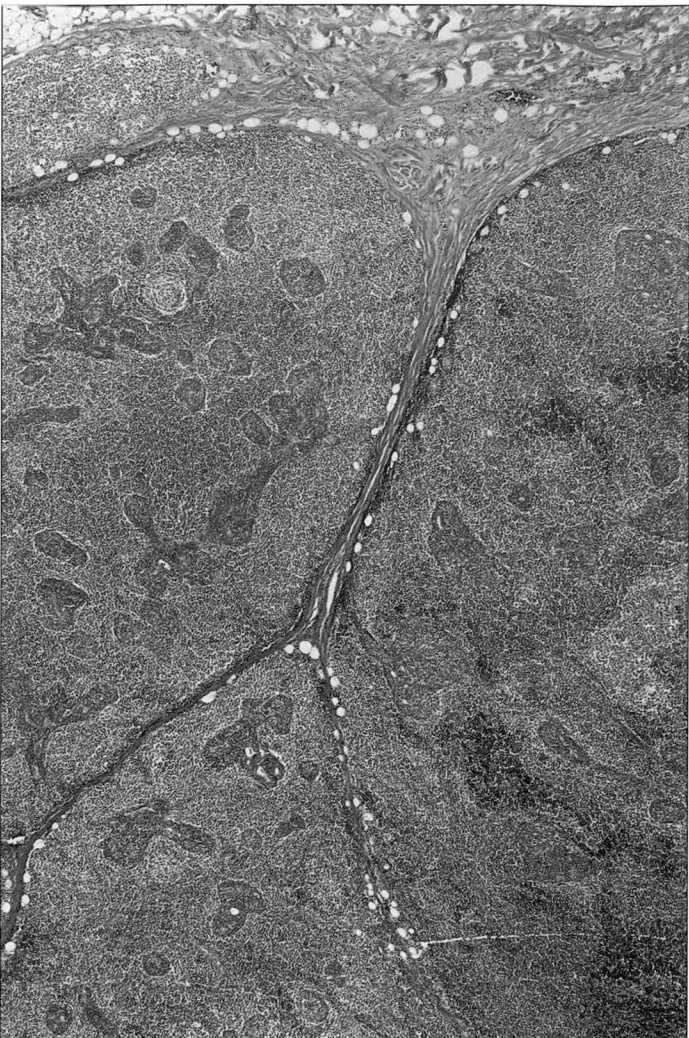

Fig. 23.66 The parenchyma of the visible portions of three lobules of parotid gland are almost entirely replaced by lymphoid tissue in this benign lymphoepithelial lesion, but the lobular architecture is preserved. Many epimyoepithelial islands are present within the lymphoid infiltrate.

material and are permeated by intermediate sized lymphocytes, which often have clear cytoplasm, so-called monocytoid B cells of mucosal associated lymphoid tissue (MALT).[869,870]

In patients with Sjögren's syndrome, the minor salivary glands rarely manifest lymphoepithelial lesions but undergo alterations, and the labial salivary gland biopsy is often used in assessment of patients for Sjögren's syndrome. The labial salivary gland biopsy is supportive but not diagnostically exclusive of other criteria for the diagnosis of Sjögren's syndrome. It is evaluated in conjunction with other clinical and laboratory parameters. In brief, the number of aggregates of 50 or more lymphocytes is counted and a 'focus score' of more than 1 per $4mm^2$ of salivary tissue is considered supportive for Sjögren's syndrome.[861]

Patients with lymphoepithelial sialadenitis or Sjögren's syndrome have a markedly increased risk of development of non-Hodgkin lymphomas.[829,871–873] In fact, it has become evident with recent investigations that many lesions formerly regarded as benign lympho-epithelial lesions manifest monoclonal proliferations of centrocyte-like B cells, and this monoclonal proliferation seems to correlate with expansion of halos of monocytoid/centrocyte-like B cells around the lymphoepithelial complexes.[846,858,859,874–876] Although the subsequent development of disseminated lymphoma is low, lesions with expansion of zones of monocytoid B cells are regarded as low-grade, extranodal marginal zone B-cell lymphomas. Lymphoepithelial complexes are as characteristic of extranodal marginal zone B-cell lymphoma as they are of lymphoepithelial sialadenitis.[829,859,874]

NECROTIZING SIALOMETAPLASIA

Necrotizing sialometaplasia is an inflammatory condition characterized by lobular coagulative necrosis of salivary gland acini, squamous metaplasia of salivary gland ducts, pseudoepitheliomatous hyperplasia of overlying mucosal epithelium, and inflammation. Local ischemia is believed to be the pathogenesis.[877,878] Traumatic injury, dental injection, denture use, adjacent cysts and tumors, surgery, and upper respiratory infection or allergy may be predisposing factors; however, a specific cause of this ischemia is unknown in most cases.[879]

Brannon et al.[879] reported 69 cases and reviewed another 115 cases in the literature. The average age is 46 years, but patients range from infants to elderly. There is a male predominance of nearly 2:1. Over three-fourths of lesions occur on the palate, and the parotid gland is affected in only about 8.5% of cases.

Clinically, necrotizing sialometaplasia usually develops as a sudden swelling that rapidly breaks down into a deep, crater-like, 1–5 cm ulcer.[880] Duration as long as six months has been reported, but the average is about three weeks. Healing after diagnosis varies from 3 to 12 weeks,[878,881] and this failure to resolve in a timely fashion often heightens concern about neoplasia. Many patients complain of pain or numbness.

Histologically, coagulative necrosis of the acini and ductal squamous metaplasia, which may be extensive, are the principal features (Fig. 23.67). Cytologically, the squamous epithelium is usually bland. The lobular architecture of the salivary gland is preserved. Inflammatory cells are frequently minimal within the necrotic lobules but prominent in the surrounding tissues. Some mucous cells usually persist. The mucosal epithelium adjacent to the ulcer is often hyperplastic. The ductal squamous metaplasia and pseudoepitheliomatous hyperplasia must be differentiated from squamous cell carcinoma and mucoepidermoid carcinoma. Features that help distinguish necrotizing sialometaplasia from these malignant neoplasms are maintenance of the lobular architecture, infarctive necrosis of salivary gland lobules, bland cytologic features, and a more intense and mixed inflammatory reaction.

No specific therapy is necessary other than reassurance of the patient of the benign nature of the lesion. Although resolution is often slow, necrotizing sialometaplasia is self-healing.

CHRONIC SCLEROSING SIALADENITIS

Chronic sclerosing sialadenitis is the most common disease of the submandibular gland and often causes tumor-like enlargement.[882,883] *Küttner tumor* is a synonym.[872,884] Recurrent pain and swelling are frequent symptoms.[885] Men are affected slightly more than women, and most patients are in the third through seventh decades of life.[885]

Sialoliths have been found in 50–83% of submandibular gland lesions.[885–889] Sialoliths develop by accretion of mineralized secretions within a salivary gland duct and are primarily calcium salts.[890] Most sialoliths are radiopaque, but up to 20% are radiolucent.[888] Disorders

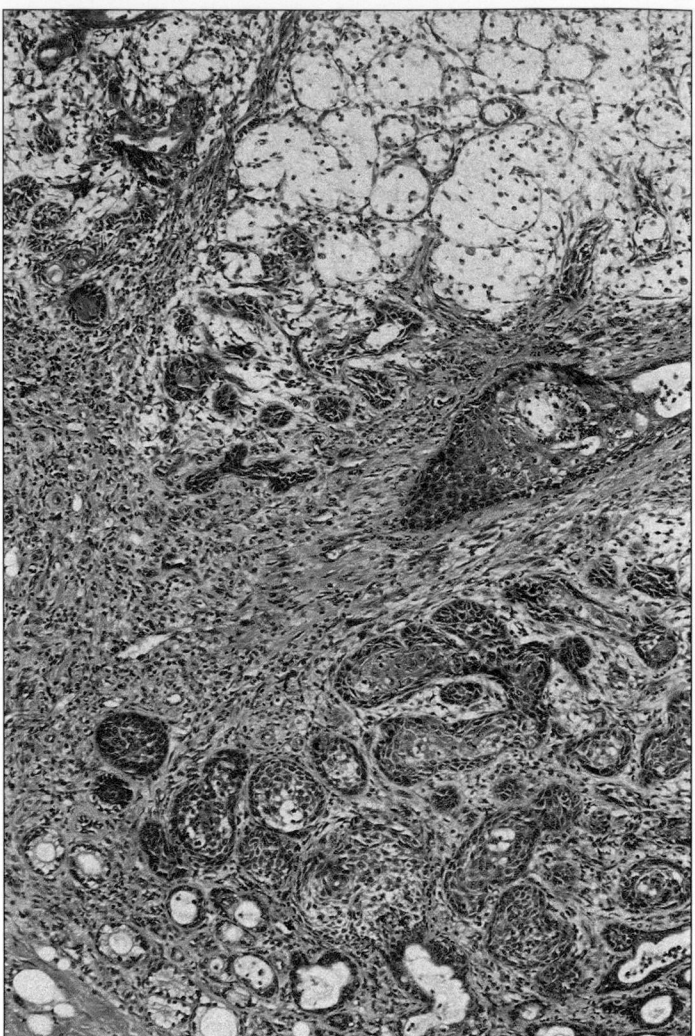

Fig. 23.67 In this necrotizing sialometaplasia of the soft palate there is squamous metaplasia of salivary ducts adjacent to necrotic mucous gland lobules (top). There is a moderately intense inflammatory cell infiltrate in the fibrous connective tissue.

of secretion and immune reactions are other pathogenic factors noted by Seifert.[872]

Histopathologic alterations of the gland vary from mild, focal, periductal chronic inflammation and fibrosis and ductal ectasia to extensive fibrosis, acinar atrophy, and ductal dilatation. The lobular architecture of the gland is usually preserved, but all lobules of the gland may not be equally affected. Lymphocytes and plasma cells predominate the infiltrate, and include lymphoid follicles in some cases (Fig. 23.68). Focal granulomas have been observed in some cases.[885,887,891] Squamous metaplasia of dilated ducts is common, and mucous cells and ciliated cells are conspicuous in some cases.[885,892] Sialoliths, which are more frequent in the extraglandular than intraglandular ducts, are typically associated with squamous metaplasia, ulceration of ductal epithelium, and marked periductal inflammation. Lymphoepithelial complexes, which are characteristic of lymphoepithelial sialadenitis, are absent.

In most cases, swelling of the gland and pain resolve after removal of the sialolith, but in about 20% of cases swelling and pain

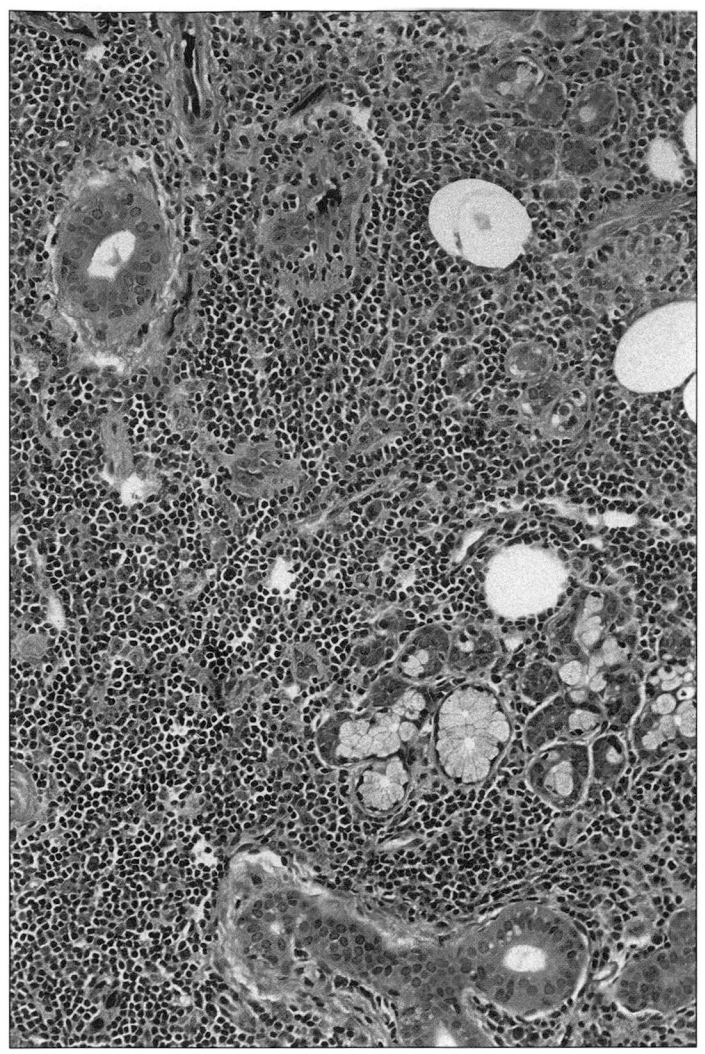

Fig. 23.68 Intense lymphocytic and plasmacytic infiltrates in this intermediate stage of chronic sclerosing sialadenitis of the submandibular gland are associated with loss of acinar tissue but persistence of ducts. In a more advanced stage fibrosis becomes prominent.

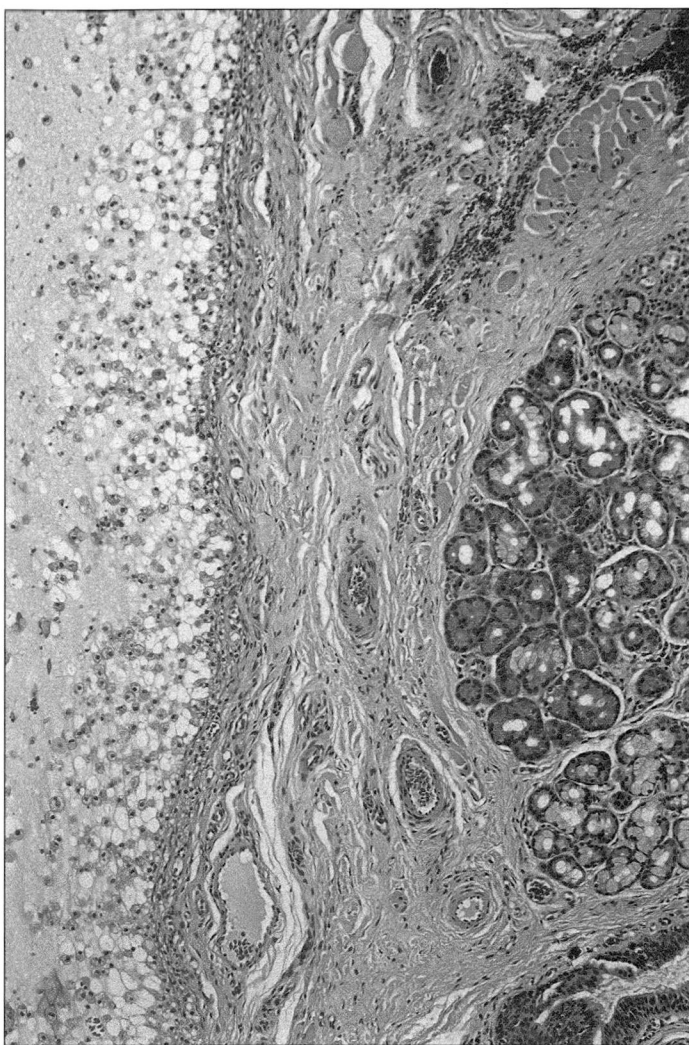

Fig. 23.69 Mucus escape reaction is a pool of mucus and hemorrhage within the lamina propria that is surrounded by inflamed fibrous tissue. Inflammatory cells have migrated into the mucus pool.

persist and necessitate excision of the gland.[893] In cases without sialolithiasis, excision of the gland is usually performed.

MUCOCELES

Mucoceles are pools of saliva within a cystic cavity and are the most common non-neoplastic lesion of salivary glands.[872] There are two types: the extravasation type and the retention type. The extravasation type results from the rupture of a salivary gland duct and secretion of saliva in the surrounding connective tissues. *Mucus escape reaction* and *mucus extravasation phenomenon* are terms used for this type of mucocele. Accidental biting of the lip is probably the most common cause.[894] In the much less common retention type, referred to as *mucous retention cyst*, saliva pools within a markedly dilated duct that forms an epithelial-lined cyst.[895,896]

About 70% of extravasation mucoceles occur in the lower lip, and most of the remainder occur in other intraoral sites.[866] Mucus retention cysts are more evenly distributed among intraoral and major salivary glands. Over two-thirds of mucus escape reactions occur in patients under 30 years old, and men are slightly more affected than women.[866,897] The peak incidence for mucus retention cysts is the seventh and eighth decades of life.

Clinically, mucoceles generally occur as rapidly developing, painless, soft and fluctuant, dome-shaped mucosal nodules that are 0.2–1.0 cm except in the floor of the mouth where they are often several centimeters in diameter and extend into the submandibular and cervical tissues. These large mucoceles of the floor of the mouth are referred to as *ranulas* or, if they extend into the cervical tissues, *plunging ranulas*. The sublingual gland is commonly the source of saliva for ranulas. Patients often describe fluctuation in size, but as lesions become organized by granulation tissue, they become firmer and more fixed.

Microscopically, the mucous escape reaction is a pool of mucus in fibrous connective tissue (Fig. 23.69) surrounded by an inflammatory reaction dominated by macrophages. Older lesions are frequently primarily granulation tissue. The mucous retention cyst has an epithelial-lined fibrous tissue around the mucus pool, and there is little inflammation as long as the epithelium is intact. The epithelium may be cuboidal, columnar, or stratified squamous.

Some superficial mucoceles rupture and spontaneously resolve, but others must be excised along with the salivary gland that supplies saliva to the mucocele. Successful cryotherapy has been reported.[898] Recurrences are common.

SALIVARY DUCT CYST

Salivary duct cyst results from marked dilatation of a salivary gland duct. Duct obstruction is considered a common cause, but it differs from mucus retention cyst by not containing a mucus plug, occurrence primarily in the parotid gland, and larger size.

In AFIP's experience, 85% of salivary duct cysts occur in the parotid gland and 10% in the submandibular gland.[866] They comprise 2–3% of parotid gland lesions.[899,900] There is no sex predilection, and the majority of patients have been over 30 years old. The cysts have been as large as 10 cm, but the majority are 1 to 3 cm.[881] They are well circumscribed, usually unilocular, and have a dense fibrous wall that often has mild to moderate chronic inflammation. The cyst is lined by stratified squamous, flattened squamous, cuboidal, or columnar epithelium, which occasionally has goblet-type mucous cells or oncocytic cells. Surgical excision is curative. A very rare condition is polycystic (dysgenetic) disease of the parotid gland in which most of the gland parenchyma is replaced by numerous dilated ducts.[901,902]

LYMPHOEPITHELIAL CYST

Similar to salivary duct cysts, salivary lymphoepithelial cysts nearly always occur in the parotid gland as unilateral and unicystic lesions, except HIV-associated cysts that are discussed separately. They comprise about 2–3% of all parotid surgical specimens. The male to female ratio is about 3:1, and the peak incidence is in the 4th decade of life.[866,881,899,903]

Microscopically, the characteristic feature is dense lymphoid tissue, usually with conspicuous germinal centers, in the wall of the cyst. The lymphoid tissue is usually well demarcated from the adjacent parotid parenchyma. These cysts typically have a more irregular luminal surface than salivary duct cysts (Fig. 23.70). The epithelial lining is usually stratified squamous, but cuboidal, columnar, or pseudostratified ciliated types also occur.[866,899,904] Unilocular form, minimal papillary configuration, and absence of oncocytic columnar cells distinguish them from Warthin's tumors. Cystic foci of metastatic squamous cell carcinoma, especially from the nasopharynx, sometimes mimics lymphoepithelial cyst, but cytologic atypia in the cyst-lining epithelial cells differentiates cystic carcinoma from lymphoepithelial cyst. Cystic lymphoepithelial complexes in lymphoepithelial sialadenitis, which may be associated with Sjögren's syndrome, are distinct from lymphoepithelial cyst and characterized by diffuse involvement of the gland and multiple lymphoepithelial complexes.

Proposed pathogenesis is that they develop either from remnants of the embryonic branchial apparatus, i.e. *branchial cleft cyst*, or, more likely, from cystic proliferation of salivary gland epithelium entrapped in intraparotid and paraparotid lymph nodes.[881,903–905] They are treated by surgical excision and usually do not recur.

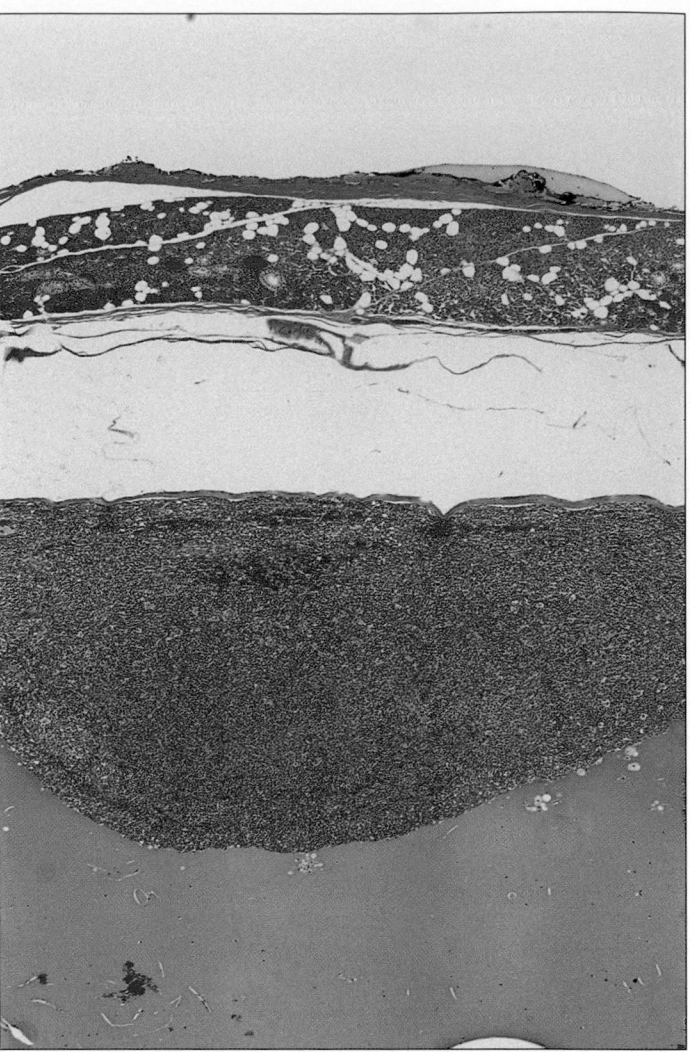

Fig. 23.70 A lymphoepithelial cyst of the parotid has an undulating, epithelial-lined luminal surface and a wall of dense lymphoid tissue that is well demarcated from the adjacent parotid parenchyma. The separation is a tissue processing artifact.

HIV-ASSOCIATED SALIVARY GLAND DISEASE (MULTIPLE LYMPHOEPITHELIAL CYSTS OF THE PAROTID GLAND)

Related to persistent generalized lymphadenopathy that is a manifestation of human immunodeficiency virus (HIV) infection is lymphoid hyperplasia with cystic ductal epithelial proliferation in the parotid glands.[866,905–910] This manifestation of HIV infection is also a component of *diffuse infiltrative lymphocytosis* syndrome.[911–913] The incidence of salivary gland involvement in HIV infection is not well known, but Schiødt et al.[914] found it to be about 5%, and Mulligan et al.[915] reported salivary gland enlargement in 4.3% of HIV-infected women. Terry et al.[907] reported that 60% of patients with lympho-epithelial lesions were HIV infected. HIV-related parotid sialadenopathy affects men over women about 7:1 and typically manifests before development of AIDS.[916] It is usually bilateral, associated with cervical lymphadenopathy, and painless, although tenderness of the glands has been described.[915]

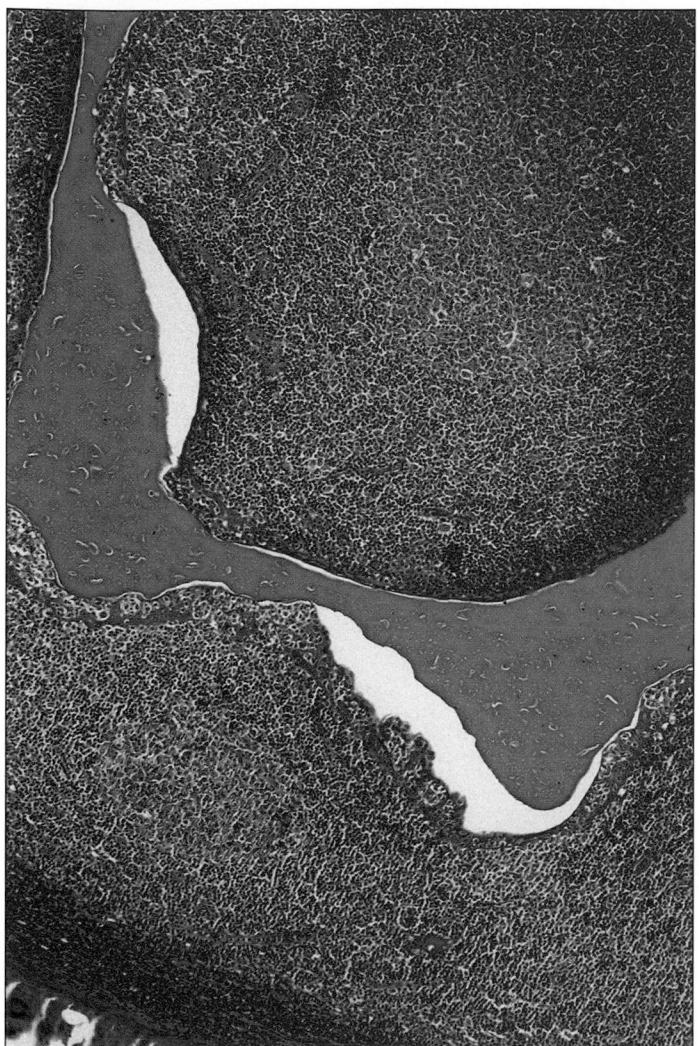

Fig. 23.71 In HIV-associated parotid gland disease, multiple irregularly shaped epithelial cysts, similar to this one, within intraparotid lymphoid tissue replace much of the parotid gland parenchyma. Lymphoid follicles often have irregular outlines, poorly defined mantle zones, and focal follicle lysis.

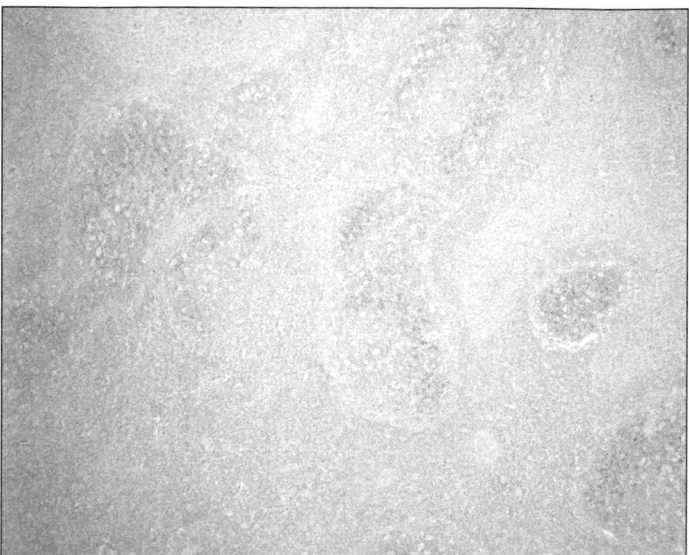

Fig. 23.72 Follicular dendritic cells are reactive with the immunostain for the p24 core antigen of HIV in HIV-associated sialadenitis.

The microscopic features of the lymphoid hyperplasia are similar to those of persistent generalized lymphadenopathy. Florid follicular hyperplasia disrupts and replaces the normal parotid parenchyma. Lymphoid follicles are frequently large and irregularly shaped, have attenuated mantle zones and follicle lysis, and contain numerous tingible-body macrophages and mitotic figures. The interfollicular lymphoid tissue contains many large histiocytes, which are often clustered, neutrophils, and plasma cells. Lymphoepithelial complexes similar to those in Sjögren's syndrome and squamous epithelial-lined cysts occur within the lymphoid proliferation (Fig. 23.71).[866,906]

Unlike patients with Sjögren's syndrome, HIV patients lack the serum autoantibodies (antinuclear antibodies, anti-SSA, anti-SSB, rheumatoid factor) typical in Sjögren's syndrome, and the parotid lymphoid proliferation is predominantly CD8 cells rather than CD4 cells.[912,917,918] The p24 core antigen of HIV can be demonstrated in the follicular dendritic cells and interfollicular histiocytes with immunohistochemistry (Fig. 23.72).[918,919]

Sialadenopathy does not appear to influence the course of HIV infection, and therapy specific for parotid disease is primarily for cosmetic reasons and includes antiviral drug therapy, surgery, radiation, and chemical sclerosis.[904,906,907,918–922] Lymphomas have developed in some cases of HIV-associated sialadenitis. These lymphomas have been both low grade (MALT type) and high grade.[923–925]

SCLEROSING POLYCYSTIC ADENOSIS

Sclerosing polycystic adenosis is a rare lesion of major salivary glands. The lesion is a reactive proliferation and degeneration of glandular elements with some features similar to those of sclerosing adenosis in the breast.[926]

Sclerosing polycystic adenoses are slow-growing masses in the parotid gland and submandibular gland (only one case). The patients have ranged in age from 12 to 63 years. There is no gender predilection. The clinical working diagnosis is usually a benign salivary gland tumor.

Grossly, the lesions are discrete, pale, rubbery nodules embedded within the salivary gland parenchyma. Microscopically, the lesions are circumscribed but unencapsulated masses composed of sclerotic and hyalinized collagenous tissue with irregularly distributed hyperplastic ductal and acinar elements in a vaguely lobular pattern that are usually accompanied by cystically ectatic ducts (Fig. 23.73). Dilated ducts frequently manifest epithelial hyperplasia that often forms transluminal bridges in a cribriform pattern. This epithelial hyperplasia sometimes surrounds eosinophilic globules, as seen in so-called collagenous spherulosis. A few ducts with apocrine-like metaplasia are often evident. The combination of fibrosis, epithelial hyperplasia, and cystic changes are reminiscent of fibrocystic changes of the breast. Some of the epithelial cells appear to be altered acinar cells because they contain large, periodic acid–Schiff-positive, intracytoplasmic granules. Unlike normal acinar cells, however, the cytoplasmic granules are intensely eosinophilic and are believed to represent altered zymogen granules.

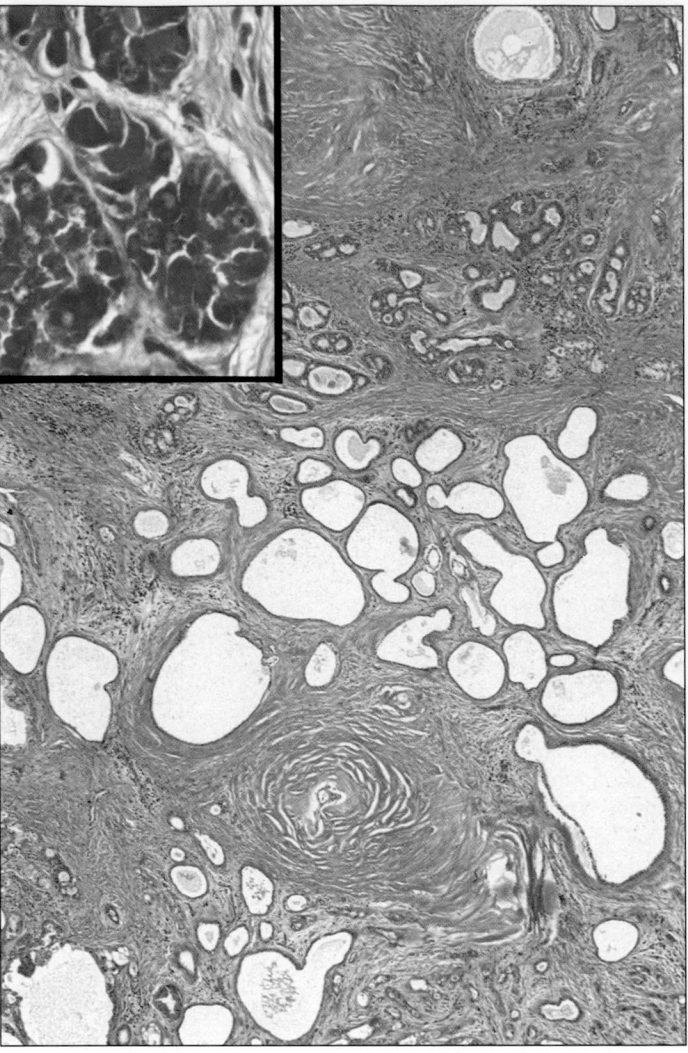

Fig. 23.73 Multiple cystic ducts, ductal hyperplasia, fibrosis with nodular sclerosis, and acinar cells with large, eosinophilic, cytoplasmic granules (inset) are characteristics of sclerosing polycystic adenosis.

A prominent feature in several of these lesions is rounded, nodular areas of dense, hyalinized collagenous sclerosis. These sclerotic nodules probably represent end-stage degeneration and sclerosis of ectatic ducts within the lesion. This conclusion is supported by observations of ballooning degeneration of the epithelium of some cystic ducts, xanthoma cell infiltrates in some degenerated ducts, and collagenous sclerosis around some xanthomatous nodules. There is a sparse to focally intense lymphocytic infiltrate associated with these lesions. Immunoreactivity of estrogen and progesterone receptors has been reported.[927]

Two patients had recurrence, but this process has a favorable prognosis. Skalova et al.[927] have described foci of ductal dysplasia in three cases of sclerosing polycystic adenosis.

REFERENCES

1. Leegaard T, Lindeman H. Salivary-gland tumours. Clinical picture and treatment. Acta Otolaryngol Suppl (Stockh) 1969; 263: 155–159.

2. Spiro RH. Salivary neoplasms: overview of a 35-year experience with 2,807 patients. Head Neck Surg 1986; 8: 177–184.

3. Spiro RH, Koss LG, Hajdu SI, et al. Tumors of minor salivary origin. A clinicopathologic study of 492 cases. Cancer 1973; 31: 117–129.

4. Abiose BO, Oyejide O, Ogunniyi J. Salivary gland tumours in Ibadan, Nigeria: a study of 295 cases. Afr J Med Med Sci 1990; 19: 195–199.

5. Hui KK, Luna MA, Batsakis JG, et al. Undifferentiated carcinomas of the major salivary glands. Oral Surg Oral Med Oral Pathol 1990; 69: 76–83.

6. Sun EC, Curtis R, Melbye M, et al. Salivary gland cancer in the United States. Cancer Epidemiol Biomarkers Prev 1999; 8: 1095–1100.

7. Ostman J, Anneroth G, Gustafsson H, et al. Malignant salivary gland tumours in Sweden 1960–1989 – an epidemiological study. Oral Oncol 1997; 33: 169–176.

8. Auclair PL, Ellis GL, Gnepp DR, et al. Salivary gland neoplasms: general considerations. In: Ellis GL, Auclair PL, Gnepp DR, eds. Surgical pathology of the salivary glands. 1st edn. Philadelphia: WB Saunders; 1991: 135–164.

9. Seifert G, Miehlke A, Haubrich J, Chilla R. Diseases of the salivary glands: diagnosis, pathology, treament, facial nerve surgery. 1st edn. Stuttgart: Georg Thieme Verlag; 1986.

10. Eneroth CM. Salivary gland tumors in the parotid gland, submandibular gland, and the palate region. Cancer 1971; 27: 1415–1418.

11. Eveson JW, Cawson RA. Salivary gland tumours. A review of 2410 cases with particular reference to histological types, site, age and sex distribution. J Pathol 1985; 146: 51–58.

12. Pinkston JA, Cole P. Incidence rates of salivary gland tumors: results from a population-based study. Otolaryngol Head Neck Surg 1999; 120: 834–840.

13. Heller KS, Attie JN, Dubner S. Accuracy of frozen section in the evaluation of salivary tumors. Am J Surg 1993; 166: 424–427.

14. Wong DS. Frozen section during parotid surgery revisited: efficacy of its applications and changing trend of indications. Head Neck 2002; 24: 191–197.

15. Frankenthaler RA, Byers RM, Luna MA, et al. Predicting occult lymph node metastasis in parotid cancer. Arch Otolaryngol Head Neck Surg 1993; 119: 517–520.

16. Kane WJ, McCaffrey TV, Olsen KD, et al. Primary parotid malignancies. A clinical and pathologic review. Arch Otolaryngol Head Neck Surg 1991; 117: 307–315.

17. Spiro RH, Thaler HT, Hicks WF, et al. The importance of clinical staging of minor salivary gland carcinoma. Am J Surg 1991; 162: 330–336.

18. Auclair PL, Goode RK, Ellis GL. Mucoepidermoid carcinoma of intraoral salivary glands. Evaluation and application of grading criteria in 143 cases. Cancer 1992; 69: 2021–2030.

19. Goode RK, Auclair PL, Ellis GL. Mucoepidermoid carcinoma of the major salivary glands: clinical and histopathologic analysis of 234 cases with evaluation of grading criteria. Cancer 1998; 82: 1217–1224.

20. Levitt SH, McHugh RB, Gómez-Marin O, et al. Clinical staging system for cancer of the salivary gland: a retrospective study. Cancer 1981; 47: 2712–2724.

21. Spiro RH, Huvos AG, Strong EW. Cancer of the parotid gland. A clinicopathologic study of 288 primary cases. Am J Surg 1975; 130: 452–459.

22. Spiro RH, Hajdu SI, Strong EW. Tumors of the submaxillary gland. Am J Surg 1976; 132: 463–468.

23. Greene FL, Page DL, Fleming ID, et al. AJCC Cancer Staging Manual. 6th edn. New York: Springer-Verlag; 2002: 69–75.

24. Spiro RH, Huvos AG, Berk R, et al. Mucoepidermoid carcinoma of salivary gland origin. A clinicopathologic study of 367 cases. Am J Surg 1978; 136: 461–468.

25. Foote FW Jr, Frazell EL. Tumors of the major salivary glands, section iv, fascicle 11, 1st series. Atlas of tumor pathology. Washington, DC: Armed Forces Institute of Pathology; 1954.

26. Seifert G, Sobin LH. Histological typing of salivary gland tumours. World Health Organization international classification of tumours. 2nd edn. Berlin: Springer-Verlag; 1991.

27. Thackray AC, Sobin LH. Histological typing of salivary gland tumours. World Health Organization. International histological classification of tumours No. 7. Geneva: The Organization; 1972.

28. Ellis GL, Auclair PL. Tumors of the salivary glands. Atlas of tumor pathology, 3rd series, fascicle 17. 1st edn. Washington, DC: Armed Forces Institute of Pathology; 1996: 27–30.

29. Luna MA. Salivary glands. In: Pilch BZ, ed. Head and neck surgical pathology. Philadelphia: Lippincott Williams & Wilkins; 2001: 284–349.

30. Pell RL. Diseases of the salivary glands. In: Barnes L, ed. Surgical pathology of the head and neck. 2nd edn. Vol. 1. New York: Marcel Dekker; 2001: 633–757.

31. Eversole L. II. Salivary gland pathology. In: Fu Y-S, Wenig BM, Abemayor E, Wenig BL, eds. Head and neck pathology with clinical correlations. New York: Churchill Livingstone; 2001: 242–292.

32. Stanley MW, Lowhagen T. Fine needle aspiration of palpable masses. Stoneham, MA, USA: Butterworth-Heinnemann; 1993.

33. Flynn MB, Wolfson SE, Thomas S, et al. Fine needle aspiration biopsy in clinical management of head and neck tumors. J Surg Oncol 1990; 44: 214–217.

34. Zakowski MF. Fine-needle aspiration cytology of tumors: diagnostic accuracy and potential pitfalls. Cancer Invest 1994; 12: 505–515.

35. Schelkun PM, Grundy WG. Fine-needle aspiration biopsy of head and neck lesions. J Oral Maxillofac Surg 1991; 49: 262–267.

36. Schwarz R, Chan NH, MacFarlane JK. Fine needle aspiration cytology in the evaluation of head and neck masses. Am J Surg 1990; 159: 482–485.

37. Heller KS, Dubner S, Chess Q, et al. Value of fine needle aspiration biopsy of salivary gland masses in clinical decision-making. Am J Surg 1992; 164: 667–670.

38. Carter MJ. Letters. J Miss State Med Assoc 1994; 35: 265.

39. Henry-Stanley MJ, Stanley MW. Processing of needle rinse material from fine-needle aspirations rarely detects malignancy not identified in smears. Diagn Cytopathol 1992; 8: 538–540.

40. O'Dwyer P, Farrar WB, James AG, et al. Needle aspiration biopsy of major salivary gland tumors. Its value. Cancer 1986; 57: 554–557.

41. Felson B. Chest roentgenology. Philadelphia: WB Saunders; 1973.

42. Stanley MW, Knoedler JP. Skeletal structures that clinically simulate lymph nodes: encounters during fine needle aspiration. Diagn Cytopathol 1993; 9: 86–88.

43. Layfield LJ, Glasgow BJ. Diagnosis of salivary gland tumors by fine-needle aspiration cytology: a review of clinical utility and pitfalls. Diagn Cytopathol 1991; 7: 267–272.

44. Layfield LJ, Glasgow BJ, DuPuis MH. Fine-needle aspiration of lymphadenopathy of suspected infectious etiology. Arch Pathol Lab Med 1985; 109: 810–812.

45. Silverman JF. Guides to clinical aspiration biopsy: Infectious and inflammatory diseases and other nonneoplastic disorders. New York: Igaku-Shoin; 1991.

46. Das DK, Gulati A, Bhatt NC, et al. Fine needle aspiration cytology of oral and pharyngeal lesions. A study of 45 cases. Acta Cytol 1993; 37: 333–342.

47. Bayramoglu H, Duzcan E, Akbulut M, et al. Infarction after fine needle aspiration biopsy of pleomorphic adenoma of the parotid gland. Acta Cytol 2001; 45: 1008–1010.

48. Gottschalk-Sabag S, Glick T. Necrosis of parotid pleomorphic adenoma following fine needle aspiration. A case report. Acta Cytol 1995; 39: 252–254.

49. Kameswaran M, Abu-Eshy S, Hamdi J. Facial palsy following fine needle aspiration biopsy of parotid hemangioma: a case report and review of the literature. Ear Nose Throat J 1991; 70: 801–803.

50. Kern SB. Necrosis of a Warthin's tumor following fine needle aspiration. Acta Cytol 1988; 32: 207–208.

51. Layfield LJ, Reznicek M, Lowe M, et al. Spontaneous infarction of a parotid gland pleomorphic adenoma. Report of a case with cytologic and radiographic overlap with a primary salivary gland malignancy. Acta Cytol 1992; 36: 381–386.

52. Li S, Baloch ZW, Tomaszewski JE, et al. Worrisome histologic alterations following fine-needle aspiration of benign parotid lesions. Arch Pathol Lab Med 2000; 124: 87–91.

53. Skalova A, Starek I, Michal M, et al. Malignancy-simulating change in parotid gland oncocytoma following fine needle aspiration. Report of 3 cases. Pathol Res Pract 1999; 195: 399–405.

54. Jones JD, Pittman DL, Sanders LR. Necrosis of thyroid nodules after fine needle aspiration. Acta Cytol 1985; 29: 29–32.

55. Davies JD, Webb AJ. Segmental lymph-node infarction after fine-needle aspiration. J Clin Pathol 1982; 35: 855–857.

56. Allen CM, Damm D, Neville B, et al. Necrosis in benign salivary gland neoplasms. Not necessarily a sign of malignant transformation. Oral Surg Oral Med Oral Pathol 1994; 78: 455–461.

57. Mukunyadzi P, Bardales RH, Palmer HE, et al. Tissue effects of salivary gland fine-needle aspiration. Does this procedure preclude accurate histologic diagnosis? Am J Clin Pathol 2000; 114: 741–745.

58. Batsakis JG. Letters to the Editor. Ann Otol Rhinol Laryngol 1993; 102: 484–485.

59. Guyot JP, Auberson S, Obradovic D, et al. Fine-needle aspiration in the diagnosis of head and neck growths: the pitfalls of false-positive diagnosis. ORL J Otorhinolaryngol Relat Spec 1993; 55: 41–44.

60. Batsakis JG, Sneige N, el-Naggar AK. Fine-needle aspiration of salivary glands: its utility and tissue effects. Ann Otol Rhinol Laryngol 1992; 101: 185–188.

61. Cohen MB, Ljung BM, Boles R. Salivary gland tumors. Fine-needle aspiration vs frozen-section diagnosis. Arch Otolaryngol Head Neck Surg 1986; 112: 867–869.

62. Layfield LJ, Tan P, Glasgow BJ. Fine-needle aspiration of salivary gland lesions. Comparison with frozen sections and histologic findings. Arch Pathol Lab Med 1987; 111: 346–353.

63. Hee CG, Perry CF. Fine-needle aspiration cytology of parotid tumours: is it useful? ANZ J Surg 2001; 71: 345–348.

64. Costas A, Castro P, Martin-Granizo R, et al. Fine needle aspiration biopsy (FNAB) for lesions of the salivary glands. Br J Oral Maxillofac Surg 2000; 38: 539–542.

65. Wong DS, Li GK. The role of fine-needle aspiration cytology in the management of parotid tumors: a critical clinical appraisal. Head Neck 2000; 22(5): 469–473.

66. Al Khafaji BM, Nestok BR, Katz RL. Fine-needle aspiration of 154 parotid masses with histologic correlation: ten-year experience at the University of Texas M.D. Anderson Cancer Center. Cancer 1998; 84: 153–159.

67. Stewart CJ, MacKenzie K, McGarry GW, et al. Fine-needle aspiration cytology of salivary gland: a review of 341 cases. Diagn Cytopathol 2000; 22: 139–146.

68. Stanley MW. Selected problems in fine needle aspiration of head and neck masses. Mod Pathol 2002; 15: 342–350.

69. Patt BS, Schaefer SD, Vuitch F. Role of fine-needle aspiration in the evaluation of neck masses. Med Clin North Am 1993; 77: 611–623.

70. Zurrida S, Alasio L, Tradati N, et al. Fine-needle aspiration of parotid masses. Cancer 1993; 72: 2306–2311.

71. Cross DL, Gansler TS, Morris RC. Fine needle aspiration and frozen section of salivary gland lesions. South Med J 1990; 83: 283–286.

72. Roland NJ, Caslin AW, Smith PA, et al. Fine needle aspiration cytology of salivary gland lesions reported immediately in a head and neck clinic. J Laryngol Otol 1993; 107: 1025–1028.

73. Megerian CA, Maniglia AJ. Parotidectomy: a ten year experience with fine needle aspiration and frozen section biopsy correlation. Ear Nose Throat J 1994; 73: 377–380.

74. Wheelis RF, Yarington CT Jr. Tumors of the salivary glands. Comparison of frozen-section diagnosis with final pathologic diagnosis. Arch Otolaryngol Head Neck Surg 1984; 110: 76–77.

75. Miller RH, Calcaterra TC, Paglia DE. Accuracy of frozen section diagnosis of parotid lesions. Ann Otol Rhinol Laryngol 1979; 88: 573–576.

76. Weinberger MS, Rosenberg WW, Meurer WT, et al. Fine-needle aspiration of parotid gland lesions. Head Neck 1992; 14: 483–487.

77. Tew S, Poole AG, Philips J. Fine-needle aspiration biopsy of parotid lesions: comparison with frozen section. Aust NZ J Surg 1997; 67: 438–441.

78. Hajdu SI, Melamed MR. Limitations of aspiration cytology in the diagnosis of primary neoplasms. Acta Cytol 1984; 28: 337–345.

79. Kline TS, Merriam JM, Shapshay SM. Aspiration biopsy cytology of the salivary gland. Am J Clin Pathol 1981; 76: 263–269.

80. Eneroth CM, Zajicek J. Aspiration biopsy cytology of salivary gland tumors. III. Morphologic studies on smears and histologic sections from 368 mixed tumors. Acta Cytol 1966; 10: 440–454.

81. Auclair PL. Tumor-associated lymphoid proliferation in the parotid gland: A potential diagnostic pitfall. Oral Surg Oral Med Oral Pathol 1994; 77: 19–26.

82. Batsakis JG, el-Naggar AK. Sebaceous lesions of salivary glands and oral cavity. Ann Otol Rhinol Laryngol 1990; 99: 416–418.

83. Hayes MM, Cameron RD, Jones EA. Sebaceous variant of mucoepidermoid carcinoma of the salivary gland. A case report with cytohistologic correlation. Acta Cytol 1993; 37: 237–241.

84. Derias NW, Chong WH, Pambakian H. Sebaceous adenoma of parotid gland – a rare tumour diagnosed by fine needle aspiration cytology. Cytopathology 1994; 5: 392–395.

85. Pai RR, Bharathi S, Naik R, et al. Unilocular cystic sebaceous lymphadenoma of the parotid gland. Indian J Pathol Microbiol 1994; 37: 327–330.

86. Weidner N, Geisinger KR, Sterling RT, et al. Benign lymphoepithelial cysts of the parotid gland. A histologic, cytologic, and ultrastructural study. Am J Clin Pathol 1986; 85: 395–401.

87. Stanley MW, Bardales RH, Beneke J, et al. Sialolithiasis. Differential diagnostic problems in fine-needle aspiration cytology. Am J Clin Pathol 1996; 106: 229–233.

88. Carson HJ, Raslan WF, Castelli MJ, et al. Tyrosine crystals in benign parotid gland cysts: report of two cases diagnosed by fine-needle aspiration biopsy with ultrastructural and histochemical evaluation. Am J Clin Pathol 1994; 102: 699–702.

89. Ramzy I, Rone R, Schantz HD. Squamous cells in needle aspirates of subcutaneous lesions: a diagnostic problem. Am J Clin Pathol 1986; 85: 319–324.

90. Sperling NM, Lin PT, Lucente FE. Cystic parotid masses in HIV infection. Head Neck 1990; 12: 337–341.

91. Mavec P, Eneroth CM, Franzen S, et al. Aspiration biopsy of salivary gland tumors. Acta Otolaryngol 1964; 58: 471–484.

92. Laucirica R, Farnum JB, Leopold SK, et al. False-positive diagnosis in fine-needle aspiration of an atypical Warthin's tumor: histochemical differential stains for cytodiagnosis. Diagn Cytopathol 1989; 5: 412–415.

93. Chen K. Letter to the editor: Aspiration cytology of metaplastic Warthin's tumor mimicking squamous cell carcinoma. Diagn Cytopathol 1991; 7: 330–331.

94. Olsen KD, Goellner JR. False-positive cytologic findings in Warthin's tumor: a report of two cases. Ear Nose Throat J 1992; 71: 417–421.

95. Guazzi A, Gabrielli M, Guadagni G. Cytologic features of a functioning parathyroid carcinoma: a case report. Acta Cytol 1982; 26: 709–713.

96. Hood IC, Qizilbash AH, Young JE, et al. Fine needle aspiration biopsy cytology of paragangliomas. Cytologic, light microscopic and ultrastructural studies of three cases. Acta Cytol 1983; 27: 651–657.

97. Leiman G. Editorial comments: Clear cell tumors of the salivary glands. Diagn Cytopathol 1993; 9: 711–712.

98. Layfield LJ, Glasgow BJ. Aspiration cytology of clear-cell lesions of the parotid gland: morphologic features and differential diagnosis. Diagn Cytopathol 1993; 9: 705–711; discussion 711–712.

99. Gattuso P, Castelli MJ, Shah PA, et al. Fine needle aspiration cytologic diagnosis of metastatic Merkel cell carcinoma in the parotid gland. Acta Cytol 1988; 32: 576–578.

100. Carrillo R, Poblet E, Rocamora A, et al. Epithelial-myoepithelial carcinoma of the salivary gland. Fine needle aspiration cytologic findings. Acta Cytol 1990; 34: 243–247.

101. Arora VK, Misra K, Bhatia A. Cytomorphologic features of the rare epithelial-myoepithelial carcinoma of the salivary gland. Acta Cytol 1990; 34: 239–242.

102. Abdul-Karim FW, Weaver MG. Needle aspiration cytology of an oncocytic carcinoma of the parotid gland. Diagn Cytopathol 1991; 7: 420–422.

103. Candel A, Gattuso P, Reddy V, et al. Is fine needle aspiration biopsy of salivary gland masses really necessary? Ear Nose Throat J 1993; 72: 485–489.

104. Henry-Stanley MJ, Beneke J, Bardales RH, et al. Fine-needle aspiration of normal tissue from enlarged salivary glands: sialosis or missed target? Diagn Cytopathol 1995; 13: 300–303.

105. Layfield LJ, Glasgow BJ, Goldstein N, et al. Lipomatous lesions of the parotid gland. Potential pitfalls in fine needle aspiration biopsy diagnosis. Acta Cytol 1991; 35: 553–556.

106. Speight PM, Tinkler S. The salivary glands: Sialosis. In: McGee JD, Isaacson PG, Wright NA, eds. Oxford textbook of pathology, pathology of systems. 9th edn. Vol. 2a. Oxford: Oxford university Press; 1992: 1080.

107. Waldron CA. Face, lips, teeth, oral soft tissue, jaws, salivary gland and neck: Enlargements related to malnutrition, hormonal distrubances, and alcoholic cirrhosis (sialosis). In: Kissane JM, ed. Anderson's pathology. 9th edn. Vol. 2. St. Louis: CV Mosby; 1990: 1128.

108. Ascoli V, Albedi FM, De Blasiis R, et al. Sialadenosis of the parotid gland: report of four cases diagnosed by fine-needle aspiration cytology. Diagn Cytopathol 1993; 9: 151–155.

109. Ellis GL, Auclair PL. Tumors of the salivary glands. Atlas of tumor pathology, 3rd series, fascicle 17. Washington, DC: Armed Forces Institute of Pathology; 1996: 39–56.

110. Waldron CA, el-Mofty SK, Gnepp DR. Tumors of the intraoral minor salivary glands: a demographic and histologic study of 426 cases. Oral Surg Oral Med Oral Pathol 1988; 66: 323–333.

111. Woods JE, Chong GC, Beahrs OH. Experience with 1,360 primary parotid tumors. Am J Surg 1975; 130: 460–462.

112. Fitzpatrick PJ, Black KM. Salivary gland tumors. J Otolaryngol 1985; 14: 296–300.

113. Eveson JW, Cawson RA. Tumours of the minor (oropharyngeal) salivary glands: a demographic study of 336 cases. J Oral Pathol 1985; 14: 500–509.

114. Isacsson G, Shear M. Intraoral salivary gland tumors: a retrospective study of 201 cases. J Oral Pathol 1983;12: 57–62.

115. Breitenecker G, Wepner F. A pleomorphic adenoma (so-called mixed tumor) in the wall of a dentigerous cyst. Oral Surg Oral Med Oral Pathol 1973; 36: 63–71.

116. Miller AS, Winnick M. Salivary gland inclusion in the anterior mandible. Report of a case with a review of the literature on aberrant salivary gland tissue and neoplasms. Oral Surg Oral Med Oral Pathol 1971; 31: 790–797.

117. Lack EE, Upton MP. Histopathologic review of salivary gland tumors in childhood. Arch Otolaryngol Head Neck Surg 1988; 114: 898–906.

118. Waldron CA. Mixed tumor (pleomorphic adenoma) and myoepithelioma. In: Ellis GL, Auclair PL, Gnepp DR, eds. Surgical pathology of the salivary glands. 1st edn. Philadelphia: WB Saunders; 1991: 165–186.

119. Ahn MS, Hayashi GM, Hilsinger RLJ, et al. Familial mixed tumors of the parotid gland. Head Neck 1999; 21: 772–775.

120. Allison RS, van der Waal I, Snow GB. Parapharyngeal tumours: a review of 23 cases. Clin Otolaryngol 1989; 14: 199–203.

121. Goodwin WJ Jr, Chandler JR. Transoral excision of lateral pharyngeal space tumors presenting intraorally. Laryngoscope 1988; 98: 266–269.

122. Blevins NH, Jackler RK, Kaplan MJ, et al. Facial paralysis due to benign parotid tumors. Arch Otolaryngol Head Neck Surg 1992; 118: 427–430.

123. O'Dwyer TP, Gullane PJ, Dardick I. A pseudo-malignant Warthin's tumor presenting with facial nerve paralysis. J Otolaryngol 1990; 19: 353–357.

124. Seifert G, Langrock I, Donath K. Pathomorphologische Subklassifikation der pleomorphen Spreicheldrüsenadenome. Analyse von 310 Parotisadenomen. HNO 1976; 24: 415–426.

125. Seifert G, Miehlke A, Haubrich J, Chilla R. Diseases of the salivary glands: diagnosis, pathology, treament, facial nerve surgery. 1st edn. Stuttgart: Georg Thieme Verlag; 1986: 19.

126. Wenig BM, Hitchcock CL, Ellis GL, et al. Metastasizing mixed tumor of salivary glands. A clinicopathologic and flow cytometric analysis. Am J Surg Pathol 1992; 16: 845–858.

127. Saku T, Cheng J, Okabe H, et al. Immunolocalization of basement membrane molecules in the stroma of salivary gland pleomorphic adenoma. J Oral Pathol Med 1990; 19: 208–214.

128. Dardick I, Ostrynski VL, Ekem JK, et al. Immunohistochemical and ultrastructural correlates of muscle-actin expression in pleomorphic adenomas and myoepitheliomas based on comparison of formalin and methanol fixation. Virchows Arch [A] 1992; 421: 95–104.

129. Dardick I, van Nostrand AW, Phillips MJ. Histogenesis of salivary gland pleomorphic adenoma (mixed tumor) with an evaluation of the role of the myoepithelial cell. Hum Pathol 1982; 13: 62–75.

130. Dardick I, van Nostrand AW. Myoepithelial cells in salivary gland tumors – revisited. Head Neck Surg 1985; 7: 395–408.

131. Erlandson RA, Cardon-Cardo C, Higgins PJ. Histogenesis of benign pleomorphic adenoma (mixed tumor) of the major salivary glands. An ultrastructural and immunohistochemical study. Am J Surg Pathol 1984; 8: 803–820.

132. Morinaga S, Nakajima T, Shimosato Y. Normal and neoplastic myoepithelial cells in salivary glands: an immunohistochemical study. Hum Pathol 1987; 18: 1218–1226.

133. Dardick I, van Nostrand AW, Jeans MT, et al. Pleomorphic adenoma, II: Ultrastructural organization of 'stromal' regions. Hum Pathol 1983; 14: 798–809.

134. Dardick I, van Nostrand AW, Jeans MT, et al. Pleomorphic adenoma, I: Ultrastructural organization of 'epithelial' regions. Hum Pathol 1983; 14: 780–797.

135. Savera AT, Gown AM, Zarbo RJ. Immunolocalization of three novel smooth muscle-specific proteins in salivary gland pleomorphic adenoma: assessment of the morphogenetic role of myoepithelium. Mod Pathol 1997; 10: 1093–1100.

136. Dardick I, Stratis M, Parks WR, et al. S-100 protein antibodies do not label normal salivary gland myoepithelium. Histogenetic implications for salivary gland tumors. Am J Pathol 1991; 138: 619–628.

137. Kas K, Voz ML, Roijer E, et al. Promoter swapping between the genes for a novel zinc finger protein and beta-catenin in pleiomorphic adenomas with t(3;8)(p21; q12) translocations. Nat Genet 1997; 15: 170–174.

138. Voz ML, Van de Ven WJ, Kas K. First insights into the molecular basis of pleomorphic adenomas of the salivary glands. Adv Dent Res 2000; 14: 81–83.

139. Gillenwater A, Hurr K, Wolf P, et al. Microsatellite alterations at chromosome 8q loci in pleomorphic adenoma. Otolaryngol Head Neck Surg 1997; 117: 448–452.

140. Debiec-Rychter M, Van Valckenborgh I, Van den Broeck C, et al. Histologic localization of PLAG1 (pleomorphic adenoma gene 1) in pleomorphic adenoma of the salivary gland: cytogenetic evidence of common origin of phenotypically diverse cells. Lab Invest 2001; 81: 1289–1297.

141. Astrom AK, Voz ML, Kas K, et al. Conserved mechanism of PLAG1 activation in salivary gland tumors with and without chromosome 8q12 abnormalities: identification of SII as a new fusion partner gene. Cancer Res 1999; 59: 918–923.

142. Yamamoto Y, Kishimoto Y, Wistuba II, et al. DNA analysis at p53 locus in carcinomas arising from pleomorphic adenomas of salivary glands: comparison of molecular study and p53 immunostaining. Pathol Int 1998; 48: 265–272.

143. Righi PD, Li YQ, Deutsch M, et al. The role of the p53 gene in the malignant transformation of pleomorphic adenomas of the parotid gland. Anticancer Res 1994; 14: 2253–2257.

144. Roijer E, Nordkvist A, Strom AK, et al. Translocation, deletion/amplification, and expression of HMGIC and MDM2 in a carcinoma ex pleomorphic adenoma. Am J Pathol 2002; 160: 433–440.

145. Junquera L, Alonso D, Sampedro A, et al. Pleomorphic adenoma of the salivary glands: prospective clinicopathologic and flow cytometric study. Head Neck 1999; 21: 652–656.

146. Curran AE, White DK, Damm DD, et al. Polymorphous low-grade adenocarcinoma versus pleomorphic adenoma of minor salivary glands: resolution of a diagnostic dilemma by immunohistochemical analysis with glial fibrillary acidic protein. Oral Surg Oral Med Oral Pathol Oral Radiol Endod 2001; 91(2): 194 –199.

147. Auclair PL, Ellis GL. Atypical features in salivary gland mixed tumors: their relationship to malignant transformation. Mod Pathol 1996; 9: 652–657.

148. Coleman H, Altini M. Intravascular tumour in intra-oral pleomorphic adenomas: a diagnostic and therapeutic dilemma. Histopathology 1999; 35: 439–444.

149. Brandwein M, Huvos AG, Dardick I, et al. Noninvasive and minimally invasive carcinoma ex mixed tumor: a clinicopathologic and ploidy study of 12 patients with major salivary tumors of low (or no?) malignant potential. Oral Surg Oral Med Oral Pathol Oral Radiol Endod 1996; 81: 655–664.

150. Ostrzega N, Cheng L, Layfield L. Glial fibrillary acid protein immunoreactivity in fine-needle aspiration of salivary gland lesions: a useful adjunct for the differential diagnosis of salivary gland neoplasms. Diagn Cytopathol 1989; 5: 145–149.

151. Takahashi H, Tsuda N, Tezuka F, et al. Immunohistochemical localization of carcinoembryonic antigen in carcinoma in pleomorphic adenoma of salivary gland: use in the diagnosis of benign and malignant lesions. Tohoku J Exp Med 1986; 149: 329–340.

152. Donovan DT, Conley JJ. Capsular significance in parotid tumor surgery: reality and myths of lateral lobectomy. Laryngoscope 1984; 94: 324–329.

153. Dykun RJ, Deitel M, Borowy ZJ, et al. Treatment of parotid neoplasms. Can J Surg 1980; 23: 14–19.

154. Myssiorek D, Ruah CB, Hybels RL. Recurrent pleomorphic adenomas of the parotid gland. Head Neck 1990; 12: 332–336.

155. Touquet R, Mackenzie IJ, Carruth JA. Management of the parotid pleomorphic adenoma, the problem of exposing tumour tissue at operation. The logical pursuit of treatment policies. Br J Oral Maxillofac Surg 1990; 28: 404–408.

156. Gleave EN, Whittaker JS, Nicholson A. Salivary tumours – experience over thirty years. Clin Otolaryngol 1979; 4: 247–257.

157. Wennmo C, Spandow O, Emgård P, et al. Pleomorphic adenomas of the parotid gland: superficial parotidectomy or limited excision? J Laryngol Otol 1988; 102: 603–605.

158. Hancock BD. Pleomorphic adenomas of the parotid: removal without rupture. Ann R Coll Surg Engl 1987; 69: 293–295.

159. Yamashita T, Tomoda K, Kumazawa T. The usefulness of partial parotidectomy for benign parotid gland tumors. A retrospective study of 306 cases. Acta Otolaryngol Suppl (Stockh) 1993; 500: 113–116.

160. Maynard JD. Management of pleomorphic adenoma of the parotid. Br J Surg 1988; 75: 305–308.

161. Hickman RE, Cawson RA, Duffy SW. The prognosis of specific types of salivary gland tumors. Cancer 1984; 54: 1620–1624.

162. Owen ER, Banerjee AK, Kissin M, et al. Complications of parotid surgery: the need for selectivity. Br J Surg 1989; 76: 1034–1035.

163. Hardingham M. Complications of superficial parotidectomy versus extracapsular lumpectomy in the treatment of benign parotid lesions (letter). J R Coll Surg Edinb 1993; 38: 180–181.

164. Dallera P, Marchetti C, Campobassi A. Local capsular dissection of parotid pleomorphic adenomas. Int J Oral Maxillofac Surg 1993; 22: 154–157.

165. Leverstein H, van de Wal J, Tiwari RM, et al. Surgical management of 246 previously untreated pleomorphic adenomas of the parotid gland. Br J Surg 1997; 84: 399–403.

166. Weber RS, Byers RM, Petit B, et al. Submandibular gland tumors. Adverse histologic factors and therapeutic implications. Arch Otolaryngol Head Neck Surg 1990; 116: 1055–1060.

167. Stanley RE, Mackenzie IJ, Maran AG. The surgical approach to recurrent pleomorphic adenoma of the parotid gland. Ann Acad Med Singapore 1984; 13: 91–95.

168. Niparko JK, Beauchamp ML, Krause CJ, et al. Surgical treatment of recurrent pleomorphic adenoma of the parotid gland. Arch Otolaryngol Head Neck Surg 1986;112: 1180–1184.

169. Samson MJ, Metson R, Wang CC, et al. Preservation of the facial nerve in the management of recurrent pleomorphic adenoma. Laryngoscope 1991; 101: 1060–1062.

170. Maran AG, Mackenzie IJ, Stanley RE. Recurrent pleomorphic adenomas of the parotid gland. Arch Otolaryngol Head Neck Surg 1984; 110: 167–171.

171. Jackson SR, Roland NJ, Clarke RW, et al. Recurrent pleomorphic adenoma. J Laryngol Otol 1993; 107: 546–549.

172. Phillips PP, Olsen KD. Recurrent pleomorphic adenoma of the parotid gland: report of 126 cases and a review of the literature. Ann Otol Rhinol Laryngol 1995; 104: 100–104.

173. Chau MN, Radden BG. A clinical-pathological study of 53 intra-oral pleomorphic adenomas. Int J Oral Maxillofac Surg 1989; 18: 158–162.

174. Stanley MW, Lowhagen T. Mucin production by pleomorphic adenomas of the parotid gland: a cytologic spectrum. Diagn Cytopathol 1990; 6: 49–52.

175. Viguer JM, Vicandi B, Jimenez-Heffernan JA, et al. Fine needle aspiration cytology of pleomorphic adenoma. An analysis of 212 cases. Acta Cytol 1997; 41: 786–794.

176. Murty DA, Sodhani P. Intranuclear inclusions in pleomorphic adenoma of salivary gland: a case report. Diagn Cytopathol 1993; 9: 194–196.

177. Bottles K, Ferrell LD, Miller TR. Tyrosine crystals in fine needle aspirates of a pleomorphic adenoma of the parotid gland. Acta Cytol 1984; 28: 490–492.

178. Cleveland DB, Cosgrove MM, Martin SE. Tyrosine-rich crystalloids in a fine needle aspirate of a polymorphous low grade adenocarcinoma of a minor salivary gland. A case report. Acta Cytol 1994; 38: 247–251.

179. Stanley MW, Horwitz CA, Bardales RH, et al. Basal cell carcinoma metastatic to the salivary glands: differential diagnosis in fine-needle aspiration cytology. Diagn Cytopathol 1997; 16: 247–252.

180. Qizilbash AH, Sianos J, Young JE, et al. Fine needle aspiration biopsy cytology of major salivary glands. Acta Cytol 1985; 29: 503–512.

181. Martin H, Janda J, Werbs M, et al. [Unusual chordoma of the neck region simulating salivary gland pleomorphic adenoma]. HNO 1990; 38: 462–464.

182. Verma K, Kapila K. Role of fine needle aspiration cytology in diagnosis of pleomorphic adenomas. Cytopathology 2002; 13: 121–127.

183. Ritland F, Lubensky I, LiVolsi VA. Polymorphous low-grade adenocarcinoma of the parotid salivary gland. Arch Pathol Lab Med 1993; 117: 1261–1263.

184. Domagala W, Halczy-Kowalik L, Weber K, et al. Coexpression of glial fibrillary acid protein, keratin and vimentin. A unique feature useful in the diagnosis of pleomorphic adenoma of the salivary gland in fine needle aspiration biopsy smears. Acta Cytol 1988; 32: 403–408.

185. Swanson PE, Pettinato G, Lillemoe TJ, et al. Gross cystic disease fluid protein-15 in salivary gland tumors. Arch Pathol Lab Med 1991; 115: 158–163.

186. Dardick I, Cavell S, Boivin M, et al. Salivary gland myoepithelioma variants. Histological, ultrastructural, and immunocytological features. Virchows Arch [A] 1989; 416: 25–42.

187. Dardick I, Thomas MJ, van Nostrand AW. Myoepithelioma – new concepts of histology and classification: a light and electron microscopic study. Ultrastruct Pathol 1989; 13: 187–224.

188. Sciubba JJ, Brannon RB. Myoepithelioma of salivary glands: report of 23 cases. Cancer 1982; 49: 562–572.

189. Lomax-Smith JD, Azzopardi JG. The hyaline cell: a distinctive feature of 'mixed' salivary tumors. Histopathology 1978; 2: 77–92.

190. Dodd LG, Caraway NP, Luna MA, et al. Myoepithelioma of the parotid. Report of a case initially examined by fine needle aspiration biopsy. Acta Cytol 1994; 38: 417–421.

191. Lopez JI, Ugalde A, Arostegui J, et al. Plasmacytoid myoepithelioma of the soft palate. Report of a case with cytologic, immunohistochemical and electron microscopic studies. Acta Cytol 2000; 44: 647–652.

192. Franquemont DW, Mills SE. Plasmacytoid monomorphic adenoma of salivary glands. Absence of myogenous differentiation and comparison to spindle cell myoepithelioma. Am J Surg Pathol 1993; 17: 146–153.

193. Erhardt CA, Vesoulis Z, Kashkari S. Fine needle aspiration cytology of cellular hemangioma of infancy. A case report. Acta Cytol 2000; 44: 1090–1094.

194. Lamelas J, Terry JH, Jr, Alfonso AE. Warthin's tumor: multicentricity and increasing incidence in women. Am J Surg 1987; 154: 347–351.

195. Fantasia JE, Miller AS. Papillary cystadenoma lymphomatosum arising in minor salivary glands. Oral Surg Oral Med Oral Pathol 1981; 52: 411–416.

196. Foulsham CK, Johnson GS, Snyder GG, et al. Immunohistopathology of papillary cystadenoma lymphomatosum (Warthin's tumor). Ann Clin Lab Sci 1984; 14: 47–63.

197. Kukreja HK, Jain HK. Adenolymphoma of submandibular salivary gland. J Laryngol Otol 1971; 85: 1201–1203.

198. Eveson JW, Cawson RA. Warthin's tumor (cystadenolymphoma) of salivary glands. A clinicopathologic investigation of 278 cases. Oral Surg Oral Med Oral Pathol 1986; 61: 256–262.

199. Li WY, Liu HC. Histopathological study of neoplasms of the salivary glands, a review of 657 cases. Chin Med J 1987; 39: 231–246.

200. Poulsen P, Jorgensen K, Grontved A. Benign and malignant neoplasms of the parotid gland: incidence and histology in the Danish County of Funen. Laryngoscope 1987; 97: 102–104.

201. Albrecht D, Arzt L. Beiträge zur Frage der Gewebsverirrung. Papilläre Cystadenome in Lymphdrüsen. Frankfurt Z Pathol 1910; 4: 47–69.

202. Snyderman C, Johnson JT, Barnes EL. Extraparotid Warthin's tumor. Otolaryngol Head Neck Surg 1986; 94: 169–175.

203. Dietert SE. Papillary cystadenoma lymphomatosum (Warthin's tumor) in patients in a general hospital over a 24-year period. Am J Clin Pathol 1975; 63: 866–875.

204. Noyek AM, Pritzker KP, Greyson ND, et al. Familial Warthin's tumor. 1. Its synchronous occurrence in mother and son. 2. Its association with cystic oncocytic metaplasia of the larynx. J Otolaryngol 1980; 9: 90–96.

205. Allegra SR. Warthin's tumor: a hypersensitivity disease? Ultrastructural, light, and immunofluorescent study. Hum Pathol 1971; 2: 403–420.

206. Hsu SM, Hsu PL, Nayak RN. Warthin's tumor: an immunohistochemical study of its lymphoid stroma. Hum Pathol 1981; 12: 251–257.

207. Hsu SM, Raine L. Warthin's tumor – epithelial cell differences. Am J Clin Pathol 1982; 77: 78–82.

208. Takezawa K, Jackson C, Gnepp DR, et al. Molecular characterization of Warthin tumor. Oral Surg Oral Med Oral Pathol Oral Radiol Endod 1998; 85: 569–575.

209. Gnepp DR, Schroeder W, Heffner D. Synchronous tumors arising in a single major salivary gland. Cancer 1989; 63: 1219–1224.

210. Ebbs SR, Webb AJ. Adenolymphoma of the parotid: aetiology, diagnosis and treatment. Br J Surg 1986; 73: 627–630.

211. Seifert G, Bull HG, Donath K. Histologic subclassification of the cystadenolymphoma of the parotid gland. Analysis of 275 cases. Virchows Arch [A] 1980; 388: 13–38.

212. Lefor AT, Ord RA. Multiple synchronous bilateral Warthin's tumors of the parotid glands with pleomorphic adenoma. Case report and review of the literature. Oral Surg Oral Med Oral Pathol 1993; 76: 319–324.

213. Foote FW Jr, Frazell EL. Tumors of the major salivary glands. Cancer 1953; 6: 1065–1133.

214. Chaudhry AP, Gorlin R. Papillary cystadenoma lymphomatosum (adenolymphoma): a review of the literature. Am J Surg 1958; 95: 923–931.

215. Kennedy TL. Warthin's tumor: a review indicating no male predominance. Laryngoscope 1983; 93: 889–891.

216. Monk JS Jr, Church JS. Warthin's tumor. A high incidence and no sex predominance in central Pennsylvania. Arch Otolaryngol Head Neck Surg 1992; 118: 477–478.

217. Yoo GH, Eisele DW, Askin FB, et al. Warthin's tumor: a 40-year experience at The Johns Hopkins Hospital. Laryngoscope 1994; 104: 799–803.

218. Pinkston JA, Cole P. Cigarette smoking and Warthin's tumor. Am J Epidemiol 1996; 144: 183–187.

219. Kotwall CA. Smoking as an etiologic factor in the development of Warthin's tumor of the parotid gland. Am J Surg 1992; 164: 646–647.

220. White RR, Arm RN, Randall P. A large Warthin's tumor of the parotid. Case report. Plast Reconstr Surg 1978; 61: 452–454.

221. Chapnik JS. The controversy of Warthin's tumor. Laryngoscope 1983; 93: 695–716.

222. Ishikawa H, Ishii Y. Evaluation of salivary gland tumors with 99mTc-pertechnetate. J Oral Maxillofac Surg 1984; 42(7): 429–434.

223. Higashi T, Murahashi H, Ikuta H, et al. Identification of Warthin's tumor with technetium-99m pertechnetate. Clin Nucl Med 1987; 12: 796–800.

224. Sostre S, Medina L, de Arellano GR. The various scintigraphic patterns of Warthin's tumor. Clin Nucl Med 1987; 12: 620–626.

225. Weinstein GS, Harvey RT, Zimmer W, et al. Technetium-99m pertechnetate salivary gland imaging: its role in the diagnosis of Warthin's tumor (clinical conference). J Nucl Med 1994; 35: 179–183.

226. Warnock GR. Papillary cystadenoma lymphomatosum (Warthin's tumor). In: Ellis GL, Auclair PL, Gnepp DR, eds. Surgical pathology of the salivary glands. 1st edn. Philadelphia: WB Saunders; 1991: 187–201.

227. Di Palma S, Simpson RH, Skalova A, et al. Metaplastic (infarcted) Warthin's tumour of the parotid gland: a possible consequence of fine needle aspiration biopsy. Histopathology 1999; 35: 432–438.

228. Damjanov I, Sneff EM, Delerme AN. Squamous cell carcinoma arising in Warthin's tumor of the parotid gland. A light, electron microscopic, and immunohistochemical study. Oral Surg Oral Med Oral Pathol 1983; 55: 286–290.

229. Morrison GA, Shaw HJ. Squamous carcinoma arising within a Warthin's tumour of the parotid gland. J Laryngol Otol 1988; 102: 1189–1191.

230. McClatchey KD, Appelblat NH, Langin JL. Carcinoma in papillary cytadenoma lymphomatosum (Warthin's tumor). Laryngoscope 1982; 92: 98–99.

231. Gunduz M, Yamanaka N, Hotomi M, et al. Squamous cell carcinoma arising in a Warthin's tumor. Auris Nasus Larynx 1999; 26: 355–360.

232. Nagao T, Sugano I, Ishida Y, et al. Mucoepidermoid carcinoma arising in Warthin's tumour of the parotid gland: report of two cases with histopathological, ultrastructural and immunohistochemical studies. Histopathology 1998; 33: 379–386.

233. Seifert G. Bilateral mucoepidermoid carcinomas arising in bilateral pre-existing Warthin's tumours of the parotid gland. Oral Oncol 1997; 33: 284–287.

234. Bengoechea O, Sánchez F, Larrínaga B, et al. Oncocytic adenocarcinoma arising in Warthin's tumor. Pathol Res Pract 1989; 185: 907–911.

235. Therkildsen MH, Christensen N, Andersen LJ, et al. Malignant Warthin's tumour: a case study. Histopathology 1992; 21: 167–171.

236. Moosavi H, Ryan C, Schwartz S, et al. Malignant adenolymphoma. Hum Pathol 1980; 11: 80–83.

237. Medeiros LJ, Rizzi R, Lardelli P, et al. Malignant lymphoma involving a Warthin's tumor: a case with immunophenotypic and gene rearrangement analysis. Hum Pathol 1990; 21: 974–977.

238. Miller R, Yanagihara ET, Dubrow AA, et al. Malignant lymphoma in the Warthin's tumor. Report of a case. Cancer 1982; 50: 2948–2950.

239. Hall G, Tesluk H, Baron S. Lymphoma arising in an adenolymphoma. Hum Pathol 1985; 16: 424–427.

240. Giardini R, Mastore M. Follicular non Hodgkin's lymphoma in adenolymphoma: report of a case. Tumori 1990; 76: 212–215.

241. Heller KS, Attie JN. Treatment of Warthin's tumor by enucleation. Am J Surg 1988; 156: 294–296.

242. Gant TD, Hovey LM, Williams C. Surgical management of parotid gland tumors. Ann Plast Surg 1981; 6: 389–392.

243. Klijanienko J, Vielh P. Fine-needle sampling of salivary gland lesions. II. Cytology and histology correlation of 71 cases of Warthin's tumor (adenolymphoma). Diagn Cytopathol 1997; 16: 221–225.

244. MacLeod CB, Frable WJ. Fine-needle aspiration biopsy of the salivary gland: Problem cases. Diagn Cytopathol 1993; 9: 216–225.

245. Gray SR, Cornog JL Jr, Seo IS. Oncocytic neoplasms of salivary glands: a report of fifteen cases including two malignant oncocytomas. Cancer 1976; 38: 1306–1317.

246. Taxy JB. Necrotizing squamous/mucinous metaplasia in oncocytic salivary gland tumors. A potential diagnostic problem. Am J Clin Pathol 1992; 97: 40–45.

247. Cohen MB, Fisher PE, Holly EA, et al. Fine needle aspiration biopsy diagnosis of mucoepidermoid carcinoma. Statistical analysis. Acta Cytol 1990; 34: 43–49.

248. Sauer T, Jebsen PW, Olsholt R. Cytologic features of papillary-cystic variant of acinic-cell adenocarcinoma: a case report. Diagn Cytopathol 1994; 10: 30–32.

249. Yu GY, Ussmueller J, Donath K. Histogenesis and development of membranous basal cell adenoma. Oral Surg Oral Med Oral Pathol Oral Radiol Endod 1998; 86: 446–451.

250. Ellis GL, Auclair PL. Tumors of the salivary glands. Atlas of tumor pathology, 3rd series, fascicle 17. 1st edn. Washington, DC: Armed Forces Institute of Pathology; 1996: 80–94.

251. Lopes MA, Kowalski LP, da Cunha SG, et al. A clinicopathologic study of 196 intraoral minor salivary gland tumours. J Oral Pathol Med 1999; 28: 264–267.

252. Ethunandan M, Pratt CA, Macpherson DW. Changing frequency of parotid gland neoplasms – analysis of 560 tumours treated in a district general hospital. Ann R Coll Surg Engl 2002; 84: 1–6.

253. Batsakis JG, Luna MA, el-Naggar AK. Basaloid monomorphic adenomas. Ann Otol Rhinol Laryngol 1991; 100: 687–690.

254. Bentz BG, Hughes CA, Ludemann JP, et al. Masses of the salivary gland region in children. Arch Otolaryngol Head Neck Surg 2000; 126: 1435–1439.

255. Orvidas LJ, Kasperbauer JL, Lewis JE, et al. Pediatric parotid masses. Arch Otolaryngol Head Neck Surg 2000; 126: 177–184.

256. Batsakis JG, Brannon RB. Dermal analogue tumours of major salivary glands. J Laryngol Otol 1981; 95: 155–164.

257. Luna MA, Tortoledo ME, Allen M. Salivary dermal analogue tumors arising in lymph nodes. Cancer 1987; 59: 1165–1169.

258. Schmidt KT, Ma A, Goldberg R, et al. Multiple adnexal tumors and a parotid basal cell adenoma. J Am Acad Dermatol 1991; 25: 960–964.

259. Jungehulsing M, Wagner M, Damm M. Turban tumour with involvement of the parotid gland. J Laryngol Otol 1999; 113: 779–783.

260. Choi HR, Batsakis JG, Callender DL, et al. Molecular analysis of chromosome 16q regions in dermal analogue tumors of salivary glands: a genetic link to dermal cylindroma? Am J Surg Pathol 2002; 26: 778–783.

261. Abiko Y, Shimono M, Hashimoto S, et al. Ultrastructure of basal cell adenoma in the parotid gland. Bull Tokyo Dent Coll 1989; 30: 145–153.

262. Takahashi H, Fujita S, Okabe H, et al. Immunohistochemical characterization of basal cell adenomas of the salivary gland. Pathol Res Pract 1991; 187: 145–156.

263. Williams SB, Ellis GL, Auclair PL. Immunohistochemical analysis of basal cell adenocarcinoma. Oral Surg Oral Med Oral Pathol 1993; 75: 64–69.

264. Nishimura T, Furukawa M, Kawahara E, et al. Differential diagnosis of pleomorphic adenoma by immunohistochemical means. J Laryngol Otol 1991; 105: 1057–1060.

265. Hamano H, Abiko Y, Hashimoto S, et al. Immunohistochemical study of basal cell adenoma in the parotid gland. Bull Tokyo Dent Coll 1990; 31: 23–31.

266. Ferreiro JA. Immunohistochemistry of basal cell adenoma of the major salivary glands. Histopathology 1994; 24: 539–542.

267. Zarbo RJ, Prasad AR, Regezi JA, et al. Salivary gland basal cell and canalicular adenomas: immunohistochemical demonstration of myoepithelial cell participation and morphogenetic considerations. Arch Pathol Lab Med 2000; 124: 401–405.

268. el-Naggar AK, Hurr K, Kagan J, et al. Genotypic alterations in benign and malignant salivary gland tumors: histogenetic and clinical implications. Am J Surg Pathol 1997; 21: 691–697.

269. Karja VJ, Syrjanen KJ, Kurvinen AK, et al. Expression and mutations of p53 in salivary gland tumours. J Oral Pathol Med 1997; 26: 217–223.

270. Luna MA, Batsakis JG, Tortoledo ME, et al. Carcinomas ex monomorphic adenoma of salivary glands. J Laryngol Otol 1989; 103: 756–759.

271. Stanley MW, Horwitz CA, Rollins SD, et al. Basal cell (monomorphic) and minimally pleomorphic adenomas of the salivary glands. Distinction from the solid (anaplastic) type of adenoid cystic carcinoma in fine-needle aspiration. Am J Clin Pathol 1996; 106: 35–41.

272. Lopez JI, Ballestin C. Fine-needle aspiration cytology of a membranous basal cell adenoma arising in an intraparotid lymph node. Diagn Cytopathol 1993; 9: 668–672.

273. Sahu K, Pai RR, Pai KP. Basal cell adenoma, solid variant, diagnosed by fine needle aspiration cytology. Acta Cytol 1999; 43: 1198–1200.

274. Galed-Placed I, Yebra-Pimentel MT. Synchronous, double parotid tumor: fine needle aspiration cytology diagnosis of the membranous basal cell adenoma component. Acta Cytol 2000; 44: 1120–1122.

275. Pisharodi LR. Basal cell adenocarcinoma of the salivary gland. Diagnosis by fine-needle aspiration cytology. Am J Clin Pathol 1995; 103: 603–608.

276. Moroz K, Ferreira C, Dhurandhar N. Fine needle aspiration of basal cell adenocarcinoma of the parotid gland. Report of a case with assessment of DNA ploidy in aspirates and tissue sections by image analysis. Acta Cytol 1996; 40: 773–778.

277. Tse GM, To EW, Yuen EH, et al. Basal cell adenocarcinoma of the salivary gland: report of a case with morphology on fine needle aspiration cytology. Acta Cytol 2001; 45: 775–778.

278. Pogrel MA. The intraoral basal cell adenoma. J Craniomaxillofac Surg 1987; 15: 372–375.

279. Gardner DG, Daley TD. The use of the terms monomorphic adenoma, basal cell adenoma, and canalicular adenoma as applied to salivary gland tumors. Oral Surg Oral Med Oral Pathol 1983; 56: 608–615.

280. Daley TD, Gardner DG, Smout MS. Canalicular adenoma: not a basal cell adenoma. Oral Surg Oral Med Oral Pathol 1984; 57: 181–188.

281. Ellis GL, Auclair PL. Tumors of the salivary glands. Atlas of tumor pathology, 3rd series, fascicle 17. 1st edn. Washington, DC: Armed Forces Institute of Pathology; 1996: 95–103.

282. Daley TD. The canalicular adenoma: considerations on differential diagnosis and treatment. J Oral Maxillofac Surg 1984; 42: 728–730.

283. Zarbo RJ, Regezi JA, Batsakis JG. S-100 protein in salivary gland tumors: an immunohistochemical study of 129 cases. Head Neck Surg 1986; 8: 268–275.

284. Ferreiro JA. Immunohistochemical analysis of salivary gland canalicular adenoma. Oral Surg Oral Med Oral Pathol 1994; 78: 761–765.

285. Huang JW, Ming Z, Shrestha P, et al. Immunohistochemical evaluation of the Ca(2+)-binding S-100 proteins S-100A1, S-100A2, S-100A4, S-100A6 and S-100B in salivary gland tumors. J Oral Pathol Med 1996; 25: 547–555.

286. Guccion JG, Redman RS. Canalicular adenoma of the buccal mucosa. An ultrastructural and histochemical study. Oral Surg Oral Med Oral Pathol 1986; 61: 173–178.

287. Harmse JL, Saleh HA, Odutoye T, et al. Recurrent canalicular adenoma of the minor salivary glands in the upper lip. J Laryngol Otol 1997; 111: 985–987.

288. Chang A, Harawi SJ. Oncocytes, oncocytosis, and oncocytic tumors. Pathol Annu 1992; 27(Pt. 1): 263–304.

289. Loreti A, Sturla M, Gentileschi S, et al. Diffuse hyperplastic oncocytosis of the parotid gland. Br J Plast Surg 2002; 55: 151–152.

290. Hartwick RW, Batsakis JG. Non-Warthin's tumor oncocytic lesions. Ann Otol Rhinol Laryngol 1990; 99: 674–677.

291. Palmer TJ, Gleeson MJ, Eveson JW, et al. Oncocytic adenomas and oncocytic hyperplasia of salivary glands: a clinicopathological study of 26 cases. Histopathology 1990; 16: 487–493.

292. Brandwein MS, Huvos AG. Oncocytic tumors of major salivary glands. A study of 68 cases with follow-up of 44 patients. Am J Surg Pathol 1991; 15: 514–528.

293. Seifert G, Miehlke A, Haubrich J, Chilla R. Diseases of the salivary glands: pathology-diagnosis-treatment-facial nerve surgery. 1st edn. New York: Georg Thieme Verlag; 1986: 171.

294. Ellis GL, Auclair PL. Tumors of the salivary glands. Atlas of tumor pathology, 3rd series, fascicle 17. 1st edn. Washington, DC: Armed Forces Institute of Pathology; 1996: 103–114.

295. Nagler RM, Laufer D. Tumors of the major and minor salivary glands: review of 25 years of experience. Anticancer Res 1997; 17: 701–707.

296. Thompson LD, Wenig BM, Ellis GL. Oncocytomas of the submandibular gland. A series of 22 cases and a review of the literature. Cancer 1996; 78: 2281–2287.

297. Kanazawa H, Furuya T, Murano A, et al. Oncocytoma of an intraoral minor salivary gland: report of a case and review of literature. J Oral Maxillofac Surg 2000; 58: 894–897.

298. Ellis GL. 'Clear cell' oncocytoma of salivary gland. Hum Pathol 1988; 19: 862–867.

299. Ellis GL. Clear cell neoplasms in salivary glands: clearly a diagnostic challenge. Ann Diagn Pathol 1998; 2: 61–78.

300. Shintaku M, Honda T. Identification of oncocytic lesions of salivary glands by anti-mitochondrial immunohistochemistry. Histopathology 1997; 31: 408–411.

301. Carlsöö B, Domeij S, Helander HF. A quantitative ultrastructural study of a parotid oncocytoma. Arch Pathol Lab Med 1979; 103: 471–474.

302. Hamed G, Shmookler BM, Ellis GL, et al. Oncocytic mucoepidermoid carcinoma of the parotid gland. Arch Pathol Lab Med 1994; 118: 313–314.

303. Avery AK, Beckstead J, Renshaw AA, et al. Use of antibodies to RCC and CD10 in the differential diagnosis of renal neoplasms. Am J Surg Pathol 2000; 24: 203–210.

304. Damm DD, White DK, Geissler RH, Jr., et al. Benign solid oncocytoma of intraoral minor salivary glands. Oral Surg Oral Med Oral Pathol 1989; 67: 84–86.

305. Kosuda S, Ishikawa M, Tamura K, et al. Iodine-131 therapy for parotid oncocytoma. J Nucl Med 1988; 29: 1126–1129.

306. Chaudhry AP, Labay GR, Yamane GM, et al. Clinico-pathologic and histogenetic study of 189 intraoral minor salivary gland tumors. J Oral Med 1984; 39: 58–78.

307. Wilson DF, MacEntree MI. Papillary cystadenoma of minor salivary gland origin. Oral Surg Oral Med Oral Pathol 1974; 915: 918.

308. Evans RW, Cruickshank AH. Epithelial tumours of the salivary glands. 1st edn. Philadelphia: WB Saunders; 1970: 19–23.

309. Auclair PL, Ellis GL, Gnepp DR. Other benign epithelial neoplasms. In: Ellis GL, Auclair PL, Gnepp DR, eds. Surgical pathology of the salivary glands. 1st edn. Philadelphia: WB Saunders; 1991: 252–268.

310. Skalova A, Leivo I, Wolf H, et al. Oncocytic cystadenoma of the parotid gland with tyrosine-rich crystals. Pathol Res Pract 2000; 196: 849–851.

311. Pahl S, Puschel W, Federspil P. Cystadenoma of the parotid gland with unusual prominent lymphoid stroma. J Laryngol Otol 1997; 111: 883–885.

312. Kerpel SM, Freedman PD, Lumerman H. The papillary cystadenoma of minor salivary gland origin. Oral Surg Oral Med Oral Pathol 1978; 46: 820–826.

313. Sher L. The papillary cystadenoma of salivary gland origin. Diastema 1982; 10: 37–41.

314. Goldman RL. Melanogenic papillary cystadenoma of the soft palate. Am J Clin Pathol 1967; 48: 49–52.

315. Linhartová A. Sebaceous glands in salivary gland tissue. Arch Pathol 1974; 98: 320–324.

316. Mesa-Chavez L. Sebaceous glands in normal and neoplastic parotid glands in respect to the origin of tumors of the salivary glands. Am J Pathol 1949; 25: 627–645.

317. Ellis GL, Auclair PL. Tumors of the salivary glands. Atlas of tumor pathology, 3rd series, fascicle 17. 1st edn. Washington, DC: Armed Forces Institute of Pathology; 1996: 130–136.

318. Gnepp DR. Sebaceous neoplasms of salivary gland origin: a review. Pathol Annu 1983; 18(Pt. 1): 71–102.

319. Hsueh C, Gonzalez-Crussi F. Sialoblastoma: a case report and review of the literature on congenital epithelial tumors of salivary gland origin. Pediatr Pathol 1992; 12: 205–214.

320. Taylor GP. Congenital epithelial tumor of the parotid – sialoblastoma. Pediatr Pathol 1988; 8: 447–452.

321. Harris MD, McKeever P, Robertson JM. Congenital tumours of the salivary gland: a case report and review. Histopathology 1990; 17: 155–157.

322. Batsakis JG, Frankenthaler R. Embryoma (sialoblastoma) of salivary glands. Ann Otol Rhinol Laryngol 1992; 101: 958–960.

323. Siddiqi SH, Solomon MP, Haller JO. Sialoblastoma and hepatoblastoma in a neonate. Pediatr Radiol 2000; 30: 349–351.

324. Green RS, Tunkel DE, Small D, et al. Sialoblastoma: association with cutaneous hamartoma (organoid nevus)? Pediatr Dev Pathol 2000; 3: 504–505.

325. Garrido A, Humphrey G, Squire RS, et al. Sialoblastoma. Br J Plast Surg 2000; 53: 697–699.

326. Brandwein M, Al-Naeif NS, Manwani D, et al. Sialoblastoma: clinicopathological/ immunohistochemical study. Am J Surg Pathol 1999; 23: 342–348.

327. Luna MA. Sialoblastoma and epithelial tumors in children: their morphologic spectrum and distribution by age. Adv Anat Pathol 1999; 6: 287–292.

328. Mostafapour SP, Folz B, Barlow D, et al. Sialoblastoma of the submandibular gland: report of a case and review of the literature. Int J Pediatr Otorhinolaryngol 2000; 53: 157–161.

329. Ortiz-Hidalgo C, de Leon-Bojorge B, Fernandez-Sobrino G, et al. Sialoblastoma: report of a congenital case with dysembryogenic alterations of the adjacent parotid gland. Histopathology 2001; 38: 79–80.

330. Simpson PR, Rutledge JC, Schaefer SD, et al. Congenital hybrid basal cell adenoma – adenoid cystic carcinoma of the salivary gland. Pediatr Pathol 1986; 6: 199–202.

331. Canalis RF, Mok MW, Fishman SM, et al. Congenital basal cell adenoma of the submandibular gland. Arch Otolaryngol Head Neck Surg 1980; 106: 284–286.

332. Alvarez-Mendoza A, Calderon-Elvir C, Carrasco-Daza D. Diagnostic and therapeutic approach to sialoblastoma: report of a case. J Pediatr Surg 1999; 34: 1875–1877.

333. Ellis GL, Auclair PL. Tumors of the salivary glands. Atlas of tumor pathology, 3rd series, fascicle 17. 1st edn. Washington, DC: Armed Forces Institute of Pathology; 1996: 155–175.

334. Spitz MR, Batsakis JG. Major salivary gland carcinoma. Descriptive epidemiology and survival of 498 patients. Arch Otolaryngol Head Neck Surg 1984; 110: 45–49.

335. Neville BW, Damm DD, Weir JC, et al. Labial salivary gland tumors. Cancer 1988; 61: 2113–2116.

336. Nascimento AG, Amaral LP, Prado LA, et al. Mucoepidermoid carcinoma of salivary glands: a clinicopathologic study of 46 cases. Head Neck Surg 1986; 8: 409–417.

337. Accetta PA, Gray GF Jr, Hunter RM, et al. Mucoepidermoid carcinoma of salivary glands. Arch Pathol Lab Med 1984; 108: 321–325.

338. Evans HL. Mucoepidermoid carcinoma of salivary glands: a study of 69 cases with special attention to histologic grading. Am J Clin Pathol 1984; 81: 696–701.

339. Olsen KD, Devine KD, Weiland LH. Mucoepidermoid carcinoma of the oral cavity. Otolaryngol Head Neck Surg 1981; 89: 783–791.

340. Melrose RJ, Abrams AM, Howell FV. Mucoepidermoid tumors of the intraoral minor salivary glands: a clinicopathologic study of 54 cases. J Oral Pathol 1973; 2: 314–325.

341. Jahan-Parwar B, Huberman RM, Donovan DT, et al. Oncocytic mucoepidermoid carcinoma of the salivary glands. Am J Surg Pathol 1999; 23: 523–529.

342. Paulino AF, Huvos AG. Oncocytic and oncocytoid tumors of the salivary glands. Semin Diagn Pathol 1999; 16: 98–104.

343. Ferreiro JA, Stylopoulos N. Oncocytic differentiation in salivary gland tumours. J Laryngol Otol 1995; 109: 569–571.

344. Dardick I, Birek C, Lingen MW, et al. Differentiation and the cytomorphology of salivary gland tumors with specific reference to oncocytic metaplasia. Oral Surg Oral Med Oral Pathol Oral Radiol Endod 1999; 88: 691–701.

345. Muller S, Barnes L, Goodurn WJ Jr. Sclerosing mucoepidermoid carcinoma of the parotid. Oral Surg Oral Med Oral Pathol Oral Radiol Endod 1997; 83: 685–690.

346. Loyola AM, de Sousa SO, Araujo NS, et al. Study of minor salivary gland mucoepidermoid carcinoma differentiation based on immunohistochemical expression of cytokeratins, vimentin and muscle-specific actin. Oral Oncol 1998; 34: 112–118.

347. Brandwein MS, Ivanov K, Wallace DI, et al. Mucoepidermoid carcinoma: a clinicopathologic study of 80 patients with special reference to histological grading. Am J Surg Pathol 2001; 25: 835–845.

348. Hanna DC, Clairmont AA. Submandibular gland tumors. Plast Reconstr Surg 1978; 61: 198–203.

349. Zhu Q, Tipoe GL, White FH. Proliferative activity as detected by immunostaining with Ki-67 and proliferating cell nuclear antigen in benign and malignant epithelial lesions of the human parotid gland. Anal Quant Cytol Histol 1999; 21: 336–342.

350. Suzuki M, Ichimiya I, Matsushita F, et al. Histological features and prognosis of patients with mucoepidermoid carcinoma of the parotid gland. J Laryngol Otol 1998; 112: 944–947.

351. Gemryd P, Lundquist PG, Tytor M, et al. Prognostic significance of DNA ploidy in mucoepidermoid carcinoma. Eur Arch Otorhinolaryngol 1997; 254: 180–185.

352. Cerilli LA, Swartzbaugh JR, Saadut R, et al. Analysis of chromosome 9p21 deletion and p16 gene mutation in salivary gland carcinomas. Hum Pathol 1999; 30: 1242–1246.

353. el-Naggar AK, Lovell M, Killary AM, et al. Genotypic characterization of a primary mucoepidermoid carcinoma of the parotid gland by cytogenetic, fluorescence in situ hybridization, and DNA ploidy analysis. Cancer Genet Cytogenet 1996; 89: 38–43.

354. el-Naggar AK, Lovell M, Killary AM, et al. A mucoepidermoid carcinoma of minor salivary gland with t(11; 19)(q21;p13.1) as the only karyotypic abnormality. Cancer Genet Cytogenet 1996; 87: 29–33.

355. Dahlenfors R, Wedell B, Rundrantz H, et al. Translocation(11;19)(q14-21;p12) in a parotid mucoepidermoid carcinoma of a child. Cancer Genet Cytogenet 1995; 79: 188.

356. Nordkvist A, Gustafsson H, Juberg-Ode M, et al. Recurrent rearrangements of 11q14-22 in mucoepidermoid carcinoma. Cancer Genet Cytogenet 1994; 74: 77–83.

357. Healey WV, Perzin KH, Smith L. Mucoepidermoid carcinoma of salivary gland origin. Classification, clinical-pathologic correlation, and results of treatment. Cancer 1970; 26: 368–388.

358. Eneroth CM, Hjertman L, Moberger G, et al. Muco-epidermoid carcinomas of the salivary glands with special reference to the possible existence of a benign variety. Acta Otolaryngol (Stockh) 1972; 73: 68–74.

359. Jensen OJ, Poulsen T, Schiødt T. Mucoepidermoid tumors of salivary glands. A long term follow-up study. APMIS 1988; 96: 421–427.

360. Garden AS, el-Naggar AK, Morrison WH, et al. Postoperative radiotherapy for malignant tumors of the parotid gland. Int J Radiat Oncol Biol Phys 1997; 37: 79–85.

361. Caselitz J, Schmitt P, Seifert G, et al. Basal membrane associated substances in human salivary glands and salivary gland tumours. Pathol Res Pract 1988; 183: 386–394.

362. Sadeghi A, Tran LM, Mark R, et al. Minor salivary gland tumors of the head and neck: treatment strategies and prognosis. Am J Clin Oncol 1993; 16: 3–8.

363. Eversole LR, Rovin S, Sabes WR. Mucoepidermoid carcinoma of minor salivary glands: report of 17 cases with follow-up. J Oral Surg 1972; 30: 107–112.

364. Frable WJ, Elzay RP. Tumors of minor salivary glands. A report of 73 cases. Cancer 1970; 25: 932–941.

365. Spiro RH. The management of salivary neoplasms: an overview. Auris Nasus Larynx 1985; 12 Suppl 2: S122–S127.

366. Kumar N, Kapila K, Verma K. Fine needle aspiration cytology of mucoepidermoid carcinoma. A diagnostic problem. Acta Cytol 1991; 35: 357–359.

367. Klijanienko J, Vielh P. Fine-needle sampling of salivary gland lesions. IV. Review of 50 cases of mucoepidermoid carcinoma with histologic correlation. Diagn Cytopathol 1997; 17: 92–98.

368. Yu GY, Ma DQ. Carcinoma of the salivary gland: a clinicopathologic study of 405 cases. Semin Surg Oncol 1987; 3: 240–244.

369. Ellis GL, Auclair PL. Tumors of the salivary glands. Atlas of tumor pathology, 3rd series, fascicle 17. 1st edn. Washington, DC: Armed Forces Institute of Pathology; 1996: 183–203.

370. van der Wal JE, Leverstein H, Snow GB, et al. Parotid gland tumors: histologic reevaluation and reclassification of 478 cases. Head Neck 1998; 20: 204–207.

371. Zbaeren P, Lehmann W, Widgren S. Acinic cell carcinoma of minor salivary gland origin. J Laryngol Otol 1991; 105: 782–785.

372. Castellanos JL, Lally ET. Acinic cell tumor of the minor salivary glands. J Oral Maxillofac Surg 1982; 40: 428–431.

373. Abrams AM, Melrose RJ. Acinic cell tumors of minor salivary gland origin. Oral Surg Oral Med Oral Pathol 1978; 46: 220–233.

374. Di Palma S, Corletto V, Lavarino C, et al. Unilateral aneuploid dedifferentiated acinic cell carcinoma associated with bilateral low-grade diploid acinic cell carcinoma of the parotid gland. Virchows Arch 1999; 434: 361–365.

375. Ellis GL, Auclair PL. Acinic cell adenocarcinoma. In: Ellis GL, Auclair PL, Gnepp DR, eds. Surgical pathology of the salivary glands. 1st edn. Philadelphia: WB Saunders; 1991: 299–317.

376. Ellis GL, Corio RL. Acinic cell adenocarcinoma. A clinicopathologic analysis of 294 cases. Cancer 1983; 52: 542–549.

377. Colmenero C, Patron M, Sierra I. Acinic cell carcinoma of the salivary glands. A review of 20 new cases. J Craniomaxillofac Surg 1991; 19: 260–266.

378. Spiro RH, Huvos AG, Strong EW. Acinic cell carcinoma of salivary origin. A clinicopathologic study of 67 cases. Cancer 1978; 41: 924–935.

379. Laskawi R, Rodel R, Zirk A, et al. Retrospective analysis of 35 patients with acinic cell carcinoma of the parotid gland. J Oral Maxillofac Surg 1998; 56 440–443.

380. Dardick I, George D, Jeans MT, et al. Ultrastructural morphology and cellular differentiation in acinic cell carcinoma. Oral Surg Oral Med Oral Pathol 1987; 63: 325–334.

381. Batsakis JG, Luna MA, el-Naggar AK. Histopathologic grading of salivary gland neoplasms: II. Acinic cell carcinomas. Ann Otol Rhinol Laryngol 1990; 99: 929–933.

382. Lewis JE, Olsen KD, Weiland LH. Acinic cell carcinoma. Clinicopathologic review. Cancer 1991; 67: 172–179.

383. Perzin KH, LiVolsi VA. Acinic cell carcinomas arising in salivary glands: a clinicopathologic study. Cancer 1979; 44: 1434–1457.

384. Chaudhry AP, Cutler LS, Leifer C, et al. Histogenesis of acinic cell carcinoma of the major and minor salivary glands. An ultrastructural study. J Pathol 1986; 148: 307–320.

385. el-Naggar AK, Batsakis JG, Luna MA, et al. DNA flow cytometry of acinic cell carcinomas of major salivary glands. J Laryngol Otol 1990; 104: 410–416.

386. Henley JD, Geary WA, Jackson CL, et al. Dedifferentiated acinic cell carcinoma of the parotid gland: a distinct rarely described entity. Hum Pathol 1997; 28: 869–873.

387. Takahashi H, Fujita S, Okabe H, et al. Distribution of tissue markers in acinic cell carcinomas of salivary gland. Pathol Res Pract 1992; 188: 692–700.

388. Hamper K, Schmitz-Watjen W, Mausch HE, et al. Multiple expression of tissue markers in mucoepidermoid carcinomas and acinic cell carcinomas of the salivary glands. Virchows Arch [A] 1989; 414: 407–413.

389. Seifert G, Caselitz J. Tumor markers in parotid gland carcinomas: immunohistochemical investigations. Cancer Detect Prev 1983; 6: 119–130.

390. Caselitz J, Seifert G, Grenner G, et al. Amylase as an additional marker of salivary gland neoplasms. An immunoperoxidase study. Pathol Res Pract 1983; 176: 276–283.

391. Egan M, Crocker J, Nar P. Localization of salivary amylase and epithelial membrane antigen in salivary gland tumours by means of immunoperoxidase and immunogold-silver techniques. J Laryngol Otol 1988; 102: 242–247.

392. Childers EL, Ellis GL, Auclair PL. An immunohistochemical analysis of anti-amylase antibody reactivity in acinic cell adenocarcinoma. Oral Surg Oral Med Oral Pathol Oral Radiol Endod 1996; 81: 691–694.

393. Heikinheimo AK, Laine MA, Ritvos OV, et al. Bone morphogenetic protein-6 is a marker of serous acinar cell differentiation in normal and neoplastic human salivary gland. Cancer Res 1999; 59: 5815–5821.

394. Fujita S, Takahashi H, Okabe H. Nucleolar organizer regions in malignant salivary gland tumors. Acta Pathol Jpn 1992; 42: 727–733.

395. Murakami M, Ohtani I, Hojo H, et al. Immunohistochemical evaluation with Ki-67: an application to salivary gland tumours. J Laryngol Otol 1992; 106: 35–38.

396. Yang L, Hashimura K, Qin C, et al. Immunoreactivity of proliferating cell nuclear antigen in salivary gland tumours: an assessment of growth potential. Virchows Arch A Pathol Anat Histopathol 1993; 422: 481–486.

397. Gandour-Edwards R, Kapadia SB, Gumerlock PH, et al. Immunolocalization of interleukin-6 in salivary gland tumors. Hum Pathol 1995; 26: 501–503.

398. Lee CH, Lee SK, Chi JG, et al. Immunohistochemical evaluation of transglutaminase C in tumours of salivary glands. Eur J Cancer B Oral Oncol 1996; 32B: 401–406.

399. Mark HF, Hanna I, Gnepp DR. Cytogenetic analysis of salivary gland type tumors. Oral Surg Oral Med Oral Pathol Oral Radiol Endod 1996; 82: 187–192.

400. Martins C, Fonseca I, Roque L, et al. Malignant salivary gland neoplasms: a cytogenetic study of 19 cases. Eur J Cancer B Oral Oncol 1996; 32B: 128–132.

401. Zhao M, Zhao QX, Saitoh M, et al. Proliferating patterns of salivary gland adenocarcinomas with the use of PCNA labeling. Anticancer Res 1996; 16: 2693–2698.

402. Doi R, Kuratate I, Okamoto E, et al. Expression of p53 oncoprotein increases intratumoral microvessel formation in human salivary gland carcinomas. J Oral Pathol Med 1999; 28: 259–263.

403. el-Naggar AK, Abdul-Karim FW, Hurr K, et al. Genetic alterations in acinic cell carcinoma of the parotid gland determined by microsatellite analysis. Cancer Genet Cytogenet 1998; 102: 19–24.

404. Nordkvist A, Roijer E, Bang G, et al. Expression and mutation patterns of p53 in benign and malignant salivary gland tumors. Int J Oncol 2000; 16 477–483.

405. Jordan R, Dardick I, Lui E, et al. Demonstration of c-erbB-2 oncogene overexpression in salivary gland neoplasms by in situ hybridization. J Oral Pathol Med 1994; 23: 226–231.

406. Kamio N. Coexpression of p53 and c-erbB-2 proteins is associated with histological type, tumour stage, and cell proliferation in malignant salivary gland tumours. Virchows Arch 1996; 428: 5–83.

407. Bang G, Donath K, Thoresen S, et al. DNA flow cytometry of reclassified subtypes of malignant salivary gland tumors. J Oral Pathol Med 1994; 23: 291–297.

408. Timon CI, Dardick I, Panzarella T, et al. Acinic cell carcinoma of salivary glands. Prognostic relevance of DNA flow cytometry and nucleolar organizer regions. Arch Otolaryngol Head Neck Surg 1994; 120: 727–733.

409. Skalova A, Leivo I, von Boguslawsky K, et al. Cell proliferation correlates with prognosis in acinic cell carcinomas of salivary gland origin. Immunohistochemical study of 30 cases using the MIB 1 antibody in formalin-fixed paraffin sections. J Pathol 1994; 173: 13–21.

410. Hellquist HB, Sundelin K, Di Bacco A, et al. Tumour growth fraction and apoptosis in salivary gland acinic cell carcinomas. Prognostic implications of Ki-67 and bcl-2 expression and of in situ end labelling (TUNEL). J Pathol 1997; 181: 323–329.

411. Guimaraes DS, Amaral AP, Prado LF, et al. Acinic cell carcinoma of salivary glands: 16 cases with clinicopathologic correlation. J Oral Pathol Med 1989; 18: 396–399.

412. Chomette G, Auriol M, Vaillant JM. Acinic cell tumors of salivary glands. Frequency and morphological study. J Biol Buccale 1984; 12: 157–169.

413. Gustafsson H, Lindholm C, Carlsöö B. DNA cytophotometry of acinic cell carcinoma and its relation to prognosis. Acta Otolaryngol (Stockh) 1987; 104: 370–376.

414. Hoffman HT, Karnell LH, Robinson RA, et al. National Cancer Data Base report on cancer of the head and neck: acinic cell carcinoma. Head Neck 1999; 21: 297–309.

415. Oliveira P, Fonseca I, Soares J. Acinic cell carcinoma of the salivary glands. A long term follow-up study of 15 cases. Eur J Surg Oncol 1992; 18: 7–15.

416. Hamper K, Mausch HE, Caselitz J, et al. Acinic cell carcinoma of the salivary glands: the prognostic relevance of DNA cytophotometry in a retrospective study of long duration (1965–1987). Oral Surg Oral Med Oral Pathol 1990; 69: 68–75.

417. Hamper K, Caselitz J, Arps H, et al. The relationship between nuclear DNA content in salivary gland tumors and prognosis. Comparison of mucoepidermoid tumors and acinic cell tumors. Arch Otorhinolaryngol 1989; 246: 328–332.

418. Clemis JD, Bland J, Fung C. Acinic cell tumors of salivary gland origin. Laryngoscope 1977; 87: 1500–1508.

419. Abrams AM, Cornyn J, Scofield HH, et al. Acinic cell adenocarcinoma of the major salivary glands: a clinicopathologic study of 77 cases. Cancer 1965; 18: 1145–1162.

420. Timon CI, Dardick I, Panzarella T, et al. Clinico-pathological predictors of recurrence for acinic cell carcinoma. Clin Otolaryngol 1995; 20: 396–401.

421. Miki H, Masuda E, Ohata S, et al. Late recurrence of acinic cell carcinoma of the parotid gland. J Med Invest 1999; 46: 213–216.

422. Hunter RM, Davis BW, Gray GF Jr, et al. Primary malignant tumors of salivary gland origin. A 52–year review. Am Surg 1983; 49: 82–89.

423. Nagel H, Laskawi R, Buter JJ, et al. Cytologic diagnosis of acinic-cell carcinoma of salivary glands. Diagn Cytopathol 1997; 16: 402–412.

424. Klijanienko J, Vielh P. Fine-needle sample of salivary gland lesions. V: Cytology of 22 cases of acinic cell carcinoma with histologic correlation. Diagn Cytopathol 1997; 17: 347–352.

425. Sheyn I, Yassin R, Seiden A, et al. Papillary-cystic variant of acinic cell carcinoma of the salivary gland diagnosed by fine needle aspiration biopsy. A case report. Acta Cytol 2000; 44: 1073–1076.

426. Auclair PL, Ellis GL. Adenocarcinoma, not otherwise specified. In: Ellis GL, Auclair PL, Gnepp DR, eds. Surgical pathology of the salivary glands. Philadelphia: WB Saunders; 1991: 318–332.

427. Spiro RH, Huvos AG, Strong EW. Adenocarcinoma of salivary origin. Clinicopathologic study of 204 patients. Am J Surg 1982; 144: 423–431.

428. Matsuba HM, Mauney M, Simpson JR, et al. Adenocarcinomas of major and minor salivary gland origin: a histopathologic review of treatment failure patterns. Laryngoscope 1988; 98: 784–788.

429. McCutcheon IE, Kitagawa RH, Sherman SI, et al. Adenocarcinoma of the salivary gland metastatic to the pituitary gland: case report. Neurosurgery 2001; 48: 1161–1165.

430. Ellis GL, Auclair PL. Tumors of the salivary glands. Atlas of tumor pathology, 3rd series, fascicle 17. 1st edn. Washington, DC: Armed Forces Institute of Pathology; 1996: 203–216.

431. Neely MM, Rohrer MD, Young SK. Tumors of minor salivary glands and the analysis of 106 cases. J Okla Dent Assoc 1996; 86: 50–52.

432. Loyola AM, de Araujo VC, de Sousa SO, et al. Minor salivary gland tumours. A retrospective study of 164 cases in a Brazilian population. Eur J Cancer B Oral Oncol 1995; 31B: 197–201.

433. Renehan A, Gleave EN, Hancock BD, et al. Long-term follow-up of over 1000 patients with salivary gland tumours treated in a single centre. Br J Surg 1996; 83: 1750–1754.

434. Sur RK, Donde B, Levin V, et al. Adenoid cystic carcinoma of the salivary glands: a review of 10 years. Laryngoscope 1997; 107: 1276–1280.

435. Nara Y, Takeuchi J, Yoshida K, et al. Immunohistochemical characterisation of extracellular matrix components of salivary gland tumours. Br J Cancer 1991; 64: 307–314.

436. Nakanishi K, Kawai T, Suzuki M, et al. Glycosaminoglycans in pleomorphic adenoma and adenoid cystic carcinoma of the salivary gland. Arch Pathol Lab Med 1990; 114: 1227–1231.

437. Toida M, Takeuchi J, Sobue M, et al. Histochemical studies on pseudocysts in adenoid cystic carcinoma of the human salivary gland. Histochem J 1985; 17: 913–924.

438. d'Ardenne AJ, Kirkpatrick P, Wells CA, et al. Laminin and fibronectin in adenoid cystic carcinoma. J Clin Pathol 1986; 39: 138–144.

439. Chen JC, Gnepp DR, Bedrossian CW. Adenoid cystic carcinoma of the salivary glands: an immunohistochemical analysis. Oral Surg Oral Med Oral Pathol 1988; 65: 316–326.

440. Loducca SV, Raitz R, Araujo NS, et al. Polymorphous low-grade adenocarcinoma and adenoid cystic carcinoma: distinct architectural composition revealed by collagen IV, laminin and their integrin ligands (alpha2beta1 and alpha3beta1). Histopathology 2000; 37: 118–123.

441. Prasad AR, Savera AT, Gown AM, et al. The myoepithelial immunophenotype in 135 benign and malignant salivary gland tumors other than pleomorphic adenoma. Arch Pathol Lab Med 1999; 123: 801–806.

442. Orenstein JM, Dardick I, van Nostrand AW. Ultrastructural similarities of adenoid cystic carcinoma and pleomorphic adenoma. Histopathology 1985; 9: 623–638.

443. Chaudhry AP, Leifer C, Cutler LS, et al. Histogenesis of adenoid cystic carcinoma of the salivary glands. Light and electronmicroscopic study. Cancer 1986; 58: 72–82.

444. Azumi N, Battifora H. The cellular composition of adenoid cystic carcinoma. An immunohistochemical study. Cancer 1987; 60: 1589–1598.

445. Chomette G, Auriol M, Vaillant JM, et al. Heterogeneity and co-expression of intermediate filament proteins in adenoid cystic carcinoma of salivary glands. Pathol Biol (Paris) 1991; 39: 110–116.

446. Gunhan O, Evren G, Demiriz M, et al. Expression of S-100 protein, epithelial membrane antigen, carcinoembryonic antigen and alpha fetoprotein in normal salivary glands and primary salivary gland tumors. J Nihon Univ Sch Dent 1992; 34: 240–248.

447. Takahashi H, Tsuda N, Fujita S, et al. Immunohistochemical investigation of vimentin, neuron-specific enolase, alpha 1-antichymotrypsin and alpha 1-antitrypsin in adenoid cystic carcinoma of the salivary gland. Acta Pathol Jpn 1990; 40: 655–664.

448. Takahashi H, Fujita S, Tsuda N, et al. Iron-binding proteins in adenoid cystic carcinoma of salivary glands: an immunohistochemical study. Tohoku J Exp Med 1991; 163: 1–16.

449. Chomette G, Auriol M, Vaillant JM, et al. An immunohistochemical study of the distribution of lysozyme, lactoferrin, alpha 1–antitrypsin and alpha 1-antichymotrypsin in salivary adenoid cystic carcinoma. Pathol Res Pract 1991; 187: 1001–1008.

450. Ozono S, Onozuka M, Sato K, et al. Immunohistochemical localization of estradiol, progesterone, and progesterone receptor in human salivary glands and salivary adenoid cystic carcinomas. Cell Struct Funct 1992; 17: 169–175.

451. Shick PC, Riordan GP, Foss RD. Estrogen and progesterone receptors in salivary gland adenoid cystic carcinoma. Oral Surg Oral Med Oral Pathol Oral Radiol Endod 1995; 80: 440–444.

452. Miller AS, Hartman GG, Chen SY, et al. Estrogen receptor assay in polymorphous low-grade adenocarcinoma and adenoid cystic carcinoma of salivary gland origin. An immunohistochemical study. Oral Surg Oral Med Oral Pathol 1994; 77: 36–40.

453. Jeannon JP, Soames JV, Bell H, et al. Immunohistochemical detection of oestrogen and progesterone receptors in salivary tumours. Clin Otolaryngol 1999; 24: 52–54.

454. Karja V, Syrjanen S, Kataja V, et al. c-erbB-2 oncogene expression in salivary gland tumours. ORL J Otorhinolaryngol Relat Spec 1994; 56: 206–212.

455. Shintani S, Funayama T, Yoshihama Y, et al. Expression of c-erbB family gene products in adenoid cystic carcinoma of salivary glands: an immunohistochemical study. Anticancer Res 1995; 15: 2623–2626.

456. Rosa JC, Felix A, Fonseca I, et al. Immunoexpression of c-erbB-2 and p53 in benign and malignant salivary neoplasms with myoepithelial differentiation. J Clin Pathol 1997; 50: 661–663.

457. Cho KJ, Lee SS, Lee YS. Proliferating cell nuclear antigen and c-erbB-2 oncoprotein expression in adenoid cystic carcinomas of the salivary glands. Head Neck 1999; 21: 414–419.

458. Gibbons MD, Manne U, Carroll WR, et al. Molecular differences in mucoepidermoid carcinoma and adenoid cystic carcinoma of the major salivary glands. Laryngoscope 2001; 111: 1373–1378.

459. Jeng YM, Lin CY, Hsu HC. Expression of the c-kit protein is associated with certain subtypes of salivary gland carcinoma. Cancer Lett 2000; 154: 107–111.

460. Stenman G, Sandros J, Dahlenfors R, et al. 6q- and loss of the Y chromosome – two common deviations in malignant human salivary gland tumors. Cancer Genet Cytogenet 1986; 22: 283–293.

461. Higashi K, Jin Y, Johansson M, et al. Rearrangement of 9p13 as the primary chromosomal aberration in adenoid cystic carcinoma of the respiratory tract. Genes Chromosom Cancer 1991; 3: 21–23.

462. Li X, Tsuji T, Wen S, et al. A fluorescence in situ hybridization (FISH) analysis with centromere-specific DNA probes of chromosomes 3 and 17 in pleomorphic adenomas and adenoid cystic carcinomas. J Oral Pathol Med 1995; 24: 398–401.

463. Johns MM, Westra WH, Califano JA, et al. Allelotype of salivary gland tumors. Cancer Res 1996; 56: 1151–1154.

464. el-Naggar AK, Lovell M, Callender DL, et al. Limited nonrandom chromosomal aberrations in a recurrent adenoid cystic carcinoma of the parotid gland. Cancer Genet Cytogenet 1999; 109: 66–69.

465. El Rifai W, Rutherford S, Knuutila S, et al. Novel DNA copy number losses in chromosome 12q12-q13 in adenoid cystic carcinoma. Neoplasia 2001; 3: 173–178.

466. Martins C, Fonseca I, Roque L, et al. Cytogenetic similarities between two types of salivary gland carcinomas: adenoid cystic carcinoma and polymorphous low-grade adenocarcinoma. Cancer Genet Cytogenet 2001; 128: 130–136.

467. Stallmach I, Zenklusen P, Komminoth P, et al. Loss of heterozygosity at chromosome 6q23-25 correlates with clinical and histologic parameters in salivary gland adenoid cystic carcinoma. Virchows Arch 2002; 440: 77–84.

468. van Heerden WF, Raubenheimer EJ. Evaluation of the nucleolar organizer region associated proteins in minor salivary gland tumors. J Oral Pathol Med 1991; 20: 291–295.

469. Fonseca I, Soares J. Adenoid cystic carcinoma: a study of nucleolar organizer regions (AgNOR) counts and their relation to prognosis. J Pathol 1993; 169: 255–258.

470. Vuhahula EA, Nikai H, Ogawa I, et al. Prognostic value of argyrophilic nucleolar organizer regions (AgNOR) count in adenoid cystic carcinoma of salivary glands. Pathol Int 1994; 44: 368–373.

471. Vuhahula EA, Nikai H, Ogawa I, et al. Correlation between argyrophilic nucleolar organizer region (AgNOR) counts and histologic grades with respect to biologic behavior of salivary adenoid cystic carcinoma. J Oral Pathol Med 1995; 24: 437–442.

472. Yamamoto Y, Itoh T, Saka T, et al. Nucleolar organizer regions in adenoid cystic carcinoma of the salivary glands. Eur Arch Otorhinolaryngol 1995; 252: 176–180.

473. Xie X, Nordgard S, Halvorsen TB, et al. Prognostic significance of nucleolar organizer regions in adenoid cystic carcinomas of the head and neck. Arch Otolaryngol Head Neck Surg 1997; 123: 615–620.

474. Skalova A, Leivo I. Cell proliferation in salivary gland tumors. Gen Diagn Pathol 1996; 142: 7–16.

475. Skalova A, Simpson RH, Lehtonen H, et al. Assessment of proliferative activity using the MIB1 antibody helps to distinguish polymorphous low grade adenocarcinoma from adenoid cystic carcinoma of salivary glands. Pathol Res Pract 1997; 193: 695–703.

476. Daniele E, Tralongo V, Morello V, et al. Pleomorphic adenoma and adenoid-cystic carcinoma of salivary glands: immunohistochemical assessment of proliferative activity in comparison with flow-cytometric study. Cell Prolif 1996; 29: 153–162.

477. Zhu Q, White FH, Tipoe GL. The assessment of proliferating cell nuclear antigen (PCNA) immunostaining in human benign and malignant epithelial lesions of the parotid gland. Oral Oncol 1997; 33: 29–35.

478. Hirabayashi S. Immunohistochemical detection of DNA topoisomerase type II alpha and Ki-67 in adenoid cystic carcinoma and pleomorphic adenoma of the salivary gland. J Oral Pathol Med 1999; 28: 131–136.

479. Trendell-Smith NJ, Oates J, Crocker J. The evaluation of salivary gland tumours using proliferating cell nuclear antigen. J Laryngol Otol 1997; 111: 551–555.

480. Takata T, Kudo Y, Zhao M, et al. Reduced expression of p27(Kip1) protein in relation to salivary adenoid cystic carcinoma metastasis. Cancer 1999; 86: 928–935.

481. Luna MA, el Naggar A, Parichatikanond P, et al. Basaloid squamous carcinoma of the upper aerodigestive tract. Clinicopathologic and DNA flow cytometric analysis. Cancer 1990; 66: 537–542.

482. Banks ER, Frierson HF Jr, Mills SE, et al. Basaloid squamous cell carcinoma of the head and neck. A clinicopathologic and immunohistochemical study of 40 cases. Am J Surg Pathol 1992; 16: 939–946.

483. Tsubochi H, Suzuki T, Suzuki S, et al. Immunohistochemical study of basaloid squamous cell carcinoma, adenoid cystic and mucoepidermoid carcinoma in the upper aerodigestive tract. Anticancer Res 2000; 20: 1205–1211.

484. Szanto PA, Luna MA, Tortoledo ME, et al. Histologic grading of adenoid cystic carcinoma of the salivary glands. Cancer 1984; 54: 1062–1069.

485. Matsuba HM, Spector GJ, Thawley SE, et al. Adenoid cystic salivary gland carcinoma. A histopathologic review of treatment failure patterns. Cancer 1986; 57: 519–524.

486. Hamper K, Lazar F, Dietel M, et al. Prognostic factors for adenoid cystic carcinoma of the head and neck: a retrospective evaluation of 96 cases. J Oral Pathol Med 1990; 19: 101–107.

487. Greiner TC, Robinson RA, Maves MD. Adenoid cystic carcinoma. A clinicopathologic study with flow cytometric analysis (see comments). Am J Clin Pathol 1989; 92: 711–720.

488. Batsakis JG, Luna MA, el-Naggar A. Histopathologic grading of salivary gland neoplasms: III. Adenoid cystic carcinomas. Ann Otol Rhinol Laryngol 1990; 99: 1007–1009.

489. Spiro RH, Huvos AG. Stage means more than grade in adenoid cystic carcinoma. Am J Surg 1992; 164: 623–628.

490. van der Wal JE, Snow GB, van der Waal I. Intraoral adenoid cystic carcinoma. The presence of perineural spread in relation to site, size, local extension, and metastatic spread in 22 cases. Cancer 1990; 66: 2031–2033.

491. Vrielinck LJ, Ostyn F, van Damme B, et al. The significance of perineural spread in adenoid cystic carcinoma of the major and minor salivary glands. Int J Oral Maxillofac Surg 1988; 17: 190–193.

492. Luna MA, el-Naggar A, Batsakis JG, et al. Flow cytometric DNA content of adenoid cystic carcinoma of submandibular gland. Correlation of histologic features and prognosis. Arch Otolaryngol Head Neck Surg 1990; 116: 1291–1296.

493. Matsuba HM, Thawley SE, Simpson JR, et al. Adenoid cystic carcinoma of major and minor salivary gland origin. Laryngoscope 1984; 94: 1316–1318.

494. Ampil FL, Misra RP. Factors influencing survival of patients with adenoid cystic carcinoma of the salivary glands. J Oral Maxillofac Surg 1987; 45: 1005–1010.

495. Simpson JR, Thawley SE, Matsuba HM. Adenoid cystic salivary gland carcinoma: treatment with irradiation and surgery. Radiology 1984; 151: 509–512.

496. Spiro RH. Distant metastasis in adenoid cystic carcinoma of salivary origin. Am J Surg 1997; 174: 495–498.

497. Franzën G, Klausen OG, Grenko RT, et al. Adenoid cystic carcinoma: DNA as a prognostic indicator. Laryngoscope 1991; 101: 669–673.

498. Eibling DE, Johnson JT, McCoy JP Jr, et al. Flow cytometric evaluation of adenoid cystic carcinoma: correlation with histologic subtype and survival. Am J Surg 1991; 162: 367–372.

499. Saka T, Yamamoto Y, Takahashi H. Comparative cytofluorometric DNA analysis of pleomorphic adenoma and adenoid cystic carcinoma of the salivary glands. Virchows Arch [Cell Pathol] 1991; 61: 255–261.

500. Nordgård S, Franzën G, Boysen M, et al. Ki-67 as a prognostic marker in adenoid cystic carcinoma assessed with the monoclonal antibody MIB1 in paraffin sections. Laryngoscope 1997; 107: 531–536.

501. Casler JD, Conley JJ. Surgical management of adenoid cystic carcinoma in the parotid gland. Otolaryngol Head Neck Surg 1992; 106: 332–338.

502. Stell PM, Cruikshank AH, Stoney PJ, et al. Adenoid cystic carcinoma: the results of radical surgery. Clin Otolaryngol 1985; 10: 205–208.

503. Hosokawa Y, Ohmori K, Kaneko M, et al. Analysis of adenoid cystic carcinoma treated by radiotherapy. Oral Surg Oral Med Oral Pathol 1992; 74: 251–255.

504. Teshima T, Inoue T, Ikeda H, et al. Radiation therapy for carcinoma of the major salivary glands. Results of conventional irradiation technique. Strahlenther Onkol 1993; 169: 486–491.

505. Sakata K, Aoki Y, Karasawa K, et al. Radiation therapy for patients of malignant salivary gland tumors with positive surgical margins. Strahlenther Onkol 1994; 170: 342–346.

506. Stelzer KJ, Laramore GE, Griffin TW, et al. Fast neutron radiotherapy. The University of Washington experience. Acta Oncol 1994; 33: 275–280.

507. Douglas JG, Laramore GE, Austin-Seymour M, et al. Neutron radiotherapy for adenoid cystic carcinoma of minor salivary glands. Int J Radiat Oncol Biol Phys 1996; 36: 87–93.

508. Krull A, Schwarz R, Engenhart R, et al. European results in neutron therapy of malignant salivary gland tumors. Bull Cancer Radiother 1996; 83 Suppl: 125–129s.

509. Krull A, Schwarz R, Brackrock S, et al. Neutron therapy in malignant salivary gland tumors: results at European centers. Recent Results Cancer Res 1998; 150: 88–99.

510. Debus J, Engenhart-Cabillic R, Kraft G, et al. The role of high-LET radiotherapy compared to conformal photon radiotherapy in adenoid cystic carcinoma. Strahlenther Onkol 1999; 175 Suppl 2: 63–65.

511. Potter R, Prott FJ, Micke O, et al. Results of fast neutron therapy of adenoid cystic carcinoma of the salivary glands. Strahlenther Onkol 1999; 175 Suppl 2: 65–68.

512. Prott FJ, Micke O, Haverkamp U, et al. Results of fast neutron therapy of adenoid cystic carcinoma of the salivary glands. Anticancer Res 2000; 20: 3743–3749.

513. Umeda M, Nishimatsu N, Yokoo S, et al. The role of radiotherapy for patients with adenoid cystic carcinoma of the salivary gland. Oral Surg Oral Med Oral Pathol Oral Radiol Endod 2000; 89: 724–729.

514. Shadaba A, Gaze MN, Grant HR. The response of adenoid cystic carcinoma to tamoxifen. J Laryngol Otol 1997; 111: 1186–1189.

515. Airoldi M, Bumma C, Bertetto O, et al. Vinorelbine treatment of recurrent salivary gland carcinomas. Bull Cancer 1998; 85: 892–894.

516. Airoldi M, Fornari G, Pedani F, et al. Paclitaxel and carboplatin for recurrent salivary gland malignancies. Anticancer Res 2000; 20: 3781–3783.

517. Airoldi M, Pedani F, Succo G, et al. Phase II randomized trial comparing vinorelbine versus vinorelbine plus cisplatin in patients with recurrent salivary gland malignancies. Cancer 2001; 91: 541–547.

518. Lee SS, Cho KJ, Jang JJ, et al. Differential diagnosis of adenoid cystic carcinoma from pleomorphic adenoma of the salivary gland on fine needle aspiration cytology. Acta Cytol 1996; 40: 1246–1252.

519. Nagel H, Hotze HJ, Laskawi R, et al. Cytologic diagnosis of adenoid cystic carcinoma of salivary glands. Diagn Cytopathol 1999; 20: 358–366.

520. Bondeson L, Lindholm K, Thorstenson S. Benign dermal eccrine cylindroma. A pitfall in the cytologic diagnosis of adenoid cystic carcinoma. Acta Cytol 1983; 27: 326–328.

521. Kapadia SB, Dusenbery D, Dekker A. Fine needle aspiration of pleomorphic adenoma and adenoid cystic carcinoma of salivary gland origin. Acta Cytol 1997; 41(2): 487–492.

522. Klijanienko J, Vielh P. Fine-needle sampling of salivary gland lesions. III. Cytologic and histologic correlation of 75 cases of adenoid cystic carcinoma: review and experience at the Institut Curie with emphasis on cytologic pitfalls. Diagn Cytopathol 1997; 17(1): 36–41.

523. Löwhagen T, Tani EM, Skoog L. Salivary glands and rare head and neck lesions. In: Bibbo M, ed. Comprehensive cytopathology. 1st edn. Philadelphia: WB Saunders; 1991: 627–634.

524. Freedman PD, Lumerman H. Lobular carcinoma of intraoral minor salivary gland origin. Report of twelve cases. Oral Surg Oral Med Oral Pathol 1983; 56: 157–165.

525. Batsakis JG, Pinkston GR, Luna MA, et al. Adenocarcinomas of the oral cavity: a clinicopathologic study of terminal duct carcinomas. J Laryngol Otol 1983; 97: 825–835.

526. Evans HL, Batsakis JG. Polymorphous low-grade adenocarcinoma of minor salivary glands. A study of 14 cases of a distinctive neoplasm. Cancer 1984; 53: 935–942.

527. Seifert G, Sobin LH. Histological classification of salivary gland tumours. World Health Organization. International histological classification of tumours. 2nd edn. Berlin: Springer-Verlag; 1991.

528. Miliauskas JR. Polymorphous low-grade (terminal duct) adenocarcinoma of the parotid gland. Histopathology 1991; 19: 555–557.

529. Katoh T, Yoshihara T, Naitoh J, et al. [A case of polymorphous adenocarcinoma in the right parotid gland]. Article in Japanese, English abstract. Gan No Rinsho 1985; 31: 861–864.

530. Haba R, Kobayashi S, Miki H, et al. Polymorphous low-grade adenocarcinoma of submandibular gland origin. Acta Pathol Jpn 1993; 43: 774–778.

531. Kemp BL, Batsakis JG, el-Naggar AK, et al. Terminal duct adenocarcinomas of the parotid gland. J Laryngol Otol 1995; 109: 466–468.

532. Puxeddu R, Puxeddu P, Parodo G, et al. Polymorphous low-grade adenocarcinoma of the parotid gland. Eur J Morphol 1998; 36 Supp: 262–266.

533. Merchant WJ, Cook MG, Eveson JW. Polymorphous low-grade adenocarcinoma of parotid gland. Br J Oral Maxillofac Surg 1996; 34: 328–330.

534. Blanchaert RH, Ord RA, Kumar D. Polymorphous low-grade adenocarcinoma of the sublingual gland. Int J Oral Maxillofac Surg 1998; 27: 115–117.

535. Ellis GL, Auclair PL. Tumors of the salivary glands. Atlas of tumor pathology, 3rd series, fascicle 17. 1st edn. Washington, DC: Armed Forces Institute of Pathology; 1996: 216–228.

536. van Heerden WF, Raubenheimer EJ. Intraoral salivary gland neoplasms: a retrospective study of seventy cases in an African population. Oral Surg Oral Med Oral Pathol 1991; 71: 579–582.

537. Vincent SD, Hammond HL, Finkelstein MW. Clinical and therapeutic features of polymorphous low-grade adenocarcinoma. Oral Surg Oral Med Oral Pathol 1994; 77: 41–47.

538. Clayton JR, Pogrel MA, Regezi JA. Simultaneous multifocal polymorphous low-grade adenocarcinoma. Report of two cases. Oral Surg Oral Med Oral Pathol Oral Radiol Endod 1995; 80: 71–77.

539. Castle JT, Thompson LD, Frommelt RA, et al. Polymorphous low grade adenocarcinoma: a clinicopathologic study of 164 cases. Cancer 1999; 86: 207–219.

540. Pelkey TJ, Mills SE. Histologic transformation of polymorphous low-grade adenocarcinoma of salivary gland. Am J Clin Pathol 1999; 111: 785–791.

541. Kelsch RD, Bhuiya T, Fuchs A, et al. Polymorphous low-grade adenocarcinoma: flow cytometric, p53, and PCNA analysis. Oral Surg Oral Med Oral Pathol Oral Radiol Endod 1997; 84: 391–399.

542. Fonseca I, Felix A, Soares J. Cell proliferation in salivary gland adenocarcinomas with myoepithelial participation. A study of 78 cases. Virchows Arch 1997; 430: 227–232.

543. Gnepp DR, el-Mofty S. Polymorphous low-grade adenocarcinoma: glial fibrillary acidic protein staining in the differential diagnosis with cellular mixed tumors. Oral Surg Oral Med Oral Pathol Oral Radiol Endod 1997; 83: 691–695.

544. Penner CR, Folpe AL, Budnick SD. C-kit expression distinguishes salivary gland adenoid cystic carcinoma from polymorphous low-grade adenocarcinoma. Mod Pathol 2002; 15: 687–691.

545. Tanaka F, Wada H, Inui K, et al. Pulmonary metastasis of polymorphous low-grade adenocarcinoma of the minor salivary gland. Thorac Cardiovasc Surg 1995; 43: 178–180.

546. Thomas KM, Cumberworth VL, McEwan J. Orbital and skin metastases in a polymorphous low grade adenocarcinoma of the salivary gland. J Laryngol Otol 1995; 109: 1222–1225.

547. Wenig BM, Gnepp DR. Polymorphous low-grade adenocarcinoma of minor salivary glands. In: Ellis GL, Auclair PL, Gnepp DR, eds. Surgical pathology of the salivary glands. 1st edn. Philadelphia: WB Saunders; 1991: 390–411.

548. Aberle AM, Abrams AM, Bowe R, et al. Lobular (polymorphous low-grade) carcinoma of minor salivary glands. A clinicopathologic study of twenty cases. Oral Surg Oral Med Oral Pathol 1985; 60: 387–395.

549. Gibbons D, Saboorian MH, Vuitch F, et al. Fine-needle aspiration findings in patients with polymorphous low grade adenocarcinoma of the salivary glands. Cancer 1999; 87: 31–36.

550. Watanabe K, Ono N, Saito K, et al. Fine-needle aspiration cytology of polymorphous low-grade adenocarcinoma of the tongue. Diagn Cytopathol 1999; 20: 167–169.

551. Ellis GL, Auclair PL. Tumors of the salivary glands. Atlas of tumor pathology, 3rd series, fascicle 17. 1st edn. Washington, DC: Armed Forces Institute of Pathology; 1996: 228–251.

552. Gnepp DR. Malignant mixed tumors of the salivary glands: a review. Pathol Annu 1993; 28 Pt 1: 279–328.

553. Eneroth CM, Zetterberg A. Malignancy in pleomorphic adenoma. A clinical and microspectrophotometric study. Acta Otolaryngol (Stockh) 1974; 77: 426–432.

554. Eneroth CM. Die Klinik der Kopfspeicheldrüsentumoren. Arch Otorhinolaryngol 1976; 213: 61–110.

555. Eneroth CM, Zetterberg A. Microspectrophotometric DNA analysis of malignant salivary gland tumours. Acta Otolaryngol (Stockh) 1974; 77: 289–294.

556. Franchi A, Moroni M, Paglierani M, et al. Expression of CD44 standard and variant isoforms in parotid gland and parotid gland tumours. J Oral Pathol Med 2001; 30: 564–568.

557. Spiro RH, Huvos AG, Strong EW. Malignant mixed tumor of salivary origin: a clinicopathologic study of 146 cases. Cancer 1977; 39: 388–396.

558. LiVolsi VA, Perzin KH. Malignant mixed tumors arising in salivary glands. I. Carcinomas arising in benign mixed tumors: a clinicopathologic study. Cancer 1977; 39: 2209–2230.

559. Ersoz C, Cetik F, Aydin O, et al. Salivary duct carcinoma ex pleomorphic adenoma: analysis of the findings in fine-needle aspiration cytology and histology. Diagn Cytopathol 1998; 19: 201–204.

560. Jacobs JC. Low grade mucoepidermoid carcinoma ex pleomorphic adenoma. A diagnostic problem in fine needle aspiration biopsy. Acta Cytol 1994; 38: 93–97.

561. Shrikhande SS, Talvalkar GV. Malignant mixed salivary gland tumors – a clinico-pathological study of 48 cases. Indian J Cancer 1979; 16: 9–12.

562. Littman CD, Alguacil-Garcia A. Clear cell carcinoma arising in pleomorphic adenoma of the salivary gland. Am J Clin Pathol 1987; 88: 239–243.

563. Tortoledo ME, Luna MA, Batsakis JG. Carcinomas ex pleomorphic adenoma and malignant mixed tumors. Histomorphologic indexes. Arch Otolaryngol Head Neck Surg 1984; 110: 172–176.

564. Yoshihara T, Tanaka M, Itoh M, et al. Carcinoma ex pleomorphic adenoma of the soft palate. J Laryngol Otol 1995; 109: 240–243.

565. Lewis JE, Olsen KD, Sebo TJ. Carcinoma ex pleomorphic adenoma: pathologic analysis of 73 cases. Hum Pathol 2001; 32(6): 596–604.

566. Felix A, Rosa-Santos J, Mendonca ME, et al. Intracapsular carcinoma ex pleomorphic adenoma. Report of a case with unusual metastatic behaviour. Oral Oncol 2002; 38: 107–110.

567. Garner SL, Robinson RA, Maves MD, et al. Salivary gland carcinosarcoma: true malignant mixed tumor. Ann Otol Rhinol Laryngol 1989; 98: 611–614.

568. Stephen J, Batsakis JG, Luna MA, et al. True malignant mixed tumors (carcinosarcoma) of salivary glands. Oral Surg Oral Med Oral Pathol 1986; 61: 597–602.

569. Toynton SC, Wilkins MJ, Cook HT, et al. True malignant mixed tumour of a minor salivary gland. J Laryngol Otol 1994; 108: 76–79.

570. Ellis GL, Auclair PL. Tumors of the salivary glands. Atlas of tumor pathology, 3rd series, fascicle 17. 1st edn. Washington, DC: Armed Forces Institute of Pathology; 1996: 238–245.

571. Kwon MY, Gu M. True malignant mixed tumor (carcinosarcoma) of parotid gland with unusual mesenchymal component: a case report and review of the literature. Arch Pathol Lab Med 2001; 125: 812–815.

572. Bleiweiss IJ, Huvos AG, Lara J, et al. Carcinosarcoma of the submandibular salivary gland. Immunohistochemical findings. Cancer 1992; 69: 2031–2035.

573. Dardick I, Hardie J, Thomas MJ, et al. Ultrastructural contributions to the study of morphological differentiation in malignant mixed (pleomorphic) tumors of salivary gland. Head Neck 1989; 11: 5–21.

574. Rumnong V, Banerjee AK, Joshi K, et al. Carcinosarcoma of parotid gland having osteosarcoma as sarcomatous component: a case report. Indian J Pathol Microbiol 1993; 36: 492–494.

575. Latkovich P, Johnson RL. Carcinosarcoma of the parotid gland: report of a case with cytohistologic and immunohistochemical findings. Arch Pathol Lab Med 1998; 122: 743–746.

576. Harada H. Histomorphological investigation regarding to malignant transformation of pleomorphic adenoma (so-called malignant mixed tumor) of the salivary gland origin: special reference to carcinosarcoma. Kurume Med J 2000; 47: 307–323.

577. Chen KT, Weinberg RA, Moseley D. Carcinosarcoma of the salivary gland. Am J Otolaryngol 1984; 5: 415–417.

578. Suzuki J, Takagi M, Okada N, et al. Carcinosarcoma of the submandibular gland. An autopsy case. Acta Pathol Jpn 1990; 40: 827–831.

579. Takata T, Nikai H, Ogawa I, et al. Ultrastructural and immunohistochemical observations of a true malignant mixed tumor (carcinosarcoma) of the tongue. J Oral Pathol Med 1990; 19: 261–265.

580. Yamashita T, Kameda N, Katayama K, et al. True malignant mixed tumor of the submandibular gland. Acta Pathol Jpn 1990; 40: 137–142.

581. Huntington HW, Dardick I. Intracranial metastasis from a malignant mixed tumor of parotid salivary gland. Ultrastruct Pathol 1985; 9: 169–173.

582. Grenko RT, Tytor M, Boeryd B. Giant-cell tumour of the salivary gland with associated carcinosarcoma. Histopathology 1993; 23: 594–595.

583. Gandour-Edwards RF, Donald PJ, Vogt PJ, et al. Carcinosarcoma (malignant mixed tumor) of the parotid: report of a case with a pure rhabdomyosarcoma component. Head Neck 1994; 16: 379–382.

584. Alvarez-Canas C, Rodilla IG. True malignant mixed tumor (carcinosarcoma) of the parotid gland. Report of a case with immunohistochemical study. Oral Surg Oral Med Oral Pathol Oral Radiol Endod 1996; 81: 454–458.

585. Morey-Mas M, Caubet-Biayna J, Gomez-Bellvert C, et al. Carcinosarcoma of the submandibular and sublingual salivary glands. A case report and review of the literature. Acta Stomatol Belg 1997; 94: 69–73.

586. Gogas J, Markopoulos C, Karydakis V, et al. Carcinosarcoma of the submandibular salivary gland. Eur J Surg Oncol 1999; 25: 333–335.

587. Bocklage T, Feddersen R. Unusual mesenchymal and mixed tumors of the salivary gland. An immunohistochemical and flow cytometric analysis of three cases. Arch Pathol Lab Med 1995; 119: 69–74.

588. Auclair PL, Langloss JM, Weiss SW, et al. Sarcomas and sarcomatoid neoplasms of the major salivary gland regions. A clinicopathologic and immunohistochemical study of 67 cases and review of the literature. Cancer 1986; 58: 1305–1315.

589. Ellis GL, Auclair PL. Tumors of the salivary glands. Atlas of tumor pathology, 3rd series, fascicle 17. 1st edn. Washington, DC: Armed Forces Institute of Pathology; 1996: 379–399.

590. Fujimura M, Sugawara T, Seki H, et al. Carcinomatous change in the cranial metastasis from a metastasizing mixed tumor of the salivary gland – case report. Neurol Med Chir (Tokyo) 1997; 37: 546–550

591. Freeman SB, Kennedy KS, Parker GS, et al. Metastasizing pleomorphic adenoma of the nasal septum. Arch Otolaryngol Head Neck Surg 1990; 116: 1331–1333.

592. Wermuth DJ, Mann CH, Odere F. Metastasizing pleomorphic adenoma arising in the soft palate. Otolaryngol Head Neck Surg 1988; 99: 505–508.

593. Pitman MB, Thor AD, Goodman ML, et al. Benign metastasizing pleomorphic adenoma of salivary gland: diagnosis of bone lesions by fine-needle aspiration biopsy. Diagn Cytopathol 1992; 8: 384–387.

594. Klijanienko J, el-Naggar AK, Servois V, et al. Clinically aggressive metastasizing pleomorphic adenoma: report of two cases. Head Neck 1997; 19: 629–633.

595. Hoorweg JJ, Hilgers FJ, Keus RB, et al. Metastasizing pleomorphic adenoma: a report of three cases. Eur J Surg Oncol 1998; 24: 452–455.

596. Gnepp DR, Wenig BM. Malignant mixed tumors. In: Ellis GL, Auclair PL, Gnepp DR, eds. Surgical pathology of the salivary glands. 1st edn. Philadelphia: WB Saunders; 1991: 350–368.

597. el-Naggar A, Batsakis JG, Kessler S. Benign metastatic mixed tumours or unrecognized salivary carcinomas? J Laryngol Otol 1988; 102: 810–812.

598. Sim DW, Maran AG, Harris D. Metastatic salivary pleomorphic adenoma. J Laryngol Otol 1990; 104 45–47.

599. Moberger JG, Eneroth CM. Malignant mixed tumors of the major salivary glands. Special reference to the histologic structure in metastases. Cancer 1968; 21: 1198–1211.

600. Jin Y, Jin C, Arheden K, et al. Unbalanced chromosomal rearrangements in a metastasizing salivary gland tumor with benign histology. Cancer Genet Cytogenet 1998; 102: 59–64.

601. Cresson DH, Goldsmith M, Askin FB, et al. Metastasizing pleomorphic adenoma with myoepithelial cell predominance. Pathol Res Pract 1990; 186: 795–800.

602. Sampson BA, Jarcho JA, Winters GL. Metastasizing mixed tumor of the parotid gland: a rare tumor with unusually rapid progression in a cardiac transplant recipient. Mod Pathol 1998; 11: 1142–1145.

603. Granger JK, Houn HY. Malignant mixed tumor (carcinosarcoma) of parotid gland diagnosed by fine-needle aspiration biopsy. Diagn Cytopathol 1991; 7: 427–432.

604. Klijanienko J, el-Naggar AK, Servois V, et al. Mucoepidermoid carcinoma ex pleomorphic adenoma: nonspecific preoperative cytologic findings in six cases. Cancer 1998; 84: 231–234.

605. Anand A, Brockie ES. Cytomorphological features of salivary duct carcinoma ex pleomorphic adenoma: diagnosis by fine-needle aspiration biopsy with histologic correlation. Diagn Cytopathol 1999; 20: 375–378.

606. Kim T, Yoon GS, Kim O, et al. Fine needle aspiration diagnosis of malignant mixed tumor (carcinosarcoma) arising in pleomorphic adenoma of the salivary gland. A case report. Acta Cytol 1998; 42: 1027–1031.

607. Goldman RL, Klein HZ. Glycogen-rich adenoma of the parotid gland. An uncommon benign clear-cell tumor resembling certain clear-cell carcinomas of salivary origin. Cancer 1972; 30: 749–754.

608. Saksela E, Tarkkanen J, Wartiovaara J. Parotid clear-cell adenoma of possible myoepithelial origin. Cancer 1972; 30: 742–748.

609. Thackray AC, Lucas RB. Tumors of the major salivary glands. Atlas of tumor pathology, 2nd series, fascicle 10. 1st edn.Washington, DC: Armed Forces Institute of Pathology; 1974: 62–63.

610. Batsakis JG, el-Naggar AK, Luna MA. Epithelial-myoepithelial carcinoma of salivary glands. Ann Otol Rhinol Laryngol 1992; 101: 540–542.

611. Corio RL, Sciubba JJ, Brannon RB, et al. Epithelial-myoepithelial carcinoma of intercalated duct origin. A clinicopathologic and ultrastructural assessment of sixteen cases. Oral Surg Oral Med Oral Pathol 1982; 53: 280–287.

612. Fonseca I, Soares J. Epithelial-myoepithelial carcinoma of the salivary glands. A study of 22 cases. Virchows Arch A Pathol Anat Histopathol 1993; 422: 389–396.

613. Simpson RH, Clarke TJ, Sarsfield PT, et al. Epithelial-myoepithelial carcinoma of salivary glands. J Clin Pathol 1991; 44: 419–423.

614. Hamper K, Brugmann M, Koppermann R, et al. Epithelial-myoepithelial duct carcinoma of salivary glands: a follow-up and cytophotometric study of 21 cases. J Oral Pathol Med 1989; 18: 299–304.

615. Ellis GL, Auclair PL. Tumors of the salivary glands. Atlas of tumor pathology, 3rd series, fascicle 17. 1st edn. Washington, DC: Armed Forces Institute of Pathology; 1996: 268–281.

616. Tralongo V, Daniele E. Epithelial-myoepithelial carcinoma of the salivary glands: a review of literature. Anticancer Res 1998; 18: 603–608.

617. Kasper HU, Mellin W, Kriegsmann J, et al. Epithelial-myoepithelial carcinoma of the salivary gland – a low grade malignant neoplasm? Report of two cases and review of the literature. Pathol Res Pract 1999; 195: 189–192.

618. Noel S, Brozna JP. Epithelial-myoepithelial carcinoma of salivary gland with metastasis to lung: report of a case and review of the literature. Head Neck 1992; 14: 401–406.

619. Collina G, Gale N, Visona A, et al. Epithelial-myoepithelial carcinoma of the parotid gland: a clinico-pathologic and immunohistochemical study of seven cases. Tumori 1991; 77: 257–263.

620. Daley TD, Wysocki GP, Smout MS, et al. Epithelial-myoepithelial carcinoma of salivary glands. Oral Surg Oral Med Oral Pathol 1984; 57: 512–519.

621. Luna MA, Ordóñez NG, Mackay B, et al. Salivary epithelial-myoepithelial carcinomas of intercalated ducts: a clinical, electron microscopic, and immunocytochemical study. Oral Surg Oral Med Oral Pathol 1985; 59: 482–490.

622. Palmer RM. Epithelial-myoepithelial carcinoma: an immunocytochemical study. Oral Surg Oral Med Oral Pathol 1985; 59: 511–515.

623. Cho KJ, el-Naggar AK, Ordóñez NG, et al. Epithelial-myoepithelial carcinoma of salivary glands. A clinicopathologic, DNA flow cytometric, and immunohistochemical study of Ki-67 and HER-2/neu oncogene. Am J Clin Pathol 1995; 103 432–437.

624. Daa T, Kashima K, Gamachi A, et al. Epithelial-myoepithelial carcinoma harboring p53 mutation. APMIS 2001; 109: 316–320.

625. Tralongo V, Rodolico V, Nagar C, et al. Epithelial-myoepithelial carcinoma of the salivary glands: a clinico-pathologic, immunohistochemical and DNA flow cytometric study of three cases. Anticancer Res 1997; 17: 761–768.

626. Luna MA, Batsakis JG, Ordóñez NG, et al. Salivary gland adenocarcinomas: a clinicopathologic analysis of three distinctive types. Semin Diagn Pathol 1987; 4: 117–135.

627. Yang GC, Soslow RA. Epithelial-myoepithelial carcinoma of the parotid. A case of ductal-predominant presentation with cytologic, histologic and ultrastructural correlations. Acta Cytol 1999; 43: 1113–1118.

628. Ng WK, Choy C, Ip P, et al. Fine needle aspiration cytology of epithelial-myoepithelial carcinoma of salivary glands. A report of three cases. Acta Cytol 1999; 43: 675–680.

629. Klijanienko J, Vielh P. Fine-needle sampling of salivary gland lesions. VII. Cytology and histology correlation of five cases of epithelial-myoepithelial carcinoma. Diagn Cytopathol 1998; 19: 405–409.

630. Shemen LJ, Huvos AG, Spiro RH. Squamous cell carcinoma of salivary gland origin. Head Neck Surg 1987; 9: 235–240.

631. Marks MW, Ryan RF, Litwin MS, et al. Squamous cell carcinoma of the parotid gland. Plast Reconstr Surg 1987; 79: 550–554.

632. Schneider AB, Favus MJ, Stachura ME, et al. Salivary gland neoplasms as a late consequence of head and neck irradiation. Ann Intern Med 1977; 87: 160–164.

633. Ju DM. Salivary gland tumors occurring after radiation of the head and neck area. Am J Surg 1968; 116: 518–523.

634. Friedman M, Levin B, Grybauskas V, et al. Malignant tumors of the major salivary glands. Otolaryngol Clin North Am 1986; 19: 625–636.

635. Gaughan RK, Olsen KD, Lewis JE. Primary squamous cell carcinoma of the parotid gland. Arch Otolaryngol Head Neck Surg 1992; 118: 798–801.

636. Sterman BM, Kraus DH, Sebek BA, et al. Primary squamous cell carcinoma of the parotid gland. Laryngoscope 1990; 100: 146–148.

637. Auclair PL, Ellis GL. Primary squamous cell carcinoma. In: Ellis GL, Auclair PL, Gnepp DR, eds. Surgical pathology of the salivary glands. 1st edn. Philadelphia: WB Saunders; 1991: 369–378.

638. Khurana VG, Mentis DH, O'Brien CJ, et al. Parotid and neck metastases from cutaneous squamous cell carcinoma of the head and neck. Am J Surg 1995; 170: 446–450.

639. Taxy JB. Squamous carcinoma in a major salivary gland: a review of the diagnostic considerations. Arch Pathol Lab Med 2001; 125: 740–745.

640. Pisani P, Krengli M, Ramponi A, et al. Metastases to parotid gland from cancers of the upper airway and digestive tract. Br J Oral Maxillofac Surg 1998; 36: 54–57.

641. Brauneis J, Laskawi R, Schröder M, et al. Plattenepithelkarzinome im Bereich der Glandula parotis. Metastase oder Primärtumor? HNO 1990; 38: 292–294.

642. Batsakis JG, McClatchey KD, Johns M, et al. Primary squamous cell carcinoma of the parotid gland. Arch Otolaryngol Head Neck Surg 1976; 102: 355–357.

643. Ridenhour CE, Spratt JS Jr. Epidermoid carcinoma of the skin involving the parotid gland. Am J Surg 1966; 112: 504–507.

644. Jecker P, Hartwein J. Metastasis to the parotid gland: is a radical surgical approach justified? Am J Otolaryngol 1996; 17: 102–105.

645. Lee S, Kim GE, Park CS, et al. Primary squamous cell carcinoma of the parotid gland. Am J Otolaryngol 2001; 22: 400–406.

646. Klijanienko J, Vielh P. Fine-needle sampling of salivary gland lesions. VI. Cytological review of 44 cases of primary salivary squamous-cell carcinoma with histological correlation. Diagn Cytopathol 1998; 18: 174–178.

647. Ogawa I, Nikai H, Takata T, et al. Clear cell tumors of minor salivary gland origin. An immunohistochemical and ultrastructural analysis. Oral Surg Oral Med Oral Pathol 1991; 72: 200–207.

648. Lattanzi DA, Polverini P, Chin DC. Glycogen-rich adenocarcinoma of a minor salivary gland. J Oral Maxillofac Surg 1985; 43: 122–124.

649. Simpson RH, Sarsfield PT, Clarke T, et al. Clear cell carcinoma of minor salivary glands. Histopathology 1990;1 7: 433–438.

650. Chen KT. Clear cell carcinoma of the salivary gland. Hum Pathol 1983; 14: 91–93.

651. Hayashi K, Ohtsuki Y, Sonobe H, et al. Glycogen-rich clear cell carcinoma arising from minor salivary glands of the uvula. A case report. Acta Pathol Jpn 1988; 38: 1227–1234.

652. Milchgrub S, Gnepp DR, Vuitch F, et al. Hyalinizing clear cell carcinoma of salivary gland. Am J Surg Pathol 1994; 18: 74–82.

653. Ellis GL, Auclair PL. Tumors of the salivary glands. Atlas of tumor pathology, 3rd series, fascicle 17. 1st edn. Washington, DC: Armed Forces Institute of Pathology; 1996: 281–289.

654. Wang B, Brandwein M, Gordon R, et al. Primary salivary clear cell tumors – a diagnostic approach: a clinicopathologic and immunohistochemical study of 20 patients with clear cell carcinoma, clear cell myoepithelial carcinoma, and epithelial-myoepithelial carcinoma. Arch Pathol Lab Med 2002; 126: 676–685.

655. Rinaldo A, McLaren KM, Boccato P, et al. Hyalinizing clear cell carcinoma of the oral cavity and of the parotid gland. ORL J Otorhinolaryngol Relat Spec 1999; 61: 48–51.

656. Uri AK, Wetmore RF, Iozzo RV. Glycogen-rich clear cell carcinoma in the tongue. A cytochemical and ultrastructural study. Cancer 1986; 57: 1803–1809.

657. Michal M, Skalova A, Simpson RH, et al. Clear cell malignant myoepithelioma of the salivary glands. Histopathology 1996; 28: 309–315.

658. Chaudhry AP, Cutler LS, Satchidanand S, et al. Glycogen-rich tumor of the oral minor salivary glands. A histochemical and ultrastructural study. Cancer 1983; 52: 105–111.

659. Mohamed AH, Cherrick HM. Glycogen-rich adenocarcinoma of minor salivary glands. A light and electron microscopic study. Cancer 1975; 36: 1057–1066.

660. Shrestha P, Yang LT, Liu BL, et al. Clear cell carcinoma of salivary glands: immunohistochemical evaluation of clear tumor cells. Anticancer Res 1994; 14: 825–836.

661. Eversole LR. On the differential diagnosis of clear cell tumours of the head and neck. Eur J Cancer B Oral Oncol 1993; 29B: 173–179.

662. Milles M, Doyle JL, Mesa M, et al. Clear cell odontogenic carcinoma with lymph node metastasis. Oral Surg Oral Med Oral Pathol 1993; 76: 82–89.

663. Berho M, Huvos AG. Central hyalinizing clear cell carcinoma of the mandible and the maxilla: a clinicopathologic study of two cases with an analysis of the literature. Hum Pathol 1999; 30: 101–105.

664. Grenevicki LF, Barker BF, Fiorella RM, et al. Clear cell carcinoma of the palate. Int J Oral Maxillofac Surg 2001; 30: 452–454.

665. Milchgrub S, Vuitch F, Saboorian MH, et al. Hyalinizing clear-cell carcinoma of salivary glands in fine-needle aspiration. Diagn Cytopathol 2000; 23: 333–337.

666. Ellis GL, Wiscovitch JG. Basal cell adenocarcinomas of the major salivary glands. Oral Surg Oral Med Oral Pathol 1990; 69: 461–469.

667. Batsakis JG, Luna MA. Basaloid salivary carcinoma. Ann Otol Rhinol Laryngol 1991; 100: 785–787.

668. Hyman BA, Scheithauer BW, Weiland LH, et al. Membranous basal cell adenoma of the parotid gland. Malignant transformation in a patient with multiple dermal cylindromas. Arch Pathol Lab Med 1988; 112: 209–211.

669. Chen KT. Carcinoma arising in monomorphic adenoma of the salivary gland. Am J Otolaryngol 1985; 6: 39–41.

670. Klima M, Wolfe K, Johnson PE. Basal cell tumors of the parotid gland. Arch Otolaryngol Head Neck Surg 1978; 104: 111–116.

671. Evans RW, Cruickshank AH. Epithelial tumours of the salivary glands. 1st edn. Philadelphia: WB Saunders; 1970: 254.

672. Muller S, Barnes L. Basal cell adenocarcinoma of the salivary glands. Report of seven cases and review of the literature. Cancer 1996; 78: 2471–2477.

673. Ellis GL, Auclair PL. Tumors of the salivary glands. Atlas of tumor pathology, 3rd series, fascicle 17. 1st edn. Washington, DC: Armed Forces Institute of Pathology; 1996: 257–267.

674. Antonescu CR, Terzakis JA. Multiple malignant cylindromas of skin in association with basal cell adenocarcinoma with adenoid cystic features of minor salivary gland. J Cutan Pathol 1997; 24: 449–453.

675. Raslan WF, Leonetti JP, Sawyer DR. Basal cell adenocarcinoma of the parotid gland: a case report with immunohistochemical, ultrastructural findings and review of the literature. J Oral Maxillofac Surg 1995; 53: 1457–1462.

676. Quddus MR, Henley JD, Affify AM, et al. Basal cell adenocarcinoma of the salivary gland: an ultrastructural and immunohistochemical study. Oral Surg Oral Med Oral Pathol Oral Radiol Endod 1999; 87: 485–492.

677. Atula T, Klemi PJ, Donath K, et al. Basal cell adenocarcinoma of the parotid gland: a case report and review of the literature. J Laryngol Otol 1993; 107: 862–864.

678. McCluggage G, Sloan J, Cameron S, et al. Basal cell adenocarcinoma of the submandibular gland. Oral Surg Oral Med Oral Pathol Oral Radiol Endod 1995; 79: 342–350.

679. Toida M, Balazs M, Mori T, et al. Analysis of genetic alterations in salivary gland tumors by comparative genomic hybridization. Cancer Genet Cytogenet 2001; 127: 34–37.

680. Wain SL, Kier R, Vollmer RT, et al. Basaloid-squamous carcinoma of the tongue, hypopharynx, and larynx: report of 10 cases. Hum Pathol 1986; 17: 1158–1166.

681. Murty GE, Welch AR, Soames JV. Basal cell adenocarcinoma of the parotid gland. J Laryngol Otol 1990; 104: 150–151.

682. Evans RW, Cruickshank AH. Epithelial tumours of the salivary glands. 1st edn. Philadelphia: WB Saunders; 1970: 58–76.

683. Batsakis JG, Luna MA. Undifferentiated carcinomas of salivary glands. Ann Otol Rhinol Laryngol 1991; 100: 82–84.

684. Nagao K, Matsuzaki O, Saiga H, et al. Histopathologic studies of undifferentiated carcinoma of the parotid gland. Cancer 1982; 50: 1572–1579.

685. O'Brien CJ, Soong SJ, Herrera GA, et al. Malignant salivary tumors – analysis of prognostic factors and survival. Head Neck Surg 1986; 9: 82–92.

686. Ellis GL, Auclair PL. Tumors of the salivary glands. Atlas of tumor pathology, 3rd series, fascicle 17. 1st edn. Washington, DC: Armed Forces Institute of Pathology; 1996: 306–311.

687. Fiade GC, Lozano RA, Garcia CT, et al. Epidemiological study of salivary gland tumours. Rev Laryngol Otol Rhinol (Bord) 1999; 120: 331–336.

688. Tsai CC, Chen CL, Hsu HC. Expression of Epstein-Barr virus in carcinomas of major salivary glands: a strong association with lymphoepithelioma-like carcinoma. Hum Pathol 1996; 27: 258–262.

689. Sheen TS, Tsai CC, Ko JY, et al. Undifferentiated carcinoma of the major salivary glands. Cancer 1997; 80: 357–363.

690. Pollock AM, Toner M, McMenamin M, et al. Absence of Epstein-Barr virus encoded RNA and latent membrane protein (LMP1) in salivary gland neoplasms. J Laryngol Otol 1999; 113: 906–908.

691. Yaku Y, Kanda T, Yoshihara T, et al. Undifferentiated carcinoma of the parotid gland. Case report with electron microscopic findings. Virchows Arch [A] 1983; 401: 89–97.

692. Balogh K, Wolbarsht RL, Federman M, et al. Carcinoma of the parotid gland with osteoclastlike giant cells. Immunohistochemical and ultrastructural observations. Arch Pathol Lab Med 1985; 109: 756–761.

693. Hayashi Y, Aoki N. Undifferentiated carcinoma of the parotid gland with bizarre giant cells. Clinicopathologic report with ultrastructural study. Acta Pathol Jpn 1983; 33: 169–176.

694. Gelb AB, van de Rijn M, Regula DP Jr, et al. Epstein-Barr virus-associated natural killer-large granular lymphocyte leukemia. Hum Pathol 1994; 25: 953–960.

695. Regis DBS, Kowalski LP, Cavalcante DA, et al. Multivariate analysis of risk factors for neck metastases in surgically treated parotid carcinomas. Arch Otolaryngol Head Neck Surg 2001; 127: 56–60.

696. North CA, Lee DJ, Piantadosi S, et al. Carcinoma of the major salivary glands treated by surgery or surgery plus postoperative radiotherapy. Int J Radiat Oncol Biol Phys 1990; 18: 1319–1326.

697. Theriault C, Fitzpatrick PJ. Malignant parotid tumors. Prognostic factors and optimum treatment. Am J Clin Oncol 1986; 9: 510–516.

698. Matsuba HM, Thawley SE, Deviveni VR, et al. High-grade malignancies of the parotid gland: effective use of planned combined surgery and irradiation. Laryngoscope 1985; 95: 1059–1063.

699. Airoldi M, Gabriele AM, Gabriele P, et al. Concomitant chemoradiotherapy followed by adjuvant chemotherapy in parotid gland undifferentiated carcinoma. Tumori 2001; 87: 14–17.

700. Ellis GL, Auclair PL. Tumors of the salivary glands. Atlas of tumor pathology, 3rd series, fascicle 17. 1st edn. Washington, DC: Armed Forces Institute of Pathology; 1996: 296–318.

701. Eversole LR, Gnepp DR, Eversole GM. Undifferentiated carcinoma. In: Ellis GL, Auclair PL, Gnepp DR, eds. Surgical pathology of the salivary glands, 1st edn. Philadelphia: WB Saunders; 1991: 422–440.

702. Gnepp DR, Corio RL, Brannon RB. Small cell carcinoma of the major salivary glands. Cancer 1986; 58: 705–714.

703. Rollins CE, Yost BA, Costa MJ, et al. Squamous differentiation in small-cell carcinoma of the parotid gland. Arch Pathol Lab Med 1995; 119: 183–185.

704. Tischler AS, Mobtaker H, Mann K, et al. Anti-lymphocyte antibody Leu-7 (HNK-1) recognizes a constituent of neuroendocrine granule matrix. J Histochem Cytochem 1986; 34: 1213–1216.

705. Michels S, Swanson PE, Robbs JA, et al. Leu-7 in small cell neoplasms. Cancer 1987; 60: 2958–2964.

706. Gould VE, Lee I, Wiedenmann B, et al. Synaptophysin: A novel marker for neurons, certain neuroendocrine cells, and their neoplasms. Hum Pathol 1986; 17: 979–983.

707. Leader M, Collins M, Patel J, et al. Antineuron specific enolase staining reactions in sarcomas and carcinomas: Its lack of neuroendocrine specificity. J Clin Pathol 1986; 39: 1186–1192.

708. Weiler R, Fischer-Colbris R, Schmid KW, et al. Immunological studies on the occurrence and properties of chromogranin A and B and secretogranin II in endocrine tumors. Am J Surg Pathol 1988; 12: 877–884.

709. Gnepp DR, Wick MR. Small cell carcinoma of the major salivary glands. An immunohistochemical study. Cancer 1990; 66: 185–192.

710. Chan JK, Suster S, Wenig BM, et al. Cytokeratin 20 immunoreactivity distinguishes Merkel cell (primary cutaneous neuroendocrine) carcinomas and salivary gland small cell carcinomas from small cell carcinomas of various sites. Am J Surg Pathol 1997; 21: 226–234.

711. Brodsky G, Rabson AB. Metastasis to the submandibular gland as the initial presentation of small cell ('oat cell') lung carcinoma. Oral Surg Oral Med Oral Pathol 1984; 58: 76–80.

712. Shalowitz JI, Cassidy C, Anders CB. Parotid metastasis of small cell carcinoma of the lung causing facial nerve paralysis. J Oral Maxillofac Surg 1988; 46: 404–406.

713. Hisa Y, Tatemoto K. Bilateral parotid gland metastases as the initial manifestation of a small cell carcinoma of the lung. Am J Otolaryngol 1998; 19: 140–143.

714. Leipzig B, Gonzales-Vitale JC. Small cell epidermoid carcinoma of salivary glands. 'Pseudo'-oat cell carcinoma. Arch Otolaryngol Head Neck Surg 1982; 108: 511–514.

715. Henke AC, Cooley ML, Hughes JH, et al. Fine-needle aspiration cytology of small-cell carcinoma of the parotid. Diagn Cytopathol 2001; 25: 126–129.

716. Moore JG, Bocklage T. Fine-needle aspiration biopsy of large-cell undifferentiated carcinoma of the salivary glands: presentation of two cases, literature review, and differential cytodiagnosis of high-grade salivary gland malignancies. Diagn Cytopathol 1998; 19: 44–50.

717. Safneck JR, Ravinsky E, Yazdi HM, et al. Fine needle aspiration biopsy findings in lymphoepithelial carcinoma of salivary gland. Acta Cytol 1997; 41: 1023–1030.

718. Cleary KR, Batsakis JG. Undifferentiated carcinoma with lymphoid stroma of the major salivary glands. Ann Otol Rhinol Laryngol 1990; 99: 236–238.

719. Batsakis JG. Pathology consultation. Carcinoma ex lymphoepithelial lesion. Ann Otol Rhinol Laryngol 1983; 92: 657–658.

720. Hamilton-Dutoit SJ, Therkildsen MH, Neilsen NH, et al. Undifferentiated carcinoma of the salivary gland in Greenlandic Eskimos: demonstration of Epstein-Barr virus DNA by in situ nucleic acid hybridization. Hum Pathol 1991; 22: 811–815.

721. Gallo O, Santucci M, Calzolari A, et al. Epstein-Barr virus (EBV) infection and undifferentiated carcinoma of the parotid gland in Caucasian patients. Acta Otolaryngol (Stockh) 1994; 114: 572–575.

722. Borg MF, Benjamin CS, Morton RP, et al. Malignant lympho-epithelial lesion of the salivary gland: a case report and review of the literature. Australas Radiol 1993; 37: 288–291.

723. Krishnamurthy S, Lanier AP, Dohan P, et al. Salivary gland cancer in Alaskan natives, 1966–1980. (Published erratum appears in Hum Pathol 1988 Mar; 19(3): 328.) Hum Pathol 1987; 18: 986–996.

724. James PD, Ellis IO. Malignant epithelial tumours associated with autoimmune sialadenitis. J Clin Pathol 1986; 39: 497–502.

725. Kott ET, Goepfert H, Ayala AG, et al. Lymphoepithelial carcinoma (malignant lymphoepithelial lesion) of the salivary glands. Arch Otolaryngol Head Neck Surg 1984; 110: 50–53.

726. Kountakis SE, SooHoo W, Maillard A. Lymphoepithelial carcinoma of the parotid gland. Head Neck 1995; 17: 445–450.

727. Chan JK, Yip TT, Tsang WY, et al. Specific association of Epstein-Barr virus with lymphoepithelial carcinoma among tumors and tumorlike lesions of the salivary gland. Arch Pathol Lab Med 1994; 118: 994–997.

728. Hamilton-Dutoit SJ, Pallesen G. Detection of Epstein-Barr virus small RNAs in routine paraffin sections using non-isotopic RNA/RNA in situ hybridization. Histopathology 1994; 25: 101–111.

729. Leung SY, Chung LP, Yuen ST, et al. Lymphoepithelial carcinoma of the salivary gland: in situ detection of Epstein-Barr virus. J Clin Pathol 1995; 48: 1022–1027.

730. Nagao T, Ishida Y, Sugano I, et al. Epstein-Barr virus-associated undifferentiated carcinoma with lymphoid stroma of the salivary gland in Japanese patients.

Comparison with benign lymphoepithelial lesion. Cancer 1996; 78: 695–703.

731. Karja V, Syrjanen K, Syrjanen S. No Epstein Barr and cytomegalovirus DNA found in salivary gland tumours. ORL J Otorhinolaryngol Relat Spec 1997; 59: 97–99.

732. Wen S, Mizugaki Y, Shinozaki F, et al. Epstein-Barr virus (EBV) infection in salivary gland tumors: lytic EBV infection in nonmalignant epithelial cells surrounded by EBV-positive T-lymphoma cells. Virology 1997; 227: 484–487.

733. Ellis GL, Auclair PL. Tumors of the salivary glands. Atlas of tumor pathology, 3rd series, fascicle 17. 1st edn. Washington, DC: Armed Forces Institute of Pathology; 1996: 311–318.

734. Albeck H, Nielsen NH, Hansen HE, et al. Epidemiology of nasopharyngeal and salivary gland carcinoma in Greenland. Arctic Med Res 1992; 51: 189–195.

735. Autio-Harmainen H, Pääkkö P, Alavaikko M, et al. Familial occurrence of malignant lymphoepithelial lesion of the parotid gland in a Finnish family with dominantly inherited trichoepithelioma. Cancer 1988; 61: 161–166.

736. Merrick Y, Albeck H, Nielsen NH, et al. Familial clustering of salivary gland carcinoma in Greenland. Cancer 1986; 57: 2097–2102.

737. Worley NK, Daroca PJ Jr. Lymphoepithelial carcinoma of the minor salivary gland. Arch Otolaryngol Head Neck Surg 1997; 123: 638–640.

738. Saw D, Lau WH, Ho JH, et al. Malignant lymphoepithelial lesion of the salivary gland. Hum Pathol 1986; 17: 914–923.

739. Kitazawa M, Ohnishi Y, Nonomura N, et al. Malignant lymphoepithelial lesion. Acta Pathol Jpn 1987; 37: 515–526.

740. Sehested M, Hainau B, Albeck H, et al. Ultrastructural investigation of anaplastic salivary gland carcinomas in Eskimos. Cancer 1985; 55: 2732–2736.

741. Wanamaker JR, Kraus DH, Biscotti CV, et al. Undifferentiated nasopharyngeal carcinoma presenting as a parotid mass. Head Neck 1994; 16: 589–593.

742. Bosch JD, Kudryk WH, Johnson GH. The malignant lymphoepithelial lesion of the salivary glands. J Otolaryngol 1988; 17: 187–190.

743. Ellis GL, Auclair PL. Tumors of the salivary glands. Atlas of tumor pathology, 3rd series, fascicle 17. 1st edn. Washington, DC: Armed Forces Institute of Pathology; 1996: 289–296.

744. Ellis GL, Auclair PL, Gnepp DR, Goode RK. Other malignant epithelial neoplasms. In: Ellis GL, Auclair PL, Gnepp DR, eds Surgical pathology of the salivary glands. 1st edn. Philadelphia: WB Saunders; 1991: 455–488.

745. Thackray AC, Lucas RB. Tumors of the major salivary glands. Atlas of tumor pathology, 2nd series, fascicle 10. Washington, DC: Armed Forces Institute of Pathology; 1974: 11–14.

746. Foss RD, Ellis GL, Auclair PL. Salivary gland cystadenocarcinomas. A clinicopathologic study of 57 cases. Am J Surg Pathol 1996; 20: 1440–1447.

747. Shteyer A, Fundoianu-Dayan D. Papillary cystic adenocarcinoma of minor salivary glands. Int J Oral Maxillofac Surg 1986; 15: 361–364.

748. Danford M, Eveson JW, Flood TR. Papillary cystadenocarcinoma of the sublingual gland presenting as a ranula. Br J Oral Maxillofac Surg 1992; 30: 270–272.

749. Chen XM. [Papillary cystadenocarcinoma of the salivary glands: clinicopathologic analysis of 22 cases]. Chinese language article, English abstract. Chung Hua Kou Chiang Hsueh Tsa Chih 1990; 25: 102–104, 126.

750. Simpson RH, Clarke TJ, Sarsfield PT, et al. Salivary duct adenocarcinoma. Histopathology 1991; 18: 229–235.

751. Hui KK, Batsakis JG, Luna MA, et al. Salivary duct adenocarcinoma: a high grade malignancy. J Laryngol Otol 1986; 100: 105–114.

752. Anderson C, Muller R, Piorkowski R, et al. Intraductal carcinoma of major salivary gland (see comments). Cancer 1992; 69: 609–614.

753. Colmenero Ruiz C, Patrón Romero M, Martín P: Salivary duct carcinoma: a report of nine cases. J Oral Maxillofac Surg 1993; 51: 641–646.

754. Delgado R, Vuitch F, Albores-Saavedra J. Salivary duct carcinoma. Cancer 1993; 72: 1503–1512.

755. Butterworth DM, Jones AW, Kotecha B. Salivary duct carcinoma: report of a case and review of the literature. Virchows Arch [A] 1992; 420: 371–374.

756. Murrah VA, Batsakis JG. Salivary duct carcinoma. Ann Otol Rhinol Laryngol 1994; 103: 244–247.

757. Ellis GL, Auclair PL. Tumors of the salivary glands. Atlas of tumor pathology, 3rd series, fascicle 17. 1st edn. Washington, DC: Armed Forces Institute of Pathology; 1996: 324–333.

758. Barnes L, Rao U, Krause J, et al. Salivary duct carcinoma. Part I. A clinicopathologic evaluation and DNA image analysis of 13 cases with review of the literature. Oral Surg Oral Med Oral Pathol 1994; 78: 64–73.

759. Felix A, el-Naggar AK, Press MF, et al. Prognostic significance of biomarkers (c-erbB-2, p53, proliferating cell nuclear antigen, and DNA content) in salivary duct carcinoma. Hum Pathol 1996; 27: 561–566.

760. Lewis JE, McKinney BC, Weiland LH, et al. Salivary duct carcinoma. Clinicopathologic and immunohistochemical review of 26 cases. Cancer 1996; 77: 223–230.

761. Brandwein MS, Jagirdar J, Patil J, et al. Salivary duct carcinoma (cribriform salivary carcinoma of excretory ducts). A clinicopathologic and immunohistochemical study of 12 cases. Cancer 1990; 65: 2307–2314.

762. Minamiguchi S, Iwasa Y, Shoji K, et al. Salivary duct carcinoma: a clinicopathologic study of three cases with a review of the literature. Pathol Int 1996; 46: 614–622.

763. Barnes L, Rao U, Contis L, et al. Salivary duct carcinoma. Part II. Immunohistochemical evaluation of 13 cases for estrogen and progesterone receptors, cathepsin D, and c-erbB-2 protein. Oral Surg Oral Med Oral Pathol 1994; 78: 74–80.

764. Hellquist HB, Karlsson MG, Nilsson C. Salivary duct carcinoma – a highly aggressive salivary gland tumour with overexpression of c-erbB-2. J Pathol 1994; 172: 35–44.

765. Kapadia SB, Barnes L. Expression of androgen receptor, gross cystic disease fluid protein, and CD44 in salivary duct carcinoma. Mod Pathol 1998; 11: 1033–1038.

766. Wick MR, Ockner DM, Mills SE, et al. Homologous carcinomas of the breasts, skin, and salivary glands. A histologic and immunohistochemical comparison of ductal mammary carcinoma, ductal sweat gland carcinoma, and salivary duct carcinoma. Am J Clin Pathol 1998; 109: 75–84.

767. Fan CY, Wang J, Barnes EL. Expression of androgen receptor and prostatic specific markers in salivary duct carcinoma: an immunohistochemical analysis of 13 cases and review of the literature. Am J Surg Pathol 2000; 24: 579–586.

768. Moriki T, Ueta S, Takahashi T, et al. Salivary duct carcinoma: cytologic characteristics and application of androgen receptor immunostaining for diagnosis. Cancer 2001; 93: 344–350.

769. James GK, Pudek M, Berean KW, et al. Salivary duct carcinoma secreting prostate-specific antigen. Am J Clin Pathol 1996; 106: 242–247.

770. Martinez-Barba E, Cortes-Guardiola JA, Minguela-Puras A, et al. Salivary duct carcinoma: clinicopathological and immunohistochemical studies. J Craniomaxillofac Surg 1997; 25: 328–334.

771. Ishii K, Nakajima T. Evaluation of malignant grade of salivary gland tumors: studies by cytofluorometric nuclear DNA analysis, histochemistry for nucleolar organizer regions and immunohistochemistry for p53. Pathol Int 1994; 44: 287–296.

772. Grenko RT, Gemryd P, Tytor M, et al. Salivary duct carcinoma. Histopathology 1995; 26: 261–266.

773. de Araújo VC, de Souza SO, Sesso A, et al. Salivary duct carcinoma: ultrastructural and histogenetic considerations. Oral Surg Oral Med Oral Pathol 1987; 63: 592–596.

774. Garland TA, Innes DJ Jr, Fechner RE. Salivary duct carcinoma: an analysis of four cases with review of literature. Am J Clin Pathol 1984; 81: 436–441.

775. Brandwein M, Biller H. Intraductal carcinoma of major salivary gland (letter; comment). Cancer 1992; 70: 1202.

776. Guzzo M, Di Palma S, Grandi C, et al. Salivary duct carcinoma: clinical characteristics and treatment strategies. Head Neck 1997; 19: 126–133.

777. Elsheikh TM, Bernacki EG Jr, Pisharodi L. Fine-needle aspiration cytology of salivary duct carcinoma. Diagn Cytopathol 1994; 11: 47–51.

778. Fyrat P, Cramer H, Feczko JD, et al. Fine-needle aspiration biopsy of salivary duct carcinoma: report of five cases. Diagn Cytopathol 1997; 16: 526–530.

779. Garcia-Bonafe M, Catala I, Tarragona J, et al. Cytologic diagnosis of salivary duct carcinoma: a review of seven cases. Diagn Cytopathol 1998; 19: 120–123.

780. Klijanienko J, Vielh P. Cytologic characteristics and histomorphologic correlations of 21 salivary duct carcinomas. Diagn Cytopathol 1998; 19: 333–337.

781. Gilcrease MZ, Guzman-Paz M, Froberg K, et al. Salivary duct carcinoma. Is a specific diagnosis possible by fine needle aspiration cytology? Acta Cytol 1998; 42: 1389–1396.

782. Khurana KK, Pitman MB, Powers CN, et al. Diagnostic pitfalls of aspiration cytology of salivary duct carcinoma. Cancer 1997; 81: 373–378.

783. Ellis GL, Auclair PL. Tumors of the salivary glands. Atlas of tumor pathology, 3rd series, fascicle 17. 1st edn. Washington, DC: Armed Forces Institute of Pathology; 1996: 318–324.

784. Goode RK, Corio RL. Oncocytic adenocarcinoma of salivary glands. Oral Surg Oral Med Oral Pathol 1988; 65: 61–66.

785. Ziegler M, Maibach EA, Ussmuller J. Malignes Onkozytom der Glandula submandibularis. Laryngol Rhinol Otol 1992; 71: 423–425.

786. Sugimoto T, Wakizono S, Uemura T, et al. Malignant oncocytoma of the parotid gland: a case report with an immunohistochemical and ultrastructural study. J Laryngol Otol 1993; 107: 69–74.

787. Ramakrishna B, Perakath B, Chandi SM. Malignant 'multinodular' oncocytoma of parotid gland – a case report and literature review. Indian J Cancer 1992; 29: 230–233.

788. Nakada M, Nishizaki K, Akagi H, et al. Oncocytic carcinoma of the submandibular gland: a case report and literature review. J Oral Pathol Med 1998; 27: 225–228.

789. Ruby SG, Kish JK. Oncocytic adenocarcinoma of minor salivary gland. An unusual glossal presentation of a minor salivary gland tumor. Pathol Res Pract 1996; 192: 856–864.

790. Lee SC, Roth LM. Malignant oncocytoma of the parotid gland. A light and electron microscopic study. Cancer 1976; 37: 1606–1614.

791. Johns ME, Regezi JA, Batsakis JG. Oncocytic neoplasms of salivary glands: an ultrastructural study. Laryngoscope 1977; 87: 862–871.

792. Gnepp DR, Brannon R. Sebaceous neoplasms of salivary gland origin. Report of 21 cases. Cancer 1984; 53: 2155–2170.

793. Ohara N, Taguchi K, Yamamoto M, et al. Sebaceous carcinoma of the submandibular gland with high-grade malignancy: report of a case. Pathol Int 1998; 48: 287–291.

794. Hill DS, Ellis GL, Gatland DJ. A unique parotid adenocarcinoma. J Laryngol Otol 2000; 114: 402–404.

795. Di Palma S, Guzzo M. Malignant myoepithelioma of salivary glands: clinicopathological features of ten

cases. Virchows Arch A Pathol Anat Histopathol 1993; 423: 389–396.

796. Ellis GL, Auclair PL. Tumors of the salivary glands. Atlas of tumor pathology, 3rd series, fascicle 17. 1st edn. Washington, DC: Armed Forces Institute of Pathology; 1996: 337–343.

797. Nagao T, Sugano I, Ishida Y, et al. Salivary gland malignant myoepithelioma: a clinicopathologic and immunohistochemical study of ten cases. Cancer 1998; 83: 1292–1299.

798. Wang J, Wu Q, Sun K, et al. Quantitative multivariate analysis of myoepithelioma and myoepithelial carcinoma. Int J Oral Maxillofac Surg 1995; 24: 153–157.

799. Alos L, Cardesa A, Bombi JA, et al. Myoepithelial tumors of salivary glands: a clinicopathologic, immunohistochemical, ultrastructural, and flow-cytometric study. Semin Diagn Pathol 1996; 13: 138–147.

800. Savera AT, Sloman A, Huvos AG, et al. Myoepithelial carcinoma of the salivary glands: a clinicopathologic study of 25 patients. Am J Surg Pathol 2000; 24: 761–774.

801. Saxe SJ, Grossniklaus HE, Someren AO. Malignant myoepithelioma after radiation for retinoblastoma (letter). Am J Ophthalmol 1992; 114: 512–513.

802. Takeda Y. Malignant myoepithelioma of minor salivary gland origin. Acta Pathol Jpn 1992; 42: 518–522.

803. de Araújo VC, de Araújo NS. Vimentin as a marker of myoepithelial cells in salivary gland tumors. Eur Arch Otorhinolaryngol 1990; 247: 252–255.

804. Herrera GA. Light microscopic, ultrastructural and immunocytochemical spectrum of malignant lacrimal and salivary gland tumors, including malignant mixed tumors (published erratum appears in Pathobiology 1991; 59(1): 56). Pathobiology 1990; 58: 312–322.

805. Singh R, Cawson RA. Malignant myoepithelial carcinoma (myoepithelioma) arising in a pleomorphic adenoma of the parotid gland. An immunohistochemical study and review of the literature. Oral Surg Oral Med Oral Pathol 1988; 66: 65–70.

806. Dardick I. Malignant myoepithelioma of parotid salivary gland. Ultrastruct Pathol 1985; 9: 163–168.

807. Crissman JD, Wirman JA, Harris A. Malignant myoepithelioma of the parotid gland. Cancer 1977; 40: 3042–3049.

808. Stromeyer FW, Haggitt RC, Nelson JF, et al. Myoepithelioma of minor salivary gland origin. Light and electron microscopical study. Arch Pathol 1975; 99: 242–245.

809. Carrillo R, el-Naggar AK, Luna MA, et al. Nucleolar organizer regions (NORs) and myoepitheliomas: a comparison with DNA content and clinical course. J Laryngol Otol 1992; 106: 616–620.

810. Ibrahim R, Bird DJ, Sieler MW. Malignant myoepithelioma of the larynx with massive metastatic spread to the liver: an ultrastructural and immunocytochemical study. Ultrastruct Pathol 1991; 15: 69–76.

811. el-Naggar A, Batsakis JG, Luna MA, et al. DNA content and proliferative activity of myoepitheliomas. J Laryngol Otol 1989; 103: 1192–1197.

812. Gerughty RM, Hennigar GR, Brown FM. Adenosquamous carcinoma of the nasal, oral and laryngeal cavities. A clinicopathologic survey of ten cases. Cancer 1968; 22: 1140–1155.

813. Siar CH, Ng KH. Adenosquamous carcinoma of the floor of the mouth and lower alveolus: a radiation-induced lesion? Oral Surg Oral Med Oral Pathol 1987; 63: 216–220.

814. Martinez-Madrigal F, Baden E, Casiraghi O, et al. Oral and pharyngeal adenosquamous carcinoma. A report of four cases with immunohistochemical studies. Eur Arch Otorhinolaryngol 1991; 248: 255–258.

815. Peel RL, Gnepp DR. Diseases of the salivary glands. In: Barnes L, ed. Surgical pathology of the head and neck. 1st edn. New York: Marcel Dekker; 1985: 533–645.

816. Ellis GL, Gnepp DR. Unusual salivary gland tumors. In: Gnepp DR, ed. Pathology of the head and neck. 1st edn. New York: Churchill Livingstone; 1988: 585–661.

817. Minic AJ, Stajcic Z. Adenosquamous carcinoma of the inferior turbinate: a case report. J Oral Maxillofac Surg 1994; 52: 764–767.

818. Ellis GL, Auclair PL. Tumors of the salivary glands. Atlas of tumor pathology, 3rd series, fascicle 17. 1st edn. Washington, DC: Armed Forces Institute of Pathology; 1996: 343–349.

819. Jones AC, Freedman PD, Kerpel SM. Oral adenoid squamous cell carcinoma: a report of three cases and review of the literature. J Oral Maxillofac Surg 1993; 51: 676–681.

820. Gleeson MJ, Bennett MH, Cawson RA. Lymphomas of salivary glands. Cancer 1986; 58: 699–704.

821. Colby TV, Dorfman RF. Malignant lymphomas involving the salivary glands. Pathol Annu 1979; 14(Pt 2): 307–324.

822. Hyman GA, Wolff M. Malignant lymphomas of the salivary glands. Review of the literature and report of 33 new cases, including four cases associated with the lymphoepithelial lesion. Am J Clin Pathol 1976; 65: 421–438.

823. Watkin GT, MacLennan KA, Hobsley M. Lymphomas presenting as lumps in the parotid region. Br J Surg 1984; 71: 701–702.

824. Schusterman MA, Granick MS, Erikson ER, et al. Lyphoma presenting as a salivary gland mass. Head Neck Surg 1988; 10: 411–415.

825. Sciubba JJ, Auclair PL, Ellis GL. Malignant lymphomas. In: Ellis GL, Auclair PL, Gnepp DR, eds. Surgical pathology of the salivary glands. Philadelphia: WB Saunders; 1991: 528–543.

826. Ellis GL, Auclair PL. Tumors of the salivary glands. Atlas of tumor pathology, 3rd series, fascicle 17. 1st edn. Washington, DC: Armed Forces Institute of Pathology; 1996: 387–399.

827. Schmid U, Helbron D, Lennert K. Primary malignant lymphomas localized in salivary glands. Histopathology 1982; 6: 673–687.

828. Burke JS. Waldeyer's ring, sinonasal region, salivary gland, thyroid gland, central nervous system, and other extranodal lymphomas and lymphoid hyperplasias. In: Knowles DM, ed. Neoplastic Hematopathology. Baltimore: Williams & Wilkins; 1992: 1047–1079.

829. Harris NL. Lymphoid proliferations of the salivary glands. Am J Clin Pathol 1999; 111: S94–S103.

830. Hew WS, Carey FA, Kernohan NM, et al. Primary T cell lymphoma of salivary gland: a report of a case and review of the literature. J Clin Pathol 2002; 55: 61–63.

831. Harris NL, Jaffe ES, Stein H, et al. A revised European-American classification of lymphoid neoplasms: a proposal from the International Lymphoma Study Group (see comments). Blood 1994; 84: 1361–1392.

832. Harris NL, Jaffe ES, Diebold J, et al. The World Health Organization classification of hematological malignancies. Report of the Clinical Advisory Committee Meeting, Airlie House, Virginia, November 1997. Mod Pathol 2000; 13: 193–207.

833. Ngan BY, Warnke RA, Wilson M, et al. Monocytoid B-cell lymphoma: a study of 36 cases. Hum Pathol 1991; 22: 409–421.

834. Shin SS, Sheibani K, Fishleder A, et al. Monocytoid B-cell lymphoma in patients with Sjögren's syndrome: a clinicopathologic study of 13 patients. Hum Pathol 1991; 22: 422–430.

835. Harris NL. Low-grade B-cell lymphoma of mucosa-associated lymphoid tissue and monocytoid B-cell lymphoma. Related entities that are distinct from other low-grade B-cell lymphomas (editorial; comment). Arch Pathol Lab Med 1993; 117: 771–775.

836. Sheibani K, Burke JS, Swartz WG, et al. Monocytoid B-cell lymphoma. Clinicopathologic study of 21 cases of a unique type of low-grade lymphoma. Cancer 1988; 62: 1531–1538.

837. Nathwani BN, Mohrmann RL, Brynes RK, et al. Monocytoid B-cell lymphomas: an assessment of diagnostic criteria and a perspective on histogenesis. Hum Pathol 1992; 23: 1061–1071.

838. Isaacson PG, Spencer J. Monocytoid B-cell lymphomas (comment). Am J Surg Pathol 1990; 14: 888–891.

839. Slovak ML, Weiss LM, Nathwani BN, et al. Cytogenetic studies of composite lymphomas: monocytoid B-cell lymphoma and other B-cell non-Hodgkin's lymphomas. Hum Pathol 1993; 24: 1086–1094.

840. Sheibani K, Sohn CC, Burke JS, et al. Monocytoid B-cell lymphoma. A novel B-cell neoplasm. Am J Pathol 1986; 124: 310–318.

841. Weiss LM. Monocytoid B-cell lymphoma (editorial; comment). Hum Pathol 1991; 22: 407–408.

842. Isaacson PG. Extranodal lymphomas: the MALT concept. Verh Dtsch Ges Pathol 1992; 76: 14–23.

843. Isaacson P, Wright DH. Extranodal malignant lymphoma arising from mucosa-associated lymphoid tissue. Cancer 1984; 53: 2515–2524.

844. Isaacson PG, Spencer J. Malignant lymphoma of mucosa-associated lymphoid tissue. Histopathology 1987; 11: 445–462.

845. Isaacson P, Wright DH. Malignant lymphoma of mucosa-associated lymphoid tissue. A distinctive type of B-cell lymphoma. Cancer 1983; 52: 1410–1416.

846. Hsi ED, Zukerberg LR, Schnitzer B, et al. Development of extrasalivary gland lymphoma in myoepithelial sialadenitis. Mod Pathol 1995; 8: 817–824.

847. Banks PM, Isaacson PG. MALT lymphomas in 1997. Where do we stand? Am J Clin Pathol 1999; 111: S75–S83.

848. Rosenstiel DB, Carroll WR, Listinsky CM. MALT lymphoma presenting as a cystic salivary gland mass. Head Neck 2001; 23: 254–258.

849. Schmid U, Lennert K, Gloor F. Immunosialadenitis (Sjögren's syndrome) and lymphoproliferation. Clin Exp Rheumatol 1989; 7: 175–180.

850. Biasi D, Caramaschi P, Ambrosetti A, et al. Mucosa-associated lymphoid tissue lymphoma of the salivary glands occurring in patients affected by Sjögren's syndrome: report of 6 cases. Acta Haematol 2001; 105: 83–88.

851. Utz GL, Swerdlow SH. Distinction of follicular hyperplasia from follicular lymphoma in B5-fixed tissues: comparison of MT2 and bcl-2 antibodies. Hum Pathol 1993; 24: 1155–1158.

852. Griesser H. Applied molecular genetics in the diagnosis of malignant non-Hodgkin's lymphoma. Diagn Mol Pathol 1993; 2: 177–191.

853. Zukerberg LR, Medeiros LJ, Ferry JA, et al. Diffuse low-grade B-cell lymphomas. Four clinically distinct subtypes defined by a combination of morphologic and immunophenotypic features. Am J Clin Pathol 1993; 100: 373–385.

854. Sundeen JT, Longo DL, Jaffe ES. CD5 expression in B-cell small lymphocytic malignancies. Am J Surg Pathol 1992; 16: 130–137.

855. Isaacson PG, Spencer J, Finn T. Primary B-cell gastric lymphoma. Hum Pathol 1986; 17: 72–82.

856. Harris NL, Isaacson PG. What are the criteria for distinguishing MALT from non-MALT lymphoma at extranodal sites? Am J Clin Pathol 1999; 111: S126–S132.

857. Fishleder A, Tubbs R, Hesse B, et al. Uniform detection of immunoglobulin-gene rearrangement in benign lymphoepithelial lesions. N Engl J Med 1987; 316: 1118–1121.

858. Diss TC, Wotherspoon AC, Speight P, et al. B-cell monoclonality, Epstein-Barr virus, and t(14;18) in myoepithelial sialadenitis and low-grade B-cell MALT lymphoma of the parotid gland. Am J Surg Pathol 1995; 19: 531–536.

859. Quintana PG, Kapadia SB, Bahler DW, et al. Salivary gland lymphoid infiltrates associated with lymphoepithelial lesions: a clinicopathologic,

immunophenotypic, and genotypic study (see comments). Hum Pathol 1997; 28: 850–861.

860. Hsi ED, Siddiqui J, Schnitzer B, et al. Analysis of immunoglobulin heavy chain gene rearrangement in myoepithelial sialadenitis by polymerase chain reaction. Am J Clin Pathol 1996; 106: 498–503.

861. Kurtin PJ. How do you distinguish benign from malignant extranodal small B-cell proliferations? Am J Clin Pathol 1999; 111: S119–S125.

862. Qin C, Pan Y, Hashimoto J, et al. Destructive processes of salivary gland parenchyma and development of epimyoepithelial islands assessed by immunohistochemistry. Arch Anat Cytol Pathol 1994; 42: 16–25.

863. Ihrler S, Zietz C, Sendelhofert A, et al. Lymphoepithelial duct lesions in Sjögren-type sialadenitis. Virchows Arch 1999; 434: 315–323.

864. Daniels TE. Benign lymphoepithelial lesion and Sjögren's syndrome. In: Ellis GL, Auclair PL, Gnepp DR, eds. Surgical pathology of the salivary glands. 1st edn. Philadelphia: WB Saunders; 1991: 83–106.

865. Manthorpe R. New criteria for diagnosing Sjögren's syndrome: a step forward? – or… Scand J Rheumatol Suppl 2001; 115: 14–20.

866. Ellis GL, Auclair PL. Tumors of the salivary glands. Atlas of tumor pathology, 3rd series, fascicle 17. 1st edn. Washington, DC: Armed Forces Institute of Pathology; 1996: 411–440.

867. Dardick I, van Nostrand AW, Rippstein P, et al. Characterization of epimyoepithelial islands in benign lymphoepithelial lesions of major salivary gland: an immunohistochemical and ultrastructural study. Head Neck Surg 1988; 10: 168–178.

868. Bridges AJ, England DM. Benign lymphoepithelial lesion: relationship to Sjögren's syndrome and evolving malignant lymphoma. Semin Arthritis Rheum 1989; 19: 201–208.

869. Andrade RE, Hagen KA, Manivel JC. Distribution and immunophenotype of the inflammatory cell population in the benign lymphoepithelial lesion (Mikulicz's disease). Hum Pathol 1988; 19: 932–941.

870. Palmer RM, Eveson JW, Gusterson BA. Epimyoepithelial islands in lymphoepithelial lesions. An immunocytochemical study. Virchows Arch A Pathol Anat Histopathol 1986; 408: 603–609.

871. Falzon M, Isaacson PG. The natural history of benign lymphoepithelial lesion of the salivary gland in which there is a monoclonal population of B cells. A report of two cases. Am J Surg Pathol 1991; 15: 59–65.

872. Seifert G. Tumour-like lesions of the salivary glands. The new WHO classification. Pathol Res Pract 1992; 188: 836–846.

873. Pisa EK, Pisa P, Kang HI, et al. High frequency of t(14;18) translocation in salivary gland lymphomas from Sjögren's syndrome patients. J Exp Med 1991; 174: 1245–1250.

874. Jordan RC, Odell EW, Speight PM. B-cell monoclonality in salivary lymphoepithelial lesions. Eur J Cancer B Oral Oncol 1996; 32B: 38–44.

875. Bahler DW, Swerdlow SH. Clonal salivary gland infiltrates associated with myoepithelial sialadenitis (Sjögren's syndrome) begin as nonmalignant antigen-selected expansions. Blood 1998; 91: 1864–1872.

876. Carbone A, Gloghini A, Ferlito A. Pathological features of lymphoid proliferations of the salivary glands: lymphoepithelial sialadenitis versus low–grade B-cell lymphoma of the MALT type. Ann Otol Rhinol Laryngol 2000; 109: 1170–1175.

877. Shigematsu H, Shigematsu Y, Noguchi Y, et al. Experimental study on necrotizing sialometaplasia of the palate in rats. Role of local anesthetic injections. Int J Oral Maxillofac Surg 1996; 25: 239–241.

878. Imbery TA, Edwards PA. Necrotizing sialometaplasia: literature review and case reports. J Am Dent Assoc 1996; 127: 1087–1092.

879. Brannon RB, Fowler CB, Hartman KS. Necrotizing sialometaplasia. A clinicopathologic study of sixty-nine cases and review of the literature. Oral Surg Oral Med Oral Pathol 1991; 72: 317–325.

880. Daudia A, Murty GE. First case of full-thickness palatal necrotizing sialometaplasia. J Laryngol Otol 2002; 116: 219–220.

881. Jensen JL. Idiopathic diseases. In: Ellis GL, Auclair PL, Gnepp DR, eds. Surgical pathology of the salivary glands. 1st edn. Philadelphia: WB Saunders; 1991: 60–82.

882. Gallina E, Gallo O, Boccuzzi S, et al. Analysis of 185 submandibular gland excisions. Acta Otorhinolaryngol Belg 1990; 44: 7–10.

883. Crabtree GM, Yarington CT. Submandibular gland excision. Laryngoscope 1988; 98: 1044–1045.

884. Chan JK. Kuttner tumor (chronic sclerosing sialadenitis) of the submandibular gland: an underrecognized entity. Adv Anat Pathol 1998; 5: 239–251.

885. Harrison JD, Epivatianos A, Bhatia SN. Role of microliths in the aetiology of chronic submandibular sialadenitis: a clinicopathological investigation of 154 cases. Histopathology 1997; 31: 237–251.

886. Kondratowicz GM, Smallman LA, Morgan DW. Clinicopathological study of myoepithelial sialadenitis and chronic sialadenitis (sialolithiasis). J Clin Pathol 1988; 41: 403–409.

887. van der Walt JD, Leake J. Granulomatous sialadenitis of the major salivary glands. A clinicopathological study of 57 cases. Histopathology 1987; 11: 131–144.

888. Isacsson G, Isberg A, Haverling M, et al. Salivary calculi and chronic sialadenitis of the submandibular gland: a radiographic and histologic study. Oral Surg Oral Med Oral Pathol 1984; 58: 622–627.

889. Bates D, O'Brien CJ, Tikaram K, et al. Parotid and submandibular sialadenitis treated by salivary gland excision. Aust NZ J Surg 1998; 68: 120–124.

890. Harrison JD, Triantafyllou A, Baldwin D, et al. Histochemical and biochemical determination of calcium in salivary glands with particular reference to chronic submandibular sialadenitis. Virchows Arch A Pathol Anat Histopathol 1993; 423: 29–32.

891. Therkildsen MH, Nielsen BA, Krogdahl A. A case of granulomatous sialadenitis of the submandibular gland. APMIS 1989; 97: 75–78.

892. Testa Riva F, Riva A, Puxeddu P. Ciliated cells in the main excretory duct of the submandibular gland in obstructive sialadenitis: a SEM and TEM study. Ultrastruct Pathol 1987; 11: 1–10.

893. Isacsson G, Lundquist PG. Salivary calculi as an aetiological factor in chronic sialadenitis of the submandibular gland. Clin Otolaryngol 1982; 7: 231–236.

894. Eveson JW. Troublesome tumours 2: borderline tumours of salivary glands. J Clin Pathol 1992; 45: 369–377.

895. Tal H, Altini M, Lemmer J. Multiple mucous retention cysts of the oral mucosa. Oral Surg Oral Med Oral Pathol 1984; 58: 692–695.

896. Koudelka BK. Obstructive disorders. In: Ellis GL, Auclair PL, Gnepp DR, eds. Surgical pathology of the salivary glands. 1st edn. Philadelphia: WB Saunders; 1991: 26–38.

897. Das S, Das AK. A review of pediatric oral biopsies from a surgical pathology service in a dental school. Pediatr Dent 1993; 15: 208–211.

898. Toida M, Ishimaru JI, Hobo N. A simple cryosurgical method for treatment of oral mucous cysts. Int J Oral Maxillofac Surg 1993; 22: 353–355.

899. Pieterse AS, Seymour AE. Parotid cysts. An analysis of 16 cases and suggested classification. Pathology 1981; 13: 225–234.

900. Cohen MN, Rao U, Shedd DP. Benign cysts of the parotid gland. J Surg Oncol 1984; 27: 85–88.

901. Brown E, August M, Pilch BZ, et al. Polycystic disease of the parotid glands. Am J Neuroradiol 1995; 16: 1128–1131.

902. Ficarra G, Sapp JP, Christensen RE, et al. Dysgenetic polycystic disease of the parotid gland: report of case. J Oral Maxillofac Surg 1996; 54: 1246–1249.

903. Fujibayashi T, Itoh H. Lymphoepithelial (so-called branchial) cyst within the parotid gland. Report of a case and review of the literature. Int J Oral Surg 1981; 10: 283–292.

904. Antoniadis K, Karakasis D, Tzarou V, et al. Benign cysts of the parotid gland. Int J Oral Maxillofac Surg 1990; 19: 139–140.

905. Cleary KR, Batsakis JG. Lymphoepithelial cysts of the parotid region: a new face on an old lesion. Ann Otol Rhinol Laryngol 1990; 99: 162–164.

906. Huang RD, Pearlman S, Friedman WH, et al. Benign cystic vs. solid lesions of the parotid gland in HIV patients. Head Neck 1991; 13: 522–527.

907. Terry JH, Loree TR, Thomas MD, et al. Major salivary gland lymphoepithelial lesions and the acquired immunodeficiency syndrome. Am J Surg 1991; 162: 324–329.

908. Shaha AR, DiMaio T, Webber C, et al. Benign lymphoepithelial lesions of the parotid. Am J Surg 1993; 166: 403–406.

909. Goldstein J, Rubin J, Silver C, et al. Radiation therapy as a treatment for benign lymphoepithelial parotid cysts in patients infected with human immunodeficiency virus-1. Int J Radiat Oncol Biol Phys 1992; 23: 1045–1050.

910. Mandel L, Reich R. HIV parotid gland lymphoepithelial cysts. Review and case reports. Oral Surg Oral Med Oral Pathol 1992; 74: 273–278.

911. Mandel L, Kim D, Uy C. Parotid gland swelling in HIV diffuse infiltrative CD8 lymphocytosis syndrome. Oral Surg Oral Med Oral Pathol Oral Radiol Endod 1998; 85: 565–568.

912. Mandel L, Hong J. HIV-associated parotid lymphoepithelial cysts. J Am Dent Assoc 1999; 130: 528–532.

913. McArthur CP, Subtil-DeOliveira A, Palmer D, et al. Characteristics of salivary diffuse infiltrative lymphocytosis syndrome in West Africa. Arch Pathol Lab Med 2000; 124: 1773–1779.

914. Schiødt M, Greenspan D, Daniels TE, et al. Parotid gland enlargement and xerostomia associated with labial sialadenitis in HIV-infected patients. J Autoimmun 1989; 2: 415–425.

915. Mulligan R, Navazesh M, Komaroff E, et al. Salivary gland disease in human immunodeficiency virus-positive women from the WIHS study. Women's Interagency HIV Study. Oral Surg Oral Med Oral Pathol Oral Radiol Endod 2000; 89: 702–709.

916. Schiødt M. HIV-associated salivary gland disease: a review. Oral Surg Oral Med Oral Pathol 1992; 73: 164–167.

917. Labouyrie E, Merlio JP, Beylot-Barry M, et al. Human immunodeficiency virus type 1 replication within cystic lymphoepithelial lesion of the salivary gland. Am J Clin Pathol 1993; 100: 41–46.

918. Chetty R, Vaithilingum M, Thejpal R. Epstein-Barr virus status and the histopathological changes of parotid gland lymphoid infiltrates in HIV-positive children. Pathology 1999; 31: 413–417.

919. Uccini S, Riva E, Antonelli G, et al. The benign cystic lymphoepithelial lesion of the parotid gland is a viral reservoir in HIV type 1-infected patients. AIDS Res Hum Retroviruses 1999; 15: 1339–1344.

920. Ferraro FJ Jr, Rush BF Jr, Ruark D, et al. Enucleation of parotid lymphoepithelial cyst in patients who are human immunodeficiency virus positive. Surg Gynecol Obstet 1993; 177: 524–526.

921. Craven DE, Duncan RA, Stram JR, et al. Response of lymphoepithelial parotid cysts to antiretroviral treatment in HIV-infected adults. Ann Intern Med 1998; 128: 455–459.

922. Lustig LR, Lee KC, Murr A, et al. Doxycycline sclerosis of benign lymphoepithelial cysts in patients infected with HIV. Laryngoscope 1998; 108: 1199–1205.

923. Joshi VV, Gagnon GA, Chadwick EG, et al. The spectrum of mucosa-associated lymphoid tissue lesions in pediatric patients infected with HIV: A clinicopathologic study of six cases. Am J Clin Pathol 1997; 107: 592–600.

924. Del B, Pretolesi F, Pontali E, et al. Possible malignant transformation of benign lymphoepithelial parotid lesions in human immunodeficiency virus-infected patients: report of three cases. Clin Infect Dis 2000; 30: 947–949.

925. Ioachim HL, Antonescu C, Giancotti F, et al. EBV-associated primary lymphomas in salivary glands of HIV-infected patients. Pathol Res Pract 1998; 194: 87–95.

926. Smith BC, Ellis GL, Slater LJ, et al. Sclerosing polycystic adenosis of major salivary glands. A clinicopathologic analysis of nine cases. Am J Surg Pathol 1996; 20: 161–170.

927. Skalova A, Michal M, Simpson RH, et al. Sclerosing polycystic adenosis of parotid gland with dysplasia and ductal carcinoma in situ. Report of three cases with immunohistochemical and ultrastructural examination. Virchows Arch 2002; 440(1): 29–35.

Index

Note:
FNA = fine needle aspiration
Page numbers followed by 'f' refer to figures; those
    followed by 't' refer to tables.
Page numbers followed by 'f' refer to figures; those
    followed by 't' refer to tables. *vs* denotes
    differential diagnosis.
5q-syndrome 636, 637f
'10% tumor', pheochromocytoma 2191
14-3-3 protein 2413
34βE12 monoclonal antibody 1792–1793, 1793f
    atypical adenomatous hyperplasia of prostate 1799,
        1800
    focal glandular atypia (prostate) 1805
    prostatic adenocarcinoma 1796, 1807–1808, 1812
    technical considerations 1812–1813

A

A103 (melan-A) reactivity 33, 35f, 286, 2188
A band, muscle 2215
ABCD features, melanoma 283
ABC technique, immunohistochemistry 31
abdominal aortic aneurysm, inflammatory 1078–1079
abdominal cysts, postoperative 146–147
Abelson proto-oncogene (c-*abl*) 632–633
abetalipoproteinemia 1380, 1380f
abnormal junction of pancreatic and bile duct (AJPBD)
    1579–1580, 1581, 1583
abnormal localization of immature precursors (ALIP)
    635, 636f
abortions 2079
    spontaneous 2079–2080, 2079t
abruptio placentae 2072
abscess 69
    amebic liver 103, 103f
    cerebral *see* cerebral abscess
    cholangitic 1494
    crypt 1388, 1389, 1395
    liver, candidal 71
    neutrophilic 199, 225
    orbital 2294
    ovary 1989
    in psoriasis vulgaris 199
    spleen 577
    subareolar, Paget's disease of nipple *vs* 457
    tubo-ovarian 143, 2040, 2041
    vitreous 2313
absorptive (columnar) cells, colon 1373
Acanthamoeba 105, 106, 2412
    encephalitis 106f
    keratitis 2301, 2302f
acantholysis 195
    Darier's disease 219
    impetigo 217
    paraneoplastic pemphigus 219f
    pemphigus vulgaris 218
acantholytic actinic keratosis 244
acantholytic dermatosis
    transient (Grover's disease) 219, 220–221, 221f
    vulvocrural area 1894
acanthoma, clear cell 242, 242f
acanthosis 195
    epidermal nevi 241, 241f
    of esophagus 1289–1290

glycogenic 1289–1290
    pseudoepitheliomatous hyperplasia 243
Accreditation Council for Graduate Medical Education
    (ACGME) 8
acetaminophen
    overdose 1513
    renal cell carcinoma association 1677
acetylcholine receptor(s) 2217
    antibodies 2227
    reduced in myasthenia gravis 2227
acetylcholine receptor protein 2214
acetylcholinesterase stain 1403f
achalasia 1284
achondroplasia 681
acid-fast stain 60, 60t, 64f, 65f, 83f
acid hematein (Formalin pigment) 15
acidic (anionic) dyes 18
acid maltase deficiency 2230–2231, 2231f, 2232f
acidophilic bodies, hepatocyte apoptosis 1476f
acidophilic degeneration 1475–1476, 1476f
acid phosphatase 610
    lysosome-associated 2231, 2232f
    skeletal muscle 2215t
acinar cell(s) 1231, 1233–1234, 1233f
    pancreatic 1326
acinar cell carcinoma
    differential diagnosis 176
    pancreas *see* pancreas
acinar hepatocellular carcinoma 1531, 1532f
acinic cell carcinoma
    lung 949, 952, 954f
    parotid gland 797, 1230
    salivary gland *see* salivary gland tumors
    sinonasal region 797
    Warthin's tumor *vs* 1219
acne keloidalis nuchae 226
acne rosacea 226, 226f
    differential diagnosis 200, 215
acoustic neuroma (eighth nerve schwannoma) 810,
    2279, 2279f, 2385
acquired immunodeficiency syndrome *see* AIDS
acral arteriovenous tumor (cutaneous arteriovenous
    hemangioma) 271, 271f
acral myxoinflammatory fibroblastic sarcoma
    (inflammatory myxohyaline tumor) 327–328,
    328f
acrochordon 264
acrodermatitis, in pseudo-Kaposi's sarcoma 370
acrolein 17
acromegaly 2093, 2099, 2100, 2109
    neuromuscular abnormalities 2233
acrospiroma 256–257, 257f
    malignant 261
    nodular 257, 259f
acrosyringeal nevus 257, 259f
acrosyringia 194, 204
ACTH
    ectopic secretion 2180–2181, 2180f, 2181f
    pituitary-dependent overproduction 2179–2180,
        2180f
        see also Cushing's disease
    plasma levels, Cushing's disease 2179
    production, medullary thyroid carcinoma 2137
    raised levels 2178–2183

thymic carcinoid 1108–1109
    stress effect 2173
ACTH stimulation test, rapid 2176
actin 2215, 2218t
    staining, gastric leiomyoma 1345
actin binding proteins 31t
actinic granuloma 213, 213f
actinic keratopathy, chronic 2303
actinic (solar) keratosis 243, 243f
    eyelid 2290
    pigmented 244, 277
    squamous cell carcinoma *vs* 246
    variants 243–244
actinic reticuloid 295
Actinomadura 74
Actinomyces 1512f
    cervical infection 1837, 1851
    pericardial lesions 1069
    tubo-ovarian abscess 143
Actinomyces israelii 61, 69–70, 1837, 2041
actinomycetes 1989
actinomycosis 69–70, 70f, 1512f
    cervicitis/cervical infection 1836t, 1837, 1850f, 1851
    fallopian tube 2041–2042
    IUD-associated 70, 143, 2041
    nasopharynx and upper respiratory tract 78
    ovary 1989, 1990f
activated charcoal, aspiration, foreign body
    bronchiolitis 908
ACTN4 gene 1610
'acute fibrinous and organizing pneumonia' (AFOP)
    882, 883f
acute interstitial nephritis 1640, 1640f
acute retinal necrosis (ARN) syndrome 2313
acute tubular necrosis (ATN) 1609f, 1630f,
    1637–1639
    pathology 1637–1638, 1638f, 1639f
adamantinoma 740, 744–746
    classic 744, 745
    dedifferentiated variant 745
    histologic patterns 745, 747f
    of long bones 1153
    osteofibrous dysplasia and 743
    radiography 745, 746f
    well-differentiated 744–745, 746
ADAMTS 13, deficiency 617
Addison's disease 113, 2110, 2175–2177
    idiopathic (autoimmune) 2175–2176, 2176f
    neuromuscular abnormalities 2233
adenine deaminase gene, mutation 113
adenoacanthoma, endometrial 1960, 1961f, 1966
adenoameloblastoma 1154
adenocarcinoma
    fetal 975–976, 978f
    metastatic 168, 173
        effusions 183
        mesothelioma *vs* 184, 185t
        primary *vs* (immunohistochemistry) 962t
    see also specific adenocarcinoma types; specific
        organs/regions
adenofibroma
    biliary 1539
    Brenner tumors 2012
    clear cell, ovary 2011

adenofibroma (cont'd)
  endometrioid, ovarian 2007, 2007f
  endometrium 1975, 1976, 1976f
  metanephric 1674
  mucinous, ovarian 2002
  serous, ovarian 1997
adenohypophysis 2093, 2094f, 2095f
  cell types 2094–2095
  cellular differentiation 2094–2096, 2096f
  development 2093–2094
  ectopic 2098
  primary tumors 2098
adenoid basal carcinoma, cervix 1876–1877, 1877f
adenoid cystic carcinoma
  breast see breast carcinoma
  ceruminous gland tumor vs 2276
  cervix 1876, 1876f
  epithelial mesothelioma pattern similar 1008
  immunohistochemistry 796t
  lacrimal gland 2298–2299, 2299f
  laryngeal 846–847, 847f
  lung see lung, carcinoma
  ovary 2014
  palate 1189
  prostate 1820
  salivary gland see salivary gland tumors
  sinonasal 794–795, 795f, 796t
  of skin 262
  trachea 846–847
  vulva 1914
adenoid squamous carcinoma, oral cavity 1176, 1176f
adenolipoma, breast 446
adenoma
  acidophil stem cell 2101, 2102–2103, 2103f
  adrenal cortex see adrenal cortex, adenoma
  alveolar 947, 947f
  ampulla of Vater 1588
  anogenital sweat glands 1897–1899, 1898f
  Bartholin's gland 1897, 1914
  basal cell, salivary gland tumors 1187, 1187f
  bile duct 1538, 1538f, 1539f
  breast see breast, adenoma
  bronchial gland 945–946, 946f, 949
  ceruminous 2276, 2276f
  ciliary epithelial 2309
  Crooke's cell adenoma 2105, 2105f
  eccrine, papillary 8, 19f, 257–258
  extrahepatic bile ducts 1584
  fallopian tube 2044, 2045f
  follicular, of thyroid 2124–2126, 2125f
  gallbladder 1578–1579
  gastric 1342–1344, 1344f, 1356
  hepatic see hepatic adenoma
  Hürthle cell 2124–2126, 2125f
  large intestine see large intestine
  Leydig cell 2185
  lung see under lung
  mammosomatotroph 2100
  middle ear 2277–2278, 2278f
  nipple see nipple, adenoma
  null cell 2106–2107, 2106f, 2107f
  papillary
    lung 949, 949f
    middle ear 2278–2279, 2279f
    renal 1673
  parathyroid see parathyroid glands, adenoma
  pituitary see pituitary adenoma
  pleomorphic
    lacrimal gland 2298, 2299f
    lung 946–947
    salivary glands see salivary gland tumors
    sinonasal 795–796, 797f
  renal see kidney, adenoma
  salivary gland see salivary gland tumors
  sebaceous 250, 251f
  Sertoli cell 1759
  signet-ring, thyroid 2126
  small intestine 1421–1422, 1422f
  thyroid see thyroid gland, adenoma

  uveal tract 2309
  vestibular glands 1899
adenoma malignum (minimal deviation
    adenocarcinoma) 1870–1871, 1871f
adenoma sebaceum 264
adenomatoid odontogenic tumor/cyst 1140f
adenomatoid tumor
  adrenal gland 2201–2202, 2201f
  fallopian tube 2044, 2045f
  odontogenic see odontogenic tumors, adenomatoid
  paratesticular region 1763–1764, 1764f
  peritoneal 1024
  pleura 1015
  thyroid gland nodules 2124
  uterus 1978, 1978f
adenomatous hyperplasia
  liver 1529
  pancreas 1570
  prostate see prostate gland
adenomatous polyposis coli gene see APC gene
adenomatous polyps
  gallbladder 1578–1579
  large intestine see familial adenomatous polyposis
    (FAP)
adenomyoepithelioma, breast 446–447, 447f
adenomyoma
  atypical polypoid, endometrial 1946, 1946f,
    1976–1977, 1977f
  cervix 1842
  endometrial 1976
  gallbladder 1578, 1578f
adenomyosis, uterine 1951–1952, 1959
adenopathy see lymphadenopathy
adenosarcoma
  cervix 1877
  endometrial 1975, 1976, 1976f
  fallopian tube 2046
  metanephric 1674
  ovary 2010
adenosis
  microglandular, breast 444, 444f
  prostate 1799–1800, 1800f, 1812
  sclerosing see sclerosing adenosis
  vagina 1923, 1923f
'adenosis tumor' 431
adenosquamous carcinoma
  breast see under breast carcinoma
  cervix 1874, 1875f
  endometrial 1960
  gallbladder 1580
  lung see lung
  oral cavity 1176
  pancreatic 1557–1558, 1558f
  salivary gland 1254–1256, 1255f
  thymic 1103
adenovirus 102
  appendiceal infection 1407, 1409
  cervicitis 1837
  hepatitis 1482, 1483f
  inclusions 102
  intestinal infection 1398
  pneumonia 876–878, 877f
adhesion proteins 31t, 167
adhesions
  peritoneal 1020
  tubo-ovarian 2041
adipocytes 195, 336
  atypical lymphocytes surrounding 293, 294f
adipose tissue
  in salivary gland FNA 1206
  in thymolipoma 1126, 1127f
adipose tissue tumors 335–347, 336t
  benign 335–341
    see also lipoma
  malignant 341–347
    see also liposarcoma
adnexal carcinoma, microcystic 252, 261, 262f
adnexal tumors, of skin see skin, adnexal
    tumors/pseudotumors

adnexal tumors of Wolffian origin
  female (FATWO) 2046, 2047, 2048f
  in ovary 1990
adrenal apoplexy 2169
adrenal capsule 2169, 2171, 2171f
  arteriopathy 2177
adrenal cortex 2169–2189
  abnormal size/shape 2174
  accessory tissue 2172–2173, 2173f
  adenoma 2177, 2178, 2178f, 2179f, 2185f
    'black' 2185, 2185f, 2186f
    calretinin staining 33, 35f
    Cushing's syndrome with 2180f, 2185, 2185f,
      2186f
    FNA biopsy 2178, 2179f
    heterotopic 2183–2185
    Melan-A staining 33, 35f
    nonhyperfunctional 2178, 2179f
    oncocytic 2185, 2187f
    primary hyperaldosteronism with (Conn's
      syndrome) 2183–2185, 2184f
  in adrenoleukodystrophy 2175
  in adrenomyeloneuropathy 2175
  agenesis 2174
  Beckwith-Wiedemann syndrome 2174, 2174f
  carcinoma 2185–2189, 2187t, 2189f
    pheochromocytoma vs 2188
  chronic insufficiency 2175–2177
    see also Addison's disease
  congenital abnormalities 2174
  congenital/familial insufficiency 2174–2175
  corticosteroid biosynthesis 2169, 2170f
  cytomegaly 2174
  developmental anatomy 2169–2170, 2171f
  fetal 2169, 2171f
  hemorrhage 2169, 2176, 2177, 2177f
  hereditary unresponsiveness 2175
  heterotopia 2172, 2173f
  histology (normal) 2169–2170, 2171f
  hyperplasia 2170
    congenital see congenital adrenal hyperplasia
      (CAH)
    diffuse and micronodular 2179, 2180f
    with hyperaldosteronism 2182–2183
    with hypercorticalism 2178–2183
    idiopathic bilateral (IHA) 2182–2183
    macronodular 2179–2180, 2181f
    macronodular with adrenal enlargement 2180f,
      2182, 2183f
    unilateral 2182
    with virilization or feminization 2183
    see also Cushing's disease; Cushing's syndrome
  incidentaloma 171, 2178, 2179f
  innervation 2171–2172
  lipid depletion 2173, 2173f
  lipid reversion 2173
  mass, incidental detection 2178, 2179f
  medullary junction 2170, 2172f
  in MEN type 1 2178
  metastases in 2176
  microcysts 2173
  micronodules 2182f
  myelolipoma 2175
  nodules 2177–2178
    benign (BACN) 171
    in congenital adrenal hyperplasia 2175
    extrusions 2170, 2172f
    pigmented 2177–2178, 2181, 2182f
  ovarian thecal metaplasia 2173–2174, 2173f
  primary pigmented nodular disease 2180f, 2181,
    2182f
  stress-related changes 2169, 2173
  in tuberculosis 2176
  tubular degeneration of cells 2173
  tumors 2183–2189
    in congenital adrenal hyperplasia 2175
    corticomedullary mixed tumor 2185
    criteria predictive of malignancy 2187, 2187t
    oncocytic 2185, 2187f

virilization and feminization with 2185
see also adrenal cortex, carcinoma
vasculature 2171
in Waterhouse-Friderichsen syndrome 2177, 2177f
adrenal cortical rests
in broad ligament 2047, 2047f
testicular/paratesticular 1735
adrenal corticomedullary junction 2170, 2172f
adrenalectomy 2178, 2183
adrenal gland 2169–2209
adenomatoid tumor 2201–2202, 2201f
average combined weight 2169, 2171f
ectopic ACTH syndrome 2181
primary pigmented nodular adrenocortical disease 2181, 2182f
cysts 2201
examination 2169
hemorrhage 2169, 2176, 2177, 2177f
infection, Cryptococcus neoformans 91f
lymphoma 2202
mass, calcified 384
melanoma 2202, 2202f
metastases in 169t, 171, 2202, 2202f
myelolipoma 2199–2200, 2201f
nodules 2177–2178
neuroblastic 2189, 2190f
regions 2169, 2169f
stress effect 2169, 2173
vasculature and innervation 2171, 2172f
see also adrenal cortex; adrenal medulla
adrenal medulla 2169, 2189–2199
corticomedullary mixed tumor 2185
developmental anatomy 2189
ganglioneuroblastoma 2194–2199
ganglioneuroma 2199, 2200f
histology (normal) 2189, 2190f
hyperplasia 2190, 2190f
'1 cm rule' 2190, 2190f
neuroblastic nodules 2189, 2190f
neuroblastoma 383, 2194–2199, 2195f
classification 2196, 2197t, 2198
grading system (low/high risk) 2196, 2198f
in situ 2195
microscopic pathology 2195–2198, 2195f, 2196f
prognostic factors and survival 2198–2199, 2198f, 2199t
stroma-rich/stroma-poor 2196, 2197f
ultrastructure and immunohistochemistry 2198, 2199f
pheochromocytoma see pheochromocytoma
adrenalmyeloneuropathy (AMN) 2175
adrenal veins 2171
adrenocorticotropic hormone see ACTH
adrenogenital syndrome see congenital adrenal hyperplasia (CAH)
adrenoleukodystrophy (ALD) 2175, 2246, 2247f
Adriamycin®, cardiotoxicity 1048
adult respiratory distress syndrome (ARDS) 872, 873–874
acute lung injury pattern, 17.16 869, 869f
lung adenocarcinoma vs 961
adult T-cell leukemia/lymphoma (ATLL) 566, 650–651
skin involvement 294
Aeromonas 101, 1395
agammaglobulinemia, X-linked (Bruton's) 113
aganglionosis (Hirschsprung's disease) 1403–1404, 1403f
age, CNS tumor differential diagnosis 2348t
age related changes
CNS neurons 2340
skeletal muscle 2217
AgNor technique see silver-stained nucleolar organizing regions (AgNORs)
agranulocytosis, bone marrow 617
AIDS 116–120
bone marrow, granulomatous changes 661–662, 661f, 662f
CMV esophagitis 1288–1289, 1289f
CNS involvement 2409–2410

CNS lymphoma 2395
Cryptococcus in vocal cord biopsy 835, 836f
cytopenia 662
effusion cytology of lymphoma 184
Hodgkin's disease and non-Hodgkin's lymphoma 662
Kaposi's sarcoma see Kaposi's sarcoma
lymph node infections 96, 96f
lymphoma 571, 662
neoplasms 121t
oral pyogenic granuloma 1181
oral vascular lesions 1186
pituitary gland involvement 2113
Pneumocystis pneumonia 88, 89, 89f, 881
progressive multifocal leukoencephalopathy 2408
renal cell carcinoma association 1677
sputum examination 866
see also HIV infection
AIDS dementia complex 2409
AIDS-related lymphoma (ARL) 571, 662
AIRE gene mutations 2176
air flow obstruction, chronic, bronchiolitis with 906–909
airspace filling (lung consolidation) 864, 866f
pattern 870, 870f
airways, conducting
anatomy 860–861, 860f
diffuse large airway lesions 911
diseases after lung transplantation 920–921
epithelium 860, 860f
small, diseases see small airways disease (SAD)
AJCC staging see American Joint Committee on Cancer (AJCC)
Alagille's syndrome 1502
Albright's hereditary osteodystrophy 267
Albright syndrome 393
fibrous dysplasia of temporal bone 2282
ossifying fibroma 1192
see also McCune–Albright syndrome
albumin 1598, 1606
Alcian blue stain 21f, 226, 229, 250
Barrett's esophagus diagnosis 1302, 1303, 1304f
cardiac amyloidosis 1047–1048, 1047f
effusions 184
fungi detection 61
goblet cells 1373
mesothelioma 1011
skeletal muscle evaluation 2215t
alcohol
carcinogenesis pathways 1168–1169
oral squamous cell carcinoma 1168–1169
alcohol abuse
chronic pancreatitis 1552
osteonecrosis 683
alcoholic cirrhosis 1493f
alcoholic foamy degeneration 1489
alcoholic hepatitis 1471f, 1490–1492, 1491f
alcoholic hyaline see Mallory bodies
alcoholic liver disease 1481, 1489–1492
iron accumulation 1505
steatosis 1489–1490
alcoholic mouth rinses 1169
alcoholic myopathy, acute 2234, 2235t
alcoholic steatohepatitis (steatonecrosis) 1490–1492
aldosterone secretion, by tumors 2183
see also hyperaldosteronism
Alexander disease 2342
Alizarin red stain 233
alkaline phosphatase
horseradish peroxidase 30
leukocyte (LAP) 633
placental see placental alkaline phosphatase (PLAP)
serum, osteosarcoma 728
skeletal muscle evaluation 2215t
alkylating agents
bladder changes due to 1719
epithelial abnormalities due to 148, 148f
tumors associated 149
allantoic duct, remnants 2066, 2066f
allergic angiitis and granulomatosis see Churg-Strauss syndrome (angiitis)

allergic bronchopulmonary aspergillosis (fungal disease) 91, 880, 880f
allergic contact dermatitis 196, 196f
allergic enterocolitis 1405
allergic granulomatosis and angiitis see Churg-Strauss syndrome (angiitis)
allergic reaction
eosinophilic colitis 1405
hypersensitivity myocarditis 1044–1045
Allison-Ghormley bodies 693
allograft injuries 129–131
perfusion injury 129–130, 130f
allograft rejection see graft rejection
all-trans-retinoic acid (ATRA) 626
alopecia 193, 201
alpha-1-antitrypsin deficiency 1508
liver involvement 1506–1508, 1507f
phenotypes 1506–1507
alpha-1-antitrypsin (AAT) globules 1491
alpha-actinin 2218t
alpha chain disease 657
alpha-enolase 2111
alpha-fetoprotein (AFP)
embryonal carcinoma 1748
hepatocellular carcinoma 1531, 1534
immature teratoma of ovary 2032, 2033
insulinoma 1573
malignant mixed germ cell tumors, ovary 2036
mediastinal embryonal carcinoma 1118
metastases of unknown primary 185
seminoma 1745
Sertoli-Leydig cell tumors 2023
yolk sac tumor of ovary 2028, 2030
yolk sac tumor of testis 1750–1751
alpha-gliadin 1374
alpha-internexin, medulloblastoma 2383
alpha-methylacyl CoA racemase (AMACR - P504S)
atypical adenomatous hyperplasia of prostate 1800
prostate atrophy vs adenocarcinoma 1796
prostatic adenocarcinoma 1813, 1813f
prostatic intraepithelial neoplasia 1803
alpha-naphthyl butyrate esterase stain 610
Alport's syndrome see hereditary nephritis of Alport
aluminium pneumoconiosis 905t
aluminium toxicity 686
alveolar adenoma, lung 947, 947f
alveolar adenoma-sclerosing hemangioma, lung 947
alveolar cell hyperplasia, atypical 956, 956f
alveolar ducts 861
alveolar lipoproteinosis 925–926, 926f
alveolar macrophages 861
alveolar rhabdomyosarcoma 356–361
chromosomal translocation 310t, 386
desmoplastic small round cell tumors vs 386
electron microscopy 360, 360f
Ewing family of tumors vs 386
microscopic features 358–359, 359f, 360f
orbital 2297
alveolar sacs 861
alveolar septal widening, bleomycin causing 885, 886f
alveolar soft part sarcoma (ASPS) 397–398, 397f, 398f
chromosomal translocation 310t
pleomorphic form 398
alveoli 861
anatomy 861
diffuse damage see diffuse alveolar damage (DAD)
alveolitis
cryptogenic fibrosing see pneumonia, usual interstitial (UIP)
extrinsic allergic see hypersensitivity pneumonitis
fibrosing, desquamative interstitial pneumonia progression 899
Alzheimer's disease 2414, 2415f
Alzheimer type II astrocytes 2342, 2343f
AMACR see alpha-methylacyl CoA racemase (AMACR - P504S)
amastia 421
amastigotes 100
ambiguous genitalia 1887

amebae, free-living 105–106
amebiasis, cerebral 2412, 2412f
amebic abscess 103, 103f
amebic dysentery 103
ameloblastic carcinoma 1153
ameloblastic fibroma 1141f, 1159–1161, 1160f
   ameloblastoma vs 1152
ameloblastic fibro-odontoma 1141f, 1161
ameloblastic fibrosarcoma 1162
ameloblastoma 1140f, 1150–1153, 1151f
   acanthomatous variant 1151, 1151f
   benign, squamous cell carcinoma in 1153
   congenital epulis of newborn and 1185
   cystogenic 1152
   desmoplastic variant 1151–1152
   differential diagnosis 1150, 1152–1153, 1160–1161
   extraosseous (peripheral) 1152
   follicular variant 1151, 1151f
   granular cell 1151, 1152f
   in situ 1150
   invasive 1150
   malignant 1153
   mandibular/maxillary 744, 1150
   melanotic (pigmented) 750–751, 751f
   microinvasive/transmural 1150
   multicystic solid central osseous form 1150, 1151, 1151f
   mural 1150
   plexiform pattern 1151, 1151f
   plexiform unicystic 1152
   unilocular cystic 1150, 1152
   variants 1152
ameloblasts 1139
amenorrhea 1989
American College of Surgeons (ACS) Commission on Cancer 4
American Fertility Society 1952, 1952t
American Gastroenterology Association (AGA) 1438
American Joint Committee on Cancer (AJCC)
   bladder tumor classification 1712, 1713t
   bone sarcoma staging 703, 703t
   breast cancer prognostic factors 489
   renal cell carcinoma staging 1672, 1673t
   soft tissue tumor trading 308
   testicular tumors classification 1741, 1742t
amianthoid fibers 377, 515
aminoethylcarbazole 32
amiodarone
   phospholipid accumulation in liver 1490, 1490f
   toxic effects 148, 961
Ammon's horn (mesial temporal sclerosis) 2405, 2405f
amnion 2064, 2067
   degenerative changes 2067, 2067f
   infections 2068, 2069
amnionic bands 2067–2068
amnion nodosum 2067, 2067f
amniotic bands 2063, 2064, 2068f
amniotic cavity 2064
amniotic membrane 2064, 2067–2068, 2067f
   in acute chorioamnionitis 2068, 2069
   development 2063–2064
   diamnionic/dichorionic (DiDi) 2075–2076, 2076f
   diamnionic/monochorionic (DiMo) 2075, 2076f
   'dividing' 2075, 2076f
   monoamnionic/monochorionic (MoMo) twin 2078, 2078f
   multiple gestation 2075
   premature rupture 2068
amphotericin B 73
ampulla, of semicircular canals 2269, 2269f
ampulla of Vater 1588–1589
   adenocarcinoma, invasive 1588
   adenoma 1588
   anatomy 1588
   endocrine tumors 1589
   gangliocytic paraganglioma 1589
   mucin oozing from 1565
amputation (traumatic) neuroma 378–379, 2245, 2246f
amylase, serum, elevated 1565

amyloid 656
   deposition 116, 117f, 118f
      CNS 2414, 2414t
      collagenous colitis 1401
      insulinoma 1573
      lymph nodes 515, 516f
      mesangium 1608f
      peripheral nerves 2247
      sites 116, 116t
   fibrils, in kidney 1631, 1632f
   globular 1519f
   in medullary thyroid carcinoma 2137, 2138f, 2139
   staining methods 16t, 20f, 656
   stromal, thymic carcinoid 1110
amyloid-β-protein 116
   cerebral amyloid angiopathy 2415f
   inclusion body myositis 2220–2221
amyloid glomerulopathy 1631, 1631f, 1632f, 1637t
amyloid myopathy 2238
amyloid neuropathy 2247
amyloidosis 116
   Addison's disease due to 2176
   AH (heavy chain-related) 656, 1631, 1631f, 1632f
   AL (light chain-related) 656, 1631, 1631f, 1632, 1632f
   bladder 1723, 1724f
   cardiac 116t, 1047–1048, 1047f
   cerebral 116t
   classification 116t
   esophagus 1291
   familial (hereditary) 116, 116t, 656, 2304
   hemodialysis-associated 116t
   heredofamilial 116t
   immunologic 116t
   intestinal 1400, 1405, 1406f
   lichen 230, 230f
   liver 1518, 1518f, 1519f
   localized (nodular) 116t
   macular 230
   microscopic colitis 1400
   in multiple myeloma 2247
   nodular 230, 230f
   pituitary involvement 2113
   pleura 1007
   primary 230, 656–657, 656f
   reactive systemic 116t
   renal involvement 656, 1631, 1631f, 1632f
   secondary (AA) 230, 656
   'senile' cardiac 116t
   skin involvement 229–231
   in Waldenström's macroglobulinemia 2247
amyloid plaques 2413
amyloid tumor
   heart 1066
   nodular, lung 968, 968f
   vocal cord 835
anabolic steroids 1517, 1518f, 1528
anaerobic bacteria, vaginal infection 1851
anal canal tumors 1455
   basaloid carcinoma 1455–1456, 1456f
   see also anus
anal carcinoma see anus
anal duct carcinoma 1456–1457, 1458f
analgesics
   acute diffuse lung disease due to 886
   overdose 886
anal gland carcinoma 1456–1457, 1458f
anal intraepithelial neoplasia 1455, 1455f
anaphylaxis, after blood transfusion 114
anaplasia (nuclear), Wilms' tumor 1666, 1667f
anaplastic lymphoma kinase (ALK) 563, 652
   anaplastic large cell lymphoma 293, 563
   gene fusion involving 332
   seminoma differential diagnosis 1775t
anaplastic tumors see individual tumor types
anastomoses, surgical, tissue alterations at 146
anatomic pathology, quality issues 9–10
ancillary studies 178, 184, 186
   see also immunohistochemistry

Andersen's disease 2232
androgen-deprivation therapy, effect on prostate gland 1821, 1821f
androgen insensitivity syndrome 1737
   germ cell tumor risk 1742
   Sertoli cell nodules 1759
androgen receptor, gene mutations 1737
anemia
   AIDS 661
   aplastic 616–617
   congenital dyserythropoietic 619
   hemolytic 663
   of hereditary red cell abnormalities 619
   hypochromic 619
   iron deficiency 1169, 1374
   megaloblastic 619
   pernicious 619
   refractory see refractory anemia (RA)
aneurysm
   by anastomosis 363
   aortic
      abdominal aorta 1078–1079
      ascending aorta 1082
      mycotic 1079
   arteriovenous 364
   atherosclerotic 1070
   cirsoid 363
   idiopathic non-inflammatory 1083
   involving ear 2275
   mesangial nodule adjacent 1629f
   muscular arteries 1082
   mycotic 1079
   nonsyphilitic infectious 1079
   racemose 363
   splenic artery 1070, 1083
aneurysmal cyst
   of bone 756–758, 757f
      chondroblastoma vs 713
      fibrous dysplasia vs 742
      fine needle aspiration 704, 758, 758f
      giant cell reparative granuloma vs 753, 758
      giant cell tumor of jaw vs 1183
      histology 757–758, 758f
      simple (unicameral) bone cyst vs 756
      solid variant 757–758
   soft tissue 391, 392f
angiitis
   Churg-Strauss see Churg-Strauss syndrome (angiitis)
   CNS 2414
angioblastoma of Nakagawa (acquired tufted hemangioma) 269, 270, 270f
angiodermatitis, in pseudo-Kaposi's sarcoma 370
angioendothelioma
   endovascular papillary (Dabska tumor) 366, 366f
   skin 273–274, 273f
   papillary intralymphatic 274
angiofibroma
   cellular, vulva 1902
   juvenile nasopharyngeal 394
   nasopharyngeal 817–818, 817f, 818f
   of skin 264–265, 265f
angiofollicular lymphoid hyperplasia see Castleman's disease
angiogenesis, metastasis mechanism 167
angioimmunoblastic (immunoblastic) lymphadenopathy 535, 663
   with dysproteinemia (AILD) 535
angioimmunoblastic (immunoblastic) lymphadenopathy-like T-cell lymphoma 565, 566f
angiokeratoma 269, 269f
   scrotum 1772
   vulva 1900, 1901, 1901f
angiokeratoma corporis diffusum universale see Fabry's disease
angioleiomyoma 349–350
angiolymphoid hyperplasia with eosinophilia 211, 271, 272f, 519
   ear involvement 2275, 2275f

angioma
    cavernous, of CNS 2415
    cherry 269, 270f
    intramuscular *see* hemangioma
    littoral cell, of spleen 582, 582f
    pulsating 363
    venous, of CNS 2415
angiomatosis 365, 365f
    bacillary *see* bacillary angiomatosis
    bacterial 1902
    CNS 2394–2395
    diffuse cystic 766
    encephalofacial (Sturge–Weber syndrome) 365, 365f
    gastrointestinal tract 1449
angiomyoadenomatous tumor, benign, renal 1695
angiomyofibroblastic stromal reaction, fallopian tube
        2040
angiomyofibroblastoma, vulva 1900
angiomyofibroblastoma-like tumor, paratesticular
        region 1764
angiomyolipoma 340
    epithelioid 1691–1692, 1692f
    kidney 970, 1690–1691, 1691f
    liver *see* liver, angiomyolipoma
    renal 970
    uterus 1978
angiomyoma 349–350, 349f
angiomyxoma
    aggressive 1764, 1917, 1917f
    paratesticular region 1764
    of skin 267
    superficial 267, 1902
    umbilical cord 2067
    vulvar 1902, 1917, 1917f
angiosarcoma 371–373
    angiolymphoid hyperplasia with eosinophilia *vs* 2275
    breast *see* breast, angiosarcoma
    cutaneous 275, 276, 276f, 372f
    of deep soft tissue 371–372
    epithelioid *see* epithelioid angiosarcoma
    epithelioid hemangioendothelioma *vs* 768
    of face and scalp (Wilson Jones) 371, 371f
    gastrointestinal tract 1449
    head and neck 818
    high-grade, epithelioid hemangioendothelioma *vs*
        768
    idiopathic cutaneous 275
    large intestine 1449
    littoral cell 582, 591
    liver 1542–1543, 1543f
    lung 973, 974f
    lymphangiosarcoma *vs* 276
    lymphedema-associated 147, 275–276, 371
    malignant peripheral nerve sheath tumor with 2258
    mesenteric 372f
    morphology 372–373, 372f
    nasopharynx 818
    papillary endothelial hyperplasia *vs* 363
    pericardial 1070
    postirradiation 276, 276f, 371, 371f
    sinonasal 818
    skeletal 769, 769f
    small intestine *see* small intestine
    spindled and epithelioid 372f, 373f
    spleen 591, 591f
    squamous cell carcinoma of skin *vs* 248
    thyroid 2141
ankylosing spondylitis 1058
ankylosis, in rheumatoid arthritis 693
Ann Arbor system 543
annular elastolytic granuloma (AEG) 213
annuloaortic ectasia 1081
anogenital sweat glands 1885
    adenocarcinoma 1914
    cysts and adenoma 1897–1899, 1898f, 1898t
anorchidism 1734–1735
anorectal area
    secondary tumors 1459
    see also anus; large intestine; rectum

anorexigen-induced disease, tricuspid valve 1059
anovulation 1950
anterior horn cell, disorders 2224–2225
anterior segment, conditions 2316
anterior synechias 2315, 2316f
anthracene cathartics 1401
anthracosis 905t
anthracycline, cardiotoxicity 1048–1049, 1049f
antibodies
    cell line and site-specific 180–182, 180t
    graft rejection mechanism 122
    see also specific antibodies
anti-CD20 (retuximab) 551, 1354
anti-CD52 551
anticipation, genetic 2237
anticytokeratins 230, 1100
antidiuretic hormone, inappropriate ectopic production
        1108
antiendomysial antibody test 1374
anti-GBM antibodies 1622
anti-GBM disease (ABMD) *see* antiglomerular
        basement membrane disease (ABMD)
antigen presentation, HLA system 120
antigen-presenting cells (APCs) 120, 122
antigen (epitope) retrieval methods 32–33, 33f
antigliadin antibody test 1374
antiglomerular basement membrane disease (ABMD)
        1622, 1654
    crescentic glomerulonephritis and 1621
    diffuse alveolar hemorrhage 884, 884f
antikeratin antibodies 230, 1100
antimesothelioma antibodies 1012
antimitochondrial antibodies (AMA) 1498
antimony pneumoconiosis 905t
anti-müllerian hormone (müllerian inhibitor substance)
        1734, 1737
antineutrophil cytoplasmic antibodies (ANCA)
    c-ANCA 1621
    glomerulonephritis 1620, 1621
    p-ANCA 1076, 1384, 1621
    Wegener's granulomatosis 1076
antinuclear antibody PM-1 2218
antioncogenes 1170
antiphospholipid syndrome 665, 1084, 1385
α1-antitrypsin deficiency *see* alpha-1-antitrypsin
        deficiency
antitubular basement membrane antibodies 1640
Antoni A tissue 2249, 2250f
    schwannoma 2249–2250, 2250f, 2251–2252, 2385,
        2386, 2386f
Antoni B tissue 2249, 2250f, 2385, 2386f
    schwannoma 2249–2250, 2250f
antral cysts 1149
antrectomy (distal gastrectomy) 1323, 1324
antrochoanal polyps 787
antrum *see* stomach, antrum
anus 1453–1459
    carcinoma 1454
    condyloma accuminatum 1444f, 1454
    extramammary Paget's disease 1458, 1458f, 1908
    intraepithelial neoplasia (carcinoma in situ) 1455,
        1455f
    melanoma 1458–1459, 1458f, 1459f
    squamous cell carcinoma 1455–1456, 1456f
        TNM staging 1456, 1457t
    squamous dysplasia 1455, 1455f
    verrucous carcinoma 1456, 1457f
aorta
    abdominal, aneurysm 1078–1079
    ascending
        diseases 1058
        dissection 1081, 1082
        inflammatory aneurysms 1082
        non-inflammatory aneurysms 1083
        surgical pathology 1082–1083
    coarctation 1082
    giant cell arteritis 1073
    medial degeneration 1081, 1082f
    mycotic aneurysms 1079

aortic arch syndrome *see* Takayasu's disease
aortic pseudoaneurysms 1083
aortic root, dilatation 1058, 1081
aortic valve 1057–1059
    acquired degenerative disease 1057f, 1058
    bicuspid 1057f, 1058, 1083
    calcific 1057, 1057f
    congenital disease 1057–1058, 1057f
    incompetence 1058
    insufficiency 1058–1059
    median raphe 1057f, 1058
    miscellaneous lesions 1058
    postinflammatory disease 1058
    replacement, indications 1057t
    stenosis 1057, 1057f, 1058
    unicuspid 1057, 1057f
aortitis
    giant cell 1082
    syphilitic 1079, 1082
APC gene 325, 1437
    fibromatosis and 320
    Gardner syndrome 325
    gastric adenocarcinoma 1359–1360
    see also familial adenomatous polyposis (FAP)
apical peridontal cysts (radicular cysts) 1146–1147
aplastic anemia 616–617
'apocrine adenosis' 431
apocrine glands
    ectopic 194
    normal histology 194
apocrine metaplastic cells, nipple discharge 425
apocrine tubulopapillary hidradenoma 258
apolipoprotein E, ε4 and ε2 alleles 2414
apoptosis 195
    in autoimmune thyroiditis 2121
    crypt cells 1402, 1403f
    hepatocytes 1475, 1476, 1476f
appendectomy 1408
'appendiceal neuroma' 1407
appendicitis
    acute 1407–1408
    chronic 1408
    Crohn's 1409
    granulomatous 1391, 1395
    idiopathic granulomatous 1409
    Yersinia 98f
appendix 1406–1410
    adenocarcinoma, metastases in ovary 2039
    anatomy 1406–1407
    conditions involving 1409–1410
    congenital and neuromuscular disorders 1407
    Crohn's disease 1390, 1391, 1409, 1409f
    cystic fibrosis 1407, 1409, 1410f
    diverticula 1407, 1409
    endometriosis 1409, 1410f
    histology (normal) 1406–1407
    infections 104, 104f, 1408–1409, 1409f
    intussusception 1407
    necrotizing arteritis 1410, 1410f
    neuroendocrine tumors 1428–1429, 1429f
    ulcerative colitis 1390, 1409
appendix epididymis 1732, 1733
appendix testis 1732, 1733, 1733f
'apple-green' birefringence 116, 118f, 515, 516f,
        1471
aqueous humor
    in glaucoma 2314
    outflow block/pathways 2314–2315, 2315f
arachnoidal cap cells
    meningothelial (syncytial) meningioma 2388–2389
    microcystic meningioma 2390
arachnoid cysts 2113, 2403
arcuate arteries 1600
areola 419, 420
argentaffin cells 16t, 1322
argon-ion laser 36–37
argyrophil cells 16t, 1832
argyrophilia, mesangial cells 1600
argyrophilic breast carcinoma 460

Arias-Stella reaction 1838, 1939f, 1946, 2043, 2044
  endocervical glands 1838, 1848
    features and gestational endometrium 1948–1949, 1949f
    postpartum/portabortal endometrium 1949
Armed Forces Institute of Pathology (AFIP) 308–309, 399, 1153, 1215, 2194, 2307
aromatase, deficiency 1736
arsenic, lung cancer etiology 935–936
arterial dissection 1080, 1080f, 1082
arterial dysplasia 1080–1081, 1081f
arterial thrombosis 1084
arteries
  elastic, vasculitis 1072–1074, 1072t
  muscular, vasculitis 1072t, 1074–1075
  pseudoaneurysms 1083, 1084f
  radiation effect 153, 153f
arteriohepatic dysplasia 1502
arteriopathy
  adrenal capsule 2177
  CADASIL 2415, 2415f
  plexogenic pulmonary 912
  segmental mediolytic 1083
arteriovenous crossing defects (AV nicking), retina 2318
arteriovenous malformations
  CNS 2415–2416, 2416f
  congenital 363
  cutaneous arteriovenous hemangioma vs 271
  diffuse, angiomatosis vs 365
  soft tissues 363
arteritis
  giant cell see giant cell arteritis
  Heubner 2407
  necrotizing, appendix 1410, 1410f
  Takayasu's see Takayasu's disease
artery-to-artery communication 2076–2077, 2076f
arthritis
  degenerative see osteoarthritis
  inflammatory 692
  rheumatoid see rheumatoid arthritis
arthropathy, traumatic and hemorrhagic 694
arthropod bites, bullous, bullous pemphigoid vs 222
arthrosis, rapidly destructive 682–683, 682f
articular cartilage 691
arylsulfatase A, deficiency 2246
asbestos bodies 902, 903f
asbestos exposure 902, 935
  Blesovsky's syndrome due to 1007, 1007f
  lung cancer etiology 935
  mesothelioma due to 1007
  parietal pleural plaque 1006, 1006f
asbestosis 896, 902–903, 935
Ascaris lumbricoides 77
ascites
  malignant 183
  ovarian epithelial tumors 1996
Asherman's syndrome 1947
'ashleaf spots' 264
Askin tumor 385, 994
aspergilloma 92, 93f
aspergillosis/Aspergillus infection 91–93
  allergic bronchopulmonary 91, 880, 880f
  cerebral/CNS 2410, 2410f
  esophagitis 1289
  intestinal 1399
  invasive 91, 92–93, 93f
  laryngeal 835
  lung infection posttransplant 920
  pneumonia 880, 880f
Aspergillus 91–93, 94f, 2410
  autofluorescence 62
  morphologic characteristics 66t
Aspergillus niger 92, 93f
aspiration
  nipple 425
  renal cysts 1665
aspiration biopsy (cytology) see fine needle aspiration (FNA) biopsy

ASPL–TFE3 fusion gene, alveolar soft part sarcoma 397
Association of Directors of Anatomic and Surgical Pathology (ADASP) 4, 9
asteroid bodies 71, 533, 2304
asteroid hyalosis 2304
asthma 911, 912f
astroblastoma 2339t, 2372
astrocytes 2349
  gray matter 2340
  histology (normal) 2340–2343, 2341f
  inclusions 2342
  processes 2340, 2341f
  radiation-induced changes 2344, 2344f
  reactive 2340–2341, 2342f
    Alzheimer type II 2342, 2343f
  white matter fibrillary 2340, 2341f
astrocytic tumors 2348–2360
  gliosarcoma 2356, 2356f, 2357f
  immunohistochemistry 2338t
  pleomorphic xanthoastrocytoma see xanthoastrocytoma, pleomorphic
  SEGA see subependymal giant cell astrocytoma (SEGA)
  see also astrocytoma; glioblastoma
astrocytoma 2348–2360
  anaplastic 2348, 2351–2352, 2351f
    crush preparations 2351, 2351f, 2352f
  circumscribed 2348, 2356
    see also astrocytoma, pilocytic
  desmoplastic infantile 2374
  diffuse 2348, 2349–2351, 2349f
    crush preparation 2330f
    pilocytic astrocytoma vs 2359
    ultrastructure 2350, 2350f
  fibrillary 2342f, 2349
  gemistocytic 2349–2350, 2349f
  genetic abnormalities 2340t
  granular cell 2350
  immunohistochemistry 2338t
  low-grade, gliosis 2342f
  pilocytic 2356–2359, 2358f
    cerebellar 2357
    crush (smear) preparations 2357–2358, 2357f, 2358f
    pituitary 2109
  protoplasmic 2350, 2350f
  retinal 2311
  subependymal giant cell 2338t, 2359–2360, 2360f
  superficial cerebral 2374
  ultrastructural characteristics 2336t
  WHO grade I see astrocytoma, pilocytic
  WHO grade II 2348, 2350, 2359
  WHO grade III 2348, 2351
    see also astrocytoma, anaplastic
  WHO grade IV 2348, 2350
    see also glioblastoma
astrocytoma-ependymoma 2370
astrocytosis, reactive see gliosis
ataxia-telangiectasia (A-T) 115, 571
atelectasis, rounded 1007, 1007f
athelia 421
atherectomy, coronary 1071
atheroembolic renal disease 1646, 1646f
atheroembolism 1084–1085
atherosclerosis 1070–1072
  accelerated, diabetic nephropathy 1629
  penetrating ulcer 1070
atherosclerotic aneurysm 1070
atherosis, acute, uteroplacental vessels 2071
atopic dermatitis 196
ATP, deficiency, mitochondrial myopathies 2229
ATPase, skeletal muscle evaluation 2215, 2215t, 2216, 2216f, 2216t
ATPase reaction 23f
atrial septum, lipomatous hypertrophy 1065, 1066f
atrophia bulbi 2314
atypical decubital fibroplasia (ischemic fasciitis) 314, 315f

'atypical lipomatous tumor' 342
atypical teratoid/rhabdoid tumor (AT/RT) 2384–2385, 2384f, 2385f
  medulloblastoma vs 2383
  ultrastructural characteristics 2337t
auditory canal see external auditory canal (EAC)
auditory placode 2267
Auerbach's plexus 1283
Auer rods 622, 623f, 626
aural polyp 2274
aural sinuses, congenital 2271
auricle see pinna (ear)
auricular chondritis 2282
aurintricarboxylic acid stain 686
autoantibodies, to desmoglein-3 219
autofluorescence 62
autoimmune blistering disorder 223
autoimmune chronic gastritis see gastritis, autoimmune chronic
autoimmune disease 113, 114t
  autoimmune chronic gastritis and 1329
  lymphoproliferative diseases with 572
  myositis in 2221–2222
  non-specific interstitial pneumonia 898
  non-specific pericarditis due to 1068
  silicone breast implants associated 142
autoimmune enteropathy 1376
autoimmune polyendocrinopathy-candidiasis-ectodermal dystrophy (APECED) 2175
autoimmune regular (AIRE) gene 2176
autoimmune thyroiditis (Hashimoto's) 2120–2122, 2121f
  fibrous variant 2121–2122, 2122f
  Riedel's disease with 2122
automated biopsy gun, breast core needle biopsy 426
automation
  cytology 44
  immunohistochemistry 36
autonomic neuropathy, diabetes 2248
autopsy pathology 3
autosomal dominant moderate hyperparathyroidism (ADMH) 2158
autosomal dominant (adult) polycystic kidney disease 1662, 1662f, 1663f, 1665, 1690
autosplenectomy 580
Avellino dystrophy 2302
avian hypersensitivity (bird fancier's lung) 890–891
avidin-based method 31
avidin biotin peroxidase complex method 31
Avitene® 140
axillary lymph nodes
  metastases, in breast cancer
    ductal carcinoma in situ 456
    medullary carcinoma 475
    metaplastic carcinoma 480
    mucinous carcinoma 473
    occult micrometastases 430
    pathologic evaluation 429–430
    as prognostic factor 486–487
    sampling extent for evaluation 429–430
    tubular breast carcinoma 471
  sampling complication 28
axolemma 2240
axons 2240–2241, 2240f
  degeneration 2240, 2241, 2241f
  regeneration 2241
  sprouting 2241, 2241f
  stretch injury 2245
  terminal 2217
azoospermia, obstructive vs nonobstructive 1738
azurophilic granules 613, 620, 622, 651
Azzopardi effect 249, 988, 989, 991f
  neuroendocrine tumors 175

B

B-72.3 1534, 1540
bacillary angiomatosis 99, 99f, 100f, 370–371
  conjunctiva 2294
  lymph nodes 514
  peliosis hepatis vs 1517

'backwash ileitis' 1389, 1395
bacteria
    diagnostic techniques 59–60
    identification by molecular methods 107, 107t
    staining methods 17t, 59–60, 62t
bacterial angiomatosis 1902
bacterial infections
    acute pyogenic 63–64
    anaerobic, vaginal infection 1851
    cervicitis 1835, 1836t
    CNS 2406–2407
    corneal 2301
    endophthalmitis 2313
    fallopian tubes 2040–2041
    hepatic granuloma 1511
    infectious endocarditis 1059, 1060
    nasopharynx/upper respiratory tract 78–79
    pneumonia 874, 875f
        atypical 875–876
    purulent pericarditis 1069
    renal transplant recipient 1653
    respiratory tract 81–83
    skeletal muscle 2222, 2222f
    skin/soft tissue/mucocutaneous 67–70
    vulvar 1889–1891
    see also specific infections
bacterial overgrowth 1377
bacterial vaginosis 1851
bagassosis 891
'bag of worms' appearance 2254, 2254f
Baker's cyst 697
Balamuthia 105
balanitis 1772
balanitis xerotica obliterans 232, 1771
balanoposthitis 1772
Balkan nephropathy 1640–1641
BALT lymphoma, lung 977–979, 978f, 979f, 981
bands of Bünger 2241
Banff classification, renal transplant rejection 1649,
        1649t
barium pneumoconiosis (baritosis) 905t
barium sulfate 138
BARN syndrome 2313
Barrett's adenocarcinoma 1309, 1312, 1314
Barrett's esophagus 1299–1312, 1300f
    anatomic landmarks 1300, 1300f, 1301f, 1303
        long segments of gastric-type mucosa 1301,
            1301f
        lower esophageal sphincter 1300–1301, 1301f
        metaplastic glands 1302, 1302f
    Barrett's adenocarcinoma vs 1314
    brush cytology 1310
    characteristics 1302–1303
    children 1302
    diagnosis and definition 1299–1302
    dysplasia in 1304–1306, 1305f, 1307f
        diagnostic problems 1306–1307
        diagnostic variability 1307
        esophagectomy 1312
        glands involved 1304, 1305f, 1308
        high-grade see below
        histology 1304–1306, 1308
        'indefinite' for 1306, 1307f
        low-grade 1305, 1305f
        overdiagnosis avoidance 1308–1309
        photodynamic therapy 1307, 1311–1312
        reactive/regenerative change vs 1306–1307
        significance and management 1310
    endoscopic/histologic diagnosis 1299–1300, 1300f,
        1303
    flow cytometry 1310
    genetic abnormalities 1310
    high-grade dysplasia in 1305–1306, 1306f, 1308f
        carcinoma vs 1308f, 1309
        endoscopic ablative therapy 1311–1312
        focal 1310
        incident vs prevalent 1310
        incorrect diagnosis 1307–1308, 1308t
        marker of unsampled carcinoma 1310

    natural history 1310–1311
    overdiagnosis 1307–1308
    histology 1302–1303
    inflamed gastric cardiac-type mucosa vs 1303,
        1305f
    metaplastic epithelium 1299, 1301, 1303f
        detection methods 1310
        glandular atypia 1306, 1306f, 1309
        glandular dysplasia 1313
        with true goblet cells 1301, 1302, 1304f
    minimum histologic requirements 1301
    neoplastic progression 1303–1304
    pathologic evaluation problems 1299, 1300t
    pseudogoblet cells 1303, 1304f
    regenerative glands, baseline atypia 1306f, 1309
    'short segment' 1301–1302
    squamous overgrowth 1309–1310
Bartholin's gland 1885, 1886f
    adenoma 1897, 1899, 1914
    carcinoma 1913–1914
    cyst 349, 1897
    enlargement 1913
Bartholin's gland duct 1885, 1886f
    cysts 1897, 1914
Bartonella henselae 78, 96, 533, 534, 1902
    confirmed using molecular methods 107, 107t
    staining 97, 97f
    see also cat-scratch disease/fever
Bartonella quintana, trench fever 99
basal cell(s)
    hyperplasia, in dermatofibroma 265, 266f
    prostate gland 1792–1793, 1793f
basal cell adenoma see salivary gland tumors
basal cell carcinoma
    of eyelid 2290
    of pinna and periauricular 2280
    of scrotum 1773
    of vulva 1912–1913, 1913f
basal cell carcinoma, of skin 244–246
    adenoid (pseudoglandular) 245, 1913
    basosquamous 244, 1913
    differential diagnosis 243, 245–246, 248, 252
    fibroepitheliomatous (of Pinkus) 245
    indeterminate 246
    infiltrative 244
    metatypical (squamoid) 244, 248, 1913
    micronodular variant 244
    'morpheaform'/'sclerosing' 244, 245f
    morphea-like, desmoplastic trichoepithelioma vs 252
    nodular form 244, 244f
    nodulocystic 244–245
    pigmented 245
    pilar (organotypical) 245
    post-irradiation 158
    superficial 244, 245f, 246
        dermatofibroma vs 265, 266f
basal cell immunostain, prostatic adenocarcinoma
        1812
basal cell nevus syndrome, fetal rhabdomyoma
        association 355, 356
basal ganglia, tumor differential diagnosis 2348t
basalis layer, endometrium 1933, 1934f
basal lamina see basement membranes
basaloid carcinoma
    anal canal tumors 1455–1456, 1456f
    ovary 2014
    see also basaloid squamous cell carcinoma
basaloid cell(s)
    basal cell carcinoma of skin 244
    canalicular adenoma 1223
    nests, vulval carcinoma 1913, 1913f
    pilomatrixoma 253, 253f
    seborrheic keratosis 242, 242f
    trichoblastoma 252, 252f
basaloid squamous cell carcinoma
    cervix 1861
    esophageal 1299
    head and neck 790–791, 791f
    laryngeal 843, 845–846

    oral cavity 439 42f
    penis 1768t, 1769f, 1770
    salivary gland see salivary gland tumors
    sinonasal region 790–791, 791f, 795, 796t
    thymic 1102, 1104f
    vulva 1911
basaloma 1945
    endometrial polyps 1943, 1945–1946, 1946f, 1956,
        1968f
basement membranes
    airways 861
    glomerular see glomerular basement membrane
    skeletal muscle 2215
    staining methods 16t
basic (cationic) dyes 18
basic fibroblastic growth factor (bFGF), gastric
        carcinoids 1350
basilar membrane (inner ear) 2269
'basket-weave pattern', parietal pleural plaque 1006,
        1006f
basophilic granules
    acute basophilic leukemia 624
    cervical squamous epithelium 1831
    medulloblastoma 2381f
basophilic mucin, prostatic adenocarcinoma 1808,
        1809f
basophil invasion, corticotrophs 2097
B cells
    dermatomyositis 2219, 2220f
    failure to produce immunoglobulins 115
    ghost cells 530–531
    lymphoma see lymphoma, B-cell
    markers and antigen detection 611t, 2027
    maturation failure 113, 114
    monocytoid 527, 533
    monocytoid proliferation 519, 520f, 527, 527f
    persistent polyclonal lymphocytosis 643
    precursor 584
    sinus hyperplasia 527, 527f
    small, lymph node mantle zone 517
    toxoplasmic lymphadenitis 519, 520f
BCG 148, 1719, 1795
bcl-1 oncogene, lymphomas 557, 1352
bcl-2 gene rearrangement/oncogene 509
    diffuse large B cell lymphoma 560
    follicular lymphoma 550
    Hodgkin's disease 540
    lung carcinoma 937
    MALT lymphoma 1352
bcl-2 protein
    basal cell carcinoma of skin 246, 252
    cutaneous MALToma 290
    follicular lymphoma 548–550, 550f
    lymphomas 518
    salivary gland lymphoma vs follicular lymphoid
        hyperplasia 1256
    splenic marginal zone lymphocytes 589
    synovial sarcoma 403
bcl-6 protein 543, 549, 560
Bcl110 oncogene, MALT lymphoma 1352
bcr/abl fusion 633
bcr gene 633
Beale ducts, intramural 1582, 1583f
Becker muscular dystrophy 2213, 2235–2236, 2235t
Becker's nevus 282
Beckwith-Wiedemann syndrome 1666
    adrenal cortex changes 2174, 2174f
    hepatoblastoma association 1536
Bednar's tumor 266
Behçet's syndrome
    inflammatory myofibroblastic pseudotumor (renal)
        1696
    intestinal involvement 1386
Bence–Jones proteinuria 654
'benign cystosarcoma phyllodes' 436
benign diffuse uveal melanocytic proliferation
        (BDUMP) syndrome 2306
benign familial pemphigus (Hailey-Hailey disease)
        220, 220f, 1894

benign fibrous histiocytoma (BFH) 739, 739f
  giant cell tumor of bone *vs* 754
  larynx 848
  sinonasal region 823
benign prostatic hyperplasia (BPH) 1798–1799
'benign recurring atypical histiocytoma' 265
benign triton tumor (neuromuscular hamartoma) 2249, 2249f
benzopyrene, lung cancer development 936
Ber-EP4 antibodies, basal cell carcinoma of skin 246
Bernatz system, thymoma classification 1096
Bertin, columns 1598
berylliosis 904
beta-2-microglobulin, accumulation 2247
beta-defensin-1 1676, 1684
betal quid, oral squamous cell carcinoma 1168
Bethesda system 7, 1832–1835
  liquid-based sample collection 1834
  recommendations (2001) 1833–1834, 1833t
  semiquantitative method 1834
  specimen adequacy 1833–1835
Betz cells 2340
Bielschowsky stain 2335t
BIGH3 gene, corneal dystrophy 2302
'big spleen' disease 1518
bile
  extravasation 1496f
  in mechanical obstruction 1497
  pigmentation in renal tubular cells 1634f
  staining and differentiation 1493
  stasis 1494
bile canaliculi 1471f, 1474
  bile plugs 1493, 1493f
bile duct(s)
  abnormal junction with pancreatic duct 1579–1580, 1581, 1583
  acinar (interlobular) 1474
  adenoma 1538, 1538f, 1539f
  cysts 1582–1583
  ductopenia 1501f
  extrahepatic *see* extrahepatic bile ducts
  hepatitis-associated lesions 1485, 1485f, 1487
  paucity 1502
  rupture 1496f
  septal 1474
  tumors 1538–1540
    benign lesions 1538–1539
    malignant lesions 1540
  vanishing, syndrome 128, 128f
  see also entries beginning biliary
bile duct-like structures 1475f
bile ductules 1474, 1475f, 1494
  cholestasis 1494, 1497f
  dilatation 1497f
  in primary biliary cirrhosis 1501
  reactive 1493–1494, 1496f
bile lake 1496f
bile plugs 1493f, 1494f
bile reflux, postgastrectomy 1338–1339
biliary adenocarcinoma 1585, 1585f, 1586
biliary adenofibroma 1539
biliary atresia 1495f
  extrahepatic 1483, 1497, 1498f
biliary cirrhosis 1497
  primary *see* primary biliary cirrhosis (PBC)
  secondary 1497, 1498f
biliary cystadenocarcinoma 1539
biliary cystadenoma 1539
  extrahepatic bile ducts 1586, 1587f
biliary epithelium
  dysplasia 1584, 1585
  normal 1583, 1585f
  reactive 1583–1584, 1585f
biliary hamartoma 1522, 1523f, 1538, 1538f
biliary obstruction, mechanical 1497, 1498f
biliary papillomatosis (BP) 1539, 1539f, 1586–1587
bilirubin, staining 20t
Billroth I procedure, gastric adenocarcinoma after 1356–1357, 1357f

Billroth II resection
  gastric adenocarcinoma after 1356–1357, 1357f
  gastric stump carcinoma 146
  reactive gastritis after 1338
biloma 1539
Binet staging system, chronic lymphocytic leukemia 642
biopsy
  aspiration *see* fine needle aspiration (FNA) biopsy
  core needle *see* core needle biopsy (CNB)
  endoscopic surgical, stomach 1324
  trauma of, iatrogenic lesions 135–136
  see also specific anatomic sites
Biosorb 139, 139f
biotin, staining in immunohistochemistry 33
Birbeck granules 287, 610, 610f, 659, 760, 760f, 2110
  airways 861
  histiocytosis of bone 690
  Langerhans cells in lymph nodes 524
  neoplastic Langerhans cells 573
bird fancier's lung (avian hypersensitivity) 890–891
Birt-Hogg-Dube syndrome 1674, 1675, 1676
bischloromethyl ether, lung cancer etiology 935–936, 989
Bismark brown stain 26
'bizarre parosteal osteochondromatous proliferation' 773–774, 773f, 774f
B-K mole syndrome 280
bladder (urinary) 1707–1724
  adenocarcinoma 1710, 1720–1721, 1720f
  amyloidosis 1723, 1724f
  anatomy 1707, 1707f
  biopsy, report 1718
  carcinoma in situ 1716, 1716f
    dysplasia *vs* 1717
    interstitial cystitis *vs* 1709
  condyloma acuminatum 1723
  congenital abnormalities 1707–1708
  diverticula 1707–1708
  dysplastic intraepithelial lesions 1716–1717, 1716f
  embryology 1707
  epithelial neoplasms 1710–1721
    classification 1712, 1712t, 1713t
    urothelial *see* urothelial neoplasms
  exstrophy 1707, 1708, 1720
  Hodgkin's disease 1723
  inflammation *see* cystitis
  interstitium, fat 1707f
  ionizing radiation effect 156–157
  leiomyosarcoma 1722, 1722f
  lymphoma 1722–1723
  malakoplakia 1710, 1710f
  mesenchymal tumors 1721–1722
  metaplasia 1709–1710
    intestinal 1709, 1710f, 1720
    nephrogenic 1709, 1710f
    squamous 1709
  metastatic tumors in 1721
  myosarcoma 1722
  non-epithelial neoplasms 1721–1723
  non-neoplastic tumorous conditions 1723
  pathologic effects of treatment 1719, 1719f
  pathologic examination methods 1724
  pheochromocytoma 1722
  poorly differentiated small cell carcinoma 1721, 1721f
  postoperative spindle cell nodule 1723, 1723f
  pseudosarcomatous fibromyxoid tumor 1723, 1723f
  rare tumors 1721
  rhabdomyosarcoma 1722, 1722f
  sarcomatoid carcinoma 177f
  signet ring adenocarcinoma 1720
  spindle cell carcinoma, iatrogenic reactions resembling 147
  squamous cell carcinoma 1710, 1719–1720, 1720f
  squamous papilloma 1723
  transitional cell (urothelial) carcinoma 1713
    chemotherapy associated 150, 1719, 1719f
    classification 1712, 1712t
    collecting duct carcinoma *vs* 1685

  with gland-like lumina 1717, 1717f
  high-grade 1715–1716, 1715f
  in situ 1711–1712, 1716, 1716f, 1717
  ionizing radiation effect 154, 156–157, 1719
  low-grade 1714–1715, 1715f
  micropapillary-type 1717–1718, 1719f
  nested type 1717, 1718f
  prognostic factors 1718
  sarcomatoid type 1717, 1718f
  spread to prostate 1820, 1820f
  variants 1717–1718
  tumors 1710–1721
  verrucous carcinoma 1720
Bladder Cancer Flow Cytometry Network 42
bladder (Wedl) cells 2300, 2300f
'bladder worms' 104
blastema
  adult nephroblastoma 1690
  Wilms' tumor 1666, 1667, 1667f, 1668f
blastoma
  pleuropulmonary 976, 1016–1017
  pulmonary 975–976, 977f
Blastomyces dermatitidis 66, 85, 85f, 2410
  differential diagnosis 85, 86f
  identification/characteristics 67t
blastomycosis 1512f
  CNS involvement 2410
  laryngeal 79–80, 835
  respiratory tract 85–86, 85f, 90, 90f
bleomycin, disease/changes due to 148, 885, 886f
blepharoplasts 2367
blepharoptosis 2290
Blesovsky's syndrome (rounded atelectasis) 1007, 1007f
blindness 2289, 2317
B lineage lymphoid precursor cells 614, 618, 640
blistering disorders *see* bullous disorders
blisters
  acantholytic 217, 218f, 218t
  intraepidermal 218–221, 218t, 220
  subcorneal 216–218, 216t, 217f
  subepidermal 221–225, 222t
  suprabasilar 219, 220
blood group antigens, mesothelioma 1013
blood–nerve barrier 2240
blood supply
  adrenal cortex 2171
  breast 420
  cervix 1831
  esophagus 1283
  fallopian tube 2039
  kidney 1600–1601
  lung 861–862
  peripheral nerves 2240
  pituitary gland 2097
  placenta 2064
  pleura 1005
  skin 194
  testis 1731
  umbilical cord 2065
  vagina 1918–1919
  vulva 1885–1886
blood transfusion, anaphylaxis after 114
blood urea nitrogen (BUN), postinfectious glomerulonephritis 1617
blood vessels
  calcification of walls 233
  ectatic 396, 396f
    acne rosacea 226
    nevus flammeus 268
  inflammatory diseases *see* vasculitis
  invasion, breast cancer 488
  medial degeneration 1081–1083
  non-inflammatory diseases 1080–1085
  traumatic diseases 1083
  see also entries beginning vascular
bloody specimens, technical problems with 21
Bloom and Richardson grading system 464, 465t
Bloom syndrome 115

blot and dot hemorrhages 2317
'blueberry muffin babies' 383
'blue bodies' 899
'blue bone' 757
blue dome appearance, mucocele 1149
blue eardrum syndrome 2274
blue nevus *see* nevus, blue
blue rubber bleb syndrome 271
B-lymphoblastic leukemia/lymphoblastic lymphoma 627
B-lymphoblasts, staining 610
B lymphocytes *see* B cells
Bodian stain 2335t
Bohn's nodules 1142
bombesin, small cell lung carcinoma 991
bone 677–699
  aneurysmal cyst *see* aneurysmal cyst
  biopsy 612
    decalcification 609–610
    metastases 170
    in oral cavity 1137
  calcified lipoma 684, 685f
  capillary hemangioma 766, 767f
  cells 680
  creeping substitution 683, 684f
  cysts
    aneurysmal *see* aneurysmal cyst, of bone
    fine needle aspiration 704
    primary 755–758
    simple (unicameral) 756, 756f
  dead, recognition 678f, 683, 683f
  density 681, 687
  deposition of abnormal metabolic products 688–689
  development 681
  developmental disturbances 681
  disappearing, disease 687
  disorders 681–690
  dysmorphogenesis 1193
  dysplasia 1193
  eosinophilic granuloma of *see* Langerhans cell histiocytosis
  epithelioid hemangioendothelioma 767–768, 768f
  examination methods 677, 679
  fiber 679
  fibrous tumors 736–746
  formation
    defect, fibrous dysplasia as 741
    sunburst (onion-skin-like) pattern 728
  formation by tumors 702t, 721–736
    benign 721, 722–726, 722f
      see also osteoblastoma; osteoma
    epidemiology 701
    malignant 705, 721
      see also osteosarcoma
    malignant *vs* benign 705
  fragments, in crush preparations of CNS 2330, 2331f
  giant-cell-rich lesions 751–755
  giant cell tumor *see* giant cell tumor, of bone
  hemangioma 765–767, 766f
  hemangiopericytoma 769–770, 770f
  hematopoietic tumors 758–763
  heterotopic calcification 684–685
  heterotopic formation 684–685
  in histiocytoses 690
  Hodgkin's lymphoma 761
  hyperparathyroid disease 686, 686f, 2151
  immature 679
  infarction (osteonecrosis) 682, 683–684, 684f
  infections 689–690
    see also osteomyelitis
  lamellar 678–679, 679f
    fibrous dysplasia 1191
  large, metastases 169–170, 169t
  leiomyoma 771
  leiomyosarcoma 771
  leukemia involvement 762, 762t
  lipoma 770
  liposarcoma 770–771
  malignant round cell tumors 747t
    see also Ewing family of tumors

maturation, arrested 813–814
metabolic disease/disturbance 679, 685–689
metastases 771–772
  infiltrating (invasive) lobular carcinoma (breast) 469
  to large bones 169–170, 169t
  osteolytic *vs* osteoblastic 170
mineral, disturbances 686
myofibroma 736, 736f, 737f
necrosis 682
neuroectodermal tumors 702t, 746–751
non-Hodgkin's lymphoma (primary) 760–761, 761f
notochordal tumors 763–765
pagetoid 680f
Paget's disease *see* Paget's disease, of bone
pain, tumors causing 702
peripheral nerve sheath tumors 771
physiology 680–681
pseudosarcomatous appearance 682, 682f
radiation-associated tumors 159–160, 727, 735
sarcoma 701, 704
  epidemiology and site 701–702, 701t
  Ewing's *see* Ewing's sarcoma
  grading and staging 703, 703t
  metastatic sarcomatoid carcinoma *vs* 772
  reporting on specimens 705
  see also chondrosarcoma
scintigraphy 704, 772
small, metastases in 171t, 173
smooth muscle tumors 771
solitary plasmacytoma 654
staining methods 677
structure 677–678
trabeculum 680, 680f
tumor-like lesions 701–783
tumors 701–706, 701t
  bone-forming *see above*
  cartilage-forming *see* cartilage tumors
  fatty 770–771
  grading and staging 703, 703t
  primary, classification 702, 702t–703t
  reactive lesions simulating 703t
  secondary *see* bone, metastases
  in soft tissue 387–391
  specimens 704–705, 705f
  see also specific tumors/tumor types (see table 702–703t)
vascular tumors 765–770
woven 679, 679f
  fibrous dysplasia 813–814, 1191
  reactive 772–773, 773f
bone island 722, 722f
bone marrow 609–674
  acute leukemia *see* leukemia, acute
  agranulocytosis 617
  in AIDS 661–662, 661f, 662f
  angioimmunoblastic (immunoblastic) lymphadenopathy 663
  aplastic anemia 616–617
  aspiration 609, 664
  biopsy
    aspiration smears *vs* 609, 664
    site 609
    stains 610
  carcinocythemia 664, 664f
  cell types 612
  cellularity 616–639
    hypercellular 618–639, 619t
      see also hyperplasia (below)
    hypocellular 616–618, 616t
  changes in bone marrow recipients 618
  chronic leukemia *see* leukemia, chronic lymphocytic
  components 612
  cytochemistry 610
  cytologic studies 609
  'damaged' 618
  'dry tap' 609, 610, 624, 644, 665
  examination 609, 614–616

failure 633
fatty 612
fibrosis 639–640, 639t
  see also myelofibrosis
foamy cells 662, 662t
granuloma
  AIDS 662
  epithelioid 661, 661f
  infectious 661, 661f
  lipid 662
granulomatous changes/diseases 660–664, 660t
  benign nonhematologic conditions 661–662, 661f
  hematologic disorders 662
  proliferative 661
hematologic disorders, markers 611t
hematopoietic to fatty ratio 612
histiocytic proliferative disorders 657–660
  see also histiocytic proliferative disorders
histoplasmosis 662f
Hodgkin's lymphoma 647
hyperplasia, neoplastic 620–630
  see also leukemia, acute; myeloproliferative syndromes
hyperplasia, non-neoplastic 618–620, 619t
  erythroid 619–620, 620f
  granulocytic 620, 633
  megakaryocytic 620, 632
  myeloid 620
  reactive 618–619, 620
hypoplastic (hypocellular) acute leukemia 618, 618f
hypoplastic myelodysplastic syndrome 617–618
immunophenotypic studies 610
infarction 665–666
Kaposi's sarcoma 665f, 666
leukoerythroblastic reaction 664
lymphocytes 612, 614, 641
lymphocytic infiltration 640–653
  lymphoproliferative 641–646, 641t
    B-cell leukemia 641–644, 642f
    hairy cell leukemia 644–646, 645f
    NK-cell and T-cell leukemia 646–647, 646f
    see also leukemia, chronic lymphocytic; lymphoma (non-Hodgkin's)
  non-neoplastic 640–641, 641t
lymphoid aggregates 640, 640f
lymphoid follicles with germinal centers 640
lymphoid nodules 640
mast cell disease 663–664, 663f
megakaryocytic hypoplasia 617
metastases in 664–665, 664f
myeloid/erythroid ratio 612
necrosis 665–666, 665f, 665t
  children 664
  fat 665
in non-Hodgkin's lymphoma 647–652
normal 612–614, 616
paroxysmal nocturnal hemoglobinuria 617
pathology 616–666
plasmacytic disorders 653–657
pluripotent stem cells 612
postchemotherapy aplasia 616f, 618
in pure red cell aplasia 617
reactive lymphohistiocytic infiltrates 640
reactive lymphoid lesions 640–641
serous (mucinous, gelatinous) degeneration 616, 616f
specimen handling and processing 609, 610, 611t
  reporting checklist 615, 615t–616t
touch preparations 609, 648
transplantation
  bone marrow changes after 618
  graft-*versus*-host disease 129, 1402
  rejection 123, 618
  veno-occlusive disease after 1516, 1516f
vascular lesions 665f, 666
bone tissue 678–679
Bordetella pertussis 95

Borrelia burgdorferi 2244
  CNS infection 2407
  erythema migrans and 207
  MALT lymphoma and, cutaneous 290
  see also Lyme disease
botryoid embryonal rhabdomyosarcoma 1587–1588,
  1588f
botryoid odontogenic cysts 1142–1143, 1142f, 1143f
botryoid rhabdomyosarcoma *see* rhabdomyosarcoma
botryoid sarcoma
  bladder 1722
  cervix 1877
  middle ear 2281
  vulva 1916–1917, 1916f, 1917f
  see also embryonal rhabdomyosarcoma
botryomycosis 70
botulism 63
Bouin's solution 17, 1733
Bourneville's syndrome, large cell calcifying Sertoli
  cell tumors 1759
Bournville disease *see* tuberous sclerosis
'bowenoid' actinic keratosis 243–244
Bowenoid papulosis 246, 1902, 1903, 1904, 1905
  penis 1771
Bowenoid reticulosis, Paget's disease *vs* 1908
Bowen's disease 246, 1902
  of nipple, Paget's disease of nipple *vs* 457
  of penis 1771, 1771f
  true *vs* squamous cell carcinoma in situ 246
  see also vulva, intraepithelial neoplasia (VIN)
Bowman's capsule 1598
Bowman's membrane 2301, 2303
Bowman's space (urinary space) 1598
brachiocephalic arteries 1080
brachytherapy, uveal melanoma 2308
brain
  abscess *see* cerebral abscess
  biopsy 2329, 2331, 2335
  cysts *see* central nervous system (CNS), cysts
  HIV infection 118–119
  metastases in 169t
  tumors *see* central nervous system (CNS), tumors
  see also entries beginning cerebral
brainstem tumors 2345
  pilocytic astrocytoma 2357
branchial apparatus
  first branchial cleft cysts 2270–2271, 2271f
  fistulas and sinuses 2270–2271
branchial arches 834
branchial cleft cysts 244, 1260, 2270–2271, 2271f
branchial cysts 1148
branching enzyme deficiency 2232
Branham's sign 363
BRCA1 mutation
  breast carcinomas 473–474, 485
  fallopian tube adenocarcinoma 2045
  serous carcinoma of ovary 2001, 2001f
BRCA2 mutation
  breast carcinomas 485
  fallopian tube adenocarcinoma 2045
  parathyroid carcinoma 2162
  serous carcinoma of ovary 2001
breast 419–504
  adenoma 437–440
    carcinoma *vs* 438
    ductal 440
    lactating 437–439, 440f, 441f
    pleomorphic 438
    tubular 437, 439f
  adenomyoepithelioma 446–447, 447f
  anatomy 420–421
  angiosarcoma 485, 486f
    differential diagnosis 446
    of parenchyma 372
    postirradiation 371, 371f
  atypical ductal hyperplasia (ADH) 424, 430t, 432,
    434f, 459f
    core needle biopsy 427
    DCIS *vs* 461

atypical hyperplasia 430t, 432–433, 434f, 459f
atypical lobular hyperplasia 432–433, 434f
  lobular carcinoma in situ *vs* 461–462
benign disorders 430–433, 430t, 433–452
  factors modifying carcinoma risk 433
  nonproliferative lesions 430–431, 430t
  proliferative lesions without atypia 430t
benign neoplasms 433–452
biopsy
  core needle 419, 421, 426–427
  excisional 427–428
  fine needle *see* breast, fine needle aspiration (FNA)
  implantation of abnormal/normal epithelium 137
  incisional 427–428
  margin evaluation 427–428
  needle localization, nonpalpable lesions 428–429
  specimen radiography 428
  see also axillary lymph nodes
blood supply 420
calcification 428, 430
chondromatous lesions 446
collagenous spherulosis 448, 448f
complex sclerosing lesion (radial scars) 445, 445f
congenital abnormalities 421
core needle biopsy 419, 421, 426–427
cysts 25, 424, 424f, 430
cytology specimens 421–433
  benign disorders 430–433
  core needle biopsy 426–427
  FNA *see* breast, fine needle aspiration (FNA)
  incisional biopsies 427–428
  needle localization biopsies 428–429
diabetic mastopathy 450–451
embryology 419–420, 419f
epithelial proliferative lesion
  with atypia 423–424, 424f
  without atypia 424, 424f, 436–437
  see also breast, proliferative lesions
epithelium inclusion in lymph node 512
fat necrosis 448–449, 449f, 450f
  after irradiation 158, 450
  after needle biopsy 135
fibroadenoma 433–436, 435f
  ancient (calcified/ossified) 434
  atypical hyperplasia in 436
  carcinoma in 436
  carcinoma *vs* 437
  cytology 436–437, 438f, 439f
  FNA 28, 424, 424f
  giant 436
  infarction 436
  intracanalicular 435, 435f
  juvenile 435
  mucinous carcinoma *vs* 473
  pericanalicular 435, 435f
  phyllodes tumor *vs* 436
fibromatosis 445
fine needle aspiration (FNA) 28, 419, 421–426
  carcinoma diagnosis 423, 423f
  carcinoma types 423, 423f, 426, 468–469
  cysts 25, 424, 424f
  diagnostic categories 423–424
  epithelial proliferative lesions 423–424, 424f
  fat necrosis 135–136, 449
  fibroadenoma *vs* carcinoma 437
  gynecomastia 453f
  limitations 426
  NCI recommendations 422, 422t
  nonproliferative (benign) lesions 431
  probabilistic approach to diagnosis 423–424, 425t
  silicone-augmented tissue 450
  sites and false-negative results 28
  specimen adequacy 421–423, 422t
  specimen processing 422–423
  stereotactic guidance 426
  thin-layer techniques 422
  tissue changes due to 138
  'triple test' 422, 437
  unremarkable category 424, 424f

foreign-body-type inflammation 449–450
granular cell tumor 445
  differential diagnosis 482, 2255
hamartoma 447, 447f
hemangioma 446, 446f
histology 419–420, 420f
hyperplasia
  atypical 430t, 432–433, 434f
  columnar cell with atypia 459f
  cystic hypersecretory 461
  ductal 431, 431f, 432f
  mild 430
  moderate or florid 431
  nodular lactational 437–439
  without atypia 430t, 431–432, 431f, 432f, 433f
  see also atypical ductal hyperplasia (above)
hypertrophy 421
implants *see* breast, prostheses/implants
inflammatory lesions 448–450
intraductal papilloma 135–136
leiomyoma 446
leukemia infiltrates 485–486
lipoma 445–446
lymphatic system 420, 421f
lymphocytic mastopathy 450–451, 452f
lymphoma infiltrates 485–486
male
  carcinoma 484
  gynecomastia 421, 451–452, 452f, 453f
  metastatic tumors in 171t, 172
metastatic tumors in 171–172, 171t, 484–485
  sclerosing epithelioid fibrosarcoma mimicking
    329–330
microcalcifications, biopsy 428
microcyst 431f
microglandular adenosis 444, 444f
mucocele-like lesion 447–448, 447f
  mucinous carcinoma *vs* 472
myofibroblastoma 316f, 317f, 447
neural lesions 446
neuroendocrine abnormalities 421
nonpalpable lesions, needle localization biopsy
  428–429
papillary apocrine change 430
papillary lesions 440–444
papilloma, intraductal 440–444, 443f, 444f
  with atypia 443
  cardinal features *vs* carcinoma 442, 442t, 443
  intraductal 439
  multiple (peripheral) 440, 443
  sclerotic 440
  solitary 440–443, 442f, 442t
papillomatosis 440
  juvenile (Swiss cheese disease) 443–444
phyllodes tumor *see* phyllodes tumor
physiology 419
precocious development 421
proliferative lesions 433–452
  with atypia 437
  without atypia 430t, 431–432, 431f, 432f, 433f
prostheses/implants
  extra-abdominal fibromatosis (desmoid) with 322
  reactions to 142, 449–450
  silicone 142, 142f, 449–450, 451f
pseudoangiomatous stromal hyperplasia 446, 446f
radial scars 444–445, 445f
radiation therapy-induced lesions 158, 450, 451f,
  452f
reactive/inflammatory lesions 448–450
sarcoidosis 450
sarcoma 436, 485
schwannoma (neurilemoma) 446
sclerosing adenosis 431, 433f, 434f, 462
sclerosing papillary proliferation (radial scars) 445,
  445f
specimens 421–433
  cytology *see* breast, cytology specimens
  frozen sections 428
  lymph nodes 429–430

mastectomy 429
pathologic evaluation 421–433
re-excision 429
see also breast, biopsy
supernumerary 421
tumors *see* breast carcinoma; *specific tumors above*
vascular lesions, 446f 446
breast carcinoma 458, 475–476, 476f
adenoid cystic carcinoma 481–482, 481f, 482f
differential diagnosis 448
adenosquamous 440
differential diagnosis 446–447
low-grade 478, 480
aneuploid, DNA analysis 38, 38f
axillary node metastases *see* axillary lymph nodes
biological markers 488–489
BRCA1 and *BRCA2* mutations 485
cancerization of lobules 461
chemotherapy, epithelial changes due to 148
clinging (clinging DCIS) 458–459, 459f
colloid (mucinous) 472–473, 472f, 473f
differential diagnosis 261
adenoma *vs* 438
fibroadenoma *vs* 437
radiation-associated changes *vs* 450
DNA diploidy 37f
DNA ploidy determination 40f
ductal carcinoma in situ (DCIS) 452–461
adenoid cystic carcinoma with 481
apocrine 459–460, 460f
biological markers 454
characteristics 458–461
classification 452–453
clinging (clinging carcinoma) 458–459, 459f
comedo type 453, 456f, 458
cribriform 448, 453, 453f, 476
cystic hypersecretory 460–461
differential diagnosis 461
ductal hyperplasia *vs* 461
endocrine (argyrophilic) 460
fibroadenoma involvement 436
fine needle aspiration 426
high-grade (poorly differentiated) 458, 462f
intermediate-grade 458
in invasive micropapillary carcinoma 477
LCIS *vs* 462
lobule involvement 461
low-grade (well differentiated) 458
in medullary carcinoma 474
in metaplastic carcinoma 478–479
microcalcifications 454–455
micropapillary 453, 454f
multicentricity, incidence 455
needle core biopsy specimen 138f
noncomedo 459–460
nuclear grading 457f
occult invasion, incidence 456
papillary 453, 460, 460f
papillary, *vs* benign intraductal papilloma 442, 442t, 443
papillary stratified spindle cell type 455f
signet ring cell 460
solid type 453, 455f, 460, 460f
tubular carcinoma with 470
see also Paget's disease, of nipple
fine needle aspiration 423, 423f, 426, 468–469
fluorescence in situ hybridization (FISH) 47f
frozen sections and false-positives 5
growth rates 486
histologic grading importance 487
HRT-associated risk 150
infiltrating carcinoma of no special type (IC-NST) 463, 477
infiltrating ductal not otherwise specified (IDC-NOS) 463
in situ with indeterminate features (CIS-IF) 462, 463
invasive 462–485, 483t
choriocarcinomatous features 483
glycogen-rich 484

lipid-rich 484
osteoclast-like giant cells 483, 484f
rare types 483–484
invasive apocrine 482, 483f
invasive cribriform 475–476, 476f
invasive (infiltrating) ductal 463–465, 464f, 466f
atypical medullary carcinoma *vs* 474
clinical course/prognosis 464–465, 487, 488
grading systems 464, 465t
granular cell tumor *vs* 2255
Her 2 neu staining 33, 34f, 46
histopathology 464, 464f, 465f
scirrhous-type 465
invasive (infiltrating) lobular 465–470
alveolar type 467, 467f
bone metastases 772
BRCA2 mutation 485
classical form 466–467, 467f, 468, 470
cytopathology 468–469, 469f
histiocytoid 468, 468f, 469
histopathology 175, 466–468, 467f
lymph node metastasis 479f
pleomorphic variant 468, 468f, 469, 470
pleural effusions 1029, 1030f
signet ring cell variant 468, 470, 485
single-file arrangement 466, 467f
solid form 467, 467f
trabecular variant 467
tubulolobular variant 468, 468f, 470
invasive micropapillary 476–477, 477f
invasive papillary 476
invasive with ductal and lobular features 470
invasive with neuroendocrine differentiation 480
lobular carcinoma in situ (LCIS) 461–462, 462f
benign lesions involved 462
DCIS *vs* 462
fibroadenoma involvement 436
infiltrating lobular carcinoma with 465
tubular carcinoma with 470
type A (classical) and type B 461
male 484
medullary 473–475, 474f, 487
atypical 474, 475
BRCA1 mutation 473–474, 485
metaplastic 477–480, 478f, 479f
chondroid differentiation 478, 478f
fibromatosis-like 479
monophasic (sarcomatoid) 479
spindle-cell differentiation 478, 478f
metastatic
to adrenal gland 2202, 2202f
to CNS 2399, 2400f
to ovary 2039
to parathyroid gland 2165
to thyroid 2141
to uveal tract 2309
micrometastases, bone marrow 664–665
mucinous 472–473, 472f, 473f
mucocele-like lesion *vs* 447
mucinous cystadenocarcinoma 484
nipple discharge exfoliative cytology 425
pleural effusions 1029, 1030f
in pregnancy and lactation 438
prognostic factors 486–489
pulmonary Langerhans cell histiocytosis with 923–924
quantitative immunohistochemistry 43
radiation-associated 160
risk, benign breast diseases 430, 430t, 433
scirrhous, radial scars *vs* 445
secretory ('juvenile') 482–483
sentinel lymph nodes *see* sentinel lymph nodes
small cell 480
surgical report contents 489
tubular 440, 470–471, 471f, 472f, 487
mammography 463
microglandular adenosis *vs* 444
'mixed' 470
radial scars *vs* 445
syringomatous adenoma of nipple *vs* 440

breath test, *Helicobacter pylori* detection 1330
Brenner tumors 1021, 2012–2013
benign 2012, 2012f
borderline 2012–2013, 2013f
malignant 2012, 2013
'metaplastic' 2012
proliferating 2012, 2013
Breslow thickness 284, 286
British Testicular Tumor Panel (BTTP) 1741
broad ligament, tumors 2047–2048
adrenal cortical rests and tumors 2047, 2047f
ependymoma 2048
epithelial cysts/tumors 2047–2048
mesenchymal tumors 2048
papillary tumors 2048
Broder's system 1859–1860
bronchi
adenoma
gland adenoma 945–946, 946f, 949
pleomorphic (benign mixed tumor) 946–947
anatomy 860
biopsy 868
carcinoma *see* lung, carcinoma
gland-forming lesions 945–962, 946t
localized diseases 935–1003
reactive cells, pulmonary carcinoid tumors *vs* 985
reactive/hyperplastic epithelium 957
bronchial brushing, lung carcinoma 939
bronchial forceps biopsy, lung carcinoma 939
bronchial gland adenoma 945–946, 946f, 949
bronchial washing, lung carcinoma 939
bronchiectasis, traction 896
bronchiolar fibrosis, neuroendocrine hyperplasia with 908, 908f
bronchioles
anatomy 860, 860f
lesions in smokers 906
loss 910, 911f
respiratory 860
terminal 861
bronchiolitis 901, 906
acute, lung transplant recipient 920
in asthma 911, 912f
cellular 906f, 909, 920
classification (etiologic) 906, 906t
constrictive (obliterative) 905, 909–910, 910f
chronic rejection of lung graft 128, 129
lung transplant recipient 920–921, 921f
rheumatoid arthritis 888, 906–907
cryptogenic 908–909
diffuse panbronchiolitis (DPB) 907, 907f
eosinophilic, lung transplant recipient 920
follicular 909, 910f
rheumatoid arthritis 888, 888f
Sjögren's syndrome 889, 889f
foreign body 908, 910
graft-*versus*-host disease (GVHD) 907
in hypersensitivity pneumonitis 890
inflammatory bowel disease-associated 908, 909f
with interstitial disease 898–899
lung transplant recipient 920–921, 921f
lymphocytic 919, 920
mineral dust 907–908
nontobacco 906–909
occlusive 909, 910, 910f
lung transplant recipient 920–921, 921f
respiratory 922, 923f
respiratory syncytial virus (RSV) 94
rheumatoid 888, 906–907
tobacco 906
in unexplained chronic air-flow obstruction 906–909
bronchiolitis obliterans 901
lung transplant recipient 920–921, 921f, 922f
bronchiolitis obliterans interstitial pneumonia 900–901, 901f
bronchiolitis obliterans organizing pneumonia (BOOP) 900–901, 901f
lung transplant recipient 920

bronchiolitis obliterans syndrome (BOS), lung transplantation 919–920
bronchiolization 922
bronchioloalveolar carcinoma (BAC) 952–958
  cytology 939, 956–958, 957f, 958f
  differential diagnosis 956, 957–958
  immunohistochemistry 182f, 954
  mucinous 955f, 956, 957f
  nonmucinous 955f, 956, 958f
  staging 937
  types A, B and C 953–954, 955f
bronchitis
  acute, lung transplant recipient 920
  chronic 911, 912f
  follicular 909, 910f
  lymphocytic, lung transplant recipient 920
bronchoalveolar lavage (BAL) 866, 939
bronchoalveolar tumor, intravascular 973–974, 974f
bronchogenic cysts
  mediastinum 1093, 1093f
  pericardial 1070
  skin 244
bronchovascular bundle 861
  sarcoidosis 892, 892f, 893f
  thickened 864f, 927
bronchus-associated lymphoid tissue (BALT) 860–861
  lymphoma, lung 977–979, 978f, 979f, 981
brown bowel syndrome 1404
Brown-Brenn stain (tissue Gram stain) 60t, 69, 2335t
'brown' fat cells 1065, 1066f
Brown-Hopps stain 59, 60t
brown tumor, of hyperparathyroidism 686, 751–752, 751f, 752f, 753, 1183, 2151
Brucella and brucellosis 101, 101f
Brunner's glands 1323–1324, 1373
  hamartoma 1420, 1420f
  hyperplasia 1396–1397, 1397f
  lesions 1420–1421
Brunn's nests 1715
  proliferations 1708
Brunsting-Perry variant of cicatricial pemphigoid 224
Bruton's agammaglobulinemia (X-linked) 113
Bruton tyrosine kinase (Btk) gene, mutation 113
'bubble gum' colloid, papillary thyroid carcinoma 2130
buccal mucosa, squamous cell carcinoma 1173
Budd–Chiari syndrome 353, 1515, 1516f
Buerger's disease (thromboangiitis obliterans) 1078, 1079f
bulla 195
bullous dermatosis of childhood 223–224, 224f
bullous disorders 216–225
  autoimmune 223
  intraepidermal blisters 218–221, 218t
  subcorneal blisters 216–218
  subepidermal 221–225, 222t
  vulva and vagina 1893t
bullous keratopathy (corneal edema) 2301, 2301f
bullous pemphigoid 222–223, 222f
  cicatricial pemphigoid *vs* 224
  vulva 1894
buphthalmos 2316
Burkitt's lymphoma 569–570
  acute lymphoblastic leukemia with 627, 627f
  atypical 570, 570f
  bone marrow 650
  classical 628
  differential diagnosis 561, 570–571
  endemic and sporadic types 569, 628
  Epstein–Barr virus (EBV) and 1453
  histology 569–570, 570f
  HIV-associated 571
  immunodeficiency-associated 569
  immunohistochemistry 1453
  intestinal involvement 1450, 1453
  lymph node granulomas 532
  oncogenes 1352
  plasmacytoid differentiation 628
  sporadic 569
  WHO classification 628

Burkitt's-type lymphoma, lymphoblastic lymphoma *vs* 569
burns, larynx and trachea 834
burr holes, bone fragments in crush preparations due to 2330–2331
bursitis 697
Buschke-Lowenstein tumor 248, 1771
'busy sign', clear cell renal cell carcinoma 1680, 1681f
byssinosis 891
'byssinosis bodies' 891

C

C1q nephropathy 1633–1634, 1634f
C3 deposits, kidney 1609–1610, 1615
C4d staining, renal transplant biopsy 1649, 1651, 1651f
CA-19-9 180
CA-125 180
CA-125 monoclonal antibody test 1996
c-abl proto-oncogene 632–633
CADASIL 2415, 2415f
cadherins
  lack, diffuse gastric adenocarcinoma 1358
  see also E-cadherin
cadmium, lung cancer etiology 936
café-au-lait pigmented macules 282, 740, 741
CAG-A *see* gastritis, autoimmune chronic
calcification
  aortic valve 1057, 1057f
  blood vessels 233
  breast *see* breast, calcification
  cardiac myxoma 1063
  dystrophic
    calcinosis cutis 233
    neuroblastoma of adrenal medulla 2195
  'eggshell' 904
  gallbladder (diffuse dystrophic) 1576
  heterotopic, of bone 684–685
  Liesgang ring 1153
  medial 1083
  mitral valve 1056
  oligodendroglioma 2361, 2361f
  ossifying fibroma 1181, 1181f
  pericardial 1019
  psammomatoid 743, 743f
  synovial sarcoma 402
calcifying aponeurotic fibroma 311–312, 311f, 312f
calcifying epithelial odontogenic tumor *see* odontogenic tumors
calcifying epithelioma of Malherbe (pilomatrixoma) 253–254, 253f
calcifying fibrous pseudotumor 317–318, 317f, 318f
  of pleura 1017, 1017f
calcifying giant cell tumor *see* chondroblastoma
calcifying intracardiac pseudoneoplasm 1066
calcifying Sertoli cell tumors 1758, 1759–1760, 1760f
calcinosis 233–234
  idiopathic tumoral 233
  metastatic 233
  vascular 1083
calcinosis cutis 233
calcinosis universalis 206
calciphylaxis 233, 233f
calcitonin, medullary thyroid carcinoma 2135, 2137
calcitonin gene-related peptide (CGRP), medullary thyroid carcinoma 2137
calcium
  homeostasis 2150–2151
    disturbances 686
  staining methods 16t
calcium binding proteins 31t
calcium channels, autoantibodies 2227
calcium-dependent adhesion molecules 1358
  see also cadherins
calcium oxalate crystal, near mycetomas 92, 93f
calcium oxalate crystalluria 1895
calcium oxalate deposits, breast 428
calcium phosphate deposits, breast 428

calcium pyrophosphate dihydrate deposition disease 688, 688f, 691
calcium-sensing receptor (CaR) 2152
  chief cell hyperplasia 2158
  gastrinoma 1573
  mutations 2158
calcofluor white stain 61, 88
calculi
  extrahepatic bile ducts 1583
  prostatic 1793
CALLA *see* CD10 (common acute lymphoblastic leukemia antigen)
Callendar classification, uveal melanoma 2306–2307, 2307f
Call-Exner bodies 1987, 2016
calponin 348, 403, 404
calretinin staining
  adrenal cortical adenoma 33, 35f
  effusions 1033
  granulosa cell tumor of ovary 2017
  mesothelioma 1012, 1012f
  sex cord-stromal tumor differential diagnosis 2017t
Calymmatobacterium granulomatis 1890
CAM 5.2 stain, hepatocellular carcinoma 1534
cambium layer, botryoid rhabdomyosarcoma 358, 359f, 820
'cambium zone' 1916
Campylobacter
  appendiceal infection 1409
  colitis 1395
Campylobacter jejuni 1390f, 2242
canalicular adenoma, salivary glands 1186, 1188, 1188f, 1222–1223, 1224f
canal of Nuck, cysts 1899
canals of Hering 1474
cancrum oris (noma) 78–79
Candida 70–71
  identification/characteristics 66t, 67t
Candida albicans 70–71
  cervical infection 1836t, 1837, 1849
  larynx and tracheal infection 835
Candida glabrata 71, 85, 1849
Candida krusei 71
Candida tropicalis 71
candidiasis/*Candida* infections 217
  CNS involvement 2410, 2411f
  disseminated, myositis 2222
  esophagitis 1289, 1289f
  intestinal 1399
  lung involvement 880
  mucosal 71f
  oral (thrush) 71
  pustular, vulvar 1891, 1891f
  vagina 1919
'candle wax dripping' appearance, pleural plaque 1006, 1006f
'cannibalism', cell 1031
cannonball metastases 170, 183
cap disease 2229
capillaries
  glomerular *see* glomerular capillaries
  pulmonary *see* pulmonary capillaries
  vasculitis 1075–1078, 1076t
capillaritis, diffuse alveolar hemorrhage 884, 884f
capillary hemangioma
  of bone 766, 767f
  juvenile 269–270, 269f
    oral cavity 1186
  lobular 269, 270, 270f
  orbital 2296–2297
  sinonasal region 817
  of skin 269, 269f
  vulva 1901
capillary telangiectasis, CNS 2415–2416
Caplan's syndrome 888
carbohydrates, staining methods 16t
carbol fuchsin method 60
carbuncle 225
Carbus' disease 1772

carcinoembryonic antigen (CEA) 179
  ampulla of Vater invasive adenocarcinoma 1588
  antibodies, liver biopsy 1470
  carcinoid tumors 1423
  cystic tumors of pancreas 1562
  epithelioid sarcoma 400
  gallbladder labeling 1576
  intrauterine/extrauterine synchronous carcinoma
    1967
  mucinous tumors of ovary 2006
  Paget's disease of nipple 457
  papillary renal cell carcinoma 1681
  polyclonal, hepatocellular carcinoma 1534
  tumors associated 179
carcinogenesis, multistage 1168, 1170
carcinogens
  esophageal squamous carcinoma 1293–1294
  lung cancer 935, 936
  oral cancer 1138
carcinoid–carcinoma composite tumors, stomach 1350
carcinoid heart disease 1059
carcinoid syndrome 1350, 1425–1426, 1689
  carcinoid heart disease 1059
  carcinoid tumor of ovary 2035
  carcinoid tumor of testis 1756
  features 1425–1426, 2035
  laryngeal carcinoid 843
  small intestinal endocrine tumors 1425–1426
carcinoid tumor(s)
  breast carcinoma with neuroendocrine features 480
  duodenum 1424, 1425f
  endobronchial 983, 984–985
  extrahepatic bile ducts 1586, 1587f
  fallopian tube 2045
  goblet cell 1429, 1429f
  kidney 1689–1690
  laryngeal 843
  lung see lung
  metastases
    in breast 484
    in ovary 2039
  of middle ear 2278
  mid-gut 23
  multifocal, small intestinal 1425f
  ovary see ovary, carcinoid tumors
  sclerotic bone metastases 772
  small intestinal 1423, 1425–1426, 1427f, 1428f
  stomach see gastric carcinoid tumors
  testis 1756
  thymus see thymus
  see also neuroendocrine tumors
carcinoid 'tumorlets' 908, 908f
carcinoma
  cytokeratin 7 and 20 expression 512t
  lymph node involvement 511
  metastatic
    in bone 771
    in bone marrow 664, 664f
    embryonal carcinoma vs 1750
    epithelioid hemangioendothelioma vs 768
    Leydig cell tumor vs 1758
    skeletal angiosarcoma vs 769
  pleomorphic rhabdomyosarcoma vs 362
  poorly differentiated, pulmonary lymphoma vs 982
  of unknown origin 511
  see also specific types of carcinoma, anatomic sites
carcinoma cuniculatum 248
carcinoma ex mixed tumor 258
carcinoma in situ see specific anatomic sites
carcinoma prostate gland, basaloid/adenoid cystic
  1820
carcinomatous meningitis, breast carcinoma 469
carcinosarcoma 1819
  cervix 1877
  endometrium 1977, 1977f, 1978f
  fallopian tube 2046
  hepatocellular 1536
  larynx 846
  lung 975, 977f

oral cavity 1177
ovary 2010, 2010f
pleomorphic rhabdomyosarcoma vs 362–363
prostatic 1819–1820, 1819f
salivary gland 1243–1244, 1244f
sinonasal region 791, 793, 793f
see also sarcomatoid carcinoma
carcinothymia 664, 664f
cardiac calcifying amorphous tumor 1066
cardiac catheterization, tumor confusion after 146
cardiac fibroma 1064
cardiac myxoma 1062, 1063–1064, 1064f, 1157
cardiac 'pheochromocytoma' 1066
cardiac rhabdomyoma 1065, 1065f
cardiac surgery, tumor confusion after 146
cardiac transplantation see heart transplantation
cardiac valves see heart valves
cardiomyopathy 1045–1048
  amyloidosis vs 1048
  dilated 1045, 1046f
  drug-induced 1048–1049
  Fabry's disease vs 1048
  histiocytoid 1048
  hypertrophic 1048, 1065
  idiopathic dilated 1045
  restrictive 1045–1047
  sarcoidosis 1045
'cardiopyloric' glands 1321
cardiovascular disease
  atherosclerosis 1070–1072
  blood vessel disease 1070–1079
  saphenous vein bypass grafts 1072
  vasculitis see vasculitis
cardiovascular system 1041–1089
  biopsy see endomyocardial biopsy
  infections 99–100
Carneiro classification, gastric adenocarcinoma 1354
Carney complex
  cutaneous myxoma in 267
  primary pigmented nodular adrenocortical disease
    2181
  superficial angiomyxoma 1902
Carney's syndrome
  blue nevus 279
  large cell calcifying Sertoli cell tumors 1759
  melanotic schwannoma in 2252–2253
  multiple lentigines 277
Carney's triad 706, 975, 1347
carnitine, deficiency 2232
carnitine palmityltransferase deficiency 2233
Carnoy's fixative 21
Carnoy's fluid 17
Caroli's disease 1521
carotenes, oral squamous cell carcinoma and 1169
carotid artery disease
  plaques 1071, 1071f
  restenosis lesions 1071, 1071f
carotid endarterectomy 1071, 1072t
carpal tunnel syndrome 697
cartilage
  articular 691, 692
  bone formation 681
  elastic 706
  fibrillated 692f
  hyaline 706
  inflammatory diseases 225–228
  malignant, in parosteal osteosarcoma 732
  myxoid 706
  necrosis, chondrodermatitis nodularis helicis 227
cartilage tumors 702t, 706–721
  benign 706–715
    see also chondroblastoma; chondroma;
      osteochondroma (exostosis)
  malignant 715–721
    see also chondrosarcoma
  in soft tissue 387–391
caruncle, urethral 1724, 1725f
CASTLE (carcinoma showing thymus-like
  differentiation) 2140, 2140f

Castleman's disease (angiofollicular lymphoid
    hyperplasia) 521–522, 980
  calcifying fibrous pseudotumor association 317
  dendritic cell tumors and 574
  differential diagnosis 522, 1101t, 1102t
    HIV-associated lymphadenopathy vs 523, 524
    thymoma vs 1098, 1099f
  hyaline vascular type 521–522, 521f, 522
    lymphoid variant 521
  mantle zones 522
  multicentric 522
  plasma cell type 522
  stromal-rich variant 522
catalyzed reporter deposition (CARD) method 32
cataracts 2299–2300
  cortical (soft) 2299, 2300f
  posterior/anterior subcapsular 2300, 2300f
  removal 2299, 2304
  senile nuclear (nuclear sclerosis) 2299
catecholamine secretion 2189, 2190f
  neuroblastoma investigation 384
β-catenin
  antibodies, solid pseudopapillary tumor of pancreas
    1568, 1569f
  mutations
    fibromatosis association 320
    gallbladder adenoma 1579
    juvenile nasal angiofibroma 394
    pulmonary blastoma 976
  nuclear
    extra-abdominal fibromatosis (desmoid) 324, 324f
    intra-abdominal fibromatosis (desmoid) 325
β-catenin/APC pathway, acinar cell carcinoma of
    pancreas 1560
caterpillar (chenille) bodies 311, 311f
catgut 144, 145f
cat-scratch disease/fever 64, 78, 96–98, 97f
  cytologic diagnosis 97–98, 97f, 534
  differential diagnosis 97, 534
  lymphadenitis 533–534, 534f
  oculoglandular 78, 78f, 2294
cavernous angioma, CNS 2415
cavernous hemangioma
  liver 1540–1541
  oral cavity 1186
  orbital 2297, 2297f
  of skin 270–271, 271f
  vulva 1901
C cells, thyroid 2119, 2134
  hyperplasia 2136, 2139
  lesions 2135–2139
    see also thyroid carcinoma, medullary
  origin and location 2135
CD1a 573, 760
CD2-associated protein (CD2AP) 1598–1599
CD3, lymphoblastic lymphoma 568
CD4, acute leukemia 631
CD4 cells see T cells, helper (CD4)
CD5 1101, 1105, 1105f
CD7, lymphoblastic lymphoma 568
CD8 lymphocytes
  cytotoxicity mechanisms 122
  graft rejection 122
  polymyositis 2219
  thymoma 1100
CD9, acute basophilic leukemia 624
CD10 (common acute lymphoblastic leukemia antigen)
    639
  benign metastasizing leiomyoma of lung 971
  clear cell renal cell carcinoma 1680
  diffuse large B cell lymphoma 560
  endometrial stromal sarcoma 1974
  endometrial-type stroma 1995
  endometrium 1934, 1934f
  follicular lymphoma 549
  lymphoblastic lymphoma 569
  solid pseudopapillary tumor of pancreas 1568, 1569f
CD14 287
CD15 631, 2012

CD17, acute basophilic leukemia 624
CD19, acute leukemia 631
CD20
  anti-CD20 (retuximab) 551, 1354
  cutaneous MALToma 290
  lymphoblastic lymphoma 569
  lymphomatoid granulomatosis 290
  small lymphocytic lymphoma 551
CD23, small lymphocytic (B-cell) 552
CD30 (Ki-1) antigen 180, 509
  anaplastic large cell lymphoma 292, 563, 564, 565f, 652
  embryonal carcinoma of ovary 2030
  Hodgkin's disease 540
  seminoma differential diagnosis 1775t
CD31
  angiosarcoma 276, 373
  epithelioid hemangioendothelioma 367
  Kaposi's sarcoma 275
CD34
  angiosarcoma 276, 373
  cardiac myxoma 1063
  choroid glioma of third ventricle 2373
  gastrointestinal stromal tumors 1345
  hepatocellular carcinoma 1534
  Kaposi's sarcoma 275
  myofibroblastoma 316, 316f
  solitary fibrous tumor 376, 377, 377f, 1900
  synovial sarcoma 403
CD38, chronic lymphocytic leukemia 643
CD43 509, 511
  lymphoblastic lymphoma 568
  small lymphocytic (B-cell) lymphoma 552, 553f
CD45 511
  anaplastic large cell lymphoma 564
  diffuse large B cell lymphoma 559–560, 560f
  lymphoma immunostaining and malpractice 13, 13f
  peripheral T-cell lymphoma 562
CD45RA, salivary gland lymphoma 1256
CD45RB 511
CD45RO, lymphomas 562, 564
CD52, antibodies 551
CD55, paroxysmal nocturnal hemoglobinuria 617
CD56 (neural-cell adhesion molecule)
  adult rhabdomyoma 355
  C-cell hyperplasia (thyroid) 2139
  peripheral T-cell lymphoma 562
CD57 (Leu-7) 181, 381
CD59, paroxysmal nocturnal hemoglobinuria 617
CD61, chronic myeloid leukemia 633
CD68 287
CD70, thymic carcinoma 1105
CD79a, cutaneous MALToma 290
CD99 (O13; MIC2)
  Ewing's sarcoma 386
  juvenile granulosa cell tumor 2018
  sex cord-stromal tumor differential diagnosis 2017t
  synovial sarcoma 403, 404
  thymoma 1101, 1101f
CD117 (c-kit)
  dysgerminoma 2028
  gastrointestinal stromal tumors 1345, 1443, 1444
  systemic mastocytosis 763
  thymic seminoma 1117, 1118f
  see also c-kit proto-oncogene
CD130, mediastinal embryonal carcinoma 1118, 1119f
CDX2 staining 33, 34f, 182
cecal red patch 1392
celiac disease 1374–1375, 1374f, 1375f, 1377
  complications 1376
  dermatitis herpetiformis and 223, 223f, 1374, 1375
  duodenal biopsy classification 1375
  lymphocytic/collagenous colitis with 1401
  lymphocytic gastritis and 1335
  lymphoma risk 1375
cell block method 21
  FNA samples for 24–25, 35
cell line antibodies 180–182, 180t

cell staining methods 16t–17t, 17–19
cellular blue nevus see nevus, blue
cellular proliferation, biological markers 2338
cellulitis 68–69, 68f
  orbital 2294
cellulose, tissue reactions to 139
'cell windows', pancreas cytopathology 1550, 1550f
'cementicles' 743
cement lines 688
cementoblastoma 1141f, 1159, 1159f, 1193
cementoblasts 1159
cemento-osseous dysplasia 1193–1194, 1194f
  periapical 1193
cementum-like material, simple (unicameral) bone cyst 756, 756f
central core myopathy 2228, 2228t
'central fibrous scar', focal nodular hyperplasia of liver 1527
central giant cell reparative granuloma (CGCRG) 814, 815
central giant cell tumor, oral cavity 1182–1183, 1182f
central nervous system (CNS) 2329–2428
  in AIDS/HIV infection 2409–2410
  angiomatosis of see hemangioblastoma, CNS
  arteriovenous malformations 2415–2416, 2416f
  cavernous angioma 2415
  chemotherapy-induced injury/effects 2344–2345
  crush preparations 2329–2331, 2330f
    artifacts 2330–2331, 2330f, 2331f
    necrotic vs hemorrhagic tissue 2329
    staining 2329
    structural changes, differential diagnosis 2332t–2334t
  cysts 2400–2404
    arachnoid 2403
    colloid 2401, 2402f, 2403f
    dermoid 2400–2401, 2402f
    endodermal origin 2401
    ependymal 2403
    epidermoid 2400, 2402f
    neurenteric (enterogenous) 2401
    pineal 2403, 2404f
    Rathke cleft 2401, 2403
  degenerative disorders 2417
  demyelinating diseases 2413, 2414f
  developmental disorders 2417
  diagnostic techniques 2331–2340
    cytogenetics and molecular diagnosis 2338, 2340
    electron microscopy 2335–2336, 2336t–2337t
    fixation/stains for light microscopy 2335, 2335t
    frozen sections and stains 2331
    immunohistochemistry 2336–2338, 2338t
    tissue microarrays 2340
  epilepsy pathology 2404–2406
  glioblastoma of see glioblastoma
  gliosarcoma 2355–2356, 2356f, 2357f
  hematomas 2416–2417
  hematopoietic lesions 2397
  histology (normal) 2340–2345
    astrocytes 2340–2343, 2341f
    choroid plexus 2344
    ependyma cells 2343, 2344f
    glia 2340–2344
    macrophage 2344
    microglia 2344
    neurons 2340, 2340f
    oligodendrocytes 2343, 2343f
    see also individual cell types
  infarcts 2417
  infectious disorders 105–106, 2406–2413
    bacterial 2406–2407
    fungal 2410–2411
    parasitic 2411–2412
    prion disorders 2412–2413, 2413f
    viral 2407–2410
  inflammatory disorders 2406, 2413–2414
  intraoperative evaluation of lesions 2329
    crush preparations see above
    fixation delays effect 2331

  frozen sections 2331, 2331f
    pitfalls 2329
    stains 2331, 2335t
  metabolic disorders 2417
  primary melanocytic lesions 2393
  radiation-induced changes 2344, 2345f
  radiation-induced tumors 160, 2344, 2348
  transmissible spongiform encephalopathies 2412–2413, 2413f
  tumor-like lesions 2403–2404
  tumors 2345–2348
    astrocytic see astrocytic tumors
    choroid plexus 2370–2372
    differential diagnosis by site/age 2348t
    embryonal see embryonal tumors of CNS
    ependymal 2364–2369
    familial tumor syndromes 2400, 2401t
    genetic abnormalities 2340t
    germ cell 2397
    glial tumors of uncertain origin 2372–2374
    granular cell tumor 2399
    immunohistochemistry 2338t–2339t
    lipoma 2404
    lymphoma see lymphoma, CNS
    meningeal 2387–2394
    metastases 2347, 2399–2400
    mixed neuronal-glial 2374–2377
    nerve sheath 2385–2387
    neuronal 2374–2377
    neuroradiologic evaluation 2345–2346, 2346t
    oligodendroglial 2360–2364
    primary 2348–2399
    radiation-associated 160, 2344, 2348
    sarcomas 2393
    of sellar region 2398–2399
    ultrastructure 2336t–2337t
    WHO classification 2346–2347, 2346t
    WHO grading 2347, 2347t
    see also individual tumor types
  vascular disorders 2414–2417
  vascular malformations 2415–2416
  vasculitis 2414
  venous angioma and varix 2415
central neurocytoma see neurocytoma, central
central nuclear (myotubular) myopathy 2228–2229, 2228t
central retinal artery, occlusion 2315f
centroblasts 547
  diffuse large B-cell lymphoma 558
  follicular lymphoma 289, 547, 548, 548f, 549f
centrocytes 547
  follicular lymphoma 289, 289f, 547, 548, 548f, 549f
c-erbB-1, oral squamous cell carcinoma 1170
c-erbB-2, salivary large cell undifferentiated carcinoma 1249
cerebellar liponeurocytoma 2376–2377, 2377f
cerebellar pilocytic astrocytoma 2357
cerebellopontine angle
  acoustic neuroma 2279
  tumor differential diagnosis by age 2348t
cerebellum
  dysplastic gangliocytoma 2374
  medulloblastoma 2379, 2380
  melanosis 2393, 2393f, 2394f
cerebral abscess 2406, 2407f
  aspergillosis 2410, 2410f
  Nocardia infection 2406
cerebral amebiasis 2412, 2412f
cerebral amyloid angiopathy 2414, 2414t, 2415f
cerebral autosomal dominant arteriopathy with subcortical infarcts and leukoencephalopathy (CADASIL) 2415, 2415f
cerebral hemispheres
  malformations 2405
  tumor differential diagnosis 2348t
  see also brain
cerebral hemorrhage 2414, 2416–2417
cerebral hernia 2271
cerebral infarction 2417

cerebrospinal fluid
  formation 2344
  malignant cells in, CNS lymphoma 2395, 2396f
ceruminous adenocarcinoma 2276
ceruminous adenomas 2276, 2276f
ceruminous gland tumors 2276, 2276f
  middle ear adenoma vs 2278
cervical intraepithelial neoplasia (CIN) 1852–1856
  atypical squamous cells of undetermined
      significance 1864–1866, 1865f
  diagnostic methods 1855
  epidemiology and risk factors 1852, 1853, 1861
  high-grade squamous intraepithelial lesion (HSIL)
      1833, 1853t
    atypical squamous cells (ASC-H) 1864, 1865,
        1865f
    cytopathology 1844t, 1862–1863, 1863f
    histology 1854, 1855f
    keratinizing dysplasia variant 1862
  low-grade squamous intraepithelial lesion (LSIL)
      1833, 1853t
    cytopathology 1861–1862, 1862f
    histology 1854, 1854f
  malignant transformation 1852
  mild dysplasia (CIN 1) 1854, 1854f
  moderate dysplasia (CIN 2) 1854, 1854f, 1855f
  progression to cervical carcinoma 1856–1857
  severe dysplasia (CIN 3) 1854, 1855f
  terminology 1853, 1853t
  vaginal intraepithelial neoplasia (VAIN) secondary
      to 1923
cervical lymph nodes, metastases 169, 169t
cervical lymphoepithelial cysts 1148
cervical ribs 1205
cervical smears 1935
  adequacy 1834–1835, 1834t
  automation 44
  Bethesda system see Bethesda system
  cell types in 1842–1843
  endometrial adenocarcinoma 1873–1874
  endometrial cells in 1871, 1872, 1873
  endometrial hyperplasia diagnosis and 1958
  herpes virus in 75, 75f
  IUDs effect 143
  neoplastic lesions 1834
  normal components 1842–1843
  radiation-associated changes 152, 152f
  squamous cells 1842–1843
  unsatisfactory 1833, 1835
  see also cervix, cytology/cytopathology
cervicitis 1835–1838, 1854–1855
  acute or chronic 1835
  follicular 1835
  granulomatous 1836t, 1837
  infectious 1835–1838, 1836t
    actinomycosis 1836t, 1837
    bacterial 1835, 1836t
    chlamydial 1835–1836, 1836t
    fungal 1836t, 1837, 1849
    parasitic 1836t, 1837
    viral 1836–1837, 1836t
  noninfectious 1835
  vesicular 1837
cervicovaginitis emphysematosa 1838
cervix 1831–1884
  actinomycosis 1836t, 1837, 1850, 1851
  adenocarcinoma
    cytology 1873, 1874f
    endometrial adenocarcinoma vs 1869, 1869t,
        1873–1874
    endometrial cells 1873, 1874f
    endometrioid 1867f, 1868, 1870f
    extrauterine 1874
    grading 1868–1869
    intestinal 1868
    invasive 1868–1870, 1869f, 1870f
    metastases, to uterus 1979
    metastatic 1874, 1875f
    microinvasive 1868, 1869f

minimal deviation (adenoma malignum)
    1870–1871, 1871f
  mucinous 1868, 1870f
  prognosis 1869–1870
  villoglandular 36, 39f, 1867, 1868
adenocarcinoma in situ 1846t, 1866–1868
  adenosquamous type 1867f
  benign lesions vs 1872–1873
  cytology 1872–1873, 1873f
  differential diagnosis 1868
  endometrioid type 1867f
  histology 1867–1868, 1867f
  villoglandular adenocarcinoma vs 36, 39f, 1867
adenoid basal carcinoma 1876–1877, 1877f
adenoid cystic carcinoma 1876, 1876f
adenomyoma 1842
adenosarcoma 1877
adenosquamous carcinoma 1874, 1875f
anatomy 1831
atrophy 1846, 1854
  atypical cells with 1866
'barrel-shaped' 1859
basal cell layer 1831, 1832
benign and reactive conditions 1835–1838
  cytopathology 1842–1848
benign glandular changes 1844–1845
  cytopathology 1871–1872
benign non-neoplastic epithelial lesions 1838–1842
benign tumor-like conditions 1838–1842
benign tumors 1842
biopsy 136
blue nevus 1842
candidal infections 1849
carcinoma in situ 1854, 1855f
carcinosarcoma 1877
cell trauma due to biopsy 136
chemotherapy-induced changes 1846, 1848f
Chlamydia trachomatis infection 1835–1836, 1836t,
    1851–1852 8t
clear cell carcinoma 1876, 1923
  microglandular hyperplasia vs 1839
columnar epithelium 1832
cryotherapy, iatrogenic lesions 144
cytology/cytopathology 1837
  atypical glandular cells 1872
  atypical squamous cells 1863–1866, 1865f, 1872,
      1873
  benign glandular changes 1844–1845, 1871–1872
  infectious diseases 1848–1852
  intermediate cells 1842, 1846
  malignant glandular lesions 1872—1874
  non-neoplastic findings 1845–1848
  normal 1842–1843
  parabasal cells 1842, 1846
  squamous cells 1842
  squamous intraepithelial lesions 1861–1864
  see also cervical smears
cytomegalovirus infection 1850f, 1852
diffuse laminar endocervical glandular hyperplasia
    1839, 1840f
dysplasia 1853
  postirradiation 154–155
  see also cervical intraepithelial neoplasia (CIN)
ectopic tissue 1841–1842
endocervical cells see endocervical cells
endocervical epithelium 1832, 1844
endocervical polyps 1841
endocervical sarcoma 1877
endometrial adenocarcinoma invasion 1960
endometriosis 1840, 1845
epithelial inclusion cysts 1840, 1841
giant cell arteritis 1837
glandular cells 1832
  atypical 1863–1866, 1865f, 1872, 1873
glassy cell carcinoma 1866f, 1875
herpes simplex infections 1836–1837, 1850f, 1851
histology (normal) 1831–1832
infectious diseases, cytopathology 1848–1852
inflammatory pseudotumor 1841

intestinal metaplasia 1838
IUD-associated changes 1846, 1848, 1848f
large cell neuroendocrine carcinoma 1875
leiomyoma 1842, 1842f
leiomyosarcoma 1877
lobular endocervical glandular hyperplasia 1839,
    1839f
lower uterine segment 1846t
lymphoepithelioma-like carcinoma 1861
malignant glandular tumors 1866–1871
  cytopathology 1872–1874
melanosis 1842
mesonephric adenocarcinoma 1877
mesonephric remnant hyperplasia 1839–1840, 1840f
microcystic endocervical adenocarcinoma 1877
microglandular hyperplasia 1838–1839, 1839f
mixed endocervical-endometrial polyps 1841
molluscum contagiosum 1850f, 1852
Nabothian cysts 1840
postoperative spindle cell nodule 1841
pregnancy-related changes 1848, 1849f
preinvasive squamous lesions see cervical
    intraepithelial neoplasia (CIN)
preneoplastic squamous lesions 1833
radiation-induced changes 154–155, 1846, 1848f
sarcoma botryoides 1877
serous adenocarcinoma 1876
signet-ring adenosquamous carcinoma 1874, 1875f
small cell carcinoma 1875–1876
squamous cell carcinoma 1856–1861
  basaloid 1861
  CIN progression 1856–1857
  cytopathology 1866, 1866f
  frankly invasive 1858–1860, 1859f
  highly differentiating keratinizing 1860
  immunosuppression/HIV and 1856
  keratinizing 1866, 1866f
  large cell 1859
  lymphatic space invasion 1858
  microinvasive 1857–1858, 1858f, 1859f
  nonkeratinizing 1866, 1866f
  papillary 1860
  papillary squamotransitional cell 1861, 1861f
  pathogenesis 1856–1857
  small cell 1859, 1860f
  spindle cell 1861
  staging 1857, 1857t
  transitional cell 1861
  verrucous carcinoma 1860
squamous hyperplasia 1838
squamous intraepithelial lesions 1853–1854
  see also cervical intraepithelial neoplasia (CIN)
squamous metaplasia 1831, 1832, 1833f, 1843,
    1844f
  atypical immature 1854
  immature 1832, 1833f, 1844t, 1854
  immature vs HSIL 1862
squamous mucosa, atrophy 1846, 1854
squamous mucosal repair 1844f, 1845–1846
squamous papilloma 1838
stratified squamous epithelium 1831–1832
  metaplastic see cervix, squamous metaplasia
  native 1831
  reparative 1845–1846
  stromal tissue 1832
transformation/transitional zone (T-zone) 1832,
    1833, 1923
transitional cell metaplasia 1838
Trichomonas vaginalis infection 1836t, 1837, 1849,
    1850f
tubal metaplasia 1838, 1844, 1846t, 1847f
tunnel clusters 1840–1841, 1841f
undifferentiated carcinoma 1876, 1876f
warty (condylomatous) 1860
see also entries beginning endocervical
Cervix Brush™ 1834
cestodes 104–105
Chagas' disease 100
chalazion 2289, 2289f, 2290

chalcosis 2312
chancre 1890
chancroid, vulva 1890
channelopathies 2233–2234, 2233f
Charcot-Böttcher crystalloids 1732
Charcot-Böttcher filaments 1759, 1760, 2024
Charcot-Leyden crystals 91, 1047
Charcot–Marie–Tooth disease 2225, 2226f, 2241, 2244–2245, 2245f
Chédiak-Higashi syndrome 115–116, 659
chemical agents
    bladder tumors and 1710–1711
    iatrogenic lesions due to 139–145
chemical gastritis 1338
chemodectoma
    lung 968–970, 970f
    middle ear 2276–2277
chemotaxins, metastases mechanism 167
chemotherapy
    bladder changes due to 1719, 1719f
    bone marrow aplasia after 616f, 618
    cervical changes 1846, 1848f
    CNS changes after 2344–2345
    esophageal squamous atypia after 1292
    histologic maturation after 149
    oligodendroglioma 2363
    osteosarcoma 735
    skin changes, graft-versus-host disease vs 204
    tumor cell lysis, bone marrow necrosis 665
    see also cytotoxic drugs
chenille (caterpillar) bodies 311, 311f
Chernobyl incident 2130
cherry angioma 269, 270f
cherry-red spots, macular 2318
cherubism 1183, 1193, 1193f
Chester–Erdheim disease 1069, 2290
chest wall hamartoma 706, 706f, 707f
chickenpox 58, 75, 221, 221f
'chicken-wire' drying artifact, goiter 2124, 2124f
'chicken-wire' fibrosis (liver) 1491, 1492f
'chicken-wire' pattern, chondroblastoma 713, 713f
chief cells 1321–1322, 2150
    aggregates 2159, 2160f
    hyperplasia 2156, 2158–2159, 2159f
    jugulotympanic paraganglioma 2277
    parathyroid adenoma 2153, 2154, 2154f
childhood fibrous tumor with psammoma bodies 317–318, 317f, 318f
children
    acute postinfectious glomerulonephritis 1617
    acute suppurative thyroiditis 2120
    adamantinomatous craniopharyngioma 2398
    anaplastic large cell lymphoma 563
    atypical teratoid/rhabdoid tumor 2384
    Barrett's esophagus 1302
    basal cell carcinoma of skin 244
    bone marrow necrosis 664
    cardiac rhabdomyoma 354
    Carney's syndrome 279
    chronic myeloid leukemia 638
    CNS tumors 2348
    condyloma acuminata 1887
    effusions, tumors with 183
    ependymoblastoma 2379
    ependymoma 2367
    focal segmental glomerulosclerosis 1612
    granuloma annulare 212
    hepatoblastoma 1536–1537, 1537f
    incontinentia pigmenti 198, 198f
    intraocular tumors 2311
    lichen nitidus 202
    medulloblastoma 2379
    medulloepithelioma 2379
    myelodysplastic syndromes 638
    myofibroma of bone 736, 737f
    otitis media 2272, 2272f
    papillary thyroid carcinoma 2130
    pilocytic astrocytoma 2357
    pleuropulmonary blastoma 976

polycystic disease of liver 1522, 1522f
    renal tumors 1665–1672
    retinoblastoma 2309–2311
    salivary acinic cell carcinoma 1230
    small round blue cell tumors 174
    spleen histology 577
    vulvar lichen sclerosus 1892
    see also entries beginning 'juvenile'; specific tumors
Chlamydia pneumoniae, pneumonia 875–876
Chlamydia trachomatis
    acute endometritis 1944
    acute salpingitis 2040
    cervicitis/cervical infection 1835–1836, 1836t, 1851
    lymphogranuloma venereum see lymphogranuloma venereum
4-chloro-1-naphthol 32
chloroacetate esterase (CAE) stain 19, 575, 610, 613, 622
chloroma see granulocytic sarcoma (chloroma)
chloromethyl ether, lung cancer etiology 935–936
chloroquine, cardiotoxicity 1049
'chocolate cysts' 1951, 1952f, 1994
cholangiocarcinoma (cholangiolar carcinoma) 1540, 1540f
    hepatocellular carcinoma with 1533, 1535–1536, 1536f
    peripheral and hilar variants 1540
cholangioles (ductules) 1474, 1475f
    see also bile ductules
cholangiolitis, acute 1478, 1486
cholangitic abscesses 1494
cholangitis
    acute 1494
    acute suppurative 1496f
    chronic nonsuppurative destructive 1499
    inflammatory pseudotumor association 1542
    primary sclerosing see primary sclerosing cholangitis (PSC)
    recurrent pyogenic (Oriental) 1583
    sclerosing 1497–1498
cholate stasis 1493
cholecystitis 1576–1577, 1577f
    acalculous 1576
    acute 1576
    chronic 1577f, 1578f
    eosinophilic 1577
    primary sclerosing cholangitis with 1577
    xanthogranulomatous 1576, 1577f
choledochal (bile duct) cysts 1582–1583
choledocholithiasis 1494, 1496f
cholelithiasis 1577
cholemic nephrosis 1634f
cholera 63
cholestasis 1492–1502
    acute injury 1493–1496
        extrahepatic biliary obstruction 1493–1494
    acute viral hepatitis 1477
    benign recurrent 1494–1495
    bile ductular 1494, 1497f
    chronic injury 1496–1497
    in cirrhosis 1521
    drug-induced 1493, 1493f, 1494, 1495t
        chronic 1502
    in graft rejection 1502
    intrahepatic 1494–1496
        in sarcoidosis 1502, 1502f
    in steatohepatitis 1491
    submassive hepatic necrosis with 1480, 1480f
cholesteatoma 2113, 2273
cholesterol clefting, dentigerous cysts 1140–1141
cholesterol crystals, polarizing microscopy 1471
cholesterol emboli, renal 1646, 1646f
cholesterol ester storage disease 1471
cholesterol granuloma, ear 2273–2274
cholesterol-lowering agents, myopathy due to 2235
cholesterolosis 1577–1578
cholesterol pericarditis 1068
chondritis, auricular 2282
chondroblastoma 712–713, 712f, 713f
    'malignant' 713

chondroblasts 712, 713, 713f
chondrodermatitis nodularis helicis 227–228, 228f, 2274, 2275f
chondroid metaplasia, peritoneum 1021
chondroid syringoma 258, 259f, 396
    vulva 1899, 1899f
chondrolipoma 336
chondroma 708–712
    enchondroma see enchondroma
    'extraskeletal, with lipoblast-like cells' 339–340
    immunohistochemistry 796t
    intracortical 712
    juxtacortical 711–712
    larynx 849, 849f
    nasal septum 816, 816f
    sinonasal 796t, 816, 816f
    soft tissue 389
    subperiosteal 711–712
chondromalacia, cystic (endochondral pseudocyst) 2281, 2281f
chondromatosis, synovial 696–697, 696f
chondromyxoid fibroma 713–715, 714f
    malignant 715
chondro-osseous lesions, benign, of skin 267
chondrosarcoma 715–721
    in carcinosarcoma 1243, 1244f
    chondroblastic 715
    chordoma vs 764, 765f
    clear cell 720–721, 721f
    conventional type 715–718, 715f, 716f, 718
    craniofacial 816–817
    dedifferentiated 718–719, 719f, 720, 721f
    development in enchondroma 711, 715f, 719f
    enchondroma vs 709, 710
    epithelioid hemangioendothelioma vs 368
    extraskeletal mesenchymal 390–391, 391f
    extraskeletal myxoid see extraskeletal myxoid chondrosarcoma (EMCs)
    grade 1 (low-grade) 715, 715f, 716–717, 719f
    grade 2 and 3 717, 717f
    grading system 716–717, 716f, 717f
    head and neck 816–817
    immunohistochemistry 796t
    intraosseous 389
    juxtacortical chondroma vs 712
    larynx 849
    Maffucci syndrome 816
    mesenchymal 390–391, 391f, 719–720, 720f, 817
        Ewing family of tumors vs 750
        solitary fibrous tumor vs 378t
    myxoid matrix in 709, 716, 717f
    osteochondroma (exostosis) vs 708
    osteochondroma with 718
    periosteal (juxtacortical) 718
    peripheral 718
    pleomorphic spindle cell sarcoma with 719, 719f
    pre-existing conditions 715, 718
    secondary 718
    sinonasal 796t, 816–817
    synovial chondromatosis vs 697
    temporal bone 2284
CHOP gene, myxoid/round cell liposarcoma 344
chorangioma 2074, 2074f
chorangiosis 2073–2074, 2074f
chordoid meningioma 2373–2374, 2391
chordoma 763–765, 763f
    chondroid 764, 765f
    chondrosarcoma vs 764, 765f
    choroid glioma of third ventricle vs 2373
    conventional 763, 763f
    dedifferentiated 764–765
    immunohistochemistry 796t
    parachordoma vs 395
    pituitary 2109
    sinonasal 796t, 813
    ultrastructure 764, 764f
chordoma periphericum (parachordoma) 394–396, 395f
chorioadenoma destruens 1949
chorioamnionitis 2064, 2068–2069, 2069f

choriocarcinoma 1115, 2080, 2083–2084, 2083f
  differential diagnosis 2031, 2083, 2087
  endometrium in 1949
  in fallopian tube 2043, 2047
  histologic maturation after chemotherapy 149
  metastatic lesions 2083
  monophasic, testis 1753
  ovarian see ovary, choriocarcinoma
  ovarian epithelial tumor with 2014
  testis see testicular tumors
  thymus 1119–1120, 1120f
chorion 2064, 2067
  infections 2068, 2069
chorionepithelioma, atypical 2084
chorion frondosum 2067
chorionic villi 2064, 2070–2074
  accelerated maturity 2071
  atrophy 2070
  avascular (hyalinization) 2073, 2074f
  infarcts 2071, 2072f
  intervillous thrombi 2073
  normal anatomy 2070
  placenta accreta 2075
chorion laeve 2067
choristoma 2404
  corneal 2303–2304
  middle ear–mastoid 2271
  neuromuscular 2249, 2249f
  phakomatous 2296
  salivary gland, of middle ear 2271
  sinonasal region 811–812, 812f
choroid
  benign nevi 2309
  hemangioma 2309
  infections 2313
  melanoma 2306, 2307f
choroid glioma of third ventricle 2373–2374, 2373f
  immunohistochemistry 2339t, 2373
  ultrastructural characteristics 2337t, 2373
choroid plexus, histology and function 2344
choroid plexus tumors 2370–2372
  benign, tissue embolizing by ventriculoperitoneal
    shunts 146
  carcinoma 2371–2372, 2372f
  immunohistochemistry 2338t
  papilloma (benign) 2371, 2371f
    papillary adenocarcinoma of ear vs 2279
  ultrastructural characteristics 2337t
chromaffin cells, adrenal medulla 2170, 2172f, 2189,
  2190f
chromaffin reaction 17
chromate fixatives 17
chromatin
  checkerboard, pancreatic endocrine neoplasm 1571,
    1571f
  clearing, in autoimmune thyroiditis 2121, 2121f
  'salt and pepper' see 'salt and pepper' chromatin
  speckled, pancreatic endocrine neoplasms 1570
  'spoked wheel' pattern 762, 762f
  stippled, Merkel cell carcinoma 249, 249f
chromatolysis, central, CNS neurons 2340
chromium, lung cancer etiology 936
chromium-containing fixatives 17
chromoblastomycosis 72, 72f
chromogen 32
chromogenic in situ hybridization (CISH) 47
chromogranin 181
  acinar cell carcinoma of pancreas 1561f
  Merkel cell carcinoma 250
  neuroblastoma 384
  pancreatic endocrine neoplasms 1571
  pheochromocytoma, 2096f 2193
  sex cord-stromal tumor differential diagnosis 2017t
chromogranin A 1322
  thymic neuroendocrine tumors 1112, 1112f
chromomycosis 67t
chromophobe cell carcinoma, renal see renal cell
  carcinoma
chromosomal abnormalities

acute leukemia 629–630, 629t
chronic idiopathic myelofibrosis 634
chronic lymphocytic leukemia 642–643
Crohn's disease 1387
detection methods 44, 44t
fibromatoses 320
hairy cell leukemia 645
malignant peripheral nerve sheath tumor 2257
multiple myeloma 655
osteosarcoma association 727–728, 728t
polycythemia vera 632
prostatic adenocarcinoma 1813–1814, 1814f
salivary adenoid cystic carcinoma 1238
spontaneous abortions 2079, 2079t
uveal malignant melanoma 2308
chromosomal microsatellite markers 1171
chromosomal translocation
  acute lymphoblastic leukemia 629
  acute myeloid leukemia 622–623, 625, 626, 629
  alveolar rhabdomyosarcoma 310t, 386
  anaplastic large cell lymphoma 564
  Burkitt's lymphoma 569, 570
  chondroid lipoma 340
  clear cell sarcoma 381
  desmoplastic small round cell tumors 386
  detection methods 44, 44t
  Ewing family of tumors 386
  Ewing's sarcoma 746–747
  follicular lymphoma 550
  follicular thyroid carcinoma 2133
  lymph node specimens 510
  lymphomas 293, 544, 544t, 649
  mantle cell lymphoma 557
  myelodysplastic syndromes 636–637
  olfactory neuroblastoma 801
  Philadelphia see Philadelphia chromosome
  soft tissue tumors 310t
  synovial sarcoma, lung 972
  t(1;19) abnormality 629
  t(2;5) abnormality 293
  t(4;11) abnormality 629–630
  t(8;14) abnormality 630
  t(8;21) abnormality 625, 625f
  t(11;14) abnormality 630
  t(12;21) abnormality 630
  t(15;17) abnormality 625
  tumors associated 44, 44t
  Waldenström's macroglobulinemia 555
  Xp11.2 renal cell carcinoma 1671, 1671f, 1682
chromosome 1p loss 2363, 2370
chromosome 3p deletion, lung cancer 937
chromosome 6q, deletion, leukemia 643
chromosome 8q24 defects, osteochondroma 707
chromosome 9p deletion, oligodendroglioma 2363
chromosome 10q deletion, oligodendroglioma 2363
chromosome 11, loss, chronic lymphocytic leukemia 643
chromosome 11p, loss of heterozygosity 1560, 1561
chromosome 12 552, 1118
chromosome 13, loss, chronic lymphocytic leukemia
  642–643
chromosome 13q, suppressor gene 642
chromosome 17q, medulloblastoma 2383
chromosome 18q, osteosarcoma and 728
chromosome 19, loss 2363, 2370
chromosome 22
  22q changes 724, 2367
  in atypical teratoid/rhabdoid tumor (AT/RT) 2385
  chronic myeloid leukemia 633
chromosomes, ring 341
chronic granulomatous disease (CGD) 115
chronic inflammatory demyelinating
  polyradiculoneuropathy (CIDP) 2239,
  2242–2243, 2243f
chronic myeloproliferative disorders (CMPDs) 631
  see also myeloproliferative syndromes
chronic obstructive pulmonary disease (COPD)
  915–916
chronic passive congestion (lung) (CPC) 915, 915f
chronic pelvic pain syndrome (CPPS) 1794

chronic tubular interstitial nephritis 1640–1641, 1641f
chronic venous insufficiency 370
chronic villitis of unknown etiology (VUE) 2063, 2068,
  2070
Churg-Strauss syndrome (angiitis) 211–212, 882,
  1076t, 1077, 1384
  intestinal 1384, 1384t, 1385f
  peripheral nerve involvement 2243
Churukian-Schenk stain 1110
cicatricial pemphigoid 224
  Brunsting-Perry variant 224
  dermatitis herpetiformis vs 223
  ocular 2303
  vaginal 1919
  vulvar 1893–1894
ciclosporin nephrotoxicity, renal transplant
  complication 1652
ciliary body, melanoma 2306, 2308
ciliary dyskinesia syndrome 911
ciliocytophthoria 58
circumcision, female 1887
cirrhosis of liver 1519–1521
  alcoholic 1491, 1493f
  in alpha-1-antitrypsin deficiency 1508
  biliary see biliary cirrhosis
  chronic hepatitis C 1485f, 1486f, 1519f, 1520f
  glomerulopathy associated 1632–1633
  hepatocellular carcinoma and 1530–1531
  high-grade dysplastic nodule and 1529–1530
  'incomplete' 1486
  liver biopsy 1467, 1519–1520, 1519f, 1520f
  macronodular 1519
    in Wilson's disease 1505, 1506f, 1507f
  micronodular 1491, 1493f, 1519
    of hemochromatosis 1504f
  preneoplastic lesions 1520
  regenerative nodules 1519
  secondary IgA nephropathy 1619–1620
Civatte bodies see colloid bodies
civil lawsuits 11
CK903 see 34βE12 monoclonal antibody
c-kit proto-oncogene
  exon 11 mutations 1348
  gastrointestinal stromal tumors 353, 1345, 1348,
    1443, 1444
  mast cell disease 664, 1380
  see also CD117 (c-kit)
Clara cells 954, 955f, 1015
Clark levels, melanoma 286
Clark's nevus 280
classical trichoepithelioma (CTE) see
  trichoepithelioma, classical
clear cell(s)
  endometrium see endometrium, clear cells
  in lymphoma 176
  in melanoma 176
  salivary gland tumors with 1246, 1247
    acinic cell carcinoma 1231, 1233f, 1235
    clear cell adenocarcinoma 1246
    epithelial-myoepithelial carcinoma 1245, 1246
clear cell acanthoma 242, 242f
clear cell adenocarcinoma
  endometrial see endometrial adenocarcinoma
  lung see lung
  salivary glands see salivary gland tumors
  urethra 1725, 1725f
  vagina 1924
clear cell adenofibroma, ovary 2011
clear cell carcinoma
  cervical 1839, 1876, 1923
  gallbladder 1580
  ovarian see ovary, clear cell carcinoma
  renal see renal cell carcinoma
  salivary glands see salivary gland tumors
  sinonasal region 808
  thymic 1102, 1104f
  vaginal 150, 1923
clear cell chondrosarcoma 720–721, 721f
clear cell eccrine adenocarcinoma (CCEA) 262

clear cell eosinophilia 1678
clear cell meningioma 2362, 2391, 2392f
clear cell papulosis, vulva, Paget's disease vs 1908
clear cell sarcoma 310t, 381–383, 381f
   cytology 382, 383f
   differential diagnosis 381–383, 1668, 1670
   kidney see kidney, clear cell sarcoma
   microscopic structure 381–382, 381f, 382f
clear cell tumors 176f
   lung (benign) 962, 963t, 964f
   metastases, differential diagnosis 175–176, 176f
   sclerosing 176
Clinical Laboratory Improvement Act (CLIA) 11–12
clitoris 1885
   hypertrophy 1887
   length 1887
clomiphene citrate, endometrial changes 1947
clonal expansion 122
clonality, analysis 48
Clonorchis sinensis 1583, 1585
Clostridium
   gas gangrene 2222
   necrotizing infection of GI tract 69, 69f
Clostridium difficile colitis 1381, 1396, 1397f
   biopsy 1388, 1396, 1396f
Clostridium perfringens 69
Clostridium septicum 69
clubbing (digital), asbestosis 902
'clue cells' 78f
c-met gene, mutations, gastric adenocarcinoma 1360
c-myb gene, acute basophilic leukemia 624
c-myc gene, oral squamous cell carcinoma 1170
coal workers' pneumoconiosis 905t, 907
coarctation of aorta 1082
Coats disease 2311, 2317
cobalt pneumoconiosis 904–905, 905f
cobblestone appearance, Crohn's disease 1391, 1391f
cocaine, talc embolization 917
Coccidioides immitis 58, 87, 87f, 2410
   differential diagnosis 85, 86
   identification/characteristics 67t
coccidioidomycosis 1512f
   CNS involvement 2410–2411
   respiratory tract 87, 87f, 90, 90f, 92f
cochlea 2269, 2269f
cochlear duct 2269, 2269f
Codman's triangle, osteosarcoma 728, 729, 729f, 730f
Codman's tumor see chondroblastoma
coin lesions 96f
COL4A5 gene, hereditary nephritis of Alport 1624
colchicine, myopathy 2234–2235, 2235t
colectomy, ulcerative colitis 1389, 1395
colitis
   'acute self-limited' 1389, 1390f, 1395
   allergic 1405
   bacterial 1389, 1395–1396
   Clostridium difficile see Clostridium difficile colitis
   collagenous 1400, 1401, 1402
   Crohn's disease 1391, 1391f
   diversion 1395
   'diverticular disease-associated' 1388, 1393
   Entamoeba histolytica 1399–1400
   eosinophilic 1405
   indeterminate 1392
   ischemic see ischemic colitis
   lymphocytic 1400, 1401
   microscopic 1400–1401
   NSAID 1402, 1402f
   pseudomembranous see pseudomembranous colitis
   radiation 1388, 1406
   ulcerative see ulcerative colitis
colitis cystica profunda 146, 155, 1457
Collaborative Ocular Melanoma Study (COMS) 2306, 2308
collagen
   alterations, keloids 231
   articular cartilage 691
   bone 677, 678
      diseases involving 686

bundle encirclement in dermatofibroma 265, 266f
degeneration, elastofibroma 311, 311f
deposition diseases, of skin 231–233
dermis 194
   in endoneurium 2240
   glomerular basement membrane 1598
   hyalinized dermal 8, 24f, 264
   necrobiotic, necrobiosis lipoidica 214
   staining methods 16t, 677
   type I 194, 1471
   type II, clear cell chondrosarcoma 721
   type III 194, 1470, 1471
   type IV 952, 1470
   type VII, dystrophic epidermolysis bullosa 225
   wiry 291, 377
collagenase 38
   type IV 167
collagenous colitis 1400, 1401, 1402
collagenous fibroma 308–309, 309f
collagenous spherulosis
   breast 448, 448f
   salivary glands 1261
collagenous sprue 1376
collagen vascular diseases
   diffuse alveolar hemorrhage with 884
   esophageal involvement 1290
   lung involvement 882–883, 887t
   myositis in 2221–2222
   vasculitis 1078
   see also individual diseases
collecting duct(s), anatomy 1600
collecting duct carcinoma 1685, 1685f, 1686f
   differential diagnosis 1682
collecting duct system 1598
College of American Pathologists (CAP) 4, 10, 1835, 2329
   Consensus Conference, breast cancer 489
'collision' tumor
   basosquamous basal cell carcinoma of skin 244
   intestinal adenocarcinoma/neuroendocrine tumors 1430
   mixed germ cell-sex cord-stromal tumors (male) 1761–1762
   odontoameloblastoma 1161
   plurihormonal pituitary adenoma 2107
   spindle cell squamous cell carcinoma of oral cavity 1177
colloidal iron stain 226, 229, 250
colloid bodies 195
   lichen planus 202, 1894
   lichen planus-like keratosis 243, 243f
   retinal exudates 2317
'colloid' carcinoma of skin 261–262
colloid cysts 2401, 2402f, 2403f
colloid milium 230, 231, 231f
colon
   adenocarcinoma
      cervical involvement 1874
      flow cytometry 38
      metastases, to liver 169t, 170–171
      metastatic, cholangiocarcinoma vs 1540
      see also colorectal adenocarcinoma
   'cathartic' 1404
   diffuse lipomatous polyposis 1450
   diverticular disease 1404–1405
   dysplasia 1441–1443, 1442f, 1443t
   histology (normal) 1373
   ischemic infarction 1386f
      see also ischemic colitis
   lymphocytic phlebitis 1079
   lymphoma 1450
   mass, histoplasmosis 84f
   mucosal prolapse 1382
   neuroendocrine tumors 1429
   pneumatosis cystoides intestinalis 1405–1406
   polyps 1419t
      electrothermal cautery, thermal artifact 137
      hyperplastic 1431–1432, 1432f
      see also large intestine, polyps

pseudo-obstruction 1404
ulcers
   Entamoeba histolytica 1400f
   NSAID-associated 1402
see also intestine; large intestine
colonic polypectomy
   colonoscopic 136
   implantation of abnormal epithelium 137
colorectal adenocarcinoma 1438–1443
   dysplasia and 1441–1443
   gene mutations 1359–1360
   in inflammatory bowel disease 1439, 1441–1443, 1443
   intramucosal 1433, 1435, 1435f
   invasion 1439, 1439f
   medullary 1440
   metastatic 2038, 2038f
      to ovary 2037–2038, 2038f
   mixed glandular/neuroendocrine 1440
   mucinous 1438–1439, 1440f
   pathologic features 1438, 1439f
   post-irradiation 159
   precursor adenomas 1438
   sarcomatoid 1440
   signet ring cell 1438–1439
   small cell 1440
   squamous cell component 1440
   subtypes 1438–1439
   undifferentiated 1440
   see also colon, adenocarcinoma
colorectal dysplasia 1441–1443, 1442f, 1443t
colorimetric in situ hybridization (CISH) methods 62
columnar cell metaplasia
   vagina 1923
   vulva 1899
columnar cell papilloma (CCP) 789, 789f, 798
comedonecrosis, salivary duct carcinoma 1252, 1252f
'comma-shaped' cells 810
common ALL antigen (CALLA) see CD10 (common acute lymphoblastic leukemia antigen)
common bile duct 1581
common cold 787
common hepatic duct 1581
common variable immunodeficiency (CVID) 114–115, 571
   small intestine in 1379, 1379f
compacta, endometrium 1933, 1934f
comparative genomic hybridization (CGH) 47
   parathyroid carcinoma 2162
   small cell lung carcinoma 992
complement activation 127, 1615
computed tomography (CT)
   bone tumors 704
   CNS tumors 2345–2346
   high-resolution see high-resolution computed tomography (HRCT)
   lung 863, 864f, 866t, 868
   lung carcinoma 936
   mesothelioma 1007–1008, 1008f
   osteosarcoma 728
   silicosis 903–904
computerized checklists, reports 7
conception, products of 2079
conceptus 2079
condyloma(ta)
   cervical 1854
   flat, condyloma acuminatum vs 1887
   regressing, condyloma acuminatum vs 1888
   scrotal 1772
   vaginal 1921
   vulvar 1887, 1887f
condyloma acuminatum 242
   anus 1444f, 1454
   bladder 1723
   giant, penis 1771
   oral cavity 1163–1164
   penis 1771
   podophyllin therapy effect 148
   squamous cell carcinoma of skin vs 246

urethra 1725
vagina 1921, 1921f
verrucous carcinoma of bladder and 1720
vulvar 1887–1888, 1887f
condyloma lata 1890
congenital abnormalities
adrenal cortex 2174
appendix 1407
bladder 1707–1708
breast 421
ear 2270–2271
esophagus 1283–1284
fallopian tube 2040
gallbladder 1576
liver 1521–1523
ovary 1988
pancreas 1551
pituitary gland 2098
testis 1734–1735
thyroid gland 2119
uterine corpus 1933
vagina 1919
vulva 1887
congenital adrenal hyperplasia (CAH) (adrenogenital
syndrome) 2174–2175
adrenocortical nodules/neoplasms 2077, 2175
male 1737, 1737f
micromastia 421
salt-losing form 2175
simple virilizing form 1736, 2175
testicular and other tumors 2175
congenital adrenal hypoplasia 2175
congenital epulis of newborn 1185
congenital fiber type disproportion 2228t, 2229
congenital heart disease, pulmonary hypertension in 912
congenital hepatic fibrosis 1521, 1521f
congenital malformations, kidney 1661
congenital nephrotic syndrome 1622–1623
congenital rests, lymph nodes 510, 512–513, 513f
congestive heart failure 1517
'congestive vasculopathy' 914–915
Congo red stain 20f, 2335t, 2414
amyloidosis 116
cardiac amyloidosis 1047–1048, 1047f
intestinal amyloidosis 1405, 1406f
lymph node amyloid 515
renal amyloidosis 1632f
skeletal muscle evaluation 2215t
conjunctiva 2292–2294
anatomy 2292
benign tumors 2292
biopsy 2292
granuloma 2294
inflammatory diseases 2294
intraepithelial neoplasia (dysplasia) 2292, 2292f
lymphoid tumors 2293–2294
melanocytic lesions 2292–2293
melanoma 2293
nevi 2292–2293
papilloma 2292
spindle cell carcinoma 2292
squamous epithelial tumors 2292
conjunctivitis, follicular or pseudomembranous 2294
connectin (titin) 2218t
connective tissue disease 697–698
non-specific interstitial pneumonia 898
see also individual diseases
connective tissue nevi 231
connective tissue proteins 31t
Conn's syndrome 2183–2185, 2184f
constipation 1404
contextual karyometry 43
continuous quality improvement (CQI) 9
continuous throughout processing method
(CTPM) 17
contraceptive creams, iatrogenic reactions 141
contraction bands, endomyocardial biopsy 1042
conus medullaris, tumor differential diagnosis by age
2348t

Cope needle biopsy, pleura 1005
copper
in liver 1474, 1505
staining 20t
Wilson's disease 1505, 1505f
core needle biopsy (CNB)
breast 419, 421, 426–427
lung carcinoma 940
Cori-Forbes disease 2232
cornea 2300–2304
conical (keratoconus) 2301
degeneration 2303
dystrophies 2302, 2302t, 2303f
edema (bullous keratopathy) 2301, 2301f
endothelial cells 2301
epithelial cells 2301
histology (normal) 2300–2301
infections 2301–2302, 2302f
melts 2302
specimens 2301
see also keratitis; keratopathy
Cornelia de Lange syndrome 2098, 2174
coronary atherectomy 1071
coronavirus, SARS-associated 95, 879
corpora amylacea 2342–2343, 2343f
corps ronds 242, 243f
corps ronds and grains
Darier's disease 219, 220f
Grover's disease 221f
corpus albicans 1988
corpus atreticum 1988
corpuscles of Erzholz 2241
corpus luteum 1987, 1988, 1988f
cystic 1991
cysts 1991, 1991f
of pregnancy 1988
corpus spongiosum 1767
cortactin 1138
cortical dysplasia 2405, 2405f
corticosteroids
biosynthesis, adrenal cortex 2169, 2170f
osteonecrosis due to 683
corticosterone methyl oxidase (CMO) 2175
corticotrophs 2096, 2097f
adenoma see pituitary adenoma
hyperplasia 2110
corticotropin-releasing hormone (CRH) 2110, 2173
ectopic secretion 2180–2181, 2180f, 2181f
corticotropin upstream transcription-binding element
(CUTE) proteins 2096
cortisol, excess 2178–2183
see also Cushing's syndrome
Corynebacterium minutissimum 1891
cotton lint, tissue reactions to 139, 139f
cotton-wool exudates 2317
cotton-wool spots 2317
coup de sabre 231
Cowden's disease 265, 1436–1437, 1676
Cowden syndrome 2374
genes and CNS features 2401t
trichilemmoma association 252, 2291
Cowdry A intranuclear inclusions
acute herpetic hepatitis 1482, 1482f
acute herpetic keratitis 2301
herpes simplex encephalitis 2408, 2408f
herpetic esophagitis 1288
Cowdry bodies, CNS neurons 2340
cow's milk protein intolerance 1376–1377, 1405
COX-2 see cyclooxygenase-2
Coxiella burnetii 82
see also Q fever
coxsackie B virus
acute hepatocellular injury 1482
epidemic pleurodynia 2222
orchitis 1767
coxsackievirus infection
myositis 2222
vulvar 1889

'cracking' artifact, hyalinizing spindle cell tumor with
giant rosettes 327
cranial arteritis see giant cell arteritis
cranial nerve palsy, in middle ear adenoma and 2277
craniofacial chondrosarcoma 816–817
craniofacial fibrous dysplasia 813–814, 1191
craniofacial osteoma 722
craniopharyngioma 2108, 2108f, 2398–2399
adamantinomatous 2108, 2398, 2398f
ameloblastoma vs 1152
immunohistochemistry 2339t
papillary 2108, 2398–2399, 2399f
ultrastructural characteristics 2337t
'crazy paving' pattern, pulmonary alveolar proteinosis
925
creatine kinase 2218t
creatinine, serum, elevated in glomerulonephritis 1617,
1621
creatinine kinase (CK), serum 2213
creeping substitution 683, 684f
Creola bodies 961, 963f
crescentic glomerulonephritis see glomerulonephritis
crescents
crescentic glomerulonephritis 1621–1622
focal proliferative/necrotizing glomerulonephritis
1620, 1620f
in malignant hypertension 1645
CREST syndrome 114t, 232
cresyl violet stain 2335t
Creutzfeldt cells 2413
Creutzfeldt–Jakob disease (CJD) 2412–2413, 2413f
variant 2413
critical care myopathy 2238
Crohn's disease 1386–1394
adenocarcinoma association 1387
appendiceal disease 1391, 1409, 1409f
appendicitis 1409
biopsy diagnosis 1387–1389, 1388f
colitis 1391, 1391f
duodenitis 1389, 1389f
duodenum in 1337f
esophagus in 1291
fistulas involving vagina 1920
fulminant 1391
granulomatous gastritis 1336
granulomatous salpingitis 2042
ileitis 1390, 1390f, 1391, 1392f
indeterminate colitis vs 1392
inflammatory polyps 1391
ovary in 1989
pathology in resection specimens 1390–1391,
1390f
small intestinal adenocarcinoma 1430–1431
stomach in 1336, 1337f
terminal ileal biopsy 1389
transmural disease 1388
ulcerative colitis vs 1388–1389
vulval involvement 1896
see also inflammatory bowel disease
Cronkhite-Canada syndrome 1437
Crooke's cell adenoma 2105, 2105f
Crooke's hyaline change 2097, 2097f, 2098f
cross-reactivity, detection of infectious agents 61–62
croup (laryngotracheobronchitis) 94
crush preparations, CNS see under central nervous
system
cryoglobulinemia 211–212, 1076t, 1636
mixed 211
cryoglobulinemic glomerulopathy 1636, 1636f, 1637f,
1637t
cryoglobulins 1636
cryotherapy, iatrogenic lesions 144
crypt(s)
abscess 1388, 1389, 1395
atrophy 1376–1377
hyperplasia 1377–1378
inflammatory bowel disease 1387–1388, 1388
normal colonic mucosa 1387
crypt cells, apoptosis 1402, 1403f

cryptitis 1388, 1389, 1395
    focal eosinophilic 1405
cryptococcosis/cryptococcal infection
    adrenal gland infection 91f
    CNS involvement 2411
    corpora amylacea vs 2342–2343
    differential diagnosis 85–86, 87
    meningeal infection 91f, 2411
    respiratory tract 86–87, 86f
Cryptococcus, in vocal cord biopsy 835, 836f
Cryptococcus neoformans 66
    differential diagnosis 85–86
    identification/characteristics 67t
    staining 61
cryptogenic bronchiolitis 908–909
cryptogenic fibrosing alveolitis see pneumonia, usual
        interstitial (UIP)
cryptogenic organizing pneumonia 900–901, 901f, 902t
cryptorchidism 1734, 1735f, 1737, 1742
Cryptosporidium parvum 1400, 1400f, 1576
C-section, endometriosis in scar 146
Curling's ulcers 1327
Cushing's disease 2108, 2179, 2180f, 2181f
    corticotroph adenomas causing 2104, 2105
    corticotroph hyperplasia causing 2110
    ectopic pituitary adenoma 2098
    in MEN type 1 2178
    neuromuscular abnormalities 2233
    steroid cell tumors of ovary 2026
Cushing's syndrome 2104, 2178–2182
    adrenal incidentaloma causing 2178
    adrenocortical adenoma with 2180f, 2185, 2185f,
        2186f
    carcinoid tumors of thymus and 1108, 1109, 1113
    in MEN type 1 2178
    pituitary-dependent transition 2182
    pulmonary carcinoid tumors and 982
Cushing's ulcers 1327
cutaneous appendages, normal histology 194
cutaneous lymphoid hyperplasia (CLH) 295
cutaneous mixed tumor (CMT) 258, 259f
cutaneous ossification 267
cutaneous T-cell lymphoma see mycosis fungoides
cyclic adenosine monophosphate (cAMP), excess,
        fibrous dysplasia of bone 741
cyclin D1 557, 1294, 2151, 2162
cyclooxygenase-2 (COX-2)
    esophageal squamous cell carcinoma 1294
    overexpression, osteoid osteoma 724
cyclophosphamide
    bladder carcinoma association 150
    effect on urine cytology 148
cyclosporine nephrotoxicity 127, 130f, 131
CYLD mutation 1220
cylindroma
    dermal ('turban tumor') 255–256, 255f
    dermal eccrine, in external auditory canal 2276
    malignant 263
    salivary gland 1236–1237
CYP11B1 gene mutations 2174, 2183
CYP21 gene, mutations 2174
cyst(s)
    adrenal gland 2201
    aneurysmal see aneurysmal cyst
    anogenital sweat glands 1897–1899, 1898f
    antral 1149
    arachnoid 2113, 2403
    Baker's 697
    Bartholin's gland see Bartholin's gland
    bone see bone, cysts
    branchial cleft 244, 1260, 2270–2271, 2271f
    bronchogenic see bronchogenic cysts
    canal of Nuck 1899
    'chocolate' 1951, 1952f, 1994
    choledochal (bile duct) 1582–1583
    ciliated, vulvar 1899
    CNS see central nervous system (CNS), cysts
    colloid 2401, 2402f, 2403f
    congenital, pancreas 1551

corpus luteum 1991, 1991f
cutaneous ciliated 244
dental (radicular) 1146–1147
dentigerous 1140–1141
dermoid see dermoid cysts
developmental, of skin 244
developmental nonodontogenic 1147
echinococcal see echinococcal cysts
ejaculatory duct 1791
endodermal origin (CNS) 2401
endometrioid 1995
enteric see bronchogenic cysts
enterogenous 2401
ependymal (glioependymal) 2403
epidermal, oral cavity 1149
epidermoid see epidermoid cyst
epithelial
    broad ligament 2047
    ovarian 1990
    vulval 1899
epithelial inclusion see epithelial inclusion cysts
eruption 1141, 1142f
esophageal 1283
extrahepatic bile ducts 1582–1583
eyelid 2290
fallopian tube 2043
first branchial cleft 2270–2271, 2271f
fissural nonodontogenic 1147
follicles 1990, 1991f
follicular (dentigerous) 1140–1141
ganglion see ganglion cysts
ganglion (mucinous nerve) see ganglion cysts
Gartner's duct 1920, 1920f
gingival 1141–1142, 1142f
granulosa lutein 1990
heart, infectious 1066
hepatic see liver, cysts
heterotopic oral gastrointestinal 1149
hybrid, pilar 254
hydatid 105, 105f
incisive canal 1147–1148
infectious, heart 1066
infundibular, of skin 254, 254f
intradermal (milia) 254
intraspinal 2401
keratin-filled (horn) see horn cysts
larynx and trachea 835
lateral periodontal 1142–1143, 1142f
lung see lung, cysts
lymphoepithelial see lymphoepithelial cysts
lymphoepithelial, of oral cavity 1148, 1148f
median palatal (mid-palatine) 1147
median raphe 244
mediastinum see mediastinum
mesenteric, postoperative 147
mesonephric 1920, 1920f
mesonephric duct 1899
mesothelial see mesothelial cysts
mucous retention 787, 1259
Müllerian duct 1791
Müllerian origin 2043
multilocular, cystic nephroma 1668, 1669f,
        1694–1695, 1695f
Nabothian 1840
nasolabial 1147f, 1148
nasopalatine duct 1147–1148
neurenteric 2401
odontogenic see odontogenic cysts
oral cavity see oral cavity
ovarian see ovary, cysts
palatine papilla 1147
pancreas 1551, 1551f
paradental 1147
paraesophageal 1093
parathyroid glands 2164–2165, 2165f
paratubal 2043
parotid gland 1260
periapical (apical periodontal) 1146–1147
pericardial 1019, 1070, 1093, 1094f

peripheral nerves see ganglion cysts
peritoneal inclusion 146
pilar 261, 2290
pilar (trichilemmal) inclusion 254, 254f
pineal 2403, 2404f
pituitary gland 2113
postoperative abdominal 146–147
primordial see odontogenic keratocyst
radicular 1142f, 1146–1147
Rathke cleft 2113, 2113f, 2401, 2403
renal 1664–1665
residual 1142f
rete ovarii 1990, 1990f
salivary ducts 1260, 1260f
salivary glands 1207t, 1260, 1260f
sebaceous, oral cavity 1149
sialo-odontogenic 1146
solitary luteinized follicular 1993, 1994f
spleen 580, 580t
subchondral, intraosseous ganglion vs 755
theca lutein see theca lutein cysts
third pharyngeal pouch 1092, 2164
third ventricle 2402f, 2403f
thymic see thymus, cysts
thyroglossal tract 1148–1149
thyroid 25, 2164
utricular 1791
vagina 1920, 1920f
vocal cords 835
wolffian duct 1899
cystadenocarcinoma
    biliary 1539
    mucinous see mucinous cystadenocarcinoma
    salivary gland see salivary gland tumors
cystadenofibroma, ovarian see ovary, cystadenofibroma
cystadenoma
    apocrine 255
    biliary 1539
    hepatobiliary, of extrahepatic bile ducts 1586, 1587f
    mucinous
        lung 958
        ovarian 2002
        pancreas 1563–1565, 1564f
    papillary, epididymis 1764, 1764f
    papillary oncocytic, salivary gland 1226
    papillary serous, ovarian 1997
    salivary gland 1226, 1226f
    serous
        biliary 1539
        ovarian 1997, 1997f
        pancreas 1562–1563, 1562t, 1565
cystectomy 1724
    reports 1719
cystic adventitial disease 1083–1084, 1085f
cystic chondromalacia (endochondral pseudocyst)
        2281, 2281f
cystic disease, kidney see kidney
cystic duct neuroma 1578
cysticercosis
    CNS involvement 2411–2412
    gastrointestinal tract 104
    muscle involvement 2223
cystic fibrosis
    appendiceal diverticula 1407, 1409
    appendix involvement 1407, 1409, 1410f
    chronic pancreatitis 1552
    fibrosing colopathy 1401
cystic fibrosis transmembrane receptor (CFTR) gene
        1552
cystic hamartoma, of renal pelvis 1695
cystic hemangioma, multilocular peritoneal inclusion
        cyst vs 1022
cystic medial changes 1081, 1082f
cystic medial necrosis 1081, 1082f, 1083
cystic mucinous tumors, lung 958–959, 959f
cystic nephroma 1668–1669
cystic odontoma 1145
cystic partially differentiated nephroblastoma
        1668–1669

cystic tumors, pancreatic *see* pancreas
cystitis 1708–1709
  eosinophilic 1709
  interstitial 1708–1709
  papillary 1708, 1708f
  polypoid 1708
  radiation 1709, 1709f
cystitis cystica 1708
cystitis glandularis 1708, 1709, 1721
cystoprostatectomy 1815
cystosarcoma, vulvar 1914
cytochrome C oxidase, skeletal muscle 2215t, 2230f
cytogenetics 44, 44t
  CNS lesions 2338, 2340
  Hodgkin's disease 539–540
  lymph node specimens 510
cytoid bodies *see* colloid bodies
cytokeratin(s) 179, 179t
  axillary lymph node analysis 430
  diagnostic work-up studies 179, 182
  differential patterns of tumors 179, 179t
  effusion immunohistochemistry 184
  endometrium 1934
  liver biopsy 1470, 1471f
  mesothelioma 1011–1012, 1011f
  prostate gland (normal) 1792–1793
  seminoma 1775t
  sex cord-stromal tumor differential diagnosis
    2017t
  staining, rhabdoid tumor of kidney 1671
  synovial sarcoma 402
  see also keratin
cytokeratin 5/6, mesothelioma 1011, 1011f
cytokeratin 7 179, 179t, 1423
  Brenner tumors 2013
  carcinomas expressing 512t
  chromophobe renal cell carcinoma 1684
  endometrioid carcinoma of ovary 2009
  hepatocellular carcinoma 1534
  lung adenocarcinoma 33, 34f
  metanephric adenoma 1674
  mucinous tumors of ovary 2006
  oncocytoma 1676
  serous tumors of ovary 2002
  squamous cell carcinoma in situ 247
cytokeratin 8 179, 1534
cytokeratin 14 1676, 1680
cytokeratin 18, hepatocellular carcinoma 1534
cytokeratin 19, thyroid carcinoma 2130, 2133
cytokeratin 20 179, 179t
  carcinomas expressing 512t
  extramammary Paget's disease 263
  Merkel cell carcinoma 250
  metastatic colorectal cancer 2038
  mucinous tumors of ovary 2006
  oncocytoma 1676
cytokines
  expressed by Hodgkin cells 540
  hematopoietic 612
  T cells 122
  therapeutic, hematologic changes after 620
cytological sampling
  breast 421–426
  stomach 1324–1325
cytology automation 44
Cytolyte 20, 21, 24
cytomegalovirus (CMV) infection 101–102
  acute cholecystitis 1576
  acute hepatocellular injury 1481, 1482f
  adrenal gland infection 2176, 2177f
  cardiac allograft infection 1051
  cervicitis/cervical infection 1837, 1850f, 1852
  chronic villitis due to 2069
  esophagitis 1288–1289, 1289f
  gastric mucosal infection 1340
  gastritis 1329, 1329f
  immunologic detection 62
  inclusions 68t, 102f, 525, 1472f, 1479f, 1482f
    'owl's eye' 2313, 2314f

intestinal infection 1398
  lymphadenitis 525
  mononucleosis hepatitis 1478–1479, 1479f
  oral squamous cell carcinoma 1170
  peripheral nerve involvement 2244, 2244f
  pneumonia 102f, 878, 879f, 973
  renal transplant complication 1652
  retinitis 2313
  vulvar infection 1889
cytometry
  bladder tumors 1712
  laser scanning 42
  see also flow cytometry; image cytometry
cytopathological and surgical pathology techniques
    15–54
  cell and tissue staining methods 16t–17t
  comparative genomic hybridization 47
  cytogenetics 44, 44t
  cytological samples 19–29
    technical problems 20–22
    see also fine needle aspiration (FNA) biopsy
  cytology automation 44
  electron microscopy 29–30, 29t
  flow cytometry *see* flow cytometry
  image cytometry 36, 42–43
  immunohistochemistry *see* immunohistochemistry
  laser scanning cytometry 42
  molecular biology 44–48
  morphometry 43
  special techniques 15t
  tissue fixation 15–17
cytopathologists
  infectious disease team 57
  interventional 3
cytopathology 3
  communication importance 4
  quality issues 9–10
  standardization 7
  training 8–9
  see also surgical pathology/pathologists
cytopenia, AIDS 662
cytoplasmic 'snouting' 430, 470, 471f, 476
cytoskeleton-associated actin binding proteins 31t
Cytospin preparations 422
cytotoxic drugs
  acute diffuse lung disease due to 885–886, 886f
  metabolism, markers 31t
  reactions to 147–151
  see also chemotherapy
cytotoxicity, graft rejection 122
cytotoxic T cells
  lymphoma 567
  see also CD8 lymphocytes
cytotrophoblast 2063, 2080
  choriocarcinoma 1120, 1753, 2031

D

Dabska tumor *see* angioendothelioma, endovascular
    papillary
Dacron®, foreign body giant cell reaction 145f
dacryoadenitis, granulomatous 2298
dacryolithiasis 2298
dacryoliths 2291
Dalen–Fuchs nodules 2312
danazol 1947, 1952
dandruff 200
Darier's disease (keratosis follicularis) 219–220
  vulvar area 1894
Darier's sign 295
'dark bodies', *Pneumocystis* pneumonia 880, 881f
'dark' neurons 2340, 2341f
daunorubicin, cardiotoxicity 1048
Davies disease 1046
DAX1 gene, mutations 2175
DCC gene, mutations 1359–1360
deafness 2267, 2270
  see also hearing, loss
debrancher enzyme deficiency 2232
decidua

ectopic 1021
  gestational 1948, 1949f
  lack 2075
decidua basalis 2071f
decidual arteriolopathy 2071
decidual cells, nests 1994
decidual nodule 1841, 1841f
decidual reaction 1021
decidual vasculopathy 2071
deciduosis
  acute appendicitis and 1409
  peritoneum 1021
'decoy' cells 1652
dedifferentiation, concept 343
deep venous thrombosis 1079
degenerative disorders, CNS 2417
degenerative joint disease, affecting inner ear 2282
Dejerine–Sottas disease 2245
dematiaceous molds 66, 66t
dementia, HIV 2409
demyelinating diseases 2413, 2414f
demyelination 2241, 2242f
  chronic inflammatory demyelinating
    polyradiculopathy 2242–2243, 2243f
  Guillain-Barr syndrome 2242
  in leprosy 2244
  oligodendrocyte injury causing 2343, 2343f
  progressive multifocal leukoencephalopathy 2408
dendritic cells 287, 573–574
  airways 861
  interdigitating 574
    neoplasms 574
    proliferation 526–527, 526f
  see also follicular dendritic cells
dendritic cell sarcoma, not otherwise specified 574
dendritic cell tumors 573–574
dendrocytes, dermal 264
Denny-Brown syndrome 2244
dense deposit disease 1615–1616, 1616f
dental caries 1146
dental cysts (radicular cysts) 1146–1147
dentate line, anal carcinoma at 1455, 1456f
dentigerous cyst 1140–1141, 1142f
dentin 1139
  dysplastic 1162
denture hyperplasia 1180
dentures
  inflammatory papillary hyperplasia and 1164
  oral squamous cell carcinoma and 1169
Denys-Drash syndrome 1666
de Quervain's disease, tendon sheath thickening 697
de Quervain's thyroiditis (subacute thyroiditis) 2120
dermal duct tumor 257
'dermal erythema multiforme' 208
dermal hypersensitivity reaction (DHR) 208
dermal stromal fibroplasia, atypical melanocytic nevus
    281
dermatitis
  allergic contact 196, 196f
  atopic 196
  dyshidrotic 197, 197f
  herpetic 221, 221f
  irritant contact 196
  nummular 196, 197f
  radiation 155
  seborrheic 200, 200f, 226
  stasis 197, 233, 370
dermatitis herpetiformis 223, 223f, 1374, 1375
dermatochalasis 2290
dermatofibroma (DF) 265, 266f
dermatofibrosarcoma, fibrosarcoma development 326
dermatofibrosarcoma protuberans (DFSP) 265, 266,
    266f
  fibrosarcoma development 325
  vulva 1916
dermatomyofibroma 265–266
dermatomyositis 206, 2219, 2219f
  autoantibodies 114t
  differential diagnosis 2220t

dermatomyositis (cont'd)
  juvenile 206
  lung involvement 883, 889
  muscle histology 2219, 2219f
  skin rash 2219
dermatopathology, terms/definitions 195
dermatophytosis 198, 198f
dermatoses
  granulomatous 212–216, 213t
  interface 202, 203–206, 203t, 222
  lichenoid 202–203, 202t
  neutrophilic 212
  psoriasiform 199–202
  spongiotic 195–199
  superficial (and deep) perivascular 206–209, 206t
dermis
  collagen thickening 231, 232, 232t
  'cracked pavement' appearance 230, 230f, 231f
  deposition disorders 228–234
  dermatoses involving 202–206, 206–209
  normal histology 194–195
  papillary 194
    edema 207, 209f, 212f
  reticular 194
    thickening 229
dermoid cysts 2400–2401, 2402f
  oral cavity 1149
  orbital 2296
  ovarian 2031
  pituitary 2113
  of skin (facial midline) 244
  of testis, teratoma of testis vs 1755
dermoids
  of cornea (solid limbal) 2303
  epibulbar 2303
Descemet's membrane 2301, 2301f
  Fuch's endothelial dystrophy 2301, 2301f
desmin 2218t
desminopathy 2228t
desmin staining
  epithelioid sarcoma 400
  gastric leiomyoma 1345
  leiomyoma 348
  myofibroblastoma 316, 317f
desmin storage myopathy 2229
desmoglein-3, autoantibodies 219
desmoid tumors 320
  abdominal 324–325
  extra-abdominal 322–324, 323f, 324f
  intra-abdominal 325
  sinonasal 822
desmoplasia, esophageal squamous cell carcinoma 1296
desmoplastic fibroma see fibroma, desmoplastic
desmoplastic small round cell tumor see small round
    cell tumors
development, of organs see embryology
developmental abnormalities
  CNS 2417
  oral cavity 1162–1163
  prostate gland 1791
developmental cysts, of skin 244
developmental nonodontogenic cysts 1147
diabetes insipidus 2110, 2345, 2397
diabetes mellitus
  granuloma annulare 212
  hepatic adenoma and 1528
  necrobiosis lipoidica in 214
  necrolytic migratory erythema with 1574
  ocular complications 2304, 2317
  pancreas transplantation 1575
  scleredema in 229
  type 1 113
diabetic mastopathy 450–451
diabetic nephropathy 1629, 1629f
diabetic neuropathy 2247–2248
diabetico-dermatogenic syndrome (DDS) 1574
diabetic ophthalmoplegia 2247
diabetic retinopathy 2317
  proliferative 2304, 2317

diagnostic competency, evaluation 10
diagnostic procedures, iatrogenic reaction 135–138
diaminobenzidine 32
diamnioci/dichorionic membrane 2075
Diamond–Blackfan syndrome 617
diaphragma sella 2093
diaphysis 678
diastase, periodic acid–Schiff (DPAS) 1011
diathermy pigment 137
diet
  gluten-free 1376
  low-fiber 1405
  oral squamous cell carcinoma and 1169
Dieterle stain 207, 875, 875f
diethylstilbestrol (DES) 150
  uterine anomalies 1933
  vaginal adenosis 1923, 1923f
  vaginal anomalies 1919
  vaginal clear cell carcinoma 1923, 1924
  vaginal intraepithelial neoplasia 1924
Diff-Quik stain 25, 26f
  CNS tissue 2331
  effusions 1026
  germ cell tumors of testis 1774
  pancreas 1549
  Papanicolaou stain vs 27, 27f
diffuse alveolar damage (DAD) 868, 872, 873, 874
  acute, in collagen vascular diseases 882–883
  causes 873t
  histology 873, 873f
  idiopathic 886–887
  'organizing'/'proliferative' phase 873, 874f
diffuse alveolar hemorrhage (DAH) 883–884, 883f, 884f
  capillaritis 884, 884f
  with collagen vascular disease 884
  diagnostic algorithm 883f
  Goodpasture's syndrome 884, 884f, 1622
  idiopathic pulmonary hemosiderosis 884, 885f
diffuse cortical necrosis (renal) 1646–1647
diffuse laminar endocervical glandular hyperplasia
    (DLEGH) 1839, 1840f
diffuse lung disease see lung, diffuse diseases
diffuse lymphoid hyperplasia (lung) 861, 900, 900f
diffuse panbronchiolitis (DPB) 907, 907f
DiGeorge anomaly 113
digital automated microscopy 43
digital papillary adenocarcinoma 258
digital papillary eccrine adenocarcinoma (DPEA) 262,
    263f
digital papillary sweat gland tumors 262
digitate dermatosis (small plaque parapsoriasis) 200, 207
diktyoma (embryonal medulloepithelioma) 2311, 2311f
Dilantin (diphenylhydantoin)
  hyperplasia, oral cavity 1180
  lymphadenopathy due to 525–526
  osteomalacia and 686
dimethylpolysiloxane 142
'dimple sign' 265
Dioctophyma renale 1665
diphenylhydantoin see Dilantin
Diphyllobothrium latum 104
direct fluorescent antibody (DFA) stains 62
direct immunofluorescence
  bullous pemphigoid 222
  cicatricial pemphigoid 224
  dermatitis herpetiformis 223
  dermatomyositis 206
  epidermolysis bullosa 225
  leukocytoclastic vasculitis 210
  lupus erythematosus 205–206
  oral cavity specimens 1138
  pemphigus foliaceus vs pemphigus erythematosus
    217–218
  porphyria cutanea tarda 224
  skin specimens 193
directional vacuum-assisted biopsy devices (VABD)
    426
direct touch preparations 58–59
Dirofilaria, respiratory tract infection 95–96, 96f

Dirofilaria immitis 96
'dirty necrosis'
  colorectal adenocarcinoma 1438, 1874
  endometrioid carcinoma 2008
  liver metastases 170–171
  metastatic colorectal cancer 2038, 2038f
disappearing bone disease (Gorham syndrome) 766
disseminated intravascular coagulation 626, 1647,
    1648f
disseminated peritoneal adenomucinosis (DPAM)
    2006, 2006f
diversion colitis 1395
diverticula (diverticulum) 1325
  appendix 1407, 1409
  bladder 1707–1708
  esophageal 1284
  gastric 1325
  Meckel's 1404
  urethra 1724–1725
diverticular disease 1404–1405
  colonic 1404–1405
  NSAID-associated 1402
  sigmoid colon 1382, 1383f
  small bowel 1404
'diverticular disease-associated colitis' 1388, 1393
diverticulosis 1395
DNA
  amplification methods 107
  content determination 39–40
  damage, carcinogens causing 1138
  extraction 45
  fluorochromes binding to 39
  hybridization 45
  methylation 48, 1438
  microarrays 48, 560
  mismatch genes 1360, 1438
  repair disorders 115, 1170, 1438
  staining methods 16t
  streaking 175
  two-color analysis, flow cytometry 38, 38f
  see also ploidy determination
DNA index
  calculation in flow cytometry 39
  laryngeal squamous cell carcinoma 842–843
DNA polymerase, antibodies 43
dog tapeworm (Echinococcus granulosus) 104, 105, 105f
Döhle bodies 620
Donovan bodies 1890
donovaniasis 1890
dopamine agonists, prolactinoma 2103
dorsal root ganglion 2239, 2240
'doughnut' cells 564f
Down syndrome 622, 1163, 1536
doxorubicin (Adriamycin®), cardiotoxicity 1048
DPC4 gene
  ampulla of Vater adenocarcinoma 1588
  gallbladder carcinoma 1581
  mucinous tumors of ovary 2006
  pancreatic carcinoma 1556, 1557f
Drash syndrome 1622
drug abuse, talc embolization 917
drug eruptions
  bullous, bullous pemphigoid vs 222
  fixed 203
  leukocytoclastic vasculitis with 209
  lichenoid 202
drug-induced conditions
  acute diffuse lung disease 884–885
  acute hepatocellular injury 1475t, 1476f, 1478
  cardiomyopathy 1048–1049
  cardiotoxicity 1048–1049, 1049f
  chronic lung reactions 889
  collagenous colitis 1401
  crypt and villous atrophy 1376
  esophagitis 1290
  gastritis 1338
  hepatic granuloma 1510, 1511f
  hypersensitivity myocarditis 1044–1045
  intestinal diseases 1401–1402

intrahepatic cholestasis 1493, 1493f, 1494, 1495t, 1502
liver injury 1472
lymphocytic colitis 1401
nephrotoxicity 128, 131, 1652
pulmonary eosinophilia 882t
pulmonary hypertension 913t
radiation recall phenomenon 151
Stevens-Johnson syndrome 203
tumors 149–150
Dubin–Johnson-like pigment 1529
Dubin-Johnson syndrome 1468, 1531
Duchenne muscular dystrophy 2213, 2235–2236, 2235f, 2236f
ductal carcinoma in situ (DCIS) see breast carcinoma
ductal eccrine adenocarcinoma (DEA) 261
ductal lavage, breast 425
ductopenia 1501f, 1502
ductules see bile ductules
Duke classification 1440
dumbbell-shaped tumors, schwannoma 2385
Duncan syndrome 115
duodenal folds, celiac disease 1374, 1374f
duodenitis 1420
    'chronic' 1396
    Crohn's 1389, 1389f
    peptic 1396–1397
duodenum
    biopsy
        celiac disease 1374, 1375
        complete villous flattening 1374–1376
        crypt and villous atrophy 1376–1377
        examination 1374
        villous flattening with crypt hyperplasia 1377–1378
    Brunner's glands 1420
    carcinoid tumor 1424, 1425f
    Crohn's disease 1337f
    endocrine tumors 193f, 1424, 1426f
    epithelium, in pancreatic FNA samples 1550–1551, 1551f
    erosion, NSAID-induced 1397
    gangliocytic paraganglioma 1447
    neuroendocrine tumors 1424
    somatostatinoma 1574
    ulcers
        diffuse antral gastritis and 1332, 1357
        gastric cancer prevention 1333
        Helicobacter pylori and 1332, 1396
        perforated, barium into peritoneal cavity by 138
        treatment 1324
    see also small intestine
Dupuytren's contracture 320, 321, 321f, 1771
'dust macule' 908
Dutcher bodies 552, 553, 649
    lymphoplasmacytic lymphoma 554, 555, 555f, 587, 587f
dwarfism, pituitary 2098, 2108
dyes, staining methods 18
dysembryoplastic neuroepithelial tumor 2374, 2375f
    immunohistochemistry 2339t
    oligodendroglioma vs 2362
dysentery, amebic 103
dyserythropoiesis 619, 661
dysfunctional uterine bleeding 1949–1950
dysgerminoma, of ovary 2027–2028, 2028f, 2029t
    arising in gonadoblastoma 2037
    mixed tumors 2036, 2037f
dyshidrotic dermatitis (eczema) 197, 197f
dyskeratoma, warty 242, 243f
dyskeratosis 195
    vulvar intraepithelial neoplasia 1894–1895, 1903, 1904
dysplasia 1579, 1579f
    definition 838, 1304, 1434, 1441, 1853
    see also specific types/sites of dysplasia
dysplasia-associated lesion or mass (DALM) 1394, 1443
dysplasia epiphysealis hemimelica 707

dysplastic gangliocytoma of cerebellum 2374
'dysplastic nevus' see melanocytic nevi
dysplastic nevus syndrome 280
dystrobrevin 2218t
dystrophin 2218t, 2235, 2236
    staining/evaluation 2236, 2236f
dystrophinopathies 2235
dystrophoglycan 2218t

E
ear 2267–2287
    accessory 2270, 2270f
    anatomy 2267–2270, 2268f, 2269f
    angiolymphoid hyperplasia with eosinophilia 2275, 2275f
    basal cell carcinoma 2280
    bone and joint diseases 2281–2284
    cholesteatoma 2273
    cholesterol granuloma 2273–2274
    congenital abnormalities 2270–2271
    cutaneous disorders 2274–2275
    embryology 2267
    external 2267, 2268f
        see also pinna (ear)
    gouty tophi 2274
    hematologic diseases involving 2284
    histology (normal) 2267–2270, 2268f, 2269f
    inflammatory and infectious diseases 2271–2274
    inner (labyrinth) see labyrinth (inner ear)
    keloids 2274
    Langerhans cell histiocytosis 2284
    melanoma 2280
    middle 2267, 2268f
        adenoma 2277–2278, 2278f
        anatomical regions 2268–2269, 2268f
        carcinoid tumors 2278
        chemodectoma 2276–2277
        embryonal rhabdomyosarcoma 2281, 2281f
        inverted papilloma (epithelial/transitional) 2277
        low-grade papillary adenocarcinoma 2278–2279, 2279f
        lymphoma 2284
        meningioma involving 2279–2280
        paraganglioma 2276–2277, 2277f
        rhabdomyosarcoma 2281, 2281f
        salivary gland choristoma 2271
        squamous cell carcinoma 2280
        tumors 2276–2278
        tympanosclerosis after inflammation 2274
    myospherulosis 2273, 2273f
    neoplasms 2276–2281
    osteosarcoma involving 2283
    in Paget's disease of bone 2283
    physiology 2270
    polyarteritis nodosa 2276
    relapsing polychondritis 2282
    vascular disorders 2275–2276
    verrucous carcinoma 2280
    Wegener's granulomatosis 2276
    see also external auditory canal (EAC)
Early Lung Cancer Action Project 936
EA solution 26
Eaton-Lambert syndrome 1108
E-cadherin
    breast carcinoma 461, 462, 462f, 467
    expression loss, metastases mechanism 167
    gastric adenocarcinoma 1360
ecchordosis physaliphora 2404
eccrine adenocarcinoma
    clear cell 262
    digital papillary 262, 263f
    ductal 261
    mucinous 261–262
eccrine adenoma, papillary 257–258, 259f
eccrine glands, normal histology 194
eccrine hidradenocarcinoma, low-grade 261
eccrine hidrocystoma, eyelid 2290
eccrine poroma/acrospiroma 256–257, 257f

eccrine spiradenoma 256, 256f
echinococcal cysts
    heart 1066
    liver 1545
    spleen 580
Echinococcus granulosus 104, 105, 105f
eclampsia, glomerulopathy associated 1637
ectocervix 1831, 1918
ectoparasites, vulvar area 1891
ectopic ACTH syndrome 2180–2181, 2180f, 2181f
ectopic gestational trophoblastic disease 2087
ectopic pregnancy see pregnancy, ectopic
ectropion 1835, 2290
eczema 195
    see also dermatitis
edema
    cornea (bullous keratopathy) 2301, 2301f
    massive ovarian 1992, 2021
    optic disc (papilledema) 2318
    papillary dermis 207, 209f, 212f
    pulmonary, 'photographic negative of' 894
efferent arterioles, kidney 1600
effusions 1025
    benign 1026–1028
        cell components 1026–1027, 1026f, 1027f
    cytology in cancer diagnosis 182–184
    cytopathology 183–184, 1025–1033
    fluid, characteristics 1026
    immunocytochemistry 184, 1032–1033, 1032f
    malignant 1026, 1028–1033
        breast cancer 1029, 1030f
        cancer cell structure 1028–1029, 1029f
        gastrointestinal cancer 1030, 1031f
        hematologic neoplasms 1031–1032, 1031f
        lung cancer 1030, 1030f
        melanoma 1030–1031, 1031f
        mesothelioma 1028, 1029, 1029f, 1032, 1032f
        ovarian cancer 1029–1030, 1030f
        pitfalls in cytological diagnosis 1033
        rare neoplasms 1032
    reactive mesothelial hyperplasia 1027, 1027f
        atypical 1027–1028, 1028f
        malignancy vs 1027–1028
    serous 183
    specimen preparation and reporting 1025–1026
    tumor types with 183–184, 184f
    see also pericardial effusions; peritoneal effusions; pleural effusions
'eggshell' calcification 904
Ehlers-Danlos syndrome 686
ejaculatory duct cysts 1791
ejaculatory ducts 1791
elastase 1, cystic tumors of pancreas 1562
elastic cartilage, cartilage-forming tumors 706
elastic tissue, staining methods 16t, 19f
elastofibroma 310–311, 311f
elderly, aortic valve degenerative disease 1057f, 1058
electrocautery, thermal artifact in tissue 137
electromyography (EMG) 2213
electron microscopy 29–30, 29t
    CNS tissue 2335–2336, 2336t–2337t
    diagnostic applications 29, 29t
    liver biopsy 1472
    renal transplant biopsy 1651, 1652f
electron probe analysis 1472
electron probe X-ray microanalysis 29
'elephant foot' cells 542
ELISA assays, celiac disease diagnosis 1374
Elschnig's pearls 2300
Elston–Ellis histologic grading system 464, 465t, 487
embedding, renal biopsy 1603
Embogold® 140, 141f
embolic disease, lung 916–917, 917f
embolizing agents, reaction to 139–140, 140f
embryoid bodies 1119
embryology
    ear 2267
    esophagus 1281

embryology (cont'd)
  gonads 1114
  larynx and trachea 834
  pancreas 1549
  parathyroid glands 2149
  penis and scrotum 1768
  pleura 1005
  prostate gland 1791
  skeletal muscle 2214–2215
  testis 1734
  thyroid gland 2119
embryoma, diffuse 1757
embryonal carcinoma 1115
  immunohistochemistry 180, 1746
  mediastinum see mediastinum
  metastatic 1776–1777, 1777f
  ovarian 2029t, 2030, 2030f
  testicular see under testicular tumors
  thymus 1118, 1118f, 1119f
embryonal medullopeithlioma (diktyoma) 2311, 2311f
embryonal rhabdomyosarcoma 356–361
  botryoid, extrahepatic bile ducts 1587–1588, 1588f
  fetal rhabdomyoma vs 356
  fibrodysplasia ossificans progressiva vs 387
  fibrous hamartoma of infancy vs 318
  genital rhabdomyoma vs 356
  histological features 358, 358f
  larynx 850
  middle ear 2281, 2281f
  necrotizing sialometaplasia with 1179
  orbital 2297
  sinonasal 820
  vagina 1925
  vulva 1916–1917, 1916f, 1917f
embryonal sarcoma 358
  liver 1544, 1544f
embryonal tumors of CNS 2377–2385
  ependymoblastoma 2368, 2379
  immunohistochemistry 2339t
  medulloblastoma see medulloblastoma
  medulloepithelioma 2379
  terminology 2378
embryonic remnants 2065–2066
embryonic rests 1990, 1990f
Emery-Dreifuss dystrophy 2236
EMG syndrome see Beckwith-Wiedemann syndrome
emperipolesis
  interface hepatitis 1485
  Rosai–Dorfman disease 288, 529, 759
emphysema, cystic lung disease vs 863–864
empty sella syndrome 2098
empyema 69
enamel, development 1139
enamel organ, cysts 1140
encephalitis
  Acanthamoeba 106f
  granulomatous amebic 2412
  herpes simplex 2407–2408, 2408f
  HIV 118–119, 119f, 2409, 2410f
  Naegleria 106
  Rasmussen 2405–2406, 2406f
  toxoplasmic 2411, 2412f
  viral 2407–2418, 2407f
encephalitis viruses, vector-transmitted 58
encephalocele 2404
  middle ear–mastoid 2271
encephalofacial angiomatosis see Sturge-Weber syndrome
encephalofacial vascular malformations 365
encephalomyopathies 2229–2230, 2230f
encephalopathies, transmissible spongiform 2412–2413, 2413f
enchondroma 708–710, 709f
  chondrosarcoma development in 711, 715f, 719f
  chondrosarcoma vs 709, 710
  digits 710, 710f
  malignant transformation 711
  multiple 708, 710–711, 710f, 711f
  solitary 708

enchondroma protuberans 709
enchondromatosis 708, 710–711, 710f, 711f
  see also Ollier's disease
endarterectomy 1071, 1072t
endarteritis, obliterative see obliterative endarteritis
endobodies 140, 141
endobronchial papillary-glandular tumor 945–946, 946f
endocarditis
  autoimmune 1060
  infectious see infectious endocarditis
  Libman-Sacks 1060
  Löffler's 1046
  nonbacterial thrombotic 1060
endocervical adenocarcinoma see cervix, adenocarcinoma
endocervical canal 1831, 1832, 1918
endocervical cells 1844, 1871
  cyclical changes 1832
  reactive changes 1872
  tubal metaplasia 1842, 1847f
  see also cervical smears
endocervical epithelium 1832, 1844
endocervical glands 1832
  malignant tumors 1866–1871, 1872–1874
endocervical glandular dysplasia (EGD) 1868
endocervical-like mucinous borderline tumors 2003–2004, 2004f
endocervical polyps 1841
endocervical sarcoma 1877
endocervix 1831, 1844
endochondral ossification 681
endochondral pseudocyst 2281, 2281f
endocrine autoimmune diseases 113
endocrine cells
  closed/'open' 1423
  gastrointestinal 1373, 1422–1423, 1423
  staining and ultrastructure 1423
endocrine tumors
  ampulla of Vater 1589
  heart 1066
  small intestinal see small intestine
  see also neuroendocrine tumors; specific sites
endodermal sinus tumors see yolk sac tumors
endolymph 2269
  excessive amount 2284
endolymphatic hydrops 2269–2270, 2284
  idiopathic (Ménière's disease) 2269–2270, 2284
endolymphatic sac tumor 2278–2279, 2279f
endometrial adenocarcinoma 1958–1968
  cervical involvement 1960
  cervical smears 1873–1874
  cilia in glands and 1943
  clear cell 1959, 1962, 1963, 1964, 1964f, 1965f, 1967
    differential diagnosis 1949
  confluent pattern 1956f
  cytopathology 1873–1874, 1874f, 1965–1967, 1965f
  desmoplastic reaction 1956f
  detection from cervical/vaginal smears 1935
  differential diagnosis 1944, 1949
    endocervical carcinoma vs 1869, 1869t
    endometrial hyperplasia vs 1955–1957, 1956f
  endometrioid 1957, 1957f, 1959–1961, 1959f, 1963
    adenoacanthoma type 1960, 1961f, 1966
    ciliated cell 1962
    cytopathology 1966
    microglandular 1962, 1963f
    mixed adenosquamous type 1960, 1961f
    ovarian carcinoma with 2009
    secretory variant 1962, 1962f
    sertoliform 1962, 1963f
    squamous differentiation 1960–1961, 1961f, 1962f, 1964, 1966
    treatment 1968
    villoglandular 1961, 1962f
    well-differentiated 1962f
    WHO classification 1960, 1960t
  extrauterine carcinoma synchronous with 1967–1968

FIGO staging 1958, 1958t, 1959
  in situ 1955, 1957
  keratin granuloma in 1989f
  metastatic 1968
    to ovary 1967, 2038
  morules, with 1960, 1961f
  mucinous 1963, 1963f, 1966–1967
  myometrial invasion 1959–1960, 1959f
  prognosis 1958–1959, 1960
  serous 1959, 1962f, 1963–1964, 1964f
    cytopathology 1967, 1967f
  specimen reporting 1968
  stromal foam cells 1956, 1956f
  stromal invasion/necrosis 1956f
  TNM classification 1958
  treatment 1968
  type 1 see endometrial adenocarcinoma, endometrioid
  type 2 1959
  variants 1961–1962, 1964
  well-differentiated 1966, 1966f
    complex hyperplasia vs 1954
  see also endometrium, carcinoma/cancer
endometrial intraepithelial neoplasia (EIN) 1955, 1957, 1957f, 1964
endometrioid adenocarcinoma
  cervix 1867f, 1868, 1870f
  ovary see ovary, endometrioid carcinoma
  of prostate 1818, 1818f
  vagina 1925
endometrioid carcinoma, fallopian tube 2045, 2046, 2046f
endometrioid cysts 1995
endometrioid stromal sarcoma, ovary 2010
endometrioma 1899
endometriosis 1951–1952, 1952t
  of appendix 1409, 1410f
  of cervix 1840, 1845
  endosalpingiosis vs 2000
  epithelial cells in peritoneal fluid 1033
  of fallopian tube 2043, 2044f
  of lymph nodes 512
  of ovary 1994–1995, 1994f, 1995f, 2007
    atypical 1952f, 1995
    clear cell carcinoma and 1995, 2012
    endometrioid carcinoma with 2008
  peritoneal lesions 1020–1021
  tumor differential diagnosis 146
  tumors associated 1951, 1967–1968
  of vagina 1899, 1918, 1920f, 1921
  vulvar 1899, 1918
endometriosis externa 1951
endometriosis interna (adenomyosis) 1951–1952
endometritis 1944–1945
  acute 1944
  chronic nongranulomatous 1945, 1945f
  granulomatous 1945
  xanthogranulomatous 1945
endometrium
  abnormal cycling 1949–1950
  adenoacanthoma 1960
  adenocarcinoma see endometrial adenocarcinoma
  adenofibroma 1975, 1976, 1976f
  adenomyoma 1976
  adenosarcoma 1975, 1976, 1976f
  anovulatory cycles 1950
  artifacts 1942–1944
  atrophy 1948f
    cystic 1948, 1948f, 1953–1954
      infertility disorders 1950
      simple 1947–1948, 1948f
  atypical polypoid adenomyoma 1946, 1946f, 1976–1977, 1977f
  biopsy 1934, 1936
    dating 1936
    dating not possible 1944–1947
    foreign body giant cell reaction 137f
  'bleeding' phase 1939, 1940f
  carcinoma/cancer 1952–1968, 1955

adenocarcinoma *see* endometrial adenocarcinoma
  differential diagnosis 1955–1957
  endometriosis and 1951
  estrogen therapy 150
  hyperplasia-atypical hyperplasia sequence 1955
  mixed adenosquamous 1960
  mixed types 1965
  post-irradiation 154, 159
  risk factors 1952–1953
  secretory 1961–1962, 1962f, 1967
  small cell 1965f
  squamous cell 1964
  tamoxifen association 150
  transitional cell 1965f
carcinosarcoma 1977, 1977f, 1978f
cells in cervical smears 1871–1872, 1873
clear cells 1936, 1937f
  gestational change 1949, 1949f
curettage 136f
  distortion of normal tissue 135, 135f
endometrioid lesions 1957
epithelial metaplasia 1942
epithelium 1933
gestational 1948–1949, 1949f, 1950f
glands 1933
  cilia 1943
  proliferative phase 1936–1937, 1936f, 1940f
  secretory phase 1937f, 1938, 1938f, 1941f
  simple hyperplasia 1953, 1953f
histology 1847f, 1933, 1934f
hyperplasia 1952–1968
  atrophy *vs* 1948
  atypical (adenomatous with atypia) 1953t, 1954–1955, 1954f, 1955f, 1958
  classification 1953t, 1955
  complex adenomatous (without atypia) 1953t, 1954, 1954f, 1955–1956, 1958
  cytologic diagnosis 1957–1958
  differential diagnosis 1955–1957
  granulosa cell tumor 2015
  in polyps 1954
  progression risk to carcinoma 1955
  secretory 1962, 1962f
  simple 1953–1954, 1953f, 1953t, 1954f, 1955, 1958
  types 1953t
iatrogenic disturbances 1946–1947, 1947f
inactive (resting) 1950
infertility disorders 1949–1950
interval (ovulatory) phase 1937
irregular shedding 1950, 1951f
luteal-phase defects 1950
menstrual phase 1939, 1940f
  cytology 1941–1942, 1942f
mesenchymal and glial metaplasias 1943–1944
metaplasia 1942–1944
  classification 1942, 1943t
metastatic tumors, to ovary 2009
mixed epithelial-stromal tumors 1975–1978, 1975t
mucinous metaplasia 1943
normal menstrual cycle 1936–1942
  see also specific phases above/below
papillary metaplasia 1943, 1943f
pathologic noncycling 1949–1950
physiologic noncycling 1947–1949
polyps 1943, 1945–1946, 1946f, 1956, 1968f
postabortal 1949
postcurettage regenerative atypia 1944, 1944f
postmenopausal 1947–1948, 1948f
postpartum 1949
predecidual (pseudodecidual) stromal reaction 1938, 1938f, 1939f
premenstrual phase 1934f, 1938, 1939f
proliferative, diagnosis 1936
proliferative phase 1936–1937, 1936f, 1937f
  cytology (normal) 1940, 1940f, 1941f
rhabdomyosarcoma 1977, 1977f
sarcoma

endometriosis and 1951
undifferentiated (high-grade stromal) 1973, 1973f, 1974f
secretory phase
  cytology (normal) 1940–1941, 1941f
  early 1937–1938, 1937f, 1938f
  late 1938, 1938f, 1939f
  mid 1938, 1938f
specimens 1936
spiral arterioles 1938, 1938f, 1939f
squamous cell carcinoma 1964
squamous metaplasia 1942
stroma 1933, 1939
  proliferative phase 1937f, 1940, 1941f
  pseudodecidual 1938, 1939f
  secretory phase 1937f, 1938f
'stromal glands' 1974
stromal nodule 1973, 1974
stromal sarcoma
  chromosomal translocation 310t
  cytology 1975, 1975f
  high-grade 1973, 1973f, 1974f
  low-grade 1973–1974, 1974f, 1975, 1975f
  metastatic 971, 971f
stromal tumors (pure) 1973–1975
subnuclear vacuoles 1937, 1937f
surface syncytial change 1943, 1943f, 1944f
tubal metaplasia (ciliary change) 1942–1943, 1943f
endomyocardial biopsy 1041–1052
  artifacts and non-specific findings 1041–1042
  cardiomyopathy 1045–1048
  contraction bands 1042
  fixation and staining 1041
  heart transplant rejection 1049–1051, 1055f
    Quilty effect 1051, 1055f
  indications 1041
  ischemic injury 1050
  myocarditis 1042–1045
  role in unexplained heart failure 1042
  sarcoidosis 1045
  specimen processing and evaluation 1041, 1041t
endomyocardial fibrosis, idiopathic 1046
endomyometriosis 1021
endomysial fibrosis 2220, 2220f
endomysium, inflammation, polymyositis 2218, 2219f
endoneurium 2240
endophthalmitis 2312–2313
  phacoanaphylactic 2300, 2300f
  vitrectomy 2304
endosalpingiosis 512, 1936
  endometriosis *vs* 2000
  epithelial cells in peritoneal fluid 1033
  peritoneal implant from ovarian serous tumor *vs* 2000
  peritoneal lesions 1020–1021
endoscope, flexible 1324, 1419
endoscopic retrograde cholangiopancreatography (ERCP) 1549
endoscopic ultrasound-guided transmucosal fine needle aspiration, stomach 1325
endoscopy, laryngeal and tracheal 833
endothelial cells
  alveolar capillary 861
  as antigen-presenting cells 122
  cornea 2301
  destruction, leukocytoclastic vasculitis 209
  epithelioid 271, 272f
  flattened, cavernous hemangioma of skin 270–271, 271f
  glomerular capillaries 1598, 1599, 1623, 1623f
  hyperplasia 1890
  immunohistochemistry, breast cancer and 487–488
endothelial hyperplasia, papillary 363, 363f, 365
endothelialitis 919
endothelial proteins 31t
endothelin-secreting (X) cells 1323
endothelium, fenestrated, glomerulus 1598
endovascular papillary angioendothelioma *see* angioendothelioma, endovascular papillary

end-stage renal disease (ESRD) 1629, 1643, 1664
'enigmatic bodies' 2097
Enneking system, soft tissue tumor trading 308
enophthalmos 2294
enostosis (bone island) 722, 722f
Entamoeba gingivalis 1838
Entamoeba hartmanni 103
Entamoeba histolytica 102–103, 1388
  cervicitis 1838
  colitis 1399–1400
  colonic ulcer 1400f
enteritis 1377
  phlegmonous 1398
  radiation 1406
Enterobacteriaceae 59, 68–69
Enterobius vermicularis
  appendiceal infection 104, 104f, 1409, 1409f
  fallopian tube infection 2042
  vulvar infection 1891
enterochromaffin (EC) cells 1322–1323, 1423
enterochromaffin-like (ECL) cells 1323, 1423
  gastric carcinoids 1348, 1350f
  hyperplasia 1348, 1349, 1349f
  hyperplasia-to-neoplasia sequence 1349
enterocolic lymphocytic phlebitis 1386, 1387f
enterocolitis
  allergic 1405
  necrotizing 1397–1398, 1398f, 1406
  neutropenic 1397
  radiation 155
enterogenous cyst 2401
enteropathy
  autoimmune 1376
  gluten-sensitive *see* celiac disease
  protein-losing 1340
enteropathy-associated T-cell lymphoma (EATL) 567, 652, 1453, 1454f
entropion, senile 2290
environmental tobacco smoking (ETS), oral carcinoma 1168
En Vision™ 31
enzymes, markers 31t
eosinophil(s)
  acute eosinophilic lung disease 881–882
  erythema nodosum 234, 234f
  in esophagus 1282f, 1285–1286, 1285t
  gastroesophageal reflux disease 1282f, 1285–1286, 1285t
  Hodgkin's disease 537
  infiltrate, polymyositis 2219
  intestinal 1373
  Langerhans cell histiocytosis 759
  subepidermal blisters 221–222, 222f, 222t
  vasculitis 211–212
eosinophilia
  allergic sinusitis 787
  graft 920
  Kimura's disease 519, 519f
  oncocytes 1218
  pleural effusions 1027
  pulmonary, drugs causing 882t
eosinophilic cholecystitis 1577
eosinophilic colitis 1405
eosinophilic cystitis 1709
eosinophilic cytoplasmic inclusions 2384
eosinophilic folliculitis 227, 227f
eosinophilic gastroenteritis 1290, 1336–1337, 1337f, 1378, 1378f
  idiopathic 1336, 1405
  inflammatory fibroid polyp and 1341
eosinophilic globules 1261, 1753
eosinophilic granuloma
  bone involvement 690, 690f
  bone marrow involvement 659–660
  lung 968, 969f
  pulmonary *see* Langerhans cell histiocytosis, pulmonary
  sinonasal 826
  skin involvement *see* Langerhans cell histiocytosis

eosinophilic granuloma (cont'd)
    solitary see Langerhans cell histiocytosis
    temporal bone 2284
    unifocal and multifocal types 659
eosinophilic microabscesses 572
'eosinophilic pleuritis' 925
eosinophilic pneumonia see pneumonia
eosin stains 26
ependymal canal 2366f
ependymal cells 2343, 2344f
ependymal cysts 2403
ependymal tumors 2364–2369
    see also ependymoma
ependymitis, granular 2343, 2344f
ependymoblastic rosettes 2379
ependymoblastoma 2368, 2379
ependymoma 2364–2367
    anaplastic 2367–2368, 2368f
        differential diagnosis 2368, 2379, 2383
    in broad ligament 2048
    cellular type 2366
    clear cell 2362, 2366–2367
    crush preparations 2364, 2365f
    ectopic 2364
    genetic abnormalities 2340t, 2367
    histology 2364–2366, 2365f
    immunohistochemistry 2338t, 2367
    lung 970
    myxopapillary 2368–2369, 2368f, 2369f
    of ovary 2036, 2036f
    papillary 2366
    pituitary 2109
    rosettes 2365–2366, 2366f
    sites 2364
    tanycytic 2359, 2367
    ultrastructural characteristics 2336t
epidemic pleurodynia 2222
epidermal growth factor receptor (EGFR) 837, 1138,
    2354
epidermal nevi 241, 241f
epidermis
    atrophy, lichen sclerosus 232
    dermatoses involving 195–202, 202–206
    histology (normal) 193–194
    hyperplasia
        chondrodermatitis nodularis helicis 227
        lichen nitidus 202, 203f
        psoriasiform 200, 201
    necrosis, leukocytoclastic vasculitis 209
    squamous hyperplasia 263
epidermodysplasia verruciformis 242
epidermoid cyst 2400, 2402f
    of bone 755
    of CNS 2400
    first branchial cleft cysts vs 2270
    of ovary 1990
    pituitary 2113
    proliferating, of thymus 1092
    scrotum 1772
    of skin 254, 254f
    teratoma of testis vs 1755, 1756f
epidermolysis bullosa 224–225
    Herlitz variant 225
epidermolysis bullosa acquisita 223, 225
epidermolysis bullosa simplex 225
epidermotropism 291, 291f, 293
epididymis 1731
    benign cystic mesothelioma 1764
    carcinoma 1765
    histology (normal) 1733
    nodular/diffuse fibrous proliferation 1763
    papillary cystadenoma 1764, 1764f
    tumors and tumor-like conditions 1763–1766
epididymo-orchitis, pyogenic 1767
epidural hemorrhage 2416
epigenetic (methylation) analysis 48
epiglottitis 834
epignathus 827
epilepsy 2405–2406

epimyoepithelial islands 1257
epineurium 2240
epiphora (excessive tearing) 2291
epiphyseal chondromatous giant cell tumor see
    chondroblastoma
epiphysis 678
epithelial atypia 1166–1167
epithelial cells
    airways 860, 860f
    glomerulus 1598–1599
    respiratory see respiratory epithelial cells
    see also specific cells/sites
epithelial downgrowth
    glaucoma 2316
    ocular surface epithelium 2312, 2313f
epithelial inclusion cysts
    cervix 1840, 1841
    ovary 1990, 1991f
    vaginal 1920
epithelial membrane antigen (EMA) 179
    adrenal gland metastases 171
    basal cell carcinoma differential diagnosis 245, 246
    effusion immunohistochemistry 184
    endometrioid carcinoma of ovary 2009
    ependymoma 2367
    epithelioid sarcoma 400
    leiomyosarcoma 352
    mesothelioma 1012–1013
    sex cord-stromal tumor differential diagnosis 2017t
    synovial sarcoma 402
    thymic neuroendocrine tumors 1112
    thymoma 1100, 1100f
    tumors associated 179
epithelial–mesenchymal interactions, oral cavity 1139
epithelial nodules, basal cell carcinoma of skin 244, 244f
epithelial tumors
    broad ligament 2047
    fallopian tube see fallopian tube
    kidney see under kidney
    lacrimal gland 2298–2299, 2299f
    larynx 842–846
    ovarian-type, in paratesticular region 1765–1766
    ovary see ovary
    paratesticular region 1765–1766
    trachea 842–846
    vagina 1921–1922
    vulval, benign 1899
    see also specific anatomic sites and tumors
epithelioid angiomyolipoma 1691–1692, 1692f
epithelioid angiosarcoma 276, 372f, 373f, 769, 769f
    epithelioid hemangioendothelioma vs 368
    epithelioid sarcoma vs 400
epithelioid-cell nevus see Spitz nevus
epithelioid cells
    malignant peripheral nerve sheath tumor 2258
    uveal malignant melanoma 2306–2307, 2307f
epithelioid fibrosarcoma, sclerosing 329–330, 330f
epithelioid glioblastoma 2354
epithelioid granuloma
    bone marrow 661, 661f
    in Crohn's disease (small intestinal) 1388, 1388f
    lung 96f
    in primary biliary cirrhosis 1500, 1501f
    splenic 579
epithelioid hemangioendothelioma 273, 366–368, 367f,
    368f
    of bone 767–768, 768f
    differential diagnosis 400, 768
    liver 1543–1544, 1543f, 1544f
    lung 973–974, 974f
    pleural 1016, 1016f, 1017f
    of skin 273
    splenic 591
epithelioid hemangioma
    of bone 766–767, 767f
    epithelioid hemangioendothelioma vs 368, 768
    pericardial 1019
    of skin see angiolymphoid hyperplasia with
        eosinophilia

epithelioid histiocytes 519, 520f, 537, 640
epithelioid leiomyoma, larynx 849
'epithelioid' leiomyosarcoma 349
epithelioid sarcoma 398–400, 399f
    epithelioid hemangioendothelioma vs 368
    hand/wrist 398, 398f
    of vulva 1918
epithelioid stromal tumor, stomach 1347
epithelioid trophoblastic tumor (ETT) 2084,
    2086–2087
epithelioma
    basosebaceous 250
    calcifying, of Malherbe (pilomatrixoma) 253–254,
        253f
    superficial with sebaceous differentiation 250
epithelioma adenoides cysticum syndrome 251
epithelioma cuniculatum pedis 248
epithelium
    changes due to cytotoxic drugs 148–149
    'collarette' 270, 1902
    implantation during biopsy 137
    radiation effects 152, 152f
    regeneration, acute erosive gastritis 1328, 1328f
    reparative, cervical 1845–1846
    Wilms' tumor element 1666, 1667, 1667f, 1668f
    see also specific anatomic sites
epitope (antigen) retrieval methods 32–33, 33f
epitympanum 2268
EPOS system, immunohistochemistry 31
Epstein–Barr virus (EBV)
    Burkitt's lymphoma and 1453
    CNS lymphoma 2395
    gastric adenocarcinoma 1361–1362
    gastric remnant cancer and 1356–1357
    hemophagocytic syndrome 527
    hepatitis 101, 102f
    Hodgkin's disease 539
    immunohistochemistry 525
    inclusions 68t
    infectious mononucleosis 101, 524f, 525,
        1478–1479, 1479f
    inflammatory pseudotumor of spleen 583
    large B-cell lymphoma 980
    lymphoepithelioma-like carcinoma of lung 965
    lymphoid proliferations associated 150
    lymphoma of lung 980, 981
    lymphomatoid granulomatosis 290
    malignant histiocytosis and 659
    oral squamous cell carcinoma 1170
    PTLD see post-transplantation lymphoproliferative
        disorders
    salivary lymphoepithelial carcinoma 1249, 1251
    smooth muscle tumors associated 353
    thymic carcinoma 1105
    vulvar infection 1889
    X-linked lymphoproliferative disease 115
Epstein's pearls 1142
epulis fissuratum 1180
Erdheim–Chester disease 1069, 2290
ergot compounds 1726
Erlenmeyer flask deformity 689
eruption cysts 1141, 1142f
erythema
    gyrate 207–208, 207f
    heliotrope 206
    necrolytic migratory, diabetes with 1574
erythema annulare centrifugum 207–208, 207f
erythema elevatum diutinum (EED) 210, 210f
erythema gyratum repens 207–208
erythema induratum 215, 235, 235f
erythema infectiosum 76
erythema migrans 207–208
erythema multiforme 203–204, 203f
    'dermal' 208
    paraneoplastic pemphigus vs 219
erythema nodosum 7/24, 234–235, 235f
erythrasma 1891
erythroblastopenia, transient, of childhood 617
erythroblasts 610, 617, 621, 622f

erythrocytosis 619, 632
erythroderma, cutaneous T-cell lymphoma 291
erythroid cells
   hyperplasia *see* bone marrow, hyperplasia
   megaloblastic 619
   megaloblastoid 619–620
   precursors, decreased/absent 617
   regeneration after chemotherapy 618
erythroid lineage, markers and antigen detection 611t
erythroleukemia 610
erythrophagocytosis 659
   malignant lymphoma with 528
   splenic red pulp 578, 578f
erythroplakia
   esophagus 1292
   oral cavity 1165, 1166f
erythroplasia of Queyrat 246, 1771, 1902
erythropoiesis 612–613, 613f
   ineffective 619
erythropoietic islands 612
erythropoietin, production, by hemangioblastoma
   2394–2395
Escherichia coli
   acute appendicitis 1408
   acute pyelonephritis 1639
   acute suppurative gastritis 1329
Escherichia coli O157:H7 infection 1382–1384,
   1384f
esophageal glands 1282
   Barrett's esophagus diagnosis 1303, 1304f
esophageal varices 1662
esophagectomy 1296–1297, 1312
esophagin, cytoplasmic 1294
esophagitis 1285–1291
   drug-induced 1290
   idiopathic eosinophilic 1286, 1286t
   infectious 1287–1290
      Aspergillus 1289
      Candida 1289, 1289f
      cytomegalovirus 1288–1289, 1289f
      fungal, mimickers 1289–1290
      herpetic 74, 74f, 1287–1288, 1288f
      rare pathogens 1290
   inflammatory cells 1282f, 1285–1286, 1285t
   'pill' 1287, 1290
   radiation-related 1288
   reflux *see* gastroesophageal reflux disease (GERD)
esophagoscopy, esophageal squamous cell carcinoma
   1296
esophagus 1281–1321
   adenocarcinoma 1312–1314, 1313f
      Barrett's esophagus progression 1303–1304, 1309,
        1312, 1314
   amyloidosis 1291
   anatomy 1281, 1301f
   atresia 1283
   Barrett's *see* Barrett's esophagus
   basaloid squamous cell carcinoma 1299
   in collagen vascular disorders 1290
   columnar-lined of Barrett's type *see* Barrett's
      esophagus
   columnar-lined of non-Barrett's type 1301, 1301f
   congenital anomalies 1283–1284
   congenital stenosis 1283
   Crohn's disease 1291
   cysts 1283
   cytology (normal) 1283
   in dermatologic disease 1290–1291
   diverticula 1284
   ectopic sebaceous glands 1289–1290
   embryology 1281
   erosions/ulcers 1286–1287, 1286f, 1287f
   erythroplakia 1292
   fibrovascular polyps 1315
   fine needle aspiration biopsy 1283
   gastrointestinal stromal tumor 1315
   glandular dysplasia 1312–1313
   glandular lesions 1299–1314
      see also Barrett's esophagus

glycogenic acanthosis 1289–1290
graft-*versus*-host disease 1291
granular cell tumor 1315
hematolymphoid tumors 1315
histology (normal) 1281–1283, 1281f
idiopathic ulceration 1290
inlet patches (islands of ectopic gastric mucosa)
   1283
lamina propria 1282–1283
leiomyoma 1314–1315
leiomyomatosis 1315
leiomyosarcoma 1315
leukoplakia 1292
lymphoepithelioma 1299
melanoma 1314
melanosis 1314
mesenchymal tumors 1314–1315
motility disorders 1284–1285
mucosa 1281–1282, 1283
   hyperemia 1285
   hyperplastic 1281f
in muscular dystrophy 1284
muscularis and adventitia 1282–1283
Paget's disease 1312
pseudodiverticulosis 1284
rings and webs 1284
salivary gland adenocarcinoma 1312
sarcomatoid carcinoma 1299
in scleroderma 1284
small cell undifferentiated carcinoma 1314
squamocolumnar junction (Z-line) 1282, 1300
squamous cell carcinoma 1293–1299, 1295f
   advanced 1296
   cytology 1297–1298, 1297f, 1298f
   dysplasia progression 1293, 1293f
   herpetic esophagitis *vs* 1288
   histopathology 1294–1296, 1296f, 1297f
   staging 1296–1297, 1297t
   variants 1298–1299
squamous cell dysplasia 1291–1292, 1291f, 1291t,
   1292–1293
   cytology 1292–1293, 1297–1298
   progression to squamous carcinoma 1293, 1293f
   reactive hyperplasia *vs* 1291–1292, 1291f, 1291t
   screening for 1298
squamous hyperplasia 1285, 1291–1292, 1291f, 1291t
squamous lesions 1292–1299
squamous papilloma 1292, 1292f
submucosa 1282–1283
traumatic disorders 1285
vascular supply and lymphatics 1283
verrucous carcinoma 1298–1299
webs 1284
essential thrombocythemia 585, 632, 633f, 635t
esthesioneuroblastoma, neuroblastoma *vs* 384–385
estrogen
   exogenous
      endometrial carcinoma risk 1952–1953
      endometrial changes 1946, 1947f
   secretion
      epithelial hyperplasia of fallopian tube 2044
      Sertoli cell tumors 2023
      thecomas 2019–2020
   therapy, endometrial carcinoma 150
estrogen receptor positivity 181
   breast cancer 488
      invasive cribriform carcinoma 476
      invasive micropapillary carcinoma 477
      invasive papillary carcinoma 476
      medullary carcinoma 475
      mucinous carcinoma 473
      tubular carcinoma 470
   endometrial adenocarcinoma 1960
ethanol, as fixative 17
ethmoidal sinuses
   adenoid cystic carcinoma 794–795
   inverted papilloma 788–789, 788f
   squamous cell carcinoma 790
   see also sinuses (paranasal)

ethylene glycol poisoning, kidney 1642–1643, 1643f
ETV6–NTRK3 gene fusion 330–331
eustachian tube, anatomy 2269
Evans sarcoma (low-grade fibromyxoid) 326–327,
   326f, 327f
Ewing, James 746
Ewing family of tumors 385, 746–750
   Askin tumor 385, 994
   differential diagnosis 747t
   soft tissue 385
   see also Ewing's sarcoma; primitive
      neuroectodermal tumors (PNET)
'Ewing-like adamantinoma' 750
Ewing's sarcoma 746–750, 748f
   atypical 386
   chromosomal translocation 310t
   differential diagnosis 747t, 750
   extraskeletal 385–386, 385f
   hematogenous osteomyelitis *vs* 690
   immunohistochemistry 749, 796t
   large cell 386
   osteosarcoma after irradiation for 159
   rosette formation 174
   sinonasal 796t, 806–807
   typical 385–386
   ultrastructure/cytology 748–749, 749f
   see also primitive neuroectodermal tumors (PNET),
      peripheral
Ewing's sarcoma gene 1024
EWS–ATF1 fusion 382, 386
EWS–ETS fusion 384
EWS–FLI1 fusion 385, 386, 747
EWS–WT1 fusion 386, 387
exaggerated placental site (EPS) 2084, 2085, 2085f
exfoliatin 218
exocytosis 195
   'misplaced' 1112, 2095, 2102
exophthalmos (ocular proptosis) 2294, 2296
exostosis *see* osteochondroma (exostosis)
'expert' testimony 10
expressed sequence tags (ESTs) 47
exstrophy 1707, 1708, 1720
EXT1 and *EXT2* genes, mutations 707
external auditory canal (EAC) 2267, 2268f
   congenital defects 2270–2271
   exostosis 2282
   inflammation 2271–2272
   osteoma 2282
   otitis externa 2271–2272
   squamous cell carcinoma 2280
extracapsular cataract extraction (ECCE) 2299
extracellular matrix
   bone marrow 612
   kidney 1600
   malignant cell invasion (metastases) 167
extrahepatic bile ducts 1581–1588
   adenocarcinoma 1585, 1587f
   adenoma 1584
   anatomy 1581
   atresia 1483, 1497, 1498f, 1583
   benign lesions 1582–1584
   benign/reactive cytology 1583–1584, 1585f
   bile plugs 1494f
   biliary papillomatosis 1586–1587
   botryoid embryonal rhabdomyosarcoma 1587–1588,
      1588f
   calculi 1583
   carcinoid tumors 1586, 1587f
   carcinoma 1585–1586, 1585f, 1587f
      cytopathology 1586, 1586f
      papillary 1585
   cystadenoma 1586, 1587f
   cysts 1582–1583
   dysplasia 1584–1585
   granular cell tumor 1583, 1584f
   hepatobiliary cystadenoma 1586, 1587f
   histology (normal) 1581–1582
   metaplasia 1584
   obstruction 1493–1494

extrahepatic bile ducts (*cont'd*)
  stent placement, strictures after 1583, 1584f
  strictures 1583, 1584f
extramedullary myeloid cell tumor (EMCT) 294, 575, 624
extraplacental membranes 2063
extraprostatic extension (EPE) 1815, 1817, 1817f
'extraskeletal chondroma with lipoblast-like cells' 339–340
extraskeletal mesenchymal chondrosarcoma 390–391, 391f
extraskeletal myxoid chondrosarcoma (EMCs) 389–390, 389f, 390f, 715
  parachordoma *vs* 395, 396
extrinsic allergic alveolitis *see* hypersensitivity pneumonitis
exudates 1025–1026
  foamy eosinophilic intra-alveolar 880–881
  mesothelial cells 1026, 1026f
eye 2289–2327
  contusion 2312
  enlargement 2316
  enucleated 2305, 2305f
  epithelial downgrowth 2312, 2313f
  hemorrhage 2304, 2312, 2317
  infections 2301–2302, 2302f, 2312
  inflammation 2312–2314
  specimens 2289
  surgery complications 2312
  trauma 2311–2312
  tumors *see* intraocular tumors
  see also specific anatomical structures
eyelid 2289–2292
  actinic keratosis 2290
  benign epidermal tumors 2289–2290
  carcinoma
    basal cell 2290
    excision 2291
    Pagetoid invasion 1887f, 2291
    sebaceous 258, 2290–2291, 2291f
    squamous cell 2291
  chalazion 2289, 2289f, 2290
  cysts 2290
  histology (normal) 2289, 2289f
  hordeolum 2289
  infections 2290
  malignant tumors 2290–2291, 2291f
  pigmented lesions 2290
  premalignant lesions 2290
  sebaceous lesions 2291
  xanthelasma 2290

F

Fabry's disease 579, 1900
  cardiac involvement 1048, 1048f
  renal involvement 1623, 1623f
face, angiosarcoma 371, 371f
facial paralysis 1208
facioscapulohumeral dystrophy 2237
factitial panniculitis 236
factor VIII-related antigen 275, 1470
factor VIII-related antigen (vWF) 275, 276, 372, 613, 1470
factor XIIIa 265, 287
faggot cells (Auer rods) 623f, 626
'fallen fragment' sign 756
fallopian tube 2039–2048
  absence 2040
  adenocarcinoma 2045–2046, 2046t
  adenomatoid tumor 2044, 2045f
  adenosarcoma 2046
  ampulla, ectopic pregnancy 2043
  anatomy 2039
  benign tumors 2044–2045
  carcinoid tumors 2045
  carcinosarcoma 2046
  cysts 2043
  ectopic pregnancy 2042–2043, 2043f
  embryological remnants 2043

endometrioid carcinoma 2045, 2046, 2046f
endometriosis 2043, 2044f
epithelial hyperplasia 2044, 2044f
epithelial tumors
  benign 2044–2045
  malignant 2045–2046
foreign body granuloma 2042
giant cell arteritis 2042
histology 2040
inflammatory diseases 2040–2042
  see also salpingitis
leiomyoma 2045
lymphoma 2047
malformations 2040
malignant tumors 2045–2047
mesenchymal tumors 2045, 2046–2047
metaplasia 2043–2044
metaplastic papillary tumor 2044
metastatic tumors 2047
mucosa 2040
necrotizing vasculitis 2042
non-neoplastic noninflammatory conditions 2042–2044
papilloma 2044
parasitic infections 2042
polyps 2044
prolapse 2040
reactive epithelium 2041
serous carcinoma 2045, 2046, 2046f
teratoma 2045
torsion 2040
vaginal mass after hysterectomy 146
false-negative diagnosis 6, 28, 1206
false-positive diagnoses 5, 28–29, 1206
familial adenomatous polyposis (FAP) 1437–1438, 1437f
  ampulla of Vater adenomas 1588
  attenuated 1438
  fibromatosis (desmoid) with 325, 1451f
  fundic gland polyps 1344, 1345f
  gastric adenomas 1343
  hepatoblastoma association 1536
  ileal pouch-anal anastomosis 1394
  nuchal fibroma association 318
  papillary thyroid carcinoma variant 2130
  small intestinal adenomas 1421–1422, 1422f
  tumors associated 325
  variants 1437–1438
familial atypical mole-melanoma syndrome 2306
familial hemophagocytic lymphohistiocytosis 528
familial high density lipoprotein deficiency 579
familial hypercalcemic hypercalciuria 2158
familial hypercholesterolemia 288
familial hypocalciuric hypercalcemia (FHH) 2158
familial isolated hyperparathyroidism (FIHP) 2158
familial Mediterranean fever 1020
familial tumor syndromes 2400, 2401t
Fanconi's syndrome 1631, 1631f, 1632
farmer's lung *see* hypersensitivity pneumonitis
fascicular atrophy 2225, 2226, 2227f
fasciculus cervicoangularis 1934
fasciitis
  cranial 312–313
  intravascular 312, 313f
  ischemic 314, 315f
  nodular *see* nodular fasciitis
  ossifying 312
  proliferative 313–314, 314f
  pseudosarcomatous 1183
fascin 540
fat, hyalinization 236, 236f
fat emboli, renal 1646, 1646f
fat necrosis
  bone marrow 665
  breast *see* breast, fat necrosis
  in erythema induratum 235
  in lipoma 337f
  scrotal 1772
  subcutaneous, of newborn 235–236, 235fg

fatty liver
  of pregnancy 1489f
  see also steatosis
fatty tumors 702t
  of bone 770–771
  see also lipoma; liposarcoma
Felty's syndrome 580
female adnexal tumors of Wolffian origin (FATWO) 2046, 2047, 2048f
female circumcision (genital mutilation) 1887
female pseudohermaphroditism 1736–1737
feminization 2183, 2185
femoral head, infarction (osteonecrosis) 683
fenfluramine–phentermine 1059
Ferguson-Smith type, keratoacanthoma 248
ferritin 612, 619
'ferruginous asbestos bodies' 902, 903f
festooning, subepidermal blister with, porphyria cutanea tarda 224, 224f
fetal distress 2067
fetal-maternal hemorrhage 2073
fetal membrane *see* amniotic membrane
fetal rhabdomyoma 355–356, 820
  classic type 355
  intermediate type 355–356
fetal thrombotic vasculopathy 2073, 2073f, 2074f
α-fetoprotein *see* alpha-fetoprotein (AFP)
fetus 2079
  compressed 2078, 2079f
  decreased movement, syndromes associated 2065
  mammary gland 419
  placental development and 2063–2064
'fetus-in-fetus' 827
fetus papyraceous 2078, 2079f
Feulgen stain 42–43
FHIT gene 937, 1678
fiberglass pneumoconiosis 905t
fibrillary glomerulopathy 1634–1635, 1635f, 1637t
'fibrillinopathy' 1081
fibrin
  deposits, conjunctiva 2294
  staining methods 16t
fibrinogen, deposits, renal 1647, 1648f
fibrinoid deposition, massive perivillous 2072–2073
fibrinoid necrosis
  polyarteritis nodosa 1074, 1075f, 2224f
  renal vessels 1611f, 1647, 1648
    malignant hypertension 1645, 1645f
  retinal vessels 2318
  uteroplacental perfusion abnormalities 2071
fibrinous pericarditis 1019, 1068, 1068f
fibrin ring granuloma 82, 1511, 1511f
fibrin tactoids 1645, 1647, 1648f
fibroadenoma, breast *see* breast, fibroadenoma
fibroblast(s) 195
  'ganglion-like' 314f
  Hodgkin's disease 537
  radiation 152, 152f
  spindle 737, 738f
  stellate 309, 309f, 1156, 1157f
fibroblastic proliferations
  benign *see* pseudosarcomatous proliferative lesions
  oral cavity 1183
  skin 263–267
fibroblastic reticular cells (FRC) 657
  tumors 657
fibroblastic sarcoma, acral myxoinflammatory 327–328, 328f
fibroblastic tumors 702t, 736–746
fibroblastoma
  desmoplastic (collagenous fibroma) 308–309, 309f
  giant cell 266
fibrocartilaginous dysplasia 742
fibrocartilaginous mesenchymoma 742
fibrodysplasia ossificans progressive (FOP) 387
fibroelastoma, papillary 1060, 1061f
fibroepithelial polyps
  adipose tissue-rich variant 264
  lung 940, 941f

of skin 8, 24f, 264
vagina 356, 1921f, 1922
vulva 356, 1899
fibrohistiocytic tumors 333–336
of indeterminate biological potential 266
fibrohistiocytic proliferations, skin 263–267
fibroid epulis 1180
fibrokeratoma, acral 265, 265f
fibroleiomyomatous hamartoma, lung 970–971, 971f
fibrolipoma 336
neural 2249, 2249f
of skin 264
vulva 1901
fibrolipomatous hamartoma of nerve 2249, 2249f
fibroma 308–312
ameloblastic *see* ameloblastic fibroma
calcifying aponeurotic 311–312, 311f, 312f
cardiac 1064
cellular, ovarian 2018
cemento-ossifying (psammomatoid ossifying) 742–743, 743f, 1192
juvenile 742–743, 743f, 813
sinonasal 813, 814f
chondromyxoid 713–715, 714f
collagenous 308–309, 309f
desmoplastic 705, 738–739, 738f
extra-abdominal fibromatosis *vs* 324
fibrous dysplasia of bone *vs* 742
oral region 1184
'irritation' (oral) 1180
juvenile aggressive 813
larynx 848
non-ossifying 737–738, 737f
giant cell tumor of bone *vs* 754
multiple 737
nuchal 318–319, 319f
odontogenic *see* odontogenic fibroma
oral cavity 1180
ossifying *see* ossifying fibroma
ovary 2018–2019, 2018f, 2020
peripheral, with calcification (oral cavity) 1181, 1181f
pleomorphic, skin 265
sclerotic 265
with sex cord elements 2018
soft 264
submesothelial 1015–1016, 1015f, 1016f
tendon sheath 309–310, 310f, 327
testis 1761
trichoblastic 252
fibromatosis 320–325
abdominal desmoid-type 1184
breast 445
classification 320–321
congenital, oral region 1184
congenital generalized 315
deep (aggressive) *see* desmoid tumors
diffuse mesenteric 1450
Gardner syndrome and 320
gastrointestinal tract 1450
infantile *see* infantile fibromatosis
intra-abdominal *see* desmoid tumors
juvenile, oral region 1184
large intestine 1450
larynx and trachea 849
low-grade fibromyxoid sarcoma *vs* 326, 327
mesenteric 325
musculoaponeurotic 322
myofibroma *vs* 316
oral cavity 1184
ovary 1992
pelvic 325
prostate 1820
superficial 320, 321–322
infantile digital 320, 322, 322f
knuckle pads 320, 322
palmar 320, 321, 321f
penile 320, 321, 322f
plantar 320, 321, 321f

fibromatosis colli 319, 319f
fibromatosis gingivae 1180
fibromuscular dysplasia 1080–1081, 1081f
fibromuscular hyperplasia 1645
fibromyxoid sarcoma, low-grade 326–327, 326f, 327f
chromosomal translocation 310t
differential diagnosis 326, 327
fibromyxoid tumor
nonossifying variant 380
ossifying 378f, 379–381, 380f
pseudosarcomatous, bladder 1723, 1723f
fibromyxoma
sinonasal 823
superficial acral 267–268, 392, 392f
fibronectin glomerulopathy 1624
fibro-odontoma, ameloblastic 1141f
fibro-osseous dysplasia 1190–1194
fibro-osseous pseudotumor (florid reactive periostitis) 772–773, 773f
of digits 387–388, 388f
fibro-osseous tumors 740–746
osteofibrous dysplasia *see* osteofibrous dysplasia
polymorphic 742
psammomatoid ossifying fibroma 742–743, 743f
see also fibrous dysplasia, of bone
fibroplasia, atypical decubital (ischemic fasciitis) 314, 315f
fibrosarcoma 325–331, 739–740
ameloblastic 1162
classic adult 325–326, 325f, 326f
CNS 2393
congenital (infantile) 330–331, 331f
adult (classic) *vs* 325
chromosomal translocation 310t
fibrodysplasia ossificans progressiva *vs* 387
fibrous hamartoma of infancy *vs* 318
differential diagnosis 325
desmoplastic fibroma *vs* 738
extra-abdominal fibromatosis (desmoid) *vs* 324
low-grade, solitary fibrous tumor *vs* 377
monophasic synovial sarcoma *vs* 404
myofibroma *vs* 316
well-differentiated, desmoplastic fibroma *vs* 739
inflammatory 331–332, 332f
inflammatory myofibroblastic tumor 331, 332, 332f
inflammatory myxohyaline tumor 327–328, 328f
larynx and trachea 849
metastases 326
myxofibrosarcoma 326, 328–329, 329f, 330f
oral region 1184
ovarian 2018–2019
radiation-associated 160
sclerosing epithelioid 329–330, 330f
sinonasal 822–823
see also fibromyxoid sarcoma
fibrothecoma, ovary 2018
fibrous cortical defects 701, 737–738
see also fibroma, non-ossifying
fibrous dysplasia 1190
of bone 393, 740–742, 741f, 742f
differential diagnosis 740, 742
craniofacial 813–814, 1191
head and neck 1191
monostotic lesion 740, 814, 1190
oral cavity 1190–1192, 1191f
ossifying fibroma *vs* 1191, 1192
polyostotic lesion 741, 742, 814, 1190, 1191
temporal bone 2282
fibrous hamartoma of infancy 318–319, 318f
fibrous histiocytoma
benign *see* benign fibrous histiocytoma (BFH); dermatofibroma (DF)
malignant *see* malignant fibrous histiocytoma (MFH)
orbital 2297
thymus, differential diagnosis 1101t, 1102t
fibrous papule 264–265, 265f
fibrous proteins, staining methods 16t

fibrous tissue tumors/fibrous tumors 308–333
benign fibroblastic/pseudosarcomatous proliferations 312–315
of bone 736–746
see also fibroma; fibro-osseous tumors; fibrosarcoma
calcifying fibrous pseudotumor 317–318, 317f, 318f
childhood with psammoma bodies (calcifying fibrous pseudotumor) 317–318, 317f, 318f
fasciitis *see* fasciitis
fibroma *see* fibroma
fibromatosis colli 319, 319f
fibrosarcoma *see* fibrosarcoma
fibrous hamartoma of infancy 318–319, 318f
lipofibromatosis 319–320, 320f
myofibroma and myofibromatosis 315–317
nuchal fibrocartilaginous tumor 319
nuchal fibroma 318–319, 319f
of peritoneum 1024
of pleura 1015–1016, 1015f, 1016f
solitary *see* solitary fibrous tumor
see also specific tumor types
fibrovascular polyps, esophageal 1315
fibroxanthoma 695
atypical 158, 248, 266–267
'field cancerization' theory 936–937
'field change' phenomenon 1711
filamentous molds 66, 66t
filaments (muscle), formation 2214
filariasis, scrotum 1772
Filobasidiella neoformans 86
filum terminale
myxopapillary ependymoma 2368
paraganglioma 2377, 2378f
tumor differential diagnosis by age 2348t
fimbriae, fallopian tube 2039
adenocarcinoma 2045
fine needle aspiration (FNA) biopsy 19, 22–29
breast *see* breast
complications 22–23, 28
rate, ovarian cysts and 138
cytopathologists' role 3
endoscopic ultrasound-guided (EUS-FNA)
pancreas 1549
stomach 1325
equipment 23, 24t
esophagus 1283
false-negative results 28
false-positive results 28–29
fixation and stains for 25–29
golden rules 29
historical background 22
immunohistochemistry samples 35
lymph nodes 507, 516
oral cavity 1137
pancreas 1549, 1550
percutaneous transabdominal, pancreas 1549
pleural 1005
preparation of surgical pathologist 6
prostate gland 1794
reporting 27–28
samples for cell blocks 24–25
smear preparation technique 24, 25t, 26f
spermatogenesis 1741
spleen 576
technique 23–24, 24t
thyroid gland 138, 2119–2120
tissue changes due to 138
transthoracic, lung carcinoma 940
tumor cell seeding 28
see also specific tumors/conditions
fingerprint myopathy 2228t, 2229
fissural nonodontogenic cysts 1147
fistulas
branchial apparatus 2270–2271
involving vagina 1920
preauricular 2271
Fite stain 60, 60t, 64, 82

fixation/fixatives 15, 17, 19, 25
  CNS tissue 2331, 2335, 2335t
  coating 20t
  for electron microscopy 29
  for endomyocardial biopsy 1041
  for flow cytometry 37
  for FNA biopsy 25–29
  for immunohistochemistry 32
  for liver biopsy 1468
  lung tissue samples 869
  methods 15–17, 19
  wet 19
    air-dried smears vs 27, 28t
Fizzera's morphologic scheme 150
FK-506 (Tacrolimus) 1652
FKHR gene, alveolar rhabdomyosarcoma 360
Fleischner's ring 2301
'flesh eating bacteria' 68
fleurettes, in retinoblastoma 2310
Flexner–Wintersteiner rosettes 801, 2310, 2310f, 2311
FLI1 antibodies 368, 373, 404
FLI1 gene, Ewing family of tumors 386
florid cemento-osseous dysplasia 1193, 1194
florid oral papillomatosis (FOP) 1163, 1175
florid reactive periostitis 772–773, 773f
flow cytometry 36–42
  Barrett's esophagus 1310
  bone marrow 610
  cell/nuclei isolation and staining 37–39
  cell quantity and analysis 39
  Consensus Conference on 36, 38
  DNA ploidy determination 36, 37, 37f, 39–40
  instrumentation 36–37
  lymph node specimens 509–510
  principle 36–37
  quality control 41–42
  samples suitable for 37
  specimen disaggregation/preanalytic
    preparation 37
  S-phase fraction (SPF) 36, 37, 40–41, 41t
  two-color DNA analysis 39, 40
flukes 105, 1540
fluorescence in situ hybridization (FISH) 35, 45, 47
  breast carcinoma 47f
  CNS tumors 2340
  lymph node specimens 510
  neuroblastoma 384
  technique 47
foam cells
  in bone marrow 662, 662t
  glomerular 1609, 1613f
  intraductal papilloma (breast) 444f
  nipple discharge 425
  stromal, endometrial adenocarcinoma 1956, 1956f
foamy casts, airspace filling pattern 870, 870f
focal nodular hyperplasia, of liver see liver
folate, deficiency 619
follicles (lymph nodes) see lymph nodes
follicles (ovarian) 1987, 1987f, 1988f
  absent 1988
  cystic 1990, 1991f
  cysts 1990, 1991f
    solitary luteinized, of puerperium 1993, 1994f
  graafian 1987
  number and degeneration 1988
  primordial 1987, 1991
follicle-stimulating hormone (FSH) 2097
follicular bronchiolitis see bronchiolitis
follicular bronchitis/bronchiolitis 909, 910f
follicular dendritic cells 573–574
  HIV-associated parotid gland disease 1261, 1261f
follicular dendritic cells (FDC) 657
follicular dendritic cell sarcoma/tumors 574
follicular infundibulum, tumors 254–255
follicular mucinosis 226–227, 227f, 292
follicular plugging 205, 205f
folliculitis
  bacterial 225–226
  eosinophilic 227, 227f

fungal 225–226
  granulomatous 226, 226f
folliculitis decalvans 226
folliculosebaceous cystic hamartoma, vulvar 1902
folliculostellate cells, pituitary 2093, 2095f
Fontana stain 1469
Fontan-Masson stain 73, 73f, 85, 86
Food and Drug Administration (FDA) 12, 35–36
forced expiratory volume (FEV$_1$) 905
Fordyce spots 194
Fordyce type, angiokeratoma 269
foreign bodies, intraocular 2312
foreign body bronchiolitis 908, 910
foreign body giant cell(s) 530f
foreign body giant cell reaction 212, 215–216, 216f
  breast 449, 449f
  calcifying odontogenic cysts 1145
  Dacron® 145f
  endometrial biopsy 137f
  muscle 2224
foreign body granuloma
  after hysterosalpingograms 138
  fallopian tube 2042
  ovary 1989
  sarcoidosis vs 215
foreign body granulomatous reaction
  breast implants 449–450
  to Teflon® 142
formaldehyde 15, 17
formalin 15, 19, 20t
  fixation for flow cytometry 37
  immunohistochemistry fixative 32
Formalin pigment (acid hematein) 15, 171
Fournier's gangrene 69, 1772
fourth ventricle, ependymoma 2364
foveolae
  hyperplasia, reactive gastritis with 1340, 1341f
  normal stomach 1321, 1322f
Fox–Fordyce disease 1895
FOXP3 (scurfin) gene 1376
fracture 678f, 682
  healing 682–683, 682f
  pathologic 682, 703
    dedifferentiated chondrosarcoma 719f
    enchondroma 709f
    Langerhans cell histiocytosis 759
    metastases in bone 772
    non-ossifying fibromas 737, 738
    osteosarcoma 728
    simple (unicameral) bone cyst 756
  stabilization 682
  stress 682
  subchondral insufficiency 682, 682f, 683
fracture callus 679f, 682, 705
fragile histidine triad gene (FHIT gene) 937, 1678
Francisella tularensis 72
Franseen needle 25
freckles (lentigo simplex) 277, 277f
freezing, skeletal muscle samples 2214
French–American–British (FAB) classification, acute
    leukemia 620, 621t
French Federation of Cancer Centers, soft tissue tumor
    grading 307, 308t
frostbite 2245
frozen sections 5–6
  artifacts 6, 2331, 2331f
  breast biopsy 5, 428
  CNS lesions 2331, 2331f
  contraindications of freezing 5
  imprint preparations vs 6
  indications 5
  larynx and trachea 833
  lymph node biopsy 507, 509, 509t
  margin adequacy for resections 5–6
  oral cavity 1137
  pancreatic carcinoma 1554, 1555f
  salivary gland tumors, FNA vs 1206
  surgical pathology reports 6
Fuch's endothelial dystrophy 2301, 2301f, 2302

Fuhrman nuclear grading
  clear cell renal cell carcinoma 1679, 1679f, 1679t
  papillary renal cell carcinoma 1681, 1682f
Fukuyama congenital muscular dystrophy 2238
Fuller's earth (aluminium silicate) pneumoconiosis 905t
fundic mucosa, inflammation 1286
fungal infections
  cervix/cervicitis 1836t, 1837, 1849
  CNS 2410–2411
  corneal 2301
  ear–temporal bone 2273
  endophthalmitis 2313
  esophagitis 1289–1290
  folliculitis 225, 226f
  granulomatous dermatoses due to 215
  hepatic granuloma 1511, 1512f
  intestinal 1399
  keratitis 2301
  lymph node involvement 533
  myositis 2222
  nasopharynx and upper respiratory tract 79–81
  pneumonia 879–881
  renal transplant recipient 1653
  respiratory tract 83–93, 835
  sclerosing mediastinitis 1128
  sinus/sinusitis 81, 787, 2295
  skin/soft tissue/mucocutaneous 70–72, 73–74
  vulvar 1891
fungi 65–66
  confirmation by molecular methods 108t
  dimorphic 66, 90–91
  staining methods 17t, 61, 62t
  types and characteristics 65–66, 66t
fungus balls 880
funisitis, necrotizing 2069
furuncle 225
Fusarium 81
FUS gene, myxoid/round cell liposarcoma 344
fusion proteins, markers 31t
FWT1 and FWT2 genes 1666

G

galectin-3, papillary thyroid carcinoma 2131
gallbladder 1576–1581
  abnormal positioning 1576
  adenoma 1578–1579
  adenomatous polyps 1578–1579
  adenomyoma 1578, 1578f
  agenesis 1576
  anatomy 1576
  benign lesions 1577–1578
  carcinoma 1579–1581
    adenomatous polyp precursor 1578–1579
    adenosquamous 1580
    clear cell 1580
    dysplasia as precursor 1579
    infiltrating adenocarcinoma 1580, 1580f, 1581f
    metaplasia to dysplasia sequence 1580
    small cell neuroendocrine 1581, 1582f
    undifferentiated 1580
    variants 1580–1581
  carcinoma in situ 1579, 1580f
    papillary 1580, 1581f
  congenital abnormalities 1576
  diffuse dystrophic calcification 1576
  dysplasia 1579, 1579f, 1580f
  epithelial heterotopia 1576
  'floating' 1576
  histology (normal) 1576
  hypoplasia 1576
  inflammation see cholecystitis
  inflammatory polyps 1577–1578
  metaplasia 1578, 1578f
  mucosa 1576
  multiseptate 1576
  porcelain 1576, 1580
gallstones 1577, 1579
Gamma–Gandy body formation 1063
gamma heavy chain disease 657

gangliocytic paraganglioma 1448f
   ampulla of Vater 1589
   duodenal 1424
   intestinal 1447–1448, 1448f
gangliocytoma 2108, 2374
   dysplastic, of cerebellum 2374
   hypothalamus 2110
   immunohistochemistry 2339t
   pituitary 2108, 2109f
ganglioglioma 2374–2376, 2375f
   anaplastic 2376
   desmoplastic infantile 2374
   immunohistochemistry 2339t
   pilocytic astrocytoma vs 2359
ganglion 697
   intraosseous 755, 755f
ganglion cells
   differentiation, neuroblastoma 2196, 2197f
   neonates 1403
   staining 2256
ganglion cysts 394, 2248
   Morton's neuroma vs 379
ganglioneuroblastoma 383–384, 2384
   adrenal medulla 2194–2199
   histologic maturation after chemotherapy 149
   proliferative fasciitis vs 313
ganglioneuroma 383–384, 2108
   adrenal medulla 2199, 2200f
   intestinal 1446–1447, 1448f
   malignant transformation in 2256
   mediastinum 2199, 2200f
   peripheral nerves 2256, 2256f
   virilizing 2199, 2200f
ganglioneuromatosis, diffuse, intestinal 1447
gangrene 68
   Fournier's 69, 1772
   gas 2222
gangrenous necrosis, intestinal 1382
Gardner syndrome 1437–1438
   APC gene mutation 325
   desmoid tumor in 325
   epidermoid cysts of skin association 254
   familial multiple leiomyoma with 348
   fibromatosis association 320, 325
   nuchal fibroma association 318
   osteoma association 722
   small intestinal adenomas 1422
'garland' pattern, metastatic colorectal cancer 2038
Gartner's duct 1839
   cyst 1920, 1920f
gas cysts, colonic pneumatosis cystoides intestinalis
      1406, 1407f
gas-forming infections 69
gas gangrene 2222
gastrectomy
   distal/total 1323, 1324
   gastric adenocarcinoma after 1356–1357, 1357f
   in gastric carcinoid tumors 1351
   partial, reactive gastritis after 1338, 1338f
   xanthelasma after 1342
gastric acid, hypersecretion 1340
gastric adenocarcinoma 1354–1361
   abundant lymphocytic infiltration with 1361–1362,
      1362f
   abundant lymphoid stroma with 1362
   autoimmune gastritis association 1330, 1356
   ciliated tumor cells with 1362
   classification schemes 1354–1355
   diffuse type 1358–1359, 1358f
      intestinal type vs 1354
      gastric dysplasia vs 1358
   intestinal type 1354, 1355–1358, 1355f
      autoimmune chronic gastritis and 1330, 1356
      cytopathology 1357–1358, 1359f
      gastric adenoma association 1356
      of gastric cardia 1357, 1357f, 1361
      multifocal atrophic gastritis and 1355–1356, 1356f
      postgastrectomy state 1356–1357, 1357f
   malpractice case 11–12, 12f

metastatic 1358f
   mucinous 1354
   pylorocardiac gland cell type 1357
   rhabdoid 1362
   signet ring see stomach, signet ring carcinoma
   staining method 21f
   TNM classification 1360, 1360t
   tubular 1354
   ulcerated, benign gastric ulcer vs 1334, 1334f,
      1356
   well differentiated papillary 1354
   see also gastric carcinoma
gastric adenoma 1342–1344, 1344f
   gastric adenocarcinoma and 1356
   neoplastic evolution 1343
gastric antral vascular ectasia (GAVE) 1339, 1340f
gastric brushing 1324, 1325
gastric carcinoid tumors 1348, 1351
   enterochromaffin-like cell 1348–1350, 1349f,
      1350f
   malignancy predictors/criteria 1351
   type I and II 1348, 1350
   type III 1350, 1351
gastric carcinoma
   duodenal ulcer protective role 1333
   gastric adenoma leading to 1343
   hyperplastic polyps vs 1343
   lymphoepithelial 1362, 1362f
   with lymphoid stroma 1361
   metastatic (hematogenous) 1362
   multifocal atrophic gastritis and 1333
   rhabdoid 1362
   signet ring see stomach, signet ring carcinoma
   see also gastric adenocarcinoma
gastric cytology 1324–1325
gastric dysplasia 1355, 1358
gastric epithelium, in pancreatic FNA samples
      1550–1551, 1551f
gastric erosions, acute gastritis 1327, 1327f
gastric juvenile polyposis syndrome 1436
gastric lymphoma see lymphoma, gastric
gastric metaplasia
   extrahepatic bile ducts 1584
   gallbladder 1578, 1578f
gastric mucosa
   cardiac type
      Barrett's esophagus vs 1303, 1305f, 1308
      fundic type vs 1301, 1301f
      see also Barrett's esophagus
   CMV infection 1340
   ectopic, esophageal islands 1283
   endoscopic surgical biopsy 1324
   Helicobacter pylori infection 1331, 1340
   inflammation 1286
   pancreatic acinar metaplasia 1326
gastric pits 1321, 1331
gastric polypectomy, endoscopic specimens 1324
gastric polyps 1342–1344
   around gastroenterostomy stomas 146
   fundic gland 1344, 1345f
   hyperplastic 1342–1344, 1343f
   inflammatory fibroid 1341, 1342f
gastric remnant cancer 1356–1357, 1357f
gastric rugae
   hypertrophy 1339–1340, 1340f
   in MALT lymphoma 1354f
gastric syphilis 1336
gastric ulcers
   benign 1333
      ulcerated carcinoma vs 1328, 1334, 1334f, 1356
   chronic 1338
   multifocal atrophic gastritis and 1333–1334
   non-Helicobacter causes 1333
   reactive gastritis 1338
   stress 1327
gastrin cells 1323, 1323f
gastrinoma 1424, 1573
gastrin-releasing peptide, esophageal squamous cell
      carcinoma 1294

gastritis
   acute 1327–1329, 1327t
      CMV infection 1329, 1329f
   acute erosive (hemorrhagic) 1327–1329, 1328f
      carcinoma vs 1328
      epithelial regeneration 1328, 1328f
      erosions and ulcers 1327, 1328, 1328f
      infectious form 1329
      noninfectious form 1327–1328
      NSAID-associated 1327, 1327f
   acute stress 1327
   acute suppurative (phlegmonous) 1327, 1329
   atrophic, trauma of biopsy 135
   atrophic type B see gastritis, multifocal atrophic
      (MAG)
   autoimmune chronic 1329–1330
      enterochromaffin-like cell carcinoids 1348, 1349,
         1349f, 1350
      gastric adenocarcinoma and 1330, 1356
   chemical 1338
   chronic 1327t, 1329–1337
      trophic see gastritis, multifocal atrophic
      Helicobacter-associated see below
      hyperplastic polyps in 1343
   classification and reporting system 1326, 1327t
   diffuse antral 1331–1332, 1332f, 1357
   diffuse corporal see gastritis, autoimmune chronic
   duodenal ulcer association 1332, 1357
   environmental see gastritis, multifocal atrophic (MAG)
   eosinophilic see eosinophilic gastroenteritis
   fundal/body gastritis see gastritis, autoimmune
      chronic
   granulomatous 1336, 1336f
   Helicobacter-associated 1330–1335, 1338, 1339,
      1375
      diffuse antral gastritis 1331–1332, 1332f
      H. heilmannii 1331
      H. pylori 1330–1335
      MALT lymphoma and 1351
      multifocal atrophic gastritis 1332–1333, 1333f,
         1355
   hypertrophic 1327t, 1339–1341
      hypersecretory gastropathy 1340–1341, 1341f
      protein-losing enteropathy 1340
   lymphocytic 1335–1336, 1335f
   multifocal atrophic (MAG) 1332–1333, 1333f, 1343f
      adenomas 1343
      gastric cancer risk 1333
      gastric ulcer and 1333–1334
      Helicobacter-associated 1332–1333, 1333f, 1355
      intestinal gastric adenocarcinoma and 1355–1356,
         1356f
   octopus sucker 1335
   pancreatic acinar metaplasia and 1326
   peptic ulcer and 1326–1342
   reactive 1327t, 1337–1339
      after partial gastrectomy 1338, 1338f
      bile reflux causing 1338–1339
      chemical (drugs) associated 1338
      gastric antral vascular ectasia 1339, 1340f
      with massive foveolar hyperplasia 1340, 1341f
      mucosal prolapse-associated conditions 1339,
         1339f
      NSAID-induced injury vs 1338
   superficial 1330, 1331, 1332f
   type A (CAG-A) see gastritis, autoimmune chronic
   type AB see gastritis, multifocal atrophic (MAG)
   varioliform 1335
gastritis cystica polyposa 146, 1338
gastritis cystica profunda 1338, 1338f
gastroenteritis
   eosinophilic see eosinophilic gastroenteritis
   viral 1377
gastroesophageal junction (GEJ) 1300
   Barrett's esophagus 1299–1300, 1300, 1300f
   gastroesophageal reflux disease and 1302
   H. pylori gastritis and 1302
   metaplastic glands 1302, 1302f
   pancreatic acinar metaplasia 1302

gastroesophageal reflux disease (GERD) 1285–1287
  adenocarcinoma of gastric cardia and 1357
  differential diagnosis 1286, 1286t, 1287, 1302
  gastrinoma and 1573
  Helicobacter pylori treatment 1335
  inflammatory cells 1282f, 1285t
gastrointestinal autonomic nerve tumors (GANT) 353, 1345
gastrointestinal carcinoma *see* gastrointestinal tract
gastrointestinal pacemaker cells 1345
gastrointestinal stromal tumors (GISTs) 1345–1348, 1346f, 1443–1445
  aggressive 1445t
  benign *vs* malignant 1444–1445, 1445t
  c-kit proto-oncogene 1345
  esophageal 1315
  extraintestinal tumors 353–354, 354f
  histology 1444, 1444f
  immunohistochemistry 1345, 1444
  intestinal 1443–1445, 1444f
  mesenteric fibromatosis *vs* 325
  mixed cell type 1444
  round cell (epithelioid) type 1347, 1444
  spindle-cell type 1444, 1444f
  stomach 1345–1348, 1347f
gastrointestinal tract
  carcinoma
    effusions 1030, 1031f
    mucinous, effusions 1030
    risk in juvenile polyposis syndrome 1436
    small intestinal 1430–1431, 1431t
    see also colon, adenocarcinoma; gastric carcinoma
  endocrine cells 1422–1423, 1423
  infections 100–105
  necrotizing infection 69, 69f
  neuromatous hyperplasia 2248–2249
  protozoal infections 102–103
  see also intestine(s); *specific anatomic regions*
gastropathy
  classification 1327t
  hypersecretory 1340–1341
  hypertrophic gastritis *see* gastritis, hypertrophic
  portal hypertensive 1339
  reactive gastritis *see* gastritis, reactive
GATA1 transcription factor, mutations 622
GATA-2, pituitary development 2095, 2097
Gaucher's cells 579, 579f, 658
Gaucher's disease 658
  bone deformity 689
  spleen 579, 579f
G-cell hyperplasia 1348
Gelfoam® 139, 140, 140f
gemistocytes, neoplastic 2352, 2353, 2354f
gene expression microarrays 47–48, 48f
  DNA 48, 560
  Hodgkin's disease 540
genital herpes 75, 75f, 1836–1837
genitalia, ambiguous 1737, 1887
genital leiomyoma 348–349, 349f
genital warts *see* condyloma accuminatum
geographic necrosis 2257, 2257f
germ cells
  primordial 1734, 1741
  testis 1732
germ cell-sex cord stromal tumors 1743t
germ cell tumors
  CNS 2339t, 2397
  diagnostic work-up 180
  ectopic gestational trophoblastic disease *vs* 2087
  extragonadal 180f
  fine needle aspiration 1773–1781
  Hodgkin's disease 540
  immunohistochemistry 1744, 1745t, 2339t
  intracranial 2397
  intratubular *see* intratubular germ cell neoplasia (IGCN)
  mediastinum *see* mediastinum
  mixed malignant (MMGCTs) 1115

mediastinum 1115, 1119, 1120, 1121f
  testis 1756–1757, 1757f, 1781
ovary *see* ovary, germ cell tumors
pituitary 2109
terminology 1114–1115
testicular *see* testicular tumors
thymus *see* thymus
yolk sac tumors *see* yolk sac tumors
germinal cell aplasia 1739–1740, 1740f
germinal centers, lymph nodes *see* lymph nodes
germinoma, intracranial 2337t, 2397
  suprasellar 2345
germinoma cells 2027, 2027f, 2028f
gestational trophoblastic disease 2080–2087
  definition 2083
  ectopic 2087
  in fallopian tube 2043, 2047
  staging 2084t
gestrinone 1947, 1952
ghost cells 235
  calcifying odontogenic cysts 1145, 1146f
giant cell(s)
  acute hepatitis with 1483, 1483f
  in cherubism 1193
  erythema induratum 235, 235f
  erythema nodosum 234, 234f
  fibroma of oral cavity 1180
  foreign body reaction *see* foreign body giant cell reaction
  foreign body type 530f, 660
  granuloma annulare 213, 213f
  of Langhans type 660
  osteoclast-type 314f, 713f
    in giant cell tumor of bone 753, 754f
    pancreatic carcinoma with 1558–1559, 1559f
  primary CNS vasculitis 2414
  pyogenic granuloma, oral cavity 1181
  Touton type 288–289, 662
    solitary xanthogranuloma 287, 287f
  vulvar squamous cell carcinoma 1911, 1911f
giant cell aortitis 1082
giant cell arteritis 1072–1073, 1072t, 1073f
  cervix 1837
  fallopian tube 2042
  'large vessel' 1073
  retinal artery occlusion 2318
giant cell carcinoma, lung 963, 965, 966f
giant cell epulis 1181–1182
giant cell fibroblastoma 266
giant cell fibroma, oral cavity 1180
giant cell glioblastoma 2355
  histology 2355, 2355f
  immunohistochemistry 2338t
  ultrastructure 2336t
giant cell granuloma
  of oral cavity, peripheral 1181–1182
  peripheral, of oral cavity 1181–1182
  reparative *see* giant cell reparative granuloma
  'true' giant cell tumor *vs* 1183
giant cell hepatitis, neonatal 1483, 1483f
giant cell interstitial pneumonia (GIP) 904–905, 905f
'giant cell lesion', bone 752
giant cell malignant fibrous histiocytoma 335, 336f
giant cell myocarditis 1044, 1044f
giant cell phlebitis 1079
giant cell reaction 752
  see also foreign body giant cell reaction
giant cell reparative granuloma 752–753, 752f, 815
  differential diagnosis 753, 758
giant-cell-rich lesions of bone 751–755
  brown tumor 751–752, 751f, 752f, 753
  giant cell reparative granuloma 752–753, 752f
  giant cell tumor *see* giant cell tumor, of bone
giant cell tumor
  of bone 753–755, 753f, 754f, 1183
    bone metastases *vs* 176–177, 772
    giant cell reparative granuloma *vs* 753
    non-ossifying fibromas *vs* 738
    sarcoma development in 755

calcifying *see* chondroblastoma
epiphyseal chondromatous *see* chondroblastoma
of jaws 1183
metastases differential diagnosis 176–177
of oral cavity
  central 1182–1183, 1182f
  peripheral 1181–1182
osteoclast-type, pancreatic carcinoma 1558–1559, 1559f
sinonasal 814–815
of tendon sheath (tenosynovial) 374–376, 375f, 695
  clear cell sarcoma *vs* 382
  diffuse 375–376, 376f
  localized 374–375, 375f
  malignant 376
giant condyloma of Buschke and Loewenstein 248, 1771
'giant fold disease' 1340
giant lymph node hyperplasia *see* Castleman's disease
giant osteoid osteoma *see* osteoblastoma
giant vertebral notochordal rests, chordoma *vs* 765
Giardia lamblia 1379f, 1400
giardiasis 1378–1379, 1379f
Giemsa stain 27, 60t, 296, 1470
  lymph node biopsy 507
gigantism 681, 2099, 2100
Gimenez stain 60t
gingiva
  granular cell tumor 1185
  pyogenic granuloma 1180–1181
  squamous cell carcinoma 1173
gingival cysts 1141–1142, 1142f
glassy cell carcinoma, cervix 1866f, 1875
glaucoma 2314–2317
  closed angle 2315, 2316f
  developmental/congenital 2316
  neovascular 2315, 2316f
  phacolytic 2300
  phacomorphic 2300
  pigmentary 2316
  primary closed angle 2315
  primary (idiopathic) open angle 2315
  secondary 2312
  secondary closed angle 2315, 2316
Gleason's grades *see* prostatic adenocarcinoma
Gleevec 610, 634
glia, normal histology 2340–2344, 2341f
gliadin 1374
glial fibers, in pilocytic astrocytoma 2357, 2357f, 2358f
glial fibrillary acidic protein (GFAP) 2336
  anaplastic astrocytoma 2351
  astrocytes 2340, 2341f
  choroid glioma of third ventricle 2373
  diffuse astrocytoma 2350
  ependymoma 2367
  folliculostellate cells (pituitary) 2093
  glioblastoma 2354
  immunoperoxidase stain 2338
  medulloblastoma 2383
  oligodendroglioma 2361, 2362
  pleomorphic adenoma of salivary gland 1210
  pleomorphic xanthoastrocytoma 2359
  subependymal giant cell astrocytoma 2360
glial tumors
  immunohistochemistry 2339t
  mixed neuronal 2337t, 2339t, 2374–2377
  ovarian 2036
  pituitary 2108–2109
  of uncertain origin 2372–2374
    astroblastoma 2339t, 2372
    choroid glioma of third ventricle *see* choroid glioma of third ventricle
    gliomatosis cerebri 2372–2373
glioblastoma 2352–2355
  circumscribed 2352
  crush preparations 2352–2353, 2352f, 2353f
  cytology 2353–2354, 2353f, 2354f
  differential diagnosis 2353, 2353f, 2354
    anaplastic oligoastrocytoma *vs* 2370

epithelioid 2354
genetic abnormalities 2340t, 2354–2355
giant cell *see* giant cell glioblastoma
immunohistochemistry 2338t, 2354
lipidized, pleomorphic xanthoastrocytoma *vs* 2359
primary/secondary 2352, 2354
small cell 2352f, 2353, 2353f, 2354, 2355
spinal cord 2352
terminology 2353
ultrastructural characteristics 2336t
WHO grade IV tumor 2348
glioblastoma multiforme 2352f, 2353, 2354f
glioma
butterfly 2352, 2360
gliosis *vs* 2341, 2342f
low-grade, microcystic change 2331f
mixed 2361, 2369–2370
anaplastic oligoastrocytoma 2370
'biphasic' 2369, 2370
immunohistochemistry 2338t
oligoastrocytoma 2369–2370
nasal 2404
optic nerve 2298
pituitary 2109
gliomatosis cerebri 2372–2373
gliomatosis peritonei 1022
glioneural tumors 2374–2377
gliosarcoma 2355–2356, 2356f, 2357f
immunohistochemistry 2338t
ultrastructural characteristics 2336t
gliosis 2340–2341, 2342f
glioma *vs* 2341, 2342f
long-standing, Rosenthal fibers *see* Rosenthal
fibers
pilocytic astrocytoma *vs* 2358–2359
globes, enucleated 2304–2306
dimensions and handling 2305, 2305f
globoid cell leukodystrophy 2246
glomangioma 272–273
glomerular basement membrane 1598, 1599f
abnormalities, diseases with 1624–1626
decreased negative charge 1622
duplication 1601–1602, 1602f, 1616f, 1647
chronic rejection of renal graft 127
immune deposits, membranous
glomerulonephropathy 1615
lamina densa, thickened 1625, 1630f
NC1 domain 1598, 1599f
protrusions (spikes) 1601–1602, 1602f, 1614,
1614f
thickened 1647
diabetic nephropathy 1629
'double-contour' 1615, 1624
thin 1609f
disease 1624–1626
glomerular capillaries
basement membrane *see* glomerular basement
membrane
double-contoured walls 1624
endothelium 1598, 1599
increased permeability 1607
'spikes' on walls 1607f
tufts, acute postinfectious glomerulonephritis 1617,
1617f
wall thickening 1606f, 1614, 1614f
light chain deposition disease 1631
membranoproliferative glomerulonephritis 1615,
1616, 1616f
membranous glomerulonephropathy 1614, 1614f,
1615
glomerular diseases 1604–1605, 1606–1637
hematuria/nephritic syndrome with 1617–1622
proteinuria/nephrotic syndrome with 1606–1617
glomerular fibrillosis 1629, 1630f
glomerular filtration 1598
rate reduced, vascular nephrosclerosis 1643–1644
'glomerular syndromes' 1604
glomerulitis, necrotizing 1645
glomeruloid bodies, Wilms' tumor 1668f

glomeruloid hemangioma 271
glomerulonephritis
ANCA-positive 1621, 1622
'chronic', lupus 1627
crescentic 1621–1622, 1648
in hereditary nephritis of Alport 1624
diffuse (global) proliferative 1607f
focal proliferative/necrotizing 1620–1621, 1620f
idiopathic 1617
membranoproliferative (mesangiocapillary)
1615–1617, 1618, 1619f, 1636
type I 1615, 1616
type II (dense deposit disease) 1615–1616, 1616f
type IIII 1615, 1616
membranous, in renal transplant 1653, 1654
mesangial proliferative 1607f, 1609f
necrotizing 1648
pauci-immune ANCA positive 1622
pauci-immune crescentic 1648
postinfectious (acute) 1609f, 1617–1618
proliferative 1616f
segmental proliferative 1607f
glomerulonephropathy, membranous (MGN)
1614–1615, 1614f
glomerulopathy
amyloid 1631, 1631f, 1632f, 1637t
cirrhosis-associated (cirrhotic) 1632–1633
collagen III (collagenofibrotic) 1624, 1624f
collapsing 1603f, 1612
cryoglobulinemic 1636, 1636f, 1637f, 1637t
eclampsia-associated 1637
fibrillary 1634–1635, 1635f, 1637t
fibrils/microtubules in 1637t
fibronectin 1624
immunotactoid 1635–1637, 1636f, 1637t
mesangiopathic (mesangial proliferative)
1608–1609, 1612f
minimal change 1606–1608, 1612f
nodular 1633f
transplant 1650, 1651f, 1653–1654, 1653f
glomerulosclerosis
collapsing glomerulopathy variant 1603f, 1612
diffuse, diabetic nephropathy 1629
focal segmental (focal sclerosis) 1608, 1609–1612,
1613f, 1640
familial 1610
secondary 1613–1614
in hypertension 1644, 1644f
nodular 1608f
diabetic nephropathy 1629, 1629f
segmental 1607f
advanced 1602, 1602f, 1607f
glomerulus
amyloid deposition 1608f
anatomy and histology 1598–1600, 1599f, 1606f
crescent 1608f
epithelial cells (podocytes) 1598–1599
infarct and necrosis 1609f
ischemic obsolescence 1644f
mesangial cells *see* mesangial cells
sclerosis/hyalinized regions 1609, 1613f
segmental necrotizing changes 1608f
subepithelial 'humps' 1617f, 1618, 1618f
glomus jugulare 819
glomus tumor
angioleiomyoma *vs* 349
immunohistochemistry 796t
'malignant' 273
of middle ear 2276–2277
of nasal cavity 796t, 819–820
of skin 272–273, 273f
glomus tympanicum 819, 2277
glossitis, median rhomboid 1162–1163
glottic carcinoma, hemilaryngectomy specimen 834
glucagon, excess 1573–1574
glucagonoma 1573–1574
glucagonoma syndrome 1574
glucocorticoid receptor gene mutation 1736
glucose-6-phosphatase deficiency 1508, 1508f

glucose metabolism abnormalities, necrobiosis
lipoidica in 214
glucose oxidase method 30
glue ear 2272
glutaraldehyde 17, 29
gluten-free diet 1376
gluten-sensitive enteropathy *see* celiac disease
glycogen
accumulation, oncocytoma 1224
cytoplasmic 250
intracytoplasmic, serous cystic tumor of pancreas
1563
lysosomal storage 2231
glycogenic acanthosis 1289–1290
glycogenoses (glycogen storage diseases) 2230–2232
cardiac involvement 1048, 1048f
hepatic adenoma and 1508, 1528
liver involvement 1508, 1508f, 1509f
type I (glucose-6-phosphatase deficiency) 1508
type II (acid maltase deficiency) 2230–2231, 2231f,
2232f
type III (debrancher enzyme deficiency) 1508, 2232
type IV (branching enzyme deficiency) 1508, 1509f,
2232
type V (McArdle's disorder) 2231–2232, 2232f
type VII (phosphofructokinase deficiency) 2232
glycoprotein membrane antigens 31t
mesothelioma 1012–1013, 1013f
tumors associated 179–180
glycoproteins, staining methods 16t
GM2-gangliosidosis type1 2318
GNAS1 gene 1192
goblet cell(s)
in Barrett's esophagus 1301, 1302, 1304f
bronchioles 860, 861f
conjunctiva 2292
metastatic colorectal cancer 2038
pseudomyxoma ovarii 2006, 2007
small intestine 1373
goblet cell carcinoid tumors 1429, 1429f
goiter 2122–2124, 2123f, 2124f
colloid 2122–2123
diffuse toxic *see* Graves' disease
dyshormonogenetic 2124
lymphadenoid *see* autoimmune thyroiditis
(Hashimoto's)
nodular 2123, 2123f, 2124f
non-neoplastic, FNA specimens 24
nontoxic/sporadic types 2122
goitrogens 2122
Goldenhar syndrome 2304
Goldner trichome 710f
Golgi bodies, 'honeycomb Golgi' 2107
Golgi tendon organ 2217
Gomori methenamine silver stain 60t, 61, 69
fungal infections of liver 1511, 1512f
liver biopsy 1469, 1511
Gomori's reticulin stain 18f
Gomori's trichrome stain 18f
skeletal muscle evaluation 2215t, 2230, 2230f
gonad, streak 1737, 1738, 1738f
gonadal deficiency, primary, male 1738
gonadal dysgenesis 1738
germ cell tumor risk 1742
mixed 1737
gonadal tumors 1738
gonadoblastoma
gonadal dysgenesis and 1742
ovary 2036 2037
in streak gonad 1737, 1738f
testicular 1737, 1761
gonadotrophs
adenoma *see* pituitary adenoma
development 2097
hyperplasia 2110
gonadotropin-releasing hormone agonists 1969
iatrogenic reaction to 151
gonocytes 1734, 1741
Goodpasture antigen 1622

Goodpasture's syndrome 1622
diffuse alveolar hemorrhage 884, 884f, 1622
Gordon-Sweet reticulin stain 18
Gorham syndrome 766
Gorlin syndrome *see* multiple endocrine neoplasia type 2b
Goseki classification, gastric adenocarcinoma 1354–1355
Gottron's papules 206
Gottron's sign 2219
gout 688–689
renal involvement 1643, 1643f
tophi 233–234, 234f, 689, 689f
ear 2274
Gower sign 2235
gp100, premelanosomes 286
G protein, fibrous dysplasia of bone 741, 742
graafian follicles 1987
graft eosinophilia 920
graft rejection
acute, pathological manifestations 122–127
acute antibody-mediated 124–127
accelerated 126–127, 127f
hyperacute 124–126
acute cellular 122–124, 123t, 1502
grading systems 125t, 126t
antibody-mediated 122
chronic 126t, 127–129
cytokine-mediated 122
effector function mechanisms 122
mechanisms 120, 122
specific/nonspecific cytotoxicity 122
see also specific organ transplantations
graft-*versus*-host disease (GVHD) 129
bronchiolitis 907
cutaneous involvement 204
esophagus 1291
intestinal 1402, 1403f
Gram stain 59, 60t, 2335t
Gram-Weigert stain 88, 88f
granular astrocytic mitoses (Creutzfeldt cells) 2413
granular cell tumor ('myoblastoma')
breast 445, 482, 2255
CNS 2399
congenital, oral cavity 1185
esophageal 1315
extrahepatic bile ducts 1583, 1584f
gastrointestinal tract 1450
gingiva 1185
laryngeal/vocal cord 848, 848f
lung 952, 954f
malignant variant 2256
oral cavity 1184–1185, 1184f
peripheral nerves 2255–2256, 2256f
pituitary 2109
Schwann cell origin 1184
vulvar 1902, 1903f
granular ependymitis 2343, 2344f
granulation tissue
laryngeal pseudotumor 834, 836
mucocele 1149
vagina 1919, 1920
granulocyte colony-stimulating factor (G-CSF) 616
granulocytic sarcoma (chloroma) 294, 575, 762
orbit 2296
of ovary 2026, 2027, 2029t
sinonasal region 825
testis involvement 1762
see also myeloid sarcoma
granulocytic series, maturation arrest 620
granulocytopenia, severe 618
granuloma 64
acne rosacea 226
actinic 213, 213f
annular elastolytic 213
bone marrow *see* bone marrow
caseating
acne rosacea 226
laryngeal and tracheal 835

caseating necrosis 82–83, 215
cholecystic (ceroid; xanthogranulomatous cholecystitis) 1576, 1577f
cholesterol, ear 2273–2274
conjunctiva 2294
Crohn's disease 1391
definition 660, 1508
'doughnut' 661
drug-induced 1510, 1511f
electrocautery, thermal artifact in tissue 137
eosinophilic *see* eosinophilic granuloma
eosinophilic of bone *see* Langerhans cell histiocytosis
epithelioid (proliferative) *see* epithelioid granuloma
fibrin ring 82, 1511, 1511f
foreign body type *see* foreign body granuloma
giant cell reparative *see* giant cell reparative granuloma
hepatic *see* hepatic granuloma
histoplasmosis 84f
intravascular pyogenic 270
keratin, ovary 1989f
lipid 141
lung 889–893
lymph nodes 532–533
Majocchi's 225, 226f
Miescher's 234
necrobiotic 400
cervix 1837
rheumatoid bronchiolitis 907
silk sutures 144
noncaseating 64f
lymph nodes 532–533
non-necrotizing, muscle 2223, 2224f
NSAID-associated 1402
of oral cavity
central giant cell 1182–1183, 1182f
pyogenic 1180–1181
plasma cell, peritoneum 1022
pulmonary hyalinizing 967–968, 968f
pulmonary veno-occlusive disease 915
pyogenic
conjunctiva 2294
mucocele *vs* 1149
oral cavity 1180–1181
sinonasal region 817
vulva 1901–1902
'pyogenic' (lobular capillary hemangioma) 269, 270, 270f
sarcoidal 214, 892f
lung 891, 892f, 893f
lymph nodes 533
in necrobiosis lipoidica 214
sarcoid-like, in Hodgkin's disease 653
in sclerosing mediastinitis 1127–1128
skeletal muscle 2223, 2224
skin involvement 212–216
spleen 578–579
stages 1508–1509
starch 139
subacute/chronic lung disease with 889–893
suppurative 533, 534f
suture 145
swimming pool 72
talc 139
granuloma annulare (GA) 212–214, 213f
epithelioid sarcoma *vs* 400
subcutaneous 213, 214
granuloma faciale 210, 211f
granuloma gravidarum 270
granuloma inguinale 1836t, 1890
granuloma pyogenicum *see* granuloma, pyogenic
granulomatosis
allergic 211–212
allergic bronchocentric 92
Langerhans cell 195, 610f
lymphomatoid, lung *see* lymphomatoid granulomatosis

Miescher's 213
necrotizing sarcoid 893
Wegener's *see* Wegener's granulomatosis
granulomatous diseases
bone marrow involvement *see* bone marrow
liver 1508–1513
portal 1514
of skin 212–216, 213t
granulomatous hypophysitis, idiopathic 2112, 2112f
granulomatous inflammation
eyelid 2289, 2289f
lung 881
peripheral nerve 2243
pleura 1006
skin 212–216, 213f
granulomatous meningitis, after iodized oil in myelography 138
granulomatous mesenteric lymphadenitis 98, 99f
granulomatous reactions 64–66, 64f
BCG immunotherapy 148
to foreign bodies *see* foreign body granulomatous reaction
starch and talc causing 139
steroid injections causing 141
granulomatous slack skin 292
granuloma venereum 1890
granulosa cells (ovary) 1987
luteinized 1988
proliferation, in pregnancy 1994, 1994f
granulosa cell tumor
ovary *see* ovary, granulosa cell tumor
testis 1759, 1760–1761, 1760f
granulosa lutein cysts 1990
Graves' disease 229, 2123, 2123f
cold nodule in 2124
thyroid cancer after 159, 2123
Graves orbitopathy 2295, 2295f
'gray zone' lesions, extrahepatic bile duct carcinoma 1586
Grenz zone
diffuse large B cell lymphoma of skin 290
leprosy 215
leukemia cutis in acute myeloid leukemia 294
prominent, granuloma faciale 210, 211f
subepidermal, Merkel cell carcinoma 249, 249f
Gridley stain 60t
Grimelius' stain 23
Grocott stain 2335t
gross cystic disease fluid protein (GCDFP) 181, 468, 482, 1213
'ground-glass' appearance, fibrous dysplasia of bone 741
'ground-glass cells' (hepatitis B) 1486–1487, 1487f
'ground-glass' nuclei 119, 120f, 1482, 1482f
Alzheimer type II astrocytes 2343f
ground-glass opacity, lung 863, 864, 866f, 890, 892
Grover's disease (transient acantholytic dermatosis) 219, 220–221, 221f
growth factors, markers 31t
growth hormone-releasing hormone (GHRH) 2110
Grzybowski type, keratoacanthoma 248
Guillain-Barré syndrome 2242, 2242f, 2243f
gumma, syphilitic 70, 1890
gynandroblastoma, ovary 2026
Gynecologic Oncology Group (GOG) 1910–1911, 1911t
gynecomastia 421, 451–452, 452f, 453f
choriocarcinoma of testis 1753
granulosa cell tumors 1760
Leydig cell tumor 1757
gyrate erythema 207–208, 207f

H

HACEK group of bacteria 1060
Haemophilus ducreyi 1890
Haemophilus influenzae, otitis media 2272
Hailey-Hailey disease (benign familial pemphigus) 220, 220f, 1894
hair, growth cycle 194

hair follicles
  embryonic 251, 251f
  inflammatory diseases 225–228
  normal 194
  primitive, pilar differentiation 252, 252f
  secondary 251, 251f
'hair germ, tumors 252, 252f
Hale's colloidal iron stain 1676, 1680, 1684
'hallmark' cells 563, 564f
Hall stain 1469, 1493
halo-like phenomenon 282
HAM-56 antibodies 287
hamartoma
  angiomyomatous, of lymph nodes 514
  biliary 1522, 1523f, 1538, 1538f
  breast 447, 447f
  Brunner's glands 1420, 1420f
  cardiac rhabdomyoma 1065, 1065f
  chest wall 706, 706f, 707f
  cystic, of renal pelvis 1695
  definition 826
  epilepsy due to 2405
  fibroleiomyomatous, lung 970–971, 971f
  fibrolipomatous, peripheral nerves 2249, 2249f
  fibrous of infancy 318–319, 318f
  folliculosebaceous cystic, vulvar 1902
  head and neck 826
  lipoadenoma 2155f
  lymphoid, vulva 1902
  mesenchymal, liver 1540, 1541f
  middle ear–mastoid 2271
  myoid 447
  neuromuscular 2249, 2249f
  omental-mesenteric myxoid 1022
  oral cavity 1186
  pulmonary 974–975, 975f, 976f
  sinonasal region 826
  spleen 582–583
  trachea 848
  vascular, of infancy 706
  vascular-cartilaginous 706
Hamazaki-Wesenberg bodies 71, 533
hand, foot and mouth disease, vulvar infection 1889
hand and wrist
  epithelioid sarcoma 398, 398f
  giant cell reparative granuloma 752
Hand–Schüller–Christian disease 289, 571, 659, 759, 826
  bone involvement 690, 2284
hantaviruses
  pneumonia 879, 880f
  respiratory tract infection 95, 95f, 99
hantavirus pulmonary syndrome 95, 95f
hard metal pneumoconiosis 904–905, 905f
'hard thermal residue' 137, 137f
Hartmann's pouch 1395, 1576
Hart's line 1885, 1886f
Hashimoto's thyroiditis see autoimmune thyroiditis
  (Hashimoto's)
Hassall's corpuscles
  absence 115
  in thymolipoma 1126
HBME-1 2130, 2133
h-caldesmon, leiomyoma 348
head and neck
  anatomy 1205
  angiosarcoma 818
  carcinoma 839
  chondrosarcoma 816–817
  fibrous dysplasia 1191
  liposarcoma 822
  osteogenic sarcoma 815
  radiation-associated tumors 158–159
  squamous cell carcinoma 789
    basaloid 790–791, 791f
    metastatic 1246
  see also salivary glands; sinonasal region
hearing, loss 2267, 2270
  conductive 2283
  Paget's disease of bone 2283

rheumatoid arthritis 2282
  sensorineural 2284
heart
  amyloidosis 1047–1048, 1047f
  failure, unexplained 1042, 1042t
  infectious cysts 1066
  inflammation see myocarditis
  left-sided disease, pulmonary venous hypertension
    914–915
  masses 1062–1067
  tumors 1062–1067
    amyloid 1066
    benign 1065–1066
    calcifying intracardiac pseudoneoplasm 1066
    endocrine tumors 1066
    fibroma 1064
    lymphoma 1067
    malignant 1066–1067
    metastatic 1067
    myxoma 1062, 1063–1064, 1064f, 1157
    rhabdomyoma 1065, 1065f
    sarcoma 1066–1067, 1067t
    soft tissue neoplasms 1066
    types and age of presentation 1063t
  see also entries beginning cardiac
heart transplantation 123f, 123t
  accelerated antibody-mediated rejection 127
  acute cellular rejection 123, 123f, 1049–1051
    general features 1049
    grades 1051f, 1052f, 1053f, 1054f
    grading scheme 125t, 1049, 1050t
    misinterpretation of biopsy 1050, 1055f
    'ongoing'/'resolving' 1049
  acute vascular rejection 1050, 1054f
  chronic rejection 127, 128, 128f
  hyperacute rejection 126f
  ischemic injury 1050
  opportunistic infections 1051
  perfusion injury of allograft 129, 130f
  Quilty effect 1051, 1055f
heart valves 1052–1061
  examination 1052–1061
  general approach 1052–1053
  papillary fibroelastoma 1060, 1061f
  photography 1053
  prosthetic 1060–1062
    bioprosthetic 1060–1061, 1061f
    mechanical 1061, 1062f
    vegetations 1059–1060, 1084
    marantic 1060
  see also individual valves
Heath-Edwards classification, pulmonary arterial
    hypertension 912
heat-induced antigen retrieval methods 32–33
heavy chain deposition disease 1631–1632, 1633f
heavy chain disease 657
heavy chain-related (AH) amyloidosis, renal 656, 1631,
    1631f, 1632f
Heck's disease 1163
Hedley's technique 37, 38t
Heffner's tumor 2278–2279, 2279f
Heinz bodies 1026
Heister's spiral valves 1576
Helicobacter heilmannii 1330, 1330f
  chronic gastritis 1331
Helicobacter pylori 1330f
  acquisition of infection 1331
  cytotoxin production and genotypes 1331
  detection tests 1330
  discovery 1330
  duodenal ulcer association 1332, 1396
  enterochromaffin-like cell proliferation 1349
  epidemiology 1330–1331
  eradication/treatment 1334
    effect on gastric disease 1334
    effect on gastric surgical pathology 1334–1335
    in gastroesophageal reflux disease 1335
  FldA protein secretion 1351–1352
  gastric adenocarcinoma and 1355

gastric lymphoma association 1332
gastric mucosal infection 1340
gastritis association 1326, 1375
  autoimmune chronic gastritis 1329, 1330
  Barrett's esophagus and/vs 1302
  chronic gastritis 1330–1335
  diffuse antral gastritis 1331–1332, 1332f
  granulomatous 1336, 1336f
  multifocal atrophic gastritis 1332–1333, 1333f,
    1335
MALT lymphoma and 290, 1351, 1354
microbiology 1330, 1331
peptic duodenitis 1396–1397
HELLP syndrome 2072
hemangioblastoma
  CNS 2394–2395, 2395f
    immunohistochemistry 2339t
    ultrastructural characteristics 2337t
  retinal 2317
hemangioendothelial sarcoma 769, 769f
hemangioendothelioma 273, 365–368
  epithelioid see epithelioid hemangioendothelioma
  hobnail, of skin 274, 274f
  infantile, liver 1541–1542, 1541f
  Kaposiform (infantile) 274, 366, 367f
  littoral cell 591
  malignant, angiosarcoma vs 818
  retiform 274, 274f, 366, 366f
  of skin 273, 274, 274f
  spindle cell 365
    of skin 272, 273, 273f
  splenic 591
  'vegetant intravascular' 362–363, 363f
hemangioma 363
  acquired tufted, of skin 269, 270, 270f
  arteriovenous
    oral cavity 1186
    of skin 271, 271f
  of bone 765–767, 766f
  breast 446, 446f
  capillary see capillary hemangioma
  cardiac 1065
  cavernous see cavernous hemangioma
  choroidal 2309
  cystic 1022
  epithelioid see epithelioid hemangioma
  glomeruloid 271
  histiocytoid see angiolymphoid hyperplasia with
    eosinophilia
  hobnail, of skin 272, 272f
  intestinal 1448–1449
  intramuscular 364, 364f
    angiomatosis vs 365
    lesions/tumors included 364
    lipoma vs 337
  juvenile 365
    see also capillary hemangioma
  kidney 1692
  laryngeal 849
  liver 1540–1541
  marrow cavity infiltration 705
  microvenular, of skin 272
  multiple primary of bone 766
  nasal septum 817
  oral cavity 1186
  orbital 2297, 2297f
  perilobular (breast) 446, 446f
  sclerosing, lung 947–949, 948f
  sinonasal region 817
  sinusoidal 271
  of skin 269–271, 270f, 271f, 272f
  spindle cell 365–366, 711
    of skin 272, 273, 273f
  spine 701
  splenic 581, 582–583, 591
  strawberry see capillary hemangioma
  targetoid hemosiderotic 370
  umbilical cord 2067
  verrucous, of skin 269, 270

hemangioma (cont'd)
  vocal cords 849
  vulva 1901
hemangiomatosis, pulmonary capillary 918, 918f
hemangiopericytoma 373–374, 373f, 374f, 2387, 2392
  of bone 769–770, 770f
    differential diagnosis 1101t, 1102t
      monophasic synovial sarcoma vs 404
      solitary fibrous tumor vs 378t
      vulvar pyogenic granuloma vs 1902
    immunohistochemistry 796t
    larynx 850
    lipomatous 374
    orbit 2297
    pulmonary 968
    sinonasal 818–819, 819f
hemangiosarcoma 371
  larynx and trachea 850
hematein 18
hematogones (lymphoid precursors) 614, 618, 640
hematoidin, staining 20t
hematologic disorders
  in bone marrow, markers 611t
  ear and temporal bone 2284
  neoplasms, effusions 1031–1032, 1031f
  see also hematopoietic tumors
hematolymphoid cells, markers 508–510, 508t–509t
hematolymphoid tumors, esophageal 1315
hematoma
  CNS 2416–2417
  retroplacental 2065, 2072, 2072f
  umbilical cord 2066–2067
hematopoiesis 613, 613f
  extramedullary 585, 1945
  failure, AIDS 661
hematopoietic growth factors 585, 612, 616
  recombinant human 612
  therapeutic, hematologic changes 620
hematopoietic lesions, CNS 2397
hematopoietic tumors 703t
  CNS 2397
    see also lymphoma, CNS
  involving bone 758–763
  renal 1693–1694
  testis 1762
  thyroid 2141
  see also leukemia; lymphoma; myeloma
hematoxylin and eosin (H&E) stain 27, 2335t
  bone specimens 704
  CNS tissue 2329, 2331
  infectious disease specimens 59, 60t, 66
  lymph node biopsy 507
  skeletal muscle 2215t
hematoxylin bodies, lupus nephritis 1628
hematuria 1605t
  familial benign 1624–1626
  IgA nephropathy 1618
  microscopic 1614, 1615
  renal metastases causing 1694
  in vasculitides 1648
hemilaryngectomy, vertical, specimens 834
hemochromatosis
  genetic 1504
    liver involvement 1503–1505, 1504f
  liver biopsy 1468, 1504f
  micronodular cirrhosis 1504f
  restrictive cardiomyopathy 1045
hemodialysis, acquired cystic disease of kidney
    1663
hemoglobinopathy 76
hemoglobin SC disease, medullary carcinoma of
    kidney 1687
hemoglobinuria 1638
hemolysis, intravascular, prolonged 619
hemolytic uremic syndrome (HUS) 1383, 1647
hemophagocytic syndrome 658–659, 658f
  familial 658–659
  infection-associated 527–528, 528, 528f, 658, 658f,
    659

hemophagocytosis
  familial 578
  infection-associated 578, 578f
  malignancy-associated 659, 659f
  peripheral T-cell lymphoma 562
  secondary 578
hemoptysis, lung carcinoma 936
hemorrhage
  adrenal cortex 2169, 2176, 2177, 2177f
  alveolar see diffuse alveolar hemorrhage (DAH)
  cerebral 2414, 2416–2417
  eye 2304, 2312, 2317
  fetal-maternal 2073
  intramedullary 616
  pulmonary 884, 884f
  retinal 2317
  into skeletal muscle 2238
  testis 1754
  vitreous 2304, 2317
hemorrhagic endovasculitis 2073, 2074f, 2080
  villous capillaries 2073
hemorrhagic fever viruses 99
hemorrhagic fever with renal syndrome 879
hemorrhagic vasculitis (HEV) 2073, 2074f
hemosiderin 619, 1493
  leukocytoclastic vasculitis 208
  pigmented villonodular synovitis 1195, 1195f
  staining 20t
  stromal deposition, hobnail hemangioma 272, 272f
hemosiderinuria 619
hemosiderosis 1504
  idiopathic pulmonary (IPH) 884, 885f
  pituitary involvement 2113
  in steatohepatitis 1491
hemotympanum, idiopathic 2274
Henoch–Schönlein purpura 1076t
  intestinal involvement 1386
  nephropathy 1618–1619, 1619f
heparinase, metastases mechanism 167
hepatic adenoma 1528–1529
  differential diagnosis 1528t, 1529, 1529t
hepatic adenomatosis 1528
hepatic carcinoma, sclerosing 1536
hepatic ducts 1581
hepatic fibrosis 1501
  in chronic hepatitis 1486
  congenital 1521, 1521f
  early pericellular ('chicken-wire') 1491, 1492f
hepatic granuloma 1508–1513
  causes 1509t, 1510
  drug-induced 1510, 1511f
  infectious 1509t, 1510–1511, 1511f, 1512, 1512f
  sarcoidosis 1509–1510, 1510f
hepatic vein thrombosis 353, 1515, 1516f
hepatic venules, terminal (central veins) 1474, 1513f,
    1514
  central–central bridging 1480
  outflow obstruction 1514–1517
  portal–central bridging 1480
hepatitis
  acute 1475–1483
    'classic' 1475–1477
      giant cell transformation 1483, 1483f
      massive necrosis 1480–1481, 1481f
      submassive necrosis 1479–1480, 1480f
      subsiding 1478, 1478f
      see also hepatocellular injury
    acute cholestatic 1478, 1478f
    acute viral 1475–1477, 1477f
    adenovirus 1482, 1483f
    alcoholic 1471f, 1490–1492, 1491f
    autoimmune 1479, 1484, 1487–1488
      chronic 1484, 1484t, 1485f, 1487–1488
    bile duct lesions associated 1485, 1485f, 1487
    chronic 1484–1489
      causes 1484, 1484t
      classification and reporting 1488–1489, 1488t
      grading 1488t
      Wilson's disease vs 1505, 1506f

  chronic active, biopsy 1467
  chronic viral 1486–1487
  diabetic 1491
  Epstein–Barr virus (EBV) 101, 102f
  fatty liver 1490–1492, 1491
  giant cell, neonatal 1483, 1483f
  herpes simplex virus (HSV) 1482, 1482f
  herpes virus 74, 75f
  idiopathic neonatal 1483
  interface 1485, 1486f, 1488t, 1501
  ischemic 1513
  mononucleosis 1478–1479, 1479f
hepatitis A 1477
  acute 1480f
  submassive necrosis 1479, 1480f
hepatitis A virus (HAV) 1475t
hepatitis B
  acute 1487
  chronic 1484, 1484t, 1486–1487
  hepatocellular carcinoma and/vs 1530–1531
hepatitis B virus (HBV) 1475t
  core antigen (HBcAg) 1487
  liver biopsy immunostaining 1471, 1472f
  surface antigen (HBsAg) 1486, 1487, 1487f
    polyarteritis nodosa 1074
hepatitis C
  bile duct lesions 1487
  chronic 1484, 1484t, 1485f, 1487, 1489
    cirrhosis in 1485f, 1486f, 1519f, 1520f
  hepatocellular carcinoma and 1530–1531
  liver biopsy immunostaining 1471
hepatitis C virus (HCV) 1475t
hepatitis D 1487
  acute submassive necrosis 1480f
  chronic 1484, 1484t, 1487
  liver biopsy immunostaining 1471
hepatitis D virus (HDV) 1475t, 1487
hepatitis E, cholestatic hepatitis 1478, 1478f
hepatitis E virus (HEV) 1475t
hepatitis viruses 1475t, 1484
hepatobiliary cystadenoma, of extrahepatic bile ducts
    1586, 1587f
hepatoblastoma 1536–1538, 1537f
  fetal type 1528t, 1537, 1537f
  macrotrabecular differentiation 1537, 1538f
  mixed types and rare variants 1537
hepatocellular adenoma see hepatic adenoma
hepatocellular carcinoma (HCC) 1530–1538
  acinar (adenoid, pseudoglandular) 1531, 1532f
  cholangiocarcinoma with 1533, 1535–1536, 1536f
  clear-cell type 176, 1533f
  cytology 1531, 1531f, 1532–1533, 1532f, 1533f, 1534f
  diagnostic attributes 1534
  differential diagnosis 1529t, 1531, 1533–1534
    adenoma vs 1528t
    angiomyolipoma vs 1529t, 1542
    borderline (dysplastic) nodules vs 1530t
    fetal type hepatoblastoma vs 1528t
    focal nodular hyperplasia vs 1528, 1528t
    macroregenerative nodules vs 1530t
    partial nodular transformation vs 1528t
  fibrolamellar variant (FLHCC) 1533, 1535, 1535f
  in hemochromatosis 1504–1505
  histologic grading/patterns 1531–1533
  immunohistochemistry 1533–1534
  macroregenerative nodules predisposing to 1529
  poorly differentiated 1534
  rare variants 1536
  scirrhous pattern 1531
  sclerosing variant 1536
  solid (compact) pattern 1531
  specimens, processing and reporting 1536
  trabecular (plate-like; sinusoidal) 1531, 1531f, 1533f
  well differentiated 1533–1534
hepatocellular-cholangiolar carcinoma 1533,
    1535–1536, 1536f
hepatocellular injury 1475–1489
  acidophilic degeneration 1475–1476, 1476f
  acute coagulative necrosis 1513

acute drug-induced 1475t, 1476f, 1478
acute necroinflammatory (hepatitis) 1475–1483
   focal coagulative necrosis 1482, 1482f
   infections causing 1481, 1482
   microabscess formation 1481–1482, 1481f
   patchy/confluent coagulative necrosis 1482, 1482f
   see also hepatitis, acute
cholestatic hepatitis 1478, 1478f
chronic necroinflammatory 1484–1489
   see also hepatitis, chronic
hepatocanalicular (mixed hepatocellular/cholestatic)
      1478
massive necrosis 1475f, 1480–1481, 1481f
mononucleosis hepatitis 1478–1479, 1479f
piecemeal necrosis 1477, 1485
submassive necrosis 1475f, 1479–1480, 1480f
see also hepatocytes
hepatocellular nodules 1527–1538
   benign nodules/lesions 1527–1530
      high-grade dysplastic 1529–1530, 1530f, 1530t
      macroregenerative (low-grade dysplastic) 1520,
         1521f, 1529–1530, 1530f, 1530t
      multiacinar regenerative 1529
      partial nodular transformation 1528t, 1529
      regenerative 1480f, 1519
      see also hepatic adenoma
   malignant lesions 1530–1538, 1537
      sampling and reporting 1537–1538
      see also hepatoblastoma; hepatocellular carcinoma
         (HCC)
   solitary necrotic nodules 1545
Hepatocyte Ab 1534
hepatocytes 1474
   apoptosis 1475, 1476, 1476f
   balloon degeneration 130f, 1476, 1477f
   cytoplasmic dissociation 1485
   degenerating 1485
   feathery degeneration 1493, 1495f
   focal nodular hyperplasia 1527, 1527f
   giant cell transformation 1483, 1483f
   injury see hepatocellular injury
   'islets' 1486
   loss, submassive necrosis 1479, 1480f
   macrovesicular steatosis 1488f, 1489
   microvesicular steatosis 1489, 1489f
   see also hepatocellular injury
hepatoid adenocarcinoma, gastric 1361, 1362
hepatoid carcinoma, ovary 2014
hepatomegaly, liver biopsy 1467
hepatoportal sclerosis 1514, 1514f
hepatorenal syndrome 1632, 1634f
HER2/neu oncogene 33, 34f
   breast carcinoma 33, 34f, 454, 461, 468, 470, 473,
      475
      importance and assays 489
      in situ hybridization 46
      osteosarcoma 735
      quantitative immunohistochemistry 43
Her2 protein, lung carcinoma 937
herald patch 197
hereditary hemorrhagic telangiectasia 1517, 2416
hereditary motor and sensory neuropathies (HMSN)
      2244–2245, 2245f
   type I (Charcot–Marie–Tooth) 2225, 2226f, 2241,
      2244–2245, 2245f
   type II 2245
   type III (Dejerine–Sottas disease) 2245
hereditary multiple exostoses 707, 708, 718
hereditary nephritis (nephropathy) of Alport
      1624–1626, 1625f
   Schönlein-Henoch purpura vs 1619
hereditary nonpolyposis colon cancer syndrome
      (HNPCC) 1438
   microsatellite instability 48
   mucinous colorectal cancer 1438–1439
   storiform pleomorphic malignant fibrous
      histiocytoma and 333
hereditary osteo-onychodysplasia (nail patella
      syndrome) 1623–1624

Hering bodies 2094f
Hermansky-Pudlak syndrome 579
hermaphroditism see intersex states
hernia
   cerebral 2271
   hiatus 1281
herpes genitalis 1836–1837, 1850f
herpes gestationis 198, 223
herpes gladiatorum 74
herpes pemphigoides, differential diagnosis 198
herpes simplex virus (HSV) 74–75
   acute erosive gastritis 1329
   adrenalitis 2176, 2176f
   cervicitis/genital infections 1836–1837, 1850f,
      1851
   effect on HPV 1836
   encephalitis 2407–2408, 2408f
   esophageal infection 1398
   esophagitis 74, 74f, 1287–1288, 1288f
   eyelid infection 2290
   female genital tract infections 75, 75f
   hepatitis 74, 75f, 1482, 1482f
   immunologic detection 62
   inclusions 68t, 878, 878f, 1837
   lymphadenitis 525, 525f
   miliary nodular pneumonia 878, 878f
   ocular infection 2313
   oral squamous cell carcinoma 1170
   pneumonia 74, 75f, 878, 878f
   skin and soft tissue infections 74–75
   staining 74
   type 1 74, 221, 1836
   type 2 74, 221, 1836, 1851
      vulvar infection 1888, 1888f
herpes viruses
   erythema multiforme 203
   laryngeal and tracheal infections 834
   vulvar infections 1888, 1888f
herpes zoster 75
   eyelid involvement 2290
   herpetic dermatitis 221, 221f
   peripheral nerve involvement 2244
   vulvar involvement 1888, 1889f
herpetic dermatitis 221, 221f
herpetic vulvitis 1888, 1888f
herringbone pattern, fibrosarcoma lesion 325, 325f
heterochromia iridium 2292
heterotypic aggregation of cells 167
Heubner arteritis 2407
HFE gene, mutations 1503
hiatus hernia 1281
hibernoma 340–341, 342f
hidradenitis suppurativa, vulvar involvement
      1890–1891, 1909
hidradenocarcinoma, low-grade eccrine 261
hidradenoma
   nodular 257, 259f
   tubulopapillary 257–258, 259f
hidradenoma papilliferum (HP) 258, 260f
   vulva 1898, 1898f
hidroacanthoma simplex 257
hidrocystoma 255, 255f
   apocrine/eccrine, eyelid 2290
high-resolution computed tomography (HRCT), lung
      863, 868
   hypersensitivity pneumonitis 889–890
   usual interstitial pneumonia 893
hilar mass, pulmonary venous hypertension 915
hillock of Doyère 2217
hilus cell rests, in fallopian tube 2043
hilus cells (ovary) 1988, 2024
   hyperplasia 1994, 2025
hilus cell tumors 2024
hip
   rapidly destructive arthrosis 682–683, 682f
   replacement/prosthesis 144, 691
hippocampal sclerosis (mesial temporal sclerosis)
      2405, 2405f
Hirschsprung's disease 1403–1404, 1403f

histiocytes 287, 657
   bone marrow 614
   ceroid 579
   CNS 2344
   in dermatopathic lymphadenopathy 526
   in effusions 1026f, 1027
   epithelioid 519, 520f, 537, 640
   with erythrophagocytosis 527, 528f
   foamy 2284
   foreign body giant cell reaction 215, 216f
   hemophagocytosis 562
   indeterminate 287
   infection-associated hemophagocytic syndrome 527,
      528f
   lamellated inclusions 1641, 1642f
      see also Michaelis-Gutman bodies
   Langerhans 660f
   lipid-laden 210, 210f
   lipofuscin pigment in 2042, 2043
   lymphoma involving ovary 2026
   non-specific sinus histiocytosis 527
   palisading
      granuloma annulare 213, 213f
      necrobiosis lipoidica 214, 214f
      rheumatoid nodule 214, 215f
   proliferation, in skin 287–289
   reactive proliferation 657
      lymph nodes 529
      neoplastic vs, of skin 287
      splenic 579
   in Rosai–Dorfman disease 528, 529, 529f, 759
   sea-blue 579, 658
   solitary xanthogranuloma 287, 287f
   in splenic red pulp 579
   tingible-body 1095, 1095f
   vacuolization 530
   with vesicular nucleus 529, 529f
   see also dendritic cells; macrophage
histiocytic medullary reticulosis 659
histiocytic proliferative disorders 657–660
   bone marrow involvement 657–660, 660
   malignant 660
   reactive 657–658
   see also hemophagocytic syndrome
histiocytic sarcoma 574–575, 575f
   malignant histiocytosis as synonym 574
   malignant histiocytosis vs 660
histiocytoid hemangioma see angiolymphoid
      hyperplasia with eosinophilia
histiocytoma, fibrous see fibrous histiocytoma
histiocytosis 690
   benign cephalic 288
   congenital self-healing 289
   familial hemophagocytic lymphohistiocytosis 528
   generalized eruptive 288
   hemophagocytic 658–659
   indeterminate cell 574
   Langerhans cell see Langerhans cell
      histiocytosis
   malignant 572, 574–575, 659, 660
      anaplastic large cell lymphoma vs 565
   nodular 288
   sinus see sinus histiocytosis
   sinus with lymphadenopathy see Rosai–Dorfman
      disease
histiocytosis X see Langerhans cell histiocytosis
histochemical stains 59
   quality control 61, 62t
   see also immunohistochemical stains; individual
      stains
histochemistry 19
   see also immunohistochemistry
Histology Activity Index 1488
Histoplasma capsulatum 84f, 2411
   identification/characteristics 67t
   respiratory tract infection 83–85, 83f
   sclerosing mediastinitis 1128
   staining 61
Histoplasma duboisii 67t, 85

histoplasmosis 1512f
  Addison's disease 2176, 2176f
  bone marrow 662f
  CNS involvement 2411
  disseminated 77f
  granulomatous gastritis 1336
  intestinal 1399, 1399f
  larynx and trachea 835
  lymph node involvement 533
  respiratory tract 83–85, 83f, 84f, 92f
    cytologic diagnosis 90–91
HIV-1 57, 67, 116
  mutations 116
  replication 117
  RNA and viremia 117
HIV-associated nephropathy (HIVAN) 1603f, 1612
HIV infection 67, 116–120
  acute 117
  anal carcinoma and 1455
  brain involvement 118–119
  cervical neoplasia and 1856
  CNS 2409–2410
  collapsing glomerulopathy 1603f, 1612
  dementia 2409
  encephalitis 118–119, 119f, 2409, 2410f
  esophagitis 1289, 1290
  histoplasmosis 84, 84f
  Kaposi's sarcoma 274
  leukoencephalopathy 119
  lymphadenopathy 117–118, 522–524, 523f
  lymph nodes 522–524, 523f
  lymphoid interstitial pneumonia (LIP) in 900
  lymphomas in 571, 662
  lymphoproliferative disease 571
  Mycobacterium avium complex infection 64, 64f, 65f
  myopathy 2223, 2223f
  neuromuscular disease 2223
  neuropathy 2244
  peripheral nerve involvement 2244
  Pneumocystis pneumonia 88, 89, 89f, 881
  pneumocystosis 88
  pulmonary hypertension in 914
  salivary gland disease 1260–1261, 1261f
  smooth muscle tumors associated 353
  spindle cell lesion 65f
  ulcer, vulvar 1889
  wasting (cachetic) syndrome 2223
  see also AIDS
'hives' 208, 209f
HLA, diffuse panbronchiolitis (DPB) association 907
HLA-DQA1*0102 genotype 1355
HLA DR3, DR4, DR5, antibodies 451
HLA system 120, 122
HMB-45
  angiomyolipoma of kidney 1691
  clear cell sarcoma 381, 382f
  melanoma 181, 286
  renal leiomyosarcoma 1693
  seminoma differential diagnosis 1775t
HMFG-2, mesothelioma 1012–1013
HMGIC-LPP fusion gene, lipoma of bone 770
hobnail cells 176
  borderline clear cell tumors, of ovary 2011
  clear cell carcinoma
    of ovary 2011
    of vagina 1925
  Dabska's tumor 273
  hobnail hemangioma 272, 272f
  retiform hemangioendothelioma 274, 274f
'hobnail' morphology, multilocular cyst (cystic nephroma) 1695
Hodgkin cells 525, 535
  characteristics 536–537
  cytokines expressed 540
  immunohistochemistry 518, 539, 539t, 540f
  mononuclear 536, 537f
Hodgkin's disease 535–541, 653t
  in AIDS 121t, 662
  of bladder 1723

of bone 761
bone marrow 647, 652–653
cell of origin 540
chronic lymphocytic leukemia transformation 644
classic form 535–541
classification 535, 536t, 538, 545t, 546t, 652
  Cotswold's staging classification 536, 536t
differential diagnosis 540–541, 555, 653, 653t
  diffuse large B-cell lymphoma *vs* 557, 561
  Kimura disease *vs* 519
  Langerhans cell histiocytosis *vs* 760
  seminoma *vs* 1775–1776, 1775t
effusions 1031
epidemiology 535–536
Epstein–Barr virus-associated 539
fibrous bands in 537, 538f
fine needle aspiration 539, 539f
histopathologic diagnosis 536–539, 536f
immunohistochemistry 518, 539–540, 539t, 541, 652
interfollicular variant 518
L&H lymphocyte predominance 541–543, 542f
  follicular lymphoma *vs* 550
  progressive transformation of germinal centers *vs* 520
liver involvement 1517
lung involvement 981
lymph node granulomas 532
lymphocyte depletion type 538
lymphocyte predominance 535, 541–543
lymphocyte-rich 535, 537, 538
  differential diagnosis 543
mixed cellularity type 537f, 538
nodular lymphocyte predominance form 535, 541–543
nodular sclerosing type 537, 537f, 538f
  differential diagnosis 540
non-Hodgkin's lymphoma with 541
recurrences 538
renal involvement 1693
sarcoid-like granulomas 653
splenic granulomas 579
splenic involvement 588, 589f
subtype determination 538
syncytial variant 538, 538f
  mediastinal lymphoma *vs* 1125, 1125f
thymus 1092
Hollande's solution 1324
Holzer (crystal violet) stain 2335t
homeobox genes, pituitary development 2093–2094
Homer Wright (pseudo)rosettes 2380, 2381f, 2383
  Flexner–Wintersteiner rosettes *vs* 2310
  neuroblastoma of adrenal medulla 2195, 2195f
  olfactory neuroblastoma 801
  primitive neuroectodermal tumors 385, 385f, 748, 748f
homotypic aggregation of cells 167
honeycomb Golgi 2207
hordeolums (styes) 2289
hormone receptors 31t
  status, breast cancer *see* estrogen receptor positivity; progesterone receptor positivity
hormone replacement therapy (HRT)
  breast cancer risk 150
  endometrial metaplasia 1943
  infiltrating (invasive) lobular carcinoma and 465
hormones
  iatrogenic lesions due to 150–151
  markers 31t
  papillary thyroid carcinoma due to 2127
horn cysts
  desmoplastic trichoepithelioma 252, 252f
  seborrheic keratosis 242, 242f
horseradish peroxidase alkaline phosphatase 30
Hortega's method, staining 2335t
host defense mechanisms 62–67, 63t
  acute inflammatory response 63–64, 63t
  granulomatous/macrophage-rich 64–66
  lymphocyte rich response 66–67
'hot tub' lung 893

Howell–Jolly bodies 619
H-*ras* oncogene, oral squamous cell carcinoma 1170
HRPT2 gene 2158, 2161, 2162
human chorionic gonadotrophin (hCG)
  choriocarcinoma 2083
  embryonal carcinoma of testis 1777
  giant cell carcinoma of lung 964
  invasive carcinoma (of breast), choriocarcinomatous 483
  malignant mixed germ cell tumors of ovary 2036
  metastases of unknown primary 185
  non-small-cell carcinoma of lung 1779f
  seminoma 1745
human herpesvirus type 6 617
human herpesvirus type 8 *see* Kaposi's sarcoma-associated herpesvirus (KSHV)
human immunodeficiency virus (HIV) *see* HIV-1; HIV infection
human papillomavirus (HPV)
  anal carcinoma 1455
  anal intraepithelial neoplasia 1455
  cervical neoplasia and 1860, 1861
    adenocarcinoma 1868
    adenocarcinoma in situ 1867
    squamous cell carcinoma 1856–1857
    squamous intraepithelial lesion 1852, 1853, 1861
  cervicitis 1836, 1837
  common warts (verruca vulgaris) 241
  condyloma accuminatum of anus 1444f, 1454
  cytopathic effect 1861
  epidermodysplasia verruciformis 242
  esophageal squamous cell carcinoma 1294
  genes and malignant transformation 1852
  head and neck carcinoma 839
  HPV-2 1163, 1889
  HPV-6 1163, 1454, 1455
  HPV-11 1454, 1455
  HPV-16 242, 1170
    anal carcinoma 1455
    cervical adenocarcinoma in situ 1867
    cervical squamous carcinoma 1860
    laryngeal and tracheal dysplasia 839
    oral cancer 1138
    squamous carcinoma of penis 1768
    verrucous carcinoma of vulva 1912
    vulvar intraepithelial neoplasia 1905
  HPV-18
    anal carcinoma 1455
    cervical adenocarcinoma in situ 1867
    cervical squamous carcinoma 1860
    oral cancer 1138
  in situ hybridization 1855, 1856f, 1888, 1888f
  laryngeal carcinoma 839
  laryngeal dysplasia 839–841
  oral squamous cell carcinoma 1170
  oral verrucous carcinoma 1174
  parakeratosis in cervical samples 1843
  smokeless tobacco leukoplakia 1165
  squamous cell carcinoma of penis 1768
  squamous papilloma of esophagus 1292, 1292f
  squamous papilloma of larynx and trachea 836–837
  squamous papilloma of lung 940
  squamous papilloma of oral cavity 1163
  verrucous carcinoma of larynx 844–845
  vulvar infection 1887–1888, 1887f, 1889
  vulvar intraepithelial neoplasia 1905
human placental lactogen (HPL) 1753
human T-cell lymphotropic virus type 1 (HTLV-1) 294, 543, 566
HUMARA assay 970
Hunner's ulcer (interstitial cystitis) 1708–1709
Hürthle cell(s) 175f, 2121, 2134, 2134f
Hürthle cell adenoma 2124–2126, 2125f, 2134, 2134f
Hürthle cell carcinoma 2121, 2134–2135, 2134f
Hutchinson's melanotic freckle 283, 284f
Hutchinson's posture 2237
hyaline arteriolosclerosis, renal 1644, 1644f
'hyaline' bodies 1476

hyaline cartilage, cartilage-forming tumors 706
hyaline casts, acute tubular necrosis 1638
hyaline globules
    clear cell carcinoma, of ovary 2012
    extracellular, Kaposi's sarcoma 275f
    intracytoplasmic
        adrenal medulla 2189, 2190f
        adrenocortical tumors 2188, 2188f
        pheochromocytoma 2191, 2192f
    tumors with 177
    yolk sac tumors of ovary 2029
hyaline membranes, diffuse alveolar damage 872, 873,
    873f
hyaline molds 65, 66t
hyaline necrosis, sclerosing 1490–1492
hyaline thrombi 1628–1629, 1636
hyalinization
    basaloid squamous cell carcinoma 790, 791f
    solitary reticulohistiocytoma 288, 288f
    Spitz nevus 279
hyalinizing granuloma, lung 967–968, 968f
hyalinizing spindle cell tumor with giant rosettes 326,
    327, 327f
hyalinosis
    glomerular 1610
    renal arteries 1611f
    renal arterioles 1644, 1644f
hyaluronic acid, pleura 1005
Hyams grading system 801, 802, 803t
hydatid cysts 105, 105f, 1066
hydatidiform moles 2080, 2081t
    choriocarcinoma after 2083
    complete 2081–2082, 2081t, 2082f
    differential diagnosis 2082–2083
    ectopic 2087
    endometrial changes 1949
    in fallopian tube 2043, 2047
    hydropic abortus vs 2080
    invasive 2083
    partial 2081, 2081t, 2082, 2082f
hydatid sand 105, 105f
hydatids of Morgagni 2043
hydrocele 1765
hydrocephalus, brain tumors 2345
hydropic abortus 2080, 2082
hydropic degeneration 195
hydrosalpinx 143, 2041, 2041f
hydroxychloroquine, cardiotoxicity 1049
11β-hydroxylase deficiency 2174
17α-hydroxylase deficiency 1737, 1737f
21-hydroxylase
    autoantibodies 2175
    deficiency 2174, 2175
hymen 1918
    imperforate 1887, 1919
hyperadrenalism see Cushing's disease
hyperaldosteronism
    adrenocortical hyperplasia with 2182–2183
    familial 2183
    primary 2182–2183
        adrenocortical adenoma causing 2183–2185
        adrenocortical carcinoma causing 2186
hyperbilirubinemia, chronic cholestatic injury 1496
hypercalcemia
    familial hypocalciuric 2158
    renal cell carcinoma 1677
    small cell carcinoma of ovary 2014–2015, 2015f
hypercalcitoninemia 2137
hypercalciuria, familial hypercalcemic 2158
hypercholesterolemia, chronic cholestatic injury 1496
hypercorticalism
    ACTH-dependent/-independent 2178, 2180f
    adrenocortical hyperplasia with 2178–2183
    autoimmune form 2181
hyperemesis gravidarum 2081
hypereosinophilic syndrome 1046–1047
hypergastrinemia 1573
    enterochromaffin-like carcinoid tumors 1348, 1349
    gastrinoma 1573

hyperplasia-to-neoplasia sequence for ECL cells
    1349
    neuroendocrine tumors associated 1348–1350
    neuroendocrine tumors not associated 1350–1351
hypergranulosis, lichen simplex chronicus 201, 201f
hyper IgM syndrome 115
hyperinsulinism of infancy 1569–1570
hyperkalemic periodic paralysis 2233, 2233f
hyperkeratosis 195
    cervical squamous epithelium 1832, 1843
    Darier's disease 219, 220f
    lichen simplex chronicus 201
    'porcelain-white' patch 232
hyperlipidemia, xanthoma and 228
hyperlipoproteinemia, staining 21f
hyperoxaluria (oxalosis), renal involvement 1642–1643
hyperparathyroidism 2151
    autosomal dominant moderate 2158
    bone changes 686, 686f, 2151
    brown tumor 686, 751–752, 751f, 752f, 753, 1183,
        2151
    familial isolated 2158
    neonatal severe 2158
    neuromuscular abnormalities 2233
    primary/tertiary 2151, 2161
    secondary 2151, 2160, 2161
    thyroid carcinoma association 159
hyperparathyroidism jaw tumor (HPT-JT) syndrome
    2151, 2158
    parathyroid carcinoma and 2161, 2162
hyperphosphatasemia 686
hyperpigmentation, vulva 1896, 1897 12t
hyperpituitarism 681
hyperplastic polyposis syndrome 1431
hyperprolactinemia 2098, 2099, 2101, 2108, 2111
hyperreactio luteinalis 1992–1993, 1993f
hypersensitivity
    avian (bird fancier's lung) 890–891
    delayed-type, graft rejection 122
    dermal reaction (DHR) 208
    drug-induced, interstitial nephritis 1640
    occupational 891
    polymorphous light eruption 206–207
    type III reaction 889
hypersensitivity myocarditis 1044–1045
hypersensitivity pneumonitis (HSP) 869–870, 870f,
    889–891
    differential diagnosis 890, 891t
    metal working fluid-associated 891
    pathology/histology 890, 890f, 890t
hypersplenism 581
hypertension
    Conn's syndrome causing 2184
    end-stage renal disease 1643
    IgA nephropathy 1618
    malignant 1643
        renal involvement 1611f, 1645, 1645f, 1647
    medial degeneration induced by 1081–1082
    pulmonary see pulmonary hypertension
    renal cell carcinoma 1677
    retinal vasospasm 2318
    vascular nephrosclerosis related to 1643–1645
hypertensive renal disease 1643–1645, 1644f
hyperthecosis, ovary 1991–1992, 1992f
hyperthermia
    lesions associated 160
    malignant 2233
hyperthyroidism
    choriocarcinoma of testis 1753
    Graves' disease 2123
    neuromuscular abnormalities 2233
    pituitary adenoma causing 2103
hypertrophic actinic keratosis 244
hypertrophic osteoarthropathy 1108
hyphema, chronic, eye 2312
hypoadrenalism see Addison's disease
hypocorticalism 2175
hypoglycemia
    fibrosarcoma 325

insulinoma 1572
    islet cell hyperplasia 1569
    neoplasm-induced, tumors causing 1572–1573
hypogonadism 1738, 1741, 2110
hypokalemic periodic paralysis 2233
hypopharynx, synovial sarcoma 850
hypophosphatasemia 686
hypophysial arteries 2097
hypophysitis
    primary 2110–2112
    secondary 2112–2113
hypopigmentation, vulva 1896, 1896t
hypopituitarism 2098, 2106, 2108, 2110, 2111
    bone maturation disturbances 681
hypoplastic acute leukemia, bone marrow 618, 618f
hypoplastic myelodysplastic syndrome, bone marrow
    617–618
hypoproteinemia, hypertrophic gastritis 1340
hypospermatogenesis 1739, 1739f
hypothalamic-pituitary-adrenal (HPA) axis 2173, 2180f
hypothalamus
    gangliocytoma 2110
    pilocytic astrocytoma 2357
hypothyroidism 2110
    bone maturation disturbances 681
    neuromuscular abnormalities 2233
    pituitary adenoma causing 2103
    Riedel's disease 2122
    subacute thyroiditis 2120
hypotympanum 2268
hypoxemia 915–916
Hyrtl anastomoses 2064
hysterectomy specimens 1934, 1935–1936
hysterosalpingograms, foreign body granuloma due to
    138
H zone (muscle) 2215

I

iatrogenic lesions 135–166
    cytotoxic drugs/immunosuppression causing 147–151
    diagnostic procedures reaction 135–138
    due to surgical procedures 146–147
    ionizing radiation causing 151–158
    physical/chemical agents reaction 139–145
    radiation-associated tumors 158–160
    resembling neoplasms 147
I band, muscle 2215
idiopathic granulomatous hypophysitis 2112, 2112f
idiopathic inflammatory orbital pseudotumor 2295,
    2295f
idiopathic pulmonary fibrosis (IPF) 895
idiopathic pulmonary hemosiderosis (IPH) 884, 885f
idiopathic thrombocytopenic purpura (ITP), spleen 580
ifosfamide, Ewing family of tumors 385
IgA see immunoglobulin A (IgA)
IgA nephropathy 1609f, 1618–1620
IgM nephropathy 1608, 1620
IgM paraproteinemia 2258
ileal pouch-anal anastomosis 1392, 1394
ileitis, Crohn's disease 1391, 1392f
ileocecectomy 1390
ileum, neuroendocrine tumors 1425
ILVEN (inflammatory linear verrucous epidermal
    nevus) 241
image cytometry (image analysis) 36, 42–43
imiquimod, basal cell carcinoma of skin 246
immune activation, graft rejection mechanism 120, 122
immune competence, oral squamous cell carcinoma
    and 1170
immune complex(es)
    acute interstitial nephritis 1640
    circulating, lupus nephritis 1626
    renal disease mediated by 1603
immune complex deposition
    crescentic glomerulonephritis 1621–1622, 1621f
    fingerprints (in lupus) 1628, 1628f
    lupus 1628, 1628f
    membranoproliferative glomerulonephritis 1615
    membranous glomerulonephropathy 1614f, 1615

immune complex deposition (cont'd)
  mesangial 1609–1610, 1619, 1628, 1628f, 1634f
  paramesangial 1619
  subendothelial (kidney) 1616f
    postinfectious glomerulonephritis 1618, 1618f
    Schönlein-Henoch purpura 1619
  subendothelial, lupus 1626f, 1628, 1628f
immune-related necrotizing polyangiitis 1077–1078
immune thrombocytopenic purpura (ITP) 587, 617, 620
immunoblasts 524
  diffuse large B-cell lymphoma 558, 560f
  hantavirus pneumonia 879
  Hodgkin's disease 537, 540
  reactive paracortical hyperplasia 524, 525
  reactive proliferation, Hodgkin's disease vs 540
  small lymphocytic lymphoma 551
immunocompromised host
  diffuse alveolar hemorrhage 884
  lung disease 867
  respiratory tract infections 81, 874
immunocytochemistry
  at ultrastructural level 30
  see also immunohistochemistry
immunocytoma 289, 554
immunodeficiency diseases 113–116, 571
  lymphoproliferative disorders in 571
  primary/secondary 571
immunofluorescence 30
  kidney and renal biopsies 1602–1603
  oral cavity specimens 1138
  renal transplant biopsy 1651
  see also direct immunofluorescence; indirect
    immunofluorescence
immunoglobulin(s)
  deposits, lupus erythematosus 205f, 206
  enzyme bridge method 30–31
  gene rearrangements
    diffuse large B cell lymphoma 560
    follicular lymphoma 550
    lymphoblastic lymphoma 569
    lymphomas 544, 544t
  markers 31t
immunoglobulin A (IgA)
  antiendomysial antibody test 1374
  circulating complexes, cirrhosis-associated
    glomerulopathy 1632
  mesangial deposits 1612f
  nephropathy 1609f, 1618–1620
  selective (isolated) deficiency 113–114
  subcorneal pustular dermatosis of Sneddon and
    Wilkinson 216
immunoglobulin G (IgG) deposits
  membranoproliferative glomerulonephritis 1615
  membranous glomerulonephropathy 1614
immunoglobulin M (IgM)
  deposits
    membranoproliferative glomerulonephritis 1615
    mesangium 1609–1610
  hyper IgM syndrome 115
  nephropathy 1608, 1620
  paraproteinemia 2258
immunohistochemical stains 35
  costs, in metastasis of unknown primary origin 169t
  for endothelial cells, breast cancer prognosis 487–488
  FDA listing of recognized stains 12
immunohistochemistry 30–36, 178
  algorithms 178
  antigen (epitope) retrieval methods 32–33, 33f
  automation and tissue microarrays 36
  background staining 33
  CNS lesions 2336–2338
  cytological samples 35
  fixative 32
  liver biopsy 1470–1471, 1471f
  lymph nodes 508–510
  marker classes 31t
  metastases 178–182, 186
  methods 30–32

panels for primary malignant tumors 509t
quantitative 43
regulatory issues (USA) 35–36
requirements for definitive diagnoses 178
result interpretation and controls 33–35
see also specific tumors and conditions
immunologically-mediated diseases 113–133
immunologic techniques, infectious disease diagnosis
  61–62
immunoperoxidase stain 1653, 1653f, 2338
immunoperoxidase techniques, hepatocellular
  carcinoma 1534
immunoproliferative small intestinal disease (IPSID)
  657, 1450, 1451
  stages, histology and immunohistochemistry 1452
immunosuppression
  cervical neoplasia and 1856
  lymphoproliferative disorders with 571–572, 572f
  reactions to 147–151
  smooth muscle tumors associated 353
  toxicity after transplantation 127, 130f, 131
immunotactoid glomerulopathy 1635–1637, 1636f, 1637t
impetigo 217, 217f
impetigo of Bockhart 225
imprint preparations 6, 21–22
incidentaloma 171, 2178, 2179f
incisive canal cysts 1147–1148
inclusion bodies, acute CMV gastritis 1329, 1329f
inclusion body myositis (IBM) 2219–2221, 2221f
  differential diagnosis 2220t
incontinentia pigmenti (IP) 198, 198f
incus 2268–2269
  degenerative joint disease affecting 2282
'Indian-file' arrangement, tumor cells 2290
indirect immunofluorescence
  bullous pemphigoid 222–223
  celiac disease diagnosis 1374
indurative mastopathy 445
infantile fibromatosis
  calcifying aponeurotic fibroma vs 311
  digital 320, 322, 322f
  fibrodysplasia ossificans progressiva vs 387
  fibrous hamartoma of infancy vs 318
infantile hemangioendothelioma
  Kaposiform 274, 366–367, 367f
  liver 1541–1542, 1541f
infantile myofibromatosis 315
infantile polyarteritis nodosa see Kawasaki disease
infantile polyposis syndrome 1436
infants
  acute leukemia 628–629
  autosomal recessive polycystic kidney disease
    1662–1663, 1663f
infarction
  bone (osteonecrosis) 682, 683–684, 684f
  bone marrow 665–666
  breast 436
  chorionic villi 2071, 2072f
  CNS 2417
  colon 1386f
  kidney 1609f, 1646
  maternal floor 2072–2073, 2073f, 2080
  pituitary gland 2113
  salivary gland tumors 1205, 1211
  skeletal muscle 2238
  testis 1754
infection-associated hemophagocytic syndrome (IAHS)
  527–528, 528, 528f, 658, 658f, 659
infection-associated hemophagocytosis, spleen 578, 578f
infections/infectious diseases 57–112
  bronchiolitis (nontobacco) 906
  diagnostic techniques 58–62
  etiologic diagnosis 58–62, 59t
    bacteria 59–60
    forgotten cultures 62
    fungi 61
    histochemical stains 59–61, 60t
    immunologic detection 61–62
    mycobacteria 60–61

parasites 61
quality control 61
rapid direct examination 58–59
viruses 61
granulomatous dermatoses due to 215
host defense mechanisms see host defense
  mechanisms
immunodeficiency diseases 113, 114, 115, 116
malabsorption due to 1378
molecular technique application 106–108
organ-based approach 67–106
see also individual anatomic regions
pathology-based team 57–58
peripheral neuropathies 2243–2244
tissue responses 63t
see also bacterial infections; fungal infections;
  parasitic infections; viral infections
infectious endocarditis 99
  culture-negative 1060
  focal proliferative/necrotizing glomerulonephritis in
    1621
  heart valve vegetations 1059–1060, 1060f
infectious mononucleosis 101
  before Hodgkin's disease 535
  spleen 578, 578f
inferior vena cava (IVC), leiomyosarcoma 352–353
infertility
  endometrial changes 1949–1950
  endometriosis and 1952
  male 1738–1741
    germ cell tumor risk 1742
  ovarian changes 1988–1989
inflammation/inflammatory diseases
  acute response to 63–64, 63t
  allografts 130–131
  cartilage 225–228
  conjunctiva 2294
  ear 2271–2274
  esophagus see esophagitis
  eye 2312–2314
  fallopian tube 2040–2042
  hair follicles 225–228
  orbit 2294–2295
  ovary 1989
  peripheral nerves 2242–2244
  skeletal muscle 2218–2224, 2218t
  skin see skin
  thyroid gland 2120
  vagina 1919–1920
  see also specific anatomic sites and diseases
inflammatory bowel disease 1386
  adenoma-like lesions 1443
  bacterial colitis vs 1389
  bronchiolitis association 908, 909f
  colorectal carcinoma 1439, 1441–1443, 1443
  colorectal signet ring cell carcinoma 1439
  dysplasia in 1393–1394, 1393f, 1394f, 1441–1443,
    1442f, 1443t
  fulminant 1391–1392
  histology 1387–1389
  indeterminate type 1392
  primary sclerosing cholangitis with 1393, 1497
  see also Crohn's disease; ulcerative colitis
inflammatory cells
  gastroesophageal reflux disease 1282f
  skin 195
inflammatory fibroid polyp, stomach 1341, 1342f
inflammatory fibrosarcoma 331–332, 332f
inflammatory fibrous hyperplasia, oral cavity 1180
inflammatory linear verrucous epidermal nevus
  (ILVEN) 241
inflammatory malignant fibrous histiocytoma 335, 336f
inflammatory myofibroblastic tumor (plasma cell
    granuloma) 331, 332, 332f
  calcifying fibrous pseudotumor and 317
  chromosomal translocation 310t
  peritoneum 1022
  sinonasal region 796t, 823–824, 824f
  see also inflammatory pseudotumor

inflammatory myxohyaline tumor 327–328, 328f
inflammatory papillary hyperplasia 1164
inflammatory pseudotumor (inflammatory
        myofibroblastic) 331, 332, 332f
    cardiac 1066
    cervix 1841
    liver 1542
    lung 966–967, 967f
    lymph nodes 515, 515f
    renal 1696
    sinonasal region 796t, 823–824, 824f
    spleen 583, 583f
influenza
    myositis 2222
    pneumonia 94, 94f, 876, 876f
influenza virus 93–94
infundibular cysts, of skin 254, 254f
infundibular neurohypophysitis 2111
inhaled irritant gases 906
inhibin 1992, 2017, 2017t
'inlet patches', in esophagus 1283
in pleural effusions
    mesothelioma 1028, 1029, 1029f
    small cell lung carcinoma 1030, 1031f
in situ hybridization 45, 46–47
    chromogenic (CISH) 47
    fluorescent see fluorescence in situ hybridization
        (FISH)
    human papillomavirus 1856f, 1857, 1888, 1888f
    lymph node specimens 510
    microorganisms 107
    at ultrastructural level 30
'insular and trabecular round cell sarcoma' 750
insulin-like growth factor II (IGF-II) 1573
insulinoma 1572–1573
integrins, loss, metastases mechanism 167
intercalary 'peg' cells, fallopian tube 2040
interface change, skin, definition 195
interface dermatoses 203–206, 203t, 222
interferon alfa, chronic myeloid leukemia 634
interferon gamma, T cells (CD4) releasing 122
interfusal fibers 2217
Intergroup Ewing's Sarcoma Study 385
Intergroup Rhabdomyosarcoma Study Group (IRSG)
        356, 357, 359, 850, 2297
interleukin-1 (IL-1), T cells secreting 122
interleukin-1 beta (IL-1 beta), intestinal gastric
        adenocarcinoma 1355
interleukin-2 (IL-2), T cells secreting 122
interleukin-3 (IL-3), T cells secreting 122
interleukin-4 (IL-4), T cells secreting 122
interlobar arteries 1600
interlobular arteries 1600
intermediate filaments, markers 31t
internal auditory canal (IAC), meatus, acoustic
        neuroma 2279, 2279f
International Agency for Research on Cancer (IARC),
        lung carcinogens 935
International Association for the Study of the Liver
        (IASL) 1488
International Consensus Committee classification of
        idiopathic interstitial pneumonia 893t
International Federation of Gynecology and Obstetrics
        (FIGO)
    cervical carcinoma 1857, 1857t
    endometrial adenocarcinoma 1958, 1958t
    gestational trophoblastic disease 2084t
    vulvar squamous cell carcinoma 1909, 1910f
International Neuroblastoma Staging System (INSS)
        383, 383t, 2196, 2197t, 2198
International Prognostic Index, lymphomas 545, 547t,
        557
International Prognostic Scoring System (IPSS),
        myelodysplastic syndromes 637, 637t
International Society for the Study of Vulvovaginal
        Disease (ISSVD) 1891–1892
International Union Against Cancer (UICC), breast
        cancer prognostic factors 489
interobserver agreement, quality management 10

interpectoral nodes (Rotter's) 420, 429
intersex states 1736–1738
    true gonadal intersex 1736, 1736t
interstitial cells of Cajal (ICC)
    colonic pseudo-obstruction 1404
    gastrointestinal stromal tumors 353, 1345
intervertebral disc, prolapsed 697–698
intestinal adenoma see small intestine
'intestinal angina' 1381
intestinal metaplasia
    bladder 1709, 1710f, 1720
    cervix 1838
    extrahepatic bile ducts 1584
    gallbladder 1578, 1579f
    stomach, staining 21f
intestinal neuronal dysplasia 1404
intestinal type adenocarcinoma, sinonasal see sinonasal
        region
intestine(s)
    adenoma see large intestine
    amyloidosis 1405, 1406f
    drug-induced diseases 1401–1402
    graft-versus-host disease 1402, 1403f
    histology (normal) 1373
    infectious diseases 1395–1400
        bacterial 1395–1398
        fungal 1399
        protozoal 1399–1400
        spirochetosis 1398
        viral 1398–1399
    inflammation
        surgical procedures associated 1394–1395
        see also colitis; duodenitis
    ionizing radiation effect 155
    ischemia 1380–1384
        acute 1381, 1381f
        mechanical causes 1382
        mucosal prolapse 1382
        nonocclusive mesenteric 1380–1381
        vascular occlusive diseases causing 1381–1382
    neuromuscular disorders 1403–1404
    perforation 1382
    pseudo-obstruction, chronic 1404
    radiation-associated tumors 159
    strictures, Crohn's disease 1391
    systemic vasculitides affecting 1384–1386
    vascular occlusion 1381–1382
    'watershed zones' 1380
    see also colon; gastrointestinal tract; large intestine;
        small intestine; individual anatomic regions
INTI gene 1671
intracerebral hematoma 2416
intracranial pressure (ICP) elevation, brain tumors
        2345, 2379, 2384
intracytoplasmic vesicle, microvillus inclusion disease
        1377f
intraepithelial layer of Dierks 1831
intraepithelial lymphocytes (IELs) 1373
    celiac disease 1374, 1375, 1375f
    diseases with/numbers 1375
    esophagus 1282, 1282f
intraepithelial lymphocytosis 1375–1376, 1401
intraepithelial neoplasia see specific types/sites
intramedullary hemorrhage 616
intraneural fibrosis 2245
intranuclear pseudoinclusions see nuclear
        pseudoinclusions
intranuclear viral inclusions see Cowdry A intranuclear
        inclusions
intraocular hemorrhage 2312
intraocular pressure, elevation 2314
intraocular tumors 2306–2311
    of childhood 2311
    melanoma see uveal malignant melanoma
    metastatic 2309
    nonpigmented 2309
    pigmented (not melanoma) 2309
    see also retinoblastoma
intraosseous ganglion 755, 755f

intrathyroidal thymoma 2140
intratubular germ cell neoplasia (IGCN) 1743–1744
    unclassified (IGCNU) 1734, 1741, 1742, 1744,
        1745f
intrauterine devices (IUDs)
    actinomycosis association 70, 143, 2041
    cervical changes 1846, 1848, 1848f
    cervicovaginal smear abnormalities 143
    chronic nongranulomatous endometritis 1945
    complications/reactions 143–144
    endometrial changes 1947
    tumors associated 143–144
intrauterine infections 2068–2070, 2080
intussusception 1382, 1407
in vitro fertilization (IVF) 1739
iodine
    deficiency 2122
    papillary thyroid carcinoma due to 2127
ionizing radiation 151
    see also radiation-induced conditions/changes
IPEX syndrome 1376
iridocyclectomy 2309
iridocyclitis, endogenous chronic nongranulomatous
        2313
iris
    juvenile xanthogranuloma 2311
    melanoma 2306, 2308
    neovascularization 2315, 2316f
'iris' lesions 203
iron
    intraocular foreign bodies 2312
    overload, liver involvement 1503–1505
    storage 612, 619
iron deficiency anemia 1169, 1374
iron pneumoconiosis 905t
irritant contact dermatitis 196
ischemic colitis
    in amyloidosis 1406f
    biopsy 1388
    necrotizing vasculitis causing 1385f
ischemic fasciitis (atypical decubital fibroplasia) 314,
        315f
ischemic heart disease, mitral regurgitation 1056
ischemic infarction, colon 1386f
islets of Langerhans 1549
    hyperplasia 1569–1570
isobutyl 2-cyanoacrylate 140, 140f
isoniazid, hepatocellular injury 1476f
Ito cells (stellate cells in liver) 1474, 1474f
itraconazole 73

J
'jack-straw' crystals 354
Jaffe–Campanacci syndrome 737, 753
Jagged 1 gene, mutations 1502
jaundice, recurrent, of pregnancy 1496
jaw(s)
    cementoblastoma 1193
    cemento-osseous dysplasia 1193–1194, 1194f
    central giant cell reparative granuloma 815
    in cherubism 1193, 1193f
    fibrous dysplasia 1190–1191
    giant cell reparative granuloma 752
    giant cell tumor (granuloma) 1183
    myxoma 1156–1157, 1157f
    ossifying fibroma 1192–1193, 1192f
        fibrous dysplasia vs 1191, 1192
    osteoblastoma 1194
    osteogenic sarcoma 815
    osteoid osteoma 1194
    osteoma 1193
    osteosarcoma 1194
    peripheral giant cell granuloma (tumor) 1182
    tumors 1194–1195
    see also mandible; maxilla
J chain 542
JC virus 68t, 75–76, 119, 2408
jejunoleitis, ulcerative 1376
jejunum, neuroendocrine tumors 1425

'jelly belly' 1025
joint disease 691–697
joint replacement 144, 691, 694–695
    failure 694f
joints 690–691
    artificial 694–695
joint tissues 690–691
Jones modified hexamine silver technique 19f
jugular bulb 2275
jugulotympanic paraganglioma 2276–2277, 2277f,
    2279
juvenile active ossifying fibroma 1192
juvenile aggressive osteoblastoma 815
juvenile capillary hemangioma 269–270, 269f, 1186
juvenile carcinoma of breast 483
juvenile dermatomyositis 206
juvenile fibroadenoma of breast 435
juvenile granulosa cell tumor 2015, 2017–2018, 2017f
    Sertoli cell tumor vs 1759
    testis 1760–1761, 1760f
    yolk sac tumor (testis) vs 1753
juvenile hemangioma 365
juvenile malignant melanoma 278
juvenile myelomonocytic leukemia (JMML) 638
juvenile nasopharyngeal angiofibroma (JNA) 394
juvenile (psammomatoid) ossifying fibroma 742–743,
    743f, 813
juvenile Paget's disease 686
juvenile papillomatosis, breast 443–444
juvenile polyposis syndrome (JPS) 1436, 1437f
juvenile xanthogranuloma 228, 287, 287f
juxta-articular myxoma (JAM) 394
juxtacortical chondroma 711–712
juxtacortical chondrosarcoma 718
juxtacortical osteosarcoma 727
juxtaglomerular apparatus 1598
    renal artery stenosis 1645, 1645f
juxtaglomerular cell tumor 1694, 1694f
juxtamedullary (cortico-medullary) region (kidney)
    1598

K

Kadish grading system 802, 803t
kala-azar 76
Kamino bodies 278, 279, 280f
Kaposiform (infantile) hemangioendothelioma 366,
    367f
    Kaposi's sarcoma vs 274, 366
Kaposi's sarcoma 274–275, 368–371
    African (endemic) form 274, 368
        lymphadenopathic variant 274
    AIDS (epidemic)-associated form 121t, 274–275,
        368–371, 369f
        differential diagnosis 370–371
        generalized form 368
        lymphangioma-like variant 369–370
        nodular stage 275, 275f, 369, 369f, 370–371,
            370f
        patch lesions (early stage) 275, 275f, 368–369,
            369f
        plaque stage 275, 275f, 369
        pleomorphic change (malignant transformation)
            370
        promontory sign 369, 369f
    bone marrow 665f, 666
    classic (European) form 274, 368
    differential diagnosis 275–276
        Castleman's disease vs 522
        HIV-associated lymphadenopathy vs 524
        Kaposiform hemangioendothelioma vs 274, 366
        oral pyogenic granuloma vs 1181
        smooth muscle tumors vs 353
        stasis dermatitis vs 197
        vulvar pyogenic granuloma vs 1902
    gastrointestinal tract 1449, 1450f
    iatrogenic 274
    immunohistochemistry 275
    immunosuppression-associated form 274, 368
    intestine 1449, 1450f

larynx 850
liver 1544
lung 973, 973f
lymph nodes 514, 514f, 515
oral cavity 1186
retiform hemangioendothelioma and 366
spleen 592
Kaposi's sarcoma-associated herpesvirus (KSHV) 274,
    368, 514, 655–656, 973
    Castleman's disease 522
Karnovsky's solution 2335
Kartagener's syndrome 911
karyorrhectic debris 209, 212, 293, 294f
Kasabach–Merritt syndrome 271, 274, 363, 366,
    367f
Kawasaki disease 1072t, 1075
    lymphadenopathy 532, 532f
Kearns–Sayre syndrome 2231t
keloids 8, 24f, 231, 231f, 264
    ear 2274
    hypertrophic scars vs 2274
    steroid injection 141
keratan sulfate 2302
keratin
    abnormal, epidermolysis bullosa 225
    accumulation, cholesteatoma 2273
    pancreatoblastoma 1561
    pleural effusions 1032, 1032f
    thymic seminoma 1118
    thymoma 1100, 1100f
    see also cytokeratin
keratin 903 (34βE12) see 34βE12 monoclonal antibody
    (start of index)
keratin-filled cysts see horn cysts
keratin flakes, epidermoid cysts of skin 254, 254f
keratinization
    'abrupt' (trichilemmal) 254, 254f, 261, 261f
    adenosquamous carcinoma of pancreas 1558
    'church spire' form 248
    esophageal squamous cell carcinoma 1295, 1296,
        1296f
    oral squamous cell carcinoma 1172
    sinonasal squamous cell carcinoma 790, 791
    thymic carcinoma 1107, 1109f
keratinocytes 193–194
    acantholytic, warty dyskeratoma 242, 243f
    atypia, squamous cell carcinoma of skin 246, 246f
    atypical, pagetoid spread 246, 246f
    'balling up' (acantholysis) 195
    ballooning degeneration 221, 1888, 1888f
    basal, atypical 220
    basal, pemphigus vulgaris 218
    cytokines produced 1138
    dying 195
        erythema multiforme 203, 203f
        graft-versus-host disease 204, 204f
        incontinentia pigmenti 198
        lichen planus 202, 202f
        lichen sclerosus 232
        lupus erythematosus 205
        pityriasis lichenoides et varioliformis acuta
            (PLEVA) 204
        subepidermal blisters 222
    excess, epidermal nevi 241, 241f
    HSV vulvitis 1888, 1888f
    maturation 194
    nuclear atypia 243, 243f
    proliferation, psoriasis 199
    in stratum granulosum (granular layer) 194
    terminal differentiation 194
    'tombstone' pattern 218, 219f
    vacuolization 241, 241f
keratin 'pearls'
    esophageal squamous cell carcinoma 1294, 1296,
        1296f, 1297, 1298f
    oral squamous cell carcinoma 1172
    sebaceous carcinoma of skin 260
    squamous cell carcinoma of skin 247, 247f
    thymoma 1099

keratin plugs, warty dyskeratoma 242, 243f
keratitis
    acanthamoeba 2301, 2302f
    acute bacterial/fungal 2301
    acute herpetic dendritic 2301–2302
    chronic herpetic stromal 2301–2302
    chronic luetic interstitial 2302
    measles 2303
keratoacanthoma 248
    eyelid 2290
    intraoral 1164
    oral cavity 1164–1165, 1175
    skin 1164
keratoconjunctivitis 129, 2294
keratoconjunctivitis sicca 2298
keratoconus (conical cornea) 2301
keratocyst, odontogenic see odontogenic keratocyst
keratohyaline granules 194
    oral verrucous carcinoma 1174, 1175f
    verruca vulgaris 241, 241f
keratopathy
    bullous (corneal edema) 2301, 2301f
    types 2303
keratoplasty, emergent penetrating 2301
keratosis
    actinic (solar) see actinic (solar) keratosis
    with atypia, laryngeal 839
    inverted follicular 2290
    lichen planus-like (benign lichenoid) 242–243
    'pigmented actinic' 277
    seborrheic see seborrheic keratosis
keratosis follicularis see Darier's disease (keratosis
    follicularis)
kerion 225
Kerley B lines 885, 915
Ketron-Goodman syndrome 292
Ki-67
    atypical pulmonary carcinoid tumors 987, 994
    basal cell carcinoma of skin 246
    Burkitt's lymphoma 570
    cervical intraepithelial neoplasia 1855, 1856f
    epithelial kidney tumors 1672
    gastrointestinal stromal tumors 1348
    lymph node evaluation 509
    parathyroid carcinoma vs adenoma 2162
    salivary gland tumors 1228, 1244–1245
    sialoblastoma 1227
    trichoepithelioma 251
kidney
    adenoma
        cortical 1673, 1673f
        metanephric 1673, 1674f
        papillary 1673
    amyloidosis 1631, 1631f, 1632, 1632f
    anatomy 1598–1601
    angiomyolipoma 970, 1690–1691, 1691f
    biopsy 1597
        communication with clinicians 1603–1604
        diffuse vs focal lesions 1603
        evaluation techniques 1601–1604, 1601f
        interpretation 1603
        percutaneous 1597
        staining 1601–1602
        transplant biopsy 1597
    blood supply 1600–1601
    carcinoid tumor 1689–1690
    cholesterol emboli 1646, 1646f
    clear cell adenocarcinoma, pulmonary metastases
        962, 964f
    clear cell sarcoma 1670, 1670f
        Wilms' tumor vs 1668, 1670
    congenital and hereditary diseases 1622–1626
    congenital malformations 1661
    cortex, anatomy 1598
    cystic diseases 1622–1626, 1662–1665, 1662f, 1663f
        acquired 1663–1664, 1664f
        aspiration of cysts 1665
        autosomal dominant (adult) polycystic 1662,
            1662f, 1663f, 1665

kidney (cont'd)
  autosomal recessive (infantile) polycystic
      1662–1663 1663f
    cytology 1665
    medullary 1664
    simple cysts 1664–1665, 1665f
  diabetes mellitus 1629, 1629f, 1630f
  diffuse cortical necrosis 1646–1647
  dysplasia 1661, 1662f
  ectopic 1661
  epithelial tumors (adults) 1672–1690
    classification 1672, 1672t
    prognostic markers 1672–1673
    see also renal cell carcinoma
  epithelioid angiomyolipoma 1691, 1692t
  fat emboli 1646, 1646f
  glomerular diseases see entries beginning
      glomerulo-; glomerular diseases
  hemangioma 1692
  hematopoietic tumors 1693–1694
  horseshoe 1661, 1689
  in hypertension 1643–1645
  hypoplasia 1661
  immune complex-mediated 1603
  infarcts 1609f, 1646
  inflammatory myofibroblastic pseudotumor
      1696–1697
  interstitium 1600
    see also renal tubular interstitium
  ionizing radiation effect 156
  juxtaglomerular cell tumors 1694–1695, 1694f
  leiomyoma 1692
  leiomyosarcoma 1692–1693, 1693f
  in lupus see lupus nephritis
  lymphoma 1672, 1690, 1693–1694, 1694f
  lymphoreticular tumors 1693–1694
  malposition 1661
  medical diseases 1597–1659
    classification 1604
    clinical syndromes 1604–1654
    communication with clinicians 1603–1604
    evaluation 1597, 1601–1604
    'full-house' staining 1627, 1633
    glomerular see glomerular diseases
    immunofluorescent evaluation 1602–1603
    light microscopy algorithms 1604t, 1605t, 1606t
    light microscopy and staining 1601–1602, 1603
  medulla 1598, 1600
  medullary carcinoma 1687, 1687f
  medullary sponge 1664
  mesenchymal tumors
    benign 1690–1692
    malignant 1692–1693
  mesoblastic nephroma see nephroma, mesoblastic
  metabolic disorders affecting 1642–1643
  metanephric neoplasms 1673–1674
  metastases in 171t, 172–173, 1694
  mixed epithelial and stromal tumors 1695, 1695f
  mucinous tubular carcinoma 1685–1686, 1686f
  'myeloma' 1630, 1630f
  nephroma see nephroma
  neuroendocrine tumors 1689–1690
  oncocytoma 1674–1676, 1675f
  pelvic 1661
  plasma cell dyscrasia-associated conditions
      1630–1632
  renal cell carcinoma see renal cell carcinoma
  renomedullary interstitial cell tumors 1695–1696
  rhabdoid tumor 1668, 1670–1671, 1671t
  sarcomas 1692–1693, 1693f
  sarcomatoid renal cell carcinoma 1688
  specimen collection 1597
  specimen handling 1603
  spindle cell tumors 1685–1686, 1686f, 1688
  surgical diseases 1661–1705
  thrombotic microangiopathies 1647–1648, 1647f
  transplantation see renal transplantation
  tubular interstitial disorders see tubular interstitial
      disorders
  tubules/tubular interstitium see renal tubular
      interstitium
  tubulocystic carcinoma 1686–1687, 1686f
  tumors
    gross techniques and reporting 1665–1666, 1672
    pediatric 1665–1672
    see also specific tumors
  vascular disorders see renal vascular disorders
  in vasculitides 1648–1649, 1648f
  weight 1598
Kiel classification (updated), lymphomas 544, 546t,
    554, 561, 1762
Kikuchi histiocytic necrotizing lymphadenitis 531–532,
    531f, 561
Kimmelstiel-Wilson lesion 1602f, 1629, 1629f
Kimura lymphadenopathy 519, 519f
Kimura's disease/tumor 271
  see also angiolymphoid hyperplasia with eosinophilia
Kinyoun stain 60, 60t
KIT protein (CD117) see CD117 (c-kit)
Klatskin tumors 1585
Klebsiella rhinoscleromatis 78
Klinefelter's syndrome 1738
  mature teratoma of mediastinum 1115
  mediastinal embryonal carcinoma 1118
  testis biopsy 1740, 1740f
Klippel-Trenaunay syndrome 365, 1085, 1692
Klippel-Trenaunay-Weber syndrome 268, 363–364
Kluver-Barrera stain 2335t
knuckle pads 320, 322
koebnerization 199, 202
koilocytes
  cervical intraepithelial neoplasia 1854
  verruca vulgaris 241, 241f
koilocytosis
  cervical sample 1842, 1843f, 1854, 1854f
  vaginal condyloma 1921
  vulval condyloma 1887, 1887f
Korean hemorrhagic fever 95
Krabbe's disease 2246
KRAS gene mutations 1586, 1588
K-ras mutations, lung cancer 937
kraurosis vulvae 232, 1892
  see also lichen sclerosus (et atrophicus)
Krukenberg tumor 469, 2038–2039, 2039f
Kugelberg–Welander disease (spinal muscular atrophy
    type III) 2226
Kulchitsky cells, neuroendocrine carcinoma arising
    from 844
Kupffer cells
  function 1476
  hyperplasia 1477, 1477f, 1478
  hypertrophy 1478, 1478f, 1479, 1481, 1513
  phospholipidosis 1490, 1490f
  polarizing microscopy 1471
kuru plaques 2413
Küttner tumor 1258
Kveim test 533

L

labeled avidin biotin (LAB) 31
labeled streptavidin biotin (LSAB) method 31
labia (majora and minora) 1885
  anomalies/disorders 1887
labyrinth (inner ear) 2269
  anatomy 2268, 2269, 2269f
  membranous 2267, 2269, 2269f
  osseous 2267, 2269
    otospongiosis 2283, 2283f
labyrinthitis 2272, 2272f
lacrimal drainage system 2291–2292
lacrimal gland 2298–2299
  adenocarcinoma 2299
  adenoid cystic carcinoma 2298–2299, 2299f
  epithelial tumors 2298–2299, 2299f
  mixed tumors 2299
  mucoepidermoid carcinoma 2298, 2299
  pleomorphic adenoma 2298, 2299f
lacrimal gland ducts, cystic dilatation 2298
lacrimal obstruction 2291
lacrimal sac, tumors 2291–2292
lacrimal stones 2291
lactation 419–420, 420f
  breast carcinoma 438
lactic dehydrogenase 1647, 2213
lactiferous ducts 419, 420f
Lactobacillus acidophilus 1851
lactotrophs 2095, 2096f
  adenomas see pituitary adenoma
  development 2094–2095
  hyperplasia 2110
Lambert-Eaton syndrome 2227
lamina lucida 194
lamina propria
  colon 1373
  esophageal 1282–1283
  small intestine 1373
  vaginal 1919
laminin, liver biopsy 1470
Langerhans cell(s) 194, 287, 289, 657, 660f, 759, 759f,
    969f
  in airways 861
  appearance 924, 924f
  characteristics 572, 573f, 2284
  in dermatopathic lymphadenopathy 526, 526f, 527
  as HIV reservoir 117
  microabscesses 196, 196f, 217
  neoplastic 573
  in paracortex of lymph node 524
Langerhans cell granulomatosis 195, 610f
Langerhans cell histiocytosis 657, 659–660, 660f,
    759–760, 759f
  bone marrow 659–660
  differential diagnosis 573
    Rosai-Dorfman disease vs 529
  disseminated see Letterer–Siwe disease
  electron microscopy 30f
  fine needle aspirates 760, 760f
  immunohistochemistry 289, 760
  Langerhans cells in 572, 573, 573f, 861
  lymph node involvement 571–573, 573f
    Kimura disease vs 519
  pituitary involvement 2110
  pulmonary 572, 922–925
    'burnt out' (resolved) 924–925, 925f
    immunohistochemistry 924f
    radiology/pathology 924–925, 924f
  sinonasal 826
  skin involvement 289, 289f
  temporal bone and ear involvement 2284
  terminology 759
Langerhans cell sarcoma 572
large cell calcifying Sertoli cell tumors (LCCSCT)
    1758, 1759–1760, 1760f
large cell neuroendocrine carcinoma (LCNEC)
  cervix 1875
  of lung 987–988, 989–990, 989f, 990f
    carcinoma of lung vs 964
    differential diagnosis 994t
  of ovary 2014
large cells, in effusions 183
large intestine
  adenocarcinoma 1434
    adenomas with 1436
    see also colorectal adenocarcinoma
  adenoma 1394, 1419t, 1432–1436, 1433f
    adenocarcinoma with 1436
    dysplastic changes 1432–1433
    flat 1434
    in inflammatory bowel disease 1443
    mixed hyperplastic polyps 1434
    as precursor for adenocarcinoma 1438
    reporting and nomenclature 1434
    serrated 1433, 1435f
    sessile 1433f
    tubular 1432, 1434f
    tubulovillous 1432
    villous 1432, 1435f

large intestine (*cont'd*)
  adenoma-carcinoma sequence 1435
  adenomatous polyposis syndromes 1436–1438
    Cronkhite-Canada syndrome 1437
    see also familial adenomatous polyposis (FAP)
  angiosarcoma 1449
  carcinoma 1419t, 1434
  diffuse lipomatous polyposis 1450
  dysplasia 1434
    dysplasia-associated lesion or mass (DALM)
      1394, 1443
    high-grade 1435, 1442, 1442f
    histology 1442, 1442f
    'indefinite' 1441
    in inflammatory bowel disease 1441–1443, 1442f,
      1443t
    low-grade 1442, 1442f
  epithelial tumors 1431–1443
    benign 1431–1432
  fibromatosis 1450
  ganglioneuroma 1446–1447
  ganglioneuromatous polyposis 1446–1447
  granular cell tumors 1450
  hamartomatous syndromes 1436–1438
    juvenile polyposis syndrome 1436, 1437f
  hyperplastic polyps 1431–1432, 1432f
    atypical 1432
    mixed adenomatous polyps 1434
  intramucosal adenocarcinoma 1433, 1435, 1435f
  leiomyoma 1445, 1446f
  leiomyomatosis 1445
  leiomyosarcoma 1445, 1447f
  lipoma 1449–1450
  liposarcoma 1449–1450
  lymphangioma 1449
  lymphoproliferative tumors 1450–1453
  mesenchymal tumors 1443–1445, 1443–1448
    see also gastrointestinal stromal tumors (GISTs)
  neurofibroma 1446
  neurofibromatosis type 1 1446
  polyps
    atypical juvenile 1436
    ganglioneuromatous 1446–1447
    hyperplastic *see above*
    juvenile 1436, 1437f
    sessile serrated 1432
    see also colon, polyps
  pseudocarcinoma 1433
  schwannoma 1446
  smooth muscle tumors 1445
  tumor-like conditions of blood vessels 1448–1450
  tumors 1419–1464
    distribution 1419t
    neural origin 1446–1448
    vascular tumors 1448–1450
  see also colon; intestine(s)
large loop excision of transformation zone (LLETZ),
    thermal artifact due to 137
laryngectomy 833
laryngitis 834–835, 835f
laryngocele 835
laryngotracheal groove 834
larynx 833–855
  adenocarcinoma 846
  adenoid cystic carcinoma 846–847, 847f
  adenoid (acantholytic) squamous cell carcinoma 846
  anatomy and histology 834
  basaloid squamous carcinoma 843, 845–846
  benign connective tissue tumors 848–849
  benign fibrous histiocytoma 848
  blastomycosis 835
  carcinoma
    carcinogens and risk factors 839, 841
    ionizing radiation effect 154, 155
    specimens and standard sections 833–834, 834f
  carcinoma ex pleomorphic adenoma 847
  carcinoma in situ 839, 840f, 841, 841f
  chondroma 849, 849f
  chondrosarcoma 849

cysts 835
dysplasia 838–839, 840f
embryology 834
embryonal rhabdomyosarcoma 850
epithelial hyperplastic lesions 838, 840f
epithelial tumors
  benign 836–838, 838f
  malignant 842–846
  surface 843
epithelioid leiomyoma (leiomyoblastoma) 849
fibroma 848
fibrosarcoma 849
fungal infections 835
future tumor research 850–851
glandular tumors (malignant/benign) 846–848
granular cell tumor 848, 848f
hemangioma 849
hemangiopericytoma 850
hemangiosarcoma 850
hyperplasia and precancerous lesions 838–842
inflammatory and degenerative conditions 834–835
intraepithelial neoplasia 839, 840f
Kaposi's sarcoma 850
keratinizing carcinoma 842, 843f
leiomyoma 848–849
leiomyosarcoma 849
liposarcoma 850
lymphangioma 849
lymphoepithelial carcinoma 846
lymphoma 843, 850
malignant fibrous histiocytoma 849, 850f
malignant tumors of connective tissue/cartilage
    849–850
melanoma 848
metastatic tumors 848
microabscess 844
myoepithelioma 847
myxoma 848
neoplasms 836–850
neuroendocrine carcinoma 843–844
neurogenic tumors 848
nodule (singer's node) 835
nonkeratinizing carcinoma 842, 843f
non-neoplastic conditions 834–836
oncocytic carcinoma 847
osteosarcoma 850
plasmacytoma 850
pleomorphic adenoma 847
primary paraganglioma 843–844
pseudosarcoma (carcinosarcoma) 846
pseudotumor 834, 835–836
relapsing polychondritis 835
rhabdomyoma 849
rheumatoid arthritis 835
salivary gland type tumors 847–848
sarcomatoid carcinoma 846
small cell carcinoma 843, 844
specimen handling 833–834
spindle cell carcinoma 846, 846f, 847f
squamous cell carcinoma 842–843, 843f
  adenoid (acantholytic) 846
  blastomycosis *vs* 79–80
  ionizing radiation effect 153–154
  molecular/genetic markers 843, 844t
  papillary 846, 1175
  spindle cell 846, 846f, 847f
squamous papilloma 836–838, 838f
surface epithelial tumors 843
synovial sarcoma 850
thermal burns 834
tuberculoid leprosy 835
tuberculosis 835
verrucous carcinoma 13, 844–, 845f
verrucous hyperplasia 845
Wegener's granulomatosis 835
see also trachea; vocal cords
laser glaucoma surgery 2316–2317
laser microprobe mass analysis (LAMMA) 30
laser scanning cytometry 42

laser therapy, thermal artifact in tissue 137
lateral periodontal cysts 1142–1143, 1142f
lateral ventricles
  ependymoma 2364
  tumor differential diagnosis 2348t
LATS antibodies 229
Lauren's classification, gastric adenocarcinoma 1354
Lawrence–Seip syndrome 1887
lawsuits, in anatomic pathology 10–13
laxatives, mucosal melanosis due to 1404
lead nephropathy, chronic 1641, 1641f
Leber's hereditary optic neuropathy 2231t
Ledderhose's disease 320
Leder stain (chloroacetate esterase; CAE) 19, 575, 610,
    613, 622
legal (medical) risks, fine needle aspiration (FNA)
    biopsy 28
Legionella micdadei 65, 875
Legionella pneumonia 81, 82f, 874–875, 875f
Legionella pneumophila 81, 82f, 875
Legionnaires disease 81, 874–875, 875f
Leigh syndrome 2231t
leiomyoblastoma 348, 351
  larynx 849
  uterine 1971
leiomyoma 347–350
  atypical, uterine 1971
  benign metastasizing, of lung 970–971, 971f
  of bone 771
  breast 446
  broad ligament 2048
  cellular, uterine 1971
  cervix 1842, 1842f
  cutaneous (pilar) 348, 348f
  of deep soft tissue 350
  degenerative change (hemorrhagic) 348
  epithelioid, uterine 1971
  esophageal 1314–1315
  fallopian tube 2045
  familial multiple 348
  gastrointestinal tract 1445, 1445f, 1446f
  genital 348–349, 349f
  hypertrophic scar *vs* 231
  immunohistochemistry 796t
  intraocular 2309
  kidney 1692
  larynx 848–849
  multiple uterine (Reed's syndrome) 348
  nipple 349
  oral cavity 1185
  ovary 2026
  prostate 1820
  round ligament 2048
  scrotal 349, 349f
  sinonasal 796t, 821
  of skin and subcutaneous tissue 347–350
  stomach 1345, 1346f
  thyroid 2140
  uterus *see* uterine corpus
  vagina 1922
  vascular (angiomyoma) 349–350, 350f
    oral cavity 1185
  vulvar 349, 1900–1901
leiomyoma cutis 348
leiomyomatosis
  esophageal 1315
  gastrointestinal tract 1445
  intravenous, uterine 1973, 1973f
  of lymph nodes 514–515
  uterine 1973
leiomyomatosis peritonealis disseminata 1021, 1973
leiomyosarcoma 349f, 350–353, 350f
  bladder 1722, 1722f
  of bone 771
  broad ligament 2048
  cervix 1877
  criteria for malignancy 352
  cutaneous/subcutaneous 352
  deep soft tissue 352

desmin expression absence 351
differential diagnosis 351–352
'epithelioid' 349, 351, 1916
esophageal 1315
gastrointestinal tract 1445
gastrointestinal wall tumors 353–354, 354f
iatrogenic reactions resembling 147
of inferior vena cava (IVC) 352–353
larynx and trachea 849
monophasic synovial sarcoma vs 404
myofibrosarcoma vs 332
myxoid, bladder 1722, 1722f
nipple 349
nodular fasciitis vs 313
paratesticular region 1766
pleomorphic soft tissue
    malignant fibrous histiocytoma vs 335
    pleomorphic rhabdomyosarcoma vs 362
poorly differentiated 334
prostate 1820, 1820f
pulmonary artery 353
rectal 1445, 1447f
renal 1692–1693, 1693f
retroperitoneal 352
sinonasal 821, 821f
stomach 1345
thyroid 2140
uterine see uterine corpus, leiomyosarcoma
vagina 1925
vascular 352–353
venous 353
vulva 1916
Leishmania 61, 76
Leishmaniasis 76
cutaneous 76, 77f
toxoplasmic lymphadenitis vs 520
visceral, hepatic granuloma 1511
Lennert's lymphoma 294
lens 2299–2300
opacification see cataracts
phacoanaphylactic endophthalmitis 2300, 2300f
pseudoexfoliation 2316
lensectomy 2304
lens epithelial cells, proliferation/fibrous metaplasia
    2300
lentigines
multiple 277
vulvar 1896–1897
lentiginous nevus, speckled 277
lentigo
solar (senile) 277
vaginal 1922
lentigo maligna 283, 284f
lentigo maligna melanoma 284–285
lentigo simplex 277, 277f
vulvar 1896–1897
leonine facies 228
LEOPARD complex 277
leprosy
borderline 533
cutaneous 66f, 215
hepatic granuloma 1511
lepromatous 215, 228, 533
lymphadenitis 533
peripheral neuropathy 2243–2244
tuberculoid 215, 533, 835, 2244
Leptothrix, cervical infection 1849
Leser-Trelat, sign 242
lethal midline granuloma (sinonasal lymphoma)
    824–826, 825t
Letterer–Siwe disease 289, 571, 659–660, 759, 826
bone involvement 690, 2284
Leu-7 (CD57) 181, 387
leukemia
acute 620–631
    alkylating agents association 149
    of ambiguous lineage 630–631
    bone marrow 620–631
    chromosomal abnormalities 629–630, 629t

classification 620, 621, 622t, 626, 627t
cytochemical/immunologic diagnosis 621, 623t
cytogenetics 620
definition 620
diagnosis 621
hypoplastic (hypocellular), bone marrow 618,
    618f
infants 628–629
mediastinal germ cell tumor with 1107
prognostic factors 630, 630t
spleen involvement 584
acute basophilic (ABL) 624
acute erythroleukemia (AEL, M6) 621t
acute lymphoblastic (ALL) 620, 627–628, 641
B-lineage 569, 628, 628t, 630–631
Burkitt's lymphoma with 627, 627f
chromosomal abnormalities 629–630, 629t
classification 627, 628t
cytogenetics/markers 628
FAB groups (L1-L3) 627
leukemia cutis 294
myeloid-associated antigens 631
Philadelphia chromosome 629
precursor B-ALL 627, 628
prognostic factors 630, 630t
testis involvement 1762
T-lineage 628, 628t, 630–631
acute megakaryoblastic (M7) 621t, 622
acute monocytic (M5) 621t
acute myeloblastic with maturation (M2) 621t, 625
acute myeloblastic without maturation (M1) 621t
acute myeloid (AML) 621–626, 640f
blast types (I-III) 621–622, 623f
childhood 628
chromosomal abnormalities 622, 626, 629, 629t
chromosomal translocations 622f, 624, 625,
    625f
classification 621, 622f, 626, 627t
cytogenetics 624, 625, 626
with dyserythropoiesis 622
essential thrombocythemia progression 632
extramedullary 575
FAB classification 620, 621t
hypocellular 621
incidence 622
with inversion 626, 626f
leukemia cutis 294
lymphoid associated antigen (Ly⁺AML) 631
M0 (minimally differentiated) 620, 621t, 623
with multilineage dysplasia 622t, 624
not otherwise categorized 621, 622t
prognostic factors 630, 630t
recurrent genetic abnormalities 622t, 624–625
therapy-related 622t, 624
acute myelomonocytic (M4) 621t, 626
acute promyelocytic (APL; M3) 621t, 623f, 625
B-cell prolymphocytic 644
bone involvement 762, 762t
bone marrow specimen processing 610
breast involvement 485–486
chronic lymphocytic (CLL)
atypical 641, 642f
B-cell (B-CLL) 641–644, 642f, 643t
chromosomal abnormalities 642–643
differential diagnosis 643, 643t
histology 642
immunology/markers 641–642
immunophenotype 549t
leukemia cutis 294
mixed 641, 642f
NK/T cells 641t
prolymphocytoid transformation 643–644
prostatic involvement 1821
small lymphocytes with prolymphocytes 641,
    642f
small lymphocytic (B-cell) lymphoma and 550
splenic involvement 585
staging systems 642
T-cell 646–647

transformation 643–644
typical 641, 642f
chronic myelogenous, splenic involvement 585
chronic myeloid (CML) 632–634, 633f
atypical 638
blastic transformation 633
children 628, 638
differential diagnosis 634, 634t, 635t
leukemia cutis 294
leukemoid reaction vs 620
phases and transformation 633
Philadelphia chromosome 629, 632–633, 634
polycythemia vera vs 632
types 1/2 638
chronic myelomonocytic 636t, 638, 639f
congenital 628–629
ear involvement 2284
effusions 1032
hairy cell 575, 576f, 644–646, 645f
differential diagnosis 645–646
splenic involvement 585, 586f
splenic marginal zone lymphoma vs 589
variants 645
hypergranular promyelocytic 625
immunohistochemistry 294–295
juvenile chronic myeloid 628, 638
juvenile myelomonocytic (JMML) 638
large granular lymphocyte 646–647, 646f
NK cell 647
T-cell 646–647
mast cell 664
microgranular promyelocytic 625
minimal residual disease 630
NK-cell 647, 647t
ovary 2026–2027
plasma cell 656, 656f
prolymphocytic 646
acute 621t, 623f, 625
B-cell 644
T-cell 646
prostatic involvement 1820–1821
pure erythroid 621
secondary 150
Sézary cell 650
T-cell 646–647, 647t
testis involvement 1762
T-prolymphocytic 646
small cell variant 646
uterine involvement 1978
leukemia cutis 294–295, 294f
leukemogenesis 629
leukemoid reaction 620
leukocoria 2309
leukocyte adhesion deficiency 116
leukocyte alkaline phosphatase (LAP) 633
leukocyte common antigen (LCA) 2017t
leukocytes, in effusions 1026–1027
leukocytoclasia 195
leukocytoclastic vasculitis (LCV) 209–210, 210f
differential diagnosis 208
drug-induced 211–212
leukocytosis 620
leukodystrophies 2246
leukoencephalopathy
HIV infection 119, 2409
progressive multifocal see progressive multifocal
    leukoencephalopathy (PML)
leukoerythroblastic reaction, bone marrow 664
leukokeratosis nicotini palati 1179
leukoplakia 1165
esophagus 1292
oral cavity 1165, 1165f, 1165t, 1166f
proliferative verrucous
    larynx 845
    oral cavity 1165
smokeless tobacco 1165
verrucous, oral cavity 1165
vulvar 1892
Leu-M1 1534, 1540

Leydig cell(s) 1732–1733, 1733f, 2024
  adenoma 2185
  embryology 1734
  hyperplasia 1758
  immunohistochemistry 2023
  in Sertoli-Leydig cell tumor 2021–2022
Leydig cell tumors
  of ovary 2024–2025, 2024f, 2025f
    hilar 2024, 2025f
    nonhilar 2024
    stromal 2024
  testis 1757–1758, 1758f
    differential diagnosis 1758
    metastatic 1757, 1758f
    Sertoli cell tumor vs 1759
L&H cells
  Hodgkin's disease 541, 542, 542f
  immunophenotype 539t, 542–543
Lhermitte-Duclos disease 2374
Libman-Sacks endocarditis 1060
Libman-Sacks vegetations 1084
lice, pubic 1891
lichen amyloidosis 230, 230f
lichen aureus 208
lichenification 195
lichen myxedematosis 228–229
lichen nitidus 202–203
lichenoid actinic keratosis 244
lichenoid dermatoses 202–203, 202t
lichenoid drug eruption 202
lichenoid dysplasia, oral cavity 1166
lichenoid keratosis 202, 242–243
lichenoid pattern 195
lichenoid vulvovaginitis 1894, 1894f
lichen planopilaris 202
lichen planus 202, 202f
  lichen sclerosus vs 233
  oral cavity 1166
  paraneoplastic pemphigus vs 219
  vagina 1919
  variants 202
  vulva 1894, 1894f
lichen planus-like keratosis 242–243
lichen sclerosus (et atrophicus) 232–233, 233f
  vulvar 1892, 1892f, 1897
    squamous cell carcinoma and 1892, 1909
    vulvar intraepithelial neoplasia with 1904
lichen scrofulosorum 215
lichen simplex chronicus 201, 201f, 232
  vulvar 1892–1893, 1893f
Liebermann-Buchardt reaction 1470
Liebow classification, idiopathic interstitial pneumonia
    893t
Liesegang deposits 1665, 1665f
Liesgang ring calcification 1153
Li-Fraumeni syndrome 1170, 2401t
light chain(s)
  (AL) amyloidosis, renal involvement 1631, 1631f,
    1632, 1632f
  kappa vs lambda, deposition 1632, 1634f
  lambda, Schönlein-Henoch purpura 1619
  nephrotoxicity 1632
light chain deposition disease 1631–1632, 1633f
light chain myeloma 655
limb girdle muscular dystrophies 2235t, 2237–2238
Lim factor 2094
LIM homeobox genes 2093–2094
limiting plate, liver 1474
linear IgA bullous dermatosis 223–224, 224f
lingual thyroid nodule (lingual thyroid gland) 1163
linitis plastica appearance, signet ring carcinoma 1359
linitis plastica carcinoma 1336, 1339
lipase, serum, elevated 1565
lipid(s)
  deposits
    corneal 2303
    lymphadenopathy due to 530
  staining methods 16t
lipid cell tumors see steroid cell tumors

lipid granuloma 141
lipid histiocytosis see Gaucher's disease
lipidoses 228
lipid pneumonia 961
lipiodol-mediated drug delivery, reactions to 140
lipoadenoma, parathyroid glands 2154–2155, 2155f
lipoblastoma 337–338, 338f
lipoblastomatosis 337
lipoblasts 336, 338f, 341, 346f, 347f
lipocytes, perisinusoidal (stellate cells) 1474, 1474f
lipofibromatosis 319–320, 320f
lipofuscin 20t, 147, 1493
  central zone of prostate 1793
  in hepatocytes 1474
lipogranuloma
  liver 1513, 1513f
  sclerosing, scrotum 1772
  splenic 579
lipogranulomatosis 530
lipohyperplasia, chief cell 2159, 2159f
lipoid nephrosis (minimal change glomerulopathy)
    1606–1608, 1612f
lipoma 336–337, 337f
  atypical 341, 342–343
  of bone 684, 685f, 770
  breast 445–446
  calcified 684, 685f
  cardiac 1066
  chondroid 339–340, 340f
  CNS 2404
  fat necrosis in 337f
  gastrointestinal tract 1449–1450
  intermuscular 336
  intramedullary 770
  intramuscular 336, 337f
  larynx 848
  multiple 337
  oral region 1184
  ossifying 770
  parosteal 336, 770
  pleomorphic 338–339, 339f, 342
  sinonasal region 822
  spindle cell 338, 338f, 339f
  superficial and deep types 336–337
  vulvar 1901
lipomatosis 337, 513
'lipomatous hemangiopericytoma' 373
lipomatous hypertrophy, atrial septum 1065, 1066f
lipomeningocele 2404
liponeurocytoma, cerebellar 2376–2377, 2377f
lipopolysaccharide 62
liposarcoma 336, 341–347
  of bone 770–771
  dedifferentiated 341, 343–344, 344f
    frequency by site 344t
    prognosis 335
  gastrointestinal 1449–1450
  larynx 850
  myxoid 344–345, 345f, 346f
    of bone 771
    chondroid lipoma vs 340
    lipoblastoma vs 338
    liposarcoma vs 342
  myxoid/round (mixed) cell type 344, 346f
    transitional type 345, 346f
  paratesticular region 1766
  pleomorphic 346–347
    of bone 771
    malignant fibrous histiocytoma vs 335
    pleomorphic rhabdomyosarcoma vs 362
    prognosis 335
  round cell 344–345, 346f
  sclerosing, pleomorphic lipoma vs 339–340
  sinonasal 822
  subtypes 341, 822
  thymoliposarcoma vs 1126
  well differentiated 341–343, 342f
    inflammatory type 342, 343f
    intra-abdominal 341

lipoma-like variant 341, 342f
lipoma vs 337
low-grade with spindle cell non-lipogenic sarcoma
    343
  sclerosing type 342
  variants 341–343
liposclerosing myxofibrous tumor 742
liposes, skeletal muscle 2232–2233
lips
  keratoacanthoma 1164
  spindle cell squamous cell carcinoma 1177
  squamous cell carcinoma 1172–1173
Listeria monocytogenes, acute villitis due to
    2069–2070, 2070f
littoral cell angioma, of spleen 582, 582f
littoral cell angiosarcoma 582, 591
liver
  abscess, candidal 71
  acini 1473–1474
  adenoma see hepatic adenoma
  adenomatous hyperplasia 1520, 1529
  alcoholic disease see alcoholic liver disease
  alpha-1 antitrypsin deficiency 1506–1508, 1507f
  amebic abscess 103, 103f
  amyloidosis 1518, 1518f, 1519f
  angiomyolipoma 1542, 1542f
    differential diagnosis 1529t, 1542
  angiosarcoma 1542–1543, 1543f
  anoxic pseudolobular necrosis 1521
  atrophy of left lobe 1514, 1515f
  biopsy 1467–1473
    artifacts 1472–1473, 1473f
    cirrhosis 1467, 1519–1520, 1519f, 1520f
    color 1468
    electron microscopy 1472
    evaluation method 1467–1473
    fixation and sectioning 1468
    follow-up, in chronic hepatitis 1489
    gross findings 1467–1468
    immunopathology 1470–1471
    immunostaining for viral antigens 1471, 1472f
    indications 1467
    microscopic examination 1468
    needle biopsy 1467
    special microscopy 1471–1472
    special stains 1468–1470, 1469f, 1470f
    wedge biopsy 1467
  carcinoma see hepatocellular carcinoma (HCC)
  cavernous hemangioma 1540–1541
  centrilobular coagulative necrosis 1513
  cholestasis see cholestasis
  chronic disease, secondary IgA nephropathy
    1619–1620
  cirrhosis see cirrhosis of liver
  copper 1474
  cysts
    infectious 1545
    simple 1538–1539
  decompensated disease, biopsy 1467
  drug-induced injury 1472
  embryonal (undifferentiated) sarcoma 1544, 1544f
  epithelioid hemangioendothelioma 1543–1544,
    1543f, 1544f
  fatty see steatosis
  fibrosis see hepatic fibrosis
  focal fatty change 1545
  focal nodular hyperplasia 1527–1528, 1527f, 1528f
    differential diagnosis 1528, 1528t
  glycogen storage disease 1508, 1508f
  granuloma see hepatic granuloma
  granulomatous diseases 1508–1513
  hepatocellular injury see hepatocellular injury
  hereditary hemorrhagic telangiectasia 1517
  histology (normal) 1473–1474
  Hodgkin's disease 1517
  infantile hemangioendothelioma 1541–1542, 1541f
  infections 100–105, 1481
  inflammatory pseudotumor 1542
  ionizing radiation effect 155–156

iron overload 1503–1505
ischemia 1513–1518
    acute 1513, 1514f
    chronic 1514
    necrosis 1513, 1514f
Kaposi's sarcoma 1544
large cell dysplasia 1530, 1531f
lipogranuloma 1513, 1513f
lobule 1473
malformations/congenital lesions 1521–1523
medical diseases 1467–1526
mesenchymal hamartoma 1540, 1541f
mesenchymal tumors 1540–1544
    benign 1540–1542
    malignant 1542–1544
metabolic diseases 1503–1508
metastases in 169t, 170–171
    carcinoid syndrome with 1426
    gastrinoma 1573
    melanoma 177f
    uveal malignant melanoma 2308
    VIPoma 1574
nodular regenerative hyperplasia 1514, 1515f
nodules see hepatocellular nodules
partial nodular transformation 1528t, 1529
polycystic disease 1521–1523, 1522f
rupture 1517
sarcoidosis 1502, 1502f
sclerosing carcinoma 1536
segmental atrophy 1514, 1515f
sinusoidal dilatation 1517, 1517f
sinusoidal diseases 1517–1518
sinusoids 1474
small cell dysplasia 1530
solitary necrotic nodules 1545
surgical diseases 1527–1547
toxemia of pregnancy 1517–1518
transplantation
    acute cellular rejection 123t, 124, 124f, 1502,
        1503f
    acute rejection grading scheme 125t
    chronic rejection 128, 128f, 1502, 1503f
    hyperacute rejection 124
    perfusion injury of allograft 130, 130f
tumor-like lesions 1538–1540
tumors
    benign 1544–1545
    ductular 1538–1540
    malignant 1545
        see also hepatoblastoma; hepatocellular
            carcinoma (HCC)
vascular disorders 1513–1518
venous outflow obstruction 1514–1517
Wilson's disease 1505–1506, 1505f
liver flukes 1540
LMP1 (EBV latent membrane-1 protein),
        lymphomatoid granulomatosis 290
lobular endocervical glandular hyperplasia, cervix
        1839, 1839f
Loeffler syndrome (simple eosinophilic pneumonia)
        214, 881, 881f
Löffler's endocardial fibrosis 1077
loop electrosurgical excision procedure (LEEP),
        thermal artifact due to 137
loss of heterozygosity (LOH) 48
    bronchioloalveolar carcinoma 953–954
    CNS tumors 2340
    follicular thyroid carcinoma 2133
    insulinoma 1573
    oligoastrocytoma 2370
    pancreatic endocrine neoplasm 1572
    papillary thyroid carcinoma 2128
Lotus tetragonolobus 1600
lovastatin 2235
lower esophageal sphincter (LES) 1281, 1301f
    anatomic landmarks 1300–1301, 1301f
    Barrett's esophagus landmark 1300
    normal and reflux 1300–1301
lower motor neuron disorders 2224–2225

low-grade intestinal-type adenocarcinoma (LGITAC),
        sinonasal region 799
low-grade nasopharyngeal papillary adenocarcinoma
        (LGNPPA), sinonasal region 807–808
low-grade papillary adenocarcinoma (LGPA)
        (sinonasal) 800, 808
lubricating creams, iatrogenic reactions 141
Ludwig's angina 69
Lugol's stain 1924
lumbar puncture, implantation of normal epithelium by
        137
lumpectomy, breast excisional biopsy 427–428
'lumpy jaw' 78
lung
    acinic cell carcinoma 949, 952, 954f
    acute diffuse disease 872–887
        diffuse alveolar damage see diffuse alveolar
            damage (DAD)
        drug and radiation reactions 884–886
        hemorrhage see diffuse alveolar hemorrhage
            (DAH)
        idiopathic alveolar damage 886–887
        infections see pneumonia
        see also adult respiratory distress syndrome
    acute eosinophilic disease 881–882, 881f, 882f
    adenocarcinoma 936, 959–962
        acinar pattern 959, 960f
        bronchioloalveolar carcinoma vs 957
        clear cell 959, 960f
        cytokeratin 7 staining 33, 34f
        cytology 960–962, 963f
        differential diagnosis 960, 961–962, 961f, 963t
        endobronchial polypoid 952, 954f
        fetal 975–976, 978f
        hepatoid variant 960, 962t
        lymphoid stroma 960, 962t
        markers in effusions 1033
        metastatic 168, 960, 963t
        metastatic to pleura 1018, 1018f
        occult, metastases in thymic region 1105, 1111,
            1113
        papillary 959, 960f
        pleural effusions 1030, 1030f
        staging 937
    adenoid cystic carcinoma 951–952, 952, 952f, 953f
    adenoma
        alveolar 947, 947f
        papillary 949, 949f
        pleomorphic 946–947
    adenosquamous cell carcinoma 937, 949–950
    in AIDS 121t
    alveolar adenoma-sclerosing hemangioma 947
    alveolar cell hyperplasia, atypical (atypical
            adenomatous) 956, 956f
    angiosarcoma 973, 974f
    benign clear cell tumor 962, 963t, 964f
    benign mixed (pleomorphic adenoma) tumor
            946–947
    biopsy
        bronchial forceps 939
        open surgical 866–867
        pattern analysis see below
        surgical 868–869
        tissue processing 868–869
        transbronchial 866, 868, 920
        video-assisted thoracoscopic 867, 867f, 868, 868f
        wedge 867
    blastoma 975–976, 977f
    blastomycosis 90, 90f
    blood supply 861–862
    bronchioloalveolar carcinoma see bronchioloalveolar
            carcinoma (BAC)
    carcinoid tumors 952, 982–986, 992f
        atypical 986–987, 987f, 988f, 992, 994, 994t
        clear cell 984, 984f
        cytology 985–986, 986f
        differential diagnosis 985–986, 994, 994t
        histology 983–984, 984f
        mucinous 984, 985f

    papillary pattern 984, 985f
    radiographic imaging 936
    ultrastructure 984–985, 985f
carcinoma
    carcinogens 935, 936
    classification 940, 940t
    clinical features 936
    cytologic diagnosis 939–940
    epidemiology 935
    etiology 935–936, 989
    FNA 940
    metastases, in breast 484
    molecular pathogenesis 936–937
    pleural effusions 1030, 1030f
    primary 940–994
    radiation-induced changes 158
    radiologic features 936
    sputum cytology 939
    staging and grading 937–939, 938t
    types included in small cell carcinoma 989
    see also specific carcinoma types (above/below)
carcinosarcoma 975, 977f
cavitation, metastases 170
cellular interstitial infiltrates, rheumatoid arthritis
        888
chemodectoma 968–970, 970f
chronic drug reactions 889
chronic thrombotic/embolic disease 916–917, 917f
    in collagen vascular diseases 887t
colloid carcinoma 959
consolidation 864, 866f
    pattern 870, 870f
cystadenoma, benign mucinous 958
cystic mucinous tumor 958–959, 959f
    borderline malignancy 958–959, 959f
cysts 863–864
    honeycomb 863
dermatomyositis and polymyositis 883, 889
diffuse alveolar damage see diffuse alveolar damage
        (DAD)
diffuse alveolar hemorrhage see diffuse alveolar
        hemorrhage (DAH)
diffuse diseases 859–934, 859t
    acute, subacute and chronic 868, 871–905
    CT patterns 866t
    differential diagnosis 859t, 867
    general concepts 862–863
    immunocompromised host 867
    miscellaneous 922–928
    multidisciplinary approach 862–863
    normal immunity with 867–868
    of small airways see small airways disease (SAD)
    terminology and diseases included 863
    see also lung, acute diffuse disease; lung,
        subacute/chronic diffuse disease
diffuse large airway lesions 911
diffuse vascular disease 911–918
    see also pulmonary hypertension
'diffuse white out' 874
end-stage disease 895
eosinophilic granuloma 968, 969f
ependymoma 970
epithelioid hemangioendothelioma 973–974, 974f
fibroepithelial polyps 940, 941f
fibroleiomyomatous hamartoma 970–971, 971f
fibrosis see pulmonary fibrosis
folded (rounded atelectasis) 1007, 1007f
giant cell carcinoma 963, 965, 966f
gland-forming lesions 945–962, 946t
    benign 945–949
    malignant 949–952
    see also specific tumors (see table 12t)
granular cell tumor 952, 954f
granulomatous inflammation 881
hamartoma 974–975, 975f, 976f
hemangioma, sclerosing 947–949, 948f
hemangiopericytoma 968
Hodgkin's disease 981
'honeycomb' 871, 871f, 895

lung (cont'd)
  'hot tub' 893
  hyalinizing granuloma 967–968, 968f
  infections 874–881
    see also pneumonia
  inflammatory pseudotumor 966–967, 967f
  intermediate carcinoma 989
  interstitial diseases 863, 915–916
  interstitium 861, 862
  ionizing radiation effect 158
  Kaposi's sarcoma 973, 973f
  Langerhans cell histiocytosis 922–925
  large cell carcinoma 962–964
    cytology 965, 965f
    giant cell variant 963, 964f, 965, 966f
    neuroendocrine 987–988, 989–990, 989f, 990f
    pleural effusions 1030
    staging 937
    undifferentiated 942
  large cell neuroendocrine carcinoma 987–988,
      989–990, 989f, 990f
    differential diagnosis 994t
  leiomyoma, benign metastasizing 970–971, 971f
  localized diseases 935–1003
  lymphangioleiomyomatosis 970, 971f
  lymphatic system 862
  lymphocytic tumor, small cell carcinoma vs 994
  lymphoepithelioma-like carcinoma 964–965, 965,
      965f
  lymphoid tumors 977–982, 978t
  lymphoma see lymphoma, lung
  lymphomatoid granulomatosis (LYG) 980–981,
      981f
  malakoplakia 968, 968f
  malignant fibrous histiocytoma 972, 972f
  meningioma 970
  meningothelial-like nodules (chemodectoma)
      968–970, 970f
  metastases in 169t, 170, 175f
    from benign chondroblastoma 713
    TTF-1 in effusions 1033
  metastatic carcinoma, in CNS 2400f
  microscopic anatomy 859–862, 860f
  miliary nodules, metastases 170
  mixed connective tissue disease 888–889
  mixed glandular papilloma 940, 941f
  monophasic synovial sarcoma 972, 973f
  mucinous cystadenocarcinoma 958, 959f
  mucoepidermoid carcinoma 949–951, 950f, 951f
    low-grade, bronchial gland adenoma vs 946, 949
  mycobacterial pseudotumor 968, 968f
  neuroendocrine carcinoma 982–994
    classification 990
    differential diagnosis 994t
    see also lung, carcinoid tumors; small cell lung
        carcinoma (SCLC)
  neuroendocrine tumors 982–994, 983t
  nodular amyloid tumor 968, 968f
  nodular lymphoid hyperplasia (pseudotumor) 977,
      979–980, 979f, 980f
  nodular scars 924
  nodules 864, 865f, 870
  non-small-cell carcinoma 937, 939, 1779f
  non-specific acute injury 868
  oat cell carcinoma see small cell lung carcinoma
      (SCLC)
  opacity/opacification 863–864
    cystic 863–864, 865f
    ground-glass 863, 864, 866f, 890, 892
    linear 863
    nodular 864, 865f, 866f
    reticular pattern 863, 865f
    septal lines 863, 865f, 885, 915
  parenchymatous diseases 863
  pattern analysis approach 869–871, 869f, 870f, 871f,
      872t
    acute injury pattern 849f, 869, 869f, 872, 872t
    airspace filling pattern 870, 870f, 872t
    cellular interstitial pattern 869–870, 870f, 872t

  fibrosis pattern 869, 869f, 872t
    honeycombing 870–871, 871f, 895
    microscopic honeycombing 871
    near normal pattern 870, 871f, 872t
    nodular 870, 872t
  pleomorphic carcinoma 971
  progressive systemic sclerosis 888
  radiology 863–865, 865t
    CT 863, 864f, 866t, 868
    patterns 866t
  reperfusion injury (reimplantation response) 919
  restrictive disease 863
  rheumatoid arthritis 882, 887–888, 887t, 888f
  rheumatoid nodules 888, 888f
  samples, handling 865–869
    techniques and clinical aspects 865–868, 867t
  sarcoidosis see sarcoidosis
  sclerosing hemangioma 947–949, 948f
  Sjögren's syndrome 889, 889f
  SLE 882–883, 889
  small cell carcinoma see small cell lung carcinoma
      (SCLC)
  solitary fibrous tumor 968, 970f
  spindle cell carcinoma 966, 966t, 971, 972f
  spindle cell sarcoma 971–972
  spindle cell tumors 965–972, 966t
    benign 966–971, 966t
    malignant 966t
  squamous cell carcinoma 936, 941–945
    basaloid variant 942, 943f
    carcinoma in situ vs 945
    clear cell variant 942, 943f
    cytology 942–945, 944f, 945f, 946f
    in situ 941, 941f, 946f
    invasive well-differentiated 942, 942f
    papillary variant 942, 942f
    pleural effusions 1030
    poorly differentiated 944, 945f
    reactive conditions vs 944–945
    small cell variant 942, 943f
    squamous papilloma vs 940
    staging 937
    well-differentiated keratinizing 943, 944f
  squamous papilloma 940, 941f
  squamous tumors 940–945
  subacute/chronic diffuse disease 887–905, 902t
    bioaerosol-associated atypical mycobacterial
        infection 893
    drug reactions 889
    with granulomas 889–893
    hypersensitivity see hypersensitivity pneumonitis
        (HSP)
    idiopathic interstitial pneumonia see pneumonia
    occupational hypersensitivity 891
    pneumoconioses see pneumoconiosis
  'sugar' (clear cell) tumors 962, 964f
  synovial sarcoma see synovial sarcoma
  transplantation 918–922
    acute cellular rejection, grading system 126t
    acute rejection 919, 919f
    airways diseases 920–921
    chronic rejection 128–129
    complications 918t, 919–921
    infections 920
    lymphoproliferative disorders after 921–922
    perfusion injury of allograft 130, 130f
    rejection grading 919–920, 920t
    sampling (transbronchial biopsy) 920
    survival rates 918
  tumors/tumor-like conditions 935–940
    biphasic pattern 974–976, 975f
    vascular patterns 973–974, 973t
  venous outflow restriction, pulmonary venous
      hypertension 914–915
lupus cells, in effusions 1027
lupus erythematosus 204–206
  bullous, dermatitis herpetiformis vs 223
  discoid 114t, 204, 236
  effusions 1027

  seborrheic dermatitis vs 200
  skin involvement 204–206
  subacute (SCLE) 205, 206
  systemic see systemic lupus erythematosus (SLE)
lupus miliaris disseminatum faciei 226
lupus nephritis 1626–1629, 1626f, 1627f
  crescentic 1626f
  diffuse proliferative 1626f, 1628f
  membranous 1626f, 1627
  mesangial proliferative 1619f, 1628, 1628f
  Schönlein-Henoch purpura vs 1619
lupus panniculitis 205, 236, 236f
lupus pernio 214
lupus profundus 205
lupus vasculitis 1076t, 1078
lupus vulgaris 215, 226
Luse body 2386
Lushka ducts 1576
luteal-phase defects 1950
luteinization 1988, 1992
luteinizing hormone (LH) 2097
luteoma of pregnancy 1992, 1993
Lutzner cells 292
Luxol fast blue stain 2335t
Lyme disease
  CNS involvement 2407
  erythema migrans 207
  peripheral nerve involvement 2244
  see also Borrelia burgdorferi
lymphadenectomy, melanoma 286
lymphadenitis 516
  benign, with prominent necrosis 530–532
  cat-scratch disease/fever 533–534, 534f
  EBV-associated 524f, 525
  granulomatous mesenteric 98, 99f
  herpes simplex 525, 525f
  infectious granulomatous 533–535
  Kikuchi histiocytic necrotizing 531–532, 531f, 561
  lepromatous 533
  lymphogranuloma venereum 535
  necrotizing granulomatous, Hodgkin's disease vs 541
  syphilitic 520
  toxoplasmic 519–520
  viral 525, 525f
  yersinial 535
lymphadenoma, cutaneous 252, 252f
lymphadenoma benigna cutis 295
lymphadenopathy
  amyloid 515
  angioimmunoblastic (immunoblastic) 535, 663
  benign, with prominent necrosis 530–532
  Castleman's disease see Castleman's disease
  deposition of exogenous lipids 530
  dermatopathic 526–527, 526f
  drug-induced 525–526
    Kimura disease vs 519
  HIV-associated 117–118, 522–524, 523f
  immunoblastic (IBL) 535
  Kawasaki disease 532, 532f
  Kimura 519 15f
  massive, sinus histiocytosis with see Rosai–Dorfman
      disease
  noninfectious granulomatous 532–533
  non-neoplastic, after chemotherapy 149
  persistent generalized (PGL) 118, 522
  postvaccinial 526
  proteinaceous (angiocentric sclerosing) 515
  reactive 516–535
    extensive necrosis 516t, 530–532
    FNA 516
    follicular 516t, 517–524
    granulomatous 516t, 532–535
    granulomatous, infectious 516t, 533–535
    granulomatous, noninfectious 516t, 532–533
    paracortical 516t, 524–527
    sinusoidal 516t, 527–530
    see also lymphadenitis; lymphoid hyperplasia
  rheumatoid 518–519
  silicone 142, 530, 530f

Sjögren's 519
  systemic lupus erythematosus 532
  tuberculosis 533
  Whipple's disease 530
lymphagocytosis 529
lymphangiectasia 1379–1380
lymphangioendothelioma, benign (acquired progressive
    lymphangioma) 370
lymphangiography dye 530
lymphangioleiomyomatosis, lung 926, 927f, 928f, 970,
    971f
  meningothelial-like nodules of lung vs 970
lymphangioma
  acquired progressive 370
  intestinal 1449, 1449f
  larynx and trachea 849
  oral cavity 1186
  orbital 2297
  renal 1672
  serous cystic tumor of pancreas vs 1563
  spleen 581–582
lymphangioma circumscriptum 268–269, 269f
lymphangiomatosis, spleen 582
lymphangiomatous papules 371
lymphangiomyomatosis 514, 514f
  uterine 1973
lymphangiosarcoma 147, 276, 371
lymphangitic carcinomatosis, pulmonary 927–928, 928f
lymphangitic metastasis 170
lymphatic channels, dilated, lymphangioma
    circumscripta 269f
lymphatic drainage
  breast 420, 421f
  cervix 1831
  esophagus 1283
  fallopian tube 2039
  lung 862
  vagina 1919
  vulva 1885
lymphatic vessels, breast cancer invasion 487–488
lymphedema 343
  chronic, angiosarcoma in 275–276
  congenital 276, 371
  postmastectomy 371
lymphedema-associated angiosarcoma 147, 275–276,
    371
lymph nodes 507–576
  amyloid deposition 515, 516f
  axillary see axillary lymph nodes
  bacillary angiomatosis 514
  benign intranodal squamous inclusions 512
  benign mesothelial inclusions 512–513
  biopsy
    excisional 507
    FNA 507, 511, 516
    frozen sections 507, 509, 509t
    metastases 511
    needle core 507
  Castleman's disease see Castleman's disease
  cat-scratch fever 97–98, 97f
  cervical, metastases 169, 169t
  congenital rests and inclusions 510, 512–513, 512f
  drug-induced lymphadenopathy 525–526
  enlargement see lymphadenopathy
  false-negative results 6
  familial hemophagocytic lymphohistiocytosis 528
  fatty replacement 337, 513
  follicles
    bone marrow 640
    enlarged 520
    in follicular lymphoma 546–547, 547f
    hemorrhage 523
    hyaline-vascular 521, 522
    hyperplasia see lymph nodes, reactive follicular
        hyperplasia
    lysis in HIV infection 522–523, 523, 523f
    polarization 517, 517f
    primary/secondary 517
    reactive 521f

germinal centers 517, 640
  in HIV infection 522, 523f
    progressive transformation 520–521, 521f, 543
  granulomatous disorders 532–535
    infectious 533–535
    noninfectious 532–533
  in hairy cell leukemia 575, 576f
  in HIV infection 522–524, 523f
  iliac and sacral 1831
  immunohistochemistry 508–510, 511
    hematolymphoid cell markers 508t–509t
    malignant tumor markers 509t
  infection-associated hemophagocytic syndrome
      527–528, 528, 528f
  in infections 96–99, 533–535
  inflammatory pseudotumor 515, 515f
  inguinal, superficial 1885
  interfollicular areas
    Castleman's disease 521
    follicular lymphoma 518, 547, 547f
  interpectoral nodes (Rotter's) 420, 429
  Kaposi's sarcoma 514, 514f, 515
  karyorrhectic debris 531, 531f, 532
  Kimura disease 519, 519f
  lymphocyte depletion, HIV infection 523, 524,
      524f
  lymphogranuloma venereum 535
  malignant lymphoma with benign
      erythrophagocytosis 528
  mantle zones 517
    Castleman's disease 522
    in HIV infection 522–523
  marginal zone 552, 553
  mediastinal, atypical mycobacterial infections 96f
  mesenchymal lesions 510, 513–515
  metastatic tumors 169, 169t, 510, 511
    endometrial adenocarcinoma 1968
    mesothelioma 1008
  monocytoid B-cell hyperplasia 527, 527f, 534
  mycobacterial infections 96, 96f
  mycobacterial pseudotumor 515
  of neck 833, 833f
    from radical neck dissection 833, 833f
  necrosis
    coagulative 530
    complete 530–531
    liquefactive 530
  neoplasms involving 572–576
    see also lymphoma
  nonhematopoietic lesions 510–516
  normal thyroid tissue in 2119
  para-aortic, ovarian serous tumors 2000–2001, 2000f
  paracortical regions 524
    eosinophilia 519, 519f
    HIV infection 523, 524, 524f
    hyperplasia 524, 524f
    peripheral T-cell lymphoma 562
  pathologic evaluation 507–510
  primary plasmacytoma 575–576
  protein deposition 515–516
  reactive follicular hyperplasia 517–518, 517f
    in Castleman's disease 522
    differential diagnosis 518, 518t
    explosive, in HIV infection 522, 523, 523f
    florid 519, 519f, 520f, 525, 534, 1261
    follicular lymphoma vs 518, 518t, 550
    non-specific 518, 520
    rheumatoid lymphadenopathy 518–519
    salivary gland lymphoma vs 1256
    toxoplasmic lymphadenitis 519–520, 520f
    viral lymphadenitis 525
    see also lymphadenitis; lymphadenopathy
  reactive lymphadenopathy see lymphadenopathy,
      reactive
  reactive paracortical hyperplasia 524, 524f
    benign 524
    drug-induced 526
    peripheral T-cell lymphoma vs 562–563
    viral lymphadenitis 525, 525f

Rosai-Dorfman disease 528–530, 529f
  sarcoidosis 533
  sclerosis 516
  sentinel see sentinel lymph nodes
  sinuses
    anaplastic large cell lymphoma 563, 564f
    histiocytic hyperplasia 525
    nodular spindle variant of vascular transformation
        513, 513f
    vascular transformation 513, 513f
  sinus histiocytosis see sinus histiocytosis
  sinus hyperplasia 527–530, 527f
  smooth muscle tumors 514–515
  supraclavicular, metastases 169, 169t
  systemic mastocytosis 576
  tuberculosis 96, 96f, 533
  undifferentiated tumors 511
  vascular neoplasms 514
  Whipple's disease 530
lymphoblasts 584
lymphocysts, formation 146–147
lymphocytes
  atypical
    anaplastic large cell lymphoma 293, 293f
    around adipocytes 293, 294f
  bone marrow 612, 614, 641
  depletion, in lymph nodes in HIV infection 523, 524,
      524f
  in effusions 1026–1027, 1033
  in esophagus 1282, 1282f, 1285t, 1286
  exocytosis, scabies 217
  in gastroesophageal reflux disease 1282f, 1285t,
      1286
  intraepithelial see intraepithelial lymphocytes (IELs)
  large granular (LGL) 646
  plasmacytoid 554, 555f
  response to infectious agents 66–67
  subepidermal blisters 222, 222t
  see also B cells; T cells
lymphocytic and histiocytic cells see L&H cells
lymphocytic bronchitis/bronchiolitis (LBB) 919, 920
lymphocytic gastritis 1335–1336, 1335f
lymphocytic hyphophysitis 113, 2111–2112, 2112f
lymphocytic infiltration
  acute cellular graft rejection 122–124
  benign, of skin 295
  malignant see lymphoma
  myocardial 1042–1044, 1043f
  perivascular 207, 207f, 232
lymphocytic interstitial pneumonia (LIP) 891t, 977
lymphocytic mastopathy 450–451, 452f
lymphocytoma cutis of Spiegler-Fendt 295
lymphocytosis
  bone marrow 641
  chronic NK cell 647
  large granular 646–647
    splenic involvement 586, 591
lymphoepithelial carcinoma
  gastric 1362, 1362f
  salivary gland 1250–1251, 1251f
lymphoepithelial cysts
  benign, lymph nodes 512
  cervical 1148
  oral cavity 1148, 1148f
  pancreas 1551, 1551f
  salivary glands 1260–1261, 1260f, 1261f
lymphoepithelial lesions (LEL)
  MALT lymphoma 1451, 1453f
  salivary gland 1256
    malignant 1250–1251, 1251f
lymphoepithelial sialadenitis see sialadenitis
lymphoepithelioma
  esophageal 1299
  nasopharyngeal 793, 1251
lymphoepithelioma-like carcinoma
  cervix 1861
  lung 964–965, 965f
  vagina 1924
  vulva 1912

lymphoglandular bodies 174, 1120, 1124–1125, 1218
lymphogranuloma venereum 99, 535, 1890, 1891f
　　cervical involvement 1836t
　　lymph node involvement 535
lymphohematopoietic growth factors 612
lymphohistiocytosis, familial hemophagocytic 528
lymphoid aggregates, lung 861
lymphoid cells
　　cerebriform 291, 291f
　　plasmacytoid features 553
lymphoid hyperplasia 115, 516
　　with germinal centers, rheumatoid arthritis 888, 888f
　　in HIV infection 118
　　localized reactive, of spleen 583
　　reactive follicular see under lymph nodes
　　see also lymphadenopathy, reactive
lymphoid interstitial pneumonia (LIP) see pneumonia
lymphoid interstitial pneumonitis (LIP) 118, 118f
lymphoid lesions, bone marrow 640
lymphoid nodules, bone marrow 640
lymphoid precursors 614, 618, 640
lymphoid tangles 1218, 1219f
lymphoid tumors
　　conjunctiva 2293–2294
　　lung 977–982, 978t
　　orbit 2296, 2296f
　　see also lymphoma
lymphoma (Hodgkin) see Hodgkin's disease
lymphoma (non-Hodgkin's) 543–570
　　acute lymphoblastic, FNA smear and staining 26f
　　adrenal gland 2202
　　adult T-cell see adult T-cell leukemia/lymphoma
　　in AIDS 121t, 571, 662
　　anaplastic large cell (ALCL) 563–565, 564f, 652
　　　　of childhood 660
　　　　embryonal carcinoma of testis vs 1777
　　　　Hodgkin's disease vs 541
　　　　immunohistochemistry 564, 565f
　　　　lymphohistiocytic 563
　　　　metastases vs 169
　　　　mycosis fungoides progression 292
　　　　pleomorphic rhabdomyosarcoma vs 362
　　　　primary cutaneous 292–293, 293f
　　　　pulmonary lymphoma vs 982
　　　　salivary large cell undifferentiated carcinoma vs 1250
　　　　seminoma vs 1775, 1775t, 1776f
　　　　testicular 1762
　　　　variants 563–564, 564f
　　angioimmunoblastic T-cell 565, 566f
　　BALT, of lung 977–979, 978f, 979f, 981
　　B-cell 543, 649–650
　　　　bone marrow in 649–650
　　　　classification 545t, 546t
　　　　follicular see lymphoma, follicular
　　　　high-grade in AIDS 121t
　　　　histiocyte-rich 543
　　　　Hodgkin's disease with 541
　　　　immunoglobulin gene rearrangements 544, 544t
　　　　immunophenotype of cells 539t
　　　　intestinal tract 1450, 1451
　　　　large cell see large B-cell (below)
　　　　marginal zone see lymphoma, marginal zone B-cell
　　　　orbital 2296, 2296f
　　　　of ovary 2026
　　　　renal 1694
　　　　sinonasal 825, 825t
　　　　of skin 288–291, 289–291
　　　　small lymphocytic see lymphoma, small lymphocytic (B-cell)
　　　　splenic involvement 586–587, 587f
　　　　T-cell and histiocyte-rich 290, 558, 559, 560f, 561
　　　　T-cell lymphoma vs 563
　　　　T-cell rich 541, 650, 981
　　benign erythrophagocytosis with 528
　　bladder 1722–1723
　　B-lymphoblastic leukemia/lymphoblastic 627
　　body-cavity-based 121t, 368

of bone 760–761, 761f
bone marrow in 647–652
bone marrow/lymph node morphologic discordance 648
breast involvement 485–486
Burkitt's see Burkitt's lymphoma
cardiac 1067
centrocytic 555, 978
　　see also lymphoma, mantle cell
chromosomal translocations 544, 544t, 649
classification systems 544, 545t, 546t
clear cells 176
clinical features 543
CNS 2395–2397, 2396f, 2397f
　　in AIDS 2409–2410
　　glioblastoma vs 2354
　　immunohistochemistry 2339t, 2396
　　involving vitreous 2304, 2305f
　　ultrastructural characteristics 2337t, 2397
coagulative necrosis of lymph nodes 530
colonic 1450
composite 544
conjunctiva 2293–2294
cutaneous non-Hodgkin's, AIDS 121t
cutaneous T-cell see mycosis fungoides (cutaneous T-cell lymphoma)
diffuse large B-cell 557–561, 559f, 560f, 650
　　AIDS 121t
　　Burkitt's lymphoma vs 570
　　coagulative necrosis of lymph nodes 530
　　differential diagnosis 541, 543, 560–561
　　follicular lymphoma transformation 545–546
　　immunoblastic 558, 559
　　immunophenotype 559–560, 560f
　　intravascular 558, 558f
　　mediastinal 557, 558, 559f, 560
　　prostatic involvement 1821, 1821f
　　rosetting type 558, 559f
　　salivary gland 1256
　　of skin 290
　　T-cell/histiocyte-rich 558, 559, 560f, 561
　　variants 557, 558
diffuse small cleaved cell see lymphoma, mantle cell
discordant 544
ear involvement 2284
effusion cytology 184
eosinophilia with, Kimura disease vs 519
epidemiology 543
Ewing family of tumors vs 386, 750
extranodal low-grade B-cell 1257
extranodal marginal-zone of MALT type see MALT lymphoma
fallopian tube 2047
fine needle aspiration biopsy 544
follicular 545–550, 648f, 649–650
　　differential diagnosis 550, 555
　　fine needle aspiration 548, 549f
　　floral variant 547, 547f
　　follicle appearance 546–547, 547f
　　grading 289, 547–548
　　immunophenotype 518, 548–550, 549t
　　in situ localization 548
　　interfollicular areas 518
　　lymphocyte predominance Hodgkin's disease vs 543
　　mantle cell lymphoma vs 550, 557
　　marginal zone B-cell lymphoma vs 554
　　progressive transformation of germinal centers vs 520
　　reactive follicular hyperplasia vs 518, 518t
　　salivary gland 1256
　　signet-ring cell variant 548, 549f
　　of skin 289, 289f
　　small cleaved cell type 548, 548f
　　small lymphocytic lymphoma vs 552
　　of spleen 587–588
　　transformation to diffuse large cell 545–546
follicular center cell, lung 980
gastric 1324, 1339, 1351

Helicobacter pylori association 1332
　　see also MALT lymphoma
granulomatous changes in bone marrow 662
hepatosplenic (γ/δ) T-cell 567, 590–591, 590f, 651
high grade 546t
histiocytic necrotizing lymphadenitis vs 532
histopathology 556, 556f
Hodgkin's disease with 541
in situ 548
intestinal tract 1450–1453
intravascular 650
Kaposi's sarcoma-associated herpesvirus (KSHV) 368
karyorrhectic debris 532
kidney 1672, 1690, 1693–1694, 1694f
Langerhans cell histiocytosis vs 760
large B-cell
　　of bone 761, 761f
　　diffuse see above
　　gene expression profiling 48
　　intravascular 290–291, 2397
　　intravascular affecting lung 980, 981f
　　Langerhans cell histiocytosis vs 760
　　of legs 290
　　lung 980, 981f
　　mediastinal 557–558, 560
　　peripheral nerves 2258, 2258f
　　splenic involvement 588, 588f
large cell
　　anaplastic see lymphoma, anaplastic large cell
　　CNS 2396f
　　effusions 1031
　　embryonal carcinoma vs 1750
　　lung 980, 980f
　　malpractice case 12–13, 13f
　　ovary 2026, 2027f
　　salivary large cell undifferentiated carcinoma vs 1250
　　splenic involvement 588, 588f
　　viral lymphadenitis vs 525
large T cell
　　lung 980
　　splenic 588, 588f
laryngeal 843, 850
Lennert's (lymphoepithelioid T-cell) 294, 565, 565f
leukemic phase 641, 648f
Leydig cell tumor vs 1758
low-grade 544, 546t
　　splenic involvement 586–587, 587f
low-grade BALT 977–979, 978f, 979f, 981
low- to intermediate- grade 552, 554, 555
lung 977–980, 982f
　　intravascular large cell 980, 981f
　　large cell 980, 980f
　　low-grade BALT 977–979, 978f, 981
lymph node granulomas 532
lymphoblastic 567–569, 568f
　　B-cell type 567, 569, 627, 650
　　Ewing family of tumors vs 750
　　mantle cell lymphoma vs 557
　　mediastinum 1122–1123, 1122f
　　precursor B-cell type 628
　　T-cell, of testis 1762
　　T-cell type 567, 568, 628, 650
　　variants 567, 568
lymphoepithelial sialadenitis and 1257
lymphoepithelioid T-cell (Lennert's) 565, 565f
lymphoid interstitial pneumonia (LIP) vs 900
lymphoplasmacytic 554–555, 649
　　immunophenotype 549t, 555
　　marginal zone B-cell lymphoma vs 554
　　small lymphocytic lymphoma vs 552
　　splenic involvement 587
MALT see MALT lymphoma
mantle cell 555–557, 649
　　anaplastic variant 556–557
　　blastic variant 557
　　blastoid variant 556, 561
　　differential diagnosis 518, 550, 554, 557, 569

immunophenotype 549t, 557
intestinal 1452–1453
lung 980
'mantle zone' pattern 556, 556f, 557
of spleen 587, 588f
translocations 557
marginal zone B-cell (nodal) 552–554, 554f, 649
differential diagnosis 527, 550, 552, 554, 555
immunophenotype 549t, 553–554
splenic 589, 590f, 649
transformation to large cell lymphoma 553
mediastinum *see* mediastinum
Mediterranean abdominal 657
metastatic 174
to bladder 1721
monoclonal gene rearrangements 544, 544t
monocytoid B-cell *see* lymphoma, marginal zone B-
cell
nasal NK/T-cell 651
NK cell 543, 561–567, 650–652
NK/T cell, extranodal 566–567
NK/T cell, sinonasal 651, 825, 825t
orbital 2296, 2296f
of ovary 2026–2027
peripheral nerves 2258, 2258f
peripheral T-cell 294, 561–563, 562f, 652
differential diagnosis 526, 555, 561, 562–563
Hodgkin's disease *vs* 541
see also mycosis fungoides
pituitary involvement 2110
plasmablastic 571
pleural effusions 1031–1032, 1031f
post-thymic T-cell 561, 650–652
post-transplantation lymphoproliferative disorders
150
primary effusion 368, 571
prostatic involvement 1820–1821, 1821f
risk in Sjögren's syndrome 1257
S-100-positive T-cell lymphoproliferative 651–652
salivary gland 1256–1257, 1256f
seminoma *vs* 1775, 1775t
sinonasal region 824–826
sinusoidal 573
small bowel, risk in celiac disease 1375, 1376
small cell, effusions 1031, 1031f
small cell carcinoma of pancreas *vs* 1575
small cleaved cell, low-grade BALT lymphoma *vs*
978
small lymphocytic (B-cell) 541, 550–552, 553f, 649
conjunctiva 2293
differential diagnosis 541, 552, 554
immunophenotype 549t, 551–552
proliferation centers 551, 551f, 555, 556
splenic involvement 586–587, 587f
transformations 550, 587
variants 551, 561
small noncleaved 570, 570f
splenic
primary 588–591
secondary 586–588
splenic marginal zone 589, 590f, 649
splenic with villous lymphocytes 589–590, 649
subcutaneous panniculitis-like T-cell 236
T-cell 543, 561–567, 651
angiocentric 566–567, 825
angioimmunoblastic 565, 566f, 652
B-cell lymphoma *vs* 563
beta-TCR gene rearrangements 544, 544t
CD30-negative 291
CD30-positive 292–293
classification 545t, 546t
cutaneous *see* mycosis fungoides
enteropathy-associated (EATL) 246 652, 1453,
1454f
hepatosplenic 567, 590–591, 590f, 651
immunophenotype of cells 539t
of intestinal tract 1450
intestinal-type 567
larynx 850

malignant histiocytosis *vs* 659
peripheral (unspecified) *see* lymphoma, peripheral
T-cell
post-transplant 150, 572
salivary gland 1256
sinonasal 825, 825t
of skin 291–292, 293–294
splenic involvement 586, 588, 588f
subcutaneous panniculitis-like 293–294, 294f,
567, 652
testicular 1762, 1762f
thymus *see* thymus
thyroid 2141
true histiocytic 574–575, 575f
true seminoma *vs* 1746
types 648
T-zone pattern 562
uterine involvement 1978
vitreous 2304, 2305f
vulva 1918
Warthin's tumor *vs* 1218, 1219
WHO classification 544, 545t
lymphomatoid granulomatosis (LYG)
lung 980–981, 981f
lymphoid interstitial pneumonia (LIP) *vs* 900
skin 290, 291f
lymphomatoid papulosis (LYP) 293, 293f
lymphomatosis, intravascular 290–291, 2397
lymphoplasmacytic endotheliitis 1890
lymphoplasmacytic proliferative disorder 555
lymphoproliferative disorders 641t
autoimmune disease with 572
HIV-associated 571
immunodeficiencies 571
immunohistochemical staining 35
intestinal 1450–1453
mast cell disease with 663
post-transplantation *see* post-transplantation
lymphoproliferative disorders
senile EBV-positive B-cell 572
see also leukemia, acute lymphoblastic (ALL);
leukemia, chronic lymphocytic (CLL)
lymphoreticular tumors, renal 1693–1694
Lynch syndrome 1 and II *see* hereditary nonpolyposis
colon cancer syndrome (HNPCC)
lysosomal storage diseases
renal involvement 1623, 1623f
splenic involvement 579, 579f
lysosome-associated acid phosphatase 2231, 2232f

M

MacCallum-Goodpasture stain 59, 60t
macrocysts, papillary eccrine adenoma 258
macromastia 421
macropapillae, digital papillary eccrine
adenocarcinoma 262, 263f
macrophage 287
alveolar 861
CNS 2344
in degenerating muscle fiber 2218, 2218f
eosinophilic pneumonia 882
foamy 267f, 288, 530f, 1567, 1568f
graft rejection 122
hemosiderin-laden 612, 1553, 1553f
diffuse alveolar hemorrhage 883, 884f
HIV infection 119
pigmented villonodular synovitis 1195, 1195f
as HIV reservoir 117, 118
Kikuchi histiocytic necrotizing lymphadenitis 531,
531f, 532
lipid-laden 228, 228f, 2250, 2251f, 2252
melanin-laden 205, 526, 526f
myelin stripping by 2242, 2243
pigment-laden, in fetal membranes 2068f
response to infectious diseases 64–66
schwannoma 2250, 2251f, 2252
tingible body 295, 650
Burkitt's lymphoma 569, 570f
follicular lymphoma 547–548

in lymph node follicles 517
thymoma 1097
'macrophage activation syndrome' 659
maculae adherentes 1111, 1112f
macular cherry-red spots 2318
macular edema 2317
macules 195
erythematous 208–209
melanotic 277
MAdCAM-1, MALT lymphoma 1352
Maffucci syndrome 271, 711
carcinoma development 711
chondrosarcoma 816
enchondroma 708, 710
juvenile granulosa cell tumor 2017
spindle cell hemangioendothelioma 365
magnesium silicate (talcosis) pneumoconiosis 905t
magnetic resonance imaging (MRI)
bone tumors 704
CNS tumors 2345–2346
osteosarcoma 728
magnetic resonance spectroscopy, skeletal muscle 2213
Majocchi's granuloma 225, 226f
major histocompatibility complex (MHC) 120
malabsorptive disorders 1373–1378
malakoplakia 1641–1642, 1642f
bladder 1710, 1710f
gastric 1341–1342
ovary 1989, 1990f
pulmonary 968, 968f
testis 1767, 1767f
vaginal 1921
malanophages 277
Malassezia furfur 67t
male adrenogenital syndrome 1737
male infertility, germ cell tumor risk 1742
male pseudohermaphroditism 1737
Malherbe, calcifying epithelioma of (pilomatrixoma)
253–254, 253f
malignant fibrous histiocytoma (MFH) 333–336
adult (classic) fibrosarcoma *vs* 325–326
angiomatoid type 333
atypical fibroxanthoma as form of 266–267
of bone 739–740, 740f
CNS 2393
giant cell 335, 336f
immunohistochemistry 796t
inflammatory (xanthomatous) 335, 336f
irradiation associated 158
larynx 849, 850f
lung 972, 972f
myxoid type 333, 347
myxofibrosarcoma 326, 328–329, 329f, 330f
orthopedic prostheses association 144
pancreas 1569f
pleomorphic rhabdomyosarcoma *vs* 361, 362f
proliferative fasciitis *vs* 313
sinonasal region 796t, 823
at site of surgery 147
storiform pleomorphic 333–335, 334f, 335f
vulva 1916
malignant hyperthermia 2233
malignant melanotic tumor of infancy 751
malignant midline reticulosis (sinonasal lymphoma)
824–826, 825t
malignant peripheral nerve sheath tumor (MPNST)
2256–2259, 2257f, 2387
angiosarcoma with 2258
chromosomal abnormalities 2257
differential diagnosis 2257–2258
biphasic synovial sarcoma *vs* 2258
cellular schwannoma *vs* 2386
clear cell sarcoma *vs* 382–383
monophasic synovial sarcoma *vs* 404
neurofibroma *vs* 2254–2255
epithelioid 382–383, 2258, 2258f
glandular differentiation 2258
immunohistochemistry 2257, 2258f
rhabdomyoblastic 2258, 2258f

malignant peripheral nerve sheath tumor (MPNST)
  (cont'd)
  sinonasal 810
  spindle cells 2257, 2257f
malignant tumors, immunohistochemistry panels 509t
malleus 2268–2269
  degenerative joint disease 2282
Mallory bodies 1471, 1471f, 1481, 1490, 1492f
  formation/components 1490, 1491f
  in primary biliary cirrhosis 1501
  ultrastructure 1492f
  in Wilson's disease 1505, 1506f
Mallory-Weiss tears 1285
Malpighian corpuscles (spleen) 577, 586
Malpighian layer (stratum spinosum) 193, 194
malpractice lawsuits 10–13
MALT lymphoma (MALToma) 657, 1332,
      1351–1354
  AIDS 121t
  B-cell 1352, 1353, 1353f
  bone marrow in 649
  classification 1352
  cutaneous 289–290, 290f
  extranodal marginal-zone (EMZL) 1352
    conjunctival 2293
    orbital 2296
  Helicobacter pylori and 1351, 1354
  high-grade, defining criteria 1353, 1353f
  histology 1352f, 1451, 1453f
  intestinal 1451
  salivary gland 1256, 1256f
  Sjögren's syndrome 889
  stomach 1451
  trachea 850
mammary duct ectasia 448
mammary gland see breast
mammary-like gland adenoma and cyst, vulva
      1897–1899, 1898f
mammography 22, 463, 466, 470
mammosomatotrophs 2094–2095
  adenoma 2100
  hyperplasia 2110
mandible
  ameloblastoma 1150
  central giant cell tumor 1182–1183, 1182f
  giant cell reparative granuloma 752
  myxoma 823
  odontogenic keratocyst 1144f
  osteoblastoma 815
  osteosarcoma 1194
mantleoma 250
MAP-2 181
Marfan syndrome 1058, 1081, 1082, 1083
  aortic root dilatation 1058
MART-1 (melan-A antibodies) 182, 286, 1691
Masaoka system 1102
massive perivillous fibrinoid deposition 2072–2073
Masson bodies 901, 901f
Masson's pseudotumor 1901f
Masson stain 1488
Masson trichrome stain 2335t
  extrahepatic biliary atresia 1498f
  kidney 1602, 1602f, 1603
  liver biopsy 1468, 1468f
mast cell(s) 663
  antigen expression 664
  bone marrow examination 614
  cutaneous mastocytosis 296, 296f
  degranulation 663
  immunohistochemistry 584
  small intestine 1373, 1373f
  spindle cell lipoma 338, 339, 339f
  staining 663–664
  systemic mastocytosis 762
mast cell disease 584
  bone marrow 663–664, 663f
  see also mastocytosis
mast cell leukemia 664
mast cell sarcoma 663

mastectomy 371, 427–428, 429
mastitis
  granulomatous, sarcoidosis vs 450
  periductal 448
  plasma cell 448, 449f
mastocytoma, solitary 295
mastocytosis 545t
  cutaneous 295–296, 296f, 663
  'malignant' 296, 584
  reactive 663
  systemic 762–763
    bone marrow 663–664, 663f
    classification 663
    lymph nodes 576
    with lymphoproliferative disorders 663
    skin involvement 296
    small intestine 1380, 1381f
    spleen 584, 584f
mastoid
  aberrant neuroglial tissue 2271
  squamous cell carcinoma 2280
mastoiditis cerebri 2271
mastopathy
  diabetic 450–451
  lymphocytic 450–451, 452f
'matchstick' crystals 354
maternal floor infarction 2072–2073, 2073f, 2080
maxilla
  ameloblastoma 1150
  giant cell reparative granuloma 752
  osteoblastoma 815
  osteosarcoma 1194
  polymorphous low-grade adenocarcinoma
      799–800
  surgical ciliated cyst 1149
maxillary antrum
  mucoepidermoid carcinoma 798–799, 799f
  squamous cell carcinoma 790, 1173
maxillary sinus
  mucous retention cyst 1149
  squamous cell carcinoma 1173
maxillofacial region, fibromatoses 1184
Max Joseph space 202
Mayer–Rokitansky–Kutner–Hauser syndrome 1919
Mayer's hematoxylin procedure 18
May-Grunwald-Geimsa stain 27
Mazabraud syndrome 741
McArdle's disorder 2231–2232, 2232f
McCune–Albright syndrome 741, 742, 2110
  oral cavity involvement 1190
  sinonasal fibrous dysplasia 814
  see also Albright syndrome
M cells 1373
McGovern modification, Clark levels, melanoma
      286
measles
  appendix infection 1408–1409
  keratitis 2303
  pneumonia 95, 95f, 876, 876f
measles virus
  inclusions 68t
  otosclerosis and 2283
  respiratory tract infection 95, 95f
Meckel's diverticulum 1404
meconium, in utero discharge 2067, 2068f
meconium aspiration syndrome 2067
medial calcification 1083
medial degeneration, blood vessels 1081–1083
median palatal (mid-palatine) cysts 1147
median raphe cyst 244
median rhomboid glossitis 1162–1163
mediastinitis, sclerosing (fibrosing) 84–85, 1127–1129,
      1128–1129, 1128f
  pulmonary hyalinizing granuloma with 967
mediastinum 1091–1134
  cystic lesions 1091–1094, 1093f, 1094f
  embryonal carcinoma 1118, 1118f, 1119f
    thymic carcinoma vs 1106t, 1107
  germ cell tumor 1120–1121, 1121f, 1122f

  acute leukemia with 1107
  mixed malignant 1115, 1120, 1121f
  non-germ cell tumors in 1120
  thymic carcinoma vs 1106, 1106t
  thymic neuroendocrine tumor vs 1113
immature teratoma 1115–1116, 1116f
lymphoma 1122–1124
  cytopathology 1124–1125, 1124f
  large B-cell 557–558, 558, 559f, 560
  large cell (not further specified) 1123–1124,
      1123f, 1124, 1125f
  lymphoblastic 567, 1122–1123, 1122f
mass
  anterior 1095, 1096f
  metastatic 180f
  pulmonary venous hypertension 915
mature teratoma 1115, 1115f, 1116f, 1121f
metastasis from occult carcinoma 1105
paraganglioma, thymic carcinoid vs 1113
pleomorphic sarcoma 1120
posterior, ganglioneuroma 2199, 2200f
primary neoplasms, thymic carcinoma vs 1106t
pseudotumor 1128
sarcoma, thymic carcinoma vs 1106t, 1107
seminoma 1116–1118, 1117f
space-occupying lesion 1116
yolk sac tumors 1119, 1119f
  see also thymus
medionecrosis 1081
medullary carcinoma
  kidney 1687, 1687f
  thyroid see thyroid carcinoma
medullary carcinoma of lymphocytic infiltration of
      stomach (MCLI) 1361
medullary cystic disease, of kidney 1664
medullary sponge kidney 1664
medullary tropism, definition 2171
medulloblastoma 2378, 2379–2383
  anaplastic type cells 2382, 2382f
  of cerebellum 2379, 2380
  classic form 2380
  crush preparations 2380, 2380f
  desmoplastic 2380, 2382f
  differential diagnosis 2383
    atypical teratoid/rhabdoid tumor vs 2385
    pilocytic astrocytoma vs 2357
  with extensive nodularity/neuronal differentiation
      2380, 2382, 2382f
  genetic abnormalities 2340t, 2383
  immunohistochemistry 2339t, 2382–2383
  irradiation late effects 159
  large cell 2382, 2382f
  medullomyoblastoma variant 2382, 2383
  melanotic 2382, 2383–2384
  ultrastructural characteristics 2337t
medulloepithelioma 2379
  embryonal 2311, 2311f
edullomyoblastoma 2382, 2383
Meesman dystrophy 2302
megakaryoblasts 613, 621
megakaryocytes 612
  aplasia/hypoplasia 617
  hyperplasia 620, 632
  markers and antigen detection 611t
  osteoclasts vs 613
megakaryopoiesis 613
megaloblastic anemia 619
megamitochondria 1472, 1491, 1492f
meibomian glands 2289
Meig's syndrome 2018
Meissner's corpuscles 195
Meissner's plexus 1283
melan-A 182
melan-A antibodies 33, 35f, 286, 2188
melanin
  incontinence, blue nevus 280f
  in primary CNS tumors 2393–2394
  staining 20t
melanoameloblastoma 750–751, 751f

melanocarcinoma 750–751, 751f
melanocyte(s) 194, 276–277
  atypical hyperplasia 283
  dendriform 2292
  dendritic processes 194, 277
  epidermal 194
  junctional 277, 278
  junctional florets 281f, 283
  migration (upward/descent) 277, 278
  multinucleated 278, 281, 283
  nesting 277, 278, 283
    vulvar nevi 1897, 1897f
  pagetoid spread 278, 282, 283, 285f
  proliferation see melanocytic proliferation/lesions
  severe dysplasia 283
  'shouldering' 281, 1897
melanocytic nevi 277
  age-related changes 277
  atypical ('dysplastic'/architecturally-disordered)
      280–281, 283
    vulvar 1897, 1897f, 1914
  compound 277–278, 278f
  incomplete excision 281
  junctional 277, 278f
  severe dysplasia 283
  types 277–282
  vulvar 1897
melanocytic proliferation/lesions 276–287, 277
  atypical, with features of Spitz nevus 279
  atypical intraepidermal 283
  benign 277
    nevi see melanocytic nevi
  histochemistry/immunohistochemistry 286
  lentiginous 277, 278f
  malignant 282–287
    see also melanoma, malignant
  oral cavity 1177–1178
  pagetoid 283
  primary, of CNS 2393
  spindle-cell pattern 278, 280f
melanocytic proteins, markers 31t
melanocytoma 2309, 2393
melanocytosis 282, 283, 2393
melanoma, malignant 282–287
  acral-lentiginous 285, 1914
  adrenal gland 2202, 2202f
  amelanotic, differential diagnosis 248, 1251
  anal 1458–1459, 1458f, 1459f
  anterior segment 2316
  borderline/indeterminate 286
  Breslow thickness 284, 286
  Clark levels 286
  clear cells 176
  clinical features 283
  CNS 2393–2394, 2394f
  congenital 750–751, 751f
  congenital nevi association 283
  conjunctival 2293
  of connective tissue see clear cell sarcoma
  dermal invasion 284
  desmoplastic 285, 285f
  diagnostic work-up 181
  differential diagnosis
    clear cell sarcoma vs 381–382, 383
    epithelioid hemangioendothelioma vs 367–368
    epithelioid sarcoma vs 400
    hepatocellular carcinoma vs 1535
    Hodgkin's disease vs 540
    melanotic schwannoma vs 2253
    pleomorphic rhabdomyosarcoma vs 362
    pulmonary lymphoma vs 982
    Spitz nevus vs 279, 280f
    squamous cell carcinoma in situ vs 247
  of ear 2280
  effusions 1030–1031, 1031f
  esophageal 1314
  eyelid 2290
  familial 283
  fine needle biopsy 511

halo change 282
immunohistochemistry 286, 796t
incidence and mortality 282–283
in situ 283, 283f
  conjunctival 2293
  differential diagnosis 281
  lentiginous 283
  metastasis risk 286
  persistence without invasion 283
invasive 283–285, 285f
juvenile 278
larynx and trachea 848
lentiginous invasive 284–285
markers 181, 381
'maturational descent' 279
metastases 177f, 286
  in bladder 1721
  in breast 484
  in CNS 2399, 2400f
  in gallbladder 1582f
  in larynx 848
  Leydig cell tumor vs 1758
  in liver 171
  in lymph nodes 511
  salivary large cell undifferentiated carcinoma vs
      1250
  seminoma vs 1746, 1775t, 1776
  in skin 285–286
  survival 185
micrometastatic, sentinel lymph node dissection
    511
microstaging 284, 286
'minimal-deviation' 285, 285f
Monsel's solution mimicking 145
neuroid 285
'nevoid' 285
nipple 457
nodular 284, 1914
oral cavity 1177–1178
of ovary see ovary
pagetoid in situ, differential diagnosis 263, 263f
pathogenesis 283
of penis 1770, 1770f
prognostic factors 286
  seminoma vs 1775t, 1776
  skeletal angiosarcoma vs 769
radial growth phase 284
regression 286, 287f
rhabdoid features 177
ring 2309, 2316
risk
  dysplastic nevus (atypical nevus) 280, 283
  in large congenital nevi 278, 283
sarcomatoid, atypical fibroxanthoma vs 267
scrotum 1773
sinonasal 796t, 804–805, 806f
of skin 284–287
of soft parts see clear cell carcinoma
spindle-cell/sarcomatoid 285
Spitzoid 279
superficial spreading 283–284, 284f
  vulvar 1914, 1915
treatment 286–287
ulceration 286
uveal tract see uveal malignant melanoma
of vagina 1925
variants 285–286
vertical growth phase 284, 284f, 285, 1914
vulvar see vulva
melanophages 1896
melanosis
  cervix 1842
  conjunctiva 2293
  esophagus 1314
  mucosal (intestinal) 1404, 1409
  neurocutaneous 2393, 2393f, 2394f
  peritoneum 1022, 2031
  precancerous 283
  primary acquired, conjunctiva 2293, 2293f

vagina 1922
  vulvar 1896, 1896f
melanosis coli 1400, 1401
melanosis coli pigment (pseudomelanin) 20t
melanotic neuroectodermal tumor of infancy 750–751,
    751f, 805–806, 1178, 1178f
  paratesticular region 1766
melanotic tumor of infancy, malignant 751
MELAS syndrome 2231t
melioidosis 1481
membranous glomerulonephropathy 1614–1615, 1614f
MEN1 gene 2151, 2158
  pancreatic endocrine neoplasm 1572
  parathyroid carcinoma 2162
  small cell lung carcinoma 992
MEN2 gene 2158
Ménétrier's disease 1332, 1340
Ménière's disease 2269–2270, 2284
meningeal fibrous histiocytoma 2359
meningeal infection, Cryptococcus neoformans 91f
meningeal tumors 2387–2394
  see also hemangiopericytoma; meningioma
meningioma 2387–2392
  of CNS
    angioblastic 2390
    angiomatous 2389–2390, 2390f
    angioplastic (malignant) 2391
    atypical 2391, 2391f
    chordoid 2373–2374, 2391
    clear cell 2362, 2391, 2392f
    of CNS 2387–2392
    'dural tail' on MRI 2387, 2387f
    ectopic 2387
    fibrous (fibroblastic) 2389, 2389f
    genetic abnormalities 2340t, 2392
    histology 2387–2388, 2388f
    immunohistochemistry 2339t, 2392
    lymphoplasmacyte-rich 2391
    meningothelial (syncytial) 2388–2389, 2389f
    metaplastic 2391
    microcystic 2390–2391, 2390f
    papillary 2392
    psammomatous 743, 2389, 2390f
    rhabdoid 2392
    schwannoma vs 2251
    secretory 2391, 2391f
    sites 2387
    transitional (mixed) 2389, 2390f
    ultrastructural characteristics 2337t
    whorl formation 2388, 2388f
  of ear 2279–2280
  of orbit 2298
  of pituitary 2109
  primary pulmonary 970
  radiation-associated 160
  of sinonasal region 811, 811f
  of temporal bone–middle ear 2279–2280
meningitis
  acute pyogenic (bacterial) 2406
  AIDS/HIV 2409
  aseptic (viral) 2407
  fungal infections causing 2411
  granulomatous, after iodized oil in myelography
      138
meningocele 2403–2404, 2404f
meningoencephalitis, primary amebic 2412
meningomyelocele 2403, 2404, 2404f
meningothelial-like nodules, lung 968–970, 970f
meningovascular neurosyphilis 2407
menopause, premature 1988
mensicus, torn 697
menstrual cycle 1950
  normal 1936–1942
mercuric chloride 17
MERFF syndrome 2231t
Merkel cell(s) 194, 248, 252
Merkel-cell carcinoma 248–250, 249f, 261
Merkel cell tumor, vulva 1913
merlin (schwannomin) 2258, 2386

mesangial cells 1599–1600
  hypercellularity 1599, 1600
    acute postinfectious glomerulonephritis 1617,
      1617f
    diffuse 1608–1609, 1612f
    in nephrotic syndrome 1608, 1612f
  interposition 1615, 1616f
  macrophage phenotype 1599
  myofibroblastic phenotype 1599
  proliferation
    glomerulopathy 1608–1609, 1612f
    lupus nephritis 1619f
    membranoproliferative glomerulonephritis 1615
  staining 1600
mesangial matrix 1599, 1600
mesangial nodules 1608f
  diabetic nephropathy 1629, 1629f
  fibrils 1629, 1630f
  light chain deposition disease 1631
  sclerotic 1602, 1602f
mesangial sclerosis 1614, 1622
mesangium 1599
  amyloid deposition 1608f
  IgA staining 1619, 1619f
  immune complex deposition 1619
mesenchymal chondrosarcoma 719–720, 720f
mesenchymal hamartoma, liver 1540, 1541f
mesenchymal tumors
  bladder 1721–1722
  broad ligament 2048
  esophagus 1314–1315
  fallopian tube 2045, 2046–2047
  gastrointestinal tract 1443–1448
  kidney 1690–1693
  liver 1540–1544
  non-meningothelial 2392–2393
  ovary 2026
  pancreas 1569, 1569f
  pituitary gland 2109–2110
  scrotum 1773
  stomach 1344–1348
  thymus 1125–1128
  thyroid gland 2140–2142
  uterine 1978
  uterus 1968–1973, 1978
mesenchymal tumors/pseudotumors, of skin 263–276
  benign chondro-osseous lesions 267
  benign myxoid lesions 267–268
  benign peripheral nerve tumors 268
  benign vascular tumors 268–273
  borderline vascular tumors 273–274
  fibrohistiocytic/fibroblastic 263–267
  malignant endothelial tumors 274–276
mesenchymoma, fibrocartilaginous 742
mesenteric cysts, postoperative 147
mesenteric ischemia, nonocclusive 1380–1381
mesenteric lymphadenitis 98, 99f
mesenteric thrombosis 1385
mesial temporal sclerosis 2405, 2405f
mesoblastic nephroma see nephroma
mesodermal stromal polyp see fibroepithelial polyps
mesonephric adenocarcinoma, cervix 1877
mesonephric carcinoma, endometrial clear cell
    adenocarcinoma as 1964
mesonephric cyst 1899, 1920, 1920f
mesonephric hyperplasia 1839–1840, 1840f
mesonephric remnant hyperplasia, cervix 1839–1840,
    1840f
mesonephroma, endometrial clear cell adenocarcinoma
    as 1964
mesothelial cells
  in effusions 1026, 1026f, 1027f
  pleural 1005, 1006, 1006f
  reactive 1006, 1006f, 1027, 1027f, 1033
  resembling adenocarcinoma 147
mesothelial cysts
  fallopian tube 2043
  pericardial 1070
mesothelial tumors

paratesticular region 1765, 1765f
  radiation-associated 160
mesothelioma
  cytoplasmic vacuoles 183–184
  localized fibrous (fibrous tumor of pleura)
    1015–1016, 1015f, 1016f
  of paratesticular region see paratesticular region
  of pericardium 1019, 1020f, 1070
  of peritoneum 1022–1023, 1022f
    deciduoid variant 1023
    well-differentiated papillary 1023–1024, 1024f
  of pleura (malignant) 146, 1007–1015
    adenocarcinoma vs 184, 185t, 1014–1015, 1014t
    classification 1008t
    clinical and radiographic features 1007–1008,
      1008f
    deciduoid 1009
    desmoplastic 1010, 1010f, 1128
    desmoplastic small round cell tumors vs 386
    diagnostic panel and antibodies 1012, 1013,
      1014t
    effusions 1028, 1029, 1029f, 1032, 1032f
    epidemiology and pathogenesis 1007
    epithelial 1008–1009
    histochemistry 1010–1011
    histology 1008–1010, 1008t
    immunodiagnosis, approach 1013–1015, 1014f
    immunohistochemistry 1011–1015, 1011f
    in situ 1009
    lymph node metastases 1008
    lymphohistiocytoid 1010, 1010f
    macroscopic features 1008, 1008f
    metastases 1019
    microcystic 1008–1009, 1009f
    mixed (biphasic) epithelial/sarcomatoid 976,
      1010, 1011f
    molecular biology 1015
    papillary, effusions 1029
    'patternless pattern' of Stout 1010, 1010f
    pleomorphic variant 1009, 1009f
    pulmonary adenocarcinoma vs 960, 961f
    radiation-associated 160
    sarcomatoid 1009–1010, 1010f, 1015
      immunohistochemistry 1011–1012, 1012f
    small cell variant 1009
    tubulopapillary 1008, 1009f
    ultrastructure 1015
    well-differentiated papillary 1009, 1009f
  uterine, benign 1978
mesothelioma cells, in effusions 1029, 1029f
mesotympanum 2268
mesovarium, torsion 1992
metabolic disease, bone 679, 685–689
metabolic disorders
  CNS 2417
  pituitary gland 2113
  spleen 579–580
metachromatic dyes 2246
metachromatic leukodystrophy 2246
metals, lung cancer etiology 936
metal working fluid-associated hypersensitivity
    pneumonitis 891
metanephric adenofibroma 1674
metanephric adenoma 1673–1674, 1674f
metanephric adenosarcoma 1674
metanephric neoplasms 1673–1674
metaphyseal fibrous defect see fibroma, non-ossifying
metaphysis 678
metaplasia, definition 1832
  see also specific types/sites
metaplastic carcinoma 1819
  see also sarcomatoid carcinoma
metaplastic papillary tumor, fallopian tube 2044
metastases 167–190
  biopsy 185–186
  cannonball 170
  clinical patterns 168
  common sites 169–171, 169t, 178t
  diagnostic approach 173–174

  differential diagnosis 167–190
  histologic/cytologic features 177–178
  immunohistochemistry 178–182
  information required by oncologist 184–185
  malignant cell invasion of extracellular matrix 167
  mechanisms 167–168
  morphologic patterns and cell types 173–178, 174f,
    178t
  primary tumor location 168
  suspected, principles in analysis 186t
  tumor cell emboli arrest/proliferation at distant sites
    167–168
  tumor-to-tumor 173
  of unknown primary origin (MUO) 168–169
    carcinomas, effusions in 183
    cell line and site-specific antibodies 180–182, 180t
    cost analysis for pathologic evaluation 168–169,
      169t
    cost of immunohistochemical stains 169
    diagnostic approach 173–174
    effusion cytology 182–184
    favorable clinical subsets 184–185, 185t
    histologic/cytologic features 177–178
    immunohistochemistry 178–182
    morphologic features 173–178, 174f, 178t
    treatment and prognosis 168, 184–185
  unusual sites 171–173, 171t
  vascular dissemination 167
  see also specific anatomic regions/cancers
methanol, as fixative 17
methenamine silver stain 2335t
methotrexate, lung disease due to 885–886, 886f
methylation, epigenetic analysis 48
methyl green-pyronine stain 507
metochromasia 18
Mibelli type, angiokeratoma 269
Michaelis-Gutman bodies 968, 969f, 1342, 1641–1642,
    1642f, 1710, 1710f
  malacoplakia of testis 1767, 1767f
  in ovary 1989
  Rhodococcus equi infections 79
  staining 79
  in vagina 1921
microabscess 195
  eosinophilic 572
  hepatic 1481–1482, 1481f
  Langerhans cells 196, 196f, 217
  larynx 844
  Munro's 199, 199f
  neutrophilic 223, 223f
  Pautrier 291, 292f
  renal tubular 1610f
  retina 2317
  stellate 532, 534
microadenoma 2104
microadenoma, pituitary 2101, 2104
microadenomatosis, pancreas, MEN type 1 1574
microangiopathic obliterative endarteritis 928
microarrays
  DNA 48, 560
  gene expression 47–48, 48f
  tissue 36, 2340
microbiologists 57
microcyst(s)
  adrenal cortex 2173
  breast 431f
  oligodendroglioma 2362f
  pilar 251
  renal tubules 1622
microcystic adnexal carcinoma (MAC) 252, 261, 262f
microcystic endocervical adenocarcinoma, cervix
    1877
'microcystic tubule disease' 1603f, 1612
microdysgenesis 2405
microglia 2344
  HIV infection 118–119
  in Rasmussen encephalitis 2406f
  reactive 2344
microglial nodules 119, 2344, 2344f

β2-microglobulin, accumulation 2247
microinvasive carcinoma, definition 1857
micromastia 421
Micromonospora vulgaris 889
micronodular pneumocyte hyperplasia 926
micropapillae, papillary endothelial 273
Micropolyspora faeni 889
microsatellite analysis 48
microsatellite instability 48
microscopic polyangiitis (polyarteritis) 1075,
    1076–1077, 1076t, 1384–1385
    appendix involvement 1410, 1410f
    intestinal 1384, 1384t, 1386f
microsporidial keratoconjunctivitis 2294
microtophi 1643
microtubule-associated protein 2, neuroblastoma 384
microtubules, peripheral nerves 2240
microvascular proliferation, definition 2350
microvilli, proximal tubules 1600
microvillus inclusion disease 1377, 1377f
microwave fixation 17
microwave-induced antigen retrieval 32, 33f
middle ear *see* ear, middle
Miescher–Melkersson–Rosenthal syndrome 1896
Miescher's granuloma/granulomatosis 213, 234
Mikulicz cells 78
milium 254
milium osteoma (osteoma cutis) 268f
milk line nevi 1897
milk ridges 419, 421
Milroy's disease 276
mineral dust bronchiolitis 907–908
mineralocorticoids 2169, 2183
Ming classification, gastric adenocarcinoma 1354
minigemistocytes 2361, 2361f
minimal change glomerulopathy 1606–1608, 1612f
minimal change nephrotic syndrome 1606–1608,
    1612f
'misplaced exocytosis' *see* exocytosis
mitochondria
    hyperplasia/hypertrophy 2230
    paracrystalline inclusions 2230, 2230f
mitochondrial myopathies 2229–2230, 2230f, 2231t
mitomycin C, bladder changes due to 1719, 1719f
mitosis-karyorrhexis index (MKI) 2196, 2198
mitotic activity 2350
mitotic figures, Wilms' tumor 1666, 1667f
mitral valve 1053–1057
    annular calcification 1056
    chronic rheumatic disease 1055–1056, 1056f
    examination 1053–1057
    insufficiency 1053
    miscellaneous lesions 1056–1057
    prolapse 1054–1055, 1056f
    regurgitation secondary to ischemic heart disease
        1056
    replacement, indications 1053, 1055t
    rheumatic disease 1055–1056
    stenosis 1053, 1055–1056
    surgical options of treatment 1053, 1054
mittelschmerz 1937
mixed connective tissue disease 114t, 1076t
    lung involvement 888–889
    muscle fiber changes 2222
mixed epithelial and stromal tumor, kidney 1695,
    1695f
mixed glioma *see* glioma
mixed malignant germ cell tumors (MMGCTs) *see*
    germ cell tumors
mixed mesodermal tumor, malignant 1819–1820,
    1977
    see also sarcomatoid carcinoma
mixed neuronal-glial tumors 2374–2377
    immunohistochemistry 2339t
    ultrastructural characteristics 2337t
mixed tumor, malignant
    salivary gland *see* salivary gland tumors
    vagina 1925
    vulva 1913

MLL gene 624, 626, 628
MMH classification, thymoma classification 1096
MOC-31 179
Modfit software 41
Mohs' technique 246, 2280, 2291
molecular biology 44–48
'moles', atypical 280
molluscum contagiosum 76
    cervix 1850f, 1852
    eyelid 2290
    vulvar 1889–1890, 1890f
Mönckeberg's medial calcification 1083
Mondor's disease 450
Mongolian spot 282
monoclonal antibodies
    anti-CD20 (retuximab) 551, 1354
    immunohistochemistry 32, 184
monoclonal gammopathy of undetermined significance
    654
monoclonal gene rearrangements 544, 544t
monoclonal immunoglobulin deposition disease 656,
    657
    renal involvement 1631–1632, 1633f
monocyte/macrophage incidental cardiac excrescent
    (MICE) 1065, 1066f
monocytes, bone marrow 613
mononeuropathy 2239, 2239t
mononeuropathy multiplex 2247
mononuclear inflammatory cell infiltrate, breast cancer
    488
monorchidism 1734–1735
monostotic solitary bone lesions 740
Monsel's solution 145, 1920
mordant 18
morgagnian globules 2299
morphea 231–232
morphometry 7, 43
Morquio's disease 686
Morton's neuroma 379, 697, 698f, 2245–2246, 2246f
morulae, cancer cells in effusions 1028–1029, 1029f
mosaicism, confined placental 2080
motor end plate *see* neuromuscular junction
motor neuron disease 2225, 2227
Mott cells 655
mouth
    floor, squamous cell carcinoma 1173
    ulcers, suppression, smoking 1386
    see also oral cavity
Movat pentachrome stain 1081, 1468, 1469f
M-protein 654, 655
MUC2, intraductal papillary mucinous neoplasms 1566
MUC5A (mucin gene product), mucinous tumors of
    ovary 2006
Mucha-Habermann disease 204, 205f
mu chain disease 657
mucicarmine method 21f, 86, 184, 261–262
mucin
    dermal 206, 206f, 213, 213f
    extracellular, staining 261–262
    gallbladder 1576
    gastric-type, in ovarian benign mucinous tumors
        2002
    genes and immunohistochemistry 180
    intraluminal wispy blue 1808, 1809f
    markers 31t
    neutral, mesothelioma 1010–1011
    peritoneal deposits 2006
    pools, pseudomyxoma ovarii 2006
    scleredema *229*, 229f
    staining methods 16t
mucinosis
    cutaneous 228–231, 228t
    follicular 226–227, 227f, 292
    papular, lichen myxedematosis 228
mucinous cystadenocarcinoma
    of breast 484
    of lung 958, 959f
mucinous cysts, spleen 580
mucinous eccrine adenocarcinoma (MEA) 261–262

mucinous tumors
    metastases differential diagnosis 177
    of ovary *see* ovary, mucinous tumors
mucocele 1149
    gallbladder 1578
    salivary gland 1259–1260, 1259f
    sinonasal 787
mucocele-like lesion, breast *see* breast, mucocele-like
    lesion
mucocutaneous lymph node syndrome *see* Kawasaki
    disease
mucocutaneous surfaces, infectious diseases 67–77
mucocytes 1247
mucoepidermoid carcinoma
    central osseous 1189
    grading 799, 800t
    lacrimal gland 2298, 2299
    lung *see* lung, carcinoma
    oral cavity 1179
    salivary gland *see* salivary gland tumors
    thyroid 2139, 2140f
mucohyaline stroma, salivary adenocarcinoma 1241,
    1242f
mucoid (mucinous) intimal hyperplasia, renal vessels
    1647
'mucoid wedge' 2096
mucopolysaccharidoses 579, 686
Mucor, intestinal infection 1399
Mucormyces, pneumonia 880
mucormycosis 80
    CNS involvement 2411
    granulomatous gastritis 1336
    sino-orbital 2294
mucosa associated lymphoid tissue (MALT)
    lymphoma *see* MALT lymphoma
    in stomach 1331–1332, 1351–1352
mucosal neuroma 2248–2249, 2249f
mucosal prolapse-associated conditions, stomach
    1339
mucositis, oral 79f
mucous cysts, vulva 1899, 1900f
mucous glands
    bronchi 860
    gallbladder 1576
mucous membranes, radiation effect 155
mucous neck cells, stomach 1322, 1323f
mucous retention cysts 787, 1259
mucus escape reaction 1259–1260, 1259f
mucus extravasation phenomenon 1259
Muir-Torre syndrome 250, 1164, 2291
Müllerian agenesis 1919
Müllerian cysts 1920
Müllerian duct cysts 1791
Müllerian epithelium, inclusion in lymph node 512,
    512f
müllerian inhibitor substance 1734, 1737
Müllerian mucinous borderline tumors 2003–2004,
    2004f
Müllerian papilloma 1922
Multicycle software 41, 41f
multidrug resistance protein (MDR-1) 630
multifilament synthetic sutures 144
'multilocular mesothelioma' 1022
multilocular peritoneal inclusion cyst (MPIC) 1021,
    1021f, 1022
multiple endocrine neoplasia (MEN) 1574–1575
    medullary thyroid carcinoma 2136
    pituitary adenoma 2098
multiple endocrine neoplasia (MEN) type 1
    1574–1575, 2098
    adrenal gland involvement 2178
    carcinoid tumors of lung and 982
    chief cell hyperplasia 2158, 2159f
    familial multiple leiomyoma with 348
    gastric carcinoids associated 1348, 1349, 1351
    glucagonoma 1573–1574
    insulinoma 1572
    parathyroid adenoma and 2151
    pituitary adenoma 2098

multiple endocrine neoplasia (MEN) type 2a 1574
  adrenal medullary hyperplasia 2190, 2190f
  medullary thyroid carcinoma and 2136, 2137
  pheochromocytoma with 2192
multiple endocrine neoplasia (MEN) type 2b 1574,
      2379, 2383
  genes and CNS features 2401t
  medullary thyroid carcinoma and 2136, 2137
  mucosal neuroma 2248
  pheochromocytoma with 2192
multiple endocrine neoplasia (MEN) type 3 2137
multiple hamartoma syndrome (Cowden's disease) 265,
      1436–1437, 1676
multiple hereditary exostoses 707, 708, 718
multiple lymphomatous polyposis 1451, 1452, 1452f
multiple myeloma 654–655
  amyloidosis 656, 2247
  brown tumor vs 751
  chromosomal abnormalities 655
  effusions 1032
  with osteosclerotic lesions 655–656
  peripheral nerve involvement 2258
  sinonasal region 826
  spleen 580
  testis involvement 1762
  WHO diagnostic criteria 655
multiple nevoid basal cell carcinoma see multiple
      endocrine neoplasia (MEN) type 2b
multiple sclerosis 2343, 2343f, 2413
multivacuolated cells, sebaceous carcinoma 258,
      260f
'mummified' cells see Hodgkin cells
mumps
  myositis 2219–2220
  orchitis 1738, 1767
Munro's microabscesses 199, 199f
muricarmine stain 2335t
muscle
  markers 31t, 1013
  skeletal see skeletal muscle
  weakness 206, 2220
muscle–eye–brain disease 2238
muscle fascicles 2216
  atrophy 2225, 2226f
muscle fibers
  abnormal mitochondria 2229–2230, 2230f
  anatomy 2215–2217
  angular atrophic esterase-positive 2220f, 2223, 2225
  atrophy 2226, 2227f
  checkerboard pattern 2216f, 2225
  congenital type disproportion 2228t, 2229
  degeneration, infections associated 2222
  degeneration and necrosis, polymyositis 2218, 2218f
  denervated 2225
  denervation atrophy 2225, 2225f
  grouping of types 2225, 2226, 2226f
  hypertrophy 2236
  necrosis 2238
  ragged red fibers 2221, 2230
  regeneration 2218, 2219f
  reinnervation 2226
  ring fibers 2237
  striations 2215, 2216f
  target and targetoid 2225
  type I (red muscle, slow twitch) 2215, 2216, 2216f
    atrophy 2237
    central core myopathy 2228
    lipid accumulation 2232
  type II (white muscle, fast twitch) 2215, 2216, 2216f
    atrophy 23f, 2222, 2224, 2227, 2234f
  variation in size 2236, 2237
  zones of staining 2225, 2226f, 2229
muscle-specific actin (MSA)
  alveolar rhabdomyosarcoma 360–361
  leiomyoma 348
  leiomyosarcoma 351–352
  mesothelioma 1013
  synovial sarcoma 403
muscle spindles 2216–2217, 2217f

muscular dystrophies 2235–2238
  autosomal dominant/recessive 2235t
  Becker 2213, 2235–2236, 2235t
  congenital 2238
  Duchenne 2213, 2235–2236, 2235t
  Emery-Dreifuss 2236
  esophageal dysmotility 1284
  facioscapulohumeral 2237
  inheritance 2235, 2235t
  limb girdle 2235t, 2237–2238
  oculopharyngeal 2237
  X-linked recessive 2235t
muscularis propria
  bladder 1707
  stomach 1321, 1346f
Musculoskeletal Tumor Society, bone sarcoma staging
      703, 704t
mushroom poisoning 1513
myasthenia gravis 2227
N-myc, oncogenes 1170, 2198, 2199
mycetoma 73–74, 91, 92, 93f
  sinus 787
MYC gene translocation, Burkitt's lymphoma 569, 570
mycobacterial infections
  atypical
    bioaerosol-associated 893
    lymph node infections 96f, 515, 533
    skin infections 215
    vulvar infection 1891
  CNS 2406, 2407f
  diagnostic techniques 60–61
  hepatic granuloma 1511
  intestinal 1398
  nasopharynx and upper respiratory tract 79
mycobacterial pseudotumor
  lung 968, 968f
  lymph nodes 515
  spindle cell, smooth muscle tumors vs 353
Mycobacterium abscessus 65, 65f
Mycobacterium avium complex 64
  CNS infections 2406
  granuloma in bone marrow 662
  in HIV infection 64, 64f, 65f
  intestinal infection 1398, 1399f
Mycobacterium avium-intracellulare 65f
  disseminated, in AIDS 1511, 1512f
  granulomatous gastritis 1336
  hepatic granuloma 1511, 1512f
  lymph node infection 530
  malabsorption due to 1378
Mycobacterium chelonae 60, 65
Mycobacterium fortuitum 60, 65
Mycobacterium leprae 215, 2243–2244
Mycobacterium tuberculosis 58
  cutaneous 215
  esophagitis 1290
  granulomatous infection of bone 690
  granulomatous salpingitis 2041, 2041f
  immunocompromised host 81
  noncaseating granuloma 64f
  pericardial fibrosis 1019
  respiratory tract infection 82–83
  vulvar infection 1891
  see also tuberculosis
Mycoplasma pneumoniae
  bronchiolitis/pneumonia 875, 906
  erythema multiforme 203
mycosis fungoides (cutaneous T-cell lymphoma)
      291–292, 566, 566f, 650
  CD30-negative 291
  CD30-positive 292–293
  digitate dermatosis as 207
  follicular mucinosis association 226, 292
  histology 291, 291f, 292f
  immunohistochemistry 291–292
  parapsoriasis variants as 207
  plaque, patch and tumor stages 291, 291f
  transformation to large cell lymphoma 566
  variants 292

myelin, stripping by macrophage 2242, 2243
myelin-associated glycoprotein (MAG) 2241
myelination, loss see demyelination
myelin bodies, acute tubular necrosis 1638, 1639f
myelin-forming cells, CNS see oligodendrocytes
myelin-like bodies, Fabry's disease 1623, 1623f
myelin sheath 2241
myeloblasts 294f, 613
myelodysplastic syndromes 635–638, 637t
  blasts types I-III 635
  cellularity 635, 636f
  classification 626, 635, 636t, 637–638, 637t
  cytogenetic abnormalities 636–637
  essential thrombocythemia progression 632
  morphologic abnormalities 625t, 636f
  with myelofibrosis 635–636
  secondary 616
  subgroups 636t
  therapy-related 622t, 624, 635
myelofibrosis 631, 639–640, 639t
  acute panmyelosis with 624
  chronic idiopathic 634–635, 635t
  myelodysplastic syndromes with 635–636
  osteosclerosis with 634
  primary/secondary 639
myeloid hyperplasia 620
myeloid metaplasia, agnogenic 584
myeloid sarcoma 575, 576f, 624
  lymphoblastic lymphoma vs 569
  see also granulocytic sarcoma
myelolipoma 340
  adrenal gland 2175, 2199–2200, 2201f
myeloma 654–655, 761–762, 762f
  epithelioid hemangioendothelioma vs 368
  indolent/light chain 655
  localized 762
  multiple see multiple myeloma
  nonsecretory/smoldering types 655
  post-transplantation lymphoproliferative disorders 150
myeloma cast nephropathy ('myeloma kidney') 1630,
      1630f
myelomonocytic cells, markers and antigen detection
      611t
myeloperoxidase 610
  antibodies 1622
  cytoplasmic (cMPO), leukemia 584, 623
  myeloid sarcoma 569
myelopoiesis 613, 613f
myeloproliferative syndromes 631–635, 635t
  chronic 584, 638
  chronic idiopathic myelofibrosis 634–635, 635t
  essential thrombocythemia 632, 633f
  polycythemia vera 631–632, 632f
myelosclerosis
  acute malignant 624
  with myeloid metaplasia 584, 585f
myoadenylate deaminase
  deficiency 2233
  skeletal muscle evaluation 2215t
myoblasts 2214
myocarditis 1042
  endomyocardial biopsy 1042–1045
  giant cell 1044, 1044f
  hypersensitivity 1044–1045
  immunohistochemistry 1043–1044
  lymphocytic 1042–1044, 1043f
  toxic 1045
myocytes, rimmed (autophagic) vacuoles 2220f, 2221f
MyoD 360
MyoD1, alveolar soft part sarcoma 397
myoepithelial carcinoma, sinonasal 796–797, 796t
myoepithelial cells 1210
  adenoid cystic carcinoma 794, 795f
  salivary pleomorphic adenoma 1210, 1211f, 1212,
      1212f, 1213f, 1214f, 1215f
myoepithelioma 446
  plasmacytoid 1214, 1216f
  salivary glands 796–797, 1187, 1213–1214, 1216f
  sinonasal 796–797

myofibrillar ATPase reaction 19
myofibrillary apparatus, proteins 2217, 2218t
myofibrils 2215
    familial myopathy with lysis of 2229
    loss in cardiomyopathies 1045, 1048
myofibroblastic proliferative lesions, benign *see* pseudosarcomatous proliferative lesions
myofibroblastic sarcoma 332
myofibroblastoma 316, 316f, 317f
    breast 316f, 317f, 447
    palisaded, of lymph node 316f, 515
    schwannoma *vs* 2251
    solitary fibrous tumor *vs* 377–378, 378t
    superficial cervicovaginal 1922
myofibroblasts 264, 824f, 861, 873
myofibroma 315–317
    of bone 736, 736f
        infantile 736, 736f, 737f
    differential diagnosis 315, 316
    solitary 315, 315f, 316f, 736
    solitary fibrous tumor *vs* 378t
myofibromatosis 315–317
myofibrosarcoma 332–333, 332f
    pleomorphic 333–334
    sinonasal region 822–823
myofilaments 2215, 2216f
myogenic tumors, oral cavity 1185
myogenin 360, 397
myogenous tumors, rhabdomyosarcoma *vs* 361t
myoglobin, alveolar rhabdomyosarcoma 360–361
myoglobinemia 2213
myoglobinuria 1638, 2213, 2222
myoglobulin casts 1638f
myolipoma 336, 340, 340f, 341f
myometrium 1933, 1934
    endometrial adenocarcinoma invasion 1959–1960, 1959f
myopathy
    acute alcoholic 2234, 2235t
    amyloid 2238
    central core 2228, 2228t
    congenital 2227–2229, 2228t
    critical care 2238
    Cushing's disease 2233
    desmin storage 2229
    distal 2238
    endocrine 2234
    familial with lysis of myofibrils 2229
    fingerprint 2228t, 2229
    HIV 2223, 2223f
    inflammatory 2218–2224, 2218t
        dermatomyositis 2219, 2219f
        inclusion body myositis 2220–2221, 2220f, 2221f
        polymyositis 2218–2219, 2218f, 2219f
        see also myositis
    mini multicore (mini core) 2229
    mitochondrial 2229–2230, 2230f
    myotubular (central nuclear) 2228–2229, 2228t
    nemaline rod 2227–2228, 2228f, 2228t
    neurogenic muscle disease *vs* 2225t
    reducing body 2228t, 2229
    spheroid body 2229
    steroid 2235
    toxic 2234–2235, 2235t
    trilaminar 2229
    tubular aggregates 2228t, 2229
    zebra body 2229
    zidovudine therapy associated 2223, 2229
myophosphorylase
    deficiency (McArdle's disorder) 2231–2232, 2232f
    skeletal muscle evaluation 2215t
myosarcoma, bladder 1722
myosin 2215, 2218t
    fetal, adult rhabdomyoma 355
myositis
    in autoimmune disorders 2221–2222
    in collagen vascular disorders 2221–2222
    focal 2224, 2225f
    granulomatous 2223–2224

inclusion body *see* inclusion body myositis (IBM)
    infectious 2222–2223, 2222f
    mumps 2219–2220
    proliferative 314
myositis ossificans 387, 684–685
    differential diagnosis 312, 388–389
myositis ossificans circumscripta 684, 685f
myositis ossificans progressiva 387, 684
myospherulosis 140–141, 141f
    ear involvement 2273, 2273f
    xanthogranulomatous pyelonephritis 1696
myotonia 2237
myotonic dystrophy 2237
myotubular (central nuclear) myopathy 2228–2229, 2228t
myotubules, formation 2214
myxedema
    generalized 229
    pretibial 228–229
myxofibroma (odontogenic myxoma) 1156–1157, 1157f, 1158
myxofibrosarcoma 326, 328–329, 329f, 330f
myxoid cartilage, cartilage-forming tumors 706
myxoid chondrosarcoma, chromosomal translocation 310t
myxoid expansion, renal vessels 1647
myxoid lesions, benign, of skin 267–268
myxoid liposarcoma, chromosomal translocation 310t
myxolipoma 336
myxoma
    of bone, jaws 1156–1157, 1157f
    cardiac 1062, 1063–1064, 1157
    cutaneous 267, 268f
    extra-abdominal fibromatosis (desmoid) *vs* 324
    eyelid 2291
    intramuscular 392–394, 393f
    juxta-articular 394
    larynx 848
    mandibular 823
    of nerve sheath 1185
    odontogenic 823, 1141f, 1156–1157, 1157f, 1158
    oral soft tissue 1157
    sinonasal 823
myxoma syndrome complex 1157
myxosarcoma, cardiac 1067

N

Nabothian cysts 1840
NADH staining, muscle fibers 2225, 2228, 2229f, 2230
NADH-TR, skeletal muscle evaluation 2215t
Naegleria, encephalitis 106
Naegleria fowleri 105, 106, 2412
nail patella syndrome, renal involvement 1623–1624
NARP syndrome 2231t
nasal cavity
    adenoid cystic carcinoma 794–795
    glioma 811–812, 812f
    glomus tumor 796t, 819–820
    inverted papilloma 788–789, 788f
    papillomas *see* Schneiderian papillomas
    polyps 787, 812f
    squamous cell carcinoma 790, 790f
    see also sinonasal region
nasal fossa, angiomatous polyps 818
nasal glial heterotopia 811–812, 812f
nasal mucosa, papillomas *see* Schneiderian papillomas
nasal septum
    chondroma 816, 816f
    hemangioma 817
    pleomorphic adenoma 795–796, 797f
    squamous cell carcinoma 789–790, 790f
nasal tip, metastases to 827
nasolabial cysts 1147f, 1148
nasopalatine duct cysts 1147–1148
nasopharyngeal congenital pleomorphic adenoma 800–801
nasopharyngeal orifice 2269
nasopharynx 787–831
    adenoid cystic carcinoma 794–795
    angiofibroma 817–818, 817f, 818f

angiosarcoma 818
    carcinoma 793–794, 793f, 1173
        immunohistochemistry 796t
        metastatic 1776, 1777f
        squamous cell 789
        transitional-type 793
        undifferentiated 154, 793, 1251
        WHO classification 793–794, 794f
    hairy polyps 826
    infections 77–81
    lymphoepithelioma 793, 1251
    see also sinonasal region
National Cancer Institute (NCI) 307, 307t, 422, 422t
National Committee for Laboratory Standards 36
natural killer (NK) cells
    blastic lymphoma/leukemia 651
    graft rejection 122
    leukemia 646–647
    lymphomas 543, 561–567, 650–652
navicular cells 1842
NC1 domain, glomerular basement membrane 1598, 1599f
NCAM (CD56), small cell lung carcinoma 991
Nebenkern formation 2095, 2102, 2103f
nebular bodies 1851
nebulin 2218t
neck dissection, radical, specimens 833
necrobiosis lipoidica 214, 214f
    differential diagnosis 213, 214, 234
necrotizing arteriolitis, malignant hypertension 1645, 1645f
necrotizing arteritis, appendix 1410, 1410f
necrotizing enterocolitis 1397–1398, 1398f, 1406
necrotizing fasciitis 68, 1772
necrotizing infections 69
necrotizing papillitis (papillary necrosis) 1641, 1642f
necrotizing sialometaplasia 1179, 1179f
necrotizing vasculitis, fallopian tube 2042
needle biopsy, breast, fat necrosis 135
needle-track seeding 138
negligence 10
Neisseria gonorrhoea 1835, 1836t, 2040
Nelson's syndrome 2047, 2104
nemaline rod myopathy 2227–2228, 2228f, 2228t
nemaline rods 2223, 2227, 2228f
nematode infections, gastrointestinal tract 104
neonates
    enteropathies 1376
    ganglion cells 1403
    gingival cysts 1141–1142
    subcutaneous fat necrosis 235–236, 235fg
nephrectomy
    renal cell carcinoma 1677
    specimen handling 1665–1666, 1672
nephrin 1598
nephritic syndrome, light microscopy diagnostic algorithm 1605t
nephritis
    acute interstitial *see* tubular interstitial nephritis
    lupus *see* lupus nephritis
    radiation 156
nephroblastoma *see* Wilms' tumor
nephroblastoma-like tumor 1756
nephroblastomatosis 1668, 1668f
nephrogenic adenoma (nephrogenic metaplasia) 1709, 1710f
nephrogenic metaplasia, bladder 1709, 1710f
nephrogenic rests 1668, 1670
nephroglomerulosis, post-irradiation 156
nephroma
    cystic 1668–1669
        multilocular cyst 1668, 1669f, 1694–1695, 1695f
    mesoblastic 1669–1670, 1669f
        adult 1695
        chromosomal translocation 310t
        ETV6–NTRK3 gene fusion 331
        Wilms' tumor *vs* 1667–1668
nephronophthisis 1664

nephrons 1598–1601
    see also glomerulus; renal tubules
nephropathia endemica 95
nephropathy
    Balkan 1640–1641
    C1q 1633–1634, 1634f
    chronic lead 1641, 1641f
    diabetic 1629, 1629f
    Henoch–Schönlein purpura 1618–1619, 1619f
    hereditary see hereditary nephritis of Alport
    HIV-associated 1603f, 1612
    IgA 1618–1620, 1619f
    IgM 1608, 1620
    membranous, de-novo after transplant 1653–1654,
        1653f
    membranous lupus 1626f, 1627
    myeloma cast ('myeloma kidney') 1630, 1630f
    postperfusion 1651
    radiation 156
    transplant 1650
nephrosclerosis
    benign 1643–1645, 1644f
    vascular, related to benign hypertension 1643–1645
nephrosis, cholemic 1634f
nephrotic syndrome 1605
    congenital 1622–1623
    diagnostic algorithms 1604t
    fibrillary glomerulopathy 1634–1635
    focal segmental glomerulosclerosis 1610
    IgM nephropathy with 1608
    membranous glomerulonephropathy causing 1614
    mesangial hypercellularity 1608–1609, 1612f
    minimal change glomerulopathy causing 1606
nerve biopsy see peripheral nerves, biopsy
nerve conduction 2241
    acute demyelinating block 2245
nerve fascicles (bundles) 2239, 2240
    traumatic neuroma 2245, 2246f
nerve fibers
    alpha, beta and gamma 2217
    classes A/B 2240
    interfusal 2217
    myelinated 2239, 2240, 2240f
    teased fiber analysis 2239, 2241f
    ultrastructure 2240–2241
    unmyelinated 2239, 2240, 2240f
nerves
    mixed sensory and motor 2239
    peripheral see peripheral nerves
nerve sheath 2241
    myxoma (neurothekeoma) 2255, 2255f
nerve sheath tumors 702t
    CNS 2385–2387
    see also malignant peripheral nerve sheath tumor
        (MPNST); schwannoma (neurilemoma)
nerve supply
    adrenal cortex 2171–2172
    skeletal muscle 2217
    skin 194
    testis 1731
    vagina 1919
    vulva 1886
nesidioblastosis 1569–1570
NeuN protein 2336, 2338
neural adhesion molecule (NCAM) see CD56 (neural-
    cell adhesion molecule)
neural sheath 2240
neural tumors
    gastrointestinal tract 1446–1448
    pituitary 2108–2109
    soft tissue 378–387
    see also specific tumors
neurenteric cysts 2401
neurilemoma see schwannoma (neurilemoma)
neurinoma see schwannoma (neurilemoma)
neuritis, localized interdigital (Morton's neuroma) 379,
    697, 698f, 2245–2246, 2246f
neuroblastic pseudorosettes see Homer Wright
    (pseudo)rosettes

neuroblastic tumors 383
    adrenal gland 2194
    see also ganglioneuroblastoma; ganglioneuroma;
        neuroblastoma
neuroblastoma 383–385
    adrenal medulla see adrenal medulla
    cerebral, supratentorial primitive neuroectodermal
        tumors vs 2384
    histologic maturation after chemotherapy 149
    international staging system 383, 383t
    metastatic 664, 750
    olfactory see olfactory neuroblastoma (ONB)
    pleomorphic rhabdomyosarcoma vs 359
    Shimada grading system 384, 384t
    synovial sarcoma vs 404
    Wilms' tumor vs 1667
neuroborreliosis 2407
neurocutaneous melanosis 2393, 2393f, 2394f
neurocysticercosis 2411–2412
neurocytoma, central 2376, 2376f, 2377f
    immunohistochemistry 2339t
    oligodendroglioma vs 2362
    ultrastructural characteristics 2337t
neurodermatitis 201
neuroectodermal tubules, in immature teratoma of
    ovary 2033, 2033f
neuroectodermal tumors
    of infancy, melanotic see melanotic neuroectodermal
        tumor of infancy
    malignant, of bone 702t, 746–751
        melanotic of infancy 750–751, 751f
        see also Ewing family of tumors
    monodermal, of ovary 2035–2036, 2036f
    olfactory neuroblastoma see olfactory neuroblastoma
        (ONB)
    primitive see primitive neuroectodermal tumors
        (PNET)
    sinonasal region 801–807
neuroendocrine abnormalities, breast 421
neuroendocrine carcinoma 1350
    large cell see large cell neuroendocrine carcinoma
        (LCNEC)
    larynx 843–844
    lymph node metastases 511
    ovary 2013, 2014
    sinonasal see sinonasal region, neuroendocrine
        carcinoma
neuroendocrine cells
    airways 860
    hyperplasia with bronchiolar fibrosis 908, 908f
    stomach 1297
neuroendocrine granules 803
neuroendocrine secretory granule matrix proteins 31t
neuroendocrine tumors
    appendix 1428–1429, 1429f
    colon and rectum 1429
    diagnostic work-up 181
    duodenum 1424
    hepatocellular carcinoma vs 1535
    kidney 1689–1690
    lung 982–994, 983t
    metastases, differential diagnosis 175
    pancreas, poorly differentiated 1575
    primary, of skin (Merkel cell carcinoma) 248–250,
        249f, 261
    prostate 1819
    small intestinal 1423–1429
    stomach 1348–1351
    thymus and mediastinum see thymus
    see also carcinoid tumor(s); neuroendocrine
        carcinoma
neuroepithelial bodies, airways 860
neuroepithelial tumors, diagnostic significance of
    rosettes 2366t
neuroepithelioma 385–386, 385f
neurofibroma 2253–2255, 2253f, 2386–2387
    bone involvement 771
    breast 446
    cardiac 1066

differential diagnosis 2254–2255
    diffuse 2254
    infiltrative growth 2253, 2253f
    intestinal 1446
    nuclear atypia in 2254, 2254f, 2255
    oral cavity 1185
    pigmented 2254
    plexiform 2254, 2254f
    radiation-associated 160
    sinonasal 810
    'with atypical features' 2255
neurofibromatosis 2258
neurofibromatosis type 1 (von Recklinghausen's
        disease) 2253, 2258, 2386–2387
    angiomyolipoma association 1690
    bone involvement 771
    café-au-lait pigmented macules 282
    dissecting osteitis 2151
    genes and CNS features 2401t
    intestinal involvement 1446
    laryngeal involvement 848
    malignant peripheral nerve sheath tumor 2256
    multiple non-ossifying fibromas 737
    pheochromocytoma with 2192
    plexiform neurofibroma involving orbit 2297–2298
    schwannomas 1185, 2249, 2250f
    somatostatinoma 1574
    uveal melanoma in 2306
neurofibromatosis type 2 2258, 2401t
    schwannomas 2249, 2250f, 2385
neurofibromin gene 2258
neurofilament protein 384, 2336, 2338
neurofilaments 2240
neurogenic atrophy 2224–2226, 2225t, 2226f
neurogenic muscle disease, myopathic disease vs 2225t
neurogenic tumors
    larynx and trachea 848
    oral cavity 1185
neuroglial heterotopia 2404
neuroglial tissue, aberrant in middle ear 2271
neurohypophysis 2093, 2094f
neurohypophysitis, infundibular 2111
neuroma
    amputation (traumatic) 378–379, 2245, 2246f
    c-fiber, oral cavity 1185
    cystic duct 1578
    Morton's (plantar) 379, 697, 698f, 2245–2246, 2246f
    mucosal 2248–2249, 2249f
    Pacinian 2246
    palisaded encapsulated 268, 268f, 2248
        oral cavity 1185
    solitary circumscribed 268, 268f
    traumatic 378–379, 2246f
        oral cavity 1185
neuromatous hyperplasia, of gastrointestinal tract
        2248–2249
neuromuscular disease/disorders
    appendix 1407
    HIV infection 2223
    intestine 1403–1404
neuromuscular junction 2217, 2217f
    disorders 2224–2238
neuronal tumors, CNS 2374–2377
neuronophagia 2344
neurons
    CNS 2340, 2340f
    'dark' 2340, 2341f
    ischemic 2340
    'red' 2340, 2341f
neuron specific enolase (NSE) 610, 1322, 2336, 2338
    adrenocortical carcinoma 2188
    neuroblastoma 384
    neuroendocrine tumors 181
    pancreatic endocrine neoplasms 1571
    skeletal muscle evaluation 2215t
    small cell lung carcinoma 991
neuropathy 2239t
    acute ascending 2239, 2239t
    amyloid 2247

autonomic 2248
chronic 2239, 2239t
chronic demyelinative 2242f, 2258
chronic progressive 2239t
chronic relapsing and remitting 2239, 2239t
diabetic 2247–2248
differential diagnosis 2239, 2239t
distal symmetrical sensory 2248
entrapment 2245
hereditary 2239, 2239t, 2241
    see also hereditary motor and sensory
        neuropathies (HMSN)
HIV-associated 2244
infectious causes 2243–2244
inflammatory 2242–2244, 2242f
metabolic 2247–2248
nutritional 2247, 2248t
paraneoplastic 2244
subacute sensory motor 2239, 2239t
toxic 2247, 2248t
uremic 2248
neuropil 384, 2196
neurosecretory granules 1571, 2193, 2193f
neurosyphilis 2407
neurothecoma, oral cavity 1185
neurothekeoma 2255, 2255f
neurotization 278
neurotrophin receptor Trk C, medulloblastoma 2383
neurotubules, peripheral nerves 2240
neutropenia 617
neutropenic enterocolitis 1397
neutrophilic dermatoses 212
neutrophilic microabscesses 223, 223f
neutrophils
    acute inflammatory response 63–64
    adult respiratory distress syndrome 874
    around Mallory bodies (satellitosis) 1490, 1492f
    in effusions 1026–1027
    in esophagus 1282f, 1285, 1285t
    gastroesophageal reflux disease 1282f, 1285, 1285t
    granules 63
    leukocytoclastic vasculitis 209, 210f
    subcorneal pustule 216
    subepidermal blisters 222, 222t, 223
    vasculitis 209–211
nevocytes
    migration mechanisms (to/from epidermis) 277, 278
    multinucleated 281
    see also melanocyte(s)
nevoid lentigo 277
nevomelanocytes 1897
nevus (nevi) 277
    acrosyringeal 257, 259f
    arising in pregnancy or adolescence 277–278
    atypical (dysplastic) see melanocytic nevi
    'balloon'-cell 282
    Becker's 282
    blue 279–280, 280f
        'cellular' 279, 1842
        cervix 1842
        conjunctiva 2292
        eyelid 2290
        hypopigmented 279
        vaginal 1923
    Clark's 280
    compound 277–278, 278f
    congenital 278, 283
        large/'giant' 278
        vulvar 1897
    conjunctival 2292–2293
    connective tissue 231, 232
    cystic compound 2292, 2293f
    deep penetrating 282, 282f
    epidermal 241, 241f
    epithelioid-cell 278
    eyelid 2290
    halo 282
    hypopigmentation around 282
    incomplete excision 281

intradermal (IDN) 278
    of Ito 282
    junctional 277, 278f, 2292
    lentiginous junctional 277
    magnocellular (melanocytoma) 2309
    melanocytic see melanocytic nevi
    milk line 1897
    organoid 194, 250, 250f, 258
    of Ota 282
    plexiform spindle cell (deep penetrating) 282, 282f
    'privileged' 277, 278
    recurrent/persistent 281–282
    speckled lentiginous 277
    spindle cell, uveal tract 2307
    Spitz (spindle-cell and epithelioid-cell) 278–279,
        279f
    'strawberry' 269–270, 269f
nevus cell see melanocyte(s); nevocytes
nevus cell inclusions, lymph nodes 513, 513f
nevus flammeus 268
nevus lipomatosus 264
nevus lipomatosus superficialis, vulva 1901
nevus of Ota 2292, 2306
nevus perstans 281–282
nevus recurrens 281–282
nevus sebaceus of Jadassohn 194, 250, 250f, 258
nevus spilus 277
NF2 mutations, mesothelioma 1015
nickel sulfide, lung cancer etiology 936
nicotine stomatitis 1166
Niemann-Pick cells 579
Niemann–Pick disease 579, 658, 1470
night pain, osteoid osteoma 702
night tourniquet paralysis 2245
NIH Consensus Conference, atypical (dysplastic) nevi
    280, 281
Nijmegen syndrome 115, 571
Nikolski sign 218, 222, 1893
nil disease (minimal change glomerulopathy)
    1606–1608, 1612f
nipple 420
    adenoma 439–440, 441f
        syringomatous 440, 442f
    aspiration 425
    discharge 425–426
    ductal lavage 425
    embryology 419
    leiomyoma 349
    leiomyosarcoma 349
    melanoma 457
    Paget's disease see Paget's disease, of nipple
    primary carcinoma 458
    sampling techniques 425–426
    scrape cytology 425
    supernumerary 421
Nissl bodies 2256, 2381f
nissle substance 2340
Nissl substance, ganglioneuroblastoma 384
nitrofurantoin, lung disease due to 885, 899
nitrosamines, esophageal squamous cell carcinoma
    1294
N-myc oncogene, neuroblastoma 384
Nocardia 74
    cerebral abscess 2406
    pneumonia 81–82, 82f, 83f
    pulmonary alveolar proteinosis 925–926
Nocardia asteroides 81–82, 901
NOD2/CARD15 gene, mutations, Crohn's disease
    1387
NOD2 protein expression, Crohn's disease 1373
nodal basin, melanoma 286
nodes of Ranvier 2241
'nodular adenosis' 431
nodular amyloid tumor, lung 968, 968f
nodular fasciitis 312–313, 312f, 313f, 314f
    differential diagnosis 313, 324
    oral cavity 1183
    oral postradiation squamous cell carcinoma vs
        1177

nodular lymphoid hyperplasia (pseudotumor), lung
    977, 979–980, 979f, 980f
nodules
    definition 195
    dermal 233
    erythematous 211, 215
    see also specific nodules/sites
noma 78–79
non-Hodgkin's lymphoma see lymphoma (non-
    Hodgkin's)
nonodontogenic cysts 1147–1149
nonsteroidal antiinflammatory drugs (NSAIDs)
    acute hemorrhagic gastritis due to 1327, 1327f
    colitis 1402, 1402f
    colonic ulcers 1402
    duodenal erosion due to 1397
    esophagitis 1290
    intestinal lesions due to 1401–1402
    reactive gastritis due to 1338
    small bowel damage 1401–1402
Nora's lesion 773–774, 773f, 774f
normoblasts 612
normokalemic periodic paralysis 2233
Northern blots 45
Norwalk agent 1377
notochordal rests 763, 765
notochordal tumors 702t, 765
    see also chordoma
Nottingham grading system 464
Nottingham Prognostic Index, breast cancer 488
NPHPH1 gene 1664
N-trk gene, papillary thyroid carcinoma 2132
nuchal fibrocartilaginous tumor 319
nuchal fibroma 318–319, 319f
nuclear anaplasia, basal cell carcinoma of skin 244
nuclear atypia 2350
nuclear bag fibers 2217
nuclear chain fibers 2217
nuclear pseudoinclusions
    giant cell glioblastoma 2355, 2355f
    meningioma 2387, 2388f, 2389f
nuclear smudging
    polyomavirus infection 1652, 1652f
    salivary mucoepidermoid carcinoma 1230, 1231f
nucleated red blood cells (NRBCs) 612
nuclei
    angular 1237, 1239f
    'cigar-shaped' 348
    'coffee-bean'-like 572, 659
    'floret-like' arrangement 339, 339f
    'ground-glass' 119, 120f, 1482, 1482f, 2343f
    knobby 650, 651f
    'Orphan Annie' (ground glass) 2128
    palisading see palisading of nuclei
    'steel-gray' 221, 221f
nucleic acid
    analysis 45
    probes 45, 46, 106–107
    staining methods 16t
nucleoli, prominence 1559, 1560, 1560f
nucleolonema 1117f, 1120
null cells 2097
    adenoma 2106–2107, 2106f, 2107f
nummular dermatitis 196, 197f
nutrition, oral squamous cell carcinoma due to 1169

O

oat cell carcinoma
    lung see small cell lung carcinoma (SCLC)
    sinonasal see sinonasal region, neuroendocrine
        carcinoma (SNEC)
    of thymus see thymus, neuroendocrine tumors
obesity, renal cell carcinoma 1677
obliterative bronchiolitis, chronic rejection of lung graft
    128, 129
obliterative endarteritis 2407
    liver allograft rejection 128, 128f
    microangiopathic 928
    villitis in syphilis 2069

occupational exposures
  lung cancer etiology 935–936
    oral squamous cell carcinoma and 1169
    sinonasal intestinal type adenocarcinoma and 807
occupational hypersensitivity 891
ochronosis, aortic stenosis 1058
OCT3/4 1744, 1745f, 1750, 1775t, 1776
OCT4 180
octreotide, gastric carcinoma tumors 1351
ocular contusion 2312
ocular evisceration 2304–2305
ocular proptosis 2294, 2296
ocular siderosis 2312
ocular specimens 2289
ocular surgery, complications 2312
ocular toxocariasis 2310
ocular trauma 2311–2312
oculodermal melanocytosis (nevus of Ota) 2292,
    2306
oculoglandular cat-scratch disease (Parinaud's) 78, 78f,
    2294
oculomotor nerve, diabetes mellitus 2247
oculopharyngeal muscular dystrophy 2237
oculoplastic procedures 2290
odontoameloblastoma 1141f, 1161–1162, 1161f
odontoblasts 1139
odontogenesis 1139, 1140f, 1141f
odontogenic carcinoma, clear cell 1153, 1247
odontogenic cysts 1139–1146
  adenomatoid see odontogenic tumors,
      adenomatoid
  botryoid 1142–1143, 1142f, 1143f
  calcifying 1142f, 1145–1146, 1145f
  carcinoma associated 1146
  classification 1139, 1139t
  dentigerous 1140–1141, 1142f
  developmental 1139, 1139t
  gingival 1141–1142, 1142f
  glandular 1146
  inflammatory 1139, 1139t, 1146–1147
  keratocysts see odontogenic keratocyst
  squamous cell carcinoma arising 1173
odontogenic epithelial rests 1141
odontogenic fibroma 1141f
  central 1158–1159, 1158f
  peripheral 1159
odontogenic keratocyst 1142f, 1143–1145, 1144f
  parakeratotic and orthokeratotic types 1144
  satellite (daughter) cysts 1144
odontogenic rests 1158f
odontogenic tumors 1149–1162
  adenomatoid 1140f, 1154–1156, 1155f
    ameloblastic fibroma vs 1161
  ameloblastic fibroma 1141f, 1159–1161, 1160f
  ameloblastic fibro-odontoma 1141f, 1161
  ameloblastic fibrosarcoma 1162
  ameloblastoma see ameloblastoma
  benign 1150t
    epithelial 1150–1156
    mesenchymal 1156–1159
  calcifying epithelial 1140f, 1153–1154, 1154f
    ameloblastic fibroma vs 1161
    clear cell variant 1154
  cementoblastoma 1141f, 1159, 1159f
  classification 1139, 1140f, 1150t
  dual (mixed) origin 1141f, 1159–1162
  epithelial 1140f, 1150–1156
  fibroma 1141f
  malignant 1150t
    nonepithelial origin, rare 1162
  mesenchymal 1141f
    benign 1156–1159
  myxoma 1141f, 1156–1157, 1157f, 1158
  odontoameloblastoma 1161–1162, 1161f
  squamous 1156
  see also specific tumors (see table page 16)
odontoma 1141f, 1162
  ameloblastic 750–751, 751f
  cystic 1145

Ofuji's syndrome 227
Ogilvie's syndrome 1404
Oil red O stain 21f, 1470, 1470f, 2335t
  skeletal muscle evaluation 2215t
OKT3, heart transplant rejection 1050
oleogranuloma 141
oleoma 141
olfactory neuroblastoma (ONB) 384–385, 801–803
  clinical features/treatment 801t, 803
  grading 801, 802, 803t
  immunohistochemistry 796t, 801
  pathology 801–803, 802f
  sinonasal neuroendocrine carcinoma and 803
oligoastrocytoma 2369–2370
  anaplastic 2370
oligodendrocytes 2343, 2343f
  'ballooned' 119, 120f
  gliofibrillary 2361
  round nuclei 2361, 2362f
oligodendroglial cells
  enlarged 2409f
  neoplastic 2361, 2361f, 2362
  see also oligodendrocytes
oligodendroglial tumors 2360–2364
oligodendroglioma 2360–2363
  anaplastic 2363–2364, 2363f
    WHO grades III/IV 2363
  calcification 2361, 2361f
  central neurocytoma vs 2376
  cytology 2361, 2361f
  genetic abnormalities 2340t, 2363
  GFAP expression status 2361, 2362
  histology 2361, 2361f, 2363
  immunohistochemistry 2338t, 2362, 2363
  pituitary 2109
  smear preparations 2360–2361, 2361f
  ultrastructural characteristics 2336t, 2362
oligohydramnios 2067
Ollier's disease 710–711, 711f
  chondrosarcoma 816
  enchondroma 708, 710, 710f, 711
  juvenile granulosa cell tumor in 2017
omental implants, ovarian serous tumors 1999–2000,
    1999f
omental-mesenteric myxoid hamartoma 1022
omphalomesenteric duct remnants 2066
onchocerciasis 2313
oncocytes 1223, 1225f, 2097, 2150
  eosinophilia 1218
  nodules 2150, 2150f
  parathyroid adenoma 2154, 2154f
  Warthin's tumor 1217–1218, 1217f, 1218f
oncocytic adrenocortical neoplasm 2185, 2187f
oncocytic cells 175f
  salivary glands 1208t, 1223, 1224
oncocytic metaplasia 1225
  parotid gland 1223–1224
oncocytic tumors, sinonasal region 797–798
oncocytoma
  adrenal cortex 2185, 2187f
  kidney 1674–1676, 1675f
    differential diagnosis 1675, 1676, 1677t
  pituitary 2106–2107, 2107f
  salivary gland see salivary gland tumors
  sinonasal region 797–798
oncocytomatosis 1674
oncocytosis (oncocytic metaplasia) 1223, 1224
oncogenes 44, 1169–1170
  markers 31t
  oral cavity disease 1138, 1169–1170
  osteosarcoma association 728t
  see also RB gene
onion bulbs, nerves 2241, 2242f, 2244, 2245, 2245f
'onion-skinning', renal arterioles 1611f, 1645
oocytes 1987
oophoritis 1989
ophthalmoplegia, diabetic 2247
Opisthorchis viverrine 1583, 1585
opportunistic infections

of CNS, in AIDS 2409–2410
  malabsorption due to 1378
optic atrophy
  ascending/descending 2319
  glaucomatous 2314, 2315f, 2318
optic chiasm, tumor differential diagnosis 2348t
optic disc
  atrophy, glaucoma 2314, 2315f
  edema (papilledema) 2318
optic nerve 2318–2319
  atrophy 2318
  examination 2305, 2306
  glioma 2298
  invasion by retinoblastoma 2310
  tumors, pilocytic astrocytoma 2357
optic neuropathy, Leber's hereditary 2231t
oral cavity 1137–1201
  adenoid squamous carcinoma 1176, 1176f
  adenosquamous carcinoma 1176
  benign epithelial lesions resembling malignant
      lesions 1178–1179
  benign reactive desmoplastic stromal reaction 1177
  biopsy
    bone 1137
    brush biopsy 1137
    reactive change in salivary glands 136, 136f
    soft tissue 1137
  bleeding 1180–1181
  bone/cartilage tumors 1194–1195
  carcinoma in situ (intraepithelial) 1167
  carcinosarcoma 1177
  cavernous hemangioma 1186
  central giant cell granuloma 1182–1183, 1182f
  central giant cell tumor 1182–1183, 1182f
  cysts 1147–1149
    lymphoepithelial 1148, 1148f
    rare nonodontogenic 1149
    see also odontogenic cysts
  developmental conditions 1162–1163
  epithelial dysplasia 1166–1167, 1167f, 1167t
  epithelial lesions 1163–1165
  erythroplakia 1165, 1166f
  etiological agents of disease 1138
  fibroma 1180
  fibromatoses 1184
  fibro-osseous dysplasia and bone lesions see jaw(s);
      specific lesions
  fibrosarcoma 1184
  giant cell fibroma 1180
  granular cell tumor 1184–1185, 1184f
  histologic/taxonomic considerations 1138–1139
  inflammatory fibrous hyperplasia 1180
  inflammatory papillary hyperplasia 1164
  inverted papilloma 1179
  keratoacanthoma 1164–1165, 1175
  leukoplakia 1165, 1165f, 1165t, 1166f
  lichen planus 1166
  lipoma 1184
  lymphatic lesions 1186
  melanocytic lesions 1177–1178
  melanoma 1177–1178
  melanotic neuroectodermal tumor of infancy 1178,
      1178f
  mesenchymal soft tissue lesions 1180–1186
  metaplastic (spindle cell squamous) 1176–1177,
      1177f
  metastatic tumors in 1179–1180
  mucoceles 1149
  mucoepidermal tumor, mucocele vs 1149
  mucoepidermoid carcinoma 1179
  myogenic tumors 1185
  myxomas 1157
  necrotizing sialometaplasia 1179, 1179f
  neurogenic tumors 1185
  nicotine stomatitis 1166
  nodular fasciitis 1183
  odontogenic lesions see entries beginning
      odontogenic
  papillary endothelial hyperplasia 1181

peripheral giant cell granuloma 1181–1182
peripheral ossifying fibroma (peripheral with
    calcification) 1181, 1181f
pleomorphic carcinoma (spindle cell squamous)
    1176–1177, 1177f
premalignant lesions 1165, 1166
pseudoepitheliomatous hyperplasia 1178–1179,
    1184
pyogenic granuloma 1180–1181
soft tissue lesions 1162–1186
specimens
    artifacts 1137–1138
    nature and handling 1137–1138
spindle cell squamous cell carcinoma 1176–1177,
    1177f, 1244
squamous cell carcinoma 1167–1177
    adenoid (acantholytic) 1175–1176
    basaloid 439 42f
    grades 1171–1172
    histologic features (invasion depth) 1171
    lymph node metastases 1171, 1172–1173
    necrotizing sialometaplasia vs 1179
    papillary (exophytic) 1170, 1171f, 1175, 1175f
    pathologic features 1171–1172, 1172f
    poorly differentiated 1172
    postradiation 1177
    sarcomatoid (polypoid) 1176–1177, 1177f
    sites 1170, 1172–1173
    staging and prognostic parameters 1170–1171,
        1171t
    subtypes 1170
    undifferentiated 1172
    variants 1173–1177
    well-differentiated 1172, 1172t, 1175
squamous papilloma 1163–1164
ulceration 1178
vascular lesions 1186
verrucous carcinoma 1173–1175, 1174f, 1175f
verrucous hyperplasia 1174
see also jaw(s); salivary glands; specific anatomic
    structures
oral contraceptives
    chronic nongranulomatous endometritis 1945
    endometrial changes 1946, 1947f
    endometrial hyperplasia/carcinoma 151, 151f
    erythema nodosum and 234
    focal nodular hyperplasia of liver and 1527
    hepatic adenoma and 1528
    intestinal ischemia associated 1381–1382
    sinusoidal dilatation after 1517, 1517f
oral intraepithelial neoplasia (OIN) 1167
orange G (OG) solution 26
orangeophilic cytoplasm 1297, 1298f
orbit 2294–2298
    abscess 2294
    capillary hemangioma 2296–2297
    cavernous hemangioma 2297, 2297f
    cellulitis 2294
    dermoid cysts 2296
    exenteration 2305
    fibrous histiocytoma 2297
    in Graves' disease 2295, 2295f
    hemangiopericytoma 2297
    idiopathic inflammatory pseudotumor 2295, 2295f
    inflammatory diseases 2294–2295
    lymphangioma 2297
    lymphoid tumors 2296, 2296f
    lymphomas 2296, 2296f
    meningioma 2298
    metastases in 171t, 173
    neural and meningeal tumors 2297–2298
    rhabdomyosarcoma 2297
    schwannoma 2298
    secondary tumors 2298
    soft tissue tumors 2297
    tumors 2296–2298
    vascular tumors 2296–2297
    vasculitides 2295
orbital bones

blowout fractures 2294
    lesions 2297
orcein stain 1468, 1486
orchiectomy, radical 1733, 1746
orchitis 1767
    granulomatous 1767, 1767f
    testicular lymphoma vs 1762
    viral 1738, 1767
oropharynx, carcinoma 1173
    squamous cell carcinoma 1173
orthokeratosis 194, 195
    actinic keratosis 243f
    hyperkeratotic, lichen planus 202
    'spiky', epidermal nevi 241, 241f
orthopedic hardware, iatrogenic lesions 144
orthopedic prostheses, tumors associated 144
    sarcoma development 702
osmium tetroxide 17
osseous dysplasia, florid (cemento-osseous) 1193–1194
osseous metaplasia, peritoneum 1021
ossicles, middle ear 2268–2269
ossification
    cutaneous 267
    endochondral 681
ossifying fasciitis, myositis ossificans vs 312
ossifying fibroma
    fibrous dysplasia vs 1191, 1192
    jaws 1192–1193, 1192f
    juvenile active 1192
    peripheral, with calcification (oral cavity) 1181,
        1181f
    sinonasal region 813, 814f
ossifying fibromyxoid tumor 378f, 379–381, 380f
ossifying renal tumor 1672
osteitis, dissecting 751, 2151
osteitis fibrosa 686
osteitis fibrosa cystica 740, 751
osteitis fibrosa cystica generalisata 2151
    see also neurofibromatosis type 1
osteitis fibrosa disseminata 1190
osteoarthritis (osteoarthrosis) 691–693, 692f
    rheumatoid arthritis vs 692–693
    synovial fluid 691, 691t
osteoblastic rimming 387
osteoblastoma 724–726, 726f
    aggressive 725, 726f
    hemorrhagic 726f
    jaws 815, 1194
    juvenile aggressive 815
    large osteoid osteoma as 723–724
    pseudomalignant 725
    sphenoethmoid 815
    subperiosteal 725f
osteoblasts 614, 680
    in osteoblastoma 725, 726f
osteochondroma (exostosis) 706–708, 707f, 708f
    chondrosarcoma vs 708
    external auditory canal 2282
    hereditary multiple 707, 708, 718
    post-radiotherapy 160
    solitary, malignant degeneration 708
osteochondromatous proliferation, parosteal 388
osteochondromyxoma of bone 706
osteoclast giant cells 713f, 814
osteoclasts 613, 680
    bone marrow examination 614
osteocytes 679, 679f, 680
osteodystrophy, Albright's hereditary 267
osteofibrous dysplasia 743, 744f, 745f
    adamantinoma and 743
    fibrous dysplasia of bone vs 742
osteogenesis imperfecta 686
osteogenic sarcoma
    head and neck and jaw 815
    stress fracture vs 682
    subtypes 815
osteoid 813
    in aneurysmal bone cyst 758f
    in osteosarcoma 733, 733f

osteoid osteoma 702, 723–724, 724, 724f, 725f
    giant see osteoblastoma
    intracortical chondroma vs 712
    jaws 1194
osteoid seam 687f
osteolipoma 336
osteolysis, myeloma 762
osteoma 722–723, 723f
    craniofacial 722
    external auditory canal (EAC) 2282
    ivory and compact types 813
    jaw 1193
    osteoid see osteoid osteoma
    sinonasal 813
osteoma cutis 233, 268f
osteomalacia 681, 686, 687f
    tumor-associated 740, 819, 819f
osteomatosis
    congenital plaque-like 267
    multiple 267, 268f
osteomyelitis 689–690
    cryptococcal 86f
    hematogenous 689
    Langerhans cell histiocytosis vs 760
    osteonecrosis complication 683
osteonecrosis 682, 683–684, 684f
osteopenia 681
osteopetrosis 681, 681f
osteopoikilosis 722, 723f
osteoporosis 681, 687, 687f
    idiopathic transient 687
    myeloma causing 762
osteosarcoma 726–736
    bone structure/pattern 721
    chondroblastic 730f, 731, 732f, 733, 734, 734f
    classification 726–727, 727t
    conventional 728–729
        cytology 733–734, 734f
        subtypes 731
    cytogenetic abnormalities 727–728, 728t
    cytology 733–735, 734f
    development in Paget's disease of bone 728
    differential diagnosis 734–735
    ear and temporal bone 2283
    epithelioid variant 732, 733
    etiology 727–728
    fibroblastic 731
    fine needle aspiration 733–735, 733f, 734f
    genetic syndromes associated 727
    giant-cell-rich variant 732
    grading 727
    gross morphology 728–731, 729f, 730f
    immunohistochemistry and ultrastructure 735
    intramedullary well differentiated 727, 728, 736
        gross morphology 730–731, 730f, 731f
        microscopic morphology 733, 733f
    jaws 1194
    larynx 850
    low-grade, differential diagnosis 738, 739, 742
    metastases 735, 736
    microscopic morphology 731–733
    mixed variant 731, 733
    osteoblastic (high-grade surface) 727, 728, 730, 731,
        731f, 735
        microscopic morphology 733
        sclerosing variant 732f
    osteoblastoma-like variant 732
    Paget's 735, 2283
    parosteal (juxtacortical well differentiated) 727, 728,
        729f, 730, 730f, 735
        cytology 735, 735f
        dedifferentiated 732
        of jaws 1194
        microscopic morphology 732, 733f
    periosteal (intermediate-grade) 727, 728, 729f, 730,
        735
        microscopic morphology 733
    pleomorphic 733
    pre-existing conditions 728

osteosarcoma (*cont'd*)
  primary, of skin 267
  prognosis 735–736
  radiation association 159, 727, 735
  radiography 728, 729f
  sarcomatoid carcinoma of prostate and 1819f, 1820
  secondary 728
  sites 727
  skip metastases 729
  small cell 731, 732f, 733, 735
    Ewing family of tumors *vs* 750
  soft tissue 388–389
  surface 727, 728
  telangiectatic 729, 730f, 731, 732f
    cytology 734, 734f
  treatment 735, 736f
otitis externa 2271–2272
otitis media 2272, 2272f
  tuberculous 2272–2273
otorrhea, bloody 2274
otosclerosis 2283, 2283f
otospongiosis 2283, 2283f
ovarian hyperstimulation syndrome 1993
ovarian remnant syndrome 1988
ovarian thecal metaplasia, adrenal cortex 2173–2174, 2173f
ovary 1987–2039
  abscess 1989
  absence 1988
  accessory/supernumerary 1988
  actinomycosis 1989, 1990f
  adenocarcinoma
    grading system 1996t
    primary *vs* secondary 2038t
  adenofibroma
    clear cell 2011
    endometrioid 2007–2008
    mucinous 2002
    serous 1997
  adenoid cystic carcinoma 2014
  adenosarcoma 2010
  anatomy and size 1987
  atrophy 1988, 1989
  basaloid carcinoma 2014
  biopsy 1988
  Brenner tumors *see* Brenner tumors
  carcinoid tumors 2035, 2035f
    immunohistochemistry 2017t
  carcinoma
    leukemia after 149
    metastases, to uterus 1979
    peritoneal effusions 1029–1030, 1030f
    see also specific carcinomas (below)
  carcinosarcoma 2010, 2010f
  choriocarcinoma 2030–2031, 2031f
    mixed tumors 2036, 2037f
  clear cell carcinoma 2011–2012
    endometriosis and 1995, 2012
    growth patterns 2011–2012, 2011f, 2012f
  clear cell tumors 2011–2012
    benign 2011
    borderline 2011, 2011f
  congenital abnormalities 1988
  cortex 1987
  in Crohn's disease 1989
  cystadenofibroma 1997
    endometrioid 2007–2008
    mucinous 2002, 2002f
    serous 1997
  cystadenoma
    mucinous 2002
    serous 1997, 1997f
  cysts 1987, 1990–1991
    benign epithelial 1990, 1991f
    benign of follicular origin 1990
    borderline mucinous tumors and 2002, 2003
    'chocolate' 1951, 1952f, 1994
    embryonic rests and 1990
    endometrioid 1995

FNA, complication rate 138
    needle-tract seeding 138
    outpouchings 2003
    pregnancy related 1992, 1993t
    serous cystadenoma and 1997, 1997f
  desmoplastic small round cell tumor 2026, 2039
  duplication 1988
  ectopic tissue 1988
  embryonal carcinoma 2029t, 2030, 2030f
  endometrioid carcinoma 2008–2009, 2008f
    borderline tumors *vs* 2008
    endometriosis in 1995
    grading systems 1996t, 2009
    immunohistochemistry 2009
    microglandular (spindle-cell) 2009
    oxyphilic variant 2009
    sertoliform pattern 2009, 2009f
    Sertoli-Leydig cell tumors *vs* 2023
    squamous/mucinous differentiation 2008, 2008f
    yolk sac tumor mixture 2009
    yolk sac tumors arising in 2028
    yolk sac tumors *vs* 2009
  endometrioid stromal sarcoma 2010
  endometrioid tumors 2007–2010
    benign 2007
    borderline 2007–2008, 2008f
    immunohistochemistry 2009–2010
    intraepithelial carcinoma with 2008
    squamous/mucinous metaplasia 2008
  endometriosis 1994–1995, 1994f, 1995f, 2007
    atypical 1952f, 1995
  enlargement 1993
  epithelial tumors 1995, 1996
    benign 1996t
    borderline 1996t
    categories 1996t
    classification 1996, 1996t
    endometrioid *see* ovary, endometrioid tumors
    grading system 1567t, 1996
    malignant 1996t, 2013–2014
    mucinous *see* ovary, mucinous tumors
    serous *see* ovary, serous tumors
    'undifferentiated carcinoma' 2013, 2015f
  failure 1988–1989
  fibroma 2018–2019, 2018f
  fibromatosis 1992
  fibrosarcoma 2018–2019
  fibrothecoma 2018
  germ cell-stromal tumors 2037
  germ cell tumors 1995, 2027–2036, 2027t
    arising in gonadoblastoma 2037
    choriocarcinoma 2030–2031, 2031f
    dysgerminoma 2027–2028, 2028f
    epithelial carcinoma with 2014
    malignant mixed 2036, 2037f
    teratoma 2031–2036
    yolk sac tumors *see* yolk sac tumors
  gonadoblastoma 2036–2037
  granulocytic sarcoma 2026, 2027, 2029t
  granulosa cell tumor 2015–2017, 2015f
    adult *vs* juvenile comparison 2018t
    cystic 2016
    immunostaining 2016–2017, 2017t
    juvenile 2015, 2017–2018, 2017f
    microfollicular pattern 2016, 2016f
  gross examination 1987
  gynandroblastoma 2026
  hepatoid carcinoma 2014
  histology (normal) 1987–1988, 1987f
  hyperreactio luteinalis 1992–1993, 1993f
  hyperthecosis 1991–1992, 1992f
  infertility and 1988–1989
  inflammatory disorders 1989
  large cell neuroendocrine carcinoma 2014
  leiomyoma 2026
  leukemia 2026–2027
  lymphoma 2026–2027, 2027f
    immunohistochemistry 2017t, 2029t

malacoplakia 1989, 1990f
  massive edema 1992, 2021
  medulla 1988
  melanoma, immunohistochemistry 2029t
  mesenchymal tumors 2026
  metastatic tumors 1995, 2002, 2037–2039
    appendiceal adenocarcinoma 2039
    breast cancer 2039
    carcinoid tumors 2039
    colorectal cancer 2037–2038, 2038f
    endometrial tumors with 1967
    immunophenotypes 2038t
  microcystic carcinoma 2009
  monodermal neuroectodermal tumors 2035–2036, 2036f
  mucinous carcinoma, of intestinal type 2004–2005, 2004f
    cribriform pattern of growth 2004, 2004f
    mural nodules 2005, 2005f
    peritoneal effusions 1029–1030, 1030f
  mucinous epithelium 2002, 2003f
  mucinous tumors 2002–2007
    benign 2002
    borderline, endocervical-like 2003–2004, 2004f
    borderline of intestinal type 2002–2003, 2003f
    immunohistochemistry 2005–2006, 2005f
    intraglandular (noninvasive) 2003
    malignant 2002, 2004–2005, 2004f
    in pseudomyxoma peritonei 2006–2007, 2006f, 2008f
  necrotic pseudoxanthomatous nodules 1989
  neuroendocrine carcinoma 2013
  non-neoplastic conditions 1988–1995
  non-neoplastic cysts and tumors 1990–1995
  papillae
    borderline seromucinous tumors 2003–2004, 2004f
    borderline serous tumors 1997, 1998f
    mucinous carcinoma 2004
  polycystic 1991, 1992f
  in pregnancy, unusual microscopic findings 1994
  pregnancy related pseudotumors and cysts 1992, 1993t
  pseudotumors, pregnancy related 1992, 1993t
  schistosomiasis 1989
  sectioning method 1987
  seromucinous adenocarcinoma 2005, 2005f, 2006
    borderline 2003–2004, 2004f
  serous adenocarcinoma, metastases to cervix 1875f
  serous carcinoma 1996–1997, 2001–2002, 2001f
    low-grade forms 2001–2002
    peritoneal effusions 1029–1030, 1030f
  serous surface papillary carcinoma 2001
  serous tumors 1996–2002
    benign 1997, 1997f
    immunohistochemistry 2002
    malignant *see* ovary, serous carcinoma
  serous tumors, borderline 1997–2001, 1997f, 1998f
    benign epithelial inclusions 2000, 2000f
    cribriform pattern 1998, 1998f
    lymph node involvement 2000–2001, 2000f
    micropapillary 1997–1998, 1998f
    peritoneal/omental implants 1999, 1999f
    serous carcinoma *vs* 1998
    stromal invasion 1998–1999, 1999f
  Sertoli cell tumors 2023, 2023f
  Sertoli-Leydig cell tumor 2017t, 2021–2023, 2022f
  sex cord-stromal tumor *see* sex cord-stromal tumors
  sex cord tumor with annular tubules (SCTAT) 2023–2024
  small cell carcinoma 2013–2014, 2017t
    of hypercalcemic type 2014–2015, 2015f
    of pulmonary type 2013–2014
  squamous cell carcinoma 2014
    arising in benign cystic teratoma 2032, 2032f
    nonteratomatous 2014
  steroid cell tumors 2025–2026, 2026f
  stromal hyperplasia 1991–1992

stromal luteoma 2025, 2025f
stromal tumors, 'unclassified' 2026
surface carcinoma, desmoplastic small round cell
    tumors vs 386
surface epithelium (OSE) 1987, 1987f
transitional cell carcinoma 2012, 2013, 2014f
tuberculosis 1989
tumor-like conditions 1993t
tumors 1995–2039
    aldosterone secretion by 2183
    endometrial tumors with 1967
    FIGO staging 1995, 1995t
    frequency 1995
    histological types 1996t
    pathological examination 1995–1996
    WHO classification 1993t
ovotestis 1736, 1736t
ovulation 1987, 2040
'owls eye' intranuclear inclusions 2313, 2314f
oxalate, acute overload, renal involvement 1643
oxalosis, renal involvement 1642–1643
oxyphilic cells see oncocytes

P

p14ARF gene mutations, mesothelioma 1015
p16 gene
    esophageal squamous cell carcinoma 1294
    gallbladder carcinoma 1581
    lung cancer 937, 992
    melanoma and 283
    mesothelioma 1015
p16(INK-4a) gene, cervical intraepithelial neoplasia 1855
p27 gene 2162
p53 gene/p53 protein 1138
    Barrett's esophagus 1310
    breast carcinoma 461, 485
    dedifferentiated chondrosarcoma 719
    diffuse astrocytoma 2351
    ductal carcinoma in situ 454
    epithelial kidney tumors 1673
    esophageal squamous cell carcinoma 1294
    gastric adenocarcinoma 1360
    intraductal papillary mucinous neoplasms 1566
    leiomyosarcoma 1970
    lung cancer 936, 937
    mesothelioma 1013, 1013f
    oral squamous cell carcinoma 1170
    pituitary carcinoma 2107
    pleomorphic adenoma of salivary gland 1210
    quantitative immunohistochemistry 43
    serous tumors of ovary 2002
    small cell lung carcinoma 992
    Wilms' tumor 1666
p57[163a], partial hydatidiform moles 2082
p190[bcr/abl] 633
p210[bcr/abl] 633
P504S see alpha-methylacyl CoA racemase (AMACR -
    P504S)
Pacinian corpuscles 195
Paget cells 425, 456, 458f
    characteristics 1906, 1907
    in normal-appearing skin 1907, 1909
Paget-like disease, secondary to urothelial neoplasia
    1908
Pagetoid invasion, sebaceous carcinoma of eyelid
    1887f, 2291
pagetoid spread
    atypical keratinocytes 246, 246f
    melanocytes 278, 282, 283, 285t
pagetoid urothelial intraepithelial neoplasia (PUIN)
    1908
pagetoid urothelial neoplasia 1908
Paget's disease
    of anus 1458, 1458f
    of bone 681, 687–688, 688f, 702
        ear and temporal bone affected 2283
        osteogenic sarcoma arising 815
        osteosarcoma development 728, 2283
        secondary chondrosarcoma 718

of breast 247
of esophagus 1312
extramammary 262–263, 263f
of nipple 425, 456–458, 457f
    anaplastic 457
    cytology 457–458, 458f
    diagnostic methods 425
    differential diagnosis 439, 457
    infiltrating ductal carcinoma presenting with 463
    mastectomy specimen examination 429
of penis and scrotum 1773
recurrent cutaneous 1909
type 1 1906
type 2 1908
type 3 1908
of urothelial origin 1908
of vulva 1905–1909
    cutaneous 1906, 1907
    immunohistochemistry 1905t, 1907, 1908
    invasive carcinoma with 1907, 1907f,
        1908–1909
    melanoma vs 1915
    pagetoid spread 1907, 1909
    secondary to rectal/anal adenocarcinoma 1908
Paget's osteosarcoma 728, 735, 2283
palate
    adenoid cystic carcinoma 1189
    necrotizing sialometaplasia 136
    polymorphous low-grade adenocarcinoma
        799–800
    squamous cell carcinoma 1173
'pale bodies', hepatocellular carcinoma 1535
'pale islands', desmoplastic medulloblastoma 2380,
    2382f, 2383
palisading myofibroblastoma of lymph nodes 2251
palisading of cells
    cat-scratch fever 96, 97f
    oligodendroglioma 2362, 2362f
palisading of nuclei
    basal cell carcinoma of skin 244
    basaloid squamous cell carcinoma 790, 791f
    leiomyoma 348
    salivary basal cell adenocarcinoma 1248
    schwannoma 2249, 2250f
    solitary circumscribed neuroma 268
    tumors with 2251
palmar fibromatosis 320, 321, 321f
pampiniform plexus 1731, 1732
    dilated/tortuous veins 1735
PAM/RARα fusion product 625
panbronchiolitis, diffuse (DPB) 907, 907f
pancreas 1549–1581
    acinar cells 1326
    acinar epithelium 1549, 1550f
    anatomy 1549
    annular 1551
    carcinoma see pancreatic carcinoma
    cell types 1549–1550, 1550f
    congenital abnormalities 1551
    congenital cyst 1551
    cystic neoplasms 1562–1569, 1562t
    cytopathology (normal) 1549–1551
        normal contaminants 1549, 1550
    development 1549
    ductal epithelium 1549, 1550f
        reactive 1552, 1552f
    dysplasia 1564
    embryology 1549
    endocrine cells 1549–1550
    endocrine hyperplasia 1569–1570
    endocrine neoplasm 1569–1575
        clear cell 1570–1571
        gastrinoma 1424, 1573
        insulinoma 1572–1573
        malignancy criteria 1571–1572, 1572f
        mixed ductal-/acinar-endocrine 1572
        nonsyndromic well-differentiated 1570–1572,
            1570f, 1571f
        pancreatic ductal adenocarcinoma vs 1557

syndromic well-differentiated 1572–1574
    see also glucagonoma
examination methods 1549, 1550f
    'normal' cells contaminating 1549, 1550–1551,
        1550f, 1551f
exocrine cells 1549
exocrine tumors, solid 1553–1562
    see also pancreatic carcinoma
fibrosis 1552
glycogen rich adenoma 1562
intraductal oncocytic papillary neoplasm (IOPNs)
    1566–1567, 1567f
intraductal papillary mucinous neoplasms (IPMNs)
    1563, 1564, 1565–1566, 1565f, 1566f
    branch duct-type 1565
    differential diagnosis 1565, 1566, 1586–1587
intraepithelial neoplasia (PanINs) 1557, 1558f
lymphoepithelial cyst 1551, 1551f
lymphoma, small cell carcinoma vs 1575
malignant fibrous histiocytoma 1569f
mesenchymal tumors 1569f
metastases in 171t, 172, 1569, 1570f
microadenomatosis 1574
microcystic adenoma 1562
mucinous cystic neoplasm 1563–1565
    'ovarian' stroma appearance 1564, 1564f
neuroendocrine carcinoma, poorly differentiated 1575
primitive neuroectodermal tumors (PNET) 1575
serous cystic neoplasm 1562–1565, 1562t, 1563f
small cell carcinoma 1575, 1575f
solid exocrine neoplasms 1553–1562
    reporting, points to include 1554t
    see also pancreatic carcinoma
solid pseudopapillary tumor 1567–1569, 1568f
    acinar cell carcinoma of pancreas vs 1560
    differential diagnosis 1557t
    immunocytochemistry 1568, 1569f
    mucinous cystic tumor vs 1565
spindle-cell neoplasms, mucinous cystic tumor with
    1565
transplantation and rejection 1575–1576
    acute cellular rejection grading 126t
    chronic rejection 129
pancreas divisum 1551
pancreatic acinar metaplasia
    of gastric mucosa 1326
    at gastroesophageal junction 1302
pancreatic carcinoma 1553–1557
    acinar cell 1559–1560, 1560f
        differential diagnosis 1557, 1557t, 1561–1562
    adenosquamous 1557–1558, 1558f
    anaplastic 1558
    colloid 1557, 1558f, 1566
    dissemination by needle-track seeding 138
    ductal adenocarcinoma 1553–1557
        differential diagnosis 1555f, 1557, 1557t
        FNA, diagnostic criteria 1554–1555
        frozen sections 1554, 1555f
        genetic alterations/markers 1556, 1557f, 1557t
        immunohistochemistry 1555–1556
        intraductal papillary mucinous neoplasm with
            1566
        invasion 1554, 1555f
        mucinous cystic tumor with 1565
        poorly/moderately differentiated 1555, 1556f
        prognosis and precursor lesions 1557, 1558f
        variants 1557–1559
        well-differentiated 1555, 1555f, 1556f
    in situ 1564
    medullary 1558
    metastases 168, 174f
        to ovary 2039
    mucinous noncystic adenocarcinoma 1557, 1558f
    nonductal solid 1559–1560
    reporting, points to include 1554t
    resection 1554
    small cell 1575, 1575f
    undifferentiated with osteoclast-like giant cells
        1558–1559, 1559f

pancreatic duct
    abnormal junction with bile duct 1579–1580, 1581, 1583
    brushings 1549
pancreatic fluid, aspiration 1549
pancreatic heterotopia 1326, 1326f
    in gastric duplication 1325, 1326f
pancreatic intraepithelial neoplasia (PanINs) 1557, 1558f
pancreaticoduodenectomy (Whipple procedure) 1554
pancreatic panniculitis 235
pancreatic pseudocysts 1553, 1553f, 1554f
pancreatitis 1551–1553
    acute 1551–1552
        in gastric duplication 1326
    acute hemorrhagic 1552
    chronic 1552–1553, 1552f
        neoplasia vs 1552, 1555f, 1557, 1572
    hereditary 1551–1552
    lymphoplasmacytic sclerosing 1553, 1553f
pancreatoblastoma 1560–1562, 1561f, 1562f
    differential diagnosis 1557t, 1561–1562
pancreticoduodenal-kidney transplant 1575
Paneth cells 1373, 1387
pangastritis see gastritis, multifocal atrophic (MAG)
panniculitis 234–236
    cytophagic histiocytic 293
    factitial 236
    lobular 235–236
    lupus 205, 236, 236f
    pancreatic 235
    septal 234–235
pannus, rheumatoid 692
panophthalmitis 2312–2313
Papanicolaou classification 1833
Papanicolaou smears 1935
    see also cervical smears
Papanicolaou Society of Cytopathology 426
Papanicolaou stain 25–26
    automation for cervical smears 44
    communication of results 4
    Diff-Quik stain vs 27, 27f
    effusions 1026
    focal nodular hyperplasia of liver 1527
    fungi 62
    genital herpes simplex infections 75
    germ cell tumors of testis 1774
    infectious disease specimens 60t
    lipoblasts in myxoid liposarcoma 347f
    rapid Pap staining method 26
    reporting standardization 7
    Romanowsky staining vs 27, 28t
'Pap' cells, squamous cell carcinoma of lung vs 944
papillae, renal 1598
    necrotizing papillitis (papillary necrosis) 1641, 1642f
papillary adenocarcinoma
    digital 258
    middle ear 2278–2279, 2279f
    sinonasal region 800, 808
papillary cystadenoma lymphomatosum see Warthin's tumor
papillary eccrine adenoma 257–258, 259f
papillary endothelial hyperplasia 362–363, 363f, 365
papillary fibroelastoma 1060, 1061f
'papillary mesenchymal bodies' 251–252
papillary oncocytic cystadenoma, Warthin's tumor vs 1216
papillary renal cell carcinoma see renal cell carcinoma
papillary squamotransitional cell carcinoma, vagina 1924
papillary tumors, metastases differential diagnosis 177
papilledema 2318
papilloma
    breast see breast, papilloma
    choroid plexus 2279, 2371, 2371f
    columnar cell (CCP) 789, 789f, 798
    conjunctiva 2292
    cutaneous 264
    exophytic

sinonasal region 787–788, 788f
    urothelial 1713, 1714f
fallopian tube 2044
fibroelastic 1060, 1061f
hirsutoid, of penis 1771
inverted (epithelial/transitional)
    middle ear 2277
    oral cavity 1179
    sinonasal region 788–789, 788f
laryngeal 836–838
Müllerian 1922
oral 1163–1164, 1179
penis 1771
Schneiderian see Schneiderian papillomas
squamous see squamous papilloma
urothelial 1713, 1713f, 1714f
vaginal 1921–1922
papillomatosis
    biliary 1539, 1539f
    diffuse squamous, lung 940
    epidermal nevi 241, 241f
    florid oral 1163
    respiratory 839–841
papovaviruses 75–76
papular acantholytic dyskeratosis, of vulva 1894–1895
papules 195
    erythematous 203, 225
    pearly penile 264, 1771
papulosquamous disorders, vulva involvement 1893t
papulosquamous eruptions 197, 200, 200f
para-amyloid 515
parabasal cells 1842, 1846
parachordoma 394–396, 395f
paracrine growth factors 167, 168
paradental cysts 1147
paraffinoma 141
paraffinoma (sclerosing lipogranuloma), scrotum 1772
paraformaldehyde 15, 17
paraganglioma
    cardiac 1066
    of filum terminale 2377, 2378f
    gangliocytic see gangliocytic paraganglioma
    immunohistochemistry 796t, 2339t
    jugulotympanic 2276–2277, 2277f, 2279
    larynx 843–844
    middle ear and temporal bone 2276–2277
    parathyroid tumors vs 2156
    sinonasal 796t, 801
    small intestinal 1447
    spinal cord 2377
    thyroid gland 2139
    ultrastructural characteristics 2337t
    zellballen pattern 176
paraimmunoblasts, small lymphocytic lymphoma 551
parainfluenza virus 68t
    myositis 2222
    respiratory tract infection 94, 94f
parakeratin plugging, oral verrucous carcinoma 1174, 1175f
parakeratosis 194, 195
    actinic keratosis 243f
    cervical squamous epithelium 1832, 1843, 1845f
    erythema annulare centrifugum 207
    lichen nitidus 202
    lichenoid dermatoses 202
    pityriasis rosea 197, 197f
    pityriasis rubra pilaris 200, 200f
    pleomorphic 1843
    psoriasis vulgaris 199
    seborrheic dermatitis 200
    secondary syphilis 201, 201f
parametrium 1831
paramyotonia congenita 2234
paranasal sinuses see sinuses (paranasal)
paraneoplastic pemphigus 219, 219f
paraneoplastic syndromes
    Lambert-Eaton syndrome 2227
    thymic carcinoma 1107
    in thymoma 1095

paraphimosis 1771–1772
parapsoriasis 207
    large plaque 207, 291
    small plaque 200, 207
parapsoriasis variegata 207
parasites, staining 61
parasitic infections
    cervicitis 1836t, 1837
    CNS 2411–2412
    confirmation using molecular methods 108t
    fallopian tubes 2042
    gastrointestinal tract 102–105
    hepatic granuloma 1512
    Kimura disease vs 519
    myositis 2223
    respiratory tract infection 95–96, 96f
    skin/soft tissue/mucocutaneous surfaces 76–77
paratesticular region
    adenomatoid tumor 1763–1764, 1764f
    aggressive angiomyxoma 1764
    epithelial tumors 1765–1766
    mesothelial hyperplasia 1765
    mesothelioma 1765, 1765f, 1766
        benign cystic 1764
        differential diagnosis 1763
        fibrous 1763
        well-differentiated papillary 1765, 1765f
    multiphenotypic tumors 1766
    nodular/diffuse fibrous proliferation 1763
    sarcomas 1766, 1766f
    tumors 1743t, 1763–1766
        benign 1763–1765
        malignant 1765–1766
    see also testis
parathyroid adenoma 1 (PRAD1) oncogene 2151
parathyroid glands 2149–2168
    adenoma 2151–2158
        atypical 2155, 2155f, 2156f
        brown tumor association 751
        cystic 2152–2153, 2153f, 2162
        cytologic features 2154, 2154f
        differential diagnosis 1113, 2156–2157
        double 2155–2156
        fibrosis areas 2163
        gross/microscopic features 2152–2154, 2152f, 2153f
        microadenoma 2152
        oncocytic 2154, 2155f
        staining of rim 2156, 2157f
        variants 2154–2155
        water-clear cell 2155
    anatomy (gross and microscopic) 2149–2150, 2149f, 2150f
    carcinoma 2151, 2161–2164
        adenoma vs 2156
        gross/microscopic features 2162–2163, 2162f, 2163f, 2164f
        metastatic 2164, 2164f
        thymic carcinoid vs 1113
    chief cells see chief cells
    clear cell hyperplasia 2160, 2160f
    cysts 25, 2164–2165, 2165f
    embryology 2149
    histology (normal) 2149–2150, 2150f
    hyperplasia 2151, 2156
        adenoma vs 2156–2157
        chief cells 2156, 2158–2159, 2159f
        clear cell (Wesserhelle) 2160, 2160f
        nodular (multiple adenomatosis) 2158
        secondary 2160–2161, 2161f
        water-clear cell 2160, 2160f
    immunohistochemistry 2150
    lipoadenoma 2154–2155, 2155f
    metastases in 2165
    nodules, oncocytic 2154
    oncocytic tumors 2156
    physiology (normal) 2150–2151
    secondary tumors 2165
    tumors, paraganglioma vs 2156

parathyroid hormone (PTH) 2150–2151
    excess see hyperparathyroidism
    intraoperative (iPTH), assays 2157–2158
    preoperative localization 2157–2158
parathyroid secretory protein see chromogranin A
parathyromatosis 146, 2159, 2160f, 2161
paraurethral (Skene's) glands 1885, 1914
parietal cells 1321
Parinaud's oculoglandular syndrome 78, 78f, 2294
Parinaud's syndrome 2345, 2378, 2397
Parkes Weber syndrome (Klippel-Trenaunay-Weber
    syndrome) 268, 363–364
parosteal osteosarcoma see osteosarcoma
parotid gland
    acinic cell carcinoma 797, 1230
    basal cell adenoma see under salivary gland tumors
    cysts 1260
    large cell undifferentiated carcinoma 1249–1250,
        1249f, 1250
    lymphoepithelial cysts 1260, 1260f
    metastatic squamous cell carcinoma 1246
    multiple lymphoepithelial cysts (in HIV infection)
        1260–1261, 1261f
    oncocytic metaplasia 1223–1224
    pleomorphic adenoma 1208
    polycystic (dysgenetic) disease 1260
    sebaceous carcinoma 1253
    sebaceous glands in 1226
    small cell undifferentiated carcinoma 1250, 1250f
    Warthin's tumor see Warthin's tumor
    see also salivary glands
paroxysmal nocturnal hemoglobinuria, bone marrow
    617
pars intermedia 2097
pars tuberalis 2097
partial nodular transformation (PNT), of liver 1528t,
    1529
parvalbumin 1676, 1684
parvovirus B19 68t, 76, 76f
    pure red cell aplasia 617, 617f
patch (cutaneous), definition 195
pathergy 212
Patterson-Kelly syndrome 1284
Pautrier microabscesses 291, 292f
PAX3 gene, alveolar rhabdomyosarcoma 360
PAX7 gene, alveolar rhabdomyosarcoma 360
PAX8 peroxisome, follicular thyroid carcinoma 2133
PCV (procarbazine/CCNU/vincristine) chemotherapy,
    oligodendroglioma 2362, 2363
'pearly penile papule' 264, 1171
Pearson syndrome 2231t
Pediatric Oncology Group, neuroblastoma staging 383,
    383t
peliosis, spleen 581, 581f
peliosis hepatis 100f, 1517, 1518f, 1529
pelvic inflammatory disease 1945
pelvic lymph nodes, in ovarian borderline serous
    tumors 2000–2001, 2000f
pelvocalyceal system 1598
pemphigoid
    benign mucous membrane 2294
    bullous see bullous pemphigoid
    cicatricial see cicatricial pemphigoid
pemphigoides gestationis 223
pemphigus
    benign familial (Hailey-Hailey disease) 220, 220f,
        1894
    paraneoplastic 219, 219f
pemphigus erythematosus 217–218, 218f
pemphigus foliaceus 217–218, 218f
pemphigus vulgaris 217, 218–219
    vagina 1919
Pemphigus vulgaris, cervicitis 1837
Penicillium marneffi 67t, 89–90
penis 1767–1773
    anatomy 1767–1768
    Bowen's disease (squamous cell carcinoma in situ)
        1771, 1771f
    condyloma accuminatum 1771

embryology 1768
extramammary Paget's disease 1773
fibromatoses 320, 321, 322f
hirsutoid papilloma (pearly papules) 264, 1771
melanoma 1770, 1770f
Peyronie's disease 1771
phimosis and paraphimosis 1768, 1771–1772
plastic induration (penile fibromatoses) 320, 321, 322f
precursor squamous cell lesions 1770–1771
pseudoepitheliomatous hyperplasia 1769–1770
rare carcinomas 1770
squamous cell carcinoma 1768–1771, 1768f
    basaloid 1768t, 1769f, 1770
    papillary not otherwise specified 1768t, 1770
    pseudohyperplastic 1769f, 1770
    sarcomatoid (spindle cell) 1770
    variants 1768t, 1770
    verrucous 1768t, 1769f, 1770
    warty/condylomatous 1768t, 1769f, 1770
squamous hyperplasia 1771
tumor-like conditions 1771
tumors 1768–1771
    primary 1770
    secondary 1770
verruciform xanthoma 1771
PEO syndrome 2231t
peptic ulcer 1340
    see also duodenum, ulcers; gastric ulcers
perfusion injury, allografts 129–130, 130f
periampullary adenocarcinoma 1557
perianal mucinous carcinoma (anal duct carcinoma)
    1456–1457, 1458f
periapical cysts (radicular cysts) 1146–1147
periappendicitis 1408
periareolar duct hyperplasia 457
periaxonal space of Klebs 2240, 2241
peribronchiolar fibrosis, chronic rejection of lung graft
    129
pericardial constriction 1068
pericardial effusions
    radiotherapy causing 1069
    tissue sampling, indications 1067
    see also effusions
pericardial lesions, miscellaneous 1069
pericardial sac 1018
    diverticulum 1019
pericardial tamponade 1069
pericardial window 1067
pericardiectomy 1067, 1068
pericardiotomy, subxiphoid 1067
pericarditis 1019
    calcific 1068, 1069f
    cholesterol 1068
    fibrinous 1019, 1068, 1068f
    granulomatous 1019
    mycobacterial 1068–1069
    non-specific 1068, 1068f
    purulent 1069
    radiation 1069
    sarcoidal 1069
    suppurative 1019
pericardium 1018–1019
    anatomy 1018
    benign tumors 1019
    calcification 1019
    congenital cysts and defects 1019
    cysts 1070
    fibrosis 1019
    neoplastic diseases 1019, 1069–1070
        mesothelioma see mesothelioma
        secondary tumors 1019
    non-neoplastic diseases 1019, 1068–1069
    plaque formation 1019
    sarcoma 1070
    surgical pathology 1067–1070
    tissue sampling, indications 1067–1068
pericellular lacunae 184
perichondrium, in osteochondroma 707, 708f
perifascicular atrophy 2219, 2219f

'periglandular cuffing', ovarian adenosarcoma 2010
periglomerular fibrosis 1644
perilymph 2269–2270
perimysium 2215, 2216
perineal body, abnormalities 1919
perineal phlegmon (Fournier's gangrene) 69, 1772
perineural pseudoinvasion, sclerosing adenosis 431
perineurinoma 2255, 2387
perineurium 2240
periodic acid-Schiff (PAS) stain 21f, 2335t
    infectious organisms 60t, 61
    kidney 1601, 1601f
    liver biopsy 1468–1469, 1469f
    mesothelioma 1011
    Pneumocystis jiroveci 88
    salivary acinic cell carcinoma 1230
    seminoma 1775
    skeletal muscle evaluation 2215t
periodic acid-Schiff (PAS) with diastase (DPAS) stain
    1468–1469
periodic acid-Schiff (PAS) with digestion (PASD)
    1533–1534
periodic paralyses 2233–2234, 2233f
periodontal ligament, widening 1194
periorchitis, nodular fibrous (reactive) 1763
periosteal chondrosarcoma 718
periosteal osteosarcoma see osteosarcoma
periosteum 678
    fracture healing 682
    reactive pseudosarcomatous lesions 772–774, 772t
        florid reactive periostitis 772–773, 773f
        Nora's lesion 773–774, 773f, 774f
periostitis
    florid reactive 387–388, 388f, 772–773, 773f
    reactive 685
peripheral giant cell granuloma (tumor), oral cavity
    1181–1182
peripheral giant cell reparative granuloma (PGCRG) 815
    see also giant cell reparative granuloma
peripheral myelin protein 22 (PMP22) 2244
peripheral nerves 2238–2259
    amyloid deposition 2247
    axons see axons
    biopsy 2238–2240
        artifacts 2239–2240
    blood supply 2240
    crush and percussion injuries 2245
    cysts see ganglion cysts
    fibrolipomatous hamartoma 2249, 2249f
    granulomatous inflammation 2243
    hereditary conditions 2246–2247
    histology (normal) 2240–2241
    hyperplasia (mucosal neuroma) 2248
    inflammatory diseases 2242–2244
    lymphoma 2258, 2258f
    pathologic processing affecting 2241
    in porphyria 2247
    in sarcoidosis 2243
    segmental demyelination/remyelination 2241, 2242f
    teased fiber analysis 2239, 2241f
    trauma 2245–2246
    tumors/tumor syndromes 2248–2259
        enign, of skin 268
        secondary 2258
        see also specific tumors
    vasculitis 2243
    see also neuropathy
peripheral nerve sheath tumors
    benign see neurofibroma; schwannoma
        (neurilemoma)
    of bone 771
    malignant see malignant peripheral nerve sheath
        tumor (MPNST)
    sinonasal region 810
peripheral neuroepithelioma see primitive
    neuroectodermal tumors (PNET), of CNS
peripheral neuropathy see neuropathy
peritoneal adenomucinosis, disseminated 1025
peritoneal carcinomatosis 184–185

peritoneal effusions
    gastrointestinal cancer 1030, 1031f
    ovarian cancer 1029–1030, 1030f
    pitfalls in cytological diagnosis 1033
    see also effusions
peritoneal implant, ovarian serous tumors 1999–2000, 1999f
peritoneal mucinous carcinomatosis (PMC) 1025, 2006
peritoneal seeding, of tumors 138
peritoneum 1019–1025
    adhesions 1020
    chondroid and osseous metaplasia 1021
    cysts
        multilocular 1021–1022, 1021f
        postoperative 146
        unilocular 1021–1022
    deciduosis 1021
    endometriosis of 1020–1021
    endosalpingiosis 1020–1021
    inflammation *see* peritonitis
    inflammatory myofibroblastic tumor (plasma cell granuloma) 1022
    leiomyomatosis peritonealis disseminata 1021
    melanosis 1022, 2031
    metaplastic conditions 1020–1021
    metastases in, breast carcinoma 469
    neoplastic diseases 1022–1025
        adenomatoid tumor 1024
        desmoplastic small round cell tumor 1024, 1025f
        localized fibrous tumor 1024
        mesothelioma *see* mesothelioma
        primary tumors 1022–1024
        secondary tumors 1025
        serous carcinoma 1023, 1023f, 1024f
    non-neoplastic diseases 1019–1020
    omental-mesenteric myxoid hamartoma 1022
    parietal 1019
    reactive fibrosis 1020
    reactive mesothelial hyperplasia 1020, 1020f
    splenosis 1022
    trophoblastic implants 1022
    visceral 1019
    Walthard rests 1021
peritonitis 1019–1020
    bacterial (primary and secondary) 1019
    chemical 2031
    colonic diverticular disease 1405
    granulomatous 1019–1020
    sclerosing (fibrosing) 1020, 2020f
        thecomas with 2020
    starch causing 139
perivascular epithelioid cell tumors (PEComas)
    benign clear cell tumor of lung 962
    of uterus 1978f
perivascular pseudorosettes
    ependymoma 2364, 2365, 2365f, 2366f
    pancreatic endocrine neoplasms 1570
perivascular serum lakes, thymoma 1098
perivascular spaces, thymoma 1098
perivascular tumors 373
Perls stain 2335t
pernicious anemia *see* gastritis, autoimmune chronic
peroxidase antiperoxidase methods 30
Perry-Romberg hemifacial atrophy 231–232
persistent generalized lymphadenopathy (PGL) 118, 522
persistent hyperplastic primary vitreous (PHPV) 2311
persistent müllerian duct syndrome 1737
persistent nodular scabetic reaction 217
persistent polyclonal B-cell lymphocytosis 643
persistent trophoblastic activity 2043
pertussis 95
Peutz-Jeghers gene *(STK11/LKB1),* intraductal papillary mucinous neoplasms (pancreas) 1566
Peutz-Jeghers syndrome 1421
    hamartomatous polyps of small intestine 1421, 1421f
    large cell calcifying Sertoli cell tumors 1759
    Sertoli cell tumor NOS 1758–1759
    sex cord tumor with annular tubules 2023–2024
    testicular tumor 1737

Peyer's patches
    hyperplasia 1395
    infection 1395
Peyronie's disease 320, 1771
P-glycoprotein 630
phacoanaphylactic endophthalmitis 2300, 2300f
phaeohyphomycosis 73, 73f
phelmonous enteritis 1398
phenacetin, renal cell carcinoma association 1677
phenylbutazone, hepatic granuloma 1510, 1511f
pheochromocytoma 2110, 2191–2194, 2191f
    '1 cm rule' 2190, 2190f
    adrenocortical carcinoma *vs* 2188
    biologic behavior 2194
    bladder involvement 1722
    'cardiac' 1066
    composite 2192–2193, 2193f
    cystic degeneration 2191, 2191f
    cytologic features 2193–2194, 2195f
    familial 2192
    microscopic pathology 2191, 2192f
    pigmented ('black') 2191, 2192f
    ultrastructure and immunophenotype 2193, 2193f
Philadelphia chromosome 629
    acute basophilic leukemia 624
    chronic myeloid leukemia 629, 632–633, 634
    lymphoblastic lymphoma 569
phimosis 1768, 1771–1772
phlebitis 1079
    enterocolic lymphocytic 1386, 1387f
    giant cell 1079
    lymphocytic, of colon 1079
    thoracoepigastric vein 450
phosphates, staining methods 16t
phosphatidyl inositol glycan class A gene 617
phosphofructokinase
    deficiency 2232
    skeletal muscle evaluation 2215t
phospholipidosis 1490, 1490f
phosphorus, homeostasis 2151
phosphotungstic acid-hematoxylin (PTAH) stain 1224, 2335t
photodynamic therapy, Barrett's esophagus dysplasia 1307, 1311–1312
photomicrographs, for external consultation 5
photopheresis, heart transplant rejection 1050
Phrygian cap 1576
phthisis bulbi 2314
phycomycosis *see* mucormycosis
phyllodes tumor 436–437, 436f
    cytology 28, 439f
    endometrial adenofibroma similar 1976
    histology 437f, 438f
physaliphorous cells, chordoma 763, 763f, 764, 764f, 2109
physical agents, iatrogenic lesions due to *see* iatrogenic lesions
picker's nodule 201
picric acid 17, 32
PIG-A gene, mutation 617
pigmentary incontinence, postinflammatory 230
pigmentation disorders, vulva 1896–1897, 1896t
pigmented actinic keratosis 244, 277
pigmented neuroectodermal tumor 384
pigmented purpuric eruptions (PPE) 208, 208f
pigmented spindle-cell nevus of reed 278, 279
pigmented villondular tenosynovitis 375–376, 376f
pigmented villonodular synovitis (PVNS) 695–696, 696f
    temporomandibular joint 1195, 1195f
pigmentosus tubae (pseudoxanthomatous salpingitis) 2042, 2042f
pigments, types and staining 19, 20t
pi granules of Reich 2241
pilar cyst
    eyelid 2290
    malignant proliferating 261
pilar (trichilemmal) inclusion cysts 254, 254f
pilar tumor, proliferating 254, 254f, 261

'piling up' of neoplastic cells, postirradiation angiosarcoma 276
pilomatrix carcinoma (PMC) 261
pilomatrixoma (pilomatricoma) 253–254, 253f
pilosebaceous duct, malformation 251
pilosebaceous unit 194
    abnormal formation 250
    benign lesions 250–255
    malignant tumors 258–261
pinch biopsies, gastric 1324, 1353
'pinch purpura' 229–230
pineal area tumors 2345, 2377
    differential diagnosis by age 2348t
    germ cell tumors 2397
    see also pinealoma
pineal cysts 2403, 2404f
pinealoma 2377–2378
    germ cell tumors 2377
    parenchymal tumors 2377–2378
pineoblastoma 2337t, 2378
    immunohistochemistry 2339t
pineocytes 2377
pineocytoma 2337t, 2377, 2378, 2378f
    immunohistochemistry 2339t
Pinkus, fibroepitheliomatous basal cell carcinoma 245
pinna (ear) 2267, 2268f
    accessory 2270
    basal cell carcinoma 2280
    congenital abnormalities 2270–2271
    cutaneous disorders 2274–2275, 2275f
    squamous cell carcinoma 2280
Pit-1 transcription factor 2094, 2098, 2099, 2100
pituitary adenoma 2098–2107
    acidophil stem cell 2101, 2102–2103, 2103f
    classification 2099, 2099t
    clinically nonfunctioning 2106–2107, 2106f, 2107, 2107f
    clinicopathological classification 2099, 2100t
    corticotroph 2107, 2179
        functioning 2104–2105, 2105f
        silent 2106
    ectopic 2098
    gonadotroph
        female type 2107
        functioning 2105–2106, 2106f
        silent 2106
    immunohistochemistry 796t
    intrasellar 2098
    lactotroph
        functioning 2101–2103, 2102f, 2103f
        silent 2106
    mammosomatotroph 2100
    metastatic tumors *vs* 2110
    plurihormonal 2107
    poorly differentiated 2107
    reticulin staining 2111f
    somatotroph
        functioning 2099–2101, 2100f, 2101f, 2110
        silent 2106
    thyrotroph
        functioning 2103–2104, 2104f
        silent 2106
pituitary dwarfism 2098, 2108
pituitary gland 2093–2117
    adenohypophysis *see* adenohypophysis
    adenoma *see* pituitary adenoma
    in AIDS 2113
    amyloid deposition 2113
    anatomy and cytology (normal) 2093–2097, 2094f
    aplasia/hypoplasia 2098
    apoplexy 2113
    blood supply 2097
    carcinoma 2107–2108
        metastatic 2108, 2110
    congenital disorders 2098
    craniopharyngioma 2108, 2108f
    cysts 2113
    duplication/dystopia 2098
    ectopic tissue 812–813

examination methodology 2093
gangliocytoma 2108, 2109f
germ cell tumors 2109
glial tumors 2108–2109
granular cell tumor ('myoblastoma') 2109
hemosiderosis 2113
hyperplasia 2110, 2111f
idiopathic granulomatous hypophysitis 2112, 2112f
infarction (ischemic necrosis) 2113
inflammation 2110–2113
lymphocytic hypophysitis 2111–2112, 2112f
lymphoid neoplasms 2110
mesenchymal tumors 2109–2110
metabolic disorders 2113
microadenoma 2101, 2104
neural tumors 2108–2109
postpartum necrosis (Sheehan's syndrome) 2113
primary tumors 2098–2110
reticulin staining 2111f
secondary hypophysitis 2112–2113
secondary tumors 2108, 2110
tumor-like lesions 2110–2113
vascular disorders 2113
vascular tumors 2113
xanthomatous hypophysitis 2112
pituitary sarcoma 160
pityriasis lichenoides chronica (PLC) 204, 207
pityriasis lichenoides et varioliformis acuta (PLEVA)
    204, 205f
pityriasis rosea 197, 197f, 207
pityriasis rubra pilaris (PRP) 200, 200f
PKD1, PKD2, PKD3 genes 1662
placenta 2063–2079
    abnormalities 2064–2065, 2064f
    accessory lobe 2064f, 2065
    battledore 2066
    bilobed 2064f, 2070
    circummarginate 2064f, 2071
    circumvallate 2064f, 2071
    confined mosaicism 2080
    development 2063–2064
    diamnionic/monochorionic (DiMo) twin 2076–2078,
        2076f
    DiDi (diamnionic/dichorionic) twin 2075–2076,
        2076f
    examination 2064–2065
    inflammation and infection 2068–2070, 2069f
    maternal floor infarction 2072–2073, 2073f, 2080
    monoamnionic/monochorionic (MoMo) twin 2078,
        2078f
    normal 2064f
    polyps 2075
    shape abnormalities 2064f, 2070–2071
    succenturiate lobe 2070
    uteroplacental perfusion abnormalities 2071–2072
    vascular lesions 2073–2074, 2073f
    velamentous cord insertion 2064f, 2066, 2066f,
        2077f
placenta accreta 2065, 2074–2075
placenta diffusa (membranacea) 2064, 2064f, 2070,
    2071
placenta increta 2074, 2075
placental abruption 2072
placental alkaline phosphatase (PLAP) 180, 1741,
    1775t, 2084
    choriocarcinoma 1753
    dysgerminoma 2028
    embryonal carcinoma of ovary 2030
    seminoma differential diagnosis 1775t, 1776
    yolk sac tumor of ovary 2030
placental disk 2063, 2070–2074
    examination 2065
placental site nodule 2084–2085, 2085f
placental site reaction, exaggerated 2084, 2085, 2085f
placental site trophoblastic nodule (decidual nodule)
    1841, 1841f
placental site trophoblastic tumor (PSTT) 2084,
    2085–2086, 2085f, 2086f
    fallopian tube 2047

placenta membranacea 2064, 2064f, 2070, 2071
placenta percreta 2075
placenta previa 2064
placenta previa accreta 2075
plague 98
plantar fibromatosis 320, 321, 321f
plantar neuroma (Morton's neuroma) 379, 697,
    2245–2246, 2246f
plaque, cutaneous, definition 195
plasmablastic cells 654
plasmablasts 522, 654–655
plasma cell(s) 653–654
    aggregation, cutaneous MALToma 290, 290f
    bone marrow 614
    Hodgkin's disease 537
    perivascular cuffing 614, 614f
    phenotype 655
    Waldenström's macroglobulinemia 555
plasma cell disorders 653–657
    neoplastic 654–657, 654t
    non-neoplastic 654
    renal conditions associated 1630–1632
plasma cell granuloma see inflammatory
        myofibroblastic tumor (plasma cell granuloma)
plasma cell infiltration, scleroderma 232, 232f
plasma cell leukemia 656, 656f
plasma cell myeloma see myeloma
plasma cell pneumonia 88, 88f
plasma cell vulvitis 1895, 1895f
plasmacytes, syringocystadenoma papilliferum 258
plasmacytic disorders 653–657
plasmacytic hyperplasia 150, 571
plasmacytoma
    bone marrow 654
    extramedullary 654, 826
    immunohistochemistry 796t
    larynx 850
    primary, of lymph nodes 575–576
    pulmonary carcinoid tumors vs 985–986
    renal involvement 1693
    solitary of bone 654
    testis involvement 1762
plasmacytosis
    rheumatoid arthritis 518–519
    splenic red pulp 585
pleomorphic adenoma, salivary gland see salivary
        gland tumors
pleomorphic adenoma gene 1 (PLAG1) 1210
pleomorphic hyalinizing angiectatic tumor (PHAT)
    396, 396f
'pleomorphic myofibrosarcoma' 333–334
pleomorphic tumors, metastases differential diagnosis
    176–177
pleomorphic xanthoastrocytoma see
        xanthoastrocytoma, pleomorphic
pleura 1005–1018
    adenocarcinoma, mesothelioma vs 1014–1015, 1014t
    adenomatoid tumor 1015
    amyloidosis 1007
    anatomy and function 1005
    calcifying fibrous pseudotumor 1017, 1017f
    Cope needle biopsy 1005
    desmoplastic small round cell tumor 1017
    development 1005
    diagnostic specimens 1005
    epithelioid hemangioendothelioma 1016, 1016f, 1017f
    inflammation 1005–1006
    localized fibrous tumor 1015–1016, 1015f, 1016f
    mesothelioma see mesothelioma
    neoplastic diseases 1007–1018
        primary tumors 1007–1015
        secondary tumors 1018, 1018f
    non-neoplastic diseases 1005–1007
    open biopsy 1005
    parietal 1005
        plaque 1006, 1006f
    plaques, asbestosis 903
    pleuropulmonary blastoma 1016–1017
    reactive mesothelial hyperplasia 1006, 1006f

rounded atelectasis 1007, 1007f
    synovial sarcoma 1017–1018
    thoracoscopic biopsy 1005
    visceral 1005
        diffuse fibrosis 1006–1007
pleural effusions
    asbestosis 902–903
    bloody 1026
    in breast carcinoma 1029, 1030f
    causes 1026
    cloudy 1026
    eosinophilia 1027
    hematologic neoplasms 1031–1032, 1031f
    immunocytochemistry 1032–1033
    leukocyte-rich 1027
    in lung cancer 1030, 1030f
    malignant 1028
    in metastatic cancers 1028
    pulmonary embolization causing 1026
    single-cell pattern 184f
    tuberculous 1027
    tumors with 183
    see also effusions
pleuritis 1005–1006
    eosinophilic 925, 1006
pleuropericardial window 1067
pleuropulmonary blastoma 1016–1017
plexogenic pulmonary arteriopathy 912
PLGA see polymorphous low-grade adenocarcinoma
    (PLGA)
plicae palmatae 1831
ploidy determination
    flow cytometry 36, 37f, 39, 40f
    image cytometry 43
Plummer-Vinson syndrome 1169, 1284
pluripotent stem cells 612, 632
PNET family of tumors see Ewing family of tumors
pneumatosis 1397, 1398f
pneumatosis cystoides intestinalis 1405–1406
Pneumococcus, acute suppurative (phlegmonous)
        gastritis 1329
pneumoconiosis 901–905
    asbestosis 896, 902–903, 935
    berylliosis 904
    cobalt 904–905, 905f
    endogenous 915
    hard metal 904–905, 905f
    less common forms 905t
    rheumatoid (Caplan's syndrome) 888
    silicosis 903–904, 905t
Pneumocystis carinii see Pneumocystis jiroveci
Pneumocystis jiroveci 81, 87–89, 661, 867, 973
    differential diagnosis 88–89
    intracystic bodies (trophozoites) 87, 89f
    lymph node involvement 533
    staining 61, 62t, 87–88
Pneumocystis pneumonia 88, 88f, 880–881, 881f
    in AIDS/HIV infection 88, 89, 89f
    detection 88, 88f, 89f, 866
    granulomatous 881, 881f
    sarcoidosis vs 893
pneumocystosis 88
pneumocytes, hyperplastic 926
pneumonia
    acute fibrinous and organizing 882, 883f
    acute interstitial (AIP) 886–887, 902t
    adenovirus 876–878, 877f
    atypical 875–876
    bacterial 874, 875f
        atypical 875–876
    cellular interstitial 898
    coronavirus 879
    cryptogenic organizing 900–901, 901, 901f, 902t
    cytomegalovirus (CMV) 102f, 878, 879f, 973
    desquamative interstitial 898–899, 899f, 923f
        differential diagnosis 902t, 925
    eosinophilic
        acute 881, 881f, 882f
        chronic 881–882, 893–894

pneumonia (cont'd)
  drugs causing 882t
  simple (Loeffler syndrome) 214, 881, 881f
  fungal 879–881
  giant cell, viral 94, 94f, 95, 95f
  giant cell interstitial (GIP) 904–905, 905f
  groups 897–898, 897f, 898f
  hantavirus 879, 880f
  herpes simplex virus (HSV) 74, 75f, 878, 878f
  herpesvirus 89
  idiopathic interstitial 894–901
    classification 893, 893t
  immunocompromised hosts 874
  influenza 94, 94f, 876
  interstitial
    in rheumatoid arthritis 887
    sarcoidosis 893
  Legionnaires disease 81, 82f, 874–875, 875f
  lipid 961
  lymphoid interstitial (LIP) 118f, 899–900, 899f, 900f
    differential diagnosis 900, 902t
    in HIV infection 118, 900
    idiopathic form 899
  measles 95, 95f, 876, 876f
  Nocardia 81–82, 82f, 83f
  non-specific interstitial 897–898, 898t
    differential diagnosis 902t
    histopathology 897–898, 897f, 897t
  organizing (OP) 882, 883f, 888
    airspace filling pattern 870, 870f
    bronchiolitis with 920
    rheumatoid arthritis 888
  parainfluenza virus 94, 94f
  Pneumocystis see Pneumocystis pneumonia
  primary plague 98
  respiratory syncytial virus (RSV) 94, 95f, 876, 877f
  Rhodococcus equi 65f
  secondary bacterial 93
  usual interstitial (UIP) 893–897, 895f, 896f
    differential diagnosis 896–897, 902t
    'fibroblastic focus' 895, 896f
    fibrosis pattern 869, 869f
    honeycombing pattern 870–871, 871f
    smooth muscle 895, 896f
    'temporal heterogeneity' 895, 896f
  varicella-zoster virus (VZV) 76f, 878–879, 879f
  viral 876–879, 876f, 876t
pneumonitis
  acute lupus 882–883
  hypersensitivity see hypersensitivity pneumonitis
  lymphoid interstitial 118, 118f
  radiation 886
pneumothorax, lymph node sampling complication 28
podocin 1610
podocytes 1598–1599
  familial focal segmental glomerulosclerosis 1610
  markers 1612
podophyllin therapy, effect on condyloma accuminatum 148
POEMS syndrome 654, 655, 762
  chronic demyelinative neuropathy in 2258
  glomeruloid hemangioma 271
  multicentric Castleman's disease with 522
poison ivy dermatitis 196
polarization, lymph node follicles 517, 517f
polarizing microscopy, liver biopsy 1470f, 1471
'polka dot' pattern, hemangioma of bone 766, 766f
polyangiitis, immune-related necrotizing 1077–1078
polyarteritis nodosa 1072t, 1074–1075, 1075
  benign cutaneous 211
  differential diagnosis 1074–1075, 1385
  ear involvement 2276
  infantile see Kawasaki disease
  inflammatory fibroid polyp association 1341
  intestinal 1384, 1384t, 1385
  localized forms 1075
  microscopic 211
  necrotizing vasculitis with fibrinoid necrosis 2224f

peripheral nerve involvement 2243
  skin involvement 211, 211f
polychondritis, relapsing
  chondrodermatitis nodularis helicis vs 227–228
  ear involvement 2282
  larynx and trachea 835
polyclonal antisera, immunohistochemistry 32, 33, 34
polyclonal B cell lymphoproliferative disorder (PBLD) 118
polycystic kidney disease
  autosomal dominant (adult) 1662, 1662f, 1663f, 1665, 1690
  autosomal recessive (infantile) 1662–1663, 1663f
polycystic liver disease 1521–1523, 1522f
polycystic ovary syndrome 1991, 1992f
polycythemia, secondary 619
polycythemia vera 585, 631–632, 632f
  differential diagnosis 635t
polyembryoma 1757, 1757f
polyethylene glycol 20
polyglactin sutures 144
polyglandular autoimmune (PGA) syndromes 2175–2176
polymastia 421
polymerase chain reaction (PCR) 45–46, 1653
  CNS tumors 2340
  lymph node specimens 510
  MALT lymphoma 1353
polymorphic reticulosis (sinonasal lymphoma) 824–826, 825t
polymorphonuclear neutrophils (PMNs) see neutrophils
polymorphous light eruption (PMLE) 206–207, 207t
polymorphous low-grade adenocarcinoma (PLGA)
  palate/maxilla 799–800
  salivary gland see salivary gland tumors
  salivary pleomorphic adenoma vs 1210, 1212–1213
polymyalgia rheumatica 1072, 2222
polymyositis 2218–2219, 2218f, 2219f
  autoantibodies 114t
  differential diagnosis 2220t
  disorders/malignancy associated 2218
  lung involvement 883, 889
  muscle fiber degeneration and necrosis 2218, 2218f
  muscle histology 2218–2219, 2218f, 2219f
polyomavirus (BK type) infection 1652
polyorchidism 1735
polyostotic fibrous dysplasia 393
polyotia 2270
polypectomy, colonoscopic 136
polypropylene sutures 144
polyps
  antrochoanal 787
  aural 2274
  colonic see colon, polyps; large intestine
  endocervical 1841
  endometrial 1943, 1945–1946, 1946f, 1956, 1968f
  esophagus 1315
  fallopian tube 2044
  fibroepithelial see fibroepithelial polyps
  gallbladder 1577–1579
  gastric see gastric polyps
  hamartomatous, small intestine 1421, 1421f
  hyperplastic, large intestine 1431–1432, 1432f
  inflammatory bowel disease 1390, 1390f, 1391
  inflammatory cloacogenic 1382
  nasal cavity 787, 812f
  nasopharynx 826
  placenta 2075
  prostatic 1725
  urethra 1725
  vaginal 356, 1922
  vocal cord 835, 837f
  vulval 356, 1899
polytetrafluoroethylene (PTFE) 142–143
polythelia 421
polyvinyl alcohol particles, intravascular emboli 140, 140f
Pompe's disease 1065

Pontiac fever 81
poorly differentiated endocrine carcinoma (PDEC) 1350, 1351
'popcorn' cells 542, 652
popliteal artery, cystic adventitial disease 1083–1084, 1085f
porocarcinoma 261
poroma 257, 257f
  eccrine 256–257, 257f
porphyria
  hepatic, UV microscopy 1472
  peripheral nerve involvement 2247
porphyria cutanea tarda 224, 224f, 225
porphyrin, staining 20t
portal granulomatous diseases 1514
portal hypertension 1662
  idiopathic (hepatoportal sclerosis) 1514, 1514f
portal tract, edema 1496f
portal vein embolization, myospherulosis after 140–141
port-wine stain 268
positron emission tomography (PET)
  bone tumors 704
  CNS tumors 2346
  lung carcinoma 936
postcapillary venules, leukocytoclastic vasculitis 209
posterior choroidal tumors
  melanoma 2306, 2308
  metastatic 2309
posterior fossa
  medulloblastoma 2379
  metastases in 2399
  tumor differential diagnosis 2348t
posterior synechias 2313–2314
postinflammatory changes, vulva 1896
postirradiation angiosarcoma 371, 371f
postmenopausal bleeding 2019
postoperative abdominal cysts 146–147
postoperative spindle cell nodule 1841
  bladder 1723, 1723f
postperfusion nephropathy 1651
post-transplantation lymphoproliferative disorders (PTLD) 150, 571–572, 572f, 1652–1653
  lung transplant 921–922
  monomorphic 571–572
  polymorphic 150, 571, 572f
Potter syndrome 1662
pouchitis 1394–1395
pouch of Douglas 1831, 1933
Power Vision System 32
PRCC/TFE3 genes 1671
preauricular pits, sinuses and fistulas 2271
predecidua 1938, 1948
predecidual (pseudodecidual) stromal reaction 1938, 1938f, 1939f
pre-eclampsia 2071f, 2072
pregnancy
  acute fatty liver 1489f
  breast carcinoma 438
  cervical changes 1848, 1849f
  choriocarcinoma after 2083
  corpus luteum of 1988
  ectopic 2042–2043, 2043f
    persistent 2087
    salpingitis isthmica nodosa 2042, 2043f
  extrachorial (extramembranous) 2071
  granuloma annulare 212
  granulosa cell proliferation 1994, 1994f
  herpes gestationis 223
  hilus cell hyperplasia 1994
  lobular capillary hemangioma 270
  luteoma of 1992, 1993
  metaplastic squamous epithelium of cervix 1832
  molar 2080–2081
    ectopic 2087
  multiple 2063, 2075–2079
  nevi arising in 277–278
  oral pyogenic granuloma 1181
  ovarian pseudotumors and cysts 1992, 1993t

ovary, unusual microscopic findings 1994
    pruritic urticarial papules and plaques 198
pregnancy-specific β1-glycoprotein (SP1) 1753
pregnancy tumor (oral pyogenic granuloma) 1181
premelanosomes 286
PreserveCyte 20, 21
preterm labor 2068
pretibial myxedema 228–229, 229, 230f
'Prevalence' microarrays 36
primary biliary cirrhosis (PBC) 1475f, 1498–1501,
        1500f, 1501
    epithelioid granuloma in 1500, 1501f
    'florid duct lesions' 1485, 1485f, 1500, 1500f
    granulomas 1510
primary central nervous system lymphomas (PCNSLs)
        see lymphoma, CNS
primary neuroendocrine tumors of skin (Merkel cell)
        248–250, 249f, 261
primary sclerosing cholangitis (PSC) 1497–1498,
        1499f, 1583, 1583f
    cholecystitis with 1577
    fibrosis after 1501
    inflammatory bowel disease with 1497
    'jigsaw' pattern 1497, 1498f
    ulcerative colitis with 1393
primary spongiosa 681, 681f
primitive neuroectodermal tumors (PNET)
    of CNS 385–386, 385f, 2378
        chromosomal translocation 310t
        immunohistochemistry 2339t
        medulloblastoma vs 2383
        neuroblastic tumors vs 383
        rhabdoid tumor of kidney and 1670
        supratentorial 2378, 2379, 2384
    immunohistochemistry 796t
    of kidney 1689
    of ovary 2035–2036, 2036f
    of pancreas 1575
    peripheral 746–750
        differential diagnosis 747t, 750
        Homer Wright rosettes 174, 385, 385f, 748, 748f
        immunohistochemistry 749
        ultrastructure/cytology 748–749, 749f
        see also Ewing's sarcoma
    sinonasal 796t, 806–807
    of soft tissues 385–386, 385f
    teratoma malignant transformation to 1755
    testis 1756
primordial follicles 1987, 1991
prion disorders, CNS involvement 2412–2413, 2413f
prismatic bodies 2246
proctectomy, ulcerative colitis 1389
proctitis, granulomatous 99
proctocolectomy 1389, 1391, 1394
proerythroblasts 612
progestational agents, endometrial changes 1946,
        1947f
progesterone receptor positivity 181
    breast cancer 488
        invasive cribriform carcinoma 476
        invasive micropapillary carcinoma 477
        invasive papillary carcinoma 476
        medullary carcinoma 475
    endometrial adenocarcinoma 1960
progestins, endometrial changes 1946, 1947f
'Prognosis' microarrays 36
progonoma see melanotic neuroectodermal tumor of
        infancy
'Progression' microarrays 36
progressive massive fibrosis 904
progressive multifocal leukoencephalopathy (PML) 75,
        76f, 2408, 2409f
    in HIV infection 119–120, 120f
progressive outer retinal necrosis (PORN) syndrome
        2313
prolactinoma 2101, 2103, 2113
proliferating cell nuclear antigen (PCNA) 1672
    basal cell carcinoma of skin 246
    epithelial kidney tumors 1672

gastrointestinal stromal tumors 1348
    laryngeal carcinoma 841
    quantitative immunohistochemistry 43
    salivary mucoepidermoid carcinoma 1228
    salivary polymorphous low-grade adenocarcinoma
        1241
proliferating cell nuclear antigen (PCNA) index 1348,
        1672
proliferation centers, small lymphocytic (B-cell)
        lymphoma 551, 551f, 555, 556
proliferative fasciitis 313–314, 314f
proliferative myositis 314
proliferative verrucous leukoplakia, differential
        diagnosis 845
prolymphocytes 551, 552f
promegakaryocytes 613
'promontory sign' 275, 275f
promyelocytes 613, 621
proopiomelanocortin (POMC) 2096
PROP-1 (prophet of Pit-1) 2094, 2098
Propionibacterium acnes 2300, 2300f
Proplast®, iatrogenic reactions 142–143
proptosis 2294, 2296
prostatectomy 1794, 1815
prostate gland 1791–1828
    adenocarcinoma see prostatic adenocarcinoma
    adenosquamous carcinoma 1819
    anatomy 1791–1794, 1792f
    androgen-deprivation therapy effect 1821, 1821f
    atrophy 1795–1797, 1796f
        adenocarcinoma vs 1795, 1796, 1797t, 1812
        classification 1795t
        hyperplastic 1796, 1796f, 1797
        proliferative inflammatory 1796, 1797
        sclerotic 1796, 1796f
        simple 1796, 1796f
    atypical adenomatous hyperplasia (adenosis)
        1799–1800, 1800f, 1812
        sclerosing 1800, 1800f
    atypical small acinar proliferation 1804–1805
    basal cell carcinoma 1820
    benign conditions (rare) 1800
    benign hyperplasia (BPH) 1798–1799
    biopsy methods 1794
    calculi 1793
    carcinoma
        benign conditions mimicked by 1822, 1822t
        in congenital adrenal hyperplasia 2175
        diagnosis from prostatic secretions 1794
        fine needle aspiration 1794, 1794f
        grading of variants 1815, 1816t
        high-grade urothelial carcinoma of bladder vs
            1716
        metastases 168, 484, 1818, 1818f
        neutrophilic infiltrates 1794
        poorly differentiated, granulomatous prostatitis vs
            1795
        prevalence 1791
        pseudoneoplasms vs 1800–1801, 1801t
        radiation-induced atypia 157
        sclerotic bone metastases 772
        sites/zones 1791
        staging (TNM) 1815–1818
        variants 1818–1820, 1819f
        see also specific carcinomas above/below
    central zone cribriform glands 1792, 1792f
    cryotherapy, iatrogenic lesions 144
    cytopathologic diagnosis 1794
    developmental abnormalities 1791
    ectopic 1810
    embryology 1791
    fibromatosis 1820
    fibromuscular stroma 1791, 1792f
    fine needle aspiration (FNA) 1794, 1794f
    focal glandular atypia 1804–1805
    functions 1793–1794
    hyperplasia 1798–1799
        atypical adenomatous see above
        'atypical basal cell' 1799

basal cell 1798–1799, 1799f, 1812
    'basal cell with prominent nucleoli' 1799
    benign 1798–1799
    cribriform (clear cell cribriform) 1799
    mesonephric remnant 1799
    post-atrophic 1796, 1796f, 1797
    sclerosing basal cell 1799
    stromal cell 1798, 1799f
    verumontanum mucosal gland 1799
immunophenotype 1792–1793
infections 1795
inflammation 1794–1795, 1795f
    see also prostatitis
intraepithelial neoplasia (PIN) 1793, 1794, 1798,
        1801–1804
    diagnosis of high-grade 1802–1804, 1809–1810
    high-grade, carcinoma risk 1803–1804
    high-grade, histology 1801–1802, 1801f, 1802f
    high-grade with outpouching 1803, 1803f
    invasion from high-grade PIN 1803, 1803f
    low-grade 1801
    PINATYP (with atypical glands) 1803
    small cell neuroendocrine 1801, 1802f
    structural patterns 1801–1802, 1801f, 1802f
ionizing radiation effect 157
leiomyoma 1820
leiomyosarcoma 1820, 1820f
leukemia 1820–1821
lymphoma 1820–1821, 1821, 1821f
metaplasia 1797–1798
    see also prostate gland, squamous metaplasia
mixed small cell carcinoma–adenocarcinoma
        1819f
mucinous metaplasia 1797–1798
neuroendocrine carcinoma 1819
normal histology 1792, 1792f, 1793f
Paneth cell-like metaplasia 1798
polyps 1725
post-atrophic hyperplasia 1796, 1796f, 1797
pseudohyperplastic carcinoma 1799
pseudoneoplasms 1800–1801, 1801t
radiation-induced changes 157, 1821, 1821f
rhabdomyosarcoma 1820
sarcoma 1820
sarcomatoid (carcinosarcoma) carcinoma
        1819–1820, 1819f
sclerotic, partial 1796
signet-ring carcinoma 1819, 1819f
size/weight 1791
small cell carcinoma 1819
spindle cell carcinoma, iatrogenic reactions
        resembling 147
squamous cell carcinoma 1815, 1819
squamous metaplasia 1794, 1797
    differential diagnosis 1798
    estrogen therapy association 151
    transitional cell metaplasia 1797, 1798f
transition zone 1791, 1792
    nodules 1798
transurethral resection effect 1821
treatment effects on 1821, 1821f
tumors
    primary (unusual) 1820
    secondary 1820–1821, 1820f
urothelial (transitional cell) carcinoma 1815, 1819
    prostatic adenocarcinoma vs 1813t
urothelium (transitional cell) 1793
    metaplasia types 1798
vasculitis 1795
xanthoma 1795
prostate-specific antigen (PSA) 1793
    immunohistochemical staining 35
prostatic acid phosphatase (PAP) 180
prostatic adenocarcinoma 1805–1815
    acinar 1819
    atrophic 1810f
        differential diagnosis 1796–1797, 1804
    benign conditions mimicked by 1822, 1822t
    bladder neck involvement 1818

prostatic adenocarcinoma (*cont'd*)
  collagenous micronodules (mucinous fibroplasia) 1811, 1811f
  crystalloids in 1809, 1809f
  diagnostic criteria 1805–1810, 1805t
    intraluminal secretions 1808–1809, 1809f
    nuclear atypia 1808, 1808f
  diagnostic methods 22
  differential diagnosis 1810
    atypical adenomatous hyperplasia *vs* 1799
    immunohistochemical markers 1812–1813
    prostatic atrophy *vs* 1795, 1796, 1797t
    prostatic hyperplasia *vs* 1799
    urothelial carcinoma *vs* 1813t
  DNA and RNA analyses 1813–1814, 1814f
  ductal (endometrioid, endometrial, papillary) 1818, 1818f
  endocrine therapy, iatrogenic reaction 151
  extraprostatic extension by 1815, 1817, 1817f
  foamy gland 1810
  Gleason grades 1805, 1806f, 1814, 1815, 1816t
  glomeruloid structures 1811, 1811f
  grading 1815
  histopathologic features 1810–1811
  immunohistochemistry 1812–1814
  lymphovascular space invasion 1811, 1811f
  metastases 1818, 1818f
    in testis 1763, 1763f
  microinvasive (early invasive) 1803
  minimal (limited) 1811–1812, 1812f
  mixed small cell–adenocarcinoma 1819f
  molecular diagnostic studies 1812–1814
  mucinous (colloid) 1818–1819
  perineural invasion 1810, 1810f, 1814
  prognostic factors and reporting 1814–1815
  pseudohyperplastic 1806, 1807f
  radiation therapy effect 154, 154f, 1821, 1821f
  small acinar 1806f
  staging (TNM) 1815–1818
  variants 1818–1820
prostatic 'capsule' 1793
prostatic specific antigen (PSA) 180
prostatitis 1794–1795
  BCG causing 1795
  classification 1794
  eosinophilic (allergic) 1794
  granulomatous 1794, 1795, 1795f, 1813
    TURP causing 1821
  infectious causes 1795
protease-induced retrieval (antigens) 32
protease inhibitors 31t
  alpha-1-antitrypsin as 1506
14-3-3 protein 2413
protein, deposition in lymph nodes 515–516
protein A-based methods 32
proteinase 3, antibodies 1622
protein gene product 9.5 1322
proteinuria
  acute postinfectious glomerulonephritis 1617
  glomerular diseases 1605
  IgA nephropathy 1618
  light microscopy diagnostic algorithms 1604t
  minimal change glomerulopathy 1606
  in vasculitides 1648
proteoglycan 678
  diseases involving 686
  staining methods 677
Proteus, acute suppurative (phlegmonous) gastritis 1329
proto-oncogenes 1169
Prototheca 72–73, 72f
protothecosis 72–73, 72f, 73f
protozoal infections
  confirmation by molecular methods 108t
  gastrointestinal tract and liver 102–103
  hepatic granuloma 1511
  intestinal 1399–1400
prurigo nodularis 201
pruritic urticarial papules and plaques of pregnancy (PUPPP) 198

Prussian blue stain, liver biopsy 1469
psammocarcinoma, peritoneal serous carcinoma 1023, 1023f
psammoma bodies 1967f
  bone fragments in crush preparations *vs* 2330
  childhood fibrous tumor (calcifying fibrous pseudotumor) 317–318, 317f, 318f
  definition 1997
  endosalpingiosis 2000
  in malignant effusions 184, 1028–1029
  melanotic schwannoma 2253
  meningioma 2251, 2387, 2388f
  oligodendroglioma 2361
  ovarian cancer 1029–1030, 1030f, 1997, 2002
  papillary renal cell carcinoma 1680–1681
  papillary thyroid carcinoma 2128
  peritoneal serous carcinoma 1023, 1023f
  pituitary adenoma 2101, 2102, 2102f, 2104
  serous endometrial adenocarcinoma 1963, 1967, 1967f
  serous tumors of ovary 1997, 2002
  sinonasal meningioma 811, 811f
psammomatoid calcifications 743, 743f
psammomatoid' ossicles 743
psammomatoid (juvenile) ossifying fibroma 742–743, 743f
pseudoacrochordons 277
pseudoactinomycotic radiate granules 1837
pseudoalcoholic liver disease 1490–1492
pseudo-ALIP 635
Pseudoallescheria boydii 94f
pseudoaneurysms
  aortic 1083
  of peripheral arteries 1083, 1084f
pseudoangiomatous stromal hyperplasia 446, 446f
pseudocarcinoma, large intestine 1433
pseudocarcinomatous hyperplasia
  fallopian tube 2041, 2044
  vulva 1902, 1903f
pseudocysts
  endochondral 2281, 2281f
  pancreatic 1553, 1553f, 1554f
pseudodecidua 1938, 1938f, 1939f, 1948
pseudodiverticulosis, esophageal 1284
pseudoepitheliomatous hyperplasia (PEH) 243
  cervix 1837
  oral cavity 1178–1179, 1184
  penis 1769–1770
  squamous cell carcinoma *vs* 80f
pseudofollicles (proliferation centers) 551, 551f, 555, 556
pseudo-Gaucher cells 96
pseudogoblet cells, Barrett's esophagus 1303, 1304f
pseudogout 688, 688f
pseudohyphae 71
pseudoinclusions
  adrenal cortex 2178, 2189
  nuclear, pheochromocytoma 2191, 2192f, 2193
  thymic neuroendocrine carcinoma 1111–1112, 1112f
'pseudoinvasion' of vascular spaces, local anesthetic in cervix 137
pseudo-Kaposi's sarcoma 370–371
pseudokoilocytosis, cervical sample 1842, 1843f
pseudolipomatosis, colonic 1406
pseudolymphoma
  gastric 1351
  renal 1694
  upper respiratory tract 835–836
pseudomalignant cells, chondromyxoid fibroma 714
pseudomeissnerian corpuscles 2254
pseudomelanin 20t
pseudomembranous colitis 1396, 1396f, 1397f
  neutropenic enterocolitis *vs* 1397
pseudomesotheliomatous adenocarcinoma 961f, 1018, 1018f
  pulmonary adenocarcinoma *vs* 960
Pseudomonas
  abscess formation 69
  autofluorescence 62
  otitis externa 2272

Pseudomonas aeruginosa
  acute appendicitis 1408
  noma due to 78–79
  vasculitis 99
'*Pseudomonas* vasculitis' 79f
pseudomyogenous tumors, rhabdomyosarcoma *vs* 361t
pseudomyxoma ovarii 2006
  acellular 2003
  cellular 2003, 2006–2007
pseudomyxoma peritonei 1025, 1025f, 2006
  disseminated peritoneal adenomucinosis 2006, 2006f
  mucinous tumors of ovary with 2002, 2006–2007, 2006f, 2008f
  peritoneal mucinous carcinomatosis 2006
  primary tumors causing 2007
pseudo-Nelson's syndrome 1109
pseudoparakeratosis, oral contraceptives and 151
pseudopelade of Brocq 202
pseudopsammoma bodies 2391
pseudopuberty, precocious 2017, 2025, 2030, 2031
pseudorosettes
  medulloblastoma 2380, 2381f
  neuroblastic *see* Homer Wright (pseudo) rosettes
  perivascular *see* perivascular pseudorosettes
pseudosarcoma 313, 314f
  of periosteum *see* periosteum
  of skin 266
pseudosarcoma botryoides *see* fibroepithelial polyps
pseudosarcomatoid carcinoma, sinonasal region 791, 793, 793f
pseudosarcomatous fibromyxoid tumor, bladder 1723, 1723f
pseudosarcomatous proliferative lesions 312–314
  atypical decubital fibroplasia (ischemic fasciitis) 314, 315f
  nodular fasciitis 312–313, 312f, 313f, 314f
  proliferative fasciitis 314f, 313–314
  proliferative myositis 314
pseudostratification, bronchioles 860
pseudosupernumerary vessel 2065
pseudotuberculosis, Peyer's patches infection 1395
pseudotumor
  bone-forming reactive *see* myositis ossificans
  calcifying fibrous 317–318, 317f, 318f
  fibrous, paratesticular 1763
  inflammatory 331, 332, 332f
    bladder 1723, 1723f
    thymic 1128
  laryngeal 834, 835–836
  mediastinum 1128
  xanthogranulomatous, vagina 1921
pseudovascular (angiectoid) spaces 266
pseudovesicles, Sweet's syndrome 212
pseudoxanthomatous change (cholate stasis) 1493, 1495f
pseudoxanthomatous nodules, necrotic 1989
pseudoxanthomatous salpingitis 2042, 2042f, 2043
psoriasiform dermatoses 199–202
psoriasis 199, 1058
psoriasis vulgaris 199–200, 199f
PTAH stain 1469
PTEN gene, mutations 252
pterygia 2303
Ptx1 and *Ptx2* 2093–2094
puberty, precocious 1536, 2109
pubic lice 1891
puerperium, solitary luteinized follicular cyst 1993, 1994f
pulmonary alveolar proteinosis (PAP) 925–926, 926f
pulmonary arterial hypertension 912–914
  chronic thromboembolic 917, 917f
  classification 913t
  concentric intimal fibrosis 912, 913f, 916
  in congenital heart disease 912
  dilatation and angiomatoid lesions 912, 914f
  eccentric intimal fibrosis 916
  intimal proliferation 912, 913f
  muscular hypertrophy 912, 913f
  necrotizing vasculitis 912, 914f

plexiform lesions 912, 914f
  primary (sporadic) 912, 916
  risk factors (drugs and toxins) 913t
  secondary 912–914, 916
pulmonary arteries 861–862, 862f
pulmonary artery leiomyosarcoma 353
pulmonary capillaries 861
  capillaritis 884, 884f
  congestion 915, 915f
  hypertension 912
pulmonary capillaritis 1076
pulmonary capillary hemangiomatosis (PCH) 918, 918f
pulmonary colloid carcinoma 959
pulmonary edema, 'photographic negative of' 894
pulmonary embolization, pleural effusions due to 1026
pulmonary fibrosis
  asbestosis 902, 903f
  idiopathic (IPFT) 895, 896
  progressive massive 904
  small airways 910–911, 911f
pulmonary hemorrhage 884, 884f
pulmonary hypertension 911–912
  arterial see pulmonary arterial hypertension
  capillary 912
  classification 913t
  pre-/postcapillary 912
  rheumatoid arthritis 887–888
pulmonary infiltrates with eosinophilia (PIE) 881,
    881f
pulmonary lymphoid hyperplasia (PLH), in HIV
    infection 118
pulmonary metastases, cavitation, chemotherapy
    association 147
pulmonary tumors see lung
pulmonary valve, disorders 1059
pulmonary vasculature, disorders affecting 918
pulmonary veins 862, 862f
pulmonary veno-occlusive disease (PVOD) 915, 916f,
    917f
pulmonary venous hypertension 914–915
  tricuspid insufficiency due to 1059
pulseless disease see Takayasu's disease
punch biopsy, skin 193
pupillary reflex, white 2309
pupil–optic (P–O) nerve segment 2306
pure red cell aplasia 617
pustular disorders 216–225
pustular psoriasis of Barber 199
pustules 195
  satellite 217
  subcorneal 216, 216f
Putt stain 60, 60t
pyelonephritis
  acute 1610f, 1639, 1639f
  chronic 1610f, 1639–1640
  xanthogranulomatous 1642, 1642f, 1696, 1696f,
      1697f
pyloric metaplasia see gastric metaplasia
pyloric sphincter 1321
pyloric stenosis, hypertrophic 1339, 1339f
pyoderma gangrenosum 212
pyometra 1944–1945
pyomyositis 2222
pyosalpinx 2040
pyrrolizidine alkaloids 1515

Q

Q fever 82
  granulomatous changes, in bone marrow 661, 661t
  hepatic granulomas 1511, 1511f
quality assessments 10
quality assurance (QA) 9, 11, 13
quality control (QC) 9, 13
  for histochemical stains 61, 62t
  infectious agent detection 61
Quilty phenomenon 130, 130f, 1051, 1055f

R

rabies virus, inclusions 68t

racemose pattern, postirradiation angiosarcoma 276,
    276f
radial scars, breast 444–445, 445f
radial sclerosing lesion, breast 445, 445f
'radiation atypia', lung 886
radiation-induced conditions/changes 151–158
  acute diffuse lung disease 884–885
  arterial changes 153, 153f
  bladder changes 156–157, 1709, 1709f
  breast changes 158, 450
  cervical changes 1846, 1848f
  CNS changes 2344, 2345f
  CNS tumors associated 2348
  colitis 155, 1388, 1406
  dermatitis 155, 233
  effect on neoplasms 153–155
  effect on normal tissue 151–152
  enteritis 1406
  enterocolitis 155
  esophagitis 1288
  iatrogenic lesions 151–158
  intestinal changes 155
  kidney changes 156
  liver changes 155–156
  lung changes 158, 989
  lung injury, chronic 886
  necrosis, CNS 2344
  nephritis/nephropathy 156
  pericarditis 1069
  pneumonitis 886
  prostate changes 157, 1821, 1821f
  salivary gland changes 155, 155f
  skin and mucous membrane changes 155
  thyroid changes 157–158
  tumors associated see radiation-induced tumors
  uterine changes 157, 157f
radiation-induced tumors 158–160
  angiosarcoma 276, 276f, 371, 371f
  bone 159–160
  breast 160
  CNS 160, 2344, 2348
  head and neck 158–159
  intestine 159
  mesothelium 160
  oral squamous cell carcinoma 1169
  osteosarcoma 159, 727, 735
  papillary thyroid carcinoma 2127
  skin 158, 276, 276f
  soft tissue 160
  squamous cell carcinoma of salivary glands 1246
  uterus 159
radiation recall phenomenon 151
radicular cysts 1142f, 1146–1147
radiographic media, iatrogenic lesions due to 138
radiography, bone tumors 704
radon, lung cancer etiology 935
ragged red fibers 2221, 2230
'raisinoid' appearance, chromophobe renal cell
    carcinoma 1683
Rai's staging system, chronic lymphocytic leukemia 642
RANKL 713, 762
ranulas 1149, 1259
  plunging 1259
rapid Pap staining method 26
rapid-urease tests 1330
Rasmussen encephalitis 2405–2406, 2406f
ras oncogene
  follicular thyroid carcinoma 2133
  gastric adenocarcinoma 1360
  Hürthle cell carcinoma 2135
  lung cancer 937
  metastasis development 168
Rathke cleft cysts 2113, 2113f, 2401, 2403
Rathke's cleft, ectopic pituitary adenoma 2098
Rathke's pouch 1152, 2093
Rathke's pouch homeobox (Rpx) protein 2093–2094
RB gene 735, 937, 992, 2309
RCC marker, chromophobe renal cell carcinoma 1684
reactive follicular hyperplasia see under lymph nodes

reactive mediastinal spindle cell pseudotumors 515
reactive mesothelial hyperplasia
  atypical, effusions 1027–1028, 1028f
  effusions in 1027, 1027f
  peritoneum 1020, 1020f
  pleura 1006, 1006f
reactive pseudosarcomatous lesions, of periosteum see
    periosteum
REAL classification, lymphomas 544, 546t, 554, 557,
    561, 824, 1256
rectal adenocarcinoma, Paget's disease secondary to
    1908
rectosigmoid, eroded polypoid hyperplasia 1382
rectum
  carcinoma see colorectal adenocarcinoma
  leiomyosarcoma 1445, 1447f
  neuroendocrine tumors 1429
  viral infections 1398–1399
red blood cells
  in effusions 1026
  nucleated (NRBCs) 612
red cells, hypoplasia/aplasia, AIDS 662
'red' neurons 2340, 2341f
reducing body myopathy 2228t, 2229
5α-reductase deficiency 1737, 1794
Reed, pigmented spindle-cell nevus of 278, 279
Reed's syndrome, familial multiple leiomyoma with 348
Reed–Sternberg cells 535, 536f, 652, 653, 761, 981
  characteristics/structure 536, 536f, 537f, 652
  in effusions 1031
  inflammatory myxohyaline tumor cells similar 328
  lymphomatoid granulomatosis 290
  variants 652, 653
Reed–Sternberg-like cells, small lymphocytic
    lymphoma 541
Reese's cancerous melanosis 2293, 2293f
refractory anemia (RA) 635, 636f, 637t
  with excess blasts (RAEB-1/-2) 636t, 637t
  with excess blasts in transformation (RAEB-T) 636t,
      638
  with ringed sideroblasts (RARS) 636f, 637t
refractory cytopenia with multilineage dysplasia 637t
refractory sprue 1376
refractory watery diarrhea, hypokalemia and
    achlorhydria (WDHA) 1574, 2193
Refsum's disease 2247
Reinke, crystals 1988
  in fallopian tube 2043
  Leydig cell tumor 1757
Reinke crystalloids 1732, 1733f
  congenital adrenal hyperplasia 2175
  hilus cell hyperplasia 1994
  Leydig cell tumor 2024
Reis–Bücklers dystrophy 2302
Reiter syndrome 1058
relapsing polychondritis see polychondritis, relapsing
remyelination 2241
renal adenoma see kidney, adenoma
renal arteries 1600
  dysplasia 1080
  fibrinoid necrosis 1611f, 1645, 1645f, 1647, 1648
  hyalinosis 1611f
  stenosis 1645–1646, 1645f
renal arterioles
  hyalinosis 1644, 1644f
  'onion-skinning' 1611f, 1645
renal biopsy see kidney, biopsy
renal cell carcinoma 1676–1689
  acquired cystic disease of kidney and 1663
  angiomyolipoma association 1690
  autosomal dominant polycystic kidney disease and
      1662
  bone metastases 771
  chromophobe 1674, 1675, 1676, 1682–1685, 1684f
    clear cell carcinoma vs 1678
    microscopic pathology 1683, 1683f, 1684f
    oncocytoma vs 1676, 1677t
  classification 1672t, 1676
  clear cell 176, 176f, 1677–1680, 1678f

renal cell carcinoma (*cont'd*)
acquired cystic disease of kidney and 1664
clear cell carcinoma of ovary *vs* 2012
cystic 1688
cytology 1680, 1680f, 1681f
differential diagnosis 1680, 1681, 1696
Fuhrman nuclear grading 1679, 1679f, 1679t
microscopic pathology 1678–1679, 1678f
sarcomatoid 1678, 1678f, 1687–1688, 1688f
clinical features 1677
collecting duct carcinoma 1682, 1685, 1685f, 1686f
cystic 1688–1689
differential diagnosis
adenoma *vs* 1673
oncocytoma *vs* 1675, 1676
xanthogranulomatous pyelonephritis 1696
epidemiology 1676–1677
metastases 1677
benign clear cell of lung *vs* 962
clear cell carcinoma of ovary *vs* 2012
clear cell eccrine adenocarcinoma *vs* 262
clear cell gallbladder carcinoma *vs* 1580
hepatocellular carcinoma *vs* 1535
to liver 171, 1535
low-grade papillary adenocarcinoma of ear *vs* 2279
to pancreas 1569, 1570f
to pleura 1018
salivary clear cell adenocarcinoma *vs* 1247
salivary epithelial-myoepithelial carcinoma *vs* 1246
salivary gland oncocytoma *vs* 1225
seminoma *vs* 1746
serous cystic tumor of pancreas *vs* 1563
sinonasal 808–810, 809f
to sinonasal tract 827
in thyroid 2141, 2141f
tumor-to-tumor 173
mucinous tubular 1685–1686, 1686f
multilocular cystic 1688, 1689f
papillary (chromophil) 1673, 1676, 1680–1682, 1689
collecting duct 1685, 1685f
cytology 1681, 1682f
differential diagnosis 1681, 1685
Fuhrman nuclear grading 1681, 1682f
pediatric 1671–1672
postneuroblastoma 1671–1672
Xp11.2 associated carcinoma 1671, 1671f, 1682
in renal dysplasia 1661
sarcomatoid 1687–1688, 1688f, 1693
sinonasal renal cell-like carcinoma *vs* 810t
spindle cell 1685–1686, 1686f
staging 1672, 1673t
treatment and outcome 1677
tubulocystic 1686–1687, 1686f
unclassified 1687
in Wilms' tumor 1667, 1671–1672
renal cell-like carcinoma, sinonasal 808–810, 809f
renal cortical adenoma 1673, 1673f
renal dialysis 686
renal diseases *see* kidney, medical diseases
renal dysplasia 1661, 1662f
renal failure
acute 1605, 1637
chronic 2160, 2161f
evaluation 1603
renal parenchyma
biopsy 1597
staining 1601
renal pelvis 1726
cystic hamartoma 1695
tumors 1726
renal pyramids 1598
renal transplantation 1649–1654
accelerated acute rejection 1649
accelerated antibody-mediated rejection 127
acute cellular rejection 123, 123t, 124f, 125t
acute interstitial rejection 1610f, 1650, 1650f
acute rejection 1649–1650, 1650f

acute vascular rejection 1650
biopsy 1597, 1651
chronic rejection 127–128, 127f, 1650
classification (Banff) of rejection 1649, 1649t
complications 1652–1654
hyperacute (cytotoxic antibodies) rejection 1649
indications for biopsy 1649
Kaposi's sarcoma, of lung 973
non-neoplastic lymphadenopathy 149
perfusion injury of allograft 129, 130f
recurrent/de novo diseases 1653–1654, 1653f
tumors associated 150
renal tubular interstitium
anatomy 1600
foamy cells 1625
red blood cells/casts in 1619
scarring 1644
striped fibrosis 1652
'thyroidization' 1610f, 1639
renal tubules
anatomy and histology 1600
bile pigmentation in cells 1634f
disorders *see* tubular interstitial disorders
distal/proximal 1600
microabscess 1610f
microcysts 1622
regeneration, in acute tubular necrosis 1638f
staining 1601–1602
renal tumors *see* kidney, tumors
renal vascular disorders 1605, 1643–1649
light microscopy diagnostic algorithm 1606t
renal vasculature
anatomy 1600–1601
fibrinoid necrosis 1611f, 1645, 1645f, 1647, 1648
renal vein thrombosis 1614
Renaut bodies 2240, 2240f, 2245
Rendu-Osler-Weber syndrome (hereditary hemorrhagic telangiectasia) 1517, 2416
reperfusion injury, lung 919
reports *see under* surgical pathology/pathologists
reserve cells 952
cervical 1832
hyperplasia 993–994
adenoid cystic carcinoma of lung *vs* 952
cervical 1832
small cell lung carcinoma *vs* 993
residual cysts 1142f
resistant ovary syndrome 1989
respiratory bronchioles, anatomy 860
respiratory bronchiolitis 922, 923f
respiratory bronchiolitis with interstitial disease (RBILD) 898–899, 922, 923f
pulmonary Langerhans cell histiocytosis *vs* 925
respiratory epithelial cells
type I 861, 863
type II 861
hyperplasia 882, 882f
respiratory epithelium 860, 860f
respiratory papillomatosis, HPV and 839–841
respiratory syncytial virus (RSV) 68t
bronchiolitis 94
pneumonia 94, 95f, 876, 877f
respiratory tract
disorders 915–916
see also lung
infections 81–96
bacterial 81–83
fungal 83–93
parasitic 95–96, 96f
viral 93–95
restriction fragment length polymorphism (RFLP) 45
rests of Malassez 1139, 1146
rests of Serres 1139, 1142
rete ovarii 1990, 1990f
rete pegs
cervical squamous epithelium 1832
loss 1892
'saw-toothing' 1894, 1894f
verrucous carcinoma of ear 2280

rete ridges
diminution, lichen myxedematosis 228
elongation
angiokeratoma 269, 269f
Darier's disease 219
squamous cell carcinoma 246
flattening
scars 231
scleroderma 232
fusion, atypical nevus 281, 281f
'in-curving' 241, 241f
oral pseudoepitheliomatous hyperplasia 1179
'saw-toothed', lichen planus 202, 202f
verrucous carcinoma, oral 1174, 1175
rete testis
adenocarcinoma 1763
anatomy 1731
tumors 1743t, 1763
RET gene 1403, 2192
reticulin, staining methods 16t, 18, 18f
reticulin fibers 1470
reticulin stain 610
liver biopsy 1468, 1469f
pituitary gland 2111f
reticuloendotheliosis, malignant *see* Rosai–Dorfman disease
reticulohistiocytoma, solitary 288, 288f
reticulohistiocytosis 288
reticuloid, actinic 295
reticulosis, pagetoid 292
retiform tubules 2021, 2022f
retina
astrocytoma 2311
atrophy
glaucomatous 2314, 2314f
inner ischemic 2314, 2315f
coagulative necrosis 2315f, 2318
cotton-wool exudates 2317
detachment (separation) 2317
dysplasia, bilateral 2311
hard exudates 2317
hemangioblastoma 2317
hemorrhage 2317
ischemia 2318
microabscess 2317
normal 2318f
vascular disease 2317–2318
vasospasm 2318
retinal anlage tumor 750–751, 751f
neuroblastoma *vs* 384
see also melanotic neuroectodermal tumor of infancy
retinal arterioles, fibrosis 2318
retinal artery, central, occlusion 2315f, 2318
retinal ganglion cells, apoptosis 2314
retinal pigment epithelium
adenocarcinoma 2309
hemorrhage under 2317
retinal-S antigen 2376, 2383
retinal vein, central, occlusion 2318
retinitis, cytomegalovirus (CMV) 2313
retinoblastoma 2309–2311
differential diagnosis 2310–2311
diffuse infiltrative 2310
endophytic 2309, 2310f
exophytic 2310
familial 2309
metastases 2310
sinonasal small cell neoplasm after 158
sporadic 2309
trilateral 2309, 2378
retinoblastoma oncogene 735, 937, 992, 2309
retinochoroiditis, toxoplasma 2313, 2314f
retinoic acid syndrome 626
retinopathy
diabetic *see* diabetic retinopathy
of prematurity (ROP) 2311
RET oncogene 2132, 2158
RET/PTC oncogene 2132
retrobulbar tumors 2294

retrolental fibroplasia (retinopathy of prematurity (ROP)) 2311
retroperitoneal fibrosis 1726
retroperitoneal leiomyosarcoma 352
retroperitoneal lymph node dissection (RPLND) 1750
retroperitoneal mass, well differentiated liposarcoma 343f
retroperitonitis, sclerosing 1127
retroplacental hematoma 2065, 2072, 2072f
retuximab (anti_CD20), MALT lymphoma treatment 1354
reverse transcriptase PCR (RT-PCR) 46, 1043
Reye's syndrome 1489
RGB color 42
rhabdoid cells 2392
rhabdoid tumor
    atypical see atypical teratoid/rhabdoid tumor (AT/RT)
    extrarenal 404–405
    gastric 1362
    of kidney 1668, 1670–1671, 1671f
    metastases differential diagnosis 177
    of soft tissue 404–405
    of vulva 1918
rhabdomyoblasts 357–358, 358f, 359f
    markers 405
rhabdomyolysis 2222
rhabdomyoma 354–356
    adult 354–355, 355f
    cardiac 354, 820
    fetal see fetal rhabdomyoma
    genital 356
    heart 1065, 1065f
    larynx 849
    sinonasal region 820
    vagina 1922
    vulva 1900–1901
    well-differentiated, congenital granular cell tumor vs 1185
rhabdomyomatosis, leptomeningeal 2404
rhabdomyosarcoma 356–363
    alveolar see alveolar rhabdomyosarcoma
    anaplastic 359–360
    bladder 1722, 1722f
    botryoid variant 357, 358, 358f, 820
        cambium layer 358, 359f, 820
    classification 356, 357t
    differential diagnosis
        Ewing's sarcoma vs 386
        extrarenal rhabdoid tumor vs 405
        fetal rhabdomyoma vs 356
        genital rhabdomyoma vs 356
        myogenous/pseudomyogenous tumors vs 361t
        proliferative fasciitis vs 313
        small round blue cell tumors vs 361t
        synovial sarcoma vs 404
    electron microscopy 30f
    embryonal see embryonal rhabdomyosarcoma
    endometrial 1977, 1977f
    histologic maturation after chemotherapy 149
    immunohistochemistry 796t
    juvenile 359
    metastatic, differential diagnosis 174–175
    middle ear 2281
    'not otherwise specified' 360
    orbit 2297
    paratesticular region 1766, 1766f
    pleomorphic 359–360, 361–362, 361f, 362f, 820–821
        differential diagnosis 362–363
        malignant fibrous histiocytoma vs 335, 361, 361f
        prognosis 335
    prostate 1820
    sinonasal 796t, 820–821
    spindle cell 356, 357, 358–359
    TNM classification 357, 357t
rheumatic heart disease
    aortic valve 1058
    mitral valve 1055–1056, 1056f
    tricuspid valve 1059

rheumatoid arthritis 693–694, 694f
    autoantibodies 114t
    hearing loss 2282
    histiocytes in effusions 1027
    intestinal involvement 1385–1386
    larynx and trachea 835
    lung involvement 882
        chronic 887–888, 887t, 888f
    lymphadenopathy 518–519
    muscle fiber changes 2222
    osteoarthritis vs 692–693
    peripheral nerve vasculitis 2243
    synovial fluid 691, 691t, 693
    synovium 693, 693f
    vasculitis 1076t, 1078
rheumatoid bronchiolitis 906–907
rheumatoid nodule 214, 215f, 694, 694f
    epithelioid sarcoma vs 400
    gouty tophi vs 233–234
    granuloma annulare vs 213
    lung 888, 888f
    necrobiosis lipoidica vs 214
rheumatoid pneumoconiosis (Caplan's syndrome) 888
rheumatoid vasculitis 1076t, 1078
rhinitis 787
rhinocerebral zygomycosis 80–81, 80f
rhinophyma 226
rhinoscleroma 78, 835
rhinosporidiosis 80, 80f
Rhinosporidium seeberi 80, 80f
rhinotomy, lateral 789
rhodanine stain 1469, 1470f, 1501
Rhodococcus equi 64, 65, 79, 79f, 81, 968
    pneumonia 65f
Richter syndrome 550, 643, 644
rickets 681
rickettsia, hepatic granulomas 1511
Rickettsia rickettsia 99
Riedel's thyroiditis (disease) 1127, 2122
Rigaud tumor 793
right ventricle, myofiber disarray in biopsy 1041
ring sideroblasts 613, 619, 636f
ringworm 198
risk management department (RMD) 11
rituximab (anti-CD20) 551, 610
river blindness 2313
RNA
    extraction/hybridization 45
    staining methods 16t
Robson staging system, renal cell carcinoma 1672
Rochalimaea henselae see Bartonella henselae
Rocky Mountain spotted fever 99
'rod cells' 2344
Rokitansky-Aschoff sinuses 1576
    rupture 1576, 1577f
Romanowsky staining 27
    bone specimens 704
    dyshormonogenetic goiter 2124, 2124f
    enchondroma 710
    focal nodular hyperplasia of liver 1527
    osteoid, in osteosarcoma 733, 733f
    Papanicolaou stain vs 27, 28t
    Pneumocystis jiroveci staining 87
    thymic lymphoma 1124, 1124f, 1125f
Rosai–Dorfman disease 335f, 528–530, 759
    differential diagnosis 334, 529–530, 573
    laryngeal involvement 850
    lymph nodes 528–530, 529f
    sinonasal involvement 826
    skin involvement 288
Rosenthal fibers 2342, 2342f
    orbital tumors 2298
    pilocytic astrocytoma 2357, 2358, 2358f
    pineal cysts 2404f
rosettes
    dysplastic, intraocular 2311
    ependymal 2365, 2366f
    Ewing's sarcoma 174

Flexner–Wintersteiner 801, 2310, 2310f, 2311
giant, hyalinizing spindle cell tumor with 326, 327, 327f
Homer Wright see Homer Wright (pseudo) rosettes
    in neuroepithelial tumors 2366t
    peripheral neuroectodermal tumor 174
    schwannoma (neurilemoma) 2251, 2251f
    thymic carcinoid 1110, 1110f
    see also perivascular pseudorosettes
rotavirus infection 1377, 1398, 1409
Roth spots 2317
round cells, in leiomyoma 348
round cell stromal tumor, stomach 1347
round cell tumors, small see small round cell tumors
round ligament 1933
    tumors 2047–2048
roundworms 104
Rpx-1 gene (Hesx-1) 2098
rubeosis iridis (iris neovascularization) 2315, 2316f
Rushton bodies 1146
Russell bodies 552, 554, 655, 979, 979f
    aural polyps 2274
    inflammatory myofibroblastic tumor 824f
    rheumatoid arthritis 693, 694
Rye classification, Hodgkin's disease 535, 536t, 537

S
S-100 protein
    adipocytes 336
    chondromyxoid fibroma 714
    clear cell chondrosarcoma 721
    clear cell sarcoma 381, 382, 382f
    CNS tumors 2336, 2338
        glioblastoma 2354
        pleomorphic xanthoastrocytoma 2359
        subependymal giant cell astrocytoma 2360
    folliculostellate cells (pituitary) 2093, 2095f
    Langerhans cell histiocytosis 760
    malignant peripheral nerve sheath tumor 2257, 2258f
    melanoma 181, 285, 286
    mesenchymal chondrosarcoma 720
    microglandular adenosis (of breast) 444
    neoplastic Langerhans cells 573
    neuroblastoma of adrenal medulla 2198
    ossifying fibromyxoid tumor 380
    pheochromocytoma 2193, 2194f
    pleomorphic adenoma of salivary gland 1210
    schwannoma (neurilemoma) 379, 2251, 2251f
    seminoma differential diagnosis 1775t
    synovial sarcoma 403
    T-cell lymphoproliferative disorder 651–652
saccule 2269, 2269f
sacrum, chordoma 763f, 765
saffranin 59
salivary ducts 1186f
    carcinoma 1252–1253, 1252f, 1255
    cysts 1260
    heterotopic 1215
'salivary gland anlage tumor' 800–801
salivary glands 1203–1277
    aberrant 834
    anatomy/histology 1186f
    benign lymphoepithelial lesion see sialadenitis, lymphoepithelial
    choristoma of middle ear 2271
    clear cell changes 1208t
    cystic changes 1208t
    cysts, FNA 1207t
    cytologic features of lesions 1208t
    duct system 1186f
    enlargement 1206
    HIV-associated disease 1260–1261, 1261f
    inflammation 1207t
    intraductal hyperplasia 1226
    ionizing radiation effect 155, 155f
    lymphoepithelial cysts 1260, 1260f
    masses, FNA evaluation 1205, 1206
    mucoceles 1259–1260, 1259f

salivary glands (cont'd)
  nodular oncocytic hyperplasia 1224
  non-neoplastic conditions 1257–1262
  oncocytic cells 1208t, 1223, 1224
  reactive change after mucosal biopsy 136, 136f
  sclerosing polycystic adenosis 1261–1262, 1262f
  sclerotic nodules 1262
  sebaceous differentiation 1208t
  tissue
    aspiration by FNA 1206
    inclusions in lymph nodes 512
  tumors see salivary gland tumors
salivary gland tumors 794–801, 1186–1190,
    1203–1257
  acinic cell carcinoma 797, 1230–1235
    clear cells 1232, 1233f, 1235
    cytopathology 1234–1235, 1234f, 1235f
    'dedifferentiated'/undifferentiated 1233
    differential diagnosis 1234, 1235
    follicular pattern 1232f, 1233
    immunohistochemistry 1234
    large granular cells 1235
    microcystic pattern 1230, 1231, 1231f
    microscopic features 1230–1234, 1231f, 1232f
    papillary-cystic pattern 1232, 1232f
    salivary duct carcinoma vs 1252
    solid pattern 1230, 1231, 1231f
  adenocarcinoma, esophageal 1312
  adenocarcinoma not otherwise specified 1235–1236,
    1236f
  adenoid cystic carcinoma 794–795, 1186,
    1189–1190, 1190, 1236–1240, 1237f
    adenosquamous carcinoma vs 1256
    basal cell adenoma vs 1221
    canalicular adenoma vs 1223
    cribriform pattern 795f, 1189f, 1237, 1238f, 1240,
      1240f
    cytopathology 1239–1240, 1240f
    differential diagnosis 1238–1239, 1240, 1241f
    epithelial-myoepithelial carcinoma vs 1246
    histologic features 795f, 1237, 1237f, 1238f,
      1239f
    pleomorphic adenoma vs 1212, 1214f, 1215f
    polymorphous low-grade adenocarcinoma vs 1242
    solid pattern 1189f, 1237, 1239f, 1240, 1240f,
      1241f
    tubular pattern 1237, 1239f
  adenosquamous carcinoma 1254–1256, 1255f
  basal cell adenocarcinoma 1248–1249, 1248f
    differential diagnosis 1221
  basal cell adenoma 1187, 1187f, 1219–1222
    adenoid cystic carcinoma vs 1221, 1240, 1241f
    basal cell adenocarcinoma vs 1248
    canalicular adenoma vs 1223
    cytopathology 1221–1222, 1222f, 1223f
    malignant transformation 1221
    membranous type 1220, 1220f, 1221
    microscopic features 1219–1220, 1220f
    small blue cell pattern 1221, 1222f, 1223f
    solid pattern 1219–1220, 1220f
    tubulotrabecular 1220, 1221f
  basaloid squamous carcinoma
    adenoid cystic carcinoma vs 1239
    adenosquamous carcinoma vs 1256
    basal cell adenocarcinoma vs 1248
  benign 1186–1188, 1207–1227
  benign epithelial 1205t
  canalicular adenoma 1186, 1188, 1188f, 1222–1223,
    1224f
  carcinoma ex lymphoepithelial lesion 1250–1251,
    1251f
  carcinoma ex mixed tumor 1243, 1243f
  carcinoma in situ 1210, 1243
  carcinosarcoma 1243–1244, 1244f
  classification 1186, 1204, 1205t
  clear cell (hyalinizing) adenocarcinoma 1246–1248,
    1247f
  clear cell carcinoma 808, 810t
  clear cell myoepithelial carcinoma 1254

clear cell oncocytoma 1246
cystadenocarcinoma 1251–1252
  salivary duct carcinoma vs 1252–1253
  salivary mucoepidermoid carcinoma vs 1228
cystadenoma 1226, 1226f
cytological features 1208t
epidemiology 1203
epidermoid carcinoma 1255
epithelial, large/small cell 1207t
epithelial-myoepithelial carcinoma 1245–1246,
    1245f
  adenoid cystic carcinoma vs 1238
  clear cell adenocarcinoma vs 1247
fine needle aspiration 1204–1206
  classification of findings 1207t
  cytologic commonalities 1206, 1207t
  normal tissue, significance 1206–1207
  tissue damage/infarction 1205, 1211
grading and staging 1203, 1204t
intracapsular carcinoma (carcinoma in situ) 1210,
    1243
intraductal carcinoma 1252–1253, 1252f
lobular carcinoma 1241
  see also salivary gland tumors, polymorphous
    low-grade adenocarcinoma
low-grade adenocarcinoma 1245
lymphomas 1256–1257, 1256f
malignant 1188–1190, 1227–1257
malignant epithelial 1205t
malignant lymphoepithelial lesion 1250–1251, 1251f
mesenchymal 1205t
metastases in 169t, 171
minimally pleomorphic adenoma 1212, 1221
mixed tumors 1243–1245
  adenoid cystic carcinoma vs 1238–1239
  irradiation associated 158–159
  metastasizing 1244–1245
  polymorphous low-grade adenocarcinoma vs 1242
  true malignant 1243–1244, 1244f
  see also pleomorphic adenoma (below)
mucoepidermoid carcinoma 798–799, 799f, 1186,
    1188–1189, 1189f, 1227–1230
  adenosquamous carcinoma vs 1256
  central osseous 1189
  clear cell adenocarcinoma vs 1247
  cystadenoma vs 1226
  cytopathology 1229–1230, 1230f, 1231f
  differential diagnosis 1228
  epithelial-myoepithelial carcinoma vs 1246
  high-grade 1189f, 1228, 1230f
  intermediate-grade 799f, 1188f, 1228, 1229f
  low-grade 1228, 1228f, 1229–1230, 1229f, 1230f
  microscopic features 1227–1228, 1228f
  salivary duct carcinoma vs 1252
myoepithelial carcinoma 1254, 1254f
myoepithelioma 796–797, 1213–1214, 1216f
  myoepithelial carcinoma vs 1254
oncocytic carcinoma 1253, 1253f
  salivary duct carcinoma vs 1252
oncocytic lesions 1223–1226
  Warthin's tumor vs 1219
oncocytic metaplasia 1223–1224, 1225
oncocytoma 1223–1226, 1225f
  clear cell 1224, 1225, 1225f
  clear cell adenocarcinoma vs 1247
pleomorphic adenoma (mixed tumor) 795–796,
    1186–1187, 1187f, 1207–1213, 1207t
  adenoid cystic carcinoma vs 1212, 1214f, 1215f
  basal cell adenoma vs 1221
  chondromyxoid matrix 1209, 1210, 1212, 1212f,
    1213f
  cytopathology 1210–1213, 1211f, 1212f, 1213f
  differential diagnosis 1210, 1211–1213
  epithelial cell elements 1208, 1209, 1210, 1212
  FNA evaluation 1206
  gross features 797f, 1208, 1208f
  immunohistochemistry 1209–1210
  infarction 1211
  malignant transformation 1210

mesenchymal-like elements 1208, 1209
microscopic features 797f, 1208–1209, 1209f
myoepithelial cells 1210, 1211f, 1212, 1212f,
    1213f
plasmacytoid myoepithelial cells 1210, 1214f
polymorphous low-grade adenocarcinoma vs
    1210, 1212–1213
prognosis and treatment 1210
spindled myoepithelial cells 1210, 1213, 1213f
polymorphous low-grade adenocarcinoma 1190,
    1190f, 1237, 1241–1243
  adenoid cystic carcinoma vs 1238
  epithelial-myoepithelial carcinoma vs 1246
  microscopic features 1241, 1241f, 1242f
sarcoma 1244
sebaceous adenoma 1226–1227
  clear cell adenocarcinoma vs 1247
sebaceous carcinoma 1253
sebaceous lymphadenocarcinoma 1253
sialoblastoma 1227, 1227f, 1248–1249, 1248f
specimens 1203
spindle cell 1207t
squamous cell carcinoma 1246, 1255
terminal duct carcinoma 1241
undifferentiated carcinoma 1249–1251
  large cell 1249–1250, 1249f, 1250
  lymphoepithelial carcinoma 1250–1251, 1251f
  small cell 1250, 1250f
Warthin's tumor see Warthin's tumor
Salmonella
  appendiceal infection 1409
  colitis 1395
  osteomyelitis 689
Salmonella typhi 101f
Salmonella typhimurium, colitis 1395
'salmon patch' 268
salpingitis
  acute 1989, 2040, 2040f
  chronic 2040–2041, 2045
  'follicular' 2041
  granulomatous 2041, 2041f, 2042
  lipoid 138
  'physiologic' 2040
  pseudoxanthomatous 2042, 2042f
  tuberculous 2041, 2041f
  xanthogranulomatous 2042
  xanthomatous 138
salpingitis isthmica nodosa 2042, 2043f
'salt and pepper' chromatin 174f
  carcinoid tumor of ovary 2035
  extramedullary myeloid cell tumor 624
  gastric carcinoids 1350
  medullary thyroid carcinoma 2138f
  neuroblastoma of adrenal medulla 2195
  neuroendocrine tumors 175
  small cell carcinoma of lung 1030
saltatory conduction 2241
salt-split skin technique 222
salvage cytology, gastric 1325
Santorini, duct 1549
saphenous vein bypass grafts 1072
sarcocystis, muscle involvement 2223, 2224f
sarcoidosis
  breast 450
  cardiomyopathy 1045
  cutaneous 214–215, 216f
  differential diagnosis 533
    acne rosacea vs 226
  endomyocardial biopsy 1045
  erythema nodosum associated 214
  granulomatous salpingitis 2042
  hepatic granuloma 1509–1510, 1510f
  hypersensitivity pneumonitis vs 891t
  interstitial pneumonia 893
  intracranial 2413–2414
  liver 1502, 1502f
  lung involvement 214, 891–893, 892f, 893f
  lymph node granulomas 533
  lymph node involvement 533

peripheral nerves 2243
skeletal muscle involvement 2223–2224
staging and radiography 891–892
trachea 835
sarcolemmal membrane 2215
sarcoma
acral myxoinflammatory fibroblastic 327–328, 328f
alveolar soft part *see* alveolar soft part sarcoma (ASPS)
bone *see* bone, sarcoma
botryoid *see* botryoid sarcoma
breast 436, 485
cardiac 1066–1067, 1067t
cervix 1877
clear cell *see* clear cell sarcoma
CNS, gliosarcoma *vs* 2356
dendritic cell not otherwise specified 574
effusions 1032
embryonal *see* embryonal sarcoma
endometrium *see* endometrium
epithelioid *see* epithelioid sarcoma
fibrodysplasia ossificans progressiva *vs* 387
fibromyxoid *see* fibromyxoid sarcoma, low-grade
fibrous dysplasia of bone transformation 742
granulocytic *see* granulocytic sarcoma (chloroma)
histiocytic, malignant histiocytosis *vs* 660
Kaposi's *see* Kaposi's sarcoma
Langerhans cell 572
low-grade, myofibroma *vs* 316
mast cell 663
mediastinum, thymic carcinoma *vs* 1106t, 1107
myeloid 569, 575, 576f, 624
myofibroblastic 822
orthopedic prostheses association 144
osteogenic *see* osteogenic sarcoma
paratesticular region 1766, 1766f
pericardial (primary) 1070
pituitary 160
pleomorphic, malignant fibrous histiocytoma *vs* 335
prostate 1820
radiation-associated 159–160
renal 1692–1693, 1693f
salivary glands 1244
spleen 592
synovial *see* synovial sarcoma
undifferentiated (embryonal) *see* embryonal sarcoma
vascular prostheses association 145
sarcoma botryoides *see* botryoid sarcoma; embryonal rhabdomyosarcoma
sarcomatoid carcinoma
esophageal 1299
penis 1770
prostate 1819–1820, 1819f
see also carcinosarcoma
sarcomatous cells, gliosarcoma 2356, 2356f, 2357f
sarcoplasmic masses 2237
Sarcoptes scabiei see scabies
SARS (severe acute respiratory syndrome) 879
SARS-associated coronavirus 95, 879
satellite cells, skeletal muscle 2216
satellitosis 286, 1490, 1492f
'saucerization' of bone 747, 748f
scabies 216–217, 1891
Norwegian 216, 217f
'scaffolding', angiosarcoma of liver 1542, 1543f
scala media 2269
scala tympani 2269
scala vestibuli 2269
scale, skin 195
scale crust 195
scalp, angiosarcoma 371, 371f
scanning electron microscopy, liver biopsy 1472, 1473f
scar(s) 231, 231f
differential diagnosis 232, 324, 2274
hypertrophic 231, 264, 2274
scarring, discoid lupus erythematosus 204
Scedosporium 81
Scedosporium apiospermum 94f
Schatzki's ring 1284

Schaumann bodies 533, 892, 893f
Schiller-Duval bodies 1119, 1119f, 1918
yolk sac tumor of ovary 2029, 2030f
yolk sac tumor of testis 1751, 1778f, 1779
Schiller's stain 1924
Schirmer's test 129
Schistosoma haematobium 105, 1837
fallopian tube infection 2042
squamous cell carcinoma of bladder 1719, 1720
squamous metaplasia of bladder 1709
urothelial tumors 1710, 1711
Schistosoma japonicum 105
Schistosoma mansoni 105, 1837
schistosomiasis 105
cervix 1837
hepatic granuloma 1512, 1513f
ovary 1989
portal granulomatous disease 1514
vulvar 1891
Schmidt–Lanterman clefts 2241
Schmidt's syndrome 2176
Schmincke tumor 793
Schnabel's cavernous optic atrophy 2318
Schneiderian mucosa 787
Schneiderian papillomas 787–789
columnar cell (oncocytic/cylindrical cell) 789, 789f, 798
exophytic (fungiform/squamous) 787–788, 788f
inverted 788–789, 788f
Schönlein-Henoch purpura *see* Henoch–Schönlein purpura
schwann cells 2241
granular cell tumor origin 1184
leprosy 2244
lipid accumulation 2246, 2247f
proliferation 2241
schwannoma (neurilemoma) 379, 2249–2252
'ancient' 350, 396, 705
Antoni A and B tissues 2249–2250, 2250f, 2251, 2385, 2386, 2386f
of bone 771
breast 446
cardiac 1066
cellular 2386
CNS 2385–2386, 2386f
immunohistochemistry 2339t
ultrastructural characteristics 2337t
differential diagnosis 2251
eighth nerve (acoustic neuroma) 810, 2279, 2279f, 2385
epithelioid 2252, 2252f
genetic abnormalities 2340t
gross features 2249, 2250f
histologic features 2249–2250, 2250f, 2251f
immunohistochemistry 2251, 2251f
intestinal 1446
location/sites 2252
melanotic (melanocytic) 2252–2253, 2253f, 2386
neurofibroma *vs* 2254
nuclear pleomorphism 2251, 2251f
oral cavity 1185
orbital 2298
pituitary 2109
plexiform 2386
plexiform growth pattern 2252, 2252f
psammomatous melanotic 2252–2253, 2386
sinonasal 810
stomach 1344–1345
schwannomatosis 2252
schwannomin (merlin) 2386
sclera 2294
scleredema 229, 229f, 232
scleroderma
autoantibodies 114t
erythema nodosum *vs* 234
esophageal dysmotility 1284
myositis 2221
renal involvement 1647

scleredema *vs* 229, 232
skin features 231–232
small bowel diverticula 1404
vasculitis 1078
scleromyxedema 228–229, 229f
sclerosing adenosis
breast 431, 433f, 434f, 462
lobular carcinoma in situ 462
prostate gland 1800, 1800f
sclerosing angiomatoid nodular transformation, spleen 581
sclerosing cholangitis 1497–1498
primary *see* primary sclerosing cholangitis (PSC)
secondary 1497
sclerosing hemangioma, lung 947–949, 948f
sclerosing mucoepidermoid carcinoma with eosinophilia, thyroid 2139, 2140f
sclerosing nephrosis, post-irradiation 156
sclerosing polycystic adenosis, salivary glands 1261–1262, 1262f
sclerotic bodies 72
scrofuloderma 215
scrotal calcinosis, 'idiopathic' 1772
scrotal leiomyoma 349, 349f
scrotal sac 1768
scrotum 1772–1773
angiokeratoma 1772
basal cell carcinoma 1773
benign tumors/tumor-like conditions 1772
epidermoid cyst 1772
extramammary Paget's disease 1773
infectious/inflammatory conditions 1772
malignant tumors 1772–1773
squamous cell carcinoma 1772–1773, 1773f
sea-blue histiocytes 579, 658
sea-blue histiocyte syndrome 658
sebaceoma 250
sebaceous adenoma
salivary gland 1226–1227, 1247
of skin 250, 251f
sebaceous carcinoma 258, 260, 260f
with basaloid features, small cell 246
eyelid 2290–2291, 2291f
salivary gland 1253
vulvar 1911
sebaceous glands
benign conditions 250
ectopic 194
esophageal 1289–1290
enlargement, nevus sebaceous 250
esophageal 1282
hyperplasia 226
neoplasms, benign 250, 251f
normal histology 194
in parotid/submandibular glands 1226
sebaceous hyperplasia 250
sebaceous lymphadenocarcinoma, salivary gland 1253
sebocytes 194
sebomatricoma 250
seborrheic dermatitis 200, 200f, 226
seborrheic keratosis 242, 242f
epidermal nevi *vs* 241
variant, eyelid 2290
secondary ion mass spectrometry (SIMS) 30
secretin injection test 1573
secretory granules 2104
matrix proteins, markers 31t
segmental arterial mediolysis 1081
segmental mediolytic arteriopathy 1083
seizure disorders, brain tumors 2345
selective IgA deficiency 113–114
self-healing carcinoma (keratoacanthoma) 1164–1165
sellar region tumors 2398–2399
hemorrhagic infarction 2113
see also craniopharyngioma
sella turcica, tumor differential diagnosis by age 2348t
semenogelin 1793
semicircular canals 2269, 2269f

seminal vesicle, prostatic adenocarcinoma invasion 1818f
seminiferous tubules 1731, 1733
    histology (normal) 1732, 1732f
seminoma 1115, 1734, 1742, 1744–1747
    anaplastic 1745
    FNA cytopathology 1774–1776, 1775f
    immunohistochemistry 180, 1746
    intratubular 1744
    mediastinum, thymic carcinoma vs 1106, 1106t
    metastatic 1774–1776, 1775f
    pure (classic) 1744–1747
        differential diagnosis 1175, 1746, 1775t
        FNA cytopathology 1774–1776, 1775f
        gross/microscopic features 1745–1746, 1746f, 1747f
        immunohistochemistry/genetics 1746, 1775t
        immunostains 1745, 1747f
        spermatocytic seminoma vs 1748
    spermatocytic 1747–1748, 1748f
        anaplastic 1748
    testicular lymphoma vs 1762
    thymus see thymus
    tigroid background/pattern
        testis 1774–1775, 1775f
        thymus 1120, 1121f
senile EBV-positive B-cell lymphoproliferative disorder 572
sentinel lymph nodes
    biopsy 429
        implantation of normal/abnormal epithelium 137
        melanoma 286–287
        Merkel cell carcinoma 250
    dissection 511
        breast cancer 137
    evaluation 429, 487
septal lines 863, 865f, 885
seromucinous borderline tumors, ovary 2003–2004, 2004f
seromucous glands, larynx and trachea 834
seronegative spondyloarthropathies, aortic insufficiency 1058
serosa, uterine 1934
serotonin 1424
serous adenocarcinoma, cervix 1876
serous carcinoma
    fallopian tube 2045, 2046, 2046f
    ovary see ovary, serous carcinoma
    peritoneum 1023, 1023f, 1024f
serous psammocarcinoma, ovary 2002
serous tumors, ovary see ovary
Sertoli cell adenoma 1759
Sertoli cell nodules 1759
Sertoli cell-only syndrome 1739–1740, 1740f
Sertoli cells 1732, 2021, 2023, 2023f
    embryology 1734
    immunohistochemistry 2023
    in Sertoli cell-only syndrome 1739–1740, 1740f
    in Sertoli cell tumors 2023
    in Sertoli-Leydig cell tumor 2021, 2022f
Sertoli cell tumors
    large cell calcifying 1758, 1759–1760, 1760f
    lipid-rich 2023, 2023f
    of ovary 2023, 2023f
    oxyphilic 2023
    seminoma vs 1746
    testis 1758–1760, 1759f
        large cell calcifying 1758, 1759–1760, 1760f
        not otherwise specified (NOS) 1758–1759
        sclerosing 1759
        well-differentiated 1759f
Sertoli-Leydig cell tumor
    immunohistochemistry 2023
    intermediate type 2021, 2021f, 2022f
    mucinous epithelium of intestinal type 2022, 2022f
    of ovary 2017t, 2021–2023, 2022f
    poorly differentiated type 2021, 2022, 2022f
    retiform tubules 2021, 2022f
    testis 1760
    well-differentiated 2021, 2021f

sesame oil, self-injection 141
SETTLE (spindle epithelial tumor with thymus-like differentiation) 2140
severe acute respiratory syndrome (SARS) 95, 879
severe combined immunodeficiency (SCID) 113, 571
Sevier-Munger stain 1110
sex cord-stromal tumors
    ovary 1995, 2015–2026
        classification 2016t
        endometrial stromal sarcoma similar 1974
        granulosa cell see granulosa cell tumor
        Leydig cell tumors 2024–2025, 2024f, 2025f
        sclerosing stromal tumor 2020–2021, 2021f
        thecoma see thecoma
    testicular 1743t, 1757–1762
        fibroma-thecoma 1761
        granulosa cell tumors 1753, 1760–1761, 1760f
        Leydig cell tumor see Leydig cell tumors
        mixed 1761, 1761f
        mixed germ cell- 1761–1762
        Sertoli cell tumor see Sertoli cell tumors
sex cord tumor with annular tubules (SCTAT) 2023–2024
    nonsyndrome 2024
    ovary 2023–2024
    Peutz-Jeghers syndrome 2023–2024
sexual abuse, children 1887, 1892
Sezary cells 291, 292
Sézary cells 650
Sézary syndrome 292, 646, 650
    cutaneous T-cell lymphoma vs 291
'shadow' cells, eosinophilic 253, 253f
'shagreen patches' 264
'shared cotyledons' 2077
Sharpey's fibers 1139
Sharpey's-like fibers 742
shave biopsy, skin 193
Sheehan's syndrome 2113
Shiga toxins 1382
Shigella, colitis 1395
Shigella dysenteriae 1382
Shimada grading system, neuroblastoma 384, 384t
    adrenal medulla 2196, 2197f, 2198
shingles see herpes zoster
'shock lung' 874
short gut syndrome 1397
shoulder, extra-abdominal fibromatosis (desmoid) 323f
'shouldering', atypical ('dysplastic'/architecturally-disordered) melanocytic nevi 281, 1897
sialadenitis 1257
    chronic sclerosing 1258–1259, 1259f
    lymphoepithelial (LESA) 1251, 1257–1258, 1257f
        salivary gland lymphoma vs 1257
    myoepithelial 1257
sialadenopathy, in HIV infection 1261
sialoadenitis, chronic 24
sialoblastoma, salivary gland 1227, 1227f, 1248–1249, 1248f
sialoliths 1258
sialometaplasia, necrotizing 1179, 1179f, 1258, 1258f
    salivary mucoepidermoid carcinoma vs 1228
sialomucins 1302
sialo-odontogenic cyst 1146
sialosis 1206
sicca syndrome 129
sickle cell disease
    bone radiographs 678f
    osteomyelitis 689
    osteonecrosis 683
    retinal ischemia 2318
    spleen 580
sickle cell trait, medullary carcinoma of kidney 1687
sideroblasts 612, 619
sideromitochondria 612
sideropenia dysphasia 1169
siderophages 918f
siderosis, ocular 2312
siderotic granules 612
sigmoid colon, diverticular disease 1405
    mucosal prolapse with 1382, 1383f

sigmoiditis 1388, 1393
signet ring carcinoma
    bladder 1720
    breast 460, 468, 470, 485
    cervix 1874, 1875f
    colorectal 1438–1439
    Krukenberg tumor 2038–2039, 2039f
    prostate 1819, 1819f
    stomach see stomach, signet ring carcinoma
signet ring cell(s), in effusions 183, 1030, 1031f
silicon dioxide 903
silicone
    breast implants 142, 142f, 449–450, 451f
    lip augmentation, reaction 147
    reactions to 142, 342
silicone lymphadenopathy 142, 530, 530f
silicosis 903–904, 905t
silicotic nodule 904, 904f
silk sutures 144, 145f
silver impregnation stains 59, 60t
silver methenamine stain 1601–1602, 1602f, 1614
silver-stained nucleolar organizing regions (AgNORs)
    salivary gland tumors 1239, 1254
    uveal melanoma 2308
simian virus 40 75–76
    choroid plexus papilloma 2371
    mesothelioma and 1007, 1015
    renal transplant recipient infection 1653
singer's node 835
single cell pattern 177, 184f
single photon-emission computed tomography (SPECT), CNS 2346
Sin Nombre virus 95
sinonasal region 787–831
    acinic cell carcinoma 797
    adenoid cystic carcinoma 794–795, 795f, 796t
    angiofibroma 817–818, 817f, 818f
    angiosarcoma 818
    benign fibrous histiocytoma 823
    capillary hemangioma 817
    carcinoma see nasopharynx, carcinoma
    chondroma 796t, 816, 816f
    chondrosarcoma 796t, 816–817
    chordoma 796t, 813
    choristomas 811–812, 812f
    clear cell carcinoma 808
    desmoid tumors 822
    ectopic pituitary 812–813
    Ewing's sarcoma 796t, 806–807
    exophytic papilloma 787–788, 788f
    fibromas 822–823
    fibromyxoma and myxoma 823
    fibrosarcoma 822–823
    giant cell tumor 814–815
    granulocytic sarcoma (chloroma) 825
    hairy polyps 826
    hamartoma 826
    hemangioma 817
    hemangiopericytoma 818–819, 819f
    inflammatory myofibroblastic tumor 796t, 823–824, 824f
    intestinal type adenocarcinoma 799, 807, 807f
        classification/grading 807, 808t, 809f
    inverted papilloma 788–789, 788f
    Langerhans cell histiocytosis 826
    leiomyoma 796t, 821
    leiomyosarcoma 821, 821f
    lipoma 822
    liposarcoma 822
    low-grade intestinal-type adenocarcinoma (LGITAC) 799
    low-grade nasopharyngeal papillary adenocarcinoma (LGNPPA) 807–808
    low-grade papillary adenocarcinoma (LGPA) 800, 808
    lymphoma 824–826, 825t
    malignant fibrous histiocytoma 796t, 823
    malignant peripheral nerve sheath tumor 810
    melanomas 796t, 804–805, 806f

meningioma 811, 811f
metastatic tumors 827
mucoepidermoid carcinoma 798–799, 799f
multiple myeloma 826
myoepithelial carcinoma 796–797, 796t
myoepithelioma 796–797
myofibrosarcoma 822–823
neuroectodermal tumors 801–807
neuroendocrine carcinoma (SNEC) 795, 801,
    803–804, 804f
  immunohistochemistry 796t, 803
  prognosis 804, 804t
neurofibroma 810
oncocytic carcinoma 798, 798f
oncocytic tumors 797–798
  benign 797–798
osseous (fibro-osseous) tumors 813–817
ossifying fibroma 813, 814f
osteoma 813
papillomas see Schneiderian papillomas
paraganglioma 796t, 801
peripheral nerve sheath tumors 796t, 810
pleomorphic adenoma 795–796, 797f
polymorphous low-grade adenocarcinoma (PLGA)
    799–800
polyps 787
primitive neuroectodermal tumors 796t, 806–807
pyogenic granuloma 817
renal cell-like carcinoma 808–810, 809f, 810t
rhabdomyoma 820
rhabdomyosarcoma 796t, 820–821
Rosai–Dorfman disease 826
schwannoma 810
small cell neoplasm, after retinoblastoma 158
solitary fibrous tumor 796t, 822–823, 822f
spindle cell carcinoma (carcinosarcoma) 791, 793,
    793f, 796t
squamous cell carcinoma 789
  basaloid 790–791, 791f, 795, 796t
teratoma (teratocarcinoma) 791, 826–827
tumor immunohistochemistry 796t
undifferentiated carcinoma (SNUC) 801, 804,
    805f
  immunohistochemistry 796t, 804
  patient outcome 805t
vascular/perivascular tumors 817–826
verrucous carcinoma 791, 792f
  see also nasal cavity; sinuses (paranasal)
sino-orbital phycomycosis 2294
sinuses (paranasal)
  branchial apparatus 2270–2271
  fungal infections, opportunistic 81
  hemangioma 817
  melanoma 805
  papillary goblet cell hyperplasia 787
  papillary hyperplasia 787
  preauricular 2271
  see also sinonasal region
sinus 'fungal ball' 787
sinus histiocytosis
  lymphoma with benign erythrophagocytosis 528
  with massive lymphadenopathy see Rosai–Dorfman
    disease
  non-specific 527
  reactive 529
  signet-ring variant 527
sinusitis 787
  allergic fungal 787, 2295
  chronic 787
Sipple's syndrome (MEN type 2a) see multiple
    endocrine neoplasia type 2a
site-specific antibodies 180–182, 180t
Sjögren's syndrome
  autoantibodies 114t
  keratoconjunctivitis sicca 2298
  low-grade BALT lymphoma 977
  lung involvement 889, 889f
  lymphadenopathy 519
  lymphoepithelial sialadenitis 1257

lymphoma risk 1257
  muscle fiber changes 2222
  peripheral nerve vasculitis 2243
skeletal angiosarcoma 769, 769f
skeletal development 681
skeletal disease 681–690
  see also bone
skeletal hemangioma 765–767, 766f
skeletal muscle 2213–2238
  age-related changes 2217
  in autoimmune disorders 2221–2222
  biopsy 23f, 2213–2214
    histochemistry, enzymes and stains 2214, 2215t
    nerve biopsy with 2239
  channelopathies 2233–2234, 2233f
  in collagen vascular disorders 2221–2222
  disorders see myopathy; myositis
  disuse atrophy 2217
  dystrophy see muscular dystrophies
  embryology 2214–2215
  fibers see muscle fibers
  foreign body giant cell reaction 2224
  freezing artifacts 2214, 2214f
  gender differences 2217
  in glycogenoses 2230–2232
  granulomas 2223, 2224
  hemorrhage into 2238
  histology (normal) 2214–2217, 2216f, 2217f
  infarction 2238
  in liposes 2232–2233
  in malignant hyperthermia 2233
  metabolic disorders 2229–2235
  myofibrillary apparatus, proteins 2217, 2218t
  nerve supply 2217
  number and dimensions 2215
  sample processing/transport 2214
  in sarcoidosis 2223–2224
  structure 2215–2217, 2216f, 2217f
  trauma 2238
  tumors 354–362
    benign 354–356
      see also rhabdomyoma
    malignant 356–363
      see also rhabdomyosarcoma
  vasculitis affecting 2224, 2224f
  weakness 2227
  see also muscle; myopathy; specific disorders
skeletal system, infections 99–100
Skene's glands 1885, 1914
skin
  adnexal tumors/pseudotumors 250–263
    basal cell carcinoma of skin vs 246
    benign pilosebaceous lesions 250–255
    benign sweat gland proliferations 255–258
    malignant pilosebaceous neoplasms 258–261
    malignant sweat gland tumors 261–263
    sweat gland carcinomas 263
    of vulva 1899, 1899t
  atrophy 195
  basal cell carcinoma see basal cell carcinoma, of skin
  basal layer 194
  biopsy, types 193
  bullous disorders 216–225
  chondro-osseous lesions 267
  clinical history 193
  collagen deposition diseases 231–233
  dermal deposition disorders 228–234
  developmental cysts 244
  dimpling 265
  diseases see dermatoses
  disorders involving ear 2274–2275
  disorders involving esophagus 1290–1291
  disorders involving vulva 1893–1896
  elliptical excisions 193
  endothelial neoplasms, malignant 274–276
  epithelial lesions 241–296
    benign proliferations 241–244
    malignant tumors 244–250
    see also nevus (nevi)

fibroblastic proliferation 263–267
  fibroepithelial polyps 8, 24f, 264
  fibrohistiocytic proliferation 263–267
  granular layer 194
  granulomatous dermatoses 212–216, 213t
  hematopoietic tumors 289–296
  histiocytic proliferations 287–289
  histology (normal) 193–195
  infectious diseases 67–77
  inflammatory cells 195
  inflammatory diseases 195–209
    epidermal and dermal processes 202–206
    predominantly dermal processes 206–209
    predominantly epidermal processes 195–202
  interface dermatoses 203–206, 203t, 222
  leiomyoma 348–350
  lichenoid dermatoses 202–203
  lymphoid infiltrates, benign 295
  lymphomas
    B-cell 289–291
    T-cell 291–292
  mast cell infiltrates 295–296
  melanocytic proliferations 276–287
    see also melanoma, malignant
  mesenchymal tumors/pseudotumors see
    mesenchymal tumors/pseudotumors
  metastases in 169t
  mucinosis 228–231, 228t
  myxoid lesions, benign 267–268
  nerve supply 194–195
  neutrophilic dermatoses 212
  non-neoplastic diseases 193–239
  peripheral nerve tumors 268
  psoriasiform dermatoses 199–202
  pustular disorders 216–225
  radiation-associated tumors 158
  radiation effect 155
  sarcoidosis 214–215, 216f
  secondary syphilis 201, 201f
  specimen preparation 193
  spongiotic dermatoses 195–199
  squamous cell carcinoma see squamous cell
    carcinoma, of skin
  superficial (and deep) perivascular dermatoses
    206–209, 206t
  tumors and tumor-like conditions 241–306
    nonmelanocytic, with melanin pigment 257
  vascular tumors
    benign 268–273
    borderline 273–274
    malignant 274–276
  vasculature 194
  vasculitides and vasculopathies 209–216
skin tags 264
'skip areas' 1388, 1392
skull
  chordoma 764, 765
  osteosarcoma involving 2283
  Paget's disease of bone 2283
sleep disordered breathing 915–916
small airways disease (SAD) 870, 871f
  definition 905
  etiologic classification 906–909, 906f
  fibrosis associated 910–911, 911f
  morphologic classification 909–911, 909t
  radiologic classification 909
small blue cells see small round blue cell(s)
small cell carcinoma
  bladder 1721, 1721f
  cervix 1875–1876
  effusions 183, 184f
  endometrial 1965f
  of hypercalcemic type (of ovary) 2014–2015,
    2015f
  immunohistochemistry 33, 35f
  kidney 1689–1690
  larynx 843, 844
  lung see small cell lung carcinoma (SCLC)
  metastatic

small cell carcinoma (*cont'd*)
    to CNS 2399
      medulloblastoma *vs* 2383
      testis 1756
    ovary *see* ovary, small cell carcinoma
    pancreas 1575, 1575f
    prostate 1819
    undifferentiated, esophageal 1314
    vagina 1924
    see also specific types/anatomic sites
small cell lung carcinoma (SCLC) 988–994, 991f
    cell trauma due to biopsy 135
    classification 989
    clinical features 936
    combined, types 990, 991f
    cytokeratin staining 33, 35f
    cytology 993–994, 993f
    differential diagnosis 992, 993–994, 994t
      adenoid cystic carcinoma of lung *vs* 952
      anaplastic, small cell squamous *vs* 942
      non-small-cell *vs* 939
      pulmonary carcinoid tumors *vs* 986
    etiology 989
    histology 989, 989f
    immunocytochemistry 991–992, 1575
    Lambert-Eaton syndrome and 2227
    metastases
      in bone marrow 664
      in ovary 2039
      pancreatic small cell carcinoma *vs* 1575
    molecular pathogenesis 937, 992
    pleural effusions 1030, 1031f
    prognosis 992
    types included 989
small intestine
    adenocarcinoma 1430–1431, 1431t
    adenoma 1421–1422, 1422f
    angiosarcoma 159, 1449
    carcinoid tumor 1423, 1427f, 1428f
    diverticula 1404
    dysplasia, grading 1422
    endocrine differentiation 1423
    endocrine tumors 1422–1430
      combined adenocarcinoma 1429–1430
      duodenum 193f, 1424, 1426f
      foregut/midgut and hindgut 1424
      metastases 1427–1428
      pathologic features 193f, 1426f, 1427
    epithelial tumors 1420–1431, 1420t
      benign 1420–1422
      malignant 1430–1431, 1431t
    fibromatosis 1450, 1451f
    ganglioneuroma 1446–1447
    hamartomatous polyps 1421, 1421f
    histology (normal) 1373
    Kaposi's sarcoma 1449, 1450f
    leiomyoma 1445, 1445f
    leiomyomatosis 1445
    leiomyosarcoma 1445
    lymphangioma 1449, 1449f
    lymphoproliferative tumors 1450–1453
    malabsorptive disorders 1373–1378
    mucosa, CDX2 staining 33, 34f
    multiple lymphomatous polyposis 1451, 1452,
      1452f
    neuroendocrine tumors 1423–1429
    neurofibroma 1446
    neurofibromatosis type 1 1446
    perforation, cytotoxic chemotherapy association 147
    schwannoma 1446
    in systemic mastocytosis 1380
    tumor-like conditions of blood vessels 1448–1450
    tumors 1419–1464
      distribution 1419
      histologic classification 1420t
      neural origin 1446–1448
    vascular tumors 1448–1450
    vasculitis 1384–1386, 1384t
    see also duodenum

smallpox virus 68t
small round blue cell(s)
    salivary basal cell adenoma 1221, 1222f, 1223f
    sinonasal teratoma 791
small round blue cell tumors 2378
    adenoid cystic carcinoma *see* adenoid cystic carcinoma
    children
      metastases in lymph nodes 511
      tumors associated 174
    Ewing's sarcoma as 385–386
    metastases, tumors associated 174
    renal, differential diagnosis 1693
    rhabdomyosarcoma *vs* 361t
small round cell(s), bone tumors 749f
small round cell tumors
    of bone 747t
      see also Ewing's sarcoma; primitive
        neuroectodermal tumors (PNET)
    desmoplastic 386–387, 386f
      chromosomal translocation 310t
      of ovary 2026, 2039
      paratesticular region 1766
      peritoneal 1024, 1025f
      pleural 1017
smear preparation technique 24, 25t, 26f
    air-dried *vs* wet-fixed 27, 28t
SMN1 gene 2226
smokeless tobacco
    carcinogens 1168
    leukoplakia 1165
    oral squamous cell carcinoma 1168
    oral verrucous carcinoma 1174
smoking
    Crohn's disease risk 1386
    laryngeal carcinoma risk 842
    lung cancer etiology 935, 989
    mouth ulcer suppression 1386
    oral squamous cell carcinoma 1168
    oral verrucous carcinoma 1174
    passive, lung cancer etiology 935
    pulmonary Langerhans cell histiocytosis with 923
    renal cell carcinoma 1676–1677
    stomatitis nicotina 1166
    ulcerative colitis risk reduced 1386
    vulvar squamous cell carcinoma 1909
smooth muscle
    airways 861
    lesions, solitary myofibroma *vs* 316
    usual interstitial pneumonia (UIP) 895, 896f
smooth muscle actin (SMA)
    chondromyxoid fibroma 714
    leiomyoma 348
    liver biopsy 1470
    mesothelioma 1013
    reactivity, collagenous fibroma 309
smooth muscle tumors 347–353, 702t
    in AIDS 121t
    benign 348–350
      see also leiomyoma
    bone involvement 771
    immunosuppression-associated 353
    intestinal 1445
    of lymph nodes 514–515
    malignant 350–353
      see also leiomyosarcoma
    uterus 1968–1973
    vulva 1916
'smudge cells' 102, 877f, 878
'soap bubble' lesion/appearance
    adamantinoma 745, 746f
    central giant cell tumor of oral cavity 1182–1183,
      1182f
    cherubism 1193
    giant cell reparative granuloma 752
    metastatic renal cell carcinoma 1570f
    papillary thyroid carcinoma variant 2130, 2131f
    simple (unicameral) bone cyst 756f
Société Internationale d'Oncologie Pédiatrique (SIOP)
    358

sodium urate crystals 691
soft part sarcoma, alveolar *see* alveolar soft part sarcoma
soft tissue
    aneurysmal cyst 391, 392f
    arteriovenous malformations 363
    deep
      angiosarcoma 371
      leiomyoma 350
      leiomyosarcoma 352
    infectious diseases 67–77
    Rosai–Dorfman disease 335f
soft tissue tumors 307–417
    adipose tissue tumors 336–348
    cartilage and bone in soft tissue 387–391
    chromosomal translocations 310t
    classification 308, 310t
    differentiation scores 308t
    fibrohistiocytic tumors 333–336
    fibrous tissue *see* fibrous tissue tumors/fibrous tumors
    grading and staging 307–308, 307t, 308t
    heart 1066
    matrix-containing 391
    miscellaneous 392–405
    neural 378–387
    orbit 2297
    perivascular 373
    radiation-associated 160
    skeletal muscle tumors 354–362
    smooth muscle tumors 347–353
    solitary fibrous tumor 376–378, 377f
    synovium-related 374–376
    TNM staging 309t
    vagina *see* vagina
    vascular tumors 362–373
    vulva 1915–1918
    see also specific tumors and tumor types
solar (actinic) keratosis *see* actinic (solar) keratosis
solitary cecal ulcer 1402
solitary fibrous tumor 376–378, 377f
    differential diagnosis 377–378, 378t
    immunohistochemistry 796t
    pleural 1015–1016, 1015f, 1016f
    sinonasal 796t, 822–823, 822f
    thyroid 2140
    vulva 1900
solitary rectal ulcer syndrome 1382
somatostatin analogue 1351, 2100–2101
somatostatin (D) cells 1323
somatostatinoma 1574
    duodenal 1424, 1426f
somatostatinoma syndrome 1574
somatotrophs 2095, 2096f
    adenoma *see* pituitary adenoma
    development 2094–2095
    hyperplasia 2110
sound and hearing 2269f, 2270
Southern blotting 45, 45t
    Hodgkin's disease 539
    lymph node specimens 510
    MALT lymphoma 1353
SOX9 expression, mesenchymal chondrosarcoma 720
Sox9 gene 1734
space of Disse 1474
space of Mall 1474
special techniques *see* cytopathological and surgical
      pathology techniques
specimens
    staining *see* staining methods
    technical problems 20–22
spermatic cord 1731
    tumors/tumor-like conditions 1763–1766
spermatocytes 1732
    maturation arrest 1739, 1740f
spermatocytic seminoma 1747–1748, 1748f
spermatocytoma 1743–1744
spermatogenesis 1732, 1734, 1735, 1739, 1739f
    abnormalities 1738
    FNA biopsy 1741
    maturation arrest 1739, 1740f

spermatogonia 1732, 1732f, 1734
spermiogenesis 1732
S-phase fraction (SPF), flow cytometry 36, 37, 40–441, 415
sphenoid sinus, angiofibroma 817–818, 817f, 818f
spherocytosis, hereditary 580
spheroid body myopathy 2229
spherulosis, collagenous, of breast 448, 448f
'spider cells' 355, 355f, 1065
spinal cord
    ependymoma 2364
    glioblastoma 2352
    paraganglioma 2377
    pilocytic astrocytoma 2357
    tumors, clinical features 2345
spinal muscular atrophies 2226–2227
    type I 2226–2227, 2226f, 2227f
    type II (intermediate) 2226
    type III 2226
spinal tumors
    differential diagnosis by age 2348t
    schwannoma 2385
spindle cell(s)
    gastrointestinal stromal tumors 1345, 1347, 1347f
    interlacing fascicles, solitary circumscribed neuroma 268
    raining-like descent 278, 280f
    uveal malignant melanoma 2306–2307, 2307f
spindle cell carcinoma 1819
    bladder 147
    conjunctiva 2292
    iatrogenic reactions resembling 147
    immunohistochemistry 796t
    larynx 846, 846f, 847f
    lung 966, 966t, 971, 972f
    metastases differential diagnosis 176
    pleomorphic, dedifferentiated chondrosarcoma with 719, 719f
    prostate gland 147
    renal 1685–1686, 1686f
    sinonasal region 791, 793, 793f, 796t
    see also sarcomatoid carcinoma
spindle cell hemangioendothelioma see hemangioendothelioma
spindle cell hemangioma see hemangioma
spindle cell lipoma 338, 338f, 339f
spindle cell nevus see Spitz nevus
spindle cell nodule, postoperative 1841
spindle cell pseudotumors
    Mycobacterium avium complex 64, 65f, 2406
    reactive mediastinal 515
spindle cell rhabdomyosarcoma 356, 358–359
spindle cell sarcoma 176
    lung 971–972
    malignant peripheral nerve sheath tumor similar 2257
spindle cell squamous cell carcinoma
    oral cavity 1176–1177, 1177f
    vulva 1912
spindle cell tumor, hemorrhagic, with amianthoid fibers 515
spine, hemangioma 701
SPINK1 gene 1552
spiradenoma
    eccrine 256, 256f
    giant vascular 256, 256f
    malignant 263
spiral arterioles, menstrual cycle 1938, 1938f, 1939f
spirochetes, staining 62t
spirochetosis, intestinal 1398
spironolactone bodies 2184f, 2185
Spitz nevus 278–279, 279f, 280f
    'malignant' 279
    melanoma vs 279, 280f
    probable/atypical 279
    sclerotic 279
spleen 576–592
    abscesses 577
    accessory 577

angiosarcoma 591, 591f
autotransplantation 577
benign tumors/proliferations 581–584
    vascular/lymphatic 581–582
biopsy 576
cysts 580, 580t
    primary (true) 580, 581f
enlargement see splenomegaly
epithelioid hemangioendothelioma 591
fine needle aspiration 576
granulomas 578–579
hamartoma 582–583
hemangioma 581, 582–583, 591
hemophagocytosis 578
histology (normal) 576–577, 577f
Hodgkin's disease 579, 588, 589f
idiopathic thrombocytopenic purpura (ITP) 580
infections 577–579
infectious mononucleosis 578, 578f
inflammatory pseudotumor 583, 583f
Kaposi's sarcoma 592
leukemia 584–586, 586t
littoral cell angioma 582, 582f
localized reactive lymphoid hyperplasia 583
lymphangioma 581–582
lymphocyte zone 577
lymphomas
    primary 588–591
    secondary 586–588, 586t
malignant tumors 584–592, 586t
marginal zone 552, 577
    reactive hyperplasia 589
metabolic diseases 579–580
metastases in 171t, 173, 175f
metastatic tumors of 592
mucinous cysts 580
nodular disease, hematopoietic malignant tumors 586t
peliosis 581, 581f
reactive follicular hyperplasia 583
reactive histiocyte proliferation 579
in red blood cell disorders 580
red pulp 577
    erythrophagocytosis 578, 578f
    fibrosis of cords 585
    hematopoietic malignant tumors 586t
    hepatosplenic γδ T-cell lymphoma 590–591, 590f
    histiocyte accumulation 579
    leukemia 584
    lymphomas 588, 589f
    marginal zone lymphoma 589, 590f
    plasmacytosis 585
rupture 577, 578, 592
sarcomas 592
sclerosing angiomatoid nodular transformation 581
sickle cell disease 580
size/weight 581, 584
specimens and processing 576
stellate fibrosis 584
systemic mastocytosis 584, 584f
trauma 577, 580
vascular tumors 591–592
white pulp 577, 577f, 583
    atrophy 578
    hematopoietic malignant tumors 586t
    Hodgkin's disease 588, 589f
    in leukemia 585
    lymphoma 586, 587, 588
'spleen in spleen' 582–583
Splendore-Hoeppli phenomenon 69, 71
splenectomy 576, 587
splenic artery, aneurysms 1070, 1083
splenic capsule, systemic mastocytosis 584
splenic cords (of Billroth) 577, 580
splenic-gonadal fusion 579
    testicular 1735, 1735f
splenoma (splenic hamartoma) 582–583
splenomegaly 576, 580
    acute leukemia 584
    hairy cell leukemia 644, 645

infectious diseases 577
infectious mononucleosis 578
    silicone causing 142
    splenic marginal zone lymphoma 589, 590f
    tropical 1518
    Waldenström's macroglobulinemia 587
splenosis 577
    peritoneum 1022
spongiform pustule of Kogoj 199, 199f
spongiosa
    endometrium 1933, 1934f
    primary/secondary of bone 681, 681f
spongiosis 195, 197f
    eosinophilic 198, 198f
    follicular 200f
    lichen simplex chronicus 201
    plasma cell vulvitis 1895f
    scabies 217
    spongiotic dermatoses 195–199, 196t
spongiotic dermatoses 195–199, 196t
Sporothrix schenckii 67t, 71–72
sprue
    collagenous 1376
    refractory sprue 1376
    tropical 1377
sputum
    cytology, lung carcinoma 939
    examination 866
    technical problems with samples 20
squamoid nests, pancreatoblastoma 1561, 1561f
squamous cell carcinoma
    acantholytic, vulvar 1911
    AIDS 121t
    basaloid see basaloid squamous cell carcinoma
    bladder 1719–1720, 1720f
    cervix see cervix
    endometrial 1964
    esophageal see under esophagus
    of external auditory canal 2280
    eyelid 2291
    flow cytometry 38
    in situ see Bowen's disease
    larynx see larynx
    lips 1172–1173, 1177
    lung see lung
    in metastasis of unknown primary origin 168
    middle ear 2280
    nasal septum/vestibule 789–790, 790f
    oral cavity see oral cavity
    ovary 2014
    pagetoid 263f
    penile see under penis
    salivary gland 1246, 1255
    scrotal 1772–1773, 1773f
    vagina 1924
    vulva see under vulva
    see also specific types and sites
squamous cell carcinoma, of skin 246–248
    adenoid (acantholytic/pseudoglandular) 247–248, 248f
    Darier's disease vs 220
    differential diagnosis 248
        atypical fibroxanthoma vs 267
        basal cell carcinoma vs 246
        epithelioid sarcoma vs 400
        lichen planus-like keratosis vs 243
    dystrophic epidermolysis bullosa with 225
    histologic subtypes 247–248
    in situ 246, 246t
        metaplastic variant 246
        pagetoid variants 246–247, 246f, 263, 263f
        variants 246–247
    invasive 247, 247f
    of pinna/ear 2280
    poorly differentiated 248
    post-irradiation 158
    pseudovascular 248
    spindle cell 247, 247f, 267
    'well-differentiated' 248

squamous cell dysplasia, esophageal *see* esophagus
squamous cell hyperplasia, vulvar 1892–1893, 1904
squamous hyperplasia, penis 1771
squamous intraepithelial lesion (SIL), of penis 1770–1771
squamous metaplasia
    amnion 2067
    bladder 1709
    endometrium 1942
    gallbladder 1578
    ionizing radiation effect 154
    oral cavity 1166, 1179f
    umbilical cord 2065
squamous papilloma
    bladder 1723
    cervix 1838
    esophagus 1292, 1292f
    larynx and trachea 836–838
    lung 940, 941f
    oral cavity 1163–1164
    vagina 1921–1922
SRY gene 1734, 1738
SSX1 and *SSX2* genes 403–404
ST1571 (Gleevec) 610, 634
'staghorn' appearance, fibroadenoma 437, 438f
'staghorn' vessels, sinonasal hemangiopericytoma 819, 820f
staining methods 16t–17t, 17–19
    background, in immunohistochemistry 33
    for FNA biopsy 25–29
    indications 6
    nuclei and cells for flow cytometry 37–39
stains
    bone marrow biopsy 610
    CNS 2331, 2335t
    kidney 1601–1602
    liver biopsy 1468–1470, 1469f, 1470f
stannosis 905t
stapes 2268–2269
    degenerative joint disease 2282
staphylococcal scalded skin syndrome 203, 218, 218f
Staphylococcus
    acute suppurative gastritis 1329
    myositis 2222
Staphylococcus aureus
    abscess formation 69, 69f
    botryomycosis 70
    cellulitis 68–69, 68f
    focal proliferative/necrotizing glomerulonephritis 1621
    hematogenous osteomyelitis 689
    impetigo 217
    infections in immunodeficiency 113, 114, 115, 116
    staphylococcal scalded skin syndrome 218
staphyloma 2294, 2303
starch, tissue reactions to 139
starch granuloma 139
'starry-sky' pattern 650
    Burkitt's lymphoma 569, 570f
    lymphoma involving ovary 2026
    reactive follicular hyperplasia 517
    thymoma 1097
stasis dermatitis 197, 233
status thymicolymphaticus 1094
steatocystoma 251
steatocystoma multiplex 251
steatocystoma uniplex 251
steatohepatitis 1489–1492
    alcoholic 1490–1492, 1491f
    early pericellular fibrosis 1492f
    nonalcoholic 1490–1492, 1491f
steatosis 1468, 1489–1492
    alcoholic liver disease 1489–1490
    in chronic hepatitis C 1486
    macrovesicular 1488f, 1489
    microvesicular 1489, 1489f
    in Wilson's disease 1505, 1505f
Steiner (silver) stain, secondary syphilis 201, 201f
Steinert's disease (myotonic dystrophy) 2237

Stein-Leventhal syndrome 1991, 1992f
    atypical endometrial hyperplasia *vs* carcinoma 1956
    endometrial carcinoma risk 1953
    endometrioid adenocarcinoma treatment 1968
stellate cells
    liver 1474, 1474f
    teeth 1139
stellate microabscesses 532, 534
'stellate reticulum' 1139, 2398
Sternberg's sarcoma 1122
steroid cell tumors
    broad ligament 2047
    ovary 2025–2026, 2026f
steroid injection, iatrogenic reaction 141
steroidogenic factor-1 (SF-1) 1734, 2097, 2106
steroids, myopathy 2235
Stevens-Johnson syndrome (SJS) 203, 2303
Stewart–Bluefarb syndrome 370
Stewart–Treves syndrome 147, 275–276, 371
St Gallen Conference on Adjuvant Therapy of Primary Breast Cancer 489
STI-571, gastrointestinal stromal tumor treatment 1348
stomach 1321–1372
    adenocarcinoma *see* gastric adenocarcinoma
    adenoma *see* gastric adenoma
    anatomic malformations 1325–1326
    anatomy and histology 1321–1323
    antrum 1321, 1322f
        adenoma 1343–1344
        neuroendocrine carcinoma 803–804, 804f
    carcinoids *see* gastric carcinoid tumors
    carcinoma *see* gastric carcinoma
    cardia 1321
        adenocarcinoma 1357, 1357f, 1361
    Crohn's disease 1336, 1337f
    cytology 1324–1325, 1359f
    diverticula 1325
    duplication 1325–1326, 1325f, 1326f
    dysplasia 1355, 1358
    endoscopic surgical biopsy 1324
    fundus 1321
    histology (normal) 1321–1323, 1322f, 1323f
    inflammation *see* gastritis
    inflammatory conditions (various) 1341–1342
    leather bottle appearance 1359
    leiomyoma 1345
    leiomyosarcoma 1345
    lesions, management 1324
    lymphoma *see* lymphoma; MALT lymphoma
    mesenchymal tumors 1344–1348
    metaplasia, staining 21f
    metastases from breast carcinoma 469
    metastatic tumors 1362
    mucosa *see* gastric mucosa
    mucosal prolapse-associated conditions 1339
    muscle 1321
    muscularis propria 1321
    neuroendocrine tumors 1348–1351
    polyps *see* gastric polyps
    resection 1323–1324
    rhabdoid carcinoma 1362
    schwannoma 1344–1345
    signet ring carcinoma 1358–1359, 1358f
        cytology 1359f
        xanthelasma *vs* 1342, 1342f
    stromal tumors *see* gastrointestinal stromal tumors (GISTs)
    tumors 1344–1362
        rare 1361–1362
    ulcers *see* gastric ulcers
stomatitis
    gangrenous (noma) 78–79
    nicotine 1166
stomatitis nicotina 1166
stool, impaction 1388
storage diseases, bone marrow in 658
storiform (pinwheel-like) growth pattern 266, 266f
'stork bite' 268
'strap' cells 354, 356

stratum basalis (basal layer) 194
stratum corneum 194
stratum cylindricum 1831, 1832
stratum granulosum (granular layer) 194
stratum intermedium 1139
stratum spinosum 194
'strawberry nevus' 269–270, 269f
'streaming' effect 1287
streptavidin-based methods 31
streptococci, group A beta-hemolytic 68, 78
Streptococcus
    acute appendicitis 1408
    acute suppurative gastritis 1329
Streptococcus pneumoniae, otitis media 2272
Streptococcus pyogenes, cellulitis 68–69, 68f
stress, adrenal gland changes 2169, 2173
stress ulcers 1327
'string of beads' 1080
stromal hyperplasia, ovarian 1991–1992
stromal luteoma, ovary 2025, 2025f
stromosis 2035
Strongyloides stercoralis 104, 104f, 1336
    hyperinfection 104f
struma lymphomatosa *see* autoimmune thyroiditis (Hashimoto's)
struma ovarii 2034–2035, 2034f
    thyroid carcinoma 2034–2035, 2034f
Sturge-Weber syndrome 2416
    angiomatosis 365, 365f
    choroidal hemangioma 2309
    facial port-wine stain 268
    renal hemangioma 1692
styes (hordeolums) 2289
subareolar abscess, Paget's disease of nipple *vs* 457
subcorneal blisters 216–218, 216t
subcorneal pustular dermatosis of Sneddon-Wilkinson 199, 216, 216f
subcutaneous fat necrosis of newborn 235–236, 235fg
subcutaneous panniculitis-like T-cell lymphoma (SPTL) 293–294, 294f
subcutaneous tissue, leiomyoma 348–350
subcutis, normal histology 195
subdural hemorrhage 2416
subendothelial immune complexes *see* immune complex deposition
subendothelial spaces, membranoproliferative glomerulonephritis 1616
subendothelial zones, expansion 1650
    chronic rejection of transplants 1651, 1651f
    thrombotic microangiopathy 1648f
subependymal giant cell astrocytoma (SEGA) 2338t, 2359–2360, 2360f
subependymoma 2369, 2369f
    immunohistochemistry 2338t
    ultrastructural characteristics 2336t
subepidermal bullous disorders 221–225
submandibular glands 1186
    chronic sclerosing sialadenitis 1259, 1259f
    cysts 1260
    mixed tumors (pleomorphic adenoma) 1210
    sebaceous glands in 1226
    see also salivary glands
subperiosteal chondroma 711–712
subpleural lines 902
subungual exostosis 773–774, 773f, 774f
succinate dehydrogenase, skeletal muscle evaluation 2215t
succinate dehydrogenase subunit B (SDHB) 2192
succinate dehydrogenase subunit D (SDHD) 2192
Sucquet-Hoyer complexes 272
Sudan black B stain 610, 620, 2335t
    skeletal muscle evaluation 2215t
Sudeck's atrophy 687
'sugar tumor' 1691
sulfomucins 1302
sulfonylurea receptor-1 (SUR-1), mutations 1570
sulfur granules 69, 70, 70f, 78, 143, 1512f, 1837, 2042

sunburst appearance
  Ewing's sarcoma 748f
  hemangioma of bone 766
sun damage/exposure
  basal cell carcinoma 244
  keratoacanthoma 248
  melanoma 283
  Merkel cell carcinoma 249
  solar (actinic) keratosis 243, 243f
  squamous cell carcinoma of skin 246
superior vena cava syndrome 989, 1109, 1123
suprabasal vesicle 1837
supraclavicular node, sampling complication 28
suprarenal apoplexy 2177
supratentorial PNET 2378, 2379, 2384
sural nerve, biopsy 2238–2240, 2240f
surfactant, lung 861
surgical diseases
  kidney 1661–1705
  liver 1527–1547
surgical pathology/pathologists 3–14
  approach to specimens 3
  autopsy pathology vs 3
  as clinical consultant 4
  communication with clinician 4, 1467, 1832–1833
  consensus diagnosis 4
  consultative role 3–4
  diagnosis and specificity 7
  diagnostic competency, evaluation 10
  false-positive diagnoses 5
  in infectious disease team 58
  interpathologist consultation 4–5
    external consultation 5
    internal consultation 4–5
    selection of consultant 4
  intraoperative consultation 5–6
  malpractice 10–13
    number of claims 11
  new adjuncts 7
  'one consultant per case' rule 4, 5
  quality issues 9–10
  recording of gross specimens 7
  reports/reporting 6–7
    computerized checklists 7
    consistency 6
    of consultant pathologist 5
    diagnostic, structure 10
    guidelines 3–4
    microscopic description debate 7
    preparation method 6
    standardization 7
    synoptic format 10
  request form and clinical information 4
  responsibilities after diagnosis 4
  role 3
  training see training
  workload of pathologists 3
surgical pathology techniques see cytopathological and
    surgical pathology techniques
surgical procedures, untoward results 146–147
  implantation of normal tissue 146
Surgifoam® 140
sustentacular cells, in jugulotympanic paraganglioma
    2277
suture granulomas 145
suture materials 144
  iatrogenic lesions due to 144–145
sweat duct
  carcinoma, sclerosing 261
  proliferation, syringoma-like 256
sweat glands
  anogenital see anogenital sweat glands
  carcinoma 262, 263
  proliferations
    benign 255–258
    malignant tumors 261–263
Sweet's syndrome 212, 212f
swimmer's ear 2272
swimmer's itch 105

'Swiss cheese' appearance, adenoid cystic carcinoma
    2299f
Swiss cheese disease 443–444
Swyer's syndrome 1738
sympathetic nervous system, embryonal tumors see
    neuroblastic tumors
sympathetic uveitis (ophthalmia) 2311–2312
synaptic cleft 2217
synaptic plasma membrane-associated proteins,
    markers 31t
synaptic vesicle proteins, markers 31t
synaptic vesicles 2217
synaptophysin 181, 1322
  adrenocortical carcinoma 2188, 2188f
  CNS lesions 2336
  medulloblastoma 2382–2383
  Merkel cell carcinoma 250
  neuroblastoma 384
  pancreatic endocrine neoplasms 1571
  thymic neuroendocrine tumors 1112
syncytial endometritis 2084
syncytial knots 2071
syncytioma 2084
syncytiotrophoblast 2063
  choriocarcinoma 1120
  increased knots 2071
syncytiotrophoblast cells
  seminoma with 1746, 1747f, 1754
  thymic seminoma 1116, 1120f
syncytiotrophoblast giant cells
  choriocarcinoma 2031
  dysgerminoma 2028, 2028f
  embryonal carcinoma of ovary 2030
  metastatic choriocarcinoma of testis 1779, 1779f
synechias
  anterior 2315, 2316f
  posterior 2313–2314
synovial chondromatosis 696–697, 696f
synovial fluid, examination/cytopathology 691, 691t
synovial hyperplasia, reactive, pigmented villondular
    tenosynovitis vs 376
synovial membrane (synovium) 690
  osteoarthritis 692f
  rheumatoid arthritis 693, 693f
  tumors 374–376
synovial sarcoma 400–404, 401f, 403f
  biphasic 400–401, 401f, 404
    lung 972
    malignant peripheral nerve sheath tumor vs
      2258
  calcification 402
  chromosomal translocation 310t
  clear cell sarcoma vs 382–383
  hemangiopericytoma vs 373
  hypopharynx 850
  monophasic (spindle cell) 401, 402f
    differential diagnosis 404
    lung 972, 973f
    mediastinum, vs thymic carcinoma 1107
  pleural 1017–1018
  poorly differentiated (PDSS) 402, 402f, 404
  solitary fibrous tumor vs 378t
synovioma, benign 695
synovitis 694–695
  crystal 691
  pigmented villonodular 695–696, 696f
synovium-related tumors 374–376
syntrophin 2218t
α-synuclein 2336, 2338
syphilis 70
  aortitis 1079, 1082
  cervicitis 1836t, 1837
  chronic villitis due to 2069, 2070f
  CNS involvement 2407
  congenital 71f, 2069, 2070f
  cutaneous involvement 201, 201f
  diagnostic methods 1890
  ear involvement 2273
  gastric 1336

  intestinal involvement 1398
  lymphadenitis 520
  primary 1890
  secondary 70f, 201, 201f, 1890
  tertiary, vulvar involvement 1890
  vulvar involvement 1889–1890
syringocystadenoma papilliferum (SCP) 258, 260f
syringofibroadenoma 257, 258f
syringoma 256, 257f
  chondroid see chondroid syringoma
  desmoplastic trichoepithelioma vs 252
  eruptive 256
  poroma vs 257, 258f
syringometaplasia 256
systemic lupus erythematosus (SLE) 204
  autoantibodies 114t
  drug-induced 114t
  intestinal 1385
  lung involvement 882–883, 889
  lymphadenopathy 532
  myositis 2222
  nephritis see lupus nephritis
  peripheral nerve vasculitis 2243
systemic sclerosis
  progressive, lung involvement 888
  see also scleroderma
SYT gene, synovial sarcoma 403
SYT–SSX chimeric RNA, synovial sarcoma 403

T
tachyzoites 103
tacrolimus, nephrotoxicity 128, 131
'tactoids' 1635, 1636f, 1645, 1647, 1648f
'tadpole' cell changes, radiation causing 152, 152f
Taenia solium 104, 2223, 2411
TAG-72 (B72.3) 179
Takayasu's disease 1072t, 1073–1074, 1082
  healing phase 1074, 1074f
talc
  embolization, lung 917
  tissue reactions to 139
talc crystals
  in portal macrophages 1484
  scanning electron microscopy 1472, 1473f
talc granulomas 139
talcosis 905t
Tamm-Horsfall protein 1630, 1639
tamoxifen
  endometrial adenosarcoma 1976
  endometrial cancer risk 150, 1953
  endometrial carcinosarcoma 1977
  endometrial changes 1947
  endometrial polyps risk 1946
  fibromatosis therapy 320
tampon ulcer 1919
Tangier's disease 579
tanycytic ependymoma see ependymoma
tapeworm infections 104–105
target fibers 2225, 2226f
targetoid fibers 2225
'targetoid' lesions 203
targetoid pattern 1190
tartrate resistant acid phosphatase (TRAP) 586
Tarui's disease 2232
tattoo, traumatic 216f
tau protein, phosphorylated 2221
Tay-Sach's disease 579, 2318
T-cell receptor (TCR)
  beta-, gene rearrangements 544, 544t, 562, 564, 569
  gamma-, gene rearrangements 591
T cells
  abnormal, epidermodysplasia verruciformis 242
  activation 120, 122
  in colon 1373
  cytokines 122
  γδ, hepatosplenic lymphoma 567, 590–591, 590f
  helper (CD4)
    cytokines 122
    defective 114

T cells (cont'd)
HIV infection 116, 117
mycosis fungoides 566
intraepithelial 1373
Kikuchi histiocytic necrotizing lymphadenitis 531, 531f, 532
lymphoma see lymphoma (non-Hodgkin's), T-cell
markers and antigen detection 568t, 611t
maturation stages 568t
in paracortex of lymph node 524
reduced numbers 113, 115
spleen 577
see also CD8 lymphocytes
teardrop cells 624
technetium-99m-labeled diphosphonate, bone tumors 704
techniques in cytopathology see cytopathological and surgical pathology techniques
teeth
development 1139
examination 1137
Teflon® paste, iatrogenic reactions 142–143
telangiectasia macularis eruptiva perstans (TMEP) 295, 296
telomerase, activation, lung cancer 937
telomerase assay, oral squamous cell carcinoma 1171
temporal arteritis see giant cell arteritis
temporal artery, age-related changes 1073
temporal artery biopsy 1073
temporal bone
chondrosarcoma 2284
eosinophilic granuloma 2284
fibrous dysplasia 2282
fungal infections 2273
Langerhans cell histiocytosis 2284
meningioma involving 2279–2280
metastases to 2281
osteosarcoma involving 2283
in Paget's disease of bone 2283
temporal lobe epilepsy 2405
temporomandibular joint
implants, Proplast® 143
pigmented villondular synovitis 1195, 1195f
tenascin deposits 1401
tendon sheath
fibroma 309–310, 310f, 327
giant cell tumor see giant cell tumor, of tendon sheath
Tenney-Parker change 2072, 2072f
tenosynovial giant cell tumor see giant cell tumor, of tendon sheath
tenosynovitis 695–696
pigmented villondular 375–376, 376f
tensor tympani 2269
teratocarcinoma
sinonasal 791
testis 1756
teratoid nephroblastoma 1672
teratoid/rhabdoid tumor, atypical see atypical teratoid/rhabdoid tumor (AT/RT)
teratoma
benign cystic
of ovary 2031–2032, 2032f, 2035
secondary malignancy in ovary 2032
fallopian tube 2045
immature (malignant) 1115
CNS, medulloepithelioma vs 2379
grading and prognosis 2033, 2034t
immunohistochemistry 2034
mediastinum 1115–1116, 1116f
metastases 2033
ovary 2032–2034, 2033f
testis 1756, 1780–1781, 1780f
mature (benign) 1115
mediastinum 1115, 1115f, 1116f
ovary 2031–2032, 2032f
testis 1754–1755, 1755f, 1780–1781, 1780f
tissues present 2031, 2032f

monodermal, of ovary 2031, 2034–2036
carcinoid tumors 2035, 2035f
neuroectodermal 2035–2036, 2036f
struma ovarii 2034–2035, 2034f
monodermal, of testis 1756
of ovary 2031–2036
renal 1672
retinoblastic 750–751, 751f
sinonasal 791
sinonasal region 826–827
testis 1754–1756, 1755f
differential diagnosis 1781
embryonal carcinoma with 1756
FNA cytopathology 1780–1781, 1780f
immature (malignant) 1756, 1780–1781, 1780f
mature (benign) 1754–1755, 1755f, 1780–1781, 1780f
pre-/postpubertal comparison 1754, 1754t
secondary malignant components 1754–1755
umbilical cord 2067
teratomatous glands, yolk sac tumor vs 1753
terminal bronchioles 861
terminal deoxynucleotidyl transferase (TdT) 557, 568, 569, 570
terminal ileal biopsy, inflammatory bowel disease 1389
testicular feminization 1794
incomplete forms 1737
testicular regression syndrome 1737
testicular tumors 1737, 1741–1763
carcinoid tumor 1756
carcinoma in situ 1741, 1743–1744
choriocarcinoma 1753–1754, 1754f
FNA cytopathology 1779–1780, 1779f
metastatic 1779–1780, 1779f
in congenital adrenal hyperplasia 2175
embryonal carcinoma 1748–1750, 1749f
anaplastic spermatocytic seminoma vs 1748
classic seminoma vs 1746
FNA cytopathology 1776–1777
metastatic, FNA cytopathology 1776–1777, 1777f
teratoma with 1756
germ cell tumors 1741–1743
choriocarcinoma see above
classification 1743t
contralateral testis 1742
embryonal carcinoma see above
fine needle aspiration 1773–1781
FNA processing/staining 1774
histogenesis 1741–1742, 1744f
histologic maturation after chemotherapy 149
intratubular see intratubular germ cell neoplasia (IGCN)
mixed 1756–1757, 1757f, 1781
risk factors/associations 1742
seminoma see seminoma
sex cord-stromal tumors mixed 1761–1762
subclassification by FNA 1774
teratoma see teratoma
hematopoietic 1762
histological classification 1741, 1743t
infectious/inflammatory conditions mimicking 1767
lymphoma 1762, 1762f
metastatic 1763, 1763f
primitive neuroectodermal tumors 1756
sex cord-stromal tumors see sex cord-stromal tumors
staging 1741, 1742t
see also paratesticular region
testis 1731–1763
absence 1734–1735
acquired abnormalities 1735–1736
anatomy 1731–1732, 1731f
biopsy 1733
infertility 1738–1741
intratubular germ cell neoplasia (IGCN) 1744
congenital abnormalities 1734–1735
descent 1734
dysgenesis 1737
ectopic 1734

embryology 1734
end-stage 1740–1741, 1741f
hemorrhagic infarction, choriocarcinoma vs 1754
histology (normal) 1732–1733, 1732f
infectious disorders 1767, 1767f
inflammatory conditions see orchitis
intersex states 1736–1738, 1736t
leukemia 1762
malakoplakia 1767, 1767f
in multiple myeloma 1762
plasmacytoma 1762
retractile 1734
specimen handling 1733
torsion 1735
tuberculosis 1767, 1767f
tumors see testicular tumors
undescended 1734, 1735f
varicocele 1735–1736
see also paratesticular region
testosterone
defective synthesis 1737
elevation, steroid cell tumors of ovary 2025–2026, 2026f
tetraploid moles 2081
thalamus, tumor differential diagnosis 2348t
thalassemia 580
theca cells
hyperplasia 1992
luteinized 1988
theca interna 1987
theca lutein cysts 1990, 1992
multiple bilateral 1992–1993, 1993f
thecoma
of ovary 2019–2020, 2019f
fibroma vs 2020
luteinized 2019–2020, 2019f
of testis 1761
thermal artifact, electrocautery/laser specimens 137
thermal therapy, tumors associated 160
Thermophylliae polyspora 889
Thiel–Behnke dystrophy 2302
ThinPrep 20, 35, 422
thioflavine T stain 116, 1631, 2335t
third ventricle
choroid glioma see choroid glioma of third ventricle
colloid cyst 2402f, 2403f
pilocytic astrocytoma 2357
tumor differential diagnosis 2348t
thoracoepigastric vein, phlebitis 450
thoracoscopic biopsy, pleura 1005
thorium dioxide (Thorotrast), tumors associated 160
thorotrast, angiosarcoma of liver 1542
Thorotrast, tumors associated 160
thrombi
acute fibrin platelet, on endocardial surface 1041
intervillous 2073
thromboangiitis obliterans 1078, 1079f
thromboaortopathy, occlusive see Takayasu's disease
thrombocythemia, essential 632, 633f, 635t
thrombocytopenia
congenital amegakaryocytic 617
X-linked 115
thrombomodulin, antibody staining, mesothelioma 1012
thrombophlebitis 1079
superficial 1079
superficial migratory 211, 1079
superficial nonmigratory 1079
thrombosis
arterial 1084
fetal vessels 2073, 2073f
thrombotic disease, lung 916–917, 917f
thrombotic microangiopathies, renal involvement 1647–1648, 1647f, 1652
thrombotic thrombocytopenic purpura (TTP) 617, 1383, 1647
thymic differentiation, tumors with 2140, 2140f
thymocytes 569, 1122
thymofibrolipoma 1126

thymohemangiolipoma 1126
thymoid hyperplasia 1092, 1094
thymolipoma 1126–1127, 1126f
thymoliposarcoma 1126–1127, 1128f
thymoma 1091, 1095–1102, 1096f
    'atypical' 1099, 1100f, 1101, 1108, 1108f
        thymic carcinoma vs 1107
    classification 1096–1097, 1097f
    cortical/medullary types 1096
    differential diagnosis 1101t, 1102t
        lymphoblastic lymphoma vs 569, 1122
        thymic carcinoid vs 1112, 1113
    ectopic 1095
    encapsulated 1095
    epithelial cells 1095–1096, 1100
    fibrous septations 1097, 1098f
    fine needle aspiration 1107, 1108f, 1109f
    immunocytochemistry 1100–1101, 1100f
    intrathyroidal 2140
    lymphocytes 1095–1096, 1097, 1100, 1107
    medullary differentiation 1098
    micronodular 1098, 1099f
    mixed lymphoepithelial 1096, 1097f
    myasthenia gravis and 2227
    organoid, thymic carcinoid vs 1113
    predominantly epithelial 1096, 1097f, 1113
    predominantly lymphocytic 1096, 1097f, 1098, 1122
    pseudosarcomatous stroma 1099, 1099f
    seminomatous 1116
    spindle-cell ('medullary') 1096, 1109f
    spindle-cell epithelial 1099, 1100f
    squamous metaplasia in 1098
    thymocytes 569
    types A-C (WHO) 1096–1097
thymomatous nodules 1095
thymus 1091–1134, 1110, 1110f
    carcinoid tumors 1108, 1109f
        atypical 1110, 1111
        cytopathology 1113–1114, 1114f
        differential diagnosis 1101t, 1102t, 1113
        immunohistochemistry 1112–1113, 1112f
        mortality and behavior 1113
        organoid growth 1110f
        special studies 1111–1113
        spindle cell growth 1101f, 1110
        thymoma vs 1112, 1113
    carcinoma 1102–1107, 1103f
        adenosquamous 1103
        basaloid squamous 1102, 1104f
        clear cell 1102, 1104f
        cytopathology 1107–1108, 1108f, 1109f
        differential diagnosis 1105–1107, 1106t
        immunohistochemistry 1105
        keratinizing/non-keratinizing squamous 1102, 1103f
        large cell lymphoma vs 1123
        lymphoepthelioma-like squamous cell 1102, 1103f, 1105, 1106
        mediastinal embryonal carcinoma vs 1118
        metastases 1107
        mucoepidermoid 1102, 1103, 1104f
        primary adenocarcinoma (not further specified) 1104, 1105f
        sarcomatoid 1102–1103, 1104f, 1105, 1109f, 1126
        ultrastructure 1104–1105
        well-differentiated, thymoma vs 1099–1100
    choriocarcinoma 1119–1120, 1120f
    cystic lesions 1091–1094
    cysts 1091–1093, 1091f, 1092f
        multilocular 1091, 1092, 1092f
        unilocular 1091, 1092
    embryonal carcinoma 1118, 1118f, 1119f, 1122f
    epithelial neoplasms 1095–1108
        cytopathology 1107–1108, 1108f, 1109f
        thymomas see thymoma
    fibrous histiocytoma, differential diagnosis 1101t, 1102t
    germ cell tumors 1114–1121
    Hodgkin's disease 1092

hyperplasia 1094–1095, 1095f
    after chemotherapy 149
    lymphoid 1094–1095
        'massive' 1094
        myasthenia gravis and 2227
        'rebound' 1094
        true vs endocrinopathy-associated 1094
    inflammatory pseudotumor 1128
    large cell lymphoma 1123–1124, 1123f
        fine needle aspiration 1124–1125, 1125f
        stromal sclerosis in 1123, 1124f
        thymic carcinoma vs 1106, 1106t
    lymphoma 1121–1124, 1124f
        cytopathology 1124–1125, 1124f
        thymic carcinoid vs 1113
        see also under mediastinum
    mesenchymal tumors 1125–1128
    metastatic tumors in 1113
    neuroendocrine tumors 1108–1114
        cytopathology 1113–1114, 1114f
        differential diagnosis 1098, 1113
        FNA 1113–1114, 1114f
        immunohistochemistry 1112–1113, 1112f
        large cell 1111, 1111f
        small cell (oat cell) 1108, 1110–1111, 1111f, 1114, 1114f
        see also thymus, carcinoid tumors
    pseudoepitheliomatous hyperplasia 1092
    seminoma 1116–1118, 1117f, 1120, 1121f
        immunohistochemistry 1116–1118, 1118f
        large cell lymphoma vs 1123
        'tigroid' pattern 1120, 1121f
    in severe combined immunodeficiency 113
    see also mediastinum
thyroglobulin expression 2130, 2135
thyroglossal duct 2119
thyroglossal tract cysts 1148–1149
thyroid carcinoma
    anaplastic 2135, 2136f
    C-cell lesions 2135–2139
    composite (papillary and medullary) 2139
    in dyshormonogenetic goiter 2124
    follicular 2132–2133, 2132f
        capsular invasion 2133
        encapsulated type 2132, 2132f
        follicular adenoma vs 2125f, 2126, 2133
        metastases 178f
        minimally invasive type 2133
        pseudocapsular invasion 2133
        in struma ovarii 2034–2035
        vascular invasion 2132, 2133
        widely invasive type 2132
    Hürthle cell 2134–2135, 2134f
    hyperparathyroidism associated 159
    immunohistochemistry 181, 181f
    insular 2135, 2136f
    irradiation associated 159
    medullary 2135–2137, 2138f
        amyloid in 2137, 2138f, 2139
        cytology 2138–2139, 2138f
        familial 2136, 2137
        familial non-MEN (FMTC) 2137
        lymph node metastases 2137
        MEN syndromes associated 2136, 2137
        micromedullary 2138
        parathyroid adenoma vs 2156
        spindle-cell morphology 2137, 2138f
    metastases
        in bone 771
        in larynx 848
    microcarcinoma 2127, 2128f, 2129
    mixed follicular and medullary tumors 2139
    mucoepidermoid 2139, 2140f
    papillary 2119, 2127–2132
        autoimmune thyroiditis vs 2121
        'bubble gum' colloid 2130
        classic/conventional variant 2127–2128, 2128f
        columnar cell 2130
        cribriform-morular variant 2130

        cytology 2130, 2131f
        diffuse sclerosing variant 2129f, 2130
        encapsulated variant 2126, 2129
        familial form 2129
        follicular cells in Graves' disease vs 2123
        follicular variant (FVPTC) 2128f, 2129, 2130, 2131f
        immunohistochemistry 2130–2131
        lymphatic spread 2128
        metastatic, differential diagnosis 957, 2279
        microcarcinoma 2127, 2128f, 2129
        nodular fasciitis-like stroma with 2130
        Papanicolaou stain vs Diff-Quik stain 27, 27f
        pediatric 2130
        sclerosis 2128
        in struma ovarii 2034, 2034f
        tall cell variant 2129–2130, 2129f, 2130, 2131f
        variants 2128–2130, 2128f
        Warthin-like variant 2129f, 2130
    poorly differentiated 2135, 2136f
        TTF-1 staining 33, 34f
    sclerosing mucoepidermoid with eosinophilia 2139, 2140f
    in struma ovarii 2034, 2034f
    well-differentiated (WDTC) 2127, 2127t
    well-differentiated follicular of 'undetermined malignant potential' 2134
thyroid eye disease see Graves' disease
thyroid gland 2119–2148
    adenoma 2124–2126, 2125f
        after irradiation 158
        follicular see below
        hyalinizing trabecular 2126, 2126f
        'signet-ring' 2126
        thymic remnants 2140
    anatomy 2119
    aplasia and hypoplasia 2119
    autoimmune disorders
        Graves' disease 2123
        see also autoimmune thyroiditis (Hashimoto's)
    benign conditions, papillary carcinoma association 2127
    carcinoma see thyroid carcinoma
    C cells see C cells, thyroid
    cystic papillary carcinoma 25
    cysts 25, 2164
    developmental anomalies 2119
    ectopic 2119
    embryology 2119
    enlargement 2122
    epithelial tumors 2127t
        benign 2124–2126, 2127t
        malignant 2126–2139, 2127t
        see also thyroid carcinoma
    epithelium inclusion in lymph node 512
    FNA biopsy 24, 2119–2120
        complication rate 138
    follicles
        in autoimmune thyroiditis 2121
        colloid accumulation 2122–2123
        hyperplasia 2122, 2123f
        involution 2122
    follicular adenoma 2124–2126, 2125f
        atypical 2126
        carcinoma vs 2125f, 2126, 2133
    follicular carcinoma see thyroid carcinoma
    follicular cells 2119, 2123
    goiter see goiter
    hematopoietic tumors 2141
    histology (normal) 2119
    inflammation 2120
        see also thyroiditis
    ionizing radiation effect 157–158
    lingual 2119
        persistent 1163
    lymphoma 2141
    mesenchymal tumors 2140–2142
    metastases in 171t, 172
    nodules 2119–2120

thyroid gland (cont'd)
    adenomatoid/hyperplastic 2124
    cold 2124
    FNA interpretation 2120
    follicular adenoma 2125, 2125f
    hyperplastic, goiter 2122, 2123
    lingual 1163
    medullary carcinoma with 2137
    solitary cold 2132
paraganglioma 2139
primary nonepithelial tumors 2140–2142
secondary tumors 2141, 2141f
solid cell nests (SCN) 2119
    hyperplasia 2121
tumors 2124–2141
    benign 2124–2126, 2127t
    classification 2127t
    thymic/branchial pouch differentiation 2140
thyroiditis 2120
    acute suppurative 2120
    autoimmune see autoimmune thyroiditis (Hashimoto's)
    chronic lymphocytic see autoimmune thyroiditis
        (Hashimoto's)
    palpation 2120, 2120f
    postpartum 2122
    Riedel's 1127, 2122
    silent 2122
    subacute (de Quervain's disease) 2120
thyroid-stimulating hormone (TSH), increased 2122
thyroid tissue
    implantation of normal tissue during surgery 146
    in struma ovarii 2034–2035, 2034f
thyroid transcription factor 1 (TTF-1) 2383
    bronchioloalveolar carcinoma 956
    effusion differential diagnosis 1033
    mesothelioma 1013–1014, 1014f
    metastatic lung cancer 1033
    pulmonary adenocarcinoma 960, 1105, 1107f
    small cell lung carcinoma 991, 1575
    struma ovarii 2034
    thyroid carcinoma staining 33, 34f, 181, 181f
thyrotoxicosis see hyperthyroidism
thyrotroph embryonic factor (TEF) 2095
thyrotrophin (TSH) 2095
thyrotrophs 2095
    adenoma see pituitary adenoma
    development 2094–2095
    hyperplasia 2110, 2111f
tight junctions 1732, 2240
tin dioxide pneumoconiosis 905t
tinea capitis 198
tinea corporis 198
tinea cruris 198
tinea manuum 198
tinea pedis 198
tinnitus 2284
tissue fillers 141
    iatrogenic reactions 141–143
tissue fixation see fixation/fixatives
tissue microarrays 36, 2340
tissue staining methods 16t–17t, 17–19
titanium dye pneumoconiosis 905t
titin (connectin) 2218t
TNM classification
    anal squamous cell carcinoma 1456, 1457t
    Barrett's adenocarcinoma 1312
    bone sarcomas 703, 703t
    colorectal cancer 1440, 1441t
    esophageal squamous cell carcinoma 1296, 1297t
    gastric adenocarcinoma 1360, 1360t
    laryngeal squamous cell carcinoma 842
    lung carcinoma 937–939, 938t
    oral squamous cell carcinoma 1170, 1171t
    prostatic carcinoma 1815–1817, 1817t
    rhabdomyosarcoma 357, 357t
    salivary gland tumors 1203, 1204t
    small intestinal adenocarcinoma 1430, 1431t
    soft tissue tumors 309t
    testicular tumors 1741, 1742t

tobacco
    chewing, oral squamous cell carcinoma 1168
    smokeless see smokeless tobacco
    see also smoking
tobacco bronchiolitis 906
Toker cells 457
toluidine blue stain 29, 296
'tombstone' appearance 1837
tongue
    developmental disorders 1162–1163
    squamous cell carcinoma 1172, 1172f
    squamous papilloma 1163
tonsils, squamous cell carcinoma 1173
tooth germ apparatus 1139
tophi, gouty see gout
topoisomerase inhibitors, leukemia after 149
torulopsis 67t
Torulopsis (Candida) glabrata 85
toxemia of pregnancy 1517–1518
toxic epidermal necrolysis (TEN) 203
toxic epidermal necrosis 203, 218
toxic megacolon, in Crohn's disease 1391
toxic shock syndrome 1919
toxins
    acute cholangitis 1494
    pulmonary hypertension due to 913t
Toxocara spp. 77, 1512
toxocariasis, ocular 2310
Toxoplasma gondii 103, 103f, 519, 2313, 2411
toxoplasmosis
    cardiac allograft infection 1051
    CNS involvement 2411
    encephalitis 2411, 2412f
    lymphadenitis 519–520
    monocytoid B-cell hyperplasia 527
    ocular 103, 2313, 2314f
TP53 gene mutations
    anaplastic astrocytoma 2352
    diffuse astrocytoma 2351
    gallbladder carcinoma 1581
    giant cell glioblastoma 2355
    glioblastoma 2354
    mucinous cystic neoplasm of pancreas 1565
    oligoastrocytoma 2370
Tpit transcription factor 2096
'trabecular carcinoma' 249
trabecular meshwork 2315f
    blocked 2316
    descemetization 2316
trachea 833–855
    adenocarcinoma 846
    adenoid cystic carcinoma 846–847
    adenoma, pleomorphic 946–947
    anatomy 834, 860
    benign epithelial neoplasms (squamous papilloma)
        836–838
        malignant degeneration 836, 837–838
        recurrence 837, 838f
    benign mixed tumor 847–848
    dysplasia 838–839
    embryology 834
    fibrosarcoma 849
    future tumor research 850–851
    glandular tumors (malignant/benign) 846–848
    hamartoma 848
    histology 834
    hyperplasia and precancerous lesions 838–842
    leiomyosarcoma 849
    lymphangioma 849
    lymphoma and plasmacytoma 850
    malignant epithelial tumors 842–846
    malignant tumors of connective tissue/cartilage
        849–850
    melanoma 848
    neoplasms 836–850
    non-neoplastic conditions 834–836
        inflammatory and degenerative 834–835
    relapsing polychondritis 835

    rheumatoid arthritis 835
    sarcoidosis 835
    specimen handling 833–834
    thermal burns 834
    tuberculosis 835
    see also larynx
tracheitis, herpetic 834
tracheobronchitis, HSV ulcerative 878, 878f
tracheoesophageal fistula 1283
tracheopathia osteochondroplastica 849
trachoma 2294, 2303
tragi, accessory 2270, 2270f
training, surgical pathology/cytopathology 8–10
    fundamentals to master 8
    goals 8
    for nonpathologists (clinical trainees) 9
transbronchial biopsy 866–867, 868
transbronchial needle aspiration (TBNA) 939–940
transcriptional profiling 47–48, 48f
transcription factors
    adenohypophysial development 2093–2094
    markers 31t
transforming growth factor-alpha (TGF-alpha) 1138
transforming growth factor-B (TGF-B) 1170, 1632
transgenic mice, pancreatic endocrine neoplasm 1572
transient acantholytic dermatosis (Grover's disease)
    219, 220–221, 221f
transient myeloproliferative disorder (TMPD) 622
transillumination of eyes 2305, 2306f
transitional cell(s) 793, 1707
transitional cell (urothelial) carcinoma
    bladder see under bladder (urinary)
    cervix 1861
    endometrial 1965f
    ovary 2012, 2013, 2014f
    paraurethral (Skene's) glands 1914
    prostate see prostate gland, urothelial (transitional
        cell) carcinoma
transitional cell epithelium see urothelium
transitional cell metaplasia, cervix 1838
transmembrane glycoproteins, markers 31t
transmissible spongiform encephalopathies 2412–2413,
    2413f
transmission electron microscopy, liver biopsy 1472
transplantation
    allograft injuries 129–131
    allograft perfusion duration 129
    graft rejection see graft rejection
    immunosuppressive drug toxicity 127, 130f
    lymphomas after 572
    lymphoproliferative diseases see post-transplantation
        lymphoproliferative disorders
    tissue (HLA) typing 124
    see also specific organs
transplant glomerulopathy 1650, 1651f
transport chain activity 2230
transpupillary thermotherapy 2308
transthoracic fine needle aspiration (TTNA) 940
transudates, definition 1025
transurethral resection, thermal artifact in tissue 137
transurethral resection of bladder tumors (TURBTs)
    1718, 1724
transurethral resection of prostate (TURP) 1794, 1821
'trapped lung' 1007
trastuzumab 489
trematode infections, gastrointestinal tract 105
trench fever 99
Treponema pallidum 70, 2407
    staining 59
Trevor's disease 707
trichilemmal carcinoma 260–261, 261f
trichilemmal (pilar) inclusion cysts 254, 254f
trichilemmal keratinization 254, 254f
trichilemmal tumor (pilar), proliferating 254, 254f
trichilemmoma 252–253, 252f
    desmoplastic form 253
    eyelid 2291
Trichinella spiralis 100, 100f, 2223, 2223f
trichinosis 100, 100f, 2223

trichoadenoma (of Nikolowski) 255, 255f
trichoblastic fibroma 252
trichoblastoma 252, 252f
trichoepithelioma
    classical 251–252, 251f
        basal cell carcinoma vs 245–246
    desmoplastic (DTE) 246, 252, 252f
trichofolliculoma 251, 251f
Trichomonas vaginalis 77, 77f, 1919
    cervical infections 1836t, 1837, 1849, 1850f
Trichophyton rubra 225
trichoptysis 1115
trichrome stain see Masson trichrome stain
tricuspid valve 1059
    anorexigen-induced disease 1059
    carcinoid disease 1059
    floppy (myxomatous degeneration) 1059
    insufficiency due to pulmonary venous hypertension
        1059
    postinflammatory (rheumatic) disease 1059
trigger finger 697, 698f
trilineage dysplasia 618
trinucleotide (CTG) repeat 2237
TriPath 422
trisomies
    alveolar soft part sarcoma 397
    frequency in spontaneous abortions 2079t
    parachordoma 396
trisomy 7 743, 1680
trisomy 8 320, 743
trisomy 11 330
trisomy 17 1680
trisomy 20 320
triton tumor
    benign (neuromuscular hamartoma) 2249, 2249f
    malignant 2258, 2258f
Tropheryma whippelii 530, 1378, 2407
trophoblast 2063, 2080
    extravillous (intermediate; transitional) 2063, 2080
        ectopic lesions 2087
        lesions 2084–2087
    lesions 2080–2087
    persistent trophoblastic activity 2043
    villous 2063, 2080
        lesions 2080–2084
trophoblastic disease, fallopian tube 2047
trophoblastic implants 1022, 2087
trophoblastic inclusions 2082, 2082f
trophoblastic pseudotumor 2084
trophoblastic tissue, residual 2087
trophoblastic tumor
    epithelioid 2084, 2086–2087
    placental site (PSTT) 2084, 2085–2086, 2085f, 2086f
trophotropism, placental shape abnormalities 2070
trophozoites 103, 106
tropical splenomegaly 1518
tropical sprue 1377
tropomyosin 2218t
troponin 2218t
Trotter's triad 793
Trousseau's syndrome 1554
Trypanosoma cruzi 100
trypsin, acinar cell carcinoma of pancreas 1561f
tryptase, antibody 614
Tsanck preparation 74, 74f, 1888
TSC-1 and TSC-2 genes 970
TSC2/PKD1 contiguous gene syndrome 1690
TTF-1 see thyroid transcription factor 1 (TTF-1)
T tubule system 2215
    periodic paralyses 2233–2234, 2233f
tubal metaplasia 1838
tubal pregnancy see pregnancy, ectopic
tubercle, tuberculosis 82, 83f
tubercles of Montgomery 420
tuberculid, papulonecrotic 215
tuberculoma, CNS 2406, 2407f
tuberculosis
    Addison's disease 2176
    cervicitis 1836t, 1837

CNS 2406, 2407f
    granulomatous gastritis 1336
    granulomatous response 64
    hepatic granuloma 1511
    larynx 835
    lymph node involvement 96, 96f, 533
    otitis media 2272–2273
    ovary 1989
    pleural effusions 1027
    pulmonary 82–83, 96f
    salpingitis 2041, 2041f
    silicosis and 903
    of testis 1767, 1767f
    trachea 835
    vulva 1891
    see also Mycobacterium tuberculosis
tuberculosis verrucosa cutis 215
tuberous sclerosis
    angiofibroma of skin 264–265, 265f
    angiomyolipoma association 1690, 1691f
    cardiac rhabdomyoma association 354
    genetics and CNS features 2401t
    lymphangioleiomyomatosis in 926
    renal cell carcinoma 1676
    renal cysts 1665
    subependymal giant cell astrocytoma and 2359, 2360
tuberous sclerosis complex genes 970
tuboendometrioid metaplasia, cervix 1838
tubo-ovarian abscess 143, 2040, 2041
tubo-ovarian adhesions 2041
tubular aggregates myopathy 2228t, 2229
tubular apocrine adenoma 258
tubular casts (renal) 1630
tubular interstitial disorders 1637–1643
    acute tubular necrosis see acute tubular necrosis
    clinical presentation 1605
    interstitial 'thyroidization' 1610f, 1639
    light microscopy diagnostic algorithm 1605t
    primary and secondary 1605
    pyelonephritis see pyelonephritis
    renal biopsy interpretation 1603
tubular interstitial nephritis
    acute 1640, 1640f
    chronic 1640–1641, 1641f
    lupus nephritis 1628, 1628f
    'tubulitis' with 1610f, 1640, 1640f
tubular interstitium see renal tubular interstitium
tubular reticular inclusions, lupus nephritis 1628, 1628f
'tubular simplification' 1638
tubulin, class III B-tubulin 2359
β-tubulin, small cell lung carcinoma 992
tubulitis (renal) 1610f, 1640, 1640f
tubulocystic carcinoma, kidney 1686–1687, 1686f
tubulofilaments, inclusion body myositis 2220f, 2221f
tubulopathy, acute 1630–1631, 1630f, 1631f
tubuloreticular inclusions, in collapsing
        glomerulopathy 1603f, 1612
Tuffstone bodies 2246
tularemia 64, 72, 98, 98f
'tumefactive fibroinflammatory lesions' 824, 1127
tumor, dissemination, by needle-track seeding 138
tumor cell islands, sebaceous carcinoma 260
tumor cell 'lakes' 257, 261
tumor cell lysis, bone marrow necrosis 665
tumor cell nests
    adenoid (acantholytic/pseudoglandular) squamous
        cell carcinoma 247, 248f
    melanoma 284
    Merkel cell carcinoma 249
tumorigenesis, multistep, theory 936–937
tumor-like lesions, CNS 2403–2404
tumor mass, persistent after chemotherapy 149
tumors
    drug-associated 149–150
    iatrogenic lesions mimicking/causing see iatrogenic
        lesions
    radiation-associated 153–155, 158–160
tumor suppressor genes
    gastric adenocarcinoma 1359–1360

markers 31t
    mutations 44
    oral cavity disease 1138
    oral squamous cell carcinoma and 1169–1170
    osteosarcoma association 728t
    see also p53 gene/p53 protein; RB gene
tunica albuginea 1731, 1731f
tunica propria 1732
tunnel clusters 1840–1841, 1841f
'turban tumor' (dermal cylindroma) 255–256, 255f
turbinates, middle, neuroendocrine carcinoma
        803–804, 804f
Turcot syndrome 2379, 2401t
Turcotte syndrome 1437–1438
Turner's syndrome 1082, 1738, 2078
twin reversed arterial perfusion (TRAP) 2078
twins 2075
    acardiac 2078, 2078f
    dizygotic 2075–2076, 2076f
    monozygotic 2075, 2076, 2078
        heterokaryotic 2078
twin-to-twin transfusion syndrome (TTTS) 2075,
        2077–2078, 2077f
tympanic cavity (tympanum) see ear, middle
tympanic membrane
    anatomy 2267–2268
    development 2267
    in middle ear adenoma 2277
tympanosclerosis 2274
tympanotomy 2275
typhlitis 1397
typhoid fever, hepatic microabscess 1481, 1481f
tyramide amplification technique (TAT) 32
tyrosinase, melanoma 286
tyrosine crystals, salivary pleomorphic adenoma 1211
Tzanck cells 1837
Tzanck preparation 74, 74f, 1888

U
ubiquitin
    antibodies, in alcoholic hepatitis 1471f, 1490
    inclusion body myositis 2221, 2221f
ulcer(s)
    colon see colon, ulcers
    Cushing's (Curling's, stress) 1327
    duodenal see duodenum, ulcers
    esophageal 1286–1287, 1286f, 1287f
    gastric see gastric ulcers
    herpetic, esophageal 1287
    mouth 1386
    penetrating atherosclerotic 1070
    rectal, solitary 1382
    skin 195
    stercoral 1388
    tampon 1919
ulcerative colitis 1386–1394
    adenocarcinoma association 1387, 1390, 1393, 1441
    appendiceal disease 1390, 1409
    atypical histologic features 1392–1393
    biopsy diagnosis 1387–1389
    clinical features 1386–1387
    Crohn's disease vs 1388–1389
    dysplasia 1393–1394, 1393f, 1394f, 1441–1443,
        1442f
    endoscopic surveillance 1442
    ileal pouch-anal anastomosis 1393, 1394
    inflammatory polyps 1390, 1390f
    patchy disease 1388, 1392
    pathology in colectomy specimens 1389–1390
    primary sclerosing cholangitis with 1393, 1497
    terminal ileal biopsy 1389
    see also inflammatory bowel disease
ulcerative jejunoileitis 1376
ulcerogingivostomatitis, necrotizing (noma) 78–79
Ulex europaeus 372, 613, 1685
ultimobranchial body rest 2121
ultrasound
    preoperative PTH localization 2157
    renal cysts 1665

ultraviolet (UV) microscopy, liver biopsy 1472
umbilical artery, single (SUA) 2065, 2075, 2078
umbilical cord 2065–2067
    anatomy 2065
    angiomyxoma 2067
    development 2063–2064
    dizygotic twins 2075–2076, 2076f
    excessively long 2065
    false knots 2066
    hematoma 2066–2067
    insertion, abnormalities 2064, 2064f, 2066, 2066f
    knot 2063
    monozygotic twins 2077, 2077f, 2078, 2078f
    pathology 2065–2067, 2066f
    persistent allantoic duct with 2066, 2066f
    short/excessive short 2065
    tumors 2067
    twist (direction, lack and excessive) 2065
uniparental disomy 2080
upper respiratory system, infections 77–81
urachal remnants, persistent 1708, 1720, 1721
urachal tract, maldevelopment 1707, 1708
uranyl acetate 29
urates, staining methods 17t
Ureaplasma urealyticum, cervicitis 1835
uremic neuropathy 2248
ureterosigmoidostomy, colonic adenocarcinoma around
    146
ureters 1726
    tumors 1726
urethra 1724–1726
    carcinoma in situ 1725
    caruncle 1724, 1725f
    clear cell adenocarcinoma 1725, 1725f
    condyloma accuminatum 1725
    diverticula 1724–1725
    fibrous polyps 1725
    polyps 1725
    prostatic 1791
    strictures 1725
    tumors 1725, 1725f
urinary bladder see bladder
urinary cytopathology 1711–1712
urinary incontinence, reaction to Teflon® paste 142
urinary tract anomalies, renal dysplasia 1661
urine, technical problems with samples 20–21
uropathy, obstructive 1605
uroplakins 1707
uroporphyrin crystals, acicular, in liver cells 1471
urothelial cell carcinoma see transitional cell carcinoma
urothelial cells, superficial 1707, 1708f
urothelial neoplasms 1710, 1713–1716
    carcinoma see transitional cell carcinoma
    classification 1712, 1712t
    Paget-like disease secondary to 1908
    papillary, of low malignant potential (PUNLMP)
        1713–1714, 1714f
    papilloma 1713, 1713f, 1719
        exophytic 1713, 1714f
    staging 1713, 1713t
urothelium 1707
    dysplastic lesions 1716–1717, 1716f
    normal 1707, 1707f
    prostate see prostate gland, urothelium
    tumor pathogenesis 1710–1711
urticaria 208, 209f
urticarial vasculitis 208, 209, 209f
urticaria pigmentosa 295, 663, 762
uterine arteries 1831
uterine artery embolization, bilateral 1969
uterine bleeding, dysfunctional 1949–1950
uterine cervix see cervix
uterine corpus 1933–1985
    adenocarcinoma see endometrial adenocarcinoma
    adenomatoid tumor 1978, 1978f
    adenomyosis 1951–1952, 1951f
    anatomy 1933–1934, 1933f
    angiomyolipoma 1978
    benign glandular inclusions 1935

    biopsies and curettages 1934–1935
        endometrial changes after 1947
    carcinoma 1958t
        see also endometrium, carcinoma/cancer
    congenital abnormalities 1933
    cytologic specimens 1935
    endometriosis see endometriosis
    endometrium see endometrium
    ionizing radiation effect 157, 157f
    leiomyoblastoma 1971
    leiomyoma 1935, 1968–1969, 1968f, 1969f
        benign metastasizing 1973
        cellular/atypical 1971, 1972f
        clear cell 1971, 1972, 1972f
        epithelioid 1971, 1972f
        intramural/cotyledonoid dissecting 1973
        multinodular hydropic 1973
        plexiform 1971, 1972
    leiomyomatosis
        diffuse 1973
        intravenous 1973, 1973f
    leiomyosarcoma 1969–1971, 1969f, 1970f, 1971f
        coagulative tumor cell necrosis 1970, 1970f
        epithelioid 1971, 1971f
        leiomyoma vs 1969t
        myxoid 1972, 1972f
    leukemia 1978
    lymphoma 1978
    mesenchymal tumors 1968–1973, 1978
    metastases to 1978–1979
    perforation, intrauterine devices 143
    perivascular epithelioid cell tumors (PEComas)
        1978f
    septate 1933
    smooth muscle tumors 1968–1973
        benign vs malignant 1970–1971
        of uncertain malignant potential 1972
        unusual/atypical 1971–1973
    specimen processing 1934–1936
    stromal sarcoma, low-grade 1951
    tumors, radiation-associated 159
uterine serosa l 1934
uteroplacental perfusion 2064
    abnormalities 2071–2072
utricle 2269, 2269f
utricular cysts 1791
uveal malignant melanoma 2306–2309
    Callendar classification 2306–2307, 2307f
    epithelioid cells 2306–2307, 2307f
    metastases 2308
    prognostic factors (cell type/size) 2308, 2308t
    ring melanoma 2309
    spindle cells (spindle A and B) types 2306–2307, 2307f
uveal tract
    hamartomatous thickening 2309
    inflammation see uveitis
    pigmented tumors 2309
        see also uveal malignant melanoma
uveitis 2313
    phacoantigenic 2300, 2300f
    sympathetic (ophthalmia) 2311–2312

V

vacuolar degeneration 195
vacuolar myelopathy, in AIDS 2409
vacuoles
    in adenocarcinomas 183
    adipocytes 336
    cytoplasmic
        in mesothelial cells in effusions 183, 1026, 1027,
            1027f
        salivary acinic cell carcinoma 1231
    glycogen in 2231, 2232f
    periodic paralyses 2233, 2233f
    rimmed (autophagic) 2220f, 2221f, 2237
    subnuclear, endometrium 1937, 1937f, 1938, 1938f
vagina 1918–1925
    adenocarcinoma 1924–1925, 1924f
        of enteric type 1925

    adenosis 1923, 1923f
        endocervical/tubal-endometrial types 1923, 1923f
    agenesis 1919
    anatomy 1918–1919
    atrophy 1919
    benign disorders/tumors 1919–1923
    benign epithelial tumors 1921–1922
    benign fibroepithelial stromal polyps 356, 1922
    benign soft tissue tumors 1922
    benign stromal tumors 1922
    blood supply 1918–1919
    bullous disorders 1893t
    clear cell adenocarcinoma 1924
    clear cell carcinoma 150, 1923
    columnar cell metaplasia 1923
    condyloma accuminatum 1921, 1921f
    congenital abnormalities 1919
    cysts 1920, 1920f
    duplication 1919
    ectopic tissues in 1922
    embryonal rhabdomyosarcoma 1925
    endometrioid adenocarcinoma 1925
    endometriosis 1899, 1920f, 1921
    fibroepithelial polyp 1921f, 1922
    fistulas involving 1920
    iatrogenic reactions resembling tumors 147
    infections 1919–1920
    inflammatory disorders 1919–1920
    innervation 1919
    intraepithelial neoplasia (VAIN) 1923–1924
    leiomyoma 1922
    leiomyosarcoma 1925
    lymphatic drainage 1919
    lymphoepithelioma-like carcinoma 1924
    malignant tumors 1923–1925
    maturation index 1919
    melanoma 1925
    melanosis 1922, 1925
    metastatic tumors in 1925
    microglandular hyperplasia 1923
    mucosa 1918
    mucosal lentiginous melanoma 1925
    Müllerian papilloma 1922
    papillary squamotransitional cell carcinoma 1924
    postoperative spindle cell nodule 1920–1921
    rhabdomyoma 1922
    small cell carcinoma 1924
    smears 1935
    soft tissue tumors 1922, 1925
        benign 1922
        malignant 1925
    squamous cell carcinoma 1924
    squamous papilloma 1921–1922
    submucosa 1919
    superficial cervicovaginal myofibroblastoma 1922
    transverse septum 1919
    tumor-like changes 1920–1921
    vascular ectasia 1919
    verrucous carcinoma 1924
    xanthogranulomatous pseudotumor 1921
    yolk sac tumors 1925
vaginal flora, bacterial vaginosis 1851
vaginitis
    bacterial 78f
    'condylomatous' 1921
vaginosis 1851
van der Waals forces 33
vanillylmandelic acid (VMA) 750, 2194, 2199
vanishing bile duct syndrome 128, 128f
varicella-zoster virus (VZV) 75
    adrenalitis 2176
    chronic villitis 2069
    CNS involvement 2410
    herpetic dermatitis 221, 221f
    inclusions 68t
    ocular infection 2313
    peripheral nerve involvement 2244
    pneumonia 76f
varicocele 1735–1736

varicose veins 1085
varix, CNS 2415
vasa nervorum 2240
vasa recta 1600–1601
vascular calcinosis 1083
vascular-cartilaginous hamartoma 706
vascular disease/lesions 1070–1079, 1083–1085
  bone marrow 665f, 666
  breast 446, 446f
  CNS 2414–2417
  diffuse pulmonary 911–918
    see also lung
  ear 2275–2276
  liver 1513–1518
  occlusive, intestinal ischemia due to 1381–1382
  pituitary gland 2113
vascular dissemination, malignant cells 167
vascular endothelial cell growth factor (VEGF), iris
    neovascularization 2315
vascular endothelial cell growth factor receptor 3
    (VEGFR3) 273, 276
vascular hamartoma of infancy 706
vascular malformations
  CNS 2415–2416
  in dysgenetic syndromes 2416
  ear 2275
vascular prostheses, sarcomas associated 145
vascular tumors 702t
  angiosarcoma see angiosarcoma
  benign, of skin 268–273
  of bone 765–770
  hemangioendothelioma see hemangioendothelioma
  hemangioma see hemangioma
  intestinal 1448–1450
  lung 973–974, 973t
  of lymph nodes 514
  orbit 2296–2297
  pituitary gland 2109–2110
  sinonasal region 817–826
  of skin see skin, vascular tumors
  of soft tissue 362–373
  spleen 591–592
  thyroid 2141
vasculitides
  granulomatous 211–212
  neutrophilic 209–211
  orbital involvement 2295
  renal involvement 1648–1649, 1648f
  skin involvement 209–216
vasculitis 209, 1072–1074
  capillaries and venules (small vessel) 1075–1078,
    1076t
  CNS 2414
  of collagen vascular disease 1078, –1078
  disorders mimicking 1079
  elastic arteries 1072–1074, 1072t
  granulomatous 211–212
  hemorrhagic 2073
  hypersensitivity 1075
  immune-mediated 1076t, 1077–1078
  infectious 1079
  leukocytoclastic see leukocytoclastic vasculitis (LCV)
  lupus 1076t, 1078
  muscular arteries 1072t, 1074–1075
  necrotizing
    axonal degeneration 2241f
    ischemic colitis due to 1385f
    muscle involvement 2224, 2224f
    pulmonary arterial hypertension 912
  neutrophilic 209–211, 210, 211
  nodular 235
  non-necrotizing, muscle involvement 2224
  pauci-immune 1076t
  peripheral nerve involvement 2243
  in prostate 1795
  renal vessels 1611f
  rheumatoid 1076t, 1078
  scleroderma 1078
  septic 209

small intestine 1384–1386, 1384t
  urticarial 208, 209, 209f
vasculopathies
  chronic allograft 127–129
  skin involvement 209–216
vasculosyncytial membrane 2064
vas deferens 1731, 1733
  obstruction 1738
vasoformative channels, interanastomosing 372f
Vater, papilla 1549
'vegetant intravascular hemangioendothelioma'
    362–363, 363f
VEGFR 3 273, 276
veins, varicose 1085
'Velcro crackles' 893
veno-occlusive disease, liver 1515, 1516f
veno-occlusive lesions, alcoholic cirrhosis 1493f
venous angioma, CNS 2415
venous drainage, testis 1731
venous hypertension, pulmonary 914–915
venous outflow tract, liver, obstruction 1514–1517
venous phlebitis, lymphoplasmacytic sclerosing
    pancreatitis 1553, 1553f
ventricles of brain, tumor differential diagnosis 2348t
ventricles of heart, hypokinetic 1065–1066
ventriculoperitoneal shunts, complications 146
venulitis, lymphoplasmacytic sclerosing pancreatitis
    1553, 1553f
Verhoeff's elastic fiber stain 19f
Verhoeff-van Gieson method 292
vermis, medulloblastoma 2380
Verner-Morrison syndrome 1574
Verocay bodies
  nuclear palisading in leiomyoma similar 348
  schwannoma 2109, 2249, 2250f, 2385, 2386f
  spindle-cell palisading mimicking 1347, 1347f
verotoxins 1382
verruca plana (plane wart) 241–242
verruca plantaris (plantar wart) 242
verruca vulgaris 241, 241f
  oral cavity 1163
verruciform xanthoma, vulva 1902
verrucous carcinoma
  anus 1456, 1457f
  bladder 1720
  cervix 1860
  ear 2280
  esophageal 1298–1299
  larynx 13, 844–, 845f
  oral cavity 1173–1175, 1174f, 1175f
  sinonasal region 791, 792f
  of skin 248
  vagina 1924
  vulva 1912, 1912f
verrucous hyperplasia
  larynx 845
  oral cavity 1174
vertebrae, 'butterfly' 1502
vertigo, Ménière's disease 2284
vesicles 195
vesicoureteral reflux 1639
vestibular apparatus 2269, 2269f, 2270
vestibular glands see Bartholin's gland
vestibular papillomas, vulva 1899, 1900f
vestibule (sinonasal), squamous cell carcinoma
    789–790, 790f
Vibrio, necrotizing inflammation 101, 101f
Vibrio cholerae 101
Vibrio vulnificus 101
Victoria blue stain 1468, 1469, 1486, 1487f
Video-assisted Thoracoscopic (VATS) biopsy technique
    867, 867f, 868, 868f
villi (small intestinal)
  atrophy pattern 1376–1377
  complete flattening pattern 1374–1376
  variable flattening with crypt hyperplasia 1377–1378
villitis
  acute 2069–2070
  chronic 2069–2070

villitis of unknown etiology (VUE), chronic 2063,
    2068, 2070
villous tissue
  accelerated maturity 2071
  anatomy 2070
  avascular 2073, 2074f
  infarcts 2071, 2072f
vimentin 179, 2218t
  choroid glioma of third ventricle 2373
  granulosa cell tumor of ovary 2016
  intrauterine/extrauterine synchronous carcinoma
    1967
  mesenchymal chondrosarcoma 720
  mesothelioma 1013
  ossifying fibromyxoid tumor 380
  rhabdoid tumor of kidney 1671
  tumors associated 179
  Wilms' tumor 1667
vinyl chloride
  liver angiosarcoma 1542
  lung cancer etiology 936
VIPoma 1574, 2193
viral antigens, immunostaining of liver biopsy 1471,
    1472f
viral exanthems 208–209
viral infections
  bronchiolitis 906
  cervicitis 1836–1837, 1836t
  CNS 2407–2410
  cornea 2301–2302
  enteritis 1377
  eyelid 2290
  hepatic granulomas 1510
  intestinal 1398–1399
  lymphocyte rich response 67
  myositis 2222
  pneumonia 876–879, 876f, 876t
  renal transplant recipient 1652–1653
  respiratory tract 93–95
  skin/soft tissue/mucocutaneous surfaces 74–76
  vulva 1887–1889
  see also specific infections and sites
virilization
  46, XX with 1736–1737
  adrenocortical hyperplasia with 2183
  adrenocortical neoplasm with 2185
  luteoma of pregnancy and 1992
  massive ovarian edema associated 1992
  Sertoli-Leydig cell tumor 2021
  steroid cell tumors, of ovary 2025
viruses
  CNS tumors associated 2348
  confirmation using molecular methods 108t
  inclusions 68t, 102, 1472f
  mimics 95
  oral cavity disease 1138
  oral squamous cell carcinoma and 1169–1170
  staining 17t, 61
  see also specific viruses
visceral larva migrans 77, 77f, 1512, 1513f
visual disturbances, brain tumors 2345
visual loss 2289, 2306
vitamin A
  storage, stellate liver cells 1474, 1474f
  veno-occlusive disease due to 1515–1516
vitamin B$_{12}$, deficiency 619
vitamin D 686, 2150
vitamin D receptor 2152
vitamins, oral squamous cell carcinoma and 1169
vitelline vessels, remnants 2066
vitiligo, vulva 1896
vitrectomy 2304
vitreitis, chronic granulomatous (idiopathic senile)
    2304
vitreoretinal neovascularization ('sea fans') 2318
vitreoretinopathy, proliferative 2304
vitreous (body)
  abscess 2313
  hemorrhage 2304, 2317

vitreous (body) (cont'd)
  infection 2312
  persistent hyperplastic primary 2311
vitreous humor 2304
  hemorrhage 2304
  lymphoma 2304, 2305f
  opacification 2304
vocal cords 834
  amyloid tumors 835
  carcinoma in situ 841f
  cysts 835
  granular cell tumor 848, 848f
  hemangioma 849
  hyperplasia and precancerous lesions 838
  inflammatory atypia 835f
  metastatic tumors in 848
  paralysis, Teflon® paste treatment 142, 143f
  plasmacytoma 850
  polyps 835, 837f
  see also larynx
voice changes 838
von Brunn, nests 1708, 1715
von Gierke's disease 579
von Hansemann cells 1767
von Hippel-Lindau disease
  genes and CNS features 2401t
  hemangioblastoma of CNS 2394
  pancreatic endocrine neoplasms 1570–1571
  papillary adenocarcinoma of middle ear 2278–2279, 2279f
  papillary cystadenoma of epididymis 1764, 1764f
  papillary tumors of broad ligament 2048
  renal cell carcinoma 1676, 1677–1678
    metastatic vs pancreatic tumor 1569
  renal cysts 1665
  serous cystic neoplasms of pancreas 1562
  tumors associated 2394
von Kossa stain 233, 686, 2335t
von Leder stain 296
von Meyenberg complexes (biliary hamartoma) 1522, 1523f, 1538, 1538f
von Recklinghausen's disease see neurofibromatosis type 1
von Recklinghausen's disease of bone (osteitis fibrosa cystica) 751
von Willebrand factor (vWF) (factor VIII-related antigen) 275, 276, 372, 613, 1470
von Zumbusch, disseminated pustular psoriasis 199
vulva 1885–1918
  adenocarcinoma 1914
  adnexal cysts and tumors 1899, 1899t
  aggressive angiomyxoma 1917, 1917f
  anatomy 1885–1886, 1885f, 1886f
  angiokeratoma 1900, 1901, 1901f
  angiomyofibroblastoma 1900
  basal cell carcinoma 1912–1913, 1913f
  benign fibroepithelial stromal polyps 356
  benign neoplasms 1897–1902
    epithelial cysts/tumors 1899
    granular cell tumor 1902, 1903f
    mammary-like gland adenoma/cyst 1897–1899, 1898f
    stromal tumors 1900, 1901f
  blood supply 1885–1886
  bullous dermatoses 1893t
  bullous disorders 1893t
  carcinoma in situ 1902
  cavernous hemangioma 1901
  cellular angiofibroma 1902
  chondroid syringoma 1899, 1899f
  cicatricial pemphigoid 1893–1894
  in Crohn's disease 1896
  cysts 1899, 1900f
  developmental abnormalities 1887
  dystrophy 1891–1892
  embryonal rhabdomyosarcoma 1916–1917, 1916f, 1917f
  endometriosis 1899, 1918
  epithelial malignant tumors 1909–1913

fibroepithelial polyps 1899
fibrolipoma 1901
folliculosebaceous cystic hamartoma 1902
hemangioma 1901
hyperplastic dystrophy 1892–1893
iatrogenic changes 1887
infectious diseases 1887–1891
innervation 1886
intraepithelial neoplasia (VIN) 1902–1906
  basaloid type 1903, 1904f
  condyloma acuminatum vs 1887–1888
  differential diagnosis 1905, 1905t, 1908
  differentiated (simplex) type 1903, 1904f
  dyskeratosis 1903, 1904
  grading 1905, 1905t
  immunohistochemistry 1905
  invasive carcinoma with 1905, 1906f
  microscopic features 1903–1904, 1903f, 1904f
  'pagetoid' type 1904
  pigmented papular lesions 1903
  skin-colored (acetowhite) lesions 1903
  squamous cell carcinoma in situ vs 246
  warty (condylomatous) type 1903, 1903f
invasive tumors 1913–1914
leiomyoma 349, 1900–1901
leiomyosarcoma 1916
lentigo simplex 1896–1897
lichen planus 1894, 1894f
lichen sclerosus see lichen sclerosus (et atrophicus)
lichen simplex chronicus 1892–1893, 1893f
lipoma 1901
lymphatic drainage 1885
lymphoepithelioma-like carcinoma 1912
lymphoid hamartoma 1902
lymphoma 1918
malignant fibrous histiocytoma 1916
melanoma 1914–1915
  immunohistochemistry 1905t
  metastatic to vagina 1925
  Paget's disease vs 1908
  types 1887f, 1914
  vulvar nevi vs 1897
melanosis 1896, 1896f
Merkel cell tumor 1913
metastatic tumors 1918
mucinous columnar cell metaplasia 1899
mucous cysts 1899, 1900f
nevi (melanocytic) 1897
  atypical 1897, 1897f, 1914
nevus lipomatosus superficialis 1901
non-infectious inflammatory lesions 1891–1893, 1893t, 1894t
Paget-like lesions 1906
Paget's disease see Paget's disease, of vulva
papular acantholytic dyskeratosis 1894–1895
papulosquamous dermatoses 1893t
pigmentary disorders 1896–1897, 1896t
pyogenic granuloma 1901–1902
rhabdomyoma 1900–1901
sebaceous carcinoma 1911
smooth muscle tumors 1916
soft tissue tumors 1915–1918
solitary fibrous tumor 1900
specimen processing 1886
spindle cell squamous cell carcinoma 1912
squamous cell carcinoma 1909–1912, 1910f
  basaloid 1911
  giant-cell 1911–1912, 1911f
  invasion pattern ('finger-like/pushing') 1910, 1910f
  lichen sclerosus and 1892, 1909
  melanoma vs 1914–1915
  TNM staging and classification 1909–1910, 1910t
  warty 1911
squamous cell hyperplasia 1892–1893, 1904
superficial angiomyxoma 1902
systemic dermatoses affecting 1893–1896
tuberculosis 1891
verrucous carcinoma 1912, 1912f
vestibular papillomas 1899, 1900f

vulvar leiomyoma 349
vulva vestibulitis syndrome 1895, 1895f
vulvectomy, partial deep 1907, 1915
vulvitis
  atrophic 1892
  herpes simplex virus (herpetic) 1888, 1888f
  plasma cell 1895, 1895f
vulvitis circumscripta plasmacellularis 1895, 1895f
vulvitis granulomatosa 1896, 1896f
vulvo-vaginal-gingival syndrome 1894
vulvovaginitis, lichenoid 1894, 1894f

W

Wagner–Meissner bodies 2254
Waldenström's macroglobulinemia 554–555, 649, 654
  amyloidosis 2247
  splenic involvement 587
Walthard rests 1021, 2043
WarthinFinkeldey cells 95, 95f, 519, 1408–1409
Warthin-Starry stain 59, 207, 1470, 2069
  Legionella 81, 82f
  syphilis 1890
Warthin's tumor 1214–1219
  cytopathology 1217–1219, 1217f, 1218f
  differential diagnosis 1216–1217
    acinic cell carcinoma vs 1219
    lymphoma vs 1218, 1219
    oncocytic lesions vs 1219
    papillary oncocytic cystadenoma vs 1216
  false-negative 1206
  FNA evaluation 1206, 1207t
  microscopic features 1216, 1216f, 1217f
  oncocytes 1217–1218, 1217f, 1218f
warts
  common (verruca vulgaris) 241, 241f
  genital see condyloma accuminatum
  plane (verruca plana) 241–242
  plantar (verruca plantaris) 242
warty dyskeratoma 242, 243f
Waterhouse-Friderichsen syndrome 2177, 2177f
Wedl (bladder) cells 2300, 2300f
Wegener's granulomatosis 1076, 1076t, 1077f
  ear involvement 2276
  intestinal 1384, 1384t, 1385
  larynx 835
  lymphomatoid granulomatosis vs 290, 981
  peripheral nerve vasculitis 2243
  polyarteritis nodosa vs 1075
  renal involvement 1648, 1648f
Werdnig–Hoffmann disease (spinal muscular atrophy type I) 2226–2227, 2226f, 2227f
Wermer's syndrome see multiple endocrine neoplasia (MEN) type 1
wet keratin, craniopharyngioma 2398
Wharton's jelly 2065
  lack 2066
Whipple procedure 1554
Whipple's disease 1378
  CNS involvement 2407
  lymphadenopathy 530
  Mycobacterium avium complex infection vs 64, 64f
Wickham's striae 202
Wiebel–Palade bodies 974
Wilms-anridia-genital anomaly-retardation (WAGR) syndrome 1666
Wilms' tumor 1666–1668, 1667f
  adults, differential diagnosis 1690
  cytology 1667, 1668f
  differential diagnosis 1667–1668, 1670, 1674
    clear cell sarcoma vs 1668, 1670
    Ewing family of tumors vs 385
    neuroblastoma vs 384
    pleomorphic rhabdomyosarcoma vs 359, 362
  histologic maturation after chemotherapy 149
  metastatic, pulmonary blastoma vs 976
  microscopic pathology 1666–1667, 1667f
  renal cell carcinoma after 1667, 1671–1672
  in renal dysplasia 1661

staging 1666, 1666t
stromal cells 1666, 1667, 1667f, 1668f
Wilms' tumor gene (WT1)
  male differentiation role 1734
  mesothelioma 1012, 1015
  serous tumors of ovary 2002
  small round cell tumor of peritoneum 1024
Wilson Jones angiosarcoma 371, 371f
Wilson's disease 1470f, 1505–1506, 1505f
'wire-loop' lesions, lupus nephritis 1626f, 1628
Wirsung, duct 1549
Wiskott-Aldrich syndrome (WAS) 115, 571
Wolbachia infection, eye 2313
wolffian duct cyst 1899
Wolman's disease 579, 1470, 1471
Woringer-Kolopp disease 292
Working Formula, lymphoma classification 544, 546t
World Health Organization (WHO) classification
  acute leukemia 621, 622t, 627
  bladder tumor 1712, 1712t
  breast cancer 462–483, 483t
  Burkitt's lymphoma 628
  CNS tumor 2346–2347, 2346t
  CNS tumor grading 2347, 2347t, 2350, 2363
  endometrial metaplasia 1942, 1943t
  endometrial mixed epithelial-stromal tumors 1975t
  endometrioid endometrial adenocarcinoma 1960, 1960t
  epithelial kidney tumor 1672, 1672t
  Hodgkin's disease 535, 536t, 538
  lupus nephritis 1626
  lymphoma 544, 545t, 554, 557, 563, 567, 569
  multiple myeloma diagnostic criteria 655
  myelodysplastic syndromes 637–638, 637t
  nasopharyngeal carcinoma 793–794, 794f
  neuroendocrine tumor 1423
  ovarian tumor 1993t
  prostatic carcinoma grading 1815
  pulmonary hypertension 913t
  salivary gland tumor 1204, 1205t
  small cell lung carcinoma 989
  thymoma 1096–1097
  vulvar intraepithelial neoplasia grading 1905, 1905t
'worry wart' 201
wrist see hand and wrist
Wuchereria bancrofti, scrotum 1772
Wyburn-Mason syndrome 2416

X

xanthelasma 228, 228f, 1342
  eyelid 2290
  signet ring carcinoma vs 1342, 1342f
  skin 288–289, 288f
xanthoastrocytoma, pleomorphic 2359, 2359f
  immunohistochemistry 2338t, 2359
  ultrastructural characteristics 2336t, 2359
xanthogranuloma
  juvenile 228, 287, 287f
    of iris 2311
    necrobiotic 288, 2290
    periocular 2290
    solitary 287, 287f
xanthogranulomatous inflammation 1710
xanthogranulomatous pseudotumor, vagina 1921
xanthogranulomatous pyelonephritis 1642, 1642f, 1696, 1696f, 1697f
xanthogranulomatous salpingitis 2042
xanthoma
  of bone 739, 739f
  eruptive 228, 288
  papular 288
  planar 228, 288
  of skin 228, 288–289
  tendinous 228, 288
  tuberous 228, 288
  verruciform 288
    penis 1771
    vulva 1902
xanthoma disseminatum 288
xanthomatous change (cholate stasis) 1493, 1495f
xanthomatous halo 287f
xanthomatous hypophysitis 2212
xanthomatous malignant fibrous histiocytoma 336, 336f
X-linked agammaglobulinemia 113
X-linked lymphoproliferative syndrome 115, 571, 659
X-linked thrombocytopenia (XLT) 115
Xp11.2 renal cell carcinoma 1671, 1671f, 1682
X-rays
  bone tumors 704, 706f
  enchondroma 708–709, 709f
X-ray spectrophotometry 1472
XX genotype with virilization 1736–1737
XY with undervirilization 1737

Y

Y chromosome
  GBY region 2037
  SRY gene 1734
yeasts 65–66
  identification 66, 67t
yellow fever, hepatocellular injury 1482, 1482f
Yersina, infections 98–99, 98f
Yersinia
  appendiceal infection 1409
  colitis 1395
  mesenteric lymphadenitis 98, 99f
Yersinia enterocolitica 98
  lymphadenitis 535
  Peyer's patches infection 1395
Yersinia pestis 98
Yersinia pseudotuberculosis 98, 535
yolk sac tumors 1115
  immunohistochemistry 2012
  mediastinum 1119, 1119f
  of ovary 2028–2030, 2029f
    in endometrioid carcinoma 2028
    endometrioid carcinoma vs 2009
    festoon/pseudopapillary pattern 2029, 2029f
    glomeruloid appearance 2029, 2030f
    mixed tumors 2036
    reticular/microcystic pattern 2029, 2029f
  testis 1750–1753, 1752f
    embryonal carcinoma vs 1750
    FNA cytopathology 1777–1779, 1778f
    metastatic 1777–1779, 1778f
    microscopic features 1751–1753
    mixed tumors 1779
    patterns/variants 1751, 1752f
    pre-/postpubertal comparison 1750–1751, 1751t
  true seminoma vs 1746
  vagina 1925
  vulval 1918
young female arteritis see Takayasu's disease

Z

ZAP-70, chronic lymphocytic leukemia 643
Z disk (band), muscle 2215, 2227
zebra body myopathy 2229
Zeis, glands of 2289
'zellballen' 1722
  cells in jugulotympanic paraganglioma 2277
  chemodectoma (meningothelial-like nodules) 970, 970f
  middle ear adenoma 2278
  paraganglioma 176
  sinonasal neuroendocrine carcinoma 803
Zenker's fixative 17
zidovudine, myopathy associated 2223, 2229
Ziehl-Neelsen stain 59, 60, 60t, 2335t
  modified 60t
Zimmermann's pericyte 819
Zimmermann's tumor 2296
Z-line (squamocolumnar junction of esophagus) 1282, 1300
Zollinger-Ellison syndrome
  duodenal biopsy pattern 1377–1378
  gastric carcinoids associated 1348, 1349, 1351
  gastrinoma 1573
  histology 1340–1341, 1341f
  hypersecretory gastropathy 1340–1341, 1341f
  MEN type 1 1574
  peptic duodenitis in 1397
  prognosis 1573
zona fasciculata 2169, 2172f
zona glomerulosa 2169, 2172f
  adrenal cortex adenoma 2185
  hyperplasia 2183, 2184f
zona reticularis 2169, 2172f
'zoning' phenomenon 387, 388f, 389
zygomycetes 66t, 81f
  upper respiratory tract infection 80–81, 80f
Zygomycetes, intestinal infection 1399
zygomycosis, rhinocerebral 80–81, 80f
zygote 2079
zymogen cells 1321
zymogen secretory granules, salivary acinic cell carcinoma 1230